Mark frequently used sections in your code book with these color-coded flags.

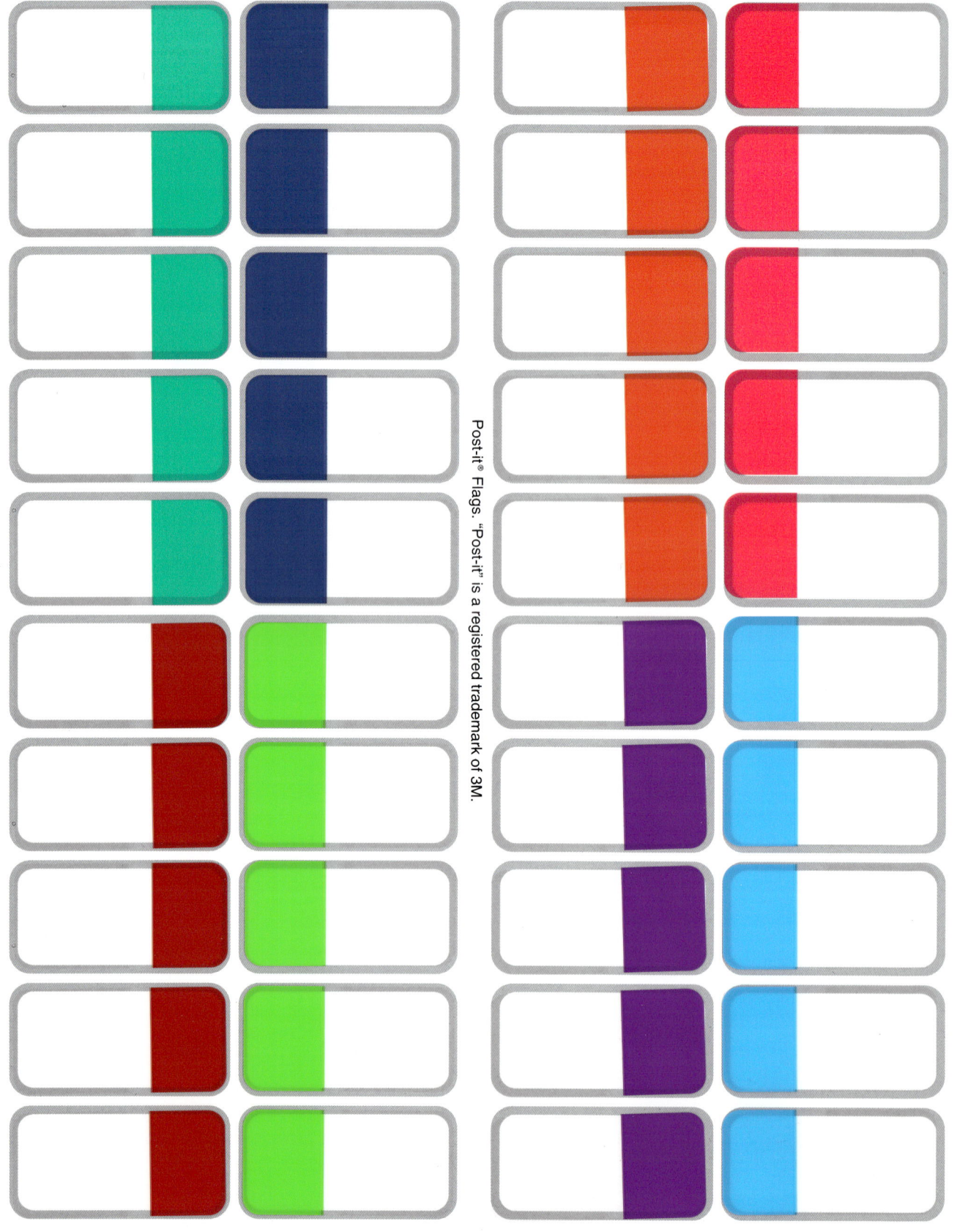

ICD-10-CM Code Book

2024

Anne B. Casto, RHIA, CCS
Consulting Editor

AHIMA
American Health Information Management Association®

Copyright © 2024 by the American Health Information Management Association. All rights reserved. Except as permitted under the Copyright Act of 1976, no part of this publication may be reproduced, stored in a retrieval system, or transmitted, in any form or by any means, electronic, photocopying, recording, or otherwise, without the prior written permission of the AHIMA, 233 North Michigan Avenue, 21st Floor, Chicago, Illinois, 60601-5809 (https://www.ahima.org/education-events/education-by-product/books/textbook-resources/reprint-permissions/).

Softbound
ISBN: 978-1-58426-944-1
eISBN: 978-1-58426-945-8
AHIMA Product No.: AC221023

Spiralbound
ISBN: 978-1-58426-946-5
AHIMA Product No.: AC221123

AHIMA Staff:
Sarah Cybulski, MA, Production Development Editor
Christine Scheid, Content Development Manager
Megan Grennan, Director, Content Production and AHIMA Press
James Pinnick, Vice President, Content and Learning Solutions

Cover image: © fatmayilmaz: iStock. Laurie Entringer

Limit of Liability/Disclaimer of Warranty: This book is sold, as is, without warranty of any kind, either express or implied. While every precaution has been taken in the preparation of this book, the publisher and author assume no responsibility for errors or omissions. Neither is any liability assumed for damages resulting from the use of the information or instructions contained herein. It is further stated that the publisher and author are not responsible for any damage or loss to your data or your equipment that results directly or indirectly from your use of this book.

The Centers for Medicare and Medicaid Services (CMS) and the National Center for Health Statistics (NCHS), two departments within the US Federal Government's Department of Health and Human Services (HHS) provide the *International Classification of Diseases, Tenth Revision, Clinical Modification* (ICD-10-CM) for coding and reporting. ICD-10-CM is the US modification to the World Health Organization's (WHO) International Classification of Diseases, Tenth Revision (ICD-10).

Coding Clinic for ICD-10-CM and ICD-10-PCS is a publication of the American Hospital Association (AHA).

Unless otherwise noted, art pieces were created by Jason Isley and Cognition Studio, Inc, and are all copyright of the American Health Information Management Association.

The websites listed in this book were current and valid as of the date of publication. However, webpage addresses and the information on them may change at any time. The user is encouraged to perform his or her own general web searches to locate any site addresses listed here that are no longer valid.

All copyrights and trademarks mentioned in this book are the possession of their respective owners. AHIMA makes no claim of ownership by mentioning products that contain such marks.

For more information about AHIMA Press publications, including updates, visit https://www.ahima.org/education-events/education-by-product/books/.

American Health Information Management Association
233 North Michigan Avenue, 21st Floor
Chicago, Illinois 60601-5809
ahima.org

Contents

About the Consulting Editor		iv
Acknowledgments		iv
Introduction		v
Index to Diseases and Injuries		1
Table of Neoplasms		347
Table of Drugs and Chemicals		369
External Cause of Injuries Index		450
Tabular List of Diseases and Injuries		486
Chapter 1	Certain Infectious and Parasitic Diseases (A00-B99)	487
Chapter 2	Neoplasms (C00-D49)	509
Chapter 3	Diseases of the Blood and Blood-Forming Organs and Certain Disorders Involving the Immune Mechanism (D50-D89)	548
Chapter 4	Endocrine, Nutritional and Metabolic Disease (E00-E89)	560
Chapter 5	Mental, Behavioral and Neurodevelopmental Disorders (F01-F99)	583
Chapter 6	Diseases of the Nervous System (G00-G99)	611
Chapter 7	Diseases of the Eye and Adnexa (H00-H59)	635
Chapter 8	Diseases of the Ear and Mastoid Process (H60-H95)	671
Chapter 9	Diseases of the Circulatory System (I00-I99)	682
Chapter 10	Diseases of the Respiratory System (J00-J99)	731
Chapter 11	Diseases of the Digestive System (K00-K95)	747
Chapter 12	Diseases of the Skin and Subcutaneous Tissue (L00-L99)	776
Chapter 13	Diseases of the Musculoskeletal System and Connective Tissue (M00-M99)	798
Chapter 14	Diseases of the Genitourinary System (N00-N99)	886
Chapter 15	Pregnancy, Childbirth and the Puerperium (O00-O9A)	912
Chapter 16	Certain Conditions Originating in the Perinatal Period (P00-P96)	950
Chapter 17	Congenital Malformations, Deformations and Chromosomal Abnormalities (Q00-Q99)	961
Chapter 18	Symptoms, Signs and Abnormal Clinical and Laboratory Findings, Not Elsewhere Classified (R00-R99)	977
Chapter 19	Injury, Poisoning and Certain Other Consequences of External Causes (S00-T88)	996
Chapter 20	External Causes of Morbidity (V00-Y99)	1230
Chapter 21	Factors Influencing Health Status and Contact with Health Services (Z00-Z99)	1305
Chapter 22	Codes for Special Purposes (U00-U85)	1341
Online Appendices:		
Appendix A:	**CC/MCC Principal Diagnosis Collections and Exclusion Lists**	1342
Appendix B:	**Hospital-Acquired Conditions (HAC) List**	1342
Appendix C:	**New ICD-10-CM Codes FY2024**	1343
Appendix D:	**Deleted ICD-10-CM Codes FY2024**	1343

About the Consulting Editor

Anne B. Casto, RHIA, CCS, is the president of Casto Consulting, LLC. Casto Consulting, LLC is a consulting firm that provides services to hospitals and other healthcare stakeholders primarily in the areas of reimbursement and coding. Casto Consulting, LLC specializes in linking coding and billing practices to positive revenue cycle outcomes. Additionally, the firm provides guidance to consulting firms, healthcare organizations and healthcare insurers regarding reimbursement methodologies and Medicare regulations.

Additionally, Ms. Casto is a lecturer in the HIMS department at The Ohio State University, School of Health and Rehabilitation Sciences. Over the past 20 years, Ms. Casto has taught numerous courses in the areas of healthcare reimbursement, coding, healthcare data trending, and coding analytics.

Prior to her current roles, Ms. Casto was the vice president of clinical information for Cleverley & Associates where she worked very closely with APC regulations and guidelines, preparing hospitals for the implementation of the Medicare OPPS. Ms. Casto was also the clinical information product manager for CHIPS/Ingenix. She joined CHIPS/Ingenix in 1998 and spent the majority of her time developing coding compliance products for the inpatient and outpatient settings.

Ms. Casto has been responsible for inpatient and outpatient coding activities in several large hospitals including Mt. Sinai Medical Center (NYC), Beth Israel Medical Center (NYC), and The Ohio State University. She has worked extensively with CMI, quality measures, physician documentation, and coding accuracy efforts at these facilities.

Ms. Casto received her degree in Health Information Management at The Ohio State University in 1995. She received her Certified Coding Specialist credential in 1998 from the American Health Information Management Association. In 2009 Ms. Casto received her ICD-10-CM/PCS Trainer certificate from AHIMA. Ms. Casto is the co-author of an AHIMA published text book entitled *Principles of Healthcare Reimbursement*. Additionally, Ms. Casto was a contributing author to the published AHIMA books: *Severity DRGs and Reimbursement; A MS-DRG Primer* and *Effective Management of Coding Services*.

Ms. Casto received the AHIMA Legacy Award, part of the FORE Triumph Awards, in 2007 which honors a significant contribution to the knowledge base of the HIM field through an insightful publication. Additionally, Ms. Casto was honored with the Ohio Health Information Management Association's Distinguished Member Award in 2008 and the Ohio Health Information Management Association's Professional Achievement Award in 2011.

Acknowledgments

Many thanks to my family for their support during this project. Thanks to Dr. Susan White, The Ohio State University; your data manipulation skills are second to none. Thanks to Drew Beverick for providing valuable insight from the student perspective. Many thanks to Linda Hyde, RHIA, and Angela Comfort, MBA, RHIA, CDIP, CCS, CCS-P, CICA, for their very thorough technical review of the book.

Introduction

ICD-10-CM History and Background

The International Classification of Diseases, Tenth Revision, Clinical Modification (ICD-10-CM) is the United Stated modification to the World Health Organization's (WHO) International Classification of Diseases, Tenth Revision (ICD-10). The WHO adopted the tenth revision in 1990. Since that time, several countries, including Australia and Canada, have developed their own modification to ICD-10 and have implemented it for use.

In 1994, the National Center for Health Statistics (NCHS) began the process of determining the viability of ICD-10 and the applicability of a clinical modification of the code set for the United States. The NCHS has made draft versions of ICD-10-CM available since 2002. NCHS continued to refine and update the code set for use in the United States while the healthcare community waited for adoption of the code set by Congress. On August 22, 2008, the long-awaited official Notice of Proposed Rule Making (NPRM) regarding the adopting of the ICD-10-CM and ICD-10-PCS classifications was published in the *Federal Register*. On January 16, 2009, the Centers for Medicare and Medicaid Services (CMS) published the Final Rule for adoption of the ICD-10-CM and ICD-10-PCS code sets udders rules, 45 CFR Parts 160 and 162 of the Health Insurance Portability and Accountability Act of 1996 (HIPAA). Within this rule, a compliance (implementation) date of October 1, 2013 was released. The compliance date was revised and ICD-10-CM was successfully implemented on October 1, 2015.

Characteristics of ICD-10-CM

ICD-10-CM far exceeds its predecessors in the number of codes provided. The disease classification has been expanded to include health-related conditions and to provide greater specificity at the seventh-character level of detail. When available, these seventh characters are not optional; they are intended for use in recording the information substantiated in the clinical record.

The ICD-10-CM/PCS Coordination and Maintenance Committee

Annual modifications are made to ICD-10-CM through the ICD-10-CM Coordination and Maintenance Committee (C&M). The Committee is made up of representatives from two US federal government agencies, the National Center for Health Statistics, and the Centers for Medicare and Medicaid Services (CMS). C&M holds meetings twice a year, which are open to the public. Modification proposals submitted to C&M for consideration are presented at the meetings for public discussion. An open comment period follows each of these meetings. Those modification proposals which are approved are incorporated into the official government version of ICD-10-CM and become effective for use on October 1 of each year.

Guidance in the Use of ICD10-CM

To code accurately, it is necessary to have a working knowledge of medical terminology and to understand the characteristics, code book terminology, and conventions of ICD-10-CM. Transforming verbal descriptions of diseases, injuries, and conditions into numerical designations (coding) is a complex activity and should not be undertaken without proper training.

Originally, coding was accomplished to provide access to health records by diagnoses and operations through retrieval for medical research education and administration. Today, medical codes are utilized to facilitate payment of health services, evaluate utilization patterns, and study the appropriateness of healthcare costs. Coding also provides the basis for epidemiological studies and research into the quality of healthcare.

Coding must be performed correctly and consistently to produce meaningful statics to aid in planning for the health needs of the nation.

Official Conventions

ICD-10-CM Official Guidelines for Coding and Reporting 2024

(October 1, 2023 - September 30, 2024)

Narrative changes appear in bold text

Items underlined have been moved within the guidelines since the 2023 version

Italics are used to indicate revisions to heading changes

The Centers for Medicare and Medicaid Services (CMS) and the National Center for Health Statistics (NCHS), two departments within the US Federal Government's Department of Health and Human Services (HHS) provide the following guidelines for coding and reporting using the International Classification of Diseases, Tenth Revision, Clinical

Modification (ICD-10-CM). These guidelines should be used as a companion document to the official version of the ICD-10-CM as published on the NCHS website. The ICD-10-CM is a morbidity classification published by the United States for classifying diagnoses and reason for visits in all healthcare settings. The ICD-10-CM is based on the ICD-10, the statistical classification of disease published by the World Health Organization (WHO).

These guidelines have been approved by the four organizations that make up the Cooperating Parties for the ICD-10-CM: the American Hospital Association (AHA), the American Health Information Management Association (AHIMA), CMS, and NCHS.

These guidelines are a set of rules that have been developed to accompany and complement the official conventions and instructions provided within the ICD-10-CM itself. The instructions and conventions of the classification take precedence over guidelines. These guidelines are based on the coding and sequencing instructions in the Tabular List and Alphabetic Index of ICD-10-CM, but provide additional instruction. Adherence to these guidelines when assigning ICD-10-CM diagnosis codes is required under the Health Insurance Portability and Accountability Act (HIPAA). The diagnosis codes (Tabular List and Alphabetic Index) have been adopted under HIPAA for all healthcare settings. A joint effort between the healthcare provider and the coder is essential to achieve complete and accurate documentation, code assignment, and reporting of diagnoses and procedures. These guidelines have been developed to assist both the healthcare provider and the coder in identifying those diagnoses that are to be reported. The importance of consistent, complete documentation in the medical record cannot be overemphasized. Without such documentation accurate coding cannot be achieved. The entire record should be reviewed to determine the specific reason for the encounter and the conditions treated.

The term encounter is used for all settings, including hospital admissions. In the context of these guidelines, the term provider is used throughout the guidelines to mean physician or any qualified healthcare practitioner who is legally accountable for establishing the patient's diagnosis. Only this set of guidelines, approved by the Cooperating Parties, is official.

The guidelines are organized into sections. Section I includes the structure and conventions of the classification and general guidelines that apply to the entire classification, and chapter-specific guidelines that correspond to the chapters as they are arranged in the classification. Section II includes guidelines for selection of principal diagnosis for non-outpatient settings. Section III includes guidelines for reporting additional diagnoses in non-outpatient settings. Section IV is for outpatient coding and reporting. It is necessary to review all sections of the guidelines to fully understand all of the rules and instructions needed to code properly.

Section I. Conventions, General Coding Guidelines and Chapter Specific Guidelines

The conventions, general guidelines and chapter-specific guidelines are applicable to all healthcare settings unless otherwise indicated. The conventions and instructions of the classification take precedence over guidelines.

A. Conventions for the ICD-10-CM

The conventions for the ICD-10-CM are the general rules for use of the classification independent of the guidelines. These conventions are incorporated within the Alphabetic Index and Tabular List of the ICD-10-CM as instructional notes.

1. The Alphabetic Index and Tabular List

The ICD-10-CM is divided into the Alphabetic Index, an alphabetical list of terms and their corresponding code, and the Tabular List, a structured list of codes divided into chapters based on body system or condition. The Alphabetic Index consists of the following parts: the Index of Diseases and Injury, the Index of External Causes of Injury, the Table of Neoplasms, and the Table of Drugs and Chemicals.

See Section I.C.2. Neoplasms

See Section I.C.19. Adverse effects, poisoning, underdosing and toxic effects

2. Format and Structure

The ICD-10-CM Tabular List contains categories, subcategories and codes. Characters for categories, subcategories and codes may be either a letter or a number. All categories are 3 characters. A three-character category that has no further subdivision is equivalent to a code. Subcategories are either 4 or 5 characters. Codes may be 3, 4, 5, 6, or 7 characters. That is, each level of subdivision after a category is a subcategory. The final level of subdivision is a code. Codes that have applicable 7th characters are still referred to as codes, not subcategories. A code that has an applicable 7th character is considered invalid without the 7th character.

The ICD-10-CM uses an indented format for ease in reference.

3. Use of Codes for Reporting Purposes

For reporting purposes only codes are permissible, not categories or subcategories, and any applicable 7th character is required.

4. **Placeholder Character**

   The ICD-10-CM utilizes a placeholder character X. The X is used as a placeholder at certain codes to allow for future expansion. An example of this is at the poisoning, adverse effect and underdosing codes, categories T36–T50. Where a placeholder exists, the X must be used in order for the code to be considered a valid code.

5. **7th Characters**

   Certain ICD-10-CM categories have applicable 7th characters. The applicable 7th character is required for all codes within the category, or as the notes in the Tabular List instruct. The 7th character must always be the 7th character in the data field. If a code that requires a 7th character is not 6 characters, a placeholder X must be used to fill in the empty characters.

6. **Abbreviations**

   a. **Alphabetic Index Abbreviations**

   NEC   "Not elsewhere classifiable"
   This abbreviation in the Alphabetic Index represents "other specified". When a specific code is not available for a condition, the Alphabetic Index directs the coder to the "other specified" code in the Tabular List.

   NOS   "Not otherwise specified"
   This abbreviation is the equivalent of unspecified.

   b. **Tabular List Abbreviations**

   NEC   "Not elsewhere classifiable"
   This abbreviation in the Tabular List represents "other specified". When a specific code is not available for a condition the Tabular List includes an NEC entry under a code to identify the code as the "other specified" code.

   NOS   "Not otherwise specified"
   This abbreviation is the equivalent of unspecified.

7. **Punctuation**

   [ ]   Brackets are used in the Tabular List to enclose synonyms, alternative wording or explanatory phrases. Brackets are used in the Alphabetic Index to identify manifestation codes.

   ( )   Parentheses are used in both the Alphabetic Index and Tabular List to enclose supplementary words that may be present or absent in the statement of a disease or procedure without affecting the code number to which it is assigned. The terms within the parentheses are referred to as nonessential modifiers. The nonessential modifiers in the Alphabetic Index to Diseases apply to subterms following a main term except when a nonessential modifier and a subentry are mutually exclusive, the subentry takes precedence. For example, in the ICD-10-CM Alphabetic Index under the main term Enteritis, "acute" is a nonessential modifier and "chronic" is a subentry. In this case, the nonessential modifier "acute" does not apply to the subentry "chronic".

   :   Colons are used in the Tabular List after an incomplete term which needs one or more of the modifiers following the colon to make it assignable to a given category.

8. **Use of "and"**

   See Section I.A.14. Use of the term "And"

9. **Other and Unspecified Codes**

   a. **"Other" Codes**

   Codes titled "other" or "other specified" are for use when the information in the medical record provides detail for which a specific code does not exist. Alphabetic Index entries with NEC in the line designate "other" codes in the Tabular List. These Alphabetic Index entries represent specific disease entities for which no specific code exists so the term is included within an "other" code.

   b. **"Unspecified" Codes**

   Codes titled "unspecified" are for use when the information in the medical record is insufficient to assign a more specific code. For those categories for which an unspecified code is not provided, the "other specified" code may represent both other and unspecified.

   See Section I.B.18 Use of Signs/Symptom/Unspecified Codes

10. **Includes Notes**

    This note appears immediately under a three character code title to further define, or give examples of, the content of the category.

11. **Inclusion Terms**

    List of terms is included under some codes. These terms are the conditions for which that code is to be used. The terms may be synonyms of the code title, or, in the case of "other specified" codes, the terms are a list of the various conditions assigned to that code. The inclusion terms are not necessarily exhaustive. Additional terms found only in the Alphabetic Index may also be assigned to a code.

12. **Excludes Notes**

    The ICD-10-CM has two types of excludes notes. Each type of note has a different definition for use but they are all similar in that they indicate that codes excluded from each other are independent of each other.

    a. **Excludes1**

    A type 1 Excludes note is a pure excludes note. It means "NOT CODED HERE!" An Excludes1 note indicates that the code excluded should never be used at the same time as the code above the Excludes1 note. An Excludes1 is used when two conditions cannot occur together, such as a congenital form versus an acquired form of the same condition.

    An exception to the Excludes1 definition is the circumstance when the two conditions are unrelated to each other. If it is not clear whether the two conditions involving an Excludes1 note are related or not, query the provider. For example, code F45.8, Other somatoform disorders, has an Exlcudes1 note for "sleep related teeth grinding (G47.63)," because "teeth grinding" is an inclusion term under F45.8. Only one of these two codes should be assigned for teeth grinding. However, psychogenic dysmenorrhea is also an inclusion term under F45.8, and a patient could have both this conditions and sleep related teeth grinding. In this case, the two conditions are clearly unrelated to each other, and do it would be appropriate to report F45.8 and G47.63 together.

    b. **Excludes2**

    A type 2 Excludes note represents "Not included here". An Excludes2 note indicates that the condition excluded is not part of the condition represented by the code, but a patient may have both conditions at the same time. When an Excludes2 note appears under a code, it is acceptable to use both the code and the excluded code together, when appropriate.

13. **Etiology/Manifestation Convention ("Code first", "Use additional code" and "In Diseases Classified Elsewhere" Notes)**

    Certain conditions have both an underlying etiology and multiple body system manifestations due to the underlying etiology. For such conditions, the ICD-10-CM has a coding convention that requires the underlying condition be sequenced first, if applicable, followed by the manifestation. Wherever such a combination exists, there is a "use additional code" note at the etiology code, and a "code first" note at the manifestation code. These instructional notes indicate the proper sequencing order of the codes, etiology followed by manifestation.

    In most cases the manifestation codes will have in the code title, "in diseases classified elsewhere." Codes with this title are a component of the etiology/manifestation convention. The code title indicates that it is a manifestation code. "In diseases classified elsewhere" codes are never permitted to be used as first-listed or principal diagnosis codes. They must be used in conjunction with an underlying condition code and they must be listed following the underlying condition. See category F02, Dementia in other diseases classified elsewhere, for an example of this convention.

    There are manifestation codes that do not have "in diseases classified elsewhere" in the title. For such codes, there is a "use additional code" note at the etiology code and a "code first" note at the manifestation code and the rules for sequencing apply.

    In addition to the notes in the Tabular List, these conditions also have a specific Alphabetic Index entry structure. In the Alphabetic Index both conditions are listed together with the etiology code first followed by the manifestation codes in brackets. The code in brackets is always to be sequenced second.

    An example of the etiology/manifestation convention is dementia with Parkinson's disease. In the Alphabetic Index, **a code from category** G20 is listed first, followed by code F02.80 or F02.81- in brackets. **A code from category G20-** represents the underlying etiology, Parkinson's disease, and must be sequenced first, whereas codes F02.80 and F02.81- represent the manifestation of dementia in diseases classified elsewhere, with or without behavioral disturbance.

    "Code first" and "Use additional code" notes are also used as sequencing rules in the classification for certain codes that are not part of an etiology/ manifestation combination.

    See Section I.B. 7. Multiple coding for a single condition.

14. **"And"**

    The word "and" should be interpreted to mean either "and" or "or" when it appears in a title.

    For example, cases of "tuberculosis of bones", "tuberculosis of joints" and "tuberculosis of bones and joints" are classified to subcategory A18.0, Tuberculosis of bones and joints.

15. **"With"**

The word "with" or "in" should be interpreted to mean "associated with" or "due to" when it appears in a code title, the Alphabetic Index (either under a main term or subterm), or an instructional note in the Tabular List. The classification presumes a causal relationship between the two conditions linked by these terms in the Alphabetic Index or Tabular List. These conditions should be coded as related even in the absence of provider documentation explicitly linking them, unless the documentation clearly states the conditions are unrelated or when another guideline exists that specifically requires a documented linkage between two conditions (e.g., sepsis guideline for "acute organ dysfunction that is not clearly associated with the sepsis"). For conditions not specifically linked by these relational terms in the classification or when a guideline requires that a linkage between two conditions be explicitly documented, provider documentation must link the conditions in order to code them as related.

The word "with" in the Alphabetic Index is sequenced immediately following the main term or subterm, not in alphabetical order.

16. **"See" and "See Also"**

The "see" instruction following a main term in the Alphabetic Index indicates that another term should be referenced. It is necessary to go to the main term referenced with the "see" note to locate the correct code.

A "see also" instruction following a main term in the Alphabetic Index instructs that there is another main term that may also be referenced that may provide additional Alphabetic Index entries that may be useful. It is not necessary to follow the "see also" note when the original main term provides the necessary code.

17. **"Code Also Note"**

A "code also" note instructs that two codes may be required to fully describe a condition, but this note does not provide sequencing direction. The sequencing depends on the circumstances of the encounter.

18. **Default Codes**

A code listed next to a main term in the ICD-10-CM Alphabetic Index is referred to as a default code. The default code represents that condition that is most commonly associated with the main term, or is the unspecified code for the condition. If a condition is documented in a medical record (for example, appendicitis) without any additional information, such as acute or chronic, the default code should be assigned.

19. **Code Assignment and Clinical Criteria**

The assignment of a diagnosis code is based on the provider's diagnostic statement that the condition exists. The provider's statement that the patient has a particular condition is sufficient. Code assignment is not based on clinical criteria used by the provider to establish the diagnosis. If there is conflicting medical record documentation, query the provider.

B. General Coding Guidelines

1. **Locating a Code in the ICD-10-CM**

To select a code in the classification that corresponds to a diagnosis or reason for visit documented in a medical record, first locate the term in the Alphabetic Index, and then verify the code in the Tabular List. Read and be guided by instructional notations that appear in both the Alphabetic Index and the Tabular List.

It is essential to use both the Alphabetic Index and Tabular List when locating and assigning a code. The Alphabetic Index does not always provide the full code. Selection of the full code, including laterality and any applicable 7th character can only be done in the Tabular List. A dash (-) at the end of an Alphabetic Index entry indicates that additional characters are required. Even if a dash is not included at the Alphabetic Index entry, it is necessary to refer to the Tabular List to verify that no 7th character is required.

2. **Level of Detail in Coding**

Diagnosis codes are to be used and reported at their highest number of characters available and to the highest level of specificity documented in the medical record.

ICD-10-CM diagnosis codes are composed of codes with 3, 4, 5, 6, or 7 characters. Codes with three characters are included in ICD-10-CM as the heading of a category of codes that may be further subdivided by the use of fourth and/or fifth characters and/or sixth characters, which provide greater detail.

A three-character code is to be used only if it is not further subdivided. A code is invalid if it has not been coded to the full number of characters required for that code, including the 7th character, if applicable.

3. **Code or Codes from A00.0–T88.9, Z00–Z99.8, U00–U85**
   The appropriate code or codes from A00.0–T88.9, Z00–Z99.8, and U00–U85 must be used to identify diagnoses, symptoms, conditions, problems, complaints or other reason(s) for the encounter/visit.

4. **Signs and Symptoms**
   Codes that describe symptoms and signs, as opposed to diagnoses, are acceptable for reporting purposes when a related definitive diagnosis has not been established (confirmed) by the provider. Chapter 18 of ICD-10-CM, Symptoms, Signs, and Abnormal Clinical and Laboratory Findings, Not Elsewhere Classified (codes R00.0–R99) contains many, but not all codes for symptoms.
   See Section I.B.18 Use of Signs/Symptom/Unspecified Codes

5. **Conditions that are an Integral Part of a Disease Process**
   Signs and symptoms that are associated routinely with a disease process should not be assigned as additional codes, unless otherwise instructed by the classification.

6. **Conditions that are not an Integral Part of a Disease Process**
   Additional signs and symptoms that may not be associated routinely with a disease process should be coded when present.

7. **Multiple Coding for a Single Condition**
   In addition to the etiology/manifestation convention that requires two codes to fully describe a single condition that affects multiple body systems, there are other single conditions that also require more than one code. "Use additional code" notes are found in the Tabular List at codes that are not part of an etiology/manifestation pair where a secondary code is useful to fully describe a condition. The sequencing rule is the same as the etiology/manifestation pair, "use additional code" indicates that a secondary code should be added, if known.

   For example, for bacterial infections that are not included in chapter 1, a secondary code from category B95, Streptococcus, Staphylococcus, and Enterococcus, as the cause of diseases classified elsewhere, or B96, Other bacterial agents as the cause of diseases classified elsewhere, may be required to identify the bacterial organism causing the infection. A "use additional code" note will normally be found at the infectious disease code, indicating a need for the organism code to be added as a secondary code.

   "Code first" notes are also under certain codes that are not specifically manifestation codes but may be due to an underlying cause. When there is a "code first" note and an underlying condition is present, the underlying condition should be sequenced first, if known.

   "Code, if applicable, any causal condition first", notes indicate that this code may be assigned as a principal diagnosis when the causal condition is unknown or not applicable. If a causal condition is known, the code for that condition should be sequenced as the principal or first-listed diagnosis.

   Multiple codes may be needed for sequela, complication codes and obstetric codes to more fully describe a condition. See the specific guidelines for these conditions for further instruction.

8. **Acute and Chronic Conditions**
   If the same condition is described as both acute (subacute) and chronic, and separate subentries exist in the Alphabetic Index at the same indentation level, code both and sequence the acute (subacute) code first.

9. **Combination Code**
   A combination code is a single code used to classify:
   - Two diagnoses, or
   - A diagnosis with an associated secondary process (manifestation)
   - A diagnosis with an associated complication

   Combination codes are identified by referring to subterm entries in the Alphabetic Index and by reading the inclusion and exclusion notes in the Tabular List.

   Assign only the combination code when that code fully identifies the diagnostic conditions involved or when the Alphabetic Index so directs. Multiple coding should not be used when the classification provides a combination code that clearly identifies all of the elements documented in the diagnosis. When the combination code lacks necessary specificity in describing the manifestation or complication, an additional code should be used as a secondary code.

10. Sequela (Late Effects)

A sequela is the residual effect (condition produced) after the acute phase of an illness or injury has terminated. There is no time limit on when a sequela code can be used. The residual may be apparent early, such as in cerebral infarction, or it may occur months or years later, such as that due to a previous injury. Examples of sequela include: scar formation resulting from a burn, deviated septum due to a nasal fracture, and infertility due to tubal occlusion from old tuberculosis. Coding of sequela generally requires two codes sequenced in the following order: The condition or nature of the sequela is sequenced first. The sequela code is sequenced second.

An exception to the above guidelines are those instances where the code for the sequela is followed by a manifestation code identified in the Tabular List and title, or the sequela code has been expanded (at the fourth, fifth or sixth, character levels) to include the manifestation(s). The code for the acute phase of an illness or injury that led to the sequela is never used with a code for the late effect.

- *See Section I.C.9. Sequelae of cerebrovascular disease*
- *See Section I.C.15. Sequelae of complication of pregnancy, childbirth and the puerperium*
- *See Section I.C.19. Application of 7th characters for Chapter 19*

11. Impending or Threatened Condition

Code any condition described at the time of discharge as "impending" or "threatened" as follows:

- If it did occur, code as confirmed diagnosis.
- If it did not occur, reference the Alphabetic Index to determine if the condition has a subentry term for "impending" or "threatened" and also reference main term entries for "Impending" and for "Threatened."
- If the subterms are listed, assign the given code.
- If the subterms are not listed, code the existing underlying condition(s) and not the condition described as impending or threatened.

12. Reporting Same Diagnosis Code More than Once

Each unique ICD-10-CM diagnosis code may be reported only once for an encounter. This applies to bilateral conditions when there are no distinct codes identifying laterality or two different conditions classified to the same ICD-10-CM diagnosis code.

13. Laterality

Some ICD-10-CM codes indicate laterality, specifying whether the condition occurs on the left, right or is bilateral. If no bilateral code is provided and the condition is bilateral, assign separate codes for both the left and right side. If the side is not identified in the medical record, assign the code for the unspecified side.

When a patient has a bilateral condition and each side is treated during separate encounters, assign the "bilateral" code (as the conditions still exists on both sides), including for the encounter to treat the first side. For the second encounter for treatment after one side has previously been treated and the condition no longer exists on that side, assign the appropriate unilateral code for the side where the conditions still exists (e.g., cataract surgery performed on each eye in separate encounters). The bilateral code would not be assigned for the subsequent encounter, as the patient no longer has the condition in the previously-treated site. If the treatment on the first side did not completely resolve the condition, then the bilateral code would still be appropriate.

When laterality is not documented by the patient's provider, code assignment for the affected side may be based on medical record documentation from other clinicians. If there is conflicting medical record documentation regarding the affected side, the patient's attending provider should be queried for clarification. Codes for "unspecified" side should rarely be used, such as when the documentation in the record is insufficient to determine the affected side and it is not possible to obtain clarification.

14. Documentation by Clinicians Other than the Patient's Provider

Code assignment is based on the documentation by **the** patient's provider (i.e., physician or other qualified healthcare practitioner legally accountable for establishing the patient's diagnosis). There are a few exceptions **when** code assignment may be based on medical record documentation from clinicians who are not the patient's provider (i.e., physician, or other qualified healthcare practitioner legally accountable for establishing the patient's diagnosis). In this context, "clinicians" other than the patient's provider refer to healthcare professionals permitted, based on regulatory or accreditation requirements or internal hospital policies, to document in a patient's official medical record.

These exceptions include codes for:

- Body Mass Index (BMI)
- Depth of non-pressure chronic ulcers
- Pressure ulcer stage

- Coma scale
- NIH stroke scale (NIHSS)
- Social determinants of health (SDOH) **classified to Chapter 21**
- Laterality
- Blood alcohol level
- Underimmunization status

This information is typically, or may be, documented by other clinicians involved in the care of the patient (e.g., a dietitian often documents the BMI, a nurse often documents the pressure ulcer stages, and an emergency medical technician often documents the coma scale). However, the associated diagnosis (such as overweight, obesity, acute stroke pressure ulcer, or a condition classifiable to category F10, Alcohol related disorders) must be documented by the patient's provider. If there is conflicting medical record documentation, either from the same clinician or different clinicians, the patient's attending provider should be queried for clarification.

The BMI, coma scale, and NIHSS codes blood alcohol level codes, and codes for social determinants of health and underimmunization status should only be reported as secondary diagnoses.

See Section I.C.21.c.17 for additional information regarding coding social determinants of health

15. Syndromes
Follow the Alphabetic Index guidance when coding syndromes. In the absence of Alphabetic Index guidance, assign codes for the documented manifestations of the syndrome. Additional codes for manifestations that are not an integral part of the disease process may also be assigned when the condition does not have a unique code.

16. Documentation of Complications of Care
Code assignment is based on the provider's documentation of the relationship between the condition and the care or procedure, unless otherwise instructed by the classification. The guideline extends to any complications of care, regardless of the chapter the code is located in. It is important to note that not all conditions that occur during or following medical care or surgery are classified as complications. There must be a cause-and-effect relationship between the care provided and the condition, and the documentation must support that the condition is clinically significant. It is not necessary for the provider to explicitly document the term "complication." For example, if the condition alters the course of the surgery as documented in the operative report, then it would be appropriate to report a complication code. Query the provider for clarification, if the documentation is not clear as to the relationship between the condition and the care or procedure.

17. Borderline Diagnosis
If the provider documents a "borderline" diagnosis at the time of discharge, the diagnosis is coded as confirmed, unless the classification provides a specific entry (e.g., borderline diabetes). If a borderline condition has a specific index entry in ICD-10-CM, it should be coded as such. Since borderline conditions are not uncertain diagnoses, no distinction is made between the care setting (inpatient versus outpatient). Whenever the documentation is unclear regarding a borderline condition, coders are encouraged to query for clarification.

18. Use of Sign/Symptom/Unspecified Codes
Sign/symptom and "unspecified" codes have acceptable, even necessary, uses. While specific diagnosis codes should be reported when they are supported by the available medical record documentation and clinical knowledge of the patient's health condition, there are instances when signs/symptoms or unspecified codes are the best choices for accurately reflecting the healthcare encounter. Each healthcare encounter should be coded to the level of certainty known for that encounter.

As stated in the introductory section of these official coding guidelines, a joint effort between the healthcare provider and the coder is essential to achieve complete and accurate documentation, code assignment, and reporting of diagnoses and procedures. The importance of consistent, complete documentation in the medical record cannot be overemphasized. Without such documentation accurate coding cannot be achieved. The entire record should be reviewed to determine the specific reason for the encounter and the conditions treated.

If a definitive diagnosis has not been established by the end of the encounter, it is appropriate to report codes for sign(s) and/or symptom(s) in lieu of a definitive diagnosis. When sufficient clinical information isn't known or available about a particular health condition to assign a more specific code, it is acceptable to report the appropriate "unspecified" code (e.g., a diagnosis of pneumonia has been determined, but not the specific type). Unspecified codes should be reported when they are the codes that most accurately reflects what is known about the patient's condition at the time of that particular encounter. It would be inappropriate to select a specific code that is not supported by the medical record documentation or conduct medically unnecessary diagnostic testing in order to determine a more specific code.

19. Coding for Healthcare Encounters in Hurricane Aftermath

a. Use of External Cause of Morbidity Codes

An external cause of morbidity code should be assigned to identify the cause of the injury(ies) incurred as a result of the hurricane. The use of external cause of morbidity codes is supplemental to the application of ICD-10-CM codes. External cause of morbidity codes are never to be recorded as a principal diagnosis (first-listed in non-inpatient settings). The appropriate injury code should be sequenced before any external cause codes. The external cause of morbidity codes capture how the injury or health condition happened (cause), the intent (unintentional or accidental; or intentional, such as suicide or assault), the place where the event occurred, the activity of the patient at the time of the event, and the person's status (e.g., civilian, military). They should not be assigned for encounters to treat hurricane victims' medical conditions when no injury, adverse effect or poisoning is involved. External cause of morbidity codes should be assigned for each encounter for care and treatment of the injury. External cause of morbidity codes may be assigned in all health care settings. For the purpose of capturing complete and accurate ICD-10-CM data in the aftermath of the hurricane, a healthcare setting should be considered as any location where medical care is provided by licensed healthcare professionals.

b. Sequencing of External Causes of Morbidity Codes

Codes for cataclysmic events, such as hurricane, take priority over all other external cause codes except child and adult abuse and terrorism and should be sequenced before other external cause of injury codes. Assign as many external cause of morbidity codes as necessary to fully explain each cause. For example, if an injury occurs as a result of a building collapse during the hurricane, external cause codes for both the hurricane and the building collapse should be assigned with the external causes code for hurricane being sequenced as the first external cause code. For injuries incurred as a direct result of the hurricane, assign the appropriate code(s) for the injuries, followed by the code X37.0-, Hurricane (with the appropriate 7th character), and any other applicable external cause of injury codes. Code X37.0- also should be assigned when an injury is incurred as a result of flooding caused by a levee breaking related to the hurricane. Code X38.-, Flood (with appropriate 7th character), should be assigned when an injury is from flooding resulting directly from the storm. Code X36.0-, Collapse of dam or man-made structure, should not be assigned when the cause of the collapse is due to the hurricane. Use of code X36.0- is limited to collapses of man-made structures due to earth surface movements, not due to storm surges directly from a hurricane.

c. Other External Causes of Morbidity Code Issues

For injuries that are not a direct result of the hurricane, such as an evacuee that has incurred an injury as a result of a motor vehicle accident, assign the appropriate external cause of morbidity code(s) to describe the cause of the injury, but do not assign code X37.0-, Hurricane. If it is not clear whether the injury was a direct result of the hurricane, assume the injury is due to the hurricane and assign code X37.0-, Hurricane, as well as any other applicable external cause of morbidity codes. In addition to code X37.0-, Hurricane, other possible applicable external cause of morbidity codes include:

- X30-, Exposure to excessive natural heat
- X31-, Exposure to excessive natural cold
- X38-, Flood

d. Use of Z codes

Z codes (other reasons for healthcare encounters) may be assigned as appropriate to further explain the reasons for presenting for healthcare services, including transfers between healthcare facilities, or provide additional information relevant to a patient encounter. The ICD-10-CM Official Guidelines for Coding and Reporting identify which codes may be assigned as principal or first-listed diagnosis only, secondary diagnosis only, or principal/first-listed or secondary (depending on the circumstances). Possible applicable Z codes include:

- Z59.0. Homelessness
- Z59.1-, Inadequate housing
- Z59.5-, Extreme poverty
- Z75.1-, Person awaiting admission to adequate facility elsewhere
- Z75.3-, Unavailability and inaccessibility of health-care facilities
- Z74.4-, Unavailability and inaccessibility of other helping agencies
- Z76.2-, Encounter for health supervision and care of other healthy infant and child
- Z99.12-, Encounter for respirator [ventilator] dependence during power failure

The external cause of morbidity codes and the Z codes listed above are not an all-inclusive list. Other codes may be applicable to the encounter based upon the documentation. Assign as many codes as necessary to fully explain each healthcare encounter. Since patient history information may be very limited, use any available documentation to assign the appropriate external cause of morbidity and Z codes.

C. Chapter-Specific Coding Guidelines

> **Consulting Editor Note**
>
> In this book the Chapter-Specific Coding Guidelines are included here and in the Tabular List of Diseases and Injuries at the beginning of the chapter for which they are applicable.
>
> Additionally, notes have been added throughout the Diagnosis and Procedure Tabular to alert the coder when the code under review is included in a chapter specific coding guideline. The user can then reference the coding guideline prior to making their final code selection. For example:
>
> **A41 Other sepsis**
>
> **Review coding guideline C.1.d**
>
> This note alerts the coder to reference the chapter specific coding guidelines (C), chapter 1, guideline d, before making the final code selection. The guidelines for chapter 1, Certain Infectious and Parasitic Diseases, is located at the beginning of Chapter 1 in the Diagnosis Tabular. Please note that the coding guideline notes may be provided at the category, sub-category, or sub-classification level, whichever is applicable to the coding guidance.

In addition to general coding guidelines, there are guidelines for specific diagnoses and/or conditions in the classification. Unless otherwise indicated, these guidelines apply to all health care settings. Please refer to Section II for guidelines on the selection of principal diagnosis.

1. Chapter 1: Certain Infectious and Parasitic Diseases (A00-B99), U07.1 U09.9

a. Human Immunodeficiency Virus (HIV) Infections

1) Code only confirmed cases

Code only confirmed cases of HIV infection/illness. This is an exception to the hospital inpatient guideline Section II, H.

In this context, "confirmation" does not require documentation of positive serology or culture for HIV; the provider's diagnostic statement that the patient is HIV positive, or has an HIV-related illness is sufficient.

2) Selection and sequencing of HIV codes

(a) Patient admitted for HIV-related condition

If a patient is admitted for an HIV-related condition, the principal diagnosis should be B20, Human immunodeficiency virus [HIV] disease followed by additional diagnosis codes for all reported HIV-related conditions.

An exception to this guideline is if the reason for admission is hemolytic-uremic syndrome associated with HIV disease. Assign code D59.31, Infection-associated hemolytic-uremic syndrome, followed by code B20, Human immunodeficiency virus [HIV] disease.

(b) Patient with HIV disease admitted for unrelated condition

If a patient with HIV disease is admitted for an unrelated condition (such as a traumatic injury), the code for the unrelated condition (e.g., the nature of injury code) should be the principal diagnosis. Other diagnoses would be B20 followed by additional diagnosis codes for all reported HIV-related conditions.

(c) Whether the patient is newly diagnosed

Whether the patient is newly diagnosed or has had previous admissions/encounters for HIV conditions is irrelevant to the sequencing decision.

(d) Asymptomatic human immunodeficiency virus

Z21, Asymptomatic human immunodeficiency virus [HIV] infection status, is to be applied when the patient without any documentation of symptoms is listed as being "HIV positive," "known HIV," "HIV test positive," or similar terminology. Do not use this code if the term "AIDS" is used or if the patient is treated for any HIV-related illness or is described as having any condition(s) resulting from his/her HIV positive status; use B20 in these cases.

(e) Patients with inconclusive HIV serology

Patients with inconclusive HIV serology, but no definitive diagnosis or manifestations of the illness, may be assigned code R75, Inconclusive laboratory evidence of human immunodeficiency virus [HIV].

(f) Previously diagnosed HIV-related illness

Patients with any known prior diagnosis of an HIV-related illness should be coded to B20. Once a patient has developed an HIV-related illness, the patient should always be assigned code B20 on every subsequent admission/encounter. Patients previously diagnosed with any HIV illness (B20) should never be assigned to R75 or Z21, Asymptomatic human immunodeficiency virus [HIV] infection status.

(g) HIV Infection in Pregnancy, Childbirth and the Puerperium

During pregnancy, childbirth or the puerperium, a patient admitted (or presenting for a health care encounter) because of an HIV-related illness should receive a principal diagnosis code of O98.7-, Human immunodeficiency [HIV] disease complicating pregnancy, childbirth and the puerperium, followed by B20 and the code(s) for the HIV-related illness(es). Codes from Chapter 15 always take sequencing priority. Patients with asymptomatic HIV infection status admitted (or presenting for a health care encounter) during pregnancy, childbirth, or the puerperium should receive codes of O98.7- and Z21.

(h) Encounters for testing for HIV

If a patient is being seen to determine his/her HIV status, use code Z11.4, Encounter for screening for human immunodeficiency virus [HIV]. Use additional codes for any associated high risk behavior.

If a patient with signs or symptoms is being seen for HIV testing, code the signs and symptoms. An additional counseling code Z71.7, Human immunodeficiency virus [HIV] counseling, may be used if counseling is provided during the encounter for the test.

When a patient returns to be informed of his/her HIV test results and the test result is negative, use code Z71.7, Human immunodeficiency virus [HIV] counseling.

If the results are positive, see previous guidelines and assign codes as appropriate.

(i) HIV managed by antiretroviral medication

If a patient with documented history of HIV disease, HIV-related illness or AIDS is currently managed on antiretroviral medications, assign code B20, Human immunodeficiency virus [HIV] disease. Code Z79.899, Other long term (current) drug therapy, may be assigned as an additional code to identify the long-term (current) use of antiretroviral medications.

(j) Encounter for HIV Prophylaxis Measures

When a patient is seen for administration of pre-exposure prophylaxis medication for HIV, assign code Z29.81, Encounter for HIV pre-exposure prophylaxis. Pre-exposure prophylaxis (PrEP) is intended to prevent infection in people who are at risk for getting HIV through sex or injection drug use. Any risk factors for HIV should also be coded.

b. Infectious agents as the cause of diseases classified to other chapters

Certain infections are classified in chapters other than Chapter 1 and no organism is identified as part of the infection code. In these instances, it is necessary to use an additional code from Chapter 1 to identify the organism. A code from category B95, Streptococcus, Staphylococcus, and Enterococcus as the cause of diseases classified to other chapters, B96, Other bacterial agents as the cause of diseases classified to other chapters, or B97, Viral agents as the cause of diseases classified to other chapters, is to be used as an additional code to identify the organism. An instructional note will be found at the infection code advising that an additional organism code is required.

c. Infections resistant to antibiotics

Many bacterial infections are resistant to current antibiotics. It is necessary to identify all infections documented as antibiotic resistant. Assign a code from category Z16, Resistance to antimicrobial drugs, following the infection code only if the infection code does not identify drug resistance.

d. Sepsis, Severe Sepsis, and Septic Shock

1) Coding of Sepsis and Severe Sepsis

(a) Sepsis

For a diagnosis of sepsis, assign the appropriate code for the underlying systemic infection. If the type of infection or causal organism is not further specified, assign code A41.9, Sepsis, unspecified organism.

A code from subcategory R65.2, Severe sepsis, should not be assigned unless severe sepsis or an associated acute organ dysfunction is documented.

(i) Negative or inconclusive blood cultures and sepsis

Negative or inconclusive blood cultures do not preclude a diagnosis of sepsis in patients with clinical evidence of the condition, however, the provider should be queried.

(ii) Urosepsis

The term urosepsis is a nonspecific term. It is not to be considered synonymous with sepsis. It has no default code in the Alphabetic Index. Should a provider use this term, he/she must be queried for clarification.

(iii) Sepsis with organ dysfunction

If a patient has sepsis and associated acute organ dysfunction or multiple organ dysfunction (MOD), follow the instructions for coding severe sepsis.

(iv) Acute organ dysfunction that is not clearly associated with the sepsis

If a patient has sepsis and an acute organ dysfunction, but the medical record documentation indicates that the acute organ dysfunction is related to a medical condition other than the sepsis, do not assign a code from subcategory R65.2, Severe sepsis. An acute organ dysfunction must be associated with the sepsis in order to assign the severe sepsis code. If the documentation is not clear as to whether an acute organ dysfunction is related to the sepsis or another medical condition, query the provider.

(b) Severe sepsis

The coding of severe sepsis requires a minimum of 2 codes: first a code for the underlying systemic infection, followed by a code from subcategory R65.2, Severe sepsis. If the causal organism is not documented, assign code A41.9, Sepsis, unspecified organism, for the infection. Additional code(s) for the associated acute organ dysfunction are also required.

Due to the complex nature of severe sepsis, some cases may require querying the provider prior to assignment of the codes.

2) Septic shock

Septic shock generally refers to circulatory failure associated with severe sepsis, and therefore, it represents a type of acute organ dysfunction.

For cases of septic shock, the code for the systemic infection should be sequenced first, followed by code R65.21, Severe sepsis with septic shock or code T81.12, Postprocedural septic shock. Any additional codes for the other acute organ dysfunctions should also be assigned. As noted in the sequencing instructions in the Tabular List, the code for septic shock cannot be assigned as a principal diagnosis.

3) Sequencing of severe sepsis

If severe sepsis is present on admission, and meets the definition of principal diagnosis, the underlying systemic infection should be assigned as principal diagnosis followed by the appropriate code from subcategory R65.2 as required by the sequencing rules in the Tabular List. A code from subcategory R65.2 can never be assigned as a principal diagnosis.

When severe sepsis develops during an encounter (it was not present on admission) the underlying systemic infection and the appropriate code from subcategory R65.2 should be assigned as secondary diagnoses.

Severe sepsis may be present on admission but the diagnosis may not be confirmed until sometime after admission. If the documentation is not clear whether severe sepsis was present on admission, the provider should be queried.

For infection-associated hemolytic-uremic syndrome with severe sepsis, see guideline I.C.1.d.9.

4) Sepsis or severe sepsis with a localized infection

If the reason for admission is both sepsis or severe sepsis and a localized infection, such as pneumonia or cellulitis, a code(s) for the underlying systemic infection should be assigned first and the code for the localized infection should be assigned as a secondary diagnosis. If the patient has severe sepsis, a code from subcategory R65.2 should also be assigned as a secondary diagnosis. If the patient is admitted with a localized infection, such as pneumonia, and sepsis/severe sepsis doesn't develop until after admission, the localized infection should be assigned first, followed by the appropriate sepsis/severe sepsis codes.

For hemolytic-uremic syndrome associated with sepsis, see guideline I.C.1.d.9.

5) Sepsis due to a postprocedural infection

(a) Documentation of causal relationship

As with all postprocedural complications, code assignment is based on the provider's documentation of the relationship between the infection and the procedure.

(b) Sepsis due to a postprocedural infection

For **sepsis** following a **postprocedural wound (surgical site) infection**, a code from T81.41, to T81.43, Infection following a procedure, or a code from O86.00 to O86.03, Infection of obstetric surgical wound, that identifies the site of the infection should be **sequenced** first, if known. Assign an additional code for sepsis following a procedure (T81.44) or sepsis following an obstetrical procedure (O86.04). Use an additional code to identify the infectious agent. If the patient has severe sepsis the appropriate code from subcategory R65.2 should also be assigned with the additional code(s) for any acute organ dysfunction.

For infections following infusion, transfusion, therapeutic injection, or immunization, a code from subcategory T80.2, Infections following infusion, transfusion, and therapeutic injection, or code T88.0-, Infection following immunization, should be coded first, followed by the code for the specific infection. If the patient has severe sepsis, the appropriate code from subcategory R65.2 should also be assigned, with the additional code(s) for any acute organ dysfunction.

- (c) **Postprocedural infection and postprocedural septic shock**

    If a postprocedural infection has resulted in postprocedural septic shock, assign the codes indicated above for sepsis due to a postprocedural infection, followed by code T81.12-, Postprocedural septic shock. Do not assign code R65.21, Severe sepsis with septic shock. Additional code(s) should be assigned for any acute organ dysfunction.

6) **Sepsis and severe sepsis associated with a noninfectious process (condition)**

    In some cases a noninfectious process (condition), such as trauma, may lead to an infection which can result in sepsis or severe sepsis. If sepsis or severe sepsis is documented as associated with a noninfectious condition, such as a burn or serious injury, and this condition meets the definition for principal diagnosis, the code for the noninfectious condition should be sequenced first, followed by the code for the resulting infection. If severe sepsis, is present a code from subcategory R65.2 should also be assigned with any associated organ dysfunction(s) codes. It is not necessary to assign a code from subcategory R65.1, Systemic inflammatory response syndrome (SIRS) of non-infectious origin, for these cases.

    If the infection meets the definition of principal diagnosis it should be sequenced before the non-infectious condition. When both the associated non-infectious condition and the infection meet the definition of principal diagnosis either may be assigned as principal diagnosis.

    Only one code from category R65, Symptoms and signs specifically associated with systemic inflammation and infection, should be assigned. Therefore, when a non-infectious condition leads to an infection resulting in severe sepsis, assign the appropriate code from subcategory R65.2, Severe sepsis. Do not additionally assign a code from subcategory R65.1, Systemic inflammatory response syndrome (SIRS) of non-infectious origin.

    See Section I.C.18. SIRS due to non-infectious process

7) **Sepsis and septic shock complicating abortion, pregnancy, childbirth, and the puerperium**

    See Section I.C.15. Sepsis and septic shock complicating abortion, pregnancy, childbirth and the puerperium

8) **Newborn sepsis**

    See Section I.C.16. f. Bacterial sepsis of Newborn

9) **Hemolytic-uremic syndrome associated with sepsis**

    If the reason for admission is hemolytic-uremic syndrome that is associated with sepsis, assign code D59.31, Infection-associated hemolytic-uremic syndrome, as the principal diagnosis. Codes for the underlying systemic infection and any other conditions (such as severe sepsis) should be assigned as secondary diagnoses.

e. **Methicillin Resistant Staphylococcus aureus (MRSA) Conditions**

1) **Selection and sequencing of MRSA codes**

    (a) **Combination codes for MRSA infection**

    When a patient is diagnosed with an infection that is due to methicillin resistant Staphylococcus aureus (MRSA), and that infection has a combination code that includes the causal organism (e.g., sepsis, pneumonia) assign the appropriate combination code for the condition (e.g., code A41.02, Sepsis due to Methicillin resistant Staphylococcus aureus or code J15.212, Pneumonia due to Methicillin resistant Staphylococcus aureus). Do not assign code B95.62, Methicillin resistant Staphylococcus aureus infection as the cause of diseases classified elsewhere, as an additional code because the combination code includes the type of infection and the MRSA organism. Do not assign a code from subcategory Z16.11, Resistance to penicillins, as an additional diagnosis.

    See Section C.1. for instructions on coding and sequencing of sepsis and severe sepsis.

    (b) **Other codes for MRSA infection**

    When there is documentation of a current infection (e.g., wound infection, stitch abscess, urinary tract infection) due to MRSA, and that infection does not have a combination code that includes the causal organism, assign the appropriate code to identify the condition along with code B95.62, Methicillin resistant Staphylococcus aureus infection as the cause of diseases classified elsewhere for the MRSA infection. Do not assign a code from subcategory Z16.11, Resistance to penicillins.

    (c) **Methicillin susceptible Staphylococcus aureus (MSSA) and MRSA colonization**

    The condition or state of being colonized or carrying MSSA or MRSA is called colonization or carriage, while an individual person is described as being colonized or being a carrier. Colonization means that MSSA or MSRA is present on or in the body without necessarily causing illness. A positive MRSA colonization test might be documented by the provider as "MRSA screen positive" or "MRSA nasal swab positive".

Assign code Z22.322, Carrier or suspected carrier of Methicillin resistant Staphylococcus aureus, for patients documented as having MRSA colonization. Assign code Z22.321, Carrier or suspected carrier of Methicillin susceptible Staphylococcus aureus, for patient documented as having MSSA colonization. Colonization is not necessarily indicative of a disease process or as the cause of a specific condition the patient may have unless documented as such by the provider.

(d) MRSA colonization and infection

If a patient is documented as having both MRSA colonization and infection during a hospital admission, code Z22.322, Carrier or suspected carrier of Methicillin resistant Staphylococcus aureus, and a code for the MRSA infection may both be assigned.

f. Zika virus infections

1) Code only confirmed cases

Code only a confirmed diagnosis of Zika virus (A92.5, Zika virus disease) as documented by the provider. This is an exception to the hospital inpatient guideline Section II, H. In this context, "confirmation" does not require documentation of the type of test performed; the provider's diagnostic statement that the condition is confirmed is sufficient. This code should be assigned regardless of the stated mode of transmission.

If the provider documents "suspected", "possible" or "provable" Zika, do not assign code A92.5. Assign a code(s) explaining the reason for encounter (such as fever, rash, or joint pain) or Z20.821, Contact with and (suspected) exposure to Zika virus.

g. Coronavirus infections

1) COVID-19 infection (infection due to SARS-CoV-2)

(a) Code only confirmed cases

Code only a confirmed diagnosis of the 2019 novel coronavirus disease (COVID-19) as documented by the provider or documentation of a positive COVID-19 test result. For a confirmed diagnosis, assign code U07.1, COVID-19. This is an exception to the hospital inpatient guideline Section II, H. In this context, "confirmation" does not require documentation of a positive test result for COVID-19; the provider's documentation that the individual has COVID-19 is sufficient.

If the provider documents "suspected," "possible," "probable," or "inconclusive" COVID-19, do not assign code U07.1. Instead, code the signs and symptoms reported.

See guideline I.C.1.g.1.g.

(b) Sequencing of codes

When COVID-19 meets the definition of principle diagnosis, code U07.1, COVID-19, should be sequenced first, followed by the appropriate codes for associated manifestations, except when another guideline requires that certain codes be sequenced first, such as obstetrics, sepsis, or transplant complications.

For a COVID-19 infection that progresses to sepsis, see Section I.C.1.d Sepsis, Severe Sepsis, and Septic Shock

See Section I.C.15.s. for COVID-19 infection in pregnancy, childbirth, and the puerperium

See Section I.C.16.h. for COVID-19 infection in newborn

For a COVID-19 infection in a lung transplant patient, see Section I.C.19.g.3.a. Transplant complications other than kidney

(c) Acute respiratory manifestations of COVID-19

When the reason for the encounter/admission is a respiratory manifestation of COVID-19, assign code U07.1, COVID-19, as the principal/first-listed diagnosis and assign code(s) for the respiratory manifestation(s) as additional diagnoses.

The following conditions are examples of common respiratory manifestations of COVID-19.

(i) Pneumonia

For a patient with pneumonia confirmed as due to COVID-19, assign codes U07.1, COVID-19, and J12.82, Pneumonia due to coronavirus disease 2019.

(ii) Acute bronchitis

For a patient with acute bronchitis confirmed as due to COVID-19, assign codes U07.1, and J20.8, Acute bronchitis due to other specified organisms.

Bronchitis not otherwise specified (NOS) due to COVID-19 should be coded using code U07.1 and J40, Bronchitis, not specified as acute or chronic.

(iii) Lower respiratory infection

If the COVID-19 is documented as being associated with lower respiratory infection, not otherwise specified (NOS), or an acute respiratory infection, NOS, codes U07.1 and J22, Unspecified acute lower respiratory infection, should be assigned.

If the COVID-19 is documented as being associated with a respiratory infection, NOS, codes U07.1 and J98.8, Other specified respiratory disorders, should be assigned.

(iv) Acute respiratory distress syndrome

For acute respiratory distress syndrome (ARDS) due to COVID-19, assign codes U07.1 and J80, Acute respiratory distress syndrome

(v) Acute respiratory failure

For acute respiratory failure due to COVID-19, assign code U07.1 and code J96.0-, Acute respiratory failure.

(d) Non-respiratory manifestations of COVID-19

When the reason for the encounter/admission is a non-respiratory manifestation (e.g., viral enteritis) of COVID-19, assign code U07.1, COVID-19, as the principal/first-listed diagnosis and assign code(s) for the manifestation(s) as additional diagnoses.

(e) Exposure to COVID-19

For asymptomatic individuals with actual or suspected exposure to COVID-19, assign code Z20.822, Contact with and (suspected) exposure to COVID-19.

For symptomatic individuals with actual or suspected exposure to COVID-19 and the infection has been ruled out, or test results are inconclusive or unknown, assign code Z20.822, Contact with and (suspected) exposure to COVID-19.

See guidelines I.C.21.c.1, Contact/Exposure, for additional guidance regarding the use of category Z20 codes.

If COVID-19 is confirmed, see guidelines I.C.1.g.1.a.

(f) Screening for COVID-19

For screening for COVID-19, including preoperative testing, assign code Z11.52, Encounter for screening for COVID-19.

(g) Signs and symptoms without definitive diagnosis of COVID-19

For patient presenting with any signs/symptoms associated with COVID-19 (such as fever, etc.) but a definitive diagnosis has not been established, assign the appropriate code(s) for each of the presenting signs and symptoms such as:

- R05.1, Acute cough, or R05.9, Cough, unspecified
- R06.02 Shortness of breath
- R50.9 Fever, unspecified

If a patient with signs/symptoms associated with COVID-19 also has an actual or suspected contact with or exposure to COVID-19, assign Z20.828, Contact with and (suspected) exposure to other viral communicable diseases, as an additional code.

(h) Asymptomatic individuals who test positive for COVID-19

For asymptomatic individuals who test positive for COVID-19, *see guideline I.C.1.g.1.a.* Although the individual is asymptomatic, the individual has tested positive and is considered to have a COVID-19 infection.

(i) Personal history of COVID-19

For patients with a history of COVID-19, assign code Z86.16, Personal history of COVID-19.

(j) Follow-up visits after COVID-19 infection has resolved

For individuals who previously had COVID-19, without residual symptom(s) or condition(s) and are being seen for follow-up evaluation, and COVID-19 test results are negative, assign codes Z09, Encounter for follow-up examination after completed treatment for conditions other than malignant neoplasm, and Z86.16, Personal history of COVID-19. For follow-up visits for individuals with symptom(s) or condition(s) related to a previous COVID-19 infection, see guideline I.C.1.g.l.m.

See Section I.C.21.c.8, Factors influencing health states and contact with health services, Follow-up

(k) Encounter for antibody testing

For an encounter for antibody testing that is not being performed to confirm a current COVID-19 infection, nor is a follow-up test after resolution of COVID-19, assign Z01.84, Encounter for antibody response examination.

Follow the applicable guidelines above if the individual is being tested to confirm a current COVID-19 infection.

For follow-up testing after a COVID-19 infection, see guideline I.C.1.g.1.j.

(l) Multisystem Inflammatory Syndrome

For individuals with multisystem inflammatory syndrome (MIS) and COVID-19, assign code U07.1, COVID-19, as the principal/first-listed diagnosis and assign code M35.81, Multisystem inflammatory syndrome, as an additional diagnosis.

If an individual with a history of COVID-19 develops MIS, assign codes M35.81, Multisystem inflammatory syndrome, and U09.9, Post COVID-19 condition, unspecified.

If an individual with a known or suspected exposure to COVID-19, and no current COVID-19 infection or history of COVID-19, develops MIS, assign codes M5.81, Muyltisystem Inflammatory Syndrome, and Z20.822, Contact with and (suspected) exposure to COVID-19.

Additional codes should be assigned for any associated complications of MIS.

(m) Post COVID-19 Condition

For sequela of COVID-19, or associated symptoms or conditions that develop following a previous COVID-19 infection, assign a code(s) for the specific symptom(s) or condition(s) related to the previous COVID-19 infection, if known, and code U09.9, Post COVID-19 condition, unspecified.

Code U09.9 should not be assigned for manifestations of an active (current) COVID-19 infection.

If a patient has a condition(s) associated with a previous COVID-19 infection and develops a new active (current) COVID-19 infection, code U09.9 may be assigned in conjunction with code U07.1, COVID-19, to identify that the patient also has a condition(s) associated with a previous COVID-19 infection. Code(s) for the specific condition(s) associated with the previous COVID-19 infection and code(s) for manifestation(s) of the new active (current) COVID-19 infection should also be assigned.

(n) Underimmunization for COVID-19 Status

Code Z28.310, Unvaccinated for COVID-19, may be assigned when the patient has not received a COVID-19 vaccine of any type. Code Z28.311, Partially vaccinated for COVID-19, may be assigned when the patient has been partially vaccinated for COVID-19 as per the recommendations of the Centers for Disease Control and Prevention (CDC) in place at the time of the encounter. For information, visit the CDC's website https://www.cdc.gov/coronavirus/2019-ncov/vaccines/.

See Section I.B.14. for underimmunization documentation by clinicians other than patient's provider.

2. Chapter 2: Neoplasms (C00-D49)
General guidelines

Chapter 2 of the ICD-10-CM contains the codes for most benign and all malignant neoplasms. Certain benign neoplasms, such as prostatic adenomas, may be found in the specific body system chapters. To properly code a neoplasm it is necessary to determine from the record if the neoplasm is benign, in-situ, malignant, or of uncertain histologic behavior. If malignant, any secondary (metastatic) sites should also be determined.

Primary malignant neoplasms overlapping site boundaries

A primary malignant neoplasm that overlaps two or more contiguous (next to each other) sites should be classified to the subcategory/code .8 ('overlapping lesion'), unless the combination is specifically indexed elsewhere. For multiple neoplasms of the same site that are not contiguous such as tumors in different quadrants of the same breast, codes for each site should be assigned.

Malignant neoplasm of ectopic tissue

Malignant neoplasms of ectopic tissue are to be coded to the site of origin mentioned, e.g., ectopic pancreatic malignant neoplasms involving the stomach are coded to malignant neoplasm of pancreas, unspecified (C25.9).

The neoplasm table in the Alphabetic Index should be referenced first. However, if the histological term is documented, that term should be referenced first, rather than going immediately to the Neoplasm Table, in order to determine which column in the Neoplasm Table is appropriate. For example, if the documentation indicates "adenoma," refer to the term in the Alphabetic Index to review the entries under this term and the instructional note to "see also neoplasm, by site, benign." The table provides the proper code based on the type of neoplasm and the site. It is important to select the proper column in the table that corresponds to the type of neoplasm. The Tabular List should then be referenced to verify that the correct code has been selected from the table and that a more specific site code does not exist.

See Section I.C.21. Factors influencing health status and contact with health services, Status, for information regarding Z15.0, codes for genetic susceptibility to cancer.

a. Admission/Encounter for treatment of primary site

If the malignancy is chiefly responsible for occasioning the patient admission/encounter and treatment is directed at the primary site, designate the primary malignancy as the principal/first-listed diagnosis.

The only exception to this guideline is if the administration of chemotherapy, immunotherapy or external beam radiation therapy is chiefly responsible for occasioning the admission/encounter. In that case, assign the appropriate Z51.-- code as the first-listed or principal diagnosis, and the underlying diagnosis or problem for which the service is being performed as a secondary diagnosis.

b. Admission/Encounter for treatment of secondary site

When a patient is admitted because of a primary neoplasm with metastasis and treatment is directed toward the secondary site only, the secondary neoplasm is designated as the principal diagnosis even though the primary malignancy is still present.

c. Coding and sequencing of complications

Coding and sequencing of complications associated with the malignancies or with the therapy thereof are subject to the following guidelines:

1) Anemia associated with malignancy

When admission/encounter is for management of an anemia associated with the malignancy, and the treatment is only for anemia, the appropriate code for the malignancy is sequenced as the principal or first-listed diagnosis followed by the appropriate code for the anemia (such as code D63.0, Anemia in neoplastic disease).

2) Anemia associated with chemotherapy, immunotherapy and radiation therapy

When the admission/encounter is for management of an anemia associated with an adverse effect of the administration of chemotherapy or immunotherapy and the only treatment is for the anemia, the anemia code is sequenced first followed by the appropriate codes for the neoplasm and the adverse effect (T45.1X5, Adverse effect of antineoplastic and immunosuppressive drugs).

When the admission/encounter is for management of an anemia associated with an adverse effect of radiotherapy, the anemia code should be sequenced first, followed by the appropriate neoplasm code and code Y84.2, Radiological procedure and radiotherapy as the cause of abnormal reaction of the patient, or of later complication, without mention of misadventure at the time of the procedure.

3) Management of dehydration due to the malignancy

When the admission/encounter is for management of dehydration due to the malignancy and only the dehydration is being treated (intravenous rehydration), the dehydration is sequenced first, followed by the code(s) for the malignancy.

4) Treatment of a complication resulting from a surgical procedure

When the admission/encounter is for treatment of a complication resulting from a surgical procedure, designate the complication as the principal or first-listed diagnosis if treatment is directed at resolving the complication.

d. Primary malignancy previously excised

When a primary malignancy has been previously excised or eradicated from its site and there is no further treatment directed to that site and there is no evidence of any existing primary malignancy at that site, a code from category Z85, Personal history of malignant neoplasm, should be used to indicate the former site of the malignancy. Any mention of extension, invasion, or metastasis to another site is coded as a secondary malignant neoplasm to that site. The secondary site may be the principal or first-listed diagnosis with the Z85 code used as a secondary code.

See section I.C.2.t. Secondary malignant neoplasm of lymphoid tissue.

e. Admissions/Encounters involving chemotherapy, immunotherapy and radiation therapy

1) Episode of care involves surgical removal of neoplasm

When an episode of care involves the surgical removal of a neoplasm, primary or secondary site, followed by adjunct chemotherapy or radiation treatment during the same episode of care, the code for the neoplasm should be assigned as principal or first-listed diagnosis.

2) Patient admission/encounter chiefly for administration of chemotherapy, immunotherapy and radiation therapy

If a patient admission/encounter is **chiefly** for the administration of chemotherapy, immunotherapy or external beam radiation therapy assign code Z51.0, Encounter for antineoplastic radiation therapy, or Z51.11, Encounter for antineoplastic chemotherapy, or Z51.12, Encounter for antineoplastic immunotherapy as the first-listed or principal diagnosis. If a patient receives more than one of these therapies during the same admission more than one of these codes may be assigned, in any sequence.

The malignancy for which the therapy is being administered should be assigned as a secondary diagnosis.

If a patient admission/encounter is for the insertion or implantation of radioactive elements (e.g., brachytherapy) the appropriate code for the malignancy is sequenced as the principal or first-listed diagnosis. Code Z51.0 should not be assigned.

3) Patient admitted for radiation therapy, chemotherapy or immunotherapy and develops complications

When a patient is admitted for the purpose of external beam radiotherapy, immunotherapy or chemotherapy and develops complications such as uncontrolled nausea and vomiting or dehydration, the principal or first-listed diagnosis is Z51.0, Encounter for antineoplastic radiation therapy, or Z51.11, Encounter for antineoplastic chemotherapy, or Z51.12, Encounter for antineoplastic immunotherapy followed by any codes for the complications.

When a patient is admitted for the purpose of insertion or implantation of radioactive elements (e.g., brachytherapy) and develops complications such as uncontrolled nausea and vomiting or dehydration, the principal or first-listed diagnosis is the appropriate code for the malignancy followed by any codes for the complications.

f. Admission/encounter to determine extent of malignancy

When the reason for admission/encounter is to determine the extent of the malignancy, or for a procedure such as paracentesis or thoracentesis, the primary malignancy or appropriate metastatic site is designated as the principal or first-listed diagnosis, even though chemotherapy or radiotherapy is administered.

g. Symptoms, signs, and abnormal findings listed in Chapter 18 associated with neoplasms

Symptoms, signs, and ill-defined conditions listed in Chapter 18 characteristic of, or associated with, an existing primary or secondary site malignancy cannot be used to replace the malignancy as principal or first-listed diagnosis, regardless of the number of admissions or encounters for treatment and care of the neoplasm.

See section I.C.21. Factors influencing health status and contact with health services, Encounter for prophylactic organ removal.

h. Admission/encounter for pain control/management

See Section I.C.6. for information on coding admission/encounter for pain control/management.

i. Malignancy in two or more noncontiguous sites

A patient may have more than one malignant tumor in the same organ. These tumors may represent different primaries or metastatic disease, depending on the site. Should the documentation be unclear, the provider should be queried as to the status of each tumor so that the correct codes can be assigned.

j. Disseminated malignant neoplasm, unspecified

Code C80.0, Disseminated malignant neoplasm, unspecified, is for use only in those cases where the patient has advanced metastatic disease and no known primary or secondary sites are specified. It should not be used in place of assigning codes for the primary site and all known secondary sites.

k. Malignant neoplasm without specification of site

Code C80.1, Malignant (primary) neoplasm, unspecified, equates to Cancer, unspecified. This code should only be used when no determination can be made as to the primary site of a malignancy. This code should rarely be used in the inpatient setting.

l. Sequencing of neoplasm codes

1) Encounter for treatment of primary malignancy

If the reason for the encounter is for treatment of a primary malignancy, assign the malignancy as the principal/first-listed diagnosis. The primary site is to be sequenced first, followed by any metastatic sites.

2) Encounter for treatment of secondary malignancy

When an encounter is for a primary malignancy with metastasis and treatment is directed toward the metastatic (secondary) site(s) only, the metastatic site(s) is designated as the principal/first-listed diagnosis. The primary malignancy is coded as an additional code.

3) Malignant neoplasm in a pregnant patient

When a pregnant woman has a malignant neoplasm, a code from subcategory O9A.1-, Malignant neoplasm complicating pregnancy, childbirth, and the puerperium, should be sequenced first, followed by the appropriate code from Chapter 2 to indicate the type of neoplasm.

4) Encounter for complication associated with a neoplasm

When an encounter is for management of a complication associated with a neoplasm, such as dehydration, and the treatment is only for the complication, the complication is coded first, followed by the appropriate code(s) for the neoplasm.

The exception to this guideline is anemia. When the admission/encounter is for management of an anemia associated with the malignancy, and the treatment is only for anemia, the appropriate code for the malignancy is sequenced as the principal or first-listed diagnosis followed by code D63.0, Anemia in neoplastic disease.

5) Complication from surgical procedure for treatment of a neoplasm

When an encounter is for treatment of a complication resulting from a surgical procedure performed for the treatment of the neoplasm, designate the complication as the principal/first-listed diagnosis. See the guideline regarding the coding of a current malignancy versus personal history to determine if the code for the neoplasm should also be assigned.

6) Pathologic fracture due to a neoplasm

When an encounter is for a pathological fracture due to a neoplasm, and the focus of treatment is the fracture, a code from subcategory M84.5, Pathological fracture in neoplastic disease, should be sequenced first, followed by the code for the neoplasm.

If the focus of treatment is the neoplasm with an associated pathological fracture, the neoplasm code should be sequenced first, followed by a code from M84.5 for the pathological fracture.

m. Current malignancy versus personal history of malignancy

When a primary malignancy has been excised but further treatment, such as an additional surgery for the malignancy, radiation therapy or chemotherapy is directed to that site, the primary malignancy code should be used until treatment is completed.

When a primary malignancy has been previously excised or eradicated from its site, there is no further treatment (of the malignancy) directed to that site, and there is no evidence of any existing primary malignancy at that site, a code from category Z85, Personal history of malignant neoplasm, should be used to indicate the former site of the malignancy.

Subcategories Z85.0-Z85.7 should only be assigned for the former site of a primary malignancy, not the site of a secondary malignancy. Codes from subcategory Z85.8-, may be assigned for the former site(s) of either a primary or secondary malignancy included in this subcategory.

See Section I.C.21. Factors influencing health status and contact with health services, History (of)

n. Leukemia, Multiple Myeloma, and Malignant Plasma Cell Neoplasms in remission versus personal history

The categories for leukemia, and category C90, Multiple myeloma and malignant plasma cell neoplasms, have codes indicating whether or not the leukemia has achieved remission. There are also codes Z85.6, Personal history of leukemia, and Z85.79, Personal history of other malignant neoplasms of lymphoid, hematopoietic and related tissues. If the documentation is unclear, as to whether the leukemia has achieved remission, the provider should be queried.

See Section I.C.21. Factors influencing health status and contact with health services, History (of)

o. Aftercare following surgery for neoplasm

See Section I.C.21. Factors influencing health status and contact with health services, Aftercare

p. Follow-up care for completed treatment of a malignancy

See Section I.C.21. Factors influencing health status and contact with health services, Follow-up

q. Prophylactic organ removal for prevention of malignancy

See Section I.C. 21, Factors influencing health status and contact with health services, Prophylactic organ removal

r. Malignant neoplasm associated with transplanted organ

A malignant neoplasm of a transplanted organ should be coded as a transplant complication. Assign first the appropriate code from category T86.-, Complications of transplanted organs and tissue, followed by code C80.2, Malignant neoplasm associated with transplanted organ. Use an additional code for the specific malignancy.

s. Breast Implant Associated Anaplastic Large Cell Lymphoma

Breast implant associated anaplastic large cell lymphoma (BIA-ALCL) is a type of lymphoma that can develop around breast implants. Assign code C84.7A, Anaplastic large cell lymphoma, ALK-negative, breast, for BIA-ALCL. Do not assign a complication code from chapter 19.

t. Secondary malignant neoplasm of lymphoid tissue

When a malignant neoplasm of lymphoid tissue metastasizes beyond the lymph nodes, a code from categories C81-C85 with a final character "9" should be assigned identifying "extranodal and solid organ sites" rather than a code for the secondary neoplasm of the affected solid organ. For example, for metastasis **diffuse large** of B-cell lymphoma to the lung, brain and left adrenal gland, assign code C83.39, Diffuse large B-cell lymphoma, extranodal and solid organ sites.

3. **Chapter 3: Diseases of the Blood and Blood-Forming Organs and Certain Disorders Involving the Immune Mechanism (D50-D89)**

    Reserved for future guideline expansion

4. **Chapter 4: Endocrine, Nutritional and Metabolic Diseases (E00-E89)**

    a. **Diabetes mellitus**

    The diabetes mellitus codes are combination codes that include the type of diabetes mellitus, the body system affected, and the complications affecting that body system. As many codes within a particular category as are necessary to describe all of the complications of the disease may be used. They should be sequenced based on the reason for a particular encounter. Assign as many codes from categories E08 – E13 as needed to identify all of the associated conditions that the patient has.

    1) **Type of diabetes**

        The age of a patient is not the sole determining factor, though most type 1 diabetics develop the condition before reaching puberty. For this reason type 1 diabetes mellitus is also referred to as juvenile diabetes.

    2) **Type of diabetes mellitus not documented**

        If the type of diabetes mellitus is not documented in the medical record the default is E11.-, Type 2 diabetes mellitus.

    3) **Diabetes mellitus and the use of insulin and oral hypoglycemics**

        If the documentation in a medical record does not indicate the type of diabetes but does indicate that the patient uses insulin, code E11-, Type 2 diabetes mellitus, should be assigned. Additional code(s) should be assigned from category Z79 to identify the long-term (current) use of insulin, oral hypoglycemic drugs, or injectable non-insulin antidiabetic, as follows:

        If the patient is treated with both oral hypoglycemic drugs and insulin, both code Z79.4, Long term (current) use of insulin, and code Z79.84, Long term (current) use of oral hypoglycemic drugs, should be assigned. If the patient is treated with both insulin and an injectable non-insulin antidiabetic drug, assign codes Z79.4, Long-term (current) use of insulin, and Z79.85, Long-term (current) use of injectable non-insulin antidiabetic drugs. If the patient is treated with both oral hypoglycemic drugs and an injectable non-insulin antidiabetic drug, assign codes Z79.84, Long-term (current) use of oral hypoglycemic drugs, and Z79.85, Long-term (current) use of injectable non-insulin antidiabetic drugs. Code Z79.4 should not be assigned if insulin is given temporarily to bring a type 2 patient's blood sugar under control during an encounter.

    4) **Diabetes mellitus in pregnancy and gestational diabetes**

        See Section I.C.15. Diabetes mellitus in pregnancy.

        See Section I.C.15. Gestational (pregnancy induced) diabetes

    5) **Complications due to insulin pump malfunction**

        (a) **Underdose of insulin due to insulin pump failure**

            An underdose of insulin due to an insulin pump failure should be assigned to a code from subcategory T85.6, Mechanical complication of other specified internal and external prosthetic devices, implants and grafts, that specifies the type of pump malfunction, as the principal or first-listed code, followed by code T38.3x6-, Underdosing of insulin and oral hypoglycemic [antidiabetic] drugs. Additional codes for the type of diabetes mellitus and any associated complications due to the underdosing should also be assigned.

        (b) **Overdose of insulin due to insulin pump failure**

            The principal or first-listed code for an encounter due to an insulin pump malfunction resulting in an overdose of insulin, should also be T85.6-, Mechanical complication of other specified internal and external prosthetic devices, implants and grafts, followed by code T38.3x1-, Poisoning by insulin and oral hypoglycemic [antidiabetic] drugs, accidental (unintentional).

    6) **Secondary diabetes mellitus**

        Codes under categories E08, Diabetes mellitus due to underlying condition, E09, Drug or chemical induced diabetes mellitus, and E13, Other specified diabetes mellitus, identify complications/manifestations associated with secondary diabetes mellitus. Secondary diabetes is always caused by another condition or event (e.g., cystic fibrosis, malignant neoplasm of pancreas, pancreatectomy, adverse effect of drug, or poisoning).

        (a) **Secondary diabetes mellitus and the use of insulin or oral hypoglycemic drugs**

            For patients with secondary diabetes mellitus who routinely use insulin or oral hypoglycemic drugs, or injectable non-insulin drugs, an additional code from category Z79 should be assigned to identify the long-term (current) use of insulin, oral hypoglycemic drugs, or non-injectable non-insulin drugs as follows:

If the patient is treated with both oral hypoglycemic drugs and insulin, both code Z79.4, Long term (current) use of insulin, and code Z79.84, Long term (current) use of oral hypoglycemic drugs, should be assigned. If the patient is treated with both insulin and an injectable non-insulin antidiabetic drug, assign codes Z79.4, Long-term (current) use of insulin, and Z79.85, Long-term (current) use of injectable non-insulin antidiabetic drugs. If the patient is treated with both oral hypoglycemic drugs and an injectable non-insulin antidiabetic drug, assign codes Z79.84, Long-term (current) use of oral hypoglycemic drugs, and Z79.85, Long-term (current) use of injectable non-insulin antidiabetic drugs. Code Z79.4 should not be assigned if insulin is given temporarily to bring a secondary diabetic patient's blood sugar under control during an encounter.

(b) Assigning and sequencing secondary diabetes codes and its causes

The sequencing of the secondary diabetes codes in relationship to codes for the cause of the diabetes is based on the Tabular List instructions for categories E08, E09 and E13.

(i) Secondary diabetes mellitus due to pancreatectomy

For postpancreatectomy diabetes mellitus (lack of insulin due to the surgical removal of all or part of the pancreas), assign code E89.1, Postprocedural hypoinsulinemia. Assign a code from category E13 and a code from subcategory Z90.41-, Acquired absence of pancreas, as additional codes.

(ii) Secondary diabetes due to drugs

Secondary diabetes may be caused by an adverse effect of correctly administered medications, poisoning or sequela of poisoning.

See section I.C.19.e for coding of adverse effects and poisoning, and section I.C.20 for external cause code reporting.

5. Chapter 5: Mental, Behavioral and Neurodevelopmental Disorders (F01-F99)

a. Pain disorders related to psychological factors

Assign code F45.41, for pain that is exclusively related to psychological disorders. As indicated by the Excludes 1 note under category G89, a code from category G89 should not be assigned with code F45.41

Code F45.42, Pain disorders with related psychological factors, should be used with a code from category G89, Pain, not elsewhere classified, if there is documentation of a psychological component for a patient with acute or chronic pain.

See Section I.C.6. Pain

b. Mental and behavioral disorders due to psychoactive substance use

1) In Remission

Selection of codes describing "in remission" for categories F10-F19, Mental and behavioral disorders due to psychoactive substance use (categories F10-F19 with -.11, -.21, -91) requires the provider's clinical judgment and are assigned only on the basis of provider documentation (as defined in the Official Guidelines for Coding and Reporting), unless otherwise instructed by the classification.

Mild substance use disorders in early or sustained remission are classified to the appropriate codes for substance abuse in remission, and moderate or severe substance use disorders in early or sustained remission are classified to the appropriate codes for substance dependence in remission.

2) Psychoactive Substance Use, Abuse And Dependence

When the provider documentation refers to use, abuse and dependence of the same substance (e.g. alcohol, opioid, cannabis, etc.), only one code should be assigned to identify the pattern of use based on the following hierarchy:

- If both use and abuse are documented, assign only the code for abuse
- If both abuse and dependence are documented, assign only the code for dependence
- If use, abuse and dependence are all documented, assign only the code for dependence
- If both use and dependence are documented, assign only the code for dependence.

3) Psychoactive Substance Use Unspecified

As with all other unspecified diagnoses, the codes for unspecified psychoactive substance use disorders (F10.9-, F11.9-, F12.9-, F13.9-, F14.9-, F15.9-, F16.9-, F18.9-, F19.9-) should only be assigned based on provider documentation and when they meet the definition of a reportable diagnosis (see Section III, Reporting Additional Diagnoses). These codes are to be used only when the psychoactive substance use is associated with a substance related disorder (chapter 5 disorders such as sexual dysfunction, sleep disorder, or a mental or behavioral disorder) or medical condition, mental or behavioral disorder, and such a relationship is documented by the provider.

4) Medical Conditions Due to Psychoactive Substance Use, Abuse and Dependence

Medical conditions due to substance use, abuse, and dependence are not classified as substance-induced disorders. Assign the diagnosis code for the medical condition as directed by the Alphabetical Index along with the appropriate psychoactive substance use, abuse or dependence code. For example, for alcoholic pancreatitis due to alcohol dependence, assign the appropriate code from subcategory K85.2, Alcohol induced acute pancreatitis, and the appropriate code from subcategory F10.2, such as code F10.20, Alcohol dependence, uncomplicated. It would not be appropriate to assign code F10.288, Alcohol dependence with other alcohol-induced disorder.

5) Blood Alcohol Level

A code from category Y90, Evidence of alcohol involvement determined by blood alcohol level, may be assigned when this information is documented and the patient's provider has documented a condition classifiable to category F10, Alcohol related disorders. The blood alcohol level does not need to be documented by the patient's provider in order for it to be coded.

See Section I.B.14. for blood alcohol level documentation by clinicians other than patient's provider.

c. Factitious Disorder

Factitious disorder imposed on self or Munchausen's syndrome is a disorder in which a person falsely reports or causes his or her own physical or psychological signs or symptoms. For patients with documented factitious disorder on self or Munchausen's syndrome, assign the appropriate code from subcategory F68.1-, Factitious disorder imposed on self.

Munchausen's syndrome by proxy (MSBP) is a disorder in which a caregiver (perpetrator) falsely reports or causes an illness or injury in another person (victim) under his or her care, such as a child, an elderly adult, or a person who has a disability. The conditions is also referred to as "factitious disorder imposed on another" or "factitious disorder by proxy." The perpetrator, not the victim, receives this diagnosis. Assign code F68.A, Factitious disorder imposed on another, to the perpetrator's record. For the victim of a patient suffering from MSBP, assign the appropriate code from categories T74, Adult and child abuse, neglect and other maltreatment, confirmed, or T76, Adult and child abuse, neglect and other maltreatment, suspected.

See Section I.C.19.f. Adult and child abuse, neglect and other maltreatment

d. Dementia

The ICD-10-CM classifies dementia (categories F01, F02, and F03) on the basis of the etiology and severity (unspecified, mild, moderate or severe). Selection of the appropriate severity level requires the provider's clinical judgment and codes should be assigned only on the basis of provider documentation (as defined in the *Official Guidelines for Coding and Reporting*), unless otherwise instructed by the classification. If the documentation does not provide information about the severity of the dementia, assign the appropriate code for unspecified severity.

If a patient is admitted to an inpatient acute care hospital or other inpatient facility setting with dementia at one severity level and it progresses to a higher severity level, assign one code for the highest severity level reported during the stay.

6. Chapter 6: Diseases of the Nervous System (G00-G99)

a. Dominant/nondominant side

Codes from category G81, Hemiplegia and hemiparesis, and subcategories, G83.1, Monoplegia of lower limb, G83.2, Monoplegia of upper limb, and G83.3, Monoplegia, unspecified, identify whether the dominant or nondominant side is affected. Should the affected side be documented, but not specified as dominant or nondominant, and the classification system does not indicate a default, code selection is as follows:

- For ambidextrous patients, the default should be dominant.
- If the left side is affected, the default is non-dominant.
- If the right side is affected, the default is dominant.

b. Pain-Category G89

1) General coding information

Codes in category G89, Pain, not elsewhere classified, may be used in conjunction with codes from other categories and chapters to provide more detail about acute or chronic pain and neoplasm-related pain, unless otherwise indicated below.

If the pain is not specified as acute or chronic, post- thoracotomy, post procedural, or neoplasm-related, do not assign codes from category G89.

A code from category G89 should not be assigned if the underlying (definitive) diagnosis is known, unless the reason for the encounter is pain control/management and not management of the underlying condition.

When an admission or encounter is for a procedure aimed at treating the underlying condition (e.g., spinal fusion, kyphoplasty), a code for the underlying condition (e.g., vertebral fracture, spinal stenosis) should be assigned as the principal diagnosis. No code from category G89 should be assigned.

(a) Category G89 Codes as Principal or First-Listed Diagnosis

Category G89 codes are acceptable as principal diagnosis or the first-listed code:

- When pain control or pain management is the reason for the admission/encounter (e.g., a patient with displaced intervertebral disc, nerve impingement and severe back pain presents for injection of steroid into the spinal canal). The underlying cause of the pain should be reported as an additional diagnosis, if known.
- When a patient is admitted for the insertion of a neurostimulator for pain control, assign the appropriate pain code as the principal or first-listed diagnosis. When an admission or encounter is for a procedure aimed at treating the underlying condition and a neurostimulator is inserted for pain control during the same admission/encounter, a code for the underlying condition should be assigned as the principal diagnosis and the appropriate pain code should be assigned as a secondary diagnosis.

(b) Use of Category G89 Codes in Conjunction with Site Specific Pain Codes

(i) Assigning Category G89 and Site-Specific Pain Codes

Codes from category G89 may be used in conjunction with codes that identify the site of pain (including codes from chapter 18) if the category G89 code provides additional information. For example, if the code describes the site of the pain, but does not fully describe whether the pain is acute or chronic, then both codes should be assigned.

(ii) Sequencing of Category G89 Codes with Site- Specific Pain Codes

The sequencing of category G89 codes with site-specific pain codes (including chapter 18 codes), is dependent on the circumstances of the encounter/admission as follows:

- If the encounter is for pain control or pain management, assign the code from category G89 followed by the code identifying the specific site of pain (e.g., encounter for pain management for acute neck pain from trauma is assigned code G89.11, Acute pain due to trauma, followed by code M54.2, Cervicalgia, to identify the site of pain).
- If the encounter is for any other reason except pain control or pain management, and a related definitive diagnosis has not been established (confirmed) by the provider, assign the code for the specific site of pain first, followed by the appropriate code from category G89.

2) Pain due to devices, implants and grafts

See Section I.C.19. Pain due to medical devices

3) Postoperative Pain

The provider's documentation should be used to guide the coding of postoperative pain, as well as *Section III. Reporting Additional Diagnoses and Section IV. Diagnostic Coding* and *Reporting in the Outpatient Setting.*

The default for post-thoracotomy and other postoperative pain not specified as acute or chronic is the code for the acute form.

Routine or expected postoperative pain immediately after surgery should not be coded.

(a) Postoperative pain not associated with specific postoperative complication

Postoperative pain not associated with a specific postoperative complication is assigned to the appropriate postoperative pain code in category G89.

(b) Postoperative pain associated with specific postoperative complication

Postoperative pain associated with a specific postoperative complication (such as painful wire sutures) is assigned to the appropriate code(s) found in Chapter 19, Injury, poisoning, and certain other consequences of external causes. If appropriate, use additional code(s) from category G89 to identify acute or chronic pain (G89.18 or G89.28).

4) Chronic pain

Chronic pain is classified to subcategory G89.2. There is no time frame defining when pain becomes chronic pain. The provider's documentation should be used to guide use of these codes.

5) Neoplasm Related Pain

Code G89.3 is assigned to pain documented as being related, associated or due to cancer, primary or secondary malignancy, or tumor. This code is assigned regardless of whether the pain is acute or chronic.

This code may be assigned as the principal or first-listed code when the stated reason for the admission/encounter is documented as pain control/pain management. The underlying neoplasm should be reported as an additional diagnosis.

When the reason for the admission/encounter is management of the neoplasm and the pain associated with the neoplasm is also documented, code G89.3 may be assigned as an additional diagnosis. It is not necessary to assign an additional code for the site of the pain.

See Section I.C.2 for instructions on the sequencing of neoplasms for all other stated reasons for the admission/encounter (except for pain control/pain management).

6) Chronic pain syndrome

Central pain syndrome (G89.0) and chronic pain syndrome (G89.4) are different than the term "chronic pain," and therefore codes should only be used when the provider has specifically documented this condition.

See Section I.C.5. Pain disorders related to psychological factors

7. Chapter 7: Diseases of the Eye and Adnexa (H00-H59)

a. Glaucoma

1) Assigning Glaucoma Codes

Assign as many codes from category H40, Glaucoma, as needed to identify the type of glaucoma, the affected eye, and the glaucoma stage.

2) Bilateral glaucoma with same type and stage

When a patient has bilateral glaucoma and both eyes are documented as being the same type and stage, and there is a code for bilateral glaucoma, report only the code for the type of glaucoma, bilateral, with the seventh character for the stage.

When a patient has bilateral glaucoma and both eyes are documented as being the same type and stage, and the classification does not provide a code for bilateral glaucoma (i.e. subcategories H40.10, H40.11 and H40.20) report only one code for the type of glaucoma with the appropriate seventh character for the stage.

3) Bilateral glaucoma stage with different types or stages

When a patient has bilateral glaucoma and each eye is documented as having a different type or stage, and the classification distinguishes laterality, assign the appropriatecode for each eye rather than the code for bilateral glaucoma.

When a patient has bilateral glaucoma and each eye is documented as having a different type, and the classification does not distinguish laterality (i.e. subcategories H40.10, H40.11 and H40.20), assign one code for each type of glaucoma with the appropriate seventh character for the stage.

When a patient has bilateral glaucoma and each eye is documented as having the same type, but different stage, and the classification does not distinguish laterality (i.e. subcategories H40.10, H40.11 and H40.20), assign a code for the type of glaucoma for each eye with the seventh character for the specific glaucoma stage documented for each eye.

4) Patient admitted with glaucoma and stage evolves during the admission

If a patient is admitted with glaucoma and the stage progresses during the admission, assign the code for highest stage documented.

5) Indeterminate stage glaucoma

Assignment of the seventh character "4" for "indeterminate stage" should be based on the clinical documentation. The seventh character "4" is used for glaucomas whose stage cannot be clinically determined. This seventh character should not be confused with the seventh character "0", unspecified, which should be assigned when there is no documentation regarding the stage of the glaucoma.

b. Blindness

If "blindness" or "low vision" of both eyes is documented but the visual impairment category is not documented, assign code H54.3, Unqualified visual loss, both eyes. If "blindness" or "low vision" in one eye is documented but the visual impairment category is not documented, assign a code from H54.6-, Unqualified visual loss, one eye. If "blindness" or "visual loss" is documented without any information about whether one or both eyes are affected, assign code H54.7, Unspecified visual loss.

8. **Chapter 8: Diseases of the Ear and Mastoid Process (H60-H95)**

   Reserved for future guideline expansion

9. **Chapter 9: Diseases of the Circulatory System (I00-I99)**

   a. **Hypertension**

   The classification presumes a causal relationship between hypertension and heart involvement and between hypertension and kidney involvement, as the two conditions are linked by the term "with" in the Alphabetic Index. These conditions should be coded as related even in the absence of provider documentation explicitly linking them, unless the documentation clearly states the conditions are unrelated.

   For hypertension and conditions not specifically linked by relational terms such as "with," "associated with" or "due to" in the classification, provider documentation must link the conditions in order to code them as related.

   1) **Hypertension with Heart Disease**

   Hypertension with heart conditions classified to I50.- or I51.4-I51.7, I51.89, I51.9, are assigned to, a code from category I11, Hypertensive heart disease. Use an additional code(s) from category I50, Heart failure, to identify the type(s) of heart failure in those patients with heart failure.

   The same heart conditions (I50.-, I51.4-I51.7, I51.89, I51.9) with hypertension are coded separately if the provider has documented they are unrelated to the hypertension. Sequence according to the circumstances of the admission/encounter.

   2) **Hypertensive Chronic Kidney Disease**

   Assign codes from category I12, Hypertensive chronic kidney disease, when both hypertension and a condition classifiable to category N18, Chronic kidney disease (CKD), are present. CKD should not be coded as hypertensive if the provider indicates the CKD is not related to the hypertension.

   The appropriate code from category N18 should be used as a secondary code with a code from category I12 to identify the stage of chronic kidney disease.

   See Section I.C.14. Chronic kidney disease.

   If a patient has hypertensive chronic kidney disease and acute renal failure, the acute renal failure should also be coded. Sequence according to the circumstances of the admission/encounter.

   3) **Hypertensive Heart and Chronic Kidney Disease**

   Assign codes from combination category I13, Hypertensive heart and chronic kidney disease, when there is hypertension with both heart and kidney involvement. If heart failure is present, assign an additional code from category I50 to identify the type of heart failure.

   The appropriate code from category N18, Chronic kidney disease, should be used as a secondary code with a code from category I13 to identify the stage of chronic kidney disease.

   See Section I.C.14. Chronic kidney disease.

   The codes in category I13, Hypertensive heart and chronic kidney disease, are combination codes that include hypertension, heart disease and chronic kidney disease. The Includes note at I13 specifies that the conditions included at I11 and I12 are included together in I13. If a patient has hypertension, heart disease and chronic kidney disease then a code from I13 should be used, not individual codes for hypertension, heart disease and chronic kidney disease, or codes from I11 or I12.

   For patients with both acute renal failure and chronic kidney disease the acute renal failure should also be coded. Sequence according to the circumstances of the admission/encounter.

   4) **Hypertensive Cerebrovascular Disease**

   For hypertensive cerebrovascular disease, first assign the appropriate code from categories I60-I69, followed by the appropriate hypertension code.

   5) **Hypertensive Retinopathy**

   Subcategory H35.0, Background retinopathy and retinal vascular changes, should be used with a code from category I10 – I15, Hypertensive disease to include the systemic hypertension. The sequencing is based on the reason for the encounter.

   6) **Hypertension, Secondary**

   Secondary hypertension is due to an underlying condition. Two codes are required: one to identify the underlying etiology and one from category I15 to identify the hypertension. Sequencing of codes is determined by the reason for admission/encounter.

7) Hypertension, Transient

Assign code R03.0, Elevated blood pressure reading without diagnosis of hypertension, unless patient has an established diagnosis of hypertension. Assign code O13.-, Gestational [pregnancy-induced] hypertension without significant proteinuria, or O14.-, Pre-eclampsia, for transient hypertension of pregnancy.

8) Hypertension, Controlled

This diagnostic statement usually refers to an existing state of hypertension under control by therapy. Assign the appropriate code from categories I10-I15, Hypertensive diseases.

9) Hypertension, Uncontrolled

Uncontrolled hypertension may refer to untreated hypertension or hypertension not responding to current therapeutic regimen. In either case, assign the appropriate code from categories I10-I15, Hypertensive diseases.

10) Hypertensive Crisis

Assign a code from category I16, Hypertensive crisis, for documented hypertensive urgency, hypertensive emergency or unspecified hypertensive crisis. Code also any identified hypertensive disease (I10-I15). The sequencing is based on the reason for the encounter.

11) Pulmonary Hypertension

Pulmonary hypertension is classified to category I27, Other pulmonary heart diseases. For secondary pulmonary hypertension (I27.1, I27.2-), code also any associated conditions or adverse effects of drugs or toxins. The sequencing is based on the reason for the encounter, except for adverse effects of drugs (See Section I.C.19.e).

12) Hypertension, Resistant

Resistant hypertension refers to blood pressure of a patient with hypertension that remains above goal in spite of the use of antihypertensive medications. Assign code I1A.0 Resistant hypertension, as an additional code when apparent treatment resistant hypertension, treatment resistant hypertension, or true resistant hypertension is documented by the provider. A code for the specific type of existing hypertension is sequenced first, if known.

b. Atherosclerotic Coronary Artery Disease and Angina

ICD-10-CM has combination codes for atherosclerotic heart disease with angina pectoris. The subcategories for these codes are I25.11, Atherosclerotic heart disease of native coronary artery with angina pectoris and I25.7, Atherosclerosis of coronary artery bypass graft(s) and coronary artery of transplanted heart with angina pectoris.

When using one of these combination codes it is not necessary to use an additional code for angina pectoris. A causal relationship can be assumed in a patient with both atherosclerosis and angina pectoris, unless the documentation indicates the angina is due to something other than the atherosclerosis.

If a patient with coronary artery disease is admitted due to an acute myocardial infarction (AMI), the AMI should be sequenced before the coronary artery disease.

See Section I.C.9. Acute myocardial infarction (AMI)

c. Intraoperative and Postprocedural Cerebrovascular Accident

Medical record documentation should clearly specify the cause- and-effect relationship between the medical intervention and the cerebrovascular accident in order to assign a code for intraoperative or postprocedural cerebrovascular accident.

Proper code assignment depends on whether it was an infarction or hemorrhage and whether it occurred intraoperatively or postoperatively. If it was a cerebral hemorrhage, code assignment depends on the type of procedure performed.

d. Sequelae of Cerebrovascular Disease

1) Category I69, Sequelae of Cerebrovascular disease

Category I69 is used to indicate conditions classifiable to categories I60-I67 as the causes of sequela (neurologic deficits), themselves classified elsewhere. These "late effects" include neurologic deficits that persist after initial onset of conditions classifiable to categories I60-I67. The neurologic deficits caused by cerebrovascular disease may be present from the onset or may arise at any time after the onset of the condition classifiable to categories I60-I67.

Codes from category I69, Sequelae of cerebrovascular disease, that specify hemiplegia, hemiparesis and monoplegia identify whether the dominant or nondominant side is affected. Should the affected side be documented, but not specified as dominant or nondominant, and the classification system does not indicate a default, code selection is as follows:

- For ambidextrous patients, the default should be dominant.
- If the left side is affected, the default is non-dominant.
- If the right side is affected, the default is dominant.

2) **Codes from category I69 with codes from I60-I67**

Codes from category I69 may be assigned on a health care record with codes from I60-I67, if the patient has a current cerebrovascular disease and deficits from an old cerebrovascular disease.

3) **Codes from category I69 and Personal history of transient ischemic attack (TIA) and cerebral infarction (Z86.73)**

Codes from category I69 should not be assigned if the patient does not have neurologic deficits.

See Section I.C.21. 4. History (of) for use of personal history codes

e. **Acute myocardial infarction (AMI)**

1) **ST elevation myocardial infarction (STEMI) and non ST elevation myocardial infarction (NSTEMI)**

The ICD-10-CM codes for type 1 acute myocardial infarction (AMI) identify the site, such as anterolateral wall or true posterior wall. Subcategories I21.0-I21.2 and code I21.3 are used for type 1 ST elevation myocardial infarction (STEMI). Code I21.4, Non-ST elevation (NSTEMI) myocardial infarction, is used for type 1 non ST elevation myocardial infarction (NSTEMI) and nontransmural MIs.

If a type 1 NSTEMI evolves to STEMI, assign the STEMI code. If a type 1 STEMI converts to NSTEMI due to thrombolytic therapy, it is still coded as STEMI.

For encounters occurring while the myocardial infarction is equal to, or less than, four weeks old, including transfers to another acute setting or a postacute setting, and the myocardial infarction meets the definition for "other diagnoses" (see Section III, Reporting Additional Diagnoses), codes from category I21 may continue to be reported. For encounters after the 4 week time frame and the patient is still receiving care related to the myocardial infarction, the appropriate aftercare code should be assigned, rather than a code from category I21. For old or healed myocardial infarctions not requiring further care, code I25.2, Old myocardial infarction, may be assigned.

2) **Acute myocardial infarction, unspecified**

Code I21.9, Acute myocardial infarction, unspecified, is the default for unspecified acute myocardial infarction or unspecified type. If only type 1 STEMI or transmural MI without the site is documented, assign code I21.3, ST elevation (STEMI) myocardial infarction of unspecified site.

3) **AMI documented as nontransmural or subendocardial but site provided**

If an AMI is documented as nontransmural or subendocardial, but the site is provided, it is still coded as a subendocardial AMI.

See Section I.C.21.3 for information on coding status post administration of tPA in a different facility within the last 24 hours.

4) **Subsequent acute myocardial infarction**

A code from category I22, Subsequent ST elevation (STEMI) and non-ST elevation (NSTEMI) myocardial infarction, is to be used when a patient who has suffered a type 1 or unspecified AMI has a new AMI within the 4 week time frame of the initial AMI. A code from category I22 must be used in conjunction with a code from category I21. The sequencing of the I22 and I21 codes depends on the circumstances of the encounter.

Do not assign code I22 for subsequent myocardial infarctions other than type 1 or unspecified. For subsequent type 2 AMI assign only code I21.A1. For subsequent type 4 or type 5 AMI, assign only code I21.A9.

If a subsequent myocardial infarction of one type occurs within 4 weeks of a myocardial infarction of a different type, assign the appropriate codes from category I21 to identify each type. Do not assign a code from I22. Codes from category I22 should only be assigned if both the initial and subsequent myocardial infarctions are type 1 or unspecified.

5) **Other Types of Myocardial Infarction**

The ICD-10-CM provides codes for different types of myocardial infarction. Type 1 myocardial infarctions are assigned to codes I21.0-I21.4.

Type 2 myocardial infarction (myocardial infarction due to demand ischemia or secondary to ischemic imbalance) is assigned to code I21.A1, Myocardial infarction type 2 with the underlying cause coded first. Do not assign code I24.8, Other forms of acute ischemic heart disease, for the demand ischemia. If a type 2 AMI is described as NSTEMI or STEMI, only assign code I21.A1. Codes I21.0-I21.4 should only be assigned for type 1 AMIs.

Acute myocardial infarctions type 3, 4a, 4b, 4c and 5 are assigned to code I21.A9, Other myocardial infarction type.

The "Code also" and "Code first" notes should be followed related to complications, and for coding of postprocedural myocardial infarctions during or following cardiac surgery.

6) **Myocardial Infarction with Coronary Microvascular Dysfunction**

Coronary microvascular dysfunction (CMD) is a condition that impacts the microvasculature by restricting microvascular flow and increasing microvascular resistance. Code I21.B, Myocardial infarction with coronary microvascular dysfunction, is assigned for myocardial infarction with coronary microvascular disease, myocardial infarction with coronary microvascular dysfunction, and myocardial infarction with non-obstructive coronary arteries (MINOCA) with microvascular disease.

10. **Chapter 10: Diseases of the Respiratory System (J00-J99), U07.0**

    a. **Chronic Obstructive Pulmonary Disease [COPD] and Asthma**

       1) **Acute exacerbation of chronic obstructive bronchitis and asthma**

          The codes in categories J44 and J45 distinguish between uncomplicated cases and those in acute exacerbation. An acute exacerbation is a worsening or a decompensation of a chronic condition. An acute exacerbation is not equivalent to an infection superimposed on a chronic condition, though an exacerbation may be triggered by an infection.

    b. **Acute Respiratory Failure**

       1) **Acute respiratory failure as principal diagnosis**

          A code from subcategory J96.0, Acute respiratory failure, or subcategory J96.2, Acute and chronic respiratory failure, may be assigned as a principal diagnosis when it is the condition established after study to be chiefly responsible for occasioning the admission to the hospital, and the selection is supported by the Alphabetic Index and Tabular List. However, chapter-specific coding guidelines (such as obstetrics, poisoning, HIV, newborn) that provide sequencing direction take precedence.

       2) **Acute respiratory failure as secondary diagnosis**

          Respiratory failure may be listed as a secondary diagnosis if it occurs after admission, or if it is present on admission, but does not meet the definition of principal diagnosis.

       3) **Sequencing of acute respiratory failure and another acute condition**

          When a patient is admitted with respiratory failure and another acute condition, (e.g., myocardial infarction, cerebrovascular accident, aspiration pneumonia), the principal diagnosis will not be the same in every situation. This applies whether the other acute condition is a respiratory or nonrespiratory condition. Selection of the principal diagnosis will be dependent on the circumstances of admission. If both the respiratory failure and the other acute condition are equally responsible for occasioning the admission to the hospital, and there are no chapter-specific sequencing rules, the guideline regarding two or more diagnoses that equally meet the definition for principal diagnosis *(Section II, C.)* may be applied in these situations.

          If the documentation is not clear as to whether acute respiratory failure and another condition are equally responsible for occasioning the admission, query the provider for clarification.

    c. **Influenza due to certain identified influenza viruses**

       Code only confirmed cases of influenza due to certain identified influenza viruses (category J09), and due to other identified influenza virus (category J10). This is an exception to the hospital inpatient guideline Section II, H. (Uncertain Diagnosis).

       In this context, "confirmation" does not require documentation of positive laboratory testing specific for avian or other novel influenza A or other identified influenza virus. However, coding should be based on the provider's diagnostic statement that the patient has avian influenza, or other novel influenza A, for category J09, or has another particular identified strain of influenza, such as H1N1 or H3N2, but not identified as novel or variant, for category J10.

       If the provider records "suspected" or "possible" or "probable" avian influenza, or novel influenza, or other identified influenza, then the appropriate influenza code from category J11, Influenza due to unidentified influenza virus, should be assigned. A code from category J09, Influenza due to certain identified influenza viruses, should not be assigned nor should a code from category J10, Influenza due to other identified influenza virus.

    d. **Ventilator associated Pneumonia**

       1) **Documentation of Ventilator associated Pneumonia**

          As with all procedural or postprocedural complications, code assignment is based on the provider's documentation of the relationship between the condition and the procedure.

          Code J95.851, Ventilator associated pneumonia, should be assigned only when the provider has documented ventilator associated pneumonia (VAP). An additional code to identify the organism (e.g., Pseudomonas aeruginosa, code B96.5) should also be assigned. Do not assign an additional code from categories J12-J18 to identify the type of pneumonia.

Code J95.851 should not be assigned for cases where the patient has pneumonia and is on a mechanical ventilator and the provider has not specifically stated that the pneumonia is ventilator-associated pneumonia. If the documentation is unclear as to whether the patient has a pneumonia that is a complication attributable to the mechanical ventilator, query the provider.

2) Ventilator associated Pneumonia Develops after Admission

A patient may be admitted with one type of pneumonia (e.g., code J13, Pneumonia due to Streptococcus pneumonia) and subsequently develop VAP. In this instance, the principal diagnosis would be the appropriate code from categories J12- J18 for the pneumonia diagnosed at the time of admission. Code J95.851, Ventilator associated pneumonia, would be assigned as an additional diagnosis when the provider has also documented the presence of ventilator associated pneumonia.

e. Vaping-related disorders

For patients presenting with condition(s) related to vaping, assign code U07.0, Vaping-related disorder, as the principal diagnosis. For lung injury due to vaping, assign only code U07.0. Assign additional codes for other manifestations, such as acute respiratory failure (subcategory J96.0-) or pneumonitis (code J68.0).

Associated respiratory signs and symptoms due to vaping, such as cough, shortness of breath, etc., are not coded separately, when a definitive diagnosis has been established. However, it would be appropriate to code separately any gastrointestinal symptoms, such as diarrhea and abdominal pain.

See Section I.C.1.g.1.c.i. for Pneumonia confirmed as due to COVID-19

11. Chapter 11: Diseases of the Digestive System (K00-K95)

Reserved for future guideline expansion

12. Chapter 12: Diseases of the Skin and Subcutaneous Tissue (L00-L99)

a. Pressure ulcer stage codes

1) Pressure ulcer stages

Codes in category L89, Pressure ulcer, identify the site and stage of the pressure ulcer.

The ICD-10-CM classifies pressure ulcer stages based on severity, which is designated by stages 1-4, deep tissue pressure injury, unspecified stage and unstageable.

Assign as many codes from category L89 as needed to identify all the pressure ulcers the patient has, if applicable.

See Section I.B.14 for pressure ulcer stage documentation by clinicians other than patient's provider.

2) Unstageable pressure ulcers

Assignment of the code for unstageable pressure ulcer (L89.--0) should be based on the clinical documentation. These codes are used for pressure ulcers whose stage cannot be clinically determined (e.g., the ulcer is covered by eschar or has been treated with a skin or muscle graft) and pressure ulcers that are documented as deep tissue injury but not documented as due to trauma. This code should not be confused with the codes for unspecified stage (L89.--9). When there is no documentation regarding the stage of the pressure ulcer, assign the appropriate code for unspecified stage (L89.--9).

If during an encounter, the stage of an unstageable pressure ulcer is revealed after debridement, assign only the code for the stage revealed following debridement.

3) Documented pressure ulcer stage

Assignment of the pressure ulcer stage code should be guided by clinical documentation of the stage or documentation of the terms found in the Alphabetic Index. For clinical terms describing the stage that are not found in the Alphabetic Index, and there is no documentation of the stage, the provider should be queried.

4) Patients admitted with pressure ulcers documented as healed

No code is assigned if the documentation states that the pressure ulcer is completely healed at the time of admission.

5) Patients admitted with pressure ulcers documented as healing

Pressure ulcers described as healing should be assigned the appropriate pressure ulcer stage code based on the documentation in the medical record. If the documentation does not provide information about the stage of the healing pressure ulcer, assign the appropriate code for unspecified stage.

If the documentation is unclear as to whether the patient has a current (new) pressure ulcer or if the patient is being treated for a healing pressure ulcer, query the provider.

For ulcers that were present on admission but healed at the time of discharge, assign the code for the site and stage of the pressure ulcer at the time of admission.

6) Patient admitted with pressure ulcer evolving into another stage during the admission

If a patient is admitted to an inpatient hospital with a pressure ulcer at one stage and it progresses to a higher stage, two separate codes should be assigned: one code for the site and stage of the ulcer on admission and a second code for the same ulcer site and the highest stage reported during the stay.

7) Pressure-induced deep tissue damage

For pressure-induced deep tissue damage or deep tissue pressure injury, assign only the appropriate code for pressure-induced deep tissue damage (L89.--6).

b. Non-Pressure Chronic Ulcers

1) Patients admitted with non-pressure ulcers documented as healed

No code is assigned if the documentation states that the non-pressure ulcer is completely healed at the time of admission.

2) Patients admitted with non-pressure ulcers documented as healing

Non-pressure ulcers described as healing should be assigned the appropriate non-pressure ulcer code based on the documentation in the medical record. If the documentation does not provide information about the severity of the healing non-pressure ulcer, assign the appropriate code unspecified severity.

If the documentation is unclear as to whether the patient has a current (new) non-pressure ulcer or if the patient is being treated for a healing non-pressure ulcer, query the provider.

For ulcers that were present on admission but healed at the time of discharge, assign the code for the site and severity of the non-pressure ulcer at the time of admission.

3) Patient admitted with non-pressure ulcer that progresses to another severity level during the admission

If a patient is admitted to an inpatient hospital with a non-pressure ulcer at one severity level and it progresses to a higher severity level, two separate codes should be assigned; one code for the site and severity level of the ulcer on admission and a second code for the same ulcer site and the highest severity level reported during the stay.

See Section I.B.14 for pressure ulcer stage documentation by clinicians other than patient's provider.

13. Chapter 13: Diseases of the Musculoskeletal System and Connective Tissue (M00-M99)

a. Site and laterality

Most of the codes within Chapter 13 have site and laterality designations. The site represents the bone, joint or the muscle involved. For some conditions where more than one bone, joint or muscle is usually involved, such as osteoarthritis, there is a "multiple sites" code available. For categories where no multiple site code is provided and more than one bone, joint or muscle is involved, multiple codes should be used to indicate the different sites involved.

1) Bone versus joint

For certain conditions, the bone may be affected at the upper or lower end, (e.g., avascular necrosis of bone, M87, Osteoporosis, M80, M81). Though the portion of the bone affected may be at the joint, the site designation will be the bone, not the joint.

b. Acute traumatic versus chronic or recurrent musculoskeletal conditions

Many musculoskeletal conditions are a result of previous injury or trauma to a site, or are recurrent conditions. Bone, joint or muscle conditions that are the result of a healed injury are usually found in chapter 13. Recurrent bone, joint or muscle conditions are also usually found in chapter 13. Any current, acute injury should be coded to the appropriate injury code from chapter 19. Chronic or recurrent conditions should generally be coded with a code from chapter 13. If it is difficult to determine from the documentation in the record which code is best to describe a condition, query the provider.

c. Coding of Pathologic Fractures

7th character A is for use as long as the patient is receiving active treatment for the fracture. While the patient may be seen by a new or different provider over the course of treatment for a pathological fracture, assignment of the 7th character is based on whether the patient is undergoing active treatment and not whether the provider is seeing the patient for the first time.

7th character, D is to be used for encounters after the patient has completed active treatment for the fracture and is receiving routine care for the fracture during the healing or recovery phase. The other 7th characters, listed under each subcategory in the Tabular List, are to be used for subsequent encounters for routine care of fractures during the healing and recovery phase as well as treatment of problems associated with the healing, such as malunions, nonunions, and sequelae.

Care for complications of surgical treatment for fracture repairs during the healing or recovery phase should be coded with the appropriate complication codes.

See Section I.C.19. Coding of traumatic fractures.

d. Osteoporosis

Osteoporosis is a systemic condition, meaning that all bones of the musculoskeletal system are affected. Therefore, site is not a component of the codes under category M81, Osteoporosis without current pathological fracture. The site codes under category M80, Osteoporosis with current pathological fracture, identify the site of the fracture, not the osteoporosis.

1) Osteoporosis without pathological fracture

Category M81, Osteoporosis without current pathological fracture, is for use for patients with osteoporosis who do not currently have a pathologic fracture due to the osteoporosis, even if they have had a fracture in the past. For patients with a history of osteoporosis fractures, status code Z87.310, Personal history of (healed) osteoporosis fracture, should follow the code from M81.

2) Osteoporosis with current pathological fracture

Category M80, Osteoporosis with current pathological fracture, is for patients who have a current pathologic fracture at the time of an encounter. The codes under M80 identify the site of the fracture. A code from category M80, not a traumatic fracture code, should be used for any patient with known osteoporosis who suffers a fracture, even if the patient had a minor fall or trauma, if that fall or trauma would not usually break a normal, healthy bone.

e. Multisystem Inflammatory Syndrome

See Section I.C.1.g.1.l for Multisystem Inflammatory Syndrome

14. Chapter 14: Diseases of the Genitourinary System (N00-N99)

a. Chronic kidney disease

1) Stages of chronic kidney disease (CKD)

The ICD-10-CM classifies CKD based on severity. The severity of CKD is designated by stages 1-5. Stage 2, code N18.2, equates to mild CKD; stage 3, code N18.3, equates to moderate CKD; and stage 4, code N18.4, equates to severe CKD. Code N18.6, End stage renal disease (ESRD), is assigned when the provider has documented end-stage-renal disease (ESRD).

If both a stage of CKD and ESRD are documented, assign code N18.6 only.

2) Chronic kidney disease and kidney transplant status

Patients who have undergone kidney transplant may still have some form of chronic kidney disease (CKD) because the kidney transplant may not fully restore kidney function. Therefore, the presence of CKD alone does not constitute a transplant complication. Assign the appropriate N18 code for the patient's stage of CKD and code Z94.0, Kidney transplant status. If a transplant complication such as failure or rejection or other transplant complication is documented, see section I.C.19.g for information on coding complications of a kidney transplant. If the documentation is unclear as to whether the patient has a complication of the transplant, query the provider.

3) Chronic kidney disease with other conditions

Patients with CKD may also suffer from other serious conditions, most commonly diabetes mellitus and hypertension. The sequencing of the CKD code in relationship to codes for other contributing conditions is based on the conventions in the Tabular List.

See I.C.9. Hypertensive chronic kidney disease.

See I.C.19. Chronic kidney disease and kidney transplant complications.

15. Chapter 15: Pregnancy, Childbirth and the Puerperium (O00-O9A)

a. General Rules for Obstetric Cases

1) Codes from chapter 15 and sequencing priority

Obstetric cases require codes from chapter 15, codes in the range O00-O9A, Pregnancy, Childbirth, and the Puerperium. Chapter 15 codes have sequencing priority over codes from other chapters. Additional codes from other chapters may be used in conjunction with chapter 15 codes to further specify conditions. Should the provider document that the pregnancy is incidental to the encounter, then code Z33.1, Pregnant state, incidental, should be used in place of any chapter 15 codes. It is the provider's responsibility to state that the condition being treated is not affecting the pregnancy.

2) Chapter 15 codes used only on the maternal record

Chapter 15 codes are to be used only on the maternal record, never on the record of the newborn.

3) Final character for trimester

The majority of codes in Chapter 15 have a final character indicating the trimester of pregnancy. The timeframes for the trimesters are indicated at the beginning of the chapter. If trimester is not a component of a code it is because the condition always occurs in a specific trimester, or the concept of trimester of pregnancy is not applicable. Certain codes have characters for only certain trimesters because the condition does not occur in all trimesters, but it may occur in more than just one.

Assignment of the final character for trimester should be based on the provider's documentation of the trimester (or number of weeks) for the current admission/encounter. This applies to the assignment of trimester for pre-existing conditions as well as those that develop during or are due to the pregnancy. The provider's documentation of the number of weeks may be used to assign the appropriate code identifying the trimester.

Whenever delivery occurs during the current admission, and there is an "in childbirth" option for the obstetric complication being coded, the "in childbirth" code should be assigned. When the classification does not provide an obstetric code with an "in childbirth" option, it is appropriate to assign a code describing the current trimester.

4) Selection of trimester for inpatient admissions that encompass more than one trimester

In instances when a patient is admitted to a hospital for complications of pregnancy during one trimester and remains in the hospital into a subsequent trimester, the trimester character for the antepartum complication code should be assigned on the basis of the trimester when the complication developed, not the trimester of the discharge. If the condition developed prior to the current admission/encounter or represents a pre-existing condition, the trimester character for the trimester at the time of the admission/encounter should be assigned.

5) Unspecified trimester

Each category that includes codes for trimester has a code for "unspecified trimester." The "unspecified trimester" code should rarely be used, such as when the documentation in the record is insufficient to determine the trimester and it is not possible to obtain clarification.

6) 7th character for Fetus Identification

Where applicable, a 7th character is to be assigned for certain categories (O31, O32, O33.3 - O33.6, O35, O36, O40, O41, O60.1, O60.2, O64, and O69) to identify the fetus for which the complication code applies.

Assign 7th character "0":

- For single gestations
- When the documentation in the record is insufficient to determine the fetus affected and it is not possible to obtain clarification.
- When it is not possible to clinically determine which fetus is affected.

7) Completed weeks of gestation

In ICD-10-CM, "completed" weeks of gestation refers to full weeks. For example, if the provider documents gestation at 39 weeks and 6 days, the code for 39 weeks of gestation should be assigned, as the patient has not yet reached 40 completed weeks.

b. Selection of OB Principal or First-listed Diagnosis

1) Routine outpatient prenatal visits

For routine outpatient prenatal visits when no complications are present, a code from category Z34, Encounter for supervision of normal pregnancy, should be used as the first-listed diagnosis. These codes should not be used in conjunction with chapter 15 codes.

2) Supervision of High-Risk Pregnancy

Codes from category O09, Supervision of high-risk pregnancy, are intended for use only during the prenatal period. For complications during the labor or delivery episode as a result of a high-risk pregnancy, assign the applicable complication codes from Chapter 15. If there are no complications during the labor or delivery episode, assign code O80, Encounter for full-term uncomplicated delivery.

For routine prenatal outpatient visits for patients with high-risk pregnancies, a code from category O09, Supervision of high-risk pregnancy, should be used as the first-listed diagnosis. Secondary chapter 15 codes may be used in conjunction with these codes if appropriate.

3) Episodes when no delivery occurs

In episodes when no delivery occurs, the principal diagnosis should correspond to the principal complication of the pregnancy which necessitated the encounter. Should more than one complication exist, all of which are treated or monitored, any of the complications codes may be sequenced first.

4) When a delivery occurs

When an obstetric patient is admitted and delivers during that admission, the condition that prompted the admission should be sequenced as the principal diagnosis. If multiple conditions prompted the admission, sequence the one most related to the delivery as the principal diagnosis. A code for any complication of the delivery should be assigned as an additional diagnosis. In cases of cesarean delivery, if the patient was admitted with a condition that resulted in the performance of a cesarean procedure, that condition should be selected as the principal diagnosis. If the reason for the admission was unrelated to the condition resulting in the cesarean delivery, the condition related to the reason for the admission should be selected as the principal diagnosis.

5) Outcome of delivery

A code from category Z37, Outcome of delivery, should be included on every maternal record when a delivery has occurred. These codes are not to be used on subsequent records or on the newborn record.

c. Pre-existing conditions versus conditions due to the pregnancy

Certain categories in Chapter 15 distinguish between conditions of the mother that existed prior to pregnancy (pre-existing) and those that are a direct result of pregnancy. When assigning codes from Chapter 15, it is important to assess if a condition was pre-existing prior to pregnancy or developed during or due to the pregnancy in order to assign the correct code.

Categories that do not distinguish between pre-existing and pregnancy- related conditions may be used for either. It is acceptable to use codes specifically for the puerperium with codes complicating pregnancy and childbirth if a condition arises postpartum during the delivery encounter.

d. Pre-existing hypertension in pregnancy

Category O10, Pre-existing hypertension complicating pregnancy, childbirth and the puerperium, includes codes for hypertensive heart and hypertensive chronic kidney disease. When assigning one of the O10 codes that includes hypertensive heart disease or hypertensive chronic kidney disease, it is necessary to add a secondary code from the appropriate hypertension category to specify the type of heart failure or chronic kidney disease.

See Section I.C.9. Hypertension.

e. Fetal Conditions Affecting the Management of the Mother

1) Codes from categories O35 and O36

Codes from categories O35, Maternal care for known or suspected fetal abnormality and damage, and O36, Maternal care for other fetal problems, are assigned only when the fetal condition is actually responsible for modifying the management of the mother, i.e., by requiring diagnostic studies, additional observation, special care, or termination of pregnancy. The fact that the fetal condition exists does not justify assigning a code from this series to the mother's record.

2) In utero surgery

In cases when surgery is performed on the fetus, a diagnosis code from category O35, Maternal care for known or suspected fetal abnormality and damage, should be assigned identifying the fetal condition. Assign the appropriate procedure code for the procedure performed.

No code from Chapter 16, the perinatal codes, should be used on the mother's record to identify fetal conditions. Surgery performed in utero on a fetus is still to be coded as an obstetric encounter.

f. HIV Infection in Pregnancy, Childbirth and the Puerperium

During pregnancy, childbirth or the puerperium, a patient admitted because of an HIV-related illness should receive a principal diagnosis from subcategory O98.7-, Human immunodeficiency [HIV] disease complicating pregnancy, childbirth and the puerperium, followed by the code(s) for the HIV-related illness(es).

Patients with asymptomatic HIV infection status admitted during pregnancy, childbirth, or the puerperium should receive codes of O98.7- and Z21, Asymptomatic human immunodeficiency virus [HIV] infection status.

g. Diabetes mellitus in pregnancy

Diabetes mellitus is a significant complicating factor in pregnancy. Pregnant women who are diabetic should be assigned a code from category O24, Diabetes mellitus in pregnancy, childbirth, and the puerperium, first, followed by the appropriate diabetes code(s) (E08- E13) from Chapter 4.

h. Long term use of insulin and oral hypoglycemics

See section I.C.4.a.3 for information on the long term use of insulin and oral hypoglycemic.

i. Gestational (pregnancy induced) diabetes

Gestational (pregnancy induced) diabetes can occur during the second and third trimester of pregnancy in patients who were not diabetic prior to pregnancy. Gestational diabetes can cause complications in the pregnancy similar to those of pre-existing diabetes mellitus. It also puts the patient at greater risk of developing diabetes after the pregnancy. Codes for gestational diabetes are in subcategory O24.4, Gestational diabetes mellitus. No other code from category O24, Diabetes mellitus in pregnancy, childbirth, and the puerperium, should be used with a code from O24.4

The codes under subcategory O24.4 include diet controlled, insulin controlled, and controlled by oral hypoglycemic drugs. If a patient with gestational diabetes is treated with both diet and insulin, only the code for insulin-controlled is required. If a patient with gestational diabetes is treated with both diet and oral hypoglycemic medications, only the code for "controlled by oral hypoglycemic drugs" is required. Code Z79.4, Long-term (current) use of insulin, Z79.84, Long-term (current) use of oral hypoglycemic drugs, and Z79.85, Long-term (current) use of injectable non-insulin antidiabetic drugs, should not be assigned with codes from subcategory O24.4.

An abnormal glucose tolerance in pregnancy is assigned a code from subcategory O99.81, Abnormal glucose complicating pregnancy, childbirth, and the puerperium.

j. Sepsis and septic shock complicating abortion, pregnancy, childbirth and the puerperium

When assigning a chapter 15 code for sepsis complicating abortion, pregnancy, childbirth, and the puerperium, a code for the specific type of infection should be assigned as an additional diagnosis. If severe sepsis is present, a code from subcategory R65.2, Severe sepsis, and code(s) for associated organ dysfunction(s) should also be assigned as additional diagnoses.

k. Puerperal sepsis

Code O85, Puerperal sepsis, should be assigned with a secondary code to identify the causal organism (e.g., for a bacterial infection, assign a code from category B95-B96, Bacterial infections in conditions classified elsewhere). A code from category A40, Streptococcal sepsis, or A41, Other sepsis, should not be used for puerperal sepsis. If applicable, use additional codes to identify severe sepsis (R65.2-) and any associated acute organ dysfunction.

Code O85 should not be assigned for sepsis following an obstetrical procedure (*See Section I.C.1.d.5b., Sepsis due to a postprocedural infection*).

l. Alcohol, tobacco and drug use during pregnancy, childbirth and the puerperium

1) Alcohol use during pregnancy, childbirth and the puerperium

Codes under subcategory O99.31, Alcohol use complicating pregnancy, childbirth, and the puerperium, should be assigned for any pregnancy case when a patient uses alcohol during the pregnancy or postpartum. A secondary code from category F10, Alcohol related disorders, should also be assigned to identify manifestations of the alcohol use.

2) Tobacco use during pregnancy, childbirth and the puerperium

Codes under subcategory O99.33, Smoking (tobacco) complicating pregnancy, childbirth, and the puerperium, should be assigned for any pregnancy case when a mother uses any type of tobacco product during the pregnancy or postpartum. A secondary code from category F17, Nicotine dependence, should also be assigned to identify the type of nicotine dependence.

3) Drug use during pregnancy, childbirth and the puerperium

Codes under subcategory O99.32, Drug use complicating pregnancy, childbirth, and the puerperium, should be assigned for any pregnancy case when a patient uses drugs during the pregnancy or postpartum. This can involve illegal drugs, or inappropriate use or abuse of prescription drugs. Secondary code(s) from categories F11-F16 and F18-F19 should also be assigned to identify manifestations of the drug use.

m. Poisoning, toxic effects, adverse effects and underdosing in a pregnant patient

A code from subcategory O9A.2, Injury, poisoning and certain other consequences of external causes complicating pregnancy, childbirth, and the puerperium, should be sequenced first, followed by the appropriate injury, poisoning, toxic effect, adverse effect or underdosing code, and then the additional code(s) that specifies the condition caused by the poisoning, toxic effect, adverse effect or underdosing.

See Section I.C.19. Adverse effects, poisoning, underdosing and toxic effects.

n. Normal Delivery, Code O80

1) Encounter for full term uncomplicated delivery

Code O80 should be assigned when a **patient** is admitted for a full-term normal delivery and delivers a single, healthy infant without any complications antepartum, during the delivery, or postpartum during the delivery episode. Code O80 is always a principal diagnosis. It is not to be used if any other code from chapter 15 is needed to describe a current complication of the antenatal, delivery, or postnatal period. Additional codes from other chapters may be used with code O80 if they are not related to or are in any way complicating the pregnancy.

2) Uncomplicated delivery with resolved antepartum complication

Code O80 may be used if the patient had a complication at some point during the pregnancy, but the complication is not present at the time of the admission for delivery.

3) Outcome of delivery for O80

Z37.0, Single live birth, is the only outcome of delivery code appropriate for use with O80.

o. The Peripartum and Postpartum Periods

1) Peripartum and Postpartum periods

The postpartum period begins immediately after delivery and continues for six weeks following delivery. The peripartum period is defined as the last month of pregnancy to five months postpartum.

2) Peripartum and postpartum complication

A postpartum complication is any complication occurring within the six-week period.

3) Pregnancy-related complications after 6 week period

Chapter 15 codes may also be used to describe pregnancy-related complications after the peripartum or postpartum period if the provider documents that a condition is pregnancy related.

4) Admission for routine postpartum care following delivery outside hospital

When the mother delivers outside the hospital prior to admission and is admitted for routine postpartum care and no complications are noted, code Z39.0, Encounter for care and examination of mother immediately after delivery, should be assigned as the principal diagnosis.

5) Pregnancy associated cardiomyopathy

Pregnancy associated cardiomyopathy, code O90.3, is unique in that it may be diagnosed in the third trimester of pregnancy but may continue to progress months after delivery. For this reason, it is referred to as peripartum cardiomyopathy. Code O90.3 is only for use when the cardiomyopathy develops as a result of pregnancy in a woman who did not have pre-existing heart disease.

p. Code O94, Sequelae of complication of pregnancy, childbirth, and the puerperium

1) Code O94

Code O94, Sequelae of complication of pregnancy, childbirth, and the puerperium, is for use in those cases when an initial complication of a pregnancy develops a sequelae requiring care or treatment at a future date.

2) After the initial postpartum period

This code may be used at any time after the initial postpartum period.

3) Sequencing of Code O94

This code, like all sequela codes, is to be sequenced following the code describing the sequelae of the complication.

q. Termination of Pregnancy and Spontaneous abortions

1) Abortion with Liveborn Fetus

When an attempted termination of pregnancy results in a liveborn fetus, assign code Z33.2, Encounter for elective termination of pregnancy and a code from category Z37, Outcome of Delivery.

2) Retained Products of Conception following an abortion

Subsequent encounters for retained products of conception following a spontaneous abortion or elective termination of pregnancy, without complications are assigned O03.4, Incomplete spontaneous, abortion without complication, or codes O07.4, Failed attempted termination of pregnancy without complication. This advice is appropriate even when the patient was discharged previously with a discharge diagnosis of complete abortion. If the patient has a specific complication associated with the spontaneous abortion or elective termination of pregnancy in addition to retained products of conception, assign the appropriate complication code (e.g., O03.-, O04.-, O07.-) instead of code O03.4 or O07.4.

3) Complications leading to abortion

Codes from Chapter 15 may be used as additional codes to identify any documented complications of the pregnancy in conjunction with codes in categories in O04, O07 and O08.

4) Hemorrhage following elective abortion

For hemorrhage post elective abortion, assign code O04.6, Delayed or excessive hemorrhage following (induced) termination of pregnancy. Do not assign code O72.1, Other immediate postpartum hemorrhage, as this code should not be assigned for post abortion conditions. Do not assign code Z33.2, Encounter for elective termination of pregnancy, when the patient experiences a complication post elective abortion.

r. Abuse in a pregnant patient

For suspected or confirmed cases of abuse of a pregnant patient, a code(s) from subcategories O9A.3, Physical abuse complicating pregnancy, childbirth, and the puerperium, O9A.4, Sexual abuse complicating pregnancy, childbirth, and the puerperium, and O9A.5, Psychological abuse complicating pregnancy, childbirth, and the puerperium, should be sequenced first, followed by the appropriate codes (if applicable) to identify any associated current injury due to physical abuse, sexual abuse, and the perpetrator of abuse.

See Section I.C.19. Adult and child abuse, neglect and other maltreatment.

s. COVID-19 infection in pregnancy, childbirth, and the puerperium

During pregnancy, childbirth or the puerperium, when COVID-19 is the reason for admission/encounter, code O98.5-, Other viral diseases complicating pregnancy, childbirth and the puerperium, should be sequenced as the principal/first-listed diagnosis, and code U07.1, COVID-19, and the appropriate codes for associated manifestation(s) should be assigned as additional diagnoses. Codes from Chapter 15 always take sequencing priority.

If the reason for admission/encounter is unrelated to COVID-19 but the patient tests positive for COVID-19 during the admission/encounter, the appropriate code for the reason for admission/encounter should be sequenced as the principal/first-listed diagnosis, and code O98.5- and U07.1, as well as the appropriate codes for associated COVID-19 manifestations, should be assigned as additional diagnoses.

16. Chapter 16: Certain Conditions Originating in the Perinatal Period (P00-P96)

For coding and reporting purposes the perinatal period is defined as before birth through the 28th day following birth. The following guidelines are provided for reporting purposes

a. General Perinatal Rules

1) Use of Chapter 16 Codes

Codes in this chapter are <u>never</u> for use on the maternal record. Codes from Chapter 15, the obstetric chapter, are never permitted on the newborn record. Chapter 16 codes may be used throughout the life of the patient if the condition is still present.

2) Principal Diagnosis for Birth Record

When coding the birth episode in a newborn record, assign a code from category Z38, Liveborn infants according to place of birth and type of delivery, as the principal diagnosis. A code from category Z38 is assigned only once, to a newborn at the time of birth. If a newborn is transferred to another institution, a code from category Z38 should not be used at the receiving hospital.

A code from category Z38 is used only on the newborn record, not on the mother's record.

3) Use of Codes from other Chapters with Codes from Chapter 16

Codes from other chapters may be used with codes from chapter 16 if the codes from the other chapters provide more specific detail. Codes for signs and symptoms may be assigned when a definitive diagnosis has not been established. If the reason for the encounter is a perinatal condition, the code from chapter 16 should be sequenced first.

4) Use of Chapter 16 Codes after the Perinatal Period

Should a condition originate in the perinatal period, and continue throughout the life of the patient, the perinatal code should continue to be used regardless of the patient's age.

5) Birth process or community acquired conditions

If a newborn has a condition that may be either due to the birth process or community acquired and the documentation does not indicate which it is, the default is due to the birth process and the code from Chapter 16 should be used. If the condition is community-acquired, a code from Chapter 16 should not be assigned.

For COVID-19 infection in a newborn, see guideline I.C.16.h

6) Code all clinically significant conditions

All clinically significant conditions noted on routine newborn examination should be coded. A condition is clinically significant if it requires:

- clinical evaluation; or
- therapeutic treatment; or
- diagnostic procedures; or
- extended length of hospital stay; or
- increased nursing care and/or monitoring; or
- has implications for future health care needs

Note: The perinatal guidelines listed above are the same as the general coding guidelines for "additional diagnoses", except for the final point regarding implications for future health care needs. Codes should be assigned for conditions that have been specified by the provider as having implications for future health care needs.

b. Observation and Evaluation of Newborns for Suspected Conditions not Found

1) Use of Z05 codes

Assign a code from category Z05, Observation and evaluation of newborns and infants for suspected **diseases and** conditions ruled out, to identify those instances when a healthy newborn is evaluated for a suspected condition/**disease** that is determined after study not to be present. Do not use a code from category Z05 when the patient **is documented to have** signs or symptoms of a suspected problem; in such cases code the sign or symptom.

2) Z05 on Other than the Birth Record

A code from category Z05 may also be assigned as a principal or first-listed code for readmissions or encounters when the code from category Z38 code no longer applies. Codes from category Z05 are fur use only for healthy newborns and infants for which no condition after study is found to be present.

3) Z05 on a birth record

A code from category Z05 is to be used as a secondary code after the code from category Z38, Liveborn infants according to place of birth and type of delivery.

c. Coding Additional Perinatal Diagnoses

1) Assigning codes for conditions that require treatment

Assign codes for conditions that require treatment or further investigation, prolong the length of stay, or require resource utilization.

2) Codes for conditions specified as having implications for future health care needs

Assign codes for conditions that have been specified by the provider as having implications for future health care needs.

Note: This guideline should not be used for adult patients.

d. Prematurity and Fetal Growth Retardation

Providers utilize different criteria in determining prematurity. A code for prematurity should not be assigned unless it is documented. Assignment of codes in categories P05, Disorders of newborn related to slow fetal growth and fetal malnutrition, and P07, Disorders of newborn related to short gestation and low birth weight, not elsewhere classified, should be based on the recorded birth weight and estimated gestational age.

When both birth weight and gestational age are available, two codes from category P07 should be assigned, with the code for birth weight sequenced before the code for gestational age.

e. Low birth weight and immaturity status

Codes from category P07, Disorders of newborn related to short gestation and low birth weight, not elsewhere classified, are for use for a child or adult who was premature or had a low birth weight as a newborn and this is affecting the patient's current health status.

See Section I.C.21. Factors influencing health status and contact with health services, Status.

f. Bacterial Sepsis of Newborn

Category P36, Bacterial sepsis of newborn, includes congenital sepsis. If a perinate is documented as having sepsis without documentation of congenital or community acquired, the default is congenital and a code from category P36 should be assigned. If the P36 code includes the causal organism, an additional code from category B95, Streptococcus, Staphylococcus, and Enterococcus as the cause of diseases classified elsewhere, or B96, Other bacterial agents as the cause of diseases classified elsewhere, should not be assigned. If the P36 code does not include the causal organism, assign an additional code from category B96. If applicable, use additional codes to identify severe sepsis (R65.2-) and any associated acute organ dysfunction.

g. Stillbirth

Code P95, Stillbirth, is only for use in institutions that maintain separate records for stillbirths. No other code should be used with P95. Code P95 should not be used on the mother's record.

h. COVID-19 Infection in Newborn

For a newborn that tests positive for COVID-19, assign code U07.1, COVID-19, and the appropriate codes for associated manifestation(s) in neonates/newborns in the absence of documentation indicating a specific type of transmission. For a newborn that tests positive for COVID-19 and the provider documents the condition was contracted in utero or during the birth process, assign codes P35.8, Other congenital viral diseases, and U07.1, COVID-19. When coding the birth episode in a newborn record, the appropriate code from category Z38, Liveborn infants according to place of birth and type of delivery, should be assigned as the principal diagnosis.

17. Chapter 17: Congenital Malformations, Deformations and Chromosomal Abnormalities (Q00-Q99)

Assign an appropriate code(s) from categories Q00-Q99, Congenital malformations, deformations, and chromosomal abnormalities when a malformation/deformation or chromosomal abnormality is documented. A malformation/deformation or chromosomal abnormality may be the principal/first-listed diagnosis on a record or a secondary diagnosis.

When a malformation/deformation or chromosomal abnormality does not have a unique code assignment, assign additional code(s) for any manifestations that may be present.

When the code assignment specifically identifies the malformation/deformation or chromosomal abnormality, manifestations that are an inherent component of the anomaly should not be coded separately. Additional codes should be assigned for manifestations that are not an inherent component.

Codes from Chapter 17 may be used throughout the life of the patient. If a congenital malformation or deformity has been corrected, a personal history code should be used to identify the history of the malformation or deformity. Although present at birth, a malformation/deformation or chromosomal abnormality may not be identified until later in life. Whenever the condition is diagnosed by the provider, it is appropriate to assign a code from codes Q00-Q99. For the birth admission, the appropriate code from category Z38, Liveborn infants, according to place of birth and type of delivery, should be sequenced as the principal diagnosis, followed by any congenital anomaly codes, Q00-Q99.

18. Chapter 18: Symptoms, Signs, and Abnormal Clinical and Laboratory Findings, Not Elsewhere Classified (R00-R99)

Chapter 18 includes symptoms, signs, abnormal results of clinical or other investigative procedures, and ill-defined conditions regarding which no diagnosis classifiable elsewhere is recorded. Signs and symptoms that point to a specific diagnosis have been assigned to a category in other chapters of the classification.

a. Use of symptom codes

Codes that describe symptoms and signs are acceptable for reporting purposes when a related definitive diagnosis has not been established (confirmed) by the provider.

b. Use of a symptom code with a definitive diagnosis code

Codes for signs and symptoms may be reported in addition to a related definitive diagnosis when the sign or symptom is not routinely associated with that diagnosis, such as the various signs and symptoms associated with complex syndromes. The definitive diagnosis code should be sequenced before the symptom code.

Signs or symptoms that are associated routinely with a disease process should not be assigned as additional codes, unless otherwise instructed by the classification.

c. Combination codes that include symptoms

ICD-10-CM contains a number of combination codes that identify both the definitive diagnosis and common symptoms of that diagnosis. When using one of these combination codes, an additional code should not be assigned for the symptom.

d. Repeated falls

Code R29.6, Repeated falls, is for use for encounters when a patient has recently fallen and the reason for the fall is being investigated.

Code Z91.81, History of falling, is for use when a patient has fallen in the past and is at risk for future falls. When appropriate, both codes R29.6 and Z91.81 may be assigned together.

e. Coma

Code R40.20, Unspecified coma, **should** be assigned **when the underlying cause of the coma is not known, or the cause is a traumatic brain injury and the coma scale is not documented in the medical record.**

Do not report codes for unspecified coma, individual or total Glasgow coma scale scores for a patient with a medically induced coma or a sedated patient.

1) Coma Scale

The coma scale codes (R40.21- to R40.24-) can be used in conjunction with traumatic brain injury codes. These codes **cannot be used with code R40.2A, Nontraumatic coma due to underlying condition. They** are primarily for use by trauma registries, but they may be used in any setting where this information is collected. The coma scale codes should be sequenced after the diagnosis code(s).

These codes, one from each subcategory, are needed to complete the scale. The 7th character indicates when the scale was recorded. The 7th character should match for all three codes.

At a minimum, report the initial score documented on presentation at your facility. This may be a score from the emergency medicine technician (EMT) or in the emergency department. If desired, a facility may choose to capture multiple coma scale scores.

Assign code R40.24, Glasgow coma scale, total score, when only the total score is documented in the medical record and not the individual score(s).

If multiple coma scores are captured within the first 24 hours after hospital admission, assign only the code for the score at the time of admission. ICD-10-CM does not classify coma scores that are reported after admission but less than 24 hours later.

See Section I.B.14 for coma scale documentation by clinicians other than the patient's provider.

f. Functional quadriplegia

GUIDELINE HAS BEEN DELETED EFFECTIVE OCTOBER 1, 2017

g. SIRS due to Non-Infectious Process

The systemic inflammatory response syndrome (SIRS) can develop as a result of certain non-infectious disease processes, such as trauma, malignant neoplasm, or pancreatitis. When SIRS is documented with a noninfectious condition, and no subsequent infection is documented, the code for the underlying condition, such as an injury, should be assigned, followed by code R65.10, Systemic inflammatory response syndrome (SIRS) of non-infectious origin without acute organ dysfunction, or code R65.11, Systemic inflammatory response syndrome (SIRS) of non-infectious origin with acute organ dysfunction. If an associated acute organ dysfunction is documented, the appropriate code(s) for the specific type of organ dysfunction(s) should be assigned in addition to code R65.11. If acute organ dysfunction is documented, but it cannot be determined if the acute organ dysfunction is associated with SIRS or due to another condition (e.g., directly due to the trauma), the provider should be queried.

h. Death NOS

Code R99, Ill-defined and unknown cause of mortality, is only for use in the very limited circumstance when a patient who has already died is brought into an emergency department or other healthcare facility and is pronounced dead upon arrival. It does not represent the discharge disposition of death.

i. NIHSS Stroke Scale

The NIH stroke scale (NIHSS) codes (R29.7--) can be used in conjunction with acute stroke codes (I60-I63) to identify the patient's neurological status and the severity of the stroke. The stroke scale codes should be sequenced after the acute stroke diagnosis code(s).

At a minimum, report the initial score documented. If desired, a facility may choose to capture multiple stroke scale scores.

See Section I.B.14 for NIHSS stroke scale documentation by clinicians other than patient's provider.

19. Chapter 19: Injury, Poisoning and Certain Other Consequences of External Causes (S00-T88)

a. Application of 7th Characters in Chapter 19

Most categories in chapter 19 have a 7th character requirement for each applicable code. Most categories in this chapter have three 7th character values (with the exception of fractures): A, initial encounter, D, subsequent encounter and S, sequela. Categories for traumatic fractures have additional 7th character values. While the patient may be seen by a new or different provider over the course of treatment for an injury, assignment of the 7th character is based on whether the patient is undergoing active treatment and not whether the provider is seeing the patient for the first time.

For complication codes, active treatment refers to treatment for the condition described by the code, even though it may be related to an earlier precipitating problem. For example, code T84.50XA, Infection and inflammatory reaction due to unspecified internal joint prosthesis, initial encounter, is used when active treatment is provided for the infection, even though the condition relates to the prosthetic device, implant or graft that was placed at a previous encounter.

7th character "A", initial encounter is used for each encounter where the patient is receiving active treatment for the condition.

7th character "D" subsequent encounter is used for encounters after the patient has completed active treatment of the condition and is receiving routine care for the condition during the healing or recovery phase.

The aftercare Z codes should not be used for aftercare for conditions such as injuries or poisonings, where 7th characters are provided to identify subsequent care. For example, for aftercare of an injury, assign the acute injury code with the 7th character "D" (subsequent encounter).

7th character "S", sequela, is for use for complications or conditions that arise as a direct result of a condition, such as scar formation after a burn. The scars are sequelae of the burn. When using 7th character "S", it is necessary to use both the injury code that precipitated the sequela and the code for the sequela itself. The "S" is added only to the injury code, not the sequela code. The 7th character "S" identifies the injury responsible for the sequela. The specific type of sequela (e.g. scar) is sequenced first, followed by the injury code.

See Section I.B.10 Sequela (Late Effects)

b. Coding of Injuries

When coding injuries, assign separate codes for each injury unless a combination code is provided, in which case the combination code is assigned. Codes from category T07, Unspecified multiple injuries should not be assigned in the inpatient setting unless information for a more specific code is not available. Traumatic injury codes (S00-T14.9) are not to be used for normal, healing surgical wounds or to identify complications of surgical wounds.

The code for the most serious injury, as determined by the provider and the focus of treatment, is sequenced first.

1) Superficial injuries

Superficial injuries such as abrasions or contusions are not coded when associated with more severe injuries of the same site.

2) Primary injury with damage to nerves/blood vessels

When a primary injury results in minor damage to peripheral nerves or blood vessels, the primary injury is sequenced first with additional code(s) for injuries to nerves and spinal cord (such as category S04), and/or injury to blood vessels (such as category S15). When the primary injury is to the blood vessels or nerves, that injury should be sequenced first.

3) Iatrogenic injuries

Injury codes from Chapter 19 should not be assigned for injuries that occur during, or as a result of, a medical intervention. Assign the appropriate complication code(s).

c. Coding of Traumatic Fractures

The principles of multiple coding of injuries should be followed in coding fractures. Fractures of specified sites are coded individually by site in accordance with both the provisions within categories S02, S12, S22, S32, S42, S49, S52, S59, S62, S72, S79, S82, S89, S92 and the level of detail furnished by medical record content.

A fracture not indicated as open or closed should be coded to closed. A fracture not indicated whether displaced or not displaced should be coded to displaced.

More specific guidelines are as follows:

1) Initial vs. Subsequent Encounter for Fractures

Traumatic fractures are coded using the appropriate 7th character for initial encounter (A, B, C) for each encounter where the patient is receiving active treatment for the fracture. The appropriate 7th character for initial encounter should also be assigned for a patient who delayed seeking treatment for the fracture or nonunion.

Fractures are coded using the appropriate 7th character for subsequent care for encounters after the patient has completed active treatment of the fracture and is receiving routine care for the fracture during the healing or recovery phase.

Care for complications of surgical treatment for fracture repairs during the healing or recovery phase should be coded with the appropriate complication codes.

Care of complications of fractures, such as malunion and nonunion, should be reported with the appropriate 7th character for subsequent care with nonunion (K, M, N,) or subsequent care with malunion (P, Q, R).

Malunion/nonunion: The appropriate 7th character for initial encounter should also be assigned for a patient who delayed seeking treatment for the fracture or nonunion.

The open fracture designations in the assignment of the 7th character for fractures of the forearm, femur and lower leg, including ankle are based on the Gustilo open fracture classification. When the Gustilo classification type is not specified for an open fracture, the 7th character for open fracture type I or II should be assigned (B, E, H, M, Q).

A code from category M80, not a traumatic fracture code, should be used for any patient with known osteoporosis who suffers a fracture, even if the patient had a minor fall or trauma, if that fall or trauma would not usually break a normal, healthy bone.

See Section I.C.13. Osteoporosis.

The aftercare Z codes should not be used for aftercare for traumatic fractures. For aftercare of a traumatic fracture, assign the acute fracture code with the appropriate 7th character.

2) Multiple fractures sequencing

Multiple fractures are sequenced in accordance with the severity of the fracture.

3) Physeal fractures

For physeal fractures, assign only the code identifying the type of physeal fracture. Do not assign a separate code to identify the specific bone that is fractured.

d. Coding of Burns and Corrosions

The ICD-10-CM makes a distinction between burns and corrosions. The burn codes are for thermal burns, except sunburns, that come from a heat source, such as a fire or hot appliance. The burn codes are also for burns resulting from electricity and radiation. Corrosions are burns due to chemicals. The guidelines are the same for burns and corrosions.

Current burns (T20-T25) are classified by depth, extent and by agent (X code). Burns are classified by depth as first degree (erythema), second degree (blistering), and third degree (full-thickness involvement). Burns of the eye and internal organs (T26-T28) are classified by site, but not by degree.

1) **Sequencing of burn and related condition codes**

   Sequence first the code that reflects the highest degree of burn when more than one burn is present.

   a. When the reason for the admission or encounter is for treatment of external multiple burns, sequence first the code that reflects the burn of the highest degree.

   b. When a patient has both internal and external burns, the circumstances of admission govern the selection of the principal diagnosis or first-listed diagnosis.

   c. When a patient is admitted for burn injuries and other related conditions such as smoke inhalation and/or respiratory failure, the circumstances of admission govern the selection of the principal or first-listed diagnosis.

2) **Burns of the same anatomic site**

   Classify burns of the same anatomic site and on the same side but of different degrees to the subcategory identifying the highest degree recorded in the diagnosis (e.g., for second and third degree burns of right thigh, assign only code T24.311-).

3) **Non-healing burns**

   Non-healing burns are coded as acute burns.

   Necrosis of burned skin should be coded as a non-healed burn.

4) **Infected Burn**

   For any documented infected burn site, use an additional code for the infection.

5) **Assign separate codes for each burn site**

   When coding burns, assign separate codes for each burn site. Category T30, Burn and corrosion, body region unspecified is extremely vague and should rarely be used.

   Codes for burns of "multiple sites" should only be assigned when the medical record documentation does not specify the individual sites.

6) **Burns and Corrosions Classified According to Extent of Body Surface Involved**

   Assign codes from category T31, Burns classified according to extent of body surface involved, or T32, Corrosions classified according to extent of body surface involved, for acute burns or corrosions when the site of the burn or corrosion is not specified or when there is a need for additional data. It is advisable to use category T31 as additional coding when needed to provide data for evaluating burn mortality, such as that needed by burn units. It is also advisable to use category T31 as an additional code for reporting purposes when there is mention of a third-degree burn involving 20 percent or more of the body surface. Codes from categories T31 and T32 should not be used for sequelae of burns or corrosions.

   Categories T31 and T32 are based on the classic "rule of nines" in estimating body surface involved: head and neck are assigned nine percent, each arm nine percent, each leg 18 percent, the anterior trunk 18 percent, posterior trunk 18 percent, and genitalia one percent. Providers may change these percentage assignments where necessary to accommodate infants and children who have proportionately larger heads than adults, and patients who have large buttocks, thighs, or abdomen that involve burns.

7) **Encounters for treatment of sequela of burns**

   Encounters for the treatment of the late effects of burns or corrosions (i.e., scars or joint contractures) should be coded with a burn or corrosion code with the 7th character "S" for sequela.

8) **Sequelae with a late effect code and current burn**

   When appropriate, both a code for a current burn or corrosion with 7th character "A" or "D" and a burn or corrosion code with 7th character "S" may be assigned on the same record (when both a current burn and sequelae of an old burn exist). Burns and corrosions do not heal at the same rate and a current healing wound may still exist with sequela of a healed burn or corrosion.

   See Section I.B.10 Sequela (Late Effects)

9) **Use of an external cause code with burns and corrosions**

   An external cause code should be used with burns and corrosions to identify the source and intent of the burn, as well as the place where it occurred.

e. Adverse Effects, Poisoning, Underdosing and Toxic Effects

Codes in categories T36-T65 are combination codes that include the substance that was taken as well as the intent. No additional external cause code is required for poisonings, toxic effects, adverse effects and underdosing codes.

1) **Do not code directly from the Table of Drugs**

   Do not code directly from the Table of Drugs and Chemicals. Always refer back to the Tabular List.

2) **Use as many codes as necessary to describe**

   Use as many codes as necessary to describe completely all drugs, medicinal or biological substances.

3) **If the same code would describe the causative agent**

   If the same code would describe the causative agent for more than one adverse reaction, poisoning, toxic effect or underdosing, assign the code only once.

4) **If two or more drugs, medicinal or biological substances**

   If two or more drugs, medicinal or biological substances are taken, code each individually unless a combination code is listed in the Table of Drugs and Chemicals.

   If multiple unspecified drugs, medicinal or biological substances were taken, assign the appropriate code from subcategory T50.91, Poisoning by, adverse effect of and underdosing of multiple unspecified drugs, medicaments and biological substances.

5) **The occurrence of drug toxicity is classified in ICD-10-CM as follows:**

   (a) **Adverse Effect**

   When coding an adverse effect of a drug that has been correctly prescribed and properly administered, assign the appropriate code for the nature of the adverse effect followed by the appropriate code for the adverse effect of the drug (T36-T50). The code for the drug should have a 5th or 6th character "5" (for example T36.0X5-) Examples of the nature of an adverse effect are tachycardia, delirium, gastrointestinal hemorrhaging, vomiting, hypokalemia, hepatitis, renal failure, or respiratory failure.

   (b) **Poisoning**

   When coding a poisoning or reaction to the improper use of a medication (e.g., overdose, wrong substance given or taken in error, wrong route of administration), first assign the appropriate code from categories T36-T50. The poisoning codes have an associated intent as their 5th or 6th character (accidental, intentional self-harm, assault and undetermined.) If the intent of the poisoning is unknown or unspecified, code the intent as accidental intent. The undetermined intent is only for use if the documentation in the record specifies that the intent cannot be determined. Use additional code(s) for all manifestations of poisonings.

   If there is also a diagnosis of abuse or dependence of the substance, the abuse or dependence is assigned as an additional code.

   Examples of poisoning include:

   (i) Error was made in drug prescription

   Errors made in drug prescription or in the administration of the drug by provider, nurse, patient, or other person.

   (ii) Overdose of a drug intentionally taken

   If an overdose of a drug was intentionally taken or administered and resulted in drug toxicity, it would be coded as a poisoning.

   (iii) Nonprescribed drug taken with correctly prescribed and properly administered drug

   If a nonprescribed drug or medicinal agent was taken in combination with a correctly prescribed and properly administered drug, any drug toxicity or other reaction resulting from the interaction of the two drugs would be classified as a poisoning.

   (iv) Interaction of drug(s) and alcohol

   When a reaction results from the interaction of a drug(s) and alcohol, this would be classified as poisoning.

   See Section I.C.4. if poisoning is the result of insulin pump malfunctions.

   (c) **Underdosing**

   Underdosing refers to taking less of a medication than is prescribed by a provider or a manufacturer's instruction. Discontinuing the use of a prescribed medication on the patient's own initiative (not directed by the patient's provider) is also classified as an underdosing. For underdosing, assign the code from categories T36-T50 (fifth or sixth character "6").

Documentation of a change in the patient's condition is not required in order to assign an underdosing code. Documentation that the patient is taking less of a medication than is prescribed or discontinued the prescribed medication is sufficient for code assignment.

Codes for underdosing should never be assigned as principal or first-listed codes. If a patient has a relapse or exacerbation of the medical condition for which the drug is prescribed because of the reduction in dose, then the medical condition itself should be coded.

Noncompliance (Z91.12-, Z91.13-, Z91.14- **and Z91.A4-**) or complication of care (Y63.6-Y63.9) codes are to be used with an underdosing code to indicate intent, if known.

(d) Toxic Effects

When a harmful substance is ingested or comes in contact with a person, this is classified as a toxic effect. The toxic effect codes are in categories T51-T65.

Toxic effect codes have an associated intent: accidental, intentional self-harm, assault and undetermined.

For Sequela (Late Effects) see Section I.B.10. Sequela

f. Adult and child abuse, neglect and other maltreatment

Sequence first the appropriate code from categories T74.- (Adult and child abuse, neglect and other maltreatment, confirmed) or T76.- (Adult and child abuse, neglect and other maltreatment, suspected) for abuse, neglect and other maltreatment, followed by any accompanying mental health or injury code(s).

If the documentation in the medical record states abuse or neglect it is coded as confirmed (T74.-). It is coded as suspected if it is documented as suspected (T76.-).

For cases of confirmed abuse or neglect an external cause code from the assault section (X92-Y09) should be added to identify the cause of any physical injuries. A perpetrator code (Y07) should be added when the perpetrator of the abuse is known. For suspected cases of abuse or neglect, do not report external cause or perpetrator code.

If a suspected case of abuse, neglect or mistreatment is ruled out during an encounter code Z04.71, Encounter for examination and observation following alleged physical adult abuse, ruled out, or code Z04.72, Encounter for examination and observation following alleged child physical abuse, ruled out, should be used, not a code from T76.

If a suspected case of alleged rape or sexual abuse is ruled out during an encounter code Z04.41, Encounter for examination and observation following alleged adult rape or code Z04.42, Encounter for examination and observation following alleged child rape, should be used, not a code from T76.

If a suspected case of forced sexual exploitation or forced labor exploitation is ruled out during an encounter, code Z04.81, Encounter for examination and observation of victim following forced sexual exploitation, or code Z04.82, Encounter for examination and observation of victim following forced labor exploitation, should be used, not a code from T76.

See Section I.C.15. Abuse in a pregnant patient.

g. Complications of care

1) General guidelines for complications of care

(a) Documentation of complications of care

See Section I.B.16. for information on documentation of complications of care.

2) Pain due to medical devices

Pain associated with devices, implants or grafts left in a surgical site (for example painful hip prosthesis) is assigned to the appropriate code(s) found in Chapter 19, Injury, poisoning, and certain other consequences of external causes. Specific codes for pain due to medical devices are found in the T code section of the ICD-10-CM. Use additional code(s) from category G89 to identify acute or chronic pain due to presence of the device, implant or graft (G89.18 or G89.28).

3) Transplant complications

(a) Transplant complications other than kidney

Codes under category T86, Complications of transplanted organs and tissues, are for use for both complications and rejection of transplanted organs. A transplant complication code is only assigned if the complication affects the function of the transplanted organ. Two codes are required to fully describe a transplant complication: the appropriate code from category T86 and a secondary code that identifies the complication.

Pre-existing conditions or conditions that develop after the transplant are not coded as complications unless they affect the function of the transplanted organs.

See I.C.21. for transplant organ removal status.

See I.C.2. for malignant neoplasm associated with transplanted organ.

See I.C.1.d.4 for sequencing of sepsis due to infection in transplanted organ

(b) Kidney transplant complications

Patients who have undergone kidney transplant may still have some form of chronic kidney disease (CKD) because the kidney transplant may not fully restore kidney function. Code T86.1- should be assigned for documented complications of a kidney transplant, such as transplant failure or rejection or other transplant complication. Code T86.1- should not be assigned for post kidney transplant patients who have chronic kidney (CKD) unless a transplant complication such as transplant failure or rejection is documented. If the documentation is unclear as to whether the patient has a complication of the transplant, query the provider.

Conditions that affect the function of the transplanted kidney, other than CKD, should be assigned a code from subcategory T86.1, Complications of transplanted organ, Kidney, and a secondary code that identifies the complication.

For patients with CKD following a kidney transplant, but who do not have a complication such as failure or rejection, *see section I.C.14. Chronic kidney disease and kidney transplant status.*

See I.C.1.d.4 for sequencing of sepsis due to infection in transplanted organ.

4) Complication codes that include the external cause

As with certain other T codes, some of the complications of care codes have the external cause included in the code. The code includes the nature of the complication as well as the type of procedure that caused the complication. No external cause code indicating the type of procedure is necessary for these codes.

5) Complications of care codes within the body system chapters

Intraoperative and postprocedural complication codes are found within the body system chapters with codes specific to the organs and structures of that body system. These codes should be sequenced first, followed by a code(s) for the specific complication, if applicable.

Complication codes from the body system chapters should be assigned for intraoperative and postprocedural complications (e.g., the appropriate complication code from chapter 9 would be assigned for a vascular intraoperative or postprocedural complication) unless the complication is specifically indexed to a T code in chapter 19.

20. Chapter 20: External Causes of Morbidity (V00-Y99)

The external causes of morbidity codes should never be sequenced as the first-listed or principal diagnosis.

External cause codes are intended to provide data for injury research and evaluation of injury prevention strategies. These codes capture how the injury or health condition happened (cause), the intent (unintentional or accidental; or intentional, such as suicide or assault), the place where the event occurred the activity of the patient at the time of the event, and the person's status (e.g., civilian, military).

There is no national requirement for mandatory ICD-10-CM external cause code reporting. Unless a provider is subject to a state-based external cause code reporting mandate or these codes are required by a particular payer, reporting of ICD-10-CM codes in Chapter 20, External Causes of Morbidity, is not required. In the absence of a mandatory reporting requirement, providers are encouraged to voluntarily report external cause codes, as they provide valuable data for injury research and evaluation of injury prevention strategies.

a. General External Cause Coding Guidelines

1) Used with any code in the range of A00.0-T88.9, Z00-Z99

An external cause code may be used with any code in the range of A00.0-T88.9, Z00-Z99, classification that represents a health condition due to an external cause. Though they are most applicable to injuries, they are also valid for use with such things as infections or diseases due to an external source, and other health conditions, such as a heart attack that occurs during strenuous physical activity.

2) External cause code used for length of treatment

Assign the external cause code, with the appropriate 7th character (initial encounter, subsequent encounter or sequela) for each encounter for which the injury or condition is being treated.

Most categories in chapter 20 have a 7th character requirement for each applicable code. Most categories in this chapter have three 7th character values: A, initial encounter, D, subsequent encounter and S, sequela. While the patient may be seen by a new or different provider over the course of treatment for an injury or condition, assignment of the 7th character for external cause should match the 7th character of the code assigned for the associated injury or condition for the encounter.

3) Use the full range of external cause codes

Use the full range of external cause codes to completely describe the cause, the intent, the place of occurrence, and if applicable, the activity of the patient at the time of the event, and the patient's status, for all injuries, and other health conditions due to an external cause.

4) **Assign as many external cause codes as necessary**

   Assign as many external cause codes as necessary to fully explain each cause. If only one external code can be recorded, assign the code most related to the principal diagnosis.

5) **The selection of the appropriate external cause code**

   The selection of the appropriate external cause code is guided by the Alphabetic Index of External Causes and by Inclusion and Exclusion notes in the Tabular List.

6) **External cause code can never be a principal diagnosis**

   An external cause code can never be a principal (first-listed) diagnosis.

7) **Combination external cause codes**

   Certain of the external cause codes are combination codes that identify sequential events that result in an injury, such as a fall which results in striking against an object. The injury may be due to either event or both. The combination external cause code used should correspond to the sequence of events regardless of which caused the most serious injury.

8) **No external cause code needed in certain circumstances**

   No external cause code from Chapter 20 is needed if the external cause and intent are included in a code from another chapter (e.g. T36.0X1- Poisoning by penicillins, accidental (unintentional)).

b. **Place of Occurrence Guideline**

Codes from category Y92, Place of occurrence of the external cause, are secondary codes for use after other external cause codes to identify the location of the patient at the time of injury or other condition.

Generally, a place of occurrent code is assigned only once, at the initial encounter for treatment. However, in the rare instance that a new injury occurs during hospitalization, an additional place of occurrence code may be assigned. No 7th characters are used for Y92.

Do not use place of occurrence code Y92.9 if the place is not stated or is not applicable.

c. **Activity Code**

Assign a code from category Y93, Activity code, to describe the activity of the patient at the time the injury or other health condition occurred.

An activity code is used only once, at the initial encounter for treatment. Only one code from Y93 should be recorded on a medical record.

The activity codes are not applicable to poisonings, adverse effects, misadventures or sequela.

Do not assign Y93.9, Unspecified activity, if the activity is not stated.

A code from category Y93 is appropriate for use with external cause and intent codes if identifying the activity provides additional information about the event.

d. **Place of Occurrence, Activity, and Status Codes Used with other External Cause Code**

When applicable, place of occurrence, activity, and external cause status codes are sequenced after the main external cause code(s). Regardless of the number of external cause codes assigned, generally there should be only one place of occurrence code, one activity code, and one external cause status code assigned to an encounter. However, in the rare instance that a new injury occurs during hospitalization, an additional place of occurrence code may be assigned.

e. **If the Reporting Format Limits the Number of External Cause Codes**

If the reporting format limits the number of external cause codes that can be used in reporting clinical data, report the code for the cause/intent most related to the principal diagnosis. If the format permits capture of additional external cause codes, the cause/intent, including medical misadventures, of the additional events should be reported rather than the codes for place, activity, or external status.

f. **Multiple External Cause Coding Guidelines**

More than one external cause code is required to fully describe the external cause of an illness or injury. The assignment of external cause codes should be sequenced in the following priority:

If two or more events cause separate injuries, an external cause code should be assigned for each cause. The first-listed external cause code will be selected in the following order:

External codes for child and adult abuse take priority over all other external cause codes.

See Section I.C.19., Child and Adult abuse guidelines.

External cause codes for terrorism events take priority over all other external cause codes except child and adult abuse.

External cause codes for cataclysmic events take priority over all other external cause codes except child and adult abuse and terrorism.

External cause codes for transport accidents take priority over all other external cause codes except cataclysmic events, child and adult abuse and terrorism.

Activity and external cause status codes are assigned following all causal (intent) external cause codes.

The first-listed external cause code should correspond to the cause of the most serious diagnosis due to an assault, accident, or self-harm, following the order of hierarchy listed above.

g. Child and Adult Abuse Guideline

Adult and child abuse, neglect and maltreatment are classified as assault. Any of the assault codes may be used to indicate the external cause of any injury resulting from the confirmed abuse.

For confirmed cases of abuse, neglect and maltreatment, when the perpetrator is known, a code from Y07, Perpetrator of maltreatment and neglect, should accompany any other assault codes.

See Section I.C.19. Adult and child abuse, neglect and other maltreatment

h. Unknown or Undetermined Intent Guideline

If the intent (accident, self-harm, assault) of the cause of an injury or other condition is unknown or unspecified, code the intent as accidental intent. All transport accident categories assume accidental intent.

1) Use of undetermined intent

External cause codes for events of undetermined intent are only for use if the documentation in the record specifies that the intent cannot be determined.

i. Sequelae (Late Effects) of External Cause Guidelines

1) Sequelae external cause codes

Sequela are reported using the external cause code with the 7th character "S" for sequela. These codes should be used with any report of a late effect or sequela resulting from a previous injury.

See Section I.B.10 Sequela (Late Effects)

2) Sequela external cause code with a related current injury

A sequela external cause code should never be used with a related current nature of injury code.

3) Use of sequela external cause codes for subsequent visits

Use a late effect external cause code for subsequent visits when a late effect of the initial injury is being treated. Do not use a late effect external cause code for subsequent visits for follow-up care (e.g., to assess healing, to receive rehabilitative therapy) of the injury when no late effect of the injury has been documented.

j. Terrorism Guidelines

1) Cause of injury identified by the Federal Government (FBI) as terrorism

When the cause of an injury is identified by the Federal Government (FBI) as terrorism, the first-listed external cause code should be a code from category Y38, Terrorism. The definition of terrorism employed by the FBI is found at the inclusion note at the beginning of category Y38. Use additional code for place of occurrence (Y92.-). More than one Y38 code may be assigned if the injury is the result of more than one mechanism of terrorism.

2) Cause of an injury is suspected to be the result of terrorism

When the cause of an injury is suspected to be the result of terrorism a code from category Y38 should not be assigned. Suspected cases should be classified as assault.

3) Code Y38.9, Terrorism, secondary effects

Assign code Y38.9, Terrorism, secondary effects, for conditions occurring subsequent to the terrorist event. This code should not be assigned for conditions that are due to the initial terrorist act.

It is acceptable to assign code Y38.9 with another code from Y38 if there is an injury due to the initial terrorist event and an injury that is a subsequent result of the terrorist event.

k. External cause status

A code from category Y99, External cause status, should be assigned whenever any other external cause code is assigned for an encounter, including an Activity code, except for the events noted below. Assign a code from category Y99, External cause status, to indicate the work status of the person at the time the event occurred. The status code indicates whether the event occurred during military activity, whether a non-military person was at work, whether an individual including a student or volunteer was involved in a non-work activity at the time of the causal event.

A code from Y99, External cause status, should be assigned, when applicable, with other external cause codes, such as transport accidents and falls. The external cause status codes are not applicable to poisonings, adverse effects, misadventures or late effects. Do not assign a code from category Y99 if no other external cause codes (cause, activity) are applicable for the encounter.

An external cause status code is used only once, at the initial encounter for treatment. Only one code from Y99 should be recorded on a medical record.

Do not assign code Y99.9, Unspecified external cause status, if the status is not stated.

21. Chapter 21: Factors Influencing Health Status and Contact with Health Services (Z00-Z99)

NOTE The chapter specific guidelines provide additional information about the use of Z codes for specified encounters.

a. Use of Z codes in any healthcare setting

Z codes are for use in any healthcare setting. Z codes may be used as either a first-listed (principal diagnosis code in the inpatient setting) or secondary code, depending on the circumstances of the encounter. Certain Z codes may only be used as first-listed or principal diagnosis.

b. Z Codes indicate a reason for an encounter or Provide Additional Information about a Patient Encounter

Z codes are not procedure codes. A corresponding procedure code must accompany a Z code to describe any procedure performed.

c. Categories of Z Codes

1) Contact/Exposure

Category Z20 indicates contact with, and suspected exposure to, communicable diseases. These codes are for patients who do not show any sign or symptom of a disease but are suspected to have been exposed to it by close personal contact with an infected individual or are in an area where a disease is epidemic.

Category Z77, Other contact with and (suspected) exposures hazardous to health, indicates contact with and suspected exposures hazardous to health.

Contact/exposure codes may be used as a first-listed code to explain an encounter for testing, or, more commonly, as a secondary code to identify a potential risk.

2) Inoculations and vaccinations

Code Z23 is for encounters for inoculations and vaccinations. It indicates that a patient is being seen to receive a prophylactic inoculation against a disease. Procedure codes are required to identify the actual administration of the injection and the type(s) of immunizations given. Code Z23 may be used as a secondary code if the inoculation is given as a routine part of preventive health care, such as a well-baby visit.

3) Status

Status codes indicate that a patient is either a carrier of a disease or has the sequelae or residual of a past disease or condition. This includes such things as the presence of prosthetic or mechanical devices resulting from past treatment. A status code is informative, because the status may affect the course of treatment and its outcome. A status code is distinct from a history code. The history code indicates that the patient no longer has the condition.

A status code should not be used with a diagnosis code from one of the body system chapters, if the diagnosis code includes the information provided by the status code. For example, code Z94.1, Heart transplant status, should not be used with a code from subcategory T86.2, Complications of heart transplant. The status code does not provide additional information. The complication code indicates that the patient is a heart transplant patient.

For encounters for weaning from a mechanical ventilator, assign a code from subcategory J96.1, Chronic respiratory failure, followed by code Z99.11, Dependence on respirator [ventilator] status.

The status Z codes/categories are:

Z14 Genetic carrier

Genetic carrier status indicates that a person carries a gene, associated with a particular disease, which may be passed to offspring who may develop that disease. The person does not have the disease and is not at risk of developing the disease.

Z15 Genetic susceptibility to disease

Genetic susceptibility indicates that a person has a gene that increases the risk of that person developing the disease.

Codes from category Z15 should not be used as principal or first-listed codes. If the patient has the condition to which he/she is susceptible, and that condition is the reason for the encounter, the code for the current condition should be sequenced first. If the patient is being seen for follow-up after completed treatment for this condition, and the condition no longer exists, a follow-up code should be sequenced first, followed by the appropriate personal history and genetic susceptibility codes. If the purpose of the encounter is genetic counseling associated with procreative management, code Z31.5, Encounter for genetic counseling, should be assigned as the first-listed code, followed by a code from category Z15. Additional codes should be assigned for any applicable family or personal history.

Z16   Resistance to antimicrobial drugs

This code indicates that a patient has a condition that is resistant to antimicrobial drug treatment. Sequence the infection code first.

Z17   Estrogen receptor status

Z18   Retained foreign body fragments

Z19   Hormone sensitivity malignancy status

Z21   Asymptomatic HIV infection status

This code indicates that a patient has tested positive for HIV but has manifested no signs or symptoms of the disease.

Z22   Carrier of infectious disease

Carrier status indicates that a person harbors the specific organisms of a disease without manifest symptoms and is capable of transmitting the infection.

Z28.3   Underimmunization status

See Section I.B.14. for underimmunization documentation by clinicians other than the patient's provider.

Z33.1   Pregnant state, incidental

This code is a secondary code only for use when the pregnancy is in no way complicating the reason for visit. Otherwise, a code from the obstetric chapter is required.

Z66   Do not resuscitate

This code may be used when it is documented by the provider that a patient is on do not resuscitate status at any time during the stay.

Z67   Blood type

Z68   Body mass index (BMI)

BMI codes should only be assigned when there is an associated, reportable diagnosis (such as obesity). Do not assign BMI codes during pregnancy.

See Section I.B.14 for BMI documentation by clinicians other than the patient's provider.

Z74.01   Bed confinement status

Z76.82   Awaiting organ transplant status

Z78   Other specified health status

Code Z78.1, Physical restraint status, may be used when it is documented by the provider that a patient has been put in restraints during the current encounter. Please note that this code should not be reported when it is documented by the provider that a patient is temporarily restrained during a procedure.

Z79   Long-term (current) drug therapy

Codes from this category indicate a patient's continuous use of a prescribed drug (including such things as aspirin therapy) for the long-term treatment of a condition or for prophylactic use. It is not for use for patients who have addictions to drugs. This subcategory is not for use of medications for detoxification or maintenance programs to prevent withdrawal symptoms in patients with drug dependence (e.g., methadone maintenance for opiate dependence). Assign the appropriate code for the drug dependence instead.

Assign a code from Z79 if the patient is receiving a medication for an extended period as a prophylactic measure (such as for the prevention of deep vein thrombosis) or as treatment of a chronic condition (such as arthritis) or a disease requiring a lengthy course of treatment (such as cancer). Do not assign a code from category Z79 for medication being administered for a brief period of time to treat an acute illness or injury (such as a course of antibiotics to treat acute bronchitis).

Z88   Allergy status to drugs, medicaments and biological substances

Except: Z88.9, Allergy status to unspecified drugs, medicaments and biological substances status

Z89   Acquired absence of limb

Z90	Acquired absence of organs, not elsewhere classified
Z91.0-	Allergy status, other than to drugs and biological substances
Z92.82	Status post administration of tPA (rtPA) in a different facility within the last 24 hours prior to admission to a current facility

Assign code Z92.82, Status post administration of tPA (rtPA) in a different facility within the last 24 hours prior to admission to current facility, as a secondary diagnosis when a patient is received by transfer into a facility and documentation indicates they were administered tissue plasminogen activator (tPA) within the last 24 hours prior to admission to the current facility.

This guideline applies even if the patient is still receiving the tPA at the time they are received into the current facility.

The appropriate code for the condition for which the tPA was administered (such as cerebrovascular disease or myocardial infarction) should be assigned first.

Code Z92.82 is only applicable to the receiving facility record and not to the transferring facility record.

Z93	Artificial opening status
Z94	Transplanted organ and tissue status
Z95	Presence of cardiac and vascular implants and grafts
Z96	Presence of other functional implants
Z97	Presence of other devices
Z98	Other postprocedural states

Assign code Z98.85, Transplanted organ removal status, to indicate that a transplanted organ has been previously removed. This code should not be assigned for the encounter in which the transplanted organ is removed. The complication necessitating removal of the transplant organ should be assigned for that encounter.

See section I.C19. for information on the coding of organ transplant complications.

Z99	Dependence on enabling machines and devices, not elsewhere classified

NOTE Categories Z89-Z90 and Z93-Z99 are for use only if there are no complications or malfunctions of the organ or tissue replaced, the amputation site or the equipment on which the patient is dependent.

4) History (of)

There are two types of history Z codes, personal and family. Personal history codes explain a patient's past medical condition that no longer exists and is not receiving any treatment, but that has the potential for recurrence, and therefore may require continued monitoring.

Family history codes are for use when a patient has a family member(s) who has had a particular disease that causes the patient to be at higher risk of also contracting the disease.

Personal history codes may be used in conjunction with follow-up codes and family history codes may be used in conjunction with screening codes to explain the need for a test or procedure. History codes are also acceptable on any medical record regardless of the reason for visit. A history of an illness, even if no longer present, is important information that may alter the type of treatment ordered.

The reason for the encounter (for example, screening or counseling) should be sequenced first and the appropriate personal and/or family history code(s) should be assigned as additional diagnos(es).

The history Z code categories are:

Z80	Family history of primary malignant neoplasm
Z81	Family history of mental and behavioral disorders
Z82	Family history of certain disabilities and chronic diseases (leading to disablement)
Z83	Family history of other specific disorders
Z84	Family history of other conditions
Z85	Personal history of malignant neoplasm
Z86	Personal history of certain other diseases
Z87	Personal history of other diseases and conditions
Z91.4-	Personal history of psychological trauma, not elsewhere classified
Z91.5	Personal history of self-harm

	Z91.81	History of falling
	Z91.82	Personal history of military deployment
	Z91.85	**Personal history of military service**
	Z92	Personal history of medical treatment
		Except: Z92.0, Personal history of contraception Except: Z92.82, Status post administration of tPA (rtPA) in a different facility within the last 24 hours prior to admission to a current facility

5) **Screening**

Screening is the testing for disease or disease precursors in seemingly well individuals so that early detection and treatment can be provided for those who test positive for the disease (e.g., screening mammogram).

The testing of a person to rule out or confirm a suspected diagnosis because the patient has some sign or symptom is a diagnostic examination, not a screening. In these cases, the sign or symptom is used to explain the reason for the test.

A screening code may be a first-listed code if the reason for the visit is specifically the screening exam. It may also be used as an additional code if the screening is done during an office visit for other health problems. A screening code is not necessary if the screening is inherent to a routine examination, such as a pap smear done during a routine pelvic examination.

Should a condition be discovered during the screening then the code for the condition may be assigned as an additional diagnosis.

The Z code indicates that a screening exam is planned. A procedure code is required to confirm that the screening was performed.

The screening Z codes/categories:

Z11	Encounter for screening for infectious and parasitic diseases
Z12	Encounter for screening for malignant neoplasms
Z13	Encounter for screening for other diseases and disorders
	Except: Z13.9, Encounter for screening, unspecified
Z36	Encounter for antenatal screening for mother

6) **Observation**

There are three observation Z code categories. They are for use in very limited circumstances when a person is being observed for a suspected condition that is ruled out. The observation codes are not for use if an injury or illness or any signs or symptoms related to the suspected condition are present. In such cases the diagnosis/symptom code is used with the corresponding external cause code.

The observation codes are primarily to be used as principal/first-listed diagnosis. An observation code may be assigned as a secondary diagnosis code when the patient is being observed for a condition that is ruled out and is unrelated to the principal/first-listed diagnosis (e.g., patient presents for treatment following injuries sustained in a motor vehicle accident and is also observed for suspected COVID-19 infection that is subsequently ruled out). Also, when the principal diagnosis is required to be a code from category Z38, Liveborn infants according to place of birth and type of delivery, then a code form category Z05, Encounter for observation and evaluation of newborn for suspected diseases and conditions ruled out, is sequenced after the Z38 code. Additional codes may be used in addition to the observation code but only if they are unrelated to the suspected condition being observed.

Codes from subcategory Z03.7, Encounter for suspected maternal and fetal conditions ruled out, may either be used as a first-listed or as an additional code assignment depending on the case. They are for use in very limited circumstances on a maternal record when an encounter is for a suspected maternal or fetal condition that is ruled out during that encounter (for example, a maternal or fetal condition may be suspected due to an abnormal test result). These codes should not be used when the condition is confirmed. In those cases, the confirmed condition should be coded. In addition, these codes are not for use if an illness or any signs or symptoms related to the suspected condition or problem are present. In such cases the diagnosis/symptom code is used.

Additional codes may be used in addition to the code from subcategory Z03.7, but only if they are unrelated to the suspected condition being evaluated.

Codes from subcategory Z03.7 may not be used for encounters for antenatal screening of mother. *See Section I.C.21. Screening.*

For encounters for suspected fetal condition that are inconclusive following testing and evaluation, assign the appropriate code from category O35, O36, O40 or O41.

The observation Z code categories:

- Z03   Encounter for medical observation for suspected diseases and conditions ruled out
- Z04   Encounter for examination and observation for other reasons
  - Except: Z04.9, Encounter for examination and observation for unspecified reason
- Z05   Encounter for observation and evaluation of newborn for suspected diseases and conditions ruled out

7) Aftercare

Aftercare visit codes cover situations when the initial treatment of a disease has been performed and the patient requires continued care during the healing or recovery phase, or for the long-term consequences of the disease. The aftercare Z code should not be used if treatment is directed at a current, acute disease. The diagnosis code is to be used in these cases. Exceptions to this rule are codes Z51.0, Encounter for antineoplastic radiation therapy, and codes from subcategory Z51.1, Encounter for antineoplastic chemotherapy and immunotherapy. These codes are to be first-listed, followed by the diagnosis code when a patient's encounter is solely to receive radiation therapy, chemotherapy, or immunotherapy for the treatment of a neoplasm. If the reason for the encounter is more than one type of antineoplastic therapy, code Z51.0 and a code from subcategory Z51.1 may be assigned together, in which case one of these codes would be reported as a secondary diagnosis.

The aftercare Z codes should also not be used for aftercare for injuries. For aftercare of an injury, assign the acute injury code with the appropriate 7th character (for subsequent encounter).

The aftercare codes are generally first-listed to explain the specific reason for the encounter. An aftercare code may be used as an additional code when some type of aftercare is provided in addition to the reason for admission and no diagnosis code is applicable. An example of this would be the closure of a colostomy during an encounter for treatment of another condition.

Aftercare codes should be used in conjunction with other aftercare codes or diagnosis codes to provide better detail on the specifics of an aftercare encounter visit, unless otherwise directed by the classification. Should a patient receive multiple types of antineoplastic therapy during the same encounter, code Z51.0, Encounter for antineoplastic radiation therapy, and codes from subcategory Z51.1, Encounter for antineoplastic chemotherapy and immunotherapy, may be used together on a record. The sequencing of multiple aftercare codes depends on the circumstances of the encounter.

Certain aftercare Z code categories need a secondary diagnosis code to describe the resolving condition or sequelae. For others, the condition is included in the code title.

Additional Z code aftercare category terms include fitting and adjustment, and attention to artificial openings.

Status Z codes may be used with aftercare Z codes to indicate the nature of the aftercare. For example code Z95.1, Presence of aortocoronary bypass graft, may be used with code Z48.812, Encounter for surgical aftercare following surgery on the circulatory system, to indicate the surgery for which the aftercare is being performed. A status code should not be used when the aftercare code indicates the type of status, such as using Z43.0, Encounter for attention to tracheostomy, with Z93.0, Tracheostomy status.

The aftercare Z category/codes:

- Z42   Encounter for plastic and reconstructive surgery following medical procedure or healed injury
- Z43   Encounter for attention to artificial openings
- Z44   Encounter for fitting and adjustment of external prosthetic device
- Z45   Encounter for adjustment and management of implanted device
- Z46   Encounter for fitting and adjustment of other devices
- Z47   Orthopedic aftercare
- Z48   Encounter for other postprocedural aftercare
- Z49   Encounter for care involving renal dialysis
- Z51   Encounter for other aftercare and medical care

8) Follow-up

The follow-up codes are used to explain continuing surveillance following completed treatment of a disease, condition, or injury. They imply that the condition has been fully treated and no longer exists. They should not be confused with aftercare codes, or injury codes with a 7th character for subsequent encounter, that explain ongoing care of a healing condition or its sequelae. Follow-up codes may be used in conjunction with history codes to provide the full picture of the healed condition and its treatment. The follow-up code is sequenced first, followed by the history code.

A follow-up code may be used to explain multiple visits. Should a condition be found to have recurred on the follow-up visit, then the diagnosis code for the condition should be assigned in place of the follow-up code.

The follow-up Z code categories:

- Z08   Encounter for follow-up examination after completed treatment for malignant neoplasm
- Z09   Encounter for follow-up examination after completed treatment for conditions other than malignant neoplasm

Codes Z08, Encounter for follow-up examination after completed treatment for malignant neoplasm, and Z09, Encounter for follow up examination after completed treatment for conditions other than malignant neoplasm, may be assigned following any type of completed treatment modality (including both medical and surgical treatments).

- Z39   Encounter for maternal postpartum care and examination

9) Donor

Codes in category Z52, Donors of organs and tissues, are used for living individuals who are donating blood or other body tissue. These codes are only for individuals donating for others, not for self-donations. They are not used to identify cadaveric donations.

10) Counseling

Counseling Z codes are used when a patient or family member receives assistance in the aftermath of an illness or injury, or when support is required in coping with family or social problems.

The counseling Z codes/categories:

- Z30.0-   Encounter for general counseling and advice on contraception
- Z31.5   Encounter for procreative genetic counseling
- Z31.6-   Encounter for general counseling and advice on procreation
- Z32.2   Encounter for childbirth instruction
- Z32.3   Encounter for childcare instruction
- Z69   Encounter for mental health services for victim and perpetrator of abuse
- Z70   Counseling related to sexual attitude, behavior and orientation
- Z71   Persons encountering health services for other counseling and medical advice, not elsewhere classified

    NOTE Code Z71.84, Encounter for health counseling related to travel, is to be used for health risk and safety counseling for future travel purposes.

    Code Z71.85, Encounter for immunization safety counseling, is to be used for counseling of the patient or caregiver regarding the safety of a vaccine. This code should not be used for the provision of general information regarding risks and potential side effects during routine encounters for the administration of vaccines.

    Code Z71.87, Encounter for pediatric-to-adult transition counseling, should be assigned when pediatric-to-adult transition counseling is the sole reason for the encounter or when this counseling is provided in addition to other services, such as treatment of a chronic condition. If both transition counseling and treatment of a medical condition are provided during the same encounter, the code(s) for the medical condition(s) treated and code Z71.87 should be assigned, with sequencing depending on the circumstances of the encounter.

- Z76.81   Expectant mother prebirth pediatrician visit

11) Encounters for Obstetrical and Reproductive Services

See Section I.C.15. Pregnancy, Childbirth, and the Puerperium, for further instruction on the use of these codes.

Z codes for pregnancy are for use in those circumstances when none of the problems or complications included in the codes from the Obstetrics chapter exist (a routine prenatal visit or postpartum care). Codes in category Z34, Encounter for supervision of normal pregnancy, are always first-listed and are not to be used with any other code from the OB chapter.

Codes in category Z3A, Weeks of gestation, may be assigned to provide additional information about the pregnancy. Category Z3A codes should not be assigned for pregnancies with abortive outcomes (categories O00-O08), elective termination of pregnancy (code Z33.2), nor for postpartum conditions, as category Z3A is not applicable to these conditions. The date of the admission should be used to determine weeks of gestation for inpatient admissions that encompass more than one gestational week.

The outcome of delivery, category Z37, should be included on all maternal delivery records. It is always a secondary code. Codes in category Z37 should not be used on the newborn record.

Z codes for family planning (contraceptive) or procreative management and counseling should be included on an obstetric record either during the pregnancy or the postpartum stage, if applicable.

Z codes/categories for obstetrical and reproductive services:

Z30	Encounter for contraceptive management
Z31	Encounter for procreative management
Z32.2	Encounter for childbirth instruction
Z32.3	Encounter for childcare instruction
Z33	Pregnant state
Z34	Encounter for supervision of normal pregnancy
Z36	Encounter for antenatal screening of mother
Z3A	Weeks of gestation
Z37	Outcome of delivery
Z39	Encounter for maternal postpartum care and examination
Z76.81	Expectant mother prebirth pediatrician visit

12) Newborns and Infants

See Section I.C.16. Newborn (Perinatal) Guidelines, for further instruction on the use of these codes.

Newborn Z codes/categories:

Z76.1	Encounter for health supervision and care of foundling
Z00.1-	Encounter for routine child health examination
Z38	Liveborn infants according to place of birth and type of delivery

13) Routine and administrative examinations

The Z codes allow for the description of encounters for routine examinations, such as, a general check-up, or, examinations for administrative purposes, such as, a pre-employment physical. The codes are not to be used if the examination is for diagnosis of a suspected condition or for treatment purposes. In such cases the diagnosis code is used. During a routine exam, should a diagnosis or condition be discovered, it should be coded as an additional code. Pre-existing and chronic conditions and history codes may also be included as additional codes as long as the examination is for administrative purposes and not focused on any particular condition.

Some of the codes for routine health examinations distinguish between "with" and "without" abnormal findings. Code assignment depends on the information that is known at the time the encounter is being coded. For example, if no abnormal findings were found during the examination, but the encounter is being coded before test results are back, it is acceptable to assign the code for "without abnormal findings." When assigning a code for "with abnormal findings," additional code(s) should be assigned to identify the specific abnormal finding(s).

Pre-operative examination and pre-procedural laboratory examination Z codes are for use only in those situations when a patient is being cleared for a procedure or surgery and no treatment is given.

The Z codes/categories for routine and administrative examinations:

Z00	Encounter for general examination without complaint, suspected or reported diagnosis
Z01	Encounter for other special examination without complaint, suspected or reported diagnosis
Z02	Encounter for administrative examination
	Except: Z02.9, Encounter for administrative examinations, unspecified
Z32.0-	Encounter for pregnancy test

14) Miscellaneous Z codes

The miscellaneous Z codes capture a number of other health care encounters that do not fall into one of the other categories. Certain of these codes identify the reason for the encounter; others are for use as additional codes that provide useful information on circumstances that may affect a patient's care and treatment.

Prophylactic Organ Removal

For encounters specifically for prophylactic removal of an organ (such as prophylactic removal of breasts due to a genetic susceptibility to cancer or a family history of cancer), the principal or first-listed code should be a code from category Z40, Encounter for prophylactic surgery, followed by the appropriate codes to identify the associated risk factor (such as genetic susceptibility or family history).

If the patient has a malignancy of one site and is having prophylactic removal at another site to prevent either a new primary malignancy or metastatic disease, a code for the malignancy should also be assigned in addition to a code from subcategory Z40.0, Encounter for prophylactic surgery for risk factors related to malignant neoplasms. A Z40.0 code should not be assigned if the patient is having organ removal for treatment of a malignancy, such as the removal of the testes for the treatment of prostate cancer.

Miscellaneous Z codes/categories:

Z28	Immunization not carried out
	Except: Z28.3, Underimmunization status
Z29	Encounter for other prophylactic measures
Z40	Encounter for prophylactic surgery
Z41	Encounter for procedures for purposes other than remedying health state
	Except: Z41.9, Encounter for procedure for purposes other than remedying health state, unspecified
Z53	Persons encountering health services for specific procedures and treatment, not carried out
Z55	Problems related to education and literacy
Z56	Problems related to employment and unemployment
Z57	Occupational exposure to risk factors
Z58	Problems related to physical environment
Z59	Problems related to housing and economic circumstances
Z60	Problems related to social environment
Z62	Problems related to upbringing
Z63	Other problems related to primary support group, including family circumstances
Z64	Problems related to certain psychosocial circumstances
Z65	Problems related to other psychosocial circumstances
Z72	Problems related to lifestyle
	Note: These codes should be assigned only when the documentation specifies that the patient has an associated problem.
Z73	Problems related to life management difficulty
	NOTE These codes should be assigned only when the documentation specifies that the patient has an associated problem.
Z74	Problems related to care provider dependency
	Except: Z74.01, Bed confinement status
Z75	Problems related to medical facilities and other health care
Z76.0	Encounter for issue of repeat prescription
Z76.3	Healthy person accompanying sick person
Z76.4	Other boarder to healthcare facility
Z76.5	Malingerer [conscious simulation]
Z91.1-	Patient's noncompliance with medical treatment and regimen
A91.A-	**Caregiver's noncompliance with patient's medical treatment and regimen**
Z91.83	Wandering in diseases classified elsewhere
Z91.84-	Oral health risk factors
Z91.89	Other specified personal risk factors, not elsewhere classified

See Section I.B.14 for Z55-Z65 Persons with potential health hazards related to socioeconomic and psychosocial circumstances, documentation by clinicians other than the patient's provider.

15) Nonspecific Z codes

Certain Z codes are so non-specific, or potentially redundant with other codes in the classification, that there can be little justification for their use in the inpatient setting. Their use in the outpatient setting should be limited to those instances when there is no further documentation to permit more precise coding. Otherwise, any sign or symptom or any other reason for visit that is captured in another code should be used.

Nonspecific Z codes/categories:

Z02.9	Encounter for administrative examinations, unspecified
Z04.9	Encounter for examination and observation for unspecified reason
Z13.9	Encounter for screening, unspecified
Z41.9	Encounter for procedure for purposes other than remedying health state, unspecified
Z52.9	Donor of unspecified organ or tissue
Z86.59	Personal history of other mental and behavioral disorders

Z88.9 Allergy status to unspecified drugs, medicaments and biological substances status
Z92.0 Personal history of contraception

16) Z Codes That May Only be Principal/First-Listed Diagnosis

The following Z codes/categories may only be reported as the principal/first-listed diagnosis, except when there are multiple encounters on the same day and the medical records for the encounters are combined:

Z00 Encounter for general examination without complaint, suspected or reported diagnosis
Except: Z00.6
Z01 Encounter for other special examination without complaint, suspected or reported diagnosis
Z02 Encounter for administrative examination
Z03 Encounter for medical observation for suspected diseases and conditions ruled out
Z04 Encounter for examination and observation for other reasons
Z33.2 Encounter for elective termination of pregnancy
Z31.81 Encounter for male factor infertility in female patient
Z31.83 Encounter for assisted reproductive fertility procedure cycle
Z31.84 Encounter for fertility preservation procedure
Z34 Encounter for supervision of normal pregnancy
Z39 Encounter for maternal postpartum care and examination
Z38 Liveborn infants according to place of birth and type of delivery
Z40 Encounter for prophylactic surgery
Z42 Encounter for plastic and reconstructive surgery following medical procedure or healed injury
Z51.0 Encounter for antineoplastic radiation therapy
Z51.1- Encounter for antineoplastic chemotherapy and immunotherapy
Z52 Donors of organs and tissues
Except: Z52.9, Donor of unspecified organ or tissue
Z76.1 Encounter for health supervision and care of foundling
Z76.2 Encounter for health supervision and care of other healthy infant and child
Z99.12 Encounter for respirator [ventilator] dependence during power failure

17) Social Determinants of Health

Social determinants of health (SDOH) codes describing social problems, conditions, or risk factors that influence a patient's health should be assigned when this information is documented in the patient's medical record. Assign as many SDOH codes as are necessary to describe all of the social problems, conditions, or risk factors documented during the current episode of care. For example, a patient who lives alone may suffer an acute injury temporarily impacting their ability to perform routine activities of daily living. When documented as such, this would support assignment of code Z60.2, Problems related to living alone. However, merely living alone, without documentation of a risk or unmet need for assistance at home, would not support assignment of code Z60.2. Documentation by a clinician (or patient-reported information that is signed off by a clinician) that the patient expressed concerns with access and availability of food would support assignment of code Z59.41, Food insecurity. Similarly, medical record documentation indicating the patient is homeless would support assignment of a code from subcategory Z59.0-, Homelessness.

For social determinants of health **classified to chapter 21**, such as information found in categories Z55-Z65, Persons with potential health hazards related to socioeconomic and psychosocial circumstances, code assignment may be based on medical record documentation from clinicians involved in the care of the patient who are not the patient's provider since this information represents social information, rather than medical diagnoses. For example, coding professionals may utilize documentation of social information from social workers, community health workers, case managers, or nurses, if their documentation is included in the official medical record.

Patient self-reported documentation may be used to assign codes for social determinants of health, as long as the patient self-reported information is signed-off by and incorporated into the medical record by either a clinician or provider.

Social determinants of health codes are located primarily in these Z code categories:

Z55 Problems related to education and literacy
Z56 Problems related to employment and unemployment
Z57 Occupational exposure to risk factors

Z58	Problems related to physical environment
Z59	Problems related to housing and economic circumstances
Z60	Problems related to social environment
Z62	Problems related to upbringing
Z63	Other problems related to primary support group, including family circumstances
Z64	Problems related to certain psychosocial circumstances
Z65	Problems related to other psychosocial circumstances

See Section I.B.14. Documentation by Clinicians Other than the Patient's Provider.

22. Chapter 22: Codes for Special Purposes (U00-U85)

U07.0	Vaping-related disorder (*see Section I.C.10.e, Vaping-related disorders*)
U07.1	COVID-19 (*see Section I.C.1.g.1., COVID-19 infection*)
U09.9	Post COVID-19 condition, unspecified (*see Section I.C.1.g.1.m*)

Section II. Selection of Principal Diagnosis

The circumstances of inpatient admission always govern the selection of principal diagnosis. The principal diagnosis is defined in the Uniform Hospital Discharge Data Set (UHDDS) as "that condition established after study to be chiefly responsible for occasioning the admission of the patient to the hospital for care."

The UHDDS definitions are used by hospitals to report inpatient data elements in a standardized manner. These data elements and their definitions can be found in the July 31, 1985, Federal Register (Vol. 50, No, 147), pp. 31038–40.

Since that time the application of the UHDDS definitions has been expanded to include all non-outpatient settings (acute care, short term, long term care and psychiatric hospitals; home health agencies; rehab facilities; nursing homes, etc). The UHDDS definitions also apply to hospice services (all levels of care).

In determining principal diagnosis, coding conventions in the ICD-10-CM, the Tabular List and Alphabetic Index take precedence over these official coding guidelines.
(See Section I.A., Conventions for the ICD-10-CM)

The importance of consistent, complete documentation in the medical record cannot be overemphasized. Without such documentation the application of all coding guidelines is a difficult, if not impossible, task.

A. Codes for Symptoms, Signs, and Ill-Defined Conditions

Codes for symptoms, signs, and ill-defined conditions from Chapter 18 are not to be used as principal diagnosis when a related definitive diagnosis has been established.

B. Two or More Interrelated Conditions, Each Potentially Meeting the Definition for Principal Diagnosis

When there are two or more interrelated conditions (such as diseases in the same ICD-10-CM chapter or manifestations characteristically associated with a certain disease) potentially meeting the definition of principal diagnosis, either condition may be sequenced first, unless the circumstances of the admission, the therapy provided, the Tabular List, or the Alphabetic Index indicate otherwise.

C. Two or More Diagnoses that Equally Meet the Definition for Principal Diagnosis

In the unusual instance when two or more diagnoses equally meet the criteria for principal diagnosis as determined by the circumstances of admission, diagnostic workup and/or therapy provided, and the Alphabetic Index, Tabular List, or another coding guidelines does not provide sequencing direction, any one of the diagnoses may be sequenced first.

D. Two or More Comparative or Contrasting Conditions

In those rare instances when two or more contrasting or comparative diagnoses are documented as "either/or" (or similar terminology), they are coded as if the diagnoses were confirmed and the diagnoses are sequenced according to the circumstances of the admission. If no further determination can be made as to which diagnosis should be principal, either diagnosis may be sequenced first.

E. A Symptom(s) Followed by Contrasting/Comparative Diagnoses

GUIDELINE HAS BEEN DELETED EFFECTIVE OCTOBER 1, 2014.

F. Original Treatment Plan not Carried out

Sequence as the principal diagnosis the condition, which after study occasioned the admission to the hospital, even though treatment may not have been carried out due to unforeseen circumstances.

G. Complications of Surgery and Other Medical Care

When the admission is for treatment of a complication resulting from surgery or other medical care, the complication code is sequenced as the principal diagnosis. If the complication is classified to the T80–T88 series and the code lacks the necessary specificity in describing the complication, an additional code for the specific complication should be assigned.

H. Uncertain Diagnosis

If the diagnosis documented at the time of discharge is qualified as "probable", "suspected", "likely", "questionable", "possible", or "still to be ruled out," "compatible with," "consistent with," or other similar terms indicating uncertainty, code the condition as if it existed or was established. The bases for these guidelines are the diagnostic workup, arrangements for further workup or observation, and initial therapeutic approach that correspond most closely with the established diagnosis.

Note: This guideline is applicable only to inpatient admissions to short-term, acute, long-term care and psychiatric hospitals.

I. Admission from Observation Unit

1. Admission Following Medical Observation

When a patient is admitted to an observation unit for a medical condition, which either worsens or does not improve, and is subsequently admitted as an inpatient of the same hospital for this same medical condition, the principal diagnosis would be the medical condition which led to the hospital admission.

2. Admission Following Post-Operative Observation

When a patient is admitted to an observation unit to monitor a condition (or complication) that develops following outpatient surgery, and then is subsequently admitted as an inpatient of the same hospital, hospitals should apply the Uniform Hospital Discharge Data Set (UHDDS) definition of principal diagnosis as "that condition established after study to be chiefly responsible for occasioning the admission of the patient to the hospital for care."

J. Admission from Outpatient Surgery

When a patient receives surgery in the hospital's outpatient surgery department and is subsequently admitted for continuing inpatient care at the same hospital, the following guidelines should be followed in selecting the principal diagnosis for the inpatient admission:

- If the reason for the inpatient admission is a complication, assign the complication as the principal diagnosis.
- If no complication, or other condition, is documented as the reason for the inpatient admission, assign the reason for the outpatient surgery as the principal diagnosis.
- If the reason for the inpatient admission is another condition unrelated to the surgery, assign the unrelated condition as the principal diagnosis.

K. Admissions/Encounters for Rehabilitation

When the purpose for the admission/encounter is rehabilitation, sequence first the code for the condition for which the service is being performed. For example, for an admission/encounter for rehabilitation for rightsided dominant hemiplegia following a cerebrovascular infarction, report code I69.351, Hemiplegia and hemiparesis following cerebral infarction affecting right dominant side, as the first-listed or principal diagnosis.

If the condition for which the rehabilitation service is being provided is no longer present, report the appropriate aftercare code as the first-listed or principal diagnosis, unless the rehabilitation service is being provided following an injury. For rehabilitation services following active treatment of an injury, assign the injury code with the appropriate seventh character for subsequent encounter as the first-listed or principal diagnosis. For example, if a patient with severe degenerative osteoarthritis of the hip, underwent hip replacement and the current encounter/admission is for rehabilitation, report code Z47.1, Aftercare following joint replacement surgery, as the first-listed or principal diagnosis. If the patient requires rehabilitation post hip replacement for right intertrochanteric femur fracture, report code S72.141D, Displaced intertrochanteric fracture of right femur, subsequent encounter for closed fracture with routine healing, as the first-listed or principal diagnosis.

See Section I.C.21.c.7, Factors influencing health states and contact with health services, Aftercare.
See Section I.C.19.a for additional information about the use of 7th characters for injury codes.

Section III. Reporting Additional Diagnoses

GENERAL RULES FOR OTHER (ADDITIONAL) DIAGNOSES

For reporting purposes the definition for "other diagnoses" is interpreted as additional **clinically significant** conditions that affect patient care in terms of requiring:

- clinical evaluation; or
- therapeutic treatment; or
- diagnostic procedures; or
- extended length of hospital stay; or
- increased nursing care and/or
- monitoring

The UHDDS item #11-b defines Other Diagnoses as "all conditions that coexist at the time of admission, that develop subsequently, or that affect the treatment received and/or the length of stay. Diagnoses that relate to an earlier episode which have no bearing on the current hospital stay are to be excluded." UHDDS definitions apply to inpatients in acute-care, short-term, long term care and psychiatric hospital setting. The UHDDS definitions are used by acute-care shortterm hospitals to report inpatient data elements in a standardized manner. These data elements and their definitions can be found in the July 31, 1985, *Federal Register* (Vol. 50, No, 147), pp. 31038–40.

Since that time the application of the UHDDS definitions has been expanded to include all nonoutpatient settings (acute-care, short-term, long-term care and psychiatric hospitals; home health agencies; rehab facilities; nursing homes, etc). The UHDDS definitions also apply to hospice services (all levels of care).

The following guidelines are to be applied in designating "other diagnoses" when neither the Alphabetic Index nor the Tabular List in ICD-10-CM provide direction. The listing of the diagnoses in the patient record is the responsibility of the attending provider.

A. Previous Conditions

If the provider has included a diagnosis in the final diagnostic statement, such as the discharge summary or the face sheet, it should ordinarily be coded. Some providers include in the diagnostic statement resolved conditions or diagnoses and status-post procedures from previous admission that have no bearing on the current stay. Such conditions are not to be reported and are coded only if required by hospital policy.

However, history codes (categories Z80–Z87) may be used as secondary codes if the historical condition or family history has an impact on current care or influences treatment.

B. Abnormal Findings

Abnormal findings (laboratory, x-ray, pathologic, and other diagnostic results) are not coded and reported unless the provider indicates their clinical significance. If the findings are outside the normal range and the attending provider has ordered other tests to evaluate the condition or prescribed treatment, it is appropriate to ask the provider whether the abnormal finding should be added.

Please note: This differs from the coding practices in the outpatient setting for coding encounters for diagnostic tests that have been interpreted by a provider.

C. Uncertain Diagnosis

If the diagnosis documented at the time of discharge is qualified as "probable", "suspected", "likely", "questionable", "possible", or "still to be ruled out," "compatible with," "consistent with," or other similar terms indicating uncertainty, code the condition as if it existed or was established. The bases for these guidelines are the diagnostic workup, arrangements for further workup or observation, and initial therapeutic approach that correspond most closely with the established diagnosis.

Note: This guideline is applicable only to inpatient admissions to short-term, acute-care, long-term care and psychiatric hospitals.

Section IV. Diagnostic Coding and Reporting Guidelines for Outpatient Services

These coding guidelines for outpatient diagnoses have been approved for use by hospitals/ providers in coding and reporting hospital-based outpatient services and provider-based office visits. Guidelines in Section I, Conventions, general coding guidelines and chapter-specific guidelines, should also be applied for outpatient services and office visits.

Information about the use of certain abbreviations, punctuation, symbols, and other conventions used in the ICD-10-CM Tabular List (code numbers and titles), can be found in Section IA of these guidelines, under "Conventions Used in the

Tabular List." Section I.B. contains general guidelines that apply to the entire classification. Section I.C. contains chapter-specific guidelines that correspond to the chapters as they are arranged in the classification. Information about the correct sequence to use in finding a code is also described in Section I.

The terms encounter and visit are often used interchangeably in describing outpatient service contacts and, therefore, appear together in these guidelines without distinguishing one from the other.

Though the conventions and general guidelines apply to all settings, coding guidelines for outpatient and provider reporting of diagnoses will vary in a number of instances from those for inpatient diagnoses, recognizing that:

The Uniform Hospital Discharge Data Set (UHDDS) definition of principal diagnosis does not apply to hospital-based outpatient services and provider-based office visits.

Coding guidelines for inconclusive diagnoses (probable, suspected, rule out, etc.) were developed for inpatient reporting and do not apply to outpatients.

A. Selection of First-Listed Condition

In the outpatient setting, the term first-listed diagnosis is used in lieu of principal diagnosis.

In determining the first-listed diagnosis the coding conventions of ICD-10-CM, as well as the general and disease specific guidelines take precedence over the outpatient guidelines.

Diagnoses often are not established at the time of the initial encounter/visit. It may take two or more visits before the diagnosis is confirmed.

The most critical rule involves beginning the search for the correct code assignment through the Alphabetic Index. Never begin searching initially in the Tabular List as this will lead to coding errors.

1. Outpatient Surgery
When a patient presents for outpatient surgery (same day surgery), code the reason for the surgery as the first-listed diagnosis (reason for the encounter), even if the surgery is not performed due to a contraindication.

2. Observation Stay
When a patient is admitted for observation for a medical condition, assign a code for the medical condition as the first-listed diagnosis.

When a patient presents for outpatient surgery and develops complications requiring admission to observation, code the reason for the surgery as the first reported diagnosis (reason for the encounter), followed by codes for the complications as secondary diagnoses.

B. Codes from A00.0–T88.9, Z00–Z99, U00–U85

The appropriate code(s) from A00.0–T88.9, Z00–Z99 **and U00–U85** must be used to identify diagnoses, symptoms, conditions, problems, complaints, or other reason(s) for the encounter/visit.

C. Accurate Reporting of ICD-10-CM Diagnosis Codes

For accurate reporting of ICD-10-CM diagnosis codes, the documentation should describe the patient's condition, using terminology which includes specific diagnoses as well as symptoms, problems, or reasons for the encounter. There are ICD-10-CM codes to describe all of these.

D. Codes that Describe Symptoms and Signs

Codes that describe symptoms and signs, as opposed to diagnoses, are acceptable for reporting purposes when a diagnosis has not been established (confirmed) by the provider. Chapter 18 of ICD-10-CM, Symptoms, Signs, and Abnormal Clinical, and Laboratory Findings Not Elsewhere Classified (codes R00–R99) contain many, but not all codes for symptoms.

E. Encounters for Circumstances Other than a Disease or Injury

ICD-10-CM provides codes to deal with encounters for circumstances other than a disease or injury. The Factors Influencing Health Status and Contact with Health Services codes (Z00–Z99) are provided to deal with occasions when circumstances other than a disease or injury are recorded as diagnosis or problems.

See Section I.C.21. Factors influencing health status and contact with health services.

F. Level of Detail in Coding

1. ICD-10-CM Codes with 3, 4, 5, 6, Or 7 Characters
ICD-10-CM is composed of codes with 3, 4, 5, 6, or 7 characters. Codes with three characters are included in ICD-10-CM as the heading of a category of codes that may be further subdivided by the use of fourth**,** fifth, sixth, or seventh characters to provide greater specificity.

2. **Use of Full Number of Characters Required for a Code**
A three-character code is to be used only if it is not further subdivided. A code is invalid if it has not been coded to the full number of characters required for that code, including the 7th character, if applicable.

3. **Highest level of specificity**
Code to the highest level of specificity when supported by the medical record documentation.

G. ICD-10-CM Code for the Diagnosis, Condition, Problem, or Other Reason for Encounter/Visit

List first the ICD-10-CM code for the diagnosis, condition, problem, or other reason for encounter/visit shown in the medical record to be chiefly responsible for the services provided. List additional codes that describe any coexisting conditions. In some cases the first-listed diagnosis may be a symptom when a diagnosis has not been established (confirmed) by the provider.

H. Uncertain Diagnosis

Do not code diagnoses documented as "probable", "suspected," "questionable," "rule out," "compatible with," "consistent with," or "working diagnosis" or other similar terms indicating uncertainty. Rather, code the condition(s) to the highest degree of certainty for that encounter/visit, such as symptoms, signs, abnormal test results, or other reason for the visit.

Please note: This differs from the coding practices used by short-term, acute-care, long-term care and psychiatric hospitals.

I. Chronic Diseases

Chronic diseases treated on an ongoing basis may be coded and reported as many times as the patient receives treatment and care for the condition(s).

J. Code All Documented Conditions that Coexist

Code all documented conditions that coexist at the time of the encounter/visit, and require or affect patient care treatment or management. Do not code conditions that were previously treated and no longer exist. However, history codes (categories Z80–Z87) may be used as secondary codes if the historical condition or family history has an impact on current care or influences treatment.

K. Patients Receiving Diagnostic Services Only

For patients receiving diagnostic services only during an encounter/visit, sequence first the diagnosis, condition, problem, or other reason for encounter/visit shown in the medical record to be chiefly responsible for the outpatient services provided during the encounter/visit. Codes for other diagnoses (e.g., chronic conditions) may be sequenced as additional diagnoses.

For encounters for routine laboratory/radiology testing in the absence of any signs, symptoms, or associated diagnosis, assign Z01.89, Encounter for other specified special examinations. If routine testing is performed during the same encounter as a test to evaluate a sign, symptom, or diagnosis, it is appropriate to assign both the Z code and the code describing the reason for the non-routine test.

For outpatient encounters for diagnostic tests that have been interpreted by a physician, and the final report is available at the time of coding, code any confirmed or definitive diagnosis(es) documented in the interpretation. Do not code related signs and symptoms as additional diagnoses.

Please note: This differs from the coding practice in the hospital inpatient setting regarding abnormal findings on test results.

L. Patients Receiving Therapeutic Services Only

For patients receiving therapeutic services only during an encounter/visit, sequence first the diagnosis, condition, problem, or other reason for encounter/visit shown in the medical record to be chiefly responsible for the outpatient services provided during the encounter/visit. Codes for other diagnoses (e.g., chronic conditions) may be sequenced as additional diagnoses.

The only exception to this rule is that when the primary reason for the admission/encounter is chemotherapy or radiation therapy, the appropriate Z code for the service is listed first, and the diagnosis or problem for which the service is being performed listed second.

M. Patients Receiving Preoperative Evaluations Only

For patients receiving preoperative evaluations only, sequence first a code from subcategory Z01.81, Encounter for pre-procedural examinations, to describe the pre-op consultations. Assign a code for the condition to describe the reason for the surgery as an additional diagnosis. Code also any findings related to the pre-op evaluation.

N. Ambulatory Surgery

For ambulatory surgery, code the diagnosis for which the surgery was performed. If the postoperative diagnosis is known to be different from the preoperative diagnosis at the time the diagnosis is confirmed, select the postoperative diagnosis for coding, since it is the most definitive.

O. Routine Outpatient Prenatal Visits

See Section I.C.15. Routine outpatient prenatal visits.

P. Encounters for General Medical Examinations with Abnormal Findings

The subcategories for encounters for general medical examinations, Z00.0- and encounter for routine child health examination, Z00.12-, provide codes for with and without abnormal findings. Should a general medical examination result in an abnormal finding, the code for general medical examination with abnormal finding should be assigned as the first-listed diagnosis. An examination with abnormal findings refers to a condition/diagnosis that is newly identified or a change in severity of a chronic condition (such as uncontrolled hypertension, or an acute exacerbation of chronic obstructive pulmonary disease) during a routine physical examination. A secondary code for the abnormal finding should also be coded.

Q. Encounters for Routine Health Screenings

See Section I.C.21. Factors influencing health status and contact with health services, Screening

Appendix I. Present on Admission Reporting Guidelines

Introduction

These guidelines are to be used as a supplement to the *ICD-10-CM Official Guidelines for Coding and Reporting* to facilitate the assignment of the Present on Admission (POA) indicator for each diagnosis and external cause of injury code reported on claim forms (UB-04 and 837 Institutional).

These guidelines are not intended to replace any guidelines in the main body of the *ICD-10-CM Official Guidelines for Coding and Reporting*. The POA guidelines are not intended to provide guidance on when a condition should be coded, but rather, how to apply the POA indicator to the final set of diagnosis codes that have been assigned in accordance with Sections I, II, and III of the official coding guidelines. Subsequent to the assignment of the ICD-10-CM codes, the POA indicator should then be assigned to those conditions that have been coded.

As stated in the Introduction to the ICD-10-CM Official Guidelines for Coding and Reporting, a joint effort between the healthcare provider and the coder is essential to achieve complete and accurate documentation, code assignment, and reporting of diagnoses and procedures. The importance of consistent, complete documentation in the medical record cannot be overemphasized. Medical record documentation from any provider involved in the care and treatment of the patient may be used to support the determination of whether a condition was present on admission or not. In the context of the official coding guidelines, the term "provider" means a physician or any qualified healthcare practitioner who is legally accountable for establishing the patient's diagnosis.

These guidelines are not a substitute for the provider's clinical judgment as to the determination of whether a condition was or was not present on admission. The provider should be queried regarding issues related to the linking of signs/symptoms, timing of test results, and the timing of findings.

Please see the CDC website for the detailed list of ICD-10-CM codes that do not require the use of a POA indicator (https://www.cdc.gov/nchs/icd/icd10cm.htm). The codes and categories on this exempt list are for circumstances regarding the healthcare encounter or factors influencing health status that do not represent a current disease or injury or that describe conditions that are always present on admission.

General Reporting Requirements

All claims involving inpatient admissions to general acute-care hospitals or other facilities that are subject to a law or regulation mandating collection of present on admission information.

Present on admission is defined as present at the time the order for inpatient admission occurs—conditions that develop during an outpatient encounter, including emergency department, observation, or outpatient surgery, are considered as present on admission.

POA indicator is assigned to principal and secondary diagnoses (as defined in Section II of the Official Guidelines for Coding and Reporting) and the external cause of injury codes.

Issues related to inconsistent, missing, conflicting or unclear documentation must still be resolved by the provider.

If a condition would not be coded and reported based on UHDDS definitions and current official coding guidelines, then the POA indicator would not be reported.

Reporting Options
- Y—Yes
- N—No
- U—Unknown
- W—Clinically undetermined
- Unreported/Not used—(Exempt from POA reporting)

Reporting Definitions
- Y = present at the time of inpatient admission
- N = not present at the time of inpatient admission
- U = documentation is insufficient to determine if condition is present on admission
- W = provider is unable to clinically determine whether condition was present on admission or not

Timeframe for POA Identification and Documentation

There is no required timeframe as to when a provider (per the definition of "provider" used in these guidelines) must identify or document a condition to be present on admission. In some clinical situations, it may not be possible for a provider to make a definitive diagnosis (or a condition may not be recognized or reported by the patient) for a period of time after admission. In some cases it may be several days before the provider arrives at a definitive diagnosis. This does not mean that the condition was not present on admission. Determination of whether the condition was present on admission or not will be based on the applicable POA guideline as identified in this document, or on the provider's best clinical judgment.

If at the time of code assignment the documentation is unclear as to whether a condition was present on admission or not, it is appropriate to query the provider for clarification.

Assigning the POA Indicator

Condition is on the "Exempt from Reporting" list
Leave the "present on admission" field blank if the condition is on the list of ICD-10-CM codes for which this field is not applicable. This is the only circumstance in which the field may be left blank.

POA Explicitly Documented
Assign "Y" for any condition the provider explicitly documents as being present on admission.

Assign "N" for any condition the provider explicitly documents as not present at the time of admission.

Conditions diagnosed prior to inpatient admission
Assign "Y" for conditions that were diagnosed prior to admission (example: hypertension, diabetes mellitus, asthma)

Conditions diagnosed during the admission but clearly present before admission
Assign "Y" for conditions diagnosed during the admission that were clearly present but not diagnosed until after admission occurred.

Diagnoses subsequently confirmed after admission are considered present on admission if at the time of admission they are documented as suspected, possible, rule out, differential diagnosis, or constitute an underlying cause of a symptom that is present at the time of admission.

Condition develops during outpatient encounter prior to inpatient admission
Assign "Y" for any condition that develops during an outpatient encounter prior to a written order for inpatient admission.

Documentation does not indicate whether condition was present on admission
Assign "U" when the medical record documentation is unclear as to whether the condition was present on admission. "U" should not be routinely assigned and used only in very limited circumstances. Coders are encouraged to query the providers when the documentation is unclear.

Documentation states that it cannot be determined whether the condition was or was not present on admission
Assign "W" when the medical record documentation indicates that it cannot be clinically determined whether or not the condition was present on admission.

Chronic condition with acute exacerbation during the admission
If a single code identifies both the chronic condition and the acute exacerbation, see POA guidelines pertaining to codes that contain multiple clinical concepts.

If a single code only identifies the chronic condition and not the acute exacerbation (e.g., acute exacerbation of chronic leukemia), assign "Y."

Conditions documented as possible, probable, suspected, or rule out at the time of discharge
If the final diagnosis contains a possible, probable, suspected, or rule out diagnosis, and this diagnosis was based on signs, symptoms or clinical findings suspected at the time of inpatient admission, assign "Y."

If the final diagnosis contains a possible, probable, suspected, or rule out diagnosis, and this diagnosis was based on signs, symptoms or clinical findings that were not present on admission, assign "N".

Conditions documented as impending or threatened at the time of discharge

If the final diagnosis contains an impending or threatened diagnosis, and this diagnosis is based on symptoms or clinical findings that were present on admission, assign "Y".

If the final diagnosis contains an impending or threatened diagnosis, and this diagnosis is based on symptoms or clinical findings that were not present on admission, assign "N".

Acute and Chronic Conditions

Assign "Y" for acute conditions that are present at time of admission and N for acute conditions that are not present at time of admission.

Assign "Y" for chronic conditions, even though the condition may not be diagnosed until after admission.

If a single code identifies both an acute and chronic condition, see the POA guidelines for codes that contain multiple clinical concepts.

Codes That Contain Multiple Clinical Concepts

Assign "N" if at least one of the clinical concepts included in the code was not present on admission (e.g., COPD with acute exacerbation and the exacerbation was not present on admission; gastric ulcer that does not start bleeding until after admission; asthma patient develops status asthmaticus after admission)

Assign "Y" if all parts of the clinical concepts included in the code were present on admission (e.g., duodenal ulcer that perforates prior to admission)

For infection codes that include the causal organism, assign "Y" if the infection (or signs of the infection) were present on admission, even though the culture results may not be known until after admission (e.g., patient is admitted with pneumonia and the provider documents pseudomonas as the causal organism a few days later).

Same Diagnosis Code for Two or More Conditions

When the same ICD-10-CM diagnosis code applies to two or more conditions during the same encounter (e.g. two separate conditions classified to the same ICD-10-CM diagnosis code):

Assign "Y" if all conditions represented by the single ICD-10-CM code were present on admission (e.g. bilateral unspecified age-related cataracts).

Assign "N" if any of the conditions represented by the single ICD-10-CM code was not present on admission (e.g. traumatic secondary and recurrent hemorrhage and seroma is assigned to a single code T79.2, but only one of the conditions was present on admission).

Obstetrical Conditions

Whether or not the patient delivers during the current hospitalization does not affect assignment of the POA indicator. The determining factor for POA assignment is whether the pregnancy complication or obstetrical condition described by the code was present at the time of admission or not.

If the pregnancy complication or obstetrical condition was present on admission (e.g., patient admitted in preterm labor), assign "Y".

If the pregnancy complication or obstetrical condition was not present on admission (e.g., 2nd degree laceration during delivery, postpartum hemorrhage that occurred during current hospitalization, fetal distress develops after admission), assign "N".

If the obstetrical code includes more than one diagnosis and any of the diagnoses identified by the code were not present on admission assign "N" (e.g., Category O11, Pre-existing hypertension with pre-eclampsia).

Perinatal Conditions

Newborns are not considered to be admitted until after birth. Therefore, any condition present at birth or that developed in utero is considered present at admission and should be assigned "Y". This includes conditions that occur during delivery (e.g., injury during delivery, meconium aspiration, exposure to streptococcus B in the vaginal canal).

Congenital Conditions and Anomalies

Assign "Y" for congenital conditions and anomalies except for categories Q00–Q99, Congenital anomalies, which are on the exempt list. Congenital conditions are always considered present on admission.

External Cause of Injury Codes

Assign "Y" for any external cause code representing an external cause of morbidity that occurred prior to inpatient admission (e.g., patient fell out of bed at home, patient fell out of bed in emergency room prior to admission).

Assign "N" for any external cause code representing an external cause of morbidity that occurred during inpatient hospitalization (e.g., patient fell out of hospital bed during hospital stay, patient experienced an adverse reaction to a medication administered after inpatient admission).

> **Consulting Editor's Note**
>
> The Official Coding Guidelines Appendix I, Present on Admission Reporting Guidelines, no longer provides a listing of Present on Admission (POA) exempt codes by category/sub-category. Instead interested parties can view a full list of the POA exempt code list via the National Center for Health Statistics webpage.
>
> Here we are providing an updated 2024 POA exempt code list by category/sub-category to be used as a reference guide for the users of this code book. Users, including educators, can use this list to provide examples of the types of codes included on the POA exempt code list.

B90–B94	Sequelae of infectious and parasitic diseases
E64	Sequelae of malnutrition and other nutritional deficiencies
I25.2	Old myocardial infarction
I69	Sequelae of cerebrovascular disease
M84.7	Nontraumatic fracture, NEC (excluding codes ending in 7th character A)
M97	Periprosthetic fracture around internal prosthetic joint (excluding codes ending in 7th character A)
O09	Supervision of high risk pregnancy
O66.5	Attempted application of vacuum extractor and forceps
O80	Encounter for full-term uncomplicated delivery
O94	Sequelae of complication of pregnancy, childbirth, and the puerperium
P00	Newborn affected by maternal conditions that may be unrelated to present pregnancy
P29.3	Persistent fetal circulation
P78.84	Gestational alloimmune liver disease
P83.8	Other specified conditions of integument specific to newborn
P91.81	Neonatal encephalopathy
P91.82-	Neonatal cerebral infarction
P91.88	Other specified disturbances of cerebral status of newborn
Q00–Q99	Congenital malformations, deformations and chromosomal abnormalities
S00–T88.9	Injury, poisoning and certain other consequences of external causes with 7th character representing subsequent encounter or sequela
V00–V09	Pedestrian injured in transport accident
	Except V00.81-, Accident with wheelchair (powered)
	V00.83-, Accident with motorized mobility scooter
V10–V19	Pedal cycle rider injured in transport accident
V20–V29	Motorcycle rider injured in transport accident
V30–V39	Occupant of three-wheeled motor vehicle injured in transport accident
V40–V49	Car occupant injured in transport accident
V50–V59	Occupant of pick-up truck or van injured in transport accident
V60–V69	Occupant of heavy transport vehicle injured in transport accident
V70–V79	Bus occupant injured in transport accident
V80–V89	Other land transport accidents
V90–V94	Water transport accidents
V95–V97	Air and space transport accidents
V98–V99	Other and unspecified transport accidents
W09	Fall on and from playground equipment (except codes ending in 7th character A)
W14	Fall from tree
W15	Fall from cliff
W16	Fall, jump or diving into water (excluding codes that end in 7th character A)

W17.0	Fall into well
W17.1	Fall into storm drain or manhole
W17.3	Fall into empty swimming pool
W17.4	Fall from dock
W17.8	Other fall from one level to another
W18.00	Striking against unspecified object with subsequent fall (excluding codes ending in 7th character A)
W18.01	Striking against sports equipment with subsequent fall
W18.02	Striking against glass with subsequent fall (except codes ending in 7th character A)
W18.09	Striking against other object with subsequent fall (except codes ending in 7th character A)
W18.1	Fall from or off toilet (except codes ending in 7th character A)
W18.2	Fall in (into) shower or empty bathtub (except codes ending in 7th character A)
W18.3	Other and unspecified fall on same level (except codes ending in 7th character A)
W18.4	Slipping, tripping and stumbling without falling (except codes ending in 7th character A)
W21	Striking against or struck by sports equipment
W22.01	Walked into wall (except codes ending in 7th character A)
W22.02	Walked into lamppost
W22.03	Walked into furniture (except codes ending in 7th character A)
W22.04	Striking against wall of swimming pool (except codes ending in 7th character A)
W22.09	Striking against other stationary object (except codes ending in 7th character A)
W22.1	Striking against or struck by automobile airbag
W22.8	Striking against or struck by other objects
W24.0	Contact with lifting devices, not elsewhere classified (except codes ending in 7th character A)
W24.1	Contact with transmission devices, NEC
W26.1–W26.9	Contact with knife, sword or dagger
W27.0	Contact with workbench
W27.1	Contact with garden tool
W27.2	Contact with scissors (except codes ending in 7th character A)
W27.3	Contact with needle (except codes ending in 7th character A)
W27.4	Contact with kitchen utensil (except codes ending in 7th character A)
W27.5	Contact with paper-cutter (except codes ending in 7th character A)
W27.8	Contact with other nonpowered hand tool
W28	Contact with powered lawn mower
W29	Contact with other powered hand tools and household machinery
W30	Contact with agricultural machinery
W31	Contact with other and unspecified machinery
W32–W34	Accidental handgun discharge and malfunction
W35–W40	Exposure to inanimate mechanical forces
W42.0	Exposure to supersonic waves
W42.9	Exposure to other noise (except codes ending in 7th character A)
W45.0	Nail entering through skin
W49	Exposure to other inanimate mechanical forces (except codes ending in 7th character A)
W52	Crushed, pushed or stepped on by crowd or human stampede
W53	Contact with rodent
W54	Contact with dog
W55	Contact with other mammals
W56	Contact with nonvenomous marine animal

W57	Bitten or stung by nonvenomous insect and other nonvenomous arthropods (except codes ending in 7th character A)
W58	Contact with crocodile or alligator
W59.01	Bitten by nonvenomous lizards (except codes ending in 7th character A)
W59.02–W59.8	Contact with other nonvenomous reptiles
W60	Contact with nonvenomous plant thorns and spines and sharp leaves
W61	Contact with birds (domestic) (wild)
W62	Contact with nonvenomous amphibians
W64	Exposure to other animate mechanical forces
W65	Accidental drowning and submersion while in bath-tub (except codes ending in 7th character A)
W67	Accidental drowning and submersion while in swimming pool (except codes ending in 7th character A)
W69	Accidental drowning and submersion while in natural water
W73	Other specified cause of accidental non-transport drowning and submersion
W74	Unspecified cause of accidental drowning and submersion
W85	Exposure to electric transmission lines (except codes ending in 7th character A)
W86	Exposure to other specified electric current (except codes ending in 7th character A)
W88	Exposure to ionizing radiation (except codes ending in 7th character A)
W89	Exposure to man-made visible and ultraviolet light
W90	Exposure to other nonionizing radiation (except codes ending in 7th character A)
W92	Exposure to excessive heat of man-made origin
W93	Exposure to excessive cold of man-made origin
W94	Exposure to high and low air pressure and changes in air pressure
W99	Exposure to other man-made environmental factors
X02	Exposure to controlled fire in building or structure (except codes ending in 7th character A)
X03	Exposure to controlled fire, not in building or structure (except codes ending in 7th character A)
X04	Exposure to ignition of highly flammable material
X30	Exposure to excessive natural heat
X31	Exposure to excessive natural cold
X32	Exposure to sunlight
X34	Earthquake (except codes ending in 7th character A)
X35	Volcanic eruption
X36	Avalanche, landslide and other earth movements (except codes ending in 7th character A)
X37	Cataclysmic storm (except codes ending in 7th character A)
X38	Flood (except codes ending in 7th character A)
X39	Exposure to other forces of nature
X50	Overexertion and strenuous or repetitive movements
X52	Prolonged stay in weightless environment
X71	Intentional self-harm by drowning and submersion (except codes ending in 7th character A) Except X71.0-, Intentional self-harm by drowning and submersion while in bath tub
X72	Intentional self-harm by handgun discharge
X73	Intentional self-harm by rifle, shotgun and larger firearm discharge
X74	Intentional self-harm by other and unspecified firearm and gun discharge
X75	Intentional self-harm by explosive material
X76	Intentional self-harm by smoke, fire and flames
X77	Intentional self-harm by steam, hot vapors and hot objects
X81	Intentional self-harm by jumping or lying in front of moving object

X82	Intentional self-harm by crashing of motor vehicle
X83	Intentional self-harm by other specified means
X92	Assault by drowning and submersion (except codes ending in 7th character A)
X93	Assault by handgun discharge (except codes ending in 7th character A)
X94	Assault by rifle, shotgun and larger firearm discharge (except codes ending in 7th character A)
X95	Assault by other and unspecified firearm and gun discharge (except codes ending in 7th character A)
X96	Assault by explosive material (except codes ending in 7th character A)
X97	Assault by smoke, fire and flames (except codes ending in 7th character A)
X98	Assault by steam, hot vapors and hot objects (except codes ending in 7th character A)
X99	Assault by sharp object (except codes ending in 7th character A)
Y00	Assault by blunt object (except codes ending in 7th character A)
Y01	Assault by pushing from high place (except codes ending in 7th character A)
Y02	Assault by pushing or placing victim in front of moving object
Y03	Assault by crashing of motor vehicle
Y04	Assault by bodily force (except codes ending in 7th character A)
Y07	Perpetrator of assault, maltreatment and neglect
Y08	Assault by other specified means
Y21	Drowning and submersion, undetermined intent
Y22	Handgun discharge, undetermined intent (except codes ending in 7th character A)
Y23	Rifle, shotgun and larger firearm discharge, undetermined intent (except codes ending in 7th character A)
Y24	Other and unspecified firearm discharge, undetermined intent (except Y24.9, Unspecified firearm discharge, undetermined intent, initial encounter)
Y30	Falling, jumping or pushed from a high place, undetermined intent
Y32	Assault by crashing of motor vehicle, undetermined intent
Y35	Legal intervention (except codes ending in 7th character A)
Y36	Operations of war
Y37	Military operations
Y38	Terrorism (except codes ending in 7th character A)
Y92	Place of occurrence of the external cause (except Y92.23-, Y92.530 and Y92.538)
Y93.12–Y93.9	Activity code
Y99	External cause status
Z00	Encounter for general examination without complaint, suspected or reported diagnosis
Z01	Encounter for other special examination without complaint, suspected or reported diagnosis
Z02	Encounter for administrative examination
Z03	Encounter for medical observation for suspected diseases and conditions ruled out
Z04.8-	Encounter for examination and observation for other specified reasons
Z05	Encounter for observation and evaluation of newborn for suspected diseases and conditions ruled out
Z08	Encounter for follow-up examination following completed treatment for malignant neoplasm
Z09	Encounter for follow-up examination after completed treatment for conditions other than malignant neoplasm
Z11	Encounter for screening for infectious and parasitic diseases
Z11.8	Encounter for screening for other infectious and parasitic diseases
Z12	Encounter for screening for malignant neoplasms
Z13	Encounter for screening for other diseases and disorders
Z14	Genetic carrier
Z15	Genetic susceptibility to disease
Z17	Estrogen receptor status

Z18	Retained foreign body fragments
Z19	Hormone sensitivity malignancy status
Z20.821	Contact with and (suspected) exposure to Zika virus
Z22	Carrier of infectious disease
Z23	Encounter for immunization
Z28	Immunization not carried out and underimmunization status
Z29	Encounter for prophylactic measures
Z30	Encounter for contraceptive management
Z31	Encounter for procreative management
Z34	Encounter for supervision of normal pregnancy
Z3A	Weeks of gestation
Z36	Encounter for antenatal screening of mother
Z37	Outcome of delivery
Z38	Liveborn infants according to place of birth and type of delivery
Z39	Encounter for maternal postpartum care and examination
Z40.3	Encounter for prophylactic removal of fallopian tube(s)
Z41	Encounter for procedures for purposes other than remedying health state
Z42	Encounter for plastic and reconstructive surgery following medical procedure or healed injury
Z43	Encounter for attention to artificial openings
Z44	Encounter for fitting and adjustment of external prosthetic device
Z45	Encounter for adjustment and management of implanted device
Z46	Encounter for fitting and adjustment of other devices
Z47	Orthopedic aftercare
Z48	Encounter for other postprocedural aftercare
Z49	Encounter for care involving renal dialysis
Z51	Encounter for other aftercare (except Z51.5, Encounter for palliative care)
Z52	Donors of organs and tissues
Z53.3	Procedure converted to open procedure
Z55	Problems related to education and literacy
Z56	Problems related to employment and unemployment
Z57	Occupational exposure to risk factors
Z58.6	Inadequate drinking-water supply
Z59	Problems related to housing and economic circumstances
Z62.813	Personal history of forced labor or sexual exploitation in childhood
Z63	Other problems related to primary support group, including family circumstances
Z64	Problems related to certain psychosocial circumstances
Z65	Problems related to other psychosocial circumstances
Z65.8	Other specified problems related to psychosocial circumstances
Z67.1–Z67.9	Blood type
Z68	Body mass index (BMI)
Z69	Encounter for mental health services for victim and perpetrator of abuse
Z70	Counseling related to sexual attitude, behavior and orientation
Z71	Persons encountering health services for other counseling and medical advice, NEC
Z72	Problems related to lifestyle
Z73	Problems related to life management difficulty
Z74.01	Bed confinement status
Z75	Problems related to medical facilities and other health care
Z76	Persons encountering health services in other circumstances

Z77.110–Z77.128	Environmental pollution and hazards in the physical environment
Z78	Other specified health status
Z79	Long-term (current) drug therapy
Z80	Family history of primary malignant neoplasm
Z81	Family history of mental and behavioral disorders
Z82	Family history of certain disabilities and chronic diseases (leading to disablement)
Z83	Family history of other specific disorders
Z84	Family history of other conditions
Z85	Personal history of primary malignant neoplasm
Z86	Personal history of certain other diseases
Z87	Personal history of other diseases and conditions
Z87.828	Personal history of other (healed) physical injury and trauma
Z87.891	Personal history of nicotine dependence
Z88	Allergy status to drugs, medicaments and biological substances
Z89	Acquired absence of limb
Z90	Acquired absence of organs, NEC
Z91	Personal risk factors, NEC
Z92	Personal history of medical treatment
Z93	Artificial opening status
Z94	Transplanted organ and tissue status
Z95	Presence of cardiac and vascular implants and grafts
Z96.82	Presence of neurostimulator
Z97	Presence of other devices
Z98	Other postprocedural states
Z99	Dependence on enabling machines and devices, not elsewhere classified

Additional Conventions

The use of symbols and color-coding has been added to this code book to alert the user to Medicare reimbursement logic and edits that are impacted by diagnosis coding. Although some third-party payers have adopted Medicare's reimbursement methodology, others have not. Therefore, it is important to review your facilities payer reporting requirements for non-Medicare payers prior to diagnosis coding.

Some codes may be included in multiple reimbursement issues and, therefore, may have more than one symbol or color-coding feature. For a quick reference review, the legend at the bottom of each page of the Tabular as well as the inside cover of the code book. The symbols and color-coding features are described in detail here.

Tabular Enhancements

In an effort to make the Tabular more user-friendly, the following symbols and color-coding features have been added. These features are indented to help the user in selecting a complete and accurate diagnosis code.

Final Character Indicator

ICD-10-CM codes range in length from 3 to 7 characters. In order for a code to be "valid" it must be listed to the fullest character length available. For example, if a fourth character is available, a three-character code is considered invalid.

To help users comply with this convention, a red plus sign (+) is listed to the left of any subcategory or subclassification code that requires an additional character. For example:

+ J45.2 Mild intermittent asthma

The assignment of the seventh character can, at times, be tricky. There are designated categories of codes that require a seventh character even though the code may not already have six characters present. For these codes, the user must insert the placeholder character of X after the code to fill any open characters prior to the seventh character.

To help users comply with this convention, in this book, the phrase **X+7th** is in red and is located to the left of the code that requires the placeholder of X and/or the seventh character. For example:

X+7th M80.00 Age-related osteoporosis with current pathological fracture

Additionally, there are six character codes that require the application of a seventh character. For these codes a placeholder X is not required. To help users differentiate these codes, in this book, the phrase **+7ᵗʰ** is in red and is located to the left of the code that requires the seventh character. For example:

+7ᵗʰ S72.021 Displaced fracture of epiphysis (separation) (upper) of right femur

Lastly, there are some codes that have only three characters. They require no further specification with additional characters and are therefore valid codes. The following note: Valid 3-character code, no further characters required is located below the code description in this book. This note alerts the coder that the three-character code is valid and can be used for reporting.

Color Identification

The Tabular section of this code book contains many instructional notes for the user. In order to help navigate the various types of instructional notes, a color-coding system has been applied:

- Category block headers are presented in dark green font.
- Category codes (three characters) are presented in blue font.
- Includes notes have a gray color bar over the **Includes**
- Excludes1 notes have a yellow color bar over the *Excludes1*
- Excludes2 notes have a bright green color bar over the *Excludes2*
- Notes have a maroon color bar over the **NOTE**
- *Use additional code* notes are presented in orange font
- *Code also* notes are presented in orange font
- *Code first* notes are presented in orange font
- Seventh character options are presented in a box and are highlighted in gray

The following excerpt from the Tabular illustrates the color-coding applied in this code book.

Disorders of bone density and structure (M80–M85)
M80 Osteoporosis with current pathological fracture
    Includes: osteoporosis with current fragility fracture
    Use additional code to identify major osseous defect, if applicable (M89.7-)
    Excludes1: collapsed vertebra NOS (M48.5)
                 pathological fracture NOS (M84.4)
                 wedging of vertebra NOS (M48.5)
    Excludes2: personal history of (healed) osteoporosis fracture (Z87.310)

The appropriate 7th character is to be added to each code from category M80:
A   initial encounter for fracture
D   subsequent encounter for fracture with routine healing
G   subsequent encounter for fracture with delayed healing
K   subsequent encounter for fracture with nonunion
P   subsequent encounter for fracture with malunion
S   sequela

Medicare Code Edits

Hospital inpatient Medicare claims paid under the Inpatient Prospective payment System (IPPS) are processed through the Medicare Code Editor (MCE) prior to payment by the Medicare administrative contractor (MAC). The code edits are intended to ensure that all claims processed by the MAC are accurate and complete. The information in this manual is based on the MCE v41.

Several of the MCE edits pertain to diagnoses. We have identified the codes included in these edits throughout the Tabular section this manual to assist users with preparing accurate and complete claims. The MCE edits included in this manual:

- Age conflict
- Sex Conflict Edit
- Manifestation codes not allowed as principal diagnosis
- Unacceptable principal diagnoses

Note: It is important to remember these edits are Medicare edits and may not apply to other third-party payers claim processing.

Age Conflict

The age conflict edit is activated when the age of the patient and the type diagnosis code reported does not match. The following symbols are used to identify the four age conflict categories.

- Newborn diagnosis age 0: This symbol appears to the left of the applicable code in the Tabular.
- Pediatric diagnosis age 0–17: This symbol appears to the left of the applicable code in the Tabular.
- Maternity diagnosis age 12–55: This symbol appears to the left of the applicable code in the Tabular.
- Adult diagnosis age 15–124: This symbol appears to the left of the applicable code in the Tabular.

Sex Conflict Edit

The sex conflict edit is activated when the sex of the patient and the diagnosis reported does not match. The following symbols are used to identify female-only and male-only diagnoses.

- ♀ Female-only diagnosis: This symbol appears to the left of the applicable code in the Tabular.
- ♂ Male-only diagnosis: This symbol appears to the left of the applicable code in the Tabular.

Manifestation Code Not Allowed as Principal Diagnosis

Manifestation codes are used to report the manifestation of an underlying disease, not to report the disease itself. Therefore, within ICD-10-CM the manifestation should not be reported as the principal diagnosis; rather it should always be reported as a secondary diagnosis.

Manifestation codes are identified with a light green color bar over the code in the Tabular. For example:

D63.0 Anemia in neoplastic disease

Unacceptable Principal Diagnosis

There are specified codes that describe a circumstance which influences an individual's health status but not a current illness or injury, or codes that are not specific manifestations but may be due to an underlying cause. These codes are considered unacceptable as a principal diagnosis.

Unacceptable principal diagnosis codes are identified with a light blue color bar over the code in the Tabular:

B60.13 Keratoconjunctivitis due to Acanthamoeba

MS-DRG Diagnosis Designations

The MS-DRG system is utilized within the IPPS to determine the unadjusted reimbursement amount for Medicare hospital inpatient claims. The MS-DRG Definitions Manual includes the logic for MS-DRG refinement and selection as well as logic based on the IPPS final rules released each August. The information in this book is based on the MS-DRG v41. *Note:* It is important to remember that these edits are Medicare edits and may not apply to other third-party payers claim processing.

CC and MCC Codes

Within the MS-DRG system, one of the refinement pathways is whether there is a complication/comorbidity (CC) or major complication/comorbidity (MCC) code reported as a secondary diagnosis. For some of the MS-DRG families, the presence of a CC or MCC allows for an MS-DRG assignment that has a higher relative weight and, therefore, a higher reimbursement amount. There are exceptions to the application of the CC or MCC codes and the exceptions are referred to as *CC Exclusions* or *MCC Exclusions*. If exclusions apply, the CC/MCC code is assigned a principal diagnosis collection. Within this collection are the codes that, when reported as principal diagnosis, excludes the CC/MCC status from the secondary diagnosis code under review. Essentially, it takes away the CC/MCC code's ability to influence the MS-DRG assignment.

Codes that are considered CC codes have a purple **CC** to the left of the code in the Tabular. The principal diagnosis collection for each CC code is provided in Appendix A. Coding professionals may review the principal diagnosis collection identified if required for the task at hand. If the code requires a seventh character, the characters that are eligible for CC status are included within Appendix A.

Codes that are considered MCC codes have a purple **MCC** to the left of the code in the Tabular. The principal diagnosis collection for each MCC code is provided in Appendix A. Coding professionals may review the principal diagnosis collection identified if required for the task at hand. If the code requires a seventh character, the characters that are eligible for MCC status are included within Appendix A.

Hospital-Acquired Conditions Related Diagnoses

As part of the Medicare Value-Based Purchasing program, CMS has implemented a Paying for Value program entitled Hospital-Acquired Conditions (HACs) Present on Admission Indicator Program. This program is designed to reduce reimbursements to facilities where the value of the medical or surgical services have been comprised due to preventable conditions. Reimbursement for admissions that meet the HAC Present on Admission Indicator Program criteria will be reduced. In this manual, the HAC-associated procedures are identified with an orange rectangle HAC with HAC. The orange rectangle is located below the code description in the code listing. If there is conditional logic for the diagnosis code, it is included in Appendix B.

AHA *Coding Clinic for ICD-10-CM and ICD-10-PCS*
The American Hospital Association began publishing coding guidance for ICD-10-CM and ICD-10-PCS in the fourth quarter of 2012. In this code book we identify diagnosis codes that are discussed in the *Coding Clinic* guidance fourth quarter 2012 through second quarter 2023. Within the Tabular the following sky-blue note alerts the coder to review the AHA *Coding Clinic* prior to assignment of the code to ensure appropriate and accurate reporting. The quarter of publication, year, and page number(s) are provided in the note.

AHA CC: 4Q; 2012; pg#-pg#

CMS Hierarchical Condition Categories Risk Adjustment System
Since 2004, Medicare has utilized the CMS Hierarchical Condition Categories (CMS-HCC) model to risk adjust within the Medicare Advantage capitation payment system. Using the CMS-HCC model Medicare uses large pools of data to predict average costs for a predetermined set of factors; one of the factors is individual disease groups. The HCC diagnosis code listing is utilized to determine the individual disease groups from Medicare claims data. Additionally, CMS-HCC model is utilized in accountable care organizations payment methodologies (inpatient and outpatient settings) and in Medicare's inpatient acute care (IPPS) value-based purchasing program. The use of the CMS-HCC model for risk adjustment within payment systems continues to grow. Therefore, it is imperative that coding professionals in all settings are familiar with the reporting of HCC diagnosis codes. The most current list of CMS-HCC model diagnosis codes are identified in this code book. The CMS-HCC model is updated each year with an effective date of January 1.

CMS-HCC diagnosis codes are identified with a lavender color bar over the code in the Tabular:

E11.21 Type 2 diabetes mellitus with diabetic nephropathy

Basic Steps in ICD-10-CM Coding

To code each disease or condition completely and accurately, the coder should:

1. Identify all main terms included in the diagnostic statement.
2. Locate each main term in the Alphabetic Index.
3. Refer to any subterms indented under the main term. The subterms form individual line entries and describe essential differences by site, etiology, or clinical type.
4. Follow the instructions (see, see also) provided in the Alphabetic Index if the needed code is not located under the first main entry consulted.
5. Verify the code selected in the Tabular List.
6. Read and be guided by any instructional terms in the Tabular List.
7. Assign codes to their highest level of specificity, up to a total of seven characters if applicable.
8. Continue coding the diagnostic statement until all the component elements are fully identified.

(*Source:* Schraffenberger, L.A. *Basic ICD-10-CM/PCS Coding*, 2020 Edition, pp. 43–44. AHIMA.)

Index to Diseases and Injuries

A

Aarskog's syndrome Q87.19
Abandonment —*see* Maltreatment
Abasia (-astasia) (hysterical) F44.4
Abderhalden-Kaufmann-Lignac syndrome (cystinosis) E72.04
Abdomen, abdominal —*see also* condition
  acute R10.0
  angina K55.1
  muscle deficiency syndrome Q79.4
Abdominalgia —*see* Pain, abdominal
Abduction contracture, hip or other joint —*see* Contraction, joint
Aberrant (congenital) —*see also* Malposition, congenital
  adrenal gland Q89.1
  artery (peripheral) Q27.8
    basilar NEC Q28.1
    cerebral Q28.3
    coronary Q24.5
    digestive system Q27.8
    eye Q15.8
    lower limb Q27.8
    precerebral Q28.1
    pulmonary Q25.79
    renal Q27.2
    retina Q14.1
    specified site NEC Q27.8
    subclavian Q27.8
    upper limb Q27.8
    vertebral Q28.1
  breast Q83.8
  endocrine gland NEC Q89.2
  hepatic duct Q44.5
  pancreas Q45.3
  parathyroid gland Q89.2
  pituitary gland Q89.2
  sebaceous glands, mucous membrane, mouth, congenital Q38.6
  spleen Q89.09
  subclavian artery Q27.8
  thymus (gland) Q89.2
  thyroid gland Q89.2
  vein (peripheral) NEC Q27.8
    cerebral Q28.3
    digestive system Q27.8
    lower limb Q27.8
    precerebral Q28.1
    specified site NEC Q27.8
    upper limb Q27.8
Aberration
  distantial —*see* Disturbance, visual
  mental F99
Abetalipoproteinemia E78.6
Abiotrophy R68.89
Ablatio, ablation
  retinae —*see* Detachment, retina
Ablepharia, ablepharon Q10.3
Abnormal, abnormality, abnormalities —*see also* Anomaly
  acid-base balance (mixed) E87.4
  albumin R77.0
  alphafetoprotein R77.2
  alveolar ridge K08.9
  anatomical relationship Q89.9
  apertures, congenital, diaphragm Q79.1
  atrial septal, specified NEC Q21.19
  auditory perception H93.29-

Abnormal, abnormality, abnormalities (*continued*)
 auditory perception (*continued*)
    diplacusis —*see* Diplacusis
    hyperacusis —*see* Hyperacusis
    recruitment —*see* Recruitment, auditory
    threshold shift —*see* Shift, auditory threshold
  autosomes Q99.9
    fragile site Q95.5
  basal metabolic rate R94.8
  biosynthesis, testicular androgen E29.1
  bleeding time R79.1
  blood amino-acid level R79.83
  blood-gas level R79.81
  blood level (of)
    cobalt R79.0
    copper R79.0
    iron R79.0
    lithium R78.89
    magnesium R79.0
    mineral NEC R79.0
    zinc R79.0
  blood pressure
    elevated R03.0
    low reading (nonspecific) R03.1
  blood sugar R73.09
  bowel sounds R19.15
    absent R19.11
    hyperactive R19.12
  brain scan R94.02
  breathing R06.9
  caloric test R94.138
  cerebrospinal fluid R83.9
    cytology R83.6
    drug level R83.2
    enzyme level R83.0
    hormones R83.1
    immunology R83.4
    microbiology R83.5
    nonmedicinal level R83.3
    specified type NEC R83.8
  chemistry, blood R79.9
    C-reactive protein R79.82
    drugs —*see* Findings, abnormal, in blood
    gas level R79.81
    minerals R79.0
    pancytopenia D61.818
    PTT R79.1
    specified NEC R79.89
    toxins —*see* Findings, abnormal, in blood
  chest sounds (friction) (rales) R09.89
  chromosome, chromosomal Q99.9
    with more than three X chromosomes, female Q97.1
    analysis result R89.8
    bronchial washings R84.8
    cerebrospinal fluid R83.8
    cervix uteri NEC R87.89
    nasal secretions R84.8
    nipple discharge R89.8
    peritoneal fluid R85.89
    pleural fluid R84.8
    prostatic secretions R86.8
    saliva R85.89
    seminal fluid R86.8
    sputum R84.8
    synovial fluid R89.8
    throat scrapings R84.8
    vagina R87.89
    vulva R87.89
    wound secretions R89.8

Abnormal, abnormality, abnormalities (*continued*)
  chromosome (*continued*)
    dicentric replacement Q93.2
    ring replacement Q93.2
    sex Q99.8
      female phenotype Q97.9
        specified NEC Q97.8
      male phenotype Q98.9
        specified NEC Q98.8
      structural male Q98.6
    specified NEC Q99.8
  clinical findings NEC R68.89
  coagulation D68.9
    newborn, transient P61.6
    profile R79.1
    time R79.1
  communication —*see* Fistula
  conjunctiva, vascular H11.41-
  coronary artery Q24.5
  cortisol-binding globulin E27.8
  course, eustachian tube Q17.8
  creatinine clearance R94.4
  cytology
    anus R85.619
      atypical squamous cells cannot exclude high grade squamous intraepithelial lesion (ASC-H) R85.611
      atypical squamous cells of undetermined significance (ASC-US) R85.610
      cytologic evidence of malignancy R85.614
      high grade squamous intraepithelial lesion (HGSIL) R85.613
      human papillomavirus (HPV) DNA test
        high risk positive R85.81
        low risk postive R85.82
      inadequate smear R85.615
      low grade squamous intraepithelial lesion (LGSIL) R85.612
      satisfactory anal smear but lacking transformation zone R85.616
      specified NEC R85.618
      unsatisfactory smear R85.615
    female genital organs —*see* Abnormal, Papanicolaou (smear)
  dark adaptation curve H53.61
  dentofacial NEC —*see* Anomaly, dentofacial
  development, developmental Q89.9
    central nervous system Q07.9
  diagnostic imaging
    abdomen, abdominal region NEC R93.5
    biliary tract R93.2
    bladder R93.41
    breast R92.8
    central nervous system NEC R90.89
    cerebrovascular NEC R90.89
    coronary circulation R93.1
    digestive tract NEC R93.3
    gastrointestinal (tract) R93.3
    genitourinary organs R93.89
    head R93.0
    heart R93.1
    intrathoracic organ NEC R93.89
    kidney R93.42-

Abnormal, abnormality, abnormalities (*continued*)
  diagnostic imaging (*continued*)
    limbs R93.6
    liver R93.2
    lung (field) R91.8
    musculoskeletal system NEC R93.7
    renal pelvis R93.41
    retroperitoneum R93.5
    site specified NEC R93.89
    skin and subcutaneous tissue R93.89
    skull R93.0
    testis R93.81-
    urinary organs specified NEC R93.49
    ureter R93.41
  direction, teeth, fully erupted M26.30
  ear ossicles, acquired NEC H74.39-
    ankylosis —*see* Ankylosis, ear ossicles
    discontinuity —*see* Discontinuity, ossicles, ear
    partial loss —*see* Loss, ossicles, ear (partial)
  Ebstein Q22.5
  echocardiogram R93.1
  echoencephalogram R90.81
  echogram —*see* Abnormal, diagnostic imaging
  electrocardiogram [ECG] [EKG] R94.31
  electroencephalogram [EEG] R94.01
  electrolyte —*see* Imbalance, electrolyte
  electromyogram [EMG] R94.131
  electro-oculogram [EOG] R94.110
  electrophysiological intracardiac studies R94.39
  electroretinogram [ERG] R94.111
  erythrocytes
    congenital, with perinatal jaundice D58.9
  feces (color) (contents) (mucus) R19.5
  finding —*see* Findings, abnormal, without diagnosis
  fluid
    amniotic —*see* Abnormal, specimen, specified
    cerebrospinal —*see* Abnormal, cerebrospinal fluid
    peritoneal —*see* Abnormal, specimen, digestive organs
    pleural —*see* Abnormal, specimen, respiratory organs
    synovial —*see* Abnormal, specimen, specified
    thorax (bronchial washings) (pleural fluid) —*see* Abnormal, specimen, respiratory organs
    vaginal —*see* Abnormal, specimen, female genital organs
  form
    teeth K00.2
    uterus —*see* Anomaly, uterus
  function studies
    auditory R94.120
    bladder R94.8
    brain R94.09

1

Abnormal, abnormality, abnormalities *(continued)*
  function studies *(continued)*
    cardiovascular R94.30
    ear R94.128
    endocrine NEC R94.7
    eye NEC R94.118
    kidney R94.4
    liver R94.5
    nervous system
      central NEC R94.09
      peripheral NEC R94.138
    pancreas R94.8
    placenta R94.8
    pulmonary R94.2
    special senses NEC R94.128
    spleen R94.8
    thyroid R94.6
    vestibular R94.121
  gait —*see* Gait
    hysterical F44.4
  gastrin secretion E16.4
  globulin R77.1
    cortisol-binding E27.8
    thyroid-binding E07.89
  glomerular, minor *(see also N00-N07 with fourth character .0)* N05.0
  glucagon secretion E16.3
  glucose tolerance (test) (non-fasting) R73.09
  gravitational (G) forces or states (effect of) T75.81
  hair (color) (shaft) L67.9
    specified NEC L67.8
  hard tissue formation in pulp (dental) K04.3
  head movement R25.0
  heart
    rate R00.9
      specified NEC R00.8
    shadow R93.1
    sounds NEC R01.2
  hemoglobin (disease) —*see also* Disease, hemoglobin D58.2
    trait —*see* Trait, hemoglobin, abnormal
  histology NEC R89.7
  immunological findings R89.4
    in serum R76.9
      specified NEC R76.8
  increase in appetite R63.2
  involuntary movement —*see* Abnormal, movement, involuntary
  jaw closure M26.51
  karyotype R89.8
  kidney function test R94.4
  knee jerk R29.2
  leukocyte (cell) (differential) NEC D72.9
  liver function test *(see also* Elevated, liver function, test) R79.89
  loss of
    height R29.890
    weight R63.4
  mammogram NEC R92.8
    calcification (calculus) R92.1
    microcalcification R92.0
  Mantoux test R76.11
  movement (disorder) —*see also* Disorder, movement
    head R25.0
    involuntary R25.9
      fasciculation R25.3
      of head R25.0
      spasm R25.2
      specified type NEC R25.8
      tremor R25.1

Abnormal, abnormality, abnormalities *(continued)*
  myoglobin (Aberdeen) (Annapolis) R89.7
  neonatal screening P09.9
    for
      congenital adrenal hyperplasia P09.2
      congenital endocrine disease P09.2
      congenital hematologic disorders P09.3
      critical congenital heart disease P09.5
      cystic fibrosis P09.4
      hemoglobinopathy P09.3
      hypothyroidism P09.2
      inborn errors of metabolism P09.1
    neonatal hearing loss P09.6
    red cell membrane defects P09.3
    sickle cell P09.3
    specified NEC P09.8
  oculomotor study R94.113
  palmar creases Q82.8
  Papanicolaou (smear)
    anus R85.619
      atypical squamous cells
        cannot exclude high grade squamous intraepithelial lesion (ASC-H) R85.611
      atypical squamous cells of undetermined significance (ASC-US) R85.610
      cytologic evidence of malignancy R85.614
      high grade squamous intraepithelial lesion (HGSIL) R85.613
      human papillomavirus (HPV) DNA test
        high risk positive R85.81
        low risk postive R85.82
      inadequate smear R85.615
      low grade squamous intraepithelial lesion (LGSIL) R85.612
      satisfactory anal smear but lacking transformation zone R85.616
      specified NEC R85.618
      unsatisfactory smear R85.615
    bronchial washings R84.6
    cerebrospinal fluid R83.6
    cervix R87.619
      atypical squamous cells
        cannot exclude high grade squamous intraepithelial lesion (ASC-H) R87.611
      atypical squamous cells of undetermined significance (ASC-US) R87.610
      cytologic evidence of malignancy R87.614
      high grade squamous intraepithelial lesion (HGSIL) R87.613
      inadequate smear R87.615
      low grade squamous intraepithelial lesion (LGSIL) R87.612
      non-atypical endometrial cells R87.618
      satisfactory cervical smear but lacking transformation zone R87.616
      specified NEC R87.618
      thin preparaton R87.619

Abnormal, abnormality, abnormalities *(continued)*
  Papanicolaou *(continued)*
    cervix *(continued)*
      unsatisfactory smear R87.615
    nasal secretions R84.6
    nipple discharge R89.6
    peritoneal fluid R85.69
    pleural fluid R84.6
    prostatic secretions R86.6
    saliva R85.69
    seminal fluid R86.6
    sites NEC R89.6
    sputum R84.6
    synovial fluid R89.6
    throat scrapings R84.6
    vagina R87.629
      atypical squamous cells
        cannot exclude high grade squamous intraepithelial lesion (ASC-H) R87.621
      atypical squamous cells of undetermined significance (ASC-US) R87.620
      cytologic evidence of malignancy R87.624
      high grade squamous intraepithelial lesion (HGSIL) R87.623
      inadequate smear R87.625
      low grade squamous intraepithelial lesion (LGSIL) R87.622
      specified NEC R87.628
      thin preparation R87.629
      unsatisfactory smear R87.625
    vulva R87.69
    wound secretions R89.6
  partial thromboplastin time (PTT) R79.1
  pelvis (bony) —*see* Deformity, pelvis
  percussion, chest (tympany) R09.89
  periods (grossly) —*see* Menstruation
  phonocardiogram R94.39
  plantar reflex R29.2
  plasma
    protein R77.9
      specified NEC R77.8
    viscosity R70.1
  pleural (folds) Q34.0
  posture R29.3
  product of conception O02.9
    specified type NEC O02.89
  prothrombin time (PT) R79.1
  pulmonary
    artery, congenital Q25.79
    function, newborn P28.89
    test results R94.2
  pulsations in neck R00.2
  pupillary H21.56-
    function (reaction) (reflex) —*see* Anomaly, pupil, function
  radiological examination —*see* Abnormal, diagnostic imaging
  red blood cell(s) (morphology) (volume) R71.8
  reflex —*see* Reflex
  renal function test R94.4
  response to nerve stimulation R94.130
  retinal correspondence H53.31
  retinal function study R94.111
  rhythm, heart —*see also* Arrhythmia
  saliva —*see* Abnormal, specimen, digestive organs
  scan
    kidney R94.4
    liver R93.2

Abnormal, abnormality, abnormalities *(continued)*
  scan *(continued)*
    thyroid R94.6
  secretion
    gastrin E16.4
    glucagon E16.3
  semen, seminal fluid —*see* Abnormal, specimen, male genital organs
  serum level (of)
    acid phosphatase R74.8
    alkaline phosphatase R74.8
    amylase R74.8
    enzymes R74.9
      specified NEC R74.8
    lipase R74.8
    triacylglycerol lipase R74.8
  shape
    gravid uterus —*see* Anomaly, uterus
  sinus venosus Q21.16
  size, tooth, teeth K00.2
  spacing, tooth, teeth, fully erupted M26.30
  specimen
    digestive organs (peritoneal fluid) (saliva) R85.9
      cytology R85.69
      drug level R85.2
      enzyme level R85.0
      histology R85.7
      hormones R85.1
      immunology R85.4
      microbiology R85.5
      nonmedicinal level R85.3
      specified type NEC R85.89
    female genital organs (secretions) (smears) R87.9
      cytology R87.69
        cervix R87.619
          human papillomavirus (HPV) DNA test
            high risk positive R87.810
            low risk positive R87.820
          inadequate (unsatisfactory) smear R87.615
          non-atypical endometrial cells R87.618
          specified NEC R87.618
        vagina R87.629
          human papillomavirus (HPV) DNA test
            high risk positive R87.811
            low risk positive R87.821
          inadequate (unsatisfactory) smear R87.625
        vulva R87.69
      drug level R87.2
      enzyme level R87.0
      histological R87.7
      hormones R87.1
      immunology R87.4
      microbiology R87.5
      nonmedicinal level R87.3
      specified type NEC R87.89
    male genital organs (prostatic secretions) (semen) R86.9
      cytology R86.6
      drug level R86.2
      enzyme level R86.0
      histological R86.7
      hormones R86.1
      immunology R86.4
      microbiology R86.5

Abnormal, abnormality, abnormalities (continued)
  specimen (continued)
    male genital organs (continued)
      nonmedicinal level R86.3
      specified type NEC R86.8
    nipple discharge —see Abnormal, specimen, specified
    respiratory organs (bronchial washings) (nasal secretions) (pleural fluid) (sputum) R84.9
      cytology R84.6
      drug level R84.2
      enzyme level R84.0
      histology R84.7
      hormones R84.1
      immunology R84.4
      microbiology R84.5
      nonmedicinal level R84.3
      specified type NEC R84.8
    specified organ, system and tissue NOS R89.9
      cytology R89.6
      drug level R89.2
      enzyme level R89.0
      histology R89.7
      hormones R89.1
      immunology R89.4
      microbiology R89.5
      nonmedicinal level R89.3
      specified type NEC R89.8
    synovial fluid —see Abnormal, specimen, specified
    thorax (bronchial washings) (pleural fluids) —see Abnormal, specimen, respiratory organs
    vagina (secretion) (smear) R87.629
    vulva (secretion) (smear) R87.69
    wound secretion —see Abnormal, specimen, specified
  spermatozoa —see Abnormal, specimen, male genital organs
  sputum (amount) (color) (odor) R09.3
  stool (color) (contents) (mucus) R19.5
    bloody K92.1
    guaiac positive R19.5
  synchondrosis Q78.8
  thermography —see also Abnormal, diagnostic imaging R93.89
  thyroid-binding globulin E07.89
  tooth, teeth (form) (size) K00.2
  toxicology (findings) R78.9
  transport protein E88.09
  tumor marker NEC R97.8
  ultrasound results —see Abnormal, diagnostic imaging
  umbilical cord complicating delivery O69.9
  urination NEC R39.198
  urine (constituents) R82.90
    bile R82.2
    cytological examination R82.89
    drugs R82.5
    fat R82.0
    glucose R81
    heavy metals R82.6
    hemoglobin R82.3
    histological examination R82.89
    ketones R82.4
    microbiological examination (culture) R82.79
    myoglobin R82.1
    positive culture R82.79
    protein —see Proteinuria

Abnormal, abnormality, abnormalities (continued)
  urine (continued)
    specified substance NEC R82.998
      chromoabnormality NEC R82.91
    substances nonmedical R82.6
  uterine hemorrhage —see Hemorrhage, uterus
  vectorcardiogram R94.39
  visually evoked potential (VEP) R94.112
  white blood cells D72.9
    specified NEC D72.89
  X-ray examination —see Abnormal, diagnostic imaging

Abnormity (any organ or part) —see Anomaly

Abocclusion M26.29
  hemolytic disease (newborn) P55.1
  incompatibility reaction ABO —see Complication(s), transfusion, incompatibility reaction, ABO

Abolition, language R48.8

Aborter, habitual or recurrent —see Loss (of), pregnancy, recurrent

Abortion (complete) (spontaneous) O03.9
  with
    retained products of conception —see Abortion, incomplete
  attempted (elective) (failed) O07.4
    complicated by O07.30
      afibrinogenemia O07.1
      cardiac arrest O07.36
      chemical damage of pelvic organ(s) O07.34
      circulatory collapse O07.31
      cystitis O07.38
      defibrination syndrome O07.1
      electrolyte imbalance O07.33
      embolism (air) (amniotic fluid) (blood clot) (fat) (pulmonary) (septic) (soap) O07.2
      endometritis O07.0
      genital tract and pelvic infection O07.0
      hemolysis O07.1
      hemorrhage (delayed) (excessive) O07.1
      infection
        genital tract or pelvic O07.0
        urinary tract O07.38
      intravascular coagulation O07.1
      laceration of pelvic organ(s) O07.34
      metabolic disorder O07.33
      oliguria O07.32
      oophoritis O07.0
      parametritis O07.0
      pelvic peritonitis O07.0
      perforation of pelvic organ(s) O07.34
      renal failure or shutdown O07.32
      salpingitis or salpingo-oophoritis O07.0
      sepsis O07.37
      shock O07.31
      specified condition NEC O07.39
      tubular necrosis (renal) O07.32

Abortion (continued)
  attempted (continued)
    complicated (continued)
      uremia O07.32
      urinary tract infection O07.38
      venous complication NEC O07.35
        embolism (air) (amniotic fluid) (blood clot) (fat) (pulmonary) (septic) (soap) O07.2
  complicated (by) (following) O03.80
    afibrinogenemia O03.6
    cardiac arrest O03.86
    chemical damage of pelvic organ(s) O03.84
    circulatory collapse O03.81
    cystitis O03.88
    defibrination syndrome O03.6
    electrolyte imbalance O03.83
    embolism (air) (amniotic fluid) (blood clot) (fat) (pulmonary) (septic) (soap) O03.7
    endometritis O03.5
    genital tract and pelvic infection O03.5
    hemolysis O03.6
    hemorrhage (delayed) (excessive) O03.6
    infection
      genital tract or pelvic O03.5
      urinary tract O03.88
    intravascular coagulation O03.6
    laceration of pelvic organ(s) O03.84
    metabolic disorder O03.83
    oliguria O03.82
    oophoritis O03.5
    parametritis O03.5
    pelvic peritonitis O03.5
    perforation of pelvic organ(s) O03.84
    renal failure or shutdown O03.82
    salpingitis or salpingo-oophoritis O03.5
    sepsis O03.87
    shock O03.81
    specified condition NEC O03.89
    tubular necrosis (renal) O03.82
    uremia O03.82
    urinary tract infection O03.88
    venous complication NEC O03.85
      embolism (air) (amniotic fluid) (blood clot) (fat) (pulmonary) (septic) (soap) O03.7
  failed —see Abortion, attempted
  habitual or recurrent N96
    with current abortion —see categories O03-O04
    without current pregnancy N96
    care in current pregnancy O26.2-
  incomplete (spontaneous) O03.4
    complicated (by) (following) O03.30
      afibrinogenemia O03.1
      cardiac arrest O03.36
      chemical damage of pelvic organ(s) O03.34
      circulatory collapse O03.31
      cystitis O03.38
      defibrination syndrome O03.1
      electrolyte imbalance O03.33
      embolism (air) (amniotic fluid) (blood clot) (fat) (pulmonary) (septic) (soap) O03.2
      endometritis O03.0

Abortion (continued)
  incomplete (continued)
    complicated (continued)
      genital tract and pelvic infection O03.0
      hemolysis O03.1
      hemorrhage (delayed) (excessive) O03.1
      infection
        genital tract or pelvic O03.0
        urinary tract O03.38
      intravascular coagulation O03.1
      laceration of pelvic organ(s) O03.34
      metabolic disorder O03.33
      oliguria O03.32
      oophoritis O03.0
      parametritis O03.0
      pelvic peritonitis O03.0
      perforation of pelvic organ(s) O03.34
      renal failure or shutdown O03.32
      salpingitis or salpingo-oophoritis O03.0
      sepsis O03.37
      shock O03.31
      specified condition NEC O03.39
      tubular necrosis (renal) O03.32
      uremia O03.32
      urinary infection O03.38
      venous complication NEC O03.35
        embolism (air) (amniotic fluid) (blood clot) (fat) (pulmonary) (septic) (soap) O03.2
  induced (encounter for) Z33.2
    complicated by O04.80
      afibrinogenemia O04.6
      cardiac arrest O04.86
      chemical damage of pelvic organ(s) O04.84
      circulatory collapse O04.81
      cystitis O04.88
      defibrination syndrome O04.6
      electrolyte imbalance O04.83
      embolism (air) (amniotic fluid) (blood clot) (fat) (pulmonary) (septic) (soap) O04.7
      endometritis O04.5
      genital tract and pelvic infection O04.5
      hemolysis O04.6
      hemorrhage (delayed) (excessive) O04.6
      infection
        genital tract or pelvic O04.5
        urinary tract O04.88
      intravascular coagulation O04.6
      laceration of pelvic organ(s) O04.84
      metabolic disorder O04.83
      oliguria O04.82
      oophoritis O04.5
      parametritis O04.5
      pelvic peritonitis O04.5
      perforation of pelvic organ(s) O04.84
      renal failure or shutdown O04.82
      salpingitis or salpingo-oophoritis O04.5
      sepsis O04.87
      shock O04.81
      specified condition NEC O04.89
      tubular necrosis (renal) O04.82

Abortion (continued)
induced (continued)
complicated (continued)
uremia O04.82
urinary tract infection O04.88
venous complication NEC O04.85
embolism (air) (amniotic fluid) (blood clot) (fat) (pulmonary) (septic) (soap) O04.7
inevitable O03.4
missed O02.1
spontaneous —see Abortion (complete) (spontaneous)
threatened O20.0
threatened (spontaneous) O20.0
tubal O00.10-
with intrauterine pregnancy O00.11-

Abortus fever A23.1

Aboulomania F60.7

Abrami's disease D59.8

Abramov-Fiedler myocarditis (acute isolated myocarditis) I40.1

Abrasion T14.8
abdomen, abdominal (wall) S30.811
alveolar process S00.512
ankle S90.51-
antecubital space —see Abrasion, elbow
anus S30.817
arm (upper) S40.81-
auditory canal —see Abrasion, ear
auricle —see Abrasion, ear
axilla —see Abrasion, arm
back, lower S30.810
breast S20.11-
brow S00.81
buttock S30.810
calf —see Abrasion, leg
canthus —see Abrasion, eyelid
cheek S00.81
internal S00.512
chest wall —see Abrasion, thorax
chin S00.81
clitoris S30.814
cornea S05.0-
costal region —see Abrasion, thorax
dental K03.1
digit(s)
foot —see Abrasion, toe
hand —see Abrasion, finger
ear S00.41-
elbow S50.31-
epididymis S30.813
epigastric region S30.811
epiglottis S10.11
esophagus (thoracic) S27.818
cervical S10.11
eyebrow —see Abrasion, eyelid
eyelid S00.21-
face S00.81
finger(s) S60.41-
index S60.41-
little S60.41-
middle S60.41-
ring S60.41-
flank S30.811
foot (except toe(s) alone) S90.81-
toe —see Abrasion, toe
forearm S50.81-
elbow only —see Abrasion, elbow
forehead S00.81
genital organs, external
female S30.816
male S30.815

Abrasion (continued)
groin S30.811
gum S00.512
hand S60.51-
head S00.91
ear —see Abrasion, ear
eyelid —see Abrasion, eyelid
lip S00.511
nose S00.31
oral cavity S00.512
scalp S00.01
specified site NEC S00.81
heel —see Abrasion, foot
hip S70.21-
inguinal region S30.811
interscapular region S20.419
jaw S00.81
knee S80.21-
labium (majus) (minus) S30.814
larynx S10.11
leg (lower) S80.81-
knee —see Abrasion, knee
upper —see Abrasion, thigh
lip S00.511
lower back S30.810
lumbar region S30.810
malar region S00.81
mammary —see Abrasion, breast
mastoid region S00.81
mouth S00.512
nail
finger —see Abrasion, finger
toe —see Abrasion, toe
nape S10.81
nasal S00.31
neck S10.91
specified site NEC S10.81
throat S10.11
nose S00.31
occipital region S00.01
oral cavity S00.512
orbital region —see Abrasion, eyelid
palate S00.512
palm —see Abrasion, hand
parietal region S00.01
pelvis S30.810
penis S30.812
perineum
female S30.814
male S30.810
periocular area —see Abrasion, eyelid
phalanges
finger —see Abrasion, finger
toe —see Abrasion, toe
pharynx S10.11
pinna —see Abrasion, ear
popliteal space —see Abrasion, knee
prepuce S30.812
pubic region S30.810
pudendum
female S30.816
male S30.815
sacral region S30.810
scalp S00.01
scapular region —see Abrasion, shoulder
scrotum S30.813
shin —see Abrasion, leg
shoulder S40.21-
skin NEC T14.8
sternal region S20.319
submaxillary region S00.81
submental region S00.81
subungual
finger(s) —see Abrasion, finger
toe(s) —see Abrasion, toe
supraclavicular fossa S10.81
supraorbital S00.81

Abrasion (continued)
temple S00.81
temporal region S00.81
testis S30.813
thigh S70.31-
thorax, thoracic (wall) S20.91
back S20.41-
front S20.31-
throat S10.11
thumb S60.31-
toe(s) (lesser) S90.416
great S90.41-
tongue S00.512
tooth, teeth (dentifrice) (habitual) (hard tissues) (occupational) (ritual) (traditional) K03.1
trachea S10.11
tunica vaginalis S30.813
tympanum, tympanic membrane —see Abrasion, ear
uvula S00.512
vagina S30.814
vocal cords S10.11
vulva S30.814
wrist S60.81-

Abrism —see Poisoning, food, noxious, plant

Abruptio placentae O45.9-
with
afibrinogenemia O45.01-
coagulation defect O45.00-
specified NEC O45.09-
disseminated intravascular coagulation O45.02-
hypofibrinogenemia O45.01-
specified NEC O45.8-

Abruption, placenta —see Abruptio placentae

Abscess (connective tissue) (embolic) (fistulous) (infective) (metastatic) (multiple) (pernicious) (pyogenic) (septic) L02.91
with
diverticular disease (intestine) K57.80
with bleeding K57.81
large intestine K57.20
with
bleeding K57.21
small intestine K57.40
with bleeding K57.41
small intestine K57.00
with
bleeding K57.01
large intestine K57.40
with bleeding K57.41
lymphangitis - code by site under Abscess
abdomen, abdominal
cavity K65.1
wall L02.211
abdominopelvic K65.1
accessory sinus —see Sinusitis
adrenal (capsule) (gland) E27.8
alveolar K04.7
with sinus K04.6
amebic A06.4
brain (and liver or lung abscess) A06.6
genitourinary tract A06.82
liver (without mention of brain or lung abscess) A06.4
lung (and liver) (without mention of brain abscess) A06.5
specified site NEC A06.89
spleen A06.89
anerobic A48.0
ankle —see Abscess, lower limb

Abscess (continued)
anorectal K61.2
antecubital space —see Abscess, upper limb
antrum (chronic) (Highmore) —see Sinusitis, maxillary
anus K61.0
apical (tooth) K04.7
with sinus (alveolar) K04.6
appendix K35.33
areola (acute) (chronic) (nonpuerperal) N61.1
puerperal, postpartum or gestational —see Infection, nipple
arm (any part) —see Abscess, upper limb
artery (wall) I77.89
atheromatous I77.2
auricle, ear —see Abscess, ear, external
axilla (region) L02.41-
lymph gland or node L04.2
back (any part, except buttock) L02.212
Bartholin's gland N75.1
with
abortion —see Abortion, by type complicated by, sepsis
ectopic or molar pregnancy O08.0
following ectopic or molar pregnancy O08.0
Bezold's —see Mastoiditis, acute
bilharziasis B65.1
bladder (wall) —see Cystitis, specified type NEC
bone (subperiosteal) —see also Osteomyelitis, specified type NEC
accessory sinus (chronic) —see Sinusitis
chronic or old —see Osteomyelitis, chronic
jaw (lower) (upper) M27.2
mastoid —see Mastoiditis, acute, subperiosteal
petrous —see Petrositis
spinal (tuberculous) A18.01
nontuberculous —see Osteomyelitis, vertebra
bowel K63.0
brain (any part) (cystic) (otogenic) G06.0
amebic (with abscess of any other site) A06.6
gonococcal A54.82
pheomycotic (chromomycotic) B43.1
tuberculous A17.81
breast (acute) (chronic) (nonpuerperal) N61.1
newborn P39.0
puerperal, postpartum, gestational —see Mastitis, obstetric, purulent
broad ligament N73.2
acute N73.0
chronic N73.1
Brodie's (localized) (chronic) M86.8X-
bronchi J98.09
buccal cavity K12.2
bulbourethral gland N34.0
bursa M71.00
ankle M71.07-
elbow M71.02-
foot M71.07-
hand M71.04-
hip M71.05-
knee M71.06-

4

Abscess (continued)
　bursa (continued)
　　multiple sites M71.09
　　pharyngeal J39.1
　　shoulder M71.01-
　　specified site NEC M71.08
　　wrist M71.03-
　buttock L02.31
　canthus —see
　　Blepharoconjunctivitis
　cartilage —see Disorder, cartilage,
　　specified type NEC
　cecum K35.33
　cerebellum, cerebellar G06.0
　　sequelae G09
　cerebral (embolic) G06.0
　　sequelae G09
　cervical (meaning neck) L02.11
　　lymph gland or node L04.0
　cervix (stump) (uteri) —see
　　Cervicitis
　cheek (external) L02.01
　　inner K12.2
　chest J86.9
　　with fistula J86.0
　　wall L02.213
　chin L02.01
　choroid —see Inflammation,
　　chorioretinal
　circumtonsillar J36
　cold (lung) (tuberculous) —see
　　also Tuberculosis, abscess, lung
　　articular —see Tuberculosis, joint
　colon (wall) K63.0
　colostomy K94.02
　conjunctiva —see Conjunctivitis,
　　acute
　cornea H16.31-
　corpus
　　cavernosum N48.21
　　luteum —see Oophoritis
　Cowper's gland N34.0
　cranium G06.0
　cul-de-sac (Douglas') (posterior)
　　—see Peritonitis, pelvic, female
　cutaneous —see Abscess, by site
　dental K04.7
　　with sinus (alveolar) K04.6
　dentoalveolar K04.7
　　with sinus K04.6
　diaphragm, diaphragmatic K65.1
　Douglas' cul-de-sac or pouch —see
　　Peritonitis, pelvic, female
　Dubois A50.59
　ear (middle) —see also Otitis,
　　media, suppurative
　　acute —see Otitis, media,
　　　suppurative, acute
　　external H60.0-
　entameboic —see Abscess, amebic
　enterostomy K94.12
　epididymis N45.4
　epidural G06.2
　　brain G06.0
　　spinal cord G06.1
　epiglottis J38.7
　epiploon, epiploic K65.1
　erysipelatous —see Erysipelas
　esophagus K20.80
　ethmoid (bone) (chronic) (sinus)
　　J32.2
　external auditory canal —see
　　Abscess, ear, external
　extradural G06.2
　　brain G06.0
　　　sequelae G09
　　spinal cord G06.1
　extraperitoneal K68.19
　eye —see Endophthalmitis,
　　purulent
　eyelid H00.03-

Abscess (continued)
　face (any part, except ear, eye and
　　nose) L02.01
　fallopian tube —see Salpingitis
　fascia M72.8
　fauces J39.1
　fecal K63.0
　femoral (region) —see Abscess,
　　lower limb
　filaria, filarial —see Infestation,
　　filarial
　finger (any) —see also Abscess,
　　hand
　　nail —see Cellulitis,
　　　finger
　foot L02.61-
　forehead L02.01
　frontal sinus (chronic) J32.1
　gallbladder K81.0
　genital organ or tract
　　female (external) N76.4
　　male N49.9
　　　multiple sites N49.8
　　　specified NEC N49.8
　gestational mammary O91.11-
　gestational subareolar O91.11-
　gingival
　　aggressive K05.20
　　　generalized K05.229
　　　　moderate K05.222
　　　　severe K05.223
　　　　slight K05.221
　　　localized K05.219
　　　　moderate K05.212
　　　　severe K05.213
　　　　slight K05.211
　gland, glandular (lymph) (acute)
　　—see Lymphadenitis, acute
　gluteal (region) L02.31
　gonorrheal —see Gonococcus
　groin L02.214
　gum
　　aggressive K05.20
　　　generalized K05.229
　　　　moderate K05.222
　　　　severe K05.223
　　　　slight K05.221
　　　localized K05.219
　　　　moderate K05.212
　　　　severe K05.213
　　　　slight K05.211
　hand L02.51-
　head NEC L02.811
　　face (any part, except ear, eye
　　　and nose) L02.01
　heart —see Carditis
　heel —see Abscess, foot
　helminthic —see Infestation,
　　helminth
　hepatic (cholangitic) (hematogenic)
　　(lymphogenic) (pylephlebitic)
　　K75.0
　　amebic A06.4
　horseshoe K61.31
　hip (region) —see Abscess, lower
　　limb
　ileocecal K35.33
　ileostomy (bud) K94.12
　iliac (region) L02.214
　　fossa K35.33
　infraclavicular (fossa) —see
　　Abscess, upper limb
　inguinal (region) L02.214
　　lymph gland or node L04.1
　intersphincteric K61.4
　intestine, intestinal NEC K63.0
　　rectal K61.1
　intra-abdominal (see also Abscess,
　　peritoneum) K65.1
　　following procedure T81.43
　　　obstetrical O86.03

Abscess (continued)
　intra-abdominal (continued)
　　postprocedural T81.43
　　retroperitoneal K68.11
　intracranial G06.0
　intramammary —see Abscess,
　　breast
　intramuscular, following procedure
　　T81.42
　　obstetrical O86.02
　intraorbital —see Abscess, orbit
　intraperitoneal K65.1
　intrasphincteric (anus) K61.4
　intraspinal G06.1
　intratonsillar J36
　ischiorectal (fossa) (specified NEC)
　　K61.39
　jaw (bone) (lower) (upper) M27.2
　joint —see Arthritis, pyogenic or
　　pyemic
　　spine (tuberculous) A18.01
　　　nontuberculous —see
　　　　Spondylopathy, infective
　kidney N15.1
　　with calculus N20.0
　　　with hydronephrosis N13.6
　　puerperal (postpartum) O86.21
　knee —see also Abscess, lower
　　limb
　　joint M00.9
　labium (majus) (minus) N76.4
　lacrimal
　　caruncle —see Inflammation,
　　　lacrimal, passages, acute
　　gland —see Dacryoadenitis
　　passages (duct) (sac) —see
　　　Inflammation, lacrimal,
　　　passages, acute
　lacunar N34.0
　larynx J38.7
　lateral (alveolar) K04.7
　　with sinus K04.6
　leg (any part) —see Abscess, lower
　　limb
　lens H27.8
　lingual K14.0
　　tonsil J36
　lip K13.0
　Littre's gland N34.0
　liver (cholangitic) (hematogenic)
　　(lymphogenic) (pylephlebitic)
　　(pyogenic) K75.0
　　amebic (due to Entamoeba
　　　histolytica) (dysenteric)
　　　(tropical) A06.4
　　　with
　　　　brain abscess (and liver or
　　　　　lung abscess) A06.6
　　　　lung abscess A06.5
　loin (region) L02.211
　lower limb L02.41-
　lumbar (tuberculous) A18.01
　　nontuberculous L02.212
　lung (miliary) (putrid) J85.2
　　with pneumonia J85.1
　　　due to specified organism (see
　　　　Pneumonia, in (due to))
　　amebic (with liver abscess)
　　　A06.5
　　　with
　　　　brain abscess A06.6
　　　　pneumonia A06.5
　lymph, lymphatic, gland or
　　node (acute) —see also
　　　Lymphadenitis, acute
　　mesentery I88.0
　malar M27.2
　mammary gland —see Abscess,
　　breast
　marginal, anus K61.0
　mastoid —see Mastoiditis, acute

Abscess (continued)
　maxilla, maxillary M27.2
　　molar (tooth) K04.7
　　　with sinus K04.6
　　premolar K04.7
　　sinus (chronic) J32.0
　mediastinum J85.3
　meibomian gland —see Hordeolum
　meninges G06.2
　mesentery, mesenteric K65.1
　mesosalpinx —see Salpingitis
　mons pubis L02.215
　mouth (floor) K12.2
　muscle —see Myositis, infective
　myocardium I40.0
　nabothian (follicle) —see Cervicitis
　nasal J32.9
　nasopharyngeal J39.1
　navel L02.216
　　newborn P38.9
　　　with mild hemorrhage P38.1
　　　without hemorrhage P38.9
　neck (region) L02.11
　　lymph gland or node L04.0
　nephritic —see Abscess, kidney
　nipple N61.1
　　associated with
　　　lactation —see Pregnancy,
　　　　complicated by
　　　pregnancy —see Pregnancy,
　　　　complicated by
　nose (external) (fossa) (septum)
　　J34.0
　　sinus (chronic) —see Sinusitis
　omentum K65.1
　operative wound T81.49
　orbit, orbital —see Cellulitis, orbit
　otogenic G06.0
　ovary, ovarian (corpus luteum)
　　—see Oophoritis
　oviduct —see Oophoritis
　palate (soft) K12.2
　　hard M27.2
　palmar (space) —see Abscess,
　　hand
　pancreas (duct) —see Pancreatitis,
　　acute
　parafrenal N48.21
　parametric, parametrium N73.2
　　acute N73.0
　　chronic N73.1
　paranephric N15.1
　parapancreatic —see Pancreatitis,
　　acute
　parapharyngeal J39.0
　pararectal K61.1
　parasinus —see Sinusitis
　parauterine —see also Disease,
　　pelvis, inflammatory N73.2
　paravaginal —see Vaginitis
　parietal region (scalp) L02.811
　parodontal —see Periodontitis,
　　aggressive, localized
　parotid (duct) (gland) K11.3
　　region K12.2
　pectoral (region) L02.213
　pelvis, pelvic
　　female —see Disease, pelvis,
　　　inflammatory
　　male, peritoneal K65.1
　penis N48.21
　　gonococcal (accessory gland)
　　　(periurethral) A54.1
　perianal K61.0
　periapical K04.7
　　with sinus (alveolar) K04.6
　periappendicular K35.33
　pericardial I30.1
　pericecal K35.33
　pericemental —see Periodontitis,
　　aggressive, localized

Abscess (continued)
  pericholecystic —see Cholecystitis, acute
  pericoronal —see Periodontitis, aggressive, localized
  peridental —see Periodontitis, aggressive, localized
  perimetric —see also Disease, pelvis, inflammatory N73.2
  perinephric, perinephritic —see Abscess, kidney
  perineum, perineal (superficial) L02.215
    urethra N34.0
  periodontal (parietal) —see Periodontitis, aggressive, localized
    apical K04.7
  periosteum, periosteal —see also Osteomyelitis, specified type NEC
    with osteomyelitis —see also Osteomyelitis, specified type NEC
      acute —see Osteomyelitis, acute
      chronic —see Osteomyelitis, chronic
  peripharyngeal J39.0
  peripleuritic J86.9
    with fistula J86.0
  periprostatic N41.2
  perirectal K61.1
  perirenal (tissue) —see Abscess, kidney
  perisinuous (nose) —see Sinusitis
  peritoneum, peritoneal (perforated) (ruptured) K65.1
    with appendicitis (see also Appendicitis) K35.33
    pelvic
      female —see Peritonitis, pelvic, female
      male K65.1
    postoperative T81.43
    puerperal, postpartum, childbirth O85
    tuberculous A18.31
  peritonsillar J36
  perityphlic K35.33
  periureteral N28.89
  periurethral N34.0
    gonococcal (accessory gland) (periurethral) A54.1
  periuterine —see also Disease, pelvis, inflammatory N73.2
  perivesical —see Cystitis, specified type NEC
  petrous bone —see Petrositis
  phagedenic NOS L02.91
    chancroid A57
  pharynx, pharyngeal (lateral) J39.1
  pilonidal L05.01
  pituitary (gland) E23.6
  pleura J86.9
    with fistula J86.0
  popliteal —see Abscess, lower limb
  postcecal K35.33
  postlaryngeal J38.7
  postnasal J34.0
  postoperative (any site) (see also Infection, postoperative wound) T81.49
    retroperitoneal K68.11
  postpharyngeal J39.0
  posttonsillar J36
  post-typhoid A01.09
  pouch of Douglas —see Peritonitis, pelvic, female
  premammary —see Abscess, breast
  prepatellar —see Abscess, lower limb

Abscess (continued)
  presacral K68.19
  prostate N41.2
    gonococcal (acute) (chronic) A54.22
  psoas muscle K68.12
  puerperal - code by site under Puerperal, abscess
  pulmonary —see Abscess, lung
  pulp, pulpal (dental) K04.01
    irreversible K04.02
    reversible K04.01
  rectovaginal septum K63.0
  rectovesical —see Cystitis, specified type NEC
  rectum K61.1
  renal —see Abscess, kidney
  retina —see Inflammation, chorioretinal
  retrobulbar —see Abscess, orbit
  retrocecal K65.1
  retrolaryngeal J38.7
  retromammary —see Abscess, breast
  retroperitoneal NEC K68.19
    postprocedural K68.11
  retropharyngeal J39.0
  retrouterine —see Peritonitis, pelvic, female
  retrovesical —see Cystitis, specified type NEC
  root, tooth K04.7
    with sinus (alveolar) K04.6
  round ligament —see also Disease, pelvis, inflammatory N73.2
  rupture (spontaneous) NOS L02.91
  sacrum (tuberculous) A18.01
    nontuberculous M46.28
  salivary (duct) (gland) K11.3
  scalp (any part) L02.811
  scapular —see Osteomyelitis, specified type NEC
  sclera —see Scleritis
  scrofulous (tuberculous) A18.2
  scrotum N49.2
  seminal vesicle N49.0
  septal, dental K04.7
    with sinus (alveolar) K04.6
  serous —see Periostitis
  shoulder (region) —see Abscess, upper limb
  sigmoid K63.0
  sinus (accessory) (chronic) (nasal) —see also Sinusitis
    intracranial venous (any) G06.0
  Skene's duct or gland N34.0
  skin —see Abscess, by site
  specified site NEC L02.818
  spermatic cord N49.1
  sphenoidal (sinus) (chronic) J32.3
  spinal cord (any part) (staphylococcal) G06.1
    tuberculous A17.81
  spine (column) (tuberculous) A18.01
    epidural G06.1
    nontuberculous —see Osteomyelitis, vertebra
  spleen D73.3
    amebic A06.89
  stitch T81.41
    following an obstetrical procedure O86.01
  subarachnoid G06.2
    brain G06.0
    spinal cord G06.1
  subareolar —see Abscess, breast
  subcecal K35.33
  subcutaneous —see also Abscess, by site
    following procedure T81.41
      obstetrical O86.01

Abscess (continued)
  subcutaneous (continued)
    pheomycotic (chromomycotic) B43.2
  subdiaphragmatic K65.1
  subdural G06.2
    brain G06.0
    sequelae G09
    spinal cord G06.1
  sub-fascial, following an obstetrical procedure O86.02
  subgaleal L02.811
  subhepatic K65.1
  sublingual K12.2
    gland K11.3
  submammary —see Abscess, breast
  submandibular (region) (space) (triangle) K12.2
    gland K11.3
  submaxillary (region) L02.01
    gland K11.3
  submental L02.01
    gland K11.3
  subperiosteal —see Osteomyelitis, specified type NEC
  subphrenic K65.1
    following an obstetrical procedure O86.03
    postoperative T81.43
  suburethral N34.0
  sudoriparous L75.8
  supraclavicular (fossa) —see Abscess, upper limb
  supralevator K61.5
  suprapelvic, acute N73.0
  suprarenal (capsule) (gland) E27.8
  sweat gland L74.8
  tear duct —see Inflammation, lacrimal, passages, acute
  temple L02.01
  temporal region L02.01
  temporosphenoidal G06.0
  tendon (sheath) M65.00
    ankle M65.07-
    foot M65.07-
    forearm M65.03-
    hand M65.04-
    lower leg M65.06-
    pelvic region M65.05-
    shoulder region M65.01-
    specified site NEC M65.08
    thigh M65.05-
    upper arm M65.02-
  testis N45.4
  thigh —see Abscess, lower limb
  thorax J86.9
    with fistula J86.0
  throat J39.1
  thumb —see also Abscess, hand
    nail —see Cellulitis, finger
  thymus (gland) E32.1
  thyroid (gland) E06.0
  toe (any) —see also Abscess, foot
    nail —see Cellulitis, toe
  tongue (staphylococcal) K14.0
  tonsil(s) (lingual) J36
  tonsillopharyngeal J36
  tooth, teeth (root) K04.7
    with sinus (alveolar) K04.6
    supporting structures NEC — see Periodontitis, aggressive, localized
  trachea J39.8
  trunk L02.219
    abdominal wall L02.211
    back L02.212
    chest wall L02.213
    groin L02.214
    perineum L02.215
    umbilicus L02.216
  tubal —see Salpingitis

Abscess (continued)
  tuberculous —see Tuberculosis, abscess
  tubo-ovarian —see Salpingo-oophoritis
  tunica vaginalis N49.1
  umbilicus L02.216
  upper
    limb L02.41-
    respiratory J39.8
  urethral (gland) N34.0
  urinary N34.0
  uterus, uterine (wall) —see also Endometritis
    ligament —see also Disease, pelvis, inflammatory N73.2
    neck —see Cervicitis
  uvula K12.2
  vagina (wall) —see Vaginitis
  vaginorectal —see Vaginitis
  vas deferens N49.1
  vermiform appendix K35.33
  vertebra (column) (tuberculous) A18.01
    nontuberculous —see Osteomyelitis, vertebra
  vesical —see Cystitis, specified type NEC
  vesico-uterine pouch —see Peritonitis, pelvic, female
  vitreous (humor) —see Endophthalmitis, purulent
  vocal cord J38.3
  von Bezold's —see Mastoiditis, acute
  vulva N76.4
  vulvovaginal gland N75.1
  web space —see Abscess, hand
  wound T81.49
  wrist —see Abscess, upper limb
Absence (of) (organ or part) (complete or partial)
  adrenal (gland) (congenital) Q89.1
    acquired E89.6
  albumin in blood E88.09
  alimentary tract (congenital) Q45.8
    upper Q40.8
  alveolar process (acquired) —see Anomaly, alveolar
  ankle (acquired) Z89.44-
  anus (congenital) Q42.3
    with fistula Q42.2
  aorta (congenital) Q25.41
  appendix, congenital Q42.8
  arm (acquired) Z89.20-
    above elbow Z89.22-
      congenital (with hand present) —see Agenesis, arm, with hand present
      and hand —see Agenesis, forearm, and hand
    below elbow Z89.21-
      congenital (with hand present) —see Agenesis, arm, with hand present
      and hand —see Agenesis, forearm, and hand
    congenital —see Defect, reduction, upper limb
    shoulder (following explantation of shoulder joint prosthesis) (joint) (with or without presence of antibiotic-impregnated cement spacer) Z89.23-
      congenital (with hand present) —see Agenesis, arm, with hand present
  artery (congenital) (peripheral) Q27.8
    brain Q28.3

Absence *(continued)*
 artery *(continued)*
  coronary Q24.5
  pulmonary Q25.79
  specified NEC Q27.8
  umbilical Q27.0
 atrial septum (congenital) Q21.19
 auditory canal (congenital) (external) Q16.1
 auricle (ear), congenital Q16.0
 bile, biliary duct, congenital Q44.5
 bladder (acquired) Z90.6
  congenital Q64.5
 bowel sounds R19.11
 brain Q00.0
  part of Q04.3
 breast(s) (and nipple(s)) (acquired) Z90.1-
  congenital Q83.8
 broad ligament Q50.6
 bronchus (congenital) Q32.4
 canaliculus lacrimalis, congenital Q10.4
 cerebellum (vermis) Q04.3
 cervix (acquired) (with uterus) Z90.710
  with remaining uterus Z90.712
  congenital Q51.5
 chin, congenital Q18.8
 cilia (congenital) Q10.3
  acquired —see Madarosis
 clitoris (congenital) Q52.6
 coccyx, congenital Q76.49
 cold sense R20.8
 congenital
  lumen —see Atresia
  organ or site NEC —see Agenesis
  septum —see Imperfect, closure
 corpus callosum Q04.0
 cricoid cartilage, congenital Q31.8
 diaphragm (with hernia), congenital Q79.1
 digestive organ(s) or tract, congenital Q45.8
  acquired NEC Z90.49
  upper Q40.8
 ductus arteriosus Q28.8
 duodenum (acquired) Z90.49
  congenital Q41.0
 ear, congenital Q16.9
  acquired H93.8-
  auricle Q16.0
  external Q16.0
  inner Q16.5
  lobe, lobule Q17.8
  middle, except ossicles Q16.4
   ossicles Q16.3
  ossicles Q16.3
 ejaculatory duct (congenital) Q55.4
 endocrine gland (congenital) NEC Q89.2
  acquired E89.89
 epididymis (congenital) Q55.4
  acquired Z90.79
 epiglottis, congenital Q31.8
 esophagus (congenital) Q39.8
  acquired (partial) Z90.49
 eustachian tube (congenital) Q16.2
 extremity (acquired) Z89.9
  congenital Q73.0
  knee (following explantation of knee joint prosthesis) (joint) (with or without presence of antibiotic-impregnated cement spacer) Z89.52-
  lower (above knee) Z89.619
   below knee Z89.51-
  upper —see Absence, arm
 eye (acquired) Z90.01
  congenital Q11.1
  muscle (congenital) Q10.3

Absence *(continued)*
 eyeball (acquired) Z90.01
 eyelid (fold) (congenital) Q10.3
  acquired Z90.01
 face, specified part NEC Q18.8
 fallopian tube(s) (acquired) Z90.79
  congenital Q50.6
 family member (causing problem in home) NEC —see also Disruption, family Z63.32
 femur, congenital —see Defect, reduction, lower limb, longitudinal, femur
 fibrinogen (congenital) D68.2
  acquired D65
 finger(s) (acquired) Z89.02-
  congenital —see Agenesis, hand
 foot (acquired) Z89.43-
  congenital —see Agenesis, foot
 forearm (acquired) —see Absence, arm, below elbow
 gallbladder (acquired) Z90.49
  congenital Q44.0
 gamma globulin in blood D80.1
  hereditary D80.0
 genital organs
  acquired (female) (male) Z90.79
  female, congenital Q52.8
   external Q52.71
   internal NEC Q52.8
  male, congenital Q55.8
 genitourinary organs, congenital NEC
  female Q52.8
  male Q55.8
 globe (acquired) Z90.01
  congenital Q11.1
 glottis, congenital Q31.8
 hand and wrist (acquired) Z89.11-
  congenital —see Agenesis, hand
 head, part (acquired) NEC Z90.09
 heat sense R20.8
 hip (following explantation of hip joint prosthesis) (joint) (with or without presence of antibiotic-impregnated cement spacer) Z89.62-
 hymen (congenital) Q52.4
 ileum (acquired) Z90.49
  congenital Q41.2
 immunoglobulin, isolated NEC D80.3
  IgA D80.2
  IgG D80.3
  IgM D80.4
 incus (acquired) —see Loss, ossicles, ear
  congenital Q16.3
 inner ear, congenital Q16.5
 intestine (acquired) (small) Z90.49
  congenital Q41.9
   specified NEC Q41.8
  large Z90.49
   congenital Q42.9
   specified NEC Q42.8
 iris, congenital Q13.1
 jejunum (acquired) Z90.49
  congenital Q41.1
 joint
  acquired
   hip (following explantation of hip joint prosthesis) (with or without presence of antibiotic-impregnated cement spacer) Z89.62-
   knee (following explantation of knee joint prosthesis) (with or without presence of antibiotic-impregnated cement spacer) Z89.52-

Absence *(continued)*
 joint *(continued)*
  acquired *(continued)*
   shoulder (following explantation of shoulder joint prosthesis) (with or without presence of antibiotic-impregnated cement spacer) Z89.23-
  congenital NEC Q74.8
 kidney(s) (acquired) Z90.5
  congenital Q60.2
   bilateral Q60.1
   unilateral Q60.0
 knee (following explantation of knee joint prosthesis) (joint) (with or without presence of antibiotic-impregnated cement spacer) Z89.52-
 labyrinth, membranous Q16.5
 larynx (congenital) Q31.8
  acquired Z90.02
 leg (acquired) (above knee) Z89.61-
  below knee (acquired) Z89.51-
  congenital —see Defect, reduction, lower limb
 lens (acquired) —see also Aphakia
  congenital Q12.3
  post cataract extraction Z98.4-
 limb (acquired) —see Absence, extremity
 lip Q38.6
 liver (congenital) Q44.79
 lung (fissure) (lobe) (bilateral) (unilateral) (congenital) Q33.3
  acquired (any part) Z90.2
 menstruation —see Amenorrhea
 muscle (congenital) (pectoral) Q79.8
  ocular Q10.3
 neck, part Q18.8
 neutrophil —see Agranulocytosis
 nipple(s) (with breast(s)) (acquired) Z90.1-
  congenital Q83.2
 nose (congenital) Q30.1
  acquired Z90.09
 organ
  of Corti, congenital Q16.5
  or site, congenital NEC Q89.8
   acquired NEC Z90.89
 osseous meatus (ear) Q16.4
 ovary (acquired)
  bilateral Z90.722
  congenital
   bilateral Q50.02
   unilateral Q50.01
  unilateral Z90.721
 oviduct (acquired)
  bilateral Z90.722
  congenital Q50.6
  unilateral Z90.721
 pancreas (congenital) Q45.0
  acquired Z90.410
   complete Z90.410
   partial Z90.411
   total Z90.410
 parathyroid gland (acquired) E89.2
  congenital Q89.2
 patella, congenital Q74.1
 penis (congenital) Q55.5
  acquired Z90.79
 pericardium (congenital) Q24.8
 pituitary gland (congenital) Q89.2
  acquired E89.3
 prostate (acquired) Z90.79
  congenital Q55.4
 pulmonary valve Q22.0
 punctum lacrimale (congenital) Q10.4
 radius, congenital —see Defect, reduction, upper limb, longitudinal, radius

Absence *(continued)*
 rectum (congenital) Q42.1
  with fistula Q42.0
  acquired Z90.49
 respiratory organ NOS Q34.9
 rib (acquired) Z90.89
  congenital Q76.6
 sacrum, congenital Q76.49
 salivary gland(s), congenital Q38.4
 scrotum, congenital Q55.29
 seminal vesicles (congenital) Q55.4
  acquired Z90.79
 septum
  atrial (congenital) Q21.19
  between aorta and pulmonary artery Q21.4
  ventricular (congenital) Q20.4
 sex chromosome
  female phenotype Q97.8
  male phenotype Q98.8
 skull bone (congenital) Q75.8
  with
   anencephaly Q00.0
   encephalocele —see Encephalocele
   hydrocephalus Q03.9
    with spina bifida —see Spina bifida, by site, with hydrocephalus
   microcephaly Q02
 spermatic cord, congenital Q55.4
 spine, congenital Q76.49
 spleen (congenital) Q89.01
  acquired Z90.81
 sternum, congenital Q76.7
 stomach (acquired) (partial) Z90.3
  congenital Q40.2
 superior vena cava, congenital Q26.8
 teeth, tooth (congenital) K00.0
  acquired (complete) K08.109
   class I K08.101
   class II K08.102
   class III K08.103
   class IV K08.104
   due to
    caries K08.139
     class I K08.131
     class II K08.132
     class III K08.133
     class IV K08.134
    periodontal disease K08.129
     class I K08.121
     class II K08.122
     class III K08.123
     class IV K08.124
   specified NEC K08.199
    class I K08.191
    class II K08.192
    class III K08.193
    class IV K08.194
   trauma K08.119
    class I K08.111
    class II K08.112
    class III K08.113
    class IV K08.114
   partial K08.409
    class I K08.401
    class II K08.402
    class III K08.403
    class IV K08.404
    due to
     caries K08.439
      class I K08.431
      class II K08.432
      class III K08.433
      class IV K08.434
     periodontal disease K08.429
      class I K08.421
      class II K08.422

Absence (continued)
teeth, tooth (continued)
acquired (continued)
partial K08.409 (continued)
due to (continued)
periodontal (continued)
class III K08.423
class IV K08.424
specified NEC K08.499
class I K08.491
class II K08.492
class III K08.493
class IV K08.494
trauma K08.419
class I K08.411
class II K08.412
class III K08.413
class IV K08.414
tendon (congenital) Q79.8
testis (congenital) Q55.0
acquired Z90.79
thumb (acquired) Z89.01-
congenital —see Agenesis, hand
thymus gland Q89.2
thyroid (gland) (acquired) E89.0
cartilage, congenital Q31.8
congenital E03.1
toe(s) (acquired) Z89.42-
with foot —see Absence, foot and ankle
congenital —see Agenesis, foot
great Z89.41-
tongue, congenital Q38.3
trachea (cartilage), congenital Q32.1
transverse aortic arch, congenital Q25.49
tricuspid valve Q22.4
umbilical artery, congenital Q27.0
upper arm and forearm with hand present, congenital —see Agenesis, arm, with hand present
ureter (congenital) Q62.4
acquired Z90.6
urethra, congenital Q64.5
uterus (acquired) Z90.710
with cervix Z90.710
with remaining cervical stump Z90.711
congenital Q51.0
uvula, congenital Q38.5
vagina, congenital Q52.0
vas deferens (congenital) Q55.4
acquired Z90.79
vein (peripheral) congenital NEC Q27.8
cerebral Q28.3
digestive system Q27.8
great Q26.8
lower limb Q27.8
portal Q26.5
precerebral Q28.1
specified site NEC Q27.8
upper limb Q27.8
vena cava (inferior) (superior), congenital Q26.8
ventricular septum Q20.4
vertebra, congenital Q76.49
von Willebrand factor, complete (near) (see also Disease, von Willebrand) D68.03
vulva, congenital Q52.71
wrist (acquired) Z89.12-

Absorbent system disease I87.8

Absorption
carbohydrate, disturbance K90.49
chemical —see Table of Drugs and Chemicals

Absorption (continued)
chemical (continued)
through placenta (newborn) P04.9
environmental substance P04.6
nutritional substance P04.5
obstetric anesthetic or analgesic drug P04.0
drug NEC —see Table of Drugs and Chemicals
addictive
through placenta (newborn) (see also Newborn, affected by, maternal, use of) P04.40
cocaine P04.41
hallucinogens P04.42
specified drug NEC P04.49
medicinal
through placenta (newborn) P04.19
through placenta (newborn) P04.19
obstetric anesthetic or analgesic drug P04.0
fat, disturbance K90.49
pancreatic K90.3
noxious substance —see Table of Drugs and Chemicals
protein, disturbance K90.49
starch, disturbance K90.49
toxic substance —see Table of Drugs and Chemicals
uremic —see Uremia

Abstinence symptoms, syndrome
alcohol F10.239
with delirium F10.231
cocaine F14.23
neonatal P96.1
nicotine —see Dependence, drug, nicotine, with, withdrawal
opioid F11.93
with dependence F11.23
psychoactive NEC F19.939
with
delirium F19.931
dependence F19.239
with
delirium F19.231
perceptual disturbance F19.232
uncomplicated F19.230
perceptual disturbance F19.932
uncomplicated F19.930
sedative F13.939
with
delirium F13.931
dependence F13.239
with
delirium F13.231
perceptual disturbance F13.232
uncomplicated F13.230
perceptual disturbance F13.932
uncomplicated F13.930
stimulant NEC F15.93
with dependence F15.23

Abulia R68.89

Abulomania F60.7

Abuse
adult —see Maltreatment, adult
as reason for
couple see king advice (including offender) Z63.0
alcohol (non-dependent) F10.10
with
anxiety disorder F10.180

Abuse (continued)
alcohol (continued)
with (continued)
intoxication F10.129
with delirium F10.121
uncomplicated F10.120
mood disorder F10.14
other specified disorder F10.188
psychosis F10.159
delusions F10.150
hallucinations F10.151
sexual dysfunction F10.181
sleep disorder F10.182
unspecified disorder F10.19
withdrawal F10.139
with
perceptual disturbance F10.132
delirium F10.131
uncomplicated F10.130
counseling and surveillance Z71.41
in remission (early) (sustained) F10.11
amphetamine (or related substance) —see also Abuse, drug, stimulant NEC
stimulant NEC F15.10
with
anxiety disorder F15.180
intoxication F15.129
with
delirium F15.121
perceptual disturbance F15.122
withdrawal F15.13
analgesics (non-prescribed) (over the counter) F55.8
antacids F55.0
antidepressants —see Abuse, drug, psychoactive NEC
anxiolytic —see Abuse, drug, sedative
barbiturates —see Abuse, drug, sedative
caffeine —see Abuse, drug, stimulant NEC
cannabis, cannabinoids —see Abuse, drug, cannabis
child —see Maltreatment, child
cocaine —see Abuse, drug, cocaine
drug NEC (non-dependent) F19.10
with sleep disorder F19.182
amphetamine type —see Abuse, drug, stimulant NEC
analgesics (non-prescribed) (over the counter) F55.8
antacids F55.0
antidepressants —see Abuse, drug, psychoactive NEC
anxiolytics —see Abuse, drug, sedative
barbiturates —see Abuse, drug, sedative
caffeine —see Abuse, drug, stimulant NEC
cannabis F12.10
with
anxiety disorder F12.180
intoxication F12.129
with
delirium F12.121
perceptual disturbance F12.122
uncomplicated F12.120
other specified disorder F12.188
psychosis F12.159
delusions F12.150
hallucinations F12.151

Abuse (continued)
drug NEC (continued)
cannabis (continued)
with (continued)
unspecified disorder F12.19
withdrawal F12.13
in remission (early) (sustained) F12.11
cocaine F14.10
with
anxiety disorder F14.180
intoxication F14.129
with
delirium F14.121
perceptual disturbance F14.122
uncomplicated F14.120
mood disorder F14.14
other specified disorder F14.188
psychosis F14.159
delusions F14.150
hallucinations F14.151
sexual dysfunction F14.181
sleep disorder F14.182
unspecified disorder F14.19
withdrawal F14.13
in remission (early) (sustained) F14.11
counseling and surveillance Z71.51
hallucinogen F16.10
with
anxiety disorder F16.180
flashbacks F16.183
intoxication F16.129
with
delirium F16.121
perceptual disturbance F16.122
uncomplicated F16.120
mood disorder F16.14
other specified disorder F16.188
perception disorder, persisting F16.183
psychosis F16.159
delusions F16.150
hallucinations F16.151
unspecified disorder F16.19
in remission (early) (sustained) F16.11
hashish —see Abuse, drug, cannabis
herbal or folk remedies F55.1
hormones F55.3
hypnotics —see Abuse, drug, sedative
inhalant F18.10
with
anxiety disorder F18.180
dementia, persisting F18.17
intoxication F18.129
with delirium F18.121
uncomplicated F18.120
mood disorder F18.14
other specified disorder F18.188
psychosis F18.159
delusions F18.150
hallucinations F18.151
unspecified disorder F18.19
in remission (early) (sustained) F18.11
laxatives F55.2
in remission (early) (sustained) F19.11
LSD —see Abuse, drug, hallucinogen
marihuana —see Abuse, drug, cannabis

Abuse *(continued)*
  drug NEC *(continued)*
    morphine type (opioids) —*see*
      Abuse, drug, opioid
    opioid F11.10
      with
        intoxication F11.129
          with
            delirium F11.121
            perceptual disturbance
              F11.122
          uncomplicated F11.120
        mood disorder F11.14
        opioid-associated amnestic
          syndrome F11.188
        other specified disorder
          F11.188
        psychosis F11.159
          delusions F11.150
          hallucinations F11.151
        sexual dysfunction F11.181
        sleep disorder F11.182
        unspecified disorder F11.19
        withdrawal F11.13
      in remission (early)
        (sustained) F11.11
    PCP (phencyclidine) (or related
      substance) —*see* Abuse, drug,
      hallucinogen
    psychoactive NEC F19.10
      with
        amnestic disorder F19.16
        anxiety disorder F19.180
        dementia F19.17
        intoxication F19.129
          with
            delirium F19.121
            perceptual disturbance
              F19.122
          uncomplicated F19.120
        mood disorder F19.14
        other specified disorder
          F19.188
        psychosis F19.159
          delusions F19.150
          hallucinations F19.151
        sexual dysfunction F19.181
        sleep disorder F19.182
        unspecified disorder F19.19
        withdrawal F19.139
          with
            perceptual disturbance
              F19.132
            delirium F19.131
            uncomplicated F19.130
    sedative, hypnotic or anxiolytic
      F13.10
      with
        anxiety disorder F13.180
        intoxication F13.129
          with delirium F13.121
          uncomplicated F13.120
        mood disorder F13.14
        other specified disorder
          F13.188
        psychosis F13.159
          delusions F13.150
          hallucinations F13.151
        sexual dysfunction F13.181
        sleep disorder F13.182
        unspecified disorder F13.19
        withdrawal F13.139
          with
            perceptual disturbance
              F13.132
            delirium F13.131
            uncomplicated F13.130
      in remission (early)
        (sustained) F13.11
    solvent —*see* Abuse, drug, inhalant
    steroids F55.3

Abuse *(continued)*
  drug NEC *(continued)*
    stimulant NEC F15.10
      with
        anxiety disorder F15.180
        intoxication F15.129
          with
            delirium F15.121
            perceptual disturbance
              F15.122
          uncomplicated F15.120
        mood disorder F15.14
        other specified disorder
          F15.188
        psychosis F15.159
          delusions F15.150
          hallucinations F15.151
        sexual dysfunction F15.181
        sleep disorder F15.182
        unspecified disorder F15.19
        withdrawal F15.13
      in remission (early)
        (sustained) F15.11
    tranquilizers —*see* Abuse, drug,
      sedative
    vitamins F55.4
  hallucinogens —*see* Abuse, drug,
    hallucinogen
  hashish —*see* Abuse, drug,
    cannabis
  herbal or folk remedies F55.1
  hormones F55.3
  hypnotic —*see* Abuse, drug,
    sedative
  inhalant —*see* Abuse, drug,
    inhalant
  laxatives F55.2
  LSD —*see* Abuse, drug,
    hallucinogen
  marihuana —*see* Abuse, drug,
    cannabis
  morphine type (opioids) —*see*
    Abuse, drug, opioid
  non-psychoactive substance NEC
    F55.8
    antacids F55.0
    folk remedies F55.1
    herbal remedies F55.1
    hormones F55.3
    laxatives F55.2
    steroids F55.3
    vitamins F55.4
  opioids —*see* Abuse, drug, opioid
  PCP (phencyclidine) (or related
    substance) —*see* Abuse, drug,
    hallucinogen
  physical (adult) (child) —*see*
    Maltreatment
  psychoactive substance —*see*
    Abuse, drug, psychoactive NEC
  psychological (adult) (child) —*see*
    Maltreatment
  sedative —*see* Abuse, drug,
    sedative
  sexual —*see* Maltreatment
  solvent —*see* Abuse, drug, inhalant
  steroids F55.3
  vitamins F55.4
Acalculia R48.8
  developmental F81.2
Acanthamebiasis (with) B60.10
  conjunctiva B60.12
  keratoconjunctivitis B60.13
  meningoencephalitis B60.11
  other specified B60.19
Acanthocephaliasis B83.8
Acanthocheilonemiasis B74.4
Acanthocytosis E78.6
Acantholysis L11.9

Acanthosis (acquired) (nigricans) L83
  benign Q82.8
  congenital Q82.8
  seborrheic L82.1
    inflamed L82.0
  tongue K14.3
Acapnia E87.3
Acarbia E87.29
Acardia, acardius Q89.8
Acardiacus amorphus Q89.8
Acardiotrophia I51.4
Acariasis B88.0
  scabies B86
Acarodermatitis (urticarioides) B88.0
Acarophobia F40.218
Acatalasemia, acatalasia E80.3
Acathisia (drug induced) G25.71
Accelerated atrioventricular conduction I45.6
Accentuation of personality traits (type A) Z73.1
Accessory (congenital)
  adrenal gland Q89.1
  anus Q43.4
  appendix Q43.4
  atrioventricular conduction I45.6
  auditory ossicles Q16.3
  auricle (ear) Q17.0
  biliary duct or passage Q44.5
  bladder Q64.79
  blood vessels NEC Q27.9
    coronary Q24.5
  bone NEC Q79.8
  breast tissue, axilla Q83.1
  carpal bones Q74.0
  cecum Q43.4
  chromosome(s) NEC (nonsex) Q92.9
    with complex rearrangements
      NEC Q92.5
      seen only at prometaphase Q92.8
    partial Q92.9
    sex
      female phenotype Q97.8
    13 —*see* Trisomy, 13
    18 —*see* Trisomy, 18
    21 —*see* Trisomy, 21
  coronary artery Q24.5
  cusp(s), heart valve NEC Q24.8
    pulmonary Q22.3
  cystic duct Q44.5
  digit(s) Q69.9
  ear (auricle) (lobe) Q17.0
  endocrine gland NEC Q89.2
  eye muscle Q10.3
  eyelid Q10.3
  face bone(s) Q75.8
  fallopian tube (fimbria) (ostium)
    Q50.6
  finger(s) Q69.0
  foreskin N47.8
  frontonasal process Q75.8
  gallbladder Q44.1
  genital organ(s)
    female Q52.8
      external Q52.79
      internal NEC Q52.8
    male Q55.8
  genitourinary organs NEC Q89.8
    female Q52.8
    male Q55.8
  hallux Q69.2
  heart Q24.8
    valve NEC Q24.8
      pulmonary Q22.3
  hepatic ducts Q44.5
  hymen Q52.4
  intestine (large) (small) Q43.4

Accessory *(continued)*
  kidney Q63.0
  lacrimal canal Q10.6
  leaflet, heart valve NEC Q24.8
  ligament, broad Q50.6
  liver Q44.79
    duct Q44.5
  lobule (ear) Q17.0
  lung (lobe) Q33.1
  muscle Q79.8
  navicular of carpus Q74.0
  nervous system, part NEC Q07.8
  nipple Q83.3
  nose Q30.8
  organ or site not listed —*see*
    Anomaly, by site
  ovary Q50.31
  oviduct Q50.6
  pancreas Q45.3
  parathyroid gland Q89.2
  parotid gland (and duct) Q38.4
  pituitary gland Q89.2
  preauricular appendage Q17.0
  prepuce N47.8
  renal arteries (multiple) Q27.2
  rib Q76.6
    cervical Q76.5
  roots (teeth) K00.2
  salivary gland Q38.4
  sesamoid bones Q74.8
    foot Q74.2
    hand Q74.0
  skin tags Q82.8
  spleen Q89.09
  sternum Q76.7
  submaxillary gland Q38.4
  tarsal bones Q74.2
  teeth, tooth K00.1
  tendon Q79.8
  thumb Q69.1
  thymus gland Q89.2
  thyroid gland Q89.2
  toes Q69.2
  tongue Q38.3
  tooth, teeth K00.1
  tragus Q17.0
  ureter Q62.5
  urethra Q64.79
  urinary organ or tract NEC Q64.8
  uterus Q51.28
  vagina Q52.10
  valve, heart NEC Q24.8
    pulmonary Q22.3
  vertebra Q76.49
  vocal cords Q31.8
  vulva Q52.79
Accident
  birth —*see* Birth, injury
  cardiac —*see* Infarct, myocardium
  cerebrovascular (ischemic) I63.9
    aborted I63.9
    chronic (old) (remote) (imaging)
      (without sequelae) Z86.73
      with residual defects -
        see Sequelae, disease,
        cerebrovascular
    embolic I63.-
    hemorrhagic —*see* Hemorrhage,
      intracranial, intracerebral
    old (without sequelae) Z86.73
      with sequelae (of) —*see*
        Sequelae, infarction, cerebral
    thrombotic I63.-
  coronary —*see* Infarct, myocardium
  craniovascular I63.9
  vascular, brain I63.9
Accidental —*see* condition
Accommodation (disorder) —*see also* condition
  hysterical paralysis of F44.89

Accommodation (continued)
  insufficiency of H52.4
  paresis —see Paresis, of accommodation
  spasm —see Spasm, of accommodation
Accouchement —see Delivery
Accreta placenta O43.21-
Accretio cordis (nonrheumatic) I31.0
Accretions, tooth, teeth K03.6
Acculturation difficulty Z60.3
Accumulation secretion, prostate N42.89
Acephalia, acephalism, acephalus, acephaly Q00.0
Acephalobrachia monster Q89.8
Acephalochirus monster Q89.8
Acephalogaster Q89.8
Acephalostomus monster Q89.8
Acephalothorax Q89.8
Acerophobia F40.298
Acetonemia R79.89
  in Type 1 diabetes E10.10
    with coma E10.11
Acetonuria R82.4
Achalasia (cardia) (esophagus) K22.0
  congenital Q39.5
  pylorus Q40.0
  sphincteral NEC K59.89
Ache(s) —see Pain
Acheilia Q38.6
Achillobursitis —see Tendinitis, Achilles
Achillodynia —see Tendinitis, Achilles
Achlorhydria, achlorhydric (neurogenic) K31.83
  anemia D50.8
  diarrhea K31.83
  psychogenic F45.8
  secondary to vagotomy K91.1
Achluophobia F40.228
Acholia K82.8
Acholuric jaundice (familial) (splenomegalic) —see also Spherocytosis
  acquired D59.8
Achondrogenesis Q77.0
Achondroplasia (osteosclerosis congenita) Q77.4
Achroma, cutis L80
Achromat (ism), achromatopsia (acquired) (congenital) H53.51
Achromia, congenital —see Albinism
Achromia parasitica B36.0
Achylia gastrica K31.89
  psychogenic F45.8
Acid
  burn —see Corrosion
  deficiency
    amide nicotinic E52
    ascorbic E54
    folic E53.8
    nicotinic E52
    pantothenic E53.8
  intoxication (see also Acidosis) E87.29
  peptic disease K30
  phosphatase deficiency E83.39
  stomach K30
    psychogenic F45.8
Acidemia (see also Acidosis) E87.20
  argininosuccinic E72.22
  isovaleric E71.110

Acidemia (continued)
  metabolic —see also Acidosis, metabolic
    newborn P19.9
      first noted before onset of labor P19.0
      first noted during labor P19.1
      noted at birth P19.2
  methylmalonic E71.120
  pipecolic E72.3
  propionic E71.121
Acidity, gastric (high) K30
  psychogenic F45.8
Acidocytopenia —see Agranulocytosis
Acidocytosis D72.10
Acidopenia —see Agranulocytosis
Acidosis (lactic) E87.20
  in Type 1 diabetes E10.10
    with coma E10.11
  kidney, tubular N25.89
  lactic E87.20
    acute E87.21
    chronic E87.22
  metabolic NEC E87.20
    acute E87.21
    chronic E87.22
    with respiratory acidosis E87.4
    hyperchloremic, of newborn P74.421
    late, of newborn P74.0
  mixed metabolic and respiratory, newborn P84
  newborn P84
  renal (hyperchloremic) (tubular) N25.89
  respiratory E87.29
    acute J96.02
    chronic J96.12
    complicated by
      metabolic
        acidosis E87.4
        alkalosis E87.4
  specified NEC E87.29
Aciduria
  specified NEC E87.29
  4-hydroxybutyric E72.81
  argininosuccinic E72.22
  gamma-hydroxybutyric E72.81
  glutaric (type I) E72.3
    type II E71.313
    type III E71.5-
  orotic (congenital) (hereditary) (pyrimidine deficiency) E79.89
    anemia D53.0
Acladiosis (skin) B36.0
Aclasis, diaphyseal Q78.6
Acleistocardia Q21.19
Aclusion —see Anomaly, dentofacial, malocclusion
Acne L70.9
  artificialis L70.8
  atrophica L70.2
  cachecticorum (Hebra) L70.8
  conglobata L70.1
  cystic L70.0
  decalvans L66.2
  excoriée (des jeunes filles) L70.5
  frontalis L70.2
  indurata L70.0
  infantile L70.4
  keloid L73.0
  lupoid L70.2
  necrotic, necrotica (miliaris) L70.2
  neonatal L70.4
  nodular L70.0
  occupational L70.8
  picker's L70.5
  pustular L70.0

Acne (continued)
  rodens L70.2
  rosacea L71.9
  specified NEC L70.8
  tropica L70.3
  varioliformis L70.2
  vulgaris L70.0
Acnitis (primary) A18.4
Acosta's disease T70.29
Acoustic —see condition
Acousticophobia F40.298
ACPO (acute colonic pseudo-obstruction) K59.81
Acquired —see also condition
  immunodeficiency syndrome (AIDS) B20
Acrania Q00.0
Acroangiodermatitis I78.9
Acroasphyxia, chronic I73.89
Acrobystitis N47.7
Acrocephalopolysyndactyly Q87.0
Acrocephalosyndactyly Q87.0
Acrocephaly Q75.009
Acrochondrohyperplasia —see Syndrome, Marfan
Acrocyanosis I73.89
  newborn P28.2
    meaning transient blue hands and feet - omit code
Acrodermatitis L30.8
  atrophicans (chronica) L90.4
  continua (Hallopeau) L40.2
  enteropathica (hereditary) E83.2
  Hallopeau's L40.2
  infantile papular L44.4
  perstans L40.2
  pustulosa continua L40.2
  recalcitrant pustular L40.2
Acrodynia —see Poisoning, mercury
Acromegaly, acromegalia E22.0
Acromelalgia I73.81
Acromicria, acromikria Q79.8
Acronyx L60.0
Acropachy, thyroid —see Thyrotoxicosis
Acroparesthesia (simple) (vasomotor) I73.89
Acropathy, thyroid —see Thyrotoxicosis
Acrophobia F40.241
Acroposthitis N47.7
Acroscleriasis, acroscleroderma, acrosclerosis —see Sclerosis, systemic
Acrosphacelus I96
Acrospiroma, eccrine —see Neoplasm, skin, benign
Acrostealgia —see Osteochondropathy
Acrotrophodynia —see Immersion
ACTH ectopic syndrome E24.3
Actinic —see condition
Actinobacillosis, actinobacillus A28.8
  mallei A24.0
  muris A25.1
Actinomyces israelii (infection) —see Actinomycosis
Actinomycetoma (foot) B47.1
Actinomycosis, actinomycotic A42.9
  with pneumonia A42.0
  abdominal A42.1

Actinomycosis, actinomycotic (continued)
  cervicofacial A42.2
  cutaneous A42.89
  gastrointestinal A42.1
  pulmonary A42.0
  sepsis A42.7
  specified site NEC A42.89
Actinoneuritis G62.82
Action, heart
  disorder I49.9
  irregular I49.9
    psychogenic F45.8
Activated protein C resistance D68.51
Activation
  mast cell (disorder) (syndrom) D89.40
    idiopathic D89.42
    monoclonal D89.41
    secondary D89.43
    specified type NEC D89.49
Active —see condition
Acute —see also condition
  abdomen R10.0
  gallbladder —see Cholecystitis, acute
Acyanotic heart disease (congenital) Q24.9
Acystia Q64.5
Adair-Dighton syndrome (brittle bones and blue sclera, deafness) Q78.0
Adamantinoblastoma —see Ameloblastoma
Adamantinoma —see also Cyst, calcifying odontogenic
  long bones C40.90
    lower limb C40.2-
    upper limb C40.0-
  malignant C41.1
    jaw (bone) (lower) C41.1
      upper C41.0
  tibial C40.2-
Adamantoblastoma —see Ameloblastoma
Adams-Stokes (-Morgagni) **disease or syndrome** I45.9
Adaption reaction —see Disorder, adjustment
Addiction —see also Dependence F19.20
  alcohol, alcoholic (ethyl) (methyl) (wood) (without remission) F10.20
    with remission F10.21
  drug —see Dependence, drug
  ethyl alcohol (without remission) F10.20
    with remission F10.21
  heroin —see Dependence, drug, opioid
  methyl alcohol (without remission) F10.20
    with remission F10.21
  methylated spirit (without remission) F10.20
    with remission F10.21
  morphine(-like substances) —see Dependence, drug, opioid
  nicotine —see Dependence, drug, nicotine
  opium and opioids —see Dependence, drug, opioid
  tobacco —see Dependence, drug, nicotine
Addisonian crisis E27.2
Addison's
  anemia (pernicious) D51.0
  disease (bronze) or syndrome E27.1
    tuberculous A18.7
  keloid L94.0

Addison-Biermer anemia
  (pernicious) D51.0
Addison-Schilder complex E71.528
Additional —see also Accessory
  chromosome(s) (see also Trisomy)
    Q99.8
    marker —see Extra, marker
      chromosomes
    sex —see Abnormal,
      chromosome, sex
    21 —see Trisomy, 21
**Adduction contracture, hip or other
  joint** —see Contraction, joint
Adenitis —see also Lymphadenitis
  acute, unspecified site L04.9
  axillary I88.9
    acute L04.2
    chronic or subacute I88.1
  Bartholin's gland N75.8
  bulbourethral gland —see
    Urethritis
  cervical I88.9
    acute L04.0
    chronic or subacute I88.1
  chancroid (Hemophilus ducreyi) A57
  chronic, unspecified site I88.1
  Cowper's gland —see Urethritis
  due to Pasteurella multocida
    (P. septica) A28.0
  epidemic, acute B27.09
  gangrenous L04.9
  gonorrheal NEC A54.89
  groin I88.9
    acute L04.1
    chronic or subacute I88.1
  infectious (acute) (epidemic) B27.09
  inguinal I88.9
    acute L04.1
    chronic or subacute I88.1
  lymph gland or node, except
    mesenteric I88.9
    acute —see Lymphadenitis, acute
    chronic or subacute I88.1
  mesenteric (acute) (chronic)
    (nonspecific) (subacute) I88.0
  parotid gland (suppurative) —see
    Sialoadenitis
  salivary gland (any) (suppurative)
    —see Sialoadenitis
  scrofulous (tuberculous) A18.2
  Skene's duct or gland —see Urethritis
  strumous, tuberculous A18.2
  subacute, unspecified site I88.1
  sublingual gland (suppurative)
    —see Sialoadenitis
  submandibular gland (suppurative)
    —see Sialoadenitis
  submaxillary gland (suppurative)
    —see Sialoadenitis
  tuberculous —see Tuberculosis,
    lymph gland
  urethral gland —see Urethritis
  Wharton's duct (suppurative) —see
    Sialoadenitis
Adenoacanthoma —see Neoplasm,
  malignant, by site
Adenoameloblastoma —see Cyst,
  calcifying odontogenic
Adenocarcinoid (tumor) —see
  Neoplasm, malignant, by site
Adenocarcinoma —see also
  Neoplasm, malignant, by site
  acidophil
    specified site —see Neoplasm,
      malignant, by site
    unspecified site C75.1
  adrenal cortical C74.0-
  alveolar —see Neoplasm, lung,
    malignant

Adenocarcinoma (continued)
  apocrine
    breast —see Neoplasm, breast,
      malignant
    in situ
      breast D05.8-
      specified site NEC —see
        Neoplasm, skin, in situ
      unspecified site D04.9
    specified site NEC —see
      Neoplasm, skin, malignant
    unspecified site C44.99
  basal cell
    specified site —see Neoplasm,
      skin, malignant
    unspecified site C08.9
  basophil
    specified site —see Neoplasm,
      malignant, by site
    unspecified site C75.1
  bile duct type C22.1
    liver C22.1
    specified site NEC —see
      Neoplasm, malignant, by site
    unspecified site C22.1
  bronchiolar —see Neoplasm, lung,
    malignant
  bronchioloalveolar —see
    Neoplasm, lung, malignant
  ceruminous C44.29-
  cervix, in situ —see also Carcinoma,
    cervix uteri, in situ D06.9
  chromophobe
    specified site —see Neoplasm,
      malignant, by site
    unspecified site C75.1
  diffuse type
    specified site —see Neoplasm,
      malignant, by site
    unspecified site C16.9
  duct
    infiltrating
      with Paget's disease —see
        Neoplasm, breast, malignant
      specified site —see Neoplasm,
        malignant, by site
      unspecified site (female) 50.91-
        male C50.92-
    specified site —see Neoplasm,
      malignant, by site
    unspecified site
      female C56.9
      male C61
  eosinophil
    specified site —see Neoplasm,
      malignant, by site
    unspecified site C75.1
  follicular
    with papillary C73
    moderately differentiated C73
    specified site —see Neoplasm,
      malignant, by site
    trabecular C73
    unspecified site C73
    well differentiated C73
  Hurthle cell C73
  in
    adenomatous
      polyposis coli C18.9
  infiltrating duct
    with Paget's disease —see
      Neoplasm, breast, malignant
    specified site —see Neoplasm,
      by site, malignant
    unspecified site (female) C50.91-
      male C50.92-
  inflammatory
    specified site —see Neoplasm,
      by site, malignant
    unspecified site (female) C50.91-
      male C50.92-

Adenocarcinoma (continued)
  intestinal type
    specified site —see Neoplasm,
      by site, malignant
    unspecified site C16.9
  intracystic papillary
  intraductal
    breast D05.1-
    noninfiltrating
      breast D05.1-
      papillary
        with invasion
          specified site —see
            Neoplasm, by site,
            malignant
          unspecified site (female)
            C50.91-
            male C50.92-
        breast D05.1-
        specified site NEC —see
          Neoplasm, in situ, by site
        unspecified site D05.1-
      specified site NEC —see
        Neoplasm, in situ, by site
      unspecified site D05.1-
    papillary
      with invasion
        specified site —see
          Neoplasm, malignant,
          by site
        unspecified site (female)
          C50.91-
          male C50.92-
      breast D05.1-
      specified site —see Neoplasm,
        in situ, by site
      unspecified site D05.1-
    specified site NEC —see
      Neoplasm, in situ, by site
    unspecified site D05.1-
  islet cell
    with exocrine, mixed
      specified site —see Neoplasm,
        malignant, by site
      unspecified site C25.9
    pancreas C25.4
    specified site NEC —see
      Neoplasm, malignant, by site
    unspecified site C25.4
  lobular
    in situ
      breast D05.0-
      specified site NEC —see
        Neoplasm, in situ, by site
      unspecified site D05.0-
    specified site —see Neoplasm,
      malignant, by site
    unspecified site (female) C50.91-
      male C50.92-
  mucoid —see also Neoplasm,
    malignant, by site
  cell
    specified site —see Neoplasm,
      malignant, by site
    unspecified site C75.1
  nonencapsulated sclerosing C73
  papillary
    with follicular C73
    follicular variant C73
    intraductal (noninfiltrating)
      with invasion
        specified site —see
          Neoplasm, malignant,
          by site
        unspecified site (female)
          C50.91-
          male C50.92-
      breast D05.1-
      specified site NEC —see
        Neoplasm, in situ, by site
      unspecified site D05.1-

Adenocarcinoma (continued)
  papillary (continued)
    serous
      specified site —see Neoplasm,
        malignant, by site
      unspecified site C56.9
  papillocystic
    specified site —see Neoplasm,
      malignant, by site
    unspecified site C56.9
  pseudomucinous
    specified site —see Neoplasm,
      malignant, by site
    unspecified site C56.9
  renal cell C64-
  sebaceous —see Neoplasm, skin,
    malignant
  serous —see also Neoplasm,
    malignant, by site
    papillary
      specified site —see Neoplasm,
        malignant, by site
      unspecified site C56.9
  sweat gland —see Neoplasm, skin,
    malignant
  water-clear cell C75.0
Adenocarcinoma-in-situ —see also
  Neoplasm, in situ, by site
  breast D05.9-
Adenofibroma
  clear cell —see Neoplasm, benign,
    by site
  endometrioid D27.9
    borderline malignancy D39.10
    malignant C56-
  mucinous
    specified site —see Neoplasm,
      benign, by site
    unspecified site D27.9
  papillary
    specified site —see Neoplasm,
      benign, by site
    unspecified site D27.9
  prostate —see Enlargement,
    enlarged, prostate
  serous
    specified site —see Neoplasm,
      benign, by site
    unspecified site D27.9
  specified site —see Neoplasm,
    benign, by site
  unspecified site D27.9
Adenofibrosis
  breast —see Fibroadenosis, breast
  endometrioid N80.00
Adenoiditis (chronic) J35.02
  with tonsillitis J35.03
  acute J03.90
    recurrent J03.91
    specified organism NEC
      J03.80
      recurrent J03.81
    staphylococcal J03.80
      recurrent J03.81
    streptococcal J03.00
      recurrent J03.01
Adenoids —see condition
Adenolipoma —see Neoplasm,
  benign, by site
**Adenolipomatosis, Launois-
  Bensaude** E88.89
Adenolymphoma
  specified site —see Neoplasm,
    benign, by site
  unspecified site D11.9
Adenoma —see also Neoplasm,
  benign, by site
  acidophil

11

Adenoma (continued)
  acidophil (continued)
    specified site —see Neoplasm, benign, by site
    unspecified site D35.2
  acidophil-basophil, mixed
    specified site —see Neoplasm, benign, by site
    unspecified site D35.2
  adrenal (cortical) D35.00
    clear cell D35.00
    compact cell D35.00
    glomerulosa cell D35.00
    heavily pigmented variant D35.00
    mixed cell D35.00
  alpha-cell
    pancreas D13.7
    specified site NEC —see Neoplasm, benign, by site
    unspecified site D13.7
  alveolar D14.30
  apocrine
    breast D24-
    specified site NEC —see Neoplasm, skin, benign, by site
    unspecified site D23.9
  basal cell D11.9
  basophil
    specified site —see Neoplasm, benign, by site
    unspecified site D35.2
  basophil-acidophil, mixed
    specified site —see Neoplasm, benign, by site
    unspecified site D35.2
  beta-cell
    pancreas D13.7
    specified site NEC —see Neoplasm, benign, by site
    unspecified site D13.7
  bile duct D13.4
    common D13.5
    extrahepatic D13.5
    intrahepatic D13.4
    specified site NEC —see Neoplasm, benign, by site
    unspecified site D13.4
  black D35.00
  bronchial D38.1
    cylindroid type —see Neoplasm, lung, malignant
  ceruminous D23.2-
  chief cell D35.1
  chromophobe
    specified site —see Neoplasm, benign, by site
    unspecified site D35.2
  colloid
    specified site —see Neoplasm, benign, by site
    unspecified site D34
  eccrine, papillary —see Neoplasm, skin, benign
  endocrine, multiple
    single specified site —see Neoplasm, uncertain behavior, by site
    two or more specified sites D44-
    unspecified site D44.9
  endometrioid —see also Neoplasm, benign
    borderline malignancy —see Neoplasm, uncertain behavior, by site
  eosinophil
    specified site —see Neoplasm, benign, by site
    unspecified site D35.2
  fetal
    specified site —see Neoplasm, benign, by site

Adenoma (continued)
  fetal (continued)
    unspecified site D34
  follicular
    specified site —see Neoplasm, benign, by site
    unspecified site D34
  hepatocellular D13.4
  Hurthle cell D34
  islet cell
    pancreas D13.7
    specified site NEC —see Neoplasm, benign, by site
    unspecified site D13.7
  liver cell D13.4
  macrofollicular
    specified site —see Neoplasm, benign, by site
    unspecified site D34
  malignant, malignum —see Neoplasm, malignant, by site
  microcystic
    pancreas D13.6
    specified site NEC —see Neoplasm, benign, by site
    unspecified site D13.6
  microfollicular
    specified site —see Neoplasm, benign, by site
    unspecified site D34
  mucoid cell
    specified site —see Neoplasm, benign, by site
    unspecified site D35.2
  multiple endocrine
    single specified site —see Neoplasm, uncertain behavior, by site
    two or more specified sites D44-
    unspecified site D44.9
  nipple D24-
  papillary —see also Neoplasm, benign, by site
    eccrine —see Neoplasm, skin, benign, by site
  Pick's tubular
    specified site —see Neoplasm, benign, by site
    unspecified site
      female D27.9
      male D29.20
  pleomorphic
    carcinoma in —see Neoplasm, salivary gland, malignant
      specified site —see Neoplasm, malignant, by site
      unspecified site C08.9
  polypoid —see also Neoplasm, benign
    adenocarcinoma in —see Neoplasm, malignant, by site
    adenocarcinoma in situ —see Neoplasm, in situ, by site
  prostate —see Neoplasm, benign, prostate
  rete cell D29.20
  sebaceous —see Neoplasm, skin, benign
  Sertoli cell
    specified site —see Neoplasm, benign, by site
    unspecified site
      female D27.9
      male D29.20
  skin appendage —see Neoplasm, skin, benign
  sudoriferous gland —see Neoplasm, skin, benign
  sweat gland —see Neoplasm, skin, benign

Adenoma (continued)
  testicular
    specified site —see Neoplasm, benign, by site
    unspecified site
      female D27.9
      male D29.20
  tubular —see also Neoplasm, benign, by site
    adenocarcinoma in —see Neoplasm, malignant, by site
    adenocarcinoma in situ —see Neoplasm, in situ, by site
  Pick's
    specified site —see Neoplasm, benign, by site
    unspecified site
      female D27.9
      male D29.20
  tubulovillous —see also Neoplasm, benign, by site
    adenocarcinoma in —see Neoplasm, malignant, by site
    adenocarcinoma in situ —see Neoplasm, in situ, by site
  villous —see Neoplasm, uncertain behavior, by site
    adenocarcinoma in —see Neoplasm, malignant, by site
    adenocarcinoma in situ —see Neoplasm, in situ, by site
  water-clear cell D35.1

Adenomatosis
  endocrine (multiple) E31.20
    single specified site —see Neoplasm, uncertain behavior, by site
  erosive of nipple D24-
  pluriendocrine —see Adenomatosis, endocrine
  pulmonary D38.1
    malignant —see Neoplasm, lung, malignant
  specified site —see Neoplasm, benign, by site
  unspecified site D12.6

Adenomatous
  goiter (nontoxic) E04.9
    with hyperthyroidism —see Hyperthyroidism, with, goiter, nodular
    toxic —see Hyperthyroidism, with, goiter, nodular

Adenomyoma —see also Neoplasm, benign, by site
  prostate —see Enlarged, prostate

Adenomyometritis N80.00

Adenomyosis (uterus) N80.03

Adenopathy (lymph gland) R59.9
  generalized R59.1
  inguinal R59.0
  localized R59.0
  mediastinal R59.0
  mesentery R59.0
  syphilitic (secondary) A51.49
  tracheobronchial R59.0
    tuberculous A15.4
      primary (progressive) A15.7
  tuberculous —see also Tuberculosis, lymph gland
    tracheobronchial A15.4
      primary (progressive) A15.7

Adenosalpingitis —see Salpingitis

Adenosarcoma —see Neoplasm, malignant, by site

Adenosclerosis I88.8

Adenosis (sclerosing) breast —see Fibroadenosis, breast

Adenovirus, as cause of disease classified elsewhere B97.0

Adentia (complete) (partial) —see Absence, teeth

Adherent —see also Adhesions
  labia (minora) N90.89
  pericardium (nonrheumatic) I31.0
    rheumatic I09.2
  placenta (with hemorrhage) O72.0
    without hemorrhage O73.0
  prepuce, newborn N47.0
  scar (skin) L90.5
  tendon in scar L90.5

Adhesions, adhesive (postinfective)
  with intestinal obstruction K56.50
    complete K56.52
    incomplete K56.51
    partial K56.51
  abdominal (wall) —see Adhesions, peritoneum
  appendix K38.8
  bile duct (common) (hepatic) K83.8
  bladder (sphincter) N32.89
  bowel —see Adhesions, peritoneum
  cardiac I31.0
    rheumatic I09.2
  cecum —see Adhesions, peritoneum
  cervicovaginal N88.1
    congenital Q52.8
    postpartal O90.89
      old N88.1
  cervix N88.1
  ciliary body NEC —see Adhesions, iris
  clitoris N90.89
  colon —see Adhesions, peritoneum
  common duct K83.8
  congenital —see also Anomaly, by site
    fingers —see Syndactylism, complex, fingers
    omental, anomalous Q43.3
    peritoneal Q43.3
    tongue (to gum or roof of mouth) Q38.3
  conjunctiva (acquired) H11.21-
    congenital Q15.8
  cystic duct K82.8
  diaphragm —see Adhesions, peritoneum
  due to foreign body —see Foreign body
  duodenum —see Adhesions, peritoneum
  ear
    middle H74.1-
  epididymis N50.89
  epidural —see Adhesions, meninges
  epiglottis J38.7
  eyelid H02.59
  female pelvis N73.6
  gallbladder K82.8
  globe H44.89
  heart I31.0
    rheumatic I09.2
  ileocecal (coil) —see Adhesions, peritoneum
  ileum —see Adhesions, peritoneum
  intestine —see also Adhesions, peritoneum
    with obstruction K56.50
      complete K56.52
      incomplete K56.51
      partial K56.51
  intra-abdominal —see Adhesions, peritoneum

Adhesions, adhesive (continued)
- iris H21.50-
  - anterior H21.51-
  - goniosynechiae H21.52-
  - posterior H21.54-
  - to corneal graft T85.898
- joint —see Ankylosis
  - knee M23.8X
  - temporomandibular M26.61-
- labium (majus) (minus), congenital Q52.5
- liver —see Adhesions, peritoneum
- lung J98.4
- mediastinum J98.59
- meninges (cerebral) (spinal) G96.12
  - congenital Q07.8
  - tuberculous (cerebral) (spinal) A17.0
- mesenteric —see Adhesions, peritoneum
- nasal (septum) (to turbinates) J34.89
- ocular muscle —see Strabismus, mechanical
- omentum —see Adhesions, peritoneum
- ovary N73.6
  - congenital (to cecum, kidney or omentum) Q50.39
- paraovarian N73.6
- pelvic (peritoneal)
  - female N73.6
    - postprocedural N99.4
  - male —see Adhesions, peritoneum
  - postpartal (old) N73.6
  - tuberculous A18.17
- penis to scrotum (congenital) Q55.8
- periappendiceal —see also Adhesions, peritoneum
- pericardium (nonrheumatic) I31.0
  - focal I31.8
  - rheumatic I09.2
  - tuberculous A18.84
- pericholecystic K82.8
- perigastric —see Adhesions, peritoneum
- periovarian N73.6
- periprostatic N42.89
- perirectal —see Adhesions, peritoneum
- perirenal N28.89
- peritoneum, peritoneal (postinfective) K66.0
  - with obstruction (intestinal) K56.50
    - complete K56.52
    - incomplete K56.51
    - partial K56.51
  - congenital Q43.3
  - pelvic, female N73.6
    - postprocedural N99.4
  - postpartal, pelvic N73.6
  - postprocedural K66.0
  - to uterus N73.6
- peritubal N73.6
- periureteral N28.89
- periuterine N73.6
- perivesical N32.89
- perivesicular (seminal vesicle) N50.89
- pleura, pleuritic J94.8
  - tuberculous NEC A15.6
- pleuropericardial J94.8
- postoperative (gastrointestinal tract) K66.0
  - with obstruction (see also Obstruction, intestine, postoperative) K91.30

Adhesions, adhesive (continued)
- postoperative (continued)
  - due to foreign body accidentally left in wound —see Foreign body, accidentally left during a procedure
  - pelvic peritoneal N99.4
  - urethra —see Stricture, urethra, postprocedural
  - vagina N99.2
- postpartal, old (vulva or perineum) N90.89
- preputial, prepuce N47.5
- pulmonary J98.4
- pylorus —see Adhesions, peritoneum
- sciatic nerve —see Lesion, nerve, sciatic
- seminal vesicle N50.89
- shoulder (joint) —see Capsulitis, adhesive
- sigmoid flexure —see Adhesions, peritoneum
- spermatic cord (acquired) N50.89
  - congenital Q55.4
- spinal canal G96.12
- stomach —see Adhesions, peritoneum
- subscapular —see Capsulitis, adhesive
- temporomandibular M26.61-
- tendinitis —see also Tenosynovitis, specified type NEC
  - shoulder —see Capsulitis, adhesive
- testis N44.8
- tongue, congenital (to gum or roof of mouth) Q38.3
  - acquired K14.8
- trachea J39.8
- tubo-ovarian N73.6
- tunica vaginalis N44.8
- uterus N73.6
  - internal N85.6
  - to abdominal wall N73.6
- vagina (chronic) N89.5
  - postoperative N99.2
- vitreomacular H43.82-
- vitreous H43.89
- vulva N90.89

Adiaspiromycosis B48.88

Adie (-Holmes) **pupil or syndrome** —see Anomaly, pupil, function, tonic pupil

Adiponecrosis neonatorum P83.88

Adiposis —see also Obesity
- cerebralis E23.6
- dolorosa E88.2

Adiposity —see also Obesity
- heart —see Degeneration, myocardial
- localized E65

Adiposogenital dystrophy E23.6

Adjustment
- disorder —see Disorder, adjustment
- implanted device —see Encounter (for), adjustment (of)
- prosthesis, external —see Fitting
- reaction —see Disorder, adjustment

Administration of tPA (rtPA) **in a different facility within the last 24 hours prior to admission to current facility** Z92.82

Admission (for) —see also Encounter (for)
- adjustment (of)
  - artificial
    - arm Z44.00-
      - complete Z44.01-
      - partial Z44.02-

Admission (continued)
- adjustment (continued)
  - artificial (continued)
    - eye Z44.2
    - leg Z44.10-
      - complete Z44.11-
      - partial Z44.12-
  - brain neuropacemaker Z46.2
    - implanted Z45.42
  - breast
    - implant Z45.81
    - prosthesis (external) Z44.3
  - colostomy belt Z46.89
  - contact lenses Z46.0
  - cystostomy device Z46.6
  - dental prosthesis Z46.3
  - device NEC
    - abdominal Z46.89
    - implanted Z45.89
      - cardiac Z45.09
        - defibrillator (with synchronous cardiac pacemaker) Z45.02
        - pacemaker (cardiac resynchronization therapy (CRT-P)) Z45.018
          - pulse generator Z45.010
        - resynchronization therapy defibrillator (CRT-D) Z45.02
      - hearing device Z45.328
        - bone conduction Z45.320
        - cochlear Z45.321
      - infusion pump Z45.1
      - nervous system Z45.49
        - CSF drainage Z45.41
        - hearing device —see Admission, adjustment, device, implanted, hearing device
        - neuropacemaker Z45.42
        - visual substitution Z45.31
      - specified NEC Z45.89
      - vascular access Z45.2
      - visual substitution Z45.31
    - nervous system Z46.2
      - implanted —see Admission, adjustment, device, implanted, nervous system
    - orthodontic Z46.4
    - prosthetic Z44.9
      - arm —see Admission, adjustment, artificial, arm
      - breast Z44.3
      - dental Z46.3
      - eye Z44.2
      - leg —see Admission, adjustment, artificial, leg
      - specified type NEC Z44.8
    - substitution
      - auditory Z46.2
        - implanted —see Admission, adjustment, device, implanted, hearing device
      - nervous system Z46.2
        - implanted —see Admission, adjustment, device, implanted, nervous system
      - visual Z46.2
        - implanted Z45.31
    - urinary Z46.6
  - hearing aid Z46.1
    - implanted —see Admission, adjustment, device, implanted, hearing device
  - ileostomy device Z46.89

Admission (continued)
- adjustment (continued)
  - intestinal appliance or device NEC Z46.89
  - neuropacemaker (brain) (peripheral nerve) (spinal cord) Z46.2
    - implanted Z45.42
  - orthodontic device Z46.4
  - orthopedic (brace) (cast) (device) (shoes) Z46.89
  - pacemaker (cardiac resynchronization therapy (CRT-P))
    - cardiac Z45.018
      - pulse generator Z45.010
    - nervous system Z46.2
      - implanted Z45.42
  - portacath (port-a-cath) Z45.2
  - prosthesis Z44.9
    - arm —see Admission, adjustment, artificial, arm
    - breast Z44.3
    - dental Z46.3
    - eye Z44.2
    - leg —see Admission, adjustment, artificial, leg
    - specified NEC Z44.8
  - spectacles Z46.0
- aftercare —see also Aftercare Z51.89
- postpartum
  - immediately after delivery Z39.0
  - routine follow-up Z39.2
- radiation therapy (antineoplastic) Z51.0
- attention to artificial opening (of) Z43.9
  - artificial vagina Z43.7
  - colostomy Z43.3
  - cystostomy Z43.5
  - enterostomy Z43.4
  - gastrostomy Z43.1
  - ileostomy Z43.2
  - jejunostomy Z43.4
  - nephrostomy Z43.6
  - specified site NEC Z43.8
    - intestinal tract Z43.4
    - urinary tract Z43.6
  - tracheostomy Z43.0
  - ureterostomy Z43.6
  - urethrostomy Z43.6
- breast augmentation or reduction Z41.1
- breast reconstruction following mastectomy Z42.1
- change of
  - dressing (nonsurgical) Z48.00
  - neuropacemaker device (brain) (peripheral nerve) (spinal cord) Z46.2
    - implanted Z45.42
  - surgical dressing Z48.01
- circumcision, ritual or routine (in absence of diagnosis) Z41.2
- clinical research investigation (control) (normal comparison) (participant) Z00.6
- contraceptive management Z30.9
- cosmetic surgery NEC Z41.1
- counseling —see also Counseling
  - dietary Z71.3
  - gestational carrier Z31.7
  - HIV Z71.7
  - human immunodeficiency virus Z71.7
  - nonattending third party Z71.0
  - procreative management NEC Z31.69
- delivery, full-term, uncomplicated O80
  - cesarean, without indication O82

13

Admission (continued)
  desensitization to allergens Z51.6
  dietary surveillance and counseling Z71.3
  ear piercing Z41.3
  examination at health care facility (adult) (see also Examination) Z00.00
    with abnormal findings Z00.01
    clinical research investigation (control) (normal comparison) (participant) Z00.6
    dental Z01.20
      with abnormal findings Z01.21
    donor (potential) Z00.5
    ear Z01.10
      with abnormal findings NEC Z01.118
    eye Z01.00
      with abnormal findings Z01.01
      following failed vision screening Z01.020
        with abnormal findings Z01.021
    general, specified reason NEC Z00.8
    hearing Z01.10
      with abnormal findings NEC Z01.118
    infant or child (over 28 days old) Z00.129
      with abnormal findings Z00.121
    postpartum checkup Z39.2
    psychiatric (general) Z00.8
      requested by authority Z04.6
    vision Z01.00
      with abnormal findings Z01.01
      following failed vision screening Z01.020
        with abnormal findings Z01.021
      infant or child (over 28 days old) Z00.129
        with abnormal findings Z00.121
  fitting (of)
    artificial
      arm —see Admission, adjustment, artificial, arm
      eye Z44.2
      leg —see Admission, adjustment, artificial, leg
    brain neuropacemaker Z46.2
      implanted Z45.42
    breast prosthesis (external) Z44.3
    colostomy belt Z46.89
    contact lenses Z46.0
    cystostomy device Z46.6
    dental prosthesis Z46.3
    dentures Z46.3
    device NEC
      abdominal Z46.89
      nervous system Z46.2
        implanted —see Admission, adjustment, device, implanted, nervous system
      orthodontic Z46.4
      prosthetic Z44.9
        breast Z44.3
        dental Z46.3
        eye Z44.2
      substitution
        auditory Z46.2
          implanted —see Admission, adjustment, device, implanted, hearing device

Admission (continued)
  fitting (continued)
    device NEC (continued)
      substitution (continued)
        nervous system Z46.2
          implanted —see Admission, adjustment, device, implanted, nervous system
        visual Z46.2
          implanted Z45.31
    hearing aid Z46.1
    ileostomy device Z46.89
    intestinal appliance or device NEC Z46.89
    neuropacemaker (brain) (peripheral nerve) (spinal cord) Z46.2
      implanted Z45.42
    orthodontic device Z46.4
    orthopedic device (brace) (cast) (shoes) Z46.89
    prosthesis Z44.9
      arm —see Admission, adjustment, artificial, arm
      breast Z44.3
      dental Z46.3
      eye Z44.2
      leg —see Admission, adjustment, artificial, leg
      specified type NEC Z44.8
    spectacles Z46.0
  follow-up examination Z09
  intrauterine device management Z30.431
    initial prescription Z30.014
  mental health evaluation Z00.8
    requested by authority Z04.6
  observation —see Observation
  Papanicolaou smear, cervix Z12.4
    for suspected malignant neoplasm Z12.4
  plastic and reconstructive surgery following medical procedure or healed injury NEC Z42.8
  plastic surgery, cosmetic NEC Z41.1
  postpartum observation
    immediately after delivery Z39.0
    routine follow-up Z39.2
  poststerilization (for restoration) Z31.0
    aftercare Z31.42
  procreative management Z31.9
  prophylactic (measure) —see also Encounter, prophylactic measures
    organ removal Z40.00
      breast Z40.01
      fallopian tube(s) Z40.03
        with ovary(s) Z40.02
      ovary(s) Z40.02
      specified organ NEC Z40.09
      testes Z40.09
    vaccination Z23
  psychiatric examination (general) Z00.8
    requested by authority Z04.6
  radiation therapy (antineoplastic) Z51.0
  reconstructive surgery following medical procedure or healed injury NEC Z42.8
  removal of
    cystostomy catheter Z43.5
    drains Z48.03
    dressing (nonsurgical) Z48.00
    implantable subdermal contraceptive Z30.46
    intrauterine contraceptive device Z30.432
    neuropacemaker (brain) (peripheral nerve) (spinal cord) Z46.2
      implanted Z45.42

Admission (continued)
  removal of (continued)
    staples Z48.02
    surgical dressing Z48.01
    sutures Z48.02
    ureteral stent Z46.6
  respirator [ventilator] use during power failure Z99.12
  restoration of organ continuity (poststerilization) Z31.0
    aftercare Z31.42
  sensitivity test —see also Test, skin allergy NEC Z01.82
    Mantoux Z11.1
  tuboplasty following previous sterilization Z31.0
    aftercare Z31.42
  vasoplasty following previous sterilization Z31.0
    aftercare Z31.42
  vision examination Z01.00
    with abnormal findings Z01.01
    following failed vision screening Z01.020
      with abnormal findings Z01.021
    infant or child (over 28 days old) Z00.129
      with abnormal findings Z00.121
  waiting period for admission to other facility Z75.1

Adnexitis (suppurative) —see Salpingo-oophoritis
Adolescent X-linked adrenoleukodystrophy E71.521
Adrenal (gland) —see condition
Adrenalism, tuberculous A18.7
Adrenalitis, adrenitis E27.8
  autoimmune E27.1
  meningococcal, hemorrhagic A39.1
Adrenarche, premature E27.0
Adrenocortical syndrome —see Cushing's, syndrome
Adrenogenital syndrome E25.9
  acquired E25.8
  congenital E25.0
  salt loss E25.0
Adrenogenitalism, congenital E25.0
Adrenoleukodystrophy E71.529
  neonatal E71.511
  X-linked E71.529
    Addison only phenotype E71.528
    Addison-Schilder E71.528
    adolescent E71.521
    adrenomyeloneuropathy E71.522
    childhood cerebral E71.520
    other specified E71.528
Adrenomyeloneuropathy E71.522
Adventitious bursa —see Bursopathy, specified type NEC
Adverse effect —see Table of Drugs and Chemicals, categories T36-T50, with 6th character 5
Advice —see Counseling
Adynamia (episodica) (hereditary) (periodic) G72.3
Aeration lung imperfect, newborn —see Atelectasis
Aerobullosis T70.3
Aerocele —see Embolism, air
Aerodermectasia
  subcutaneous (traumatic) T79.7
Aerodontalgia T70.29
Aeroembolism T70.3
Aerogenes capsulatus infection A48.0

Aero-otitis media T70.0
Aerophagy, aerophagia (psychogenic) F45.8
Aerophobia F40.228
Aerosinusitis T70.1
Aerotitis T70.0
Affection —see Disease
Afibrinogenemia (see also Defect, coagulation) D68.8
  acquired D65
  congenital D68.2
  following ectopic or molar pregnancy O08.1
  in abortion —see Abortion, by type, complicated by, afibrinogenemia
  puerperal O72.3
African
  sleeping sickness B56.9
  tick fever A68.1
  trypanosomiasis B56.9
    gambian B56.0
    rhodesian B56.1
Aftercare (see also Care) Z51.89
  following surgery (for) (on)
    amputation Z47.81
    attention to
      drains Z48.03
      dressings (nonsurgical) Z48.00
        surgical Z48.01
      sutures Z48.02
    circulatory system Z48.812
    delayed (planned) wound closure Z48.1
    digestive system Z48.815
    explantation of joint prosthesis (staged procedure)
      hip Z47.32
      knee Z47.33
      shoulder Z47.31
    genitourinary system Z48.816
    joint replacement Z47.1
    neoplasm Z48.3
    nervous system Z48.811
    oral cavity Z48.814
    organ transplant
      bone marrow Z48.290
      heart Z48.21
      heart-lung Z48.280
      kidney Z48.22
      liver Z48.23
      lung Z48.24
      multiple organs NEC Z48.288
      specified NEC Z48.298
    orthopedic NEC Z47.89
    planned wound closure Z48.1
    removal of internal fixation device Z47.2
    respiratory system Z48.813
    scoliosis Z47.82
    sense organs Z48.810
    skin and subcutaneous tissue Z48.817
    specified body system
      circulatory Z48.812
      digestive Z48.815
      genitourinary Z48.816
      nervous Z48.811
      oral cavity Z48.814
      respiratory Z48.813
      sense organs Z48.810
      skin and subcutaneous tissue Z48.817
      teeth Z48.814
    specified NEC Z48.89
    spinal Z47.89
    teeth Z48.814
  fracture - code to fracture with seventh character D

Aftercare (continued)
  involving
    removal of
      drains Z48.03
      dressings (nonsurgical) Z48.00
      staples Z48.02
      surgical dressings Z48.01
      sutures Z48.02
    neuropacemaker (brain) (peripheral nerve) (spinal cord) Z46.2
    implanted Z45.42
  orthopedic NEC Z47.89
  postprocedural —*see* Aftercare, following surgery

After-cataract —*see* Cataract, secondary

Agalactia (primary) O92.3
  elective, secondary or therapeutic O92.5

Agammaglobulinemia (acquired (secondary)) (nonfamilial) D80.1
  with
    immunoglobulin-bearing B-lymphocytes D80.1
    lymphopenia D81.9
  autosomal recessive (Swiss type) D80.0
  Bruton's X-linked D80.0
  common variable (CVAgamma) D80.1
  congenital sex-linked D80.0
  hereditary D80.0
  lymphopenic D81.9
  Swiss type (autosomal recessive) D80.0
  X-linked (with growth hormone deficiency) (Bruton) D80.0

Aganglionosis (bowel) (colon) Q43.1

Age (old) —*see* Senility

Agenesis
  adrenal (gland) Q89.1
  alimentary tract (complete) (partial) NEC Q45.8
    upper Q40.8
  anus, anal (canal) Q42.3
    with fistula Q42.2
  aorta Q25.41
  appendix Q42.8
  arm (complete) Q71.0-
    with hand present Q71.1-
  artery (peripheral) Q27.9
    brain Q28.3
    coronary Q24.5
    pulmonary Q25.79
    specified NEC Q27.8
    umbilical Q27.0
  auditory (canal) (external) Q16.1
  auricle (ear) Q16.0
  bile duct or passage Q44.5
  bladder Q64.5
  bone Q79.9
  brain Q00.0
    part of Q04.3
  breast (with nipple present) Q83.8
    with absent nipple Q83.0
  bronchus Q32.4
  canaliculus lacrimalis Q10.4
  carpus —*see* Agenesis, hand
  cartilage Q79.9
  cecum Q42.8
  cerebellum Q04.3
  cervix Q51.5
  chin Q18.8
  cilia Q10.3
  circulatory system, part NOS Q28.9
  clavicle Q74.0

Agenesis (continued)
  clitoris Q52.6
  coccyx Q76.49
  colon Q42.9
    specified NEC Q42.8
  corpus callosum Q04.0
  cricoid cartilage Q31.8
  diaphragm (with hernia) Q79.1
  digestive organ(s) or tract (complete) (partial) NEC Q45.8
    upper Q40.8
  ductus arteriosus Q28.8
  duodenum Q41.0
  ear Q16.9
    auricle Q16.0
    lobe Q17.8
  ejaculatory duct Q55.4
  endocrine (gland) NEC Q89.2
  epiglottis Q31.8
  esophagus Q39.8
  eustachian tube Q16.2
  eye Q11.1
    adnexa Q15.8
  eyelid (fold) Q10.3
  face
    bones NEC Q75.8
    specified part NEC Q18.8
  fallopian tube Q50.6
  femur —*see* Defect, reduction, lower limb, longitudinal, femur
  fibula —*see* Defect, reduction, lower limb, longitudinal, fibula
  finger (complete) (partial) —*see* Agenesis, hand
  foot (and toes) (complete) (partial) Q72.3-
  forearm (with hand present) —*see* Agenesis, arm, with hand present and hand Q71.2-
  gallbladder Q44.0
  gastric Q40.2
  genitalia, genital (organ(s))
    female Q52.8
      external Q52.71
      internal NEC Q52.8
    male Q55.8
  glottis Q31.8
  hair Q84.0
  hand(and fingers) (complete) (partial) Q71.3-
  heart Q24.8
    valve NEC Q24.8
      pulmonary Q22.0
  hepatic Q44.79
  humerus —*see* Defect, reduction, upper limb
  hymen Q52.4
  ileum Q41.2
  incus Q16.3
  intestine (small) Q41.9
    large Q42.9
      specified NEC Q42.8
  iris (dilator fibers) Q13.1
  jaw M26.09
  jejunum Q41.1
  kidney(s) (partial) Q60.2
    bilateral Q60.1
    unilateral Q60.0
  labium (majus) (minus) Q52.71
  labyrinth, membranous Q16.5
  lacrimal apparatus Q10.4
  larynx Q31.8
  leg (complete) Q72.0-
    with foot present Q72.1-
    lower leg (with foot present) —*see* Agenesis, leg, with foot present and foot Q72.2-
  lens Q12.3
  limb (complete) Q73.0
    lower —*see* Agenesis, leg
    upper —*see* Agenesis, arm

Agenesis (continued)
  lip Q38.0
  liver Q44.79
  lung (fissure) (lobe) (bilateral) (unilateral) Q33.3
  mandible, maxilla M26.09
  metacarpus —*see* Agenesis, hand
  metatarsus —*see* Agenesis, foot
  muscle Q79.8
    eyelid Q10.3
    ocular Q15.8
  musculoskeletal systemNEC Q79.8
  nail(s) Q84.3
  neck, part Q18.8
  nerve Q07.8
  nervous system, part NEC Q07.8
  nipple Q83.2
  nose Q30.1
  nuclear Q07.8
  organ
    of Corti Q16.5
    or site not listed —*see* Anomaly, by site
  osseous meatus (ear) Q16.1
  ovary
    bilateral Q50.02
    unilateral Q50.01
  oviduct Q50.6
  pancreas Q45.0
  parathyroid (gland) Q89.2
  parotid gland(s) Q38.4
  patella Q74.1
  pelvic girdle (complete) (partial) Q74.2
  penis Q55.5
  pericardium Q24.8
  pituitary (gland) Q89.2
  prostate Q55.4
  punctum lacrimale Q10.4
  radioulnar —*see* Defect, reduction, upper limb
  radius —*see* Defect, reduction, upper limb, longitudinal, radius
  rectum Q42.1
    with fistula Q42.0
  renal Q60.2
    bilateral Q60.1
    unilateral Q60.0
  respiratory organ NEC Q34.8
  rib Q76.6
  roof of orbit Q75.8
  round ligament Q52.8
  sacrum Q76.49
  salivary gland Q38.4
  scapula Q74.0
  scrotum Q55.29
  seminal vesicles Q55.4
  septum
    atrial Q21.19
    between aorta and pulmonary artery Q21.4
    ventricular Q20.4
  shoulder girdle (complete) (partial) Q74.0
  skull (bone) Q75.8
    with
      anencephaly Q00.0
      encephalocele —*see* Encephalocele
      hydrocephalus Q03.9
        with spina bifida —*see* Spina bifida, by site, with hydrocephalus
      microcephaly Q02
  spermatic cord Q55.4
  spinal cord Q06.0
  spine Q76.49
  spleen Q89.01
  sternum Q76.7
  stomach Q40.2

Agenesis (continued)
  submaxillary gland(s) (congenital) Q38.4
  tarsus —*see* Agenesis, foot
  tendon Q79.8
  testicle Q55.0
  thymus (gland) Q89.2
  thyroid (gland) E03.1
    cartilage Q31.8
  tibia —*see* Defect, reduction, lower limb, longitudinal, tibia
  tibiofibular —*see* Defect, reduction, lower limb, specified type NEC
  toe (and foot) (complete) (partial) —*see* Agenesis, foot
  tongue Q38.3
  trachea (cartilage) Q32.1
  ulna —*see* Defect, reduction, upper limb, longitudinal, ulna
  upper limb —*see* Agenesis, arm
  ureter Q62.4
  urethra Q64.5
  urinary tract NEC Q64.8
  uterus Q51.0
  uvula Q38.5
  vagina Q52.0
  vas deferens Q55.4
  vein(s) (peripheral) Q27.9
    brain Q28.3
    great NEC Q26.8
    portal Q26.5
    vena cava (inferior) (superior) Q26.8
  vermis of cerebellum Q04.3
  vertebra Q76.49
  vulva Q52.71

Ageusia R43.2

Agitated —*see* condition

Agitation R45.1

Aglossia (congenital) Q38.3

Aglossia-adactylia syndrome Q87.0

Aglycogenosis E74.00

Agnosia (body image) (other senses) (tactile) R48.1
  developmental F88
  verbal R48.1
    auditory R48.1
      developmental F80.2
    developmental F80.2
  visual (object) R48.3

Agoraphobia F40.00
  with panic disorder F40.01
  without panic disorder F40.02

Agrammatism R48.8

Agranulocytopenia —*see* Agranulocytosis

Agranulocytosis (chronic) (cyclical) (genetic) (infantile) (periodic) (pernicious) —*see also* Neutropenia D70.9
  congenital D70.0
  cytoreductive cancer chemotherapy sequela D70.1
  drug-induced D70.2
    due to cytoreductive cancer chemotherapy D70.1
  due to infection D70.3
  secondary D70.4
    drug-induced D70.2
    due to cytoreductive cancer chemotherapy D70.1

Agraphia (absolute) R48.8
  with alexia R48.0
  developmental F81.81

Ague (dumb) —*see* Malaria

Agyria Q04.3

Ahumada-del Castillo syndrome E23.0
Aichomophobia F40.298
AIDS (related complex) B20
Ailment heart —*see* Disease, heart
Ailurophobia F40.218
AIN —*see* Neoplasia, intraepithelial, anal
Ainhum (disease) L94.6
AIPHI (acute idiopathic pulmonary hemorrhage in infants (over 28 days old)) R04.81
Air
  anterior mediastinum J98.2
  compressed, disease T70.3
  conditioner lung or pneumonitis J67.7
  embolism (artery) (cerebral) (any site) T79.0
    with ectopic or molar pregnancy O08.2
    due to implanted device NEC —*see* Complications, by site and type, specified NEC
    following
      abortion —*see* Abortion by type, complicated by, embolism
      ectopic or molar pregnancy O08.2
    infusion, therapeutic injection or transfusion T80.0
    in pregnancy, childbirth or puerperium —*see* Embolism, obstetric
    traumatic T79.0
  hunger, psychogenic F45.8
  rarefied, effects of —*see* Effect, adverse, high altitude
  sickness T75.3
Airplane sickness T75.3
Akathisia (drug-induced) (treatment-induced) G25.71
  neuroleptic induced (acute) G25.71
  tardive G25.71
Akinesia R29.898
Akinetic mutism R41.89
Akureyri's disease G93.39
Alactasia, congenital E73.0
Alagille (-Watson) syndrome Q44.71
Alastrim B03
Albers-Schönberg syndrome Q78.2
Albert's syndrome —*see* Tendinitis, Achilles
Albinism, albino E70.30
  with hematologic abnormality E70.339
    Chédiak-Higashi syndrome E70.330
    Hermansky-Pudlak syndrome E70.331
    other specified E70.338
  I E70.320
  II E70.321
  ocular E70.319
    autosomal recessive E70.311
    other specified E70.318
    X-linked E70.310
  oculocutaneous E70.329
    other specified E70.328
    tyrosinase (ty) negative E70.320
    tyrosinase (ty) positive E70.321
  other specified E70.39
Albinismus E70.30
Albright (-McCune) (-Sternberg) syndrome Q78.1

Albuminous —*see* condition
Albuminuria, albuminuric (acute) (chronic) (subacute) (*see also* Proteinuria) R80.9
  complicating pregnancy —*see* Proteinuria, gestational
  with
    gestational hypertension —*see* Pre-eclampsia
    pre-existing hypertension —*see* Hypertension, complicating pregnancy, pre-existing, with, pre-eclampsia
  gestational —*see* Proteinuria, gestational
  with
    gestational hypertension —*see* Pre-eclampsia
    pre-existing hypertension —*see* Hypertension, complicating pregnancy, pre-existing, with, pre-eclampsia
  orthostatic R80.2
  postural R80.2
  pre-eclamptic —*see* Pre-eclampsia
  scarlatinal A38.8
Albuminurophobia F40.298
Alcaptonuria E70.29
Alcohol, alcoholic, alcohol-induced
  addiction (without remission) F10.20
    with remission F10.21
  amnestic disorder, persisting F10.96
    with dependence F10.26
  anxiety disorder F10.980
  bipolar and related disorder F10.94
  brain syndrome, chronic F10.97
    with dependence F10.27
  cardiopathy I42.6
  counseling and surveillance Z71.41
    family member Z71.42
  delirium (acute) (tremens) (withdrawal) F10.921
    with intoxication F10.921
    in
      abuse F10.121
      dependence F10.221
  abuse F10.131
    with intoxication F10.121
  dependence (acute) (tremens) (withdrawal) F10.231
    with intoxication F10.221
  use, unspecified F10.931
    with intoxication F10.921
  dementia F10.97
    with dependence F10.27
  depressive disorder F10.94
    with dependence F10.27
  deterioration F10.97
  hallucinosis (acute) F10.951
    in
      abuse F10.151
      dependence F10.251
  insanity F10.959
  intoxication (acute) (without dependence) F10.129
    with
      delirium F10.121
      dependence F10.229
        with delirium F10.221
        uncomplicated F10.220
    uncomplicated F10.120
  jealousy F10.988
  Korsakoff's, Korsakov's, Korsakow's F10.26
  liver K70.9
    acute —*see* Disease, liver, alcoholic, hepatitis

Alcohol, alcoholic, alcohol-induced
(continued)
  major neurocognitive disorder, amnestic-confabulatory type F10.96
  major neurocognitive disorder, nonamnestic-confabulatory type F10.97
  mania (acute) (chronic) F10.959
  mild neurocognitive disorder F10.988
  paranoia, paranoid (type) psychosis F10.950
  pellagra E52
  poisoning, accidental (acute) NEC —*see* Table of Drugs and Chemicals, alcohol, poisoning
  psychosis —*see* Psychosis, alcoholic
  psychotic disorder F10.959
  sexual dysfunction F10.981
  sleep disorder F10.982
  withdrawal (without convulsions) F10.239
    with delirium F10.231
Alcoholism (chronic) (without remission) F10.20
  with
    psychosis —*see* Psychosis, alcoholic
    remission F10.21
  Korsakov's F10.96
    with dependence F10.26
Alder (-Reilly) anomaly or syndrome (leukocyte granulation) D72.0
Aldosteronism E26.9
  familial (type I) E26.02
  glucocorticoid-remediable E26.02
  primary (due to (bilateral) adrenal hyperplasia) E26.09
  primary NEC E26.09
  secondary E26.1
  specified NEC E26.89
Aldosteronoma D44.10
Aldrich (-Wiskott) syndrome (eczema-thrombocytopenia) D82.0
Alektorophobia F40.218
Aleppo boil B55.1
Aleukemic —*see* condition
Aleukia
  congenital D70.0
  hemorrhagica D61.9
    congenital D61.09
  splenica D73.1
Alexia R48.0
  developmental F81.0
  secondary to organic lesion R48.0
Algoneurodystrophy M89.00
  ankle M89.07-
  foot M89.07-
  forearm M89.03-
  hand M89.04-
  lower leg M89.06-
  multiple sites M89.0-
  shoulder M89.01-
  specified site NEC M89.08
  thigh M89.05-
  upper arm M89.02-
Algophobia F40.298
Alienation, mental —*see* Psychosis
Alkalemia E87.3
Alkalosis E87.3
  metabolic E87.3
    with respiratory acidosis E87.4
    of newborn P74.41
  respiratory E87.3

Alkaptonuria E70.29
Allen-Masters syndrome N83.8
Allergy, allergic (reaction) (to) T78.40
  air-borne substance NEC (rhinitis) J30.89
  alveolitis (extrinsic) J67.9
    due to
      Aspergillus clavatus J67.4
      Cryptostroma corticale J67.6
      organisms (fungal, thermophilic actinomycete) growing in ventilation (air conditioning) systems J67.7
    specified type NEC J67.8
  anaphylactic reaction or shock T78.2
  angioneurotic edema T78.3
  animal (dander) (epidermal) (hair) (rhinitis) J30.81
  bee sting (anaphylactic shock) —*see* Toxicity, venom, arthropod, bee
  biological —*see* Allergy, drug
  colitis (*see also* Colitis, allergic) K52.29
  dander (animal) (rhinitis) J30.81
  dandruff (rhinitis) J30.81
  dental restorative material (existing) K08.55
  dermatitis —*see* Dermatitis, contact, allergic
  diathesis —*see* History, allergy
  drug, medicament & biological (any) (external) (internal) T78.40
    correct substance properly administered —*see* Table of Drugs and Chemicals, by drug, adverse effect
    wrong substance given or taken NEC (by accident) —*see* Table of Drugs and Chemicals, by drug, poisoning
  due to pollen J30.1
  dust (house) (stock) (rhinitis) J30.89
    with asthma —*see* Asthma, allergic extrinsic
  eczema —*see* Dermatitis, contact, allergic
  epidermal (animal) (rhinitis) J30.81
  feathers (rhinitis) J30.89
  food (any) (ingested) NEC T78.1
    anaphylactic shock —*see* Shock, anaphylactic, due to food
    dermatitis —*see* Dermatitis, due to, food
    dietary counseling and surveillance Z71.3
    in contact with skin L23.6
    rhinitis J30.5
    status (without reaction) Z91.018
      beef Z91.014
      lamb Z91.014
      eggs Z91.012
      mammalian meats Z91.04
      milk products Z91.011
      peanuts Z91.010
      pork Z91.014
      red meats Z91.04
      seafood Z91.013
      specified NEC Z91.018
  gastrointestinal —*see also* specific type of allergic reaction
    meaning colitis (*see also* Colitis, allergic) K52.29
    meaning gastroenteritis (*see also* Gastroenteritis, allergic) K52.29
    meaning other adverse food reaction not elsewhere classified T78.1
  grain J30.1

Allergy, allergic (continued)
　grass (hay fever) (pollen) J30.1
　　asthma —see Asthma, allergic
　　　extrinsic
　hair (animal) (rhinitis) J30.81
　history (of) —see History, allergy
　horse serum —see Allergy, serum
　inhalant (rhinitis) J30.89
　　pollen J30.1
　kapok (rhinitis) J30.89
　medicine —see Allergy, drug
　milk protein (see also Allergy,
　　food) Z91.011
　　anaphylactic reaction T78.07
　　dematitis L27.2
　　enterocolitis syndrome K52.21
　　enteropathy K52.22
　　gastroenteritis K52.29
　　gastroesophageal reflux (see also
　　　Reaction, adverse, food) K21.9
　　　with esophagitis (without
　　　　bleeding) K21.00
　　　　with bleeding K21.01
　　proctocolitis K52.29
　nasal, seasonal due to pollen J30.1
　pneumonia J82.89
　pollen (any) (hay fever) J30.1
　　asthma —see Asthma, allergic
　　　extrinsic
　primrose J30.1
　primula J30.1
　proctocolitis K52.29
　purpura D69.0
　ragweed (hay fever) (pollen) J30.1
　　asthma —see Asthma, allergic
　　　extrinsic
　rose (pollen) J30.1
　seasonal NEC J30.2
　Senecio jacobae (pollen) J30.1
　serum (see also Reaction, serum)
　　T80.69
　　anaphylactic shock T80.59
　shock (anaphylactic) T78.2
　　due to
　　　administration of blood and
　　　　blood products T80.51
　　　adverse effect of correct
　　　　medicinal substance
　　　　properly administered
　　　　T88.6
　　　immunization T80.52
　　　serum NEC T80.59
　　　vaccination T80.52
　specific NEC T78.49
　tree (any) (hay fever) (pollen) J30.1
　　asthma —see Asthma, allergic
　　　extrinsic
　upper respiratory J30.9
　urticaria L50.0
　vaccine —see Allergy, serum
　wheat —see Allergy, food

Allescheriasis B48.2

Alligator skin disease Q80.9

Allocheiria, allochiria R20.8

Almeida's disease —see
　Paracoccidioidomycosis

Alopecia (hereditaria) (seborrheica)
　L65.9
　androgenic L64.9
　　drug-induced L64.0
　　specified NEC L64.8
　areata L63.9
　　ophiasis L63.2
　　specified NEC L63.8
　　totalis L63.0
　　universalis L63.1
　cicatricial L66.9
　　specified NEC L66.8
　circumscripta L63.9

Alopecia (continued)
　congenital, congenitalis Q84.0
　due to cytotoxic drugs NEC L65.8
　mucinosa L65.2
　postinfective NEC L65.8
　postpartum L65.0
　premature L64.8
　specific (syphilitic) A51.32
　specified NEC L65.8
　syphilitic (secondary) A51.32
　totalis (capitis) L63.0
　universalis (entire body) L63.1
　X-ray L58.1

Alpers' disease G31.81

Alpine sickness T70.29

Alport syndrome Q87.81

**ALTE (apparent life threatening
　event) in newborn and infant**
　R68.13

Alteration (of), **Altered**
　awareness
　　transient R40.4
　　unintended under general
　　　anesthesia, during procedure
　　　T88.53
　mental status R41.82
　pattern of family relationships
　　affecting child Z62.898
　sensation
　　following
　　　cerebrovascular disease I69.998
　　　　cerebral infarction I69.398
　　　　intracerebral hemorrhage
　　　　　I69.198
　　　　nontraumatic intracranial
　　　　　hemorrhage NEC I69.298
　　　　specified disease NEC
　　　　　I69.898
　　　　subarachnoid hemorrhage
　　　　　I69.098

Alternating —see condition

Altitude, high (effects) —see Effect,
　adverse, high altitude

Aluminosis (of lung) J63.0

Alveolitis
　allergic (extrinsic) —see
　　Pneumonitis, hypersensitivity
　due to
　　Aspergillus clavatus J67.4
　　Cryptostroma corticale J67.6
　fibrosing (cryptogenic) (idiopathic)
　　J84.112
　jaw M27.3
　sicca dolorosa M27.3

Alveolus, alveolar —see condition

Alymphocytosis D72.810
　thymic (with immunodeficiency)
　　D82.1

Alymphoplasia, thymic D82.1

Alzheimer's disease or sclerosis —
　see Disease, Alzheimer's

Amastia (with nipple present) Q83.8
　with absent nipple Q83.0

Amathophobia F40.228

Amaurosis (acquired) (congenital) —
　see also Blindness
　fugax G45.3
　hysterical F44.6
　Leber's congenital H35.50
　uremic —see Uremia

Amaurotic idiocy (infantile)
　(juvenile) (late) E75.4

Amaxophobia F40.248

Ambiguous genitalia Q56.4

Amblyopia (congenital) (ex anopsia)
　(partial) (suppression) H53.00-
　anisometropic —see Amblyopia,
　　refractive
　deprivation H53.01-
　hysterical F44.6
　nocturnal —see also Blindness, night
　　vitamin A deficiency E50.5
　refractive H53.02-
　strabismic H53.03-
　suspect H53.04-
　tobacco H53.8
　toxic NEC H53.8
　uremic —see Uremia

Ameba, amebic (histolytica) —see
　also Amebiasis
　abscess (liver) A06.4

Amebiasis A06.9
　with abscess —see Abscess, amebic
　acute A06.0
　chronic (intestine) A06.1
　　with abscess —see Abscess,
　　　amebic
　cutaneous A06.7
　cutis A06.7
　cystitis A06.81
　genitourinary tract NEC A06.82
　hepatic —see Abscess, liver, amebic
　intestine A06.0
　nondysenteric colitis A06.2
　skin A06.7
　specified site NEC A06.89

Ameboma (of intestine) A06.3

Amelia Q73.0
　lower limb —see Agenesis, leg
　upper limb —see Agenesis, arm

Ameloblastoma —see also Cyst,
　calcifying odontogenic
　long bones C40.9-
　　lower limb C40.2-
　　upper limb C40.0-
　malignant C41.1
　　jaw (bone) (lower) C41.1
　　upper C41.0
　tibial C40.2-

Amelogenesis imperfecta K00.5
　nonhereditaria (segmentalis) K00.4

Amenorrhea N91.2
　hyperhormonal E28.8
　primary N91.0
　secondary N91.1

Amentia —see Disability,intellectual
　Meynert's (nonalcoholic) F04

American
　leishmaniasis B55.2
　mountain tick fever A93.2

Ametropia —see Disorder, refraction

**AMH (asymptomatic microscopic
　hematuria)** R31.21

Amianthosis J61

Amimia R48.8

Amino-acid disorder E72.9
　anemia D53.0

Aminoacidopathy E72.9

Aminoaciduria E72.9

Amnes(t)ic syndrome
　(post-traumatic) F04
　induced by
　　alcohol F10.96
　　　with dependence F10.26
　　psychoactive NEC F19.96
　　　with
　　　　abuse F19.16
　　　　dependence F19.26
　　sedative F13.96
　　　with dependence F13.26

Amnesia R41.3
　anterograde R41.1
　auditory R48.8
　dissociative F44.0
　　with dissociative fugue F44.1
　hysterical F44.0
　postictal in epilepsy —see
　　Epilepsy
　psychogenic F44.0
　retrograde R41.2
　transient global G45.4

Amnion, amniotic —see condition

Amnionitis —see Pregnancy,
　complicated by

Amok F68.8

Amoral traits F60.89

**Amphetamine (or other stimulant)
　-induced**
　anxiety disorder F15.980
　bipolar and related disorder F15.94
　delirium F15.921
　depressive disorder F15.94
　obsessive-compulsive and related
　　disorder F15.988
　psychotic disorder F15.959
　sexual dysfunction F15.981
　sleep disorder F15.982
　stimulant withdrawal F15.23

Ampulla
　lower esophagus K22.89
　phrenic K22.89

Amputation —see also Absence, by
　site, acquired
　neuroma (postoperative)
　　(traumatic) —see Complications,
　　amputation stump, neuroma
　stump (surgical)
　　abnormal, painful, or with
　　　complication (late) —see
　　　Complications, amputation
　　　stump
　　healed or old NOS Z89.9
　traumatic (complete) (partial)
　　arm (upper) (complete) S48.91-
　　　at
　　　　elbow S58.01-
　　　　　partial S58.02-
　　　　shoulder joint (complete)
　　　　　S48.01-
　　　　　partial S48.02-
　　　between
　　　　elbow and wrist (complete)
　　　　　S58.11-
　　　　　partial S58.12-
　　　　shoulder and elbow
　　　　　(complete) S48.11-
　　　　　partial S48.12-
　　　partial S48.92-
　　breast (complete) S28.21-
　　　partial S28.22-
　　clitoris (complete) S38.211
　　　partial S38.212
　　ear (complete) S08.11-
　　　partial S08.12-
　　finger (complete)
　　　(metacarpophalangeal)
　　　S68.11-
　　　index S68.11-
　　　little S68.11-
　　　middle S68.11-
　　　partial S68.12-
　　　　index S68.12-
　　　　little S68.12-
　　　　middle S68.12-
　　　　ring S68.12-
　　　ring S68.11-
　　　thumb —see Amputation,
　　　　traumatic, thumb

Amputation (continued)
　traumatic (continued)
　　finger (continued)
　　　transphalangeal (complete)
　　　　S68.61-
　　　　　index S68.61-
　　　　　little S68.61-
　　　　　middle S68.61-
　　　　　partial S68.62-
　　　　　　index S68.62-
　　　　　　little S68.62-
　　　　　　middle S68.62-
　　　　　　ring S68.62-
　　　　　ring S68.61-
　　foot (complete) S98.91-
　　　at ankle level S98.01-
　　　　partial S98.02-
　　　midfoot S98.31-
　　　　partial S98.32-
　　　partial S98.92-
　　forearm (complete) S58.91-
　　　at elbow level (complete)
　　　　S58.01-
　　　　　partial S58.02-
　　　between elbow and wrist
　　　　(complete) S58.11-
　　　　　partial S58.12-
　　　partial S58.92-
　　genital organ(s) (external)
　　　female (complete) S38.211
　　　　partial S38.212
　　　male
　　　　penis (complete) S38.221
　　　　　partial S38.222
　　　　scrotum (complete) S38.231
　　　　　partial S38.232
　　　　testes (complete) S38.231
　　　　　partial S38.232
　　hand (complete) (wrist level)
　　　S68.41-
　　　finger(s) alone —see
　　　　Amputation, traumatic,
　　　　finger
　　　partial S68.42-
　　　thumb alone —see
　　　　Amputation, traumatic,
　　　　thumb
　　　transmetacarpal (complete)
　　　　S68.71-
　　　　partial S68.72-
　　head
　　　ear —see Amputation,
　　　　traumatic, ear
　　　nose (partial) S08.812
　　　　complete S08.811
　　　part S08.89
　　　　scalp S08.0
　　hip (and thigh) (complete)
　　　S78.91-
　　　at hip joint (complete) S78.01-
　　　　partial S78.02-
　　　between hip and knee
　　　　(complete) S78.11-
　　　　partial S78.12-
　　　partial S78.92-
　　labium (majus) (minus)
　　　(complete) S38.21-
　　　　partial S38.21-
　　leg (lower) S88.91-
　　　at knee level S88.01-
　　　　partial S88.02-
　　　between knee and ankle
　　　　S88.11-
　　　　partial S88.12-
　　　partial S88.92-
　　nose (partial) S08.812
　　　complete S08.811
　　penis (complete) S38.221
　　　partial S38.222
　　scrotum (complete) S38.231
　　　partial S38.232

Amputation (continued)
　traumatic (continued)
　　shoulder —see Amputation,
　　　traumatic, arm
　　　at shoulder joint —see
　　　　Amputation, traumatic, arm,
　　　　at shoulder joint
　　testes (complete) S38.231
　　　partial S38.232
　　thigh —see Amputation,
　　　traumatic, hip
　　thorax, part of S28.1
　　　breast —see Amputation,
　　　　traumatic, breast
　　thumb (complete)
　　　(metacarpophalangeal)
　　　S68.01-
　　　partial S68.02-
　　　transphalangeal (complete)
　　　　S68.51-
　　　　partial S68.52-
　　toe (lesser) S98.13-
　　　great S98.11-
　　　　partial S98.12-
　　　more than one S98.21-
　　　　partial S98.22-
　　　partial S98.14-
　　vulva (complete) S38.211
　　　partial S38.212

Amputee (bilateral) (old)
　Z89.9

Amsterdam dwarfism Q87.19

Amusia R48.8
　developmental F80.89

Amyelencephalus, amyelencephaly
　Q00.0

Amyelia Q06.0

Amygdalitis —see Tonsillitis

Amygdalolith J35.8

Amyloid heart (disease)
　E85.4 [I43]

Amyloidosis (generalized) (primary)
　E85.9
　with lung involvement
　　E85.4 [J99]
　familial E85.2
　genetic E85.2
　heart E85.4 [I43]
　hemodialysis-associated E85.3
　liver E85.4 [K77]
　light chain (AL) E85.81
　localized E85.4
　neuropathic heredofamilial
　　E85.1
　non-neuropathic heredofamilial
　　E85.0
　organ limited E85.4
　Portuguese E85.1
　pulmonary E85.4 [J99]
　secondary systemic E85.3
　senile systemic (SSA) E85.82
　skin (lichen) (macular)
　　E85.4 [L99]
　specified NEC E85.89
　subglottic E85.4 [J99]
　wild-type transthyretin-related
　　(ATTR) E85.82

Amylopectinosis (brancher enzyme
　deficiency) E74.03

Amylophagia —see Pica

Amyoplasia congenita Q79.8

Amyotonia M62.89
　congenita G70.2

**Amyotrophia, amyotrophy,
　amyotrophic** G71.8
　congenita Q79.8

**Amyotrophia, amyotrophy,
　amyotrophic** (continued)
　diabetic —see Diabetes,
　　amyotrophy
　lateral sclerosis G12.21
　neuralgic G54.5
　spinal progressive G12.25

Anacidity, gastric K31.83
　psychogenic F45.8

Anaerosis of newborn P28.89

Analbuminemia E88.09

Analgesia —see Anesthesia

Analphalipoproteinemia E78.6

Anaphylactic
　purpura D69.0
　shock or reaction —see Shock,
　　anaphylactic

Anaphylactoid shock or reaction
　—see Shock, anaphylactic

**Anaphylactoid syndrome of
　pregnancy** O88.01-

Anaphylaxis —see Shock,
　anaphylactic

Anaplasia cervix —see also
　Dysplasia, cervix N87.9

Anaplasmosis
　[A. phagocytophilum]
　(transfusion transmitted) A79.82
　human A77.49

Anarthria R47.1

Anasarca R60.1
　cardiac —see Failure, heart,
　　congestive
　lung J18.2
　newborn P83.2
　nutritional E43
　pulmonary J18.2
　renal N04.9

Anastomosis
　aneurysmal —see Aneurysm
　arteriovenous ruptured brain I60.8
　　intracerebral I61.8
　　intraparenchymal I61.8
　　intraventricular I61.5
　　subarachnoid I60.8
　intestinal K63.89
　　complicated NEC K91.89
　　　involving urinary tract
　　　　N99.89
　retinal and choroidal vessels
　　(congenital) Q14.8

Anatomical narrow angle
　H40.03-

Ancylostoma, ancylostomiasis
　(braziliense) (caninum)
　(ceylanicum) (duodenale) B76.0
　Necator americanus B76.1

Andersen's disease (glycogen
　storage) E74.09

Anderson-Fabry disease E75.21

Andes disease T70.29

Andrews' disease (bacterid)
　L08.89

Androblastoma
　benign
　　specified site —see Neoplasm,
　　　benign, by site
　　unspecified site
　　　female D27.9
　　　male D29.20
　malignant
　　specified site —see Neoplasm,
　　　malignant, by site

Androblastoma (continued)
　malignant (continued)
　　unspecified site
　　　female C56.9
　　　male C62.90
　specified site —see Neoplasm,
　　uncertain behavior, by site
　tubular
　　with lipid storage
　　　specified site —see Neoplasm,
　　　　benign, by site
　　　unspecified site
　　　　female D27.9
　　　　male D29.20
　　specified site —see Neoplasm,
　　　benign, by site
　　unspecified site
　　　female D27.9
　　　male D29.20
　unspecified site
　　female D39.10
　　male D40.10

Androgen insensitivity syndrome
　—see also Syndrome, androgen
　insensitivity E34.50

Androgen resistance syndrome
　—see also Syndrome, androgen
　insensitivity E34.50

Android pelvis Q74.2
　with disproportion (fetopelvic)
　　O33.3
　causing obstructed labor O65.3

Androphobia F40.290

Anectasis, pulmonary (newborn)
　—see Atelectasis

Anemia (essential) (general)
　(hemoglobin deficiency) (infantile)
　(primary) (profound) D64.9
　with (due to) (in)
　　disorder of
　　　anaerobic glycolysis D55.29
　　　pentose phosphate pathway
　　　　D55.1
　　koilonychia D50.9
　achlorhydric D50.8
　achrestic D53.1
　Addison (-Biermer) (pernicious)
　　D51.0
　agranulocytic —see
　　Agranulocytosis
　amino-acid-deficiency D53.0
　aplastic D61.9
　　congenital D61.09
　　drug-induced D61.1
　　due to
　　　drugs D61.1
　　　external agents NEC D61.2
　　　infection D61.2
　　　radiation D61.2
　　idiopathic D61.3
　　red cell (pure) D60.9
　　　chronic D60.0
　　　congenital D61.01
　　　specified type NEC D60.8
　　　transient D60.1
　　specified type NEC D61.89
　　toxic D61.2
　aregenerative
　　congenital D61.09
　asiderotic D50.9
　atypical (primary) D64.9
　Baghdad spring D55.0
　Balantidium coli A07.0
　Biermer's (pernicious) D51.0
　blood loss (chronic) D50.0
　　acute D62
　bothriocephalus B70.0 [D63.8]
　brickmaker's B76.9 [D63.8]

Anemia (continued)
  cerebral I67.89
  childhood D58.9
  chlorotic D50.8
  chronic
    blood loss D50.0
    hemolytic D58.9
      idiopathic D59.9
    simple D53.9
  chronica congenita aregenerativa D61.09
  combined system disease NEC D51.0 [G32.0]
    due to dietary vitamin B12 deficiency D51.3 [G32.0]
  complicating pregnancy, childbirth or puerperium —see Pregnancy, complicated by (management affected by), anemia
  congenital P61.4
    aplastic D61.09
    due to isoimmunization NOS P55.9
    dyserythropoietic, dyshematopoietic D64.4
    following fetal blood loss P61.3
    Heinz body D58.2
    hereditary hemolytic NOS D58.9
    pernicious D51.0
    spherocytic D58.0
  Cooley's (erythroblastic) D56.1
  cytogenic D51.0
  deficiency D53.9
    2, 3 diphosphoglycurate mutase D55.29
    2, 3 PG D55.29
    6 phosphogluconate dehydrogenase D55.1
    6-PGD D55.1
    amino-acid D53.0
    combined B12 and folate D53.1
    enzyme D55.9
      drug-induced (hemolytic) D59.2
      glucose-6-phosphate dehydrogenase (G6PD) D55.0
      glycolytic D55.29
      nucleotide metabolism D55.3
      related to hexose monophosphate (HMP) shunt pathway NEC D55.1
      specified type NEC D55.8
    erythrocytic glutathione D55.1
    folate D52.9
      dietary D52.0
      drug-induced D52.1
    folic acid D52.9
      dietary D52.0
      drug-induced D52.1
    G SH D55.1
    GGS-R D55.1
    glucose-6-phosphate dehydrogenase D55.0
    glutathione reductase D55.1
    glyceraldehyde phosphate dehydrogenase D55.29
    G6PD D55.0
    hexokinase D55.29
    iron D50.9
      secondary to blood loss (chronic) D50.0
    nutritional D53.9
      with
        poor iron absorption D50.8
        specified deficiency NEC D53.8
    phosphofructo-aldolase D55.29
    phosphoglycerate kinase D55.29
    PK D55.21
    protein D53.0

Anemia (continued)
  deficiency (continued)
    pyruvate kinase D55.21
    transcobalamin II D51.2
    triose-phosphate isomerase D55.29
    vitamin B12 NOS D51.9
      dietary D51.3
      due to
        intrinsic factor deficiency D51.0
        selective vitamin B12 malabsorption with proteinuria D51.1
      pernicious D51.0
      specified type NEC D51.8
  Diamond-Blackfan (congenital hypoplastic) D61.01
  dibothriocephalus B70.0 [D63.8]
  dimorphic D53.1
  diphasic D53.1
  Diphyllobothrium (Dibothriocephalus) B70.0 [D63.8]
  due to (in) (with)
    antineoplastic chemotherapy D64.81
    blood loss (chronic) D50.0
      acute D62
    chemotherapy, antineoplastic D64.81
    chronic disease classified elsewhere NEC D63.8
    chronic kidney disease D63.1
    deficiency
      amino-acid D53.0
      copper D53.8
      folate (folic acid) D52.9
        dietary D52.0
        drug-induced D52.1
      molybdenum D53.8
      protein D53.0
      zinc D53.8
    dietary vitamin B12 deficiency D51.3
    disorder of
      glutathione metabolism D55.1
      nucleotide metabolism D55.3
    drug —see Anemia, by type —see also Table of Drugs and Chemicals
    end stage renal disease D63.1
    enzyme disorder D55.9
    fetal blood loss P61.3
    fish tapeworm (D.latum) infestation B70.0 [D63.8]
    hemorrhage (chronic) D50.0
      acute D62
    impaired absorption D50.9
    loss of blood (chronic) D50.0
      acute D62
    myxedema E03.9 [D63.8]
    Necator americanus B76.1 [D63.8]
    prematurity P61.2
    selective vitamin B12 malabsorption with proteinuria D51.1
    transcobalamin II deficiency D51.2
  Dyke-Young type (secondary) (symptomatic) D59.19
  dyserythropoietic (congenital) D64.4
  dyshematopoietic (congenital) D64.4
  Egyptian B76.9 [D63.8]
  elliptocytosis —see Elliptocytosis
  enzyme-deficiency, drug-induced D59.2
  epidemic —see also Ancylostomiasis B76.9 [D63.8]

Anemia (continued)
  erythroblastic
    familial D56.1
    newborn (see also Disease, hemolytic) P55.9
    of childhood D56.1
  erythrocytic glutathione deficiency D55.1
  erythropoietin-resistant anemia (EPO resistant anemia) D63.1
  Faber's (achlorhydric anemia) D50.9
  factitious (self-induced blood letting) D50.0
  familial erythroblastic D56.1
  Fanconi's (congenital pancytopenia) D61.09
  favism D55.0
  fish tapeworm (D. latum) infestation B70.0 [D63.8]
  folate (folic acid) deficiency D52.9
  glucose-6-phosphate dehydrogenase (G6PD) deficiency D55.0
  glutathione-reductase deficiency D55.1
  goat's milk D52.0
  granulocytic —see Agranulocytosis
  Heinz body, congenital D58.2
  hemolytic D58.9
    acquired D59.9
      with hemoglobinuria NEC D59.6
      autoimmune NEC D59.19
      infectious D59.4
      specified type NEC D59.8
      toxic D59.4
    acute D59.9
      due to enzyme deficiency specified type NEC D55.8
      Lederer's D59.19
    autoimmune D59.10
      cold D59.12
      drug-induced D59.0
      mixed D59.13
      warm D59.11
    chronic D58.9
      idiopathic D59.9
    cold type (primary) (secondary) (symptomatic) D59.12
    congenital (spherocytic) —see Spherocytosis
    due to
      cardiac conditions D59.4
      drugs (nonautoimmune) D59.2
        autoimmune D59.0
      enzyme disorder D55.9
        drug-induced D59.2
      presence of shunt or other internal prosthetic device D59.4
    familial D58.9
    hereditary D58.9
      due to enzyme disorder D55.9
        specified type NEC D55.8
      specified type NEC D58.8
    idiopathic (chronic) D59.9
    mechanical D59.4
    microangiopathic D59.4
    mixed type (primary) (secondary) (symptomatic) D59.13
    nonautoimmune D59.4
      drug-induced D59.2
    nonspherocytic
      congenital or hereditary NEC D55.8
        glucose-6-phosphate dehydrogenase deficiency D55.0
        pyruvate kinase deficiency D55.21

Anemia (continued)
  hemolytic (continued)
    nonspherocytic (continued)
      congenital or hereditary (continued)
        type
          I D55.1
          II D55.29
      type
        I D55.1
        II D55.29
    primary
      autoimmune
        cold type D59.12
        mixed type D59.13
        warm type D59.11
    secondary D59.4
      autoimmune
        cold type D59.12
        mixed type D59.13
        warm type D59.11
    specified (hereditary) type NEC D58.8
    Stransky-Regala type (see also Hemoglobinopathy) D58.8
    symptomatic D59.4
      autoimmune
        cold type D59.12
        mixed type D59.13
        warm type D59.11
    toxic D59.4
    warm type (primary) (secondary) (symptomatic) D59.11
  hemorrhagic (chronic) D50.0
    acute D62
  Herrick's D57.1
  hexokinase deficiency D55.29
  hookworm B76.9 [D63.8]
  hypochromic (idiopathic) (microcytic) (normoblastic) D50.9
    due to blood loss (chronic) D50.0
      acute D62
    familial sex-linked D64.0
    pyridoxine-responsive D64.3
    sideroblastic, sex-linked D64.0
  hypoplasia, red blood cells D61.9
    congenital or familial D61.01
  hypoplastic (idiopathic) D61.9
    congenital or familial (of childhood) D61.01
  hypoproliferative (refractive) D61.9
  idiopathic D64.9
    aplastic D61.3
    hemolytic, chronic D59.9
  in (due to) (with)
    chronic kidney disease D63.1
    end stage renal disease D63.1
    failure, kidney (renal) D63.1
    neoplastic disease (see also Neoplasm) D63.0
  intertropical —see also Ancylostomiasis D63.8
  iron deficiency D50.9
    secondary to blood loss (chronic) D50.0
      acute D62
    specified type NEC D50.8
  Joseph-Diamond-Blackfan (congenital hypoplastic) D61.01
  Lederer's (hemolytic) D59.19
  leukoerythroblastic D61.82
  macrocytic D53.9
    nutritional D52.0
    tropical D52.8
  malarial (see also Malaria) B54 [D63.8]
  malignant (progressive) D51.0
  malnutrition D53.9
  marsh (see also Malaria) B54 [D63.8]

19

Anemia (continued)
　Mediterranean (with other hemoglobinopathy) D56.9
　megaloblastic D53.1
　　combined B12 and folate deficiency D53.1
　　hereditary D51.1
　　nutritional D52.0
　　orotic aciduria D53.0
　　refractory D53.1
　　specified type NEC D53.1
　megalocytic D53.1
　microcytic (hypochromic) D50.9
　　due to blood loss (chronic) D50.0
　　　acute D62
　　familial D56.8
　microdrepanocytosis D57.40
　microelliptopoikilocytic (Rietti-Greppi- Micheli) D56.9
　miner's B76.9 *[D63.8]*
　myelodysplastic D46.9
　myelofibrosis D75.81
　myelogenous D64.89
　myelopathic D64.89
　myelophthisic D61.82
　myeloproliferative D47.Z9
　newborn P61.4
　　due to
　　　ABO (antibodies, isoimmunization, maternal/ fetal incompatibility) P55.1
　　　Rh (antibodies, isoimmunization, maternal/ fetal incompatibility) P55.0
　　following fetal blood loss P61.3
　　posthemorrhagic (fetal) P61.3
　nonspherocytic hemolytic —*see* Anemia, hemolytic, nonspherocytic
　normocytic (infectional) D64.9
　　due to blood loss (chronic) D50.0
　　　acute D62
　　myelophthisic D61.82
　nutritional (deficiency) D53.9
　　with
　　　poor iron absorption D50.8
　　　specified deficiency NEC D53.8
　　megaloblastic D52.0
　of prematurity P61.2
　oroticaciduric (congenital) (hereditary) D53.0
　osteosclerotic D64.89
　ovalocytosis (hereditary) —*see* Elliptocytosis
　paludal (*see also* Malaria) B54 *[D63.8]*
　pernicious (congenital) (malignant) (progressive) D51.0
　pleochromic D64.89
　　of sprue D52.8
　posthemorrhagic (chronic) D50.0
　　acute D62
　　newborn P61.3
　postoperative (postprocedural)
　　due to (acute) blood loss D62
　　　chronic blood loss D50.0
　　specified NEC D64.89
　postpartum O90.81
　pressure D64.89
　progressive D64.9
　　malignant D51.0
　　pernicious D51.0
　protein-deficiency D53.0
　pseudoleukemica infantum D64.89
　pure red cell D60.9
　　congenital D61.01
　pyridoxine-responsive D64.3
　pyruvate kinase deficiency D55.21

Anemia (continued)
　refractory D46.4
　　with
　　　excess of blasts D46.20
　　　　1(RAEB 1) D46.21
　　　　2(RAEB 2) D46.22
　　　　in transformation (RAEB T) —*see* Leukemia, acute myeloblastic
　　　hemochromatosis D46.1
　　　sideroblasts (ring) (RARS) D46.1
　　megaloblastic D53.1
　　sideroblastic D46.1
　　sideropenic D50.9
　　without ring sideroblasts, so stated D46.0
　　without sideroblasts without excess of blasts D46.0
　Rietti-Greppi-Micheli D56.9
　scorbutic D53.2
　secondary to
　　blood loss (chronic) D50.0
　　　acute D62
　　hemorrhage (chronic) D50.0
　　　acute D62
　semiplastic D61.89
　sickle-cell —*see* Disease, sickle-cell
　sideroblastic D64.3
　　hereditary D64.0
　　hypochromic, sex-linked D64.0
　　pyridoxine-responsive NEC D64.3
　　refractory D46.1
　　secondary (due to)
　　　disease D64.1
　　　drugs and toxins D64.2
　　specified type NEC D64.3
　sideropenic (refractory) D50.9
　　due to blood loss (chronic) D50.0
　　　acute D62
　simple chronic D53.9
　specified type NEC D64.89
　spherocytic (hereditary) —*see* Spherocytosis
　splenic D64.89
　splenomegalic D64.89
　stomatocytosis D58.8
　syphilitic (acquired) (late) A52.79 *[D63.8]*
　target cell D64.89
　thalassemia D56.9
　thrombocytopenic —*see* Thrombocytopenia
　toxic D61.2
　tropical B76.9 *[D63.8]*
　　macrocytic D52.8
　tuberculous A18.89 *[D63.8]*
　vegan D51.3
　vitamin
　　B6-responsive D64.3
　　B12 deficiency (dietary)
　　　pernicious D51.0
　von Jaksch's D64.89
　Witts' (achlorhydric anemia) D50.8

Anemophobia F40.228

Anencephalus, anencephaly Q00.0

Anergasia —*see* Psychosis, organic

Anesthesia, anesthetic R20.0
　complication or reaction NEC (*see also* Complications, anesthesia) T88.59
　　due to
　　　correct substance properly administered —*see* Table of Drugs and Chemicals, by drug, adverse effect

Anesthesia, anesthetic (continued)
　complication or reaction (continued)
　　due to (continued)
　　　overdose or wrong substance given —*see* Table of Drugs and Chemicals, by drug, poisoning
　　unintended awareness under general anesthesia during procedure T88.53
　　personal history of Z92.84
　cornea H18.81-
　dissociative F44.6
　functional (hysterical) F44.6
　hyperesthetic, thalamic G89.0
　hysterical F44.6
　local skin lesion R20.0
　sexual (psychogenic) F52.1
　shock (due to) T88.2
　skin R20.0
　testicular N50.9

Anetoderma (maculosum) (of) L90.8
　Jadassohn-Pellizzari L90.2
　Schweniger-Buzzi L90.1

Aneurin deficiency E51.9

Aneurysm (anastomotic) (artery) (cirsoid) (diffuse) (false) (fusiform) (multiple) (saccular) I72.9
　abdominal (aorta) I71.40
　　infrarenal I71.43
　　　ruptured I71.33
　　juxtarenal I71.42
　　　ruptured I71.32
　　pararenal I71.41
　　　ruptured I71.31
　　ruptured I71.30
　　syphilitic A52.01
　aorta, aortic (nonsyphilitic) I71.9
　　abdominal I71.40
　　　dissecting - *see* Dissection, aorta, abdominal
　　　ruptured I71.30
　　arch I71.22
　　　ruptured I71.12
　　arteriosclerotic I71.9
　　　ruptured I71.8
　　ascending I71.21
　　　ruptured I71.11
　　congenital Q25.43
　　descending I71.9
　　　abdominal I71.40
　　　　ruptured I71.30
　　　ruptured I71.8
　　　thoracic I71.23
　　　　ruptured I71.13
　　dissecting - *see* Dissection, aorta
　　root Q25.43
　　ruptured I71.8
　　sinus, congenital Q25.43
　　syphilitic A52.01
　　thoracic I71.20
　　　ruptured I71.10
　　thoracoabdominal I71.60
　　　paravisceral I71.62
　　　　ruptured I71.52
　　　ruptured I71.50
　　　supraceliac I71.61
　　　　ruptured I71.51
　　thorax, thoracic I71.20
　　　arch I71.22
　　　　ruptured I71.12
　　　ascending I71.21
　　　　ruptured I71.11
　　　descending I71.23
　　　　ruptured I71.13
　　　ruptured I71.10
　　　arch I71.12
　　　　ascending I71.11
　　　　descending I71.13
　　　root Q25.43

Aneurysm (continued)
　aorta, aortic (continued)
　　transverse I71.22
　　　ruptured I71.12
　　valve (heart) (*see also* Endocarditis, aortic) I35.8
　arteriosclerotic I72.9
　　cerebral I67.1
　　　ruptured —*see* Hemorrhage, intracranial, subarachnoid
　arteriovenous (congenital) —*see also* Malformation, arteriovenous
　　acquired I77.0
　　brain I67.1
　　　ruptured —*see* Aneurysm, arteriovenous, brain, ruptured
　　coronary I25.41
　　pulmonary I28.0
　brain Q28.2
　　ruptured I60.8
　　intracerebral I61.8
　　intraparenchymal I61.8
　　intraventricular I61.5
　　subarachnoid I60.8
　peripheral —*see* Malformation, arteriovenous, peripheral
　precerebral vessels Q28.0
　specified site NEC —*see also* Malformation, arteriovenous
　　acquired I77.0
　basal —*see* Aneurysm, brain
　basilar (trunk) I72.5
　berry (congenital) (nonruptured) I67.1
　　ruptured I60.7
　brain I67.1
　　arteriosclerotic I67.1
　　　ruptured —*see* Hemorrhage, intracranial, subarachnoid
　　arteriovenous (congenital) (nonruptured) Q28.2
　　acquired I67.1
　　　ruptured —*see* Aneurysm, arteriovenous, brain, ruptured I60.8-
　　ruptured —*see* Aneurysm, arteriovenous, brain, ruptured I60.8-
　　berry (congenital) (nonruptured) I67.1
　　　ruptured (*see also* Hemorrhage, intracranial, subarachnoid) I60.7
　　congenital Q28.3
　　　ruptured I60.7
　　meninges I67.1
　　　ruptured I60.8
　　miliary (congenital) (nonruptured) I67.1
　　　ruptured (*see also* Hemorrhage, intracranial, subarachnoid) I60.7
　　mycotic I67.1
　　　with endocarditis —*see also* Endocarditis
　　ruptured —*see* Hemorrhage, intracranial, subarachnoid
　　syphilitic (hemorrhage) A52.05
　cardiac (false) (*see also* Aneurysm, heart) I25.3
　carotid artery (common) (external) I72.0
　　internal (intracranial) I67.1
　　　extracranial portion I72.0
　　ruptured into brain I60.0-
　　syphilitic A52.09
　　　intracranial A52.05
　cavernous sinus I67.1
　　arteriovenous (congenital) (nonruptured) Q28.3
　　ruptured I60.8

Aneurysm (continued)
  celiac I72.8
  central nervous system, syphilitic A52.05
  cerebral —see Aneurysm, brain
  chest —see Aneurysm, thorax
  circle of Willis I67.1
    congenital Q28.3
      ruptured I60.6
    ruptured I60.6
  common iliac artery I72.3
  congenital (peripheral) Q27.8
    aorta (root) (sinus) Q25.43
    brain Q28.3
      ruptured I60.7
    coronary Q24.5
    digestive system Q27.8
    lower limb Q27.8
    pulmonary Q25.79
    retina Q14.1
    specified site NEC Q27.8
    upper limb Q27.8
  conjunctiva —see Abnormality, conjunctiva, vascular
  conus arteriosus —see Aneurysm, heart
  coronary (arteriosclerotic) (artery) I25.41
    arteriovenous, congenital Q24.5
    congenital Q24.5
    ruptured —see Infarct, myocardium
    syphilitic A52.06
    vein I25.89
  cylindroid (aorta) I71.9
    ruptured I71.8
    syphilitic A52.01
  ductus arteriosus Q25.0
  endocardial, infective (any valve) I33.0
  femoral (artery) (ruptured) I72.4
  gastroduodenal I72.8
  gastroepiploic I72.8
  heart (wall) (chronic or with a stated duration of over 4 weeks) I25.3
    valve —see Endocarditis
  hepatic I72.8
  iliac (common) (artery) (ruptured) I72.3
  infective I72.9
    endocardial (any valve) I33.0
  innominate (nonsyphilitic) I72.8
    syphilitic A52.09
  interauricular septum —see Aneurysm, heart
  interventricular septum —see Aneurysm, heart
  intrathoracic (nonsyphilitic) (see also Aneurysm, aorta, thorax) I71.20
    ruptured (see also Aneurysm, aorta, thorax, ruptured) I71.10
    syphilitic A52.01
  lower limb I72.4
  lung (pulmonary artery) I28.1
  mediastinal (nonsyphilitic) I72.8
    syphilitic A52.09
  miliary (congenital) I67.1
    ruptured —see Hemorrhage, intracerebral, subarachnoid, intracranial
  mitral (heart) (valve) I34.89
  mural —see Aneurysm, heart
  mycotic I72.9
    endocardial (any valve) I33.0
    ruptured, brain —see Hemorrhage, intracerebral, subarachnoid
  myocardium —see Aneurysm, heart
  neck I72.0
  pancreaticoduodenal I72.8
  patent ductus arteriosus Q25.0
  peripheral NEC I72.8
    congenital Q27.8
      digestive system Q27.8

Aneurysm (continued)
  peripheral NEC (continued)
    congenital (continued)
      lower limb Q27.8
      specified site NEC Q27.8
      upper limb Q27.8
  popliteal (artery) (ruptured) I72.4
  precerebral
    congenital (nonruptured) Q28.1
    specified site, NEC I72.5
  pulmonary I28.1
    arteriovenous Q25.72
      acquired I28.0
    syphilitic A52.09
    valve (heart) —see Endocarditis, pulmonary
  racemose (peripheral) I72.9
    congenital —see Aneurysm, congenital
  radial I72.1
  Rasmussen NEC A15.0
  renal (artery) I72.2
  retina —see also Disorder, retina, microaneurysms
    congenital Q14.1
    diabetic —see E08-E13 with .3-
  sinus of Valsalva Q25.43
  specified NEC I72.8
  spinal (cord) I72.8
    syphilitic (hemorrhage) A52.09
  splenic I72.8
  subclavian (artery) (ruptured) I72.8
    syphilitic A52.09
  superior mesenteric I72.8
  syphilitic (aorta) A52.01
    central nervous system A52.05
    congenital (late) A50.54 [I79.0]
    spine, spinal A52.09
  thoracoabdominal (aorta) I71.60
    ruptured I71.50
    syphilitic A52.01
  thorax, thoracic (aorta) (arch) (nonsyphilitic) —see Aneurysm, aorta, thorax
    ruptured —see Aneurysm, aorta, thorax, ruptured
    syphilitic A52.01
  traumatic (complication) (early), specified site —see Injury, blood vessel
  tricuspid (heart) (valve) I07.8
  ulnar I72.1
  upper limb (ruptured) I72.1
  valve, valvular —see Endocarditis
  venous (see also Varix) I86.8
    congenital Q27.8
      digestive system Q27.8
      lower limb Q27.8
      specified site NEC Q27.8
      upper limb Q27.8
  ventricle —see Aneurysm, heart
  vertebral artery I72.6
  visceral NEC I72.8

Angelman syndrome Q93.51

Anger R45.4

Angiectasis, angiectopia I99.8

Angiitis I77.6
  allergic granulomatous M30.1
  hypersensitivity M31.0
  necrotizing M31.9
    specified NEC M31.8
  nervous system, granulomatous I67.7

Angina (attack) (cardiac) (chest) (heart) (pectoris) (syndrome) (vasomotor) I20.9

Angina (continued)
  with
    atherosclerotic heart disease —see Arteriosclerosis, coronary (artery),
    coronary microvascular disease I20.81
    coronary microvascular dysfunction I20.81
    documented spasm I20.1
  abdominal K55.1
  accelerated —see Angina, unstable
  agranulocytic —see Agranulocytosis
  angiospastic —see Angina, with documented spasm
  aphthous B08.5
  crescendo —see Angina, unstable
  croupous J05.0
  cruris I73.9
  de novo effort —see Angina, unstable
  diphtheritic, membranous A36.0
  equivalent I20.89
  exudative, chronic J37.0
  following acute myocardial infarction I23.7
  gangrenous diphtheritic A36.0
  intestinal K55.1
  Ludovici K12.2
  Ludwig's K12.2
  malignant diphtheritic A36.0
  membranous J05.0
    diphtheritic A36.0
    Vincent's A69.1
  mesenteric K55.1
  monocytic —see Mononucleosis, infectious
  of effort —see Angina, specified NEC
  phlegmonous J36
    diphtheritic A36.0
  post-infarctional I23.7
  pre-infarctional —see Angina, unstable
  Prinzmetal —see Angina, with documented spasm
  progressive —see Angina, unstable
  pseudomembranous A69.1
  pultaceous, diphtheritic A36.0
  refractory I20.2
  spasm-induced —see Angina, with documented spasm
  specified NEC I20.89
  stable I20.89
  stenocardia —see Angina, specified NEC
  stridulous, diphtheritic A36.2
  tonsil J36
  trachealis J05.0
  unstable I20.0
  variant —see Angina, with documented spasm
  Vincent's A69.1
  worsening effort —see Angina, unstable

Angioblastoma —see Neoplasm, connective tissue, uncertain behavior

Angiocholecystitis —see Cholecystitis, acute

Angiocholitis —see also Cholecystitis, acute K83.09

Angiodysgenesis spinalis G95.19

Angiodysplasia (cecum) (colon) K55.20
  with bleeding K55.21
  duodenum (and stomach) K31.819
    with bleeding K31.811
  stomach (and duodenum) K31.819
    with bleeding K31.811

Angioedema (allergic) (any site) (with urticaria) T78.3
  episodic, with eosinophilia D72.118
  hereditary D84.1

Angioendothelioma —see Neoplasm, uncertain behavior, by site
  benign D18.00
    intra-abdominal D18.03
    intracranial D18.02
    skin D18.01
    specified site NEC D18.09
  bone —see Neoplasm, bone, malignant
  Ewing's —see Neoplasm, bone, malignant

Angioendotheliomatosis C85.8-

Angiofibroma —see also Neoplasm, benign, by site
  juvenile
    specified site —see Neoplasm, benign, by site
    unspecified site D10.6

Angiohemophilia (A) (B) —see Disease, von Willebrand

Angioid streaks (choroid) (macula) (retina) H35.33

Angiokeratoma —see Neoplasm, skin, benign
  corporis diffusum E75.21

Angioleiomyoma —see Neoplasm, connective tissue, benign

Angiolipoma —see also Lipoma
  infiltrating —see Lipoma

Angioma —see also Hemangioma, by site
  capillary I78.1
  hemorrhagicum hereditaria I78.0
  intra-abdominal D18.03
  intracranial D18.02
  malignant —see Neoplasm, connective tissue, malignant
  plexiform D18.00
    intra-abdominal D18.03
    intracranial D18.02
    skin D18.01
    specified site NEC D18.09
  senile I78.1
  serpiginosum L81.7
  skin D18.01
  specified site NEC D18.09
  spider I78.1
  stellate I78.1
  venous Q28.3

Angiomatosis Q82.8
  bacillary A79.89
  encephalotrigeminal Q85.89
  hemorrhagic familial I78.0
  hereditary familial I78.0
  liver K76.4

Angiomyolipoma —see Lipoma

Angiomyoliposarcoma —see Neoplasm, connective tissue, malignant

Angiomyoma —see Neoplasm, connective tissue, benign

Angiomyosarcoma —see Neoplasm, connective tissue, malignant

Angiomyxoma —see Neoplasm, connective tissue, uncertain behavior

Angioneurosis F45.8

Angioneurotic edema (allergic) (any site) (with urticaria) T78.3
  hereditary D84.1

21

Angiopathia, angiopathy I99.9
- cerebral I67.9
  - amyloid E85.4 [I68.0]
- diabetic (peripheral) —see Diabetes, angiopathy
- peripheral I73.9
  - diabetic —see Diabetes, angiopathy
  - specified type NEC I73.89
- retinae syphilitica A52.05
- retinalis (juvenilis)
  - diabetic —see Diabetes, retinopathy
  - proliferative —see Retinopathy, proliferative

Angiosarcoma —see also Neoplasm, connective tissue, malignant
- liver C22.3

Angiosclerosis —see Arteriosclerosis

Angiospasm (peripheral) (traumatic) (vessel) (see also Vasospasm) I73.9
- brachial plexus G54.0
- cerebral G45.9
- cervical plexus G54.2
- nerve
  - arm —see Mononeuropathy, upper limb
    - axillary G54.0
    - median —see Lesion, nerve, median
    - ulnar —see Lesion, nerve, ulnar
  - axillary G54.0
  - leg —see Mononeuropathy, lower limb
  - median —see Lesion, nerve, median
  - plantar —see Lesion, nerve, plantar
  - ulnar —see Lesion, nerve, ulnar

Angiospastic disease or edema I73.9

Angiostrongyliasis
- due to
  - Parastrongylus
    - cantonensis B83.2
    - costaricensis B81.3
- intestinal B81.3

Anguillulosis —see Strongyloidiasis

Angulation
- cecum —see Obstruction, intestine
- coccyx (acquired) (see also subcategory) M43.8
  - congenital NEC Q76.49
- femur (acquired) —see also Deformity, limb, specified type NEC, thigh
  - congenital Q74.2
- intestine (large) (small) —see Obstruction, intestine
- sacrum (acquired) (see also subcategory) M43.8
  - congenital NEC Q76.49
- sigmoid (flexure) —see Obstruction, intestine
- spine —see Dorsopathy, deforming, specified NEC
- tibia (acquired) —see also Deformity, limb, specified type NEC, lower leg
  - congenital Q74.2
- ureter N13.5
  - with infection N13.6
- wrist (acquired) —see also Deformity, limb, specified type NEC, forearm
  - congenital Q74.0

Angulus infectiosus (lips) K13.0

Anhedonia R45.84
- sexual F52.0

Anhidrosis L74.4

Anhydration E86.0

Anhydremia E86.0

Anidrosis L74.4

Aniridia (congenital) Q13.1

Anisakiasis (infection) (infestation) B81.0

Anisakis larvae infestation B81.0

Aniseikonia H52.32

Anisocoria (pupil) H57.02
- congenital Q13.2

Anisocytosis R71.8

Anisometropia (congenital) H52.31

Ankle —see condition

Ankyloblepharon (eyelid) (acquired)
—see also Blepharophimosis
- filiforme (adnatum) (congenital) Q10.3
- total Q10.3

Ankyloglossia Q38.1

Ankylosis (fibrous) (osseous) (joint) M24.60
- ankle M24.67-
- arthrodesis status Z98.1
- cricoarytenoid (cartilage) (joint) (larynx) J38.7
- dental K03.5
- ear ossicles H74.31-
- elbow M24.62-
- foot M24.67-
- hand M24.64-
- hip M24.65-
- incostapedial joint (infectional) —see Ankylosis, ear ossicles
- jaw (temporomandibular) M26.61-
- knee M24.66-
- lumbosacral (joint) M43.27
- postoperative (status) Z98.1
- produced by surgical fusion, status Z98.1
- sacro-iliac (joint) M43.28
- shoulder M24.61-
- specified site NEC M24.69
- spine (joint) —see also Fusion, spine
  - spondylitic —see Spondylitis, ankylosing
- surgical Z98.1
- temporomandibular M26.61-
- tooth, teeth (hard tissues) K03.5
- wrist M24.63-

Ankylostoma —see Ancylostoma

Ankylostomiasis —see Ancylostomiasis

Ankylurethria —see Stricture, urethra

Annular —see also condition
- detachment, cervix N88.8
- organ or site, congenital NEC —see Distortion
- pancreas (congenital) Q45.1

Anoctaminopathy G71.035

Anodontia (complete) (partial) (vera) K00.0
- acquired K08.10

Anomaly, anomalous (congenital) (unspecified type) Q89.9
- abdominal wall NEC Q79.59
- acoustic nerve Q07.8
- adrenal (gland) Q89.1
- Alder (-Reilly) (leukocyte granulation) D72.0
- alimentary tract Q45.9
  - upper Q40.9

Anomaly, anomalous (continued)
- alveolar M26.70
  - hyperplasia M26.79
    - mandibular M26.72
    - maxillary M26.71
  - hypoplasia M26.79
    - mandibular M26.74
    - maxillary M26.73
  - ridge (process) M26.79
  - specified NEC M26.79
- ankle (joint) Q74.2
- anus Q43.9
- aorta (arch) NEC Q25.40
  - coarctation (preductal) (postductal) Q25.1
- aortic cusp or valve Q23.9
- appendix Q43.8
- apple peel syndrome Q41.1
- aqueduct of Sylvius Q03.0
  - with spina bifida —see Spina bifida, with hydrocephalus
- arm Q74.0
- arteriovenous NEC
  - coronary Q24.5
  - gastrointestinal Q27.33
    - acquired —see Angiodysplasia
- artery (peripheral) Q27.9
  - basilar NEC Q28.1
  - cerebral Q28.3
  - coronary Q24.5
  - digestive system Q27.8
  - eye Q15.8
  - great Q25.9
    - specified NEC Q25.8
  - lower limb Q27.8
  - peripheral Q27.9
    - specified NEC Q27.8
  - pulmonary NEC Q25.79
  - renal Q27.2
  - retina Q14.1
  - specified site NEC Q27.8
  - subclavian Q27.8
    - origin Q25.48
  - umbilical Q27.0
  - upper limb Q27.8
  - vertebral NEC Q28.1
- aryteno-epiglottic folds Q31.8
- atrial
  - bands or folds Q20.8
  - septa Q21.10
- atrioventricular
  - excitation I45.6
  - septum Q21.0
- auditory canal Q17.8
- auricle
  - ear Q17.8
    - causing impairment of hearing Q16.9
  - heart Q20.8
- Axenfeld's Q15.0
- back Q89.9
- band
  - atrial Q20.8
  - heart Q24.8
  - ventricular Q24.8
- Bartholin's duct Q38.4
- biliary duct or passage Q44.5
- bladder Q64.70
  - absence Q64.5
  - diverticulum Q64.6
  - exstrophy Q64.10
    - cloacal Q64.12
    - extroversion Q64.19
    - specified type NEC Q64.19
    - supravesical fissure Q64.11
  - neck obstruction Q64.31
  - specified type NEC Q64.79
- bone Q79.9
  - arm Q74.0
  - face Q75.9
  - leg Q74.2

Anomaly, anomalous (continued)
- bone (continued)
  - pelvic girdle Q74.2
  - shoulder girdle Q74.0
  - skull Q75.9
    - with
      - anencephaly Q00.0
      - encephalocele —see Encephalocele
      - hydrocephalus Q03.9
        - with spina bifida —see Spina bifida, by site, with hydrocephalus
      - microcephaly Q02
- brain (multiple) Q04.9
  - vessel Q28.3
- breast Q83.9
- broad ligament Q50.6
- bronchus Q32.4
- bulbus cordis Q21.9
- bursa Q79.9
- canal of Nuck Q52.4
- canthus Q10.3
- capillary Q27.9
- cardiac Q24.9
  - chambers Q20.9
    - specified NEC Q20.8
  - septal closure Q21.9
    - specified NEC Q21.8
  - valve NEC Q24.8
    - pulmonary Q22.3
- cardiovascular system Q28.8
- carpus Q74.0
- caruncle, lacrimal Q10.6
- cascade stomach Q40.2
- cauda equina Q06.3
- cecum Q43.9
- cerebral Q04.9
  - vessels Q28.3
- cervix Q51.9
- Chédiak-Higashi (-Steinbrinck) (congenital gigantism of peroxidase granules) E70.330
- cheek Q18.9
- chest wall Q67.8
  - bones Q76.9
- chin Q18.9
- chordae tendineae Q24.8
- choroid Q14.3
  - plexus Q07.8
- chromosomes, chromosomal Q99.9
  - D (1) —see condition, chromosome 13
  - E (3) —see condition, chromosome 18
  - G —see condition, chromosome 21
  - sex
    - female phenotype Q97.8
    - gonadal dysgenesis (pure) Q99.1
    - Klinefelter's Q98.4
    - male phenotype Q98.9
    - Turner's Q96.9
  - specified NEC Q99.8
- cilia Q10.3
- circulatory system Q28.9
- clavicle Q74.0
- clitoris Q52.6
- coccyx Q76.49
- colon Q43.9
- common duct Q44.5
- communication
  - coronary artery Q24.5
  - left ventricle with right atrium Q21.0
- concha (ear) Q17.3
- connection
  - portal vein Q26.5
  - pulmonary venous Q26.4
    - partial Q26.3
    - total Q26.2
  - renal artery with kidney Q27.2

Anomaly, anomalous *(continued)*
- cornea (shape) Q13.4
- coronary artery or vein Q24.5
- cranium —*see* Anomaly, skull
- cricoid cartilage Q31.8
- cystic duct Q44.5
- dental
  - alveolar —*see* Anomaly, alveolar
  - arch relationship M26.20
    - specified NEC M26.29
- dentofacial M26.9
  - alveolar —*see* Anomaly, alveolar
  - dental arch relationship M26.20
    - specified NEC M26.29
  - functional M26.50
    - specified NEC M26.59
  - jaw-cranial base relationship M26.10
    - asymmetry M26.12
      - maxillary M26.11
    - specified type NEC M26.19
  - jaw size M26.00
    - macrogenia M26.05
    - mandibular
      - hyperplasia M26.03
      - hypoplasia M26.04
    - maxillary
      - hyperplasia M26.01
      - hypoplasia M26.02
    - microgenia M26.06
    - specified type NEC M26.09
  - malocclusion M26.4
    - dental arch relationship NEC M26.29
    - jaw-cranial base relationship —*see* Anomaly, dentofacial, jaw-cranial base relationship
    - jaw size —*see* Anomaly, dentofacial, jaw size
  - specified type NEC M26.89
  - temporomandibular joint M26.60 -
    - adhesions M26.61 -
    - ankylosis M26.61 -
    - arthralgia M26.62 -
    - articular disc M26.63 -
    - specified type NEC M26.69
  - tooth position, fully erupted M26.30
    - specified NEC M26.39
- dermatoglyphic Q82.8
- diaphragm (apertures) NEC Q79.1
- digestive organ(s) or tract Q45.9
  - lower Q43.9
  - upper Q40.9
- distance, interarch (excessive) (inadequate) M26.25
- distribution, coronary artery Q24.5
- ductus
  - arteriosus Q25.0
  - botalli Q25.0
- duodenum Q43.9
- dura (brain) Q04.9
  - spinal cord Q06.9
- ear (external) Q17.9
  - causing impairment of hearing Q16.9
  - inner Q16.5
  - middle (causing impairment of hearing) Q16.4
  - ossicles Q16.3
- Ebstein's (heart) (tricuspid valve) Q22.5
- ectodermal Q82.9
- Eisenmenger's (ventricular septal defect) Q21.8
- ejaculatory duct Q55.4
- elbow Q74.0
- endocrine gland NEC Q89.2
- epididymis Q55.4

Anomaly, anomalous *(continued)*
- epiglottis Q31.8
- esophagus Q39.9
- eustachian tube Q17.8
- eye Q15.9
  - anterior segment Q13.9
    - specified NEC Q13.89
  - posterior segment Q14.9
    - specified NEC Q14.8
  - ptosis (eyelid) Q10.0
  - specified NEC Q15.8
- eyebrow Q18.8
- eyelid Q10.3
  - ptosis Q10.0
- face Q18.9
  - bone(s) Q75.9
- fallopian tube Q50.6
- fascia Q79.9
- femur NEC Q74.2
- fibula NEC Q74.2
- finger Q74.0
- fixation, intestine Q43.3
- flexion (joint) NOS Q74.9
  - hip or thigh Q65.89
- foot NEC Q74.2
  - varus (congenital) Q66.3-
- foramen
  - Botalli Q21.12
  - ovale Q21.12
- forearm Q74.0
- forehead Q75.8
- form, teeth K00.2
- fovea centralis Q14.1
- frontal bone —*see* Anomaly, skull
- gallbladder (position) (shape) (size) Q44.1
- Gartner's duct Q52.4
- gastrointestinal tract Q45.9
- genitalia, genital organ(s) or system
  - female Q52.9
    - external Q52.70
    - internal NOS Q52.9
  - male Q55.9
    - hydrocele P83.5
    - specified NEC Q55.8
- genitourinary NEC
  - female Q52.9
  - male Q55.9
- Gerbode Q21.0
- glottis Q31.8
- granulation or granulocyte, genetic (constitutional) (leukocyte) D72.0
- gum Q38.6
- gyri Q07.9
- hair Q84.2
- hand Q74.0
- hard tissue formation in pulp K04.3
- head —*see* Anomaly, skull
- heart Q24.9
  - auricle Q20.8
  - bands or folds Q24.8
  - fibroelastosis cordis I42.4
  - obstructive NEC Q22.6
  - patent ductus arteriosus (Botalli) Q25.0
  - septum Q21.9
    - auricular Q21.19
    - interatrial Q21.19
    - interventricular Q21.0
      - with pulmonary stenosis or atresia, dextraposition of aorta and hypertrophy of right ventricle Q21.3
    - specified NEC Q21.8
    - ventricular Q21.0
      - with pulmonary stenosis or atresia, dextraposition of aorta and hypertrophy of right ventricle Q21.3

Anomaly, anomalous *(continued)*
- heart *(continued)*
  - tetralogy of Fallot Q21.3
  - valve NEC Q24.8
    - aortic
      - bicuspid valve Q23.1
      - insufficiency Q23.1
      - stenosis Q23.0
        - subaortic Q24.4
    - mitral
      - insufficiency Q23.3
      - stenosis Q23.2
    - pulmonary Q22.3
      - atresia Q22.0
      - insufficiency Q22.2
      - stenosis Q22.1
        - infundibular Q24.3
        - subvalvular Q24.3
    - tricuspid
      - atresia Q22.4
      - stenosis Q22.4
  - ventricle Q20.8
- heel NEC Q74.2
- Hegglin's D72.0
- hemianencephaly Q00.0
- hemicephaly Q00.0
- hemicrania Q00.0
- hepatic duct Q44.5
- hip NEC Q74.2
- hourglass stomach Q40.2
- humerus Q74.0
- hydatid of Morgagni
  - female Q50.5
  - male (epididymal) Q55.4
    - testicular Q55.29
- hymen Q52.4
- hypersegmentation of neutrophils, hereditary D72.0
- hypophyseal Q89.2
- ileocecal (coil) (valve) Q43.9
- ileum Q43.9
- ilium NEC Q74.2
- integument Q84.9
  - specified NEC Q84.8
- interarch distance (excessive) (inadequate) M26.25
- intervertebral cartilage or disc Q76.49
- intestine (large) (small) Q43.9
  - with anomalous adhesions, fixation or malrotation Q43.3
- iris Q13.2
- ischium NEC Q74.2
- jaw —*see* Anomaly, dentofacial
  - alveolar —*see* Anomaly, alveolar
- jaw-cranial base relationship —*see* Anomaly, dentofacial, jaw-cranial base relationship
- jejunum Q43.8
- joint Q74.9
  - specified NEC Q74.8
- Jordan's D72.0
- kidney(s) (calyx) (pelvis) Q63.9
  - artery Q27.2
  - specified NEC Q63.8
- Klippel-Feil (brevicollis) Q76.1
- knee Q74.1
- labium (majus) (minus) Q52.70
- labyrinth, membranous Q16.5
- lacrimal apparatus or duct Q10.6
- larynx, laryngeal (muscle) Q31.9
  - web (bed) Q31.0
- lens Q12.9
- leukocytes, genetic D72.0
  - granulation (constitutional) D72.0
- lid (fold) Q10.3
- ligament Q79.9
  - broad Q50.6
  - round Q52.8
- limb Q74.9

Anomaly, anomalous *(continued)*
- limb *(continued)*
  - lower NEC Q74.2
    - reduction deformity —*see* Defect, reduction, lower limb
  - upper Q74.0
- lip Q38.0
- liver Q44.70
  - duct Q44.5
- lower limb NEC Q74.2
- lumbosacral (joint) (region) Q76.49
  - kyphosis —*see* Kyphosis, congenital
  - lordosis —*see* Lordosis, congenital
- lung (fissure) (lobe) Q33.9
- mandible —*see* Anomaly, dentofacial
- maxilla —*see* Anomaly, dentofacial
- May (-Hegglin) D72.0
- meatus urinarius NEC Q64.79
- meningeal bands or folds Q07.9
  - constriction of Q07.8
  - spinal Q06.9
- meninges Q07.9
  - cerebral Q04.8
  - spinal Q06.9
- meningocele Q05.9
- mesentery Q45.9
- metacarpus Q74.0
- metatarsus NEC Q74.2
- middle ear Q16.4
  - ossicles Q16.3
- mitral (leaflets) (valve) Q23.9
  - insufficiency Q23.3
  - specified NEC Q23.8
  - stenosis Q23.2
- mouth Q38.6
- Müllerian —*see also* Anomaly, by site
  - uterus NEC Q51.818
- multiple NEC Q89.7
- muscle Q79.9
  - eyelid Q10.3
- musculoskeletal system, except limbs Q79.9
- myocardium Q24.8
- nail Q84.6
- narrowness, eyelid Q10.3
- nasal sinus (wall) Q30.8
- neck (any part) Q18.9
- nerve Q07.9
  - acoustic Q07.8
  - optic Q07.8
- nervous system (central) Q07.9
- nipple Q83.9
- nose, nasal (bones) (cartilage) (septum) (sinus) Q30.9
  - specified NEC Q30.8
- ocular muscle Q15.8
- omphalomesenteric duct Q43.0
- opening, pulmonary veins Q26.4
- optic
  - disc Q14.2
  - nerve Q07.8
- opticociliary vessels Q13.2
- orbit (eye) Q10.7
- organ Q89.9
  - of Corti Q16.5
- origin
  - artery
    - innominate Q25.48
    - pulmonary Q25.79
    - renal Q27.2
    - subclavian Q25.48
- osseous meatus (ear) Q16.1
- ovary Q50.39
- oviduct Q50.6
- palate (hard) (soft) NEC Q38.5
- pancreas or pancreatic duct Q45.3
- papillary muscles Q24.8

Anomaly, anomalous (continued)
  parathyroid gland Q89.2
  paraurethral ducts Q64.79
  parotid (gland) Q38.4
  patella Q74.1
  Pelger-Huët (hereditary hyposegmentation) D72.0
  pelvic girdle NEC Q74.2
  pelvis (bony) NEC Q74.2
    rachitic E64.3
  penis (glans) Q55.69
  pericardium Q24.8
  peripheral vascular system Q27.9
  Peter's Q13.4
  pharynx Q38.8
  pigmentation L81.9
    congenital Q82.8
  pituitary (gland) Q89.2
  pleural (folds) Q34.0
  portal vein Q26.5
    connection Q26.5
  position, tooth, teeth, fully erupted M26.30
    specified NEC M26.39
  precerebral vessel Q28.1
  prepuce Q55.69
  prostate Q55.4
  pulmonary Q33.9
    artery NEC Q25.79
    valve Q22.3
      atresia Q22.0
      insufficiency Q22.2
      specified type NEC Q22.3
      stenosis Q22.1
        infundibular Q24.3
        subvalvular Q24.3
    venous connection Q26.4
      partial Q26.3
      total Q26.2
  pupil Q13.2
    function H57.00
      anisocoria H57.02
      Argyll Robertson pupil H57.01
      miosis H57.03
      mydriasis H57.04
      specified type NEC H57.09
      tonic pupil H57.05-
  pylorus Q40.3
  radius Q74.0
  rectum Q43.9
  reduction (extremity) (limb)
    femur (longitudinal) —see Defect, reduction, lower limb, longitudinal, femur
    fibula (longitudinal) —see Defect, reduction, lower limb, longitudinal, fibula
    lower limb —see Defect, reduction, lower limb
    radius (longitudinal) —see Defect, reduction, upper limb, longitudinal, radius
    tibia (longitudinal) —see Defect, reduction, lower limb, longitudinal, tibia
    ulna (longitudinal) —see Defect, reduction, upper limb, longitudinal, ulna
    upper limb —see Defect, reduction, upper limb
  refraction —see Disorder, refraction
  renal Q63.9
    artery Q27.2
    pelvis Q63.9
      specified NEC Q63.8
  respiratory system Q34.9
    specified NEC Q34.8
  retina Q14.1
  rib Q76.6
    cervical Q76.5

Anomaly, anomalous (continued)
  Rieger's Q13.81
  rotation —see Malrotation
    hip or thigh Q65.89
  round ligament Q52.8
  sacroiliac (joint) NEC Q74.2
  sacrum NEC Q76.49
    kyphosis —see Kyphosis, congenital
    lordosis —see Lordosis, congenital
  saddle nose, syphilitic A50.57
  salivary duct or gland Q38.4
  scapula Q74.0
  scrotum —see Malformation, testis and scrotum
  sebaceous gland Q82.9
  seminal vesicles Q55.4
  sense organs NEC Q07.8
  sex chromosomes NEC —see also Anomaly, chromosomes
    female phenotype Q97.8
    male phenotype Q98.9
  shoulder (girdle) (joint) Q74.0
  sigmoid (flexure) Q43.9
  simian crease Q82.8
  sinus of Valsalva Q25.49
  skeleton generalized Q78.9
  skin (appendage) Q82.9
  skull Q75.9
    with
      anencephaly Q00.0
      encephalocele —see Encephalocele
      hydrocephalus Q03.9
        with spina bifida —see Spina bifida, by site, with hydrocephalus
      microcephaly Q02
  specified organ or site NEC Q89.8
  spermatic cord Q55.4
  spine, spinal NEC Q76.49
    column NEC Q76.49
      kyphosis —see Kyphosis, congenital
      lordosis —see Lordosis, congenital
    cord Q06.9
    nerve root Q07.8
  spleen Q89.09
    agenesis Q89.01
  stenonian duct Q38.4
  sternum NEC Q76.7
  stomach Q40.3
  submaxillary gland Q38.4
  tarsus NEC Q74.2
  tendon Q79.9
  testis —see Malformation, testis and scrotum
  thigh NEC Q74.2
  thorax (wall) Q67.8
    bony Q76.9
  throat Q38.8
  thumb Q74.0
  thymus gland Q89.2
  thyroid (gland) Q89.2
    cartilage Q31.8
  tibia NEC Q74.2
    saber A50.56
  toe Q74.2
  tongue Q38.3
  tooth, teeth K00.9
    eruption K00.6
    position, fully erupted M26.30
    spacing, fully erupted M26.30
  trachea (cartilage) Q32.1
  tragus Q17.9
  tricuspid (leaflet) (valve) Q22.9
    atresia or stenosis Q22.4
    Ebstein's Q22.5

Anomaly, anomalous (continued)
  Uhl's (hypoplasia of myocardium, right ventricle) Q24.8
  ulna Q74.0
  umbilical artery Q27.0
  union
    cricoid cartilage and thyroid cartilage Q31.8
    thyroid cartilage and hyoid bone Q31.8
    trachea with larynx Q31.8
  upper limb Q74.0
  urachus Q64.4
  ureter Q62.8
    obstructive NEC Q62.39
      cecoureterocele Q62.32
      orthotopic ureterocele Q62.31
  urethra Q64.70
    absence Q64.5
    double Q64.74
    fistula to rectum Q64.73
    obstructive Q64.39
      stricture Q64.32
    prolapse Q64.71
    specified type NEC Q64.79
  urinary tract Q64.9
  uterus Q51.9
    with only one functioning horn Q51.4
  uvula Q38.5
  vagina Q52.4
  valleculae Q31.8
  valve (heart) NEC Q24.8
    coronary sinus Q24.5
    inferior vena cava Q24.8
    pulmonary Q22.3
    sinus coronario Q24.5
    venae cavae inferioris Q24.8
  vas deferens Q55.4
  vascular Q27.9
    brain Q28.3
    ring Q25.45
  vein(s) (peripheral) Q27.9
    brain Q28.3
    cerebral Q28.3
    coronary Q24.5
    developmental Q28.3
    great Q26.9
      specified NEC Q26.8
  vena cava (inferior) (superior) Q26.9
  venous —see Anomaly, vein(s)
  venous return Q26.8
  ventricular
    bands or folds Q24.8
    septa Q21.0
  vertebra Q76.49
    kyphosis —see Kyphosis, congenital
    lordosis —see Lordosis, congenital
  vesicourethral orifice Q64.79
  vessel(s) Q27.9
    optic papilla Q14.2
    precerebral Q28.1
  vitelline duct Q43.0
  vitreous body or humor Q14.0
  vulva Q52.70
  wrist (joint) Q74.0

Anomia R48.8

Anonychia (congenital) Q84.3
  acquired L60.8

Anophthalmos, anophthalmus (congenital) (globe) Q11.1
  acquired Z90.01

Anopia, anopsia H53.46-
  quadrant H53.46-

Anorchia, anorchism, anorchidism Q55.0

Anorexia R63.0
  hysterical F44.89
  nervosa F50.00
    atypical F50.9
    binge-eating type F50.2
      with purging F50.02
    restricting type F50.01

Anorgasmy, psychogenic (female) F52.31
  male F52.32

Anosmia R43.0
  hysterical F44.6
  postinfectional J39.8

Anosognosia R41.89

Anosteoplasia Q78.9

Anovulatory cycle N97.0

Anoxemia R09.02
  newborn P84

Anoxia (pathological) R09.02
  altitude T70.29
  cerebral G93.1
    complicating
      anesthesia (general) (local) or other sedation T88.59
        in labor and delivery O74.3
        in pregnancy O29.21-
        postpartum, puerperal O89.2
      delivery (cesarean) (instrumental) O75.4
      during a procedure G97.81
    newborn P84
    resulting from a procedure G97.82
  due to
    drowning T75.1
    high altitude T70.29
  heart —see Insufficiency, coronary
  intrauterine P84
  myocardial —see Insufficiency, coronary
  newborn P84
  spinal cord G95.11
  systemic (by suffocation) (low content in atmosphere) —see Asphyxia, traumatic

Anteflexion —see Anteversion

Antenatal
  care (normal pregnancy) Z34.90
  screening (encounter for) of mother (see also Encounter, antenatal screening) Z36.9

Antepartum —see condition

Anterior —see condition

Antero-occlusion M26.220

Anteversion
  cervix —see Anteversion, uterus
  femur (neck), congenital Q65.89
  uterus, uterine (cervix) (postinfectional) (postpartal, old) N85.4
    congenital Q51.818
    in pregnancy or childbirth —see Pregnancy, complicated by

Anthophobia F40.228

Anthracosilicosis J60

Anthracosis (lung) (occupational) J60
  lingua K14.3

Anthrax A22.9
  with pneumonia A22.1
  cerebral A22.8
  colitis A22.2
  cutaneous A22.0
  gastrointestinal A22.2

Anthrax *(continued)*
　inhalation A22.1
　intestinal A22.2
　meningitis A22.8
　pulmonary A22.1
　respiratory A22.1
　sepsis A22.7
　specified manifestation NEC A22.8
Anthropoid pelvis Q74.2
　with disproportion (fetopelvic) O33.0
Anthropophobia F40.10
　generalized F40.11
Antibodies, maternal (blood group) —*see* Isoimmunization, affecting management of pregnancy
　anti-D —*see* Isoimmunization, affecting management of pregnancy, Rh
　newborn P55.0
Antibody
　anticardiolipin R76.0
　　with
　　　hemorrhagic disorder D68.312
　　　hypercoagulable state D68.61
　antiphosphatidylglycerol R76.0
　　with
　　　hemorrhagic disorder D68.312
　　　hypercoagulable state D68.61
　antiphosphatidylinositol R76.0
　　with
　　　hemorrhagic disorder D68.312
　　　hypercoagulable state D68.61
　antiphosphatidylserine R76.0
　　with
　　　hemorrhagic disorder D68.312
　　　hypercoagulable state D68.61
　antiphospholipid R76.0
　　with
　　　hemorrhagic disorder D68.312
　　　hypercoagulable state D68.61
Anticardiolipin syndrome D68.61
Anticoagulant, circulating (intrinsic) (*see also* Disorder, hemorrhagic) D68.318
　drug-induced (extrinsic) (*see also* Disorder, hemorrhagic) D68.32
　iatrogenic D68.32
Antidiuretic hormone syndrome E22.2
Antimonial cholera —*see* Poisoning, antimony
Antiphospholipid
　antibody
　　with hemorrhagic disorder D68.312
　　syndrome D68.61
Antisocial personality F60.2
Antithrombinemia —*see* Circulating anticoagulants
Antithromboplastinemia D68.318
Antithromboplastinogenemia D68.318
Antitoxin complication or reaction —*see* Complications, vaccination
Antlophobia F40.228
Antritis J32.0
　maxilla J32.0
　　acute J01.00
　　　recurrent J01.01
　stomach K29.50
　　with bleeding K29.51
Antrum, antral —*see* condition
Anuria R34
　calculous (impacted) (recurrent) (*see also* Calculus, urinary) N20.9

Anuria *(continued)*
　following
　　abortion —*see* Abortion by type complicated by, renal failure
　　ectopic or molar pregnancy O08.4
　newborn P96.0
　postprocedural N99.0
　postrenal N13.8
　puerperal O90.49
　traumatic (following crushing) T79.5
Anus, anal —*see* condition
Anusitis K62.89
Anxiety F41.9
　depression F41.8
　episodic paroxysmal F41.0
　generalized F41.1
　hysteria F41.8
　neurosis F41.1
　panic type F41.0
　reaction F41.1
　separation, abnormal (of childhood) F93.0
　specified NEC F41.8
　state F41.1
Aorta, aortic —*see* condition
Aortectasia —*see* Ectasia, aorta
　with aneurysm —*see* Aneurysm, aorta
Aortitis (nonsyphilitic) (calcific) I77.6
　arteriosclerotic I70.0
　Doehle-Heller A52.02
　luetic A52.02
　rheumatic —*see* Endocarditis, acute, rheumatic
　specific (syphilitic) A52.02
　syphilitic A52.02
　　congenital A50.54 *[I79.1]*
Apathetic thyroid storm —*see* Thyrotoxicosis
Apathy R45.3
Apeirophobia F40.228
Apepsia K30
　psychogenic F45.8
Aperistalsis, esophagus K22.0
Apertognathia M26.29
Apert's syndrome Q87.0
Aphagia R13.0
　psychogenic F50.9
Aphakia (acquired) (postoperative) H27.0-
　congenital Q12.3
Aphasia (amnestic) (global) (nominal) (semantic) (syntactic) R47.01
　acquired, with epilepsy (Landau-Kleffner syndrome) —*see* Epilepsy, specified NEC
　auditory (developmental) F80.2
　developmental (receptive type) F80.2
　　expressive type F80.1
　　Wernicke's F80.2
　following
　　cerebrovascular disease I69.920
　　　cerebral infarction I69.320
　　　intracerebral hemorrhage I69.120
　　　nontraumatic intracranial hemorrhage NEC I69.220
　　　specified disease NEC I69.820
　　　subarachnoid hemorrhage I69.020
　primary progressive (*see also* Dementia, in, diseases specified elsewhere) G31.01 *[F02.80]*
　　with behavioral disturbance (*see also* Dementia, in, diseases specified elsewhere) G31.01 *[F02.81-]*

Aphasia *(continued)*
　progressive isolated (*see also* Dementia, in, diseases specified elsewhere) G31.01 *[F02.80]*
　　with behavioral disturbance (*see also* Dementia, in, diseases specified elsewhere) G31.01 *[F02.81-]*
　sensory F80.2
　syphilis, tertiary A52.19
　Wernicke's (developmental) F80.2
Aphonia (organic) R49.1
　hysterical F44.4
　psychogenic F44.4
Aphthae, aphthous —*see also* condition
　Bednar's K12.0
　cachectic K14.0
　epizootic B08.8
　fever B08.8
　oral (recurrent) K12.0
　stomatitis (major) (minor) K12.0
　thrush B37.0
　ulcer (oral) (recurrent) K12.0
　　genital organ(s) NEC
　　　female N76.6
　　　male N50.89
　　larynx J38.7
Apical —*see* condition
Apiphobia F40.218
Aplasia —*see also* Agenesis
　abdominal muscle syndrome Q79.4
　alveolar process (acquired) —*see* Anomaly, alveolar
　　congenital Q38.6
　aorta (congenital) Q25.41
　axialis extracorticalis (congenita) E75.29
　bone marrow (myeloid) D61.9
　　congenital D61.01
　brain Q00.0
　　part of Q04.3
　bronchus Q32.4
　cementum K00.4
　cerebellum Q04.3
　cervix (congenital) Q51.5
　congenital pure red cell D61.01
　corpus callosum Q04.0
　cutis congenita Q84.8
　erythrocyte congenital D61.01
　extracortical axial E75.29
　eye Q11.1
　fovea centralis (congenital) Q14.1
　gallbladder, congenital Q44.0
　iris Q13.1
　labyrinth, membranous Q16.5
　limb (congenital) Q73.8
　　lower —*see* Defect, reduction, lower limb
　　upper —*see* Agenesis, arm
　lung, congenital (bilateral) (unilateral) Q33.3
　pancreas Q45.0
　parathyroid-thymic D82.1
　Pelizaeus-Merzbacher E75.27
　penis Q55.5
　prostate Q55.4
　red cell (with thymoma) D60.9
　　acquired D60.9
　　　due to drugs D60.9
　　adult D60.9
　　chronic D60.0
　　congenital D61.01
　　constitutional D61.01
　　due to drugs D60.9
　　hereditary D61.01
　　of infants D61.01
　　primary D61.01
　　pure D61.01
　　　due to drugs D60.9

Aplasia *(continued)*
　red cell *(continued)*
　　specified type NEC D60.8
　　transient D60.1
　round ligament Q52.8
　skin Q84.8
　spermatic cord Q55.4
　spleen Q89.01
　testicle Q55.0
　thymic, with immunodeficiency D82.1
　thyroid (congenital) (with myxedema) E03.1
　uterus Q51.0
　ventral horn cell Q06.1
Apnea, apneic (of) (spells) R06.81
　newborn P28.40
　　central P28.41
　　mixed P28.43
　　obstructive P28.42
　　sleep
　　　primary P28.30
　　　　central P28.31
　　　　mixed P28.33
　　　　obstructive P28.32
　　　　specified NEC P28.39
　　specified NEC P28.49
　prematurity P28.49
　sleep G47.30
　　central (primary) G47.31
　　　idiopathic G47.31
　　　in conditions classified elsewhere G47.37
　　obstructive (adult) (pediatric) G47.33
　　　hypopnea G47.33
　　primary central G47.31
　　specified NEC G47.39
Apneumatosis, newborn P28.0
Apocrine metaplasia (breast) —*see* Dysplasia, mammary, specified type NEC
Apophysitis (bone) —*see also* Osteochondropathy
　calcaneus M92.8
　juvenile M92.9
Apoplectiform convulsions (cerebral ischemia) I67.82
Apoplexia, apoplexy, apoplectic
　adrenal A39.1
　heart (auricle) (ventricle) —*see* Infarct, myocardium
　heat T67.01
　hemorrhagic (stroke) —*see* Hemorrhage, intracranial
　meninges, hemorrhagic —*see* Hemorrhage, intracranial, subarachnoid
　uremic N18.9 *[I68.8]*
Appearance
　bizarre R46.1
　specified NEC R46.89
　very low level of personal hygiene R46.0
Appendage
　epididymal (organ of Morgagni) Q55.4
　intestine (epiploic) Q43.8
　preauricular Q17.0
　testicular (organ of Morgagni) Q55.29
Appendicitis (pneumococcal) (retrocecal) K37
　with
　　gangrene K35.891
　　　with localized peritonitis K35.31
　　perforation NOS K35.32

25

Appendicitis (continued)
  with (continued)
    peritoneal abscess K35.33
    peritonitis NEC K35.33
      generalized K35.209
        with
          abscess K35.219
            with perforation or rupture K35.211
            following rupture or perforation of appendix NOS K35.211
            without perforation or rupture K35.210
          perforation or rupture K35.201
          following rupture or perforation of appendix NOS K35.201
          without rupture or perforation of appendix K35.200
    localized K35.30
      with
        gangrene K35.31
        perforation K35.32
          and abscess K35.33
        rupture (with localized peritonitis) K35.32
  acute (catarrhal) (fulminating) (obstructive) (retrocecal) (suppurative) K35.80
    with
      gangrene K35.891
      peritoneal abscess K35.33
      peritonitis NEC K35.33
        generalized K35.209
          with
            abscess K35.219
              with perforation or rupture K35.211
              following rupture or perforation of appendix NOS K35.211
              without perforation or rupture K35.210
            perforation or rupture K35.201
            following rupture or perforation of appendix NOS K35.201
            without rupture or perforation of appendix K35.200
      localized K35.30
        with
          gangrene K35.31
          perforation K35.32
            and abscess K35.33
    specified NEC K35.890
      with gangrene K35.891
      with localized peritonitis K35.31
  amebic A06.89
  chronic (recurrent) K36
  exacerbation —see Appendicitis, with, gangrene
  gangrenous —see Appendicitis, acute
  healed (obliterative) K36
  interval K36
  neurogenic K36
  obstructive K36
  recurrent K36
  relapsing K36

Appendicitis (continued)
  ruptured NOS (with localized peritonitis) K35.32
  subacute (adhesive) K36
  subsiding K36
  suppurative —see Appendicitis, acute
  tuberculous A18.32
Appendicopathia oxyurica B80
Appendix, appendicular —see also condition
  epididymis Q55.4
  Morgagni
    female Q50.5
    male (epididymal) Q55.4
    testicular Q55.29
  testis Q55.29
Appetite
  depraved —see Pica
  excessive R63.2
  lack or loss (see also Anorexia) R63.0
    nonorganic origin F50.89
    psychogenic F50.89
  perverted (hysterical) —see Pica
Apple peel syndrome Q41.1
Apprehension state F41.1
Apprehensiveness, abnormal F41.9
Approximal wear K03.0
Apraxia (classic) (ideational) (ideokinetic) (ideomotor) (motor) (verbal) R48.2
  following
    cerebrovascular disease I69.990
      cerebral infarction I69.390
      intracerebral hemorrhage I69.190
      nontraumatic intracranial hemorrhage NEC I69.290
      specified disease NEC I69.890
      subarachnoid hemorrhage I69.090
  oculomotor, congenital H51.8
Aptyalism K11.7
Apudoma —see Neoplasm, uncertain behavior, by site
Aqueous misdirection H40.83-
Arabicum elephantiasis —see Infestation, filarial
Arachnitis —see Meningitis
Arachnodactyly —see Syndrome, Marfan
Arachnoiditis (acute) (adhesive) (basal) (brain) (cerebrospinal) —see Meningitis
Arachnophobia F40.210
Arboencephalitis, Australian A83.4
Arborization block (heart) I45.5
ARC (AIDS-related complex) B20
Arch
  aortic Q25.49
  bovine Q25.49
Arches —see condition
Arcuate uterus Q51.810
Arcuatus uterus Q51.810
Arcus (cornea) senilis —see Degeneration, cornea, senile
Arc-welder's lung J63.4
Areflexia R29.2
Areola —see condition

Argentaffinoma —see also Neoplasm, uncertain behavior, by site
  malignant —see Neoplasm, malignant, by site
  syndrome E34.0
Argininemia E72.21
Arginosuccinic aciduria E72.22
Argyll Robertson phenomenon, pupil or syndrome (syphilitic) A52.19
  atypical H57.09
  nonsyphilitic H57.09
Argyria, argyriasis
  conjunctival H11.13-
  from drug or medicament —see Table of Drugs and Chemicals, by substance
Argyrosis, conjunctival H11.13-
Arhinencephaly Q04.1
Ariboflavinosis E53.0
Arm —see condition
Arnold-Chiari disease, obstruction or syndrome (type II) Q07.00
  with
    hydrocephalus Q07.02
      with spina bifida Q07.03
    spina bifida Q07.01
      with hydrocephalus Q07.03
  type III —see Encephalocele
  type IV Q04.8
Aromatic amino-acid metabolism disorder E70.9
  specified NEC E70.89
Arousals, confusional G47.51
Arrest, arrested
  cardiac I46.9
    complicating
      abortion —see Abortion, by type, complicated by, cardiac arrest
      anesthesia (general) (local) or other sedation —see Table of Drugs and Chemicals, by drug,
      in labor and delivery O74.2
      in pregnancy O29.11-
      postpartum, puerperal O89.1
      delivery (cesarean) (instrumental) O75.4
    due to
      cardiac condition I46.2
      specified condition NEC I46.8
    intraoperative I97.71-
    newborn P29.81
    personal history, successfully resuscitated Z86.74
    postprocedural I97.12-
    obstetric procedure O75.4
  cardiorespiratory —see Arrest, cardiac
  circulatory —see Arrest, cardiac
  deep transverse O64.0
  development or growth
    bone —see Disorder, bone, development or growth
    child R62.50
    tracheal rings Q32.1
  epiphyseal
    complete
      femur M89.15-
      humerus M89.12-
      tibia M89.16-
      ulna M89.13-
    forearm M89.13-
      specified NEC M89.13-
      ulna —see Arrest, epiphyseal, by type, ulna

Arrest, arrested (continued)
  epiphyseal (continued)
    lower leg M89.16-
      specified NEC M89.168
      tibia —see Arrest, epiphyseal, by type, tibia
    partial
      femur M89.15-
      humerus M89.12-
      tibia M89.16-
      ulna M89.13-
    specified NEC M89.18
  granulopoiesis —see Agranulocytosis
  growth plate —see Arrest, epiphyseal
  heart —see Arrest, cardiac
  legal, anxiety concerning Z65.3
  physeal —see Arrest, epiphyseal
  respiratory R09.2
    newborn P28.81
  sinus I45.5
  spermatogenesis (complete) —see Azoospermia
    incomplete —see Oligospermia
  transverse (deep) O64.0
Arrhenoblastoma
  benign
    specified site —see Neoplasm, benign, by site
    unspecified site
      female D27.9
      male D29.20
  malignant
    specified site —see Neoplasm, malignant, by site
    unspecified site
      female C56.9
      male C62.90
  specified site —see Neoplasm, uncertain behavior, by site
  unspecified site
    female D39.10
    male D40.10
Arrhythmia (auricle)(cardiac) (juvenile)(nodal) (reflex) (supraventricular)(transitory) (ventricle) I49.9
  block I45.9
  extrasystolic I49.49
  newborn
    bradycardia P29.12
    occurring before birth P03.819
      before onset of labor P03.810
      during labor P03.811
    tachycardia P29.11
  psychogenic F45.8
  sinus I49.8
  specified NEC I49.8
  vagal R55
  ventricular re-entry I47.0
Arrillaga-Ayerza syndrome (pulmonary sclerosis with pulmonary hypertension) I27.0
Arsenical pigmentation L81.8
  from drug or medicament —see Table of Drugs and Chemicals
Arsenism —see Poisoning, arsenic
Arterial —see condition
Arteriofibrosis — see Arteriosclerosis
Arteriolar sclerosis —see Arteriosclerosis
Arteriolith —see Arteriosclerosis
Arteriolitis I77.6
  necrotizing, kidney I77.5
  renal —see Hypertension, kidney

Arteriolosclerosis —*see* Arteriosclerosis

Arterionephrosclerosis —*see* Hypertension, kidney

Arteriopathy I77.9
- cerebral autosomal dominant, with subcortical infarcts and leukoencephalopathy (CADASIL) I67.850

Arteriosclerosis, arteriosclerotic (diffuse) (obliterans) (of) (senile) (with calcification) I70.90
- with
  - chronic limb-threatening ischemia —*see* Arteriosclerosis, with critical limb ischemia
  - critical limb ischemia
    - bypass graft I70.329
      - autologous vein graft I70.429
        - leg I70.429
          - with
            - gangrene (and intermittent claudication, rest pain, and ulcer) I70.469
            - rest pain (and intermittent claudication) I70.429
          - bilateral I70.423
            - with
              - gangrene (and intermittent claudication, rest pain, and ulcer) I70.463
              - rest pain (and intermittent claudication) I70.423
          - left I70.422
            - with
              - gangrene (and intermittent claudication, rest pain, and ulcer) I70.462
              - rest pain (and intermittent claudication) I70.422
              - ulceration (and intermittent claudication and rest pain) I70.449
                - ankle I70.443
                - calf I70.442
                - foot site NEC I70.445
                - heel I70.444
                - lower leg NEC I70.448
                - mid foot I70.444
                - thigh I70.441
          - right I70.421
            - with
              - gangrene (and intermittent claudication, rest pain, and ulcer) I70.461
              - rest pain (and intermittent claudication) I70.421

Arteriosclerosis, arteriosclerotic *(continued)*
- with *(continued)*
  - critical limb ischemia *(continued)*
    - bypass graft *(continued)*
      - autologous vein graft *(continued)*
        - leg *(continued)*
          - right *(continued)*
            - with *(continued)*
              - ulceration (and intermittent claudication and rest pain) I70.439
                - ankle I70.433
                - calf I70.432
                - foot site NEC I70.435
                - heel I70.434
                - lower leg NEC I70.438
                - mid foot I70.434
                - thigh I70.431
      - leg I70.329
        - with
          - gangrene (and intermittent claudication, rest pain, and ulcer) I70.369
          - rest pain (and intermittent claudication) I70.329
        - bilateral I70.323
          - with
            - gangrene (and intermittent claudication, rest pain, and ulcer) I70.363
            - rest pain (and intermittent claudication) I70.323
        - left I70.322
          - with
            - gangrene (and intermittent claudication, rest pain, and ulcer) I70.362
            - rest pain (and intermittent claudication) I70.322
            - ulceration (and intermittent claudication and rest pain) I70.349
              - ankle I70.343
              - calf I70.342
              - foot site NEC I70.345
              - heel I70.344
              - lower leg NEC I70.348
              - mid foot I70.344
              - thigh I70.341
        - right I70.321
          - with
            - gangrene (and intermittent claudication, rest pain, and ulcer) I70.361
            - rest pain (and intermittent claudication) I70.321

Arteriosclerosis, arteriosclerotic *(continued)*
- with *(continued)*
  - critical limb ischemia *(continued)*
    - bypass graft *(continued)*
      - leg *(continued)*
        - right I70.321
          - with *(continued)*
            - ulceration (and intermittent claudication and rest pain) I70.339
              - ankle I70.333
              - calf I70.332
              - foot site NEC I70.335
              - heel I70.334
              - lower leg NEC I70.338
              - mid foot I70.334
              - thigh I70.331
      - nonautologous biological graft I70.529
        - leg I70.529
          - with
            - gangrene (and intermittent claudication, rest pain, and ulcer) I70.569
            - rest pain (and intermittent claudication) I70.529
          - bilateral I70.523
            - with
              - gangrene (and intermittent claudication, rest pain, and ulcer) I70.563
              - rest pain (and intermittent claudication) I70.523
          - left I70.522
            - with
              - gangrene (and intermittent claudication, rest pain, and ulcer) I70.562
              - rest pain (and intermittent claudication) I70.522
              - ulceration (and intermittent claudication and rest pain) I70.549
                - ankle I70.543
                - calf I70.542
                - foot site NEC I70.545
                - heel I70.544
                - lower leg NEC I70.548
                - mid foot I70.544
                - thigh I70.541
          - right I70.521
            - with
              - gangrene (and intermittent claudication, rest pain, and ulcer) I70.561
              - rest pain (and intermittent claudication) I70.521

Arteriosclerosis, arteriosclerotic *(continued)*
- with *(continued)*
  - critical limb ischemia *(continued)*
    - bypass graft *(continued)*
      - nonbiological graft *(continued)*
        - leg *(continued)*
          - right *(continued)*
            - with *(continued)*
              - ulceration (and intermittent claudication and rest pain) I70.539
                - ankle I70.533
                - calf I70.532
                - foot site NEC I70.535
                - heel I70.534
                - lower leg NEC I70.538
                - mid foot I70.534
                - thigh I70.531
      - nonbiological graft I70.629
        - leg I70.629
          - with
            - gangrene (and intermittent claudication, rest pain, and ulcer) I70.669
            - rest pain (and intermittent claudication) I70.629
          - bilateral I70.623
            - with
              - gangrene (and intermittent claudication, rest pain, and ulcer) I70.663
              - rest pain (and intermittent claudication) I70.623
          - left I70.622
            - with
              - gangrene (and intermittent claudication, rest pain, and ulcer) I70.662
              - rest pain (and intermittent claudication) I70.622
              - ulceration (and intermittent claudication and rest pain) I70.649
                - ankle I70.643
                - calf I70.642
                - foot site NEC I70.645
                - heel I70.644
                - lower leg NEC I70.648
                - mid foot I70.644
                - thigh I70.641
          - right I70.621
            - with
              - gangrene (and intermittent claudication, rest pain, and ulcer) I70.661

Arteriosclerosis, arteriosclerotic
(continued)
  with *(continued)*
    critical limb ischemia *(continued)*
      bypass graft *(continued)*
        nonbiological graft *(continued)*
          leg *(continued)*
            right *(continued)*
              with *(continued)*
                rest pain (and intermittent claudication) I70.621
                ulceration (and intermittent claudication and rest pain) I70.639
                  ankle I70.633
                  calf I70.632
                  foot site NEC I70.635
                  heel I70.634
                  lower leg NEC I70.638
                  mid foot I70.634
                  thigh I70.631
        specified graft NEC I70.729
          leg I70.729
            with
              gangrene (and intermittent claudication, rest pain, and ulcer) I70.769
              rest pain (and intermittent claudication) I70.729
            bilateral I70.723
              with
                gangrene (and intermittent claudication, rest pain, and ulcer) I70.763
                rest pain (and intermittent claudication) I70.723
            left I70.722
              with
                gangrene (and intermittent claudication, rest pain, and ulcer) I70.762
                rest pain (and intermittent claudication) I70.722
                ulceration (and intermittent claudication and rest pain) I70.749
                  ankle I70.743
                  calf I70.742
                  foot site NEC I70.745
                  heel I70.744
                  lower leg NEC I70.748
                  mid foot I70.744
                  thigh I70.741

Arteriosclerosis, arteriosclerotic
(continued)
  with *(continued)*
    critical limb ischemia *(continued)*
      bypass graft *(continued)*
        specified graft *(continued)*
          leg *(continued)*
            right I70.721
              with
                gangrene (and intermittent claudication, rest pain, and ulcer) I70.761
                rest pain (and intermittent claudication) I70.721
                ulceration (and intermittent claudication and rest pain) I70.739
                  ankle I70.733
                  calf I70.732
                  foot site NEC I70.735
                  heel I70.734
                  lower leg NEC I70.738
                  mid foot I70.734
                  thigh I70.731
          leg I70.229
            with
              gangrene (and intermittent claudication, rest pain, and ulcer) I70.269
              rest pain (and intermittent claudication) I70.229
            bilateral I70.223
              with
                gangrene (and intermittent claudication, rest pain, and ulcer) I70.263
                rest pain (and intermittent claudication) I70.223
            left I70.222
              with
                gangrene (and intermittent claudication, rest pain, and ulcer) I70.262
                rest pain (and intermittent claudication) I70.222
                ulceration (and intermittent claudication and rest pain) I70.249
                  ankle I70.243
                  calf I70.242
                  foot site NEC I70.245
                  heel I70.244
                  lower leg NEC I70.248
                  mid foot I70.244
                  thigh I70.241

Arteriosclerosis, arteriosclerotic
(continued)
  with *(continued)*
    critical limb ischemia *(continued)*
      bypass graft *(continued)*
        leg *(continued)*
          right I70.221
            with
              gangrene (and intermittent claudication, rest pain, and ulcer) I70.261
              rest pain (and intermittent claudication) I70.221
              ulceration (and intermittent claudication and rest pain) I70.239
                ankle I70.233
                calf I70.232
                foot site NEC I70.235
                heel I70.234
                lower leg NEC I70.238
                mid foot I70.234
                thigh I70.231
    aorta I70.0
    arteries of extremities —*see* Arteriosclerosis, extremities
    with
      chronic limb-threatening ischemia —*see* Arteriosclerosis, with critical limb ischemia
      critical limb ischemia —*see* Arteriosclerosis, with clinical limb ischemia
    brain I67.2
      with infarction —*see* Occlusion, artery, brain or cerebral, with infarction
    bypass graft
      with
        chronic limb-threatening ischemia —*see* Arteriosclerosis, with critical limb ischemia
        critical limb ischemia —*see* Arteriosclerosis, with clinical limb ischemia
      coronary —*see* Arteriosclerosis, coronary, bypass graft
      extremities —*see* Arteriosclerosis, extremities, bypass graft
    cardiac —*see* Disease, heart, ischemic, atherosclerotic
    cardiopathy —*see* Disease, heart, ischemic, atherosclerotic
    cardiorenal —*see* Hypertension, cardiorenal
    cardiovascular —*see* Disease, heart, ischemic, atherosclerotic
    carotid (*see also* Occlusion, artery, carotid) I65.2-
    central nervous system I67.2
      with infarction —*see* Occlusion, artery, cerebral or precerebral, with infarction
    cerebral I67.2
      with infarction —*see* Occlusion, artery, brain or cerebral, with infarction
    cerebrovascular I67.2
      with infarction —*see* Occlusion, artery, brain or cerebral, with infarction

Arteriosclerosis, arteriosclerotic
(continued)
  coronary (artery) I25.10
    due to
      calcified coronary lesion (severely) I25.84
      lipid rich plaque I25.83
    bypass graft I25.810
      with
        angina pectoris I25.709
          with documented spasm I25.701
          refractory I25.702
          specified type NEC I25.708
          unstable I25.700
        ischemic chest pain I25.709
      autologous artery I25.810
        with
          angina pectoris I25.729
            with documented spasm I25.721
            refractory I25.722
            specified type I25.728
            unstable I25.720
          ischemic chest pain I25.729
      autologous vein I25.810
        with
          angina pectoris I25.719
            with documented spasm I25.711
            refractory I25.712
            specified type I25.718
            unstable I25.710
          ischemic chest pain I25.719
      nonautologous biological I25.810
        with
          angina pectoris I25.739
            with documented spasm I25.731
            refractory I25.732
            specified type I25.738
            unstable I25.730
          ischemic chest pain I25.739
      specified type NEC I25.810
        with
          angina pectoris I25.799
            with documented spasm I25.791
            refractory I25.792
            specified type I25.798
            unstable I25.790
          ischemic chest pain I25.799
    native vessel
      with
        angina pectoris I25.119
          with documented spasm I25.111
          refractory I25.112
          specified type NEC I25.118
          unstable I25.110
        ischemic chest pain I25.119
    transplanted heart I25.811
      bypass graft I25.812
        with
          angina pectoris I25.769
            with documented spasm I25.761
            refractory I25.762
            specified type I25.768
            unstable I25.760
          ischemic chest pain I25.769

Arteriosclerosis, arteriosclerotic
(continued)
  coronary *(continued)*
    transplanted heart *(continued)*
      native coronary artery I25.811
        with
          angina pectoris I25.759
            with documented
              spasm I25.751
            refractory I25.752
            specified type I25.758
            unstable I25.750
          ischemic chest pain
            I25.759
  extremities (native arteries)
    I70.209
    with
      chronic limb-threatening
        ischemia —*see*
        Arteriosclerosis, with
        critical limb ischemia
      critical limb ischemia —*see*
        Arteriosclerosis, with
        clinical limb ischemia
    bypass graft I70.309
      with
        chronic limb-threatening
          ischemia —*see*
          Arteriosclerosis, with
          critical limb ischemia
        critical limb ischemia —*see*
          Arteriosclerosis, with
          clinical limb ischemia
      autologous vein graft
        I70.409
        leg I70.409
          with
            gangrene (and
              intermittent
              claudication, rest
              pain and ulcer)
              I70.469
            intermittent
              claudication
              I70.419
            rest pain (and
              intermittent
              claudication)
              I70.429
        bilateral I70.403
          with
            gangrene (and
              intermittent
              claudication,
              rest
              pain and ulcer)
              I70.463
            intermittent
              claudication
              I70.413
            rest pain (and
              intermittent
              claudication)
              I70.423
          specified type NEC
            I70.493
        left I70.402
          with
            gangrene (and
              intermittent
              claudication, rest
              pain and ulcer)
              I70.462
            intermittent
              claudication
              I70.412
            rest pain (and
              intermittent
              claudication)
              I70.422

Arteriosclerosis, arteriosclerotic
(continued)
  extremities *(continued)*
    bypass graft *(continued)*
      autologous vein graft
        (continued)
        leg *(continued)*
          left *(continued)*
            with *(continued)*
              ulceration (and
                intermittent
                claudication and
                rest pain) I70.449
                ankle I70.443
                calf I70.442
                foot site NEC
                  I70.445
                heel I70.444
                lower leg NEC
                  I70.448
                midfoot I70.444
                thigh I70.441
            specified type NEC
              I70.492
          right I70.401
            with
              gangrene (and
                intermittent
                claudication, rest
                pain and ulcer)
                I70.461
              intermittent
                claudication
                I70.411
              rest pain (and
                intermittent
                claudication)
                I70.421
              ulceration (and
                intermittent
                claudication and
                rest pain) I70.439
                ankle I70.433
                calf I70.432
                foot site NEC
                  I70.435
                heel I70.434
                lower leg NEC
                  I70.438
                midfoot I70.434
                thigh I70.431
            specified type NEC
              I70.491
        specified type NEC
          I70.499
      specified NEC I70.408
        with
          gangrene (and
            intermittent
            claudication, rest pain
            and ulcer) I70.468
          intermittent
            claudication
            I70.418
          rest pain (and
            intermittent
            claudication)
            I70.428
          ulceration (and
            intermittent
            claudication and rest
            pain) I70.45
        specified type NEC
          I70.498
      leg I70.309
        with
          gangrene (and
            intermittent
            claudication, rest pain
            and ulcer) I70.369

Arteriosclerosis, arteriosclerotic
(continued)
  extremities *(continued)*
    bypass graft *(continued)*
      leg *(continued)*
        with *(continued)*
          intermittent claudication
            I70.319
          rest pain (and intermittent
            claudication) I70.329
        bilateral I70.303
          with
            gangrene (and
              intermittent
              claudication, rest pain
              and ulcer) I70.363
            intermittent
              claudication I70.313
            rest pain (and
              intermittent
              claudication)
              I70.323
          specified type NEC
            I70.393
        left I70.302
          with
            gangrene (and
              intermittent
              claudication, rest
              pain and ulcer)
              I70.362
            intermittent
              claudication I70.312
            rest pain (and
              intermittent
              claudication)
              I70.322
            ulceration (and
              intermittent
              claudication and rest
              pain) I70.349
              ankle I70.343
              calf I70.342
              foot site NEC
                I70.345
              heel I70.344
              lower leg NEC
                I70.348
              midfoot I70.344
              thigh I70.341
          specified type NEC
            I70.392
        right I70.301
          with
            gangrene (and
              intermittent
              claudication, rest
              pain and ulcer)
              I70.361
            intermittent
              claudication I70.311
            rest pain (and
              intermittent
              claudication)
              I70.321
            ulceration (and
              intermittent
              claudication and rest
              pain) I70.339
              ankle I70.333
              calf I70.332
              foot site NEC
                I70.335
              heel I70.334
              lower leg NEC
                I70.338
              midfoot I70.334
              thigh I70.331
          specified type NEC
            I70.391
        specified type NEC I70.399

Arteriosclerosis, arteriosclerotic
(continued)
  extremities *(continued)*
    bypass graft *(continued)*
      nonautologous biological graft
        I70.509
        leg I70.509
          with
            gangrene (and
              intermittent
              claudication, rest
              pain and ulcer)
              I70.569
            intermittent
              claudication
              I70.519
            rest pain (and
              intermittent
              claudication)
              I70.529
        bilateral I70.503
          with
            gangrene (and
              intermittent
              claudication, rest
              pain and ulcer)
              I70.563
            intermittent
              claudication
              I70.513
            rest pain (and
              intermittent
              claudication)
              I70.523
          specified type NEC
            I70.593
        left I70.502
          with
            gangrene (and
              intermittent
              claudication, rest
              pain and ulcer)
              I70.562
            intermittent
              claudication
              I70.512
            rest pain (and
              intermittent
              claudication)
              I70.522
            ulceration (and
              intermittent
              claudication and
              rest pain)
              I70.549
              ankle I70.543
              calf I70.542
              foot site NEC
                I70.545
              heel I70.544
              lower leg NEC
                I70.548
              midfoot
                I70.544
              thigh I70.541
          specified type NEC
            I70.592
        right I70.501
          with
            gangrene (and
              intermittent
              claudication, rest
              pain and ulcer)
              I70.561
            intermittent
              claudication
              I70.511
            rest pain (and
              intermittent
              claudication)
              I70.521

Arteriosclerosis, arteriosclerotic
(continued)
  extremities *(continued)*
    bypass graft *(continued)*
      nonbiological graft
        (continued)
        leg *(continued)*
          right *(continued)*
            with *(continued)*
              ulceration (and
                  intermittent
                  claudication and
                  rest pain) I70.539
                ankle I70.533
                calf I70.532
                foot site NEC
                  I70.535
                heel I70.534
                lower leg NEC
                  I70.538
                midfoot I70.534
                thigh I70.531
              specified type NEC
                I70.591
          specified type NEC
            I70.599
      specified NEC I70.508
        with
          gangrene (and
              intermittent
              claudication, rest pain
              and ulcer) I70.568
          intermittent
              claudication I70.518
          rest pain (and
              intermittent
              claudication)
              I70.528
          ulceration (and
              intermittent
              claudication and rest
              pain) I70.55
          specified type NEC
            I70.598
      nonbiological graft I70.609
        leg I70.609
          with
            gangrene (and
                intermittent
                claudication, rest pain
                and ulcer) I70.669
            intermittent
                claudication I70.619
            rest pain (and
                intermittent
                claudication)
                I70.629
            bilateral I70.603
              with
                gangrene (and
                    intermittent
                    claudication, rest
                    pain and ulcer)
                    I70.663
                intermittent
                    claudication
                    I70.613
                rest pain(and
                    intermittent
                    claudication)
                    I70.623
                specified type NEC
                  I70.693
            left I70.602
              with
                gangrene (and
                    intermittent
                    claudication, rest
                    pain and ulcer)
                    I70.662

Arteriosclerosis, arteriosclerotic
(continued)
  extremities *(continued)*
    bypass graft *(continued)*
      nonbiological graft *(continued)*
        leg *(continued)*
          left *(continued)*
            with *(continued)*
              intermittent
                  claudication
                  I70.612
              rest pain (and
                  intermittent
                  claudication)
                  I70.622
              ulceration (and
                  intermittent
                  claudication
                  and rest pain)
                  I70.649
                ankle I70.643
                calf I70.642
                foot site NEC
                  I70.645
                heel I70.644
                lower leg NEC
                  I70.648
                midfoot I70.644
                thigh I70.641
              specified type NEC
                I70.692
            right I70.601
              with
                gangrene (and
                    intermittent
                    claudication, rest
                    pain and ulcer)
                    I70.661
                intermittent
                    claudication
                    I70.611
                rest pain (and
                    intermittent
                    claudication)
                    I70.621
                ulceration (and
                    intermittent
                    claudication and
                    rest pain) I70.639
                  ankle I70.633
                  calf I70.632
                  foot site NEC
                    I70.635
                  heel I70.634
                  lower leg NEC
                    I70.638
                  midfoot I70.634
                  thigh I70.631
                specified type NEC
                  I70.691
            specified type NEC
              I70.699
        specified NEC I70.608
          with
            gangrene (and
                intermittent
                claudication, rest
                pain and ulcer)
                I70.668
            intermittent
                claudication I70.618
            rest pain (and
                intermittent
                claudication)
                I70.628
            ulceration (and
                intermittent
                claudication and rest
                pain) I70.65
            specified type NEC
              I70.698

Arteriosclerosis, arteriosclerotic
(continued)
  extremities *(continued)*
    bypass graft *(continued)*
      specified graft NEC
        I70.709
        leg I70.709
          with
            gangrene (and
                intermittent
                claudication, rest
                pain and ulcer)
                I70.769
            intermittent
                claudication
                I70.719
            rest pain (and
                intermittent
                claudication)
                I70.729
          bilateral I70.703
            with
              gangrene (and
                  intermittent
                  claudication, rest
                  pain and ulcer)
                  I70.763
              intermittent
                  claudication
                  I70.713
              rest pain (and
                  intermittent
                  claudication)
                  I70.723
              specified type NEC
                I70.793
          left I70.702
            with
              gangrene (and
                  intermittent
                  claudication, rest
                  pain and ulcer)
                  I70.762
              intermittent
                  claudication
                  I70.712
              rest pain (and
                  intermittent
                  claudication)
                  I70.722
              ulceration (and
                  intermittent
                  claudication
                  and rest pain)
                  I70.749
                ankle I70.743
                calf I70.742
                foot site NEC
                  I70.745
                heel I70.744
                lower leg NEC
                  I70.748
                midfoot I70.744
                thigh I70.741
              specified type NEC
                I70.792
          right I70.701
            with
              gangrene (and
                  intermittent
                  claudication, rest
                  pain and ulcer)
                  I70.761
              intermittent
                  claudication
                  I70.711
              rest pain (and
                  intermittent
                  claudication)
                  I70.721

Arteriosclerosis, arteriosclerotic
(continued)
  extremities *(continued)*
    bypass graft *(continued)*
      specified graft NEC
        (continued)
        leg *(continued)*
          right *(continued)*
            with *(continued)*
              ulceration (and
                  intermittent
                  claudication and
                  rest pain) I70.739
                ankle I70.733
                calf I70.732
                foot site NEC
                  I70.735
                heel I70.734
                lower leg NEC
                  I70.738
                midfoot I70.734
                thigh I70.731
              specified type NEC
                I70.791
          specified type NEC
            I70.799
      specified NEC I70.708
        with
          gangrene (and
              intermittent
              claudication, rest
              pain and ulcer)
              I70.768
          intermittent
              claudication
              I70.718
          rest pain (and
              intermittent
              claudication)
              I70.728
          ulceration (and
              intermittent
              claudication and rest
              pain) I70.75
          specified type NEC
            I70.798
    spcified NEC I70.308
      with
        gangrene (and
            intermittent
            claudication, rest pain
            and ulcer) I70.368
        intermittent claudication
            I70.318
        rest pain (and intermittent
            claudication) I70.328
        ulceration (and
            intermittent
            claudication and rest
            pain) I70.35
        specified type NEC I70.398
    leg I70.209
      with
        gangrene (and intermittent
            claudication, rest pain
            and ulcer) I70.269
        intermittent claudication
            I70.219
        rest pain (and intermittent
            claudication) I70.229
      bilateral I70.203
        with
          gangrene (and intermittent
              claudication, rest pain
              and ulcer) I70.263
          intermittent claudication
              I70.213
          rest pain (and intermittent
              claudication) I70.223
          specified type NEC
            I70.293

Arteriosclerosis, arteriosclerotic *(continued)*
  extremities *(continued)*
    leg *(continued)*
      left I70.202
        with
          gangrene (and intermittent claudication, rest pain and ulcer) I70.262
          intermittent claudication I70.212
          rest pain (and intermittent claudication) I70.222
          ulceration (and intermittent claudication and rest pain) I70.249
            ankle I70.243
            calf I70.242
            foot site NEC I70.245
            heel I70.244
            lower leg NEC I70.248
            midfoot I70.244
            thigh I70.241
          specified type NEC I70.292
      right I70.201
        with
          gangrene (and intermittent claudication, rest pain and ulcer) I70.261
          intermittent claudication I70.211
          rest pain (and intermittent claudication) I70.221
          ulceration (and intermittent claudication and rest pain) I70.239
            ankle I70.233
            calf I70.232
            foot site NEC I70.235
            heel I70.234
            lower leg NEC I70.238
            midfoot I70.234
            thigh I70.231
          specified type NEC I70.291
        specified type NEC I70.299
      specified site NEC I70.208
        with
          gangrene (and intermittent claudication, rest pain and ulcer) I70.268
          intermittent claudication I70.218
          rest pain (and intermittent claudication) I70.228
          ulceration (and intermittent claudication and rest pain) I70.25
          specified type NEC I70.298
  generalized I70.91
  heart (disease) —*see* Arteriosclerosis, coronary (artery)
  kidney —*see* Hypertension, kidney
  medial —*see* Arteriosclerosis, extremities
  mesenteric (artery) K55.1
  Mönckeberg's —*see* Arteriosclerosis, extremities
  myocarditis I51.4
  peripheral (of extremities) —*see* Arteriosclerosis, extremities
  pulmonary (idiopathic) I27.0
  renal (arterioles) —*see also* Hypertension, kidney
    artery I70.1
  retina (vascular) I70.8 *[H35.0]*-
  specified artery NEC I70.8
  spinal (cord) G95.19

Arteriosclerosis, arteriosclerotic *(continued)*
  vertebral (artery) I67.2
    with infarction —*see* Occlusion, artery, vertebral, with infarction

Arteriospasm I73.9

Arteriovenous —*see* condition

Arteritis I77.6
  allergic M31.0
  aorta (nonsyphilitic) I77.6
    syphilitic A52.02
  aortic arch M31.4
  brachiocephalic M31.4
  brain I67.7
    syphilitic A52.04
  cerebral I67.7
    in
      diseases classified elsewhere I68.2
      systemic lupus erythematosus M32.19
    listerial A32.89
    syphilitic A52.04
    tuberculous A18.89
  coronary (artery) I25.89
    rheumatic I01.8
      chronic I09.89
    syphilitic A52.06
  cranial (left) (right), giant cell M31.6
  deformans —*see* Arteriosclerosis
  giant cell NEC M31.6
    with polymyalgia rheumatica M31.5
  necrosing or necrotizing M31.9
    specified NEC M31.8
  nodosa M30.0
  obliterans —*see* Arteriosclerosis
  pulmonary I28.8
  rheumatic —*see* Fever, rheumatic
  senile —*see* Arteriosclerosis
  suppurative I77.2
  syphilitic (general) A52.09
    brain A52.04
    coronary A52.06
    spinal A52.09
  temporal, giant cell M31.6
  young female aortic arch syndrome M31.4

Artery, arterial —*see also* condition
  abscess I77.89
  single umbilical Q27.0

Arthralgia (allergic) —*see also* Pain, joint
  in caisson disease T70.3
  temporomandibular M26.62-

Arthritis, arthritic (acute) (chronic) (nonpyogenic) (subacute) M19.90
  allergic —*see* Arthritis, specified form NEC
  ankylosing (crippling) (spine) —*see also* Spondylitis, ankylosing
    sites other than spine —*see* Arthritis, specified form NEC
  atrophic —*see* Osteoarthritis
    spine —*see* Spondylitis, ankylosing
  back —*see* Spondylopathy, inflammatory
  blennorrhagic (gonococcal) A54.42
  Charcot's —*see* Arthropathy, neuropathic
    diabetic —*see* Diabetes, arthropathy, neuropathic
    syringomyelic G95.0
  chylous (filarial) (*see also* category M01) B74.9

Arthritis, arthritic *(continued)*
  climacteric (any site) NEC —*see* Arthritis, specified form NEC
  crystal (-induced) —*see* Arthritis, in, crystals
  deformans —*see* Osteoarthritis
  degenerative —*see* Osteoarthritis
  due to or associated with
    acromegaly E22.0
    brucellosis —*see* Brucellosis
    caisson disease T70.3
    diabetes —*see* Diabetes, arthropathy
    dracontiasis (*see also* category M01) B72
    enteritis NEC
      regional —*see* Enteritis, regional
    erysipelas (*see also* category M01) A46
    erythema
      epidemic A25.1
      nodosum L52
    filariasis NOS B74.9
    glanders A24.0
    helminthiasis (*see also* category M01) B83.9
    hemophilia D66 *[M36.2]*
    Henoch-(Schönlein) purpura D69.0 *[M36.4]*
    human parvovirus (*see also* category M01) B97.6
    infectious disease NEC M01
    leprosy (*see also* category M01) —*see also* Leprosy A30.9
    Lyme disease A69.23
    mycobacteria (*see also* category M01) A31.8
    parasitic disease NEC (*see also* category M01) B89
    paratyphoid fever (*see also* category M01) (*see also* Fever, paratyphoid) A01.4
    rat bite fever (*see also* category M01) A25.1
    regional enteritis —*see* Enteritis, regional
    respiratory disorder NOS J98.9
    serum sickness (*see also* Reaction, serum) T80.69
    syringomyelia G95.0
    typhoid fever A01.04
  epidemic erythema A25.1
  febrile —*see* Fever, rheumatic
  gonococcal A54.42
  gouty (acute) —*see* Gout
  in (due to)
    acromegaly (*see also* subcategory M14.8-) E22.0
    amyloidosis (*see also* subcategory M14.8-) E85.4
    bacterial disease (*see also* subcategory M01) A49.9
    Behçet's syndrome M35.2
    caisson disease (*see also* subcategory M14.8-) T70.3
    coliform bacilli (Escherichia coli) —*see* Arthritis, in, pyogenic organism NEC
    crystals M11.9
      dicalcium phosphate —*see* Arthritis, in, crystals, specified type NEC
      hydroxyapatite M11.0-
      pyrophosphate —*see* Arthritis, in, crystals, specified type NEC
      specified type NEC M11.80
        ankle M11.87-
        elbow M11.82-
        foot joint M11.87-

Arthritis, arthritic *(continued)*
  in *(continued)*
    crystals *(continued)*
      specified type *(continued)*
        hand joint M11.84-
        hip M11.85-
        knee M11.86-
        multiple sites M11.8-
        shoulder M11.81-
        vertebrae M11.88
        wrist M11.83-
    dermatoarthritis, lipoid E78.81
    dracontiasis (dracunculiasis) (*see also* category M01) B72
    endocrine disorder NEC (*see also* subcategory M14.8-) E34.9
    enteritis, infectious NEC (*see also* category M01) A09
      specified organism NEC (*see also* category M01) A08.8
    erythema
      multiforme (*see also* subcategory M14.8-) L51.9
      nodosum (*see also* subcategory M14.8-) L52
    facet joint (*see also* Spondylosis) M47.819
    gout —*see* Gout
    helminthiasis NEC (*see also* category M01) B83.9
    hemochromatosis (*see also* subcategory M14.8-) E83.118
    hemoglobinopathy NEC D58.2 *[M36.3]*
    hemophilia NEC D66 *[M36.2]*
    Hemophilus influenzae M00.8- *[B96.2]*
    Henoch (-Schönlein) purpura D69.0 *[M36.4]*
    hyperparathyroidism NEC (*see also* subcategory M14.8-) E21.3
    hypersensitivity reaction NEC T78.49 *[M36.4]*
    hypogammaglobulinemia (*see also* subcategory M14.8-) D80.1
    hypothyroidism NEC (*see also* subcategory M14.8-) E03.9
    infection —*see* Arthritis, pyogenic or pyemic
      spine —*see* Spondylopathy, infective
    infectious disease NEC M01
    leprosy (*see also* category M01) A30.9
    leukemia NEC C95.9- *[M36.1]*
    lipoid dermatoarthritis E78.81
    Lyme disease A69.23
    Mediterranean fever, familial (*see also* subcategory M14.8-) M04.1
    Meningococcus A39.83
    metabolic disorder NEC (*see also* subcategory M14.8-) E88.9
    multiple myelomatosis C90.0- *[M36.1]*
    mumps B26.85
    mycosis NEC (*see also* category M01) B49
    myelomatosis (multiple) C90.0- *[M36.1]*
    neurological disorder NEC G98.0
    ochronosis (*see also* subcategory M14.8-) E70.29
    O'nyong-nyong (*see also* category M01) A92.1
    parasitic disease NEC (*see also* category M01) B89

Arthritis, arthritic (continued)
  in (continued)
    paratyphoid fever (see also category M01) A01.4
    Pseudomonas —see Arthritis, pyogenic, bacterial NEC
    psoriasis L40.50
    pyogenic organism NEC —see Arthritis, pyogenic, bacterial NEC
    Reiter's disease —see Reiter's disease
    respiratory disorder NEC (see also subcategory M14.8-) J98.9
    reticulosis, malignant (see also subcategory M14.8-) C86.0
    rubella B06.82
    Salmonella (arizonae) (cholerae-suis) (enteritidis) (typhimurium) A02.23
    sarcoidosis D86.86
    specified bacteria NEC —see Arthritis, pyogenic, bacterial NEC
    sporotrichosis B42.82
    syringomyelia G95.0
    thalassemia NEC D56.9 [M36.3]
    tuberculosis —see Tuberculosis, arthritis
    typhoid fever A01.04
    urethritis, Reiter's —see Reiter's disease
    viral disease NEC (see also category M01) B34.9
  infectious or infective —see also Arthritis, pyogenic or pyemic
    spine —see Spondylopathy, infective
  juvenile M08.90
    with systemic onset —see Still's disease
    ankle M08.97-
    elbow M08.92-
    foot joint M08.97-
    hand joint M08.94-
    hip M08.95-
    knee M08.96-
    multiple site M08.99
    pauciarticular M08.40
      ankle M08.47-
      elbow M08.42-
      foot joint M08.47-
      hand joint M08.44-
      hip M08.45-
      knee M08.46-
      shoulder M08.41-
      specified site NEC M08.4A
      vertebrae M08.48
      wrist M08.43-
    psoriatic L40.54
    rheumatoid —see Arthritis, rheumatoid, juvenile
    shoulder M08.91-
    specified site NEC M08.9A
    specified type NEC M08.80
      ankle M08.87-
      elbow M08.82-
      foot joint M08.87-
      hand joint M08.84-
      hip M08.85-
      knee M08.86-
      multiple site M08.89
      shoulder M08.81-
      specified joint NEC M08.88
      vertebrae M08.88
      wrist M08.83-
    vertebra M08.98
    wrist M08.93-

Arthritis, arthritic (continued)
  meaning osteoarthritis —see Osteoarthritis
  meningococcal A39.83
  menopausal (any site) NEC —see Arthritis, specified form NEC
  mutilans (psoriatic) L40.52
  mycotic NEC (see also category M01) B49
  neuropathic (Charcot) —see Arthropathy, neuropathic
    diabetic —see Diabetes, arthropathy, neuropathic
    nonsyphilitic NEC G98.0
    syringomyelic G95.0
  ochronotic (see also subcategory M14.8-) E70.29
  palindromic (any site) —see Rheumatism, palindromic
  pneumococcal M00.10
    ankle M00.17-
    elbow M00.12-
    foot joint —see Arthritis, pneumococcal, ankle
    hand joint M00.14-
    hip M00.15-
    knee M00.16-
    multiple site M00.19
    shoulder M00.11-
    vertebra M00.18
    wrist M00.13-
  postdysenteric —see Arthropathy, postdysenteric
  postmeningococcal A39.84
  postrheumatic, chronic —see Arthropathy, postrheumatic, chronic
  primary progressive —see also Arthritis, specified form NEC
    spine —see Spondylitis, ankylosing
  psoriatic L40.50
  purulent (any site except spine) — see Arthritis, pyogenic or pyemic
    spine —see Spondylopathy, infective
  pyogenic or pyemic (any site except spine) M00.9
    bacterial NEC M00.80
      ankle M00.87-
      elbow M00.82-
      foot joint —see Arthritis, pyogenic, bacterial NEC, ankle
      hand joint M00.84-
      hip M00.85-
      knee M00.86-
      multiple site M00.89
      shoulder M00.81-
      vertebra M00.88
      wrist M00.83-
    pneumococcal —see Arthritis, pneumococcal
    spine —see Spondylopathy, infective
    staphylococcal —see Arthritis, staphylococcal
    streptococcal —see Arthritis, streptococcal NEC
    pneumococcal —see Arthritis, pneumococcal
  reactive —see Reiter's disease
  rheumatic —see also Arthritis, rheumatoid
    acute or subacute —see Fever, rheumatic
  rheumatoid M06.9
    with
      carditis —see Rheumatoid, carditis

Arthritis, arthritic (continued)
  rheumatoid (continued)
    with (continued)
      endocarditis —see Rheumatoid, carditis
      heart involvement NEC —see Rheumatoid, carditis
      lung involvement —see Rheumatoid, lung
      myocarditis —see Rheumatoid, carditis
      myopathy —see Rheumatoid, myopathy
      pericarditis —see Rheumatoid, carditis
      polyneuropathy —see Rheumatoid, polyneuropathy
      rheumatoid factor —see Arthritis, rheumatoid, seropositive
      splenoadenomegaly and leukopenia —see Felty's syndrome
      vasculitis —see Rheumatoid, vasculitis
      visceral involvement NEC —see Rheumatoid, arthritis, with involvement of organs NEC
    juvenile (with or without rheumatoid factor) M08.00
      with systemic onset —see Still's disease
      ankle M08.07-
      elbow M08.02-
      foot joint M08.07-
      hand joint M08.04-
      hip M08.05-
      knee M08.06-
      multiple site M08.09
      shoulder M08.01-
      specified site NEC M08.0A
      vertebra M08.08
      wrist M08.03-
    seronegative M06.00
      ankle M06.07-
      elbow M06.02-
      foot joint M06.07-
      hand joint M06.04-
      hip M06.05-
      knee M06.06-
      multiple site M06.09
      shoulder M06.01-
      specified site NEC M06.0A
      vertebra M06.08
      wrist M06.03-
    seropositive M05.9
      specified NEC M05.80
        ankle M05.87-
        elbow M05.82-
        foot joint M05.87-
        hand joint M05.84-
        hip M05.85-
        knee M05.86-
        multiple sites M05.89
        shoulder M05.81-
        specified site NEC M05.8A
        vertebra —see Spondylitis, ankylosing
        wrist M05.83-
      without organ involvement M05.70
        ankle M05.77-
        elbow M05.72-
        foot joint M05.77-
        hand joint M05.74-
        hip M05.75-
        knee M05.76-
        multiple sites M05.79
        shoulder M05.71-
        specified site NEC M05.7A

Arthritis, arthritic (continued)
  rheumatoid (continued)
    seropositive (continued)
      without organ involvement (continued)
        vertebra —see Spondylitis, ankylosing
        wrist M05.73-
    specified type NEC M06.80
      ankle M06.87-
      elbow M06.82-
      foot joint M06.87-
      hand joint M06.84-
      hip M06.85-
      knee M06.86-
      multiple site M06.89
      shoulder M06.81-
      specified site NEC M06.8A
      vertebra M06.88
      wrist M06.83-
    spine —see Spondylitis, ankylosing
  rubella B06.82
  scorbutic (see also subcategory M14.8-) E54
  senile or senescent —see Osteoarthritis
  septic (any site except spine) —see Arthritis, pyogenic or pyemic
    spine —see Spondylopathy, infective
  serum (nontherapeutic) (therapeutic) —see Arthropathy, postimmunization
  specified form NEC M13.80
    ankle M13.87-
    elbow M13.82-
    foot joint M13.87-
    hand joint M13.84-
    hip M13.85-
    knee M13.86-
    multiple site M13.89
    shoulder M13.81-
    specified joint NEC M13.88
    wrist M13.83-
  spine —see also Spondylosis
    infectious or infective NEC — see Spondylopathy, infective
    Marie-Strümpell —see Spondylitis, ankylosing
    pyogenic —see Spondylopathy, infective
    rheumatoid —see Spondylitis, ankylosing
    traumatic (old) —see Spondylopathy, traumatic
  tuberculous A18.01
  staphylococcal M00.00
    ankle M00.07-
    elbow M00.02-
    foot joint —see Arthritis, staphylococcal, ankle
    hand joint M00.04-
    hip M00.05-
    knee M00.06-
    multiple site M00.09
    shoulder M00.01-
    vertebra M00.08
    wrist M00.03-
  streptococcal NEC M00.20
    ankle M00.27-
    elbow M00.22-
    foot joint —see Arthritis, streptococcal, ankle
    hand joint M00.24-
    hip M00.25-
    knee M00.26-
    multiple site M00.29
    shoulder M00.21-
    vertebra M00.28
    wrist M00.23-

Arthritis, arthritic *(continued)*
   suppurative —*see* Arthritis, pyogenic or pyemic
   syphilitic (late) A52.16
      congenital A50.55 *[M12.80]*
   syphilitica deformans (Charcot) A52.16
   temporomandibular M26.64-
   toxic of menopause (any site) —*see* Arthritis, specified form NEC
   transient —*see* Arthropathy, specified form NEC
   traumatic (chronic) —*see* Arthropathy, traumatic
   tuberculous A18.02
      spine A18.01
   uratic —*see* Gout
   urethritica (Reiter's) —*see* Reiter's disease
   vertebral —*see* Spondylopathy, inflammatory
   villous (any site) —*see* Arthropathy, specified form NEC

Arthrocele —*see* Effusion, joint
Arthrodesis status Z98.1
Arthrodynia —*see also* Pain, joint
Arthrodysplasia Q74.9
Arthrofibrosis, joint —*see* Ankylosis
Arthrogryposis (congenital) Q68.8
   multiplex congenita Q74.3
Arthrokatadysis M24.7
Arthropathy —*see also* Arthritis M12.9
   Charcot's —*see* Arthropathy, neuropathic
      diabetic —*see* Diabetes, arthropathy, neuropathic
      syringomyelic G95.0
   cricoarytenoid J38.7
   crystal (-induced) —*see* Arthritis, in, crystals
   diabetic NEC —*see* Diabetes, arthropathy
   distal interphalangeal, psoriatic L40.51
   enteropathic M07.60
      ankle M07.67-
      elbow M07.62-
      foot joint M07.67-
      hand joint M07.64-
      hip M07.65-
      knee M07.66-
      multiple site M07.69
      shoulder M07.61-
      vertebra M07.68
      wrist M07.63-
   facet joint (*see* Spondylosis) M47.819
   following intestinal bypass M02.00
      ankle M02.07-
      elbow M02.02-
      foot joint M02.07-
      hand joint M02.04-
      hip M02.05-
      knee M02.06-
      multiple site M02.09
      shoulder M02.01-
      vertebra M02.08
      wrist M02.03-
   gouty —*see also* Gout
      in (due to)
         Lesch-Nyhan syndrome E79.1 *[M14.8-]*
         sickle-cell disorders D57- *[M14.8-]*

Arthropathy *(continued)*
   hemophilic NEC D66 *[M36.2]*
      in (due to)
         hyperparathyroidism NEC E21.3 *[M14.8-]*
         metabolic disease NOS E88.9 *[M14.8-]*
   in (due to)
      acromegaly E22.0 *[M14.8-]*
      amyloidosis E85.4 *[M14.8-]*
      blood disorder NOS D75.9 *[M36.3]*
      diabetes —*see* Diabetes, arthropathy
      endocrine disease NOS E34.9 *[M14.8-]*
      erythema
         multiforme L51.9 *[M14.8-]*
         nodosum L52 *[M14.8-]*
      hemochromatosis E83.118 *[M14.8-]*
      hemoglobinopathy NEC D58.2 *[M36.3]*
      hemophilia NEC D66 *[M36.2]*
      Henoch-Schönlein purpura D69.0 *[M36.4]*
      hyperthyroidism E05.90 *[M14.8-]*
      hypothyroidism E03.9 *[M14.8-]*
      infective endocarditis I33.0 *[M12.80]*
      leukemia NEC C95.9- *[M36.1]*
      malignant histiocytosis C96.A *[M36.1]*
      metabolic disease NOS E88.9 *[M14.8-]*
      multiple myeloma C90.0- *[M36.1]*
      neoplastic disease NOS (*see also* Neoplasm) D49.9 *[M36.1]*
      nutritional deficiency (*see also* subcategory M14.8-) E63.9
      psoriasis NOS L40.50
      sarcoidosis D86.86
      syphilis (late) A52.77
         congenital A50.55 *[M12.80]*
      thyrotoxicosis (*see also* subcategory M14.8-) E05.90
      ulcerative colitis K51.90 *[M07.60]*
      viral hepatitis (postinfectious) NEC B19.9 *[M12.80]*
      Whipple's disease (*see also* subcategory M14.8-) K90.81
   Jaccoud —*see* Arthropathy, postrheumatic, chronic
   juvenile —*see* Arthritis, juvenile
      psoriatic L40.54
   mutilans (psoriatic) L40.52
   neuropathic (Charcot) M14.60
      ankle M14.67-
      diabetic —*see* Diabetes, arthropathy, neuropathic
      elbow M14.62-
      foot joint M14.67-
      hand joint M14.64-
      hip M14.65-
      knee M14.66-
      multiple site M14.69
      nonsyphilitic NEC G98.0
      shoulder M14.61-
      syringomyelic G95.0
      vertebra M14.68
      wrist M14.63-
   osteopulmonary —*see* Osteoarthropathy, hypertrophic, specified NEC
   postdysenteric M02.10
      ankle M02.17-
      elbow M02.12-
      foot joint M02.17-
      hand joint M02.14-
      hip M02.15-
      knee M02.16-

Arthropathy *(continued)*
   postdysenteric *(continued)*
      multiple site M02.19
      shoulder M02.11-
      vertebra M02.18
      wrist M02.13-
   postimmunization M02.20
      ankle M02.27-
      elbow M02.22-
      foot joint M02.27-
      hand joint M02.24-
      hip M02.25-
      knee M02.26-
      multiple site M02.29
      shoulder M02.21-
      vertebra M02.28
      wrist M02.23-
   postinfectious NEC B99 *[M12.80]*
      in (due to)
         enteritis due to Yersinia enterocolitica A04.6 *[M12.80]*
         syphilis A52.77
         viral hepatitis NEC B19.9 *[M12.80]*
   postrheumatic, chronic (Jaccoud) M12.00
      ankle M12.07-
      elbow M12.02-
      foot joint M12.07-
      hand joint M12.04-
      hip M12.05-
      knee M12.06-
      multiple site M12.09
      shoulder M12.01-
      specified joint NEC M12.08
      vertebrae M12.08
      wrist M12.03-
   psoriatic NEC L40.59
      interphalangeal, distal L40.51
   reactive M02.9
      in (due to)
         infective endocarditis I33.0 *[M02.9]*
      specified type NEC M02.80
         ankle M02.87-
         elbow M02.82-
         foot joint M02.87-
         hand joint M02.84-
         hip M02.85-
         knee M02.86-
         multiple site M02.89
         shoulder M02.81-
         vertebra M02.88
         wrist M02.83-
   specified form NEC M12.80
      ankle M12.87-
      elbow M12.82-
      foot joint M12.87-
      hand joint M12.84-
      hip M12.85-
      knee M12.86-
      multiple site M12.89
      shoulder M12.81-
      specified joint NEC M12.88
      vertebrae M12.88
      wrist M12.83-
   syringomyelic G95.0
   tabes dorsalis A52.16
   tabetic A52.16
   temporomandibular joint M26.65-
   transient —*see* Arthropathy, specified form NEC
   traumatic M12.50
      ankle M12.57-
      elbow M12.52-
      foot joint M12.57-
      hand joint M12.54-
      hip M12.55-
      knee M12.56-
      multiple site M12.59
      shoulder M12.51-

Arthropathy *(continued)*
   traumatic *(continued)*
      specified joint NEC M12.58
      vertebrae M12.58
      wrist M12.53-

Arthropyosis —*see* Arthritis, pyogenic or pyemic
Arthrosis (deformans) (degenerative) (localized) —*see also* Osteoarthritis M19.90
   spine —*see* Spondylosis
Arthus' phenomenon or reaction T78.41
   due to
      drug —*see* Table of Drugs and Chemicals, by drug
Articular —*see* condition
Articulation, reverse (teeth) M26.24
Artificial
   insemination complication —*see* Complications, artificial, fertilization
   opening status (functioning) (without complication) Z93.9
      anus (colostomy) Z93.3
      colostomy Z93.3
      cystostomy Z93.50
         appendico-vesicostomy Z93.52
         cutaneous Z93.51
         specified NEC Z93.59
      enterostomy Z93.4
      gastrostomy Z93.1
      ileostomy Z93.2
      intestinal tract NEC Z93.4
      jejunostomy Z93.4
      nephrostomy Z93.6
      specified site NEC Z93.8
      tracheostomy Z93.0
      ureterostomy Z93.6
      urethrostomy Z93.6
      urinary tract NEC Z93.6
      vagina Z93.8
   vagina status Z93.8
Arytenoid —*see* condition
Asadollahi-Rauch syndrome Q87.85
Asbestosis (occupational) J61
ASC-H (atypical squamous cells cannot exclude high grade squamous intraepithelial lesion on cytologic smear)
   anus R85.611
   cervix R87.611
   vagina R87.621
ASC-US (atypical squamous cells of undetermined significance on cytologic smear)
   anus R85.610
   cervix R87.610
   vagina R87.620
Ascariasis B77.9
   with
      complications NEC B77.89
      intestinal complications B77.0
      pneumonia, pneumonitis B77.81
Ascaridosis, ascaridiasis —*see* Ascariasis
Ascaris (infection) (infestation) (lumbricoides) —*see* Ascariasis
Ascending —*see* condition
Aschoff's bodies —*see* Myocarditis, rheumatic

33

Ascites (abdominal) R18.8
  cardiac (*see also* Failure, heart, right) I50.810
  chylous (nonfilarial) I89.8
    filarial —*see* Infestation, filarial
  due to
    cirrhosis, alcoholic K70.31
    hepatitis
      alcoholic K70.11
        chronic active K71.51
      S. japonicum B65.2
  heart (*see also* Failure, heart, right) I50.810
  malignant R18.0
  pseudochylous R18.8
  syphilitic A52.74
  tuberculous A18.31
Aseptic —*see* condition
Asherman's syndrome N85.6
Asialia K11.7
Asiatic cholera —*see* Cholera
Asimultagnosia (simultanagnosia) R48.3
Askin's tumor —*see* Neoplasm, connective tissue, malignant
Asocial personality F60.2
Asomatognosia R41.4
Aspartylglucosaminuria E77.1
Asperger's disease or syndrome F84.5
Aspergilloma —*see* Aspergillosis
Aspergillosis (with pneumonia) B44.9
  bronchopulmonary, allergic B44.81
  disseminated B44.7
  generalized B44.7
  pulmonary NEC B44.1
    allergic B44.81
    invasive B44.0
  specified NEC B44.89
  tonsillar B44.2
Aspergillus (flavus) (fumigatus) (infection) (terreus) —*see* Aspergillosis
Aspermatogenesis —*see* Azoospermia
Aspermia (testis) —*see* Azoospermia
Asphyxia, asphyxiation (by) R09.01
  antenatal P84
  birth P84
  bunny bag —*see* Asphyxia, due to, mechanical threat to breathing, trapped in bed clothes
  crushing S28.0
  drowning T75.1
  gas, fumes, or vapor —*see* Table of Drugs and Chemicals
  inhalation —*see* Inhalation
  intrauterine P84
  local I73.00
    with gangrene I73.01
  mucus —*see also* Foreign body, respiratory tract, causing asphyxiation
  newborn P84
  pathological R09.01
  postnatal P84
    mechanical —*see* Asphyxia, due to, mechanical threat to breathing
  prenatal P84
  reticularis R23.1
  strangulation —*see* Asphyxia, due to, mechanical threat to breathing
  submersion T75.1

Asphyxia, asphyxiation (*continued*)
  traumatic T71.9
    due to
      crushed chest S28.0
      foreign body (in) —*see* Foreign body, respiratory tract, causing asphyxia
      low oxygen content of ambient air T71.20
        due to
          being trapped in low oxygen environment T71.29
            in car trunk T71.221
              circumstances undetermined T71.224
              done with intent to harm by
                another person T71.223
                self T71.222
            in refrigerator T71.231
              circumstances undetermined T71.234
              done with intent to harm by
                another person T71.233
                self T71.232
          cave-in T71.21
      mechanical threat to breathing (accidental) T71.191
        circumstances undetermined T71.194
        done with intent to harm by
          another person T71.193
          self T71.192
        hanging T71.161
          circumstances undetermined T71.164
          done with intent to harm by
            another person T71.163
            self T71.162
        plastic bag T71.121
          circumstances undetermined T71.124
          done with intent to harm by
            another person T71.123
            self T71.122
        smothering
          in furniture T71.151
            circumstances undetermined T71.154
            done with intent to harm by
              another person T71.153
              self T71.152
          under
            another person's body T71.141
              circumstances undetermined T71.144
              done with intent to harm T71.143
            pillow T71.111
              circumstances undetermined T71.114
              done with intent to harm by
                another person T71.113
                self T71.112

Asphyxia, asphyxiation (*continued*)
  traumatic (*continued*)
    due to (*continued*)
      mechanical threat to breathing (*continued*)
        trapped in bed clothes T71.131
          circumstances undetermined T71.134
          done with intent to harm by
            another person T71.133
            self T71.132
  vomiting, vomitus —*see* Foreign body, respiratory tract, causing asphyxia
Aspiration
  amniotic (clear) fluid (newborn) P24.10
    with
      pneumonia (pneumonitis) P24.11
      respiratory symptoms P24.11
  blood
    newborn (without respiratory symptoms) P24.20
      with
        pneumonia (pneumonitis) P24.21
        respiratory symptoms P24.21
    specified age NEC —*see* Foreign body, respiratory tract
  bronchitis J69.0
  food or foreign body —*see* Foreign body, by site
  liquor (amnii) (newborn) P24.10
    with
      pneumonia (pneumonitis) P24.11
      respiratory symptoms P24.11
  meconium (newborn) (without respiratory symptoms) P24.00
    with
      pneumonitis (pneumonitis) P24.01
      respiratory symptoms P24.01
  milk (newborn) (without respiratory symptoms) P24.30
    with
      pneumonia (pneumonitis) P24.31
      respiratory symptoms P24.31
    specified age NEC —*see* Foreign body, respiratory tract
  mucus —*see also* Foreign body, by site, causing asphyxia
    newborn P24.10
      with
        pneumonia (pneumonitis) P24.11
        respiratory symptoms P24.11
  neonatal P24.9
    specific NEC (without respiratory symptoms) P24.80
      with
        pneumonia (pneumonitis) P24.81
        respiratory symptoms P24.81
  newborn P24.9
    specific NEC (without respiratory symptoms) P24.80
      with
        pneumonia (pneumonitis) P24.81
        respiratory symptoms P24.81

Aspiration (*continued*)
  pneumonia J69.0
  pneumonitis J69.0
  syndrome of newborn —*see* Aspiration, by substance, with pneumonia
  vernix caseosa (newborn) P24.80
    with
      pneumonia (pneumonitis) P24.81
      respiratory symptoms P24.81
  vomitus —*see also* Foreign body, respiratory tract
    newborn (without respiratory symptoms) P24.30
      with
        pneumonia (pneumonitis) P24.31
        respiratory symptoms P24.31
Asplenia (congenital) Q89.01
  postsurgical Z90.81
Assam fever B55.0
Assault, sexual —*see* Maltreatment
Assmann's focus NEC A15.0
Astasia(-abasia) (hysterical) F44.4
Asteatosis cutis L85.3
Astereognosia, astereognosis R48.1
Asterixis R27.8
  in liver disease K71.3
Asteroid hyalitis —*see* Deposit, crystalline
Asthenia, asthenic R53.1
  cardiac (*see also* Failure, heart) I50.9
    psychogenic F45.8
  cardiovascular (*see also* Failure, heart) I50.9
    psychogenic F45.8
  heart (*see also* Failure, heart) I50.9
    psychogenic F45.8
  hysterical F44.4
  myocardial (*see also* Failure, heart) I50.9
    psychogenic F45.8
  nervous F48.8
  neurocirculatory F45.8
  neurotic F48.8
    psychogenic F48.8
  psychoneurotic F48.8
  psychophysiologic F48.8
  reaction (psychophysiologic) F48.8
  senile R54
Asthenopia —*see also* Discomfort, visual
  hysterical F44.6
  psychogenic F44.6
Asthenospermia —*see* Abnormal, specimen, male genital organs
Asthma, asthmatic (bronchial) (catarrh) (spasmodic) J45.909
  with
    chronic obstructive bronchitis J44.89
      with
        acute lower respiratory infection J44.0
        exacerbation (acute) J44.1

Asthma, asthmatic *(continued)*
with *(continued)*
chronic obstructive pulmonary disease J44.89
with
acute lower respiratory infection J44.0
exacerbation (acute) J44.1
exacerbation (acute) J45.901
hay fever —*see* Asthma, allergic extrinsic
rhinitis, allergic —*see* Asthma, allergic extrinsic
status asthmaticus J45.902
allergic extrinsic J45.909
with
exacerbation (acute) J45.901
status asthmaticus J45.902
atopic —*see* Asthma, allergic extrinsic
cardiac —*see* Failure, ventricular, left
cardiobronchial I50.1
childhood J45.909
with
exacerbation (acute) J45.901
status asthmaticus J45.902
chronic obstructive J44.89
with
acute lower respiratory infection J44.0
exacerbation (acute) J44.1
collier's J60
cough variant J45.991
detergent J69.8
due to
detergent J69.8
inhalation of fumes J68.3
eosinophilic J82.83
extrinsic, allergic —*see* Asthma, allergic extrinsic
grinder's J62.8
hay —*see* Asthma, allergic extrinsic
heart I50.1
idiosyncratic —*see* Asthma, nonallergic
intermittent (mild) J45.20
with
exacerbation (acute) J45.21
status asthmaticus J45.22
intrinsic, nonallergic —*see* Asthma, nonallergic
Kopp's E32.8
late-onset J45.909
with
exacerbation (acute) J45.901
status asthmaticus J45.902
mild intermittent J45.20
with
exacerbation (acute) J45.21
status asthmaticus J45.22
mild persistent J45.30
with
exacerbation (acute) J45.31
status asthmaticus J45.32
Millar's (laryngismus stridulus) J38.5
miner's J60
mixed J45.909
with
exacerbation (acute) J45.901
status asthmaticus J45.902
moderate persistent J45.40
with
exacerbation (acute) J45.41
status asthmaticus J45.42
nervous —*see* Asthma, nonallergic
nonallergic (intrinsic) J45.909
with
exacerbation (acute) J45.901
status asthmaticus J45.902

Asthma, asthmatic *(continued)*
persistent
mild J45.30
with
exacerbation (acute) J45.31
status asthmaticus J45.32
moderate J45.40
with
exacerbation (acute) J45.41
status asthmaticus J45.42
severe J45.50
with
exacerbation (acute) J45.51
status asthmaticus J45.52
platinum J45.998
pneumoconiotic NEC J64
potter's J62.8
predominantly allergic J45.909
psychogenic F54
pulmonary eosinophilic J82.83
red cedar J67.8
Rostan's I50.1
sandblaster's J62.8
sequoiosis J67.8
severe persistent J45.50
with
exacerbation (acute) J45.51
status asthmaticus J45.52
specified NEC J45.998
stonemason's J62.8
thymic E32.8
tuberculous —*see* Tuberculosis, pulmonary
Wichmann's (laryngismus stridulus) J38.5
wood J67.8

Astigmatism (compound) (congenital) H52.20-
irregular H52.21-
regular H52.22-

Astraphobia F40.220

Astroblastoma
specified site —*see* Neoplasm, malignant, by site
unspecified site C71.9

Astrocytoma (cystic)
anaplastic
specified site —*see* Neoplasm, malignant, by site
unspecified site C71.9
fibrillary
specified site —*see* Neoplasm, malignant, by site
unspecified site C71.9
fibrous
specified site —*see* Neoplasm, malignant, by site
unspecified site C71.9
gemistocytic
specified site —*see* Neoplasm, malignant, by site
unspecified site C71.9
juvenile
specified site —*see* Neoplasm, malignant, by site
unspecified site C71.9
pilocytic
specified site —*see* Neoplasm, malignant, by site
unspecified site C71.9
piloid
specified site —*see* Neoplasm, malignant, by site
unspecified site C71.9
protoplasmic
specified site —*see* Neoplasm, malignant, by site
unspecified site C71.9
specified site NEC —*see* Neoplasm, malignant, by site

Astrocytoma *(continued)*
subependymal D43.2
giant cell
specified site —*see* Neoplasm, uncertain behavior, by site
unspecified site D43.2
specified site —*see* Neoplasm, uncertain behavior, by site
unspecified site D43.2
unspecified site C71.9

Astroglioma
specified site —*see* Neoplasm, malignant, by site
unspecified site C71.9

Asymbolia R48.8

Asymmetry —*see also* Distortion
between native and reconstructed breast N65.1
face Q67.0
jaw (lower) —*see* Anomaly, dentofacial, jaw-cranial base relationship, asymmetry

Asynergia, asynergy R27.8
ventricular I51.89

Asystole (heart) —*see* Arrest, cardiac

At risk
for
dental caries Z91.849
high Z91.843
low Z91.841
moderate Z91.842
feeling loneliness Z65.8
social isolation Z91.89
falling Z91.81

Ataxia, ataxy, ataxic R27.0
acute R27.8
autosomal recessive Friedreich G11.11
brain (hereditary) G11.9
cerebellar (hereditary) G11.9
with defective DNA repair G11.3
alcoholic G31.2
early-onset G11.10
with
essential tremor G11.19
myoclonus [Hunt's ataxia] G11.19
retained tendon reflexes G11.19
in
alcoholism G31.2
myxedema E03.9 *[G13.2]*
neoplastic disease (*see also* Neoplasm) D49.9 *[G32.81]*
specified disease NEC G32.81
late-onset (Marie's) G11.2
cerebral (hereditary) G11.9
congenital nonprogressive G11.0
family, familial —*see* Ataxia, hereditary
following
cerebrovascular disease I69.993
cerebral infarction I69.393
intracerebral hemorrhage I69.193
nontraumatic intracranial hemorrhage NEC I69.293
specified disease NEC I69.893
subarachnoid hemorrhage I69.093
Friedreich's (heredofamilial) (cerebellar) (spinal) (with retained reflexes) G11.11
gait R26.0
hysterical F44.4
general R27.8
gluten M35.9 *[G32.81]*
with celiac disease K90.0 *[G32.81]*

Ataxia, ataxy, ataxic *(continued)*
hereditary G11.9
with neuropathy G60.2
cerebellar —*see* Ataxia, cerebellar
spastic G11.4
specified NEC G11.8
spinal (Friedreich's) G11.11
heredofamilial —*see* Ataxia, hereditary
Hunt's G11.19
hysterical F44.4
locomotor (progressive) (syphilitic) (partial) (spastic) A52.11
diabetic —*see* Diabetes, ataxia
Marie's (cerebellar) (heredofamilial) (late- onset) G11.2
nonorganic origin F44.4
nonprogressive, congenital G11.0
psychogenic F44.4
Roussy-Lévy G60.0
Sanger-Brown's (hereditary) G11.2
spastic hereditary G11.4
spinal
hereditary (Friedreich's) G11.11
progressive (syphilitic) A52.11
spinocerebellar, X-linked recessive G11.19
telangiectasia (Louis-Bar) G11.3

Ataxia-telangiectasia (Louis-Bar) G11.3

Atelectasis (massive) (partial) (pressure) (pulmonary) J98.11
newborn P28.10
due to resorption P28.11
partial P28.19
primary P28.0
secondary P28.19
primary (newborn) P28.0
tuberculous —*see* Tuberculosis, pulmonary

Atelocardia Q24.9

Atelomyelia Q06.1

Atheroembolism
of
extremities
lower I75.02-
upper I75.01-
kidney I75.81
specified NEC I75.89

Atheroma, atheromatous —*see also* Arteriosclerosis I70.90
aorta, aortic I70.0
valve —*see also* Endocarditis, aortic I35.8
aorto-iliac I70.0
artery —*see* Arteriosclerosis
basilar (artery) I67.2
carotid (artery) (common) (internal) I67.2
cerebral (arteries) I67.2
coronary (artery) I25.10
with angina pectoris —*see* Arteriosclerosis, coronary (artery),
degeneration —*see* Arteriosclerosis
heart, cardiac —*see* Disease, heart, ischemic, atherosclerotic
mitral (valve) I34.89
myocardium, myocardial —*see* Disease, heart, ischemic, atherosclerotic
pulmonary valve (heart) (*see also* Endocarditis, pulmonary) I37.8
tricuspid (heart) (valve) I36.8
valve, valvular —*see* Endocarditis
vertebral (artery) I67.2

Atheromatosis —*see* Arteriosclerosis

35

Atherosclerosis —see also
 Arteriosclerosis
 coronary
  artery I25.10
   with angina pectoris —see
     Arteriosclerosis, coronary
     (artery),
   due to
    calcified coronary lesion
     (severely) I25.84
    lipid rich plaque I25.83
  transplanted heart I25.811
   bypass graft I25.812
    with angina pectoris —see
     Arteriosclerosis, coronary
     (artery),
   native coronary artery I25.811
    with angina pectoris —see
     Arteriosclerosis, coronary
     (artery),

Athetosis (acquired) R25.8
 bilateral (congenital) G80.3
 congenital (bilateral) (double) G80.3
 double (congenital) G80.3
 unilateral R25.8

Athlete's
 foot B35.3
 heart I51.7

Athrepsia E41

Athyrea (acquired) —see also
  Hypothyroidism
 congenital E03.1

Atonia, atony, atonic
 bladder (sphincter) (neurogenic)
  N31.2
 capillary I78.8
 cecum K59.89
  psychogenic F45.8
 colon —see Atony, intestine
 congenital P94.2
 esophagus K22.89
 intestine K59.89
  psychogenic F45.8
 stomach K31.89
  neurotic or psychogenic F45.8
 uterus (during labor) O62.2
  with hemorrhage (postpartum)
   O72.1
  postpartum (with hemorrhage)
   O72.1
   without hemorrhage O75.89

Atopy —see History, allergy

Atransferrinemia, congenital E88.09

Atresia, atretic
 alimentary organ or tract NEC Q45.8
  upper Q40.8
 ani, anus, anal (canal) Q42.3
  with fistula Q42.2
 aorta (ring) Q25.29
 aortic (orifice) (valve) Q23.0
  arch Q25.21
  congenital with hypoplasia of
   ascending aorta and defective
   development of left ventricle
   (with mitral stenosis) Q23.4
  in hypoplastic left heart
   syndrome Q23.4
 aqueduct of Sylvius Q03.0
  with spina bifida —see Spina
   bifida, with hydrocephalus
 artery NEC Q27.8
  cerebral Q28.3
  coronary Q24.5
  digestive system Q27.8
  eye Q15.8
  lower limb Q27.8
  pulmonary Q25.5
  specified site NEC Q27.8
  umbilical Q27.0
  upper limb Q27.8

Atresia, atretic (continued)
 auditory canal (external) Q16.1
 bile duct (common) (congenital)
  (hepatic) Q44.2
  acquired —see Obstruction, bile
   duct
 bladder (neck) Q64.39
  obstruction Q64.31
 bronchus Q32.4
 cecum Q42.8
 cervix (acquired) N88.2
  congenital Q51.828
   in pregnancy or childbirth —see
    Anomaly, cervix, in pregnancy
    or childbirth
    causing obstructed labor
     O65.5
 choana Q30.0
 colon Q42.9
  specified NEC Q42.8
 common duct Q44.2
 cricoid cartilage Q31.8
 cystic duct Q44.2
  acquired K82.8
   with obstruction K82.0
 digestive organs NEC Q45.8
 duodenum Q41.0
 ear canal Q16.1
 ejaculatory duct Q55.4
 epiglottis Q31.8
 esophagus Q39.0
  with tracheoesophageal fistula
   Q39.1
 eustachian tube Q17.8
 fallopian tube (congenital) Q50.6
  acquired N97.1
 follicular cyst N83.0-
 foramen of
  Luschka Q03.1
   with spina bifida —see Spina
    bifida, with hydrocephalus
  Magendie Q03.1
   with spina bifida —see Spina
    bifida, with hydrocephalus
 gallbladder Q44.1
 genital organ
  external
   female Q52.79
   male Q55.8
  internal
   female Q52.8
   male Q55.8
 glottis Q31.8
 gullet Q39.0
  with tracheoesophageal fistula
   Q39.1
 heart valve NEC Q24.8
  pulmonary Q22.0
  tricuspid Q22.4
 hymen Q52.3
  acquired (postinfective)
   N89.6
 ileum Q41.2
 intestine (small) Q41.9
  large Q42.9
   specified NEC Q42.8
 iris, filtration angle Q15.0
 jejunum Q41.1
 lacrimal apparatus Q10.4
 larynx Q31.8
 meatus urinarius Q64.33
 mitral valve Q23.2
  in hypoplastic left heart
   syndrome Q23.4
 nares (anterior) (posterior) Q30.0
 nasopharynx Q34.8
 nose, nostril Q30.0
  acquired J34.89
 organ or site NEC Q89.8
 osseous meatus (ear) Q16.1

Atresia, atretic (continued)
 oviduct (congenital) Q50.6
  acquired N97.1
 parotid duct Q38.4
  acquired K11.8
 pulmonary (artery) Q25.5
  valve Q22.0
 pulmonic Q22.0
 pupil Q13.2
 rectum Q42.1
  with fistula Q42.0
 salivary duct Q38.4
  acquired K11.8
 sublingual duct Q38.4
  acquired K11.8
 submandibular duct Q38.4
  acquired K11.8
 submaxillary duct Q38.4
  acquired K11.8
 thyroid cartilage Q31.8
 trachea Q32.1
 tricuspid valve Q22.4
 ureter Q62.10
  pelvic junction Q62.11
  vesical orifice Q62.12
 ureteropelvic junction Q62.11
 ureterovesical orifice Q62.12
 urethra (valvular) Q64.39
  stricture Q64.32
 urinary tract NEC Q64.8
 uterus Q51.818
  acquired N85.8
 vagina (congenital) Q52.4
  acquired (postinfectional)
   (senile) N89.5
 vas deferens Q55.3
 vascular NEC Q27.8
  cerebral Q28.3
  digestive system Q27.8
  lower limb Q27.8
  specified site NEC Q27.8
  upper limb Q27.8
 vein NEC Q27.8
  digestive system Q27.8
  great Q26.8
  lower limb Q27.8
  portal Q26.5
  pulmonary Q26.4
   partial Q26.3
   total Q26.2
  specified site NEC Q27.8
  upper limb Q27.8
 vena cava (inferior) (superior) Q26.8
 vesicourethral orifice Q64.31
 vulva Q52.79
  acquired N90.5

Atrichia, atrichosis —see Alopecia

Atrophia —see also Atrophy
 cutis senilis L90.8
  due to radiation L57.8
 gyrata of choroid and retina H31.23
 senilis R54
  dermatological L90.8
   due to radiation (nonionizing)
    (solar) L57.8
 unguium L60.3
  congenita Q84.6

Atrophie blanche (en plaque)
 (de Milian) L95.0

Atrophoderma, atrophodermia (of)
 L90.9
 diffusum (idiopathic) L90.4
 maculatum L90.8
  et striatum L90.8
   due to syphilis A52.79
   syphilitic A51.39
 neuriticum L90.8
 Pasini and Pierini L90.3
 pigmentosum Q82.1

Atrophoderma, atrophodermia (of)
 (continued)
 reticulatum symmetricum faciei
  L66.4
 senile L90.8
  due to radiation (nonionizing)
   (solar) L57.8
 vermiculata (cheeks) L66.4

Atrophy, atrophic (of)
 adrenal (capsule) (gland) E27.49
  primary (autoimmune) E27.1
 alveolar process or ridge
  (edentulous) K08.20
 anal sphincter (disuse) N81.84
 appendix K38.8
 arteriosclerotic —see Arteriosclerosis
 bile duct (common) (hepatic) K83.8
 bladder N32.89
  neurogenic N31.8
 blanche (en plaque) (of Milian)
  L95.0
 bone (senile) NEC —see also
   Disorder, bone, specified type
   NEC
  due to
   tabes dorsalis (neurogenic)
    A52.11
 brain (cortex) (progressive) G31.9
  frontotemporal circumscribed
   (see also Dementia, in,
   diseases specified elsewhere)
   G31.01 [F02.80]
   with behavioral disturbance
    (see also Dementia,
    in, diseases specified
    elsewhere) G31.01 [F02.81-]
  senile NEC G31.1
 breast N64.2
  obstetric —see Disorder, breast,
   specified type NEC
 buccal cavity K13.79
 cardiac —see Degeneration,
  myocardial
 cartilage (infectional) (joint) —see
  Disorder, cartilage, specified
  NEC
 cerebellar —see Atrophy, brain
 cerebral —see Atrophy, brain
 cervix (mucosa) (senile) (uteri)
  N88.8
  menopausal N95.8
 Charcot-Marie-Tooth G60.0
 choroid (central) (macular)
  (myopic) (retina) H31.10-
  diffuse secondary H31.12-
  gyrate H31.23
  senile H31.11-
 ciliary body —see Atrophy, iris
 conjunctiva (senile) H11.89
 corpus cavernosum N48.89
 cortical —see Atrophy, brain
 cystic duct K82.8
 Déjérine-Thomas G23.8
 disuse NEC —see Atrophy, muscle
 Duchenne-Aran G12.21
 ear H93.8-
 edentulous alveolar ridge K08.20
 endometrium (senile) N85.8
  cervix N88.8
 enteric K63.89
 epididymis N50.89
 eyeball —see Disorder, globe,
  degenerated condition, atrophy
 eyelid (senile) —see Disorder,
  eyelid, degenerative
 facial (skin) L90.9
 fallopian tube (senile) N83.32-
  with ovary N83.33-
 fascioscapulohumeral (Landouzy-
  Déjérine) G71.02

Atrophy, atrophic (continued)
  fatty, thymus (gland) E32.8
  gallbladder K82.8
  gastric K29.40
    with bleeding K29.41
  gastrointestinal K63.89
  glandular I89.8
  globe H44.52-
  gum -see Recession, gingival
  hair L67.8
  heart (brown) —see Degeneration, myocardial
  hemifacial Q67.4
    Romberg G51.8
  infantile E41
    paralysis, acute —see Poliomyelitis, paralytic
  intestine K63.89
  iris (essential) (progressive) H21.26-
    specified NEC H21.29
  kidney (senile) (terminal) (see also Sclerosis, renal) N26.1
    congenital or infantile Q60.5
      bilateral Q60.4
      unilateral Q60.3
    hydronephrotic —see Hydronephrosis
  lacrimal gland (primary) H04.14-
    secondary H04.15-
  Landouzy-Déjérine G71.02
  laryngitis, infective J37.0
  larynx J38.7
  Leber's optic (hereditary) H47.22
  lip K13.0
  liver (yellow) K72.90
    with coma K72.91
    acute, subacute K72.00
      with coma K72.01
    chronic K72.10
      with coma K72.11
  lung (senile) J98.4
  macular (dermatological) L90.8
    syphilitic, skin A51.39
      striated A52.79
  mandible (edentulous) K08.20
    minimal K08.21
    moderate K08.22
    severe K08.23
  maxilla K08.20
    minimal K08.24
    moderate K08.25
    severe K08.26
  muscle, muscular (diffuse) (general) (idiopathic) (primary) M62.50
    ankle M62.57-
    back M62.5A9
      cervical M62.5A0
      lumbosacral M62.5A2
      thoracic M62.5A1
    Duchenne-Aran G12.21
    foot M62.57-
    forearm M62.53-
    hand M62.54-
    infantile spinal G12.0
    lower leg M62.56-
    multiple sites M62.59
    myelopathic —see Atrophy, muscle, spinal
    myotonic G71.11
    neuritic G58.9
    neurogenic (peroneal) (progressive) G60.0
    pelvic (disuse) N81.84
    peroneal G60.0
    progressive (bulbar) G12.21
      adult G12.1
      infantile (spinal) G12.0
      spinal G12.25
        adult G12.1
        infantile G12.0

Atrophy, atrophic (continued)
  muscle, muscular (continued)
    pseudohypertrophic G71.02
    shoulder region M62.51-
    specified site NEC M62.58
    spinal G12.9
      adult form G12.1
      Aran-Duchenne G12.21
      childhood form, type II G12.1
      distal G12.1
      hereditary NEC G12.1
      infantile, type I (Werdnig-Hoffmann) G12.0
      juvenile form, type III (Kugelberg- Welander) G12.1
      progressive G12.25
      scapuloperoneal form G12.1
      specified NEC G12.8
    syphilitic A52.78
    thigh M62.55-
    upper arm M62.52-
  myocardium —see Degeneration, myocardial
  myometrium (senile) N85.8
    cervix N88.8
  myopathic NEC —see Atrophy, muscle
  myotonia G71.11
  nail L60.3
  nasopharynx J31.1
  nerve —see also Disorder, nerve
    abducens —see Strabismus, paralytic, sixth nerve
    accessory G52.8
    acoustic or auditory H93.3
    cranial G52.9
      eighth (auditory) H93.3
      eleventh (accessory) G52.8
      fifth (trigeminal) G50.8
      first (olfactory) G52.0
      fourth (trochlear) —see Strabismus, paralytic, fourth nerve
      second (optic) H47.20
      sixth (abducens) —see Strabismus, paralytic, sixth nerve
      tenth (pneumogastric) (vagus) G52.2
      third (oculomotor) —see Strabismus, paralytic, third nerve
      twelfth (hypoglossal) G52.3
    hypoglossal G52.3
    oculomotor —see Strabismus, paralytic, third nerve
    olfactory G52.0
    optic (papillomacular bundle)
      syphilitic (late) A52.15
        congenital A50.44
    pneumogastric G52.2
    trigeminal G50.8
    trochlear —see Strabismus, paralytic, fourth nerve
    vagus (pneumogastric) G52.2
  neurogenic, bone, tabetic A52.11
  nutritional E43
    with marasmus E41
  old age R54
  olivopontocerebellar G23.8
  optic (nerve) H47.20
    glaucomatous H47.23-
    hereditary H47.22
    primary H47.21-
    specified type NEC H47.29-
    syphilitic (late) A52.15
      congenital A50.44
  orbit H05.31-
  ovary (senile) N83.31-
    with fallopian tube N83.33-

Atrophy, atrophic (continued)
  oviduct (senile) —see Atrophy, fallopian tube
  palsy, diffuse (progressive) G12.22
  pancreas (duct) (senile) K86.89
  parotid gland K11.0
  pelvic muscle N81.84
  penis N48.89
  pharynx J39.2
  pluriglandular E31.8
    autoimmune E31.0
  polyarthritis M15.9
  prostate N42.89
  pseudohypertrophic (muscle) G71.02
  renal (see also Sclerosis, renal) N26.1
  retina, retinal (postinfectional) H35.89
  rhinitis J31.0
  salivary gland K11.0
  scar L90.5
  sclerosis, lobar (of brain) (see also Dementia, in, diseases specified elsewhere) G31.09 [F02.80]
    with behavioral disturbance (see also Dementia, in, diseases specified elsewhere) G31.09 [F02.81-]
  scrotum N50.89
  seminal vesicle N50.89
  senile R54
    due to radiation (nonionizing) (solar) L57.8
  skin (patches) (spots) L90.9
    degenerative (senile) L90.8
    due to radiation (nonionizing) (solar) L57.8
    senile L90.8
  spermatic cord N50.89
  spinal (acute) (cord) G95.89
    muscular —see Atrophy, muscle, spinal
    paralysis G12.20
      acute —see Poliomyelitis, paralytic
      meaning progressive muscular atrophy G12.25
  spine (column) —see Spondylopathy, specified NEC
  spleen (senile) D73.0
  stomach K29.40
    with bleeding K29.41
  striate (skin) L90.6
    syphilitic A52.79
  subcutaneous L90.9
  sublingual gland K11.0
  submandibular gland K11.0
  submaxillary gland K11.0
  Sudeck's —see Algoneurodystrophy
  suprarenal (capsule) (gland) E27.49
    primary E27.1
  systemic affecting central nervous system
    in
      myxedema E03.9 [G13.2]
      neoplastic disease (see also Neoplasm) D49.9 [G13.1]
      specified disease NEC G13.8
  tarso-orbital fascia, congenital Q10.3
  testis N50.0
  thenar, partial —see Syndrome, carpal tunnel
  thymus (fatty) E32.8
  thyroid (gland) (acquired) E03.4
    with cretinism E03.1
    congenital (with myxedema) E03.1
  tongue (senile) K14.8
    papillae K14.4

Atrophy, atrophic (continued)
  trachea J39.8
  tunica vaginalis N50.89
  turbinate J34.89
  tympanic membrane (nonflaccid) H73.82-
    flaccid H73.81-
  upper respiratory tract J39.8
  uterus, uterine (senile) N85.8
    cervix N88.8
    due to radiation (intended effect) N85.8
      adverse effect or misadventure N99.89
  vagina (senile) N95.2
  vas deferens N50.89
  vascular I99.8
  vertebra (senile) —see Spondylopathy, specified NEC
  vulva (senile) N90.5
  Werdnig-Hoffmann G12.0
  yellow —see Failure, hepatic

Attack, attacks
  with alteration of consciousness (with automatisms) —see Epilepsy, localization-related, symptomatic, with complex partial seizures
  Adams-Stokes I45.9
  akinetic —see Epilepsy, generalized, specified NEC
  angina —see Angina
  atonic —see Epilepsy, generalized, specified NEC
  benign shuddering G25.83
  cataleptic —see Catalepsy
  sp
  coronary —see Infarct, myocardium
  cyanotic, newborn P28.2
  drop NEC R55
  epileptic —see Epilepsy
  heart —see infarct, myocardium
  hysterical F44.9
  jacksonian —see Epilepsy, localization-related, symptomatic, with simple partial seizures
  myocardium, myocardial —see Infarct, myocardium
  myoclonic —see Epilepsy, generalized, specified NEC
  panic F41.0
  psychomotor —see Epilepsy, localization-related, symptomatic, with complex partial seizures
  salaam —see Epilepsy, spasms
  schizophreniform, brief F23
  shuddering, benign G25.83
  Stokes-Adams I45.9
  syncope R55
  transient ischemic (TIA) G45.9
    specified NEC G45.8
  unconsciousness R55
    hysterical F44.89
  vasomotor R55
  vasovagal (paroxysmal) (idiopathic) R55
  without alteration of consciousness —see Epilepsy, localization-related, symptomatic, with simple partial seizures

Attention (to)
  artificial
    opening (of) Z43.9
      digestive tract NEC Z43.4
        colon Z43.3
        ilium Z43.2
        stomach Z43.1

Attention (continued)
  artificial (continued)
    opening (of) Z43.9 (continued)
      specified NEC Z43.8
      trachea Z43.0
      urinary tract NEC Z43.6
        cystostomy Z43.5
        nephrostomy Z43.6
        ureterostomy Z43.6
        urethrostomy Z43.6
      vagina Z43.7
    colostomy Z43.3
    cystostomy Z43.5
    deficit disorder or syndrome F98.8
      with hyperactivity —*see* Disorder, attention-deficit hyperactivity
    gastrostomy Z43.1
    ileostomy Z43.2
    jejunostomy Z43.4
    nephrostomy Z43.6
    surgical dressings Z48.01
    sutures Z48.02
    tracheostomy Z43.0
    ureterostomy Z43.6
    urethrostomy Z43.6

Attrition
  gum -*see* Recession, gingival
  tooth, teeth (excessive) (hard tissues) K03.0

Atypical, atypism —*see also* condition
  cells (on cytological smear) (endocervical) (endometrial) (glandular)
    cervix R87.619
    vagina R87.629
  cervical N87.9
  endometrium N85.9
    hyperplasia N85.00
  parenting situation Z62.9

Auditory —*see* condition

Aujeszky's disease B33.8

Aurantiasis, cutis E67.1

Auricle, auricular —*see also* condition
  cervical Q18.2

Auriculotemporal syndrome G50.8

Austin Flint murmur (aortic insufficiency) I35.1

Australian
  Q fever A78
  X disease A83.4

Autism, autistic (childhood) (infantile) F84.0
  atypical F84.9
  spectrum disorder F84.0

Autodigestion R68.89

Autoerythrocyte sensitization (syndrome) D69.2

Autographism L50.3

Autoimmune
  disease (systemic) M35.9
  inhibitors to clotting factors D68.311
  lymphoproliferative syndrome [ALPS] D89.82
  thyroiditis E06.3

Autointoxication R68.89

Automatism G93.89
  with temporal sclerosis G93.81

Automatism (continued)
  epileptic —*see* Epilepsy, localization-related, symptomatic, with complex partial seizures
  paroxysmal, idiopathic —*see* Epilepsy, localization-related, symptomatic, with complex partial seizures

Autonomic, autonomous
  bladder (neurogenic) N31.2
  hysteria seizure F44.5

Autosensitivity, erythrocyte D69.2

Autosensitization, cutaneous L30.2

Autosome —*see* condition by chromosome involved

Autotopagnosia R48.1

Autotoxemia R68.89

Autumn —*see* condition

Avellis' syndrome G46.8

Aversion
  oral R63.39
    newborn P92.-
    nonorganic origin F98.2
  sexual F52.1

Aviator's
  disease or sickness —*see* Effect, adverse, high altitude
  ear T70.0

Avitaminosis (multiple) (*see also* Deficiency, vitamin) E56.9
  B E53.9
    with
      beriberi E51.11
      pellagra E52
  B2 E53.0
  B6 E53.1
  B12 E53.8
  D E55.9
    with rickets E55.0
  G E53.0
  K E56.1
  nicotinic acid E52

AVNRT (atrioventricular nodal re-entrant tachycardia) I47.19

AVRT (atrioventricular nodal re-entrant tachycardia) I47.19

Avulsion (traumatic)
  blood vessel —*see* Injury, blood vessel
  bone —*see* Fracture, by site
  cartilage —*see also* Dislocation, by site
    symphyseal (inner), complicating delivery O71.6
  external site other than limb —*see* Wound, open, by site
  eye S05.7-
  head (intracranial)
    external site NEC S08.89
    scalp S08.0
  internal organ or site —*see* Injury, by site
  joint —*see also* Dislocation, by site
  capsule —*see* Sprain, by site
  kidney S37.06-
  ligament —*see* Sprain, by site
  limb —*see also* Amputation, traumatic, by site
    skin and subcutaneous tissue —*see* Wound, open, by site
  muscle —*see* Injury, muscle
  nerve (root) —*see* Injury, nerve
  scalp S08.0
  skin and subcutaneous tissue —*see* Wound, open, by site

Avulsion (continued)
  spleen S36.032
  symphyseal cartilage (inner), complicating delivery O71.6
  tendon —*see* Injury, muscle
  tooth S03.2

Awareness of heart beat R00.2

Axenfeld's
  anomaly or syndrome Q15.0
  degeneration (calcareous) Q13.4

Axilla, axillary —*see also* condition
  breast Q83.1

Axonotmesis —*see* Injury, nerve

Ayerza's disease or syndrome (pulmonary artery sclerosis with pulmonary hypertension) I27.0

Azoospermia (organic) N46.01
  due to
    drug therapy N46.021
    efferent duct obstruction N46.023
    infection N46.022
    radiation N46.024
    specified cause NEC N46.029
    systemic disease N46.025

Azotemia R79.89
  meaning uremia N19

Aztec ear Q17.3

Azygos
  continuation inferior vena cava Q26.8
  lobe (lung) Q33.1

B

Baastrup's disease —*see* Kissing spine

Babesiosis B60.00
  due to
    Babesia
      divergens B60.03
      duncani B60.02
      KO-1 B60.09
      microti B60.01
      MO-1 B60.03
      species
        unspecified B60.00
      venatorum B60.09
    specified NEC B60.09

Babington's disease (familial hemorrhagic telangiectasia) I78.0

Babinski's syndrome A52.79

Baby
  crying constantly R68.11
  floppy (syndrome) P94.2

Bacillary —*see* condition

Bacilluria R82.71

Bacillus —*see also* Infection, bacillus
  abortus infection A23.1
  anthracis infection A22.9
  coli infection —*see also* Escherichia coli B96.20
  Flexner's A03.1
  mallei infection A24.0
  Shiga's A03.0
  suipestifer infection —*see* Infection, salmonella

Back —*see* condition

Backache (postural) M54.9
  sacroiliac M53.3
  specified NEC M54.89

Backflow —*see* Reflux

Backward reading (dyslexia) F81.0

Bacteremia R78.81
  with sepsis —*see* Sepsis

Bactericholia —*see* Cholecystitis, acute

Bacterid, bacteride (pustular) L40.3

Bacterium, bacteria, bacterial
  agent NEC, as cause of disease classified elsewhere B96.89
  in blood —*see* Bacteremia
  in urine —*see* Bacteriuria

Bacteriuria, bacteruria R82.71
  asymptomatic R82.71

Bacteroides
  fragilis, as cause of disease classified elsewhere B96.6

Bad
  heart —*see* Disease, heart
  trip
    due to drug abuse —*see* Abuse, drug, hallucinogen
    due to drug dependence —*see* Dependence, drug, hallucinogen

Baelz's disease (cheilitis glandularis apostematosa) K13.0

Baerensprung's disease (eczema marginatum) B35.6

Bagasse disease or pneumonitis J67.1

Bagassosis J67.1

Baker's cyst —*see* Cyst, Baker's

Bakwin-Krida syndrome (metaphyseal dysplasia) Q78.5

Balancing side interference M26.56

Balanitis (circinata) (erosiva) (gangrenosa) (phagedenic) (vulgaris) N48.1
  amebic A06.82
  candidal B37.42
  due to Haemophilus ducreyi A57
  gonococcal (acute) (chronic) A54.23
  xerotica obliterans N48.0

Balanoposthitis N47.6
  gonococcal (acute) (chronic) A54.23
  ulcerative (specific) A63.8

Balanorrhagia —*see* Balanitis

Balantidiasis, balantidiosis A07.0

Bald tongue K14.4

Baldness —*see also* Alopecia
  male-pattern —*see* Alopecia, androgenic

Balkan grippe A78

Balloon disease —*see* Effect, adverse, high altitude

Balo's disease (concentric sclerosis) G37.5

Bamberger-Marie disease —*see* Osteoarthropathy, hypertrophic, specified type NEC

Bancroft's filariasis B74.0

Band(s)
  adhesive —*see* Adhesions, peritoneum
  anomalous or congenital —*see also* Anomaly, by site
    heart (atrial) (ventricular) Q24.8
    intestine Q43.3
    omentum Q43.3
  cervix N88.1
  constricting, congenital Q79.8
  gallbladder (congenital) Q44.1

Band(s) *(continued)*
 intestinal (adhesive) —*see* Adhesions, peritoneum
 obstructive
  intestine K56.50
   complete K56.52
   incomplete K56.51
   partial K56.51
  peritoneum K56.50
   complete K56.52
   incomplete K56.51
   partial K56.51
 periappendiceal, congenital Q43.3
 peritoneal (adhesive) —*see* Adhesions, peritoneum
 uterus N73.6
  internal N85.6
 vagina N89.5

Bandemia D72.825

Bandl's ring (contraction), **complicating delivery** O62.4

Bangkok hemorrhagic fever A91

Bang's disease (brucella abortus) A23.1

Bankruptcy (anxiety concerning) Z59.86

Bannister's disease T78.3
 hereditary D84.1

Banti's disease or syndrome (with cirrhosis) (with portal hypertension) K76.6

Bar, median, prostate —*see* Enlargement, enlarged, prostate

Barcoo disease or rot —*see* Ulcer, skin

Barlow's disease E54

Barodontalgia T70.29

Baron Münchausen syndrome —*see* Disorder, factitious

Barosinusitis T70.1

Barotitis T70.0

Barotrauma T70.29
 odontalgia T70.29
 otitic T70.0
 sinus T70.1

Barraquer (-Simons) **disease or syndrome** (progressive lipodystrophy) E88.1

Barré-Guillain disease or syndrome G61.0

Barré-Liéou syndrome (posterior cervical sympathetic) M53.0

Barrel chest M95.4

Barrett's
 disease —*see* Barrett's, esophagus
 esophagus K22.70
  with dysplasia K22.719
   high grade K22.711
   low grade K22.710
  without dysplasia K22.70
 syndrome —*see* Barrett's, esophagus
 ulcer K22.10
  with bleeding K22.11
  without bleeding K22.10

Bársony (-Polgár) (-Teschendorf) **syndrome** (corkscrew esophagus) K22.4

Bartholinitis (suppurating) N75.8
 gonococcal (acute) (chronic) (with abscess) A54.1

Barth syndrome E78.71

Bartonellosis A44.9
 cutaneous A44.1
 mucocutaneous A44.1
 specified NEC A44.8
 systemic A44.0

Barton's fracture S52.56-

Bartter's syndrome E26.81

Basal —*see* condition

Basan's (hidrotic) **ectodermal dysplasia** Q82.4

Baseball finger —*see* Dislocation, finger

Basedow's disease (exophthalmic goiter) —*see* Hyperthyroidism, with, goiter

Basic —*see* condition

Basilar —*see* condition

Bason's (hidrotic) **ectodermal dysplasia** Q82.4

Basopenia —*see* Agranulocytosis

Basophilia D72.824

Basophilism (cortico-adrenal) (Cushing's) (pituitary) E24.0

Bassen-Kornzweig disease or syndrome E78.6

Bat ear Q17.5

Bateman's
 disease B08.1
 purpura (senile) D69.2

Bathing cramp T75.1

Bathophobia F40.248

Batten (-Mayou) **disease** E75.4
 retina E75.4 *[H36.89]*

Batten-Steinert syndrome G71.11

Battered —*see* Maltreatment

Battey Mycobacterium infection A31.0

Battle exhaustion F43.0

Battledore placenta O43.19-

Baumgarten-Cruveilhier cirrhosis, disease or syndrome K74.69

Bauxite fibrosis (of lung) J63.1

Bayle's disease (general paresis) A52.17

Bazin's disease (primary) (tuberculous) A18.4

Beach ear —*see* Swimmer's, ear

Beaded hair (congenital) Q84.1

Béal conjunctivitis or syndrome B30.2

Beard's disease (neurasthenia) F48.8

Beat(s)
 atrial, premature I49.1
 ectopic I49.49
 elbow —*see* Bursitis, elbow
 escaped, heart I49.49
 hand —*see* Bursitis, hand
 knee —*see* Bursitis, knee
 premature I49.40
  atrial I49.1
  auricular I49.1
  supraventricular I49.1

Beau's
 disease or syndrome —*see* Degeneration, myocardial
 lines (transverse furrows on fingernails) L60.4

Bechterev's syndrome —*see* Spondylitis, ankylosing

Beck's syndrome (anterior spinal artery occlusion) I65.8

Becker's
 cardiomyopathy I42.8
 disease
  idiopathic mural endomyocardial disease I42.3
  myotonia congenita, recessive form G71.12
 dystrophy G71.01
 pigmented hairy nevus D22.5

Beckwith-Wiedemann syndrome Q87.3

Bed confinement status Z74.01

Bed sore —*see* Ulcer, pressure, by site

Bedbug bite(s) —*see* Bite(s), by site, superficial, insect

Bedclothes, asphyxiation or suffocation by —*see* Asphyxia, traumatic, due to, mechanical, trapped

Bednar's
 aphthae K12.0
 tumor —*see* Neoplasm, malignant, by site

Bedridden Z74.01

Bed-sharing, infant Z72.823

Bedsore —*see* Ulcer, pressure, by site

Bedwetting —*see* Enuresis

Bee sting (with allergic or anaphylactic shock) —*see* Toxicity, venom, arthropod, bee

Beer drinker's heart (disease) I42.6

Begbie's disease (exophthalmic goiter) —*see* Hyperthyroidism, with, goiter

Behavior
 antisocial
  adult Z72.811
  child or adolescent Z72.810
 disorder, disturbance —*see* Disorder, conduct
 disruptive —*see* Disorder, conduct
 drug seeking Z76.5
 inexplicable R46.2
 marked evasiveness R46.5
 obsessive-compulsive R46.81
 overactivity R46.3
 poor responsiveness R46.4
 self-damaging(life-style) Z72.89
 sleep-incompatible Z72.821
 slowness R46.4
 specified NEC R46.89
 strange (and inexplicable) R46.2
 suspiciousness R46.5
 type A pattern Z73.1
 undue concern or preoccupation with stressful events R46.6
 verbosity and circumstantial detail obscuring reason for contact R46.7

Behçet's disease or syndrome M35.2

Behr's disease —*see* Degeneration, macula

Beigel's disease or morbus (white piedra) B36.2

Bejel A65

Bekhterev's syndrome —*see* Spondylitis, ankylosing

Belching —*see* Eructation

Bell's
 mania F30.8
 palsy, paralysis G51.0
  infant or newborn P11.3
 spasm G51.3-

Bence Jones albuminuria or proteinuria NEC R80.3

Bends T70.3

Benedikt's paralysis or syndrome G46.3

Benign —*see also* condition
 prostatic hyperplasia —*see* Hyperplasia, prostate

Bennett's fracture (displaced) S62.21-

Benson's disease —*see* Deposit, crystalline

Bent
 back (hysterical) F44.4
 nose M95.0
  congenital Q67.4

Bereavement (uncomplicated) Z63.4

Bergeron's disease (hysterical chorea) F44.4

Berger's disease —*see* Nephropathy, IgA

Beriberi (dry) E51.11
 heart (disease) E51.12
 polyneuropathy E51.11
 wet E51.12
  involving circulatory system E51.11

Berlin's disease or edema (traumatic) S05.8X-

Berlock (berloque) **dermatitis** L56.2

Bernard-Horner syndrome G90.2

Bernard-Soulier disease or thrombopathia D69.1

Bernhardt (-Roth) **disease** —*see* Mononeuropathy, lower limb, meralgia paresthetica

Bernheim's syndrome —*see* Failure, heart, right

Bertielliasis B71.8

Berylliosis (lung) J63.2

Besnier-Boeck (-Schaumann) **disease** —*see* Sarcoidosis

Besnier's
 lupus pernio D86.3
 prurigo L20.0

Bestiality F65.89

Best's disease H35.50

Beta-mercaptolactate-cysteine disulfiduria E72.09

Betalipoproteinemia, broad or floating E78.2

Betting and gambling Z72.6
 pathological (compulsive) F63.0

Bezoar T18.9
 intestine T18.3
 stomach T18.2

Bezold's abscess —*see* Mastoiditis, acute

Bianchi's syndrome R48.8

Bicornate or bicornis uterus Q51.3
 in pregnancy or childbirth O34.00
  causing obstructed labor O65.5

Bicuspid aortic valve Q23.1

Biedl-Bardet syndrome Q87.83

Bielschowsky (-Jansky) **disease** E75.4

Biermer's (pernicious) **anemia or disease** D51.0

Biett's disease L93.0

Bifid (congenital)
    apex, heart Q24.8
    clitoris Q52.6
    kidney Q63.8
    nose Q30.2
    patella Q74.1
    scrotum Q55.29
    toe NEC Q74.2
    tongue Q38.3
    ureter Q62.8
    uterus Q51.3
    uvula Q35.7

Biforis uterus (suprasimplex) Q51.3

Bifurcation (congenital)
    gallbladder Q44.1
    kidney pelvis Q63.8
    renal pelvis Q63.8
    rib Q76.6
    tongue, congenital Q38.3
    trachea Q32.1
    ureter Q62.8
    urethra Q64.74
    vertebra Q76.49

Big spleen syndrome D73.1

Bigeminal pulse R00.8

Bilateral —see condition

Bile
    duct —see condition
    pigments in urine R82.2

Bilharziasis —see also Schistosomiasis
    chyluria B65.0
    cutaneous B65.3
    galacturia B65.0
    hematochyluria B65.0
    intestinal B65.1
    lipemia B65.9
    lipuria B65.0
    oriental B65.2
    piarhemia B65.9
    pulmonary NOS B65.9 [J99]
        pneumonia B65.9 [J17]
    tropical hematuria B65.0
    vesical B65.0

Biliary —see condition

Bilirubin metabolism disorder E80.7
    specified NEC E80.6

Bilirubinemia, familial nonhemolytic E80.4

Bilirubinuria R82.2

Biliuria R82.2

Bilocular stomach K31.2

Binswanger's disease I67.3

Biparta, bipartite
    carpal scaphoid Q74.0
    patella Q74.1
    vagina Q52.10

BI-RADS —see Breast, Imaging Reporting and Data System

Bird
    face Q75.8
    fancier's disease or lung J67.2

Birt-Hogg-Dube syndrome Q87.89

Birth
    complications in mother —see Delivery, complicated
    compression during NOS P15.9
    defect —see Anomaly

Birth
    immature (less than 37 completed weeks) —see Preterm, newborn
        extremely (less than 28 completed weeks) —see Immaturity, extreme
    inattention, at or after —see Maltreatment, child, neglect
    injury NOS P15.9
        basal ganglia P11.1
        brachial plexus NEC P14.3
        brain (compression) (pressure) P11.2
        central nervous system NOS P11.9
        cerebellum P11.1
        cerebral hemorrhage P10.1
        external genitalia P15.5
        eye P15.3
        face P15.4
        fracture
            bone P13.9
                specified NEC P13.8
            clavicle P13.4
            femur P13.2
            humerus P13.3
            long bone, except femur P13.3
            radius and ulna P13.3
            skull P13.0
            spine P11.5
            tibia and fibula P13.3
        intracranial P11.2
            laceration or hemorrhage P10.9
                specified NEC P10.8
        intraventricular hemorrhage P10.2
        laceration
            brain P10.1
            by scalpel P15.8
            peripheral nerve P14.9
        liver P15.0
        meninges
            brain P11.1
            spinal cord P11.5
        nerve
            brachial plexus P14.3
            cranial NEC (except facial) P11.4
            facial P11.3
            peripheral P14.9
            phrenic (paralysis) P14.2
        paralysis
            facial nerve P11.3
            spinal P11.5
        penis P15.5
        rupture
            spinal cord P11.5
        scalp P12.9
        scalpel wound P15.8
        scrotum P15.5
        skull NEC P13.1
            fracture P13.0
        specified type NEC P15.8
        spinal cord P11.5
        spine P11.5
        spleen P15.1
        sternomastoid (hematoma) P15.2
        subarachnoid hemorrhage P10.3
        subcutaneous fat necrosis P15.6
        subdural hemorrhage P10.0
        tentorial tear P10.4
        testes P15.5
        vulva P15.5
    lack of care, at or after —see Maltreatment, child, neglect
    neglect, at or after —see Maltreatment, child, neglect
    palsy or paralysis, newborn, NOS (birth injury) P14.9
    premature (infant) —see Preterm, newborn
    shock, newborn P96.89
    trauma —see Birth, injury

Birth (continued)
    weight
        low (2499 grams or less) —see Low, birthweight
            extremely (999 grams or less) —see Low, birthweight, extreme
        4000 grams to 4499 grams P08.1
        4500 grams or more P08.0

Birthmark Q82.5

Bisalbuminemia E88.09

Biskra's button B55.1

Bite(s) (animal) (human)
    abdomen, abdominal
        wall S31.159
            with penetration into peritoneal cavity S31.659
            epigastric region S31.152
                with penetration into peritoneal cavity S31.652
            left
                lower quadrant S31.154
                    with penetration into peritoneal cavity S31.654
                upper quadrant S31.151
                    with penetration into peritoneal cavity S31.651
            periumbilic region S31.155
                with penetration into peritoneal cavity S31.655
            right
                lower quadrant S31.153
                    with penetration into peritoneal cavity S31.653
                upper quadrant S31.150
                    with penetration into peritoneal cavity S31.650
            superficial NEC S30.871
                insect S30.861
    alveolar (process) —see Bite, oral cavity
    amphibian (venomous) —see Venom, bite, amphibian
    animal —see also Bite, by site
        venomous —see Venom
    ankle S91.05-
        superficial NEC S90.57-
            insect S90.56-
    antecubital space —see Bite, elbow
    anus S31.835
        superficial NEC S30.877
            insect S30.867
    arm (upper) S41.15-
        lower —see Bite, forearm
        superficial NEC S40.87-
            insect S40.86-
    arthropod NEC —see Venom, bite, arthropod
    auditory canal (external) (meatus) —see Bite, ear
    auricle, ear —see Bite, ear
    axilla —see Bite, arm
    back —see also Bite, thorax, back
        lower S31.050
            with penetration into retroperitoneal space S31.051
            superficial NEC S30.870
                insect S30.860
    bedbug —see Bite(s), by site, superficial, insect
    breast S21.05-
        superficial NEC S20.17-
            insect S20.16-
    brow —see Bite, head, specified site NEC

Bite (continued)
    buttock S31.805
        left S31.825
        right S31.815
        superficial NEC S30.870
            insect S30.860
    calf —see Bite, leg
    canaliculus lacrimalis —see Bite, eyelid
    canthus, eye —see Bite, eyelid
    centipede —see Toxicity, venom, arthropod, centipede
    cheek (external) S01.45-
        superficial NEC S00.87
            insect S00.86
        internal —see Bite, oral cavity
    chest wall —see Bite, thorax
    chigger B88.0
    chin —see Bite, head, specified site NEC
    clitoris —see Bite, vulva
    costal region —see Bite, thorax
    digit(s)
        hand —see Bite, finger
        toe —see Bite, toe
    ear (canal) (external) S01.35-
        superficial NEC S00.47-
            insect S00.46-
    elbow S51.05-
        superficial NEC S50.37-
            insect S50.36-
    epididymis —see Bite, testis
    epigastric region —see Bite, abdomen
    epiglottis —see Bite, neck, specified site NEC
    esophagus, cervical S11.25
        superficial NEC S10.17
            insect S10.16
    eyebrow —see Bite, eyelid
    eyelid S01.15-
        superficial NEC S00.27-
            insect S00.26-
    face NEC —see Bite, head, specified site NEC
    finger(s) S61.259
        with
            damage to nail S61.359
        index S61.258
            with
                damage to nail S61.358
            left S61.251
                with
                    damage to nail S61.351
            right S61.250
                with
                    damage to nail S61.350
            superficial NEC S60.478
                insect S60.46-
        little S61.25-
            with
                damage to nail S61.35-
            superficial NEC S60.47-
                insect S60.46-
        middle S61.25-
            with
                damage to nail S61.35-
            superficial NEC S60.47-
                insect S60.46-
        ring S61.25-
            with
                damage to nail S61.35-
            superficial NEC S60.47-
                insect S60.46-
        superficial NEC S60.479
            insect S60.469
        thumb —see Bite, thumb
    flank —see Bite, abdomen, wall
    flea —see Bite, by site, superficial, insect

Bite (*continued*)
 foot (except toe(s) alone) S91.35-
  superficial NEC S90.87-
   insect S90.86-
  toe —*see* Bite, toe
 forearm S51.85-
  elbow only —*see* Bite, elbow
  superficial NEC S50.87-
   insect S50.86-
 forehead —*see* Bite, head, specified site NEC
 genital organs, external
  female S31.552
   superficial NEC S30.876
    insect S30.866
   vagina and vulva —*see* Bite, vulva
  male S31.551
   penis —*see* Bite, penis
   scrotum —*see* Bite, scrotum
   superficial NEC S30.875
    insect S30.865
   testes —*see* Bite, testis
 groin —*see* Bite, abdomen, wall
 gum —*see* Bite, oral cavity
 hand S61.45-
  finger —*see* Bite, finger
  superficial NEC S60.57-
   insect S60.56-
  thumb —*see* Bite, thumb
 head S01.95
  cheek —*see* Bite, cheek
  ear —*see* Bite, ear
  eyelid —*see* Bite, eyelid
  lip —*see* Bite, lip
  nose —*see* Bite, nose
  oral cavity —*see* Bite, oral cavity
  scalp —*see* Bite, scalp
  specified site NEC S01.85
   superficial NEC S00.87
    insect S00.86
  superficial NEC S00.97
   insect S00.96
  temporomandibular area —*see* Bite, cheek
 heel —*see* Bite, foot
 hip S71.05-
  superficial NEC S70.27-
   insect S70.26-
 hymen S31.45
 hypochondrium —*see* Bite, abdomen, wall
 hypogastric region —*see* Bite, abdomen, wall
 inguinal region —*see* Bite, abdomen, wall
 insect —*see* Bite, by site, superficial, insect
 instep —*see* Bite, foot
 interscapular region —*see* Bite, thorax, back
 jaw —*see* Bite, head, specified site NEC
 knee S81.05-
  superficial NEC S80.27-
   insect S80.26-
 labium (majus) (minus) —*see* Bite, vulva
 lacrimal duct —*see* Bite, eyelid
 larynx S11.015
  superficial NEC S10.17
   insect S10.16
 leg (lower) S81.85-
  ankle —*see* Bite, ankle
  foot —*see* Bite, foot
  knee —*see* Bite, knee
  superficial NEC S80.87-
   insect S80.86-
  toe —*see* Bite, toe
  upper —*see* Bite, thigh

Bite (*continued*)
 lip S01.551
  superficial NEC S00.571
   insect S00.561
 lizard (venomous) —*see* Venom, bite, reptile
 loin —*see* Bite, abdomen, wall
 lower back —*see* Bite, back, lower
 lumbar region —*see* Bite, back, lower
 malar region —*see* Bite, head, specified site NEC
 mammary —*see* Bite, breast
 marine animals (venomous) —*see* Toxicity, venom, marine animal
 mastoid region —*see* Bite, head, specified site NEC
 mouth —*see* Bite, oral cavity
 nail
  finger —*see* Bite, finger
  toe —*see* Bite, toe
 nape —*see* Bite, neck, specified site NEC
 nasal (septum) (sinus) —*see* Bite, nose
 nasopharynx —*see* Bite, head, specified site NEC
 neck S11.95
  involving
   cervical esophagus —*see* Bite, esophagus, cervical
   larynx —*see* Bite, larynx
   pharynx —*see* Bite, pharynx
   thyroid gland S11.15
   trachea —*see* Bite, trachea
  specified site NEC S11.85
   superficial NEC S10.87
    insect S10.86
  superficial NEC S10.97
   insect S10.96
  throat S11.85
   superficial NEC S10.17
    insect S10.16
 nose (septum) (sinus) S01.25
  superficial NEC S00.37
   insect S00.36
 occipital region —*see* Bite, scalp
 oral cavity S01.552
  superficial NEC S00.572
   insect S00.562
 orbital region —*see* Bite, eyelid
 palate —*see* Bite, oral cavity
 palm —*see* Bite, hand
 parietal region —*see* Bite, scalp
 pelvis S31.050
  with penetration into retroperitoneal space S31.051
  superficial NEC S30.870
   insect S30.860
 penis S31.25
  superficial NEC S30.872
   insect S30.862
 perineum
  female —*see* Bite, vulva
  male —*see* Bite, pelvis
 periocular area (with or without lacrimal passages) —*see* Bite, eyelid
 phalanges
  finger —*see* Bite, finger
  toe —*see* Bite, toe
 pharynx S11.25
  superficial NEC S10.17
   insect S10.16
 pinna —*see* Bite, ear
 poisonous —*see* Venom
 popliteal space —*see* Bite, knee
 prepuce —*see* Bite, penis
 pubic region —*see* Bite, abdomen, wall
 rectovaginal septum —*see* Bite, vulva
 red bug B88.0

Bite (*continued*)
 reptile NEC —*see also* Venom, bite, reptile
  nonvenomous —*see* Bite, by site
  snake —*see* Venom, bite, snake
 sacral region —*see* Bite, back, lower
 sacroiliac region —*see* Bite, back, lower
 salivary gland —*see* Bite, oral cavity
 scalp S01.05
  superficial NEC S00.07
   insect S00.06
 scapular region —*see* Bite, shoulder
 scrotum S31.35
  superficial NEC S30.873
   insect S30.863
 sea-snake (venomous) —*see* Toxicity, venom, snake, sea snake
 shin —*see* Bite, leg
 shoulder S41.05-
  superficial NEC S40.27-
   insect S40.26-
 snake —*see also* Venom, bite, snake
  nonvenomous —*see* Bite, by site
 spermatic cord —*see* Bite, testis
 spider (venomous) —*see* Toxicity, venom, spider
  nonvenomous —*see* Bite, by site, superficial, insect
 sternal region —*see* Bite, thorax, front
 submaxillary region —*see* Bite, head, specified site NEC
 submental region —*see* Bite, head, specified site NEC
 subungual
  finger(s) —*see* Bite, finger
  toe —*see* Bite, toe
 superficial —*see* Bite, by site, superficial
 supraclavicular fossa S11.85
 supraorbital —*see* Bite, head, specified site NEC
 temple, temporal region —*see* Bite, head, specified site NEC
 temporomandibular area —*see* Bite, cheek
 testis S31.35
  superficial NEC S30.873
   insect S30.863
 thigh S71.15-
  superficial NEC S70.37-
   insect S70.36-
 thorax, thoracic (wall) S21.95
  back S21.25-
   with penetration into thoracic cavity S21.45-
  breast —*see* Bite, breast
  front S21.15-
   with penetration into thoracic cavity S21.35-
  superficial NEC S20.97
   back S20.47-
   front S20.37-
   insect S20.96
    back S20.46-
    front S20.36-
 throat —*see* Bite, neck, throat
 thumb S61.05-
  with
   damage to nail S61.15-
  superficial NEC S60.37-
   insect S60.36-
 thyroid S11.15
  superficial NEC S10.87
   insect S10.86
 toe(s) S91.15-
  with
   damage to nail S91.25-
  great S91.15-
   with
    damage to nail S91.25-

Bite (*continued*)
 toe(s) (*continued*)
  lesser S91.15-
   with
    damage to nail S91.25-
  superficial NEC S90.47-
   great S90.47-
   insect S90.46-
    great S90.46-
 tongue S01.552
 trachea S11.025
  superficial NEC S10.17
   insect S10.16
 tunica vaginalis —*see* Bite, testis
 tympanum, tympanic membrane —*see* Bite, ear
 umbilical region S31.155
 uvula —*see* Bite, oral cavity
 vagina —*see* Bite, vulva
 venomous —*see* Venom
 vocal cords S11.035
  superficial NEC S10.17
   insect S10.16
 vulva S31.45
  superficial NEC S30.874
   insect S30.864
 wrist S61.55-
  superficial NEC S60.87-
   insect S60.86-

Biting, cheek or lip K13.1

Biventricular failure (heart) I50.82

Björck (-Thorson) **syndrome** (malignant carcinoid) E34.0

Black
 death A20.9
 eye S00.1-
 hairy tongue K14.3
 heel (foot) S90.3-
 lung (disease) J60
 palm (hand) S60.22-

Blackfan-Diamond anemia or syndrome (congenital hypoplastic anemia) D61.01

Blackhead L70.0

Blackout R55

Bladder —*see* condition

Blast (air) (hydraulic) (immersion) (underwater)
 blindness S05.8X-
 injury
  abdomen or thorax —*see* Injury, by site
  ear (acoustic nerve trauma) —*see* Injury, nerve, acoustic, specified type NEC
 syndrome NEC T70.8

Blastoma —*see* Neoplasm, malignant, by site
 pulmonary —*see* Neoplasm, lung, malignant

Blastomycosis, blastomycotic B40.9
 Brazilian —*see* Paracoccidioidomycosis
 cutaneous B40.3
 disseminated B40.7
 European —*see* Cryptococcosis
 generalized B40.7
 keloidal B48.0
 North American B40.9
 primary pulmonary B40.0
 pulmonary B40.2
  acute B40.0
  chronic B40.1
 skin B40.3

41

Blastomycosis, blastomycotic (continued)
South American —see Paracoccidioidomycosis
specified NEC B40.89

Bleb(s) R23.8
emphysematous (lung) (solitary) J43.9
endophthalmitis H59.43
filtering (vitreous), after glaucoma surgery Z98.83
inflamed (infected), postprocedural H59.40
stage 1 H59.41
stage 2 H59.42
stage 3 H59.43
lung (ruptured) J43.9
congenital —see Atelectasis
newborn P25.8
subpleural (emphysematous) J43.9

Blebitis, postprocedural H59.40
stage 1 H59.41
stage 2 H59.42
stage 3 H59.43

Bleeder (familial) (hereditary) —see Hemophilia

Bleeding —see also Hemorrhage
anal K62.5
anovulatory N97.0
atonic, following delivery O72.1
capillary I78.8
puerperal O72.2
contact (postcoital) N93.0
due to uterine subinvolution N85.3
ear —see Otorrhagia
excessive, associated with menopausal onset N92.4
familial —see Defect, coagulation
following intercourse N93.0
gastrointestinal K92.2
hemorrhoids —see Hemorrhoids
intermenstrual (regular) N92.3
irregular N92.1
intraoperative —see Complication, intraoperative, hemorrhage
irregular N92.6
menopausal N92.4
newborn, intraventricular —see Newborn, affected by, hemorrhage, intraventricular
nipple N64.59
nose R04.0
ovulation N92.3
perimenopausal N92.4
pre-pubertal vaginal N93.1
postclimacteric N95.0
postcoital N93.0
postmenopausal N95.0
postoperative —see Complication, postprocedural, hemorrhage
preclimacteric N92.4
puberty (excessive, with onset of menstrual periods) N92.2
rectum, rectal K62.5
newborn P54.2
tendencies —see Defect, coagulation
throat R04.1
tooth socket (post-extraction) K91.840
umbilical stump P51.9
uterus, uterine NEC N93.9
climacteric N92.4
dysfunctional or functional N93.8
menopausal N92.4
preclimacteric or premenopausal N92.4
unrelated to menstrual cycle N93.9

Bleeding (continued)
vagina, vaginal (abnormal) N93.9
dysfunctional or functional N93.8
newborn P54.6
pre-pubertal N93.1
vicarious N94.89

Blennorrhagia, blennorrhagic —see Gonorrhea

Blennorrhea (acute) (chronic) —see also Gonorrhea
inclusion (neonatal) (newborn) P39.1
lower genitourinary tract (gonococcal) A54.00
neonatorum (gonococcal ophthalmia) A54.31

Blepharelosis —see Entropion

Blepharitis (angularis) (ciliaris) (eyelid) (marginal) (nonulcerative) H01.009
herpes zoster B02.39
left H01.006
lower H01.005
upper H01.004
upper and lower H01.00B
right H01.003
lower H01.002
upper H01.001
upper and lower H01.00A
squamous H01.029
left H01.026
lower H01.025
upper H01.024
upper and lower H01.02B
right H01.023
lower H01.022
upper H01.021
upper and lower H01.02A
ulcerative H01.019
left H01.016
lower H01.015
upper H01.014
upper and lower H01.01B
right H01.013
lower H01.012
upper H01.011
upper and lower H01.01A

Blepharochalasis H02.30
congenital Q10.0
left H02.36
lower H02.35
upper H02.34
right H02.33
lower H02.32
upper H02.31

Blepharoclonus H02.59

Blepharoconjunctivitis H10.50-
angular H10.52-
contact H10.53-
ligneous H10.51-

Blepharophimosis (eyelid) H02.529
congenital Q10.3
left H02.526
lower H02.525
upper H02.524
right H02.523
lower H02.522
upper H02.521

Blepharoptosis H02.40-
congenital Q10.0
mechanical H02.41-
myogenic H02.42-
neurogenic H02.43-
paralytic H02.43-

Blepharopyorrhea, gonococcal A54.39

Blepharospasm G24.5
drug induced G24.01

Blighted ovum O02.0

Blind —see also Blindness
bronchus (congenital) Q32.4
loop syndrome K90.2
congenital Q43.8
sac, fallopian tube (congenital) Q50.6
spot, enlarged —see Defect, visual field, localized, scotoma, blind spot area
tract or tube, congenital NEC —see Atresia, by site

Blindness (acquired) (congenital) (both eyes) H54.0X-
blast S05.8X-
color —see Deficiency, color vision
concussion S05.8X-
cortical H47.619
left brain H47.612
right brain H47.611
day H53.11
due to injury (current episode) S05.9-
sequelae -- code to injury with seventh character S
eclipse (total) —see Retinopathy, solar
emotional (hysterical) F44.6
face H53.16
hysterical F44.6
legal (both eyes) (USA definition) H54.8
mind R48.8
night H53.60
abnormal dark adaptation curve H53.61
acquired H53.62
congenital H53.63
specified type NEC H53.69
vitamin A deficiency E50.5
one eye (other eye normal) H54.40
left (normal vision on right) H54.42-
low vision on right H54.12-
low vision, other eye H54.10
right (normal vision on left) H54.41-
low vision on left H54.11-
psychic R48.8
river B73.01
snow —see Photokeratitis
sun, solar —see Retinopathy, solar
transient —see Disturbance, vision, subjective, loss, transient
traumatic (current episode) S05.9-
word (developmental) F81.0
acquired R48.0
secondary to organic lesion R48.0

Blister (nonthermal)
abdominal wall S30.821
alveolar process S00.522
ankle S90.52-
antecubital space —see Blister, elbow
anus S30.827
arm (upper) S40.82-
auditory canal —see Blister, ear
auricle —see Blister, ear
axilla —see Blister, arm
back, lower S30.820
beetle dermatitis L24.89
breast S20.12-
brow S00.82
calf —see Blister, leg
canthus —see Blister, eyelid
cheek S00.82
internal S00.522
chest wall —see Blister, thorax
chin S00.82
costal region —see Blister, thorax

Blister (continued)
digit(s)
foot —see Blister, toe
hand —see Blister, finger
due to burn —see Burn, by site, second degree
ear S00.42-
elbow S50.32-
epiglottis S10.12
esophagus, cervical S10.12
eyebrow —see Blister, eyelid
eyelid S00.22-
face S00.82
fever B00.1
finger(s) S60.429
index S60.42-
little S60.42-
middle S60.42-
ring S60.42-
foot (except toe(s) alone) S90.82-
toe —see Blister, toe
forearm S50.82-
elbow only —see Blister, elbow
forehead S00.82
fracture - omit code
genital organ
female S30.826
male S30.825
gum S00.522
hand S60.52-
head S00.92
ear —see Blister, ear
eyelid —see Blister, eyelid
lip S00.521
nose S00.32
oral cavity S00.522
scalp S00.02
specified site NEC S00.82
heel —see Blister, foot
hip S70.22-
interscapular region S20.429
jaw S00.82
knee S80.22-
larynx S10.12
leg (lower) S80.82-
knee —see Blister, knee
upper —see Blister, thigh
lip S00.521
malar region S00.82
mammary —see Blister, breast
mastoid region S00.82
mouth S00.522
multiple, skin, nontraumatic R23.8
nail
finger —see Blister, finger
toe —see Blister, toe
nasal S00.32
neck S10.92
specified site NEC S10.82
throat S10.12
nose S00.32
occipital region S00.02
oral cavity S00.522
orbital region —see Blister, eyelid
palate S00.522
palm —see Blister, hand
parietal region S00.02
pelvis S30.820
penis S30.822
periocular area —see Blister, eyelid
phalanges
finger —see Blister, finger
toe —see Blister, toe
pharynx S10.12
pinna —see Blister, ear
popliteal space —see Blister, knee
scalp S00.02
scapular region —see Blister, shoulder

Blister (continued)
scrotum S30.823
shin —see Blister, leg
shoulder S40.22-
sternal region S20.329
submaxillary region S00.82
submental region S00.82
subungual
finger(s) —see Blister, finger
toe(s) —see Blister, toe
supraclavicular fossa S10.82
supraorbital S00.82
temple S00.82
temporal region S00.82
testis S30.823
thermal —see Burn, by site, second degree
thigh S70.32-
thorax, thoracic (wall) S20.92
back S20.42-
front S20.32-
throat S10.12
thumb S60.32-
toe(s) S90.42-
great S90.42-
tongue S00.522
trachea S10.12
tympanum, tympanic membrane —see Blister, ear
upper arm —see Blister, arm (upper)
uvula S00.522
vagina S30.824
vocal cords S10.12
vulva S30.824
wrist S60.82-

Bloating R14.0

Bloch-Sulzberger disease or syndrome Q82.3

Block, blocked
alveolocapillary J84.10
arborization (heart) I45.5
arrhythmic I45.9
atrioventricular (incomplete) (partial) I44.30
with atrioventricular dissociation I44.2
complete I44.2
congenital Q24.6
congenital Q24.6
first degree I44.0
second degree (types I and II) I44.1
specified NEC I44.39
third degree I44.2
types I and II I44.1
auriculoventricular —see Block, atrioventricular
bifascicular (cardiac) I45.2
bundle-branch (complete) (false) (incomplete) I45.4
bilateral I45.2
left I44.7
with right bundle branch block I45.2
hemiblock I44.60
anterior I44.4
posterior I44.5
incomplete I44.7
with right bundle branch block I45.2
right I45.10
with
left bundle branch block I45.2
left fascicular block I45.2
specified NEC I45.19
Wilson's type I45.19
cardiac I45.9
conduction I45.9
complete I44.2

Block, blocked (continued)
fascicular (left) I44.60
anterior I44.4
posterior I44.5
right I45.0
specified NEC I44.69
foramen Magendie (acquired) G91.1
congenital Q03.1
with spina bifida —see Spina bifida, by site, with hydrocephalus
heart I45.9
bundle branch I45.4
bilateral I45.2
complete (atrioventricular) I44.2
congenital Q24.6
first degree (atrioventricular) I44.0
second degree (atrioventricular) I44.1
specified type NEC I45.5
third degree (atrioventricular) I44.2
hepatic vein I82.0
intraventricular (nonspecific) I45.4
bundle branch
bilateral I45.2
kidney N28.9
postcystoscopic or postprocedural N99.0
Mobitz (types I and II) I44.1
myocardial —see Block, heart
nodal I45.5
organ or site, congenital NEC —see Atresia, by site
portal (vein) I81
second degree (types I and II) I44.1
sinoatrial I45.5
sinoauricular I45.5
third degree I44.2
trifascicular I45.3
tubal N97.1
vein NOS I82.90
Wenckebach (types I and II) I44.1

Blockage —see Obstruction

Blocq's disease F44.4

Blood
constituents, abnormal R78.9
disease D75.9
donor —see Donor, blood
dyscrasia D75.9
with
abortion —see Abortion, by type, complicated by, hemorrhage
ectopic pregnancy O08.1
molar pregnancy O08.1
following ectopic or molar pregnancy O08.1
newborn P61.9
puerperal, postpartum O72.3
flukes NEC —see Schistosomiasis
in
feces K92.1
occult R19.5
urine —see Hematuria
mole O02.0
occult in feces R19.5
pressure
decreased, due to shock following injury T79.4
examination only Z01.30
fluctuating I99.8
high —see Hypertension
borderline R03.0
incidental reading, without diagnosis of hypertension R03.0

Blood (continued)
pressure (continued)
low —see also Hypotension
incidental reading, without diagnosis of hypotension R03.1
spitting —see Hemoptysis
staining cornea —see Pigmentation, cornea, stromal
transfusion
reaction or complication —see Complications, transfusion
type
A (Rh positive) Z67.10
Rh negative Z67.11
AB (Rh positive) Z67.30
Rh negative Z67.31
B (Rh positive) Z67.20
Rh negative Z67.21
O (Rh positive) Z67.40
Rh negative Z67.41
Rh (positive) Z67.90
negative Z67.91
vessel rupture —see Hemorrhage
vomiting —see Hematemesis

Blood-forming organs, disease D75.9

Bloodgood's disease —see Mastopathy, cystic

Bloom (-Machacek) (-Torre) syndrome Q82.8

Blount disease or osteochondrosis M92.51-

Blue
baby Q24.9
diaper syndrome E72.09
dome cyst (breast) —see Cyst, breast
dot cataract Q12.0
nevus D22.9
sclera Q13.5
with fragility of bone and deafness Q78.0
toe syndrome I75.02-

Blueness —see Cyanosis

Blues, postpartal O90.6
baby O90.6

Blurring, visual H53.8

Blushing (abnormal) (excessive) R23.2

BMI —see Body, mass index

Boarder, hospital NEC Z76.4
accompanying sick person Z76.3
healthy infant or child Z76.2
foundling Z76.1

Bockhart's impetigo L01.02

Bodechtel-Guttman disease (subacute sclerosing panencephalitis) A81.1

Boder-Sedgwick syndrome (ataxia-telangiectasia) G11.3

Body, bodies
Aschoff's —see Myocarditis, rheumatic
asteroid, vitreous —see Deposit, crystalline
cytoid (retina) —see Occlusion, artery, retina
drusen (degenerative) (macula) (retinal) —see also Degeneration, macula, drusen
optic disc —see Drusen, optic disc
foreign —see Foreign body

Body, bodies (continued)
loose
joint, except knee —see Loose, body, joint
knee M23.4-
sheath, tendon —see Disorder, tendon, specified type NEC
mass index (BMI)
adult
19.9 or less Z68.1
20.0-20.9 Z68.20
21.0-21.9 Z68.21
22.0-22.9 Z68.22
23.0-23.9 Z68.23
24.0-24.9 Z68.24
25.0-25.9 Z68.25
26.0-26.9 Z68.26
27.0-27.9 Z68.27
28.0-28.9 Z68.28
29.0-29.9 Z68.29
30.0-30.9 Z68.30
31.0-31.9 Z68.31
32.0-32.9 Z68.32
33.0-33.9 Z68.33
34.0-34.9 Z68.34
35.0-35.9 Z68.35
36.0-36.9 Z68.36
37.0-37.9 Z68.37
38.0-38.9 Z68.38
39.0-39.9 Z68.39
40.0-44.9 Z68.41
45.0-49.9 Z68.42
50.0-59.9 Z68.43
60.0-69.9 Z68.44
70 and over Z68.45
pediatric
5th percentile to less than 85th percentile for age Z68.52
85th percentile to less than 95th percentile for age Z68.53
greater than or equal to ninety-fifth percentile for age Z68.54
less than fifth percentile for age Z68.51
Mooser's A75.2
rice —see also Loose, body, joint
knee M23.4-
rocking F98.4

Boeck's
disease or sarcoid —see Sarcoidosis
lupoid (miliary) D86.3

Boerhaave's syndrome (spontaneous esophageal rupture) K22.3

Boggy
cervix N88.8
uterus N85.8

Boil —see also Furuncle, by site
Aleppo B55.1
Baghdad B55.1
Delhi B55.1
lacrimal
gland —see Dacryoadenitis
passages (duct) (sac) —see Inflammation, lacrimal, passages, acute
Natal B55.1
orbit, orbital —see Abscess, orbit
tropical B55.1

Bold hives —see Urticaria

Bombé, iris —see Membrane, pupillary

Bone —see condition

Bonnevie-Ullrich syndrome (see also Turner's syndrome) Q87.19

Bonnier's syndrome —see subcategory H81.8
Bonvale dam fever T73.3
Bony block of joint —see Ankylosis
BOOP (bronchiolitis obliterans organized pneumonia) J84.89
Borderline
  diabetes mellitus R73.03
  hypertension R03.0
  osteopenia M85.8-
  pelvis, with obstruction during labor O65.1
  personality F60.3
Borna disease A83.9
Bornholm disease B33.0
Boston exanthem A88.0
Botalli, ductus (patent) (persistent) Q25.0
Bothriocephalus latus infestation B70.0
Botulism (foodborne intoxication) A05.1
  infant A48.51
  non-foodborne A48.52
  wound A48.52
Bouba —see Yaws
Bouchard's nodes (with arthropathy) M15.2
Bouffée délirante F23
Bouillaud's disease or syndrome (rheumatic heart disease) I01.9
Bourneville's disease Q85.1
Boutonniere deformity (finger) —see Deformity, finger, boutonniere
Bouveret (-Hoffmann) syndrome (paroxysmal tachycardia) I47.9
Bovine heart —see Hypertrophy, cardiac
Bowel —see condition
Bowen's
  dermatosis (precancerous) —see Neoplasm, skin, in situ
  disease —see Neoplasm, skin, in situ
  epithelioma —see Neoplasm, skin, in situ
  type
    epidermoid carcinoma-in-situ —see Neoplasm, skin, in situ
    intraepidermal squamous cell carcinoma —see Neoplasm, skin, in situ
Bowing
  femur —see also Deformity, limb, specified type NEC, thigh
    congenital Q68.3
  fibula —see also Deformity, limb, specified type NEC, lower leg
    congenital Q68.4
  forearm —see Deformity, limb, specified type NEC, forearm
  leg(s), long bones, congenital Q68.5
  radius —see Deformity, limb, specified type NEC, forearm
  tibia —see also Deformity, limb, specified type NEC, lower leg
    congenital Q68.4
Bowleg(s) (acquired) M21.16-
  congenital Q68.5
  rachitic E64.3
Boyd's dysentery A03.2

Brachial —see condition
Brachycardia R00.1
Brachycephaly, non-deformational Q75.022
Bradley's disease A08.19
Bradyarrhythmia, cardiac I49.8
Bradycardia (sinoatrial) (sinus) (vagal) R00.1
  neonatal P29.12
  reflex G90.09
  tachycardia syndrome I49.5
Bradykinesia R25.8
Bradypnea R06.89
Bradytachycardia I49.5
Brailsford's disease or osteochondrosis —see Osteochondrosis, juvenile, radius
Brain —see also condition
  death G93.82
  syndrome —see Syndrome, brain
Branched-chain amino-acid disorder E71.2
Branchial —see condition
  cartilage, congenital Q18.2
Branchiogenic remnant (in neck) Q18.0
Brandt's syndrome (acrodermatitis enteropathica) E83.2
Brash (water) R12
Bravais-jacksonian epilepsy —see Epilepsy, localization-related, symptomatic, with simple partial seizures
Braxton Hicks contractions —see False, labor
Brazilian leishmaniasis B55.2
BRBPR K62.5
Break, retina (without detachment) H33.30-
  with retinal detachment —see Detachment, retina
  horseshoe tear H33.31-
  multiple H33.33-
  round hole H33.32-
Breakdown
  device, graft or implant —see also Complications, by site and type, mechanical T85.618
    arterial graft NEC —see Complication, cardiovascular device, mechanical, vascular
    breast (implant) T85.41
    catheter NEC T85.618
      cystostomy T83.010
      dialysis (renal) T82.41
        intraperitoneal T85.611
      Hopkins T83.018
      ileostomy T83.018
      infusion NEC T82.514
        cranial T85.610
        epidural T85.610
        intrathecal T85.610
        spinal T85.610
        subarachnoid T85.610
        subdural T85.610
      nephrostomy T83.012
      urethral indwelling T83.011
      urinary NEC T83.018
      urostomy T83.018

Breakdown (continued)
  device, graft or implant (continued)
    electronic (electrode) (pulse generator) (stimulator)
      bone T84.310
      cardiac T82.119
        electrode T82.110
        pulse generator T82.111
        specified type NEC T82.118
      nervous system —see Complication, prosthetic device, mechanical, electronic nervous system stimulator
      urinary —see Complication, genitourinary, device, urinary, mechanical
    fixation, internal (orthopedic) NEC —see Complication, fixation device, mechanical
    gastrointestinal —see Complications, prosthetic device, mechanical, gastrointestinal device
    genital NEC T83.418
      intrauterine contraceptive device T83.31
      penile prosthesis (cylinder) (implanted) (pump) (resevoir) T83.410
      testicular prosthesis T83.411
    heart NEC —see Complication, cardiovascular device, mechanical
    intrathecal infusion pump T85.615
    joint prosthesis —see Complications..., joint prosthesis, internal, mechanical, by site
    nervous system, specified device NEC T85.615
    ocular NEC —see Complications, prosthetic device, mechanical, ocular device
    orthopedic NEC —see Complication, orthopedic, device, mechanical
    specified NEC T85.618
    subcutaneous device pocket
      nervous system prosthetic device, implant, or graft T85.890
      other internal prosthetic device, implant or graft T85.898
    sutures, permanent T85.612
      used in bone repair —see Complications, fixation device, internal (orthopedic), mechanical
    urinary NEC T83.118
      graft T83.21
      sphincter, implanted T83.111
      stent (ileal conduit) (nephroureteral) T83.113
      ureteral indwelling T83.112
    vascular NEC —see Complication, cardiovascular device, mechanical
    ventricular intracranial shunt T85.01
  nervous F48.8
  perineum O90.1
  respirator J95.850
    specified NEC J95.859
    ventilator J95.850
    specified NEC J95.859

Breast —see also condition
  buds E30.1
    in newborn P96.89
  dense R92.3-
  Imaging Reporting and Data System (BI-RADS) : A R92.31-
  Imaging Reporting and Data System (BI-RADS) : B R92.32-
  Imaging Reporting and Data System (BI-RADS) : C R92.33-
  Imaging Reporting and Data System (BI-RADS) : D R92.34-
  Imaging Reporting and Data System (BI-RADS) : 1 R92.31-
  Imaging Reporting and Data System (BI-RADS) : 2 R92.32-
  Imaging Reporting and Data System (BI-RADS) : 3 R92.33-
  Imaging Reporting and Data System (BI-RADS) : 4 R92.34-
  nodule (see also Lump, breast) N63.0
Breath
  foul R19.6
  holder, child R06.89
  holding spell R06.89
  shortness R06.02
Breathing
  labored —see Hyperventilation
  mouth R06.5
    causing malocclusion M26.5
  periodic R06.3
    high altitude G47.32
Breathlessness R06.81
Breda's disease —see Yaws
Breech presentation (mother) O32.1
  causing obstructed labor O64.1
  footling O32.8
    causing obstructed labor O64.8
  incomplete O32.8
    causing obstructed labor O64.8
Breisky's disease N90.4
Brennemann's syndrome I88.0
Brenner
  tumor (benign) D27.9
    borderline malignancy D39.1-
    malignant C56
    proliferating D39.1-
Bretonneau's disease or angina A36.0
Breus' mole O02.0
Brevicollis Q76.49
Brickmakers' anemia B76.9 *[D63.8]*
Bridge, myocardial Q24.5
Bright red blood per rectum (BRBPR) K62.5
Bright's disease —see also Nephritis
  arteriosclerotic —see Hypertension, kidney
Brill (-Zinsser) disease (recrudescent typhus) A75.1
Brill-Symmers' disease C82.90
Brion-Kayser disease —see Fever, parathyroid
Briquet's disorder or syndrome F45.0
Brissaud's
  infantilism or dwarfism E23.0
  motor-verbal tic F95.2
Brittle
  bones disease Q78.0
  nails L60.3
    congenital Q84.6

Broad —see also condition
  beta disease E78.2
  ligament laceration syndrome N83.8
Broad- or floating-betalipoproteinemia E78.2
Brock's syndrome (atelectasis due to enlarged lymph nodes) J98.19
Brocq-Duhring disease (dermatitis herpetiformis) L13.0
Brodie's abscess or disease M86.8X-
Broken
  arches —see also Deformity, limb, flat foot
  arm (meaning upper limb) —see Fracture, arm
  back —see Fracture, vertebra
  bone —see Fracture
  implant or internal device —see Complications, by site and type, mechanical
  leg (meaning lower limb) —see Fracture, leg
  nose S02.2
  tooth, teeth —see Fracture, tooth
Bromhidrosis, bromidrosis L75.0
Bromidism, bromism G92.8
  due to
    correct substance properly administered —see Table of Drugs and Chemicals, by drug, adverse effect
    overdose or wrong substance given or taken —see Table of Drugs and Chemicals, by drug, poisoning
  chronic (dependence) F13.20
Bromidrosiphobia F40.298
Bronchi, bronchial
  —see condition
Bronchiectasis (cylindrical) (diffuse) (fusiform) (localized) (saccular) J47.9
  with
    acute
      bronchitis J47.0
      lower respiratory infection J47.0
    exacerbation (acute) J47.1
  congenital Q33.4
  tuberculous NEC —see Tuberculosis, pulmonary
Bronchiolectasis —see Bronchiectasis
Bronchiolitis (acute) (infective) (subacute) J21.9
  with
    bronchospasm or obstruction J21.9
    influenza, flu or grippe —see Influenza, with, respiratory manifestations NEC
  chemical (chronic) J68.4
    acute J68.0
  chronic (fibrosing) (obliterative) J44.89
    obliterative J44.81
  due to
    external agent —see Bronchitis, acute, due to
    human metapneumovirus J21.1
    respiratory syncytial virus (RSV) J21.0
    specified organism NEC J21.8
  fibrosa obliterans J44.81

Bronchiolitis (continued)
  influenzal —see Influenza, with, respiratory manifestations NEC
  obliterans (see also Bronchiolitis, obliterative) J44.81
    syndrome J44.81
    with organizing pneumonia (BOOP) J84.89
  obliterative (chronic) (subacute) (see also Bronchiolitis, obliterans) J44.81
    due to chemicals, gases, fumes or vapors (inhalation) (see also Disease, respiratory, chronic, due to chemicals, gases, fumes or vapors) J44.81
    due to fumes or vapors (see also Disease, respiratory, chronic, due to chemicals, gases, fumes or vapors) J44.81
  respiratory, interstitial lung disease J84.115
Bronchitis (diffuse) (fibrinous) (hypostatic) (infective) (membranous) J40
  with
    influenza, flu or grippe —see Influenza, with, respiratory manifestations NEC
    obstruction (airway) (lung) J44.89
    tracheitis (15 years of age and above) J40
      acute or subacute J20.9
      chronic J42
      under 15 years of age J20.9
  acute or subacute (with bronchospasm or obstruction) J20.9
    with
      bronchiectasis J47.0
      chronic obstructive pulmonary disease J44.0
    chemical (due to gases, fumes or vapors) J68.0
    due to
      fumes or vapors J68.0
      Haemophilus influenzae J20.1
      Mycoplasma pneumoniae J20.0
      radiation J70.0
      specified organism NEC J20.8
      Streptococcus J20.2
      virus
        coxsackie J20.3
        echovirus J20.7
        parainfluenzae J20.4
        respiratory syncytial (RSV) J20.5
        rhinovirus J20.6
    viral NEC J20.8
  allergic (acute) J45.909
    with
      exacerbation (acute) J45.901
      status asthmaticus J45.902
  arachidic T17.528
  aspiration (due to food and vomit) J69.0
  asthmatic J45.9
    chronic J44.89
      with
        acute lower respiratory infection J44.0
        exacerbation (acute) J44.1
  capillary —see Pneumonia, broncho

Bronchitis (continued)
  caseous (tuberculous) A15.5
  Castellani's A69.8
  catarrhal (15 years of age and above) J40
    acute —see Bronchitis, acute
    chronic J41.0
    under 15 years of age J20.9
  chemical (acute) (subacute) J68.0
    chronic (see also Disease, respiratory, chronic, due to chemicals, gases, fumes or vapors) J42
    due to fumes or vapors (see also Disease, respiratory, chronic, due to chemicals, gases, fumes or vapors) J42
    chronic J68.4
  chronic J42
    with
      airways obstruction J44.89
      tracheitis (chronic) J42
      asthmatic (obstructive) J44.89
    catarrhal J41.0
    chemical (due to fumes or vapors) (see also Disease, respiratory, chronic, due to chemicals, gases, fumes or vapors) J42
    due to
      chemicals, gases, fumes or vapors (inhalation) (see also Disease, respiratory, chronic, due to chemicals, gases, fumes or vapors) J42
      radiation J70.1
      tobacco smoking J41.0
    emphysematous J44.89
    mucopurulent J41.1
    non-obstructive J41.0
    obliterans —see Bronchiolitis, obliterans
    obstructive J44.89
    purulent J41.1
    simple J41.0
  croupous —see Bronchitis, acute
  due to gases, fumes or vapors (chemical) J68.0
  emphysematous (obstructive) J44.89
  exudative —see Bronchitis, acute
  fetid J41.1
  grippal —see Influenza, with, respiratory manifestations NEC
  in those under 15 years age —see Bronchitis, acute
    chronic —see Bronchitis, chronic
  influenzal —see Influenza, with, respiratory manifestations NEC
  mixed simple and mucopurulent J41.8
  moulder's J62.8
  mucopurulent (chronic) (recurrent) J41.1
    acute or subacute J20.9
    simple (mixed) J41.8
  obliterans (chronic) —see Bronchiolitis, obliterans
  obstructive (chronic) (diffuse) J44.89
  pituitous J41.1
  pneumococcal, acute or subacute J20.2
  pseudomembranous, acute or subacute —see Bronchitis, acute

Bronchitis (continued)
  purulent (chronic) (recurrent) J41.1
    acute or subacute —see Bronchitis, acute
  putrid J41.1
  senile (chronic) J42
  simple and mucopurulent (mixed) J41.8
  smokers' J41.0
  spirochetal NEC A69.8
  subacute —see Bronchitis, acute
  suppurative (chronic) J41.1
    acute or subacute —see Bronchitis, acute
  tuberculous A15.5
  under 15 years of age —see Bronchitis, acute
    chronic —see Bronchitis, chronic
  viral NEC, acute or subacute —see also Bronchitis, acute J20.8
Bronchoalveolitis J18.0
Bronchoaspergillosis B44.1
Bronchocele meaning goiter E04.0
Broncholithiasis J98.09
  tuberculous NEC A15.5
Bronchomalacia J98.09
  congenital Q32.2
Bronchomycosis NOS B49 [J99]
  candidal B37.1
Bronchopleuropneumonia —see Pneumonia, broncho
Bronchopneumonia —see Pneumonia, broncho
Bronchopneumonitis —see Pneumonia, broncho
Bronchopulmonary —see condition
Bronchopulmonitis —see Pneumonia, broncho
Bronchorrhagia (see Hemoptysis)
Bronchorrhea J98.09
  acute J20.9
  chronic (infective) (purulent) J42
Bronchospasm (acute) J98.01
  with
    bronchiolitis, acute J21.9
    bronchitis, acute (conditions in J20) —see Bronchitis, acute
  due to external agent —see condition, respiratory, acute, due to
  exercise induced J45.990
Bronchospirochetosis A69.8
  Castellani A69.8
Bronchostenosis J98.09
Bronchus —see condition
Brontophobia F40.220
Bronze baby syndrome P83.88
Brooke's tumor —see Neoplasm, skin, benign
Brown enamel of teeth (hereditary) K00.5
Brown's sheath syndrome H50.61-
Brown-Séquard disease, paralysis or syndrome G83.81

45

Bruce sepsis A23.0
Brucellosis (infection) A23.9
  abortus A23.1
  canis A23.3
  dermatitis A23.9
  melitensis A23.0
  mixed A23.8
  sepsis A23.9
    melitensis A23.0
    specified NEC A23.8
  suis A23.2
Bruck-de Lange disease Q87.19
Bruck's disease —*see* Deformity, limb
BRUE (brief resolved unexplained event) R68.13
Brugsch's syndrome Q82.8
Bruise (skin surface intact) —*see also* Contusion
  with
    open wound —*see* Wound, open
    internal organ —*see* Injury, by site
  newborn P54.5
  scalp, due to birth injury, newborn P12.3
  umbilical cord O69.5
Bruit (arterial) R09.89
  cardiac R01.1
Brush burn —*see* Abrasion, by site
Bruton's X-linked agammaglobulinemia D80.0
Bruxism
  psychogenic F45.8
  sleep related G47.63
Bubbly lung syndrome P27.0
Bubo I88.8
  blennorrhagic (gonococcal) A54.89
  chancroidal A57
  climatic A55
  due to Haemophilus ducreyi A57
  gonococcal A54.89
  indolent (nonspecific) I88.8
  inguinal (nonspecific) I88.8
    chancroidal A57
    climatic A55
    due to H. ducreyi A57
  infective I88.8
  scrofulous (tuberculous) A18.2
  soft chancre A57
  suppurating —*see* Lymphadenitis, acute
  syphilitic (primary) A51.0
    congenital A50.07
  tropical A55
  virulent (chancroidal) A57
Bubonic plague A20.0
Bubonocele —*see* Hernia, inguinal
Buccal —*see* condition
Buchanan's disease or osteochondrosis M91.0
Buchem's syndrome (hyperostosis corticalis) M85.2
Bucket-handle fracture or tear
  (semilunar cartilage) —*see* Tear, meniscus
Budd-Chiari syndrome (hepatic vein thrombosis) I82.0

Budgerigar fancier's disease or lung J67.2
Buds
  breast E30.1
    in newborn P96.89
Buerger's disease (thromboangiitis obliterans) I73.1
Bulbar —*see* condition
Bulbus cordis (left ventricle) (persistent) Q21.8
Bulimia (nervosa) F50.2
  atypical F50.9
  normal weight F50.9
Bulky
  stools R19.5
  uterus N85.2
Bulla (e) R23.8
  lung (emphysematous) (solitary) J43.9
  newborn P25.8
Bullet wound —*see also* Puncture
  fracture - code as Fracture, by site
  internal organ —*see* Injury, by site
Bundle
  branch block (complete) (false) (incomplete) —*see* Block, bundle-branch
  of His —*see* condition
Bunion M21.61-
  tailor's M21.62-
Bunionette M21.62-
Buphthalmia, buphthalmos (congenital) Q15.0
Burdwan fever B55.0
Bürger-Grütz disease or syndrome E78.3
Buried
  penis (congenital) Q55.64
    acquired N48.83
  roots K08.3
Burke's syndrome K86.89
Burkholderia
  cepacia A49.8
  mallei A24.0
  pseudomallei —*see* Melioidosis
Burkitt
  cell leukemia C91.0-
  lymphoma (malignant) C83.7-
    small noncleaved, diffuse C83.7-
    spleen C83.77
    undifferentiated C83.7-
  tumor C83.7-
  type
    acute lymphoblastic leukemia C91.0-
    undifferentiated C83.7-
Burn (electricity) (flame) (hot gas, liquid or hot object) (radiation) (steam) (thermal) T30.0
  abdomen, abdominal (muscle) (wall) T21.02
    first degree T21.12
    second degree T21.22
    third degree T21.32
  above elbow T22.039
    first degree T22.139
    left T22.032
      first degree T22.132
      second degree T22.232
      third degree T22.332

Burn (*continued*)
  above elbow (*continued*)
    right T22.031
      first degree T22.131
      second degree T22.231
      third degree T22.331
    second degree T22.239
    third degree T22.339
  acid (caustic) (external) (internal)
    —*see* Corrosion, by site
  alimentary tract NEC T28.2
    esophagus T28.1
    mouth T28.0
    pharynx T28.0
  alkaline (caustic) (external) (internal)
    —*see* Corrosion, by site
  ankle T25.019
    first degree T25.119
    left T25.012
      first degree T25.112
      second degree T25.212
      third degree T25.312
    multiple with foot —*see* Burn, lower, limb, multiple, ankle and foot
    right T25.011
      first degree T25.111
      second degree T25.211
      third degree T25.311
    second degree T25.219
    third degree T25.319
  anus —*see* Burn, buttock
  arm (lower) (upper) —*see* Burn, upper, limb
  axilla T22.049
    first degree T22.149
    left T22.042
      first degree T22.142
      second degree T22.242
      third degree T22.342
    right T22.041
      first degree T22.141
      second degree T22.241
      third degree T22.341
    second degree T22.249
    third degree T22.349
  back (lower) T21.04
    first degree T21.14
    second degree T21.24
    third degree T21.34
    upper T21.03
      first degree T21.13
      second degree T21.23
      third degree T21.33
  blisters - code as Burn, second degree, by site
  breast(s) —*see* Burn, chest wall
  buttock(s) T21.05
    first degree T21.15
    second degree T21.25
    third degree T21.35
  calf T24.039
    first degree T24.139
    left T24.032
      first degree T24.132
      second degree T24.232
      third degree T24.332
    right T24.031
      first degree T24.131
      second degree T24.231
      third degree T24.331
    second degree T24.239
    third degree T24.339
  canthus (eye) —*see* Burn, eyelid
  caustic acid or alkaline —*see* Corrosion, by site
  cervix T28.3
  cheek T20.06
    first degree T20.16
    second degree T20.26
    third degree T20.36

Burn (*continued*)
  chemical (acids) (alkalines) (caustics) (external) (internal)
    —*see* Corrosion, by site
  chest wall T21.01
    first degree T21.11
    second degree T21.21
    third degree T21.31
  chin T20.03
    first degree T20.13
    second degree T20.23
    third degree T20.33
  colon T28.2
  conjunctiva (and cornea) —*see* Burn, cornea
  cornea (and conjunctiva) T26.1-
    chemical —*see* Corrosion, cornea
  corrosion (external) (internal)
    —*see* Corrosion, by site
  deep necrosis of underlying tissue - code as Burn, third degree, by site
  dorsum of hand T23.069
    first degree T23.169
    left T23.062
      first degree T23.162
      second degree T23.262
      third degree T23.362
    right T23.061
      first degree T23.161
      second degree T23.261
      third degree T23.361
    second degree T23.269
    third degree T23.369
  due to ingested chemical agent
    —*see* Corrosion, by site
  ear (auricle) (external) (canal) T20.01
    first degree T20.11
    second degree T20.21
    third degree T20.31
  elbow T22.029
    first degree T22.129
    left T22.022
      first degree T22.122
      second degree T22.222
      third degree T22.322
    right T22.021
      first degree T22.121
      second degree T22.221
      third degree T22.321
    second degree T22.229
    third degree T22.329
  epidermal loss - code as Burn, second degree, by site
  erythema, erythematous - code as Burn, first degree, by site
  esophagus T28.1
  extent (percentage of body surface)
    less than 10 percent T31.0
    10-19 percent T31.10
      with 0-9 percent third degree burns T31.10
      with 10-19 percent third degree burns T31.11
    20-29 percent T31.20
      with 0-9 percent third degree burns T31.20
      with 10-19 percent third degree burns T31.21
      with 20-29 percent third degree burns T31.22
    30-39 percent T31.30
      with 0-9 percent third degree burns T31.30
      with 10-19 percent third degree burns T31.31
      with 20-29 percent third degree burns T31.32
      with 30-39 percent third degree burns T31.33

Burn *(continued)*
　extent *(continued)*
　　40-49 percent T31.40
　　　with 0-9 percent third degree burns T31.40
　　　with 10-19 percent third degree burns T31.41
　　　with 20-29 percent third degree burns T31.42
　　　with 30-39 percent third degree burns T31.43
　　　with 40-49 percent third degree burns T31.44
　　50-59 percent T31.50
　　　with 0-9 percent third degree burns T31.50
　　　with 10-19 percent third degree burns T31.51
　　　with 20-29 percent third degree burns T31.52
　　　with 30-39 percent third degree burns T31.53
　　　with 40-49 percent third degree burns T31.54
　　　with 50-59 percent third degree burns T31.55
　　60-69 percent T31.60
　　　with 0-9 percent third degree burns T31.60
　　　with 10-19 percent third degree burns T31.61
　　　with 20-29 percent third degree burns T31.62
　　　with 30-39 percent third degree burns T31.63
　　　with 40-49 percent third degree burns T31.64
　　　with 50-59 percent third degree burns T31.65
　　　with 60-69 percent third degree burns T31.66
　　70-79 percent T31.70
　　　with 0-9 percent third degree burns T31.70
　　　with 10-19 percent third degree burns T31.71
　　　with 20-29 percent third degree burns T31.72
　　　with 30-39 percent third degree burns T31.73
　　　with 40-49 percent third degree burns T31.74
　　　with 50-59 percent third degree burns T31.75
　　　with 60-69 percent third degree burns T31.76
　　　with 70-79 percent third degree burns T31.77
　　80-89 percent T31.80
　　　with 0-9 percent third degree burns T31.80
　　　with 10-19 percent third degree burns T31.81
　　　with 20-29 percent third degree burns T31.82
　　　with 30-39 percent third degree burns T31.83
　　　with 40-49 percent third degree burns T31.84
　　　with 50-59 percent third degree burns T31.85
　　　with 60-69 percent third degree burns T31.86
　　　with 70-79 percent third degree burns T31.87
　　　with 80-89 percent third degree burns T31.88

Burn *(continued)*
　extent *(continued)*
　　90 percent or more T31.90
　　　with 0-9 percent third degree burns T31.90
　　　with 10-19 percent third degree burns T31.91
　　　with 20-29 percent third degree burns T31.92
　　　with 30-39 percent third degree burns T31.93
　　　with 40-49 percent third degree burns T31.94
　　　with 50-59 percent third degree burns T31.95
　　　with 60-69 percent third degree burns T31.96
　　　with 70-79 percent third degree burns T31.97
　　　with 80-89 percent third degree burns T31.98
　　　with 90 percent or more third degree burns T31.99
　extremity —*see* Burn, limb
　eye(s) and adnexa T26.4-
　　with resulting rupture and destruction of eyeball T26.2-
　　conjunctival sac —*see* Burn, cornea
　　cornea —*see* Burn, cornea
　　lid —*see* Burn, eyelid
　　periocular area —*see* Burn, eyelid
　　specified site NEC T26.3-
　eyeball —*see* Burn, eye
　eyelid(s) T26.0-
　　chemical —*see* Corrosion, eyelid
　face —*see* Burn, head
　finger T23.029
　　first degree T23.129
　　left T23.022
　　　first degree T23.122
　　　second degree T23.222
　　　third degree T23.322
　　multiple sites (without thumb) T23.039
　　　with thumb T23.049
　　　　first degree T23.149
　　　　left T23.042
　　　　　first degree T23.142
　　　　　second degree T23.242
　　　　　third degree T23.342
　　　　right T23.041
　　　　　first degree T23.141
　　　　　second degree T23.241
　　　　　third degree T23.341
　　　　second degree T23.249
　　　　third degree T23.349
　　　first degree T23.139
　　　left T23.032
　　　　first degree T23.132
　　　　second degree T23.232
　　　　third degree T23.332
　　　right T23.031
　　　　first degree T23.131
　　　　second degree T23.231
　　　　third degree T23.331
　　　second degree T23.239
　　　third degree T23.339
　　right T23.021
　　　first degree T23.121
　　　second degree T23.221
　　　third degree T23.321
　　second degree T23.229
　　third degree T23.329
　flank —*see* Burn, abdominal wall
　foot T25.029
　　first degree T25.129
　　left T25.022
　　　first degree T25.122
　　　second degree T25.222
　　　third degree T25.322

Burn *(continued)*
　foot *(continued)*
　　multiple with ankle —*see* Burn, lower, limb, multiple, ankle and foot
　　right T25.021
　　　first degree T25.121
　　　second degree T25.221
　　　third degree T25.321
　　second degree T25.229
　　third degree T25.329
　forearm T22.019
　　first degree T22.119
　　left T22.012
　　　first degree T22.112
　　　second degree T22.212
　　　third degree T22.312
　　right T22.011
　　　first degree T22.111
　　　second degree T22.211
　　　third degree T22.311
　　second degree T22.219
　　third degree T22.319
　forehead T20.06
　　first degree T20.16
　　second degree T20.26
　　third degree T20.36
　fourth degree - code as Burn, third degree, by site
　friction —*see* Burn, by site
　from swallowing caustic or corrosive substance NEC —*see* Corrosion, by site
　full thickness skin loss - code as Burn, third degree, by site
　gastrointestinal tract NEC T28.2
　　from swallowing caustic or corrosive substance T28.7
　genital organs
　　external
　　　female T21.07
　　　　first degree T21.17
　　　　second degree T21.27
　　　　third degree T21.37
　　　male T21.06
　　　　first degree T21.16
　　　　second degree T21.26
　　　　third degree T21.36
　　internal T28.3
　　　from caustic or corrosive substance T28.8
　groin —*see* Burn, abdominal wall
　hand(s) T23.009
　　back —*see* Burn, dorsum of hand
　　finger —*see* Burn, finger
　　first degree T23.109
　　left T23.002
　　　first degree T23.102
　　　second degree T23.202
　　　third degree T23.302
　　multiple sites with wrist T23.099
　　　first degree T23.199
　　　left T23.092
　　　　first degree T23.192
　　　　second degree T23.292
　　　　third degree T23.392
　　　right T23.091
　　　　first degree T23.191
　　　　second degree T23.291
　　　　third degree T23.391
　　　second degree T23.299
　　　third degree T23.399
　　palm —*see* Burn, palm
　　right T23.001
　　　first degree T23.101
　　　second degree T23.201
　　　third degree T23.301
　　second degree T23.209
　　third degree T23.309
　　thumb —*see* Burn, thumb

Burn *(continued)*
　head (and face) (and neck) T20.00
　　cheek —*see* Burn, cheek
　　chin —*see* Burn, chin
　　ear —*see* Burn, ear
　　eye(s) only —*see* Burn, eye
　　first degree T20.10
　　forehead —*see* Burn, forehead
　　lip —*see* Burn, lip
　　multiple sites T20.09
　　　first degree T20.19
　　　second degree T20.29
　　　third degree T20.39
　　neck —*see* Burn, neck
　　nose —*see* Burn, nose
　　scalp —*see* Burn, scalp
　　second degree T20.20
　　third degree T20.30
　hip(s) —*see* Burn, thigh
　inhalation —*see* Burn, respiratory tract
　　caustic or corrosive substance (fumes) —*see* Corrosion, respiratory tract
　internal organ(s) T28.40
　　alimentary tract T28.2
　　　esophagus T28.1
　　eardrum T28.41
　　esophagus T28.1
　　from caustic or corrosive substance (swallowing) NEC —*see* Corrosion, by site
　　genitourinary T28.3
　　mouth T28.0
　　pharynx T28.0
　　respiratory tract —*see* Burn, respiratory tract
　　specified organ NEC T28.49
　interscapular region —*see* Burn, back, upper
　intestine (large) (small) T28.2
　knee T24.029
　　first degree T24.129
　　left T24.022
　　　first degree T24.122
　　　second degree T24.222
　　　third degree T24.322
　　right T24.021
　　　first degree T24.121
　　　second degree T24.221
　　　third degree T24.321
　　second degree T24.229
　　third degree T24.329
　labium (majus) (minus) —*see* Burn, genital organs, external, female
　lacrimal apparatus, duct, gland or sac —*see* Burn, eye, specified site NEC
　larynx T27.0
　　with lung T27.1
　leg(s) (lower) (upper) —*see* Burn, lower, limb
　lightning —*see* Burn, by site
　limb(s)
　　lower (except ankle or foot alone) —*see* Burn, lower, limb
　　upper —*see* Burn, upper limb
　lip(s) T20.02
　　first degree T20.12
　　second degree T20.22
　　third degree T20.32
　lower
　　back —*see* Burn, back
　　limb T24.009
　　　ankle —*see* Burn, ankle
　　　calf —*see* Burn, calf
　　　first degree T24.109
　　　foot —*see* Burn, foot
　　　hip —*see* Burn, thigh

Burn *(continued)*
  lower *(continued)*
    limb *(continued)*
      knee —*see* Burn, knee
      left T24.002
        first degree T24.102
        second degree T24.202
        third degree T24.302
      multiple sites, except ankle and foot T24.099
        ankle and foot T25.099
          first degree T25.199
          left T25.092
            first degree T25.192
            second degree T25.292
            third degree T25.392
          right T25.091
            first degree T25.191
            second degree T25.291
            third degree T25.391
          second degree T25.299
          third degree T25.399
        first degree T24.199
        left T24.092
          first degree T24.192
          second degree T24.292
          third degree T24.392
        right T24.091
          first degree T24.191
          second degree T24.291
          third degree T24.391
        second degree T24.299
        third degree T24.399
      right T24.001
        first degree T24.101
        second degree T24.201
        third degree T24.301
      second degree T24.209
      thigh —*see* Burn, thigh
      third degree T24.309
      toe —*see* Burn, toe
  lung (with larynx and trachea) T27.1
  mouth T28.0
  neck T20.07
    first degree T20.17
    second degree T20.27
    third degree T20.37
  nose (septum) T20.04
    first degree T20.14
    second degree T20.24
    third degree T20.34
  ocular adnexa —*see* Burn, eye
  orbit region —*see* Burn, eyelid
  palm T23.059
    first degree T23.159
    left T23.052
      first degree T23.152
      second degree T23.252
      third degree T23.352
    right T23.051
      first degree T23.151
      second degree T23.251
      third degree T23.351
    second degree T23.259
    third degree T23.359
  partial thickness - code as Burn, by site, second degree
  pelvis —*see* Burn, trunk
  penis —*see* Burn, genital organs, external, male
  perineum
    female —*see* Burn, genital organs, external, female
    male —*see* Burn, genital organs, external, male
  periocular area —*see* Burn, eyelid
  pharynx T28.0
  rectum T28.2

Burn *(continued)*
  respiratory tract T27.3
    larynx —*see* Burn, larynx
    specified part NEC T27.2
    trachea —*see* Burn, trachea
  sac, lacrimal —*see* Burn, eye, specified site NEC
  scalp T20.05
    first degree T20.15
    second degree T20.25
    third degree T20.35
  scapular region T22.069
    first degree T22.169
    left T22.062
      first degree T22.162
      second degree T22.262
      third degree T22.362
    right T22.061
      first degree T22.161
      second degree T22.261
      third degree T22.361
    second degree T22.269
    third degree T22.369
  sclera —*see* Burn, eye, specified site NEC
  scrotum —*see* Burn, genital organs, external, male
  shoulder T22.059
    first degree T22.159
    left T22.052
      first degree T22.152
      second degree T22.252
      third degree T22.352
    right T22.051
      first degree T22.151
      second degree T22.251
      third degree T22.351
    second degree T22.259
    third degree T22.359
  stomach T28.2
  temple —*see* Burn, head
  testis —*see* Burn, genital organs, external, male
  thigh T24.019
    first degree T24.119
    left T24.012
      first degree T24.112
      second degree T24.212
      third degree T24.312
    right T24.011
      first degree T24.111
      second degree T24.211
      third degree T24.311
    second degree T24.219
    third degree T24.319
  thorax (external) —*see* Burn, trunk
  throat (meaning pharynx) T28.0
  thumb(s) T23.019
    first degree T23.119
    left T23.012
      first degree T23.112
      second degree T23.212
      third degree T23.312
    multiple sites with fingers T23.049
      first degree T23.149
      left T23.042
        first degree T23.142
        second degree T23.242
        third degree T23.342
      right T23.041
        first degree T23.141
        second degree T23.241
        third degree T23.341
      second degree T23.249
      third degree T23.349
    right T23.011
      first degree T23.111
      second degree T23.211
      third degree T23.311

Burn *(continued)*
  thumb(s) *(continued)*
    second degree T23.219
    third degree T23.319
  toe T25.039
    first degree T25.139
    left T25.032
      first degree T25.132
      second degree T25.232
      third degree T25.332
    right T25.031
      first degree T25.131
      second degree T25.231
      third degree T25.331
    second degree T25.239
    third degree T25.339
  tongue T28.0
  tonsil(s) T28.0
  trachea T27.0
    with lung T27.1
  trunk T21.00
    abdominal wall —*see* Burn, abdominal wall
    anus —*see* Burn, buttock
    axilla —*see* Burn, upper limb
    back —*see* Burn, back
    breast —*see* Burn, chest wall
    buttock —*see* Burn, buttock
    chest wall —*see* Burn, chest wall
    first degree T21.10
    flank —*see* Burn, abdominal wall
    genital
      female —*see* Burn, genital organs, external, female
      male —*see* Burn, genital organs, external, male
    groin —*see* Burn, abdominal wall
    interscapular region —*see* Burn, back, upper
    labia —*see* Burn, genital organs, external, female
    lower back —*see* Burn, back
    penis —*see* Burn, genital organs, external, male
    perineum
      female —*see* Burn, genital organs, external, female
      male —*see* Burn, genital organs, external, male
    scapula region —*see* Burn, scapular region
    scrotum —*see* Burn, genital organs, external, male
    second degree T21.20
    specified site NEC T21.09
      first degree T21.19
      second degree T21.29
      third degree T21.39
    testes —*see* Burn, genital organs, external, male
    third degree T21.30
    upper back —*see* Burn, back, upper
    vulva —*see* Burn, genital organs, external, female
  unspecified site with extent of body surface involved specified
    less than 10 percent T31.0
    10-19 percent (0-9 percent third degree) T31.10
      with 10-19 percent third degree T31.11
    20-29 percent (0-9 percent third degree) T31.20
      with
        10-19 percent third degree T31.21
        20-29 percent third degree T31.22

Burn *(continued)*
  unspecified site with extent of body surface involved specified *(continued)*
    30-39 percent (0-9 percent third degree) T31.30
      with
        10-19 percent third degree T31.31
        20-29 percent third degree T31.32
        30-39 percent third degree T31.33
    40-49 percent (0-9 percent third degree) T31.40
      with
        10-19 percent third degree T31.41
        20-29 percent third degree T31.42
        30-39 percent third degree T31.43
        40-49 percent third degree T31.44
    50-59 percent (0-9 percent third degree) T31.50
      with
        10-19 percent third degree T31.51
        20-29 percent third degree T31.52
        30-39 percent third degree T31.53
        40-49 percent third degree T31.54
        50-59 percent third degree T31.55
    60-69 percent (0-9 percent third degree) T31.60
      with
        10-19 percent third degree T31.61
        20-29 percent third degree T31.62
        30-39 percent third degree T31.63
        40-49 percent third degree T31.64
        50-59 percent third degree T31.65
        60-69 percent third degree T31.66
    70-79 percent (0-9 percent third degree) T31.70
      with
        10-19 percent third degree T31.71
        20-29 percent third degree T31.72
        30-39 percent third degree T31.73
        40-49 percent third degree T31.74
        50-59 percent third degree T31.75
        60-69 percent third degree T31.76
        70-79 percent third degree T31.77
    80-89 percent (0-9 percent third degree) T31.80
      with
        10-19 percent third degree T31.81
        20-29 percent third degree T31.82
        30-39 percent third degree T31.83
        40-49 percent third degree T31.84

Burn (continued)
  unspecified site with extent of body surface involved specified (continued)
    80-89 percent (continued)
      with (continued)
        50-59 percent third degree T31.85
        60-69 percent third degree T31.86
        70-79 percent third degree T31.87
        80-89 percent third degree T31.88
    90 percent or more (0-9 percent third degree) T31.90
      with
        10-19 percent third degree T31.91
        20-29 percent third degree T31.92
        30-39 percent third degree T31.93
        40-49 percent third degree T31.94
        50-59 percent third degree T31.95
        60-69 percent third degree T31.96
        70-79 percent third degree T31.97
        80-89 percent third degree T31.98
        90-99 percent third degree T31.99
  upper limb T22.00
    above elbow —see Burn, above elbow
    axilla —see Burn, axilla
    elbow —see Burn, elbow
    first degree T22.10
    forearm —see Burn, forearm
    hand —see Burn, hand
    interscapular region —see Burn, back, upper
    multiple sites T22.099
      first degree T22.199
      left T22.092
        first degree T22.192
        second degree T22.292
        third degree T22.392
      right T22.091
        first degree T22.191
        second degree T22.291
        third degree T22.391
      second degree T22.299
      third degree T22.399
    scapular region —see Burn, scapular region
    second degree T22.20
    shoulder —see Burn, shoulder
    third degree T22.30
    wrist —see Burn, wrist
  uterus T28.3
  vagina T28.3
  vulva —see Burn, genital organs, external, female
  wrist T23.079
    first degree T23.179
    left T23.072
      first degree T23.172
      second degree T23.272
      third degree T23.372
    multiple sites with hand T23.099
      first degree T23.199
      left T23.092
        first degree T23.192
        second degree T23.292
        third degree T23.392

Burn (continued)
  wrist (continued)
    multiple sites with hand (continued)
      right T23.091
        first degree T23.191
        second degree T23.291
        third degree T23.391
      second degree T23.299
      third degree T23.399
    right T23.071
      first degree T23.171
      second degree T23.271
      third degree T23.371
    second degree T23.279
    third degree T23.379

Burnett's syndrome E83.52

Burning
  feet syndrome E53.9
  sensation R20.8
  tongue K14.6

Burn-out (state) Z73.0

Burns' disease or osteochondrosis —see Osteochondrosis, juvenile, ulna

Bursa —see condition

Bursitis M71.9
  Achilles —see Tendinitis, Achilles
  adhesive —see Bursitis, specified NEC
  ankle —see Enthesopathy, lower limb, ankle, specified type NEC
  calcaneal —see Enthesopathy, foot, specified type NEC
  collateral ligament, tibial —see Bursitis, tibial collateral
  due to use, overuse, pressure —see also Disorder, soft tissue, due to use, specified type NEC
    specified NEC —see Disorder, soft tissue, due to use, specified NEC
  Duplay's M75.0
  elbow NEC M70.3-
    olecranon M70.2-
  finger —see Disorder, soft tissue, due to use, specified type NEC, hand
  foot —see Enthesopathy, foot, specified type NEC
  gonococcal A54.49
  gouty —see Gout
  hand M70.1-
  hip NEC M70.7-
    trochanteric M70.6-
  infective NEC M71.10
    abscess —see Abscess, bursa
    ankle M71.17-
    elbow M71.12-
    foot M71.17-
    hand M71.14-
    hip M71.15-
    knee M71.16-
    multiple sites M71.19
    shoulder M71.11-
    specified site NEC M71.18
    wrist M71.13-
  ischial —see Bursitis, hip
  knee NEC M70.5-
    prepatellar M70.4-
  occupational NEC —see also Disorder, soft tissue, due to, use
  olecranon —see Bursitis, elbow, olecranon
  pharyngeal J39.1
  popliteal —see Bursitis, knee
  prepatellar M70.4-
  radiohumeral M70.3-
  rheumatoid M06.20
    ankle M06.27-
    elbow M06.22-

Bursitis (continued)
  rheumatoid (continued)
    foot joint M06.27-
    hand joint M06.24-
    hip M06.25-
    knee M06.26-
    multiple site M06.29
    shoulder M06.21-
    vertebra M06.28
    wrist M06.23-
  scapulohumeral —see Bursitis, shoulder
  semimembranous muscle (knee) —see Bursitis, knee
  shoulder M75.5-
    adhesive —see Capsulitis, adhesive
  specified NEC M71.50
    ankle M71.57-
    due to use, overuse or pressure —see Disorder, soft tissue, due to, use
    elbow M71.52-
    foot M71.57-
    hand M71.54-
    hip M71.55-
    knee M71.56-
    shoulder —see Bursitis, shoulder
    specified site NEC M71.58
    tibial collateral M76.4-
    wrist M71.53-
  subacromial —see Bursitis, shoulder
  subcoracoid —see Bursitis, shoulder
  subdeltoid —see Bursitis, shoulder
  syphilitic A52.78
  Thornwaldt, Tornwaldt J39.2
  tibial collateral M76.4-
  toe —see Enthesopathy, foot, specified type NEC
  trochanteric (area) —see Bursitis, hip, trochanteric
  wrist —see Bursitis, hand

Bursopathy M71.9
  specified type NEC M71.80
    ankle M71.87-
    elbow M71.82-
    foot M71.87-
    hand M71.84-
    hip M71.85-
    knee M71.86-
    multiple sites M71.89
    shoulder M71.81-
    specified site NEC M71.88
    wrist M71.83-

Burst stitches or sutures
  (complication of surgery) T81.31
  external operation wound T81.31
  internal operation wound T81.32

Buruli ulcer A31.1

Bury's disease L95.1

Buschke's
  disease —see Cryptococcosis by site
  scleredema —see Sclerosis, systemic

Busse-Buschke disease —see Cryptococcosis by site

Buttock —see condition

Button
  Biskra B55.1
  Delhi B55.1
  oriental B55.1

Buttonhole deformity (finger) —see Deformity, finger, boutonniere

Bwamba fever A92.8

Byssinosis J66.0

Bywaters' syndrome T79.5

C

Cachexia E43
  cancerous R64
  cardiac —see Disease, heart
  dehydration E86.0
  due to
    malnutrition (see also Malnutrition, severe) E88.A
    underlying condition E88.A
  exophthalmic —see Hyperthyroidism
  heart —see Disease, heart
  hypophyseal E23.0
  hypopituitary E23.0
  lead —see Poisoning, lead
  malignant R64
  marsh —see Malaria
  nervous F48.8
  old age R54
  paludal —see Malaria
  pituitary E23.0
  pulmonary R64
  renal N28.9
  saturnine —see Poisoning, lead
  senile R54
  Simmonds' E23.0
  splenica D73.0
  strumipriva E03.4
  tuberculous NEC —see Tuberculosis

CADASIL (cerebral autosomal dominant arteriopathy with subcortical infarcts and leukoencephalopathy) I67.850

Café, au lait spots L81.3

Caffeine-induced
  anxiety disorder F15.980
  sleep disorder F15.982

Caffey's syndrome Q78.8

Caisson disease T70.3

Cake kidney Q63.1

Caked breast (puerperal, postpartum) O92.79

Calabar swelling B74.3

Calcaneal spur —see Spur, bone, calcaneal

Calcaneo-apophysitis M92.8

Calcareous —see condition

Calcicosis J62.8

Calciferol (vitamin D) **deficiency** E55.9
  with rickets E55.0

Calcification
  adrenal (capsule) (gland) E27.49
    tuberculous E35 [B90.8]
  aorta I70.0
  artery (annular) —see Arteriosclerosis
  auricle (ear) —see Disorder, pinna, specified type NEC
  basal ganglia G23.8
  bladder N32.89
    due to Schistosoma hematobium B65.0
  brain (cortex) —see Calcification, cerebral
  bronchus J98.09
  bursa M71.40
    ankle M71.47-
    elbow M71.42-
    foot M71.47-
    hand M71.44-
    hip M71.45-

Calcification (continued)
  bursa (continued)
    knee M71.46-
    multiple sites M71.49
    shoulder M75.3-
    specified site NEC M71.48
    wrist M71.43-
  cardiac —see Degeneration, myocardial
  cerebral (cortex) G93.89
    artery I67.2
  cervix (uteri) N88.8
  choroid plexus G93.89
  conjunctiva —see Concretion, conjunctiva
  corpora cavernosa (penis) N48.89
  cortex (brain) —see Calcification, cerebral
  dental pulp (nodular) K04.2
  dentinal papilla K00.4
  fallopian tube N83.8
  falx cerebri G96.198
  gallbladder K82.8
  general E83.59
  heart —see also Degeneration, myocardial
    valve —see also Endocarditis
      mitral —see Calcification, mitral
  idiopathic infantile arterial (IIAC) Q28.8
  intervertebral cartilage or disc (postinfective) —see Disorder, disc, specified NEC
  intracranial —see Calcification, cerebral
  joint —see Disorder, joint, specified type NEC
  kidney N28.89
    tuberculous N29 [B90.1]
  larynx (senile) J38.7
  lens —see Cataract, specified NEC
  lung (active) (postinfectional) J98.4
    tuberculous B90.9
  lymph gland or node (postinfectional) I89.8
    tuberculous (see also Tuberculosis, lymph gland) B90.8
  mammographic R92.1
  massive (paraplegic) —see Myositis, ossificans, in, quadriplegia
  medial —see Arteriosclerosis, extremities
  meninges (cerebral) (spinal) G96.198
  metastatic E83.59
  mitral (valve)
    annular I34.81
      nonrheumatic I34.81
      rheumatic I05.8
    annulus I34.81
      nonrheumatic I34.81
      rheumatic I05.8
  Mönckeberg's —see Arteriosclerosis, extremities
  muscle M61.9
    due to burns —see Myositis, ossificans, in, burns
    paralytic —see Myositis, ossificans, in, quadriplegia
    specified type NEC M61.40
      ankle M61.47-
      foot M61.47-
      forearm M61.43-
      hand M61.44-
      lower leg M61.46-
      multiple sites M61.49
      pelvic region M61.45-
      shoulder region M61.41-
      specified site NEC M61.48
      thigh M61.45-
      upper arm M61.42-

Calcification (continued)
  myocardium, myocardial —see Degeneration, myocardial
  ovary N83.8
  pancreas K86.89
  penis N48.89
  periarticular —see Disorder, joint, specified type NEC
  pericardium —see also Pericarditis I31.1
  pineal gland E34.8
  pleura J94.8
    postinfectional J94.8
    tuberculous NEC B90.9
  pulpal (dental) (nodular) K04.2
  sclera H15.89
  spleen D73.89
  subcutaneous L94.2
  suprarenal (capsule) (gland) E27.49
  tendon (sheath) —see also Tenosynovitis, specified type NEC
    with bursitis, synovitis or tenosynovitis —see Tendinitis, calcific
  trachea J39.8
  ureter N28.89
  uterus N85.8
  vitreous —see Deposit, crystalline

Calcified —see Calcification

Calcinosis (interstitial) (tumoral) (universalis) E83.59
  with Raynaud's phenomenon, esophageal dysfunction, sclerodactyly, telangiectasia (CREST syndrome) M34.1
  circumscripta (skin) L94.2
  cutis L94.2

Calciphylaxis —see also Calcification, by site E83.59

Calcium
  deposits —see Calcification, by site
  metabolism disorder E83.50
  salts or soaps in vitreous —see Deposit, crystalline

Calciuria R82.994

Calculi —see Calculus

Calculosis, intrahepatic —see Calculus, bile duct

Calculus, calculi, calculous
  ampulla of Vater —see Calculus, bile duct
  anuria (impacted) (recurrent) —see also Calculus, urinary N20.9
  appendix K38.1
  bile duct (common) (hepatic) K80.50
    with
      calculus of gallbladder —see Calculus, gallbladder and bile duct
      cholangitis K80.30
        with
          cholecystitis —see Calculus, bile duct, with cholecystitis
          obstruction K80.31
        acute K80.32
          with
            chronic cholangitis K80.36
              with obstruction K80.37
            obstruction K80.33

Calculus, calculi, calculous (continued)
  bile duct (continued)
    with
      cholangitis (continued)
        chronic K80.34
          with
            acute cholangitis K80.36
              with obstruction K80.37
            obstruction K80.35
        cholecystitis (with cholangitis) K80.40
          with obstruction K80.41
          acute K80.42
            with
              chronic cholecystitis K80.46
                with obstruction K80.47
              obstruction K80.43
            chronic K80.44
              with
                acute cholecystitis K80.46
                  with obstruction K80.47
                obstruction K80.45
        obstruction K80.51
    biliary —see also Calculus, gallbladder
    specified NEC K80.80
      with obstruction K80.81
  bilirubin, multiple —see Calculus, gallbladder
  bladder (encysted) (impacted) (urinary) (diverticulum) N21.0
  bronchus J98.09
  calyx (kidney) (renal) —see Calculus, kidney
  cholesterol (pure) (solitary) —see Calculus, gallbladder
  common duct (bile) —see Calculus, bile duct
  conjunctiva —see Concretion, conjunctiva
  cystic N21.0
    duct —see Calculus, gallbladder
  dental (subgingival) (supragingival) K03.6
  diverticulum
    bladder N21.0
    kidney N20.0
  epididymis N50.89
  gallbladder K80.20
    with
      bile duct calculus —see Calculus, gallbladder and bile duct
      cholecystitis K80.10
        with obstruction K80.11
        acute K80.00
          with
            chronic cholecystitis K80.12
              with obstruction K80.13
            obstruction K80.01
        chronic K80.10
          with
            acute cholecystitis K80.12
              with obstruction K80.13
            obstruction K80.11
      specified NEC K80.18
        with obstruction K80.19
      obstruction K80.21

Calculus, calculi, calculous (continued)
  gallbladder and bile duct K80.70
    with
      cholecystitis K80.60
        with obstruction K80.61
        acute K80.62
          with
            chronic cholecystitis K80.66
              with obstruction K80.67
            obstruction K80.63
          chronic K80.64
            with
              acute cholecystitis K80.66
                with obstruction K80.67
              obstruction K80.65
      obstruction K80.71
  hepatic (duct) —see Calculus, bile duct
  hepatobiliary K80.80
    with obstruction K80.81
  ileal conduit N21.8
  intestinal (impaction) (obstruction) K56.49
  kidney (impacted) (multiple) (pelvis) (recurrent) (staghorn) N20.0
    with calculus, ureter N20.2
    congenital Q63.8
  lacrimal passages —see Dacryolith
  liver (impacted) —see Calculus, bile duct
  lung J98.4
  mammographic R92.1
  nephritic (impacted) (recurrent) —see Calculus, kidney
  nose J34.89
  pancreas (duct) K86.89
  parotid duct or gland K11.5
  pelvis, encysted —see Calculus, kidney
  prostate N42.0
  pulmonary J98.4
  pyelitis (impacted) (recurrent) N20.0
    with hydronephrosis N13.6
  pyelonephritis (impacted) (recurrent) N20
    with hydronephrosis N13.6
  renal (impacted) (recurrent) —see Calculus, kidney
  salivary (duct) (gland) K11.5
  seminal vesicle N50.89
  staghorn —see Calculus, kidney
  Stensen's duct K11.5
  stomach K31.89
  sublingual duct or gland K11.5
    congenital Q38.4
  submandibular duct, gland or region K11.5
  submaxillary duct, gland or region K11.5
  suburethral N21.8
  tonsil J35.8
  tooth, teeth (subgingival) (supragingival) K03.6
  tunica vaginalis N50.89
  ureter (impacted) (recurrent) N20.1
    with calculus, kidney N20.2
      with hydronephrosis N13.2
        with infection N13.6
  ureteropelvic junction N20.1
  urethra (impacted) N21.1
  urinary (duct) (impacted) (passage) (tract) N20.9
    with hydronephrosis N13.2
      with infection N13.6
    in (due to)

Calculus, calculi, calculous (continued)
　urinary (continued)
　　lower N21.9
　　　specified NEC N21.8
　　vagina N89.8
　　vesical (impacted) N21.0
　　Wharton's duct K11.5
　　xanthine E79.82 [N22]
Calicectasis N28.89
Caliectasis N28.89
California
　disease B38.9
　encephalitis A83.5
Caligo cornea —see Opacity, cornea, central
Callositas, callosity (infected) L84
Callus (infected) L84
　bone —see Osteophyte
　　excessive, following fracture - code as Sequelae of fracture
CALME (childhood asymmetric labium majus enlargement) N90.61
Calorie deficiency or malnutrition (see also Malnutrition) E46
Calpainopathy (primary) G71.032
　autosomal dominant G71.031
　autosomal recessive G71.032
Calvé-Perthes disease —see Legg-Calvé-Perthes disease
Calvé's disease —see Osteochondrosis, juvenile, spine
Calvities —see Alopecia, androgenic
Cameroon fever —see Malaria
Camptocormia (hysterical) F44.4
Camurati-Engelmann syndrome Q78.3
Canal —see also condition
　atrioventricular Q21.20
　　common Q21.23
　　incomplete Q21.21
　　intermediate Q21.22
　　partial Q21.21
　　transitional Q21.22
Canaliculitis (lacrimal) (acute) (subacute) H04.33-
　Actinomyces A42.89
　chronic H04.42-
Canavan disease E75.28
Canceled procedure (surgical) Z53.9
　because of
　　contraindication Z53.09
　　　smoking Z53.01
　　left against medical advice (AMA) Z53.29
　　patient's decision Z53.20
　　　for reasons of belief or group pressure Z53.1
　　　specified reason NEC Z53.29
　　specified reason NEC Z53.8
Cancer —see also Neoplasm, by site, malignant
　bile duct type liver C22.1
　blood —see Leukemia
　breast (see also Neoplasm, breast, malignant) C50.91-
　　hepatocellular C22.0
　lung (see also Neoplasm, lung, malignant) C34.90-
　ovarian (see also Neoplasm, ovary, malignant) C56.9-
　unspecified site (primary) C80.1
Cancer (o)**phobia** F45.29

Cancerous —see Neoplasm, malignant, by site
Cancrum oris A69.0
Candidiasis, candidal B37.9
　balanitis B37.42
　bronchitis B37.1
　cheilitis B37.83
　congenital P37.5
　cystitis B37.41
　disseminated B37.7
　endocarditis B37.6
　enteritis B37.82
　esophagitis B37.81
　intertrigo B37.2
　lung B37.1
　meningitis B37.5
　mouth B37.0
　nails B37.2
　neonatal P37.5
　onychia B37.2
　oral B37.0
　osteomyelitis B37.89
　otitis externa B37.84
　paronychia B37.2
　perionyxis B37.2
　pneumonia B37.1
　proctitis B37.82
　pulmonary B37.1
　pyelonephritis B37.49
　sepsis B37.7
　skin B37.2
　specified site NEC B37.89
　stomatitis B37.0
　systemic B37.7
　urethritis B37.41
　urogenital site NEC B37.49
　vagina (acute) B37.31
　　chronic (recurrent) B37.32
　vulva (acute) B37.31
　　chronic (recurrent) B37.32
　vulvovaginitis (acute) B37.31
　　chronic (recurrent) B37.32
Candidid L30.2
Candidosis —see Candidiasis
Candiru infection or infestation B88.8
Canities (premature) L67.1
　congenital Q84.2
Canker (mouth) (sore) K12.0
　rash A38.9
Cannabinosis J66.2
Cannabis induced
　anxiety disorder F12.980
　psychotic disorder F12.959
　sleep disorder F12.988
Canton fever A75.9
Cantrell's syndrome Q87.89
Capillariasis (intestinal) B81.1
　hepatic B83.8
Capillary —see condition
Caplan's syndrome —see Rheumatoid, lung
Capsule —see condition
Capsulitis (joint) —see also Enthesopathy
　adhesive (shoulder) M75.0-
　hepatic K65.8
　labyrinthine —see Otosclerosis, specified NEC
　thyroid E06.9
Caput
　crepitus Q75.8
　medusae I86.8
　succedaneum P12.81
Car sickness T75.3

Carapata (disease) A68.0
Carate —see Pinta
Carbon lung J60
Carbuncle L02.93
　abdominal wall L02.231
　anus K61.0
　auditory canal, external —see Abscess, ear, external
　auricle ear —see Abscess, ear, external
　axilla L02.43-
　back (any part) L02.232
　breast N61.1
　buttock L02.33
　cheek (external) L02.03
　chest wall L02.233
　chin L02.03
　corpus cavernosum N48.21
　ear (any part) (external) (middle) —see Abscess, ear, external
　external auditory canal —see Abscess, ear, external
　eyelid —see Abscess, eyelid
　face NEC L02.03
　femoral (region) —see Carbuncle, lower limb
　finger —see Carbuncle, hand
　flank L02.231
　foot L02.63-
　forehead L02.03
　genital —see Abscess, genital
　gluteal (region) L02.33
　groin L02.234
　hand L02.53-
　head NEC L02.831
　heel —see Carbuncle, foot
　hip —see Carbuncle, lower limb
　kidney —see Abscess, kidney
　knee —see Carbuncle, lower limb
　labium (majus) (minus) N76.4
　lacrimal
　　gland —see Dacryoadenitis
　　passages (duct) (sac) —see Inflammation, lacrimal, passages, acute
　leg —see Carbuncle, lower limb
　lower limb L02.43-
　malignant A22.0
　navel L02.236
　neck L02.13
　nose (external) (septum) J34.0
　orbit, orbital —see Abscess, orbit
　palmar (space) —see Carbuncle, hand
　partes posteriores L02.33
　pectoral region L02.233
　penis N48.21
　perineum L02.235
　pinna —see Abscess, ear, external
　popliteal —see Carbuncle, lower limb
　scalp L02.831
　seminal vesicle N49.0
　shoulder —see Carbuncle, upper limb
　specified site NEC L02.838
　temple (region) L02.03
　thumb —see Carbuncle, hand
　toe —see Carbuncle, foot
　trunk L02.239
　　abdominal wall L02.231
　　back L02.232
　　chest wall L02.233
　　groin L02.234
　　perineum L02.235
　　umbilicus L02.236
　umbilicus L02.236
　upper limb L02.43-
　urethra N34.0
　vulva N76.4

Carbunculus —see Carbuncle
Carcinoid (tumor) —see Tumor, carcinoid
Carcinoidosis E34.0
Carcinoma (malignant) —see also Neoplasm, by site, malignant
　acidophil
　　specified site —see Neoplasm, malignant, by site
　　unspecified site C75.1
　acidophil-basophil, mixed
　　specified site —see Neoplasm, malignant, by site
　　unspecified site C75.1
　adnexal (skin) —see Neoplasm, skin, malignant
　adrenal cortical C74.0-
　alveolar —see Neoplasm, lung, malignant
　　cell —see Neoplasm, lung, malignant
　ameloblastic C41.1
　　upper jaw (bone) C41.0
　apocrine
　　breast —see Neoplasm, breast, malignant
　　specified site NEC —see Neoplasm, skin, malignant
　　unspecified site C44.99
　basal cell (pigmented) (see also Neoplasm, skin, malignant) C44.91
　　fibro-epithelial —see Neoplasm, skin, malignant
　　morphea —see Neoplasm, skin, malignant
　　multicentric —see Neoplasm, skin, malignant
　basaloid
　basal-squamous cell, mixed —see Neoplasm, skin, malignant
　basophil
　　specified site —see Neoplasm, malignant, by site
　　unspecified site C75.1
　basophil-acidophil, mixed
　　specified site —see Neoplasm, malignant, by site
　　unspecified site C75.1
　basosquamous —see Neoplasm, skin, malignant
　bile duct
　　with hepatocellular, mixed C22.0
　　liver C22.1
　　specified site NEC —see Neoplasm, malignant, by site
　　unspecified site C22.1
　branchial or branchiogenic C10.4
　bronchial or bronchogenic —see Neoplasm, lung, malignant
　bronchiolar —see Neoplasm, lung, malignant
　bronchioloalveolar —see Neoplasm, lung, malignant
　C cell
　　specified site —see Neoplasm, malignant, by site
　　unspecified site C73
　ceruminous C44.29-
　cervix uteri
　　in situ D06.9
　　　endocervix D06.0
　　　exocervix D06.1
　　　specified site NEC D06.7
　chorionic
　　specified site —see Neoplasm, malignant, by site
　　unspecified site
　　　female C58
　　　male C62.90

Carcinoma (*continued*)
  chromophobe
    specified site —*see* Neoplasm,
      malignant,
      by site
    unspecified site C75.1
  cloacogenic
    specified site —*see* Neoplasm,
      malignant,
      by site
    unspecified site C21.2
  diffuse type
    specified site —*see* Neoplasm,
      malignant, by site
    unspecified site C16.9
  duct (cell)
    with Paget's disease —*see*
      Neoplasm, breast, malignant
    infiltrating
      with lobular carcinoma
        (in situ)
        specified site —*see*
          Neoplasm, malignant,
          by site
        unspecified site (female)
          C50.91-
          male C50.92-
      specified site —*see* Neoplasm,
        malignant, by site
      unspecified site (female)
        C50.91-
        male C50.92-
  ductal
    with lobular
      specified site —*see* Neoplasm,
        malignant, by site
      unspecified site (female)
        C50.91-
        male C50.92-
  ductular, infiltrating
    specified site —*see* Neoplasm,
      malignant, by site
    unspecified site (female) C50.91-
      male C50.92-
  embryonal
    liver C22.7
  endometrioid
    specified site —*see* Neoplasm,
      malignant, by site
    unspecified site
      female C56.9
      male C61
  eosinophil
    specified site —*see* Neoplasm,
      malignant, by site
    unspecified site C75.1
  epidermoid —*see also* Neoplasm,
    skin malignant
    in situ, Bowen's type —*see*
      Neoplasm, skin, in situ
  fibroepithelial, basal cell —*see*
    Neoplasm, skin, malignant
  follicular
    with papillary (mixed) C73
    moderately differentiated C73
    pure follicle C73
    specified site —*see* Neoplasm,
      malignant, by site
    trabecular C73
    unspecified site C73
    well differentiated C73
  generalized, with unspecified
    primary site C80.0
  glycogen-rich —*see* Neoplasm,
    breast, malignant
  granulosa cell C56-
  hepatic cell C22.0
  hepatocellular C22.0
    with bile duct, mixed C22.0
      fibrolamellar C22.0
  hepatocholangiolitic C22.0
  Hurthle cell C73

Carcinoma (*continued*)
  in
    adenomatous
      polyposis coli C18.9
    pleomorphic adenoma
      —*see* Neoplasm, salivary
      glands, malignant
    situ —*see* Carcinoma-in-situ
  infiltrating
    duct
      with lobular
        specified site —*see*
          Neoplasm, malignant,
          by site
        unspecified site (female)
          C50.91-
          male C50.92-
      with Paget's disease —*see*
        Neoplasm, breast, malignant
      specified site —*see* Neoplasm,
        malignant
      unspecified site (female)
        C50.91-
        male C50.92-
    ductular
      specified site —*see* Neoplasm,
        malignant
      unspecified site (female)
        C50.91-
        male C50.92-
    lobular
      specified site —*see* Neoplasm,
        malignant
      unspecified site (female)
        C50.91-
        male C50.92-
  inflammatory
    specified site —*see* Neoplasm,
      malignant
    unspecified site (female)
      C50.91-
      male C50.92-
  intestinal type
    specified site —*see* Neoplasm,
      malignant, by site
    unspecified site C16.9
  intracystic
    noninfiltrating —*see* Neoplasm,
      in situ, by site
  intraductal (noninfiltrating)
    with Paget's disease —*see*
      Neoplasm, breast, malignant
    breast D05.1-
    papillary
      with invasion
        specified site —*see*
          Neoplasm, malignant,
          by site
        unspecified site (female)
          C50.91-
          male C50.92-
      breast D05.1-
      specified site NEC —*see*
        Neoplasm, in situ, by
        site
      unspecified site (female)
        D05.1-
    specified site NEC —*see*
      Neoplasm, in situ, by site
    unspecified site (female)
      D05.1-
  intraepidermal —*see* Neoplasm,
    in situ
    squamous cell, Bowen's type
      —*see* Neoplasm, skin, in situ
  intraepithelial —*see* Neoplasm, in
    situ, by site
    squamous cell —*see* Neoplasm,
      in situ, by site
  intraosseous C41.1
    upper jaw (bone) C41.0

Carcinoma (*continued*)
  islet cell
    with exocrine, mixed
      specified site —*see* Neoplasm,
        malignant, by site
      unspecified site C25.9
    pancreas C25.4
    specified site NEC —*see*
      Neoplasm, malignant, by site
    unspecified site C25.4
  juvenile, breast —*see* Neoplasm,
    breast, malignant
  large cell
    small cell
      specified site —*see* Neoplasm,
        malignant, by site
      unspecified site C34.90
  Leydig cell (testis)
    specified site —*see* Neoplasm,
      malignant, by site
    unspecified site
      female C56.9
      male C62.90
  lipid-rich (female) C50.91-
    male C50.92-
  liver cell C22.0
  liver NEC C22.7
  lobular (infiltrating)
    with intraductal
      specified site —*see* Neoplasm,
        malignant, by site
      unspecified site (female)
        C50.91-
        male C50.92-
    noninfiltrating
      breast D05.0-
      specified site NEC —*see*
        Neoplasm, in situ, by site
      unspecified site D05.0-
    specified site —*see* Neoplasm,
      malignant, by site
    unspecified site (female) C50.91-
      male C50.92-
  medullary
    with
      amyloid stroma
        specified site —*see*
          Neoplasm, malignant,
          by site
        unspecified site C73
      lymphoid stroma
        specified site —*see*
          Neoplasm, malignant,
          by site
        unspecified site (female)
          C50.91-
          male C50.92-
  Merkel cell C4A.9
    anal margin C4A.51
    anal skin C4A.51
    canthus C4A.1-
    ear and external auricular canal
      C4A.2-
    external auricular canal C4A.2-
    eyelid, including canthus C4A.1-
    face C4A.30
      specified NEC C4A.39
    hip C4A.7-
    lip C4A.0
    lower limb, including hip C4A.7-
    neck C4A.4
    nodal presentation C7B.1
    nose C4A.31
    overlapping sites C4A.8
    perianal skin C4A.51
    scalp C4A.4
    secondary C7B.1
    shoulder C4A.6-
    skin of breast C4A.52
    trunk NEC C4A.59

Carcinoma (*continued*)
  Merkel cell (*continued*)
    upper limb, including shoulder
      C4A.6-
    visceral metastatic C7B.1
  metastatic —*see* Neoplasm,
    secondary, by site
  metatypical —*see* Neoplasm, skin,
    malignant
  morphea, basal cell —*see*
    Neoplasm, skin, malignant
  mucoid
    cell
      specified site —*see* Neoplasm,
        malignant, by site
      unspecified site C75.1
  neuroendocrine —*see also* Tumor,
    neuroendocrine
    high grade, any site C7A.1
    poorly differentiated, any site
      C7A.1
  nonencapsulated sclerosing C73
  noninfiltrating
    intracystic —*see* Neoplasm, in
      situ, by site
    intraductal
      breast D05.1-
      papillary
        breast D05.1-
        specified site NEC —*see*
          Neoplasm, in situ, by site
        unspecified site D05.1-
      specified site —*see* Neoplasm,
        in situ, by site
      unspecified site D05.1-
    lobular
      breast D05.0-
      specified site NEC —*see*
        Neoplasm, in situ, by site
      unspecified site (female)
        D05.0-
  oat cell
    specified site —*see* Neoplasm,
      malignant, by site
    unspecified site C34.90
  odontogenic C41.1
    upper jaw (bone) C41.0
  papillary
    with follicular (mixed) C73
    follicular variant C73
    intraductal (noninfiltrating)
      with invasion
        specified site —*see*
          Neoplasm, malignant,
          by site
        unspecified site (female)
          C50.91-
          male C50.92-
      breast D05.1-
      specified site NEC —*see*
        Neoplasm, in situ, by site
      unspecified site D05.1-
    serous
      specified site —*see* Neoplasm,
        malignant, by site
      surface
        specified site —*see*
          Neoplasm, malignant,
          by site
        unspecified site C56.9
      unspecified site C56.9
  papillocystic
    specified site —*see* Neoplasm,
      malignant, by site
    unspecified site C56.9
  parafollicular cell
    specified site —*see* Neoplasm,
      malignant, by site
    unspecified site C73
  pilomatrix —*see* Neoplasm, skin,
    malignant

Carcinoma *(continued)*
  pseudomucinous
    specified site —*see* Neoplasm, malignant, by site
    unspecified site C56.9
  renal cell C64-
  Schmincke —*see* Neoplasm, nasopharynx, malignant
  Schneiderian
    specified site —*see* Neoplasm, malignant, by site
    unspecified site C30.0
  sebaceous —*see* Neoplasm, skin, malignant
  secondary —*see also* Neoplasm, secondary, by site
    Merkel cell C7B.1
  secretory, breast —*see* Neoplasm, breast, malignant
  serous
    papillary
      specified site —*see* Neoplasm, malignant, by site
      unspecified site C56.9
    surface, papillary
      specified site —*see* Neoplasm, malignant, by site
      unspecified site C56.9
  Sertoli cell
    specified site —*see* Neoplasm, malignant, by site
    unspecified site C62.90
      female C56.9
      male C62.90
  skin appendage —*see* Neoplasm, skin, malignant
  small cell
    fusiform cell
      specified site —*see* Neoplasm, malignant, by site
      unspecified site C34.90
    intermediate cell
      specified site —*see* Neoplasm, malignant, by site
      unspecified site C34.90
    large cell
      specified site —*see* Neoplasm, malignant, by site
      unspecified site C34.90
  solid
    with amyloid stroma
      specified site —*see* Neoplasm, malignant, by site
      unspecified site C73
    microinvasive
      specified site —*see* Neoplasm, malignant, by site
      unspecified site C53.9
  sweat gland —*see* Neoplasm, skin, malignant
  theca cell C56.-
  thymic C37
  unspecified site (primary) C80.1
  water-clear cell C75.0

Carcinoma-in-situ —*see also* Neoplasm, in situ, by site
  breast NOS D05.9-
    specified type NEC D05.8-
  epidermoid —*see also* Neoplasm, in situ, by site
    with questionable stromal invasion
      cervix D06.9
      specified site NEC —*see* Neoplasm, in situ, by site
      unspecified site D06.9
    Bowen's type —*see* Neoplasm, skin, in situ
  intraductal
    breast D05.1-

Carcinoma-in-situ *(continued)*
  intraductal *(continued)*
    specified site NEC —*see* Neoplasm, in situ, by site
    unspecified site D05.1-
  lobular
    with
      infiltrating duct
        breast (female) C50.91-
          male C50.92-
        specified site NEC —*see* Neoplasm, malignant
        unspecified site (female) C50.91-
          male C50.92-
      intraductal
        breast D05.8-
        specified site NEC —*see* Neoplasm, in situ, by site
        unspecified site (female) D05.8-
    breast D05.0-
    specified site NEC —*see* Neoplasm, in situ, by site
    unspecified site D05.0-
  squamous cell —*see also* Neoplasm, in situ, by site
    with questionable stromal invasion
      cervix D06.9
      specified site NEC —*see* Neoplasm, in situ, by site
      unspecified site D06.9

Carcinomaphobia F45.29

Carcinomatosis C80.0
  peritonei C78.6
  unspecified site (primary) (secondary) C80.0

Carcinosarcoma —*see* Neoplasm, malignant, by site
  embryonal —*see* Neoplasm, malignant, by site

Cardia, cardial —*see* condition

Cardiac —*see also* condition
  death, sudden —*see* Arrest, cardiac
  pacemaker
    in situ Z95.0
    management or adjustment Z45.018
  tamponade I31.4

Cardialgia —*see* Pain, precordial

Cardiectasis —*see* Hypertrophy, cardiac

Cardiochalasia K21.9

Cardiomalacia I51.5

Cardiomegalia glycogenica diffusa E74.02 *[143]*

Cardiomegaly —*see also* Hypertrophy, cardiac
  congenital Q24.8
  glycogen E74.02 *[143]*
  idiopathic I51.7

Cardiomyoliposis I51.5

Cardiomyopathy (familial) (idiopathic) I42.9
  alcoholic I42.6
  amyloid E85.4 *[143]*
    transthyretin-related (ATTR) familial E85.4 *[143]*
  arteriosclerotic —*see* Disease, heart, ischemic, atherosclerotic
  beriberi E51.12
  cobalt-beer I42.6
  congenital I42.4
  congestive I42.0
  constrictive NOS I42.5
  dilated I42.0

Cardiomyopathy *(continued)*
  due to
    alcohol I42.6
    beriberi E51.12
    cardiac glycogenosis E74.02 *[143]*
    drugs I42.7
    external agents NEC I42.7
    Friedreich's ataxia G11.11
    myotonia atrophica G71.11 *[143]*
    progressive muscular dystrophy (*see also* Dystrophy, muscular, by type) G71.09 *[143]*
  glycogen storage E74.02 *[143]*
  hypertensive —*see* Hypertension, heart
  hypertrophic (nonobstructive) I42.2
    obstructive I42.1
      congenital Q24.8
  in
    Chagas' disease (chronic) B57.2
      acute B57.0
    sarcoidosis D86.85
  ischemic I25.5
  metabolic E88.9 *[143]*
    thyrotoxic E05.90 *[143]*
      with thyroid storm E05.91 *[143]*
  newborn I42.8
    congenital I42.4
  non-ischemic (*see also* by cause) I42.8
  nutritional E63.9 *[143]*
    beriberi E51.12
  obscure of Africa I42.8
  peripartum O90.3
  postpartum O90.3
  restrictive NEC I42.5
  rheumatic I09.0
  secondary I42.9
  specified NEC I42.8
  stress induced I51.81
  takotsubo I51.81
  thyrotoxic E05.90 *[143]*
    with thyroid storm E05.91 *[143]*
  toxic NEC I42.7
  transthyretin-related (ATTR) familial amyloid E85.4
  tuberculous A18.84
  viral B33.24

Cardionephritis —*see* Hypertension, cardiorenal

Cardionephropathy —*see* Hypertension, cardiorenal

Cardionephrosis —*see* Hypertension, cardiorenal

Cardiopathia nigra I27.0

Cardiopathy —*see also* Disease, heart I51.9
  idiopathic I42.9
  mucopolysaccharidosis E76.3 *[152]*

Cardiopericarditis —*see* Pericarditis

Cardiophobia F45.29

Cardiorenal —*see* condition

Cardiorrhexis —*see* Infarct, myocardium

Cardiosclerosis —*see* Disease, heart, ischemic, atherosclerotic

Cardiosis —*see* Disease, heart

Cardiospasm (esophagus) (reflex) (stomach) K22.0
  congenital Q39.5
  with megaesophagus Q39.5

Cardiostenosis —*see* Disease, heart

Cardiosymphysis I31.0

Cardiovascular —*see* condition

Carditis (acute) (bacterial) (chronic) (subacute) I51.89
  meningococcal A39.50

Carditis *(continued)*
  rheumatic —*see* Disease, heart, rheumatic
  rheumatoid —*see* Rheumatoid, carditis
  viral B33.20

Care (of) (for) (following)
  child (routine) Z76.2
  family member (handicapped) (sick)
    creating problem for family Z63.6
    provided away from home for holiday relief Z75.5
    unavailable, due to
      absence (person rendering care) (sufferer) Z74.2
      inability (any reason) of person rendering care Z74.2
  foundling Z76.1
  holiday relief Z75.5
  improper —*see* Maltreatment
  lack of (at or after birth) (infant) —*see* Maltreatment, child, neglect
  lactating mother Z39.1
  palliative Z51.5
  postpartum
    immediately after delivery Z39.0
    routine follow-up Z39.2
  respite Z75.5
  unavailable, due to
    absence of person rendering care Z74.2
    inability (any reason) of person rendering care Z74.2
  well-baby Z76.2

Caries
  bone NEC A18.03
  dental (dentino enamel junction) (early in childhood) (of dentine) (pre-eruptive) (recurrent) (to the pulp) K02.9
    arrested (coronal) (root) K02.3
    chewing surface
      limited to enamel K02.51
      penetrating into dentin K02.52
      penetrating into pulp K02.53
    coronal surface
      chewing surface
        limited to enamel K02.51
        penetrating into dentin K02.52
        penetrating into pulp K02.53
      pit and fissure surface
        limited to enamel K02.51
        penetrating into dentin K02.52
        penetrating into pulp K02.53
      smooth surface
        limited to enamel K02.61
        penetrating into dentin K02.62
        penetrating into pulp K02.63
    pit and fissure surface
      limited to enamel K02.51
      penetrating into dentin K02.52
      penetrating into pulp K02.53
    primary, cervical origin K02.52
    root K02.7
    smooth surface
      limited to enamel K02.61
      penetrating into dentin K02.62
      penetrating into pulp K02.63
  external meatus —*see* Disorder, ear, external, specified type NEC
  hip (tuberculous) A18.02

Caries *(continued)*
  initial (tooth)
    chewing surface K02.51
    pit and fissure surface K02.51
    smooth surface K02.61
  knee (tuberculous) A18.02
  labyrinth —*see* subcategory H83.8
  limb NEC (tuberculous) A18.03
  mastoid process (chronic) —*see* Mastoiditis, chronic tuberculous A18.03
  middle ear —*see* subcategory H74.8
  nose (tuberculous) A18.03
  orbit (tuberculous) A18.03
  ossicles, ear —*see* Abnormal, ear ossicles
  petrous bone —*see* Petrositis
  root (dental) (tooth) K02.7
  sacrum (tuberculous) A18.01
  spine, spinal (column) (tuberculous) A18.01
  syphilitic A52.77
    congenital (early) A50.02 *[M90.80]*
  tooth, teeth —*see* Caries, dental
  tuberculous A18.03
  vertebra (column) (tuberculous) A18.01

Carious teeth —*see* Caries, dental

Carneous mole O02.0

Carnitine insufficiency E71.40

Carotenemia (dietary) E67.1

Carotenosis (cutis) (skin) E67.1

Carotid body or sinus syndrome G90.01

Carotidynia G90.01

Carpal tunnel syndrome —*see* Syndrome, carpal tunnel

Carpenter's syndrome Q87.0

Carpopedal spasm —*see* Tetany

Carr-Barr-Plunkett syndrome Q97.1

Carrier (suspected) of
  Acinetobacter baumannii Z22.349
    carbapenem-resistant Z22.340
    carbapenem-sensitive Z22.341
  amebiasis Z22.1
  bacterial disease NEC Z22.39
    diphtheria Z22.2
    intestinal infectious NEC Z22.1
      typhoid Z22.0
    meningococcal Z22.31
    sexually transmitted Z22.4
    specified NEC Z22.39
    staphylococcal (Methicillin susceptible) Z22.321
      Methicillin resistant Z22.322
    streptococcal Z22.338
      group B Z22.330
        complicating pregnancy or delivery O99.82-
    typhoid Z22.0
  cholera Z22.1
  diphtheria Z22.2
  E. coli (Escherichia coli) Z22.35-
  Enterobacterales Z22.359
    carbapenem-resistant Z22.350
    carbapenem-sensitive Z22.358
    Enterobacterales, specified type NEC Z22.358
    ESBL-producing Z22.358
    extended-spectrum beta-lactamase producing Z22.358
  gastrointestinal pathogens NEC Z22.1

Carrier *(continued)*
  genetic Z14.8
    cystic fibrosis Z14.1
    hemophilia A (asymptomatic) Z14.01
      symptomatic Z14.02
  gestational, pregnant Z33.1
  gonorrhea Z22.4
  HAA (hepatitis Australian-antigen) B18.8
  HB (c)(s)-AG B18.1
  hepatitis (viral) B18.9
    Australia-antigen (HAA) B18.8
    B surface antigen (HBsAg) B18.1
      with acute delta-(super) infection B17.0
    C B18.2
    specified NEC B18.8
  human T-cell lymphotropic virus type-1(HTLV-1) infection Z22.6
  infectious organism Z22.9
    specified NEC Z22.8
  K. pneumoniae (Klebsiella pneumoniae) Z22.35-
  meningococci Z22.31
  Salmonella typhosa Z22.0
  serum hepatitis —*see* Carrier, hepatitis
  staphylococci (Methicillin susceptible) Z22.321
    Methicillin resistant Z22.322
  streptococci Z22.338
    group B Z22.330
      complicating pregnancy or delivery O99.82-
  syphilis Z22.4
  typhoid Z22.0
  venereal disease NEC Z22.4

Carrion's disease A44.0

Carter's relapsing fever (Asiatic) A68.1

Cartilage —*see* condition

Caruncle (inflamed)
  conjunctiva (acute) —*see* Conjunctivitis, acute
  labium (majus) (minus) N90.89
  lacrimal —*see* Inflammation, lacrimal, passages
  myrtiform N89.8
  urethral (benign) N36.2

Cascade stomach K31.2

Caseation lymphatic gland (tuberculous) A18.2

Cassidy (-Scholte) **syndrome** (malignant carcinoid) E34.0

Castellani's disease A69.8

Castration, traumatic, male S38.231

Casts in urine R82.998

Cat
  cry syndrome Q93.4
  ear Q17.3
  eye syndrome Q92.8

Catabolism, senile R54

Catalepsy (hysterical) F44.2
  schizophrenic F20.2

Cataplexy (idiopathic) —*see* - Narcolepsy

Cataract (cortical) (immature) (incipient) H26.9
  with
    neovascularization —*see* Cataract, complicated
  age-related —*see* Cataract, senile
  anterior
    and posterior axial embryonal Q12.0
    pyramidal Q12.0

Cataract *(continued)*
  associated with
    galactosemia E74.21 *[H28]*
    myotonic disorders G71.19 *[H28]*
  blue Q12.0
  central Q12.0
  cerulean Q12.0
  complicated H26.20
    with
      neovascularization H26.21-
      ocular disorder H26.22-
      glaucomatous flecks H26.23-
  congenital Q12.0
  coraliform Q12.0
  coronary Q12.0
  crystalline Q12.0
  diabetic —*see* Diabetes, cataract
  drug-induced H26.3-
  due to
    ocular disorder —*see* Cataract, complicated
    radiation H26.8
  electric H26.8
  extraction status Z98.4-
  glass-blower's H26.8
  heat ray H26.8
  heterochromic —*see* Cataract, complicated
  hypermature —*see* Cataract, senile, morgagnian type
  in (due to)
    chronic iridocyclitis —*see* Cataract, complicated
    diabetes —*see* Diabetes, cataract
    endocrine disease E34.9 *[H28]*
    eye disease —*see* Cataract, complicated
    hypoparathyroidism E20.9 *[H28]*
    malnutrition-dehydration E46 *[H28]*
    metabolic disease E88.9 *[H28]*
    myotonic disorders G71.19 *[H28]*
    nutritional disease E63.9 *[H28]*
  infantile —*see* Cataract, presenile
  irradiational —*see* Cataract, specified NEC
  juvenile —*see* Cataract, presenile
  malnutrition-dehydration E46 *[H28]*
  morgagnian —*see* Cataract, senile, morgagnian type
  myotonic G71.19 *[H28]*
  myxedema E03.9 *[H28]*
  nuclear
    embryonal Q12.0
    sclerosis —*see* Cataract, senile, nuclear
  presenile H26.00-
    combined forms H26.06-
    cortical H26.01-
      lamellar —*see* Cataract, presenile, cortical
    nuclear H26.03-
    specified NEC H26.09
    subcapsular polar (anterior) H26.04-
      posterior H26.05-
    zonular —*see* Cataract, presenile, cortical
  secondary H26.40
    Soemmering's ring H26.41-
    specified NEC H26.49-
    to eye disease —*see* Cataract, complicated
  senile H25.9
    brunescens —*see* Cataract, senile, nuclear
    combined forms H25.81-

Cataract *(continued)*
  senile *(continued)*
    coronary —*see* Cataract, senile, incipient
    cortical H25.01-
    hypermature —*see* Cataract, senile, morgagnian type
    incipient (mature) (total) H25.09-
      cortical —*see* Cataract, senile, cortical
      subcapsular —*see* Cataract, senile, subcapsular
    morgagnian type (hypermature) H25.2-
    nuclear (sclerosis) H25.1-
    polar subcapsular (anterior) (posterior) —*see* Cataract, senile, incipient
    punctate —*see* Cataract, senile, incipient
    specified NEC H25.89
    subcapsular polar (anterior) H25.03-
      posterior H25.04-
  snowflake —*see* Diabetes, cataract
  specified NEC H26.8
  toxic —*see* Cataract, drug-induced
  traumatic H26.10-
    localized H26.11-
    partially resolved H26.12-
    total H26.13-
  zonular (perinuclear) Q12.0

Cataracta —*see also* Cataract
  brunescens —*see* Cataract, senile, nuclear
  centralis pulverulenta Q12.0
  cerulea Q12.0
  complicata —*see* Cataract, complicated
  congenita Q12.0
  coralliformis Q12.0
  coronaria Q12.0
  diabetic —*see* Diabetes, cataract
  membranacea
    accreta —*see* Cataract, secondary
    congenita Q12.0
  nigra —*see* Cataract, senile, nuclear
  sunflower —*see* Cataract, complicated

Catarrh, catarrhal (acute) (febrile) (infectious) (inflammation) —*see also* condition J00
  bronchial —*see* Bronchitis
  chest —*see* Bronchitis
  chronic J31.0
  due to congenital syphilis A50.03
  enteric —*see* Enteritis
  eustachian H68.009
  fauces —*see* Pharyngitis
  gastrointestinal —*see* Enteritis
  gingivitis K05.00
    nonplaque induced K05.01
    plaque induced K05.00
  hay —*see* Fever, hay
  intestinal —*see* Enteritis
  larynx, chronic J37.0
  liver B15.9
    with hepatic coma B15.0
  lung —*see* Bronchitis
  middle ear, chronic —*see* Otitis, media, nonsuppurative, chronic, serous
  mouth K12.1
  nasal (chronic) —*see* Rhinitis
  nasobronchial J31.1
  nasopharyngeal (chronic) J31.1
    acute J00

Catarrh, catarrhal *(continued)*
  pulmonary —*see* Bronchitis
  spring (eye) (vernal) —*see*
    Conjunctivitis, acute, atopic
  summer (hay) —*see* Fever, hay
  throat J31.2
  tubotympanal —*see also* Otitis,
    media, nonsuppurative
    chronic —*see* Otitis, media,
      nonsuppurative, chronic,
      serous
Catatonia (schizophrenic) F20.2
Catatonic
  disorder due to known physiologic
    condition F06.1
  schizophrenia F20.2
  stupor R40.1
Cat-scratch —*see also* Abrasion
  disease or fever A28.1
Cauda equina —*see* condition
Cauliflower ear M95.1-
Causalgia (upper limb) G56.4-
  lower limb G57.7-
Cause
  external, general effects T75.89
Caustic burn —*see* Corrosion, by site
Cavare's disease (familial periodic
  paralysis) G72.3
Cave-in, injury
  crushing (severe) —*see* Crush
  suffocation —*see* Asphyxia,
    traumatic, due to low oxygen,
    due to cave-in
Cavernitis (penis) N48.29
Cavernositis N48.29
Cavernous —*see* condition
Cavitation of lung —*see also*
  Tuberculosis, pulmonary
  nontuberculous J98.4
Cavities, dental —*see* Caries, dental
Cavity
  lung —*see* Cavitation of lung
  optic papilla Q14.2
  pulmonary —*see* Cavitation of lung
Cavovarus foot, congenital Q66.1-
Cavus foot (congenital) Q66.7-
  acquired —*see* Deformity, limb,
    foot, specified NEC
Cazenave's disease L10.2
CDKL5 (Cyclin-Dependent Kinase-
  Like 5 Deficiency Disorder) G40.42
Cecitis K52.9
  with perforation, peritonitis, or
    rupture K65.8
Cecoureterocele Q62.32
Cecum —*see* condition
Celiac
  artery compression syndrome I77.4
  disease (with steatorrhea) K90.0
  infantilism K90.0
Cell(s), cellular —*see also* condition
  in urine R82.998
Cellulitis (diffuse) (phlegmonous)
  (septic) (suppurative) L03.90
  abdominal wall L03.311
  anaerobic A48.0
  ankle —*see* Cellulitis, lower limb
  anus K61.0
  arm —*see* Cellulitis, upper limb
  auricle (ear) —*see* Cellulitis, ear
  axilla L03.11-

Cellulitis *(continued)*
  back (any part) L03.312
  breast (acute) (nonpuerperal)
    (subacute) N61.0
    nipple N61.0
  broad ligament
    acute N73.0
  buttock L03.317
  cervical (meaning neck) L03.221
  cervix (uteri) —*see* Cervicitis
  cheek (external) L03.211
    internal K12.2
  chest wall L03.313
  chronic L03.90
  clostridial A48.0
  corpus cavernosum N48.22
  digit
    finger —*see* Cellulitis, finger
    toe —*see* Cellulitis, toe
  Douglas' cul-de-sac or pouch
    acute N73.0
  drainage site (following operation)
    T81.49
  ear (external) H60.1-
  eosinophilic (granulomatous) L98.3
  erysipelatous —*see* Erysipelas
  external auditory canal —*see*
    Cellulitis, ear
  eyelid —*see* Abscess, eyelid
  face NEC L03.211
  finger (intrathecal) (periosteal)
    (subcutaneous) (subcuticular)
    L03.01-
  foot —*see* Cellulitis, lower limb
  gangrenous —*see* Gangrene
  genital organ NEC
    female (external) N76.4
    male N49.9
      multiple sites N49.8
      specified NEC N49.8
  gluteal (region) L03.317
  gonococcal A54.89
  groin L03.314
  hand —*see* Cellulitis, upper limb
  head NEC L03.811
    face (any part, except ear, eye
      and nose) L03.211
  heel —*see* Cellulitis, lower limb
  hip —*see* Cellulitis, lower limb
  jaw (region) L03.211
  knee —*see* Cellulitis, lower limb
  labium (majus) (minus) —*see*
    Vulvitis
  lacrimal passages —*see*
    Inflammation, lacrimal, passages
  larynx J38.7
  leg —*see* Cellulitis, lower limb
  lip K13.0
  lower limb L03.11-
    toe —*see* Cellulitis, toe
  mouth (floor) K12.2
  multiple sites, so stated L03.90
  nasopharynx J39.1
  navel L03.316
    newborn P38.9
      with mild hemorrhage P38.1
      without hemorrhage P38.9
  neck (region) L03.221
  nipple (acute) (nonpuerperal)
    (subacute) N61.0
  nose (septum) (external) J34.0
  orbit, orbital H05.01-
  palate (soft) K12.2
  pectoral (region) L03.313
  pelvis, pelvic (chronic)
    female —*see also* Disease,
      pelvis, inflammatory N73.2
      acute N73.0
    following ectopic or molar
      pregnancy O08.0
    male K65.0

Cellulitis *(continued)*
  penis N48.22
  perineal, perineum L03.315
  periorbital L03.213
  perirectal K61.1
  peritonsillar J36
  periurethral N34.0
  periuterine (*see also* Disease pelvis,
    inflammatory) N73.2
    acute N73.0
  pharynx J39.1
  preseptal L03.213
  rectum K61.1
  retroperitoneal K68.9
  round ligament
    acute N73.0
  scalp (any part) L03.811
  scrotum N49.2
  seminal vesicle N49.0
  shoulder —*see* Cellulitis, upper limb
  specified site NEC L03.818
  submandibular (region) (space)
    (triangle) K12.2
    gland K11.3
  submaxillary (region) K12.2
    gland K11.3
  thigh —*see* Cellulitis, lower limb
  thumb (intrathecal) (periosteal)
    (subcutaneous) (subcuticular)
    —*see* Cellulitis, finger
  toe (intrathecal) (periosteal)
    (subcutaneous) (subcuticular)
    L03.03-
  tonsil J36
  trunk L03.319
    abdominal wall L03.311
    back (any part) L03.312
    buttock L03.317
    chest wall L03.313
    groin L03.314
    perineal, perineum L03.315
    umbilicus L03.316
  tuberculous (primary) A18.4
  umbilicus L03.316
  upper limb L03.11-
    axilla —*see* Cellulitis, axilla
    finger —*see* Cellulitis, finger
    thumb —*see* Cellulitis, finger
  vaccinal T88.0
  vocal cord J38.3
  vulva —*see* Vulvitis
  wrist —*see* Cellulitis, upper limb
Cementoblastoma, benign —*see*
  Cyst, calcifying odontogenic
Cementoma —*see* Cyst, calcifying
  odontogenic
Cementoperiostitis —*see* Periodontitis
Cementosis K03.4
**Central auditory processing
  disorder** H93.25
Central pain syndrome G89.0
Cephalematocele, cephalhematocele
  newborn P52.8
  birth injury P10.8
  traumatic —*see* Hematoma, brain
Cephalematoma, cephalhematoma
  (calcified)
  newborn (birth injury) P12.0
  traumatic —*see* Hematoma, brain
Cephalgia, cephalalgia —*see also*
  Headache
  histamine G44.009
    intractable G44.001
    not intractable G44.009
  trigeminal autonomic (TAC) NEC
    G44.099
    intractable G44.091
    not intractable G44.099

Cephalic —*see* condition
Cephalitis —*see* Encephalitis
Cephalocele —*see* Encephalocele
Cephalomenia N94.89
Cephalopelvic —*see* condition
Cerclage (with cervical
  incompetence) **in pregnancy** —*see*
  Incompetence, cervix, in pregnancy
Cerebellitis —*see* Encephalitis
Cerebellum, cerebellar —*see* condition
Cerebral —*see* condition
Cerebritis —*see* Encephalitis
Cerebro-hepato-renal syndrome
  Q87.89
Cerebromalacia —*see* Softening,
  brain
  sequelae of cerebrovascular disease
    I69.398
Cerebroside lipidosis E75.22
Cerebrospasticity (congenital) G80.1
Cerebrospinal —*see* condition
Cerebrum —*see* condition
Ceroid-lipofuscinosis, neuronal
  E75.4
Cerumen (accumulation) (impacted)
  H61.2-
Cervical —*see also* condition
  auricle Q18.2
  dysplasia in pregnancy —*see*
    Abnormal, cervix, in pregnancy
    or childbirth
  erosion in pregnancy —*see*
    Abnormal, cervix, in pregnancy
    or childbirth
  fibrosis in pregnancy —*see*
    Abnormal, cervix, in pregnancy
    or childbirth
  fusion syndrome Q76.1
  rib Q76.5
  shortening (complicating
    pregnancy) O26.87-
Cervicalgia M54.2
Cervicitis (acute) (atrophic) (chronic)
  (nonvenereal) (senile) (subacute)
  (with ulceration) N72
  with
    abortion —*see* Abortion, by type
      complicated by genital tract
      and pelvic infection
    ectopic pregnancy O08.0
    molar pregnancy O08.0
  chlamydial A56.09
  gonococcal A54.03
  herpesviral A60.03
  puerperal (postpartum) O86.11
  syphilitic A52.76
  trichomonal A59.09
  tuberculous A18.16
Cervicocolpitis (emphysematosa)
  (*see also* Cervicitis) N72
Cervix —*see* condition
**Cesarean delivery, previous,
  affecting management of
  pregnancy** O34.219
  classical (vertical) scar O34.212
  isthmocele (non-pregnant state)
    N85.A
    maternal care for O34.22
  low transverse scar O34.211
  mid-transverse T incision O34.218
  scar
    defect (non-pregnant state) N85.A
    maternal care for O34.22
    specified type NEC O34.218

55

Céstan (-Chenais) **paralysis or syndrome** G46.3
Céstan-Raymond syndrome I65.8
Cestode infestation B71.9
  specified type NEC B71.8
Cestodiasis B71.9
Chabert's disease A22.9
Chacaleh E53.8
Chafing L30.4
Chagas' (-Mazza) **disease** (chronic) B57.2
  with
    cardiovascular involvement NEC B57.2
    digestive system involvement B57.30
      megacolon B57.32
      megaesophagus B57.31
      other specified B57.39
    megacolon B57.32
    megaesophagus B57.31
    myocarditis B57.2
    nervous system involvement B57.40
      meningitis B57.41
      meningoencephalitis B57.42
      other specified B57.49
    specified organ involvement NEC B57.5
  acute (with) B57.1
    cardiovascular NEC B57.0
    myocarditis B57.0
Chagres fever B50.9
Chairridden Z74.09
Chalasia (cardiac sphincter) K21.9
Chalazion H00.19
  left H00.16
    lower H00.15
    upper H00.14
  right H00.13
    lower H00.12
    upper H00.11
Chalcosis —see also Disorder, globe, degenerative, chalcosis
  cornea —see Deposit, cornea
  crystalline lens —see Cataract, complicated
  retina H35.89
Chalicosis (pulmonum) J62.8
Chancre (any genital site) (hard) (hunterian) (mixed) (primary) (seronegative) (seropositive) (syphilitic) A51.0
  congenital A50.07
  conjunctiva NEC A51.2
  Ducrey's A57
  extragenital A51.2
  eyelid A51.2
  lip A51.2
  nipple A51.2
  Nisbet's A57
  of
    carate A67.0
    pinta A67.0
    yaws A66.0
  palate, soft A51.2
  phagedenic A57
  simple A57
  soft A57
    bubo A57
    palate A51.2
  urethra A51.0
  yaws A66.1
Chancroid (anus) (genital) (penis) (perineum) (rectum) (urethra) (vulva) A57

Chandler's disease (osteochondritis dissecans, hip) —see Osteochondritis, dissecans, hip
Change(s) (in) (of) —see also Removal
  arteriosclerotic —see Arteriosclerosis
  bone —see also Disorder, bone
    diabetic —see Diabetes, bone change
  bowel habit R19.4
  cardiorenal (vascular) —see Hypertension, cardiorenal
  cardiovascular —see Disease, cardiovascular
  circulatory I99.9
  cognitive (mild) (organic) R41.89
  color, tooth, teeth
    during formation K00.8
    posteruptive K03.7
  contraceptive device Z30.433
  corneal membrane H18.30
    Bowman's membrane fold or rupture H18.31-
    Descemet's membrane fold H18.32-
    rupture H18.33-
  coronary —see Disease, heart, ischemic
  degenerative, spine or vertebra —see Spondylosis
  dental pulp, regressive K04.2
  dressing (nonsurgical) Z48.00
    surgical Z48.01
  heart —see Disease, heart
  hip joint —see Derangement, joint, hip
  hyperplastic larynx J38.7
  hypertrophic
    nasal sinus J34.89
    turbinate, nasal J34.3
    upper respiratory tract J39.8
  indwelling catheter Z46.6
  inflammatory —see also Inflammation
    sacroiliac M46.1
  job, anxiety concerning Z56.1
  joint —see Derangement, joint
  life —see Menopause
  mental status R41.82
  minimal (glomerular) (see also N00-N07 with fourth character .0) N05.0
  myocardium, myocardial —see Degeneration, myocardial
  of life —see Menopause
  pacemaker Z45.018
    pulse generator Z45.010
  personality (enduring) F68.8
    due to (secondary to)
      general medical condition F07.0
      secondary (nonspecific) F60.89
  regressive, dental pulp K04.2
  renal —see Disease, renal
  retina H35.9
    myopic (see also Myopia, degenerative) H44.2-
  sacroiliac joint M53.3
  senile (see also condition) R54
  sensory R20.8
  skin R23.9
    acute, due to ultraviolet radiation L56.9
      specified NEC L56.8
    chronic, due to nonionizing radiation L57.9
      specified NEC L57.8
    cyanosis R23.0
    flushing R23.2
    pallor R23.1
    petechiae R23.3
    specified change NEC R23.8
    swelling —see Mass, localized
    texture R23.4

Change (continued)
  trophic
    arm —see Mononeuropathy, upper limb
    leg —see Mononeuropathy, lower limb
  vascular I99.9
  vasomotor I73.9
  voice R49.9
    psychogenic F44.4
    specified NEC R49.8
Changing sleep-work schedule, affecting sleep G47.26
Changuinola fever A93.1
Chapping skin T69.8
Charcot-Marie-Tooth disease, paralysis or syndrome G60.0
Charcot's
  arthropathy —see Arthropathy, neuropathic
  cirrhosis K74.3
  disease (tabetic arthropathy) A52.16
  joint (disease) (tabetic) A52.16
    diabetic —see Diabetes, with, arthropathy
    syringomyelic G95.0
  syndrome (intermittent claudication) I73.9
CHARGE association Q89.8
Charley-horse (quadriceps) M62.831
  traumatic (quadriceps) S76.11-
Charlouis' disease —see Yaws
Cheadle's disease E54
Checking (of)
  cardiac pacemaker (battery) (electrode(s)) Z45.018
    pulse generator Z45.010
  implantable subdermal contraceptive Z30.46
  intrauterine contraceptive device Z30.431
  wound Z48.0-
    due to injury - code to Injury, by site, using appropriate seventh character for subsequent encounter
    postoperative —see Aftercare
Check-up —see Examination
Chédiak-Higashi (-Steinbrinck) **syndrome** (congenital gigantism of peroxidase granules) E70.330
Cheek —see condition
Cheese itch B88.0
Cheese-washer's lung J67.8
Cheese-worker's lung J67.8
Cheilitis (acute) (angular) (catarrhal) (chronic) (exfoliative) (gangrenous) (glandular) (infectional) (suppurative) (ulcerative) (vesicular) K13.0
  actinic (due to sun) L56.8
    other than from sun L59.8
  candidal B37.83
Cheilodynia K13.0
Cheiloschisis —see Cleft, lip
Cheilosis (angular) K13.0
  with pellagra E52
  due to
    vitamin B2(riboflavin) deficiency E53.0
Cheiromegaly M79.89
Cheiropompholyx L30.1
Cheloid —see Keloid
Chemical burn —see Corrosion, by site

Chemodectoma —see Paraganglioma, nonchromaffin
Chemosis, conjunctiva —see Edema, conjunctiva
Chemotherapy (session) (for)
  cancer Z51.11
  neoplasm Z51.11
Cherubism M27.8
Chest —see condition
Cheyne-Stokes breathing (respiration) R06.3
Chiari's
  disease or syndrome (hepatic vein thrombosis) I82.0
  malformation
    type I G93.5
    type II —see Spina bifida
  net Q24.8
Chicago disease B40.9
Chickenpox —see Varicella
Chiclero ulcer or sore B55.1
Chigger (infestation) B88.0
Chignon (disease) B36.8
  newborn (from vacuum extraction) (birth injury) P12.1
Chilaiditi's syndrome (subphrenic displacement, colon) Q43.3
Chilblain(s) (lupus) T69.1
Child
  custody dispute Z65.3
Childbirth —see Delivery
Childhood
  cerebral X-linked adrenoleukodystrophy E71.520
  period of rapid growth Z00.2
Chill(s) R68.83
  with fever R50.9
  congestive in malarial regions B54
  without fever R68.83
Chilomastigiasis A07.8
Chimera 46,XX/46,XY Q99.0
Chin —see condition
Chinese dysentery A03.9
Chionophobia F40.228
Chitral fever A93.1
Chlamydia, chlamydial A74.9
  cervicitis A56.09
  conjunctivitis A74.0
  cystitis A56.01
  endometritis A56.11
  epididymitis A56.19
  female
    pelvic inflammatory disease A56.11
    pelviperitonitis A56.11
  orchitis A56.19
  peritonitis A74.81
  pharyngitis A56.4
  proctitis A56.3
  psittaci (infection) A70
  salpingitis A56.11
  sexually-transmitted infection NEC A56.8
  specified NEC A74.89
  urethritis A56.01
  vulvovaginitis A56.02
Chlamydiosis —see Chlamydia
Chloasma (skin) (idiopathic) (symptomatic) L81.1
  eyelid H02.719
    hyperthyroid E05.90 [H02.719]
    with thyroid storm E05.91 [H02.719]

Chloasma *(continued)*
  eyelid *(continued)*
    left H02.716
      lower H02.715
      upper H02.714
    right H02.713
      lower H02.712
      upper H02.711
Chloroma C92.3-
Chlorosis D50.9
  Egyptian B76.9 *[D63.8]*
  miner's B76.9 *[D63.8]*
Chlorotic anemia D50.8
Chocolate cyst (ovary) N80.10-
Choked
  disc or disk —*see* Papilledema
  on food, phlegm, or vomitus NOS
    —*see* Foreign body, by site
  while vomiting NOS —*see* Foreign
    body, by site
Chokes (resulting from bends) T70.3
Choking sensation R09.89
Cholangiectasis K83.8
Cholangiocarcinoma
  with hepatocellular carcinoma,
    combined C22.0
  liver C22.1
  specified site NEC —*see*
    Neoplasm, malignant, by site
  unspecified site C22.1
Cholangiohepatitis K83.8
  due to fluke infestation B66.1
Cholangiohepatoma C22.0
Cholangiolitis (acute) (chronic)
  (extrahepatic) (gangrenous)
  (intrahepatic) K83.09
  paratyphoidal —*see* Fever,
    paratyphoid
  typhoidal A01.09
Cholangioma D13.4
  malignant —*see*
    Cholangiocarcinoma
Cholangitis (ascending) (primary)
  (recurrent) (sclerosing) (secondary)
  (stenosing) (suppurative) K83.09
  with calculus, bile duct —*see*
    Calculus, bile duct, with
    cholangitis
  chronic nonsuppurative destructive
    K74.3
  primary K83.09
    sclerosing K83.01
  sclerosing K83.09
Cholecystectasia K82.8
Cholecystitis K81.9
  with
    calculus, stones in
      bile duct (common) (hepatic)
        —*see* Calculus, bile duct,
        with cholecystitis
      cystic duct —*see* Calculus,
        gallbladder, with
        cholecystitis
      gallbladder —*see* Calculus,
        gallbladder, with
        cholecystitis
    choledocholithiasis —*see*
      Calculus, bile duct, with
      cholecystitis
    cholelithiasis —*see* Calculus,
      gallbladder, with cholecystitis
  gangrene of gallbladder
    K82.A1
  perforation of gallbladder
    K82.A2

Cholecystitis *(continued)*
  acute (emphysematous)
    (gangrenous) (suppurative)
    K81.0
    with
      calculus, stones in
        cystic duct —*see* Calculus,
          gallbladder, with
          cholecystitis, acute
        gallbladder —*see* Calculus,
          gallbladder, with
          cholecystitis, acute
      choledocholithiasis —*see*
        Calculus, bile duct, with
        cholecystitis, acute
      cholelithiasis —*see*
        Calculus, gallbladder, with
        cholecystitis, acute
    chronic cholecystitis K81.2
      with gallbladder calculus
        K80.12
        with obstruction K80.13
  chronic K81.1
    with acute cholecystitis K81.2
      with gallbladder calculus
        K80.12
        with obstruction K80.13
  emphysematous (acute) —*see*
    Cholecystitis, acute
  gangrenous —*see* Cholecystitis,
    acute
  paratyphoidal, current A01.4
  suppurative —*see* Cholecystitis,
    acute
  typhoidal A01.09
Cholecystolithiasis —*see* Calculus,
  gallbladder
Choledochitis (suppurative) K83.09
Choledocholith —*see* Calculus, bile
  duct
Choledocholithiasis (common duct)
  (hepatic duct) —*see* Calculus, bile
  duct
  cystic —*see* Calculus, gallbladder
  typhoidal A01.09
Cholelithiasis (cystic duct)
  (gallbladder) (impacted) (multiple)
  —*see* Calculus, gallbladder
  bile duct (common) (hepatic) —*see*
    Calculus, bile duct
  hepatic duct —*see* Calculus,
    bile duct
  specified NEC K80.80
    with obstruction K80.81
Cholemia —*see also* Jaundice
  familial (simple) (congenital) E80.4
  Gilbert's E80.4
Choleperitoneum, choleperitonitis
  K65.3
Cholera (Asiatic) (epidemic)
  (malignant) A00.9
  antimonial —*see* Poisoning,
    antimony
  classical A00.0
  due to Vibrio cholerae 01 A00.9
    biovar cholerae A00.0
    biovar eltor A00.1
  el tor A00.1
Cholerine —*see* Cholera
Cholestasis NEC K83.1
  with hepatocyte injury K71.0
  due to total parenteral nutrition
    (TPN) K76.89
  pure K71.0

Cholesteatoma (ear) (middle) (with
  reaction) H71.9-
  attic H71.0-
  external ear (canal) H60.4-
  mastoid H71.2-
  postmastoidectomy cavity
    (recurrent) —*see* Complications,
    postmastoidectomy, recurrent
    cholesteatoma
  recurrent (postmastoidectomy)
    —*see* Complications,
    postmastoidectomy, recurrent
    cholesteatoma
  tympanum H71.1-
Cholesteatosis, diffuse H71.3-
Cholesteremia E78.00
Cholesterin in vitreous —*see*
  Deposit, crystalline
Cholesterol
  deposit
    retina H35.89
    vitreous —*see* Deposit, crystalline
  elevated (high) E78.00
    with elevated (high) triglycerides
      E78.2
    screening for Z13.220
  imbibition of gallbladder K82.4
Cholesterolemia (essential) (pure)
  E78.00
  familial E78.01
  hereditary E78.01
Cholesterolosis, cholesterosis
  (gallbladder) K82.4
  cerebrotendinous E75.5
Cholocolic fistula K82.3
Choluria R82.2
Chondritis M94.8X9
  aurical H61.03-
  costal (Tietze's) M94.0
  external ear H61.03-
  patella, posttraumatic —*see*
    Chondromalacia, patella
  pinna H61.03-
  purulent M94.8X-
  tuberculous NEC A18.02
    intervertebral A18.01
Chondroblastoma —*see also*
  Neoplasm, bone, benign
  malignant —*see* Neoplasm, bone,
    malignant
Chondrocalcinosis M11.20
  ankle M11.27-
  elbow M11.22-
  familial M11.10
    ankle M11.17-
    elbow M11.12-
    foot joint M11.17-
    hand joint M11.14-
    hip M11.15-
    knee M11.16-
    multiple site M11.19
    shoulder M11.11-
    vertebrae M11.18
    wrist M11.13-
  foot joint M11.27-
  hand joint M11.24-
  hip M11.25-
  knee M11.26-
  multiple site M11.29
  shoulder M11.21-
  vertebrae M11.28
  specified type NEC M11.20
    ankle M11.27-
    elbow M11.22-
    foot joint M11.27-
    hand joint M11.24-
    hip M11.25-

Chondrocalcinosis *(continued)*
  specified type *(continued)*
    knee M11.26-
    multiple site M11.29
    shoulder M11.21-
    vertebrae M11.28
    wrist M11.23-
  wrist M11.23-
**Chondrodermatitis nodularis
  helicis or anthelicis** —*see*
  Perichondritis, ear
Chondrodysplasia Q78.9
  with hemangioma Q78.4
  calcificans congenita Q77.3
  fetalis Q77.4
  metaphyseal (Jansen's)
    (McKusick's) (Schmid's) Q78.8
  punctata Q77.3
**Chondrodystrophy,
  chondrodystrophia** (familial)
  (fetalis) (hypoplastic) Q78.9
  calcificans congenita Q77.3
  myotonic (congenital) G71.13
  punctata Q77.3
Chondroectodermal dysplasia
  Q77.6
Chondrogenesis imperfecta Q77.4
Chondrolysis M94.35-
Chondroma —*see also* Neoplasm,
  cartilage, benign
  juxtacortical —*see* Neoplasm,
    bone, benign
  periosteal —*see* Neoplasm, bone,
    benign
Chondromalacia (systemic) M94.20
  acromioclavicular joint M94.21-
  ankle M94.27-
  elbow M94.22-
  foot joint M94.27-
  glenohumeral joint M94.21-
  hand joint M94.24-
  hip M94.25-
  knee M94.26-
    patella M22.4-
  multiple sites M94.29
  patella M22.4-
  rib M94.28
  sacroiliac joint M94.259
  shoulder M94.21-
  sternoclavicular joint M94.21-
  vertebral joint M94.28
  wrist M94.23-
Chondromatosis —*see also* Neoplasm,
  cartilage, uncertain behavior
  internal Q78.4
Chondromyxosarcoma —*see*
  Neoplasm, cartilage, malignant
Chondro-osteodysplasia
  (Morquio-Brailsford type) E76.219
Chondro-osteodystrophy E76.29
Chondro-osteoma —*see* Neoplasm,
  bone, benign
Chondropathia tuberosa M94.0
Chondrosarcoma —*see* Neoplasm,
  cartilage, malignant
  juxtacortical —*see* Neoplasm,
    bone, malignant
  mesenchymal —*see* Neoplasm,
    connective tissue, malignant
  myxoid —*see* Neoplasm, cartilage,
    malignant
Chordee (nonvenereal) N48.89
  congenital Q54.4
  gonococcal A54.09

Chorditis (fibrinous) (nodosa) (tuberosa) J38.2

Chordoma —*see* Neoplasm, vertebral (column), malignant

Chorea (chronic) (gravis) (posthemiplegic) (senile) (spasmodic) G25.5
- with
  - heart involvement I02.0
    - active or acute (conditions in I01-) I02.0
      - rheumatic I02.9
        - with valvular disorder I02.0
    - rheumatic heart disease (chronic) (inactive) (quiescent) - code to rheumatic heart condition involved
- drug-induced G25.4
- habit F95.8
- hereditary G10
- Huntington's G10
- hysterical F44.4
- minor I02.9
  - with heart involvement I02.0
- progressive G25.5
  - hereditary G10
- rheumatic (chronic) I02.9
  - with heart involvement I02.0
- Sydenham's I02.9
  - with heart involvement —*see* Chorea, with rheumatic heart disease
- nonrheumatic G25.5

Choreoathetosis (paroxysmal) G25.5

Chorioadenoma (destruens) D39.2

Chorioamnionitis O41.12-

Chorioangioma D26.7

Choriocarcinoma —*see* Neoplasm, malignant, by site
- combined with
  - embryonal carcinoma —*see* Neoplasm, malignant, by site
  - other germ cell elements —*see* Neoplasm, malignant, by site
  - teratoma —*see* Neoplasm, malignant, by site
- specified site —*see* Neoplasm, malignant, by site
- unspecified site
  - female C58
  - male C62.90

Chorioencephalitis (acute) (lymphocytic) (serous) A87.2

Chorioepithelioma —*see* Choriocarcinoma

Choriomeningitis (acute) (lymphocytic) (serous) A87.2

Chorionepithelioma —*see* Choriocarcinoma

Chorioretinitis —*see also* Inflammation, chorioretinal
- disseminated —*see also* Inflammation, chorioretinal, disseminated
  - in neurosyphilis A52.19
- Egyptian B76.9 *[D63.8]*
- focal —*see also* Inflammation, chorioretinal, focal
- histoplasmic B39.9 *[H32]*
- in (due to)
  - histoplasmosis B39.9 *[H32]*
  - syphilis (secondary) A51.43
    - late A52.71
  - toxoplasmosis (acquired) B58.01
    - congenital (active) P37.1 *[H32]*
  - tuberculosis A18.53

Chorioretinitis (*continued*)
- juxtapapillary, juxtapapillaris —*see* Inflammation, chorioretinal, focal, juxtapapillary
- leprous A30.9 *[H32]*
- miner's B76.9 *[D63.8]*
- progressive myopia (degeneration) (*see also* Myopia, degenerative) H44.2-
- syphilitic (secondary) A51.43
  - congenital (early) A50.01 *[H32]*
    - late A50.32
  - late A52.71
- tuberculous A18.53

Choroid —*see* condition

Choroideremia H31.21

Choroiditis —*see* Chorioretinitis

Choroidopathy —*see* Disorder, choroid

Choroidoretinitis —*see* Chorioretinitis

Choroidoretinopathy, central serous —*see* Chorioretinopathy, central serous

Christian-Weber disease M35.6

Christmas disease D67

Chromaffinoma —*see also* Neoplasm, benign, by site
- malignant —*see* Neoplasm, malignant, by site

Chromatopsia —*see* Deficiency, color vision

Chromhidrosis, chromidrosis L75.1

Chromoblastomycosis —*see* Chromomycosis

Chromoconversion R82.91

Chromomycosis B43.9
- brain abscess B43.1
- cerebral B43.1
- cutaneous B43.0
- skin B43.0
- specified NEC B43.8
- subcutaneous abscess or cyst B43.2

Chromophytosis B36.0

Chromosome —*see* condition by chromosome involved
- D (1) —*see* condition, chromosome 13
- E (3) —*see* condition, chromosome 18
- G —*see* condition, chromosome 21

Chromotrichomycosis B36.8

Chronic —*see* condition
- fracture —*see* Fracture, pathological

Churg-Strauss syndrome M30.1

Chyle cyst, mesentery I89.8

Chylocele (nonfilarial) I89.8
- filarial (*see also* Infestation, filarial) B74.9 *[N51]*
- tunica vaginalis N50.89
  - filarial (*see also* Infestation, filarial) B74.9 *[N51]*

Chylomicronemia (fasting) (with hyperprebetalipoproteinemia) E78.3

Chylopericardium I31.39
- acute I30.9

Chylothorax (nonfilarial) J94.0
- filarial (*see also* Infestation, filarial) B74.9 *[J91.8]*

Chylous —*see* condition

Chyluria (nonfilarial) R82.0
- due to
  - bilharziasis B65.0
  - Brugia (malayi) B74.1
    - timori B74.2
  - schistosomiasis (bilharziasis) B65.0
  - Wuchereria (bancrofti) B74.0
- filarial —*see* Infestation, filarial

Cicatricial (deformity) —*see* Cicatrix

Cicatrix (adherent) (contracted) (painful) (vicious) (*see also* Scar) L90.5
- adenoid (and tonsil) J35.8
- alveolar process M26.79
- anus K62.89
- auricle —*see* Disorder, pinna, specified type NEC
- bile duct (common) (hepatic) K83.8
- bladder N32.89
- bone —*see* Disorder, bone, specified type NEC
- brain G93.89
- cervix (postoperative) (postpartal) N88.1
- common duct K83.8
- cornea H17.9
  - tuberculous A18.59
- duodenum (bulb), obstructive K31.5
- esophagus K22.2
- eyelid —*see* Disorder, eyelid function
- hypopharynx J39.2
- lacrimal passages —*see* Obstruction, lacrimal
- larynx J38.7
- lung J98.4
- middle ear H74.8
- mouth K13.79
- muscle M62.89
  - with contracture —*see* Contraction, muscle NEC
- nasopharynx J39.2
- palate (soft) K13.79
- penis N48.89
- pharynx J39.2
- prostate N42.89
- rectum K62.89
- retina —*see* Scar, chorioretinal
- semilunar cartilage —*see* Derangement, meniscus
- seminal vesicle N50.89
- skin L90.5
  - infected L08.89
  - postinfective L90.5
  - tuberculous B90.8
- specified site NEC L90.5
- throat J39.2
- tongue K14.8
- tonsil (and adenoid) J35.8
- trachea J39.8
- tuberculous NEC B90.9
- urethra N36.8
- uterus N85.8
- vagina N89.8
  - postoperative N99.2
- vocal cord J38.3
- wrist, constricting (annular) L90.5

CIDP (chronic inflammatory demyelinating polyneuropathy) G61.81

CIN —*see* Neoplasia, intraepithelial, cervix

CINCA (chronic infantile neurological, cutaneous and articular syndrome) M04.2

Cinchonism —*see* Deafness, ototoxic
- correct substance properly administered —*see* Table of Drugs and Chemicals, by drug, adverse effect
- overdose or wrong substance given or taken —*see* Table of Drugs and Chemicals, by drug, poisoning

Circle of Willis —*see* condition

Circular —*see* condition

Circulating anticoagulants (*see also* Disorder, hemorrhagic) D68.318
- due to drugs (*see also* Disorder, hemorrhagic) D68.32
- following childbirth O72.3

Circulation
- collateral, any site I99.8
- defective (lower extremity) I99.9
  - congenital Q28.9
- embryonic Q28.9
- failure (peripheral) R57.9
  - newborn P29.89
- fetal, persistent P29.38
- heart, incomplete Q28.9

Circulatory system —*see* condition

Circulus senilis (cornea) —*see* Degeneration, cornea, senile

Circumcision (in absence of medical indication) (ritual) (routine) Z41.2

Circumscribed —*see* condition

Circumvallate placenta O43.11-

Cirrhosis, cirrhotic (hepatic) (liver) K74.60
- alcoholic K70.30
  - with ascites K70.31
- atrophic —*see* Cirrhosis, liver
- Baumgarten-Cruveilhier K74.69
- biliary (cholangiolitic) (cholangitic) (hypertrophic) (obstructive) (pericholangiolitic) K74.5
  - due to
    - Clonorchiasis B66.1
    - flukes B66.3
  - primary K74.3
  - secondary K74.4
- cardiac (of liver) K76.1
- Charcot's K74.3
- cholangiolitic, cholangitic, cholostatic (primary) K74.3
- congestive K76.1
- Cruveilhier-Baumgarten K74.69
- cryptogenic (liver) K74.69
- due to
  - hepatolenticular degeneration E83.01
  - Wilson's disease E83.01
  - xanthomatosis E78.2
- fatty K76.0
  - alcoholic K70.0
- Hanot's (hypertrophic) K74.3
- hepatic —*see* Cirrhosis, liver
- hypertrophic K74.3
- Indian childhood K74.69
- kidney —*see* Sclerosis, renal
- Laennec's K70.30
  - with ascites K70.31
  - alcoholic K70.30
    - with ascites K70.31
  - nonalcoholic K74.69
- liver K74.60
  - alcoholic K70.30
    - with ascites K70.31
  - fatty K70.0
  - congenital P78.81
  - syphilitic A52.74
- lung (chronic) J84.10

Cirrhosis, cirrhotic *(continued)*
  macronodular K74.69
    alcoholic K70.30
      with ascites K70.31
  micronodular K74.69
    alcoholic K70.30
      with ascites K70.31
  mixed type K74.69
  monolobular K74.3
  nephritis —*see* Sclerosis, renal
  nutritional K74.69
    alcoholic K70.30
      with ascites K70.31
  obstructive —*see* Cirrhosis, biliary
  ovarian N83.8
  pancreas (duct) K86.89
  pigmentary E83.110
  portal K74.69
    alcoholic K70.30
      with ascites K70.31
  postnecrotic K74.69
    alcoholic K70.30
      with ascites K70.31
  pulmonary J84.10
  renal —*see* Sclerosis, renal
  spleen D73.2
  stasis K76.1
  Todd's K74.3
  unilobar K74.3
  xanthomatous (biliary) K74.5
    due to xanthomatosis (familial) (metabolic) (primary) E78.2
Cistern, subarachnoid R93.0
Citrullinemia E72.23
Citrullinuria E72.23
Civatte's disease or poikiloderma L57.3
CLAD —*see* Dysfunction, chronic, lung allograft
Clam digger's itch B65.3
Clammy skin R23.1
Clap —*see* Gonorrhea
Clarke-Hadfield syndrome (pancreatic infantilism) K86.89
Clark's paralysis G80.9
Clastothrix L67.8
Claude Bernard-Horner syndrome G90.2
  traumatic —*see* Injury, nerve, cervical sympathetic
Claude's disease or syndrome G46.3
Claudication (intermittent) I73.9
  cerebral (artery) G45.9
  spinal cord (arteriosclerotic) G95.19
    syphilitic A52.09
  venous (axillary) I87.8
Claudicatio venosa intermittens I87.8
Claustrophobia F40.240
Clavus (infected) L84
Clawfoot (congenital) Q66.89
  acquired —*see* Deformity, limb, clawfoot
Clawhand (acquired) —*see also* Deformity, limb, clawhand
  congenital Q68.1
Clawtoe (congenital) Q66.89
  acquired —*see* Deformity, toe, specified NEC
Clay eating —*see* Pica
Cleansing of artificial opening —*see* Attention to, artificial, opening
Cleft (congenital) —*see also* Imperfect, closure
  alveolar process M26.79

Cleft *(continued)*
  branchial (persistent) Q18.2
    cyst Q18.0
    fistula Q18.0
    sinus Q18.0
  cricoid cartilage, posterior Q31.8
  foot Q72.7
  hand Q71.6
  lip (unilateral) Q36.9
    with cleft palate Q37.9
      hard Q37.1
        with soft Q37.5
      soft Q37.3
        with hard Q37.5
    bilateral Q36.0
      with cleft palate Q37.8
        hard Q37.0
          with soft Q37.4
        soft Q37.2
          with hard Q37.4
    median Q36.1
  nose Q30.2
  palate Q35.9
    with cleft lip (unilateral) Q37.9
      bilateral Q37.8
    hard Q35.1
      with
        cleft lip (unilateral) Q37.1
          bilateral Q37.0
        soft Q35.5
          with cleft lip (unilateral) Q37.5
            bilateral Q37.4
    medial Q35.5
    soft Q35.3
      with
        cleft lip (unilateral) Q37.3
          bilateral Q37.2
        hard Q35.5
          with cleft lip (unilateral) Q37.5
            bilateral Q37.4
  penis Q55.69
  scrotum Q55.29
  thyroid cartilage Q31.8
  uvula Q35.7
Cleidocranial dysostosis Q74.0
Cleptomania F63.2
Clicking hip (newborn) R29.4
Climacteric (female) —*see also* Menopause
  arthritis (any site) NEC —*see* Arthritis, specified form NEC
  depression (single episode) F32.89
    recurrent episode F33.8
  melancholia (single episode) F32.89
    recurrent episode F33.8
  male (symptoms) (syndrome) NEC N50.89
  paranoid state F22
  polyarthritis NEC —*see* Arthritis, specified form NEC
  symptoms (female) N95.1
Clinical research investigation (clinical trial) (control subject) (normal comparison) (participant) Z00.6
Clitoris —*see* condition
Cloaca (persistent) Q43.7
Clonorchiasis, clonorchis infection (liver) B66.1
Clonus R25.8
Closed bite M26.29
Clostridium (C.) **perfringens, as cause of disease classified elsewhere** B96.7

Closure
  congenital, nose Q30.0
  cranial sutures, premature Q75.009
  defective or imperfect NEC —*see* Imperfect, closure
  fistula, delayed —*see* Fistula
  foramen ovale, imperfect Q21.12
  hymen N89.6
  interauricular septum, defective Q21.19
  interventricular septum, defective Q21.0
  lacrimal duct —*see also* Stenosis, lacrimal, duct
    congenital Q10.5
  nose (congenital) Q30.0
    acquired M95.0
  of artificial opening —*see* Attention to, artificial, opening
  primary angle, without glaucoma damage H40.06-
  vagina N89.5
  valve —*see* Endocarditis
  vulva N90.5
Clot (blood) —*see also* Embolism
  artery (obstruction) (occlusion) —*see* Embolism
  bladder N32.89
  brain (intradural or extradural) —*see* Occlusion, artery, cerebral
  circulation I74.9
  heart —*see also* Infarct, myocardium
    not resulting in infarction I51.3
  vein —*see* Thrombosis
Clouded state R40.1
  epileptic —*see* Epilepsy, specified NEC
  paroxysmal —*see* Epilepsy, specified NEC
Cloudy antrum, antra J32.0
Clouston's (hidrotic) **ectodermal dysplasia** Q82.4
Cloverleaf skull Q75.051
Clubbed nail pachydermoperiostosis M89.40 *[L62]*
Clubbing of finger(s) (nails) R68.3
Clubfinger R68.3
  congenital Q68.1
Clubfoot (congenital) Q66.89
  acquired —*see* Deformity, limb, clubfoot
  equinovarus Q66.0-
  paralytic —*see* Deformity, limb, clubfoot
Clubhand (congenital) (radial) Q71.4-
  acquired —*see* Deformity, limb, clubhand
Clubnail R68.3
  congenital Q84.6
Clump, kidney Q63.1
Clumsiness, clumsy child syndrome F82
Cluttering F80.81
Clutton's joints A50.51 *[M12.80]*
Coagulation, intravascular (diffuse) (disseminated) —*see also* Defibrination syndrome
  complicating abortion —*see* Abortion, by type, complicated by, intravascular coagulation
  COVID-19 associated (*see also* COVID-19) D65
  following ectopic or molar pregnancy O08.1

Coagulopathy —*see also* Defect, coagulation
  consumption D65
  intravascular D65
    newborn P60
Coalition
  calcaneo-scaphoid Q66.89
  tarsal Q66.89
Coalminer's
  elbow —*see* Bursitis, elbow, olecranon
  lung or pneumoconiosis J60
Coalworker's lung or pneumoconiosis J60
Coarctation
  aorta (preductal) (postductal) Q25.1
  pulmonary artery Q25.71
Coated tongue K14.3
Coats' disease (exudative retinopathy) —*see* Retinopathy, exudative
Cocaine-induced
  anxiety disorder F14.980
  bipolar and related disorder F14.94
  depressive disorder F14.94
  obsessive-compulsive and related disorder F14.988
  psychotic disorder F14.959
  sleep disorder F14.982
  sexual dysfunction F14.981
Cocainism —*see* Disorder, cocaine use
Coccidioidomycosis B38.9
  cutaneous B38.3
  disseminated B38.7
  generalized B38.7
  meninges B38.4
  prostate B38.81
  pulmonary B38.2
    acute B38.0
    chronic B38.1
  skin B38.3
  specified NEC B38.89
Coccidioidosis —*see* Coccidioidomycosis
Coccidiosis (intestinal) A07.3
Coccydynia, coccygodynia M53.3
Coccyx —*see* condition
Cochin-China diarrhea K90.1
Cockayne's syndrome Q87.19
Cocked up toe —*see* Deformity, toe, specified NEC
Cock's peculiar tumor L72.3
Codman's tumor —*see* Neoplasm, bone, benign
Coenurosis B71.8
Coffee-worker's lung J67.8
Cogan's syndrome H16.32-
  oculomotor apraxia H51.8
Coitus, painful (female) N94.10
  male N53.12
  psychogenic F52.6
Cold J00
  with influenza, flu, or grippe —*see* Influenza, with, respiratory manifestations NEC
  agglutinin disease or hemoglobinuria (chronic) D59.12
  bronchial —*see* Bronchitis
  chest —*see* Bronchitis
  common (head) J00

Cold *(continued)*
　effects of T69.9
　　specified effect NEC T69.8
　excessive, effects of T69.9
　　specified effect NEC T69.8
　exhaustion from T69.8
　exposure to T69.9
　　specified effect NEC T69.8
　head J00
　injury syndrome (newborn) P80.0
　on lung —*see* Bronchitis
　rose J30.1
　sensitivity, auto-immune D59.12
　symptoms J00
　virus J00

Coldsore B00.1

Colibacillosis A49.8
　as the cause of other disease (*see also* Escherichia coli) B96.20
　generalized (*see also* Sepsis, Escherichia coli) A41.51

Colic (bilious) (infantile) (intestinal) (recurrent) (spasmodic) R10.83
　abdomen R10.83
　　psychogenic F45.8
　appendix, appendicular K38.8
　bile duct —*see* Calculus, bile duct
　biliary —*see* Calculus, bile duct
　common duct —*see* Calculus, bile duct
　cystic duct —*see* Calculus, gallbladder
　Devonshire NEC —*see* Poisoning, lead
　gallbladder —*see* Calculus, gallbladder
　gallstone —*see* Calculus, gallbladder
　　gallbladder or cystic duct —*see* Calculus, gallbladder
　hepatic (duct) —*see* Calculus, bile duct
　hysterical F45.8
　kidney N23
　lead NEC —*see* Poisoning, lead
　mucous K58.9
　　with diarrhea K58.0
　　psychogenic F54
　nephritic N23
　painter's NEC —*see* Poisoning, lead
　pancreas K86.89
　psychogenic F45.8
　renal N23
　saturnine NEC —*see* Poisoning, lead
　ureter N23
　urethral N36.8
　　due to calculus N21.1
　uterus NEC N94.89
　　menstrual —*see* Dysmenorrhea
　worm NOS B83.9

Colicystitis —*see* Cystitis

Colitis (acute) (catarrhal) (chronic) (noninfective) (hemorrhagic) (*see also* Enteritis) K52.9
　allergic K52.29
　　with
　　　food protein-induced enterocolitis syndrome K52.21
　　　proctocolitis K52.29
　amebic (acute) (*see also* Amebiasis) A06.0
　　nondysenteric A06.2
　anthrax A22.2
　bacillary —*see* Infection, Shigella
　balantidial A07.0
　Clostridium difficile
　　not specified as recurrent A04.72
　　recurrent A04.71

Colitis *(continued)*
　coccidial A07.3
　collagenous K52.831
　cystica superficialis K52.89
　dietary counseling and surveillance (for) Z71.3
　dietetic (*see also* Colitis, allergic) K52.29
　drug-induced K52.1
　due to radiation K52.0
　eosinophilic K52.82
　food hypersensitivity (*see also* Colitis, allergic) K52.29
　giardial A07.1
　granulomatous —*see* Enteritis, regional, large intestine
　indeterminate, so stated K52.3
　infectious —*see* Enteritis, infectious
　ischemic K55.9
　　acute (subacute) (*see also* Ischemia, intestine, acute) K55.039
　　chronic K55.1
　　due to mesenteric artery insufficiency K55.1
　　fulminant (acute) (*see also* Ischemia, intestine, acute) K55.039
　left sided K51.50
　　with
　　　abscess K51.514
　　　complication K51.519
　　　　specified NEC K51.518
　　　fistula K51.513
　　　obstruction K51.512
　　　rectal bleeding K51.511
　lymphocytic K52.832
　membranous
　　psychogenic F54
　microscopic K52.839
　　specified NEC K52.838
　mucous —*see* Syndrome, irritable, bowel
　　psychogenic F54
　noninfective K52.9
　　specified NEC K52.89
　polyposa —*see* Polyp, colon, inflammatory
　protozoal A07.9
　pseudomembranous
　　not specified as recurrent A04.72
　　recurrent A04.71
　pseudomucinous —*see* Syndrome, irritable, bowel
　regional —*see* Enteritis, regional, large intestine
　　infectious A09
　segmental —*see* Enteritis, regional, large intestine
　septic —*see* Enteritis, infectious
　spastic K58.9
　　with diarrhea K58.0
　　psychogenic F54
　staphylococcal A04.8
　　foodborne A05.0
　subacute ischemic (*see also* Ischemia, intestine, acute) K55.039
　thromboulcerative (*see also* Ischemia, intestine, acute) K55.039
　toxic NEC K52.1
　　due to Clostridium difficile
　　　not specified as recurrent A04.72
　　　recurrent A04.71
　transmural —*see* Enteritis, regional, large intestine
　trichomonal A07.8
　tuberculous (ulcerative) A18.32

Colitis *(continued)*
　ulcerative (chronic) K51.90
　　with
　　　complication K51.919
　　　　abscess K51.914
　　　　fistula K51.913
　　　　obstruction K51.912
　　　　rectal bleeding K51.911
　　　　specified complication NEC K51.918
　　enterocolitis —*see* Enterocolitis, ulcerative
　　ileocolitis —*see* Ileocolitis, ulcerative
　　mucosal proctocolitis —*see* Proctocolitis, mucosal
　　proctitis —*see* Proctitis, ulcerative
　　pseudopolyposis —*see* Polyp, colon, inflammatory
　　psychogenic F54
　　rectosigmoiditis —*see* Rectosigmoiditis, ulcerative
　　specified type NEC K51.80
　　　with
　　　　complication K51.819
　　　　　abscess K51.814
　　　　　fistula K51.813
　　　　　obstruction K51.812
　　　　　rectal bleeding K51.811
　　　　　specified complication NEC K51.818

Collagenosis, collagen disease (nonvascular) (vascular) M35.9
　cardiovascular I42.8
　reactive perforating L87.1
　specified NEC M35.89

Collapse R55
　adrenal E27.2
　cardiorespiratory R57.0
　cardiovascular R57.0
　　newborn P29.89
　circulatory (peripheral) R57.9
　　during or after labor and delivery O75.1
　　following ectopic or molar pregnancy O08.3
　　newborn P29.89
　during or after labor and delivery O75.1
　resulting from a procedure, not elsewhere classified T81.10
　external ear canal —*see* Stenosis, external ear canal
　general R55
　heart —*see* Disease, heart
　heat T67.1
　hysterical F44.89
　labyrinth, membranous (congenital) Q16.5
　lung (massive) (*see also* Atelectasis) J98.19
　　pressure due to anesthesia (general) (local) or other sedation T88.2
　　　during labor and delivery O74.1
　　　in pregnancy O29.02-
　　　postpartum, puerperal O89.09
　myocardial —*see* Disease, heart
　nervous F48.8
　neurocirculatory F45.8
　nose M95.0
　postoperative T81.10
　pulmonary (*see also* Atelectasis) J98.19
　　newborn —*see* Atelectasis
　trachea J39.8
　tracheobronchial J98.09

Collapse *(continued)*
　valvular —*see* Endocarditis
　vascular (peripheral) R57.9
　　during or after labor and delivery O75.1
　　following ectopic or molar pregnancy O08.3
　　newborn P29.89
　vertebra M48.50-
　　cervical region M48.52-
　　cervicothoracic region M48.53-
　　in (due to)
　　　neoplasm (metastasis) M84.58-
　　　osteoporosis (*see also* Osteoporosis) M80.88
　　　　cervical region M80.88
　　　　cervicothoracic region M80.88
　　　　lumbar region M80.88
　　　　lumbosacral region M80.88
　　　　multiple sites M80.88
　　　　occipito-atlanto-axial region M80.88
　　　　sacrococcygeal region M80.88
　　　　thoracic region M80.88
　　　　thoracolumbar region M80.88
　　specified disease NEC M48.50-
　　　cervical region M48.52-
　　　cervicothoracic region M48.53-
　　　lumbar region M48.56-
　　　lumbosacral region M48.57-
　　　occipito-atlanto-axial region M48.51-
　　　sacrococcygeal region M48.58-
　　　thoracic region M48.54-
　　　thoracolumbar region M48.55-
　　lumbar region M48.56-
　　lumbosacral region M48.57-
　　occipito-atlanto-axial region M48.51-
　　sacrococcygeal region M48.58-
　　thoracic region M48.54-
　　thoracolumbar region M48.55-

Collateral —*see also* condition
　circulation (venous) I87.8
　dilation, veins I87.8

Colles' fracture S52.53-

Collet (-Sicard) **syndrome** G52.7

Collier's asthma or lung J60

Collodion baby Q80.2

Colloid nodule (of thyroid) (cystic) E04.1

Coloboma (iris) Q13.0
　eyelid Q10.3
　fundus Q14.8
　lens Q12.2
　optic disc (congenital) Q14.2
　　acquired H47.31-

Coloenteritis —*see* Enteritis

Colon —*see* condition

Colonization
　MRSA (Methicillin resistant Staphylococcus aureus) Z22.322
　MSSA (Methicillin susceptible Staphylococcus aureus) Z22.321
　status —*see* Carrier (suspected) of

Coloptosis K63.4

Color blindness —*see* Deficiency, color vision

Colostomy
  attention to Z43.3
  fitting or adjustment Z46.89
  malfunctioning K94.03
  status Z93.3

Colpitis (acute) —*see* Vaginitis

Colpocele N81.5

Colpocystitis —*see* Vaginitis

Colpospasm N94.2

Column, spinal, vertebral —*see* condition

Coma R40.20
  with
    motor response (none) R40.231
      abnormal R40.233
      abnormal extensor posturing to pain or noxious stimuli (<2 years of age) R40.232
      abnormal flexure posturing to pain or noxious stimuli (0-5 years of age) R40.233
      extension R40.232
      extensor posturing to pain or noxious stimuli (2-5 years of age) R40.232
      flexion/decorticate posturing (<2 years of age) R40.233
      flexion withdrawal R40.234
      localizes pain (2-5 years of age) R40.235
      normal or spontaneous movement (<2 years of age) R40.236
      obeys commands (2-5 years of age) R40.236
      score of
        1 R40.231
        2 R40.232
        3 R40.233
        4 R40.234
        5 R40.235
        6 R40.236
      withdraws from pain or noxious stimuli (0-5 years of age) R40.234
      withdraws to touch (<2 years of age) R40.235
    opening of eyes (never) R40.211
      in response to pain R40.212
      sound R40.213
      score of
        1 R40.211
        2 R40.212
        3 R40.213
        4 R40.214
      spontaneous R40.214
    verbal response (none) R40.221
      confused conversation R40.224
      cooing or babbling or crying appropriately (<2 years of age) R40.225
      inappropriate crying or screaming (<2 years of age) R40.223
      inappropriate words (2-5 years of age) R40.224
      incomprehensible sounds (2-5 years of age) R40.222
      incomprehensible words R40.222
      irritable cries (<2 years of age) R40.224
      moans/grunts to pain; restless (<2 years of age) R40.222
      oriented R40.225
      score of
        1 R40.221
        2 R40.222

Coma (*continued*)
  with
    verbal response (*continued*)
      score of (*continued*)
        3 R40.223
        4 R40.224
        5 R40.225
      screaming (2-5 years of age) R40.223
      uses appropriate words (2-5 years of age) R40.225
  eclamptic —*see* Eclampsia
  epileptic —*see* Epilepsy
  Glasgow, scale score —*see* Glasgow coma scale
  hepatic —*see* Failure, hepatic, by type, with coma
  hyperglycemic (diabetic) —*see* Diabetes, by type, with hyperosmolarity, with coma
  hyperosmolar (diabetic) —*see* Diabetes, by type, with hyperosmolarity, with coma
  hypoglycemic (diabetic) —*see* Diabetes, by type, with hypoglycemia, with coma
    nondiabetic E15
  in diabetes —*see* Diabetes, coma
  insulin-induced —*see* Coma, hypoglycemic
  ketoacidotic (diabetic) —*see* Diabetes, by type, with ketoacidosis, with coma
  myxedematous E03.5
  newborn P91.5
  nontraumatic, due to underlying condition R40.2A
  persistent vegetative state R40.3
  secondary R40.2A
  specified NEC, without documented Glasgow coma scale score, or with partial Glasgow coma scale score reported R40.244

Comatose —*see* Coma

Combat fatigue F43.0

Combined —*see* condition

Comedo, comedones (giant) L70.0

Comedocarcinoma —*see also* Neoplasm, breast, malignant
  noninfiltrating
    breast D05.8-
    specified site —*see* Neoplasm, in situ, by site
    unspecified site D05.8-

Comedomastitis —*see* Ectasia, mammary duct

Comminuted fracture - code as Fracture, closed

Common
  arterial trunk Q20.0
  atrioventricular canal Q21.23
  atrium Q21.19
  cold (head) J00
  truncus (arteriosus) Q20.0
  variable immunodeficiency —*see* Immunodeficiency, common variable
  ventricle Q20.4

Commotio, commotion (current)
  brain —*see* Injury, intracranial, concussion
  cerebri —*see* Injury, intracranial, concussion
  retinae S05.8X-
  spinal cord —*see* Injury, spinal cord, by region
  spinalis —*see* Injury, spinal cord, by region

Communication
  between
    base of aorta and pulmonary artery Q21.4
    left ventricle and right atrium Q20.5
    pericardial sac and pleural sac Q34.8
    pulmonary artery and pulmonary vein, congenital Q25.72
  congenital between uterus and digestive or urinary tract Q51.7

Compartment syndrome (deep) (posterior) (traumatic) T79.A0
  abdomen T79.A3
  lower extremity (hip, buttock, thigh, leg, foot, toes) T79.A2
  nontraumatic
    abdomen M79.A3
    lower extremity (hip, buttock, thigh, leg, foot, toes) M79.A2-
    specified site NEC M79.A9
    upper extremity (shoulder, arm, forearm, wrist, hand, fingers) M79.A1-
  specified site NEC T79.A9
  upper extremity (shoulder, arm, forearm, wrist, hand, fingers) T79.A1

Compensation
  failure —*see* Disease, heart
  neurosis, psychoneurosis —*see* Disorder, factitious

Complaint —*see also* Disease
  bowel, functional K59.9
    psychogenic F45.8
  intestine, functional K59.9
    psychogenic F45.8
  kidney —*see* Disease, renal
  miners' J60

Complete —*see* condition

Complex
  Addison-Schilder E71.528
  cardiorenal —*see* Hypertension, cardiorenal
  Costen's M26.69
  disseminated mycobacterium avium- intracellulare (DMAC) A31.2
  Eisenmenger's (ventricular septal defect) I27.83
  hypersexual F52.8
  jumped process, spine —*see* Dislocation, vertebra
  primary, tuberculous A15.7
  Schilder-Addison E71.528
  subluxation (vertebral) M99.19
    abdomen M99.19
    acromioclavicular M99.17
    cervical region M99.11
    cervicothoracic M99.11
    costochondral M99.18
    costovertebral M99.18
    head region M99.10
    hip M99.15
    lower extremity M99.16
    lumbar region M99.13
    lumbosacral M99.13
    occipitocervical M99.10
    pelvic region M99.15
    pubic M99.15
    rib cage M99.18
    sacral region M99.14
    sacrococcygeal M99.14
    sacroiliac M99.14
    specified NEC M99.19
    sternochondral M99.18
    sternoclavicular M99.17
    thoracic region M99.12

Complex (*continued*)
  subluxation (*continued*)
    thoracolumbar M99.12
    upper extremity M99.17
  Taussig-Bing (transposition, aorta and overriding pulmonary artery) Q20.1

Complication(s) (from) (of)
  accidental puncture or laceration during a procedure (of) —*see* Complications, intraoperative (intraprocedural), puncture or laceration
  amputation stump (surgical) (late) NEC T87.9
    dehiscence T87.81
    infection or inflammation T87.40
      lower limb T87.4-
      upper limb T87.4-
    necrosis T87.50
      amputation stump (surgical)
        lower limb T87.5-
        upper limb T87.5-
    neuroma T87.30
      lower limb T87.3-
      upper limb T87.3-
    specified type NEC T87.89
  anastomosis (and bypass) —*see also* Complications, prosthetic device or implant
    intestinal (internal) NEC K91.89
      involving urinary tract N99.89
    urinary tract (involving intestinal tract) N99.89
    vascular —*see* Complications, cardiovascular device or implant
  anesthesia, anesthetic (*see also* Anesthesia, complication) T88.59
    general, unintended awareness during procedure T88.53
    unintended awareness under general anesthesia during procedure T88.53
    brain, postpartum, puerperal O89.2
    cardiac
      in
        labor and delivery O74.2
        pregnancy O29.19-
      postpartum, puerperal O89.1
    central nervous system
      in
        labor and delivery O74.3
        pregnancy O29.29-
      postpartum, puerperal O89.2
    difficult or failed intubation T88.4
      in pregnancy O29.6-
    failed sedation (conscious) (moderate) during procedure T88.52
    hyperthermia, malignant T88.3
    hypothermia T88.51
    intubation failure T88.4
    malignant hyperthermia T88.3
    pulmonary
      in
        labor and delivery O74.1
        pregnancy NEC O29.09-
      postpartum, puerperal O89.09
    shock T88.2
    spinal and epidural
      in
        labor and delivery NEC O74.6
          headache O74.5
        pregnancy NEC O29.5X-
      postpartum, puerperal NEC O89.5
        headache O89.4

Complication *(continued)*
  anti-reflux device —*see* Complications, esophageal anti-reflux device
  aortic (bifurcation) graft —*see* Complications, graft, vascular
  aortocoronary (bypass) graft —*see* Complications, coronary artery (bypass) graft
  aortofemoral (bypass) graft —*see* Complications, extremity artery (bypass) graft
  arteriovenous
    fistula, surgically created T82.9
      embolism T82.818
      fibrosis T82.828
      hemorrhage T82.838
      infection or inflammation T82.7
      mechanical
        breakdown T82.510
        displacement T82.520
        leakage T82.530
        malposition T82.520
        obstruction T82.590
        perforation T82.590
        protrusion T82.590
      pain T82.848
      specified type NEC T82.898
      stenosis T82.858
      thrombosis T82.868
    shunt, surgically created T82.9
      embolism T82.818
      fibrosis T82.828
      hemorrhage T82.838
      infection or inflammation T82.7
      mechanical
        breakdown T82.511
        displacement T82.521
        leakage T82.531
        malposition T82.521
        obstruction T82.591
        perforation T82.591
        protrusion T82.591
      pain T82.848
      specified type NEC T82.898
      stenosis T82.858
      thrombosis T82.868
  arthroplasty —*see* Complications, joint prosthesis
  artificial
    fertilization or insemination N98.9
      attempted introduction (of)
        embryo in embryo transfer N98.3
        ovum following in vitro fertilization N98.2
      hyperstimulation of ovaries N98.1
      infection N98.0
      specified NEC N98.8
    heart T82.9
      embolism T82.817
      fibrosis T82.827
      hemorrhage T82.837
      infection or inflammation T82.7
      mechanical
        breakdown T82.512
        displacement T82.522
        leakage T82.532
        malposition T82.522
        obstruction T82.592
        perforation T82.592
        protrusion T82.592
      pain T82.847
      specified type NEC T82.897
      stenosis T82.857
      thrombosis T82.867

Complication *(continued)*
  artificial *(continued)*
    opening
      cecostomy —*see* Complications, colostomy
      colostomy —*see* Complications, colostomy
      cystostomy —*see* Complications, cystostomy
      enterostomy —*see* Complications, enterostomy
      gastrostomy —*see* Complications, gastrostomy
      ileostomy —*see* Complications, enterostomy
      jejunostomy —*see* Complications, enterostomy
      nephrostomy —*see* Complications, stoma, urinary tract
      tracheostomy —*see* Complications, tracheostomy
      ureterostomy —*see* Complications, stoma, urinary tract
      urethrostomy —*see* Complications, stoma, urinary tract
  balloon implant or device
    gastrointestinal T85.9
      embolism T85.818
      fibrosis T85.828
      hemorrhage T85.838
      infection and inflammation T85.79
      pain T85.848
      specified type NEC T85.898
      stenosis T85.858
      thrombosis T85.868
    vascular (counterpulsation) T82.9
      embolism T82.818
      fibrosis T82.828
      hemorrhage T82.838
      infection or inflammation T82.7
      mechanical
        breakdown T82.513
        displacement T82.523
        leakage T82.533
        malposition T82.523
        obstruction T82.593
        perforation T82.593
        protrusion T82.593
      pain T82.848
      specified type NEC T82.898
      stenosis T82.858
      thrombosis T82.868
  bariatric procedure
    gastric band procedure K95.09
      infection K95.01
    specified procedure NEC K95.89
      infection K95.81
  bile duct implant (prosthetic) T85.9
    embolism T85.818
    fibrosis T85.828
    hemorrhage T85.838
    infection and inflammation T85.79
    mechanical
      breakdown T85.510
      displacement T85.520
      malfunction T85.510
      malposition T85.520
      obstruction T85.590
      perforation T85.590
      protrusion T85.590
      specified NEC T85.590
    pain T85.848
    specified type NEC T85.898

Complication *(continued)*
  bile duct implant *(continued)*
    stenosis T85.858
    thrombosis T85.868
  bladder device (auxiliary) —*see* Complications, genitourinary, device or implant, urinary system
  bleeding (postoperative) —*see* Complication, postoperative, hemorrhage
    intraoperative —*see* Complication, intraoperative, hemorrhage
  blood vessel graft —*see* Complications, graft, vascular
  bone
    device NEC T84.9
      embolism T84.81
      fibrosis T84.82
      hemorrhage T84.83
      infection or inflammation T84.7
      mechanical
        breakdown T84.318
        displacement T84.328
        malposition T84.328
        obstruction T84.398
        perforation T84.398
        protrusion T84.398
      pain T84.84
      specified type NEC T84.89
      stenosis T84.85
      thrombosis T84.86
    graft —*see* Complications, graft, bone
    growth stimulator (electrode) —*see* Complications, electronic stimulator device, bone
    marrow transplant —*see* Complications, transplant, bone, marrow
  brain neurostimulator (electrode) —*see* Complications, electronic stimulator device, brain
  breast implant (prosthetic) T85.9
    capsular contracture T85.44
    embolism T85.818
    fibrosis T85.828
    hemorrhage T85.838
    infection and inflammation T85.79
    mechanical
      breakdown T85.41
      displacement T85.42
      leakage T85.43
      malposition T85.42
      obstruction T85.49
      perforation T85.49
      protrusion T85.49
      specified NEC T85.49
    pain T85.848
    specified type NEC T85.898
    stenosis T85.858
    thrombosis T85.868
  bypass —*see also* Complications, prosthetic device or implant
    aortocoronary —*see* Complications, coronary artery (bypass) graft
    arterial —*see also* Complications, graft, vascular
      extremity —*see* Complications, extremity artery (bypass) graft
  cardiac —*see also* Disease, heart
    device, implant or graft T82.9
      embolism T82.817
      fibrosis T82.827
      hemorrhage T82.837
      infection or inflammation T82.7
      valve prosthesis T82.6

Complication *(continued)*
  cardiac *(continued)*
    device, implant or graft *(continued)*
      mechanical
        breakdown T82.519
          specified device NEC T82.518
        displacement T82.529
          specified device NEC T82.528
        leakage T82.539
          specified device NEC T82.538
        malposition T82.529
          specified device NEC T82.528
        obstruction T82.599
          specified device NEC T82.598
        perforation T82.599
          specified device NEC T82.598
        protrusion T82.599
          specified device NEC T82.598
      pain T82.847
      specified type NEC T82.897
      stenosis T82.857
      thrombosis T82.867
  cardiovascular device, graft or implant T82.9
    aortic graft —*see* Complications, graft, vascular
    arteriovenous
      fistula, artificial —*see* Complication, arteriovenous, fistula, surgically created
      shunt —*see* Complication, arteriovenous, shunt, surgically created
    artificial heart —*see* Complication, artificial, heart
    balloon (counterpulsation) device —*see* Complication, balloon implant, vascular
    carotid artery graft —*see* Complications, graft, vascular
    coronary bypass graft —*see* Complication, coronary artery (bypass) graft
    dialysis catheter (vascular) —*see* Complication, catheter, dialysis
    electronic T82.9
      electrode T82.9
        embolism T82.817
        fibrosis T82.827
        hemorrhage T82.837
        infection T82.7
        mechanical
          breakdown T82.110
          displacement T82.120
          leakage T82.190
          obstruction T82.190
          perforation T82.190
          protrusion T82.190
          specified type NEC T82.190
        pain T82.847
        specified NEC T82.897
        stenosis T82.857
        thrombosis T82.867
      embolism T82.817
      fibrosis T82.827
      hemorrhage T82.837
      infection T82.7
      mechanical
        breakdown T82.119
        displacement T82.129
        leakage T82.199
        obstruction T82.199

Complication *(continued)*
  cardiovascular device, graft or implant *(continued)*
    electronic *(continued)*
      mechanical *(continued)*
        perforation T82.199
        protrusion T82.199
        specified type NEC T82.199
      pain T82.847
    pulse generator T82.9
      embolism T82.817
      fibrosis T82.827
      hemorrhage T82.837
      infection T82.7
      mechanical
        breakdown T82.111
        displacement T82.121
        leakage T82.191
        obstruction T82.191
        perforation T82.191
        protrusion T82.191
        specified type NEC T82.191
      pain T82.847
      specified NEC T82.897
      stenosis T82.857
      thrombosis T82.867
    specified condition NEC T82.897
    specified device NEC T82.9
      embolism T82.817
      fibrosis T82.827
      hemorrhage T82.837
      infection T82.7
      mechanical
        breakdown T82.118
        displacement T82.128
        leakage T82.198
        obstruction T82.198
        perforation T82.198
        protrusion T82.198
        specified type NEC T82.198
      pain T82.847
      specified NEC T82.897
      stenosis T82.857
      thrombosis T82.867
    stenosis T82.857
    thrombosis T82.867
  extremity artery graft —*see* Complication, extremity artery (bypass) graft
  femoral artery graft —*see* Complication, extremity artery (bypass) graft
  heart-lung transplant —*see* Complication, transplant, heart, with lung
  heart
    transplant —*see* Complication, transplant, heart
    valve —*see* Complication, prosthetic device, heart valve
      graft —*see* Complication, heart, valve, graft
  infection or inflammation T82.7
  umbrella device —*see* Complication, umbrella device, vascular
  vascular graft (or anastomosis) —*see* Complication, graft, vascular
  carotid artery (bypass) graft —*see* Complications, graft, vascular
  catheter (device) NEC —*see also* Complications, prosthetic device or implant
    cranial infusion
      infection and inflammation T85.735

Complication *(continued)*
  catheter (device) NEC *(continued)*
    cranial infusion *(continued)*
      mechanical
        breakdown T85.610
        displacement T85.620
        leakage T85.630
        malfunction T85.690
        malposition T85.620
        obstruction T85.690
        perforation T85.690
        protrusion T85.690
        specified NEC T85.690
    cystostomy T83.9
      embolism T83.81
      fibrosis T83.82
      hemorrhage T83.83
      infection and inflammation T83.510
      mechanical
        breakdown T83.010
        displacement T83.020
        leakage T83.030
        malposition T83.020
        obstruction T83.090
        perforation T83.090
        protrusion T83.090
        specified NEC T83.090
      pain T83.84
      specified type NEC T83.89
      stenosis T83.85
      thrombosis T83.86
    dialysis (vascular) T82.9
      embolism T82.818
      fibrosis T82.828
      hemorrhage T82.838
      infection and inflammation T82.7
      intraperitoneal —*see* Complications, catheter, intraperitoneal
      mechanical
        breakdown T82.41
        displacement T82.42
        leakage T82.43
        malposition T82.42
        obstruction T82.49
        perforation T82.49
        protrusion T82.49
      pain T82.848
      specified type NEC T82.898
      stenosis T82.858
      thrombosis T82.868
    epidural infusion T85.9
      embolism T85.810
      fibrosis T85.820
      hemorrhage T85.830
      infection and inflammation T85.735
      mechanical
        breakdown T85.610
        displacement T85.620
        leakage T85.630
        malfunction T85.690
        malposition T85.620
        obstruction T85.690
        perforation T85.690
        protrusion T85.690
        specified NEC T85.690
      pain T85.840
      specified type NEC T85.890
      stenosis T85.850
      thrombosis T85.860
    intraperitoneal dialysis T85.9
      embolism T85.818
      fibrosis T85.828
      hemorrhage T85.838
      infection and inflammation T85.735
      mechanical
        breakdown T85.611
        displacement T85.621

Complication *(continued)*
  catheter (device) NEC *(continued)*
    intraperitoneal dialysis *(continued)*
      mechanical *(continued)*
        leakage T85.631
        malfunction T85.611
        malposition T85.621
        obstruction T85.691
        perforation T85.691
        protrusion T85.691
        specified NEC T85.691
      pain T85.848
      specified type NEC T85.898
      stenosis T85.858
      thrombosis T85.868
    intrathecal infusion
      infection and inflammation T85.735
      mechanical
        breakdown T85.610
        displacement T85.620
        leakage T85.630
        malfunction T85.690
        malposition T85.620
        obstruction T85.690
        perforation T85.690
        protrusion T85.690
        specified NEC T85.690
    intravenous infusion T82.9
      embolism T82.818
      fibrosis T82.828
      hemorrhage T82.838
      infection or inflammation T82.7
      mechanical
        breakdown T82.514
        displacement T82.524
        leakage T82.534
        malposition T82.524
        obstruction T82.594
        perforation T82.594
        protrusion T82.594
      pain T82.848
      specified type NEC T82.898
      stenosis T82.858
      thrombosis T82.868
    spinal infusion
      infection and inflammation T85.735
      mechanical
        breakdown T85.610
        displacement T85.620
        leakage T85.630
        malfunction T85.690
        malposition T85.620
        obstruction T85.690
        perforation T85.690
        protrusion T85.690
        specified NEC T85.690
    subarachnoid infusion
      infection and inflammation T85.735
      mechanical
        breakdown T85.610
        displacement T85.620
        leakage T85.630
        malfunction T85.690
        malposition T85.620
        obstruction T85.690
        perforation T85.690
        protrusion T85.690
        specified NEC T85.690
    subdural infusion T85.9
      embolism T85.810
      fibrosis T85.820
      hemorrhage T85.830
      infection and inflammation T85.735
      mechanical
        breakdown T85.610
        displacement T85.620
        leakage T85.630

Complication *(continued)*
  catheter (device) NEC *(continued)*
    subdural infusion *(continued)*
      mechanical *(continued)*
        malfunction T85.690
        malposition T85.620
        obstruction T85.690
        perforation T85.690
        protrusion T85.690
        specified NEC T85.690
      pain T85.840
      specified type NEC T85.890
      stenosis T85.850
      thrombosis T85.860
    urethral T83.9
      displacement T83.028
      embolism T83.81
      fibrosis T83.82
      hemorrhage T83.83
      indwelling
        breakdown T83.011
        displacement T83.021
        infection and inflammation T83.511
        leakage T83.031
        specified complication NEC T83.091
      infection and inflammation T83.511
      leakage T83.038
      malposition T83.028
      mechanical
        breakdown T83.011
      obstruction (mechanical) T83.091
      pain T83.84
      perforation T83.091
      protrusion T83.091
      specified type NEC T83.091
      stenosis T83.85
      thrombosis T83.86
    urinary NEC
      breakdown T83.018
      displacement T83.028
      infection and inflammation T83.518
      leakage T83.038
      specified complication NEC T83.098
  cecostomy (stoma) —*see* Complications, colostomy
  cesarean delivery wound NEC O90.89
    disruption O90.0
    hematoma O90.2
    infection (following delivery) O86.00
  chemotherapy (antineoplastic) NEC T88.7
  chimeric antigen receptor (CAR-T) cell therapy T80.82
  chin implant (prosthetic) —*see* Complication, prosthetic device or implant, specified NEC
  circulatory system I99.8
    intraoperative I97.88
    postprocedural I97.89
      following cardiac surgery (*see also* Infarct, myocardium, associated with revascularization procedure) I97.19-
      postcardiotomy syndrome I97.0
    hypertension I97.3
    lymphedema after mastectomy I97.2
    postcardiotomy syndrome I97.0

Complication (*continued*)
  circulatory system (*continued*)
    postprocedural (*continued*)
      seroma —*see* Complications, postprocedural, seroma (of), mastoid process
      specified NEC I97.89
  colostomy (stoma) K94.00
    hemorrhage K94.01
    infection K94.02
    malfunction K94.03
    mechanical K94.03
    specified complication NEC K94.09
  contraceptive device, intrauterine —*see* Complications, intrauterine, contraceptive device
  cord (umbilical) —*see* Complications, umbilical cord
  corneal graft —*see* Complications, graft, cornea
  coronary artery (bypass) graft T82.9
    atherosclerosis —*see* Arteriosclerosis, coronary (artery)
    embolism T82.817
    fibrosis T82.827
    hemorrhage T82.837
    infection and inflammation T82.7
    mechanical
      breakdown T82.211
      displacement T82.212
      leakage T82.213
      malposition T82.212
      obstruction T82.218
      perforation T82.218
      protrusion T82.218
      specified NEC T82.218
    pain T82.847
    specified type NEC T82.898
    stenosis T82.857
    thrombosis T82.867
  counterpulsation device (balloon), intra- aortic —*see* Complications, balloon implant, vascular
  cystostomy (stoma) N99.518
    catheter —*see* Complications, catheter, cystostomy
    hemorrhage N99.510
    infection N99.511
    malfunction N99.512
    specified type NEC N99.518
  delivery (*see also* Complications, obstetric) O75.9
    procedure (instrumental) (manual) (surgical) O75.4
    specified NEC O75.89
  dialysis (peritoneal) (renal) —*see also* Complications, infusion
    catheter (vascular) —*see* Complication, catheter, dialysis
      peritoneal, intraperitoneal —*see* Complications, catheter, intraperitoneal
  dorsal column (spinal) neurostimulator —*see* Complications, electronic stimulator device, spinal cord
  drug NEC T88.7
  ear procedure —*see also* Disorder, ear
    intraoperative H95.88
      hematoma —*see* Complications, intraoperative, hemorrhage (hematoma) (of), ear
      hemorrhage —*see* Complications, intraoperative, hemorrhage (hematoma) (of), ear

Complication (*continued*)
  ear procedure (*continued*)
    intraoperative (*continued*)
      laceration —*see* Complications, intraoperative, puncture or laceration..., ear
      specified NEC H95.88
    postoperative H95.89
      external ear canal stenosis H95.81-
      hematoma —*see* Complications, postprocedural, hematoma (of), ear
      hemorrhage —*see* Complications, postprocedural, hemorrhage (of), ear
      postmastoidectomy —*see* Complications, postmastoidectomy
      specified NEC H95.89
      seroma — *see* Complications, postprocedural, seroma (of), mastoid process
  ectopic pregnancy O08.9
    damage to pelvic organs O08.6
    embolism O08.2
    genital infection O08.0
    hemorrhage (delayed) (excessive) O08.1
    metabolic disorder O08.5
    renal failure O08.4
    shock O08.3
    specified type NEC O08.0
    venous complication NEC O08.7
  electronic stimulator device
    bladder (urinary) —*see* Complications, electronic stimulator device, urinary
    bone T84.9
      breakdown T84.310
      displacement T84.320
      embolism T84.81
      fibrosis T84.82
      hemorrhage T84.83
      infection or inflammation T84.7
      malfunction T84.310
      malposition T84.320
      mechanical NEC T84.390
      obstruction T84.390
      pain T84.84
      perforation T84.390
      protrusion T84.390
      specified type NEC T84.89
      stenosis T84.85
      thrombosis T84.86
    brain T85.9
      embolism T85.810
      fibrosis T85.820
      hemorrhage T85.830
      infection and inflammation T85.731
      mechanical
        breakdown T85.110
        displacement T85.120
        leakage T85.190
        malposition T85.120
        obstruction T85.190
        perforation T85.190
        protrusion T85.190
        specified NEC T85.190
      pain T85.840
      specified type NEC T85.890
      stenosis T85.850
      thrombosis T85.860
    cardiac (defibrillator) (pacemaker) —*see* Complications, cardiovascular device or implant, electronic

Complication (*continued*)
  electronic stimulator device (*continued*)
    generator (brain) (gastric) (peripheral) (sacral) (spinal)
      breakdown T85.113
      displacement T85.123
      leakage T85.193
      malposition T85.123
      obstruction T85.193
      perforation T85.193
      protrusion T85.193
      specified NEC T85.193
    muscle T84.9
      breakdown T84.418
      displacement T84.428
      embolism T84.81
      fibrosis T84.82
      hemorrhage T84.83
      infection or inflammation T84.7
      mechanical NEC T84.498
      pain T84.84
      specified type NEC T84.89
      stenosis T84.85
      thrombosis T84.86
    nervous system T85.9
      brain —*see* Complications, electronic stimulator device, brain
      cranial nerve —*see* Complications, electronic stimulator device, peripheral nerve
      embolism T85.810
      fibrosis T85.820
      gastric nerve —*see* Complications, electronic stimulator device, peripheral nerve
      hemorrhage T85.830
      infection and inflammation T85.738
      mechanical
        breakdown T85.118
        displacement T85.128
        leakage T85.199
        malposition T85.128
        obstruction T85.199
        perforation T85.199
        protrusion T85.199
        specified NEC T85.199
      pain T85.840
      peripheral nerve —*see* Complications, electronic stimulator device, peripheral nerve
      sacral nerve —*see* Complications, electronic stimulator device, peripheral nerve
      specified type NEC T85.890
      spinal cord —*see* Complications, electronic stimulator device, spinal cord
      stenosis T85.850
      thrombosis T85.860
      vagal nerve —*see* Complications, electronic stimulator device, peripheral nerve
    peripheral nerve T85.9
      embolism T85.810
      fibrosis T85.820
      hemorrhage T85.830
      infection and inflammation T85.732

Complication (*continued*)
  electronic stimulator device (*continued*)
    peripheral nerve (*continued*)
      mechanical
        breakdown T85.111
        displacement T85.121
        leakage T85.191
        malposition T85.121
        obstruction T85.191
        perforation T85.191
        protrusion T85.191
        specified NEC T85.191
      pain T85.840
      specified type NEC T85.890
      stenosis T85.850
      thrombosis T85.860
    spinal cord T85.9
      embolism T85.810
      fibrosis T85.820
      hemorrhage T85.830
      infection and inflammation T85.733
      mechanical
        breakdown T85.112
        displacement T85.122
        leakage T85.192
        malposition T85.122
        obstruction T85.192
        perforation T85.192
        protrusion T85.192
        specified NEC T85.192
      pain T85.840
      specified type NEC T85.890
      stenosis T85.850
      thrombosis T85.860
    urinary T83.9
      embolism T83.81
      fibrosis T83.82
      hemorrhage T83.83
      infection and inflammation T83.598
      mechanical
        breakdown T83.110
        displacement T83.120
        malposition T83.120
        perforation T83.190
        protrusion T83.190
        specified NEC T83.190
      pain T83.84
      specified type NEC T83.89
      stenosis T83.85
      thrombosis T83.86
  electroshock therapy T88.9
    specified NEC T88.8
  endocrine E34.9
    postprocedural
      adrenal hypofunction E89.6
      hypoinsulinemia E89.1
      hypoparathyroidism E89.2
      hypopituitarism E89.3
      hypothyroidism E89.0
      ovarian failure E89.40
        asymptomatic E89.40
        symptomatic E89.41
      specified NEC E89.89
      testicular hypofunction E89.5
  endodontic treatment NEC M27.59
  enterostomy (stoma) K94.10
    hemorrhage K94.11
    infection K94.12
    malfunction K94.13
    mechanical K94.13
    specified complication NEC K94.19
  episiotomy, disruption O90.1
  esophageal anti-reflux device T85.9
    embolism T85.818
    fibrosis T85.828
    hemorrhage T85.838

Complication (continued)
  esophageal anti-reflux device (continued)
    infection and inflammation T85.79
    mechanical
      breakdown T85.511
      displacement T85.521
      malfunction T85.511
      malposition T85.521
      obstruction T85.591
      perforation T85.591
      protrusion T85.591
      specified NEC T85.591
    pain T85.848
    specified type NEC T85.898
    stenosis T85.858
    thrombosis T85.868
  esophagostomy K94.30
    hemorrhage K94.31
    infection K94.32
    malfunction K94.33
    mechanical K94.33
    specified complication NEC K94.39
  extracorporeal circulation T80.90
  extremity artery (bypass) graft T82.9
    arteriosclerosis —see Arteriosclerosis, extremities, bypass graft
    embolism T82.818
    fibrosis T82.828
    hemorrhage T82.838
    infection and inflammation T82.7
    mechanical
      breakdown T82.318
        femoral artery T82.312
      displacement T82.328
        femoral artery T82.322
      leakage T82.338
        femoral artery T82.332
      malposition T82.328
        femoral artery T82.322
      obstruction T82.398
        femoral artery T82.392
      perforation T82.398
        femoral artery T82.392
      protrusion T82.398
        femoral artery T82.392
    pain T82.848
    specified type NEC T82.898
    stenosis T82.858
    thrombosis T82.868
  eye H57.9
    corneal graft —see Complications, graft, cornea
    implant (prosthetic) T85.9
      embolism T85.818
      fibrosis T85.828
      hemorrhage T85.838
      infection and inflammation T85.79
      mechanical
        breakdown T85.318
        displacement T85.328
        leakage T85.398
        malposition T85.328
        obstruction T85.398
        perforation T85.398
        protrusion T85.398
        specified NEC T85.398
      pain T85.848
      specified type NEC T85.898
      stenosis T85.858
      thrombosis T85.868
    intraocular lens —see Complications, intraocular lens
    orbital prosthesis —see Complications, orbital prosthesis

Complication (continued)
  female genital N94.9
    device, implant or graft NEC —see Complications, genitourinary, device or implant, genital tract
  femoral artery (bypass) graft —see Complication, extremity artery (bypass) graft
  fixation device, internal (orthopedic) T84.9
    infection and inflammation T84.60
      arm T84.61-
        humerus T84.61-
        radius T84.61-
        ulna T84.61-
      leg T84.629
        femur T84.62-
        fibula T84.62-
        tibia T84.62-
      specified site NEC T84.69
      spine T84.63
    mechanical
      breakdown
        limb T84.119
          carpal T84.210
          femur T84.11-
          fibula T84.11-
          humerus T84.11-
          metacarpal T84.210
          metatarsal T84.213
          phalanx
            foot T84.213
            hand T84.210
          radius T84.11-
          tarsal T84.213
          tibia T84.11-
          ulna T84.11-
        specified bone NEC T84.218
        spine T84.216
      displacement
        limb T84.129
          carpal T84.220
          femur T84.12-
          fibula T84.12-
          humerus T84.12-
          metacarpal T84.220
          metatarsal T84.223
          phalanx
            foot T84.223
            hand T84.220
          radius T84.12-
          tarsal T84.223
          tibia T84.12-
          ulna T84.12-
        specified bone NEC T84.228
        spine T84.226
      malposition —see Complications, fixation device, internal, mechanical, displacement
      obstruction —see Complications, fixation device, internal, mechanical, specified type NEC
      perforation —see Complications, fixation device, internal, mechanical, specified type NEC
      protrusion —see Complications, fixation device, internal, mechanical, specified type NEC
      specified type NEC
        limb T84.199
          carpal T84.290
          femur T84.19-

Complication (continued)
  fixation device, internal (continued)
    mechanical (continued)
      specified type NEC (continued)
        limb (continued)
          fibula T84.19-
          humerus T84.19-
          metacarpal T84.290
          metatarsal T84.293
          phalanx
            foot T84.293
            hand T84.290
          radius T84.19-
          tarsal T84.293
          tibia T84.19-
          ulna T84.19-
        specified bone NEC T84.298
        vertebra T84.296
      specified type NEC T84.89
        embolism T84.81
        fibrosis T84.82
        hemorrhage T84.83
        pain T84.84
        specified complication NEC T84.89
        stenosis T84.85
        thrombosis T84.86
  following
    acute myocardial infarction NEC I23.8
      aneurysm (false) (of cardiac wall) (of heart wall) (ruptured) I23.3
      angina I23.7
      atrial
        septal defect I23.1
        thrombosis I23.6
      cardiac wall rupture I23.3
      chordae tendinae rupture I23.4
      defect
        septal
          atrial (heart) I23.1
          ventricular (heart) I23.2
      hemopericardium I23.0
      papillary muscle rupture I23.5
      rupture
        cardiac wall I23.3
          with hemopericardium I23.0
        chordae tendineae I23.4
        papillary muscle I23.5
      specified NEC I23.8
      thrombosis
        atrium I23.6
        auricular appendage I23.6
        ventricle (heart) I23.6
      ventricular
        septal defect I23.2
        thrombosis I23.6
    ectopic or molar pregnancy O08.9
      cardiac arrest O08.81
      sepsis O08.82
      specified type NEC O08.89
      urinary tract infection O08.83
    termination of pregnancy —see Abortion
  gastrointestinal K92.9
    bile duct prosthesis —see Complications, bile duct implant
    esophageal anti-reflux device —see Complications, esophageal anti-reflux device
    postoperative
      colostomy —see Complications, colostomy
      dumping syndrome K91.1

Complication (continued)
  gastrointestinal (continued)
    postoperative (continued)
      enterostomy —see Complications, enterostomy
      gastrostomy —see Complications, gastrostomy
      malabsorption NEC K91.2
      obstruction (see also Obstruction, intestine, postoperative) K91.30
      postcholecystectomy syndrome K91.5
      specified NEC K91.89
      vomiting after GI surgery K91.0
    prosthetic device or implant
      bile duct prosthesis —see Complications, bile duct implant
      esophageal anti-reflux device —see Complications, esophageal anti-reflux device
      specified type NEC
        embolism T85.818
        fibrosis T85.828
        hemorrhage T85.838
        mechanical
          breakdown T85.518
          displacement T85.528
          malfunction T85.518
          malposition T85.528
          obstruction T85.598
          perforation T85.598
          protrusion T85.598
          specified NEC T85.598
        pain T85.848
        specified complication NEC T85.898
        stenosis T85.858
        thrombosis T85.868
  gastrostomy (stoma) K94.20
    hemorrhage K94.21
    infection K94.22
    malfunction K94.23
    mechanical K94.23
    specified complication NEC K94.29
  genitourinary
    device or implant T83.9
      genital tract T83.9
        infection or inflammation T83.69
        intrauterine contraceptive device —see Complications, intrauterine, contraceptive device
        mechanical —see Complications, by device, mechanical
        mesh —see Complications, prosthetic device or implant, mesh
        penile prosthesis —see Complications, prosthetic device, penile
        specified type NEC T83.89
          embolism T83.81
          fibrosis T83.82
          hemorrhage T83.83
          pain T83.84
          specified complication NEC T83.89
          stenosis T83.85
          thrombosis T83.86
        vaginal mesh —see Complications, prosthetic device or implant mesh

65

Complication *(continued)*
  genitourinary *(continued)*
    device or implant *(continued)*
      urinary system T83.9
        cystostomy catheter —*see*
          Complication, catheter,
          cystostomy
        electronic stimulator —*see*
          Complications, electronic
          stimulator device,
          urinary
        indwelling urethral catheter
          —*see* Complications,
          catheter, urethral,
          indwelling
        infection or inflammation
          T83.598
          indwelling urethral
            catheter T83.511
        kidney transplant —*see*
          Complication, transplant,
          kidney
        organ graft —*see*
          Complication, graft,
          urinary organ
        specified type NEC T83.89
          embolism T83.81
          fibrosis T83.82
          hemorrhage T83.83
          mechanical T83.198
            breakdown T83.118
            displacement T83.128
            malfunction T83.118
            malposition T83.128
            obstruction T83.198
            perforation T83.198
            protrusion T83.198
            specified NEC T83.198
        sphincter implant —*see*
          Complications, implant,
          urinary sphincter
        sphincter, implanted T83.191
        stent (ileal conduit)
          (nephroureteral) T83.193
          pain T83.84
          specified complication
            NEC T83.89
          stenosis T83.85
          thrombosis T83.86
        ureteral indwelling
          T83.192
    postprocedural
      pelvic peritoneal adhesions
        N99.4
      renal failure N99.0
      specified NEC N99.89
      stoma —*see* Complications,
        stoma, urinary tract
      urethral stricture —*see*
        Stricture, urethra,
        postprocedural
    vaginal
      adhesions N99.2
      vault prolapse N99.3
  graft (bypass) (patch) —*see also*
    Complications, prosthetic device
    or implant
    aorta —*see* Complications, graft,
      vascular
    arterial —*see* Complication,
      graft, vascular
    bone T86.839
      failure T86.831
      infection T86.832
      mechanical T84.318
        breakdown T84.318
        displacement T84.328
        protrusion T84.398
        specified type NEC T84.398
      rejection T86.830
      specified type NEC T86.838

Complication *(continued)*
  graft *(continued)*
    carotid artery —*see*
      Complications, graft, vascular
    cornea T86.849-
      failure T86.841-
      infection T86.842-
      mechanical T85.398
        breakdown T85.318
        displacement T85.328
        protrusion T85.398
        specified type NEC
          T85.398-
      rejection T86.840-
      retroprosthetic membrane
        T85.398
      specified type NEC T86.848-
    femoral artery (bypass) —*see*
      Complication, extremity artery
      (bypass) graft
    genital organ or tract —*see*
      Complications, genitourinary,
      device or implant, genital
      tract
    muscle T84.9
      breakdown T84.410
      displacement T84.420
      embolism T84.81
      fibrosis T84.82
      hemorrhage T84.83
      infection and inflammation
        T84.7
      mechanical NEC
        T84.490
      pain T84.84
      specified type NEC
        T84.89
      stenosis T84.85
      thrombosis T84.86
    nerve —*see* Complication,
      prosthetic device or implant,
      specified NEC
    skin —*see* Complications,
      prosthetic device or implant,
      skin graft
    tendon T84.9
      breakdown T84.410
      displacement T84.420
      embolism T84.81
      fibrosis T84.82
      hemorrhage T84.83
      infection and inflammation
        T84.7
      mechanical NEC T84.490
      pain T84.84
      specified type NEC T84.89
      stenosis T84.85
      thrombosis T84.86
    urinary organ T83.9
      embolism T83.81
      fibrosis T83.82
      hemorrhage T83.83
      infection and inflammation
        T83.598
        indwelling urethral catheter
          T83.511
      mechanical
        breakdown T83.21
        displacement T83.22
        erosion T83.24
        exposure T83.25
        leakage T83.23
        malposition T83.22
        obstruction T83.29
        perforation T83.29
        protrusion T83.29
        specified NEC T83.29
      pain T83.84
      specified type NEC T83.89
      stenosis T83.85
      thrombosis T83.86

Complication *(continued)*
  graft *(continued)*
    vascular T82.9
      embolism T82.818
      femoral artery —*see*
        Complication, extremity
        artery (bypass) graft
      fibrosis T82.828
      hemorrhage T82.838
      mechanical
        breakdown T82.319
          aorta (bifurcation)
            T82.310
          carotid artery
            T82.311
          specified vessel NEC
            T82.318
        displacement T82.329
          aorta (bifurcation)
            T82.320
          carotid artery T82.321
          specified vessel NEC
            T82.328
        leakage T82.339
          aorta (bifurcation)
            T82.330
          carotid artery T82.331
          specified vessel NEC
            T82.338
        malposition T82.329
          aorta (bifurcation)
            T82.320
          carotid artery T82.321
          specified vessel NEC
            T82.328
        obstruction T82.399
          aorta (bifurcation)
            T82.390
          carotid artery T82.391
          specified vessel NEC
            T82.398
        perforation T82.399
          aorta (bifurcation)
            T82.390
          carotid artery T82.391
          specified vessel NEC
            T82.398
        protrusion T82.399
          aorta (bifurcation)
            T82.390
          carotid artery T82.391
          specified vessel NEC
            T82.398
      pain T82.848
      specified complication NEC
        T82.898
      stenosis T82.858
      thrombosis T82.868
  heart I51.9
    assist device
      infection and inflammation
        T82.7
    following acute myocardial
      infarction —*see*
      Complications, following,
      acute myocardial infarction
    postoperative —*see*
      Complications, circulatory
      system
    transplant —*see* Complication,
      transplant, heart
      and lung(s) —*see*
        Complications, transplant,
        heart, with lung
    valve
      graft (biological) T82.9
        embolism T82.817
        fibrosis T82.827
        hemorrhage T82.837
        infection and inflammation
          T82.7

Complication *(continued)*
  heart *(continued)*
    valve *(continued)*
      graft *(continued)*
        mechanical T82.228
          breakdown T82.221
          displacement T82.222
          leakage T82.223
          malposition T82.222
          obstruction T82.228
          perforation T82.228
          protrusion T82.228
        pain T82.847
        specified type NEC T82.897
        stenosis T82.857
        thrombosis T82.867
      prosthesis T82.9
        embolism T82.817
        fibrosis T82.827
        hemorrhage T82.837
        infection or inflammation
          T82.6
        mechanical T82.09
          breakdown T82.01
          displacement T82.02
          leakage T82.03
          malposition T82.02
          obstruction T82.09
          perforation T82.09
          protrusion T82.09
        pain T82.847
        specified type NEC
          T82.897
          mechanical T82.09
          stenosis T82.857
          thrombosis T82.867
  hematoma
    intraoperative —*see*
      Complication, intraoperative,
      hemorrhage
    postprocedural —*see*
      Complication, postprocedural,
      hematoma
  hemodialysis —*see* Complications,
    dialysis
  hemorrhage
    intraoperative —*see*
      Complication, intraoperative,
      hemorrhage
    postprocedural —*see*
      Complication, postprocedural,
      hemorrhage
  IEC (immune effector cellular)
    therapy T80.82
  ileostomy (stoma) —*see*
    Complications, enterostomy
  immune effector cellular (IEC)
    therapy T80.82
  immunization (procedure) —*see*
    Complications, vaccination
  implant —*see also* Complications,
    by site and type
    urinary sphincter T83.9
      embolism T83.81
      fibrosis T83.82
      hemorrhage T83.83
      infection and inflammation
        T83.591
      mechanical
        breakdown T83.111
        displacement T83.121
        leakage T83.191
        malposition T83.121
        obstruction T83.191
        perforation T83.191
        protrusion T83.191
        specified NEC T83.191
      pain T83.84
      specified type NEC T83.89
      stenosis T83.85
      thrombosis T83.86

Complication (*continued*)
  infusion (procedure) T80.90
    air embolism T80.0
    blood —*see* Complications, transfusion
    catheter —*see* Complications, catheter
    infection T80.29
    pump —*see* Complications, cardiovascular, device or implant
    sepsis T80.29
    serum reaction (*see also* Reaction, serum) T80.69
      anaphylactic shock (*see also* Shock, anaphylactic) T80.59
    specified type NEC T80.89
  inhalation therapy NEC T81.81
  injection (procedure) T80.90
    drug reaction —*see* Reaction, drug
    infection T80.29
    sepsis T80.29
    serum (prophylactic) (therapeutic) —*see* Complications, vaccination
    specified type NEC T80.89
    vaccine (any) —*see* Complications, vaccination
  inoculation (any) —*see* Complications, vaccination
  insulin pump
    infection and inflammation T85.72
    mechanical
      breakdown T85.614
      displacement T85.624
      leakage T85.633
      malposition T85.624
      obstruction T85.694
      perforation T85.694
      protrusion T85.694
      specified NEC T85.694
  intestinal pouch NEC K91.858
  intraocular lens (prosthetic) T85.9
    embolism T85.818
    fibrosis T85.828
    hemorrhage T85.838
    infection and inflammation T85.79
    mechanical
      breakdown T85.21
      displacement T85.22
      malposition T85.22
      obstruction T85.29
      perforation T85.29
      protrusion T85.29
      specified NEC T85.29
    pain T85.848
    specified type NEC T85.898
    stenosis T85.858
    thrombosis T85.868
  intraoperative (intraprocedural)
    cardiac arrest —*see also* Infarct, myocardium, associated with revascularization procedure
      during cardiac surgery I97.710
      during other surgery I97.711
    cardiac functional disturbance NEC —*see also* Infarct, myocardium, associated with revascularization procedure
      during cardiac surgery I97.790
      during other surgery I97.791
    hemorrhage (hematoma) (of)
      circulatory system organ or structure
        during cardiac bypass I97.411

Complication (*continued*)
  intraoperative (*continued*)
    hemorrhage (*continued*)
      circulatory system organ or structure (*continued*)
        during cardiac catheterization I97.410
        during other circulatory system procedure I97.418
        during other procedure I97.42
      digestive system organ
        during procedure on digestive system K91.61
        during procedure on other organ K91.62
      ear
        during procedure on ear and mastoid process H95.21
        during procedure on other organ H95.22
      endocrine system organ or structure
        during procedure on endocrine system organ or structure E36.01
        during procedure on other organ E36.02
      eye and adnexa
        during ophthalmic procedure H59.11-
        during other procedure H59.12-
      genitourinary organ or structure
        during procedure on genitourinary organ or structure N99.61
        during procedure on other organ N99.62
      mastoid process
        during procedure on ear and mastoid process H95.21
        during procedure on other organ H95.22
      musculoskeletal structure
        during musculoskeletal surgery M96.810
        during non-orthopedic surgery M96.811
        during orthopedic surgery M96.810
      nervous system
        during a nervous system procedure G97.31
        during other procedure G97.32
      respiratory system
        during other procedure J95.62
        during procedure on respiratory system organ or structure J95.61
      skin and subcutaneous tissue
        during a dermatologic procedure L76.01
        during a procedure on other organ L76.02
      spleen
        during a procedure on other organ D78.02
        during a procedure on the spleen D78.01
    puncture or laceration (accidental) (unintentional) (of)
      brain
        during a nervous system procedure G97.48
        during other procedure G97.49

Complication (*continued*)
  intraoperative (*continued*)
    puncture or laceration (*continued*)
      circulatory system organ or structure
        during circulatory system procedure I97.51
        during other procedure I97.52
      digestive system
        during procedure on digestive system K91.71
        during procedure on other organ K91.72
      ear
        during procedure on ear and mastoid process H95.31
        during procedure on other organ H95.32
      endocrine system organ or structure
        during procedure on endocrine system organ or structure E36.11
        during procedure on other organ E36.12
      eye and adnexa
        during ophthalmic procedure H59.21-
        during other procedure H59.22-
      genitourinary organ or structure
        during procedure on genitourinary organ or structure N99.71
        during procedure on other organ N99.72
      mastoid process
        during procedure on ear and mastoid process H95.31
        during procedure on other organ H95.32
      musculoskeletal structure
        during musculoskeletal surgery M96.820
        during non-orthopedic surgery M96.821
        during orthopedic surgery M96.820
      nervous system
        during a nervous system procedure G97.48
        during other procedure G97.49
      respiratory system
        during other procedure J95.72
        during procedure on respiratory system organ or structure J95.71
      skin and subcutaneous tissue
        during a dermatologic procedure L76.11
        during a procedure on other organ L76.12
      spleen
        during a procedure on other organ D78.12
        during a procedure on the spleen D78.11
    specified NEC
      circulatory system I97.88
      digestive system K91.81
      ear H95.88
      endocrine system E36.8
      eye and adnexa H59.88
      genitourinary system N99.81
      mastoid process H95.88
      musculoskeletal structure M96.89
      nervous system G97.81
      respiratory system J95.88

Complication (*continued*)
  intraoperative (*continued*)
    specified NEC (*continued*)
      skin and subcutaneous tissue L76.81
      spleen D78.81
  intraperitoneal catheter (dialysis) (infusion) —*see* Complication(s), catheter, intraperitoneal dialysis
  intrathecal infusion pump
    infection and inflammation T85.738
    mechanical
      breakdown T85.615
      displacement T85.625
      leakage T85.635
      malfunction T85.695
      malposition T85.625
      obstruction T85.695
      perforation T85.695
      protrusion T85.695
      specified NEC T85.695
  intrauterine
    contraceptive device
      embolism T83.81
      fibrosis T83.82
      hemorrhage T83.83
      infection and inflammation T83.69
      mechanical
        breakdown T83.31
        displacement T83.32
        malposition T83.32
        obstruction T83.39
        perforation T83.39
        protrusion T83.39
        specified NEC T83.39
      pain T83.84
      specified type NEC T83.89
      stenosis T83.85
      thrombosis T83.86
    procedure (fetal), to newborn P96.5
  jejunostomy (stoma) —*see* Complications, enterostomy
  joint prosthesis, internal T84.9
    breakage (fracture) T84.01-
    dislocation T84.02-
    fracture T84.01-
    infection or inflammation T84.50
      hip T84.5-
      knee T84.5-
      specified joint NEC T84.59
    instability T84.02-
    malposition —*see* Complications, joint prosthesis, mechanical, displacement
    mechanical
      breakage, broken T84.01-
      dislocation T84.02-
      displacement T84.02-
      fracture T84.01-
      instability T84.02-
      leakage —*see* Complications, joint prosthesis, mechanical, specified NEC
      loosening T84.039
        hip T84.03-
        knee T84.03-
        specified joint NEC T84.038
      obstruction —*see* Complications, joint prosthesis, mechanical, specified NEC

Complication (continued)
  joint prosthesis, internal (continued)
    mechanical (continued)
      perforation —see Complications, joint prosthesis, mechanical, specified NEC
      osteolysis T84.059
        hip T84.05-
        knee T84.05-
        other specified joint T84.058
        periprosthetic osteolysis, by site T84.05-
      protrusion —see Complications, joint prosthesis, mechanical, specified NEC
      specified complication NEC T84.099
        hip T84.09-
        knee T84.09-
        other specified joint T84.098
      subluxation T84.02-
      wear of articular bearing surface T84.069
        hip T84.06-
        knee T84.06-
        other specified joint T84.068
    specified joint NEC T84.89
      embolism T84.81
      fibrosis T84.82
      hemorrhage T84.83
      pain T84.84
      specified complication NEC T84.89
      stenosis T84.85
      thrombosis T84.86
    subluxation T84.02-
  kidney transplant —see Complications, transplant, kidney
  labor O75.9
    specified NEC O75.89
  liver transplant (immune or nonimmune) —see Complications, transplant, liver
  lumbar puncture G97.1
    cerebrospinal fluid leak G97.0
    headache or reaction G97.1
  lung transplant —see Complications, transplant, lung
    and heart —see Complications, transplant, lung, with heart
  male genital N50.9
    device, implant or graft —see Complications, genitourinary, device or implant, genital tract
    postprocedural or postoperative —see Complications, genitourinary, postprocedural
    specified NEC N99.89
  mastoid (process) procedure
    intraoperative H95.88
      hematoma —see Complications, intraoperative, hemorrhage (hematoma) (of), mastoid process
      hemorrhage —see Complications, intraoperative, hemorrhage (hematoma) (of), mastoid process
      laceration —see Complications, intraoperative, puncture or laceration..., mastoid process
      specified NEC H95.88

Complication (continued)
  mastoid (continued)
    postmastoidectomy —see Complications, postmastoidectomy
    postoperative H95.89
      external ear canal stenosis H95.81-
      hematoma —see Complications..., postprocedural, hematoma (of), mastoid process
      hemorrhage —see Complications..., postprocedural, hemorrhage (of), mastoid process
      postmastoidectomy —see Complications, postmastoidectomy
      seroma —see Complications, postprocedureal, seroma (of), mastoid process
      specified NEC H95.89
  mastoidectomy cavity —see Complications, postmastoidectomy
  mechanical —see Complications, by site and type, mechanical
  medical procedures (see also Complication(s), intraoperative) T88.9
  metabolic E88.9
    postoperative E89.89
      specified NEC E89.89
  molar pregnancy NOS O08.9
    damage to pelvic organs O08.6
    embolism O08.2
    genital infection O08.0
    hemorrhage (delayed) (excessive) O08.1
    metabolic disorder O08.5
    renal failure O08.4
    shock O08.3
    specified type NEC O08.0
    venous complication NEC O08.7
  musculoskeletal system —see also Complication, intraoperative (intraprocedural), by site
    device, implant or graft NEC —see Complications, orthopedic, device or implant
    internal fixation (nail) (plate) (rod) —see Complications, fixation device, internal
    joint prosthesis —see Complications, joint prosthesis
    postoperative (postprocedural) M96.89
      with osteoporosis —see Osteoporosis
      fracture following insertion of device —see Fracture, following insertion of orthopedic implant, joint prosthesis or bone plate
      joint instability after prosthesis removal M96.89
      lordosis M96.4
      postlaminectomy syndrome NEC M96.1
      kyphosis M96.3
      pseudarthrosis M96.0
      specified complication NEC M96.89
    post radiation M96.89
      kyphosis M96.2
      scoliosis M96.5
      specified complication NEC M96.89

Complication (continued)
  nephrostomy (stoma) —see Complications, stoma, urinary tract, external NEC
  nervous system G98.8
    central G96.9
    device, implant or graft —see also Complication, prosthetic device or implant, specified NEC
      electronic stimulator (electrode(s)) —see Complications, electronic stimulator device
      specified NEC
        infection and inflammation T85.738
        mechanical T85.695
          breakdown T85.615
          displacement T85.625
          leakage T85.635
          malfunction T85.695
          malposition T85.625
          obstruction T85.695
          perforation T85.695
          protrusion T85.695
          specified NEC T85.695
      ventricular shunt —see Complications, ventricular shunt
    electronic stimulator (electrode(s)) —see Complications, electronic stimulator device
    postprocedural G97.82
      intracranial hypotension G97.2
      specified NEC G97.82
      spinal fluid leak G97.0
  newborn, due to intrauterine (fetal) procedure P96.5
  nonabsorbable (permanent) sutures —see Complication, sutures, permanent
  obstetric O75.9
    procedure (instrumental) (manual) (surgical) specified NEC O75.4
    specified NEC O75.89
    surgical wound NEC O90.89
      hematoma O90.2
      infection O86.00
  ocular lens implant —see Complications, intraocular lens
  ophthalmologic
    postprocedural bleb —see Blebitis
  orbital prosthesis T85.9
    embolism T85.818
    fibrosis T85.828
    hemorrhage T85.838
    infection and inflammation T85.79
    mechanical
      breakdown T85.31-
      displacement T85.32-
      malposition T85.32-
      obstruction T85.39-
      perforation T85.39-
      protrusion T85.39-
      specified NEC T85.39-
    pain T85.848
    specified type NEC T85.898
    stenosis T85.858
    thrombosis T85.868
  organ or tissue transplant (partial) (total) —see Complications, transplant
  orthopedic —see also Disorder, soft tissue

Complication (continued)
  orthopedic (continued)
    device or implant T84.9
      bone
        device or implant —see Complication, bone, device NEC
        graft —see Complication, graft, bone
        breakdown T84.418
        displacement T84.428
        electronic bone stimulator —see Complications, electronic stimulator device, bone
        embolism T84.81
        fibrosis T84.82
        fixation device —see Complication, fixation device, internal
        hemorrhage T84.83
        infection or inflammation T84.7
        joint prosthesis —see Complication, joint prosthesis, internal
        malfunction T84.418
        malposition T84.428
        mechanical NEC T84.498
        muscle graft —see Complications, graft, muscle
        obstruction T84.498
        pain T84.84
        perforation T84.498
        protrusion T84.498
        specified complication NEC T84.89
        stenosis T84.85
        tendon graft —see Complications, graft, tendon
        thrombosis T84.86
      fracture (following insertion of device) —see Fracture, following insertion of orthopedic implant, joint prosthesis or bone plate
    postprocedural M96.89
      fracture —see Fracture, following insertion of orthopedic implant, joint prosthesis or bone plate
      postlaminectomy syndrome NEC M96.1
      kyphosis M96.3
      lordosis M96.4
      postradiation
        kyphosis M96.2
        scoliosis M96.5
      pseudarthrosis post-fusion M96.0
      specified type NEC M96.89
  pacemaker (cardiac) —see Complications, cardiovascular device or implant, electronic
  pancreas transplant —see Complications, transplant, pancreas
  penile prosthesis (implant) —see Complications, prosthetic device, penile
  perfusion NEC T80.90
  perineal repair (obstetrical) NEC O90.89
    disruption O90.1
    hematoma O90.2
    infection (following delivery) O86.09
  phototherapy T88.9
    specified NEC T88.8

Complication (continued)
    postmastoidectomy NEC H95.19-
        cyst, mucosal H95.13-
        granulation H95.12-
        inflammation, chronic H95.11-
        recurrent cholesteatoma H95.0-
    postoperative —see Complications, postprocedural
        circulatory —see Complications, circulatory system
        ear —see Complications, ear
        endocrine —see Complications, endocrine
        eye —see Complications, eye
        lumbar puncture G97.1
            cerebrospinal fluid leak G97.0
        nervous system (central) (peripheral) —see Complications, nervous system
        respiratory system —see Complications, respiratory system
    postprocedural —see also Complications, surgical procedure
        cardiac arrest —see also Infarct, myocardium, associated with revascularization procedure
            following cardiac surgery I97.120
            following other surgery I97.121
        cardiac functional disturbance NEC —see also Infarct, myocardium, associated with revascularization procedure
            following cardiac surgery I97.190
            following other surgery I97.191
        cardiac insufficiency
            following cardiac surgery I97.110
            following other surgery I97.111
        chorioretinal scars following retinal surgery H59.81-
        following cataract surgery
            cataract (lens) fragments H59.02-
            cystoid macular edema H59.03-
            specified NEC H59.09-
            vitreous (touch) syndrome H59.01-
        heart failure
            following cardiac surgery I97.130
            following other surgery I97.131
        hematoma (of)
            circulatory system organ or structure
                following cardiac bypass I97.631
                following cardiac catheterization I97.630
                following other circulatory system procedure I97.638
                following other procedure I97.621
            digestive system
                following procedure on digestive system K91.870
                following procedure on other organ K91.871
            ear
                following other procedure H95.52
                following procedure on ear and mastoid process H95.51

Complication (continued)
    postprocedural (continued)
        hematoma (continued)
            endocrine system
                following endocrine system procedure E89.820
                following other procedure E89.821
            eye and adnexa
                following ophthalmic procedure H59.33-
                following other procedure H59.34-
            genitourinary organ or structure
                following procedure on genitourinary organ or structure N99.840
                following procedure on other organ N99.841
            mastoid process
                following other procedure H95.52
                following procedure on ear and mastoid process H95.51
            musculoskeletal structure
                following musculoskeletal surgery M96.840
                following non-orthopedic surgery M96.841
                following orthopedic surgery M96.840
            nervous system
                following nervous system procedure G97.61
                following other procedure G97.62
            respiratory system
                following other procedure J95.861
                following procedure on respiratory system organ or structure J95.860
            skin and subcutaneous tissue
                following dematologic procedure L76.31
                following procedure on other organ L76.32
            spleen
                following procedure on other organ D78.32
                following procedure on the spleen D78.31
        hemorrhage (of)
            circulatory system organ or structure
                following cardiac bypass I97.611
                following cardiac catheterization I97.610
                following other circulatory system procedure I97.618
                following other procedure I97.620
            digestive system
                following procedure on digestive system K91.840
                following procedure on other organ K91.841
            ear
                following other procedure H95.42
                following procedure on ear and mastoid process H95.41
            endocrine system
                following endocrine system procedure E89.810
                following other procedure E89.811

Complication (continued)
    postprocedural (continued)
        hemorrhage (continued)
            eye and adnexa
                following ophthalmic procedure H59.31-
                following other procedure H59.32-
            genitourinary organ or structure
                following procedure on genitourinary organ or structure N99.820
                following procedure on other organ N99.821
            mastoid process
                following other procedure H95.42
                following procedure on ear and mastoid process H95.41
            musculoskeletal structure
                following musculoskeletal surgery M96.830
                following non-orthopedic surgery M96.831
                following orthopedic surgery M96.830
            nervous system
                following nervous system procedure G97.51
                following other procedure G97.52
            respiratory system
                following other procedure J95.831
                following procedure on respiratory system organ or structure J95.830
            skin and subcutaneous tissue
                following dermatologic procedure L76.21
                following a procedure on other organ L76.22
            spleen
                following procedure on other organ D78.22
                following procedure on the spleen D78.21
        seroma (of)
            circulatory system organ or structure
                following cardiac bypass I97.641
                following cardiac catheterization I97.640
                following other circulatory system procedure I97.648
                following other procedure I97.622
            digestive system
                following procedure on digestive system K91.872
                following procedure on other organ K91.873
            ear
                following other procedure H95.54
                following procedure on ear and mastoid process H95.53
            endocrine system
                following endocrine system procedure E89.822
                following other procedure E89.823
            eye and adnexa
                following ophthalmic procedure H59.35-
                following other procedure H59.36-

Complication (continued)
    postprocedural (continued)
        seroma (continued)
            genitourinary organ or structure
                following procedure on genitourinary organ or structure N99.842
                following procedure on other organ N99.843
            mastoid process
                following other procedure H95.54
                following procedure on ear and mastoid process H95.53
            musculoskeletal structure
                following musculoskeletal surgery M96.842
                following non-orthopedic surgery M96.843
                following orthopedic surgery M96.842
            nervous system
                following nervous system procedure G97.63
                following other procedure G97.64
            respiratory system
                following other procedure J95.863
                following procedure on respiratory system organ or structure J95.862
            skin and subcutaneous tissue
                following dematologic procedure L76.33
                following procedure on other organ L76.34
            spleen
                following procedure on other organ D78.34
                following procedure on the spleen D78.33
        specified NEC
            circulatory system I97.89
            digestive K91.89
            ear H95.89
            endocrine E89.89
            eye and adnexa H59.89
            genitourinary N99.89
            mastoid process H95.89
            metabolic E89.89
            musculoskeletal structure M96.89
            nervous system G97.82
            respiratory system J95.89
            skin and subcutaneous tissue L76.82
            spleen D78.89
    pregnancy NEC —see Pregnancy, complicated by
    prosthetic device or implant T85.9
        bile duct —see Complications, bile duct implant
        breast —see Complications, breast implant
        bulking agent
            ureteral
                erosion T83.714
                exposure T83.724
            urethral
                erosion T83.713
                exposure T83.723
        cardiac and vascular NEC —see Complications, cardiovascular device or implant
        corneal transplant —see Complications, graft, cornea

Complication (*continued*)
  prosthetic device or implant (*continued*)
    electronic nervous system stimulator —*see* Complications, electronic stimulator device
    epidural infusion catheter —*see* Complications, catheter, epidural
    esophageal anti-reflux device — *see* Complications, esophageal anti-reflux device
    genital organ or tract —*see* Complications, genitourinary, device or implant, genital tract
      specified NEC T83.79
    heart valve —*see* Complications, heart, valve, prosthesis
    infection or inflammation T85.79
      intestine transplant T86.852
      liver transplant T86.43
      lung transplant T86.812
      pancreas transplant T86.892
      skin graft T86.822
    intraocular lens —*see* Complications, intraocular lens
    intraperitoneal (dialysis) catheter —*see* Complication(s), catheter, intraperitoneal dialysis
    joint —*see* Complications, joint prosthesis, internal
    mechanical NEC T85.698
      dialysis catheter (vascular) —*see also* Complication, catheter, dialysis, mechanical
        peritoneal —*see* Complication(s), catheter, intraperitoneal, dialysis
      gastrointestinal device T85.598
      ocular device T85.398
      subdural (infusion) catheter T85.690
      suture, permanent T85.692
        that for bone repair — *see* Complications, fixation device, internal (orthopedic), mechanical
      ventricular shunt
        breakdown T85.01
        displacement T85.02
        leakage T85.03
        malposition T85.02
        obstruction T85.09
        perforation T85.09
        protrusion T85.09
        specified NEC T85.09
    mesh
      erosion (to surrounding organ or tissue) T83.718
        vaginal (into pelvic floor muscles) T83.711
        urethral (into pelvic floor muscles) T83.712
      exposure (into surrounding organ or tissue) T83.728
        vaginal (into vagina) (through vaginal wall) T83.721
        urethral (through urethral wall) T83.722
    orbital —*see* Complications, orbital prosthesis
    penile T83.9
      embolism T83.81
      fibrosis T83.82
      hemorrhage T83.83
      infection and inflammation T83.61

Complication (*continued*)
  prosthetic device or implant (*continued*)
    penile (*continued*)
      mechanical
        breakdown T83.410
        displacement T83.420
        leakage T83.490
        malposition T83.420
        obstruction T83.490
        perforation T83.490
        protrusion T83.490
        specified NEC T83.490
      pain T83.848
      specified type NEC T83.89
      stenosis T83.85
      thrombosis T83.86
    prosthetic materials NEC
      erosion (to surrounding organ or tissue) T83.718
      exposure (into surrounding organ or tissue) T83.728
    skin graft T86.829
      artificial skin or decellularized allodermis
        embolism T85.818
        fibrosis T85.828
        hemorrhage T85.838
        infection and inflammation T85.79
        mechanical
          breakdown T85.613
          displacement T85.623
          malfunction T85.613
            malposition T85.623
            obstruction T85.693
            perforation T85.693
            protrusion T85.693
            specified NEC T85.693
        pain T85.848
        specified type NEC T85.898
        stenosis T85.858
        thrombosis T85.868
      failure T86.821
      infection T86.822
      rejection T86.820
      specified NEC T86.828
    sling
      urethral (female) (male)
        erosion T83.712
        exposure T83.722
    specified NEC T85.9
      embolism T85.818
      fibrosis T85.828
      hemorrhage T85.838
      infection and inflammation T85.79
      mechanical
        breakdown T85.618
        displacement T85.628
        leakage T85.638
        malfunction T85.618
        malposition T85.628
        obstruction T85.698
        perforation T85.698
        protrusion T85.698
        specified NEC T85.698
      pain T85.848
      specified type NEC T85.898
      stenosis T85.858
      thrombosis T85.868
    subdural infusion catheter —*see* Complications, catheter, subdural
    sutures —*see* Complications, sutures
    urinary organ or tract NEC —*see* Complications, genitourinary, device or implant, urinary system

Complication (*continued*)
  prosthetic device or implant (*continued*)
    vascular —*see* Complications, cardiovascular device, graft or implant
    ventricular shunt —*see* Complications, ventricular shunt (device)
  puerperium —*see* Puerperal
  puncture, spinal G97.1
    cerebrospinal fluid leak G97.0
    headache or reaction G97.1
  pyelogram N99.89
  radiation
    kyphosis M96.2
    scoliosis M96.5
  reattached
    extremity (infection) (rejection)
      lower T87.1X-
      upper T87.0X-
    specified body part NEC T87.2
  reconstructed breast
    asymmetry between native and reconstructed breast N65.1
    deformity N65.0
    disproportion between native and reconstructed breast N65.1
    excess tissue N65.0
    misshappen N65.0
  reimplant NEC —*see also* Complications, prosthetic device or implant
    limb (infection) (rejection) —*see* Complications, reattached, extremity
    organ (partial) (total) —*see* Complications, transplant
    prosthetic device NEC —*see* Complications, prosthetic device
  renal N28.9
    allograft —*see* Complications, transplant, kidney
    dialysis —*see* Complications, dialysis
  respirator
    mechanical J95.850
    specified NEC J95.859
  respiratory system J98.9
    device, implant or graft —*see* Complication, prosthetic device or implant, specified NEC
    lung transplant —*see* Complications, prosthetic device or implant, lung transplant
    postoperative J95.89
      air leak J95.812
      Mendelson's syndrome (chemical pneumonitis) J95.4
      pneumothorax J95.811
      pulmonary insufficiency (acute) (after nonthoracic surgery) J95.2
        chronic J95.3
        following thoracic surgery J95.1
      respiratory failure (acute) J95.821
        acute and chronic J95.822
      specified NEC J95.89
      subglottic stenosis J95.5
      tracheostomy complication —*see* Complications, tracheostomy
    therapy T81.89
  sedation during labor and delivery O74.9
    cardiac O74.2
    central nervous system O74.3
    pulmonary NEC O74.1

Complication (*continued*)
  sedation during labor and delivery (*continued*)
  shunt —*see also* Complications, prosthetic device or implant
    arteriovenous —*see* Complications, arteriovenous, shunt
    ventricular (communicating) —*see* Complications, ventricular shunt
  skin
    graft T86.829
      failure T86.821
      infection T86.822
      rejection T86.820
      specified type NEC T86.828
  spinal
    anesthesia —*see* Complications, anesthesia, spinal
    catheter (epidural) (subdural) —*see* Complications, catheter
    puncture or tap G97.1
      cerebrospinal fluid leak G97.0
      headache or reaction G97.1
  stent
    bile duct —*see* Complications, bile duct prosthesis
    ureteral indwelling
      breakdown T83.112
      displacement T83.122
      leakage T83.192
      malposition T83.122
      obstruction T83.192
      perforation T83.192
      protrusion T83.192
      specified NEC T83.192
    urinary NEC (ileal conduit) (nephroureteral) T83.193
      embolism T83.81
      fibrosis T83.82
      hemorrhage T83.83
      infection and inflammation T83.593
      mechanical
        breakdown T83.113
        displacement T83.123
        leakage T83.193
        malposition T83.123
        obstruction T83.193
        perforation T83.193
        protrusion T83.193
        specified NEC T83.193
      pain T83.84
      specified type NEC T83.89
      stenosis T83.85
      thrombosis T83.86
    vascular
      end stent stenosis —*see* Restenosis, stent
      in stent stenosis —*see* Restenosis, stent
  stoma
    digestive tract
      colostomy —*see* Complications, colostomy
      enterostomy —*see* Complications, enterostomy
      esophagostomy —*see* Complications, esophagostomy
      gastrostomy —*see* Complications, gastrostomy
    urinary tract N99.528
      continent N99.538
        hemorrhage N99.530
        herniation N99.533
        infection N99.531
        malfunction N99.532
        specified type NEC N99.538

Complication (continued)
   stoma (continued)
      urinary tract (continued)
         continent (continued)
            stenosis N99.534
            cystostomy —see
               Complications, cystostomy
            external NOS N99.528
            hemorrhage N99.520
            herniation N99.523
            incontinent N99.528
               hemorrhage N99.520
               herniation N99.523
               infection N99.521
               malfunction N99.522
               specified type NEC N99.528
               stenosis N99.524
            infection N99.521
            malfunction N99.522
            specified type NEC N99.528
            stenosis N99.524
   stomach banding —see
      Complication(s), bariatric procedure
   stomach stapling —see
      Complication(s), bariatric procedure
   surgical material, nonabsorbable
      —see Complication, suture, permanent
   surgical procedure (on) T81.9
      amputation stump (late) —see
         Complications, amputation stump
      cardiac —see Complications, circulatory system
      cholesteatoma, recurrent
         —see Complications, postmastoidectomy, recurrent cholesteatoma
      circulatory (early) —see
         Complications, circulatory system
      digestive system —see
         Complications, gastrointestinal
      dumping syndrome (postgastrectomy) K91.1
      ear —see Complications, ear
      elephantiasis or lymphedema I97.89
         postmastectomy I97.2
      emphysema (surgical) T81.82
      endocrine —see Complications, endocrine
      eye —see Complications, eye
      fistula (persistent postoperative) T81.83
      foreign body inadvertently left in wound (sponge) (suture) (swab) —see Foreign body, accidentally left during a procedure
      gastrointestinal —see
         Complications, gastrointestinal
      genitourinary NEC N99.89
      hematoma
         intraoperative —see
            Complication, intraoperative, hemorrhage
         postprocedural —
            see Complication, postprocedural, hematoma
      hemorrhage
         intraoperative —see
            Complication, intraoperative, hemorrhage

Complication (continued)
   surgical procedure (continued)
      hemorrhage (continued)
         postprocedural —
            see Complication, postprocedural, hemorrhage
      hepatic failure K91.82
      hyperglycemia (postpancreatectomy) E89.1
      hypoinsulinemia (postpancreatectomy) E89.1
      hypoparathyroidism (postparathyroidectomy) E89.2
      hypopituitarism (posthypophysectomy) E89.3
      hypothyroidism (post-thyroidectomy) E89.0
      intestinal obstruction (see also Obstruction, intestine, postoperative) K91.30
      intracranial hypotension following ventricular shunting (ventriculostomy) G97.2
      lymphedema I97.89
         postmastectomy I97.2
      malabsorption (postsurgical) NEC K91.2
         osteoporosis —see
            Osteoporosis, postsurgical malabsorption
      mastoidectomy cavity NEC
         —see Complications, postmastoidectomy
      metabolic E89.89
         specified NEC E89.89
      musculoskeletal —see
         Complications, musculoskeletal system
      nervous system (central) (peripheral) —see
         Complications, nervous system
      ovarian failure E89.40
         asymptomatic E89.40
         symptomatic E89.41
      peripheral vascular —see
         Complications, surgical procedure, vascular
      postcardiotomy syndrome I97.0
      postcholecystectomy syndrome K91.5
      postcommissurotomy syndrome I97.0
      postgastrectomy dumping syndrome K91.1
      postlaminectomy syndrome NEC M96.1
         kyphosis M96.3
      postmastectomy lymphedema syndrome I97.2
      postmastoidectomy
         cholesteatoma —see
            Complications, postmastoidectomy, recurrent cholesteatoma
      postvagotomy syndrome K91.1
      postvalvulotomy syndrome I97.0
      pulmonary insufficiency (acute) J95.2
         chronic J95.3
         following thoracic surgery J95.1
      reattached body part —see
         Complications, reattached
      respiratory —see Complications, respiratory system
      shock (hypovolemic) T81.19
      spleen (postoperative) D78.89
         intraoperative D78.81

Complication (continued)
   surgical procedure (continued)
      stitch abscess T81.41
      subglottic stenosis (postsurgical) J95.5
      testicular hypofunction E89.5
      transplant —see Complications, organ or tissue transplant
      urinary NEC N99.89
      vaginal vault prolapse (posthysterectomy) N99.3
      vascular (peripheral)
         artery T81.719
            mesenteric T81.710
            renal T81.711
            specified NEC T81.718
         vein T81.72
      wound infection T81.49
   suture, permanent (wire) NEC T85.9
      with repair of bone —see
         Complications, fixation device, internal
      embolism T85.818
      fibrosis T85.828
      hemorrhage T85.838
      infection and inflammation T85.79
      mechanical
         breakdown T85.612
         displacement T85.622
         malfunction T85.612
         malposition T85.622
         obstruction T85.692
         perforation T85.692
         protrusion T85.692
         specified NEC T85.692
      pain T85.848
      specified type NEC T85.898
      stenosis T85.858
      thrombosis T85.868
   tracheostomy J95.00
      granuloma J95.09
      hemorrhage J95.01
      infection J95.02
      malfunction J95.03
      mechanical J95.03
      obstruction J95.03
      specified type NEC J95.09
      tracheo-esophageal fistula J95.04
   transfusion (blood) (lymphocytes) (plasma) T80.92
      air embolism T80.0
      circulatory overload E87.71
      febrile nonhemolytic transfusion reaction R50.84
      hemolysis T80.89
      hemochromatosis E83.111
      hemolytic reaction (antigen unspecified) T80.919
      incompatibility reaction (antigen unspecified) T80.919
         ABO T80.30
            delayed serologic (DSTR) T80.39
            hemolytic transfusion reaction (HTR) (unspecified time after transfusion) T80.319
               acute (AHTR) (less than 24 hours after transfusion) T80.310
               delayed (DHTR) (24 hours or more after transfusion) T80.311
            specified NEC T80.39
         acute (antigen unspecified) T80.910
         delayed (antigen unspecified) T80.911

Complication (continued)
   transfusion (continued)
      incompatibility reaction (continued)
         delayed serologic (DSTR) T80.89
         Non-ABO (minor antigens (Duffy) (K) (Kell) (Kidd) (Lewis) (M) (N) (P) (S)) T80.A0
            delayed serologic (DSTR) T80.A9
            hemolytic transfusion reaction (HTR) (unspecified time after transfusion) T80.A19
               acute (AHTR) (less than 24 hours after transfusion) T80.A10
               delayed (DHTR) (24 hours or more after transfusion) T80.A11
            specified NEC T80.A9
         Rh (antigens (C) (c) (D) (E) (e)) (factor) T80.40
            delayed serologic (DSTR) T80.49
            hemolytic transfusion reaction (HTR) (unspecified time after transfusion) T80.419
            hemolytic transfusion acute (AHTR) (less than 24 hours after transfusion) T80.410
               delayed (DHTR) (24 hours or more after transfusion) T80.411
            specified NEC T80.49
      infection T80.29
         acute T80.22
      reaction NEC T80.89
      sepsis T80.29
      shock T80.89
   transplant T86.90
      bone T86.839
         failure T86.831
         infection T86.832
         rejection T86.830
         specified type NEC T86.838
      bone marrow T86.00
         failure T86.02
         infection T86.03
         rejection T86.01
         specified type NEC T86.09
      cornea T86.849-
         failure T86.841-
         infection T86.842-
         rejection T86.840-
         specified type NEC T86.848-
      failure T86.92
      heart T86.20
         with lung T86.30
         cardiac allograft vasculopathy T86.290
         failure T86.32
         infection T86.33
         rejection T86.31
         specified type NEC T86.39
      failure T86.22
      infection T86.23
      rejection T86.21
      specified type NEC T86.298
   infection T86.93
   intestine T86.859
      failure T86.851
      infection T86.852
      rejection T86.850
      specified type NEC T86.858

71

Complication (continued)
 transplant (continued)
  kidney T86.10
   failure T86.12
   infection T86.13
   rejection T86.11
   specified type NEC T86.19
  liver T86.40
   failure T86.42
   infection T86.43
   rejection T86.41
   specified type NEC T86.49
  lung T86.819
   with heart T86.30
    failure T86.32
    infection T86.33
    rejection T86.31
    specified type NEC T86.39
   failure T86.811
   infection T86.812
   rejection T86.810
   specified type NEC T86.818
  malignant neoplasm C80.2
  pancreas T86.899
   failure T86.891
   infection T86.892
   rejection T86.890
   specified type NEC T86.898
  peripheral blood stem cells T86.5
  post-transplant lymphoproliferative disorder (PTLD) D47.Z1
  rejection T86.91
  skin T86.829
   failure T86.821
   infection T86.822
   rejection T86.820
   specified type NEC T86.828
  specified
   tissue T86.899
    failure T86.891
    infection T86.892
    rejection T86.890
    specified type NEC T86.898
   type NEC T86.99
  stem cell (from peripheral blood) (from umbilical cord) T86.5
  umbilical cord stem cells T86.5
 trauma (early) T79.9
  specified NEC T79.8
 ultrasound therapy NEC T88.9
 umbilical cord NEC
  complicating delivery O69.9
   specified NEC O69.89
 umbrella device, vascular T82.9
  embolism T82.818
  fibrosis T82.828
  hemorrhage T82.838
  infection or inflammation T82.7
  mechanical
   breakdown T82.515
   displacement T82.525
   leakage T82.535
   malposition T82.525
   obstruction T82.595
   perforation T82.595
   protrusion T82.595
  pain T82.848
  specified type NEC T82.898
  stenosis T82.858
  thrombosis T82.868
 urethral catheter —see Complications, catheter, urethral, indwelling
 vaccination T88.1
  anaphylaxis NEC T80.52
  arthropathy —see Arthropathy, postimmunization

Complication (continued)
 vaccination (continued)
  cellulitis T88.0
  encephalitis or encephalomyelitis G04.02
  infection (general) (local) NEC T88.0
  meningitis G03.8
  myelitis G04.02
  protein sickness T80.62
  rash T88.1
  reaction (allergic) T88.1
   serum T80.62
  sepsis T88.0
  serum intoxication, sickness, rash, or other serum reaction NEC T80.62
   anaphylactic shock T80.52
  shock (allergic) (anaphylactic) T80.52
  vaccinia (generalized) (localized) T88.1
 vas deferens device or implant —see Complications, genitourinary, device or implant, genital tract
 vascular I99.9
  device or implant T82.9
   embolism T82.818
   fibrosis T82.828
   hemorrhage T82.838
   infection or inflammation T82.7
   mechanical
    breakdown T82.519
     specified device NEC T82.518
    displacement T82.529
     specified device NEC T82.528
    leakage T82.539
     specified device NEC T82.538
    malposition T82.529
     specified device NEC T82.528
    obstruction T82.599
     specified device NEC T82.598
    perforation T82.599
     specified device NEC T82.598
    protrusion T82.599
     specified device NEC T82.598
   pain T82.848
   specified type NEC T82.898
   stenosis T82.858
   thrombosis T82.868
  dialysis catheter —see Complication, catheter, dialysis
  following infusion, therapeutic injection or transfusion T80.1
  graft T82.9
   embolism T82.818
   fibrosis T82.828
   hemorrhage T82.838
   mechanical
    breakdown T82.319
     aorta (bifurcation) T82.310
     carotid artery T82.311
     specified vessel NEC T82.318
    displacement T82.329
     aorta (bifurcation) T82.320
     carotid artery T82.321
     specified vessel NEC T82.328

Complication (continued)
 vascular (continued)
  graft (continued)
   mechanical (continued)
    leakage T82.339
     aorta (bifurcation) T82.330
     carotid artery T82.331
     femoral artery T82.332
     specified vessel NEC T82.338
    malposition T82.329
     aorta (bifurcation) T82.320
     carotid artery T82.321
     specified vessel NEC T82.328
    obstruction T82.399
     aorta (bifurcation) T82.390
     carotid artery T82.391
     specified vessel NEC T82.398
    perforation T82.399
     aorta (bifurcation) T82.390
     carotid artery T82.391
     specified vessel NEC T82.398
    protrusion T82.399
     aorta (bifurcation) T82.390
     carotid artery T82.391
     specified vessel NEC T82.398
   pain T82.848
   specified complication NEC T82.898
   stenosis T82.858
   thrombosis T82.868
  postoperative —see Complications, postoperative, circulatory
 vena cava device (filter) (sieve) (umbrella) —see Complications, umbrella device, vascular
 ventilation therapy NEC T81.81
 ventilator
  mechanical J95.850
   specified NEC J95.859
 ventricular (communicating) shunt (device) T85.9
  embolism T85.810
  fibrosis T85.820
  hemorrhage T85.830
  infection and inflammation T85.730
  mechanical
   breakdown T85.01
   displacement T85.02
   leakage T85.03
   malposition T85.02
   obstruction T85.09
   perforation T85.09
   protrusion T85.09
   specified NEC T85.09
  pain T85.840
  specified type NEC T85.890
  stenosis T85.850
  thrombosis T85.860
 wire suture, permanent (implanted) —see Complications, suture, permanent

Compressed air disease T70.3
Compression
 with injury - code by Nature of injury
 artery I77.1
  celiac, syndrome I77.4
 brachial plexus G54.0

Compression (continued)
 brain (stem) G93.5
  due to
   contusion (diffuse) (see also Injury, intracranial, diffuse) S06.A0
    with herniation S06.A1
    focal (see also Injury, intracranial, focal) S06.A0
     with herniation S06.A1
   injury NEC (see also Injury, intracranial, diffuse) S06.A0
  nontraumatic G93.5
  traumatic (see also Injury, intracranial, diffuse) S06.A0
   with herniation S06.A1
 bronchus J98.09
 cauda equina G83.4
 celiac (artery) (axis) I77.4
 cerebral —see Compression, brain
 cervical plexus G54.2
 cord
  spinal —see Compression, spinal
  umbilical —see Compression, umbilical cord
 cranial nerve G52.9
  eighth H93.3
  eleventh G52.8
  fifth G50.8
  first G52.0
  fourth —see Strabismus, paralytic, fourth nerve
  ninth G52.1
  second —see Disorder, nerve, optic
  seventh G51.8
  sixth —see Strabismus, paralytic, sixth nerve
  tenth G52.2
  third —see Strabismus, paralytic, third nerve
  twelfth G52.3
 diver's squeeze T70.3
 during birth (newborn) P15.9
 esophagus K22.2
 eustachian tube —see Obstruction, eustachian tube, cartilagenous
 facies Q67.1
 fracture
  nontraumatic NOS —see Collapse, vertebra
  pathological —see Fracture, pathological
  traumatic —see Fracture, traumatic
 heart —see Disease, heart
 intestine —see Obstruction, intestine
 laryngeal nerve, recurrent G52.2
  with paralysis of vocal cords and larynx J38.00
   bilateral J38.02
   unilateral J38.01
 lumbosacral plexus G54.1
 lung J98.4
 lymphatic vessel I89.0
 medulla —see Compression, brain
 nerve (see also Disorder, nerve) G58.9
  arm NEC —see Mononeuropathy, upper limb
  axillary G54.0
  cranial —see Compression, cranial nerve
  leg NEC —see Mononeuropathy, lower limb

Compression (continued)
nerve (continued)
median (in carpal tunnel) —see Syndrome, carpal tunnel
optic —see Disorder, nerve, optic
plantar —see Lesion, nerve, plantar
posterior tibial (in tarsal tunnel) —see Syndrome, tarsal tunnel
root or plexus NOS (in) G54.9
intervertebral disc disorder NEC —see Disorder, disc, with, radiculopathy
with myelopathy —see Disorder, disc, with, myelopathy
neoplastic disease —see also Neoplasm D49.9 [G55]
spondylosis —see Spondylosis, with radiculopathy
sciatic (acute) —see Lesion, nerve, sciatic
sympathetic G90.8
traumatic —see Injury, nerve
ulnar —see Lesion, nerve, ulnar
upper extremity NEC —see Mononeuropathy, upper limb
spinal (cord) G95.20
by displacement of intervertebral disc NEC —see also Disorder, disc, with, myelopathy
nerve root NOS G54.9
due to displacement of intervertebral disc NEC —see Disorder, disc, with, radiculopathy
with myelopathy —see Disorder, disc, with, myelopathy
specified NEC G95.29
spondylogenic (cervical) (lumbar, lumbosacral) (thoracic) —see Spondylosis, with myelopathy NEC
anterior —see Syndrome, anterior, spinal artery, compression
traumatic —see Injury, spinal cord, by region
subcostal nerve (syndrome) —see Mononeuropathy, upper limb, specified NEC
sympathetic nerve NEC G90.8
syndrome T79.5
trachea J39.8
ulnar nerve (by scar tissue) —see Lesion, nerve, ulnar
umbilical cord
complicating delivery O69.2
cord around neck O69.1
prolapse O69.0
specified NEC O69.2
ureter N13.5
vein I87.1
vena cava (inferior) (superior) I87.1

Compulsion, compulsive
gambling F63.0
neurosis F42.8
personality F60.5
states F42.8
swearing F42.8
in Gilles de la Tourette's syndrome F95.2
tics and spasms F95.9

Concato's disease (pericardial polyserositis) A19.9
nontubercular I31.1

Concato's disease (continued)
pleural —see Pleurisy, with effusion
Concavity chest wall M95.4
Concealed penis Q55.64
Concern (normal) about sick person in family Z63.6
Concrescence (teeth) K00.2
Concretio cordis I31.1
rheumatic I09.2
Concretion —see also Calculus
appendicular K38.1
canaliculus —see Dacryolith
clitoris N90.89
conjunctiva H11.12-
eyelid —see Disorder, eyelid, specified type NEC
lacrimal passages —see Dacryolith
prepuce (male) N47.8
salivary gland (any) K11.5
seminal vesicle N50.89
tonsil J35.8
Concussion (brain) (cerebral) (current) S06.0X9
with
loss of consciousness
30 minutes or less S06.0X1
brief S06.0X1
status unknown S06.0XA
unspecified duration S06.0X9
no loss of consciousness S06.0X0
blast (air) (hydraulic) (immersion) (underwater)
abdomen or thorax —see Injury, blast, by site
ear with acoustic nerve injury —see Injury, nerve, acoustic, specified type NEC
cauda equina S34.3
conus medullaris S34.02
ocular S05.8X-
spinal (cord)
cervical S14.0
lumbar S34.01
sacral S34.02
thoracic S24.0
syndrome F07.81
without loss of consciousness S06.0X0
Condition —see also Disease
post COVID-19 U09.9
Conditions arising in the perinatal period —see Newborn, affected by
Conduct disorder —see Disorder, conduct
Condyloma A63.0
acuminatum A63.0
gonorrheal A54.09
latum A51.31
syphilitic A51.31
congenital A50.07
venereal, syphilitic A51.31
Conflagration —see also Burn
asphyxia (by inhalation of gases, fumes or vapors) (see also Table of Drugs and Chemicals) T59.9-
Conflict (with) —see also Discord
family Z73.9
grandparent-child Z62.831
group home staff-child Z62.833
kinship-care child Z62.831
marital Z63.0
involving divorce or estrangement Z63.5
non-parental relative legal guardian-child Z62.831
non-parental relative-child Z62.831

Conflict (continued)
non-relative guardian-child Z62.832
other relative-child Z62.831
parent-child Z62.820
parent-adopted child Z62.821
parent-biological child Z62.820
parent-foster child Z62.822
parent-step child Z62.823
social role NEC Z73.5
Confluent —see condition
Confusion, confused R41.0
epileptic F05
mental state (psychogenic) F44.89
psychogenic F44.89
reactive (from emotional stress, psychological trauma) F44.89
Confusional arousals G47.51
Congelation T69.9
Congenital —see also condition
aortic septum Q25.49
intrinsic factor deficiency D51.0
malformation —see Anomaly
Congestion, congestive
bladder N32.89
bowel K63.89
brain G93.89
breast N64.59
bronchial J98.09
catarrhal J31.0
chest R09.89
chill, malarial —see Malaria
circulatory NEC I99.8
duodenum K31.89
eye —see Hyperemia, conjunctiva
facial, due to birth injury P15.4
general R68.89
glottis J37.0
heart —see Failure, heart, congestive
hepatic K76.1
hypostatic (lung) —see Edema, lung
intestine K63.89
kidney N28.89
labyrinth —see subcategory H83.8
larynx J37.0
liver K76.1
lung R09.89
active or acute —see Pneumonia
malaria, malarial —see Malaria
nasal R09.81
nose R09.81
orbit, orbital —see also Exophthalmos
inflammatory (chronic) —see Inflammation, orbit
ovary N83.8
pancreas K86.89
pelvic, female N94.89
pleural J94.8
prostate (active) N42.1
pulmonary —see Congestion, lung
renal N28.89
retina H35.81
seminal vesicle N50.1
spinal cord G95.19
spleen (chronic) D73.2
stomach K31.89
trachea —see Tracheitis
urethra N36.8
uterus N85.8
with subinvolution N85.3
venous (passive) I87.8
viscera R68.89
Congestive —see Congestion
Conical
cervix (hypertrophic elongation) N88.4
cornea —see Keratoconus
teeth K00.2

Conjoined twins Q89.4
Conjugal maladjustment Z63.0
involving divorce or estrangement Z63.5
Conjunctiva —see condition
Conjunctivitis (staphylococcal) (streptococcal) NOS H10.9
Acanthamoeba B60.12
acute H10.3-
atopic H10.1-
mucopurulent H10.02-
follicular H10.01-
chemical (see also Corrosion, cornea) H10.21-
pseudomembranous H10.22-
serous except viral H10.23-
viral —see Conjunctivitis, viral
toxic H10.21-
adenoviral (acute) (follicular) B30.1
allergic (acute) —see Conjunctivitis, acute, atopic
chronic H10.45
vernal H10.44
anaphylactic —see Conjunctivitis, acute, atopic
Apollo B30.3
atopic (acute) —see Conjunctivitis, acute, atopic
Béal's B30.2
blennorrhagic (gonococcal) (neonatorum) A54.31
chemical (acute) (see also Corrosion, cornea) H10.21-
chlamydial A74.0
due to trachoma A71.1
neonatal P39.1
chronic (nodosa) (petrificans) (phlyctenular) H10.40-
allergic H10.45
vernal H10.44
follicular H10.43-
giant papillary H10.41-
simple H10.42-
vernal H10.44
coxsackievirus 24 B30.3
diphtheritic A36.86
due to
dust —see Conjunctivitis, acute, atopic
filariasis B74.9
mucocutaneous leishmaniasis B55.2
enterovirus type 70 (hemorrhagic) B30.3
epidemic (viral) B30.9
hemorrhagic B30.3
gonococcal (neonatorum) A54.31
granular (trachomatous) A71.1
sequelae (late effect) B94.0
hemorrhagic (acute) (epidemic) B30.3
herpes zoster B02.31
in (due to)
Acanthamoeba B60.12
adenovirus (acute) (follicular) B30.1
Chlamydia A74.0
coxsackievirus 24 B30.3
diphtheria A36.86
enterovirus type 70 (hemorrhagic) B30.3
filariasis B74.9
gonococci A54.31
herpes (simplex) virus B00.53
zoster B02.31
infectious disease NEC B99
meningococci A39.89
mucocutaneous leishmaniasis B55.2
rosacea H10.82-

Conjunctivitis (continued)
in (continued)
syphilis (late) A52.71
zoster B02.31
inclusion A74.0
infantile P39.1
gonococcal A54.31
Koch-Weeks' —see Conjunctivitis, acute, mucopurulent
light —see Conjunctivitis, acute, atopic
ligneous —see Blepharoconjunctivitis, ligneous
meningococcal A39.89
mucopurulent —see Conjunctivitis, acute, mucopurulent
neonatal P39.1
gonococcal A54.31
Newcastle B30.8
of Béal B30.2
parasitic
filariasis B74.9
mucocutaneous leishmaniasis B55.2
Parinaud's H10.89
petrificans H10.89
rosacea H10.82-
specified NEC H10.89
swimming-pool B30.1
trachomatous A71.1
acute A71.0
sequelae (late effect) B94.0
traumatic NEC H10.89
tuberculous A18.59
tularemic A21.1
tularensis A21.1
viral B30.9
due to
adenovirus B30.1
enterovirus B30.3
specified NEC B30.8

Conjunctivochalasis H11.82-

Connective tissue —see condition

Conn's syndrome E26.01

Conradi (-Hunermann) **disease** Q77.3

Consanguinity Z84.3
counseling Z71.89

Conscious simulation (of illness) Z76.5

Consecutive —see condition

Consolidation lung (base) —see Pneumonia, lobar

Constipation (atonic) (neurogenic) (simple) (spastic) K59.00
chronic K59.09
idiopathic K59.04
drug-induced K59.03
functional K59.04
outlet dysfunction K59.02
psychogenic F45.8
slow transit K59.01
specified NEC K59.09

Constitutional —see also condition
substandard F60.7

Constitutionally substandard F60.7

Constriction —see also Stricture
auditory canal —see Stenosis, external ear canal
bronchial J98.09
duodenum K31.5
esophagus K22.2
external
abdomen, abdominal (wall) S30.841
alveolar process S00.542
ankle S90.54-
antecubital space —see Constriction, external, forearm

Constriction (continued)
external (continued)
arm (upper) S40.84-
auricle —see Constriction, external, ear
axilla —see Constriction, external, arm
back, lower S30.840
breast S20.14-
brow S00.84
buttock S30.840
calf —see Constriction, external, leg
canthus —see Constriction, external, eyelid
cheek S00.84
internal S00.542
chest wall —see Constriction, external, thorax
chin S00.84
clitoris S30.844
costal region —see Constriction, external, thorax
digit(s)
foot —see Constriction, external, toe
hand —see Constriction, external, finger
ear S00.44-
elbow S50.34-
epididymis S30.843
epigastric region S30.841
esophagus, cervical S10.14
eyebrow —see Constriction, external, eyelid
eyelid S00.24-
face S00.84
finger(s) S60.44-
index S60.44-
little S60.44-
middle S60.44-
ring S60.44-
flank S30.841
foot (except toe(s) alone) S90.84-
toe —see Constriction, external, toe
forearm S50.84-
elbow only —see Constriction, external, elbow
forehead S00.84
genital organs, external
female S30.846
male S30.845
groin S30.841
gum S00.542
hand S60.54-
head S00.94
ear —see Constriction, external, ear
eyelid —see Constriction, external, eyelid
lip S00.541
nose S00.34
oral cavity S00.542
scalp S00.04
specified site NEC S00.84
heel —see Constriction, external, foot
hip S70.24-
inguinal region S30.841
interscapular region S20.449
jaw S00.84
knee S80.24-
labium (majus) (minus) S30.844
larynx S10.14
leg (lower) S80.84-
knee —see Constriction, external, knee
upper —see Constriction, external, thigh

Constriction (continued)
external (continued)
lip S00.541
lower back S30.840
lumbar region S30.840
malar region S00.84
mammary —see Constriction, external, breast
mastoid region S00.84
mouth S00.542
nail
finger —see Constriction, external, finger
toe —see Constriction, external, toe
nasal S00.34
neck S10.94
specified site NEC S10.84
throat S10.14
nose S00.34
occipital region S00.04
oral cavity S00.542
orbital region —see Constriction, external, eyelid
palate S00.542
palm —see Constriction, external, hand
parietal region S00.04
pelvis S30.840
penis S30.842
perineum
female S30.844
male S30.840
periocular area —see Constriction, external, eyelid
phalanges
finger —see Constriction, external, finger
toe —see Constriction, external, toe
pharynx S10.14
pinna —see Constriction, external, ear
popliteal space —see Constriction, external, knee
prepuce S30.842
pubic region S30.840
pudendum
female S30.846
male S30.845
sacral region S30.840
scalp S00.04
scapular region —see Constriction, external, shoulder
scrotum S30.843
shin —see Constriction, external, leg
shoulder S40.24-
sternal region S20.349
submaxillary region S00.84
submental region S00.84
subungual
finger(s) —see Constriction, external, finger
toe(s) —see Constriction, external, toe
supraclavicular fossa S10.84
supraorbital S00.84
temple S00.84
temporal region S00.84
testis S30.843
thigh S70.34-
thorax, thoracic (wall) S20.94
back S20.44-
front S20.34-
throat S10.14
thumb S60.34-
toe(s) (lesser) S90.44-
great S90.44-
tongue S00.542

Constriction (continued)
external (continued)
trachea S10.14
tunica vaginalis S30.843
uvula S00.542
vagina S30.844
vulva S30.844
wrist S60.84-
gallbladder —see Obstruction, gallbladder
intestine —see Obstruction, intestine
larynx J38.6
congenital Q31.8
specified NEC Q31.8
subglottic Q31.1
organ or site, congenital NEC —see Atresia, by site
prepuce (acquired) (congenital) N47.1
pylorus (adult hypertrophic) K31.1
congenital or infantile Q40.0
newborn Q40.0
ring dystocia (uterus) O62.4
spastic —see also Spasm
ureter N13.5
ureter N13.5
with infection N13.6
urethra —see Stricture, urethra
visual field (peripheral) (functional) —see Defect, visual field

Constrictive —see condition

Consultation
medical —see Counseling, medical
religious Z71.81
specified reason NEC Z71.89
spiritual Z71.81
without complaint or sickness Z71.9
feared complaint unfounded Z71.1
specified reason NEC Z71.89

Consumption —see Tuberculosis

Contact (with) —see also Exposure (to)
acariasis Z20.7
AIDS virus Z20.6
air pollution Z77.110
algae and algae toxins Z77.121
algae bloom Z77.121
anthrax Z20.810
aromatic amines Z77.020
aromatic (hazardous) compounds NEC Z77.028
aromatic dyes NOS Z77.028
arsenic Z77.010
asbestos Z77.090
bacterial disease NEC Z20.818
benzene Z77.021
blue-green algae bloom Z77.121
body fluids (potentially hazardous) Z77.21
brown tide Z77.121
chemicals (chiefly nonmedicinal) (hazardous) NEC Z77.098
cholera Z20.09
chromium compounds Z77.018
communicable disease Z20.9
bacterial NEC Z20.818
specified NEC Z20.89
viral NEC Z20.828
Zika virus Z20.821
coronavirus (disease) (novel) 2019 Z20.822
COVID-19 Z20.822
cyanobacteria bloom Z77.121
dyes Z77.098
Escherichia coli (E. coli) Z20.01
fiberglass —see Table of Drugs and Chemicals, fiberglass
German measles Z20.4
gonorrhea Z20.2
hazardous metals NEC Z77.018

Contact (continued)
  hazardous substances NEC Z77.29
  hazards in the physical environment NEC Z77.128
  hazards to health NEC Z77.9
  HIV Z20.6
  HTLV-III/LAV Z20.6
  human immunodeficiency virus (HIV) Z20.6
  infection Z20.9
    specified NEC Z20.89
  infestation (parasitic) NEC Z20.7
  intestinal infectious disease NEC Z20.09
    Escherichia coli (E. coli) Z20.01
  lead Z77.011
  meningococcus Z20.811
  mold (toxic) Z77.120
  nickel dust Z77.018
  noise Z77.122
  parasitic disease Z20.7
  pediculosis Z20.7
  pfiesteria piscicida Z77.121
  poliomyelitis Z20.89
  pollution
    air Z77.110
    environmental NEC Z77.118
    soil Z77.112
    water Z77.111
  polycyclic aromatic hydrocarbons Z77.028
  positive maternal group B streptococcus P00.82
  rabies Z20.3
  radiation, naturally occurring NEC Z77.123
  radon Z77.123
  red tide (Florida) Z77.121
  rubella Z20.4
  SARS-CoV-2 Z20.822
  sexually-transmitted disease Z20.2
  smallpox (laboratory) Z20.89
  syphilis Z20.2
  tuberculosis Z20.1
  uranium Z77.012
  varicella Z20.820
  venereal disease Z20.2
  viral disease NEC Z20.828
  viral hepatitis Z20.5
  water pollution Z77.111
  Zika virus Z20.821
Contamination, food —see Intoxication, foodborne
Contraception, contraceptive
  advice Z30.09
  counseling Z30.09
  device (intrauterine) (in situ) Z97.5
    causing menorrhagia T83.83
    checking Z30.431
    complications —see Complications, intrauterine, contraceptive device
    in place Z97.5
    initial prescription Z30.014
    reinsertion Z30.433
    removal Z30.432
    replacement Z30.433
  emergency (postcoital) Z30.012
  initial prescription Z30.019
    barrier Z30.018
    diaphragm Z30.018
    injectable Z30.013
    intrauterine device Z30.014
    pills Z30.011
    postcoital (emergency) Z30.012
    specified type NEC Z30.018
    subdermal implantable Z30.017
    transdermal patch hormonal Z30.016
    vaginal ring hormonal Z30.015

Contraception, contraceptive (continued)
  maintenance Z30.40
    barrier Z30.49
    diaphragm Z30.49
    examination Z30.8
    injectable Z30.42
    intrauterine device Z30.431
    pills Z30.41
    specified type NEC Z30.49
    subdermal implantable Z30.46
    transdermal patch hormonal Z30.45
    vaginal ring hormonal Z30.44
  management Z30.9
    specified NEC Z30.8
  postcoital (emergency) Z30.012
  prescription Z30.019
    repeat Z30.40
  sterilization Z30.2
  surveillance (drug) —see Contraception, maintenance

Contraction(s), contracture, contracted
  Achilles tendon —see also Short, tendon, Achilles
    congenital Q66.89
  amputation stump (surgical) (flexion) (late) (next proximal joint) T87.89
  anus K59.89
  bile duct (common) (hepatic) K83.8
  bladder N32.89
    neck or sphincter N32.0
  bowel, cecum, colon or intestine, any part —see Obstruction, intestine
  Braxton Hicks —see False, labor
  breast implant, capsular T85.44
  bronchial J98.09
  burn (old) —see Cicatrix
  cervix —see Stricture, cervix
  cicatricial —see Cicatrix
  conjunctiva, trachomatous, active A71.1
    sequelae (late effect) B94.0
  Dupuytren's M72.0
  eyelid —see Disorder, eyelid function
  fascia (lata) (postural) M72.8
    Dupuytren's M72.0
    palmar M72.0
    plantar M72.2
  finger NEC —see also Deformity, finger
    congenital Q68.1
    joint —see Contraction, joint, hand
  flaccid —see Contraction, paralytic
  gallbladder K82.0
  heart valve —see Endocarditis
  hip —see Contraction, joint, hip
  hourglass
    bladder N32.89
      congenital Q64.79
    gallbladder K82.0
      congenital Q44.1
    stomach K31.89
      congenital Q40.2
      psychogenic F45.8
    uterus (complicating delivery) O62.4
  hysterical F44.4
  internal os —see Stricture, cervix
  joint (abduction) (acquired) (adduction) (flexion) (rotation) M24.50
    ankle M24.57-
      congenital NEC Q68.8
      hip Q65.89

Contraction(s), contracture, contracted (continued)
  joint (continued)
    elbow M24.52-
    foot joint M24.57-
    hand joint M24.54-
    hip M24.55-
      congenital Q65.89
    hysterical F44.4
    knee M24.56-
    shoulder M24.51-
    specified site NEC M24.59
    wrist M24.53-
  kidney (granular) (secondary) N26.9
    congenital Q63.8
    hydronephritic —see Hydronephrosis
    Page N26.2
    pyelonephritic —see Pyelitis, chronic
    tuberculous A18.11
  ligament —see also Disorder, ligament
    congenital Q79.8
  muscle (postinfective) (postural) NEC M62.40
    with contracture of joint —see Contraction, joint
    ankle M62.47-
    congenital Q79.8
      sternocleidomastoid Q68.0
    extraocular —see Strabismus
    eye (extrinsic) —see Strabismus
    foot M62.47-
    forearm M62.43-
    hand M62.44-
    hysterical F44.4
    ischemic (Volkmann's) T79.6
    lower leg M62.46-
    multiple sites M62.49
    pelvic region M62.45-
    posttraumatic —see Strabismus, paralytic
    psychogenic F45.8
      conversion reaction F44.4
    shoulder region M62.41-
    specified site NEC M62.48
    thigh M62.45-
    upper arm M62.42-
  neck —see Torticollis
  ocular muscle —see Strabismus
  organ or site, congenital NEC —see Atresia, by site
  outlet (pelvis) —see Contraction, pelvis
  palmar fascia M72.0
  paralytic
    joint —see Contraction, joint
    muscle —see also Contraction, muscle NEC
      ocular —see Strabismus, paralytic
  pelvis (acquired) (general) M95.5
    with disproportion (fetopelvic) O33.1
      causing obstructed labor O65.1
    inlet O33.2
    mid-cavity O33.3
    outlet O33.3
  plantar fascia M72.2
  premature
    atrium I49.1
    auriculoventricular I49.49
    heart I49.49
    junctional I49.2
    supraventricular I49.1
    ventricular I49.3
  prostate N42.89

Contraction(s), contracture, contracted (continued)
  pylorus NEC —see also Pylorospasm
    psychogenic F45.8
  rectum, rectal (sphincter) K59.89
  ring (Bandl's) (complicating delivery) O62.4
  scar —see Cicatrix
  spine —see Dorsopathy, deforming
  sternocleidomastoid (muscle), congenital Q68.0
  stomach K31.89
    hourglass K31.89
      congenital Q40.2
      psychogenic F45.8
    psychogenic F45.8
  tendon (sheath) M62.40
    with contracture of joint —see Contraction, joint
    Achilles —see Short, tendon, Achilles
    ankle M62.47-
      Achilles —see Short, tendon, Achilles
    foot M62.47-
    forearm M62.43-
    hand M62.44-
    lower leg M62.46-
    multiple sites M62.49
    neck M62.48
    pelvic region M62.45-
    shoulder region M62.41-
    specified site NEC M62.48
    thigh M62.45-
    thorax M62.48
    trunk M62.48
    upper arm M62.42-
  toe —see Deformity, toe, specified NEC

Contraction(s), contracture,
  ureterovesical orifice (postinfectional) N13.5
    with infection N13.6
  urethra —see also Stricture, urethra
    orifice N32.0
  uterus N85.8
    abnormal NEC O62.9
    clonic (complicating delivery) O62.4
    dyscoordinate (complicating delivery) O62.4
    hourglass (complicating delivery) O62.4
    hypertonic O62.4
    hypotonic NEC O62.2
    inadequate
      primary O62.0
      secondary O62.1
    incoordinate (complicating delivery) O62.4
    poor O62.2
    tetanic (complicating delivery) O62.4
  vagina (outlet) N89.5
  vesical N32.89
    neck or urethral orifice N32.0
  visual field —see Defect, visual field, generalized
  Volkmann's (ischemic) T79.6

Contusion (skin surface intact) T14.8
  abdomen, abdominal (muscle) (wall) S30.1
  adnexa, eye NEC S05.8X-
  adrenal gland S37.812
  alveolar process S00.532
  ankle S90.0-
  antecubital space —see Contusion, forearm
  anus S30.3

Contusion (continued)
arm (upper) S40.02-
  lower (with elbow) —see Contusion, forearm
auditory canal —see Contusion, ear
auricle —see Contusion, ear
axilla —see Contusion, arm, upper
back —see also Contusion, thorax, back
  lower S30.0
bile duct S36.13
bladder S37.22
bone NEC T14.8
brain (diffuse) —see Injury, intracranial, diffuse
  focal —see Injury, intracranial, focal
brainstem S06.38-
breast S20.0-
broad ligament S37.892
brow S00.83
buttock S30.0
canthus, eye S00.1-
cauda equina S34.3
cerebellar, traumatic S06.37-
cerebral S06.33-
  left side S06.32-
  right side S06.31-
cheek S00.83
  internal S00.532
chest (wall) —see Contusion, thorax
chin S00.83
clitoris S30.23
colon —see Injury, intestine, large, contusion
common bile duct S36.13
conjunctiva S05.1-
  with foreign body (in conjunctival sac) —see Foreign body, conjunctival sac
conus medullaris (spine) S34.139
cornea —see Contusion, eyeball
  with foreign body —see Foreign body, cornea
corpus cavernosum S30.21
cortex (brain) (cerebral) —see Injury, intracranial, diffuse
  focal —see Injury, intracranial, focal
costal region —see Contusion, thorax
cystic duct S36.13
diaphragm S27.802
duodenum S36.420
ear S00.43-
elbow S50.0-
  with forearm —see Contusion, forearm
epididymis S30.22
epigastric region S30.1
epiglottis S10.0
esophagus (thoracic) S27.812
  cervical S10.0
eyeball S05.1-
eyebrow S00.1-
eyelid (and periocular area) S00.1-
face NEC S00.83
fallopian tube S37.529
  bilateral S37.522
  unilateral S37.521
femoral triangle S30.1
finger(s) S60.00
  with damage to nail (matrix) S60.10
  index S60.02-
    with damage to nail S60.12-
  little S60.05-
    with damage to nail S60.15-
  middle S60.03-
    with damage to nail S60.13-
  ring S60.04-
    with damage to nail S60.14-
  thumb —see Contusion, thumb

Contusion (continued)
flank S30.1
foot (except toe(s) alone) S90.3-
  toe —see Contusion, toe
forearm S50.1-
  elbow only —see Contusion, elbow
forehead S00.83
gallbladder S36.122
genital organs, external
  female S30.202
  male S30.201
globe (eye) —see Contusion, eyeball
groin S30.1
gum S00.532
hand S60.22-
  finger(s) —see Contusion, finger
  wrist —see Contusion, wrist
head S00.93
  ear —see Contusion, ear
  eyelid —see Contusion, eyelid
  lip S00.531
  nose S00.33
  oral cavity S00.532
  scalp S00.03
  specified part NEC S00.83
heart (see also Injury, heart) S26.91
heel —see Contusion, foot
hepatic duct S36.13
hip S70.0-
ileum S36.428
iliac region S30.1
inguinal region S30.1
interscapular region S20.229
intra-abdominal organ S36.92
  colon —see Injury, intestine, large, contusion
  liver S36.112
  pancreas —see Contusion, pancreas
  rectum S36.62
  small intestine —see Injury, intestine, small, contusion
  specified organ NEC S36.892
  spleen —see Contusion, spleen
  stomach S36.32
iris (eye) —see Contusion, eyeball
jaw S00.83
jejunum S36.428
kidney S37.01-
  major (greater than 2 cm) S37.02-
  minor (less than 2 cm) S37.01-
knee S80.0-
labium (majus) (minus) S30.23
lacrimal apparatus, gland or sac S05.8X-
larynx S10.0
leg (lower) S80.1-
  knee —see Contusion, knee
lens —see Contusion, eyeball
lip S00.531
liver S36.112
lower back S30.0
lumbar region S30.0
lung S27.329
  bilateral S27.322
  unilateral S27.321
malar region S00.83
mastoid region S00.83
membrane, brain —see Injury, intracranial, diffuse
  focal —see Injury, intracranial, focal
mesentery S36.892
mesosalpinx S37.892
mouth S00.532
muscle —see Contusion, by site
nail
  finger —see Contusion, finger, with damage to nail
  toe —see Contusion, toe, with damage to nail

Contusion (continued)
nasal S00.33
neck S10.93
  specified site NEC S10.83
  throat S10.0
nerve —see Injury, nerve
newborn P54.5
nose S00.33
occipital
  lobe (brain) —see Injury, intracranial, diffuse
    focal —see Injury, intracranial, focal
  region (scalp) S00.03
orbit (region) (tissues) S05.1-
ovary S37.429
  bilateral S37.422
  unilateral S37.421
palate S00.532
pancreas S36.229
  body S36.221
  head S36.220
  tail S36.222
parietal
  lobe (brain) —see Injury, intracranial, diffuse
    focal —see Injury, intracranial, focal
  region (scalp) S00.03
pelvic organ S37.92
  adrenal gland S37.812
  bladder S37.22
  fallopian tube —see Contusion, fallopian tube
  kidney —see Contusion, kidney
  ovary —see Contusion, ovary
  prostate S37.822
  specified organ NEC S37.892
  ureter S37.12
  urethra S37.32
  uterus S37.62
pelvis S30.0
penis S30.21
perineum
  female S30.23
  male S30.0
periocular area S00.1-
peritoneum S36.81
periurethral tissue —see Contusion, urethra
pharynx S10.0
pinna —see Contusion, ear
popliteal space —see Contusion, knee
prepuce S30.21
prostate S37.822
pubic region S30.1
pudendum
  female S30.202
  male S30.201
quadriceps femoris —see Contusion, thigh
rectum S36.62
retroperitoneum S36.892
round ligament S37.892
sacral region S30.0
scalp S00.03
  due to birth injury P12.3
scapular region —see Contusion, shoulder
sclera —see Contusion, eyeball
scrotum S30.22
seminal vesicle S37.892
shoulder S40.01-
skin NEC T14.8
small intestine —see Injury, intestine, small, contusion
spermatic cord S30.22
spinal cord —see Injury, spinal cord, by region
  cauda equina S34.3
  conus medullaris S34.139

Contusion (continued)
spleen S36.029
  major S36.021
  minor S36.020
sternal region S20.219
stomach S36.32
subconjunctival S05.1-
subcutaneous NEC T14.8
submaxillary region S00.83
submental region S00.83
subperiosteal NEC T14.8
subungual
  finger —see Contusion, finger, with damage to nail
  toe —see Contusion, toe, with damage to nail
supraclavicular fossa S10.83
supraorbital S00.83
suprarenal gland S37.812
temple (region) S00.83
temporal
  lobe (brain) —see Injury, intracranial, diffuse
    focal —see Injury, intracranial, focal
  region S00.83
testis S30.22
thigh S70.1-
thorax (wall) S20.20
  back S20.22-
  front S20.21-
throat S10.0
thumb S60.01-
  with damage to nail S60.11-
toe(s) (lesser) S90.12-
  with damage to nail S90.22-
  great S90.11-
    with damage to nail S90.21-
tongue S00.532
trachea (cervical) S10.0
  thoracic S27.52
tunica vaginalis S30.22
tympanum, tympanic membrane —see Contusion, ear
ureter S37.12
urethra S37.32
urinary organ NEC S37.892
uterus S37.62
uvula S00.532
vagina S30.23
vas deferens S37.892
vesical S37.22
vocal cord(s) S10.0
vulva S30.23
wrist S60.21-

Conus (congenital) (any type) Q14.8
cornea —see Keratoconus
medullaris syndrome G95.81

Conversion hysteria, neurosis or reaction F44.9

Converter, tuberculosis (test reaction) R76.11

Conviction (legal), **anxiety concerning** Z65.0
with imprisonment Z65.1

Convulsions (idiopathic) (see also Seizure(s)) R56.9
apoplectiform (cerebral ischemia) I67.82
dissociative F44.5
epileptic —see Epilepsy
epileptiform, epileptoid —see Seizure, epileptiform
ether (anesthetic) —see Table of Drugs and Chemicals, by drug
febrile R56.00
  with status epilepticus G40.901
  complex R56.01
    with status epilepticus G40.901
  simple R56.00

Convulsions (continued)
  hysterical F44.5
  infantile P90
    epilepsy —see Epilepsy
  jacksonian —see Epilepsy,
    localization-related, symptomatic,
    with simple partial seizures
  myoclonic G25.3
  newborn P90
  obstetrical (nephritic) (uremic)
    —see Eclampsia
  paretic A52.17
  post traumatic R56.1
  psychomotor —see Epilepsy,
    localization-related,
    symptomatic, with complex
    partial seizures
  recurrent R56.9
  reflex R25.8
  scarlatinal A38.8
  tetanus, tetanic —see Tetanus
  thymic E32.8

Convulsive —see also Convulsions

Cooley's anemia D56.1

Coolie itch B76.9

Cooper's
  disease —see Mastopathy, cystic
  hernia —see Hernia, abdomen,
    specified site NEC

Copra itch B88.0

Coprophagy F50.89

Coprophobia F40.298

Coproporphyria, hereditary E80.29

Cor
  biloculare Q20.8
  bovis, bovinum —see Hypertrophy,
    cardiac
  pulmonale I27.81
    acute I26.09
      without pulmonary embolism
        I27.81
    chronic I27.81
      with chronic pulmonary
        embolism I27.82
  triatriatum, triatrium Q24.2
  triloculare Q20.8
    biatrium Q20.4
    biventriculare Q21.19

Corbus' disease (gangrenous
  balanitis) N48.1

Cord —see also condition
  around neck
    complicating delivery O69.81
      with compression O69.1
  bladder G95.89
    tabetic A52.19

Cordis ectopia Q24.8

Corditis (spermatic) N49.1

Corectopia Q13.2

Cori's disease (glycogen storage)
  E74.03

Corkhandler's disease or lung J67.3

Corkscrew esophagus K22.4

Corkworker's disease or lung J67.3

Corn (infected) L84

Cornea —see also condition
  donor Z52.5
  plana Q13.4

Cornelia de Lange syndrome Q87.19

Cornu cutaneum L85.8

Cornual gestation or pregnancy
  O00.80
  with intrauterine pregnancy O00.81

Coronary (artery) —see condition

Coronavirus (infection)
  2019 (see also COVID-19)
    U07.1
  as cause of disease classified
    elsewhere B97.29
  coronavirus-19 (see also
    COVID-19) U07.1
  COVID-19 (see also COVID-19)
    U07.1
  SARS-associated B97.21

Corpora —see also condition
  amylacea, prostate N42.89
  cavernosa —see condition

Corpulence —see Obesity

Corpus —see condition

Corrected transposition
  Q20.5

Corrosion (injury) (acid) (caustic)
  (chemical) (lime) (external)
  (internal) T30.4
  abdomen, abdominal (muscle)
    (wall) T21.42
    first degree T21.52
    second degree T21.62
    third degree T21.72
  above elbow T22.439
    first degree T22.539
    left T22.432
      first degree T22.532
      second degree T22.632
      third degree T22.732
    right T22.431
      first degree T22.531
      second degree T22.631
      third degree T22.731
    second degree T22.639
    third degree T22.739
  alimentary tract NEC T28.7
  ankle T25.419
    first degree T25.519
    left T25.412
      first degree T25.512
      second degree T25.612
      third degree T25.712
    multiple with foot —see
      Corrosion, lower, limb,
      multiple, ankle and foot
    right T25.411
      first degree T25.511
      second degree T25.611
      third degree T25.711
    second degree T25.619
    third degree T25.719
  anus —see Corrosion, buttock
  arm(s) (meaning upper limb(s)) —
    see Corrosion, upper limb
  axilla T22.449
    first degree T22.549
    left T22.442
      first degree T22.542
      second degree T22.642
      third degree T22.742
    right T22.441
      first degree T22.541
      second degree T22.641
      third degree T22.741
    second degree T22.649
    third degree T22.749
  back (lower) T21.44
    first degree T21.54
    second degree T21.64
    third degree T21.74
    upper T21.43
      first degree T21.53
      second degree T21.63
      third degree T21.73
  blisters - code as Corrosion, second
    degree, by site
  breast(s) —see Corrosion, chest
    wall

Corrosion (continued)
  buttock(s) T21.45
    first degree T21.55
    second degree T21.65
    third degree T21.75
  calf T24.439
    first degree T24.539
    left T24.432
      first degree T24.532 sickle-
        cell D57.00
      second degree T24.632
      third degree T24.732
    right T24.431
      first degree T24.531
      second degree T24.631
      third degree T24.731
    second degree T24.639
    third degree T24.739
  canthus (eye) —see Corrosion,
    eyelid
  cervix T28.8
  cheek T20.46
    first degree T20.56
    second degree T20.66
    third degree T20.76
  chest wall T21.41
    first degree T21.51
    second degree T21.61
    third degree T21.71
  chin T20.43
    first degree T20.53
    second degree T20.63
    third degree T20.73
  colon T28.7
  conjunctiva (and cornea) —see
    Corrosion, cornea
  cornea (and conjunctiva)
    T26.6-
  deep necrosis of underlying tissue -
    code as Corrosion, third degree,
    by site
  dorsum of hand T23.469
    first degree T23.569
    left T23.462
      first degree T23.562
      second degree T23.662
      third degree T23.762
    right T23.461
      first degree T23.561
      second degree T23.661
      third degree T23.761
    second degree T23.669
    third degree T23.769
  ear (auricle) (external) (canal)
    T20.41
    drum T28.91
    first degree T20.51
    second degree T20.61
    third degree T20.71
  elbow T22.429
    first degree T22.529
    left T22.422
      first degree T22.522
      second degree T22.622
      third degree T22.722
    right T22.421
      first degree T22.521
      second degree T22.621
      third degree T22.721
    second degree T22.629
    third degree T22.729
  entire body —see Corrosion,
    multiple body regions
  epidermal loss - code as Corrosion,
    second degree, by site
  epiglottis T27.4
  erythema, erythematous -
    code as Corrosion, first degree,
    by site
  esophagus T28.6

Corrosion (continued)
  extent (percentage of body
    surface)
    less than 10 percent T32.0
    10-19 percent (0-9 percent third
      degree) T32.10
      with 10-19 percent third
        degree T32.11
    20-29 percent (0-9 percent third
      degree) T32.20
      with
        10-19 percent third degree
          T32.21
        20-29 percent third degree
          T32.22
    30-39 percent (0-9 percent third
      degree) T32.30
      with
        10-19 percent third degree
          T32.31
        20-29 percent third degree
          T32.32
        30-39 percent third degree
          T32.33
    40-49 percent (0-9 percent third
      degree) T32.40
      with
        10-19 percent third degree
          T32.41
        20-29 percent third degree
          T32.42
        30-39 percent third degree
          T32.43
        40-49 percent third degree
          T32.44
    50-59 percent (0-9 percent third
      degree) T32.50
      with
        10-19 percent third degree
          T32.51
        20-29 percent third degree
          T32.52
        30-39 percent third degree
          T32.53
        40-49 percent third degree
          T32.54
        50-59 percent third degree
          T32.55
    60-69 percent (0-9 percent third
      degree) T32.60
      with
        10-19 percent third degree
          T32.61
        20-29 percent third degree
          T32.62
        30-39 percent third degree
          T32.63
        40-49 percent third degree
          T32.64
        50-59 percent third degree
          T32.65
        60-69 percent third degree
          T32.66
    70-79 percent (0-9 percent third
      degree) T32.70
      with
        10-19 percent third degree
          T32.71
        20-29 percent third degree
          T32.72
        30-39 percent third degree
          T32.73
        40-49 percent third degree
          T32.74
        50-59 percent third degree
          T32.75
        60-69 percent third degree
          T32.76
        70-79 percent third degree
          T32.77

Corrosion (continued)
extent (continued)
80-89 percent (0-9 percent third degree) T32.80
with
10-19 percent third degree T32.81
20-29 percent third degree T32.82
30-39 percent third degree T32.83
40-49 percent third degree T32.84
50-59 percent third degree T32.85
60-69 percent third degree T32.86
70-79 percent third degree T32.87
80-89 percent third degree T32.88
90 percent or more (0-9 percent third degree) T32.90
with
10-19 percent third degree T32.91
20-29 percent third degree T32.92
30-39 percent third degree T32.93
40-49 percent third degree T32.94
50-59 percent third degree T32.95
60-69 percent third degree T32.96
70-79 percent third degree T32.97
80-89 percent third degree T32.98
90-99 percent third degree T32.99
extremity —see Corrosion, limb
eye(s) and adnexa T26.9-
with resulting rupture and destruction of eyeball T26.7-
conjunctival sac —see Corrosion, cornea
cornea —see Corrosion, cornea
lid —see Corrosion, eyelid
periocular area —see Corrosion, eyelid
specified site NEC T26.8-
eyeball —see Corrosion, eye
eyelid(s) T26.5-
face —see Corrosion, head
finger T23.429
first degree T23.529
left T23.422
first degree T23.522
second degree T23.622
third degree T23.722
multiple sites (without thumb) T23.439
with thumb T23.449
first degree T23.549
left T23.442
first degree T23.542
second degree T23.642
third degree T23.742
right T23.441
first degree T23.541
second degree T23.641
third degree T23.741
second degree T23.649
third degree T23.749
first degree T23.539
left T23.432
first degree T23.532
second degree T23.632
third degree T23.732

Corrosion (continued)
finger (continued)
multiple sites (continued)
right T23.431
first degree T23.531
second degree T23.631
third degree T23.731
second degree T23.639
third degree T23.739
right T23.421
first degree T23.521
second degree T23.621
third degree T23.721
second degree T23.629
third degree T23.729
flank —see Corrosion, abdomen
foot T25.429
first degree T25.529
left T25.422
first degree T25.522
second degree T25.622
third degree T25.722
multiple with ankle —see Corrosion, lower, limb, multiple, ankle and foot
right T25.421
first degree T25.521
second degree T25.621
third degree T25.721
second degree T25.629
third degree T25.729
forearm T22.419
first degree T22.519
left T22.412
first degree T22.512
second degree T22.612
third degree T22.712
right T22.411
first degree T22.511
second degree T22.611
third degree T22.711
second degree T22.619
third degree T22.719
forehead T20.46
first degree T20.56
second degree T20.66
third degree T20.76
fourth degree - code as Corrosion, third degree, by site
full thickness skin loss - code as Corrosion, third degree, by site
gastrointestinal tract NEC T28.7
genital organs
external
female T21.47
first degree T21.57
second degree T21.67
third degree T21.77
male T21.46
first degree T21.56
second degree T21.66
third degree T21.76
internal T28.8
groin —see Corrosion, abdominal wall
hand(s) T23.409
back —see Corrosion, dorsum of hand
finger —see Corrosion, finger
first degree T23.509
left T23.402
first degree T23.502
second degree T23.602
third degree T23.702
multiple sites with wrist T23.499
first degree T23.599
left T23.492
first degree T23.592
second degree T23.692
third degree T23.792
right T23.491
first degree T23.591

Corrosion (continued)
hand(s) (continued)
multiple sites with wrist (continued)
right (continued)
second degree T23.691
third degree T23.791
second degree T23.699
third degree T23.799
palm —see Corrosion, palm
right T23.401
first degree T23.501
second degree T23.601
third degree T23.701
second degree T23.609
third degree T23.709
thumb —see Corrosion, thumb
head (and face) (and neck) T20.40
cheek —see Corrosion, cheek
chin —see Corrosion, chin
ear —see Corrosion, ear
eye(s) only —see Corrosion, eye
first degree T20.50
forehead —see Corrosion, forehead
lip —see Corrosion, lip
multiple sites T20.49
first degree T20.59
second degree T20.69
third degree T20.79
neck —see Corrosion, neck
nose —see Corrosion, nose
scalp —see Corrosion, scalp
second degree T20.60
third degree T20.70
hip(s) —see Corrosion, lower, limb
inhalation —see Corrosion, respiratory tract
internal organ(s) (see also Corrosion, by site) T28.90
alimentary tract T28.7
esophagus T28.6
esophagus T28.6
genitourinary T28.8
mouth T28.5
pharynx T28.5
specified organ NEC T28.99
interscapular region —see Corrosion, back, upper
intestine (large) (small) T28.7
knee T24.429
first degree T24.529
left T24.422
first degree T24.522
second degree T24.622
third degree T24.722
right T24.421
first degree T24.521
second degree T24.621
third degree T24.721
second degree T24.629
third degree T24.729
labium (majus) (minus) —see Corrosion, genital organs, external, female
lacrimal apparatus, duct, gland or sac —see Corrosion, eye, specified site NEC
larynx T27.4
with lung T27.5
leg(s) (meaning lower limb(s)) —see Corrosion, lower limb
limb(s)
lower —see Corrosion, lower, limb
upper —see Corrosion, upper limb
lip(s) T20.42
first degree T20.52
second degree T20.62
third degree T20.72
lower
back —see Corrosion, back

Corrosion (continued)
lower (continued)
limb T24.409
ankle —see Corrosion, ankle
calf —see Corrosion, calf
first degree T24.509
foot —see Corrosion, foot
knee —see Corrosion, knee
left T24.402
first degree T24.502
second degree T24.602
third degree T24.702
multiple sites, except ankle and foot T24.499
ankle and foot T25.499
first degree T25.599
left T25.492
first degree T25.592
second degree T25.692
third degree T25.792
right T25.491
first degree T25.591
second degree T25.691
third degree T25.791
second degree T25.699
third degree T25.799
first degree T24.599
left T24.492
first degree T24.592
second degree T24.692
third degree T24.792
right T24.491
first degree T24.591
second degree T24.691
third degree T24.791
second degree T24.699
third degree T24.799
right T24.401
first degree T24.501
second degree T24.601
third degree T24.701
second degree T24.609
hip —see Corrosion, thigh
thigh —see Corrosion, thigh
third degree T24.709
lung (with larynx and trachea) T27.5
mouth T28.5
neck T20.47
first degree T20.57
second degree T20.67
third degree T20.77
nose (septum) T20.44
first degree T20.54
second degree T20.64
third degree T20.74
ocular adnexa —see Corrosion, eye
orbit region —see Corrosion, eyelid
palm T23.459
first degree T23.559
left T23.452
first degree T23.552
second degree T23.652
third degree T23.752
right T23.451
first degree T23.551
second degree T23.651
third degree T23.751
second degree T23.659
third degree T23.759
partial thickness - code as Corrosion, unspecified degree, by site
pelvis —see Corrosion, trunk
penis —see Corrosion, genital organs, external, male
perineum
female —see Corrosion, genital organs, external, female
male —see Corrosion, genital organs, external, male

Corrosion *(continued)*
  periocular area —*see* Corrosion, eyelid
  pharynx T28.5
  rectum T28.7
  respiratory tract T27.7
    larynx —*see* Corrosion, larynx
    specified part NEC T27.6
    trachea —*see* Corrosion, larynx
  sac, lacrimal —*see* Corrosion, eye, specified site NEC
  scalp T20.45
    first degree T20.55
    second degree T20.65
    third degree T20.75
  scapular region T22.469
    first degree T22.569
    left T22.462
      first degree T22.562
      second degree T22.662
      third degree T22.762
    right T22.461
      first degree T22.561
      second degree T22.661
      third degree T22.761
    second degree T22.669
    third degree T22.769
  sclera —*see* Corrosion, eye, specified site NEC
  scrotum —*see* Corrosion, genital organs, external, male
  shoulder T22.459
    first degree T22.559
    left T22.452
      first degree T22.552
      second degree T22.652
      third degree T22.752
    right T22.451
      first degree T22.551
      second degree T22.651
      third degree T22.751
    second degree T22.659
    third degree T22.759
  stomach T28.7
  temple —*see* Corrosion, head
  testis —*see* Corrosion, genital organs, external, male
  thigh T24.419
    first degree T24.519
    left T24.412
      first degree T24.512
      second degree T24.612
      third degree T24.712
    right T24.411
      first degree T24.511
      second degree T24.611
      third degree T24.711
    second degree T24.619
    third degree T24.719
  thorax (external) —*see* Corrosion, trunk
  throat (meaning pharynx) T28.5
  thumb(s) T23.419
    first degree T23.519
    left T23.412
      first degree T23.512
      second degree T23.612
      third degree T23.712
    multiple sites with fingers T23.449
      first degree T23.549
      left T23.442
        first degree T23.542
        second degree T23.642
        third degree T23.742
      right T23.441
        first degree T23.541
        second degree T23.641
        third degree T23.741
      second degree T23.649
      third degree T23.749

Corrosion *(continued)*
  thumb(s) *(continued)*
    right T23.411
      first degree T23.511
      second degree T23.611
      third degree T23.711
    second degree T23.619
    third degree T23.719
  toe T25.439
    first degree T25.539
    left T25.432
      first degree T25.532
      second degree T25.632
      third degree T25.732
    right T25.431
      first degree T25.531
      second degree T25.631
      third degree T25.731
    second degree T25.639
    third degree T25.739
  tongue T28.5
  tonsil(s) T28.5
  total body —*see* Corrosion, multiple body regions
  trachea T27.4
    with lung T27.5
  trunk T21.40
    abdominal wall —*see* Corrosion, abdominal wall
    anus —*see* Corrosion, buttock
    axilla —*see* Corrosion, upper limb
    back —*see* Corrosion, back
    breast —*see* Corrosion, chest wall
    buttock —*see* Corrosion, buttock
    chest wall —*see* Corrosion, chest wall
    first degree T21.50
    flank —*see* Corrosion, abdominal wall
    genital
      female —*see* Corrosion, genital organs, external, female
      male —*see* Corrosion, genital organs, external, male
    groin —*see* Corrosion, abdominal wall
    interscapular region —*see* Corrosion, back, upper
    labia —*see* Corrosion, genital organs, external, female
    lower back —*see* Corrosion, back
    penis —*see* Corrosion, genital organs, external, male
    perineum
      female —*see* Corrosion, genital organs, external, female
      male —*see* Corrosion, genital organs, external, male
    scapular region —*see* Corrosion, upper limb
    scrotum —*see* Corrosion, genital organs, external, male
    second degree T21.60
    shoulder —*see* Corrosion, upper limb
    specified site NEC T21.49
      first degree T21.59
      second degree T21.69
      third degree T21.79
    testes —*see* Corrosion, genital organs, external, male
    third degree T21.70
    upper back —*see* Corrosion, back, upper
    vagina T28.8
    vulva —*see* Corrosion, genital organs, external, female

Corrosion *(continued)*
  unspecified site with extent of body surface involved specified
    less than 10 percent T32.0
    10-19 percent (0-9 percent third degree) T32.10
      with 10-19 percent third degree T32.11
    20-29 percent (0-9 percent third degree) T32.20
      with
        10-19 percent third degree T32.21
        20-29 percent third degree T32.22
    30-39 percent (0-9 percent third degree) T32.30
      with
        10-19 percent third degree T32.31
        20-29 percent third degree T32.32
        30-39 percent third degree T32.33
    40-49 percent (0-9 percent third degree) T32.40
      with
        10-19 percent third degree T32.41
        20-29 percent third degree T32.42
        30-39 percent third degree T32.43
        40-49 percent third degree T32.44
    50-59 percent (0-9 percent third degree) T32.50
      with
        10-19 percent third degree T32.51
        20-29 percent third degree T32.52
        30-39 percent third degree T32.53
        40-49 percent third degree T32.54
        50-59 percent third degree T32.55
    60-69 percent (0-9 percent third degree) T32.60
      with
        10-19 percent third degree T32.61
        20-29 percent third degree T32.62
        30-39 percent third degree T32.63
        40-49 percent third degree T32.64
        50-59 percent third degree T32.65
        60-69 percent third degree T32.66
    70-79 percent (0-9 percent third degree) T32.70
      with
        10-19 percent third degree T32.71
        20-29 percent third degree T32.72
        30-39 percent third degree T32.73
        40-49 percent third degree T32.74
        50-59 percent third degree T32.75
        60-69 percent third degree T32.76
        70-79 percent third degree T32.77

Corrosion *(continued)*
  unspecified site with extent of body surface involved specified *(continued)*
    80-89 percent (0-9 percent third degree) T32.80
      with
        10-19 percent third degree T32.81
        20-29 percent third degree T32.82
        30-39 percent third degree T32.83
        40-49 percent third degree T32.84
        50-59 percent third degree T32.85
        60-69 percent third degree T32.86
        70-79 percent third degree T32.87
        80-89 percent third degree T32.88
    90 percent or more (0-9 percent third degree) T32.90
      with
        10-19 percent third degree T32.91
        20-29 percent third degree T32.92
        30-39 percent third degree T32.93
        40-49 percent third degree T32.94
        50-59 percent third degree T32.95
        60-69 percent third degree T32.96
        70-79 percent third degree T32.97
        80-89 percent third degree T32.98
        90-99 percent third degree T32.99
  upper limb (axilla) (scapular region) T22.40
    above elbow —*see* Corrosion, above elbow
    axilla —*see* Corrosion, axilla
    elbow —*see* Corrosion, elbow
    first degree T22.50
    forearm —*see* Corrosion, forearm
    hand —*see* Corrosion, hand
    interscapular region —*see* Corrosion, back, upper
    multiple sites T22.499
      first degree T22.599
      left T22.492
        first degree T22.592
        second degree T22.692
        third degree T22.792
      right T22.491
        first degree T22.591
        second degree T22.691
        third degree T22.791
      second degree T22.699
      third degree T22.799
    scapular region —*see* Corrosion, scapular region
    second degree T22.60
    shoulder —*see* Corrosion, shoulder
    third degree T22.70
    wrist —*see* Corrosion, hand
  uterus T28.8
  vagina T28.8
  vulva —*see* Corrosion, genital organs, external, female

Corrosion (continued)
  wrist T23.479
    first degree T23.579
    left T23.472
      first degree T23.572
      second degree T23.672
      third degree T23.772
    multiple sites with hand T23.499
      first degree T23.599
      left T23.492
        first degree T23.592
        second degree T23.692
        third degree T23.792
      right T23.491
        first degree T23.591
        second degree T23.691
        third degree T23.791
      second degree T23.699
      third degree T23.799
    right T23.471
      first degree T23.571
      second degree T23.671
      third degree T23.771
    second degree T23.679
    third degree T23.779
Corrosive burn —see Corrosion
Corsican fever —see Malaria
Cortical —see condition
Cortico-adrenal —see condition
Coryza (acute) J00
  with grippe or influenza —see
    Influenza, with, respiratory
    manifestations NEC
  syphilitic
    congenital (chronic) A50.05
Co-sleeping, child-caregiver
  Z72.823
Costen's syndrome or complex
  M26.69
Costiveness —see Constipation
Costochondritis M94.0
Cotard's syndrome F22
Cot death R99
Cotia virus B08.8
Cotton wool spots (retinal) H35.81
Cotungo's disease —see Sciatica
Cough (affected) (epidemic)
    (nervous) R05.9
  with hemorrhage —see
    Hemoptysis
  acute R05.1
  bronchial R05.8
    with grippe or influenza —see
      Influenza, with, respiratory
      manifestations NEC
  chronic R05.3
  functional F45.8
  hysterical F45.8
  laryngeal, spasmodic R05.8
  paroxysmal, due to Bordetella
    pertussis (without pneumonia)
    A37.00
    with pneumonia A37.01
  persistent R05.3
  psychogenic F45.8
  refractory R05.3
  specified NEC R05.8
  smokers' J41.0
  subacute R05.2
  syncope R05.4
  tea taster's B49
  unexplained R05.3
Counseling (for) Z71.9
  abuse NEC
    perpetrator Z69.82
    victim Z69.81
  alcohol abuser Z71.41
    family Z71.42

Counseling (continued)
  child abuse
    nonparental
      perpetrator Z69.021
      victim Z69.020
    parental
      perpetrator Z69.011
      victim Z69.010
  consanguinity Z71.89
  contraceptive Z30.09
  dietary Z71.3
  drug abuser Z71.51
    family member Z71.52
  exercise Z71.82
  family Z71.89
  fertility preservation (prior to
      cancer therapy) (prior to removal
      of gonads) Z31.62
  for non-attending third party Z71.0
    related to sexual behavior or
      orientation Z70.2
  genetic
    nonprocreative Z71.83
    procreative NEC Z31.5
  gestational carrier Z31.7
  health (advice) (education)
      (instruction) —see Counseling,
      medical
    risk for travel (international) Z71.84
  human immunodeficiency virus
      (HIV) Z71.7
  immunization safety Z71.85
  impotence Z70.1
  insulin pump use Z46.81
  medical (for) Z71.9
    boarding school resident Z59.3
    consanguinity Z71.89
    feared complaint and no disease
      found Z71.1
    human immunodeficiency virus
      (HIV) Z71.7
    institutional resident Z59.3
    on behalf of another Z71.0
      related to sexual behavior or
        orientation Z70.2
    person living alone (see also
      Consultation, specified reason
      NEC) Z60.2
    specified reason NEC Z71.89
  natural family planning
    procreative Z31.61
    to avoid pregnancy Z30.02
  pediatric-to-adult transition
    Z71.87
  perpetrator (of)
    abuse NEC Z69.82
    child abuse
      non-parental Z69.021
      parental Z69.011
    rape NEC Z69.82
    spousal abuse Z69.12
  procreative NEC Z31.69
    fertility preservation (prior to
      cancer therapy) (prior to
      removal of gonads) Z31.62
    using natural family planning
      Z31.61
  promiscuity Z70.1
  rape victim Z69.81
  religious Z71.81
  safety for travel (international)
    Z71.84
  sex, sexual (related to) Z70.9
    attitude(s) Z70.0
    behavior or orientation Z70.1
    combined concerns Z70.3
    non-responsiveness Z70.1
    on behalf of third party Z70.2
    specified reason NEC Z70.8
  socioeconomic factors Z71.88
  specified reason NEC Z71.89

Counseling (continued)
  spiritual Z71.81
  spousal abuse (perpetrator) Z69.12
    victim Z69.11
  substance abuse Z71.89
    alcohol Z71.41
    drug Z71.51
    tobacco Z71.6
  tobacco use Z71.6
  travel (international) Z71.84
  use (of)
    insulin pump Z46.81
  vaccine product safety Z71.85
  victim (of)
    abuse Z69.81
    child abuse
      by parent Z69.010
      non-parental Z69.020
    rape NEC Z69.81
Coupled rhythm R00.8
Couvelaire syndrome or uterus
    (complicating delivery) O45.8X-
COVID-19 U07.1
  condition post U09.9
  contact (with) Z20.822
  exposure (to) Z20.822
  history of (personal) Z86.16
  long (haul) U09.9
  partially vaccinated (for) Z28.311
  pneumonia J12.82
  screening Z11.52
  sequelae (post acute) U09.9
  unvaccinated (for) Z28.310
Cowperitis —see Urethritis
Cowper's gland —see condition
Cowpox B08.010
  due to vaccination T88.1
Coxa
  magna M91.4-
  plana M91.2-
  valga (acquired) —see also
      Deformity, limb, specified type
      NEC, thigh
    congenital Q65.81
    sequelae (late effect) of rickets
      E64.3
  vara (acquired) —see also Deformity,
      limb, specified type NEC, thigh
    congenital Q65.82
    sequelae (late effect) of rickets
      E64.3
Coxalgia, coxalgic (nontuberculous)
    —see also Pain, joint, hip
  tuberculous A18.02
Coxitis —see Monoarthritis, hip
Coxsackie (virus) (infection) B34.1
  as cause of disease classified
    elsewhere B97.11
  carditis B33.20
  central nervous system NEC A88.8
  endocarditis B33.21
  enteritis A08.39
  meningitis (aseptic) A87.0
  myocarditis B33.22
  pericarditis B33.23
  pharyngitis B08.5
  pleurodynia B33.0
  specific disease NEC B33.8
Crabs, meaning pubic lice B85.3
Crack baby P04.41
Cracked nipple N64.0
  associated with
    lactation O92.13
    pregnancy O92.11-
    puerperium O92.12
Cracked tooth K03.81
Cradle cap L21.0

Craft neurosis F48.8
Cramp(s) R25.2
  abdominal —see Pain, abdominal
  bathing T75.1
  colic R10.83
    psychogenic F45.8
  due to immersion T75.1
  fireman T67.2
  heat T67.2
  immersion T75.1
  intestinal —see Pain, abdominal
    psychogenic F45.8
  leg, sleep related G47.62
  limb (lower) (upper) NEC R25.2
    sleep related G47.62
  linotypist's F48.8
    organic G25.89
  muscle (limb) (general) R25.2
    due to immersion T75.1
    psychogenic F45.8
  occupational (hand) F48.8
    organic G25.89
  salt-depletion E87.1
  sleep related, leg G47.62
  stoker's T67.2
  swimmer's T75.1
  telegrapher's F48.8
    organic G25.89
  typist's F48.8
    organic G25.89
  uterus N94.89
    menstrual —see Dysmenorrhea
  writer's F48.8
    organic G25.89
Cranial —see condition
Craniocleidodysostosis Q74.0
Craniofenestria (skull) Q75.8
Craniolacunia (skull) Q75.8
Craniopagus Q89.4
Craniopathy, metabolic M85.2
Craniopharyngeal —see condition
Craniopharyngioma D44.4
Craniorachischisis (totalis) Q00.1
Cranioschisis Q75.8
Craniostenosis Q75.009
Craniosynostosis Q75.009
  bilateral Q75.002
  coronal Q75.029
    bilateral Q75.022
    unilateral Q75.021
  lambdoid Q75.049
    bilateral Q75.042
    unilateral Q75.041
  metopic Q75.03
  multi-suture, specified NEC Q75.058
  sagittal Q75.01
  single-suture, specified NEC Q75.08
  unilateral Q75.001
Craniotabes (cause unknown) M83.8
  neonatal P96.3
  rachitic E64.3
  syphilitic A50.56
Cranium —see condition
Craw-craw —see Onchocerciasis
Creaking joint —see Derangement,
    joint, specified type NEC
Creeping
  eruption B76.9
  palsy or paralysis G12.22
Crenated tongue K14.8
Creotoxism A05.9
Crepitus
  caput Q75.8
  joint —see Derangement, joint,
    specified type NEC

Crescent or conus choroid, congenital Q14.3
CREST syndrome M34.1
Cretin, cretinism (congenital) (endemic) (nongoitrous) (sporadic) E00.9
  pelvis
    with disproportion (fetopelvic) O33.0
      causing obstructed labor O65.0
  type
    hypothyroid E00.1
    mixed E00.2
    myxedematous E00.1
    neurological E00.0
Creutzfeldt-Jakob disease or syndrome (with dementia) A81.00
  familial A81.09
  iatrogenic A81.09
  specified NEC A81.09
  sporadic A81.09
  variant (vCJD) A81.01
Crib death R99
Cribriform hymen Q52.3
Cri-du-chat syndrome Q93.4
Crigler-Najjar disease or syndrome E80.5
Crime, victim of Z65.4
Crimean hemorrhagic fever A98.0
Criminalism F60.2
Crisis
  abdomen R10.0
  acute reaction F43.0
  addisonian E27.2
  adrenal (cortical) E27.2
  celiac K90.0
  Dietl's N13.8
  emotional —see also Disorder, adjustment
    acute reaction to stress F43.0
    specific to childhood and adolescence F93.8
  glaucomatocyclitic —see Glaucoma, secondary, inflammation
  heart —see Failure, heart
  nitritoid I95.2
    correct substance properly administered —see Table of Drugs and Chemicals, by drug, adverse effect
    overdose or wrong substance given or taken —see Table of Drugs and Chemicals, by drug, poisoning
  oculogyric H51.8
    psychogenic F45.8
  Pel's (tabetic) A52.11
  psychosexual identity F64.2
  renal N28.0
  sickle-cell (see also Disease, sickle-cell, by type, with crisis) D57.00
    with
      acute chest syndrome D57.01
      cerebral vascular involvement D57.03
      complication specified NEC D57.09
      pain (vaso-occlusive) D57.00
      splenic sequestration D57.02
  state (acute reaction) F43.0
  tabetic A52.11
  thyroid —see Thyrotoxicosis with thyroid storm
  thyrotoxic —see Thyrotoxicosis with thyroid storm
Crocq's disease (acrocyanosis) I73.89

Crohn's disease —see Enteritis, regional
Crooked septum, nasal J34.2
Cross syndrome E70.328
Crossbite (anterior) (posterior) M26.24
Cross-eye —see Strabismus, convergent concomitant
Croup, croupous (catarrhal) (infectious) (inflammatory) (nondiphtheritic) J05.0
  bronchial J20.9
  diphtheritic A36.2
  false J38.5
  spasmodic J38.5
    diphtheritic A36.2
  stridulous J38.5
    diphtheritic A36.2
Crouzon's disease Q75.1
Crowding, tooth, teeth, fully erupted M26.31
CRST syndrome M34.1
Cruchet's disease A85.8
Cruelty in children —see also Disorder, conduct
Crural ulcer —see Ulcer, lower limb
Crush, crushed, crushing T14.8
  abdomen S38.1
  ankle S97.0-
  arm (upper) (and shoulder) S47.-
  axilla —see Crush, arm
  back, lower S38.1
  buttock S38.1
  cheek S07.0
  chest S28.0
  cranium S07.1
  ear S07.0
  elbow S57.0-
  extremity
    lower
      ankle —see Crush, ankle
      below knee —see Crush, leg
      foot —see Crush, foot
      hip —see Crush, hip
      knee —see Crush, knee
      thigh —see Crush, thigh
      toe —see Crush, toe
    upper
      below elbow S67.9-
      elbow —see Crush, elbow
      finger —see Crush, finger
      forearm —see Crush, forearm
      hand —see Crush, hand
      thumb —see Crush, thumb
      upper arm —see Crush, arm
      wrist —see Crush, wrist
  face S07.0
  finger(s) S67.1-
    with hand (and wrist) —see Crush, hand, specified site NEC
    index S67.19-
    little S67.19-
    middle S67.19-
    ring S67.19-
    thumb —see Crush, thumb
  foot S97.8-
    toe —see Crush, toe
  forearm S57.8-
  genitalia, external
    female S38.002
      vagina S38.03
      vulva S38.03
    male S38.001
      penis S38.01
      scrotum S38.02
      testis S38.02

Crush, crushed, crushing (continued)
  hand (except fingers alone) S67.2-
    with wrist S67.4-
  head S07.9
    specified NEC S07.8
  heel —see Crush, foot
  hip S77.0-
    with thigh S77.2-
  internal organ (abdomen, chest, or pelvis) NEC T14.8
  knee S87.0-
  labium (majus) (minus) S38.03
  larynx S17.0
  leg (lower) S87.8-
    knee —see Crush, knee
  lip S07.0
  lower
    back S38.1
    leg —see Crush, leg
  neck S17.9
  nerve —see Injury, nerve
  nose S07.0
  pelvis S38.1
  penis S38.01
  scalp S07.8
  scapular region —see rush, arm
  scrotum S38.02
  severe, unspecified site T14.8
  shoulder (and upper arm) —see Crush, arm
  skull S07.1
  syndrome (complication of trauma) T79.5
  testis S38.02
  thigh S77.1-
    with hip S77.2-
  throat S17.8
  thumb S67.0-
    with hand (and wrist) —see Crush, hand, specified site NEC
  toe(s) S97.10-
    great S97.11-
    lesser S97.12-
  trachea S17.0
  vagina S38.03
  vulva S38.03
  wrist S67.3-
    with hand S67.4-
Crusta lactea L21.0
Crusts R23.4
Crutch paralysis —see Injury, brachial plexus
Cruveilhier-Baumgarten cirrhosis, disease or syndrome K74.69
Cruveilhier's atrophy or disease G12.8
Crying (constant) (continuous) (excessive)
  child, adolescent, or adult R45.83
  infant (baby) (newborn) R68.11
Cryofibrinogenemia D89.2
Cryoglobulinemia (essential) (idiopathic) (mixed) (primary) (purpura) (secondary) (vasculitis) D89.1
  with lung involvement D89.1 [J99]
Cryptitis (anal) (rectal) K62.89
Cryptococcosis, cryptococcus (infection) (neoformans) B45.9
  bone B45.3
  cerebral B45.1
  cutaneous B45.2
  disseminated B45.7
  generalized B45.7
  meningitis B45.1
  meningocerebralis B45.1

Cryptococcosis, cryptococcus (continued)
  osseous B45.3
  pulmonary B45.0
  skin B45.2
  specified NEC B45.8
Cryptopapillitis (anus) K62.89
Cryptophthalmos Q11.2
  syndrome Q87.0
Cryptorchid, cryptorchism, cryptorchidism Q53.9
  bilateral Q53.20
    abdominal Q53.211
    perineal Q53.22
  unilateral Q53.10
    abdominal Q53.111
    perineal Q53.12
Cryptosporidiosis A07.2
  hepatobiliary B88.8
  respiratory B88.8
Cryptostromosis J67.6
Crystalluria R82.998
Cubitus
  congenital Q68.8
  valgus (acquired) M21.0-
    congenital Q68.8
    sequelae (late effect) of rickets E64.3
  varus (acquired) M21.1-
    congenital Q68.8
    sequelae (late effect) of rickets E64.3
Cultural deprivation or shock Z60.3
Curling esophagus K22.4
Curling's ulcer —see Ulcer, peptic, acute
Curschmann (-Batten) (-Steinert) **disease or syndrome** G71.11
Curse, Ondine's —see Apnea, sleep
Curvature
  organ or site, congenital NEC —see Distortion
  penis (lateral) Q55.61
  Pott's (spinal) A18.01
  radius, idiopathic, progressive (congenital) Q74.0
  spine (acquired) (angular) (idiopathic) (incorrect) (postural) —see Dorsopathy, deforming
    congenital Q67.5
    due to or associated with
      Charcot-Marie-Tooth disease (see also subcategory M49.8) G60.0
      osteitis
        deformans M88.88
        fibrosa cystica (see also subcategory M49.8) E21.0
      tuberculosis (Pott's curvature) A18.01
    sequelae (late effect) of rickets E64.3
    tuberculous A18.01
Cushingoid due to steroid therapy E24.2
  correct substance properly administered —see Table of Drugs and Chemicals, by drug, adverse effect
  overdose or wrong substance given or taken —see Table of Drugs and Chemicals, by drug, poisoning

Cushing's
  syndrome or disease E24.9
    drug-induced E24.2
    iatrogenic E24.2
    pituitary-dependent E24.0
    specified NEC E24.8
  ulcer —see Ulcer, peptic, acute

Cusp, Carabelli - omit code

Cut (external) —see also Laceration
  muscle —see Injury, muscle

Cutaneous —see also condition
  hemorrhage R23.3
  larva migrans B76.9

Cutis —see also condition
  hyperelastica Q82.8
    acquired L57.4
  laxa (hyperelastica) —see
    Dermatolysis
  marmorata R23.8
  osteosis L94.2
  pendula —see Dermatolysis
  rhomboidalis nuchae L57.2
  verticis gyrata Q82.8
    acquired L91.8

Cyanosis R23.0
  due to
    patent foramen botalli Q21.12
    persistent foramen ovale Q21.12
  enterogenous D74.8
  paroxysmal digital —see
    Raynaud's disease
    with gangrene I73.01
  retina, retinal H35.89

Cyanotic heart disease I24.9
  congenital Q24.9

Cycle
  anovulatory N97.0
  menstrual, irregular N92.6

Cyclencephaly Q04.9

Cyclical vomiting, in migraine, (see
  also Vomiting, cyclical) G43.A0
  psychogenic F50.89

Cyclitis (see also Iridocyclitis) H20.9
  chronic —see Iridocyclitis, chronic
  Fuchs' heterochromic H20.81-

Cyclitis
  granulomatous —see Iridocyclitis,
    chronic
  lens-induced —see Iridocyclitis,
    lens-induced
  posterior H30.2-

Cycloid personality F34.0

Cyclophoria H50.54

Cyclopia, cyclops Q87.0

Cyclopism Q87.0

Cyclosporiasis A07.4

Cyclothymia F34.0

Cyclothymic personality F34.0

Cyclotropia H50.41-

Cylindroma —see also Neoplasm,
  malignant, by site
  eccrine dermal —see Neoplasm,
    skin, benign
  skin —see Neoplasm, skin, benign

Cylindruria R82.998

Cynanche
  diphtheritic A36.2
  tonsillaris J36

Cynophobia F40.218

Cynorexia R63.2

Cyphosis —see Kyphosis

Cyprus fever —see Brucellosis

Cyst (colloid) (mucous) (simple)
  (retention)
  adenoid (infected) J35.8
  aneurysmal M27.49
  adrenal gland E27.8
    congenital Q89.1
  air, lung J98.4
  allantoic Q64.4
  alveolar process (jaw bone) M27.40
  amnion, amniotic O41.8X-
  anterior
    chamber (eye) —see Cyst, iris
    nasopalatine K09.1
  antrum J34.1
  anus K62.89
  apical (tooth) (periodontal) K04.8
  appendix K38.8
  arachnoid, brain (acquired) G93.0
    congenital Q04.6
  arytenoid J38.7
  Baker's M71.2-
    ruptured M66.0
    tuberculous A18.02
  Bartholin's gland N75.0
  bile duct (common) (hepatic) K83.5
  bladder (multiple) (trigone) N32.89
  blue dome (breast) —see Cyst,
    breast
  bone (local) NEC M85.60
    aneurysmal M85.50
      ankle M85.57-
      foot M85.57-
      forearm M85.53-
      hand M85.54-
      jaw M27.49
      lower leg M85.56-
      multiple site M85.59
      neck M85.58
      rib M85.58
      shoulder M85.51-
      skull M85.58
      specified site NEC M85.58
      thigh M85.55-
      toe M85.57-
      upper arm M85.52-
      vertebra M85.58
    solitary M85.40
      ankle M85.47-
      fibula M85.46-
      foot M85.47-
      hand M85.44-
      humerus M85.42-
      jaw M27.49
      neck M85.48
      pelvis M85.45-
      radius M85.43-
      rib M85.48
      shoulder M85.41-
      skull M85.48
      specified site NEC M85.48
      tibia M85.46-
      toe M85.47-
      ulna M85.43-
      vertebra M85.48
    specified type NEC M85.60
      ankle M85.67-
      foot M85.67-
      forearm M85.63-
      hand M85.64-
      jaw M27.40
        developmental
          (nonodontogenic) K09.1
        odontogenic K09.0
        latent M27.0
      lower leg M85.66-
      multiple site M85.69
      neck M85.68
      rib M85.68
      shoulder M85.61-

Cyst (continued)
  bone (continued)
    specified type (continued)
      skull M85.68
      specified site NEC M85.68
      thigh M85.65-
      toe M85.67-
      upper arm M85.62-
      vertebra M85.68
  brain (acquired) G93.0
    congenital Q04.6
    hydatid B67.99 [G94]
    third ventricle (colloid),
      congenital Q04.6
  branchial (cleft) Q18.0
  branchiogenic Q18.0
  breast (benign) (blue dome)
    (pedunculated) (solitary) N60.0-
    involution —see Dysplasia,
      mammary, specified type NEC
    sebaceous —see Dysplasia,
      mammary, specified type NEC
  broad ligament (benign) N83.8
  bronchogenic (mediastinal)
    (sequestration) J98.4
    congenital Q33.0
  buccal K09.8
  bulbourethral gland N36.8
  bursa, bursal NEC M71.30
    with rupture —see Rupture,
      synovium
    ankle M71.37-
    elbow M71.32-
    foot M71.37-
    hand M71.34-
    hip M71.35-
    multiple sites M71.39
    pharyngeal J39.2
    popliteal space —see Cyst, Baker's
    shoulder M71.31-
    specified site NEC M71.38
    wrist M71.33-
  calcifying odontogenic D16.5
    upper jaw (bone) (maxilla) D16.4
  canal of Nuck (female) N94.89
    congenital Q52.4
  canthus —see Cyst, conjunctiva
  carcinomatous —see Neoplasm,
    malignant, by site
  cauda equina G95.89
  cavum septi pellucidi —see Cyst,
    brain
  celomic (pericardium) Q24.8
  cerebellopontine (angle) —see
    Cyst, brain
  cerebellum —see Cyst, brain
  cerebral —see Cyst, brain
  cervical lateral Q18.0
  cervix NEC N88.8
    embryonic Q51.6
    nabothian N88.8
  chiasmal optic NEC —see
    Disorder, optic, chiasm
  chocolate (ovary) N80.10-
  choledochus, congenital Q44.4
  chorion O41.8X-
  choroid plexus G93.0
    congenital Q04.6
  ciliary body —see Cyst, iris
  clitoris N90.7
  colon K63.89
  common (bile) duct K83.5
  congenital NEC Q89.8
    adrenal gland Q89.1
    epiglottis Q31.8
    esophagus Q39.8
    fallopian tube Q50.4
    kidney Q61.00
      more than one (multiple) Q61.02
        specified as polycystic Q61.3
          adult type Q61.2

Cyst (continued)
  congenital (continued)
    kidney (continued)
      more than one (continued)
        specified as polycystic
          (continued)
          infantile type NEC
            Q61.19
            collecting duct dilation
              Q61.11
        solitary Q61.01
    larynx Q31.8
    liver Q44.6
    lung Q33.0
    mediastinum Q34.1
    ovary Q50.1
    oviduct Q50.4
    periurethral (tissue) Q64.79
    prepuce Q55.69
    salivary gland (any) Q38.4
    sublingual Q38.6
    submaxillary gland Q38.6
    thymus (gland) Q89.2
    tongue Q38.3
    ureterovesical orifice Q62.8
    vulva Q52.79
  conjunctiva H11.44-
  cornea H18.89-
  corpora quadrigemina G93.0
  corpus
    albicans N83.29-
    luteum (hemorrhagic) (ruptured)
      N83.1-
  Cowper's gland (benign) (infected)
    N36.8
  cranial meninges G93.0
  craniobuccal pouch E23.6
  craniopharyngeal pouch E23.6
  cystic duct K82.8
  Cysticercus —see Cysticercosis
  Dandy-Walker Q03.1
    with spina bifida —see Spina
      bifida
  dental (root) K04.8
    developmental K09.0
    eruption K09.0
    primordial K09.0
  dentigerous (mandible) (maxilla)
    K09.0
  dermoid —see Neoplasm, benign,
    by site
    with malignant transformation
      C56.-
    implantation
      external area or site (skin)
        NEC L72.0
      iris —see Cyst, iris,
        implantation
      vagina N89.8
      vulva N90.7
    mouth K09.8
    oral soft tissue K09.8
    sacrococcygeal —see Cyst,
      pilonidal
  developmental K09.1
    odontogenic K09.0
    oral region (nonodontogenic)
      K09.1
  ovary, ovarian Q50.1
  dura (cerebral) G93.0
    spinal G96.198
  ear (external) Q18.1
  echinococcal —see Echinococcus
  embryonic
    cervix uteri Q51.6
    fallopian tube Q50.4
    vagina Q52.4
  endometrium, endometrial (uterus)
    N85.8
  ectopic —see Endometriosis
  enterogenous Q43.8

Cyst *(continued)*
  epidermal, epidermoid (inclusion)
    (see also Cyst, skin) L72.0
    mouth K09.8
    oral soft tissue K09.8
  epididymis N50.3
  epiglottis J38.7
  epiphysis cerebri E34.8
  epithelial (inclusion) L72.0
  epoophoron Q50.5
  eruption K09.0
  esophagus K22.89
  ethmoid sinus J34.1
  external female genital organs NEC
      N90.7
  eye NEC H57.89
    congenital Q15.8
  eyelid (sebaceous) H02.829
    infected —*see* Hordeolum
    left H02.826
      lower H02.825
      upper H02.824
    right H02.823
      lower H02.822
      upper H02.821
  fallopian tube N83.8
    congenital Q50.4
  fimbrial (twisted) Q50.4
  fissural (oral region) K09.1
  follicle (graafian) (hemorrhagic)
      N83.0-
    nabothian N88.8
  follicular (atretic) (hemorrhagic)
      (ovarian) N83.0-
    dentigerous K09.0
    odontogenic K09.0
    skin L72.9
      specified NEC L72.8
  frontal sinus J34.1
  gallbladder K82.8
  ganglion —*see* Ganglion
  Gartner's duct Q52.4
  gingiva K09.0
  gland of Moll —*see* Cyst, eyelid
  globulomaxillary K09.1
  graafian follicle (hemorrhagic)
      N83.0-
  granulosal lutein (hemorrhagic)
      N83.1-
  hemangiomatous D18.00
    intra-abdominal D18.03
    intracranial D18.02
    skin D18.01
    specified site NEC D18.09
  hemorrhagic M27.49
  hydatid *(see also* Echinococcus)
      B67.90
    brain B67.99 *[G94]*
    liver *(see also* Cyst, liver,
      hydatid) B67.8
    lung NEC B67.99 *[J99]*
    Morgagni
      female Q50.5
      male (epididymal) Q55.4
        testicular Q55.29
    specified site NEC B67.99
  hymen N89.8
    embryonic Q52.4
  hypopharynx J39.2
  hypophysis, hypophyseal (duct)
      (recurrent) E23.6
    cerebri E23.6
  implantation (dermoid)
    external area or site (skin) NEC
        L72.0
    iris —*see* Cyst, iris,
        implantation
    vagina N89.8
    vulva N90.7
  incisive canal K09.1

Cyst *(continued)*
  inclusion (epidermal) (epithelial)
      (epidermoid) (squamous) L72.0
    not of skin - code under Cyst,
        by site
  intestine (large) (small) K63.89
  intracranial —*see* Cyst, brain
  intraligamentous —*see also*
      Disorder, ligament
    knee —*see* Derangement, knee
  intrasellar E23.6
  iris H21.309
    exudative H21.31-
    idiopathic H21.30-
    implantation H21.32-
    parasitic H21.33-
    pars plana (primary) H21.34-
      exudative H21.35-
  jaw (bone) M27.40
    aneurysmal M27.49
    developmental (odontogenic)
        K09.0
    fissural K09.1
    hemorrhagic M27.49
    traumatic M27.49
  joint NEC —*see* Disorder, joint,
      specified type NEC
  kidney N28.1
    acquired N28.1
    calyceal —*see* Hydronephrosis
    congenital Q61.00
      more than one (multiple) Q61.02
      specified as polycystic Q61.3
        adult type (autosomal
            dominant) Q61.2
        infantile type (autosomal
            recessive) NEC Q61.19
          collecting duct dilation
              Q61.11
    pyelogenic —*see*
        Hydronephrosis
    simple N28.1
    solitary (single) N28.1
      acquired N28.1
      congenital Q61.01
  labium (majus) (minus) N90.7
    sebaceous N90.7
  lacrimal —*see also* Disorder,
      lacrimal system, specified NEC
    gland H04.13-
    passages or sac —*see* Disorder,
        lacrimal system, specified NEC
  larynx J38.7
  lateral periodontal K09.0
  lens H27.8
    congenital Q12.8
  lip (gland) K13.0
  liver (idiopathic) (simple) K76.89
    congenital Q44.6
    hydatid B67.8
      granulosus B67.0
      multilocularis B67.5
  lung J98.4
    congenital Q33.0
    giant bullous J43.9
  lutein N83.1-
  lymphangiomatous D18.1
  lymphoepithelial, oral soft tissue
      K09.8
  macula —*see* Degeneration,
      macula, hole
  malignant —*see* Neoplasm,
      malignant, by site
  mammary gland —*see* Cyst, breast
  mandible M27.40
    dentigerous K09.0
    radicular K04.8
  maxilla M27.40
    dentigerous K09.0
    radicular K04.8
  medial, face and neck Q18.8

Cyst *(continued)*
  median
    anterior maxillary K09.1
    palatal K09.1
  mediastinum, congenital Q34.1
  meibomian (gland) —*see*
      Chalazion
    infected —*see* Hordeolum
  membrane, brain G93.0
  meninges (cerebral) G93.0
    spinal G96.198
  meniscus, knee —*see* Derangement,
      knee, meniscus, cystic
  mesentery, mesenteric K66.8
    chyle I89.8
  mesonephric duct
    female Q50.5
    male Q55.4
  milk N64.89
  Morgagni (hydatid)
    female Q50.5
    male (epididymal) Q55.4
      testicular Q55.29
  mouth K09.8
  Müllerian duct Q50.4
    appendix testis Q55.29
    cervix Q51.6
    fallopian tube Q50.4
    female Q50.4
    male Q55.29
    prostatic utricle Q55.4
    vagina (embryonal) Q52.4
  multilocular (ovary) D39.10
    benign —*see* Neoplasm, benign,
        by site
  myometrium N85.8
  nabothian (follicle) (ruptured)
      N88.8
  nasoalveolar K09.1
  nasolabial K09.1
  nasopalatine (anterior) (duct) K09.1
  nasopharynx J39.2
  neoplastic —*see* Neoplasm,
      uncertain behavior, by site
    benign —*see* Neoplasm, benign,
        by site
  nerve root
    cervical G96.191
    lumbar G96.191
    sacral G96.191
    thoracic G96.191
  nervous system NEC G96.89
  neuroenteric (congenital) Q06.8
  nipple —*see* Cyst, breast
  nose (turbinates) J34.1
    sinus J34.1
  odontogenic, developmental K09.0
  omentum (lesser) K66.8
    congenital Q45.8
  ora serrata —*see* Cyst, retina, ora
      serrata
  oral
    region K09.9
      developmental
          (nonodontogenic) K09.1
      specified NEC K09.8
    soft tissue K09.9
      specified NEC K09.8
  orbit H05.81-
  ovary, ovarian (twisted) N83.20-
    adherent N83.20-
    chocolate N80.10-
    corpus
      albicans N83.29-
      luteum (hemorrhagic) N83.1-
    dermoid D27.9
    developmental Q50.1
    due to failure of involution NEC
        N83.20-
    endometrial N80.10-

Cyst *(continued)*
  ovary, ovarian *(continued)*
    follicular (graafian)
        (hemorrhagic) N83.0-
    hemorrhagic N83.20-
      in pregnancy or childbirth
          O34.8-
        with obstructed labor O65.5
    multilocular D39.10
    pseudomucinous D27.9
    retention N83.29-
    serous N83.20-
    specified NEC N83.29-
    theca lutein (hemorrhagic)
        N83.1-
    tuberculous A18.18
  oviduct N83.8
  palate (median) (fissural) K09.1
  palatine papilla (jaw) K09.1
  pancreas, pancreatic (hemorrhagic)
      (true) K86.2
    congenital Q45.2
    false K86.3
  paralabral
    hip M24.85-
    shoulder S43.43-
  paramesonephric duct Q50.4
    female Q50.4
    male Q55.29
  paranephric N28.1
  paraphysis, cerebri, congenital
      Q04.6
  parasitic B89
  parathyroid (gland) E21.4
  paratubal N83.8
  paraurethral duct N36.8
  paroophoron Q50.5
  parotid gland K11.6
  parovarian Q50.5
  pelvis, female N94.89
    in pregnancy or childbirth O34.8-
      causing obstructed labor O65.5
  penis (sebaceous) N48.89
  periapical K04.8
  pericardial (congenital) Q24.8
    acquired (secondary) I31.8
  pericoronal K09.0
  perineural G96.191
  periodontal K04.8
    lateral K09.0
  peripelvic (lymphatic) N28.1
  peritoneum K66.8
    chylous I89.8
  periventricular, acquired, newborn
      P91.1
  pharynx (wall) J39.2
  pilar L72.11
  pilonidal (infected) (rectum)
      L05.91
    with abscess L05.01
    malignant C44.59-
  pituitary (duct) (gland) E23.6
  placenta O43.19-
  pleura J94.8
  popliteal —*see* Cyst, Baker's
  porencephalic Q04.6
    acquired G93.0
  postanal (infected) —*see* Cyst,
      pilonidal
  postmastoidectomy cavity
      (mucosal) —*see* Complications,
      postmastoidectomy, cyst
  preauricular Q18.1
  prepuce N47.4
    congenital Q55.69
  primordial (jaw) K09.0
  prostate N42.83
  pseudomucinous (ovary) D27.9
  pupillary, miotic H21.27-
  radicular (residual) K04.8
  radiculodental K04.8

Cyst (continued)
- ranular K11.8
- Rathke's pouch E23.6
- rectum (epithelium) (mucous) K62.89
- renal —see Cyst, kidney
- residual (radicular) K04.8
- retention (ovary) N83.29-
  - salivary gland K11.6
- retina H33.19-
  - ora serrata H33.11-
  - parasitic H33.12-
- retroperitoneal K68.9
- sacrococcygeal (dermoid) —see Cyst, pilonidal
- salivary gland or duct (mucous extravasation or retention) K11.6
- Sampson's N80.10-
- sclera H15.89
- scrotum L72.9
- sebaceous L72.3
- sebaceous (duct) (gland) L72.3
  - breast —see Dysplasia, mammary, specified type NEC
  - eyelid —see Cyst, eyelid
  - genital organ NEC
    - female N94.89
    - male N50.89
  - scrotum L72.3
- semilunar cartilage (knee) (multiple) —see Derangement, knee, meniscus, cystic
- seminal vesicle N50.89
- serous (ovary) N83.20-
- sinus (accessory) (nasal) J34.1
- Skene's gland N36.8
- skin L72.9
  - breast —see Dysplasia, mammary, specified type NEC
  - epidermal, epidermoid L72.0
  - epithelial L72.0
  - eyelid —see Cyst, eyelid
  - genital organ NEC
    - female N90.7
    - male N50.89
  - inclusion L72.0
  - scrotum L72.9
  - sebaceous L72.3
  - sweat gland or duct L74.8
- solitary
  - bone —see Cyst, bone, solitary
  - jaw M27.40
  - kidney N28.1
- spermatic cord N50.89
- sphenoid sinus J34.1
- spinal meninges G96.198
- spleen NEC D73.4
  - congenital Q89.09
  - hydatid (see also Echinococcus) B67.99 [D77]
- Stafne's M27.0
- subarachnoid intrasellar R93.0
- subcutaneous, pheomycotic (chromomycotic) B43.2
- subdural (cerebral) G93.0
  - spinal cord G96.198
- sublingual gland K11.6
- submandibular gland K11.6
- submaxillary gland K11.6
- suburethral N36.8
- suprarenal gland E27.8
- suprasellar —see Cyst, brain
- sweat gland or duct L74.8
- synovial —see also Cyst, bursa
  - ruptured —see Rupture, synovium
- Tarlov G96.191
- tarsal —see Chalazion
- tendon (sheath) —see Disorder, tendon, specified type NEC
- testis N44.2
  - tunica albuginea N44.1

Cyst (continued)
- theca lutein (ovary) N83.1-
- Thornwaldt's J39.2
- thymus (gland) E32.8
- thyroglossal duct (infected) (persistent) Q89.2
- thyrolingual duct (infected) (persistent) Q89.2
- thyroid (gland) E04.1
- tongue K14.8
- tonsil J35.8
- tooth —see Cyst, dental
- Tornwaldt's J39.2
- trichilemmal (proliferating) L72.12
- trichodermal L72.12
- tubal (fallopian) N83.8
  - inflammatory —see Salpingitis, chronic
- tubo-ovarian N83.8
  - inflammatory N70.13
- tunica
  - albuginea testis N44.1
  - vaginalis N50.89
- turbinate (nose) J34.1
- Tyson's gland N48.89
- urachus, congenital Q64.4
- ureter N28.89
- ureterovesical orifice N28.89
- urethra, urethral (gland) N36.8
- uterine ligament N83.8
- uterus (body) (corpus) (recurrent) N85.8
  - embryonic Q51.818
    - cervix Q51.6
- vagina, vaginal (implantation) (inclusion) (squamous cell) (wall) N89.8
  - embryonic Q52.4
- vallecula, vallecular (epiglottis) J38.7
- vesical (orifice) N32.89
- vitreous body H43.89
- vulva (implantation) (inclusion) N90.7
  - congenital Q52.79
  - sebaceous gland N90.7
- vulvovaginal gland N90.7
- wolffian
  - female Q50.5
  - male Q55.4

Cystadenocarcinoma —see Neoplasm, malignant, by site
- bile duct C22.1
- endometrioid —see Neoplasm, malignant, by site
  - specified site —see Neoplasm, malignant, by site
  - unspecified site
    - female C56.9
    - male C61
- mucinous
  - papillary
    - specified site —see Neoplasm, malignant, by site
    - unspecified site C56.9
  - specified site —see Neoplasm, malignant, by site
  - unspecified site C56.9
- papillary
  - mucinous
    - specified site —see Neoplasm, malignant, by site
    - unspecified site C56.9
  - pseudomucinous
    - specified site —see Neoplasm, malignant, by site
    - unspecified site C56.9
  - serous
    - specified site —see Neoplasm, malignant, by site
    - unspecified site C56.9

Cystadenocarcinoma (continued)
- papillary (continued)
  - specified site —see Neoplasm, malignant, by site
  - unspecified site C56.9
- pseudomucinous
  - papillary
    - specified site —see Neoplasm, malignant, by site
    - unspecified site C56.9
  - specified site —see Neoplasm, malignant, by site
  - unspecified site C56.9
- serous
  - papillary
    - specified site —see Neoplasm, malignant, by site
    - unspecified site C56.9
  - specified site —see Neoplasm, malignant, by site
  - unspecified site C56.9

Cystadenofibroma
- clear cell —see Neoplasm, benign, by site
- endometrioid D27.9
  - borderline malignancy D39.1-
  - malignant C56.-
- mucinous
  - specified site —see Neoplasm, benign, by site
  - unspecified site D27.9
- serous
  - specified site —see Neoplasm, benign, by site
  - unspecified site D27.9
- specified site —see Neoplasm, benign, by site
- unspecified site D27.9

Cystadenoma —see also Neoplasm, benign, by site
- bile duct D13.4
- endometrioid —see Neoplasm, benign, by site
  - borderline malignancy —see Neoplasm, uncertain behavior, by site
- malignant —see Neoplasm, malignant, by site
- mucinous
  - borderline malignancy
    - ovary C56.-
    - specified site NEC —see Neoplasm, uncertain behavior, by site
    - unspecified site C56.9
  - papillary
    - borderline malignancy
      - ovary C56.-
      - specified site NEC —see Neoplasm, uncertain behavior, by site
      - unspecified site C56.9
    - specified site —see Neoplasm, benign, by site
    - unspecified site D27.9
  - specified site —see Neoplasm, benign, by site
  - unspecified site D27.9
- papillary
  - borderline malignancy
    - ovary C56.-
    - specified site NEC —see Neoplasm, uncertain behavior, by site
    - unspecified site C56.9
  - lymphomatosum
    - specified site —see Neoplasm, benign, by site
    - unspecified site D11.9

Cystadenoma (continued)
- papillary (continued)
  - mucinous
    - borderline malignancy
      - ovary C56.-
      - specified site NEC —see Neoplasm, uncertain behavior, by site
      - unspecified site C56.9
    - specified site —see Neoplasm, benign, by site
    - unspecified site D27.9
  - pseudomucinous
    - borderline malignancy
      - ovary C56.-
      - specified site NEC —see Neoplasm, uncertain behavior, by site
      - unspecified site C56.9
    - specified site —see Neoplasm, benign, by site
    - unspecified site D27.9
  - serous
    - borderline malignancy
      - ovary C56.-
      - specified site NEC —see Neoplasm, uncertain behavior, by site
      - unspecified site C56.9
    - specified site —see Neoplasm, benign, by site
    - unspecified site D27.9
  - specified site —see Neoplasm, benign, by site
  - unspecified site D27.9
- pseudomucinous
  - borderline malignancy
    - ovary C56.-
    - specified site NEC —see Neoplasm, uncertain behavior, by site
    - unspecified site C56.9
  - papillary
    - borderline malignancy
      - ovary C56.-
      - specified site NEC —see Neoplasm, uncertain behavior, by site
      - unspecified site C56.9
    - specified site —see Neoplasm, benign, by site
    - unspecified site D27.9
  - specified site —see Neoplasm, benign, by site
  - unspecified site D27.9
- serous
  - borderline malignancy
    - ovary C56.-
    - specified site NEC —see Neoplasm, uncertain behavior, by site
    - unspecified site C56.9
  - papillary
    - borderline malignancy
      - ovary C56.-
      - specified site NEC —see Neoplasm, uncertain behavior, by site
      - unspecified site C56.9
    - specified site —see Neoplasm, benign, by site
    - unspecified site D27.9
  - specified site —see Neoplasm, benign, by site
  - unspecified site D27.9

Cystathionine synthase deficiency E72.11

Cystathioninemia E72.19

Cystathioninuria E72.19

Cystic —*see also* condition
  breast (chronic) —*see* Mastopathy, cystic
  corpora lutea (hemorrhagic) N83.1-
  duct —*see* condition
  eyeball (congenital) Q11.0
  fibrosis —*see* Fibrosis, cystic
  kidney (congenital) Q61.9
    adult type Q61.2
    infantile type NEC Q61.19
      collecting duct dilatation Q61.11
    medullary Q61.5
  liver, congenital Q44.6
  lung disease J98.4
    congenital Q33.0
  mastitis, chronic —*see* Mastopathy, cystic
  medullary, kidney Q61.5
  meniscus —*see* Derangement, knee, meniscus, cystic
  ovary N83.20-
Cysticercosis, cysticerciasis B69.9
  with
    epileptiform fits B69.0
    myositis B69.81
  brain B69.0
  central nervous system B69.0
  cerebral B69.0
  ocular B69.1
  specified NEC B69.89
Cysticercus cellulose infestation —*see* Cysticercosis
Cystinosis (malignant) E72.04
Cystinuria E72.01
Cystitis (exudative) (hemorrhagic) (septic) (suppurative) N30.90
  with
    fibrosis —*see* Cystitis, chronic, interstitial
    hematuria N30.91
    leukoplakia —*see* Cystitis, chronic, interstitial
    malakoplakia —*see* Cystitis, chronic, interstitial
    metaplasia —*see* Cystitis, chronic, interstitial
    prostatitis N41.3
  acute N30.00
    with hematuria N30.01
    of trigone N30.30
      with hematuria N30.31
  allergic —*see* Cystitis, specified type NEC
  amebic A06.81
  bilharzial B65.9 [N33]
  blennorrhagic (gonococcal) A54.01
  bullous —*see* Cystitis, specified type NEC
  calculus N21.0
  chlamydial A56.01
  chronic N30.20
    with hematuria N30.21
    interstitial N30.10
      with hematuria N30.11
    of trigone N30.30
      with hematuria N30.31
    specified NEC N30.20
      with hematuria N30.21
  cystic (a) —*see* Cystitis, specified type NEC
  diphtheritic A36.85
  echinococcal
    granulosus B67.39
    multilocularis B67.69
  emphysematous —*see* Cystitis, specified type NEC
  encysted —*see* Cystitis, specified type NEC

Cystitis (*continued*)
  eosinophilic —*see* Cystitis, specified type NEC
  follicular —*see* Cystitis, of trigone
  gangrenous —*see* Cystitis, specified type NEC
  glandularis —*see* Cystitis, specified type NEC
  gonococcal A54.01
  incrusted —*see* Cystitis, specified type NEC
  interstitial (chronic) —*see* Cystitis, chronic, interstitial
  irradiation N30.40
    with hematuria N30.41
  irritation —*see* Cystitis, specified type NEC
  malignant —*see* Cystitis, specified type NEC
  of trigone N30.30
    with hematuria N30.31
  panmural —*see* Cystitis, chronic, interstitial
  polyposa —*see* Cystitis, specified type NEC
  prostatic N41.3
  puerperal (postpartum) O86.22
  radiation —*see* Cystitis, irradiation
  specified type NEC N30.80
    with hematuria N30.81
  subacute —*see* Cystitis, chronic
  submucous —*see* Cystitis, chronic, interstitial
  syphilitic (late) A52.76
  trichomonal A59.03
  tuberculous A18.12
  ulcerative —*see* Cystitis, chronic, interstitial
Cystocele (-urethrocele)
  female N81.10
    with prolapse of uterus —*see* Prolapse, uterus
    lateral N81.12
    midline N81.11
    paravaginal N81.12
  in pregnancy or childbirth O34.8-
    causing obstructed labor O65.5
  male N32.89
Cystolithiasis N21.0
Cystoma —*see also* Neoplasm, benign, by site
  endometrial, ovary N80.10-
  mucinous
    specified site —*see* Neoplasm, benign, by site
    unspecified site D27.9
  serous
    specified site —*see* Neoplasm, benign, by site
    unspecified site D27.9
  simple (ovary) N83.29-
Cystoplegia N31.2
Cystoptosis N32.89
Cystopyelitis —*see* Pyelonephritis
Cystorrhagia N32.89
Cystosarcoma phyllodes D48.6-
  benign D24-
  malignant —*see* Neoplasm, breast, malignant
Cystostomy
  attention to Z43.5
  complication —*see* Complications, cystostomy
  status Z93.50
    appendico-vesicostomy Z93.52
    cutaneous Z93.51
    specified NEC Z93.59

Cystourethritis —*see* Urethritis
Cystourethrocele —*see also* Cystocele
  female N81.10
    with uterine prolapse —*see* Prolapse, uterus
    lateral N81.12
    midline N81.11
    paravaginal N81.12
  male N32.89
Cytomegalic inclusion disease
  congenital P35.1
Cytomegalovirus infection B25.9
Cytomycosis (reticuloendothelial) B39.4
Cytopenia D75.9
  refractory
    with multilineage dysplasia D46.A
    and ring sideroblasts (RCMD RS) D46.B
Czerny's disease (periodic hydrarthrosis of the knee) —*see* Effusion, joint, knee

D

Daae (-Finsen) **disease** (epidemic pleurodynia) B33.0
Da Costa's syndrome F45.8
Dabney's grip B33.0
Dacryoadenitis, dacryadenitis H04.00-
  acute H04.01-
  chronic H04.02-
Dacryocystitis H04.30-
  acute H04.32-
  chronic H04.41-
  neonatal P39.1
  phlegmonous H04.31-
  syphilitic A52.71
    congenital (early) A50.01
  trachomatous, active A71.1
    sequelae (late effect) B94.0
Dacryocystoblenorrhea —*see* Inflammation, lacrimal, passages, chronic
Dacryocystocele —*see* Disorder, lacrimal system, changes
Dacryolith, dacryolithiasis H04.51-
Dacryoma —*see* Disorder, lacrimal system, changes
Dacryopericystitis —*see* Dacryocystitis
Dacryops H04.11-
Dacryostenosis —*see also* Stenosis, lacrimal
  congenital Q10.5
Dactylitis
  bone —*see* Osteomyelitis
  sickle-cell D57.00
    Hb C D57.219
    Hb SS D57.00
    specified NEC D57.819
  skin L08.9
  syphilitic A52.77
  tuberculous A18.03
Dactylolysis spontanea (ainhum) L94.6
Dactylosymphysis Q70.9
  fingers —*see* Syndactylism, complex, fingers
  toes —*see* Syndactylism, complex, toes

Damage
  arteriosclerotic —*see* Arteriosclerosis
  brain (nontraumatic) G93.9
    anoxic, hypoxic G93.1
      resulting from a procedure G97.82
    child NEC G80.9
    due to birth injury P11.2
  cardiorenal (vascular) —*see* Hypertension, cardiorenal
  cerebral NEC —*see* Damage, brain
  coccyx, complicating delivery O71.6
  coronary —*see* Disease, heart, ischemic
  deep tissue, pressure-induced —*see also* L89 with final character .6
  eye, birth injury P15.3
  liver (nontraumatic) K76.9
    alcoholic K70.9
    due to drugs —*see* Disease, liver, toxic
    toxic —*see* Disease, liver, toxic
  lung
    dabbing (related) U07.0
    electronic cigarette (related) U07.0
    vaping (associated) (device) (product) (use) U07.0
  medication T88.7
  organ
    dabbing (related) U07.0
    electronic cigarette (related) U07.0
    vaping (associated) (device) (product) (use) U07.0
  pelvic
    joint or ligament, during delivery O71.6
    organ NEC
      during delivery O71.5
      following ectopic or molar pregnancy O08.6
  renal —*see* Disease, renal
  subendocardium, subendocardial —*see* Degeneration, myocardial
  vascular I99.9
Dana-Putnam syndrome (subacute combined sclerosis with pernicious anemia) —*see* Degeneration, combined
Danbolt (-Cross) **syndrome** (acrodermatitis enteropathica) E83.2
Dandruff L21.0
Dandy-Walker syndrome Q03.1
  with spina bifida —*see* Spina bifida
Danlos' syndrome (*see also* Syndrome, Ehlers-Danlos) Q79.60
Darier (-White) **disease** (congenital) Q82.8
  meaning erythema annulare centrifugum L53.1
Darier-Roussy sarcoid D86.3
Darling's disease or histoplasmosis B39.4
Darwin's tubercle Q17.8
Dawson's (inclusion body) **encephalitis** A81.1
De Beurmann (-Gougerot) **disease** B42.1
De la Tourette's syndrome F95.2
De Lange's syndrome Q87.19
De Morgan's spots (senile angiomas) I78.1

85

De Quervain's
disease (tendon sheath) M65.4
syndrome E34.51
thyroiditis (subacute granulomatous thyroiditis) E06.1

De Toni-Fanconi (-Debré) **syndrome** E72.09
with cystinosis E72.04

Dead
fetus, retained (mother) O36.4
early pregnancy O02.1
labyrinth H83.2
ovum, retained O02.0

Deaf nonspeaking NEC H91.3

Deafmutism (acquired) (congenital) NEC H91.3
hysterical F44.6
syphilitic, congenital (see also subcategory H94.8) A50.09

Deafness (acquired) (complete) (hereditary) (partial) H91.9-
with blue sclera and fragility of bone Q78.0
auditory fatigue —see Deafness, specified type NEC
aviation T70.0
nerve injury —see Injury, nerve, acoustic, specified type NEC
boilermaker's —see subcategory H83.3
central —see Deafness, sensorineural
conductive H90.2
and sensorineural
mixed H90.8
bilateral H90.6
bilateral H90.0
unilateral H90.1-
with restricted hearing on the contralateral side H90.A-
congenital H90.5
with blue sclera and fragility of bone Q78.0
due to toxic agents —see Deafness, ototoxic
emotional (hysterical) F44.6
functional (hysterical) F44.6
high frequency H91.9-
hysterical F44.6
low frequency H91.9-
mental R48.8
mixed conductive and sensorineural H90.8
bilateral H90.6
unilateral H90.7-
nerve —see Deafness, sensorineural
neural —see Deafness, sensorineural
noise-induced —see also subcategory H83.3
nerve injury —see Injury, nerve, acoustic, specified type NEC
nonspeaking H91.3
ototoxic H91.0
perceptive —see Deafness, sensorineural
psychogenic (hysterical) F44.6
sensorineural H90.5
and conductive
mixed H90.8
bilateral H90.6
bilateral H90.3
unilateral H90.4-
with restricted hearing on the contralateral side H90.A-
sensory —see Deafness, sensorineural
specified type NEC H91.8
sudden (idiopathic) H91.2-
syphilitic A52.15

Deafness (continued)
transient ischemic H93.01-
traumatic —see Injury, nerve, acoustic, specified type NEC
word (developmental) H93.25

Death (cause unknown) (of) (unexplained) (unspecified cause) R99
brain G93.82
cardiac (sudden) (with successful resuscitation) - see Arrest, cardiac
family history of Z82.41
personal history of Z86.74
family member (assumed) Z63.4

Debility (chronic) (general) (nervous) R53.81
congenital or neonatal NOS P96.9
nervous R53.81
old age R54
senile R54

Débove's disease (splenomegaly) R16.1

Debt, burdensome Z59.86

Decalcification
bone —see Osteoporosis
teeth K03.89

Decapsulation, kidney N28.89

Decay
dental —see Caries, dental
senile R54
tooth, teeth —see Caries, dental

Deciduitis (acute)
following ectopic or molar pregnancy O08.0

Decline (general) —see Debility
cognitive, age-associated R41.81

Decompensation
cardiac (acute) (chronic) —see Disease, heart
cardiovascular —see Disease, cardiovascular
heart —see Disease, heart
hepatic —see Failure, hepatic
myocardial (acute) (chronic) —see Disease, heart
respiratory J98.8

Decompression sickness T70.3

Decrease (d)
absolute neutrophile count —see Neutropenia
blood
platelets —see Thrombocytopenia
pressure R03.1
due to shock following injury T79.4
operation T81.19
estrogen E28.39
postablative E89.40
asymptomatic E89.40
symptomatic E89.41
fragility of erythrocytes D58.8
function
lipase (pancreatic) K90.3
ovary in hypopituitarism E23.0
parenchyma of pancreas K86.89
pituitary (gland) (anterior) (lobe) E23.0
posterior (lobe) E23.0
functional activity R68.89
glucose R73.09
hematocrit R71.0
hemoglobin R71.0
leukocytes D72.819
specified NEC D72.818
libido R68.82

Decrease (continued)
lymphocytes D72.810
platelets D69.6
respiration, due to shock following injury T79.4
sexual desire R68.82
tear secretion NEC —see Syndrome, dry eye
tolerance
fat K90.49
glucose R73.09
pancreatic K90.3
salt and water E87.8
vision NEC H54.7
white blood cell count D72.819
specified NEC D72.818

Decubitus (ulcer) —see Ulcer, pressure, by site
cervix N86

Deepening acetabulum —see Derangement, joint, specified type NEC, hip

Defect, defective Q89.9
3-beta-hydroxysteroid dehydrogenase E25.0
11-hydroxylase E25.0
21-hydroxylase E25.0
abdominal wall, congenital Q79.59
antibody immunodeficiency D80.9
aorticopulmonary septum Q21.4
atrial septal Q21.10
coronary sinus Q21.13
following acute myocardial infarction (current complication) I23.1
ostium primum type (type I) Q21.20
with
common atrioventricular valves and moderate or larger inlet VSD Q21.23
separate atrioventricular valves Q21.21
and small or restrictive inlet VSD Q21.22
ostium secundum type (patent persistent) (type II) Q21.11
sinus venosus Q21.16
inferior Q21.15
superior Q21.14
specified NEC Q21.19
vena cava type
inferior Q21.15
superior Q21.14
atrioventricular
canal Q21.20
septal
common Q21.23
complete Q21.23
incomplete Q21.21
intermediate Q21.22
partial Q21.21
transitional Q21.22
unspecified as to partial or complete Q21.20
septum Q21.20
auricular septal Q21.10
bilirubin excretion NEC E80.6
biosynthesis, androgen (testicular) E29.1
bulbar septum Q21.0
catalase E80.3
cell membrane receptor complex (CR3) D71
circulation I99.9
congenital Q28.9
newborn Q28.9
coagulation (factor) (see also Deficiency, factor) D68.9

Defect, defective (continued)
coagulation (factor) (continued)
with
COVID-19 associated coagulopathy D68.8
ectopic pregnancy O08.1
molar pregnancy O08.1
acquired D68.4
antepartum with hemorrhage —see Hemorrhage, antepartum, with coagulation defect
due to
liver disease D68.4
vitamin K deficiency D68.4
hereditary NEC D68.2
intrapartum O67.0
newborn, transient P61.6
postpartum O99.13
with hemorrhage O72.3
specified type NEC D68.8
complement system D84.1
conduction (heart) I45.9
bone —see Deafness, conductive
congenital, organ or site not listed —see Anomaly, by site
coronary sinus Q21.13
cushion, endocardial Q21.20
common Q21.23
incomplete Q21.21
intermediate Q21.22
transitional Q21.22
degradation, glycoprotein E77.1
dental bridge, crown, fillings —see Defect, dental restoration
dental restoration K08.50
specified NEC K08.59
dentin (hereditary) K00.5
Descemet's membrane, congenital Q13.89
developmental —see also Anomaly
cauda equina Q06.3
diaphragm
with elevation, eventration or hernia —see Hernia, diaphragm
congenital Q79.1
with hernia Q79.0
gross (with hernia) Q79.0
ectodermal, congenital Q82.9
Eisenmenger's Q21.8
enzyme
catalase E80.3
peroxidase E80.3
esophagus, congenital Q39.9
extensor retinaculum M62.89
fibrin polymerization D68.2
filling
bladder R93.41
kidney R93.42-
renal pelvis R93.41
stomach R93.3
ureter R93.41
urinary organs, specified NEC R93.49
GABA (gamma aminobutyric acid) metabolic E72.81
Gerbode Q21.0
glucose transport, blood-brain barrier E74.810
glycoprotein degradation E77.1
Hageman (factor) D68.2
hearing —see Deafness
high grade F70
home, technical, preventing adequate care Z59.19
interatrial septal Q21.19
interauricular septal Q21.19
interventricular septal Q21.0
with dextroposition of aorta, pulmonary stenosis and hypertrophy of right ventricle Q21.3

Defect, defective *(continued)*
  interventricular septal *(continued)*
    in tetralogy of Fallot Q21.3
  intervertebral annular fibrosis *(see also* Disease, intervertebral disc, by site)* M51.9
    lumbar M51.A0
      large M51.A2
      small M51.A1
    lumbosacral M51.A3
      large M51.A5
      small M51.A4
  learning (specific) —*see* Disorder, learning
  lymphocyte function antigen-1 (LFA-1) D84.0
  lysosomal enzyme, post-translational modification E77.0
  major osseous M89.70
    ankle M89.77-
    carpus M89.74-
    clavicle M89.71-
    femur M89.75-
    fibula M89.76-
    fingers M89.74-
    foot M89.77-
    forearm M89.73-
    hand M89.74-
    humerus M89.72-
    lower leg M89.76-
    metacarpus M89.74-
    metatarsus M89.77-
    multiple sites M89.79
    pelvic region M89.75-
    pelvis M89.75-
    radius M89.73-
    scapula M89.71-
    shoulder region M89.71-
    specified NEC M89.78
    tarsus M89.77-
    thigh M89.75-
    tibia M89.76-
    toes M89.77-
    ulna M89.73-
  mental —*see* Disability, intellectual
  modification, lysosomal enzymes, post-translational E77.0
  obstructive, congenital
    renal pelvis Q62.39
    ureter Q62.39
      atresia —*see* Atresia, ureter
      cecoureterocele Q62.32
      megaureter Q62.2
      orthotopic ureterocele Q62.31
  osseous, major M89.70
    ankle M89.77-
    carpus M89.74-
    clavicle M89.71-
    femur M89.75-
    fibula M89.76-
    fingers M89.74-
    foot M89.77-
    forearm M89.73-
    hand M89.74-
    humerus M89.72-
    lower leg M89.76-
    metacarpus M89.74-
    metatarsus M89.77-
    multiple sites M89.9
    pelvic region M89.75-
    pelvis M89.75-
    radius M89.73-
    scapula M89.71-
    shoulder region M89.71-
    specified NEC M89.78
    tarsus M89.77-
    thigh M89.75-
    tibia M89.76-
    toes M89.77-
    ulna M89.73-

Defect, defective *(continued)*
  osteochondral NEC *(see also* Deformity*)* M95.8
  ostium
    primum Q21.20
    secundum Q21.11
  peroxidase E80.3
  placental blood supply —*see* Insufficiency, placental
  platelets, qualitative D69.1
    constitutional —*see* Disease, von Willebrand
  postural NEC, spine —*see* Dorsopathy, deforming
  qualitative, of von Willebrand factor
    with
      decreased platelet adhesion and selective deficiency of high-molecular-weight multimers *(see also* Disease, von Willebrand*)* D68.020
      defective platelet adhesion with a normal size distribution of von Willebrand factor multimers *(see also* Disease, von Willebrand*)* D68.022
      defective von Willebrand factor to factor VIII binding *(see also* Disease, von Willebrand*)* D68.023
      high-molecular-weight von Willebrand factor loss *(see also* Disease, von Willebrand*)* D68.021
      hyper-adhesive forms *(see also* Disease, von Willebrand*)* D68.021
      increased affinity for platelet glycoprotein Ib *(see also* Disease, von Willebrand*)* D68.021
      markedly decreased affinity for factor VIII *(see also* Disease, von Willebrand*)* D68.023
    in von Willebrand factor function, with no further subtyping *(see also* Disease, von Willebrand*)* D68.029
  reduction
    limb Q73.8
      lower Q72.9-
        absence —*see* Agenesis, leg
          foot —*see* Agenesis, foot
        longitudinal
          femur Q72.4-
          fibula Q72.6-
          tibia Q72.5-
        specified type NEC Q72.89-
        split foot Q72.7-
      specified type NEC Q73.8
      upper Q71.9-
        absence —*see* Agenesis, arm
          forearm —*see* Agenesis, forearm
          hand —*see* Agenesis, hand
        lobster-claw hand Q71.6-
        longitudinal
          radius Q71.4-
          ulna Q71.5-
        specified type NEC Q71.89-
    renal pelvis Q63.8
      obstructive Q62.39
    respiratory system, congenital Q34.9
  restoration, dental K08.50
    specified NEC K08.59

Defect, defective *(continued)*
  retinal nerve bundle fibers H35.89
  septal (heart) NOS Q21.9
    acquired (atrial) (auricular) (ventricular) (old) I51.0
    atrial *(see also* Defect, atrial septal*)* Q21.10
      concurrent with acute myocardial infarction —*see* Infarct, myocardium
      following acute myocardial infarction (current complication) I23.1
    ventricular *(see also* Defect, ventricular septal*)* Q21.0
    sinus venosus *(see also* Defect, atrial septal, sinus venosus*)* Q21.16
  speech —*see* disorder speech
    developmental F80.9
    specified NEC R47.89
  Taussig-Bing (aortic transposition and overriding pulmonary artery) Q20.1
  teeth, wedge K03.1
  vascular (local) I99.9
    congenital Q27.9
  ventricular septal Q21.0
    concurrent with acute myocardial infarction —*see* Infarct, myocardium
    following acute myocardial infarction (current complication) I23.2
    in tetralogy of Fallot Q21.3
  vision NEC H54.7
  visual field H53.40
    bilateral
      heteronymous H53.47
      homonymous H53.46-
    generalized contraction H53.48-
    localized
      arcuate H53.43-
      scotoma (central area) H53.41-
        blind spot area H53.42-
      sector H53.43-
      specified type NEC H53.45-
  voice R49.9
    specified NEC R49.8
  wedge, tooth, teeth (abrasion) K03.1

Deferentitis N49.1
  gonorrheal (acute) (chronic) A54.23

Defibrination (syndrome) D65
  antepartum —*see* Hemorrhage, antepartum, with coagulation defect, disseminated intravascular coagulation
  following ectopic or molar pregnancy O08.1
  intrapartum O67.0
  newborn P60
  postpartum O72.3

Deficiency, deficient
  3-beta hydroxysteroid dehydrogenase E25.0
  5-alpha reductase (with male pseudohermaphroditism) E29.1
  11-hydroxylase E25.0
  21-hydroxylase E25.0
  AADC (aromatic L-amino acid decarboxylase) E70.81
  abdominal muscle syndrome Q79.4
  accelerator globulin (Ac G) (blood) D68.2
  AC globulin (congenital) (hereditary) D68.2
    acquired D68.4

Deficiency, deficient *(continued)*
  acid phosphatase E83.39
  acid sphingomyelinase (ASMD) E75.249
    type
      A E75.240
      A/B E75.244
      B E75.241
  activating factor (blood) D68.2
  ADA2 (adenosine deaminase 2) D81.32
  adenosine deaminase (ADA) D81.30
    with severe combined immuno-deficiency (SCID) D81.32
    partial (type 1) D81.39
    specified NEC D81.39
    type 1 (without SCID) (without severe combined immunodeficiency) D81.39
    type 2 D81.32
  aldolase (hereditary) E74.19
  alpha-1-antitrypsin E88.01
  amino-acids E72.9
  anemia —*see* Anemia
  aneurin E51.9
  antibody with
    hyperimmunoglobulinemia D80.6
    near-normal immunoglobins D80.6
  antidiuretic hormone E23.2
  anti-hemophilic
    factor (A) D66
      B D67
      C D68.1
    globulin (AHG) NEC D66
  antithrombin (antithrombin III) D68.59
  aromatic L-amino acid decarboxylase (AADC) E70.81
  ascorbic acid E54
  attention (disorder) (syndrome) F98.8
    with hyperactivity —*see* Disorder, attention-deficit hyperactivity
  autoprothrombin
    I D68.2
    II D67
    C D68.2
  beta-glucuronidase E76.29
  biotin E53.8
  biotin-dependent carboxylase D81.819
  biotinidase D81.810
  brancher enzyme (amylopectinosis) E74.03
  calciferol E55.9
    with
      adult osteomalacia M83.8
      rickets —*see* Rickets
  calcium (dietary) E58
  calorie, severe E43
    with marasmus E41
      and kwashiorkor E42
  cardiac —*see* Insufficiency, myocardial
  carnitine E71.40
    due to
      hemodialysis E71.43
      inborn errors of metabolism E71.42
      Valproic acid therapy E71.43
    iatrogenic E71.43
    muscle palmityltransferase E71.314
    primary E71.41
    secondary E71.448
  carotene E50.9
  central nervous system G96.89

87

Deficiency, deficient (continued)
ceruloplasmin (Wilson) E83.01
choline E53.8
Christmas factor D67
chromium E61.4
chronic neurovisceral acid
 sphingomyelinase E75.244
chronic visceral acid
 sphingomyelinase E75.241
clotting (blood) (see also Deficiency,
 coagulation factor) D68.9
clotting factor NEC (hereditary)
 (see also Deficiency, factor)
 D68.2
coagulation NOS D68.9
 with
  ectopic pregnancy O08.1
  molar pregnancy O08.1
 acquired (any) D68.4
 antepartum hemorrhage —see
  Hemorrhage, antepartum, with
  coagulation defect
 clotting factor NEC (see also
  Deficiency, factor) D68.2
 due to
  hyperprothrombinemia D68.4
  liver disease D68.4
  vitamin K deficiency D68.4
 newborn, transient P61.6
 postpartum O72.3
 specified NEC D68.8
cognitive F09
color vision H53.50
 achromatopsia H53.51
 acquired H53.52
 deuteranomaly H53.53
 protanomaly H53.54
 specified type NEC H53.59
 tritanomaly H53.55
combined glucocorticoid and
 mineralocorticoid E27.49
contact factor D68.2
copper (nutritional) E61.0
corticoadrenal E27.40
 primary E27.1
craniofacial axis Q75.009
cyanocobalamin E53.8
C1 esterase inhibitor (C1-INH) D84.1
debrancher enzyme (limit
 dextrinosis) E74.03
dehydrogenase
 long chain/very long chain acyl
  CoA E71.310
 medium chain acyl CoA E71.311
 short chain acyl CoA E71.312
diet E63.9
dihydropyrimidine dehydrogenase
 (DPD) E88.89
disaccharidase E73.9
edema —see Malnutrition, severe
endocrine E34.9
energy-supply —see Malnutrition
enzymes, circulating NEC E88.09
ergosterol E55.9
 with
  adult osteomalacia M83.8
  rickets —see Rickets
essential fatty acid (EFA) E63.0
eye movements
 saccadic H55.81
 smooth pursuit H55.82
factor —see also Deficiency,
 coagulation
 Hageman D68.2
 I (congenital) (hereditary) D68.2
 II (congenital) (hereditary) D68.2
 IX (congenital) (functional)
  (hereditary) (with functional
  defect) D67
 multiple (congenital) D68.8
  acquired D68.4

Deficiency, deficient (continued)
factor (continued)
 V (congenital) (hereditary) D68.2
 VII (congenital) (hereditary) D68.2
 VIII (congenital) (functional)
  (hereditary) (with functional
  defect) D66
  with vascular defect —see
   Disease, von Willebrand
 X (congenital) (hereditary) D68.2
 XI (congenital) (hereditary) D68.1
 XII (congenital) (hereditary) D68.2
 XIII (congenital) (hereditary) D68.2
femoral, proximal focal (congenital)
 —see Defect, reduction, lower
 limb, longitudinal, femur
fibrin-stabilizing factor (congenital)
 (hereditary) D68.2
 acquired D68.4
fibrinase D68.2
fibrinogen (congenital) (hereditary)
 D68.2
 acquired D65
folate E53.8
folic acid E53.8
foreskin N47.3
fructokinase E74.11
fructose 1,6-diphosphatase
 E74.19
fructose-1-phosphate aldolase
 E74.19
GABA (gamma aminobutyric acid)
 transaminase E72.81
GABA-T (gamma aminobutyric
 acid transaminase) E72.81
galactokinase E74.29
galactose-1-phosphate uridyl
 transferase E74.29
gammaglobulin in blood D80.1
 hereditary D80.0
glass factor D68.2
glucocorticoid E27.49
 mineralocorticoid E27.49
glucose-6-phosphatase E74.01
glucose-6-phosphate
 dehydrogenase
  anemia D55.0
  without anemia D75.A
glucose transporter protein type 1
 E74.810
glucuronyl transferase E80.5
Glut1 E74.810
glycogen synthetase E74.09
gonadotropin (isolated) E23.0
growth hormone (idiopathic)
 (isolated) E23.0
Hageman factor D68.2
hemoglobin D64.9
hepatophosphorylase E74.09
homogentisate 1,2-dioxygenase
 E70.29
hormone
 anterior pituitary (partial) NEC
  E23.0
  growth E23.0
 growth (isolated) E23.0
 pituitary E23.0
 testicular E29.1
hypoxanthine-(guanine)-
 phosphoribosyltransferase (HG-
 PRT) (total H-PRT) E79.1
immunity D84.9
 cell-mediated D84.89
  with thrombocytopenia and
   eczema D82.0
 combined D81.9
 humoral D80.9
 IgA (secretory) D80.2
 IgG D80.3
 IgM D80.4
immuno —see Immunodeficiency

Deficiency, deficient (continued)
immunoglobulin, selective
 A (IgA) D80.2
 G (IgG) (subclasses) D80.3
 M (IgM) D80.4
infantile neurovisceral acid
 sphingomyelinase E75.240
inositol (B complex) E53.8
intrinsic
 factor (congenital) D51.0
 sphincter N36.42
  with urethral hypermobility
   N36.43
iodine E61.8
 congenital syndrome —see
  Syndrome, iodine-deficiency,
  congenital
iron E61.1
 anemia D50.9
kalium E87.6
kappa-light chain D80.8
labile factor (congenital)
 (hereditary) D68.2
 acquired D68.4
lacrimal fluid (acquired) —see also
 Syndrome, dry eye
 congenital Q10.6
lactase
 congenital E73.0
 secondary E73.1
Laki-Lorand factor D68.2
LCAD (long chain acyl CoA
 dehydrogenase deficiency)
 E71.310
lecithin cholesterol acyltransferase
 E78.6
lipocaic K86.89
lipoprotein (familial) (high density)
 E78.6
liver phosphorylase E74.09
lysosomal alpha-1, 4 glucosidase
 E74.02
lysosome-associated membrane
 protein 2 [LAMP2] E74.05
magnesium E61.2
MCAD (medium chain acyl CoA
 dehydrogenase deficiency)
 E71.311
major histocompatibility complex
 class I D81.6
 class II D81.7
manganese E61.3
menadione (vitamin K) E56.1
 newborn P53
mental (familial) (hereditary) —see
 Disability, intellectual
methylenetetrahydrofolate
 reductase (MTHFR) E72.12
mevalonate kinase M04.1
mineral NEC E61.8
mineralocorticoid E27.49
 with glucocorticoid E27.49
molybdenum (nutritional) E61.5
moral F60.2
multiple nutrient elements E61.7
multiple sulfatase (MSD) E75.26
muscle
 carnitine (palmityltransferase)
  E71.314
 phosphofructokinase E74.09
myoadenylate deaminase E79.2
myocardial —see Insufficiency,
 myocardial
myophosphorylase E74.04
NADH diaphorase or reductase
 (congenital) D74.0
NADH-methemoglobin reductase
 (congenital) D74.0
natrium E87.1
niacin (amide) (-tryptophan) E52
nicotinamide E52

Deficiency, deficient (continued)
nicotinic acid E52
number of teeth —see Anodontia
nutrient element E61.9
 multiple E61.7
 specified NEC E61.8
nutrition, nutritional (see also
 Nutrition deficient) E63.9
 sequelae —see Sequelae,
  nutritional deficiency
 specified NEC E63.8
of interleukin 1 receptor antagonist
 [DIRA] M04.8
ornithine transcarbamylase E72.4
ovarian E28.39
oxygen —see Anoxia
pantothenic acid E53.8
parathyroid (gland) E20.9
perineum (female) N81.89
phenylalanine hydroxylase E70.1
phosphoenolpyruvate
 carboxykinase E74.4
phosphofructokinase E74.19
phosphomannomutase E74.818
phosphomannose isomerase E74.818
phosphomannosyl mutase E74.818
phosphorylase kinase, liver
 E74.09
pituitary hormone (isolated) E23.0
plasma thromboplastin
 antecedent (PTA) D68.1
 component (PTC) D67
plasminogen (type 1) (type 2)
 E88.02
platelet NEC D69.1
 constitutional —see Disease, von
  Willebrand
polyglandular E31.8
 autoimmune E31.0
potassium (K) E87.6
prepuce N47.3
proaccelerin (congenital)
 (hereditary) D68.2
 acquired D68.4
proconvertin factor (congenital)
 (hereditary) D68.2
 acquired D68.4
protein (see also Malnutrition)
 E46
 anemia D53.0
 C D68.59
 S D68.59
prothrombin (congenital)
 (hereditary) D68.2
 acquired D68.4
Prower factor D68.2
pseudocholinesterase E88.09
PTA (plasma thromboplastin
 antecedent) D68.1
PTC (plasma thromboplastin
 component) D67
purine nucleoside phosphorylase
 (PNP) D81.5
pyracin (alpha) (beta) E53.1
pyridoxal E53.1
pyridoxamine E53.1
pyridoxine (derivatives) E53.1
pyruvate
 carboxylase E74.4
 dehydrogenase E74.4
riboflavin (vitamin B2) E53.0
salt E87.1
SCAD (short chain acyl CoA
 dehydrogenase deficiency)
 E71.312
secretion
 ovary E28.39
 salivary gland (any) K11.7
 urine R34
selenium (dietary) E59
serum antitrypsin, familial E88.01

Deficiency, deficient (continued)
  short stature homeobox gene (SHOX)
    with
      dyschondrosteosis Q78.8
      short stature (idiopathic)
        E34.328
      Turner's syndrome Q96.9
  sodium (Na) E87.1
  SPCA (factor VII) D68.2
  sphincter, intrinsic N36.42
    with urethral hypermobility N36.43
  stable factor (congenital)
    (hereditary) D68.2
    acquired D68.4
  Stuart-Prower (factor X) D68.2
  succinic semialdehyde
    dehydrogenase E72.81
  sucrase E74.39
  sulfatase E75.26
  sulfite oxidase E72.19
  thiamin, thiaminic (chloride) E51.9
    beriberi (dry) E51.11
      wet E51.12
  thrombokinase D68.2
    newborn P53
  thyroid (gland) —see
    Hypothyroidism
  tocopherol E56.0
  tooth bud K00.0
  transcobalamine II (anemia) D51.2
  vanadium E61.6
  vascular I99.9
  vasopressin E23.2
  vertical ridge K06.8
  viosterol —see Deficiency,
    calciferol
  vitamin (multiple) NOS E56.9
    A E50.9
      with
        Bitot's spot (corneal) E50.1
        follicular keratosis E50.8
        keratomalacia E50.4
        manifestations NEC E50.8
        night blindness E50.5
        scar of cornea,
          xerophthalmic E50.6
        xeroderma E50.8
        xerophthalmia E50.7
        xerosis
          conjunctival E50.0
            and Bitot's spot E50.1
          cornea E50.2
            and ulceration E50.3
      sequelae E64.1
    B (complex) NOS E53.9
      with
        beriberi (dry) E51.11
          wet E51.12
        pellagra E52
    B1 NOS E51.9
      beriberi (dry) E51.11
        with circulatory system
          manifestations E51.11
        wet E51.12
    B12 E53.8
    B2 (riboflavin) E53.0
    B6 E53.1
    C E54
      sequelae E64.2
    D E55.9
      with
        adult osteomalacia M83.8
        rickets —see Rickets
      25-hydroxylase E83.32
    E E56.0
    folic acid E53.8
    G E53.0
    group B E53.9
      specified NEC E53.8
    H (biotin) E53.8
    K E56.1
      of newborn P53

Deficiency, deficient (continued)
  vitamin (continued)
    nicotinic E52
    P E56.8
    PP (pellagra-preventing) E52
    specified NEC E56.8
    thiamin E51.9
      beriberi —see Beriberi
    VLCAD (very long chain acyl
      CoA dehydrogenase deficiency)
      E71.310
    von Willebrand factor
      partial quantitative (see also
        Disease, von Willebrand)
        D68.01
      total quantitative (see also
        Disease, von Willebrand)
        D68.03
    zinc, dietary E60

Deficit —see also Deficiency
  attention and concentration
    R41.840
    disorder —see Attention, deficit
    following
      cerebral infarction I69.310
      cerebrovascular disease
        I69.910
        specified disease NEC
          I69.810
      nontraumatic
        intracerebral hemorrhage
          I69.110
        specified intracranial
          hemorrhage NEC I69.210
        subarachnoid hemorrhage
          I69.010
  cognitive
    communication R41.841
    emotional
      following
        cerebral infarction I69.315
        cerebrovascular disease
          I69.915
          specified disease NEC
            I69.815
        nontramantic
          intracerebral hemorrhage
            I69.115
          specified intracranial
            hemorrhage NEC
            I69.215
          subarachnoid hemorrhage
            I69.015
    following
      cerebral infarction I69.319
      cerebrovascular disease I69.919
        specified disease NEC
          I69.819
      nontraumatic
        intracerebral hemorrhage
          I69.119
        specified intracranial
          hemorrhage NEC I69.219
        subarachnoid hemorrhage
          I69.019
    social
      following
        cerebral infarction I69.315
        cerebrovascular disease
          I69.915
          specified disease NEC
            I69.815
        nontraumatic
          intracerebral hemorrhage
            I69.115
          specified intracranial
            hemorrhage NEC
            I69.215
          subarachnoid hemorrhage
            I69.015

Deficit (continued)
  cognitive NEC R41.89
    following
      cerebral infarction I69.318
      cerebrovascular disease
        I69.918
        specified disease NEC
          I69.818
      nontraumatic
        intracerebral hemorrhage
          I69.118
        specified intracarnial
          hemorrhage NEC I69.218
        subarachnoid hemorrhage
          I69.018
  concentration R41.840
  executive function R41.844
    following
      cerebral infarction I69.314
      cerebrovascular disease
        I69.914
        specified disease NEC
          I69.814
      nontraumatic
        intracerebral hemorrhage
          I69.114
        specified intracranial
          hemorrhage NEC I69.214
        subarachnoid hemorrhage
          I69.014
  frontal lobe R41.844
    following
      cerebral infarction I69.314
      cerebrovascular disease
        I69.914
        specified disease NEC
          I69.814
      nontraumatic
        intracerebral hemorrhage
          I69.114
        specified intracranial
          hemorrhage NEC
          I69.214
        subarachnoid hemorrhage
          I69.014
  memory
    following
      cerebral infarction I69.311
      cerebrovascular disease
        I69.911
        specified disease NEC
          I69.811
      nontraumatic
        intracerebral hemorrhage
          I69.111
        specified intracranial
          hemorrhage NEC I69.211
        subarachnoid hemorrhage
          I69.011
  neurologic NEC R29.818
    ischemic
      reversible (RIND) I63.9
      prolonged (PRIND) I63.9
  oxygen R09.02
  prolonged reversible ischemic
    neurologic (PRIND) I63.9
  psychomotor R41.843
    following
      cerebral infarction I69.313
      cerebrovascular disease
        I69.913
        specified disease NEC
          I69.813
      nontraumatic
        intracerebral hemorrhage
          I69.113
        specified intracranial
          hemorrhage NEC I69.213
        subarachnoid hemorrhage
          I69.013

Deficit (continued)
  visuospatial R41.842
    following
      cerebral infarction I69.312
      cerebrovascular disease I69.912
        specified disease NEC
          I69.812
      nontraumatic
        intracerebral hemorrhage
          I69.112
        specified intracranial
          hemorrhage NEC I69.212
        subarachnoid hemorrhage
          I69.012

Deflection
  radius —see Deformity, limb,
    specified type NEC, forearm
  septum (acquired) (nasal) (nose)
    J34.2
  spine —see Curvature, spine
  turbinate (nose) J34.2

Defluvium
  capillorum —see Alopecia
  ciliorum —see Madarosis
  unguium L60.8

Deformity Q89.9
  abdomen, congenital Q89.9
  abdominal wall
    acquired M95.8
    congenital Q79.59
  acquired (unspecified site) M95.9
  adrenal gland Q89.1
  alimentary tract, congenital Q45.9
    upper Q40.9
  ankle (joint) (acquired) —see also
    Deformity, limb, lower leg
    abduction —see Contraction,
      joint, ankle
    congenital Q68.8
    contraction —see Contraction,
      joint, ankle
    specified type NEC —see
      Deformity, limb, foot,
      specified NEC
  anus (acquired) K62.89
    congenital Q43.9
  aorta (arch) (congenital) Q25.40
    acquired I77.89
  aortic
    arch, acquired I77.89
    cusp or valve (congenital) Q23.8
      acquired (see also
        Endocarditis, aortic) I35.8
  arm (acquired) (upper) —see also
    Deformity, limb, upper arm
    congenital Q68.8
    forearm —see Deformity, limb,
      forearm
  artery (congenital) (peripheral)
    NOS Q27.9
    acquired I77.89
    coronary (acquired) I25.9
      congenital Q24.5
    umbilical Q27.0
  atrial septal (see also Defect, atrial
    septal) Q21.10
  auditory canal (external)
    (congenital) —see also
    Malformation, ear, external
    acquired —see Disorder, ear,
      external, specified type NEC
  auricle
    ear (congenital) —see also
      Malformation, ear, external
    acquired —see Disorder,
      pinna, deformity
  back —see Dorsopathy, deforming
  bile duct (common) (congenital)
    (hepatic) Q44.5
    acquired K83.8

Deformity (continued)
- biliary duct or passage (congenital) Q44.5
  - acquired K83.8
- bladder (neck) (trigone) (sphincter) (acquired) N32.89
  - congenital Q64.79
- bone (acquired) NOS M95.9
  - congenital Q79.9
  - turbinate M95.0
- brain (congenital) Q04.9
  - acquired G93.89
  - reduction Q04.3
- breast (acquired) N64.89
  - congenital Q83.9
  - reconstructed N65.0
- bronchus (congenital) Q32.4
  - acquired NEC J98.09
- bursa, congenital Q79.9
- canaliculi (lacrimalis) (acquired) —see also Disorder, lacrimal system, changes
  - congenital Q10.6
- canthus, acquired —see Disorder, eyelid, specified type NEC
- capillary (acquired) I78.8
- cardiovascular system, congenital Q28.9
- caruncle, lacrimal (acquired) —see also Disorder, lacrimal system, changes
  - congenital Q10.6
- cascade, stomach K31.2
- cecum (congenital) Q43.9
  - acquired K63.89
- cerebral, acquired G93.89
  - congenital Q04.9
- cervix (uterus) (acquired) NEC N88.8
  - congenital Q51.9
- cheek (acquired) M95.2
  - congenital Q18.9
- chest (acquired) (wall) M95.4
  - congenital Q67.8
  - sequelae (late effect) of rickets E64.3
- chin (acquired) M95.2
  - congenital Q18.9
- choroid (congenital) Q14.3
  - acquired H31.8
  - plexus Q07.8
    - acquired G96.198
- cicatricial —see Cicatrix
- cilia, acquired —see Disorder, eyelid, specified type NEC
- clavicle (acquired) M95.8
  - congenital Q68.8
- clitoris (congenital) Q52.6
  - acquired N90.89
- clubfoot —see Clubfoot
- coccyx (acquired) M43.8
- colon (congenital) Q43.9
  - acquired K63.89
- concha (ear), congenital —see also Malformation, ear, external
  - acquired —see Disorder, pinna, deformity
- cornea (acquired) H18.70
  - congenital Q13.4
  - descemetocele —see Descemetocele
  - ectasia —see Ectasia, cornea
  - specified NEC H18.79-
  - staphyloma —see Staphyloma, cornea
- coronary artery (acquired) I25.9
  - congenital Q24.5
- cranium (acquired) —see Deformity, skull
- cricoid cartilage (congenital) Q31.8
  - acquired J38.7

Deformity (continued)
- cystic duct (congenital) Q44.5
  - acquired K82.8
- Dandy-Walker Q03.1
  - with spina bifida —see Spina bifida
- diaphragm (congenital) Q79.1
  - acquired J98.6
- digestive organ NOS Q45.9
- ductus arteriosus Q25.0
- duodenal bulb K31.89
- duodenum (congenital) Q43.9
  - acquired K31.89
- dura —see Deformity, meninges
- ear (acquired) —see also Disorder, pinna, deformity
  - congenital (external) Q17.9
    - internal Q16.5
    - middle Q16.4
      - ossicles Q16.3
    - ossicles Q16.3
- ectodermal (congenital) NEC Q84.9
- ejaculatory duct (congenital) Q55.4
  - acquired N50.89
- elbow (joint) (acquired) —see also Deformity, limb, upper arm
  - congenital Q68.8
  - contraction —see Contraction, joint, elbow
- endocrine gland NEC Q89.2
- epididymis (congenital) Q55.4
  - acquired N50.89
- epiglottis (congenital) Q31.8
  - acquired J38.7
- esophagus (congenital) Q39.9
  - acquired K22.89
- eustachian tube (congenital) NEC Q17.8
- eye, congenital Q15.9
- eyebrow (congenital) Q18.8
- eyelid (acquired) —see also Disorder, eyelid, specified type NEC
  - congenital Q10.3
- face (acquired) M95.2
  - congenital Q18.9
- fallopian tube, acquired N83.8
- femur (acquired) —see Deformity, limb, specified type NEC, thigh
- fetal
  - with fetopelvic disproportion O33.7
  - causing obstructed labor O66.3
- finger (acquired) M20.00-
  - boutonniere M20.02-
  - congenital Q68.1
  - flexion contracture —see Contraction, joint, hand
  - mallet finger M20.01-
  - specified NEC M20.09-
  - swan-neck M20.03-
- flexion (joint) (acquired) (see also Deformity, limb, flexion) M21.20
  - congenital NOS Q74.9
    - hip Q65.89
- foot (acquired) —see also Deformity, limb, lower leg
  - cavovarus (congenital) Q66.1-
  - congenital NOS Q66.9-
    - specified type NEC Q66.89
  - specified type NEC —see Deformity, limb, foot, specified NEC
  - valgus (congenital) Q66.6
    - acquired —see Deformity, valgus, ankle
  - varus (congenital) NEC Q66.3-
    - acquired —see Deformity, varus, ankle

Deformity (continued)
- forearm (acquired) —see also Deformity, limb, forearm
  - congenital Q68.8
- forehead (acquired) M95.2
  - congenital Q75.8
- frontal bone (acquired) M95.2
  - congenital Q75.8
- gallbladder (congenital) Q44.1
  - acquired K82.8
- gastrointestinal tract (congenital) NOS Q45.9
  - acquired K63.89
- genitalia, genital organ(s) or system NEC
  - female (congenital) Q52.9
    - acquired N94.89
    - external Q52.70
  - male (congenital) Q55.9
    - acquired N50.89
- globe (eye) (congenital) Q15.8
  - acquired H44.89
- gum, acquired NEC K06.8
- hand (acquired) —see Deformity, limb, hand
  - congenital Q68.1
- head (acquired) M95.2
  - congenital Q75.8
- heart (congenital) Q24.9
  - septum Q21.9
    - auricular (see also Defect, atrial septal) Q21.10
    - ventricular Q21.0
  - valve (congenital) NEC Q24.8
    - acquired —see Endocarditis
- heel (acquired) —see Deformity, foot
- hepatic duct (congenital) Q44.5
  - acquired K83.8
- hip (joint) (acquired) —see also Deformity, limb, thigh
  - congenital Q65.9
  - due to (previous) juvenile osteochondrosis —see Coxa, plana
  - flexion —see Contraction, joint, hip
- hourglass —see Contraction, hourglass
- humerus (acquired) M21.82-
  - congenital Q74.0
- hypophyseal (congenital) Q89.2
- ileocecal (coil) (valve) (acquired) K63.89
  - congenital Q43.9
- ileum (congenital) Q43.9
  - acquired K63.89
- ilium (acquired) M95.5
  - congenital Q74.2
- integument (congenital) Q84.9
- intervertebral cartilage or disc (acquired) —see Disorder, disc, specified NEC
- intestine (large) (small) (congenital) NOS Q43.9
  - acquired K63.89
- intrinsic minus or plus (hand) —see Deformity, limb, specified type NEC, forearm
- iris (acquired) H21.89
  - congenital Q13.2
- ischium (acquired) M95.5
  - congenital Q74.2
- jaw (acquired) (congenital) M26.9
- joint (acquired) NEC M21.90
  - congenital Q68.8
  - elbow M21.92-
  - hand M21.94-
  - hip M21.95-
  - knee M21.96-
  - shoulder M21.92-
  - wrist M21.93-

Deformity (continued)
- kidney(s) (calyx) (pelvis) (congenital) Q63.9
  - acquired N28.89
  - artery (congenital) Q27.2
    - acquired I77.89
- Klippel-Feil (brevicollis) Q76.1
- knee (acquired) NEC —see also Deformity, limb, lower leg
  - congenital Q68.2
- labium (majus) (minus) (congenital) Q52.79
  - acquired N90.89
- lacrimal passages or duct (congenital) NEC Q10.6
  - acquired —see Disorder, lacrimal system, changes
- larynx (muscle) (congenital) Q31.8
  - acquired J38.7
  - web (glottic) Q31.0
- leg (upper) (acquired) NEC —see also Deformity, limb, thigh
  - congenital Q68.8
  - lower leg —see Deformity, limb, lower leg
- lens (acquired) H27.8
  - congenital Q12.9
- lid (fold) (acquired) —see also Disorder, eyelid, specified type NEC
  - congenital Q10.3
- ligament (acquired) —see Disorder, ligament
  - congenital Q79.9
- limb (acquired) M21.90
  - clawfoot M21.53-
  - clawhand M21.51-
    - congenital Q68.1
  - clubfoot M21.54-
  - clubhand M21.52-
  - congenital, except reduction deformity Q74.9
  - flat foot M21.4-
  - flexion M21.20
    - ankle M21.27-
    - elbow M21.22-
    - finger M21.24-
    - hip M21.25-
    - knee M21.26-
    - shoulder M21.21-
    - toe M21.27-
    - wrist M21.23-
  - foot
    - claw —see Deformity, limb, clawfoot
    - club —see Deformity, limb, clubfoot
    - drop M21.37-
    - flat —see Deformity, limb, flat foot
    - specified NEC M21.6X-
  - forearm M21.93-
  - hand M21.94-
  - lower leg M21.96-
  - specified type NEC M21.80
    - forearm M21.83-
    - lower leg M21.86-
    - thigh M21.85-
    - upper arm M21.82-
  - thigh M21.95-
  - unequal length M21.70
    - short site is
      - femur M21.75-
      - fibula M21.76-
      - humerus M21.72-
      - radius M21.73-
      - tibia M21.76-
      - ulna M21.73-
  - upper arm M21.92-
  - valgus —see Deformity, valgus

Deformity (continued)
  limb (continued)
    varus —see Deformity, varus
    wrist drop M21.33-
  lip (acquired) NEC K13.0
    congenital Q38.0
  liver (congenital) Q44.70
    acquired K76.89
  lumbosacral (congenital) (joint)
    (region) Q76.49
    acquired M43.8
    kyphosis —see Kyphosis,
      congenital
    lordosis —see Lordosis,
      congenital
  lung (congenital) Q33.9
    acquired J98.4
  lymphatic system, congenital Q89.9
  Madelung's (radius) Q74.0
  mandible (acquired) (congenital)
    M26.9
  maxilla (acquired) (congenital) M26.9
  meninges or membrane
    (congenital) Q07.9
    cerebral Q04.8
      acquired G96.198
    spinal cord (congenital) Q06.-
      acquired G96.198
  metacarpus (acquired) —see
    Deformity, limb, forearm
    congenital Q74.0
  metatarsus (acquired) —see
    Deformity, foot
    congenital Q66.9-
  middle ear (congenital) Q16.4
    ossicles Q16.3
  mitral (leaflets) (valve) I05.8
    parachute Q23.2
    stenosis, congenital Q23.2
  mouth (acquired) K13.79
    congenital Q38.6
  multiple, congenital NEC Q89.7
  muscle (acquired) M62.89
    congenital Q79.9
      sternocleidomastoid Q68.0
  musculoskeletal system (acquired)
    M95.9
    congenital Q79.9
    specified NEC M95.8
  nail (acquired) L60.8
    congenital Q84.6
  nasal —see Deformity, nose
  neck (acquired) M95.3
    congenital Q18.9
      sternocleidomastoid Q68.0
  nervous system (congenital) Q07.9
  nipple (congenital) Q83.9
    acquired N64.89
  nose (acquired) (cartilage) M95.0
    bone (turbinate) M95.0
    congenital Q30.9
      bent or squashed Q67.4
    saddle M95.0
      syphilitic A50.57
    septum (acquired) J34.2
      congenital Q30.8
    sinus (wall) (congenital) Q30.8
      acquired M95.0
    syphilitic (congenital) A50.57
      late A52.73
  ocular muscle (congenital) Q10.3
    acquired —see Strabismus,
      mechanical
  opticociliary vessels (congenital)
    Q13.2
  orbit (eye) (acquired) H05.30
    atrophy —see Atrophy, orbit
    congenital Q10.7
    due to
      bone disease NEC H05.32-
      trauma or surgery H05.33-

Deformity (continued)
  orbit (continued)
    enlargement —see Enlargement,
      orbit
    exostosis —see Exostosis, orbit
  organ of Corti (congenital) Q16.5
  ovary (congenital) Q50.39
    acquired N83.8
  oviduct, acquired N83.8
  palate (congenital) Q38.5
    acquired M27.8
    cleft (congenital) —see Cleft,
      palate
  pancreas (congenital) Q45.3
    acquired K86.89
  parathyroid (gland) Q89.2
  parotid (gland) (congenital) Q38.4
    acquired K11.8
  patella (acquired) —see Disorder,
    patella, specified NEC
  pelvis, pelvic (acquired) (bony)
    M95.5
    with disproportion (fetopelvic)
      O33.0
      causing obstructed labor
        O65.0
    congenital Q74.2
    rachitic sequelae (late effect)
      E64.3
  penis (glans) (congenital) Q55.69
    acquired N48.89
  pericardium (congenital) Q24.8
    acquired —see Pericarditis
  pharynx (congenital) Q38.8
    acquired J39.2
  pinna, acquired —see also
    Disorder, pinna, deformity
    congenital Q17.9
  pituitary (congenital) Q89.2
  posture —see Dorsopathy, deforming
  prepuce (congenital) Q55.69
    acquired N47.8
  prostate (congenital) Q55.4
    acquired N42.89
  pupil (congenital) Q13.2
    acquired —see Abnormality,
      pupillary
  pylorus (congenital) Q40.3
    acquired K31.89
  rachitic (acquired), old or healed
    E64.3
  radius (acquired) —see also
    Deformity, limb, forearm
    congenital Q68.8
  rectum (congenital) Q43.9
    acquired K62.89
  reduction (extremity) (limb),
    congenital (see also condition
    and site) Q73.8
    brain Q04.3
    lower —see Defect, reduction,
      lower limb
    upper —see Defect, reduction,
      upper limb
  renal —see Deformity, kidney
  respiratory system (congenital)
    Q34.9
  rib (acquired) M95.4
    congenital Q76.6
      cervical Q76.5
  rotation (joint) (acquired) —see
    Deformity, limb, specified site
    NEC
    congenital Q74.9
    hip —see Deformity, limb,
      specified type NEC, thigh
      congenital Q65.89
  sacroiliac joint (congenital) Q74.2
    acquired —see subcategory M43.8
  sacrum (acquired) —see
    subcategory M43.8

Deformity (continued)
  saddle
    back —see Lordosis
    nose M95.0
      syphilitic A50.57
  salivary gland or duct (congenital)
    Q38.4
    acquired K11.8
  scapula (acquired) M95.8
    congenital Q68.8
  scrotum (congenital) —see also
    Malformation, testis and scrotum
    acquired N50.89
  seminal vesicles (congenital) Q55.4
    acquired N50.89
  septum, nasal (acquired) J34.2
  shoulder (joint) (acquired) —see
    Deformity, limb, upper arm
    congenital Q74.0
    contraction —see Contraction,
      joint, shoulder
  sigmoid (flexure) (congenital) Q43.9
    acquired K63.89
  skin (congenital) Q82.9
  skull (acquired) M95.2
    congenital Q75.8
    with
      anencephaly Q00.0
      encephalocele —see
        Encephalocele
      hydrocephalus Q03.9
        with spina bifida —see
          Spina bifida, by site,
          with hydrocephalus
      microcephaly Q02
  soft parts, organs or tissues (of
    pelvis)
    in pregnancy or childbirth NEC
      O34.8-
      causing obstructed labor O65.5
  spermatic cord (congenital) Q55.4
    acquired N50.89
    torsion —see Torsion,
      spermatic cord
  spinal —see Dorsopathy, deforming
    column (acquired) —see
      Dorsopathy, deforming
    congenital Q67.5
    cord (congenital) Q06.9
      acquired G95.89
    nerve root (congenital) Q07.9
  spine (acquired) —see also
    Dorsopathy, deforming
    congenital Q67.5
    rachitic E64.3
    specified NEC —see
      Dorsopathy, deforming,
      specified NEC
  spleen
    acquired D73.89
    congenital Q89.09
  Sprengel's (congenital) Q74.0
  sternocleidomastoid (muscle),
    congenital Q68.0
  sternum (acquired) M95.4
    congenital NEC Q76.7
  stomach (congenital) Q40.3
    acquired K31.89
  submandibular gland (congenital)
    Q38.4
  submaxillary gland (congenital)
    Q38.4
    acquired K11.8
  talipes —see Talipes
  testis (congenital) —see also
    Malformation, testis and scrotum
    acquired N44.8
    torsion —see Torsion, testis
  thigh (acquired) —see also
    Deformity, limb, thigh
    congenital NEC Q68.8

Deformity (continued)
  thorax (acquired) (wall) M95.4
    congenital Q67.8
    sequelae of rickets E64.3
  thumb (acquired) —see also
    Deformity, finger
    congenital NEC Q68.1
  thymus (tissue) (congenital) Q89.2
  thyroid (gland) (congenital) Q89.2
    cartilage Q31.8
      acquired J38.7
  tibia (acquired) —see also
    Deformity, limb, specified type
    NEC, lower leg
    congenital NEC Q68.8
    saber (syphilitic) A50.56
  toe (acquired) M20.6-
    congenital Q66.9-
    hallux rigidus M20.2-
    hallux valgus M20.1-
    hallux varus M20.3-
    hammer toe M20.4-
    specified NEC M20.5X-
  tongue (congenital) Q38.3
    acquired K14.8
  tooth, teeth K00.2
  trachea (rings) (congenital) Q32.1
    acquired J39.8
  transverse aortic arch (congenital)
    Q25.49
  tricuspid (leaflets) (valve) I07.8
    atresia or stenosis Q22.4
    Ebstein's Q22.5
  trunk (acquired) M95.8
    congenital Q89.9
  ulna (acquired) —see also
    Deformity, limb, forearm
    congenital NEC Q68.8
  urachus, congenital Q64.4
  ureter (opening) (congenital) Q62.8
    acquired N28.89
  urethra (congenital) Q64.79
    acquired N36.8
  urinary tract (congenital) Q64.9
    urachus Q64.4
  uterus (congenital) Q51.9
    acquired N85.8
  uvula (congenital) Q38.5
  vagina (acquired) N89.8
    congenital Q52.4
  valgus NEC M21.00
    ankle M21.07-
    elbow M21.02-
    hip M21.05-
    knee M21.06-
  valve, valvular (congenital) (heart)
    Q24.8
    acquired —see Endocarditis
  varus NEC M21.10
    ankle M21.17-
    elbow M21.12-
    hip M21.15
    knee M21.16-
    tibia —see Osteochondrosis,
      juvenile, tibia
  vas deferens (congenital) Q55.4
    acquired N50.89
  vein (congenital) Q27.9
    great Q26.9
  vertebra —see Dorsopathy,
    deforming
  vertical talus (congenital) Q66.80
    left foot Q66.82
    right foot Q66.81
  vesicourethral orifice (acquired)
    N32.89
    congenital NEC Q64.79
  vessels of optic papilla (congenital)
    Q14.2
  visual field (contraction) —see
    Defect, visual field

Deformity (continued)
vitreous body, acquired H43.89
vulva (congenital) Q52.79
acquired N90.89
wrist (joint) (acquired) —see also Deformity, limb, forearm
congenital Q68.8
contraction —see Contraction, joint, wrist

Degeneration, degenerative
adrenal (capsule) (fatty) (gland) (hyaline) (infectional) E27.8
amyloid (see also Amyloidosis) E85.9
anterior cornua, spinal cord G12.29
anterior labral S43.49-
aorta, aortic I70.0
fatty I77.89
aortic valve (heart) —see Endocarditis, aortic
arteriovascular —see Arteriosclerosis
artery, arterial (atheromatous) (calcareous) —see also Arteriosclerosis
cerebral, amyloid E85.4 [I68.0]
medial —see Arteriosclerosis, extremities
articular cartilage NEC —see Derangement, joint, articular cartilage, by site
atheromatous —see Arteriosclerosis
basal nuclei or ganglia G23.9
specified NEC G23.8
bone NEC —see Disorder, bone, specified type NEC
brachial plexus G54.0
brain (cortical) (progressive) G31.9
alcoholic G31.2
arteriosclerotic I67.2
childhood G31.9
specified NEC G31.89
cystic G31.89
congenital Q04.6
in
alcoholism G31.2
beriberi E51.2
cerebrovascular disease I67.9
congenital hydrocephalus Q03.9
with spina bifida —see also Spina bifida
Fabry-Anderson disease E75.21
Gaucher's disease E75.22
Hunter's syndrome E76.1
lipidosis
cerebral E75.4
generalized E75.6
mucopolysaccharidosis —see Mucopolysaccharidosis
myxedema E03.9 [G32.89]
neoplastic disease (see also Neoplasm) D49.6 [G32.89]
Niemann-Pick disease E75.249 [G32.89]
sphingolipidosis E75.3 [G32.89]
vitamin B12 deficiency E53.8 [G32.89]
senile NEC G31.1
breast N64.89
Bruch's membrane —see Degeneration, choroid
capillaries (fatty) I78.8
amyloid E85.89 [I79.8]
cardiac —see also Degeneration, myocardial
valve, valvular —see Endocarditis
cardiorenal —see Hypertension, cardiorenal
cardiovascular —see also Disease, cardiovascular
renal —see Hypertension, cardiorenal

Degeneration, degenerative (continued)
cerebellar NOS G31.9
alcoholic G31.2
primary (hereditary) (sporadic) G11.9
cerebral —see Degeneration, brain
cerebrovascular I67.9
due to hypertension I67.4
cervical plexus G54.2
cervix N88.8
due to radiation (intended effect) N88.5
adverse effect or misadventure N99.89
chamber angle H21.21-
changes, spine or vertebra —see Spondylosis
chorioretinal —see also Degeneration, choroid
hereditary H31.20
choroid (colloid) (drusen) H31.10-
atrophy —see Atrophy, choroidal
hereditary —see Dystrophy, choroidal, hereditary
ciliary body H21.22-
cochlear H83.8
combined (spinal cord) (subacute) E53.8 [G32.0]
with anemia (pernicious) D51.0 [G32.0]
due to dietary vitamin B12 deficiency D51.3 [G32.0]
in (due to)
vitamin B12 deficiency E53.8 [G32.0]
anemia D51.9 [G32.0]
conjunctiva H11.10
concretions —see Concretion, conjunctiva
deposits —see Deposit, conjunctiva
pigmentations —see Pigmentation, conjunctiva
pinguecula —see Pinguecula
xerosis —see Xerosis, conjunctiva
cornea H18.40
calcerous H18.43
band keratopathy H18.42-
familial, hereditary —see Dystrophy, cornea
hyaline (of old scars) H18.49
keratomalacia —see Keratomalacia
nodular H18.45-
peripheral H18.46-
senile H18.41-
specified type NEC H18.49
cortical (cerebellar) (parenchymatous) G31.89
alcoholic G31.2
diffuse, due to arteriopathy I67.2
corticobasal G31.85
cutis L98.8
amyloid E85.4 [L99]
dental pulp K04.2
disc disease —see Degeneration, intervertebral disc, by site
dorsolateral (spinal cord) —see Degeneration, combined
extrapyramidal G25.9
eye, macular —see also Degeneration, macula
congenital or hereditary —see Dystrophy, retina
facet joints —see Spondylosis
fatty
liver NEC K76.0
alcoholic K70.0

Degeneration, degenerative (continued)
grey matter (brain) (Alpers') G31.81
heart —see also Degeneration, myocardial
amyloid E85.4 [I43]
atheromatous —see Disease, heart, ischemic, atherosclerotic
ischemic —see Disease, heart, ischemic
hepatolenticular (Wilson's) E83.01
hepatorenal K76.7
hyaline (diffuse) (generalized)
localized —see Degeneration, by site
infrapatellar fat pad M79.4
intervertebral disc NOS
with
myelopathy —see Disorder, disc, with, myelopathy
radiculitis or radiculopathy —see Disorder, disc, with, radiculopathy
cervical, cervicothoracic —see Disorder, disc, cervical, degeneration
with
myelopathy —see Disorder, disc, cervical, with myelopathy
neuritis, radiculitis or radiculopathy —see Disorder, disc, cervical, with neuritis
lumbar region M51.36
with
myelopathy M51.06
neuritis, radiculitis, radiculopathy or sciatica M51.16
lumbosacral region M51.37
with
neuritis, radiculitis, radiculopathy or sciatica M51.17
sacrococcygeal region M53.3
thoracic region M51.34
with
myelopathy M51.04
neuritis, radiculitis, radiculopathy M51.14
thoracolumbar region M51.35
with
myelopathy M51.05
neuritis, radiculitis, radiculopathy M51.15
intestine, amyloid E85.4
iris (pigmentary) H21.23-
ischemic —see Ischemia
joint disease —see Osteoarthritis
kidney N28.89
amyloid E85.4 [N29]
cystic, congenital Q61.9
fatty N28.89
polycystic Q61.3
adult type (autosomal dominant) Q61.2
infantile type (autosomal recessive) NEC Q61.19
collecting duct dilatation Q61.11
Kuhnt-Junius (see also Degeneration, macula) H35.32-
lens —see Cataract
lenticular (familial) (progressive) (Wilson's) (with cirrhosis of liver) E83.01
liver (diffuse) NEC K76.89
amyloid E85.4 [K77]
cystic K76.89
congenital Q44.6

Degeneration, degenerative (continued)
liver (continued)
fatty NEC K76.0
alcoholic K70.0
hypertrophic K76.89
parenchymatous, acute or subacute K72.00
with coma K72.01
pigmentary K76.89
toxic (acute) K71.9
lung J98.4
lymph gland I89.8
hyaline I89.8
macula, macular (acquired) (age-related) (senile) H35.30
angioid streaks H35.33
atrophic age-related H35.31-
congenital or hereditary —see Dystrophy, retina
cystoid H35.35-
dry age-related H35.31-
drusen H35.36-
exudative H35.32-
hole H35.34-
nonexudative H35.31-
puckering H35.37-
toxic H35.38-
wet age-related H35.32-
membranous labyrinth, congenital (causing impairment of hearing) Q16.5
meniscus —see Derangement, meniscus
mitral —see Insufficiency, mitral
Mönckeberg's —see Arteriosclerosis, extremities
motor centers, senile G31.1
multi-system G90.3
mural —see Degeneration, myocardial
muscle (fatty) (fibrous) (hyaline) (progressive) M62.89
heart —see Degeneration, myocardial
myelin, central nervous system G37.9
myocardial, myocardium (fatty) (hyaline) (senile) I51.5
with rheumatic fever (conditions in I00) I09.0
active, acute or subacute I01.2
with chorea I02.0
inactive or quiescent (with chorea) I09.0
hypertensive —see Hypertension, heart
rheumatic —see Degeneration, myocardial, with rheumatic fever
syphilitic A52.06
nasal sinus (mucosa) J32.9
frontal J32.1
maxillary J32.0
nerve —see Disorder, nerve
nervous system G31.9
alcoholic G31.2
amyloid E85.4 [G99.8]
autonomic G90.9
fatty G31.89
specified NEC G31.89
nipple N64.89
olivopontocerebellar (hereditary) (familial) G23.8
osseous labyrinth —see subcategory H83.8
ovary N83.8
cystic N83.20-
microcystic N83.20-
pallidal pigmentary (progressive) G23.0

Degeneration, degenerative (continued)
- pancreas K86.89
  - tuberculous A18.83
- penis N48.89
- pigmentary (diffuse) (general)
  - localized —see Degeneration, by site
  - pallidal (progressive) G23.0
- pineal gland E34.8
- pituitary (gland) E23.6
- popliteal fat pad M79.4
- posterolateral (spinal cord) —see Degeneration, combined
- pulmonary valve (heart) I37.8
- pulp (tooth) K04.2
- pupillary margin H21.24-
- renal —see Degeneration, kidney
- retina H35.9
  - hereditary (cerebroretinal) (congenital) (juvenile) (macula) (peripheral) (pigmentary) —see Dystrophy, retina
  - Kuhnt-Junius (see also Degeneration, macula) H35.32-
  - macula (cystic) (exudative) (hole) (nonexudative) (pseudohole) (senile) (toxic) —see Degeneration, macula
  - peripheral H35.40
    - lattice H35.41-
    - microcystoid H35.42-
    - paving stone H35.43-
    - secondary
      - pigmentary H35.45-
      - vitreoretinal H35.46-
    - senile reticular H35.44-
  - pigmentary (primary) —see also Dystrophy, retina
  - secondary —see Degeneration, retina, peripheral, secondary
  - posterior pole —see Degeneration, macula
- saccule, congenital (causing impairment of hearing) Q16.5
- senile R54
  - brain G31.1
  - cardiac, heart or myocardium —see Degeneration, myocardial
  - motor centers G31.1
  - vascular —see Arteriosclerosis
- sinus (cystic) —see also Sinusitis
  - polypoid J33.1
- skin L98.8
  - amyloid E85.4 *[L99]*
  - colloid L98.8
- spinal (cord) G31.89
  - amyloid E85.4 *[G32.89]*
  - combined (subacute) —see Degeneration, combined
  - dorsolateral —see Degeneration, combined
  - familial NEC G31.89
  - fatty G31.89
  - funicular —see Degeneration, combined
  - posterolateral —see Degeneration, combined
  - subacute combined —see Degeneration, combined
  - tuberculous A17.81
- spleen D73.0
  - amyloid E85.4 *[D77]*
- stomach K31.89
- striatonigral G23.2
- suprarenal (capsule) (gland) E27.8
- synovial membrane (pulpy) —see Disorder, synovium, specified type NEC

Degeneration, degenerative (continued)
- tapetoretinal —see Dystrophy, retina
- thymus (gland) E32.8
  - fatty E32.8
- thyroid (gland) E07.89
- tricuspid (heart) (valve) I07.9
- tuberculous NEC —see Tuberculosis
- turbinate J34.89
- uterus (cystic) N85.8
- vascular (senile) —see Arteriosclerosis
  - hypertensive —see Hypertension
- vitreoretinal, secondary —see Degeneration, retina, peripheral, secondary, vitreoretinal
- vitreous (body) H43.81-
- Wallerian —see Disorder, nerve
- Wilson's hepatolenticular E83.01

Deglutition
- paralysis R13.0
  - hysterical F44.4
- pneumonia J69.0

Degos' disease I77.89

Dehiscence (of)
- amputation stump T87.81
- cesarean wound O90.0
- closure of
  - cornea T81.31
  - craniotomy T81.32
  - fascia (muscular) (superficial) T81.32
  - internal organ or tissue T81.32
  - laceration (external) (internal) T81.33
  - ligament T81.32
  - mucosa T81.31
  - muscle or muscle flap T81.32
  - ribs or rib cage T81.32
  - skin and subcutaneous tissue (full-thickness) (superficial) T81.31
  - skull T81.32
  - sternum (sternotomy) T81.32
  - tendon T81.32
  - traumatic laceration (external) (internal) T81.33
- episiotomy O90.1
- operation wound NEC T81.31
  - external operation wound (superficial) T81.31
  - internal operation wound (deep) T81.32
- perineal wound (postpartum) O90.1
- traumatic injury wound repair T81.33
- wound T81.30
  - traumatic repair T81.33

Dehydration E86.0
- newborn P74.1

Déjérine-Roussy syndrome G89.0

Déjérine-Sottas disease or neuropathy (hypertrophic) G60.0

Déjérine-Thomas atrophy G23.8

Delay, delayed
- any plane in pelvis
  - complicating delivery O66.9
- birth or delivery NOS O63.9
- closure, ductus arteriosus (Botalli) P29.38
- coagulation —see Defect, coagulation
- conduction (cardiac) (ventricular) I45.9
- delivery, second twin, triplet, etc O63.2
- development R62.50
  - global F88
  - intellectual (specific) F81.9

Delay, delayed (continued)
- development (continued)
  - language F80.9
    - due to hearing loss F80.4
  - learning F81.9
  - milestone R62.0
  - pervasive F84.9
  - physiological R62.50
    - specified stage NEC R62.0
  - reading F81.0
  - sexual E30.0
  - speech F80.9
    - due to hearing loss F80.4
  - spelling F81.81
- ejaculation F52.32
- gastric emptying K30
- menarche E30.0
- menstruation (cause unknown) N91.0
- milestone R62.0
- passage of meconium (newborn) P76.0
- primary respiration P28.9
- puberty (constitutional) E30.0
- separation of umbilical cord P96.82
- sexual maturation, female E30.0
- sleep phase syndrome G47.21
- union, fracture —see Fracture, by site
- vaccination Z28.9

Deletion(s)
- autosome Q93.9
  - identified by fluorescence in situ hybridization (FISH) Q93.89
  - identified by in situ hybridization (ISH) Q93.89
- chromosome
  - with complex rearrangements NEC Q93.7
  - part of NEC Q93.59
  - seen only at prometaphase Q93.89
  - short arm
    - 4 Q93.3
    - 5p Q93.4
    - 22q11.2 Q93.81
  - specified NEC Q93.89
- long arm chromosome 18 or 21 Q93.89
  - with complex rearrangements NEC Q93.7
- microdeletions NEC Q93.88

Delhi boil or button B55.1

Delinquency (juvenile) (neurotic) F91.8
- group Z72.810

Delinquent immunization status Z28.3

Delirium, delirious (acute or subacute) (not alcohol- or drug-induced) (with dementia) R41.0
- alcoholic (acute) (tremens) (withdrawal) F10.921
  - with intoxication F10.921
    - in
      - abuse F10.121
      - dependence F10.221
- due to (secondary to)
  - alcohol
    - intoxication F10.921
      - in
        - abuse F10.121
        - dependence F10.221
    - withdrawal F10.231
  - amphetamine intoxication F15.921
    - in
      - abuse F15.121
      - dependence F15.221
  - anxiolytic
    - intoxication F13.921
      - in
        - abuse F13.121
        - dependence F13.221
    - withdrawal F13.231

Delirium, delirious (continued)
- due to (continued)
  - cannabis intoxication (acute) F12.921
    - in
      - abuse F12.121
      - dependence F12.221
  - cocaine intoxication (acute) F14.921
    - in
      - abuse F14.121
      - dependence F14.221
  - general medical condition F05
  - hallucinogen intoxication F16.921
    - in
      - abuse F16.121
      - dependence F16.221
  - hypnotic
    - intoxication F13.921
      - in
        - abuse F13.121
        - dependence F13.221
    - withdrawal F13.231
  - inhalant intoxication (acute) F18.921
    - in
      - abuse F18.121
      - dependence F18.221
  - multiple etiologies F05
  - opioid intoxication (acute) F11.921
    - in
      - abuse F11.121
      - dependence F11.221
  - other (or unknown) substance F19.921
  - phencyclidine intoxication (acute) F16.921
    - in
      - abuse F16.121
      - dependence F16.221
  - psychoactive substance NEC intoxication (acute) F19.921
    - in
      - abuse F19.121
      - dependence F19.221
  - sedative
    - intoxication F13.921
      - in
        - abuse F13.121
        - dependence F13.221
    - withdrawal F13.231
  - unknown etiology R41.0
- exhaustion F43.0
- hysterical F44.89
- postprocedural (postoperative) F05
- puerperal F05
- thyroid —see Thyrotoxicosis with thyroid storm
- traumatic —see Injury, intracranial
- tremens (alcohol-induced) F10.231
  - sedative-induced F13.231

Delivery (childbirth) (labor)
- arrested active phase O62.1
- cesarean (for)
  - abnormal
    - pelvis (bony) (deformity) (major) NEC with disproportion (fetopelvic) O33.0
      - with obstructed labor O65.0
    - presentation or position O32.9
  - abruptio placentae (see also Abruptio placentae) O45.9-
  - acromion presentation O32.2
  - atony, uterus O62.2
  - breech presentation O32.1
    - incomplete O32.8
  - brow presentation O32.3

Delivery (continued)
  cesarean (continued)
    cephalopelvic disproportion O33.9
    cerclage O34.3-
    chin presentation O32.3
    cicatrix of cervix O34.4-
    contracted pelvis (general)
      inlet O33.2
      outlet O33.3
    cord presentation or prolapse O69.0
    cystocele O34.8-
    deformity (acquired) (congenital)
      pelvic organs or tissues NEC O34.8-
      pelvis (bony) NEC O33.0
    disproportion NOS O33.9
    eclampsia —see Eclampsia
    face presentation O32.3
    failed
      forceps O66.5
      induction of labor O61.9
        instrumental O61.1
        mechanical O61.1
        medical O61.0
        specified NEC O61.8
        surgical O61.1
      trial of labor NOS O66.40
        following previous cesarean delivery O66.41
      vacuum extraction O66.5
      ventouse O66.5
    fetal-maternal hemorrhage O43.01-
    hemorrhage (intrapartum) O67.9
      with coagulation defect O67.0
      specified cause NEC O67.8
    high head at term O32.4
    hydrocephalic fetus O33.6
    incarceration of uterus O34.51-
    incoordinate uterine action O62.4
    increased size, fetus O33.5
    inertia, uterus O62.2
      primary O62.0
      secondary O62.1
    isthmocele O34.22
    lateroversion, uterus O34.59-
    mal lie O32.9
    malposition
      fetus O32.9
      pelvic organs or tissues NEC O34.8-
      uterus NEC O34.59-
    malpresentation NOS O32.9
    oblique presentation O32.2
    occurring after 37 completed weeks of gestation but before 39 completed weeks gestation due to (spontaneous) onset of labor O75.82
    oversize fetus O33.5
    pelvic tumor NEC O34.8-
    placenta previa O44.0-
      complete O44.0-
        with hemorrhage O44.1-
    placental insufficiency O36.51-
    planned, occurring after 37 completed weeks of gestation but before 39 completed weeks gestation due to (spontaneous) onset of labor O75.82
    polyp, cervix O34.4-
      causing obstructed labor O65.5
    poor dilatation, cervix O62.0
    pre-eclampsia O14.94
      mild O14.04
      moderate O14.04
      severe O14.14
        with hemolysis, elevated liver enzymes and low platelet count (HELLP) O14.24

Delivery (continued)
  cesarean (continued)
    previous
      cesarean delivery O34.219
        classical (vertical) O34.212
        isthmocele O34.22
        low transverse scar O34.211
        mid-transverse T incision O34.218
        scar
          defect (isthmocele) O34.22
          specified type NEC O34.218
      surgery (to)
        cervix O34.4-
        gynecological NEC O34.8-
        rectum O34.7-
        uterus O34.29
        vagina O34.6-
    prolapse
      arm or hand O32.2
      uterus O34.52-
    prolonged labor NOS O63.9
    rectocele O34.8-
    retroversion
      uterus O34.53-
    rigid
      cervix O34.4-
      pelvic floor O34.8-
      perineum O34.7-
      vagina O34.6-
      vulva O34.7-
    sacculation, pregnant uterus O34.59-
    scar(s)
      cervix O34.4-
      cesarean delivery O34.219
        classical (vertical) O34.212
        isthmocele O34.22
        low transverse O34.211
        mid-transverse T incision O34.218
        scar
          defect (isthmocele) O34.22
          specified type NEC O34.218
      defect (isthmocele) O34.22
      transmural uterine O34.29
      uterus O34.29
    Shirodkar suture in situ O34.3-
    shoulder presentation O32.2
    stenosis or stricture, cervix O34.4-
    streptococcus group B (GBS) carrier state O99.824
    transmural uterine scar O34.29
    transverse presentation or lie O32.2
    tumor, pelvic organs or tissues NEC O34.8-
      cervix O34.4-
    umbilical cord presentation or prolapse O69.0
    without indication O82
  completely normal case O80
  complicated O75.9
    by
      abnormal, abnormality (of)
        forces of labor O62.9
          specified type NEC O62.8
        glucose O99.814
        uterine contractions NOS O62.9
      abruptio placentae (see also Abruptio placentae) O45.9-
      abuse
        physical O9A.32
        psychological O9A.52
        sexual O9A.42

Delivery (continued)
  complicated (continued)
    by (continued)
      adherent placenta O72.0
        without hemorrhage O73.0
      alcohol use O99.314
      anemia (pre-existing) O99.02
      anesthetic death O74.8
      annular detachment of cervix O71.3
      atony, uterus O62.2
      attempted vacuum extraction and forceps O66.5
      Bandl's ring O62.4
      bariatric surgery status O99.844
      biliary tract disorder O26.62
      bleeding —see Delivery, complicated by, hemorrhage
      blood disorder NEC O99.12
      cervical dystocia (hypotonic) O62.2
        primary O62.0
        secondary O62.1
      circulatory system disorder O99.42
      compression of cord (umbilical) NEC O69.2
      condition NEC O99.892
      contraction, contracted ring O62.4
      cord (umbilical)
        around neck
          with compression O69.1
          without compression O69.81
        bruising O69.5
        complication O69.9
          specified NEC O69.89
        compression NEC O69.2
        entanglement O69.2
          without compression O69.82
        hematoma O69.5
        presentation O69.0
        prolapse O69.0
        short O69.3
        thrombosis (vessels) O69.5
        vascular lesion O69.5
      Couvelaire uterus O45.8X-
      damage to (injury to) NEC
        perineum O71.82
        periurethral tissue O71.82
        vulva O71.82
      delay following rupture of membranes (spontaneous) —see Pregnancy, complicated by, premature rupture of membranes
      depressed fetal heart tones O76
      diabetes O24.92
        gestational
          diabetes O24.429
            diet controlled O24.420
            insulin (and diet) controlled O24.424
            oral drug controlled (antidiabetic) (hypoglycemic) O24.425
          edema O12.04
            with proteinuria O12.24
          proteinuria O12.14
        pre-existing O24.32
          specified NEC O24.82
          type 1 O24.02
          type 2 O24.12
      diastasis recti (abdominis) O71.89

Delivery (continued)
  complicated (continued)
    by (continued)
      dilatation
        bladder O66.8
        cervix incomplete, poor or slow O62.0
      disease NEC O99.892
      disruptio uteri —see Delivery, complicated by, rupture, uterus
      drug use O99.324
      dysfunction, uterus NOS O62.9
        hypertonic O62.4
        hypotonic O62.2
          primary O62.0
          secondary O62.1
        incoordinate O62.4
      eclampsia O15.1
      embolism (pulmonary) —see Embolism, obstetric
      endocrine, nutritional or metabolic disease NEC O99.284
      failed
        attempted vaginal birth after previous cesarean delivery O66.41
        induction of labor O61.9
          instrumental O61.1
          mechanical O61.1
          medical O61.0
          specified NEC O61.8
          surgical O61.1
        trial of labor O66.40
      female genital mutilation O65.5
      fetal
        abnormal acid-base balance O68
        acidemia O68
        acidosis O68
        alkalosis O68
        death, early O02.1
        deformity O66.3
        heart rate or rhythm (abnormal) (non-reassuring) O76
        hypoxia O77.8
        stress O77.9
          due to drug administration O77.1
          electrocardiographic evidence of O77.8
          specified NEC O77.8
          ultrasound evidence of O77.8
      fever during labor O75.2
      gastric banding status O99.844
      gastric bypass status O99.844
      gastrointestinal disease NEC O99.62
      gestational
        diabetes O24.429
          diet controlled O24.420
          insulin (and diet) controlled O24.424
          oral drug controlled (antidiabetic) (hypoglycemic) O24.425
        edema O12.04
          with proteinuria O12.14
        proteinuria O12.14
      gonorrhea O98.22
      hematoma O71.7
        ischial spine O71.7
        pelvic O71.7
        vagina O71.7
        vulva or perineum O71.7

94

Delivery (continued)
  complicated (continued)
    by (continued)
      hemorrhage (uterine) O67.9
        associated with
          afibrinogenemia O67.0
          coagulation defect O67.0
          hyperfibrinolysis O67.0
          hypofibrinogenemia O67.0
        due to
          low implantation of placenta O44.5-
          low-lying placenta O44.5-
          placenta previa O44.1-
            marginal O44.3-
            partial O44.3-
          premature separation of placenta (normally implanted) (see also Abruptio placentae) O45.9-
          retained placenta O72.0
          uterine leiomyoma O67.8
        placenta NEC O67.8
        postpartum NEC (atonic) (immediate) O72.1
          with retained or trapped placenta O72.0
          delayed O72.2
          secondary O72.2
          third stage O72.0
      hourglass contraction, uterus O62.4
      hypertension, hypertensive (pre-existing) —see Hypertension, complicated by, childbirth (labor)
      hypotension O26.5-
      incomplete dilatation (cervix) O62.0
      incoordinate uterus contractions O62.4
      inertia, uterus O62.2
        during latent phase of labor O62.0
        primary O62.0
        secondary O62.1
      infection (maternal) O98.92
        carrier state NEC O99.834
        gonorrhea O98.22
        human immunodeficiency virus (HIV) O98.72
        sexually transmitted NEC O98.32
        specified NEC O98.82
        syphilis O98.12
        tuberculosis O98.02
        viral hepatitis O98.42
        viral NEC O98.52
      injury (to mother) (see also Delivery, complicated by, damage to) O71.9
        nonobstetric O9A.22
          caused by abuse —see Delivery, complicated by, abuse
      intrauterine fetal death, early O02.1
      inversion, uterus O71.2
      laceration (perineal) O70.9
        anus (sphincter) O70.4
          with third degree laceration (see also Delivery, complicated, by, laceration, perineum, third degree) O70.20
            with mucosa O70.3
          without third degree laceration O70.4

Delivery (continued)
  complicated (continued)
    by (continued)
      laceration (continued)
        bladder (urinary) O71.5
        bowel O71.5
        cervix (uteri) O71.3
        fourchette O70.0
        hymen O70.0
        labia O70.0
        pelvic
          floor O70.1
          organ NEC O71.5
        perineum, perineal O70.9
          first degree O70.0
          fourth degree O70.3
          muscles O70.1
          second degree O70.1
          skin O70.0
          slight O70.0
          third degree O70.20
            with
              both external anal sphincter (EAS) and internal anal sphincter (IAS) torn (IIIc) O70.23
              less than 50% of external anal sphincter (EAS) thickness torn (IIIa) O70.21
              more than 50% of external anal sphincter (EAS) thickness torn (IIIb) O70.22
            IIIa O70.21
            IIIb O70.22
            IIIc O70.23
        peritoneum (pelvic) O71.5
        rectovaginal (septum) (without perineal laceration) O71.4
          with perineum (see also Delivery, complicated, by, laceration, perineum, third degree) O70.20
            with anal or rectal mucosa O70.3
        specified NEC O71.89
        sphincter ani —see Delivery, complicated, by, laceration, anus (sphincter)
        urethra O71.5
        uterus O71.81
          before labor O71.81
        vagina, vaginal (deep) (high) (without perineal laceration) O71.4
          with perineum O70.0
          muscles, with perineum O70.1
        vulva O70.0
      liver disorder O26.62
      malignancy O9A.12
      malnutrition O25.2
      malposition, malpresentation placenta O44.0-
        with hemorrhage O44.1-
        uterus or cervix O65.5
        without obstruction (see also Delivery, complicated by, obstruction) O32.9
          breech O32.1
          compound O32.6
          face (brow) (chin) O32.3
          footling O32.8
          high head O32.4
          oblique O32.2

Delivery (continued)
  complicated (continued)
    by (continued)
      malposition, malpresentation (continued)
        without obstruction (continued)
          specified NEC O32.8
          transverse O32.2
          unstable lie O32.0
      meconium in amniotic fluid O77.0
      mental disorder NEC O99.344
      metrorrhexis —see Delivery, complicated by, rupture, uterus
      nervous system disorder O99.354
      obesity (pre-existing) O99.214
      obesity surgery status O99.844
      obstetric trauma O71.9
        specified NEC O71.89
      obstructed labor
        due to
          breech (complete) (frank) presentation O64.1
            incomplete O64.8
          brow presentation O64.3
          buttock presentation O64.1
          chin presentation O64.2
          compound presentation O64.5
          contracted pelvis O65.1
          deep transverse arrest O64.0
          deformed pelvis O65.0
          dystocia (fetal) O66.9
            due to
              conjoined twins O66.3
              fetal
                abnormality NEC O66.3
                ascites O66.3
                hydrops O66.3
                meningomyelocele O66.3
                sacral teratoma O66.3
                tumor O66.3
              hydrocephalic fetus O66.3
              shoulder O66.0
          face presentation O64.2
          fetopelvic disproportion O65.4
          footling presentation O64.8
          impacted shoulders O66.0
          incomplete rotation of fetal head O64.0
          large fetus O66.2
          locked twins O66.1
          malposition O64.9
            specified NEC O64.8
          malpresentation O64.9
            specified NEC O64.8
          multiple fetuses NEC O66.6
          pelvic
            abnormality (maternal) O65.9
              organ O65.5
              specified NEC O65.8
            contraction
              inlet O65.2
              mid-cavity O65.3
              outlet O65.3
          persistent (position)
            occipitoiliac O64.0
            occipitoposterior O64.0

Delivery (continued)
  complicated (continued)
    by (continued)
      obstructed labor (continued)
        due to (continued)
          persistent (continued)
            occipitosacral O64.0
            occipitotransverse O64.0
          prolapsed arm O64.4
          shoulder presentation O64.4
          specified NEC O66.8
      pathological retraction ring, uterus O62.4
      penetration, pregnant uterus by instrument O71.1
      perforation —see Delivery, complicated by, laceration
      placenta, placental
        ablatio (see also Abruptio placentae) O45.9-
        abnormality O43.9-
          specified NEC O43.89-
        abruptio (see also Abruptio placentae) O45.9-
        accreta O43.21-
        adherent (with hemorrhage) O72.0
          without hemorrhage O73.0
        detachment (premature) (see also Abruptio placentae) O45.9-
        disorder O43.9-
          specified NEC O43.89-
        hemorrhage NEC O67.8
        increta O43.22-
        low (implantation) (lying) O44.4-
          with hemorrhage O44.5-
        malformation O43.10-
        malposition O44.0-
          with hemorrhage O44.1-
        percreta O43.23-
        previa (central) (complete) (lateral) (total) O44.0-
          with hemorrhage O44.1-
          marginal O44.2-
            with hemorrhage O44.3-
          partial O44.2-
            with hemorrhage O44.3-
        retained (with hemorrhage) O72.0
          without hemorrhage O73.0
        separation (premature) O45.9-
          specified NEC O45.8X-
        vicious insertion O44.1-
      precipitate labor O62.3
      premature rupture, membranes (see also Pregnancy, complicated by, premature rupture of membranes) O42.90
      prolapse
        arm or hand O32.2
        cord (umbilical) O69.0
        foot or leg O32.8
        uterus O34.52-
      prolonged labor O63.9
        first stage O63.0
        second stage O63.1
      protozoal disease (maternal) O98.62
      respiratory disease NEC O99.52
      retained membranes or portions of placenta O72.2
        without hemorrhage O73.1
      retarded birth O63.9

95

Delivery (continued)
  complicated (continued)
    by (continued)
      retention of secundines (with hemorrhage) O72.0
        without hemorrhage O73.0
        partial O72.2
          without hemorrhage O73.1
      rupture
        bladder (urinary) O71.5
        cervix O71.3
        pelvic organ NEC O71.5
        urethra O71.5
        uterus (during or after labor) O71.1
          before labor O71.0-
      separation, pubic bone (symphysis pubis) O71.6
      shock O75.1
      shoulder presentation O64.4
      skin disorder NEC O99.72
      spasm, cervix O62.4
      stenosis or stricture, cervix O65.5
      streptococcus group B (GBS) carrier state O99.824
      subluxation of symphysis (pubis) O26.72
      syphilis (maternal) O98.12
      tear —see Delivery, complicated by, laceration
      tetanic uterus O62.4
      trauma (obstetrical) (see also Delivery, complicated by, damage to) O71.9
        non-obstetric O9A.22
        periurethral O71.82
        specified NEC O71.89
      tuberculosis (maternal) O98.02
      tumor, pelvic organs or tissues NEC O65.5
      umbilical cord around neck
        with compression O69.1
        without compression O69.81
      uterine inertia O62.2
        during latent phase of labor O62.0
        primary O62.0
        secondary O62.1
      vasa previa O69.4
      velamentous insertion of cord O43.12-
      specified complication NEC O75.89
  delayed NOS O63.9
    following rupture of membranes
      artificial O75.5
    second twin, triplet, etc. O63.2
  forceps, low following failed vacuum extraction O66.5
  missed (at or near term) O36.4
  normal O80
  obstructed —see Delivery, complicated by, obstructed labor
  precipitate O62.3
  preterm (see also Pregnancy, complicated by, preterm labor) O60.10
  spontaneous O80
  term pregnancy NOS O80
  uncomplicated O80
  vaginal, following previous
    cesarean delivery O34.219
    classical (vertical) scar O34.212
    low transverse scar O34.211
    mid-transverse T incision O34.218
    scar
      defect (isthmocele) O34.22
      specified type NEC O34.218

Delusions (paranoid) —see Disorder, delusional

Dementia (degenerative (primary)) (old age) (persisting) (unspecified severity) (without behavioral disturbance, psychotic disturbance, mood disturbance, and anxiety) F03.90
  with
    aberrant motor behavior (exit-seeking) (pacing) (restlessness) (rocking) F03.911
    agitation F03.911
    anxiety F03.94
    behavioral disturbances (sexual disinhibition) (sleep disturbance) (social disinhibition) F03.918
      specified NEC F03.918
    Lewy bodies (see also Dementia, in, diseases specified elsewhere) G31.83 [F02.80]
      with behavioral disturbance (see also Dementia, in, diseases specified elsewhere) G31.83 [F02.81-]
    mood disturbance (anhedonia) (apathy) (depression) F03.93
    Parkinsonism (see also Dementia, in, diseases specified elsewhere) G20.C [F02.80]
      with behavioral disturbance (see also Dementia, in, diseases specified elsewhere) G20.C [F02.81-]
    Parkinson's disease (see also Dementia, in, diseases specified elsewhere) G20.A1 [F02.80]
      with behavioral disturbance (see also Dementia, in, diseases specified elsewhere) G20.A1 [F02.81-]
    psychotic disturbance (delusional state) (hallucinations) (paranoia) (suspiciousness) F03.92
    verbal or physical behaviors (anger) (aggression) (combativeness) (profanity) (shouting) (threatening) (violence) F03.911
  alcoholic F10.97
    with dependence F10.27
  Alzheimer's type —see Disease, Alzheimer's
  arteriosclerotic —see Dementia, vascular
  atypical, Alzheimer's type —see Disease, Alzheimer's, specified NEC
  congenital —see Disability, intellectual
  frontal (lobe) (see also Dementia, in, diseases specified elsewhere) G31.09 [F02.80]
    with behavioral disturbance (see also Dementia, in, diseases specified elsewhere) G31.09 [F02.81-]
  frontotemporal G31.09 [F02.80]
    with behavioral disturbance G31.09 [F02.81]
  specified NEC (see also Dementia, in, diseases specified elsewhere) G31.09 [F02.80]
    with behavioral disturbance (see also Dementia, in, diseases specified elsewhere) G31.09 [F02.81-]

Dementia (continued)
  in (due to)
    alcohol F10.97
      with dependence F10.27
    Alzheimer's disease —see Disease, Alzheimer's
    arteriosclerotic brain disease —see Dementia, vascular
    cerebral lipidoses (see also Dementia, in, diseases specified elsewhere) E75.- [F02.80]
      with behavioral disturbance (see also Dementia, in, diseases specified elsewhere) E75.- [F02.81-]
    Creutzfeldt-Jakob disease —see also Creutzfeldt-Jakob disease or syndrome (with dementia) A81.00
    diseases specified elsewhere (unspecified severity) (without behavioral disturbance, psychotic disturbance, mood disturbance, and anxiety) F02.80
      with
        aberrant motor behavior (exit-seeking) (pacing) (restlessness) (rocking) F02.811
        agitation F02.811
        anxiety F02.84
        behavioral disturbances (sexual disinhibition) (sleep disturbance) (social disinhibition) F02.818
          specified NEC F02.818
        mood disturbance (anhedonia) (apathy) (depression) F02.83
        psychotic disturbance (delusional state) (hallucinations) (paranoia) (suspiciousness) F02.82
        verbal or physical behaviors (anger) (aggression) (combativeness) (profanity) (shouting) (threatening) (violence) F02.811
    mild F02.A0
      with
        aberrant motor behavior (exit-seeking) (pacing) (restlessness) (rocking) F02.A11
        agitation F02.A11
        anxiety F02.A4
        behavioral disturbances (sexual disinhibition) (sleep disturbance) (social disinhibition) F02.A18
          specified NEC F02.A18
        mood disturbance (anhedonia) (apathy) (depression) F02.A3
        psychotic disturbance (delusional state) (hallucinations) (paranoia) (suspiciousness) F02.A2
        verbal or physical behaviors (anger) (aggression) (combativeness) (profanity) (shouting) (threatening) (violence) F02.A11

Dementia (continued)
  in (continued)
    moderate F02.B0
      with
        aberrant motor behavior (exit-seeking) (pacing) (restlessness) (rocking) F02.B11
        agitation F02.B11
        anxiety F02.B4
        behavioral disturbances (sexual disinhibition) (sleep disturbance) (social disinhibition) F02.B18
          specified NEC F02.B18
        mood disturbance (anhedonia) (apathy) (depression) F02.B3
        psychotic disturbance (delusional state) (hallucinations) (paranoia) (suspiciousness) F02.B2
        verbal or physical behaviors (anger) (aggression) (combativeness) (profanity) (shouting) (threatening) (violence) F02.B11
    severe F02.C0
      with
        aberrant motor behavior (exit-seeking) (pacing) (restlessness) (rocking) F02.C11
        agitation F02.C11
        anxiety F02.C4
        behavioral disturbances (sexual disinhibition) (sleep disturbance) (social disinhibition) F02.C18
          specified NEC F02.C18
        mood disturbance (anhedonia) (apathy) (depression) F02.C3
        psychotic disturbance (delusional state) (hallucinations) (paranoia) (suspiciousness) F02.C2
        verbal or physical behaviors (anger) (aggression) (combativeness) (profanity) (shouting) (threatening) (violence) F02.C11
    epilepsy (see also Dementia, in, diseases specified elsewhere) G40.- [F02.80]
      with behavioral disturbance (see also Dementia, in, diseases specified elsewhere) G40.- [F02.81-]
    hepatolenticular degeneration (see also Dementia, in, diseases specified elsewhere) E83.01 [F02.80]
      with behavioral disturbance (see also Dementia, in, diseases specified elsewhere) E83.01 [F02.81-]
    human immunodeficiency virus (HIV) disease (see also Dementia, in, diseases specified elsewhere) B20 [F02.80]
      with behavioral disturbance (see also Dementia, in, diseases specified elsewhere) B20 [F02.81-]

Dementia (*continued*)
in (*continued*)
- Huntington's disease or chorea (*see also* Dementia, in, diseases specified elsewhere) G10 *[F02.80]*
  - with behavioral disturbance (*see also* Dementia, in, diseases specified elsewhere) G10 *[F02.81-]*
- hypercalcemia (*see also* Dementia, in, diseases specified elsewhere) E83.52 *[F02.80]*
  - with behavioral disturbance (*see also* Dementia, in, diseases specified elsewhere) E83.52 *[F02.81-]*
- hypothyroidism, acquired (*see also* Dementia, in, diseases specified elsewhere) E03.9 *[F02.80]*
  - with behavioral disturbance (*see also* Dementia, in, diseases specified elsewhere) E03.9 *[F02.81-]*
  - due to iodine deficiency (*see also* Dementia, in, diseases specified elsewhere) E01.8 *[F02.80]*
    - with behavioral disturbance (*see also* Dementia, in, diseases specified elsewhere) E01.8 *[F02.81-]*
- inhalants F18.97
  - with dependence F18.27
- multiple
  - etiologies F03
  - sclerosis (*see also* Dementia, in, diseases specified elsewhere) G35 *[F02.80]*
    - with behavioral disturbance (*see also* Dementia, in, diseases specified elsewhere) G35 *[F02.81-]*
- neurosyphilis (*see also* Dementia, in, diseases specified elsewhere) A52.17 *[F02.80-]*
  - with behavioral disturbance (*see also* Dementia, in, diseases specified elsewhere) A52.17 *[F02.81-]*
  - juvenile (*see also* Dementia, in, diseases specified elsewhere) A50.49 *[F02.80]*
    - with behavioral disturbance (*see also* Dementia, in, disease specified elsewhere) A50.49 *[F02.81-]*
- niacin deficiency (*see also* Dementia, in, diseases specified elsewhere) E52 *[F02.80]*
  - with behavioral disturbance (*see also* Dementia, in, diseases specified elsewhere) E52 *[F02.81-]*
- paralysis agitans (*see also* Dementia, in, diseases specified elsewhere) G20.C *[F02.80]*
  - with behavioral disturbance (*see also* Dementia, in, diseases specified elsewhere) G20.C *[F02.81-]*
- Parkinson's disease (*see also* Dementia, in, diseases specified elsewhere) G20.A1 *[F02.80]*

Dementia (*continued*)
in (*continued*)
- pellagra (*see also* Dementia, in, diseases specified elsewhere) E52 *[F02.80]*
  - with behavioral disturbance (*see also* Dementia, in, diseases specified elsewhere) E52 *[F02.81-]*
- Pick's (*see also* Dementia, in, diseases specified elsewhere) G31.01 *[F02.80]*
  - with behavioral disturbance (*see also* Dementia, in, diseases specified elsewhere) G31.01 *[F02.81-]*
- polyarteritis nodosa (*see also* Dementia, in, diseases specified elsewhere) M30.0 *[F02.80]*
  - with behavioral disturbance (*see also* Dementia, in, diseases specified elsewhere) M30.0 *[F02.81-]*
- psychoactive drug F19.97
  - with dependence F19.27
  - inhalants F18.97
    - with dependence F18.27
  - sedatives, hypnotics or anxiolytics F13.97
    - with dependence F13.27
- sedatives, hypnotics or anxiolytics F13.97
  - with dependence F13.27
- systemic lupus erythematosus (*see also* Dementia, in, diseases specified elsewhere) M32.- *[F02.80]*
  - with behavioral disturbance (*see also* Dementia, in, diseases specified elsewhere) M32.- *[F02.81-]*
- trypanosomiasis
  - African (*see also* Dementia, in, diseases specified elsewhere) B56.9 *[F02.80]*
    - with behavioral disturbance (*see also* Dementia, in, diseases specified elsewhere) B56.9 *[F02.81-]*
- unknown etiology F03-
- vitamin B12 deficiency (*see also* Dementia, in, diseases specified elsewhere) E53.8 *[F02.80]*
  - with behavioral disturbance (*see also* Dementia, in, diseases specified elsewhere) E53.8 *[F02.81-]*
- volatile solvents F18.97
  - with dependence F18.27
infantile, infantilis F84.3
Lewy body (*see also* Dementia, in, diseases specified elsewhere) G31.83 *[F02.80]*
  - with behavioral disturbance (*see also* Dementia, in, diseases specified elsewhere) G31.83 *[F02.81-]*
mild F03.A0
  with
    aberrant motor behavior (exit-seeking) (pacing) (restlessness) (rocking) F03.A11
    agitation F03.A11
    anxiety F03.A4

Dementia (*continued*)
mild (*continued*)
  with (*continued*)
    behavioral disturbances (sexual disinhibition) (sleep disturbance) (social disinhibition) F03.A18
      specified NEC F03.A18
    mood disturbance (anhedonia) (apathy) (depression) F03.A3
    psychotic disturbance (delusional state) (hallucinations) (paranoia) (suspiciousness) F03.A2
    verbal or physical behaviors (anger) (aggression) (combativeness) (profanity) (shouting) (threatening) (violence) F03.A11
moderate F03.B0
  with
    aberrant motor behavior (exit-seeking) (pacing) (restlessness) (rocking) F03.B11
    agitation F03.B11
    anxiety F03.B4
    behavioral disturbances (sexual disinhibition) (sleep disturbance) (social disinhibition) F03.B18
      specified NEC F03.B18
    mood disturbance (anhedonia) (apathy) (depression) F03.B3
    psychotic disturbance (delusional state) (hallucinations) (paranoia) (suspiciousness) F03.B2
    verbal or physical behaviors (anger) (aggression) (combativeness) (profanity) (shouting) (threatening) (violence) F03.B11
multi-infarct —*see* Dementia, vascular
paralytica, paralytic (syphilitic) (*see also* Dementia, in, diseases specified elsewhere) A52.17 *[F02.80]*
  with behavioral disturbance (*see also* Dementia, in, diseases specified elsewhere) A52.17 *[F02.81-]*
  juvenilis A50.45
paretic A52.17
praecox —*see* Schizophrenia
presenile F03
  Alzheimer's type —*see* Disease, Alzheimer's, early onset
primary degenerative F03
progressive, syphilitic A52.17
senile F03
  with acute confusional state F05
  Alzheimer's type —*see* Disease, Alzheimer's, late onset
  depressed or paranoid type F03
severe F03.C0
  with
    aberrant motor behavior (exit-seeking) (pacing) (restlessness) (rocking) F03.C11
    agitation F03.C11
    anxiety F03.C4
    behavioral disturbances (sexual disinhibition) (sleep disturbance) (social disinhibition) F03.C18
      specified NEC F03.C18

Dementia (*continued*)
severe (*continued*)
  with (*continued*)
    mood disturbance (anhedonia) (apathy) (depression) F03.C3
    psychotic disturbance (delusional state) (hallucinations) (paranoia) (suspiciousness) F03.C2
    verbal or physical behaviors (anger) (aggression) (combativeness) (profanity) (shouting) (threatening) (violence) F03.C11
vascular (acute onset) (mixed) (multi-infarct) (subcortical) (unspecified severity) (without behavioral disturbance, psychotic disturbance, mood disturbance, and anxiety) F01.50
  with
    aberrant motor behavior (exit-seeking) (pacing) (restlessness) (rocking) F01.511
    agitation F01.511
    anxiety F01.54
    behavioral disturbances (sleep disturbance) (sexual disinhibition) (social disinhibition) F01.518
      specified NEC F01.518
    mood disturbance (anhedonia) (apathy) (depression) F01.53
    psychotic disturbance (delusional state) (hallucinations) (paranoia) (suspiciousness) F01.52
    verbal or physical behaviors (anger) (aggression) (combativeness) (profanity) (shouting) (threatening) (violence) F01.511
  mild F01.A0
    with
      aberrant motor behavior (exit-seeking) (pacing) (restlessness) (rocking) F01.A11
      agitation F01.A11
      anxiety F01.A4
      behavioral disturbances (sleep disturbance) (sexual disinhibition) (social disinhibition) F01.A18
        specified NEC F01.A18
      mood disturbance (anhedonia) (apathy) (depression) F01.A3
      psychotic disturbance (delusional state) (hallucinations) (paranoia) (suspiciousness) F01.A2
      verbal or physical behaviors (anger) (aggression) (combativeness) (profanity) (shouting) (threatening) (violence) F01.A11
  moderate F01.B0
    with
      aberrant motor behavior (exit-seeking) (pacing) (restlessness) (rocking) F01.B11
      agitation F01.B11
      anxiety F01.B4

Dementia *(continued)*
vascular *(continued)*
moderate *(continued)*
with *(continued)*
behavioral disturbances
(sleep disturbance)
(sexual disinhibition)
(social disinhibition)
F01.B18
specified NEC F01.B18
mood disturbance
(anhedonia) (apathy)
(depression) F01.B3
psychotic disturbance
(delusional state)
(hallucinations)
(paranoia)
(suspiciousness)
F01.B2
verbal or physical behaviors
(anger) (aggression)
(combativeness)
(profanity) (shouting)
(threatening)(violence)
F01.B11
severe F01.C0
with
aberrant motor behavior
(exit-seeking) (pacing)
(restlessness) (rocking)
F01.C11
agitation F01.C11
anxiety F01.C4
behavioral disturbances
(sleep disturbance)
(sexual disinhibition)
(social disinhibition)
F01.C18
specified NEC
F01.C18
mood disturbance
(anhedonia) (apathy)
(depression) F01.C3
psychotic disturbance
(delusional state)
(hallucinations)
(paranoia)
(suspiciousness)
F01.C2
verbal or physical behaviors
(anger) (aggression)
(combativeness)
(profanity) (shouting)
(threatening)(violence)
F01.C11
Demineralization, bone —see Osteoporosis
Demodex folliculorum (infestation) B88.0
Demophobia F40.248
Demoralization R45.3
Demyelination, demyelinization
central nervous system G37.9
specified NEC G37.89
corpus callosum (central) G37.1
disseminated, acute G36.9
specified NEC G36.8
global G35
in optic neuritis G36.0
Dengue (classical) (fever) A90
hemorrhagic A91
sandfly A93.1
Dennie-Marfan syphilitic syndrome A50.45
Dens evaginatus, in dente or invaginatus K00.2
Dense breasts (see also Density, breast) R92.30

Density
breast R92.30
mammographic
extreme R92.34-
fatty tissue R92.31-
fibroglandular R92.32-
heterogeneous R92.33-
increased, bone (disseminated) (generalized) (spotted) —see Disorder, bone, density and structure, specified type NEC
low R92.30
lung (nodular) J98.4
Dental —see also condition
examination Z01.20
with abnormal findings Z01.21
restoration
aesthetically inadequate or displeasing K08.56
defective K08.50
specified NEC K08.59
failure of marginal integrity K08.51
failure of periodontal anatomical integrity K08.54
Dentia praecox K00.6
Denticles (pulp) K04.2
Dentigerous cyst K09.0
Dentin
irregular (in pulp) K04.3
opalescent K00.5
secondary (in pulp) K04.3
sensitive K03.89
Dentinogenesis imperfecta K00.5
Dentinoma —see Cyst, calcifying odontogenic
Dentition (syndrome) K00.7
delayed K00.6
difficult K00.7
precocious K00.6
premature K00.6
retarded K00.6
Dependence (on) (syndrome) F19.20
with remission F19.21
alcohol (ethyl) (methyl) (without remission) F10.20
with
amnestic disorder, persisting F10.26
anxiety disorder F10.280
dementia, persisting F10.27
intoxication F10.229
with delirium F10.221
uncomplicated F10.220
mood disorder F10.24
psychotic disorder F10.259
with
delusions F10.250
hallucinations F10.251
remission F10.21
sexual dysfunction F10.281
sleep disorder F10.282
specified disorder NEC F10.288
withdrawal F10.239
with
delirium F10.231
perceptual disturbance F10.232
uncomplicated F10.230
counseling and surveillance Z71.41
in remission F10.21
amobarbital —see Dependence, drug, sedative
amphetamine(s) (type) —see Dependence, drug, stimulant NEC

Dependence *(continued)*
amytal (sodium) —see Dependence, drug, sedative
analgesic NEC F55.8
anesthetic (agent) (gas) (general) (local) NEC —see Dependence, drug, psychoactive NEC
anxiolytic NEC —see Dependence, drug, sedative
barbital(s) —see Dependence, drug, sedative
barbiturate(s) (compounds) (drugs classifiable to T42) —see Dependence, drug, sedative
benzedrine —see Dependence, drug, stimulant NEC
bhang —see Dependence, drug, cannabis
bromide(s) NEC —see Dependence, drug, sedative
caffeine —see Dependence, drug, stimulant NEC
cannabis (sativa) (indica) (resin) (derivatives) (type) —see Dependence, drug, cannabis
chloral (betaine) (hydrate) —see Dependence, drug, sedative
chlordiazepoxide —see Dependence, drug, sedative
coca (leaf) (derivatives) —see Dependence, drug, cocaine
cocaine —see Dependence, drug, cocaine
codeine —see Dependence, drug, opioid
combinations of drugs F19.20
dagga —see Dependence, drug, cannabis
demerol —see Dependence, drug, opioid
dexamphetamine —see Dependence, drug, stimulant NEC
dexedrine —see Dependence, drug, stimulant NEC
dextromethorphan —see Dependence, drug, opioid
dextromoramide —see Dependence, drug, opioid
dextro-nor-pseudo-ephedrine —see Dependence, drug, stimulant NEC
dextrorphan —see Dependence, drug, opioid
diazepam —see Dependence, drug, sedative
dilaudid —see Dependence, drug, opioid
D-lysergic acid diethylamide —see Dependence, drug, hallucinogen
drug NEC F19.20
with sleep disorder F19.282
cannabis F12.20
with
anxiety disorder F12.280
intoxication F12.229
with
delirium F12.221
perceptual disturbance F12.222
uncomplicated F12.220
other specified disorder F12.288
psychosis F12.259
delusions F12.250
hallucinations F12.251
unspecified disorder F12.29
withdrawal F12.23
in remission F12.21
cocaine F14.20
with
anxiety disorder F14.280

Dependence *(continued)*
drug NEC *(continued)*
cocaine *(continued)*
with *(continued)*
intoxication F14.229
with
delirium F14.221
perceptual disturbance F14.222
uncomplicated F14.220
mood disorder F14.24
other specified disorder F14.288
psychosis F14.259
delusions F14.250
hallucinations F14.251
sexual dysfunction F14.281
sleep disorder F14.282
unspecified disorder F14.29
withdrawal F14.23
in remission F14.21
withdrawal symptoms in newborn P96.1
counseling and surveillance Z71.51
hallucinogen F16.20
with
anxiety disorder F16.280
flashbacks F16.283
intoxication F16.229
with delirium F16.221
uncomplicated F16.220
mood disorder F16.24
other specified disorder F16.288
perception disorder, persisting F16.283
psychosis F16.259
delusions F16.250
hallucinations F16.251
unspecified disorder F16.29
in remission F16.21
in remission F19.21
inhalant F18.20
with
anxiety disorder F18.280
dementia, persisting F18.27
intoxication F18.229
with delirium F18.221
uncomplicated F18.220
mood disorder F18.24
other specified disorder F18.288
psychosis F18.259
delusions F18.250
hallucinations F18.251
unspecified disorder F18.29
in remission F18.21
nicotine F17.200
with disorder F17.209
in remission F17.201
specified disorder NEC F17.208
withdrawal F17.203
chewing tobacco F17.220
with disorder F17.229
in remission F17.221
specified disorder NEC F17.228
withdrawal F17.223
cigarettes F17.210
with disorder F17.219
in remission F17.211
specified disorder NEC F17.218
withdrawal F17.213
specified product NEC F17.290
with disorder F17.299
remission F17.291
specified disorder NEC F17.298
withdrawal F17.293

Dependence (continued)
  drug NEC (continued)
    opioid F11.20
      with
        intoxication F11.229
          with
            delirium F11.221
            perceptual disturbance F11.222
          uncomplicated F11.220
        mood disorder F11.24
        opioid-associated amnestic syndrome F11.288
        other specified disorder F11.288
        psychosis F11.259
          delusions F11.250
          hallucinations F11.251
        sexual dysfunction F11.281
        sleep disorder F11.282
        unspecified disorder F11.29
        withdrawal F11.23
      in remission F11.21
    psychoactive NEC F19.20
      with
        amnestic disorder F19.26
        anxiety disorder F19.280
        dementia F19.27
        intoxication F19.229
          with
            delirium F19.221
            perceptual disturbance F19.222
          uncomplicated F19.220
        mood disorder F19.24
        other specified disorder F19.288
        psychosis F19.259
          delusions F19.250
          hallucinations F19.251
        sexual dysfunction F19.281
        sleep disorder F19.282
        unspecified disorder F19.29
        withdrawal F19.239
          with
            delirium F19.231
            perceptual disturbance F19.232
          uncomplicated F19.230
      in remission F19.21
    sedative, hypnotic or anxiolytic F13.20
      with
        amnestic disorder F13.26
        anxiety disorder F13.280
        dementia, persisting F13.27
        intoxication F13.229
          with delirium F13.221
          uncomplicated F13.220
        mood disorder F13.24
        other specified disorder F13.288
        psychosis F13.259
          delusions F13.250
          hallucinations F13.251
        sexual dysfunction F13.281
        sleep disorder F13.282
        unspecified disorder F13.29
        withdrawal F13.239
          with
            delirium F13.231
            perceptual disturbance F13.232
          uncomplicated F13.230
      in remission F13.21
    stimulant NEC F15.20
      with
        anxiety disorder F15.280

Dependence (continued)
  drug NEC (continued)
    stimulant NEC (continued)
      with (continued)
        intoxication F15.229
          with
            delirium F15.221
            perceptual disturbance F15.222
          uncomplicated F15.220
        mood disorder F15.24
        other specified disorder F15.288
        psychosis F15.259
          delusions F15.250
          hallucinations F15.251
        sexual dysfunction F15.281
        sleep disorder F15.282
        unspecified disorder F15.29
        withdrawal F15.23
      in remission F15.21
  ethyl
    alcohol (without remission) F10.20
      with remission F10.21
    bromide —see Dependence, drug, sedative
    carbamate F19.20
    chloride F19.20
    morphine —see Dependence, drug, opioid
  ganja —see Dependence, drug, cannabis
  glue (airplane) (sniffing) —see Dependence, drug, inhalant
  glutethimide —see Dependence, drug, sedative
  hallucinogenics —see Dependence, drug, hallucinogen
  hashish —see Dependence, drug, cannabis
  hemp —see Dependence, drug, cannabis
  heroin (salt) (any) —see Dependence, drug, opioid
  hypnotic NEC —see Dependence, drug, sedative
  Indian hemp —see Dependence, drug, cannabis
  inhalants —see Dependence, drug, inhalant
  khat —see Dependence, drug, stimulant NEC
  laudanum —see Dependence, drug, opioid
  LSD(-25) (derivatives) —see Dependence, drug, hallucinogen
  luminal —see Dependence, drug, sedative
  lysergic acid —see Dependence, drug, hallucinogen
  maconha —see Dependence, drug, cannabis
  marihuana —see Dependence, drug, cannabis
  meprobamate —see Dependence, drug, sedative
  mescaline —see Dependence, drug, hallucinogen
  methadone —see Dependence, drug, opioid
  methamphetamine(s) —see Dependence, drug, stimulant NEC
  methaqualone —see Dependence, drug, sedative
  methyl
    alcohol (without remission) F10.20
      with remission F10.21

Dependence (continued)
  methyl (continued)
    bromide —see Dependence, drug, sedative
    morphine —see Dependence, drug, opioid
    phenidate —see Dependence, drug, stimulant NEC
    sulfonal —see Dependence, drug, sedative
  morphine (sulfate) (sulfite) (type) —see Dependence, drug, opioid
  narcotic (drug) NEC —see Dependence, drug, opioid
  nembutal —see Dependence, drug, sedative
  neraval —see Dependence, drug, sedative
  neravan —see Dependence, drug, sedative
  neurobarb —see Dependence, drug, sedative
  nicotine —see Dependence, drug, nicotine
  nitrous oxide F19.20
  nonbarbiturate sedatives and tranquilizers with similar effect —see Dependence, drug, sedative
  on
    artificial heart (fully implantable) (mechanical) Z95.812
    aspirator Z99.0
    care provider (because of) Z74.9
      impaired mobility Z74.09
      need for
        assistance with personal care Z74.1
        continuous supervision Z74.3
        no other household member able to render care Z74.2
        specified reason NEC Z74.8
    machine Z99.89
      enabling NEC Z99.89
      specified type NEC Z99.89
    renal dialysis (hemodialysis) (peritoneal) Z99.2
    respirator Z99.11
    ventilator Z99.11
    wheelchair Z99.3
  opiate —see Dependence, drug, opioid
  opioids —see Dependence, drug, opioid
  opium (alkaloids) (derivatives) (tincture) —see Dependence, drug, opioid
  oxygen (long-term) (supplemental) Z99.81
  paraldehyde —see Dependence, drug, sedative
  paregoric —see Dependence, drug, opioid
  PCP (phencyclidine) (or related substance) —see Dependence, drug, hallucinogen
  pentobarbital —see Dependence, drug, sedative
  pentobarbitone (sodium) —see Dependence, drug, sedative
  pentothal —see Dependence, drug, sedative
  peyote —see Dependence, drug, hallucinogen
  phencyclidine (PCP) (or related substance) —see Dependence, drug, hallucinogen
  phenmetrazine —see Dependence, drug, stimulant NEC

Dependence (continued)
  phenobarbital —see Dependence, drug, sedative
  polysubstance F19.20
  psilocibin, psilocin, psilocyn, psilocyline —see Dependence, drug, hallucinogen
  psychostimulant NEC —see Dependence, drug, stimulant NEC
  secobarbital —see Dependence, drug, sedative
  seconal —see Dependence, drug, sedative
  sedative NEC —see Dependence, drug, sedative
  specified drug NEC —see Dependence, drug
  stimulant NEC —see Dependence, drug, stimulant NEC
  substance NEC —see Dependence, drug
  supplemental oxygen Z99.81
  tobacco —see Dependence, drug, nicotine
    counseling and surveillance Z71.6
  tranquilizer NEC —see Dependence, drug, sedative
  vitamin B6 E53.1
  volatile solvents —see Dependence, drug, inhalant

Dependency
  care-provider Z74.9
  passive F60.7
  reactions (persistent) F60.7

Depersonalization (in neurotic state) (neurotic) (syndrome) F48.1

Depletion
  extracellular fluid E86.9
  plasma E86.1
  potassium E87.6
    nephropathy N25.89
  salt or sodium E87.1
    causing heat exhaustion or prostration T67.4
    nephropathy N28.9
  volume NOS E86.9

Deployment (current) (military) status Z56.82
  in theater or in support of military war, peacekeeping and humanitarian operations Z56.82
  personal history of Z91.82
    military war, peacekeeping and humanitarian deployment (current or past conflict) Z91.82
  returned from Z91.82

Depolarization, premature I49.40
  atrial I49.1
  junctional I49.2
  specified NEC I49.49
  ventricular I49.3

Deposit
  bone in Boeck's sarcoid D86.89
  calcareous, calcium —see Calcification
  cholesterol
    retina H35.89
    vitreous (body) (humor) —see Deposit, crystalline
  conjunctiva H11.11-
  cornea H18.00-
    argentous H18.02-
    due to metabolic disorder H18.03-
    Kayser-Fleischer ring H18.04-
    pigmentation —see Pigmentation, cornea

99

Deposit *(continued)*
  crystalline, vitreous (body) (humor) H43.2-
  hemosiderin in old scars of cornea —*see* Pigmentation, cornea, stromal
  metallic in lens —*see* Cataract, specified NEC
  skin R23.8
  tooth, teeth (betel) (black) (green) (materia alba) (orange) (tobacco) K03.6
  urate, kidney —*see* Calculus, kidney

Depraved appetite —*see* Pica

Depressed
  HDL cholesterol E78.6

Depression (acute) (mental) F32.A
  agitated (single episode) F32.2
  anaclitic —*see* Disorder, adjustment
  anxiety F41.8
    persistent F34.1
  arches —*see also* Deformity, limb, flat foot
  atypical (single episode) F32.89
    recurrent episode F33.8
  basal metabolic rate R94.8
  bone marrow D75.89
  central nervous system R09.2
  cerebral R29.818
    newborn P91.4
  cerebrovascular I67.9
  chest wall M95.4
  climacteric (single episode) F32.89
    recurrent episode F33.8
  endogenous (without psychotic symptoms) F33.2
    with psychotic symptoms F33.3
  functional activity R68.89
  hysterical F44.89
  involutional (single episode) F32.89
    recurrent episode F33.8
  major F32.9
    with psychotic symptoms F32.3
    recurrent —*see* Disorder, depressive, recurrent
  manic-depressive —*see* Disorder, depressive, recurrent
  masked (single episode) F32.89
  medullary G93.89
  menopausal (single episode) F32.89
    recurrent episode F33.8
  metatarsus —*see* Depression, arches
  monopolar F33.9
  nervous F34.1
  neurotic F34.1
  nose M95.0
  postnatal NOS F53.0
  postpartum NOS F53.0
  post-psychotic of schizophrenia F32.89
  post-schizophrenic F32.89
  psychogenic (reactive) (single episode) F32.9
  psychoneurotic F34.1
  psychotic (single episode) F32.3
    recurrent F33.3
  reactive (psychogenic) (single episode) F32.9
    psychotic (single episode) F32.3
  recurrent —*see* Disorder, depressive, recurrent
  respiratory center G93.89
  seasonal —*see* Disorder, depressive, recurrent
  senile F03
  severe, single episode F32.2

Depression *(continued)*
  situational F43.21
  skull Q67.4
  specified NEC (single episode) F32.89
  sternum M95.4
  visual field —*see* Defect, visual field
  vital (recurrent) (without psychotic symptoms) F33.2
    with psychotic symptoms F33.3
    single episode F32.2

Deprivation
  cultural Z60.3
  effects NOS T73.9
    specified NEC T73.8
  emotional NEC Z65.8
    affecting infant or child —*see* Maltreatment, child, psychological
  food T73.0
  material due to limited financial resources, specified NEC Z59.87
  articular cartilage,
  protein —*see* Malnutrition
  sleep Z72.820
  social Z60.4
    affecting infant or child —*see* Maltreatment, child, psychological
  specified NEC T73.8
  vitamins —*see* Deficiency, vitamin
  water T73.1

Derangement
  ankle (internal) —*see* Derangement, joint, articular cartilage, ankle
  cartilage (articular) NEC —*see* Derangement, joint, articular cartilage, by site
    recurrent —*see* Dislocation, recurrent
  cruciate ligament, anterior, current injury —*see* Sprain, knee, cruciate, anterior
  elbow (internal) —*see* Derangement, joint, articular cartilage, elbow
  hip (joint) (internal) (old) —*see* Derangement, joint, articular cartilage, hip
  joint (internal) M24.9
    ankylosis —*see* Ankylosis
    articular cartilage M24.10
      ankle M24.17-
      elbow M24.12-
      foot M24.17-
      hand M24.14-
      hip M24.15-
      knee NEC M23.9-
      loose body —*see* Loose, body
      shoulder M24.11-
      specified site NEC M24.19
      wrist M24.13-
    contracture —*see* Contraction, joint
    current injury —*see also* Dislocation
      knee, meniscus or cartilage —*see* Tear, meniscus
    dislocation
      pathological —*see* Dislocation, pathological
      recurrent —*see* Dislocation, recurrent
    knee —*see* Derangement, knee
    ligament —*see* Disorder, ligament
    loose body —*see* Loose, body
    recurrent —*see* Dislocation, recurrent

Derangement *(continued)*
  joint *(continued)*
    specified type NEC M24.80
      ankle M24.87-
      elbow M24.82-
      foot joint M24.87-
      hand joint M24.84-
      hip M24.85-
      shoulder M24.81-
      specified site NEC M24.89
      wrist M24.83-
      temporomandibular M26.69
  knee (recurrent) M23.9-
    ligament disruption, spontaneous M23.60-
      anterior cruciate M23.61-
      capsular M23.67-
      instability, chronic M23.5-
      lateral collateral M23.64-
      medial collateral M23.63-
      posterior cruciate M23.62-
    loose body M23.4-
    meniscus M23.30-
      cystic M23.00-
        lateral M23.002
          anterior horn M23.04-
          posterior horn M23.05-
          specified NEC M23.06-
        medial M23.005
          anterior horn M23.01-
          posterior horn M23.02-
          specified NEC M23.03-
      degenerate —*see* Derangement, knee, meniscus, specified NEC
      detached —*see* Derangement, knee, meniscus, specified NEC
      due to old tear or injury M23.20-
        lateral M23.20-
          anterior horn M23.24-
          posterior horn M23.25-
          specified NEC M23.26-
        medial M23.20-
          anterior horn M23.21-
          posterior horn M23.22-
          specified NEC M23.23-
      retained —*see* Derangement, knee, meniscus, specified NEC
      specified NEC M23.30-
        lateral M23.30-
          anterior horn M23.34-
          posterior horn M23.35-
          specified NEC M23.36-
        medial M23.30-
          anterior horn M23.31-
          posterior horn M23.32-
          specified NEC M23.33-
    old M23.8X-
    specified NEC —*see* subcategory M23.8
  low back NEC —*see* Dorsopathy, specified NEC
  meniscus —*see* Derangement, knee, meniscus
  mental —*see* Psychosis
  patella, specified NEC —*see* Disorder, patella, derangement NEC
  semilunar cartilage (knee) —*see* Derangement, knee, meniscus, specified NEC
  shoulder (internal) —*see* Derangement, joint, shoulder

Dercum's disease E88.2

Derealization (neurotic) F48.1

Dermal —*see* condition

Dermaphytid —*see* Dermatophytosis

Dermatitis (eczematous) L30.9
  ab igne L59.0
  acarine B88.0
  actinic (due to sun) L57.8
    other than from sun L59.8
  allergic —*see* Dermatitis, contact, allergic
  ambustionis, due to burn or scald —*see* Burn
  amebic A06.7
  ammonia L22
  arsenical (ingested) L27.8
  artefacta L98.1
    psychogenic F54
  atopic L20.9
    psychogenic F54
    specified NEC L20.89
  autoimmune progesterone L30.8
  berlock, berloque L56.2
  blastomycotic B40.3
  blister beetle L24.89
  bullous, bullosa L13.9
    mucosynechial, atrophic L12.1
    seasonal L30.8
    specified NEC L13.8
  calorica L59.0
    due to burn or scald —*see* Burn
  caterpillar L24.89
  cercarial B65.3
  combustionis L59.0
    due to burn or scald —*see* Burn
  congelationis T69.1
  contact (occupational) L25.9
    allergic L23.9
      due to
        adhesives L23.1
        cement L23.5
        chemical products NEC L23.5
        chromium L23.0
        cosmetics L23.2
        dander (cat) (dog) L23.81
        drugs in contact with skin L23.3
        dyes L23.4
        food in contact with skin L23.6
        hair (cat) (dog) L23.81
        insecticide L23.5
        metals L23.0
        nickel L23.0
        plants, non-food L23.7
        plastic L23.5
        rubber L23.5
        specified agent NEC L23.89
    due to
      cement L25.3
      chemical products NEC L25.3
      cosmetics L25.0
      dander (cat) (dog) L23.81
      drugs in contact with skin L25.1
      dyes L25.2
      food in contact with skin L25.4
      hair (cat) (dog) L23.81
      plants, non-food L25.5
      specified agent NEC L25.8
    irritant L24.9
      due to
        body fluids L24.A0
          feces L24.A2
          incontinence (dual) (fecal) (urinary) L24.A2
          saliva L24.A1
          urine L24.A2
          wound exudate L24.A9
        exudate L24.A9
        friction L24.A0
          specified NEC L24.A9
        cement L24.5

Dermatitis (continued)
- contact (continued)
  - irritant (continued)
    - due to (continued)
      - chemical products NEC L24.5
      - cosmetics L24.3
      - detergents L24.0
      - drugs in contact with skin L24.4
      - food in contact with skin L24.6
      - oils and greases L24.1
      - plants, non-food L24.7
      - solvents L24.2
      - specified agent NEC L24.89
    - related to
      - colostomy L24.B3
      - endotracheal tube L24.A9
      - enterocutaneous fistula L24.B3
      - gastrostomy L24.B1
      - ileostomy L24.B3
      - jejunostomy L24.B1
      - saliva or spit fistula L24.B1
      - stoma or fistula L24.B0
        - digestive L24.B1
        - fecal or urinary L24.B3
        - respiratory L24.B2
      - tracheostomy L24.B2
- contusiformis L52
- desquamative L30.8
- diabetic —*see* E08-E13 with .620
- diaper L22
- diphtheritica A36.3
- dry skin L85.3
- due to
  - acetone (contact) (irritant) L24.2
  - acids (contact) (irritant) L24.5
  - adhesive(s) (allergic) (contact) (plaster) L23.1
    - irritant L24.5
  - alcohol (irritant) (skin contact) (substances in category T51) L24.2
    - taken internally L27.8
  - alkalis (contact) (irritant) L24.5
  - arsenic (ingested) L27.8
  - carbon disulfide (contact) (irritant) L24.2
  - caustics (contact) (irritant) L24.5
  - cement (contact) L25.3
  - cereal (ingested) L27.2
  - chemical(s) NEC L25.3
    - taken internally L27.8
  - chlorocompounds L24.2
  - chromium (contact) (irritant) L24.81
  - coffee (ingested) L27.2
  - cold weather L30.8
  - cosmetics (contact) L25.0
    - allergic L23.2
    - irritant L24.3
  - cyclohexanes L24.2
  - dander (cat) (dog) L23.81
  - Demodex species B88.0
  - Dermanyssus gallinae B88.0
  - detergents (contact) (irritant) L24.0
  - dichromate L24.81
  - drugs and medicaments
    - (generalized) (internal use) L27.0
    - external —*see* Dermatitis, due to, drugs, in contact with skin
    - in contact with skin L25.1
      - allergic L23.3
      - irritant L24.4
    - localized skin eruption L27.1
    - specified substance —*see* Table of Drugs and Chemicals
  - dyes (contact) L25.2
    - allergic L23.4
    - irritant L24.89

Dermatitis (continued)
- due to (continued)
  - epidermophytosis —*see* Dermatophytosis
  - esters L24.2
  - external irritant NEC L24.9
  - exudate (wound fluids) L24.A9
  - fish (ingested) L27.2
  - flour (ingested) L27.2
  - food (ingested) L27.2
    - in contact with skin L25.4
  - fruit (ingested) L27.2
  - furs (allergic) (contact) L23.81
  - glues —*see* Dermatitis, due to, adhesives
  - glycols L24.2
  - greases NEC (contact) (irritant) L24.1
  - hair (cat) (dog) L23.81
  - hot
    - objects and materials —*see* Burn
    - weather or places L59.0
  - hydrocarbons L24.2
  - infrared rays L59.8
  - ingestion, ingested substance L27.9
    - chemical NEC L27.8
    - drugs and medicaments —*see* Dermatitis, due to, drugs
    - food L27.2
    - specified NEC L27.8
  - insecticide in contact with skin L24.5
  - internal agent L27.9
    - drugs and medicaments (generalized) —*see* Dermatitis, due to, drugs
    - food L27.2
  - irradiation —*see* Dermatitis, due to, radioactive substance
  - ketones L24.2
  - lacquer tree (allergic) (contact) L23.7
  - light (sun) NEC L57.8
    - acute L56.8
    - other L59.8
  - Liponyssoides sanguineus B88.0
  - low temperature L30.8
  - meat (ingested) L27.2
  - metals, metal salts (contact) (irritant) L24.81
  - milk (ingested) L27.2
  - nickel (contact) (irritant) L24.81
  - nylon (contact) (irritant) L24.5
  - oils NEC (contact) (irritant) L24.1
  - paint solvent (contact) (irritant) L24.2
  - petroleum products (contact) (irritant) (substances in T52.0) L24.2
  - plants NEC (contact) L25.5
    - allergic L23.7
    - irritant L24.7
  - plasters (adhesive) (any) (allergic) (contact) L23.1
    - irritant L24.5
  - plastic (contact) L25.3
  - preservatives (contact) —*see* Dermatitis, due to, chemical, in contact with skin
  - primrose (allergic) (contact) L23.7
  - primula (allergic) (contact) L23.7
  - radiation L59.8
    - nonionizing (chronic exposure) L57.8
    - sun NEC L57.8
      - acute L56.8
  - radioactive substance L58.9
    - acute L58.0
    - chronic L58.1

Dermatitis (continued)
- due to (continued)
  - radium L58.9
    - acute L58.0
    - chronic L58.1
  - ragweed (allergic) (contact) L23.7
  - Rhus (allergic) (contact) (diversiloba) (radicans) (toxicodendron) (venenata) (verniciflua) L23.7
  - rubber (contact) L24.5
  - Senecio jacobaea (allergic) (contact) L23.7
  - solvents (contact) (irritant) (substances in categories T52) L24.2
  - specified agent NEC (contact) L25.8
    - allergic L23.89
    - irritant L24.89
  - sunshine NEC L57.8
    - acute L56.8
  - tetrachlorethylene (contact) (irritant) L24.2
  - toluene (contact) (irritant) L24.2
  - turpentine (contact) L24.2
  - ultraviolet rays (sun NEC) (chronic exposure) L57.8
    - acute L56.8
  - vaccine or vaccination L27.0
    - specified substance —*see* Table of Drugs and Chemicals
  - varicose veins —*see* Varix, leg, with, inflammation
  - X-rays L58.9
    - acute L58.0
    - chronic L58.1
- dyshydrotic L30.1
- dysmenorrheica N94.6
- escharotica —*see* Burn
- exfoliative, exfoliativa (generalized) L26
  - neonatorum L00
- eyelid (*see also* Dermatosis, eyelid) H01.9
  - allergic H01.119
    - left H01.116
      - lower H01.115
      - upper H01.114
    - right H01.113
      - lower H01.112
      - upper H01.111
  - contact —*see* Dermatitis, eyelid, allergic
  - due to
    - Demodex species B88.0
    - herpes (zoster) B02.39
      - simplex B00.59
  - eczematous H01.139
    - left H01.136
      - lower H01.135
      - upper H01.134
    - right H01.133
      - lower H01.132
      - upper H01.131
  - specified NEC H01.8
- facta, factitia, factitial L98.1
  - psychogenic F54
- flexural NEC L20.82
- friction L30.4
- fungus B36.9
  - specified type NEC B36.8
- gangrenosa, gangrenous infantum L08.0
- harvest mite B88.0
- heat L59.0
- herpesviral, vesicular (ear) (lip) B00.1

Dermatitis (continued)
- herpetiformis (bullous) (erythematous) (pustular) (vesicular) L13.0
  - juvenile L12.2
  - senile L12.0
- hiemalis L30.8
- hypostatic, hypostatica —*see* Varix, leg, with, inflammation
- infectious eczematoid L30.3
- infective L30.3
- irritant —*see* Dermatitis, contact, irritant
- Jacquet's (diaper dermatitis) L22
- Leptus B88.0
- lichenified NEC L28.0
- medicamentosa (generalized) (internal use) —*see* Dermatitis, due to drugs
- mite B88.0
- multiformis L13.0
  - juvenile L12.2
- napkin L22
- neurotica L13.0
- nummular L30.0
- papillaris capillitii L73.0
- pellagrous E52
- perioral L71.0
- photocontact L56.2
- polymorpha dolorosa L13.0
- pruriginosa L13.0
- pruritic NEC L30.8
- psychogenic F54
- purulent L08.0
- pustular
  - contagious B08.02
  - subcorneal L13.1
- pyococcal L08.0
- pyogenica L08.0
- repens L40.2
- Ritter's (exfoliativa) L00
- Schamberg's L81.7
- schistosome B65.3
- seasonal bullous L30.8
- seborrheic L21.9
  - infantile L21.1
  - specified NEC L21.8
- sensitization NOS L23.9
- septic L08.0
- solare L57.8
- specified NEC L30.8
- stasis I87.2
  - with
    - varicose ulcer —*see* Varix, leg, with ulcer, with inflammation
    - Varicose veins —*see* Varix, leg, with, inflammation
  - due to postthrombotic syndrome —*see* Syndrome, postthrombotic
- suppurative L08.0
- traumatic NEC L30.4
- trophoneurotica L13.0
- ultraviolet (sun) (chronic exposure) L57.8
  - acute L56.8
- varicose —*see* Varix, leg, with, inflammation
- vegetans L10.1
- verrucosa B43.0
- vesicular, herpesviral B00.1

Dermatoarthritis, lipoid E78.81

Dermatochalasis, eyelid H02.839
- left H02.836
  - lower H02.835
  - upper H02.834
- right H02.833
  - lower H02.832
  - upper H02.831

Dermatofibroma (lenticulare) —see
Neoplasm, skin, benign
protuberans —see Neoplasm, skin,
uncertain behavior
Dermatofibrosarcoma (pigmented)
(protuberans) —see Neoplasm,
skin, malignant
Dermatographia L50.3
Dermatolysis (exfoliativa)
(congenital) Q82.8
acquired L57.4
eyelids —see Blepharochalasis
palpebrarum —see Blepharochalasis
senile L57.4
Dermatomegaly NEC Q82.8
Dermatomucosomyositis (see also
Dermatomyositis) M33.10
with
myopathy M33.12
respiratory involvement M33.11
specified organ involvement
NEC M33.19
Dermatomycosis B36.9
furfuracea B36.0
specified type NEC B36.8
Dermatomyositis (acute) (chronic)
—see also Dermatopolymyositis
adult (see also Dematomyositis,
specified NEC) M33.10
in (due to) neoplastic disease (see
also Neoplasm) D49.9 [M36.0]
juvenile M33.00
with
myopathy M33.02
respiratory involvement M33.01
specified organ involvement
NEC M33.09
without myopathy M33.03
amyopathic M33.03
specified NEC M33.10
with
myopathy M33.12
respiratory involvement
M33.11
specified organ involvement
NEC M33.19
without myopathy M33.13
amyopathic M33.13
Dermatoneuritis of children —see
Poisoning, mercury
Dermatophilosis A48.8
Dermatophytid L30.2
Dermatophytide —see
Dermatophytosis
Dermatophytosis (epidermophyton)
(infection) (Microsporum) (tinea)
(Trichophyton) B35.9
beard B35.0
body B35.4
capitis B35.0
corporis B35.4
deep-seated B35.8
disseminated B35.8
foot B35.3
granulomatous B35.8
groin B35.6
hand B35.2
nail B35.1
perianal (area) B35.6
scalp B35.0
specified NEC B35.8
Dermatopolymyositis M33.90
with
myopathy M33.92
respiratory involvement M33.91
specified organ involvement
NEC M33.99

Dermatopolymyositis (continued)
without myopathy M33.93
amyopathic M33.93
in neoplastic disease (see also
Neoplasm) D49.9 [M36.0]
juvenile M33.00
with
myopathy M33.02
respiratory involvement M33.01
specified organ involvement
NEC M33.09
amyopathic M33.03
without myopathy M33.03
specified NEC M33.10
amyopathic M33.13
myopathy M33.12
respiratory involvement M33.11
specified organ involvement
NEC M33.19
without myopathy M33.13
Dermatopolyneuritis —see
Poisoning, mercury
Dermatorrhexis (see also Syndrome,
Ehlers-Danlos) Q79.60
acquired L57.4
Dermatosclerosis —see also
Scleroderma
localized L94.0
Dermatosis L98.9
Andrews' L08.89
Bowen's —see Neoplasm, skin,
in situ
bullous L13.9
specified NEC L13.8
exfoliativa L26
eyelid (noninfectious) (see also
Dermatitis, eyelid) H01.9
discoid lupus erythematosus
—see Lupus, erythematosus,
eyelid
xeroderma —see Xeroderma,
acquired, eyelid
factitial L98.1
febrile neutrophilic L98.2
gonococcal A54.89
herpetiformis L13.0
juvenile L12.2
linear IgA L13.8
menstrual NEC L98.8
neutrophilic, febrile L98.2
occupational —see Dermatitis,
contact
papulosa nigra L82.1
pigmentary L81.9
progressive L81.7
Schamberg's L81.7
psychogenic F54
purpuric, pigmented L81.7
pustular, subcorneal L13.1
transient acantholytic L11.1
Dermographia, dermographism L50.3
Dermoid (cyst) —see also Neoplasm,
benign, by site
with malignant transformation C56-
due to radiation (nonionizing) L57.8
Dermopathy
infiltrative with thyrotoxicosis
—see Thyrotoxicosis
nephrogenic fibrosing L90.8
Dermophytosis —see Dermatophytosis
Descemetocele H18.73-
Descemet's membrane —see condition
Descending —see condition
Descensus uteri —see Prolapse, uterus
Desert
rheumatism B38.0
sore —see Ulcer, skin

Desertion (newborn) —see
Maltreatment
Desmoid (extra-abdominal) (tumor)
—see Neoplasm, connective tissue,
uncertain behavior
abdominal wall D48.113
back D48.117
buttock D48.116
chest wall D48.111
extremity
lower D48.116
upper D48.115
head and neck D48.110
intraabdominal D48.114
intrathoracic D48.112
pelvic cavity D48.114
pelvic girdle D48.116
peritoneal D48.114
retroperitoneal D48.114
shoulder girdle D48.115
site unspecified D48.119
specified site NEC D48.118
Despondency F32.A
Desquamation, skin R23.4
Destruction, destructive —see also
Damage
articular facet —see also
Derangement, joint, specified
type NEC
knee M23.8X-
vertebra —see Spondylosis
bone —see also Disorder, bone,
specified type NEC
syphilitic A52.77
joint —see also Derangement,
joint, specified type NEC
sacroiliac M53.3
rectal sphincter K62.89
septum (nasal) J34.89
tuberculous NEC —see Tuberculosis
tympanum, tympanic membrane
(nontraumatic) —see Disorder,
tympanic membrane, specified
NEC
vertebral disc —see Degeneration,
intervertebral disc
Destructiveness —see also Disorder,
conduct
adjustment reaction —see Disorder,
adjustment
Desultory labor O62.2
Detachment
cartilage —see Sprain
cervix, annular N88.8
complicating delivery O71.3
choroid (old) (postinfectional)
(simple) (spontaneous) H31.40-
hemorrhagic H31.41-
serous H31.42-
ligament —see Sprain
meniscus (knee) —see also
Derangement, knee, meniscus,
specified NEC
current injury —see Tear, meniscus
due to old tear or injury —see
Derangement, knee, meniscus,
due to old tear
retina (without retinal break)
(serous) H33.2-
with retinal:
break H33.00-
giant H33.03-
multiple H33.02-
single H33.01-
dialysis H33.04-
pigment epithelium —see
Degeneration, retina,
separation of layers, pigment
epithelium detachment

Detachment (continued)
retina (continued)
rhegmatogenous —see
Detachment, retina, with
retinal, break
specified NEC H33.8
total H33.05-
traction H33.4-
vitreous (body) H43.81
Detergent asthma J69.8
Deterioration
epileptic F06.8
general physical R53.81
heart, cardiac —see Degeneration,
myocardial
mental —see Psychosis
myocardial, myocardium —see
Degeneration, myocardial
senile (simple) R54
Deuteranomaly (anomalous
trichromat) H53.53
Deuteranopia (complete)
(incomplete) H53.53
Development
abnormal, bone Q79.9
arrested R62.50
bone —see Arrest, development
or growth, bone
child R62.50
due to malnutrition E45
defective, congenital —see also
Anomaly, by site
cauda equina Q06.3
left ventricle Q24.8
in hypoplastic left heart
syndrome Q23.4
valve Q24.8
pulmonary Q22.3
delayed —see also Delay,
development R62.50
arithmetical skills F81.2
language (skills) (expressive) F80.1
learning skill F81.9
mixed skills F88
motor coordination F82
reading F81.0
specified learning skill NEC
F81.89
speech F80.9
spelling F81.81
written expression F81.81
imperfect, congenital —see also
Anomaly, by site
heart Q24.9
lungs Q33.6
incomplete
bronchial tree Q32.4
organ or site not listed —see
Hypoplasia, by site
respiratory system Q34.9
sexual, precocious NEC E30.1
tardy, mental (see also Disability,
intellectual) F79
Developmental —see condition
testing, infant or child —see
Examination, child
Devergie's disease (pityriasis rubra
pilaris) L44.0
Deviation (in)
conjugate palsy (eye) (spastic) H51.0
esophagus (acquired) K22.89
eye, skew H51.8
midline (jaw) (teeth) (dental arch)
M26.29
specified site NEC —see
Malposition
nasal septum J34.2
congenital Q67.4

Deviation (continued)
  opening and closing of the mandible M26.53
  organ or site, congenital NEC —see Malposition, congenital
  septum (nasal) (acquired) J34.2
    congenital Q67.4
  sexual F65.9
    bestiality F65.89
    erotomania F52.8
    exhibitionism F65.2
    fetishism, fetishistic F65.0
      transvestism F65.1
    frotteurism F65.81
    masochism F65.51
    multiple F65.89
    necrophilia F65.89
    nymphomania F52.8
    pederosis F65.4
    pedophilia F65.4
    sadism, sadomasochism F65.52
    satyriasis F52.8
    specified type NEC F65.89
    transvestism F64.1
    voyeurism F65.3
  teeth, midline M26.29
  trachea J39.8
  ureter, congenital Q62.61

Device
  cerebral ventricle (communicating) in situ Z98.2
  contraceptive —see Contraceptive, device
  drainage, cerebrospinal fluid, in situ Z98.2

Devic's disease G36.0

Devil's
  grip B33.0
  pinches (purpura simplex) D69.2

Devitalized tooth K04.99

Devonshire colic —see Poisoning, lead

Dextraposition, aorta Q20.3
  in tetralogy of Fallot Q21.3

Dextrinosis, limit (debrancher enzyme deficiency) E74.03

Dextrocardia (true) Q24.0
  with
    complete transposition of viscera Q89.3
    situs inversus Q89.3

Dextrotransposition, aorta Q20.3

d-glycericacidemia E72.59

Dhat syndrome F48.8

Dhobi itch B35.6

Di George's syndrome D82.1

Di Guglielmo's disease C94.0-

Diabetes, diabetic (mellitus) (sugar) E11.9
  with
    amyotrophy E11.44
    arthropathy NEC E11.618
    autonomic (poly)neuropathy E11.43
    cataract E11.36
    Charcot's joints E11.610
    chronic kidney disease E11.22
    circulatory complication NEC E11.59
    coma due to
      hyperosmolarity E11.01
      hypoglycemia E11.641
      ketoacidosis E11.11
    complication E11.8
      specified NEC E11.69
    dermatitis E11.620
    foot ulcer E11.621
    gangrene E11.52

Diabetes, diabetic (continued)
  with (continued)
    gastroparalysis E11.43
    gastroparesis E11.43
    glomerulonephrosis, intracapillary E11.21
    glomerulosclerosis, intercapillary E11.21
    hyperglycemia E11.65
    hyperosmolarity E11.00
      with coma E11.01
    hypoglycemia E11.649
      with coma E11.641
    ketoacidosis E11.10
      with coma E11.11
    kidney complications NEC E11.29
    Kimmelstiel-Wilson disease E11.21
    loss of protective sensation (LOPS) —see Diabetes, by type, with neuropathy
    mononeuropathy E11.41
    myasthenia E11.44
    necrobiosis lipoidica E11.620
    nephropathy E11.21
    neuralgia E11.42
    neurologic complication NEC E11.49
    neuropathic arthropathy E11.610
    neuropathy E11.40
    ophthalmic complication NEC E11.39
    oral complication NEC E11.638
    osteomyelitis E11.69
    periodontal disease E11.630
    peripheral angiopathy E11.51
      with gangrene E11.52
    polyneuropathy E11.42
    renal complication NEC E11.29
    renal tubular degeneration E11.29
    retinopathy E11.319
      with macular edema E11.311
      resolved following treatment E11.37
      nonproliferative E11.329
        with macular edema E11.321
        mild E11.329
          with macular edema E11.321
        moderate E11.339
          with macular edema E11.331
        severe E11.349
          with macular edema E11.341
          with
            combined traction retinal detachment and rhegmatogenous retinal detachment E11.354
            macular edema E11.351
            stable proliferative diabetic retinopathy E11.355
            traction retinal detachment involving the macula E11.352
            traction retinal detachment no involving the macula E11.353
      proliferative E11.359
        with
          combined traction retinal detachment and rhegmatogenous retinal detachment E11.354
          macular edema E11.351

Diabetes, diabetic (continued)
  with (continued)
    retinopathy (continued)
      proliferative (continued)
        with (continued)
          stable proliferative diabetic retinopathy E11.355
          traction retinal detachment involving the macula E11.352
          traction retinal detachement not involving the macula E11.353
    skin complication NEC E11.628
    skin ulcer NEC E11.622
  brittle —see Diabetes, type 1
  bronzed E83.110
  complicating pregnancy —see Pregnancy, complicated by, diabetes
  dietary counseling and surveillance Z71.3
  due to
    autoimmune process —see Diabetes, type 1
    immune mediated pancreatic islet beta-cell destruction —see Diabetes, type 1
    pancreatectomy —see Diabetes, specified type, NEC
  due to drug or chemical E09.9
    with
      amyotrophy E09.44
      arthropathy NEC E09.618
      autonomic (poly)neuropathy E09.43
      cataract E09.36
      Charcot's joints E09.610
      chronic kidney disease E09.22
      circulatory complication NEC E09.59
      complication E09.8
        specified NEC E09.69
      dermatitis E09.620
      foot ulcer E09.621
      gangrene E09.52
      gastroparalysis E09.43
      gastroparesis E09.43
      glomerulonephrosis, intracapillary E09.21
      glomerulosclerosis, intercapillary E09.21
      hyperglycemia E09.65
      hyperosmolarity E09.00
        with coma E09.01
      hypoglycemia E09.649
        with coma E09.11
      ketoacidosis E09.10
        with coma E09.11
      kidney complications NEC E09.29
      Kimmelstiel-Wilson disease E09.21
      mononeuropathy E09.41
      myasthenia E09.44
      necrobiosis lipoidica E09.620
      nephropathy E09.21
      neuralgia E09.42
      neurologic complication NEC E09.49
      neuropathic arthropathy E09.610
      neuropathy E09.40
      ophthalmic complication NEC E09.39
      oral complication NEC E09.638
      periodontal disease E09.630

Diabetes, diabetic (continued)
  due to drug or chemical (continued)
    with (continued)
      peripheral angiopathy E09.51
        with gangrene E09.52
      polyneuropathy E09.42
      renal complication NEC E09.29
      renal tubular degeneration E09.29
      retinopathy E09.319
        with macular edema E09.311
        resolved following treatment E09.37
        nonproliferative E09.329
          with macular edema E09.321
          mild E09.329
            with macular edema E09.321
          moderate E09.339
            with macular edema E09.331
          severe E09.349
            with macular edema E09.341
        proliferative E09.359
          with
            combined traction retinal detachment and rhegmatogenous retinal detachment E09.354
            macular edema E09.351
            stable proliferative diabetic retinopathy E09.355
            traction retinal detachment involving the macula E09.352
            traction retinal detachment not involving the macula E09.353
      skin complication NEC E09.628
      skin ulcer NEC E09.622
  due to underlying condition E08.9
    with
      amyotrophy E08.44
      arthropathy NEC E08.618
      autonomic (poly)neuropathy E08.43
      cataract E08.36
      Charcot's joints E08.610
      chronic kidney disease E08.22
      circulatory complication NEC E08.59
      complication E08.8
        specified NEC E08.69
      dermatitis E08.620
      foot ulcer E08.621
      gangrene E08.52
      gastroparalysis E08.43
      gastroparesis E08.43
      glomerulonephrosis, intracapillary E08.21
      glomerulosclerosis, intercapillary E08.21
      hyperglycemia E08.65
      hyperosmolarity E08.00
        with coma E08.01
      hypoglycemia E08.649
        with coma E08.641
      ketoacidosis E08.10
        with coma E08.11
      kidney complications NEC E08.29

Diabetes, diabetic *(continued)*
  due to underlying condition *(continued)*
    with *(continued)*
      Kimmelstiel-WIlson disease E08.21
      mononeuropathy E08.41
      myasthenia E08.44
      necrobiosis lipoidica E08.620
      nephropathy E08.21
      neuralgia E08.42
      neurologic complication NEC E08.49
      neuropathic arthropathy E08.610
      neuropathy E08.40
      ophthalmic complication NEC E08.39
      oral complication NEC E08.638
      periodontal disease E08.630
      peripheral angiopathy E08.51
        with gangrene E08.52
      polyneuropathy E08.42
      renal complication NEC E08.29
      renal tubular degeneration E08.29
      retinopathy E08.319
        with macular edema E08.311
        resolved following treatment E08.37
        nonproliferative E08.329
          with macular edema E08.321
          mild E08.329
            with macular edema E08.321
          moderate E08.339
            with macular edema E08.331
          severe E08.349
            with macular edema E08.341
        proliferative E08.359
          with
            combined traction retinal detachment and rhegmatogenous retinal detachment E08.354
            macular edema E08.351
            stable proliferative diabetic retinopathy E08.355
            traction retinal detachment involving the macula E08.352
            traction retinal detachment not involving the macula E08.353
      skin complication NEC E08.628
      skin ulcer NEC E08.622
  gestational (in pregnancy) O24.419
    affecting newborn P70.0
    diet controlled O24.410
    in childbirth O24.429
      diet controlled O24.420
      insulin (and diet) controlled O24.424
      oral drug controlled (antidiabetic) (hypoglycemic) O24.425
    oral drug controlled (antidiabetic) (hypoglycemic) O24.415

Diabetes, diabetic *(continued)*
  gestational *(continued)*
    insulin (and diet) controlled O24.414
    puerperal O24.439
      diet controlled O24.430
      insulin (and diet) controlled O24.434
      oral drug controlled (antidiabetic) (hypoglycemic) O24.435
  hepatogenous E13.9
  idiopathic —*see* Diabetes, type 1
  inadequately controlled —*see* Diabetes, by type, with hyperglycemia
  insipidus E23.2
    nephrogenic N25.1
    pituitary E23.2
    vasopressin resistant N25.1
  insulin dependent - code to type of diabetes
  juvenile-onset —*see* Diabetes, type 1
  ketosis-prone —*see* Diabetes, type 1
  latent R73.03
  neonatal (transient) P70.2
  non-insulin dependent - code to type of diabetes
  out of control —*see* Diabetes, by type, with hyperglycemia
  phosphate E83.39
  poorly controlled —*see* Diabetes, by type, with hyperglycemia
  postpancreatectomy —*see* Diabetes, specified type NEC
  postprocedural —*see* Diabetes, specified type NEC
  secondary diabetes mellitus NEC —*see* Diabetes, specified type NEC
  specified type NEC E13.9
    with
      amyotrophy E13.44
      arthropathy NEC E13.618
      autonomic (poly)neuropathy E13.43
      cataract E13.36
      Charcot's joints E13.610
      chronic kidney disease E13.22
      circulatory complication NEC E13.59
      complication E13.8
        specified NEC E13.69
      dermatitis E13.620
      foot ulcer E13.621
      gangrene E13.52
      gastroparalysis E13.43
      gastroparesis E13.43
      glomerulonephrosis, intracapillary E13.21
      glomerulosclerosis, intercapillary E13.21
      hyperglycemia E13.65
      hyperosmolarity E13.00
        with coma E13.01
      hypoglycemia E13.649
        with coma E13.641
      ketoacidosis E13.10
        with coma E13.11
      kidney complications NEC E13.29
      Kimmelstiel-Wilson disease E13.21
      mononeuropathy E13.41
      myasthenia E13.44
      necrobiosis lipoidica E13.620
      nephropathy E13.21
      neuralgia E13.42
      neurologic complication NEC E13.49

Diabetes, diabetic *(continued)*
  specified type *(continued)*
    with *(continued)*
      neuropathic arthropathy E13.610
      neuropathy E13.40
      ophthalmic complication NEC E13.39
      oral complication NEC E13.638
      periodontal disease E13.630
      peripheral angiopathy E13.51
        with gangrene E13.52
      polyneuropathy E13.42
      renal complication NEC E13.29
      renal tubular degeneration E13.29
      retina, hemorrhage E13.39
      retinopathy E13.319
        with macular edema E13.311
        resolved following treatment E13.37
        nonproliferative E13.329
          with macular edema E13.321
          mild E13.329
            with macular edema E13.321
          moderate E13.339
            with macular edema E13.331
          severe E13.349
            with macular edema E13.341
        proliferative E13.359
          with
            combined traction retinal detachment and rhegmatogenous retinal detachment E13.354
            macular edema E13.351
            stable proliferative diabetic retinopathy E13.355
            traction retinal detachment involving the macula E13.352
            traction retinal detachment not involving the macula E13.353
      skin complication NEC E13.628
      skin ulcer NEC E13.622
  steroid-induced —*see* Diabetes, due to, drug or chemical
  type 1 E10.9
    with
      amyotrophy E10.44
      arthropathy NEC E10.618
      autonomic (poly)neuropathy E10.43
      cataract E10.36
      Charcot's joints E10.610
      chronic kidney disease E10.22
      circulatory complication NEC E10.59
      coma due to
        hypoglycemia E10.641
        ketoacidosis E10.11
      complication E10.8
        specified NEC E10.69
      dermatitis E10.620
      foot ulcer E10.621
      gangrene E10.52
      gastroparalysis E10.43

Diabetes, diabetic *(continued)*
  type 1 *(continued)*
    with *(continued)*
      gastroparesis E10.43
      glomerulonephrosis, intracapillary E10.21
      glomerulosclerosis, intercapillary E10.21
      hyperglycemia E10.65
      hypoglycemia E10.649
        with coma E10.641
      ketoacidosis E10.10
        with coma E10.11
      kidney complications NEC E10.29
      Kimmelstiel-Wilson disease E10.21
      mononeuropathy E10.41
      myasthenia E10.44
      necrobiosis lipoidica E10.620
      nephropathy E10.21
      neuralgia E10.42
      neurologic complication NEC E10.49
      neuropathic arthropathy E10.610
      neuropathy E10.40
      ophthalmic complication NEC E10.39
      oral complication NEC E10.638
      osteomyelitis E10.69
      periodontal disease E10.630
      peripheral angiopathy E10.51
        with gangrene E10.52
      polyneuropathy E10.42
      renal complication NEC E10.29
      renal tubular degeneration E10.29
      retinopathy E10.319
        with macular edema E10.311
        resolved following treatment E10.37
        nonproliferative E10.329
          with macular edema E10.321
          mild E10.329
            with macular edema E10.321
          moderate E10.339
            with macular edema E10.331
          severe E10.349
            with macular edema E10.341
        proliferative E10.359
          with
            combined traction retinal detachment and rhegmatogenous retinal detachment E10.354
            with
              macular edema E10.351
              stable proliferative diabetic retinopathy E10.355
              traction retinal detachment involving the macula E10.352
              traction retinal detachment not involving the macula E10.353
      skin complication NEC E10.628
      skin ulcer NEC E10.622

Diabetes, diabetic (continued)
  type 2 E11.9
    with
      amyotrophy E11.44
      arthropathy NEC E11.618
      autonomic (poly)neuropathy
        E11.43
      cataract E11.36
      Charcot's joints E11.610
      chronic kidney disease
        E11.22
      circulatory complication NEC
        E11.59
      coma due to
        hyperosmolarity E11.01
        hypoglycemia E11.641
        ketoacidosis E11.1-
      complication E11.8
        specified NEC E11.69
      dermatitis E11.620
      foot ulcer E11.621
      gangrene E11.52
      gastroparalysis E11.43
      gastroparesis E11.43
      glomerulonephrosis,
        intracapillary E11.21
      glomerulosclerosis,
        intercapillary E11.21
      hyperglycemia E11.65
      hyperosmolarity E11.00
        with coma E11.01
      hypoglycemia E11.649
        with coma E11.641
      ketoacidosis E11.10
        with coma E11.11
      kidney complications NEC
        E11.29
      Kimmelstiel-Wilson disease
        E11.21
      mononeuropathy E11.41
      myasthenia E11.44
      necrobiosis lipoidica
        E11.620
      nephropathy E11.21
      neuralgia E11.42
      neurologic complication NEC
        E11.49
      neuropathic arthropathy
        E11.610
      neuropathy E11.40
      ophthalmic complication NEC
        E11.39
      oral complication NEC
        E11.638
      osteomyelitis E11.69
      periodontal disease E11.630
      peripheral angiopathy
        E11.51
        with gangrene E11.52
      polyneuropathy E11.42
      renal complication NEC
        E11.29
      renal tubular degeneration
        E11.29
      retinopathy E11.319
        with macular edema
          E11.311
        resolved following
          treatment E11.37
        nonproliferative E11.329
          with macular edema
            E11.321
          mild E11.329
            with macular edema
              E11.321
          moderate E11.339
            with macular edema
              E11.331
          severe E11.349
            with macular edema
              E11.341

Diabetes, diabetic (continued)
  type (continued)
    with (continued)
      retinopathy (continued)
        proliferative E11.359
          with
            combined traction
              retinal detachment
              and rhegmatogenous
              retinal detachment
              E11.354
            macular edema E11.351
            stable proliferative
              diabetic retinopathy
              E11.355
            traction retinal
              detachment
              involving the macula
              E11.352
            traction retinal
              detachment not
              involving the macula
              E11.353
      skin complication NEC E11.628
      skin ulcer NEC E11.622
  uncontrolled
    meaning
    hyperglycemia —see Diabetes, by
      type, with, hyperglycemia
    hypoglycemia —see Diabetes, by
      type, with, hypoglycemia

Diacyclothrombopathia D69.1
Diagnosis deferred R69
Dialysis (intermittent) (treatment)
  noncompliance (with) Z91.158
    due to financial hardship Z91.151
  renal (hemodialysis) (peritoneal),
    status Z99.2
  retina, retinal —see Detachment,
    retina, with retinal, dialysis
Diamond-Blackfan anemia
  (congenital hypoplastic) D61.01
Diamond-Gardener syndrome
  (autoerythrocyte sensitization)
  D69.2
Diaper rash L22
Diaphoresis (excessive) R61
Diaphragm —see condition
Diaphragmalgia R07.1
Diaphragmatitis, diaphragmitis
  J98.6
Diaphysial aclasis Q78.6
Diaphysitis —see Osteomyelitis,
  specified type NEC
Diarrhea, diarrheal (disease)
  (infantile) (inflammatory) R19.7
  achlorhydric K31.83
  allergic K52.29
    due to
      colitis —see Colitis, allergic
      enteritis —see Enteritis, allergic
  amebic (see also Amebiasis) A06.0
    with abscess —see Abscess,
      amebic
    acute A06.0
    chronic A06.1
    nondysenteric A06.2
  bacillary —see Dysentery, bacillary
  balantidial A07.0
  cachectic NEC K52.89
  Chilomastix A07.8
  choleriformis A00.1
  chronic (noninfectious) K52.9
  coccidial A07.3
  Cochin-China K90.1
    strongyloidiasis B78.0

Diarrhea, diarrheal (continued)
  Dientamoeba A07.8
  dietetic (see also Diarrhea, allergic)
    K52.29
  drug-induced K52.1
  due to
    bacteria A04.9
      specified NEC A04.8
    Campylobacter A04.5
    Capillaria philippinensis B81.1
    Clostridium difficile
      not specified as recurrent
        A04.72
      recurrent A04.71
    Clostridium perfringens (C) (F)
      A04.8
    Cryptosporidium A07.2
    drugs K52.1
    Escherichia coli A04.4
      enteroaggregative A04.4
      enterohemorrhagic A04.3
      enteroinvasive A04.2
      enteropathogenic A04.0
      enterotoxigenic A04.1
      specified NEC A04.4
    food hypersensitivity (see also
      Diarrhea, allergic) K52.29
    Necator americanus B76.1
    S. japonicum B65.2
    specified organism NEC A08.8
      bacterial A04.8
      viral A08.39
    Staphylococcus A04.8
    Trichuris trichiuria B79
    virus —see Enteritis, viral
    Yersinia enterocolitica A04.6
  dysenteric A09
  endemic A09
  epidemic A09
  flagellate A07.9
  Flexner's (ulcerative) A03.1
  functional K59.1
    following gastrointestinal
      surgery K91.89
    psychogenic F45.8
  Giardia lamblia A07.1
  giardial A07.1
  hill K90.1
  infectious A09
  malarial —see Malaria
  mite B88.0
  mycotic NEC B49
  neonatal (noninfectious) P78.3
  nervous F45.8
  neurogenic K59.1
  noninfectious K52.9
  postgastrectomy K91.1
  postvagotomy K91.1
  protozoal A07.9
    specified NEC A07.8
  psychogenic F45.8
  specified
    bacterium NEC A04.8
    virus NEC A08.39
  strongyloidiasis B78.0
  toxic K52.1
  trichomonal A07.8
  tropical K90.1
  tuberculous A18.32
  viral —see Enteritis, viral
Diastasis
  cranial bones M84.88
    congenital NEC Q75.8
  joint (traumatic) —see Dislocation
  muscle M62.00
    ankle M62.07-
    congenital Q79.8
    foot M62.07-
    forearm M62.03-
    hand M62.04-

Diastasis (continued)
  muscle (continued)
    lower leg M62.06-
    pelvic region M62.05-
    shoulder region M62.01-
    specified site NEC M62.08
    thigh M62.05-
    upper arm M62.02-
  recti (abdomen)
    complicating delivery O71.89
    congenital Q79.59
Diastema, tooth, teeth, fully erupted
  M26.32
Diastematomyelia Q06.2
Diataxia, cerebral G80.4
Diathesis
  allergic —see History, allergy
  bleeding (familial) D69.9
  cystine (familial) E72.00
  gouty —see Gout
  hemorrhagic (familial) D69.9
    newborn NEC P53
  spasmophilic R29.0
Diaz's disease or osteochondrosis
  (juvenile) (talus) —see
  Osteochondrosis, juvenile, tarsus
Dibothriocephalus,
  dibothriocephaliasis (latus)
  (infection) (infestation) B70.0
  larval B70.1
Dicephalus, dicephaly Q89.4
Dichotomy, teeth K00.2
Dichromat, dichromatopsia
  (congenital) —see Deficiency,
  color vision
Dichuchwa A65
Dicroceliasis B66.2
Didelphia, didelphys —see Double
  uterus
Didymytis N45.1
  with orchitis N45.3
Dietary
  inadequacy or deficiency E63.9
  surveillance and counseling Z71.3
Dietl's crisis N13.8
Dieulafoy lesion (hemorrhagic)
  duodenum K31.82
  esophagus K22.89
  intestine (colon) K63.81
  stomach K31.82
Difficult, difficulty (in)
  acculturation Z60.3
  feeding R63.30
    elderly R63.39
    infant NOS R63.39
    newborn P92.9
      breast P92.5
      specified NEC P92.8
    nonorganic (infant or child)
      F98.29
    specified NEC R63.39
  intubation, in anesthesia T88.4
  mechanical, gastroduodenal stoma
    K91.89
    causing obstruction (see also
      Obstruction, intestine,
      postoperative) K91.30
  micturition
    need to immediately re-void
      R39.191
    position dependent R39.192
    specified NEC R39.198
  reading (developmental) F81.0
    secondary to emotional disorders
      F93.9

Difficult, difficulty (continued)
spelling (specific) F81.81
with reading disorder F81.89
due to inadequate teaching Z55.8
swallowing —see Dysphagia
understanding
health related information Z55.6
medication instructions Z55.6
walking R26.2
work
conditions NEC Z56.5
schedule Z56.3

Diffuse —see condition

DiGeorge's syndrome (thymic hypoplasia) D82.1

Digestive —see condition

Dihydropyrimidine dehydrogenase disease (DPD) E88.89

Diktyoma —see Neoplasm, malignant, by site

Dilaceration, tooth K00.4

Dilatation
anus K59.89
venule —see Hemorrhoids
aorta (focal) (general) —see Ectasia, aorta
with aneurysm —see Aneurysm, aorta
congenital Q25.44
artery —see Aneurysm
bladder (sphincter) N32.89
congenital Q64.79
blood vessel I99.8
bronchial J47.9
with
exacerbation (acute) J47.1
lower respiratory infection J47.0
calyx N28.89
due to obstruction —see Hydronephrosis
capillaries I78.8
cardiac (acute) (chronic) —see also Hypertrophy, cardiac
congenital Q24.8
valve NEC Q24.8
pulmonary Q22.3
valve —see Endocarditis
cavum septi pellucidi Q06.8
cervix (uteri) —see also Incompetency, cervix
incomplete, poor, slow
complicating delivery O62.0
colon K59.39
congenital Q43.1
psychogenic F45.8
toxic K59.31
common duct (acquired) K83.8
congenital Q44.5
cystic duct (acquired) K82.8
congenital Q44.5
duct, mammary —see Ectasia, mammary duct
duodenum K59.89
esophagus K22.89
congenital Q39.5
due to achalasia K22.0
eustachian tube, congenital Q17.8
gallbladder K82.8
gastric —see Dilatation, stomach
heart (acute) (chronic) —see also Hypertrophy, cardiac
congenital Q24.8
valve —see Endocarditis
ileum K59.89
psychogenic F45.8
jejunum K59.89
psychogenic F45.8

Dilatation (continued)
kidney (calyx) (collecting structures) (cystic) (parenchyma) (pelvis) (idiopathic) N28.89
due to obstruction —see Hydronephrosis
lacrimal passages or duct —see Disorder, lacrimal system, changes
lymphatic vessel I89.0
mammary duct —see Ectasia, mammary duct
Meckel's diverticulum (congenital) Q43.0
malignant —see Table of Neoplasms, small intestine, malignant
myocardium (acute) (chronic) —see Hypertrophy, cardiac
organ or site, congenital NEC —see Distortion
pancreatic duct K86.89
pericardium —see Pericarditis
pharynx J39.2
prostate N42.89
pulmonary
artery (idiopathic) I28.8
valve, congenital Q22.3
pupil H57.04
rectum K59.39
saccule, congenital Q16.5
salivary gland (duct) K11.8
sphincter ani K62.89
stomach K31.89
acute K31.0
psychogenic F45.8
submaxillary duct K11.8
trachea, congenital Q32.1
ureter (idiopathic) N28.82
congenital Q62.2
due to obstruction N13.4
urethra (acquired) N36.8
vasomotor I73.9
vein I86.8
ventricular, ventricle (acute) (chronic) —see also Hypertrophy, cardiac
cerebral, congenital Q04.8
venule NEC I86.8
vesical orifice N32.89

Dilated, dilation —see Dilatation

Diminished, diminution
hearing (acuity) —see Deafness
sense or sensation (cold) (heat) (tactile) (vibratory) R20.8
vision NEC H54.7
vital capacity R94.2

Diminuta taenia B71.0

Dimitri-Sturge-Weber disease Q85.89

Dimple
congenital sacral Q82.6
parasacral Q82.6
pilonidal or postanal —see Cyst, pilonidal

Dioctophyme renalis (infection) (infestation) B83.8

Dipetalonemiasis B74.4

Diphallus Q55.69

Diphtheria, diphtheritic
(gangrenous) (hemorrhagic) A36.9
carrier (suspected) Z22.2
cutaneous A36.3
faucial A36.0
infection of wound A36.3
laryngeal A36.2
myocarditis A36.81
nasal, anterior A36.89
nasopharyngeal A36.1
neurological complication A36.89
pharyngeal A36.0

Diphtheria, diphtheritic (continued)
specified site NEC A36.89
tonsillar A36.0

Diphyllobothriasis (intestine) B70.0
larval B70.1

Diplacusis H93.22-

Diplegia (upper limbs) G83.0
congenital (cerebral) G80.8
facial G51.0
lower limbs G82.20
spastic G80.1

Diplococcus, diplococcal —see condition

Diplopia H53.2

Dipsomania F10.20
with
psychosis —see Psychosis, alcoholic
remission F10.21

Dipylidiasis B71.1

DIRA (deficiency of interleukin 1 receptor antagonist) M04.8

Direction, teeth, abnormal, fully erupted M26.30

Dirofilariasis B74.8

Dirt-eating child F98.3

Disability, disabilities
heart —see Disease, heart
intellectual F79
with
autistic features F84.9
pathogenic CHAMP1 (genetic) (variant) F78.A9
pathogenic HNRNPH2 (genetic) (variant) F78.A9
pathogenic SATB2 (genetic) (variant) F78.A9
pathogenic SETBP1 (genetic) (variant) F78.A9
pathogenic STXBP1 (genetic) (variant) F78.A9
pathogenic SYNGAP1 (genetic) (variant) F78.A1
autosomal dominant F78.A9
autosomal recessive F78.A9
genetic related F78.A9
with
pathogenic CHAMP1 (variant) F78.A9
pathogenic HNRNPH2 (variant) F78.A9
pathogenic SATB2 (variant) F78.A9
pathogenic SETBP1 (variant) F78.A9
pathogenic STXBP1 (variant) F78.A9
pathogenic SYNGAP1 (variant) F78.A1
specified NEC F78.A9
SYNGAP1-related F78.A1
in
autosomal dominant mental retardation F78.A9
autosomal recessive mental retardation F78.A9
SATB2-associated syndrome F78.A9
SETBP1 disorder F78.A9
STXBP1 encephalopathy
with epilepsy (see also Encephalopathy; and see also Epilepsy) F78.A9
X-linked mental retardation (syndromic) (Bain type) F78.A9

Disability, disabilities (continued)
intellectual (continued)
mild (I.Q.50-69) F70
moderate (I.Q.35-49) F71
profound (I.Q. under 20) F73
severe (I.Q.20-34) F72
specified level NEC F78.A9
SYNGAP1-related F78.A1
X-linked (syndromic) (Bain type) F78.A9
knowledge acquisition F81.9
learning F81.9
limiting activities Z73.6
spelling, specific F81.81

Disappearance of family member Z63.4

Disarticulation —see Amputation
meaning traumatic amputation —see Amputation, traumatic

Discharge (from)
abnormal finding in —see Abnormal, specimen
breast (female) (male) N64.52
diencephalic autonomic idiopathic —see Epilepsy, specified NEC
ear —see also Otorrhea
blood —see Otorrhagia
excessive urine R35.89
nipple N64.52
penile R36.9
postnasal R09.82
prison, anxiety concerning Z65.2
urethral R36.9
without blood R36.0
hematospermia R36.1
vaginal N89.8

Discitis, diskitis M46.40
cervical region M46.42
cervicothoracic region M46.43
lumbar region M46.46
lumbosacral region M46.47
multiple sites M46.49
occipito-atlanto-axial region M46.41
pyogenic —see Infection, intervertebral disc, pyogenic
sacrococcygeal region M46.48
thoracic region M46.44
thoracolumbar region M46.45

Discoid
meniscus (congenital) Q68.6
semilunar cartilage (congenital) —see Derangement, knee, meniscus, specified NEC

Discoloration
nails L60.8
teeth (posteruptive) K03.7
during formation K00.8

Discomfort
chest R07.89
visual H53.14-

Discontinuity, ossicles, ear H74.2-

Discord (with)
boss Z56.4
classmates Z55.4
counselor Z64.4
employer Z56.4
family Z63.8
fellow employees Z56.4
in-laws Z63.1
landlord Z59.2
lodgers Z59.2
neighbors Z59.2
probation officer Z64.4
social worker Z64.4
teachers Z55.4
workmates Z56.4

Discordant connection
- atrioventricular (congenital) Q20.5
- ventriculoarterial Q20.3

Discrepancy
- centric occlusion maximum intercuspation M26.55
- leg length (acquired) —*see* Deformity, limb, unequal length
  - congenital —*see* Defect, reduction, lower limb
- uterine size date O26.84-

Discrimination
- ethnic Z60.5
- political Z60.5
- racial Z60.5
- religious Z60.5
- sex Z60.5

Disease, diseased —*see also* Syndrome
- absorbent system I87.8
- acid-peptic K30
- Acosta's T70.29
- Adams-Stokes (-Morgagni) (syncope with heart block) I45.9
- Addison's anemia (pernicious) D51.0
- adenoids (and tonsils) J35.9
- adrenal (capsule) (cortex) (gland) (medullary) E27.9
  - hyperfunction E27.0
  - specified NEC E27.8
- ainhum L94.6
- airway
  - obstructive, chronic J44.9
    - due to
      - cotton dust J66.0
      - specific organic dusts NEC J66.8
  - reactive —*see* Asthma
- akamushi (scrub typhus) A75.3
- Albers-Schönberg (marble bones) Q78.2
- Albert's —*see* Tendinitis, Achilles
- Alexander G31.86
- alimentary canal K63.9
- alligator-skin Q80.9
  - acquired L85.0
- alpha heavy chain C88.3
- alpine T70.29
- altitude T70.20
- alveolar ridge
  - edentulous K06.9
    - specified NEC K06.8
- alveoli, teeth K08.9
- Alzheimer's (*see also* Dementia, in, diseases specified elsewhere) G30.9 [F02.80]
  - with behavioral disturbance (*see also* Dementia, in, diseases specified elsewhere) G30.9 [F02.81-]
  - early onset (*see also* Dementia, in, diseases specified elsewhere) G30.0 [F02.80]
    - with behavioral disturbance (*see also* Dementia, in, diseases specified elsewhere) G30.0 [F02.81-]
  - late onset (*see also* Dementia, in, diseases specified elsewhere) G30.1 [F02.80]
    - with behavioral disturbance (*see also* Dementia, in, diseases specified elsewhere) G30.1 [F02.81-]
  - specified NEC (*see also* Dementia, in, diseases specified elsewhere) G30.8 [F02.80]

Disease, diseased *(continued)*
- Alzheimer's *(continued)*
  - specified NEC *(continued)*
    - with behavioral disturbance (*see also* Dementia, in, diseases specified elsewhere) G30.8 [F02.81-]
- amyloid —*see* Amyloidosis
- Andersen's (glycogenosis IV) E74.09
- Andes T70.29
- Andrews' (bacterid) L08.89
- angiospastic I73.9
  - cerebral G45.9
  - vein I87.8
- anterior
  - chamber H21.9
  - horn cell G12.29
- antiglomerular basement membrane (anti-GBM) antibody M31.0
  - tubulo-interstitial nephritis N12
- Antopol E74.05
- antral —*see* Sinusitis, maxillary
- anus K62.9
  - specified NEC K62.89
- aorta (nonsyphilitic) I77.9
  - syphilitic NEC A52.02
- aortic (heart) (valve) I35.9
  - rheumatic I06.9
- Apollo B30.3
- aponeuroses —*see* Enthesopathy
- appendix K38.9
  - specified NEC K38.8
- aqueous (chamber) H21.9
- Arnold-Chiari —*see* Arnold-Chiari disease
- arterial —*see also* Disease, artery I77.9
  - occlusive —*see also* Occlusion, by site
    - due to stricture or stenosis I77.1
  - peripheral I73.9
- arteriocardiorenal —*see* Hypertension, cardiorenal
- arteriolar (generalized) (obliterative) I77.9
- arteriorenal —*see* Hypertension, kidney
- arteriosclerotic —*see also* Arteriosclerosis
  - cardiovascular —*see* Disease, heart, ischemic, atherosclerotic
  - coronary (artery) —*see* Disease, heart, ischemic, atherosclerotic
  - heart —*see* Disease, heart, ischemic, atherosclerotic
- artery (*see also* Disease, arterial) I77.9
  - cerebral I67.9
  - coronary I25.10
    - with angina pectoris —*see* Arteriosclerosis, coronary (artery)
  - peripheral I73.9
- arthropod-borne NOS (viral) A94
  - specified type NEC A93.8
- atticoantral, chronic H66.20
  - left H66.22
    - with right H66.23
  - right H66.21
    - with left H66.23
- auditory canal —*see* Disorder, ear, external
- auricle, ear NEC —*see* Disorder, pinna
- Australian X A83.4

Disease, diseased *(continued)*
- autoimmune (systemic) NOS M35.9
  - hemolytic D59.10
    - cold type (primary) (secondary) (symptomatic) D59.12
    - drug-induced D59.0
    - mixed type (primary) (secondary) (symptomatic) D59.13
    - warm type (primary) (secondary) (symptomatic) D59.11
  - thyroid E06.3
- autoinflammatory M04.9
  - NOD2-associated M04.8
  - specified type NEC M04.8
- aviator's —*see* Effect, adverse, high altitude
- Ayerza's (pulmonary artery sclerosis with pulmonary hypertension) I27.0
- Babington's (familial hemorrhagic telangiectasia) I78.0
- bacterial A49.9
  - specified NEC A48.8
  - zoonotic A28.9
    - specified type NEC A28.8
- Baelz's (cheilitis glandularis apostematosa) K13.0
- bagasse J67.1
- balloon —*see* Effect, adverse, high altitude
- Bang's (brucella abortus) A23.1
- Bannister's T78.3
- barometer makers' —*see* Poisoning, mercury
- Barraquer (-Simons') (progressive lipodystrophy) E88.1
- Barrett's —*see* Barrett's, esophagus
- Bartholin's gland N75.9
- basal ganglia G25.9
  - degenerative G23.9
    - specified NEC G23.8
  - specified NEC G25.89
- Basedow's (exophthalmic goiter) —*see* Hyperthyroidism, with, goiter (diffuse)
- Bateman's B08.1
- Batten-Steinert G71.11
- Battey A31.0
- Beard's (neurasthenia) F48.8
- Becker
  - idiopathic mural endomyocardial I42.3
  - myotonia congenita G71.12
- Begbie's (exophthalmic goiter) —*see* Hyperthyroidism, with, goiter (diffuse)
- behavioral, organic F07.9
- Beigel's (white piedra) B36.2
- Benson's —*see* Deposit, crystalline
- Bernard-Soulier (thrombopathy) D69.1
- Bernhardt (-Roth) —*see* Mononeuropathy, lower limb, meralgia paresthetica
- Biermer's (pernicious anemia) D51.0
- bile duct (common) (hepatic) K83.9
  - with calculus, stones —*see* Calculus, bile duct
  - specified NEC K83.8
- biliary (tract) K83.9
  - specified NEC K83.8
- Billroth's —*see* Spina bifida
- bird fancier's J67.2
- black lung J60

Disease, diseased *(continued)*
- bladder N32.9
  - in (due to)
    - schistosomiasis (bilharziasis) B65.0 [N33]
  - specified NEC N32.89
- bleeder's D66
- blood D75.9
  - forming organs D75.9
  - vessel I99.9
- Bloodgood's —*see* Mastopathy, cystic
- Blount M92.51-
- Bodechtel-Guttmann (subacute sclerosing panencephalitis) A81.1
- bone —*see also* Disorder, bone
  - aluminum M83.4
  - fibrocystic NEC
    - jaw M27.49
- bone-marrow D75.9
- Borna A83.9
- Bornholm (epidemic pleurodynia) B33.0
- Bouchard's (myopathic dilatation of the stomach) K31.0
- Bouillaud's (rheumatic heart disease) I01.9
- Bourneville (-Brissaud) (tuberous sclerosis) Q85.1
- Bouveret (-Hoffmann) (paroxysmal tachycardia) I47.9
- bowel K63.9
  - functional K59.9
    - psychogenic F45.8
- brain G93.9
  - arterial, artery I67.9
  - arteriosclerotic I67.2
  - congenital Q04.9
  - degenerative —*see* Degeneration, brain
  - inflammatory —*see* Encephalitis
  - organic G93.9
    - arteriosclerotic I67.2
  - parasitic NEC B71.9 [G94]
  - senile NEC G31.1
  - specified NEC G93.89
- breast —*see also* Disorder, breast N64.9
  - cystic (chronic) —*see* Mastopathy, cystic
  - fibrocystic —*see* Mastopathy, cystic
  - Paget's
    - female, unspecified side C50.91-
    - male, unspecified side C50.92-
  - specified NEC N64.89
- Breda's —*see* Yaws
- Bretonneau's (diphtheritic malignant angina) A36.0
- Bright's —*see* Nephritis
  - arteriosclerotic —*see* Hypertension, kidney
- Brill's (recrudescent typhus) A75.1
- Brill-Zinsser (recrudescent typhus) A75.1
- Brion-Kayser —*see* Fever, paratyphoid
- broad
  - beta E78.2
  - ligament (noninflammatory) N83.9
    - inflammatory —*see* Disease, pelvis, inflammatory
    - specified NEC N83.8

107

Disease, diseased (continued)
  Brocq-Duhring (dermatitis herpetiformis) L13.0
  Brocq's
    meaning
      dermatitis herpetiformis L13.0
      prurigo L28.2
  bronchopulmonary J98.4
  bronchus NEC J98.09
  bronze Addison's E27.1
    tuberculous A18.7
  budgerigar fancier's J67.2
  bullous L13.9
    chronic of childhood L12.2
    specified NEC L13.8
  Buerger's (thromboangiitis obliterans) I73.1
  Bürger-Grütz (essential familial hyperlipemia) E78.3
  bursa —see Bursopathy
  caisson T70.3
  California —see Coccidioidomycosis
  Canavan E75.28
  capillaries I78.9
    specified NEC I78.8
  Carapata A68.0
  cardiac —see Disease, heart
  cardiopulmonary, chronic I27.9
  cardiorenal (hepatic) (hypertensive) (vascular) —see Hypertension, cardiorenal
  cardiovascular (atherosclerotic) I25.10
    with angina pectoris —see Arteriosclerosis, coronary (artery)
    congenital Q28.9
    newborn P29.9
      specified NEC P29.89
    hypertensive —see Hypertension, heart
    renal (hypertensive) —see Hypertension, cardiorenal
    syphilitic (asymptomatic) A52.00
  cartilage —see Disorder, cartilage
  Castellani's A69.8
  Castleman (unicentric) (multicentric) D47.Z2
    HHV-8-associated (see also Herpesvirus, human, 8) D47.Z2
  cat-scratch A28.1
  Cavare's (familial periodic paralysis) G72.3
  cecum K63.9
  celiac (adult) (infantile) (with steatorrhea) K90.0
  cellular tissue L98.9
  central core G71.29
  cerebellar, cerebellum —see Disease, brain
  cerebral —see also Disease, brain
    degenerative —see Degeneration, brain
  cerebrospinal G96.9
  cerebrovascular I67.9
    acute I67.89
      embolic I63.4-
      thrombotic I63.3-
    arteriosclerotic I67.2
    hereditary NEC I67.858
    specified NEC I67.89
  cervix (uteri) (noninflammatory) N88.9
    inflammatory —see Cervicitis
    specified NEC N88.8
  Chabert's A22.9

Disease, diseased (continued)
  Chandler's (osteochondritis dissecans, hip) —see Osteochondritis, dissecans, hip
  Charlouis —see Yaws
  Chédiak-Steinbrinck (-Higashi) (congenital gigantism of peroxidase granules) E70.330
  chest J98.9
  Chiari's (hepatic vein thrombosis) I82.0
  Chicago B40.9
  Chignon B36.8
  chigo, chigoe B88.1
  childhood granulomatous D71
  Chinese liver fluke B66.1
  chlamydial A74.9
    specified NEC A74.89
  cholecystic K82.9
  choroid H31.9
    specified NEC H31.8
  Christmas D67
  chronic bullous of childhood L12.2
  chylomicron retention E78.3
  ciliary body H21.9
    specified NEC H21.89
  circulatory (system) NEC I99.8
    newborn P29.9
    syphilitic A52.00
      congenital A50.54
  coagulation factor deficiency (congenital) —see Defect, coagulation
  coccidioidal —see Coccidioidomycosis
  cold
    agglutinin or hemoglobinuria D59.12
      paroxysmal D59.6
    hemagglutinin (chronic) D59.12
  collagen NOS (nonvascular) (vascular) M35.9
    specified NEC M35.89
  colon K63.9
    functional K59.9
      congenital Q43.2
    ischemic (see also Ischemia, intestine, acute) K55.039
  colonic inflammatory bowel, unclassified (IBDU) K52.3
  combined system —see Degeneration, combined
  compressed air T70.3
  Concato's (pericardial polyserositis) A19.9
    nontubercular I31.1
    pleural —see Pleurisy, with effusion
  conjunctiva H11.9
    chlamydial A74.0
    specified NEC H11.89
    viral B30.9
      specified NEC B30.8
  connective tissue, systemic (diffuse) M35.9
    in (due to)
      hypogammaglobulinemia D80.1 [M36.8]
      ochronosis E70.29 [M36.8]
    specified NEC M35.89
  Conor and Bruch's (boutonneuse fever) A77.1
  Cooper's —see Mastopathy, cystic
  Cori's (glycogenosis III) E74.03
  corkhandler's or corkworker's J67.3
  cornea H18.9
    specified NEC H18.89-

Disease, diseased (continued)
  coronary (artery) —see Disease, heart, ischemic, atherosclerotic
    congenital Q24.5
    microvascular
      with
        angina pectoris I20.81
        myocardial infarction I21.B
      acute I24.81
      chronic I25.85
    ostial, syphilitic (aortic) (mitral) (pulmonary) A52.03
  corpus cavernosum N48.9
    specified NEC N48.89
  Cotugno's —see Sciatica
  COVID-19 U07.1
  coxsackie (virus) NEC B34.1
  cranial nerve NOS G52.9
  Creutzfeldt-Jakob —see Creutzfeldt-Jakob disease or syndrome
  Crocq's (acrocyanosis) I73.89
  Crohn's —see Enteritis, regional
  Curschmann G71.11
  cystic
    breast (chronic) —see Mastopathy, cystic
    kidney, congenital Q61.9
    liver, congenital Q44.6
    lung J98.4
      congenital Q33.0
  cytomegalic inclusion (generalized) B25.9
    with pneumonia B25.0
    congenital P35.1
  cytomegaloviral B25.9
    specified NEC B25.8
  Czerny's (periodic hydrarthrosis of the knee) —see Effusion, joint, knee
  Daae (-Finsen) (epidemic pleurodynia) B33.0
  Danon E74.05
  Darling's —see Histoplasmosis capsulati
  Débove's (splenomegaly) R16.1
  deer fly —see Tularemia
  Degos' I77.89
  demyelinating, demyelinizating (nervous system) G37.9
    multiple sclerosis G35
    specified NEC G37.89
  dense deposit (see also N00-N07 with fourth character .6) N05.6
  deposition, hydroxyapatite — see Disease, hydroxyapatite deposition
  de Quervain's (tendon sheath) M65.4
    thyroid (subacute granulomatous thyroiditis) E06.1
  Devergie's (pityriasis rubra pilaris) L44.0
  Devic's G36.0
  diaphorase deficiency D74.0
  diaphragm J98.6
  diarrheal, infectious NEC A09
  digestive system K92.9
    specified NEC K92.89
  disc, degenerative —see Degeneration, intervertebral disc
  discogenic —see also Displacement, intervertebral disc NEC
    with myelopathy —see Disorder, disc, with, myelopathy
  diverticular —see Diverticula
  Dubois (thymus) A50.59 [E35]
  Duchenne-Griesinger G71.01

Disease, diseased (continued)
  Duchenne's
    muscular dystrophy G71.01
    pseudohypertrophy, muscles G71.01
  ductless glands E34.9
  Duhring's (dermatitis herpetiformis) L13.0
  duodenum K31.9
    specified NEC K31.89
  Dupré's (meningism) R29.1
  Dupuytren's (muscle contracture) M72.0
  Durand-Nicholas-Favre (climatic bubo) A55
  Duroziez's (congenital mitral stenosis) Q23.2
  ear —see Disorder, ear
  Eberth's —see Fever, typhoid
  Ebola (virus) A98.4
  Ebstein's heart Q22.5
  Echinococcus —see Echinococcus
  echovirus NEC B34.1
  Eddowes' (brittle bones and blue sclera) Q78.0
  edentulous (alveolar) ridge K06.9
    specified NEC K06.8
  Edsall's T67.2
  Eichstedt's (pityriasis versicolor) B36.0
  Eisenmenger's (irreversible) I27.83
  Ellis-van Creveld (chondroectodermal dysplasia) Q77.6
  end stage renal (ESRD) N18.6
    due to hypertension I12.0
  endocrine glands or system NEC E34.9
  endomyocardial (eosinophilic) I42.3
  English (rickets) E55.0
  enteroviral, enterovirus NEC B34.1
    central nervous system NEC A88.8
  epidemic B99.9
    specified NEC B99.8
  epididymis N50.9
  Erb (-Landouzy) G71.02
  Erdheim-Chester (ECD) E88.89
  esophagus K22.9
    functional K22.4
    psychogenic F45.8
    specified NEC K22.89
  Eulenburg's (congenital paramyotonia) G71.19
  eustachian tube —see Disorder, eustachian tube
  external
    auditory canal —see Disorder, ear, external
    ear —see Disorder, ear, external
  extrapyramidal G25.9
    specified NEC G25.89
  eye H57.9
    anterior chamber H21.9
    inflammatory NEC H57.89
    muscle (external) —see Strabismus
    specified NEC H57.89
    syphilitic —see Oculopathy, syphilitic
  eyeball H44.9
    specified NEC H44.89
  eyelid —see Disorder, eyelid
    specified NEC —see Disorder, eyelid, specified type NEC
  eyeworm of Africa B74.3
  facial nerve (seventh) G51.9
    newborn (birth injury) P11.3

Disease, diseased (continued)
Fahr (of brain) G23.8
Fahr Volhard (of kidney) I12.-
fallopian tube (noninflammatory) N83.9
  inflammatory —see Salpingo-oophoritis
  specified NEC N83.8
familial periodic paralysis G72.3
Fanconi's (congenital pancytopenia) D61.09
fascia NEC —see also Disorder, muscle
  inflammatory —see Myositis
  specified NEC M62.89
Fauchard's (periodontitis) —see Periodontitis
Favre-Durand-Nicolas (climatic bubo) A55
Fede's K14.0
Feer's —see Poisoning, mercury
female pelvic inflammatory —see also Disease, pelvis, inflammatory N73.9
  syphilitic (secondary) A51.42
  tuberculous A18.17
Fernels' (aortic aneurysm) I71.9
fibrocaseous of lung —see Tuberculosis, pulmonary
fibrocystic —see Fibrocystic disease
Fiedler's (leptospiral jaundice) A27.0
fifth B08.3
file-cutter's —see Poisoning, lead
fish-skin Q80.9
  acquired L85.0
Flajani (-Basedow) (exophthalmic goiter) —see Hyperthyroidism, with, goiter (diffuse)
flax-dresser's J66.1
fluke —see Infestation, fluke
foot and mouth B08.8
foot process N04.9
Forbes' (glycogenosis III) E74.03
Fordyce-Fox (apocrine miliaria) L75.2
Fordyce's (ectopic sebaceous glands) (mouth) Q38.6
Forestier's (rhizomelic pseudopolyarthritis) M35.3
  meaning ankylosing hyperostosis —see Hyperostosis, ankylosing
Fothergill's
  neuralgia —see Neuralgia, trigeminal
  scarlatina anginosa A38.9
Fournier (gangrene) N49.3
  female N76.82
  vagina and vulva N76.82
fourth B08.8
Fox (-Fordyce) (apocrine miliaria) L75.2
Francis' —see Tularemia
Franklin C88.2
Frei's (climatic bubo) A55
Friedreich's
  combined systemic or ataxia G11.11
  myoclonia G25.3
frontal sinus —see Sinusitis, frontal
fungus NEC B49
Gaisböck's (polycythemia hypertonica) D75.1
gallbladder K82.9
  calculus —see Calculus, gallbladder
  cholecystitis —see Cholecystitis
  cholesterolosis K82.4
  fistula —see Fistula, gallbladder

Disease, diseased (continued)
gallbladder (continued)
  hydrops K82.1
  obstruction —see Obstruction, gallbladder
  perforation K82.2
  specified NEC K82.8
gamma heavy chain C88.2
Gamna's (siderotic splenomegaly) D73.2
Gamstorp's (adynamia episodica hereditaria) G72.3
Gandy-Nanta (siderotic splenomegaly) D73.2
ganister J62.8
gastric —see Disease, stomach
gastroesophageal reflux (GERD) K21.9
  with esophagitis (without bleeding) K21.00
    with bleeding K21.01
gastrointestinal (tract) K92.9
  amyloid E85.4
  functional K59.9
    psychogenic F45.8
  specified NEC K92.89
Gee (-Herter) (-Heubner) (-Thaysen) (nontropical sprue) K90.0
genital organs
  female N94.9
  male N50.9
Gerhardt's (erythromelalgia) I73.81
Gibert's (pityriasis rosea) L42
Gierke's (glycogenosis I) E74.01
Gilles de la Tourette's (motor-verbal tic) F95.2
gingiva K06.9
  plaque induced K05.00
  specified NEC K06.8
gland (lymph) I89.9
Glanzmann's (hereditary hemorrhagic thrombasthenia) D69.1
glass-blower's (cataract) —see Cataract, specified NEC
  salivary gland hypertrophy K11.1
Glisson's —see Rickets
globe H44.9
  specified NEC H44.89
glomerular —see also Glomerulonephritis
  with edema —see Nephrosis
  acute —see Nephritis, acute
  chronic —see Nephritis, chronic
  minimal change N05.0
  rapidly progressive N01.9
glycogen storage E74.00
  Andersen's E74.09
  Cori's E74.03
  Forbes' E74.03
  generalized E74.00
  glucose-6-phosphatase deficiency E74.01
  heart E74.02 [143]
  hepatorenal E74.09
  Hers' E74.09
  liver and kidney E74.09
  lysosomal E74.02
    with acid maltase deficiency E74.02
    without acid maltase deficiency E74.05
  McArdle's E74.04
  muscle phosphofructokinase E74.09
  myocardium E74.02 [143]
  Pompe's E74.02
  Tauri's E74.09

Disease, diseased (continued)
glycogen storage (continued)
  type 0 E74.09
  type I E74.01
  type II E74.02
  type IIB E74.05
  type III E74.03
  type IV E74.09
  type V E74.04
  type VI-XI E74.09
  Von Gierke's E74.01
Goldstein's (familial hemorrhagic telangiectasia) I78.0
gonococcal NOS A54.9
graft-versus-host (GVH) D89.813
  acute D89.810
  acute on chronic D89.812
  chronic D89.811
grainhandler's J67.8
granulomatous (childhood) (chronic) D71
Graves' (exophthalmic goiter) —see Hyperthyroidism, with, goiter (diffuse)
Griesinger's —see Ancylostomiasis
Grisel's M43.6
Gruby's (tinea tonsurans) B35.0
Guillain-Barré G61.0
Guinon's (motor-verbal tic) F95.2
gum K06.9
gynecological N94.9
H (Hartnup's) E72.02
Haff —see Poisoning, mercury
Hageman (congenital factor XII deficiency) D68.2
hair (color) (shaft) L67.9
  follicles L73.9
    specified NEC L73.8
Hamman's (spontaneous mediastinal emphysema) J98.2
hand, foot and mouth B08.4
Hansen's —see Leprosy
Hantavirus, with pulmonary manifestations B33.4
  with renal manifestations A98.5
Harada's H30.81-
Hartnup (pellagra-cerebellar ataxia-renal aminoaciduria) E72.02
Hart's (pellagra-cerebellar ataxia-renal aminoaciduria) E72.02
Hashimoto's (struma lymphomatosa) E06.3
Hb —see Disease, hemoglobin
heart (organic) I51.9
  with
    pulmonary edema (acute) —see also Failure, ventricular, left I50.1
    rheumatic fever (conditions in I00)
      active I01.9
        with chorea I02.0
        specified NEC I01.8
      inactive or quiescent (with chorea) I09.9
        specified NEC I09.89
  amyloid E85.4 [143]
  aortic (valve) I35.9
  arteriosclerotic or sclerotic (senile) —see Disease, heart, ischemic, atherosclerotic
  artery, arterial —see Disease, heart, ischemic, atherosclerotic
  beer drinkers' I42.6
  beriberi (wet) E51.12
  black I27.0
  congenital Q24.9
    cyanotic Q24.9
    specified NEC Q24.8

Disease, diseased (continued)
heart (continued)
  coronary —see Disease, heart, ischemic
  cryptogenic I51.9
  fibroid —see Myocarditis
  functional I51.89
    psychogenic F45.8
  glycogen storage E74.02 [143]
  gonococcal A54.83
  hypertensive —see Hypertension, heart
  hyperthyroid —see also Hyperthyroidism E05.90 [143]
    with thyroid storm E05.91 [143]
  ischemic (chronic or with a stated duration of over 4 weeks) I25.9
    atherosclerotic (of) I25.10
      with angina pectoris —see Arteriosclerosis, coronary (artery)
      coronary artery bypass graft —see Arteriosclerosis, coronary (artery), cardiomyopathy I25.5
    diagnosed on ECG or other special investigation, but currently presenting no symptoms I25.6
    silent I25.6
    specified form NEC
      acute I24.89
      chronic I25.89
  kyphoscoliotic I27.1
  meningococcal A39.50
    endocarditis A39.51
    myocarditis A39.52
    pericarditis A39.53
  mitral I05.9
    specified NEC I05.8
  muscular —see Degeneration, myocardial
  psychogenic (functional) F45.8
  pulmonary (chronic) I27.9
    in schistosomiasis B65.9 [152]
    specified NEC I27.89
  rheumatic (chronic) (inactive) (old) (quiescent) (with chorea) I09.9
    active or acute I01.9
      with chorea (acute) (rheumatic) (Sydenham's) I02.0
    specified NEC I09.89
  senile —see Myocarditis
  syphilitic A52.06
    aortic A52.03
      aneurysm A52.01
    congenital A50.54 [152]
  thyrotoxic (see also Thyrotoxicosis) E05.90 [143]
    with thyroid storm E05.91 [143]
  valve, valvular (obstructive) (regurgitant) —see also Endocarditis
    congenital NEC Q24.8
      pulmonary Q22.3
  vascular —see Disease, cardiovascular
heavy chain NEC C88.2
  alpha C88.3
  gamma C88.2
  mu C88.2

109

Disease, diseased (continued)
- Hebra's
  - pityriasis
    - maculata et circinata L42
    - rubra pilaris L44.0
  - prurigo L28.2
- hematopoietic organs D75.9
- hemoglobin or Hb
  - abnormal (mixed) NEC D58.2
    - with thalassemia D56.9
  - AS genotype D57.3
  - Bart's D56.0
  - C (Hb-C) D58.2
    - with other abnormal hemoglobin NEC D58.2
    - elliptocytosis D58.1
    - Hb-S D57.2-
    - sickle-cell D57.2-
    - thalassemia D56.8
  - Constant Spring D58.2
  - D(Hb-D) D58.2
  - E(Hb-E) D58.2
  - E-beta thalassemia D56.5
  - elliptocytosis D58.1
  - H(Hb-H) (thalassemia) D56.0
    - with other abnormal hemoglobin NEC D56.9
    - Constant Spring D56.0
  - I thalassemia D56.9
  - M D74.0
  - S or SS D57.1
    - with
      - acute chest syndrome D57.01
      - cerebral vascular involvement D57.03
      - crisis (painful) D57.00
        - with complication specified NEC D57.09
      - pain (vaso-occlusive) D57.00
      - splenic sequestration D57.02
    - beta plus D57.44
      - with
        - acute chest syndrome D57.451
        - cerebral vascular involvement D57.453
        - crisis D57.459
          - with specified complication NEC D57.458
          - pain (vaso-occlusive) D57.459
          - splenic sequestration D57.452
      - without crisis D57.44
    - beta zero D57.42
      - with
        - acute chest syndrome D57.431
        - cerebral vascular involvement D57.433
        - crisis D57.439
          - with specified complication NEC D57.438
          - pain (vaso-occlusive) D57.439
          - splenic sequestration D57.432
      - without crisis D57.42

Disease, diseased (continued)
- hemoglobin or Hb (continued)
  - S or SS (continued)
    - SC D57.2-
    - SD D57.8-
    - SE D57.8-
    - spherocytosis D58.0
    - unstable, hemolytic D58.2
  - hemolytic (newborn) P55.9
    - autoimmune D59.10
      - cold type (primary) (secondary) (symptomatic) D59.12
      - mixed type (primary) (secondary) (symptomatic) D59.13
      - warm type (primary) (secondary) (symptomatic) D59.11
    - drug-induced D59.0
    - due to or with
      - incompatibility
        - ABO (blood group) P55.1
        - blood (group) (Duffy) (K) (Kell) (Kidd) (Lewis) (M) (S) NEC P55.8
        - Rh (blood group) (factor) P55.0
      - Rh negative mother P55.0
    - specified type NEC P55.8
    - unstable hemoglobin D58.2
  - hemorrhagic D69.9
    - newborn P53
  - Henoch (-Schönlein) (purpura nervosa) D69.0
  - hepatic —*see* Disease, liver
  - hepatobiliary K83.9
    - toxic K71.9
  - hepatolenticular E83.01
  - heredodegenerative NEC
    - spinal cord G95.89
  - herpesviral, disseminated B00.7
  - Hers' (glycogenosis VI) E74.09
  - Herter (-Gee) (-Heubner) (nontropical sprue) K90.0
  - Heubner-Herter (nontropical sprue) K90.0
  - high fetal gene or hemoglobin thalassemia D56.9
  - Hildenbrand's —*see* Typhus
  - hip (joint) M25.9
    - congenital Q65.89
    - suppurative M00.9
    - tuberculous A18.02
  - His (-Werner) (trench fever) A79.0
  - Hodgson's (*see also* Aneurysm, aorta, thorax) I71.20
    - ruptured (*see also* Aneurysm, aorta, thorax, ruptured) I71.10
  - Holla —*see* Spherocytosis
  - hookworm B76.9
    - specified NEC B76.8
  - host-versus-graft D89.813
    - acute D89.810
    - acute on chronic D89.812
    - chronic D89.811
  - human immunodeficiency virus (HIV) B20
  - Hunt's (herpetic geniculate ganglionitis) (neuralgia) B02.21
    - dyssynergia cerebellaris myoclonica G11.19
  - Huntington's G10
    - with dementia (*see also* Dementia, in, diseases specified elsewhere) G10 [F02.80]
  - Hutchinson's (cheiropompholyx) —*see* Hutchinson's disease

Disease, diseased (continued)
- hyaline (diffuse) (generalized)
  - membrane (lung) (newborn) P22.0
    - adult J80
- hydatid —*see* Echinococcus
- hydroxyapatite deposition M11.00
  - ankle M11.07-
  - elbow M11.02-
  - foot joint M11.07-
  - hand joint M11.04-
  - hip M11.05-
  - knee M11.06-
  - multiple site M11.09
  - shoulder M11.01-
  - vertebra M11.08
  - wrist M11.03-
- hyperkinetic —*see* Hyperkinesia
- hypertensive —*see* Hypertension
- hypophysis E23.7
- Iceland G93.39
- I-cell E77.0
- IgG4-related D89.84
- immune D89.9
- immunoglobulin G4-related D89.84
- immunoproliferative (malignant) C88.9
  - small intestinal C88.3
  - specified NEC C88.8
- inclusion B25.9
  - salivary gland B25.9
- infectious, infective B99.9
  - congenital P37.9
    - specified NEC P37.8
    - viral P35.9
      - specified type NEC P35.8
  - specified NEC B99.8
- inflammatory
  - penis N48.29
    - abscess N48.21
    - cellulitis N48.22
  - prepuce N47.7
    - balanoposthitis N47.6
  - tubo-ovarian —*see* Salpingo-oophoritis
- intervertebral disc —*see also* Disorder, disc
  - with myelopathy —*see* Disorder, disc, with, myelopathy
  - cervical, cervicothoracic —*see* Disorder, disc, cervical
    - with
      - myelopathy —*see* Disorder, disc, cervical, with myelopathy
      - neuritis, radiculitis or radiculopathy —*see* Disorder, disc, cervical, with neuritis
      - specified NEC —*see* Disorder, disc, cervical, specified type NEC
  - lumbar (with)
    - myelopathy M51.06
    - neuritis, radiculitis, radiculopathy or sciatica M51.16
    - specified NEC M51.86
  - lumbosacral (with)
    - neuritis, radiculitis, radiculopathy or sciatica M51.17
    - specified NEC M51.87
  - specified NEC —*see* Disorder, disc, specified NEC
  - thoracic (with)
    - myelopathy M51.04
    - neuritis, radiculitis or radiculopathy M51.14
    - specified NEC M51.84

Disease, diseased (continued)
- intervertebral disc (continued)
  - thoracolumbar (with)
    - myelopathy M51.05
    - neuritis, radiculitis or radiculopathy M51.15
    - specified NEC M51.85
- intestine K63.9
  - functional K59.9
    - psychogenic F45.8
    - specified NEC K59.89
  - organic K63.9
  - protozoal A07.9
  - specified NEC K63.89
- iris H21.9
  - specified NEC H21.89
- iron metabolism or storage E83.10
- island (scrub typhus) A75.3
- itai-itai —*see* Poisoning, cadmium
- Jakob-Creutzfeldt —*see* Creutzfeldt-Jakob disease or syndrome
- jaw M27.9
  - fibrocystic M27.49
  - specified NEC M27.8
- jigger B88.1
- joint —*see also* Disorder, joint
  - Charcot's —*see* Arthropathy, neuropathic (Charcot)
  - degenerative —*see* Osteoarthritis
    - multiple M15.9
    - spine —*see* Spondylosis
  - facet joint (*see also* Spondylosis) M47.819
  - hypertrophic —*see* Osteoarthritis
  - sacroiliac M53.3
  - specified NEC —*see* Disorder, joint, specified type NEC
  - spine NEC —*see* Dorsopathy
  - suppurative —*see* Arthritis, pyogenic or pyemic
- Jourdain's (acute gingivitis) K05.00
  - nonplaque induced K05.01
  - plaque induced K05.00
- Kaschin-Beck (endemic polyarthritis) M12.10
  - ankle M12.17-
  - elbow M12.12-
  - foot joint M12.17-
  - hand joint M12.14-
  - hip M12.15-
  - knee M12.16-
  - multiple site M12.19
  - shoulder M12.11-
  - vertebra M12.18
  - wrist M12.13-
- Katayama B65.2
- Kedani (scrub typhus) A75.3
- Keshan E59
- kidney (functional) (pelvis) N28.9
  - chronic N18.9
    - hypertensive —*see* Hypertension, kidney
    - stage 1 N18.1
    - stage 2(mild) N18.2
    - stage 3(moderate) N18.30
    - stage 3a N18.31
    - stage 3b N18.32
    - stage 4(severe) N18.4
    - stage 5 N18.5
  - complicating pregnancy —*see* Pregnancy, complicated by, renal disease
  - cystic (congenital) Q61.9
  - diabetic —*see* E08-E13 with .22
  - fibrocystic (congenital) Q61.8

Disease, diseased (continued)
  kidney (continued)
    hypertensive —see Hypertension, kidney
    in (due to)
      schistosomiasis (bilharziasis) B65.9 [N29]
    multicystic Q61.4
    polycystic Q61.3
      adult type Q61.2
      childhood type NEC Q61.19
        collecting duct dilatation Q61.11
  Kimmelstiel (-Wilson) (intercapillary polycystic) (congenital) glomerulosclerosis) —see E08-E13 with .21
  Kimura D21.9
    specified site (see Neoplasm, connective tissue benign)
  Kinnier Wilson's (hepatolenticular degeneration) E83.01
  kissing —see Mononucleosis, infectious
  Klebs' (see also Glomerulonephritis) N05.-
  Klippel-Feil (brevicollis) Q76.1
  Köhler-Pellegrini-Stieda (calcification, knee joint) —see Bursitis, tibial collateral
  Kok Q89.8
  König's (osteochondritis dissecans) —see Osteochondritis, dissecans
  Korsakoff's (nonalcoholic) F04
    alcoholic F10.96
      with dependence F10.26
  Kostmann's (infantile genetic agranulocytosis) D70.0
  kuru A81.81
  Kyasanur Forest A98.2
  labyrinth, ear —see Disorder, ear, inner
  lacrimal system —see Disorder, lacrimal system
  Lafora body (see also Epilepsy, progressive, Lafora) G40.C09
  Lancereaux-Mathieu (leptospiral jaundice) A27.0
  Landry's G61.0
  Larrey-Weil (leptospiral jaundice) A27.0
  larynx J38.7
  legionnaires' A48.1
    nonpneumonic A48.2
  Lenegre's I44.2
  lens H27.9
    specified NEC H27.8
  Lev's (acquired complete heart block) I44.2
  Lewy body (dementia) (see also Dementia, in, diseases specified elsewhere) G31.83 [F02.80]
    with behavioral disturbance (see also Dementia, in, diseases specified elsewhere) G31.83 [F02.81-]
  Lichtheim's (subacute combined sclerosis with pernicious anemia) D51.0
  Lightwood's (renal tubular acidosis) N25.89
  Lignac's (cystinosis) E72.04
  lip K13.0
  lipid-storage E75.6
    specified NEC E75.5
  Lipschütz's N76.6
  liver (chronic) (organic) K76.9
    alcoholic (chronic) K70.9
      acute —see Disease, liver, alcoholic, hepatitis

Disease, diseased (continued)
  liver (continued)
    alcoholic (continued)
      cirrhosis K70.30
        with ascites K70.31
      failure K70.40
        with coma K70.41
      fatty liver K70.0
      fibrosis K70.2
      hepatitis K70.10
        with ascites K70.11
      sclerosis K70.2
    cystic, congenital Q44.6
    drug-induced (idiosyncratic) (toxic) (predictable) (unpredictable) —see Disease, liver, toxic
    end stage K72.1-
      with coma K72.11
      due to hepatitis —see Hepatitis
    fatty, nonalcoholic (NAFLD) K76.0
      alcoholic K70.0
    fibrocystic (congenital) Q44.6
    fluke
      Chinese B66.1
      oriental B66.1
      sheep B66.3
    gestational alloimmune (GALD) P78.84
    glycogen storage E74.09 [K77]
    in (due to)
      schistosomiasis (bilharziasis) B65.9 [K77]
    inflammatory K75.9
      alcoholic K70.1
      specified NEC K75.89
    polycystic (congenital) Q44.6
    toxic K71.9
      with
        cholestasis K71.0
        cirrhosis (liver) K71.7
        fibrosis (liver) K71.7
        focal nodular hyperplasia K71.8
        hepatic granuloma K71.8
        hepatic necrosis K71.10
          with coma K71.11
        hepatitis NEC K71.6
          acute K71.2
          chronic
            active K71.50
              with ascites K71.51
            lobular K71.4
            persistent K71.3
          lupoid K71.50
            with ascites K71.51
        peliosis hepatis K71.8
        veno-occlusive disease (VOD) of liver K71.8
    veno-occlusive K76.5
  Lobo's (keloid blastomycosis) B48.0
  Lobstein's (brittle bones and blue sclera) Q78.0
  Ludwig's (submaxillary cellulitis) K12.2
  lumbosacral region M53.87
  lung J98.4
    black J60
    congenital Q33.9
    cystic J98.4
      congenital Q33.0
    dabbing (related) U07.0
    electronic cigarette (related) U07.0
    fibroid (chronic) —see Fibrosis, lung

Disease, diseased (continued)
  lung (continued)
    fluke B66.4
      oriental B66.4
    in
      amyloidosis E85.4 [J99]
      sarcoidosis D86.0
      Sjögren's syndrome M35.02
      systemic
        lupus erythematosus M32.13
        sclerosis M34.81
    interstitial J84.9
      with progressive fibrotic phenotype, in diseases classified elsewhere J84.170
      drug-induced —see Disorder, lung, interstitial, drug-induced
      of childhood, specified NEC J84.848
        drug-induced —see Disorder, lung, interstitial, drug-induced
      respiratory bronchiolitis J84.115
      specified NEC J84.89
    obstructive (chronic) J44.9
      with
        acute
          bronchitis J44.0
          exacerbation NEC J44.1
          lower respiratory infection J44.0
        alveolitis, allergic J67.9
        asthma J44.9
        bronchiectasis J47.9
          with
            exacerbation (acute) J47.1
            lower respiratory infection J47.0
        bronchitis J44.89
          with
            exacerbation (acute) J44.1
            lower respiratory infection J44.0
        emphysema J43.9
        hypersensitivity pneumonitis J67.9
      decompensated J44.1
        with
          exacerbation (acute) J44.1
    polycystic J98.4
      congenital Q33.0
    rheumatoid (diffuse) (interstitial) —see Rheumatoid, lung
    vaping (associated) (device) (product) (use) U07.0
  Lutembacher's (atrial septal defect with mitral stenosis) Q21.19
  Lyme A69.20
  lymphatic (gland) (system) (channel) (vessel) I89.9
  lymphoproliferative D47.9
    specified NEC D47.Z9
    T-gamma D47.Z9
    X-linked D82.3
  Magitot's M27.2
  malarial —see Malaria
  malignant —see also Neoplasm, malignant, by site
  Manson's B65.1
  maple bark J67.6
  maple-syrup-urine E71.0
  Marburg (virus) A98.3
  Marion's (bladder neck obstruction) N32.0

Disease, diseased (continued)
  Marsh's (exophthalmic goiter) —see Hyperthyroidism, with, goiter (diffuse)
  mastoid (process) —see Disorder, ear, middle
  Mathieu's (leptospiral jaundice) A27.0
  Maxcy's A75.2
  McArdle (-Schmid-Pearson) (glycogenosis V) E74.04
  mediastinum J98.59
  medullary center (idiopathic) (respiratory) G93.89
  Meige's (chronic hereditary edema) Q82.0
  meningococcal —see Infection, meningococcal
  mental F99
    organic F09
  mesenchymal M35.9
  mesenteric embolic (see also Ischemia, intestine, acute) K55.039
  metabolic, metabolism E88.9
    bilirubin E80.7
  metal-polisher's J62.8
  metastatic (see also Neoplasm, secondary, by site) C79.4.9
  microvascular - code to condition
  microvillus
    atrophy Q43.8
    inclusion (MVD) Q43.8
  middle ear —see Disorder, ear, middle
  Mikulicz' (dryness of mouth, absent or decreased lacrimation) K11.8
  Milroy's (chronic hereditary edema) Q82.0
  Minamata —see Poisoning, mercury
  minicore G71.29
  Minor's G95.19
  Minot's (hemorrhagic disease, newborn) P53
  Minot-von Willebrand-Jürgens (angiohemophilia) —see Disease, von Willebrand
  Mitchell's (erythromelalgia) I73.81
  mitral (valve) I05.9
    nonrheumatic I34.9
  mixed connective tissue M35.1
  MOG antibody G37.81
  moldy hay J67.0
  Monge's T70.29
  Morgagni-Adams-Stokes (syncope with heart block) I45.9
  Morgagni's (syndrome) (hyperostosis frontalis interna) M85.2
  Morton's (with metatarsalgia) —see Lesion, nerve, plantar
  Morvan's G60.8
  motor neuron (bulbar) (mixed type) (spinal) G12.20
    amyotrophic lateral sclerosis G12.21
    familial G12.24
    progressive bulbar palsy G12.22
    specified NEC G12.29
  moyamoya I67.5
  mu heavy chain disease C88.2
  multicore G71.29
  multiminicore G71.29
  muscle —see also Disorder, muscle
    inflammatory —see Myositis
    ocular (external) —see Strabismus

Disease, diseased *(continued)*
- musculoskeletal system, soft tissue —*see also* Disorder, soft tissue
  - specified NEC —*see* Disorder, soft tissue, specified type NEC
- mushroom workers' J67.5
- mycotic B49
- myelin oligodendrocyte glycoprotein antibody G37.81
- myelodysplastic (*see also* Syndrome, myelodysplasia) C94.6
- myelodysplastic/myeloproliferative neoplasm, unclassifiable C94.6
- myeloproliferative, D47.1
  - chronic D47.1
  - not classified C94.6
  - specified NEC C94.6
  - unclassifiable C94.6
- myocardium, myocardial (*see also* Degeneration, myocardial) I51.5
  - primary (idiopathic) I42.9
- myoneural G70.9
- Naegeli's D69.1
- nails L60.9
  - specified NEC L60.8
- Nairobi (sheep virus) A93.8
- nasal J34.9
- nemaline body G71.21
- nerve —*see* Disorder, nerve
- nervous system G98.8
  - autonomic G90.9
  - central G96.9
    - specified NEC G96.89
  - congenital Q07.9
  - parasympathetic G90.9
  - specified NEC G98.8
  - sympathetic G90.9
  - vegetative G90.9
- neuromuscular system G70.9
- Newcastle B30.8
- Nicolas (-Durand)-Favre (climatic bubo) A55
- nipple N64.9
  - Paget's C50.01-
    - female C50.01-
    - male C50.02-
- Nishimoto (-Takeuchi) I67.5
- nonarthropod-borne NOS (viral) B34.9
  - enterovirus NEC B34.1
- nonautoimmune hemolytic D59.4
  - drug-induced D59.2
- Nonne-Milroy-Meige (chronic hereditary edema) Q82.0
- nose J34.9
- nucleus pulposus —*see* Disorder, disc
- nutritional E63.9
- oast-house-urine E72.19
- ocular
  - herpesviral B00.50
  - zoster B02.30
- obliterative vascular I77.1
- Ohara's —*see* Tularemia
- Opitz's (congestive splenomegaly) D73.2
- Oppenheim-Urbach (necrobiosis lipoidica diabeticorum) —*see* E08-E13 with .620
- optic nerve NEC —*see* Disorder, nerve, optic
- orbit —*see* Disorder, orbit
- organ
  - dabbing (related) U07.0
  - electronic cigarette (related) U07.0
  - vaping (associated) (device) (product) (use) U07.0

Disease, diseased *(continued)*
- Oriental liver fluke B66.1
- Oriental lung fluke B66.4
- Ormond's N13.5
- Oropouche virus A93.0
- Osler-Rendu (familial hemorrhagic telangiectasia) I78.0
- osteofibrocystic E21.0
- Otto's M24.7
- outer ear —*see* Disorder, ear, external
- ovary (noninflammatory) N83.9
  - cystic N83.20-
  - inflammatory —*see* Salpingo-oophoritis
  - polycystic E28.2
  - specified NEC N83.8
- Owren's (congenital) —*see* Defect, coagulation
- p110d-activating mutation causing senescent T cells, lymphadenopathy, and immunodeficiency [PASLI] D81.82
- pancreas K86.9
  - cystic K86.2
  - fibrocystic E84.9
  - specified NEC K86.89
- panvalvular I08.9
  - specified NEC I08.8
- parametrium (noninflammatory) N83.9
- parasitic B89
  - cerebral NEC B71.9 *[G94]*
  - intestinal NOS B82.9
  - mouth B37.0
  - skin NOS B88.9
  - specified type —*see* Infestation
  - tongue B37.0
- parathyroid (gland) E21.5
  - specified NEC E21.4
- Parkinson's G20.A1
  - with dyskinesia
    - with
      - fluctuations G20.B2
      - OFF episodes G20.B2
    - without mention of
      - fluctuations G20.B1
      - OFF episodes G20.B1
  - without dyskinesia
    - with
      - fluctuations G20.A2
      - OFF episodes G20.A2
    - without mention of
      - fluctuations G20.A1
      - OFF episodes G20.A1
- parodontal K05.6
- Parrot's (syphilitic osteochondritis) A50.02
- Parry's (exophthalmic goiter) —*see* Hyperthyroidism, with, goiter (diffuse)
- Parson's (exophthalmic goiter) —*see* Hyperthyroidism, with, goiter (diffuse)
- Paxton's (white piedra) B36.2
- pearl-worker's —*see* Osteomyelitis, specified type NEC
- Pellegrini-Stieda (calcification, knee joint) —*see* Bursitis, tibial collateral
- pelvis, pelvic
  - female NOS N94.9
    - specified NEC N94.89
  - gonococcal (acute) (chronic) A54.24
  - inflammatory (female) N73.9
    - acute N73.0
    - chlamydial A56.11
    - chronic N73.1

Disease, diseased *(continued)*
- pelvis, pelvic *(continued)*
  - inflammatory *(continued)*
    - specified NEC N73.8
    - syphilitic (secondary) A51.42
      - late A52.76
    - tuberculous A18.17
  - organ, female N94.9
  - peritoneum, female NEC N94.89
- penis N48.9
  - inflammatory N48.29
    - abscess N48.21
    - cellulitis N48.22
  - specified NEC N48.89
- periapical tissues NOS K04.90
- periodontal K05.6
  - specified NEC K05.5
- periosteum —*see* Disorder, bone, specified type NEC
- peripheral
  - arterial I73.9
  - autonomic nervous system G90.9
  - nerves —*see* Polyneuropathy
  - vascular NOS I73.9
    - in diabetes mellitus —*see* Diabetes, by type, with peripheral angiopathy
- peritoneum K66.9
  - pelvic, female NEC N94.89
  - specified NEC K66.8
- persistent mucosal (middle ear) H66.20
  - left H66.22
    - with right H66.23
  - right H66.21
    - with left H66.23
- Petit's —*see* Hernia, abdomen, specified site NEC
- pharynx J39.2
  - specified NEC J39.2
- Phocas' —*see* Mastopathy, cystic
- photochromogenic (acid-fast bacilli) (pulmonary) A31.0
  - nonpulmonary A31.9
- Pick's (*see also* Dementia, in, diseases specified elsewhere) G31.01 *[F02.80]*
  - with behavioral disturbance (*see also* Dementia, in, diseases specified elsewhere) G31.01 *[F02.81-]*
  - brain (*see also* Dementia, in, diseases specified elsewhere) G31.01 *[F02.80]*
    - with behavioral disturbance (*see also* Dementia, in, diseases specified elsewhere) G31.01 *[F02.81-]*
  - of pericardium (pericardial pseudocirrhosis of liver) I31.1
- pigeon fancier's J67.2
- pineal gland E34.8
- pink —*see* Poisoning, mercury
- Pinkus' (lichen nitidus) L44.1
- pinworm B80
- Piry virus A93.8
- pituitary (gland) E23.7
- pituitary-snuff-taker's J67.8
- pleura (cavity) J94.9
  - specified NEC J94.8
- pneumatic drill (hammer) T75.21
- Pollitzer's (hidradenitis suppurativa) L73.2
- polycystic
  - kidney or renal Q61.3
    - adult type Q61.2
    - childhood type NEC Q61.19
      - collecting duct dilatation Q61.11
  - liver or hepatic Q44.6

Disease, diseased *(continued)*
- polycystic *(continued)*
  - lung or pulmonary J98.4
    - congenital Q33.0
  - ovary, ovaries E28.2
  - spleen Q89.09
- polyethylene T84.05-
- Pompe's (glycogenosis II) E74.02
- Posadas-Wernicke B38.9
- Potain's (pulmonary edema) —*see* Edema, lung
- prepuce N47.8
  - inflammatory N47.7
    - balanoposthitis N47.6
- Pringle's (tuberous sclerosis) Q85.1
- prion, central nervous system A81.9
  - specified NEC A81.89
- prostate N42.9
  - specified NEC N42.89
- protozoal B64
  - acanthamebiasis —*see* Acanthamebiasis
  - African trypanosomiasis —*see* African trypanosomiasis
  - babesiosis (*see also* Babesiosis) B60.00
  - Chagas disease —*see* Chagas disease
  - intestine, intestinal A07.9
  - leishmaniasis —*see* Leishmaniasis
  - malaria —*see* Malaria
  - naegleriasis B60.2
  - pneumocystosis B59
  - specified organism NEC B60.8
  - toxoplasmosis —*see* Toxoplasmosis
- pseudo-Hurler's E77.0
- psychiatric F99
- psychotic —*see* Psychosis
- Puente's (simple glandular cheilitis) K13.0
- puerperal (*see also* Puerperal) O90.89
- pulmonary —*see also* Disease, lung
  - artery I28.9
  - chronic obstructive J44.9
    - with
      - acute bronchitis J44.0
      - exacerbation (acute) J44.1
      - lower respiratory infection (acute) J44.0
    - decompensated J44.1
      - with
        - exacerbation (acute) J44.1
  - heart I27.9
    - specified NEC I27.89
  - hypertensive (vascular) (*see also* Hypertension, pulmonary) I27.20
    - primary (idiopathic) I27.0
  - valve I37.9
    - rheumatic I09.89
- pulp (dental) NOS K04.90
- pulseless M31.4
- Putnam's (subacute combined sclerosis with pernicious anemia) D51.0
- Pyle (-Cohn) (metaphyseal dysplasia) Q78.5
- ragpicker's or ragsorter's A22.1
- Raynaud's —*see* Raynaud's disease
- reactive airway —*see* Asthma
- Reclus' (cystic) —*see* Mastopathy, cystic
- rectum K62.9
  - specified NEC K62.89

Disease, diseased (continued)
Refsum's (heredopathia atactica polyneuritiformis) G60.1
renal (functional) (pelvis) (see also Disease, kidney) N28.9
  with
    edema —see Nephrosis
    glomerular lesion —see Glomerulonephritis
      with edema —see Nephrosis
    interstitial nephritis N12
  acute N28.9
  chronic (see also Disease, kidney, chronic) N18.9
  cystic, congenital Q61.9
  diabetic —see E08-E13 with .22
  end-stage (failure) N18.6
    due to hypertension I12.0
  fibrocystic (congenital) Q61.8
  hypertensive —see Hypertension, kidney
  lupus M32.14
  phosphate-losing (tubular) N25.0
  polycystic (congenital) Q61.3
    adult type Q61.2
    childhood type NEC Q61.19
      collecting duct dilatation Q61.11
  rapidly progressive N01.9
  subacute N01.9
Rendu-Osler-Weber (familial hemorrhagic telangiectasia) I78.0
renovascular (arteriosclerotic) —see Hypertension, kidney
respiratory (tract) J98.9
  acute or subacute NOS J06.9
    due to
      chemicals, gases, fumes or vapors (inhalation) J68.3
      external agent J70.9
        specified NEC J70.8
      radiation J70.0
      smoke inhalation J70.5
    noninfectious J39.8
  chronic NOS J98.9
    due to
      chemicals, gases, fumes or vapors J68.4
      external agent J70.9
        specified NEC J70.8
      radiation J70.1
  newborn P27.9
    specified NEC P27.8
  due to
    chemicals, gases, fumes or vapors J68.9
      acute or subacute NEC J68.3
      chronic J68.4
    external agent J70.9
      specified NEC J70.8
  newborn P28.9
    specified type NEC P28.89
  upper J39.9
    acute or subacute J06.9
    noninfectious NEC J39.8
    specified NEC J39.8
    streptococcal J06.9
retina, retinal H35.9
  Batten's or Batten-Mayou E75.4 [H36.89]
  specified NEC H35.89
  rheumatoid —see Arthritis, rheumatoid
rickettsial NOS A79.9
  specified type NEC A79.89
Riga (-Fede) (cachectic aphthae) K14.0
Riggs' (compound periodontitis) —see Periodontitis
Ritter's L00

Disease, diseased (continued)
Rivalta's (cervicofacial actinomycosis) A42.2
Robles' (onchocerciasis) B73.01
rod body G71.21
Roger's (congenital interventricular septal defect) Q21.0
Rosenthal's (factor XI deficiency) D68.1
Rossbach's (hyperchlorhydria) K31.89
  psychogenic F45.8
Ross River B33.1
Rotes Quérol —see Hyperostosis, ankylosing
Roth (-Bernhardt) —see Mononeuropathy, lower limb, meralgia paresthetica
Runeberg's (progressive pernicious anemia) D51.0
sacroiliac NEC M53.3
salivary gland or duct K11.9
  inclusion B25.9
  specified NEC K11.8
  virus B25.9
sandworm B76.9
Schimmelbusch's —see Mastopathy, cystic
Schmorl's —see Schmorl's disease or nodes
Schönlein (-Henoch) (purpura rheumatica) D69.0
Schottmüller's —see Fever, paratyphoid
Schultz's (agranulocytosis) —see Agranulocytosis
Schwalbe-Ziehen-Oppenheim G24.1
Schwartz-Jampel G71.13
sclera H15.9
  specified NEC H15.89
scrofulous (tuberculous) A18.2
scrotum N50.9
sebaceous glands L73.9
semilunar cartilage, cystic —see also Derangement, knee, meniscus, cystic
seminal vesicle N50.9
serum NEC (see also Reaction, serum) T80.69
sexually transmitted A64
  anogenital
    herpesviral infection —see Herpes, anogenital
    warts A63.0
  chancroid A57
  chlamydial infection —see Chlamydia
  gonorrhea —see Gonorrhea
  granuloma inguinale A58
  specified organism NEC A63.8
  syphilis —see Syphilis
  trichomoniasis —see Trichomoniasis
Sézary C84.1-
shimamushi (scrub typhus) A75.3
shipyard B30.0
sickle-cell D57.1
  with
    acute chest syndrome D57.01
    cerebral vascular involvement D57.03
    crisis (painful) D57.00
      with
        complication specified NEC D57.09
        dactylitis D57.04
    dactylitis D57.04
    pain (vaso-occlusive) D57.00
    priapism D57.09
    splenic sequestration D57.02

Disease, diseased (continued)
sickle-cell (continued)
  elliptocytosis D57.8-
  Hb-C D57.20
    with
      acute chest syndrome D57.211
      cerebral vascular involvement D57.213
      crisis D57.219
        with
          dactylitis D57.214
          specified complication NEC D57.218
      dactylitis D57.214
      pain (vaso-occlusive) D57.219
      priapism D57.218
      splenic sequestration D57.212
    without crisis D57.20
  Hb-SD D57.80
    with
      acute chest syndrome D57.811
      cerebral vascular involvement D57.813
      crisis D57.819
        with
          complication specified NEC D57.818
          dactylitis D57.814
      dactylitis D57.814
      pain (vaso-occlusive) D57.819
      splenic sequestration D57.812
    without crisis D57.80
  Hb-SE D57.80
    with
      acute chest syndrome D57.811
      cerebral vascular involvement D57.813
      crisis D57.819
        with
          complication specified NEC D57.818
          dactylitis D57.814
      dactylitis D57.814
      pain (vaso-occlusive) D57.819
      splenic sequestration D57.812
    without crisis D57.80
  specified NEC D57.80
    with
      acute chest syndrome D57.811
      cerebral vascular involvement D57.813
      crisis D57.819
        with
          complication specified NEC D57.818
          dactylitis D57.814
      dactylitis D57.814
      pain (vaso-occlusive) D57.819
      splenic sequestration D57.812
    without crisis D57.80
  spherocytosis D57.80
    with
      acute chest syndrome D57.811
      cerebral vascular involvement D57.813

Disease, diseased (continued)
sickle-cell (continued)
  spherocytosis (continued)
    with (continued)
      crisis D57.819
        with complication specified NEC D57.818
        pain (vaso-occlusive) D57.819
        splenic sequestration D57.812
      without crisis D57.80
  thalassemia D57.40
    with
      acute chest syndrome D57.411
        with dactylitis D57.414
        with specified complication NEC D57.418
      cerebral vascular involvement D57.413
      crisis D57.419
        with specified complication NEC D57.418
      dactylitis D57.414
      pain (vaso-occlusive) D57.419
      splenic sequestration D57.412
    beta plus D57.44
      with
        acute chest syndrome D57.451
          with dactylitis D57.454
        cerebral vascular involvement D57.453
        crisis D57.459
          with specified complication NEC D57.458
        dactylitis D57.454
        pain (vaso-occlusive) D57.459
        splenic sequestration D57.452
      without crisis D57.44
    beta zero D57.42
      with
        acute chest syndrome D57.431
          with dactylitis D57.434
        cerebral vascular involvement D57.433
        crisis D57.439
          with specified complication NEC D57.438
        dactylitis D57.434
        pain (vaso-occlusive) D57.439
        splenic sequestration D57.432
      without crisis D57.42
silo-filler's J68.8
  bronchitis J68.0
  pneumonitis J68.0
  pulmonary edema J68.1
simian B B00.4
Simons' (progressive lipodystrophy) E88.1
sin nombre virus B33.4
sinus —see Sinusitis
Sirkari's B55.0
sixth B08.20
  due to human herpesvirus 6 B08.21
  due to human herpesvirus 7 B08.22

Disease, diseased (continued)
- skin L98.9
  - due to metabolic disorder NEC E88.9 [L99]
  - specified NEC L98.8
- slim (HIV) B20
- small vessel I73.9
- Sneddon-Wilkinson (subcorneal pustular dermatosis) L13.1
- South African creeping B88.0
- spinal (cord) G95.9
  - congenital Q06.9
  - specified NEC G95.89
- spine —see also Spondylopathy
  - joint —see Dorsopathy
  - tuberculous A18.01
- spinocerebellar (hereditary) G11.9
  - specified NEC G11.8
- spleen D73.9
  - amyloid E85.4 [D77]
  - organic D73.9
  - polycystic Q89.09
  - postinfectional D73.89
- sponge-diver's —see Toxicity, venom, marine animal, sea anemone
- Startle Q89.8
- Steinert's G71.11
- Sticker's (erythema infectiosum) B08.3
- Stieda's (calcification, knee joint) —see Bursitis, tibial collateral
- Stokes' (exophthalmic goiter) —see Hyperthyroidism, with, goiter (diffuse)
- Stokes-Adams (syncope with heart block) I45.9
- stomach K31.9
  - functional, psychogenic F45.8
  - specified NEC K31.89
- stonemason's J62.8
- storage
  - glycogen —see Disease, glycogen storage
  - mucopolysaccharide —see Mucopolysaccharidosis
- striatopallidal system NEC G25.89
- Stuart-Prower (congenital factor X deficiency) D68.2
- Stuart's (congenital factor X deficiency) D68.2
- subcutaneous tissue —see Disease, skin
- supporting structures of teeth K08.9
  - specified NEC K08.89
- suprarenal (capsule) (gland) E27.9
  - hyperfunction E27.0
  - specified NEC E27.8
- sweat glands L74.9
  - specified NEC L74.8
- Sweeley-Klionsky E75.21
- Swift (-Feer) —see Poisoning, mercury
- swimming-pool granuloma A31.1
- Sylvest's (epidemic pleurodynia) B33.0
- sympathetic nervous system G90.9
- synovium —see Disorder, synovium
- syphilitic —see Syphilis
- systemic tissue mast cell D47.02
- tanapox (virus) B08.71
- Tangier E78.6
- Tarral-Besnier (pityriasis rubra pilaris) L44.0
- Tauri's E74.09
- tear duct —see Disorder, lacrimal system
- tendon, tendinous —see also Disorder, tendon
  - nodular —see Trigger finger

Disease, diseased (continued)
- terminal vessel I73.9
- testis N50.9
- thalassemia Hb-S —see Disease, sickle-cell, thalassemia
- Thaysen-Gee (nontropical sprue) K90.0
- Thomsen G71.12
- throat J39.2
  - septic J02.0
- thromboembolic —see Embolism
- thymus (gland) E32.9
  - specified NEC E32.8
- thyroid (gland) E07.9
  - heart (see also Hyperthyroidism) E05.90 [I43]
    - with thyroid storm E05.91 [I43]
  - specified NEC E07.89
- Tietze's M94.0
- tongue K14.9
  - specified NEC K14.8
- tonsils, tonsillar (and adenoids) J35.9
- tooth, teeth K08.9
  - hard tissues K03.9
    - specified NEC K03.89
  - pulp NEC K04.99
  - specified NEC K08.89
- Tourette's F95.2
- trachea NEC J39.8
- tricuspid I07.9
  - nonrheumatic I36.9
- triglyceride-storage E75.5
- trophoblastic —see Mole, hydatidiform
- tsutsugamushi A75.3
- tube (fallopian) (noninflammatory) N83.9
  - inflammatory —see Salpingitis
  - specified NEC N83.8
- tuberculous NEC —see Tuberculosis
- tubo-ovarian (noninflammatory) N83.9
  - inflammatory —see Salpingo-oophoritis
  - specified NEC N83.8
- tubotympanic, chronic —see Otitis, media, suppurative, chronic, tubotympanic
- tubulo-interstitial N15.9
  - specified NEC N15.8
- tympanum —see Disorder, tympanic membrane
- Uhl's Q24.8
- Underwood's (sclerema neonatorum) P83.0
- Unverricht (-Lundborg) —see Epilepsy, generalized, idiopathic
- Urbach-Oppenheim (necrobiosis lipoidica diabeticorum) —see E08-E13 with .620
- ureter N28.9
  - in (due to)
    - schistosomiasis (bilharziasis) B65.0 [N29]
- urethra N36.9
  - specified NEC N36.8
- urinary (tract) N39.9
  - bladder N32.9
    - specified NEC N32.89
  - specified NEC N39.8
- uterus (noninflammatory) N85.9
  - infective —see Endometritis
  - inflammatory —see Endometritis
  - specified NEC N85.8
- uveal tract (anterior) H21.9
  - posterior H31.9

Disease, diseased (continued)
- vagabond's B85.1
- vagina, vaginal (noninflammatory) N89.9
  - inflammatory NEC N76.89
  - specified NEC N89.8
- valve, valvular I38
  - multiple I08.9
    - specified NEC I08.8
- van Creveld-von Gierke (glycogenosis I) E74.01
- vas deferens N50.9
- vascular I99.9
  - arteriosclerotic —see Arteriosclerosis
  - ciliary body NEC —see Disorder, iris, vascular
  - hypertensive —see Hypertension
  - iris NEC —see Disorder, iris, vascular
  - obliterative I77.1
    - peripheral I73.9
  - occlusive I99.8
    - peripheral (occlusive) I73.9
      - in diabetes mellitus —see E08-E13 with .51
- vasomotor I73.9
- vasospastic I73.9
- vein I87.9
- venereal (see also Disease, sexually transmitted) A64
  - chlamydial NEC A56.8
    - anus A56.3
    - genitourinary NOS A56.2
    - pharynx A56.4
    - rectum A56.3
  - fifth A55
  - sixth A55
  - specified nature or type NEC A63.8
- vertebra, vertebral —see also Spondylopathy
  - disc —see Disorder, disc
- vibration —see Vibration, adverse effects
- viral, virus (see also Disease, by type of virus) B34.9
  - arbovirus NOS A94
  - arthropod-borne NOS A94
  - congenital P35.9
    - specified NEC P35.8
  - Hanta (with renal manifestations) (Dobrava) (Puumala) (Seoul) A98.5
    - with pulmonary manifestations (Andes) (Bayou) (Bermejo) (Black Creek Canal) (Choclo) (Juquitiba) (Laguna negra) (Lechiguanas) (New York) (Oran) (Sin nombre) B33.4
  - Hantaan (Korean hemorrhagic fever) A98.5
  - human immunodeficiency (HIV) B20
  - Kunjin A83.4
  - nonarthropod-borne NOS B34.9
  - Powassan A84.81
  - Rocio (encephalitis) A83.6
  - Sin nombre (Hantavirus) (cardio)-pulmonary syndrome) B33.4
  - Tahyna B33.8
  - vesicular stomatitis A93.8
- vitreous H43.9
  - specified NEC H43.89
- vocal cord J38.3
- Volkmann's, acquired T79.6
- von Eulenburg's (congenital paramyotonia) G71.19

Disease, diseased (continued)
- von Gierke's (glycogenosis I) E74.01
- von Graefe's —see Strabismus, paralytic, ophthalmoplegia, progressive
- von Willebrand (-Jürgens) (angiohemophilia) D68.00
  - acquired D68.04
  - platelet-type D68.09
  - pseudo D68.09
  - specified NEC D68.09
  - type 1 D68.01
  - type 1C D68.01
  - type 2 D68.029
    - type 2A D68.020
    - type 2B D68.021
    - type 2M D68.022
    - type 2N D68.023
  - type 3 D68.03
- Vrolik's (osteogenesis imperfecta) Q78.0
- vulva (noninflammatory) N90.9
  - inflammatory NEC N76.89
  - specified NEC N90.89
- Wallgren's (obstruction of splenic vein with collateral circulation) I87.8
- Wassilieff's (leptospiral jaundice) A27.0
- wasting NEC E88.A
  - due to
    - malnutrition E43
      - with marasmus E41
    - underlying condition E88.A
- Waterhouse-Friderichsen A39.1
- Wegner's (syphilitic osteochondritis) A50.02
- Weil's (leptospiral jaundice of lung) A27.0
- Weir Mitchell's (erythromelalgia) I73.81
- Werdnig-Hoffmann G12.0
- Werner's E31.21
- Werner-His (trench fever) A79.0
- Werner-Schultz (neutropenic splenomegaly) D73.81
- Wernicke-Posadas B38.9
- whipworm B79
- white blood cells D72.9
  - specified NEC D72.89
- white matter R90.82
- white-spot, meaning lichen sclerosus et atrophicus L90.0
  - penis N48.0
  - vulva N90.4
- Wilkie's K55.1
- Wilkinson-Sneddon (subcorneal pustular dermatosis) L13.1
- Willis' —see Diabetes
- Wilson's (hepatolenticular degeneration) E83.01
- woolsorter's A22.1
- yaba monkey tumor B08.72
- yaba pox (virus) B08.72
- Zika virus A92.5
  - congenital P35.4
- zoonotic, bacterial A28.9
  - specified type NEC A28.8

Disfigurement (due to scar) L90.5

Disgerminoma —see Dysgerminoma

DISH (diffuse idiopathic skeletal hyperostosis) —see Hyperostosis, ankylosing

Disinsertion, retina —see Detachment, retina

Dislocatable hip, congenital Q65.6

Dislocation (articular)
　with fracture —see Fracture
　acromioclavicular (joint) S43.10-
　　with displacement
　　　100%-200% S43.12-
　　　　more than 200% S43.13-
　　　inferior S43.14-
　　　posterior S43.15-
　ankle S93.0-
　astragalus —see Dislocation,
　　ankle
　atlantoaxial S13.121
　atlantooccipital S13.111
　atloidooccipital S13.111
　breast bone S23.29
　capsule, joint - code by site under
　　Dislocation
　carpal (bone) —see Dislocation,
　　wrist
　carpometacarpal (joint) NEC S63.05-
　　thumb S63.04-
　cartilage (joint) - code by site under
　　Dislocation
　cervical spine (vertebra) —see
　　Dislocation, vertebra, cervical
　chronic —see Dislocation,
　　recurrent
　clavicle —see Dislocation,
　　acromioclavicular joint
　coccyx S33.2
　congenital NEC Q68.8
　coracoid —see Dislocation,
　　shoulder
　costal cartilage S23.29
　costochondral S23.29
　cricoarytenoid articulation
　　S13.29
　cricothyroid articulation S13.29
　dorsal vertebra —see Dislocation,
　　vertebra, thoracic
　ear ossicle —see Discontinuity,
　　ossicles, ear
　elbow S53.10-
　　congenital Q68.8
　　pathological —see Dislocation,
　　　pathological NEC, elbow
　　radial head alone —see
　　　Dislocation, radial head
　　recurrent —see Dislocation,
　　　recurrent, elbow
　　traumatic S53.10-
　　　anterior S53.11-
　　　lateral S53.14-
　　　medial S53.13-
　　　posterior S53.12-
　　　specified type NEC S53.19-
　eye, nontraumatic —see Luxation,
　　globe
　eyeball, nontraumatic —see
　　Luxation, globe
　femur
　　distal end —see Dislocation,
　　　knee
　　proximal end —see Dislocation,
　　　hip
　fibula
　　distal end —see Dislocation,
　　　ankle
　　proximal end —see Dislocation,
　　　knee
　finger S63.25-
　　index S63.25-
　　interphalangeal S63.27-
　　　distal S63.29-
　　　　index S63.29-
　　　　little S63.29-
　　　　middle S63.29-
　　　　ring S63.29-
　　　index S63.27-
　　　little S63.27-
　　　middle S63.27-

Dislocation (continued)
　finger (continued)
　　interphalangeal (continued)
　　　proximal S63.28-
　　　　index S63.28-
　　　　little S63.28-
　　　　middle S63.28-
　　　　ring S63.28-
　　　ring S63.27-
　　little S63.25-
　　metacarpophalangeal S63.26-
　　　index S63.26-
　　　little S63.26-
　　　middle S63.26-
　　　ring S63.26-
　　middle S63.25-
　　recurrent —see Dislocation,
　　　recurrent, finger
　　ring S63.25-
　　thumb —see Dislocation, thumb
　foot S93.30-
　　recurrent —see Dislocation,
　　　recurrent, foot
　　specified site NEC S93.33-
　　tarsal joint S93.31-
　　tarsometatarsal joint S93.32-
　　toe —see Dislocation, toe
　fracture —see Fracture
　glenohumeral (joint) —see
　　Dislocation, shoulder
　glenoid —see Dislocation, shoulder
　habitual —see Dislocation,
　　recurrent
　hip S73.00-
　　anterior S73.03-
　　　obturator S73.02-
　　central S73.04-
　　congenital (total) Q65.2
　　　bilateral Q65.1
　　　partial Q65.5
　　　　bilateral Q65.4
　　　　unilateral Q65.3-
　　　unilateral Q65.0-
　　developmental M24.85-
　　pathological —see Dislocation,
　　　pathological NEC, hip
　　posterior S73.01-
　　recurrent —see Dislocation,
　　　recurrent, hip
　humerus, proximal end —see
　　Dislocation, shoulder
　incomplete —see Subluxation,
　　by site
　incus —see Discontinuity, ossicles,
　　ear
　infracoracoid —see Dislocation,
　　shoulder
　innominate (pubic junction) (sacral
　　junction) S33.39
　　acetabulum —see Dislocation,
　　　hip
　interphalangeal (joint(s))
　　finger S63.279
　　　distal S63.29-
　　　　index S63.29-
　　　　little S63.29-
　　　　middle S63.29-
　　　　ring S63.29-
　　　index S63.27-
　　　little S63.27-
　　　middle S63.27-
　　　proximal S63.28-
　　　　index S63.28-
　　　　little S63.28-
　　　　middle S63.28-
　　　　ring S63.28-
　　　ring S63.27-
　　foot or toe —see Dislocation,
　　　toe
　　thumb S63.12-
　jaw (cartilage) (meniscus) S03.0-

Dislocation (continued)
　joint prosthesis —see
　　Complications, joint prosthesis,
　　mechanical, displacement,
　　by site
　knee S83.106
　　cap —see Dislocation, patella
　　congenital Q68.2
　　old M23.8X-
　　patella —see Dislocation,
　　　patella
　　pathological —see Dislocation,
　　　pathological NEC, knee
　　proximal tibia
　　　anteriorly S83.11-
　　　laterally S83.14-
　　　medially S83.13-
　　　posteriorly S83.12-
　　recurrent —see also Derangement,
　　　knee, specified NEC
　　specified type NEC S83.19-
　lacrimal gland H04.16-
　lens (complete) H27.10
　　anterior H27.12-
　　congenital Q12.1
　　ocular implant —see
　　　Complications, intraocular lens
　　partial H27.11-
　　posterior H27.13-
　　traumatic S05.8X-
　ligament - code by site under
　　Dislocation
　lumbar (vertebra) —see
　　Dislocation, vertebra, lumbar
　lumbosacral (vertebra) —see also
　　Dislocation, vertebra, lumbar
　　congenital Q76.49
　mandible S03.0-
　meniscus (knee) —see Tear, meniscus
　　other sites - code by site under
　　　Dislocation
　metacarpal (bone)
　　distal end —see Dislocation,
　　　finger
　　proximal end S63.06-
　metacarpophalangeal (joint)
　　finger S63.26-
　　　index S63.26-
　　　little S63.26-
　　　middle S63.26-
　　　ring S63.26-
　　thumb S63.11-
　metatarsal (bone) —see
　　Dislocation, foot
　metatarsophalangeal (joint(s))
　　—see Dislocation, toe
　midcarpal (joint) S63.03-
　midtarsal (joint) —see Dislocation,
　　foot
　neck S13.20
　　specified site NEC S13.29
　　vertebra —see Dislocation,
　　　vertebra, cervical
　nose (septal cartilage) S03.1
　occipitoatloid S13.111
　old —see Derangement, joint,
　　specified type NEC
　ossicles, ear —see Discontinuity,
　　ossicles, ear
　partial —see Subluxation, by site
　patella S83.006
　　congenital Q74.1
　　lateral S83.01-
　　recurrent (nontraumatic)
　　　M22.0-
　　　incomplete M22.1-
　　specified type NEC S83.09-
　pathological NEC M24.30
　　ankle M24.37-
　　elbow M24.32-
　　foot joint M24.37-

Dislocation (continued)
　pathological NEC (continued)
　　hand joint M24.34-
　　hip M24.35-
　　knee M24.36-
　　lumbosacral joint —see
　　　subcategory M53.2
　　pelvic region —see Dislocation,
　　　pathological, hip
　　sacroiliac —see subcategory
　　　M53.2
　　shoulder M24.31-
　　specified site NEC M24.39
　　wrist M24.33-
　pelvis NEC S33.30
　　specified NEC S33.39
　phalanx
　　finger or hand —see Dislocation,
　　　finger
　　foot or toe —see Dislocation,
　　　toe
　prosthesis, internal —see
　　Complications, prosthetic device,
　　by site, mechanical
　radial head S53.006
　　anterior S53.01-
　　posterior S53.02-
　　specified type NEC S53.09-
　radiocarpal (joint) S63.02-
　radiohumeral (joint) —see
　　Dislocation, radial head
　radioulnar (joint)
　　distal S63.01-
　　proximal —see Dislocation,
　　　elbow
　radius
　　distal end —see Dislocation,
　　　wrist
　　proximal end —see Dislocation,
　　　radial head
　recurrent M24.40
　　ankle M24.47-
　　elbow M24.42-
　　finger M24.44-
　　foot joint M24.47-
　　hand joint M24.44-
　　hip M24.45-
　　knee M24.46-
　　　patella —see Dislocation,
　　　　patella, recurrent
　　patella —see Dislocation,
　　　patella, recurrent
　　sacroiliac —see subcategory
　　　M53.2
　　shoulder M24.41-
　　specified site NEC M24.49
　　toe M24.47-
　　vertebra (see also subcategory)
　　　M43.5
　　　atlantoaxial M43.4
　　　　with myelopathy M43.3
　　wrist M24.43-
　rib (cartilage) S23.29
　sacrococcygeal S33.2
　sacroiliac (joint) (ligament)
　　S33.2
　　congenital Q74.2
　　recurrent M53.2
　sacrum S33.2
　scaphoid (bone) (hand) (wrist)
　　—see Dislocation, wrist
　　foot —see Dislocation, foot
　scapula —see Dislocation,
　　shoulder, girdle, scapula
　semilunar cartilage, knee —see
　　Tear, meniscus
　septal cartilage (nose) S03.1
　septum (nasal) (old) J34.2
　sesamoid bone - code by site under
　　Dislocation

Dislocation (continued)
  shoulder (blade) (ligament) (joint)
      (traumatic) S43.006
    acromioclavicular —see
        Dislocation, acromioclavicular
    chronic —see Dislocation,
        recurrent, shoulder
    congenital Q68.8
    girdle S43.30-
      scapula S43.31-
      specified site NEC S43.39-
    humerus S43.00-
      anterior S43.01-
      inferior S43.03-
      posterior S43.02-
    pathological —see Dislocation,
        pathological NEC,
        shoulder
    recurrent —see Dislocation,
        recurrent, shoulder
    specified type NEC S43.08-
  spine
    cervical —see Dislocation,
        vertebra, cervical
    congenital Q76.49
    due to birth trauma P11.5
    lumbar —see Dislocation,
        vertebra, lumbar
    thoracic —see Dislocation,
        vertebra, thoracic
  spontaneous —see Dislocation,
      pathological
  sternoclavicular (joint) S43.206
    anterior S43.21-
    posterior S43.22-
  sternum S23.29
  subglenoid —see Dislocation,
      shoulder
  symphysis pubis S33.4
  talus —see Dislocation, ankle
  tarsal (bone(s)) (joint(s)) —see
      Dislocation, foot
  tarsometatarsal (joint(s)) —see
      Dislocation, foot
  temporomandibular (joint) S03.0-
  thigh, proximal end —see
      Dislocation, hip
  thorax S23.20
    specified site NEC S23.29
    vertebra —see Dislocation,
        vertebra
  thumb S63.10-
    interphalangeal joint —see
        Dislocation, interphalangeal
        (joint), thumb
    metacarpophalangeal
        joint —see Dislocation,
        metacarpophalangeal (joint),
        thumb
  thyroid cartilage S13.29
  tibia
    distal end —see Dislocation,
        ankle
    proximal end —see Dislocation,
        knee
  tibiofibular (joint)
    distal —see Dislocation, ankle
    superior —see Dislocation, knee
  toe(s) S93.106
    great S93.10-
      interphalangeal joint S93.11-
      metatarsophalangeal joint
          S93.12-
    interphalangeal joint S93.119
    lesser S93.106
      interphalangeal joint S93.11-
      metatarsophalangeal joint
          S93.12-
    metatarsophalangeal joint
        S93.12-
  tooth S03.2

Dislocation (continued)
  trachea S23.29
  ulna
    distal end S63.07-
    proximal end —see Dislocation,
        elbow
  ulnohumeral (joint) —see
      Dislocation, elbow
  vertebra (articular process) (body)
      (traumatic)
    cervical S13.101
      atlantoaxial joint S13.121
      atlantooccipital joint
          S13.111
      atloidooccipital joint
          S13.111
      joint between
        C0 and C1 S13.111
        C1 and C2 S13.121
        C2 and C3 S13.131
        C3 and C4 S13.141
        C4 and C5 S13.151
        C5 and C6 S13.161
        C6 and C7 S13.171
        C7 and T1 S13.181
      occipitoatloid joint S13.111
    congenital Q76.49
    lumbar S33.101
      joint between
        L1 and L2 S33.111
        L2 and L3 S33.121
        L3 and L4 S33.131
        L4 and L5 S33.141
    nontraumatic —see
        Displacement, intervertebral
        disc
    partial —see Subluxation,
        by site
    recurrent NEC —see
        subcategory M43.5
    thoracic S23.101
      joint between
        T1 and T2 S23.111
        T2 and T3 S23.121
        T3 and T4 S23.123
        T4 and T5 S23.131
        T5 and T6 S23.133
        T6 and T7 S23.141
        T7 and T8 S23.143
        T8 and T9 S23.151
        T9 and T10 S23.153
        T10 and T11 S23.161
        T11 and T12 S23.163
        T12 and L1 S23.171
  wrist (carpal bone) S63.006
    carpometacarpal joint —see
        Dislocation, carpometacarpal
        (joint)
    distal radioulnar joint —see
        Dislocation, radioulnar (joint),
        distal
    metacarpal bone, proximal
        —see Dislocation, metacarpal
        (bone), proximal end
    midcarpal —see Dislocation,
        midcarpal (joint)
    radiocarpal joint —see
        Dislocation, radiocarpal (joint)
    recurrent —see Dislocation,
        recurrent, wrist
    specified site NEC S63.09-
    ulna —see Dislocation, ulna,
        distal end
  xiphoid cartilage S23.29

Disorder (of) —see also Disease
  acantholytic L11.9
    specified NEC L11.8
  acute
    psychotic —see Psychosis, acute
    stress F43.0
  adjustment (grief) F43.20

Disorder (continued)
  adjustment (continued)
    with
      anxiety F43.22
        with depressed mood F43.23
      conduct disturbance F43.24
        with emotional disturbance
            F43.25
      depressed mood F43.21
        with anxiety F43.23
      other specified symptom F43.29
  adrenal (capsule) (gland)
      (medullary) E27.9
    specified NEC E27.8
  adrenogenital (see also
      Adrenogenital syndrome) E25.9
    drug-induced E25.8
    iatrogenic E25.8
    idiopathic E25.8
  adult personality (and behavior) F69
    specified NEC F68.8
  affective (mood) —see Disorder,
      mood
  aggressive, unsocialized F91.1
  alcohol-related F10.99
    with
      amnestic disorder, persisting
          F10.96
      anxiety disorder F10.980
      dementia, persisting F10.97
      intoxication F10.929
        with delirium F10.921
        uncomplicated F10.920
      mood disorder F10.94
      other specified F10.988
      psychotic disorder F10.959
        with
          delusions F10.950
          hallucinations F10.951
      sexual dysfunction F10.981
      sleep disorder F10.982
  alcohol use
    mild F10.10
      with
        alcohol-induced
          anxiety disorder F10.180
          bipolar and related
              disorder F10.14
          depressive disorder
              F10.14
          psychotic disorder F10.159
          sexual dysfunction
              F10.181
          sleep disorder F10.182
        alcohol intoxication F10.129
          delirium F10.121
        in remission (early)
            (sustained) F10.11
    moderate or severe F10.20
      with
        alcohol-induced
          anxiety disorder F10.280
          bipolar and related
              disorder F10.24
          depressive disorder
              F10.24
          major neurocognitive
              disorder, amnestic-
              confabulatory type
              F10.26
          major neurocognitive
              disorder, nonamnestic-
              confabulatory type
              F10.27
          mild neurocognitive
              disorder F10.288
          psychotic disorder
              F10.259
          sexual dysfunction
              F10.281
          sleep disorder F10.282

Disorder (continued)
  alcohol use (continued)
    moderate or severe (continued)
      with (continued)
        alcohol intoxication F10.229
          delirium F10.221
        in remission (early)
            (sustained) F10.21
  allergic —see Allergy
  alveolar NEC J84.09
  amino-acid
    cystathioninuria E72.19
    cystinosis E72.04
    cystinuria E72.01
    glycinuria E72.09
    homocystinuria E72.11
    metabolism —see Disturbance,
        metabolism, amino-acid
        specified NEC E72.89
    neonatal, transitory P74.8
    renal transport NEC E72.09
    transport NEC E72.09
  amnesic, amnestic
    alcohol-induced F10.96
      with dependence F10.26
    due to (secondary to) general
        medical condition F04
    psychoactive NEC-induced
        F19.96
      with
        abuse F19.16
        dependence F19.26
    sedative, hypnotic or anxiolytic-
        induced F13.96
      with dependence F13.26
  amphetamine-type substance use
    mild F15.10
      in remission (early)
          (sustained) F15.11
    moderate F15.20
      in remission (early)
          (sustained) F15.21
    severe 15.20
      in remission (early)
          (sustained) F15.21
  use
    mild F15.10
      with
        amphetamine (or other
            stimulant) -induced
            anxiety disorder
                F15.180
            bipolar and related
                disorder F15.14
            depressive disorder F15.14
            obsessive-compulsive
                and related disorder
                F15.188
            psychotic disorder F15.159
            sexual dysfunction
                F15.181
        amphetamine, cocaine,
            or other stimulant
            intoxication
            with perceptual
                disturbances F15.122
            without perceptual
                disturbances F15.129
        intoxication delirium F15.121
      in remission (early)
          (sustained) F15.11
    moderate or severe
      with
        amphetamine (or other
            stimulant) -induced
            anxiety disorder F15.280
            bipolar and related
                disorder F15.14
            depressive disorder
                F15.24

Disorder *(continued)*
  use *(continued)*
    moderate or severe *(continued)*
      with *(continued)*
        amphetamine *(continued)*
          obsessive-compulsive
            and related disorder
            F15.288
          psychotic disorder
            F15.259
          sexual dysfunction
            F15.281
        amphetamine, cocaine,
          or other stimulant
          intoxication
          with perceptual
            disturbances F15.222
          without perceptual
            disturbances F15.229
        intoxication delirium
          F15.221
anaerobic glycolysis with anemia
  D55.29
anxiety F41.9
  due to (secondary to)
    alcohol F10.980
      in
        abuse F10.980
        dependence F10.280
    amphetamine F15.980
      in
        abuse F15.180
        dependence F15.280
    anxiolytic F13.980
      in
        abuse F13.180
        dependence F13.280
    caffeine F15.980
      in
        abuse F15.180
        dependence F15.280
    cannabis F12.980
      in
        abuse F12.180
        dependence F12.280
    cocaine F14.980
      in
        abuse F14.180
        dependence F14.180
    general medical condition
      F06.4
    hallucinogen F16.980
      in
        abuse F16.180
        dependence F16.280
    hypnotic F13.980
      in
        abuse F13.180
        dependence F13.280
    inhalant F18.980
      in
        abuse F18.180
        dependence F18.280
    phencyclidine F16.980
      in
        abuse F16.180
        dependence F16.280
    psychoactive substance NEC
      F19.980
      in
        abuse F19.180
        dependence F19.280
    sedative F13.980
      in
        abuse F13.180
        dependence F13.280
    volatile solvents F18.980
      in
        abuse F18.180
        dependence F18.280
  generalized F41.1

Disorder *(continued)*
  anxiety *(continued)*
    illness F45.21
    mixed
      with depression (mild)
        F41.8
      specified NEC F41.3
    organic F06.4
    phobic F40.9
      of childhood F40.8
    specified NEC F41.8
  aortic valve —*see* Endocarditis,
    aortic
  aromatic amino-acid metabolism
    E70.9
    specified NEC E70.89
  arteriole NEC I77.89
  artery NEC I77.89
  articulation —*see* Disorder, joint
  attachment (childhood)
    disinhibited F94.2
    reactive F94.1
  attention-deficit hyperactivity
    (adolescent) (adult) (child)
    F90.0
    combined
      presentation F90.2
      type F90.2
    hyperactive
      impulsive presentation
        F90.1
      type F90.1
    inattentive
      presentation F90.0
      type F90.0
    specified type NEC F90.8
  attention-deficit without
    hyperactivity (adolescent) (adult)
    (child) F98.8
  auditory processing (central)
    H93.25
  autistic F84.0
  autoimmune D89.89
  autonomic nervous system G90.9
    specified NEC G90.8
  autism spectrum F84.0
  avoidant
    child or adolescent F40.10
    restrictive food intake F50.82
  balance
    acid-base E87.8
      mixed E87.4
    electrolyte E87.8
    fluid NEC E87.8
  behavioral (disruptive) —*see*
    Disorder, conduct
  bereavement, persistent complex
    F43.81
  beta-amino-acid metabolism
    E72.89
  bile acid and cholesterol
    metabolism E78.70
    Barth syndrome E78.71
    other specified E78.79
    Smith-Lemli-Opitz syndrome
      E78.72
  bilirubin excretion E80.6
  binge eating F50.81
  binocular
    movement H51.9
      convergence
        excess H51.12
        insufficiency H51.11
      internuclear ophthalmoplegia
        —*see* Ophthalmoplegia,
        internuclear
      palsy of conjugate gaze
        H51.0
      specified type NEC H51.8
    vision NEC —*see* Disorder,
      vision, binocular

Disorder *(continued)*
  bipolar (I) (seasonal) (type 1)
    F31.9
    and related due to a known
      physiological condition
      with
        manic features F06.33
        manic- or hypomanic-like
          episodes F06.33
        mixed features F06.34
    current (or most recent)
      episode
      depressed F31.9
        with psychotic features
          F31.5
        without psychotic features
          F31.30
          mild F31.31
          moderate F31.32
          severe (without psychotic
            features) F31.4
          with psychotic features
            F31.5
      hypomanic F31.0
      manic F31.9
        with psychotic features
          F31.2
        without psychotic features
          F31.10
          mild F31.11
          moderate F31.12
          severe (without psychotic
            features) F31.13
          with psychotic features
            F31.2
      mixed F31.60
        mild F31.61
        moderate F31.62
        severe (without psychotic
          features) F31.63
        with psychotic features
          F31.64
      severe depression (without
        psychotic features)
        F31.4
        with psychotic features
          F31.5
    in remission (currently)
      F31.70
      in full remission
        most recent episode
          depressed F31.76
          hypomanic F31.72
          manic F31.74
          mixed F31.78
      in partial remission
        most recent episode
          depressed F31.75
          hypomanic F31.71
          manic F31.73
          mixed F31.77
    specified NEC F31.89
    II (type 2) F31.81
    organic F06.30
    single manic episode F30.9
      mild F30.11
      moderate F30.12
      severe (without psychotic
        symptoms) F30.13
      with psychotic symptoms
        F30.2
  bladder N32.9
    functional NEC N31.9
    in schistosomiasis B65.0
      [N33]
    specified NEC N32.89
  bleeding D68.9
  blood D75.9
    in congenital early syphilis
      A50.09 [D77]
  body dysmorphic F45.22

Disorder *(continued)*
  bone M89.9
    continuity M84.9
      specified type NEC
        M84.80
        ankle M84.87-
        fibula M84.86-
        foot M84.87-
        hand M84.84-
        humerus M84.82-
        neck M84.88
        pelvis M84.859
        radius M84.83-
        rib M84.88
        shoulder M84.81-
        skull M84.88
        thigh M84.85-
        tibia M84.86-
        ulna M84.83-
        vertebra M84.88
    density and structure M85.9
      cyst —*see also* Cyst, bone,
        specified type NEC
        aneurysmal —*see* Cyst,
          bone, aneurysmal
        solitary —*see* Cyst, bone,
          solitary
      diffuse idiopathic skeletal
        hyperostosis —*see*
        Hyperostosis, ankylosing
      fibrous dysplasia (monostotic)
        —*see* Dysplasia, fibrous,
        bone
      fluorosis —*see* Fluorosis,
        skeletal
      hyperostosis of skull
        M85.2
      osteitis condensans —*see*
        Osteitis, condensans
      specified type NEC M85.8-
        ankle M85.87-
        foot M85.87-
        forearm M85.83-
        hand M85.84-
        lower leg M85.86-
        multiple sites M85.89
        neck M85.88
        rib M85.88
        shoulder M85.81-
        skull M85.88
        thigh M85.85-
        upper arm M85.82-
        vertebra M85.88
    development and growth NEC
      M89.20
      carpus M89.24-
      clavicle M89.21-
      femur M89.25-
      fibula M89.26-
      finger M89.24-
      humerus M89.22-
      ilium M89.28
      ischium M89.28
      metacarpus M89.24-
      metatarsus M89.27-
      multiple sites M89.29
      neck M89.28
      radius M89.23-
      rib M89.28
      scapula M89.21-
      skull M89.28
      tarsus M89.27-
      tibia M89.26-
      toe M89.27-
      ulna M89.23-
      vertebra M89.28
    specified type NEC M89.8X-
  brachial plexus G54.0
  branched-chain amino-acid
    metabolism E71.2
    specified NEC E71.19

Disorder (continued)
  breast N64.9
    agalactia —see Agalactia
    associated with
      lactation O92.70
        specified NEC O92.79
      pregnancy O92.20
        specified NEC O92.29
      puerperium O92.20
        specified NEC O92.29
    cracked nipple —see Cracked nipple
    galactorrhea —see Galactorrhea
    hypogalactia O92.4
    lactation disorder NEC O92.79
    mastitis —see Mastitis
    nipple infection —see Infection, nipple
    retracted nipple —see Retraction, nipple
    specified type NEC N64.89
  Briquet's F45.0
  bullous, in diseases classified elsewhere L14
  caffeine use
    mild
      with
        caffeine-induced
          anxiety disorder F15.180
          sleep disorder F15.182
    moderate or severe
      with
        caffeine-induced
          anxiety disorder F15.280
          sleep disorder F15.282
  cannabis use
    mild F12.10
      with
        cannabis-induced
          anxiety disorder F12.180
          psychotic disorder F12.159
          sleep disorder F12.188
        cannabis intoxication
          delirium F12.121
          with perceptual disturbances F12.122
          without perceptual disturbances F12.129
        in remission (early) (sustained) F12.11
    moderate or severe F12.20
      with
        cannabis-induced
          anxiety disorder F12.280
          psychotic disorder F12.259
          sleep disorder F12.288
        cannabis intoxication
          with perceptual disturbances F12.222
          without perceptual disturbances F12.229
          delirium F12.221
        in remission (early) (sustained) F12.21
  carbohydrate
    absorption, intestinal NEC E74.39
    metabolism (congenital) E74.9
      specified NEC E74.89
  cardiac, functional I51.89
  carnitine metabolism E71.40
  cartilage M94.9
    articular NEC —see Derangement, joint, articular cartilage
    chondrocalcinosis —see Chondrocalcinosis

Disorder (continued)
  cartilage (continued)
    specified type NEC M94.8X-
      articular —see Derangement, joint, articular cartilage
      multiple sites M94.8X0
  catatonia (due to known physiological condition) (with another mental disorder) F06.1
  catatonic
    due to (secondary to) known physiological condition F06.1
    organic F06.1
  central auditory processing H93.25
  cervical
    region NEC M53.82
    root (nerve) NEC G54.2
  character NOS F60.9
  childhood disintegrative NEC F84.3
  cholesterol and bile acid metabolism E78.70
    Barth syndrome E78.71
    other specified E78.79
    Smith-Lemli-Opitz syndrome E78.72
  choroid H31.9
    atrophy —see Atrophy, choroid
    degeneration —see Degeneration, choroid
    detachment —see Detachment, choroid
    dystrophy —see Dystrophy, choroid
    hemorrhage —see Hemorrhage, choroid
    rupture —see Rupture, choroid
    scar —see Scar, chorioretinal
    solar retinopathy —see Retinopathy, solar
    specified type NEC H31.8
  ciliary body —see Disorder, iris
    degeneration —see Degeneration, ciliary body
  coagulation (factor) (see also Defect, coagulation) D68.9
    newborn, transient P61.6
  cocaine use
    mild F14.10
      with
        amphetamine, cocaine, or other stimulant intoxication
          with perceptual disturbances F14.122
          without perceptual disturbances F14.129
        cocaine-induced
          anxiety disorder F14.180
          bipolar and related disorder F14.14
          depressive disorder F14.14
          obsessive-compulsive and related disorder F14.188
          psychotic disorder F14.159
          sexual dysfunction F14.181
          sleep disorder F14.182
        cocaine intoxication
          delirium F14.121
        in remission (early) (sustained) F14.11

Disorder (continued)
  cocaine use (continued)
    moderate or severe
      with
        amphetamine, cocaine, or other stimulant intoxication
          with perceptual disturbances F14.222
          without perceptual disturbances F14.229
        cocaine-induced
          anxiety disorder F14.280
          bipolar and related disorder F14.24
          depressive disorder F14.24
          obsessive-compulsive and related disorder F14.288
          psychotic disorder F14.259
          sexual dysfunction F14.281
          sleep disorder F14.282
        cocaine intoxication
          delirium F14.221
        in remission (early) (sustained) F14.21
  coccyx NEC M53.3
  cognitive F09
    due to (secondary to) general medical condition F09
    persisting R41.89
      due to
        alcohol F10.97
          with dependence F10.27
        anxiolytics F13.97
          with dependence F13.27
        hypnotics F13.97
          with dependence F13.27
        sedatives F13.97
          with dependence F13.27
        specified substance NEC F19.97
          with
            abuse F19.17
            dependence F19.27
  communication F80.9
    social pragmatic F80.82
  conduct (childhood) F91.9
    adjustment reaction —see Disorder, adjustment
    adolescent onset type F91.2
    childhood onset type F91.1
    compulsive F63.9
    confined to family context F91.0
    depressive F91.8
    group type F91.2
    hyperkinetic —see Disorder, attention-deficit hyperactivity
    oppositional defiance F91.3
    socialized F91.2
    solitary aggressive type F91.1
    specified NEC F91.8
    unsocialized (aggressive) F91.1
  conduction, heart I45.9
  congenital glycosylation (CDG) E74.89
  conjunctiva H11.9
    infection —see Conjunctivitis
  connective tissue, localized L94.9
    specified NEC L94.8
  conversion (functional neurological symptom disorder)
    with
      abnormal movement F44.4
      anesthesia or sensory loss F44.6

Disorder (continued)
  conversion (continued)
    with (continued)
      attacks or seizures F44.5
      mixed symptoms F44.7
      special sensory symptoms F44.6
      speech symptoms F44.4
      swallowing symptoms F44.4
      weakness or paralysis F44.4
  convulsive (secondary) —see Convulsions
  cornea H18.9
    deformity —see Deformity, cornea
    degeneration —see Degeneration, cornea
    deposits —see Deposit, cornea
    due to contact lens H18.82-
      specified as edema —see Edema, cornea
    edema —see Edema, cornea
    keratitis —see Keratitis
    keratoconjunctivitis —see Keratoconjunctivitis
    membrane change —see Change, corneal membrane
    neovascularization —see Neovascularization, cornea
    scar —see Opacity, cornea
    specified type NEC H18.89-
    ulcer —see Ulcer, cornea
  corpus cavernosum N48.9
  cranial nerve —see Disorder, nerve, cranial
  Cyclin-Dependent Kinase-Like 5 Deficiency (CDKL5) G40.42
  cyclothymic F34.0
  defiant oppositional F91.3
  delusional (persistent) (systematized) F22
    induced F24
  depersonalization F48.1
  depressive F32.A
    due to known physiological condition
      with
        depressive features F06.31
        major depressive-like episode F06.32
        mixed features F06.34
    major F32.9
      with psychotic symptoms F32.3
      in remission (full) F32.5
        partial F32.4
      recurrent F33.9
        with psychotic features F33.3
      single episode F32.9
        mild F32.0
        moderate F32.1
        severe (without psychotic symptoms) F32.2
          with psychotic symptoms F32.3
    organic F06.31
    persistent F34.1
    recurrent F33.9
      current episode
        mild F33.0
        moderate F33.1
        severe (without psychotic symptoms) F33.2
          with psychotic symptoms F33.3
      in remission F33.40
        full F33.42
        partial F33.41
      specified NEC F33.8

Disorder *(continued)*
  depressive *(continued)*
    single episode —*see* Episode, depressive
    specified NEC F32.89
  developmental F89
    arithmetical skills F81.2
    coordination (motor) F82
    expressive writing F81.81
    language F80.9
      expressive F80.1
      mixed receptive and expressive F80.2
      receptive type F80.2
      specified NEC F80.89
    learning F81.9
      arithmetical F81.2
      reading F81.0
    mixed F88
    motor coordination or function F82
    pervasive F84.9
      specified NEC F84.8
    phonological F80.0
    reading F81.0
    scholastic skills —*see also* Disorder, learning
      mixed F81.89
    specified NEC F88
    speech F80.9
      articulation F80.0
      specified NEC F80.89
    written expression F81.81
  diaphragm J98.6
  digestive (system) K92.9
    newborn P78.9
      specified NEC P78.89
    postprocedural —*see* Complication, gastrointestinal
    psychogenic F45.8
  disc (intervertebral) M51.9
    with
      myelopathy
        cervical region M50.00
        cervicothoracic region M50.03
        high cervical region M50.01
        lumbar region M51.06
        mid-cervical region M50.020
        sacrococcygeal region M53.3
        thoracic region M51.04
        thoracolumbar region M51.05
      radiculopathy
        cervical region M50.10
        cervicothoracic region M50.13
        high cervical region M50.11
        lumbar region M51.16
        lumbosacral region M51.17
        mid-cervical region M50.120
        sacrococcygeal region M53.3
        thoracic region M51.14
        thoracolumbar region M51.15
    cervical M50.90
      with
        myelopathy M50.00
          C2-C3 M50.01
          C3-C4 M50.01
          C4-C5 M50.021
          C5-C6 M50.022
          C6-C7 M50.023
          C7-T1 M50.03
          cervicothoracic region M50.03

Disorder *(continued)*
  disc *(continued)*
    cervical *(continued)*
      with *(continued)*
        myelopathy *(continued)*
          high cervical region M50.01
          mid-cervical region M50.020
        neuritis, radiculitis or radiculopathy M50.10
          C2-C3 M50.11
          C3-C4 M50.11
          C4-C5 M50.121
          C5-C6 M50.122
          C6-C7 M50.123
          C7-T1 M50.13
          cervicothoracic region M50.13
          high cervical region M50.11
          mid-cervical region M50.120
        C2-C3 M50.91
        C3-C4 M50.91
        C4-C5 M50.921
        C5-C6 M50.922
        C6-C7 M50.923
        C7-T1 M50.93
        cervicothoracic region M50.93
      degeneration M50.30
        C2-C3 M50.31
        C3-C4 M50.31
        C4-C5 M50.321
        C5-C6 M50.322
        C6-C7 M50.323
        C7-T1 M50.33
        cervicothoracic region M50.33
        high cervical region M50.31
        mid-cervical region M50.320
      displacement M50.20
        C2-C3 M50.21
        C3-C4 M50.21
        C4-C5 M50.221
        C5-C6 M50.222
        C6-C7 M50.223
        C7-T1 M50.23
        cervicothoracic region M50.23
        high cervical region M50.21
        mid-cervical region M50.220
      high cervical region M50.91
      mid-cervical region M50.920
      specified type NEC M50.80
        C2-C3 M50.81
        C3-C4 M50.81
        C4-C5 M50.821
        C5-C6 M50.822
        C6-C7 M50.823
        C7-T1 M50.83
        cervicothoracic region M50.83
        high cervical region M50.81
        mid-cervical region M50.820
    specified NEC
      lumbar region M51.86
      lumbosacral region M51.87
      sacrococcygeal region M53.3
      thoracic region M51.84
      thoracolumbar region M51.85
  disinhibited attachment (childhood) F94.2
  disintegrative, childhood NEC F84.3
  disruptive F91.9
    mood dysregulation F34.81
    specified NEC F91.8

Disorder *(continued)*
  disruptive behavior —*see* Disorder, conduct
  dissocial personality F60.2
  dissociative F44.9
    affecting
      motor function F44.4
        and sensation F44.7
      sensation F44.6
        and motor function F44.7
    brief reactive F43.0
    due to (secondary to) general medical condition F06.8
    mixed F44.7
    organic F06.8
    other specified NEC F44.89
  double heterozygous sickling —*see* Disease, sickle-cell
  dream anxiety F51.5
  drug induced hemorrhagic D68.32
  drug related F19.99
    abuse —*see* Abuse, drug
    dependence —*see* Dependence, drug
  dysmorphic body F45.22
  dysthymic F34.1
  ear H93.9-
    bleeding —*see* Otorrhagia
    deafness —*see* Deafness
    degenerative H93.09-
    discharge —*see* Otorrhea
    external H61.9-
      auditory canal stenosis —*see* Stenosis, external ear canal
      exostosis —*see* Exostosis, external ear canal
      impacted cerumen —*see* Impaction, cerumen
      otitis —*see* Otitis, externa
      perichondritis —*see* Perichondritis, ear
      pinna —*see* Disorder, pinna
      specified type NEC H61.89-
        in diseases classified elsewhere H62.8X-
    inner H83.9-
      vestibular dysfunction —*see* Disorder, vestibular function
    middle H74.9-
      adhesive H74.1-
      ossicle —*see* Abnormal, ear ossicles
      polyp —*see* Polyp, ear (middle)
      specified NEC, in diseases classified elsewhere H75.8-
    postprocedural —*see* Complications, ear, procedure
    specified NEC, in diseases classified elsewhere H94.8-
  eating (adult) (psychogenic) F50.9
    anorexia —*see* Anorexia
    binge F50.81
    bulimia F50.2
    child F98.29
      pica F98.3
      rumination disorder F98.21
    pica F50.89
      childhood F98.3
    specified NEC F50.89
  electrolyte (balance) NEC E87.8
    with
      abortion —*see* Abortion by type complicated by specified condition NEC
      ectopic pregnancy O08.5
      molar pregnancy O08.5

Disorder *(continued)*
  electrolyte *(continued)*
    acidosis (lactic) (metabolic) E87.20
      acute E87.21
      chronic E87.22
      respiratory E87.29
      specified NEC E87.29
    alkalosis (metabolic) (respiratory) E87.3
  elimination, transepidermal L87.9
    specified NEC L87.8
  emotional (persistent) F34.9
    of childhood F93.9
      specified NEC F93.8
  endocrine E34.9
    postprocedural E89.89
    specified NEC E89.89
  erectile (male) (organic) *(see also* Dysfunction, sexual, male, erectile) N52.9
    nonorganic F52.21
  erythematous —*see* Erythema
  esophagus K22.9
    functional K22.4
    psychogenic F45.8
  eustachian tube H69.9-
    infection —*see* Salpingitis, eustachian
    obstruction —*see* Obstruction, eustachian tube
    patulous —*see* Patulous, eustachian tube
    specified NEC H69.8-
  exhibitionistic F65.2
  extrapyramidal G25.9
    in diseases classified elsewhere —*see* category G26
    specified type NEC G25.89
  eye H57.9
    postprocedural —*see* Complication, postprocedural, eye
  eyelid H02.9
    cyst —*see* Cyst, eyelid
    degenerative H02.70
      chloasma —*see* Chloasma, eyelid
      madarosis —*see* Madarosis
      specified type NEC H02.79
      vitiligo —*see* Vitiligo, eyelid
      xanthelasma —*see* Xanthelasma
    dermatochalasis —*see* Dermatochalasis
    edema —*see* Edema, eyelid
    elephantiasis —*see* Elephantiasis, eyelid
    foreign body, retained —*see* Foreign body, retained, eyelid
    function H02.59
      abnormal innervation syndrome —*see* Syndrome, abnormal innervation
      blepharochalasis —*see* Blepharochalasis
      blepharoclonus —*see* Blepharoclonus
      blepharophimosis —*see* Blepharophimosis
      blepharoptosis —*see* Blepharoptosis
      lagophthalmos —*see* Lagophthalmos
      lid retraction —*see* Retraction, lid

119

Disorder (continued)
  eyelid (continued)
    hypertrichosis —see
      Hypertrichosis, eyelid
    specified type NEC H02.89
    vascular H02.879
      left H02.876
        lower H02.875
        upper H02.874
      right H02.873
        lower H02.872
        upper H02.871
  factitious
    by proxy F68.A
    imposed on another F68.A
    imposed on self F68.10
      with predominantly
        psychological symptoms
          F68.11
          with physical symptoms
            F68.13
        physical symptoms
          F68.12
          with psychological
            symptoms F68.13
  factor, coagulation —see Defect,
    coagulation
  fatty acid
    metabolism E71.30
      specified NEC E71.39
      oxidation
        LCAD E71.310
        MCAD E71.311
        SCAD E71.312
        specified deficiency NEC
          E71.318
  feeding (infant or child) (see also
    Disorder, eating) R63.30
    or eating disorder F50.9
    pediatric
      acute R63.31
      chronic R63.32
    specified NEC F50.9
  feigned (with obvious motivation)
    Z76.5
    without obvious motivation
      —see Disorder, factitious
  female
    hypoactive sexual desire
      F52.0
    orgasmic F52.31
    sexual interest/arousal F52.22
  fetishistic F65.0
  fibroblastic M72.9
    specified NEC M72.8
  fluency
    adult onset F98.5
    childhood onset F80.81
    following
      cerebral infarction I69.323
      cerebrovascular disease
        I69.923
        specified disease NEC
          I69.823
      intracerebral hemorrhage
        I69.123
      nontraumatic intracranial
        hemorrhage NEC
        I69.223
      subarachnoid hemorrhage
        I69.023
    in conditions classified elsewhere
      R47.82
  fluid balance E87.8
  follicular (skin) L73.9
    specified NEC L73.8
  frotteuristic F65.81
  fructose metabolism E74.10
    essential fructosuria E74.11
    fructokinase deficiency E74.11

Disorder (continued)
  fructose metabolism (continued)
    fructose-1, 6-diphosphatase
      deficiency E74.19
    hereditary fructose intolerance
      E74.12
    other specified E74.19
  functional polymorphonuclear
    neutrophils D71
  gallbladder, biliary tract and
    pancreas in diseases classified
    elsewhere K87
  gambling F63.0
  gamma aminobutyric acid (GABA)
    metabolism E72.81
  gamma-glutamyl cycle E72.89
  gastric (functional) K31.9
    motility K30
    psychogenic F45.8
    secretion K30
  gastrointestinal (functional) NOS
    K92.9
    newborn P78.9
    psychogenic F45.8
  gender-identity or -role F64.9
    childhood F64.2
    effect on relationship F66
    of adolescence or adulthood
      F64.0
      nontranssexual F64.8
    specified NEC F64.8
    uncertainty F66
  gender incongruence F64.9
    in adolescents and adults F64.0
    of childhood F64.2
  genito-pelvic pain penetration
    F52.6
  genitourinary system
    female N94.9
    male N50.9
    psychogenic F45.8
  globe H44.9
    degenerated condition
      H44.50
      absolute glaucoma H44.51-
      atrophy H44.52-
      leucocoria H44.53-
    degenerative H44.30
      chalcosis H44.31-
      myopia (see also Myopia,
        degenerative) H44.2-
      siderosis H44.32-
      specified type NEC H44.39-
    endophthalmitis —see
      Endophthalmitis
    foreign body, retained —see
      Foreign body, intraocular, old,
      retained
    hemophthalmos —see
      Hemophthalmos
    hypotony H44.40
      due to
        ocular fistula H44.42-
        specified disorder NEC
          H44.43-
      flat anterior chamber
        H44.41-
      primary H44.44-
    luxation —see Luxation, globe
    specified type NEC H44.89
  glomerular (in) N05.9
    amyloidosis E85.4 [N08]
    cryoglobulinemia D89.1 [N08]
    disseminated intravascular
      coagulation D65 [N08]
    Fabry's disease E75.21 [N08]
    familial lecithin cholesterol
      acyltransferase deficiency
      E78.6 [N08]
    Goodpasture's syndrome
      M31.0

Disorder (continued)
  glomerular (continued)
    hemolytic-uremic syndrome
      —see Syndrome, hemolytic-
      uremic
    Henoch (-Schönlein) purpura
      D69.0 [N08]
    malariae malaria B52.0
    microscopic polyangiitis M31.7
      [N08]
    multiple myeloma C90.0-
      [N08]
    mumps B26.83
    schistosomiasis B65.9 [N08]
    sepsis NEC A41.- [N08]
      streptococcal A40.- [N08]
    sickle-cell disorders D57.- [N08]
    strongyloidiasis B78.9 [N08]
    subacute bacterial endocarditis
      I33.0 [N08]
    syphilis A52.75
    systemic lupus erythematosus
      M32.14
    thrombotic thrombocytopenic
      purpura M31.19 [N08]
    Waldenström macroglobulinemia
      C88.0 [N08]
    Wegener's granulomatosis M31.31
  gluconeogenesis E74.4
  glucosaminoglycan metabolism
    —see Disorder, metabolism,
    glucosaminoglycan
  glucose transport E74.819
    specified NEC E74.818
  glycine metabolism E72.50
    d-glycericacidemia E72.59
    hyperhydroxyprolinemia E72.59
    hyperoxaluria R82.992
      primary E72.53
    hyperprolinemia E72.59
    non-ketotic hyperglycinemia
      E72.51
    oxalosis E72.53
    oxaluria E72.53
    sarcosinemia E72.59
    trimethylaminuria E72.52
  glycoprotein metabolism E77.9
    specified NEC E77.8
  grief
    complicated F43.81
    prolonged F43.81
  habit (and impulse) F63.9
    involving sexual behavior NEC
      F65.9
    specified NEC F63.89
  hallucinogen use
    mild F16.10
      with
        hallucinogen-induced
          anxiety disorder F16.180
          bipolar and related
            disorder F16.14
          depressive disorder
            F16.14
          psychotic disorder F16.159
        hallucinogen intoxication
          delirium F16.121
        other hallucinogen
          intoxication F16.129
      in remission (early)
        (sustained) F16.11
    moderate or severe F16.20
      with
        hallucinogen-induced
          anxiety disorder F16.280
          bipolar and related
            disorder F16.24
          depressive disorder F16.24
          psychotic disorder
            F16.259

Disorder (continued)
  hallucinogen use (continued)
    moderate or severe (continued)
      with (continued)
        hallucinogen intoxication
          delirium F16.221
        other hallucinogen
          intoxication F16.229
      in remission (early)
        (sustained) F16.21
  heart action I49.9
  hematological D75.9
    newborn (transient) P61.9
    specified NEC P61.8
  hematopoietic organs D75.9
  hemorrhagic NEC D69.9
    drug-induced D68.32
    due to
      extrinsic circulating
        anticoagulants D68.32
      increase in
        anti-IIa D68.32
        anti-Xa D68.32
      intrinsic
        circulating anticoagulants
          D68.318
        increase in
          antithrombin D68.318
          anti-VIIIa D68.318
          anti-IXa D68.318
          anti-XIa D68.318
    following childbirth O72.3
  hemostasis —see Defect, coagulation
  histidine metabolism E70.40
    histidinemia E70.41
    other specified E70.49
  hoarding F42.3
  hyperkinetic —see Disorder,
    attention-deficit hyperactivity
  hyperleucine-isoleucinemia E71.19
  hypervalinemia E71.19
  hypoactive sexual desire F52.0
  hypochondriacal F45.20
    body dysmorphic F45.22
    neurosis F45.21
    other specified F45.29
  identity
    dissociative F44.81
    illness anxiety F45.21
    of childhood F93.8
  immune mechanism (immunity)
    D89.9
    specified type NEC D89.89
  impaired renal tubular function N25.9
    specified NEC N25.89
  impulse (control) F63.9
  inflammatory
    pelvic, in diseases classified
      elsewhere —see category N74
    penis N48.29
      abscess N48.21
      cellulitis N48.22
  inhalant use
    mild F18.10
      with
        inhalant-induced
          anxiety disorder F18.180
          depressive disorder
            F18.14
          major neurocognitive
            disorder F18.17
          mild neurocognitive
            disorder F18.188
          psychotic disorder
            F18.159
        inhalant intoxication
          F18.129
        inhalant intoxication
          delirium F18.121
      in remission (early)
        (sustained) F18.11

Disorder *(continued)*
- inhalant use *(continued)*
  - moderate or severe F18.20
    - with
      - inhalant-induced
        - anxiety disorder F18.280
        - depressive disorder F18.24
        - major neurocognitive disorder F18.27
        - mild neurocognitive disorder F18.288
        - psychotic disorder F18.259
      - inhalant intoxication F18.229
      - inhalant intoxication delirium F18.221
    - in remission (early) (sustained) F18.21
- integument, newborn P83.9
  - specified NEC P83.88
- intermittent explosive F63.81
- internal secretion pancreas —*see* Increased, secretion, pancreas, endocrine
- intestine, intestinal
  - carbohydrate absorption NEC E74.39
    - postoperative K91.2
  - functional NEC K59.9
    - postoperative K91.89
  - psychogenic F45.8
  - vascular K55.9
    - chronic K55.1
    - specified NEC K55.8
- intraoperative (intraprocedural) —*see* Complications, intraoperative
- involuntary emotional expression (IEED) F48.2
- iris H21.9
  - adhesions —*see* Adhesions, iris
  - atrophy —*see* Atrophy, iris
  - chamber angle recession —*see* Recession, chamber angle
  - cyst —*see* Cyst, iris
  - degeneration —*see* Degeneration, iris
  - in diseases classified elsewhere H22
  - iridodialysis —*see* Iridodialysis
  - iridoschisis —*see* Iridoschisis
  - miotic pupillary cyst —*see* Cyst, pupillary
  - pupillary
    - abnormality —*see* Abnormality, pupillary
    - membrane —*see* Membrane, pupillary
  - specified type NEC H21.89
  - vascular NEC H21.1X-
- iron metabolism E83.10
  - specified NEC E83.19
- isovaleric acidemia E71.110
- jaw, developmental M27.0
  - temporomandibular (*see* Anomaly, dentofacial, temporomandibular joint) M26.60-
- joint M25.9
  - derangement —*see* Derangement, joint
  - effusion —*see* Effusion, joint
  - fistula —*see* Fistula, joint
  - hemarthrosis —*see* Hemarthrosis
  - instability —*see* Instability, joint
  - osteophyte —*see* Osteophyte
  - pain —*see* Pain, joint
  - psychogenic F45.8

Disorder *(continued)*
- joint *(continued)*
  - specified type NEC M25.80
    - ankle M25.87-
    - elbow M25.82-
    - foot joint M25.87-
    - hand joint M25.84-
    - hip M25.85-
    - knee M25.86-
    - shoulder M25.81-
    - wrist M25.83-
  - stiffness —*see* Stiffness, joint
- ketone metabolism E71.32
- kidney N28.9
  - functional (tubular) N25.9
  - in
    - schistosomiasis B65.9 *[N29]*
  - tubular function N25.9
    - specified NEC N25.89
- lacrimal system H04.9
  - changes H04.69
    - fistula —*see* Fistula, lacrimal
  - gland H04.19
    - atrophy —*see* Atrophy, lacrimal gland
    - cyst —*see* Cyst, lacrimal, gland
    - dacryops —*see* Dacryops
    - dislocation —*see* Dislocation, lacrimal gland
    - dry eye syndrome —*see* Syndrome, dry eye
    - infection —*see* Dacryoadenitis
    - granuloma —*see* Granuloma, lacrimal
    - inflammation —*see* Inflammation, lacrimal
    - obstruction —*see* Obstruction, lacrimal
  - specified NEC H04.89
- lactation NEC O92.79
- language (developmental) F80.9
  - expressive F80.1
  - mixed receptive and expressive F80.2
  - receptive F80.2
- late luteal phase dysphoric N94.89
- learning (specific) F81.9
  - acalculia R48.8
  - alexia R48.0
  - mathematics F81.2
  - reading F81.0
  - specified
    - with impairment in
      - mathematics F81.2
      - reading F81.0
      - written expression F81.81
    - specified NEC F81.89
    - spelling F81.81
    - written expression F81.81
- lens H27.9
  - aphakia —*see* Aphakia
  - cataract —*see* Cataract
  - dislocation —*see* Dislocation, lens
  - specified type NEC H27.8
- ligament M24.20
  - ankle M24.27-
  - attachment, spine —*see* Enthesopathy, spinal
  - elbow M24.22-
  - foot joint M24.27-
  - hand joint M24.24-
  - hip M24.25-
  - knee —*see* Derangement, knee, specified NEC
  - shoulder M24.21-
  - specified site NEC M24.29
  - vertebra M24.28
  - wrist M24.23-

Disorder *(continued)*
- ligamentous attachments —*see also* Enthesopathy
  - spine —*see* Enthesopathy, spinal
- lipid
  - metabolism, congenital E78.9
  - storage E75.6
    - specified NEC E75.5
- lipoprotein
  - deficiency (familial) E78.6
  - metabolism E78.9
    - specified NEC E78.89
- liver K76.9
  - malarial B54 *[K77]*
- low back —*see also* Dorsopathy, specified NEC
- lumbosacral
  - plexus G54.1
  - root (nerve) NEC G54.4
- lung, interstitial, drug-induced J70.4
  - acute J70.2
  - chronic J70.3
  - dabbing (related) U07.0
  - e-cigarette (related) U07.0
  - electronic cigarette (related) U07.0
  - vaping (associated) (device) (product) (related) (use) U07.0
- lymphoproliferative, post-transplant (PTLD) D47.Z1
- lysine and hydroxylysine metabolism E72.3
- male
  - erectile (organic) (*see also* Dysfunction, sexual, male, erectile) N52.9
    - nonorganic F52.21
  - hypoactive sexual desire F52.0
  - orgasmic F52.32
- major neurocognitive (*see also* Dementia, in (due to)) F03-
- manic F30.9
  - organic F06.33
- mast cell activation —*see* Activation, mast cell
- mastoid —*see also* Disorder, ear, middle
  - postprocedural —*see* Complications, ear, procedure
- meninges, specified type NEC G96.198
- meniscus —*see* Derangement, knee, meniscus
- menopausal N95.9
  - specified NEC N95.8
- menstrual N92.6
  - psychogenic F45.8
  - specified NEC N92.5
- mental (or behavioral) (nonpsychotic) F99
  - due to (secondary to)
    - amphetamine
      - due to drug abuse —*see* Abuse, drug, stimulant
      - due to drug dependence —*see* Dependence, drug, stimulant
    - brain disease, damage and dysfunction F09
    - caffeine use
      - due to drug abuse —*see* Abuse, drug, stimulant
      - due to drug dependence —*see* Dependence, drug, stimulant
    - cannabis use
      - due to drug abuse —*see* Abuse, drug, cannabis
      - due to drug dependence —*see* Dependence, drug, cannabis

Disorder *(continued)*
- mental *(continued)*
  - due to *(continued)*
    - general medical condition F09
    - sedative or hypnotic use
      - due to drug abuse —*see* Abuse, drug, sedative
      - due to drug dependence —*see* Dependence, drug, sedative
    - tobacco (nicotine) use —*vsee* Dependence, drug, nicotine
  - following organic brain damage F07.9
    - frontal lobe syndrome F07.0
    - personality change F07.0
    - postconcussional syndrome F07.81
    - specified NEC F07.89
  - infancy, childhood or adolescence F98.9
  - neurotic —*see* Neurosis
  - organic or symptomatic F09
  - presenile, psychotic F03
  - problem NEC
  - psychoneurotic —*see* Neurosis
  - psychotic —*see* Psychosis
  - puerperal F53.0
  - senile, psychotic NEC F03
- metabolic, amino acid, transitory, newborn P74.8
- metabolism NOS E88.9
  - amino-acid E72.9
    - aromatic E70.9
      - albinism —*see* Albinism
      - histidine E70.40
        - histidinemia E70.41
        - other specified E70.49
      - hyperphenylalaninemia E70.1
        - classical phenylketonuria E70.0
      - other specified E70.89
      - tryptophan E70.5
      - tyrosine E70.20
        - hypertyrosinemia E70.21
        - other specified E70.29
    - branched chain E71.2
      - 3-methylglutaconic aciduria E71.111
      - hyperleucine-isoleucinemia E71.19
      - hypervalinemia E71.19
      - isovaleric acidemia E71.110
      - maple syrup urine disease E71.0
      - methylmalonic acidemia E71.120
      - organic aciduria NEC E71.118
      - other specified E71.19
      - proprionate NEC E71.128
      - proprionic acidemia E71.121
    - glycine E72.50
      - d-glycericacidemia E72.59
      - hyperhydroxyprolinemia E72.59
      - hyperoxaluria R82.992
        - primary E72.53
      - hyperprolinemia E72.59
      - non-ketotic hyperglycinemia E72.51
      - other specified E72.59
      - sarcosinemia E72.59
      - trimethylaminuria E72.52
    - hydroxylysine E72.3
    - lysine E72.3
    - ornithine E72.4

Disorder (continued)
- metabolism NOS (continued)
  - amino-acid (continued)
    - other specified E72.89
      - beta-amino acid E72.89
      - gamma-glutamyl cycle E72.89
    - straight-chain E72.89
    - sulfur-bearing E72.10
      - homocystinuria E72.11
      - methylenetetrahydrofolate reductase deficiency E72.12
    - other specified E72.19
  - bile acid and cholesterol metabolism E78.70
  - bilirubin E80.7
    - specified NEC E80.6
  - calcium E83.50
    - hypercalcemia E83.52
    - hypocalcemia E83.51
    - other specified E83.59
  - carbohydrate E74.9
    - specified NEC E74.89
  - cholesterol and bile acid metabolism E78.70
  - congenital E88.9
  - copper E83.00
    - Wilson's disease E83.01
    - specified type NEC E83.09
  - cystinuria E72.01
  - fructose E74.10
  - galactose E74.20
  - glucosaminoglycan E76.9
    - mucopolysaccharidosis —see Mucopolysaccharidosis
    - specified NEC E76.8
  - glutamine E72.89
  - glycine E72.50
  - glycogen storage (hepatorenal) E74.09
  - glycoprotein E77.9
    - specified NEC E77.8
  - glycosaminoglycan E76.9
    - specified NEC E76.8
  - in labor and delivery O75.89
  - iron E83.10
  - isoleucine E71.19
  - leucine E71.19
  - lipoid E78.9
  - lipoprotein E78.9
    - specified NEC E78.89
  - magnesium E83.40
    - hypermagnesemia E83.41
    - hypomagnesemia E83.42
    - other specified E83.49
  - mineral E83.9
    - specified NEC E83.89
  - mitochondrial E88.40
    - MELAS syndrome E88.41
    - MERRF syndrome (myoclonic epilepsy associated with ragged-red fibers) E88.42
    - other specified E88.49
    - tRNA synthetases E88.43
  - ornithine E72.4
  - phosphatases E83.30
  - phosphorus E83.30
    - acid phosphatase deficiency E83.39
    - hypophosphatasia E83.39
    - hypophosphatemia E83.39
      - familial E83.31
    - other specified E83.39
    - pseudovitamin D deficiency E83.32
  - plasma protein NEC E88.09
  - porphyrin —see Porphyria
  - postprocedural E89.89
    - specified NEC E89.89

Disorder (continued)
- metabolism NOS (continued)
  - purine E79.9
    - specified NEC E79.89
  - pyrimidine E79.9
    - specified NEC E79.89
  - pyruvate E74.4
  - serine E72.89
  - sodium E87.8
  - specified NEC E88.89
  - threonine E72.89
  - valine E71.19
  - zinc E83.2
- methylmalonic acidemia E71.120
- micturition NEC (see also Difficulty, micturition) R39.198
  - feeling of incomplete emptying R39.14
  - hesitancy R39.11
  - poor stream R39.12
  - psychogenic F45.8
  - split stream R39.13
  - straining R39.16
  - urgency R39.15
- mild neurocognitive G31.84
  - due to known physiological condition (without behavioral disturbance) F06.70
    - with behavioral disturbance F06.71
- mitochondrial metabolism E88.40
- mitral (valve) —see Endocarditis, mitral
- mixed
  - anxiety and depressive F41.8
  - of scholastic skills (developmental) F81.89
  - receptive expressive language F80.2
- mood F39
  - bipolar —see Disorder, bipolar
  - depressive —see Disorder, depressive
  - due to (secondary to)
    - alcohol F10.94
    - amphetamine F15.94
      - in
        - abuse F15.14
        - dependence F15.24
    - anxiolytic F13.94
      - in
        - abuse F13.14
        - dependence F13.24
    - cocaine F14.94
      - in
        - abuse F14.14
        - dependence F14.24
    - general medical condition F06.30
    - hallucinogen F16.94
      - in
        - abuse F16.14
        - dependence F16.24
    - hypnotic F13.94
      - in
        - abuse F13.14
        - dependence F13.24
    - inhalant F18.94
      - in
        - abuse F18.14
        - dependence F18.24
    - opioid F11.94
      - in
        - abuse F11.14
        - dependence F11.24
    - phencyclidine (PCP) F16.94
      - in
        - abuse F16.14
        - dependence F16.24

Disorder (continued)
- mood (continued)
  - due to (continued)
    - physiological condition F06.30
      - with
        - depressive features F06.31
        - major depressive-like episode F06.32
        - manic features F06.33
        - mixed features F06.34
    - psychoactive substance NEC F19.94
      - in
        - abuse F19.14
        - dependence F19.24
    - sedative F13.94
      - in
        - abuse F13.14
        - dependence F13.24
    - volatile solvents F18.94
      - in
        - abuse F18.14
        - dependence F18.24
  - manic episode F30.9
    - with psychotic symptoms F30.2
    - in remission (full) F30.4
      - partial F30.3
    - specified type NEC F30.8
    - without psychotic symptoms F30.10
      - mild F30.11
      - moderate F30.12
      - severe F30.13
  - organic F06.30
    - right hemisphere F07.89
  - persistent F34.9
    - cyclothymia F34.0
    - dysthymia F34.1
    - specified type NEC F34.89
  - recurrent F39
  - right hemisphere organic F07.89
- movement G25.9
  - drug-induced G25.70
    - akathisia G25.71
    - specified NEC G25.79
  - hysterical F44.4
  - in diseases classified elsewhere —see category G26
  - periodic limb G47.61
    - sleep related G47.61
  - specified NEC G25.89
  - sleep related NEC G47.69
  - stereotyped F98.4
  - treatment-induced G25.9
- multiple personality F44.81
- muscle M62.9
  - attachment, spine —see Enthesopathy, spinal
  - in trichinellosis —see Trichinellosis, with muscle disorder
  - psychogenic F45.8
  - specified type NEC M62.89
- tone, newborn P94.9
  - specified NEC P94.8
- muscular
  - attachments —see also Enthesopathy
    - spine —see Enthesopathy, spinal
  - urethra N36.44
- musculoskeletal system, soft tissue —see Disorder, soft tissue
  - postprocedural M96.89
  - psychogenic F45.8
- myoneural G70.9
  - due to lead G70.1
  - specified NEC G70.89
  - toxic G70.1

Disorder (continued)
- myotonic NEC G71.19
- nail, in diseases classified elsewhere L62
- neck region NEC —see Dorsopathy, specified NEC
- neonatal onset multisystemic inflammatory (NOMID) M04.2
- nerve G58.9
  - abducent NEC —see Strabismus, paralytic, sixth nerve
  - accessory G52.8
  - acoustic —see subcategory H93.3
  - auditory —see subcategory H93.3
  - auriculotemporal G50.8
  - axillary G54.0
  - cerebral —see Disorder, nerve, cranial
  - cranial G52.9
    - eighth —see subcategory H93.3
    - eleventh G52.8
    - fifth G50.9
    - first G52.0
    - fourth NEC —see Strabismus, paralytic, fourth nerve
    - multiple G52.7
    - ninth G52.1
    - second NEC —see Disorder, nerve, optic
    - seventh NEC G51.8
    - sixth NEC —see Strabismus, paralytic, sixth nerve
    - specified NEC G52.8
    - tenth G52.2
    - third NEC —see Strabismus, paralytic, third nerve
    - twelfth G52.3
  - entrapment —see Neuropathy, entrapment
  - facial G51.9
    - specified NEC G51.8
  - femoral —see Lesion, nerve, femoral
  - glossopharyngeal NEC G52.1
  - hypoglossal G52.3
  - intercostal G58.0
  - lateral
    - cutaneous of thigh —see Mononeuropathy, lower limb, meralgia paresthetica
    - popliteal —see Lesion, nerve, popliteal
  - lower limb —see Mononeuropathy, lower limb
  - medial popliteal —see Lesion, nerve, popliteal, medial
  - median NEC —see Lesion, nerve, median
  - multiple G58.7
  - oculomotor NEC —see Strabismus, paralytic, third nerve
  - olfactory G52.0
  - optic NEC H47.09-
    - hemorrhage into sheath —see Hemorrhage, optic nerve
    - ischemic H47.01-
  - peroneal —see Lesion, nerve, popliteal
  - phrenic G58.8
  - plantar —see Lesion, nerve, plantar
  - pneumogastric G52.2
  - posterior tibial —see Syndrome, tarsal tunnel
  - radial —see Lesion, nerve, radial
  - recurrent laryngeal G52.2
  - root G54.9
    - cervical G54.2
    - lumbosacral G54.1
    - specified NEC G54.8
    - thoracic G54.3

Disorder *(continued)*
- nerve *(continued)*
  - sciatic NEC —*see* Lesion, nerve, sciatic
  - specified NEC G58.8
    - lower limb —*see* Mononeuropathy, lower limb, specified NEC
    - upper limb —*see* Mononeuropathy, upper limb, specified NEC
  - sympathetic G90.9
  - tibial —*see* Lesion, nerve, popliteal, medial
  - trigeminal G50.9
    - specified NEC G50.8
  - trochlear NEC —*see* Strabismus, paralytic, fourth nerve
  - ulnar —*see* Lesion, nerve, ulnar
  - upper limb —*see* Mononeuropathy, upper limb
  - vagus G52.2
- nervous system G98.8
  - autonomic (peripheral) G90.9
    - specified NEC G90.8
  - central G96.9
    - specified NEC G96.89
  - parasympathetic G90.9
    - specified NEC G98.8
  - sympathetic G90.9
  - vegetative G90.9
- neurocognitive R41.9
  - with Lewy bodies (*see also* Dementia, in, diseases specified elsewhere) G31.83 [F02.-]
  - frontotemporal, specified NEC (*see also* Dementia, in, diseases specified elsewhere) G31.09 [F02.-]
  - major (*see also* Dementia) F03.-
    - due to vascular disease - *see* Dementia, vascular
      - mild - *see* Dementia, vascular, mild
      - moderate - *see* Dementia, vascular, moderate
      - severe - *see* Dementia, vascular, severe
    - in (due to) (other diseases classified elsewhere) (*see also* Dementia, in (due to)) F02.80
      - with
        - aggressive behavior (*see also* Dementia, in (due to)) F02.81-
        - combative behavior (*see also* Dementia, in (due to)) F02.81-
          - violent behavior (*see also* Dementia, in (due to)) F02.81-
  - mild (of uncertain or unknown etiology) (*see also* Disorder, mild neurocognitive) G31.84
- neurodevelopment F89
  - specified NEC F88
- neurohypophysis NEC E23.3
- neurological NEC R29.818
- neuromuscular G70.9
  - hereditary NEC G71.9
  - specified NEC G70.89
  - toxic G70.1
- neurotic F48.9
  - specified NEC F48.8
- neutrophil, polymorphonuclear D71
- nicotine use —*see* Dependence, drug, nicotine
- nightmare F51.5

Disorder *(continued)*
- non-rapid eye movement sleep arousal
  - sleep terror type F51.4
  - sleepwalking type F51.3
- nose J34.9
  - specified NEC J34.89
- obsessive-compulsive F42.9
  - and related disorder due to a known physiological condition F06.8
- odontogenesis NOS K00.9
- opioid use
  - with
    - opioid-induced psychotic disorder F11.959
      - with
        - delusions F11.950
        - hallucinations F11.951
  - due to drug abuse —*see* Abuse, drug, opioid
  - due to drug dependence —*see* Dependence, drug, opioid
  - mild F11.10
    - with
      - opioid-induced
        - anxiety disorder F11.188
        - depressive disorder F11.14
        - sexual dysfunction F11.181
      - opioid intoxication
        - with perceptual disturbances F11.122
        - delirium F11.121
        - without perceptual disturbances F11.129
    - in remission (early) (sustained) F11.11
  - moderate or severe F11.20
    - with
      - opioid-induced
        - anxiety disorder F11.288
        - anxiety disorder F11.988
        - depressive disorder F11.24
        - depressive disorder F11.94
        - sexual dysfunction F11.281
        - sexual dysfunction F11.981
      - opioid intoxication
        - with perceptual disturbances F11.222
        - delirium F11.221
        - without perceptual disturbances F11.229
    - in remission (early) (sustained) F11.21
- oppositional defiant F91.3
- optic
  - chiasm H47.49
    - due to
      - inflammatory disorder H47.41
      - neoplasm H47.42
      - vascular disorder H47.43
  - disc H47.39-
    - coloboma —*see* Coloboma, optic disc
    - drusen —*see* Drusen, optic disc
    - pseudopapilledema —*see* Pseudopapilledema
  - radiations —*see* Disorder, visual, pathway
  - tracts —*see* Disorder, visual, pathway
- orbit H05.9
  - cyst —*see* Cyst, orbit
  - deformity —*see* Deformity, orbit

Disorder *(continued)*
- orbit H05.9 *(continued)*
  - edema —*see* Edema, orbit
  - enophthalmos —*see* Enophthalmos
  - exophthalmos —*see* Exophthalmos
  - hemorrhage —*see* Hemorrhage, orbit
  - inflammation —*see* Inflammation, orbit
  - myopathy —*see* Myopathy, extraocular muscles
  - retained foreign body —*see* Foreign body, orbit, old
  - specified type NEC H05.89
- organic
  - anxiety F06.4
  - catatonic F06.1
  - delusional F06.2
  - dissociative F06.8
  - emotionally labile (asthenic) F06.8
  - mood (affective) F06.30
  - schizophrenia-like F06.2
- orgasmic (female) F52.31
  - male F52.32
- ornithine metabolism E72.4
- overanxious F41.1
  - of childhood F93.8
- pain
  - with related psychological factors F45.42
  - exclusively related to psychological factors F45.41
  - genito-pelvic penetration disorder F52.6
- pancreatic internal secretion E16.9
  - specified NEC E16.8
- panic F41.0
  - with agoraphobia F40.01
- papulosquamous L44.9
  - in diseases classified elsewhere L45
  - specified NEC L44.8
- paranoid F22
  - induced F24
  - shared F24
- paraphilic F65.9
  - specified NEC F65.89
- parathyroid (gland) E21.5
  - specified NEC E21.4
- parietoalveolar NEC J84.09
- paroxysmal, mixed R56.9
- patella M22.9-
  - chondromalacia —*see* Chondromalacia, patella
  - derangement NEC M22.3X-
  - recurrent
    - dislocation —*see* Dislocation, patella, recurrent
    - subluxation —*see* Dislocation, patella, recurrent, incomplete
  - specified NEC M22.8X-
- patellofemoral M22.2X-
- pedophilic F65.4
- pentose phosphate pathway with anemia D55.1
- perception, due to hallucinogens F16.983
  - in
    - abuse F16.183
    - dependence F16.283
- peripheral nervous system NEC G64
- peroxisomal E71.50
  - biogenesis
    - neonatal adrenoleukodystrophy E71.511
    - specified disorder NEC E71.518
    - Zellweger syndrome E71.510

Disorder *(continued)*
- peroxisomal E71.50 *(continued)*
  - rhizomelic chondrodysplasia punctata E71.540
  - specified form NEC E71.548
    - group 1 E71.518
    - group 2 E71.53
    - group 3 E71.542
  - X-linked adrenoleukodystrophy E71.529
    - adolescent E71.521
    - adrenomyeloneuropathy E71.522
    - childhood E71.520
    - specified form NEC E71.528
  - Zellweger-like syndrome E71.541
- persistent (somatoform) pain F45.41
  - affective (mood) F34.9
- personality —*see also* Personality F60.9
  - affective F34.0
  - aggressive F60.3
  - amoral F60.2
  - anankastic F60.5
  - antisocial F60.2
  - anxious F60.6
  - asocial F60.2
  - asthenic F60.7
  - avoidant F60.6
  - borderline F60.3
  - change (secondary) due to general medical condition F07.0
  - compulsive F60.5
  - cyclothymic F34.0
  - dependent (passive) F60.7
  - depressive F34.1
  - dissocial F60.2
  - emotional instability F60.3
  - expansive paranoid F60.0
  - explosive F60.3
  - following organic brain damage F07.9
  - histrionic F60.4
  - hyperthymic F34.0
  - hypothymic F34.1
  - hysterical F60.4
  - immature F60.89
  - inadequate F60.7
  - labile F60.3
  - mixed (nonspecific) F60.89
  - moral deficiency F60.2
  - narcissistic F60.81
  - negativistic F60.89
  - obsessional F60.5
  - obsessive (-compulsive) F60.5
  - organic F07.9
  - overconscientious F60.5
  - paranoid F60.0
  - passive (-dependent) F60.7
  - passive-aggressive F60.89
  - pathological NEC F60.9
  - pseudosocial F60.2
  - psychopathic F60.2
  - schizoid F60.1
  - schizotypal F21
  - self-defeating F60.7
  - specified NEC F60.89
  - type A F60.5
  - unstable (emotional) F60.3
- pervasive, developmental F84.9
- phencyclidine use
  - mild F16.10
    - with
      - phencyclidine-induced
        - anxiety disorder F16.180
        - bipolar and related disorder F16.14
        - depressive disorder F16.14
        - psychotic disorder F16.159

123

Disorder (continued)
  phencyclidine use (continued)
    mild (continued)
      with (continued)
        phencyclidine intoxication F16.129
        phencyclidine intoxication delirium F16.121
      in remission (early) (sustained) F16.11
    moderate or severe F16.20
      with
        phencyclidine-induced
          anxiety disorder F16.280
          bipolar and related disorder F16.24
          depressive disorder F16.24
          psychotic disorder F16.259
        phencyclidine intoxication F16.229
        phencyclidine intoxication delirium F16.221
      in remission (early) (sustained) F16.21
  phobic anxiety, childhood F40.8
  phosphate-losing tubular N25.0
  pigmentation L81.9
    choroid, congenital Q14.3
    diminished melanin formation L81.6
    iron L81.8
    specified NEC L81.8
  pinna (noninfective) H61.10-
    deformity, acquired H61.11-
    hematoma H61.12-
    perichondritis —see Perichondritis, ear
    specified type NEC H61.19-
  pituitary gland E23.7
    iatrogenic (postprocedural) E89.3
    specified NEC E23.6
  platelet-activating anti-PF4, specified NEC D75.84
  platelets D69.1
  plexus G54.9
    specified NEC G54.8
  polymorphonuclear neutrophils D71
  porphyrin metabolism —see Porphyria
  postconcussional F07.81
  posthallucinogen perception F16.983
    in
      abuse F16.183
      dependence F16.283
  postmenopausal N95.9
    specified NEC N95.8
  postprocedural (postoperative) —see Complications, postprocedural
  post-transplant lymphoproliferative D47.Z1
  post-traumatic stress (PTSD) F43.10
    acute F43.11
    chronic F43.12
  premenstrual dysphoric (PMDD) F32.81
  prepuce N47.8
  propionic acidemia E71.121
  prostate N42.9
    specified NEC N42.89
  psychogenic NOS (see also condition) F45.9
    anxiety F41.8
    appetite F50.9
    asthenic F48.8
    cardiovascular (system) F45.8
    compulsive F42.8
    cutaneous F54
    depressive F32.9
    digestive (system) F45.8
    dysmenorrheic F45.8

Disorder (continued)
  psychogenic NOS (continued)
    dyspneic F45.8
    endocrine (system) F54
    eye NEC F45.8
    feeding —see Disorder, eating
    functional NEC F45.8
    gastric F45.8
    gastrointestinal (system) F45.8
    genitourinary (system) F45.8
    heart (function) (rhythm) F45.8
    hyperventilatory F45.8
    hypochondriacal —see Disorder, hypochondriacal
    intestinal F45.8
    joint F45.8
    learning F81.9
    limb F45.8
    lymphatic (system) F45.8
    menstrual F45.8
    micturition F45.8
    monoplegic NEC F44.4
    motor F44.4
    muscle F45.8
    musculoskeletal F45.8
    neurocirculatory F45.8
    obsessive F42.8
    occupational F48.8
    organ or part of body NEC F45.8
    paralytic NEC F44.4
    phobic F40.9
    physical NEC F45.8
    rectal F45.8
    respiratory (system) F45.8
    rheumatic F45.8
    sexual (function) F52.9
    skin (allergic) (eczematous) F54
    sleep F51.9
    specified part of body NEC F45.8
    stomach F45.8
  psychological F99
    associated with
      disease classified elsewhere F54
      sexual
        development F66
        relationship F66
        uncertainty about gender identity F64.9
  psychomotor NEC F44.4
    hysterical F44.4
  psychoneurotic —see also Neurosis
    mixed NEC F48.8
  psychophysiologic —see Disorder, somatoform
  psychosexual F65.9
    development F66
    identity of childhood F64.2
  psychosomatic NOS —see Disorder, somatoform
    multiple F45.0
    undifferentiated F45.1
  psychotic —see Psychosis
    transient (acute) F23
  puberty E30.9
    specified NEC E30.8
  pulmonary (valve) —see Endocarditis, pulmonary
  purine metabolism E79.9
  pyrimidine metabolism E79.9
  pyruvate metabolism E74.4
  reactive attachment (childhood) F94.1
  reading R48.0
    developmental (specific) F81.0
  receptive language F80.2
  receptor, hormonal, peripheral (see also Syndrome, androgen insensitivity) E34.50
  recurrent brief depressive F33.8
  reflex R29.2

Disorder (continued)
  refraction H52.7
    aniseikonia H52.32
    anisometropia H52.31
    astigmatism —see Astigmatism
    hypermetropia —see Hypermetropia
    myopia —see Myopia
    presbyopia H52.4
    specified NEC H52.6
  relationship F68.8
    due to sexual orientation F66
  REM sleep behavior G47.52
  renal function, impaired (tubular) N25.9
  resonance R49.9
    specified NEC R49.8
  respiratory function, impaired —see also Failure, respiration
    postprocedural —see Complication, postoperative, respiratory system
    psychogenic F45.8
  retina H35.9
    angioid streaks H35.33
    changes in vascular appearance H35.01-
    degeneration —see Degeneration, retina
    dystrophy (hereditary) —see Dystrophy, retina
    edema H35.81
    hemorrhage —see Hemorrhage, retina
    ischemia H35.82
    macular degeneration —see Degeneration, macula
    microaneurysms H35.04-
    microvascular abnormality NEC H35.09
    neovascularization —see Neovascularization, retina
    retinopathy —see Retinopathy
    separation of layers H35.70
      central serous chorioretinopathy H35.71-
      pigment epithelium detachment (serous) H35.72-
        hemorrhagic H35.73-
    specified type NEC H35.89
    telangiectasis —see Telangiectasis, retina
    vasculitis —see Vasculitis, retina
  retroperitoneal K68.9
  right hemisphere organic affective F07.89
  rumination (infant or child) F98.21
  sacrum, sacrococcygeal NEC M53.3
  schizoaffective F25.9
    bipolar type F25.0
    depressive type F25.1
    manic type F25.0
    mixed type F25.0
    specified NEC F25.8
  schizoid of childhood F84.5
  schizophrenia spectrum and other psychotic disorder F29
    specified NEC F28
  schizophreniform F20.81
    brief F23
  schizotypal (personality) F21
  seasonal affective, recurrent episodes F33.-
  secretion, thyrocalcitonin E07.0
  sedative, hypnotic, or anxiolytic-induced
    mild F13.10
      with
        sedative, hypnotic, or anxiolytic-induced
          anxiety disorder F13.180

Disorder (continued)
  sedative, hypnotic, or anxiolytic-induced (continued)
    mild (continued)
      with (continued)
        sedative, hypnotic, or anxiolytic-induced (continued)
          bipolar and related disorder F13.14
          depressive disorder F13.14
          psychotic disorder F13.159
          sexual dysfunction F13.181
        sedative, hypnotic, or anxiolytic intoxication F13.129
        sedative, hypnotic, or anxiolytic intoxication delirium F13.121
      in remission (early) (sustained) F13.11
    moderate or severe F13.20
      with
        sedative, hypnotic, or anxiolytic-induced
          anxiety disorder F13.280
          bipolar and related disorder F13.24
          depressive disorder F13.24
          major neurocognitive disorder F13.27
          mild neurocognitive disorder F13.288
          psychotic disorder F13.259
          sexual dysfunction F13.281
        sedative, hypnotic, or anxiolytic intoxication F13.229
        sedative, hypnotic, or anxiolytic intoxication delirium F13.221
      in remission (early) (sustained) F13.21
  seizure (see also Epilepsy) G40.909
    intractable G40.919
      with status epilepticus G40.911
  semantic pragmatic F80.89
    with autism F84.0
  sense of smell R43.1
    psychogenic F45.8
  separation anxiety, of childhood F93.0
  sexual
    arousal, female F52.22
    aversion F52.1
    function, psychogenic F52.9
    interest/arousal, female F52.22
    masochism F65.51
    maturation F66
    nonorganic F52.9
    preference (see also Deviation, sexual) F65.9
      fetishistic transvestism F65.1
    relationship F66
    sadism F65.52
  shyness, of childhood and adolescence F40.10
  sibling rivalry F93.8
  sickle-cell (sickling) (homozygous) —see Disease, sickle-cell
    heterozygous D57.3
    specified type NEC D57.8-
    trait D57.3
  sinus (nasal) J34.9
    specified NEC J34.89

Disorder *(continued)*
  skin L98.9
    atrophic L90.9
      specified NEC L90.8
    granulomatous L92.9
      specified NEC L92.8
    hypertrophic L91.9
      specified NEC L91.8
    infiltrative NEC L98.6
    newborn P83.9
      specified NEC P83.88
    picking F42.4
    psychogenic (allergic) (eczematous) F54
  sleep G47.9
    breathing-related —*see* Apnea, sleep
    circadian rhythm G47.20
      advance sleep phase type G47.22
      delayed sleep phase type G47.21
      due to
        alcohol
          abuse F10.182
          dependence F10.282
          use F10.982
        amphetamines
          abuse F15.182
          dependence F15.282
          use F15.982
        caffeine
          abuse F15.182
          dependence F15.282
          use F15.982
        cocaine
          abuse F14.182
          dependence F14.282
          use F14.982
        drug NEC
          abuse F19.182
          dependence F19.282
          use F19.982
        opioid
          abuse F11.182
          dependence F11.282
          use F11.982
        psychoactive substance NEC
          abuse F19.182
          dependence F19.282
          use F19.982
        sedative, hypnotic, or anxiolytic
          abuse F13.182
          dependence F13.282
          use F13.982
        stimulant NEC
          abuse F15.182
          dependence F15.282
          use F15.982
      free running type G47.24
      in conditions classified elsewhere G47.27
      irregular sleep wake type G47.23
      jet lag type G47.25
      non-24-hour sleep-wake type G47.24
      shift work type G47.26
      specified NEC G47.29
    due to
      alcohol
        abuse F10.182
        dependence F10.282
        use F10.982
      amphetamine
        abuse F15.182
        dependence F15.282
        use F15.982

Disorder *(continued)*
  sleep *(continued)*
    due to *(continued)*
      anxiolytic
        abuse F13.182
        dependence F13.282
        use F13.982
      caffeine
        abuse F15.182
        dependence F15.282
        use F15.982
      cocaine
        abuse F14.182
        dependence F14.282
        use F14.982
      drug NEC
        abuse F19.182
        dependence F19.282
        use F19.982
      hypnotic
        abuse F13.182
        dependence F13.282
        use F13.982
      opioid
        abuse F11.182
        dependence F11.282
        use F11.982
      psychoactive substance NEC
        abuse F19.182
        dependence F19.282
        use F19.982
      sedative
        abuse F13.182
        dependence F13.282
        use F13.982
      stimulant NEC
        abuse F15.182
        dependence F15.282
        use F15.982
    emotional F51.9
    excessive somnolence —*see* Hypersomnia
    hypersomnia type —*see* Hypersomnia
    initiating or maintaining —*see* Insomnia
    nightmares F51.5
    nonorganic F51.9
      specified NEC F51.8
    parasomnia type G47.50
      specified NEC G47.8
    terrors F51.4
    walking F51.3
  sleep-wake pattern or schedule — (*see also* Disorder, sleep, circadian rhythm) G47.9
    specified NEC G47.8
  social
    anxiety (of childhood) F40.10
      generalized F40.11
    functioning in childhood F94.9
      specified NEC F94.8
    pragmatic F80.82
  soft tissue M79.9
    ankle M79.9
    due to use, overuse and pressure M70.90
      ankle M70.97-
      bursitis —*see* Bursitis
      foot M70.97-
      forearm M70.93-
      hand M70.94-
      lower leg M70.96-
      multiple sites M70.99
      pelvic region M70.95-
      shoulder region M70.91-
      specified site NEC M70.98
      specified type NEC M70.80
        ankle M70.87-
        foot M70.87-
        forearm M70.83-

Disorder *(continued)*
  soft tissue *(continued)*
    due to use, overuse and pressure *(continued)*
      specified type NEC *(continued)*
        hand M70.84-
        lower leg M70.86-
        multiple sites M70.89
        pelvic region M70.85-
        shoulder region M70.81-
        specified site NEC M70.88
        thigh M70.85-
        upper arm M70.82-
      thigh M70.95-
      upper arm M70.92-
    foot M79.9
    forearm M79.9
    hand M79.9
    lower leg M79.9
    multiple sites M79.9
    occupational —*see* Disorder, soft tissue, due to use, overuse and pressure
    pelvic region M79.9
    shoulder region M79.9
    specified type NEC M79.89
    thigh M79.9
    upper arm M79.9
  somatic symptom F45.1
  somatization F45.0
  somatoform F45.9
    pain (persistent) F45.41
    somatization (multiple) (long-lasting) F45.0
    specified NEC F45.8
    undifferentiated F45.1
  somnolence, excessive —*see* Hypersomnia
  specific
    arithmetical F81.2
    developmental, of motor F82
    reading F81.0
    speech and language F80.9
    spelling F81.81
    written expression F81.81
  speech R47.9
    articulation (functional) (specific) F80.0
    developmental F80.9
    specified NEC R47.89
  speech-sound F80.0
  spelling (specific) F81.81
  spine —*see also* Dorsopathy
    ligamentous or muscular attachments, peripheral —*see* Enthesopathy, spinal
    specified NEC —*see* Dorsopathy, specified NEC
  stereotyped, habit or movement F98.4
  stimulant use (other) (unspecified)
    mild F15.10
      in remission (early) (sustained) F15.11
    moderate or severe F15.20
      in remission (early) (sustained) F15.21
  stomach (functional) —*see* Disorder, gastric
  stress F43.9
    acute F43.0
    post-traumatic F43.10
      acute F43.11
      chronic F43.12
  substance use (other) (unknown)
    mild F19.10
      with substance-induced
        anxiety disorder F19.180
        bipolar and related disorder F19.14
        depressive disorder F19.14

Disorder *(continued)*
  substance use *(continued)*
    mild *(continued)*
      with substance-induced *(continued)*
        major neurocognitive disorder F19.17
        mild neurocognitive disorder F19.188
        obsessive-compulsive and related disorder F19.188
        sexual dysfunction F19.181
        substance intoxication F19.129
        substance intoxication delirium F19.121
    moderate or severe F19.20
      with substance-induced
        anxiety disorder F19.280
        bipolar and related disorder F19.24
        depressive disorder F19.24
        major neurocognitive disorder F19.27
        mild neurocognitive disorder F19.288
        obsessive-compulsive and related disorder F19.288
        sexual dysfunction F19.281
    in remission (early) (sustained) F19.21
    substance intoxication F19.229
    substance intoxication delirium F19.221
  sulfur-bearing amino-acid metabolism E72.10
  sweat gland (eccrine) L74.9
    apocrine L75.9
      specified NEC L75.8
    specified NEC L74.8
  synovium M67.90
    acromioclavicular M67.91-
    ankle M67.97-
    elbow M67.92-
    foot M67.97-
    forearm M67.93-
    hand M67.94-
    hip M67.95-
    knee M67.96-
    multiple sites M67.99
    rupture —*see* Rupture, synovium
    shoulder M67.91-
    specified type NEC M67.80
      acromioclavicular M67.81-
      ankle M67.87-
      elbow M67.82-
      foot M67.87-
      hand M67.84-
      hip M67.85-
      knee M67.86-
      multiple sites M67.89
      wrist M67.83-
    synovitis —*see* Synovitis
    upper arm M67.92-
    wrist M67.93-
  temperature regulation, newborn P81.9
    specified NEC P81.8
  temporomandibular joint M26.60-
  tendon M67.90
    acromioclavicular M67.91-
    ankle M67.97-
    contracture —*see* Contracture, tendon
    elbow M67.92-
    foot M67.97-
    forearm M67.93-
    hand M67.94-
    hip M67.95-
    knee M67.96-
    multiple sites M67.99

Disorder (continued)
  tendon (continued)
    rupture —see Rupture, tendon
    shoulder M67.91-
    specified type NEC M67.80
      acromioclavicular M67.81-
      ankle M67.87-
      elbow M67.82-
      foot M67.87-
      hand M67.84-
      hip M67.85-
      knee M67.86-
      multiple sites M67.89
      trunk M67.88
      wrist M67.83-
    synovitis —see Synovitis
    tendinitis —see Tendinitis
    tenosynovitis —see Tenosynovitis
    trunk M67.98
    upper arm M67.92-
    wrist M67.93-
  thoracic root (nerve) NEC G54.3
  thyrocalcitonin hypersecretion E07.0
  thyroid (gland) E07.9
    function NEC, neonatal, transitory P72.2
    iodine-deficiency related E01.8
    specified NEC E07.89
  tic —see Tic
  tobacco use
    chewing tobacco (mild) (moderate) (severe)
      in remission (early) (sustained) F17.221
    cigarettes (mild) (moderate) (severe)
      in remission (early) (sustained) F17.211
    mild F17.200
      in remission (early) (sustained) F17.201
    moderate F17.200
      in remission (early) (sustained) F17.201
    severe F17.200
      in remission (early) (sustained) F17.201
    specified product NEC (mild) (moderate) (severe)
      in remission (early) (sustained) F17.291
  tooth K08.9
    development K00.9
      specified NEC K00.8
    eruption K00.6
  Tourette's F95.2
  trance and possession F44.89
  transvestic F65.1
  trauma and stressor-related NOS F43.9
    other specified F43.89
    unspecified F43.9
  tricuspid (valve) —see Endocarditis, tricuspid
  tryptophan metabolism E70.5
  tubular, phosphate-losing N25.0
  tubulo-interstitial (in)
    brucellosis A23.9 [N16]
    cystinosis E72.04
    diphtheria A36.84
    glycogen storage disease E74.00 [N16]
    leukemia NEC C95.9- [N16]
    lymphoma NEC C85.9- [N16]
    mixed cryoglobulinemia D89.1 [N16]
    multiple myeloma C90.0- [N16]
    Salmonella infection A02.25
    sarcoidosis D86.84
    sepsis A41.9 [N16]
      streptococcal A40.9 [N16]

Disorder (continued)
  tubulo-interstitial (continued)
    systemic lupus erythematosus M32.15
    toxoplasmosis B58.83
    transplant rejection T86.91 [N16]
    Wilson's disease E83.01 [N16]
  tubulo-renal function, impaired N25.9
    specified NEC N25.89
  tympanic membrane H73.9-
    atrophy —see Atrophy, tympanic membrane
    infection —see Myringitis
    perforation —see Perforation, tympanum
    specified NEC H73.89-
  unsocialized aggressive F91.1
  urea cycle metabolism E72.20
    argininemia E72.21
    arginosuccinic aciduria E72.22
    citrullinemia E72.23
    ornithine transcarbamylase deficiency E72.4
    other specified E72.29
  ureter (in) N28.9
    schistosomiasis B65.0 [N29]
    tuberculosis A18.11
  urethra N36.9
    specified NEC N36.8
  urinary system N39.9
    specified NEC N39.8
  valve, heart
    aortic —see Endocarditis, aortic
    mitral —see Endocarditis, mitral
    pulmonary —see Endocarditis, pulmonary
    rheumatic
      aortic —see Endocarditis, aortic, rheumatic
      mitral —see Endocarditis, mitral
      pulmonary —see Endocarditis, pulmonary, rheumatic
      tricuspid —see Endocarditis, tricuspid
    tricuspid —see Endocarditis, tricuspid
  vestibular function H81.9-
    specified NEC —see subcategory H81.8
    in diseases classified elsewhere H82.-
    vertigo —see Vertigo
  vision, binocular H53.30
    abnormal retinal correspondence H53.31
    diplopia H53.2
    fusion with defective stereopsis H53.32
    simultaneous perception H53.33
    suppression H53.34
  visual
    cortex
      blindness H47.619
        left brain H47.612
        right brain H47.611
        due to
          inflammatory disorder H47.629
            left brain H47.622
            right brain H47.621
          neoplasm H47.639
            left brain H47.632
            right brain H47.631
          vascular disorder H47.649
            left brain H47.642
            right brain H47.641
    pathway H47.9

Disorder (continued)
  visual (continued)
    pathway (continued)
      due to
        inflammatory disorder H47.51-
        neoplasm H47.52-
        vascular disorder H47.53-
    optic chiasm —see Disorder, optic, chiasm
  vitreous body H43.9
    crystalline deposits —see Deposit, crystalline
    degeneration —see Degeneration, vitreous
    hemorrhage —see Hemorrhage, vitreous
    opacities —see Opacity, vitreous
    prolapse —see Prolapse, vitreous
    specified type NEC H43.89
  voice R49.9
    specified type NEC R49.8
  volatile solvent use
    due to drug abuse —see Abuse, drug, inhalant
    due to drug dependence —see Dependence, drug, inhalant
  voyeuristic F65.3
  white blood cells D72.9
    specified NEC D72.89
  withdrawing, child or adolescent F40.10

Disorientation R41.0

Displacement, displaced
  acquired traumatic of bone, cartilage, joint, tendon NEC —see Dislocation
  adrenal gland (congenital) Q89.1
  appendix, retrocecal (congenital) Q43.8
  auricle (congenital) Q17.4
  bladder (acquired) N32.89
    congenital Q64.19
  brachial plexus (congenital) Q07.8
  brain stem, caudal (congenital) Q04.8
  canaliculus (lacrimalis), congenital Q10.6
  cardia through esophageal hiatus (congenital) Q40.1
  cerebellum, caudal (congenital) Q04.8
  cervix —see Malposition, uterus
  colon (congenital) Q43.3
  device, implant or graft (see also Complications, by site and type, mechanical) T85.628
    arterial graft NEC —see Complication, cardiovascular device, mechanical, vascular
    breast (implant) T85.42
    catheter NEC T85.628
      dialysis (renal) T82.42
        intraperitoneal T85.621
      infusion NEC T82.524
        spinal (epidural) (subdural) T85.620
      urinary
        cystostomy T83.020
        Hopkins T83.028
        ileostomy T83.028
        indwelling T83.021
        nephrostomy T83.022
        specified NEC T83.028
        urostomy T83.028
    electronic (electrode) (pulse generator) (stimulator) —see Complication, electronic stimulator

Displacement, displaced (continued)
  device, implant or graft (continued)
    fixation, internal (orthopedic) NEC —see Complication, fixation device, mechanical
    gastrointestinal —see Complications, prosthetic device, mechanical, gastrointestinal device
    genital NEC T83.428
      intrauterine contraceptive device (string) T83.32
      penile prosthesis (cylinder) (implanted) (pump) (resevoir) T83.420
      testicular prosthesis T83.421
    heart NEC —see Complication, cardiovascular device, mechanical
    joint prosthesis —see Complications, joint prosthesis, mechanical
    ocular —see Complications, prosthetic device, mechanical, ocular device
    orthopedic NEC —see Complication, orthopedic, device or graft, mechanical
    specified NEC T85.628
    urinary NEC T83.128
      graft T83.22
      sphincter, implanted T83.121
      stent (ileal conduit) (nephroureteral) T83.123
      ureteral indwelling T83.122
    vascular NEC —see Complication, cardiovascular device, mechanical
    ventricular intracranial shunt T85.02
  electronic stimulator
    bone T84.320
    cardiac —see Complications, cardiac device, electronic
    nervous system —see Complication, prosthetic device, mechanical, electronic nervous system stimulator
    urinary —see Complications, electronic stimulator, urinary
  esophageal mucosa into cardia of stomach, congenital Q39.8
  esophagus (acquired) K22.89
    congenital Q39.8
  eyeball (acquired) (lateral) (old) —see Displacement, globe
    congenital Q15.8
    current —see Avulsion, eye
  fallopian tube (acquired) N83.4-
    congenital Q50.6
    opening (congenital) Q50.6
  gallbladder (congenital) Q44.1
  gastric mucosa (congenital) Q40.2
  globe (acquired) (old) (lateral) H05.21-
    current —see Avulsion, eye
  heart (congenital) Q24.8
    acquired I51.89
  hymen (upward) (congenital) Q52.4
  intervertebral disc NEC
    with myelopathy —see Disorder, disc, with, myelopathy
    cervical, cervicothoracic (with) M50.20
      myelopathy —see Disorder, disc, cervical, with myelopathy
      neuritis, radiculitis or radiculopathy —see Disorder, disc, cervical, with neuritis

Displacement, displaced (continued)
  intervertebral disc NEC (continued)
    due to trauma —see Dislocation, vertebra
    lumbar region M51.26
      with
        myelopathy M51.06
        neuritis, radiculitis, radiculopathy or sciatica M51.16
    lumbosacral region M51.27
      with
        neuritis, radiculitis, radiculopathy or sciatica M51.17
    sacrococcygeal region M53.3
    thoracic region M51.24
      with
        myelopathy M51.04
        neuritis, radiculitis, radiculopathy M51.14
    thoracolumbar region M51.25
      with
        myelopathy M51.05
        neuritis, radiculitis, radiculopathy M51.15
  intrauterine device (string) T83.32
  kidney (acquired) N28.83
    congenital Q63.2
  lachrymal, lacrimal apparatus or duct (congenital) Q10.6
  lens, congenital Q12.1
  macula (congenital) Q14.1
  Meckel's diverticulum Q43.0
    malignant —see Table of Neoplasms, small intestine, malignant
  nail (congenital) Q84.6
    acquired L60.8
  opening of Wharton's duct in mouth Q38.4
  organ or site, congenital NEC —see Malposition, congenital
  ovary (acquired) N83.4-
    congenital Q50.39
      free in peritoneal cavity (congenital) Q50.39
      into hernial sac N83.4-
  oviduct (acquired) N83.4-
    congenital Q50.6
  parathyroid (gland) E21.4
  parotid gland (congenital) Q38.4
  punctum lacrimale (congenital) Q10.6
  sacro-iliac (joint) (congenital) Q74.2
    current injury S33.2
    old —see subcategory M53.2
  salivary gland (any) (congenital) Q38.4
  spleen (congenital) Q89.09
  stomach, congenital Q40.2
  sublingual duct Q38.4
  tongue (downward) (congenital) Q38.3
  tooth, teeth, fully erupted M26.30
    horizontal M26.33
    vertical M26.34
  trachea (congenital) Q32.1
  ureter or ureteric opening or orifice (congenital) Q62.62
  uterine opening of oviducts or fallopian tubes Q50.6
  uterus, uterine —see Malposition, uterus
  ventricular septum Q21.0
    with rudimentary ventricle Q20.4

Disproportion
  between native and reconstructed breast N65.1
  fiber-type G71.20
    congenital G71.29

Disruptio uteri —see Rupture, uterus
Disruption (of)
  ciliary body NEC H21.89
  closure of
    cornea T81.31
    craniotomy T81.32
    fascia (muscular) (superficial) T81.32
    internal organ or tissue T81.32
    laceration (external) (internal) T81.33
    ligament T81.32
    mucosa T81.31
    muscle or muscle flap T81.32
    ribs or rib cage T81.32
    skin and subcutaneous tissue (full-thickness) (superficial) T81.31
    skull T81.32
    sternum (sternotomy) T81.32
    tendon T81.32
    traumatic laceration (external) (internal) T81.33
  family Z63.8
    due to
      absence of family member due to military deployment Z63.31
      absence of family member NEC Z63.32
      alcoholism and drug addiction in family Z63.72
      bereavement Z63.4
      death (assumed) or disappearance of family member Z63.4
      divorce or separation Z63.5
      drug addiction in family Z63.72
      return of family member from military deployment (current or past conflict) Z63.71
      stressful life events NEC Z63.79
  iris NEC H21.89
  ligament(s) —see also Sprain
    knee
      current injury —see Dislocation, knee
      old (chronic) —see Derangement, knee, ligament, instability, chronic
      spontaneous NEC —see Derangement, knee, disruption ligament
  ossicular chain —see Discontinuity, ossicles, ear
  pelvic ring (stable) S32.810
    unstable S32.811
  wound T81.30
    episiotomy O90.1
    operation T81.31
      cesarean O90.0
      external operation wound (superficial) T81.31
      internal operation wound (deep) T81.32
    perineal (obstetric) O90.1
    traumatic injury repair T81.33
    traumatic injury wound repair T81.33

Dissatisfaction with
  employment Z56.9
  school environment Z55.4

Dissecting —see condition
Dissection
  aorta I71.00

Dissection (continued)
  aorta (continued)
    abdominal I71.02
    thoracic I71.019
      aortic arch I71.011
      ascending aorta I71.010
      descending thoracic aorta I71.012
    thoracoabdominal I71.03
  artery I77.70
    basilar (trunk) I77.75
    carotid I77.71
    cerebral (nonruptured) I67.0
      ruptured —see Hemorrhage, intracranial, subarachnoid
    coronary I25.42
    extremity
      lower I77.77
      upper I77.76
    iliac I77.72
    precerebral
      congenital (nonruptured) Q28.1
      specified site NEC I77.75
    renal I77.73
    specified NEC I77.79
    vertebral I77.74
  precerebral artery, congenital (nonruptured) Q28.1
  Heartland A93.8
  traumatic —see Wound, open, by site
  vascular I99.8
  wound —see Wound, open

Disseminated —see condition

Dissociation
  auriculoventricular or atrioventricular (AV) (any degree) (isorhythmic) I45.89
    with heart block I44.2
  interference I45.89

Dissociative reaction, state F44.9

Dissolution, vertebra —see Osteoporosis

Distension, distention
  abdomen R14.0
  bladder N32.89
  cecum K63.89
  colon K63.89
  gallbladder K82.8
  intestine K63.89
  kidney N28.89
  liver K76.89
  seminal vesicle N50.89
  stomach K31.89
    acute K31.0
    psychogenic F45.8
  ureter —see Dilatation, ureter
  uterus N85.8

Distoma hepaticum infestation B66.3

Distomiasis B66.9
  bile passages B66.3
  hemic B65.9
  hepatic B66.3
    due to Clonorchis sinensis B66.1
  intestinal B66.5
  liver B66.3
    due to Clonorchis sinensis B66.1
  lung B66.4
  pulmonary B66.4

Distomolar (fourth molar) K00.1

Disto-occlusion (Division I) (Division II) M26.212

Distortion(s) (congenital)
  adrenal (gland) Q89.1
  arm NEC Q68.8
  bile duct or passage Q44.5
  bladder Q64.79
  brain Q04.9

Distortion (continued)
  cervix (uteri) Q51.9
  chest (wall) Q67.8
    bones Q76.8
  clavicle Q74.0
  clitoris Q52.6
  coccyx Q76.49
  common duct Q44.5
  coronary Q24.5
  cystic duct Q44.5
  ear (auricle) (external) Q17.3
    inner Q16.5
    middle Q16.4
      ossicles Q16.3
  endocrine NEC Q89.2
  eustachian tube Q17.8
  eye (adnexa) Q15.8
  face bone(s) NEC Q75.8
  fallopian tube Q50.6
  femur NEC Q68.8
  fibula NEC Q68.8
  finger(s) Q68.1
  foot Q66.9-
  genitalia, genital organ(s)
    female Q52.8
      external Q52.79
      internal NEC Q52.8
  gyri Q04.8
  hand bone(s) Q68.1
  heart (auricle) (ventricle) Q24.8
    valve (cusp) Q24.8
  hepatic duct Q44.5
  humerus NEC Q68.8
  hymen Q52.4
  intrafamilial communications Z63.8
  jaw NEC M26.89
  labium (majus) (minus) Q52.79
  leg NEC Q68.8
  lens Q12.8
  liver Q44.79
  lumbar spine Q76.49
    with disproportion O33.8
      causing obstructed labor O65.0
  lumbosacral (joint) (region) Q76.49
    kyphosis —see Kyphosis, congenital
    lordosis —see Lordosis, congenital
  nerve Q07.8
  nose Q30.8
  organ
    of Corti Q16.5
    or site not listed —see Anomaly, by site
  ossicles, ear Q16.3
  oviduct Q50.6
  pancreas Q45.3
  parathyroid (gland) Q89.2
  pituitary (gland) Q89.2
  radius NEC Q68.8
  sacroiliac joint Q74.2
  sacrum Q76.49
  scapula Q74.0
  shoulder girdle Q74.0
  skull bone(s) NEC Q75.8
    with
      anencephalus Q00.0
      encephalocele —see Encephalocele
      hydrocephalus Q03.9
        with spina bifida —see Spina bifida, with hydrocephalus
      microcephaly Q02
  spinal cord Q06.8
  spine Q76.49
    kyphosis —see Kyphosis, congenital
    lordosis —see Lordosis, congenital

Distortion (continued)
   spleen Q89.09
   sternum NEC Q76.7
   thorax (wall) Q67.8
      bony Q76.8
   thymus (gland) Q89.2
   thyroid (gland) Q89.2
   tibia NEC Q68.8
   toe(s) Q66.9-
   tongue Q38.3
   trachea (cartilage) Q32.1
   ulna NEC Q68.8
   ureter Q62.8
   urethra Q64.79
      causing obstruction Q64.39
   uterus Q51.9
   vagina Q52.4
   vertebra Q76.49
      kyphosis —*see* Kyphosis,
         congenital
      lordosis —*see* Lordosis,
         congenital
   visual —*see also* Disturbance,
      vision
      shape and size H53.15
   vulva Q52.79
   wrist (bones) (joint) Q68.8

Distress
   abdomen —*see* Pain, abdominal
   acute respiratory R06.03
      syndrome (adult) (child) J80
   epigastric R10.13
   fetal P84
      complicating pregnancy —*see*
         Stress, fetal
   gastrointestinal (functional) K30
      psychogenic F45.8
   intestinal (functional) NOS K59.9
      psychogenic F45.8
   maternal, during labor and delivery
      O75.0
   relationship, with spouse or
      intimate partner Z63.0
   respiratory (adult) (child) R06.03
      newborn P22.9
         specified NEC P22.8
      orthopnea R06.01
      psychogenic F45.8
      shortness of breath R06.02
      specified type NEC R06.09

Distribution vessel, atypical Q27.9
   coronary artery Q24.5
   precerebral Q28.1

Distichiasis L68.8

Disturbance(s) —*see also* Disease
   absorption K90.9
      calcium E58
      carbohydrate K90.49
      fat K90.49
         pancreatic K90.3
      protein K90.49
      starch K90.49
      vitamin —*see* Deficiency, vitamin
   acid-base equilibrium E87.8
      mixed E87.4
   activity and attention (with
      hyperkinesis) —*see* Disorder,
      attention-deficit hyperactivity
   amino acid transport E72.00
   assimilation, food K90.9
   auditory nerve, except deafness
      —*see* subcategory H93.3
   behavior —*see* Disorder, conduct
   blood clotting (mechanism) (*see*
      also Defect, coagulation) D68.9
   cerebral
      nerve —*see* Disorder, nerve,
         cranial
      status, newborn P91.9
         specified NEC P91.88

Disturbance (continued)
   circulatory I99.9
   conduct (*see also* Disorder,
      conduct) F91.9
      adjustment reaction —*see*
         Disorder, adjustment
      compulsive F63.9
      disruptive F91.9
      hyperkinetic —*see* Disorder,
         attention-deficit hyperactivity
      socialized F91.2
      specified NEC F91.8
      unsocialized F91.1
   coordination R27.8
   cranial nerve —*see* Disorder, nerve,
      cranial
   deep sensibility —*see* Disturbance,
      sensation
   digestive K30
      psychogenic F45.8
   electrolyte —*see also* Imbalance,
      electrolyte
      newborn, transitory P74.49
         hyperammonemia P74.6
         hyperchloremia P74.421
         hyperchloremic metabolic
            acidosis P74.421
         hypochloremia P74.422
         potassium balance
            hyperkalemia P74.31
            hypokalemia P74.32
         sodium balance
            hypernatremia P74.21
            hyponatremia P74.22
         specified type NEC P74.49
   emotions specific to childhood and
      adolescence F93.9
      with
         anxiety and fearfulness NEC
            F93.8
         elective mutism F94.0
         oppositional disorder F91.3
         sensitivity (withdrawal)
            F40.10
         shyness F40.10
         social withdrawal F40.10
         involving relationship problems
            F93.8
      mixed F93.8
      specified NEC F93.8
   endocrine (gland) E34.9
      neonatal, transitory P72.9
         specified NEC P72.8
   equilibrium R42
   fructose metabolism E74.10
   gait —*see* Gait
      hysterical F44.4
      psychogenic F44.4
   gastrointestinal (functional) K30
      psychogenic F45.8
   habit, child F98.9
   hearing, except deafness and
      tinnitus —*see* Abnormal,
      auditory perception
   heart, functional (conditions in
      I44-I50)
      due to presence of (cardiac)
         prosthesis I97.19-
      postoperative I97.89
         cardiac surgery (*see also*
            Infarct, myocardium,
            associated with
            revascularization procedure)
            I97.19-
   hormones E34.9
   innervation uterus (parasympathetic)
      (sympathetic) N85.8
   keratinization NEC
      gingiva K05.10
         nonplaque induced K05.11
         plaque induced K05.10

Disturbance (continued)
   keratinization NEC (continued)
      lip K13.0
      oral (mucosa) (soft tissue)
         K13.29
      tongue K13.29
   learning (specific) —*see* Disorder,
      learning
   memory —*see* Amnesia
      mild, following organic brain
         damage F06.8
   mental F99
      associated with diseases
         classified elsewhere F54
   metabolism E88.9
      with
         abortion —*see* Abortion, by
            type with other specified
            complication
         ectopic pregnancy O08.5
         molar pregnancy O08.5
      amino-acid E72.9
         aromatic E70.9
         branched-chain E71.2
         straight-chain E72.89
         sulfur-bearing E72.10
      ammonia E72.20
      arginine E72.21
      arginosuccinic acid E72.22
      carbohydrate E74.9
      cholesterol E78.9
      citrulline E72.23
      cystathionine E72.19
      general E88.9
      glutamine E72.89
      histidine E70.40
      homocystine E72.19
      hydroxylysine E72.3
      in labor or delivery O75.89
      iron E83.10
      lipoid E78.9
      lysine E72.3
      methionine E72.19
      neonatal, transitory P74.9
         calcium and magnesium P71.9
            specified type NEC P71.8
         carbohydrate metabolism
            P70.9
            specified type NEC P70.8
         specified NEC P74.8
      ornithine E72.4
      phosphate E83.39
      sodium NEC E87.8
      threonine E72.89
      tryptophan E70.5
      tyrosine E70.20
      urea cycle E72.20
   motor R29.2
   nervous, functional R45.0
   neuromuscular mechanism (eye),
      due to syphilis A52.15
   nutritional E63.9
   nail L60.3
   ocular motion H51.9
      psychogenic F45.8
   oculogyric H51.8
      psychogenic F45.8
   oculomotor H51.9
      psychogenic F45.8
   olfactory nerve R43.1
   optic nerve NEC —*see* Disorder,
      nerve, optic
   oral epithelium, including tongue
      NEC K13.29
   perceptual due to
      alcohol withdrawal F10.232
      amphetamine intoxication
         F15.922
         in
            abuse F15.122
            dependence F15.222

Disturbance (continued)
   perceptual due to (continued)
      anxiolytic withdrawal F13.232
      cannabis intoxication (acute)
         F12.922
         in
            abuse F12.122
            dependence F12.222
      cocaine intoxication (acute)
         F14.922
         in
            abuse F14.122
            dependence F14.222
      hypnotic withdrawal F13.232
      opioid intoxication (acute)
         F19.122
      phencyclidine intoxication
         (acute) F16.122
      sedative withdrawal F13.232
   personality (pattern) (trait) —*see
      also* Disorder, personality F60.9
      following organic brain damage
         F07.9
   polyglandular E31.9
      specified NEC E31.8
   potassium balance, newborn
      hyperkalemia P74.31
      hypokalemia P74.32
   psychogenic F45.9
   psychomotor F44.4
   psychophysical visual H53.16
   pupillary —*see* Anomaly, pupil,
      function
   reflex R29.2
   rhythm, heart I49.9
   salivary secretion K11.7
   sensation (cold) (heat)
      (localization) (tactile
      discrimination) (texture)
      (vibratory) NEC R20.9
      hysterical F44.6
      skin R20.9
         anesthesia R20.0
         hyperesthesia R20.3
         hypoesthesia R20.1
         paresthesia R20.2
         specified type NEC R20.8
      smell R43.9
         and taste (mixed) R43.8
         anosmia R43.0
         parosmia R43.1
         specified NEC R43.8
      taste R43.9
         and smell (mixed) R43.8
         parageusia R43.2
         specified NEC R43.8
   sensory —*see* Disturbance,
      sensation
   situational (transient) —*see also*
      Disorder, adjustment
      acute F43.0
   sleep G47.9
      nonorganic origin F51.9
   smell —*see* Disturbance, sensation,
      smell
   sociopathic F60.2
   sodium balance, newborn
      hypernatremia P74.21
      hyponatremia P74.22
   speech R47.9
      developmental F80.9
      specified NEC R47.89
   stomach (functional) K31.9
   sympathetic (nerve) G90.9
   taste —*see* Disturbance, sensation,
      taste
   temperature
      regulation, newborn P81.9
         specified NEC P81.8
      sense R20.8
         hysterical F44.6

Disturbance (continued)
- tooth
  - eruption K00.6
  - formation K00.4
  - structure, hereditary NEC K00.5
- touch —see Disturbance, sensation
- vascular I99.9
  - arteriosclerotic —see Arteriosclerosis
- vasomotor I73.9
- vasospastic I73.9
- vision, visual H53.9
  - following
    - cerebral infarction I69.398
    - cerebrovascular disease I69.998
      - specified NEC I69.898
    - intracerebral hemorrhage I69.198
    - nontraumatic intracranial hemorrhage NEC I69.298
    - specified disease NEC I69.898
    - subarachnoid hemorrhage I69.098
  - psychophysical H53.16
  - specified NEC H53.8
  - subjective H53.10
    - day blindness H53.11
    - discomfort H53.14-
    - distortions of shape and size H53.15
    - loss
      - sudden H53.13-
      - transient H53.12-
    - specified type NEC H53.19
- voice R49.9
  - psychogenic F44.4
  - specified NEC R49.8

Diuresis R35.89

Diver's palsy, paralysis or squeeze T70.3

Diverticulitis (acute) K57.92
- bladder —see Cystitis
- ileum —see Diverticulitis, intestine, small
- intestine K57.92
  - with
    - abscess, perforation K57.80
      - with bleeding K57.81
    - bleeding K57.93
  - congenital Q43.8
  - large K57.32
    - with
      - abscess, perforation K57.20
        - with bleeding K57.21
      - bleeding K57.33
      - small intestine K57.52
        - with
          - abscess, perforation K57.40
            - with bleeding K57.41
          - bleeding K57.53
  - small K57.12
    - with
      - abscess, perforation K57.00
        - with bleeding K57.01
      - bleeding K57.13
      - large intestine K57.52
        - with
          - abscess, perforation K57.40
            - with bleeding K57.41
          - bleeding K57.53

Diverticulosis K57.90
- with bleeding K57.91

Diverticulosis (continued)
- large intestine K57.30
  - with
    - bleeding K57.31
    - small intestine K57.50
      - with bleeding K57.51
- small intestine K57.10
  - with
    - bleeding K57.11
    - large intestine K57.50
      - with bleeding K57.51

Diverticulum, diverticula (multiple) K57.90
- appendix (noninflammatory) K38.2
- bladder (sphincter) N32.3
  - congenital Q64.6
- bronchus (congenital) Q32.4
  - acquired J98.09
- calyx, calyceal (kidney) N28.89
- cardia (stomach) K31.4
- cecum —see Diverticulosis, intestine, large
  - congenital Q43.8
- colon —see Diverticulosis, intestine, large
  - congenital Q43.8
- duodenum —see Diverticulosis, intestine, small
  - congenital Q43.8
- epiphrenic (esophagus) K22.5
- esophagus (congenital) Q39.6
  - acquired (epiphrenic) (pulsion) (traction) K22.5
- eustachian tube —see Disorder, eustachian tube, specified NEC
- fallopian tube N83.8
- gastric K31.4
- heart (congenital) Q24.8
- ileum —see Diverticulosis, intestine, small
- jejunum —see Diverticulosis, intestine, small
- kidney (pelvis) (calyces) N28.89
  - with calculus —see Calculus, kidney
- Meckel's (displaced) (hypertrophic) Q43.0
  - malignant —see Table of Neoplasms, small intestine, malignant
- midthoracic K22.5
- organ or site, congenital NEC —see Distortion
- pericardium (congenital) (cyst) Q24.8
  - acquired I31.8
- pharyngoesophageal (congenital) Q39.6
  - acquired K22.5
- pharynx (congenital) Q38.7
- rectosigmoid —see Diverticulosis, intestine, large
  - congenital Q43.8
- rectum —see Diverticulosis, intestine, large
- Rokitansky's K22.5
- seminal vesicle N50.89
- sigmoid —see Diverticulosis, intestine, large
  - congenital Q43.8
- stomach (acquired) K31.4
  - congenital Q40.2
- trachea (acquired) J39.8
- ureter (acquired) N28.89
  - congenital Q62.8
- ureterovesical orifice N28.89
- urethra (acquired) N36.1
  - congenital Q64.79
- ventricle, left (congenital) Q24.8

Diverticulum, diverticula (continued)
- vesical N32.3
  - congenital Q64.6
- Zenker's (esophagus) K22.5

Division
- cervix uteri (acquired) N88.8
- glans penis Q55.69
- labia minora (congenital) Q52.79
- ligament (partial or complete) (current) —see also Sprain
  - with open wound —see Wound, open
- muscle (partial or complete) (current) —see also Injury, muscle
  - with open wound —see Wound, open
- nerve (traumatic) —see Injury, nerve
- spinal cord —see Injury, spinal cord, by region
- vein I87.8

Divorce, causing family disruption Z63.5

Dix-Hallpike neurolabyrinthitis —see Neuronitis, vestibular

Dizziness R42
- hysterical F44.89
- psychogenic F45.8

DMAC (disseminated mycobacterium avium-intracellulare complex) A31.2

DNR (do not resuscitate) Z66

Doan-Wiseman syndrome (primary splenic neutropenia) —see Agranulocytosis

Doehle-Heller aortitis A52.02

Dog bite —see Bite

Dohle body panmyelopathic syndrome D72.0

Dolichocephaly Q67.2
- non-deformational Q75.01

Dolichocolon Q43.8

Dolichostenomelia —see Syndrome, Marfan

Donohue's syndrome E34.8

Donor (organ or tissue) Z52.9
- blood (whole) Z52.000
  - autologous Z52.010
  - specified component (lymphocytes) (platelets) NEC Z52.008
    - autologous Z52.018
    - specified donor NEC Z52.098
  - specified donor NEC Z52.090
  - stem cells Z52.001
    - autologous Z52.011
    - specified donor NEC Z52.091
- bone Z52.20
  - autologous Z52.21
  - marrow Z52.3
  - specified type NEC Z52.29
- cornea Z52.5
- egg (Oocyte) Z52.819
  - age 35 and over Z52.812
    - anonymous recipient Z52.812
    - designated recipient Z52.813
  - under age 35 Z52.810
    - anonymous recipient Z52.810
    - designated recipient Z52.811
- kidney Z52.4
- liver Z52.6
- lung Z52.89
- lymphocyte —see Donor, blood, specified components NEC

Donor (continued)
- Oocyte —see Donor, egg
- platelets Z52.008
- potential, examination of Z00.5
- semen Z52.89
- skin Z52.10
  - autologous Z52.11
  - specified type NEC Z52.19
- specified organ or tissue NEC Z52.89
- sperm Z52.89

Donovanosis A58

Dorsalgia M54.9
- psychogenic F45.41
- specified NEC M54.89

Dorsopathy M53.9
- deforming M43.9
  - specified NEC —see subcategory M43.8
- specified NEC M53.80
  - cervical region M53.82
  - cervicothoracic region M53.83
  - lumbar region M53.86
  - lumbosacral region M53.87
  - occipito-atlanto-axial region M53.81
  - sacrococcygeal region M53.88
  - thoracic region M53.84
  - thoracolumbar region M53.85

Double
- albumin E88.09
- aortic arch Q25.45
- auditory canal Q17.8
- auricle (heart) Q20.8
- bladder Q64.79
- cervix Q51.820
  - with doubling of uterus (and vagina) Q51.10
    - with obstruction Q51.11
- inlet ventricle Q20.4
- kidney with double pelvis (renal) Q63.0
- meatus urinarius Q64.75
- monster Q89.4
- outlet
  - left ventricle Q20.2
  - right ventricle Q20.1
- pelvis (renal) with double ureter Q62.5
- tongue Q38.3
- ureter (one or both sides) Q62.5
  - with double pelvis (renal) Q62.5
- urethra Q64.74
- urinary meatus Q64.75
- uterus Q51.28
  - with
    - doubling of cervix (and vagina) Q51.10
      - with obstruction Q51.11
    - complete Q51.21
    - in pregnancy or childbirth O34.0-
      - causing obstructed labor O65.5
    - partial Q51.22
    - specified NEC Q51.28
- vagina Q52.10
  - with doubling of uterus (and cervix) Q51.10
    - with obstruction Q51.11
- vision H53.2
- vulva Q52.79

Doubled up Z59.01

Douglas' pouch, cul-de-sac —see condition

Down syndrome Q90.9
- meiotic nondisjunction Q90.0
- mitotic nondisjunction Q90.1
- mosaicism Q90.1
- translocation Q90.2

129

DPD (dihydropyrimidine dehydrogenase deficiency) E88.89
Dracontiasis B72
Dracunculiasis, dracunculosis B72
Dream state, hysterical F44.89
Dreschlera (hawaiiensis) (infection) B43.8
Drepanocytic anemia —see Disease, sickle-cell
Dresbach's syndrome (elliptocytosis) D58.1
Dressler's syndrome I24.1
Drift, ulnar —see Deformity, limb, specified type NEC, forearm
Drinking (alcohol)
  excessive, to excess NEC (without dependence) F10.10
    habitual (continual) (without remission) F10.20
      with remission F10.21
Drip, postnasal (chronic) R09.82
  due to
    allergic rhinitis —see Rhinitis, allergic
    common cold J00
    gastroesophageal reflux —see Reflux, gastroesophageal
    nasopharyngitis —see Nasopharyngitis
    other know condition - code to condition
    sinusitis —see Sinusitis
Droop
  facial R29.810
    cerebrovascular disease I69.992
      cerebral infarction I69.392
      intracerebral hemorrhage I69.192
      nontraumatic intracranial hemorrhage NEC I69.292
      specified disease NEC I69.892
      subarachnoid hemorrhage I69.092
Drop (in)
  attack NEC R55
  finger —see Deformity, finger
  foot —see Deformity, limb, foot, drop
  hematocrit (precipitous) R71.0
  hemoglobin R71.0
  toe —see Deformity, toe, specified NEC
  wrist —see Deformity, limb, wrist drop
Dropped heart beats I45.9
Dropsy, dropsical —see also Hydrops
  abdomen R18.8
  brain —see Hydrocephalus
  cardiac, heart —see Failure, heart, congestive
  gangrenous —see Gangrene
  heart —see Failure, heart, congestive
  kidney —see Nephrosis
  lung —see Edema, lung
  newborn due to isoimmunization P56.0
  pericardium —see Pericarditis
Drowned, drowning (near) T75.1
Drowsiness R40.0
Drug
  abuse counseling and surveillance Z71.51

Drug (continued)
  addiction —see Dependence
  dependence —see Dependence
  habit —see Dependence
  harmful use —see Abuse, drug
  induced fever R50.2
  overdose —see Table of Drugs and Chemicals, by drug, poisoning
  poisoning —see Table of Drugs and Chemicals, by drug, poisoning
  resistant organism infection (see also Resistant, organism, to, drug) Z16.30
  therapy
    long term (current) (prophylactic) —see Therapy, drug long-term (current) (prophylactic)
    short term - omit code
  wrong substance given or taken in error —see Table of Drugs and Chemicals, by drug, poisoning
Drunkenness (without dependence) F10.129
  acute in alcoholism F10.229
  chronic (without remission) F10.20
    with remission F10.21
  pathological (without dependence) F10.129
    with dependence F10.229
  sleep F51.9
Drusen
  macula (degenerative) (retina) —see Degeneration, macula, drusen
  optic disc H47.32-
Dry, dryness —see also condition
  larynx J38.7
  mouth R68.2
    due to dehydration E86.0
  nose J34.89
  socket (teeth) M27.3
  throat J39.2
DSAP L56.5
Duane's syndrome H50.81-
Dubin-Johnson disease or syndrome E80.6
Dubois' disease (thymus gland) A50.59 [E35]
Dubowitz' syndrome Q87.19
Duchenne-Aran muscular atrophy G12.21
Duchenne-Griesinger disease G71.01
Duchenne's
  disease or syndrome
    motor neuron disease G12.22
    muscular dystrophy G71.01
    locomotor ataxia (syphilitic) A52.11
  paralysis
    birth injury P14.0
    due to or associated with
      motor neuron disease G12.22
      muscular dystrophy G71.01
Ducrey's chancre A57
Duct, ductus —see condition
Duhring's disease (dermatitis herpetiformis) L13.0
Dullness, cardiac (decreased) (increased) R01.2
Dumb ague —see Malaria
Dumbness —see Aphasia
Dumdum fever B55.0
Dumping syndrome (postgastrectomy) K91.1

Duodenitis (nonspecific) (peptic) K29.80
  with bleeding K29.81
  erosive —see Ulcer, duodenum
Duodenocholangitis —see Cholangitis
Duodenum, duodenal —see condition
Duplay's bursitis or periarthritis M75.0
Duplication, duplex —see also Accessory
  alimentary tract Q45.8
  anus Q43.4
  appendix (and cecum) Q43.4
  biliary duct (any) Q44.5
  bladder Q64.79
  cecum (and appendix) Q43.4
  cervix Q51.820
  chromosome NEC —see also Trisomy
    with complex rearrangements NEC Q92.5
    seen only at prometaphase Q92.8
  cystic duct Q44.5
  digestive organs Q45.8
  esophagus Q39.8
  frontonasal process Q75.8
  intestine (large) (small) Q43.4
  kidney Q63.0
  liver Q44.79
  pancreas Q45.3
  penis Q55.69
  respiratory organs NEC Q34.8
  salivary duct Q38.4
  spinal cord (incomplete) Q06.2
  stomach Q40.2
Dupré's disease (meningism) R29.1
Dupuytren's contraction or disease M72.0
Durand-Nicolas-Favre disease A55
Duroziez's disease (congenital mitral stenosis) Q23.2
Durotomy (inadvertent) (incidental) G97.41
Dutton's relapsing fever (West African) A68.1
Dwarfism (see also Stature, short) E34.328
  achondroplastic Q77.4
  congenital (see also Short, stature) E34.328
  constitutional E34.31
  hypochondroplastic Q77.4
  hypophyseal E23.0
  infantile (see also Short, stature) E34.328
  Laron-type (see also Short, stature) E34.321
  Lorain (-Levi) type E23.0
  metatropic Q77.8
  nephrotic-glycosuric (with hypophosphatemic rickets) E72.09
  nutritional E45
  pancreatic K86.89
  pituitary E23.0
  renal N25.0
  thanatophoric Q77.1
Dyke-Young anemia (secondary) (symptomatic) D59.19
Dysacusis —see Abnormal, auditory perception
Dysadrenocortism E27.9
  hyperfunction E27.0
Dysarthria R47.1
  following
    cerebral infarction I69.322

Dysarthria (continued)
  following (continued)
    cerebrovascular disease I69.922
      specified disease NEC I69.822
    intracerebral hemorrhage I69.122
    nontraumatic intracranial hemorrhage NEC I69.222
    subarachnoid hemorrhage I69.022
Dysautonomia (familial) G90.1
Dysbarism T70.3
Dysbasia R26.2
  angiosclerotica intermittens I73.9
  hysterical F44.4
  lordotica (progressiva) G24.1
  nonorganic origin F44.4
  psychogenic F44.4
Dysbetalipoproteinemia (familial) E78.2
Dyscalculia R48.8
  developmental F81.2
Dyschezia K59.00
Dyschondroplasia (with hemangiomata) Q78.4
Dyschromia (skin) L81.9
Dyscollagenosis M35.9
Dyscranio-pygo-phalangy Q87.0
Dyscrasia
  blood (with) D75.9
    antepartum hemorrhage —see Hemorrhage, antepartum, with coagulation defect
    newborn P61.9
      specified type NEC P61.8
    intrapartum hemorrhage O67.0
    puerperal, postpartum O72.3
  polyglandular, pluriglandular E31.9
Dysendocrinism E34.9
Dysentery, dysenteric (catarrhal) (diarrhea) (epidemic) (hemorrhagic) (infectious) (sporadic) (tropical) A09
  abscess, liver A06.4
  amebic (see also Amebiasis) A06.0
    with abscess —see Abscess, amebic
    acute A06.0
    chronic A06.1
  arthritis (see also category M01) A09
  bacillary (see also category M01) A03.9
  bacillary A03.9
    arthritis (see also category M01) A03.9
    Boyd A03.2
    Flexner A03.1
    Schmitz (-Stutzer) A03.0
    Shiga (-Kruse) A03.0
    Shigella A03.9
      boydii A03.2
      dysenteriae A03.0
      flexneri A03.1
      group A A03.0
      group B A03.1
      group C A03.2
      group D A03.3
      sonnei A03.3
      specified type NEC A03.8
    Sonne A03.3
    specified type NEC A03.8
  balantidial A07.0
  Balantidium coli A07.0
  Boyd's A03.2
  candidal B37.82
  Chilomastix A07.8

Dysentery, dysenteric (continued)
  Chinese A03.9
  coccidial A07.3
  Dientamoeba (fragilis) A07.8
  Embadomonas A07.8
  Entamoeba, entamebic —see Dysentery, amebic
  Flexner-Boyd A03.2
  Flexner's A03.1
  Giardia lamblia A07.1
  Hiss-Russell A03.1
  Lamblia A07.1
  leishmanial B55.0
  malarial —see Malaria
  metazoal B82.0
  monilial B37.82
  protozoal A07.9
  Salmonella A02.0
  schistosomal B65.1
  Schmitz (-Stutzer) A03.0
  Shiga (-Kruse) A03.0
  Shigella NOS —see Dysentery, bacillary
  Sonne A03.3
  strongyloidiasis B78.0
  trichomonal A07.8
  viral —see also Enteritis, viral A08.4

Dysequilibrium R42

Dysesthesia R20.8
  hysterical F44.6

Dysferlinopathy G71.033

Dysfibrinogenemia (congenital) D68.2

Dysfunction
  adrenal E27.9
    hyperfunction E27.0
  autonomic
    due to alcohol G31.2
    somatoform F45.8
  bladder N31.9
    neurogenic NOS —see Dysfunction, bladder, neuromuscular
    neuromuscular NOS N31.9
      atonic (motor) (sensory) N31.2
      autonomous N31.2
      flaccid N31.2
      nonreflex N31.2
      reflex N31.1
      specified NEC N31.8
      uninhibited N31.0
  bleeding, uterus N93.8
  cerebral G93.89
  chronic
    coronary microvascular I25.85
    lung allograft J4A.9
      mixed J4A.0
      specified NEC J4A.8
  colon K59.9
    psychogenic F45.8
  colostomy K94.03
  coronary microvascular I25.85
    with
      angina pectoris I20.81
      myocardial infarction I21.B
    acute I24.81
    chronic I25.85
  cystic duct K82.8
  cystostomy (stoma) —see Complications, cystostomy
  ejaculatory N53.19
    anejaculatory orgasm N53.13
    painful N53.12
    premature F52.4
    retarded N53.11
  endocrine NOS E34.9
  endometrium N85.8
  enterostomy K94.13
  erectile —see Dysfunction, sexual, male, erectile

Dysfunction (continued)
  feeding, pediatric
    acute R63.31
    chronic R63.32
  gallbladder K82.8
  gastrostomy (stoma) K94.23
  gland, glandular NOS E34.9
    meibomian, of eyelid —see Dysfunction, meibomian gland
  heart I51.89
  hemoglobin D75.89
  hepatic K76.89
  hypophysis E23.7
  hypothalamic NEC E23.3
  ileostomy (stoma) K94.13
  jejunostomy (stoma) K94.13
  kidney —see Disease, renal
  labyrinthine —see subcategory H83.2
  left ventricular, following sudden emotional stress I51.81
  liver K76.89
  male —see Dysfunction, sexual, male
  meibomian gland, of eyelid H02.889
    left H02.886
      lower H02.885
      upper H02.884
      upper and lower eyelids H02.88B
    right H02.883
      lower H02.882
      upper H02.881
      upper and lower eyelids H02.88A
  orgasmic (female) F52.31
    male F52.32
  ovary E28.9
    specified NEC E28.8
  papillary muscle I51.89
  parathyroid E21.4
  physiological NEC R68.89
    psychogenic F59
  pineal gland E34.8
  pituitary (gland) E23.3
  platelets D69.1
  polyglandular E31.9
    specified NEC E31.8
  psychophysiologic F59
  psychosexual F52.9
    with
      dyspareunia F52.6
      premature ejaculation F52.4
      vaginismus F52.5
  pylorus K31.9
  rectum K59.9
    psychogenic F45.8
  reflex (sympathetic) —see Syndrome, pain, complex regional I
  segmental —see Dysfunction, somatic
  senile R54
  sexual (due to) R37
    alcohol F10.981
    amphetamine F15.981
      in
        abuse F15.181
        dependence F15.281
    anxiolytic F13.981
      in
        abuse F13.181
        dependence F13.281
    cocaine F14.981
      in
        abuse F14.181
        dependence F14.281
    excessive sexual drive F52.8
    failure of genital response (male) F52.21
      female F52.22

Dysfunction (continued)
  sexual (continued)
    female N94.9
      aversion F52.1
      dyspareunia N94.10
        psychogenic F52.6
      frigidity F52.22
      nymphomania F52.8
      orgasmic F52.31
      psychogenic F52.9
        aversion F52.1
        dyspareunia F52.6
        frigidity F52.22
        nymphomania F52.8
        orgasmic F52.31
        vaginismus F52.5
      vaginismus N94.2
        psychogenic F52.5
    hypnotic F13.981
      in
        abuse F13.181
        dependence F13.281
    inhibited orgasm (female) F52.31
      male F52.32
    lack
      of sexual enjoyment F52.1
      or loss of sexual desire F52.0
    male N53.9
      anejaculatory orgasm N53.13
      ejaculatory N53.19
        painful N53.12
        premature F52.4
        retarded N53.11
      erectile N52.9
        drug induced N52.2
        due to
          disease classified elsewhere N52.1
          drug N52.2
        postoperative (postprocedural) N52.39
          following
            cryotherapy N52.37
            interstitial seed therapy N52.36
            prostate ablative therapy N52.37
            prostatectomy N52.34
              radical N52.31
            radical cystectomy N52.32
            radiation therapy N52.35
            ultrasound ablative therapy N52.37
            urethral surgery N52.33
        psychogenic F52.21
        specified cause NEC N52.8
        vasculogenic
          arterial insufficiency N52.01
            with corporo-venous occlusive N52.03
          corporo-venous occlusive N52.02
            with arterial insufficiency N52.03
      impotence —see Dysfunction, sexual, male, erectile
      psychogenic F52.9
        aversion F52.1
        erectile F52.21
        orgasmic F52.32
        premature ejaculation F52.4
        satyriasis F52.8
        specified type NEC F52.8
      specified type NEC N53.8
    nonorganic F52.9
      specified NEC F52.8

Dysfunction (continued)
  sexual (continued)
    opioid F11.981
      in
        abuse F11.181
        dependence F11.281
    orgasmic dysfunction (female) F52.31
      male F52.32
    premature ejaculation F52.4
    psychoactive substances NEC F19.981
      in
        abuse F19.181
        dependence F19.281
    psychogenic F52.9
    sedative F13.981
      in
        abuse F13.181
        dependence F13.281
    sexual aversion F52.1
    vaginismus (nonorganic) (psychogenic) F52.5
  sinoatrial node I49.5
  somatic M99.09
    abdomen M99.09
    acromioclavicular M99.07
    cervical region M99.01
    cervicothoracic M99.01
    costochondral M99.08
    costovertebral M99.08
    head region M99.00
    hip M99.05
    lower extremity M99.06
    lumbar region M99.03
    lumbosacral M99.03
    occipitocervical M99.00
    pelvic region M99.05
    pubic M99.05
    rib cage M99.08
    sacral region M99.04
    sacrococcygeal M99.04
    sacroiliac M99.04
    specified NEC M99.09
    sternochondral M99.08
    sternoclavicular M99.07
    thoracic region M99.02
    thoracolumbar M99.02
    upper extremity M99.07
  somatoform autonomic F45.8
  stomach K31.89
    psychogenic F45.8
  suprarenal E27.9
    hyperfunction E27.0
  symbolic R48.9
    specified type NEC R48.8
  temporomandibular (joint) M26.69
    joint-pain syndrome M26.62-
  testicular (endocrine) E29.9
    specified NEC E29.8
  thymus E32.9
  thyroid E07.9
  ureterostomy (stoma) —see Complications, stoma, urinary tract
  urethrostomy (stoma) —see Complications, stoma, urinary tract
  uterus, complicating delivery O62.9
    hypertonic O62.4
    hypotonic O62.2
      primary O62.0
      secondary O62.1
  ventricular I51.9
    with congestive heart failure (see also Failure, heart) I50.9
    left, reversible, following sudden emotional stress I51.81

131

Dysgenesis
 gonadal (due to chromosomal
    anomaly) Q96.9
  pure Q99.1
 renal Q60.5
  bilateral Q60.4
  unilateral Q60.3
 reticular D72.0
 tidal platelet D69.3

Dysgerminoma
 specified site —see Neoplasm,
   malignant, by site
 unspecified site
  female C56.9
  male C62.90

Dysgeusia R43.2

Dysgraphia R27.8

Dyshidrosis, dysidrosis L30.1

Dyskaryotic cervical smear R87.619

Dyskeratosis L85.8
 cervix —see Dysplasia, cervix
 congenital Q82.8
 uterus NEC N85.8

Dyskinesia G24.9
 biliary (cystic duct or gallbladder)
   K82.8
 drug induced
  orofacial G24.01
 esophagus K22.4
 hysterical F44.4
 intestinal K59.89
 nonorganic origin F44.4
 orofacial (idiopathic) G24.4
  drug induced G24.01
 psychogenic F44.4
 subacute, drug induced G24.01
 tardive G24.01
  neuroleptic induced G24.01
 trachea J39.8
 tracheobronchial J98.09

Dyslalia (developmental) F80.0

Dyslexia R48.0
 developmental F81.0

Dyslipidemia E78.5
 depressed HDL cholesterol E78.6
 elevated fasting triglycerides E78.1

Dysmaturity —see also Light for dates
 pulmonary (newborn) (Wilson-
   Mikity) P27.0

Dysmenorrhea (essential)
    (exfoliative) N94.6
 congestive (syndrome) N94.6
 primary N94.4
 psychogenic F45.8
 secondary N94.5

Dysmetabolic syndrome X E88.810

Dysmetria R27.8

Dysmorphism (due to)
 alcohol Q86.0
 exogenous cause NEC Q86.8
 hydantoin Q86.1
 warfarin Q86.2

Dysmorphophobia (nondelusional)
   F45.22
 delusional F22

Dysnomia R47.01

Dysorexia R63.0
 psychogenic F50.89

Dysostosis
 cleidocranial, cleidocranialis Q74.0
 craniofacial Q75.1
 Fairbank's (idiopathic familial
   generalized osteophytosis) Q78.9
 mandibulofacial (incomplete) Q75.4
 multiplex E76.01
 oculomandibular Q75.5

Dyspareunia (female) N94.10
 deep N94.12
 male N53.12
 nonorganic F52.6
 psychogenic F52.6
 secondary N94.19
 specified NEC N94.19
 superficial (introital) N94.11

Dyspepsia R10.13
 atonic K30
 functional (allergic) (congenital)
   (gastrointestinal) (occupational)
   (reflex) K30
 intestinal K59.89
 nervous F45.8
 neurotic F45.8
 psychogenic F45.8

Dysphagia R13.10
 cervical R13.19
 following
  cerebral infarction I69.391
  cerebrovascular disease I69.991
   specified NEC I69.891
  intracerebral hemorrhage I69.191
  nontraumatic intracranial
    hemorrhage NEC I69.291
  specified disease NEC I69.891
  subarachnoid hemorrhage I69.091
 functional (hysterical) F45.8
 hysterical F45.8
 nervous (hysterical) F45.8
 neurogenic R13.19
 oral phase R13.11
 oropharyngeal phase R13.12
 pharyngeal phase R13.13
 pharyngoesophageal phase R13.14
 psychogenic F45.8
 sideropenic D50.1
 spastica K22.4
 specified NEC R13.19

Dysphagocytosis, congenital D71

Dysphasia R47.02
 developmental
  expressive type F80.1
  receptive type F80.2
 following
  cerebrovascular disease I69.921
   cerebral infarction I69.321
   intracerebral hemorrhage
     I69.121
   nontraumatic intracranial
     hemorrhage NEC I69.221
   specified disease NEC I69.821
   subarachnoid hemorrhage
     I69.021

Dysphonia R49.0
 functional F44.4
 hysterical F44.4
 psychogenic F44.4
 spastica J38.3

Dysphoria
 gender F64.9
  in
   adolescence and adulthood
     F64.0
   children F64.2
 postpartal O90.6
 specified NEC F64.8

Dyspituitarism E23.3

Dysplasia —see also Anomaly
 acetabular, congenital Q65.89
 alveolar capillary, with vein
   misalignment J84.843
 anus (histologically confirmed)
    (mild) (moderate) K62.82
  severe D01.3
 arrhythmogenic right ventricular
    I42.8
 arterial, fibromuscular I77.3

Dysplasia (continued)
 asphyxiating thoracic (congenital)
    Q77.2
 brain Q07.9
 bronchopulmonary, perinatal P27.1
 cervix (uteri) N87.9
  mild N87.0
  moderate N87.1
  severe D06.9
 chondroectodermal Q77.6
 colon D12.6
 craniometaphyseal Q78.8
 dentinal K00.5
 diaphyseal, progressive Q78.3
 dystrophic Q77.5
 ectodermal (anhidrotic)
    (congenital) (hereditary) Q82.4
  hydrotic Q82.8
 epithelial, uterine cervix —see
   Dysplasia, cervix
 eye (congenital) Q11.2
 fibrous
  bone NEC (monostotic) M85.00
   ankle M85.07-
   foot M85.07-
   forearm M85.03-
   hand M85.04-
   lower leg M85.06-
   multiple site M85.09
   neck M85.08
   rib M85.08
   shoulder M85.01-
   skull M85.08
   specified site NEC M85.08
   thigh M85.05-
   toe M85.07-
   upper arm M85.02-
   vertebra M85.08
  diaphyseal, progressive Q78.3
  jaw M27.8
  polyostotic Q78.1
 florid osseous —see also Cyst,
   calcifying odontogenic
 high grade, focal D12.6
 hip, congenital Q65.89
 joint, congenital Q74.8
 kidney Q61.4
  multicystic Q61.4
 leg Q74.2
 lung, congenital (not associated
    with short gestation) Q33.6
 mammary (gland) (benign) N60.9-
  cyst (solitary) —see Cyst,
    breast
  cystic —see Mastopathy, cystic
  duct ectasia —see Ectasia,
    mammary duct
  fibroadenosis —see
    Fibroadenosis, breast
  fibrosclerosis —see
    Fibrosclerosis, breast
  specified type NEC N60.8-
 metaphyseal Q78.5
  specified NEC N42.39
 muscle Q79.8
 oculodentodigital Q87.0
 periapical (cemental) (cemento-
    osseous) —see Cyst, calcifying
    odontogenic
 periosteum —see Disorder, bone,
   specified type NEC
 polyostotic fibrous Q78.1
 prostate (see also Neoplasia,
    intraepithelial, prostate) N42.30
  severe D07.5
  specified NEC N42.39
 renal Q61.4
  multicystic Q61.4
 retinal, congenital Q14.1
 right ventricular, arrhythmogenic
    I42.8

Dysplasia (continued)
 septo-optic Q04.4
 skin L98.8
 spinal cord Q06.1
 spondyloepiphyseal Q77.7
 thymic, with immunodeficiency
    D82.1
 vagina N89.3
  mild N89.0
  moderate N89.1
  severe NEC D07.2
 vulva N90.3
  mild N90.0
  moderate N90.1
  severe NEC D07.1

Dysplasminogenemia E88.02

Dyspnea (nocturnal) (paroxysmal)
   R06.00
 asthmatic (bronchial) J45.909
  with
   exacerbation (acute) J45.901
   bronchitis J45.909
    with
     exacerbation (acute)
       J45.901
     status asthmaticus
       J45.902
   chronic J44.89
    status asthmaticus J45.902
 cardiac —see Failure,
   ventricular, left
 cardiac —see Failure, ventricular,
   left
 functional F45.8
 hyperventilation R06.4
 hysterical F45.8
 newborn P28.89
 orthopnea R06.01
 psychogenic F45.8
 shortness of breath R06.02
 specified type NEC R06.09
 transfusion-associated [TAD] J95.87

Dyspraxia R27.8
 developmental (syndrome) F82

Dysproteinemia E88.09

Dysreflexia, autonomic G90.4

Dysrhythmia
 cardiac I49.9
  newborn
   bradycardia P29.12
    occurring before birth P03.819
     before onset of labor
       P03.810
     during labor P03.811
   tachycardia P29.11
  postoperative I97.89
 cerebral or cortical —see Epilepsy

Dyssomnia —see Disorder, sleep

Dyssynergia
 biliary K83.8
 bladder sphincter N36.44
 cerebellaris myoclonica (Hunt's
   ataxia) G11.19

Dysthymia F34.1

Dysthyroidism E07.9

Dystocia O66.9
 affecting newborn P03.1
 cervical (hypotonic) O62.2
  affecting newborn P03.6
  primary O62.0
  secondary O62.1
 contraction ring O62.4
 fetal O66.9
  abnormality NEC O66.3
  conjoined twins O66.3
  oversize O66.2
 maternal O66.9

Dystocia (continued)
  positional O64.9
  shoulder (girdle) O66.0
    causing obstructed labor O66.0
  uterine NEC O62.4

Dystonia G24.9
  cervical G24.3
  deformans progressiva G24.1
  drug induced NEC G24.09
    acute G24.02
    specified NEC G24.09
  familial G24.1
  idiopathic G24.1
    familial G24.1
    nonfamilial G24.2
    orofacial G24.4
  lenticularis G24.8
  musculorum deformans G24.1
  neuroleptic induced (acute) G24.02
  orofacial (idiopathic) G24.4
  oromandibular G24.4
    due to drug G24.01
  specified NEC G24.8
  torsion (familial) (idiopathic) G24.1
    acquired G24.8
    genetic G24.1
  symptomatic (nonfamilial) G24.2

Dystonic movements R25.8

Dystrophy, dystrophia
  adiposogenital E23.6
  autosomal recessive, childhood type, muscular dystrophy resembling Duchenne or Becker G71.01
  Becker's type G71.01
  cervical sympathetic G90.2
  choroid (hereditary) H31.20
    central areolar H31.22
    choroideremia H31.21
    gyrate atrophy H31.23
    specified type NEC H31.29
  cornea (hereditary) H18.50-
    endothelial H18.51-
    epithelial H18.52-
    granular H18.53-
    lattice H18.54-
    macular H18.55-
    specified type NEC H18.59-
  Duchenne's type G71.01
  due to malnutrition E45
  Erb's G71.02
  Fuchs' H18.51-
  Gower's muscular G71.01
  hair L67.8
  infantile neuraxonal G31.89
  Landouzy-Déjérine G71.02
  Leyden-Möbius (*see also* Dystrophy, muscular, limb-girdle, by type) G71.039
    meaning Limb girdle muscular dystrophy NOS G71.039
    meaning Limb girdle muscular dystrophy, other specified type, - *see by type*
    meaning Limb girdle muscular dystrophy, specified type NEC G71.038
    meaning Limb girdle muscular dystrophy type 2A (autosomal recessive) G71.032
  muscular G71.00
    autosomal recessive, childhood type, muscular dystrophy resembling Duchenne or Becker G71.01
    benign (Becker type) G71.01
      scapuloperoneal with early contractures [Emery-Dreifuss] G71.09

Dystrophy, dystrophia (continued)
  muscular (continued)
    congenital (hereditary) (progressive) (with specific morphological abnormalities of the muscle fiber) G71.09
      myotonic G71.11
    distal G71.09
    Duchenne type G71.01
    Emery-Dreifuss G71.09
    Erb type G71.02
    facioscapulohumeral G71.02
    Gower's G71.01
    hereditary (progressive) (*see also* Dystrophy, muscular, by type) G71.09
    Landouzy-Déjérine type G71.02
    limb-girdle G71.039
      alpha-sarcoglycan-related G71.0341
      anoctamin-5-related
        autosomal recessive (R12) G71.035
      autosomal recessive NEC G71.038
      beta-sarcoglycan-related G71.0342
      calpain-3-related G71.032
        autosomal dominant G71.031
        autosomal recessive G71.032
      collagen VI related
        autosomal dominant G71.031
        autosomal recessive G71.038
      D1 (autosomal dominant) G71.031
      D2 (autosomal dominant) G71.031
      D3 (autosomal dominant) G71.031
      D4 (autosomal dominant) G71.031
      D5 (autosomal dominant) G71.031
      delta-sarcoglycan-related G71.0349
      due to
        alpha sarcoglycan dysfunction G71.0341
        anoctamin-5 dysfunction G71.035
        beta sarcoglycan dysfunction G71.0342
        fukutin related protein dysfunction G71.038
        sarcoglycan dysfunction, specified NEC G71.0349
      FKRP-related autosomal recessive G71.038
      gamma-sarcoglycan-related G71.0349
      R1 (autosomal recessive) G71.032
      R2 (autosomal recessive) G71.033
      R3 (autosomal recessive) G71.0341
      R4 (autosomal recessive) G71.0342
      R5 (autosomal recessive) G71.0349
      R6 (autosomal recessive) G71.0349
      R7 (autosomal recessive) G71.038
      R8 (autosomal recessive) G71.038
      R9 (autosomal recessive) G71.038
      R10 (autosomal recessive) G71.038

Dystrophy, dystrophia (continued)
  muscular (continued)
    limb-girdle (continued)
      R11 (autosomal recessive) G71.038
      R12 (autosomal recessive) G71.035
      R13 (autosomal recessive) G71.038
      R14 (autosomal recessive) G71.038
      R15 (autosomal recessive) G71.038
      R16 (autosomal recessive) G71.038
      R17 (autosomal recessive) G71.038
      R18 (autosomal recessive) G71.038
      R19 (autosomal recessive) G71.038
      R20 (autosomal recessive) G71.038
      R21 (autosomal recessive) G71.038
      R22 (autosomal recessive) G71.038
      R23 (autosomal recessive) G71.038
      R24 (autosomal recessive) G71.038
      type 1 (autosomal dominant) G71.031
      type 1A (autosomal dominant) G71.031
      type 1B (autosomal dominant) G71.031
      type 1C (autosomal dominant) G71.031
      type 1E (autosomal dominant) G71.031
      type 1H (autosomal dominant) G71.031
      type 1I (autosomal dominant) G71.031
      type 2 (autosomal recessive) G71.038
        specified NEC G71.038
      type 2A (autosomal recessive) G71.032
      type 2B (autosomal recessive) G71.033
      type 2C (autosomal recessive) G71.0349
      type 2D (autosomal recessive) G71.0341
      type 2E (autosomal recessive) G71.0342
      type 2F (autosomal recessive) G71.0349
      type 2I (autosomal recessive) G71.038
      type 2L (autosomal recessive) G71.035
    myotonic G71.11
    progressive (hereditary) (*see also* Dystrophy, muscular, by type) G71.09
      Charcot-Marie (-Tooth) type G60.0
    pseudohypertrophic (infantile) G71.01
    scapulohumeral G71.02
    scapuloperoneal G71.09
    severe (Duchenne type) G71.01
    specified type NEC G71.09
  myocardium, myocardial —*see* Degeneration, myocardial
  nail L60.3
    congenital Q84.6

Dystrophy, dystrophia (continued)
  nutritional E45
  ocular G71.09
  oculocerebrorenal E72.03
  oculopharyngeal G71.09
  ovarian N83.8
  polyglandular E31.8
  reflex (neuromuscular) (sympathetic) —*see* Syndrome, pain, complex regional I
  retinal (hereditary) H35.50
    in
      lipid storage disorders E75.6 [H36.89]
      systemic lipidoses E75.6 [H36.89]
    involving
      pigment epithelium H35.54
      sensory area H35.53
    pigmentary H35.52
    vitreoretinal H35.51
  Salzmann's nodular —*see* Degeneration, cornea, nodular
  scapuloperoneal G71.09
  skin NEC L98.8
  sympathetic (reflex) —*see* Syndrome, pain, complex regional I
    cervical G90.2
  tapetoretinal H35.54
  thoracic, asphyxiating Q77.2
  unguium L60.3
    congenital Q84.6
  vitreoretinal H35.51
  vulva N90.4
  yellow (liver) —*see* Failure, hepatic

Dysuria R30.0
  psychogenic F45.8

E

Eales' disease H35.06-

Ear —*see also* condition
  piercing Z41.3
  tropical NEC B36.9 [H62.40]
    in
      aspergillosis B44.89
      candidiasis B37.84
      moniliasis B37.84
  wax (impacted) H61.20
    left H61.22
      with right H61.23
    right H61.21
      with left H61.23

Earache —*see subcategory* H92.0

Early satiety R68.81

Eaton-Lambert syndrome —*see* Syndrome, Lambert-Eaton

Eberth's disease (typhoid fever) A01.00

Ebola virus disease A98.4

Ebstein's anomaly or syndrome (heart) Q22.5

Eccentro-osteochondrodysplasia E76.29

Ecchondroma —*see* Neoplasm, bone, benign

Ecchondrosis D48.0

Ecchymosis R58
  conjunctiva —*see* Hemorrhage, conjunctiva
  eye (traumatic) —*see* Contusion, eyeball
  eyelid (traumatic) —*see* Contusion, eyelid
  newborn P54.5
  spontaneous R23.3
  traumatic —*see* Contusion

Echinococciasis —*see* Echinococcus

Echinococcosis —see Echinococcus
Echinococcus (infection) B67.90
- granulosus B67.4
  - bone B67.2
  - liver B67.0
  - lung B67.1
  - multiple sites B67.32
  - specified site NEC B67.39
  - thyroid B67.31
- liver NOS B67.8
  - granulosus B67.0
  - multilocularis B67.5
- lung NEC B67.99
  - granulosus B67.1
  - multilocularis B67.69
- multilocularis B67.7
  - liver B67.5
  - multiple sites B67.61
  - specified site NEC B67.69
- specified site NEC B67.99
  - granulosus B67.39
  - multilocularis B67.69
- thyroid NEC B67.99
  - granulosus B67.31
  - multilocularis B67.69 *[E35]*

Echinorhynchiasis B83.8
Echinostomiasis B66.8
Echolalia R48.8
Echovirus, as cause of disease classified elsewhere B97.12
Eclampsia, eclamptic (coma) (convulsions) (delirium) (with hypertension) **NEC** O15.9
- complicating
  - labor and delivery O15.1
  - postpartum O15.2
  - pregnancy O15.0-
  - puerperal O15.2

Economic circumstances affecting care Z59.9
Economo's disease A85.8
Ectasia, ectasis
- annuloaortic I35.8
- aorta I77.819
  - with aneurysm —see Aneurysm, aorta
  - abdominal I77.811
  - thoracic I77.810
  - thoracoabdominal I77.812
- breast —see Ectasia, mammary duct
- capillary I78.8
- cornea H18.71-
- gastric antral vascular (GAVE) K31.819
  - with hemorrhage K31.811
  - without hemorrhage K31.819
- mammary duct N60.4-
- salivary gland (duct) K11.8
- sclera —see Sclerectasia

Ecthyma L08.0
- contagiosum B08.02
- gangrenosum L08.0
- infectiosum B08.02

Ectocardia Q24.8
Ectodermal dysplasia (anhidrotic) Q82.4
Ectodermosis erosiva pluriorificialis L51.1
Ectopic, ectopia (congenital)
- abdominal viscera Q45.8
  - due to defect in anterior abdominal wall Q79.59
- ACTH syndrome E24.3
- adrenal gland Q89.1
- anus Q43.5
- atrial beats I49.1

Ectopic, ectopia *(continued)*
- beats I49.49
  - atrial I49.1
  - ventricular I49.3
- bladder Q64.10
- bone and cartilage in lung Q33.5
- brain Q04.8
- breast tissue Q83.8
- cardiac Q24.8
- cerebral Q04.8
- cordis Q24.8
- endometrium —see Endometriosis
- gastric mucosa Q40.2
- gestation —see Pregnancy, by site
- heart Q24.8
- hormone secretion NEC E34.2
- kidney (crossed) (pelvis) Q63.2
- lens, lentis Q12.1
- mole —see Pregnancy, by site
- organ or site NEC —see Malposition, congenital
- pancreas Q45.3
- pregnancy —see Pregnancy, ectopic
- pupil —see Abnormality, pupillary
- renal Q63.2
- sebaceous glands of mouth Q38.6
- spleen Q89.09
- testis Q53.00
  - bilateral Q53.02
  - unilateral Q53.01
- thyroid Q89.2
- tissue in lung Q33.5
- ureter Q62.63
- ventricular beats I49.3
- vesicae Q64.10

Ectromelia Q73.8
- lower limb —see Defect, reduction, limb, lower, specified type NEC
- upper limb —see Defect, reduction, limb, upper, specified type NEC

Ectropion H02.109
- cervix N86
  - with cervicitis N72
- congenital Q10.1
- eyelid H02.109
  - cicatricial H02.119
    - left H02.116
      - lower H02.115
      - upper H02.114
    - right H02.113
      - lower H02.112
      - upper H02.111
  - congenital Q10.1
  - left H02.106
    - lower H02.105
    - upper H02.104
  - mechanical H02.129
    - left H02.126
      - lower H02.125
      - upper H02.124
    - right H02.123
      - lower H02.122
      - upper H02.121
  - paralytic H02.159
    - left H02.156
      - lower H02.155
      - upper H02.154
    - right H02.153
      - lower H02.152
      - upper H02.151
  - right H02.103
    - lower H02.102
    - upper H02.101
  - senile H02.139
    - left H02.136
      - lower H02.135
      - upper H02.134
    - right H02.133
      - lower H02.132
      - upper H02.131

Ectropion *(continued)*
- eyelid *(continued)*
  - spastic H02.149
    - left H02.146
      - lower H02.145
      - upper H02.144
    - right H02.143
      - lower H02.142
      - upper H02.141
- iris H21.89
- lip (acquired) K13.0
  - congenital Q38.0
- urethra N36.8
- uvea H21.89

Eczema (acute) (chronic) (erythematous) (fissum) (rubrum) (squamous) —see also Dermatitis L30.9
- contact —see Dermatitis, contact
- dyshydrotic L30.1
- external ear —see Otitis, externa, acute, eczematoid
- flexural L20.82
- herpeticum B00.0
- hypertrophicum L28.0
- hypostatic —see Varix, leg, with, inflammation
- impetiginous L01.1
- infantile (due to any substance) L20.83
  - intertriginous L21.1
  - seborrheic L21.1
- intertriginous NEC L30.4
  - infantile L21.1
- intrinsic (allergic) L20.84
- lichenified NEC L28.0
- marginatum (hebrae) B35.6
- pustular L30.3
- stasis I87.2
  - with varicose veins —see Varix, leg, with, inflammation
- vaccination, vaccinatum T88.1
- varicose —see Varix, leg, with, inflammation

Eczematid L30.2

Eddowes (-Spurway) **syndrome** Q78.0

Edema, edematous (infectious) (pitting) (toxic) R60.9
- with nephritis —see Nephrosis
- allergic T78.3
- amputation stump (surgical) (sequelae (late effect)) T87.89
- angioneurotic (allergic) (any site) (with urticaria) T78.3
  - hereditary D84.1
- angiospastic I73.9
- Berlin's (traumatic) S05.8X-
- brain (cytotoxic) (vasogenic) G93.6
  - due to birth injury P11.0
  - newborn (anoxia or hypoxia) P52.4
    - birth injury P11.0
  - traumatic —see Injury, intracranial, cerebral edema
- cardiac —see Failure, heart, congestive
- cardiovascular —see Failure, heart, congestive
- cerebral —see Edema, brain
- cerebrospinal —see Edema, brain
- cervix (uteri) (acute) N88.8
  - puerperal, postpartum O90.89
- chronic hereditary Q82.0
- circumscribed, acute T78.3
  - hereditary D84.1
- conjunctiva H11.42-
- cornea H18.2-
  - idiopathic H18.22-
  - secondary H18.23-
    - due to contact lens H18.21-

Edema, edematous *(continued)*
- due to
  - lymphatic obstruction I89.0
  - salt retention E87.0
- epiglottis —see Edema, glottis
- essential, acute T78.3
  - hereditary D84.1
- extremities, lower —see Edema, legs
- eyelid NEC H02.849
  - left H02.846
    - lower H02.845
    - upper H02.844
  - right H02.843
    - lower H02.842
    - upper H02.841
- familial, hereditary Q82.0
- famine —see Malnutrition, severe
- generalized R60.1
- glottis, glottic, glottidis (obstructive) (passive) J38.4
  - allergic T78.3
    - hereditary D84.1
- heart —see Failure, heart, congestive
- heat T67.7
- hereditary Q82.0
- inanition —see Malnutrition, severe
- intracranial G93.6
- iris H21.89
- joint —see Effusion, joint
- larynx —see Edema, glottis
- legs R60.0
  - due to venous obstruction I87.1
  - hereditary Q82.0
- localized R60.0
  - due to venous obstruction I87.1
- lower limbs —see Edema, legs
- lung J81.1
  - with heart condition or failure —see Failure, ventricular, left
  - newborn P29.0
  - acute J81.0
  - chemical (acute) J68.1
    - chronic J68.1
  - chronic J81.1
  - due to
    - chemicals, gases, fumes or vapors (inhalation) J68.1
    - external agent J70.9
      - specified NEC J70.8
    - radiation J70.1
  - due to
    - chemicals, fumes or vapors (inhalation) J68.1
    - external agent J70.9
      - specified NEC J70.8
    - high altitude T70.29
    - near drowning T75.1
    - radiation J70.0
  - meaning failure, left ventricle I50.1
- lymphatic I89.0
  - due to mastectomy I97.2
- macula H35.81
  - cystoid, following cataract surgery —see Complications, postprocedural, following cataract surgery
  - diabetic —see Diabetes, by type, with, retinopathy, with macular edema
- malignant —see Gangrene, gas
- Milroy's Q82.0
- nasopharynx J39.2
- newborn P83.30
  - hydrops fetalis —see Hydrops, fetalis
  - specified NEC P83.39
- nutritional —see also Malnutrition, severe
  - with dyspigmentation, skin and hair E40

Edema, edematous (continued)
optic disc or nerve —see Papilledema
orbit H05.22-
pancreas K86.89
papilla, optic —see Papilledema
penis N48.89
periodic T78.3
hereditary D84.1
pharynx J39.2
pulmonary —see Edema, lung
Quincke's T78.3
hereditary D84.1
renal —see Nephrosis
retina H35.81
diabetic —see Diabetes, by type, with, retinopathy, with macular edema
salt E87.0
scrotum N50.89
seminal vesicle N50.89
spermatic cord N50.89
spinal (cord) (vascular) (nontraumatic) G95.19
starvation —see Malnutrition, severe
stasis —see Hypertension, venous, (chronic)
subglottic —see Edema, glottis
supraglottic —see Edema, glottis
testis N44.8
tunica vaginalis N50.89
vas deferens N50.89
vulva (acute) N90.89

Edentulism —see Absence, teeth, acquired

Edsall's disease T67.2

Educational handicap Z55.9
less than a high school diploma Z55.5
no general equivalence degree (GED) Z55.5
specified NEC Z55.8

Edward's syndrome —see Trisomy, 18

Effect, adverse
abnormal gravitational (G) forces or states T75.81
abuse —see Maltreatment
air pressure T70.9
specified NEC T70.8
altitude (high) —see Effect, adverse, high altitude
anesthesia (see also Anesthesia) T88.59
in labor and delivery O74.9
local, toxic
in labor and delivery O74.4
in pregnancy NEC O29.3-
postpartum, puerperal O89.3
postpartum, puerperal O89.9
specified NEC T88.59
in labor and delivery O74.8
postpartum, puerperal O89.8
spinal and epidural T88.59
headache T88.59
in labor and delivery O74.5
postpartum, puerperal O89.4
specified NEC
in labor and delivery O74.6
postpartum, puerperal O89.5
antitoxin —see Complications, vaccination
atmospheric pressure T70.9
due to explosion T70.8
high T70.3
low —see Effect, adverse, high altitude
specified effect NEC T70.8
biological, correct substance properly administered —see Effect, adverse, drug

Effect, adverse (continued)
blood (derivatives) (serum) (transfusion) —see Complications, transfusion
chemical substance —see Table of Drugs and Chemicals
cold (temperature) (weather) T69.9
chilblains T69.1
frostbite —see Frostbite
specified effect NEC T69.8
drugs and medicaments T88.7
specified drug —see Table of Drugs and Chemicals, by drug, adverse effect
specified effect - code to condition
electric current, electricity (shock) T75.4
burn —see Burn
exertion (excessive) T73.3
exposure —see Exposure
external cause NEC T75.89
foodstuffs T78.1
allergic reaction —see Allergy, food
causing anaphylaxis —see Shock, anaphylactic, due to food
noxious —see Poisoning, food, noxious
gases, fumes, or vapors T59.9-
specified agent —see Table of Drugs and Chemicals
glue (airplane) sniffing
due to drug abuse —see Abuse, drug, inhalant
due to drug dependence —see Dependence, drug, inhalant
heat —see Heat
high altitude NEC T70.29
anoxia T70.29
on
ears T70.0
sinuses T70.1
polycythemia D75.1
high pressure fluids T70.4
hot weather —see Heat
hunger T73.0
immersion, foot —see Immersion
immunization —see Complications, vaccination
immunological agents —see Complications, vaccination
infrared (radiation) (rays) NOS T66
dermatitis or eczema L59.8
infusion —see Complications, infusion
lack of care of infants —see Maltreatment, child
lightning —see Lightning
medical care T88.9
specified NEC T88.8
medicinal substance, correct, properly administered —see Effect, adverse, drug
motion T75.3
noise, on inner ear —see subcategory H83.3
overheated places —see Heat
psychosocial, of work environment Z56.5
radiation (diagnostic) (infrared) (natural source) (therapeutic) (ultraviolet) (X-ray) NOS T66
dermatitis or eczema —see Dermatitis, due to radiation
fibrosis of lung J70.1
pneumonitis J70.0
pulmonary manifestations
acute J70.0
chronic J70.1
skin L59.9

Effect, adverse (continued)
radioactive substance NOS
dermatitis or eczema —see Radiodermatitis
reduced temperature T69.9
immersion foot or hand —see Immersion
specified effect NEC T69.8
serum NEC (see also Reaction, serum) T80.69
specified NEC T78.8
external cause NEC T75.89
strangulation —see Asphyxia, traumatic
submersion T75.1
thirst T73.1
toxic —see Toxicity
transfusion —see Complications, transfusion
ultraviolet (radiation) (rays) NOS T66
burn —see Burn
dermatitis or eczema —see Dermatitis, due to, ultraviolet rays
acute L56.8
vaccine (any) —see Complications, vaccination
vibration —see Vibration, adverse effects
water pressure NEC T70.9
specified NEC T70.8
weightlessness T75.82
whole blood —see Complications, transfusion
work environment Z56.5

Effect(s) (of) (from) —see Effect, adverse NEC

Effects, late —see Sequelae

Effluvium
anagen L65.1
telogen L65.0

Effort syndrome (psychogenic) F45.8

Effusion
amniotic fluid —see Pregnancy, complicated by, premature rupture of membranes
brain (serous) G93.6
bronchial —see Bronchitis
cerebral G93.6
cerebrospinal —see also Meningitis
vessel G93.6
chest —see Effusion, pleura
chylous, chyliform (pleura) J94.0
intracranial G93.6
joint M25.40
ankle M25.47-
elbow M25.42-
foot joint M25.47-
hand joint M25.44-
hip M25.45-
knee M25.46-
shoulder M25.41-
specified joint NEC M25.48
wrist M25.43-
malignant pleural J91.0
meninges —see Meningitis
pericardium, pericardial (noninflammatory) I31.39
acute —see Pericarditis, acute
malignant, in disease classified elsewhere I31.31
specified type, NEC I31.39
peritoneal (chronic) R18.8
pleura, pleurisy, pleuritic, pleuropericardial J90
chylous, chyliform J94.0
due to systemic lupus erythematosis M32.13

Effusion (continued)
pleura, pleurisy, pleuritic (continued)
in conditions classified elsewhere J91.8
influenzal —see Influenza, with, respiratory manifestations NEC
malignant J91.0
newborn P28.89
tuberculous NEC A15.6
primary (progressive) A15.7
spinal —see Meningitis
thorax, thoracic —see Effusion, pleura

Egg shell nails L60.3
congenital Q84.6

EGPA (eosinophilic granulomatosis with polyangitis) M30.1

Egyptian splenomegaly B65.1

Ehrlichiosis A77.40
due to
E. chafeensis A77.41
E. ewingii A77.49
E. muris euclairensis A77.49
E. sennetsu A79.81
specified organism NEC A77.49

Ehlers-Danlos syndrome (see also Syndrome, Ehlers-Danlos) Q79.60

Eichstedt's disease B36.0

Eisenmenger's
complex or syndrome I27.83
defect Q21.8

Ejaculation
delayed F52.32
painful N53.12
premature F52.4
retarded N53.11
retrograde N53.14
semen, painful N53.12
psychogenic F52.6

Ekbom's syndrome (restless legs) G25.81

Ekman's syndrome (brittle bones and blue sclera) Q78.0

Elastic skin Q82.8
acquired L57.4

Elastofibroma —see Neoplasm, connective tissue, benign

Elastoma (juvenile) Q82.8
Miescher's L87.2

Elastomyofibrosis I42.4

Elastosis
actinic, solar L57.8
atrophicans (senile) L57.4
perforans serpiginosa L87.2
senilis L57.4

Elbow —see condition

Electric current, electricity, effects (concussion) (fatal) (nonfatal) (shock) T75.4
burn —see Burn

Electric feet syndrome E53.8

Electrocution T75.4
from electroshock gun (taser) T75.4

Electrolyte imbalance E87.8
with
abortion —see Abortion by type, complicated by, electrolyte imbalance
ectopic pregnancy O08.5
molar pregnancy O08.5

Elephantiasis (nonfilarial) I89.0
arabicum —see Infestation, filarial
bancroftian B74.0
congenital (any site) (hereditary) Q82.0

135

Elephantiasis (continued)
  due to
    Brugia (malayi) B74.1
      timori B74.2
    mastectomy I97.2
    Wuchereria (bancrofti) B74.0
  eyelid H02.859
    left H02.856
      lower H02.855
      upper H02.854
    right H02.853
      lower H02.852
      upper H02.851
  filarial, filariensis —see Infestation, filarial
  glandular I89.0
  graecorum A30.9
  lymphangiectatic I89.0
  lymphatic vessel I89.0
    due to mastectomy I97.2
  scrotum (nonfilarial) I89.0
  streptococcal I89.0
  surgical I97.89
    postmastectomy I97.2
  telangiectodes I89.0
  vulva (nonfilarial) N90.89

Elevated, elevation
  alanine transaminase (ALT) R74.01
  ALT (alanine transaminase) R74.01
  antibody titer R76.0
  aspartate transaminase (AST) R74.01
  AST (aspartate transaminase) R74.01
  basal metabolic rate R94.8
  blood pressure —see also Hypertension
    reading (incidental) (isolated) (nonspecific), no diagnosis of hypertension R03.0
  blood sugar R73.9
  body temperature (of unknown origin) R50.9
  C-reactive protein (CRP) R79.82
  cancer antigen 125 [CA 125] R97.1
  carcinoembryonic antigen [CEA] R97.0
  cholesterol E78.00
    with high triglycerides E78.2
  conjugate, eye H51.0
  diaphragm, congenital Q79.1
  erythrocyte sedimentation rate R70.0
  fasting glucose R73.01
  fasting triglycerides E78.1
  finding on laboratory examination —see Findings, abnormal, inconclusive, without diagnosis, by type of exam
  GFR (glomerular filtration rate) —see Findings, abnormal, inconclusive, without diagnosis, by type of exam
  glucose tolerance (oral) R73.02
  immunoglobulin level R76.8
  indoleacetic acid R82.5
  lactic acid dehydrogenase (LDH) level R74.02
  leukocytes D72.829
  lipoprotein a (Lp(a)) level E78.41
  liver function
    study R94.5
    test R79.89
      alkaline phosphatase R74.8
      aminotransferase R74.01
      bilirubin R17
      hepatic enzyme R74.8
      lactate dehydrogenase R74.02
  Lp(a) (lipoprotein(a)) E78.41
  lymphocytes D72.820
  prostate specific antigen [PSA] R97.20

Elevated, elevation (continued)
  Rh titer —see Complication(s), transfusion, incompatibility reaction, Rh (factor)
  scapula, congenital Q74.0
  sedimentation rate R70.0
  SGOT R74.01
  SGPT R74.01
  transaminase level R74.01
  triglycerides E78.1
    with high cholesterol E78.2
  troponin R79.89
  tumor associated antigens [TAA] NEC R97.8
  tumor specific antigens [TSA] NEC R97.8
  urine level of
    catecholamine R82.5
    indoleacetic acid R82.5
    17-ketosteroids R82.5
    steroids R82.5
    vanillylmandelic acid (VMA) R82.5
  venous pressure I87.8
  white blood cell count D72.829
    specified NEC D72.828

Elliptocytosis (congenital) (hereditary) D58.1
  Hb C (disease) D58.1
  hemoglobin disease D58.1
  sickle-cell (disease) D57.8-
    trait D57.3

Ellison-Zollinger syndrome E16.4

Ellis-van Creveld syndrome (chondroectodermal dysplasia) Q77.6

Elongated, elongation (congenital) —see also Distortion
  bone Q79.9
  cervix (uteri) Q51.828
    acquired N88.4
    hypertrophic N88.4
  colon Q43.8
  common bile duct Q44.5
  cystic duct Q44.5
  frenulum, penis Q55.69
  labia minora (acquired) N90.69
  ligamentum patellae Q74.1
  petiolus (epiglottidis) Q31.8
  tooth, teeth K00.2
  uvula Q38.6

Eltor cholera A00.1

Emaciation R64
  due to malnutrition E43

Embadomoniasis A07.8

Embedded tooth, teeth K01.0
  root only K08.3

Embolic —see condition

Embolism (multiple) (paradoxical) I74.9
  air (any site) (traumatic) T79.0
    following
      abortion —see Abortion by type complicated by embolism
      ectopic pregnancy O08.2
    infusion, therapeutic injection or transfusion T80.0
    molar pregnancy O08.2
    procedure NEC
      artery T81.719
        mesenteric T81.710
        renal T81.711
        specified NEC T81.718
      vein T81.72
    in pregnancy, childbirth or puerperium —see Embolism, obstetric

Embolism (continued)
  amniotic fluid (pulmonary) —see also Embolism, obstetric
    following
      abortion —see Abortion by type complicated by embolism
      ectopic pregnancy O08.2
      molar pregnancy O08.2
  aorta, aortic I74.10
    abdominal I74.09
      saddle I74.01
    bifurcation I74.09
    saddle I74.01
    thoracic I74.11
  artery I74.9
    auditory, internal I65.8
    basilar —see Occlusion, artery, basilar
    carotid (common) (internal) —see Occlusion, artery, carotid
    cerebellar (anterior inferior) (posterior inferior) (superior) I66.3
    cerebral —see Occlusion, artery, cerebral
    choroidal (anterior) I65.8
    communicating posterior I65.8
    coronary —see also Infarct, myocardium
      not resulting in infarction I24.0
    extremity I74.4
      lower I74.3
      upper I74.2
    hypophyseal I65.8
    iliac I74.5
    limb I74.4
      lower I74.3
      upper I74.2
    mesenteric (with gangrene) (see also Ischemia, intestine, acute) K55.059
    ophthalmic —see Occlusion, artery, retina
    peripheral I74.4
    pontine I65.8
    precerebral —see Occlusion, artery, precerebral
    pulmonary —see Embolism, pulmonary
    renal N28.0
    retinal —see Occlusion, artery, retina
    septic I76
    specified NEC I74.8
    vertebral —see Occlusion, artery, vertebral
  basilar (artery) I65.1
  blood clot
    following
      abortion —see Abortion by type complicated by embolism
      ectopic or molar pregnancy O08.2
    in pregnancy, childbirth or puerperium —see Embolism, obstetric
  brain —see also Occlusion, artery, cerebral
    following
      abortion —see Abortion by type complicated by embolism
      ectopic or molar pregnancy O08.2
    puerperal, postpartum, childbirth —see Embolism, obstetric
  capillary I78.8
  cardiac —see also Infarct, myocardium
    not resulting in infarction I51.3

Embolism (continued)
  carotid (artery) (common) (internal) —see Occlusion, artery, carotid
  cavernous sinus (venous) —see Embolism, intracranial venous sinus
  cerebral —see Occlusion, artery, cerebral
  cholesterol —see Atheroembolism
  coronary (artery or vein) (systemic) —see Occlusion, coronary
  due to device, implant or graft —see also Complications, by site and type, specified NEC
    arterial graft NEC T82.818
    breast (implant) T85.818
    catheter NEC T85.818
      dialysis (renal) T82.818
        intraperitoneal T85.818
      infusion NEC T82.818
        spinal (epidural) (subdural) T85.810
      urinary (indwelling) T83.81
    electronic (electrode) (pulse generator) (stimulator)
      bone T84.81
      cardiac T82.817
      nervous system (brain) (peripheral nerve) (spinal) T85.810
      urinary T83.81
    fixation, internal (orthopedic) NEC T84.81
    gastrointestinal (bile duct) (esophagus) T85.818
    genital NEC T83.81
    heart (graft) (valve) T82.817
    joint prosthesis T84.81
    ocular (corneal graft) (orbital implant) T85.818
    orthopedic (bone graft) NEC T86.838
    specified NEC T85.818
    urinary (graft) NEC T83.81
    vascular NEC T82.818
    ventricular intracranial shunt T85.810
  extremities
    lower —see Embolism, vein, lower extremity
    arterial I74.3
    upper I74.2
  eye H34.9
  fat (cerebral) (pulmonary) (systemic) T79.1
    following
      abortion —see Abortion by type complicated by embolism
      ectopic or molar pregnancy O08.2
    complicating delivery —see Embolism, obstetric
    following
      abortion —see Abortion by type complicated by embolism
      ectopic or molar pregnancy O08.2
    infusion, therapeutic injection or transfusion
      air T80.0
  heart (fatty) —see also Infarct, myocardium
    not resulting in infarction I51.3
  hepatic (vein) I82.0
  in pregnancy, childbirth or puerperium —see Embolism, obstetric

Embolism (continued)
   intestine (artery) (vein) (with
     gangrene) (*see also* Ischemia,
     intestine, acute) K55.039
   intracranial —*see also* Occlusion,
     artery, cerebral
     venous sinus (any) G08
       nonpyogenic I67.6
   intraspinal venous sinuses or veins
     G08
     nonpyogenic G95.19
   kidney (artery) N28.0
   lateral sinus (venous) —*see*
     Embolism, intracranial, venous
     sinus
   leg —*see* Embolism, vein, lower
     extremity
     arterial I74.3
   longitudinal sinus (venous) —*see*
     Embolism, intracranial, venous
     sinus
   lung (massive) —*see* Embolism,
     pulmonary
   meninges I66.8
   mesenteric (artery) (vein) (with
     gangrene) (*see also* Ischemia,
     intestine, acute) K55.059
   obstetric (in) (pulmonary)
     childbirth O88.22
       air O88.02
       amniotic fluid O88.12
       blood clot O88.22
       fat O88.82
       pyemic O88.32
       septic O88.32
       specified type NEC O88.82
     pregnancy O88.21-
       air O88.01-
       amniotic fluid O88.11-
       blood clot O88.21-
       fat O88.81-
       pyemic O88.31-
       septic O88.31-
       specified type NEC O88.81-
     puerperal O88.23
       air O88.03
       amniotic fluid O88.13
       blood clot O88.23
       fat O88.83
       pyemic O88.33
       septic O88.33
       specified type NEC O88.83
   ophthalmic —*see* Occlusion, artery,
     retina
   penis N48.81
   peripheral artery NOS I74.4
   pituitary E23.6
   popliteal (artery) I74.3
   portal (vein) I81
   postoperative, postprocedural
     artery T81.719
       mesenteric T81.710
       renal T81.711
       specified NEC T81.718
     vein T81.72
   precerebral artery —*see* Occlusion,
     artery, precerebral
   puerperal —*see* Embolism,
     obstetric
   pulmonary (acute) (artery) (vein)
     I26.99
     with acute cor pulmonale
       I26.09
     chronic I27.82
     following
       abortion —*see* Abortion
         by type complicated by
          embolism
       ectopic or molar pregnancy
         O08.2
     healed or old Z86.711

Embolism (continued)
   pulmonary (continued)
     in pregnancy, childbirth or
       puerperium —*see* Embolism,
       obstetric
     multiple subsegmental without
       acute cor pulmonale
       I26.94
     personal history of Z86.711
     saddle I26.92
       with acute cor pulmonale
         I26.02
     septic I26.90
       with acute cor pulmonale I26.01
     single subsegmental without
       acute cor pulmonale I26.93
     subsegmental NOS I26.93
   pyemic (multiple) I76
     following
       abortion —*see* Abortion
         by type complicated by
          embolism
       ectopic or molar pregnancy
         O08.2
     Hemophilus influenzae A41.3
     pneumococcal A40.3
       with pneumonia J13
     puerperal, postpartum, childbirth
       (any organism) —*see*
       Embolism, obstetric
     specified organism NEC A41.89
     staphylococcal A41.2
     streptococcal A40.9
   renal (artery) N28.0
     vein I82.3
   retina, retinal —*see* Occlusion,
     artery, retina
   saddle
     abdominal aorta I74.01
     pulmonary artery I26.92
       with acute cor pulmonale
         I26.02
   septic (arterial) I76
     complicating abortion
       —*see* Abortion, by type,
       complicated by, embolism
     sinus —*see* Embolism, intracranial,
       venous sinus
   soap complicating abortion —*see*
     Abortion, by type, complicated
     by, embolism
   spinal cord G95.19
     pyogenic origin G06.1
   spleen, splenic (artery) I74.8
   upper extremity I74.2
   vein (acute) I82.90
     antecubital I82.61-
       chronic I82.71-
     axillary I82.A1-
       chronic I82.A2-
     basilic I82.61-
       chronic I82.71-
     brachial I82.62-
       chronic I82.72-
     brachiocephalic (innominate)
       I82.290
       chronic I82.291
     calf, muscle I82.46-
       chronic I82.56-
     cephalic I82.61-
       chronic I82.71-
     chronic I82.91
     deep (DVT) I82.40-
       calf I82.4Z-
         chronic I82.5Z-
       lower leg I82.4Z-
         chronic I82.5Z-
       thigh I82.4Y-
         chronic I82.5Y-
       upper leg I82.4Y
         chronic I82.5y-

Embolism (continued)
   vein (continued)
     femoral I82.41-
       chronic I82.51-
     gastrocnemial I82.46-
       chronic I82.56-
     iliac (iliofemoral) I82.42-
       chronic I82.52-
     innominate I82.290
       chronic I82.291
     internal jugular I82.C1-
       chronic I82.C2-
     lower extremity
       deep I82.40-
         chronic I82.50-
         specified NEC I82.49-
           chronic NEC I82.59-
       distal
         deep I82.4Z-
       proximal
         deep I82.4Y-
           chronic I82.5Y-
       superficial I82.81-
     peroneal I82.45-
       chronic I82.55-
     popliteal I82.43-
       chronic I82.53-
     radial I82.62-
       chronic I82.72-
     renal I82.3
     saphenous (greater) (lesser) I82.81-
     soleal I82.46-
       chronic I82.56-
     specified NEC I82.890
       chronic NEC I82.891
     subclavian I82.B1-
       chronic I82.B2-
     thoracic NEC I82.290
       chronic I82.291
     tibial I82.44-
       chronic I82.54-
     ulnar I82.62-
       chronic I82.72-
     upper extremity I82.60-
       chronic I82.70-
       deep I82.62-
         chronic I82.72-
       superficial I82.61-
         chronic I82.71-
     vena cava
       inferior (acute) I82.220
         chronic I82.221
       superior (acute) I82.210
         chronic I82.211
   venous sinus G08
   vessels of brain —*see* Occlusion,
     artery, cerebral

Embolus —*see* Embolism

Embryoma —*see also* Neoplasm,
   uncertain behavior, by site
   benign —*see* Neoplasm, benign,
     by site
   kidney C64.-
   liver C22.0
   malignant —*see also* Neoplasm,
     malignant, by site
     kidney C64.-
     liver C22.0
     testis C62.9-
       descended (scrotal) C62.1-
       undescended C62.0-
   testis C62.9-
     descended (scrotal) C62.1-
     undescended C62.0-

Embryonic
   circulation Q28.9
   heart Q28.9
   vas deferens Q55.4

Embryopathia NOS Q89.9

Embryotoxon Q13.4

Emesis —*see* Vomiting

Emotional lability R45.86

Emotionality, pathological F60.3

Emotogenic disease —*see* Disorder,
   psychogenic

Emphysema (atrophic) (bullous)
   (chronic) (interlobular) (lung)
   (obstructive) (pulmonary) (senile)
   (vesicular) J43.9
   cellular tissue (traumatic) T79.7
     surgical T81.82
   centrilobular J43.2
   compensatory J98.3
   congenital (interstitial) P25.0
   conjunctiva H11.89
   connective tissue (traumatic) T79.7
     surgical T81.82
   due to chemicals, gases, fumes
     or vapors (*see also* Disease,
     respiratory, chronic, due to
     chemicals, gases, fumes or
     vapors) J43.-
   eyelid(s) —*see* Disorder, eyelid,
     specified type NEC
     surgical T81.82
     traumatic T79.7
   interstitial J98.2
     congenital P25.0
     perinatal period P25.0
   laminated tissue T79.7
     surgical T81.82
   mediastinal J98.2
     newborn P25.2
   orbit, orbital —*see* Disorder, orbit,
     specified type NEC
   panacinar J43.1
   panlobular J43.1
   specified NEC J43.8
   subcutaneous (traumatic) T79.7
     nontraumatic J98.2
     postprocedural T81.82
     surgical T81.82
   surgical T81.82
   thymus (gland) (congenital) E32.8
   traumatic (subcutaneous) T79.7
   unilateral J43.0

Empty nest syndrome Z60.0

Empyema (acute) (chest) (double)
   (pleura) (supradiaphragmatic)
   (thorax) J86.9
   with fistula J86.0
   accessory sinus (chronic) —*see*
     Sinusitis
   antrum (chronic) —*see* Sinusitis,
     maxillary
   brain (any part) —*see* Abscess,
     brain
   ethmoidal (chronic) (sinus) —*see*
     Sinusitis, ethmoidal
   extradural —*see* Abscess, extradural
   frontal (chronic) (sinus) —*see*
     Sinusitis, frontal
   gallbladder K81.0
   mastoid (process) (acute) —*see*
     Mastoiditis, acute
   maxilla, maxillary M27.2
     sinus (chronic) —*see* Sinusitis,
       maxillary
   nasal sinus (chronic) —*see* Sinusitis
   sinus (accessory) (chronic) (nasal)
     —*see* Sinusitis
   sphenoidal (sinus) (chronic) —*see*
     Sinusitis, sphenoidal
   subarachnoid —*see* Abscess,
     extradural
   subdural —*see* Abscess, subdural
   tuberculous A15.6

Empyema (continued)
  ureter —see Ureteritis
  ventricular —see Abscess, brain
En coup de sabre lesion L94.1
Enamel pearls K00.2
Enameloma K00.2
Enanthema, viral B09
Encephalitis (chronic) (hemorrhagic) (idiopathic) (nonepidemic) (spurious) (subacute) G04.90
  acute (see also Encephalitis, viral) A86
    disseminated G04.00
      infectious G04.01
      noninfectious G04.81
      postimmunization (postvaccination) G04.02
      postinfectious G04.01
    inclusion body A85.8
    necrotizing hemorrhagic G04.30
      postimmunization G04.32
      postinfectious G04.31
      specified NEC G04.39
  arboviral, arbovirus NEC A85.2
  arthropod-borne NEC (viral) A85.2
  Australian A83.4
  California (virus) A83.5
  Central European (tick-borne) A84.1
  Czechoslovakian A84.1
  Dawson's (inclusion body) A81.1
  diffuse sclerosing A81.1
  disseminated, acute G04.00
  due to
    cat scratch disease A28.1
    human immunodeficiency virus (HIV) disease B20 [G05.3]
    malaria —see Malaria
    rickettsiosis —see Rickettsiosis
    smallpox inoculation G04.02
    typhus —see Typhus
  Eastern equine A83.2
  endemic (viral) A86
  epidemic NEC (viral) A86
  equine (acute) (infectious) (viral) A83.9
    Eastern A83.2
    Venezuelan A92.2
    Western A83.1
  Far Eastern (tick-borne) A84.0
  following vaccination or other immunization procedure G04.02
  herpes zoster B02.0
  herpesviral B00.4
    due to herpesvirus 6 B10.01
    due to herpesvirus 7 B10.09
    specified NEC B10.09
  Ilheus (virus) A83.8
  inclusion body A81.1
  in (due to)
    actinomycosis A42.82
    adenovirus A85.1
    African trypanosomiasis B56.9 [G05.3]
    Chagas' disease (chronic) B57.42
    cytomegalovirus B25.8
    enterovirus A85.0
    herpes (simplex) virus B00.4
      due to herpesvirus 6 B10.01
      due to herpesvirus 7 B10.09
      specified NEC B10.09
    infectious disease NEC B99 [G05.3]
    influenza —see Influenza, with, encephalopathy
    listeriosis A32.12
    measles B05.0
    mumps B26.2
    naegleriasis B60.2

Encephalitis (continued)
  in (continued)
    parasitic disease NEC B89 [G05.3]
    poliovirus A80.9 [G05.3]
    rubella B06.01
    syphilis
      congenital A50.42
      late A52.14
    systemic lupus erythematosus M32.19 [G05.3]
    toxoplasmosis (acquired) B58.2
      congenital P37.1
    tuberculosis A17.82
    zoster B02.0
  infectious (acute) (virus) NEC A86
  Japanese (B type) A83.0
  La Crosse A83.5
  lead —see Poisoning, lead
  lethargica (acute) (infectious) A85.8
  louping ill A84.89
  lupus erythematosus, systemic M32.19 [G05.3]
  lymphatica A87.2
  Mengo A85.8
  meningococcal A39.81
  Murray Valley A83.4
  otitic NEC H66.40 [G05.3]
  parasitic NOS B71.9
  periaxial G37.0
  periaxialis (concentrica) (diffuse) G37.5
  postchickenpox B01.11
  postexanthematous NEC B09
  postimmunization G04.02
  postinfectious NEC G04.01
  postmeasles B05.0
  postvaccinal G04.02
  postvaricella B01.11
  postviral NEC A86
  Powassan A84.81
  Rasmussen G04.81
  Rio Bravo A85.8
  Russian
    autumnal A83.0
    spring-summer (taiga) A84.0
  saturnine —see Poisoning, lead
  specified NEC G04.81
  St. Louis A83.3
  subacute sclerosing A81.1
  summer A83.0
  suppurative G04.81
  tick-borne A84.9
  Torula, torular (cryptococcal) B45.1
  toxic NEC G92.8
  trichinosis B75 [G05.3]
  type
    B A83.0
    C A83.3
  van Bogaert's A81.1
  Venezuelan equine A92.2
  Vienna A85.8
  viral, virus A86
    arthropod-borne NEC A85.2
      mosquito-borne A83.9
        Australian X disease A83.4
        California virus A83.5
        Eastern equine A83.2
        Japanese (B type) A83.0
        Murray Valley A83.4
        specified NEC A83.8
        St. Louis A83.3
        type B A83.0
        type C A83.3
        Western equine A83.1
      tick-borne A84.9
        biundulant A84.1
        central European A84.1
        Czechoslovakian A84.1
        diphasic meningoencephalitis A84.1

Encephalitis (continued)
  viral, virus (continued)
    arthropod-borne (continued)
      tick-borne (continued)
        Far Eastern A84.0
        Russian spring-summer (taiga) A84.0
        specified NEC A84.89
      specified type NEC A85.8
    tick-borne, specified NEC A84.89
    Western equine A83.1
Encephalocele Q01.9
  frontal Q01.0
  nasofrontal Q01.1
  occipital Q01.2
  specified NEC Q01.8
Encephalocystocele —see Encephalocele
Encephaloduroarterio-myosynangiosis (EDAMS) I67.5
Encephalomalacia (brain) (cerebellar) (cerebral) —see Softening, brain
Encephalomeningitis —see Meningoencephalitis
Encephalomeningocele —see Encephalocele
Encephalomeningomyelitis —see Meningoencephalitis
Encephalomyelitis —see also Encephalitis G04.90
  acute disseminated G04.00
    infectious G04.01
    noninfectious G04.81
    postimmunization G04.02
    postinfectious G04.01
  acute necrotizing hemorrhagic G04.30
    postimmunization G04.32
    postinfectious G04.31
    specified NEC G04.39
  equine A83.9
    Eastern A83.2
    Venezuelan A92.2
    Western A83.1
  in diseases classified elsewhere G05.3
  myalgic G93.32
    chronic fatigue syndrome [ME/CFS] G93.32
  postchickenpox B01.11
  postinfectious NEC G04.01
  postmeasles B05.0
  postvaccinal G04.02
  postvaricella B01.11
  rubella B06.01
  specified NEC G04.81
  Venezuelan equine A92.2
Encephalomyelocele —see Encephalocele
Encephalomyelomeningitis —see Meningoencephalitis
Encephalomyelopathy G96.9
Encephalomyeloradiculitis (acute) G61.0
Encephalomyeloradiculoneuritis (acute) (Guillain-Barré) G61.0
Encephalomyeloradiculopathy G96.9
Encephalopathia hyperbilirubinemica, newborn P57.9
  due to isoimmunization (conditions in P55) P57.0

Encephalopathy (acute) G93.40
  acute necrotizing hemorrhagic G04.30
    postimmunization G04.32
    postinfectious G04.31
    specified NEC G04.39
  alcoholic G31.2
  anoxic —see Damage, brain, anoxic
  arteriosclerotic I67.2
  centrolobar progressive (Schilder) G37.0
  congenital Q07.9
  degenerative, in specified disease NEC G32.89
  demyelinating callosal G37.1
  due to
    drugs (see also Table of Drugs and Chemicals) G92.8
    hepatic (without coma) K76.82
    hyperbilirubinemic, newborn P57.9
      due to isoimmunization (conditions in P55) P57.0
  hypertensive I67.4
  hypoglycemic E16.2
  hypoxic —see Damage, brain, anoxic
  hypoxic ischemic P91.60
    mild P91.61
    moderate P91.62
    severe P91.63
  in (due to) (with)
    birth injury P11.1
    hyperinsulinism E16.1 [G94]
    influenza —see Influenza, with, encephalopathy
    lack of vitamin (see also Deficiency, vitamin) E56.9 [G32.89]
    neoplastic disease (see also Neoplasm) D49.9 [G13.1]
    serum (see also Reaction, serum) T80.69
    syphilis A52.17
    trauma (postconcussional) F07.81
      current injury —see Injury, intracranial
    vaccination G04.02
  lead —see Poisoning, lead
  metabolic G93.41
    drug induced G92.8
    toxic G92.8
  myoclonic, early, symptomatic —see Epilepsy, generalized, specified NEC
  necrotizing, subacute (Leigh) G31.82
  neonatal P91.819
    in diseases classified elsewhere P91.811
  pellagrous E52 [G32.89]
  portal-systemic K76.82
  postcontusional F07.81
    current injury —see Injury, intracranial, diffuse
  posthypoglycemic (coma) E16.1 [G94]
  postradiation G93.89
  saturnine —see Poisoning, lead
  septic G93.41
  specified NEC G93.49
  spongioform, subacute (viral) A81.09
  toxic G92.9
    metabolic G92.8
  traumatic (postconcussional) F07.81
    current injury —see Injury, intracranial
  vitamin B deficiency NEC E53.9 [G32.89]
    vitamin B1 E51.2
  Wernicke's E51.2

Encephalorrhagia —*see* Hemorrhage, intracranial, intracerebral

Encephalosis, posttraumatic F07.81

Enchondroma —*see also* Neoplasm, bone, benign

Enchondromatosis (cartilaginous) (multiple) Q78.4

Encopresis R15.9
- functional F98.1
- nonorganic origin F98.1
- psychogenic F98.1

Encounter (with health service) (for) Z76.89
- adjustment and management (of)
  - breast implant Z45.81
  - implanted device NEC Z45.89
  - myringotomy device (stent) (tube) Z45.82
  - neurostimulator (brain) (gastric) (peripheral nerve) (sacral nerve) (spinal cord) (vagus nerve) Z45.42
- administrative purpose only Z02.9
  - examination for
    - adoption Z02.82
    - armed forces Z02.3
    - child welfare Z02.84
    - disability determination Z02.71
    - driving license Z02.4
    - employment Z02.1
    - insurance Z02.6
    - medical certificate NEC Z02.79
    - paternity testing Z02.81
    - residential institution admission Z02.2
    - school admission Z02.0
    - sports Z02.5
    - specified reason NEC Z02.89
- aftercare —*see* Aftercare
- antenatal screening Z36.9
  - cervical length Z36.86
  - chromosomal anomalies Z36.0
  - congenital cardiac abnormalities Z36.83
  - elevated maternal serum alphafetoprotein level Z36.1
  - fetal growth retardation Z36.4
  - fetal lung maturity Z36.84
  - fetal macrosomia Z36.88
  - hydrops fetalis Z36.81
  - intrauterine growth restriction (IUGR)/small-for-dates Z36.4
  - isoimmunization Z36.5
  - large-for-dates Z36.88
  - malformations Z36.3
  - non-visualized anatomy on a previous scan Z36.2
  - nuchal translucency Z36.82
  - raised alphafetoprotein level Z36.1
  - risk of pre-term labor Z36.86
  - specified type NEC Z36.89
  - specified follow-up NEC Z36.2
  - specified genetic defects NEC Z36.8A
  - Streptococcus B Z36.85
  - suspected anomaly Z36.3
  - uncertain dates Z36.87
- assisted reproductive fertility procedure cycle Z31.83
- blood typing Z01.83
  - Rh typing Z01.83
- breast augmentation or reduction Z41.1
- breast implant exchange (different material) (different size) Z45.81
- breast reconstruction following mastectomy Z42.1

Encounter (continued)
- check-up —*see* Examination
- chemotherapy for neoplasm Z51.11
- child welfare screening exam Z02.84
- colonoscopy, screening Z12.11
- counseling —*see* Counseling
- delivery, full-term, uncomplicated O80
  - cesarean, without indication O82
- desensitization to allergens Z51.6
- ear piercing Z41.3
- examination —*see* Examination
- expectant parent(s) (adoptive)
  - pre-birth pediatrician visit Z76.81
- fertility preservation procedure (prior to cancer therapy) (prior to removal of gonads) Z31.84
- fitting (of) —*see* Fitting (and adjustment) (of)
- genetic
  - counseling
    - nonprocreative Z71.83
    - procreative Z31.5
  - testing —*see* Test, genetic
- hearing conservation and treatment Z01.12
- HIV
  - pre-exposure prophylaxis Z29.81
  - PrEP Z29.81
- immunotherapy for neoplasm Z51.12
- in vitro fertilization cycle Z31.83
- instruction (in)
  - childbirth Z32.2
  - child care (postpartal) (prenatal) Z32.3
  - natural family planning
    - procreative Z31.61
    - to avoid pregnancy Z30.02
- insulin pump titration Z46.81
- joint prosthesis insertion following prior explantation of joint prosthesis (staged procedure)
  - hip Z47.32
  - knee Z47.33
  - shoulder Z47.31
- laboratory (as part of a general medical examination) Z00.00
  - with abnormal findings Z00.01
- mental health services (for)
  - abuse NEC
    - perpetrator Z69.82
    - victim Z69.81
  - child abuse
    - nonparental
      - perpetrator Z69.021
      - victim Z69.020
    - parental
      - perpetrator Z69.011
      - victim Z69.010
  - child neglect
    - nonparental
      - perpetrator Z69.021
      - victim Z69.020
    - parental
      - perpetrator Z69.011
      - victim Z69.010
  - child psychological abuse
    - nonparental
      - perpetrator Z69.021
      - victim Z69.020
    - parental
      - perpetrator Z69.011
      - victim Z69.010
  - child sexual abuse
    - nonparental
      - perpetrator Z69.021
      - victim Z69.020
    - parental
      - perpetrator Z69.011
      - victim Z69.010

Encounter (continued)
- mental health services (continued)
  - non-spousal adult abuse
    - perpetrator Z69.82
    - victim Z69.81
  - spousal or parter
    - abuse
      - perpetrator Z69.12
      - victim Z69.11
    - neglect
      - perpetrator Z69.12
      - victim Z69.11
    - psychological abuse
      - perpetrator Z69.12
      - victim Z69.11
    - violence
      - perpetrator (physical) (sexual) Z69.12
      - victim (physical) Z69.11
        - sexual Z69.81
- observation (for) (ruled out)
  - alarm, without findings
    - apnea Z03.83
    - bradycardia Z03.83
    - oximeter Z03.83
  - condition suspected related to home physiologic monitoring device Z03.83
  - newborn Z05.81
    - apnea alarm Z05.81
    - bradycardia alarm Z05.81
    - malfunction of home cardiorespiratory monitor Z05.81
    - non-specific findings home physiologic monitoring device Z05.81
    - pulse oximeter alarm without findings Z05.81
  - exposure to (suspected)
    - anthrax Z03.810
    - biological agent NEC Z03.818
  - malfunction of home cardiorespiratory monitor Z03.83
  - non-specific findings home physiologic monitoring device Z03.83
- pediatrician visit, by expectant parent(s) (adoptive) Z76.81
- placental sample (taken vaginally) (*see also* Encounter, antenatal screening) Z36.9
- plastic and reconstructive surgery following medical procedure or healed injury NEC Z42.8
- postoperative —*see* Aftercare
- pregnancy
  - supervision of —*see* Pregnancy, supervision of
  - test Z32.00
    - result negative Z32.02
    - result positive Z32.01
- procreative management and counseling for gestational carrier Z31.7
- prophylactic measures Z29.9
  - antivenin Z29.12
  - fluoride administration Z29.3
  - HIV pre-exposure Z29.81
  - immunotherapy for respiratory syncytial virus (RSV) Z29.11
  - rabies immune globulin Z29.14
  - Rho (D) immune globulin Z29.13
  - specified NEC Z29.89
- radiation therapy (antineoplastic) Z51.0
- radiological (as part of a general medical examination) Z00.00
  - with abnormal findings Z00.01

Encounter (continued)
- reconstructive surgery following medical procedure or healed injury NEC Z42.8
- removal (of) —*see also* Removal
  - artificial
    - arm Z44.00-
      - complete Z44.01-
      - partial Z44.02-
    - eye Z44.2-
    - leg Z44.10-
      - complete Z44.11-
      - partial Z44.12-
  - breast implant Z45.81
    - tissue expander (with or without synchronous insertion of permanent implant) Z45.81
  - device Z46.9
    - specified NEC Z46.89
  - external
    - fixation device - code to fracture with seventh character D
    - prosthesis, prosthetic device Z44.9
      - breast Z44.3-
      - specified NEC Z44.8
  - implanted device NEC Z45.89
  - insulin pump Z46.81
  - internal fixation device Z47.2
  - myringotomy device (stent) (tube) Z45.82
  - nervous system device NEC Z46.2
    - brain neuropacemaker Z46.2
    - visual substitution device Z46.2
      - implanted Z45.31
  - non-vascular catheter Z46.82
  - orthodontic device Z46.4
  - stent
    - ureteral Z46.6
  - urinary device Z46.6
- repeat cervical smear to confirm findings of recent normal smear following initial abnormal smear Z01.42
- respirator [ventilator] use during power failure Z99.12
- Rh typing Z01.83
- screening —*see* Screening
- specified NEC Z76.89
- sterilization Z30.2
- suspected condition, ruled out
  - amniotic cavity and membrane Z03.71
  - cervical shortening Z03.75
  - fetal anomaly Z03.73
  - fetal growth Z03.74
  - maternal and fetal conditions NEC Z03.79
  - oligohydramnios Z03.71
  - placental problem Z03.72
  - polyhydramnios Z03.71
- suspected exposure (to), ruled out
  - anthrax Z03.810
  - biological agents NEC Z03.818
- termination of pregnancy, elective Z33.2
- testing —*see* Test
- therapeutic drug level monitoring Z51.81
- titration, insulin pump Z46.81
- to determine fetal viability of pregnancy O36.80
- training
  - insulin pump Z46.81
- X-ray of chest (as part of a general medical examination) Z00.00
  - with abnormal findings Z00.01

Encystment —*see* Cyst

Endarteritis (bacterial, subacute)
(infective) I77.6
  brain I67.7
  cerebral or cerebrospinal I67.7
  deformans —see Arteriosclerosis
  embolic —see Embolism
  obliterans —see also Arteriosclerosis
    pulmonary I28.8
  pulmonary I28.8
  retina —see Vasculitis, retina
  senile —see Arteriosclerosis
  syphilitic A52.09
    brain or cerebral A52.04
    congenital A50.54 [I79.8]
  tuberculous A18.89
Endemic —see condition
Endocarditis (chronic) (marantic)
  (nonbacterial) (thrombotic)
  (valvular) I38
  with rheumatic fever (conditions
    in I00)
    active —see Endocarditis, acute,
      rheumatic
    inactive or quiescent (with
      chorea) I09.1
  acute or subacute I33.9
    infective I33.0
    rheumatic (aortic) (mitral)
      (pulmonary) (tricuspid) I01.1
      with chorea (acute) (rheumatic)
        (Sydenham's) I02.0
  aortic (heart) (nonrheumatic)
    (valve) I35.8
    with
      mitral disease I08.0
        with tricuspid (valve)
          disease I08.3
          active or acute I01.1
            with chorea (acute)
              (rheumatic)
              (Sydenham's) I02.0
          rheumatic fever (conditions
            in I00)
            active —see Endocarditis,
              acute, rheumatic
            inactive or quiescent (with
              chorea) I06.9
        tricuspid (valve) disease I08.2
          with mitral (valve) disease
            I08.3
    acute or subacute I33.9
    arteriosclerotic I35.8
    rheumatic I06.9
      with mitral disease I08.0
        with tricuspid (valve)
          disease I08.3
          active or acute I01.1
            with chorea (acute)
              (rheumatic)
              (Sydenham's) I02.0
          active or acute I01.1
            with chorea (acute)
              (rheumatic)
              (Sydenham's) I02.0
          specified NEC I06.8
    specified cause NEC I35.8
    syphilitic A52.03
  arteriosclerotic I38
  atypical verrucous (Libman-Sacks)
    M32.11
  bacterial (acute) (any valve)
    (subacute) I33.0
  candidal B37.6
  congenital Q24.8
  constrictive I33.0
  Coxiella burnetii A78 [I39]
  Coxsackie B33.21
  due to
    prosthetic cardiac valve T82.6
    Q fever A78 [I39]

Endocarditis (continued)
  due to (continued)
    Serratia marcescens I33.0
    typhoid (fever) A01.02
  gonococcal A54.83
  infectious or infective (acute) (any
    valve) (subacute) I33.0
  lenta (acute) (any valve) (subacute)
    I33.0
  Libman-Sacks M32.11
  listerial A32.82
  Löffler's I42.3
  malignant (acute) (any valve)
    (subacute) I33.0
  meningococcal A39.51
  mitral (chronic) (double) (fibroid)
    (heart) (inactive) (valve) (with
    chorea) I05.9
    with
      aortic (valve) disease I08.0
        with tricuspid (valve)
          disease I08.3
          active or acute I01.1
            with chorea (acute)
              (rheumatic)
              (Sydenham's) I02.0
        rheumatic fever (conditions
          in I00)
          active —see Endocarditis,
            acute, rheumatic
          inactive or quiescent (with
            chorea) I05.9
        tricuspid (valve) disease
          I08.1
          with aortic (valve) disease
            I08.3
      active or acute I01.1
        with chorea (acute)
          (rheumatic) (Sydenham's)
          I02.0
      bacterial I33.0
    arteriosclerotic I34.89
    nonrheumatic I34.89
      acute or subacute I33.9
    specified NEC I05.8
  monilial B37.6
  multiple valves I08.9
    specified disorders I08.8
  mycotic (acute) (any valve)
    (subacute) I33.0
  pneumococcal (acute) (any valve)
    (subacute) I33.0
  pulmonary (chronic) (heart) (valve)
    I37.8
    with rheumatic fever (conditions
      in I00)
      active —see Endocarditis,
        acute, rheumatic
      inactive or quiescent (with
        chorea) I09.89
        with aortic, mitral or
          tricuspid disease
          I08.8
      acute or subacute I33.9
        rheumatic I01.1
          with chorea (acute)
            (rheumatic) (Sydenham's)
            I02.0
      arteriosclerotic I37.8
      congenital Q22.2
      rheumatic (chronic) (inactive)
        (with chorea) I09.89
        active or acute I01.1
          with chorea (acute)
            (rheumatic) (Sydenham's)
            I02.0
      syphilitic A52.03
    purulent (acute) (any valve)
      (subacute) I33.0
    Q fever A78 [I39]

Endocarditis (continued)
  rheumatic (chronic) (inactive) (with
    chorea) I09.1
    active or acute (aortic) (mitral)
      (pulmonary) (tricuspid) I01.1
      with chorea (acute)
        (rheumatic) (Sydenham's)
        I02.0
  rheumatoid —see Rheumatoid,
    carditis
  septic (acute) (any valve)
    (subacute) I33.0
  streptococcal (acute) (any valve)
    (subacute) I33.0
  subacute —see Endocarditis, acute
  suppurative (acute) (any valve)
    (subacute) I33.0
  syphilitic A52.03
  toxic I33.9
  tricuspid (chronic) (heart) (inactive)
    (rheumatic) (valve) (with chorea)
    I07.9
    with
      aortic (valve) disease I08.2
      mitral (valve) disease I08.3
      mitral (valve) disease I08.1
        aortic (valve) disease I08.3
      rheumatic fever (conditions
        in I00)
        active —see Endocarditis,
          acute, rheumatic
        inactive or quiescent (with
          chorea) I07.8
      active or acute I01.1
        with chorea (acute) (rheumatic)
          (Sydenham's) I02.0
      arteriosclerotic I36.8
      nonrheumatic I36.8
        acute or subacute I33.9
      specified cause, except rheumatic
        I36.8
  tuberculous —see Tuberculosis,
    endocarditis
  typhoid A01.02
  ulcerative (acute) (any valve)
    (subacute) I33.0
  vegetative (acute) (any valve)
    (subacute) I33.0
  verrucous (atypical) (nonbacterial)
    (nonrheumatic) M32.11
Endocardium, endocardial —see
  also condition
  cushion defect Q21.20
Endocervicitis —see also Cervicitis
  due to intrauterine (contraceptive)
    device T83.69
  hyperplastic N72
Endocrine —see condition
Endocrinopathy, pluriglandular E31.9
Endodontic
  overfill M27.52
  underfill M27.53
Endodontitis K04.01
  irreversible K04.02
  reversible K04.01
Endomastoiditis —see Mastoiditis
Endometrioma N80.12-
Endometriosis N80.9
  abdomen, abdominal N80.C0
    specified site, NEC N80.C9
    wall N80.C19
      fascia and muscular layers
        N80.C11
      subcutaneous tissue N80.C10
      unspecified depth N80.C19
  appendix N80.549
    deep N80.542
    superficial N80.541

Endometriosis (continued)
  bladder (unspecified depth)
    N80.8A0
    deep N80.A2
    superficial N80.A1
  bowel N80.50
  broad ligament N80.3C
  cardiothoracic space N80.B6
  cecum N80.539
    deep N80.532
    superficial N80.531
  cervix N80.0-
  colon N80.559
    descending N80.559
      deep N80.552
      superficial N80.551
    sigmoid N80.529
      deep N80.522
      superficial N80.521
    transverse N80.559
      deep N80.552
      superficial N80.551
  cul-de-sac (Douglas')
    anterior (unspecified depth)
      N80.319
      deep N80.312
      superficial N80.311
    posterior (unspecified depth)
      N80.329
      deep N80.322
      superficial N80.321
  deep
    involving muscular wall of
      fallopian tube N80.22
    retrocervical N80.02
  diaphragm N80.B39
    deep N80.B32
    superficial N80.B31
    unspecified depth N80.B39
  exocervix N80.01
  extra-pelvic abdominal peritoneum
    N80.C4
  fallopian tube (unspecified depth)
    N80.20-
    deep N80.22-
    superficial N80.21-
  female genital organ NEC N80.8
  gallbladder N80.8
  in scar of skin N80.6
  inguinal canal N80.C3
  internal N80.02
  intestine N80.50
    small N80.569
      deep (multifocal) N80.562
      superficial N80.561
  lung N80.B2
  mediastinal space N80.B5
  myometrium N80.03
  nerve
    femoral N80.D6
    obturator N80.D3
    pelvic N80.D0
      splanchnic N80.D1
    pudendal N80.D5
    retroperitoneum, NEC N80.D9
    sacral splanchnic N80.D1
    sciatic N80.D4
    specified, NEC N80.D9
  ovary (unspecified depth)
    N80.10-
    deep N80.12-
    superficial N80.11-
  parametrium N80.399
  pelvic
    brim N80.38-
      deep N80.37-
      superficial N80.36-
    peritoneum N80.30
      specified sites, NEC N80.399
        deep N80.392
        superficial N80.391

Endometriosis (continued)
  pelvic (continued)
    sidewall N80.35-
      deep N80.34-
      superficial N80.33-
  pericardial space N80.B4
  peritoneal (pelvic) N80.30
  pleura N80.B1
  rectovaginal septum N80.40
    with involvement of vagina N80.42
    without involvement of vagina N80.41
  rectum N80.519
    deep (multifocal) N80.512
    superficial N80.511
  retroperitoneum N80.30
  round ligament N80.3C9
  sacral nerve roots N80.D2
  skin (scar) N80.6
  specified site NEC N80.8
  stromal D39.0
  thorax N80.B-
  umbilicus N80.8C2
  ureter N80.A69
    deep N80.A5-
    extrinsic N80.A4-
    intrinsic N80.A5-
    superficial N80.A4-
    unspecified depth N80.A6-
  uterosacral ligament(s) N80.3C-
    deep N80.3B-
    superficial N80.3A-
  uterus N80.00
    deep N80.02
    internal N80.02
    superficial N80.01
  vagina N80.42
  vulva N80.8

Endometritis (decidual) (nonspecific) (purulent) (senile) (atrophic) (suppurative) N71.9
  with ectopic pregnancy O08.0
  acute N71.0
  blenorrhagic (gonococcal) (acute) (chronic) A54.24
  cervix, cervical (with erosion or ectropion) —*see also* Cervicitis hyperplastic N72
  chlamydial A56.11
  chronic N71.1
  following
    abortion —*see* Abortion by type complicated by genital infection
    ectopic or molar pregnancy O08.0
  gonococcal, gonorrheal (acute) (chronic) A54.24
  hyperplastic (*see also* Hyperplasia, endometrial) N85.00-
    cervix N72
  puerperal, postpartum, childbirth O86.12
  subacute N71.0
  tuberculous A18.17

Endometrium —*see* condition

Endomyocardiopathy, South African I42.3

Endomyocarditis —*see* Endocarditis

Endomyofibrosis I42.3

Endomyometritis —*see* Endometritis

Endopericarditis —*see* Endocarditis

Endoperineuritis —*see* Disorder, nerve

Endophlebitis —*see* Phlebitis

Endophthalmia —*see* Endophthalmitis, purulent

Endophthalmitis (acute) (infective) (metastatic) (subacute) H44.009
  bleb associated H59.4 —*see also* Bleb, inflamed (infected), postprocedural
  gonorrheal A54.39
  in (due to)
    cysticercosis B69.1
    onchocerciasis B73.01
    toxocariasis B83.0
  panuveitis —*see* Panuveitis
  parasitic H44.12-
  purulent H44.00-
    panophthalmitis —*see* Panophthalmitis
    vitreous abscess H44.02-
  specified NEC H44.19
  sympathetic —*see* Uveitis, sympathetic

Endosalpingioma D28.2

Endosalpingiosis N94.89

Endosteitis —*see* Osteomyelitis

Endothelioma, bone —*see* Neoplasm, bone, malignant

Endotheliosis (hemorrhagic infectional) D69.8

Endotoxemia - code to condition

Endotrachelitis —*see* Cervicitis

Engelmann (-Camurati) **syndrome** Q78.3

English disease —*see* Rickets

Engman's disease L30.3

Engorgement
  breast N64.59
    newborn P83.4
    puerperal, postpartum O92.79
  lung (passive) —*see* Edema, lung
  pulmonary (passive) —*see* Edema, lung
  stomach K31.89
  venous, retina —*see* Occlusion, retina, vein, engorgement

Enlargement, enlarged —*see also* Hypertrophy
  adenoids J35.2
    with tonsils J35.3
  alveolar ridge K08.89
    congenital —*see* Anomaly, alveolar
  apertures of diaphragm (congenital) Q79.1
  gingival K06.1
  heart, cardiac —*see* Hypertrophy, cardiac
  labium majus, childhood asymmetric (CALME) N90.61
  lacrimal gland, chronic H04.03-
  liver —*see* Hypertrophy, liver
  lymph gland or node R59.9
    generalized R59.1
    localized R59.0
  orbit H05.34-
  organ or site, congenital NEC —*see* Anomaly, by site
  parathyroid (gland) E21.0
  pituitary fossa R93.0
  prostate N40.0
    with lower urinary tract symptoms (LUTS) N40.1
      nodular N40.3
    nodular N40.2
      with lower urinary tract symptoms (LUTS) N40.3
      without lower urinary tract symtpoms (LUTS) N40.0
    nodular N40.2

Enlargement, enlarged (continued)
  sella turcica R93.0
  spleen —*see* Splenomegaly
  thymus (gland) (congenital) E32.0
  thyroid (gland) —*see* Goiter
  tongue K14.8
  tonsils J35.1
    with adenoids J35.3
  uterus N85.2
  vestibular aqueduct A16.5

Enophthalmos H05.40-
  due to
    orbital tissue atrophy H05.41-
    trauma or surgery H05.42-

Enostosis M27.8

Entamebic, entamebiasis —*see* Amebiasis

Entanglement
  umbilical cord(s) O69.82
    with compression O69.2
    around neck
      other, with compression O69.2
      other, without compression O69.82
      with compression O69.1
      without compression O69.81
    of twins in monoamniotic sac O69.2
    without compression O69.82

Enteralgia —*see* Pain, abdominal

Enteric —*see* condition

Enteritis (acute) (diarrheal) (hemorrhagic) (noninfective) K52.9
  adenovirus A08.2
  aertrycke infection A02.0
  allergic K52.29
    with
      eosinophilic gastritis or gastroenteritis K52.81
      food protein-induced entercolitis syndrome K52.21
      food protein-induced enteropathy K52.22
      FPIES K52.21
  amebic (acute) A06.0
    with abscess —*see* Abscess, amebic
    chronic A06.1
      with abscess —*see* Abscess, amebic
      nondysenteric A06.2
    nondysenteric A06.2
  astrovirus A08.32
  bacillary NOS A03.9
  bacterial A04.9
    specified NEC A04.8
  calicivirus A08.31
  candidal B37.82
  Chilomastix A07.8
  choleriformis A00.1
  chronic (noninfectious) K52.9
    ulcerative —*see* Colitis, ulcerative
  cicatrizing (chronic) —*see* Enteritis, regional, small intestine
  Clostridium
    botulinum (food poisoning) A05.1
    difficile
      not specified as recurrent A04.72
      recurrent A04.71
  coccidial A07.3
  coxsackie virus A08.39

Enteritis (continued)
  dietetic (*see also* Enteritis, allergic) K52.29
  drug-induced K52.1
  due to
    astrovirus A08.32
    calicivirus A08.31
    coxsackie virus A08.39
    drugs K52.1
    echovirus A08.39
    enterovirus NEC A08.39
    food hypersensitivity (*see also* Enteritis, allergic) K52.29
    infectious organism (bacterial) (viral) —*see* Enteritis, infectious
    torovirus A08.39
    Yersinia enterocolitica A04.6
  echovirus A08.39
  eltor A00.1
  enterovirus NEC A08.39
  eosinophilic K52.81
  epidemic (infectious) A09
  fulminant (*see also* Ischemia, intestine acute) K55.019
  gangrenous —*see* Enteritis, infectious
  giardial A07.1
  infectious NOS A09
    due to
      adenovirus A08.2
      Aerobacter aerogenes A04.8
      Arizona (bacillus) A02.0
      bacteria NOS A04.9
        specified NEC A04.8
      Campylobacter A04.5
      Clostridium difficile
        not specified as recurrent A04.72
        recurrent A04.71
      Clostridium perfringens A04.8
      Enterobacter aerogenes A04.8
      enterovirus A08.39
      Escherichia coli A04.4
        enteroaggregative A04.4
        enterohemorrhagic A04.3
        enteroinvasive A04.2
        enteropathogenic A04.0
        enterotoxigenic A04.1
        specified NEC A04.4
      specified
        bacteria NEC A04.8
        virus NEC A08.39
      Staphylococcus A04.8
      virus NEC A08.4
        specified type NEC A08.39
      Yersinia enterocolitica A04.6
    specified organism NEC A08.8
  influenzal —*see* Influenza, with, digestive manifestations
  ischemic K55.9
    acute (*see also* Ischemia, intestine acute) K55.019
    chronic K55.1
  microsporidial A07.8
  mucomembranous, myxomembranous —*see* Syndrome, irritable bowel
  mucous —*see* Syndrome, irritable bowel
  necroticans A05.2
  necrotizing of newborn —*see* Enterocolitis, necrotizing, in newborn
  neurogenic —*see* Syndrome, irritable bowel
  newborn necrotizing —*see* Enterocolitis, necrotizing, in newborn
  noninfectious K52.9

141

Enteritis (continued)
  norovirus A08.11
  parasitic NEC B82.9
  paratyphoid (fever) —see Fever, paratyphoid
  protozoal A07.9
    specified NEC A07.8
  radiation K52.0
  regional (of) K50.90
    with
      complication K50.919
        abscess K50.914
        fistula K50.913
        intestinal obstruction K50.912
        rectal bleeding K50.911
        specified complication NEC K50.918
    colon —see Enteritis, regional, large intestine
    duodenum —see Enteritis, regional, small intestine
    ileum —see Enteritis, regional, small intestine
    jejunum —see Enteritis, regional, small intestine
    large bowel —see Enteritis, regional, large intestine
    large intestine (colon) (rectum) K50.10
      with
        complication K50.119
          abscess K50.114
          fistula K50.113
          intestinal obstruction K50.112
          rectal bleeding K50.111
          small intestine (duodenum) (ileum) (jejunum) involvement K50.80
            with
              complication K50.819
                abscess K50.814
                fistula K50.813
                intestinal obstruction K50.812
                rectal bleeding K50.811
                specified complication NEC K50.818
          specified complication NEC K50.118
    rectum —see Enteritis, regional, large intestine
    small intestine (duodenum) (ileum) (jejunum) K50.00
      with
        complication K50.019
          abscess K50.014
          fistula K50.013
          intestinal obstruction K50.012
          large intestine (colon) (rectum) involvement K50.80
            with
              complication K50.819
                abscess K50.814
                fistula K50.813
                intestinal obstruction K50.812
                rectal bleeding K50.811
                specified complication NEC K50.818

Enteritis (continued)
  regional (continued)
    small intestine (continued)
      with (continued)
        complication (continued)
          rectal bleeding K50.011
          specified complication NEC K50.018
  rotaviral A08.0
  Salmonella, salmonellosis (arizonae) (cholerae-suis) (enteritidis) (typhimurium) A02.0
  segmental —see Enteritis, regional
  septic A09
  Shigella —see Infection, Shigella
  small round structured NEC A08.19
  spasmodic, spastic —see Syndrome, irritable bowel
  staphylococcal A04.8
    due to food A05.0
  torovirus A08.39
  toxic NEC K52.1
    due to Clostridium difficile
      not specified as recurrent A04.72
      recurrent A04.71
  trichomonal A07.8
  tuberculous A18.32
  typhosa A01.00
  ulcerative (chronic) —see Colitis, ulcerative
  viral A08.4
    adenovirus A08.2
    enterovirus A08.39
    Rotavirus A08.0
    small round structured NEC A08.19
    specified NEC A08.39
    virus specified NEC A08.39

Enterobiasis B80

Enterobius vermicularis (infection) (infestation) B80

Enterocele —see also Hernia, abdomen
  pelvic, pelvis (acquired) (congenital) N81.5
  vagina, vaginal (acquired) (congenital) NEC N81.5

Enterocolitis (see also Enteritis) K52.9
  due to Clostridium difficile
    not specified as recurrent A04.72
    recurrent A04.71
  fulminant ischemic (see also Ischemia, intestine acute) K55.059
  granulomatous —see Enteritis, regional
  hemorrhagic (acute) (see also Ischemia, intestine acute) K55.059
    chronic K55.1
  infectious NEC A09
  ischemic K55.9
  necrotizing K55.30
    with
      perforation K55.33
      pneumatosis K55.32
        and perforation K55.33
    due to Clostridium difficile
      not specified as recurrent A04.72
      recurrent A04.71
    in newborn P77.9
      stage 1 (without pneumatosis, without perforation) P77.1
      stage 2 (with pneumatosis, without perforation) P77.2
      stage 3 (with pneumatosis, with perforation) P77.3

Enterocolitis (continued)
  necrotizing (continued)
    in non-newborn K55.30
      stage 1 (without pneumatosis, without perforation) K55.31
      stage 2 (with pneumatosis, without perforation) K55.32
      stage 3 (with pneumatosis, with perforation) K55.33
      without pneumatosis or perforation K55.31
    noninfectious K52.9
    newborn —see Enterocolitis, necrotizing, in newborn
    pseudomembranous (newborn)
      not specified as recurrent A04.72
      recurrent A04.71
    radiation K52.0
      newborn —see Enterocolitis, necrotizing, in newborn
    ulcerative (chronic) —see Pancolitis, ulcerative (chronic)

Enterogastritis —see Enteritis

Enteropathy K63.9
  celiac-gluten-sensitive K90.0
    non-celiac K90.41
  food protein-induced K52.22
  hemorrhagic, terminal (see also Ischemia, intestine, acute) K55.059
  protein-losing K90.49

Enteroperitonitis —see Peritonitis

Enteroptosis K63.4

Enterorrhagia K92.2

Enterospasm —see also Syndrome, irritable, bowel
  psychogenic F45.8

Enterostenosis (see also Obstruction, intestine specified NEC) K56.699

Enterostomy
  complication —see Complication, enterostomy
  status Z93.4

Enterovirus, as cause of disease classified elsewhere B97.10
  coxsackievirus B97.11
  echovirus B97.12
  other specified B97.19

Enthesopathy (peripheral) M77.9
  Achilles tendinitis —see Tendinitis, Achilles
  ankle and tarsus M77.5-
    specified type NEC —see Enthesopathy, foot, specified type NEC
  anterior tibial syndrome M76.81-
  calcaneal spur —see Spur, bone, calcaneal
  elbow region M77.8
    lateral epicondylitis —see Epicondylitis, lateral
    medial epicondylitis —see Epicondylitis, medial
  foot NEC M77.8
    metatarsalgia —see Metatarsalgia
    specified type NEC M77.5-
  forearm M77.8
  gluteal tendinitis —see Tendinitis, gluteal
  hand M77.8
  hip —see Enthesopathy, lower limb, specified type NEC
  iliac crest spur —see Spur, bone, iliac crest
  iliotibial band syndrome —see Syndrome, iliotibial band

Enthesopathy (continued)
  knee —see Enthesopathy, lower limb, lower leg, specified type NEC
  lateral epicondylitis —see Epicondylitis, lateral
  lower limb (excluding foot) M76.9
    Achilles tendinitis —see Tendinitis, Achilles
    ankle and tarsus M77.5-
      specified type NEC —see Enthesopathy, foot, specified type NEC
    anterior tibial syndrome M76.81-
    gluteal tendinitis —see Tendinitis, gluteal
    iliac crest spur —see Spur, bone, iliac crest
    iliotibial band syndrome —see Syndrome, iliotibial band
    patellar tendinitis —see Tendinitis, patellar
    pelvic region —see Enthesopathy, lower limb, specified type NEC
    peroneal tendinitis —see Tendinitis, peroneal
    posterior tibial syndrome M76.82-
    psoas tendinitis —see Tendinitis, psoas
    specified type NEC M76.89-
    tibial collateral bursitis —see Bursitis, tibial collateral
  medial epicondylitis —see Epicondylitis, medial
  metatarsalgia —see Metatarsalgia
  multiple sites M77.8
  patellar tendinitis —see Tendinitis, patellar
  pelvis M77.8
  periarthritis of wrist —see Periarthritis, wrist
  peroneal tendinitis —see Tendinitis, peroneal
  posterior tibial syndrome M76.82-
  psoas tendinitis —see Tendinitis, psoas
  shoulder M77.8
  shoulder region —see Lesion, shoulder
  specified type NEC M77.8
  spinal M46.00
    cervical region M46.02
    cervicothoracic region M46.03
    lumbar region M46.06
    lumbosacral region M46.07
    multiple sites M46.09
    occipito-atlanto-axial region M46.01
    sacrococcygeal region M46.08
    thoracic region M46.04
    thoracolumbar region M46.05
  tibial collateral bursitis —see Bursitis, tibial collateral
  upper arm M77.8
  wrist and carpus NEC M77.8
    calcaneal spur —see Spur, bone, calcaneal
    periarthritis of wrist —see Periarthritis, wrist

Entomophobia F40.218

Entomophthoromycosis B46.8

Entrance, air into vein —see Embolism, air

Entrapment
  muscle
    eye
      extraocular H50.68-
        oblique
          inferior H50.62-
          superior H50.66-

Entrapment (continued)
  muscle (continued)
    rectus
      inferior H50.63-
      lateral H50.64-
      medial H50.65-
      superior H50.67-
  nerve —see Neuropathy, entrapment
Entropion (eyelid) (paralytic) H02.009
  cicatricial H02.019
    left H02.016
      lower H02.015
      upper H02.014
    right H02.013
      lower H02.012
      upper H02.011
  congenital Q10.2
  left H02.006
    lower H02.005
    upper H02.004
  mechanical H02.029
    left H02.026
      lower H02.025
      upper H02.024
    right H02.023
      lower H02.022
      upper H02.021
  right H02.003
    lower H02.002
    upper H02.001
  senile H02.039
    left H02.036
      lower H02.035
      upper H02.034
    right H02.033
      lower H02.032
      upper H02.031
  spastic H02.049
    left H02.046
      lower H02.045
      upper H02.044
    right H02.043
      lower H02.042
      upper H02.041
Enucleated eye (traumatic, current) S05.7-
Enuresis R32
  functional F98.0
  habit disturbance F98.0
  nocturnal N39.44
    psychogenic F98.0
  nonorganic origin F98.0
  psychogenic F98.0
Eosinopenia —see Agranulocytosis
Eosinophilia (allergic) (idiopathic) (secondary) D72.10
  with
    angiolymphoid hyperplasia (ALHE) D18.01
  familial D71.19
  hereditary D72.19
  in diseases classified elsewhere D72.18
  infiltrative —see Eosinophilia, pulmonary
  Löffler's J82.89
  peritoneal —see Peritonitis, eosinophilic
  pulmonary NEC J82.89
    acute J82.82
    asthmatic J82.83
    chronic J82.81
  specified NEC D72.19
  tropical (pulmonary) J82.89
Eosinophilia-myalgia syndrome M35.89

Ependymitis (acute) (cerebral) (chronic) (granular) —see Encephalomyelitis
Ependymoblastoma
  specified site —see Neoplasm, malignant, by site
  unspecified site C71.9
Ependymoma (epithelial) (malignant)
  anaplastic
    specified site —see Neoplasm, malignant, by site
    unspecified site C71.9
  benign
    specified site —see Neoplasm, benign, by site
    unspecified site D33.2
  myxopapillary D43.2
    specified site —see Neoplasm, uncertain behavior, by site
    unspecified site D43.2
  papillary D43.2
    specified site —see Neoplasm, uncertain behavior, by site
    unspecified site D43.2
  specified site —see Neoplasm, malignant, by site
  unspecified site C71.9
Ependymopathy G93.89
Ephelis, ephelides L81.2
Epiblepharon (congenital) Q10.3
Epicanthus, epicanthic fold (eyelid) (congenital) Q10.3
Epicondylitis (elbow)
  lateral M77.1-
  medial M77.0-
Epicystitis —see Cystitis
Epidemic —see condition
Epidermidalization, cervix —see Dysplasia, cervix
Epidermis, epidermal —see condition
Epidermodysplasia verruciformis B07.8
Epidermolysis
  bullosa (congenital) Q81.9
    acquired L12.30
      drug-induced L12.31
      specified cause NEC L12.35
    dystrophica Q81.2
    letalis Q81.1
    simplex Q81.0
    specified NEC Q81.8
  necroticans combustiformis L51.2
  due to drug —see Table of Drugs and Chemicals, by drug
Epidermophytid —see Dermatophytosis
Epidermophytosis (infected) —see Dermatophytosis
Epididymis —see condition
Epididymitis (acute) (nonvenereal) (recurrent) (residual) N45.1
  with orchitis N45.3
  blennorrhagic (gonococcal) A54.23
  caseous (tuberculous) A18.15
  chlamydial A56.19
  filarial (see also Infestation, filarial) B74.9 [N51]
  gonococcal A54.23
  syphilitic A52.76
  tuberculous A18.15
Epididymo-orchitis (see also Epididymitis) N45.3
Epidural —see condition

Epigastrium, epigastric —see condition
Epigastrocele —see Hernia, ventral
Epiglottis —see condition
Epiglottitis, epiglottiditis (acute) J05.10
  with obstruction J05.11
  chronic J37.0
Epignathus Q89.4
Epilepsia partialis continua (see also Kozhevnikof's epilepsy) G40.1-
Epilepsy, epileptic, epilepsia (attack) (cerebral) (convulsion) (fit) (seizure) G40.909

> Note: the following terms are to be considered equivalent to intractable: pharmacoresistant (pharmacologically resistant), treatment resistant, refractory (medically) and poorly controlled

  with
    complex partial seizures —see Epilepsy, localization-related, symptomatic, with complex partial seizures
    grand mal seizures on awakening —see Epilepsy, generalized, specified NEC
    myoclonic absences —see Epilepsy, generalized, specified NEC
    myoclonic-astatic seizures —see Epilepsy, generalized, specified NEC
    simple partial seizures —see Epilepsy, localization-related, symptomatic, with simple partial seizures
  akinetic —see Epilepsy, generalized, specified NEC
  benign childhood with
    centrotemporal EEG spikes —see Epilepsy, localization-related, idiopathic
  benign myoclonic in infancy G 40.80-
  Bravais-jacksonian —see Epilepsy, localization-related, symptomatic, with simple partial seizures
  childhood
    with occipital EEG paroxysms —see Epilepsy, localization-related, idiopathic
    absence G40.A09
      intractable G40.A19
        with status epilepticus G40.A11
        without status epilepticus G40.A19
      not intractable G40.A09
        with status epilepticus G40.A01
        without status epilepticus G40.A09
  climacteric —see Epilepsy, specified NEC
  cysticercosis B69.0
  deterioration (mental) F06.8
  due to syphilis A52.19
  focal —see Epilepsy, localization-related, symptomatic, with simple partial seizures
  generalized
    idiopathic G40.309
      intractable G40.319
        with status epilepticus G40.311
        without status epilepticus G40.319

Epilepsy, epileptic, epilepsia (continued)
  generalized (continued)
    idiopathic (continued)
      not intractable G40.309
        with status epilepticus G40.301
        without status epilepticus G40.309
    specified NEC G40.409
      intractable G40.419
        with status epilepticus G40.411
        without status epilepticus G40.419
      not intractable G40.409
        with status epilepticus G40.401
        without status epilepticus G40.409
  impulsive petit mal —see Epilepsy, juvenile myoclonic
  intractable G40.919
    with status epilepticus G40.911
    without status epilepticus G40.919
  juvenile absence G40.A09
    intractable G40.A19
      with status epilepticus G40.A11
      without status epilepticus G40.A19
    not intractable G40.A09
      with status epilepticus G40.A01
      without status epilepticus G40.A09
  juvenile myoclonic G40.B09
    intractable G40.B19
      with status epilepticus G40.B11
      without status epilepticus G40.B19
    not intractable G40.B09
      with status epilepticus G40.B01
      without status epilepticus G40.B09
  Lafora progressive myoclonus (see also Epilepsy, progressive, Lafora) G40.C09
  localization-related (focal) (partial)
    idiopathic G40.009
      with seizures of localized onset G40.009
        intractable G40.019
          with status epilepticus G40.011
          without status epilepticus G40.019
        not intractable G40.009
          with status epilepticus G40.001
          without status epilepticus G40.009
    symptomatic
      with complex partial seizures G40.209
        intractable G40.219
          with status epilepticus G40.211
          without status epilepticus G40.219
        not intractable G40.209
          with status epilepticus G40.201
          without status epilepticus G40.209
      with simple partial seizures G40.109
        intractable G40.119
          with status epilepticus G40.111
          without status epilepticus G40.119

Epilepsy, epileptic, epilepsia (continued)
  localization-related (continued)
    symptomatic (continued)
      with simple partial seizures (continued)
        not intractable G40.109
          with status epilepticus G40.101
          without status epilepticus G40.109
  myoclonus, myoclonic —see also Epilepsy, generalized, specified NEC
    progressive —see also Epilepsy, generalized, idiopathic
      Lafora G40.C09
        intractable G40.C19
          with status epilepticus G40.C11
          without status epilepticus G40.C19
        not intractable G40.C09
          with status epilepticus G40.C01
          without status epilepticus G40.C09
    type 1 - see Epilepsy, generalized, idiopathic
    type 2 - see Epilepsy, myoclonus, progressive, Lafora
    severe, in infancy (SMEI) G40.83-
  not intractable G40.909
    with status epilepticus G40.901
    without status epilepticus G40.909
  on awakening —see Epilepsy, generalized, specified NEC
  parasitic NOS B71.9 [G94]
  partial —see Epilepsy, localization-related, symptomatic, with simple partial seizures
  partialis continua (see also Kozhevnikof's epilepsy) G40.1-
  peripheral —see Epilepsy, specified NEC
  polymorphic, in infancy (PMEI) G40.83-
  procursiva —see Epilepsy, localization-related, symptomatic, with simple partial seizures
  progressive (familial) myoclonic —see Epilepsy, myoclonus, progressive
    Lafora (see also Epilepsy, progressive, Lafora) G40.C09
  reflex —see Epilepsy, specified NEC
  related to
    alcohol G40.509
      not intractable G40.509
        with status epilepticus G40.501
        without status epilepticus G40.509
    drugs G40.509
      not intractable G40.509
        with status epilepticus G40.501
        without status epilepticus G40.509
    external causes G40.509
      not intractable G40.509
        with status epilepticus G40.501
        without status epilepticus G40.509

Epilepsy, epileptic, epilepsia (continued)
  related to (continued)
    hormonal changes G40.509
      not intractable G40.509
        with status epilepticus G40.501
        without status eplepticus G40.509
    sleep deprivation G40.509
      not intractable G40.509
        with status epilepticus G40.501
        without status eplepticus G40.509
    stress G40.509
      not intractable G40.509
        with status epilepticus G40.501
        without status eplepticus G40.509
  somatomotor —see Epilepsy, localization-related, symptomatic, with simple partial seizures
  somatosensory —see Epilepsy, localization-related, symptomatic, with simple partial seizures
  spasms G40.822
    intractable G40.824
      with status epilepticus G40.823
      without status epilepticus G40.824
    not intractable G40.822
      with status epilepticus G40.821
      without status epilepticus G40.822
  specified NEC G40.802
    intractable G40.804
      with status epilepticus G40.803
      without status epilepticus G40.804
    not intractable G40.802
      with status epilepticus G40.801
      without status epilepticus G40.802
  syndromes
    generalized
      idiopathic G40.309
        intractable G40.319
          with status epilepticus G40.311
          without status epilepticus G40.319
        not intractable G40.309
          with status epilepticus G40.301
          without status epilepticus G40.309
      specified NEC G40.409
        intractable G40.419
          with status epilepticus G40.411
          without status epilepticus G40.419
        not intractable G40.409
          with status epilepticus G40.401
          without status epilepticus G40.409
    localization-related (focal) (partial)
      idiopathic G40.009
        with seizures of localized onset G40.009

Epilepsy, epileptic, epilepsia (continued)
  syndromes (continued)
    localization-related (continued)
      idiopathic (continued)
        with seizures of localized (continued)
          intractable G40.019
            with status epilepticus G40.011
            without status epilepticus G40.019
          not intractable G40.009
            with status epilepticus G40.001
            without status epilepticus G40.009
      symptomatic
        with complex partial seizures G40.209
          intractable G40.219
            with status epilepticus G40.211
            without status epilepticus G40.219
          not intractable G40.209
            with status epilepticus G40.201
            without status epilepticus G40.209
        with simple partial seizures G40.109
          intractable G40.119
            with status epilepticus G40.111
            without status epilepticus G40.119
          not intractable G40.109
            with status epilepticus G40.101
            without status epilepticus G40.109
      specified NEC G40.802
        intractable G40.804
          with status epilepticus G40.803
          without status epilepticus G40.804
        not intractable G40.802
          with status epilepticus G40.801
          without status epilepticus G40.802
  tonic (-clonic) —see Epilepsy, generalized, specified NEC
  twilight F05
  uncinate (gyrus) —see Epilepsy, localization-related, symptomatic, with complex partial seizures
  Unverricht (-Lundborg) (familial myoclonic) —see Epilepsy, generalized, idiopathic
  visceral —see Epilepsy, specified NEC
  visual —see Epilepsy, specified NEC

Epiloia Q85.1

Epimenorrhea N92.0

Epipharyngitis —see Nasopharyngitis

Epiphora H04.20-
  due to
    excess lacrimation H04.21-
    insufficient drainage H04.22-

Epiphyseal arrest —see Arrest, epiphyseal

Epiphyseolysis, epiphysiolysis —see Osteochondropathy

Epiphysitis —see also Osteochondropathy
  juvenile M92.9
  syphilitic (congenital) A50.02

Epiplocele —see Hernia, abdomen

Epiploitis —see Peritonitis

Epiplosarcomphalocele —see Hernia, umbilicus

Episcleritis (suppurative) H15.10-
  in (due to)
    syphilis A52.71
    tuberculosis A18.51
  nodular H15.12-
  periodica fugax H15.11-
    angioneurotic —see Edema, angioneurotic
  syphilitic (late) A52.71
  tuberculous A18.51

Episode
  affective, mixed F39
  depersonalization (in neurotic state) F48.1
  depressive F32.A
    major F32.9
      mild F32.0
      moderate F32.1
      severe (without psychotic symptoms) F32.2
        with psychotic symptoms F32.3
    recurrent F33.9
      brief F33.8
    specified NEC F32.89
  hypomanic F30.8
  manic F30.9
    with
      psychotic symptoms F30.2
      remission (full) F30.4
        partial F30.3
    other specified F30.8
    recurrent F31.89
    without psychotic symptoms F30.10
      mild F30.11
      moderate F30.12
      severe (without psychotic symptoms) F30.13
        with psychotic symptoms F30.2
  psychotic F23
    organic F06.8
  schizophrenic (acute) NEC, brief F23

Epispadias (female) (male) Q64.0

Episplenitis D73.89

Epistaxis (multiple) R04.0
  hereditary I78.0
  vicarious menstruation N94.89

Epithelioma (malignant) —see also Neoplasm, malignant, by site
  adenoides cysticum —see Neoplasm, skin, benign
  basal cell —see Neoplasm, skin, malignant
  benign —see Neoplasm, benign, by site
  Bowen's —see Neoplasm, skin, in situ
  calcifying, of Malherbe —see Neoplasm, skin, benign
  external site —see Neoplasm, skin, malignant
  intraepidermal, Jadassohn —see Neoplasm, skin, benign
  squamous cell —see Neoplasm, malignant, by site

Epitheliomatosis pigmented Q82.1
Epitheliopathy, multifocal placoid pigment H30.14-
Epithelium, epithelial —*see* condition
Epituberculosis (with atelectasis) (allergic) A15.7
Eponychia Q84.6
Epstein's
  nephrosis or syndrome —*see* Nephrosis
  pearl K09.8
Epulis (gingiva) (fibrous) (giant cell) K06.8
Equinia A24.0
Equinovarus (congenital) (talipes) Q66.0-
  acquired —*see* Deformity, limb, clubfoot
Equivalent
  convulsive (abdominal) —*see* Epilepsy, specified NEC
  epileptic (psychic) —*see* Epilepsy, localization-related, symptomatic, with complex partial seizures
Erb (-Duchenne) **paralysis** (birth injury) (newborn) P14.0
Erb-Goldflam disease or syndrome G70.00
  with exacerbation (acute) G70.01
  in crisis G70.01
Erb's
  disease G71.02
  palsy, paralysis (brachial) (birth) (newborn) P14.0
    spinal (spastic) syphilitic A52.17
  pseudohypertrophic muscular dystrophy G71.02
Erdheim's syndrome (acromegalic macrospondylitis) E22.0
Erection, painful (persistent) —*see* Priapism
Ergosterol deficiency (vitamin D) E55.9
  with
    adult osteomalacia M83.8
    rickets —*see* Rickets
Ergotism —*see also* Poisoning, food, noxious, plant
  from ergot used as drug (migraine therapy) —*see* Table of Drugs and Chemicals
Erosio interdigitalis blastomycetica B37.2
Erosion
  artery I77.2
    without rupture I77.89
  bone —*see* Disorder, bone, density and structure, specified NEC
  bronchus J98.09
  cameron —*see* Ulcer, stomach
  cartilage (joint) —*see* Disorder, cartilage, specified type NEC
  cervix (uteri) (acquired) (chronic) (congenital) N86
    with cervicitis N72
  cornea (nontraumatic) —*see* Ulcer, cornea
    recurrent H18.83-
    traumatic —*see* Abrasion, cornea
  dental (idiopathic) (occupational) (due to diet, drugs or vomiting) K03.2
  duodenum, postpyloric —*see* Ulcer, duodenum

Erosion *(continued)*
  esophagus K22.10
    with bleeding K22.11
  gastric —*see* Ulcer, stomach
  gastrojejunal —*see* Ulcer, gastrojejunal
  implanted mesh —*see* Complications, prosthetic device or implant, mesh
  intestine K63.3
  lymphatic vessel I89.8
  pylorus, pyloric (ulcer) —*see* Ulcer, stomach
  spine, aneurysmal A52.09
  stomach —*see* Ulcer, stomach
  subcutaneous device pocket
    nervous system prosthetic device, implant, or graft T85.890
    other internal prosthetic device, implant, or graft T85.898
  teeth (idiopathic) (occupational) (due to diet, drugs or vomiting) K03.2
  urethra N36.8
  uterus N85.8
Erotomania F52.8
Error
  metabolism, inborn -- se Disorder, metabolism
  refractive —*see* Disorder, refraction
Eructation R14.2
  nervous or psychogenic F45.8
Eruption
  creeping B76.9
  drug (generalized) (taken internally) L27.0
    fixed L27.1
    in contact with skin —*see* Dermatitis, due to drugs
    localized L27.1
  Hutchinson, summer L56.4
  Kaposi's varicelliform B00.0
  napkin L22
  polymorphous light (sun) L56.4
  recalcitrant pustular L13.8
  ringed R23.8
  skin (nonspecific) R21
    creeping (meaning hookworm) B76.9
    due to inoculation/vaccination (generalized) (*see also* Dermatitis, due to, vaccine) L27.0
      localized L27.1
    erysipeloid A26.0
    feigned L98.1
    Kaposi's varicelliform B00.0
    lichenoid L28.0
    meaning dermatitis —*see* Dermatitis
    toxic NEC L53.0
  tooth, teeth, abnormal (incomplete) (late) (premature) (sequence) K00.6
  vesicular R23.8
Erysipelas (gangrenous) (infantile) (newborn) (phlegmonous) (suppurative) A46
  external ear A46 *[H62.40]*
  puerperal, postpartum O86.89
Erysipeloid A26.9
  cutaneous (Rosenbach's) A26.0
  disseminated A26.8
  sepsis A26.7
  specified NEC A26.8
Erythema, erythematous (infectional) (inflammation) L53.9
  ab igne L59.0

Erythema, erythematous *(continued)*
  annulare (centrifugum) (rheumaticum) L53.1
  arthriticum epidemicum A25.1
  brucellum —*see* Brucellosis
  chronic figurate NEC L53.3
  chronicum migrans (Borrelia burgdorferi) A69.20
  diaper L22
  due to
    chemical NEC L53.0
      in contact with skin L24.5
    drug (internal use) —*see* Dermatitis, due to, drugs
  elevatum diutinum L95.1
  endemic E52
  epidemic, arthritic A25.1
  figuratum perstans L53.3
  gluteal L22
  heat - code by site under Burn, first degree
  ichthyosiforme congenitum bullous Q80.3
  in diseases classified elsewhere L54
  induratum (nontuberculous) L52
    tuberculous A18.4
  infectiosum B08.3
  intertrigo L30.4
  iris L51.9
  marginatum L53.2
    in (due to) acute rheumatic fever I00
  medicamentosum —*see* Dermatitis, due to, drugs
  migrans A26.0
    chronicum A69.20
    tongue K14.1
  multiforme (major) (minor) L51.9
    bullous, bullosum L51.1
    conjunctiva L51.1
    nonbullous L51.0
    pemphigoides L12.0
    specified NEC L51.8
  napkin L22
  neonatorum P83.88
    toxic P83.1
  nodosum L52
    tuberculous A18.4
  palmar L53.8
  pernio T69.1
  rash, newborn P83.88
  scarlatiniform (recurrent) (exfoliative) L53.8
  solare L55.0
  specified NEC L53.8
  toxic, toxicum NEC L53.0
    newborn P83.1
  tuberculous (primary) A18.4
Erythematous, erythematosus —*see* condition
Erythermalgia (primary) I73.81
Erythralgia I73.81
Erythrasma L08.1
Erythredema (polyneuropathy) —*see* Poisoning, mercury
Erythremia (acute) C94.0-
  chronic D45
  secondary D75.1
Erythroblastopenia —*see also* Aplasia, red cell D60.9
  congenital D61.01
Erythroblastophthisis D61.09
Erythroblastosis (fetalis) (newborn) P55.9
  due to

Erythroblastosis *(continued)*
  due to *(continued)*
    ABO (antibodies) (incompatibility) (isoimmunization) P55.1
    Rh (antibodies) (incompatibility) (isoimmunization) P55.0
Erythrocyanosis (crurum) I73.89
Erythrocythemia —*see* Erythremia
Erythrocytosis (megalosplenic) (secondary) D75.1
  familial D75.0
  oval, hereditary —*see* Elliptocytosis
  secondary D75.1
  stress D75.1
Erythroderma (secondary) (*see also* Erythema) L53.9
  bullous ichthyosiform, congenital Q80.3
  desquamativum L21.1
  ichthyosiform, congenital (bullous) Q80.3
  neonatorum P83.88
  psoriaticum L40.8
Erythrodysesthesia, palmar plantar (PPE) L27.1
Erythrogenesis imperfecta D61.09
Erythroleukemia C94.0-
Erythromelalgia I73.81
Erythrophagocytosis D75.89
Erythrophobia F40.298
Erythroplakia, oral epithelium, and tongue K13.29
Erythroplasia (Queyrat) D07.4
  specified site —*see* Neoplasm, skin, in situ
  unspecified site D07.4
Escherichia coli (E. coli), as cause of disease classified elsewhere B96.20
  non-O157 Shiga toxin-producing (with known O group) B96.22
  non-Shiga toxin-producing B96.29
  O157 B96.21
  O157 with confirmation of Shiga toxin when H antigen is unknown, or is not H7 B96.21
  O157:H-(nonmotile) with confirmation of Shiga toxin B96.21
  O157:H7 with or without confirmation of Shiga toxin-production B96.21
  Shiga toxin-producing (with unspecified O group) (STEC) B96.23
  specified NEC B96.29
Esophagismus K22.4
Esophagitis (acute) (alkaline) (chemical) (chronic) (infectional) (necrotic) (peptic) (postoperative) (without bleeding) K20.90
  with bleeding K20.91
  candidal B37.81
  due to gastrointestinal reflux disease (without bleeding) K21.00
    with bleeding K21.01
  eosinophilic K20.0
  reflux K21.00
    with bleeding K21.01
  specified NEC (without bleeding) K20.80
    with bleeding K21.81
  tuberculous A18.83
  ulcerative K22.10
    with bleeding K22.11

145

Esophagocele K22.5
Esophagomalacia K22.89
Esophagospasm K22.4
Esophagostenosis K22.2
Esophagostomiasis B81.8
Esophagotracheal —*see* condition
Esophagus —*see* condition
Esophoria H50.51
 convergence, excess H51.12
 divergence, insufficiency H51.8
Esotropia —*see* Strabismus, convergent concomitant
Espundia B55.2
Essential —*see* condition
Esthesioneuroblastoma C30.0
Esthesioneurocytoma C30.0
Esthesioneuroepithelioma C30.0
Esthiomene A55
Estivo-autumnal malaria (fever) B50.9
Estrangement (marital) Z63.5
 parent-child NEC Z62.890
Estriasis —*see* Myiasis
Ethanolism —*see* Alcoholism
Etherism —*see* Dependence, drug, inhalant
Ethmoid, ethmoidal —*see* condition
Ethmoiditis (chronic) (nonpurulent) (purulent) —*see also* Sinusitis, ethmoidal
 influenzal —*see* Influenza, with, respiratory manifestations NEC
 Woakes' J33.1
Ethylism —*see* Alcoholism
Eulenburg's disease (congenital paramyotonia) G71.19
Eumycetoma B47.0
Eunuchoidism E29.1
 hypogonadotropic E23.0
European blastomycosis —*see* Cryptococcosis
Eustachian —*see* condition
Evaluation (for) (of)
 development state
  adolescent Z00.3
  period of
   delayed growth in childhood Z00.70
    with abnormal findings Z00.71
   rapid growth in childhood Z00.2
  puberty Z00.3
 growth and developmental state (period of rapid growth) Z00.2
  delayed growth Z00.70
   with abnormal findings Z00.71
 mental health (status) Z00.8
 requested by authority Z04.6
 period of
  delayed growth in childhood Z00.70
   with abnormal findings Z00.71
  rapid growth in childhood Z00.2
 suspected condition —*see* Observation
Evans syndrome D69.41
Event
 apparent life threatening in newborn and infact (ALTE) R68.13
 brief resolved unexplained event (BRUE) R68.13

Eventration —*see also* Hernia, ventral
 colon into chest —*see* Hernia, diaphragm
 diaphragm (congenital) Q79.1
Eversion
 bladder N32.89
 cervix (uteri) N86
  with cervicitis N72
 foot NEC —*see also* Deformity, valgus, ankle
  congenital Q66.6
 punctum lacrimale (postinfectional) (senile) H04.52-
 ureter (meatus) N28.89
 urethra (meatus) N36.8
 uterus N81.4
Evidence
 cytologic
  of malignancy on anal smear R85.614
  of malignancy on cervical smear R87.614
  of malignancy on vaginal smear R87.624
Evisceration
 birth injury P15.8
 traumatic NEC
  eye —*see* Enucleated eye
Evulsion —*see* Avulsion
Ewing's sarcoma or tumor —*see* Neoplasm, bone, malignant
Examination (for) (following) (general) (of) (routine) Z00.00
 with abnormal findings Z00.01
 abuse, physical (alleged), ruled out
  adult Z04.71
  child Z04.72
 adolescent (development state) Z00.3
 alleged rape or sexual assault (victim), ruled out
  adult Z04.41
  child Z04.42
 allergy Z01.82
 annual (adult) (periodic) (physical) Z00.00
  with abnormal findings Z00.01
  gynecological Z01.419
   with abnormal findings Z01.411
 antibody response Z01.84
 blood —*see* Examination, laboratory
 blood pressure Z01.30
  with abnormal findings Z01.31
 cancer staging —*see* Neoplasm, malignant, by site
 cervical Papanicolaou smear Z12.4
  as part of routine gynecological examination Z01.419
   with abnormal findings Z01.411
 child (over 28 days old) Z00.129
  with abnormal findings Z00.121
  under 28 days old —*see* Newborn, examination
 clinical research control or normal comparison (control) (participant) Z00.6
 contraceptive (drug) maintenance (routine) Z30.8
  device (intrauterine) Z30.431
 dental Z01.20
  with abnormal findings Z01.21
 developmental —*see* Examination, child
 donor (potential) Z00.5
 ear Z01.10
  with abnormal findings NEC Z01.118
 eye Z01.00
  with abnormal findings Z01.01

Examination (*continued*)
 eye (*continued*)
  following failed vision screening Z01.020
   with abnormal findings Z01.021
 following
  accident NEC Z04.3
   transport Z04.1
   work Z04.2
  assault, alleged, ruled out
   adult Z04.71
   child Z04.72
  motor vehicle accident Z04.1
  treatment (for) Z09
   combined NEC Z09
    fracture Z09
    malignant neoplasm Z08
   malignant neoplasm Z08
   mental disorder Z09
   specified condition NEC Z09
 follow-up (routine) (following) Z09
  chemotherapy NEC Z09
   malignant neoplasm Z08
  fracture Z09
  malignant neoplasm Z08
  postpartum Z39.2
  psychotherapy Z09
  radiotherapy NEC Z09
   malignant neoplasm Z08
  surgery NEC Z09
   malignant neoplasm Z08
 forced sexual exploitation Z04.81
 forced labor exploitation Z04.82
 gynecological Z01.419
  with abnormal findings Z01.411
  for contraceptive maintenance Z30.8
 health —*see* Examination, medical
 hearing Z01.10
  with abnormal findings NEC Z01.118
  following failed hearing screening Z01.110
  infant or child (over 28 days old) Z00.129
   with abnormal findings Z00.121
 immunity status testing Z01.84
 laboratory (as part of a general medical examination) Z00.00
  with abnormal findings Z00.01
  preprocedural Z01.812
 lactating mother Z39.1
 medical (adult) (for) (of) Z00.00
  with abnormal findings Z00.01
  administrative purpose only Z02.9
   specified NEC Z02.89
  admission to
   armed forces Z02.3
   old age home Z02.2
   prison Z02.89
   residential institution Z02.2
   school Z02.0
    following illness or medical treatment Z02.0
   summer camp Z02.89
  adoption Z02.82
  blood alcohol or drug level Z02.83
  camp (summer) Z02.89
  clinical research, normal subject (control) (participant) Z00.6
  control subject in clinical research (normal comparison) (participant) Z00.6
  donor (potential) Z00.5
  driving license Z02.4
  general (adult) Z00.00
   with abnormal findings Z00.01
  immigration Z02.89

Examination (*continued*)
 medical (*continued*)
  insurance purposes Z02.6
  marriage Z02.89
  medicolegal reasons NEC Z04.89
  naturalization Z02.89
  participation in sport Z02.5
  paternity testing Z02.81
  population survey Z00.8
  pre-employment Z02.1
  pre-operative —*see* Examination, pre-procedural
  pre-procedural
   cardiovascular Z01.810
   respiratory Z01.811
   specified NEC Z01.818
  preschool children
   for admission to school Z02.0
  prisoners
   for entrance into prison Z02.89
  recruitment for armed forces Z02.3
  specified NEC Z00.8
  sport competition Z02.5
 medicolegal reason NEC Z04.89
  following
   forced sexual exploitation Z04.81
   forced labor exploitation Z04.82
 newborn —*see* Newborn, examination
 pelvic (annual) (periodic) Z01.419
  with abnormal findings Z01.411
 period of rapid growth in childhood Z00.2
 periodic (adult) (annual) (routine) Z00.00
  with abnormal findings Z00.01
 physical (adult) (*see also* Examination, medical) Z00.00
  sports Z02.5
 postpartum
  immediately after delivery Z39.0
  routine follow-up Z39.2
 prenatal (normal pregnancy) (*see also* Pregnancy, normal) Z34.9-
 pre-chemotherapy (antineoplastic) Z01.818
 pre-procedural (pre-operative)
  cardiovascular Z01.810
  laboratory Z01.812
  respiratory Z01.811
  specified NEC Z01.818
 prior to chemotherapy (antineoplastic) Z01.818
 psychiatric NEC Z00.8
  follow-up not needing further care Z09
  requested by authority Z04.6
 radiological (as part of a general medical examination) Z00.00
  with abnormal findings Z00.01
 repeat cervical smear to confirm findings of recent normal smear following initial abnormal smear Z01.42
 skin (hypersensitivity) Z01.82
 special (*see also* Examination, by type) Z01.89
  specified type NEC Z01.89
 specified type or reason NEC Z04.89
 teeth Z01.20
  with abnormal findings Z01.21
 urine —*see* Examination, laboratory
 vision Z01.00
  with abnormal findings Z01.01

Examination (continued)
  vision (continued)
    following failed vision screening
      Z01.020
      with abnormal findings
        Z01.021
    infant or child (over 28 days old)
      Z00.129
      with abnormal findings Z00.121

Exanthem, exanthema —see also
  Rash
  with enteroviral vesicular stomatitis
    B08.4
  Boston A88.0
  epidemic with meningitis A88.0
    [G02]
  subitum B08.20
    due to human herpesvirus 6
      B08.21
    due to human herpesvirus 7
      B08.22
  viral, virus B09
    specified type NEC B08.8

Excess, excessive, excessively
  alcohol level in blood R78.0
  androgen (ovarian) E28.1
  attrition, tooth, teeth K03.0
  carotene, carotin (dietary) E67.1
  cold, effects of T69.9
    specified effect NEC T69.8
  convergence H51.12
  crying
    in child, adolescent, or adult
      R45.83
    in infant R68.11
  development, breast N62
  divergence H51.8
  drinking (alcohol) NEC (without
    dependence) F10.10
    habitual (continual) (without
      remission) F10.20
  eating R63.2
  estrogen E28.0
  fat —see also Obesity
    in heart —see Degeneration,
      myocardial
    localized E65
  foreskin N47.8
  gas R14.0
  glucagon E16.3
  heat —see Heat
  intermaxillary vertical dimension
    of fully erupted teeth M26.37
  interocclusal distance of fully
    erupted teeth M26.37
  kalium E87.5
  large
    colon K59.39
      congenital Q43.8
      infant P08.0
    organ or site, congenital NEC
      —see Anomaly, by site
  long
    organ or site, congenital NEC
      —see Anomaly, by site
  menstruation (with regular cycle)
    N92.0
    with irregular cycle N92.1
  napping Z72.821
  natrium E87.0
  number of teeth K00.1
  nutrient (dietary) NEC R63.2
  potassium (K) E87.5
  salivation K11.7
  secretion —see also Hypersecretion
    milk O92.6
    sputum R09.3
    sweat R61
  sexual drive F52.8
  short

Excess, excessive, excessively
  (continued)
  short (continued)
    organ or site, congenital NEC
      —see Anomaly, by site
    umbilical cord in labor or
      delivery O69.3
  skin L98.7
    and subcutaneous tissue L98.7
    eyelid (acquired) —see
      Blepharochalasis
      congenital Q10.3
  sodium (Na) E87.0
  spacing of fully erupted teeth
    M26.32
  sputum R09.3
  sweating R61
  thirst R63.1
    due to deprivation of water T73.1
  transportation time Z59.82
  tuberosity of jaw M26.07
  vitamin
    A (dietary) E67.0
      administered as drug
        (prolonged intake) —see
        Table of Drugs and
        Chemicals, vitamins,
        adverse effect
      overdose or wrong substance
        given or taken —see Table
        of Drugs and Chemicals,
        vitamins, poisoning
    D (dietary) E67.3
      administered as drug
        (prolonged intake) —see
        Table of Drugs and
        Chemicals, vitamins,
        adverse effect
      overdose or wrong substance
        given or taken —see Table
        of Drugs and Chemicals,
        vitamins, poisoning
  weight
    gain R63.5
    loss R63.4

**Excitability, abnormal, under
  minor stress** (personality disorder)
  F60.3

Excitation
  anomalous atrioventricular I45.6
  psychogenic F30.8
  reactive (from emotional stress,
    psychological trauma) F30.8

Excitement
  hypomanic F30.8
  manic F30.9
  mental, reactive (from emotional
    stress, psychological trauma)
    F30.8
  state, reactive (from emotional stress,
    psychological trauma) F30.8

Excoriation (traumatic) —see also
  Abrasion
  neurotic L98.1
  skin picking disorder F42.4

Exfoliation
  due to erythematous conditions
    according to extent of body
      surface involved L49.0
      10-19 percent of body surface
        L49.1
      20-29 percent of body surface
        L49.2
      30-39 percent of body surface
        L49.3
      40-49 percent of body surface
        L49.4
      50-59 percent of body surface
        L49.5

Exfoliation (continued)
  due to erythematous conditions
    according to extent of body
      surface involved L49.0
      (continued)
      60-69 percent of body surface
        L49.6
      70-79 percent of body surface
        L49.7
      80-89 percent of body surface
        L49.8
      90-99 percent of body surface
        L49.9
      less than 10 percent of body
        surface L49.0
  teeth, due to systemic causes K08.0

Exfoliative —see condition

Exhaustion, exhaustive (physical
  NEC) R53.83
  battle F43.0
  cardiac —see Failure, heart
  delirium F43.0
  due to
    cold T69.8
    excessive exertion T73.3
    exposure T73.2
    neurasthenia F48.8
  heart —see Failure, heart
  heat (see also Heat, exhaustion)
    T67.5
    due to
      salt depletion T67.4
      water depletion T67.3
  maternal, complicating delivery
    O75.81
  mental F48.8
  myocardium, myocardial —see
    Failure, heart
  nervous F48.8
  old age R54
  psychogenic F48.8
  psychosis F43.0
  senile R54
  vital NEC Z73.0

Exhibitionism F65.2

Exocervicitis —see Cervicitis

Exomphalos Q79.2
  meaning hernia —see Hernia,
    umbilicus

Exophoria H50.52
  convergence, insufficiency H51.11
  divergence, excess H51.8

Exophthalmos H05.2-
  congenital Q15.8
  constant NEC H05.24-
  displacement, globe —see
    Displacement, globe
  due to thyrotoxicosis
    (hyperthyroidism) —see
    Hyperthyroidism, with, goiter
    (diffuse)
  dysthyroid —see Hyperthyroidism,
    with, goiter (diffuse)
  goiter —see Hyperthyroidism,
    with, goiter (diffuse)
  intermittent NEC H05.25-
  malignant —see Hyperthyroidism,
    with, goiter (diffuse)
  orbital
    edema —see Edema, orbit
    hemorrhage —see Hemorrhage,
      orbit
  pulsating NEC H05.26-
  thyrotoxic, thyrotropic —see
    Hyperthyroidism, with, goiter
    (diffuse)

Exploitation
  labor
    confirmed

Exploitation (continued)
  labor (continued)
    confirmed (continued)
      adult forced T74.61
      child forced T74.62
    suspected
      adult forced T76.61
      child forced T76.62
  sexual
    confirmed
      adult forced T74.51
      child forced T74.52
    suspected
      adult forced T76.51
      child forced T76.52

Exostosis —see also Disorder, bone
  cartilaginous —see Neoplasm,
    bone, benign
  congenital (multiple) Q78.6
  external ear canal H61.81-
  gonococcal A54.49
  jaw (bone) M27.8
  multiple, congenital Q78.6
  orbit H05.35-
  osteocartilaginous —see Neoplasm,
    bone, benign
  syphilitic A52.77

Exotropia —see Strabismus,
  divergent concomitant

Explanation of
  investigation finding Z71.2
  medication Z71.89

Exposure (to) (see also Contact,
  with) T75.89
  acariasis Z20.7
  AIDS virus Z20.6
  air pollution Z77.110
  algae and algae toxins Z77.121
  algae bloom Z77.121
  anthrax Z20.810
  aromatic amines Z77.020
  aromatic (hazardous) compounds
    NEC Z77.028
  aromatic dyes NOS Z77.028
  arsenic Z77.010
  asbestos Z77.090
  bacterial disease NEC Z20.818
  benzene Z77.021
  blue-green algae bloom Z77.121
  body fluids (potentially hazardous)
    Z77.21
  brown tide Z77.121
  chemicals (chiefly nonmedicinal)
    (hazardous) NEC Z77.098
  cholera Z20.09
  chromium compounds Z77.018
  cold, effects of T69.9
    specified effect NEC T69.8
  communicable disease Z20.9
    bacterial NEC Z20.818
    specified NEC Z20.89
    viral NEC Z20.828
    Zika virus Z20.821
  coronavirus (disease) (novel) 2019
    Z20.822
  COVID-19 Z20.822
  cyanobacteria bloom Z77.121
  disaster Z65.5
  discrimination Z60.5
  dyes Z77.098
  effects of T73.9
  environmental tobacco smoke
    (acute) (chronic) Z77.22
  Escherichia coli (E. coli) Z20.01
  exhaustion due to T73.2
  fiberglass —see Table of Drugs and
    Chemicals, fiberglass
  German measles Z20.4
  gonorrhea Z20.2
  hazardous metals NEC Z77.018

147

Exposure (continued)
hazardous substances NEC Z77.29
hazards in the physical environment NEC Z77.128
hazards to health NEC Z77.9
human immunodeficiency virus (HIV) Z20.6
human T-lymphotropic virus type-1 (HTLV-1) Z20.89
implanted
- mesh —see Complications, prosthetic device or implant, mesh
- prosthetic materials NEC —see Complications, prosthetic materials NEC

infestation (parasitic) NEC Z20.7
intestinal infectious disease NEC Z20.09
- Escherichia coli (E. coli) Z20.01

lead Z77.011
meningococcus Z20.811
mold (toxic) Z77.120
nickel dust Z77.018
noise Z77.122
occupational
- air contaminants NEC Z57.39
- dust Z57.2
- environmental tobacco smoke Z57.31
- extreme temperature Z57.6
- noise Z57.0
- radiation Z57.1
- risk factors Z57.9
  - specified NEC Z57.8
- toxic agents (gases) (liquids) (solids) (vapors) in agriculture Z57.4
- toxic agents (gases) (liquids) (solids) (vapors) in industry NEC Z57.5
- vibration Z57.7

parasitic disease NEC Z20.7
pediculosis Z20.7
persecution Z60.5
pfiesteria piscicida Z77.121
poliomyelitis Z20.89
polycyclic aromatic hydrocarbons Z77.028
pollution
- air Z77.110
- environmental NEC Z77.118
- soil Z77.112
- water Z77.111

prenatal (drugs) (toxic chemicals) —see Newborn, affected by, noxious substances transmitted via placenta or breast milk
rabies Z20.3
radiation, naturally occurring NEC Z77.123
radon Z77.123
red tide (Florida) Z77.121
rubella Z20.4
SARS-CoV-2 Z20.822
second hand tobacco smoke (acute) (chronic) Z77.22
- in the perinatal period P96.81

sexually-transmitted disease Z20.2
smallpox (laboratory) Z20.89
syphilis Z20.2
terrorism Z65.4
torture Z65.4
tuberculosis Z20.1
uranium Z77.012
varicella Z20.820
venereal disease Z20.2
viral disease NEC Z20.828
war Z65.5
water pollution Z77.111
Zika virus Z20.821

Exsanguination —see Hemorrhage
Exstrophy
abdominal contents Q45.8
bladder Q64.10
- cloacal Q64.12
- specified type NEC Q64.19
- supravesical fissure Q64.11

Extensive —see condition
Extra (see also Accessory marker chromosomes) (normal individual) Q92.61
- in abnormal individual Q92.62
- rib Q76.6
- cervical Q76.5

Extrasystoles (supraventricular) I49.49
- atrial I49.1
- auricular I49.1
- junctional I49.2
- ventricular I49.3

Extrauterine gestation or pregnancy —see Pregnancy, by site
Extravasation
blood R58
chyle into mesentery I89.8
pelvicalyceal N13.8
pyelosinus N13.8
urine (from ureter) R39.0
vesicant agent
- antineoplastic chemotherapy T80.810
- other agent NEC T80.818

Extremity —see condition, limb
Extrophy —see Exstrophy
Extroversion
bladder Q64.19
uterus N81.4
- complicating delivery O71.2
- postpartal (old) N81.4

Extruded tooth (teeth) M26.34
Extrusion
breast implant (prosthetic) T85.42
eye implant (globe) (ball) T85.328
intervertebral disc —see Displacement, intervertebral disc
ocular lens implant (prosthetic) —see Complications, intraocular lens
vitreous —see Prolapse, vitreous

Exudate
causing irritant dermatitis L24.A9
pleural —see Effusion, pleura
retina H35.89
wound fluids causing irritant dermatitis L24.A9

Exudative —see condition
Eye, eyeball, eyelid —see condition
Eyestrain —see Disturbance, vision, subjective
Eyeworm disease of Africa B74.3

F

Faber's syndrome (achlorhydric anemia) D50.9
Fabry (-Anderson) **disease** E75.21
Facet syndrome M47.89-
Faciocephalalgia, autonomic (see also Neuropathy, peripheral, autonomic) G90.09
Factor(s)
psychic, associated with diseases classified elsewhere F54

Factor(s) (continued)
psychological
- affecting physical conditions F54 or behavioral
  - affecting general medical condition F54
  - associated with disorders or diseases classified elsewhere F54

Fahr disease (of brain) G23.8
Fahr Volhard disease (of kidney) I12.-
Failure, failed
abortion —see Abortion, attempted
aortic (valve) I35.8
- rheumatic I06.8
attempted abortion —see Abortion, attempted
biventricular I50.82
- due to left heart failure I50.814
bone marrow —see Anemia, aplastic
cardiac —see Failure, heart
cardiorenal (chronic) (see also Failure, renal, and Failure, heart) I50.9
- hypertensive I13.2
cardiorespiratory (see also Failure, heart) R09.2
cardiovascular (chronic) —see Failure, heart
cerebrovascular I67.9
cervical dilatation in labor O62.0
circulation, circulatory (peripheral) R57.9
- newborn P29.89
compensation —see Disease, heart
compliance with medical treatment or regimen —see Noncompliance
congestive —see Failure, heart, congestive
dental implant (endosseous) M27.69
- due to
  - failure of dental prosthesis M27.63
  - lack of attached gingiva M27.62
  - occlusal trauma (poor prosthetic design) M27.62
  - parafunctional habits M27.62
  - periodontal infection (peri-implantitis) M27.62
  - poor oral hygiene M27.62
- osseointegration M27.61
  - due to
    - complications of systemic disease M27.61
    - poor bone quality M27.61
  - iatrogenic M27.61
- post-osseointegration
  - biological M27.62
  - due to complications of systemic disease M27.62
  - iatrogenic M27.62
  - mechanical M27.63
- pre-integration M27.61
- pre-osseointegration M27.61
- specified NEC M27.69
descent of head (at term) of pregnancy (mother) O32.4
endosseous dental implant —see Failure, dental implant
engagement of head (term of pregnancy) (mother) O32.4
erection (penile) (see also Dysfunction, sexual, male, erectile) N52.9
- nonorganic F52.21

Failure, failed (continued)
examination(s), anxiety concerning Z55.2
expansion terminal respiratory units (newborn) (primary) P28.0
forceps NOS (with subsequent cesarean delivery) O66.5
gain weight (child over 28 days old) R62.51
- adult R62.7
- newborn P92.6
genital response (male) F52.21
- female F52.22
heart (acute) (senile) (sudden) I50.9
- with
  - acute pulmonary edema —see Failure, ventricular, left
  - decompensation I50.9
    - with
      - normal ejection fraction I50.33
      - preserved ejection fraction I50.33
      - reduced ejection fraction I50.23
        - with diastolic dysfunction I50.43
      - combined systolic and diastolic I50.43
      - diastolic I50.33
      - right I50.813
      - systolic I50.23
  - dilatation —see Disease, heart
  - hypertension —see Hypertension, heart
  - normal ejection fraction —see Failure, heart diastolic
  - preserved ejection fraction —see Failure, heart diastolic
  - reduced ejection fraction —see Failure, heart systolic
- arteriosclerotic I70.90
- biventricular I50.82
  - due to left heart failure I50.814
- combined left-right sided I50.82
  - due to left heart failure I50.814
- compensated (see also Failure, heart, by type as diastolic or systolic, chronic) I50.9
- complicating
  - anesthesia (general) (local) or other sedation
    - in labor and delivery O74.2
    - in pregnancy O29.12-
    - postpartum, puerperal O89.1
  - delivery (cesarean) (instrumental) O75.4
- congestive I50.9
  - with rheumatic fever (conditions in I00)
    - active I01.8
    - inactive or quiescent (with chorea) I09.81
  - newborn P29.0
  - rheumatic (chronic) (inactive) (with chorea) I09.81
    - active or acute I01.8
      - with chorea I02.0
- decompensated (see also Failure, heart, by type as diastolic or systolic, acute and chronic) I50.9
- degenerative —see Degeneration, myocardial

Failure, failed (continued)
  heart (continued)
    diastolic (congestive) (left ventricular) I50.30
      acute (congestive) I50.31
        and (on) chronic (congestive) I50.33
      chronic (congestive) I50.32
        and (on) acute (congestive) I50.33
      combined with systolic (congestive) I50.40
        acute (congestive) I50.41
          and (on) chronic (congestive) I50.43
        chronic (congestive) I50.42
          and (on) acute (congestive) I50.43
      due to presence of cardiac prosthesis I97.13-
      end stage (see also Failure, heart, by type as diastolic or systolic, chronic) I50.84
    following cardiac surgery I97.13-
    high output NOS I50.83
    hypertensive —see Hypertension, heart
    left (ventricular) —see also Failure, ventricular, left
      combined diastolic and systolic —see Failure, heart, diastolic, combined with systolic
      diastolic —see Failure, heart, diastolic
      systolic —see Failure, heart, systolic
    low output (syndrome) NOS I50.9
    newborn P29.0
    organic —see Disease, heart
    peripartum O90.3
    postprocedural I97.13-
    rheumatic (chronic) (inactive) I09.9
    right (isolated) I50.810
      acute I50.811
        and (on) chronic I50.813
      chronic I50.812
        and acute I50.813
      secondary to left heart failure I50.814
    specified NEC I50.89
    Note: heart failure stages A, B, C and D are based on the American College of Cardiology and American Heart Association stages of heart failure, which complement and should not be confused with the New York Heart Association Classification of Heart Failure, into Class I, Class II, Class III and Class IV
    stage A Z91.89
    stage B (see also Failure, heart, by type as diastolic or systolic) I50.9
    stage C (see also Failure, heart, by type as diastolic or systolic) I50.9
    stage D (see also Failure, heart, by type as diastolic or systolic, chronic) I50.84
    systolic (congestive) (left ventricular) I50.20
      acute (congestive) I50.21
        and (on) chronic (congestive) I50.23
      chronic (congestive) I50.22
        and (on) acute (congestive) I50.23

Failure, failed (continued)
  heart (continued)
    systolic (continued)
      combined with diastolic (congestive) I50.40
        acute (congestive) I50.41
          and (on) chronic (congestive) I50.43
        chronic (congestive) I50.42
          and (on) acute (congestive) I50.43
    thyrotoxic (see also Thyrotoxicosis) E05.90 [I43]
      with
        high output (see also Thyrotoxicosis) I50.83
        thyroid storm E05.91 [I43]
          high output (see also Thyrotoxicosis) I50.83
    valvular —see Endocarditis
  hepatic K72.90
    with coma K72.91
    acute or subacute K72.00
      with coma K72.01
      due to drugs K71.10
        with coma K71.11
    alcoholic (acute) (chronic) (subacute) K70.40
      with coma K70.41
    chronic K72.10
      with coma K72.11
      due to drugs (acute) (subacute) (chronic) K71.10
        with coma K71.11
    due to drugs (acute) (subacute) (chronic) K71.10
      with coma K71.11
    end stage K72.10
      with coma K72.11
    postprocedural K91.82
  hepatorenal K76.7
  induction (of labor) O61.9
    abortion —see Abortion, attempted by
    oxytocic drugs O61.0
    prostaglandins O61.0
    instrumental O61.1
    mechanical O61.1
    medical O61.0
    specified NEC O61.8
    surgical O61.1
  intestinal failure K90.83
  intubation during anesthesia T88.4
    in pregnancy O29.6-
    labor and delivery O74.7
    postpartum, puerperal O89.6
  involution, thymus (gland) E32.0
  kidney (see also Disease, kidney, chronic) N19
    acute (see also Failure, renal, acute) N17.9-
    diabetic —see E08-E13 with .22
  lactation (complete) O92.3
    partial O92.4
  Leydig's cell, adult E29.1
  liver —see Failure, hepatic
  menstruation at puberty N91.0
  mitral I05.8
  myocardial, myocardium (see also Failure, heart) I50.9
    chronic (see also Failure, heart, congestive) I50.9
    congestive (see also Failure, heart, congestive) I50.9
  newborn screening — see Abnormal, neonatal screening
  neonatal congenital heart disease P09.5
  orgasm (female) (psychogenic) F52.31
    male F52.32

Failure, failed (continued)
  ovarian (primary) E28.39
  iatrogenic E89.40
    asymptomatic E89.40
    symptomatic E89.41
  postprocedural (postablative) (postirradiation) (postsurgical) E89.40
    asymptomatic E89.40
    symptomatic E89.41
  ovulation causing infertility N97.0
  polyglandular, autoimmune E31.0
  prosthetic joint implant —see Complications, joint prosthesis, mechanical, breakdown, by site
  renal N19
    with
      tubular necrosis (acute) N17.0
    acute N17.9
      with
        cortical necrosis N17.1
        medullary necrosis N17.2
        tubular necrosis N17.0
      specified NEC N17.8
    chronic N18.9
      hypertensive —see Hypertension, kidney
    congenital P96.0
    end stage (chronic) N18.6
      due to hypertension I12.0
    following
      abortion —see Abortion by type complicated by specified condition NEC
      crushing T79.5
      ectopic or molar pregnancy O08.4
      labor and delivery (acute) O90.49
    hypertensive —see Hypertension, kidney
    postprocedural N99.0
  respiration, respiratory J96.90
    with
      hypercarbia J96.92
      hypercapnia J96.92
      hypoxia J96.91
    acute J96.00
      with
        hypercarbia J96.02
        hypercapnia J96.02
        hypoxia J96.01
    center G93.89
    acute and (on) chronic J96.20
      with
        hypercarbia J96.22
        hypercapnia J96.22
        hypoxia J96.21
    chronic J96.10
      with
        hypercarbia J96.12
        hypercapnia J96.12
        hypoxia J96.11
    newborn P28.5
    postprocedural (acute) J95.821
      acute and chronic J95.822
  rotation
    cecum Q43.3
    colon Q43.3
    intestine Q43.3
    kidney Q63.2
  sedation (conscious) (moderate)
    during procedure T88.52
    history of Z92.83

Failure, failed (continued)
  segmentation —see also Fusion
    fingers —see Syndactylism, complex, fingers
    vertebra Q76.49
      with scoliosis Q76.3
  seminiferous tubule, adult E29.1
  senile (general) R54
  sexual arousal (male) F52.21
    female F52.22
  testicular endocrine function E29.1
  to thrive (child over 28 days old) R62.51
    adult R62.7
    newborn P92.6
  transplant T86.92
    bone T86.831
      marrow T86.02
    cornea T86.841-
    heart T86.22
      with lung(s) T86.32
    intestine T86.851
    kidney T86.12
    liver T86.42
    lung(s) T86.811
      with heart T86.32
    pancreas T86.891
    skin (allograft) (autograft) T86.821
    specified organ or tissue NEC T86.891
    stem cell (peripheral blood) (umbilical cord) T86.5
  trial of labor (with subsequent cesarean delivery) O66.40
    following previous cesarean delivery O66.41
  tubal ligation N99.89
  urinary —see Disease, kidney, chronic
  vacuum extraction NOS (with subsequent cesarean delivery) O66.5
  vasectomy N99.89
  ventouse NOS (with subsequent cesarean delivery) O66.5
  ventricular (see also Failure, heart) I50.9
    left (see also Failure, heart) I50.1
      with rheumatic fever (conditions in I00)
        active I01.8
          with chorea I02.0
        inactive or quiescent (with chorea) I09.81
      rheumatic (chronic) (inactive) (with chorea) I09.81
        active or acute I01.8
          with chorea I02.0
    right —see Failure, heart, right
  vital centers, newborn P91.88

Fainting (fit) R55

Fallen arches —see Deformity, limb, flat foot

Falling, falls (repeated) R29.6
  any organ or part —see Prolapse

Fallopian
  insufflation Z31.41
  tube —see condition

Fallot's
  pentalogy Q21.8
  tetrad or tetralogy Q21.3
  triad or trilogy Q22.3

False —see also condition
  croup J38.5
  joint —see Nonunion, fracture

False (continued)
  labor (pains) O47.9
    at or after 37 completed weeks of gestation O47.1
    before 37 completed weeks of gestation O47.0-
  passage, urethra (prostatic) N36.5
  pregnancy F45.8
Family, familial —see also condition
  disruption Z63.8
    involving divorce or separation Z63.5
  Li-Fraumeni (syndrome) Z15.01
  planning advice Z30.09
  problem Z63.9
    specified NEC Z63.8
  retinoblastoma C69.2-
Famine (effects of) T73.0
  edema —see Malnutrition, severe
Fanconi (-de Toni) (-Debré) **syndrome** E72.09
  with cystinosis E72.04
Fanconi's anemia (congenital pancytopenia) D61.09
Farber's disease or syndrome E75.29
Farcy A24.0
Farmer's
  lung J67.0
  skin L57.8
Farsightedness —see Hypermetropia
Fascia —see condition
Fasciculation R25.3
Fasciitis M72.9
  diffuse (eosinophilic) M35.4
  infective M72.8
    necrotizing M72.6
  necrotizing M72.6
  nodular M72.4
  perirenal (with ureteral obstruction) N13.5
    with infection N13.6
  plantar M72.2
  specified NEC M72.8
  traumatic (old) M72.8
    current - code by site under Sprain
Fascioliasis B66.3
Fasciolopsis, fasciolopsiasis (intestinal) B66.5
Fascioscapulohumeral myopathy G71.02
Fast pulse R00.0
Fat
  embolism —see Embolism, fat
  excessive —see also Obesity
    in heart —see Degeneration, myocardial
  in stool R19.5
  localized (pad) E65
    heart —see Degeneration, myocardial
    knee M79.4
    retropatellar M79.4
  necrosis
    breast N64.1
    mesentery K65.4
    omentum K65.4
  pad E65
    knee M79.4
Fatigue R53.83
  auditory deafness —see Deafness
  chronic R53.82
  combat F43.0

Fatigue (continued)
  general R53.83
    psychogenic F48.8
  heat (transient) T67.6
  muscle M62.89
  myocardium —see Failure, heart
  neoplasm-related R53.0
  nervous, neurosis F48.8
  operational F48.8
  psychogenic (general) F48.8
  senile R54
  voice R49.8
Fatness —see Obesity
Fatty —see also condition
  apron E65
  degeneration —see Degeneration, fatty
  heart (enlarged) —see Degeneration, myocardial
  liver NEC K76.0
    alcoholic K70.0
    nonalcoholic K76.0
  necrosis —see Degeneration, fatty
Fauces —see condition
Fauchard's disease (periodontitis) —see Periodontitis
Faucitis J02.9
Favism (anemia) D55.0
Favus —see Dermatophytosis
Fazio-Londe disease or syndrome G12.1
Fear complex or reaction F40.9
Fear of —see Phobia
Feared complaint unfounded Z71.1
Febris, febrile —see also Fever
  flava (see also Fever, yellow) A95.9
  melitensis A23.0
  pestis —see Plague
  recurrens —see Fever, relapsing
  rubra A38.9
Fecal
  incontinence R15.9
  smearing R15.1
  soiling R15.1
  urgency R15.2
Fecalith (impaction) K56.41
  appendix K38.1
  congenital P76.8
Fede's disease K14.0
Feeble rapid pulse due to shock following injury T79.4
Feeble-minded F70
Feeding
  difficulties R63.30
  problem (elderly) (infant) R63.39
    newborn P92.9
      specified NEC P92.8
    nonorganic (adult) —see Disorder, eating
Feeling (of)
  foreign body in throat R09.89
Feer's disease —see Poisoning, mercury
Feet —see condition
Feigned illness Z76.5
Feil-Klippel syndrome (brevicollis) Q76.1
Feinmesser's (hidrotic) **ectodermal dysplasia** Q82.4
Felinophobia F40.218

Felon —see also Cellulitis, digit
  with lymphangitis —see Lymphangitis, acute, digit
Felty's syndrome M05.00
  ankle M05.07-
  elbow M05.02-
  foot joint M05.07-
  hand joint M05.04-
  hip M05.05-
  knee M05.06-
  multiple site M05.09
  shoulder M05.01-
  vertebra —see Spondylitis, ankylosing
  wrist M05.03-
Female genital cutting status —see Female genital mutilation status (FGM)
Female genital mutilation status (FGM) N90.810
  specified NEC N90.818
  type I (clitorectomy status) N90.811
  type II (clitorectomy with excision of labia minora status) N90.812
  type III (infibulation status) N90.813
  type IV N90.818
Femur, femoral —see condition
Fenestration, fenestrated —see also Imperfect, closure
  aortico-pulmonary Q21.4
  atrial septum Q21.11
  cusps, heart valve NEC Q24.8
    pulmonary Q22.3
  pulmonic cusps Q22.3
Fernell's disease (aortic aneurysm) I71.9
Fertile eunuch syndrome E23.0
Fetid
  breath R19.6
  sweat L75.0
Fetishism F65.0
  transvestic F65.1
Fetus, fetal —see also condition
  alcohol syndrome (dysmorphic) Q86.0
  compressus O31.0-
  hydantoin syndrome Q86.1
  lung tissue P28.0
  papyraceous O31.0-
Fever (inanition) (of unknown origin) (persistent) (with chills) (with rigor) R50.9
  abortus A23.1
  Aden (dengue) A90
  African tick bite A77.8
  African tick-borne A68.1
  American
    mountain (tick) A93.2
    spotted A77.0
  aphthous B08.8
  arbovirus, arboviral A94
    hemorrhagic A94
    specified NEC A93.8
  Argentinian hemorrhagic A96.0
  Assam B55.0
  Australian Q A78
  Bangkok hemorrhagic A91
  Barmah forest A92.8
  Bartonella A44.0
  bilious, hemoglobinuric B50.8
  blackwater B50.8
  blister B00.1
  Bolivian hemorrhagic A96.1
  Bonvale dam T73.3
  boutonneuse A77.1
  brain —see Encephalitis

Fever (continued)
  Brazilian purpuric A48.4
  breakbone A90
  Bullis A77.0
  Bunyamwera A92.8
  Burdwan B55.0
  Bwamba A92.8
  Cameroon —see Malaria
  Canton A75.9
  catarrhal (acute) J00
    chronic J31.0
  cat-scratch A28.1
  Central Asian hemorrhagic A98.0
  cerebral —see Encephalitis
  cerebrospinal meningococcal A39.0
  Chagres B50.9
  Chandipura A92.8
  Changuinola A93.1
  Charcot's (biliary) (hepatic) (intermittent) —see Calculus, bile duct
  Chikungunya (viral) (hemorrhagic) A92.0
  Chitral A93.1
  Colombo —see Fever, paratyphoid
  Colorado tick (virus) A93.2
  congestive (remittent) —see Malaria
  Congo virus A98.0
  continued malarial B50.9
  Corsican —see Malaria
  Crimean-Congo hemorrhagic A98.0
  Cyprus —see Brucellosis
  dandy A90
  deer fly —see Tularemia
  dengue (virus) A90
    hemorrhagic A91
    sandfly A93.1
  desert B38.0
  drug induced R50.2
  due to
    conditions classified elsewhere R50.81
    heat T67.01
  enteric A01.00
  enteroviral exanthematous (Boston exanthem) A88.0
  ephemeral (of unknown origin) R50.9
  epidemic hemorrhagic A98.5
  erysipelatous —see Erysipelas
  estivo-autumnal (malarial) B50.9
  famine A75.0
  five day A79.0
  following delivery O86.4
  Fort Bragg A27.89
  gastroenteric A01.00
  gastromalarial —see Malaria
  Gibraltar —see Brucellosis
  glandular —see Mononucleosis, infectious
  Guama (viral) A92.8
  Haverhill A25.1
  hay (allergic) J30.1
    with asthma (bronchial) J45.909
      with
        exacerbation (acute) J45.901
        status asthmaticus J45.902
    due to
      allergen other than pollen J30.89
      pollen, any plant or tree J30.1
  heat (effects) T67.01
  hematuric, bilious B50.8
  hemoglobinuric (malarial) (bilious) B50.8

150

Fever (continued)
  hemorrhagic (arthropod-borne)
    NOS A94
      with renal syndrome A98.5
    arenaviral A96.9
      specified NEC A96.8
    Argentinian A96.0
    Bangkok A91
    Bolivian A96.1
    Central Asian A98.0
    Chikungunya A92.0
    Crimean-Congo A98.0
    dengue (virus) A91
    epidemic A98.5
    Junin (virus) A96.0
    Korean A98.5
    Kyasanur forest A98.2
    Machupo (virus) A96.1
    mite-borne A93.8
    mosquito-borne A92.8
    Omsk A98.1
    Philippine A91
    Russian A98.5
    Singapore A91
    Southeast Asia A91
    Thailand A91
    tick-borne NEC A93.8
    viral A99
      specified NEC A98.8
  hepatic —see Cholecystitis
  herpetic —see Herpes
  icterohemorrhagic A27.0
  Indiana A93.8
  infective B99.9
    specified NEC B99.8
  intermittent (bilious) —see also
      Malaria
    of unknown origin R50.9
    pernicious B50.9
  iodide R50.2
  Japanese river A75.3
  jungle —see also Malaria
    yellow A95.0
  Junin (virus) hemorrhagic A96.0
  Katayama B65.2
  kedani A75.3
  Kenya (tick) A77.1
  Kew Garden A79.1
  Korean hemorrhagic A98.5
  Lassa A96.2
  Lone Star A77.0
  Machupo (virus) hemorrhagic
      A96.1
  malaria, malarial —see Malaria
  Malta A23.9
  Marseilles A77.1
  marsh —see Malaria
  Mayaro (viral) A92.8
  Mediterranean (see also
      Brucellosis) A23.9
    familial M04.1
    tick A77.1
  meningeal —see Meningitis
  Meuse A79.0
  Mexican A75.2
  mianeh A68.1
  miasmatic —see Malaria
  mosquito-borne (viral) A92.9
    hemorrhagic A92.8
  mountain (see also Brucellosis)
    meaning Rocky Mountain
      spotted fever A77.0
    tick (American) (Colorado)
      (viral) A93.2
  Mucambo (viral) A92.8
  mud A27.9
  Neapolitan —see Brucellosis
  neutropenic D70.9
  newborn P81.9
    environmental P81.0
  Nine-Mile A78

Fever (continued)
  non-exanthematous tick A93.2
  North Asian tick-borne A77.2
  Omsk hemorrhagic A98.1
  O'nyong-nyong (viral) A92.1
  Oropouche (viral) A93.0
  Oroya A44.0
  pacific coast tick A77.8
  paludal —see Malaria
  Panama (malarial) B50.9
  Pappataci A93.1
  paratyphoid A01.4
    A A01.1
    B A01.2
    C A01.3
  parrot A70
  periodic (Mediterranean) M04.1
  persistent (of unknown origin)
      R50.9
  petechial A39.0
  pharyngoconjunctival B30.2
  Philippine hemorrhagic A91
  phlebotomus A93.1
  Piry (virus) A93.8
  Pixuna (viral) A92.8
  Plasmodium ovale B53.0
  polioviral (nonparalytic) A80.4
  Pontiac A48.2
  postimmunization R50.83
  postoperative R50.82
    due to infection T81.40
  posttransfusion R50.84
  postvaccination R50.83
  presenting with conditions
      classified elsewhere R50.81
  pretibial A27.89
  puerperal O86.4
  Q A78
  quadrilateral A78
  quartan (malaria) B52.9
  Queensland (coastal) (tick) A77.3
  quintan A79.0
  rabbit —see Tularemia
  rat-bite A25.9
    due to
      Spirillum A25.0
      Streptobacillus moniliformis
          A25.1
  recurrent —see Fever, relapsing
  relapsing (Borrelia) A68.9
    Carter's (Asiatic) A68.1
    Dutton's (West African) A68.1
    Koch's A68.9
    louse-borne A68.0
    Novy's
      louse-borne A68.0
      tick-borne A68.1
    Obermeyer's (European) A68.0
    tick-borne A68.1
  remittent (bilious) (congestive)
      (gastric) —see Malaria
  rheumatic (active) (acute) (chronic)
      (subacute) I00
    with central nervous system
        involvement I02.9
    active with heart involvement
        —see category I01
    inactive or quiescent with
      cardiac hypertrophy I09.89
      carditis I09.9
      endocarditis I09.1
        aortic (valve) I06.9
          with mitral (valve)
              disease I08.0
        mitral (valve) I05.9
          with aortic (valve)
              disease I08.0
        pulmonary (valve) I09.89
        tricuspid (valve) I07.8
      heart disease NEC I09.89

Fever (continued)
  rheumatic (continued)
    inactive or quiescent with
        (continued)
      heart failure (congestive)
          (conditions in category I50.)
          I09.81
      left ventricular failure (conditions
          in I50.1-I50.4-) I09.81
      myocarditis, myocardial
          degeneration (conditions in
          I51.4) I09.0
      pancarditis I09.9
      pericarditis I09.2
  Rift Valley (viral) A92.4
  Rocky Mountain spotted A77.0
  rose J30.1
  Ross River B33.1
  Russian hemorrhagic A98.5
  San Joaquin (Valley) B38.0
  sandfly A93.1
  Sao Paulo A77.0
  scarlet A38.9
  seven day (leptospirosis) (autumnal)
      (Japanese) A27.89
    dengue A90
  shin-bone A79.0
  Singapore hemorrhagic A91
  solar A90
  Songo A98.5
  sore B00.1
  South African tick-bite A68.1
  Southeast Asia hemorrhagic A91
  spinal —see Meningitis
  spirillary A25.0
  splenic —see Anthrax
  spotted A77.9
    American A77.0
    Brazilian A77.0
    cerebrospinal meningitis A39.0
    Colombian A77.0
    due to Rickettsia
      africae (African tick bite
          fever) A77.8
      australis A77.3
      conorii A77.1
      parkeri A77.8
      rickettsii A77.0
      sibirica A77.2
      specified type NEC A77.8
    Ehrlichiosis A77.40
      due to
        E. chafeensis A77.41
        specified organism NEC
            A77.49
    Rocky Mountain A77.0
  steroid R50.2
  streptobacillary A25.1
  subtertian B50.9
  Sumatran mite A75.3
  sun A90
  swamp A27.9
  swine A02.8
  sylvatic, yellow A95.0
  Tahyna B33.8
  tertian —see Malaria, tertian
  Thailand hemorrhagic A91
  thermic T67.01
  three-day A93.1
  tick
    American mountain A93.2
    Colorado A93.2
    Kemerovo A93.8
    Mediterranean A77.1
    mountain A93.2
    nonexanthematous A93.2
    Quaranfil A93.8
  tick-bite NEC A93.8
  tick-borne (hemorrhagic) NEC A93.8
  trench A79.0
  tsutsugamushi A75.3

Fever (continued)
  typhogastric A01.00
  typhoid (abortive) (hemorrhagic)
      (intermittent) (malignant) A01.00
    complicated by
      arthritis A01.04
      heart involvement A01.02
      meningitis A01.01
      osteomyelitis A01.05
      pneumonia A01.03
      specified NEC A01.09
  typhomalarial —see Malaria
  typhus —see Typhus (fever)
  undulant —see Brucellosis
  unknown origin R50.9
  uveoparotid D86.89
  valley B38.0
  Venezuelan equine A92.2
  vesicular stomatitis A93.8
  viral hemorrhagic —see Fever,
      hemorrhagic, by type of virus
  Volhynian A79.0
  Wesselsbron (viral) A92.8
  West
    African B50.8
    Nile (viral) A92.30
      with
        complications NEC A92.39
        cranial nerve disorders
            A92.32
        encephalitis A92.31
        encephalomyelitis A92.31
        neurologic manifestation
            NEC A92.32
        optic neuritis A92.32
        polyradiculitis A92.32
  Whitmore's —see Melioidosis
  Wolhynian A79.0
  worm B83.9
  yellow A95.9
    jungle A95.0
    sylvatic A95.0
    urban A95.1
  Zika virus A92.5
Fibrillation
  atrial or auricular (established) I48.91
    chronic I48.20
      persistent I48.19
    paroxysmal I48.0
    permanent I48.21
    persistent (chronic) (NOS)
        (other) I48.19
    longstanding I48.11
  cardiac I49.8
  heart I49.8
  muscular M62.89
  ventricular I49.01
Fibrin
  ball or bodies, pleural (sac) J94.1
  chamber, anterior (eye) (gelatinous
      exudate) —see Iridocyclitis,
      acute
Fibrinogenolysis —see Fibrinolysis
Fibrinogenopenia D68.8
  acquired D65
  congenital D68.2
Fibrinolysis (hemorrhagic) (acquired)
    D65
  antepartum hemorrhage —see
      Hemorrhage, antepartum, with
      coagulation defect
  following
    abortion —see Abortion by type
      complicated by hemorrhage
    ectopic or molar pregnancy
        O08.1
  intrapartum O67.0
  newborn, transient P60
  postpartum O72.3

151

Fibrinopenia (hereditary) D68.2
  acquired D68.4
Fibrinopurulent —*see* condition
Fibrinous —*see* condition
Fibroadenoma
  cellular intracanalicular D24-
  giant D24-
  intracanalicular
    cellular D24-
      giant D24-
      specified site —*see* Neoplasm, benign, by site
      unspecified site D24-
  juvenile D24-
  pericanalicular
    specified site —*see* Neoplasm, benign, by site
    unspecified site D24-
  phyllodes D24-
  prostate D29.1
  specified site NEC —*see* Neoplasm, benign, by site
  unspecified site D24-
Fibroadenosis, breast (chronic) (cystic) (diffuse) (periodic) (segmental) N60.2-
Fibroangioma —*see also* Neoplasm, benign, by site
  juvenile
    specified site —*see* Neoplasm, benign, by site
    unspecified site D10.6
Fibrochondrosarcoma —*see* Neoplasm, cartilage, malignant
Fibrocystic
  disease —*see also* Fibrosis, cystic
  breast —*see* Mastopathy, cystic
  jaw M27.49
  kidney (congenital) Q61.8
  liver Q44.6
  pancreas E84.9
  kidney (congenital) Q61.8
Fibrodysplasia ossificans progressiva —*see* Myositis, ossificans, progressiva
Fibroelastosis (cordis) (endocardial) (endomyocardial) I42.4
Fibroid (tumor) —*see also* Neoplasm, connective tissue, benign
  disease, lung (chronic) —*see* Fibrosis, lung
  heart (disease) —*see* Myocarditis
  in pregnancy or childbirth O34.1-
    causing obstructed labor O65.5
  induration, lung (chronic) —*see* Fibrosis, lung
  lung —*see* Fibrosis, lung
  pneumonia (chronic) —*see* Fibrosis, lung
  uterus (*see also* Leiomyoma, uterus) D25.9
Fibrolipoma —*see* Lipoma
Fibroliposarcoma —*see* Neoplasm, connective tissue, malignant
Fibroma —*see also* Neoplasm, connective tissue, benign
  ameloblastic —*see* Cyst, calcifying odontogenic
  bone (nonossifying) —*see* Disorder, bone, specified type NEC
    ossifying —*see* Neoplasm, bone, benign
  cementifying —*see* Neoplasm, bone, benign

Fibroma (*continued*)
  chondromyxoid —*see* Neoplasm, bone, benign
  desmoplastic —*see* Neoplasm, connective tissue, uncertain behavior
  durum —*see* Neoplasm, connective tissue, benign
  fascial —*see* Neoplasm, connective tissue, benign
  invasive —*see* Neoplasm, connective tissue, uncertain behavior
  molle —*see* Lipoma
  myxoid —*see* Neoplasm, connective tissue, benign
  nasopharynx, nasopharyngeal (juvenile) D10.6
  nonosteogenic (nonossifying) —*see* Dysplasia, fibrous
  odontogenic (central) —*see* Cyst, calcifying odontogenic
  ossifying —*see* Neoplasm, bone, benign
  periosteal —*see* Neoplasm, bone, benign
  soft —*see* Lipoma
Fibromatosis M72.9
  abdominal —*see* Neoplasm, connective tissue, uncertain behavior
  aggressive —*see* Neoplasm, connective tissue, uncertain behavior
  congenital generalized —*see* Neoplasm, connective tissue, uncertain behavior
  Dupuytren's M72.0
  gingival K06.1
  palmar (fascial) M72.0
  plantar (fascial) M72.2
  pseudosarcomatous (proliferative) (subcutaneous) M72.4
  retroperitoneal D48.3
  specified NEC M72.8
Fibromyalgia M79.7
Fibromyoma —*see also* Neoplasm, connective tissue, benign
  uterus (corpus) —*see also* Leiomyoma, uterus
    in pregnancy or childbirth —*see* Fibroid, in pregnancy or childbirth
    causing obstructed labor O65.5
Fibromyositis M79.7
Fibromyxolipoma D17.9
Fibromyxoma —*see* Neoplasm, connective tissue, benign
Fibromyxosarcoma —*see* Neoplasm, connective tissue, malignant
Fibro-odontoma, ameloblastic —*see* Cyst, calcifying odontogenic
Fibro-osteoma —*see* Neoplasm, bone, benign
Fibroplasia, retrolental H35.17-
Fibropurulent —*see* condition
Fibrosarcoma —*see also* Neoplasm, connective tissue, malignant
  ameloblastic C41.1
    upper jaw (bone) C41.0
  congenital —*see* Neoplasm, connective tissue, malignant
  fascial —*see* Neoplasm, connective tissue, malignant
  infantile —*see* Neoplasm, connective tissue, malignant

Fibrosarcoma (*continued*)
  odontogenic C41.1
    upper jaw (bone) C41.0
  periosteal —*see* Neoplasm, bone, malignant
Fibrosclerosis
  breast N60.3-
  multifocal M35.5
  penis (corpora cavernosa) N48.6
Fibrosis, fibrotic
  adrenal (gland) E27.8
  amnion O41.8X-
  anal papillae K62.89
  arteriocapillary —*see* Arteriosclerosis
  bladder N32.89
    interstitial —*see* Cystitis, chronic, interstitial
    localized submucosal —*see* Cystitis, chronic, interstitial
    panmural —*see* Cystitis, chronic, interstitial
  breast —*see* Fibrosclerosis, breast
  capillary (*see also* Arteriosclerosis) I70.90
    lung (chronic) —*see* Fibrosis, lung
  cardiac —*see* Myocarditis
  cervix N88.8
  chorion O41.8X-
  corpus cavernosum (sclerosing) N48.6
  cystic (of pancreas) E84.9
    with
      distal intestinal obstruction syndrome E84.19
      fecal impaction E84.19
      intestinal manifestations NEC E84.19
      pulmonary manifestations E84.0
      specified manifestations NEC E84.8
  due to device, implant or graft (*see also* Complications, by site and type, specified) NEC T85.828
    arterial graft NEC T82.828
    breast (implant) T85.828
    catheter NEC T85.828
      dialysis (renal) T82.828
        intraperitoneal T85.828
      infusion NEC T82.828
        spinal (epidural) (subdural) T85.820
      urinary (indwelling) T83.82
    electronic (electrode) (pulse generator) (stimulator)
      bone T84.82
      cardiac T82.827
      nervous system (brain) (peripheral nerve) (spinal) T85.820
      urinary T83.82
    fixation, internal (orthopedic) NEC T84.82
    gastrointestinal (bile duct) (esophagus) T85.828
    genital NEC T83.82
    heart NEC T82.827
    joint prosthesis T84.82
    ocular (corneal graft) (orbital implant) NEC T85.828
    orthopedic NEC T84.82
    specified NEC T85.828
    urinary NEC T83.82
    vascular NEC T82.828
    ventricular intracranial shunt T85.820
  ejaculatory duct N50.89
  endocardium —*see* Endocarditis
  endomyocardial (tropical) I42.3
  epididymis N50.89
  eye muscle —*see* Strabismus, mechanical

Fibrosis, fibrotic (*continued*)
  heart —*see* Myocarditis
  hepatic —*see* Fibrosis, liver
  hepatolienal (portal hypertension) K76.6
  hepatosplenic (portal hypertension) K76.6
  infrapatellar fat pad M79.4
  intrascrotal N50.89
  kidney N26.9
  liver K74.00
    with sclerosis K74.2
    advanced K74.02
    alcoholic K70.2
    early K74.01
    stage
      F1 or F2 K74.01
      F3 K74.02
  lung (atrophic) (chronic) (confluent) (massive) (perialveolar) (peribronchial) J84.10
    with
      anthracosilicosis J60
      anthracosis J60
      asbestosis J61
      bagassosis J67.1
      bauxite J63.1
      berylliosis J63.2
      byssinosis J66.0
      calcicosis J62.8
      chalicosis J62.8
      dust reticulation J64
      farmer's lung J67.0
      ganister disease J62.8
      graphite J63.3
      pneumoconiosis NOS J64
      siderosis J63.4
      silicosis J62.8
    capillary J84.10
    congenital P27.8
    diffuse (idiopathic) J84.10
      chemicals, gases, fumes or vapors (inhalation) (*see also* Disease, respiratory, chronic, due to chemicals, gases, fumes or vapors) J84.10
    interstitial J84.10
      acute J84.114
    talc J62.0
    following radiation J70.1
    idiopathic J84.112
    postinflammatory J84.10
    silicotic J62.8
    tuberculous —*see* Tuberculosis, pulmonary
  lymphatic gland I89.8
  median bar —*see* Hyperplasia, prostate
  mediastinum (idiopathic) J98.59
  meninges G96.198
  myocardium, myocardial —*see* Myocarditis
  ovary N83.8
  oviduct N83.8
  pancreas K86.89
  penis NEC N48.6
  pericardium I31.0
  perineum, in pregnancy or childbirth O34.7-
    causing obstructed labor O65.5
  pleura J94.1
  popliteal fat pad M79.4
  prostate (chronic) —*see* Hyperplasia, prostate
  pulmonary (*see also* Fibrosis, lung) J84.10
    congenital P27.8
    idiopathic J84.112
  rectal sphincter K62.89

Fibrosis, fibrotic (continued)
  retroperitoneal K68.2
    with infection N13.6
    idiopathic (with ureteral obstruction) N13.5
  sclerosing mesenteric (idiopathic) K65.4
  scrotum N50.89
  seminal vesicle N50.89
  senile R54
  skin L90.5
  spermatic cord N50.89
  spleen D73.89
    in schistosomiasis (bilharziasis) B65.9 [D77]
  subepidermal nodular —see Neoplasm, skin, benign
  submucous (oral) (tongue) K13.5
  testis N44.8
    chronic, due to syphilis A52.76
  thymus (gland) E32.8
  tongue, submucous K13.5
  tunica vaginalis N50.89
  uterus (non-neoplastic) N85.8
  vagina N89.8
  valve, heart —see Endocarditis
  vas deferens N50.89
  vein I87.8

Fibrositis (periarticular) M79.7
  nodular, chronic (Jaccoud's) (rheumatoid) —see Arthropathy, postrheumatic, chronic

Fibrothorax J94.1

Fibrotic —see Fibrosis

Fibrous —see condition

Fibroxanthoma —see also Neoplasm, connective tissue, benign
  atypical —see Neoplasm, connective tissue, uncertain behavior
  malignant —see Neoplasm, connective tissue, malignant

Fibroxanthosarcoma —see Neoplasm, connective tissue, malignant

Fiedler's
  disease (icterohemorrhagic leptospirosis) A27.0
  myocarditis (acute) I40.1

Fifth disease B08.3
  venereal A55

Filaria, filarial, filariasis —see Infestation, filarial

Filatov's disease —see Mononucleosis, infectious

File-cutter's disease —see Poisoning, lead

Filling defect
  biliary tract R93.2
  bladder R93.41
  duodenum R93.3
  gallbladder R93.2
  gastrointestinal tract R93.3
  intestine R93.3
  kidney R93.42-
  stomach R93.3
  ureter R93.41
  urinary organs, specified NEC R93.49

Fimbrial cyst Q50.4

Financial problem affecting care NOS Z59.9
  bankruptcy Z59.89
  foreclosure on loan Z59.89
    home loan Z59.81-
  strain Z59.86

Findings, abnormal, inconclusive, without diagnosis —see also Abnormal
  17-ketosteroids, elevated R82.5
  acetonuria R82.4
  alcohol in blood R78.0
  anisocytosis R71.8
  antenatal screening of mother O28.9
    biochemical O28.1
    chromosomal O28.5
    cytological O28.2
    genetic O28.5
    hematological O28.0
    radiological O28.4
    specified NEC O28.8
    ultrasonic O28.3
  antibody titer, elevated R76.0
  anticardiolipin antibody R76.0
  antiphosphatidylglycerol antibody R76.0
  antiphosphatidylinositol antibody R76.0
  antiphosphatidylserine antibody R76.0
  antiphospholipid antibody R76.0
  bacteriuria R82.71
  bicarbonate E87.8
  bile in urine R82.2
  blood sugar R73.09
    high R73.9
    low (transient) E16.2
  body fluid or substance, specified NEC R88.8
  casts, urine R82.998
  catecholamines R82.5
  cells, urine R82.998
  chloride E87.8
  cholesterol E78.9
    high E78.00
      with high triglycerides E78.2
  chyluria R82.0
  cloudy
    dialysis effluent R88.0
    urine R82.90
  creatinine clearance R94.4
  crystals, urine R82.998
  culture
    blood R78.81
    positive —see Positive, culture
  echocardiogram R93.1
  electrolyte level, urinary R82.998
  function study NEC R94.8
    bladder R94.8
    endocrine NEC R94.7
      thyroid R94.6
    kidney R94.4
    liver R94.5
    pancreas R94.8
    placenta R94.8
    pulmonary R94.2
    spleen R94.8
  gallbladder, nonvisualization R93.2
  glucose (tolerance test) (non-fasting) R73.09
  glycosuria R81
  heart
    shadow R93.1
    sounds R01.2
  hematinuria R82.3
  hematocrit drop (precipitous) R71.0
  hemoglobinuria R82.3
  human papillomavirus (HPV) DNA test positive
    cervix
      high risk R87.810
      low risk R87.820
    vagina
      high risk R87.811
      low risk R87.821

Findings, abnormal, inconclusive, without diagnosis (continued)
  in blood (of substance not normally found in blood) R78.9
    addictive drug NEC R78.4
    alcohol (excessive level) R78.0
    cocaine R78.2
    hallucinogen R78.3
    heavy metals (abnormal level) R78.79
    lead R78.71
    lithium (abnormal level) R78.89
    opiate drug R78.1
    psychotropic drug R78.5
    specified substance NEC R78.89
    steroid agent R78.6
  indoleacetic acid, elevated R82.5
  ketonuria R82.4
  lactic acid dehydrogenase (LDH) R74.02
  liver function test (see also Elevated, liver function, test) R79.89
  mammogram NEC R92.8
    calcification (calculus) R92.1
    inconclusive result R92.2
    microcalcification R92.0
  mediastinal shift R93.89
  melanin, urine R82.998
  myoglobinuria R82.1
  neonatal screening —see Abnormal, neonatal screening
  newborn screens, state mandated —see Abnormal, neonatal screening
  nonvisualization of gallbladder R93.2
  odor of urine NOS R82.90
  Papanicolaou cervix R87.619
    non-atypical endometrial cells R87.618
  pneumoencephalogram R93.0
  poikilocytosis R71.8
  potassium (deficiency) E87.6
    excess E87.5
  PPD R76.11
  radiologic (X-ray) R93.89
    abdomen R93.5
    biliary tract R93.2
    breast R92.8
    gastrointestinal tract R93.3
    genitourinary organs R93.89
    head R93.0
    inconclusive due to excess body fat of patient R93.9
    intrathoracic organs NEC R93.1
    musculoskeletal
      limbs R93.6
      other than limbs R93.7
    placenta R93.89
    retroperitoneum R93.5
    skin R93.89
    skull R93.0
    subcutaneous tissue R93.89
    testis R93.81-
  red blood cell (count) (morphology) (sickling) (volume) R71.8
  scan NEC R94.8
    bladder R94.8
    bone R94.8
    kidney R94.4
    liver R93.2
    lung R94.2
    pancreas R94.8
    placental R94.8
    spleen R94.8
    thyroid R94.6
  sedimentation rate, elevated R70.0
  SGOT R74.01
  SGPT R74.01

Findings, abnormal, inconclusive, without diagnosis (continued)
  sodium (deficiency) E87.1
    excess E87.0
  specified body fluid NEC R88.8
  stress test R94.39
  thyroid (function) (metabolic rate) (scan) (uptake) R94.6
  transaminase (level) R74.01
  triglycerides E78.9
    high E78.1
      with high cholesterol E78.2
  tuberculin skin test (without active tuberculosis) R76.11
  urine R82.90
    acetone R82.4
    bacteria R82.71
    bile R82.2
    casts or cells R82.998
    chyle R82.0
    culture positive R82.79
    glucose R81
    hemoglobin R82.3
    ketone R82.4
    sugar R81
    vanillylmandelic acid (VMA), elevated R82.5
  vectorcardiogram (VCG) R94.39
  ventriculogram R93.0
  white blood cell (count) (differential) (morphology) D72.9
  xerography R92.8

Finger —see condition

Fire, Saint Anthony's —see Erysipelas

Fire-setting
  pathological (compulsive) F63.1

Fish hook stomach K31.89

Fishmeal-worker's lung J67.8

Fissure, fissured
  anus, anal K60.2
    acute K60.0
    chronic K60.1
    congenital Q43.8
  ear, lobule, congenital Q17.8
  epiglottis (congenital) Q31.8
  larynx J38.7
    congenital Q31.8
  lip K13.0
    congenital —see Cleft, lip
  nipple N64.0
    associated with
      lactation O92.13
      pregnancy O92.11-
      puerperium O92.12
  nose Q30.2
  palate (congenital) —see Cleft, palate
  skin R23.4
  spine (congenital) —see also Spina bifida
    with hydrocephalus —see Spina bifida, by site, with hydrocephalus
  tongue (acquired) K14.5
    congenital Q38.3

Fistula (cutaneous) L98.8
  abdomen (wall) K63.2
    bladder N32.2
    intestine NEC K63.2
    ureter N28.89
    uterus N82.5
  abdominorectal K63.2
  abdominosigmoidal K63.2
  abdominothoracic J86.0
  abdominouterine N82.5
    congenital Q51.7
  abdominovesical N32.2

153

Fistula (continued)
  accessory sinuses —see Sinusitis
  actinomycotic —see Actinomycosis
  alveolar antrum —see Sinusitis, maxillary
  alveolar process K04.6
  anorectal K60.5
  antrobuccal —see Sinusitis, maxillary
  antrum —see Sinusitis, maxillary
  anus, anal (recurrent) (infectional) K60.3
    congenital Q43.6
      with absence, atresia and stenosis Q42.2
    tuberculous A18.32
  aorta-duodenal I77.2
  appendix, appendicular K38.3
  arteriovenous (acquired) (nonruptured) I77.0
    brain I67.1
      congenital Q28.2
        ruptured —see Fistula, arteriovenous, brain, ruptured
        ruptured I60.8
          intracerebral I61.8
          intraparenchymal I61.8
          Intraventricular I61.5
          subarachnoid I60.8
      cerebral —see Fistula, arteriovenous, brain
      congenital (peripheral) —see also Malformation, arteriovenous
        brain Q28.2
          ruptured —see Fistula, arteriovenous, brain, ruptured
        coronary Q24.5
        pulmonary Q25.72
      coronary I25.41
        congenital Q24.5
      pulmonary I28.0
        congenital Q25.72
      surgically created (for dialysis) Z99.2
        complication —see Complication, arteriovenous, fistula, surgically created
        traumatic —see Injury, blood vessel
    artery I77.2
    aural (mastoid) —see Mastoiditis, chronic
    auricle —see also Disorder, pinna, specified type NEC
      congenital Q18.1
    Bartholin's gland N82.8
    bile duct (common) (hepatic) K83.3
      with calculus, stones (see also Calculus, bile duct) K83.3
    biliary (tract) —see Fistula, bile duct
    bladder (sphincter) NEC (see also Fistula, vesico-) N32.2
      into seminal vesicle N32.2
    bone —see also Disorder, bone, specified type NEC
      with osteomyelitis, chronic — see Osteomyelitis, chronic, with draining sinus
    brain G93.89
      arteriovenous (acquired) (see also Fistula, arteriovenous, brain) I67.1
        congenital Q28.2
    branchial (cleft) Q18.0
    branchiogenous Q18.0

Fistula (continued)
  breast N61.0
    puerperal, postpartum or gestational, due to mastitis (purulent) —see Mastitis, obstetric, purulent
  bronchial J86.0
  bronchocutaneous, bronchomediastinal, bronchopleural, bronchopleuromediastinal (infective) J86.0
    tuberculous NEC A15.5
  bronchoesophageal J86.0
    congenital Q39.2
      with atresia of esophagus Q39.1
  bronchovisceral J86.0
  buccal cavity (infective) K12.2
  cecosigmoidal K63.2
  cecum K63.2
  cerebrospinal (fluid) G96.08
  cervical, lateral Q18.1
  cervicoaural Q18.1
  cervicosigmoidal N82.4
  cervicovesical N82.1
  cervix N82.8
  chest (wall) J86.0
  cholecystenteric —see Fistula, gallbladder
  cholecystocolic —see Fistula, gallbladder
  cholecystocolonic —see Fistula, gallbladder
  cholecystoduodenal —see Fistula, gallbladder
  cholecystogastric —see Fistula, gallbladder
  cholecystointestinal —see Fistula, gallbladder
  choledochoduodenal —see Fistula, bile duct
  cholocolic K82.3
  coccyx —see Sinus, pilonidal
  colon K63.2
  colostomy K94.09
  colovesical N32.1
  common duct —see Fistula, bile duct
  congenital, site not listed —see Anomaly, by site
  coronary, arteriovenous I25.41
    congenital Q24.5
  costal region J86.0
  cul-de-sac, Douglas' N82.8
  cystic duct —see also Fistula, gallbladder
    congenital Q44.5
  dental K04.6
  diaphragm J86.0
  duodenum K31.6
  ear (external) (canal) —see Disorder, ear, external, specified type NEC
  enterocolic K63.2
  enterocutaneous K63.2
  enterouterine N82.4
    congenital Q51.7
  enterovaginal N82.4
    congenital Q52.2
    large intestine N82.3
    small intestine N82.2
  enterovesical N32.1
  epididymis N50.89
    tuberculous A18.15
  esophagobronchial J86.0
    congenital Q39.2
      with atresia of esophagus Q39.1
  esophagocutaneous K22.89
  esophagopleural-cutaneous J86.0

Fistula (continued)
  esophagotracheal J86.0
    congenital Q39.2
      with atresia of esophagus Q39.1
  esophagus K22.89
    congenital Q39.2
      with atresia of esophagus Q39.1
  ethmoid —see Sinusitis, ethmoidal
  eyeball (cornea) (sclera) —see Disorder, globe, hypotony
  eyelid H01.8
  fallopian tube, external N82.5
  fecal K63.2
    congenital Q43.6
    from periapical abscess K04.6
  frontal sinus —see Sinusitis, frontal
  gallbladder K82.3
    with calculus, cholelithiasis, stones —see Calculus, gallbladder
  gastric K31.6
  gastrocolic K31.6
    congenital Q40.2
    tuberculous A18.32
  gastroenterocolic K31.6
  gastroesophageal K31.6
  gastrojejunal K31.6
  gastrojejunocolic K31.6
  genital tract (female) N82.9
    specified NEC N82.8
    to intestine NEC N82.4
    to skin N82.5
  hepatic artery-portal vein, congenital Q26.6
  hepatopleural J86.0
  hepatopulmonary J86.0
  ileorectal or ileosigmoidal K63.2
  ileovaginal N82.2
  ileovesical N32.1
  ileum K63.2
  in ano K60.3
    tuberculous A18.32
  inner ear (labyrinth) H83.1
  intestine NEC K63.2
  intestinocolonic (abdominal) K63.2
  intestinoureteral N28.89
  intestinouterine N82.4
  intestinovaginal N82.4
    large intestine N82.3
    small intestine N82.2
  intestinovesical N32.1
  ischiorectal (fossa) K61.39
  jejunum K63.2
  joint M25.10
    ankle M25.17-
    elbow M25.12-
    foot joint M25.17-
    hand joint M25.14-
    hip M25.15-
    knee M25.16-
    shoulder M25.11-
    specified joint NEC M25.18
    tuberculous —see Tuberculosis, joint
    vertebrae M25.18
    wrist M25.13-
  kidney N28.89
  labium (majus) (minus) N82.8
  labyrinth H83.1
  lacrimal (gland) (sac) H04.61-
  lacrimonasal duct —see Fistula, lacrimal
  laryngotracheal, congenital Q34.8
  larynx J38.7
  lip K13.0
    congenital Q38.0
  lumbar, tuberculous A18.01

Fistula (continued)
  lung J86.0
  lymphatic I89.8
  mammary (gland) N61.0
  mastoid (process) (region) —see Mastoiditis, chronic
  maxillary J32.0
  medial, face and neck Q18.8
  mediastinal J86.0
  mediastinobronchial J86.0
  mediastinocutaneous J86.0
  middle ear H74.8
  mouth K12.2
  nasal J34.89
    sinus —see Sinusitis
  nasopharynx J39.2
  nipple N64.0
  nose J34.89
  oral (cutaneous) K12.2
    maxillary J32.0
    nasal (with cleft palate) —see Cleft, palate
  orbit, orbital —see Disorder, orbit, specified type NEC
  oroantral J32.0
  oviduct, external N82.5
  palate (hard) M27.8
  pancreatic K86.89
  pancreaticoduodenal K86.89
  parotid (gland) K11.4
    region K12.2
  penis N48.89
  perianal K60.3
  pericardium (pleura) (sac) —see Pericarditis
  pericecal K63.2
  perineorectal K60.4
  perineosigmoidal K63.2
  perineum, perineal (with urethral involvement) NEC N36.0
    tuberculous A18.13
    ureter N28.89
  perirectal K60.4
    tuberculous A18.32
  peritoneum K65.9
  pharyngoesophageal J39.2
  pharynx J39.2
    branchial cleft (congenital) Q18.0
  pilonidal (infected) (rectum) —see Sinus, pilonidal
  pleura, pleural, pleurocutaneous, pleuroperitoneal J86.0
    tuberculous NEC A15.6
  pleuropericardial I31.8
  portal vein-hepatic artery, congenital Q26.6
  postauricular H70.81-
  postoperative, persistent T81.83
    specified site —see Fistula, by site
  preauricular (congenital) Q18.1
  prostate N42.89
  pulmonary J86.0
    arteriovenous I28.0
      congenital Q25.72
    tuberculous —see Tuberculosis, pulmonary
  pulmonoperitoneal J86.0
  rectolabial N82.4
  rectosigmoid (intercommunicating) K63.2
  rectoureteral N28.89
  rectourethral N36.0
    congenital Q64.73
  rectouterine N82.4
    congenital Q51.7
  rectovaginal N82.3
    congenital Q52.2
    tuberculous A18.18

Fistula (continued)
  rectovesical N32.1
    congenital Q64.79
  rectovesicovaginal N82.3
  rectovulval N82.4
    congenital Q52.79
  rectum (to skin) K60.4
    congenital Q43.6
      with absence, atresia and stenosis Q42.0
    tuberculous A18.32
  renal N28.89
  retroauricular —see Fistula, postauricular
  salivary duct or gland (any) K11.4
    congenital Q38.4
  scrotum (urinary) N50.89
    tuberculous A18.15
  semicircular canals H83.1
  sigmoid K63.2
    to bladder N32.1
  sinus —see Sinusitis
  skin L98.8
    to genital tract (female) N82.5
  splenocolic D73.89
  stercoral K63.2
  stomach K31.6
  sublingual gland K11.4
  submandibular gland K11.4
  submaxillary (gland) K11.4
    region K12.2
  thoracic J86.0
    duct I89.8
  thoracoabdominal J86.0
  thoracogastric J86.0
  thoracointestinal J86.0
  thorax J86.0
  thyroglossal duct Q89.2
  thyroid E07.89
  trachea, congenital (external) (internal) Q32.1
  tracheoesophageal J86.0
    congenital Q39.2
      with atresia of esophagus Q39.1
    following tracheostomy J95.04
  traumatic arteriovenous —see Injury, blood vessel, by site
  tuberculous - code by site under Tuberculosis
  typhoid A01.09
  umbilicourinary Q64.8
  urachus, congenital Q64.4
  ureter (persistent) N28.89
  ureteroabdominal N28.89
  ureterorectal N28.89
  ureterosigmoido-abdominal N28.89
  ureterovaginal N82.1
  ureterovesical N32.2
  urethra N36.0
    congenital Q64.79
    tuberculous A18.13
  urethroperineal N36.0
  urethroperineovesical N32.2
  urethrorectal N36.0
    congenital Q64.73
  urethroscrotal N50.89
  urethrovaginal N82.1
  urethrovesical N32.2
  urinary (tract) (persistent) (recurrent) N36.0
  uteroabdominal N82.5
    congenital Q51.7
  uteroenteric, uterointestinal N82.4
    congenital Q51.7
  uterorectal N82.4
    congenital Q51.7
  uteroureteric N82.1
  uterourethral Q51.7
  uterovaginal N82.8

Fistula (continued)
  uterovesical N82.1
    congenital Q51.7
  uterus N82.8
  vagina (postpartal) (wall) N82.8
  vaginocutaneous (postpartal) N82.5
  vaginointestinal NEC N82.4
    large intestine N82.3
    small intestine N82.2
  vaginoperineal N82.5
  vasocutaneous, congenital Q55.7
  vesical NEC N32.2
  vesicoabdominal N32.2
  vesicocervicovaginal N82.1
  vesicocolic N32.1
  vesicocutaneous N32.2
  vesicoenteric N32.1
  vesicointestinal N32.1
  vesicometrorectal N82.4
  vesicoperineal N32.2
  vesicorectal N32.1
    congenital Q64.79
  vesicosigmoidal N32.1
  vesicosigmoidovaginal N82.3
  vesicoureteral N32.2
  vesicoureterovaginal N82.1
  vesicourethral N32.2
  vesicourethrorectal N32.1
  vesicouterine N82.1
    congenital Q51.7
  vesicovaginal N82.0
  vulvorectal N82.4
    congenital Q52.79

Fit R56.9
  epileptic —see Epilepsy
  fainting R55
  hysterical F44.5
  newborn P90

Fitting (and adjustment) (of)
  artificial
    arm —see Admission, adjustment, artificial, arm
    breast Z44.3
    eye Z44.2
    leg —see Admission, adjustment, artificial, leg
  automatic implantable cardiac defibrillator (with synchronous cardiac pacemaker) Z45.02
  brain neuropacemaker Z46.2
    implanted Z45.42
  cardiac defibrillator —see Fitting (and adjustment) (of), automatic implantable cardiac defibrillator
  catheter, non-vascular Z46.82
  colostomy belt Z46.89
  contact lenses Z46.0
  CRT-D (resynchronization therapy defibrillator) Z45.02
  CRT-P (cardiac resynchronization therapy pacemaker) Z45.018
    pulse generator Z45.010
  cystostomy device Z46.6
  defibrillator, cardiac —see Fitting (and adjustment) (of), automatic implantable cardiac defibrillator
  dentures Z46.3
  device NOS Z46.9
    abdominal Z46.89
    gastrointestinal NEC Z46.59
    implanted NEC Z45.89
    nervous system Z46.2
      implanted —see Admission, adjustment, device, implanted, nervous system
    orthodontic Z46.4
    orthoptic Z46.0
    orthotic Z46.89

Fitting (continued)
  device (continued)
    prosthetic (external) Z44.9
      breast Z44.3
      dental Z46.3
      eye Z44.2
      specified NEC Z44.8
    specified NEC Z46.89
    substitution
      auditory Z46.2
        implanted —see Admission, adjustment, device, implanted, hearing device
      nervous system Z46.2
        implanted —see Admission, adjustment, device, implanted, nervous system
      visual Z46.2
        implanted Z45.31
    urinary Z46.6
  gastric lap band Z46.51
  gastrointestinal appliance NEC Z46.59
  glasses (reading) Z46.0
  hearing aid Z46.1
  ileostomy device Z46.89
  insulin pump Z46.81
  intestinal appliance NEC Z46.89
  myringotomy device (stent) (tube) Z45.82
  neuropacemaker Z46.2
    implanted Z45.42
  non-vascular catheter Z46.82
  orthodontic device Z46.4
  orthopedic device (brace) (cast) (corset) (shoes) Z46.89
  pacemaker (cardiac) (cardiac resynchronization therapy (CRT-P)) Z45.018
    nervous system (brain) (peripheral nerve) (spinal cord) Z46.2
      implanted Z45.42
    pulse generator Z45.010
  portacath (port-a-cath) Z45.2
  prosthesis (external) Z44.9
    arm —see Admission, adjustment, artificial, arm
    breast Z44.3
    dental Z46.3
    eye Z44.2
    leg —see Admission, adjustment, artificial, leg
    specified NEC Z44.8
  spectacles Z46.0
  wheelchair Z46.89

Fitzhugh-Curtis syndrome
  due to
    Chlamydia trachomatis A74.81
    Neisseria gonorrhorea (gonococcal peritonitis) A54.85

Fitz's syndrome (acute hemorrhagic pancreatitis) (see also Pancreatitis, acute) K85.80

Fixation
  joint —see Ankylosis
  larynx J38.7
  stapes —see Ankylosis, ear ossicles
    deafness —see Deafness, conductive
  uterus (acquired) —see Malposition, uterus
  vocal cord J38.3

Flabby ridge K06.8

Flaccid —see also condition
  palate, congenital Q38.5

Flail
  chest S22.5
    associated with chest compression and cardiopulmonary resuscitation M96.A4
    newborn (birth injury) P13.8
  joint (paralytic) M25.20
    ankle M25.27-
    elbow M25.22-
    foot joint M25.27-
    hand joint M25.24-
    hip M25.25-
    knee M25.26-
    shoulder M25.21-
    specified joint NEC M25.28
    wrist M25.23-

Flajani's disease —see Hyperthyroidism, with, goiter (diffuse)

Flap, liver K71.3

Flashbacks (residual to hallucinogen use) F16.283

Flat
  affect R45.89
  chamber (eye) —see Disorder, globe, hypotony, flat anterior chamber
  chest, congenital Q67.8
  foot (acquired) (fixed type) (painful) (postural) —see also Deformity, limb, flat foot
    congenital (rigid) (spastic (everted)) Q66.5-
    rachitic sequelae (late effect) E64.3
  organ or site, congenital NEC —see Anomaly, by site
  pelvis M95.5
    with disproportion (fetopelvic) O33.0
      causing obstructed labor O65.0
    congenital Q74.2

Flatau-Schilder disease G37.0

Flatback syndrome M40.30
  lumbar region M40.36
  lumbosacral region M40.37
  thoracolumbar region M40.35

Flattening
  head, femur M89.8X5
  hip —see Coxa, plana
  lip (congenital) Q18.8
  nose (congenital) Q67.4
    acquired M95.0

Flatulence R14.3
  psychogenic F45.8

Flatus R14.3
  vaginalis N89.8

Flax-dresser's disease J66.1

Flea bite —see Injury, bite, by site, superficial, insect

Flecks, glaucomatous (subcapsular) —see Cataract, complicated

Fleischer (-Kayser) **ring** (cornea) H18.04-

Fleshy mole O02.0

Flexibilitas cerea —see Catalepsy

Flexion
  amputation stump (surgical) T87.89
  cervix —see Malposition, uterus
  contracture, joint —see Contraction, joint
  deformity, joint (see also Deformity, limb, flexion) M21.20
    hip, congenital Q65.89
  uterus —see also Malposition, uterus
    lateral —see Lateroversion, uterus

Flexner-Boyd dysentery A03.2
Flexner's dysentery A03.1
Flexure —see Flexion
Flint murmur (aortic insufficiency) I35.1
Floater, vitreous —see Opacity, vitreous
Floating
   cartilage (joint) —see also Loose, body, joint
      knee —see Derangement, knee, loose body
   gallbladder, congenital Q44.1
   kidney N28.89
      congenital Q63.8
   spleen D73.89
Flooding N92.0
Floor —see condition
Floppy
   baby syndrome (nonspecific) P94.2
   iris syndrome (intraoperative) (IFIS) H21.81
   nonrheumatic mitral valve syndrome I34.1
Flu —see also Influenza
   avian (see also Influenza, due to, identified novel influenza A virus) J09.X2
   bird (see also Influenza, due to, identified novel influenza A virus) J09.X2
   intestinal NEC A08.4
   swine (viruses that normally cause infections in pigs) (see also Influenza, due to, identified novel influenza A virus) J09.X2
Fluctuating blood pressure I99.8
Fluid
   abdomen R18.8
   chest J94.8
   heart —see Failure, heart, congestive
   joint —see Effusion, joint
   loss (acute) E86.9
   lung —see Edema, lung
   overload E87.70
      specified NEC E87.79
   peritoneal cavity R18.8
   pleural cavity J94.8
   retention R60.9
Flukes NEC —see also Infestation, fluke
   blood NEC —see Schistosomiasis
   liver B66.3
Fluor (vaginalis) N89.8
   trichomonal or due to Trichomonas (vaginalis) A59.00
Fluorosis
   dental K00.3
   skeletal M85.10
      ankle M85.17-
      foot M85.17-
      forearm M85.13-
      hand M85.14-
      lower leg M85.16-
      multiple site M85.19
      neck M85.18
      rib M85.18
      shoulder M85.11-
      skull M85.18
      specified site NEC M85.18
      thigh M85.15-
      toe M85.17-
      upper arm M85.12-
      vertebra M85.18
Flush syndrome E34.0

Flushing R23.2
   menopausal N95.1
Flutter
   atrial or auricular I48.92
      atypical I48.4
      type I I48.3
      type II I48.4
      typical I48.3
   heart I49.8
      atrial or auricular I48.92
         atypical I48.4
         type I I48.3
         type II I48.4
         typical I48.3
      ventricular I49.02
   ventricular I49.02
FNHTR (febrile nonhemolytic transfusion reaction) R50.84
Fochier's abscess - code by site under Abscess
Focus, Assmann's —see Tuberculosis, pulmonary
Fogo selvagem L10.3
Foix-Alajouanine syndrome G95.19
Fold, folds (anomalous) —see also Anomaly, by site
   Descemet's membrane —see Change, corneal membrane, Descemet's, fold
   epicanthic Q10.3
   heart Q24.8
Folie à deux F24
Follicle
   cervix (nabothian) (ruptured) N88.8
   graafian, ruptured, with hemorrhage N83.0-
   nabothian N88.8
Follicular —see condition
Folliculitis (superficial) L73.9
   abscedens et suffodiens L66.3
   cyst N83.0-
   decalvans L66.2
   deep —see Furuncle, by site
   gonococcal (acute) (chronic) A54.01
   keloid, keloidalis L73.0
   pustular L01.02
   ulerythematosa reticulata L66.4
Folliculome lipidique
   specified site —see Neoplasm, benign, by site
   unspecified site
      female D27.9
      male D29.20
Følling's disease E70.0
Follow-up —see Examination, follow-up
Fong's syndrome (hereditary osteo-onychodysplasia) Q87.2
Food
   allergy L27.2
   asphyxia (from aspiration or inhalation) —see Foreign body, by site
   choked on —see Foreign body, by site
   deprivation T73.0
      specified kind of food NEC E63.8
   insecurity Z59.41
   intoxication —see Poisoning, food
   lack of T73.0
   poisoning —see Poisoning, food
   rejection NEC —see Disorder, eating

Food (continued)
   strangulation or suffocation —see Foreign body, by site
   toxemia —see Poisoning, food
Foot —see condition
Foramen ovale (nonclosure) (patent) (persistent) Q21.12
Forbes' glycogen storage disease E74.03
Fordyce-Fox disease L75.2
Fordyce's disease (mouth) Q38.6
Forearm —see condition
Foreclosure on loan Z59.89
Foreign body
   with
      laceration —see Laceration, by site, with foreign body
      puncture wound —see Puncture, by site, with foreign body
   accidentally left following a procedure T81.509
      aspiration T81.506
         resulting in
            adhesions T81.516
            obstruction T81.526
            perforation T81.536
            specified complication NEC T81.596
      cardiac catheterization T81.505
         resulting in
            acute reaction T81.60
               aseptic peritonitis T81.61
               specified NEC T81.69
   accidentally left following a
      adhesions T81.515
         obstruction T81.525
         perforation T81.535
         specified complication NEC T81.595
      causing
         acute reaction T81.60
            aseptic peritonitis T81.61
            specified complication NEC T81.69
         adhesions T81.519
         aseptic peritonitis T81.61
         obstruction T81.529
         perforation T81.539
         specified complication NEC T81.599
      endoscopy T81.504
         resulting in
            adhesions T81.514
            obstruction T81.524
            perforation T81.534
            specified complication NEC T81.594
      immunization T81.503
         resulting in
            adhesions T81.513
            obstruction T81.523
            perforation T81.533
            specified complication NEC T81.593
      infusion T81.501
         resulting in
            adhesions T81.511
            obstruction T81.521
            perforation T81.531
            specified complication NEC T81.591
      injection T81.503
         resulting in
            adhesions T81.513
            obstruction T81.523
            perforation T81.533
            specified complication NEC T81.593

Foreign body (continued)
   accidentally left following a adhesions (continued)
      kidney dialysis T81.502
         resulting in
            adhesions T81.512
            obstruction T81.522
            perforation T81.532
            specified complication NEC T81.592
      packing removal T81.507
         resulting in
            acute reaction T81.60
               aseptic peritonitis T81.61
               specified NEC T81.69
            adhesions T81.517
            obstruction T81.527
            perforation T81.537
            specified complication NEC T81.597
      puncture T81.506
         resulting in
            adhesions T81.516
            obstruction T81.526
            perforation T81.536
            specified complication NEC T81.596
      specified procedure NEC T81.508
         resulting in
            acute reaction T81.60
               aseptic peritonitis T81.61
               specified NEC T81.69
            adhesions T81.518
            obstruction T81.528
            perforation T81.538
            specified complication NEC T81.598
      surgical operation T81.500
         resulting in
            acute reaction T81.60
               aseptic peritonitis T81.61
               specified NEC T81.69
            adhesions T81.510
            obstruction T81.520
            perforation T81.530
            specified complication NEC T81.590
      transfusion T81.501
         resulting in
            adhesions T81.511
            obstruction T81.521
            perforation T81.531
            specified complication NEC T81.591
   alimentary tract T18.9
   anus T18.5
   colon T18.4
   esophagus —see Foreign body, esophagus
   mouth T18.0
   multiple sites T18.8
   rectosigmoid (junction) T18.5
   rectum T18.5
   small intestine T18.3
   specified site NEC T18.8
   stomach T18.2
   anterior chamber (eye) S05.5-
   auditory canal —see Foreign body, entering through orifice, ear
   bronchus T17.508
      causing
         asphyxiation T17.500
            food (bone) (seed) T17.520
            gastric contents (vomitus) T17.510
            specified type NEC T17.590
         injury NEC T17.508
            food (bone) (seed) T17.528
            gastric contents (vomitus) T17.518
            specified type NEC T17.598

Foreign body *(continued)*
- canthus —*see* Foreign body, conjunctival sac
- ciliary body (eye) S05.5-
- conjunctival sac T15.1-
- cornea T15.0-
- entering through orifice
  - accessory sinus T17.0
  - alimentary canal T18.9
    - multiple parts T18.8
    - specified part NEC T18.8
  - alveolar process T18.0
  - antrum (Highmore's) T17.0
  - anus T18.5
  - appendix T18.4
  - auditory canal —*see* Foreign body, entering through orifice, ear
  - auricle —*see* Foreign body, entering through orifice, ear
  - bladder T19.1
  - bronchioles —*see* Foreign body, respiratory tract, specified site NEC
  - bronchus (main) —*see* Foreign body, bronchus
  - buccal cavity T18.0
  - canthus (inner) —*see* Foreign body, conjunctival sac
  - cecum T18.4
  - cervix (canal) (uteri) T19.3
  - colon T18.4
  - conjunctival sac —*see* Foreign body, conjunctival sac
  - cornea —*see* Foreign body, cornea
  - digestive organ or tract NOS T18.9
    - multiple parts T18.8
    - specified part NEC T18.8
  - duodenum T18.3
  - ear (external) T16.-
  - esophagus —*see* Foreign body, esophagus
  - eye (external) NOS T15.9-
    - conjunctival sac —*see* Foreign body, conjunctival sac
    - cornea —*see* Foreign body, cornea
    - specified part NEC T15.8-
  - eyeball —*see also* Foreign body, entering through orifice, eye, specified part NEC
    - with penetrating wound —*see* Puncture, eyeball
  - eyelid —*see also* Foreign body, conjunctival sac
    - with
      - laceration —*see* Laceration, eyelid, with foreign body
      - puncture —*see* Puncture, eyelid, with foreign body
      - superficial injury —*see* Foreign body, superficial, eyelid
  - gastrointestinal tract T18.9
    - multiple parts T18.8
    - specified part NEC T18.8
  - genitourinary tract T19.9
    - multiple parts T19.8
    - specified part NEC T19.8
  - globe —*see* Foreign body, entering through orifice, eyeball
  - gum T18.0
  - Highmore's antrum T17.0
  - hypopharynx —*see* Foreign body, pharynx
  - ileum T18.3
  - intestine (small) T18.3
    - large T18.4

Foreign body *(continued)*
- entering through orifice *(continued)*
  - lacrimal apparatus (punctum) —*see* Foreign body, entering through orifice, eye, specified part NEC
  - large intestine T18.4
  - larynx —*see* Foreign body, larynx
  - lung —*see* Foreign body, respiratory tract, specified site NEC
  - maxillary sinus T17.0
  - mouth T18.0
  - nasal sinus T17.0
  - nasopharynx —*see* Foreign body, pharynx
  - nose (passage) T17.1
  - nostril T17.1
  - oral cavity T18.0
  - palate T18.0
  - penis T19.4
  - pharynx —*see* Foreign body, pharynx
  - piriform sinus —*see* Foreign body, pharynx
  - rectosigmoid (junction) T18.5
  - rectum T18.5
  - respiratory tract —*see* Foreign body, respiratory tract
  - sinus (accessory) (frontal) (maxillary) (nasal) T17.0
    - piriform —*see* Foreign body, pharynx
  - small intestine T18.3
  - stomach T18.2
  - suffocation by —*see* Foreign body, by site
  - tear ducts or glands —*see* Foreign body, entering through orifice, eye, specified part NEC
  - throat —*see* Foreign body, pharynx
  - tongue T18.0
  - tonsil, tonsillar (fossa) —*see* Foreign body, pharynx
  - trachea —*see* Foreign body, trachea
  - ureter T19.8
  - urethra T19.0
  - uterus (any part) T19.3
  - vagina T19.2
  - vulva T19.2
- esophagus T18.108
  - causing
    - injury NEC T18.108
      - food (bone) (seed) T18.128
      - gastric contents (vomitus) T18.118
      - specified type NEC T18.198
    - tracheal compression T18.100
      - food (bone) (seed) T18.120
      - gastric contents (vomitus) T18.110
      - specified type NEC T18.190
- feeling of, in throat R09.89
- fragment —*see* Retained, foreign body fragments (type of)
- genitourinary tract T19.9
  - bladder T19.1
  - multiple parts T19.8
  - penis T19.4
  - specified site NEC T19.8
  - urethra T19.0
  - uterus T19.3
    - IUD Z97.5
  - vagina T19.2
    - contraceptive device Z97.5
  - vulva T19.2

Foreign body *(continued)*
- granuloma (old) (soft tissue) —*see also* Granuloma, foreign body
  - skin L92.3
- in
  - laceration —*see* Laceration, by site, with foreign body
  - puncture wound —*see* Puncture, by site, with foreign body
  - soft tissue (residual) M79.5
- inadvertently left in operation wound —*see* Foreign body, accidentally left during a procedure
- ingestion, ingested NOS T18.9
- inhalation or inspiration —*see* Foreign body, by site
- internal organ, not entering through a natural orifice - code as specific injury with foreign body
- intraocular S05.5-
  - old, retained (nonmagnetic) H44.70-
    - anterior chamber H44.71-
    - ciliary body H44.72-
    - iris H44.72-
    - lens H44.73-
    - magnetic H44.60-
      - anterior chamber H44.61-
      - ciliary body H44.62-
      - iris H44.62-
      - lens H44.63-
      - posterior wall H44.64-
      - specified site NEC H44.69-
      - vitreous body H44.65-
    - posterior wall H44.74-
    - specified site NEC H44.79-
    - vitreous body H44.75-
- iris —*see* Foreign body, intraocular
- lacrimal punctum —*see* Foreign body, entering through orifice, eye, specified part NEC
- larynx T17.308
  - causing
    - asphyxiation T17.300
      - food (bone) (seed) T17.320
      - gastric contents (vomitus) T17.310
      - specified type NEC T17.390
    - injury NEC T17.308
      - food (bone) (seed) T17.328
      - gastric contents (vomitus) T17.318
      - specified type NEC T17.398
- lens —*see* Foreign body, intraocular
- ocular muscle S05.4-
  - old, retained —*see* Foreign body, orbit, old
- old or residual
  - soft tissue (residual) M79.5
- operation wound, left accidentally —*see* Foreign body, accidentally left during a procedure
- orbit S05.4-
  - old, retained H05.5-
- pharynx T17.208
  - causing
    - asphyxiation T17.200
      - food (bone) (seed) T17.220
      - gastric contents (vomitus) T17.210
      - specified type NEC T17.290
    - injury NEC T17.208
      - food (bone) (seed) T17.228
      - gastric contents (vomitus) T17.218
      - specified type NEC T17.298

Foreign body *(continued)*
- respiratory tract T17.908
  - bronchioles —*see* Foreign body, respiratory tract, specified site NEC
  - bronchus —*see* Foreign body, bronchus
  - causing
    - asphyxiation T17.900
      - food (bone) (seed) T17.920
      - gastric contents (vomitus) T17.910
      - specified type NEC T17.990
    - injury NEC T17.908
      - food (bone) (seed) T17.928
      - gastric contents (vomitus) T17.918
      - specified type NEC T17.998
  - larynx —*see* Foreign body, larynx
  - lung —*see* Foreign body, respiratory tract, specified site NEC
  - multiple parts —*see* Foreign body, respiratory tract, specified site NEC
  - nasal sinus T17.0
  - nasopharynx —*see* Foreign body, pharynx
  - nose T17.1
  - nostril T17.1
  - pharynx —*see* Foreign body, pharynx
  - specified site NEC T17.808
    - causing
      - asphyxiation T17.800
        - food (bone) (seed) T17.820
        - gastric contents (vomitus) T17.810
        - specified type NEC T17.890
      - injury NEC T17.808
        - food (bone) (seed) T17.828
        - gastric contents (vomitus) T17.818
        - specified type NEC T17.898
  - throat —*see* Foreign body, pharynx
  - trachea —*see* Foreign body, trachea
- retained (old) (nonmagnetic) (in)
  - anterior chamber (eye) —*see* Foreign body, intraocular, old, retained, anterior chamber
    - magnetic —*see* Foreign body, intraocular, old, retained, magnetic, anterior chamber
  - ciliary body —*see* Foreign body, intraocular, old, retained, ciliary body
    - magnetic —*see* Foreign body, intraocular, old, retained, magnetic, ciliary body
  - eyelid H02.819
    - left H02.816
      - lower H02.815
      - upper H02.814
    - right H02.813
      - lower H02.812
      - upper H02.811
  - fragments —*see* Retained, foreign body fragments (type of)
  - globe —*see* Foreign body, intraocular, old, retained
    - magnetic —*see* Foreign body, intraocular, old, retained, magnetic

Foreign body *(continued)*
  retained *(continued)*
    intraocular —*see* Foreign body, intraocular, old, retained
      magnetic —*see* Foreign body, intraocular, old, retained, magnetic
    iris —*see* Foreign body, intraocular, old, retained, iris
      magnetic —*see* Foreign body, intraocular, old, retained, magnetic, iris
    lens —*see* Foreign body, intraocular, old, retained, lens
      magnetic —*see* Foreign body, intraocular, old, retained, magnetic, lens
    muscle —*see* Foreign body, retained, soft tissue
    orbit —*see* Foreign body, orbit, old
    posterior wall of globe —*see* Foreign body, intraocular, old, retained, posterior wall
      magnetic —*see* Foreign body, intraocular, old, retained, magnetic, posterior wall
    retrobulbar —*see* Foreign body, orbit, old, retrobulbar
    soft tissue M79.5
    vitreous —*see* Foreign body, intraocular, old, retained, vitreous body
      magnetic —*see* Foreign body, intraocular, old, retained, magnetic, vitreous body
  retina S05.5-
  sensation —*see* Sensation, foreign body
  superficial, without open wound
    abdomen, abdominal (wall) S30.851
    alveolar process S00.552
    ankle S90.55-
    antecubital space —*see* Foreign body, superficial, forearm
    anus S30.857
    arm (upper) S40.85-
    auditory canal —*see* Foreign body, superficial, ear
    auricle —*see* Foreign body, superficial, ear
    axilla —*see* Foreign body, superficial, arm
    back, lower S30.850
    breast S20.15-
    brow S00.85
    buttock S30.850
    calf —*see* Foreign body, superficial, leg
    canthus —*see* Foreign body, superficial, eyelid
    cheek S00.85
      internal S00.552
    chest wall —*see* Foreign body, superficial, thorax
    chin S00.85
    clitoris S30.854
    costal region —*see* Foreign body, superficial, thorax
    digit(s)
      hand —*see* Foreign body, superficial, finger
      foot —*see* Foreign body, superficial, toe
    ear S00.45-
    elbow S50.35-
    epididymis S30.853
    epigastric region S30.851
    epiglottis S10.15
    esophagus, cervical S10.15

Foreign body *(continued)*
  superficial, without open wound *(continued)*
    eyebrow —*see* Foreign body, superficial, eyelid
    eyelid S00.25-
    face S00.85
    finger(s) S60.459
      index S60.45-
      little S60.45-
      middle S60.45-
      ring S60.45-
    flank S30.851
    foot (except toe(s) alone) S90.85-
      toe —*see* Foreign body, superficial, toe
    forearm S50.85-
      elbow only —*see* Foreign body, superficial, elbow
    forehead S00.85
    genital organs, external
      female S30.856
      male S30.855
    groin S30.851
    gum S00.552
    hand S60.55-
    head S00.95
      ear —*see* Foreign body, superficial, ear
      eyelid —*see* Foreign body, superficial, eyelid
      lip S00.551
      nose S00.35
      oral cavity S00.552
      scalp S00.05
      specified site NEC S00.85
    heel —*see* Foreign body, superficial, foot
    hip S70.25-
    inguinal region S30.851
    interscapular region S20.459
    jaw S00.85
    knee S80.25-
    labium (majus) (minus) S30.854
    larynx S10.15
    leg (lower) S80.85-
      knee —*see* Foreign body, superficial, knee
      upper —*see* Foreign body, superficial, thigh
    lip S00.551
    lower back S30.850
    lumbar region S30.850
    malar region S00.85
    mammary —*see* Foreign body, superficial, breast
    mastoid region S00.85
    mouth S00.552
    nail
      finger —*see* Foreign body, superficial, finger
      toe —*see* Foreign body, superficial, toe
    nape S10.85
    nasal S00.35
    neck S10.95
      specified site NEC S10.85
      throat S10.15
    nose S00.35
    occipital region S00.05
    oral cavity S00.552
    orbital region —*see* Foreign body, superficial, eyelid
    palate S00.552
    palm —*see* Foreign body, superficial, hand
    parietal region S00.05
    pelvis S30.850
    penis S30.852

Foreign body *(continued)*
  superficial, without open wound *(continued)*
    perineum
      female S30.854
      male S30.850
    periocular area —*see* Foreign body, superficial, eyelid
    phalanges
      finger —*see* Foreign body, superficial, finger
      toe —*see* Foreign body, superficial, toe
    pharynx S10.15
    pinna —*see* Foreign body, superficial, ear
    popliteal space —*see* Foreign body, superficial, knee
    prepuce S30.852
    pubic region S30.850
    pudendum
      female S30.856
      male S30.855
    sacral region S30.850
    scalp S00.05
    scapular region —*see* Foreign body, superficial, shoulder
    scrotum S30.853
    shin —*see* Foreign body, superficial, leg
    shoulder S40.25-
    sternal region S20.359
    submaxillary region S00.85
    submental region S00.85
    subungual
      finger(s) —*see* Foreign body, superficial, finger
      toe(s) —*see* Foreign body, superficial, toe
    supraclavicular fossa S10.85
    supraorbital S00.85
    temple S00.85
    temporal region S00.85
    testis S30.853
    thigh S70.35-
    thorax, thoracic (wall) S20.95
      back S20.45-
      front S20.35-
    throat S10.15
    thumb S60.35-
    toe(s) (lesser) S90.456
      great S90.45-
    tongue S00.552
    trachea S10.15
    tunica vaginalis S30.853
    tympanum, tympanic membrane —*see* Foreign body, superficial, ear
    uvula S00.552
    vagina S30.854
    vocal cords S10.15
    vulva S30.854
    wrist S60.85-
  swallowed T18.9
  trachea T17.408
    causing
      asphyxiation T17.400
        food (bone) (seed) T17.420
        gastric contents (vomitus) T17.410
        specified type NEC T17.490
      injury NEC T17.408
        food (bone) (seed) T17.428
        gastric contents (vomitus) T17.418
        specified type NEC T17.498
  type of fragment —*see* Retained, foreign body fragments (type of)
  vitreous (humor) S05.5-

Forestier's disease (rhizomelic pseudopolyarthritis) M35.3
  meaning ankylosing hyperostosis —*see* Hyperostosis, ankylosing

Formation
  hyalin in cornea —*see* Degeneration, cornea
  sequestrum in bone (due to infection) —*see* Osteomyelitis, chronic
  valve
    colon, congenital Q43.8
    ureter (congenital) Q62.39

Formication R20.2

Fort Bragg fever A27.89

Fossa —*see also* condition
  pyriform —*see* condition

Foster-Kennedy syndrome H47.14-

Fothergill's
  disease (trigeminal neuralgia) —*see also* Neuralgia, trigeminal
  scarlatina anginosa A38.9

Foul breath R19.6

Foundling Z76.1

Fournier disease or gangrene N49.3
  female N76.82
  vagina and vulva N76.82

Fourth
  cranial nerve —*see* condition
  molar K00.1

Foville's (peduncular) **disease or syndrome** G46.3

Fox (Fordyce) **disease** (apocrine miliaria) L75.2

FPIES (food protein-induced enterocolitis syndrome) K52.21

Fracture, burst —*see* Fracture, traumatic, by site

Fracture, chronic —*see* Fracture, pathological, by site

Fracture, insufficiency —*see* Fracture, pathologic, by site

Fracture, nontraumatic, NEC
  atypical
    femur M84.750-
      complete
        oblique M84.759
          left side M84.758
          right side M84.757
        transverse M84.756
          left side M84.755
          right side M84.754
      incomplete M84.753
        left side M84.752
        right side M84.751

Fracture, pathological (pathologic) —*see also* Fracture, traumatic M84.40
  ankle M84.47-
  carpus M84.44-
  clavicle M84.41-
  compression (not due to trauma) (*see also* Collapse, vertebra) M48.50-
  dental implant M27.63
  dental restorative material K08.539
    with loss of material K08.531
    without loss of material K08.530
  due to
    neoplastic disease NEC (*see also* Neoplasm) M84.50
      ankle M84.57-
      carpus M84.54-
      clavicle M84.51-

Fracture, pathological *(continued)*
  due to *(continued)*
    neoplastic disease NEC *(continued)*
      femur M84.55-
      fibula M84.56-
      finger M84.54-
      hip M84.559
      humerus M84.52-
      ilium M84.550
      ischium M84.550
      metacarpus M84.54-
      metatarsus M84.57-
      neck M84.58
      pelvis M84.550
      radius M84.53-
      rib M84.58
      scapula M84.51-
      skull M84.58
      specified site NEC M84.58
      tarsus M84.57-
      tibia M84.56-
      toe M84.57-
      ulna M84.53-
      vertebra M84.58
    osteoporosis M80.00
      disuse —*see* Osteoporosis, specified type NEC, with pathological fracture
      drug-induced —*see* Osteoporosis, drug induced, with pathological fracture
      idiopathic —*see* Osteoporosis, specified type NEC, with pathological fracture
      postmenopausal —*see* Osteoporosis, postmenopausal, with pathological fracture
      postoophorectomy —*see* Osteoporosis, postoophorectomy, with pathological fracture
      postsurgical malabsorption —*see* Osteoporosis, specified type NEC, with pathological fracture
      specified cause NEC —*see* Osteoporosis, specified type NEC, with pathological fracture
    specified disease NEC M84.60
      ankle M84.67-
      carpus M84.64-
      clavicle M84.61-
      femur M84.65-
      fibula M84.66-
      finger M84.64-
      hip M84.65-
      humerus M84.62-
      ilium M84.650
      ischium M84.650
      metacarpus M84.64-
      metatarsus M84.67-
      neck M84.68
      radius M84.63-
      rib M84.68
      scapula M84.61-
      skull M84.68
      tarsus M84.67-
      tibia M84.66-
      toe M84.67-
      ulna M84.63-
      vertebra M84.68
  femur M84.45-
  fibula M84.46-
  finger M84.44-
  hip M84.459
  humerus M84.42-
  ilium M84.454
  ischium M84.454

Fracture, pathological *(continued)*
  joint prosthesis —*see* Complications, joint prosthesis, mechanical, breakdown, by site
    periprosthetic —*see* Fracture, pathological, periprosthetic
  metacarpus M84.44-
  metatarsus M84.47-
  neck M84.48
  pelvis M84.454
  periprosthetic M97.9
    ankle M97.2-
    elbow M97.4-
    finger M97.8
    hip M97.0-
    knee M97.1-
    other specified joint M97.8
    shoulder M97.3-
    spinal joint M97.8
    toe joint M97.8
    wrist joint M97.8
  radius M84.43-
  restorative material (dental) K08.539
    with loss of material K08.531
    without loss of material K08.530
  rib M84.48
  scapula M84.41-
  skull M84.48
  tarsus M84.47-
  tibia M84.46-
  toe M84.47-
  ulna M84.43-
  vertebra M84.48

Fracture, traumatic (abduction) (adduction) (separation) *(see also* Fracture, pathological) T14.8
  acetabulum S32.40-
    column
      anterior (displaced) (iliopubic) S32.43-
        nondisplaced S32.436
      posterior (displaced) (ilioischial) S32.443
        nondisplaced S32.44-
    dome (displaced) S32.48-
      nondisplaced S32.48
    specified NEC S32.49-
    transverse (displaced) S32.45-
      with associated posterior wall fracture (displaced) S32.46-
        nondisplaced S32.46-
      nondisplaced S32.45-
    wall
      anterior (displaced) S32.41-
        nondisplaced S32.41-
      medial (displaced) S32.47-
        nondisplaced S32.47-
      posterior (displaced) S32.42-
        with associated transverse fracture (displaced) S32.46-
          nondisplaced S32.46-
        nondisplaced S32.42-
  acromion —*see* Fracture, scapula, acromial process
  ankle S82.899
    bimalleolar (displaced) S82.84-
      nondisplaced S82.84-
    lateral malleolus only (displaced) S82.6-
      nondisplaced S82.6-
    medial malleolus (displaced) S82.5-
      associated with Maisonneuve's fracture —*see* Fracture, Maisonneuve's
      nondisplaced S82.5-

Fracture, traumatic *(continued)*
  ankle *(continued)*
    talus —*see* Fracture, tarsal, talus
    trimalleolar (displaced) S82.85-
      nondisplaced S82.85-
  arm (upper) —*see also* Fracture, humerus, shaft
    humerus —*see* Fracture, humerus
    radius —*see* Fracture, radius
    ulna —*see* Fracture, ulna
  associated with chest compression and cardiopulmonary resuscitation M96.A9
  astragalus —*see* Fracture, tarsal, talus
  atlas —*see* Fracture, neck, cervical vertebra, first
  axis —*see* Fracture, neck, cervical vertebra, second
  back —*see* Fracture, vertebra
  Barton's —*see* Barton's fracture
  base of skull —*see* Fracture, skull, base
  basicervical (basal) (femoral) S72.0
  Bennett's —*see* Bennett's fracture
  bimalleolar —*see* Fracture, ankle, bimalleolar
  blow-out S02.3-
  bone NEC T14.8
    birth injury P13.9
    following insertion of orthopedic implant, joint prosthesis or bone plate —*see* Fracture, following insertion of orthopedic implant, joint prosthesis or bone plate
    in (due to) neoplastic disease NEC —*see* Fracture, pathological, due to, neoplastic disease
    pathological (cause unknown) —*see* Fracture, pathological
  breast bone —*see* Fracture, sternum
  bucket handle (semilunar cartilage) —*see* Tear, meniscus
  buckle —*see* Fracture, by site, torus
  burst —*see* Fracture, traumatic, by site
  calcaneus —*see* Fracture, tarsal, calcaneus
  carpal bone(s) S62.10-
    capitate (displaced) S62.13-
      nondisplaced S62.13-
    cuneiform —*see* Fracture, carpal bone, triquetrum
    hamate (body) (displaced) S62.143
      hook process (displaced) S62.15-
        nondisplaced S62.15-
      nondisplaced S62.14-
    larger multangular —*see* Fracture, carpal bones, trapezium
    lunate (displaced) S62.12-
      nondisplaced S62.12-
    navicular S62.00-
      distal pole (displaced) S62.01-
        nondisplaced S62.01-
      middle third (displaced) S62.02-
        nondisplaced S62.02-
      proximal third (displaced) S62.03-
        nondisplaced S62.03-
      volar tuberosity —*see* Fracture, carpal bones, navicular, distal pole
    os magnum —*see* Fracture, carpal bones, capitate

Fracture, traumatic *(continued)*
  carpal bone(s) *(continued)*
    pisiform (displaced) S62.16-
      nondisplaced S62.16-
    semilunar —*see* Fracture, carpal bones, lunate
    smaller multangular —*see* Fracture, carpal bones, trapezoid
    trapezium (displaced) S62.17-
      nondisplaced S62.17-
    trapezoid (displaced) S62.18-
      nondisplaced S62.18-
    triquetrum (displaced) S62.11-
      nondisplaced S62.11-
    unciform —*see* Fracture, carpal bones, hamate
  cervical —*see* Fracture, vertebra, cervical
  clavicle S42.00-
    acromial end (displaced) S42.03-
      nondisplaced S42.03-
    birth injury P13.4
    lateral end —*see* Fracture, clavicle, acromial end
    shaft (displaced) S42.02-
      nondisplaced S42.02-
    sternal end (anterior) (displaced) S42.01-
      nondisplaced S42.01-
      posterior S42.01-
  coccyx S32.2
  collapsed —*see* Collapse, vertebra
  collar bone —*see* Fracture, clavicle
  Colles' —*see* Colles' fracture
  coronoid process —*see* Fracture, ulna, upper end, coronoid process
  corpus cavernosum penis S39.840
  costochondral cartilage S23.41
  costochondral, costosternal junction —*see* Fracture, rib
  cranium —*see* Fracture, skull
  cricoid cartilage S12.8
  cuboid (ankle) —*see* Fracture, tarsal, cuboid
  cuneiform
    foot —*see* Fracture, tarsal, cuneiform
    wrist —*see* Fracture, carpal, triquetrum
  delayed union —*see* Delay, union, fracture
  dental restorative material K08.539
    with loss of material K08.531
    without loss of material K08.530
  due to
    birth injury —*see* Birth, injury, fracture
    osteoporosis —*see* Osteoporosis, with fracture
  Dupuytren's —*see* Fracture, ankle, lateral malleolus
  elbow S42.40-
  ethmoid (bone) (sinus) —*see* Fracture, skull, base
  face bone S02.92
  fatigue —*see also* Fracture, stress
    vertebra M48.40
      cervical region M48.42
      cervicothoracic region M48.43
      lumbar region M48.46
      lumbosacral region M48.47
      occipito-atlanto-axial region M48.41
      sacrococcygeal region M48.48
      thoracic region M48.44
      thoracolumbar region M48.45

Fracture, traumatic (continued)
femur, femoral S72.9-
  basicervical (basal) S72.0
  birth injury P13.2
  capital epiphyseal S79.01-
  condyles, epicondyles —see
    Fracture, femur, lower end
  distal end —see Fracture, femur,
    lower end
  epiphysis
    head —see Fracture, femur,
      upper end, epiphysis
    lower —see Fracture, femur,
      lower end, epiphysis
    upper —see Fracture, femur,
      upper end, epiphysis
  following insertion of implant,
    prosthesis or plate M96.66-
  head —see Fracture, femur,
    upper end, head
  intertrochanteric —see Fracture,
    femur, trochanteric
  intratrochanteric —see Fracture,
    femur, trochanteric
  lower end S72.40-
    condyle (displaced) S72.41-
      lateral (displaced) S72.42-
        nondisplaced S72.42-
      medial (displaced) S72.43-
        nondisplaced S72.43-
      nondisplaced S72.41-
    epiphysis (displaced)
      S72.44-
      nondisplaced S72.44-
    physeal S79.10-
      Salter-Harris
        Type I S79.11-
        Type II S79.12-
        Type III S79.13-
        Type IV S79.14-
        specified NEC S79.19-
    specified NEC S72.49-
    supracondylar (displaced)
      S72.45-
      with intracondylar
        extension (displaced)
        S72.46-
        nondisplaced S72.46-
      nondisplaced S72.45-
    torus S72.47-
  neck —see Fracture, femur,
    upper end, neck
  pertrochanteric —see Fracture,
    femur, trochanteric
  shaft (lower third) (middle third)
    (upper third) S72.30-
    comminuted (displaced)
      S72.35-
      nondisplaced S72.35-
    oblique (displaced) S72.33-
      nondisplaced S72.33-
    segmental (displaced) S72.36-
      nondisplaced S72.36-
    specified NEC S72.39-
    spiral (displaced) S72.34-
      nondisplaced S72.34-
    transverse (displaced) S72.32-
      nondisplaced S72.32-
  specified site NEC S72.8
  subcapital (displaced) S72.01-
  subtrochanteric (region) (section)
    (displaced) S72.2-
    nondisplaced S72.2-
  transcervical —see Fracture,
    femur, midcervical
  transtrochanteric —see Fracture,
    femur, trochanteric
  trochanteric S72.10-
    apophyseal (displaced)
      S72.13-
      nondisplaced S72.13-

Fracture, traumatic (continued)
femur, femoral (continued)
  trochanteric (continued)
    greater trochanter (displaced)
      S72.11-
      nondisplaced S72.11-
    intertrochanteric (displaced)
      S72.14-
      nondisplaced S72.14-
    lesser trochanter (displaced)
      S72.12-
      nondisplaced S72.12-
  upper end S72.00-
    apophyseal (displaced)
      S72.13-
      nondisplaced S72.13-
    cervicotrochanteric —see
      Fracture, femur, upper end,
      neck, base
    epiphysis (displaced)
      S72.02-
      nondisplaced S72.02-
    head S72.05-
      articular (displaced)
        S72.06-
        nondisplaced S72.06-
      specified NEC S72.09-
    intertrochanteric (displaced)
      S72.14-
      nondisplaced S72.14-
    intracapsular S72.01-
    midcervical (displaced)
      S72.03-
      nondisplaced S72.03-
    neck S72.00-
      base (displaced) S72.04-
        nondisplaced S72.04-
      specified NEC S72.09-
    pertrochanteric —see
      Fracture, femur, upper end,
      trochanteric
    physeal S79.00-
      Salter-Harris type I S79.01-
      specified NEC S79.09-
    subcapital (displaced) S72.01-
    subtrochanteric (displaced)
      S72.2-
      nondisplaced S72.2-
    transcervical —see Fracture,
      femur, midcervical
    trochanteric S72.10-
      greater (displaced) S72.11-
        nondisplaced S72.11-
      lesser (displaced) S72.12-
        nondisplaced S72.12-
fibula (shaft) (styloid) S82.40-
  comminuted (displaced) S82.45-
    nondisplaced S82.45-
  following insertion of implant,
    prosthesis or plate M96.67-
  involving ankle or malleolus
    —see Fracture, fibula, lateral
    malleolus
  lateral malleolus (displaced)
    S82.6-
    nondisplaced S82.6-
  lower end
    physeal S89.30-
      Salter-Harris
        Type I S89.31-
        Type II S89.32-
        specified NEC S89.39-
    specified NEC S82.83-
    torus S82.82-
  oblique (displaced) S82.43-
    nondisplaced S82.43-
  segmental (displaced) S82.46-
    nondisplaced S82.46-
  specified NEC S82.49-
  spiral (displaced) S82.44-
    nondisplaced S82.44-

Fracture, traumatic (continued)
fibula (continued)
  transverse (displaced)
    S82.42-
    nondisplaced S82.42-
  upper end
    physeal S89.20-
      Salter-Harris
        Type I S89.21-
        Type II S89.22-
        specified NEC S89.29-
    specified NEC S82.83-
    torus S82.81-
finger (except thumb) S62.60-
  distal phalanx (displaced)
    S62.63-
    nondisplaced S62.66-
  index S62.60-
    distal phalanx (displaced)
      S62.63-
      nondisplaced S62.66-
    middle phalanx (displaced)
      S62.62-
      nondisplaced S62.65-
    proximal phalanx (displaced)
      S62.61-
      nondisplaced S62.64-
  little S62.60-
    distal phalanx (displaced)
      S62.63-
      nondisplaced S62.66-
    middle phalanx (displaced)
      S62.62-
      nondisplaced S62.65-
    proximal phalanx (displaced)
      S62.61-
      nondisplaced S62.64-
  middle phalanx (displaced)
    S62.62-
    nondisplaced S62.65-
  middle S62.60-
    distal phalanx (displaced)
      S62.63-
      nondisplaced S62.66-
    middle phalanx (displaced)
      S62.62-
      nondisplaced S62.65-
    proximal phalanx (displaced)
      S62.61-
      nondisplaced S62.64-
  proximal phalanx (displaced)
    S62.61-
    nondisplaced S62.64-
  ring S62.60-
    distal phalanx (displaced)
      S62.63-
      nondisplaced S62.66-
    middle phalanx (displaced)
      S62.62-
      nondisplaced S62.65-
    proximal phalanx (displaced)
      S62.61-
      nondisplaced S62.64-
  thumb —see Fracture, thumb
following insertion (intraoperative)
  (postoperative) of orthopedic
  implant, joint prosthesis or bone
  plate M96.69
  femur M96.66-
  fibula M96.67-
  humerus M96.62-
  pelvis M96.65
  radius M96.63-
  specified bone NEC M96.69
  tibia M96.67-
  ulna M96.63-
foot S92.90-
  astragalus —see Fracture, tarsal,
    talus
  calcaneus —see Fracture, tarsal,
    calcaneus

Fracture, traumatic (continued)
foot (continued)
  cuboid —see Fracture, tarsal,
    cuboid
  cuneiform —see Fracture, tarsal,
    cuneiform
  metatarsal —see Fracture,
    metatarsal
  navicular —see Fracture, tarsal,
    navicular
  sesamoid S92.81-
  specified NEC S92.81-
  talus —see Fracture, tarsal, talus
  tarsal —see Fracture, tarsal
  toe —see Fracture, toe
forearm S52.9-
  radius —see Fracture, radius
  ulna —see Fracture, ulna
fossa (anterior) (middle) (posterior)
  S02.19
fragility —see Fracture,
  pathological, due to
  osteoporosis
frontal (bone) (skull) S02.0
  sinus S02.19
glenoid (cavity) (scapula) —see
  Fracture, scapula, glenoid cavity
greenstick —see Fracture, by site
hallux —see Fracture, toe, great
hand S62.9-
  carpal —see Fracture, carpal
    bone
  finger (except thumb) —see
    Fracture, finger
  metacarpal —see Fracture,
    metacarpal
  navicular (scaphoid) (hand)
    —see Fracture, carpal bone,
    navicular
  thumb —see Fracture, thumb
healed or old
  with complications - code by
    Nature of the complication
heel bone —see Fracture, tarsal,
  calcaneus
Hill-Sachs S42.29-
hip —see Fracture, femur, neck
humerus S42.30-
  anatomical neck —see Fracture,
    humerus, upper end
  articular process —see Fracture,
    humerus, lower end
  capitellum —see Fracture,
    humerus, lower end, condyle,
    lateral
  distal end —see Fracture,
    humerus, lower end
  epiphysis
    lower —see Fracture,
      humerus, lower end,
      physeal
    upper —see Fracture,
      humerus, upper end,
      physeal
  external condyle —see Fracture,
    humerus, lower end, condyle,
    lateral
  following insertion of
    implant, prosthesis or plate
    M96.62-
  great tuberosity —see Fracture,
    humerus, upper end, greater
    tuberosity
  intercondylar —see Fracture,
    humerus, lower end
  internal epicondyle —see
    Fracture, humerus, lower end,
    epicondyle, medial
  lesser tuberosity —see Fracture,
    humerus, upper end, lesser
    tuberosity

160

Fracture, traumatic (*continued*)
- humerus (*continued*)
  - lower end S42.40-
    - condyle
      - lateral (displaced) S42.45-
        - nondisplaced S42.45-
      - medial (displaced) S42.46-
        - nondisplaced S42.46-
    - epicondyle
      - lateral (displaced) S42.43-
        - nondisplaced S42.43-
      - medial (displaced) S42.44-
        - incarcerated S42.44-
        - nondisplaced S42.44-
    - physeal S49.10-
      - Salter-Harris
        - Type I S49.11-
        - Type II S49.12-
        - Type III S49.13-
        - Type IV S49.14-
      - specified NEC S49.19-
    - specified NEC (displaced) S42.49-
      - nondisplaced S42.49-
    - supracondylar (simple) (displaced) S42.41-
      - with intercondylar fracture — *see* Fracture, humerus, lower end
      - comminuted (displaced) S42.42-
        - nondisplaced S42.42-
      - nondisplaced S42.41-
    - torus S42.48-
    - transcondylar (displaced) S42.47-
      - nondisplaced S42.47-
  - proximal end —*see* Fracture, humerus, upper end
  - shaft S42.30-
    - comminuted (displaced) S42.35-
      - nondisplaced S42.35-
    - greenstick S42.31-
    - oblique (displaced) S42.33-
      - nondisplaced S42.33-
    - segmental (displaced) S42.36-
      - nondisplaced S42.36-
    - specified NEC S42.39-
    - spiral (displaced) S42.34-
      - nondisplaced S42.34-
    - transverse (displaced) S42.32-
      - nondisplaced S42.32-
  - supracondylar —*see* Fracture, humerus, lower end
  - surgical neck —*see* Fracture, humerus, upper end, surgical neck
  - trochlea —*see* Fracture, humerus, lower end, condyle, medial
  - tuberosity —*see* Fracture, humerus, upper end
  - upper end S42.20-
    - anatomical neck —*see* Fracture, humerus, upper end, specified NEC
    - articular head —*see* Fracture, humerus, upper end, specified NEC
    - epiphysis —*see* Fracture, humerus, upper end, physeal
    - greater tuberosity (displaced) S42.25-
      - nondisplaced S42.25-
    - lesser tuberosity (displaced) S42.26-
      - nondisplaced S42.26-

Fracture, traumatic (*continued*)
- humerus (*continued*)
  - upper end (*continued*)
    - physeal S49.00-
      - Salter-Harris
        - Type I S49.01-
        - Type II S49.02-
        - Type III S49.03-
        - Type IV S49.04-
      - specified NEC S49.09-
    - specified NEC (displaced) S42.29-
      - nondisplaced S42.29-
    - surgical neck (displaced) S42.21-
      - four-part S42.24-
        - nondisplaced S42.21-
      - three-part S42.23-
      - two-part (displaced) S42.22-
        - nondisplaced S42.22-
    - torus S42.27-
    - transepiphyseal —*see* Fracture, humerus, upper end, physeal
- hyoid bone S12.8
- ilium S32.30-
  - with disruption of pelvic ring — *see* Disruption, pelvic ring
  - avulsion (displaced) S32.31-
    - nondisplaced S32.31-
  - specified NEC S32.39-
- impaction, impacted - code as Fracture, by site
- innominate bone —*see* Fracture, ilium
- instep —*see* Fracture, foot
- ischium S32.60-
  - with disruption of pelvic ring — *see* Disruption, pelvic ring
  - avulsion (displaced) S32.61-
    - nondisplaced S32.61-
  - specified NEC S32.69-
- jaw (bone) (lower) —*see* Fracture, mandible
  - upper —*see* Fracture, maxilla
- joint prosthesis —*see* Complications, joint prosthesis, mechanical, breakdown, by site
  - periprosthetic —*see* Fracture, traumatic, periprosthetic
- knee cap —*see* Fracture, patella
- larynx S12.8
- late effects —*see* Sequelae, fracture
- leg (lower) S82.9-
  - ankle —*see* Fracture, ankle
  - femur —*see* Fracture, femur
  - fibula —*see* Fracture, fibula
  - malleolus —*see* Fracture, ankle
  - patella —*see* Fracture, patella
  - specified site NEC S82.89-
  - tibia —*see* Fracture, tibia
- lumbar spine —*see* Fracture, vertebra, lumbar
- lumbosacral spine S32.9
- Maisonneuve's (displaced) S82.86-
  - nondisplaced S82.86-
- malar bone —*see also* Fracture, maxilla S02.400
  - left side S02.40B
  - right side S02.40A
- malleolus —*see* Fracture, ankle
- malunion —*see* Fracture, by site
- mandible (lower jaw (bone)) S02.609
  - alveolus S02.67-
  - angle (of jaw) S02.65-
  - body, unspecified S02.600
    - left side S02.602
    - right side S02.601

Fracture, traumatic (*continued*)
- mandible (*continued*)
  - condylar process S02.61-
  - coronoid process S02.63-
  - ramus, unspecified S02.64-
  - specified site NEC S02.69
  - subcondylar process S02.62-
  - symphysis S02.66
- manubrium (sterni) S22.21
  - dissociation from sternum S22.23
- march —*see* Fracture, traumatic, stress, by site
- maxilla, maxillary (bone) (sinus) (superior) (upper jaw) S02.401
  - alveolus S02.42
  - inferior —*see* Fracture, mandible
  - LeFort I S02.411
  - LeFort II S02.412
  - LeFort III S02.413
  - left side S02.40D
  - right side S02.40C
- metacarpal S62.309
  - base (displaced) S62.319
    - nondisplaced S62.349
  - fifth S62.30-
    - base (displaced) S62.31-
      - nondisplaced S62.34-
    - neck (displaced) S62.33-
      - nondisplaced S62.36-
    - shaft (displaced) S62.32-
      - nondisplaced S62.35-
    - specified NEC S62.398
  - first S62.20-
    - base NEC (displaced) S62.23-
      - nondisplaced S62.23-
    - Bennett's —*see* Bennett's fracture
    - neck (displaced) S62.25-
      - nondisplaced S62.25-
    - shaft (displaced) S62.24-
      - nondisplaced S62.24-
    - specified NEC S62.29-
  - fourth S62.30-
    - base (displaced) S62.31-
      - nondisplaced S62.34-
    - neck (displaced) S62.33-
      - nondisplaced S62.36-
    - shaft (displaced) S62.32-
      - nondisplaced S62.35-
    - specified NEC S62.39-
  - neck (displaced) S62.33-
    - nondisplaced S62.36-
  - Rolando's —*see* Rolando's fracture
  - second S62.30-
    - base (displaced) S62.31-
      - nondisplaced S62.34-
    - neck (displaced) S62.33-
      - nondisplaced S62.36-
    - shaft (displaced) S62.32-
      - nondisplaced S62.35-
    - specified NEC S62.39-
  - shaft (displaced) S62.32-
    - nondisplaced S62.35-
  - third S62.30-
    - base (displaced) S62.31-
      - nondisplaced S62.34-
    - neck (displaced) S62.33-
      - nondisplaced S62.36-
    - shaft (displaced) S62.32-
      - nondisplaced S62.35-
    - specified NEC S62.39-
  - specified NEC S62.399
- metaphyseal —*see* Fracture, traumatic, by site, shaft
- metastatic —*see* Fracture, pathological, due to, neoplastic disease —*see also* Neoplasm

Fracture, traumatic (*continued*)
- metatarsal bone S92.30-
  - fifth (displaced) S92.35-
    - nondisplaced S92.35-
  - first (displaced) S92.31-
    - nondisplaced S92.31-
  - fourth (displaced) S92.34-
    - nondisplaced S92.34-
  - physeal S99.10-
    - Salter-Harris
      - Type I S99.11-
      - Type II S99.12-
      - Type III S99.13-
      - Type IV S99.14-
    - specified NEC S99.19-
  - second (displaced) S92.32-
    - nondisplaced S92.32-
  - third (displaced) S92.33-
    - nondisplaced S92.33-
- Monteggia's —*see* Monteggia's fracture
- multiple
  - hand (and wrist) NEC —*see* Fracture, by site
  - ribs —*see* Fracture, rib, multiple
- nasal (bone(s)) S02.2
- navicular (scaphoid) (foot) —*see also* Fracture, tarsal, navicular
  - hand —*see* Fracture, carpal, navicular
- neck S12.9
  - cervical vertebra S12.9
    - fifth (displaced) S12.400
      - nondisplaced S12.401
      - specified type NEC (displaced) S12.490
        - nondisplaced S12.491
    - first (displaced) S12.000
      - burst (stable) S12.01
        - unstable S12.02
      - lateral mass (displaced) S12.040
        - nondisplaced S12.041
      - nondisplaced S12.001
      - posterior arch (displaced) S12.030
        - nondisplaced S12.031
      - specified type NEC (displaced) S12.090
        - nondisplaced S12.091
    - fourth (displaced) S12.300
      - nondisplaced S12.301
      - specified type NEC (displaced) S12.390
        - nondisplaced S12.391
    - second (displaced) S12.100
      - nondisplaced S12.101
      - dens (anterior) (displaced) (type II) S12.110
        - nondisplaced S12.112
      - posterior S12.111
      - specified type NEC (displaced) S12.120
        - nondisplaced S12.121
      - specified type NEC (displaced) S12.190
        - nondisplaced S12.191
    - seventh (displaced) S12.600
      - nondisplaced S12.601
      - specified type NEC (displaced) S12.690
        - non displaced S12.691
    - sixth (displaced) S12.500
      - nondisplaced S12.501
      - specified type NEC (displaced) S12.590
        - non displaced S12.591

Fracture, traumatic (continued)
  neck (continued)
    cervical vertebra (continued)
      third (displaced) S12.200
        nondisplaced S12.201
        specified type NEC
          (displaced) S12.290
            non displaced S12.291
    hyoid bone S12.8
    larynx S12.8
    specified site NEC S12.8
    thyroid cartilage S12.8
    trachea S12.8
  neoplastic NEC —see Fracture, pathological, due to, neoplastic disease
  neural arch —see Fracture, vertebra
  newborn —see Birth, injury, fracture
  nontraumatic —see Fracture, pathological
  nonunion —see Nonunion, fracture
  nose, nasal (bone) (septum) S02.2
  occiput —see Fracture, skull, base, occiput
  odontoid process —see Fracture, neck, cervical vertebra, second
  olecranon (process) (ulna) —see Fracture, ulna, upper end, olecranon process
  orbit, orbital (bone) (region) S02.85
    floor (blow-out) S02.3-
    roof S02.12-
      wall S02.85
        lateral S02.84-
        medial S02.83-
  os
    calcis —see Fracture, tarsal, calcaneus
    magnum —see Fracture, carpal, capitate
    pubis —see Fracture, pubis
  palate S02.8-
  parietal bone (skull) S02.0
  patella S82.00-
    comminuted (displaced) S82.04-
      nondisplaced S82.04-
    longitudinal (displaced) S82.02-
      nondisplaced S82.02-
    osteochondral (displaced) S82.01-
      nondisplaced S82.01-
    specified NEC S82.09-
    transverse (displaced) S82.03-
      nondisplaced S82.03-
  pedicle (of vertebral arch) —see Fracture, vertebra
  pelvis, pelvic (bone) S32.9
    acetabulum —see Fracture, acetabulum
    circle —see Disruption, pelvic ring
    following insertion of implant, prosthesis or plate M96.65
    ilium —see Fracture, ilium
    ischium —see Fracture, ischium
    multiple
      with disruption of pelvic ring (circle) —see Disruption, pelvic ring
      without disruption of pelvic ring (circle) S32.82
    pubis —see Fracture, pubis
    specified site NEC S32.89
    sacrum —see Fracture, sacrum
  periprosthetic, around internal prosthetic joint M97.9
    ankle M97.2-
    elbow M97.4-
    finger M97.8
    hip M97.0-

Fracture, traumatic (continued)
  periprosthetic, around internal prosthetic joint (continued)
    knee M97.1-
    shoulder M97.3-
    specified joint NEC M97.8
    spine M97.8
    toe M97.8
    wrist M97.8
  phalanx
    foot —see Fracture, toe
    hand —see Fracture, finger
  pisiform —see Fracture, carpal, pisiform
  pond —see Fracture, skull
  prosthetic device, internal —see Complications, prosthetic device, by site, mechanical
  pubis S32.50-
    with disruption of pelvic ring —see Disruption, pelvic ring
    specified site NEC S32.59-
    superior rim S32.51-
  radius S52.9-
    distal end —see Fracture, radius, lower end
    following insertion of implant, prosthesis or plate M96.63-
    head —see Fracture, radius, upper end, head
    lower end S52.50-
      Barton's —see Barton's fracture
      Colles' —see Colles' fracture
      extraarticular NEC S52.55-
      intraarticular NEC S52.57-
      physeal S59.20-
        Salter-Harris
          Type I S59.21-
          Type II S59.22-
          Type III S59.23-
          Type IV S59.24-
        specified NEC S59.29-
      Smith's —see Smith's fracture
      specified NEC S52.59-
      styloid process (displaced) S52.51-
        nondisplaced S52.51-
      torus S52.52-
    neck —see Fracture, radius, upper end
    proximal end —see Fracture, radius, upper end
    shaft S52.30-
      bent bone S52.38-
      comminuted (displaced) S52.35-
        nondisplaced S52.35-
      Galeazzi's —see Galeazzi's fracture
      greenstick S52.31-
      oblique (displaced) S52.33-
        nondisplaced S52.33-
      segmental (displaced) S52.36-
        nondisplaced S52.36-
      specified NEC S52.39-
      spiral (displaced) S52.34-
        nondisplaced S52.34-
      transverse (displaced) S52.32-
        nondisplaced S52.32-
    upper end S52.10-
      head (displaced) S52.12-
        nondisplaced S52.12-
      neck (displaced) S52.13-
        nondisplaced S52.13-
      specified NEC S52.18-

Fracture, traumatic (continued)
  radius (continued)
    upper end (continued)
      physeal S59.10-
        Salter-Harris
          Type I S59.11-
          Type II S59.12-
          Type III S59.13-
          Type IV S59.14-
        specified NEC S59.19-
      torus S52.11-
  ramus
    inferior or superior, pubis —see Fracture, pubis
    mandible —see Fracture, mandible
  restorative material (dental) K08.539
    with loss of material K08.531
    without loss of material K08.530
  rib S22.3-
    with flail chest —see Flail, chest
    associated with chest compression and cardiopulmonary resuscitation M96.A2
    multiple S22.4-
      with flail chest —see Flail, chest
      associated with chest compression and cardiopulmonary resuscitation M96.A3
  root, tooth —see Fracture, tooth
  sacrum S32.10
    specified NEC S32.19
    Type
      1 S32.14
      2 S32.15
      3 S32.16
      4 S32.17
    Zone
      I S32.119
        displaced (minimally) S32.111
        severely S32.112
        nondisplaced S32.110
      II S32.129
        displaced (minimally) S32.121
        severely S32.122
        nondisplaced S32.120
      III S32.139
        displaced (minimally) S32.131
        severely S32.132
        nondisplaced S32.130
  scaphoid (hand) —see also Fracture, carpal, navicular
    foot —see Fracture, tarsal, navicular
  scapula S42.10-
    acromial process (displaced) S42.12-
      nondisplaced S42.12-
    body (displaced) S42.11-
      nondisplaced S42.11-
    coracoid process (displaced) S42.13-
      nondisplaced S42.13-
    glenoid cavity (displaced) S42.14-
      nondisplaced S42.14-
    neck (displaced) S42.15-
      nondisplaced S42.15-
    specified NEC S42.19-
  semilunar bone, wrist —see Fracture, carpal, lunate
  sequelae —see Sequelae, fracture

Fracture, traumatic (continued)
  sesamoid bone
    hand —see Fracture, carpal
    foot S92.81-
    other —see Fracture, traumatic, by site
  shepherd's —see Fracture, tarsal, talus
  shoulder (girdle) S42.9-
    blade —see Fracture, scapula
  sinus (ethmoid) (frontal) S02.19
  skull S02.91
    base S02.10-
      occiput S02.119
        condyle S02.113
          type I S02.110
            left side S02.11B
            right side S02.11A
          type II S02.111
            left side S02.11D
            right side S02.11C
          type III S02.112
            left side S02.11F
            right side S02.11E
          specified NEC S02.118
            left side S02.11H
            right side S02.11G
        specified NEC S02.19
      birth injury P13.0
      frontal bone S02.0
      parietal bone S02.0
      specified site NEC S02.8-
      temporal bone S02.19
      vault S02.0
    Smith's —see Smith's fracture
    sphenoid (bone) (sinus) S02.19
    spine —see Fracture, vertebra
    spinous process —see Fracture, vertebra
    spontaneous (cause unknown) —see Fracture, pathological
    stave (of thumb) —see Fracture, metacarpal, first
    sternum S22.20
      with flail chest —see Flail, chest
      associated with chest compression and cardiopulmonary resuscitation M96.A1
      body S22.22
      manubrium S22.21
      xiphoid (process) S22.24
        associated with chest compression and cardiopulmonary resuscitation M96.A1
    stress M84.30
      ankle M84.37-
      carpus M84.34-
      clavicle M84.31-
      femoral neck M84.359
      femur M84.35-
      fibula M84.36-
      finger M84.34-
      hip M84.359
      humerus M84.32-
      ilium M84.350
      ischium M84.350
      metacarpus M84.34-
      metatarsus M84.37-
      neck —see Fracture, fatigue, vertebra
      pelvis M84.350
      radius M84.33-
      rib M84.38
      scapula M84.31-
      skull M84.38
      tarsus M84.37-

Fracture, traumatic (continued)
  stress (continued)
    tibia M84.36-
    toe M84.37-
    ulna M84.33-
    vertebra —see Fracture, fatigue, vertebra
  supracondylar, elbow —see Fracture, humerus, lower end, supracondylar
  symphysis pubis —see Fracture, pubis
  talus (ankle bone) —see Fracture, tarsal, talus
  tarsal bone(s) S92.20-
    astragalus —see Fracture, tarsal, talus
    calcaneus S92.00-
      anterior process (displaced) S92.02-
        nondisplaced S92.02-
      body (displaced) S92.01-
        nondisplaced S92.01-
      extraarticular NEC (displaced) S92.05-
        nondisplaced S92.05-
      intraarticular (displaced) S92.06-
        nondisplaced S92.06-
      physeal S99.00-
        Salter-Harris
          Type I S99.01-
          Type II S99.02-
          Type III S99.03-
          Type IV S99.04-
          specified NEC S99.09-
      tuberosity (displaced) S92.04-
        avulsion (displaced) S92.03-
          nondisplaced S92.03-
        nondisplaced S92.04-
    cuboid (displaced) S92.21-
      nondisplaced S92.21-
    cuneiform
      intermediate (displaced) S92.23-
        nondisplaced S92.23-
      lateral (displaced) S92.22-
        nondisplaced S92.22-
      medial (displaced) S92.24-
        nondisplaced S92.24-
    navicular (displaced) S92.25-
      nondisplaced S92.25-
    scaphoid —see Fracture, tarsal, navicular
    talus S92.10-
      avulsion (displaced) S92.15-
        nondisplaced S92.15-
      body (displaced) S92.12-
        nondisplaced S92.12-
      dome (displaced) S92.14-
        nondisplaced S92.14-
      head (displaced) S92.12-
        nondisplaced S92.12-
      lateral process (displaced) S92.14-
        nondisplaced S92.14-
      neck (displaced) S92.11-
        nondisplaced S92.11-
      posterior process (displaced) S92.13-
        nondisplaced S92.13-
      specified NEC S92.19-
  temporal bone (styloid) S02.19
  thorax (bony) S22.9
    with flail chest —see Flail, chest
    rib S22.3-
      multiple S22.4-
        with flail chest —see Flail, chest

Fracture, traumatic (continued)
  thorax (continued)
    sternum S22.20
      body S22.22
      manubrium S22.21
      xiphoid process S22.24
        associated with chest compression and cardiopulmonary resuscitation M96.A1
    vertebra (displaced) S22.009
      burst (stable) S22.001
        unstable S22.002
      eighth S22.069
        burst (stable) S22.061
          unstable S22.062
        specified type NEC S22.068
        wedge compression S22.060
      eleventh S22.089
        burst (stable) S22.081
          unstable S22.082
        specified type NEC S22.088
        wedge compression S22.080
      fifth S22.059
        burst (stable) S22.051
          unstable S22.052
        specified type NEC S22.058
        wedge compression S22.050
      first S22.019
        burst (stable) S22.011
          unstable S22.012
        specified type NEC S22.018
        wedge compression S22.010
      fourth S22.049
        burst (stable) S22.041
          unstable S22.042
        specified type NEC S22.048
        wedge compression S22.040
      ninth S22.079
        burst (stable) S22.071
          unstable S22.072
        specified type NEC S22.078
        wedge compression S22.070
      nondisplaced S22.001
      second S22.029
        burst (stable) S22.021
          unstable S22.022
        specified type NEC S22.028
        wedge compression S22.020
      seventh S22.069
        burst (stable) S22.061
          unstable S22.062
        specified type NEC S22.068
        wedge compression S22.060
      sixth S22.059
        burst (stable) S22.051
          unstable S22.052
        specified type NEC S22.058
        wedge compression S22.050
      specified type NEC S22.008
      tenth S22.079
        burst (stable) S22.071
          unstable S22.072
        specified type NEC S22.078
        wedge compression S22.070
      third S22.039
        burst (stable) S22.031
          unstable S22.032

Fracture, traumatic (continued)
  thorax (continued)
    vertebra (continued)
      third (continued)
        specified type NEC S22.038
        wedge compression S22.030
      twelfth S22.089
        burst (stable) S22.081
          unstable S22.082
        specified type NEC S22.088
        wedge compression S22.080
      wedge compression S22.000
  thumb S62.50-
    distal phalanx (displaced) S62.52-
      nondisplaced S62.52-
    proximal phalanx (displaced) S62.51-
      nondisplaced S62.51-
  thyroid cartilage S12.8
  tibia (shaft) S82.20-
    comminuted (displaced) S82.25-
      nondisplaced S82.25-
    condyles —see Fracture, tibia, upper end
    distal end —see Fracture, tibia, lower end
    epiphysis
      lower —see Fracture, tibia, lower end
      upper —see Fracture, tibia, upper end
    following insertion of implant, prosthesis or plate M96.67-
    head (involving knee joint) —see Fracture, tibia, upper end
    intercondyloid eminence —see Fracture, tibia, upper end
    involving ankle or malleolus —see Fracture, ankle, medial malleolus
    lower end S82.30-
      physeal S89.10-
        Salter-Harris
          Type I S89.11-
          Type II S89.12-
          Type III S89.13-
          Type IV S89.14-
          specified NEC S89.19-
      pilon (displaced) S82.87-
        nondisplaced S82.87-
      specified NEC S82.39-
      torus S82.31-
    malleolus —see Fracture, ankle, medial malleolus
    oblique (displaced) S82.23-
      nondisplaced S82.23-
    pilon —see Fracture, tibia, lower end, pilon
    proximal end —see Fracture, tibia, upper end
    segmental (displaced) S82.26-
      nondisplaced S82.26-
    specified NEC S82.29-
    spine —see Fracture, tibia, upper end, spine
    spiral (displaced) S82.24-
      nondisplaced S82.24-
    transverse (displaced) S82.22-
      nondisplaced S82.22-
    tuberosity —see Fracture, tibia, upper end, tuberosity
    upper end S82.10-
      bicondylar (displaced) S82.14-
        nondisplaced S82.14-

Fracture, traumatic (continued)
  tibia (continued)
    upper end (continued)
      lateral condyle (displaced) S82.12-
        nondisplaced S82.12-
      medial condyle (displaced) S82.13-
        nondisplaced S82.13-
      physeal S89.00-
        Salter-Harris
          Type I S89.01-
          Type II S89.02-
          Type III S89.03-
          Type IV S89.04-
          specified NEC S89.09-
      plateau —see Fracture, tibia, upper end, bicondylar
      spine (displaced) S82.11-
        nondisplaced S82.11-
      torus S82.16-
      specified NEC S82.19-
      tuberosity (displaced) S82.15-
        nondisplaced S82.15-
  toe S92.91-
    great (displaced) S92.40-
      distal phalanx (displaced) S92.42-
        nondisplaced S92.42-
      nondisplaced S92.40-
      proximal phalanx (displaced) S92.41-
        nondisplaced S92.41-
      specified NEC S92.49-
    lesser (displaced) S92.50-
      distal phalanx (displaced) S92.53-
        nondisplaced S92.53-
      middle phalanx (displaced) S92.52-
        nondisplaced S92.52-
      nondisplaced S92.50-
      proximal phalanx (displaced) S92.51-
        nondisplaced S92.51-
      specified NEC S92.59-
    physeal
      phalanx S99.20-
        Salter-Harris
          Type I S99.21-
          Type II S99.22-
          Type III S99.23-
          Type IV S99.24-
          specified NEC S99.29-
  tooth (root) S02.5
  trachea (cartilage) S12.8
  transverse process —see Fracture, vertebra
  trapezium or trapezoid bone —see Fracture, carpal
  trimalleolar —see Fracture, ankle, trimalleolar
  triquetrum (cuneiform of carpus) —see Fracture, carpal, triquetrum
  trochanter —see Fracture, femur, trochanteric
  tuberosity (external) —see Fracture, traumatic, by site
  ulna (shaft) S52.20-
    bent bone S52.28-
    coronoid process —see Fracture, ulna, upper end, coronoid process
    distal end —see Fracture, ulna, lower end
    following insertion of implant, prosthesis or plate M96.63-
    head S52.60-

163

Fracture, traumatic (*continued*)
    ulna (*continued*)
        lower end S52.60-
            physeal S59.00-
                Salter-Harris
                    Type I S59.01-
                    Type II S59.02-
                    Type III S59.03-
                    Type IV S59.04-
                specified NEC S59.09-
            specified NEC S52.69-
            styloid process (displaced) S52.61-
                nondisplaced S52.61-
            torus S52.62-
        proximal end —*see* Fracture, ulna, upper end
        shaft S52.20-
            comminuted (displaced) S52.25-
                nondisplaced S52.25-
            greenstick S52.21-
            Monteggia's —*see* Monteggia's fracture
            oblique (displaced) S52.23-
                nondisplaced S52.23-
            segmental (displaced) S52.26-
                nondisplaced S52.26-
            specified NEC S52.29-
            spiral (displaced) S52.24-
                nondisplaced S52.24-
            transverse (displaced) S52.22-
                nondisplaced S52.22-
        upper end S52.00-
            coronoid process (displaced) S52.04-
                nondisplaced S52.04-
            olecranon process (displaced) S52.02-
                with intraarticular extension S52.03-
                nondisplaced S52.02-
                    with intraarticular extension S52.03-
            specified NEC S52.09-
            torus S52.01-
    unciform —*see* Fracture, carpal, hamate
    vault of skull S02.0
    vertebra, vertebral (arch) (body) (column) (neural arch) (pedicle) (spinous process) (transverse process)
        atlas —*see* Fracture, neck, cervical vertebra, first
        axis —*see* Fracture, neck, cervical vertebra, second
        cervical (teardrop) S12.9
            axis —*see* Fracture, neck, cervical vertebra, second
            first (atlas) —*see* Fracture, neck, cervical vertebra, first
            second (axis) —*see* Fracture, neck, cervical vertebra, second
        chronic M84.48
        coccyx S32.2
        dorsal —*see* Fracture, thorax, vertebra
        lumbar S32.009
            burst (stable) S32.001
                unstable S32.002
            fifth S32.059
                burst (stable) S32.051
                    unstable S32.052
                specified type NEC S32.058
                wedge compression S32.050
            first S32.019
                burst (stable) S32.011
                    unstable S32.012
                specified type NEC S32.018
                wedge compression S32.010

Fracture, traumatic (*continued*)
    vertebra, vertebral (*continued*)
        lumbar (*continued*)
            fourth S32.049
                burst (stable) S32.041
                    unstable S32.042
                specified type NEC S32.048
                wedge compression S32.040
            second S32.029
                burst (stable) S32.021
                    unstable S32.022
                specified type NEC S32.028
                wedge compression S32.020
            specified type NEC S32.008
            third S32.039
                burst (stable) S32.031
                    unstable S32.032
                specified type NEC S32.038
                wedge compression S32.030
            wedge compression S32.000
        metastatic —*see* Collapse, vertebra, in, specified disease NEC —*see also* Neoplasm
        newborn (birth injury) P11.5
        sacrum S32.10
            specified NEC S32.19
            Type
                1 S32.14
                2 S32.15
                3 S32.16
                4 S32.17
            Zone
                I S32.119
                    displaced (minimally) S32.111
                        severely S32.112
                    nondisplaced S32.110
                II S32.129
                    displaced (minimally) S32.121
                        severely S32.122
                    nondisplaced S32.120
                III S32.139
                    displaced (minimally) S32.131
                        severely S32.132
                    nondisplaced S32.130
        thoracic —*see* Fracture, thorax, vertebra
    vertex S02.0
    vomer (bone) S02.2
    wrist S62.10-
        carpal —*see* Fracture, carpal bone
        navicular (scaphoid) (hand) — *see* Fracture, carpal, navicular
    xiphisternum, xiphoid (process) S22.24
        associated with chest compression and cardiopulmonary resuscitation M96.A1
    zygoma S02.402
        left side S02.40F
        right side S02.40E

Fragile, fragility
    autosomal site Q95.5
    bone, congenital (with blue sclera) Q78.0
    capillary (hereditary) D69.8
    hair L67.8
    nails L60.3
    non-sex chromosome site Q95.5
    X chromosome Q99.2

Fragilitas
    crinium L67.8
    ossium (with blue sclerae) (hereditary) Q78.0
    unguium L60.3
        congenital Q84.6

Fragments, cataract (lens), following cataract surgery H59.02-
    retained foreign body —*see* Retained, foreign body fragments (type of)

Frailty (frail) R54
    mental R41.81

Frambesia, frambesial (tropica) —*see also* Yaws
    initial lesion or ulcer A66.0
    primary A66.0

Frambeside
    gummatous A66.4
    of early yaws A66.2

Frambesioma A66.1

Franceschetti-Klein (-Wildervanck) **disease or syndrome** Q75.4

Francis' disease —*see* Tularemia

Franklin disease C88.2

Frank's essential thrombocytopenia D69.3

Fraser's syndrome Q87.0

Freckle(s) L81.2
    malignant melanoma in —*see* Melanoma
    melanotic (Hutchinson's) —*see* Melanoma, in situ
    retinal D49.81

Frederickson's hyperlipoproteinemia, type
    I and V E78.3
    IIA E78.00
    IIB and III E78.2
    IV E78.1

Freeman Sheldon syndrome Q87.0

Freezing (*see also* Effect, adverse, cold) T69.9

Freiberg's disease (infraction of metatarsal head or osteochondrosis) —*see* Osteochondrosis, juvenile, metatarsus

Frei's disease A55

Fremitus, friction, cardiac R01.2

Frenum, frenulum
    external os Q51.828
    tongue (shortening) (congenital) Q38.1

Frequency micturition (nocturnal) R35.0
    psychogenic F45.8

Frey's syndrome
    auriculotemporal G50.8
    hyperhidrosis L74.52

Friction
    burn —*see* Burn, by site
    fremitus, cardiac R01.2
    precordial R01.2
    sounds, chest R09.89

Friderichsen-Waterhouse syndrome or disease A39.1

Friedländer's B (bacillus) **NEC** (*see also* condition) A49.8

Friedreich's
    ataxia G11.11
    combined systemic disease G11.11
    facial hemihypertrophy Q67.4
    sclerosis (cerebellum) (spinal cord) G11.11

Frigidity F52.22

Fröhlich's syndrome E23.6

Frontal —*see also* condition
    lobe syndrome F07.0

Frostbite (superficial) T33.90
    with
        partial thickness skin loss —*see* Frostbite (superficial), by site
        tissue necrosis T34.90
    abdominal wall T33.3
        with tissue necrosis T34.3
    ankle T33.81-
        with tissue necrosis T34.81-
    arm T33.4-
        with tissue necrosis T34.4-
        finger(s) —*see* Frostbite, finger
        hand —*see* Frostbite, hand
        wrist —*see* Frostbite, wrist
    ear T33.01-
        with tissue necrosis T34.01-
    face T33.09
        with tissue necrosis T34.09
    finger T33.53-
        with tissue necrosis T34.53-
    foot T33.82-
        with tissue necrosis T34.82-
    hand T33.52-
        with tissue necrosis T34.52-
    head T33.09
        with tissue necrosis T34.09
        ear —*see* Frostbite, ear
        nose —*see* Frostbite, nose
    hip (and thigh) T33.6-
        with tissue necrosis T34.6-
    knee T33.7-
        with tissue necrosis T34.7-
    leg T33.9-
        with tissue necrosis T34.9-
        ankle —*see* Frostbite, ankle
        foot —*see* Frostbite, foot
        knee —*see* Frostbite, knee
        lower T33.7-
            with tissue necrosis T34.7-
        thigh —*see* Frostbite, hip
        toe —*see* Frostbite, toe
    limb
        lower T33.99
            with tissue necrosis T34.99
        upper —*see* Frostbite, arm
    neck T33.1
        with tissue necrosis T34.1
    nose T33.02
        with tissue necrosis T34.02
    pelvis T33.3
        with tissue necrosis T34.3
    specified site NEC T33.99
        with tissue necrosis T34.99
    thigh —*see* Frostbite, hip
    thorax T33.2
        with tissue necrosis T34.2
    toes T33.83-
        with tissue necrosis T34.83-
    trunk T33.99
        with tissue necrosis T34.99
    wrist T33.51-
        with tissue necrosis T34.51-

Frotteurism F65.81

Frozen —*see also* Effect, adverse, cold T69.9
    pelvis (female) N94.89
        male K66.8
    shoulder —*see* Capsulitis, adhesive

Fructokinase deficiency E74.11

Fructose 1,6 diphosphatase deficiency E74.19

Fructosemia (benign) (essential) E74.12

Fructosuria (benign) (essential) E74.11
Fuchs'
 black spot (myopic) (see also Myopia, degenerative) H44.2-
 dystrophy (corneal endothelium) H18.51-
 heterochromic cyclitis —see Cyclitis, Fuchs' heterochromic
Fucosidosis E77.1
Fugue R68.89
 dissociative F44.1
 hysterical (dissociative) F44.1
 postictal in epilepsy —see Epilepsy
 reaction to exceptional stress (transient) F43.0
Fulminant, fulminating —see condition
Functional —see also condition
 bleeding (uterus) N93.8
Functioning, intellectual, borderline R41.83
Fundus —see condition
Fungemia NOS B49
Fungus, fungous
 cerebral G93.89
 disease NOS B49
 infection —see Infection, fungus
Funiculitis (acute) (chronic) (endemic) N49.1
 gonococcal (acute) (chronic) A54.23
 tuberculous A18.15
Funnel
 breast (acquired) M95.4
  congenital Q67.6
  sequelae (late effect) of rickets E64.3
 chest (acquired) M95.4
  congenital Q67.6
  sequelae (late effect) of rickets E64.3
 pelvis (acquired) M95.5
  with disproportion (fetopelvic) O33.3
   causing obstructed labor O65.3
  congenital Q74.2
FUO (fever of unknown origin) R50.9
Furfur L21.0
 microsporon B36.0
Furrier's lung J67.8
Furrowed K14.5
 nail(s) (transverse) L60.4
  congenital Q84.6
 tongue K14.5
  congenital Q38.3
Furuncle L02.92
 abdominal wall L02.221
 ankle —see Furuncle, lower limb
 anus K61.0
 antecubital space —see Furuncle, upper limb
 arm —see Furuncle, upper limb
 auditory canal, external —see Abscess, ear, external
 auricle (ear) —see Abscess, ear, external
 axilla (region) L02.42-
 back (any part) L02.222
 breast N61.1
 buttock L02.32
 cheek (external) L02.02

Furuncle (continued)
 chest wall L02.223
 chin L02.02
 corpus cavernosum N48.21
 ear, external —see Abscess, ear, external
 external auditory canal —see Abscess, ear, external
 eyelid —see Abscess, eyelid
 face L02.02
 femoral (region) —see Furuncle, lower limb
 finger —see Furuncle, hand
 flank L02.221
 foot L02.62-
 forehead L02.02
 gluteal (region) L02.32
 groin L02.224
 hand L02.52-
 head L02.821
  face L02.02
 hip —see Furuncle, lower limb
 kidney —see Abscess, kidney
 knee —see Furuncle, lower limb
 labium (majus) (minus) N76.4
 lacrimal
  gland —see Dacryoadenitis
  passages (duct) (sac) —see Inflammation, lacrimal, passages, acute
 leg (any part) —see Furuncle, lower limb
 lower limb L02.42-
 malignant A22.0
 mouth K12.2
 navel L02.226
 neck L02.12
 nose J34.0
 orbit, orbital —see Abscess, orbit
 palmar (space) —see Furuncle, hand
 partes posteriores L02.32
 pectoral region L02.223
 penis N48.21
 perineum L02.225
 pinna —see Abscess, ear, external
 popliteal —see Furuncle, lower limb
 prepatellar —see Furuncle, lower limb
 scalp L02.821
 seminal vesicle N49.0
 shoulder —see Furuncle, upper limb
 specified site NEC L02.828
 submandibular K12.2
 temple (region) L02.02
 thumb —see Furuncle, hand
 toe —see Furuncle, foot
 trunk L02.229
  abdominal wall L02.221
  back L02.222
  chest wall L02.223
  groin L02.224
  perineum L02.225
  umbilicus L02.226
 umbilicus L02.226
 upper limb L02.42-
 vulva N76.4
Furunculosis —see Furuncle
Fused —see Fusion, fused
Fusion, fused (congenital)
 astragaloscaphoid Q74.2
 atria Q21.19
 auditory canal Q16.1
 auricles, heart Q21.19
 binocular with defective stereopsis H53.32
 bone Q79.8
 cervical spine M43.22

Fusion, fused (continued)
 choanal Q30.0
 commissure, mitral valve Q23.2
 cusps, heart valve NEC Q24.8
  mitral Q23.2
  pulmonary Q22.1
  tricuspid Q22.4
 ear ossicles Q16.3
 fingers Q70.0-
 hymen Q52.3
 joint (acquired) —see also Ankylosis
  congenital Q74.8
 kidneys (incomplete) Q63.1
 labium (majus) (minus) Q52.5
 larynx and trachea Q34.8
 limb, congenital Q74.8
  lower Q74.2
  upper Q74.0
 lobes, lung Q33.8
 lumbosacral (acquired) M43.27
  arthrodesis status Z98.1
  congenital Q76.49
  postprocedural status Z98.1
 nares, nose, nasal, nostril(s) Q30.0
 organ or site not listed —see Anomaly, by site
 ossicles Q79.9
  auditory Q16.3
 pulmonic cusps Q22.1
 ribs Q76.6
 sacroiliac (joint) (acquired) M43.28
  arthrodesis status Z98.1
  congenital Q74.2
  postprocedural status Z98.1
 spine (acquired) NEC M43.20
  arthrodesis status Z98.1
  cervical region M43.22
  cervicothoracic region M43.23
  congenital Q76.49
  lumbar M43.26
  lumbosacral region M43.27
  occipito-atlanto-axial region M43.21
  postoperative status Z98.1
  sacrococcygeal region M43.28
  thoracic region M43.24
  thoracolumbar region M43.25
 sublingual duct with submaxillary duct at opening in mouth Q38.4
 testes Q55.1
 toes Q70.2-
 tooth, teeth K00.2
 trachea and esophagus Q39.8
 twins Q89.4
 vagina Q52.4
 ventricles, heart Q21.0
 vertebra (arch) —see Fusion, spine
 vulva Q52.5
Fusospirillosis (mouth) (tongue) (tonsil) A69.1
Fussy baby R68.12

G

Gain in weight (abnormal) (excessive) —see also Weight, gain
Gaisböck's disease (polycythemia hypertonica) D75.1
Gait abnormality R26.9
 ataxic R26.0
 falling R29.6
 hysterical (ataxic) (staggering) F44.4

Gait abnormality (continued)
 paralytic R26.1
 spastic R26.1
 specified type NEC R26.89
 staggering R26.0
 unsteadiness R26.81
 walking difficulty NEC R26.2
Galactocele (breast) N64.89
 puerperal, postpartum O92.79
Galactokinase deficiency E74.29
Galactophoritis N61.0
 gestational, puerperal, postpartum O91.2-
Galactorrhea O92.6
 not associated with childbirth N64.3
Galactosemia (classic) (congenital) E74.21
Galactosuria E74.29
Galacturia R82.0
 schistosomiasis (bilharziasis) B65.0
GALD (gestational alloimmune liver disease) P78.84
Galeazzi's fracture S52.37-
Galen's vein —see condition
Galeophobia F40.218
Gall duct —see condition
Gallbladder —see also condition
 acute K81.0
Gallop rhythm R00.8
Gallstone (colic) (cystic duct) (gallbladder) (impacted) (multiple) —see also Calculus, gallbladder
 with
  cholecystitis —see Calculus, gallbladder, with cholecystitis
  bile duct (common) (hepatic) —see Calculus, bile duct
  causing intestinal obstruction K56.3
 specified NEC K80.80
  with obstruction K80.81
Gambling Z72.6
 pathological (compulsive) F63.0
Gammopathy (of undetermined significance [MGUS]) D47.2
 associated with lymphoplasmacytic dyscrasia D47.2
 monoclonal D47.2
 polyclonal D89.0
Gamna's disease (siderotic splenomegaly) D73.1
Gamophobia F40.298
Gampsodactylia (congenital) Q66.7-
Gamstorp's disease (adynamia episodica hereditaria) G72.3
Gandy-Nanta disease (siderotic splenomegaly) D73.1
Gang
 membership offenses Z72.810
Gangliocytoma D36.10
Ganglioglioma —see Neoplasm, uncertain behavior, by site
Ganglion (compound) (diffuse) (joint) (tendon (sheath)) M67.40
 ankle M67.47-
 foot M67.47-
 forearm M67.43-
 hand M67.44-
 lower leg M67.46-

Ganglion (continued)
multiple sites M67.49
of yaws (early) (late) A66.6
pelvic region M67.45-
periosteal —see Periostitis
shoulder region M67.41-
specified site NEC M67.48
thigh region M67.45-
tuberculous A18.09
upper arm M67.42-
wrist M67.43-

Ganglioneuroblastoma —see Neoplasm, nerve, malignant

Ganglioneuroma D36.10
malignant —see Neoplasm, nerve, malignant

Ganglioneuromatosis D36.10

Ganglionitis
fifth nerve —see Neuralgia, trigeminal
gasserian (postherpetic) (postzoster) B02.21
geniculate G51.1
newborn (birth injury) P11.3
postherpetic, postzoster B02.21
herpes zoster B02.21
postherpetic geniculate B02.21

Gangliosidosis E75.10
GM1 E75.19
GM2 E75.00
other specified E75.09
Sandhoff disease E75.01
Tay-Sachs disease E75.02
GM3 E75.19
mucolipidosis IV E75.11

Gangosa A66.5

Gangrene, gangrenous (connective tissue) (dropsical) (dry) (moist) (skin) (ulcer) —see also Necrosis I96
with diabetes (mellitus) —see Diabetes, with, gangrene
abdomen (wall) I96
alveolar M27.3
appendix K35.80
with
peritonitis, localized —see also Appendicitis K35.31
arteriosclerotic (general) (senile) —see Arteriosclerosis, extremities, with, gangrene
auricle I96
Bacillus welchii A48.0
bladder (infectious) —see Cystitis, specified type NEC
bowel, cecum, or colon —see Gangrene, intestine
Clostridium perfringens or welchii A48.0
cornea H18.89-
corpora cavernosa N48.29
noninfective N48.89
cutaneous, spreading I96
decubital —see Ulcer, pressure, by site
diabetic (any site) —see Diabetes, with, gangrene
epidemic —see Poisoning, food, noxious, plant
epididymis (infectional) N45.1
erysipelas —see Erysipelas

Gangrene, gangrenous (continued)
emphysematous —see Gangrene, gas
extremity (lower) (upper) I96
Fournier N49.3
female N76.82
vagina and vulva N76.82
fusospirochetal A69.0
gallbladder —see Cholecystitis, acute
gas (bacillus) A48.0
following
abortion —see Abortion by type complicated by infection
ectopic or molar pregnancy O08.0
glossitis K14.0
hernia —see Hernia, by site, with gangrene
intestine, intestinal (hemorrhagic) (massive) (see also Infarct, intestine) K55.069
with
mesenteric embolism (see also Infarct, intestine) K55.069
obstruction —see Obstruction, intestine
laryngitis J04.0
limb (lower) (upper) I96
lung J85.0
spirochetal A69.8
lymphangitis I89.1
Meleney's (synergistic) —see Ulcer, skin
mesentery (see also Infarct, intestine) K55.069
with
embolism (see also Infarct, intestine) K55.069
intestinal obstruction —see Obstruction, intestine
mouth A69.0
ovary —see Oophoritis
pancreas —see Pancreatitis, acute
penis N48.29
noninfective N48.89
perineum I96
pharynx —see also Pharyngitis
Vincent's A69.1
presenile I73.1
progressive synergistic —see Ulcer, skin
pulmonary J85.0
pulpal (dental) K04.1
quinsy J36
Raynaud's (symmetric gangrene) I73.01
retropharyngeal J39.2
scrotum N49.3
noninfective N50.89
senile (atherosclerotic) —see Arteriosclerosis, extremities, with, gangrene
spermatic cord N49.1
noninfective N50.89
spine I96
spirochetal NEC A69.8
spreading cutaneous I96
stomatitis A69.0
symmetrical I73.01
testis (infectional) N45.2
noninfective N44.8
throat —see also Pharyngitis
diphtheritic A36.0
Vincent's A69.1
thyroid (gland) E07.89
tooth (pulp) K04.1

Gangrene, gangrenous (continued)
tuberculous NEC —see Tuberculosis
tunica vaginalis N49.1
noninfective N50.89
umbilicus I96
uterus —see Endometritis
uvulitis K12.2
vas deferens N49.1
noninfective N50.89
vulva N76.82

Ganister disease J62.8

Ganser's syndrome (hysterical) F44.89

Gardner-Diamond syndrome (autoerythrocyte sensitization) D69.2

Gargoylism E76.01

Garré's disease, osteitis (sclerosing), **osteomyelitis** —see Osteomyelitis, specified type NEC

Garrod's pad, knuckle M72.1

Gartner's duct
cyst Q52.4
persistent Q50.6

Gas R14.3
asphyxiation, inhalation, poisoning, suffocation NEC —see Table of Drugs and Chemicals
excessive R14.0
gangrene A48.0
following
abortion —see Abortion by type complicated by infection
ectopic or molar pregnancy O08.0
on stomach R14.0
pains R14.1

Gastralgia —see also Pain, abdominal

Gastrectasis K31.0
psychogenic F45.8

Gastric —see condition

Gastrinoma
malignant
pancreas C25.4
specified site NEC —see Neoplasm, malignant, by site
unspecified site C25.4
specified site —see Neoplasm, uncertain behavior
unspecified site D37.9

Gastritis (simple) K29.70
with bleeding K29.71
acute (erosive) K29.00
with bleeding K29.01
alcoholic K29.20
with bleeding K29.21
allergic K29.60
with bleeding K29.61
atrophic (chronic) K29.40
with bleeding K29.41
chronic (antral) (fundal) K29.50
with bleeding K29.51
atrophic K29.40
with bleeding K29.41
superficial K29.30
with bleeding K29.31
dietary counseling and surveillance Z71.3
due to diet deficiency E63.9
eosinophilic K52.81
giant hypertrophic K29.60
with bleeding K29.61

Gastritis (continued)
granulomatous K29.60
with bleeding K29.61
hypertrophic (mucosa) K29.60
with bleeding K29.61
nervous F54
spastic K29.60
with bleeding K29.61
specified NEC K29.60
with bleeding K29.61
superficial chronic K29.30
with bleeding K29.31
tuberculous A18.83
viral NEC A08.4

Gastrocarcinoma —see Neoplasm, malignant, stomach

Gastrocolic —see condition

Gastrodisciasis, gastrodiscoidiasis B66.8

Gastroduodenitis K29.90
with bleeding K29.91
virus, viral A08.4
specified type NEC A08.39

Gastrodynia —see Pain, abdominal

Gastroenteritis (acute) (chronic) (noninfectious) (see also Enteritis) K52.9
allergic K52.29
with
eosinophilic gastritis or gastroenteritis K52.81
food protein-induced enterocolitis syndrome K52.21
food protein-induced enteropathy K52.22
dietetic (see also Gastroenteritis, allergic) K52.29
drug-induced K52.1
due to
Cryptosporidium A07.2
drugs K52.1
food poisoning —see Intoxication, foodborne
radiation K52.0
eosinophilic K52.81
epidemic (infectious) A09
food hypersensitivity (see also Gastroenteritis, allergic) K52.29
infectious —see Enteritis, infectious
influenzal —see Influenza, with gastroenteritis
noninfectious K52.9
specified NEC K52.89
rotaviral A08.0
Salmonella A02.0
toxic K52.1
viral NEC A08.4
acute infectious A08.39
type Norwalk A08.11
infantile (acute) A08.39
Norwalk agent A08.11
rotaviral A08.0
severe of infants A08.39
specified type NEC A08.39

Gastroenteropathy (see also Gastroenteritis) K52.9
acute, due to Norwalk agent A08.11
acute, due to Norovirus A08.11
infectious A09

Gastroenteroptosis K63.4

Gastroesophageal laceration-hemorrhage syndrome K22.6

Gastrointestinal —*see* condition
Gastrojejunal —*see* condition
Gastrojejunitis (*see also* Enteritis) K52.9
Gastrojejunocolic —*see* condition
Gastroliths K31.89
Gastromalacia K31.89
Gastroparalysis K31.84
  diabetic —*see* Diabetes, gastroparalysis
Gastroparesis K31.84
  diabetic —*see* Diabetes, by type, with gastroparesis
Gastropathy K31.9
  congestive portal (*see also*, Hypertension, portal) K31.89
  erythematous K29.70
  exudative K90.89
  portal hypertensive (*see also*, Hypertension, portal) K31.89
  specified NEC K31.89
Gastroptosis K31.89
Gastrorrhagia K92.2
  psychogenic F45.8
Gastroschisis (congenital) Q79.3
Gastrospasm (neurogenic) (reflex) K31.89
  neurotic F45.8
  psychogenic F45.8
Gastrostaxis —*see* Gastritis, with bleeding
Gastrostenosis K31.89
Gastrostomy
  attention to Z43.1
  status Z93.1
Gastrosuccorrhea (continuous) (intermittent) K31.89
  neurotic F45.8
  psychogenic F45.8
Gatophobia F40.218
Gaucher's disease or splenomegaly (adult) (infantile) E75.22
Gee (-Herter) (-Thaysen) **disease** (nontropical sprue) K90.0
Gélineau's syndrome G47.419
  with cataplexy G47.411
Gemination, tooth, teeth K00.2
Gemistocytoma
  specified site —*see* Neoplasm, malignant, by site
  unspecified site C71.9
General, generalized —*see* condition
Genetic
  carrier (status)
    cystic fibrosis Z14.1
    hemophilia A (asymptomatic) Z14.01
      symptomatic Z14.02
    specified NEC Z14.8
  susceptibility to disease NEC Z15.89
    malignant neoplasm Z15.09
      breast Z15.01
      endometrium Z15.04
      ovary Z15.02
      prostate Z15.03
      specified NEC Z15.09
    multiple endocrine neoplasia Z15.81
Genital —*see* condition

Genito-anorectal syndrome A55
Genitourinary system —*see* condition
Genu
  congenital Q74.1
  extrorsum (acquired) —*see also* Deformity, varus, knee
    congenital Q74.1
    sequelae (late effect) of rickets E64.3
  introrsum (acquired) —*see also* Deformity, valgus, knee
    congenital Q74.1
    sequelae (late effect) of rickets E64.3
  rachitic (old) E64.3
  recurvatum (acquired) —*see also* Deformity, limb, specified type NEC, lower leg
    congenital Q68.2
    sequelae (late effect) of rickets E64.3
  valgum (acquired) (knock-knee) M21.06-
    congenital Q74.1
    sequelae (late effect) of rickets E64.3
  varum (acquired) (bowleg) M21.16-
    congenital Q74.1
    sequelae (late effect) of rickets E64.3
Geographic tongue K14.1
Geophagia —*see* Pica
Geotrichosis B48.3
  stomatitis B48.3
Gephyrophobia F40.242
Gerbode defect Q21.0
GERD (gastroesophageal reflux disease) K21.9
Gerhardt's
  disease (erythromelalgia) I73.81
  syndrome (vocal cord paralysis) J38.00
    bilateral J38.02
    unilateral J38.01
German measles —*see also* Rubella
  exposure to Z20.4
Germinoblastoma (diffuse) C85.9-
  follicular C82.9-
Germinoma —*see* Neoplasm, malignant, by site
Gerontoxon —*see* Degeneration, cornea, senile
Gerstmann-Sträussler-Scheinker syndrome (GSS) A81.82
Gerstmann's syndrome R48.8
  developmental F81.2
Gestation (period) —*see also* Pregnancy
  ectopic —*see* Pregnancy, by site
  multiple O30.9-
    greater than quadruplets —*see* Pregnancy, multiple (gestation), specified NEC
    specified NEC —*see* Pregnancy, multiple (gestation), specified NEC
Gestational
  mammary abscess O91.11-
  purulent mastitis O91.11-
  subareolar abscess O91.11-

Ghon tubercle, primary infection A15.7
Ghost
  teeth K00.4
  vessels (cornea) H16.41-
Ghoul hand A66.3
Gianotti-Crosti disease L44.4
Giant
  cell
    epulis K06.8
    peripheral granuloma K06.8
  esophagus, congenital Q39.5
  kidney, congenital Q63.3
  urticaria T78.3
    hereditary D84.1
Giardiasis A07.1
Gibert's disease or pityriasis L42
Giddiness R42
  hysterical F44.89
  psychogenic F45.8
Gierke's disease (glycogenosis I) E74.01
Gigantism (cerebral) (hypophyseal) (pituitary) E22.0
  constitutional E34.4
Gilbert's disease or syndrome E80.4
Gilchrist's disease B40.9
Gilford-Hutchinson disease E34.8
Gilles de la Tourette's disease or syndrome (motor-verbal tic) F95.2
Gingivitis K05.10
  acute (catarrhal) K05.00
    necrotizing A69.1
    nonplaque induced K05.01
    plaque induced K05.00
  chronic (desquamative) (hyperplastic) (simple marginal) (pregnancy associated) (ulcerative) K05.10
    nonplaque induced K05.11
    plaque induced K05.10
  expulsiva —*see* Periodontitis
  necrotizing ulcerative (acute) A69.1
  pellagrous E52
    acute necrotizing A69.1
  Vincent's A69.1
Gingivoglossitis K14.0
Gingivopericementitis —*see* Periodontitis
Gingivosis —*see* Gingivitis, chronic
Gingivostomatitis K05.10
  herpesviral B00.2
  necrotizing ulcerative (acute) A69.1
Gland, glandular —*see* condition
Glanders A24.0
Glanzmann (-Naegeli) **disease or thrombasthenia** D69.1
Glasgow coma scale
  total score
    3-8 R40.243
    9-12 R40.242
    13-15 R40.241
Glass-blower's disease (cataract) —*see* Cataract, specified NEC
Glaucoma H40.9
  with
    increased episcleral venous pressure H40.81-
    pseudoexfoliation of lens —*see* Glaucoma, open angle, primary, capsular

Glaucoma (*continued*)
  absolute H44.51-
  angle-closure (primary) H40.20-
    acute (attack) (crisis) H40.21-
    chronic H40.22-
    intermittent H40.23-
    residual stage H40.24-
  borderline H40.00-
  capsular (with pseudoexfoliation of lens) —*see* Glaucoma, open angle, primary, capsular
  childhood Q15.0
  closed angle —*see* Glaucoma, angle-closure
  congenital Q15.0
  corticosteroid-induced —*see* Glaucoma, secondary, drugs
  hypersecretion H40.82-
  in (due to)
    amyloidosis E85.4 [H42]
    aniridia Q13.1 [H42]
    concussion of globe —*see* Glaucoma, secondary, trauma
    dislocation of lens —*see* Glaucoma, secondary
    disorder of lens NEC —*see* Glaucoma, secondary
    drugs —*see* Glaucoma, secondary, drugs
    endocrine disease NOS E34.9 [H42]
    eye
      inflammation —*see* Glaucoma, secondary, inflammation
      trauma —*see* Glaucoma, secondary, trauma
    hypermature cataract —*see* Glaucoma, secondary
    iridocyclitis —*see* Glaucoma, secondary, inflammation
    lens disorder —*see* Glaucoma, secondary,
    Lowe's syndrome E72.03 [H42]
    metabolic disease NOS E88.9 [H42]
    ocular disorders NEC —*see* Glaucoma, secondary
    onchocerciasis B73.02
    pupillary block —*see* Glaucoma, secondary
    retinal vein occlusion —*see* Glaucoma, secondary
    Rieger's anomaly Q13.81 [H42]
    rubeosis of iris —*see* Glaucoma, secondary
    tumor of globe —*see* Glaucoma, secondary
  infantile Q15.0
  low tension —*see* Glaucoma, open angle, primary, low-tension
  malignant H40.83-
  narrow angle —*see* Glaucoma, angle-closure
  newborn Q15.0
  noncongestive (chronic) —*see* Glaucoma, open angle
  nonobstructive —*see* Glaucoma, open angle
  obstructive —*see also* Glaucoma, angle-closure
    due to lens changes —*see* Glaucoma, secondary
  open angle H40.10-
    primary H40.11-
      capsular (with pseudoexfoliation of lens) H40.14-

Glaucoma *(continued)*
  open angle *(continued)*
    primary *(continued)*
      low-tension H40.12-
      pigmentary H40.13-
      residual stage H40.15-
    phacolytic —see Glaucoma, secondary
    pigmentary —see Glaucoma, open angle, primary, pigmentary
    postinfectious —see Glaucoma, secondary, inflammation
  secondary (to) H40.5-
    drugs H40.6-
    inflammation H40.4-
    trauma H40.3-
  simple (chronic) H40.11-
  simplex H40.11-
  specified type NEC H40.89
  suspect H40.00-
  syphilitic A52.71
  traumatic —see also Glaucoma, secondary, trauma
    newborn (birth injury) P15.3
  tuberculous A18.59

Glaucomatous flecks (subcapsular) —see Cataract, complicated

Glazed tongue K14.4

Gleet (gonococcal) A54.01

Glénard's disease K63.4

Glioblastoma (multiforme)
  with sarcomatous component
    specified site —see Neoplasm, malignant, by site
    unspecified site C71.9
  giant cell
    specified site —see Neoplasm, malignant, by site
    unspecified site C71.9
  specified site —see Neoplasm, malignant, by site
  unspecified site C71.9

Glioma (malignant)
  astrocytic
    specified site —see Neoplasm, malignant, by site
    unspecified site C71.9
  mixed
    specified site —see Neoplasm, malignant, by site
    unspecified site C71.9
  nose Q30.8
  specified site NEC —see Neoplasm, malignant, by site
  subependymal D43.2
    specified site —see Neoplasm, uncertain behavior, by site
    unspecified site D43.2
  unspecified site C71.9

Gliomatosis cerebri C71.0

Glioneuroma —see Neoplasm, uncertain behavior, by site

Gliosarcoma
  specified site —see Neoplasm, malignant, by site
  unspecified site C71.9

Gliosis (cerebral) G93.89
  spinal G95.89

Glisson's disease —see Rickets

Globinuria R82.3

Globus (hystericus) F45.8

Glomangioma D18.00
  intra-abdominal D18.03
  intracranial D18.02

Glomangioma *(continued)*
  skin D18.01
  specified site NEC D18.09

Glomangiomyoma D18.00
  intra-abdominal D18.03
  intracranial D18.02
  skin D18.01
  specified site NEC D18.09

Glomangiosarcoma —see Neoplasm, connective tissue, malignant

Glomerular
  disease in syphilis A52.75
  nephritis —see Glomerulonephritis

Glomerulitis —see Glomerulonephritis

Glomerulonephritis (see also Nephritis) N05.9
  with
    C3
      glomerulonephritis N05.A
      glomerulopathy N05.A
        with dense deposit disease N05.6
    edema —see Nephrosis
    minimal change N05.0
    minor glomerular abnormality N05.0
  acute N00.9
  chronic N03.9
  crescentic (diffuse) NEC (see also N00-N07 with fourth character .7) N05.7
  dense deposit (see also N00-N07 with fourth character .6) N05.6
  diffuse
    crescentic (see also N00-N07 with fourth character .7) N05.7
    endocapillary proliferative (see also N00-N07 with fourth character .4) N05.4
    membranous (see also N00-N07 with fourth character .2) N05.2
    mesangial proliferative (see also N00-N07 with fourth character .3) N05.3
    mesangiocapillary (see also N00-N07 with fourth character .5) N05.5
    sclerosing N18.9
  endocapillary proliferative (diffuse) NEC (see also N00-N07 with fourth character .4) N05.4
  extracapillary NEC (see also N00-N07 with fourth character .7) N05.7
  focal (and segmental) (see also N00-N07 with fourth character .1) N05.1
  hypocomplementemic —see Glomerulonephritis, membranoproliferative
  IgA —see Nephropathy, IgA
  immune complex (circulating) NEC N05.8
  in (due to)
    amyloidosis E85.4 [N08]
    bilharziasis B65.9 [N08]
    cryoglobulinemia D89.1 [N08]
    defibrination syndrome D65 [N08]
    diabetes mellitus —see Diabetes, glomerulosclerosis
    disseminated intravascular coagulation D65 [N08]
    Fabry (-Anderson) disease E75.21 [N08]
    Goodpasture's syndrome M31.0

Glomerulonephritis *(continued)*
  in *(continued)*
    hemolytic-uremic syndrome - see Syndrome, hemolytic-uremic
    Henoch (-Schönlein) purpura D69.0 [N08]
    lecithin cholesterol acyltransferase deficiency E78.6 [N08]
    microscopic polyangiitis M31.7 [N08]
    multiple myeloma C90.0- [N08]
    Plasmodium malariae B52.0
    schistosomiasis B65.9 [N08]
    sepsis A41.9 [N08]
      streptococcal A40- [N08]
    sickle-cell disorders D57.- [N08]
    strongyloidiasis B78.9 [N08]
    subacute bacterial endocarditis I33.0 [N08]
    syphilis (late) congenital A50.59 [N08]
    systemic lupus erythematosus M32.14
    thrombotic thrombocytopenic purpura M31.19 [N08]
    typhoid fever A01.09
    Waldenström macroglobulinemia C88.0 [N08]
    Wegener's granulomatosis M31.31
  latent or quiescent N03.9
  lobular, lobulonodular —see Glomerulonephritis, membranoproliferative
  membranoproliferative (diffuse) (type 1 or 3) (see also N00-N07 with fourth character .5) N05.5
    dense deposit (type 2) NEC (see also N00-N07 with fourth character .6) N05.6
  membranous (diffuse) NEC (see also N00-N07 with fourth character .2) N05.2
  mesangial
    IgA/IgG —see Nephropathy, IgA
    proliferative (diffuse) NEC (see also N00-N07 with fourth character .3) N05.3
  mesangiocapillary (diffuse) NEC (see also N00-N07 with fourth character .5) N05.5
  necrotic, necrotizing NEC (see also N00-N07 with fourth character .8) N05.8
  nodular —see Glomerulonephritis, membranoproliferative
  poststreptococcal NEC N05.9
    acute N00.9
    chronic N03.9
    rapidly progressive N01.9
  proliferative NEC (see also N00-N07 with fourth character .8) N05.8
    diffuse (lupus) M32.14
  rapidly progressive N01.9
  sclerosing, diffuse N18.9
  specified pathology NEC (see also N00-N07 with fourth character .8) N05.8
  subacute N01.9

Glomerulopathy —see Glomerulonephritis

Glomerulosclerosis —see also Sclerosis, renal
  intercapillary (nodular) (with diabetes) —see Diabetes, glomerulosclerosis
  intracapillary —see Diabetes, glomerulosclerosis

Glossagra K14.6

Glossalgia K14.6

Glossitis (chronic superficial) (gangrenous) (Moeller's) K14.0
  areata exfoliativa K14.1
  atrophic K14.4
  benign migratory K14.1
  cortical superficial, sclerotic K14.0
  Hunter's D51.0
  interstitial, sclerous K14.0
  median rhomboid K14.2
  pellagrous E52
  superficial, chronic K14.0

Glossocele K14.8

Glossodynia K14.6
  exfoliativa K14.4

Glossoncus K14.8

Glossopathy K14.9

Glossophytia K14.3

Glossoplegia K14.8

Glossoptosis K14.8

Glossopyrosis K14.6

Glossotrichia K14.3

Glossy skin L90.8

Glottis —see condition

Glottitis —see also Laryngitis J04.0

Glucagonoma
  pancreas
    benign D13.7
    malignant C25.4
    uncertain behavior D37.8
  specified site NEC
    benign —see Neoplasm, benign, by site
    malignant —see Neoplasm, malignant, by site
    uncertain behavior —see Neoplasm, uncertain behavior, by site
  unspecified site
    benign D13.7
    malignant C25.4
    uncertain behavior D37.8

Glucoglycinuria E72.51

Glucose-galactose malabsorption E74.39

Glue
  ear —see Otitis, media, nonsuppurative, chronic, mucoid
  sniffing (airplane) —see Abuse, drug, inhalant
    dependence —see Dependence, drug, inhalant

GLUT1 deficiency syndrome 1, infantile onset E74.810

GLUT1 deficiency syndrome 2, childhood onset E74.810

Glutaric aciduria E72.3

Glycinemia E72.51

Glycinuria (renal) (with ketosis) E72.09

Glycogen
  infiltration —see Disease, glycogen storage

Glycogen (continued)
storage disease —see Disease, glycogen storage
Glycogenosis (diffuse) (generalized) —see also Disease, glycogen storage
cardiac E74.02 [I43]
diabetic, secondary —see Diabetes, glycogenosis, secondary
pulmonary interstitial J84.842
Glycopenia E16.2
Glycosuria R81
renal (familial) E74.818
Gnathostoma spinigerum (infection) (infestation), gnathostomiasis (wandering swelling) B83.1
Goiter (plunging) (substernal) E04.9
with
hyperthyroidism (recurrent) —see Hyperthyroidism, with, goiter
thyrotoxicosis —see Hyperthyroidism, with, goiter
adenomatous —see Goiter, nodular
cancerous C73
congenital (nontoxic) E03.0
diffuse E03.0
parenchymatous E03.0
transitory, with normal functioning P72.0
cystic E04.2
due to iodine-deficiency E01.1
due to
enzyme defect in synthesis of thyroid hormone E07.1
iodine-deficiency (endemic) E01.2
dyshormonogenetic (familial) E07.1
endemic (iodine-deficiency) E01.2
diffuse E01.0
multinodular E01.1
exophthalmic —see Hyperthyroidism, with, goiter
iodine-deficiency (endemic) E01.2
diffuse E01.0
multinodular E01.1
nodular E01.1
lingual Q89.2
lymphadenoid E06.3
malignant C73
multinodular (cystic) (nontoxic) E04.2
toxic or with hyperthyroidism E05.20
with thyroid storm E05.21
neonatal NEC P72.0
nodular (nontoxic) (due to) E04.9
with
hyperthyroidism E05.20
with thyroid storm E05.21
thyrotoxicosis E05.20
with thyroid storm E05.21
endemic E01.1
iodine-deficiency E01.1
sporadic E04.9
toxic E05.20
with thyroid storm E05.21
nontoxic E04.9
diffuse (colloid) E04.0
multinodular E04.2
simple E04.0
specified NEC E04.8
uninodular E04.1

Goiter (continued)
simple E04.0
toxic —see Hyperthyroidism, with, goiter
uninodular (nontoxic) E04.1
toxic or with hyperthyroidism E05.10
with thyroid storm E05.11
Goiter-deafness syndrome E07.1
Goldberg syndrome Q89.8
Goldberg-Maxwell syndrome E34.51
Goldblatt's hypertension or kidney I70.1
Goldenhar (-Gorlin) **syndrome** Q87.0
Goldflam-Erb disease or syndrome G70.00
with exacerbation (acute) G70.01
in crisis G70.01
Goldscheider's disease Q81.8
Goldstein's disease (familial hemorrhagic telangiectasia) I78.0
Golfer's elbow —see Epicondylitis, medial
Gonadoblastoma
specified site —see Neoplasm, uncertain behavior, by site
unspecified site
female D39.10
male D40.10
Gonecystitis —see Vesiculitis
Gongylonemiasis B83.8
Goniosynechiae —see Adhesions, iris, goniosynechiae
Gonococcemia A54.86
Gonococcus, gonococcal (disease) (infection) (see also condition) A54.9
anus A54.6
bursa, bursitis A54.49
conjunctiva, conjunctivitis (neonatorum) A54.31
endocardium A54.83
eye A54.30
conjunctivitis A54.31
iridocyclitis A54.32
keratitis A54.33
newborn A54.31
other specified A54.39
fallopian tubes (acute) (chronic) A54.24
genitourinary (organ) (system) (tract) (acute)
lower A54.00
with abscess (accessory gland) (periurethral) A54.1
upper (see also condition) A54.29
heart A54.83
iridocyclitis A54.32
joint A54.42
lymphatic (gland) (node) A54.89
meninges, meningitis A54.81
musculoskeletal A54.40
arthritis A54.42
osteomyelitis A54.43
other specified A54.49
spondylopathy A54.41
pelviperitonitis A54.24
pelvis (acute) (chronic) A54.24
pharynx A54.5
proctitis A54.6

Gonococcus, gonococcal (continued)
pyosalpinx (acute) (chronic) A54.24
rectum A54.6
skin A54.89
specified site NEC A54.89
tendon sheath A54.49
throat A54.5
urethra (acute) (chronic) A54.01
with abscess (accessory gland) (periurethral) A54.1
vulva (acute) (chronic) A54.02
Gonocytoma
specified site —see Neoplasm, uncertain behavior, by site
unspecified site
female D39.10
male D40.10
Gonorrhea (acute) (chronic) A54.9
Bartholin's gland (acute) (chronic) (purulent) A54.02
with abscess (accessory gland) (periurethral) A54.1
bladder A54.01
cervix A54.03
conjunctiva, conjunctivitis (neonatorum) A54.31
contact Z20.2
Cowper's gland (with abscess) A54.1
exposure to Z20.2
fallopian tube (acute) (chronic) A54.24
kidney (acute) (chronic) A54.21
lower genitourinary tract A54.00
with abscess (accessory gland) (periurethral) A54.1
ovary (acute) (chronic) A54.24
pelvis (acute) (chronic) A54.24
female pelvic inflammatory disease A54.24
penis A54.09
prostate (acute) (chronic) A54.22
seminal vesicle (acute) (chronic) A54.23
specified site not listed (see also Gonococcus) A54.89
spermatic cord (acute) (chronic) A54.23
urethra A54.01
with abscess (accessory gland) (periurethral) A54.1
vagina A54.02
vas deferens (acute) (chronic) A54.23
vulva A54.02
Goodall's disease A08.19
Goodpasture's syndrome M31.0
Gopalan's syndrome (burning feet) E53.0
Gorlin-Chaudry-Moss syndrome Q87.0
Gottron's papules L94.4
Gougerot's syndrome (trisymptomatic) L81.7
Gougerot-Blum syndrome (pigmented purpuric lichenoid dermatitis) L81.7
Gougerot-Carteaud disease or syndrome (confluent reticulate papillomatosis) L83
Gouley's syndrome (constrictive pericarditis) I31.1
Goundou A66.6

Gout, gouty (acute) (attack) (flare) (see also Gout, chronic) M10.9
drug-induced M10.20
ankle M10.27-
elbow M10.22-
foot joint M10.27-
hand joint M10.24-
hip M10.25-
knee M10.26-
multiple site M10.29
shoulder M10.21-
vertebrae M10.28
wrist M10.23-
idiopathic M10.00
ankle M10.07-
elbow M10.02-
foot joint M10.07-
hand joint M10.04-
hip M10.05-
knee M10.06-
multiple site M10.09
shoulder M10.01-
vertebrae M10.08
wrist M10.03-
in (due to) renal impairment M10.30
ankle M10.37-
elbow M10.32-
foot joint M10.37-
hand joint M10.34-
hip M10.35-
knee M10.36-
multiple site M10.39
shoulder M10.31-
vertebrae M10.38
wrist M10.33-
lead-induced M10.10
ankle M10.17-
elbow M10.12-
foot joint M10.17-
hand joint M10.14-
hip M10.15-
knee M10.16-
multiple site M10.19
shoulder M10.11-
vertebrae M10.18
wrist M10.13-
primary —see Gout, idiopathic
saturnine —see Gout, lead-induced
secondary NEC M10.40
ankle M10.47-
elbow M10.42-
foot joint M10.47-
hand joint M10.44-
hip M10.45-
knee M10.46-
multiple site M10.49
shoulder M10.41-
vertebrae M10.48
wrist M10.43-
syphilitic (see also subcategory M14.8-) A52.77
tophi —see Gout, chronic
Gout, chronic (see also Gout, gouty) M1A.9
drug-induced M1A.20
ankle M1A.27-
elbow M1A.22-
foot joint M1A.27-
hand joint M1A.24-
hip M1A.25-
knee M1A.26-
multiple site M1A.29-
shoulder M1A.21-
vertebrae M1A.28
wrist M1A.23-
idiopathic M1A.00
ankle M1A.07-
elbow M1A.02-

Gout, chronic (continued)
  idiopathic (continued)
    foot joint M1A.07-
    hand joint M1A.04-
    hip M1A.05-
    knee M1A.06-
    multiple site M1A.09
    shoulder M1A.01-
    vertebrae M1A.08
    wrist M1A.03-
  in (due to) renal impairment M1A.30
    ankle M1A.37-
    elbow M1A.32-
    foot joint M1A.37-
    hand joint M1A.34-
    hip M1A.35-
    knee M1A.36-
    multiple site M1A.39
    shoulder M1A.31-
    vertebrae M1A.38
    wrist M1A.33-
  lead-induced M1A.10
    ankle M1A.17-
    elbow M1A.12-
    foot joint M1A.17-
    hand joint M1A.14-
    hip M1A.15-
    knee M1A.16-
    multiple site M1A.19
    shoulder M1A.11-
    vertebrae M1A.18
    wrist M1A.13-
  primary —see Gout, chronic, idiopathic
  saturnine —see Gout, chronic, lead-induced
  secondary NEC M1A.40
    ankle M1A.47-
    elbow M1A.42-
    foot joint M1A.47-
    hand joint M1A.44-
    hip M1A.45-
    knee M1A.46-
    multiple site M1A.49
    shoulder M1A.41-
    vertebrae M1A.48
    wrist M1A.43-
  syphilitic (see also subcategory M14.8-) A52.77
  tophi M1A.9

Gower's
  muscular dystrophy G71.01
  syndrome (vasovagal attack) R55

Gradenigo's syndrome —see Otitis, media, suppurative, acute

Graefe's disease —see Strabismus, paralytic, ophthalmoplegia, progressive

Graft-versus-host disease D89.813
  acute D89.810
  acute on chronic D89.812
  chronic D89.811

Grainhandler's disease or lung J67.8

Grain mite (itch) B88.0

Grand mal —see Epilepsy, generalized, specified NEC

Grand multipara status only (not pregnant) Z64.1
  pregnant —see Pregnancy, complicated by, grand multiparity

Granite worker's lung J62.8

Granular —see also condition
  inflammation, pharynx J31.2
  kidney (contracting) —see Sclerosis, renal
  liver K74.69

Granulation tissue (abnormal) (excessive) L92.9
  postmastoidectomy cavity —see Complications, postmastoidectomy, granulation

Granulocytopenia (primary) (malignant) —see Agranulocytosis

Granuloma L92.9
  abdomen K66.8
    from residual foreign body L92.3
    pyogenicum L98.0
  actinic L57.5
  annulare (perforating) L92.0
  apical K04.5
  aural —see Otitis, externa, specified NEC
  beryllium (skin) L92.3
  bone
    eosinophilic C96.6
    from residual foreign body —see Osteomyelitis, specified type NEC
    lung C96.6
  brain (any site) G06.0
    schistosomiasis B65.9 [G07]
  canaliculus lacrimalis —see Granuloma, lacrimal
  candidal (cutaneous) B37.2
  cerebral (any site) G06.0
  coccidioidal (primary) (progressive) B38.7
    lung B38.1
    meninges B38.4
  colon K63.89
  conjunctiva H11.22-
  dental K04.5
  ear, middle —see Cholesteatoma
  eosinophilic C96.6
    bone C96.6
    lung C96.6
    oral mucosa K13.4
    skin L92.2
  eyelid H01.8
  facial (e) L92.2
  foreign body (in soft tissue) NEC M60.20
    ankle M60.27-
    foot M60.27-
    forearm M60.23-
    hand M60.24-
    in operation wound —see Foreign body, accidentally left during a procedure
    lower leg M60.26-
    pelvic region M60.25-
    shoulder region M60.21-
    skin L92.3
    specified site NEC M60.28
    subcutaneous tissue L92.3
    thigh M60.25-
    upper arm M60.22-
  gangraenescens M31.2
  genito-inguinale A58
  giant cell (central) (reparative) (jaw) M27.1
  gingiva (peripheral) K06.8
  gland (lymph) I88.8
  hepatic NEC K75.3
    in (due to)
      berylliosis J63.2 [K77]
      sarcoidosis D86.89
  Hodgkin C81.9-
  ileum K63.89

Granuloma (continued)
  infectious B99.9
    specified NEC B99.8
  inguinale (Donovan) (venereal) A58
  intestine NEC K63.89
  intracranial (any site) G06.0
  intraspinal (any part) G06.1
  iridocyclitis —see Iridocyclitis, chronic
  jaw (bone) (central) M27.1
    reparative giant cell M27.1
  kidney (see also Infection, kidney) N15.8
  lacrimal H04.81-
  larynx J38.7
  lethal midline (faciale(e)) M31.2
  liver NEC —see Granuloma, hepatic
  lung (infectious) —see also Fibrosis, lung
    coccidioidal B38.1
    eosinophilic C96.6
  Majocchi's B35.8
  malignant (facial(e)) M31.2
  mandible (central) M27.1
  midline (lethal) M31.2
  monilial (cutaneous) B37.2
  nasal sinus —see Sinusitis
  operation wound T81.89
    foreign body —see Foreign body, accidentally left during a procedure
    stitch T81.89
    talc —see Foreign body, accidentally left during a procedure
  oral mucosa K13.4
  orbit, orbital H05.11-
  paracoccidioidal B41.8
  penis, venereal A58
  periapical K04.5
  peritoneum K66.8
    due to ova of helminths NOS (see also Helminthiasis) B83.9 [K67]
  postmastoidectomy cavity —see Complications, postmastoidectomy, recurrent cholesteatoma
  prostate N42.89
  pudendi (ulcerating) A58
  pulp, internal (tooth) K03.3
  pyogenic, pyogenicum (of) (skin) L98.0
    gingiva K06.8
    maxillary alveolar ridge K04.5
    oral mucosa K13.4
  rectum K62.89
  reticulohistiocytic D76.3
  rubrum nasi L74.8
  Schistosoma —see Schistosomiasis
  septic (skin) L98.0
  silica (skin) L92.3
  sinus (accessory) (infective) (nasal) —see Sinusitis
  skin L92.9
    from residual foreign body L92.3
    pyogenicum L98.0
  spine
    syphilitic (epidural) A52.19
    tuberculous A18.01
  stitch (postoperative) T81.89
  suppurative (skin) L98.0
  swimming pool A31.1
  talc —see also Granuloma, foreign body

Granuloma (continued)
  talc (continued)
    in operation wound —see Foreign body, accidentally left during a procedure
  telangiectaticum (skin) L98.0
  tracheostomy J95.09
  trichophyticum B35.8
  tropicum A66.4
  umbilical P83.81
  umbilicus P83.81
  urethra N36.8
  uveitis —see Iridocyclitis, chronic
  vagina A58
  venereum A58
  vocal cord J38.3

Granulomatosis L92.9
  with polyangiitis M31.3-
  eosinophilic, with polyangiitis [EGPA] M30.1
  lymphoid C83.8-
  miliary (listerial) A32.89
  necrotizing, respiratory M31.30
  progressive septic D71
  specified NEC L92.8
  Wegener's M31.30
    with renal involvement M31.31

Granulomatous tissue (abnormal) (excessive) L92.9

Granulosis rubra nasi L74.8

Graphite fibrosis (of lung) J63.3

Graphospasm F48.8
  organic G25.89

Grating scapula M89.8X1

Gravel (urinary) —see Calculus, urinary

Graves' disease —see Hyperthyroidism, with, goiter

Gravis —see condition

Grawitz tumor C64.-

Gray syndrome (newborn) P93.0

Grayness, hair (premature) L67.1
  congenital Q84.2

Green sickness D50.8

Greenfield's disease
  meaning
    concentric sclerosis (encephalitis periaxialis concentrica) G37.5
    metachromatic leukodystrophy E75.25

Greenstick fracture - code as Fracture, by site

Grey syndrome (newborn) P93.0

Grief F43.21
  complicated F43.81
  prolonged F43.81
  reaction (see also Disorder, adjustment) F43.20

Griesinger's disease B76.0

Grinder's lung or pneumoconiosis J62.8

Grinding, teeth
  psychogenic F45.8
  sleep related G47.63

Grip
  Dabney's B33.0
  devil's B33.0

Grippe, grippal —see also Influenza
  Balkan A78
  summer, of Italy A93.1

Grisel's disease M43.6

Groin —see condition

Grooved tongue K14.5
Ground itch B76.9
Grover's disease or syndrome L11.1
Growing pains, children R29.898
Growth (fungoid) (neoplastic) (new) —*see also* Neoplasm
  adenoid (vegetative) J35.8
  benign —*see* Neoplasm, benign, by site
  malignant —*see* Neoplasm, malignant, by site
  rapid, childhood Z00.2
  secondary —*see* Neoplasm, secondary, by site
Gruby's disease B35.0
Gubler-Millard paralysis or syndrome G46.3
Guerin-Stern syndrome Q74.3
Guardianship by non-parental relative Z62.23
Guidance, insufficient anterior (occlusal) M26.54
Guillain-Barré disease or syndrome G61.0
  sequelae G65.0
Guinea worms (infection) (infestation) B72
Guinon's disease (motor-verbal tic) F95.2
Gull's disease E03.4
Gum —*see* condition
Gumboil K04.7
  with sinus K04.6
Gumma (syphilitic) A52.79
  artery A52.09
    cerebral A52.04
  bone A52.77
    of yaws (late) A66.6
  brain A52.19
  cauda equina A52.19
  central nervous system A52.3
  ciliary body A52.71
  congenital A50.59
  eyelid A52.71
  heart A52.06
  intracranial A52.19
  iris A52.71
  kidney A52.75
  larynx A52.73
  leptomeninges A52.19
  liver A52.74
  meninges A52.19
  myocardium A52.06
  nasopharynx A52.73
  neurosyphilitic A52.3
  nose A52.73
  orbit A52.71
  palate (soft) A52.79
  penis A52.76
  pericardium A52.06
  pharynx A52.73
  pituitary A52.79
  scrofulous (tuberculous) A18.4
  skin A52.79
  specified site NEC A52.79
  spinal cord A52.19
  tongue A52.79
  tonsil A52.73
  trachea A52.73
  tuberculous A18.4
  ulcerative due to yaws A66.4
  ureter A52.75
  yaws A66.4
    bone A66.6

Gunn's syndrome Q07.8
Gunshot wound —*see also* Puncture, open
  fracture - code as Fracture, by site
  internal organs —*see* Injury, by site
Gynandrism Q56.0
Gynandroblastoma
  specified site —*see* Neoplasm, uncertain behavior, by site
  unspecified site
    female D39.10
    male D40.10
Gynecological examination (periodic) (routine) Z01.419
  with abnormal findings Z01.411
Gynecomastia N62
Gynephobia F40.291
Gyrate scalp Q82.8

H

H (Hartnup's) disease E72.02
Haas' disease or osteochondrosis (juvenile) (head of humerus) —*see* Osteochondrosis, juvenile, humerus
H-ABC (hypomyelination with atrophy of the basal ganglia and cerebellum) G23.3
Habit, habituation
  bad sleep Z72.821
  chorea F95.8
  disturbance, child F98.9
  drug —*see* Dependence, drug
  irregular sleep Z72.821
  laxative F55.2
  spasm —*see* Tic
  tic —*see* Tic
Haemophilus (H.) influenzae, as cause of disease classified elsewhere B96.3
Haff disease —*see* Poisoning, mercury
Hageman's factor defect, deficiency or disease D68.2
Haglund's disease or osteochondrosis (juvenile) (os tibiale externum) —*see* Osteochondrosis, juvenile, tarsus
Hailey-Hailey disease Q82.8
Hair —*see also* condition
  plucking F63.3
    in stereotyped movement disorder F98.4
  tourniquet syndrome —*see also* Constriction, external, by site
    finger S60.44-
    penis S30.842
    thumb S60.34-
    toe S90.44-
Hairball in stomach T18.2
Hair-pulling, pathological (compulsive) F63.3
Hairy black tongue K14.3
Half vertebra Q76.49
Halitosis R19.6
Hallerman-Streiff syndrome Q87.0
Hallervorden-Spatz disease G23.0
Hallopeau's acrodermatitis or disease L40.2

Hallucination R44.3
  auditory R44.0
  gustatory R44.2
  olfactory R44.2
  specified NEC R44.2
  tactile R44.2
  visual R44.1
Hallucinosis (chronic) F28
  alcoholic (acute) F10.951
    in
      abuse F10.151
      dependence F10.251
  drug-induced F19.951
    cannabis F12.951
    cocaine F14.951
    hallucinogen F16.951
    in
      abuse F19.151
        cannabis F12.151
        cocaine F14.151
        hallucinogen F16.151
        inhalant F18.151
        opioid F11.151
        sedative, anxiolytic or hypnotic F13.151
        stimulant NEC F15.151
      dependence F19.251
        cannabis F12.251
        cocaine F14.251
        hallucinogen F16.251
        inhalant F18.251
        opioid F11.251
        sedative, anxiolytic or hypnotic F13.251
        stimulant NEC F15.251
    inhalant F18.951
    opioid F11.951
    sedative, anxiolytic or hypnotic F13.951
    stimulant NEC F15.951
  organic F06.0
Hallux
  deformity (acquired) NEC M20.5X-
  limitus M20.5X-
  malleus (acquired) NEC M20.3-
  rigidus (acquired) M20.2-
    congenital Q74.2
    sequelae (late effect) of rickets E64.3
  valgus (acquired) M20.1-
    congenital Q66.6
  varus (acquired) M20.3-
    congenital Q66.3-
Halo, visual H53.19
Hamartoma, hamartoblastoma Q85.9
  epithelial (gingival), odontogenic, central or peripheral —*see* Cyst, calcifying odontogenic
Hamartosis Q85.9
Hamman-Rich syndrome J84.114
Hammer toe (acquired) **NEC** —*see also* Deformity, toe, hammer toe
  congenital Q66.89
  sequelae (late effect) of rickets E64.3
Hand —*see* condition
Hand-foot syndrome L27.1
Handicap, handicapped
  educational Z55.9
    specified NEC Z55.8
Hand-Schüller-Christian disease or syndrome C96.5
Hanging (asphyxia) (strangulation) (suffocation) —*see* Asphyxia, traumatic, due to mechanical threat

Hangnail —*see also* Cellulitis, digit
  with lymphangitis —*see* Lymphangitis, acute, digit
Hangover (alcohol) F10.129
Hanhart's syndrome Q87.0
Hanot-Chauffard (-Troisier) **syndrome** E83.19
Hanot's cirrhosis or disease K74.3
Hansen's disease —*see* Leprosy
Hantaan virus disease (Korean hemorrhagic fever) A98.5
Hantavirus disease (with renal manifestations) (Dobrava) (Puumala) (Seoul) A98.5
  with pulmonary manifestations (Andes) (Bayou) (Bermejo) (Black Creek Canal) (Choclo) (Juquitiba) (Laguna negra) (Lechiguanas) (New York) (Oran) (Sin nombre) B33.4
Happy puppet syndrome Q93.51
Harada's disease or syndrome H30.81-
Hardening
  artery —*see* Arteriosclerosis
  brain G93.89
Hardship, material, due to limited financial resources, specified NEC Z59.87
Harelip (complete) (incomplete) —*see* Cleft, lip
Harlequin (newborn) Q80.4
Harley's disease D59.6
Harmful use (of)
  alcohol F10.10
  anxiolytics —*see* Abuse, drug, sedative
  cannabinoids —*see* Abuse, drug, cannabis
  cocaine —*see* Abuse, drug, cocaine
  drug —*see* Abuse, drug
  hallucinogens —*see* Abuse, drug, hallucinogen
  hypnotics —*see* Abuse, drug, sedative
  opioids —*see* Abuse, drug, opioid
  PCP (phencyclidine) —*see* Abuse, drug, hallucinogen
  sedatives —*see* Abuse, drug, sedative
  stimulants NEC —*see* Abuse, drug, stimulant
Harris' lines —*see* Arrest, epiphyseal
Hartnup's disease E72.02
Harvester's lung J67.0
Harvesting ovum for in vitro fertilization Z31.83
Hashimoto's disease or thyroiditis E06.3
Hashitoxicosis (transient) E06.3
Hassal-Henle bodies or warts (cornea) H18.49
Haut mal —*see* Epilepsy, generalized, specified NEC
Haverhill fever A25.1
Hay fever (*see also* Fever, hay) J30.1
Hayem-Widal syndrome D59.8
Haygarth's nodes M15.8
Haymaker's lung J67.0
Hb (abnormal)
  Bart's disease D56.0
  disease —*see* Disease, hemoglobin
  trait —*see* Trait

171

Head —see condition

Headache R51.9
- with
  - orthostatic component NEC R51.0
  - positional component NEC R51.0
- allergic NEC G44.89
- associated with sexual activity G44.82
- cervicogenic G44.86
- chronic daily R51.9
- cluster G44.009
  - chronic G44.029
    - intractable G44.021
    - not intractable G44.029
  - episodic G44.019
    - intractable G44.011
    - not intractable G44.019
  - intractable G44.001
  - not intractable G44.009
- cough (primary) G44.83
- daily chronic R51.9
- drug-induced NEC G44.40
  - intractable G44.41
  - not intractable G44.40
- exertional (primary) G44.84
- histamine G44.009
  - intractable G44.001
  - not intractable G44.009
- hypnic G44.81
- lumbar puncture G97.1
- medication overuse G44.40
  - intractable G44.41
  - not intractable G44.40
- menstrual —see Migraine, menstrual
- migraine (type) (see also Migraine) G43.909
- nasal septum R51.9
- neuralgiform, short lasting unilateral, with conjunctival injection and tearing (SUNCT) G44.059
  - intractable G44.051
  - not intractable G44.059
- new daily persistent (NDPH) G44.52
- orgasmic G44.82
- periodic syndromes in adults and children G43.C0
  - with refractory migraine G43.C1
    - intractable G43.C1
    - not intractable G43.C0
  - without refractory migraine G43.C0
- postspinal puncture G97.1
- post-traumatic G44.309
  - acute G44.319
    - intractable G44.311
    - not intractable G44.319
  - chronic G44.329
    - intractable G44.321
    - not intractable G44.329
  - intractable G44.301
  - not intractable G44.309
- pre-menstrual —see Migraine, menstrual
- preorgasmic G44.82
- primary
  - cough G44.83
  - exertional G44.84
  - stabbing G44.85
  - thunderclap G44.53
- rebound G44.40
  - intractable G44.41
  - not intractable G44.40
- short lasting unilateral
  - neuralgiform, with conjunctival injection and tearing (SUNCT) G44.059
    - intractable G44.051
    - not intractable G44.059
- specified syndrome NEC G44.89

Headache (continued)
- spinal and epidural anesthesia - induced T88.59
  - in labor and delivery O74.5
  - in pregnancy O29.4-
  - postpartum, puerperal O89.4
- spinal fluid loss (from puncture) G97.1
- stabbing (primary) G44.85
- tension (-type) G44.209
  - chronic G44.229
    - intractable G44.221
    - not intractable G44.229
  - episodic G44.219
    - intractable G44.211
    - not intractable G44.219
  - intractable G44.201
  - not intractable G44.209
- thunderclap (primary) G44.53
- vascular NEC G44.1

Healthy
- infant
  - accompanying sick mother Z76.3
  - receiving care Z76.2
- person accompanying sick person Z76.3

Hearing examination Z01.10
- with abnormal findings NEC Z01.118
- following failed hearing screening Z01.110
- for hearing conservation and treatment Z01.12
- infant or child (over 28 days old) Z00.129
  - with abnormal finding Z00.121

Heart —see condition

Heart beat
- abnormality R00.9
  - specified NEC R00.8
- awareness R00.2
- rapid R00.0
- slow R00.1

Heartburn R12
- psychogenic F45.8

Heartland virus disease A93.8

Heat (effects) T67.9
- apoplexy T67.01
- burn (see also Burn) L55.9
- collapse T67.1
- cramps T67.2
- dermatitis or eczema L59.0
- edema T67.7
- erythema - code by site under Burn, first degree
- excessive T67.9
  - specified effect NEC T67.8
- exhaustion T67.5
  - anhydrotic T67.3
  - due to
    - salt (and water) depletion T67.4
    - water depletion T67.3
      - with salt depletion T67.4
- fatigue (transient) T67.6
- fever T67.01
- hyperpyrexia T67.01
- prickly L74.0
- prostration —see Heat, exhaustion
- pyrexia T67.01
- rash L74.0
- specified effect NEC T67.8
- stroke T67.01
  - exertional T67.02
  - specified NEC T67.09
- sunburn —see Sunburn
- syncope T67.1

Heavy-for-dates NEC (infant) (4000g to 4499g) P08.1
- exceptionally (4500g or more) P08.0

Hebephrenia, hebephrenic (schizophrenia) F20.1

Heberden's disease or nodes (with arthropathy) M15.1

Hebra's
- pityriasis L26
- prurigo L28.2

Heel —see condition

Heerfordt's disease D86.89

Hegglin's anomaly or syndrome D72.0

Heilmeyer-Schoner disease D45

Heine-Medin disease A80.9

Heinz body anemia, congenital D58.2

Heliophobia F40.228

Heller's disease or syndrome F84.3

HELLP syndrome (hemolysis, elevated liver enzymes and low platelet count) O14.2-
- complicating
  - childbirth O14.24
  - puerperium O14.25

Helminthiasis —see also Infestation, helminth
- Ancylostoma B76.0
- intestinal B82.0
  - mixed types (types classifiable to more than one of the titles B65.0-B81.3 and B81.8) B81.4
  - specified type NEC B81.8
- mixed types (intestinal) (types classifiable to more than one of the titles B65.0-B81.3 and B81.8) B81.4
- Necator (americanus) B76.1
- specified type NEC B83.8

Heloma L84

Hemangioblastoma —see Neoplasm, connective tissue, uncertain behavior
- malignant —see Neoplasm, connective tissue, malignant

Hemangioendothelioma —see also Neoplasm, uncertain behavior, by site
- benign D18.00
  - intra-abdominal D18.03
  - intracranial D18.02
  - skin D18.01
  - specified site NEC D18.09
- bone (diffuse) —see Neoplasm, bone, malignant
- epithelioid —see also Neoplasm, uncertain behavior, by site
  - malignant —see Neoplasm, malignant, by site
- malignant —see Neoplasm, connective tissue, malignant

Hemangiofibroma —see Neoplasm, benign, by site

Hemangiolipoma —see Lipoma

Hemangioma D18.00
- arteriovenous D18.00
  - intra-abdominal D18.03
  - intracranial D18.02
  - skin D18.01
  - specified site NEC D18.09

Hemangioma (continued)
- capillary I78.1
  - intra-abdominal D18.03
  - intracranial D18.02
  - skin D18.01
  - specified site NEC D18.09
- cavernous D18.00
  - intra-abdominal D18.03
  - intracranial D18.02
  - skin D18.01
  - specified site NEC D18.09
- epithelioid D18.00
  - intra-abdominal D18.03
  - intracranial D18.02
  - skin D18.01
  - specified site NEC D18.09
- histiocytoid D18.00
  - intra-abdominal D18.03
  - intracranial D18.02
  - skin D18.01
  - specified site NEC D18.09
- infantile D18.00
  - intra-abdominal D18.03
  - intracranial D18.02
  - skin D18.01
  - specified site NEC D18.09
- intra-abdominal D18.03
- intracranial D18.02
- intramuscular D18.00
  - intra-abdominal D18.03
  - intracranial D18.02
  - skin D18.01
  - specified site NEC D18.09
- intrathoracic structures D18.09
- juvenile D18.00
- malignant —see Neoplasm, connective tissue, malignant
- plexiform D18.00
  - intra-abdominal D18.03
  - intracranial D18.02
  - skin D18.01
  - specified site NEC D18.09
- racemose D18.00
  - intra-abdominal D18.03
  - intracranial D18.02
  - skin D18.01
  - specified site NEC D18.09
- sclerosing —see Neoplasm, skin, benign
- simplex D18.00
  - intra-abdominal D18.03
  - intracranial D18.02
  - skin D18.01
  - specified site NEC D18.09
- skin D18.01
- specified site NEC D18.09
- venous D18.00
  - intra-abdominal D18.03
  - intracranial D18.02
  - skin D18.01
  - specified site NEC D18.09
- verrucous keratotic D18.00
  - intra-abdominal D18.03
  - intracranial D18.02
  - skin D18.01
  - specified site NEC D18.09

Hemangiomatosis (systemic) I78.8
- involving single site —see Hemangioma

Hemangiopericytoma —see also Neoplasm, connective tissue, uncertain behavior
- benign —see Neoplasm, connective tissue, benign
- malignant —see Neoplasm, connective tissue, malignant

Hemangiosarcoma —see Neoplasm, connective tissue, malignant

Hemarthrosis (nontraumatic) M25.00
  ankle M25.07-
  elbow M25.02-
  foot joint M25.07-
  hand joint M25.04-
  hip M25.05-
  in hemophilic arthropathy —see
      Arthropathy, hemophilic
  knee M25.06-
  shoulder M25.01-
  specified joint NEC M25.08
  traumatic —see Sprain, by site
  vertebrae M25.08
  wrist M25.03-
Hematemesis K92.0
  with ulcer - code by site under
      Ulcer, with hemorrhage K27.4
  newborn, neonatal P54.0
      due to swallowed maternal blood
          P78.2
Hematidrosis L74.8
Hematinuria —see also
    Hemoglobinuria
  malarial B50.8
Hematobilia K83.8
Hematocele
  female NEC N94.89
      with ectopic pregnancy
          O00.90
          with intrauterine pregnancy
              O00.91
      ovary N83.8
  male N50.1
Hematochezia (see also Melena)
    K92.1
Hematochyluria —see also
    Infestation, filarial
  schistosomiasis (bilharziasis) B65.0
Hematocolpos (with hematometra or
    hematosalpinx) N89.7
Hematocornea —see Pigmentation,
    cornea, stromal
Hematogenous —see condition
Hematoma (traumatic) (skin surface
    intact) —see also Contusion
  with
      injury of internal organs —see
          Injury, by site
      open wound —see Wound, open
  amputation stump (surgical) (late)
      T87.89
  aorta, dissecting I71.00
      abdominal I71.02
      thoracic (see also Dissection,
          aorta, thoracic) I71.019
      thoracoabdominal I71.03
  aortic intramural —see Dissection,
      aorta
  arterial (complicating trauma) —
      see Injury, blood vessel, by site
  auricle —see Contusion, ear
      nontraumatic —see Disorder,
          pinna, hematoma
  birth injury NEC P15.8
  brain (traumatic)
      with
          cerebral laceration or
              contusion (diffuse) —see
              Injury, intracranial, diffuse
              focal —see Injury,
                  intracranial, focal
      cerebellar, traumatic S06.37-
      newborn NEC P52.4
          birth injury P10.1
      intracerebral, traumatic —
          see Injury, intracranial,
              intracerebral hemorrhage

Hematoma (continued)
  brain (continued)
      nontraumatic —see Hemorrhage,
          intracranial
      subarachnoid, arachnoid,
          traumatic —see Injury,
              intracranial, subarachnoid
              hemorrhage
      subdural, traumatic —see
          Injury, intracranial, subdural
          hemorrhage
  breast (nontraumatic) N64.89
  broad ligament (nontraumatic) N83.7
      traumatic S37.892
  cerebellar, traumatic S06.37-
  cerebral —see Hematoma, brain
  cerebrum S06.36-
      left S06.35-
      right S06.34-
  cesarean delivery wound O90.2
  complicating delivery (perineal)
      (pelvic) (vagina) (vulva) O71.7
  corpus cavernosum (nontraumatic)
      N48.89
  epididymis (nontraumatic) N50.1
  epidural (traumatic) —see Injury,
      intracranial, epidural hemorrhage
      spinal —see Injury, spinal cord,
          by region
  episiotomy O90.2
  face, birth injury P15.4
  genital organ NEC (nontraumatic)
      female (nonobstetric) N94.89
          traumatic S30.202
      male N50.1
          traumatic S30.201
  internal organs —see Injury, by site
  intracerebral, traumatic —see
      Injury, intracranial, intracerebral
      hemorrhage
  intraoperative —see Complications,
      intraoperative, hemorrhage
  labia (nontraumatic) (nonobstetric)
      N90.89
  liver (subcapsular) (nontraumatic)
      K76.89
      birth injury P15.0
  mediastinum —see Injury,
      intrathoracic
  mesosalpinx (nontraumatic) N83.7
      traumatic S37.898
  muscle - code by site under
      Contusion
  nontraumatic
      muscle M79.81
      soft tissue M79.81
  obstetrical surgical wound O90.2
  orbit, orbital (nontraumatic) —see
      also Hemorrhage, orbit
      traumatic —see Contusion, orbit
  pelvis (female) (nontraumatic)
      (nonobstetric) N94.89
      obstetric O71.7
      traumatic —see Injury, by site
  penis (nontraumatic) N48.89
      birth injury P15.5
  perianal (nontraumatic) K64.5
  perineal S30.23
      complicating delivery O71.7
  perirenal —see Injury, kidney
  peritoneal K66.1
  pinna —see Contusion, ear
      nontraumatic —see Disorder,
          pinna, hematoma
  placenta O43.89-
  postoperative (postprocedural)
      —see Complication,
      postprocedural, hematoma
  retroperitoneal (nontraumatic)
      K68.3
      traumatic S36.892

Hematoma (continued)
  scrotum, superficial S30.22
      birth injury P15.5
  seminal vesicle (nontraumatic) N50.1
      traumatic S37.892
  spermatic cord (traumatic) S37.892
      nontraumatic N50.1
  spinal (cord) (meninges) —see also
      Injury, spinal cord, by region
      newborn (birth injury) P11.5
  spleen D73.5
      intraoperative —see
          Complications, intraoperative,
          hemorrhage, spleen
      postprocedural (postoperative)
          —see Complications,
          postprocedural, hemorrhage,
          spleen
  sternocleidomastoid, birth injury
      P15.2
  sternomastoid, birth injury P15.2
  subarachnoid (traumatic) —see
      Injury, intracranial, subarachnoid
      hemorrhage
      newborn (nontraumatic) P52.5
          due to birth injury P10.3
      nontraumatic —see Hemorrhage,
          intracranial, subarachnoid
  subdural (traumatic) —see
      Injury, intracranial, subdural
      hemorrhage
      newborn (localized) P52.8
          birth injury P10.0
      nontraumatic —see Hemorrhage,
          intracranial, subdural
      superficial, newborn P54.5
  testis (nontraumatic) N50.1
      birth injury P15.5
  tunica vaginalis (nontraumatic) N50.1
  umbilical cord, complicating
      delivery O69.5
  uterine ligament (broad)
      (nontraumatic) N83.7
      traumatic S37.892
  vagina (ruptured) (nontraumatic)
      N89.8
      complicating delivery O71.7
  vas deferens (nontraumatic) N50.1
      traumatic S37.892
  vitreous —see Hemorrhage, vitreous
  vulva (nontraumatic) (nonobstetric)
      N90.89
      complicating delivery O71.7
      newborn (birth injury) P15.5
Hematometra N85.7
  with hematocolpos N89.7
Hematomyelia (central) G95.19
  newborn (birth injury) P11.5
  traumatic T14.8
Hematomyelitis G04.90
Hematoperitoneum —see
    Hemoperitoneum
Hematophobia F40.230
Hematopneumothorax (see
    Hemothorax)
Hematopoiesis, cyclic D70.4
Hematoporphyria —see Porphyria
Hematorachis, hematorrhachis
    G95.19
  newborn (birth injury) P11.5
Hematosalpinx N83.6
  with
      hematocolpos N89.7
      hematometra N85.7
          with hematocolpos N89.7
  infectional —see Salpingitis
Hematospermia R36.1

Hematothorax (see Hemothorax)
Hematuria R31.9
  due to sulphonamide, sulfonamide
      —see Table of Drugs and
      Chemicals, by drug
  benign (familial) (of childhood) —
      see also Hematuria, idiopathic
      essential microscopic R31.1
  endemic (see also Schistosomiasis)
      B65.0
  gross R31.0
  idiopathic N02.9
      with glomerular lesion
          C3
              glomerulonepritis N02.A
              glomerulopathy N02.A
                  with dense deposit
                      disease N02.6
          crescentic (diffuse)
              glomerulonephritis N02.7
          dense deposit disease N02.6
          endocapillary proliferative
              glomerulonephritis N02.4
          focal and segmental hyalinosis
              or sclerosis N02.1
          membranoproliferative
              (diffuse) N02.5
          membranous (diffuse) N02.2
          mesangial proliferative
              (diffuse) N02.3
          mesangiocapillary (diffuse)
              N02.5
          minor abnormality N02.0
          proliferative NEC N02.8
          specified pathology NEC N02.8
  intermittent —see Hematuria,
      idiopathic
  malarial B50.8
  microscopic NEC (with symptoms)
      R31.29
      asymptomatic R31.21
      benign essential R31.1
  paroxysmal —see also Hematuria,
      idiopathic
      nocturnal D59.5
  persistent —see Hematuria,
      idiopathic
  recurrent —see Hematuria,
      idiopathic
  tropical (see also Schistosomiasis)
      B65.0
  tuberculous A18.13
Hemeralopia (day blindness) H53.11
  vitamin A deficiency E50.5
Hemi-akinesia R41.4
Hemianalgesia R20.0
Hemianencephaly Q00.0
Hemianesthesia R20.0
Hemianopia, hemianopsia
    (heteronymous) H53.47
  homonymous H53.46-
  syphilitic A52.71
Hemiathetosis R25.8
Hemiatrophy R68.89
  cerebellar G31.9
  face, facial, progressive (Romberg)
      G51.8
  tongue K14.8
Hemiballism (us) G25.5
Hemicardia Q24.8
Hemicephalus, hemicephaly Q00.0
Hemichorea G25.5
Hemicolitis, left —see Colitis, left sided
Hemicrania
  congenital malformation Q00.0
  continua G44.51

173

Hemicrania (continued)
  meaning migraine (see also Migraine) G43.909
  paroxysmal G44.039
    chronic G44.049
      intractable G44.041
      not intractable G44.049
    episodic G44.039
      intractable G44.031
      not intractable G44.039
    intractable G44.031
    not intractable G44.039

Hemidystrophy —see Hemiatrophy

Hemiectromelia Q73.8

Hemihypalgesia R20.8

Hemihypesthesia R20.1

Hemi-inattention R41.4

Hemimegalencephaly Q04.5

Hemimelia Q73.8
  lower limb —see Defect, reduction, lower limb, specified type NEC
  upper limb —see Defect, reduction, upper limb, specified type NEC

Hemiparalysis —see Hemiplegia

Hemiparesis —see Hemiplegia

Hemiparesthesia R20.2

Hemiparkinsonism G20.C

Hemiplegia G81.9-
  alternans facialis G83.89
  ascending NEC G81.90
    spinal G95.89
  congenital (cerebral) G80.8
    spastic G80.2
  embolic (current episode) I63.4-
  flaccid G81.0-
  following
    cerebrovascular disease I69.959
      cerebral infarction I69.35-
      intracerebral hemorrhage I69.15-
      nontraumatic intracranial hemorrhage NEC I69.25-
      specified disease NEC I69.85-
      stroke NOS I69.35-
      subarachnoid hemorrhage I69.05-
  hysterical F44.4
  newborn NEC P91.88
    birth injury P11.9
  spastic G81.1-
    congenital G80.2
  thrombotic (current episode) I63.3-

Hemisection, spinal cord —see Injury, spinal cord, by region

Hemispasm (facial) R25.2

Hemisporosis B48.8

Hemitremor R25.1

Hemivertebra Q76.49
  failure of segmentation with scoliosis Q76.3
  fusion with scoliosis Q76.3

Hemochromatosis E83.119
  with refractory anemia D46.1
  due to repeated red blood cell transfusion E83.111
  hereditary (primary) E83.110
  neonatal P78.84
  primary E83.110
  specified NEC E83.118

Hemoglobin —see also condition
  abnormal (disease) —see Disease, hemoglobin
  AS genotype D57.3
  Constant Spring D58.2

Hemoglobin (continued)
  E-beta thalassemia D56.5
  fetal, hereditary persistence (HPFH) D56.4
  H Constant Spring D56.0
  low NOS D64.9
  S (Hb S), heterozygous D57.3

Hemoglobinemia D59.9
  due to blood transfusion T80.89
  paroxysmal D59.6
    nocturnal D59.5

Hemoglobinopathy (mixed) D58.2
  with thalassemia D56.8
  sickle-cell D57.1
    with thalassemia D57.40
      with
        acute chest syndrome D57.411
        cerebral vascular involvement D57.413
        crisis (painful) D57.419
          with specified complication NEC D57.418
        pain (vaso-occlusive) D57.419
        splenic sequestration D57.412
      without crisis D57.40

Hemoglobinuria R82.3
  with anemia, hemolytic, acquired (chronic) NEC D59.6
  cold (paroxysmal) (with Raynaud's syndrome) D59.6
    agglutinin D59.12
  due to exertion or hemolysis NEC D59.6
  intermittent D59.6
  malarial B50.8
  march D59.6
  nocturnal (paroxysmal) D59.5
  paroxysmal (cold) D59.6
    nocturnal D59.5

Hemolymphangioma D18.1

Hemolysis
  intravascular
    with
      abortion —see Abortion, by type, complicated by, hemorrhage
      ectopic or molar pregnancy O08.1
      hemorrhage
        antepartum —see Hemorrhage, antepartum, with coagulation defect
        intrapartum (see also Hemorrhage, complicating, delivery) O67.0
        postpartum O72.3
  neonatal (excessive) P58.9
    specified NEC P58.8

Hemolytic —see condition

Hemopericardium I31.2
  following acute myocardial infarction (current complication) I23.0
  newborn P54.8
  traumatic —see Injury, heart, with hemopericardium

Hemoperitoneum K66.1
  infectional K65.9
  traumatic S36.899
    with open wound —see Wound, open, with penetration into peritoneal cavity

Hemophilia (classical) (familial) (hereditary) D66
  A D66
  B D67

Hemophilia (continued)
  C D68.1
  acquired D68.311
  autoimmune D68.311
  calcipriva (see also Defect, coagulation) D68.4
  nonfamilial (see also Defect, coagulation) D68.4
  secondary D68.311
  vascular —see Disease, von Willebrand

Hemophthalmos H44.81-

Hemopneumothorax —see also Hemothorax
  traumatic S27.2

Hemoptysis R04.2
  newborn P26.9
  tuberculous —see Tuberculosis, pulmonary

Hemorrhage, hemorrhagic (concealed) R58
  abdomen R58
  accidental antepartum —see Hemorrhage, antepartum
  acute idiopathic pulmonary, in infants R04.81
  adenoid J35.8
  adrenal (capsule) (gland) E27.49
    medulla E27.8
    newborn P54.4
  after delivery —see Hemorrhage, postpartum
  alveolar
    lung, newborn P26.8
    process K08.89
  alveolus K08.89
  amputation stump (surgical) T87.89
  anemia (chronic) D50.0
    acute D62
  antepartum (with) O46.90
    with coagulation defect O46.00-
      afibrinogenemia O46.01-
      disseminated intravascular coagulation O46.02-
      hypofibrinogenemia O46.01-
      specified defect NEC O46.09-
    before 20 weeks gestation O20.9
      specified type NEC O20.8
      threatened abortion O20.0
    due to
      abruptio placenta (see also Abuptio placentae) O45.9-
      leiomyoma, uterus —see Hemorrhage, antepartum, specified cause NEC
      placenta previa O44.1-
    specified cause NEC O46.8X-
  anus (sphincter) K62.5
  apoplexy (stroke) —see Hemorrhage, intracranial, intracerebral
  arachnoid —see Hemorrhage, intracranial, subarachnoid
  artery R58
  brain —see Hemorrhage, intracranial, intracerebral
  basilar (ganglion) I61.0
  bladder N32.89
  bowel K92.2
    newborn P54.3
  brain (miliary) (nontraumatic) —see Hemorrhage, intracranial, intracerebral
    due to
      birth injury P10.1
      syphilis A52.05
    epidural or extradural (traumatic) —see Injury, intracranial, epidural hemorrhage
    newborn P52.4
      birth injury P10.1

Hemorrhage, hemorrhagic (continued)
  brain (continued)
    subarachnoid —see Hemorrhage, intracranial, subarachnoid
    subdural —see Hemorrhage, intracranial, subdural
  brainstem (nontraumatic) I61.3
    traumatic S06.38-
  breast N64.59
  bronchial tube —see Hemorrhage, lung
  bronchopulmonary —see Hemorrhage, lung
  bronchus —see Hemorrhage, lung
  bulbar I61.5
  capillary I78.8
    primary D69.8
  cecum K92.2
  cerebellar, cerebellum (nontraumatic) I61.4
    newborn P52.6
    traumatic S06.37-
  cerebral, cerebrum —see also Hemorrhage, intracranial, intracerebral
    newborn (anoxic) P52.4
      birth injury P10.1
    lobe I61.1
  cerebromeningeal I61.8
  cerebrospinal —see Hemorrhage, intracranial, intracerebral
  cervix (uteri) (stump) NEC N88.8
  chamber, anterior (eye) —see Hyphema
  childbirth —see Hemorrhage, complicating, delivery
  choroid H31.30-
    expulsive H31.31-
  ciliary body —see Hyphema
  cochlea —see subcategory H83.8
  colon K92.2
  complicating
    abortion —see Abortion, by type, complicated by, hemorrhage
    delivery O67.9
      associated with coagulation defect (afibrinogenemia) (DIC) (hyperfibrinolysis) O67.0
      specified cause NEC O67.8
    surgical procedure —see Hemorrhage, intraoperative
  conjunctiva H11.3-
    newborn P54.8
  cord, newborn (stump) P51.9
  corpus luteum (ruptured) cyst N83.1-
  cortical (brain) I61.1
  cranial —see Hemorrhage, intracranial
  cutaneous R23.3
    due to autosensitivity, erythrocyte D69.2
    newborn P54.5
  delayed
    following ectopic or molar pregnancy O08.1
    postpartum O72.2
  diathesis (familial) D69.9
  disease D69.9
    newborn P53
    specified type NEC D69.8
  due to or associated with afibrinogenemia or other coagulation defect (conditions in categories D65-D69)
    antepartum —see Hemorrhage, antepartum, with coagulation defect
    intrapartum O67.0
  dental implant M27.61

Hemorrhage, hemorrhagic *(continued)*
  due to or associated with *(continued)*
    device, implant or graft *(see also* Complications, by site and type, specified NEC) T85.838
      arterial graft NEC T82.838
      breast T85.838
      catheter NEC T85.838
        dialysis (renal) T82.838
          intraperitoneal T85.838
        infusion NEC T82.838
          spinal (epidural) (subdural) T85.830
        urinary (indwelling) T83.83
      electronic (electrode) (pulse generator) (stimulator)
        bone T84.83
        cardiac T82.837
        nervous system (brain) (peripheral nerve) (spinal) T85.830
        urinary T83.83
      fixation, internal (orthopedic) NEC T84.83
      gastrointestinal (bile duct) (esophagus) T85.838
      genital NEC T83.83
      heart NEC T82.837
      joint prosthesis T84.83
      ocular (corneal graft) (orbital implant) NEC T85.838
      orthopedic NEC T84.83
        bone graft T86.838
      specified NEC T85.838
      urinary NEC T83.83
      vascular NEC T82.838
      ventricular intracranial shunt T85.830
  duodenum, duodenal K92.2
    ulcer —*see* Ulcer, duodenum, with hemorrhage
  dura mater —*see* Hemorrhage, intracranial, subdural
  endotracheal —*see* Hemorrhage, lung
  epicranial subaponeurotic (massive), birth injury P12.2
  epidural (traumatic) —*see also* Injury, intracranial, epidural hemorrhage
    nontraumatic I62.1
  esophagus K22.89
    varix I85.01
      secondary I85.11
  excessive, following ectopic gestation (subsequent episode) O08.1
  extradural (traumatic) —*see* Injury, intracranial, epidural hemorrhage
    birth injury P10.8
    newborn (anoxic) (nontraumatic) P52.8
    nontraumatic I62.1
  eye NEC H57.89
    fundus —*see* Hemorrhage, retina
    lid —*see* Disorder, eyelid, specified type NEC
  fallopian tube N83.6
  fibrinogenolysis —*see* Fibrinolysis
  fibrinolytic (acquired) —*see* Fibrinolysis
  from
    ear (nontraumatic) —*see* Otorrhagia
    tracheostomy stoma J95.01
  fundus, eye —*see* Hemorrhage, retina
  funis —*see* Hemorrhage, umbilicus, cord

Hemorrhage, hemorrhagic *(continued)*
  gastric —*see* Hemorrhage, stomach
  gastroenteric K92.2
    newborn P54.3
  gastrointestinal (tract) K92.2
    newborn P54.3
  genital organ, male N50.1
  genitourinary (tract) NOS R31.9
  gingiva K06.8
  globe (eye) —*see* Hemophthalmos
  graafian follicle cyst (ruptured) N83.0-
  gum K06.8
  heart I51.89
  hypopharyngeal (throat) R04.1
  intermenstrual (regular) N92.3
    irregular N92.1
  internal (organs) NEC R58
    capsule I61.0
    ear H83.8
    newborn P54.8
  intestine K92.2
    newborn P54.3
  intra-abdominal R58
  intra-alveolar (lung), newborn P26.8
  intracerebral (nontraumatic) —*see* Hemorrhage, intracranial, intracerebral
  intracranial (nontraumatic) I62.9
    birth injury P10.9
    epidural, nontraumatic I62.1
    extradural, nontraumatic I62.1
    newborn P52.9
      specified NEC P52.8
    intracerebral (nontraumatic) (in) I61.9
      brain stem I61.3
      cerebellum I61.4
      newborn P52.4
        birth injury P10.1
      hemisphere I61.2
        cortical (superficial) I61.1
        subcortical (deep) I61.0
      intraoperative
        during a nervous system procedure G97.31
        during other procedure G97.32
      intraventricular I61.5
      multiple localized I61.6
      postprocedural
        following a nervous system procedure G97.51
        following other procedure G97.52
      specified NEC I61.8
      superficial I61.1
      traumatic (diffuse) —*see* Injury, intracranial, diffuse
        focal —*see* Injury, intracranial, focal
    subarachnoid (nontraumatic) (from) I60.9
      newborn P52.5
        birth injury P10.3
      intracranial (cerebral) artery I60.7
        anterior communicating I60.2
        basilar I60.4
        carotid siphon and bifurcation I60.0-
        communicating I60.7
          anterior I60.2
          posterior I60.3-
        middle cerebral I60.1-
        posterior communicating I60.3-

Hemorrhage, hemorrhagic *(continued)*
  intracranial *(continued)*
    subarachnoid *(continued)*
      intracranial artery *(continued)*
        specified artery NEC I60.6
        vertebral I60.5-
      specified NEC I60.8
      traumatic S06.6X-
    subdural (nontraumatic) I62.00
      acute I62.01
      birth injury P10.0
      chronic I62.03
      newborn (anoxic) (hypoxic) P52.8
        birth injury P10.0
      spinal G95.19
      subacute I62.02
      traumatic —*see* Injury, intracranial, subdural hemorrhage
    traumatic —*see* Injury, intracranial, focal brain injury
  intramedullary NEC G95.19
  intraocular —*see* Hemophthalmos
  intraoperative, intraprocedural —*see* Complication, hemorrhage (hematoma), intraoperative (intraprocedural), by site
  intrapartum —*see* Hemorrhage, complicating, delivery
  intrapelvic
    female N94.89
    male K66.1
  intraperitoneal K66.1
  intrapontine I61.3
  intraprocedural —*see* Complication, hemorrhage (hematoma), intraoperative (intraprocedural), by site
  intrauterine N85.7
    complicating delivery (*see also* Hemorrhage, complicating, delivery) O67.9
    postpartum —*see* Hemorrhage, postpartum
  intraventricular I61.5
    newborn (nontraumatic) (*see also* Newborn, affected by, hemorrhage) P52.3
      due to birth injury P10.2
      grade
        1 P52.0
        2 P52.1
        3 P52.21
        4 P52.22
  intravesical N32.89
  iris (postinfectional) (postinflammatory) (toxic) —*see* Hyphema
  joint (nontraumatic) —*see* Hemarthrosis
  kidney N28.89
  knee (joint) (nontraumatic) —*see* Hemarthrosis, knee
  labyrinth —*see* subcategory H83.8
  lenticular striate artery I61.0
  ligature, vessel —*see* Hemorrhage, postoperative
  liver K76.89
  lung R04.89
    newborn P26.9
      massive P26.1
      specified NEC P26.8
    tuberculous —*see* Tuberculosis, pulmonary
  massive umbilical, newborn P51.0
  mediastinum —*see* Hemorrhage, lung
  medulla I61.3

Hemorrhage, hemorrhagic *(continued)*
  membrane (brain) I60.8
    spinal cord —*see* Hemorrhage, spinal cord
  meninges, meningeal (brain) (middle) I60.8
    spinal cord —*see* Hemorrhage, spinal cord
  mesentery K66.1
  metritis —*see* Endometritis
  mouth K13.79
  mucous membrane NEC R58
    newborn P54.8
  muscle M62.89
  nail (subungual) L60.8
  nasal turbinate R04.0
    newborn P54.8
  navel, newborn P51.9
  newborn P54.9
    specified NEC P54.8
  nipple N64.59
  nose R04.0
    newborn P54.8
  omentum K66.1
  optic nerve (sheath) H47.02-
  orbit, orbital H05.23-
  ovary NEC N83.8
  oviduct N83.6
  pancreas K86.89
  parathyroid (gland) (spontaneous) E21.4
  parturition —*see* Hemorrhage, complicating, delivery
  penis N48.89
  pericardium, pericarditis I31.2
  peritoneum, peritoneal K66.1
  peritonsillar tissue J35.8
    due to infection J36
  petechial R23.3
    due to autosensitivity, erythrocyte D69.2
  pituitary (gland) E23.6
  pleura —*see* Hemorrhage, lung
  polioencephalitis, superior E51.2
  polymyositis —*see* Polymyositis
  pons, pontine I61.3
  posterior fossa (nontraumatic) I61.8
    newborn P52.6
  postmenopausal N95.0
  postnasal R04.0
  postoperative —*see* Complications, postprocedural, hemorrhage, by site
  postpartum NEC (following delivery of placenta) O72.1
    delayed or secondary O72.2
    retained placenta O72.0
    third stage O72.0
  pregnancy —*see* Hemorrhage, antepartum
  preretinal —*see* Hemorrhage, retina
  prostate N42.1
  puerperal —*see* Hemorrhage, postpartum
    delayed or secondary O72.2
  pulmonary R04.89
    newborn P26.9
      massive P26.1
      specified NEC P26.8
    tuberculous —*see* Tuberculosis, pulmonary
  purpura (primary) D69.3
  rectum (sphincter) K62.5
    newborn P54.2
  recurring, following initial hemorrhage at time of injury T79.2
  renal N28.89
  respiratory passage or tract R04.9
    specified NEC R04.89

Hemorrhage, hemorrhagic (continued)
retina, retinal (vessels) H35.6-
  diabetic —see Microaneurysm, retinal, diabetic
retroperitoneal K68.3
scalp R58
scrotum N50.1
secondary (nontraumatic) R58
  following initial hemorrhage at time of injury T79.2
seminal vesicle N50.1
skin R23.3
  newborn P54.5
slipped umbilical ligature P51.8
spermatic cord N50.1
spinal (cord) G95.19
  newborn (birth injury) P11.5
spleen D73.5
  intraoperative —see Complications, intraoperative, hemorrhage, spleen
  postprocedural —see Complications, postprocedural, hemorrhage, spleen
stomach K92.2
  newborn P54.3
  ulcer —see Ulcer, stomach, with hemorrhage
subarachnoid (nontraumatic) —see Hemorrhage, intracranial, subarachnoid
subconjunctival —see also Hemorrhage, conjunctiva
  birth injury P15.3
subcortical (brain) I61.0
subcutaneous R23.3
subdiaphragmatic R58
subdural (acute) (nontraumatic) —see Hemorrhage, intracranial, subdural
subependymal
  newborn P52.0
    with intraventricular extension P52.1
      and intracerebral extension P52.22
subgaleal P12.2
subhyaloid —see Hemorrhage, retina
subperiosteal —see Disorder, bone, specified type NEC
subretinal —see Hemorrhage, retina
subtentorial —see Hemorrhage, intracranial, subdural
subungual L60.8
suprarenal (capsule) (gland) E27.49
  newborn P54.4
tentorium (traumatic) NEC —see Hemorrhage, brain
  newborn (birth injury) P10.4
testis N50.1
third stage (postpartum) O72.0
thorax —see Hemorrhage, lung
throat R04.1
thymus (gland) E32.8
thyroid (cyst) (gland) E07.89
tongue K14.8
tonsil J35.8
trachea —see Hemorrhage, lung
tracheobronchial R04.89
  newborn P26.0
traumatic - code to specific injury
  cerebellar —see Hemorrhage, brain
  intracranial —see Hemorrhage, brain
  recurring or secondary (following initial hemorrhage at time of injury) T79.2

Hemorrhage, hemorrhagic (continued)
tuberculous NEC (see also Tuberculosis, pulmonary) A15.0
tunica vaginalis N50.1
ulcer - code by site under Ulcer, with hemorrhage K27.4
umbilicus, umbilical
  cord
    after birth, newborn P51.9
    complicating delivery O69.5
  newborn P51.9
    massive P51.0
    slipped ligature P51.8
  stump P51.9
urethra (idiopathic) N36.8
uterus, uterine (abnormal) N93.9
  climacteric N92.4
  complicating delivery —see Hemorrhage, complicating, delivery
  dysfunctional or functional N93.8
  intermenstrual (regular) N92.3
    irregular N92.1
  postmenopausal N95.0
  postpartum —see Hemorrhage, postpartum
  preclimacteric or premenopausal N92.4
  prepubertal N93.8
  pubertal N92.2
vagina (abnormal) N93.9
  newborn P54.6
vas deferens N50.1
vasa previa O69.4
ventricular I61.5
vesical N32.89
viscera NEC R58
  newborn P54.8
vitreous (humor) (intraocular) H43.1-
vulva N90.89

Hemorrhoids (bleeding) (without mention of degree) K64.9
1st degree (grade/stage I) (without prolapse outside of anal canal) K64.0
2nd degree (grade/stage II) (that prolapse with straining but retract spontaneously) K64.1
3rd degree (grade/stage III) (that prolapse with straining and require manual replacement back inside anal canal) K64.2
4th degree (grade/stage IV) (with prolapsed tissue that cannot be manually replaced) K64.3
complicating
  pregnancy O22.4
  puerperium O87.2
external K64.4
  with
    thrombosis K64.5
internal (without mention of degree) K64.8
prolapsed K64.8
skin tags
  anus K64.4
  residual K64.4
specified NEC K64.8
strangulated (see also Hemorrhoids, by degree) K64.8
thrombosed (see also Hemorrhoids, by degree) K64.5
ulcerated (see also Hemorrhoids, by degree) K64.8

Hemosalpinx N83.6
with
  hematocolpos N89.7

Hemosalpinx (continued)
with (continued)
  hematometra N85.7
    with hematocolpos N89.7

Hemosiderosis (dietary) E83.19
pulmonary, idiopathic E83.1- [J84.03]
transfusion T80.89

Hemothorax (bacterial) (nontuberculous) J94.2
newborn P54.8
traumatic S27.1
  with pneumothorax S27.2
tuberculous NEC A15.6

Henoch (-Schönlein) disease or syndrome (purpura) D69.0

Henpue, henpuye A66.6

Hepar lobatum (syphilitic) A52.74

Hepatalgia K76.89

Hepatitis K75.9
acute B17.9
  with coma K72.01
  with hepatic failure —see Failure, hepatic
  alcoholic —see Hepatitis, alcoholic
  infectious B17.9
  non-viral K72.0
  viral B17.9
alcoholic (acute) (chronic) K70.10
  with ascites K70.11
amebic —see Abscess, liver, amebic
anicteric,(viral) —see Hepatitis, viral
antigen-associated (HAA) —see Hepatitis, B
Australia-antigen (positive) —see Hepatitis, B
autoimmune K75.4
B B19.10
  with hepatic coma B19.11
  acute B16.9
    with
      delta-agent (coinfection) (without hepatic coma) B16.1
        with hepatic coma B16.0
      hepatic coma (without delta-agent coinfection) B16.2
  chronic B18.1
    with delta-agent B18.0
bacterial NEC K75.89
C (viral) B19.20
  with hepatic coma B19.21
  acute B17.10
    with hepatic coma B17.11
  chronic B18.2
catarrhal (acute) B15.9
  with hepatic coma B15.0
cholangiolitic K75.89
cholestatic K75.89
chronic K73.9
  active NEC K73.2
  lobular NEC K73.1
  persistent NEC K73.0
  specified NEC K73.8
cytomegaloviral B25.1
due to ethanol (acute) (chronic) —see Hepatitis, alcoholic
epidemic B15.9
  with hepatic coma B15.0
fulminant NEC (viral) —see Hepatitis, viral
granulomatous NEC K75.3
herpesviral B00.81

Hepatitis (continued)
history of
  B Z86.19
  C Z86.19
homologous serum —see Hepatitis, viral, type B
in (due to)
  mumps B26.81
  toxoplasmosis (acquired) B58.1
    congenital (active) P37.1 [K77]
infectious, infective B15.9
  acute (subacute) B17.9
  chronic B18.9
inoculation —see Hepatitis, viral, type B
interstitial (chronic) K74.69
ischemia, ischemic K72.00
lupoid NEC K75.4
malignant NEC (with hepatic failure) K72.90
  with coma K72.91
neonatal (idiopathic) (toxic) P59.29
neonatal giant cell P59.29
newborn P59.29
postimmunization —see Hepatitis, viral, type B
post-transfusion —see Hepatitis, viral, type B
reactive, nonspecific K75.2
serum —see Hepatitis, viral, type B
shock K72.00
specified type NEC
  with hepatic failure —see Failure, hepatic
syphilitic (late) A52.74
  congenital (early) A50.08 [K77]
    late A50.59 [K77]
  secondary A51.45
toxic (see also Disease, liver, toxic) K71.6
tuberculous A18.83
viral, virus B19.9
  with hepatic coma B19.0
  acute B17.9
  chronic B18.9
    specified NEC B18.8
  type
    B B18.1
      with delta-agent B18.0
    C B18.2
congenital P35.3
coxsackie B33.8 [K77]
cytomegalic inclusion B25.1
in remission, any type - code to Hepatitis, chronic, by type
non-A, non-B B17.8
specified type NEC (with or without coma) B17.8
type
  A B15.9
    with hepatic coma B15.0
  B B19.10
    with hepatic coma B19.11
    acute B16.9
      with
        delta-agent (coinfection) (without hepatic coma) B16.1
          with hepatic coma B16.0
        hepatic coma (without delta-agent coinfection) B16.2
    chronic B18.1
      with delta-agent B18.0
  C B19.20
    with hepatic coma B19.21
    acute B17.10
      with hepatic coma B17.11
    chronic B18.2

Hepatitis (continued)
 viral, virus (continued)
  type (continued)
   E B17.2
   non-A, non-B B17.8
Hepatization lung (acute) —see Pneumonia, lobar
Hepatoblastoma C22.2
Hepatocarcinoma C22.0
Hepatocholangiocarcinoma C22.0
Hepatocholangioma, benign D13.4
Hepatocholangitis K75.89
Hepatolenticular degeneration E83.01
Hepatoma (malignant) C22.0
 benign D13.4
 embryonal C22.0
Hepatomegaly —see also Hypertrophy, liver
 with splenomegaly R16.2
 congenital Q44.79
 in mononucleosis
  gammaherpesviral B27.09
  infectious specified NEC B27.89
Hepatoptosis K76.89
Hepatorenal syndrome following labor and delivery O90.41
Hepatosis K76.89
Hepatosplenomegaly R16.2
 hyperlipemic (Bürger-Grütz type) E78.3 [K77]
Hereditary —see condition
Hereditary alpha tryptasemia (syndrome) D89.44
Heredodegeneration, macular —see Dystrophy, retina
Heredopathia atactica polyneuritiformis G60.1
Heredosyphilis —see Syphilis, congenital
Herlitz' syndrome Q81.1
Hermansky-Pudlak syndrome E70.331
Hermaphrodite, hermaphroditism (true) Q56.0
 46,XX with streak gonads Q99.1
 46,XX/46,XY Q99.0
 46,XY with streak gonads Q99.1
 chimera 46,XX/46,XY Q99.0
Hernia, hernial (acquired) (recurrent) K46.9
 with
  gangrene —see Hernia, by site, with, gangrene
  incarceration —see Hernia, by site, with, obstruction
  irreducible —see Hernia, by site, with, obstruction
  obstruction —see Hernia, by site, with, obstruction
  strangulation —see Hernia, by site, with, obstruction
 abdomen, abdominal K46.9
  with
   gangrene (and obstruction) K46.1
   obstruction K46.0
  femoral —see Hernia, femoral
  incisional —see Hernia, incisional
  inguinal —see Hernia, inguinal

Hernia, hernial (continued)
 abdomen, abdominal (continued)
  specified site NEC K45.8
   with
    gangrene (and obstruction) K45.1
    obstruction K45.0
  umbilical —see Hernia, umbilical
  wall —see Hernia, ventral
 appendix —see Hernia, abdomen
 bladder (mucosa) (sphincter)
  congenital (female) (male) Q79.51
  female —see Cystocele
  male N32.89
 brain, congenital —see Encephalocele
 cartilage, vertebra —see Displacement, intervertebral disc
 cerebral, congenital —see also Encephalocele
  endaural Q01.8
 ciliary body (traumatic) S05.2-
 colon —see Hernia, abdomen
 Cooper's —see Hernia, abdomen, specified site NEC
 crural —see Hernia, femoral
 diaphragm, diaphragmatic K44.9
  with
   gangrene (and obstruction) K44.1
   obstruction K44.0
  congenital Q79.0
 direct (inguinal) —see Hernia, inguinal
 diverticulum, intestine —see Hernia, abdomen
 double (inguinal) —see Hernia, inguinal, bilateral
 due to adhesions (with obstruction) K56.50
 epigastric (see also Hernia, ventral) K43.9
 esophageal hiatus —see Hernia, hiatal
 external (inguinal) —see Hernia, inguinal
 fallopian tube N83.4-
 fascia M62.89
 femoral K41.90
  with
   gangrene (and obstruction) K41.40
    not specified as recurrent K41.40
    recurrent K41.41
   obstruction K41.30
    not specified as recurrent K41.30
    recurrent K41.31
  bilateral K41.20
   with
    gangrene (and obstruction) K41.10
     not specified as recurrent K41.10
     recurrent K41.11
    obstruction K41.00
     not specified as recurrent K41.00
     recurrent K41.01
   not specified as recurrent K41.20
   recurrent K41.21
  unilateral K41.90
   with
    gangrene (and obstruction) K41.40
     not specified as recurrent K41.40

Hernia, hernial (continued)
 femoral (continued)
  unilateral (continued)
   with (continued)
    gangrene (continued)
     recurrent K41.41
    obstruction K41.30
     not specified as recurrent K41.30
     recurrent K41.31
   not specified as recurrent K41.90
   recurrent K41.91
  not specified as recurrent K41.90
  recurrent K41.91
 foramen magnum G93.5
  congenital Q01.8
 funicular (umbilical) —see also Hernia, umbilicus
  spermatic (cord) —see Hernia, inguinal
 gastrointestinal tract —see Hernia, abdomen
 Hesselbach's —see Hernia, femoral, specified site NEC
 hiatal (esophageal) (sliding) K44.9
  with
   gangrene (and obstruction) K44.1
   obstruction K44.0
  congenital Q40.1
 hypogastric —see Hernia, ventral
 incarcerated —see also Hernia, by site, with obstruction
  with gangrene —see Hernia, by site, with gangrene
 incisional K43.2
  with
   gangrene (and obstruction) K43.1
   obstruction K43.0
 indirect (inguinal) —see Hernia, inguinal
 inguinal (direct) (external) (funicular) (indirect) (internal) (oblique) (scrotal) (sliding) K40.90
  with
   gangrene (and obstruction) K40.40
    not specified as recurrent K40.40
    recurrent K40.41
   obstruction K40.30
    not specified as recurrent K40.30
    recurrent K40.31
  not specified as recurrent K40.90
  recurrent K40.91
  bilateral K40.20
   with
    gangrene (and obstruction) K40.10
     not specified as recurrent K40.10
     recurrent K40.11
    obstruction K40.00
     not specified as recurrent K40.00
     recurrent K40.01
   not specified as recurrent K40.20
   recurrent K40.21
  unilateral K40.90
   with
    gangrene (and obstruction) K40.40
     not specified as recurrent K40.40
     recurrent K40.41

Hernia, hernial (continued)
 inguinal (continued)
  unilateral (continued)
   with (continued)
    obstruction K40.30
     not specified as recurrent K40.30
     recurrent K40.31
    not specified as recurrent K40.90
    recurrent K40.91
  internal —see also Hernia, abdomen
   inguinal —see Hernia, inguinal
   interstitial —see Hernia, abdomen
  intervertebral cartilage or disc — see Displacement, intervertebral disc
  intestine, intestinal —see Hernia, by site
  intra-abdominal —see Hernia, abdomen
  iris (traumatic) S05.2-
  irreducible —see also Hernia, by site, with obstruction
   with gangrene —see Hernia, by site, with gangrene
  ischiatic —see Hernia, abdomen, specified site NEC
  ischiorectal —see Hernia, abdomen, specified site NEC
  lens (traumatic) S05.2-
  linea (alba) (semilunaris) —see Hernia, ventral
  Littre's —see Hernia, abdomen
  lumbar —see Hernia, abdomen, specified site NEC
  lung (subcutaneous) J98.4
  mediastinum J98.59
  mesenteric (internal) —see Hernia, abdomen
  midline —see Hernia, ventral
  muscle (sheath) M62.89
  nucleus pulposus —see Displacement, intervertebral disc
  oblique (inguinal) —see Hernia, inguinal
  obstructive —see also Hernia, by site, with obstruction
   with gangrene —see Hernia, by site, with gangrene
  obturator —see Hernia, abdomen, specified site NEC
  omental —see Hernia, abdomen
  ovary N83.4-
  oviduct N83.4-
  paraesophageal —see also Hernia, diaphragm
   congenital Q40.1
  parastomal K43.5
   with
    gangrene (and obstruction) K43.4
    obstruction K43.3
  paraumbilical —see Hernia, umbilicus
  perineal —see Hernia, abdomen, specified site NEC
  Petit's —see Hernia, abdomen, specified site NEC
  postoperative —see Hernia, incisional
  pregnant uterus —see Abnormal, uterus in pregnancy or childbirth
  prevesical N32.89
  properitoneal —see Hernia, abdomen, specified site NEC
  pudendal —see Hernia, abdomen, specified site NEC
  rectovaginal N81.6

Hernia, hernial (continued)
retroperitoneal —see Hernia, abdomen, specified site NEC
Richter's —see Hernia, abdomen, with obstruction
Rieux's, Riex's —see Hernia, abdomen, specified site NEC
sac condition (adhesion) (dropsy) (inflammation) (laceration) (suppuration) - code by site under Hernia
sciatic —see Hernia, abdomen, specified site NEC
scrotum, scrotal —see Hernia, inguinal
sliding (inguinal) —see also Hernia, inguinal
hiatus —see Hernia, hiatal
spigelian —see Hernia, ventral
spinal —see Spina bifida
strangulated —see also Hernia, by site, with obstruction
with gangrene —see Hernia, by site, with gangrene
subxiphoid —see Hernia, ventral
supra-umbilicus —see Hernia, ventral
tendon —see Disorder, tendon, specified type NEC
Treitz's (fossa) —see Hernia, abdomen, specified site NEC
tunica vaginalis Q55.29
umbilicus, umbilical K42.9
  with
    gangrene (and obstruction) K42.1
    obstruction K42.0
ureter N28.89
urethra, congenital Q64.79
urinary meatus, congenital Q64.79
uterus N81.4
  pregnant —see Abnormal, uterus in pregnancy or childbirth
vaginal (anterior) (wall) —see Cystocele
Velpeau's —see Hernia, femoral
ventral K43.9
  with
    gangrene (and obstruction) K43.7
    obstruction K43.6
  recurrent —see Hernia, incisional
  incisional K43.2
    with
      gangrene (and obstruction) K43.1
      obstruction K43.0
  specified NEC K43.9
    with
      gangrene (and obstruction) K43.7
      obstruction K43.6
vesical
  congenital (female) (male) Q79.51
  female —see Cystocele
  male N32.89
vitreous (into wound) S05.2-
  into anterior chamber —see Prolapse, vitreous
Herniation —see also Hernia
brain (stem) G93.5
  nontraumatic G93.5
  traumatic S06.A1
    cerebellar S06.A1
    subfalcine (cingulate) S06.A1
    tonsillar S06.A1
    transtentorial (central) (upward cerebellar) S06.A1
    uncal S06.A1

Herniation (continued)
cerebral G93.5
  nontraumatic G93.5
  traumatic S06.A1
mediastinum J98.59
nucleus pulposus —see Displacement, intervertebral disc
Herpangina B08.5
Herpes, herpesvirus, herpetic B00.9
anogenital A60.9
  perianal skin A60.1
  rectum A60.1
  urogenital tract A60.00
    cervix A60.03
    male genital organ NEC A60.02
    penis A60.01
    specified site NEC A60.09
    vagina A60.04
    vulva A60.04
blepharitis (zoster) B02.39
  simplex B00.59
circinatus B35.4
  bullosus L12.0
conjunctivitis (simplex) B00.53
  zoster B02.31
cornea B02.33
encephalitis B00.4
  due to herpesvirus 6 B10.01
  due to herpesvirus 7 B10.09
  specified NEC B10.09
eye (zoster) B02.30
  simplex B00.50
eyelid (zoster) B02.39
  simplex B00.59
facialis B00.1
febrilis B00.1
geniculate ganglionitis B02.21
genital, genitalis A60.00
  female A60.09
  male A60.02
gestational, gestationis O26.4-
gingivostomatitis B00.2
human B00.9
  1 —see Herpes, simplex
  2 —see Herpes, simplex
  3 —see Varicella
  4 —see Mononucleosis, Epstein-Barr (virus)
  5 —see Disease, cytomegalic inclusion (generalized)
  6
    encephalitis B10.01
    specified NEC B10.81
  7
    encephalitis B10.09
    specified NEC B10.82
  8 B10.89
infection NEC B10.89
  Kaposi's sarcoma associated B10.89
iridocyclitis (simplex) B00.51
  zoster B02.32
iris (vesicular erythema multiforme) L51.9
iritis (simplex) B00.51
Kaposi's sarcoma associated B10.89
keratitis (simplex) (dendritic) (disciform) (interstitial) B00.52
  zoster (interstitial) B02.33
keratoconjunctivitis (simplex) B00.52
  zoster B02.33
labialis B00.1
lip B00.1
meningitis (simplex) B00.3
  zoster B02.1
ophthalmicus (zoster) NEC B02.30
  simplex B00.50

Herpes, herpesvirus, herpetic (continued)
penis A60.01
perianal skin A60.1
pharyngitis, pharyngotonsillitis B00.2
rectum A60.1
scrotum A60.02
sepsis B00.7
simplex B00.9
  complicated NEC B00.89
  congenital P35.2
  conjunctivitis B00.53
  external ear B00.1
  eyelid B00.59
  hepatitis B00.81
  keratitis (interstitial) B00.52
  myleitis B00.82
  specified complication NEC B00.89
  visceral B00.89
stomatitis B00.2
tonsurans B35.0
visceral B00.89
vulva A60.04
whitlow B00.89
zoster (see also condition) B02.9
  auricularis B02.21
  complicated NEC B02.8
  conjunctivitis B02.31
  disseminated B02.7
  encephalitis B02.0
  eye (lid) B02.39
  geniculate ganglionitis B02.21
  keratitis (interstitial) B02.33
  meningitis B02.1
  myelitis B02.24
  neuritis, neuralgia B02.29
  ophthalmicus NEC B02.30
  oticus B02.21
  polyneuropathy B02.23
  specified complication NEC B02.8
  trigeminal neuralgia B02.22
Herpesvirus (human) —see Herpes
Herpetophobia F40.218
Herrick's anemia —see Disease, sickle-cell
Hers' disease E74.09
Herter-Gee syndrome K90.0
Herxheimer's reaction R68.89
Hesitancy
of micturition R39.11
urinary R39.11
Hesselbach's hernia —see Hernia, femoral, specified site NEC
Heterochromia (congenital) Q13.2
cataract —see Cataract, complicated
cyclitis (Fuchs) —see Cyclitis, Fuchs' heterochromic
hair L67.1
iritis —see Cyclitis, Fuchs' heterochromic
retained metallic foreign body (nonmagnetic) —see Foreign body, intraocular, old, retained
magnetic —see Foreign body, intraocular, old, retained, magnetic
uveitis —see Cyclitis, Fuchs' heterochromic
Heterophoria —see Strabismus, heterophoria
Heterophyes, heterophyiasis (small intestine) B66.8

Heterotopia, heterotopic —see also Malposition, congenital
cerebralis Q04.8
Heterotropia —see Strabismus
Heubner-Herter disease K90.0
Hexadactylism Q69.9
HGSIL (cytology finding) (high grade squamous intraepithelial lesion on cytologic smear) (Pap smear finding)
anus R85.613
cervix R87.613
  biopsy (histology) finding —see Neoplasia, intraepithelial, cervix, grade II or grade III
vagina R87.623
  biopsy (histology) finding —see Neoplasia, intraepithelial, vagina, grade II or grade III
Hibernoma —see Lipoma
Hiccup, hiccough R06.6
epidemic B33.0
psychogenic F45.8
Hidden penis (congenital) Q55.64
acquired N48.83
Hidradenitis (axillaris) (suppurative) L73.2
Hidradenoma (nodular) —see also Neoplasm, skin, benign
clear cell —see Neoplasm, skin, benign
papillary —see Neoplasm, skin, benign
Hidrocystoma —see Neoplasm, skin, benign
High
altitude effects T70.20
  anoxia T70.29
  on
    ears T70.0
    sinuses T70.1
  polycythemia D75.1
arch
  foot Q66.7-
  palate, congenital Q38.5
arterial tension —see Hypertension
basal metabolic rate R94.8
blood pressure —see also Hypertension
  borderline R03.0
  reading (incidental) (isolated) (nonspecific), without diagnosis of hypertension R03.0
cholesterol E78.00
  with high triglycerides E78.2
diaphragm (congenital) Q79.1
expressed emotional level within family Z63.8
head at term O32.4
palate, congenital Q38.5
risk
  infant NEC Z76.2
  sexual behavior (heterosexual) Z72.51
    bisexual Z72.53
    homosexual Z72.52
scrotal testis, testes
  bilateral Q53.23
  unilateral Q53.13
temperature (of unknown origin) R50.9
thoracic rib Q76.6
triglycerides E78.1
  with high cholesterol E78.2
Hildenbrand's disease A75.0

Hilum —see condition

Hip —see condition

Hippel's disease Q85.83

Hippophobia F40.218

Hippus H57.09

Hirschsprung's disease or megacolon Q43.1

Hirsutism, hirsuties L68.0

Hirudiniasis
　external B88.3
　internal B83.4

Hiss-Russell dysentery A03.1

Histidinemia, histidinuria E70.41

Histiocytoma —see also Neoplasm, skin, benign
　fibrous —see also Neoplasm, skin, benign
　　atypical —see Neoplasm, connective tissue, uncertain behavior
　　malignant —see Neoplasm, connective tissue, malignant

Histiocytosis D76.3
　acute differentiated progressive C96.0
　Langerhans' cell NEC C96.6
　　multifocal X
　　　multisystemic (disseminated) C96.0
　　　unisystemic C96.5
　　pulmonary, adult (adult PLCH) J84.82
　　unifocal (X) C96.6
　lipid, lipoid D76.3
　　essential E75.29
　malignant C96.A
　mononuclear phagocytes NEC D76.1
　　Langerhans' cells C96.6
　non-Langerhans cell D76.3
　polyostotic sclerosing D76.3
　sinus, with massive lymphadenopathy D76.3
　syndrome NEC D76.3
　X NEC C96.6
　　acute (progressive) C96.0
　　chronic C96.6
　　multifocal C96.5
　　multisystemic C96.0
　　unifocal C96.6

Histoplasmosis B39.9
　with pneumonia NEC B39.2
　African B39.5
　American —see Histoplasmosis, capsulati
　capsulati B39.4
　　disseminated B39.3
　　generalized B39.3
　　pulmonary B39.2
　　　acute B39.0
　　　chronic B39.1
　Darling's B39.4
　duboisii B39.5
　lung NEC B39.2

History
　family (of) —see also History, personal (of)
　　alcohol abuse Z81.1
　　allergy NEC Z84.89
　　anemia Z83.2
　　arthritis Z82.61
　　asthma Z82.5
　　blindness Z82.1
　　cardiac death (sudden) Z82.41
　　carrier of genetic disease Z84.81
　　chromosomal anomaly Z82.79
　　chronic
　　　disabling disease NEC Z82.8
　　　lower respiratory disease Z82.5

History (continued)
　family (continued)
　　colonic polyps Z83.719
　　　adenomatous and serrated Z83.710
　　　hyperplastic Z83.711
　　　inflammatory Z83.718
　　　specified, NEC Z83.718
　　　tubular adenoma Z83.710
　　　tubulovillous adenoma Z83.710
　　　villous adenoma Z83.710
　　congenital malformations and deformations Z82.79
　　　polycystic kidney Z82.71
　　consanguinity Z84.3
　　deafness Z82.2
　　diabetes mellitus Z83.3
　　disability NEC Z82.8
　　disease or disorder (of)
　　　allergic NEC Z84.89
　　　behavioral NEC Z81.8
　　　blood and blood-forming organs Z83.2
　　　cardiovascular NEC Z82.49
　　　chronic disabling NEC Z82.8
　　　digestive Z83.79
　　　ear NEC Z83.52
　　　elevated lipoprotein (a) (Lp(a)) Z83.430
　　　endocrine NEC Z83.49
　　　eye NEC Z83.518
　　　　glaucoma Z83.511
　　　familial hypercholesterolemia Z83.42
　　　genitourinary NEC Z84.2
　　　glaucoma Z83.511
　　　hematological Z83.2
　　　immune mechanism Z83.2
　　　infectious NEC Z83.1
　　　ischemic heart Z82.49
　　　kidney Z84.1
　　　lipoprotein metabolism Z83.438
　　　mental NEC Z81.8
　　　metabolic Z83.49
　　　musculoskeletal NEC Z82.69
　　　neurological NEC Z82.0
　　　nutritional Z83.49
　　　parasitic NEC Z83.1
　　　psychiatric NEC Z81.8
　　　respiratory NEC Z83.6
　　　skin and subcutaneous tissue NEC Z84.0
　　　specified NEC Z84.89
　　drug abuse NEC Z81.3
　　elevated lipoprotein (a) (Lp(a)) Z83.430
　　epilepsy Z82.0
　　familial hypercholesterolemia Z83.42
　　genetic disease carrier Z84.81
　　glaucoma Z83.511
　　hearing loss Z82.2
　　human immunodeficiency virus (HIV) infection Z83.0
　　Huntington's chorea Z82.0
　　hyperlipidemia, familial combined Z83.438
　　intellectual disability Z81.0
　　leukemia Z80.6
　　lipidemia NEC Z83.438
　　malignant neoplasm (of) NOS Z80.9
　　　bladder Z80.52
　　　breast Z80.3
　　　bronchus Z80.1
　　　digestive organ Z80.0
　　　gastrointestinal tract Z80.0
　　　genital organ Z80.49
　　　　ovary Z80.41
　　　　prostate Z80.42
　　　　specified organ NEC Z80.49

History (continued)
　family (continued)
　　malignant neoplasm (of) (continued)
　　　genital organ (continued)
　　　　testis Z80.43
　　　hematopoietic NEC Z80.7
　　　intrathoracic organ NEC Z80.2
　　　kidney Z80.51
　　　lung Z80.1
　　　lymphatic NEC Z80.7
　　　ovary Z80.41
　　　prostate Z80.42
　　　respiratory organ NEC Z80.2
　　　specified site NEC Z80.8
　　　testis Z80.43
　　　trachea Z80.1
　　　urinary organ or tract Z80.59
　　　　bladder Z80.52
　　　　kidney Z80.51
　　mental
　　　disorder NEC Z81.8
　　multiple endocrine neoplasia (MEN) syndrome Z83.41
　　osteoporosis Z82.62
　　polycystic kidney Z82.71
　　polyps (colon) (see also History, family, colonic polyps) Z83.719
　　psychiatric disorder Z81.8
　　psychoactive substance abuse NEC Z81.3
　　respiratory condition NEC Z83.6
　　　asthma and other lower respiratory conditions Z82.5
　　self-harmful behavior Z81.8
　　SIDS (sudden infant death syndrome) Z84.82
　　skin condition Z84.0
　　specified condition NEC Z84.89
　　stroke (cerebrovascular) Z82.3
　　substance abuse NEC Z81.4
　　　alcohol Z81.1
　　　drug NEC Z81.3
　　　psychoactive NEC Z81.3
　　　tobacco Z81.2
　　sudden
　　　cardiac death Z82.41
　　　infant death syndrome (SIDS) Z84.82
　　tobacco abuse Z81.2
　　violence, violent behavior Z81.8
　　visual loss Z82.1
　personal (of) —see also History, family (of)
　　abuse
　　　adult Z91.419
　　　　financial Z91.413
　　　　forced labor or sexual exploitation Z91.42
　　　　intimate partner Z91.414
　　　　physical and sexual Z91.410
　　　　psychological Z91.411
　　　childhood Z62.819
　　　　financial Z62.814
　　　　forced labor or sexual exploitation in childhood Z62.813
　　　　intimate partner Z62.815
　　　　physical Z62.810
　　　　psychological Z62.811
　　　　sexual Z62.810
　　　in adolescence —see History, personal, abuse, childhood
　　alcohol dependence F10.21
　　allergy (to) Z88.9
　　　analgesic agent NEC Z88.6
　　　anesthetic Z88.4
　　　antibiotic agent NEC Z88.1
　　　anti-infective agent NEC Z88.3
　　　contrast media Z91.041

History (continued)
　personal (continued)
　　allergy (continued)
　　　drugs, medicaments and biological substances Z88.9
　　　　specified NEC Z88.8
　　　food Z91.018
　　　　additives Z91.02
　　　　beef Z91.014
　　　　eggs Z91.012
　　　　lamb Z91.014
　　　　mammalian meats Z91.014
　　　　milk products Z91.011
　　　　peanuts Z91.010
　　　　pork Z91.014
　　　　red meats Z91.014
　　　　seafood Z91.013
　　　　specified food NEC Z91.018
　　　insect Z91.038
　　　　bee Z91.030
　　　latex Z91.040
　　　medicinal agents Z88.9
　　　　specified NEC Z88.8
　　　narcotic agent NEC Z88.5
　　　nonmedicinal agents Z91.048
　　　penicillin Z88.0
　　　serum Z88.7
　　　specified NEC Z91.09
　　　sulfonamides Z88.2
　　　vaccine Z88.7
　　anaphylactic shock Z87.892
　　anaphylaxis Z87.892
　　behavioral disorders Z86.59
　　benign carcinoid tumor Z86.012
　　benign neoplasm Z86.018
　　　carcinoid Z86.012
　　　brain Z86.011
　　　colonic polyps Z86.010
　　brain injury (traumatic) Z87.820
　　breast implant removal Z98.86
　　calculi, renal Z87.442
　　cancer —see History, personal (of), malignant neoplasm (of)
　　cardiac arrest (death), successfully resuscitated Z86.74
　　CAR-T (Chimeric Antigen Receptor T-cell) therapy Z92.850
　　cellular therapy Z92.859
　　　specified NEC Z92.858
　　cerebral infarction without residual deficit Z86.73
　　certain (corrected) conditions arising in the perinatal period, specified NEC Z87.68
　　cervical dysplasia Z87.410
　　chemotherapy for neoplastic condition Z92.21
　　childhood abuse —see History, personal (of), abuse
　　Chimeric Antigen Receptor T-cell (CAR-T) therapy Z92.850
　　cleft lip (corrected) Z87.730
　　cleft palate (corrected) Z87.730
　　cloaca, persistent Z87.732
　　cloacal malformations Z87.732
　　collapsed vertebra (healed) Z87.311
　　　due to osteoporosis Z87.310
　　combat and operational stress reaction Z86.51
　　congenital malformation (corrected) Z87.798
　　circulatory system (corrected) Z87.74
　　diaphragmatic hernia Z87.760
　　digestive system (corrected) NEC Z87.738
　　ear (corrected) Z87.721
　　eye (corrected) Z87.720
　　face and neck (corrected) Z87.790

History (continued)
  personal (continued)
    congenital malformation (continued)
      gastroschisis Z87.761
      genitourinary system (corrected) NEC Z87.718
      heart (corrected) Z87.74
      integument (corrected) Z87.768
      limb(s) (corrected) Z87.768
      malformations
        abdominal wall Z87.763
        diaphragm NEC Z87.760
        integument Z87.768
        limbs Z87.768
        musculoskeletal system Z87.768
        prune belly Z87.762
      musculoskeletal system (corrected) Z87.768
      neck (corrected) Z87.790
      nervous system (corrected) NEC Z87.728
      respiratory system (corrected) Z87.75
      sense organs (corrected) NEC Z87.728
      specified NEC Z87.798
    contraception Z92.0
    coronavirus (disease) (novel) 2019 Z86.16
    COVID-19 Z86.16
    deployment (military) Z91.82
    diabetic foot ulcer Z86.31
    disease or disorder (of) Z87.898
      blood and blood-forming organs Z86.2
      circulatory system Z86.79
        specified condition NEC Z86.79
      connective tissue NEC Z87.39
      digestive system Z87.19
        colonic polyp Z86.010
        peptic ulcer disease Z87.11
        specified condition NEC Z87.19
      ear Z86.69
      endocrine Z86.39
        diabetic foot ulcer Z86.31
        gestational diabetes Z86.32
        specified type NEC Z86.39
      eye Z86.69
      genital (track) system NEC
        female Z87.42
        male Z87.438
      hematological Z86.2
      Hodgkin Z85.71
      immune mechanism Z86.2
      infectious Z86.19
        coronavrius (disease) (novel) 2019 Z86.16
        COVID-19 Z86.16
        malaria Z86.13
        Methicillin resistant Staphylococcus aureus (MRSA) Z86.14
        poliomyelitis Z86.12
        SARS-CoV2 Z86.16
        specified NEC Z86.19
        tuberculosis Z86.11
      mental NEC Z86.59
      metabolic Z86.39
        diabetic foot ulcer Z86.31
        gestational diabetes Z86.32
        specified type NEC Z86.39
      musculoskeletal NEC Z87.39
      nervous system Z86.69
      nutritional Z86.39
      parasitic Z86.19
      respiratory system NEC Z87.09
      sense organs Z86.69

History (continued)
  personal (continued)
    disease or disorder (continued)
      skin Z87.2
      specified site or type NEC Z87.898
      subcutaneous tissue Z87.2
      trophoblastic Z87.59
      urinary system NEC Z87.448
    drug dependence —see Dependence, drug, by type, in remission
    drug therapy
      antineoplastic chemotherapy Z92.21
      estrogen Z92.23
      immunosuppression Z92.25
      inhaled steroids Z92.240
      monoclonal drug Z92.22
      specified NEC Z92.29
      steroid Z92.241
      systemic steroids Z92.241
    dysplasia
      cervical (mild) (moderate) Z87.410
        severe (grade III) Z86.001
      prostatic Z87.430
      vaginal (mild) (moderate) Z87.411
        severe (grade III) Z86.002
      vulvar (mild) (moderate) Z87.412
        severe (grade III) Z86.002
    embolism (venous) Z86.718
      pulmonary Z86.711
    encephalitis Z86.61
    estrogen therapy Z92.23
    extracorporeal membrane oxygenation (ECMO) Z92.81
    failed moderate sedation Z92.83
    failed conscious sedation Z92.83
    fall, falling Z91.81
    forced labor or sexual exploitation Z91.42
      in childhood Z62.813
    fracture (healed)
      fatigue Z87.312
      fragility Z87.310
      osteoporosis Z87.310
      pathological NEC Z87.311
      stress Z87.312
      traumatic Z87.81
    gene therapy Z92.86
    gestational diabetes Z86.32
    hepatitis
      B Z86.19
      C Z86.19
    Hodgkin disease Z85.71
    hyperthermia, malignant Z88.4
    hypospadias (corrected) Z87.710
    hysterectomy Z90.710
    immunosuppression therapy Z92.25
    in situ neoplasm
      breast Z86.000
      cervix uteri Z86.001
      digestive organs, specified NEC Z86.004
      esophagus Z86.003
      genital organs, specified NEC Z86.002
      melanoma Z86.006
      middle ear Z86.005
      oral cavity Z86.003
      respiratory system Z86.005
      skin Z86.007
      specified NEC Z86.008
      stomach Z86.003
    infection NEC Z86.19
      central nervous system Z86.61
      coronavrius (disease) (novel) 2019 Z86.16

History (continued)
  personal (continued)
    infection (continued)
      COVID-19 Z86.16
      latent tuberculosis Z86.15
      Methicillin resistant Staphylococcus aureus (MRSA) Z86.14
      SARS-CoV2 Z86.16
      urinary (recurrent) (tract) Z87.440
    injury NEC Z87.828
    in utero procedure during pregnancy Z98.870
    in utero procedure while a fetus Z98.871
    irradiation Z92.3
    kidney stones Z87.442
    latent tuberculosis infection Z86.15
    leukemia Z85.6
    lymphoma (non-Hodgkin) Z85.72
    malignant melanoma (skin) Z85.820
    malignant neoplasm (of) Z85.9
      accessory sinuses Z85.22
      anus NEC Z85.048
        carcinoid Z85.040
      bladder Z85.51
      bone Z85.830
      brain Z85.841
      breast Z85.3
      bronchus NEC Z85.118
        carcinoid Z85.110
      carcinoid —see History, personal (of), malignant neoplasm, by site, carcinioid
      cervix Z85.41
      colon NEC Z85.038
        carcinoid Z85.030
      digestive organ Z85.00
        specified NEC Z85.09
      endocrine gland NEC Z85.858
      epididymis Z85.48
      esophagus Z85.01
      eye Z85.840
      gastrointestinal tract —see History, malignant neoplasm, digestive organ
      genital organ
        female Z85.40
          specified NEC Z85.44
        male Z85.45
          specified NEC Z85.49
      hematopoietic NEC Z85.79
      intrathoracic organ Z85.20
      kidney NEC Z85.528
        carcinoid Z85.520
      large intestine NEC Z85.038
        carcinoid Z85.030
      larynx Z85.21
      liver Z85.05
      lung NEC Z85.118
        carcinoid Z85.110
      mediastinum Z85.29
      Merkel cell Z85.821
      middle ear Z85.22
      nasal cavities Z85.22
      nervous system NEC Z85.848
      oral cavity Z85.819
        specified site NEC Z85.818
      ovary Z85.43
      pancreas Z85.07
      pharynx Z85.819
        specified site NEC Z85.818
      pelvis Z85.53
      pleura Z85.29
      prostate Z85.46
      rectosigmoid junction NEC Z85.048
        carcinoid Z85.040

History (continued)
  personal (continued)
    malignant neoplasm (of) (continued)
      rectum NEC Z85.048
        carcinoid Z85.040
      respiratory organ Z85.20
      sinuses, accessory Z85.22
      skin NEC Z85.828
        melanoma Z85.820
        Merkel cell Z85.821
      small intestine NEC Z85.068
        carcinoid Z85.060
      soft tissue Z85.831
      specified site NEC Z85.89
      stomach NEC Z85.028
        carcinoid Z85.020
      testis Z85.47
      thymus NEC Z85.238
        carcinoid Z85.230
      thyroid Z85.850
      tongue Z85.810
      trachea Z85.12
      ureter Z85.54
      urinary organ or tract Z85.50
        specified NEC Z85.59
      uterus Z85.42
    maltreatment Z91.89
    medical treatment NEC Z92.89
    melanoma Z85.820
      in situ Z86.006
      malignant (skin) Z85.820
    meningitis Z86.61
    mental disorder Z86.59
    Merkel cell carcinoma (skin) Z85.821
    Methicillin resistant Staphylococcus aureus (MRSA) Z86.14
    military deployment Z91.82
    military service Z91.85
    military war, peacekeeping and humanitarian deployment (current or past conflict) Z91.82
    myocardial infarction (old) I25.2
    necrotizing enterocolitis of newborn (corrected) Z87.61
    neglect (in)
      adult Z91.412
      childhood Z62.812
    neoplasia
      anal intraepithelial, III [AIN] Z86.004
      high-grade prostatic intraepithelial, III [HGPIN III] Z86.002
      vaginal intraepithelial, III [VAIN III] Z86.002
      vulvar intraepithelial, III [VIN III] Z86.002
    neoplasm
      benign Z86.018
        brain Z86.011
        colon polyp Z86.010
      in situ
        breast Z86.000
        cervix uteri Z86.001
        digestive organs, specified NEC Z86.004
        esophagus Z86.003
        genital organs, specified NEC Z86.002
        melanoma Z86.006
        middle ear Z86.005
        oral cavity Z86.003
        respiratory system Z86.005
        skin Z86.007
        specified NEC Z86.008
        stomach Z86.003

History (continued)
　personal (continued)
　　neoplasm (continued)
　　　malignant —see History of, malignant neoplasm
　　　uncertain behavior Z86.03
　　nephrotic syndrome Z87.441
　　nicotine dependence Z87.891
　　noncompliance with medical treatment or regimen —see Noncompliance
　　nutritional deficiency Z86.39
　　obstetric complications Z87.59
　　　childbirth Z87.59
　　　pregnancy Z87.59
　　　pre-term labor Z87.51
　　　puerperium Z87.59
　　osteoporosis fractures Z87.31
　　parasuicide (attempt) Z91.51
　　physical trauma NEC Z87.828
　　　self-harm or suicide attempt Z91.51
　　poisoning NEC Z91.89
　　　self-harm or suicide attempt Z91.51
　　poor personal hygiene Z91.89
　　pneumonia (recurrent) Z87.01
　　preterm labor Z87.51
　　prolonged reversible ischemic neurologic deficit (PRIND) Z86.73
　　procedure during pregnancy Z98.870
　　procedure while a fetus Z98.871
　　prostatic dysplasia Z87.430
　　psychological
　　　abuse
　　　　adult Z91.411
　　　　child Z62.811
　　　trauma, specified NEC Z91.49
　　radiation therapy Z92.3
　　removal
　　　implant
　　　　breast Z98.86
　　renal calculi Z87.442
　　respiratory condition NEC Z87.09
　　retained foreign body fully removed Z87.821
　　risk factors NEC Z91.89
　　SARS-CoV2 infection Z86.16
　　self-harm
　　　nonsuicidal Z91.52
　　　suicidal Z91.51
　　self-inflicted injury without suicidal intent Z91.52
　　self-injury
　　　nonsuicidal Z91.52
　　self-mutilation Z91.52
　　self-poisoning attempt Z91.51
　　sex reassignment Z87.890
　　sleep-wake cycle problem Z72.821
　　specified NEC Z87.898
　　steroid therapy (systemic) Z92.241
　　　inhaled Z92.240
　　stroke without residual deficits Z86.73
　　substance abuse NEC F10-F19
　　sudden cardiac arrest Z86.74
　　sudden cardiac death successfully resuscitated Z86.74
　　suicidal behavior Z91.51
　　suicide attempt Z91.51
　　surgery NEC Z98.890
　　　with uterine scar Z98.891
　　　sex reassignment Z87.890
　　　transplant —see Transplant
　　thrombophlebitis Z86.72
　　thrombosis (venous) Z86.718
　　　pulmonary Z86.711

History (continued)
　personal (continued)
　　tobacco dependence Z87.891
　　tracheoesophageal
　　　atresia Z87.731
　　　fistula Z87.731
　　transient ischemic attack (TIA) without residual deficits Z86.73
　　trauma (physical) NEC Z87.828
　　　psychological NEC Z91.49
　　　self-harm Z91.51
　　traumatic brain injury Z87.820
　　tuberculosis, latent infection Z86.15
　　unhealthy sleep-wake cycle Z72.821
　　unintended awareness under general anesthesia Z92.84
　　urinary calculi Z87.442
　　urinary (recurrent) (tract) infection(s) Z87.440
　　uterine scar from previous surgery Z98.891
　　vaginal dysplasia Z87.411
　　venous thrombosis or embolism Z86.718
　　　pulmonary Z86.711
　　vulvar dysplasia Z87.412
His-Werner disease A79.0
HIV (see also Human, immunodeficiency virus) B20
　laboratory evidence (nonconclusive) R75
　positive, seropositive Z21
　nonconclusive test (in infants) R75
Hives (bold) —see Urticaria
Hoarseness R49.0
Hobo Z59.00
Hodgkin disease —see Lymphoma, Hodgkin
Hodgson's (see also Aneurysm, aorta, thorax) I71.20
　ruptured (see also Aneurysm, aorta, thorax, ruptured) I71.10
Hoffa-Kastert disease E88.89
Hoffa's disease E88.89
Hoffmann-Bouveret syndrome I47.9
Hoffmann's syndrome E03.9 [G73.7]
Hole (round)
　macula H35.34-
　retina (without detachment) —see Break, retina, round hole
　　with detachment —see Detachment, retina, with retinal, break
Holiday relief care Z75.5
Hollenhorst's plaque —see Occlusion, artery, retina
Hollow foot (congenital) Q66.7-
　acquired —see Deformity, limb, foot, specified NEC
Holoprosencephaly Q04.2
Holt-Oram syndrome Q87.2
Homelessness Z59.00
　sheltered Z59.01
　unsheltered Z59.02
Homesickness —see Disorder, adjustment
Homocysteinemia R79.83
Homocystinemia R79.83
Homocystinuria E72.11
Homogentisate 1,2-dioxygenase deficiency E70.29

Homologous serum hepatitis (prophylactic) (therapeutic) —see Hepatitis, viral, type B
Honeycomb lung J98.4
　congenital Q33.0
Hooded
　clitoris Q52.6
　penis Q55.69
Hookworm (disease) (infection) (infestation) B76.9
　with anemia B76.9 [D63.8]
　specified NEC B76.8
Hordeolum (eyelid) (externum) (recurrent) H00.019
　internum H00.029
　　left H00.026
　　　lower H00.025
　　　upper H00.024
　　right H00.023
　　　lower H00.022
　　　upper H00.021
　left H00.016
　　lower H00.015
　　upper H00.014
　right H00.013
　　lower H00.012
　　upper H00.011
Horn
　cutaneous L85.8
　nail L60.2
　congenital Q84.6
Horner (-Claude Bernard) **syndrome** G90.2
　traumatic —see Injury, nerve, cervical sympathetic
Horseshoe kidney (congenital) Q63.1
Horton's headache or neuralgia G44.099
　intractable G44.091
　not intractable G44.099
Hospital hopper syndrome —see Disorder, factitious
Hospitalism in children —see Disorder, adjustment
Hostility R45.5
　towards child Z62.3
Hot flashes
　menopausal N95.1
Hourglass (contracture) —see also Contraction, hourglass
　stomach K31.89
　　congenital Q40.2
　　stricture K31.2
Household, housing circumstance affecting care Z59.9
　specified NEC Z59.89
Housemaid's knee —see Bursitis, prepatellar
HSCT-TMA (hematopoietic stem cell transplantation-associated thrombotic microangiopathy) M31.11
Hudson (-Ståhli) **line** (cornea) —see Pigmentation, cornea, anterior
Human
　bite (open wound) —see also Bite
　　intact skin surface —see Bite, superficial
　　herpesvirus —see Herpes
　immunodeficiency virus (HIV) disease (infection) B20
　　asymptomatic status Z21
　　contact Z20.6
　　counseling Z71.7

Human (continued)
　immunodeficiency virus (continued)
　　dementia (see also Dementia, in, diseases specified elsewhere) B20 [F02.80]
　　　with behavioral disturbance (see also Dementia, in, diseases specified elsewhere) B20 [F02.81-]
　　exposure to Z20.6
　　laboratory evidence R75
　　type-2(HIV 2) as cause of disease classified elsewhere B97.35
　papillomavirus (HPV)
　　DNA test positive
　　　high risk
　　　　cervix R87.810
　　　　vagina R87.811
　　　low risk
　　　　cervix R87.820
　　　　vagina R87.821
　　screening for Z11.51
　T-cell lymphotropic virus
　　type-1(HTLV-I) infection B33.3
　　　as cause of disease classified elsewhere B97.33
　　　carrier Z22.6
　　type-2(HTLV-II) as cause of disease classified elsewhere B97.34
Humidifier lung or pneumonitis J67.7
Humiliation (experience) **in childhood** Z62.898
Humpback (acquired) —see Kyphosis
Hunchback (acquired) —see Kyphosis
Hunger T73.0
　air, psychogenic F45.8
Hungry bone syndrome E83.81
Hunner's ulcer —see Cystitis, chronic, interstitial
Hunter's
　glossitis D51.0
　syndrome E76.1
Huntington's disease or chorea G10
　with dementia (see also Dementia, in, diseases specified elsewhere) G10 [F02.80]
　　with behavioral disturbance (see also Dementia, in, diseases specified elsewhere) G10 [F02.81-]
Hunt's
　disease or syndrome (herpetic geniculate ganglionitis) B02.21
　dyssynergia cerebellaris myoclonica G11.19
　neuralgia B02.21
Hurler (-Scheie) **disease or syndrome** E76.02
Hurst's disease G36.1
Hurthle cell
　adenocarcinoma C73
　adenoma D34
　carcinoma C73
　tumor D34
Hutchinson-Boeck disease or syndrome —see Sarcoidosis
Hutchinson-Gilford disease or syndrome E34.8
Hutchinson's
　disease, meaning
　　angioma serpiginosum L81.7
　　pompholyx (cheiropompholyx) L30.1
　　prurigo estivalis L56.4
　　summer eruption or summer prurigo L56.4

Hutchinson's (continued)
  melanotic freckle —see Melanoma, in situ
    malignant melanoma in —see Melanoma
  teeth or incisors (congenital syphilis) A50.52
  triad (congenital syphilis) A50.53

Hyalin plaque, sclera, senile H15.89

Hyaline membrane (disease) (lung) (pulmonary) (newborn) P22.0

Hyalinosis
  cutis (et mucosae) E78.89
  focal and segmental (glomerular) (see also N00-N07 with fourth character .1) N05.1

Hyalitis, hyalosis, asteroid —see also Deposit, crystalline
  syphilitic (late) A52.71

Hydatid
  cyst or tumor —see Echinococcus
  mole —see Hydatidiform mole
  Morgagni
    female Q50.5
    male (epididymal) Q55.4
      testicular Q55.29

Hydatidiform mole (benign) (complicating pregnancy) (delivered) (undelivered) O01.9
  classical O01.0
  complete O01.0
  incomplete O01.1
  invasive D39.2
  malignant D39.2
  partial O01.1

Hydatidosis —see Echinococcus

Hydradenitis (axillaris) (suppurative) L73.2

Hydradenoma —see Hidradenoma

Hydramnios O40.-

Hydrancephaly, hydranencephaly Q04.3
  with spina bifida —see Spina bifida, with hydrocephalus

Hydrargyrism NEC —see Poisoning, mercury

Hydrarthrosis —see also Effusion, joint
  gonococcal A54.42
  intermittent M12.40
    ankle M12.47-
    elbow M12.42-
    foot joint M12.47-
    hand joint M12.44-
    hip M12.45-
    knee M12.46-
    multiple site M12.49
    shoulder M12.41-
    specified joint NEC M12.48
    wrist M12.43-
  of yaws (early) (late) (see also subcategory M14.8-) A66.6
  syphilitic (late) A52.77
    congenital A50.55 [M12.80]

Hydremia D64.89

Hydrencephalocele (congenital) —see Encephalocele

Hydrencephalomeningocele (congenital) —see Encephalocele

Hydroa R23.8
  aestivale L56.4
  vacciniforme L56.4

Hydroadenitis (axillaris) (suppurative) L73.2

Hydrocalycosis —see Hydronephrosis

Hydrocele (spermatic cord) (testis) (tunica vaginalis) N43.3
  canal of Nuck N94.89
  communicating N43.2
    congenital P83.5
  congenital P83.5
  encysted N43.0
  female NEC N94.89
  infected N43.1
  newborn P83.5
  round ligament N94.89
  specified NEC N43.2
  spinalis —see Spina bifida
  vulva N90.89

Hydrocephalus (acquired) (external) (internal) (malignant) (recurrent) G91.9
  aqueduct Sylvius stricture Q03.0
  causing disproportion O33.6
    with obstructed labor O66.3
  communicating G91.0
  congenital (external) (internal) Q03.9
    with spina bifida Q05.4
      cervical Q05.0
      dorsal Q05.1
      lumbar Q05.2
      lumbosacral Q05.2
      sacral Q05.3
      thoracic Q05.1
      thoracolumbar Q05.1
    specified NEC Q03.8
  due to toxoplasmosis (congenital) P37.1
  foramen Magendie block (acquired) G91.1
    congenital (see also Hydrocephalus, congenital) Q03.1
  in (due to)
    infectious disease NEC B89 [G91.4]
    neoplastic disease NEC (see also Neoplasm) G91.4
    parasitic disease B89 [G91.4]
  newborn Q03.9
    with spina bifida —see Spina bifida, with hydrocephalus
  noncommunicating G91.1
  normal pressure G91.2
    secondary G91.0
  obstructive G91.1
  otitic G93.2
  post-traumatic NEC G91.3
  secondary G91.4
    post-traumatic G91.3
  specified NEC G91.8
  syphilitic, congenital A50.49

Hydrocolpos (congenital) N89.8

Hydrocystoma —see Neoplasm, skin, benign

Hydroencephalocele (congenital) —see Encephalocele

Hydroencephalomeningocele (congenital) —see Encephalocele

Hydrohematopneumothorax —see Hemothorax

Hydromeningitis —see Meningitis

Hydromeningocele (spinal) —see also Spina bifida
  cranial —see Encephalocele

Hydrometra N85.8

Hydrometrocolpos N89.8

Hydromicrocephaly Q02

Hydromphalos (since birth) Q45.8

Hydromyelia Q06.4

Hydromyelocele —see Spina bifida

Hydronephrosis (atrophic) (early) (functionless) (intermittent) (primary) (secondary) NEC N13.30
  with
    infection N13.6
    obstruction (by) (of)
      renal calculus N13.2
        with infection N13.6
      ureteral NEC N13.1
        with infection N13.6
      calculus N13.2
        with infection N13.6
      ureteropelvic junction (congenital) Q62.11
        acquired N13.0
          with infection N13.6
      ureteral stricture NEC N13.1
        with infection N13.6
  congenital Q62.0
  due to acquired occlusion of ureteropelvic junction N13.0
  specified type NEC N13.39
  tuberculous A18.11

Hydropericarditis —see Pericarditis

Hydropericardium —see Pericarditis

Hydroperitoneum R18.8

Hydrophobia —see Rabies

Hydrophthalmos Q15.0

Hydropneumohemothorax —see Hemothorax

Hydropneumopericarditis —see Pericarditis

Hydropneumopericardium —see Pericarditis

Hydropneumothorax J94.8
  traumatic —see Injury, intrathoracic, lung
  tuberculous NEC A15.6

Hydrops R60.9
  abdominis R18.8
  articulorum intermittens —see Hydrarthrosis, intermittent
  cardiac —see Failure, heart, congestive
  causing obstructed labor (mother) O66.3
  endolymphatic H81.0-
  fetal —see Pregnancy, complicated by, hydrops, fetalis
  fetalis P83.2
    due to
      ABO isoimmunization P56.0
      alpha thalassemia D56.0
      hemolytic disease P56.90
        specified NEC P56.99
      isoimmunization (ABO) (Rh) P56.0
      other specified nonhemolytic disease NEC P83.2
      Rh incompatibility P56.0
    during pregnancy —see Pregnancy, complicated by, hydrops, fetalis
  gallbladder K82.1
  joint —see Effusion, joint
  labyrinth H81.0-
  newborn (idiopathic) P83.2
    due to
      ABO isoimmunization P56.0
      alpha thalassemia D56.0
      hemolytic disease P56.90
        specified NEC P56.99
      isoimmunization (ABO) (Rh) P56.0
      Rh incompatibility P56.0
  nutritional —see Malnutrition, severe
  pericardium —see Pericarditis

Hydrops (continued)
  pleura —see Hydrothorax
  spermatic cord —see Hydrocele

Hydropyonephrosis N13.6

Hydrorachis Q06.4

Hydrorrhea (nasal) J34.89
  pregnancy —see Rupture, membranes, premature

Hydrosadenitis (axillaris) (suppurative) L73.2

Hydrosalpinx (fallopian tube) (follicularis) N70.11

Hydrothorax (double) (pleura) J94.8
  chylous (nonfilarial) I89.8
  filarial (see also Infestation, filarial) B74.9 [J91.8]
  traumatic —see Injury, intrathoracic
  tuberculous NEC (non primary) A15.6

Hydroureter (see also Hydronephrosis) N13.4
  with infection N13.6
  congenital Q62.39

Hydroureteronephrosis —see Hydronephrosis

Hydrourethra N36.8

Hydroxykynureninuria E70.89

Hydroxylysinemia E72.3

Hydroxyprolinemia E72.59

Hygiene, sleep
  abuse Z72.821
  inadequate Z72.821
  poor Z72.821

Hygroma (congenital) (cystic) D18.1
  praepatellare, prepatellar —see Bursitis, prepatellar
  subdural —see Leak, cerebrospinal fluid

Hymen —see condition

Hymenolepis, hymenolepiasis (diminuta) (infection) (infestation) (nana) B71.0

Hypalgesia R20.8

Hyperacidity (gastric) K31.89
  psychogenic F45.8

Hyperactive, hyperactivity F90.9
  basal cell, uterine cervix —see Dysplasia, cervix
  bowel sounds R19.12
  cervix epithelial (basal) —see Dysplasia, cervix
  child F90.9
    attention deficit —see Disorder, attention-deficit hyperactivity
  detrusor muscle N32.81
  gastrointestinal K31.89
    psychogenic F45.8
  nasal mucous membrane J34.3
  stomach K31.89
  thyroid (gland) —see Hyperthyroidism

Hyperacusis H93.23-

Hyperadrenalism E27.5

Hyperadrenocorticism E24.9
  congenital E25.0
  iatrogenic E24.2
    correct substance properly administered —see Table of Drugs and Chemicals, by drug, adverse effect
    overdose or wrong substance given or taken —see Table of Drugs and Chemicals, by drug, poisoning

Hyperadrenocorticism *(continued)*
  not associated with Cushing's
    syndrome E27.0
  pituitary-dependent E24.0
Hyperaldosteronism E26.9
  familial (type I) E26.02
  glucocorticoid-remediable E26.02
  primary (due to (bilateral) adrenal
    hyperplasia) E26.09
  primary NEC E26.09
  secondary E26.1
  specified NEC E26.89
Hyperalgesia R20.8
Hyperalimentation R63.2
  carotene, carotin E67.1
  specified NEC E67.8
  vitamin
    A E67.0
    D E67.3
Hyperaminoaciduria
  arginine E72.21
  cystine E72.01
  lysine E72.3
  ornithine E72.4
Hyperammonemia (congenital)
  E72.20
Hyperazotemia —*see* Uremia
Hyperbetalipoproteinemia (familial)
  E78.00
  with prebetalipoproteinemia E78.2
Hyperbicarbonatemia P74.41
Hyperbilirubinemia
  constitutional E80.6
  familial conjugated E80.6
  neonatal (transient) —*see* Jaundice,
    newborn
**Hypercalcemia, hypocalciuric,
  familial** E83.52
Hypercalciuria, idiopathic R82.994
Hypercapnia R06.89
  newborn P84
Hypercarotenemia (dietary) E67.1
Hypercementosis K03.4
Hyperchloremia E87.8
Hyperchlorhydria K31.89
  neurotic F45.8
  psychogenic F45.8
Hypercholesterinemia —*see*
  Hypercholesterolemia
Hypercholesterolemia (essential)
  (primary) (pure) E78.00
  with hyperglyceridemia,
    endogenous E78.2
    dietary counseling and surveillance
      Z71.3
  familial E78.01
  hereditary E78.01
Hyperchylia gastrica, psychogenic
  F45.8
Hyperchylomicronemia (familial)
  (primary) E78.3
  with hyperbetalipoproteinemia E78.3
Hypercoagulable (state) D68.59
  activated protein C resistance
    D68.51
  antithrombin (III) deficiency D68.59
  factor V Leiden mutation D68.51
  primary NEC D68.59
  protein C deficiency D68.59
  protein S deficiency D68.59
  prothrombin gene mutation D68.52
  secondary D68.69
  specified NEC D68.69

Hypercoagulation (state) D68.59
**Hypercorticalism, pituitary-
  dependent** E24.0
Hypercorticosolism —*see* Cushing's,
  syndrome
Hypercorticosteronism E24.2
  correct substance properly
    administered —*see* Table of
    Drugs and Chemicals, by drug,
    adverse effect
  overdose or wrong substance given
    or taken —*see* Table of Drugs and
    Chemicals, by drug, poisoning
Hypercortisonism E24.2
  correct substance properly
    administered —*see* Table of
    Drugs and Chemicals, by drug,
    adverse effect
  overdose or wrong substance
    given or taken —*see* Table of
    Drugs and Chemicals, by drug,
    poisoning
Hyperekplexia Q89.8
Hyperelectrolytemia E87.8
Hyperemesis R11.10
  with nausea R11.2
  gravidarum (mild) O21.0
    with
      carbohydrate depletion O21.1
      dehydration O21.1
      electrolyte imbalance O21.1
      metabolic disturbance O21.1
      severe (with metabolic
        disturbance) O21.1
  projectile R11.12
  psychogenic F45.8
Hyperemia (acute) (passive) R68.89
  anal mucosa K62.89
  bladder N32.89
  cerebral I67.89
  conjunctiva H11.43-
  ear internal, acute H83.0
  enteric K59.89
  eye —*see* Hyperemia, conjunctiva
  eyelid (active) (passive) —*see*
    Disorder, eyelid, specified type
    NEC
  intestine K59.89
  iris —*see* Disorder, iris, vascular
  kidney N28.89
  labyrinth H83.0
  liver (active) K76.89
  lung (passive) —*see* Edema, lung
  pulmonary (passive) —*see* Edema,
    lung
  renal N28.89
  retina H35.89
  stomach K31.89
Hyperesthesia (body surface) R20.3
  larynx (reflex) J38.7
    hysterical F44.89
  pharynx (reflex) J39.2
    hysterical F44.89
Hyperestrogenism (drug-induced)
  (iatrogenic) E28.0
Hyperexplexia Q89.8
Hyperfibrinolysis —*see* Fibrinolysis
Hyperfructosemia E74.19
Hyperfunction
  adrenal cortex, not associated with
    Cushing's syndrome E27.0
    medulla E27.5
      adrenomedullary E27.5
    virilism E25.9
      congenital E25.0

Hyperfunction *(continued)*
  ovarian E28.8
  pancreas K86.89
  parathyroid (gland) E21.3
  pituitary (gland) (anterior) E22.9
    specified NEC E22.8
  polyglandular E31.1
  testicular E29.0
Hypergammaglobulinemia D89.2
  polyclonal D89.0
  Waldenström D89.0
Hypergastrinemia E16.4
Hyperglobulinemia R77.1
Hyperglycemia, hyperglycemic
  (transient) R73.9
  coma —*see* Diabetes, by type, with
    coma
  postpancreatectomy E89.1
Hyperglyceridemia (endogenous)
  (essential) (familial) (hereditary)
  (pure) E78.1
  mixed E78.3
Hyperglycinemia (non-ketotic) E72.51
Hypergonadism
  ovarian E28.8
  testicular (primary) (infantile) E29.0
Hyperheparinemia D68.32
Hyperhidrosis, hyperidrosis R61
  focal
    primary L74.519
      axilla L74.510
      face L74.511
      palms L74.512
      soles L74.513
    secondary L74.52
  generalized R61
  localized
    primary L74.519
      axilla L74.510
      face L74.511
      palms L74.512
      soles L74.513
    secondary L74.52
  psychogenic F45.8
  secondary R61
    focal L74.52
Hyperhistidinemia E70.41
Hyperhomocysteinemia E72.11
Hyperhydroxyprolinemia E72.59
Hyperinsulinism (functional) E16.1
  with
    coma (hypoglycemic) E15
    encephalopathy E16.1 *[G94]*
  ectopic E16.1
  therapeutic misadventure (from
    administration of insulin) T38.3
Hyperkalemia E87.5
Hyperkeratosis (*see also* Keratosis)
  L85.9
  cervix N88.0
  due to yaws (early) (late) (palmar
    or plantar) A66.3
  follicularis Q82.8
    penetrans (in cutem) L87.0
  palmoplantaris climacterica L85.1
  pinta A67.1
  senile (with pruritus) L57.0
  universalis congenita Q80.8
  vocal cord J38.3
  vulva N90.4
Hyperkinesia, hyperkinetic (disease)
  (reaction) (syndrome) (childhood)
  (adolescence) —*see also* Disorder,
  attention-deficit hyperactivity
  heart I51.89

Hyperleucine-isoleucinemia E71.19
Hyperlipemia, hyperlipidemia
  E78.5
  combined E78.2
    familial E78.49
  group
    A E78.00
    B E78.1
    C E78.2
    D E78.3
  mixed E78.2
  specified NEC E78.49
Hyperlipidosis E75.6
  hereditary NEC E75.5
Hyperlipoproteinemia E78.5
  Fredrickson's type
    I E78.3
    IIa E78.00
    IIb E78.2
    III E78.2
    IV E78.1
    V E78.3
  low-density-lipoprotein-type (LDL)
    E78.00
  very-low-density-lipoprotein-type
    (VLDL) E78.1
Hyperlucent lung, unilateral
  J43.0
Hyperlysinemia E72.3
Hypermagnesemia E83.41
  neonatal P71.8
Hypermenorrhea N92.0
Hypermethioninemia E72.19
Hypermetropia (congenital) H52.0-
Hypermobility, hypermotility
  cecum —*see* Syndrome, irritable
    bowel
  coccyx —*see* subcategory M53.2
  colon —*see* Syndrome, irritable
    bowel
    psychogenic F45.8
  ileum K58.9
  intestine (*see also* Syndrome,
    irritable bowel) K58.9
    psychogenic F45.8
  meniscus (knee) —*see*
    Derangement, knee, meniscus
  scapula —*see* Instability, joint,
    shoulder
  stomach K31.89
    psychogenic F45.8
  syndrome M35.7
  urethra N36.41
    with intrinsic sphincter
      deficiency N36.43
Hypernasality R49.21
Hypernatremia E87.0
Hypernephroma C64.-
Hyperopia —*see* Hypermetropia
Hyperorexia nervosa F50.2
Hyperornithinemia E72.4
Hyperosmia R43.1
Hyperosmolality (*see also*, Diabetes,
  by type, with hyperosmolarity)
  E87.0
Hyperostosis (monomelic) —*see
  also* Disorder, bone, density and
  structure, specified NEC
  ankylosing (spine) M48.10
    cervical region M48.12
    cervicothoracic region M48.13
    lumbar region M48.16
    lumbosacral region M48.17
    multiple sites M48.19

183

Hyperostosis (continued)
  occipito-atlanto-axial region
      M48.11
    sacrococcygeal region M48.18
    thoracic region M48.14
    thoracolumbar region M48.15
  cortical (skull) M85.2
    infantile M89.8X-
  frontal, internal of skull M85.2
  interna frontalis M85.2
  skeletal, diffuse idiopathic —see
      Hyperostosis, ankylosing
  skull M85.2
    congenital Q75.8
  vertebral, ankylosing —see
      Hyperostosis, ankylosing
Hyperovarism E28.8
Hyperoxaluria R82.992
  primary E72.53
Hyperparathyroidism E21.3
  primary E21.0
  secondary (renal) N25.81
    non-renal E21.1
  specified NEC E21.2
  tertiary E21.2
Hyperpathia R20.8
Hyperperistalsis R19.2
  psychogenic F45.8
Hyperpermeability, capillary I78.8
Hyperphagia R63.2
Hyperphenylalaninemia NEC E70.1
Hyperphoria (alternating) H50.53
Hyperphosphatemia E83.39
Hyperpiesis, hyperpiesia —see
    Hypertension
Hyperpigmentation —see also
    Pigmentation
  melanin NEC L81.4
  postinflammatory L81.0
Hyperpinealism E34.8
Hyperpituitarism E22.9
Hyperplasia, hyperplastic
  adenoids J35.2
  adrenal (capsule) (cortex) (gland)
      E27.8
    with
      sexual precocity (male) E25.9
        congenital E25.0
      virilism, adrenal E25.9
        congenital E25.0
      virilization (female) E25.9
        congenital E25.0
    congenital E25.0
      salt-losing E25.0
  adrenomedullary E27.5
  angiolymphoid, eosinophilia
      (ALHE) D18.01
  appendix (lymphoid) K38.0
  artery, fibromuscular I77.3
  bone —see also Hypertrophy, bone
    marrow D75.89
  breast —see also Hypertrophy,
      breast
    atypical, atypia N60.9-
      ductal N60.9-
      lobular N60.9-
  C-cell, thyroid E07.0
  cementation (tooth) (teeth) K03.4
  cervical gland R59.0
  cervix (uteri) (basal cell)
      (endometrium) (polypoid) —see
      also Dysplasia, cervix
    congenital Q51.828
  clitoris, congenital Q52.6
  denture K06.2
  endocervicitis N72

Hyperplasia, hyperplastic (continued)
  endometrium, endometrial
      (adenomatous) (cystic)
      (glandular) (glandular-cystic)
      (polypoid) N85.00
    with atypia N85.02
    benign N85.01
    cervix —see Dysplasia, cervix
    complex (without atypia) N85.01
    simple (without atypia) N85.01
  epithelial L85.9
    focal, oral, including tongue
        K13.29
    nipple N62
    skin L85.9
    tongue K13.29
    vaginal wall N89.3
  erythroid D75.89
  fibromuscular of artery (carotid)
      (renal) I77.3
  genital
    female NEC N94.89
    male N50.89
  gingiva K06.1
  glandularis cystica uteri
      (interstitialis) (see also
      Hyperplasia, endometrial)
      N85.00-
  gum K06.1
  hymen, congenital Q52.4
  irritative, edentulous (alveolar)
      K06.2
  jaw M26.09
    alveolar M26.79
      lower M26.03
        alveolar M26.72
      upper M26.01
        alveolar M26.71
  kidney (congenital) Q63.3
  labia N90.69
    epithelial N90.3
  liver (congenital) Q44.79
    nodular, focal K76.89
  lymph gland or node R59.9
  mandible, mandibular M26.03
    alveolar M26.72
    unilateral condylar M27.8
  maxilla, maxillary M26.01
    alveolar M26.71
  myometrium, myometrial
      N85.2
  neuroendocrine cell, of infancy
      J84.841
  nose
    lymphoid J34.89
    polypoid J33.9
  oral mucosa (irritative) K13.6
  organ or site, congenital NEC
      —see Anomaly, by site
  ovary N83.8
  palate, papillary (irritative)
      K13.6
  pancreatic islet cells E16.9
    alpha E16.8
      with excess
        gastrin E16.4
        glucagon E16.3
    beta E16.1
  parathyroid (gland) E21.0
  pharynx (lymphoid) J39.2
  prostate (adenofibromatous) N40.0
    with lower urinary tract
        symptoms (LUTS)
        N40.1
      nodular N40.3
    nodular N40.2
      with lower urinary tract
          symptoms (LUTS) N40.3
    without lower urinary tract
        symptoms (LUTS) N40.0
      nodular N40.2

Hyperplasia, hyperplastic (continued)
  renal artery I77.89
  reticulo-endothelial (cell)
      D75.89
  salivary gland (any) K11.1
  Schimmelbusch's —see
      Mastopathy, cystic
  suprarenal capsule (gland)
      E27.8
  thymus (gland) (persistent)
      E32.0
  thyroid (gland) —see Goiter
  tonsils (faucial) (infective) (lingual)
      (lymphoid) J35.1
    with adenoids J35.3
  unilateral condylar M27.8
  uterus, uterine N85.2
    endometrium (glandular) (see
        also Hyperplasia, endometrial)
        N85.00-
  vulva N90.69
    epithelial N90.3
Hyperpnea —see Hyperventilation
Hyperpotassemia E87.5
Hyperprebetalipoproteinemia
    (familial) E78.1
Hyperprolactinemia E22.1
Hyperprolinemia (type I) (type II)
    E72.59
Hyperproteinemia E88.09
**Hyperprothrombinemia, causing
    coagulation factor deficiency**
    D68.4
Hyperpyrexia R50.9
  heat (effects) T67.01
  malignant, due to anesthetic
      T88.3
  rheumatic —see Fever, rheumatic
  unknown origin R50.9
Hyper-reflexia R29.2
Hypersalivation K11.7
Hypersecretion
  ACTH (not associated with
      Cushing's syndrome) E27.0
    pituitary E24.0
  adrenaline E27.5
  adrenomedullary E27.5
  androgen (testicular) E29.0
    ovarian (drug-induced)
        (iatrogenic) E28.1
  calcitonin E07.0
  catecholamine E27.5
  corticoadrenal E24.9
  cortisol E24.9
  epinephrine E27.5
  estrogen E28.0
  gastric K31.89
    psychogenic F45.8
  gastrin E16.4
  glucagon E16.3
  hormone(s)
    ACTH (not associated with
        Cushing's syndrome)
        E27.0
      pituitary E24.0
    antidiuretic E22.2
    growth E22.0
    intestinal NEC E34.1
    ovarian androgen E28.1
    pituitary E22.9
    testicular E29.0
    thyroid stimulating E05.80
      with thyroid storm
          E05.81
  insulin —see Hyperinsulinism
  lacrimal glands —see Epiphora
  medulloadrenal E27.5
  milk O92.6

Hypersecretion (continued)
  ovarian androgens E28.1
  salivary gland (any) K11.7
  thyrocalcitonin E07.0
  upper respiratory J39.8
**Hypersegmentation, leukocytic,
    hereditary** D72.0
**Hypersensitive, hypersensitiveness,
    hypersensitivity** —see also
    Allergy
  carotid sinus G90.01
  colon —see Irritable, colon
  drug T88.7
  gastrointestinal K52.29
    immediate K52.29
    psychogenic F45.8
  labyrinth H83.2
  pain R20.8
  pneumonitis —see Pneumonitis,
      allergic
  reaction T78.40
  upper respiratory tract NEC
      J39.3
Hypersomnia (organic) G47.10
  due to
    alcohol
      abuse F10.182
      dependence F10.282
      use F10.982
    amphetamines
      abuse F15.182
      dependence F15.282
      use F15.982
    caffeine
      abuse F15.182
      dependence F15.282
      use F15.982
    cocaine
      abuse F14.182
      dependence F14.282
      use F14.982
    drug NEC
      abuse F19.182
      dependence F19.282
      use F19.982
    medical condition G47.14
    mental disorder F51.13
    opioid
      abuse F11.182
      dependence F11.282
      use F11.982
    psychoactive substance NEC
      abuse F19.182
      dependence F19.282
      use F19.982
    sedative, hypnotic, or anxiolytic
      abuse F13.182
      dependence F13.282
      use F13.982
    stimulant NEC
      abuse F15.182
      dependence F15.282
      use F15.982
  idiopathic G47.11
    with long sleep time G47.11
    without long sleep time G47.12
  menstrual related G47.13
  nonorganic origin F51.11
    specified NEC F51.19
  not due to a substance or known
      physiological condition F51.11
    specified NEC F51.19
  primary F51.11
  recurrent G47.13
  specified NEC G47.19
Hypersplenia, hypersplenism D73.1
Hyperstimulation, ovaries
  (associated with induced ovulation)
      N98.1

Hypersusceptibility —see Allergy
Hypertelorism (ocular) (orbital) Q75.2
Hypertension, hypertensive
(accelerated) (benign) (essential)
(idiopathic) (malignant) (systemic)
I10
  with
    heart failure (congestive) I11.0
    heart involvement (conditions in
      I50.- or I51.4- I51.7, I51.89,
      I51.9 due to hypertension)
      —see Hypertension, heart
    kidney involvement —see
      Hypertension, kidney
  benign, intracranial G93.2
  borderline R03.0
  cardiorenal (disease) I13.10
    with heart failure I13.0
      with stage 1 through stage 4
        chronic kidney disease I13.0
      with stage 5 or end stage renal
        disease I13.2
    without heart failure I13.10
      with stage 1 through stage
        4 chronic kidney disease
        I13.10
      with stage 5 or end stage renal
        disease I13.11
  cardiovascular
    disease (arteriosclerotic)
      (sclerotic) —see
      Hypertension, heart
    renal (disease) —see
      Hypertension, cardiorenal
  chronic venous —see
    Hypertension, venous (chronic)
  complicating
    childbirth (labor) O16.4
      pre-existing O10.92
        with
          heart disease O12.12
            with renal disease
              O10.32
          pre-eclampsia O11.4
          renal disease O10.22
            with heart disease
              O10.32
          essential O10.02
      secondary O10.42
    pregnancy O16.-
      with edema (see also Pre-
        eclampsia) O14.9-
      gestational (pregnancy
        induced) (without
        proteinuria) O13.-
        with proteinuria O14.9-
          mild pre-eclampsia
            O14.0-
          moderate pre-eclampsia
            O14.0-
          severe pre-eclampsia
            O14.1-
            with hemolysis,
              elevated liver
              enzymes and low
              platelet count
              (HELLP) O14.2-
      pre-existing O10.91-
        with
          heart disease O10.11-
            with renal disease
              O10.31-
          pre-eclampsia —see
            category O11
          renal disease O10.21-
            with heart disease
              O10.31-
          essential O10.01-
          secondary O10.41-
          transient O13.-

Hypertension, hypertensive
(continued)
complicating (continued)
    puerperium, pre-existing O16.5
      pre-existing
        with
          heart disease O10.13
            with renal disease
              O10.33
          pre-eclampsia O11.5
          renal disease O10.23
            with heart disease
              O10.33
          essential O10.03
      pregnancy-induced O13.9
      secondary O10.43
  crisis I16.9
  due to
    endocrine disorders I15.2
    pheochromocytoma I15.2
    renal disorders NEC I15.1
      arterial I15.0
    renovascular disorders I15.0
    specified disease NEC I15.8
  emergency I16.1
  encephalopathy I67.4
  gestational (without significant
    proteinuria) (pregnancy-induced)
    (transient) O13.-
    with significant proteinuria —see
      Pre-eclampsia
    complicating
      delivery O13.4
      puerperium O13.5
  Goldblatt's I70.1
  heart (disease) (conditions in
    I51.4-I51.9 due to hypertension)
    I11.9
    with
      heart failure (congestive) I11.0
      kidney disease (chronic) —see
        Hypertension, cardiorenal
  intracranial, benign G93.2
  kidney I12.9
    with
      heart disease —see
        Hypertension, cardiorenal
      stage 5 chronic kidney disease
        (CKD) or end stage renal
        disease (ESRD) I12.0
      stage 1 through stage 4
        chronic kidney disease
        I12.9
  lesser circulation I27.0
  maternal O16.-
  newborn P29.2
    pulmonary (persistent) P29.30
  ocular H40.05-
  pancreatic duct - code to
    underlying condition
    with chronic pancreatitis K86.1
  portal (due to chronic liver disease)
    (idiopathic) K76.6
    gastropathy K31.89
    in (due to) schistosomiasis
      (bilharziasis) B65.9 [K77]
  postoperative I97.3
  psychogenic F45.8
  pulmonary I27.20
    with
      cor pulmonale (chronic)
        I27.29
        acute I26.09
      right heart ventricular strain/
        failure I27.29
        acute I26.09
      right to left shunt related to
        congenital heart disease
        I27.83
      unclear multifactorial
        mechanisms I27.29

Hypertension, hypertensive
(continued)
pulmonary (continued)
    arterial (associated) (drug-
      induced) (toxin-induced) I27.21
    chronic thromboembolic I27.24
    due to
      hematologic disorders I27.29
      kyphoscoliotic heart disease
        I27.1
      left heart disease I27.22
      lung diseases and hypoxia
        I27.23
      metabolic disorders I27.29
      specified systemic disorders
        NEC I27.29
    group 1 (associated) (drug-
      induced) (toxin-induced) I27.21
    group 2 I27.22
    group 3 I27.23
    group 4 I27.24
    group 5 I27.29
    of newborn (persistent) P29.30
    secondary
      arterial I27.21
      specified NEC I27.29
    primary (idiopathic) I27.0
  renal —see Hypertension, kidney
  renovascular I15.0
  resistant (apparent treatment)
    (treatment) (true) I1A.0
  secondary NEC I15.9
    due to
      endocrine disorders I15.2
      pheochromocytoma I15.2
      renal disorders NEC I15.1
        arterial I15.0
      renovascular disorders I15.0
      specified NEC I15.8
  transient R03.0
  of pregnancy O13.-
  urgency I16.0
  venous (chronic)
    due to
      deep vein thrombosis —see
        Syndrome, postthrombotic
    idiopathic I87.309
      with
        inflammation I87.32-
          with ulcer I87.33-
        specified complication NEC
          I87.39-
        ulcer I87.31-
          with inflammation
            I87.33-
      asymptomatic I87.30-

Hypertensive urgency —see
Hypertension

Hyperthecosis ovary E28.8

Hyperthermia (of unknown origin)
—see also Hyperpyrexia
malignant, due to anesthesia T88.3
newborn P81.9
  environmental P81.0

Hyperthyroid (recurrent) —see
Hyperthyroidism

Hyperthyroidism (latent) (pre-adult)
(recurrent) E05.90
  with
    goiter (diffuse) E05.00
      with thyroid storm E05.01
    nodular (multinodular) E05.20
      with thyroid storm E05.21
    uninodular E05.10
      with thyroid storm
        E05.11
    storm E05.91
  due to ectopic thyroid tissue E05.30
    with thyroid storm E05.31

Hyperthyroidism (continued)
  neonatal, transitory P72.1
  specified NEC E05.80
    with thyroid storm E05.81

**Hypertony, hypertonia,
hypertonicity**
  bladder N31.8
  congenital P94.1
  stomach K31.89
  psychogenic F45.8
  uterus, uterine (contractions)
    (complicating delivery)
    O62.4

Hypertrichosis L68.9
  congenital Q84.2
  eyelid H02.869
    left H02.866
      lower H02.865
      upper H02.864
    right H02.863
      lower H02.862
      upper H02.861
  lanuginosa Q84.2
    acquired L68.1
  localized L68.2
  specified NEC L68.8

Hypertriglyceridemia, essential
E78.1

Hypertrophy, hypertrophic
  adenofibromatous, prostate
    —see Enlargement, enlarged,
    prostate
  adenoids (infective) J35.2
    with tonsils J35.3
  adrenal cortex E27.8
  alveolar process or ridge —see
    Anomaly, alveolar
  anal papillae K62.89
  artery I77.89
    congenital NEC Q27.8
      digestive system Q27.8
      lower limb Q27.8
      specified site NEC Q27.8
      upper limb Q27.8
  auricular —see Hypertrophy,
    cardiac
  Bartholin's gland N75.8
  bile duct (common) (hepatic)
    K83.8
  bladder (sphincter) (trigone)
    N32.89
  bone M89.30
    carpus M89.34-
    clavicle M89.31-
    femur M89.35-
    fibula M89.36-
    finger M89.34-
    humerus M89.32-
    ilium M89.38
    ischium M89.38
    metacarpus M89.34-
    metatarsus M89.37-
    multiple sites M89.39
    neck M89.38
    pubic ramus M89.38
    radius M89.33-
    rib M89.38
    scapula M89.31-
    skull M89.38
    tarsus M89.37-
    tibia M89.36-
    toe M89.37-
    ulna M89.33-
    vertebra M89.38
  brain G93.89
  breast N62
    cystic —see Mastopathy, cystic
    newborn P83.4
    pubertal, massive N62

185

Hypertrophy, hypertrophic *(continued)*
  breast *(continued)*
    puerperal, postpartum —*see* Disorder, breast, specified type NEC
    senile (parenchymatous) N62
  cardiac (chronic) (idiopathic) I51.7
    with rheumatic fever (conditions in I00)
      active I01.8
      inactive or quiescent (with chorea) I09.89
    congenital NEC Q24.8
    fatty —*see* Degeneration, myocardial
    hypertensive —*see* Hypertension, heart
    rheumatic (with chorea) I09.89
      active or acute I01.8
        with chorea I02.0
      valve —*see* Endocarditis
  cartilage —*see* Disorder, cartilage, specified type NEC
  cecum —*see* Megacolon
  cervix (uteri) N88.8
    congenital Q51.828
    elongation N88.4
  clitoris (cirrhotic) N90.89
    congenital Q52.6
  colon —*see also* Megacolon
    congenital Q43.2
  conjunctiva, lymphoid H11.89
  corpora cavernosa N48.89
  cystic duct K82.8
  duodenum K31.89
  endometrium (glandular) *(see also* Hyperplasia, endometrial) N85.00-
    cervix N88.8
  epididymis N50.89
  esophageal hiatus (congenital) Q79.1
    with hernia —*see* Hernia, hiatal
  eyelid —*see* Disorder, eyelid, specified type NEC
  facet joint *(see also* Spondylosis) M47.819
  fat pad E65
    knee (infrapatellar) (popliteal) (prepatellar) (retropatellar) M79.4
  foot (congenital) Q74.2
  frenulum, frenum (tongue) K14.8
    lip K13.0
  gallbladder K82.8
  gastric mucosa K29.60
    with bleeding K29.61
  gland, glandular R59.9
    generalized R59.1
    localized R59.0
  gum (mucous membrane) K06.1
  heart (idiopathic) —*see also* Hypertrophy, cardiac
    valve *(see also* Endocarditis) I38
  hemifacial Q67.4
  hepatic —*see* Hypertrophy, liver
  hiatus (esophageal) Q79.1
  hilus gland R59.0
  hymen, congenital Q52.4
  ileum K63.89
  intestine NEC K63.89
  jejunum K63.89
  kidney (compensatory) N28.81
    congenital Q63.3
  labium (majus) (minus) N90.60
  ligament —*see* Disorder, ligament
  lingual tonsil (infective) J35.1
    with adenoids J35.3
  lip K13.0
    congenital Q18.6
  liver R16.0
    acute K76.89
    cirrhotic —*see* Cirrhosis, liver

Hypertrophy, hypertrophic *(continued)*
  liver *(continued)*
    congenital Q44.79
    fatty —*see* Fatty, liver
  lymph, lymphatic gland R59.9
    generalized R59.1
    localized R59.0
    tuberculous —*see* Tuberculosis, lymph gland
  mammary gland —*see* Hypertrophy, breast
  Meckel's diverticulum (congenital) Q43.0
    malignant —*see* Table of Neoplasms, small intestine, malignant
  median bar —*see* Hyperplasia, prostate
  meibomian gland —*see* Chalazion
  meniscus, knee, congenital Q74.1
  metatarsal head —*see* Hypertrophy, bone, metatarsus
  metatarsus —*see* Hypertrophy, bone, metatarsus
  mucous membrane
    alveolar ridge K06.2
    gum K06.1
    nose (turbinate) J34.3
  muscle M62.89
  muscular coat, artery I77.89
  myocardium —*see also* Hypertrophy, cardiac
    idiopathic I42.2
  myometrium N85.2
  nail L60.2
    congenital Q84.5
  nasal J34.89
    alae J34.89
    bone J34.89
    cartilage J34.89
    mucous membrane (septum) J34.3
    sinus J34.89
    turbinate J34.3
  nasopharynx, lymphoid (infectional) (tissue) (wall) J35.2
  nipple N62
  organ or site, congenital NEC —*see* Anomaly, by site
  ovary N83.8
  palate (hard) M27.8
    soft K13.79
  pancreas, congenital Q45.3
  parathyroid (gland) E21.0
  parotid gland K11.1
  penis N48.89
  pharyngeal tonsil J35.2
  pharynx J39.2
    lymphoid (infectional) (tissue) (wall) J35.2
  pituitary (anterior) (fossa) (gland) E23.6
  prepuce (congenital) N47.8
    female N90.89
  prostate —*see* Enlargement, enlarged, prostate
    congenital Q55.4
  pseudomuscular *(see also* Dystrophy, muscular, by type, if applicable) G71.09
  pylorus (adult) (muscle) (sphincter) K31.1
    congenital or infantile Q40.0
  rectal, rectum (sphincter) K62.89
  rhinitis (turbinate) J31.0
  salivary gland (any) K11.1
    congenital Q38.4
  scaphoid (tarsal) —*see* Hypertrophy, bone, tarsus
  scar L91.0
  scrotum N50.89

Hypertrophy, hypertrophic *(continued)*
  seminal vesicle N50.89
  sigmoid —*see* Megacolon
  skin L91.9
    specified NEC L91.8
  spermatic cord N50.89
  spleen —*see* Splenomegaly
  spondylitis —*see* Spondylosis
  stomach K31.89
  sublingual gland K11.1
  submandibular gland K11.1
  suprarenal cortex (gland) E27.8
  synovial NEC M67.20
    acromioclavicular M67.21-
    ankle M67.27-
    elbow M67.22-
    foot M67.27-
    hand M67.24-
    hip M67.25-
    knee M67.26-
    multiple sites M67.29
    specified site NEC M67.28
    wrist M67.23-
  tendon —*see* Disorder, tendon, specified type NEC
  testis N44.8
    congenital Q55.29
  thymic, thymus (gland) (congenital) E32.0
  thyroid (gland) —*see* Goiter
  toe (congenital) Q74.2
    acquired —*see also* Deformity, toe, specified NEC
  tongue K14.8
    congenital Q38.2
    papillae (foliate) K14.3
  tonsils (faucial) (infective) (lingual) (lymphoid) J35.1
    with adenoids J35.3
  tunica vaginalis N50.89
  ureter N28.89
  urethra N36.8
  uterus N85.2
    neck (with elongation) N88.4
    puerperal O90.89
  uvula K13.79
  vagina N89.8
  vas deferens N50.89
  vein I87.8
  ventricle, ventricular (heart) —*see also* Hypertrophy, cardiac
    congenital Q24.8
    in tetralogy of Fallot Q21.3
  verumontanum N36.8
  vocal cord J38.3
  vulva N90.60
    stasis (nonfilarial) N90.69
Hypertropia H50.2-
Hypertyrosinemia E70.21
Hyperuricemia (asymptomatic) E79.0
Hyperuricosuria R82.993
Hypervalinemia E71.19
Hyperventilation (tetany) R06.4
  hysterical F45.8
  psychogenic F45.8
  syndrome F45.8
Hypervitaminosis (dietary) NEC E67.8
  A E67.0
    administered as drug (prolonged intake) —*see* Table of Drugs and Chemicals, vitamins, adverse effect
    overdose or wrong substance given or taken —*see* Table of Drugs and Chemicals, vitamins, poisoning
  B6 E67.2

Hypervitaminosis *(continued)*
  D E67.3
    administered as drug (prolonged intake) —*see* Table of Drugs and Chemicals, vitamins, adverse effect
    overdose or wrong substance given or taken —*see* Table of Drugs and Chemicals, vitamins, poisoning
  K E67.8
    administered as drug (prolonged intake) —*see* Table of Drugs and Chemicals, vitamins, adverse effect
    overdose or wrong substance given or taken —*see* Table of Drugs and Chemicals, vitamins, poisoning
Hypervolemia E87.70
  specified NEC E87.79
Hypesthesia R20.1
  cornea —*see* Anesthesia, cornea
Hyphema H21.0-
  traumatic S05.1-
Hypoacidity, gastric K31.89
  psychogenic F45.8
Hypoadrenalism, hypoadrenia E27.40
  primary E27.1
  tuberculous A18.7
Hypoadrenocorticism E27.40
  pituitary E23.0
  primary E27.1
Hypoalbuminemia E88.09
Hypoaldosteronism E27.40
Hypoalphalipoproteinemia E78.6
Hypobarism T70.29
Hypobaropathy T70.29
Hypobetalipoproteinemia (familial) E78.6
Hypocalcemia E83.51
  autosomal dominant E20.810
    type 1 (ADH1) E20.810
    type 2 (ADH2) E20.810
  dietary E58
  neonatal P71.1
    due to cow's milk P71.0
  phosphate-loading (newborn) P71.1
Hypochloremia E87.8
Hypochlorhydria K31.89
  neurotic F45.8
  psychogenic F45.8
Hypochondria, hypochondriac, hypochondriasis (reaction) F45.21
  sleep F51.03
Hypochondrogenesis Q77.0
Hypochondroplasia Q77.4
Hypochromasia, blood cells D50.8
Hypocitraturia R82.991
Hypodontia —*see* Anodontia
Hypoeosinophilia D72.89
Hypoesthesia R20.1
Hypofibrinogenemia D68.8
  acquired D65
  congenital (hereditary) D68.2
Hypofunction
  adrenocortical E27.40
    drug-induced E27.3
    postprocedural E89.6
    primary E27.1
  adrenomedullary, postprocedural E89.6
  cerebral R29.818

Hypofunction *(continued)*
  corticoadrenal NEC E27.40
  intestinal K59.89
  labyrinth H83.2
  ovary E28.39
  pituitary (gland) (anterior) E23.0
  testicular E29.1
    postprocedural (postsurgical) (postirradiation) (iatrogenic) E89.5
Hypogalactia O92.4
Hypogammaglobulinemia *(see also* Agammaglobulinemia) D80.1
  hereditary D80.0
  nonfamilial D80.1
  transient, of infancy D80.7
Hypogenitalism *(congenital)* —*see* Hypogonadism
Hypoglossia Q38.3
Hypoglycemia *(spontaneous)* E16.2
  coma E15
    diabetic —*see* Diabetes, by type, with hypoglycemia, with coma
  diabetic —*see* Diabetes, hypoglycemia
  dietary counseling and surveillance Z71.3
  drug-induced E16.0
    with coma (nondiabetic) E15
  due to insulin E16.0
    with coma (nondiabetic) E15
      therapeutic misadventure —*see* subcategory T38.3
  functional, nonhyperinsulinemic E16.1
  iatrogenic E16.0
    with coma (nondiabetic) E15
Hypoglycemia *(continued)*
  in infant of diabetic mother P70.1
    gestational diabetes P70.0
  infantile E16.1
  leucine-induced E71.19
  neonatal (transitory) P70.4
    iatrogenic P70.3
  reactive (not drug-induced) E16.1
  transitory neonatal P70.4
Hypogonadism
  female E28.39
  hypogonadotropic E23.0
  male E29.1
  ovarian (primary) E28.39
  pituitary E23.0
  testicular (primary) E29.1
Hypohidrosis, hypoidrosis L74.4
Hypoinsulinemia, postprocedural E89.1
Hypokalemia E87.6
Hypoleukocytosis —*see* Agranulocytosis
Hypolipoproteinemia *(alpha) (beta)* E78.6
Hypomagnesemia E83.42
  neonatal P71.2
Hypomania, hypomanic reaction F30.8
Hypomenorrhea —*see* Oligomenorrhea
Hypometabolism R63.8
Hypomotility
  gastrointestinal (tract) K31.89
    psychogenic F45.8
  intestine K59.89
    psychogenic F45.8
  stomach K31.89
    psychogenic F45.8

Hypomyelination - hypogonadotropic hypogonadism - hypodontia G11.5
Hypomyelination with atrophy of the basal ganglia and cerebellum (H-ABC) G23.3
Hyponasality R49.22
Hyponatremia E87.1
Hypo-osmolality E87.1
Hypo-ovarianism, hypo-ovarism E28.39
Hypoparathyroidism E20.9
  autoimmune E20.812
  due to impaired parathyroid hormone secretion, unspecified E20.819
  familial E20.89
    isolated E20.818
  idiopathic E20.0
  neonatal, transitory P71.4
  postprocedural E89.2
  secondary, in diseases classified elsewhere E20.811
  specified NEC E20.89
    due to impaired parathyroid hormone secretion E20.818
Hypoperfusion *(in)*
  newborn P96.89
Hypopharyngitis —*see* Laryngopharyngitis
Hypophoria H50.53
Hypophosphatemia, hypophosphatasia *(acquired) (congenital) (renal)* E83.39
  familial E83.31
Hypophyseal, hypophysis —*see also* condition
  dwarfism E23.0
  gigantism E22.0
Hypopiesis —*see* Hypotension
Hypopinealism E34.8
Hypopituitarism *(juvenile)* E23.0
  drug-induced E23.1
  due to
    hypophysectomy E89.3
    radiotherapy E89.3
  iatrogenic NEC E23.1
  postirradiation E89.3
  postpartum O99.285
  postprocedural E89.3
Hypoplasia, hypoplastic
  adrenal (gland), congenital Q89.1
  alimentary tract, congenital Q45.8
    upper Q40.8
  anus, anal (canal) Q42.3
    with fistula Q42.2
  aorta, aortic Q25.42
    ascending, in hypoplastic left heart syndrome Q23.4
    valve Q23.1
      in hypoplastic left heart syndrome Q23.4
  areola, congenital Q83.8
  arm (congenital) —*see* Defect, reduction, upper limb
  artery (peripheral) Q27.8
    brain (congenital) Q28.3
    coronary Q24.5
    digestive system Q27.8
    lower limb Q27.8
    pulmonary Q25.79
      functional, unilateral J43.0
    retinal (congenital) Q14.1
    specified site NEC Q27.8
    umbilical Q27.0
    upper limb Q27.8

Hypoplasia, hypoplastic *(continued)*
  auditory canal Q17.8
    causing impairment of hearing Q16.9
  biliary duct or passage Q44.5
  bone NOS Q79.9
    face Q75.8
    marrow D61.9
      megakaryocytic D69.49
    skull —*see* Hypoplasia, skull
  brain Q02
    gyri Q04.3
    part of Q04.3
  breast (areola) N64.82
  bronchus Q32.4
  cardiac Q24.8
  carpus —*see* Defect, reduction, upper limb, specified type NEC
  cartilage hair Q78.8
  cecum Q42.8
  cementum K00.4
  cephalic Q02
  cerebellum Q04.3
  cervix (uteri), congenital Q51.821
  clavicle (congenital) Q74.0
  coccyx Q76.49
  colon Q42.9
    specified NEC Q42.8
  corpus callosum Q04.0
  cricoid cartilage Q31.2
  digestive organ(s) or tract NEC Q45.8
    upper (congenital) Q40.8
  ear (auricle) (lobe) Q17.2
    middle Q16.4
  enamel of teeth (neonatal) (postnatal) (prenatal) K00.4
  endocrine (gland) NEC Q89.2
  endometrium N85.8
  epididymis (congenital) Q55.4
  epiglottis Q31.2
  erythroid, congenital D61.01
  esophagus (congenital) Q39.8
  eustachian tube Q17.8
  eye Q11.2
  eyelid (congenital) Q10.3
  face Q18.8
    bone(s) Q75.8
  femur (congenital) —*see* Defect, reduction, lower limb, specified type NEC
  fibula (congenital) —*see* Defect, reduction, lower limb, specified type NEC
  finger (congenital) —*see* Defect, reduction, upper limb, specified type NEC
  focal dermal Q82.8
  foot —*see* Defect, reduction, lower limb, specified type NEC
  gallbladder Q44.0
  genitalia, genital organ(s)
    female, congenital Q52.8
      external Q52.79
      internal NEC Q52.8
    in adiposogenital dystrophy E23.6
  glottis Q31.2
  hair Q84.2
  hand (congenital) —*see* Defect, reduction, upper limb, specified type NEC
  heart Q24.8
  humerus (congenital) —*see* Defect, reduction, upper limb, specified type NEC
  intestine (small) Q41.9
    large Q42.9
      specified NEC Q42.8

Hypoplasia, hypoplastic *(continued)*
  jaw M26.09
    alveolar M26.79
    lower M26.04
      alveolar M26.74
    upper M26.02
      alveolar M26.73
  kidney(s) Q60.5
    bilateral Q60.4
    unilateral Q60.3
  labium (majus) (minus), congenital Q52.79
  larynx Q31.2
  left heart syndrome Q23.4
  leg (congenital) —*see* Defect, reduction, lower limb
  limb Q73.8
    lower (congenital) —*see* Defect, reduction, lower limb
    upper (congenital) —*see* Defect, reduction, upper limb
  liver Q44.79
  lung (lobe) (not associated with short gestation) Q33.6
    associated with immaturity, low birth weight, prematurity, or short gestation P28.0
  mammary (areola), congenital Q83.8
  mandible, mandibular M26.04
    alveolar M26.74
    unilateral condylar M27.8
  maxillary M26.02
    alveolar M26.73
  medullary D61.9
  megakaryocytic D69.49
  metacarpus —*see* Defect, reduction, upper limb, specified type NEC
  metatarsus —*see* Defect, reduction, lower limb, specified type NEC
  muscle Q79.8
  nail(s) Q84.6
  nose, nasal Q30.1
  optic nerve H47.03-
  osseous meatus (ear) Q17.8
  ovary, congenital Q50.39
  pancreas Q45.0
  parathyroid (gland) Q89.2
  parotid gland Q38.4
  patella Q74.1
  pelvis, pelvic girdle Q74.2
  penis (congenital) Q55.62
  peripheral vascular system Q27.8
    digestive system Q27.8
    lower limb Q27.8
    specified site NEC Q27.8
    upper limb Q27.8
  pituitary (gland) (congenital) Q89.2
  pulmonary (not associated with short gestation) Q33.6
    artery, functional J43.0
    associated with short gestation P28.0
  radioulnar —*see* Defect, reduction, upper limb, specified type NEC
  radius —*see* Defect, reduction, upper limb
  rectum Q42.1
    with fistula Q42.0
  respiratory system NEC Q34.8
  rib Q76.6
  right heart syndrome Q22.6
  sacrum Q76.49
  scapula Q74.0
  scrotum Q55.1
  shoulder girdle Q74.0
  skin Q82.8
  skull (bone) Q75.8
    with
      anencephaly Q00.0

Hypoplasia, hypoplastic (continued)
  skull (continued)
    with (continued)
      encephalocele —see Encephalocele
      hydrocephalus Q03.9
        with spina bifida —see Spina bifida, by site, with hydrocephalus
      microcephaly Q02
  spinal (cord) (ventral horn cell) Q06.1
  spine Q76.49
  sternum Q76.7
  tarsus —see Defect, reduction, lower limb, specified type NEC
  testis Q55.1
  thymic, with immunodeficiency D82.1
  thymus (gland) Q89.2
    with immunodeficiency D82.1
  thyroid (gland) E03.1
    cartilage Q31.2
  tibiofibular (congenital) —see Defect, reduction, lower limb, specified type NEC
  toe —see Defect, reduction, lower limb, specified type NEC
  tongue Q38.3
  Turner's K00.4
  ulna (congenital) —see Defect, reduction, upper limb
  umbilical artery Q27.0
  unilateral condylar M27.8
  ureter Q62.8
  uterus, congenital Q51.811
  vagina Q52.4
  vascular NEC peripheral Q27.8
    brain Q28.3
    digestive system Q27.8
    lower limb Q27.8
    specified site NEC Q27.8
    upper limb Q27.8
  vein(s) (peripheral) Q27.8
    brain Q28.3
    digestive system Q27.8
    great Q26.8
    lower limb Q27.8
    specified site NEC Q27.8
    upper limb Q27.8
  vena cava (inferior) (superior) Q26.8
  vertebra Q76.49
  vulva, congenital Q52.79
  zonule (ciliary) Q12.8
Hypoplasminogenemia E88.02
Hypopnea, obstructive sleep apnea G47.33
Hypopotassemia E87.6
Hypoproconvertinemia, congenital (hereditary) D68.2
Hypoproteinemia E77.8
Hypoprothrombinemia (congenital) (hereditary) (idiopathic) D68.2
  acquired D68.4
  newborn, transient P61.6
Hypoptyalism K11.7
Hypopyon (eye) (anterior chamber) —see Iridocyclitis, acute, hypopyon
Hypopyrexia R68.0
Hyporeflexia R29.2
Hyposecretion
  ACTH E23.0
  antidiuretic hormone E23.2
  ovary E28.39
  salivary gland (any) K11.7
  vasopressin E23.2

Hyposegmentation, leukocytic, hereditary D72.0
Hyposiderinemia D50.9
Hypospadias Q54.9
  balanic Q54.0
  coronal Q54.0
  glandular Q54.0
  penile Q54.1
  penoscrotal Q54.2
  perineal Q54.3
  specified NEC Q54.8
Hypospermatogenesis —see Oligospermia
Hyposplenism D73.0
Hypostasis pulmonary, passive —see Edema, lung
Hypostatic —see condition
Hyposthenuria N28.89
Hypotension (arterial) (constitutional) I95.9
  chronic I95.89
  due to (of) hemodialysis I95.3
  drug-induced I95.2
  iatrogenic I95.89
  idiopathic (permanent) I95.0
  intracranial G96.810
    following
      lumbar cerebrospinal fluid shunting G97.83
      specified procedure NEC G97.84
      ventricular shunting (ventriculostomy) G97.2
    specified NEC G96.819
    spontaneous G96.811
  intra-dialytic I95.3
  maternal, syndrome (following labor and delivery) O26.5-
  neurogenic, orthostatic G90.3
  orthostatic (chronic) I95.1
    due to drugs I95.2
    neurogenic G90.3
  postoperative I95.81
  postural I95.1
  specified NEC I95.89
Hypothermia (accidental) T68
  due to anesthesia, anesthetic T88.51
  low environmental temperature T68
  neonatal P80.9
    environmental (mild) NEC P80.8
    mild P80.8
    severe (chronic) (cold injury syndrome) P80.0
    specified NEC P80.8
  not associated with low environmental temperature R68.0
Hypothyroidism (acquired) E03.9
  autoimmune —see Thyroiditis, autoimmune
  congenital (without goiter) E03.1
    with goiter (diffuse) E03.0
  due to
    exogenous substance NEC E03.2
    iodine-deficiency, acquired E01.8
      subclinical E02
    irradiation therapy E89.0
    medicament NEC E03.2
    P-aminosalicylic acid (PAS) E03.2
    phenylbutazone E03.2
    resorcinol E03.2
    sulfonamide E03.2
    surgery E89.0
    thiourea group drugs E03.2
  iatrogenic NEC E03.2
  iodine-deficiency (acquired) E01.8
    congenital —see Syndrome, iodine- deficiency, congenital
    subclinical E02

Hypothyroidism (continued)
  neonatal, transitory P72.2
  postinfectious E03.3
  postirradiation E89.0
  postprocedural E89.0
  postsurgical E89.0
  specified NEC E03.8
  subclinical, iodine-deficiency related E02
Hypotonia, hypotonicity, hypotony
  bladder N31.2
  congenital (benign) P94.2
  eye —see Disorder, globe, hypotony
Hypotrichosis —see Alopecia
Hypotropia H50.2-
Hypoventilation R06.89
  congenital central alveolar G47.35
  sleep related
    idiopathic nonobstructive alveolar G47.34
    in conditions classified elsewhere G47.36
Hypovitaminosis —see Deficiency, vitamin
Hypovolemia E86.1
  surgical shock T81.19
  traumatic (shock) T79.4
Hypoxemia R09.02
  newborn P84
  sleep related, in conditions classified elsewhere G47.36
Hypoxia (see also Anoxia) R09.02
  cerebral, during a procedure NEC G97.81
    postprocedural NEC G97.82
  intrauterine P84
  myocardial —see Insufficiency, coronary
  newborn P84
  sleep-related G47.34
Hypsarhythmia —see Epilepsy, generalized, specified NEC
Hysteralgia, pregnant uterus O26.89-
Hysteria, hysterical (conversion) (dissociative state) F44.9
  anxiety F41.8
  convulsions F44.5
  psychosis, acute F44.9
Hysteroepilepsy F44.5

I

IBDU (colonic inflammatory bowel disease unclassified) K52.3
ICANS (immune effector cell-associated neurotoxicity syndrome) —see Syndrome, immue effector cell-associated neurotoxicity
Ichthyoparasitism due to Vandellia cirrhosa B88.8
Ichthyosis (congenital) Q80.9
  acquired L85.0
  fetalis Q80.4
  hystrix Q80.8
  lamellar Q80.2
  lingual K13.29
  palmaris and plantaris Q82.8
  simplex Q80.0
  vera Q80.8
  vulgaris Q80.0
  X-linked Q80.1
Ichthyotoxism —see Poisoning, fish
  bacterial —see Intoxication, foodborne

Icteroanemia, hemolytic (acquired) D59.9
  congenital —see Spherocytosis
Icterus —see also Jaundice
  conjunctiva R17
  newborn P59.9
  gravis, newborn P55.0
  hematogenous (acquired) D59.9
  hemolytic (acquired) D59.9
    congenital —see Spherocytosis
  hemorrhagic (acute) (leptospiral) (spirochetal) A27.0
    newborn P53
  infectious B15.9
    with hepatic coma B15.0
    leptospiral A27.0
    spirochetal A27.0
  neonatorum —see Jaundice, newborn
  spirochetal A27.0
Ictus solaris, solis T67.01
Ideation
  homicidal R45.850
  suicidal R45.851
Identity disorder (child) F64.9
  gender role F64.2
  psychosexual F64.2
Id reaction (due to bacteria) L30.2
Idioglossia F80.0
Idiopathic —see condition
Idiot, idiocy (congenital) F73
  amaurotic (Bielschowsky (-Jansky)) (family) (infantile (late)) (juvenile (late)) (Vogt-Spielmeyer) E75.4
  microcephalic Q02
IgE asthma J45.909
IIAC (idiopathic infantile arterial calcification) Q28.8
Ileitis (chronic) (noninfectious) —see also Enteritis K52.9
  backwash —see Pancolitis, ulcerative (chronic)
  infectious A09
  regional (ulcerative) —see Enteritis, regional, small intestine
  segmental —see Enteritis, regional
  terminal (ulcerative) —see Enteritis, regional, small intestine
Ileocolitis (see also Enteritis) K52.9
  regional —see Enteritis, regional
  infectious A09
  ulcerative K51.0-
Ileostomy
  attention to Z43.2
  malfunctioning K94.13
  status Z93.2
  with complication —see Complications, enterostomy
Ileotyphus —see Typhoid
Ileum —see condition
Ileus (bowel) (colon) (inhibitory) (intestine) K56.7
  adynamic K56.0
  due to gallstone (in intestine) K56.3
  duodenal (chronic) K31.5
  gallstone K56.3
  mechanical NEC (see also Obstruction, intestine, specified NEC) K56.699
  meconium P76.0
    in cystic fibrosis E84.11
    meaning meconium plug (without cystic fibrosis) P76.0

Ileus (continued)
  myxedema K59.89
  neurogenic K56.0
    Hirschsprung's disease or megacolon Q43.1
  newborn
    due to meconium P76.0
      in cystic fibrosis E84.11
      meaning meconium plug (without cystic fibrosis) P76.0
    transitory P76.1
  obstructive (see also Obstruction, intestine, specified NEC) K56.699
  paralytic K56.0
  postoperative K91.89
Iliac —see condition
Iliotibial band syndrome M76.3-
Illiteracy Z55.0
  health Z55.6
Illness (see also Disease) R69
  manic-depressive —see Disorder, bipolar
Imbalance R26.89
  autonomic G90.8
  constituents of food intake E63.1
  electrolyte E87.8
    with
      abortion —see Abortion by type, complicated by, electrolyte imbalance
      molar pregnancy O08.5
    due to hyperemesis gravidarum O21.1
    following ectopic or molar pregnancy O08.5
    neonatal, transitory NEC P74.49
      potassium
        hyperkalemia P74.31
        hypokalemia P74.32
      sodium
        hypernatremia P74.21
        hyponatremia P74.22
  endocrine E34.9
  eye muscle NOS H50.9
  hormone E34.9
  hysterical F44.4
  labyrinth H83.2
  posture R29.3
  protein-energy —see Malnutrition
  sympathetic G90.8
Imbecile, imbecility (I.Q.35-49) F71
Imbedding, intrauterine device T83.39
Imbibition, cholesterol (gallbladder) K82.4
Imbrication, teeth,, fully erupted M26.30
Imerslund (-Gräsbeck) **syndrome** D51.1
Immature —see also Immaturity
  birth (less than 37 completed weeks) —see Preterm, newborn
    extremely (less than 28 completed weeks) —see Immaturity, extreme
  personality F60.89
Immaturity (less than 37 completed weeks) —see also Preterm, newborn
  extreme of newborn (less than 28 completed weeks of gestation) (less than 196 completed days of gestation) (unspecified weeks of gestation) P07.20

Immaturity (continued)
  extreme of newborn (continued)
    gestational age
      23 completed weeks (23 weeks, 0 days through 23 weeks, 6 days) P07.22
      24 completed weeks (24 weeks, 0 days through 24 weeks, 6 days) P07.23
      25 completed weeks (25 weeks, 0 days through 25 weeks, 6 days) P07.24
      26 completed weeks (26 weeks, 0 days through 26 weeks, 6 days) P07.25
      27 completed weeks (27 weeks, 0 days through 27 weeks, 6 days) P07.26
      less than 23 completed weeks P07.21
  fetus or infant light-for-dates —see Light-for-dates
  lung, newborn P28.0
  organ or site NEC —see Hypoplasia
  pulmonary, newborn P28.0
  reaction F60.89
  sexual (female) (male), after puberty E30.0
Immersion T75.1
  hand T69.01-
  foot T69.02-
Immobile, immobility
  complete, due to severe physical disability or frailty R53.2
  intestine K59.89
  syndrome (paraplegic) M62.3
Immune reconstitution (inflammatory) **syndrome [IRIS]** D89.3
Immunization —see also Vaccination
  ABO —see Incompatibility, ABO in newborn P55.1
  appropriate for age
    child (over 28 days old) Z00.129
      with abnormal findings Z00.121
  complication —see Complications, vaccination
  encounter for Z23
  not done (not carried out) -see also Underimmunization status Z28.9
    because (of)
      acute illness of patient Z28.01
      allergy to vaccine (or component) Z28.04
      caregiver refusal Z28.82
      chronic illness of patient Z28.02
      contraindication NEC Z28.09
      delay in delivery of vaccine Z28.83
      group pressure Z28.1
      guardian refusal Z28.82
      immune compromised state of patient Z28.03
      lack of availability of vaccine Z28.83
      manufacturer delay of vaccine Z28.83
      parent refusal Z28.82
      patient's belief Z28.1
      patient had disease being vaccinated against Z28.81
      patient refusal Z28.21
      religious beliefs of patient Z28.1
      specified reason NEC Z28.89
        of patient Z28.29
      unavailability of vaccine Z28.83
      unspecified patient reason Z28.20

Immunization (continued)
  partial -see also Underimmunization status for COVID-19 Z28.311
  Rh factor
    affecting management of pregnancy NEC O36.09-
      anti-D antibody O36.01-
    from transfusion —see Complication(s), transfusion, incompatibility reaction, Rh (factor)
Immunocompromised NOS D84.9
Immunocytoma C83.0-
Immunodeficiency D84.9
  with
    adenosine-deaminase deficiency (see also Deficiency, adenosine deaminase) D81.30
    antibody defects D80.9
      specified type NEC D80.8
    hyperimmunoglobulinemia D80.6
    increased immunoglobulin M (IgM) D80.5
    major defect D82.9
      specified type NEC D82.8
    partial albinism D82.8
    short-limbed stature D82.2
    thrombocytopenia and eczema D82.0
  antibody with
    hyperimmunoglobulinemia D80.6
    near-normal immunoglobulins D80.6
  autosomal recessive, Swiss type D80.0
  combined D81.9
    biotin-dependent carboxylase D81.819
      biotinidase D81.810
      holocarboxylase synthetase D81.818
      specified type NEC D81.818
    severe (SCID) D81.9
      with
        low or normal B-cell numbers D81.2
        low T- and B-cell numbers D81.1
        reticular dysgenesis D81.0
    specified type NEC D81.89
  common variable D83.9
    with
      abnormalities of B-cell numbers and function D83.0
      autoantibodies to B- or T-cells D83.2
      immunoregulatory T-cell disorders D83.1
    specified type NEC D83.8
  due to
    conditions classified elsewhere D84.81
    drugs D84.821
    external causes D84.822
    medication (current or past) D84.821
  following hereditary defective response to Epstein-Barr virus (EBV) D82.3
  selective, immunoglobulin
    A (IgA) D80.2
    G (IgG) (subclasses) D80.3
    M (IgM) D80.4
  severe combined (SCID) D81.9
    due to adenosine deaminase deficiency D81.31
  specified type NEC D84.89
  X-linked, with increased IgM D80.5
Immunodeficient NOS D84.9

Immunosuppressed NOS D84.9
Immunotherapy (encounter for)
  antineoplastic Z51.12
Impaction, impacted
  bowel, colon, rectum (see also Impaction, fecal) K56.49
    by gallstone K56.3
  calculus —see Calculus
  cerumen (ear) (external) H61.2-
  cuspid —see Impaction, tooth
  dental (same or adjacent tooth) K01.1
  fecal, feces K56.41
  fracture —see Fracture, by site
  gallbladder —see Calculus, gallbladder
  gallstone(s) —see Calculus, gallbladder
    bile duct (common) (hepatic) —see Calculus, bile duct
    cystic duct —see Calculus, gallbladder
    in intestine, with obstruction (any part) K56.3
  intestine (calculous) NEC —see also Impaction, fecal K56.49
    gallstone, with ileus K56.3
  intrauterine device (IUD) T83.39
  molar —see Impaction, tooth
  shoulder, causing obstructed labor O66.0
  tooth, teeth K01.1
  turbinate J34.89
Impaired, impairment (function)
  auditory discrimination —see Abnormal, auditory perception
  cognitive, mild, of uncertain or unknown etiology G31.84
  dual sensory Z73.82
  fasting glucose R73.01
  glucose tolerance (oral) R73.02
  hearing —see Deafness
  heart —see Disease, heart
  kidney N28.9
    disorder resulting from N25.9
    specified NEC N25.89
  liver K72.90
    with coma K72.91
  mastication K08.89
  mild cognitive G31.84
    of uncertain or unknown etiology G31.84
  mild neurocognitive
    due to known physiological condition (without behavioral disturbance) F06.70
      with behavioral disturbance F06.71
  mobility
    ear ossicles —see Ankylosis, ear ossicles
    requiring care provider Z74.09
  myocardium, myocardial —see Insufficiency, myocardial
  rectal sphincter R19.8
  renal (acute) (chronic) N28.9
    disorder resulting from N25.9
    specified NEC N25.89
  vision NEC H54.7
    both eyes H54.3
Impediment, speech (see also Disorder, speech) R47.9
  psychogenic (childhood) F98.8
  slurring R47.81
  specified NEC R47.89
Impending
  coronary syndrome I20.0
  delirium tremens F10.239
  myocardial infarction I20.0

Imperception auditory (acquired)
—see also Deafness
congenital H93.25

Imperfect
aeration, lung (newborn) NEC
—see Atelectasis
closure (congenital)
  alimentary tract NEC Q45.8
    lower Q43.8
    upper Q40.8
  atrioventricular ostium Q21.20
  atrium (secundum) Q21.11
  branchial cleft NOS Q18.2
    cyst Q18.0
    fistula Q18.0
    sinus Q18.0
  choroid Q14.3
  cricoid cartilage Q31.8
  cusps, heart valve NEC Q24.8
    pulmonary Q22.3
  ductus
    arteriosus Q25.0
    Botalli Q25.0
  ear drum (causing impairment of hearing) Q16.4
  esophagus with communication to bronchus or trachea Q39.1
  eyelid Q10.3
  foramen
    botalli Q21.12
    ovale Q21.12
  genitalia, genital organ(s) or system
    female Q52.8
      external Q52.79
      internal NEC Q52.8
    male Q55.8
  glottis Q31.8
  interatrial ostium or septum Q21.19
  interauricular ostium or septum Q21.19
  interventricular ostium or septum Q21.0
  larynx Q31.8
  lip —see Cleft, lip
  nasal septum Q30.3
  nose Q30.2
  omphalomesenteric duct Q43.0
  optic nerve entry Q14.2
  organ or site not listed —see Anomaly, by site
  ostium
    interatrial Q21.19
    interauricular Q21.19
    interventricular Q21.0
  palate —see Cleft, palate
  preauricular sinus Q18.1
  retina Q14.1
  roof of orbit Q75.8
  sclera Q13.5
  septum
    aorticopulmonary Q21.4
    atrial (secundum) Q21.19
    between aorta and pulmonary artery Q21.4
    heart Q21.9
    interatrial (secundum) Q21.19
    interauricular (secundum) Q21.19
    interventricular Q21.0
      in tetralogy of Fallot Q21.3
    nasal Q30.3
    ventricular Q21.0
      with pulmonary stenosis or atresia, dextraposition of aorta, and hypertrophy of right ventricle Q21.3
      in tetralogy of Fallot Q21.3

Imperfect (continued)
closure (continued)
  skull Q75.009
    with
      anencephaly Q00.0
      encephalocele —see Encephalocele
      hydrocephalus Q03.9
        with spina bifida —see Spina bifida, by site, with hydrocephalus
      microcephaly Q02
  spine (with meningocele) —see Spina bifida
  trachea Q32.1
  tympanic membrane (causing impairment of hearing) Q16.4
  uterus Q51.818
  vitelline duct Q43.0
erection —see Dysfunction, sexual, male, erectile
fusion —see Imperfect, closure
inflation, lung (newborn) —see Atelectasis
posture R29.3
rotation, intestine Q43.3
septum, ventricular Q21.0

Imperfectly descended testis —see Cryptorchid

Imperforate (congenital) —see also Atresia
anus Q42.3
  with fistula Q42.2
cervix (uteri) Q51.828
esophagus Q39.0
  with tracheoesophageal fistula Q39.1
hymen Q52.3
jejunum Q41.1
pharynx Q38.8
rectum Q42.1
  with fistula Q42.0
urethra Q64.39
vagina Q52.4

Impervious (congenital) —see also Atresia
anus Q42.3
  with fistula Q42.2
bile duct Q44.2
esophagus Q39.0
  with tracheoesophageal fistula Q39.1
intestine (small) Q41.9
  large Q42.9
    specified NEC Q42.8
rectum Q42.1
  with fistula Q42.0
ureter —see Atresia, ureter
urethra Q64.39

Impetiginization of dermatoses L01.1

Impetigo (any organism) (any site) (circinate) (contagiosa) (simplex) (vulgaris) L01.00
Bockhart's L01.02
bullous, bullosa L01.03
external ear L01.00 [H62.40]
follicularis L01.02
furfuracea L30.5
herpetiformis L40.1
  nonobstetrical L40.1
neonatorum L01.03
nonbullous L01.01
specified type NEC L01.09
ulcerative L01.09

Impingement (on teeth)
joint —see Disorder, joint, specified type NEC
soft tissue
  anterior M26.81
  posterior M26.82

Implant, endometrial N80.9

Implantation
anomalous —see Anomaly, by site
  ureter Q62.63
cyst
  external area or site (skin) NEC L72.0
  iris —see Cyst, iris, implantation
  vagina N89.8
  vulva N90.7
dermoid (cyst) —see Implantation, cyst

Impotence (sexual) N52.9
counseling Z70.1
organic origin (see also Dysfunction, sexual, male, erectile) N52.9
psychogenic F52.21

Impression, basilar Q75.8

Imprisonment, anxiety concerning Z65.1

Improper care (child) (newborn) —see Maltreatment

Improperly tied umbilical cord (causing hemorrhage) P51.8

Impulsiveness (impulsive) R45.87

Inability to
comply with dietary regimen Z91.118
swallow —see Aphagia

Inaccessible, inaccessibility
health care NEC Z75.3
  due to
    waiting period Z75.2
      for admission to facility elsewhere Z75.1
    other helping agencies Z75.4
    transportation Z59.82

Inactive —see condition

Inadequate, inadequacy
aesthetics of dental restoration K08.56
biologic, constitutional, functional, or social F60.7
development
  child R62.50
  genitalia
    after puberty NEC E30.0
    congenital
      female Q52.8
        external Q52.79
        internal Q52.8
      male Q55.8
  lungs Q33.6
    associated with short gestation P28.0
  organ or site not listed —see Anomaly, by site
diet (causing nutritional deficiency) E63.9
drinking-water supply Z58.6
eating habits Z72.4
environment, household Z59.11
family support Z63.8
food (supply) NEC Z59.48
  hunger effects T73.0
functional F60.7
household care, due to
  family member
    handicapped or ill Z74.2
    on vacation Z75.5
    temporarily away from home Z74.2
  technical defects in home Z59.19
  temporary absence from home of person rendering care Z74.2
housing Z59.10
  environmental temperature Z59.11
  heating Z59.11
  space Z59.19

Inadequate, inadequacy (continued)
housing (continued)
  specified NEC Z59.19
  utilities Z59.12
income (financial) Z59.6
intrafamilial communication Z63.8
material resources due to limited financial resources, specified NEC Z59.87
mental —see Disability, intellectual
parental supervision or control of child Z62.0
personality F60.7
pulmonary
  function R06.89
    newborn P28.5
  ventilation, newborn P28.5
sample of cytologic smear
  anus R85.615
  cervix R87.615
  vagina R87.625
social F60.7
  insurance Z59.7
  skills NEC Z73.4
  social support Z60.8
supervision of child by parent Z62.0
teaching affecting education Z55.8
transportation Z59.82
welfare support Z59.7

Inanition R64
with edema —see Malnutrition, severe
due to
  deprivation of food T73.0
  malnutrition —see Malnutrition
fever R50.9

Inappropriate
change in quantitative human chorionic gonadotropin (hCG) in early pregnancy O02.81
diet or eating habits Z72.4
level of quantitative human chorionic gonadotropin (hCG) for gestational age in early pregnancy O02.81
secretion
  antidiuretic hormone (ADH) (excessive) E22.2
    deficiency E23.2
  pituitary (posterior) E22.2
sinus tachycardia, so stated (IST) I47.11

Inattention at or after birth —see Neglect

Incarceration, incarcerated
enterocele K46.0
  gangrenous K46.1
epiplocele K46.0
  gangrenous K46.1
exomphalos K42.0
  gangrenous K42.1
hernia —see also Hernia, by site, with obstruction
  with gangrene —see Hernia, by site, with gangrene
iris, in wound —see Injury, eye, laceration, with prolapse
lens, in wound —see Injury, eye, laceration, with prolapse
omphalocele K42.0
prison, anxiety concerning Z65.1
rupture —see Hernia, by site
sarcoepiplocele K46.0
  gangrenous K46.1
sarcoepiplomphalocele K42.0
  with gangrene K42.1
uterus N85.8
  gravid O34.51-
    causing obstructed labor O65.5

Incised wound
  external —see Laceration
  internal organs —see Injury, by site

Incision, incisional
  hernia K43.2
    with
      gangrene (and obstruction) K43.1
      obstruction K43.0
    surgical, complication —see Complications, surgical procedure
    traumatic
      external —see Laceration
      internal organs —see Injury, by site

Inclusion
  azurophilic leukocytic D72.0
  blennorrhea (neonatal) (newborn) P39.1
  gallbladder in liver (congenital) Q44.1

Incompatibility
  ABO
    affecting management of pregnancy O36.11-
      anti-A sensitization O36.11-
      anti-B sensitization O36.19-
      specified NEC O36.19-
    infusion or transfusion reaction —see Complication(s), transfusion, incompatibility reaction, ABO
    newborn P55.1
  blood (group) (Duffy) (K) (Kell) (Kidd) (Lewis) (M) (S) NEC
    affecting management of pregnancy O36.11-
      anti-A sensitization O36.11-
      anti-B sensitization O36.19-
    infusion or transfusion reaction T80.89
    newborn P55.8
  divorce or estrangement Z63.5
  Rh (blood group) (factor) Z31.82
    affecting management of pregnancy NEC O36.09-
      anti-D antibody O36.01-
    infusion or transfusion reaction —see Complication(s), transfusion, incompatibility reaction, Rh (factor)
    newborn P55.0
  rhesus —see Incompatibility, Rh

Incompetency, incompetent, incompetence
  annular
    aortic (valve) —see Insufficiency, aortic
    mitral (valve) I34.0
    pulmonary valve (heart) I37.1
  aortic (valve) —see Insufficiency, aortic
  cardiac valve —see Endocarditis
  cervix, cervical (os) N88.3
    in pregnancy O34.3-
  chronotropic I45.89
    with
      autonomic dysfunction G90.8
      ischemic heart disease I25.89
      left ventricular dysfunction I51.89
      sinus node dysfunction I49.8
  esophagogastric (junction) (sphincter) K22.0
  mitral (valve) —see Insufficiency, mitral
  pelvic fundus N81.89
  pubocervical tissue N81.82
  pulmonary valve (heart) I37.1
    congenital Q22.3

Incompetency, incompetent, incompetence *(continued)*
  rectovaginal tissue N81.83
  tricuspid (annular) (valve) —see Insufficiency, tricuspid
  valvular —see Endocarditis
    congenital Q24.8
  vein, venous (saphenous) (varicose) —see Varix, leg

Incomplete —see also condition
  atrioventricular
    canal Q21.21
    septal defect Q21.21
  bladder, emptying R33.9
  defecation R15.0
  endocardial cushion defect Q21.21
  expansion lungs (newborn) NEC —see Atelectasis
  rotation, intestine Q43.3

Inconclusive
  diagnostic imaging due to excess body fat of patient R93.9
  findings on diagnostic imaging of breast NEC R92.8
  mammogram R92.2

Incontinence R32
  anal sphincter R15.9
  coital N39.491
  feces R15.9
    nonorganic origin F98.1
  insensible (urinary) N39.42
  overflow N39.490
  postural (urinary) N39.492
  psychogenic F45.8
  rectal R15.9
  reflex N39.498
  stress (female) (male) N39.3
    and urge N39.46
  urethral sphincter R32
  urge N39.41
    and stress (female) (male) N39.46
  urine (urinary) R32
    continuous N39.45
    due to cognitive impairment, or severe physical disability or immobility R39.81
    functional R39.81
    insensible N39.42
    mixed (stress and urge) N39.46
    nocturnal N39.44
    nonorganic origin F98.0
    overflow N39.490
    post dribbling N39.43
    postural N39.492
    reflex N39.498
    specified NEC N39.498
    stress (female) (male) N39.3
      and urge N39.46
    total N39.498
    unaware N39.42
    urge N39.41
      and stress (female) (male) N39.46

Incontinentia pigmenti Q82.3

Incoordinate, incoordination
  esophageal-pharyngeal (newborn) —see Dysphagia
  muscular R27.8
  uterus (action) (contractions) (complicating delivery) O62.4

Increase, increased
  abnormal, in development R63.8
  androgens (ovarian) E28.1
  anticoagulants (antithrombin) (anti-VIIIa) (anti-IXa) (anti-Xa) (anti-XIa) —see Circulating anticoagulants
  cold sense R20.8
  estrogen E28.0

Increase, increased *(continued)*
  function
    adrenal
      cortex —see Cushing's, syndrome
      medulla E27.5
    pituitary (gland) (anterior) (lobe) E22.9
      posterior E22.2
  heat sense R20.8
  intracranial pressure (benign) G93.2
  permeability, capillaries I78.8
  pressure, intracranial G93.2
  secretion
    gastrin E16.4
    glucagon E16.3
    pancreas, endocrine E16.9
      growth hormone-releasing hormone E16.8
      pancreatic polypeptide E16.8
      somatostatin E16.8
      vasoactive-intestinal polypeptide E16.8
  sphericity, lens Q12.4
  splenic activity D73.1
  venous pressure I87.8
    portal K76.6

Increta placenta O43.22-

Incrustation, cornea, foreign body (lead) (zinc) —see Foreign body, cornea

Incyclophoria H50.54

Incyclotropia —see Cyclotropia

Indeterminate sex Q56.4

India rubber skin Q82.8

Indigestion (acid) (bilious) (functional) K30
  catarrhal K31.89
  due to decomposed food NOS A05.9
  nervous F45.8
  psychogenic F45.8

Indirect —see condition

Induratio penis plastica N48.6

Induration, indurated
  brain G93.89
  breast (fibrous) N64.51
    puerperal, postpartum O92.29
  broad ligament N83.8
  chancre
    anus A51.1
    congenital A50.07
    extragenital NEC A51.2
  corpora cavernosa (penis) (plastic) N48.6
  liver (chronic) K76.89
  lung (black) (chronic) (fibroid) —see also Fibrosis, lung J84.10
    essential brown J84.03
  penile (plastic) N48.6
  phlebitic —see Phlebitis
  skin R23.4

Inebriety (without dependence) —see Alcohol, intoxication

Inefficiency, kidney N28.9

Inelasticity, skin R23.4

Inequality, leg (length) (acquired) —see also Deformity, limb, unequal length
  congenital —see Defect, reduction, lower limb
  lower leg —see Deformity, limb, unequal length

Inertia
  bladder (neurogenic) N31.2
  stomach K31.89
    psychogenic F45.8

Inertia *(continued)*
  uterus, uterine during labor O62.2
    during latent phase of labor O62.0
    primary O62.0
    secondary O62.1
  vesical (neurogenic) N31.2

Infancy, infantile, infantilism —see also condition
  celiac K90.0
  genitalia, genitals (after puberty) E30.0
  Herter's (nontropical sprue) K90.0
  intestinal K90.0
  Lorain E23.0
  pancreatic K86.89
  pelvis M95.5
    with disproportion (fetopelvic) O33.1
      causing obstructed labor O65.1
  pituitary E23.0
  renal N25.0
  uterus —see Infantile, genitalia

Infant(s) —see also Infancy
  excessive crying R68.11
  irritable child R68.12
  lack of care —see Neglect
  liveborn (singleton) Z38.2
    born in hospital Z38.00
      by cesarean Z38.01
    born outside hospital Z38.1
    multiple NEC Z38.8
      born in hospital Z38.68
        by cesarean Z38.69
      born outside hospital Z38.7
    quadruplet Z38.8
      born in hospital Z38.63
        by cesarean Z38.64
      born outside hospital Z38.7
    quintuplet Z38.8
      born in hospital Z38.65
        by cesarean Z38.66
      born outside hospital Z38.7
    triplet Z38.8
      born in hospital Z38.61
        by cesarean Z38.62
      born outside hospital Z38.7
    twin Z38.5
      born in hospital Z38.30
        by cesarean Z38.31
      born outside hospital Z38.4
  of diabetic mother (syndrome of) P70.1
    gestational diabetes P70.0

Infantile —see also condition
  genitalia, genitals E30.0
  os, uterine E30.0
  penis E30.0
  testis E29.1
  uterus E30.0

Infantilism —see Infancy

Infarct, infarction
  adrenal (capsule) (gland) E27.49
  appendices epiploicae (see also Infarct, intestine) K55.069
  bowel (see also Infarct, intestine) K55.0 069
  brain (stem) —see Infarct, cerebral
  breast N64.89
  brewer's (kidney) N28.0
  cardiac —see Infarct, myocardium
  cerebellar —see Infarct, cerebral
  cerebral (acute) —see also Occlusion, artery cerebral or precerebral, with infarction I63.9-
    aborted I63.9
    chronic (imaging) (old) (remote) (without sequelae) Z86.73
      with residual defects —see Sequelae, disease, cerebrovascular

Infarct, infarction (continued)
  cerebral (acute) (continued)
    cortical I63.9
    due to
      cerebral venous thrombosis, nonpyogenic I63.6
      embolism
        cerebral arteries I63.4-
        precerebral arteries I63.1-
      occlusion NEC
        cerebral arteries I63.5-
        precerebral arteries I63.2-
        small artery I63.81
      stenosis NEC
        cerebral arteries I63.5-
        precerebral arteries I63.2-
        small artery I63.81
      thrombosis
        cerebral artery I63.3-
        precerebral artery I63.0-
    intraoperative
      during cardiac surgery I97.810
      during other surgery I97.811
    neonatal P91.82-
    perinatal (arterial ischemic) P91.82-
    postprocedural
      following cardiac surgery I97.820
      following other surgery I97.821
    specified NEC I63.89
  colon (acute) (agnogenic) (embolic) (hemorrhagic) (nonocclusive) (nonthrombotic) (occlusive) (segmental) (thrombotic) (with gangrene) (see also Infarct, intestine) K55.049
  coronary artery —see Infarct, myocardium
  embolic —see Embolism
  fallopian tube N83.8
  gallbladder K82.8
  heart —see Infarct, myocardium
  hepatic K76.3
  hypophysis (anterior lobe) E23.6
  impending (myocardium) I20.0
  intestine (acute) (agnogenic) (embolic) (hemorrhagic) (nonocclusive) (nonthrombotic) (occlusive) (thrombotic) (with gangrene) K55.069
    diffuse K55.062
    focal K55.061
    large K55.049
      diffuse K55.042
      focal K55.041
    small K55.029
      diffuse K55.029
      focal K55.021
  kidney N28.0
  lacunar I63.81
  liver K76.3
  lung (embolic) (thrombotic) —see Embolism, pulmonary
  lymph node I89.8
  mesentery, mesenteric (embolic) (thrombotic) (with gangrene) (see also Infarct, intestine) K55.069
  muscle (ischemic) M62.20
    ankle M62.27-
    foot M62.27-
    forearm M62.23-
    hand M62.24-
    lower leg M62.26-
    pelvic region M62.25-
    shoulder region M62.21-
    specified site NEC M62.28
    thigh M62.25-
    upper arm M62.22-

Infarct, infarction (continued)
  myocardium, myocardial (acute) (with stated duration of 4 weeks or less) I21.9
    with
      coronary microvascular disease I21.B
      coronary microvascular dysfunction I21.B
      nonobstructive coronary arteries [MINOCA] with microvascular disease I21.B
    associated with revascularization procedure I21.A9
    diagnosed on ECG, but presenting no symptoms I25.2
    due to
      demand ischemia I21.A1
      ischemic imbalance I21.A1
    healed or old I25.2
    intraoperative —see also Infarct, myocardium, associated with revascularization procedure
      during cardiac surgery I97.790
      during other surgery I97.791
    non-Q wave I21.4
    non-ST elevation (NSTEMI) I21.4
      subsequent I22.2
    nontransmural I21.4
    past (diagnosed on ECG or other investigation, but currently presenting no symptoms) I25.2
    postprocedural —see also Infarct, myocardium, associated with revascularization procedure
      following cardiac surgery (see also Infarct, myocardium, type 4 or type 5) I97.190
      following other surgery I97.191
    Q wave (see also, Infarct, myocardium, ST elevation, by site) I21.3
    secondary to
      demand ischemia I21.A1
      ischemic imbalance I21.A1
    ST elevation (STEMI) I21.3
      anterior (anteroapical) (anterolateral) (anteroseptal) (Q wave) (wall) I21.09
        subsequent I22.0
      inferior (diaphragmatic) (inferolateral) (inferoposterior) (wall) NEC I21.19
        subsequent I22.1
      inferoposterior transmural (Q wave) I21.11
      involving
        coronary artery of anterior wall NEC I21.09
        coronary artery of inferior wall NEC I21.19
        diagonal coronary artery I21.02
        left anterior descending coronary artery I21.02
        left circumflex coronary artery I21.21
        left main coronary artery I21.01
        oblique marginal coronary artery I21.21
        right coronary artery I21.11
      lateral (apical-lateral) (basal-lateral) (high) I21.29
        subsequent I22.8
      posterior (posterobasal) (posterolateral) (posteroseptal) (true) I21.29
        subsequent I22.8

Infarct, infarction (continued)
  myocardium, myocardial (continued)
    ST elevation (continued)
      septal I21.29
        subsequent I22.8
      specified NEC I21.29
        subsequent I22.8
      subsequent I22.9
    subsequent (recurrent) (reinfarction) I22.9
      anterior (anteroapical) (anterolateral) (anteroseptal) (wall) I22.0
      diaphragmatic (wall) I22.1
      inferior (diaphragmatic) (inferolateral) (inferoposterior) (wall) I22.1
      lateral (apical-lateral) (basal-lateral) (high) I22.8
      non-ST elevation (NSTEMI) I22.2
      posterior (posterobasal) (posterolateral) (posteroseptal) (true) I22.8
      septal I22.8
      specified NEC I22.8
      ST elevation I22.9
        anterior (anteroapical) (anterolateral) (anteroseptal) (wall) I22.0
        inferior (diaphragmatic) (inferolateral) (inferoposterior) (wall) I22.1
        specified NEC I22.8
      subendocardial I22.2
      transmural I22.9
        anterior (anteroapical) (anterolateral) (anteroseptal) (wall) I22.0
      transmural
        diaphragmatic (wall) I22.1
        inferior (diaphragmatic) (inferolateral) (inferoposterior) (wall) I22.1
        lateral (apical-lateral) (basal-lateral) (high) I22.8
        posterior (posterobasal) (posterolateral) (posteroseptal) (true) I22.8
        specified NEC I22.8
      type 1 (see also Infarction, myocardial, subsequent, by site, or by ST elevation or non-ST elevation) I22.9
      type 2 I21.A1
      type 3 I21.A9
      type 4 I21.A9
      type 5 I21.A9
    syphilitic A52.06
    transmural (see also, Infarct, myocardium, ST elevation, by site) I21.3
      anterior (anteroapical) (anterolateral) (anteroseptal) (Q wave) (wall) NEC I21.09
      inferior (diaphragmatic) (inferolateral) (inferoposterior) (Q wave) (wall) NEC I21.19
      inferoposterior (Q wave) I21.11
      lateral (apical-lateral) (basal-lateral) (high) NEC I21.29
      posterior (posterobasal) (posterolateral) (posteroseptal) (true) NEC I21.29
      septal NEC I21.29
      specified NEC I21.29

Infarct, infarction (continued)
  myocardium, myocardial (continued)
    type 1 (see also Infarction, myocardial, by site, or by ST elevation or non-ST elevation) I21.9
    type 2 I21.A1
    type 3 I21.A9
    type 4 (a) (b) (c) I21.A9
    type 5 I21.A9
  nontransmural I21.4
  omentum (see also Infarct, intestine) K55.069
  ovary N83.8
  pancreas K86.89
  papillary muscle —see Infarct, myocardium
  parathyroid gland E21.4
  pituitary (gland) E23.6
  placenta O43.81-
  prostate N42.89
  pulmonary (artery) (vein) (hemorrhagic) —see Embolism, pulmonary
  renal (embolic) (thrombotic) N28.0
  retina, retinal (artery) —see Occlusion, artery, retina
  spinal (cord) (acute) (embolic) (nonembolic) G95.11
  spleen D73.5
    embolic or thrombotic I74.8
  subendocardial (acute) (nontransmural) I21.4
  suprarenal (capsule) (gland) E27.49
  testis N50.1
  thrombotic —see also Thrombosis
    artery, arterial —see Embolism
  thyroid (gland) E07.89
  ventricle (heart) —see Infarct, myocardium

Infecting —see condition

Infection, infected, infective
  (opportunistic) B99.9
  with
    drug resistant organism —see Resistance (to), drug —see also specific organism
    lymphangitis —see Lymphangitis
    organ dysfunction (acute) R65.20
      with septic shock R65.21
  abscess (skin)- code by site under Abscess
  Absidia —see Mucormycosis
  Acanthamoeba —see Acanthamebiasis
  Acanthocheilonema (perstans) (streptocerca) B74.4
  accessory sinus (chronic) —see Sinusitis
  achorion —see Dermatophytosis
  Acinetobacter baumannii, as cause of disease classified elsewhere B96.83
  Acremonium falciforme B47.0
  acromioclavicular M00.9
  Actinobacillus (actinomycetem-comitans) A28.8
    mallei A24.0
    muris A25.1
  Actinomadura B47.1
  Actinomyces (israelii) (see also Actinomycosis) A42.9
  Actinomycetales —see Actinomycosis
  actinomycotic NOS —see Actinomycosis
  adenoid (and tonsil) J03.90
    chronic J35.02

Infection, infected, infective *(continued)*
  adenovirus NEC
    as cause of disease classified elsewhere B97.0
    unspecified nature or site B34.0
  aerogenes capsulatus A48.0
  aertrycke —*see* Infection, salmonella
  alimentary canal NOS —*see* Enteritis, infectious
  Allescheria boydii B48.2
  Alternaria B48.8
  alveolus, alveolar (process) K04.7
  Ameba, amebic (histolytica) —*see* Amebiasis
  amniotic fluid, sac or cavity O41.10-
    chorioamnionitis O41.12-
    placentitis O41.14-
  amputation stump (surgical) —*see* Complication, amputation stump, infection
  Ancylostoma (duodenalis) B76.0
  Anisakiasis, Anisakis larvae B81.0
  anthrax —*see* Anthrax
  antrum (chronic) —*see* Sinusitis, maxillary
  anus, anal (papillae) (sphincter) K62.89
  arbovirus (arbor virus) A94
    specified type NEC A93.8
  artificial insemination N98.0
  Ascaris lumbricoides —*see* Ascariasis
  Ascomycetes B47.0
  Aspergillus (flavus) (fumigatus) (terreus) —*see* Aspergillosis
  atypical
    acid-fast (bacilli) —*see* Mycobacterium, atypical
    mycobacteria —*see* Mycobacterium, atypical
    virus A81.9
      specified type NEC A81.89
  auditory meatus (external) —*see* Otitis, externa, infective
  auricle (ear) —*see* Otitis, externa, infective
  axillary gland (lymph) L04.2
  Bacillus A49.9
    abortus A23.1
    anthracis —*see* Anthrax
    Ducrey's (any location) A57
    Flexner's A03.1
    Friedländer's NEC A49.8
    gas (gangrene) A48.0
    mallei A24.0
    melitensis A23.0
    paratyphoid, paratyphosus A01.4
      A A01.1
      B A01.2
      C A01.3
    Shiga (-Kruse) A03.0
    suipestifer —*see* Infection, salmonella
    swimming pool A31.1
    typhosa A01.00
    welchii —*see* Gangrene, gas
  bacterial NOS A49.9
    as cause of disease classified elsewhere B96.89
      Acinetobacter baumannii B96.83
      Bacteroides fragilis [B. fragilis] B96.6
      Clostridium perfringens [C. perfringens] B96.7

Infection, infected, infective *(continued)*
  bacterial *(continued)*
    as cause of disease classified elsewhere *(continued)*
      Cronobacter (sakazakii) B96.89
      Enterobacter sakazakii B96.89
      Enterococcus B95.2
      Escherichia coli [E. coli] —*see also* Escherichia coli B96.20
      Helicobacter pylori [H.pylori] B96.81
      Hemophilus influenzae [H. influenzae] B96.3
      Klebsiella pneumoniae [K. pneumoniae] B96.1
      Mycoplasma pneumoniae [M. pneumoniae] B96.0
      Proteus (mirabilis) (morganii) B96.4
      Pseudomonas (aeruginosa) (mallei) (pseudomallei) B96.5
      Staphylococcus B95.8
        aureus (methicillin susceptible) (MSSA) B95.61
          methicillin resistant (MRSA) B95.62
        specified NEC B95.7
      Streptococcus B95.5
        group A B95.0
        group B B95.1
        pneumoniae B95.3
        specified NEC B95.4
      Vibrio vulnificus B96.82
    specified NEC A48.8
  Bacterium
    paratyphosum A01.4
      A A01.1
      B A01.2
      C A01.3
    typhosum A01.00
  Bacteroides NEC A49.8
    fragilis, as cause of disease classified elsewhere B96.6
  Balantidium coli A07.0
  Bartholin's gland N75.8
  Basidiobolus B46.8
  bile duct (common) (hepatic) —*see* Cholangitis
  bladder —*see* Cystitis
  Blastomyces, blastomycotic —*see also* Blastomycosis
    brasiliensis —*see* Paracoccidioidomycosis
    dermatitidis —*see* Blastomycosis
    European —*see* Cryptococcosis
    Loboi B48.0
    North American B40.9
    South American —*see* Paracoccidioidomycosis
  bleb, postprocedure —*see* Blebitis
  bone —*see* Osteomyelitis
  Bordetella —*see* Whooping cough
  Borrelia bergdorfi A69.20
  brain (*see also* Encephalitis) G04.90
    membranes —*see* Meningitis
    septic G06.0
    meninges —*see* Meningitis, bacterial
  branchial cyst Q18.0
  breast —*see* Mastitis
  bronchus —*see* Bronchitis
  Brucella A23.9
    abortus A23.1

Infection, infected, infective *(continued)*
  Brucella *(continued)*
    canis A23.3
    melitensis A23.0
    mixed A23.8
    specified NEC A23.8
    suis A23.2
  Brugia (malayi) B74.1
    timori B74.2
  bursa —*see* Bursitis, infective
  buttocks (skin) L08.9
  Campylobacter, intestinal A04.5
    as cause of disease classified elsewhere B96.81
  Candida (albicans) (tropicalis) —*see* Candidiasis
  candiru B88.8
  Capillaria (intestinal) B81.1
    hepatica B83.8
    philippinensis B81.1
  cartilage —*see* Disorder, cartilage, specified type NEC
  catheter-related bloodstream (CRBSI) T80.211
  cat liver fluke B66.0
  cellulitis - code by site under Cellulitis
  central line-associated T80.219
    bloodstream (CLABSI) T80.211
    specified NEC T80.218
  Cephalosporium falciforme B47.0
  cerebrospinal —*see* Meningitis
  cervical gland (lymph) L04.0
  cervix —*see* Cervicitis
  cesarean delivery wound (puerperal) O86.00
  cestodes —*see* Infestation, cestodes
  chest J22
  Chilomastix (intestinal) A07.8
  Chlamydia, chlamydial A74.9
    anus A56.3
    genitourinary tract A56.2
      lower A56.00
        specified NEC A56.19
    lymphogranuloma A55
    pharynx A56.4
    psittaci A70
    rectum A56.3
    sexually transmitted NEC A56.8
  cholera —*see* Cholera
  Cladosporium
    bantianum (brain abscess) B43.1
    carrionii B43.0
    castellanii B36.1
    trichoides (brain abscess) B43.1
    werneckii B36.1
  Clonorchis (sinensis) (liver) B66.1
  Clostridium NEC
    bifermentans A48.0
    botulinum (food poisoning) A05.1
      infant A48.51
      wound A48.52
    difficile
      as cause of disease classified elsewhere B96.89
      foodborne (disease)
        not specified as recurrent A04.72
        recurrent A04.71
      gas gangrene A48.0
      necrotizing enterocolitis
        not specified as recurrent A04.72
        recurrent A04.71
      sepsis A41.4
    gas-forming NEC A48.0
    histolyticum A48.0
    novyi, causing gas gangrene A48.0

Infection, infected, infective *(continued)*
  Clostridium *(continued)*
    oedematiens A48.0
    perfringens
      as cause of disease classified elsewhere B96.7
      due to food A05.2
      foodborne (disease) A05.2
      gas gangrene A48.0
      sepsis A41.4
    septicum, causing gas gangrene A48.0
    sordellii, causing gas gangrene A48.0
    welchii
      as cause of disease classified elsewhere B96.7
      foodborne (disease) A05.2
      gas gangrene A48.0
      necrotizing enteritis A05.2
      sepsis A41.4
  Coccidioides (immitis) —*see* Coccidioidomycosis
  colon —*see* Enteritis, infectious
  colostomy K94.02
  common duct —*see* Cholangitis
  congenital P39.9
    Candida (albicans) P37.5
    cytomegalovirus P35.1
    hepatitis, viral P35.3
    herpes simplex P35.2
    infectious or parasitic disease P37.9
      specified NEC P37.8
    listeriosis (disseminated) P37.2
    malaria NEC P37.4
      falciparum P37.3
    Plasmodium falciparum P37.3
    poliomyelitis P35.8
    rubella P35.0
    skin P39.4
    toxoplasmosis (acute) (subacute) (chronic) P37.1
    tuberculosis P37.0
    urinary (tract) P39.3
    vaccinia P35.8
    virus P35.9
      specified type NEC P35.8
  Conidiobolus B46.8
  coronavirus-2019 U07.1
  coronavirus NEC B34.2
    as cause of disease classified elsewhere B97.29
    severe acute respiratory syndrome (SARS associated) B97.21
  corpus luteum —*see* Salpingo-oophoritis
  Corynebacterium diphtheriae —*see* Diphtheria
  cotia virus B08.8
  COVID-19 (*see also* COVID-19) U07.1
  Coxiella burnetii A78
  coxsackie —*see* Coxsackie
  Cronobacter (sakazakii) B96.89
    as cause of disease classified elsewhere B96.89
    generalized A41.59
  Cryptococcus neoformans —*see* Cryptococcosis
  Cryptosporidium A07.2
  Cunninghamella —*see* Mucormycosis
  cyst —*see* Cyst
  cystic duct (*see also* Cholecystitis) K81.9
  Cysticercus cellulosae —*see* Cysticercosis

193

Infection, infected, infective *(continued)*
  cytomegalovirus, cytomegaloviral B25.9
    congenital P35.1
    maternal, maternal care for (suspected) damage to fetus O35.3
    mononucleosis B27.10
      with
        complication NEC B27.19
        meningitis B27.12
        polyneuropathy B27.11
  delta-agent (acute), in hepatitis B carrier B17.0
  dental (pulpal origin) K04.7
  Deuteromycetes B47.0
  Dicrocoelium dendriticum B66.2
  Dipetalonema (perstans) (streptocerca) B74.4
  diphtherial —see Diphtheria
  Diphyllobothrium (adult) (latum) (pacificum) B70.0
    larval B70.1
  Diplogonoporus (grandis) B71.8
  Dipylidium caninum B67.4
  Dirofilaria B74.8
  Drechslera (hawaiiensis) B43.8
  Dracunculus medinensis B72
  Ducrey Haemophilus (any location) A57
  due to or resulting from
    artificial insemination N98.0
    Babesia
      divergens (-like) strain B60.03
      duncani (-type) species B60.02
      microti B60.01
      species
        specified NEC B60.09
    central venous catheter T80.219
      bloodstream T80.211
      exit or insertion site T80.212
      localized T80.212
      port or reservoir T80.212
      specified NEC T80.218
      tunnel T80.212
    device, implant or graft *(see also* Complications, by site and type, infection or inflammation) T85.79
      arterial graft NEC T82.7
      breast (implant) T85.79
      catheter NEC T85.79
        dialysis (renal) T82.7
          central line T80.211
          intraperitoneal T85.71
        infusion NEC T82.7
          cranial T85.735
          intrathecal T85.735
          spinal (epidural) (subdural) T85.735
          subarachnoid T85.735
        urinary T83.518
          cystostomy T83.510
          Hopkins T83.518
          ileostomy T83.518
          nephrostomy T83.512
          specified NEC T83.518
          urethral indwelling T83.511
          urostomy T83.518
      electronic (electrode) (pulse generator) (stimulator)
        bone T84.7
        cardiac T82.7
        nervous system T85.738
          brain T85.731
          cranial nerve T85.732
          gastric nerve T85.732
          generator pocket T85.734
          neurostimulator generator T85.734

Infection, infected, infective *(continued)*
  due to or resulting from *(continued)*
    device, implant or graft *(continued)*
      electronic *(continued)*
        nervous system *(continued)*
          peripheral nerve T85.732
          sacral nerve T85.732
          spinal cord T85.733
          vagal nerve T85.732
        urinary T83.590
      fixation, internal (orthopedic) NEC —see Complication, fixation device, infection
      gastrointestinal (bile duct) (esophagus) T85.79
        neurostimulator electrode (lead) T85.732
      genital NEC T83.69
      heart NEC T82.7
        valve (prosthesis) T82.6
        graft T82.7
      joint prosthesis —see Complication, joint prosthesis, infection
      ocular (corneal graft) (orbital implant) NEC T85.79
      orthopedic NEC T84.7
      penile (cylinder) (pump) (resevoir) T83.61
      specified NEC T85.79
      testicular T83.62
      urinary NEC T83.598
        ileal conduit stent T83.593
        implanted neurostimulation T83.590
        implanted sphincter T83.591
        indwelling ureteral stent T83.592
        nephroureteral stent T83.593
        specified stent NEC T83.593
      vascular NEC T82.7
      ventricular intracranial (communicating) shunt T85.730
    Hickman catheter T80.219
      bloodstream T80.211
      localized T80.212
      specified NEC T80.218
    immunization or vaccination T88.0
    infusion, injection or transfusion NEC T80.29
      acute T80.22
    injury NEC - code by site under Wound, open
    peripherally inserted central catheter (PICC) T80.219
      bloodstream T80.211
      localized T80.212
      specified NEC T80.218
    portacath (port-a-cath) T80.219
      bloodstream T80.211
      localized T80.212
      specified NEC T80.218
    protozoa of the order Piroplasmida NEC B60.09
    pulmonary artery catheter —see Infection, due to or resulting from, central venous catheter
    surgery T81.40
    Swan Ganz catheter —see Infection, due to or resulting from, central venous catheter
    triple lumen catheter T80.219
      bloodstream T80.211
      localized T80.212
      specified NEC T80.218

Infection, infected, infective *(continued)*
  due to or resulting from *(continued)*
    umbilical venous catheter T80.219
      bloodstream T80.211
      localized T80.212
      specified NEC T80.218
  during labor NEC O75.3
  ear (middle) —see also Otitis media
    external —see Otitis, externa, infective
    inner —see subcategory H83.0
  Eberthella typhosa A01.00
  Echinococcus —see Echinococcus
  echovirus
    as cause of disease classified elsewhere B97.12
    unspecified nature or site B34.1
  endocardium I33.0
  endocervix —see Cervicitis
  Entamoeba —see Amebiasis
  enteric —see Enteritis, infectious
  Enterobacter sakazakii B96.89
  Enterobius vermicularis B80
  enterostomy K94.12
  enterovirus B34.1
    as cause of disease classified elsewhere B97.10
    coxsackievirus B97.11
    echovirus B97.12
    specified NEC B97.19
  Entomophthora B46.8
  Epidermophyton —see Dermatophytosis
  epididymis —see Epididymitis
  episiotomy (puerperal) O86.09
  Erysipelothrix (insidiosa) (rhusiopathiae) —see Erysipeloid
  erythema infectiosum B08.3
  Escherichia (E.) coli NEC A49.8
    as cause of disease classified elsewhere (*see also* Escherichia coli) B96.20
    congenital P39.8
      sepsis P36.4
    generalized A41.51
    intestinal —see Enteritis, infectious, due to, Escherichia coli
  ethmoidal (chronic) (sinus) —see Sinusitis, ethmoidal
  eustachian tube (ear) —see Salpingitis, eustachian
  external auditory canal (meatus) NEC —see Otitis, externa, infective
  eye (purulent) —see Endophthalmitis, purulent
  eyelid —see Inflammation, eyelid
  fallopian tube —see Salpingo-oophoritis
  Fasciola (gigantica) (hepatica) (indica) B66.3
  Fasciolopsis (buski) B66.5
  filarial —see Infestation, filarial
  finger (skin) L08.9
    nail L03.01-
      fungus B35.1
  fish tapeworm B70.0
    larval B70.1
  flagellate, intestinal A07.9
  fluke —see Infestation, fluke
  focal
    teeth (pulpal origin) K04.7
    tonsils J35.01
  Fonsecaea (compactum) (pedrosoi) B43.0
  food —see Intoxication, foodborne
  foot (skin) L08.9
    dermatophytic fungus B35.3
  Francisella tularensis —see Tularemia

Infection, infected, infective *(continued)*
  frontal (sinus) (chronic) —see Sinusitis, frontal
  fungus NOS B49
    beard B35.0
    dermatophytic —see Dermatophytosis
    foot B35.3
    groin B35.6
    hand B35.2
    nail B35.1
    pathogenic to compromised host only B48.8
    perianal (area) B35.6
    scalp B35.0
    skin B36.9
      foot B35.3
      hand B35.2
    toenails B35.1
  Fusarium B48.8
  gallbladder —see Cholecystitis
  gas bacillus —see Gangrene, gas
  gastrointestinal —see Enteritis, infectious
  generalized NEC —see Sepsis
  generator pocket, implanted electronic neurostimulator T85.734
  genital organ or tract
    female —see Disease, pelvis, inflammatory
    male N49.9
      multiple sites N49.8
      specified NEC N49.8
  Ghon tubercle, primary A15.7
  Giardia lamblia A07.1
  gingiva (chronic) K05.10
    acute K05.00
      nonplaque induced K05.01
      plaque induced K05.00
    nonplaque induced K05.11
    plaque induced K05.10
  glanders A24.0
  glenosporopsis B48.0
  Gnathostoma (spinigerum) B83.1
  Gongylonema B83.8
  gonococcal —see Gonococcus
  gram-negative bacilli NOS A49.9
  guinea worm B72
  gum (chronic) K05.10
    acute K05.00
      nonplaque induced K05.01
      plaque induced K05.00
    nonplaque induced K05.11
    plaque induced K05.10
  Haemophilus —see Infection, Hemophilus
  heart —see Carditis
  Helicobacter pylori A04.8
    as cause of disease classified elsewhere B96.81
  helminths B83.9
    intestinal B82.0
      mixed (types classifiable to more than one of the titles B65.0-B81.3 and B81.8) B81.4
      specified type NEC B81.8
    specified type NEC B83.8
  Hemophilus
    aegyptius, systemic A48.4
    ducrey (any location) A57
    influenzae NEC A49.2
      as cause of disease classified elsewhere B96.3
      generalized A41.3
  herpes (simplex) —see also Herpes
    congenital P35.2
    disseminated B00.7
    zoster B02.9
  herpesvirus, herpesviral —see Herpes

Infection, infected, infective *(continued)*
  hip (joint) NEC M00.9
    due to internal joint prosthesis
      left T84.52
      right T84.51
    skin NEC L08.9
  Heterophyes (heterophyes) B66.8
  Histoplasma —*see* Histoplasmosis
    American B39.4
    capsulatum B39.4
  hookworm B76.9
  human
    papilloma virus A63.0
    T-cell lymphotropic virus
      type-1(HTLV-1) B33.3
  hydrocele N43.0
  Hymenolepis B71.0
  hypopharynx —*see* Pharyngitis
  inguinal (lymph) glands L04.1
    due to soft chancre A57
  intervertebral disc, pyogenic
    M46.30
    cervical region M46.32
    cervicothoracic region M46.33
    lumbar region M46.36
    lumbosacral region M46.37
    multiple sites M46.39
    occipito-atlanto-axial region
      M46.31
    sacrococcygeal region M46.38
    thoracic region M46.34
    thoracolumbar region M46.35
  intestine, intestinal —*see* Enteritis,
    infectious
    specified NEC A08.8
  intra-amniotic affecting newborn
    NEC P39.2
  intrauterine inflammation O41.12-
  Isospora belli or hominis A07.3
  Japanese B encephalitis A83.0
  jaw (bone) (lower) (upper) M27.2
  joint NEC M00.9
    due to internal joint prosthesis
      T84.50
  kidney (cortex) (hematogenous)
    N15.9
    with calculus N20.0
      with hydronephrosis N13.6
    following ectopic gestation O08.83
    pelvis and ureter (cystic) N28.85
    puerperal (postpartum) O86.21
    specified NEC N15.8
  Klebsiella (K.) pneumoniae NEC
    A49.8
    as cause of disease classified
      elsewhere B96.1
  knee (joint) NEC M00.9
    joint M00.9
    due to internal joint prosthesis
      left T84.54
      right T84.53
    skin L08.9
  Koch's —*see* Tuberculosis
  labia (majora) (minora) (acute)
    —*see* Vulvitis
  lacrimal
    gland —*see* Dacryoadenitis
    passages (duct) (sac) —*see*
      Inflammation, lacrimal,
      passages
  lancet fluke B66.2
  larynx NEC J38.7
  leg (skin) NOS L08.9
  Legionella pneumophila A48.1
    nonpneumonic A48.2
  Leishmania —*see also*
    Leishmaniasis
    aethiopica B55.1
    braziliensis B55.2
    chagasi B55.0

Infection, infected, infective *(continued)*
  Leishmania *(continued)*
    donovani B55.0
    infantum B55.0
    major B55.1
    mexicana B55.1
    tropica B55.1
  lentivirus, as cause of disease
    classified elsewhere B97.31
  Leptosphaeria senegalensis B47.0
  Leptospira interrogans A27.9
    autumnalis A27.89
    canicola A27.89
    hebdomadis A27.89
    icterohaemorrhagiae A27.0
    pomona A27.89
    specified type NEC A27.89
  leptospirochetal NEC —*see*
    Leptospirosis
  Listeria monocytogenes —*see also*
    Listeriosis
    congenital P37.2
  Loa loa B74.3
    with conjunctival infestation
      B74.3
    eyelid B74.3
  Loboa loboi B48.0
  local, skin (staphylococcal)
    (streptococcal) L08.9
    abscess - code by site under
      Abscess
    cellulitis - code by site under
      Cellulitis
    specified NEC L08.89
    ulcer —*see* Ulcer, skin
  Loefflerella mallei A24.0
  lung (*see also* Pneumonia) J18.9
    atypical Mycobacterium A31.0
    spirochetal A69.8
    tuberculous —*see* Tuberculosis,
      pulmonary
    virus —*see* Pneumonia, viral
  lymph gland —*see also*
    Lymphadenitis, acute
    mesenteric I88.0
  lymphoid tissue, base of tongue
    or posterior pharynx, NEC
    (chronic) J35.03
  Madurella (grisea) (mycetomii)
    B47.0
  major
    following ectopic or molar
      pregnancy O08.0
    puerperal, postpartum, childbirth
      O85
  Malassezia furfur B36.0
  Malleomyces
    mallei A24.0
    pseudomallei (whitmori) —*see*
      Melioidosis
  mammary gland N61.0
  Mansonella (ozzardi) (perstans)
    (streptocerca) B74.4
  mastoid —*see* Mastoiditis
  maxilla, maxillary M27.2
    sinus (chronic) —*see* Sinusitis,
      maxillary
  mediastinum J98.51
  Medina (worm) B72
  meibomian cyst or gland —*see*
    Hordeolum
  meninges —*see* Meningitis,
    bacterial
  meningococcal (*see also* condition)
    A39.9
    adrenals A39.1
    brain A39.81
    cerebrospinal A39.0
    conjunctiva A39.89
    endocardium A39.51

Infection, infected, infective *(continued)*
  meningococcal *(continued)*
    heart A39.50
      endocardium A39.51
      myocardium A39.52
      pericardium A39.53
    joint A39.83
    meninges A39.0
    meningococcemia A39.4
      acute A39.2
      chronic A39.3
    myocardium A39.52
    pericardium A39.53
    retrobulbar neuritis A39.82
    specified site NEC A39.89
  mesenteric lymph nodes or glands
    NEC I88.0
  Metagonimus B66.8
  metatarsophalangeal M00.9
  methicillin
    resistant Staphylococcus aureus
      (MRSA) A49.02
    susceptible Staphylococcus
      aureus (MSSA) A49.01
  Microsporum, microsporic —*see*
    Dermatophytosis
  mixed flora (bacterial) NEC A49.8
  Monilia —*see* Candidiasis
  Monosporium apiospermum B48.2
  mouth, parasitic B37.0
  Mucor —*see* Mucormycosis
  muscle NEC —*see* Myositis,
    infective
  mycelium NOS B49
  mycetoma B47.9
    actinomycotic NEC B47.1
    mycotic NEC B47.0
  Mycobacterium, mycobacterial
    —*see* Mycobacterium
  Mycoplasma NEC A49.3
    pneumoniae, as cause of disease
      classified elsewhere B96.0
  mycotic NOS B49
    pathogenic to compromised host
      only B48.8
    skin NOS B36.9
  myocardium NEC I40.0
  nail (chronic)
    with lymphangitis —*see*
      Lymphangitis, acute, digit
    finger L03.01-
      fungus B35.1
    ingrowing L60.0
    toe L03.03-
      fungus B35.1
  nasal sinus (chronic) —*see*
    Sinusitis
  nasopharynx —*see*
    Nasopharyngitis
  navel L08.82
  Necator americanus B76.1
  Neisseria —*see* Gonococcus
  Neotestudina rosatii B47.0
  newborn P39.9
    vintra-amniotic NEC P39.2
    skin P39.4
    specified type NEC P39.8
  nipple N61.0
    associated with
      lactation O91.03
      pregnancy O91.01-
      puerperium O91.02
  Nocardia —*see* Nocardiosis
  obstetrical surgical wound
    (puerperal) O86.00
    incisional site
      deep O86.02
      superficial O86.01
    organ and space site O86.03
    surgical site specified NEC O86.09

Infection, infected, infective *(continued)*
  Oesophagostomum (apiostomum)
    B81.8
  Oestrus ovis —*see* Myiasis
  Oidium albicans B37.9
  Onchocerca (volvulus) —*see*
    Onchocerciasis
  oncovirus, as cause of disease
    classified elsewhere B97.32
  operation wound T81.49
  Opisthorchis (felineus) (viverrini)
    B66.0
  orbit, orbital —*see* Inflammation,
    orbit
  orthopoxvirus NEC B08.09
  ovary —*see* Salpingo-oophoritis
  Oxyuris vermicularis B80
  pancreas (acute) —*see* Pancreatitis,
    acute
    abscess —*see* Pancreatitis, acute
    specified NEC (*see also*
      Pancreatitis, acute) K85.80
  papillomavirus, as cause of disease
    classified elsewhere B97.7
  papovavirus NEC B34.4
  Paracoccidioides brasiliensis —*see*
    Paracoccidioidomycosis
  Paragonimus (westermani) B66.4
  parainfluenza virus B34.8
  parameningococcus NOS A39.9
  parapoxvirus B08.60
    specified NEC B08.69
  parasitic B89
  Parastrongylus
    cantonensis B83.2
    costaricensis B81.3
  paratyphoid A01.4
    Type A A01.1
    Type B A01.2
    Type C A01.3
  paraurethral ducts N34.2
  parotid gland —*see* Sialoadenitis
  parvovirus NEC B34.3
    as cause of disease classified
      elsewhere B97.6
  Pasteurella NEC A28.0
    multocida A28.0
    pestis —*see* Plague
    pseudotuberculosis A28.0
    septica (cat bite) (dog bite)
      A28.0
    tularensis —*see* Tularemia
  pelvic, female —*see* Disease,
    pelvis, inflammatory
  Penicillium (marneffei) B48.4
  penis (glans) (retention) NEC
    N48.29
  periapical K04.5
  peridental, periodontal K05.20
    generalized —*see* Periodontitis,
      aggressive, generalized
    localized —*see* Periodontitis,
      aggressive, localized
  perinatal period P39.9
    specified type NEC P39.8
  perineal repair (puerperal) O86.09
  periorbital —*see* Inflammation,
    orbit
  perirectal K62.89
  perirenal —*see* Infection, kidney
  peritoneal —*see* Peritonitis
  periureteral N28.89
  Petriellidium boydii B48.2
  pharynx —*see also* Pharyngitis
    coxsackievirus B08.5
    posterior, lymphoid (chronic)
      J35.03
  Phialophora
    gougerotii (subcutaneous abscess
      or cyst) B43.2

195

Infection, infected, infective *(continued)*
  Phialophora *(continued)*
    jeanselmei (subcutaneous abscess or cyst) B43.2
    verrucosa (skin) B43.0
  Piedraia hortae B36.3
  pinta A67.9
    intermediate A67.1
    late A67.2
    mixed A67.3
    primary A67.0
  pinworm B80
  pityrosporum furfur B36.0
  pleuro-pneumonia-like organism (PPLO) NEC A49.3
    as cause of disease classified elsewhere B96.0
  pneumococcus, pneumococcal NEC A49.1
    as cause of disease classified elsewhere B95.3
    generalized (purulent) A40.3
      with pneumonia J13
  Pneumocystis carinii (pneumonia) B59
  Pneumocystis jiroveci (pneumonia) B59
  port or reservoir T80.212
  postoperative T81.40
  postoperative wound T81.49
    surgical site
      deep incisional T81.42
      organ and space T81.43
      specified NEC T81.49
      superficial incisional T81.41
  postprocedural T81.40
  postvaccinal T88.0
  prepuce NEC N47.7
    with penile inflammation N47.6
  prion —*see* Disease, prion, central nervous system
  prostate (capsule) —*see* Prostatitis
  Proteus (mirabilis) (morganii) (vulgaris) NEC A49.8
    as cause of disease classified elsewhere B96.4
  protozoal NEC B64
    intestinal A07.9
      specified NEC A07.8
    specified NEC B60.8
  Pseudallescheria boydii B48.2
  Pseudomonas NEC A49.8
    as cause of disease classified elsewhere B96.5
    generalized A41.52
    mallei A24.0
    pneumonia J15.1
    pseudomallei —*see* Melioidosis
  puerperal O86.4
    genitourinary tract NEC O86.89
    major or generalized O85
    minor O86.4
    specified NEC O86.89
  pulmonary —*see* Infection, lung
  purulent —*see* Abscess
  Pyrenochaeta romeroi B47.0
  Q fever A78
  rectum (sphincter) K62.89
  renal —*see also* Infection, kidney
    pelvis and ureter (cystic) N28.85
  reovirus, as cause of disease classified elsewhere B97.5
  respiratory (tract) NEC J98.8
    acute J22
    chronic J98.8
      influenzal (upper) (acute) —*see* Influenza, with, respiratory manifestations NEC

Infection, infected, infective *(continued)*
  respiratory *(continued)*
    lower (acute) J22
      chronic —*see* Bronchitis, chronic
    rhinovirus J00
    syncytial virus (RSV) —*see* Infection, virus, respiratory syncytial (RSV)
    upper (acute) NOS J06.9
      chronic J39.8
      streptococcal J06.9
      viral NOS J06.9
        due to respiratory syncytial virus (RSV) J06.9 [B97.4]
  resulting from
    presence of internal prosthesis, implant, graft —*see* Complications, by site and type, infection
  retortamoniasis A07.8
  retroperitoneal NEC K68.9
  retrovirus B33.3
    as cause of disease classified elsewhere B97.30
      human immunodeficiency, type 2(HIV 2) B97.35
      T-cell lymphotropic type I (HTLV-I) B97.33
        type II (HTLV-II) B97.34
      lentivirus B97.31
      oncovirus B97.32
      specified NEC B97.39
  Rhinosporidium (*seeberi*) B48.1
  rhinovirus
    as cause of disease classified elsewhere B97.89
    unspecified nature or site B34.8
  Rhizopus —*see* Mucormycosis
  rickettsial NOS A79.9
  roundworm (large) NEC B82.0
    Ascariasis (*see also* Ascariasis) B77.9
  rubella —*see* Rubella
  Saccharomyces —*see* Candidiasis
  salivary duct or gland (any) —*see* Sialoadenitis
  Salmonella (aertrycke) (arizonae) (callinarum) (cholerae-suis) (enteritidis) (suipestifer) (typhimurium) A02.9
    with
      (gastro)enteritis A02.0
      sepsis A02.1
      specified manifestation NEC A02.8
    due to food (poisoning) A02.9
    hirschfeldii A01.3
    localized A02.20
      arthritis A02.23
      meningitis A02.21
      osteomyelitis A02.24
      pneumonia A02.22
      pyelonephritis A02.25
      specified NEC A02.29
    paratyphi A01.4
      A A01.1
      B A01.2
      C A01.3
    schottmuelleri A01.2
    typhi, typhosa —*see* Typhoid
  Sarcocystis A07.8
  SARS-Cov-2 —*see* Infection, COVID-19
  scabies B86
  Schistosoma —*see* Infestation, Schistosoma
  scrotum (acute) NEC N49.2

Infection, infected, infective *(continued)*
  seminal vesicle —*see* Vesiculitis
  septic
    localized, skin —*see* Abscess
  Serratia NEC A49.8
    as cause of disease classified elsewhere B96.89
    generalized A41.53
  sheep liver fluke B66.3
  Shigella A03.9
    boydii A03.2
    dysenteriae A03.0
    flexneri A03.1
    group
      A A03.0
      B A03.1
      C A03.2
      D A03.3
    Schmitz (-Stutzer) A03.0
    schmitzii A03.0
    shigae A03.0
    sonnei A03.3
    specified NEC A03.8
  shoulder (joint) NEC M00.9
    due to internal joint prosthesis T84.59
    skin NEC L08.9
  sinus (accessory) (chronic) (nasal) —*see also* Sinusitis
    pilonidal —*see* Sinus, pilonidal
    skin NEC L08.89
  Skene's duct or gland —*see* Urethritis
  skin (local) (staphylococcal) (streptococcal) L08.9
    abscess - code by site under Abscess
    cellulitis - code by site under Cellulitis
    due to fungus B36.9
      specified type NEC B36.8
    mycotic B36.9
      specified type NEC B36.8
    newborn P39.4
    ulcer —*see* Ulcer, skin
  slow virus A81.9
    specified NEC A81.89
  Sparganum (mansoni) (proliferum) (baxteri) B70.1
  specific —*see also* Syphilis
    to perinatal period —*see* Infection, congenital
  specified NEC B99.8
  spermatic cord NEC N49.1
  sphenoidal (sinus) —*see* Sinusitis, sphenoidal
  spinal cord NOS —*see also* Myelitis G04.91
    abscess G06.1
    meninges —*see* Meningitis
    streptococcal G04.89
  Spirillum A25.0
  spirochetal NOS A69.9
    lung A69.8
    specified NEC A69.8
  Spirometra larvae B70.1
  spleen D73.89
  Sporotrichum, Sporothrix (schenckii) —*see* Sporotrichosis
  staphylococcal, unspecified site
    aureus (methicillin susceptible) (MSSA) A49.01
      methicillin resistant (MRSA) A49.02
    as cause of disease classified elsewhere B95.8
      aureus (methicillin susceptible) (MSSA) B95.61
      methicillin resistant (MRSA) B95.62
      specified NEC B95.7

Infection, infected, infective *(continued)*
  staphylococcal, unspecified site *(continued)*
    food poisoning A05.0
    generalized (purulent) A41.2
    pneumonia —*see* Pneumonia, staphylococcal
  Stellantchasmus falcatus B66.8
  streptobacillus moniliformis A25.1
  streptococcal NEC A49.1
    as cause of disease classified elsewhere B95.5
    B genitourinary complicating
      childbirth O98.82
      pregnancy O98.81-
      puerperium O98.83
    congenital
      sepsis P36.10
        group B P36.0
        specified NEC P36.19
    generalized (purulent) A40.9
  Streptomyces B47.1
  Strongyloides (stercoralis) —*see* Strongyloidiasis
  stump (amputation) (surgical) —*see* Complication, amputation stump, infection
  subcutaneous tissue, local L08.9
  suipestifer —*see* Infection, salmonella
  swimming pool bacillus A31.1
  Taenia —*see* Infestation, Taenia
  Taeniarhynchus saginatus B68.1
  tapeworm —*see* Infestation, tapeworm
  tendon (sheath) —*see* Tenosynovitis, infective NEC
  Ternidens diminutus B81.8
  testis —*see* Orchitis
  threadworm B80
  throat —*see* Pharyngitis
  thyroglossal duct K14.8
  toe (skin) L08.9
    cellulitis L03.03-
      fungus B35.1
    nail L03.03-
      fungus B35.1
  tongue NEC K14.0
    parasitic B37.0
  tonsil (and adenoid) (faucial) (lingual) (pharyngeal) —*see* Tonsillitis
  tooth, teeth K04.7
    periapical K04.7
    peridental, periodontal K05.20
      generalized —*see* Periodontitis, aggressive, generalized
      localized —*see* Periodontitis, aggressive, localized
    pulp K04.01
      irreversible K04.02
      reversible K04.01
    socket M27.3
  TORCH —*see* Infection, congenital without active infection P00.2
  Torula histolytica —*see* Cryptococcosis
  Toxocara (canis) (cati) (felis) B83.0
  Toxoplasma gondii —*see* Toxoplasma
  trachea, chronic J42
  trematode NEC —*see* Infestation, fluke
  trench fever A79.0
  Treponema pallidum —*see* Syphilis
  Trichinella (spiralis) B75
  Trichomonas A59.9
    cervix A59.09

Infection, infected, infective (continued)
Trichomonas (continued)
  intestine A07.8
  prostate A59.02
  specified site NEC A59.8
  urethra A59.03
  urogenitalis A59.00
  vagina A59.01
  vulva A59.01
Trichophyton, trichophytic —see Dermatophytosis
Trichosporon (beigelii) cutaneum B36.2
Trichostrongylus B81.2
Trichuris (trichiura) B79
Trombicula (irritans) B88.0
Trypanosoma
  brucei
    gambiense B56.0
    rhodesiense B56.1
  cruzi —see Chagas' disease
  tubal —see Salpingo-oophoritis
tuberculous
  latent (LTBI) Z22.7
  NEC —see Tuberculosis
tubo-ovarian —see Salpingo-oophoritis
tunnel T80.212
tunica vaginalis N49.1
tympanic membrane NEC —see Myringitis
typhoid (abortive) (ambulant) (bacillus) —see Typhoid
typhus A75.9
  flea-borne A75.2
  mite-borne A75.3
  recrudescent A75.1
  tick-borne A77.9
    African A77.1
    North Asian A77.2
umbilicus L08.82
ureter —see Ureteritis
urethra —see Urethritis
urinary (tract) N39.0
  bladder —see Cystitis
  complicating
    pregnancy O23.4-
      specified type NEC O23.3-
  kidney —see Infection, kidney
  newborn P39.3
  puerperal (postpartum) O86.20
  tuberculous A18.13
  urethra —see Urethritis
uterus, uterine —see Endometritis
vaccination T88.0
vaccinia not from vaccination B08.011
vagina (acute) —see Vaginitis
varicella B01.9
varicose veins —see Varix
vas deferens NEC N49.1
vesical —see Cystitis
Vibrio
  cholerae A00.0
    El Tor A00.1
  parahaemolyticus (food poisoning) A05.3
  vulnificus
    as cause of disease classified elsewhere B96.82
    foodborne intoxication A05.5
Vincent's (gum) (mouth) (tonsil) A69.1
virus, viral NOS B34.9
  adenovirus
    as cause of disease classified elsewhere B97.0
    unspecified nature or site B34.0

Infection, infected, infective (continued)
virus, viral NOS (continued)
  arborvirus, arbovirus arthropod-borne A94
  as cause of disease classified elsewhere B97.89
    adenovirus B97.0
    coronavirus B97.29
      SARS-associated B97.21
    coxsackievirus B97.11
    echovirus B97.12
    enterovirus B97.10
      coxsackievirus B97.11
      echovirus B97.12
      specified NEC B97.19
    human
      immunodeficiency, type 2 (HIV 2) B97.35
      T-cell lymphotropic,
        type I (HTLV-I) B97.33
        type II (HTLV-II) B97.34
    metapneumovirus B97.81
    papillomavirus B97.7
    parvovirus B97.6
    reovirus B97.5
    respiratory syncytial (RSV) —see Infection, virus, respiratory syncytial (RSV)
    retrovirus B97.30
      human
        immunodeficiency, type 2 (HIV 2) B97.35
        T-cell lymphotropic,
          type I (HTLV-I) B97.33
          type II (HTLV-II) B97.34
      lentivirus B97.31
      oncovirus B97.32
      specified NEC B97.39
    specified NEC B97.89
  central nervous system A89
    atypical A81.9
      specified NEC A81.89
    enterovirus NEC A88.8
      meningitis A87.0
    slow virus A81.9
      specified NEC A81.89
    specified NEC A88.8
  chest J98.8
  cotia B08.8
  COVID-19 U07.1
  coxsackie (see also Infection, coxsackie) B34.1
    as cause of disease classified elsewhere B97.11
  ECHO
    as cause of disease classified elsewhere B97.12
    unspecified nature or site B34.1
  encephalitis, tick-borne A84.9
  enterovirus, as cause of disease classified elsewhere B97.10
    coxsackievirus B97.11
    echovirus B97.12
    specified NEC B97.19
  exanthem NOS B09
  human papilloma as cause of disease classified elsewhere B97.7
  human metapneumovirus as cause of disease classified elsewhere B97.81
  intestine —see Enteritis, viral
  respiratory syncytial (RSV)
    as cause of disease classified elsewhere B97.4
    bronchiolitis J21.0

Infection, infected, infective (continued)
virus, viral NOS (continued)
  respiratory syncytial (continued)
    bronchitis J20.5
    bronchopneumonia J12.1
    otitis media H65.- [B97.4]
    pneumonia J12.1
    upper respiratory infection J06.9 [B97.4]
  rhinovirus
    as cause of disease classified elsewhere B97.89
    unspecified nature or site B34.8
  slow A81.9
    specified NEC A81.89
  specified type NEC B33.8
    as cause of disease classified elsewhere B97.89
    unspecified nature or site B34.8
  unspecified nature or site B34.9
  West Nile —see Virus, West Nile
  vulva (acute) —see Vulvitis
West Nile —see Virus, West Nile
whipworm B79
worms B83.9
  specified type NEC B83.8
Wuchereria (bancrofti) B74.0
  malayi B74.1
yatapoxvirus B08.70
  specified NEC B08.79
yeast (see also Candidiasis) B37.9
yellow fever —see Fever, yellow
Yersinia
  enterocolitica (intestinal) A04.6
  pestis —see Plague
  pseudotuberculosis A28.2
Zeis' gland —see Hordeolum
Zika virus A92.5
  congenital P35.4
zoonotic bacterial NOS A28.9
Zopfia senegalensis B47.0

Infective, infectious —see condition

Infertility
female N97.9
  age-related N97.8
  associated with
    anovulation N97.0
    cervical (mucus) disease or anomaly N88.3
    congenital anomaly
      cervix N88.3
      fallopian tube N97.1
      uterus N97.2
      vagina N97.8
    dysmucorrhea N88.3
    fallopian tube disease or anomaly N97.1
    pituitary-hypothalamic origin E23.0
    specified origin NEC N97.8
    Stein-Leventhal syndrome E28.2
    uterine disease or anomaly N97.2
    vaginal disease or anomaly N97.8
  due to
    cervical anomaly N88.3
    fallopian tube anomaly N97.1
    ovarian failure E28.39
    Stein-Leventhal syndrome E28.2
    uterine anomaly N97.2
    vaginal anomaly N97.8
    nonimplantation N97.2

Infertility (continued)
female (continued)
  origin
    cervical N88.3
    tubal (block) (occlusion) (stenosis) N97.1
    uterine N97.2
    vaginal N97.8
  male N46.9
    azoospermia N46.01
      extratesticular cause N46.029
        drug therapy N46.021
        efferent duct obstruction N46.023
        infection N46.022
        radiation N46.024
        specified cause NEC N46.029
        systemic disease N46.025
    oligospermia N46.11
      extratesticular cause N46.129
        drug therapy N46.121
        efferent duct obstruction N46.123
        infection N46.122
        radiation N46.124
        specified cause NEC N46.129
        systemic disease N46.125
    specified type NEC N46.8

Infestation B88.9
Acanthocheilonema (perstans) (streptocerca) B74.4
Acariasis B88.0
  demodex folliculorum B88.0
  sarcoptes scabiei B86
  trombiculae B88.0
Agamofilaria streptocerca B74.4
Ancylostoma, ankylostoma (braziliense) (caninum) (ceylanicum) (duodenale) B76.0
  americanum B76.1
  new world B76.1
Anisakis larvae, anisakiasis B81.0
arthropod NEC B88.2
Ascaris lumbricoides —see Ascariasis
Balantidium coli A07.0
beef tapeworm B68.1
Bothriocephalus (latus) B70.0
  larval B70.1
broad tapeworm B70.0
  larval B70.1
Brugia (malayi) B74.1
  timori B74.2
candiru B88.8
Capillaria
  hepatica B83.8
  philippinensis B81.1
cat liver fluke B66.0
cestodes B71.9
  diphyllobothrium —see Infestation, diphyllobothrium
  dipylidiasis B71.1
  hymenolepiasis B71.0
  specified type NEC B71.8
chigger B88.0
chigo, chigoe B88.1
Clonorchis (sinensis) (liver) B66.1
coccidial A07.3
crab-lice B85.3
Cysticercus cellulosae —see Cysticercosis
Demodex (folliculorum) B88.0
Dermanyssus gallinae B88.0
Dermatobia (hominis) —see Myiasis
Dibothriocephalus (latus) B70.0
  larval B70.1

197

Infestation (*continued*)
- Dicrocoelium dendriticum B66.2
- Diphyllobothrium (adult) (latum) (intestinal) (pacificum) B70.0
  - larval B70.1
- Diplogonoporus (grandis) B71.8
- Dipylidium caninum B67.4
- Distoma hepaticum B66.3
- dog tapeworm B67.4
- Dracunculus medinensis B72
- dragon worm B72
- dwarf tapeworm B71.0
- Echinococcus —*see* Echinococcus
- Echinostomum ilocanum B66.8
- Entamoeba (histolytica) —*see* Infection, Ameba
- Enterobius vermicularis B80
- eyelid
  - in (due to)
    - leishmaniasis B55.1
    - loiasis B74.3
    - onchocerciasis B73.09
    - phthiriasis B85.3
    - parasitic NOS B89
- eyeworm B74.3
- Fasciola (gigantica) (hepatica) (indica) B66.3
- Fasciolopsis (buski) (intestine) B66.5
- filarial B74.9
  - bancroftian B74.0
  - conjunctiva B74.9
  - due to
    - Acanthocheilonema (perstans) (streptocerca) B74.4
    - Brugia (malayi) B74.1
      - timori B74.2
    - Dracunculus medinensis B72
    - guinea worm B72
    - loa loa B74.3
    - Mansonella (ozzardi) (perstans) (streptocerca) B74.4
    - Onchocerca volvulus B73.00
      - eye B73.00
      - eyelid B73.09
    - Wuchereria (bancrofti) B74.0
  - Malayan B74.1
  - ozzardi B74.4
  - specified type NEC B74.8
- fish tapeworm B70.0
  - larval B70.1
- fluke B66.9
  - blood NOS —*see* Schistosomiasis
  - cat liver B66.0
  - intestinal B66.5
  - liver (sheep) B66.3
    - cat B66.0
    - Chinese B66.1
    - due to clonorchiasis B66.1
    - oriental B66.1
  - lancet B66.2
  - lung (oriental) B66.4
  - sheep liver B66.3
  - specified type NEC B66.8
- fly larvae —*see* Myiasis
- Gasterophilus (intestinalis) —*see* Myiasis
- Gastrodiscoides hominis B66.8
- Giardia lamblia A07.1
- Gnathostoma (spinigerum) B83.1
- Gongylonema B83.8
- guinea worm B72
- helminth B83.9
  - angiostrongyliasis B83.2
    - intestinal B81.3
  - gnathostomiasis B83.1
  - hirudiniasis, internal B83.4

Infestation (*continued*)
- helminth (*continued*)
  - intestinal B82.0
    - angiostrongyliasis B81.3
    - anisakiasis B81.0
    - ascariasis —*see* Ascariasis
    - capillariasis B81.1
    - cysticercosis —*see* Cysticercosis
    - diphyllobothriasis —*see* Infestation, diphyllobothriasis
    - dracunculiasis B72
    - echinococcus —*see* Echinococcosis
    - enterobiasis B80
    - filariasis —*see* Infestation, filarial
    - fluke —*see* Infestation, fluke
    - hookworm —*see* Infestation, hookworm
    - mixed (types classifiable to more than one of the titles B65.0-B81.3 and B81.8) B81.4
    - onchocerciasis —*see* Onchocerciasis
    - schistosomiasis —*see* Infestation, schistosoma
    - specified
      - cestode NEC —*see* Infestation, cestode
      - type NEC B81.8
    - strongyloidiasis —*see* Strongyloidiasis
    - taenia —*see* Infestation, taenia
    - trichinellosis B75
    - trichostrongyliasis B81.2
    - trichuriasis B79
  - specified type NEC B83.8
  - syngamiasis B83.3
  - visceral larva migrans B83.0
- Heterophyes (heterophyes) B66.8
- hookworm B76.9
  - ancylostomiasis B76.0
  - necatoriasis B76.1
  - specified type NEC B76.8
- Hymenolepis (diminuta) (nana) B71.0
- intestinal NEC B82.9
- leeches (aquatic) (land) —*see* Hirudiniasis
- Leishmania —*see* Leishmaniasis
- lice, louse —*see* Infestation, Pediculus
- Linguatula B88.8
- Liponyssoides sanguineus B88.0
- Loa loa B74.3
  - conjunctival B74.3
  - eyelid B74.3
- louse —*see* Infestation, Pediculus
- maggots —*see* Myiasis
- Mansonella (ozzardi) (perstans) (streptocerca) B74.4
- Medina (worm) B72
- Metagonimus (yokogawai) B66.8
- microfilaria streptocerca —*see* Onchocerciasis
  - eye B73.00
  - eyelid B73.09
- mites B88.9
  - scabic B86
- Monilia (albicans) —*see* Candidiasis
- mouth B37.0
- Necator americanus B76.1
- nematode NEC (intestinal) B82.0
  - Ancylostoma B76.0
  - conjunctiva NEC B83.9
  - Enterobius vermicularis B80
  - Gnathostoma spinigerum B83.1
  - physaloptera B80

Infestation (*continued*)
- nematode (*continued*)
  - specified NEC B81.8
  - trichostrongylus B81.2
  - trichuris (trichuria) B79
- Oesophagostomum (apiostomum) B81.8
- Oestrus ovis (*see also* Myiasis) B87.9
- Onchocerca (volvulus) —*see* Onchocerciasis
- Opisthorchis (felineus) (viverrini) B66.0
- orbit, parasitic NOS B89
- Oxyuris vermicularis B80
- Paragonimus (westermani) B66.4
- parasite, parasitic B89
  - eyelid B89
  - intestinal NOS B82.9
  - mouth B37.0
  - skin B88.9
  - tongue B37.0
- Parastrongylus
  - cantonensis B83.2
  - costaricensis B81.3
- Pediculus B85.2
  - body B85.1
  - capitis (humanus) (any site) B85.0
  - corporis (humanus) (any site) B85.1
  - head B85.0
  - mixed (classifiable to more than one of the titles B85.0-B85.3) B85.4
  - pubis (any site) B85.3
- Pentastoma B88.8
- pest Z50.19
- Phthirus (pubis) (any site) B85.3
  - with any infestation classifiable to B85.0-B85.2 B85.4
- pinworm B80
- pork tapeworm (adult) B68.0
- protozoal NEC B64
  - intestinal A07.9
    - specified NEC A07.8
  - specified NEC B60.8
- pubic, louse B85.3
- rat tapeworm B71.0
- red bug B88.0
- roundworm (large) NEC B82.0
  - Ascariasis (*see also* Ascariasis) B77.9
- sandflea B88.1
- Sarcoptes scabiei B86
- scabies B86
- Schistosoma B65.9
  - bovis B65.8
  - cercariae B65.3
  - haematobium B65.0
  - intercalatum B65.8
  - japonicum B65.2
  - mansoni B65.1
  - mattheei B65.8
  - mekongi B65.8
  - specified type NEC B65.8
  - spindale B65.8
- screw worms —*see* Myiasis
- skin NOS B88.9
- Sparganum (mansoni) (proliferum) (baxteri) B70.1
  - larval B70.1
- specified type NEC B88.8
- Spirometra larvae B70.1
- Stellantchasmus falcatus B66.8
- Strongyloides stercoralis —*see* Strongyloidiasis
- Taenia B68.9
  - diminuta B71.0
  - echinococcus —*see* Echinococcus

Infestation (*continued*)
- Taenia (*continued*)
  - mediocanellata B68.1
  - nana B71.0
  - saginata B68.1
  - solium (intestinal form) B68.0
    - larval form —*see* Cysticercosis
- Taeniarhynchus saginatus B68.1
- tapeworm B71.9
  - beef B68.1
  - broad B70.0
    - larval B70.1
  - dog B67.4
  - dwarf B71.0
  - fish B70.0
    - larval B70.1
  - pork B68.0
  - rat B71.0
- Ternidens diminutus B81.8
- Tetranychus molestissimus B88.0
- threadworm B80
- tongue B37.0
- Toxocara (canis) (cati) (felis) B83.0
- trematode(s) NEC —*see* Infestation, fluke
- Trichinella (spiralis) B75
- Trichocephalus B79
- Trichomonas —*see* Trichomoniasis
- Trichostrongylus B81.2
- Trichuris (trichiura) B79
- Trombicula (irritans) B88.0
- Tunga penetrans B88.1
- Uncinaria americana B76.1
- Vandellia cirrhosa B88.8
- whipworm B79
- worms B83.9
  - intestinal B82.0
- Wuchereria (bancrofti) B74.0

Infiltrate, infiltration
- amyloid (generalized) (localized) —*see* Amyloidosis
- calcareous NEC R89.7
  - localized —*see* Degeneration, by site
- calcium salt R89.7
- cardiac
  - fatty —*see* Degeneration, myocardial
  - glycogenic E74.02 [I43]
- corneal —*see* Edema, cornea
- eyelid —*see* Inflammation, eyelid
- glycogen, glycogenic —*see* Disease, glycogen storage
- heart, cardiac
  - fatty —*see* Degeneration, myocardial
  - glycogenic E74.02 [I43]
- inflammatory in vitreous H43.89
- kidney N28.89
- leukemic —*see* Leukemia
- liver K76.89
  - fatty —*see* Fatty, liver NEC
  - glycogen (*see also* Disease, glycogen storage) E74.03 [K77]
- lung R91.8
  - eosinophilic —*see* Eosinophilia, pulmonary
- lymphatic (*see also* Leukemia, lymphatic) C91.9-
  - gland I88.9
- muscle, fatty M62.89
- myocardium, myocardial
  - fatty —*see* Degeneration, myocardial
  - glycogenic E74.02 [I43]
- on chest x-ray R91.8
- pulmonary R91.8
  - with eosinophilia —*see* Eosinophilia, pulmonary
- skin (lymphocytic) L98.6
- thymus (gland) (fatty) E32.8

Infiltrate, infiltration (continued)
  urine R39.0
  vesicant agent
    antineoplastic chemotherapy T80.810
    other agent NEC T80.818
  vitreous body H43.89
Infirmity R68.89
  senile R54
Inflammation, inflamed, inflammatory (with exudation)
  abducent (nerve) —see Strabismus, paralytic, sixth nerve
  accessory sinus (chronic) —see Sinusitis
  adrenal (gland) E27.8
  alveoli, teeth M27.3
    scorbutic E54
  anal canal, anus K62.89
  antrum (chronic) —see Sinusitis, maxillary
  appendix —see Appendicitis
  arachnoid —see Meningitis
  areola N61.0
    puerperal, postpartum or gestational —see Infection, nipple
  areolar tissue NOS L08.9
  artery —see Arteritis
  auditory meatus (external) —see Otitis, externa
  Bartholin's gland N75.8
  bile duct (common) (hepatic) or passage —see Cholangitis
  bladder —see Cystitis
  bone —see Osteomyelitis
  brain —see also Encephalitis
    membrane —see Meningitis
  breast N61.0
    puerperal, postpartum, gestational —see Mastitis, obstetric
  broad ligament —see Disease, pelvis, inflammatory
  bronchi —see Bronchitis
  catarrhal J00
  cecum —see Appendicitis
  cerebral —see also Encephalitis
    membrane —see Meningitis
  cerebrospinal
    meningococcal A39.0
  cervix (uteri) —see Cervicitis
  chest J98.8
  chorioretinal H30.9-
    cyclitis —see Cyclitis
    disseminated H30.10-
      generalized H30.13-
      peripheral H30.12-
      posterior pole H30.11-
    epitheliopathy —see Epitheliopathy
    focal H30.00-
      juxtapapillary H30.01-
      macular H30.04-
      paramacular —see Inflammation, chorioretinal, focal, macular
      peripheral H30.03-
      posterior pole H30.02-
    specified type NEC H30.89-
  choroid —see Inflammation, chorioretinal
  chronic, postmastoidectomy cavity —see Complications, postmastoidectomy, inflammation
  colon —see Enteritis
  connective tissue (diffuse) NEC —see Disorder, soft tissue, specified type NEC

Inflammation, inflamed, inflammatory (continued)
  cornea —see Keratitis
  corpora cavernosa N48.29
  cranial nerve —see Disorder, nerve, cranial
  Douglas' cul-de-sac or pouch (chronic) N73.0
  due to device, implant or graft —see also Complications, by site and type, infection or inflammation
    arterial graft T82.7
    breast (implant) T85.79
    catheter T85.79
      dialysis (renal) T82.7
        intraperitoneal T85.71
      infusion T82.7
        cranial T85.735
        intrathecal T85.735
        spinal (epidural) (subdural) T85.735
        subarachnoid T85.735
      urinary T83.51
        cystostomy T83.510
        Hopkins T83.518
        ileostomy T83.518
        nephrostomy T83.512
        specified NEC T83.518
        urethral indwelling T83.511
        urostomy T83.518
    electronic (electrode) (pulse generator) (stimulator)
      bone T84.7
      cardiac T82.7
      nervous system T85.738
        brain T85.731
        cranial nerve T85.732
        gastric nerve T85.732
        neurostimulator generator T85.734
        peripheral nerve T85.732
        sacral nerve T85.732
        spinal cord T85.733
        vagal nerve T85.732
      urinary T83.590
    fixation, internal (orthopedic) NEC —see Complication, fixation device, infection
    gastrointestinal (bile duct) (esophagus) T85.79
      neurostimulator electrode (lead) T85.732
    genital NEC T83.69
    heart NEC T82.7
      valve (prosthesis) T82.6
        graft T82.7
    joint prosthesis —see Complication, joint prosthesis, infection
    ocular (corneal graft) (orbital implant) NEC T85.79
    orthopedic NEC T84.7
    penile (cylinder) (pump) (resevoir) T83.61
    specified NEC T85.79
    testicular T83.62
    urinary NEC T83.598
      ileal conduit stent T83.593
      implanted neurostimulation T83.590
      implanted sphincter T83.591
      indwelling ureteral stent T83.592
      nephroureteral stent T83.593
      specified stent NEC T83.593
    vascular NEC T82.7
    ventricular intracranial (communicating) shunt T85.730

Inflammation, inflamed, inflammatory (continued)
  duodenum K29.80
    with bleeding K29.81
  dura mater —see Meningitis
  ear (middle) —see also Otitis, media
    external —see Otitis, externa
    inner —see subcategory H83.0
  epididymis —see Epididymitis
  esophagus —see Esophagitis
  ethmoidal (sinus) (chronic) —see Sinusitis, ethmoidal
  eustachian tube (catarrhal) —see Salpingitis, eustachian
  eyelid H01.9
    abscess —see Abscess, eyelid
    blepharitis —see Blepharitis
    chalazion —see Chalazion
    dermatosis (noninfectious) —see Dermatosis, eyelid
    hordeolum —see Hordeolum
    specified NEC H01.8
  fallopian tube —see Salpingo-oophoritis
  fascia —see Myositis
  follicular, pharynx J31.2
  frontal (sinus) (chronic) —see Sinusitis, frontal
  gallbladder —see Cholecystitis
  gastric —see Gastritis
  gastrointestinal —see Enteritis
  genital organ (internal) (diffuse)
    female —see Disease, pelvis, inflammatory
    male N49.9
      multiple sites N49.8
      specified NEC N49.8
  gland (lymph) —see Lymphadenitis
  glottis —see Laryngitis
  granular, pharynx J31.2
  gum K05.10
    nonplaque induced K05.11
    plaque induced K05.10
  heart —see Carditis
  hepatic duct —see Cholangitis
  ileoanal (internal) pouch K91.850
  ileum —see also Enteritis
    regional or terminal —see Enteritis, regional
  intestine (any part) —see Enteritis
  intestinal pouch K91.850
  jaw (acute) (bone) (chronic) (lower) (suppurative) (upper) M27.2
  joint NEC —see Arthritis
    sacroiliac M46.1
  kidney —see Nephritis
  knee (joint) M13.169
    tuberculous A18.02
  labium (majus) (minus) —see Vulvitis
  lacrimal
    gland —see Dacryoadenitis
    passages (duct) (sac) —see also Dacryocystitis
      canaliculitis —see Canaliculitis, lacrimal
  larynx —see Laryngitis
  leg NOS L08.9
  lip K13.0
  liver (capsule) —see also Hepatitis
    chronic K73.9
    suppurative K75.0
  lung (acute) —see also Pneumonia
    chronic J98.4
  lymph gland or node —see Lymphadenitis
  lymphatic vessel —see Lymphangitis
  maxilla, maxillary M27.2
    sinus (chronic) —see Sinusitis, maxillary

Inflammation, inflamed, inflammatory (continued)
  membranes of brain or spinal cord —see Meningitis
  meninges —see Meningitis
  mouth K12.1
  muscle —see Myositis
  myocardium —see Myocarditis
  nasal sinus (chronic) —see Sinusitis
  nasopharynx —see Nasopharyngitis
  navel L08.82
  nerve NEC —see Neuritis
  nipple N61.0
    puerperal, postpartum or gestational —see Infection, nipple
  nose —see Rhinitis
  oculomotor (nerve) —see Strabismus, paralytic, third nerve
  optic nerve —see Neuritis, optic
  orbit (chronic) H05.10
    acute H05.00
      abscess —see Abscess, orbit
      cellulitis —see Cellulitis, orbit
      osteomyelitis —see Osteomyelitis, orbit
      periostitis —see Periostitis, orbital
      tenonitis —see Tenonitis, eye
    granuloma —see Granuloma, orbit
    myositis —see Myositis, orbital
  ovary —see Salpingo-oophoritis
  oviduct —see Salpingo-oophoritis
  pancreas (acute) —see Pancreatitis
  parametrium N73.0
  parotid region L08.9
  pelvis, female —see Disease, pelvis, inflammatory
  penis (corpora cavernosa) N48.29
  perianal K62.89
  pericardium —see Pericarditis
  perineum (female) (male) L08.9
  perirectal K62.89
  peritoneum —see Peritonitis
  periuterine —see Disease, pelvis, inflammatory
  perivesical —see Cystitis
  petrous bone (acute) (chronic) —see Petrositis
  pharynx (acute) —see Pharyngitis
  pia mater —see Meningitis
  pleura —see Pleurisy
  polyp, colon (see also Polyp, colon, inflammatory) K51.40
  prostate —see Prostatitis
    specified type NEC N41.8
  rectosigmoid —see Rectosigmoiditis
  rectum (see also Proctitis) K62.89
  respiratory, upper (see also Infection, respiratory, upper) J06.9
    acute, due to radiation J70.0
    chronic, due to external agent —see condition, respiratory, chronic, due to
    due to
      chemicals, gases, fumes or vapors (inhalation) J68.2
      radiation J70.1
  retina —see Chorioretinitis
  retrocecal —see Appendicitis
  retroperitoneal —see Peritonitis
  salivary duct or gland (any) (suppurative) —see Sialoadenitis
  scorbutic, alveoli, teeth E54
  scrotum N49.2

Inflammation, inflamed, inflammatory (continued)
- seminal vesicle —see Vesiculitis
- sigmoid —see Enteritis
- sinus —see Sinusitis
- Skene's duct or gland —see Urethritis
- skin L08.9
- spermatic cord N49.1
- sphenoidal (sinus) —see Sinusitis, sphenoidal
- spinal
  - cord —see Encephalitis
  - membrane —see Meningitis
  - nerve —see Disorder, nerve
- spine —see Spondylopathy, inflammatory
- spleen (capsule) D73.89
- stomach —see Gastritis
- subcutaneous tissue L08.9
- suprarenal (gland) E27.8
- synovial —see Tenosynovitis
- tendon (sheath) NEC —see Tenosynovitis
- testis —see Orchitis
- throat (acute) —see Pharyngitis
- thymus (gland) E32.8
- thyroid (gland) —see Thyroiditis
- tongue K14.0
- tonsil —see Tonsillitis
- trachea —see Tracheitis
- trochlear (nerve) —see Strabismus, paralytic, fourth nerve
- tubal —see Salpingo-oophoritis
- tuberculous NEC —see Tuberculosis
- tubo-ovarian —see Salpingo-oophoritis
- tunica vaginalis N49.1
- tympanic membrane —see Tympanitis
- umbilicus, umbilical L08.82
- uterine ligament —see Disease, pelvis, inflammatory
- uterus (catarrhal) —see Endometritis
- uveal tract (anterior) NOS —see also Iridocyclitis
  - posterior —see Chorioretinitis
- vagina —see Vaginitis
- vas deferens N49.1
- vein —see also Phlebitis
  - intracranial or intraspinal (septic) G08
  - thrombotic I80.9
    - leg —see Phlebitis, leg
    - lower extremity —see Phlebitis, leg
- vocal cord J38.3
- vulva —see Vulvitis
- Wharton's duct (suppurative) —see Sialoadenitis

Inflation, lung, imperfect (newborn) —see Atelectasis

Influenza (bronchial) (epidemic) (respiratory (upper)) (unidentified influenza virus) J11.1
- with
  - digestive manifestations J11.2
  - encephalopathy J11.81
  - enteritis J11.2
  - gastroenteritis J11.2
  - gastrointestinal manifestations J11.2
  - laryngitis J11.1
  - myocarditis J11.82
  - otitis media J11.83
  - pharyngitis J11.1
  - pneumonia J11.00
    - specified type J11.08

Influenza (continued)
- with (continued)
  - respiratory manifestations NEC J11.1
  - specified manifestation NEC J11.89
- A (non-novel) J10-
- A/H5N1 (see also Influenza, due to, identified novel influenza A virus) J09.X2
- avian (see also Influenza, due to, identified novel influenza A virus) J09.X2
- B J10-
- bird (see also Influenza, due to, identified novel influenza A virus) J09.X2
- C J10-
- due to
  - avian (see also Influenza, due to, identified novel influenza A virus) J09.X2
  - identified influenza virus NEC J10.1
    - with
      - digestive manifestations J10.2
      - encephalopathy J10.81
      - enteritis J10.2
      - gastroenteritis J10.2
      - gastrointestinal manifestations J10.2
      - laryngitis J10.1
      - myocarditis J10.82
      - otitis media J10.83
      - pharyngitis J10.1
      - pneumonia (unspecified type) J10.00
        - with same identified influenza virus J10.01
        - specified type NEC J10.08
      - respiratory manifestations NEC J10.1
      - specified manifestation NEC J10.89
  - identified novel influenza A virus J09.X2
    - with
      - digestive manifestations J09.X3
      - encephalopathy J09.X9
      - enteritis J09.X3
      - gastroenteritis J09.X3
      - gastrointestinal manifestations J09.X3
      - laryngitis J09.X2
      - myocarditis J09.X9
      - otitis media J09.X9
      - pharyngitis J09.X2
      - pneumonia J09.X1
      - respiratory manifestations NEC J09.X2
      - specified manifestation NEC J09.X9
      - upper respiratory symptoms J09.X2
  - novel (2009) H1N1 influenza (see also Influenza, due to, identified novel influenza A virus) NEC J10.1
  - novel influenza A/H1N1 (see also Influenza, due to, identified novel influenza A virus) NEC J10.1
  - of other animal origin, not bird or swine (see also Influenza, due to, identified novel influenza A virus) J09.X2
  - swine (viruses that normally cause infections in pigs) (see also Influenza, due to, identified novel influenza A virus) J09.X2

Influenza-like disease —see Influenza
Influenzal —see Influenza
Infraction, Freiberg's (metatarsal head) —see Osteochondrosis, juvenile, metatarsus
Infraeruption of tooth (teeth) M26.34
Infusion complication, misadventure, or reaction —see Complications, infusion

Ingestion
- chemical —see Table of Drugs and Chemicals, by substance, poisoning
- drug or medicament
  - correct substance properly administered —see Table of Drugs and Chemicals, by drug, adverse effect
  - overdose or wrong substance given or taken —see Table of Drugs and Chemicals, by drug, poisoning
- foreign body —see Foreign body, alimentary tract
- multiple drug —see Table of Drugs and Chemicals, multiple
- tularemia A21.3

Ingrowing
- hair (beard) L73.1
- nail (finger) (toe) L60.0

Inguinal —see also condition
- testicle Q53.9
  - bilateral Q53.212
  - unilateral Q53.112

Inhalant-induced
- anxiety disorder F18.980
- depressive disorder F18.94
- major neurocognitive disorder F18.97
- mild neurocognitive disorder F18.988
- psychotic disorder F18.959

Inhalation
- anthrax A22.1
- flame T27.3
- food or foreign body —see Foreign body, by site
- gases, fumes, or vapors T59.9-
  - specified agent NEC —see Table of Drugs and Chemicals, by substance T59.89-
- liquid or vomitus —see Asphyxia
- meconium (newborn) P24.00
  - with
    - pneumonia (pneumonitis) P24.01
    - with respiratory symptoms P24.01
- mucus —see Asphyxia, mucus
- oil or gasoline (causing suffocation) —see Foreign body, by site
- smoke T59.81-
  - with respiratory conditions J70.5
  - due to chemicals, gases, fumes and vapors J68.9
- steam (see also Burn, respiratory tract) T59.9-
- stomach contents or secretions —see Foreign body, by site
  - due to anesthesia (general) (local) or other sedation T88.59
    - in labor and delivery O74.0
    - in pregnancy O29.01-
    - postpartum, puerperal O89.01

Inhibition, orgasm
- female F52.31
- male F52.32

Inhibitor, systemic lupus erythematosus (presence of) D68.62

Iniencephalus, iniencephaly Q00.2

Injection, traumatic jet (air) (industrial) (water) (paint or dye) T70.4

Injury (see also specified injury type) T14.90
- abdomen, abdominal S39.91
  - blood vessel —see Injury, blood vessel, abdomen
  - cavity —see Injury, intra-abdominal
  - contusion S30.1
  - internal —see Injury, intra-abdominal
  - intra-abdominal organ —see Injury, intra-abdominal
  - nerve —see Injury, nerve, abdomen
  - open —see Wound, open, abdomen
  - specified NEC S39.81
  - superficial —see Injury, superficial, abdomen
- Achilles tendon S86.00-
  - laceration S86.02-
  - specified type NEC S86.09-
  - strain S86.01-
- acoustic, resulting in deafness —see Injury, nerve, acoustic
- adrenal (gland) S37.819
  - contusion S37.812
  - laceration S37.813
  - specified type NEC S37.818
- alveolar (process) S09.93
- ankle S99.91-
  - contusion —see Contusion, ankle
  - dislocation —see Dislocation, ankle
  - fracture —see Fracture, ankle
  - nerve —see Injury, nerve, ankle
  - open —see Wound, open, ankle
  - specified type NEC S99.81-
  - sprain —see Sprain, ankle
  - superficial —see Injury, superficial, ankle
- anterior chamber, eye —see Injury, eye, specified site NEC
- anus —see Injury, abdomen
- aorta (thoracic) S25.00
  - abdominal S35.00
    - laceration (minor) (superficial) S35.01
    - major S35.02
    - specified type NEC S35.09
  - laceration (minor) (superficial) S25.01
    - major S25.02
  - specified type NEC S25.09
- arm (upper) S49.9-
  - blood vessel —see Injury, blood vessel, arm
  - contusion —see Contusion, arm, upper
  - fracture —see Fracture, humerus
  - lower —see Injury, forearm
  - muscle —see Injury, muscle, shoulder
  - nerve —see Injury, nerve, arm
  - open —see Wound, open, arm
  - specified type NEC S49.8-
  - superficial —see Injury, superficial, arm

Injury *(continued)*
- artery (complicating trauma) —*see also* Injury, blood vessel, by site
  - cerebral or meningeal —*see* Injury, intracranial
- auditory canal (external) (meatus) S09.91
- auricle, auris, ear S09.91
- axilla —*see* Injury, shoulder
- back —*see* Injury, back, lower
- bile duct S36.13
- birth —*see also* Birth, injury P15.9
- bladder (sphincter) S37.20
  - at delivery O71.5
  - contusion S37.22
  - laceration S37.23
  - obstetrical trauma O71.5
  - specified type NEC S37.29
- blast (air) (hydraulic) (immersion) (underwater) NEC T14.8
  - acoustic nerve trauma —*see* Injury, nerve, acoustic
  - bladder —*see* Injury, bladder
  - brain —*see* Concussion
    - primary, specified NEC S06.8A-
  - colon —*see* Injury, intestine, large, blast injury
  - ear (primary) S09.31-
    - secondary S09.39-
  - generalized T70.8
  - lung —*see* Injury, intrathoracic, lung, blast injury
  - multiple body organs T70.8
  - peritoneum S36.81
  - rectum S36.61
  - retroperitoneum S36.898
  - small intestine S36.419
    - duodenum S36.410
    - specified site NEC S36.418
  - specified
    - intra-abdominal organ NEC S36.898
    - pelvic organ NEC S37.899
- blood vessel NEC T14.8
  - abdomen S35.9-
    - aorta —*see* Injury, aorta, abdominal
    - celiac artery —*see* Injury, blood vessel, celiac artery
    - iliac vessel —*see* Injury, blood vessel, iliac
    - laceration S35.91
    - mesenteric vessel —*see* Injury, mesenteric
    - portal vein —*see* Injury, blood vessel, portal vein
    - renal vessel —*see* Injury, blood vessel, renal
    - specified vessel NEC S35.8X-
    - splenic vessel —*see* Injury, blood vessel, splenic
    - vena cava —*see* Injury, vena cava, inferior
  - ankle —*see* Injury, blood vessel, foot
  - aorta (abdominal) (thoracic) —*see* Injury, aorta
  - arm (upper) NEC S45.90-
    - forearm —*see* Injury, blood vessel, forearm
    - laceration S45.91-
    - specified
      - site NEC S45.80-
        - laceration S45.81-
        - specified type NEC S45.89-
      - type NEC S45.99-
    - superficial vein S45.30-
      - laceration S45.31-
      - specified type NEC S45.39-

Injury *(continued)*
- blood vessel NEC *(continued)*
  - axillary
    - artery S45.00-
      - laceration S45.01-
      - specified type NEC S45.09-
    - vein S45.20-
      - laceration S45.21-
      - specified type NEC S45.29-
  - azygos vein —*see* Injury, blood vessel, thoracic, specified site NEC
  - brachial
    - artery S45.10-
      - laceration S45.11-
      - specified type NEC S45.19-
    - vein S45.20-
      - laceration S45.219
      - specified type NEC S45.29-
  - carotid artery (common) (external) (internal, extracranial) S15.00-
    - internal, intracranial S06.8
    - laceration (minor) (superficial) S15.01-
      - major S15.02-
    - specified type NEC S15.09-
  - celiac artery S35.219
    - branch S35.299
      - laceration (minor) (superficial) S35.291
        - major S35.292
      - specified NEC S35.298
    - laceration (minor) (superficial) S35.211
      - major S35.212
    - specified type NEC S35.218
  - cerebral —*see* Injury, intracranial
  - deep plantar —*see* Injury, blood vessel, plantar artery
  - digital (hand) —*see* Injury, blood vessel, finger
  - dorsal
    - artery (foot) S95.00-
      - laceration S95.01-
      - specified type NEC S95.09-
    - vein (foot) S95.20-
      - laceration S95.21-
      - specified type NEC S95.29-
  - due to accidental laceration during procedure —*see* Laceration, accidental complicating surgery
  - extremity —*see* Injury, blood vessel, limb
  - femoral
    - artery (common) (superficial) S75.00-
      - laceration (minor) (superficial) S75.01-
        - major S75.02-
      - specified type NEC S75.09-
    - vein (hip level) (thigh level) S75.10-
      - laceration (minor) (superficial) S75.11-
        - major S75.12-
      - specified type NEC S75.19-
  - finger S65.50-
    - index S65.50-
      - laceration S65.51-
      - specified type NEC S65.59-
    - laceration S65.51-
    - little S65.50-
      - laceration S65.51-
      - specified type NEC S65.59-
    - middle S65.50-
      - laceration S65.51-
      - specified type NEC S65.59-
    - specified type NEC S65.59-

Injury *(continued)*
- blood vessel NEC *(continued)*
  - finger *(continued)*
    - thumb —*see* Injury, blood vessel, thumb
  - foot S95.90-
    - dorsal
      - artery —*see* Injury, blood vessel, dorsal, artery
      - vein —*see* Injury, blood vessel, dorsal, vein
    - laceration S95.91-
    - plantar artery —*see* Injury, blood vessel, plantar artery
    - specified
      - site NEC S95.80-
        - laceration S95.81-
        - specified type NEC S95.89-
      - specified type NEC S95.99-
  - forearm S55.90-
    - laceration S55.91-
    - radial artery —*see* Injury, blood vessel, radial artery
    - specified
      - site NEC S55.80-
        - laceration S55.81-
        - specified type NEC S55.89-
      - type NEC S55.99-
    - ulnar artery —*see* Injury, blood vessel, ulnar artery
    - vein S55.20-
      - laceration S55.21-
      - specified type NEC S55.29-
  - gastric
    - artery —*see* Injury, mesenteric, artery, branch
    - vein —*see* Injury, blood vessel, abdomen
  - gastroduodenal artery —*see* Injury, mesenteric, artery, branch
  - greater saphenous vein (lower leg level) S85.30-
    - hip (and thigh) level S75.20-
      - laceration (minor) (superficial) S75.21-
        - major S75.22-
      - specified type NEC S75.29-
    - laceration S85.31-
    - specified type NEC S85.39-
  - hand (level) S65.90-
    - finger —*see* Injury, blood vessel, finger
    - laceration S65.91-
    - palmar arch —*see* Injury, blood vessel, palmar arch
    - radial artery —*see* Injury, blood vessel, radial artery, hand
    - specified
      - site NEC S65.80-
        - laceration S65.81-
        - specified type NEC S65.89-
      - type NEC S65.99-
    - thumb —*see* Injury, blood vessel, thumb
    - ulnar artery —*see* Injury, blood vessel, ulnar artery, hand
  - head S09.0
    - intracranial —*see* Injury, intracranial
    - multiple S09.0
  - hepatic
    - artery —*see* Injury, mesenteric, artery
    - vein —*see* Injury, vena cava, inferior

Injury *(continued)*
- blood vessel NEC *(continued)*
  - hip S75.90-
    - femoral artery —*see* Injury, blood vessel, femoral, artery
    - femoral vein —*see* Injury, blood vessel, femoral, vein
    - greater saphenous vein —*see* Injury, blood vessel, greater saphenous, hip level
    - laceration S75.91-
    - specified
      - site NEC S75.80-
        - laceration S75.81-
        - specified type NEC S75.89-
      - type NEC S75.99-
  - hypogastric (artery) (vein) —*see* Injury, blood vessel, iliac
  - iliac S35.5-
    - artery S35.51-
    - specified vessel NEC S35.5-
    - uterine vessel —*see* Injury, blood vessel, uterine
    - vein S35.51-
  - innominate —*see* Injury, blood vessel, thoracic, innominate
  - intercostal (artery) (vein) —*see* Injury, blood vessel, thoracic, intercostal
  - jugular vein (external) S15.20-
    - internal S15.30-
      - laceration (minor) (superficial) S15.31-
        - major S15.32-
      - specified type NEC S15.39-
    - laceration (minor) (superficial) S15.21-
      - major S15.22-
    - specified type NEC S15.29-
  - leg (level) (lower) S85.90-
    - greater saphenous —*see* Injury, blood vessel, greater saphenous
    - laceration S85.91-
    - lesser saphenous —*see* Injury, blood vessel, lesser saphenous
    - peroneal artery —*see* Injury, blood vessel, peroneal artery
    - popliteal
      - artery —*see* Injury, blood vessel, popliteal, artery
      - vein —*see* Injury, blood vessel, popliteal, vein
    - specified
      - site NEC S85.80-
        - laceration S85.81-
        - specified type NEC S85.89-
      - type NEC S85.99-
    - thigh —*see* Injury, blood vessel, hip
    - tibial artery —*see* Injury, blood vessel, tibial artery
  - lesser saphenous vein (lower leg level) S85.40-
    - laceration S85.41-
    - specified type NEC S85.49-
  - limb
    - lower —*see* Injury, blood vessel, leg
    - upper —*see* Injury, blood vessel, arm
  - lower back —*see* Injury, blood vessel, abdomen
  - specified NEC —*see* Injury, blood vessel, abdomen, specified, site NEC

Injury *(continued)*
  blood vessel NEC *(continued)*
    mammary (artery) (vein) —*see* Injury, blood vessel, thoracic, specified site NEC
    mesenteric (inferior) (superior)
      artery —*see* Injury, mesenteric, artery
      vein —*see* Injury, mesenteric, vein
    neck S15.9
      specified site NEC S15.8
    ovarian (artery) (vein) —*see* subcategory S35.8
    palmar arch (superficial) S65.20-
      deep S65.30-
        laceration S65.31-
        specified type NEC S65.39-
      laceration S65.21-
      specified type NEC S65.29-
    pelvis —*see* Injury, blood vessel, abdomen, specified NEC —*see* Injury, blood vessel, abdomen, specified, site NEC
    peroneal artery S85.20-
      laceration S85.21-
      specified type NEC S85.29-
    plantar artery (deep) (foot) S95.10-
      laceration S95.11-
      specified type NEC S95.19-
    popliteal
      artery S85.00-
        laceration S85.01-
        specified type NEC S85.09-
      vein S85.50-
        laceration S85.51-
        specified type NEC S85.59-
    portal vein S35.319
      laceration S35.311
      specified type NEC S35.318
    precerebral —*see* Injury, blood vessel, neck
    pulmonary (artery) (vein) —*see* Injury, blood vessel, thoracic, pulmonary
    radial artery (forearm level) S55.10-
      hand and wrist (level) S65.10-
        laceration S65.11-
        specified type NEC S65.19-
      laceration S55.11-
      specified type NEC S55.19-
    renal
      artery S35.40-
        laceration S35.41-
        specified NEC S35.49-
      vein S35.40-
        laceration S35.41-
        specified NEC S35.49-
    saphenous vein (greater) (lower leg level) —*see* Injury, blood vessel, greater saphenous
      hip and thigh level —*see* Injury, blood vessel, greater saphenous, hip level
      lesser —*see* Injury, blood vessel, lesser saphenous
    shoulder
      specified NEC —*see* Injury, blood vessel, arm, specified site NEC
    superficial vein —*see* Injury, blood vessel, arm, superficial vein
    specified NEC T14.8
    splenic
      artery —*see* Injury, blood vessel, celiac artery, branch

Injury *(continued)*
  blood vessel NEC *(continued)*
    splenic *(continued)*
      vein S35.329
        laceration S35.321
        specified NEC S35.328
    subclavian —*see* Injury, blood vessel, thoracic, innominate
    thigh —*see* Injury, blood vessel, hip
    thoracic S25.90
      aorta S25.00
        laceration (minor) (superficial) S25.01
          major S25.02
        specified type NEC S25.09
      azygos vein —*see* Injury, blood vessel, thoracic, specified, site NEC
      innominate
        artery S25.10-
          laceration (minor) (superficial) S25.11-
            major S25.12-
          specified type NEC S25.19-
        vein S25.30-
          laceration (minor) (superficial) S25.31-
            major S25.32-
          specified type NEC S25.39-
      intercostal S25.50-
        laceration S25.51-
        specified type NEC S25.59-
      laceration S25.91
      mammary vessel —*see* Injury, blood vessel, thoracic, specified, site NEC
      pulmonary S25.40-
        laceration (minor) (superficial) S25.41-
          major S25.42-
        specified type NEC S25.49-
      specified
        site NEC S25.80-
          laceration S25.81-
          specified type NEC S25.89-
        type NEC S25.99
      subclavian —*see* Injury, blood vessel, thoracic, innominate
      vena cava (superior) S25.20
        laceration (minor) (superficial) S25.21
          major S25.22
        specified type NEC S25.29
    thumb S65.40-
      laceration S65.41-
      specified type NEC S65.49-
    tibial artery S85.10-
      anterior S85.13-
        laceration S85.14-
        specified injury NEC S85.15-
      laceration S85.11-
      posterior S85.16-
        laceration S85.17-
        specified injury NEC S85.18-
      specified injury NEC S85.12-
    ulnar artery (forearm level) S55.00-
      hand and wrist (level) S65.00-
        laceration S65.01-
        specified type NEC S65.09-
      laceration S55.01-
      specified type NEC S55.09-

Injury *(continued)*
  blood vessel NEC *(continued)*
    upper arm (level) —*see* Injury, blood vessel, arm
      superficial vein —*see* Injury, blood vessel, arm, superficial vein
    uterine S35.5-
      artery S35.53-
      vein S35.53-
    vena cava —*see* Injury, vena cava
    vertebral artery S15.10-
      laceration (minor) (superficial) S15.11-
        major S15.12-
      specified type NEC S15.19-
    wrist (level) —*see* Injury, blood vessel, hand
  brachial plexus S14.3
    newborn P14.3
  brain (traumatic) S06.9-
    diffuse (axonal) S06.2X-
    focal S06.30-
  brainstem S06.38-
  breast NOS S29.9
  broad ligament —*see* Injury, pelvic organ, specified site NEC
  bronchus, bronchi —*see* Injury, intrathoracic, bronchus
  brow S09.90
  buttock S39.92
  canthus, eye S05.90
  cardiac plexus —*see* Injury, nerve, thorax, sympathetic
  cauda equina S34.3
  cavernous sinus —*see* Injury, intracranial
  cecum —*see* Injury, colon
  celiac ganglion or plexus —*see* Injury, nerve, lumbosacral, sympathetic
  cerebellum —*see* Injury, intracranial
  cerebral —*see* Injury, intracranial
  cervix (uteri) —*see* Injury, uterus
  cheek (wall) S09.93
  chest —*see* Injury, thorax
  childbirth (newborn) —*see also* Birth, injury
    maternal NEC O71.9
  chin S09.93
  choroid (eye) —*see* Injury, eye, specified site NEC
  clitoris S39.94
  coccyx —*see also* Injury, back, lower
    complicating delivery O71.6
  colon —*see* Injury, intestine, large
  common bile duct —*see* Injury, liver
  conjunctiva (superficial) —*see* Injury, eye, conjunctiva
  conus medullaris —*see* Injury, spinal, sacral
  cord
    spermatic (pelvic region) S37.898
      scrotal region S39.848
    spinal —*see* Injury, spinal cord, by region
  cornea —*see* Injury, eye, specified site NEC
    abrasion —*see* Injury, eye, cornea, abrasion
  cortex (cerebral) —*see also* Injury, intracranial
    visual —*see* Injury, nerve, optic
  costal region NEC S29.9
  costochondral NEC S29.9

Injury *(continued)*
  cranial
    cavity —*see* Injury, intracranial
    nerve —*see* Injury, nerve, cranial
  crushing —*see* Crush
  cutaneous sensory nerve
  cystic duct —*see* Injury, liver
  deep tissue —*see* Contusion, by site
    meaning pressure ulcer —*see* Ulcer, pressure L89 with final character .6
  delivery (newborn) P15.9
    maternal NEC O71.9
  Descemet's membrane —*see* Injury, eyeball, penetrating
  diaphragm —*see* Injury, intrathoracic, diaphragm
  duodenum —*see* Injury, intestine, small, duodenum
  ear (auricle) (external) (canal) S09.91
    abrasion —*see* Abrasion, ear
    bite —*see* Bite, ear
    blister —*see* Blister, ear
    bruise —*see* Contusion, ear
    contusion —*see* Contusion, ear
    external constriction —*see* Constriction, external, ear
    hematoma —*see* Hematoma, ear
    inner —*see* Injury, ear, middle
    laceration —*see* Laceration, ear
    middle S09.30-
      blast —*see* Injury, blast, ear
      specified NEC S09.39-
    puncture —*see* Puncture, ear
    superficial —*see* Injury, superficial, ear
  eighth cranial nerve (acoustic or auditory) —*see* Injury, nerve, acoustic
  elbow S59.90-
    contusion —*see* Contusion, elbow
    dislocation —*see* Dislocation, elbow
    fracture —*see* Fracture, ulna, upper end
    open —*see* Wound, open, elbow
    specified NEC S59.80-
    sprain —*see* Sprain, elbow
    superficial —*see* Injury, superficial, elbow
  eleventh cranial nerve (accessory) —*see* Injury, nerve, accessory
  epididymis S39.94
  epigastric region S39.91
  epiglottis NEC S19.89
  esophageal plexus —*see* Injury, nerve, thorax, sympathetic
  esophagus (thoracic part) —*see also* Injury, intrathoracic, esophagus
    cervical NEC S19.85
  eustachian tube S09.30-
  eye S05.9-
    avulsion S05.7-
    ball —*see* Injury, eyeball
    conjunctiva S05.0-
    cornea
      abrasion S05.0-
      laceration S05.3-
        with prolapse S05.2-
    lacrimal apparatus S05.8X-
    orbit penetration S05.4-
    specified site NEC S05.8X-

Injury (continued)
  eyeball S05.8X-
    contusion S05.1-
    penetrating S05.6-
      with
        foreign body S05.5-
        prolapse or loss of
          intraocular tissue S05.2-
        without prolapse or loss of
          intraocular tissue S05.3-
    specified type NEC S05.8-
  eyebrow S09.93
  eyelid S09.93
    abrasion —see Abrasion, eyelid
    contusion —see Contusion,
      eyelid
    open —see Wound, open, eyelid
  face S09.93
  fallopian tube S37.509
    bilateral S37.502
      blast injury S37.512
      contusion S37.522
      laceration S37.532
      specified type NEC S37.592
    blast injury (primary) S37.519
      bilateral S37.512
      secondary —see Injury,
        fallopian tube, specified
        type NEC
      unilateral S37.511
    contusion S37.529
      bilateral S37.522
      unilateral S37.521
    laceration S37.539
      bilateral S37.532
      unilateral S37.531
    specified type NEC S37.599
      bilateral S37.592
      unilateral S37.591
    unilateral S37.501
      blast injury S37.511
      contusion S37.521
      laceration S37.531
      specified type NEC S37.591
  fascia —see Injury, muscle
  fifth cranial nerve (trigeminal) —
    see Injury, nerve, trigeminal
  finger (nail) S69.9-
    blood vessel —see Injury, blood
      vessel, finger
    contusion —see Contusion,
      finger
    dislocation —see Dislocation,
      finger
    fracture —see Fracture, finger
    muscle —see Injury, muscle,
      finger
    nerve —see Injury, nerve, digital,
      finger
    open —see Wound, open, finger
    specified NEC S69.8-
    sprain —see Sprain, finger
    superficial —see Injury,
      superficial, finger
  first cranial nerve (olfactory) —see
    Injury, nerve, olfactory
  flank —see Injury, abdomen
  foot S99.92-
    blood vessel —see Injury, blood
      vessel, foot
    contusion —see Contusion, foot
    dislocation —see Dislocation,
      foot
    fracture —see Fracture, foot
    muscle —see Injury, muscle,
      foot
    open —see Wound, open, foot
    specified type NEC S99.82-
    sprain —see Sprain, foot
    superficial —see Injury,
      superficial, foot

Injury (continued)
  forceps NOS P15.9
  forearm S59.91-
    blood vessel —see Injury, blood
      vessel, forearm
    contusion —see Contusion,
      forearm
    fracture —see Fracture, forearm
    muscle —see Injury, muscle,
      forearm
    nerve —see Injury, nerve,
      forearm
    open —see Wound, open,
      forearm
    specified NEC S59.81-
    superficial —see Injury,
      superficial, forearm
  forehead S09.90
  fourth cranial nerve (trochlear)
    —see Injury, nerve, trochlear
  gallbladder S36.129
    contusion S36.122
    laceration S36.123
    specified NEC S36.128
  ganglion
    celiac, coeliac —see Injury,
      nerve, lumbosacral,
      sympathetic
    gasserian —see Injury, nerve,
      trigeminal
    stellate —see Injury, nerve,
      thorax, sympathetic
    thoracic sympathetic —see
      Injury, nerve, thorax,
      sympathetic
  gasserian ganglion —see Injury,
    nerve, trigeminal
  gastric artery —see Injury, blood
    vessel, celiac artery, branch
  gastroduodenal artery —see Injury,
    blood vessel, celiac artery, branch
  gastrointestinal tract —see Injury,
    intra-abdominal
    with open wound into abdominal
      cavity —see Wound, open,
      with penetration into
      peritoneal cavity
    colon —see Injury, intestine,
      large
    rectum —see Injury, intestine,
      large, rectum
      with open wound into
        abdominal cavity S36.61
    specified site NEC —see Injury,
      intra-abdominal, specified,
      site NEC
    stomach —see Injury, stomach
    small intestine —see Injury,
      intestine, small
  genital organ(s)
    external S39.94
      specified NEC S39.848
    internal S37.90
      fallopian tube —see Injury,
        fallopian tube
      ovary —see Injury, ovary
      prostate —see Injury,
        prostate
      seminal vesicle —see Injury,
        pelvis, organ, specified site
        NEC
      uterus —see Injury, uterus
      vas deferens —see Injury,
        pelvis, organ, specified site
        NEC
    obstetrical trauma O71.9
  gland
    lacrimal laceration —see Injury,
      eye, specified site NEC
    salivary S09.93
    thyroid NEC S19.84

Injury (continued)
  globe (eye) S05.90
    specified NEC S05.8X-
  groin —see Injury, abdomen
  gum S09.90
  hand S69.9-
    blood vessel —see Injury, blood
      vessel, hand
    contusion —see Contusion, hand
    fracture —see Fracture, hand
    muscle —see Injury, muscle,
      hand
    nerve —see Injury, nerve, hand
    open —see Wound, open, hand
    specified NEC S69.8-
    sprain —see Sprain, hand
    superficial —see Injury,
      superficial, hand
  head S09.90
    with loss of consciousness
      S06.9-
    specified NEC S09.8
  heart (traumatic) S26.90
    with hemopericardium S26.00
      contusion S26.01
      laceration (mild) S26.020
        moderate S26.021
        major S26.022
      specified type NEC S26.09
    contusion S26.91
    laceration S26.92
    nontraumatic (acute) (chronic)
      (non-ischemic) I5A
    specified type NEC S26.99
    without hemopericardium
      S26.10
      contusion S26.11
      laceration S26.12
      specified type NEC S26.19
  heel —see Injury, foot
  hepatic
    artery —see Injury, blood vessel,
      celiac artery, branch
    duct —see Injury, liver
    vein —see Injury, vena cava,
      inferior
  hip S79.91-
    blood vessel —see Injury, blood
      vessel, hip
    contusion —see Contusion, hip
    dislocation —see Dislocation,
      hip
    fracture —see Fracture, femur,
      neck
    muscle —see Injury, muscle, hip
    nerve —see Injury, nerve, hip
    open —see Wound, open, hip
    sprain —see Sprain, hip
    superficial —see Injury,
      superficial, hip
    specified NEC S79.81-
  hymen S39.94
  hypogastric
    blood vessel —see Injury, blood
      vessel, iliac
    plexus —see Injury, nerve,
      lumbosacral, sympathetic
  ileum —see Injury, intestine,
    small
  iliac region S39.91
  instrumental (during surgery)
    —see Laceration, accidental
    complicating surgery
    birth injury —see Birth, injury
    nonsurgical —see Injury, by site
    obstetrical O71.9
      bladder O71.5
      cervix O71.3
      high vaginal O71.4
      perineal NOS O70.9
      urethra O71.5

Injury (continued)
  instrumental (continued)
    obstetrical (continued)
      uterus O71.5
        with rupture or perforation
          O71.1
  internal T14.8
    aorta —see Injury, aorta
    bladder (sphincter) —see Injury,
      bladder
      with
        ectopic or molar pregnancy
          O08.6
        following ectopic or molar
          pregnancy O08.6
        obstetrical trauma O71.5
    bronchus, bronchi —see Injury,
      intrathoracic, bronchus
    cecum —see Injury, intestine,
      large
    cervix (uteri) —see also Injury,
      uterus
      with ectopic or molar
        pregnancy O08.6
      following ectopic or molar
        pregnancy O08.6
      obstetrical trauma O71.3
    chest —see Injury, intrathoracic
    gastrointestinal tract —see
      Injury, intra-abdominal
    heart —see Injury, heart
    intestine NEC —see Injury,
      intestine
    intrauterine —see Injury, uterus
    mesentery —see Injury,
      intra-abdominal, specified,
      site NEC
    pelvis, pelvic (organ) S37.90
      following ectopic or molar
        pregnancy (subsequent
        episode) O08.6
      obstetrical trauma NEC O71.5
        rupture or perforation O71.1
      specified NEC S39.83
    rectum —see Injury, intestine,
      large, rectum
    stomach —see Injury, stomach
    ureter —see Injury, ureter
    urethra (sphincter) following
      ectopic or molar pregnancy
      O08.6
    uterus —see Injury, uterus
  interscapular area —see Injury,
    thorax
  intestine
    large S36.509
      ascending (right) S36.500
        blast injury (primary)
          S36.510
          secondary S36.590
        contusion S36.520
        laceration S36.530
        specified type NEC S36.590
      blast injury (primary) S36.519
        ascending (right) S36.510
        descending (left) S36.512
        rectum S36.61
        sigmoid S36.513
        specified site NEC S36.518
        transverse S36.511
      contusion S36.529
        ascending (right) S36.520
        descending (left) S36.522
        rectum S36.62
        sigmoid S36.523
        specified site NEC S36.528
        transverse S36.521
      descending (left) S36.502
        blast injury (primary)
          S36.512
          secondary S36.592

203

Injury (*continued*)
  intestine (*continued*)
    large (*continued*)
      descending (*continued*)
        blast injury (primary) (*continued*)
          contusion S36.522
          laceration S36.532
          specified type NEC S36.592
      laceration S36.539
      ascending (right) S36.530
      descending (left) S36.532
      rectum S36.63
      sigmoid S36.533
      specified site NEC S36.538
      transverse S36.531
     rectum S36.60
      blast injury (primary) S36.61
        secondary S36.69
      contusion S36.62
      laceration S36.63
      specified type NEC S36.69
     sigmoid S36.503
      blast injury (primary) S36.513
        secondary S36.593
      contusion S36.523
      laceration S36.533
      specified type NEC S36.593
     specified
      site NEC S36.508
        blast injury (primary) S36.518
          secondary S36.598
        contusion S36.528
        laceration S36.538
        specified type NEC S36.598
      type NEC S36.599
        ascending (right) S36.590
        descending (left) S36.592
        rectum S36.69
        sigmoid S36.593
        specified site NEC S36.598
        transverse S36.591
     transverse S36.501
      blast injury (primary) S36.511
        secondary S36.591
      contusion S36.521
      laceration S36.531
      specified type NEC S36.591
    small S36.409
     blast injury (primary) S36.419
      duodenum S36.410
      secondary S36.499
        duodenum S36.490
        specified site NEC S36.498
      specified site NEC S36.418
     contusion S36.429
      duodenum S36.420
      specified site NEC S36.428
     duodenum S36.400
      blast injury (primary) S36.410
        secondary S36.490
      contusion S36.420
      laceration S36.430
      specified NEC S36.490
     laceration S36.439
      duodenum S36.430
      specified site NEC S36.438
     specified
      type NEC S36.499
        duodenum S36.490
        specified site NEC S36.498
      site NEC S36.408

Injury (*continued*)
  intra-abdominal S36.90
    adrenal gland —*see* Injury, adrenal gland
    bladder —*see* Injury, bladder
    colon —*see* Injury, intestine, large
    contusion S36.92
    fallopian tube —*see* Injury, fallopian tube
    gallbladder —*see* Injury, gallbladder
    intestine —*see* Injury, intestine
    laceration S36.93
    liver —*see* Injury, liver
    kidney —*see* Injury, kidney
    ovary —*see* Injury, ovary
    pancreas —*see* Injury, pancreas
    pelvic NOS S37.90
    peritoneum —*see* Injury, intra-abdominal, specified, site NEC
    prostate —*see* Injury, prostate
    rectum —*see* Injury, intestine, large, rectum
    retroperitoneum —*see* Injury, intra-abdominal, specified, site NEC
    seminal vesicle —*see* Injury, pelvis, organ, specified site NEC
    small intestine —*see* Injury, intestine, small
    specified
      site NEC S36.899
        contusion S36.892
        laceration S36.893
        specified type NEC S36.898
      type NEC S36.99
      pelvic S37.90
        specified
          site NEC S37.899
            specified type NEC S37.898
        type NEC S37.99
    spleen —*see* Injury, spleen
    stomach —*see* Injury, stomach
    ureter —*see* Injury, ureter
    urethra —*see* Injury, urethra
    uterus —*see* Injury, uterus
    vas deferens —*see* Injury, pelvis, organ, specified site NEC
  intracranial (traumatic) (*see also*, if applicable, Compression, brain, traumatic) S06.9-
    cerebellar hemorrhage, traumatic —*see* Injury, intracranial, focal
    cerebral edema, traumatic S06.1X-
      diffuse S06.1X-
      focal S06.1X-
    diffuse (axonal) S06.2X-
    epidural hemorrhage (traumatic) S06.4X-
    focal brain injury S06.30-
      contusion —*see* Contusion, cerebral
      laceration —*see* Laceration, cerebral
    intracerebral hemorrhage, traumatic S06.36-
      left side S06.35-
      right side S06.34-
    specified NEC S06.89-
    subarachnoid hemorrhage, traumatic S06.6X-
    subdural hemorrhage, traumatic S06.5X-
  intraocular —*see* Injury, eyeball, penetrating

Injury (*continued*)
  intrathoracic S27.9
    bronchus S27.409
      bilateral S27.402
      blast injury (primary) S27.419
        bilateral S27.412
        secondary —*see* Injury, intrathoracic, bronchus, specified type NEC
        unilateral S27.411
      contusion S27.429
        bilateral S27.422
        unilateral S27.421
      laceration S27.439
        bilateral S27.432
        unilateral S27.431
      specified type NEC S27.499
        bilateral S27.492
        unilateral S27.491
      unilateral S27.401
    diaphragm S27.809
      contusion S27.802
      laceration S27.803
      specified type NEC S27.808
    esophagus (thoracic) S27.819
      contusion S27.812
      laceration S27.813
      specified type NEC S27.818
    heart —*see* Injury, heart
    hemopneumothorax S27.2
    hemothorax S27.1
    lung S27.309
      aspiration J69.0
      bilateral S27.302
      blast injury (primary) S27.319
        bilateral S27.312
        secondary —*see* Injury, intrathoracic, lung, specified type NEC
        unilateral S27.311
      contusion S27.329
        bilateral S27.322
        unilateral S27.321
      laceration S27.339
        bilateral S27.332
        unilateral S27.331
      specified type NEC S27.399
        bilateral S27.392
        unilateral S27.391
      unilateral S27.301
    pleura S27.60
      laceration S27.63
      specified type NEC S27.69
    pneumothorax S27.0
    specified organ NEC S27.899
      contusion S27.892
      laceration S27.893
      specified type NEC S27.898
    thoracic duct —*see* Injury, intrathoracic, specified organ NEC
    thymus gland —*see* Injury, intrathoracic, specified organ NEC
    trachea, thoracic S27.50
      blast (primary) S27.51
      contusion S27.52
      laceration S27.53
      specified type NEC S27.59
  iris —*see* Injury, eye, specified site NEC
    penetrating —*see* Injury, eyeball, penetrating
  jaw S09.93
  jejunum —*see* Injury, intestine, small
  joint NOS T14.8
    old or residual —*see* Disorder, joint, specified type NEC
  kidney S37.00-
    acute (nontraumatic) N17.9

Injury (*continued*)
  kidney (*continued*)
    contusion —*see* Contusion, kidney
    laceration —*see* Laceration, kidney
    specified NEC S37.09-
  knee S89.9-
    contusion —*see* Contusion, knee
    dislocation —*see* Dislocation, knee
    meniscus (lateral) (medial) —*see* Sprain, knee, specified site NEC
      old injury or tear —*see* Derangement, knee, meniscus, due to old injury
    open —*see* Wound, open, knee
    specified NEC S89.8-
    sprain —*see* Sprain, knee
    superficial —*see* Injury, superficial, knee
  labium (majus) (minus) S39.94
  labyrinth, ear S09.30-
  lacrimal apparatus, duct, gland, or sac —*see* Injury, eye, specified site NEC
  larynx NEC S19.81
  leg (lower) S89.9-
    blood vessel —*see* Injury, blood vessel, leg
    contusion —*see* Contusion, leg
    fracture —*see* Fracture, leg
    muscle —*see* Injury, muscle, leg
    nerve —*see* Injury, nerve, leg
    open —*see* Wound, open, leg
    specified NEC S89.8-
    superficial —*see* Injury, superficial, leg
  lens, eye —*see* Injury, eye, specified site NEC
    penetrating —*see* Injury, eyeball, penetrating
  limb NEC T14.8
  lip S09.93
  liver S36.119
    contusion S36.112
    laceration S36.113
      major (stellate) S36.116
      minor S36.114
      moderate S36.115
    specified NEC S36.118
  lower back S39.92
    specified NEC S39.82
  lumbar, lumbosacral (region) S39.92
    plexus —*see* Injury, lumbosacral plexus
  lumbosacral plexus S34.4
  lung —*see also* Injury, intrathoracic, lung
    aspiration J69.0
    dabbing (related) U07.0
    electronic cigarette (related) U07.0
    EVALI - [e-cigarette, or vaping product use associated] U07.0
    transfusion-related (TRALI) J95.84
    vaping (associated) (device) (product) (use) V07.0
  lymphatic thoracic duct —*see* Injury, intrathoracic, specified organ NEC
  malar region S09.93
  mastoid region S09.90
  maxilla S09.93
  mediastinum —*see* Injury, intrathoracic, specified organ NEC
  membrane, brain —*see* Injury, intracranial

Injury *(continued)*
  meningeal artery —*see* Injury, intracranial, subdural hemorrhage
  meninges (cerebral) —*see* Injury, intracranial
  mesenteric
    artery
      branch S35.299
        laceration (minor) (superficial) S35.291
          major S35.292
        specified NEC S35.298
      inferior S35.239
        laceration (minor) (superficial) S35.231
          major S35.232
        specified NEC S35.238
      superior S35.229
        laceration (minor) (superficial) S35.221
          major S35.222
        specified NEC S35.228
      plexus (inferior) (superior) —*see* Injury, nerve, lumbosacral, sympathetic
    vein
      inferior S35.349
        laceration S35.341
        specified NEC S35.348
      superior S35.339
        laceration S35.331
        specified NEC S35.338
  mesentery —*see* Injury, intra-abdominal, specified site NEC
  mesosalpinx —*see* Injury, pelvic organ, specified site NEC
  middle ear S09.30-
  midthoracic region NOS S29.9
  mouth S09.93
  multiple NOS T07
  muscle (and fascia) (and tendon)
    abdomen S39.001
      laceration S39.021
      specified type NEC S39.091
      strain S39.011
    abductor
      thumb, forearm level —*see* Injury, muscle, thumb, abductor
    adductor
      thigh S76.20-
        laceration S76.22-
        specified type NEC S76.29-
        strain S76.21-
    ankle —*see* Injury, muscle, foot
    anterior muscle group, at leg level (lower) S86.20-
      laceration S86.22-
      specified type NEC S86.29-
      strain S86.21-
    arm (upper) —*see* Injury, muscle, shoulder
    biceps (parts NEC) S46.20-
      laceration S46.22-
      long head S46.10-
        laceration S46.12-
        strain S46.11-
        specified type NEC S46.19-
      specified type NEC S46.29-
      strain S46.21-
    extensor
      finger(s) (other than thumb) —*see* Injury, muscle, finger by site, extensor
      forearm level, specified NEC —*see* Injury, muscle, forearm, extensor
      thumb —*see* Injury, muscle, thumb, extensor

Injury *(continued)*
  muscle *(continued)*
    extensor *(continued)*
      toe (large) (ankle level) (foot level) —*see* Injury, muscle, toe, extensor
    finger
      extensor (forearm level) S56.40-
        hand level S66.309
          laceration S66.329
          specified type NEC S66.399
          strain S66.319
        laceration S56.429
        specified type NEC S56.499
        strain S56.419
      flexor (forearm level) S56.10-
        hand level S66.109
          laceration S66.129
          specified type NEC S66.199
          strain S66.119
        laceration S56.129
        specified type NEC S56.199
        strain S56.119
      intrinsic S66.509
        laceration S66.529
        specified type NEC S66.599
        strain S66.519
      index
        extensor (forearm level)
          hand level S66.308
            laceration S66.32-
            specified type NEC S66.39-
            strain S66.31-
          specified type NEC S56.492-
        flexor (forearm level)
          hand level S66.108
            laceration S66.12-
            specified type NEC S66.19-
            strain S66.11-
          specified type NEC S56.19-
          strain S56.11-
        intrinsic S66.50-
          laceration S66.52-
          specified type NEC S66.59-
          strain S66.51-
      little
        extensor (forearm level)
          hand level S66.30-
            laceration S66.32-
            specified type NEC S66.39-
            strain S66.31-
          laceration S56.42-
          specified type NEC S56.49-
          strain S56.41-
        flexor (forearm level)
          hand level S66.10-
            laceration S66.12-
            specified type NEC S66.19-
            strain S66.11-
          laceration S56.12-
          specified type NEC S56.19-
          strain S56.11-
        intrinsic S66.50-
          laceration S66.52-
          specified type NEC S66.59-
          strain S66.51-

Injury *(continued)*
  muscle *(continued)*
    finger *(continued)*
      middle
        extensor (forearm level)
          hand level S66.30-
            laceration S66.32-
            specified type NEC S66.39-
            strain S66.31-
          laceration S56.42-
          specified type NEC S56.49-
          strain S56.41-
        flexor (forearm level)
          hand level S66.10-
            laceration S66.12-
            specified type NEC S66.19-
            strain S66.11-
          laceration S56.12-
          specified type NEC S56.19-
          strain S56.11-
        intrinsic S66.50-
          laceration S66.52-
          specified type NEC S66.59-
          strain S66.51-
      ring
        extensor (forearm level)
          hand level S66.30-
            laceration S66.32-
            specified type NEC S66.39-
            strain S66.31-
          laceration S56.42-
          specified type NEC S56.49-
          strain S56.41-
        flexor (forearm level)
          hand level S66.10-
            laceration S66.12-
            specified type NEC S66.19-
            strain S66.11-
          laceration S56.12-
          specified type NEC S56.19-
          strain S56.11-
        intrinsic S66.50-
          laceration S66.52-
          specified type NEC S66.59-
          strain S66.51-
    flexor
      finger(s) (other than thumb) —*see* Injury, muscle, finger
      forearm level, specified NEC —*see* Injury, muscle, forearm, flexor
      thumb —*see* Injury, muscle, thumb, flexor
      toe (long) (ankle level) (foot level) —*see* Injury, muscle, toe, flexor
    foot S96.90-
      intrinsic S96.20-
        laceration S96.22-
        specified type NEC S96.29-
        strain S96.21-
      laceration S96.92-
      long extensor, toe —*see* Injury, muscle, toe, extensor
      long flexor, toe —*see* Injury, muscle, toe, flexor

Injury *(continued)*
  muscle *(continued)*
    foot *(continued)*
      specified
        site NEC S96.80-
          laceration S96.82-
          specified type NEC S96.89-
          strain S96.81-
        type NEC S96.99-
      strain S96.91-
    forearm (level) S56.90-
      extensor S56.50-
        laceration S56.52-
        specified type NEC S56.59-
        strain S56.51-
      flexor S56.20-
        laceration S56.22-
        specified type NEC S56.29-
        strain S56.21-
      laceration S56.92-
      specified S56.99-
        site NEC S56.80-
          laceration S56.82-
          strain S56.81-
          type NEC S56.89-
      strain S56.91-
    hand (level) S66.90-
      laceration S66.92-
      specified
        site NEC S66.80-
          laceration S66.82-
          specified type NEC S66.89-
          strain S66.81-
        type NEC S66.99-
      strain S66.91-
    head S09.10
      laceration S09.12
      specified type NEC S09.19
      strain S09.11
    hip NEC S76.00-
      laceration S76.02-
      specified type NEC S76.09-
      strain S76.01-
    intrinsic
      ankle and foot level —*see* Injury, muscle, foot, intrinsic
      finger (other than thumb) —*see* Injury, muscle, finger by site, intrinsic
      foot (level) —*see* Injury, muscle, foot, intrinsic
      thumb —*see* Injury, muscle, thumb, intrinsic
    leg (level) (lower) S86.90-
      Achilles tendon —*see* Injury, Achilles tendon
      anterior muscle group —*see* Injury, muscle, anterior muscle group
      laceration S86.92-
      peroneal muscle group —*see* Injury, muscle, peroneal muscle group
      posterior muscle group —*see* Injury, muscle, posterior muscle group, leg level
      specified
        site NEC S86.80-
          laceration S86.82-
          specified type NEC S86.89-
          strain S86.81-
        type NEC S86.99-
      strain S86.91-
    long
      extensor toe, at ankle and foot level —*see* Injury, muscle, toe, extensor

205

Injury (continued)
  muscle (continued)
    long (continued)
      flexor, toe, at ankle and foot level —see Injury, muscle, toe, flexor
      head, biceps —see Injury, muscle, biceps, long head
    lower back S39.002
      laceration S39.022
      specified type NEC S39.092
      strain S39.012
    neck (level) S16.9
      laceration S16.2
      specified type NEC S16.8
      strain S16.1
    pelvis S39.003
      laceration S39.023
      specified type NEC S39.093
      strain S39.013
    peroneal muscle group, at leg level (lower) S86.30-
      laceration S86.32-
      specified type NEC S86.39-
      strain S86.31-
    posterior muscle (group)
      leg level (lower) S86.10-
        laceration S86.12-
        specified type NEC S86.19-
        strain S86.11-
      thigh level S76.30-
        laceration S76.32-
        specified type NEC S76.39-
        strain S76.31-
    quadriceps (thigh) S76.10-
      laceration S76.12-
      specified type NEC S76.19-
      strain S76.11-
    shoulder S46.90-
      laceration S46.92-
      rotator cuff —see Injury, rotator cuff
      specified site NEC S46.80-
        laceration S46.82-
        strain S46.81-
        specified type NEC S46.89-
      strain S46.91-
      specified type NEC S46.99-
    thigh NEC (level) S76.90-
      adductor —see Injury, muscle, adductor, thigh
      laceration S76.92-
      posterior muscle (group) —see Injury, muscle, posterior muscle, thigh level
      quadriceps —see Injury, muscle, quadriceps
      specified
        site NEC S76.80-
          laceration S76.82-
          specified type NEC S76.89-
          strain S76.81-
        type NEC S76.99-
      strain S76.91-
    thorax (level) S29.009
      back wall S29.002
      front wall S29.001
      laceration S29.029
        back wall S29.022
        front wall S29.021
      specified type NEC S29.099
        back wall S29.092
        front wall S29.091
      strain S29.019
        back wall S29.012
        front wall S29.011

Injury (continued)
  muscle (continued)
    thumb
      abductor (forearm level) S56.30-
        laceration S56.32-
        specified type NEC S56.39-
        strain S56.31-
      extensor (forearm level) S56.30-
        hand level S66.20-
          laceration S66.22-
          specified type NEC S66.29-
          strain S66.21-
        laceration S56.32-
        specified type NEC S56.39-
        strain S56.31-
      flexor (forearm level) S56.00-
        hand level S66.00-
          laceration S66.02-
          specified type NEC S66.09-
          strain S66.01-
        laceration S56.02-
        specified type NEC S56.09-
        strain S56.01-
        wrist level —see Injury, muscle, thumb, flexor, hand level
      intrinsic S66.40-
        laceration S66.42-
        specified type NEC S66.49-
        strain S66.41-
    toe —see also Injury, muscle, foot
      extensor, long S96.10-
        laceration S96.12-
        specified type NEC S96.19-
        strain S96.11-
      flexor, long S96.00-
        laceration S96.02-
        specified type NEC S96.09-
        strain S96.01-
    triceps S46.30-
      laceration S46.32-
      specified type NEC S46.39-
      strain S46.31-
    wrist (and hand) level —see Injury, muscle, hand
  musculocutaneous nerve —see Injury, nerve, musculocutaneous
  myocardial (acute) (chronic) (non-ischemic) (non-traumatic) I5A
    traumatic —see Injury, heart
  myocardium —see also Injury, heart
    non-traumatic —see also Injury, myocardial
  nape —see Injury, neck
  nasal (septum) (sinus) S09.92
  nasopharynx S09.92
  neck S19.9
    specified NEC S19.80
      specified site NEC S19.89
  nerve NEC T14.8
    abdomen S34.9
      peripheral S34.6
      specified site NEC S34.8
    abducens S04.4-
      contusion S04.4-
      laceration S04.4-
      specified type NEC S04.4-
    abducent —see Injury, nerve, abducens
    accessory S04.7-
      contusion S04.7-
      laceration S04.7-
      specified type NEC S04.7-
    acoustic S04.6-
      contusion S04.6-
      laceration S04.6-
      specified type NEC S04.6-

Injury (continued)
  nerve NEC (continued)
    ankle S94.9-
      cutaneous sensory S94.3-
      specified site NEC —see subcategory S94.8
    anterior crural, femoral —see Injury, nerve, femoral
    arm (upper) S44.9-
      axillary —see Injury, nerve, axillary
      cutaneous —see Injury, nerve, cutaneous, arm
      median —see Injury, nerve, median, upper arm
      musculocutaneous —see Injury, nerve, musculocutaneous
      radial —see Injury, nerve, radial, upper arm
      specified site NEC S44.8
      ulnar —see Injury, nerve, ulnar, arm
    auditory —see Injury, nerve, acoustic
    axillary S44.3-
    brachial plexus —see Injury, brachial plexus
    cervical sympathetic S14.5
    cranial S04.9
      contusion S04.9
      eighth (acoustic or auditory) —see Injury, nerve, acoustic
      eleventh (accessory) —see Injury, nerve, accessory
      fifth (trigeminal) —see Injury, nerve, trigeminal
      first (olfactory) —see Injury, nerve, olfactory
      fourth (trochlear) —see Injury, nerve, trochlear
      laceration S04.9
      ninth (glossopharyngeal) —see Injury, nerve, glossopharyngeal
      second (optic) —see Injury, nerve, optic
      seventh (facial) —see Injury, nerve, facial
      sixth (abducent) —see Injury, nerve, abducens
      specified
        nerve NEC S04.89-
          contusion S04.89-
          laceration S04.89-
          specified type NEC S04.89-
        type NEC S04.9
      tenth (pneumogastric or vagus) —see Injury, nerve, vagus
      third (oculomotor) —see Injury, nerve, oculomotor
      twelfth (hypoglossal) —see Injury, nerve, hypoglossal
    cutaneous sensory
      ankle (level) S94.3-
      arm (upper) (level) S44.5-
      foot (level) —see Injury, nerve, cutaneous sensory, ankle
      forearm (level) S54.3-
      hip (level) S74.2-
      leg (lower level) S84.2-
      shoulder (level) —see Injury, nerve, cutaneous sensory, arm
      thigh (level) —see Injury, nerve, cutaneous sensory, hip
    deep peroneal —see Injury, nerve, peroneal, foot

Injury (continued)
  nerve NEC (continued)
    digital
      finger S64.4-
        index S64.49-
        little S64.49-
        middle S64.49-
        ring S64.49-
      thumb S64.3-
      toe —see Injury, nerve, ankle, specified site NEC
    eighth cranial (acoustic or auditory) —see Injury, nerve, acoustic
    eleventh cranial (accessory) —see Injury, nerve, accessory
    facial S04.5-
      contusion S04.5-
      laceration S04.5-
      newborn P11.3
      specified type NEC S04.5-
    femoral (hip level) (thigh level) S74.1-
    fifth cranial (trigeminal) —see Injury, nerve, trigeminal
    finger (digital) —see Injury, nerve, digital, finger
    first cranial (olfactory) —see Injury, nerve, olfactory
    foot S94.9-
      cutaneous sensory S94.3-
      deep peroneal S94.2-
      lateral plantar S94.0-
      medial plantar S94.1-
      specified site NEC —see subcategory S94.8
    forearm (level) S54.9-
      cutaneous sensory —see Injury, nerve, cutaneous sensory, forearm
      median —see Injury, nerve, median
      radial —see Injury, nerve, radial
      specified site NEC —see subcategory S54.8
      ulnar —see Injury, nerve, ulnar
    fourth cranial (trochlear) —see Injury, nerve, trochlear
    glossopharyngeal S04.89-
      specified type NEC S04.89-
    hand S64.9-
      median —see Injury, nerve, median, hand
      radial —see Injury, nerve, radial, hand
      specified NEC —see subcategory S64.8
      ulnar —see Injury, nerve, ulnar, hand
    hip (level) S74.9-
      cutaneous sensory —see Injury, nerve, cutaneous sensory, hip
      femoral —see Injury, nerve, femoral
      sciatic —see Injury, nerve, sciatic
      specified site NEC S74.8
    hypoglossal S04.89-
      specified type NEC S04.89-
    lateral plantar S94.0-
    leg (lower) S84.9-
      cutaneous sensory —see Injury, nerve, cutaneous sensory, leg
      peroneal —see Injury, nerve, peroneal
      specified site NEC —see subcategory S84.8
      tibial —see Injury, nerve, tibial
      upper —see Injury, nerve, thigh

Injury (continued)
nerve NEC (continued)
lower
back —see Injury, nerve, abdomen, specified site NEC
peripheral —see Injury, nerve, abdomen, peripheral
limb —see Injury, nerve, leg
lumbar spinal - see Injury, spinal, lumbar
peripheral S34.6
root S34.21
sympathetic S34.5
lumbar plexus —see Injury, nerve, lumbosacral, sympathetic
lumbosacral
plexus —see Injury, nerve, lumbosacral, sympathetic
sympathetic S34.5
medial plantar S94.1-
median (forearm level) S54.1-
hand (level) S64.1-
upper arm (level) S44.1-
wrist (level) —see Injury, nerve, median, hand
musculocutaneous S44.4-
musculospiral (upper arm level) —see Injury, nerve, radial, upper arm
neck S14.9
peripheral S14.4
specified site NEC S14.8
sympathetic S14.5
ninth cranial (glossopharyngeal) —see Injury, nerve, glossopharyngeal
oculomotor S04.1-
contusion S04.1-
laceration S04.1-
specified type NEC S04.1-
olfactory S04.81-
specified type NEC S04.81-
optic S04.01-
contusion S04.01-
laceration S04.01-
specified type NEC S04.01-
pelvic girdle —see Injury, nerve, hip
pelvis —see Injury, nerve, abdomen, specified site NEC
peripheral —see Injury, nerve, abdomen, peripheral
peripheral NEC T14.8
abdomen —see Injury, nerve, abdomen, peripheral
lower back —see Injury, nerve, abdomen, peripheral
neck —see Injury, nerve, neck, peripheral
pelvis —see Injury, nerve, abdomen, peripheral
specified NEC T14.8
peroneal (lower leg level) S84.1-
foot S94.2-
plexus
brachial —see Injury, brachial plexus
celiac, coeliac —see Injury, nerve, lumbosacral, sympathetic
mesenteric, inferior —see Injury, nerve, lumbosacral, sympathetic
sacral —see Injury, lumbosacral plexus
spinal
brachial —see Injury, brachial plexus
lumbosacral —see Injury, lumbosacral plexus

Injury (continued)
nerve NEC (continued)
pneumogastric —see Injury, nerve, vagus
radial (forearm level) S54.2-
hand (level) S64.2-
upper arm (level) S44.2-
wrist (level) —see Injury, nerve, radial, hand
root —see Injury, nerve, spinal, root
sacral plexus —see Injury, lumbosacral plexus
sacral spinal - see Injury, spinal, sacral
peripheral S34.6
root S34.22
sympathetic S34.5
sciatic (hip level) (thigh level) S74.0-
second cranial (optic) —see Injury, nerve, optic
seventh cranial (facial) —see Injury, nerve, facial
shoulder —see Injury, nerve, arm
sixth cranial (abducent) —see Injury, nerve, abducens
spinal
plexus —see Injury, nerve, plexus, spinal
root
cervical S14.2
dorsal S24.2
lumbar S34.21
sacral S34.22
thoracic —see Injury, nerve, spinal, root, dorsal
splanchnic —see Injury, nerve, lumbosacral, sympathetic
sympathetic NEC —see Injury, nerve, lumbosacral, sympathetic
cervical —see Injury, nerve, cervical sympathetic
tenth cranial (pneumogastric or vagus) —see Injury, nerve, vagus
thigh (level) —see Injury, nerve, hip
cutaneous sensory —see Injury, nerve, cutaneous sensory, hip
femoral —see Injury, nerve, femoral
sciatic —see Injury, nerve, sciatic
specified NEC —see Injury, nerve, hip
third cranial (oculomotor) —see Injury, nerve, oculomotor
thorax S24.9
peripheral S24.3
specified site NEC S24.8
sympathetic S24.4
thumb, digital —see Injury, nerve, digital, thumb
tibial (lower leg level) (posterior) S84.0-
toe —see Injury, nerve, ankle
trigeminal S04.3-
contusion S04.3-
laceration S04.3-
specified type NEC S04.3-
trochlear S04.2-
contusion S04.2-
laceration S04.2-
specified type NEC S04.2-
twelfth cranial (hypoglossal) —see Injury, nerve, hypoglossal
ulnar (forearm level) S54.0-
arm (upper) (level) S44.0-
hand (level) S64.0-

Injury (continued)
nerve NEC (continued)
ulnar (continued)
wrist (level) —see Injury, nerve, ulnar, hand
vagus S04.89-
specified type NEC S04.89-
wrist (level) —see Injury, nerve, hand
ninth cranial nerve (glossopharyngeal) —see Injury, nerve, glossopharyngeal
nose (septum) S09.92
obstetrical O71.9
specified NEC O71.89
occipital (region) (scalp) S09.90
lobe —see Injury, intracranial
optic chiasm S04.02
optic radiation S04.03-
optic tract and pathways S04.03-
orbit, orbital (region) —see Injury, eye
penetrating (with foreign body) —see Injury, eye, orbit, penetrating
specified NEC —see Injury, eye, specified site NEC
ovary, ovarian S37.409
bilateral S37.402
contusion S37.422
laceration S37.432
specified type NEC S37.492
blood vessel —see Injury, blood vessel, ovarian
contusion S37.429
bilateral S37.422
unilateral S37.421
laceration S37.439
bilateral S37.432
unilateral S37.431
specified type NEC S37.499
bilateral S37.492
unilateral S37.491
unilateral S37.401
contusion S37.421
laceration S37.431
specified type NEC S37.491
palate (hard) (soft) S09.93
pancreas S36.209
body S36.201
contusion S36.221
laceration S36.231
major S36.261
minor S36.241
moderate S36.251
specified type NEC S36.291
contusion S36.229
head S36.200
contusion S36.220
laceration S36.230
major S36.260
minor S36.240
moderate S36.250
specified type NEC S36.290
laceration S36.239
major S36.269
minor S36.249
moderate S36.259
specified type NEC S36.299
tail S36.202
contusion S36.222
laceration S36.232
major S36.262
minor S36.242
moderate S36.252
specified type NEC S36.292
parietal (region) (scalp) S09.90
lobe —see Injury, intracranial
patellar ligament (tendon) S76.10-
laceration S76.12-
specified NEC S76.19-

Injury (continued)
patellar ligament (continued)
strain S76.11-
pelvis, pelvic (floor) S39.93
complicating delivery O70.1
joint or ligament, complicating delivery O71.6
organ S37.90
with ectopic or molar pregnancy O08.6
complication of abortion —see Abortion
contusion S37.92
following ectopic or molar pregnancy O08.6
laceration S37.93
obstetrical trauma NEC O71.5
specified
site NEC S37.899
contusion S37.892
laceration S37.893
specified type NEC S37.898
type NEC S37.99
specified NEC S39.83
penis S39.94
perineum S39.94
peritoneum S36.81
laceration S36.893
periurethral tissue —see Injury, urethra
complicating delivery O71.82
phalanges
foot —see Injury, foot
hand —see Injury, hand
pharynx NEC S19.85
pleura —see Injury, intrathoracic, pleura
plexus
brachial —see Injury, brachial plexus
cardiac —see Injury, nerve, thorax, sympathetic
celiac, coeliac —see Injury, nerve, lumbosacral, sympathetic
esophageal —see Injury, nerve, thorax, sympathetic
hypogastric —see Injury, nerve, lumbosacral, sympathetic
lumbar, lumbosacral —see Injury, lumbosacral plexus
mesenteric —see Injury, nerve, lumbosacral, sympathetic
pulmonary —see Injury, nerve, thorax, sympathetic
postcardiac surgery (syndrome) I97.0
prepuce S39.94
pressure
injury —see Ulcer, pressure, by site
prostate S37.829
contusion S37.822
laceration S37.823
specified type NEC S37.828
pubic region S39.94
pudendum S39.94
pulmonary plexus —see Injury, nerve, thorax, sympathetic
rectovaginal septum NEC S39.83
rectum —see Injury, intestine, large, rectum
retina —see Injury, eye, specified site NEC
penetrating —see Injury, eyeball, penetrating
retroperitoneal —see Injury, intra-abdominal, specified site NEC
rotator cuff (muscle(s)) (tendon(s)) S46.00-

Injury *(continued)*
  rotator cuff *(continued)*
    laceration S46.02-
    specified type NEC S46.09-
    strain S46.01-
  round ligament —*see* Injury, pelvic organ, specified site NEC
  sacral plexus —*see* Injury, lumbosacral plexus
  salivary duct or gland S09.93
  scalp S09.90
    newborn (birth injury) P12.9
      due to monitoring (electrode) (sampling incision) P12.4
      specified NEC P12.89
        caput succedaneum P12.81
  scapular region —*see* Injury, shoulder
  sclera —*see* Injury, eye, specified site NEC
    penetrating —*see* Injury, eyeball, penetrating
  scrotum S39.94
  second cranial nerve (optic) —*see* Injury, nerve, optic
  self-inflicted, without suicidal intent R45.88
  seminal vesicle —*see* Injury, pelvic organ, specified site NEC
  seventh cranial nerve (facial) —*see* Injury, nerve, facial
  shoulder S49.9-
    blood vessel —*see* Injury, blood vessel, arm
    contusion —*see* Contusion, shoulder
    dislocation —*see* Dislocation, shoulder
    fracture —*see* Fracture, shoulder
  shoulder S49.9-
    muscle —*see* Injury, muscle, shoulder
    nerve —*see* Injury, nerve, shoulder
    open —*see* Wound, open, shoulder
    specified type NEC S49.8-
    sprain —*see* Sprain, shoulder girdle
    superficial —*see* Injury, superficial, shoulder
  sinus
    cavernous —*see* Injury, intracranial
    nasal S09.92
  sixth cranial nerve (abducent) —*see* Injury, nerve, abducens
  skeleton, birth injury P13.9
    specified part NEC P13.8
  skin NEC T14.8
    surface intact —*see* Injury, superficial
  skull NEC S09.90
  specified NEC T14.8
  spermatic cord (pelvic region) S37.898
    scrotal region S39.848
  spinal (cord)
    cervical (neck) S14.109
      anterior cord syndrome S14.139
        C1 level S14.131
        C2 level S14.132
        C3 level S14.133
        C4 level S14.134
        C5 level S14.135
        C6 level S14.136
        C7 level S14.137
        C8 level S14.138

Injury *(continued)*
  spinal *(continued)*
    cervical *(continued)*
      Brown-Séquard syndrome S14.149
        C1 level S14.141
        C2 level S14.142
        C3 level S14.143
        C4 level S14.144
        C5 level S14.145
        C6 level S14.146
        C7 level S14.147
        C8 level S14.148
      C1 level S14.101
      C2 level S14.102
      C3 level S14.103
      C4 level S14.104
      C5 level S14.105
      C6 level S14.106
      C7 level S14.107
      C8 level S14.108
      central cord syndrome S14.129
        C1 level S14.121
        C2 level S14.122
        C3 level S14.123
        C4 level S14.124
        C5 level S14.125
        C6 level S14.126
        C7 level S14.127
        C8 level S14.128
      complete lesion S14.119
        C1 level S14.111
        C2 level S14.112
        C3 level S14.113
        C4 level S14.114
        C5 level S14.115
        C6 level S14.116
        C7 level S14.117
        C8 level S14.118
      concussion S14.0
      edema S14.0
      incomplete lesion specified NEC S14.159
        C1 level S14.151
        C2 level S14.152
        C3 level S14.153
        C4 level S14.154
        C5 level S14.155
        C6 level S14.156
        C7 level S14.157
        C8 level S14.158
      posterior cord syndrome S14.159
        C1 level S14.151
        C2 level S14.152
        C3 level S14.153
        C4 level S14.154
        C5 level S14.155
        C6 level S14.156
        C7 level S14.157
        C8 level S14.158
    dorsal —*see* Injury, spinal, thoracic
    lumbar S34.109
      complete lesion S34.119
        L1 level S34.111
        L2 level S34.112
        L3 level S34.113
        L4 level S34.114
        L5 level S34.115
      concussion S34.01
      edema S34.01
      incomplete lesion S34.129
        L1 level S34.121
        L2 level S34.122
        L3 level S34.123
        L4 level S34.124
        L5 level S34.125
      L1 level S34.101
      L2 level S34.102
      L3 level S34.103

Injury *(continued)*
  spinal *(continued)*
    lumbar *(continued)*
      L4 level S34.104
      L5 level S34.105
    nerve root NEC
      cervical —*see* Injury, nerve, spinal, root, cervical
      dorsal —*see* Injury, nerve, spinal, root, dorsal
      lumbar S34.21
      sacral S34.22
      thoracic —*see* Injury, nerve, spinal, root, dorsal
    plexus
      brachial —*see* Injury, brachial plexus
      lumbosacral —*see* Injury, lumbosacral plexus
    sacral S34.139
      complete lesion S34.131
      incomplete lesion S34.132
    thoracic S24.109
      anterior cord syndrome S24.139
        T1 level S24.131
        T2-T6 level S24.132
        T7-T10 level S24.133
        T11-T12 level S24.134
      Brown-Séquard syndrome S24.149
        T1 level S24.141
        T2-T6 level S24.142
        T7-T10 level S24.143
        T11-T12 level S24.144
      complete lesion S24.119
        T1 level S24.111
        T2-T6 level S24.112
        T7-T10 level S24.113
        T11-T12 level S24.114
      concussion S24.0
      edema S24.0
      incomplete lesion specified NEC S24.159
        T1 level S24.151
        T2-T6 level S24.152
        T7-T10 level S24.153
        T11-T12 level S24.154
      posterior cord syndrome S24.159
        T1 level S24.151
        T2-T6 level S24.152
        T7-T10 level S24.153
        T11-T12 level S24.154
      T1 level S24.101
      T2-T6 level S24.102
      T7-T10 level S24.103
      T11-T12 level S24.104
  splanchnic nerve —*see* Injury, nerve, lumbosacral, sympathetic
  spleen S36.00
    contusion S36.029
      major S36.021
      minor S36.020
    laceration S36.039
      major (massive) (stellate) S36.032
      moderate S36.031
      superficial (capsular) (minor) S36.030
    specified type NEC S36.09
  splenic artery —*see* Injury, blood vessel, celiac artery, branch
  stellate ganglion —*see* Injury, nerve, thorax, sympathetic
  sternal region S29.9
  stomach S36.30
    contusion S36.32
    laceration S36.33
    specified type NEC S36.39

Injury *(continued)*
  subconjunctival —*see* Injury, eye, conjunctiva
  subcutaneous NEC T14.8
  submaxillary region S09.93
  submental region S09.93
  subungual
    fingers —*see* Injury, hand
    toes —*see* Injury, foot
  superficial NEC T14.8
    abdomen, abdominal (wall) S30.92
      abrasion S30.811
      bite S30.871
        insect S30.861
      contusion S30.1
      external constriction S30.841
      foreign body S30.851
    abrasion —*see* Abrasion, by site
    adnexa, eye NEC —*see* Injury, eye, specified site NEC
    alveolar process —*see* Injury, superficial, oral cavity
    ankle S90.91-
      abrasion —*see* Abrasion, ankle
      blister —*see* Blister, ankle
      bite —*see* Bite, ankle
      contusion —*see* Contusion, ankle
      external constriction —*see* Constriction, external, ankle
      foreign body —*see* Foreign body, superficial, ankle
    anus S30.98
    arm (upper) S40.92-
      abrasion —*see* Abrasion, arm
      bite —*see* Bite, superficial, arm
      blister —*see* Blister, arm (upper)
      contusion —*see* Contusion, arm
      external constriction —*see* Constriction, external, arm
      foreign body —*see* Foreign body, superficial, arm
    auditory canal (external) (meatus) —*see* Injury, superficial, ear
    auricle —*see* Injury, superficial, ear
    axilla —*see* Injury, superficial, arm
    back —*see also* Injury, superficial, thorax, back
      lower S30.91
        abrasion S30.810
        contusion S30.0
        external constriction S30.840
        superficial
          bite NEC S30.870
            insect S30.860
          foreign body S30.850
      bite NEC —*see* Bite, superficial NEC, by site
      blister —*see* Blister, by site
    breast S20.10-
      abrasion —*see* Abrasion, breast
      bite —*see* Bite, superficial, breast
      contusion —*see* Contusion, breast
      external constriction —*see* Constriction, external, breast
      foreign body —*see* Foreign body, superficial, breast

Injury (*continued*)
superficial NEC (*continued*)
- brow —*see* Injury, superficial, head, specified NEC
- buttock S30.91
- calf —*see* Injury, superficial, leg
- canthus, eye —*see* Injury, superficial, periocular area
- cheek (external) —*see* Injury, superficial, head, specified NEC
  - internal —*see* Injury, superficial, oral cavity
- chest wall —*see* Injury, superficial, thorax
- chin —*see* Injury, superficial, head NEC
- clitoris S30.95
- conjunctiva —*see* Injury, eye, conjunctiva
  - with foreign body (in conjunctival sac) —*see* Foreign body, conjunctival sac
- contusion —*see* Contusion, by site
- costal region —*see* Injury, superficial, thorax
- digit(s)
  - hand —*see* Injury, superficial, finger
- ear (auricle) (canal) (external) S00.40-
  - abrasion —*see* Abrasion, ear
  - bite —*see* Bite, superficial, ear
  - contusion —*see* Contusion, ear
  - external constriction —*see* Constriction, external, ear
  - foreign body —*see* Foreign body, superficial, ear
- elbow S50.90-
  - abrasion —*see* Abrasion, elbow
  - bite —*see* Bite, superficial, elbow
  - blister —*see* Blister, elbow
  - contusion —*see* Contusion, elbow
  - external constriction —*see* Constriction, external, elbow
  - foreign body —*see* Foreign body, superficial, elbow
- epididymis S30.94
- epigastric region S30.92
- epiglottis —*see* Injury, superficial, throat
- esophagus
  - cervical —*see* Injury, superficial, throat
- external constriction —*see* Constriction, external, by site
- extremity NEC T14.8
- eyeball NEC —*see* Injury, eye, specified site NEC
- eyebrow —*see* Injury, superficial, periocular area
- eyelid S00.20-
  - abrasion —*see* Abrasion, eyelid
  - bite —*see* Bite, superficial, eyelid
  - contusion —*see* Contusion, eyelid
  - external constriction —*see* Constriction, external, eyelid
  - foreign body —*see* Foreign body, superficial, eyelid

Injury (*continued*)
superficial NEC (*continued*)
- face NEC —*see* Injury, superficial, head, specified NEC
- finger(s) S60.949
  - abrasion —*see* Abrasion, finger
  - bite —*see* Bite, superficial, finger
  - blister —*see* Blister, finger
  - contusion —*see* Contusion, finger
  - external constriction —*see* Constriction, external, finger
  - foreign body —*see* Foreign body, superficial, finger
  - insect bite —*see* Bite, by site, superficial, insect
  - index S60.94-
  - little S60.94-
  - middle S60.94-
  - ring S60.94-
- flank S30.92
- foot S90.92-
  - abrasion —*see* Abrasion, foot
  - bite —*see* Bite, foot
  - blister —*see* Blister, foot
  - contusion —*see* Contusion, foot
  - external constriction —*see* Constriction, external, foot
  - foreign body —*see* Foreign body, superficial, foot
- forearm S50.91-
  - abrasion —*see* Abrasion, forearm
  - bite —*see* Bite, forearm, superficial
  - blister —*see* Blister, forearm
  - contusion —*see* Contusion, forearm
  - elbow only —*see* Injury, superficial, elbow
  - external constriction —*see* Constriction, external, forearm
  - foreign body —*see* Foreign body, superficial, forearm
- forehead —*see* Injury, superficial, head NEC
- foreign body —*see* Foreign body, superficial
- genital organs, external
  - female S30.97
  - male S30.96
- globe (eye) —*see* Injury, eye, specified site NEC
- groin S30.92
- gum —*see* Injury, superficial, oral cavity
- hand S60.92-
  - abrasion —*see* Abrasion, hand
  - bite —*see* Bite, superficial, hand
  - contusion —*see* Contusion, hand
  - external constriction —*see* Constriction, external, hand
  - foreign body —*see* Foreign body, superficial, hand
- head S00.90
  - ear —*see* Injury, superficial, ear
  - eyelid —*see* Injury, superficial, eyelid
  - nose S00.30
  - oral cavity S00.502
  - scalp S00.00

Injury (*continued*)
superficial NEC (*continued*)
- head (*continued*)
  - specified site NEC S00.80
- heel —*see* Injury, superficial, foot
- hip S70.91-
  - abrasion —*see* Abrasion, hip
  - bite —*see* Bite, superficial, hip
  - blister —*see* Blister, hip
  - contusion —*see* Contusion, hip
  - external constriction —*see* Constriction, external, hip
  - foreign body —*see* Foreign body, superficial, hip
- iliac region —*see* Injury, superficial, abdomen
- inguinal region —*see* Injury, superficial, abdomen
- insect bite —*see* Bite, by site, superficial, insect
- interscapular region —*see* Injury, superficial, thorax, back
- jaw —*see* Injury, superficial, head, specified NEC
- knee S80.91-
  - abrasion —*see* Abrasion, knee
  - bite —*see* Bite, superficial, knee
  - blister —*see* Blister, knee
  - contusion —*see* Contusion, knee
  - external constriction —*see* Constriction, external, knee
  - foreign body —*see* Foreign body, superficial, knee
- labium (majus) (minus) S30.95
- lacrimal (apparatus) (gland) (sac) —*see* Injury, eye, specified site NEC
- larynx —*see* Injury, superficial, throat
- leg (lower) S80.92-
  - abrasion —*see* Abrasion, leg
  - bite —*see* Bite, superficial, leg
  - contusion —*see* Contusion, leg
  - external constriction —*see* Constriction, external, leg
  - foreign body —*see* Foreign body, superficial, leg
  - knee —*see* Injury, superficial, knee
- limb NEC T14.8
- lip S00.501
- lower back S30.91
- lumbar region S30.91
- malar region —*see* Injury, superficial, head, specified NEC
- mammary —*see* Injury, superficial, breast
- mastoid region —*see* Injury, superficial, head, specified NEC
- mouth —*see* Injury, superficial, oral cavity
- muscle NEC T14.8
- nail NEC T14.8
  - finger —*see* Injury, superficial, finger
  - toe —*see* Injury, superficial, toe
- nasal (septum) —*see* Injury, superficial, nose
- neck S10.90
  - specified site NEC S10.80
- nose (septum) S00.30
- occipital region —*see* Injury, superficial, scalp

Injury (*continued*)
superficial NEC (*continued*)
- oral cavity S00.502
- orbital region —*see* Injury, superficial, periocular area
- palate —*see* Injury, superficial, oral cavity
- palm —*see* Injury, superficial, hand
- parietal region —*see* Injury, superficial, scalp
- pelvis S30.91
  - girdle —*see* Injury, superficial, hip
- penis S30.93
- perineum
  - female S30.95
  - male S30.91
- periocular area S00.20-
  - abrasion —*see* Abrasion, eyelid
  - bite —*see* Bite, superficial, eyelid
  - contusion —*see* Contusion, eyelid
  - external constriction —*see* Constriction, external, eyelid
  - foreign body —*see* Foreign body, superficial, eyelid
- phalanges
  - finger —*see* Injury, superficial, finger
  - toe —*see* Injury, superficial, toe
- pharynx —*see* Injury, superficial, throat
- pinna —*see* Injury, superficial, ear
- popliteal space —*see* Injury, superficial, knee
- prepuce S30.93
- pubic region S30.91
- pudendum
  - female S30.97
  - male S30.96
- sacral region S30.91
- scalp S00.00
- scapular region —*see* Injury, superficial, shoulder
- sclera —*see* Injury, eye, specified site NEC
- scrotum S30.94
- shin —*see* Injury, superficial, leg
- shoulder S40.91-
  - abrasion —*see* Abrasion, shoulder
  - bite —*see* Bite, superficial, shoulder
  - blister —*see* Blister, shoulder
  - contusion —*see* Contusion, shoulder
  - external constriction —*see* Constriction, external, shoulder
  - foreign body —*see* Foreign body, superficial, shoulder
- skin NEC T14.8
- sternal region —*see* Injury, superficial, thorax, front
- subconjunctival —*see* Injury, eye, specified site NEC
- subcutaneous NEC T14.8
- submaxillary region —*see* Injury, superficial, head, specified NEC
- submental region —*see* Injury, superficial, head, specified NEC

Injury *(continued)*
  superficial NEC *(continued)*
    subungual
      finger(s) —*see* Injury, superficial, finger
      toe(s) —*see* Injury, superficial, toe
    supraclavicular fossa —*see* Injury, superficial, neck
    supraorbital —*see* Injury, superficial, head, specified NEC
    temple —*see* Injury, superficial, head, specified NEC
    temporal region —*see* Injury, superficial, head, specified NEC
    testis S30.94
    thigh S70.92-
      abrasion —*see* Abrasion, thigh
      bite —*see* Bite, superficial, thigh
      blister —*see* Blister, thigh
      contusion —*see* Contusion, thigh
      external constriction —*see* Constriction, external, thigh
      foreign body —*see* Foreign body, superficial, thigh
    thorax, thoracic (wall) S20.90
      abrasion —*see* Abrasion, thorax
      back S20.40-
      bite —*see* Bite, thorax, superficial
      blister —*see* Blister, thorax
      contusion —*see* Contusion, thorax
      external constriction —*see* Constriction, external, thorax
      foreign body —*see* Foreign body, superficial, thorax
      front S20.30-
    throat S10.10
      abrasion S10.11
      bite S10.17
        insect S10.16
      blister S10.12
      contusion S10.0
      external constriction S10.14
      foreign body S10.15
    thumb S60.93-
      abrasion —*see* Abrasion, thumb
      bite —*see* Bite, superficial, thumb
      blister —*see* Blister, thumb
      contusion —*see* Contusion, thumb
      external constriction —*see* Constriction, external, thumb
      foreign body —*see* Foreign body, superficial, thumb
      insect bite —*see* Bite, by site, superficial, insect
      specified type NEC S60.39-
    toe(s) S90.93-
      abrasion —*see* Abrasion, toe
      bite —*see* Bite, toe
      blister —*see* Blister, toe
      contusion —*see* Contusion, toe
      external constriction —*see* Constriction, external, toe
      foreign body —*see* Foreign body, superficial, toe
      great S90.93-

Injury *(continued)*
  superficial NEC *(continued)*
    tongue —*see* Injury, superficial, oral cavity
    tooth, teeth —*see* Injury, superficial, oral cavity
    trachea S10.10
    tunica vaginalis S30.94
    tympanum, tympanic membrane —*see* Injury, superficial, ear
    uvula —*see* Injury, superficial, oral cavity
    vagina S30.95
    vocal cords —*see* Injury, superficial, throat
    vulva S30.95
    wrist S60.91-
  supraclavicular region —*see* Injury, neck
  supraorbital S09.93
  suprarenal gland (multiple) —*see* Injury, adrenal
  surgical complication (external or internal site) —*see* Laceration, accidental complicating surgery
  temple S09.90
  temporal region S09.90
  tendon —*see also* Injury, muscle, by site
    abdomen —*see* Injury, muscle, abdomen
    Achilles —*see* Injury, Achilles tendon
    lower back —*see* Injury, muscle, lower back
    pelvic organs —*see* Injury, muscle, pelvis
  tenth cranial nerve (pneumogastric or vagus) —*see* Injury, nerve, vagus
  testis S39.94
  thigh S79.92-
    blood vessel —*see* Injury, blood vessel, hip
    contusion —*see* Contusion, thigh
    fracture —*see* Fracture, femur
    muscle —*see* Injury, muscle, thigh
    nerve —*see* Injury, nerve, thigh
    open —*see* Wound, open, thigh
    specified NEC S79.82-
    superficial —*see* Injury, superficial, thigh
  third cranial nerve (oculomotor) —*see* Injury, nerve, oculomotor
  thorax, thoracic S29.9
    blood vessel —*see* Injury, blood vessel, thorax
    cavity —*see* Injury, intrathoracic
    dislocation —*see* Dislocation, thorax
    external (wall) S29.9
      contusion —*see* Contusion, thorax
      nerve —*see* Injury, nerve, thorax
      open —*see* Wound, open, thorax
      specified NEC S29.8
      sprain —*see* Sprain, thorax
      superficial —*see* Injury, superficial, thorax
    fracture —*see* Fracture, thorax
    internal —*see* Injury, intrathoracic
    intrathoracic organ —*see* Injury, intrathoracic
    sympathetic ganglion —*see* Injury, nerve, thorax, sympathetic
  throat *(see also* Injury, neck) S19.9

Injury *(continued)*
  thumb S69.9-
    blood vessel —*see* Injury, blood vessel, thumb
    contusion —*see* Contusion, thumb
    dislocation —*see* Dislocation, thumb
    fracture —*see* Fracture, thumb
    muscle —*see* Injury, muscle, thumb
    nerve —*see* Injury, nerve, digital, thumb
    open —*see* Wound, open, thumb
    specified NEC S69.8-
    sprain —*see* Sprain, thumb
    superficial —*see* Injury, superficial, thumb
  thymus (gland) —*see* Injury, intrathoracic, specified organ NEC
  thyroid (gland) NEC S19.84
  toe S99.92-
    contusion —*see* Contusion, toe
    dislocation —*see* Dislocation, toe
    fracture —*see* Fracture, toe
    muscle —*see* Injury, muscle, toe
    open —*see* Wound, open, toe
    specified type NEC S99.82-
    sprain —*see* Sprain, toe
    superficial —*see* Injury, superficial, toe
  tongue S09.93
  tonsil S09.93
  tooth S09.93
  trachea (cervical) NEC S19.82
    thoracic —*see* Injury, intrathoracic, trachea, thoracic
  transfusion-related acute lung (TRALI) J95.84
  tunica vaginalis S39.94
  twelfth cranial nerve (hypoglossal) —*see* Injury, nerve, hypoglossal
  ureter S37.10
    contusion S37.12
    laceration S37.13
    specified type NEC S37.19
  urethra (sphincter) S37.30
    at delivery O71.5
    contusion S37.32
    laceration S37.33
    specified type NEC S37.39
  urinary organ S37.90
    contusion S37.92
    laceration S37.93
    specified
      site NEC S37.899
        contusion S37.892
        laceration S37.893
        specified type NEC S37.898
      type NEC S37.99
  uterus, uterine S37.60
    with ectopic or molar pregnancy O08.6
    blood vessel —*see* Injury, blood vessel, iliac
    contusion S37.62
    laceration S37.63
      cervix at delivery O71.3
    rupture associated with obstetrics —*see* Rupture, uterus
    specified type NEC S37.69
  uvula S09.93
  vagina S39.93
    abrasion S30.814
    bite S31.45
      insect S30.864
      superficial NEC S30.874
    contusion S30.23
    crush S38.03

Injury *(continued)*
  vagina *(continued)*
    during delivery —*see* Laceration, vagina, during delivery
    external constriction S30.844
    insect bite S30.864
    laceration S31.41
      with foreign body S31.42
    open wound S31.40
    puncture S31.43
      with foreign body S31.44
    superficial S30.95
      foreign body S30.854
  vas deferens —*see* Injury, pelvic organ, specified site NEC
  vascular NEC T14.8
  vein —*see* Injury, blood vessel
  vena cava (superior) S25.20
    inferior S35.10
      laceration (minor) (superficial) S35.11
      major S35.12
      specified type NEC S35.19
    laceration (minor) (superficial) S25.21
      major S25.22
    specified type NEC S25.29
  vesical (sphincter) —*see* Injury, bladder
  visual cortex S04.04-
  vitreous (humor) S05.90
    specified NEC S05.8X-
  vocal cord NEC S19.83
  vulva S39.94
    abrasion S30.814
    bite S31.45
      insect S30.864
      superficial NEC S30.874
    contusion S30.23
    crush S38.03
    during delivery —*see* Laceration, perineum, female, during delivery
    external constriction S30.844
    insect bite S30.864
    laceration S31.41
      with foreign body S31.42
    open wound S31.40
    puncture S31.43
      with foreign body S31.44
    superficial S30.95
      foreign body S30.854
  whiplash (cervical spine) S13.4
  wrist S69.9-
    blood vessel —*see* Injury, blood vessel, hand
    contusion —*see* Contusion, wrist
    dislocation —*see* Dislocation, wrist
    fracture —*see* Fracture, wrist
    muscle —*see* Injury, muscle, hand
    nerve —*see* Injury, nerve, hand
    open —*see* Wound, open, wrist
    specified NEC S69.8-
    sprain —*see* Sprain, wrist
    superficial —*see* Injury, superficial, wrist

Inoculation —*see also* Vaccination
  complication or reaction —*see* Complications, vaccination

Insanity, insane —*see also* Psychosis
  adolescent —*see* Schizophrenia
  confusional F28
    acute or subacute F05
  delusional F22
  senile F03

Insect
bite —*see* Bite, by site, superficial, insect
venomous, poisoning NEC (by) —*see* Venom, arthropod

Insecurity
financial Z59.86
food Z59.41
transportation Z59.82

Insensitivity
adrenocorticotropin hormone (ACTH) E27.49
androgen E34.50
  complete E34.51
  partial E34.52

Insertion
cord (umbilical) lateral or velamentous O43.12-
intrauterine contraceptive device (encounter for) —*see* Intrauterine contraceptive device

Insolation (sunstroke) T67.01

Insomnia (organic) G47.00
adjustment F51.02
adjustment disorder F51.02
behavioral, of childhood Z73.819
  combined type Z73.812
  limit setting type Z73.811
  sleep-onset association type Z73.810
childhood Z73.819
chronic F51.04
  somatized tension F51.04
conditioned F51.04
due to
  alcohol
    abuse F10.182
    dependence F10.282
    use F10.982
  amphetamines
    abuse F15.182
    dependence F15.282
    use F15.982
  anxiety disorder F51.05
  caffeine
    abuse F15.182
    dependence F15.282
    use F15.982
  cocaine
    abuse F14.182
    dependence F14.282
    use F14.982
  depression F51.05
  drug NEC
    abuse F19.182
    dependence F19.282
    use F19.982
  medical condition G47.01
  mental disorder NEC F51.05
  opioid
    abuse F11.182
    dependence F11.282
    use F11.982
  psychoactive substance NEC
    abuse F19.182
    dependence F19.282
    use F19.982
  sedative, hypnotic, or anxiolytic
    abuse F13.182
    dependence F13.282
    use F13.982
  stimulant NEC
    abuse F15.182
    dependence F15.282
    use F15.982
fatal familial (FFI) A81.83
idiopathic F51.01
learned F51.3
nonorganic origin F51.01

Insomnia *(continued)*
not due to a substance or known physiological condition F51.01
  specified NEC F51.09
paradoxical F51.03
primary F51.01
psychiatric F51.05
psychophysiologic F51.04
related to psychopathology F51.05
short-term F51.02
specified NEC G47.09
stress-related F51.02
transient F51.02
without objective findings F51.02

Inspiration
food or foreign body —*see* Foreign body, by site
mucus —*see* Asphyxia, mucus

Inspissated bile syndrome (newborn) P59.1

Instability
emotional (excessive) F60.3
housing
  housed Z59.819
    with risk of homelessness Z59.811
  homelessness in past 12 months Z59.812
joint (post-traumatic) M25.30
  ankle M25.37-
  due to old ligament injury —*see* Disorder, ligament
  elbow M25.32-
  flail —*see* Flail, joint
  foot M25.37-
  hand M25.34-
  hip M25.35-
  knee M25.36-
  lumbosacral M53.2
  prosthesis —*see* Complications, joint prosthesis, mechanical, displacement, by site
  sacroiliac M53.2
  secondary to
    old ligament injury —*see* Disorder, ligament
    removal of joint prosthesis M96.89
  shoulder (region) M25.31-
  specified site NEC M25.39
  spine M53.2
  wrist M25.33-
knee (chronic) M23.5-
lumbosacral M53.2
nervous F48.8
personality (emotional) F60.3
spine —*see* Instability, joint, spine
vasomotor R55

Institutional syndrome (childhood) F94.2

Institutionalization, affecting child Z62.22
disinhibited attachment F94.2

Insufficiency, insufficient
accommodation, old age H52.4
adrenal (gland) E27.40
  primary E27.1
adrenocortical E27.40
  drug-induced E27.3
  iatrogenic E27.3
  primary E27.1
anatomic crown height K08.89
anterior (occlusal) guidance M26.54
anus K62.89

Insufficiency, insufficient *(continued)*
aortic (valve) I35.1
  with
    mitral (valve) disease I08.0
      with tricuspid (valve) disease I08.3
    stenosis I35.2
    tricuspid (valve) disease I08.2
      with mitral (valve) disease I08.3
  congenital Q23.1
  rheumatic I06.1
    with
      mitral (valve) disease I08.0
        with tricuspid (valve) disease I08.3
      stenosis I06.2
        with mitral (valve) disease I08.0
          with tricuspid (valve) disease I08.3
      tricuspid (valve) disease I08.2
        with mitral (valve) disease I08.3
  specified cause NEC I35.1
  syphilitic A52.03
arterial I77.1
  basilar G45.0
  carotid (hemispheric) G45.1
  cerebral I67.81
  coronary (acute or subacute) I24.89
  mesenteric K55.1
  peripheral I73.9
  precerebral (multiple) (bilateral) G45.2
  vertebral G45.0
arteriovenous I99.8
biliary K83.8
cardiac —*see also* Insufficiency, myocardial
  due to presence of (cardiac) prosthesis I97.11-
  postprocedural I97.11-
cardiorenal, hypertensive I13.2
cardiovascular —*see* Disease, cardiovascular
cerebrovascular (acute) I67.81
  with transient focal neurological signs and symptoms G45.8
circulatory NEC I99.8
  newborn P29.89
clinical crown height K08.89
convergence H51.11
coronary (acute or subacute) I24.89
  chronic or with a stated duration of over 4 weeks I25.89
corticoadrenal E27.40
  primary E27.1
dietary E63.9
divergence H51.8
food T73.0
gastroesophageal K22.89
gonadal
  ovary E28.39
  testis E29.1
heart —*see also* Insufficiency, myocardial
  newborn P29.0
  valve —*see* Endocarditis
hepatic —*see* Failure, hepatic
idiopathic autonomic G90.09
interocclusal distance of fully erupted teeth (ridge) M26.36
kidney N28.9
  acute N28.9
  chronic N18.9
lacrimal (secretion) H04.12-
  passages —*see* Stenosis, lacrimal

Insufficiency, insufficient *(continued)*
liver —*see* Failure, hepatic
lung —*see* Insufficiency, pulmonary
mental (congenital) —*see* Disability, intellectual
mesenteric K55.1
mitral (valve) I34.0
  with
    aortic valve disease I08.0
      with tricuspid (valve) disease I08.3
    obstruction or stenosis I05.2
      with aortic valve disease I08.0
    tricuspid (valve) disease I08.1
      with aortic (valve) disease I08.3
  congenital Q23.3
  rheumatic I05.1
    with
      aortic valve disease I08.0
        with tricuspid (valve) disease I08.3
      obstruction or stenosis I05.2
        with aortic valve disease I08.0
          with tricuspid (valve) disease I08.3
      tricuspid (valve) disease I08.1
        with aortic (valve) disease I08.3
    active or acute I01.1
      with chorea, rheumatic (Sydenham's) I02.0
  specified cause, except rheumatic I34.0
muscle —*see also* Disease, muscle
heart —*see* Insufficiency, myocardial
ocular NEC H50.9
myocardial, myocardium (with arteriosclerosis) *(see also* Failure, heart) I50.9
  with
    rheumatic fever (conditions in I00) I09.0
      active, acute or subacute I01.2
        with chorea I02.0
      inactive or quiescent (with chorea) I09.0
  congenital Q24.8
  hypertensive —*see* Hypertension, heart
  newborn P29.0
  rheumatic I09.0
    active, acute, or subacute I01.2
  syphilitic A52.06
nourishment *(see also* Nutrition deficient) T73.0
pancreatic K86.89
  exocrine K86.81
parathyroid (gland) E20.9
peripheral vascular (arterial) I73.9
pituitary E23.0
placental (mother) O36.51-
platelets D69.6
prenatal care affecting management of pregnancy O09.3-
progressive pluriglandular E31.0
pulmonary J98.4
  acute, following surgery (nonthoracic) J95.2
    thoracic J95.1
  chronic, following surgery J95.3
  following
    shock J98.4
    trauma J98.4

Insufficiency, insufficient (continued)
  pulmonary (continued)
    newborn P28.89
    valve I37.1
      with stenosis I37.2
      congenital Q22.2
      rheumatic I09.89
        with aortic, mitral or tricuspid (valve) disease I08.8
  pyloric K31.89
  renal (acute) N28.9
    chronic N18.9
  respiratory R06.89
    newborn P28.5
  rotation —see Malrotation
  sleep syndrome F51.12
  social insurance Z59.7
  suprarenal E27.40
    primary E27.1
  tarso-orbital fascia, congenital Q10.3
  testis E29.1
  thyroid (gland) (acquired) E03.9
    congenital E03.1
  tricuspid (valve) (rheumatic) I07.1
    with
      aortic (valve) disease I08.2
        with mitral (valve) disease I08.3
      mitral (valve) disease I08.1
        with aortic (valve) disease I08.3
      obstruction or stenosis I07.2
        with aortic (valve) disease I08.2
          with mitral (valve) disease I08.3
    congenital Q22.8
    nonrheumatic I36.1
      with stenosis I36.2
  urethral sphincter R32
  valve, valvular (heart) I38
    aortic —see Insufficiency, aortic (valve)
    congenital Q24.8
    mitral —see Insufficiency, mitral (valve)
    pulmonary —see Insufficiency, pulmonary valve
    tricuspid —see Insufficiency, tricuspid (valve)
  vascular I99.8
    intestine K55.9
      acute (see also Ischemia, intestine, acute) K55.059
    mesenteric K55.1
    peripheral I73.9
    renal —see Hypertension, kidney
  velopharyngeal
    acquired K13.79
    congenital Q38.8
  venous (chronic) (peripheral) I87.2
  ventricular —see Insufficiency, myocardial
  welfare support Z59.7
Insufflation, fallopian Z31.41
Insular —see condition
Insulinoma
  pancreas
    benign D13.7
    malignant C25.4
    uncertain behavior D37.8
  specified site
    benign —see Neoplasm, by site, benign
    malignant —see Neoplasm, by site, malignant

Insulinoma (continued)
  specified site (continued)
    uncertain behavior —see Neoplasm, by site, uncertain behavior
  unspecified site
    benign D13.7
    malignant C25.4
    uncertain behavior D37.8
Insuloma —see Insulinoma
Interference
  balancing side M26.56
  non-working side M26.56
Intermenstrual —see condition
Intermittent —see condition
Internal —see condition
Interrogation
  cardiac defibrillator (automatic) (implantable) Z45.02
  cardiac pacemaker Z45.018
  cardiac (event) (loop) recorder Z45.09
  infusion pump (implanted) (intrathecal) Z45.1
  neurostimulator Z46.2
Interruption
  aortic arch Q25.21
  bundle of His I44.30
  phase-shift, sleep cycle —see Disorder, sleep, circadian rhythm
  sleep phase-shift, or 24 hour sleep-wake cycle —see Disorder, sleep, circadian rhythm
Interstitial —see condition
Intertrigo L30.4
  labialis K13.0
Intervertebral disc —see condition
Intestine, intestinal —see condition
Intolerance
  carbohydrate K90.49
  disaccharide, hereditary E73.0
  fat NEC K90.49
    pancreatic K90.3
  food K90.49
    dietary counseling and surveillance Z71.3
  fructose E74.10
    hereditary E74.12
  glucose (-galactose) E74.39
  gluten K90.41
  lactose E73.9
    specified NEC E73.8
  lysine E72.3
  milk NEC K90.49
    lactose E73.9
  orthostatic, chronic G90.A
  protein K90.49
  starch NEC K90.49
  sucrose (-isomaltose) E74.31
Intoxicated NEC (without dependence) —see Alcohol, intoxication
Intoxication
  acid (see also Acidosis) E87.29
  alcoholic (acute) (without dependence) —see Alcohol, intoxication
  alimentary canal K52.1
  amphetamine (without dependence) —see also Abuse, drug, stimulant, with intoxication
    with dependence —see Dependence, drug, stimulant, with intoxication

Intoxication (continued)
  amphetamine (continued)
    stimulant NEC F15.10
      with
        anxiety disorder F15.180
        intoxication F15.129
          with
            delirium F15.121
            perceptual disturbance F15.122
  anxiolytic (acute) (without dependence) —see Abuse, drug, sedative, with intoxication
    with dependence —see Dependence, drug, sedative, with intoxication
  caffeine F15.929
    with
      abuse —see Abuse, drug, cannabis, with intoxication
      dependence —see Dependence, drug, cannabis, with intoxication
  cannabinoids (acute) (without dependence) —see Use, cannabis, with intoxication
    with
      abuse —see Abuse, drug, cannabis, with intoxication
      dependence —see Dependence, drug, cannabis, with intoxication
  chemical —see Table of Drugs and Chemicals
    via placenta or breast milk —see - Absorption, chemical, through placenta
  cocaine (acute) (without dependence) —see Abuse, drug, cocaine, with intoxication
    with dependence —see Dependence, drug, cocaine, with intoxication
  drug
    acute (without dependence) —see Abuse, drug, by type with intoxication
      with dependence —see Dependence, drug, by type with intoxication
    addictive
      via placenta or breast milk —see Absorption, drug, addictive, through placenta
    newborn P93.8
      gray baby syndrome P93.0
    overdose or wrong substance given or taken —see Table of Drugs and Chemicals, by drug, poisoning
  enteric K52.1
  foodborne A05.9
    bacterial A05.9
    classical (Clostridium botulinum) A05.1
    due to
      Bacillus cereus A05.4
      bacterium A05.9
        specified NEC A05.8
      Clostridium
        botulinum A05.1
        perfringens A05.2
        welchii A05.2

Intoxication (continued)
  foodborne (continued)
    due to (continued)
      Salmonella A02.9
        with
          (gastro)enteritis A02.0
          localized infection(s) A02.20
            arthritis A02.23
            meningitis A02.21
            osteomyelitis A02.24
            pneumonia A02.22
            pyelonephritis A02.25
            specified NEC A02.29
          sepsis A02.1
          specified manifestation NEC A02.8
      Staphylococcus A05.0
      Vibrio
        parahaemolyticus A05.3
        vulnificus A05.5
    enterotoxin, staphylococcal A05.0
    noxious —see Poisoning, food, noxious
  gastrointestinal K52.1
  hallucinogenic (without dependence) —see Abuse, drug, hallucinogen, with intoxication
    with dependence —see Dependence, drug, hallucinogen, with intoxication
  hepatocerebral intoxication K76.82
  hypnotic (acute) (without dependence) —see Abuse, drug, sedative, with intoxication
    with dependence —see Dependence, drug, sedative, with intoxication
  inhalant (acute) (without dependence) —see Abuse, drug, inhalant, with intoxication
    with dependence —see Dependence, drug, inhalant, with intoxication
  meaning
    inebriation F10
    poisoning —see Table of Drugs and Chemicals
  methyl alcohol (acute) (without dependence) —see Alcohol, intoxication
  opioid (acute) (without dependence) —see Abuse, drug, opioid, with intoxication
    with dependence —see Dependence, drug, opioid, with intoxication
  pathologic NEC (without dependence) —see Alcohol, intoxication
  phencyclidine (without dependence) —see Abuse, drug, hallucinogen, with intoxication
    with dependence —see Dependence, drug, hallucinogen, with intoxication
  potassium (K) E87.5
  psychoactive substance NEC (without dependence) —see Abuse, drug, psychoactive NEC, with intoxication
    with dependence —see Dependence, drug, psychoactive NEC, with intoxication

Intoxication *(continued)*
  sedative (acute) (without dependence) —*see* Abuse, drug, sedative, with intoxication
    with dependence —*see* Dependence, drug, sedative, with intoxication
  serum (*see also* Reaction, serum) T80.69
  uremic —*see* Uremia
  volatile solvents (acute) (without dependence) —*see* Abuse, drug, inhalant, with intoxication
    with dependence —*see* Dependence, drug, inhalant, with intoxication
  water E87.79
Intraabdominal testis, testes
  bilateral Q53.211
  unilateral Q53.111
Intracranial —*see* condition
Intrahepatic gallbladder Q44.1
Intraligamentous —*see* condition
Intrathoracic —*see also* condition
  kidney Q63.2
Intrauterine contraceptive device
  checking Z30.431
  insertion Z30.430
    immediately following removal Z30.433
  in situ Z97.5
  management Z30.431
  reinsertion Z30.433
  removal Z30.432
  replacement Z30.433
  retention in pregnancy O26.3-
Intraventricular —*see* condition
Intrinsic deformity —*see* Deformity
Intubation, difficult or failed T88.4
Intumescence, lens (eye) (cataract) —*see* Cataract
Intussusception (bowel) (colon) (enteric) (ileocecal) (ileocolic) (intestine) (rectum) K56.1
  appendix K38.8
  congenital Q43.8
  ureter (with obstruction) N13.5
Invagination (bowel, colon, intestine or rectum) K56.1
Inversion
  albumin-globulin (A-G) ratio E88.09
  bladder N32.89
  cecum —*see* Intussusception
  cervix N88.8
  chromosome in normal individual Q95.1
  circadian rhythm —*see* Disorder, sleep, circadian rhythm
  nipple N64.59
    congenital Q83.8
    gestational —*see* Retraction, nipple
    puerperal, postpartum —*see* Retraction, nipple
  nyctohemeral rhythm —*see* Disorder, sleep, circadian rhythm
  optic papilla Q14.2
  organ or site, congenital NEC —*see* Anomaly, by site
  sleep rhythm —*see* Disorder, sleep, circadian rhythm
  testis (congenital) Q55.29
  uterus (chronic) (postinfectional) (postpartal, old) N85.5
    postpartum O71.2

Inversion *(continued)*
  vagina (posthysterectomy) N99.3
  ventricular Q20.5
Investigation (*see also* Examination) Z04.9
  clinical research subject (control) (normal comparison) (participant) Z00.6
Involuntary movement, abnormal R25.9
Involution, involutional —*see also* condition
  breast, cystic —*see* Dysplasia, mammary, specified type NEC
  depression (single episode) F32.89
    recurrent episode F33.9
  melancholia (single episode) F32.89
    recurrent episode F33.8
  ovary, senile —*see* Atrophy, ovary
  thymus failure E32.8
I.Q.
  under 20 F73
  20-34 F72
  35-49 F71
  50-69 F70
IRDS (type I) P22.0
  type II P22.1
Irideremia Q13.1
Iridis rubeosis —*see* Disorder, iris, vascular
Iridochoroiditis (panuveitis) —*see* Panuveitis
Iridocyclitis H20.9
  acute H20.0-
    hypopyon H20.05-
    primary H20.01-
    recurrent H20.02-
    secondary (noninfectious) H20.04-
      infectious H20.03-
  chronic H20.1-
    due to allergy —*see* Iridocyclitis, acute, secondary
    endogenous —*see* Iridocyclitis, acute, primary
    Fuchs' —*see* Cyclitis, Fuchs' heterochromic
    gonococcal A54.32
    granulomatous —*see* Iridocyclitis, chronic
    herpes, herpetic (simplex) B00.51
      zoster B02.32
    hypopyon —*see* Iridocyclitis, acute, hypopyon
    in (due to)
      ankylosing spondylitis M45.9
      gonococcal infection A54.32
      herpes (simplex) virus B00.51
        zoster B02.32
      infectious disease NOS B99
      parasitic disease NOS B89 [H22]
      sarcoidosis D86.83
      syphilis A51.43
      tuberculosis A18.54
      zoster B02.32
    lens-induced H20.2-
    nongranulomatous —*see* Iridocyclitis, acute
    recurrent —*see* Iridocyclitis, acute, recurrent

Iridocyclitis *(continued)*
  rheumatic —*see* Iridocyclitis, chronic
  subacute —*see* Iridocyclitis, acute
  sympathetic —*see* Uveitis, sympathetic
  syphilitic (secondary) A51.43
  tuberculous (chronic) A18.54
  Vogt-Koyanagi H20.82-
Iridocyclochoroiditis (panuveitis) —*see* Panuveitis
Iridodialysis H21.53-
Iridodonesis H21.89
Iridoplegia (complete) (partial) (reflex) H57.09
Iridoschisis H21.25-
Iris —*see also* condition
  bombé —*see* Membrane, pupillary
Iritis —*see also* Iridocyclitis
  chronic —*see* Iridocyclitis, chronic
  diabetic —*see* E08-E13 with .39
  due to
    herpes simplex B00.51
    leprosy A30.9 [H22]
  gonococcal A54.32
  gouty (*see also* Gout, by type) M10.9 [H22]
  granulomatous —*see* Iridocyclitis, chronic
  lens induced —*see* Iridocyclitis, lens-induced
  papulosa (syphilitic) A52.71
  rheumatic —*see* Iridocyclitis, chronic
  syphilitic (secondary) A51.43
    congenital (early) A50.01
    late A52.71
  tuberculous A18.54
Iron —*see* condition
Iron-miner's lung J63.4
Irradiated enamel (tooth, teeth) K03.89
Irradiation effects, adverse T66
Irreducible, irreducibility —*see* condition
Irregular, irregularity
  action, heart I49.9
  alveolar process K08.89
  bleeding N92.6
  breathing R06.89
  contour of cornea (acquired) —*see* Deformity, cornea
    congenital Q13.4
  contour, reconstructed breast N65.0
  dentin (in pulp) K04.3
  eye movements H55.89
    nystagmus —*see* Nystagmus
    deficient
      saccadic H55.81
      smooth H55.82
  labor O62.2
  menstruation (cause unknown) N92.6
  periods N92.6
  prostate N42.9
  pupil —*see* Abnormality, pupillary
  reconstructed breast N65.0
  respiratory R06.89

Irregular, irregularity *(continued)*
  septum (nasal) J34.2
  shape, organ or site, congenital NEC —*see* Distortion
  sleep-wake pattern (rhythm) G47.23
Irritable, irritability R45.4
  bladder N32.89
  bowel (syndrome) K58.9
    with
      constipation K58.1
      diarrhea K58.0
      mixed K58.2
      psychogenic F45.8
      specified NEC K58.8
  bronchial —*see* Bronchitis
  cerebral, in newborn P91.3
  colon (*see also* Irritable, bowel) K58.9
    with diarrhea K58.0
    psychogenic F45.8
  duodenum K59.89
  heart (psychogenic) F45.8
  hip —*see* Derangement, joint, specified type NEC, hip
  ileum K59.89
  infant R68.12
  jejunum K59.89
  rectum K59.89
  stomach K31.89
    psychogenic F45.8
  sympathetic G90.8
  urethra N36.8
Irritation
  anus K62.89
  axillary nerve G54.0
  bladder N32.89
  brachial plexus G54.0
  bronchial —*see* Bronchitis
  cervical plexus G54.2
  cervix —*see* Cervicitis
  choroid, sympathetic —*see* Endophthalmitis
  cranial nerve —*see* Disorder, nerve, cranial
  gastric K31.89
    psychogenic F45.8
  globe, sympathetic —*see* Uveitis, sympathetic
  labyrinth —*see* subcategory H83.2
  lumbosacral plexus G54.1
  meninges (traumatic) —*see* Injury, intracranial
    nontraumatic —*see* Meningismus
  nerve —*see* Disorder, nerve
  nervous R45.0
  penis N48.89
  perineum NEC L29.3
  peripheral autonomic nervous system G90.8
  peritoneum —*see* Peritonitis
  pharynx J39.2
  plantar nerve —*see* Lesion, nerve, plantar
  spinal (cord) (traumatic) —*see also* Injury, spinal cord, by region
    nerve G58.9
      root NEC —*see* Radiculopathy
    nontraumatic —*see* Myelopathy
  stomach K31.89
    psychogenic F45.8
  sympathetic nerve NEC G90.8
  ulnar nerve —*see* Lesion, nerve, ulnar
  vagina N89.8

213

Ischemia, ischemic I99.8
  brain —see Ischemia, cerebral
  bowel (transient)
    acute (see also Ischemia, intestine, acute) K55.019
      diffuse K55.012
      focal K55.011
    chronic K55.1
    due to mesenteric artery insufficiency K55.1
  cardiac (see Disease, heart, ischemic)
  cardiomyopathy I25.5
  cerebral (chronic) (generalized) I67.82
    arteriosclerotic I67.2
    intermittent G45.9
    newborn P91.0
    recurrent focal G45.8
    transient G45.9
  colon chronic (due to mesenteric artery insufficiency) K55.1
  coronary —see Disease, heart, ischemic
  demand (coronary) (see also Angina) I24.89
    with myocardial infarction I21.A1
      resulting in myocardial infarction I21.A1
  heart (chronic or with a stated duration of over 4 weeks) I25.9
    acute or with a stated duration of 4 weeks or less I24.9
    subacute I24.9
  infarction, muscle —see Infarct, muscle
  intestine (large) (small) (transient) K55.9
    acute K55.059
    diffuse K55.052
    focal K55.051
    large K55.039
      diffuse K55.032
      focal K55.031
    small K55.019
      diffuse K55.012
      focal K55.011
    chronic K55.1
    due to mesenteric artery insufficiency K55.1
  kidney N28.0
  limb, critical —see Arteriosclerosis, with critical limb ischemia
  limb-threatening, chronic —see Arteriosclerosis, with critical limb ischemia
  mesenteric, acute (see also Ischemia, intestine, acute) K55.059
  muscle, traumatic T79.6
  myocardium, myocardial (chronic or with a stated duration of over 4 weeks) I25.9
    acute, without myocardial infarction I51.3
    silent (asymptomatic) I25.6
    transient of newborn P29.4
  renal N28.0
  retina, retinal —see Occlusion, artery, retina
  small bowel
    acute K55.019
      diffuse K55.012
      focal K55.011

Ischemia, ischemic (continued)
  small bowel (continued)
    chronic K55.1
    due to mesenteric artery insufficiency K55.1
  spinal cord G95.11
  subendocardial —see Insufficiency, coronary
  supply (coronary) (see also Angina) I25.9
  due to vasospasm I20.1
Ischial spine —see condition
Ischialgia —see Sciatica
Ischiopagus Q89.4
Ischium, ischial —see condition
Ischuria R34
Iselin's disease or osteochondrosis —see Osteochondrosis, juvenile, metatarsus
Islands of
  parotid tissue in
    lymph nodes Q38.6
    neck structures Q38.6
  submaxillary glands in
    fascia Q38.6
    lymph nodes Q38.6
    neck muscles Q38.6
Islet cell tumor, pancreas D13.7
Isoimmunization NEC —see also Incompatibility
  affecting management of pregnancy (ABO) (with hydrops fetalis) O36.11-
    anti-A sensitization O36.11-
    anti-B sensitization O36.19-
    anti-c sensitization O36.09-
    anti-C sensitization O36.09-
    anti-e sensitization O36.09-
    anti-E sensitization O36.09-
    Rh NEC O36.09-
      anti-D antibody O36.01-
    specified NEC O36.19-
  newborn P55.9
    with
      hydrops fetalis P56.0
      kernicterus P57.0
    ABO (blood groups) P55.1
    Rhesus (Rh) factor P55.0
    specified type NEC P55.8
Isolation, isolated
  dwelling Z59.89
  family Z63.79
  social Z60.4
Isoleucinosis E71.19
Isomerism atrial appendages (with asplenia or polysplenia) Q20.6
Isosporiasis, isosporosis A07.3
Isovaleric acidemia E71.110
Issue of
  medical certificate Z02.79
    for disability determination Z02.71
  repeat prescription (appliance) (glasses) (medicinal substance, medicament, medicine) Z76.0
  contraception —see Contraception
IST (inappropriate sinus tachycardia, so stated) I47.11
Itch, itching —see also Pruritus
  baker's L23.6
  barber's B35.0
  bricklayer's L24.5
  cheese B88.0
  clam digger's B65.3
  coolie B76.9
  copra B88.0
  dew B76.9

Itch, itching (continued)
  dhobi B35.6
  filarial —see Infestation, filarial
  grain B88.0
  grocer's B88.0
  ground B76.9
  harvest B88.0
  jock B35.6
  Malabar B35.5
    beard B35.0
    foot B35.3
    scalp B35.0
  meaning scabies B86
  Norwegian B86
  perianal L29.0
  poultrymen's B88.0
  sarcoptic B86
  scabies B86
  scrub B88.0
  straw B88.0
  swimmer's B65.3
  water B76.9
  winter L29.8
Ivemark's syndrome (asplenia with congenital heart disease) Q89.01
Ivory bones Q78.2
Ixodiasis NEC B88.8

J

Jaccoud's syndrome —see Arthropathy, postrheumatic, chronic
Jackson's
  membrane Q43.3
  paralysis or syndrome G83.89
  veil Q43.3
Jacquet's dermatitis (diaper dermatitis) L22
Jadassohn-Pellizari's disease or anetoderma L90.2
Jadassohn's
  blue nevus —see Nevus
  intraepidermal epithelioma —see Neoplasm, skin, benign
Jaffe-Lichtenstein (-Uehlinger) **syndrome** —see Dysplasia, fibrous, bone NEC
Jakob-Creutzfeldt disease or syndrome —see Creutzfeldt-Jakob disease or syndrome
Jaksch-Luzet disease D64.89
Jamaican
  neuropathy G92.8
  paraplegic tropical ataxic-spastic syndrome G92.8
Janet's disease F48.8
Janiceps Q89.4
Jansky-Bielschowsky amaurotic idiocy E75.4
Japanese
  B-type encephalitis A83.0
  river fever A75.3
Jaundice (yellow) R17
  acholuric (familial) (splenomegalic) —see also Spherocytosis
    acquired D59.8
  breast-milk (inhibitor) P59.3
  catarrhal (acute) B15.9
    with hepatic coma B15.0
  cholestatic (benign) R17

Jaundice (continued)
  due to or associated with delayed conjugation P59.8
    associated with (due to) preterm delivery P59.0
  preterm delivery P59.0
  epidemic (catarrhal) B15.9
    with hepatic coma B15.0
    leptospiral A27.0
    spirochetal A27.0
  familial nonhemolytic (congenital) (Gilbert) E80.4
  Crigler-Najjar E80.5
  febrile (acute) B15.9
    with hepatic coma B15.0
    leptospiral A27.0
    spirochetal A27.0
  hematogenous D59.9
  hemolytic (acquired) D59.9
    congenital —see Spherocytosis
  hemorrhagic (acute) (leptospiral) (spirochetal) A27.0
  infectious (acute) (subacute) B15.9
    with hepatic coma B15.0
    leptospiral A27.0
    spirochetal A27.0
  leptospiral (hemorrhagic) A27.0
  malignant (without coma) K72.90
    with coma K72.91
  newborn P59.9
    due to or associated with
      ABO
        antibodies P55.1
        incompatibility, maternal/fetal P55.1
        isoimmunization P55.1
      absence or deficiency of enzyme system for bilirubin conjugation (congenital) P59.8
      bleeding P58.1
      breast milk inhibitors to conjugation P59.3
        associated with preterm delivery P59.0
      bruising P58.0
      Crigler-Najjar syndrome E80.5
      delayed conjugation P59.8
        associated with preterm delivery P59.0
      drugs or toxins
        given to newborn P58.42
        transmitted from mother P58.41
      excessive hemolysis P58.9
        due to
          bleeding P58.1
          bruising P58.0
          drugs or toxins
            given to newborn P58.42
            transmitted from mother P58.41
          infection P58.2
          polycythemia P58.3
          swallowed maternal blood P58.5
          specified type NEC P58.8
      galactosemia E74.21
      Gilbert syndrome E80.4
      hemolytic disease P55.9
        ABO isoimmunization P55.1

Jaundice (continued)
  newborn (continued)
    due to or associated with (continued)
      hemolytic disease (continued)
        Rh isoimmunization P55.0
          specified NEC P55.8
      hepatocellular damage P59.20
        specified NEC P59.29
      hereditary hemolytic anemia P58.8
      hypothyroidism, congenital E03.1
      incompatibility, maternal/fetal NOS P55.9
      infection P58.2
      inspissated bile syndrome P59.1
      isoimmunization NOS P55.9
      mucoviscidosis E84.9
      polycythemia P58.3
      preterm delivery P59.0
      Rh
        antibodies P55.0
        incompatibility, maternal/fetal P55.0
        isoimmunization P55.0
      specified cause NEC P59.8
      swallowed maternal blood P58.5
      spherocytosis (congenital) D58.0
    neonatal —see Jaundice, newborn
    nonhemolytic congenital familial (Gilbert) E80.4
    nuclear, newborn (see also Kernicterus of newborn) P57.9
  obstructive (see also Obstruction, bile duct) K83.1
  post-immunization —see Hepatitis, viral, type, B
  post-transfusion —see Hepatitis, viral, type, B
  regurgitation (see also Obstruction, bile duct) K83.1
  serum (homologous) (prophylactic) (therapeutic) —see Hepatitis, viral, type, B
  spirochetal (hemorrhagic) A27.0
  symptomatic R17
    newborn P59.9
Jaw —see condition
Jaw-winking phenomenon or syndrome Q07.8
Jealousy
  alcoholic F10.988
  childhood F93.8
  sibling F93.8
Jejunitis —see Enteritis
Jejunostomy status Z93.4
Jejunum, jejunal —see condition
Jensen's disease —see Inflammation, chorioretinal, focal, juxtapapillary
Jerks, myoclonic G25.3
Jervell-Lange-Nielsen syndrome I45.81
Jeune's disease Q77.2
Jigger disease B88.1
Job's syndrome (chronic granulomatous disease) D71
Joint —see also condition
  mice —see Loose, body, joint
  knee M23.4-
Jordan's anomaly or syndrome D72.0

Joseph-Diamond-Blackfan anemia (congenital hypoplastic) D61.01
Jungle yellow fever A95.0
Jüngling's disease —see Sarcoidosis
Juvenile —see condition

K

Kahler's disease C90.0-
Kakke E51.11
Kala-azar B55.0
Kallmann's syndrome E23.0
Kanner's syndrome (autism) —see Psychosis, childhood
Kaposi's
  dermatosis (xeroderma pigmentosum) Q82.1
  lichen ruber L44.0
    acuminatus L44.0
  sarcoma
    colon C46.4
    connective tissue C46.1
    gastrointestinal organ C46.4
    lung C46.5-
    lymph node (multiple) C46.3
    palate (hard) (soft) C46.2
    rectum C46.4
    skin (multiple sites) C46.0
    specified site NEC C46.7
    stomach C46.4
    unspecified site C46.9
  varicelliform eruption B00.0
    vaccinia T88.1
Kartagener's syndrome or triad (sinusitis, bronchiectasis, situs inversus) Q89.3
Karyotype
  with abnormality except iso (Xq) Q96.2
  45,X Q96.0
  46,X
    iso (Xq) Q96.1
  46,XX Q98.3
    with streak gonads Q50.32
    hermaphrodite (true) Q99.1
    male Q98.3
  46,XY
    with streak gonads Q56.1
    female Q97.3
    hermaphrodite (true) Q99.1
  47,XXX Q97.0
  47,XXY Q98.0
  47,XYY Q98.5
Kaschin-Beck disease —see Disease, Kaschin-Beck
Katayama's disease or fever B65.2
Kawasaki's syndrome M30.3
Kayser-Fleischer ring (cornea) (pseudosclerosis) H18.04-
Kaznelson's syndrome (congenital hypoplastic anemia) D61.01
Kearns-Sayre syndrome H49.81-
Kedani fever A75.3
Kelis L91.0
Kelly (-Patterson) **syndrome** (sideropenic dysphagia) D50.1

Keloid, cheloid L91.0
  acne L73.0
  Addison's L94.0
  cornea —see Opacity, cornea
  Hawkin's L91.0
  scar L91.0
Keloma L91.0
Kenya fever A77.1
Keratectasia —see also Ectasia, cornea
  congenital Q13.4
Keratinization of alveolar ridge mucosa
  excessive K13.23
  minimal K13.22
Keratinized residual ridge mucosa
  excessive K13.23
  minimal K13.22
Keratitis (nodular) (nonulcerative) (simple) (zonular) H16.9
  with ulceration (central) (marginal) (perforated) (ring) —see Ulcer, cornea
  actinic —see Photokeratitis
  arborescens (herpes simplex) B00.52
  areolar H16.11-
  bullosa H16.8
  deep H16.309
    specified type NEC H16.399
  dendritic (a) (herpes simplex) B00.52
  disciform (is) (herpes simplex) B00.52
    varicella B01.81
  filamentary H16.12-
  gonococcal (congenital or prenatal) A54.33
  herpes, herpetic (simplex) B00.52
    zoster B02.33
  in (due to)
    acanthamebiasis B60.13
    adenovirus B30.0
    exanthema (see also Exanthem) B09
    herpes (simplex) virus B00.52
    measles B05.81
    syphilis A50.31
    tuberculosis A18.52
    zoster B02.33
  interstitial (nonsyphilitic) H16.30-
    diffuse H16.32-
    herpes, herpetic (simplex) B00.52
      zoster B02.33
    sclerosing H16.33-
    specified type NEC H16.39-
    syphilitic (congenital) (late) A50.31
    tuberculous A18.52
  macular H16.11-
  nummular H16.11-
  oyster shuckers' H16.8
  parenchymatous —see Keratitis, interstitial
  petrificans H16.8
  postmeasles B05.81
  punctata
    leprosa A30.9 [H16.14-]
    syphilitic (profunda) A50.31
  punctate H16.14-
  purulent H16.8
  rosacea L71.8
  sclerosing H16.33-
  specified type NEC H16.8

Keratitis (continued)
  stellate H16.11-
  striate H16.11-
  superficial H16.10-
    with conjunctivitis —see Keratoconjunctivitis
    due to light —see Photokeratitis
  suppurative H16.8
  syphilitic (congenital) (prenatal) A50.31
  trachomatous A71.1
    sequelae B94.0
  tuberculous A18.52
  vesicular H16.8
  xerotic (see also Keratomlacia) H16.8
    vitamin A deficiency E50.4
Keratoacanthoma L85.8
Keratocele —see Descemetocele
Keratoconjunctivitis H16.20-
  Acanthamoeba B60.13
  adenoviral B30.0
  epidemic B30.0
  exposure H16.21-
  herpes, herpetic (simplex) B00.52
    zoster B02.33
  in exanthema (see also Exanthem) B09
  infectious B30.0
  lagophthalmic —see Keratoconjunctivitis, specified type NEC
  neurotrophic H16.23-
  phlyctenular H16.25-
  postmeasles B05.81
  shipyard B30.0
  sicca (Sjogren's) M35.0-
    not Sjogren's H16.22-
  specified type NEC H16.29-
  tuberculous (phlyctenular) A18.52
  vernal H16.26-
Keratoconus H18.60-
  congenital Q13.4
  stable H18.61-
  unstable H18.62-
Keratocyst (dental) (odontogenic) —see Cyst, calcifying odontogenic
Keratoderma, keratodermia (congenital) (palmaris et plantaris) (symmetrical) Q82.8
  acquired L85.1
    in diseases classified elsewhere L86
  climactericum L85.1
  gonococcal A54.89
  gonorrheal A54.89
  punctata L85.2
  Reiter's —see Reiter's disease
Keratodermatocele —see Descemetocele
Keratoglobus H18.79
  congenital Q15.8
    with glaucoma Q15.0
Keratohemia —see Pigmentation, cornea, stromal
Keratoiritis —see also Iridocyclitis
  syphilitic A50.39
  tuberculous A18.54
Keratoma L57.0
  palmaris and plantaris hereditarium Q82.8
  senile L57.0

Keratomalacia H18.44-
vitamin A deficiency E50.4
Keratomegaly Q13.4
Keratomycosis B49
nigrans, nigricans (palmaris) B36.1
Keratopathy H18.9
band H18.42-
bullous H18.1-
bullous (aphakic), following cataract surgery H59.01-
Keratoscleritis, tuberculous A18.52
Keratosis L57.0
actinic L57.0
arsenical L85.8
congenital, specified NEC Q80.8
female genital NEC N94.89
follicularis Q82.8
acquired L11.0
congenita Q82.8
et parafollicularis in cutem penetrans L87.0
spinulosa (decalvans) Q82.8
vitamin A deficiency E50.8
gonococcal A54.89
lichenoid L82.0
male genital (external) N50.89
nigricans L83
obturans, external ear (canal) —see Cholesteatoma, external ear
palmaris et plantaris (inherited) (symmetrical) Q82.8
acquired L85.1
penile N48.89
pharynx J39.2
pilaris, acquired L85.8
punctata (palmaris et plantaris) L85.2
scrotal N50.89
seborrheic L82.1
inflamed L82.0
senile L57.0
solar L57.0
tonsillaris J35.8
vagina N89.4
vegetans Q82.8
vitamin A deficiency E50.8
vocal cord J38.3
Kerato-uveitis —see Iridocyclitis
Kerunoparalysis T75.09
Kerion (celsi) B35.0
Kernicterus of newborn (not due to isoimmunization) P57.9
due to isoimmunization (conditions in P55.0-P55.9) P57.0
specified type NEC P57.8
Keshan disease E59
Ketoacidosis E87.29
diabetic —see Diabetes, by type, with ketoacidosis
Ketonuria R82.4
Ketosis NEC E88.89
diabetic —see Diabetes, by type, with ketoacidosis
Kew Garden fever A79.1
Kidney —see condition
Kienböck's disease —see also Osteochondrosis, juvenile, hand, carpal lunate
adult M93.1
Kimmelstiel (-Wilson) **disease** —see Diabetes, Kimmelstiel (-Wilson) disease

Kimura disease D21.9
specified site —see Neoplasm, connective tissue benign
Kink, kinking
artery I77.1
hair (acquired) L67.8
ileum or intestine —see Obstruction, intestine
Lane's —see Obstruction, intestine
organ or site, congenital NEC —see Anomaly, by site
ureter (pelvic junction) N13.5
with
hydronephrosis N13.1
with infection N13.6
pyelonephritis (chronic) N11.1
congenital Q62.39
vein(s) I87.8
caval I87.1
peripheral I87.1
Kinnier Wilson's disease (hepatolenticular degeneration) E83.01
Kissing spine M48.20
cervical region M48.22
cervicothoracic region M48.23
lumbar region M48.26
lumbosacral region M48.27
occipito-atlanto-axial region M48.21
thoracic region M48.24
thoracolumbar region M48.25
Klatskin's tumor C24.0
Klauder's disease A26.8
Klebs' disease (see also Glomerulonephritis) N05.-
Klebsiella (K.) **pneumoniae, as cause of disease classified elsewhere** B96.1
Kleeblattschaedel skull Q75.051
Klein (e)-**Levin syndrome** G47.13
Kleptomania F63.2
Klinefelter's syndrome Q98.4
karyotype 47,XXY Q98.0
male with more than two X chromosomes Q98.1
Klippel-Feil deficiency, disease, or syndrome (brevicollis) Q76.1
Klippel's disease I67.2
Klippel-Trenaunay (-Weber) **syndrome** Q87.2
Klumpke (-Déjerine) palsy, paralysis (birth) (newborn) P14.1
Knee —see condition
Knock knee (acquired) M21.06-
congenital Q74.1
Knot(s)
intestinal, syndrome (volvulus) K56.2
surfer S89.8-
umbilical cord (true) O69.2
Knotting (of)
hair L67.8
intestine K56.2
Knuckle pad (Garrod's) M72.1
Koch's
infection —see Tuberculosis
relapsing fever A68.9
Koch-Weeks' conjunctivitis —see Conjunctivitis, acute, mucopurulent
Köebner's syndrome Q81.8
Köenig's disease (osteochondritis dissecans) —see Osteochondritis, dissecans

Köhler-Pellegrini-Steida disease or syndrome (calcification, knee joint) —see Bursitis, tibial collateral
Köhler's disease
patellar —see Osteochondrosis, juvenile, patella
tarsal navicular —see Osteochondrosis, juvenile, tarsus
Koilonychia L60.3
congenital Q84.6
Kojevnikov's, epilepsy —see Kozhevnikof's epilepsy
Koplik's spots B05.9
Kopp's asthma E32.8
Korsakoff's (Wernicke) disease, psychosis or syndrome (alcoholic) F10.96
with dependence F10.26
drug-induced
due to drug abuse —see Abuse, drug, by type, with amnestic disorder
due to drug dependence —see Dependence, drug, by type, with amnestic disorder
nonalcoholic F04
Korsakov's disease, psychosis or syndrome —see Korsakoff's disease
Korsakow's disease, psychosis or syndrome —see Korsakoff's disease
Kostmann's disease or syndrome (infantile genetic agranulocytosis) —see Agranulocytosis
Kozhevnikof's epilepsy G40.109
intractable G40.119
with status epilepticus G40.111
without status epilepticus G40.119
not intractable G40.109
with status epilepticus G40.101
without status epilepticus G40.109
Krabbe's
disease E75.23
syndrome, congenital muscle hypoplasia Q79.8
Kraepelin-Morel disease —see Schizophrenia
Kraft-Weber-Dimitri disease Q85.89
Kraurosis
ani K62.89
penis N48.0
vagina N89.8
vulva N90.4
Kreotoxism A05.9
Krukenberg's
spindle —see Pigmentation, cornea, posterior
tumor C79.6-
Kufs' disease E75.4
Kugelberg-Welander disease G12.1
Kuhnt-Junius degeneration (see also Degeneration, macula) H35.32 -
Kümmell's disease or spondylitis —see Spondylopathy, traumatic
Kupffer cell sarcoma C22.3
Kuru A81.81

Kussmaul's
disease M30.0
respiration E87.29
in diabetic acidosis —see Diabetes, by type, with ketoacidosis
Kwashiorkor E40
marasmic, marasmus type E42
Kyasanur Forest disease A98.2
Kyphoscoliosis, kyphoscoliotic (acquired) (see also Scoliosis) M41.9
congenital Q67.5
heart (disease) I27.1
sequelae of rickets E64.3
tuberculous A18.01
Kyphosis, kyphotic (acquired) M40.209
cervical region M40.202
cervicothoracic region M40.203
congenital Q76.419
cervical region Q76.412
cervicothoracic region Q76.413
occipito-atlanto-axial region Q76.411
thoracic region Q76.414
thoracolumbar region Q76.415
Morquio-Brailsford type (spinal) (see also subcategory M49.8) E76.219
postlaminectomy M96.3
postradiation therapy M96.2
postural (adolescent) M40.00
cervicothoracic region M40.03
thoracic region M40.04
thoracolumbar region M40.05
secondary NEC M40.10
cervical region M40.12
cervicothoracic region M40.13
thoracic region M40.14
thoracolumbar region M40.15
sequelae of rickets E64.3
specified type NEC M40.299
cervical region M40.292
cervicothoracic region M40.293
thoracic region M40.294
thoracolumbar region M40.295
syphilitic, congenital A50.56
thoracic region M40.204
thoracolumbar region M40.205
tuberculous A18.01
Kyrle disease L87.0

L

Labia, labium —see condition
Labile
blood pressure R09.89
vasomotor system I73.9
Labioglossal paralysis G12.29
Labium leporinum —see Cleft, lip
Labor —see Delivery
Labored breathing —see Hyperventilation
Labyrinthitis (circumscribed) (destructive) (diffuse) (inner ear) (latent) (purulent) (suppurative) —see also subcategory H83.0
syphilitic A52.79
Laceration
with abortion —see Abortion, by type, complicated by laceration of pelvic organs
abdomen, abdominal

Laceration (*continued*)
  abdomen, abdominal (*continued*)
    wall S31.119
      with
        foreign body S31.129
          penetration into peritoneal
            cavity S31.619
              with foreign body
                S31.629
    epigastric region S31.112
      with
        foreign body S31.122
          penetration into
            peritoneal cavity
              S31.612
                with foreign body
                  S31.622
    left
      lower quadrant S31.114
        with
          foreign body S31.124
            penetration into
              peritoneal cavity
                S31.614
                  with foreign body
                    S31.624
      upper quadrant S31.111
        with
          foreign body S31.121
            penetration into
              peritoneal cavity
                S31.611
                  with foreign body
                    S31.621
    periumbilic region S31.115
      with
        foreign body S31.125
          penetration into
            peritoneal cavity
              S31.615
                with foreign body
                  S31.625
    right
      lower quadrant S31.113
        with
          foreign body S31.123
            penetration into
              peritoneal cavity
                S31.613
                  with foreign body
                    S31.623
      upper quadrant S31.110
        with
          foreign body S31.120
            penetration into
              peritoneal cavity
                S31.610
                  with foreign body
                    S31.620
  accidental, complicating
    surgery —*see* Complications,
      surgical, accidental puncture or
      laceration
  Achilles tendon S86.02-
  adrenal gland S37.813
  alveolar (process) —*see*
    Laceration, oral cavity
  ankle S91.01-
    with
      foreign body S91.02-
  antecubital space —*see* Laceration,
    elbow
  anus (sphincter) S31.831
    with
      ectopic or molar pregnancy
        O08.6
      foreign body S31.832
    complicating delivery —*see*
      Delivery, complicated,
      by, laceration, anus
      (sphincter)

Laceration (*continued*)
  anus (*continued*)
    following ectopic or molar
      pregnancy O08.6
    nontraumatic, nonpuerperal
      —*see* Fissure, anus
  arm (upper) S41.11-
    with foreign body S41.12-
    lower —*see* Laceration,
      forearm
  auditory canal (external) (meatus)
    —*see* Laceration, ear
  auricle, ear —*see* Laceration,
    ear
  axilla —*see* Laceration, arm
  back —*see also* Laceration, thorax,
    back
    lower S31.010
      with
        foreign body S31.020
          with penetration into
            retroperitoneal space
              S31.021
          penetration into
            retroperitoneal space
              S31.011
  bile duct S36.13
  bladder S37.23
    with ectopic or molar pregnancy
      O08.6
    following ectopic or molar
      pregnancy O08.6
    obstetrical trauma O71.5
  blood vessel —*see* Injury, blood
    vessel
  bowel —*see also* Laceration,
    intestine
    with ectopic or molar pregnancy
      O08.6
    complicating abortion
      —*see* Abortion, by type,
      complicated by, specified
      condition NEC
    following ectopic or molar
      pregnancy O08.6
    obstetrical trauma O71.5
  brain (any part) (cortex) (diffuse)
    (membrane) —*see also* Injury,
    intracranial, diffuse
    during birth P10.8
      with hemorrhage P10.1
    focal —*see* Injury, intracranial,
      focal brain injury
  brainstem S06.38-
  breast S21.01-
    with foreign body S21.02-
  broad ligament S37.893
    with ectopic or molar pregnancy
      O08.6
    following ectopic or molar
      pregnancy O08.6
    laceration syndrome N83.8
    obstetrical trauma O71.6
    syndrome (laceration) N83.8
  buttock S31.801
    with foreign body S31.802
    left S31.821
      with foreign body S31.822
    right S31.811
      with foreign body S31.812
  calf —*see* Laceration, leg
  canaliculus lacrimalis —*see*
    Laceration, eyelid
  canthus, eye —*see* Laceration,
    eyelid
  capsule, joint —*see* Sprain
  causing eversion of cervix uteri
    (old) N86
  central (perineal), complicating
    delivery O70.9
  cerebellum, traumatic S06.37-

Laceration (*continued*)
  cerebral S06.33-
    left side S06.32-
      during birth P10.8
        with hemorrhage P10.1
      right side S06.31-
  cervix (uteri)
    with ectopic or molar pregnancy
      O08.6
    following ectopic or molar
      pregnancy O08.6
    nonpuerperal, nontraumatic N88.1
    obstetrical trauma (current) O71.3
    old (postpartal) N88.1
    traumatic S37.63
  cheek (external) S01.41-
    with foreign body S01.42-
    internal —*see* Laceration, oral
      cavity
  chest wall —*see* Laceration, thorax
  chin —*see* Laceration, head,
    specified site NEC
  chordae tendinae NEC I51.1
    concurrent with acute
      myocardial infarction —*see*
      Infarct, myocardium
    following acute myocardial
      infarction (current
      complication) I23.4
  clitoris —*see* Laceration, vulva
  colon —*see* Laceration, intestine,
    large, colon
  common bile duct S36.13
  cortex (cerebral) —*see* Injury,
    intracranial, diffuse
  costal region —*see* Laceration,
    thorax
  cystic duct S36.13
  diaphragm S27.803
  digit(s)
    hand —*see* Laceration, finger
    foot —*see* Laceration, toe
  duodenum S36.430
  ear (canal) (external) S01.31-
    with foreign body S01.32-
    drum S09.2-
  elbow S51.01-
    with
      foreign body S51.02-
  epididymis —*see* Laceration, testis
  epigastric region —*see* Laceration,
    abdomen, wall, epigastric region
  esophagus K22.89
    traumatic
      cervical S11.21
        with foreign body S11.22
      thoracic S27.813
  eye (ball) S05.3-
    with prolapse or loss of
      intraocular tissue S05.2-
    penetrating S05.6-
  eyebrow —*see* Laceration, eyelid
  eyelid S01.11-
    with foreign body S01.12-
  face NEC —*see* Laceration, head,
    specified site NEC
  fallopian tube S37.539
    bilateral S37.532
    unilateral S37.531
  finger(s) S61.219
    with
      damage to nail S61.319
        with
          foreign body S61.329
      foreign body S61.229
    index S61.218
      with
        damage to nail S61.318
          with
            foreign body S61.328
          foreign body S61.228

Laceration (*continued*)
  finger(s) (*continued*)
    index (*continued*)
      left S61.211
        with
          damage to nail S61.311
            with
              foreign body
                S61.321
          foreign body S61.221
      right S61.210
        with
          damage to nail S61.310
            with
              foreign body
                S61.320
          foreign body S61.220
    little S61.218
      with
        damage to nail S61.318
          with
            foreign body S61.328
        foreign body S61.228
      left S61.217
        with
          damage to nail S61.317
            with
              foreign body
                S61.327
          foreign body S61.227
      right S61.216
        with
          damage to nail S61.316
            with
              foreign body
                S61.326
          foreign body S61.226
    middle S61.218
      with
        damage to nail S61.318
          with
            foreign body S61.328
        foreign body S61.228
      left S61.213
        with
          damage to nail S61.313
            with
              foreign body
                S61.323
          foreign body S61.223
      right S61.212
        with
          damage to nail S61.312
            with
              foreign body
                S61.322
          foreign body S61.222
    ring S61.218
      with
        damage to nail S61.318
          with
            foreign body S61.328
        foreign body S61.228
      left S61.215
        with
          damage to nail S61.315
            with
              foreign body
                S61.325
          foreign body S61.225
      right S61.214
        with
          damage to nail S61.314
            with
              foreign body
                S61.324
          foreign body S61.224
  flank S31.119
    with foreign body S31.129
  foot (except toe(s) alone) S91.319
    with foreign body S91.329

Laceration (*continued*)
  foot (*continued*)
    left S91.312
      with foreign body S91.322
    right S91.311
      with foreign body S91.321
    toe —*see* Laceration, toe
  forearm S51.819
    with
      foreign body S51.829
    elbow only —*see* Laceration, elbow
    left S51.812
      with
        foreign body S51.822
    right S51.811
      with
        foreign body S51.821
  forehead S01.81
    with foreign body S01.82
  fourchette O70.0
    with ectopic or molar pregnancy O08.6
    complicating delivery O70.0
    following ectopic or molar pregnancy O08.6
  gallbladder S36.123
  genital organs, external
    female S31.512
      with foreign body S31.522
      vagina —*see* Laceration, vagina
      vulva —*see* Laceration, vulva
    male S31.511
      with foreign body S31.521
      penis —*see* Laceration, penis
      scrotum —*see* Laceration, scrotum
      testis —*see* Laceration, testis
  groin —*see* Laceration, abdomen, wall
  gum —*see* Laceration, oral cavity
  hand S61.419
    with
      foreign body S61.429
    finger —*see* Laceration, finger
    left S61.412
      with
        foreign body S61.422
    right S61.411
      with
        foreign body S61.421
    thumb —*see* Laceration, thumb
  head S01.91
    with foreign body S01.92
    cheek —*see* Laceration, cheek
    ear —*see* Laceration, ear
    eyelid —*see* Laceration, eyelid
    lip —*see* Laceration, lip
    nose —*see* Laceration, nose
    oral cavity —*see* Laceration, oral cavity
    scalp S01.01
      with foreign body S01.02
    specified site NEC S01.81
      with foreign body S01.82
    temporomandibular area —*see* Laceration, cheek
  heart —*see* Injury, heart, laceration
  heel —*see* Laceration, foot
  hepatic duct S36.13
  hip S71.019
    with foreign body S71.029
    left S71.012
      with foreign body S71.022
    right S71.011
      with foreign body S71.021
  hymen —*see* Laceration, vagina

Laceration (*continued*)
  hypochondrium —*see* Laceration, abdomen, wall
  hypogastric region —*see* Laceration, abdomen, wall
  ileum S36.438
  inguinal region —*see* Laceration, abdomen, wall
  instep —*see* Laceration, foot
  internal organ —*see* Injury, by site
  interscapular region —*see* Laceration, thorax, back
  intestine
    large
      colon S36.539
        ascending S36.530
        descending S36.532
        sigmoid S36.533
        specified site NEC S36.538
      rectum S36.63
        transverse S36.531
    small S36.439
      duodenum S36.430
      specified site NEC S36.438
  intra-abdominal organ S36.93
    intestine —*see* Laceration, intestine
    liver —*see* Laceration, liver
    pancreas —*see* Laceration, pancreas
    peritoneum S36.81
    specified site NEC S36.893
    spleen —*see* Laceration, spleen
    stomach —*see* Laceration, stomach
  intracranial NEC —*see also* Injury, intracranial, diffuse
    birth injury P10.9
  jaw —*see* Laceration, head, specified site NEC
  jejunum S36.438
  joint capsule —*see* Sprain, by site
  kidney S37.03-
    major (greater than 3 cm) (massive) (stellate) S37.06-
    minor (less than 1 cm) S37.04-
    moderate (1 to 3 cm) S37.05-
    multiple S37.06-
  knee S81.01-
    with foreign body S81.02-
  labium (majus) (minus) —*see* Laceration, vulva
  lacrimal duct —*see* Laceration, eyelid
  large intestine —*see* Laceration, intestine, large
  larynx S11.011
    with foreign body S11.012
  leg (lower) S81.819
    with foreign body S81.829
    foot —*see* Laceration, foot
    knee —*see* Laceration, knee
    left S81.812
      with foreign body S81.822
    right S81.811
      with foreign body S81.821
    upper —*see* Laceration, thigh
  ligament —*see* Sprain
  lip S01.511
    with foreign body S01.521
  liver S36.113
    major (stellate) S36.116
    minor S36.114
    moderate S36.115
  loin —*see* Laceration, abdomen, wall
  lower back —*see* Laceration, back, lower
  lumbar region —*see* Laceration, back, lower

Laceration (*continued*)
  lung S27.339
    bilateral S27.332
    unilateral S27.331
  malar region —*see* Laceration, head, specified site NEC
  mammary —*see* Laceration, breast
  mastoid region —*see* Laceration, head, specified site NEC
  meninges —*see* Injury, intracranial, diffuse
  meniscus —*see* Tear, meniscus
  mesentery S36.893
  mesosalpinx S37.893
  mouth —*see* Laceration, oral cavity
  muscle —*see* Injury, muscle, by site, laceration
  nail
    finger —*see* Laceration, finger, with damage to nail
    toe —*see* Laceration, toe, with damage to nail
  nasal (septum) (sinus) —*see* Laceration, nose
  nasopharynx —*see* Laceration, head, specified site NEC
  neck S11.91
    with foreign body S11.92
    involving
      cervical esophagus S11.21
        with foreign body S11.22
      larynx —*see* Laceration, larynx
      pharynx —*see* Laceration, pharynx
      thyroid gland —*see* Laceration, thyroid gland
      trachea —*see* Laceration, trachea
    specified site NEC S11.81
      with foreign body S11.82
  nerve —*see* Injury, nerve
  nose (septum) (sinus) S01.21
    with foreign body S01.22
  ocular NOS S05.3-
    adnexa NOS S01.11-
  oral cavity S01.512
    with foreign body S01.522
  orbit (eye) —*see* Wound, open, ocular, orbit
  ovary S37.439
    bilateral S37.432
    unilateral S37.431
  palate —*see* Laceration, oral cavity
  palm —*see* Laceration, hand
  pancreas S36.239
    body S36.231
      major S36.261
      minor S36.241
      moderate S36.251
    head S36.230
      major S36.260
      minor S36.240
      moderate S36.250
    major S36.269
    minor S36.249
    moderate S36.259
    tail S36.232
      major S36.262
      minor S36.242
      moderate S36.252
  pelvic S31.010
    with
      foreign body S31.020
      penetration into retroperitoneal cavity S31.021
    penetration into retroperitoneal cavity S31.011
    floor —*see also* Laceration, back, lower

Laceration (*continued*)
  pelvic (*continued*)
    floor (*continued*)
      with ectopic or molar pregnancy O08.6
      complicating delivery O70.1
      following ectopic or molar pregnancy O08.6
      old (postpartal) N81.89
    organ S37.93
      with ectopic or molar pregnancy O08.6
      adrenal gland S37.813
      bladder S37.23
      fallopian tube —*see* Laceration, fallopian tube
      following ectopic or molar pregnancy O08.6
      kidney —*see* Laceration, kidney
      obstetrical trauma O71.5
      ovary —*see* Laceration, ovary
      prostate S37.823
      specified site NEC S37.893
      ureter S37.13
      urethra S37.33
      uterus S37.63
  penis S31.21
    with foreign body S31.22
  perineum
    female S31.41
      with
        ectopic or molar pregnancy O08.6
        foreign body S31.42
      during delivery O70.9
        first degree O70.0
        fourth degree O70.3
        second degree O70.1
        third degree (*see also* Delivery, complicated, by, laceraton, perineum, third degree) O70.20
      old (postpartal) N81.89
      postpartal N81.89
      secondary (postpartal) O90.1
    male S31.119
      with foreign body S31.129
  periocular area (with or without lacrimal passages) —*see* Laceration, eyelid
  peritoneum S36.893
  periumbilic region —*see* Laceration, abdomen, wall, periumbilic
  periurethral tissue —*see* Laceration, urethra
  phalanges
    finger —*see* Laceration, finger
    toe —*see* Laceration, toe
  pharynx S11.21
    with foreign body S11.22
  pinna —*see* Laceration, ear
  popliteal space —*see* Laceration, knee
  prepuce —*see* Laceration, penis
  prostate S37.823
  pubic region S31.119
    with foreign body S31.129
  pudendum —*see* Laceration, genital organs, external
  rectovaginal septum —*see* Laceration, vagina
  rectum S36.63
  retroperitoneum S36.893
  round ligament S37.893
  sacral region —*see* Laceration, back, lower
  sacroiliac region —*see* Laceration, back, lower

Laceration (*continued*)
  salivary gland —*see* Laceration, oral cavity
  scalp S01.01
    with foreign body S01.02
  scapular region —*see* Laceration, shoulder
  scrotum S31.31
    with foreign body S31.32
  seminal vesicle S37.893
  shin —*see* Laceration, leg
  shoulder S41.019
    with foreign body S41.029
    left S41.012
      with foreign body S41.022
    right S41.011
      with foreign body S41.021
  small intestine —*see* Laceration, intestine, small
  spermatic cord —*see* Laceration, testis
  spinal cord (meninges) —*see also* Injury, spinal cord, by region
    due to injury at birth P11.5
    newborn (birth injury) P11.5
  spleen S36.039
    major (massive) (stellate) S36.032
    moderate S36.031
    superficial (minor) S36.030
  sternal region —*see* Laceration, thorax, front
  stomach S36.33
  submaxillary region —*see* Laceration, head, specified site NEC
  submental region —*see* Laceration, head, specified site NEC
  subungual
    finger(s) —*see* Laceration, finger, with damage to nail
    toe(s) —*see* Laceration, toe, with damage to nail
  suprarenal gland —*see* Laceration, adrenal gland
  temple, temporal region —*see* Laceration, head, specified site NEC
  temporomandibular area —*see* Laceration, cheek
  tendon —*see* Injury, muscle, by site, laceration
    Achilles S86.02-
  tentorium cerebelli —*see* Injury, intracranial, diffuse
  testis S31.31
    with foreign body S31.32
  thigh S71.11-
    with foreign body S71.12-
  thorax, thoracic (wall) S21.91
    with foreign body S21.92
      back S21.22-
        with penetration into thoracic cavity S21.42-
      front S21.12-
        with penetration into thoracic cavity S21.32-
    back S21.21-
      with
        foreign body S21.22-
          with penetration into thoracic cavity S21.42-
        penetration into thoracic cavity S21.41-
    breast —*see* Laceration, breast
    front S21.11-
      with
        foreign body S21.12-
          with penetration into thoracic cavity S21.32-
        penetration into thoracic cavity S21.31-

Laceration (*continued*)
  thumb S61.019
    with
      damage to nail S61.119
        with
          foreign body S61.129
      foreign body S61.029
    left S61.012
      with
        damage to nail S61.112
          with
            foreign body S61.122
        foreign body S61.022
    right S61.011
      with
        damage to nail S61.111
          with
            foreign body S61.121
        foreign body S61.021
  thyroid gland S11.11
    with foreign body S11.12
  toe(s) S91.119
    with
      damage to nail S91.219
        with
          foreign body S91.229
      foreign body S91.129
    great S91.113
      with
        damage to nail S91.213
          with
            foreign body S91.223
        foreign body S91.123
      left S91.112
        with
          damage to nail S91.212
            with
              foreign body S91.222
          foreign body S91.122
      right S91.111
        with
          damage to nail S91.211
            with
              foreign body S91.221
          foreign body S91.121
    lesser S91.116
      with
        damage to nail S91.216
          with
            foreign body S91.226
        foreign body S91.126
      left S91.115
        with
          damage to nail S91.215
            with
              foreign body S91.225
          foreign body S91.125
      right S91.114
        with
          damage to nail S91.214
            with
              foreign body S91.224
          foreign body S91.124
  tongue —*see* Laceration, oral cavity
  trachea S11.021
    with foreign body S11.022
  tunica vaginalis —*see* Laceration, testis
  tympanum, tympanic membrane —*see* Laceration, ear, drum
  umbilical region S31.115
    with foreign body S31.125
  ureter S37.13
  urethra S37.33
    with or following ectopic or molar pregnancy O08.6
    obstetrical trauma O71.5
  urinary organ NEC S37.893
  uterus S37.63
    with ectopic or molar pregnancy O08.6

Laceration (*continued*)
  uterus (*continued*)
    following ectopic or molar pregnancy O08.6
    nonpuerperal, nontraumatic N85.8
    obstetrical trauma NEC O71.81
    old (postpartal) N85.8
  uvula —*see* Laceration, oral cavity
  vagina S31.41
    with
      ectopic or molar pregnancy O08.6
      foreign body S31.42
    during delivery O71.4
      with perineal laceration —*see* Laceration, perineum, female, during delivery
    following ectopic or molar pregnancy O08.6
    nonpuerperal, nontraumatic N89.8
    old (postpartal) N89.8
  vas deferens S37.893
  vesical —*see* Laceration, bladder
  vocal cords S11.031
    with foreign body S11.032
  vulva S31.41
    with
      ectopic or molar pregnancy O08.6
      foreign body S31.42
    complicating delivery O70.0
    following ectopic or molar pregnancy O08.6
    nonpuerperal, nontraumatic N90.89
    old (postpartal) N90.89
  wrist S61.519
    with
      foreign body S61.529
    left S61.512
      with
        foreign body S61.522
    right S61.511
      with
        foreign body S61.521

Lack of
  achievement in school Z55.3
  adequate
    food Z59.48
    intermaxillary vertical dimension of fully erupted teeth M26.36
    sleep Z72.820
  air conditioning Z59.11
  appetite (*see* Anorexia) R63.0
  awareness R41.9
  basic services in physical environment Z58.81
  care
    in home Z74.2
    of infant (at or after birth) T76.02
      confirmed T74.02
  cognitive functions R41.9
  coordination R27.9
    ataxia R27.0
    specified type NEC R27.8
  development (physiological) R62.50
    failure to thrive (child over 28 days old) R62.51
      adult R62.7
      newborn P92.6
    short stature R62.52
    specified type NEC R62.59
  electricity services Z59.12
  emotional support Z60.8
  energy R53.83
  financial resources Z59.6
  food Z59.48

Lack of (*continued*)
  gas services Z59.12
  growth R62.52
  heating Z59.11
  housing (permanent) (temporary) Z59.00
    adequate Z59.10
  learning experiences in childhood Z62.898
  leisure time (affecting life-style) Z73.2
  material resources, due to limited financial resources, specified NEC Z59.87
  memory —*see also* Amnesia
    mild, following organic brain damage F06.8
  oil service Z59.12
  ovulation N97.0
  parental supervision or control of child Z62.0
  person able to render necessary care Z74.2
  physical exercise Z72.3
  play experience in childhood Z62.898
  posterior occlusal support M26.57
  relaxation (affecting life-style) Z73.2
  safe drinking water Z58.6
  sexual
    desire F52.0
    enjoyment F52.1
  shelter Z59.02
  sleep (adequate) Z72.820
  supervision of child by parent Z62.0
  support, posterior occlusal M26.57
  transportation Z59.82
  water T73.1
    safe drinking Z58.6
    services Z59.12

Lacrimal —*see* condition

Lacrimation, abnormal —*see* Epiphora

Lacrimonasal duct —*see* condition

Lactate, elevated —*see* Acidosis, lactic

Lactation, lactating (breast) (puerperal, postpartum)
  associated
    cracked nipple O92.13
    retracted nipple O92.03
  defective O92.4
  disorder NEC O92.79
  excessive O92.6
  failed (complete) O92.3
    partial O92.4
  mastitis NEC —*see* Mastitis, obstetric
  mother (care and/or examination) Z39.1
  nonpuerperal N64.3

Lacticemia, excessive (*see also* Acidosis) E87.20

Lacunar skull Q75.8

Laennec's cirrhosis K70.30
  with ascites K70.31
  nonalcoholic K74.69

Lafora disease (*see also* Epilepsy, progressive, Lafora) G40.C09

Lag, lid (nervous) —*see* Retraction, lid

Lagophthalmos (eyelid) (nervous) H02.209
  bilateral, upper and lower eyelids H02.20C
  cicatricial H02.219
    bilateral, upper and lower eyelids H02.21C
    left H02.216
      lower H02.215
      upper H02.214
      upper and lower eyelids H02.21B

Lagophthalmos (continued)
  cicatricial (continued)
    right H02.213
      lower H02.212
      upper H02.211
      upper and lower eyelids H02.21A
    keratoconjunctivitis —see Keratoconjunctivitis
    left H02.206
      lower H02.205
      upper H02.204
      upper and lower eyelids H02.20B
  mechanical H02.229
    bilateral, upper and lower eyelids H02.22C
    left H02.226
      lower H02.225
      upper H02.224
      upper and lower eyelids H02.22B
    right H02.223
      lower H02.222
      upper H02.221
      upper and lower eyelids H02.22A
  paralytic H02.239
    bilateral, upper and lower eyelids H02.23C
    left H02.236
      lower H02.235
      upper H02.234
      upper and lower eyelids H02.23B
    right H02.233
      lower H02.232
      upper H02.231
      upper and lower eyelids H02.23A
    right H02.203
      lower H02.202
      upper H02.201
      upper and lower eyelids H02.20A

Laki-Lorand factor deficiency —see Defect, coagulation, specified type NEC

Lalling F80.0

Lambert-Eaton syndrome —see Syndrome, Lambert-Eaton

Lambliasis, lambliosis A07.1

Landau-Kleffner syndrome —see Epilepsy, specified NEC

Landouzy-Déjérine dystrophy or facioscapulohumeral atrophy G71.02

Landouzy's disease (icterohemorrhagic leptospirosis) A27.0

Landry-Guillain-Barré, syndrome or paralysis G61.0

Landry's disease or paralysis G61.0

Lane's
  band Q43.3
  kink —see Obstruction, intestine
  syndrome K90.2

Langdon Down syndrome —see Trisomy, 21

Lapsed immunization schedule status Z28.39

Large
  baby (regardless of gestational age) (4000g to 4499g) P08.1
  ear, congenital Q17.1
  physiological cup Q14.2
  stature R68.89

Large-for-dates NEC (infant) (4000g to 4499g) P08.1
  affecting management of pregnancy O36.6-
  exceptionally (4500g or more) P08.0

Larsen-Johansson disease orosteochondrosis —see Osteochondrosis, juvenile, patella

Larsen's syndrome (flattened facies and multiple congenital dislocations) Q74.8

Larva migrans
  cutaneous B76.9
    Ancylostoma B76.0
  visceral B83.0

Laryngeal —see condition

Laryngismus (stridulus) J38.5
  congenital P28.89
  diphtheritic A36.2

Laryngitis (acute) (edematous) (fibrinous) (infective) (infiltrative) (malignant) (membranous) (phlegmonous) (pneumococcal) (pseudomembranous) (septic) (subglottic) (suppurative) (ulcerative) J04.0
  with
    influenza, flu, or grippe —see Influenza, with, laryngitis
    tracheitis (acute) —see Laryngotracheitis
  atrophic J37.0
  catarrhal J37.0
  chronic J37.0
    with tracheitis (chronic) J37.1
  diphtheritic A36.2
  due to external agent —see Inflammation, respiratory, upper, due to
  Hemophilus influenzae J04.0
  H. influenzae J04.0
  hypertrophic J37.0
  influenzal —see Influenza, with, respiratory manifestations NEC
  obstructive J05.0
  sicca J37.0
  spasmodic J05.0
    acute J04.0
  streptococcal J04.0
  stridulous J05.0
  syphilitic (late) A52.73
    congenital A50.59 [J99]
      early A50.03 [J99]
  tuberculous A15.5
  Vincent's A69.1

Laryngocele (congenital) (ventricular) Q31.3

Laryngofissure J38.7
  congenital Q31.8

Laryngomalacia (congenital) Q31.5

Laryngopharyngitis (acute) J06.0
  chronic J37.0
  due to external agent —see Inflammation, respiratory, upper, due to

Laryngoplegia J38.00
  bilateral J38.02
  unilateral J38.01

Laryngoptosis J38.7

Laryngospasm J38.5

Laryngostenosis J38.6

Laryngotracheitis (acute) (Infectional) (infective) (viral) J04.2
  atrophic J37.1
  catarrhal J37.1

  chronic J37.1
  diphtheritic A36.2
  due to external agent —see Inflammation, respiratory, upper, due to
  Hemophilus influenzae J04.2
  hypertrophic J37.1
  influenzal —see Influenza, with, respiratory manifestations NEC
  pachydermic J38.7
  sicca J37.1
  spasmodic J38.5
    acute J05.0
  streptococcal J04.2
  stridulous J38.5
  syphilitic (late) A52.73
    congenital A50.59 [J99]
      early A50.03 [J99]
  tuberculous A15.5
  Vincent's A69.1

Laryngotracheobronchitis —see Bronchitis

Larynx, laryngeal —see condition

Lassa fever A96.2

Lassitude —see Weakness

Late
  talker R62.0
  walker R62.0

Late effect(s) —see Sequelae

Latent —see condition

LTBI (latent tuberculosis infection) Z22.7

Laterocession —see Lateroversion

Lateroflexion —see Lateroversion

Lateroversion
  cervix —see Lateroversion, uterus
  uterus, uterine (cervix) (postinfectional) (postpartal, old) N85.4
    congenital Q51.818
    in pregnancy or childbirth O34.59-

Lathyrism —see Poisoning, food, noxious, plant

Launois' syndrome (pituitary gigantism) E22.0

Launois-Bensaude adenolipomatosis E88.89

Laurence-Moon syndrome Q87.84

Lax, laxity —see also Relaxation
  ligament (ous) —see also Disorder, ligament
    familial M35.7
    knee —see Derangement, knee
  skin (acquired) L57.4
    congenital Q82.8

Laxative habit F55.2

Lazy leukocyte syndrome D70.8

Lead miner's lung J63.6

Leak, leakage
  air NEC J93.82
    postprocedural J95.812
  amniotic fluid —see Rupture, membranes, premature
  blood (microscopic), fetal, into maternal circulation affecting management of pregnancy —see Pregnancy, complicated by
  cerebrospinal fluid G96.00
    cranial
      postoperative G96.08
      specified NEC G96.08

Leak, leakage (continued)
  cerebrospinal fluid (continued)
    cranial (continued)
      spontaneous G96.01
      traumatic G96.08
    from spinal (lumbar) puncture G97.0
    spinal
      postoperative G96.09
      post-traumatic G96.09
      specified NEC G96.09
      spontaneous G96.02
    spontaneous
      from
        skull base G96.01
        spine G96.02
  CSF —see Leak, cerebrospinal fluid
  device, implant or graft —see also Complications, by site and type, mechanical
    arterial graft NEC —see Complication, vascular, graft, mechanical, leakage T82.838
    breast (implant) T85.43
    catheter NEC T85.638
      urinary T83.038
        cystostomy T83.030
        Hopkins T83.038
        ileostomy T83.038
        indwelling T83.031
        nephrostomy T83.032
        specified NEC T83.038
        urostomy T83.038
    dialysis (renal) T82.43
      intraperitoneal T85.631
    infusion NEC T82.534
      spinal (epidural) (subdural) T85.630
    gastrointestinal —see Complications, prosthetic device, mechanical, gastrointestinal device
    genital NEC T83.498
      penile prosthesis (cylinder) (implanted) (pump) (resevoir) T83.490
      testicular prosthesis T83.491
    heart NEC —see Complication, cardiovascular device, mechanical
    joint prosthesis —see Complications, joint prosthesis, mechanical, specified NEC, by site
    ocular NEC —see Complications, prosthetic device, mechanical, ocular device
    orthopedic NEC —see Complication, orthopedic, device, mechanical
    persistent air J93.82
    specified NEC T85.638
    urinary NEC —see also Complication, genitourinary, device, urinary, mechanical graft T83.23
    vascular NEC —see Complication, cardiovascular device, mechanical
    ventricular intracranial shunt T85.03
  urine —see Incontinence

Leaky heart —see Endocarditis

Learning defect (specific) F81.9

Leather bottle stomach C16.9

Leber's
  congenital amaurosis H35.50
  optic atrophy (hereditary) H47.22

Lederer's anemia D59.19
Leeches (external) —see Hirudiniasis
Leg —see condition
Legg (-Calvé)-Perthes disease, syndrome or osteochondrosis M91.1-
Legionellosis A48.1
  nonpneumonic A48.2
Legionnaires'
  disease A48.1
    nonpneumonic A48.2
  pneumonia A48.1
Leigh's disease G31.82
Leiner's disease L21.1
Leiofibromyoma —see Leiomyoma
Leiomyoblastoma —see Neoplasm, connective tissue, benign
Leiomyofibroma —see also Neoplasm, connective tissue, benign
  uterus (cervix) (corpus) D25.9
Leiomyoma —see also Neoplasm, connective tissue, benign
  bizarre —see Neoplasm, connective tissue, benign
  cellular —see Neoplasm, connective tissue, benign
  epithelioid —see Neoplasm, connective tissue, benign
  uterus (cervix) (corpus) D25.9
    intramural D25.1
    submucous D25.0
    subserosal D25.2
  vascular —see Neoplasm, connective tissue, benign
Leiomyoma, leiomyomatosis (intravascular) —see Neoplasm, connective tissue, uncertain behavior
Leiomyosarcoma —see also Neoplasm, connective tissue, malignant
  epithelioid —see Neoplasm, connective tissue, malignant
  myxoid —see Neoplasm, connective tissue, malignant
Leishmaniasis B55.9
  American (mucocutaneous) B55.2
    cutaneous B55.1
  Asian Desert B55.1
  Brazilian B55.2
  cutaneous (any type) B55.1
  dermal —see also Leishmaniasis, cutaneous
    post-kala-azar B55.0
  eyelid B55.1
  infantile B55.0
  Mediterranean B55.0
  mucocutaneous (American) (New World) B55.2
  naso-oral B55.2
  nasopharyngeal B55.2
  old world B55.1
  tegumentaria diffusa B55.1
  visceral B55.0
Leishmanoid, dermal —see also Leishmaniasis, cutaneous
  post-kala-azar B55.0
Lenegre's disease I44.2
Lengthening, leg —see Deformity, limb, unequal length
Lennert's lymphoma —see Lymphoma, Lennert's

Lennox-Gastaut syndrome G40.812
  intractable G40.814
    with status epilepticus G40.813
    without status epilepticus G40.814
  not intractable G40.812
    with status epilepticus G40.811
    without status epilepticus G40.812
Lens —see condition
Lenticonus (anterior) (posterior) (congenital) Q12.8
Lenticular degeneration, progressive E83.01
Lentiglobus (posterior) (congenital) Q12.8
Lentigo (congenital) L81.4
  maligna —see also Melanoma, in situ
    melanoma —see Melanoma
Lentivirus, as cause of disease classified elsewhere B97.31
Leontiasis
  ossium M85.2
  syphilitic (late) A52.78
    congenital A50.59
Lepothrix A48.8
Lepra —see Leprosy
Leprechaunism E34.8
Leprosy A30.-
  with muscle disorder A30.9 [M63.80]
    ankle A30.9 [M63.87-]
    foot A30.9 [M63.87-]
    forearm A30.9 [M63.83-]
    hand A30.9 [M63.84-]
    lower leg A30.9 [M63.86-]
    multiple sites A30.9 [M63.89]
    pelvic region A30.9 [M63.85-]
    shoulder region A30.9 [M63.81-]
    specified site NEC A30.9 [M63.88]
    thigh A30.9 [M63.85-]
    upper arm A30.9 [M63.82-]
  anesthetic A30.9
  BB A30.3
  BL A30.4
  borderline (infiltrated) (neuritic) A30.3
    lepromatous A30.4
    tuberculoid A30.2
  BT A30.2
  dimorphous (infiltrated) (neuritic) A30.3
  I A30.0
  indeterminate (macular) (neuritic) A30.0
  lepromatous (diffuse) (infiltrated) (macular) (neuritic) (nodular) A30.5
  LL A30.5
  macular (early) (neuritic) (simple) A30.9
  maculoanesthetic A30.9
  mixed A30.3
  neural A30.9
  nodular A30.5
  primary neuritic A30.3
  specified type NEC A30.8
  TT A30.1
  tuberculoid (major) (minor) A30.1
Leptocytosis, hereditary D56.9
Leptomeningitis (chronic) (circumscribed) (hemorrhagic) (nonsuppurative) —see Meningitis
Leptomeningopathy G96.198

Leptospiral —see condition
Leptospirochetal —see condition
Leptospirosis A27.9
  canicola A27.89
  due to Leptospira interrogans serovar icterohaemorrhagiae A27.0
  icterohemorrhagica A27.0
  pomona A27.89
  Weil's disease A27.0
Leptus dermatitis B88.0
Leriche's syndrome (aortic bifurcation occlusion) I74.09
Leri's pleonosteosis Q78.8
Leri-Weill syndrome Q77.8
Lermoyez' syndrome —see Vertigo, peripheral NEC
Lesch-Nyhan syndrome E79.1
Leser-Trélat disease L82.1
  inflamed L82.0
Lesion(s) (nontraumatic)
  abducens nerve —see Strabismus, paralytic, sixth nerve
  alveolar process K08.9
  angiocentric immunoproliferative D47.Z9
  anorectal K62.9
  aortic (valve) I35.9
  auditory nerve —see subcategory H93.3
  basal ganglion G25.9
  bile duct —see Disease, bile duct
  biomechanical M99.9
    specified type NEC M99.89
      abdomen M99.89
      acromioclavicular M99.87
      cervical region M99.81
      cervicothoracic M99.81
      costochondral M99.88
      costovertebral M99.88
      head region M99.80
      hip M99.85
      lower extremity M99.86
      lumbar region M99.83
      lumbosacral M99.83
      occipitocervical M99.80
      pelvic region M99.85
      pubic M99.85
      rib cage M99.88
      sacral region M99.84
      sacrococcygeal M99.84
      sacroiliac M99.84
      specified NEC M99.89
      sternochondral M99.88
      sternoclavicular M99.87
      thoracic region M99.82
      thoracolumbar M99.82
      upper extremity M99.87
  bladder N32.9
  bone —see Disorder, bone
  brachial plexus G54.0
  brain G93.9
    congenital Q04.9
    vascular I67.9
      degenerative I67.9
      hypertensive I67.4
  buccal cavity K13.79
  calcified —see Calcification
  cameron —see Ulcer, stomach
  canthus —see Disorder, eyelid
  carate —see Pinta, lesions
  cardia K31.9
  cardiac (see also Disease, heart) I51.9
    congenital Q24.9
    valvular —see Endocarditis
  cauda equina G83.4
  cecum K63.9
  cerebral —see Lesion, brain

Lesion (continued)
  cerebrovascular I67.9
    degenerative I67.9
    hypertensive I67.4
  cervical (nerve) root NEC G54.2
  chiasmal —see Disorder, optic, chiasm
  chorda tympani G51.8
  coin, lung R91.1
  colon K63.9
  combined periodontic - endodontic K05.5
  congenital —see Anomaly, by site
  conjunctiva H11.9
  conus medullaris —see Injury, conus medullaris
  coronary artery —see Ischemia, heart
  cranial nerve G52.9
    eighth —see Disorder, ear
    eleventh G52.9
    fifth G50.9
    first G52.0
    fourth —see Strabismus, paralytic, fourth nerve
    seventh G51.9
    sixth —see Strabismus, paralytic, sixth nerve
    tenth G52.2
    twelfth G52.3
  cystic —see Cyst
  degenerative —see Degeneration
  duodenum K31.9
  edentulous (alveolar) ridge, associated with trauma, due to traumatic occlusion K06.2
  en coup de sabre L94.1
  eyelid —see Disorder, eyelid
  gasserian ganglion G50.8
  gastric K31.9
  gastroduodenal K31.9
  gastrointestinal K63.9
  gingiva, associated with trauma K06.2
  glomerular
    focal and segmental (see also N00-N07 with fourth character .1) N05.1
    minimal change (see also N00-N07 with fourth character .0) N05.0
  heart (organic) —see Disease, heart
  hyperchromic, due to pinta (carate) A67.1
  hyperkeratotic —see Hyperkeratosis
  hypothalamic E23.7
  ileocecal K63.9
  ileum K63.9
  iliohypogastric nerve G57.8-
  inflammatory —see Inflammation
  intestine K63.9
  intracerebral —see Lesion, brain
  intrachiasmal (optic) —see Disorder, optic, chiasm
  intracranial, space-occupying R90.0
  joint —see Disorder, joint
    sacroiliac (old) M53.3
  keratotic —see Keratosis
  kidney —see Disease, renal
  laryngeal nerve (recurrent) G52.2
  lip K13.0
  liver K76.9
  lumbosacral
    plexus G54.1
    root (nerve) NEC G54.4
  lung (coin) R91.1
  maxillary sinus J32.0
  mitral I05.9

Lesion (continued)
  Morel-Lavallée —see Hematoma, by site
  motor cortex NEC G93.89
  mouth K13.79
  nerve G58.9
    femoral G57.2-
    median G56.1-
      carpal tunnel syndrome —see Syndrome, carpal tunnel
    plantar G57.6-
    popliteal (lateral) G57.3-
      medial G57.4-
    radial G56.3-
    sciatic G57.0-
    spinal —see Injury, nerve, spinal
    ulnar G56.2-
  nervous system, congenital Q07.9
  nonallopathic —see Lesion, biomechanical
  nose (internal) J34.89
  obstructive —see Obstruction
  obturator nerve G57.8-
  oral mucosa K13.70
  organ or site NEC —see Disease, by site
  osteolytic —see Osteolysis
  peptic K27.9
  periodontal, due to traumatic occlusion K05.5
  pharynx J39.2
  pigment, pigmented (skin) L81.9
  pinta —see Pinta, lesions
  polypoid —see Polyp
  prechiasmal (optic) —see Disorder, optic, chiasm
  primary (see also Syphilis, primary) A51.0
    carate A67.0
    pinta A67.0
    yaws A66.0
  pulmonary J98.4
    valve I37.9
  pylorus K31.9
  rectosigmoid K63.9
  retina, retinal H35.9
  sacroiliac (joint) (old) M53.3
  salivary gland K11.9
    benign lymphoepithelial K11.8
  saphenous nerve G57.8-
  sciatic nerve G57.0-
  secondary —see Syphilis, secondary
  shoulder (region) M75.9-
    specified NEC M75.8-
  sigmoid K63.9
  sinus (accessory) (nasal) J34.89
  skin L98.9
    suppurative L08.0
  SLAP S43.43-
  spinal cord G95.9
    congenital Q06.9
  spleen D73.89
  stomach K31.9
  superior glenoid labrum S43.43-
  syphilitic —see Syphilis
  tertiary —see Syphilis, tertiary
  thoracic root (nerve) NEC G54.3
  tonsillar fossa J35.9
  tooth, teeth K08.9
    white spot
      chewing surface K02.51
      pit and fissure surface K02.51
      smooth surface K02.61
  traumatic —see specific type of injury by site
  tricuspid (valve) I07.9
    nonrheumatic I36.9

Lesion (continued)
  trigeminal nerve G50.9
  ulcerated or ulcerative —see Ulcer, skin
  uterus N85.9
  vagina N89.8
  vagus nerve G52.2
  valvular —see Endocarditis
  vascular I99.9
    affecting central nervous system I67.9
    following trauma NEC T14.8
    umbilical cord, complicating delivery O69.5
  vulva N90.89
  warty —see Verruca
  white spot (tooth)
    chewing surface K02.51
    pit and fissure surface K02.51
    smooth surface K02.61

Lethargic —see condition

Less than a high school diploma Z55.5

Lethargy R53.83

Letterer-Siwe's disease C96.0

Leukemia, leukemic C95.9-
  acute basophilic C94.8-
  acute bilineal C95.0-
  acute erythroid C94.0-
  acute lymphoblastic C91.0-
  acute megakaryoblastic C94.2-
  acute megakaryocytic C94.2-
  acute mixed lineage C95.0-
  acute monoblastic (monoblastic/monocytic) C93.0-
  acute monocytic (monoblastic/monocytic) C93.0-
  acute myeloblastic (minimal differentiation) (with maturation) C92.0-
  acute myeloid, NOS C92.0-
    with
      11q23-abnormality C92.6-
      dysplasia of remaining hematopoesis and/or myelodysplastic disease in its history C92.A-
      multilineage dysplasia C92.A-
      variation of MLL-gene C92.6-
    M6 (a)(b) C94.0-
    M7 C94.2-
  acute myelomonocytic C92.5-
  acute promyelocytic C92.4-
  adult T-cell (HTLV-1-associated) (acute variant) (chronic variant) (lymphomatoid variant) (smouldering variant) C91.5-
  aggressive NK-cell C94.8-
  AML (1/ETO) (M0) (M1) (M2) (without a FAB classification) C92.0-
  AML M3 C92.4-
  AML M4 (Eo with inv (16) or t (16;16)) C92.5-
  AML M5 C93.0-
  AML M5a C93.0-
  AML M5b C93.0-
  AML Me with t (15;17) and variants C92.4-
  atypical chronic myeloid, BCR/ABL-negative C92.2-
  biphenotypic acute C95.0-
  blast cell C95.0-
  Burkitt-type, mature B-cell C91.A-
  chronic eosinophilic (see also Syndrome, hypereosinophilic, myeloid) C94.8-
  chronic lymphocytic, of B-cell type C91.1-

Leukemia, leukemic (continued)
  chronic monocytic C93.1-
  chronic myelogenous (Philadelphia chromosome (Ph1) positive) (t (9;22) (q34;q11) (with crisis of blast cells) C92.1-
  chronic myeloid, BCR/ABL-positive C92.1-
    atypical, BCR/ABL-negative C92.2-
  chronic myelomonocytic C93.1-
  chronic neutrophilic D47.1
  CMML (-1) (-2) (with eosinophilia) C93.1-
  granulocytic (see also Category C92) C92.9-
  hairy cell C91.4-
  juvenile myelomonocytic C93.3-
  lymphoid C91.9-
    specified NEC C91.Z-
  mast cell C94.3-
  mature B-cell, Burkitt-type C91.A-
  monocytic (subacute) C93.9-
    specified NEC C93.Z-
  myelogenous (see also Category C92) C92.9-
  myeloid C92.9-
    specified NEC C92.Z-
  plasma cell C90.1-
  plasmacytic C90.1-
  prolymphocytic
    of B-cell type C91.3-
    of T-cell type C91.6-
  specified NEC C94.8-
  stem cell, of unclear lineage C95.0-
  subacute lymphocytic C91.9-
  T-cell large granular lymphocytic C91.Z-
  unspecified cell type C95.9-
    acute C95.0-
    chronic C95.1-

Leukemoid reaction (see also Reaction, leukemoid) D72.823-

Leukoaraiosis (hypertensive) I67.81

Leukoariosis —see Leukoaraiosis

Leukocoria —see Disorder, globe, degenerated condition, leucocoria

Leukocytopenia D72.819

Leukocytosis D72.829
  eosinophilic D72.19

Leukoderma, leukodermia NEC L81.5
  syphilitic A51.39
    late A52.79

Leukodystrophy G31.80
  with vanishing white matter disease G11.6
  LMNB1-related autosomal dominant G90.B
  metachromatic E75.25
  pol III-related G11.5

Leukoedema, oral epithelium K13.29

Leukoencephalitis G04.81
  acute (subacute) hemorrhagic G36.1
  postimmunization or postvaccinal G04.02
  postinfectious G04.01
  subacute sclerosing A81.1
  van Bogaert's (sclerosing) A81.1

Leukoencephalopathy (see also Encephalopathy) G93.49
  with calcifications and cysts G93.43
  adult-onset, with axonal spheroids (and pigmented glia) G93.44
  Binswanger's I67.3
  heroin vapor G92.8

Leukoencephalopathy (continued)
  megaloencephalic, with subcortical cysts G93.42
  metachromatic E75.25
  multifocal (progressive) A81.2
  postimmunization and postvaccinal G04.02
  progressive multifocal A81.2
  reversible, posterior G93.6
  van Bogaert's (sclerosing) A81.1
  vascular, progressive I67.3

Leukoerythroblastosis D75.9

Leukokeratosis —see also Leukoplakia
  mouth K13.21
  nicotina palati K13.24
  oral mucosa K13.21
  tongue K13.21
  vocal cord J38.3

Leukokraurosis vulva (e) N90.4

Leukoma (cornea) —see also Opacity, cornea
  adherent H17.0-
  interfering with central vision —see Opacity, cornea, central

Leukomalacia, cerebral, newborn P91.2
  periventricular P91.2

Leukomelanopathy, hereditary D72.0

Leukonychia (punctata) (striata) L60.8
  congenital Q84.4

Leukopathia unguium L60.8
  congenital Q84.4

Leukopenia D72.819
  basophilic D72.818
  chemotherapy (cancer) induced D70.1
  congenital D70.0
  cyclic D70.0
  drug induced NEC D70.2
  due to cytoreductive cancer chemotherapy D70.1
  eosinophilic D72.818
  familial D70.0
  infantile genetic D70.0
  malignant D70.9
  periodic D70.0
  transitory neonatal P61.5

Leukopenic —see condition

Leukoplakia
  anus K62.89
  bladder (postinfectional) N32.89
  buccal K13.21
  cervix (uteri) N88.0
  esophagus K22.89
  gingiva K13.21
  hairy (oral mucosa) (tongue) K13.3
  kidney (pelvis) N28.89
  larynx J38.7
  lip K13.21
  mouth K13.21
  oral epithelium, including tongue (mucosa) K13.21
  palate K13.21
  pelvis (kidney) N28.89
  penis (infectional) N48.0
  rectum K62.89
  syphilitic (late) A52.79
  tongue K13.21
  ureter (postinfectional) N28.89
  urethra (postinfectional) N36.8
  uterus N85.8
  vagina N89.4
  vocal cord J38.3
  vulva N90.4

Leukorrhea N89.8
  due to Trichomonas (vaginalis) A59.00
  trichomonal A59.00
Leukosarcoma C85.9-
Levocardia (isolated) Q24.1
  with situs inversus Q89.3
Levotransposition Q20.5
Lev's disease or syndrome (acquired complete heart block) I44.2
Levulosuria —see Fructosuria
Levurid L30.2
Lewy body (ies) (disease) G31.83
Leyden-Möbius dystrophy —see Dystrophy, Leyden-Möbius
Leydig cell
  carcinoma
    specified site —see Neoplasm, malignant, by site
    unspecified site
      female C56.9
      male C62.9-
  tumor
    benign
      specified site —see Neoplasm, benign, by site
      unspecified site
        female D27.-
        male D29.2-
    malignant
      specified site —see Neoplasm, malignant, by site
      unspecified site
        female C56.-
        male C62.9-
    specified site —see Neoplasm, uncertain behavior, by site
    unspecified site
      female D39.1-
      male D40.1-
Leydig-Sertoli cell tumor
  specified site —see Neoplasm, benign, by site
  unspecified site
    female D27.-
    male D29.2-
LGMD —see Dystrophy, muscular, limb-girdle
LGSIL (Low grade squamous intraepithelial lesion on cytologic smear of)
  anus R85.612
  cervix R87.612
  vagina R87.622
Liar, pathologic F60.2
Libido
  decreased R68.82
Libman-Sacks disease M32.11
Lice (infestation) B85.2
  body (Pediculus corporis) B85.1
  crab B85.3
  head (Pediculus capitis) B85.0
  mixed (classifiable to more than one of the titles B85.0-B85.3) B85.4
  pubic (Phthirus pubis) B85.3
Lichen L28.0
  albus L90.0
    penis N48.0
    vulva N90.4
  amyloidosis E85.4 *[L99]*
  atrophicus L90.0
    penis N48.0
    vulva N90.4

Lichen (continued)
  congenital Q82.8
  myxedematosus L98.5
  nitidus L44.1
  pilaris Q82.8
    acquired L85.8
  planopilaris L66.1
  planus (chronicus) L43.9
    annularis L43.8
    bullous L43.1
    follicular L66.1
    hypertrophic L43.0
    moniliformis L44.3
    of Wilson L43.9
    specified NEC L43.8
    subacute (active) L43.3
    tropicus L43.3
  ruber
    acuminatus L44.0
    moniliformis L44.3
    planus L43.9
  sclerosus (et atrophicus) L90.0
    penis N48.0
    vulva N90.4
  scrofulosus (primary) (tuberculous) A18.4
  simplex (chronicus) (circumscriptus) L28.0
  striatus L44.2
  urticatus L28.2
Lichenification L28.0
Lichenoid keratosis —see Keratosis, lichenoid
Lichenoides tuberculosis (primary) A18.4
Lichtheim's disease or syndrome D51.0
Lien migrans D73.89
Ligament —see condition
Light
  for gestational age —see Light for dates
  headedness R42
Light-for-dates (infant) P05.00
  with weight of
    499 grams or less P05.01
    500-749 grams P05.02
    750-999 grams P05.03
    1000-1249 grams P05.04
    1250-1499 grams P05.05
    1500-1749 grams P05.06
    1750-1999 grams P05.07
    2000-2499 grams P05.08
    2500 grams and over P05.09
  and small-for-dates —see Small for dates
  affecting management of pregnancy O36.59-
  specified NEC P05.09
Lightning (effects) (stroke) (struck by) T75.00
  burn —see Burn
  foot E53.8
  shock T75.01
  specified effect NEC T75.09
Lightwood-Albright syndrome N25.89
Lightwood's disease or syndrome (renal tubular acidosis) N25.89
Lignac (-de Toni) (-Fanconi) (-Debré) **disease or syndrome** E72.09
  with cystinosis E72.04
Ligneous thyroiditis E06.5
Likoff's syndrome I20.89

Limb —see condition
Limbic epilepsy personality syndrome F07.0
Limitation, limited
  activities due to disability Z73.6
  cardiac reserve —see Disease, heart
  eye muscle duction, traumatic —see Strabismus, mechanical
  mandibular range of motion M26.52
Lindau (-von Hippel) **disease** Q85.83
Line(s)
  Beau's L60.4
  Harris' —see Arrest, epiphyseal
  Hudson's (cornea) —see Pigmentation, cornea, anterior
  Stähli's (cornea) —see Pigmentation, cornea, anterior
Linea corneae senilis —see Change, cornea, senile
Lingua
  geographica K14.1
  nigra (villosa) K14.3
  plicata K14.5
  tylosis K13.29
Lingual —see condition
Linguatulosis B88.8
Linitis (gastric) **plastica** C16.9
Lip —see condition
Lipedema —see Edema
Lipemia —see also Hyperlipidemia
  retina, retinalis E78.3
Lipidosis E75.6
  cerebral (infantile) (juvenile) (late) E75.4
  cerebroretinal E75.4
  cerebroside E75.22
  cholesterol (cerebral) E75.5
  glycolipid E75.21
  hepatosplenomegalic E78.3
  sphingomyelin —see Niemann-Pick disease or syndrome
  sulfatide E75.29
Lipoadenoma —see Neoplasm, benign, by site
Lipoblastoma —see Lipoma
Lipoblastomatosis —see Lipoma
Lipochondrodystrophy E76.01
Lipodermatosclerosis (see also Insufficiency, venous) M79.3
  with
    varicose veins —see Varix, leg, with, inflammation
      ulcerated —see Varix, leg, with, ulcer, with inflammation by site
    ulcerated —see Ulcer, by site
Lipochrome histiocytosis (familial) D71
Lipodystrophia progressiva E88.1
Lipodystrophy (progressive) E88.1
  insulin E88.1
  intestinal K90.81
  mesenteric K65.4
Lipofibroma —see Lipoma
Lipofuscinosis, neuronal (with ceroidosis) E75.4
Lipogranuloma, sclerosing L92.8
Lipogranulomatosis E78.89
Lipoid —see also condition
  histiocytosis D76.3
    essential E75.29

Lipoid (continued)
  nephrosis N04.9
  proteinosis of Urbach E78.89
Lipoidemia —see Hyperlipidemia
Lipoidosis —see Lipidosis
Lipoma D17.9
  fetal D17.9
  fat cell D17.9
  infiltrating D17.9
  intramuscular D17.9
  pleomorphic D17.9
  site classification
    arms (skin) (subcutaneous) D17.2-
    connective tissue D17.30
      intra-abdominal D17.5
      intrathoracic D17.4
      peritoneum D17.79
      retroperitoneum D17.79
      specified site NEC D17.39
      spermatic cord D17.6
    face (skin) (subcutaneous) D17.0
    genitourinary organ NEC D17.72
    head (skin) (subcutaneous) D17.0
    intra-abdominal D17.5
    intrathoracic D17.4
    kidney D17.71
    legs (skin) (subcutaneous) D17.2-
    neck (skin) (subcutaneous) D17.0
    peritoneum D17.79
    retroperitoneum D17.79
    skin D17.30
      specified site NEC D17.39
    spermatic cord D17.6
    subcutaneous D17.30
      specified site NEC D17.39
    trunk (skin) (subcutaneous) D17.1
  unspecified D17.9
  spindle cell D17.9
Lipomatosis E88.2
  dolorosa (Dercum) E88.2
  fetal —see Lipoma
  Launois-Bensaude E88.89
Lipomyoma —see Lipoma
Lipomyxoma —see Lipoma
Lipomyxosarcoma —see Neoplasm, connective tissue, malignant
Lipoprotein metabolism disorder E78.9
Lipoproteinemia E78.5
  broad-beta E78.2
  floating-beta E78.2
  hyper-pre-beta E78.1
Liposarcoma —see also Neoplasm, connective tissue, malignant
  dedifferentiated —see Neoplasm, connective tissue, malignant
  differentiated type —see Neoplasm, connective tissue, malignant
  embryonal —see Neoplasm, connective tissue, malignant
  mixed type —see Neoplasm, connective tissue, malignant
  myxoid —see Neoplasm, connective tissue, malignant
  pleomorphic —see Neoplasm, connective tissue, malignant
  round cell —see Neoplasm, connective tissue, malignant
  well differentiated type —see Neoplasm, connective tissue, malignant

Liposynovitis prepatellaris E88.89
Lipping, cervix N86
Lipschütz disease or ulcer N76.6
Lipuria R82.0
  schistosomiasis (bilharziasis) B65.0
Lisping F80.0
Lissauer's paralysis A52.17
Lissencephalia, lissencephaly Q04.3
Listeriosis, listerellosis A32.9
  congenital (disseminated) P37.2
  cutaneous A32.0
  neonatal, newborn (disseminated) P37.2
  oculoglandular A32.81
  specified NEC A32.89
Lithemia E79.0
Lithiasis —see Calculus
Lithosis J62.8
Lithuria R82.998
Litigation, anxiety concerning Z65.3
Little leaguer's elbow —see Epicondylitis, medial
Little's disease G80.9
Littre's
  gland —see condition
  hernia —see Hernia, abdomen
Littritis —see Urethritis
Livedo (annularis) (racemosa) (reticularis) R23.1
Liver —see condition
Living alone (problems with) Z60.2
  with handicapped person Z74.2
Living in a shelter (motel) (scattered site housing) (temporary or transitional living situation) Z59.01
Lloyd's syndrome —see Adenomatosis, endocrine
Loa loa, loaiasis, loasis B74.3
Lobar —see condition
Lobomycosis B48.0
Lobo's disease B48.0
Lobotomy syndrome F07.0
Lobstein (-Ekman) **disease or syndrome** Q78.0
Lobster-claw hand Q71.6-
Lobulation (congenital) —see also Anomaly, by site
  kidney, Q63.1
  liver, abnormal Q44.79
  spleen Q89.09
Lobule, lobular —see condition
Local, localized —see condition
Locked-in state G83.5
Locked twins causing obstructed labor O66.1
Locking
  joint —see Derangement, joint, specified type NEC
    knee —see Derangement, knee
Lockjaw —see Tetanus
Löffler's
  endocarditis I42.3
  eosinophilia J82.89
  pneumonia J82.89
  syndrome (eosinophilic pneumonitis) J82.89

Loiasis (with conjunctival infestation) (eyelid) B74.3
Lone Star fever A77.0
Loneliness R45.89
Long
  COVID (-19) (see also COVID-19) U09.9
  labor O63.9
    first stage O63.0
    second stage O63.1
  QT syndrome I45.81
Long-term (current) (prophylactic)
  drug therapy (use of)
  5-fluorouracil Z79.631
  6-mercaptopurine Z79.631
  adalimumab Z79.620
  agents affecting estrogen receptors and estrogen levels NEC Z79.818
  alkylating agent Z79.630
  anastrozole (Arimidex) Z79.811
  antibiotics Z79.2
    short-term use - omit code
  anticoagulants Z79.01
  antidiabetic drugs, injectable, non-insulin Z79.85
  anti-inflammatory, non-steroidal (NSAID) Z79.1
  antimetabolite agent Z79.631
  antiplatelet Z79.02
  antithrombotics Z79.02
  antitumor antibiotic Z79.632
  apremilast Z79.61
  aromatase inhibitors Z79.811
  aspirin Z79.82
  azathioprine Z79.624
  birth control pill or patch Z79.3
  bisphosphonates Z79.83
  bleomycin Z79.632
  calcineurin inhibitor Z79.621
  chlorambucil Z79.630
  cisplatin Z79.630
  contraceptive, oral Z79.3
  cyclophosphamide Z79.630
  cyclosporine Z79.621
  cytarabine Z79.631
  doxorubicin Z79.632
  drug, specified NEC Z79.899
  estrogen receptor downregulators Z79.818
  etanercept Z79.620
  etoposide Z79.634
  Evista Z79.810
  exemestane (Aromasin) Z79.811
  Fareston Z79.810
  fulvestrant (Faslodex) Z79.818
  gonadotropin-releasing hormone (GnRH) agonist Z79.818
  goserelin acetate (Zoladex) Z79.818
  hormone replacement Z79.890
  hydroxyurea Z79.64
  immunomodulators, unspecified Z79.60
    specified NEC Z79.69
  immunomodulatory imide drug Z79.61
  immunosuppressants, unspecified Z79.60
    specified NEC Z79.69
  immunosuppressive biologic Z79.620
  infliximab Z79.620
  inhibitors of nucleotide synthesis Z79.624
  insulin Z79.4
  irinotecan Z79.634
  Janus kinase inhibitor Z79.622
  lenalidomide Z79.61
  letrozole (Femara) Z79.811

Long-term (continued)
  leuprolide acetate (leuprorelin) (Lupron) Z79.818
  mammalian target of rapamycin (mTOR) inhibitor Z79.623
  megestrol acetate (Megace) Z79.818
  methadone for pain management Z79.891
  mitomycin C Z79.632
  mitotic inhibitor Z79.633
  monoclonal antibodies Z79.620
  myelosuppressive agent Z79.64
  Nolvadex Z79.810
  non-insulin antidiabetic drug, injectable Z79.899
  non-steroidal anti-inflammatories (NSAID) Z79.1
  omycophenolate Z79.624
  opiate analgesic Z79.891
  oral
    antidiabetic Z79.84
    contraceptive Z79.3
    hypoglycemic Z79.84
  paclitaxel Z79.633
  plant alkaloids Z79.633
  pomalidomide Z79.61
  purine synthesis (IMDH) inhibitors Z79.624
  raloxifene (Evista) Z79.810
  selective estrogen receptor modulators (SERMs) Z79.810
  sirolimus Z79.623
  steroids
    inhaled Z79.51
    systemic Z79.52
  tacrolimus Z79.621
  tamoxifen (Nolvadex) Z79.810
  tofacitinib Z79.622
  topoisomerase inhibitor Z79.634
  topotecan Z79.634
  toremifene (Fareston) Z79.810
  vinblastine Z79.633
  vincristine Z79.633
Longitudinal stripes or grooves, nails L60.8
  congenital Q84.6
Loop
  intestine —see Volvulus
  vascular on papilla (optic) Q14.2
Loose —see also condition
  body
    joint M24.00
      ankle M24.07-
      elbow M24.02-
      hand M24.04-
      hip M24.05-
      knee M23.4-
      shoulder (region) M24.01-
      specified site NEC M24.08
      vertebra M24.08
      temporomandibular M24.08
      toe M24.07-
      wrist M24.03-
    knee M23.4-
    sheath, tendon —see Disorder, tendon, specified type NEC
  cartilage —see Loose, body, joint
  skin and subcutaneous tissue (following bariatric surgery weight loss) (following dietary weight loss) L98.7
  tooth, teeth K08.89

Loosening
  aseptic
    joint prosthesis —see Complications, joint prosthesis, mechanical, loosening, by site
  epiphysis —see Osteochondropathy
  mechanical
    joint prosthesis —see Complications, joint prosthesis, mechanical, loosening, by site
Looser-Milkman (-Debray) **syndrome** M83.8
Lop ear (deformity) Q17.3
Lorain (-Levi) **short stature syndrome** E23.0
Lordosis M40.50
  acquired —see Lordosis, specified type NEC
  congenital Q76.429
    lumbar region Q76.426
    lumbosacral region Q76.427
    sacral region Q76.428
    sacrococcygeal region Q76.428
    thoracolumbar region Q76.425
  lumbar region M40.56
  lumbosacral region M40.57
  postsurgical M96.4
  postural —see Lordosis, specified type NEC
  rachitic (late effect) (sequelae) E64.3
  sequelae of rickets E64.3
  specified type NEC M40.40
    lumbar region M40.46
    lumbosacral region M40.47
    thoracolumbar region M40.45
  thoracolumbar region M40.55
  tuberculous A18.01
Loss (of)
  appetite (see also Anorexia) R63.0
    hysterical F50.89
    nonorganic origin F50.89
    psychogenic F50.89
  blood —see Hemorrhage
  bone —see Loss, substance of, bone
  control, sphincter, rectum R15.9
    nonorganic origin F98.1
  consciousness, transient R55
    traumatic —see Injury, intracranial
  elasticity, skin R23.4
  family (member) in childhood Z62.898
  fluid (acute) E86.9
  function of labyrinth H83.2
  hair, nonscarring —see Alopecia
  hearing —see also Deafness
    central NOS H90.5
    conductive H90.2
      bilateral H90.0
      unilateral
        with
          restricted hearing on the contralateral side H90.A1-
          unrestricted hearing on the contralateral side H90.1-
    mixed conductive and sensorineural hearing loss H90.8
      bilateral H90.6

Loss *(continued)*
 hearing *(continued)*
  mixed conductive and
   sensorineural hearing loss
   H90.8 *(continued)*
    unilateral
     with
      restricted hearing on the
       contralateral side
       H90.A3-
      unrestricted hearing on
       the contralateral side
       H90.7-
  neural NOS H90.5
  perceptive NOS H90.5
  sensorineural NOS H90.5
   bilateral H90.3
   unilateral
    with
     restricted hearing on the
      contralateral side H90.
      A2-
     unrestricted hearing on
      the contralateral side
      H90.4-
  sensory NOS H90.5
 height R29.890
 limb or member, traumatic, current
  —*see* Amputation, traumatic
 love relationship in childhood
  Z62.898
 memory —*see also* Amnesia
  mild, following organic brain
   damage F06.8
 mind —*see* Psychosis
 occlusal vertical dimension of fully
  erupted teeth M26.37
 organ or part —*see* Absence, by
  site, acquired
 ossicles, ear (partial) H74.32-
 parent in childhood Z63.4
 pregnancy, recurrent N96
  care in current pregnancy
   O26.2-
  without current pregnancy
   N96
 recurrent pregnancy —*see* Loss,
  pregnancy, recurrent
 self-esteem, in childhood Z62.898
 sense of
  smell —*see* Disturbance,
   sensation, smell
  taste —*see* Disturbance,
   sensation, taste
  touch R20.8
 sensory R44.9
  dissociative F44.6
 sexual desire F52.0
 sight (acquired) (complete)
  (congenital) —*see* Blindness
 substance of
  bone —*see* Disorder, bone,
   density and structure, specified
   NEC
   horizontal alveolar K06.3
  cartilage —*see* Disorder,
   cartilage, specified type
   NEC
   auricle (ear) —*see* Disorder,
    pinna, specified type NEC
 vitreous (humor) H15.89
 tooth, teeth —*see* Absence, teeth,
  acquired
 vision, visual H54.7
  both eyes H54.3
  one eye H54.60
   left (normal vision on right)
    H54.62
   right (normal vision on left)
    H54.61

Loss *(continued)*
 vision *(continued)*
  specified as blindness —*see*
   Blindness
  subjective
   sudden H53.13-
   transient H53.12-
 vitreous —*see* Prolapse, vitreous
 voice —*see* Aphonia
 weight (abnormal) (cause
  unknown) R63.4
Louis-Bar syndrome (ataxia-
 telangiectasia) G11.3
Louping ill (encephalitis) A84.89
Louse, lousiness —*see* Lice
Low
 achiever, school Z55.3
 back syndrome M54.50
 basal metabolic rate R94.8
 birthweight (2499 grams or less)
  P07.10
  with weight of
   1000-1249 grams P07.14
   1250-1499 grams P07.15
   1500-1749 grams P07.16
   1750-1999 grams P07.17
   2000-2499 grams P07.18
  extreme (999 grams or less)
   P07.00
   with weight of
    499 grams or less P07.01
    500-749 grams P07.02
    750-999 grams P07.03
  for gestational age —*see* Light
   for dates
 blood pressure —*see also*
  Hypotension
  reading (incidental) (isolated)
   (nonspecific) R03.1
 cardiac reserve —*see* Disease, heart
 function —*see also* Hypofunction
  kidney N28.9
 hematocrit D64.9
 hemoglobin D64.9
 income Z59.6
 level of literacy Z55.0
 lying
  kidney N28.89
  organ or site, congenital —*see*
   Malposition, congenital
 output syndrome (cardiac) —*see*
  Failure, heart
 platelets (blood) —*see*
  Thrombocytopenia
 reserve, kidney N28.89
 salt syndrome E87.1
 self esteem R45.81
 set ears Q17.4
 vision H54.2X-
  one eye (other eye normal) H54.50
   left (normal vision on right)
    category 1 H54.52A1
    category 2 H54.52A2
    other eye blind —*see*
     Blindness
   right (normal vision on left)
    category 1 H54.511A
    category 2 H54.512A
 von Willebrand factor R79.1
Low-density-lipoprotein-type (LDL)
 hyperlipoproteinemia E78.00
Lowe's syndrome E72.03
Lown-Ganong-Levine syndrome I45.6
LSD reaction (acute) (without
 dependence) F16.90
 with dependence F16.20
L-shaped kidney Q63.8

Ludwig's angina or disease K12.2
Lues (venerea), **luetic** —*see* Syphilis
Luetscher's syndrome (dehydration)
 E86.0
Lumbago, lumbalgia M54.50
 with sciatica M54.4-
  due to intervertebral disc
   disorder M51.17
 due to displacement, intervertebral
  disc M51.27
  with sciatica M51.17
Lumbar —*see* condition
**Lumbarization, vertebra,
 congenital** Q76.49
Lumbermen's itch B88.0
Lump —*see also* Mass
 breast N63.0
  axillary tail
   left N63.32
   right N63.31
  left
   lower inner quadrant N63.24
   lower outer quadrant N63.23
   overlapping quadrants N63.25
   unspecified quadrant N63.20
   upper inner quadrant N63.22
   upper outer quadrant N63.21
  right
   lower inner quadrant N63.14
   lower outer quadrant N63.13
   overlapping quadrants N63.15
   unspecified quadrant N63.10
   upper inner quadrant N63.12
   upper outer quadrant N63.11
  subareolar
   left N63.42
   right N63.41
Lunacy —*see* Psychosis
Lung —*see* condition
Lupoid (miliary) **of Boeck** D86.3
Lupus
 anticoagulant D68.62
  with
   hemorrhagic disorder D68.312
   hypercoagulable state D68.62
  finding without diagnosis R76.0
 discoid (local) L93.0
 erythematosus (discoid) (local) L93.0
  disseminated —*see* Lupus,
   erythematosus, systemic
  eyelid H01.129
   left H01.126
    lower H01.125
    upper H01.124
   right H01.123
    lower H01.122
    upper H01.121
  profundus L93.2
  specified NEC L93.2
  subacute cutaneous L93.1
  systemic M32.9
   with organ or system
    involvement M32.10
    endocarditis M32.11
    lung M32.13
    pericarditis M32.12
    renal (glomerular) M32.14
     tubulo-interstitial M32.15
    specified organ or system
     NEC M32.19
   drug-induced M32.0
   inhibitor (presence of) D68.62
    with
     hemorrhagic disorder
      D68.312
     hypercoagulable state
      D68.62

Lupus *(continued)*
 erythematosus *(continued)*
  systemic *(continued)*
   inhibitor *(continued)*
    finding without diagnosis
     R76.0
   specified NEC M32.8
  exedens A18.4
  hydralazine M32.0
   correct substance properly
    administered —*see* Table
    of Drugs and Chemicals, by
    drug, adverse effect
   overdose or wrong substance
    given or taken —*see* Table
    of Drugs and Chemicals, by
    drug, poisoning
  nephritis (chronic) M32.14
  nontuberculous, not disseminated
   L93.0
  panniculitis L93.2
  pernio (Besnier) D86.3
  systemic —*see* Lupus,
   erythematosus, systemic
  tuberculous A18.4
   eyelid A18.4
  vulgaris A18.4
   eyelid A18.4
Luteinoma D27.-
Lutembacher's disease or syndrome
 (atrial septal defect with mitral
 stenosis) Q21.19
Luteoma D27.-
Lutz (-Splendore-de
 Almeida) **disease** —*see*
 Paracoccidioidomycosis
Luxation —*see also* Dislocation
 eyeball (nontraumatic) —*see*
  Luxation, globe
  birth injury P15.3
 globe, nontraumatic H44.82-
 lacrimal gland —*see* Dislocation,
  lacrimal gland
 lens (old) (partial)
  (spontaneous)
  congenital Q12.1
  syphilitic A50.39
Lycanthropy F22
Lyell's syndrome L51.2
 due to drug L51.2
  correct substance properly
   administered —*see* Table
   of Drugs and Chemicals, by
   drug, adverse effect
  overdose or wrong substance
   given or taken —*see* Table
   of Drugs and Chemicals, by
   drug, poisoning
Lyme disease A69.20
Lymph
 gland or node —*see* condition
 scrotum —*see* Infestation, filarial
Lymphadenitis I88.9
 with ectopic or molar pregnancy
  O08.0
 acute L04.9
  axilla L04.2
  face L04.0
  head L04.0
  hip L04.3
  limb
   lower L04.3
   upper L04.2
  neck L04.0
  shoulder L04.2
  specified site NEC L04.8
  trunk L04.1

225

Lymphadenitis (continued)
anthracosis (occupational) J60
any site, except mesenteric I88.9
chronic I88.1
subacute I88.1
breast
gestational —see Mastitis, obstetric
puerperal, postpartum (nonpurulent) O91.22
chancroidal (congenital) A57
chronic I88.1
mesenteric I88.0
due to
Brugia (malayi) B74.1
timori B74.2
chlamydial lymphogranuloma A55
diphtheria (toxin) A36.89
lymphogranuloma venereum A55
Wuchereria bancrofti B74.0
following ectopic or molar pregnancy O08.0
gonorrheal A54.89
infective —see Lymphadenitis, acute
mesenteric (acute) (chronic) (nonspecific) (subacute) I88.0
due to Salmonella typhi A01.09
tuberculous A18.39
mycobacterial A31.8
purulent —see Lymphadenitis, acute
pyogenic —see Lymphadenitis, acute
regional, nonbacterial I88.8
septic —see Lymphadenitis, acute
subacute, unspecified site I88.1
suppurative —see Lymphadenitis, acute
syphilitic (early) (secondary) A51.49
late A52.79
tuberculous —see Tuberculosis, lymph gland
venereal (chlamydial) A55

Lymphadenoid goiter E06.3

Lymphadenopathy (generalized) R59.1
angioimmunoblastic, with dysproteinemia (AILD) C86.5
due to toxoplasmosis (acquired) B58.89
congenital (acute) (subacute) (chronic) P37.1
localized R59.0
syphilitic (early) (secondary) A51.49

Lymphadenosis R59.1

Lymphangiectasis I89.0
conjunctiva H11.89
postinfectional I89.0
scrotum I89.0

Lymphangiectatic elephantiasis, nonfilarial I89.0

Lymphangioendothelioma D18.1
malignant —see Neoplasm, connective tissue, malignant

Lymphangioleiomyomatosis J84.81

Lymphangioma D18.1
capillary D18.1
cavernous D18.1
cystic D18.1
malignant —see Neoplasm, connective tissue, malignant

Lymphangiomyoma D18.1

Lymphangiomyomatosis J84.81

Lymphangiosarcoma —see Neoplasm, connective tissue, malignant

Lymphangitis I89.1
with
abscess - code by site under Abscess
cellulitis - code by site under Cellulitis
ectopic or molar pregnancy O08.0
acute L03.91
abdominal wall L03.321
ankle —see Lymphangitis, acute, lower limb
arm —see Lymphangitis, acute, upper limb
auricle (ear) —see Lymphangitis, acute, ear
axilla L03.12-
back (any part) L03.322
buttock L03.327
cervical (meaning neck) L03.222
cheek (external) L03.212
chest wall L03.323
digit
finger —see Lymphangitis, acute, finger
toe —see Lymphangitis, acute, toe
ear (external) H60.1-
external auditory canal —see Lymphangitis, acute, ear
eyelid —see Abscess, eyelid
face NEC L03.212
finger (intrathecal) (periosteal) (subcutaneous) (subcuticular) L03.02-
foot —see Lymphangitis, acute, lower limb
gluteal (region) L03.327
groin L03.324
hand —see Lymphangitis, acute, upper limb
head NEC L03.891
face (any part, except ear, eye and nose) L03.212
heel —see Lymphangitis, acute, lower limb
hip —see Lymphangitis, acute, lower limb
jaw (region) L03.212
knee —see Lymphangitis, acute, lower limb
leg —see Lymphangitis, acute, lower limb
lower limb L03.12-
toe —see Lymphangitis, acute, toe
navel L03.326
neck (region) L03.222
orbit, orbital —see Cellulitis, orbit
pectoral (region) L03.323
perineal, perineum L03.325
scalp (any part) L03.891
shoulder —see Lymphangitis, acute, upper limb
specified site NEC L03.898
thigh —see Lymphangitis, acute, lower limb
thumb (intrathecal) (periosteal) (subcutaneous) (subcuticular) —see Lymphangitis, acute, finger
toe (intrathecal) (periosteal) (subcutaneous) (subcuticular) L03.04-
trunk L03.329
abdominal wall L03.321
back (any part) L03.322
buttock L03.327
chest wall L03.323
groin L03.324
perineal, perineum L03.325
umbilicus L03.326

Lymphangitis (continued)
acute (continued)
umbilicus L03.326
upper limb L03.12-
axilla —see Lymphangitis, acute, axilla
finger —see Lymphangitis, acute, finger
thumb —see Lymphangitis, acute, finger
wrist —see Lymphangitis, acute, upper limb
breast
gestational —see Mastitis, obstetric
chancroidal A57
chronic (any site) I89.1
due to
Brugia (malayi) B74.1
timori B74.2
Wuchereria bancrofti B74.0
following ectopic or molar pregnancy O08.89
penis
acute N48.29
gonococcal (acute) (chronic) A54.09
puerperal, postpartum, childbirth O86.89
strumous, tuberculous A18.2
subacute (any site) I89.1
tuberculous —see Tuberculosis, lymph gland

Lymphatic (vessel) —see condition

Lymphatism E32.8

Lymphectasia I89.0

Lymphedema (acquired) —see also Elephantiasis
congenital Q82.0
hereditary (chronic) (idiopathic) Q82.0
postmastectomy I97.2
praecox I89.0
secondary I89.0
surgical NEC I97.89
postmastectomy (syndrome) I97.2

Lymphoblastic —see condition

Lymphoblastoma (diffuse) —see Lymphoma, lymphoblastic (diffuse)
giant follicular —see Lymphoma, lymphoblastic (diffuse)
macrofollicular —see Lymphoma, lymphoblastic (diffuse)

Lymphocele I89.8

Lymphocytic
chorioencephalitis (acute) (serous) A87.2
choriomeningitis (acute) (serous) A87.2
meningoencephalitis A87.2

Lymphocytoma, benign cutis L98.8

Lymphocytopenia D72.810

Lymphocytosis (symptomatic) D72.820
infectious (acute) B33.8

Lymphoepithelioma —see Neoplasm, malignant, by site

Lymphogranuloma (malignant) —see also Lymphoma, Hodgkin
chlamydial A55
inguinale A55
venereum (any site) (chlamydial) (with stricture of rectum) A55

Lymphogranulomatosis (malignant) —see also Lymphoma, Hodgkin
benign (Boeck's sarcoid) (Schaumann's) D86.1

Lymphohistiocytosis, hemophagocytic (familial) D76.1

Lymphoid —see condition

Lymphoma (of) (malignant) C85.90
adult T-cell (HTLV-1-associated) (acute variant) (chronic variant) (lymphomatoid variant) (smouldering variant) C91.5-
anaplastic large cell
ALK-negative C84.7-
ALK-positive C84.6-
breast implant associated (BIA-ALCL) C84.7A
CD30-positive C84.6-
primary cutaneous C86.6
angioimmunoblastic T-cell C86.5
BALT C88.4
B-cell C85.1-
B-precursor C83.5-
blastic NK-cell C86.4
blastic plasmacytoid dendritic cell neoplasm (BPDCN) C86.4
blastic plasmacytoid dendritic cell neoplasm (BPDCN) C86.4
bronchial-associated lymphoid tissue [BALT-lymphoma] C88.4
Burkitt (atypical) C83.7-
Burkitt-like C83.7-
centrocytic C83.1-
cutaneous follicle center C82.6-
cutaneous T-cell C84.A-
diffuse follicle center C82.5-
diffuse large cell C83.3-
anaplastic C83.3-
B-cell C83.3-
diffuse large cell C83.3-
CD30-positive C83.3-
centroblastic C83.3-
immunoblastic C83.3-
plasmablastic C83.3-
subtype not specified C83.3-
T-cell rich C83.3-
enteropathy-type (associated) (intestinal) T-cell C86.2
extranodal NK/T-cell, nasal type C86.0
extranodal marginal zone B-cell lymphoma of mucosa-associated lymphoid tissue [MALT-lymphoma] C88.4
follicular C82.9-
grade
I C82.0-
II C82.1-
III C82.2-
IIIa C82.3-
IIIb C82.4-
specified NEC C82.8-
hepatosplenic T-cell (alpha-beta) (gamma-delta) C86.1
histiocytic C85.9-
true C96.A
Hodgkin C81.9-
lymphocyte-rich (classical) C81.4-
lymphocyte depleted (classical) C81.3-
mixed cellularity (classical) C81.2-
nodular sclerosis (classical) C81.1-
specified NEC (classical) C81.7-
nodular
lymphocyte predominant C81.0-
sclerosis (classical) C81.1-

Lymphoma *(continued)*
  intravascular large B-cell C83.8-
  Lennert's C84.4-
  lymphoblastic B-cell C83.5-
  lymphoblastic (diffuse) C83.5-
  lymphoblastic T-cell C83.5-
  lymphoepithelioid C84.4-
  lymphoplasmacytic C83.0-
    with IgM-production C88.0
  MALT C88.4
  mantle cell C83.1-
  mature T-cell NEC C84.4-
  mature T/NK-cell C84.9-
    specified NEC C84.Z-
  mediastinal (thymic) large B-cell C85.2-
  Mediterranean C88.3
  mucosa-associated lymphoid tissue [MALT-lymphoma] C88.4
  NK/T cell C84.9-
  nodal marginal zone C83.0-
  non-follicular (diffuse) C83.9-
    specified NEC C83.8-
  non-Hodgkin *(see also* Lymphoma, by type) C85.9-
    specified NEC C85.8-
  non-leukemic variant of B-CLL C83.0-
  peripheral T-cell, NEC C84.4-
  primary cutaneous
    anaplastic large cell C86.6
    CD30-positive large T-cell C86.6
  primary effusion B-cell C83.8-
  SALT C88.4
  skin-associated lymphoid tissue [SALT-lymphoma] C88.4
  small cell B-cell C83.0-
  splenic marginal zone C83.0-
  subcutaneous panniculitis-like T-cell C86.3
  T-precursor C83.5-
  true histiocytic C96.A

Lymphomatosis —*see* Lymphoma

Lymphopathia venereum, veneris A55

Lymphopenia D72.810

Lymphoplasmacytic leukemia —*see* Leukemia, chronic lymphocytic, B-cell type

Lymphoproliferation, X-linked disease D82.3

Lymphoreticulosis, benign (of inoculation) A28.1

Lymphorrhea I89.8

Lymphosarcoma (diffuse) *(see also* Lymphoma) C85.9-

Lymphostasis I89.8

Lypemania —*see* Melancholia

Lysine and hydroxylysine metabolism disorder E72.3

Lyssa —*see* Rabies

M

Macacus ear Q17.3

Maceration, wet feet, tropical (syndrome) T69.02-

MacLeod's syndrome J43.0

Macrocephalia, macrocephaly Q75.3

Macrocheilia, macrochilia (congenital) Q18.6

Macrocolon *(see also* Megacolon) Q43.1

Macrocornea Q15.8
  with glaucoma Q15.0

Macrocytic —*see* condition

Macrocytosis D75.89

Macrodactylia, macrodactylism (fingers) (thumbs) Q74.0
  toes Q74.2

Macrodontia K00.2

Macrogenia M26.05

Macrogenitosomia (adrenal) (male) (praecox) E25.9
  congenital E25.0

Macroglobulinemia (idiopathic) (primary) C88.0
  monoclonal (essential) D47.2
  Waldenström C88.0

Macroglossia (congenital) Q38.2
  acquired K14.8

Macrognathia, macrognathism (congenital) (mandibular) (maxillary) M26.09

Macrogyria (congenital) Q04.8

Macrohydrocephalus —*see* Hydrocephalus

Macromastia —*see* Hypertrophy, breast

Macrophthalmos Q11.3
  in congenital glaucoma Q15.0

Macropsia H53.15

Macrosigmoid K59.39
  congenital Q43.2

Macrospondylitis, acromegalic E22.0

Macrostomia (congenital) Q18.4

Macrotia (external ear) (congenital) Q17.1

Macula
  cornea, corneal —*see* Opacity, cornea
  degeneration (atrophic) (exudative) (senile) —*see also* Degeneration, macula
  hereditary —*see* Dystrophy, retina

Maculae ceruleae B85.1

Maculopathy, toxic —*see* Degeneration, macula, toxic

Madarosis (eyelid) H02.729
  left H02.726
    lower H02.725
    upper H02.724
  right H02.723
    lower H02.722
    upper H02.721

Madelung's
  deformity (radius) Q74.0
  disease
    radial deformity Q74.0
    symmetrical lipomas, neck E88.89

Madness —*see* Psychosis

Madura
  foot B47.9
    actinomycotic B47.1
    mycotic B47.0

Maduromycosis B47.0

Maffucci's syndrome Q78.4

Magnesium metabolism disorder —*see* Disorder, metabolism, magnesium

Main en griffe (acquired) —*see also* Deformity, limb, clawhand
  congenital Q68.1

Maintenance (encounter for)
  antineoplastic chemotherapy Z51.11
  antineoplastic radiation therapy Z51.0
  methadone F11.20

Majocchi's
  disease L81.7
  granuloma B35.8

Major —*see* condition

Malabar itch (any site) B35.5

Malabsorption K90.9
  calcium K90.89
  carbohydrate K90.49
  disaccharide E73.9
  fat K90.49
  galactose E74.20
  glucose (-galactose) E74.39
  intestinal K90.9
    specified NEC K90.89
  isomaltose E74.31
  lactose E73.9
  methionine E72.19
  monosaccharide E74.39
  postgastrectomy K91.2
  postsurgical K91.2
  protein K90.49
  starch K90.49
  sucrose E74.39
  syndrome K90.9
    postsurgical K91.2

Malacia, bone (adult) M83.9
  juvenile —*see* Rickets

Malacoplakia
  bladder N32.89
  pelvis (kidney) N28.89
  ureter N28.89
  urethra N36.8

Malacosteon, juvenile —*see* Rickets

Maladaptation —*see* Maladjustment

Maladie de Roger Q21.0

Maladjustment
  conjugal Z63.0
    involving divorce or estrangement Z63.5
  educational Z55.4
  family Z63.9
  marital Z63.0
    involving divorce or estrangement Z63.5
  occupational NEC Z56.89
  simple, adult —*see* Disorder, adjustment
  situational —*see* Disorder, adjustment
  social Z60.9
    due to
      acculturation difficulty Z60.3
      discrimination and persecution (perceived) Z60.5
      exclusion and isolation Z60.4
      life-cycle (phase of life) transition Z60.0
      rejection Z60.4
      specified reason NEC Z60.8

Malaise R53.81

Malakoplakia —*see* Malacoplakia

Malaria, malarial (fever) B54
  with
    blackwater fever B50.8
    hemoglobinuric (bilious) B50.8
  hemoglobinuria B50.8
  accidentally induced (therapeutically) - code by type under Malaria
  algid B50.9
  cerebral B50.0 *[G94]*
  clinically diagnosed (without parasitological confirmation) B54
  congenital NEC P37.4
    falciparum P37.3
  congestion, congestive B54
  continued (fever) B50.9
  estivo-autumnal B50.9
  falciparum B50.9
    with complications NEC B50.8
      cerebral B50.0 *[G94]*
      severe B50.8
    hemorrhagic B54
  malariae B52.9
    with
      complications NEC B52.8
      glomerular disorder B52.0
  malignant (tertian) —*see* Malaria, falciparum
  mixed infections - code to first listed type in B50-B53
  ovale B53.0
  parasitologically confirmed NEC B53.8
  pernicious, acute —*see* Malaria, falciparum
  Plasmodium (P.)
    falciparum NEC —*see* Malaria, falciparum
    malariae NEC B52.9
      with Plasmodium
        falciparum (and or vivax) —*see* Malaria, falciparum
        vivax —*see also* Malaria, vivax
        and falciparum —*see* Malaria, falciparum
    ovale B53.0
      with Plasmodium malariae —*see also* Malaria, malariae
      and vivax —*see also* Malaria, vivax
      and falciparum —*see* Malaria, falciparum
    simian B53.1
      with Plasmodium malariae —*see also* Malaria, malariae
      and vivax —*see also* Malaria, vivax
      and falciparum —*see* Malaria, falciparum
    vivax NEC B51.9
      with Plasmodium falciparum —*see* Malaria, falciparum
  quartan —*see* Malaria, malariae
  quotidian —*see* Malaria, falciparum
  recurrent B54
  remittent B54
  specified type NEC (parasitologically confirmed) B53.8
  spleen B54
  subtertian (fever) —*see* Malaria, falciparum
  tertian (benign) —*see also* Malaria, vivax
    malignant B50.9

Malaria, malarial (continued)
  tropical B50.9
  typhoid B54
  vivax B51.9
    with
      complications NEC B51.8
      ruptured spleen B51.0
Malassimilation K90.9
Malassez's disease (cystic) N50.89
Mal de los pintos —see Pinta
Mal de mer T75.3
Maldescent, testis Q53.9
  bilateral Q53.20
    abdominal Q53.211
    perineal Q53.22
  unilateral Q53.10
    abdominal Q53.111
    perineal Q53.12
Maldevelopment —see also
  Anomaly
  brain Q07.9
  colon Q43.9
  hip Q74.2
    congenital dislocation Q65.2
      bilateral Q65.1
      unilateral Q65.0-
  mastoid process Q75.8
  middle ear Q16.4
    except ossicles Q16.4
    ossicles Q16.3
  ossicles Q16.3
  spine Q76.49
  toe Q74.2
Male type pelvis Q74.2
  with disproportion (fetopelvic) O33.3
    causing obstructed labor O65.3
Malformation (congenital) —see also Anomaly
  adrenal gland Q89.1
  affecting multiple systems with skeletal changes NEC Q87.5
  alimentary tract Q45.9
    specified type NEC Q45.8
    upper Q40.9
      specified type NEC Q40.8
  aorta Q25.40
    absence Q25.41
    aneurysm, congenital Q25.43
    aplasia Q25.41
    atresia Q25.29
      aortic arch Q25.21
    coarctation (preductal) (postductal) Q25.1
    dilatation, congenital Q25.44
    hypoplasia Q25.42
    patent ductus arteriosus Q25.0
    specified type NEC Q25.49
    stenosis Q25.1
      supravalvular Q25.3
  aortic valve Q23.9
    specified NEC Q23.8
  arteriovenous, aneurysmatic (congenital) Q27.30
    brain Q28.2
      ruptured I60.8
        intracerebral I61.8
        intraparenchymal I61.8
        intraventricular I61.5
        subarachnoid I60.8
    cerebral (see also Malformation, arteriovenous, brain) Q28.2
    peripheral Q27.30
      digestive system —see Angiodysplasia
        congenital Q27.33
      lower limb Q27.32

Malformation (continued)
  arteriovenous, aneurysmatic (continued)
    peripheral (continued)
      other specified site Q27.39
      renal vessel Q27.34
      upper limb Q27.31
    precerebral vessels (nonruptured) Q28.0
  auricle
    ear (congenital) Q17.3
      acquired H61.119
        left H61.112
          with right H61.113
        right H61.111
          with left H61.113
  bile duct Q44.5
  bladder Q64.79
    aplasia Q64.5
    diverticulum Q64.6
    exstrophy —see Exstrophy, bladder
    neck obstruction Q64.31
  bone Q79.9
    face Q75.9
      specified type NEC Q75.8
    skull Q75.9
      specified type NEC Q75.8
  brain (multiple) Q04.9
    arteriovenous Q28.2
    specified type NEC Q04.8
  branchial cleft Q18.2
  breast Q83.9
    specified type NEC Q83.8
  broad ligament Q50.6
  bronchus Q32.4
  bursa Q79.9
  cardiac
    chambers Q20.9
      specified type NEC Q20.8
    septum Q21.9
      specified type NEC Q21.8
  cerebral Q04.9
    vessels Q28.3
  cervix uteri Q51.9
    specified type NEC Q51.828
  Chiari
    Type I G93.5
    Type II Q07.01
  choroid (congenital) Q14.3
    plexus Q07.8
  circulatory system Q28.9
  cochlea Q16.5
  cornea Q13.4
  coronary vessels Q24.5
  corpus callosum (congenital) Q04.0
  diaphragm Q79.1
  digestive system NEC, specified type NEC Q45.8
  dura Q07.9
    brain Q04.9
    spinal Q06.9
  ear Q17.9
    causing impairment of hearing Q16.9
    external Q17.9
      accessory auricle Q17.0
      causing impairment of hearing Q16.9
        absence of
          auditory canal Q16.1
          auricle Q16.0
      macrotia Q17.1
      microtia Q17.2
      misplacement Q17.4
      misshapen NEC Q17.3
      prominence Q17.5
      specified type NEC Q17.8

Malformation (continued)
  ear (continued)
    inner Q16.5
    middle Q16.4
      absence of eustachian tube Q16.2
      ossicles (fusion) Q16.3
    ossicles Q16.3
    specified type NEC Q17.8
  epididymis Q55.4
  esophagus Q39.9
    specified type NEC Q39.8
  eye Q15.9
    lid Q10.3
    specified NEC Q15.8
  fallopian tube Q50.6
  genital organ —see Anomaly, genitalia
  great
    artery Q25.9
      aorta —see Malformation, aorta
      pulmonary artery —see Malformation, pulmonary, artery
      specified type NEC Q25.8
    vein Q26.9
      anomalous
        portal venous connection Q26.5
        pulmonary venous connection Q26.4
          partial Q26.3
          total Q26.2
      persistent left superior vena cava Q26.1
      portal vein-hepatic artery fistula Q26.6
      specified type NEC Q26.8
      vena cava stenosis, congenital Q26.0
  gum Q38.6
  hair Q84.2
  heart Q24.9
    specified type NEC Q24.8
  integument Q84.9
    specified type NEC Q84.8
  internal ear Q16.5
  intestine Q43.9
    specified type NEC Q43.8
  iris Q13.2
  joint Q74.9
    ankle Q74.2
    lumbosacral Q76.49
    sacroiliac Q74.2
    specified type NEC Q74.8
  kidney Q63.9
    accessory Q63.0
    giant Q63.3
    horseshoe Q63.1
    hydronephrosis Q62.0
    malposition Q63.2
    specified type NEC Q63.8
  lacrimal apparatus Q10.6
  lip Q38.0
  lingual Q38.3
  liver Q44.70
  lung Q33.9
  meninges or membrane (congenital) Q07.9
    cerebral Q04.8
    spinal (cord) Q06.9
  middle ear Q16.4
    ossicles Q16.3
  mitral valve Q23.9
    specified NEC Q23.8
  Mondini's (congenital) (malformation, cochlea) Q16.5
  mouth (congenital) Q38.6
  multiple types NEC Q89.7
  musculoskeletal system Q79.9

Malformation (continued)
  myocardium Q24.8
  nail Q84.6
  nervous system (central) Q07.9
  nose Q30.9
    specified type NEC Q30.8
  optic disc Q14.2
  orbit Q10.7
  ovary Q50.39
  palate Q38.5
  parathyroid gland Q89.2
  pelvic organs or tissues NEC
    in pregnancy or childbirth O34.8-
      causing obstructed labor O65.5
  penis Q55.69
    aplasia Q55.5
    curvature (lateral) Q55.61
    hypoplasia Q55.62
  pericardium Q24.8
  peripheral vascular system Q27.9
    specified type NEC Q27.8
  pharynx Q38.8
  precerebral vessels Q28.1
  prostate Q55.4
  pulmonary
    arteriovenous Q25.72
    artery Q25.9
      atresia Q25.5
      specified type NEC Q25.79
      stenosis Q25.6
    valve Q22.3
  renal artery Q27.2
  respiratory system Q34.9
  retina Q14.1
  scrotum —see Malformation, testis and scrotum
  seminal vesicles Q55.4
  sense organs NEC Q07.9
  skin Q82.9
  specified NEC Q89.8
  spinal
    cord Q06.9
    nerve root Q07.8
  spine Q76.49
    kyphosis —see Kyphosis, congenital
    lordosis —see Lordosis, congenital
  spleen Q89.09
  stomach Q40.3
    specified type NEC Q40.2
  teeth, tooth K00.9
  tendon Q79.9
  testis and scrotum Q55.20
    aplasia Q55.0
    hypoplasia Q55.1
    polyorchism Q55.21
    retractile testis Q55.22
    scrotal transposition Q55.23
    specified NEC Q55.29
  throat Q38.8
  thorax, bony Q76.9
  thyroid gland Q89.2
  tongue (congenital) Q38.3
    hypertrophy Q38.2
    tie Q38.1
  trachea Q32.1
  tricuspid valve Q22.9
    specified type NEC Q22.8
  umbilical cord NEC (complicating delivery) O69.89
  umbilicus Q89.9
  ureter Q62.8
    agenesis Q62.4
    duplication Q62.5
    malposition —see Malposition, congenital, ureter

Malformation (continued)
  ureter (continued)
    obstructive defect —see Defect, obstructive, ureter
    vesico-uretero-renal reflux Q62.7
  urethra Q64.79
    aplasia Q64.5
    duplication Q64.74
    posterior valves Q64.2
    prolapse Q64.71
    stricture Q64.32
  urinary system Q64.9
  uterus Q51.9
    specified type NEC Q51.818
  vagina Q52.4
  vascular system, peripheral Q27.9
  vas deferens Q55.4
    atresia Q55.3
  venous —see Anomaly, vein(s)
  vulva Q52.70

Malfunction —see also Dysfunction
  cardiac electronic device T82.119
    electrode T82.110
    pulse generator T82.111
    specified type NEC T82.118
  catheter device NEC T85.618
    cystostomy T83.010
    dialysis (renal) (vascular) T82.41
      intraperitoneal T85.611
    infusion NEC T82.514
      cranial (see also Complication(s), catheter, cranial infusion, mechanical) T85.690
      epidural (see also Complication(s), catheter, cranial infusion, mechanical) T85.690
      intrathecal (see also Complication(s), catheter, cranial infusion, mechanical) T85.690
      spinal (see also Complication(s), catheter, cranial infusion, mechanical) T85.690
      subarachnoid (see also Complication(s), catheter, cranial infusion, mechanical) T85.690
      subdural (see also Complication(s), catheter, cranial infusion, mechanical) T85.690
    urinary (see also Breakdown, device, catheter), T83.018
  colostomy K94.03
    valve K94.03
  cystostomy (stoma) N99.512
    catheter T83.010
  enteric stoma K94.13
  enterostomy K94.13
  esophagostomy K94.33
  gastroenteric K31.89
  gastrostomy K94.23
  ileostomy K94.13
    valve K94.13
  intrathecal infusion pump T85.615
  jejunostomy K94.13
  nervous system device, implant or graft, specified NEC T85.615
  pacemaker —see Malfunction, cardiac electronic device
  prosthetic device, internal —see Complications, prosthetic device, by site, mechanical
  tracheostomy J95.03

Malfunction (continued)
  urinary device NEC —see Complication, genitourinary, device, urinary, mechanical
  valve
    colostomy K94.03
    heart T82.09
    ileostomy K94.13
  vascular graft or shunt NEC —see Complication, cardiovascular device, mechanical, vascular
  ventricular (communicating shunt) T85.01

Malherbe's tumor —see Neoplasm, skin, benign

Malibu disease L98.8

Malignancy —see also Neoplasm, malignant, by site
  unspecified site (primary) C80.1

Malignant —see condition

Malingerer, malingering Z76.5

Mallet finger (acquired) —see Deformity, finger, mallet finger
  congenital Q74.0
  sequelae of rickets E64.3

Malleus A24.0

Mallory's bodies R89.7

Mallory-Weiss syndrome K22.6

Malnutrition E46
  degree
    first E44.1
      mild (protein) E44.1
      moderate (protein) E44.0
    second E44.0
    severe (protein-energy) E43
      intermediate form E42
        with
          kwashiorkor E42
          marasmus E41
    third E43
  following gastrointestinal surgery K91.2
  intrauterine
    light-for-dates —see Light for dates
    small-for-dates —see Small for dates
  lack of care, or neglect (child) (infant) T76.02
    confirmed T74.02
  malignant E40
  protein E46
    calorie E46
      mild E44.1
      moderate E44.0
      severe E43
        intermediate form E42
          with
            kwashiorkor (and marasmus) E42
            marasmus E41
    energy E46
      mild E44.1
      moderate E44.0
      severe E43
        intermediate form E42
          with
            kwashiorkor (and marasmus) E42
            marasmus E41
  severe (protein-energy) E43
    with
      kwashiorkor (and marasmus) E42
      marasmus E41

Malocclusion (teeth) M26.4
  Angle's M26.219
    class I M26.211
    class II M26.212
    class III M26.213
  due to
    abnormal swallowing M26.59
    mouth breathing M26.59
    tongue, lip or finger habits M26.59
  temporomandibular (joint) M26.69

Malposition
  cervix —see Malposition, uterus
  congenital
    adrenal (gland) Q89.1
    alimentary tract Q45.8
      lower Q43.8
      upper Q40.8
    aorta Q25.49
    appendix Q43.8
    arterial trunk Q20.0
    artery (peripheral) Q27.8
      coronary Q24.5
      digestive system Q27.8
      lower limb Q27.8
      pulmonary Q25.79
      specified site NEC Q27.8
      upper limb Q27.8
    auditory canal Q17.8
      causing impairment of hearing Q16.9
    auricle (ear) Q17.4
      causing impairment of hearing Q16.9
      cervical Q18.2
    biliary duct or passage Q44.5
    bladder (mucosa) —see Exstrophy, bladder
    brachial plexus Q07.8
    brain tissue Q04.8
    breast Q83.8
    bronchus Q32.4
    cecum Q43.8
    clavicle Q74.0
    colon Q43.8
    digestive organ or tract NEC Q45.8
      lower Q43.8
      upper Q40.8
    ear (auricle) (external) Q17.4
      ossicles Q16.3
    endocrine (gland) NEC Q89.2
    epiglottis Q31.8
    eustachian tube Q17.8
    eye Q15.8
    facial features Q18.8
    fallopian tube Q50.6
    finger(s) Q68.1
      supernumerary Q69.0
    foot Q66.9-
    gallbladder Q44.1
    gastrointestinal tract Q45.8
    genitalia, genital organ(s) or tract
      female Q52.8
        external Q52.79
        internal NEC Q52.8
      male Q55.8
    glottis Q31.8
    hand Q68.1
    heart Q24.8
      dextrocardia Q24.0
        with complete transposition of viscera Q89.3
    hepatic duct Q44.5
    hip (joint) Q65.89
    intestine (large) (small) Q43.8
      with anomalous adhesions, fixation or malrotation Q43.3
    joint NEC Q68.8
    kidney Q63.2
    larynx Q31.8

Malposition (continued)
  congenital (continued)
    limb Q68.8
      lower Q68.8
      upper Q68.8
    liver Q44.79
    lung (lobe) Q33.8
    nail(s) Q84.6
    nerve Q07.8
    nervous system NEC Q07.8
    nose, nasal (septum) Q30.8
    organ or site not listed —see Anomaly, by site
    ovary Q50.39
    pancreas Q45.3
    parathyroid (gland) Q89.2
    patella Q74.1
    peripheral vascular system Q27.8
    pituitary (gland) Q89.2
    respiratory organ or system NEC Q34.8
    rib (cage) Q76.6
      supernumerary in cervical region Q76.5
    scapula Q74.0
    shoulder Q74.0
    spinal cord Q06.8
    spleen Q89.09
    sternum NEC Q76.7
    stomach Q40.2
    symphysis pubis Q74.2
    thymus (gland) Q89.2
    thyroid (gland) (tissue) Q89.2
      cartilage Q31.8
    toe(s) Q66.9-
      supernumerary Q69.2
    tongue Q38.3
    trachea Q32.1
    ureter Q62.60
      deviation Q62.61
      displacement Q62.62
      ectopia Q62.63
      specified type NEC Q62.69
    uterus Q51.818
    vein(s) (peripheral) Q27.8
      great Q26.8
    vena cava (inferior) (superior) Q26.8
  device, implant or graft (see also Complications, by site and type, mechanical) T85.628
    arterial graft NEC —see Complication, cardiovascular device, mechanical, vascular
    breast (implant) T85.42
    catheter NEC T85.628
      cystostomy T83.020
      dialysis (renal) T82.42
        intraperitoneal T85.621
      infusion NEC T82.524
        spinal (epidural) (subdural) T85.620
      urinary (see also Displacement, device, catheter, urinary), T83.028
    electronic (electrode) (pulse generator) (stimulator)
      bone T84.320
      cardiac T82.129
        electrode T82.120
        pulse generator T82.121
        specified type NEC T82.128
      nervous system —see Complication, prosthetic device, mechanical, electronic nervous system stimulator
    urinary —see Complication, genitourinary, device, urinary, mechanical

Malposition (continued)
  device, implant or graft (continued)
    fixation, internal (orthopedic)
      NEC —see Complication,
      fixation device, mechanical
    gastrointestinal —see
      Complications, prosthetic
      device, mechanical,
      gastrointestinal device
    genital NEC T83.428
      intrauterine contraceptive
        device (string) T83.32
      penile prosthesis (cylinder)
        (implanted) (pump)
        (resevoir) T83.420
      testicular prosthesis T83.421
    heart NEC —see Complication,
      cardiovascular device,
      mechanical
    joint prosthesis —see
      Complication, joint prosthesis,
      mechanical
    ocular NEC —see Complications,
      prosthetic device, mechanical,
      ocular device
    orthopedic NEC —see
      Complication, orthopedic,
      device, mechanical
    specified NEC T85.628
    urinary NEC —see also
      Complication, genitourinary,
      device, urinary, mechanical
      graft T83.22
    vascular NEC —see
      Complication, cardiovascular
      device, mechanical
    ventricular intracranial shunt
      T85.02
  fetus —see Pregnancy, complicated
    by (management affected by),
    presentation, fetal
  gallbladder K82.8
  gastrointestinal tract, congenital
    Q45.8
  heart, congenital NEC Q24.8
  joint prosthesis —see
    Complications, joint prosthesis,
    mechanical, displacement, by site
  stomach K31.89
    congenital Q40.2
  tooth, teeth, fully erupted M26.30
  uterus (acute) (acquired) (adherent)
    (asymptomatic) (postinfectional)
    (postpartal, old) N85.4
    anteflexion or anteversion N85.4
      congenital Q51.818
    flexion N85.4
      lateral —see Lateroversion,
        uterus
    inversion N85.5
    lateral (flexion) (version) —see
      Lateroversion, uterus
    in pregnancy or childbirth —
      see subcategory O34.5
    retroflexion or retroversion —see
      Retroversion, uterus

Malposture R29.3

Malrotation
  cecum Q43.3
  colon Q43.3
  intestine Q43.3
  kidney Q63.2

Maltreatment
  adult
    abandonment
      confirmed T74.01
      suspected T76.01
    bullying
      confirmed T74.31
      suspected T76.31

Maltreatment (continued)
  adult (continued)
    confirmed T74.91
    financial
      confirmed T74.A1
      suspected T76.31
    history of Z91.419
    intimidation (through social media)
      confirmed T74.31
      suspected T76.31
    neglect
      confirmed T74.01
      suspected T76.01
    physical abuse
      confirmed T74.11
      suspected T76.11
    psychological abuse
      confirmed T74.31
      suspected T76.31
      history of Z91.411
    sexual abuse
      confirmed T74.21
      suspected T76.21
    suspected T76.91
    threatened abuse (harm) (physical
      violence) (sexual abuse)
      confirmed T74.31
      suspected T76.31
  child
    abandonment
      confirmed T74.02
      suspected T76.02
    bullying
      confirmed T74.32
      suspected T76.32
    confirmed T74.92
    financial
      confirmed T74.A2
      suspected T76.A2
    history of —see History,
      personal (of), abuse
    intimidation (through social media)
      confirmed T74.32
      suspected T76.32
    neglect
      confirmed T74.02
      history of —see History,
        personal (of), abuse
      suspected T76.02
    physical abuse
      confirmed T74.12
      history of —see History,
        personal (of), abuse
      suspected T76.12
    psychological abuse
      confirmed T74.32
      history of —see History,
        personal (of), abuse
      suspected T76.32
    sexual abuse
      confirmed T74.22
      history of —see History,
        personal (of), abuse
      suspected T76.22
    suspected T76.92
    threatened abuse (harm)
      (physical violence) (sexual
      abuse)
      confirmed T74.32
      suspected T76.32
  personal history of Z91.89

Malta fever —see Brucellosis

Maltworker's lung J67.4

Malunion, fracture —see Fracture, by site

Mammillitis N61.0
  puerperal, postpartum O91.02

Mammitis —see Mastitis

Mammogram (examination) Z12.39
  routine Z12.31

Mammoplasia N62

Management (of)
  bone conduction hearing device
    (implanted) Z45.320
  cardiac pacemaker NEC Z45.018
  cerebrospinal fluid drainage device
    Z45.41
  cochlear device (implanted) Z45.321
  contraceptive Z30.9
    specified NEC Z30.8
  implanted device Z45.9
    specified NEC Z45.89
  infusion pump Z45.1
  procreative Z31.9
    male factor infertility in female
      Z31.81
    specified NEC Z31.89
  prosthesis (external) (see also
    Fitting) Z44.9
    implanted Z45.9
      specified NEC Z45.89
  renal dialysis catheter Z49.01
  vascular access device Z45.2

Mangled —see specified injury by site

Mania (monopolar) —see also
  Disorder, mood, manic episode
  with psychotic symptoms F30.2
  without psychotic symptoms F30.10
    mild F30.11
    moderate F30.12
    severe F30.13
  Bell's F30.8
  chronic (recurrent) F31.89
  hysterical F44.89
  puerperal F30.8
  recurrent F31.89

Manic depression F31.9

Manic-depressive insanity, psychosis, or syndrome —see Disorder, bipolar

Mannosidosis E77.1

Mansonelliasis, mansonellosis B74.4

Manson's
  disease B65.1
  schistosomiasis B65.1

Manual —see condition

Maple-bark-stripper's lung (disease) J67.6

Maple-syrup-urine disease E71.0

Marable's syndrome (celiac artery compression) I77.4

Marasmus E41
  due to malnutrition E41
  intestinal E41
  nutritional E41
  senile R54
  tuberculous NEC —see Tuberculosis

Marble
  bones Q78.2
  skin R23.8

Marburg virus disease A98.3

March
  fracture —see Fracture, traumatic, stress, by site
  hemoglobinuria D59.6

Marchesani (-Weill) **syndrome** Q87.0

Marchiafava (-Bignami) **syndrome or disease** G37.1

Marchiafava-Micheli syndrome D59.5

Marcus Gunn's syndrome Q07.8

Marfan syndrome —see Syndrome, Marfan

Marie-Bamberger disease —see Osteoarthropathy, hypertrophic, specified NEC

Marie-Charcot-Tooth neuropathic muscular atrophy G60.0

Marie's
  cerebellar ataxia (late-onset) G11.2
  disease or syndrome (acromegaly) E22.0

Marie-Strümpell arthritis, disease or spondylitis —see Spondylitis, ankylosing

Marion's disease (bladder neck obstruction) N32.0

Marital conflict Z63.0

Mark
  port wine Q82.5
  raspberry Q82.5
  strawberry Q82.5
  stretch L90.6
  tattoo L81.8

Marker heterochromatin —see Extra, marker chromosomes

Maroteaux-Lamy syndrome (mild) (severe) E76.29

Marrow (bone)
  arrest D61.9
  poor function D75.89

Marseilles fever A77.1

Marsh fever —see Malaria

Marshall's (hidrotic) **ectodermal dysplasia** Q82.4

Marsh's disease (exophthalmic goiter) E05.00
  with storm E05.01

Masculinization (female) **with adrenal hyperplasia** E25.9
  congenital E25.0

Masculinovoblastoma D27.-

Masochism (sexual) F65.51

Mason's lung J62.8

Mass
  abdominal R19.00
    epigastric R19.06
    generalized R19.07
    left lower quadrant R19.04
    left upper quadrant R19.02
    periumbilic R19.05
    right lower quadrant R19.03
    right upper quadrant R19.01
    specified site NEC R19.09
  breast (see also Lump, breast) N63.0
  chest R22.2
  cystic —see Cyst
  ear H93.8-
  head R22.0
  intra-abdominal (diffuse)
    (generalized) —see Mass, abdominal
  kidney N28.89
  liver R16.0
  localized (skin) R22.9
    chest R22.2
    head R22.0
    limb
      lower R22.4-
      upper R22.3-
    neck R22.1
    trunk R22.2

Mass (continued)
 lung R91.8
 malignant —see Neoplasm, malignant, by site
 neck R22.1
 pelvic (diffuse) (generalized) —see Mass, abdominal
 specified organ NEC —see Disease, by site
 splenic R16.1
 substernal thyroid —see Goiter
 superficial (localized) R22.9
 umbilical (diffuse) (generalized) R19.09

Massive —see condition

Mast cell
 disease, systemic tissue D47.02
 neoplasm
  malignant C96.20
   specified type NEC C96.29
  of uncertain behavior NEC D47.09
 leukemia C94.3-
 sarcoma C96.22
 tumor D47.09

Mastalgia N64.4

Masters-Allen syndrome N83.8

Mastitis (acute) (diffuse) (nonpuerperal) (subacute) N61.0
 with abscess N61.1
 chronic (cystic) —see Mastopathy, cystic
 cystic (Schimmelbusch's type) —see Mastopathy, cystic
 fibrocystic —see Mastopathy, cystic
 granulomatous N61.2-
 infective N61.0
  newborn P39.0
 interstitial, gestational or puerperal —see Mastitis, obstetric
 neonatal (noninfective) P83.4
  infective P39.0
 obstetric (interstitial) (nonpurulent)
  associated with
   lactation O91.23
   pregnancy O91.21-
   puerperium O91.22
  purulent
   associated with
    lactation O91.13
    pregnancy O91.11-
    puerperium O91.12
 periductal —see Ectasia, mammary duct
 phlegmonous —see Mastopathy, cystic
 plasma cell —see Ectasia, mammary duct
 without abscess N61.0

Mastocytoma (extracutaneous) D47.09
 malignant C96.29
 solitary D47.01

Mastocytosis D47.09
 aggressive systemic C96.21
 cutaneous (diffuse) (maculopapular) D47.01
  congenital Q82.2
  of neonatal onset Q82.2
  of newborn onset Q82.2
 indolent systemic D47.02
 isolated bone marrow D47.02
 malignant C96.29
 systemic (indolent) (smoldering)
  with an associated hematological non-mast cell lineage disease (SM-AHNMD) D47.02

Mastodynia N64.4

Mastoid —see condition

Mastoidalgia —see subcategory H92.0

Mastoiditis (coalescent) (hemorrhagic) (suppurative) H70.9-
 acute, subacute H70.00-
  complicated NEC H70.09-
  subperiosteal H70.01-
 chronic (necrotic) (recurrent) H70.1-
 in (due to)
  infectious disease NEC B99 [H75.0-]
  parasitic disease NEC B89 [H75.0-]
  tuberculosis A18.03
 petrositis —see Petrositis
 postauricular fistula —see Fistula, postauricular
 specified NEC H70.89-
 tuberculous A18.03

Mastopathy, mastopathia N64.9
 chronica cystica —see Mastopathy, cystic
 cystic (chronic) (diffuse) N60.1-
  with epithelial proliferation N60.3-
 diffuse cystic —see Mastopathy, cystic
 estrogenic, oestrogenica N64.89
 ovarian origin N64.89

Mastoplasia, mastoplastia N62

Masturbation (excessive) F98.8

Maternal care (for) —see Pregnancy (complicated by) (management affected by)

Matheiu's disease (leptospiral jaundice) A27.0

Mauclaire's disease or osteochondrosis —see Osteochondrosis, juvenile, hand, metacarpal

Maxcy's disease A75.2

Maxilla, maxillary —see condition

May (-Hegglin) **anomaly or syndrome** D72.0

McArdle (-Schmid) (-Pearson) **disease** (glycogen storage) E74.04

McCune-Albright syndrome Q78.1

McQuarrie's syndrome (idiopathic familial hypoglycemia) E16.2

Meadow's syndrome Q86.1

Measles (black) (hemorrhagic) (suppressed) B05.9
 with
  complications NEC B05.89
  encephalitis B05.0
  intestinal complications B05.4
  keratitis (keratoconjunctivitis) B05.81
  meningitis B05.1
  otitis media B05.3
  pneumonia B05.2
 French —see Rubella
 German —see Rubella
 Liberty —see Rubella

Meatitis, urethral —see Urethritis

Meatus, meatal —see condition

Meat-wrappers' asthma J68.9

ME/CFS (myalgic encephalomyelitis/chronic fatigue syndrome) G93.32

Meckel-Gruber syndrome Q61.9

Meckel's diverticulitis, diverticulum (displaced) (hypertrophic) Q43.0
 malignant —see Table of Neoplasms, small intestine, malignant

Meconium
 ileus, newborn P76.0
  in cystic fibrosis E84.11
  meaning meconium plug (without cystic fibrosis) P76.0
 obstruction, newborn P76.0
  due to fecaliths P76.0
  in mucoviscidosis E84.11
 peritonitis P78.0
 plug syndrome (newborn) NEC P76.0

MED13L (mediator complex subunit 13L) **syndrome** Q87.85

Median —see also condition
 arcuate ligament syndrome I77.4
 bar (prostate) (vesical orifice) —see Hyperplasia, prostate
 rhomboid glossitis K14.2

Mediastinal shift R93.89

Mediastinitis (acute) (chronic) J98.51
 syphilitic A52.73
 tuberculous A15.8

Mediastinopericarditis —see also Pericarditis
 acute I30.9
 adhesive I31.0
 chronic I31.8
  rheumatic I09.2

Mediastinum, mediastinal —see condition

Mediator complex subunit 13L (MED13L) **syndrome** Q87.85

Medicine poisoning —see Table of Drugs and Chemicals, by drug, poisoning

Mediterranean
 fever —see Brucellosis
  familial M04.1
  tick A77.1
 kala-azar B55.0
 leishmaniasis B55.0
 tick fever A77.1

Medulla —see condition

Medullary cystic kidney Q61.5

Medullated fibers
 optic (nerve) Q14.8
 retina Q14.1

Medulloblastoma
 desmoplastic C71.6
 specified site —see Neoplasm, malignant, by site
 unspecified site C71.6

Medulloepithelioma —see also Neoplasm, malignant, by site
 teratoid —see Neoplasm, malignant, by site

Medullomyoblastoma
 specified site —see Neoplasm, malignant, by site
 unspecified site C71.6

Meekeren-Ehlers-Danlos syndrome (see also Syndrome, Ehlers-Danlos) Q79.69

Megacolon (acquired) (functional) (not Hirschsprung's disease) (in) K59.39
 Chagas' disease B57.32
 congenital, congenitum (aganglionic) Q43.1
 Hirschsprung's (disease) Q43.1
 toxic NEC K59.31
  due to Clostridium difficile
   not specified as recurrent A04.72
   recurrent A04.71

Megaesophagus (functional) K22.0
 congenital Q39.5
 in (due to) Chagas' disease B57.31

Megalencephaly Q04.5

Megalerythema (epidemic) B08.3

Megaloappendix Q43.8

Megalocephalus, megalocephaly NEC Q75.3

Megalocornea Q15.8
 with glaucoma Q15.0

Megalocytic anemia D53.1

Megalodactylia (fingers) (thumbs) (congenital) Q74.0
 toes Q74.2

Megaloduodenum Q43.8

Megaloesophagus (functional) K22.0
 congenital Q39.5

Megalogastria (acquired) K31.89
 congenital Q40.2

Megalophthalmos Q11.3

Megalopsia H53.15

Megalosplenia —see Splenomegaly

Megaloureter N28.82
 congenital Q62.2

Megarectum K62.89

Megasigmoid K59.39
 congenital Q43.2

Megaureter N28.82
 congenital Q62.2

Megavitamin-B6 syndrome E67.2

Megrim —see Migraine

Meibomian
 cyst, infected —see Hordeolum
 gland —see condition
 sty, stye —see Hordeolum

Meibomitis —see Hordeolum

Meige-Milroy disease (chronic hereditary edema) Q82.0

Meige's syndrome Q82.0

Melalgia, nutritional E53.8

Melancholia F32.A
 climacteric (single episode) F32.89
  recurrent episode F33.8
 hypochondriac F45.29
 intermittent (single episode) F32.89
  recurrent episode F33.8
 involutional (single episode) F32.89
  recurrent episode F33.8
 menopausal (single episode) F32.89
  recurrent episode F33.8
 puerperal F32.89
 reactive (emotional stress or trauma) F32.3
 recurrent F33.9
 senile F03
 stuporous (single episode) F32.89
  recurrent episode F33.8

Melanemia R79.89

Melanoameloblastoma —see Neoplasm, bone, benign

Melanoblastoma —see Melanoma

Melanocarcinoma —see Melanoma

Melanocytoma, eyeball D31.9-

Melanocytosis, neurocutaneous Q82.8

Melanoderma, melanodermia L81.4

Melanodontia, infantile K03.89

Melanodontoclasia K03.89

Melanoepithelioma —see Melanoma

Melanoma (malignant) C43.9
 acral lentiginous, malignant —see Melanoma, skin, by site
 amelanotic —see Melanoma, skin, by site

Melanoma (continued)
 balloon cell —see Melanoma, skin, by site
 benign —see Nevus
 desmoplastic, malignant —see Melanoma, skin, by site
 epithelioid cell —see Melanoma, skin, by site
  with spindle cell, mixed —see Melanoma, skin, by site
 in
  giant pigmented nevus —see Melanoma, skin, by site
  Hutchinson's melanotic freckle —see Melanoma, skin, by site
  junctional nevus —see Melanoma, skin, by site
  precancerous melanosis —see Melanoma, skin, by site
 in situ D03.9
  abdominal wall D03.59
  ala nasi D03.39
  ankle D03.7-
  anus, anal (margin) (skin) D03.51
  arm D03.6-
  auditory canal D03.2-
  auricle (ear) D03.2-
  auricular canal (external) D03.2-
  axilla, axillary fold D03.59
  back D03.59
  breast D03.52
  brow D03.39
  buttock D03.59
  canthus (eye) D03.1-
  cheek (external) D03.39
  chest wall D03.59
  chin D03.39
  choroid D03.8
  conjunctiva D03.8
  ear (external) D03.2-
  external meatus (ear) D03.2-
  eye D03.8
  eyebrow D03.39
  eyelid (lower) (upper) D03.1-
  face D03.30
   specified NEC D03.39
  female genital organ (external) NEC D03.8
  finger D03.6-
  flank D03.59
  foot D03.7-
  forearm D03.6-
  forehead D03.39
  foreskin D03.8
  gluteal region D03.59
  groin D03.59
  hand D03.6-
  heel D03.7-
  helix D03.2-
  hip D03.7-
  interscapular region D03.59
  iris D03.8
  jaw D03.39
  knee D03.7-
  labium (majus) (minus) D03.8
  lacrimal gland D03.8
  leg D03.7-
  lip (lower) (upper) D03.0
  lower limb NEC D03.7-
  male genital organ (external) NEC D03.8
  nail D03.9
   finger D03.6-
   toe D03.7-
  neck D03.4
  nose (external) D03.39
  orbit D03.8
  penis D03.8

Melanoma (continued)
 in situ (continued)
  perianal skin D03.51
  perineum D03.51
  pinna D03.2-
  popliteal fossa or space D03.7-
  prepuce D03.8
  pudendum D03.8
  retina D03.8
  retrobulbar D03.8
  scalp D03.4
  scrotum D03.8
  shoulder D03.6-
  specified site NEC D03.8
  submammary fold D03.52
  temple D03.39
  thigh D03.7-
  toe D03.7-
  trunk NEC D03.59
  umbilicus D03.59
  upper limb NEC D03.6-
  vulva D03.8
 juvenile —see Nevus
 malignant, of soft parts except skin —see Neoplasm, connective tissue, malignant
 metastatic
  breast C79.81
  genital organ C79.82
  specified site NEC C79.89
 neurotropic, malignant —see Melanoma, skin, by site
 nodular —see Melanoma, skin, by site
 regressing, malignant —see Melanoma, skin, by site
 skin C43.9
  abdominal wall C43.59
  ala nasi C43.31
  ankle C43.7-
  anus, anal (skin) C43.51
  arm C43.6-
  auditory canal (external) C43.2-
  auricle (ear) C43.2-
  auricular canal (external) C43.2-
  axilla, axillary fold C43.59
  back C43.59
  breast (female) (male) C43.52
  brow C43.39
  buttock C43.59
  canthus (eye) C43.1-
  cheek (external) C43.39
  chest wall C43.59
  chin C43.39
  ear (external) C43.2-
  elbow C43.6-
  external meatus (ear) C43.2-
  eyebrow C43.39
  eyelid (lower) (upper) C43.1-
  face C43.30
   specified NEC C43.39
  female genital organ (external) NEC C51.9
  finger C43.6-
  flank C43.59
  foot C43.7-
  forearm C43.6-
  forehead C43.39
  foreskin C60.0
  glabella C43.39
  gluteal region C43.59
  groin C43.59
  hand C43.6-
  heel C43.7-
  helix C43.2-
  hip C43.7-
  interscapular region C43.59
  jaw (external) C43.39
  knee C43.7-

Melanoma (continued)
 skin (continued)
  labium C51.9
   majus C51.0
   minus C51.1
  leg C43.7-
  lip (lower) (upper) C43.0
  lower limb NEC C43.7-
  male genital organ (external) NEC C63.9
  nail
   finger C43.6-
   toe C43.7-
  nasolabial groove C43.39
  nates C43.59
  neck C43.4
  nose (external) C43.31
  overlapping site C43.8
  palpebra C43.1-
  penis C60.9
  perianal skin C43.51
  perineum C43.51
  pinna C43.2-
  popliteal fossa or space C43.7-
  prepuce C60.0
  pudendum C51.9
  scalp C43.4
  scrotum C63.2
  shoulder C43.6-
  skin NEC C43.9
  submammary fold C43.52
  temple C43.39
  thigh C43.7-
  toe C43.7-
  trunk NEC C43.59
  umbilicus C43.59
  upper limb NEC C43.6-
  vulva C51.9
   overlapping sites C51.8
 spindle cell
  with epithelioid, mixed —see Melanoma, skin, by site
  type A C69.4-
  type B C69.4-
 superficial spreading —see Melanoma, skin, by site

Melanosarcoma —see also Melanoma
 epithelioid cell —see Melanoma

Melanosis L81.4
 addisonian E27.1
  tuberculous A18.7
 adrenal E27.1
 colon K63.89
 conjunctiva —see Pigmentation, conjunctiva
 cornea (presenile) (senile) —see also Pigmentation, cornea
  congenital Q13.4
 eye NEC H57.89
  congenital Q15.8
 lenticularis progressiva Q82.1
 liver K76.89
 precancerous —see also Melanoma, in situ
  malignant melanoma in —see Melanoma
 Riehl's L81.4
 sclera H15.89
  congenital Q13.89
 suprarenal E27.1
 tar L81.4
 toxic L81.4

Melanuria R82.998

MELAS syndrome E88.41

Melasma L81.1
 adrenal (gland) E27.1
 suprarenal (gland) E27.1

Melena K92.1
 with ulcer - code by site under Ulcer, with hemorrhage K27.4
 due to swallowed maternal blood P78.2
 newborn, neonatal P54.1
  due to swallowed maternal blood P78.2

Meleney's
 gangrene (cutaneous) —see Ulcer, skin
 ulcer (chronic undermining) —see Ulcer, skin

Melioidosis A24.9
 acute A24.1
 chronic A24.2
 fulminating A24.1
 pneumonia A24.1
 pulmonary (chronic) A24.2
  acute A24.1
  subacute A24.2
 sepsis A24.1
 specified NEC A24.3
 subacute A24.2

Melitensis, febris A23.0

Melkersson (-Rosenthal) **syndrome** G51.2

Mellitus, diabetes —see Diabetes

Melorheostosis (bone) —see Disorder, bone, density and structure, specified NEC

Meloschisis Q18.4

Melotia Q17.4

Membrana
 capsularis lentis posterior Q13.89
 epipapillaris Q14.2

Membranacea placenta O43.19-

Membranaceous uterus N85.8

Membrane(s), **membranous** —see also condition
 cyclitic —see Membrane, pupillary
 folds, congenital —see Web
 Jackson's Q43.3
 over face of newborn P28.9
 premature rupture —see Rupture, membranes, premature
 pupillary H21.4-
  persistent Q13.89
 retained (with hemorrhage) (complicating delivery) O72.2
  without hemorrhage O73.1
 secondary cataract —see Cataract, secondary
 unruptured (causing asphyxia) —see Asphyxia, newborn
 vitreous —see Opacity, vitreous, membranes and strands

Membranitis —see Chorioamnionitis

Memory disturbance, lack or loss —see also Amnesia
 mild, following organic brain damage F06.8

Menadione deficiency E56.1

Menarche
 delayed E30.0
 precocious E30.1

Mendacity, pathologic F60.2

Mendelson's syndrome (due to anesthesia) J95.4
 in labor and delivery O74.0
 in pregnancy O29.01-
 obstetric O74.0
 postpartum, puerperal O89.01

Ménétrier's disease or syndrome K29.60
- with bleeding K29.61

Ménière's disease, syndrome or vertigo H81.0-

Meninges, meningeal —*see* condition

Meningioma —*see also* Neoplasm, meninges, benign
- angioblastic —*see* Neoplasm, meninges, benign
- angiomatous —*see* Neoplasm, meninges, benign
- atypical —*see* Neoplasm, meninges, uncertain behavior
- endotheliomatous —*see* Neoplasm, meninges, benign
- fibroblastic —*see* Neoplasm, meninges, benign
- fibrous —*see* Neoplasm, meninges, benign
- hemangioblastic —*see* Neoplasm, meninges, benign
- hemangiopericytic —*see* Neoplasm, meninges, benign
- malignant —*see* Neoplasm, meninges, malignant
- meningiothelial —*see* Neoplasm, meninges, benign
- meningotheliomatous —*see* Neoplasm, meninges, benign
- mixed —*see* Neoplasm, meninges, benign
- multiple —*see* Neoplasm, meninges, uncertain behavior
- papillary —*see* Neoplasm, meninges, uncertain behavior
- psammomatous —*see* Neoplasm, meninges, benign
- syncytial —*see* Neoplasm, meninges, benign
- transitional —*see* Neoplasm, meninges, benign

Meningiomatosis (diffuse) —*see* Neoplasm, meninges, uncertain behavior

Meningism —*see* Meningismus

Meningismus (infectional) (pneumococcal) R29.1
- due to serum or vaccine R29.1
- influenzal —*see* Influenza, with, manifestations NEC

Meningitis (basal) (basic) (brain) (cerebral) (cervical) (congestive) (diffuse) (hemorrhagic) (infantile) (membranous) (metastatic) (nonspecific) (pontine) (progressive) (simple) (spinal) (subacute) (sympathetic) (toxic) G03.9
- abacterial G03.0
- actinomycotic A42.81
- adenoviral A87.1
- arbovirus A87.8
- aseptic (acute) G03.0
- bacterial G00.9
  - Escherichia coli (E. coli) G00.8
  - Friedländer (bacillus) G00.8
  - gram-negative G00.9
  - H. influenzae G00.0
  - Klebsiella G00.8
  - pneumococcal G00.1
  - specified organism NEC G00.8
  - staphylococcal G00.3
  - streptococcal (acute) G00.2
- benign recurrent (Mollaret) G03.2
- candidal B37.5
- caseous (tuberculous) A17.0

Meningitis (continued)
- cerebrospinal A39.0
- chronic NEC G03.1
- clear cerebrospinal fluid NEC G03.0
- coxsackievirus A87.0
- cryptococcal B45.1
- diplococcal (gram positive) A39.0
- echovirus A87.0
- enteroviral A87.0
- eosinophilic B83.2
- epidemic NEC A39.0
- Escherichia coli (E. coli) G00.8
- fibrinopurulent G00.9
  - specified organism NEC G00.8
- Friedländer (bacillus) G00.8
- gonococcal A54.81
- gram-negative cocci G00.9
- gram-positive cocci G00.9
- Haemophilus (influenzae) G00.0
- H. influenzae G00.0
- in (due to)
  - adenovirus A87.1
  - African trypanosomiasis B56.9 *[G02]*
  - anthrax A22.8
  - bacterial disease NEC A48.8 *[G01]*
  - Chagas' disease (chronic) B57.41
  - chickenpox B01.0
  - coccidioidomycosis B38.4
  - Diplococcus pneumoniae G00.1
  - enterovirus A87.0
  - herpes (simplex) virus B00.3
    - zoster B02.1
  - infectious mononucleosis B27.92
  - leptospirosis A27.81
  - Listeria monocytogenes A32.11
  - Lyme disease A69.21
  - measles B05.1
  - mumps (virus) B26.1
  - neurosyphilis (late) A52.13
  - parasitic disease NEC B89 *[G02]*
  - poliovirus A80.9 *[G02]*
  - preventive immunization, inoculation or vaccination G03.8
  - rubella B06.02
  - Salmonella infection A02.21
  - specified cause NEC G03.8
  - Streptococcal pneumoniae G00.1
  - typhoid fever A01.01
  - varicella B01.0
  - viral disease NEC A87.8
  - whooping cough A37.90
  - zoster B02.1
- infectious G00.9
- influenzal (H. influenzae) G00.0
- Klebsiella G00.8
- leptospiral (aseptic) A27.81
- lymphocytic (acute) (benign) (serous) A87.2
- meningococcal A39.0
- Mima polymorpha G00.8
- Mollaret (benign recurrent) G03.2
- monilial B37.5
- mycotic NEC B49 *[G02]*
- Neisseria A39.0
- nonbacterial G03.0
- nonpyogenic NEC G03.0
- ossificans G96.198
- pneumococcal streptococcus pneumoniae G00.1
- poliovirus A80.9 *[G02]*
- postmeasles B05.1
- purulent G00.9
  - specified organism NEC G00.8
- pyogenic G00.9
  - specified organism NEC G00.8

Meningitis (continued)
- Salmonella (arizonae) (Cholerae-Suis) (enteritidis) (typhimurium) A02.21
- septic G00.9
  - specified organism NEC G00.8
- serosa circumscripta NEC G03.0
- serous NEC G93.2
- specified organism NEC G00.8
- sporotrichosis B42.81
- staphylococcal G00.3
- sterile G03.0
- Streptococcal (acute) G00.2
  - pneumoniae G00.1
- suppurative G00.9
  - specified organism NEC G00.8
- syphilitic (late) (tertiary) A52.13
  - acute A51.41
  - congenital A50.41
  - secondary A51.41
- Torula histolytica (cryptococcal) B45.1
- traumatic (complication of injury) T79.8
- tuberculous A17.0
- typhoid A01.01
- viral NEC A87.9
- Yersinia pestis A20.3

Meningocele (spinal) —*see also* Spina bifida
- with hydrocephalus —*see* Spina bifida, by site, with hydrocephalus
- acquired (traumatic) G96.198
- cerebral —*see* Encephalocele

Meningocerebritis —*see* Meningoencephalitis

Meningococcemia A39.4
- acute A39.2
- chronic A39.3

Meningococcus, meningococcal —*see also* condition A39.9
- adrenalitis, hemorrhagic A39.1
- carrier (suspected) of Z22.31
- meningitis (cerebrospinal) A39.0

Meningoencephalitis (see also Encephalitis) G04.90
- acute NEC (*see also* Encephalitis, viral) A86
- bacterial NEC G04.2
- California A83.5
- diphasic A84.1
- eosinophilic B83.2
- epidemic A39.81
- herpesviral, herpetic B00.4
  - due to herpesvirus 6 B10.01
  - due to herpesvirus 7 B10.09
  - specified NEC B10.09
- in (due to)
  - blastomycosis NEC B40.81
  - diseases classified elsewhere G05.3
  - free-living amebae B60.2
  - Hemophilus influenzae (H .influenzae) G00.0
  - herpes B00.4
    - due to herpesvirus 6 B10.01
    - due to herpesvirus 7 B10.09
    - specified NEC B10.09
  - H. influenzae G00.0
  - Lyme disease A69.22
  - mercury —*see* subcategory T56.1
  - mumps B26.2
  - Naegleria (amebae) (organisms) (fowleri) B60.2
  - Parastrongylus cantonensis B83.2
  - toxoplasmosis (acquired) B58.2
    - congenital P37.1

Meningoencephalitis (continued)
- infectious (acute) (viral) A86
- influenzal (H. influenzae) G00.0
- Listeria monocytogenes A32.12
- lymphocytic (serous) A87.2
- mumps B26.2
- parasitic NEC B89 *[G05.3]*
- pneumococcal G04.2
- primary amebic B60.2
- specific (syphilitic) A52.14
- specified organism NEC G04.81
- staphylococcal G04.2
- streptococcal G04.2
- syphilitic A52.14
- toxic NEC G92.8
  - due to mercury —*see* subcategory T56.1
- tuberculous A17.82
- virus NEC A86

Meningoencephalocele —*see also* Encephalocele
- syphilitic A52.19
- congenital A50.49

Meningoencephalomyelitis —*see also* Meningoencephalitis
- acute NEC (viral) A86
  - disseminated G04.00
    - postimmunization or postvaccination G04.02
    - postinfectious G04.01
- due to
  - actinomycosis A42.82
  - Torula B45.1
  - Toxoplasma or toxoplasmosis (acquired) B58.2
    - congenital P37.1
- postimmunization or postvaccination G04.02

Meningoencephalomyelopathy G96.9

Meningoencephalopathy G96.9

Meningomyelitis —*see also* Meningoencephalitis
- bacterial NEC G04.2
- blastomycotic NEC B40.81
- cryptococcal B45.1
- in diseases classified elsewhere G05.4
- meningococcal A39.81
- syphilitic A52.14
- tuberculous A17.82

Meningomyelocele —*see also* Spina bifida
- syphilitic A52.19

Meningomyeloneuritis —*see* Meningoencephalitis

Meningoradiculitis —*see* Meningitis

Meningovascular —*see* condition

Menkes' disease or syndrome E83.09
- meaning maple-syrup-urine disease E71.0

Menometrorrhagia N92.1

Menopause, menopausal
- (asymptomatic) (state) Z78.0
- arthritis (any site) NEC —*see* Arthritis, specified form NEC
- bleeding N92.4
- depression (single episode) F32.89
  - agitated (single episode) F32.2
    - recurrent episode F33.9
  - psychotic (single episode) F32.89
    - recurrent episode F33.8
  - recurrent episode F33.9
- melancholia (single episode) F32.89
  - recurrent episode F33.8

Menopause, menopausal *(continued)*
  paranoid state F22
  postirradiation (postprocedural)
    asymptomatic E89.40
    symptomatic E89.41
  premature E28.319
    asymptomatic E28.319
      postirradiation E89.40
      postsurgical E89.40
    symptomatic E28.310
      postirradiation E89.41
      postsurgical E89.41
  psychosis NEC F28
  symptomatic N95.1
  toxic polyarthritis NEC —*see* Arthritis, specified form NEC

Menorrhagia (primary) N92.0
  climacteric N92.4
    menopausal N92.4
  menopausal N92.4
  perimenopausal N92.4
  postclimacteric N95.0
  postmenopausal N95.0
  preclimacteric or premenopausal N92.4
  pubertal (menses retained) N92.2

Menostaxis N92.0

Menses, retention N94.89

Menstrual —*see* Menstruation

Menstruation
  absent —*see* Amenorrhea
  anovulatory N97.0
  cycle, irregular N92.6
  delayed N91.0
  disorder N93.9
    psychogenic F45.8
  during pregnancy O20.8
  excessive (with regular cycle) N92.0
    with irregular cycle N92.1
    at puberty N92.2
  frequent N92.0
  infrequent —*see* Oligomenorrhea
  irregular N92.6
    specified NEC N92.5
  latent N92.5
  membranous N92.5
  painful (*see also* Dysmenorrhea) N94.6
    primary N94.4
    psychogenic F45.8
    secondary N94.5
  passage of clots N92.0
  precocious E30.1
  protracted N92.5
  rare —*see* Oligomenorrhea
  retained N94.89
  retrograde N92.5
  scanty —*see* Oligomenorrhea
  suppression N94.89
  vicarious (nasal) N94.89

Mental —*see also* condition
  deficiency —*see* Disability, intellectual
  deterioration —*see* Psychosis
  disorder —*see* Disorder, mental
  exhaustion F48.8
  insufficiency (congenital) —*see* Disability, intellectual
  observation without need for further medical care Z03.89
  retardation —*see* Disability, intellectual
  subnormality —*see* Disability, intellectuall
  upset —*see* Disorder, mental

Meralgia paresthetica G57.1-

Mercurial —*see* condition

Mercurialism —*see* subcategory T56.1

MERRF syndrome (myoclonic epilepsy associated with ragged-red fiber) E88.42

Merkel cell tumor —*see* Carcinoma, Merkel cell

Merocele —*see* Hernia, femoral

Meromelia
  lower limb —*see* Defect, reduction, lower limb
    intercalary
      femur —*see* Defect, reduction, lower limb, specified type NEC
      tibiofibular (complete) (incomplete) —*see* Defect, reduction, lower limb
  upper limb —*see* Defect, reduction, upper limb
    intercalary, humeral, radioulnar —*see* Agenesis, arm, with hand present

Merzbacher-Pelizaeus disease E75.27

Mesaortitis —*see* Aortitis

Mesarteritis —*see* Arteritis

Mesencephalitis —*see* Encephalitis

Mesenchymoma —*see also* Neoplasm, connective tissue, uncertain behavior
  benign —*see* Neoplasm, connective tissue, benign
  malignant —*see* Neoplasm, connective tissue, malignant

Mesenteritis
  retractile K65.4
  sclerosing K65.4

Mesentery, mesenteric —*see* condition

Mesiodens, mesiodentes K00.1

Mesio-occlusion M26.213

Mesocolon —*see* condition

Mesonephroma (malignant) —*see* Neoplasm, malignant, by site
  benign —*see* Neoplasm, benign, by site

Mesophlebitis —*see* Phlebitis

Mesostromal dysgenesia Q13.89

Mesothelioma (malignant) C45.9
  benign
    mesentery D19.1
    mesocolon D19.1
    omentum D19.1
    peritoneum D19.1
    pleura D19.0
    specified site NEC D19.7
    unspecified site D19.9
  biphasic C45.9
    benign
      mesentery D19.1
      mesocolon D19.1
      omentum D19.1
      peritoneum D19.1
      pleura D19.0
      specified site NEC D19.7
      unspecified site D19.9
  cystic D48.4
  epithelioid C45.9
    benign
      mesentery D19.1
      mesocolon D19.1
      omentum D19.1
      peritoneum D19.1

Mesothelioma *(continued)*
  epithelioid *(continued)*
    benign *(continued)*
      pleura D19.0
      specified site NEC D19.7
      unspecified site D19.9
  fibrous C45.9
    benign
      mesentery D19.1
      mesocolon D19.1
      omentum D19.1
      peritoneum D19.1
      pleura D19.0
      specified site NEC D19.7
      unspecified site D19.9
  site classification
    liver C45.7
    lung C45.7
    mediastinum C45.7
    mesentery C45.1
    mesocolon C45.1
    omentum C45.1
    pericardium C45.2
    peritoneum C45.1
    pleura C45.0
      parietal C45.0
    retroperitoneum C45.7
    specified site NEC C45.7
  unspecified C45.9

Metabolic syndrome E88.810

Metagonimiasis B66.8

Metagonimus infestation (intestine) B66.8

Metal
  pigmentation L81.8
  polisher's disease J62.8

Metamorphopsia H53.15

Metaplasia
  apocrine (breast) —*see* Dysplasia, mammary, specified type NEC
  cervix (squamous) —*see* Dysplasia, cervix
  endometrium (squamous) (uterus) N85.8
  esophagus K22.7-
  gastric intestinal K31.A0
    with dysplasia K31.A29
      high grade K31.A22
      low grade K31.A21
    indefinite for dysplasia K31.A0
    without dysplasia K31.A19
      involving
        antrum K31.A11
        body (corpus) K31.A12
        cardia K31.A14
        fundus K31.A13
        multiple sites K31.A15
  kidney (pelvis) (squamous) N28.89
  myelogenous D73.1
  myeloid (agnogenic) (megakaryocytic) D73.1
  spleen D73.1
  squamous cell, bladder N32.89

Metastasis, metastatic
  abscess —*see* Abscess
  calcification E83.59
  cancer
    from specified site —*see* Neoplasm, malignant, by site
    to specified site —*see* Neoplasm, secondary, by site
  deposits (in) —*see* Neoplasm, secondary, by site
  disease (*see also* Neoplasm, secondary, by site) C79.9
  spread (to) —*see* Neoplasm, secondary, by site

Metastrongyliasis B83.8

Metatarsalgia M77.4-
  anterior G57.6-
  Morton's G57.6-

Metatarsus, metatarsal —*see also* condition
  adductus, congenital Q66.22-
  valgus (abductus), congenital Q66.6
  varus (congenital) Q66.22-
    primus Q66.21-

Methadone use —*see* Use, opioid

Methemoglobinemia D74.9
  acquired (with sulfhemoglobinemia) D74.8
  congenital D74.0
  enzymatic (congenital) D74.0
  Hb M disease D74.0
  hereditary D74.0
  toxic D74.8

Methemoglobinuria —*see* Hemoglobinuria

Methioninemia E72.19

Methylmalonic acidemia E71.120

Metritis (catarrhal) (hemorrhagic) (septic) (suppurative) —*see also* Endometritis
  cervical —*see* Cervicitis

Metropathia hemorrhagica N93.8

Metroperitonitis —*see* Peritonitis, pelvic, female

Metrorrhagia N92.1
  climacteric N92.4
  menopausal N92.4
  perimenopausal N92.4
  postpartum NEC (atonic) (following delivery of placenta) O72.1
    delayed or secondary O72.2
  preclimacteric or premenopausal N92.4
  psychogenic F45.8

Metrorrhexis —*see* Rupture, uterus

Metrosalpingitis N70.91

Metrostaxis N93.8

Metrovaginitis —*see* Endometritis

Meyer-Schwickerath and Weyers syndrome Q87.0

Meynert's amentia (nonalcoholic) F04
  alcoholic F10.96
    with dependence F10.26

Mibelli's disease (porokeratosis) Q82.8

Mice, joint —*see* Loose, body, joint knee M23.4-

Micrencephalon, micrencephaly Q02

Microalbuminuria R80.9

Microaneurysm, retinal —*see also* Disorder, retina, microaneurysms
  diabetic —*see* E08-E13 with .31

Microangiopathy (peripheral) I73.9
  thrombotic M31.10
    hematopoietic stem cell transplantation-associated [HSCT-TMA] M31.11

Microcalcifications, breast R92.0

Microcephalus, microcephalic, microcephaly Q02
  due to toxoplasmosis (congenital) P37.1

Microcheilia Q18.7

Microcolon (congenital) Q43.8
Microcornea (congenital) Q13.4
Microcytic —*see* condition
Microdeletions NEC Q93.88
Microdontia K00.2
Microdrepanocytosis D57.40
  with
    acute chest syndrome D57.411
    cerebral vascular involvement D57.413
    crisis (painful) D57.419
      with specified complication NEC D57.418
    pain (vaso-occlusive) D57.419
    splenic sequestration D57.412
Microembolism
  atherothrombotic —*see* Atheroembolism
  retinal —*see* Occlusion, artery, retina
Microencephalon Q02
Microfilaria streptocerca infestation —*see* Onchocerciasis
Microgastria (congenital) Q40.2
Microgenia M26.06
Microgenitalia, congenital
  female Q52.8
  male Q55.8
Microglioma —*see* Lymphoma, non-Hodgkin, specified NEC
Microglossia (congenital) Q38.3
Micrognathia, micrognathism (congenital) (mandibular) (maxillary) M26.09
Microgyria (congenital) Q04.3
Microinfarct of heart —*see* Insufficiency, coronary
Microlentia (congenital) Q12.8
Microlithiasis, alveolar, pulmonary J84.02
Micromastia N64.82
Micromyelia (congenital) Q06.8
Micropenis Q55.62
Microphakia (congenital) Q12.8
Microphthalmos, microphthalmia (congenital) Q11.2
  due to toxoplasmosis P37.1
Micropsia H53.15
Microscopic polyangiitis (polyarteritis) M31.7
Microsporidiosis B60.8
  intestinal A07.8
Microsporon furfur infestation B36.0
Microsporosis —*see also* Dermatophytosis
  nigra B36.1
Microstomia (congenital) Q18.5
Microtia (congenital) (external ear) Q17.2
Microtropia H50.40
Microvillus inclusion disease (MVD) (MVID) Q43.8
Micturition
  disorder NEC (*see also* Difficulty, micturition) R39.198
    psychogenic F45.8
  frequency R35.0
    psychogenic F45.8
  hesitancy R39.11
  incomplete emptying R39.14
  nocturnal R35.1

Micturition (continued)
  painful R30.9
    dysuria R30.0
    psychogenic F45.8
    tenesmus R30.1
  poor stream R39.12
  position dependent R39.192
  split stream R39.13
  straining R39.16
  urgency R39.15
Mid plane —*see* condition
Middle
  ear —*see* condition
  lobe (right) syndrome J98.19
Miescher's elastoma L87.2
Mietens' syndrome Q87.2
Migraine (idiopathic) G43.909
  with refractory migraine G43.919
    with status migrainosus G43.911
    without status migrainosus G43.919
  with aura (acute-onset) (prolonged) (typical) (without headache) G43.109
    with refractory migraine G43.119
      with status migrainosus G43.111
      without status migrainosus G43.119
    chronic G43.E09
      with refractory migraine G43.E19
        with status migrainosus G43.E11
        without status migrainosus G43.E19
      intractable
        with status migrainosus G43.E11
        without status migrainosus G43.E19
      not intractable
        with status migrainosus G43.E01
        without status migrainosus G43.E09
      without refractory migraine G43.E09
        with status migrainosus G43.E01
        without status migrainosus G43.E09
    intractable G43.119
      with status migrainosus G43.111
      without status migrainosus G43.119
    not intractable G43.109
      with status migrainosus G43.101
      without status migrainosus G43.109
    persistent G43.509
      with cerebral infarction G43.609
        with refractory migraine G43.619
          with status migrainosus G43.611
          without status migrainosus G43.619
        intractable G43.619
          with status migrainosus G43.611
          without status migrainosus G43.619
        not intractable G43.609
          with status migrainosus G43.601
          without status migrainosus G43.609

Migraine (continued)
  with aura (continued)
    persistent (continued)
      without cerebral infarction (continued)
        without refractory migraine G43.609
          with status migrainosus G43.601
          without status migrainosus G43.609
      without cerebral infarction G43.509
        with refractory migraine G43.519
          with status migrainosus G43.511
          without status migrainosus G43.519
        intractable G43.519
          with status migrainosus G43.511
          without status migrainosus G43.519
        not intractable G43.509
          with status migrainosus G43.501
          without status migrainosus G43.509
        without refractory migraine G43.509
          with status migrainosus G43.501
          without status migrainosus G43.509
    without mention of refractory migraine G43.109
      with status migrainosus G43.101
      without status migrainosus G43.109
  abdominal G43.D0
    with refractory migraine G43.D1
    intractable G43.D1
    not intractable G43.D0
    without refractory migraine G43.D0
  basilar —*see* Migraine, with aura
  classical —*see* Migraine, with aura
  common —*see* Migraine, without aura
  complicated G43.109
  equivalents —*see* Migraine, with aura
  familiar —*see* Migraine, hemiplegic
  hemiplegic G43.409
    with refractory migraine G43.419
      with status migrainosus G43.411
      without status migrainosus G43.419
    intractable G43.419
      with status migrainosus G43.411
      without status migrainosus G43.419
    not intractable G43.409
      with status migrainosus G43.401
      without status migrainosus G43.409
    without refractory migraine G43.409
      with status migrainosus G43.401
      without status migrainosus G43.409
  intractable G43.919
    with status migrainosus G43.911
    without status migrainosus G43.919

Migraine (continued)
  menstrual G43.829
    with refractory migraine G43.839
      with status migrainosus G43.831
      without status migrainosus G43.839
    intractable G43.839
      with status migrainosus G43.831
      without status migrainosus G43.839
    not intractable G43.829
      with status migrainosus G43.821
      without status migrainosus G43.829
    without refractory migraine G43.829
      with status migrainosus G43.821
      without status migrainosus G43.829
  menstrually related —*see* Migraine, menstrual
  not intractable G43.909
    with status migrainosus G43.901
    without status migrainosus G43.919
  ophthalmoplegic G43.B0
    with refractory migraine G43.B1
    intractable G43.B1
    not intractable G43.B0
    without refractory migraine G43.B0
  persistent aura (with, without) cerebral infarction —*see* Migraine, with aura, persistent
  preceded or accompanied by transient focal neurological phenomena —*see* Migraine, with aura
  pre-menstrual —*see* Migraine, menstrual
  pure menstrual —*see* Migraine, menstrual
  retinal —*see* Migraine, with aura
  specified NEC G43.809
    intractable G43.819
      with status migrainosus G43.811
      without status migrainosus G43.819
    not intractable G43.809
      with status migrainosus G43.801
      without status migrainosus G43.809
  sporadic —*see* Migraine, hemiplegic
  transformed —*see* Migraine, without aura, chronic
  triggered seizures —*see* Migraine, with aura
  without aura G43.009
    with refractory migraine G43.019
      with status migrainosus G43.011
      without status migrainosus G43.019
    chronic G43.709
      with refractory migraine G43.719
        with status migrainosus G43.711
        without status migrainosus G43.719

Migraine (continued)
　without aura (continued)
　　chronic (continued)
　　　intractable
　　　　with status migrainosus
　　　　　G43.711
　　　　without status migrainosus
　　　　　G43.719
　　　not intractable
　　　　with status migrainosus
　　　　　G43.701
　　　　without status migrainosus
　　　　　G43.709
　　　without refractory migraine
　　　　G43.709
　　　　with status migrainosus
　　　　　G43.701
　　　　without status migrainosus
　　　　　G43.709
　　intractable
　　　with status migrainosus G43.011
　　　without status migrainosus
　　　　G43.019
　　not intractable
　　　with status migrainosus G43.001
　　　without status migrainosus
　　　　G43.009
　　without mention of refractory
　　　migraine G43.009
　　　with status migrainosus
　　　　G43.001
　　　without status migrainosus
　　　　G43.009
　　without refractory migraine
　　　G43.909
　　　with status migrainosus
　　　　G43.901
　　　without status migrainosus
　　　　G43.909
Migrant, social Z59.00
Migration, anxiety concerning Z60.3
Migratory, migrating —see also
　condition
　person Z59.00
　testis Q55.29
Mikity-Wilson disease or syndrome
　P27.0
Mikulicz' disease or syndrome
　K11.8
Miliaria L74.3
　alba L74.1
　apocrine L75.2
　crystallina L74.1
　profunda L74.2
　rubra L74.0
　tropicalis L74.2
Miliary —see condition
Milium L72.0
　colloid L57.8
Milk
　crust L21.0
　excessive secretion O92.6
　poisoning —see Poisoning, food,
　　noxious
　retention O92.79
　sickness —see Poisoning, food,
　　noxious
　spots I31.0
Milk-alkali disease or syndrome
　E83.52
Milk-leg (deep vessels)
　(nonpuerperal) —see Embolism,
　vein, lower extremity
　complicating pregnancy O22.3-
　puerperal, postpartum, childbirth
　　O87.1

Milkman's disease or syndrome
　M83.8
Milky urine —see Chyluria
Millard-Gubler (-Foville) **paralysis or syndrome** G46.3
Millar's asthma J38.5
Miller Fisher syndrome G61.0
Mills' disease —see Hemiplegia
Millstone maker's pneumoconiosis
　J62.8
Milroy's disease (chronic hereditary edema) Q82.0
Minamata disease T56.1
Miners' asthma or lung J60
Minkowski-Chauffard syndrome
　—see Spherocytosis
Minor —see condition
Minor's disease (hematomyelia)
　G95.19
Minot's disease (hemorrhagic disease), **newborn** P53
Minot-von Willebrand-Jurgens disease or syndrome
　(angiohemophilia) —see Disease,
　von Willebrand
Minus (and plus) hand (intrinsic)
　—see Deformity, limb, specified
　type NEC, forearm
Miosis (pupil) H57.03
Mirizzi's syndrome (hepatic duct stenosis) K83.1
Mirror writing F81.0
MIS-A M35.81
MIS-C M35.81
Misadventure (of) (prophylactic) (therapeutic) (see also Complications) T88.9
　administration of insulin (by accident) T38.3
　infusion —see Complications, infusion
　local applications (of fomentations, plasters, etc.) T88.9
　burn or scald —see Burn
　specified NEC T88.8
　medical care (early) (late) T88.9
　　adverse effect of drugs or chemicals —see Table of Drugs and Chemicals
　　burn or scald —see Burn
　　specified NEC T88.8
　specified NEC T88.8
　surgical procedure (early) (late)
　　—see Complications, surgical procedure
　transfusion —see Complications, transfusion
　vaccination or other immunological procedure — see Complications, vaccination
Miscarriage O03.9
Misdirection, aqueous H40.83-
Misperception, sleep state F51.02
Misplaced, misplacement
　ear Q17.4
　kidney (acquired) N28.89
　　congenital Q63.2
　organ or site, congenital NEC
　　—see Malposition, congenital
Missed
　abortion O02.1
　delivery O36.4

Missing —see also Absence
　string of intrauterine contraceptive device T83.32
Misuse of drugs F19.99
Mitchell's disease (erythromelalgia)
　I73.81
Mite(s) (infestation) B88.9
　diarrhea B88.0
　grain (itch) B88.0
　hair follicle (itch) B88.0
　in sputum B88.0
Mitral —see condition
Mittelschmerz N94.0
Mixed —see condition
MMN (multifocal motor neuropathy) G61.82
MNGIE (Mitochondrial Neurogastrointestinal Encephalopathy) **syndrome** E88.49
Mobile, mobility
　cecum Q43.3
　excessive —see Hypermobility
　gallbladder, congenital Q44.1
　kidney N28.89
　organ or site, congenital NEC
　　—see Malposition, congenital
Mobitz heart block (atrioventricular)
　I44.1
Moebius, Möbius
　disease (ophthalmoplegic migraine)
　　—see Migraine, ophthalmoplegic
　syndrome Q87.0
　　congenital oculofacial paralysis (with other anomalies) Q87.0
　　ophthalmoplegic migraine —see Migraine, ophthalmoplegic
Moeller's glossitis K14.0
MOGAD (myelin oligodendrocyte glycoprotein antibody disease)
　G37.81
Mohr's syndrome (Types I and II)
　Q87.0
Mola destruens D39.2
Molar pregnancy O02.0
Molarization of premolars K00.2
Molding, head (during birth) - omit code
Mole (pigmented) —see also
　Nevus
　blood O02.0
　Breus' O02.0
　cancerous —see Melanoma
　carneous O02.0
　destructive D39.2
　fleshy O02.0
　hydatid, hydatidiform (benign) (complicating pregnancy) (delivered) (undelivered) O01.9
　　classical O01.0
　　complete O01.0
　　incomplete O01.1
　　invasive D39.2
　　malignant D39.2
　　partial O01.1
　intrauterine O02.0
　invasive (hydatidiform) D39.2
　malignant
　　meaning
　　　malignant hydatidiform mole D39.2
　　　melanoma —see Melanoma
　nonhydatidiform O02.0

Mole (continued)
　nonpigmented —see Nevus
　pregnancy NEC O02.0
　skin —see Nevus
　tubal O00.10-
　　with intrauterine pregnancy O00.11-
　vesicular —see Mole, hydatidiform
Molimen, molimina (menstrual)
　N94.3
Molluscum contagiosum
　(epitheliale) B08.1
Mönckeberg's arteriosclerosis, disease, or sclerosis —see
　Arteriosclerosis, extremities
Mondini's malformation (cochlea)
　Q16.5
Mondor's disease I80.8
Monge's disease T70.29
Monilethrix (congenital) Q84.1
Moniliasis (see also Candidiasis)
　B37.9
　neonatal P37.5
Monitoring (encounter for)
　therapeutic drug level Z51.81
Monkey malaria B53.1
Monkeypox B04
Monoarthritis M13.10
　ankle M13.17-
　elbow M13.12-
　foot joint M13.17-
　hand joint M13.14-
　hip M13.15-
　knee M13.16-
　shoulder M13.11-
　wrist M13.13-
Monoblastic —see condition
Monochromat (ism),
　monochromatopsia (acquired) (congenital) H53.51
Monocytic —see condition
Monocytopenia D72.818
Monocytosis (symptomatic)
　D72.821
Monomania —see Psychosis
Mononeuritis G58.9
　cranial nerve —see Disorder, nerve, cranial
　femoral nerve G57.2-
　lateral
　　cutaneous nerve of thigh G57.1-
　　popliteal nerve G57.3-
　lower limb G57.9-
　　specified nerve NEC G57.8-
　medial popliteal nerve G57.4-
　median nerve G56.1-
　multiplex G58.7
　plantar nerve G57.6-
　posterior tibial nerve G57.5-
　radial nerve G56.3-
　sciatic nerve G57.0-
　specified NEC G58.8
　tibial nerve G57.4-
　ulnar nerve G56.2-
　upper limb G56.9-
　　specified nerve NEC G56.8-
　vestibular —see subcategory H93.3
Mononeuropathy G58.9
　carpal tunnel syndrome —see Syndrome, carpal tunnel

Mononeuropathy (continued)
  diabetic NEC —see E08-E13
    with .41
  femoral nerve —see Lesion, nerve, femoral
  ilioinguinal nerve G57.8-
  in diseases classified elsewhere
    —see category G59
  intercostal G58.0
  lower limb G57.9-
    causalgia —see Causalgia, lower limb
    femoral nerve —see Lesion, nerve, femoral
    meralgia paresthetica G57.1-
    plantar nerve —see Lesion, nerve, plantar
    popliteal nerve —see Lesion, nerve, popliteal
    sciatic nerve —see Lesion, nerve, sciatic
    specified NEC G57.8-
    tarsal tunnel syndrome —see Syndrome, tarsal tunnel
  median nerve —see Lesion, nerve, median
  multiplex G58.7
  obturator nerve G57.8-
  popliteal nerve —see Lesion, nerve, popliteal
  radial nerve —see Lesion, nerve, radial
  saphenous nerve G57.8-
  specified NEC G58.8
  tarsal tunnel syndrome —see Syndrome, tarsal tunnel
  tuberculous A17.83
  ulnar nerve —see Lesion, nerve, ulnar
  upper limb G56.9-
    carpal tunnel syndrome —see Syndrome, carpal tunnel
    causalgia —see Causalgia
    median nerve —see Lesion, nerve, median
    radial nerve —see Lesion, nerve, radial
    specified site NEC G56.8-
    ulnar nerve —see Lesion, nerve, ulnar

Mononucleosis, infectious B27.90
  with
    complication NEC B27.99
    meningitis B27.92
    polyneuropathy B27.91
  cytomegaloviral B27.10
    with
      complication NEC B27.19
      meningitis B27.12
      polyneuropathy B27.11
  Epstein-Barr (virus) B27.00
    with
      complication NEC B27.09
      meningitis B27.02
      polyneuropathy B27.01
  gammaherpesviral B27.00
    with
      complication NEC B27.09
      meningitis B27.02
      polyneuropathy B27.01
  specified NEC B27.80
    with
      complication NEC B27.89
      meningitis B27.82
      polyneuropathy B27.81

Monoparesis —see Monoplegia

Monoplegia G83.3-
  congenital (cerebral) G80.8
    spastic G80.1
  embolic (current episode) I63.4-
  following
    cerebrovascular disease
      cerebral infarction
        lower limb I69.34-
        upper limb I69.33-
      intracerebral hemorrhage
        lower limb I69.14-
        upper limb I69.13-
      lower limb I69.94-
      nontraumatic intracranial hemorrhage NEC
        lower limb I69.24-
        upper limb I69.23-
      specified disease NEC
        lower limb I69.84-
        upper limb I69.83-
      stroke NOS
        lower limb I69.34-
        upper limb I69.33-
      subarachnoid hemorrhage
        lower limb I69.04-
        upper limb I69.03-
      upper limb I69.93-
  hysterical (transient) F44.4
  lower limb G83.1-
  psychogenic (conversion reaction) F44.4
  thrombotic (current episode) I63.3-
  transient R29.818
  upper limb G83.2-

Monorchism, monorchidism Q55.0

Monosomy (see also Deletion, chromosome) Q93.9
  specified NEC Q93.89
  whole chromosome
    meiotic nondisjunction Q93.0
    mitotic nondisjunction Q93.1
    mosaicism Q93.1
  X Q96.9

Monster, monstrosity (single) Q89.7
  acephalic Q00.0
  twin Q89.4

Monteggia's fracture (-dislocation) S52.27-

Mooren's ulcer (cornea) —see Ulcer, cornea, Mooren's

Moore's syndrome —see Epilepsy, specified NEC

Mooser-Neill reaction A75.2

Mooser's bodies A75.2

Morbidity not stated or unknown R69

Morbilli —see Measles

Morbus —see also Disease
  angelicus, anglorum E55.0
  Beigel B36.2
  caducus —see Epilepsy
  celiacus K90.0
  comitialis —see Epilepsy
  cordis (see also Disease, heart) I51.9
    valvulorum —see Endocarditis
  coxae senilis M16.9
    tuberculous A18.02
  hemorrhagicus neonatorum P53
  maculosus neonatorum P54.5

Morel (-Stewart) (-Morgagni) **syndrome** M85.2

Morel-Kraepelin disease —see Schizophrenia

Morel-Moore syndrome M85.2

Morgagni's
  cyst, organ, hydatid, or appendage
    female Q50.5
    male (epididymal) Q55.4
      testicular Q55.29
  syndrome M85.2

Morgagni-Stokes-Adams syndrome I45.9

Morgagni-Stewart-Morel syndrome M85.2

Morgagni-Turner (-Albright) **syndrome** Q96.9

Moria F07.0

Moron (I.Q.50-69) F70

Morphea L94.0

Morphinism (without remission) F11.20
  with remission F11.21

Morphinomania (without remission) F11.20
  with remission F11.21

Morquio (-Ullrich) (-Brailsford) **disease or syndrome** —see Mucopolysaccharidosis

Mortification (dry) (moist) —see Gangrene

Morton's metatarsalgia (neuralgia) (neuroma) (syndrome) G57.6-

Morvan's disease or syndrome G60.8

Mosaicism, mosaic (autosomal) (chromosomal)
  45,X/other cell lines NEC with abnormal sex chromosome Q96.4
  45,X/46,XX Q96.3
  sex chromosome
    female Q97.8
      lines with various numbers of X chromosomes Q97.2
    male Q98.7
    XY Q96.3

Moschowitz' disease M31.19

Mother yaw A66.0

Motion sickness (from travel, any vehicle) (from roundabouts or swings) T75.3

Mottled, mottling, teeth (enamel) (endemic) (nonendemic) K00.3

Mounier-Kuhn syndrome Q32.4
  with bronchiectasis J47.9
    exacerbation (acute) J47.1
    lower respiratory infection J47.0
  acquired J98.09
    with bronchiectasis J47.9
      with
        exacerbation (acute) J47.1
        lower respiratory infection J47.0

Mountain
  sickness T70.29
    with polycythemia, acquired (acute) D75.1
  tick fever A93.2

Mouse, joint —see Loose, body, joint
  knee M23.4-

Mouth —see condition

Movable
  coccyx —see subcategory M53.2

Movable (continued)
  kidney N28.89
    congenital Q63.8
  spleen D73.89

Movements, dystonic R25.8

Moyamoya disease I67.5

MRSA (Methicillin resistant Staphylococcus aureus)
  infection A49.02
    as the cause of diseases classified elsewhere B95.62
  sepsis A41.02

MSD (multiple sulfatase deficiency) E75.26

MSSA (Methicillin susceptible Staphylococcus aureus)
  infection A49.01
    as the cause of diseases classified elsewhere B95.61
  sepsis A41.01

Mucha-Habermann disease L41.0

Mucinosis (cutaneous) (focal) (papular) (reticular erythematous) (skin) L98.5
  oral K13.79

Mucocele
  appendix K38.8
  buccal cavity K13.79
  gallbladder K82.1
  lacrimal sac, chronic H04.43-
  nasal sinus J34.1
  nose J34.1
  salivary gland (any) K11.6
  sinus (accessory) (nasal) J34.1
  turbinate (bone) (middle) (nasal) J34.1
  uterus N85.8

Mucolipidosis
  I E77.1
  II, III E77.0
  IV E75.11

Mucopolysaccharidosis E76.3
  beta-gluduronidase deficiency E76.29
  cardiopathy E76.3 [I52]
  Hunter's syndrome E76.1
  Hurler's syndrome E76.01
  Hurler-Scheie syndrome E76.02
  Maroteaux-Lamy syndrome E76.29
  Morquio syndrome E76.219
    A E76.210
    B E76.211
    classic E76.210
  Sanfilippo syndrome E76.22
  Scheie's syndrome E76.03
  specified NEC E76.29
  type
    I
      Hurler's syndrome E76.01
      Hurler-Scheie syndrome E76.02
      Scheie's syndrome E76.03
    II E76.1
    III E76.22
    IV E76.219
    IVA E76.210
    IVB E76.211
    VI E76.29
    VII E76.29

Mucormycosis B46.5
  cutaneous B46.3
  disseminated B46.4
  gastrointestinal B46.2
  generalized B46.4
  pulmonary B46.0
  rhinocerebral B46.1
  skin B46.3
  subcutaneous B46.3

Mucositis (ulcerative) K12.30
  due to drugs NEC K12.32
  gastrointestinal K92.81
  mouth (oral) (oropharyngeal)
    K12.30
    due to antineoplastic therapy
      K12.31
    due to drugs NEC K12.32
    due to radiation K12.33
    specified NEC K12.39
    viral K12.39
  nasal J34.81
  oral cavity —*see* Mucositis, mouth
  oral soft tissues —*see* Mucositis, mouth
  vagina and vulva N76.81
Mucositis necroticans agranulocytica —*see* Agranulocytosis
Mucous —*see also* condition
  patches (syphilitic) A51.39
    congenital A50.07
Mucoviscidosis E84.9
  with meconium obstruction E84.11
Mucus
  asphyxia or suffocation —*see* Asphyxia, mucus
  in stool R19.5
  plug —*see* Asphyxia, mucus
Muguet B37.0
Mulberry molars (congenital syphilis) A50.52
Müllerian mixed tumor
  specified site —*see* Neoplasm, malignant, by site
  unspecified site C54.9
Multicystic kidney (development) Q61.4
Multiparity (grand) Z64.1
  affecting management of pregnancy, labor and delivery (supervision only) O09.4-
  requiring contraceptive management —*see* Contraception
Multipartita placenta O43.19-
Multiple, multiplex —*see also* condition
  digits (congenital) Q69.9
  endocrine neoplasia —*see* Neoplasia, endocrine, multiple (MEN)
  personality F44.81
Multisystem inflammatory syndrome (in adult) (in children) M35.81
Mumps B26.9
  arthritis B26.85
  complication NEC B26.89
  encephalitis B26.2
  hepatitis B26.81
  meningitis (aseptic) B26.1
  meningoencephalitis B26.2
  myocarditis B26.82
  oophoritis B26.89
  orchitis B26.0
  pancreatitis B26.3
  polyneuropathy B26.84
Mumu —*see also* Infestation, filarial B74.9 *[N51]*
Münchhausen's syndrome —*see* Disorder, factitious
Münchmeyer's syndrome —*see* Myositis, ossificans, progressiva
Mural —*see* condition

Murmur (cardiac) (heart) (organic) R01.1
  abdominal R19.15
  aortic (valve) —*see* Endocarditis, aortic
  benign R01.0
  diastolic —*see* Endocarditis
  Flint I35.1
  functional R01.0
  Graham Steell I37.1
  innocent R01.0
  mitral (valve) —*see* Insufficiency, mitral
  nonorganic R01.0
  presystolic, mitral —*see* Insufficiency, mitral
  pulmonic (valve) I37.8
  systolic R01.1
  tricuspid (valve) I07.9
  valvular —*see* Endocarditis
Murri's disease (intermittent hemoglobinuria) D59.6
Muscle, muscular —*see also* condition
  carnitine (palmityltransferase) deficiency E71.314
Musculoneuralgia —*see* Neuralgia
Mushroom-workers'(pickers') **disease or lung** J67.5
Mushrooming hip —*see* Derangement, joint, specified NEC, hip
Mutation(s)
  factor V Leiden D68.51
  surfactant, of lung J84.83
  prothrombin gene D68.52
Mutism —*see also* Aphasia
  deaf (acquired) (congenital) NEC H91.3
  elective (adjustment reaction) (childhood) F94.0
  hysterical F44.4
  selective (childhood) F94.0
MVD (microvillus inclusion disease) Q43.8
MVID (microvillus inclusion disease) Q43.8
Myalgia M79.10
  auxiliary muscles, head and neck M79.12
  epidemic (cervical) B33.0
  mastication muscle M79.11
  site specified NEC M79.18
  traumatic NEC T14.8
Myasthenia G70.9
  congenital G70.2
  cordis —*see* Failure, heart
  developmental G70.2
  gravis G70.00
    with exacerbation (acute) G70.01
    in crisis G70.01
    neonatal, transient P94.0
    pseudoparalytica G70.00
      with exacerbation (acute) G70.01
      in crisis G70.01
  stomach, psychogenic F45.8
  syndrome
    in
      diabetes mellitus —*see* E08-E13 with .44
      neoplastic disease (*see also* Neoplasm) D49.9 *[G73.3]*
      pernicious anemia D51.0 *[G73.3]*
      thyrotoxicosis E05.90 *[G73.3]*
        with thyroid storm E05.91 *[G73.3]*

Myasthenic M62.81
Mycelium infection B49
Mycetismus —*see* Poisoning, food, noxious, mushroom
Mycetoma B47.9
  actinomycotic B47.1
  bone (mycotic) B47.9 *[M90.80]*
  eumycotic B47.0
  foot B47.9
    actinomycotic B47.1
    mycotic B47.0
  madurae NEC B47.9
    mycotic B47.0
  maduromycotic B47.0
    mycotic B47.0
  nocardial B47.1
Mycobacteriosis —*see* Mycobacterium
Mycobacterium, mycobacterial (infection) A31.9
  anonymous A31.9
  atypical A31.9
    cutaneous A31.1
    pulmonary A31.0
      tuberculous —*see* Tuberculosis, pulmonary
    specified site NEC A31.8
  avium (intracellulare complex) A31.0
  balnei A31.1
  Battey A31.0
  chelonei A31.8
  cutaneous A31.1
  extrapulmonary systemic A31.8
  fortuitum A31.8
  intracellulare (Battey bacillus) A31.0
  kansasii (yellow bacillus) A31.0
  kakaferifu A31.8
  kasongo A31.8
  leprae (*see also* Leprosy) A30.9
  luciflavum A31.1
  marinum (M. balnei) A31.1
  nonspecific —*see* Mycobacterium, atypical
  pulmonary (atypical) A31.0
    tuberculous —*see* Tuberculosis, pulmonary
  scrofulaceum A31.8
  simiae A31.8
  systemic, extrapulmonary A31.8
  szulgai A31.8
  terrae A31.8
  triviale A31.8
  tuberculosis (human, bovine) —*see* Tuberculosis
  ulcerans A31.1
  xenopi A31.8
Mycoplasma (M.) **pneumoniae, as cause of disease classified elsewhere** B96.0
Mycosis, mycotic B49
  cutaneous NEC B36.9
  ear B36.9
    in
      aspergillosis B44.89
      candidiasis B37.84
      moniliasis B37.84
  fungoides (extranodal) (solid organ) C84.0-
  mouth B37.0
  nails B35.1
  opportunistic B48.8
  skin NEC B36.9
  specified NEC B48.8
  stomatitis B37.0
  vagina, vaginitis (candidal) B37.31
    chronic (recurrent) B37.32
Mydriasis (pupil) H57.04

Myelatelia Q06.1
Myelinolysis, pontine, central G37.2
Myelitis (acute) (ascending) (childhood) (chronic) (descending) (diffuse) (disseminated) (idiopathic) (pressure) (progressive) (spinal cord) (subacute) (*see also* Encephalitis) G04.91
  flaccid G04.82
  herpes simplex B00.82
  herpes zoster B02.24
  in diseases classified elsewhere G05.4
  necrotizing, subacute G37.4
  optic neuritis in G36.0
  postchickenpox B01.12
  postherpetic B02.24
  postimmunization G04.02
  postinfectious NEC G04.89
  postvaccinal G04.02
  specified NEC G04.89
  syphilitic (transverse) A52.14
  toxic G92.9
  transverse (in demyelinating diseases of central nervous system) G37.3
  tuberculous A17.82
  varicella B01.12
Myeloblastic —*see* condition
Myeloblastoma
  granular cell —*see also* Neoplasm, connective tissue
    malignant —*see* Neoplasm, connective tissue, malignant
  tongue D10.1
Myelocele —*see* Spina bifida
Myelocystocele —*see* Spina bifida
Myelocytic —*see* condition
Myelodysplasia D46.9
  specified NEC D46.Z
  spinal cord (congenital) Q06.1
Myelodysplastic syndrome (*see also* Syndrome, myelodysplastic) D46.9
  with
    5q deletion D46.C
    isolated del (5q) chromosomal abnormality D46.C
  specified NEC D46.Z
Myeloencephalitis —*see* Encephalitis
Myelofibrosis D75.81
  with myeloid metaplasia D47.4
  acute C94.4-
  idiopathic (chronic) D47.4
  primary D47.1
  secondary D75.81
    in myeloproliferative disease D47.4
Myelogenous —*see* condition
Myeloid —*see* condition
Myelokathexis D70.9
Myeloleukodystrophy E75.29
Myelolipoma —*see* Lipoma
Myeloma (multiple) C90.0-
  monostotic C90.3
    plasma cell C90.0-
  plasma cell C90.0-
  solitary (*see also* Plasmacytoma, solitary) C90.3-
Myelomalacia G95.89
Myelomatosis C90.0-
Myelomeningitis —*see* Meningoencephalitis

Myelomeningocele (spinal cord)
—see Spina bifida
Myelo-osteo-musculodysplasia hereditaria Q79.8
Myelopathic
  anemia D64.89
  muscle atrophy —see Atrophy, muscle, spinal
  pain syndrome G89.0
Myelopathy (spinal cord) G95.9
  drug-induced G95.89
  in (due to)
    degeneration or displacement, intervertebral disc NEC —see Disorder, disc, with, myelopathy
    disease classified elsewhere G99.2
    infection —see Encephalitis
    intervertebral disc disorder —see also Disorder, disc, with, myelopathy
    mercury —see subcategory T56.1
    neoplastic disease (see also Neoplasm) D49.9 [G99.2]
    pernicious anemia D51.0 [G99.2]
    spondylosis —see Spondylosis, with myelopathy NEC
  necrotic (subacute) (vascular) G95.19
  radiation-induced G95.89
  spondylogenic NEC —see Spondylosis, with myelopathy NEC
  toxic G95.89
  transverse, acute G37.3
  vascular G95.19
  vitamin B12 E53.8 [G32.0]
Myelophthisis D61.82
Myeloradiculitis G04.91
Myeloradiculodysplasia (spinal) Q06.1
Myelosarcoma C92.3-
Myelosclerosis D75.89
  with myeloid metaplasia D47.4
  disseminated, of nervous system G35
  megakaryocytic D47.4
    with myeloid metaplasia D47.4
Myelosis
  acute C92.0-
  aleukemic C92.9-
  chronic D47.1
  erythremic (acute) C94.0-
  megakaryocytic C94.2-
  nonleukemic D72.828
  subacute C92.9-
Myiasis (cavernous) B87.9
  aural B87.4
  creeping B87.0
  cutaneous B87.0
  dermal B87.0
  ear (external) (middle) B87.4
  eye B87.2
  genitourinary B87.81
  intestinal B87.82
  laryngeal B87.3
  nasopharyngeal B87.3
  ocular B87.2
  orbit B87.2
  skin B87.0
  specified site NEC B87.89
  traumatic B87.1
  wound B87.1
Myoadenoma, prostate —see Hyperplasia, prostate

Myoblastoma
  granular cell —see also Neoplasm, connective tissue, benign
    malignant —see Neoplasm, connective tissue, malignant
  tongue D10.1
Myocardial —see condition
Myocardiopathy (congestive) (constrictive) (familial) (hypertrophic nonobstructive) (idiopathic) (infiltrative) (obstructive) (primary) (restrictive) (sporadic) (see also Cardiomyopathy) I42.9
  alcoholic I42.6
  cobalt-beer I42.6
  glycogen storage E74.02 [I43]
  hypertrophic obstructive I42.1
  in (due to)
    beriberi E51.12
    cardiac glycogenosis E74.02 [I43]
    Friedreich's ataxia G11.11 [I43]
    myotonia atrophica G71.11 [I43]
    progressive muscular dystrophy (see also Dystrophy, muscular, by type) G71.09 [I43]
  obscure (African) I42.8
  secondary I42.9
  thyrotoxic E05.90 [I43]
    with storm E05.91 [I43]
  toxic NEC I42.7
Myocarditis (with arteriosclerosis) (chronic) (fibroid) (interstitial) (old) (progressive) (senile) I51.4
  with
    rheumatic fever (conditions in I00) I09.0
      active —see Myocarditis, acute, rheumatic
      inactive or quiescent (with chorea) I09.0
  active I40.9
    rheumatic I01.2
      with chorea (acute) (rheumatic) (Sydenham's) I02.0
  acute or subacute (interstitial) I40.9
    due to
      streptococcus (beta-hemolytic) I01.2
    idiopathic I40.1
    rheumatic I01.2
      with chorea (acute) (rheumatic) (Sydenham's) I02.0
    specified NEC I40.8
  aseptic of newborn B33.22
  bacterial (acute) I40.0
  Coxsackie (virus) B33.22
  diphtheritic A36.81
  eosinophilic I40.1
  epidemic of newborn (Coxsackie) B33.22
  Fiedler's (acute) (isolated) I40.1
  giant cell (acute) (subacute) I40.1
  gonococcal A54.83
  granulomatous (idiopathic) (isolated) (nonspecific) I40.1
  hypertensive —see Hypertension, heart
  idiopathic (granulomatous) I40.1
  in (due to)
    diphtheria A36.81
    epidemic louse-borne typhus A75.0 [I41]
    Lyme disease A69.29
    sarcoidosis D86.85
    scarlet fever A38.1
    toxoplasmosis (acquired) B58.81
    typhoid A01.02
    typhus NEC A75.9 [I41]

Myocarditis (continued)
  infective I40.0
  influenzal —see Influenza, with, myocarditis
  isolated (acute) I40.1
  meningococcal A39.52
  mumps B26.82
  nonrheumatic, active I40.9
  parenchymatous I40.9
  pneumococcal I40.0
  rheumatic (chronic) (inactive) (with chorea) I09.0
    active or acute I01.2
      with chorea (acute) (rheumatic) (Sydenham's) I02.0
    rheumatoid —see Rheumatoid, carditis
  septic I40.0
  staphylococcal I40.0
  suppurative I40.0
  syphilitic (chronic) A52.06
  toxic I40.8
    rheumatic —see Myocarditis, acute, rheumatic
  tuberculous A18.84
  typhoid A01.02
  valvular —see Endocarditis
  virus, viral I40.0
    of newborn (Coxsackie) B33.22
Myocardium, myocardial —see condition
Myocardosis —see Cardiomyopathy
Myoclonus, myoclonic, myoclonia (familial) (essential) (multifocal) (simplex) G25.3
  drug-induced G25.3
  epilepsy (see also Epilepsy, generalized, specified NEC) G40.4-
    familial (progressive) —see Epilepsy, myoclonus
    Lafora —see Epilepsy, myoclonus, progressive, Lafora
  epileptica (see also Epilepsy, myoclonus) G40.409
    with status epilepticus G40.401
  facial G51.3-
  familial progressive G25.3
    epilepsy —see Epilepsy, myoclonus, progressive
  Friedreich's G25.3
  jerks G25.3
  massive G25.3
  palatal G25.3
  pharyngeal G25.3
Myocytolysis I51.5
Myodiastasis —see Diastasis, muscle
Myoendocarditis —see Endocarditis
Myoepithelioma —see Neoplasm, benign, by site
Myofasciitis (acute) —see Myositis
Myofibroma —see also Neoplasm, connective tissue, benign
  uterus (cervix) (corpus) —see Leiomyoma
Myofibromatosis D48.19
  infantile Q89.8
Myofibrosis M62.89
  heart —see Myocarditis
  scapulohumeral —see Lesion, shoulder, specified NEC
Myofibrositis M79.7
  scapulohumeral —see Lesion, shoulder, specified NEC
Myoglobulinuria, myoglobinuria (primary) R82.1

Myokymia, facial G51.4
Myolipoma —see Lipoma
Myoma —see also Neoplasm, connective tissue, benign
  malignant —see Neoplasm, connective tissue, malignant
  prostate D29.1
  uterus (cervix) (corpus) —see Leiomyoma
Myomalacia M62.89
Myometritis —see Endometritis
Myometrium —see condition
Myonecrosis, clostridial A48.0
Myopathy G72.9
  acute
    necrotizing G72.81
    quadriplegic G72.81
  alcoholic G72.1
  benign congenital G71.20
  central core G71.29
  centronuclear G71.228
    autosomal (dominant) (recessive) G71.228
    other specified NEC G71.228
  congenital (benign) G71.20
  critical illness G72.81
  distal G71.09
  drug-induced G72.0
  endocrine NEC E34.9 [G73.7]
  extraocular muscles H05.82-
  facioscapulohumeral G71.02
  hereditary G71.9
    specified NEC G71.8
  hyaline body G71.29
  immune NEC G72.49
  in (due to)
    Addison's disease E27.1 [G73.7]
    alcohol G72.1
    amyloidosis E85.0 [G73.7]
    cretinism E00.9 [G73.7]
    Cushing's syndrome E24.9 [G73.7]
    drugs G72.0
    endocrine disease NEC E34.9 [G73.7]
    giant cell arteritis M31.6 [G73.7]
    glycogen storage disease E74.00 [G73.7]
    hyperadrenocorticism E24.9 [G73.7]
    hyperparathyroidism NEC E21.3 [G73.7]
    hypoparathyroidism E20.9 [G73.7]
    hypopituitarism E23.0 [G73.7]
    hypothyroidism E03.9 [G73.7]
    infectious disease NEC B99 [G73.7]
    lipid storage disease E75.6 [G73.7]
    metabolic disease NEC E88.9 [G73.7]
    myxedema E03.9 [G73.7]
    parasitic disease NEC B89 [G73.7]
    polyarteritis nodosa M30.0 [G73.7]
    rheumatoid arthritis —see Rheumatoid, myopathy
    sarcoidosis D86.87
    scleroderma M34.82
    sicca syndrome M35.03
    Sjögren's syndrome M35.03
    systemic lupus erythematosus M32.19
    thyrotoxicosis (hyperthyroidism) E05.90 [G73.7]
      with thyroid storm E05.91 [G73.7]
    toxic agent NEC G72.2
  inflammatory NEC G72.49

239

Myopathy *(continued)*
  intensive care (ICU) G72.81
  limb-girdle —*see* Dystrophy, muscular, limb-girdle
  mitochondrial NEC G71.3
  Miyoshi, type 3 G71.035
  myosin storage G71.29
  myotubular (centronuclear) G71.220
    X-linked G71.220
  mytonic, proximal (PROMM) G71.11
  nemaline G71.21
  ocular G71.09
  oculopharyngeal G71.09
  of critical illness G72.81
  primary G71.9
    specified NEC G71.8
  progressive NEC G72.89
  proximal myotonic (PROMM) G71.11
  rod (body) G71.21
  scapulohumeral G71.02
  specified NEC G72.89
  toxic G72.2

Myopericarditis —*see also* Pericarditis
  chronic rheumatic I09.2

Myopia (axial) (congenital) H52.1-
  degenerative (malignant) H44.20
    with
      choroidal neovascularization H44.2A-
      foveoschisis H44.2D-
      macular hole H44.2B-
      retinal detachment H44.2C-
      specified maculopathy NEC H44.2E-
    bilateral H44.23
    left eye H44.22
    right eye H44.21
  malignant (*see also* Myopia, degenerative) H44.2-
  pernicious (*see also* Myopia, degenerative) H44.2-
  progressive high (degenerative) (*see also* Myopia, degenerative) H44.2-

Myosarcoma —*see* Neoplasm, connective tissue, malignant

Myosis (pupil) H57.03
  stromal (endolymphatic) D39.0

Myositis M60.9
  clostridial A48.0
  due to posture —*see* Myositis, specified type NEC
  epidemic B33.0
  fibrosa or fibrous (chronic), Volkmann's T79.6
  foreign body granuloma —*see* Granuloma, foreign body
  in (due to)
    bilharziasis B65.9 *[M63.8-]*
    cysticercosis B69.81
    leprosy A30.9 *[M63.8-]*
    mycosis B49 *[M63.8-]*
    sarcoidosis D86.87
    schistosomiasis B65.9 *[M63.8-]*
    syphilis
      late A52.78
      secondary A51.49
    toxoplasmosis (acquired) B58.82
    trichinellosis B75 *[M63.8-]*
    tuberculosis A18.09
  inclusion body [IBM] G72.41
  infective M60.009
    arm M60.002
      left M60.001
      right M60.000
    leg M60.005
      left M60.004
      right M60.003

Myositis *(continued)*
  infective *(continued)*
    lower limb M60.005
      ankle M60.07-
      foot M60.07-
      lower leg M60.06-
      thigh M60.05-
      toe M60.07-
    multiple sites M60.09
    specified site NEC M60.08
    upper limb M60.002
      finger M60.04-
      forearm M60.03-
      hand M60.04-
      shoulder region M60.01-
      upper arm M60.02-
  interstitial M60.10
    ankle M60.17-
    foot M60.17-
    forearm M60.13-
    hand M60.14-
    lower leg M60.16-
    multiple sites M60.19
    shoulder region M60.11-
    specified site NEC M60.18
    thigh M60.15-
    upper arm M60.12-
  mycotic B49 *[M63.8-]*
  orbital, chronic H05.12-
  ossificans or ossifying (circumscripta) —*see also* Ossification, muscle, specified NEC
    in (due to)
      burns M61.30
        ankle M61.37-
        foot M61.37-
        forearm M61.33-
        hand M61.34-
        lower leg M61.36-
        multiple sites M61.39
        pelvic region M61.35-
        shoulder region M61.31-
        specified site NEC M61.38
        thigh M61.35-
        upper arm M61.32-
      quadriplegia or paraplegia M61.20
        ankle M61.27-
        foot M61.27-
        forearm M61.23-
        hand M61.24-
        lower leg M61.26-
        multiple sites M61.29
        pelvic region M61.25-
        shoulder region M61.21-
        specified site NEC M61.28
        thigh M61.25-
        upper arm M61.22-
    progressiva M61.10
      ankle M61.17-
      finger M61.14-
      foot M61.17-
      forearm M61.13-
      hand M61.14-
      lower leg M61.16-
      multiple sites M61.19
      pelvic region M61.15-
      shoulder region M61.11-
      specified site NEC M61.18
      thigh M61.15-
      toe M61.17-
      upper arm M61.12-
    traumatica M61.00
      ankle M61.07-
      foot M61.07-
      forearm M61.03-
      hand M61.04-
      lower leg M61.06-

Myositis *(continued)*
  ossificans or ossifying *(continued)*
    traumatica *(continued)*
      multiple sites M61.09
      pelvic region M61.05-
      shoulder region M61.01-
      specified site NEC M61.08
      thigh M61.05-
      upper arm M61.02-
  purulent —*see* Myositis, infective
  specified type NEC M60.80
    ankle M60.87-
    foot M60.87-
    forearm M60.83-
    hand M60.84-
    lower leg M60.86-
    multiple sites M60.89
    pelvic region M60.85-
    shoulder region M60.81-
    specified site NEC M60.88
    thigh M60.85-
    upper arm M60.82-
  suppurative —*see* Myositis, infective
  traumatic (old) —*see* Myositis, specified type NEC

Myospasia impulsiva F95.2

Myotonia (acquisita) (intermittens) M62.89
  atrophica G71.11
  chondrodystrophic G71.13
  congenita (acetazolamide responsive) (dominant) (recessive) G71.12
  drug-induced G71.14
  dystrophica G71.11
  fluctuans G71.19
  levior G71.12
  permanens G71.19
  symptomatic G71.19

Myotonic pupil —*see* Anomaly, pupil, function, tonic pupil

Myriapodiasis B88.2

Myringitis H73.2-
  with otitis media —*see* Otitis, media
  acute H73.00-
    bullous H73.01-
    specified NEC H73.09-
  bullous —*see* Myringitis, acute, bullous
  chronic H73.1-

Mysophobia F40.228

Mytilotoxism —*see* Poisoning, fish

Myxadenitis labialis K13.0

Myxedema (adult) (idiocy) (infantile) (juvenile) (*see also* Hypothyroidism) E03.9
  circumscribed E05.90
    with storm E05.91
  coma E03.5
  congenital E00.1
  cutis L98.5
  localized (pretibial) E05.90
    with storm E05.91
  papular L98.5

Myxochondrosarcoma —*see* Neoplasm, cartilage, malignant

Myxofibroma —*see* Neoplasm, connective tissue, benign
  odontogenic —*see* Cyst, calcifying odontogenic

Myxofibrosarcoma —*see* Neoplasm, connective tissue, malignant

Myxolipoma D17.9

Myxoliposarcoma —*see* Neoplasm, connective tissue, malignant

Myxoma —*see also* Neoplasm, connective tissue, benign
  nerve sheath —*see* Neoplasm, nerve, benign
  odontogenic —*see* Cyst, calcifying odontogenic

Myxosarcoma —*see* Neoplasm, connective tissue, malignant

N

Naegeli's
  disease Q82.8
  leukemia, monocytic C93.1-

Naegleriasis (with meningoencephalitis) B60.2

Naffziger's syndrome G54.0

Naga sore —*see* Ulcer, skin

Nägele's pelvis M95.5
  with disproportion (fetopelvic) O33.0
    causing obstructed labor O65.0

Nail —*see also* condition
  biting F98.8
  patella syndrome Q87.2

Nanism, nanosomia —*see* Dwarfism

Nanophyetiasis B66.8

Nanukayami A27.89

Napkin rash L22

Narcolepsy G47.419
  with cataplexy G47.411
  in conditions classified elsewhere G47.429
    with cataplexy G47.421

Narcosis R06.89

Narcotism —*see* Dependence

NARP (Neuropathy, Ataxia and Retinitis pigmentosa) **syndrome** E88.49

Narrow
  anterior chamber angle H40.03-
  gingival width (of periodontal soft tissue) K05.5
  pelvis —*see* Contraction, pelvis

Narrowing —*see also* Stenosis
  artery I77.1
    auditory, internal I65.8
    basilar —*see* Occlusion, artery, basilar
    carotid —*see* Occlusion, artery, carotid
    cerebellar —*see* Occlusion, artery, cerebellar
    cerebral —*see* Occlusion artery, cerebral
    choroidal —*see* Occlusion, artery, precerebral, specified NEC
    communicating posterior —*see* Occlusion, artery, precerebral, specified NEC
    coronary —*see also* Disease, heart, ischemic, atherosclerotic
      congenital Q24.5
        syphilitic A50.54 *[I52]*
      due to syphilis NEC A52.06
    hypophyseal —*see* Occlusion, artery, precerebral, specified NEC
    pontine —*see* Occlusion, artery, precerebral, specified NEC

Narrowing (continued)
   artery (continued)
      precerebral —see Occlusion, artery, precerebral
      vertebral —see Occlusion, artery, vertebral
   auditory canal (external) —see Stenosis, external ear canal
   eustachian tube —see Obstruction, eustachian tube
   eyelid —see Disorder, eyelid function
   larynx J38.6
   mesenteric artery (see also Ischemia, intestine, acute) K55.059
   palate M26.89
   palpebral fissure —see Disorder, eyelid function
   ureter N13.5
      with infection N13.6
   urethra —see Stricture, urethra

Narrowness, abnormal, eyelid Q10.3

Nasal —see condition

Nasolachrymal, nasolacrimal —see condition

Nasopharyngeal —see also condition
   pituitary gland Q89.2
   torticollis M43.6

Nasopharyngitis (acute) (infective) (streptococcal) (subacute) J00
   chronic (suppurative) (ulcerative) J31.1

Nasopharynx, nasopharyngeal —see condition

Natal tooth, teeth K00.6

Nausea (without vomiting) R11.0
   with vomiting R11.2
   gravidarum —see Hyperemesis, gravidarum
   marina T75.3
   navalis T75.3

Navel —see condition

Neapolitan fever —see Brucellosis

Near drowning T75.1

Nearsightedness —see Myopia

Near-syncope R55

Nebula, cornea —see Opacity, cornea

Necator americanus infestation B76.1

Necatoriasis B76.1

Neck —see condition

Necrobiosis R68.89
   lipoidica NEC L92.1
      with diabetes —see E08-E13 with .620

Necrolysis, toxic epidermal L51.2
   due to drug
      correct substance properly administered —see Table of Drugs and Chemicals, by drug, adverse effect
      overdose or wrong substance given or taken —see Table of Drugs and Chemicals, by drug, poisoning

Necrophilia F65.89

Necrosis, necrotic (ischemic) —see also Gangrene
   adrenal (capsule) (gland) E27.49

Necrosis, necrotic (continued)
   amputation stump (surgical) (late) T87.50
      arm T87.5-
      leg T87.5-
   antrum J32.0
   aorta (hyaline) —see also Aneurysm, aorta
      cystic medial —see Dissection, aorta
   artery I77.5
   bladder (aseptic) (sphincter) N32.89
   bone —see also Osteonecrosis M87.9
      aseptic or avascular —see Osteonecrosis
      idiopathic M87.00
      ethmoid J32.2
      jaw M27.2
      tuberculous —see Tuberculosis, bone
   brain I67.89
   breast (aseptic) (fat) (segmental) N64.1
   bronchus J98.09
   central nervous system NEC I67.89
   cerebellar I67.89
   cerebral I67.89
   colon (see also Infarct, intestine) K55.049
   cornea H18.89-
   cortical (acute) (renal) N17.1
   cystic medial (aorta) —see Dissection, aorta
   dental pulp K04.1
   esophagus K22.89
   ethmoid (bone) J32.2
   eyelid —see Disorder, eyelid, degenerative
   fat, fatty (generalized) —see also Disorder, soft tissue, specified type NEC
      abdominal wall K65.4
      breast (aseptic) (segmental) N64.1
      localized —see Degeneration, by site, fatty
      mesentery K65.4
      omentum K65.4
      pancreas K86.89
      peritoneum K65.4
      skin (subcutaneous), newborn P83.0
      subcutaneous, due to birth injury P15.6
   gallbladder —see Cholecystitis, acute
   heart —see Infarct, myocardium
   hip, aseptic or avascular —see Osteonecrosis, by type, femur
   intestine (acute) (hemorrhagic) (massive) (see also Infarct, intestine) K55.069
   jaw M27.2
   kidney (bilateral) N28.0
      acute N17.9
      cortical (acute) (bilateral) N17.1
         with ectopic or molar pregnancy O08.4
      medullary (bilateral) (in acute renal failure) (papillary) N17.2
      papillary (bilateral) (in acute renal failure) N17.2
      tubular N17.0
         with ectopic or molar pregnancy O08.4

Necrosis, necrotic (continued)
   kidney (continued)
      tubular (continued)
         complicating
            abortion —see Abortion, by type, complicated by, tubular necrosis
            ectopic or molar pregnancy O08.4
            pregnancy —see Pregnancy, complicated by, diseases of, specified type or system NEC
         following ectopic or molar pregnancy O08.4
         traumatic T79.5
   larynx J38.7
   liver (with hepatic failure) (cell) —see Failure, hepatic
      hemorrhagic, central K76.2
   lung J85.0
   lymphatic gland —see Lymphadenitis, acute
   mammary gland (fat) (segmental) N64.1
   mastoid (chronic) —see Mastoiditis, chronic
   medullary (acute) (renal) N17.2
   mesentery (see also Infarct, intestine) K55.069
      fat K65.4
   mitral valve —see Insufficiency, mitral
   myocardium, myocardial —see Infarct, myocardium
   nose J34.0
   omentum (with mesenteric infarction) (see also Infarct, intestine) K55.069
      fat K65.4
   orbit, orbital —see Osteomyelitis, orbit
   ossicles, ear —see Abnormal, ear ossicles
   ovary N70.92
   pancreas (aseptic) (duct) (fat) K86.89
      acute (infective) —see Pancreatitis, acute
      infective —see Pancreatitis, acute
   papillary (acute) (renal) N17.2
   perineum N90.89
   peritoneum (with mesenteric infarction) (see also Infarct, intestine) K55.069
      fat K65.4
   pharynx J02.9
      in granulocytopenia —see Neutropenia
      Vincent's A69.1
   phosphorus —see subcategory T54.2
   pituitary (gland) E23.0
      postpartum O99.285
      Sheehan O99.285
   pressure —see Ulcer, pressure, by site
   pulmonary J85.0
   pulp (dental) K04.1
   radiation —see Necrosis, by site
   radium —see Necrosis, by site
   renal —see Necrosis, kidney
   sclera H15.89
   scrotum N50.89
   skin or subcutaneous tissue NEC I96
   spine, spinal (column) —see also Osteonecrosis, by type, vertebra
      cord G95.19
   spleen D73.5
   stomach K31.89

Necrosis, necrotic (continued)
   stomatitis (ulcerative) A69.0
   subcutaneous fat, newborn P83.88
   subendocardial (acute) I21.4
      chronic I25.89
   suprarenal (capsule) (gland) E27.49
   testis N50.89
   thymus (gland) E32.8
   tonsil J35.8
   trachea J39.8
   tuberculous NEC —see Tuberculosis
   tubular (acute) (anoxic) (renal) (toxic) N17.0
      postprocedural N99.0
   vagina N89.8
   vertebra —see also Osteonecrosis, by type, vertebra
      tuberculous A18.01
   vulva N90.89
   X-ray —see Necrosis, by site

Necrospermia —see Infertility, male

Need (for)
   care provider because (of)
      assistance with personal care Z74.1
      continuous supervision required Z74.3
      impaired mobility Z74.09
      no other household member able to render care Z74.2
      specified reason NEC Z74.8
   immunization —see Vaccination
   vaccination —see Vaccination

Neglect
   adult
      confirmed T74.01
      history of Z91.412
      suspected T76.01
   child (childhood)
      confirmed T74.02
      history of Z62.812
      suspected T76.02
   emotional, in childhood Z62.898
   hemispatial R41.4
   left-sided R41.4
   sensory R41.4
   visuospatial R41.4

Neisserian infection NEC —see Gonococcus

Nelaton's syndrome G60.8

Nelson's syndrome E24.1

Nematodiasis (intestinal) B82.0
   Ancylostoma B76.0

Neonatal —see also Newborn
   acne L70.4
   bradycardia P29.12
   tachycardia P29.11
   screening, abnormal findings on —see Abnormal, neonatal screening
   tooth, teeth K00.6

Neonatorum —see condition

Neoplasia
   endocrine, multiple (MEN) E31.20
      type I E31.21
      type IIA E31.22
      type IIB E31.23

241

Neoplasia (continued)
- intraepithelial (histologically confirmed)
  - anal (AIN) (histologically confirmed) K62.82
    - grade I K62.82
    - grade II K62.82
    - severe D01.3
  - cervical glandular (histologically confirmed) D06.9
  - cervix (uteri) (CIN) (histologically confirmed) N87.9
    - glandular D06.9
    - grade I N87.0
    - grade II N87.1
    - grade III (severe dysplasia) (see also Carcinoma, cervix uteri, in situ) D06.9
  - prostate (histologically confirmed) (PIN) N42.31
    - grade I N42.31
    - grade II N42.31
    - grade III (severe dysplasia) D07.5
  - vagina (histologically confirmed) (VAIN) N89.3
    - grade I N89.0
    - grade II N89.1
    - grade III (severe dysplasia) D07.2
  - vulva (histologically confirmed) (VIN) N90.3
    - grade I N90.0
    - grade II N90.1
    - grade III (severe dysplasia) D07.1

Neoplasm, neoplastic —see also Table of Neoplasms
- lipomatous, benign —see Lipoma
- malignant mast cell C96.20
  - specified type NEC C96.29
- mast cell, of uncertain behavior NEC D47.09
- myelodysplastic/myeloproliferative, unclassifiable C94.6

Neovascularization
- ciliary body —see Disorder, iris, vascular
- cornea H16.40-
  - deep H16.44-
  - ghost vessels —see Ghost, vessels
  - localized H16.43-
  - pannus —see Pannus
- iris —see Disorder, iris, vascular
- retina H35.05-

Nephralgia N23

Nephritis, nephritic (albuminuric) (azotemic) (congenital) (disseminated) (epithelial) (familial) (focal) (granulomatous) (hemorrhagic) (infantile) (nonsuppurative, excretory) (uremic) N05.9
- with
  - C3
    - glomerulonephritis N05.A
    - glomerulopathy N05.A
      - with dense deposit disease N05.6
    - dense deposit disease N05.6
  - diffuse
    - crescentic glomerulonephritis N05.7
    - endocapillary proliferative glomerulonephritis N05.4

Nephritis, nephritic (continued)
- with (continued)
  - diffuse (continued)
    - membranous glomerulonephritis N05.2
    - mesangial proliferative glomerulonephritis N05.3
    - mesangiocapillary glomerulonephritis N05.5
  - edema —see Nephrosis
  - focal and segmental glomerular lesions N05.1
  - foot process disease N04.9
  - glomerular lesion
    - diffuse sclerosing N05.8
    - hypocomplementemic —see Nephritis, membranoproliferative
  - IgA —see Nephropathy, IgA
  - lobular, lobulonodular —see Nephritis, membranoproliferative
  - nodular —see Nephritis, membranoproliferative
  - lesion of glomerulonephritis, proliferative N05.8
  - renal necrosis N05.9
  - minor glomerular abnormality N05.0
  - specified morphological changes NEC N05.8
- acute N00.9
  - with
    - C3
      - glomerulonephritis N00.A
      - glomerulopathy N00.A
        - with dense deposit disease N00.6
      - dense deposit disease N00.6
    - diffuse
      - crescentic glomerulonephritis N00.7
      - endocapillary proliferative glomerulonephritis N00.4
      - membranous glomerulonephritis N00.2
      - mesangial proliferative glomerulonephritis N00.3
      - mesangiocapillary glomerulonephritis N00.5
    - focal and segmental glomerular lesions N00.1
    - minor glomerular abnormality N00.0
    - specified morphological changes NEC N00.8
- amyloid E85.4 [N08]
- antiglomerular basement membrane (anti-GBM) antibody NEC
  - in Goodpasture's syndrome M31.0
- antitubular basement membrane (tubulo-interstitial) NEC N12
  - toxic —see Nephropathy, toxic
- arteriolar —see Hypertension, kidney
- arteriosclerotic —see Hypertension, kidney
- ascending —see Nephritis, tubulo-interstitial
- atrophic N03.9
- Balkan (endemic) N15.0
- calculous, calculus —see Calculus, kidney
- cardiac —see Hypertension, kidney
- cardiovascular —see Hypertension, kidney
- chronic N03.9
  - with
    - C3
      - glomerulonephritis N03.A

Nephritis, nephritic (continued)
- chronic (continued)
  - with (continued)
    - C3 (continued)
      - glomerulopathy N03.A
        - with dense deposit disease N03.6
      - dense deposit disease N03.6
    - diffuse
      - crescentic glomerulonephritis N03.7
      - endocapillary proliferative glomerulonephritis N03.4
      - membranous glomerulonephritis N03.2
      - mesangial proliferative glomerulonephritis N03.3
      - mesangiocapillary glomerulonephritis N03.5
    - focal and segmental glomerular lesions N03.1
    - minor glomerular abnormality N03.0
    - specified morphological changes NEC N03.8
  - arteriosclerotic —see Hypertension, kidney
- cirrhotic N26.9
- complicating pregnancy O26.83-
- croupous N00.9
- degenerative —see Nephrosis
- diffuse sclerosing N05.8
- due to
  - diabetes mellitus —see E08-E13 with .21
  - subacute bacterial endocarditis I33.0
  - systemic lupus erythematosus (chronic) M32.14
  - typhoid fever A01.09
- gonococcal (acute) (chronic) A54.21
- hypocomplementemic —see Nephritis, membranoproliferative
- IgA —see Nephropathy, IgA
- immune complex (circulating) NEC N05.8
- infective —see Nephritis, tubulo-interstitial
- interstitial —see Nephritis, tubulo-interstitial
- lead N14.3
- membranoproliferative (diffuse) (type 1 or 3) (see also N00-N07 with fourth character .5) N05.5
  - type 2 (see also N00-N07 with fourth character .6) N05.6
- minimal change N05.0
- necrotic, necrotizing NEC (see also N00-N07 with fourth character .8) N05.8
- nephrotic —see Nephrosis
- nodular —see Nephritis, membranoproliferative
- polycystic Q61.3
  - adult type Q61.2
  - autosomal
    - dominant Q61.2
    - recessive NEC Q61.19
  - childhood type NEC Q61.19
  - infantile type NEC Q61.19
- poststreptococcal N05.9
  - acute N00.9
  - chronic N03.9
  - rapidly progressive N01.9
- proliferative NEC (see also N00-N07 with fourth character .8) N05.8
- purulent —see Nephritis, tubulo-interstitial

Nephritis, nephritic (continued)
- rapidly progressive N01.9
  - with
    - C3
      - glomerulonephritis N01.A
      - glomerulopathy N01.A
        - with dense deposit disease N01.6
      - dense deposit disease N01.6
    - diffuse
      - crescentic glomerulonephritis N01.7
      - endocapillary proliferative glomerulonephritis N01.4
      - membranous glomerulonephritis N01.2
      - mesangial proliferative glomerulonephritis N01.3
      - mesangiocapillary glomerulonephritis N01.5
    - focal and segmental glomerular lesions N01.1
    - minor glomerular abnormality N01.0
    - specified morphological changes NEC N01.8
- salt losing or wasting NEC N28.89
- saturnine N14.3
- sclerosing, diffuse N05.8
- septic —see Nephritis, tubulo-interstitial
- specified pathology NEC (see also N00-N07 with fourth character .8) N05.8
- subacute N01.9
- suppurative —see Nephritis, tubulo-interstitial
- syphilitic (late) A52.75
  - congenital A50.59 [N08]
  - early (secondary) A51.44
- toxic —see Nephropathy, toxic
- tubal, tubular —see Nephritis, tubulo-interstitial
- tuberculous A18.11
- tubulo-interstitial (in) N12
  - acute (infectious) N10
  - chronic (infectious) N11.9
    - nonobstructive N11.8
    - reflux-associated N11.0
    - obstructive N11.1
    - specified NEC N11.8
  - due to
    - brucellosis A23.9 [N16]
    - cryoglobulinemia D89.1 [N16]
    - glycogen storage disease E74.00 [N16]
  - Sjögren's syndrome M35.04
- vascular —see Hypertension, kidney
- war N00.9

Nephroblastoma (epithelial) (mesenchymal) C64-

Nephrocalcinosis E83.59 [N29]

Nephrocystitis, pustular —see Nephritis, tubulo-interstitial

Nephrolithiasis (congenital) (pelvis) (recurrent) —see also Calculus, kidney

Nephroma C64-
- mesoblastic D41.0-

Nephronephritis —see Nephrosis

Nephronophthisis Q61.5

Nephropathia epidemica A98.5

Nephropathy —see also Nephritis N28.9
- with
  - edema —see Nephrosis

Nephropathy (continued)
with (continued)
glomerular lesion —see
Glomerulonephritis
amyloid, hereditary E85.0
analgesic N14.0
with medullary necrosis, acute
N17.2
Balkan (endemic) N15.0
chemical —see Nephropathy,
toxic
contrast-induced N14.11
contrast medium, radiography
N14.11
diabetic —see E08-E13 with .21
drug-induced N14.2
contrast-induced N14.11
specified NEC N14.19
focal and segmental hyalinosis or
sclerosis N02.1
heavy metal-induced N14.3
hereditary NEC N07.9
with
C3
glomerulonephritis N07.A
glomerulopathy N07.A
with dense deposit
disease N07.6
dense deposit disease N07.6
diffuse
crescentic
glomerulonephritis N07.7
endocapillary proliferative
glomerulonephritis N07.4
membranous
glomerulonephritis N07.2
mesangial proliferative
glomerulonephritis N07.3
mesangiocapillary
glomerulonephritis N07.5
focal and segmental
glomerular lesions N07.1
minor glomerular abnormality
N07.0
specified morphological
changes NEC N07.8
hypercalcemic N25.89
hypertensive —see Hypertension,
kidney
hypokalemic (vacuolar) N25.89
IgA N02.B-
with glomerular lesion N02.B1
focal and segmental hyalinosis
or sclerosis N02.B2
membranoproliferative
(diffuse) N02.B3
membranous (diffuse) N02.B4
mesangial proliferative
(diffuse) N02.B5
mesangiocapillary (diffuse)
N02.B6
proliferative NEC N02.B9
specified pathology NEC
N02.B9
lead N14.3
membranoproliferative (diffuse)
N02.5
membranous (diffuse) N06.20
with
nephrotic syndrome N04.20
primary N04.21
secondary N04.22
idiopathic, with nephrotic
syndrome N04.21
primary N06.21
with nephrotic syndrome
N04.21
secondary N06.22
with nephrotic syndrome
N04.22

Nephropathy (continued)
mesangial (IgA/IgG) —see
Nephropathy, IgA
proliferative (diffuse) N02.3
mesangiocapillary (diffuse) N02.5
obstructive N13.8
phenacetin N17.2
phosphate-losing N25.0
potassium depletion N25.89
pregnancy-related O26.83-
proliferative NEC (see also N00-N07
with fourth character .8) N05.8
protein-losing N25.89
saturnine N14.3
sickle-cell D57.- [N08]
toxic NEC N14.4
due to
drugs N14.2
analgesic N14.0
specified NEC N14.19
heavy metals N14.3
vasomotor N17.0
water-losing N25.89

Nephroptosis N28.83

Nephropyosis —see Abscess, kidney

Nephrorrhagia N28.89

Nephrosclerosis (arteriolar)
(arteriosclerotic) (chronic) (hyaline)
—see also Hypertension, kidney
hyperplastic —see Hypertension,
kidney
senile N26.9

Nephrosis, nephrotic (Epstein's)
(syndrome) (congenital) N04.9
with
foot process disease N04.9
glomerular lesion N04.1
hypocomplementemic N04.5
acute N04.9
anoxic —see Nephrosis, tubular
chemical —see Nephrosis, tubular
cholemic K76.7
diabetic —see E08-E13 with .21
Finnish type (congenital) Q89.8
hemoglobin N10
hemoglobinuric —see Nephrosis,
tubular
in
amyloidosis E85.4 [N08]
diabetes mellitus —see E08-E13
with .21
epidemic hemorrhagic fever A98.5
malaria (malariae) B52.0
ischemic —see Nephrosis, tubular
lipoid N04.9
lower nephron —see Nephrosis,
tubular
malarial (malariae) B52.0
minimal change N04.0
myoglobin N10
necrotizing —see Nephrosis, tubular
osmotic (sucrose) N25.89
radiation N04.9
syphilitic (late) A52.75
toxic —see Nephrosis, tubular
tubular (acute) N17.0
postprocedural N99.0
radiation N04.9

Nephrosonephritis, hemorrhagic
(endemic) A98.5

Nephrostomy
attention to Z43.6
status Z93.6

Nerve —see also condition
injury —see Injury, nerve, by body
site

Nerves R45.0

Nervous (see also condition) R45.0
heart F45.8
stomach F45.8
tension R45.0

Nervousness R45.0

Nesidioblastoma
pancreas D13.7
specified site NEC —see
Neoplasm, benign, by site
unspecified site D13.7

Nettleship's syndrome —see
Urticaria pigmentosa

Neumann's disease or syndrome
L10.1

Neuralgia, neuralgic (acute) M79.2
accessory (nerve) G52.8
acoustic (nerve) H93.3
auditory (nerve) H93.3
ciliary G44.009
intractable G44.001
not intractable G44.009
cranial
nerve —see also Disorder,
nerve, cranial
fifth or trigeminal —see
Neuralgia, trigeminal
postherpetic, postzoster
B02.29
ear —see subcategory H92.0
facialis vera G51.1
Fothergill's —see Neuralgia,
trigeminal
glossopharyngeal (nerve) G52.1
Horton's G44.099
intractable G44.091
not intractable G44.099
Hunt's B02.21
hypoglossal (nerve) G52.3
infraorbital —see Neuralgia,
trigeminal
malarial —see Malaria
migrainous G44.009
intractable G44.001
not intractable G44.009
Morton's G57.6-
nerve, cranial —see Disorder,
nerve, cranial
nose G52.0
occipital M54.81
olfactory G52.0
penis N48.9
perineum R10.2
postherpetic NEC B02.29
trigeminal B02.22
pubic region R10.2
scrotum R10.2
Sluder's G44.89
specified nerve NEC G58.8
spermatic cord R10.2
sphenopalatine (ganglion) G90.09
trifacial —see Neuralgia, trigeminal
trigeminal G50.0
postherpetic, postzoster B02.22
vagus (nerve) G52.2
writer's F48.8
organic G25.89

Neurapraxia —see Injury, nerve

Neurasthenia F48.8
cardiac F45.8
gastric F45.8
heart F45.8

Neurilemmoma —see also
Neoplasm, nerve, benign
acoustic (nerve) D33.3
malignant —see also Neoplasm,
nerve, malignant
acoustic (nerve) C72.4-

Neurilemmosarcoma —see
Neoplasm, nerve, malignant

Neurinoma —see Neoplasm, nerve,
benign

Neurinomatosis —see Neoplasm,
nerve, uncertain behavior

Neuritis (rheumatoid) M79.2
abducens (nerve) —see Strabismus,
paralytic, sixth nerve
accessory (nerve) G52.8
acoustic (nerve) (see also
subcategory) H93.3
in (due to)
infectious disease NEC B99
[H94.0-]
parasitic disease NEC B89
[H94.0-]
syphilitic A52.15
alcoholic G62.1
with psychosis —see Psychosis,
alcoholic
amyloid, any site E85.4 [G63]
auditory (nerve) —see subcategory
H93.3
brachial —see Radiculopathy
due to displacement,
intervertebral disc —see
Disorder, disc, cervical, with
neuritis
cranial nerve
due to Lyme disease A69.22
eighth or acoustic or auditory
H93.3
eleventh or accessory G52.8
fifth or trigeminal G50.-
first or olfactory G52.0
fourth or trochlear —see
Strabismus, paralytic, fourth
nerve
second or optic —see Neuritis,
optic
seventh or facial G51.8
newborn (birth injury) P11.3
sixth or abducent —see Strabismus,
paralytic, sixth nerve
tenth or vagus G52.2
third or oculomotor —see
Strabismus, paralytic, third nerve
twelfth or hypoglossal G52.3
Déjérine-Sottas G60.0
diabetic (mononeuropathy) —see
E08-E13 with .41
polyneuropathy —see E08-E13
with .42
due to
beriberi E51.11
displacement, prolapse or
rupture, intervertebral disc
—see Disorder, disc, with,
radiculopathy
herniation, nucleus pulposus
M51.9 [G55]
endemic E51.11
facial G51.8
newborn (birth injury) P11.3
general —see Polyneuropathy
geniculate ganglion G51.1
due to herpes (zoster) B02.21
gouty (see also Gout, by type)
M10.9 [G63]
hypoglossal (nerve) G52.3
ilioinguinal (nerve) G57.9-
infectious (multiple) NEC G61.0
interstitial hypertrophic progressive
G60.0
lumbar M54.16
lumbosacral M54.17
multiple —see also Polyneuropathy
endemic E51.11
infective, acute G61.0

Neuritis (continued)
  multiplex endemica E51.11
  nerve root —see Radiculopathy
  oculomotor (nerve) —see Strabismus, paralytic, third nerve
  olfactory nerve G52.0
  optic (nerve) (hereditary) (sympathetic) H46.9
    with demyelination G36.0
    in myelitis G36.0
    nutritional H46.2
    papillitis —see Papillitis, optic
    retrobulbar H46.1-
    specified type NEC H46.8
    toxic H46.3
  peripheral (nerve) G62.9
    multiple —see Polyneuropathy
    single —see Mononeuritis
  pneumogastric (nerve) G52.2
  postherpetic, postzoster B02.29
  progressive hypertrophic interstitial G60.0
  retrobulbar —see also Neuritis, optic, retrobulbar
    in (due to)
      late syphilis A52.15
      meningococcal infection A39.82
    meningococcal A39.82
    syphilitic A52.15
  sciatic (nerve) —see also Sciatica
    due to displacement of intervertebral disc —see Disorder, disc, with, radiculopathy
  serum (see also Reaction, serum) T80.69
  shoulder-girdle G54.5
  specified nerve NEC G58.8
  spinal (nerve) root —see Radiculopathy
  syphilitic A52.15
  thenar (median) G56.1-
  thoracic M54.14
  toxic NEC G62.2
  trochlear (nerve) —see Strabismus, paralytic, fourth nerve
  vagus (nerve) G52.2

Neuroastrocytoma —see Neoplasm, uncertain behavior, by site

Neuroavitaminosis E56.9 *[G99.8]*

Neuroblastoma
  olfactory C30.0
  specified site —see Neoplasm, malignant, by site
  unspecified site C74.90

Neurochorioretinitis —see Chorioretinitis

Neurocirculatory asthenia F45.8

Neurocysticercosis B69.0

Neurocytoma —see Neoplasm, benign, by site

Neurodermatitis (circumscribed) (circumscripta) (local) L28.0
  atopic L20.81
  diffuse (Brocq) L20.81
  disseminated L20.81

Neuroencephalomyelopathy, optic G36.0

Neuroepithelioma —see also Neoplasm, malignant, by site
  olfactory C30.0

Neurofibroma —see also Neoplasm, nerve, benign
  melanotic —see Neoplasm, nerve, benign

Neurofibroma (continued)
  multiple —see Neurofibromatosis
  plexiform —see Neoplasm, nerve, benign

Neurofibromatosis (multiple) (nonmalignant) Q85.00
  acoustic Q85.02
  malignant —see Neoplasm, nerve, malignant
  specified NEC Q85.09
  type 1 (von Recklinghausen) Q85.01
  type 2 Q85.02

Neurofibrosarcoma —see Neoplasm, nerve, malignant

Neurogenic —see also condition
  bladder (see also Dysfunction bladder, neuromuscular) N31.9
    cauda equina syndrome G83.4
  bowel NEC K59.2
  heart F45.8

Neuroglioma —see Neoplasm, uncertain behavior, by site

Neurolabyrinthitis (of Dix and Hallpike) —see Neuronitis, vestibular

Neurolathyrism —see Poisoning, food, noxious, plant

Neuroleprosy A30.9

Neuroma —see also Neoplasm, nerve, benign
  acoustic (nerve) D33.3
  amputation (stump) (traumatic) (surgical complication) (late) T87.3-
    arm T87.3-
    leg T87.3-
  digital (toe) G57.6-
  interdigital G58.8
    lower limb (toe) G57.8-
    upper limb G56.8-
  intermetatarsal G57.8-
  Morton's G57.6-
  nonneoplastic
    arm G56.9-
    leg G57.9-
    lower extremity G57.9-
    upper extremity G56.9-
  optic (nerve) D33.3
  plantar G57.6-
  plexiform —see Neoplasm, nerve, benign
  surgical (nonneoplastic)
    arm G56.9-
    leg G57.9-
    lower extremity G57.9-
    upper extremity G56.9-

Neuromyalgia —see Neuralgia

Neuromyasthenia (epidemic) (postinfectious) G93.39

Neuromyelitis G36.9
  ascending G61.0
  optica G36.0

Neuromyopathy G70.9
  paraneoplastic (see also, Neoplasm, by site, if known) D49.9 *[G13.0]*

Neuromyotonia (Isaacs) G71.19

Neuronevus —see Nevus

Neuronitis G58.9
  ascending (acute) G57.2-
  vestibular H81.2-

Neuroparalytic —see condition

Neuropathy, neuropathic G62.9
  acute motor G62.81

Neuropathy, neuropathic (continued)
  alcoholic G62.1
    with psychosis —see Psychosis, alcoholic
  arm G56.9-
  autonomic, peripheral —see Neuropathy, peripheral, autonomic
  axillary G56.9-
  bladder N31.9
    atonic (motor) (sensory) N31.2
    autonomous N31.2
    flaccid N31.2
    nonreflex N31.2
    reflex N31.1
    uninhibited N31.0
  brachial plexus G54.0
  cervical plexus G54.2
  chronic
    progressive segmentally demyelinating G62.89
    relapsing demyelinating G62.89
  Déjérine-Sottas G60.0
  diabetic —see E08-E13 with .40
    mononeuropathy —see E08-E13 with .41
    polyneuropathy —see E08-E13 with .42
  entrapment G58.9
    iliohypogastric nerve G57.8-
    ilioinguinal nerve G57.8-
    lateral cutaneous nerve of thigh G57.1-
    median nerve G56.0-
    obturator nerve G57.8-
    peroneal nerve G57.3-
    posterior tibial nerve G57.5-
    saphenous nerve G57.8-
    ulnar nerve G56.2-
  facial nerve G51.9
  hereditary G60.9
    motor and sensory (types I-IV) G60.0
    sensory G60.8
    specified NEC G60.8
  hypertrophic G60.0
    Charcot-Marie-Tooth G60.0
    -Sottas G60.0
    interstitial progressive G60.0
    of infancy G60.0
    Refsum G60.1
  idiopathic G60.9
    progressive G60.3
    specified NEC G60.8
  in association with hereditary ataxia G60.2
  intercostal G58.0
  ischemic —see Disorder, nerve
  Jamaica (ginger) G62.2
  leg NEC G57.9-
  lower extremity G57.9-
  lumbar plexus G54.1
  median nerve G56.1-
  motor and sensory —see also Polyneuropathy
    hereditary (types I-IV) G60.0
  multifocal motor (MMN) G61.82
  multiple (acute) (chronic) —see Polyneuropathy
  optic (nerve) —see also Neuritis, optic
    ischemic H47.01-
  paraneoplastic (sensorial) (Denny Brown) (see also, Neoplasm, by site, if known) D49.9 *[G13.0]*
  peripheral (nerve) (see also Polyneuropathy) G62.9
    autonomic G90.9
      idiopathic G90.09
      in (due to)
        amyloidosis E85.4 *[G99.0]*
        diabetes mellitus —see E08-E13 with .43

Neuropathy, neuropathic (continued)
  peripheral (continued)
    autonomic (continued)
      in (continued)
        endocrine disease NEC E34.9 *[G99.0]*
        gout M10.00 *[G99.0]*
        hyperthyroidism E05.90 *[G99.0]*
          with thyroid storm E05.91 *[G99.0]*
        metabolic disease NEC E88.9 *[G99.0]*
    idiopathic G60.9
      progressive G60.3
    in (due to)
      antitetanus serum G62.0
      arsenic G62.2
      drugs NEC G62.0
      lead G62.2
      organophosphate compounds G62.2
      toxic agent NEC G62.2
    plantar nerves G57.6-
    progressive
      hypertrophic interstitial G60.0
      inflammatory G62.81
    radicular NEC —see Radiculopathy
    sacral plexus G54.1
    sciatic G57.0-
    serum G61.1
    toxic NEC G62.2
    trigeminal sensory G50.8
    ulnar nerve G56.2-
    uremic N18.9 *[G63]*
    vitamin B12 E53.8 *[G63]*
      with anemia (pernicious) D51.0 *[G63]*
      due to dietary deficiency D51.3 *[G63]*

Neurophthisis —see also Disorder, nerve
  peripheral, diabetic —see E08-E13 with .42

Neuroretinitis —see Chorioretinitis

Neuroretinopathy, hereditary optic H47.22

Neurosarcoma —see Neoplasm, nerve, malignant

Neurosclerosis —see Disorder, nerve

Neurosis, neurotic F48.9
  anankastic F42.8
  anxiety (state) F41.1
    panic type F41.0
  asthenic F48.8
  bladder F45.8
  cardiac (reflex) F45.8
  cardiovascular F45.8
  character F60.9
  colon F45.8
  compensation F68.10
  compulsive, compulsion F42.8
  conversion F44.9
  craft F48.8
  cutaneous F45.8
  depersonalization F48.1
  depressive (reaction) (type) F34.1
  environmental F48.8
  excoriation L98.1
  fatigue F48.8
  functional —see Disorder, somatoform
  gastric F45.8
  gastrointestinal F45.8
  heart F45.8
  hypochondriacal F45.21
  hysterical F44.9
  incoordination F45.8
    larynx F45.8
    vocal cord F45.8

Neurosis, neurotic *(continued)*
- intestine F45.8
- larynx (sensory) F45.8
  - hysterical F44.4
- mixed NEC F48.8
- musculoskeletal F45.8
- obsessional F42.8
- obsessive-compulsive F42.8
- occupational F48.8
- ocular NEC F45.8
- organ —*see* Disorder, somatoform
- pharynx F45.8
- phobic F40.9
- posttraumatic (situational) F43.10
  - acute F43.11
  - chronic F43.12
- psychasthenic (type) F48.8
- railroad F48.8
- rectum F45.8
- respiratory F45.8
- rumination F45.8
- sexual F65.9
- situational F48.8
- social F40.10
  - generalized F40.11
- specified type NEC F48.8
- state F48.9
  - with depersonalization episode F48.1
- stomach F45.8
- traumatic F43.10
  - acute F43.11
  - chronic F43.12
- vasomotor F45.8
- visceral F45.8
- war F48.8

Neurospongioblastosis diffusa Q85.1

Neurosyphilis (arrested) (early) (gumma) (late) (latent) (recurrent) (relapse) A52.3
- with ataxia (cerebellar) (locomotor) (spastic) (spinal) A52.19
- aneurysm (cerebral) A52.05
- arachnoid (adhesive) A52.13
- arteritis (any artery) (cerebral) A52.04
- asymptomatic A52.2
- congenital A50.40
- dura (mater) A52.13
- general paresis A52.17
- hemorrhagic A52.05
- juvenile (asymptomatic) (meningeal) A50.40
- leptomeninges (aseptic) A52.13
- meningeal, meninges (adhesive) A52.13
- meningitis A52.13
- meningovascular (diffuse) A52.13
- optic atrophy A52.15
- parenchymatous (degenerative) A52.19
- paresis, paretic A52.17
  - juvenile A50.45
- remission in (sustained) A52.3
- serological (without symptoms) A52.2
- specified nature or site NEC A52.19
- tabes, tabetic (dorsalis) A52.11
  - juvenile A50.45
- taboparesis A52.17
  - juvenile A50.45
- thrombosis (cerebral) A52.05
- vascular (cerebral) NEC A52.05

Neurothekeoma —*see* Neoplasm, nerve, benign

Neurotic —*see* Neurosis

Neurotoxemia —*see* Toxemia

Neuroclusion M26.211

Neutropenia, neutropenic (chronic) (genetic) (idiopathic) (immune) (infantile) (malignant) (pernicious) (splenic) D70.9
- congenital (primary) D70.0
- cyclic D70.4
- cytoreductive cancer chemotherapy sequela D70.1
- drug-induced D70.2
  - due to cytoreductive cancer chemotherapy D70.1
- due to infection D70.3
- fever D70.9
- neonatal, transitory (isoimmune) (maternal transfer) P61.5
- periodic D70.4
- secondary (cyclic) (periodic) (splenic) D70.4
  - drug-induced D70.2
    - due to cytoreductive cancer chemotherapy D70.1
- specified NEC D70.8
- toxic D70.8

Neutrophilia, hereditary giant D72.0

Nevocarcinoma —*see* Melanoma

Nevus D22.9
- achromic —*see* Neoplasm, skin, benign
- amelanotic —*see* Neoplasm, skin, benign
- angiomatous D18.00
  - intra-abdominal D18.03
  - intracranial D18.02
  - skin D18.01
  - specified site NEC D18.09
- araneus I78.1
- balloon cell —*see* Neoplasm, skin, benign
- bathing trunk D48.5
- blue —*see* Neoplasm, skin, benign
  - cellular —*see* Neoplasm, skin, benign
  - giant —*see* Neoplasm, skin, benign
  - Jadassohn's —*see* Neoplasm, skin, benign
  - malignant —*see* Melanoma
- capillary D18.00
  - intra-abdominal D18.03
  - intracranial D18.02
  - skin D18.01
  - specified site NEC D18.09
- cavernous D18.00
  - intra-abdominal D18.03
  - intracranial D18.02
  - skin D18.01
  - specified site NEC D18.09
- cellular —*see* Neoplasm, skin, benign
  - blue —*see* Neoplasm, skin, benign
- choroid D31.3-
- comedonicus Q82.5
- conjunctiva D31.0-
- dermal —*see* Neoplasm, skin, benign
  - with epidermal nevus —*see* Neoplasm, skin, benign
- dysplastic —*see* Neoplasm, skin, benign
- eye D31.9-
- flammeus Q82.5
- hemangiomatous D18.00
  - intra-abdominal D18.03
  - intracranial D18.02
  - skin D18.01
  - specified site NEC D18.09
- iris D31.4-
- lacrimal gland D31.5-
- lymphatic D18.1

Nevus *(continued)*
- magnocellular
  - specified site —*see* Neoplasm, benign, by site
  - unspecified site D31.40
- malignant —*see* Melanoma
- meaning hemangioma D18.00
  - intra-abdominal D18.03
  - intracranial D18.02
  - skin D18.01
  - specified site NEC D18.09
- mouth (mucosa) D10.30
  - specified site NEC D10.39
  - white sponge Q38.6
- multiplex Q85.1
- non-neoplastic I78.1
- oral mucosa D10.30
  - specified site NEC D10.39
  - white sponge Q38.6
- orbit D31.6-
- pigmented
  - giant (*see also* Neoplasm, skin, uncertain behavior) D48.5
    - malignant melanoma in —*see* Melanoma
- portwine Q82.5
- retina D31.2-
- retrobulbar D31.6-
- sanguineous Q82.5
- senile I78.1
- skin D22.9
  - abdominal wall D22.5
  - ala nasi D22.39
  - ankle D22.7-
  - anus, anal D22.5
  - arm D22.6-
  - auditory canal (external) D22.2-
  - auricle (ear) D22.2-
  - auricular canal (external) D22.2-
  - axilla, axillary fold D22.5
  - back D22.5
  - breast D22.5
  - brow D22.39
  - buttock D22.5
  - canthus (eye) D22.1-
  - cheek (external) D22.39
  - chest wall D22.5
  - chin D22.39
  - ear (external) D22.2-
  - external meatus (ear) D22.2-
  - eyebrow D22.39
  - eyelid (lower) (upper) D22.1-
  - face D22.30
    - specified NEC D22.39
  - female genital organ (external) NEC D28.0
  - finger D22.6-
  - flank D22.5
  - foot D22.7-
  - forearm D22.6-
  - forehead D22.39
  - foreskin D29.0
  - genital organ (external) NEC
    - female D28.0
    - male D29.9
  - gluteal region D22.5
  - groin D22.5
  - hand D22.6-
  - heel D22.7-
  - helix D22.2-
  - hip D22.7-
  - interscapular region D22.5
  - jaw D22.39
  - knee D22.7-
  - labium (majus) (minus) D28.0
  - leg D22.7-
  - lip (lower) (upper) D22.0
  - lower limb D22.7-
  - male genital organ (external) D29.9

Nevus *(continued)*
- skin *(continued)*
  - nail D22.9
    - finger D22.6-
    - toe D22.7-
  - nasolabial groove D22.39
  - nates D22.5
  - neck D22.4
  - nose (external) D22.39
  - palpebra D22.1-
  - penis D29.0
  - perianal skin D22.5
  - perineum D22.5
  - pinna D22.2-
  - popliteal fossa or space D22.7-
  - prepuce D29.0
  - pudendum D28.0
  - scalp D22.4
  - scrotum D29.4
  - shoulder D22.6-
  - submammary fold D22.5
  - temple D22.39
  - thigh D22.7-
  - toe D22.7-
  - trunk NEC D22.5
  - umbilicus D22.5
  - upper limb D22.6-
  - vulva D28.0
  - specified site NEC —*see* Neoplasm, by site, benign
- spider I78.1
- stellar I78.1
- strawberry Q82.5
- Sutton's benign D22.9
- unius lateris Q82.5
- Unna's Q82.5
- vascular Q82.5
- verrucous Q82.5

Newborn (infant) (liveborn) (singleton) Z38.2
- acne L70.4
- abstinence syndrome P96.1
- affected by
  - abnormalities of membranes P02.9
    - specified NEC P02.8
  - abruptio placenta P02.1
  - amino-acid metabolic disorder, transitory P74.8
  - amniocentesis (while in utero) P00.6
  - amnionitis P02.78
  - apparent life threatening event (ALTE) R68.13
  - bleeding (into)
    - cerebral cortex P52.22
    - germinal matrix P52.0
    - ventricles P52.1
  - breech delivery P03.0
  - cardiac arrest P29.81
  - cardiomyopathy I42.8
    - congenital I42.4
  - cerebral ischemia P91.0
  - Cesarean delivery P03.4
  - chemotherapy agents P04.11
  - chorioamnionitis P02.78
  - cocaine (crack) P04.41
  - complications of labor and delivery P03.9
    - specified NEC P03.89
  - compression of umbilical cord NEC P02.5
  - contracted pelvis P03.1
  - cyanosis P28.2
  - delivery P03.9
    - Cesarean P03.4
    - forceps P03.2
    - vacuum extractor P03.3

Newborn (continued)
  affected by (continued)
    drugs of addiction P04.40
      cocaine P04.41
      hallucinogens P04.42
      specified drug NEC P04.49
    environmental chemicals P04.6
    entanglement (knot) in umbilical cord P02.5
    fetal (intrauterine)
      growth retardation P05.9
      inflammatory response syndrome (FIRS) P02.70
      malnutrition not light or small for gestational age P05.2
    FIRS (fetal inflammatory response syndrome) P02.70
    forceps delivery P03.2
    heart rate abnormalities
      bradycardia P29.12
      intrauterine P03.819
        before onset of labor P03.810
        during labor P03.811
      tachycardia P29.11
    hemorrhage (antepartum) P02.1
      cerebellar (nontraumatic) P52.6
      intracerebral (nontraumatic) P52.4
      intracranial (nontraumatic) P52.9
        specified NEC P52.8
      intraventricular (nontraumatic) P52.3
        grade 1 P52.0
        grade 2 P52.1
        grade 3 P52.21
        grade 4 P52.22
      posterior fossa (nontraumatic) P52.6
      subarachnoid (nontraumatic) P52.5
      subependymal P52.0
        with intracerebral extension P52.22
        with intraventricular extension P52.1
          with enlargment of ventricles P52.21
        without intraventricular extension P52.0
    hypoxic ischemic encephalopathy [HIE] P91.60
      mild P91.61
      moderate P91.62
      severe P91.63
    induction of labor P03.89
    intestinal perforation P78.0
    intrauterine (fetal) blood loss P50.9
      due to (from)
        cut end of co-twin cord P50.5
        hemorrhage into
          co-twin P50.3
          maternal circulation P50.4
        placenta P50.2
        ruptured cord blood P50.1
        vasa previa P50.0
      specified NEC P50.8
    intrauterine (fetal) hemorrhage P50.9
    intrauterine (in utero) procedure P96.5
    malpresentation (malposition) NEC P03.1
    maternal (complication of) (use of)
      alcohol P04.3
      amphetamines P04.16
      analgesia (maternal) P04.0
      anesthesia (maternal) P04.0

Newborn (continued)
  affected by (continued)
    maternal (continued)
      anticonvulsants P04.13
      antidepressants P04.15
      antineoplastic chemotherapy P04.11
      anxiolytics P04.1A
      blood loss P02.1
      cannabis P04.81
      circulatory disease P00.3
      condition P00.9
        specified NEC P00.89
      cytotoxic drugs P04.12
      delivery P03.9
        Cesarean P03.4
        forceps P03.2
        vacuum extractor P03.3
      diabetes mellitus (pre-existing) P70.1
      disorder P00.9
        specified NEC P00.89
      drugs (addictive) (illegal) NEC P04.49
      ectopic pregnancy P01.4
      gestational diabetes P70.0
      group B streptococcus (GBS) colonization (positive) P00.82
      hemorrhage P02.1
      hypertensive disorder P00.0
      incompetent cervix P01.0
      infectious disease P00.2
      injury P00.5
      labor and delivery P03.9
      malpresentation before labor P01.7
      maternal death P01.6
      medical procedure P00.7
      medication P04.19
        specified type NEC P04.18
      multiple pregnancy P01.5
      nutritional disorder P00.4
      oligohydramnios P01.2
      opiates P04.14
        administered for procedures during pregnancy or labor and delivery P04.0
      parasitic disease P00.2
      periodontal disease P00.81
      placenta previa P02.0
      polyhydramnios P01.3
      precipitate delivery P03.5
      pregnancy P01.9
        specified P01.8
      premature rupture of membranes P01.1
      renal disease P00.1
      respiratory disease P00.3
      sedative-hypnotics P04.17
      surgical procedure P00.6
      tranquilizers administered for procedures during pregnancy or labor and delivery P04.0
      urinary tract disease P00.1
      uterine contraction (abnormal) P03.6
    meconium peritonitis P78.0
    medication (legal) (maternal use) (prescribed) P04.19
    membrane abnormalities P02.9
      specified NEC P02.8
    membranitis P02.78
    methamphetamine(s) P04.49
    mixed metabolic and respiratory acidosis P84
    neonatal abstinence syndrome P96.1
    noxious substances transmitted via placenta or breast milk P04.9
      cannabis P04.81
      specified NEC P04.89

Newborn (continued)
  affected by (continued)
    nutritional supplements P04.5
    placenta previa P02.0
    placental
      abnormality (functional) (morphological) P02.20
        specified NEC P02.29
      dysfunction P02.29
      infarction P02.29
      insufficiency P02.29
      separation NEC P02.1
      transfusion syndromes P02.3
    placentitis P02.78
    precipitate delivery P03.5
    prolapsed cord P02.4
    respiratory arrest P28.81
    slow intrauterine growth P05.9
    tobacco P04.2
    twin to twin transplacental transfusion P02.3
    umbilical cord (tightly) around neck P02.5
    umbilical cord condition P02.60
      short cord P02.69
      specified NEC P02.69
    uterine contractions (abnormal) P03.6
    vasa previa P02.69
      from intrauterine blood loss P50.0
  apnea (see also Apnea, newborn) P28.40
    primary (see also Apnea, newborn, sleep, primary) P28.30
    obstructive P28.42
    sleep (central) (obstructive) (primary) (see also Apnea, newborn, sleep, primary) P28.30
  born in hospital Z38.00
    by cesarean Z38.01
  born outside hospital Z38.1
  breast buds P96.89
  breast engorgement P83.4
  check-up —see Newborn, examination
  convulsion P90
  dehydration P74.1
  examination
    8 to 28 days old Z00.111
    under 8 days old Z00.110
  fever P81.9
    environmentally-induced P81.0
  hyperbilirubinemia P59.9
    of prematurity P59.0
  hypernatremia P74.21
  hyponatremia P74.22
  infection P39.9
    candidal P37.5
    specified NEC P39.8
    urinary tract P39.3
  jaundice P59.9
    due to
      breast milk inhibitor P59.3
      hepatocellular damage P59.20
        specified NEC P59.29
      preterm delivery P59.0
    of prematurity P59.0
    specified NEC P59.8
  late metabolic acidosis P74.0
  mastitis P39.0
    infective P39.0
    noninfective P83.4
  multiple born NEC Z38.8
    born in hospital Z38.68
      by cesarean Z38.69
    born outside hospital Z38.7
  omphalitis P38.9
    with mild hemorrhage P38.1
    without hemorrhage P38.9

Newborn (continued)
  post-term P08.21
  prolonged gestation (over 42 completed weeks) P08.22
  quadruplet Z38.8
    born in hospital Z38.63
      by cesarean Z38.64
    born outside hospital Z38.7
  quintuplet Z38.8
    born in hospital Z38.65
      by cesarean Z38.66
    born outside hospital Z38.7
  seizure P90
  sepsis (congenital) P36.9
    due to
      anaerobes NEC P36.5
      Escherichia coli P36.4
      Staphylococcus P36.30
        aureus P36.2
        specified NEC P36.39
      Streptococcus P36.10
        group B P36.0
        specified NEC P36.19
    specified NEC P36.8
  triplet Z38.8
    born in hospital Z38.61
      by cesarean Z38.62
    born outside hospital Z38.7
  twin Z38.5
    born in hospital Z38.30
      by cesarean Z38.31
    born outside hospital Z38.4
  vomiting P92.09
    bilious P92.01
  weight check Z00.111
Newcastle conjunctivitis or disease B30.8
Nezelof's syndrome (pure alymphocytosis) D81.4
Niacin (amide) **deficiency** E52
Nicolas (-Durand)-**Favre disease** A55
Nicotine —see Tobacco
Nicotinic acid deficiency E52
Niemann-Pick disease or syndrome E75.249
  specified NEC E75.248
  type
    A E75.240
    A/B E75.244
    B E75.241
    C E75.242
    D E75.243
Night
  blindness —see Blindness, night
  sweats R61
  terrors (child) F51.4
Nightmares (REM sleep type) F51.5
NIHSS (National Institutes of Health Stroke Scale) score R29.7-
Nipple —see condition
Nisbet's chancre A57
Nishimoto (-Takeuchi) **disease** I67.5
Nitritoid crisis or reaction —see Crisis, nitritoid
Nitrosohemoglobinemia D74.8
Njovera A65
No general equivalence degree (GED) Z55.5
Nocardiosis, nocardiasis A43.9
  cutaneous A43.1
  lung A43.0
  pneumonia A43.0
  pulmonary A43.0
  specified site NEC A43.8

Nocturia R35.1
  psychogenic F45.8
Nocturnal —see condition
Nodal rhythm I49.8
Node(s) —see also Nodule
  Bouchard's (with arthropathy) M15.2
  Haygarth's M15.8
  Heberden's (with arthropathy) M15.1
  larynx J38.7
  lymph —see condition
  milker's B08.03
  Osler's I33.0
  Schmorl's —see Schmorl's disease
  singer's J38.2
  teacher's J38.2
  tuberculous —see Tuberculosis, lymph gland
  vocal cord J38.2
Nodule(s), **nodular**
  actinomycotic —see Actinomycosis
  breast NEC (see also Lump, breast) N63.0
  colloid (cystic), thyroid E04.1
  cutaneous —see Swelling, localized
  endometrial (stromal) D26.1
  Haygarth's M15.8
  inflammatory —see Inflammation
  juxta-articular
    syphilitic A52.77
    yaws A66.7
  larynx J38.7
  lung, solitary (subsegmental branch of the bronchial tree) R91.1
    multiple R91.8
  milker's B08.03
  prostate N40.2
    with lower urinary tract symptoms (LUTS) N40.3
    without lower urinary tract symptoms (LUTS) N40.2
  pulmonary, solitary (subsegmental branch of the bronchial tree) R91.1
  retrocardiac R09.89
  rheumatoid M06.30
    ankle M06.37-
    elbow M06.32-
    foot joint M06.37-
    hand joint M06.34-
    hip M06.35-
    knee M06.36-
    multiple site M06.39
    shoulder M06.31-
    vertebra M06.38
    wrist M06.33-
  scrotum (inflammatory) N49.2
  singer's J38.2
  solitary, lung (subsegmental branch of the bronchial tree) R91.1
    multiple R91.8
  subcutaneous —see Swelling, localized
  teacher's J38.2
  thyroid (cold) (gland) (nontoxic) E04.1
    with thyrotoxicosis E05.20
      with thyroid storm E05.21
    toxic or with hyperthyroidism E05.20
      with thyroid storm E05.21
  vocal cord J38.2
Noma (gangrenous) (hospital) (infective) A69.0
  auricle I96
  mouth A69.0
  pudendi N76.89
  vulvae N76.89
Nomad, nomadism Z59.00

NOMID (neonatal onset multisystemic inflammatory disorder) M04.2
Non-accidental trauma —see Abuse, physical
Nonadherence to medical treatment, specified NEC Z91.199
  due to
    financial hardship Z91.190
    specified reason NEC Z91.198
Nonautoimmune hemolytic anemia D59.4
  drug-induced D59.2
Nonclosure —see also Imperfect, closure
  ductus arteriosus (Botallo's) Q25.0
  foramen
    botalli Q21.12
    ovale Q21.12
Noncompliance Z91.199
  with
    dietary regimen Z91.119
      due to
        financial hardship Z91.110
        specified reason NEC Z91.118
    dialysis Z91.158
      due to financial hardship Z91.151
    medical treatment, specified NEC Z91.199
      due to
        financial hardship Z91.190
        specified reason NEC Z91.198
    medication regimen NEC Z91.141
      due to financial hardship Z91.151
    underdosing (see also Table of Drugs and Chemicals, categories T36-T50, with final character 6) Z91.148
      intentional NEC Z91.128
        by caregiver
          due to
            financial hardship Z91.A20
            specified reason NEC Z91.A28
        due to financial hardship of patient Z91.120
      unintentional NEC Z91.138
        by caregiver Z91.A3
        due to patient's age related debility Z91.130
    renal dialysis Z91.15
      due to financial hardship Z91.151
  caregiver
    with patient's
      dietary regimen
        due to
          financial hardship Z91.A10
          specified reason NEC Z91.A18
      medical treatment and regimen
        due to financial hardship Z91.A91
        specified reason NEC Z91.A98
      medication regimen
        due to financial hardship Z91.A41
        specified reason NEC Z91.A48

Noncompliance (continued)
  caregiver (continued)
    with patient's (continued)
      renal dialysis
        due to financial hardship Z91.A51
        specified reason NEC Z91.A58
Nondescent (congenital) —see also Malposition, congenital
  cecum Q43.3
  colon Q43.3
  testicle Q53.9
    bilateral Q53.20
      abdominal Q53.211
      perineal Q53.22
    unilateral Q53.10
      abdominal Q53.111
      perineal Q53.12
Nondevelopment
  brain Q02
    part of Q04.3
  heart Q24.8
  organ or site, congenital NEC —see Hypoplasia
Nonengagement
  head NEC O32.4
    in labor, causing obstructed labor O64.8
Nonexanthematous tick fever A93.2
Nonexpansion, lung (newborn) P28.0
Nonfunctioning
  cystic duct (see also Disease, gallbladder) K82.8
  gallbladder (see also Disease, gallbladder) K82.8
  kidney N28.9
  labyrinth H83.2
Non-Hodgkin lymphoma NEC —see Lymphoma, non-Hodgkin
Non-working side interference M26.56
Nonimplantation, ovum N97.2
Noninsufflation, fallopian tube N97.1
Non-ketotic hyperglycinemia E72.51
Nonne-Milroy syndrome Q82.0
Nonovulation N97.0
Nonpatent fallopian tube N97.1
Non-palpable testicle(s)
  bilateral R39.84
  unilateral R39.83
Nonpneumatization, lung NEC P28.0
Nonrotation —see Malrotation
Nonsecretion, urine —see Anuria
Nonunion
  fracture —see Fracture, by site
  joint, following fusion or arthrodesis M96.0
  organ or site, congenital NEC —see Imperfect, closure
  symphysis pubis, congenital Q74.2
Nonvisualization, gallbladder R93.2
Nonvital, nonvitalized tooth K04.99
Noonan's syndrome Q87.19
Normocytic anemia (infectional) **due to blood loss** (chronic) D50.0
  acute D62
Norrie's disease (congenital) Q15.8
North American blastomycosis B40.9
Norwegian itch B86
Nose, nasal —see condition
Nosebleed R04.0

Nose-picking F98.8
Nosomania F45.21
Nosophobia F45.22
Nostalgia F43.20
Notch of iris Q13.2
Notching nose, congenital (tip) Q30.2
Nothnagel's
  syndrome —see Strabismus, paralytic, third nerve
  vasomotor acroparesthesia I73.89
Novy's relapsing fever A68.9
  louse-borne A68.0
  tick-borne A68.1
Noxious
  foodstuffs, poisoning by —see Poisoning, food, noxious, plant
  substances transmitted through placenta or breast milk P04.9
Nucleus pulposus —see condition
Numbness R20.0
Nuns' knee —see Bursitis, prepatellar
Nursemaid's elbow S53.03-
Nutcracker esophagus K22.4
Nutmeg liver K76.1
Nutrient element deficiency E61.9
  specified NEC E61.8
Nutrition deficient or insufficient (see also Malnutrition) E63.9
  due to
    insufficient food T73.0
    lack of
      care (child) T76.02
        adult T76.01
      food T73.0
    specific element deficiency —see Nutrient element deficiency, or by element
  sequelae —see Sequelae, nutritional deficiency
  specified NEC E63.8
Nutritional stunting E45
Nyctalopia (night blindness) —see Blindness, night
Nycturia R35.1
  psychogenic F45.8
Nymphomania F52.8
Nystagmus H55.00
  benign paroxysmal —see Vertigo, benign paroxysmal
  central positional H81.4
  congenital H55.01
  dissociated H55.04
  latent H55.02
  miners' H55.09
  positional
    benign paroxysmal H81.4
    central H81.4
  specified form NEC H55.09
  visual deprivation H55.03

O

Obermeyer's relapsing fever (European) A68.0
Obesity E66.9
  with alveolar hypoventilation E66.2
  adrenal E27.8
  complicating
    childbirth O99.214
    pregnancy O99.21-
    puerperium O99.215

247

Obesity (continued)
constitutional E66.8
dietary counseling and surveillance Z71.3
drug-induced E66.1
  drug E66.1
  excess calories E66.09
    morbid E66.01
    severe E66.01
endocrine E66.8
endogenous E66.8
exogenous E66.09
familial E66.8
glandular E66.8
hypothyroid —see Hypothyroidism
hypoventilation syndrome (OHS) E66.2
morbid E66.01
  with
    alveolar hypoventilation E66.2
    obesity hypoventilation syndrome (OHS) E66.2
    due to excess calories E66.01
nutritional E66.09
pituitary E23.6
severe E66.01
specified type NEC E66.8

Oblique —see condition

Obliteration
appendix (lumen) K38.8
artery I77.1
bile duct (noncalculous) K83.1
common duct (noncalculous) K83.1
cystic duct —see Obstruction, gallbladder
disease, arteriolar I77.1
endometrium N85.8
eye, anterior chamber —see Disorder, globe, hypotony
fallopian tube N97.1
lymphatic vessel I89.0
  due to mastectomy I97.2
organ or site, congenital NEC —see Atresia, by site
ureter N13.5
  with infection N13.6
urethra —see Stricture, urethra
vein I87.8
vestibule (oral) K08.89

Observation (following) (for) (without need for further medical care) Z04.9
accident NEC Z04.3
  at work Z04.2
  transport Z04.1
adverse effect of drug Z03.6
alleged rape or sexual assault (victim), ruled out
  adult Z04.41
  child Z04.42
criminal assault Z04.89
development state
  adolescent Z00.3
  period of rapid growth in childhood Z00.2
  puberty Z00.3
disease, specified NEC Z03.89
following work accident Z04.2
forced sexual exploitation Z04.81
forced labor exploitation Z04.82
growth and development state —see Observation, development state
injuries (accidental) NEC —see also Observation, accident
newborn (for)
  suspected condition, related to exposure from the mother or birth process —see Newborn, affected by, maternal

Observation (continued)
newborn (continued)
  suspected condition, related to exposure from the mother or birth process (continued)
    ruled out Z05.9
      cardiac Z05.0
      connective tissue Z05.73
      gastrointestinal Z05.5
      genetic Z05.41
      genitourinary Z05.6
      immunologic Z05.43
      infectious Z05.1
      metabolic Z05.42
      mesculoskeletal Z05.72
      neurological Z05.2
      respiratory Z05.3
      skin and subcutaneous tissue Z05.71
      specified condition NEC Z05.89
postpartum
  immediately after delivery Z39.0
  routine follow-up Z39.2
pregnancy (normal) (without complication) Z34.9-
  high risk O09.9-
suicide attempt, alleged NEC Z03.89
  self-poisoning Z03.6
suspected, ruled out —see also Suspected condition, ruled out
  abuse, physical
    adult Z04.71
    child Z04.72
  accident at work Z04.2
  adult battering victim Z04.71
  child battering victim Z04.72
  condition NEC Z03.89
    newborn (see also Observation, newborn (for), suspected condition, ruled out) Z05.9
  drug poisoning or adverse effect Z03.6
  exposure (to)
    anthrax Z03.810
    biological agent NEC Z03.818
  foreign body
    aspirated (inhaled) Z03.822
    ingested Z03.821
    inserted (injected), in (eye) (orifice) (skin) Z03.823
  inflicted injury NEC Z03.89
  suicide attempt, alleged Z03.89
    self-poisoning Z03.6
  toxic effects from ingested substance (drug) (poison) Z03.6
toxic effects from ingested substance (drug) (poison) Z03.6

Obsession, obsessional state F42.8
mixed thoughts and acts F42.2

Obsessive-compulsive neurosis or reaction F42.8

Obstetric embolism, septic —see Embolism, obstetric, septic

Obstetrical trauma (complicating delivery) O71.9
with or following ectopic or molar pregnancy O08.6
specified type NEC O71.89

Obstipation —see Constipation

Obstruction, obstructed, obstructive
airway J98.8
  with
    allergic alveolitis J67.9

Obstruction, obstructed, obstructive (continued)
airway (continued)
  with (continued)
    asthma J45.909
      with
        exacerbation (acute) J45.901
        status asthmaticus J45.902
    bronchiectasis J47.9
      with
        exacerbation (acute) J47.1
        lower respiratory infection J47.0
    bronchitis (chronic) J44.89
    emphysema J43.9
    chronic J44.9
      with
        allergic alveolitis —see Pneumonitis, hypersensitivity
        bronchiectasis J47.9
          with
            exacerbation (acute) J47.1
            lower respiratory infection J47.0
    due to
      foreign body —see Foreign body, by site, causing asphyxia
      inhalation of fumes or vapors J68.9
    laryngospasm J38.5
ampulla of Vater K83.1
aortic (heart) (valve) —see Stenosis, aortic
aortoiliac I74.09
aqueduct of Sylvius G91.1
  congenital Q03.0
    with spina bifida —see Spina bifida, by site, with hydrocephalus
Arnold-Chiari —see Arnold-Chiari disease
artery (see also Atherosclerosis, artery) I70.9
  basilar (complete) (partial) —see Occlusion, artery, basilar
  carotid (complete) (partial) —see Occlusion, artery, carotid
  cerebellar —see Occlusion, artery, cerebellar
  cerebral (anterior) (middle) (posterior) —see Occlusion, artery, cerebral
  precerebral —see Occlusion, artery, precerebral
  renal N28.0
  retinal NEC —see Occlusion, artery, retina
  stent —see Restenosis, stent
  vertebral (complete) (partial) —see Occlusion, artery, vertebral
band (intestinal) (see also Obstruction, intestine, specified NEC) K56.699
bile duct or passage (common) (hepatic) (noncalculous) K83.1
  with calculus K80.51
  congenital (causing jaundice) Q44.3
biliary (duct) (tract) K83.1
  gallbladder K82.0
bladder-neck (acquired) N32.0
  congenital Q64.31
  due to hyperplasia (hypertrophy) of prostate —see Hyperplasia, prostate
bowel —see Obstruction, intestine

Obstruction, obstructed, obstructive (continued)
bronchus J98.09
canal, ear —see Stenosis, external ear canal
cardia K22.2
caval veins (inferior) (superior) I87.1
cecum —see Obstruction, intestine
circulatory I99.8
colon —see Obstruction, intestine
common duct (noncalculous) K83.1
coronary (artery) —see Occlusion, coronary
cystic duct —see also Obstruction, gallbladder
  with calculus K80.21
device, implant or graft (see also Complications, by site and type, mechanical) T85.698
  arterial graft NEC —see Complication, cardiovascular device, mechanical, vascular
  catheter NEC T85.628
    cystostomy T83.090
    dialysis (renal) T82.49
      intraperitoneal T85.691
    Hopkins T83.098
    ileostomy T83.098
    infusion NEC T82.594
      spinal (epidural) (subdural) T85.690
    nephrostomy T83.092
    urethral indwelling T83.091
    urinary T83.098
    urostomy T83.098
  due to infection T85.79
  gastrointestinal —see Complications, prosthetic device, mechanical, gastrointestinal device
  genital NEC T83.498
    intrauterine contraceptive device T83.39
    penile prosthesis (cylinder) (implanted) (pump) (resevoir) T83.490
    testicular prosthesis T83.491
  heart NEC —see Complication, cardiovascular device, mechanical
  joint prosthesis —see Complications, joint prosthesis, mechanical, specified NEC, by site
  orthopedic NEC —see Complication, orthopedic, device, mechanical
  specified NEC T85.628
  urinary NEC —see also Complication, genitourinary, device, urinary, mechanical
  graft T83.29
  vascular NEC —see Complication, cardiovascular device, mechanical
  ventricular intracranial shunt T85.09
due to foreign body accidentally left in operative wound T81.529
duodenum K31.5
ejaculatory duct N50.89
esophagus K22.2
eustachian tube (complete) (partial) H68.10-
  cartilagenous (extrinsic) H68.13-
  intrinsic H68.12-
  osseous H68.11-

Obstruction, obstructed, obstructive (continued)
fallopian tube (bilateral) N97.1
fecal K56.41
  with hernia —see Hernia, by site, with obstruction
foramen of Monro (congenital) Q03.8
  with spina bifida —see Spina bifida, by site, with hydrocephalus
foreign body —see Foreign body
gallbladder K82.0
  with calculus, stones K80.21
  congenital Q44.1
gastric outlet K31.1
gastrointestinal —see Obstruction, intestine
hepatic K76.89
  duct (noncalculous) K83.1
hepatobiliary K83.1
ileum —see Obstruction, intestine
iliofemoral (artery) I74.5
intestine K56.609
  complete K56.601
  incomplete K56.600
  partial K56.600
  with
    adhesions (intestinal) (peritoneal) K56.50
      complete K56.52
      incomplete K56.51
      partial K56.51
  adynamic K56.0
  by gallstone K56.3
  congenital (small) Q41.9
    large Q42.9
    specified part NEC Q42.8
  neurogenic K56.0
    Hirschsprung's disease or megacolon Q43.1
  newborn P76.9
    due to
      fecaliths P76.8
      inspissated milk P76.2
      meconium (plug) P76.0
        in mucoviscidosis E84.11
      specified NEC P76.8
  postoperative K91.30
    complete K91.32
    incomplete K91.31
    partial K91.31
  reflex K56.0
  specified NEC K56.699
    complete K56.691
    incomplete K56.690
    partial K56.690
  volvulus K56.2
intracardiac ball valve prosthesis T82.09
jejunum —see Obstruction, intestine
joint prosthesis —see Complications, joint prosthesis, mechanical, specified NEC, by site
kidney (calices) (see also Hydronephrosis) N28.89
labor —see Delivery
lacrimal (passages) (duct)
  by
    dacryolith —see Dacryolith
    stenosis —see Stenosis, lacrimal
  congenital Q10.5
  neonatal H04.53-
lacrimonasal duct —see Obstruction, lacrimal
lacteal, with steatorrhea K90.2
laryngitis —see Laryngitis

Obstruction, obstructed, obstructive (continued)
larynx NEC J38.6
  congenital Q31.8
lung J98.4
  disease, chronic J44.9
lymphatic I89.0
meconium (plug)
  newborn P76.0
    due to fecaliths P76.0
    in mucoviscidosis E84.11
mitral —see Stenosis, mitral
nasal J34.89
nasolacrimal duct —see also Obstruction, lacrimal
  congenital Q10.5
nasopharynx J39.2
nose J34.89
organ or site, congenital NEC —see Atresia, by site
pancreatic duct K86.89
parotid duct or gland K11.8
pelviureteric junction N13.5
  with hydronephrosis N13.0
  congenital Q62.39
pharynx J39.2
portal (circulation) (vein) I81
prostate —see also Hyperplasia, prostate
  valve (urinary) N32.0
pulmonary valve (heart) I37.0
pyelonephritis (chronic) N11.1
pylorus
  adult K31.1
  congenital or infantile Q40.0
rectosigmoid —see Obstruction, intestine
rectum K62.4
renal (see also Hydronephrosis) N28.89
  outflow N13.8
  pelvis, congenital Q62.39
respiratory J98.8
  chronic J44.9
retinal (vessels) H34.9
salivary duct (any) K11.8
  with calculus K11.5
sigmoid —see Obstruction, intestine
sinus (accessory) (nasal) J34.89
Stensen's duct K11.8
stomach NEC K31.89
  acute K31.0
  congenital Q40.2
  due to pylorospasm K31.3
submandibular duct K11.8
submaxillary gland K11.8
  with calculus K11.5
thoracic duct I89.0
thrombotic —see Thrombosis
trachea J39.8
tracheostomy airway J95.03
tricuspid (valve) —see Stenosis, tricuspid
upper respiratory, congenital Q34.8
ureter (functional) (pelvic junction) NEC N13.5
  with
    hydronephrosis N13.1
      with infection N13.6
    congenital Q62.39
    pyelonephritis (chronic) N11.1
  congenital Q62.39
  due to calculus —see Calculus, ureter
urethra NEC N36.8
  congenital Q64.39

Obstruction, obstructed, obstructive (continued)
urinary (moderate) N13.9
  due to hyperplasia (hypertrophy) of prostate —see Hyperplasia, prostate
  organ or tract (lower) N13.9
  prostatic valve N32.0
  specified NEC N13.8
uropathy N13.9
uterus N85.8
vagina N89.5
valvular —see Endocarditis
vein, venous I87.1
  caval (inferior) (superior) I87.1
  thrombotic —see Thrombosis
vena cava (inferior) (superior) I87.1
vesical NEC N32.0
vesicourethral orifice N32.0
  congenital Q64.31
vessel NEC I99.8
  stent —see Restenosis, stent

Obturator —see condition

Occlusal wear, teeth K03.0

Occlusio pupillae —see Membrane, pupillary

Occlusion, occluded
anus K62.4
  congenital Q42.3
    with fistula Q42.2
aortoiliac (chronic) I74.09
aqueduct of Sylvius G91.1
  congenital Q03.0
    with spina bifida —see Spina bifida, by site, with hydrocephalus
artery (see also Atherosclerosis, artery) I70.9
  auditory, internal I65.8
  basilar I65.1
    with
      infarction I63.22
        due to
          embolism I63.12
          thrombosis I63.02
  brain or cerebral I66.9
    with infarction (due to) I63.5-
      embolism I63.4-
      thrombosis I63.3-
  carotid I65.2-
    with
      infarction I63.23-
        due to
          embolism I63.13-
          thrombosis I63.03-
  cerebellar (anterior inferior) (posterior inferior) (superior) I66.3
    with infarction I63.54-
      due to
        embolism I63.44-
        thrombosis I63.34-
  cerebral I66.9
    with infarction I63.50
      due to
        embolism I63.40
          specified NEC I63.49
        thrombosis I63.30
          specified NEC I63.39
    anterior I66.1-
      with infarction I63.52-
        due to
          embolism I63.42-
          thrombosis I63.32-
    middle I66.0-
      with infarction I63.51-
        due to
          embolism I63.41-
          thrombosis I63.31-

Occlusion, occluded (continued)
artery (continued)
  cerebral (continued)
    posterior I66.2-
      with infarction I63.53-
        due to
          embolism I63.43-
          thrombosis I63.33-
    specified NEC I66.8
      with infarction I63.59
        due to
          embolism I63.4-
          thrombosis I63.3-
  choroidal (anterior) —see Occlusion, artery, precerebral, specified NEC
  communicating posterior —see Occlusion, artery, precerebral, specified NEC
  complete
    coronary I25.82
    extremities I70.92
  coronary (acute) (thrombotic) (without myocardial infarction) I24.0
    with myocardial infarction —see Infarction, myocardium
    chronic total I25.82
    complete I25.82
    healed or old I25.2
    total (chronic) I25.82
  hypophyseal —see Occlusion, artery, precerebral, specified NEC
  iliac I74.5
  lower extremities due to stenosis or stricture I77.1
  mesenteric (embolic) (thrombotic) (see also Infarct, intestine) K55.069
  perforating —see Occlusion, artery, cerebral, specified NEC
  peripheral I77.9
    thrombotic or embolic I74.4
  pontine —see Occlusion, artery, precerebral, specified NEC
  precerebral I65.9
    with infarction I63.20
      specified NEC I63.29
      due to
        embolism I63.10
          specified NEC I63.19
        thrombosis I63.09
          specified NEC I63.09
    basilar —see Occlusion, artery, basilar
    carotid —see Occlusion, artery, carotid
    puerperal O88.23
    specified NEC I65.8
      with infarction I63.29
        due to
          embolism I63.19
          thrombosis I63.09
    vertebral —see Occlusion, artery, vertebral
  renal N28.0
  retinal
    central H34.1-
    partial H34.21-
    branch H34.23-
    transient H34.0-
  spinal —see Occlusion, artery, precerebral, vertebral
  total (chronic)
    coronary I25.82
    extremities I70.92

Occlusion, occluded (continued)
artery (continued)
vertebral I65.0-
with
infarction I63.21-
due to
embolism I63.11-
thrombosis I63.01-
basilar artery —see Occlusion, artery, basilar
bile duct (common) (hepatic) (noncalculous) K83.1
bowel —see Obstruction, intestine
carotid (artery) (common) (internal) —see Occlusion, artery, carotid
centric (of teeth) M26.59
maximum intercuspation discrepancy M26.55
cerebellar (artery) —see Occlusion, artery, cerebellar
cerebral (artery) —see Occlusion, artery, cerebral
cerebrovascular —see also Occlusion, artery, cerebral
with infarction I63.5-
cervical canal —see Stricture, cervix
cervix (uteri) —see Stricture, cervix
choanal Q30.0
choroidal (artery) —see Occlusion, artery, precerebral, specified NEC
colon —see Obstruction, intestine
communicating posterior artery —see Occlusion, artery, precerebral, specified NEC
coronary (artery) (vein) (thrombotic) —see also Infarct, myocardium
chronic total I25.82
healed or old I25.2
not resulting in infarction I24.0
total (chronic) I25.82
cystic duct —see Obstruction, gallbladder
embolic —see Embolism
fallopian tube N97.1
congenital Q50.6
gallbladder —see also Obstruction, gallbladder
congenital (causing jaundice) Q44.1
gingiva, traumatic K06.2
hymen N89.6
congenital Q52.3
hypophyseal (artery) —see Occlusion, artery, precerebral, specified NEC
iliac artery I74.5
intestine —see Obstruction, intestine
lacrimal passages —see Obstruction, lacrimal
lung J98.4
lymph or lymphatic channel I89.0
mammary duct N64.89
mesenteric artery (embolic) (thrombotic) (see also Infarct, intestine) K55.069
nose J34.89
congenital Q30.0
organ or site, congenital NEC —see Atresia, by site
oviduct N97.1
congenital Q50.6
peripheral arteries
due to stricture or stenosis I77.1
upper extremity I74.2

Occlusion, occluded (continued)
pontine (artery) —see Occlusion, artery, precerebral, specified NEC
posterior lingual, of mandibular teeth M26.29
precerebral artery —see Occlusion, artery, precerebral
punctum lacrimale —see Obstruction, lacrimal
pupil —see Membrane, pupillary
pylorus, adult (see also Stricture, pylorus) K31.1
renal artery N28.0
retina, retinal
artery —see Occlusion, artery, retinal
vein (central) H34.81-
engorgement H34.82-
tributary H34.83-
vessels H34.9
spinal artery —see Occlusion, artery, precerebral, vertebral
teeth (mandibular) (posterior lingual) M26.29
thoracic duct I89.0
thrombotic —see Thrombosis, artery
traumatic
edentulous (alveolar) ridge K06.2
gingiva K06.2
periodontal K05.5
tubal N97.1
ureter (complete) (partial) N13.5
congenital Q62.10
ureteropelvic junction N13.5
congenital Q62.11
ureterovesical orifice N13.5
congenital Q62.12
urethra —see Stricture, urethra
uterus N85.8
vagina N89.5
vascular NEC I99.8
vein —see Thrombosis
retinal —see Occlusion, retinal, vein
vena cava (inferior) (superior) —see Embolism, vena cava
ventricle (brain) NEC G91.1
vertebral (artery) —see Occlusion, artery, vertebral
vessel (blood) I99.8
vulva N90.5
Occult
blood in feces (stools) R19.5
Occupational
problems NEC Z56.89
Ochlophobia —see Agoraphobia
Ochronosis (endogenous) E70.29
Ocular muscle —see condition
Oculogyric crisis or disturbance H51.8
psychogenic F45.8
Oculomotor syndrome H51.9
Oculopathy
syphilitic NEC A52.71
congenital
early A50.01
late A50.30
early (secondary) A51.43
late A52.71
Oddi's sphincter spasm K83.4
Odontalgia K08.89
Odontoameloblastoma —see Cyst, calcifying odontogenic
Odontoclasia K03.89
Odontodysplasia, regional K00.4

Odontogenesis imperfecta K00.5
Odontoma (ameloblastic) (complex) (compound) (fibroameloblastic) —see Cyst, calcifying odontogenic
Odontomyelitis (closed) (open) K04.01
irreversible K04.02
reversible K04.01
Odontorrhagia K08.89
Odontosarcoma, ameloblastic C41.1
upper jaw (bone) C41.0
Oestriasis —see Myiasis
Oguchi's disease H53.63
Ohara's disease —see Tularemia
OHS (obesity hypoventilation syndrome) E66.2
Oidiomycosis —see Candidiasis
Oidium albicans infection —see Candidiasis
Old age (without mention of debility) R54
dementia F03
Old (previous) **myocardial infarction** I25.2
Olfactory —see condition
Oligemia —see Anemia
Oligoastrocytoma
specified site —see Neoplasm, malignant, by site
unspecified site C71.9
Oligocythemia D64.9
Oligodendroblastoma
specified site —see Neoplasm, malignant
unspecified site C71.9
Oligodendroglioma
anaplastic type
specified site —see Neoplasm, malignant, by site
unspecified site C71.9
specified site —see Neoplasm, malignant, by site
unspecified site C71.9
Oligodontia —see Anodontia
Oligoencephalon Q02
Oligohidrosis L74.4
Oligohydramnios O41.0-
Oligohydrosis L74.4
Oligomenorrhea N91.5
primary N91.3
secondary N91.4
Oligophrenia —see also Disability, intellectual
phenylpyruvic E70.0
Oligospermia N46.11
due to
drug therapy N46.121
efferent duct obstruction N46.123
infection N46.122
radiation N46.124
specified cause NEC N46.129
systemic disease N46.125
Oligotrichia —see Alopecia
Oliguria R34
with, complicating or following ectopic or molar pregnancy O08.4
postprocedural N99.0
puerperal O90.49

Ollier's disease Q78.4
Omentitis —see Peritonitis
Omenocele —see Hernia, abdomen, specified site NEC
Omentum, omental —see condition
Omphalitis (congenital) (newborn) P38.9
with mild hemorrhage P38.1
without hemorrhage P38.9
not of newborn L08.82
tetanus A33
Omphalocele Q79.2
Omphalomesenteric duct, persistent Q43.0
Omphalorrhagia, newborn P51.9
Omsk hemorrhagic fever A98.1
Onanism (excessive) F98.8
Onchocerciasis, onchocercosis B73.1
with
eye disease B73.00
endophthalmitis B73.01
eyelid B73.09
glaucoma B73.02
specified NEC B73.09
eye NEC B73.00
eyelid B73.09
Oncocytoma —see Neoplasm, benign, by site
Oncovirus, as cause of disease classified elsewhere B97.32
Ondine's curse —see Apnea, sleep
Oneirophrenia F23
Onychauxis L60.2
congenital Q84.5
Onychia —see also Cellulitis, digit
with lymphangitis —see Lymphangitis, acute, digit
candidal B37.2
dermatophytic B35.1
Onychitis —see also Cellulitis, digit
with lymphangitis —see Lymphangitis, acute, digit
Onychocryptosis L60.0
Onychodystrophy L60.3
congenital Q84.6
Onychogryphosis, onychogryposis L60.2
Onycholysis L60.1
Onychomadesis L60.8
Onychomalacia L60.3
Onychomycosis (finger) (toe) B35.1
Onycho-osteodysplasia Q87.2
Onychophagia F98.8
Onychophosis L60.8
Onychoptosis L60.8
Onychorrhexis L60.3
congenital Q84.6
Onychoschizia L60.3
Onyxis (finger) (toe) L60.0
Onyxitis —see also Cellulitis, digit
with lymphangitis —see Lymphangitis, acute, digit
Oophoritis (cystic) (infectional) (interstitial) N70.92
with salpingitis N70.93
acute N70.02
with salpingitis N70.03

Oophoritis (continued)
  chronic N70.12
    with salpingitis N70.13
  complicating abortion —see
    Abortion, by type, complicated
    by, oophoritis
Oophorocele N83.4-
Opacity, opacities
  cornea H17.-
    central H17.1-
    congenital Q13.3
    degenerative —see
      Degeneration, cornea
    hereditary —see Dystrophy,
      cornea
    inflammatory —see Keratitis
    minor H17.81-
    peripheral H17.82-
  cornea
    sequelae of trachoma (healed)
      B94.0
    specified NEC H17.89
  enamel (teeth) (fluoride)
    (nonfluoride) K00.3
  lens —see Cataract
  snowball —see Deposit,
    crystalline
  vitreous (humor) NEC H43.39-
    congenital Q14.0
    membranes and strands H43.31-
Opalescent dentin (hereditary) K00.5
Open, opening
  abnormal, organ or site, congenital
    —see Imperfect, closure
  angle with
    borderline
      findings
        high risk H40.02-
        low risk H40.01-
      intraocular pressure H40.00-
    cupping of discs H40.01-
    glaucoma (primary) —see
      Glaucoma, open angle
  bite
    anterior M26.220
    posterior M26.221
  false —see Imperfect, closure
  margin on tooth restoration
    K08.51
  restoration margins of tooth K08.51
  wound —see Wound, open
Operational fatigue F48.8
Operative —see condition
Operculitis —see Periodontitis
Operculum —see Break, retina
Ophiasis L63.2
Ophthalmia (see also Conjunctivitis)
    H10.9
  actinic rays —see Photokeratitis
  allergic (acute) —see
    Conjunctivitis, acute, atopic
  blennorrhagic (gonococcal)
    (neonatorum) A54.31
  diphtheritic A36.86
  Egyptian A71.1
  electrica —see Photokeratitis
  gonococcal (neonatorum)
    A54.31
  metastatic —see Endophthalmitis,
    purulent
  migraine —see Migraine,
    ophthalmoplegic
  neonatorum, newborn P39.1
    gonococcal A54.31
  nodosa H16.24-
  purulent —see Conjunctivitis,
    acute, mucopurulent

Ophthalmia (continued)
  spring —see Conjunctivitis, acute,
    atopic
  sympathetic —see Uveitis,
    sympathetic
Ophthalmitis —see Ophthalmia
Ophthalmocele (congenital)
    Q15.8
Ophthalmoneuromyelitis G36.0
Ophthalmoplegia —see also
    Strabismus, paralytic
  anterior internuclear —see
    Ophthalmoplegia, internuclear
  ataxia-areflexia G61.0
  diabetic —see E08-E13 with .39
  exophthalmic E05.00
    with thyroid storm E05.01
  external H49.88-
    progressive H49.4-
      with pigmentary retinopathy
        —see Kearns-Sayre
        syndrome
      total H49.3-
  internal (complete) (total) H52.51-
  internuclear H51.2-
  migraine —see Migraine,
    ophthalmoplegic
  Parinaud's H49.88-
  progressive external —see
    Ophthalmoplegia, external,
    progressive
  supranuclear, progressive G23.1
  total (external) —see
    Ophthalmoplegia, external, total
Opioid(s)
  abuse —see Abuse, drug, opioids
  dependence —see Dependence,
    drug, opioids
  induced, without use disorder
    anxiety disorder F11.988
    delirium F11.921
    depressive disorder F11.94
    sexual dysfunction F11.981
    sleep disorder F11.982
Opisthognathism M26.09
Opisthorchiasis (felineus) (viverrini)
    B66.0
Opitz' disease D73.2
Opiumism —see Dependence, drug,
    opioid
Oppenheim's disease G70.2
Oppenheim-Urbach disease
    (necrobiosis lipoidica
    diabeticorum) —see E08-E13 with
    .620
Optic nerve —see condition
Orbit —see condition
Orchioblastoma C62.9-
Orchitis (gangrenous) (nonspecific)
    (septic) (suppurative) N45.2
  blennorrhagic (gonococcal) (acute)
    (chronic) A54.23
  chlamydial A56.19
  filarial —see also Infestation,
    filarial B74.9 [N51]
  gonococcal (acute) (chronic) A54.23
  mumps B26.0
  syphilitic A52.76
  tuberculous A18.15
Orf (virus disease) B08.02
Organic —see also condition
  brain syndrome F09
  heart —see Disease, heart
  mental disorder F09
  psychosis F09

Orgasm
  anejaculatory N53.13
Oriental
  bilharziasis B65.2
  schistosomiasis B65.2
Orifice —see condition
Origin of both great vessels from right ventricle Q20.1
Ormond's disease (with ureteral
    obstruction) N13.5
  with infection N13.6
Ornithine metabolism disorder E72.4
Ornithinemia (Type I) (Type II) E72.4
Ornithosis A70
Orotaciduria, oroticaciduria
    (congenital) (hereditary)
    (pyrimidine deficiency) E79.89
  anemia D53.0
Orthodontics
  adjustment Z46.4
  fitting Z46.4
Orthopnea R06.01
Orthopoxvirus B08.09
Os, uterus —see condition
Osgood-Schlatter disease or osteochondrosis M92.52-
Osler (-Weber)-**Rendu disease** I78.0
Osler's nodes I33.0
Osmidrosis L75.0
Osseous —see condition
Ossification
  artery —see Arteriosclerosis
  auricle (ear) —see Disorder, pinna,
    specified type NEC
  bronchial J98.09
  cardiac —see Degeneration,
    myocardial
  cartilage (senile) —see Disorder,
    cartilage, specified type NEC
  coronary (artery) —see Disease,
    heart, ischemic, atherosclerotic
  diaphragm J98.6
  ear, middle —see Otosclerosis
  falx cerebri G96.198
  fontanel, premature Q75.009
  heart —see also Degeneration,
    myocardial
  valve —see Endocarditis
  larynx J38.7
  ligament —see Disorder, tendon,
    specified type NEC
    posterior longitudinal —see
      Spondylopathy, specified
      NEC
  meninges (cerebral) (spinal)
    G96.198
  multiple, eccentric centers —see
    Disorder, bone, development or
    growth
  muscle —see also Calcification,
    muscle
    due to burns —see Myositis,
      ossificans, in, burns
    paralytic —see Myositis,
      ossificans, in, quadriplegia
    progressive —see Myositis,
      ossificans, progressiva
    specified NEC M61.50
      ankle M61.57-
      foot M61.57-
      forearm M61.53-
      hand M61.54-
      lower leg M61.56-
      multiple sites M61.59

Ossification (continued)
  muscle (continued)
    specified (continued)
      pelvic region M61.55-
      shoulder region M61.51-
      specified site NEC M61.58
      thigh M61.55-
      upper arm M61.52-
    traumatic —see Myositis,
      ossificans, traumatica
  myocardium, myocardial —see
    Degeneration, myocardial
  penis N48.89
  periarticular —see Disorder, joint,
    specified type NEC
  pinna —see Disorder, pinna,
    specified type NEC
  rider's bone —see Ossification,
    muscle, specified NEC
  sclera H15.89
  subperiosteal, post-traumatic M89.8X-
  tendon —see Disorder, tendon,
    specified type NEC
  trachea J39.8
  tympanic membrane —see
    Disorder, tympanic membrane,
    specified NEC
  vitreous (humor) —see Deposit,
    crystalline
Osteitis —see also Osteomyelitis
  alveolar M27.3
  condensans M85.30
    ankle M85.37-
    foot M85.37-
    forearm M85.33-
    hand M85.34-
    lower leg M85.36-
    multiple site M85.39
    neck M85.38
    rib M85.38
    shoulder M85.31-
    skull M85.38
    specified site NEC M85.38
    thigh M85.35-
    toe M85.37-
    upper arm M85.32-
    vertebra M85.38
  deformans (see also Paget's
    disease, bone) M88.9
    in (due to)
      malignant neoplasm of bone (see
        also, Neoplasm, malignant,
        by site) C41.9 [M90.60]
      neoplastic disease (see also
        Neoplasm, by type and site)
        D49.9 [M90.60]
        carpus D49.2 [M90.64-]
        clavicle D49.2 [M90.61-]
        femur D49.2 [M90.65-]
        fibula D49.2 [M90.66-]
        finger D49.2 [M90.64-]
        humerus D49.2 [M90.62-]
        ilium D49.2 [M90.68-]
        ischium D49.2 [M90.68-]
        metacarpus D49.2 [M90.64-]
        metatarsus D49.2 [M90.67-]
        multiple sites D49.89
          [M90.69]
        neck D49.2 [M90.68]
        pubic ramus D49.2
          [M90.68]
        radius D49.2 [M90.63-]
        rib D49.2 [M90.68]
        scapula D49.2 [M90.61-]
        skull D49.2 [M90.68]
        tarsus D49.2 [M90.67-]
        tibia D49.2 [M90.66-]
        toe D49.2 [M90.67-]
        ulna D49.2 [M90.63-]
        vertebra D49.2 [M90.68]

Osteitis (continued)
  deformans (continued)
    skull M88.0
    specified NEC —see Paget's disease, bone, by site
    vertebra M88.1
  due to yaws A66.6
  fibrosa NEC —see Cyst, bone, by site
    circumscripta —see Dysplasia, fibrous, bone NEC
    cystica (generalisata) E21.0
    disseminata Q78.1
    osteoplastica E21.0
  fragilitans Q78.0
  Garré's (sclerosing) —see Osteomyelitis, specified type NEC
  jaw (acute) (chronic) (lower) (suppurative) (upper) M27.2
  parathyroid E21.0
  petrous bone (acute) (chronic) —see Petrositis
  sclerotic, nonsuppurative —see Osteomyelitis, specified type NEC
  tuberculosa A18.09
    cystica D86.89
    multiplex cystoides D86.89

Osteoarthritis M19.90
  ankle M19.07-
    post-traumatic M19.17-
    primary M19.07-
    secondary M19.27-
  elbow M19.02-
    post-traumatic M19.12-
    primary M19.02-
    secondary M19.22-
  foot joint M19.07-
    post-traumatic M19.17-
    primary M19.07-
    secondary M19.27-
  generalized (multiple joints) M15.9
    erosive M15.4
    primary M15.0
    specified NEC M15.8
  hand joint M19.04-
    first carpometacarpal joint M18.9
      post-traumatic —see Osteoarthritis, post-traumatic NEC, hand joint, first carpometacarpal joint
      primary —see Osteoarthritis, primary, hand joint, first carpometacarpal joint
      secondary —see Osteoarthritis, secondary, hand joint, first carpometacarpal joint
    post-traumatic M19.14-
    primary M19.04-
    secondary M19.24-
  hip M16.9
    bilateral M16.0
      due to hip dysplasia M16.2
      post-traumatic M16.4
      secondary M16.6
    due to hip dysplasia (unilateral) M16.3-
      bilateral M16.2
    post-traumatic —see Osteoarthritis, post-traumatic, hip
    primary M16.1-
      bilateral M16.0
    secondary —see Osteoarthritis, secondary, hip
    unilateral M16.1-
      due to hip dysplasia M16.3-

Osteoarthritis (continued)
  hip (continued)
    unilateral (continued)
      post-traumatic M16.5-
      primary M16.1-
      secondary NEC M16.7
  interphalangeal
    distal (Heberden) M15.1
    proximal (Bouchard) M15.2
  knee M17.9
    bilateral M17.0
      post-traumatic M17.2
      secondary M17.4
    post-traumatic —see Osteoarthritis, post-traumatic, knee
    primary M17.1-
      bilateral M17.0
    secondary —see Osteoarthritis, secondary, knee
    unilateral M17.1-
      post-traumatic M17.3-
      primary M17.1-
      secondary NEC M17.5
  post-traumatic NEC M19.92
    ankle M19.17-
    elbow M19.12-
    foot joint M19.17-
    hand joint M19.14-
      first carpometacarpal joint M18.3-
        bilateral M18.2
    hip M16.5-
      bilateral M16.4
    knee M17.3-
      bilateral M17.2
    shoulder M19.11-
    specified site NEC M19.19
    wrist M19.13-
  primary M19.91
    ankle M19.07-
    elbow M19.02-
    foot joint M19.07-
    hand joint M19.04-
      first carpometacarpal joint M18.1-
        bilateral M18.0
    hip M16.1-
      bilateral M16.0
    knee M17.1-
      bilateral M17.0
    multiple sites M15.9
    shoulder M19.01-
    specified site NEC M19.09
    spine —see Spondylosis
    wrist M19.03-
  secondary M19.93
    ankle M19.27-
    elbow M19.22-
    foot joint M19.27-
    hand joint M19.24-
      first carpometacarpal joint M18.5-
        bilateral M18.4
    hip M16.7-
      bilateral M16.6
    knee M17.5-
      bilateral M17.4
    multiple M15.3
    shoulder M19.21-
    specified site NEC M19.29
    spine —see Spondylosis
    wrist M19.23-
  shoulder M19.01-
    post-traumatic M19.11-
    primary M19.01-
    secondary M19.21-
  specified site NEC M19.09
  spine —see Spondylosis

Osteoarthritis (continued)
  wrist M19.03-
    first carpometacarpal joint —see Osteoarthritis, hand joint, first carpometacarpal joint
    post-traumatic M19.13-
    primary M19.03-
    secondary M19.23-

Osteoarthropathy (hypertrophic) M19.90
  ankle —see Osteoarthritis, primary, ankle
  elbow —see Osteoarthritis, primary, elbow
  foot joint —see Osteoarthritis, primary, foot
  hand joint —see Osteoarthritis, primary, hand joint
  knee joint —see Osteoarthritis, primary, knee
  multiple site —see Osteoarthritis, primary, multiple joint
  pulmonary —see also Osteoarthropathy, specified type NEC
    hypertrophic —see Osteoarthropathy, hypertrophic, specified type NEC
  secondary hypertrophic —see Osteoarthropathy, specified type NEC
  shoulder —see Osteoarthritis, primary, shoulder
  specified joint NEC —see Osteoarthritis, primary, specified joint NEC
  specified type NEC M89.40
    carpus M89.44-
    clavicle M89.41-
    femur M89.45-
    fibula M89.46-
    finger M89.44-
    humerus M89.42-
    ilium M89.48
    ischium M89.48
    metacarpus M89.44-
    metatarsus M89.47-
    multiple sites M89.49
    neck M89.48
    pubic ramus M89.48
    radius M89.43-
    rib M89.48
    scapula M89.41-
    skull M89.48
    tarsus M89.47-
    tibia M89.46-
    toe M89.47-
    ulna M89.43-
    vertebra M89.48
  secondary —see Osteoarthropathy, specified type NEC
  spine —see Spondylosis
  wrist —see Osteoarthritis, primary, wrist

Osteoarthrosis (degenerative) (hypertrophic) (joint) —see also Osteoarthritis
  deformans alkaptonurica E70.29 [M36.8]
  erosive M15.4
  generalized M15.9
    primary M15.0
  polyarticular M15.9
  spine —see Spondylosis

Osteoblastoma —see Neoplasm, bone, benign
  aggressive —see Neoplasm, bone, uncertain behavior

Osteochondroarthrosis deformans endemica —see Disease, Kaschin-Beck

Osteochondritis —see also Osteochondropathy, by site
  Brailsford's —see Osteochondrosis, juvenile, radius
  dissecans M93.20
    ankle M93.27-
    elbow M93.22-
    foot M93.27-
    hand M93.24-
    hip M93.25-
    knee M93.26-
    multiple sites M93.29
    shoulder joint M93.21-
    specified site NEC M93.28
    wrist M93.23-
  juvenile M92.9
    patellar —see Osteochondrosis, juvenile, patella
  syphilitic (congenital) (early) A50.02 [M90.80]
    ankle A50.02 [M90.87-]
    elbow A50.02 [M90.82-]
    foot A50.02 [M90.87-]
    forearm A50.02 [M90.83-]
    hand A50.02 [M90.84-]
    hip A50.02 [M90.85-]
    knee A50.02 [M90.86-]
    multiple sites A50.02 [M90.89]
    shoulder joint A50.02 [M90.81-]
    specified site NEC A50.02 [M90.88]

Osteochondrodysplasia Q78.9
  with defects of growth of tubular bones and spine Q77.9
  specified NEC Q77.8
  specified NEC Q78.8

Osteochondrodystrophy E78.9

Osteochondrolysis —see Osteochondritis, dissecans

Osteochondroma —see Neoplasm, bone, benign

Osteochondromatosis D16.9
  syndrome Q78.4

Osteochondromyxosarcoma —see Neoplasm, bone, malignant

Osteochondropathy M93.90
  ankle M93.97-
  elbow M93.92-
  foot M93.97-
  hand M93.94-
  hip M93.95-
  Kienböck's disease of adults M93.1
  knee M93.96-
  multiple joints M93.99
  osteochondritis dissecans —see Osteochondritis, dissecans
  osteochondrosis —see Osteochondrosis
  shoulder region M93.91-
  slipped upper femoral epiphysis —see Slipped, epiphysis, upper femoral
  specified joint NEC M93.98
  specified type NEC M93.80
    ankle M93.87-
    elbow M93.82-
    foot M93.87-
    hand M93.84-
    hip M93.85-
    knee M93.86-
    multiple joints M93.89
    shoulder region M93.81-
    specified joint NEC M93.88
    wrist M93.83-

Osteochondropathy *(continued)*
  syphilitic, congenital
    early A50.02 *[M90.80]*
    late A50.56 *[M90.80]*
  wrist M93.93-

Osteochondrosarcoma —*see* Neoplasm, bone, malignant

Osteochondrosis —*see also* Osteochondropathy, by site
  acetabulum (juvenile) M91.0
  adult —*see* Osteochondropathy, specified type NEC, by site
  astragalus (juvenile) —*see* Osteochondrosis, juvenile, tarsus
  Blount M92.51-
  Buchanan's M91.0
  Burns' —*see* Osteochondrosis, juvenile, ulna
  calcaneus (juvenile) —*see* Osteochondrosis, juvenile, tarsus
  capitular epiphysis (femur) (juvenile) —*see* Legg-Calvé-Perthes disease
  carpal (juvenile) (lunate) (scaphoid) —*see* Osteochondrosis, juvenile, hand, carpal lunate
    adult M93.1
  coxae juvenilis —*see* Legg-Calvé-Perthes disease
  deformans juvenilis, coxae —*see* Legg-Calvé-Perthes disease
  Diaz's —*see* Osteochondrosis, juvenile, tarsus
  dissecans (knee) (shoulder) —*see* Osteochondritis, dissecans
  femoral capital epiphysis (juvenile) —*see* Legg-Calvé-Perthes disease
  femur (head), juvenile —*see* Legg-Calvé-Perthes disease
  fibula (juvenile) —*see* Osteochondrosis, juvenile, fibula
  foot NEC (juvenile) M92.8
  Freiberg's —*see* Osteochondrosis, juvenile, metatarsus
  Haas' (juvenile) —*see* Osteochondrosis, juvenile, humerus
  Haglund's —*see* Osteochondrosis, juvenile, tarsus
  hip (juvenile) —*see* Legg-Calvé-Perthes disease
  humerus (capitulum) (head) (juvenile) —*see* Osteochondrosis, juvenile, humerus
  ilium, iliac crest (juvenile) M91.0
  ischiopubic synchondrosis M91.0
  Iselin's —*see* Osteochondrosis, juvenile, metatarsus
  juvenile, juvenilis M92.9
    after congenital dislocation of hip reduction —*see* Osteochondrosis, juvenile, hip, specified NEC
    arm —*see* Osteochondrosis, juvenile, upper limb NEC
    capitular epiphysis (femur) —*see* Legg-Calvé-Perthes disease
    clavicle, sternal epiphysis —*see* Osteochondrosis, juvenile, upper limb NEC
    coxae —*see* Legg-Calvé-Perthes disease
    deformans M92.9
    fibula M92.50-
    foot NEC M92.8
    hand M92.20-
      carpal lunate M92.21-
      metacarpal head M92.22-
      specified site NEC M92.29-

Osteochondrosis *(continued)*
  juvenile, juvenilis *(continued)*
    head of femur —*see* Legg-Calvé-Perthes disease
    hip and pelvis M91.9-
      coxa plana —*see* Coxa, plana
      femoral head —*see* Legg-Calvé-Perthes disease
      pelvis M91.0
      pseudocoxalgia —*see* Pseudocoxalgia
      specified NEC M91.8-
    humerus M92.0-
    limb
      lower NEC M92.8
      upper NEC —*see* Osteochondrosis, juvenile, upper limb NEC
    medial cuneiform bone —*see* Osteochondrosis, juvenile, tarsus
    metatarsus M92.7-
    patella M92.4-
    radius M92.1-
    specified
      site NEC M92.8
      type NEC M92.8
        tibia and fibula M92.59-
    spine M42.00
      cervical region M42.02
      cervicothoracic region M42.03
      lumbar region M42.06
      lumbosacral region M42.07
      multiple sites M42.09
      occipito-atlanto-axial region M42.01
      sacrococcygeal region M42.08
      thoracic region M42.04
      thoracolumbar region M42.05
    tarsus M92.6-
    tibia M92.50-
      proximal M92.51-
      tubercle M92.52-
    ulna M92.1-
    upper limb NEC M92.3-
    vertebra (body) (epiphyseal plates) (Calvé's) (Scheuermann's) —*see* Osteochondrosis, juvenile, spine
  Kienböck's —*see* Osteochondrosis, juvenile, hand, carpal lunate
    adult M93.1
  Köhler's
    patellar —*see* Osteochondrosis, juvenile, patella
    tarsal navicular —*see* Osteochondrosis, juvenile, tarsus
  Legg-Perthes (-Calvé) (-Waldenström) —*see* Legg-Calvé-Perthes disease
  limb
    lower NEC (juvenile) M92.8
      tibia and fibula M92.59-
    upper NEC (juvenile) —*see* Osteochondrosis, juvenile, upper limb NEC
  lunate bone (carpal) (juvenile) —*see also* Osteochondrosis, juvenile, hand, carpal lunate
    adult M93.1
  Mauclaire's —*see* Osteochondrosis, juvenile, hand, metacarpal
  metacarpal (head) (juvenile) —*see* Osteochondrosis, juvenile, hand, metacarpal
  metatarsus (fifth) (head) (juvenile) (second) —*see* Osteochondrosis, juvenile, metatarsus
  navicular (juvenile) —*see* Osteochondrosis, juvenile, tarsus

Osteochondrosis *(continued)*
  os
    calcis (juvenile) —*see* Osteochondrosis, juvenile, tarsus
    tibiale externum (juvenile) —*see* Osteochondrosis, juvenile, tarsus
  Osgood-Schlatter M92.52-
  Panner's —*see* Osteochondrosis, juvenile, humerus
  patellar center (juvenile) (primary) (secondary) —*see* Osteochondrosis, juvenile, patella
  pelvis (juvenile) M91.0
  Pierson's M91.0
  radius (head) (juvenile) —*see* Osteochondrosis, juvenile, radius
  Scheuermann's —*see* Osteochondrosis, juvenile, spine
  Sever's —*see* Osteochondrosis, juvenile, tarsus
  Sinding-Larsen —*see* Osteochondrosis, juvenile, patella
  spine M42.9
    adult M42.10
      cervical region M42.12
      cervicothoracic region M42.13
      lumbar region M42.16
      lumbosacral region M42.17
      multiple sites M42.19
      occipito-atlanto-axial region M42.11
      sacrococcygeal region M42.18
      thoracic region M42.14
      thoracolumbar region M42.15
    juvenile —*see* Osteochondrosis, juvenile, spine
  symphysis pubis (juvenile) M91.0
  syphilitic (congenital) A50.02
  talus (juvenile) —*see* Osteochondrosis, juvenile, tarsus
  tarsus (navicular) (juvenile) —*see* Osteochondrosis, juvenile, tarsus
  tibia (proximal) (tubercle) (juvenile) —*see* Osteochondrosis, juvenile, tibia
  tuberculous —*see* Tuberculosis, bone
  ulna (lower) (juvenile) —*see* Osteochondrosis, juvenile, ulna
  van Neck's M91.0
  vertebral —*see* Osteochondrosis, spine

Osteoclastoma D48.0
  malignant —*see* Neoplasm, bone, malignant

Osteodynia —*see* Disorder, bone, specified type NEC

Osteodystrophy Q78.9
  azotemic N25.0
  congenital Q78.9
  parathyroid, secondary E21.1
  renal N25.0

Osteofibroma —*see* Neoplasm, bone, benign

Osteofibrosarcoma —*see* Neoplasm, bone, malignant

Osteogenesis imperfecta Q78.0

Osteogenic —*see* condition

Osteolysis M89.50
  carpus M89.54-
  clavicle M89.51-
  femur M89.55-
  fibula M89.56-
  finger M89.54-
  humerus M89.52-
  ilium M89.58
  ischium M89.58
  joint prosthesis (periprosthetic) —*see* Complications, joint prosthesis, mechanical, periprosthetic, osteolysis, by site
  metacarpus M89.54-
  metatarsus M89.57-
  multiple sites M89.59
  neck M89.58
  periprosthetic —*see* Complications, joint prosthesis, mechanical, periprosthetic, osteolysis, by site
  pubic ramus M89.58
  radius M89.53-
  rib M89.58
  scapula M89.51-
  skull M89.58
  tarsus M89.57-
  tibia M89.56-
  toe M89.57-
  ulna M89.53-
  vertebra M89.58

Osteoma —*see also* Neoplasm, bone, benign
  osteoid —*see also* Neoplasm, bone, benign
    giant —*see* Neoplasm, bone, benign

Osteomalacia M83.9
  adult M83.9
    drug-induced NEC M83.5
    due to
      malabsorption (postsurgical) M83.2
      malnutrition M83.3
    specified NEC M83.8
  aluminium-induced M83.4
  infantile —*see* Rickets
  juvenile —*see* Rickets
  oncogenic E83.89
  pelvis M83.8
  puerperal M83.0
  senile M83.1
  vitamin-D-resistant in adults E83.31 *[M90.8-]*
    carpus E83.31 *[M90.84-]*
    clavicle E83.31 *[M90.81-]*
    femur E83.31 *[M90.85-]*
    fibula E83.31 *[M90.86-]*
    finger E83.31 *[M90.84-]*
    humerus E83.31 *[M90.82-]*
    ilium E83.31 *[M90.88]*
    ischium E83.31 *[M90.88]*
    metacarpus E83.31 *[M90.84-]*
    metatarsus E83.31 *[M90.87-]*
    multiple sites E83.31 *[M90.89]*
    neck E83.31 *[M90.88]*
    pubic ramus E83.31 *[M90.88]*
    radius E83.31 *[M90.83-]*
    rib E83.31 *[M90.88]*
    scapula E83.31 *[M90.819]*
    skull E83.31 *[M90.88]*
    tarsus E83.31 *[M90.879]*
    tibia E83.31 *[M90.869]*
    toe E83.31 *[M90.879]*
    ulna E83.31 *[M90.839]*
    vertebra E83.31 *[M90.88]*

Osteomyelitis (general) (infective) (localized) (neonatal) (purulent) (septic) (staphylococcal) (streptococcal) (suppurative) (with periostitis) M86.9
acute M86.10
- carpus M86.14-
- clavicle M86.11-
- femur M86.15-
- fibula M86.16-
- finger M86.14-
- hematogenous M86.00
  - carpus M86.04-
  - clavicle M86.01-
  - femur M86.05-
  - fibula M86.06-
  - finger M86.04-
  - humerus M86.02-
  - ilium M86.08
  - ischium M86.08
  - mandible M27.2
  - metacarpus M86.04-
  - metatarsus M86.07-
  - multiple sites M86.09
  - neck M86.08
  - orbit H05.02-
  - petrous bone —see Petrositis
  - radius M86.03-
  - rib M86.08
  - scapula M86.01-
  - skull M86.08
  - tarsus M86.07-
  - tibia M86.06-
  - toe M86.07-
  - ulna M86.03-
  - vertebra —see Osteomyelitis, vertebra
- humerus M86.12-
- ilium M86.18
- ischium M86.18
- mandible M27.2
- metacarpus M86.14-
- metatarsus M86.17-
- multiple sites M86.19
- neck M86.18
- orbit H05.02-
- petrous bone —see Petrositis
- radius M86.13-
- rib M86.18
- scapula M86.11-
- skull M86.18
- tarsus M86.17-
- tibia M86.16-
- toe M86.17-
- ulna M86.13-
- vertebra —see Osteomyelitis, vertebra

chronic (or old) M86.60
- with draining sinus M86.40
  - carpus M86.44-
  - clavicle M86.41-
  - femur M86.45-
  - fibula M86.46-
  - finger M86.44-
  - humerus M86.42-
  - ilium M86.48
  - ischium M86.48
  - mandible M27.2
  - metacarpus M86.44-
  - metatarsus M86.47-
  - multiple sites M86.49
  - neck M86.48
  - orbit H05.02-
  - petrous bone —see Petrositis
  - pubic ramus M86.48
  - radius M86.43-
  - rib M86.48
  - scapula M86.41-
  - skull M86.48
  - tarsus M86.47-

Osteomyelitis *(continued)*
chronic *(continued)*
- with draining sinus *(continued)*
  - tibia M86.46-
  - toe M86.47-
  - ulna M86.43-
  - vertebra —see Osteomyelitis, vertebra
- carpus M86.64-
- clavicle M86.61-
- femur M86.65-
- fibula M86.66-
- finger M86.64-
- hematogenous NEC M86.50
  - carpus M86.54-
  - clavicle M86.51-
  - femur M86.55-
  - fibula M86.56-
  - finger M86.54-
  - humerus M86.52-
  - ilium M86.58
  - ischium M86.58
  - mandible M27.2
  - metacarpus M86.54-
  - metatarsus M86.57-
  - multifocal M86.30
    - carpus M86.34-
    - clavicle M86.31-
    - femur M86.35-
    - fibula M86.36-
    - finger M86.34-
    - humerus M86.32-
    - ilium M86.38
    - ischium M86.38
    - metacarpus M86.34-
    - metatarsus M86.37-
    - multiple sites M86.39
    - neck M86.38
    - pubic ramus M86.38
    - radius M86.33-
    - rib M86.38
    - scapula M86.31-
    - skull M86.38
    - tarsus M86.37-
    - tibia M86.36-
    - toe M86.37-
    - ulna M86.33-
    - vertebra —see Osteomyelitis, vertebra
  - multiple sites M86.59
  - neck M86.58
  - orbit H05.02-
  - petrous bone —see Petrositis
  - pubic ramus M86.58
  - radius M86.53-
  - rib M86.58
  - scapula M86.51-
  - skull M86.58
  - tarsus M86.57-
  - tibia M86.56-
  - toe M86.57-
  - ulna M86.53-
  - vertebra —see Osteomyelitis, vertebra
- humerus M86.62-
- ilium M86.659
- ischium M86.659
- mandible M27.2
- metacarpus M86.64-
- metatarsus M86.67-
- multifocal —see Osteomyelitis, chronic, hematogenous, multifocal
- multiple sites M86.69
- neck M86.68
- orbit H05.02-
- petrous bone —see Petrositis
- radius M86.63-
- rib M86.68
- scapula M86.61-

Osteomyelitis *(continued)*
chronic *(continued)*
- skull M86.68
- tarsus M86.67-
- tibia M86.66-
- toe M86.67-
- ulna M86.63-
- vertebra —see Osteomyelitis, vertebra
echinococcal B67.2
Garr's —see Osteomyelitis, specified type NEC
in diabetes mellitus —see E08-E13 with .69
jaw (acute) (chronic) (lower) (neonatal) (suppurative) (upper) M27.2
nonsuppurating —see Osteomyelitis, specified type NEC
orbit H05.02-
petrous bone —see Petrositis
Salmonella (arizonae) (choleraesuis) (enteritidis) (typhimurium) A02.24
sclerosing, nonsuppurative —see Osteomyelitis, specified type NEC
specified type NEC (see also subcategory) M86.8X-
- mandible M27.2
- orbit H05.02-
- petrous bone —see Petrositis
- vertebra —see Osteomyelitis, vertebra
subacute M86.20
- carpus M86.24-
- clavicle M86.21-
- femur M86.25-
- fibula M86.26-
- finger M86.24-
- humerus M86.22-
- mandible M27.2
- metacarpus M86.24-
- metatarsus M86.27-
- multiple sites M86.29
- neck M86.28
- orbit H05.02-
- petrous bone —see Petrositis
- radius M86.23-
- rib M86.28
- scapula M86.21-
- skull M86.28
- tarsus M86.27-
- tibia M86.26-
- toe M86.27-
- ulna M86.23-
- vertebra —see Osteomyelitis, vertebra
syphilitic A52.77
- congenital (early) A50.02 *[M90.80]*
tuberculous —see Tuberculosis, bone
typhoid A01.05
vertebra M46.20
- cervical region M46.22
- cervicothoracic region M46.23
- lumbar region M46.26
- lumbosacral region M46.27
- occipito-atlanto-axial region M46.21
- sacrococcygeal region M46.28
- thoracic region M46.24
- thoracolumbar region M46.25

Osteomyelofibrosis D47.4

Osteomyelosclerosis D75.89

Osteonecrosis M87.9
due to
- drugs —see Osteonecrosis, secondary, due to, drugs
- trauma —see Osteonecrosis, secondary, due to, trauma

Osteonecrosis *(continued)*
idiopathic aseptic M87.00
- ankle M87.07-
- carpus M87.03-
- clavicle M87.01-
- femur M87.05-
- fibula M87.06-
- finger M87.04-
- humerus M87.02-
- ilium M87.050
- ischium M87.050
- metacarpus M87.04-
- metatarsus M87.07-
- multiple sites M87.09
- neck M87.08
- pelvis M87.050
- pubic ramus M87.050
- radius M87.03-
- rib M87.08
- scapula M87.01-
- skull M87.08
- tarsus M87.07-
- tibia M87.06-
- toe M87.07-
- ulna M87.03-
- vertebra M87.08
secondary NEC M87.30
- carpus M87.33-
- clavicle M87.31-
- due to
  - drugs M87.10
    - carpus M87.13-
    - clavicle M87.11-
    - femur M87.15-
    - fibula M87.16-
    - finger M87.14-
    - humerus M87.12-
    - ilium M87.150
    - ischium M87.150
    - jaw M87.180
    - metacarpus M87.14-
    - metatarsus M87.17-
    - multiple sites M87.19
    - neck M87.18
    - pubic ramus M87.150
    - radius M87.13-
    - rib M87.18
    - scapula M87.11-
    - skull M87.18
    - tarsus M87.17-
    - tibia M87.16-
    - toe M87.17-
    - ulna M87.13-
    - vertebra M87.18
  - hemoglobinopathy NEC D58.2 *[M90.50]*
    - carpus D58.2 *[M90.54-]*
    - clavicle D58.2 *[M90.51-]*
    - femur D58.2 *[M90.55-]*
    - fibula D58.2 *[M90.56-]*
    - finger D58.2 *[M90.54-]*
    - humerus D58.2 *[M90.52-]*
    - ilium D58.2 *[M90.58]*
    - ischium D58.2 *[M90.58]*
    - metacarpus D58.2 *[M90.54-]*
    - metatarsus D58.2 *[M90.57-]*
    - multiple sites D58.2 *[M90.58]*
    - neck D58.2 *[M90.58]*
    - pubic ramus D58.2 *[M90.58]*
    - radius D58.2 *[M90.53-]*
    - rib D58.2 *[M90.58]*
    - scapula D58.2 *[M90.51-]*
    - skull D58.2 *[M90.58]*
    - tarsus D58.2 *[M90.57-]*
    - tibia D58.2 *[M90.56-]*

Osteonecrosis (continued)
secondary NEC (continued)
due to (continued)
hemoglobinopathy
NEC (continued)
toe D58.2 [M90.57-]
ulna D58.2 [M90.53-]
vertebra D58.2 [M90.58]
trauma (previous) M87.20
carpus M87.23-
clavicle M87.21-
femur M87.25-
fibula M87.26-
finger M87.24-
humerus M87.22-
ilium M87.250
ischium M87.250
metacarpus M87.24-
metatarsus M87.27-
multiple sites M87.29
neck M87.28
pubic ramus M87.250
radius M87.23-
rib M87.28
scapula M87.21-
skull M87.28
tarsus M87.27-
tibia M87.26-
toe M87.27-
ulna M87.23-
vertebra M87.28
femur M87.35-
fibula M87.36-
finger M87.34-
humerus M87.32-
ilium M87.350
in
caisson disease T70.3 [M90.50]
carpus T70.3 [M90.54-]
clavicle T70.3 [M90.51-]
femur T70.3 [M90.55-]
fibula T70.3 [M90.56-]
finger T70.3 [M90.54-]
humerus T70.3 [M90.52-]
ilium T70.3 [M90.58]
ischium T70.3 [M90.58]
metacarpus T70.3 [M90.54-]
metatarsus T70.3 [M90.57-]
multiple sites T70.3 [M90.59]
neck T70.3 [M90.58]
pubic ramus T70.3 [M90.58]
radius T70.3 [M90.53-]
rib T70.3 [M90.58]
scapula T70.3 [M90.51-]
skull T70.3 [M90.58]
tarsus T70.3 [M90.57-]
tibia T70.3 [M90.56-]
toe T70.3 [M90.57-]
ulna T70.3 [M90.53-]
vertebra T70.3 [M90.58]
ischium M87.350
metacarpus M87.34-
metatarsus M87.37-
multiple site M87.39
neck M87.38
pubic ramus M87.350
radius M87.33-
rib M87.38
scapula M87.319
skull M87.38
tarsus M87.379
tibia M87.366
toe M87.379
ulna M87.33-
vertebra M87.38
specified type NEC M87.80
carpus M87.83-
clavicle M87.81-
femur M87.85-
fibula M87.86-
finger M87.84-

Osteonecrosis (continued)
specified type NEC (continued)
humerus M87.82-
ilium M87.850
ischium M87.850
metacarpus M87.84-
metatarsus M87.87-
multiple sites M87.89
neck M87.88
pubic ramus M87.850
radius M87.83-
rib M87.88
scapula M87.81-
skull M87.88
tarsus M87.87-
tibia M87.86-
toe M87.87-
ulna M87.83-
vertebra M87.88

Osteo-onycho-arthro-dysplasia Q87.2

Osteo-onychodysplasia, hereditary Q87.2

Osteopathia condensans disseminata Q78.8

Osteopathy —see also Osteomyelitis, Osteonecrosis, Osteoporosis
after poliomyelitis M89.60
carpus M89.64-
clavicle M89.61-
femur M89.65-
fibula M89.66-
finger M89.64-
humerus M89.62-
ilium M89.68
ischium M89.68
metacarpus M89.64-
metatarsus M89.67-
multiple sites M89.69
neck M89.68
pubic ramus M89.68
radius M89.63-
rib M89.68
scapula M89.61-
skull M89.68
tarsus M89.67-
tibia M89.66-
toe M89.67-
ulna M89.63-
vertebra M89.68
in (due to)
renal osteodystrophy N25.0
specified diseases classified elsewhere M90.8

Osteopenia M85.8-
borderline M85.8-

Osteoperiostitis —see Osteomyelitis, specified type NEC

Osteopetrosis (familial) Q78.2

Osteophyte M25.70
ankle M25.77-
elbow M25.72-
foot joint M25.77-
hand joint M25.74-
hip M25.75-
knee M25.76-
shoulder M25.71-
spine M25.78
vertebrae M25.78
wrist M25.73-

Osteopoikilosis Q78.8

Osteoporosis (female) (male) M81.0
with current pathological fracture M80.00
age-related M81.0
with current pathologic fracture M80.00
carpus M80.04-

Osteoporosis (continued)
age-related (continued)
with current pathologic
clavicle M80.01-
femur M80.05-
fibula M80.06-
finger M80.04-
hip M80.05-
humerus M80.02-
ilium M80.0A
ischium M80.0A
metacarpus M80.04-
metatarsus M80.07-
pelvis M80.0B-
pubis ramus M80.0A
radius M80.03-
rib(s) M80.0A
scapula M80.01-
specified site NEC M80.0A
tarsus M80.07-
tibia M80.06-
toe M80.07-
ulna M80.03-
vertebra M80.08
disuse M81.8
with current pathological fracture M80.80
carpus M80.84-
clavicle M80.81-
femur M80.85-
fibula M80.86-
finger M80.84-
hip M80.85-
humerus M80.82-
ilium M80.8A
ischium M80.8A
metacarpus M80.84-
metatarsus M80.87-
pelvis M80.8B-
pubis ramus M80.8A
radius M80.83-
scapula M80.81-
specified site NEC M80.8A
tarsus M80.87-
tibia M80.86-
toe M80.87-
ulna M80.83-
vertebra M80.88
drug-induced —see Osteoporosis, specified type NEC
idiopathic —see Osteoporosis, specified type NEC
involutional —see Osteoporosis, age-related
Lequesne M81.6
localized M81.6
postmenopausal M81.0
with pathological fracture M80.00
carpus M80.04-
clavicle M80.01-
femur M80.05
fibula M80.06-
finger M80.04-
hip M80.05
humerus M80.02-
ilium M80.0A
ischium M80.0A
metacarpus M80.04-
metatarsus M80.07-
pelvis M80.0B-
pubis ramus M80.0A
radius M80.03-
scapula M80.01-
specified site NEC M80.0A
tarsus M80.07-
tibia M80.06-
toe M80.07-
ulna M80.03-
vertebra M80.08

Osteoporosis (continued)
postoophorectomy —see Osteoporosis, specified type NEC
postsurgical malabsorption —see Osteoporosis, specified type NEC
post-traumatic —see Osteoporosis, specified type NEC
senile —see Osteoporosis, age-related
specified type NEC M81.8
with pathological fracture M80.80
carpus M80.84-
clavicle M80.81-
femur M80.85
fibula M80.86-
finger M80.84-
hip M80.85
humerus M80.82-
ilium M80.8A
ischium M80.8A
metacarpus M80.84-
metatarsus M80.87-
pelvis M80.8B-
pubis ramus M80.8A
radius M80.83-
scapula M80.81-
specified site NEC M80.8A
tarsus M80.87-
tibia M80.86-
toe M80.87-
ulna M80.83-
vertebra M80.88

Osteopsathyrosis (idiopathica) Q78.0

Osteoradionecrosis, jaw (acute) (chronic) (lower) (suppurative) (upper) M27.2

Osteosarcoma (any form) —see Neoplasm, bone, malignant

Osteosclerosis Q78.2
acquired M85.8-
congenita Q77.4
fragilitas (generalisata) Q78.2
myelofibrosis D75.81

Osteosclerotic anemia D64.89

Osteosis
cutis L94.2
renal fibrocystic N25.0

Österreicher-Turner syndrome Q87.2

Ostium
atrioventriculare commune Q21.23
primum (arteriosum) (defect) (persistent) Q21.20
secundum (arteriosum) (defect) (patent) (persistent) Q21.11

Ostrum-Furst syndrome Q75.8

Otalgia —see subcategory H92.0

Otitis (acute) H66.90
with effusion —see also Otitis, media, nonsuppurative
purulent —see Otitis, media, suppurative
adhesive H74.1
chronic —see also Otitis, media, chronic
with effusion —see also Otitis, media, nonsuppurative, chronic
externa H60.9-
abscess —see Abscess, ear, external
acute (noninfective) H60.50-
actinic H60.51-
chemical H60.52-
contact H60.53-
eczematoid H60.54-
infective —see Otitis, externa, infective
reactive H60.55-
specified NEC H60.59-

Otitis (continued)
  externa (continued)
    cellulitis —see Cellulitis, ear
    chronic H60.6-
    diffuse —see Otitis, externa, infective, diffuse
    hemorrhagic —see Otitis, externa, infective, hemorrhagic
    in (due to)
      aspergillosis B44.89
      candidiasis B37.84
      erysipelas A46 [H62.40]
      herpes (simplex) virus infection B00.1
        zoster B02.8
      impetigo L01.00 [H62.40]
      infectious disease NEC B99 [H62.4-]
      mycosis NEC B36.9 [H62.40]
      parasitic disease NEC B89 [H62.40]
      viral disease NEC B34.9 [H62.40]
      zoster B02.8
    infective NEC H60.39-
      abscess —see Abscess, ear, external
      cellulitis —see Cellulitis, ear
      diffuse H60.31-
      hemorrhagic H60.32-
      swimmer's ear —see Swimmer's, ear
    malignant H60.2-
    mycotic NEC B36.9 [H62.40]
      in
        aspergillosis B44.89
        candidiasis B37.84
        moniliasis B37.84
    necrotizing —see Otitis, externa, malignant
    Pseudomonas aeruginosa —see Otitis, externa, malignant
    reactive —see Otitis, externa, acute, reactive
    specified NEC —see subcategory H60.8
    tropical NEC B36.9 [H62.40]
      in
        aspergillosis B44.89
        candidiasis B37.84
        moniliasis B37.84
  insidiosa —see Otosclerosis
  interna —see subcategory H83.0
  media (hemorrhagic) (staphylococcal) (streptococcal) H66.9-
    with effusion (nonpurulent) —see Otitis, media, nonsuppurative
    acute, subacute H66.90
      allergic —see Otitis, media, nonsuppurative, acute, allergic
      exudative —see Otitis, media, suppurative, acute
      mucoid —see Otitis, media, nonsuppurative, acute
      necrotizing —see also Otitis, media, suppurative, acute
        in
          measles B05.3
          scarlet fever A38.0
      nonsuppurative NEC —see Otitis, media, nonsuppurative, acute
      purulent —see Otitis, media, suppurative, acute

Otitis (continued)
  media (continued)
    acute, subacute (continued)
      sanguinous —see Otitis, media, nonsuppurative, acute
      secretory —see Otitis, media, nonsuppurative, acute, serous
      seromucinous —see Otitis, media, nonsuppurative, acute
      serous —see Otitis, media, nonsuppurative, acute, serous
      suppurative —see Otitis, media, suppurative, acute
    allergic —see Otitis, media, nonsuppurative
    catarrhal —see Otitis, media, nonsuppurative
    chronic H66.90
      with effusion (nonpurulent) —see Otitis, media, nonsuppurative, chronic
      allergic —see Otitis, media, nonsuppurative, chronic, allergic
      benign suppurative —see Otitis, media, suppurative, chronic, tubotympanic
      catarrhal —see Otitis, media, nonsuppurative, chronic, serous
      exudative —see Otitis, media, nonsuppurative, chronic
      mucinous —see Otitis, media, nonsuppurative, chronic, mucoid
      mucoid —see Otitis, media, nonsuppurative, chronic, mucoid
      nonsuppurative NEC —see Otitis, media, nonsuppurative, chronic
      purulent —see Otitis, media, suppurative, chronic
      secretory —see Otitis, media, nonsuppurative, chronic, mucoid
      seromucinous —see Otitis, media, nonsuppurative, chronic
      serous —see Otitis, media, nonsuppurative, chronic, serous
      suppurative —see Otitis, media, suppurative, chronic
      transudative —see Otitis, media, nonsuppurative, chronic, mucoid
    exudative —see Otitis, media, suppurative
    in (due to) (with)
      influenza —see Influenza, with, otitis media
      measles B05.3
      scarlet fever A38.0
      tuberculosis A18.6
      viral disease NEC B34.- [H67.-]
    mucoid —see Otitis, media, nonsuppurative

Otitis (continued)
  media (continued)
    nonsuppurative H65.9-
      acute or subacute NEC H65.19-
        allergic H65.11-
          recurrent H65.11-
        recurrent H65.19-
        secretory —see Otitis, media, nonsuppurative, serous
        serous H65.0-
          recurrent H65.0-
      chronic H65.49-
        allergic H65.41-
        mucoid H65.3-
        serous H65.2-
    postmeasles B05.3
    purulent —see Otitis, media, suppurative
    secretory —see Otitis, media, nonsuppurative
    seromucinous —see Otitis, media, nonsuppurative
    serous —see Otitis, media, nonsuppurative
    suppurative H66.4-
      acute H66.00-
        with rupture of ear drum H66.01-
        recurrent H66.00-
          with rupture of ear drum H66.01-
      chronic (see also subcategory) H66.3
        atticoantral H66.2-
        benign —see Otitis, media, suppurative, chronic, tubotympanic
        tubotympanic H66.1-
      transudative —see Otitis, media, nonsuppurative
    tuberculous A18.6
Otocephaly Q18.2
Otolith syndrome —see subcategory H81.8
Otomycosis (diffuse) NEC B36.9 [H62.40]
  in
    aspergillosis B44.89
    candidiasis B37.84
    moniliasis B37.84
Otoporosis —see Otosclerosis
Otorrhagia (nontraumatic) H92.2-
  traumatic - code by Type of injury
Otorrhea H92.1-
  cerebrospinal (fluid) G96.01
    postoperative G96.08
    specified NEC G96.08
    spontaneous G96.01
    traumatic G96.08
Otosclerosis (general) H80.9-
  cochlear (endosteal) H80.2-
  involving
    otic capsule —see Otosclerosis, cochlear
    oval window
      nonobliterative H80.0-
      obliterative H80.1-
    round window —see Otosclerosis, cochlear
  nonobliterative —see Otosclerosis, involving, oval window, nonobliterative
  obliterative —see Otosclerosis, involving, oval window, obliterative
  specified NEC H80.8-
Otospongiosis —see Otosclerosis

Otto's disease or pelvis M24.7
Outcome of delivery Z37.9
  multiple births Z37.9
    all liveborn Z37.50
      quadruplets Z37.52
      quintuplets Z37.53
      sextuplets Z37.54
      specified number NEC Z37.59
      triplets Z37.51
    all stillborn Z37.7
    some liveborn Z37.60
      quadruplets Z37.62
      quintuplets Z37.63
      sextuplets Z37.64
      specified number NEC Z37.69
      triplets Z37.61
  single NEC Z37.9
    liveborn Z37.0
    stillborn Z37.1
  twins NEC Z37.9
    both liveborn Z37.2
    both stillborn Z37.4
    one liveborn, one stillborn Z37.3
Outlet —see condition
Ovalocytosis (congenital) (hereditary) —see Elliptocytosis
Ovarian —see Condition
Ovariocele N83.4-
Ovaritis (cystic) —see Oophoritis
Ovary, ovarian —see also condition
  resistant syndrome E28.39
  vein syndrome N13.8
Overactive —see also Hyperfunction
  adrenal cortex NEC E27.0
  bladder N32.81
  hypothalamus E23.3
  thyroid —see Hyperthyroidism
Overactivity R46.3
  child —see Disorder, attention-deficit hyperactivity
Overbite (deep) (excessive) (horizontal) (vertical) M26.29
Overbreathing —see Hyperventilation
Overconscientious personality vF60.5
Overdevelopment —see Hypertrophy
Overdistension —see Distension
Overdose, overdosage (drug) —see Table of Drugs and Chemicals, by drug, poisoning
Overeating R63.2
  nonorganic origin F50.89
  psychogenic F50.89
Overexertion (effects) (exhaustion) T73.3
Overexposure (effects) T73.9
  exhaustion T73.2
Overfeeding —see Overeating
  newborn P92.4
Overfill, endodontic M27.52
Overgrowth
  bacterial
    small intestinal K63.8219
      fungal K63.822
      hydrogen-subtype K63.8211
      hydrogen sulfide-subtype K63.8212
  bone —see Hypertrophy, bone
  intestinal methanogen K63.829
Overhanging of dental restorative material (unrepairable) K08.52

Overheated (places) (effects) —*see* Heat

Overjet (excessive horizontal) M26.23

Overlaid, overlying (suffocation) —*see* Asphyxia, traumatic, due to mechanical threat

Overlap, excessive horizontal (teeth) M26.23

Overlapping toe (acquired) — *see also* Deformity, toe, specified NEC
  congenital (fifth toe) Q66.89

Overload
  circulatory, due to transfusion (blood) (blood components) (TACO) E87.71
  fluid E87.70
    due to transfusion (blood) (blood components) E87.71
    specified NEC E87.79
  iron, due to repeated red blood cell transfusions E83.111
  potassium (K) E87.5
  sodium (Na) E87.0

Overnutrition —*see* Hyperalimentation

Overproduction —*see also* Hypersecretion
  ACTH E27.0
  catecholamine E27.5
  growth hormone E22.0

Overprotection, child by parent Z62.1

Overriding
  aorta Q25.49
  finger (acquired) —*see* Deformity, finger
    congenital Q68.1
  toe (acquired) —*see also* Deformity, toe, specified NEC
    congenital Q66.89

Overstrained R53.83
  heart —*see* Hypertrophy, cardiac

Overuse, muscle NEC M70.8-

Overweight E66.3

Overworked R53.83

Oviduct —*see* condition

Ovotestis Q56.0

Ovulation (cycle)
  failure or lack of N97.0
  pain N94.0

Ovum —*see* condition

Owren's disease or syndrome (parahemophilia) D68.2

Ox heart —*see* Hypertrophy, cardiac

Oxalosis E72.53

Oxaluria E72.53

Oxycephaly, oxycephalic Q75.009
  syphilitic, congenital A50.02

Oxyuriasis B80

Oxyuris vermicularis (infestation) B80

Ozena J31.0

P

Pachyderma, pachydermia L85.9
  larynx (verrucosa) J38.7

Pachydermatocele (congenital) Q82.8

Pachydermoperiostosis —*see also* Osteoarthropathy, hypertrophic, specified type NEC
  clubbed nail M89.40 *[L62]*

Pachygyria Q04.3

Pachymeningitis (adhesive) (basal) (brain) (cervical) (chronic) (circumscribed) (external) (fibrous) (hemorrhagic) (hypertrophic) (internal) (purulent) (spinal) (suppurative) —*see* Meningitis

Pachyonychia (congenital) Q84.5

Pacinian tumor —*see* Neoplasm, skin, benign

Pad, knuckle or Garrod's M72.1

Paget-Schroetter syndrome I82.890

Paget's disease
  with infiltrating duct carcinoma — *see* Neoplasm, breast, malignant
  bone M88.9
    carpus M88.84-
    clavicle M88.81-
    femur M88.85-
    fibula M88.86-
    finger M88.84-
    humerus M88.82-
    ilium M88.88
    in neoplastic disease —*see* Osteitis, deformans, in neoplastic disease
    ischium M88.88
    metacarpus M88.84-
    metatarsus M88.87-
    multiple sites M88.89
    neck M88.88
    pubic ramus M88.88
    radius M88.83-
    rib M88.88
    scapula M88.81-
    skull M88.0
    specified NEC M88.88
    tarsus M88.87-
    tibia M88.86-
    toe M88.87-
    ulna M88.83-
    vertebra M88.1
  breast (female) C50.01-
    male C50.02-
  extramammary —*see also* Neoplasm, skin, malignant
    anus C21.0
    margin C44.590
    skin C44.590
  intraductal carcinoma —*see* Neoplasm, breast, malignant
  malignant —*see* Neoplasm, skin, malignant
    breast (female) C50.01-
      male C50.02-
    unspecified site (female) C50.01-
      male C50.02-
  mammary —*see* Paget's disease, breast
  nipple —*see* Paget's disease, breast
  osteitis deformans —*see* Paget's disease, bone

Pain(s) (*see also* Painful) R52
  abdominal R10.9
    colic R10.83
    generalized R10.84
      with acute abdomen R10.0
    lower R10.30
      left quadrant R10.32
      pelvic or perineal R10.2
      periumbilical R10.33
      right quadrant R10.31

Pain(s) (*continued*)
  abdominal (*continued*)
    rebound —*see* Tenderness, abdominal, rebound
    severe with abdominal rigidity R10.0
    tenderness —*see* Tenderness, abdominal
    upper R10.10
      epigastric R10.13
      left quadrant R10.12
      right quadrant R10.11
  acute R52
    due to trauma G89.11
    neoplasm related G89.3
    postprocedural NEC G89.18
    post-thoracotomy G89.12
    specified by site - code to Pain, by site
  adnexa (uteri) R10.2
  anginoid —*see* Pain, precordial
  anus K62.89
  arm —*see* Pain, limb, upper
  axillary (axilla) M79.62-
  back (postural) M54.9
  bladder R39.89
    associated with micturition —*see* Micturition, painful
    chronic R39.82
  bone —*see* Disorder, bone, specified type NEC
  breast N64.4
  broad ligament R10.2
  cancer associated (acute) (chronic) G89.3
  cecum —*see* Pain, abdominal
  cervicobrachial M53.1
  chest (central) R07.9
    anterior wall R07.89
    atypical R07.89
    ischemic I20.9
    musculoskeletal R07.89
    non-cardiac R07.89
    on breathing R07.1
    pleurodynia R07.81
    precordial R07.2
    wall (anterior) R07.89
  chronic G89.29
    associated with significant psychosocial dysfunction G89.4
    due to trauma G89.21
    neoplasm related G89.3
    postoperative NEC G89.28
    postprocedural NEC G89.28
    post-thoracotomy G89.22
    specified NEC G89.29
  coccyx M53.3
  colon —*see* Pain, abdominal
  coronary —*see* Angina
  costochondral R07.1
  diaphragm R07.1
  due to cancer G89.3
  due to device, implant or graft (*see also* Complications, by site and type, specified NEC) T85.848
    arterial graft NEC T82.848
    breast (implant) T85.848
    catheter NEC T85.848
      dialysis (renal) T82.848
        intraperitoneal T85.848
      infusion NEC T82.848
        spinal (epidural) (subdural) T85.840
      urinary (indwelling) T83.84

Pain(s) (*continued*)
  due to device, implant or graft (*continued*)
    electronic (electrode) (pulse generator) (stimulator)
      bone T84.84
      cardiac T82.847
      nervous system (brain) (peripheral nerve) (spinal) T85.840
      urinary T83.84
    fixation, internal (orthopedic) NEC T84.84
    gastrointestinal (bile duct) (esophagus) T85.848
    genital NEC T83.84
    heart NEC T82.847
    infusion NEC T85.848
    joint prosthesis T84.84
    ocular (corneal graft) (orbital implant) NEC T85.848
    orthopedic NEC T84.84
    specified NEC T85.848
    urinary NEC T83.84
    vascular NEC T82.848
    ventricular intracranial shunt T85.840
  due to malignancy (primary) (secondary) G89.3
  ear —*see* subcategory H92.0
  epigastric, epigastrium R10.13
  eye —*see* Pain, ocular
  face, facial R51.9
    atypical G50.1
  female genital organs NEC N94.89
  finger —*see* Pain, limb, upper
  flank —*see* Pain, abdominal
  foot —*see* Pain, limb, lower
  gallbladder K82.9
  gas (intestinal) R14.1
  gastric —*see* Pain, abdominal
  generalized NOS R52
  genital organ
    female N94.89
    male N50.89
  groin —*see* Pain, abdominal, lower
  hand —*see* Pain, limb, upper
  head —*see* Headache
  heart —*see* Pain, precordial
  infra-orbital —*see* Neuralgia, trigeminal
  intercostal R07.82
  intermenstrual N94.0
  jaw R68.84
  joint M25.50
    ankle M25.57-
    elbow M25.52-
    finger M25.54-
    foot M25.57-
    hand M25.54-
    hip M25.55-
    knee M25.56-
    shoulder M25.51-
    specified site NEC M25.59
    toe M25.57-
    wrist M25.53-
  kidney N23
  laryngeal R07.0
  leg —*see* Pain, limb, lower
  limb M79.609
    lower M79.60-
      foot M79.67-
      lower leg M79.66-
      thigh M79.65-
      toe M79.67-
    upper M79.60-
      axilla M79.62-
      finger M79.64-
      forearm M79.63-
      hand M79.64-
      upper arm M79.62-

257

Pain(s) *(continued)*
  loin M54.50
  low back M54.50
    specified NEC M54.59
      vertebral end plate M54.51
      vertebrogenic M54.51
    lumbar region M54.50
      vertebral end plate M54.51
      vertebrogenic M54.51
  mandibular R68.84
  mastoid —*see* subcategory H92.0
  maxilla R68.84
  menstrual *(see also* Dysmenorrhea) N94.6
  metacarpophalangeal (joint) —*see* Pain, joint, hand
  metatarsophalangeal (joint) —*see* Pain, joint, foot
  mouth K13.79
  muscle —*see* Myalgia
  musculoskeletal *(see also* Pain, by site)* M79.18
  myofascial M79.18
  nasal J34.89
  nasopharynx J39.2
  neck NEC M54.2
  nerve NEC —*see* Neuralgia
  neuromuscular —*see* Neuralgia
  nose J34.89
  ocular H57.1-
  ophthalmic —*see* Pain, ocular
  orbital region —*see* Pain, ocular
  ovary N94.89
  over heart —*see* Pain, precordial
  ovulation N94.0
  pelvic (female) R10.2
  penis N48.89
  pericardial —*see* Pain, precordial
  perineal, perineum R10.2
  pharynx J39.2
  pleura, pleural, pleuritic R07.81
  postoperative NOS G89.18
  postprocedural NOS G89.18
  post-thoracotomy G89.12
  precordial (region) R07.2
  premenstrual N94.3
  psychogenic (persistent) (any site) F45.41
  radicular (spinal) —*see* Radiculopathy
  rectum K62.89
  respiration R07.1
  retrosternal R07.2
  rheumatoid, muscular —*see* Myalgia
  rib R07.81
  root (spinal) —*see* Radiculopathy
  round ligament (stretch) R10.2
  sacroiliac M53.3
  sciatic —*see* Sciatica
  scrotum N50.82
  seminal vesicle N50.89
  shoulder M25.51-
  spermatic cord N50.89
  spinal root —*see* Radiculopathy
  spine M54.9
    cervical M54.2
    low back M54.50
      with sciatica M54.4-
    thoracic M54.6
  stomach —*see* Pain, abdominal
  substernal R07.2
  temporomandibular (joint) M26.62-
  testis N50.81-
  thoracic spine M54.6
    with radicular and visceral pain M54.14
  throat R07.0
  tibia —*see* Pain, limb, lower
  toe —*see* Pain, limb, lower
  tongue K14.6

Pain(s) *(continued)*
  tooth K08.89
  trigeminal —*see* Neuralgia, trigeminal
  tumor associated G89.3
  ureter N23
  urinary (organ) (system) N23
  uterus NEC N94.89
  vagina R10.2
  vertebral end plate —*see* Pain, vertebrogenic
  vertebrogenic M54.89
    low back M54.51
    lumbar M54.51
    syndrome M54.89
  vesical R39.89
    associated with micturition —*see* Micturition, painful
  vulva R10.2
Painful —*see also* Pain
  coitus
    female N94.10
    male N53.12
    psychogenic F52.6
  ejaculation (semen) N53.12
    psychogenic F52.6
  erection —*see* Priapism
  feet syndrome E53.8
  joint replacement (hip) (knee) T84.84
  menstruation —*see* Dysmenorrhea
    psychogenic F45.8
  micturition —*see* Micturition, painful
  respiration R07.1
  scar NEC L90.5
  wire sutures T81.89
Painter's colic —*see* subcategory T56.0
Palate —*see* condition
Palatoplegia K13.79
Palatoschisis —*see* Cleft, palate
Palilalia R48.8
Palliative care Z51.5
Pallor R23.1
  optic disc, temporal —*see* Atrophy, optic
Palmar —*see also* condition
  fascia —*see* condition
Palpable
  cecum K63.89
  kidney N28.89
  ovary N83.8
  prostate N42.9
  spleen —*see* Splenomegaly
Palpitations (heart) R00.2
  psychogenic F45.8
Palsy *(see also* Paralysis) G83.9
  atrophic diffuse (progressive) G12.22
  Bell's —*see also* Palsy, facial
    newborn P11.3
  brachial plexus NEC G54.0
    newborn (birth injury) P14.3
  brain —*see* Palsy, cerebral
  bulbar (progressive) (chronic) G12.22
    of childhood (Fazio-Londe) G12.1
    pseudo NEC G12.29
    supranuclear (progressive) G23.1
  cerebral (congenital) G80.9
    ataxic G80.4
    athetoid G80.3
    choreathetoid G80.3
    diplegic G80.8
      spastic G80.1

Palsy *(continued)*
  cerebral (congenital) *(continued)*
    dyskinetic G80.3
      athetoid G80.3
      choreathetoid G80.3
      distonic G80.3
    dystonic G80.3
    hemiplegic G80.8
      spastic G80.2
    mixed G80.8
    monoplegic G80.8
      spastic G80.1
    paraplegic G80.8
      spastic G80.1
    quadriplegic G80.8
      spastic G80.0
    spastic G80.1
      diplegic G80.1
      hemiplegic G80.2
      monoplegic G80.1
      quadriplegic G80.0
      specified NEC G80.1
      tetrapelgic G80.0
    specified NEC G80.8
    syphilitic A52.12
      congenital A50.49
    tetraplegic G80.8
      spastic G80.0
  cranial nerve —*see also* Disorder, nerve, cranial
    multiple G52.7
      in
        infectious disease B99 *[G53]*
        neoplastic disease *(see also* Neoplasm) D49.9 *[G53]*
        parasitic disease B89 *[G53]*
        sarcoidosis D86.82
  creeping G12.22
  diver's T70.3
  Erb's P14.0
  facial G51.0
    newborn (birth injury) P11.3
  glossopharyngeal G52.1
  Klumpke (-Déjérine) P14.1
  lead —*see* subcategory T56.0
  median nerve (tardy) G56.1-
  nerve G58.9
    specified NEC G58.8
  peroneal nerve (acute) (tardy) G57.3-
  progressive supranuclear G23.1
  pseudobulbar NEC G12.29
  radial nerve (acute) G56.3-
  seventh nerve —*see also* Palsy, facial
    newborn P11.3
  shaking —*see* Parkinsonism
  spastic (cerebral) (spinal) G80.1
  ulnar nerve (tardy) G56.2-
  wasting G12.29
Paludism —*see* Malaria
Panangiitis M30.0
Panaris, panaritium —*see also* Cellulitis, digit
  with lymphangitis —*see* Lymphangitis, acute, digit
Panarteritis nodosa M30.0
  brain or cerebral I67.7
Pancake heart R93.1
  with cor pulmonale (chronic) I27.81
Pancarditis (acute) (chronic) I51.89
  rheumatic I09.89
    active or acute I01.8

Pancoast's syndrome or tumor C34.1-
Pancolitis —*see also* Colitis
  ulcerative (chronic) K51.00
    with
      complication K51.019
        abscess K51.014
        fistula K51.013
        obstruction K51.012
        rectal bleeding K51.011
        specified complication NEC K51.018
Pancreas, pancreatic —*see* condition
Pancreatitis (annular) (apoplectic) (calcareous) (edematous) (hemorrhagic) (malignant) (subacute) (suppurative) K85.90
  with necrosis (uninfected) K85.91
    infected K85.92
  acute (without necrosis or infection) K85.90
    with necrosis (uninfected) K85.91
      infected K85.92
  alcohol induced (without necrosis or infection) K85.20
    with necrosis (uninfected) K85.21
      infected K85.22
  biliary (without necrosis or infection) K85.10
    with necrosis (uninfected) K85.11
      infected K85.12
  drug induced (without necrosis or infection) K85.30
    with necrosis (uninfected) K85.31
      infected K85.32
  gallstone (without necrosis or infection) K85.10
    with necrosis (uninfected) K85.11
      infected K85.12
  idiopathic (without necrosis or infection) K85.00
    with necrosis (uninfected) K85.01
      infected K85.02
  specified NEC (without necrosis or infection) K85.80
    with necrosis (uninfected) K85.81
      infected K85.82
  chronic (infectious) K86.1
    alcohol-induced K86.0
    recurrent K86.1
    relapsing K86.1
  cystic (chronic) K86.1
  cytomegaloviral B25.2
  fibrous (chronic) K86.1
  gangrenous —*see* Pancreatitis, acute
  gallstone (without necrosis or infection) K85.10
    with necrosis (uninfected) K85.11
      infected K85.12
  interstitial (chronic) K86.1
  acute *(see also* Pancreatitis, acute) K85.80
  mumps B26.3
  recurrent
    acute —*see* Pancreatitis, acute
    by type
    chronic K86.1

Pancreatitis (continued)
 relapsing, chronic K86.1
 syphilitic A52.74
Pancreatoblastoma —see Neoplasm, pancreas, malignant
Pancreolithiasis K86.89
Pancytolysis D75.89
Pancytopenia (acquired) D61.818
 with
  malformations D61.09
  myelodysplastic syndrome —see Syndrome, myelodysplastic
 antineoplastic chemotherapy induced D61.810
 congenital D61.09
 drug-induced NEC D61.811
PANDAS (pediatric autoimmune neuropsychiatric disorders associated with streptococcal infections syndrome) D89.89
Panencephalitis, subacute, sclerosing A81.1
Panhematopenia D61.9
 congenital D61.09
 constitutional D61.09
 splenic, primary D73.1
Panhemocytopenia D61.9
 congenital D61.09
 constitutional D61.09
Panhypogonadism E29.1
Panhypopituitarism E23.0
 prepubertal E23.0
Panic (attack) (state) F41.0
 reaction to exceptional stress (transient) F43.0
Panmyelopathy, familial, constitutional D61.09
Panmyelophthisis D61.82
 congenital D61.09
Panmyelosis (acute) (with myelofibrosis) C94.4-
Panner's disease —see Osteochondrosis, juvenile, humerus
Panneuritis endemica E51.11
Panniculitis (nodular) (nonsuppurative) M79.3
 back M54.00
  cervical region M54.02
  cervicothoracic region M54.03
  lumbar region M54.06
  lumbosacral region M54.07
  multiple sites M54.09
  occipito-atlanto-axial region M54.01
  sacrococcygeal region M54.08
  thoracic region M54.04
  thoracolumbar region M54.05
 lupus L93.2
 mesenteric K65.4
 neck M54.02
  cervicothoracic region M54.03
  occipito-atlanto-axial region M54.01
 relapsing M35.6
Panniculus adiposus (abdominal) E65
Pannus (allergic) (cornea) (degenerativus) (keratic) H16.42-
 abdominal (symptomatic) E65
 trachomatosus, trachomatous (active) A71.1
Panophthalmitis H44.01-

Pansinusitis (chronic) (hyperplastic) (nonpurulent) (purulent) J32.4
 acute J01.40
  recurrent J01.41
 tuberculous A15.8
Pansynostosis Q75.052
Panuveitis (sympathetic) H44.11-
Panvalvular disease I08.9
 specified NEC I08.8
PAPA (pyogenic arthritis, pyoderma gangrenosum, and acne syndrome) M04.8
Papanicolaou smear, cervix Z12.4
 as part of routine gynecological examination Z01.419
  with abnormal findings Z01.411
 for suspected neoplasm Z12.4
 nonspecific abnormal finding R87.619
 routine Z01.419
  with abnormal findings Z01.411
Papilledema (choked disc) H47.10
 associated with
  decreased ocular pressure H47.12
  increased intracranial pressure H47.11
  retinal disorder H47.13
 Foster-Kennedy syndrome H47.14-
Papillitis H46.00
 anus K62.89
 chronic lingual K14.4
 necrotizing, kidney N17.2
 optic H46.0-
 rectum K62.89
 renal, necrotizing N17.2
 tongue K14.0
Papilloma —see also Neoplasm, benign, by site
 basal cell L82.1
  inflamed L82.0
 acuminatum (female) (male) (anogenital) A63.0
 benign pinta (primary) A67.0
 bladder (urinary) (transitional cell) D41.4
 choroid plexus (lateral ventricle) (third ventricle) D33.0
  anaplastic C71.5
  fourth ventricle D33.1
  malignant C71.5
 renal pelvis (transitional cell) D41.1-
  benign D30.1-
 Schneiderian
  specified site —see Neoplasm, benign, by site
  unspecified site D14.0
 serous surface
  borderline malignancy
   specified site —see Neoplasm, uncertain behavior, by site
   unspecified site D39.10
  specified site —see Neoplasm, benign, by site
  unspecified site D27.9
 transitional (cell)
  bladder (urinary) D41.4
   inverted type —see Neoplasm, uncertain behavior, by site
  renal pelvis D41.1-
  ureter D41.2-
 ureter (transitional cell) D41.2-
  benign D30.2-
 urothelial —see Neoplasm, uncertain behavior, by site
 villous —see Neoplasm, uncertain behavior, by site

Papilloma (continued)
 villous (continued)
  adenocarcinoma in —see Neoplasm, malignant, by site
  in situ —see Neoplasm, in situ
 yaws, plantar or palmar A66.1
Papillomata, multiple, of yaws A66.1
Papillomatosis —see also Neoplasm, benign, by site
 confluent and reticulated L83
 cystic, breast —see Mastopathy, cystic
 ductal, breast —see Mastopathy, cystic
 intraductal (diffuse) —see Neoplasm, benign, by site
 subareolar duct D24-
Papillomavirus, as cause of disease classified elsewhere B97.7
Papillon-Léage and Psaume syndrome Q87.0
Papule(s) R23.8
 carate (primary) A67.0
 fibrous, of nose D22.39
 Gottron's L94.4
 pinta (primary) A67.0
Papulosis
 lymphomatoid C86.6
 malignant I77.89
Papyraceous fetus O31.0-
Para-albuminemia E88.09
Paracephalus Q89.7
Parachute mitral valve Q23.2
Paracoccidioidomycosis B41.9
 disseminated B41.7
 generalized B41.7
 mucocutaneous-lymphangitic B41.8
 pulmonary B41.0
 specified NEC B41.8
 visceral B41.8
Paradentosis K05.4
Paraffinoma T88.8
Paraganglioma D44.7
 adrenal D35.0-
  malignant C74.1-
 aortic body D44.7
  malignant C75.5
 carotid body D44.6
  malignant C75.4
 chromaffin —see also Neoplasm, benign, by site
  malignant —see Neoplasm, malignant, by site
 extra-adrenal D44.7
  malignant C75.5
   specified site —see Neoplasm, malignant, by site
   unspecified site C75.5
  specified site —see Neoplasm, uncertain behavior, by site
  unspecified site D44.7
 gangliocytic D13.2
  specified site —see Neoplasm, benign, by site
  unspecified site D13.2
 glomus jugulare D44.7
  malignant C75.5
 jugular D44.7
 malignant C75.5
  specified site —see Neoplasm, malignant, by site
  unspecified site C75.5

Paraganglioma (continued)
 nonchromaffin D44.7
  malignant C75.5
   specified site —see Neoplasm, malignant, by site
   unspecified site C75.5
  specified site —see Neoplasm, uncertain behavior, by site
  unspecified site D44.7
 parasympathetic D44.7
  specified site —see Neoplasm, uncertain behavior, by site
  unspecified site D44.7
  specified site —see Neoplasm, uncertain behavior, by site
 sympathetic D44.7
  specified site —see Neoplasm, uncertain behavior, by site
  unspecified site D44.7
 unspecified site D44.7
Parageusia R43.2
 psychogenic F45.8
Paragonimiasis B66.4
Paragranuloma, Hodgkin —see Lymphoma, Hodgkin, specified NEC
Parahemophilia (see also Defect, coagulation) D68.2
Parakeratosis R23.4
 variegata L41.0
Paralysis, paralytic (complete) (incomplete) G83.9
 with
  syphilis A52.17
 abducens, abducent (nerve) —see Strabismus, paralytic, sixth nerve
 abductor, lower extremity G57.9-
 accessory nerve G52.8
 accommodation —see also Paresis, of accommodation
  hysterical F44.89
 acoustic nerve (except Deafness) —see subcategory H93.3
 agitans (see also Parkinsonism) G20.C
  arteriosclerotic G21.4
 alternating (oculomotor) G83.89
 amyotrophic G12.21
 ankle G57.9-
 anus (sphincter) K62.89
 arm —see Monoplegia, upper limb
 ascending (spinal), acute G61.0
 association G12.29
 asthenic bulbar G70.00
  with exacerbation (acute) G70.01
  in crisis G70.01
 ataxic (hereditary) G11.9
  general (syphilitic) A52.17
 atrophic G58.9
  infantile, acute —see Poliomyelitis, paralytic
  progressive G12.22
  spinal (acute) —see Poliomyelitis, paralytic
 axillary G54.0
 Babinski-Nageotte's G83.89
 Bell's G51.0
  newborn P11.3
 Benedikt's G46.3
 birth injury P14.9
  spinal cord P11.5
 bladder (neurogenic) (sphincter) N31.2
 bowel, colon or intestine K56.0
 brachial plexus G54.0
  birth injury P14.3
  newborn (birth injury) P14.3

Paralysis, paralytic *(continued)*
　brain G83.9
　　diplegia G83.0
　　triplegia G83.89
　bronchial J98.09
　Brown-Séquard G83.81
　bulbar (chronic) (progressive) G12.22
　　infantile —*see* Poliomyelitis, paralytic
　　poliomyelitic —*see* Poliomyelitis, paralytic
　　pseudo G12.29
　bulbospinal G70.00
　　with exacerbation (acute) G70.01
　　in crisis G70.01
　cardiac (*see also* Failure, heart) I50.9
　cerebrocerebellar, diplegic G80.1
　cervical
　　plexus G54.2
　　sympathetic G90.09
　Céstan-Chenais G46.3
　Charcot-Marie-Tooth type G60.0
　Clark's G80.9
　colon K56.0
　compressed air T70.3
　compression
　　arm G56.9-
　　leg G57.9-
　　lower extremity G57.9-
　　upper extremity G56.9-
　congenital (cerebral) —*see* Palsy, cerebral
　conjugate movement (gaze) (of eye) H51.0
　　cortical (nuclear) (supranuclear) H51.0
　cordis —*see* Failure, heart
　cranial or cerebral nerve G52.9
　creeping G12.22
　crossed leg G83.89
　crutch —*see* Injury, brachial plexus
　deglutition R13.0
　　hysterical F44.4
　dementia A52.17
　descending (spinal) NEC G12.29
　diaphragm (flaccid) J98.6
　　due to accidental dissection of phrenic nerve during procedure —*see* Puncture, accidental complicating surgery
　digestive organs NEC K59.89
　diplegic —*see* Diplegia
　divergence (nuclear) H51.8
　diver's T70.3
　Duchenne's
　　birth injury P14.0
　　due to or associated with motor neuron disease G12.22
　　muscular dystrophy G71.01
　due to intracranial or spinal birth injury —*see* Palsy, cerebral
　embolic (current episode) I63.4-
　Erb (-Duchenne) (birth) (newborn) P14.0
　Erb's syphilitic spastic spinal A52.17
　esophagus K22.89
　eye muscle (extrinsic) H49.9
　　intrinsic —*see also* Paresis, of accommodation
　facial (nerve) G51.0
　　birth injury P11.3
　　congenital P11.3
　　following operation NEC —*see* Puncture, accidental complicating surgery
　　newborn (birth injury) P11.3
　familial (recurrent) (periodic) G72.3
　　spastic G11.4

Paralysis, paralytic *(continued)*
　fauces J39.2
　finger G56.9-
　gait R26.1
　gastric nerve (nondiabetic) G52.2
　gaze, conjugate H51.0
　general (progressive) (syphilitic) A52.17
　　juvenile A50.45
　glottis J38.00
　　bilateral J38.02
　　unilateral J38.01
　gluteal G54.1
　Gubler (-Millard) G46.3
　hand —*see* Monoplegia, upper limb
　heart —*see* Arrest, cardiac
　hemiplegic —*see* Hemiplegia
　hyperkalemic periodic (familial) G72.3
　hypoglossal (nerve) G52.3
　hypokalemic periodic G72.3
　hysterical F44.4
　ileus K56.0
　infantile (*see also* Poliomyelitis, paralytic) A80.30
　　bulbar —*see* Poliomyelitis, paralytic
　　cerebral —*see* Palsy, cerebral
　　spastic —*see* Palsy, cerebral, spastic
　　infective —*see* Poliomyelitis, paralytic
　inferior nuclear G83.9
　internuclear —*see* Ophthalmoplegia, internuclear
　intestine K56.0
　iris H57.09
　　due to diphtheria (toxin) A36.89
　ischemic, Volkmann's (complicating trauma) T79.6
　Jackson's G83.89
　jake —*see* Poisoning, food, noxious, plant
　Jamaica ginger (jake) G62.2
　juvenile general A50.45
　Klumpke (-Déjérine) (birth) (newborn) P14.1
　labioglossal (laryngeal) (pharyngeal) G12.29
　Landry's G61.0
　laryngeal nerve (recurrent) (superior) (unilateral) J38.00
　　bilateral J38.02
　　unilateral J38.01
　larynx J38.00
　　bilateral J38.02
　　due to diphtheria (toxin) A36.2
　　unilateral J38.01
　lateral G12.23
　lead —*see* subcategory T56.0
　left side —*see* Hemiplegia
　leg G83.1-
　　both —*see* Paraplegia
　　crossed G83.89
　　hysterical F44.4
　　psychogenic F44.4
　　transient or transitory R29.818
　　　traumatic NEC —*see* Injury, nerve, leg
　levator palpebrae superioris —*see* Blepharoptosis, paralytic
　limb —*see* Monoplegia
　lip K13.0
　Lissauer's A52.17
　lower limb —*see* Monoplegia, lower limb
　　both —*see* Paraplegia
　lung J98.4
　median nerve G56.1-
　medullary (tegmental) G83.89

Paralysis, paralytic *(continued)*
　mesencephalic NEC G83.89
　　tegmental G83.89
　middle alternating G83.89
　Millard-Gubler-Foville G46.3
　monoplegic —*see* Monoplegia
　motor G83.9
　muscle, muscular NEC G72.89
　　due to nerve lesion G58.9
　　eye (extrinsic) H49.9
　　　intrinsic —*see* Paresis, of accommodation
　　　oblique —*see* Strabismus, paralytic, fourth nerve
　　iris sphincter H21.9
　　ischemic (Volkmann's) (complicating trauma) T79.6
　　progressive G12.21
　　progressive, spinal G12.25
　　pseudohypertrophic G71.02
　　spinal progressive G12.25
　musculocutaneous nerve G56.9-
　musculospiral G56.9-
　nerve —*see also* Disorder, nerve
　　abducent —*see* Strabismus, paralytic, sixth nerve
　　accessory G52.8
　　auditory (except Deafness) —*see* subcategory H93.3
　　birth injury P14.9
　　cranial or cerebral G52.9
　　facial G51.0
　　　birth injury P11.3
　　　congenital P11.3
　　　newborn (birth injury) P11.3
　　fourth or trochlear —*see* Strabismus, paralytic, fourth nerve
　　newborn (birth injury) P14.9
　　oculomotor —*see* Strabismus, paralytic, third nerve
　　phrenic (birth injury) P14.2
　　radial G56.3-
　　seventh or facial G51.0
　　　newborn (birth injury) P11.3
　　sixth or abducent —*see* Strabismus, paralytic, sixth nerve
　　syphilitic A52.15
　　third or oculomotor —*see* Strabismus, paralytic, third nerve
　　trigeminal G50.9
　　trochlear —*see* Strabismus, paralytic, fourth nerve
　　ulnar G56.2-
　normokalemic periodic G72.3
　ocular H49.9
　　alternating G83.89
　oculofacial, congenital (Moebius) Q87.0
　oculomotor (external bilateral) (nerve) —*see* Strabismus, paralytic, third nerve
　palate (soft) K13.79
　paratrigeminal G50.9
　periodic (familial) (hyperkalemic) (hypokalemic) (myotonic) (normokalemic) (potassium sensitive) (secondary) G72.3
　peripheral autonomic nervous system —*see* Neuropathy, peripheral, autonomic
　peroneal (nerve) G57.3-
　pharynx J39.2
　phrenic nerve G56.8-
　plantar nerve(s) G57.6-
　pneumogastric nerve G52.2
　poliomyelitis (current) —*see* Poliomyelitis, paralytic

Paralysis, paralytic *(continued)*
　popliteal nerve G57.3-
　postepileptic transitory G83.84
　progressive (atrophic) (bulbar) (spinal) G12.22
　　general A52.17
　　infantile acute —*see* Poliomyelitis, paralytic
　　supranuclear G23.1
　pseudobulbar G12.29
　pseudohypertrophic (muscle) (*see also* Dystrophy, muscular, by type, if applicable) G71.09
　psychogenic F44.4
　quadriceps G57.9-
　quadriplegic —*see* Tetraplegia
　radial nerve G56.3-
　rectus muscle (eye) H49.9
　recurrent isolated sleep G47.53
　respiratory (muscle) (system) (tract) R06.81
　　center NEC G93.89
　　congenital P28.89
　　newborn P28.89
　right side —*see* Hemiplegia
　saturnine —*see* subcategory T56.0
　sciatic nerve G57.0-
　senile G83.9
　shaking —*see* Parkinsonism
　shoulder G56.9-
　sleep, recurrent isolated G47.53
　spastic G83.9
　　cerebral —*see* Palsy, cerebral, spastic
　　congenital (cerebral) —*see* Palsy, cerebral, spastic
　　familial G11.4
　　hereditary G11.4
　　quadriplegic G80.0
　　syphilitic (spinal) A52.17
　sphincter, bladder —*see* Paralysis, bladder
　spinal (cord) G83.9
　　accessory nerve G52.8
　　acute —*see* Poliomyelitis, paralytic
　　ascending acute G61.0
　　atrophic (acute) —*see also* Poliomyelitis, paralytic
　　　spastic, syphilitic A52.17
　　congenital NEC —*see* Palsy, cerebral
　　infantile —*see* Poliomyelitis, paralytic
　　hereditary G95.89
　　progressive G12.21
　　　muscle G12.25
　　sequelae NEC G83.89
　sternomastoid G52.8
　stomach K31.84
　　diabetic —*see* Diabetes, by type, with gastroparesis
　　nerve G52.2
　　　diabetic —*see* Diabetes, by type, with gastroparesis
　stroke —*see* Infarct, brain
　subcapsularis G56.8-
　supranuclear (progressive) G23.1
　sympathetic G90.8
　　cervical G90.09
　　nervous system —*see* Neuropathy, peripheral, autonomic
　syndrome G83.9
　　specified NEC G83.89
　syphilitic spastic spinal (Erb's) A52.17
　thigh G57.9-
　throat J39.2
　　diphtheritic A36.0
　　muscle J39.2

Paralysis, paralytic (continued)
  thrombotic (current episode) I63.3-
  thumb G56.9-
  tick —see Toxicity, venom, arthropod, specified NEC
  Todd's (postepileptic transitory paralysis) G83.84
  toe G57.6-
  tongue K14.8
  transient R29.5
    arm or leg NEC R29.818
    traumatic NEC —see Injury, nerve
  trapezius G52.8
  traumatic, transient NEC —see Injury, nerve
  trembling —see Parkinsonism
  triceps brachii G56.9-
  trigeminal nerve G50.9
  trochlear (nerve) —see Strabismus, paralytic, fourth nerve
  ulnar nerve G56.2-
  upper limb —see Monoplegia, upper limb
  uremic N18.9 [G99.8]
  uveoparotitic D86.89
  uvula K13.79
    postdiphtheritic A36.0
  vagus nerve G52.2
  vasomotor NEC G90.8
  velum palati K13.79
  vesical —see Paralysis, bladder
  vestibular nerve (except Vertigo) —see subcategory H93.3
  vocal cords J38.00
    bilateral J38.02
    unilateral J38.01
  Volkmann's (complicating trauma) T79.6
  wasting G12.29
  Weber's G46.3
  wrist G56.9-

Paramedial urethrovesical orifice Q64.79

Paramenia N92.6

Parametritis (see also Disease, pelvis, inflammatory) N73.2
  acute N73.0
  complicating abortion —see Abortion, by type, complicated by, parametritis

Parametrium, parametric —see condition

Paramnesia —see Amnesia

Paramolar K00.1

Paramyloidosis E85.89

Paramyoclonus multiplex G25.3

Paramyotonia (congenita) G71.19

Parangi —see Yaws

Paranoia (querulans) F22
  senile F03

Paranoid
  dementia (senile) F03
    praecox —see Schizophrenia
  personality F60.0
  psychosis (climacteric) (involutional) (menopausal) F22
    psychogenic (acute) F23
    senile F03
  reaction (acute) F23
    chronic F22
  schizophrenia F20.0
  state (climacteric) (involutional) (menopausal) (simple) F22
    senile F03
  tendencies F60.0

Paranoid (continued)
  traits F60.0
  trends F60.0
  type, psychopathic personality F60.0

Paraparesis —see Paraplegia

Paraphasia R47.02

Paraphilia F65.9

Paraphimosis (congenital) N47.2
  chancroidal A57

Paraphrenia, paraphrenic (late) F22
  schizophrenia F20.0

Paraplegia (lower) G82.20
  ataxic —see Degeneration, combined, spinal cord
  complete G82.21
  congenital (cerebral) G80.8
    spastic G80.1
  familial spastic G11.4
  functional (hysterical) F44.4
  hereditary, spastic G11.4
  hysterical F44.4
  incomplete G82.22
  Pott's A18.01
  psychogenic F44.4
  spastic
    Erb's spinal, syphilitic A52.17
    hereditary G11.4
    tropical G04.1
  syphilitic (spastic) A52.17
  traumatic
    current injury - code to injury with seventh character A
    sequela of previous injury - code to injury with seventh character S
  tropical spastic G04.1

Parapoxvirus B08.60
  specified NEC B08.69

Paraproteinemia D89.2
  benign (familial) D89.2
  monoclonal D47.2
  secondary to malignant disease D47.2

Parapsoriasis L41.9
  en plaques L41.4
  guttata L41.1
  large plaque L41.4
  retiform, retiformis L41.5
  small plaque L41.3
  specified NEC L41.8
  varioliformis (acuta) L41.0

Parasitic —see also condition
  disease NEC B89
  stomatitis B37.0
  sycosis (beard) (scalp) B35.0
  twin Q89.4

Parasitism B89
  intestinal B82.9
  skin B88.9
  specified —see Infestation

Parasitophobia F40.218

Parasomnia G47.50
  due to
    alcohol
      abuse F10.182
      dependence F10.282
      use F10.982
    amphetamines
      abuse F15.182
      dependence F15.282
      use F15.982
    caffeine
      abuse F15.182
      dependence F15.282
      use F15.982

Parasomnia (continued)
  due to (continued)
    cocaine
      abuse F14.182
      dependence F14.282
      use F14.982
    drug NEC
      abuse F19.182
      dependence F19.282
      use F19.982
    opioid
      abuse F11.182
      dependence F11.282
      use F11.982
    psychoactive substance NEC
      abuse F19.182
      dependence F19.282
      use F19.982
    sedative, hypnotic, or anxiolytic
      abuse F13.182
      dependence F13.282
      use F13.982
    stimulant NEC
      abuse F15.182
      dependence F15.282
      use F15.982
  in conditions classified elsewhere G47.54
  nonorganic origin F51.8
  organic G47.50
  specified NEC G47.59

Paraspadias Q54.9

Paraspasmus facialis G51.8

Parasuicide (attempt)
  history of (personal) Z91.51
    in family Z81.8

Parathyroid gland —see condition

Parathyroid tetany E20.9

Paratrachoma A74.0

Paratyphilitis —see Appendicitis

Paratyphoid (fever) —see Fever, paratyphoid

Paratyphus —see Fever, paratyphoid

Paraurethral duct Q64.79

Paraurethritis —see also Urethritis
  gonococcal (acute) (chronic) (with abscess) A54.1

Paravaccinia NEC B08.04

Paravaginitis —see Vaginitis

Parencephalitis —see also Encephalitis
  sequelae G09

Parent-child conflict —see Conflict, parent-child
  estrangement NEC Z62.890

Paresis —see also Paralysis
  accommodation —see Paresis, of accommodation
  Bernhardt's G57.1-
  bladder (sphincter) —see also Paralysis, bladder
    tabetic A52.17
  bowel, colon or intestine K56.0
  extrinsic muscle, eye H49.9
  general (progressive) (syphilitic) A52.17
    juvenile A50.45
  heart —see Failure, heart
  insane (syphilitic) A52.17
  juvenile (general) A50.45
  of accommodation H52.52-
  peripheral progressive (idiopathic) G60.3
  pseudohypertrophic (see also Dystrophy, muscular, by type, if applicable) G71.09
  senile G83.9

Paresis (continued)
  syphilitic (general) A52.17
    congenital A50.45
  vesical NEC N31.2

Paresthesia (see also Disturbance, sensation, skin) R20.2
  Bernhardt G57.1-

Paretic —see condition

Parinaud's
  conjunctivitis H10.89
  oculoglandular syndrome H10.89
  ophthalmoplegia H49.88-

Parkinsonism (idiopathic) (primary) G20.C
  with neurogenic orthostatic hypotension (symptomatic) G90.3
  arteriosclerotic G21.4
  dementia (see also Dementia, in, diseases specified elsewhere) G20.C [F02.80]
    with behavioral disturbance (see also Dementia, in, diseases specified elsewhere) G20.C [F02.81-]
  due to
    drugs NEC G21.19
      neuroleptic G21.11
  medication-induced NEC G21.19
  neuroleptic induced G21.11
  postencephalitic G21.3
  secondary G21.9
    due to
      arteriosclerosis G21.4
      drugs NEC G21.19
        neuroleptic G21.11
      encephalitis G21.3
      external agents NEC G21.2
      syphilis A52.19
    specified NEC G21.8
  syphilitic A52.19
  treatment-induced NEC G21.19
  vascular G21.4

Parkinson's disease, syndrome or tremor —see Parkinsonism

Parodontitis —see Periodontitis

Parodontosis K05.4

Paronychia —see also Cellulitis, digit
  with lymphangitis —see Lymphangitis, acute, digit
  candidal (chronic) B37.2
  tuberculous (primary) A18.4

Parorexia (psychogenic) F50.89

Parosmia R43.1
  psychogenic F45.8

Parotid gland —see condition

Parotitis, parotiditis (allergic) (nonspecific toxic) (purulent) (septic) (suppurative) —see also Sialoadenitis
  epidemic —see Mumps
  infectious —see Mumps
  postoperative K91.89
  surgical K91.89

Parrot fever A70

Parrot's disease (early congenital syphilitic pseudoparalysis) A50.02

Parry-Romberg syndrome G51.8

Parry's disease or syndrome E05.00
  with thyroid storm E05.01

Pars planitis —see Cyclitis

Parsonage (-Aldren)-**Turner syndrome** G54.5**

Parson's disease (exophthalmic goiter) E05.00
 with thyroid storm E05.01
Particolored infant Q82.8
Parturition —see Delivery
Parulis K04.7
 with sinus K04.6
Parvovirus, as cause of disease classified elsewhere B97.6
Pasini and Pierini's atrophoderma L90.3
Passage
 false, urethra N36.5
 meconium (newborn) during delivery P03.82
 of sounds or bougies —see Attention to, artificial, opening
Passive —see condition
 smoking Z77.22
Past due on rent or mortgage Z59.81-
Pasteurella septica A28.0
Pasteurellosis —see Infection, Pasteurella
PAT (paroxysmal atrial tachycardia) I47.19
Patau's syndrome —see Trisomy, 13
Patches
 mucous (syphilitic) A51.39
  congenital A50.07
 smokers' (mouth) K13.24
Patellar —see condition
Patent —see also Imperfect, closure
 canal of Nuck Q52.4
 cervix N88.3
 ductus arteriosus or Botallo's Q25.0
 foramen
  botalli Q21.12
  ovale Q21.12
 interauricular septum Q21.19
 interventricular septum Q21.0
 omphalomesenteric duct Q43.0
 os (uteri) —see Patent, cervix
 ostium secundum (type II) Q21.11
 urachus Q64.4
 vitelline duct Q43.0
Paterson (-Brown) (-Kelly) **syndrome or web** D50.1
Pathologic, pathological —see also condition
 asphyxia R09.01
 fire-setting F63.1
 gambling F63.0
 ovum O02.0
 resorption, tooth K03.3
 stealing F63.2
Pathology (of) —see Disease
 periradicular, associated with previous endodontic treatment NEC M27.59
Pattern, sleep-wake, irregular G47.23
Patulous —see also Imperfect, closure (congenital)
 alimentary tract Q45.8
  lower Q43.8
  upper Q40.8
 eustachian tube H69.0-
Pause, sinoatrial I49.5
Paxton's disease B36.2
Pearl(s)
 enamel K00.2
 Epstein's K09.8

Pearl-worker's disease —see Osteomyelitis, specified type NEC
Pectenosis K62.4
Pectoral —see condition
Pectus
 carinatum (congenital) Q67.7
  acquired M95.4
   rachitic sequelae (late effect) E64.3
 excavatum (congenital) Q67.6
  acquired M95.4
   rachitic sequelae (late effect) E64.3
 recurvatum (congenital) Q67.6
Pedatrophia E41
Pederosis F65.4
Pediatric inflammatory multisystem syndrome M35.81
Pediculosis (infestation) B85.2
 capitis (head-louse) (any site) B85.0
 corporis (body-louse) (any site) B85.1
 eyelid B85.0
 mixed (classifiable to more than one of the titles B85.0-B85.3) B85.4
 pubis (pubic louse) (any site) B85.3
 vestimenti B85.1
 vulvae B85.3
Pediculus (infestation) —see Pediculosis
Pedophilia F65.4
Peg-shaped teeth K00.2
Pelade —see Alopecia, areata
Pelger-Huët anomaly or syndrome D72.0
Peliosis (rheumatica) D69.0
 hepatis K76.4
  with toxic liver disease K71.8
Pelizaeus-Merzbacher disease E75.27
Pellagra (alcoholic) E52
 with
  polyneuropathy E52 [G63]
Pellagra-cerebellar-ataxia-renal aminoaciduria syndrome E72.02
Pellegrini (-Stieda) **disease or syndrome** —see Bursitis, tibial collateral
Pellizzi's syndrome E34.8
Pel's crisis A52.11
Pelvic —see also condition
 examination (periodic) (routine) Z01.419
  with abnormal findings Z01.411
 kidney, congenital Q63.2
Pelviolithiasis —see Calculus, kidney
Pelviperitonitis —see also Peritonitis, pelvic
 gonococcal A54.24
 puerperal O85
Pelvis —see condition or type
Pemphigoid L12.9
 benign, mucous membrane L12.1
 bullous L12.0
 cicatricial L12.1
 juvenile L12.2
 ocular L12.1
 specified NEC L12.8
Pemphigus L10.9
 benign familial (chronic) Q82.8
 Brazilian L10.3
 circinatus L13.0

Pemphigus (continued)
 conjunctiva L12.1
 drug-induced L10.5
 erythematosus L10.4
 foliaceous L10.2
 gangrenous —see Gangrene
 neonatorum L01.03
 ocular L12.1
 paraneoplastic L10.81
 specified NEC L10.89
 syphilitic (congenital) A50.06
 vegetans L10.1
 vulgaris L10.0
 wildfire L10.3
Pendred's syndrome E07.1
Pendulous
 abdomen, in pregnancy —see Pregnancy, complicated by, abnormal, pelvic organs or tissues NEC
 breast N64.89
Penetrating wound —see also Puncture
 with internal injury —see Injury, by site
 eyeball —see Puncture, eyeball
 orbit (with or without foreign body) —see Puncture, orbit
 uterus by instrument with or following ectopic or molar pregnancy O08.6
Penicillosis B48.4
Penis —see condition
Penitis N48.29
Pentalogy of Fallot Q21.8
Pentasomy X syndrome Q97.1
Pentosuria (essential) E74.89
Percreta placenta O43.23-
Peregrinating patient —see Disorder, factitious
Perforation, perforated (nontraumatic) (of)
 accidental during procedure (blood vessel) (nerve) (organ) —see Complication, accidental puncture or laceration
 antrum —see Sinusitis, maxillary
 appendix K35.32
  with localized peritonitis K35.32
 atrial septum, multiple Q21.19
 attic, ear —see Perforation, tympanum, attic
 bile duct (common) (hepatic) K83.2
 cystic K82.2
 bladder (urinary)
  with or following ectopic or molar pregnancy O08.6
  obstetrical trauma O71.5
  traumatic S37.29
   at delivery O71.5
 bowel K63.1
  with or following ectopic or molar pregnancy O08.6
  newborn P78.0
  obstetrical trauma O71.5
  traumatic —see Laceration, intestine
 broad ligament N83.8
  with or following ectopic or molar pregnancy O08.6
  obstetrical trauma O71.6

Perforation, perforated (continued)
 by
  device, implant or graft (see also Complications, by site and type, mechanical) T85.628
   arterial graft NEC —see Complication, cardiovascular device, mechanical, vascular
   breast (implant) T85.49
   catheter NEC T85.698
    cystostomy T83.090
    dialysis (renal) T82.49
     intraperitoneal T85.691
    infusion NEC T82.594
     spinal (epidural) (subdural) T85.690
    urinary (see also Complications, catheter, urinary) T83.098
   electronic (electrode) (pulse generator) (stimulator)
    bone T84.390
    cardiac T82.199
     electrode T82.190
     pulse generator T82.191
     specified type NEC T82.198
    nervous system —see Complication, prosthetic device, mechanical, electronic nervous system stimulator
    urinary —see Complication, genitourinary, device, urinary, mechanical
   fixation, internal (orthopedic) NEC —see Complication, fixation device, mechanical
   gastrointestinal —see Complications, prosthetic device, mechanical, gastrointestinal device
   genital NEC T83.498
    intrauterine contraceptive device T83.39
    penile prosthesis T83.490
   heart NEC —see Complication, cardiovascular device, mechanical
   joint prosthesis —see Complications, joint prosthesis, mechanical, specified NEC, by site
   ocular NEC —see Complications, prosthetic device, mechanical, ocular device
   orthopedic NEC —see Complication, orthopedic, device, mechanical
   specified NEC T85.628
   urinary NEC —see also Complication, genitourinary, device, urinary, mechanical
    graft T83.29
   vascular NEC —see Complication, cardiovascular device, mechanical
   ventricular intracranial shunt T85.09
 foreign body left accidentally in operative wound T81.539
 instrument (any) during a procedure, accidental —see Puncture, accidental complicating surgery
cecum K35.32
 with localized peritonitis K35.32

Perforation, perforated (continued)
cervix (uteri) N88.8
with or following ectopic or molar pregnancy O08.6
obstetrical trauma O71.3
colon K63.1
newborn P78.0
obstetrical trauma O71.5
traumatic —see Laceration, intestine, large
common duct (bile) K83.2
cornea (due to ulceration) —see Ulcer, cornea, perforated
cystic duct K82.2
diverticulum (intestine) K57.80
with bleeding K57.81
large intestine K57.20
with
bleeding K57.21
small intestine K57.40
with bleeding K57.41
small intestine K57.00
with
bleeding K57.01
large intestine K57.40
with bleeding K57.41
ear drum —see Perforation, tympanum
esophagus K22.3
ethmoidal sinus —see Sinusitis, ethmoidal
frontal sinus —see Sinusitis, frontal
gallbladder K82.2
heart valve —see Endocarditis
ileum K63.1
newborn P78.0
obstetrical trauma O71.5
traumatic —see Laceration, intestine, small
instrumental, surgical (accidental) (blood vessel) (nerve) (organ) —see Puncture, accidental complicating surgery
intestine NEC K63.1
with ectopic or molar pregnancy O08.6
newborn P78.0
obstetrical trauma O71.5
traumatic —see Laceration, intestine
ulcerative NEC K63.1
newborn P78.0
jejunum, jejunal K63.1
obstetrical trauma O71.5
traumatic —see Laceration, intestine, small
ulcer —see Ulcer, gastrojejunal, with perforation
joint prosthesis —see Complications, joint prosthesis, mechanical, specified NEC, by site
mastoid (antrum) (cell) —see Disorder, mastoid, specified NEC
maxillary sinus —see Sinusitis, maxillary
membrana tympani —see Perforation, tympanum
nasal
septum J34.89
congenital Q30.3
syphilitic A52.73
sinus J34.89
congenital Q30.8
due to sinusitis —see Sinusitis
palate (see also Cleft, palate) Q35.9
syphilitic A52.79
palatine vault (see also Cleft, palate, hard) Q35.1
syphilitic A52.79
congenital A50.59

Perforation, perforated (continued)
pars flaccida (ear drum) —see Perforation, tympanum, attic
pelvic
floor S31.030
with
ectopic or molar pregnancy O08.6
penetration into retroperitoneal space S31.031
retained foreign body S31.040
with penetration into retroperitoneal space S31.041
following ectopic or molar pregnancy O08.6
obstetrical trauma O70.1
organ S37.99
adrenal gland S37.818
bladder —see Perforation, bladder
fallopian tube S37.599
bilateral S37.592
unilateral S37.591
kidney S37.09-
obstetrical trauma O71.5
ovary S37.499
bilateral S37.492
unilateral S37.491
prostate S37.828
specified organ NEC S37.898
ureter —see Perforation, ureter
urethra —see Perforation, urethra
uterus —see Perforation, uterus
perineum —see Laceration, perineum
pharynx J39.2
rectum K63.1
newborn P78.0
obstetrical trauma O71.5
traumatic S36.63
root canal space due to endodontic treatment M27.51
sigmoid K63.1
newborn P78.0
obstetrical trauma O71.5
traumatic S36.533
sinus (accessory) (chronic) (nasal) J34.89
sphenoidal sinus —see Sinusitis, sphenoidal
surgical (accidental) (by instrument) (blood vessel) (nerve) (organ) —see Puncture, accidental complicating surgery
traumatic
external —see Puncture
eye —see Puncture, eyeball
internal organ —see Injury, by site
tympanum, tympanic (membrane) (persistent post-traumatic) (postinflammatory) H72.9-
attic H72.1-
multiple —see Perforation, tympanum, multiple
total —see Perforation, tympanum, total
central H72.0-
multiple —see Perforation, tympanum, multiple
total —see Perforation, tympanum, total
marginal NEC —see subcategory H72.2
multiple H72.81-

Perforation, perforated (continued)
tympanum, tympanic (continued)
pars flaccida —see Perforation, tympanum, attic
total H72.82-
traumatic, current episode S09.2-
typhoid, gastrointestinal —see Typhoid
ulcer —see Ulcer, by site, with perforation
ureter N28.89
traumatic S37.19
urethra N36.8
with ectopic or molar pregnancy O08.6
following ectopic or molar pregnancy O08.6
obstetrical trauma O71.5
traumatic S37.39
at delivery O71.5
uterus
with ectopic or molar pregnancy O08.6
by intrauterine contraceptive device T83.39
following ectopic or molar pregnancy O08.6
obstetrical trauma O71.1
traumatic S37.69
obstetric O71.1
uvula K13.79
syphilitic A52.79
vagina
obstetrical trauma O71.4
other trauma —see Puncture, vagina

Periadenitis mucosa necrotica recurrens K12.0

Periappendicitis (acute) —see Appendicitis

Periarteritis nodosa (disseminated) (infectious) (necrotizing) M30.0

Periarthritis (joint) —see also Enthesopathy
Duplay's M75.0-
gonococcal A54.42
humeroscapularis —see Capsulitis, adhesive
scapulohumeral —see Capsulitis, adhesive
shoulder —see Capsulitis, adhesive
wrist M77.2-

Periarthrosis (angioneural) —see Enthesopathy

Pericapsulitis, adhesive (shoulder) —see Capsulitis, adhesive

Pericarditis (with decompensation) (with effusion) I31.9
with rheumatic fever (conditions in I00)
active —see Pericarditis, rheumatic
inactive or quiescent I09.2
acute (hemorrhagic) (nonrheumatic) (Sicca) I30.9
with chorea (acute) (rheumatic) (Sydenham's) I02.0
benign I30.8
nonspecific I30.0
rheumatic I01.0
with chorea (acute) (Sydenham's) I02.0
adhesive or adherent (chronic) (external) (internal) I31.0
acute —see Pericarditis, acute
rheumatic I09.2

Pericarditis (continued)
bacterial (acute) (subacute) (with serous or seropurulent effusion) I30.1
calcareous I31.1
cholesterol (chronic) I31.8
acute I30.9
chronic (nonrheumatic) I31.9
rheumatic I09.2
constrictive (chronic) I31.1
coxsackie B33.23
fibrinocaseous (tuberculous) A18.84
fibrinopurulent I30.1
fibrinous I30.8
fibrous I31.0
gonococcal A54.83
idiopathic I30.0
in systemic lupus erythematosus M32.12
infective I30.1
meningococcal A39.53
neoplastic (chronic) I31.8
acute I30.9
obliterans, obliterating I31.0
plastic I31.0
pneumococcal I30.1
postinfarction I24.1
purulent I30.1
rheumatic (active) (acute) (with effusion) (with pneumonia) I01.0
with chorea (acute) (rheumatic) (Sydenham's) I02.0
chronic or inactive (with chorea) I09.2
rheumatoid —see Rheumatoid, carditis
septic I30.1
serofibrinous I30.8
staphylococcal I30.1
streptococcal I30.1
suppurative I30.1
syphilitic A52.06
tuberculous A18.84
uremic N18.9 *[I32]*
viral I30.1

Pericardium, pericardial —see condition

Pericellulitis —see Cellulitis

Pericementitis (chronic) (suppurative) —see also Periodontitis
acute K05.20
generalized —see Periodontitis, aggressive, generalized
localized —see Periodontitis, aggressive, localized

Perichondritis
auricle —see Perichondritis, ear
bronchus J98.09
ear (external) H61.00-
acute H61.01-
chronic H61.02-
external auditory canal —see Perichondritis, ear
larynx J38.7
syphilitic A52.73
typhoid A01.09
nose J34.89
pinna —see Perichondritis, ear
trachea J39.8

Periclasia K05.4

Pericoronitis —see Periodontitis

Pericystitis N30.90
with hematuria N30.91

263

Peridiverticulitis (intestine) K57.92
  cecum —*see* Diverticulitis, intestine, large
  colon —*see* Diverticulitis, intestine, large
  duodenum —*see* Diverticulitis, intestine, small
  intestine —*see* Diverticulitis, intestine
  jejunum —*see* Diverticulitis, intestine, small
  rectosigmoid —*see* Diverticulitis, intestine, large
  rectum —*see* Diverticulitis, intestine, large
  sigmoid —*see* Diverticulitis, intestine, large

Periendocarditis —*see* Endocarditis

Periepididymitis N45.1

Perifolliculitis L01.02
  abscedens, caput, scalp L66.3
  capitis, abscedens (et suffodiens) L66.3
  superficial pustular L01.02

Perihepatitis K65.8

Perilabyrinthitis (acute) —*see* subcategory H83.0

Perimeningitis —*see* Meningitis

Perimetritis —*see* Endometritis

Perimetrosalpingitis —*see* Salpingo-oophoritis

Perineocele N81.81

Perinephric, perinephritic —*see* condition

Perinephritis —*see also* Infection, kidney
  purulent —*see* Abscess, kidney

Perineum, perineal —*see* condition

Perineuritis NEC —*see* Neuralgia

Periodic —*see* condition

Periodontitis (chronic) (complex) (compound) (local) (simplex) K05.30
  acute K05.20
    generalized K05.229
      moderate K05.222
      severe K05.223
      slight K05.221
    localized K05.219
      moderate K05.212
      severe K05.213
      slight K05.211
  aggressive K05.20
    generalized K05.229
      moderate K05.222
      severe K05.223
      slight K05.221
    localized K05.219
      moderate K05.212
      severe K05.213
      slight K05.211
  apical K04.5
    acute (pulpal origin) K04.4
  generalized K05.329
    moderate K05.322
    severe K05.323
    slight K05.321
  localized K05.319
    moderate K05.312
    severe K05.313
    slight K05.311

Periodontoclasia K05.4

Periodontosis (juvenile) K05.4

Periods —*see also* Menstruation
  heavy N92.0
  irregular N92.6
  shortened intervals (irregular) N92.1

Perionychia —*see also* Cellulitis, digit
  with lymphangitis —*see* Lymphangitis, acute, digit

Perioophoritis —*see* Salpingo-oophoritis

Periorchitis N45.2

Periosteum, periosteal —*see* condition

Periostitis (albuminosa) (circumscribed) (diffuse) (infective) (monomelic) —*see also* Osteomyelitis
  alveolar M27.3
  alveolodental M27.3
  dental M27.3
  gonorrheal A54.43
  jaw (lower) (upper) M27.2
  orbit H05.03-
  syphilitic A52.77
    congenital (early) A50.02 [M90.80]
    secondary A51.46
  tuberculous —*see* Tuberculosis, bone
  yaws (hypertrophic) (early) (late) A66.6 [M90.80]

Periostosis (hyperplastic) —*see also* Disorder, bone, specified type NEC
  with osteomyelitis —*see* Osteomyelitis, specified type NEC

Peripartum
  cardiomyopathy O90.3

Periphlebitis —*see* Phlebitis

Periproctitis K62.89

Periprostatitis —*see* Prostatitis

Perirectal —*see* condition

Perirenal —*see* condition

Perisalpingitis —*see* Salpingo-oophoritis

Perisplenitis (infectional) D73.89

Peristalsis, visible or reversed R19.2

Peritendinitis —*see* Enthesopathy

Peritoneum, peritoneal —*see* condition

Peritonitis (adhesive) (bacterial) (fibrinous) (hemorrhagic) (idiopathic) (localized) (perforative) (primary) (with adhesions) (with effusion) K65.9
  with or following
    abscess K65.1
    appendicitis
      with perforation or rupture K35.32
      generalized (*see also* Appendicitis) K35.209
      localized (*see also* Appendicitis) K35.30
    diverticular disease (intestine) K57.80
      with bleeding K57.81
      large intestine K57.20
        with
          bleeding K57.21
          small intestine K57.40
            with bleeding K57.41
      small intestine K57.00
        with
          bleeding K57.01
          large intestine K57.40
            with bleeding K57.41
    ectopic or molar pregnancy O08.0
  acute (generalized) K65.0

Peritonitis *(continued)*
  aseptic T81.61
  bile, biliary K65.3
  chemical T81.61
  chlamydial A74.81
  complicating abortion —*see* Abortion, by type, complicated by, pelvic peritonitis
  congenital P78.1
  chronic proliferative K65.8
  diaphragmatic K65.0
  diffuse K65.0
  diphtheritic A36.89
  disseminated K65.0
  due to
    bile K65.3
    foreign
      body or object accidentally left during a procedure (instrument) (sponge) (swab) T81.599
      substance accidentally left during a procedure (chemical) (powder) (talc) T81.61
    talc T81.61
    urine K65.8
  eosinophilic K65.8
    acute K65.0
  fibrocaseous (tuberculous) A18.31
  fibropurulent K65.0
  following ectopic or molar pregnancy O08.0
  general (ized) K65.0
  gonococcal A54.85
  meconium (newborn) P78.0
  neonatal P78.1
    meconium P78.0
  pancreatic K65.0
  paroxysmal, familial E85.0
    benign E85.0
  pelvic
    female N73.5
      acute N73.3
      chronic N73.4
        with adhesions N73.6
    male K65.0
  periodic, familial E85.0
  proliferative, chronic K65.8
  puerperal, postpartum, childbirth O85
  purulent K65.0
  septic K65.0
  specified NEC K65.8
  spontaneous bacterial K65.2
  subdiaphragmatic K65.0
  subphrenic K65.0
  suppurative K65.0
  syphilitic A52.74
    congenital (early) A50.08 [K67]
  talc T81.61
  tuberculous A18.31
  urine K65.8

Peritonsillar —*see* condition

Peritonsillitis J36

Perityphlitis (*see also* Cecitis) K37

Periureteritis N28.89

Periurethral —*see* condition

Periurethritis (gangrenous) —*see* Urethritis

Periuterine —*see* condition

Perivaginitis —*see* Vaginitis

Perivasculitis, retinal H35.06-

Perivasitis (chronic) N49.1

Perivesiculitis (seminal) —*see* Vesiculitis

Perlèche NEC K13.0
  due to
    candidiasis B37.83
    moniliasis B37.83
    riboflavin deficiency E53.0
    vitamin B2 (riboflavin) deficiency E53.0

Pernicious —*see* condition

Pernio, perniosis T69.1

Perpetrator (of abuse) —*see* Index to External Causes of Injury, Perpetrator

Persecution
  delusion F22
  social Z60.5

Perseveration (tonic) R48.8

Persistence, persistent (congenital)
  anal membrane Q42.3
    with fistula Q42.2
  arteria stapedia Q16.3
  atrioventricular canal Q21.20
  branchial cleft NOS Q18.2
    cyst Q18.0
    fistula Q18.0
    sinus Q18.0
  bulbus cordis in left ventricle Q21.8
  canal of Cloquet Q14.0
  capsule (opaque) Q12.8
  cilioretinal artery or vein Q14.8
  cloaca Q43.7
  communication —*see* Fistula, congenital
  convolutions
    aortic arch Q25.46
    fallopian tube Q50.6
    oviduct Q50.6
    uterine tube Q50.6
  double aortic arch Q25.45
  ductus arteriosus (Botalli) Q25.0
  fetal
    circulation P29.38
    form of cervix (uteri) Q51.828
    hemoglobin, hereditary (HPFH) D56.4
  foramen
    Botalli Q21.12
    ovale Q21.12
  Gartner's duct Q52.4
  hemoglobin, fetal (hereditary) (HPFH) D56.4
  hyaloid
    artery (generally incomplete) Q14.0
    system Q14.8
  hymen, in pregnancy or childbirth —*see* Pregnancy, complicated by, abnormal, vulva
  lanugo Q84.2
  left
    posterior cardinal vein Q26.8
    root with right arch of aorta Q25.49
    superior vena cava Q26.1
  Meckel's diverticulum Q43.0
    malignant —*see* Table of Neoplasms, small intestine, malignant
  mucosal disease (middle ear) —*see* Otitis, media, suppurative, chronic, tubotympanic
  nail(s), anomalous Q84.6
  omphalomesenteric duct Q43.0
  organ or site not listed —*see* Anomaly, by site
  ostium
    atrioventriculare commune Q21.23
    primum Q21.20
    secundum Q21.11

Persistence, persistent *(continued)*
  ovarian rests in fallopian tube Q50.6
  pancreatic tissue in intestinal tract Q43.8
  primary (deciduous)
    teeth K00.6
    vitreous hyperplasia Q14.0
  pupillary membrane Q13.89
  right aortic arch Q25.47
  rhesus (Rh) titer —*see* Complication(s), transfusion, incompatibility reaction, Rh (factor)
  sinus
    urogenitalis
      female Q52.8
      male Q55.8
    venosus with imperfect incorporation in right auricle Q26.8
  thymus (gland) (hyperplasia) E32.0
  thyroglossal duct Q89.2
  thyrolingual duct Q89.2
  truncus arteriosus or communis Q20.0
  tunica vasculosa lentis Q12.2
  umbilical sinus Q64.4
  urachus Q64.4
  vitelline duct Q43.0

Person (with)
  admitted for clinical research, as a control subject (normal comparison) (participant) Z00.6
  awaiting admission to adequate facility elsewhere Z75.1
  concern (normal) about sick person in family Z63.6
  consulting on behalf of another Z71.0
  feigning illness Z76.5
  living (in)
    alone Z60.2
    boarding school Z59.3
    residential institution Z59.3
    without
      adequate housing
        air conditioning Z59.11
        environmental temperature Z59.11
        heating Z59.11
        space Z59.19
      housing (permanent) (temporary) Z59.00
      person able to render necessary care Z74.2
      shelter Z59.02
  on waiting list Z75.1
  sick or handicapped in family Z63.6

Personality (disorder) F60.9
  accentuation of traits (type A pattern) Z73.1
  affective F34.0
  aggressive F60.3
  amoral F60.2
  anacastic, anankastic F60.5
  antisocial F60.2
  anxious F60.6
  asocial F60.2
  asthenic F60.7
  avoidant F60.6
  borderline F60.3
  change due to organic condition (enduring) F07.0
  compulsive F60.5
  cycloid F34.0
  cyclothymic F34.0
  dependent F60.7
  depressive F34.1
  dissocial F60.2
  dual F44.81

Personality *(continued)*
  eccentric F60.89
  emotionally unstable F60.3
  expansive paranoid F60.0
  explosive F60.3
  fanatic F60.0
  haltlose type F60.89
  histrionic F60.4
  hyperthymic F34.0
  hypothymic F34.1
  hysterical F60.4
  immature F60.89
  inadequate F60.7
  labile (emotional) F60.3
  mixed (nonspecific) F60.89
  morally defective F60.2
  multiple F44.81
  narcissistic F60.81
  obsessional F60.5
  obsessive (-compulsive) F60.5
  organic F07.0
  overconscientious F60.5
  paranoid F60.0
  passive (-dependent) F60.7
  passive-aggressive F60.89
  pathologic F60.9
  pattern defect or disturbance F60.9
  pseudopsychopathic (organic) F07.0
  pseudoretarded (organic) F07.0
  psychoinfantile F60.4
  psychoneurotic NEC F60.89
  psychopathic F60.2
  querulant F60.0
  sadistic F60.89
  schizoid F60.1
  self-defeating F60.89
  sensitive paranoid F60.0
  sociopathic (amoral) (antisocial) (asocial) (dissocial) F60.2
  specified NEC F60.89
  type A Z73.1
  unstable (emotional) F60.3

Perthes' disease —*see* Legg-Calvé-Perthes disease

Pertussis (see also Whooping cough) A37.90

Perversion, perverted
  appetite F50.89
    psychogenic F50.89
  function
    pituitary gland E23.2
      posterior lobe E22.2
  sense of smell and taste R43.8
    psychogenic F45.8
  sexual —*see* Deviation, sexual

Pervious, congenital —*see also* Imperfect, closure
  ductus arteriosus Q25.0

Pes (congenital) —*see also* Talipes
  acquired —*see also* Deformity, limb, foot, specified NEC
    planus —*see* Deformity, limb, flat foot
  adductus Q66.89
  cavus Q66.7-
  deformity NEC, acquired —*see* Deformity, limb, foot, specified NEC
  planus (acquired) (any degree) —*see also* Deformity, limb, flat foot
    rachitic sequelae (late effect) E64.3
  valgus Q66.6

Pest, pestis —*see* Plague

Petechia, petechiae R23.3
  newborn P54.5

Petechial typhus A75.9

Peter's anomaly Q13.4

Petit mal seizure —*see* Epilepsy, childhood, absence

Petit's hernia —*see* Hernia, abdomen, specified site NEC

Petrellidosis B48.2

Petrositis H70.20-
  acute H70.21-
  chronic H70.22-

Peutz-Jeghers disease or syndrome Q85.89

Peyronie's disease N48.6

PFAPA (periodic fever, aphthous stomatitis, pharyngitis, and adenopathy syndrome) M04.8

Pfeiffer's disease —*see* Mononucleosis, infectious

Phagedena (dry) (moist) (sloughing) —*see also* Gangrene
  geometric L88
  penis N48.29
  tropical —*see* Ulcer, skin
  vulva N76.6

Phagedenic —*see* condition

Phakoma H35.89

Phakomatosis (*see also* specific eponymous syndromes) Q85.9
  Bourneville's Q85.1
  specified NEC Q85.89

Phantom limb syndrome (without pain) G54.7
  with pain G54.6

Pharyngeal pouch syndrome D82.1

Pharyngitis (acute) (catarrhal)(gangrenous) (infective) (malignant) (membranous) (phlegmonous) (pseudomembranous) (simple) (subacute) (suppurative) (ulcerative) (viral) J02.9
  with influenza, flu, or grippe —*see* Influenza, with, pharyngitis
  aphthous B08.5
  atrophic J31.2
  chlamydial A56.4
  chronic (atrophic) (granular) (hypertrophic) J31.2
  coxsackievirus B08.5
  diphtheritic A36.0
  enteroviral vesicular B08.5
  follicular (chronic) J31.2
  fusospirochetal A69.1
  gonococcal A54.5
  granular (chronic) J31.2
  herpesviral B00.2
  hypertrophic J31.2
  infectional, chronic J31.2
  influenzal —*see* Influenza, with, respiratory manifestations NEC
  lymphonodular, acute (enteroviral) B08.8
  pneumococcal J02.8
  purulent J02.9
  putrid J02.9
  septic J02.0
  sicca J31.2
  specified organism NEC J02.8
  staphylococcal J02.8
  streptococcal J02.0
  syphilitic, congenital (early) A50.03
  tuberculous A15.8
  vesicular, enteroviral B08.5
  viral NEC J02.8

Pharyngoconjunctivitis, viral B30.2

Pharyngolaryngitis (acute) J06.0
  chronic J37.0

Pharyngoplegia J39.2

Pharyngotonsillitis, herpesviral B00.2

Pharyngotracheitis, chronic J42

Pharynx, pharyngeal —*see* condition

Phelan-McDermid syndrome Q93.52

Phencyclidine-induced
  anxiety disorder F16.980
  bipolar and related disorder F16.94
  depressive disorder F16.94
  psychotic disorder F16.959

Phenomenon
  Arthus' —*see* Arthus' phenomenon
  jaw-winking Q07.8
  lupus erythematosus (LE) cell M32.9
  Raynaud's (secondary) I73.00
    with gangrene I73.01
  vasomotor R55
  vasospastic I73.9
  vasovagal R55
  Wenckebach's I44.1

Phenylketonuria E70.1
  classical E70.0
  maternal E70.1

Pheochromoblastoma
  specified site —*see* Neoplasm, malignant, by site
  unspecified site C74.10

Pheochromocytoma
  malignant
    specified site —*see* Neoplasm, malignant, by site
    unspecified site C74.10
  specified site —*see* Neoplasm, benign, by site
  unspecified site D35.00

Pheohyphomycosis —*see* Chromomycosis

Pheomycosis —*see* Chromomycosis

Phimosis (congenital) (due to infection) N47.1
  chancroidal A57

Phlebectasia —*see also* Varix
  congenital Q27.4

Phlebitis (infective) (pyemic) (septic) (suppurative) I80.9
  antepartum —*see* Thrombophlebitis, antepartum
  blue —*see* Phlebitis, leg, deep
  breast, superficial I80.8
  calf muscular vein (NOS) I80.25-
  cavernous (venous) sinus —*see* Phlebitis, intracranial (venous) sinus
  cerebral (venous) sinus —*see* Phlebitis, intracranial (venous) sinus
  chest wall, superficial I80.8
  cranial (venous) sinus —*see* Phlebitis, intracranial (venous) sinus
  deep (vessels) —*see* Phlebitis, leg, deep
  due to implanted device —*see* Complications, by site and type, specified NEC
  during or resulting from a procedure T81.72
  femoral vein (superficial) I80.1-
  femoropopliteal vein I80.0-
  gastrocnemial vein I80.25-

Phlebitis (continued)
   gestational —see Phlebopathy, gestational
   hepatic veins I80.8
   iliac vein (common) (external) (internal) I80.21-
   iliofemoral —see Phlebitis, femoral vein
   intracranial (venous) sinus (any) G08
     nonpyogenic I67.6
   intraspinal venous sinuses and veins G08
     nonpyogenic G95.19
   lateral (venous) sinus —see Phlebitis, intracranial (venous) sinus
   leg I80.3
     antepartum —see Thrombophlebitis, antepartum
     deep (vessels) NEC I80.20-
       iliac I80.21-
       popliteal vein I80.22-
       specified vessel NEC I80.29-
       tibial vein (anterior) (posterior) I80.23-
     femoral vein (superficial) I80.1-
     superficial (vessels) I80.0-
   longitudinal sinus —see Phlebitis, intracranial (venous) sinus
   lower limb —see Phlebitis, leg
   migrans, migrating (superficial) I82.1
   pelvic
     with ectopic or molar pregnancy O08.0
     following ectopic or molar pregnancy O08.0
     puerperal, postpartum O87.1
   peroneal vein I80.24-
   popliteal vein —see Phlebitis, leg, deep, popliteal
   portal (vein) K75.1
   postoperative T81.72
   pregnancy —see Thrombophlebitis, antepartum
   puerperal, postpartum, childbirth O87.0
     deep O87.1
     pelvic O87.1
     superficial O87.0
   retina —see Vasculitis, retina
   saphenous (accessory) (great) (long) (small) —see Phlebitis, leg, superficial
   sinus (meninges) —see Phlebitis, intracranial (venous) sinus
   soleal vein I80.25-
   specified site NEC I80.8
   syphilitic A52.09
   tibial vein —see Phlebitis, leg, deep, tibial
   ulcerative I80.9
     leg —see Phlebitis, leg
   umbilicus I80.8
   uterus (septic) —see Endometritis
   varicose (leg) (lower limb) —see Varix, leg, with, inflammation

Phlebofibrosis I87.8

Phleboliths I87.8

Phlebopathy,
   gestational O22.9-
   puerperal O87.9

Phlebosclerosis I87.8

Phlebothrombosis —see also Thrombosis
   antepartum —see Thrombophlebitis, antepartum

Phlebothrombosis (continued)
   pregnancy —see Thrombophlebitis, antepartum
   puerperal —see Thrombophlebitis, puerperal

Phlebotomus fever A93.1

Phlegmasia
   alba dolens O87.1
     nonpuerperal —see Phlebitis, femoral vein
   cerulea dolens —see Phlebitis, leg, deep

Phlegmon —see Abscess

Phlegmonous —see condition

Phlyctenulosis (allergic) (keratoconjunctivitis) (nontuberculous) —see also Keratoconjunctivitis
   cornea —see Keratoconjunctivitis
   tuberculous A18.52

Phobia, phobic F40.9
   animal F40.218
     spiders F40.210
   examination F40.298
   reaction F40.9
   simple F40.298
   social F40.10
     generalized F40.11
   specific (isolated) F40.298
     animal F40.218
       spiders F40.210
     blood F40.230
       injection F40.231
       injury F40.233
     men F40.290
     natural environment F40.228
       thunderstorms F40.220
     situational F40.248
       bridges F40.242
       closed in spaces F40.240
       flying F40.243
       heights F40.241
     specified focus NEC F40.298
     transfusion F40.231
     women F40.291
   specified NEC F40.8
     medical care NEC F40.232
   state F40.9

Phocas' disease —see Mastopathy, cystic

Phocomelia Q73.1
   lower limb —see Agenesis, leg, with foot present
   upper limb —see Agenesis, arm, with hand present

Phoria H50.50

Phosphate-losing tubular disorder N25.0

Phosphatemia E83.39

Phosphaturia E83.39

Photodermatitis (sun) L56.8
   chronic L57.8
   due to drug L56.8
   light other than sun L59.8

Photokeratitis H16.13-

Photophobia H53.14-

Photophthalmia —see Photokeratitis

Photopsia H53.19

Photoretinitis —see Retinopathy, solar

Photosensitivity, photosensitization (sun) **skin** L56.8
   light other than sun L59.8

Phrenitis —see Encephalitis

Phrynoderma (vitamin A deficiency) E50.8

Phthiriasis (pubis) B85.3
   with any infestation classifiable to B85.0-B85.2 [B85.4]

Phthirus infestation —see Phthiriasis

Phthisis —see also Tuberculosis
   bulbi (infectional) —see Disorder, globe, degenerated condition, atrophy
   eyeball (due to infection) —see Disorder, globe, degenerated condition, atrophy

PHTS Q85.81

Phycomycosis —see Zygomycosis

Physalopteriasis B81.8

Physical restraint status Z78.1

Phytobezoar T18.9
   intestine T18.3
   stomach T18.2

Pian —see Yaws

Pianoma A66.1

Pica F50.89
   in adults F50.89
   infant or child F98.3

Picking, nose F98.8

Pick-Niemann disease —see Niemann-Pick disease or syndrome

Pick's
   cerebral atrophy (see also Dementia, in, diseases specified elsewhere) G31.01 [F02.80]
     with behavioral disturbance (see also Dementia, in, diseases specified elsewhere) G31.01 [F02.81-]
   disease or syndrome (brain) (see also Dementia, in, diseases specified elsewhere) G31.01 [F02.80]
     with behavioral disturbance (see also Dementia, in, diseases specified elsewhere) G31.01 [F02.81-]
     brain (see also Dementia, in, diseases specified elsewhere) G31.01 [F02.80]
       with behavioral disturbance (see also Dementia, in, diseases specified elsewhere) G31.01 [F02.81-]
     pericardium (pericardial pseudocirrhosis of liver) I31.1
   syndrome
     brain (see also Dementia, in, diseases specified elsewhere) G31.01 [F02.80]
       with behavioral disturbance (see also Dementia, in, diseases specified elsewhere) G31.01 [F02.81-]
     of heart (pericardial pseudocirrhosis of liver) I31.1

Pickwickian syndrome E66.2

Piebaldism E70.39

Piedra (beard) (scalp) B36.8
   black B36.3
   white B36.2

Pierre Robin deformity or syndrome Q87.0

Pierson's disease or osteochondrosis M91.0

Pig-bel A05.2

Pigeon
   breast or chest (acquired) M95.4
     congenital Q67.7
       rachitic sequelae (late effect) E64.3
   breeder's disease or lung J67.2
   fancier's disease or lung J67.2
   toe —see Deformity, toe, specified NEC

Pigmentation (abnormal) (anomaly) L81.9
   conjunctiva H11.13-
   cornea (anterior) H18.01-
     posterior H18.05-
     stromal H18.06-
   diminished melanin formation NEC L81.6
   iron L81.8
   lids, congenital Q82.8
   limbus corneae —see Pigmentation, cornea
   metals L81.8
   optic papilla, congenital Q14.2
   retina, congenital (grouped) (nevoid) Q14.1
   scrotum, congenital Q82.8
   tattoo L81.8

Piles (see also Hemorrhoids) K64.9

Pili
   annulati or torti (congenital) Q84.1
   incarnati L73.1

Pill roller hand (intrinsic) —see Parkinsonism

Pilomatrixoma —see Neoplasm, skin, benign
   malignant —see Neoplasm, skin, malignant

Pilonidal —see condition

Pimple R23.8

PIMS M35.81

PIN —see Neoplasia, intraepithelial, prostate

Pinched nerve —see Neuropathy, entrapment

Pindborg tumor —see Cyst, calcifying odontogenic

Pineal body or gland —see condition

Pinealoblastoma C75.3

Pinealoma D44.5
   malignant C75.3

Pineoblastoma C75.3

Pineocytoma D44.5

Pinguecula H11.15-

Pingueculitis H10.81-

Pinhole meatus (see also Stricture, urethra) N35.919

Pink
   disease —see subcategory T56.1
   eye —see Conjunctivitis, acute, mucopurulent

Pinkus' disease (lichen nitidus) L44.1

Pinpoint
   meatus —see Stricture, urethra
   os (uteri) —see Stricture, cervix

Pins and needles R20.2

Pinta A67.9
  cardiovascular lesions A67.2
  chancre (primary) A67.0
  erythematous plaques A67.1
  hyperchromic lesions A67.1
  hyperkeratosis A67.1
  lesions A67.9
    cardiovascular A67.2
    hyperchromic A67.1
    intermediate A67.1
    late A67.2
    mixed A67.3
    primary A67.0
    skin (achromic) (cicatricial)
        (dyschromic) A67.2
      hyperchromic A67.1
      mixed (achromic and
          hyperchromic) A67.3
    papule (primary) A67.0
    skin lesions (achromic) (cicatricial)
        (dyschromic) A67.2
      hyperchromic A67.1
      mixed (achromic and
          hyperchromic) A67.3
  vitiligo A67.2
Pintids A67.1
Pinworm (disease) (infection)
    (infestation) B80
Piroplasmosis (*see also* Babesiosis)
    B60.00
  specified NEC B60.09
Pistol wound —*see* Gunshot wound
Pitchers' elbow —*see* Derangement,
    joint, specified type NEC, elbow
Pithecoid pelvis Q74.2
  with disproportion (fetopelvic) O33.0
    causing obstructed labor O65.0
Pithiatism F48.8
Pitted —*see* Pitting
Pitting (*see also* Edema) R60.9
  lip R60.0
  nail L60.8
  teeth K00.4
Pituitary gland —*see* condition
Pituitary-snuff-taker's disease J67.8
Pityriasis (capitis) L21.0
  alba L30.5
  circinata (et maculata) L42
  furfuracea L21.0
  Hebra's L26
  lichenoides L41.0
    chronica L41.1
    et varioliformis (acuta) L41.0
  maculata (et circinata) L30.5
  nigra B36.1
  pilaris, Hebra's L44.0
  rosea L42
  rotunda L44.8
  rubra (Hebra) pilaris L44.0
  simplex L30.5
  specified type NEC L30.5
  streptogenes L30.5
  versicolor (scrotal) B36.0
Placenta, placental —*see*
    Pregnancy, complicated by (care
    of) (management affected by),
    specified condition
Placentitis O41.14-
Plagiocephaly Q67.3
  non-deformational
    anterior Q75.021
    posterior Q75.04-
Plague A20.9
  abortive A20.8
  ambulatory A20.8

Plague (*continued*)
  asymptomatic A20.8
  bubonic A20.0
  cellulocutaneous A20.1
  cutaneobubonic A20.1
  lymphatic gland A20.0
  meningitis A20.3
  pharyngeal A20.8
  pneumonic (primary) (secondary)
      A20.2
  pulmonary, pulmonic A20.2
  septicemic A20.7
  tonsillar A20.8
    septicemic A20.7
Planning, family
  contraception Z30.9
  procreation Z31.69
Plaque(s)
  artery, arterial —*see*
      Arteriosclerosis
  calcareous —*see* Calcification
  coronary, lipid rich I25.83
  epicardial I31.8
  erythematous, of pinta A67.1
  Hollenhorst's —*see* Occlusion,
      artery, retina
  lipid rich, coronary I25.83
  pleural (without asbestos) J92.9
    with asbestos J92.0
  tongue K13.29
Plasmacytoma C90.3-
  extramedullary C90.2-
  medullary C90.0-
  solitary C90.3-
Plasmacytopenia D72.818
Plasmacytosis D72.822
Plaster ulcer —*see* Ulcer, pressure,
    by site
Plateau iris syndrome (post-
    iridectomy) (postprocedural)
    (without glaucoma) H21.82
  with glaucoma H40.22-
Platybasia Q75.8
Platyonychia (congenital) Q84.6
  acquired L60.8
Platypelloid pelvis M95.5
  with disproportion (fetopelvic) O33.0
    causing obstructed labor O65.0
  congenital Q74.2
Platyspondylisis Q76.49
Plaut (-Vincent) **disease** (*see also*
    Vincent's) A69.1
Plethora R23.2
  newborn P61.1
Pleura, pleural —*see* condition
Pleuralgia R07.81
Pleurisy (acute) (adhesive) (chronic)
    (costal) (diaphragmatic) (double)
    (dry) (fibrinous) (fibrous)
    (interlobar) (latent) (plastic)
    (primary) (residual) (sicca) (sterile)
    (subacute) (unresolved) R09.1
  with
    adherent pleura J86.0
    effusion J90
      chylous, chyliform J94.0
      tuberculous (non primary) A15.6
        primary (progressive) A15.7
    tuberculosis —*see* Pleurisy,
        tuberculous (non primary)
  encysted —*see* Pleurisy, with effusion
  exudative —*see* Pleurisy, with
      effusion
  fibrinopurulent, fibropurulent —*see*
      Pyothorax
  hemorrhagic —*see* Hemothorax
  pneumococcal J90

Pleurisy (*continued*)
  purulent —*see* Pyothorax
  septic —*see* Pyothorax
  serofibrinous —*see* Pleurisy, with
      effusion
  seropurulent —*see* Pyothorax
  serous —*see* Pleurisy, with effusion
  staphylococcal J86.9
  streptococcal J90
  suppurative —*see* Pyothorax
  traumatic (post) (current) —*see*
      Injury, intrathoracic, pleura
  tuberculous (with effusion) (non
      primary) A15.6
    primary (progressive) A15.7
Pleuritis sicca —*see* Pleurisy
Pleurobronchopneumonia —*see*
    Pneumonia, broncho-
Pleurodynia R07.81
  epidemic B33.0
  viral B33.0
Pleuropericarditis —*see also*
    Pericarditis
  acute I30.9
Pleuropneumonia (acute) (bilateral)
    (double) (septic) (*see also*
    Pneumonia) J18.8
  chronic —*see* Fibrosis, lung
Pleuro-pneumonia-like-organism
    (PPLO), as cause of disease
    classified elsewhere B96.0
Pleurorrhea —*see* Pleurisy, with
    effusion
Plexitis, brachial G54.0
Plica
  polonica B85.0
  syndrome, knee M67.5-
  tonsil J35.8
Plicated tongue K14.5
Plug
  bronchus NEC J98.09
  meconium (newborn) NEC
      syndrome P76.0
  mucus —*see* Asphyxia, mucus
Plumbism —*see* subcategory T56.0
Plummer's disease E05.20
  with thyroid storm E05.21
Plummer-Vinson syndrome D50.1
Pluricarential syndrome of infancy
    E40
Plus (and minus) hand (intrinsic)
    —*see* Deformity, limb, specified
    type NEC, forearm
PMEI (polymorphic epilepsy in
    infancy) G40.83-
Pneumathemia —*see* Air, embolism
Pneumatic hammer (drill)
    syndrome T75.21
Pneumatocele (lung) J98.4
  intracranial G93.89
  tension J98.8
Pneumatosis
  cystoides intestinalis K63.89
  intestinalis K63.89
  peritonei K66.8
Pneumaturia R39.89
Pneumoblastoma —*see* Neoplasm,
    lung, malignant
Pneumocephalus G93.89
Pneumococcemia A40.3
Pneumococcus, pneumococcal —*see*
    condition

Pneumoconiosis (due to) (inhalation
    of) J64
  with tuberculosis (any type in A15)
      J65
  aluminum J63.0
  asbestos J61
  bagasse, bagassosis J67.1
  bauxite J63.1
  beryllium J63.2
  coal miners' (simple) J60
  coalworkers' (simple) J60
  collier's J60
  cotton dust J66.0
  diatomite (diatomaceous earth) J62.8
  dust
    inorganic NEC J63.6
    lime J62.8
    marble J62.8
    organic NEC J66.8
  fumes or vapors (from silo) J68.9
  graphite J63.3
  grinder's J62.8
  kaolin J62.8
  mica J62.8
  millstone maker's J62.8
  mineral fibers NEC J61
  miner's J60
  moldy hay J67.0
  potter's J62.8
  rheumatoid —*see* Rheumatoid, lung
  sandblaster's J62.8
  silica, silicate NEC J62.8
    with carbon J60
  stonemason's J62.8
  talc (dust) J62.0
Pneumocystis carinii pneumonia B59
Pneumocystis jiroveci (pneumonia)
    B59
Pneumocystosis (with pneumonia)
    B59
Pneumohemopericardium I31.2
Pneumohemothorax J94.2
  traumatic S27.2
Pneumohydropericardium —*see*
    Pericarditis
Pneumohydrothorax —*see*
    Hydrothorax
Pneumomediastinum J98.2
  congenital or perinatal P25.2
Pneumomycosis B49 *[J99]*
Pneumonia (acute) (double)
    (migratory) (purulent) (septic)
    (unresolved) J18.9
  with
    lung abscess J85.1
      due to specified organism —
          see Pneumonia, in (due to)
    influenza —*see* Influenza, with,
        pneumonia
  2019 (novel) coronavirus J12.82
  adenoviral J12.0
  adynamic J18.2
  alba A50.04
  allergic (*see also* Pneumonitis,
      hypersensitivity) J82.89
  alveolar —*see* Pneumonia, lobar
  anaerobes J15.8
  anthrax A22.1
  apex, apical —*see* Pneumonia,
      lobar
  Ascaris B77.81
  aspiration J69.0
    due to
      aspiration of microorganisms
          bacterial J15.9
          viral J12.9
      food (regurgitated) J69.0

Pneumonia *(continued)*
  aspiration *(continued)*
    due to *(continued)*
      gastric secretions J69.0
      milk (regurgitated) J69.0
      oils, essences J69.1
      solids, liquids NEC J69.8
      vomitus J69.0
    newborn P24.81
      amniotic fluid (clear) P24.11
      blood P24.21
      liquor (amnii) P24.11
      meconium P24.01
      milk P24.31
      mucus P24.11
      food (regurgitated) P24.31
      specified NEC P24.81
      stomach contents P24.31
    postprocedural J95.4
  atypical NEC J18.9
  bacillus J15.9
    specified NEC J15.8
  bacterial J15.9
    specified NEC J15.8
  Bacteroides (fragilis) (oralis) (melaninogenicus) J15.8
  basal, basic, basilar—*see* Pneumonia, by type
  bronchiolitis obliterans organized (BOOP) J84.89
  broncho-, bronchial (confluent) (croupous) (diffuse) (disseminated) (hemorrhagic) (involving lobes) (lobar) (terminal) J18.0
    allergic (*see also* Pneumonitis, hypersensitivity) J82.89
    aspiration—*see* Pneumonia, aspiration
    bacterial J15.9
      specified NEC J15.8
    chronic—*see* Fibrosis, lung
    diplococcal J13
    Eaton's agent J15.7
    Escherichia coli (E. coli) J15.5
    Friedländer's bacillus J15.0
    Hemophilus influenzae J14
    hypostatic J18.2
    inhalation—*see also* Pneumonia, aspiration
      due to fumes or vapors (chemical) J68.0
      of oils or essences J69.1
    Klebsiella (pneumoniae) J15.0
    lipid, lipoid J69.1
      endogenous J84.89
    Mycoplasma (pneumoniae) J15.7
    pleuro-pneumonia-like-organisms (PPLO) J15.7
    pneumococcal J13
    Proteus J15.69
    Pseudomonas J15.1
    Serratia marcescens J15.69
    specified organism NEC J16.8
    staphylococcal—*see* Pneumonia, staphylococcal
    streptococcal NEC J15.4
      group B J15.3
      pneumoniae J13
    viral, virus—*see* Pneumonia, viral
  Butyrivibrio (fibriosolvens) J15.8
  Candida B37.1
  caseous—*see* Tuberculosis, pulmonary
  catarrhal—*see* Pneumonia, broncho
  chlamydial J16.0
    congenital P23.1
  cholesterol J84.89
  cirrhotic (chronic)—*see* Fibrosis, lung
  Clostridium (haemolyticum) (novyi) J15.8

Pneumonia *(continued)*
  confluent—*see* Pneumonia, broncho
  congenital (infective) P23.9
    due to
      bacterium NEC P23.6
      Chlamydia P23.1
      Escherichia coli P23.4
      Haemophilus influenzae P23.6
      infective organism NEC P23.8
      Klebsiella pneumoniae P23.6
      Mycoplasma P23.6
      Pseudomonas P23.5
      Staphylococcus P23.2
      Streptococcus (except group B) P23.6
        group B P23.3
      viral agent P23.0
    specified NEC P23.8
  coronavirus (novel) (disease) 2019 J12.82
  COVID-19 J12.82
  croupous—*see* Pneumonia, lobar
  cryptogenic organizing J84.116
  cytomegalic inclusion B25.0
  cytomegaloviral B25.0
  deglutition—*see* Pneumonia, aspiration
  desquamative interstitial J84.117
  diffuse—*see* Pneumonia, broncho
  diplococcal, diplococcus (broncho-) (lobar) J13
  disseminated (focal)—*see* Pneumonia, broncho
  Eaton's agent J15.7
  embolic, embolism—*see* Embolism, pulmonary
  Enterobacter J15.69
  eosinophilic J82.81
    acute J82.82
    chronic J82.81
  Escherichia coli (E. coli) J15.5
  Eubacterium J15.8
  fibrinous—*see* Pneumonia, lobar
  fibroid, fibrous (chronic)—*see* Fibrosis, lung
  Friedländer's bacillus J15.0
  Fusobacterium (nucleatum) J15.8
  gangrenous J85.0
  giant cell (measles) B05.2
  gonococcal A54.84
  gram-negative bacteria NEC J15.69
    anaerobic B01.2
  Hemophilus influenzae (broncho) (lobar) J14
  human metapneumovirus J12.3
  hypostatic (broncho) (lobar) J18.2
  in (due to)
    Acinetobacter baumannii J15.61
    actinomycosis A42.0
    adenovirus J12.0
    anthrax A22.1
    ascariasis B77.81
    aspergillosis B44.9
    Bacillus anthracis A22.1
    Bacterium anitratum J15.69
    candidiasis B37.1
    chickenpox B01.2
    Chlamydia J16.0
      neonatal P23.1
    coccidioidomycosis B38.2
      acute B38.0
      chronic B38.1
    cytomegalovirus disease B25.0
    Diplococcus (pneumoniae) J13
    Eaton's agent J15.7
    Enterobacter J15.69
    Escherichia coli (E. coli) J15.5
    Friedländer's bacillus J15.0
    fumes and vapors (chemical) (inhalation) J68.0
    gonorrhea A54.84

Pneumonia *(continued)*
  in *(continued)*
    Hemophilus influenzae (H. influenzae) J14
    Herellea J15.69
    histoplasmosis B39.2
      acute B39.0
      chronic B39.1
    human metapneumovirus J12.3
    Klebsiella (pneumoniae) J15.0
    measles B05.2
    Mycoplasma (pneumoniae) J15.7
    nocardiosis, nocardiasis A43.0
    ornithosis A70
    parainfluenza virus J12.2
    pleuro-pneumonia-like-organism (PPLO) J15.7
    pneumococcus J13
    pneumocystosis (Pneumocystis carinii) (Pneumocystis jiroveci) B59
    Proteus J15.69
    Pseudomonas NEC J15.1
      pseudomallei A24.1
    psittacosis A70
    Q fever A78
    respiratory syncytial virus (RSV) J12.1
    rheumatic fever I00 [J17]
    rubella B06.81
    Salmonella (infection) A02.22
      typhi A01.03
    schistosomiasis B65.9 [J17]
    Serratia marcescens J15.69
    specified
      bacterium NEC J15.8
      organism NEC J16.8
    spirochetal NEC A69.8
    Staphylococcus J15.20
      aureus (methicillin susceptible) (MSSA) J15.211
        methicillin resistant (MRSA) J15.212
      specified NEC J15.29
    Streptococcus J15.4
      group B J15.3
      pneumoniae J13
      specified NEC J15.4
    toxoplasmosis B58.3
    tularemia A21.2
    typhoid (fever) A01.03
    varicella B01.2
    virus—*see* Pneumonia, viral
    whooping cough A37.91
      due to
        Bordetella parapertussis A37.11
        Bordetella pertussis A37.01
        specified NEC A37.81
    Yersinia pestis A20.2
  inhalation of food or vomit—*see* Pneumonia, aspiration
  interstitial J84.9
    chronic J84.111
    desquamative J84.117
    due to
      collagen vascular disease J84.178
      known underlying cause J84.178
    idiopathic NOS J84.111
    in disease classified elsewhere J84.178
    lymphocytic (due to collagen vascular disease) (in diseases classified elsewhere) J84.178
    lymphoid J84.2
    non-specific J84.89
      due to
        collagen vascular disease J84.178
        known underlying cause J84.178

Pneumonia *(continued)*
  interstitial *(continued)*
    non-specific *(continued)*
      idiopathic J84.113
      in diseases classified elsewhere J84.178
    plasma cell B59
    pseudomonas J15.1
    usual J84.112
      due to collagen vascular disease J84.178
      idiopathic J84.112
      in diseases classified elsewhere J84.178
  Klebsiella (pneumoniae) J15.0
  lipid, lipoid (exogenous) J69.1
    endogenous J84.89
  lobar (disseminated) (double) (interstitial) J18.1
    bacterial J15.9
      specified NEC J15.8
    chronic—*see* Fibrosis, lung
    Escherichia coli (E. coli) J15.5
    Friedländer's bacillus J15.0
    Hemophilus influenzae J14
    hypostatic J18.2
    Klebsiella (pneumoniae) J15.0
    pneumococcal J13
    Proteus J15.69
    Pseudomonas J15.1
    specified organism NEC J16.8
    staphylococcal—*see* Pneumonia, staphylococcal
    streptococcal NEC J15.4
    Streptococcus pneumoniae J13
    viral, virus—*see* Pneumonia, viral
  lobular—*see* Pneumonia, broncho
  Löffler's J82.89
  lymphoid interstitial J84.2
  massive—*see* Pneumonia, lobar
  meconium P24.01
  MRSA (Methicillin resistant Staphylococcus aureus) J15.212
  MSSA (methicillin susceptible Staphylococcus aureus) J15.211
  multilobar—*see* Pneumonia, by type
  Mycoplasma (pneumoniae) J15.7
  necrotic J85.0
  neonatal P23.9
    aspiration—*see* Aspiration, by substance, with pneumonia
  nitrogen dioxide J68.0
  organizing J84.89
    due to
      collagen vascular disease J84.178
      known underlying cause J84.178
    in diseases classified elsewhere J84.178
  orthostatic J18.2
  parainfluenza virus J12.2
  parenchymatous—*see* Fibrosis, lung
  passive J18.2
  patchy—*see* Pneumonia, broncho
  Peptococcus J15.8
  Peptostreptococcus J15.8
  plasma cell (of infants) B59
  pleurolobar—*see* Pneumonia, lobar
  pleuro-pneumonia-like organism (PPLO) J15.7
  pneumococcal (broncho) (lobar) J13
  Pneumocystis (carinii) (jiroveci) B59
  postinfectional NEC B99 [J17]
  postmeasles B05.2
  Proteus J15.69
  Pseudomonas J15.1
  psittacosis A70
  radiation J70.0

Pneumonia (continued)
  respiratory syncytial virus (RSV)
      J12.1
  resulting from a procedure J95.89
  rheumatic I00 *[J17]*
  Salmonella (arizonae) (choleraesuis) (enteritidis) (typhimurium)
      A02.22
    typhi A01.03
    typhoid fever A01.03
  SARS-associated coronavirus
      J12.81
  SARS-CoV-2 J12.82
  segmented, segmental —*see*
      Pneumonia, broncho-
  Serratia marcescens J15.69
  specified NEC J18.8
    bacterium NEC J15.8
    organism NEC J16.8
    virus NEC J12.89
  spirochetal NEC A69.8
  staphylococcal (broncho) (lobar)
      J15.20
    aureus (methicillin susceptible)
        (MSSA) J15.211
      methicillin resistant (MRSA)
          J15.212
    specified NEC J15.29
  static, stasis J18.2
  streptococcal NEC (broncho)
      (lobar) J15.4
    group
      A J15.4
      B J15.3
    specified NEC J15.4
  Streptococcus pneumoniae J13
  syphilitic, congenital (early)
      A50.04
  traumatic (complication) (early)
      (secondary) T79.8
  tuberculous (any) —*see*
      Tuberculosis, pulmonary
  tularemic A21.2
  varicella B01.2
  Veillonella J15.8
  ventilator associated J95.851
  viral, virus (broncho) (interstitial)
      (lobar) J12.9
    adenoviral J12.0
    congenital P23.0
    human metapneumovirus J12.3
    parainfluenza J12.2
    respiratory syncytial (RSV) J12.1
    SARS-associated coronavirus
        J12.81
    specified NEC J12.89
  white (congenital) A50.04

Pneumonic —*see* condition

Pneumonitis (acute) (primary)
    (*see also* Pneumonia) J98.4
  air-conditioner J67.7
  allergic (due to) J67.9
    organic dust NEC J67.8
    red cedar dust J67.8
    sequoiosis J67.8
    wood dust J67.8
  aspiration J69.0
    due to
      anesthesia J95.4
        during
          labor and delivery O74.0
          pregnancy O29.01-
          puerperium O89.01
      fumes or gases J68.0
      obstetric O74.0
  chemical (due to gases, fumes or
      vapors) (inhalation) J68.0
    due to anesthesia J95.4
  cholesterol J84.89
  crack (cocaine) J68.0

Pneumonitis (continued)
  chronic —*see* Fibrosis, lung
  congenital rubella P35.0
  due to
    beryllium J68.0
    cadmium J68.0
    crack (cocaine) J68.0
    detergent J69.8
    fluorocarbon-polymer J68.0
    food, vomit (aspiration) J69.0
    fumes or vapors J68.0
    gases, fumes or vapors
        (inhalation) J68.0
    inhalation
      blood J69.8
      essences J69.1
      food (regurgitated), milk,
          vomit J69.0
      oils, essences J69.1
      saliva J69.0
      solids, liquids NEC J69.8
    manganese J68.0
    nitrogen dioxide J68.0
    oils, essences J69.1
    solids, liquids NEC J69.8
    toxoplasmosis (acquired) B58.3
      congenital P37.1
    vanadium J68.0
    ventilator J95.851
  eosinophilic J82.81
    acute J82.82
    chronic J82.81
  hypersensitivity J67.9
    air conditioner lung J67.7
    bagassosis J67.1
    bird fancier's lung J67.2
    farmer's lung J67.0
    maltworker's lung J67.4
    maple bark-stripper's lung J67.6
    mushroom worker's lung J67.5
    specified organic dust NEC J67.8
    suberosis J67.3
  interstitial (chronic) J84.89
    acute J84.114
    lymphoid J84.2
    non-specific J84.89
      idiopathic J84.113
  lymphoid, interstitial J84.2
  meconium P24.01
  noninfectious J98.4
  postanesthetic J95.4
    correct substance properly
        administered —*see* Table
        of Drugs and Chemicals, by
        drug, adverse effect
    in labor and delivery O74.0
    in pregnancy O29.01-
    obstetric O74.0
    overdose or wrong substance
        given or taken (by accident)
        —*see* Table of Drugs and
        Chemicals, by drug, poisoning
    postpartum, puerperal O89.01
  postoperative J95.4
    obstetric O74.0
  radiation J70.0
  rubella, congenital P35.0
  specified NEC J98.4
  ventilation (air-conditioning) J67.7
  ventilator associated J95.851
  wood-dust J67.8

Pneumonoconiosis —*see*
    Pneumoconiosis

Pneumoparotid K11.8

Pneumopathy NEC J98.4
  alveolar J84.09
  due to organic dust NEC J66.8
  parietoalveolar J84.09

Pneumopericarditis —*see also*
    Pericarditis
  acute I30.9

Pneumopericardium —*see also*
    Pericarditis
  congenital P25.3
  newborn P25.3
  traumatic (post) —*see* Injury, heart

Pneumophagia (psychogenic) F45.8

Pneumopleurisy, pneumopleuritis
    (*see also* Pneumonia) J18.8

Pneumopyopericardium I30.1

Pneumopyothorax —*see*
    Pyopneumothorax
  with fistula J86.0

Pneumorrhagia —*see also*
    Hemorrhage, lung
  tuberculous —*see* Tuberculosis,
      pulmonary

Pneumothorax NOS J93.9
  acute J93.83
  chronic J93.81
  congenital P25.1
  perinatal period P25.1
  postprocedural J95.811
  specified NEC J93.83
  spontaneous NOS J93.83
    newborn P25.1
    primary J93.11
    secondary J93.12
    tension J93.0
  tense valvular, infectional J93.0
  tension (spontaneous) J93.0
  traumatic S27.0
    with hemothorax S27.2
  tuberculous —*see* Tuberculosis,
      pulmonary

Podagra (*see also* Gout) M10.9

Podencephalus Q01.9

Poikilocytosis R71.8

Poikiloderma L81.6
  Civatte's L57.3
  congenital Q82.8
  vasculare atrophicans L94.5

Poikilodermatomyositis M33.10
  with
    myopathy M33.12
    respiratory involvement
        M33.11
    specified organ involvement
        NEC M33.19
  amyopathic M33.13
  without myopathy M33.13

Pointed ear (congenital) Q17.3

**Poison ivy, oak, sumac or other
plant dermatitis** (allergic)
    (contact) L23.7

Poisoning (acute) —*see also* Table of
    Drugs and Chemicals
  algae and toxins T65.82-
  Bacillus B (aertrycke) (cholera
      (suis)) (paratyphosus)
      (suipestifer) A02.9
    botulinus A05.1
  bacterial toxins A05.9
  berries, noxious —*see* Poisoning,
      food, noxious, berries
  botulism A05.1
  ciguatera fish T61.0-
  Clostridium botulinum A05.1
  death-cap (Amanita phalloides)
      (Amanita verna) —*see* Poisoning,
      food, noxious, mushrooms
  drug —*see* Table of Drugs and
      Chemicals, by drug, poisoning

Poisoning (continued)
  epidemic, fish (noxious) —*see*
      Poisoning, seafood
    bacterial A05.9
  fava bean D55.0
  fish (noxious) T61.9-
    bacterial —*see* Intoxication,
        foodborne, by agent
    ciguatera fish —*see* Poisoning,
        ciguatera fish
    scombroid fish —*see* Poisoning,
        scombroid fish
    specified type NEC T61.77-
  food NEC A05.9
    bacterial —*see* Intoxication,
        foodborne, by agent
    due to
      Bacillus (aertrycke)
          (choleraesuis)
          (paratyphosus) (suipestifer)
          A02.9
        botulinus A05.1
      Clostridium (perfringens)
          (Welchii) A05.2
      salmonella (aertrycke)
          (callinarum) (choleraesuis)
          (enteritidis) (paratyphi)
          (suipestifer) A02.9
        with
          gastroenteritis A02.0
          sepsis A02.1
      staphylococcus A05.0
      Vibrio
        parahaemolyticus A05.3
        vulnificus A05.5
    noxious or naturally toxic
        T62.9-
      berries —*see* subcategory
          T62.1-
      fish —*see* Poisoning, seafood
      mushrooms —*see* subcategory
          T62.0X-
      plants NEC —*see* subcategory
          T62.2X-
      seafood —*see* Poisoning,
          seafood
      specified NEC T62.8X-
  ichthyotoxism —*see* Poisoning,
      seafood
  kreotoxism, food A05.9
  latex T65.81-
  lead T56.0-
  mushroom —*see* Poisoning, food,
      noxious, mushroom
  mussels —*see also* Poisoning,
      shellfish
    bacterial —*see* Intoxication,
        foodborne, by agent
  nicotine (tobacco) T65.2-
  noxious foodstuffs —*see*
      Poisoning, food, noxious
  plants, noxious —*see* Poisoning,
      food, noxious, plants NEC
  ptomaine —*see* Poisoning, food
  radiation J70.0
  Salmonella (arizonae) (choleraesuis) (enteritidis) (typhimurium)
      A02.9
  scombroid fish T61.1-
  seafood (noxious) T61.9-
    bacterial —*see* Intoxication,
        foodborne, by agent
    fish —*see* Poisoning, fish
    shellfish —*see* Poisoning, shellfish
    specified NEC —*see* subcategory
        T61.8X-
  shellfish (amnesic) (azaspiracid)
      (diarrheic) (neurotoxic)
      (noxious) (paralytic) T61.78-
    bacterial —*see* Intoxication,
        foodborne, by agent

Poisoning *(continued)*
  shellfish *(continued)*
    ciguatera mollusk —*see*
      Poisoning, ciguatera fish
  specified substance NEC T65.891
  Staphylococcus, food A05.0
  tobacco (nicotine) T65.2-
  water E87.79
Poker spine —*see* Spondylitis, ankylosing
Poland syndrome Q79.8
Polioencephalitis (acute) (bulbar) A80.9
  inferior G12.22
  influenzal —*see* Influenza, with, encephalopathy
  superior hemorrhagic (acute) (Wernicke's) E51.2
  Wernicke's E51.2
Polioencephalomyelitis (acute) (anterior) A80.9
  with beriberi E51.2
Polioencephalopathy, superior hemorrhagic E51.2
  with
    beriberi E51.11
    pellagra E52
Poliomeningoencephalitis —*see* Meningoencephalitis
Poliomyelitis (acute) (anterior) (epidemic) A80.9
  with paralysis (bulbar) —*see* Poliomyelitis, paralytic
  abortive A80.4
  ascending (progressive) —*see* Poliomyelitis, paralytic
  bulbar (paralytic) —*see* Poliomyelitis, paralytic
  congenital P35.8
  nonepidemic A80.9
  nonparalytic A80.4
  paralytic A80.30
    specified NEC A80.39
    vaccine-associated A80.0
    wild virus
      imported A80.1
      indigenous A80.2
  spinal, acute A80.9
Poliosis (eyebrow) (eyelashes) L67.1
  circumscripta, acquired L67.1
Pollakiuria R35.0
  psychogenic F45.8
Pollinosis J30.1
Pollitzer's disease L73.2
Polyadenitis —*see also* Lymphadenitis
  malignant A20.0
Polyalgia M79.89
Polyangiitis M30.0
  microscopic M31.7
  overlap syndrome M30.8
Polyarteritis
  microscopic M31.7
  nodosa M30.0
    with lung involvement M30.1
    juvenile M30.2
    related condition NEC M30.8
Polyarthralgia —*see* Pain, joint
Polyarthritis, polyarthropathy (*see also* Arthritis) M13.0
  due to or associated with other specified conditions —*see* Arthritis
  epidemic (Australian) (with exanthema) B33.1
  infective —*see* Arthritis, pyogenic or pyemic

Polyarthritis, polyarthropathy *(continued)*
  inflammatory M06.4
  juvenile (chronic) (seronegative) M08.3
  migratory M13.8-
  rheumatic, acute —*see* Fever, rheumatic
Polyarthrosis M15.9
  post-traumatic M15.3
  primary M15.0
  specified NEC M15.8
Polycarential syndrome of infancy E40
Polychondritis (atrophic) (chronic) —*see also* Disorder, cartilage, specified type NEC
  relapsing M94.1
Polycoria Q13.2
Polycystic (disease)
  degeneration, kidney Q61.3
    autosomal dominant (adult type) Q61.2
    autosomal recessive (infantile type) NEC Q61.19
  kidney Q61.3
    autosomal
      dominant Q61.2
      recessive NEC Q61.19
    autosomal dominant (adult type) Q61.2
    autosomal recessive (childhood type) NEC Q61.19
    infantile type NEC Q61.19
  liver Q44.6
  lung J98.4
    congenital Q33.0
  ovary, ovaries E28.2
  spleen Q89.09
Polycythemia (secondary) D75.1
  acquired D75.1
  benign (familial) D75.0
  due to
    donor twin P61.1
    erythropoietin D75.1
    fall in plasma volume D75.1
    high altitude D75.1
    maternal-fetal transfusion P61.1
    stress D75.1
  emotional D75.1
  erythropoietin D75.1
  familial (benign) D75.0
  Gaisböck's (hypertonica) D75.1
  high altitude D75.1
  hypertonica D75.1
  hypoxemic D75.1
  neonatorum P61.1
  nephrogenous D75.1
  relative D75.1
  secondary D75.1
  spurious D75.1
  stress D75.1
  vera D45
Polycytosis cryptogenica D75.1
Polydactylism, polydactyly Q69.9
  toes Q69.2
Polydipsia R63.1
Polydystrophy, pseudo-Hurler E77.0
Polyembryoma —*see* Neoplasm, malignant, by site
Polyglandular
  deficiency E31.0
  dyscrasia E31.9
  dysfunction E31.9
  syndrome E31.8

Polyhydramnios O40.-
Polymastia Q83.1
Polymenorrhea N92.0
Polymyalgia M35.3
  arteritica, giant cell M31.5
  rheumatica M35.3
    with giant cell arteritis M31.5
Polymyositis (acute) (chronic) (hemorrhagic) M33.20
  with
    myopathy M33.22
    respiratory involvement M33.21
    skin involvement —*see* Dermatopolymyositis
    specified organ involvement NEC M33.29
  ossificans (generalisata) (progressiva) —*see* Myositis, ossificans, progressiva
Polyneuritis, polyneuritic —*see also* Polyneuropathy
  acute (post-)infective G61.0
  alcoholic G62.1
  cranialis G52.7
  demyelinating, chronic inflammatory (CIDP) G61.81
  diabetic —*see* Diabetes, polyneuropathy
  diphtheritic A36.83
  due to lack of vitamin NEC E56.9 *[G63]*
  endemic E51.11
  erythredema —*see* subcategory T56.1
  febrile, acute G61.0
  hereditary ataxic G60.1
  idiopathic, acute G61.0
  infective (acute) G61.0
  inflammatory, chronic demyelinating (CIDP) G61.81
  nutritional E63.9 *[G63]*
  postinfective (acute) G61.0
  specified NEC G62.89
Polyneuropathy (peripheral) G62.9
  alcoholic G62.1
  amyloid (Portuguese) E85.1 *[G63]*
    transthyretin-related (ATTR) familial E85.1 *[G63]*
  arsenical G62.2
  critical illness G62.81
  demyelinating, chronic inflammatory (CIDP) G61.81
  diabetic —*see* Diabetes, polyneuropathy
  drug-induced G62.0
  hereditary G60.9
    specified NEC G60.8
  idiopathic G60.9
    progressive G60.3
  in (due to)
    alcohol G62.1
      sequelae G65.2
    amyloidosis, familial (Portuguese) E85.1 *[G63]*
    antitetanus serum G61.1
    arsenic G62.2
      sequelae G65.2
    avitaminosis NEC E56.9 *[G63]*
    beriberi E51.11
    collagen vascular disease NEC M35.9 *[G63]*
    deficiency (of)
      B (-complex) vitamins E53.9 *[G63]*
      vitamin B6 E53.1 *[G63]*
    diabetes —*see* Diabetes, polyneuropathy

Polyneuropathy *(continued)*
  in *(continued)*
    diphtheria A36.83
    drug or medicament G62.0
      correct substance properly administered —*see* Table of Drugs and Chemicals, by drug, adverse effect
      overdose or wrong substance given or taken —*see* Table of Drugs and Chemicals, by drug, poisoning
    endocrine disease NEC E34.9 *[G63]*
    herpes zoster B02.23
    hypoglycemia E16.2 *[G63]*
    infectious
      disease NEC B99 *[G63]*
      mononucleosis B27.91
    lack of vitamin NEC E56.9 *[G63]*
    lead G62.2
      sequelae G65.2
    leprosy A30.9 *[G63]*
    Lyme disease A69.22
    metabolic disease NEC E88.9 *[G63]*
    microscopic polyangiitis M31.7 *[G63]*
    mumps B26.84
    neoplastic disease (*see also* Neoplasm) D49.9 *[G63]*
    nutritional deficiency NEC E63.9 *[G63]*
    organophosphate compounds G62.2
      sequelae G65.2
    parasitic disease NEC B89 *[G63]*
    pellagra E52 *[G63]*
    polyarteritis nodosa M30.0
    porphyria E80.20 *[G63]*
    radiation G62.82
    rheumatoid arthritis —*see* Rheumatoid, polyneuropathy
    sarcoidosis D86.89
    serum G61.1
    syphilis (late) A52.15
      congenital A50.43
    systemic
      connective tissue disorder M35.9 *[G63]*
      lupus erythematosus M32.19
    toxic agent NEC G62.2
      sequelae G65.2
    transthyretin-related (ATTR) familial amyloid E85.1
  inflammatory G61.9
    chronic demyelinating (CIDP) G61.81
    sequelae G65.1
    specified NEC G61.89
  lead G62.2
    sequelae G65.2
  nutritional NEC E63.9 *[G63]*
  postherpetic (zoster) B02.23
  progressive G60.3
  radiation-induced G62.82
  sensory (hereditary) (idiopathic) G60.8
  specified NEC G62.89
  syphilitic (late) A52.15
    congenital A50.43
    triorthocresyl phosphate G62.2
      sequelae G65.2
    tuberculosis A17.89
    uremia N18.9 *[G63]*

Polyneuropathy (continued)
  syphilitic (continued)
    vitamin B12 deficiency E53.8 [G63]
      with anemia (pernicious) D51.0 [G63]
        due to dietary deficiency D51.3 [G63]
  zoster B02.23
Polyopia H53.8
Polyorchism, polyorchidism Q55.21
Polyosteoarthritis (see also Osteoarthritis, generalized) M15.9-
  post-traumatic M15.3
  specified NEC M15.8
Polyostotic fibrous dysplasia Q78.1
Polyotia Q17.0
Polyp, polypus
  accessory sinus J33.8
  adenocarcinoma in —see Neoplasm, malignant, by site
  adenocarcinoma in situ in —see Neoplasm, in situ, by site
  adenoid tissue J33.0
  adenomatous —see also Neoplasm, benign, by site
    adenocarcinoma in —see Neoplasm, malignant, by site
    adenocarcinoma in situ in —see Neoplasm, in situ, by site
    carcinoma in —see Neoplasm, malignant, by site
    carcinoma in situ in —see Neoplasm, in situ, by site
    multiple —see Neoplasm, benign
      adenocarcinoma in —see Neoplasm, malignant, by site
      adenocarcinoma in situ in —see Neoplasm, in situ, by site
  antrum J33.8
  anus, anal (canal) K62.0
  Bartholin's gland N84.3
  bladder D41.4
  carcinoma in —see Neoplasm, malignant, by site
  carcinoma in situ in —see Neoplasm, in situ, by site
  cecum D12.0
  cervix (uteri) N84.1
    in pregnancy or childbirth —see Pregnancy, complicated by, abnormal, cervix
    mucous N84.1
    nonneoplastic N84.1
  choanal J33.0
  cholesterol K82.4
  clitoris N84.3
  colon K63.5
    adenomatous D12.6
      ascending D12.2
      cecum D12.0
      descending D12.4
      sigmoid D12.5
      transverse D12.3
    ascending K63.5
    cecum K63.5
    descending K63.5
    hyperplastic, (any site) K63.5
    inflammatory K51.40
      with
        abscess K51.414
        complication K51.419
          specified NEC K51.418
        fistula K51.413
        intestinal obstruction K51.412
        rectal bleeding K51.411

Polyp, polypus (continued)
  colon (continued)
    sigmoid K63.5
    transverse K63.5
  corpus uteri N84.0
  dental K04.01
    irreversible K04.02
    reversible K04.01
  duodenum K31.7
  ear (middle) H74.4-
  endometrium N84.0
  esophageal K22.81
  esophagogastric junction K22.82
  ethmoidal (sinus) J33.8
  fallopian tube N84.8
  female genital tract N84.9
    specified NEC N84.8
  frontal (sinus) J33.8
  gallbladder K82.4
  gingiva, gum K06.8
  labia, labium (majus) (minus) N84.3
  larynx (mucous) J38.1
    adenomatous D14.1
  malignant —see Neoplasm, malignant, by site
  maxillary (sinus) J33.8
  middle ear —see Polyp, ear (middle)
  myometrium N84.0
  nares
    anterior J33.9
    posterior J33.0
  nasal (mucous) J33.9
    cavity J33.0
    septum J33.0
  nasopharyngeal J33.0
  nose (mucous) J33.9
  oviduct N84.8
  pharynx J39.2
  placenta O90.89
  prostate —see Enlargement, enlarged, prostate
  pudenda, pudendum N84.3
  pulpal (dental) K04.01
    irreversible K04.02
    reversible K04.01
  rectum (nonadenomatous) K62.1
    adenomatous —see Polyp, adenomatous
  septum (nasal) J33.0
  sinus (accessory) (ethmoidal) (frontal) (maxillary) (sphenoidal) J33.8
  sphenoidal (sinus) J33.8
  stomach K31.7
    adenomatous D13.1
  tube, fallopian N84.8
  turbinate, mucous membrane J33.8
  umbilical, newborn P83.6
  ureter N28.89
  urethra N36.2
  uterus (body) (corpus) (mucous) N84.0
    cervix N84.1
    in pregnancy or childbirth —see Pregnancy, complicated by, tumor, uterus
  vagina N84.2
  vocal cord (mucous) J38.1
  vulva N84.3
Polyphagia R63.2
Polyploidy Q92.7
Polypoid —see condition
Polyposis —see also Polyp
  adenomatous D13.91
  coli (adenomatous) D12.6
    adenocarcinoma in C18.9
    adenocarcinoma in situ in —see Neoplasm, in situ, by site
    carcinoma in C18.9
  colon (adenomatous) D12.6

Polyposis (continued)
  familial D12.6
    adenocarcinoma in situ in —see Neoplasm, in situ, by site
    adenomatous D13.91
  intestinal D12.6
    adenomatous D13.91
  malignant lymphomatous C83.1-
  multiple, adenomatous (see also Neoplasm, benign) D36.9
Polyradiculitis —see Polyneuropathy
Polyradiculoneuropathy (acute) (postinfective) (segmentally demyelinating) G61.0
Polyserositis
  due to pericarditis I31.1
  pericardial I31.1
  periodic, familial E85.0
  tuberculous A19.9
    acute A19.1
    chronic A19.8
Polysplenia syndrome Q89.09
Polysyndactyly (see also Syndactylism, syndactyly) Q70.4
Polytrichia L68.3
Polyunguia Q84.6
Polyuria R35.89
  nocturnal R35.81
  psychogenic F45.8
  specified NEC R35.89
Pompe's disease (glycogen storage) E74.02
Pompholyx L30.1
Poncet's disease (tuberculous rheumatism) A18.09
Pond fracture —see Fracture, skull
Ponos B55.0
Pons, pontine —see condition
Poor
  aesthetic of existing restoration of tooth K08.56
  contractions, labor O62.2
  gingival margin to tooth restoration K08.51
  personal hygiene R46.0
  prenatal care, affecting management of pregnancy —see Pregnancy, complicated by, insufficient, prenatal care
  sucking reflex (newborn) R29.2
  urinary stream R39.12
  vision NEC H54.7
Poradenitis, nostras inguinalis or venerea A55
Porencephaly (congenital) (developmental) (true) Q04.6
  acquired G93.0
  nondevelopmental G93.0
  traumatic (post) F07.89
Porocephaliasis B88.8
Porokeratosis Q82.8
Poroma, eccrine —see Neoplasm, skin, benign
Porphyria (South African) E80.20
  acquired E80.20
  acute intermittent (hepatic) (Swedish) E80.21
  cutanea tarda (hereditary) (symptomatic) E80.1
  due to drugs E80.20
    correct substance properly administered —see Table of Drugs and Chemicals, by drug, adverse effect

Porphyria (continued)
  due to drugs (continued)
    overdose or wrong substance given or taken —see Table of Drugs and Chemicals, by drug, poisoning
  erythropoietic (congenital) (hereditary) E80.0
  hepatocutaneous type E80.1
  secondary E80.20
  toxic NEC E80.20
  variegata E80.20
Porphyrinuria —see Porphyria
Porphyruria —see Porphyria
Portal —see condition
Port wine nevus, mark, or stain Q82.5
Posadas-Wernicke disease B38.9
Positive
  culture (nonspecific)
    blood R78.81
    bronchial washings R84.5
    cerebrospinal fluid R83.5
    cervix uteri R87.5
    nasal secretions R84.5
    nipple discharge R89.5
    nose R84.5
      staphylococcus (Methicillin susceptible) Z22.321
        Methicillin resistant Z22.322
    peritoneal fluid R85.5
    pleural fluid R84.5
    prostatic secretions R86.5
    saliva R85.5
    seminal fluid R86.5
    sputum R84.5
    synovial fluid R89.5
    throat scrapings R84.5
    urine R82.79
    vagina R87.5
    vulva R87.5
    wound secretions R89.5
  PPD (skin test) R76.11
  serology for syphilis A53.0
    false R76.8
    with signs or symptoms - code as Syphilis, by site and stage
  skin test, tuberculin (without active tuberculosis) R76.11
  test, human immunodeficiency virus (HIV) R75
  VDRL A53.0
    with signs or symptoms - code by site and stage under Syphilis A53.9
  Wassermann reaction A53.0
Postcardiotomy syndrome I97.0
Postcaval ureter Q62.62
Postcholecystectomy syndrome K91.5
Postclimacteric bleeding N95.0
Postcommissurotomy syndrome I97.0
Postconcussional syndrome F07.81
Postcontusional syndrome F07.81
Postcricoid region —see condition
Post COVID-19 condition, unspecified U09.9
Post-dates (40-42 weeks) (pregnancy) (mother) O48.0
  more than 42 weeks gestation O48.1
Postencephalitic syndrome F07.89

271

Posterior —see condition
Posterolateral sclerosis (spinal cord) —see Degeneration, combined
Postexanthematous —see condition
Postfebrile —see condition
Postgastrectomy dumping syndrome K91.1
Posthemiplegic chorea —see Monoplegia
Posthemorrhagic anemia (chronic) D50.0
  acute D62
  newborn P61.3
Postherpetic neuralgia (zoster) B02.29
  trigeminal B02.22
Posthitis N47.7
Postimmunization complication or reaction —see Complications, vaccination
Postinfectious —see condition
Postlaminectomy syndrome NEC M96.1
Postleukotomy syndrome F07.0
Postmastectomy lymphedema (syndrome) I97.2
Postmaturity, postmature (over 42 weeks)
  maternal (over 42 weeks gestation) O48.1
  newborn P08.22
Postmeasles complication NEC — see also condition B05.89
Postmenopausal
  endometrium (atrophic) N95.8
    suppurative (see also Endometritis) N71.9
  osteoporosis —see Osteoporosis, postmenopausal
Postnasal drip R09.82
  due to
    allergic rhinitis —see Rhinitis, allergic
    common cold J00
    gastroesophageal reflux —see Reflux, gastroesophageal
    nasopharyngitis —see Nasopharyngitis
    other know condition - code to condition
    sinusitis —see Sinusitis
Postnatal —see condition
Postoperative (postprocedural) —see also Complication, postoperative
  pneumothorax, therapeutic Z98.3
  state NEC Z98.890
  visit —see Aftercare
  wound check —see Aftercare
Postpancreatectomy hyperglycemia E89.1
Postpartum —see Puerperal
Postphlebitic syndrome —see Syndrome, postthrombotic
Postpoliomyelitic —see also condition
  osteopathy —see Osteopathy, after poliomyelitis
Postpolio (myelitic) **syndrome** G14

Postprocedural —see also Postoperative
  hypoinsulinemia E89.1
Postschizophrenic depression F32.89
Postsurgery status —see also Status (post)
  pneumothorax, therapeutic Z98.3
Post-term (40-42 weeks) (pregnancy) (mother) O48.0
  infant P08.21
  more than 42 weeks gestation (mother) O48.1
Post-traumatic brain syndrome, nonpsychotic F07.81
Post-typhoid abscess A01.09
Postures, hysterical F44.2
Postvaccinal reaction or complication —see Complications, vaccination
Postvalvulotomy syndrome I97.0
Potain's
  disease (pulmonary edema) —see Edema, lung
  syndrome (gastrectasis with dyspepsia) K31.0
POTS (postural orthostatic tachycardia syndrome) G90.A
Potter's
  asthma J62.8
  facies Q60.6
  lung J62.8
  syndrome (with renal agenesis) Q60.6
Pott's
  curvature (spinal) A18.01
  disease or paraplegia A18.01
  spinal curvature A18.01
  tumor, puffy —see Osteomyelitis, specified type NEC
Pouch
  bronchus Q32.4
  Douglas' —see condition
  esophagus, esophageal, congenital Q39.6
    acquired K22.5
  gastric K31.4
  Hartmann's K82.8
  pharynx, pharyngeal (congenital) Q38.7
Pouchitis K91.850
Poultrymen's itch B88.0
Poverty NEC Z59.6
  extreme Z59.5
Poxvirus NEC B08.8
Prader-Willi syndrome Q87.11
Prader-Willi-like syndrome Q87.19
Preauricular appendage or tag Q17.0
Prebetalipoproteinemia (acquired) (essential) (familial) (hereditary) (primary) (secondary) E78.1
  with chylomicronemia E78.3
Precipitate labor or delivery O62.3
Preclimacteric bleeding (menorrhagia) N92.4
Precocious
  adrenarche E30.1
  menarche E30.1
  menstruation E30.1
  pubarche E30.1
  puberty E30.1
    central E22.8
  sexual development NEC E30.1
  thelarche E30.8

Precocity, sexual (constitutional) (cryptogenic) (female) (idiopathic) (male) E30.1
  with adrenal hyperplasia E25.9
    congenital E25.0
Precordial pain R07.2
Predeciduous teeth K00.2
Prediabetes, prediabetic R73.03
  complicating
    pregnancy —see Pregnancy, complicated by, diseases of, specified type or system NEC
    puerperium O99.893
Predislocation status of hip at birth Q65.6
Pre-eclampsia O14.9-
  with pre-existing hypertension —see Hypertension, complicating pregnancy, pre-existing, with, pre-eclampsia
  complicating
    childbirth O14.94
    puerperium O14.95
  mild O14.0-
    complicating
      childbirth O14.04
      puerperium O14.05
  moderate O14.0-
    complicating
      childbirth O14.04
      puerperium O14.05
  severe O14.1-
    with hemolysis, elevated liver enzymes and low platelet count (HELLP) O14.2-
      complicating
        childbirth O14.24
        puerperium O14.25
    complicating
      childbirth O14.14
      puerperium O14.15
Pre-eruptive color change, teeth, tooth K00.8
Pre-excitation atrioventricular conduction I45.6
Preglaucoma H40.00-
Pregnancy (single) (uterine) —see also Delivery and Puerperal Z33.1

> Note: The Tabular must be reviewed for assignment of the appropriate character indicating the trimester of the pregnancy
> Note: The Tabular must be reviewed for assignment of appropriate seventh character for multiple gestation codes in Chapter 15

abdominal (ectopic) O00.00
  with intrauterine pregnancy O00.01
  with viable fetus O36.7-
ampullar O00.10-
  with intrauterine pregnancy O00.11-
biochemical O02.81
broad ligament O00.80
  with intrauterine pregnancy O00.81
cervical O00.80
  with intrauterine pregnancy O00.81
chemical O02.81
complicated NOS O26.9-

Pregnancy (continued)
  complicated by (care of) (management affected by)
    abnormal, abnormality
      cervix O34.4-
        causing obstructed labor O65.5
      cord (umbilical) O69.9
      fetal heart rate or rhythm O36.83-
      findings on antenatal screening of mother O28.9
        biochemical O28.1
        cytological O28.2
        chromosomal O28.5
        genetic O28.5
        hematological O28.0
        radiological O28.4
        specified NEC O28.8
        ultrasonic O28.3
      glucose (tolerance) NEC O99.810
      pelvic organs O34.9-
        specified NEC O34.8-
          causing obstructed labor O65.5
      pelvis (bony) (major) NEC O33.0
      perineum O34.7-
      position
        placenta O44.0
          with hemorrhage O44.1-
        uterus O34.59-
      uterus O34.59-
        causing obstructed labor O65.5
        congenital O34.0-
      vagina O34.6-
        causing obstructed labor O65.5
      vulva O34.7-
        causing obstructed labor O65.5
    abruptio placentae —see Abruptio placentae
    abscess or cellulitis
      bladder O23.1-
      breast O91.11-
      genital organ or tract O23.9-
    abuse
      physical O9A.31-
      psychological O9A.51-
      sexual O9A.41-
    adverse effect anesthesia O29.9-
      aspiration pneumonitis O29.01-
      cardiac arrest O29.11-
      cardiac complication NEC O29.19-
      cardiac failure O29.12-
      central nervous system complication NEC O29.29-
      cerebral anoxia O29.21-
      failed or difficult intubation O29.6-
      inhalation of stomach contents or secretions NOS O29.01-
      local, toxic reaction O29.3X
      Mendelson's syndrome O29.01-
      pressure collapse of lung O29.02-
      pulmonary complications NEC O29.09-
      specified NEC O29.8X-
      spinal and epidural type NEC O29.5X
        induced headache O29.4-

Pregnancy (continued)
  complicated by (continued)
   albuminuria (see also
     Proteinuria, gestational)
     O12.1-
   alcohol use O99.31-
   amnionitis O41.12-
   anaphylactoid syndrome of
     pregnancy O88.01-
   anemia (conditions in D50-D64)
     (pre-existing) O99.01-
     complicating the puerperium
       O99.03
   antepartum hemorrhage O46.9-
     with coagulation defect —see
       Hemorrhage, antepartum,
       with coagulation defect
     specified NEC O46.8X-
   appendicitis O99.61-
   atrophy (yellow) (acute) liver
     (subacute) O26.61-
   bariatric surgery status O99.84-
   bicornis or bicornuate uterus
     O34.0-
   biliary tract problems O26.61-
   breech presentation O32.1
   cardiovascular diseases
     (conditions in I00-I09,
     I20-I52, I70-I99) O99.41-
   cerebrovascular disorders
     (conditions in I60-I69)
     O99.41-
   cervical shortening O26.87-
   cervicitis O23.51-
   cesarean scar defect (isthmocele)
     O34.22
   chloasma (gravidarum) O26.89-
   cholestasis (intrahepatic)
     O26.64-
   cholecystitis O99.61-
   chorioamnionitis O41.12-
   circulatory system disorder
     (conditions in I00-I09,
     I20-I99, O99.41-)
   compound presentation O32.6
   conjoined twins O30.02-
   connective system disorders
     (conditions in M00-M99)
     O99.891
   contracted pelvis (general)
     O33.1
     inlet O33.2
     outlet O33.3
   convulsions (eclamptic) (uremic)
     (see also Eclampsia) O15.9-
   cracked nipple O92.11-
   cystitis O23.1-
   cystocele O34.8-
   death of fetus (near term) O36.4
     early pregnancy O02.1
     of one fetus or more in
       multiple gestation O31.2-
   deciduitis O41.14-
   decreased fetal movement
     O36.81-
   dental problems O99.61-
   diabetes (mellitus) O24.91-
     gestational (pregnancy
       induced) —see Diabetes,
       gestational
     pre-existing O24.31-
       specified NEC O24.81-
       type 1 O24.01-
       type 2 O24.11-
   digestive system disorders
     (conditions in K00-K93)
     O99.61-
   diseases of —see Pregnancy,
     complicated by, specified body
     system disease
     biliary tract O26.61-

Pregnancy (continued)
  complicated by (continued)
   diseases of (continued)
     blood NEC (conditions in
       D65-D77) O99.11-
     liver O26.61-
     specified NEC O99.891
   disorders of —see Pregnancy,
     complicated by, specified body
     system disorder
     amniotic fluid and membranes
       O41.9-
       specified NEC O41.8X-
     biliary tract O26.61-
     ear and mastoid process
       (conditions in H60-H95)
       O99.891
     eye and adnexa (conditions in
       H00-H59) O99.891
     liver O26.61-
     skin (conditions in L00-L99)
       O99.71-
     specified NEC O99.891
   displacement, uterus NEC
     O34.59-
     causing obstructed labor
       O65.5
   disproportion (due to) O33.9
     fetal (ascites) (hydrops)
       (meningomyelocele)
       (sacral teratoma) (tumor)
       deformities NEC O33.7
     generally contracted pelvis
       O33.1
     hydrocephalic fetus O33.6
     inlet contraction of pelvis
       O33.2
     mixed maternal and fetal
       origin O33.4
     specified NEC O33.8
   double uterus O34.0-
     causing obstructed labor
       O65.5
   drug use (conditions in F11-F19)
     O99.32-
   eclampsia, eclamptic (coma)
     (convulsions) (delirium)
     (nephritis) (uremia) (see also
     Eclampsia) O15.-
   ectopic pregnancy —see
     Pregnancy, ectopic
   edema O12.0-
     with
       gestational hypertension,
         mild (see also Pre-
         eclampsia) O14.0-
       proteinuria O12.2-
   effusion, amniotic fluid —see
     Pregnancy, complicated
     by, premature rupture of
     membranes
   elderly
     multigravida O09.52-
     primigravida O09.51-
   embolism (see also Embolism,
     obstetric, pregnancy) O88.-
   endocrine diseases NEC O99.28-
   endometritis O86.12
   excessive weight gain O26.0-
   exhaustion O26.81-
     during labor and delivery
       O75.81
   face presentation O32.3
   failed induction of labor O61.9
     instrumental O61.1
     mechanical O61.1
     medical O61.0
     specified NEC O61.8
     surgical O61.1
   failed or difficult intubation for
     anesthesia O29.6-

Pregnancy (continued)
  complicated by (continued)
   false labor (pains) O47.9
     at or after 37 completed weeks
       of pregnancy O47.1
     before 37 completed weeks of
       pregnancy O47.0-
   fatigue O26.81-
     during labor and delivery O75.81
   fatty metamorphosis of liver
     O26.61-
   female genital mutilation O34.8-
     [N90.81-]
   fetal (maternal care for)
     abnormality or damage O35.9
       acid-base balance O68
       specified type NEC O35.8
     acidemia O68
     acidosis O68
     agenesis of corpus callosum
       O35.01
     alkalosis O68
     anemia and thrombocytopenia
       O36.82-
     anencephaly O35.02
     bradycardia O36.83-
     cardiac anomalies O35.B
     central nervous system
       malformation or damage
       O35.00
       specified type NEC O35.09
     choroid plexus cysts O35.03
     chromosomal abnormality
       (conditions in Q90-Q99)
       O35.10
       sex chromosome O35.15
       specified NEC O35.19
       Trisomy 13 O35.11
       Trisomy 18 O35.12
       Trisomy 21 O35.13
       Turner Syndrome O35.14
     conjoined twins O30.02-
     damage from
       amniocentesis O35.7
       biopsy procedures O35.7
       drug addiction O35.5
       hematological investigation
         O35.7
       intrauterine contraceptive
         device O35.7
       maternal
         alcohol addiction O35.4
         cytomegalovirus
           infection O35.3
         disease NEC O35.8
         drug addiction O35.5
         listeriosis O35.8
         rubella O35.3
         toxoplasmosis O35.8
         viral infection O35.3
       medical procedure NEC
         O35.7
       radiation O35.6
     death (near term) O36.4
       early pregnancy O02.1
     decreased movement O36.81-
     depressed heart rate tones
       O36.83-
     disproportion due to deformity
       (fetal) O33.7
     encephalocele O35.04
     excessive growth (large for
       dates) O36.6-
     facial anomalies O35.A
     gastrointestinal anomalies
       O35.D
     genitourinary anomalies
       O35.E
     growth retardation O36.59-
       light for dates O36.59-
       small for dates O36.59-

Pregnancy (continued)
  complicated by (continued)
   fetal (maternal care for)
     (continued)
     heart rate irregularity
       (abnormal variability)
       (bradycardia)
       (decelerations)
       (tachycardia) O36.83-
     hereditary disease O35.2
     holoprosencephaly O35.05
     hydrocephalus O35.06
     hydrocephaly O35.06
     intrauterine death O36.4
     microcephaly O35.07
     musculoskeletal anomalies
       lower extremities O35.H
       trunk O35.F
       upper extremities O35.G
     non-reassuring heart rate or
       rhythm O36.83-
     poor growth O36.59-
       light for dates O36.59-
       small for dates O36.59-
     problem O36.9-
       specified NEC O36.89-
     pulmonary anomalies O35.C
     reduction (elective) O31.3-
     selective termination O31.3-
     spina bifida O35.08
     thrombocytopenia O36.82-
   fibroid (tumor) (uterus) O34.1-
   fissure of nipple O92.11-
   gallstones O99.61-
   gastric banding status O99.84-
   gastric bypass status O99.84-
   genital herpes (asymptomatic)
     (history of) (inactive) O98.3-
   genital tract infection O23.9-
   glomerular diseases (conditions
     in N00-N07) O26.83-
     with hypertension,
       pre-existing —see
       Hypertension, complicating,
       pregnancy, pre-existing,
       with, renal disease
   gonorrhea O98.21-
   grand multiparity O09.4
   habitual aborter —see
     Pregnancy, complicated by,
     recurrent pregnancy loss
   HELLP syndrome (hemolysis,
     elevated liver enzymes and
     low platelet count) O14.2-
   hemorrhage
     antepartum —see
       Hemorrhage, antepartum
     before 20 completed weeks
       gestation O20.9
       specified NEC O20.8
     due to premature separation,
       placenta (see also Abruptio
       placentae) O45.9-
     early O20.9
       specified NEC O20.8
     threatened abortion O20.0
   hemorrhoids O22.4-
   hepatitis (viral) O98.41-
   herniation of uterus O34.59-
   high
     head at term O32.4
     risk —see Supervision (of)
       (for), high-risk
   history of in utero procedure
     during previous pregnancy
     O09.82-
   HIV O98.71-
   human immunodeficiency virus
     (HIV) disease O98.71-
   hydatidiform mole (see also
     Mole, hydatidiform) O01.9-

273

Pregnancy (*continued*)
  complicated by (*continued*)
    hydramnios O40.-
    hydrocephalic fetus (disproportion) O33.6
    hydrops
      amnii O40.-
      fetalis O36.2-
        associated with isoimmunization (*see also* Pregnancy, complicated by, isoimmunization) O36.11-
    hydrorrhea O42.90
    hyperemesis (gravidarum) (mild) (*see also* Hyperemesis, gravidarum) O21.0-
    hypertension —*see* Hypertension, complicating pregnancy
    hypertensive
      heart and renal disease, pre-existing —*see* Hypertension, complicating, pregnancy, pre-existing, with, heart disease, with renal disease
      heart disease, pre-existing —*see* Hypertension, complicating, pregnancy, pre-existing, with, heart disease
      renal disease, pre-existing —*see* Hypertension, complicating, pregnancy, pre-existing, with, renal disease
    hypotension O26.5-
    immune disorders NEC (conditions in D80-D89) O99.11-
    incarceration, uterus O34.51-
    incompetent cervix O34.3-
    inconclusive fetal viability O36.80
    infection(s) O98.91-
      amniotic fluid or sac O41.10-
      bladder O23.1-
      carrier state NEC O99.830
        streptococcus B O99.820
      genital organ or tract O23.9-
        specified NEC O23.59-
      genitourinary tract O23.9-
      gonorrhea O98.21-
      hepatitis (viral) O98.41-
      HIV O98.71-
      human immunodeficiency virus (HIV) O98.71-
      intrauterine O41.12
      kidney O23.0-
      nipple O91.01-
      parasitic disease O98.91-
        specified NEC O98.81-
      protozoal disease O98.61-
      sexually transmitted NEC O98.31-
      specified type NEC O98.81-
      syphilis O98.11-
      tuberculosis O98.01-
      urethra O23.2-
      urinary (tract) O23.4-
        specified NEC O23.3-
      viral disease O98.51-
    inflammation
      intrauterine O41.12
    injury or poisoning (conditions in S00-T88) O9A.21-
      due to abuse
        physical O9A.31-
        psychological O9A.51-
        sexual O9A.41-
    insufficient
      prenatal care O09.3-
      weight gain O26.1-
    insulin resistance O26.89

Pregnancy (*continued*)
  complicated by (*continued*)
    intrauterine fetal death (near term) O36.4
      early pregnancy O02.1
      multiple gestation (one fetus or more) O31.2-
    isoimmunization O36.11-
      anti-A sensitization O36.11-
      anti-B sensitization O36.19-
      Rh O36.09-
        anti-D antibody O36.01-
      specified NEC O36.19-
    laceration of uterus NEC O71.81
    malformation
      central nervous system O35.00
        specified type NEC O35.09
      placenta, placental (vessel) O43.10-
        specified NEC O43.19-
      uterus (congenital) O34.0-
    malnutrition (conditions in E40-E46) O25.1-
    maternal hypotension syndrome O26.5-
    mental disorders (conditions in F01-F09, F20-F52 and F54-F99) O99.34-
      alcohol use O99.31-
      drug use O99.32-
      smoking O99.33-
    mentum presentation O32.3
    metabolic disorders O99.28-
    missed
      abortion O02.1
      delivery O36.4
    multiple gestations O30.9-
      conjoined twins O30.02-
      specified number of multiples NEC —*see* Pregnancy, multiple (gestation), specified NEC
      quadruplet —*see* Pregnancy, quadruplet
      specified complication NEC O31.8X-
      triplet —*see* Pregnancy, triplet
      twin —*see* Pregnancy, twin
    musculoskeletal condition (conditions is M00-M99) O99.891
    necrosis, liver (conditions in K72) O26.61-
    neoplasm
      benign
        cervix O34.4-
        corpus uteri O34.1-
        uterus O34.1-
      malignant O9A.11-
    nephropathy NEC O26.83-
    nervous system condition (conditions in G00-G99) O99.35-
    nutritional diseases NEC O99.28-
    obesity (pre-existing) O99.21-
    obesity surgery status O99.84-
    oblique lie or presentation O32.2
    older mother —*see* Pregnancy, complicated by, elderly
    oligohydramnios O41.0-
      with premature rupture of membranes (*see also* Pregnancy, complicated by, premature rupture of membranes) O42.-

Pregnancy (*continued*)
  complicated by (*continued*)
    onset (spontaneous) of labor after 37 completed weeks of gestation but before 39 completed weeks gestation, with delivery by (planned) cesarean section O75.82
    oophoritis O23.52-
    overdose, drug (*see also* Table of Drugs and Chemicals, by drug, poisoning) O9A.21-
    oversize fetus O33.5
    papyraceous fetus O31.0-
    pelvic inflammatory disease O99.891
    periodontal disease O99.61-
    peripheral neuritis O26.82-
    peritoneal (pelvic) adhesions O99.891
    phlebitis O22.9-
    phlebopathy O22.9-
    phlebothrombosis (superficial) O22.2-
      deep O22.3-
    placenta accreta O43.21-
    placenta increta O43.22-
    placenta percreta O43.23-
    placenta previa O44.0-
      complete O44.0-
        with hemorrhage O44.1-
      marginal O44.2-
        with hemorrhage O44.3-
      partial O44.2-
        with hemorrhage O44.3-
    placental disorder O43.9-
      specified NEC O43.89-
    placental dysfunction O43.89-
    placental infarction O43.81-
    placental insufficiency O36.51-
    placental transfusion syndromes
      fetomaternal O43.01-
      fetus to fetus O43.02-
      maternofetal O43.01-
    placentitis O41.14-
    pneumonia O99.51-
    poisoning (*see also* Table of Drugs and Chemicals) O9A.21-
    polyhydramnios O40-
    polymorphic eruption of pregnancy O26.86
    poor obstetric history NEC O09.29-
    postmaturity (post-term) (40 to 42 weeks) O48.0
      more than 42 completed weeks gestation (prolonged) O48.1
    pre-eclampsia O14.9-
      mild O14.0-
      moderate O14.0-
      severe O14.1-
        with hemolysis, elevated liver enzymes and low platelet count (HELLP) O14.2-
    premature labor —*see* Pregnancy, complicated by, preterm labor
    premature rupture of membranes O42.90
      full-term, unspecified as to length of time between rupture and onset of labor O42.92
      with onset of labor
        within 24 hours O42.00
        at or after 37 weeks gestation, onset of labor within 24 hours of rupture O42.02
        pre-term (before 37 completed weeks of gestation) O42.01-

Pregnancy (*continued*)
  complicated by (*continued*)
    premature rupture of membranes (*continued*)
      with onset of labor (*continued*)
        after 24 hours O42.10
        at or after 37 weeks gestation, onset of labor more than 24 hours following rupture O42.12
        pre-term (before 37 completed weeks of gestation) O42.11-
      at or after 37 weeks gestation, unspecified as to length of time between rupture and onset of labor O42.92
      pre-term (before 37 completed weeks of gestation) O42.91-
    premature separation of placenta (*see also* Abruptio placentae) O45.9-
    presentation, fetal —*see* Delivery, complicated by, malposition
    preterm delivery O60.10
    preterm labor
      with delivery O60.10
        preterm O60.10
        term O60.20
      second trimester
        with term delivery O60.22
        without delivery O60.02
        with preterm delivery
          second trimester O60.12
          third trimester O60.13
      third trimester
        with term delivery O60.23
        without delivery O60.03
        with third trimester preterm delivery O60.14
      without delivery O60.00
        second trimester O60.02
        third trimester O60.03
    previous history of —*see* Pregnancy, supervision of, high-risk
    prolapse, uterus O34.52-
    proteinuria (gestational) (*see also* Proteinuria, gestational) O12.1-
      with edema O12.2-
    pruritic urticarial papules and plaques of pregnancy (PUPPP) O26.86
    pruritus (neurogenic) O26.89-
    psychosis or psychoneurosis (puerperal) F53.1
    ptyalism O26.89-
    PUPPP (pruritic urticarial papules and plaques of pregnancy) O26.86
    pyelitis O23.0-
    recurrent pregnancy loss O26.2-
    renal disease or failure NEC O26.83-
      with secondary hypertension, pre-existing —*see* Hypertension, complicating, pregnancy, pre-existing, secondary
      hypertensive, pre-existing —*see* Hypertension, complicating, pregnancy, pre-existing, with, renal disease
    respiratory condition (conditions in J00-J99) O99.51-

Pregnancy (continued)
   complicated by (continued)
      retained, retention
         dead ovum O02.0
         intrauterine contraceptive device O26.3-
      retroversion, uterus O34.53-
      Rh immunization, incompatibility or sensitization NEC O36.09-
         anti-D antibody O36.01-
      rupture
         amnion (premature) (see also Pregnancy, complicated by, premature rupture of membranes) O42-
         membranes (premature) (see also Pregnancy, complicated by, premature rupture of membranes) O42-
         uterus (during labor) O71.1
            before onset of labor O71.0-
      salivation (excessive) O26.89-
      salpingitis O23.52-
      salpingo-oophoritis O23.52-
      sepsis (conditions in A40, A41) O98.81-
      size date discrepancy (uterine) O26.84-
      skin condition (conditions in L00-L99) O99.71-
      smoking (tobacco) O99.33-
      social problem O09.7-
      specified condition NEC O26.89-
      spotting O26.85-
      streptococcus group B (GBS) carrier state O99.820
      subluxation of symphysis (pubis) O26.71-
      syphilis (conditions in A50-A53) O98.11-
      threatened
         abortion O20.0
         labor O47.9
            at or after 37 completed weeks of gestation O47.1
            before 37 completed weeks of gestation O47.0-
      thrombophlebitis (superficial) O22.2-
      thrombosis O22.9-
         cerebral venous O22.5-
         cerebrovenous sinus O22.5-
         deep O22.3-
      tobacco use disorder (smoking) O99.33-
      torsion of uterus O34.59-
      toxemia O14.9-
      transverse lie or presentation O32.2
      tuberculosis (conditions in A15-A19) O98.01-
      tumor (benign)
         cervix O34.4-
            malignant O9A.11-
         uterus O34.1-
      unstable lie O32.0
      upper respiratory infection O99.51-
      urethritis O23.2-
      uterine size date discrepancy O26.84-
      vaginitis or vulvitis O23.59-
      varicose veins (lower extremities) O22.0-
         genitals O22.1-
         legs O22.0-
         perineal O22.1-
         vaginal or vulval O22.1-
      venereal disease NEC (conditions in A63.8) O98.31-
      venous disorders O22.9-
         specified NEC O22.8X-

Pregnancy (continued)
   complicated by (continued)
      viral diseases (conditions in A80-B09, B25-B34) O98.51-
      very young mother —see Pregnancy, complicated by, young mother
      vomiting O21.9
         due to diseases classified elsewhere O21.8
         hyperemesis gravidarum (mild) (see also Hyperemesis, gravidarum) O21.0-
         late (occurring after 20 weeks of gestation) O21.2
      young mother
         multigravida O09.62-
         primigravida O09.61-
   concealed O09.3-
   continuing following
      elective fetal reduction of one or more fetus O31.3-
      intrauterine death of one or more fetus O31.2-
      spontaneous abortion of one or more fetus O31.1-
   cornual O00.80
      with intrauterine pregnancy O00.81
   ectopic (ruptured) O00.90
      with intrauterine pregnancy O00.91
      abdominal O00.00
         with
            intrauterine pregnancy O00.01
            viable fetus O36.7-
      cervical O00.80
         with intrauterine pregnancy O00.81
      complicated (by) O08.9
         afibrinogenemia O08.1
         cardiac arrest O08.81
         chemical damage of pelvic organ(s) O08.6
         circulatory collapse O08.3
         defibrination syndrome O08.1
         electrolyte imbalance O08.5
         embolism (amniotic fluid) (blood clot) (pulmonary) (septic) O08.2
         endometritis O08.0
         genital tract and pelvic infection O08.0
         hemorrhage (delayed) (excessive) O08.1
         infection
            genital tract or pelvic O08.0
            kidney O08.83
            urinary tract O08.83
         intravascular coagulation O08.1
         laceration of pelvic organ(s) O08.6
         metabolic disorder O08.5
         oliguria O08.4
         oophoritis O08.0
         parametritis O08.0
         pelvic peritonitis O08.0
         perforation of pelvic organ(s) O08.6
         renal failure or shutdown O08.4
         salpingitis or salpingo-oophoritis O08.0
         sepsis O08.82
         shock O08.83
            septic O08.82
         specified condition NEC O08.89
         tubular necrosis (renal) O08.4
         uremia O08.4
         urinary infection O08.83
         venous complication NEC O08.7
            embolism O08.2

Pregnancy (continued)
   ectopic (continued)
      cornual O00.80
         with intrauterine pregnancy O00.81
      intraligamentous O00.80
         with intrauterine pregnancy O00.81
      mural O00.80
         with intrauterine pregnancy O00.81
      ovarian O00.20-
         with intrauterine pregnancy O00.21-
      specified site NEC O00.80
         with intrauterine pregnancy O00.81
      tubal (ruptured) O00.10-
         with intrauterine pregnancy O00.11-
   examination (normal) Z34.9-
      high-risk —see Pregnancy, supervision of, high-risk
      first Z34.0-
      specified Z34.8-
   extrauterine —see Pregnancy, ectopic
   fallopian O00.10-
      with intrauterine pregnancy O00.11-
   false F45.8
   gestational carrier Z33.3
   heptachorionic, hepta-amniotic (septuplets) O30.83-
   hexachorionic, hexa-amniotic (septuplets) O30.83-
   hidden O09.3-
   high-risk —see Pregnancy, supervision of, high-risk
   incidental finding Z33.1
   interstitial O00.80
      with intrauterine pregnancy O00.81
   intraligamentous O00.80
      with intrauterine pregnancy O00.81
   intramural O00.80
      with intrauterine pregnancy O00.81
   intraperitoneal O00.00
      with intrauterine pregnancy O00.01
   isthmian O00.10-
      with intrauterine pregnancy O00.11-
   mesometric (mural) O00.80
      with intrauterine pregnancy O00.81
   molar NEC O02.0
      complicated (by) O08.9
         afibrinogenemia O08.1
         cardiac arrest O08.81
         chemical damage of pelvic organ(s) O08.6
         circulatory collapse O08.3
         defibrination syndrome O08.1
         electrolyte imbalance O08.5
         embolism (amniotic fluid) (blood clot) (pulmonary) (septic) O08.2
         endometritis O08.0
         genital tract and pelvic infection O08.0
         hemorrhage (delayed) (excessive) O08.1
         infection
            genital tract or pelvic O08.0
            kidney O08.83
            urinary tract O08.83

Pregnancy (continued)
   molar NEC (continued)
      complicated (continued)
         intravascular coagulation O08.1
         laceration of pelvic organ(s) O08.6
         metabolic disorder O08.5
         oliguria O08.4
         oophoritis O08.0
         parametritis O08.0
         pelvic peritonitis O08.0
         perforation of pelvic organ(s) O08.6
         renal failure or shutdown O08.4
         salpingitis or salpingo-oophoritis O08.0
         sepsis O08.82
         shock O08.3
            septic O08.82
         specified condition NEC O08.89
         tubular necrosis (renal) O08.4
         uremia O08.4
         urinary infection O08.83
         venous complication NEC O08.7
            embolism O08.2
      hydatidiform (see also Mole, hydatidiform) O01.9-
   multiple (gestation) O30.9-
      greater than quadruplets —see Pregnancy, multiple (gestation), specified NEC
      specified NEC O30.80-
         with
            two or more monoamniotic fetuses O30.82-
            two or more monochorionic fetuses O30.81-
            number of chorions and amnions are both equal to the number of fetuses O30.83-
            two or more monoamniotic fetuses O30.82-
            two or more monochorionic fetuses O30.81-
            unable to determine number of placenta and number of amniotic sacs O30.89-
            unspecified number of placenta and unspecified number of amniotic sacs O30.80-
   mural O00.80
      with intrauterine pregnancy O00.81
   normal (supervision of) Z34.9-
      high-risk —see Pregnancy, supervision of, high-risk
      first Z34.0-
      specified Z34.8-
   ovarian O00.20-
      with intrauterine pregnancy O00.21-
   pentachorionic, penta-amniotic (quintuplets) O30.83-
   postmature (40 to 42 weeks) O48.0
      more than 42 weeks gestation O48.1
   post-term (40 to 42 weeks) O48.0
   prenatal care only Z34.9-
      high-risk —see Pregnancy, supervision of, high-risk
      first Z34.0-
      specified Z34.8-
   prolonged (more than 42 weeks gestation) O48.1

Pregnancy (continued)
- quadruplet O30.20-
  - with
    - two or more monoamniotic fetuses O30.22-
    - two or more monochorionic fetuses O30.21-
  - quadrachorionic/quadra-amniotic O30.23-
  - two or more monoamniotic fetuses O30.22-
  - two or more monochorionic fetuses O30.21-
  - unable to determine number of placenta and number of amniotic sacs O30.29-
  - unspecified number of placenta and unspecified number of amniotic sacs O30.20-
- quintuplet —*see* Pregnancy, multiple (gestation), specified NEC
- sextuplet —*see* Pregnancy, multiple (gestation), specified NEC
- supervision of
  - concealed pregnancy O09.3-
  - elderly mother
    - multigravida O09.52-
    - primigravida O09.51-
  - hidden pregnancy O09.3-
  - high-risk O09.9-
    - due to (history of)
      - ectopic pregnancy O09.1-
      - elderly —*see* Pregnancy, supervision, elderly mother
      - grand multiparity O09.4
      - infertility O09.0-
      - insufficient prenatal care O09.3-
      - in utero procedure during previous pregnancy O09.82-
      - in vitro fertilization O09.81-
      - molar pregnancy O09.A-
      - multiple previous pregnancies O09.4-
      - older mother —*see* Pregnancy, supervision of, elderly mother
      - poor reproductive or obstetric history NEC O09.29-
      - pre-term labor O09.21-
      - previous neonatal death O09.29-
      - social problems O09.7-
      - specified NEC O09.89-
      - very young mother —*see* Pregnancy, supervision, young mother
  - resulting from in vitro fertilization O09.81-
  - normal Z34.9-
    - first Z34.0-
    - specified NEC Z34.8-
  - young mother
    - multigravida O09.62-
    - primigravida O09.61-
- triplet O30.10-
  - with
    - two or more monoamniotic fetuses O30.12-
    - two or more monochorionic fetuses O30.11-
  - trichorionic/triamniotic O30.13-
  - two or more monoamniotic fetuses O30.12-
  - two or more monochorionic fetuses O30.11-

Pregnancy (continued)
- triplet (continued)
  - unable to determine number of placenta and number of amniotic sacs O30.19-
  - unspecified number of placenta and unspecified number of amniotic sacs O30.10-
- tubal (with abortion) (with rupture) O00.10-
  - with intrauterine pregnancy O00.11-
- twin O30.00-
  - conjoined O30.02-
  - dichorionic/diamniotic (two placenta, two amniotic sacs) O30.04-
  - monochorionic/diamniotic (one placenta, two amniotic sacs) O30.03-
  - monochorionic/monoamniotic (one placenta, one amniotic sac) O30.01-
  - unable to determine number of placenta and number of amniotic sacs O30.09-
  - unspecified number of placenta and unspecified number of amniotic sacs O30.00-
- unwanted Z64.0
- weeks of gestation
  - 8 weeks Z3A.08
  - 9 weeks Z3A.09
  - 10 weeks Z3A.10
  - 11 weeks Z3A.11
  - 12 weeks Z3A.12
  - 13 weeks Z3A.13
  - 14 weeks Z3A.14
  - 15 weeks Z3A.15
  - 16 weeks Z3A.16
  - 17 weeks Z3A.17
  - 18 weeks Z3A.18
  - 19 weeks Z3A.19
  - 20 weeks Z3A.20
  - 21 weeks Z3A.21
  - 22 weeks Z3A.22
  - 23 weeks Z3A.23
  - 24 weeks Z3A.24
  - 25 weeks Z3A.25
  - 26 weeks Z3A.26
  - 27 weeks Z3A.27
  - 28 weeks Z3A.28
  - 29 weeks Z3A.29
  - 30 weeks Z3A.30
  - 31 weeks Z3A.31
  - 32 weeks Z3A.32
  - 33 weeks Z3A.33
  - 34 weeks Z3A.34
  - 35 weeks Z3A.35
  - 36 weeks Z3A.36
  - 37 weeks Z3A.37
  - 38 weeks Z3A.38
  - 39 weeks Z3A.39
  - 40 weeks Z3A.40
  - 41 weeks Z3A.41
  - 42 weeks Z3A.42
  - greater than 42 weeks Z3A.49
  - less than 8 weeks Z3A.01
  - not specified Z3A.00

Preiser's disease —*see* Osteonecrosis, secondary, due to, trauma, metacarpus

Pre-kwashiorkor —*see* Malnutrition, severe

Preleukemia (syndrome) D46.9

Preluxation, hip, congenital Q65.6

Premature —*see also* condition
- adrenarche E27.0
- aging E34.8

Premature (continued)
- beats I49.40
  - atrial I49.1
  - auricular I49.1
  - supraventricular I49.1
- birth NEC —*see* Preterm, newborn
- closure, foramen ovale Q21.8
- contraction
  - atrial I49.1
  - atrioventricular I49.2
  - auricular I49.1
  - auriculoventricular I49.49
  - heart (extrasystole) I49.49
  - junctional I49.2
  - ventricular I49.3
- delivery (*see also* Pregnancy, complicated by, preterm labor) O60.10
- ejaculation F52.4
- infant NEC —*see* Preterm, newborn
  - light-for-dates —*see* Light for dates
- labor —*see* Pregnancy, complicated by, preterm labor
- lungs P28.0
- menopause E28.319
  - asymptomatic E28.319
  - symptomatic E28.310
- newborn
  - extreme (less than 28 completed weeks) —*see* Immaturity, extreme
  - less than 37 completed weeks —*see* Preterm, newborn
- puberty E30.1
- rupture membranes or amnion —*see* Pregnancy, complicated by, premature rupture of membranes
- senility E34.8
- thelarche E30.8
- ventricular systole I49.3

Prematurity NEC (less than 37 completed weeks) —*see* Preterm, newborn
- extreme (less than 28 completed weeks) —*see* Immaturity, extreme

Premenstrual
- dysphoric disorder (PMDD) F32.81
- tension (syndrome) N94.3

Premolarization, cuspids K00.2

Prenatal
- care, normal pregnancy —*see* Pregnancy, normal
- screening of mother (*see also* Encounter, antenatal screening) Z36.9
- teeth K00.6

Preparatory care for subsequent treatment NEC
- for dialysis Z49.01
  - peritoneal Z49.02

Prepartum —*see* condition

Preponderance, left or right ventricular I51.7

Prepuce —*see* condition

PRES (posterior reversible encephalopathy syndrome) I67.83

Presbycardia R54

Presbycusis, presbyacusia H91.1-

Presbyesophagus K22.89

Presbyophrenia F03

Presbyopia H52.4

Prescription of contraceptives
- (initial) Z30.019
- barrier Z30.018

Prescription of contraceptives (continued)
- diaphragm Z30.018
- emergency (postcoital) Z30.012
- implantable subdermal Z30.017
- injectable Z30.013
- intrauterine contraceptive device Z30.014
- pills Z30.011
- postcoital (emergency) Z30.012
- repeat Z30.40
  - barrier Z30.49
  - diaphragm Z30.49
  - implantable subdermal Z30.46
  - injectable Z30.42
  - pills Z30.41
  - specified type NEC Z30.49
  - transdermal patch hormonal Z30.45
  - vaginal ring hormonal Z30.44
- specified type NEC Z30.018
  - transdermal patch hormonal Z30.016
  - vaginal ring hormonal Z30.015

Presence (of)
- ankle-joint implant (functional) (prosthesis) Z96.66-
- aortocoronary (bypass) graft Z95.1
- arterial-venous shunt (dialysis) Z99.2
- artificial
  - eye (globe) Z97.0
  - heart (fully implantable) (mechanical) Z95.812
    - valve Z95.2
  - larynx Z96.3
  - lens (intraocular) Z96.1
  - limb (complete) (partial) Z97.1-
    - arm Z97.1-
      - bilateral Z97.15
    - leg Z97.1-
      - bilateral Z97.16
- audiological implant (functional) Z96.29
- bladder implant (functional) Z96.0
- bone
  - conduction hearing device Z96.29
  - implant (functional) NEC Z96.7
  - joint (prosthesis) —*see* Presence, joint implant
- cardiac
  - defibrillator (functional) (with synchronous cardiac pacemaker) Z95.810
  - implant or graft Z95.9
    - specified type NEC Z95.818
  - pacemaker Z95.0
  - resynchronization therapy
    - defibrillator Z95.810
    - pacemaker Z95.0
- cardioverter-defibrillator (ICD) Z95.810
- cerebrospinal fluid drainage device Z98.2
- cochlear implant (functional) Z96.21
- contact lens (es) Z97.3
- coronary artery graft or prosthesis Z95.5
- CRT-D (cardiac resynchronization therapy defibrillator) Z95.810
- CRT-P (cardiac resynchronization therapy pacemaker) Z95.0
- CSF shunt Z98.2
- dental prosthesis device Z97.2
- dentures Z97.2
- device (external) NEC Z97.8
  - cardiac NEC Z95.818
  - heart assist Z95.811
  - implanted (functional) Z96.9
    - specified NEC Z96.89
  - prosthetic Z97.8

Presence (continued)
  ear implant Z96.20
    cochlear implant Z96.21
    myringotomy tube Z96.22
    specified type NEC Z96.29
  elbow-joint implant (functional) (prosthesis) Z96.62-
  endocrine implant (functional) NEC Z96.49
  eustachian tube stent or device (functional) Z96.29
  external hearing-aid or device Z97.4
  finger-joint implant (functional) (prosthetic) Z96.69-
  functional implant Z96.9
    specified NEC Z96.89
  graft
    cardiac NEC Z95.818
    vascular NEC Z95.828
  hearing-aid or device (external) Z97.4
    implant (bone) (cochlear) (functional) Z96.21
  heart assist device Z95.811
  heart valve implant (functional) Z95.2
    prosthetic Z95.2
    specified type NEC Z95.4
    xenogenic Z95.3
  hip-joint implant (functional) (prosthesis) Z96.64-
  ICD (cardioverter-defibrillator) Z95.810
  implanted device (artificial) (functional) (prosthetic) Z96.9
    automatic cardiac defibrillator (with synchronous cardiac pacemaker) Z95.810
    cardiac pacemaker Z95.0
    cochlear Z96.21
    dental Z96.5
    heart Z95.812
    heart valve Z95.2
      prosthetic Z95.2
      specified NEC Z95.4
      xenogenic Z95.3
    insulin pump Z96.41
    intraocular lens Z96.1
    joint Z96.60
      ankle Z96.66-
      elbow Z96.62-
      finger Z96.69-
      hip Z96.64-
      knee Z96.65-
      shoulder Z96.61-
      specified NEC Z96.698
      wrist Z96.63-
    larynx Z96.3
    myringotomy tube Z96.22
    otological Z96.20
      cochlear Z96.21
      eustachian stent Z96.29
      myringotomy Z96.22
      specified NEC Z96.29
      stapes Z96.29
    skin Z96.81
    skull plate Z96.7
    specified NEC Z96.89
    urogenital Z96.0
  insulin pump (functional) Z96.41
  intestinal bypass or anastomosis Z98.0
  intraocular lens (functional) Z96.1
  intrauterine contraceptive device (IUD) Z97.5
  intravascular implant (functional) (prosthetic) NEC Z95.9
    coronary artery Z95.5
    defibrillator (with synchronous cardiac pacemaker) Z95.810
    peripheral vessel (with angioplasty) Z95.820

Presence (continued)
  joint implant (prosthetic) (any) Z96.60
    ankle —see Presence, ankle joint implant
    elbow —see Presence, elbow joint implant
    finger —see Presence, finger joint implant
    hip —see Presence, hip joint implant
    knee —see Presence, knee joint implant
    shoulder —see Presence, shoulder joint implant
    specified joint NEC Z96.698
    wrist —see Presence, wrist joint implant
  knee-joint implant (functional) (prosthesis) Z96.65-
  laryngeal implant (functional) Z96.3
  mandibular implant (dental) Z96.5
  myringotomy tube(s) Z96.22
  neurostimulator (brain) (gastric) (peripheral nerve) (sacral nerve) (spinal cord) (vagus nerve) Z96.82
  orthopedic-joint implant (prosthetic) (any) —see Presence, joint implant
  otological implant (functional) Z96.29
  shoulder-joint implant (functional) (prosthesis) Z96.61-
  skull-plate implant Z96.7
  spectacles Z97.3
  stapes implant (functional) Z96.29
  systemic lupus erythematosus [SLE] inhibitor D68.62
  tendon implant (functional) (graft) Z96.7
  tooth root(s) implant Z96.5
  ureteral stent Z96.0
  urethral stent Z96.0
  urogenital implant (functional) Z96.0
  vascular implant or device Z95.9
    access port device Z95.828
    specified type NEC Z95.828
  wrist-joint implant (functional) (prosthesis) Z96.63-

Presenile —see also condition
  dementia F03
  premature aging E34.8

Presentation, fetal —see Delivery, complicated by, malposition

Prespondylolisthesis (congenital) Q76.2

Pressure
  area, skin —see Ulcer, pressure, by site
  brachial plexus G54.0
  brain G93.5
    injury at birth NEC P11.1
  cerebral —see Pressure, brain
  chest R07.89
  cone, tentorial G93.5
  hyposystolic —see also Hypotension
    incidental reading, without diagnosis of hypotension R03.1
  increased
    intracranial benign, G93.2
      injury at birth P11.0
    intraocular H40.05-
  injury —see Ulcer, pressure, by site
  lumbosacral plexus G54.1
  mediastinum J98.59
  necrosis (chronic) —see Ulcer, pressure, by site

Pressure (continued)
  parental, inappropriate (excessive) Z62.6
  sore (chronic) —see Ulcer, pressure, by site
  spinal cord G95.20
  ulcer (chronic) —see Ulcer, pressure, by site
  venous, increased I87.8

Pre-syncope R55

Preterm
  delivery (see also Pregnancy, complicated by, preterm labor) O60.10
  labor —see Pregnancy, complicated by, preterm labor
  newborn (infant) P07.30
    gestational age
      28 completed weeks (28 weeks, 0 days through 28 weeks, 6 days) P07.31
      29 completed weeks (29 weeks, 0 days through 29 weeks, 6 days) P07.32
      30 completed weeks (30 weeks, 0 days through 30 weeks, 6 days) P07.33
      31 completed weeks (31 weeks, 0 days through 31 weeks, 6 days) P07.34
      32 completed weeks (32 weeks, 0 days through 32 weeks, 6 days) P07.35
      33 completed weeks (33 weeks, 0 days through 33 weeks, 6 days) P07.36
      34 completed weeks (34 weeks, 0 days through 34 weeks, 6 days) P07.37
      35 completed weeks (35 weeks, 0 days through 35 weeks, 6 days) P07.38
      36 completed weeks (36 weeks, 0 days through 36 weeks, 6 days) P07.39

Previa
  placenta (total) (without hemorrhage) O44.0-
    with hemorrhage O44.1-
    complete O44.0-
      with hemorrhage O44.1-
    low (see also Delivery, complicated, by, placenta, low) O44.4-
      with hemorrhage O44.5-
    marginal O44.2-
      with hemorrhage O44.3-
    partial O44.2-
      with hemorrhage O44.3-
  vasa O69.4

Priapism N48.30
  due to
    disease classified elsewhere N48.32
    drug N48.33
    specified cause NEC N48.39
    trauma N48.31

Prickling sensation (skin) R20.2

Prickly heat L74.0

Primary —see condition

Primigravida
  elderly, affecting management of pregnancy, labor and delivery (supervision only) —see Pregnancy, complicated by, elderly, primigravida

Primigravida (continued)
  older, affecting management of pregnancy, labor and delivery (supervision only) —see Pregnancy, complicated by, elderly, primigravida
  very young, affecting management of pregnancy, labor and delivery (supervision only) —see Pregnancy, complicated by, young mother, primigravida

Primipara
  elderly, affecting management of pregnancy, labor and delivery (supervision only) —see Pregnancy, complicated by, elderly, primigravida
  older, affecting management of pregnancy, labor and delivery (supervision only) —see Pregnancy, complicated by, elderly, primigravida
  very young, affecting management of pregnancy, labor and delivery (supervision only) —see Pregnancy, complicated by, young mother, primigravida

Primus varus Q66.21-

PRIND (Prolonged reversible ischemic neurologic deficit) I63.9

Pringle's disease (tuberous sclerosis) Q85.1

Prinzmetal angina I20.1

Prizefighter ear —see Cauliflower ear

Problem (with) (related to)
  academic Z55.8
  acculturation Z60.3
  adjustment (to)
    change of job Z56.1
    life-cycle transition Z60.0
    pension Z60.0
    retirement Z60.0
  adopted child Z62.821
  alcoholism in family Z63.72
  atypical parenting situation Z62.9
  bankruptcy Z59.89
  behavioral (adult) F69
    drug seeking Z76.5
  birth of sibling affecting child Z62.898
  care (of)
    provider dependency Z74.9
      specified NEC Z74.8
    sick or handicapped person in family or household Z63.6
  child
    abuse (affecting the child) —see Maltreatment, child
    custody or support proceedings Z65.3
    in
      care of non-parental family member Z62.23
      custody of
        grandparent Z62.23
        non-parental relative Z62.23
        non-relative guardian Z62.24
      foster care Z62.21
      kinship care Z62.23
      welfare
        custody Z62.21
        guardianship Z62.21
    leaving living situation without permission Z62.892
    living in
      group home Z62.22
      orphanage Z62.22

Problem *(continued)*
  child-rearing Z62.9
    specified NEC Z62.898
  communication (developmental) F80.9
  completing medical forms Z55.6
  conflict or discord (with)
    boss Z56.4
    classmates Z55.4
    counselor Z64.4
    employer Z56.4
    family Z63.9
      specified NEC Z63.8
    probation officer Z64.4
    social worker Z64.4
    teachers Z55.4
    workmates Z56.4
  conviction in legal proceedings Z65.0
    with imprisonment Z65.1
  counselor Z64.4
  creditors Z59.89
  digestive K92.9
  drug addict in family Z63.72
  ear —*see* Disorder, ear
  economic Z59.9
    affecting care Z59.9
    specified NEC Z59.89
    strain Z59.86
  education Z55.9
    specified NEC Z55.8
  employment Z56.9
    change of job Z56.1
    discord Z56.4
    environment Z56.5
    sexual harassment Z56.81
    specified NEC Z56.89
    stress NEC Z56.6
    stressful schedule Z56.3
    threat of job loss Z56.2
    unemployment Z56.0
  enuresis, child F98.0
  eye H57.9
  failed examinations (school) Z55.2
  falling Z91.81
  family (*see also* Disruption, family) Z63.9-
    specified NEC Z63.8
  feeding (elderly) (infant) NOS R63.39
    newborn P92.9
      breast P92.5
      overfeeding P92.4
      slow P92.2
      specified NEC P92.8
      underfeeding P92.3
    nonorganic F50.89
  finance Z59.9
    specified NEC Z59.89
  foreclosure on loan Z59.89
  foster child Z62.822
  frightening experience(s) in childhood Z62.898
  genital NEC
    female N94.9
    male N50.9
  health care Z75.9
    specified NEC Z75.8
  health literacy Z55.6
  hearing —*see* Deafness
  homelessness Z59.00
  housing Z59.9
    inadequate Z59.10
    isolated Z59.89
    specified NEC Z59.89
  identity (of childhood) F93.8
  illegitimate pregnancy (unwanted) Z64.0
  illiteracy Z55.0
  impaired mobility Z74.09
  imprisonment or incarceration Z65.1

Problem *(continued)*
  inadequate teaching affecting education Z55.8
  inappropriate (excessive) parental pressure Z62.6
  influencing health status NEC Z78.9
  in-law Z63.1
  institutionalization, affecting child Z62.22
  intrafamilial communication Z63.8
  jealousy, child F93.8
  landlord Z59.2
  language (developmental) F80.9
  learning (developmental) F81.9
  legal Z65.3
    conviction without imprisonment Z65.0
    imprisonment Z65.1
    release from prison Z65.2
  life-management Z73.9
    specified NEC Z73.89
  life-style Z72.9
    gambling Z72.6
    high-risk sexual behavior (heterosexual) Z72.51
      bisexual Z72.53
      homosexual Z72.52
    inappropriate eating habits Z72.4
    self-damaging behavior NEC Z72.89
    specified NEC Z72.89
    tobacco use Z72.0
  literacy Z55.9
    low level Z55.0
    specified NEC Z55.8
  living alone Z60.2
  lodgers Z59.2
  loss of love relationship in childhood Z62.898
  marital Z63.0
    involving
      divorce Z63.5
      estrangement Z63.5
      gender identity F66
  mastication K08.89
  medical
    care, within family Z63.6
    facilities Z75.9
      specified NEC Z75.8
  mental F48.9
  money Z59.86
  multiparity Z64.1
  negative life events in childhood Z62.9
    altered pattern of family relationships Z62.898
    frightening experience Z62.898
    loss of
      love relationship Z62.898
      self-esteem Z62.898
    physical abuse (alleged) —*see* Maltreatment, child
    removal from home Z62.29
    specified event NEC Z62.898
  neighbor Z59.2
  neurological NEC R29.818
  new step-parent affecting child Z62.898
  none (feared complaint unfounded) Z71.1
  occupational NEC Z56.89
  parent-child —*see* Conflict, parent-child
  personal hygiene Z91.89
  personality F69
  phase-of-life transition, adjustment Z60.0
  presence of sick or disabled person in family or household Z63.79
    needing care Z63.6

Problem *(continued)*
  primary support group (family) Z63.9
    specified NEC Z63.8
  probation officer Z64.4
  psychiatric F99
  psychosexual (development) F66
  psychosocial Z65.9
    religious or spiritual Z65.8
    specified NEC Z65.8
  related to physical environment, specified NEC Z58.89
  relationship Z63.9
    childhood F93.8
  release from prison Z65.2
    religious or spiritual Z65.8
  removal from home affecting child Z62.29
  seeking and accepting known hazardous and harmful
    behavioral or psychological interventions Z65.8
    chemical, nutritional or physical interventions Z65.8
  sexual function (nonorganic) F52.9
  sight H54.7
  sleep disorder, child F51.9
  smell —*see* Disturbance, sensation, smell
  social
    environment Z60.9
      specified NEC Z60.8
    exclusion and rejection Z60.4
    worker Z64.4
  speech R47.9
    developmental F80.9
    specified NEC R47.89
  swallowing —*see* Dysphagia
  taste —*see* Disturbance, sensation, taste
  tic, child F95.0
  underachievement in school Z55.3
  unemployment Z56.0
    threatened Z56.2
  unwanted pregnancy Z64.0
  upbringing Z62.9
    specified NEC Z62.898
  urinary N39.9
  voice production R47.89
  work schedule (stressful) Z56.3
Procedure (surgical)
  converted
    arthroscopic to open Z53.33
    laparoscopic to open Z53.31
    specified procedure NEC to open Z53.39
    thoracoscopic to open Z53.32
  for purpose other than remedying health state Z41.9
    specified NEC Z41.8
  not done Z53.9
    because of
      administrative reasons Z53.8
      contraindication Z53.09
        smoking Z53.01
      patient's decision Z53.20
        for reasons of belief or group pressure Z53.1
        left against medical advice (AMA) Z53.29
        left without being seen Z53.21
        specified reason NEC Z53.29
      specified reason NEC Z53.8
Procidentia (uteri) N81.3
Proctalgia K62.89
  fugax K59.4
  spasmodic K59.4
Proctitis K62.89
  amebic (acute) A06.0
  chlamydial A56.3
  gonococcal A54.6

Proctitis *(continued)*
  granulomatous —*see* Enteritis, regional, large intestine
  herpetic A60.1
  radiation K62.7
  tuberculous A18.32
  ulcerative (chronic) K51.20
    with
      complication K51.219
        abscess K51.214
        fistula K51.213
        obstruction K51.212
        rectal bleeding K51.211
        specified NEC K51.218
Proctocele
  female (without uterine prolapse) N81.6
    with uterine prolapse N81.2
      complete N81.3
  male K62.3
Proctocolitis
  allergic K52.29
  food-induced eosinophilic K52.29
  food protein-induced K52.29
  mild protein-induced K52.29
  mucosal —*see* Rectosigmoiditis, ulcerative
Proctoptosis K62.3
Proctorrhagia K62.5
Proctosigmoiditis K63.89
  ulcerative (chronic) —*see* Rectosigmoiditis, ulcerative
Proctospasm K59.4
  psychogenic F45.8
Profichet's disease —*see* Disorder, soft tissue, specified type NEC
Progeria E34.8
Prognathism (mandibular) (maxillary) M26.19
Progonoma (melanotic) —*see* Neoplasm, benign, by site
Progressive —*see* condition
Prolactinoma
  specified site —*see* Neoplasm, benign, by site
  unspecified site D35.2
Prolapse, prolapsed
  anus, anal (canal) (sphincter) K62.2
  arm or hand O32.2
    causing obstructed labor O64.4
  bladder (mucosa) (sphincter) (acquired)
    congenital Q79.4
    female —*see* Cystocele
    male N32.89
  breast implant (prosthetic) T85.49
  cecostomy K94.09
  cecum K63.4
  cervix, cervical (hypertrophied) N81.2
    anterior lip, obstructing labor O65.5
    congenital Q51.828
    postpartal, old N81.2
    stump N81.85
  ciliary body (traumatic) —*see* Laceration, eye (ball), with prolapse or loss of interocular tissue
  colon (pedunculated) K63.4
  colostomy K94.09
  disc (intervertebral) —*see* Displacement, intervertebral disc
  eye implant (orbital) T85.398
    lens (ocular) —*see* Complications, intraocular lens

Prolapse, prolapsed *(continued)*
  fallopian tube N83.4-
  gastric (mucosa) K31.89
  genital, female N81.9
    specified NEC N81.89
  globe, nontraumatic —*see*
    Luxation, globe
  ileostomy bud K94.19
  intervertebral disc —*see*
    Displacement, intervertebral disc
  intestine (small) K63.4
  iris (traumatic) —*see* Laceration,
    eye (ball), with prolapse or loss
    of interocular tissue
    nontraumatic H21.89
  kidney N28.83
    congenital Q63.2
  laryngeal muscles or ventricle J38.7
  liver K76.89
  meatus urinarius N36.8
  mitral (valve) I34.1
  ocular lens implant —*see*
    Complications, intraocular lens
  organ or site, congenital NEC
    —*see* Malposition, congenital
  ovary N83.4-
  pelvic floor, female N81.89
  perineum, female N81.89
  rectum (mucosa) (sphincter) K62.3
    due to trichuris trichuria B79
  spleen D73.89
  stomach K31.89
  umbilical cord
    complicating delivery O69.0
  urachus, congenital Q64.4
  ureter N28.89
    with obstruction N13.5
      with infection N13.6
  ureterovesical orifice N28.89
  urethra (acquired) (infected)
    (mucosa) N36.8
    congenital Q64.71
  urinary meatus N36.8
    congenital Q64.72
  uterovaginal N81.4
    complete N81.3
    incomplete N81.2
  uterus (with prolapse of vagina) N81.4
    complete N81.3
    congenital Q51.818
    first degree N81.2
    in pregnancy or childbirth —*see*
      Pregnancy, complicated by,
      abnormal, uterus
    incomplete N81.2
    postpartal (old) N81.4
    second degree N81.2
    third degree N81.3
  uveal (traumatic) —*see* Laceration,
    eye (ball), with prolapse or loss
    of interocular tissue
  vagina (anterior) (wall) —*see*
    Cystocele
    with prolapse of uterus N81.4
      complete N81.3
      incomplete N81.2
    posterior wall N81.6
    posthysterectomy N99.3
  vitreous (humor) H43.0-
    in wound —*see* Laceration, eye
      (ball), with prolapse or loss of
      interocular tissue
  womb —*see* Prolapse, uterus

Prolapsus, female N81.9
  specified NEC N81.89

Proliferation(s)
  primary cutaneous CD30-positive
    large T-cell C86.6
  prostate, atypical small acinar
    N42.32

Proliferative —*see* condition

Prolonged, prolongation (of)
  bleeding (time) (idiopathic) R79.1
  coagulation (time) R79.1
  gestation (over 42 completed
    weeks)
    mother O48.1
    newborn P08.22
  interval I44.0
  labor O63.9
    first stage O63.0
    second stage O63.1
  partial thromboplastin time (PTT)
    R79.1
  pregnancy (more than 42 weeks
    gestation) O48.1
  prothrombin time R79.1
  QT interval R94.31
  uterine contractions in labor O62.4

Prominence, prominent
  auricle (congenital) (ear) Q17.5
  ischial spine or sacral
    promontory
    with disproportion (fetopelvic)
      O33.0
      causing obstructed labor O65.0
  nose (congenital) acquired M95.0

Promiscuity —*see* High, risk, sexual
  behavior

Pronation
  ankle —*see* Deformity, limb, foot,
    specified NEC
  foot —*see also* Deformity, limb,
    foot, specified NEC
    congenital Q74.2

Prophylactic
  administration of
    antibiotics, long-term Z79.2
      short-term use - omit code
    drug (*see also* Long-term
      (current) drug therapy (use
      of)) Z79.899-
    medication Z79.899
  organ removal (for neoplasia
    management) Z40.00
    breast Z40.01
    fallopian tube(s) Z40.03
      with ovary(s) Z40.02
    ovary(s) Z40.02
    specified site NEC Z40.09
  surgery Z40.9
    for risk factors related to
      malignant neoplasm —*see*
      Prophylactic, organ removal
    specified NEC Z40.8
  vaccination Z23

Propionic acidemia E71.121

Proptosis (ocular) —*see also*
  Exophthalmos
  thyroid —*see* Hyperthyroidism,
    with goiter

Prosecution, anxiety concerning
  Z65.3

Prosopagnosia R48.3

Prostadynia N42.81

Prostate, prostatic —*see* condition

Prostatism —*see* Hyperplasia,
  prostate

Prostatitis (congestive) (suppurative)
  (with cystitis) N41.9
  acute N41.0
  cavitary N41.8
  chronic N41.1
  diverticular N41.8
  due to Trichomonas (vaginalis)
    A59.02
  fibrous N41.1

Prostatitis *(continued)*
  gonococcal (acute) (chronic)
    A54.22
  granulomatous N41.4
  hypertrophic N41.1
  subacute N41.1
  trichomonal A59.02
  tuberculous A18.14

Prostatocystitis N41.3

Prostatorrhea N42.89

Prostatosis N42.82

Prostration R53.83
  heat —*see also* Heat, exhaustion
    anhydrotic T67.3
    due to
      salt (and water) depletion
        T67.4
      water depletion T67.3
  nervous F48.8
  senile R54

Protanomaly (anomalous trichromat)
  H53.54

Protanopia (complete) (incomplete)
  H53.54

Protection (against) (from) —*see*
  Prophylactic

Protein
  deficiency NEC —*see* Malnutrition
  malnutrition —*see* Malnutrition
  sickness (*see also* Reaction, serum)
    T80.69

Proteinemia R77.9

Proteinosis
  alveolar (pulmonary) J84.01
  lipid or lipoid (of Urbach) E78.89

Proteinuria R80.9
  Bence Jones R80.3
  complicating pregnancy —*see*
    Proteinuria, gestational
  gestational
    complicating
      childbirth O12.14
      pregnancy O12.1-
        with edema O12.2-
      puerperium O12.15
  idiopathic R80.0
  isolated R80.0
    with glomerular lesion N06.9
      C3
      glomerulonephritis N06.A
      glomerulopathy N06.A
        with dense deposit
          disease N06.6
      dense deposit disease N06.6
      diffuse
        crescentic
          glomerulonephritis N06.7
        endocapillary proliferative
          glomerulonephritis N06.4
        mesangiocapillary
          glomerulonephritis N06.5
      focal and segmental hyalinosis
        or sclerosis N06.1
      membranous (diffuse)
        (*see also* Nephropathy,
        membranous) N06.20
        with diffuse membranous
          glomerulonephritis
          N06.29
      mesangial proliferative
        (diffuse) N06.3
      minimal change N06.0
      specified pathology NEC N06.8
  orthostatic R80.2
    with glomerular lesion —*see*
      Proteinuria, isolated, with
      glomerular lesion

Proteinuria *(continued)*
  persistent R80.1
    with glomerular lesion —*see*
      Proteinuria, isolated, with
      glomerular lesion
  postural R80.2
    with glomerular lesion —*see*
      Proteinuria, isolated, with
      glomerular lesion
  pre-eclamptic —*see* Pre-eclampsia
  puerperal O12.15
  specified type NEC R80.8

Proteolysis, pathologic D65

Proteus (mirabilis) (morganii), **as
cause of disease classified
elsewhere** B96.4

Prothrombin gene mutation
  D68.52

Protoporphyria, erythropoietic E80.0

Protozoal —*see also* condition
  disease B64
    specified NEC B60.8

Protrusion, protrusio
  acetabuli M24.7
  acetabulum (into pelvis) M24.7
  device, implant or graft (*see also*
    Complications, by site and type,
    mechanical) T85.698
    arterial graft NEC —*see*
      Complication, cardiovascular
      device, mechanical, vascular
    breast (implant) T85.49
    catheter NEC T85.698
      cystostomy T83.090
      dialysis (renal) T82.49
        intraperitoneal T85.691
      infusion NEC T82.594
        spinal (epidural) (subdural)
          T85.690
      urinary (*see also*
        Complications, catheter,
        urinary), T83.098
    electronic (electrode) (pulse
      generator) (stimulator)
      bone T84.390
      nervous system —*see*
        Complication, prosthetic
        device, mechanical,
        electronic nervous system
        stimulator
    fixation, internal (orthopedic)
      NEC —*see* Complication,
      fixation device, mechanical
    gastrointestinal —*see*
      Complications, prosthetic
      device, mechanical,
      gastrointestinal device
    genital NEC T83.498
      intrauterine contraceptive
        device T83.39
      penile prosthesis (cylinder)
        (implanted) (pump)
        (resevoir) T83.490
      testicular prosthesis T83.491
    heart NEC —*see* Complication,
      cardiovascular device,
      mechanical
    joint prosthesis —*see*
      Complications, joint
      prosthesis, mechanical,
      specified NEC, by site
    ocular NEC —*see* Complications,
      prosthetic device, mechanical,
      ocular device
    orthopedic NEC —*see*
      Complication, orthopedic,
      device, mechanical
    specified NEC T85.628

279

Protrusion, protrusio (continued)
  device, implant or graft (continued)
    urinary NEC —see also
      Complication, genitourinary, device, urinary, mechanical graft T83.29
    vascular NEC —see
      Complication, cardiovascular device, mechanical
    ventricular intracranial shunt T85.09
  intervertebral disc —see
    Displacement, intervertebral disc
  joint prosthesis —see
    Complications, joint prosthesis, mechanical, specified NEC, by site
  nucleus pulposus —see
    Displacement, intervertebral disc

Prune belly (syndrome) Q79.4

Prurigo (ferox) (gravis) (Hebrae) (Hebra's) (mitis) (simplex) L28.2
  Besnier's L20.0
  estivalis L56.4
  nodularis L28.1
  psychogenic F45.8

Pruritus, pruritic (essential) L29.9
  ani, anus L29.0
    psychogenic F45.8
  anogenital L29.3
    psychogenic F45.8
  due to onchocerca volvulus B73.1
  gravidarum —see Pregnancy, complicated by, specified pregnancy-related condition NEC
  hiemalis L29.8
  neurogenic (any site) F45.8
  perianal L29.0
  psychogenic (any site) F45.8
  scroti, scrotum L29.1
    psychogenic F45.8
  senile, senilis L29.8
  specified NEC L29.8
    psychogenic F45.8
  Trichomonas A59.9
  vulva, vulvae L29.2
    psychogenic F45.8

Pseudarthrosis, pseudoarthrosis
  (bone) —see Nonunion, fracture
  clavicle, congenital Q74.0
  joint, following fusion or arthrodesis M96.0

Pseudoaneurysm —see Aneurysm

Pseudoangioma I81

Pseudoangina (pectoris) —see Angina

Pseudoarteriosus Q28.8

Pseudoarthrosis —see Pseudarthrosis

Pseudobulbar affect (PBA) F48.2

Pseudochromhidrosis L67.8

Pseudocirrhosis, liver, pericardial I31.1

Pseudocowpox B08.03

Pseudocoxalgia M91.3-

Pseudocroup J38.5

Pseudo-Cushing's syndrome, alcohol-induced E24.4

Pseudocyesis F45.8

Pseudocyst
  lung J98.4
  pancreas K86.3
  retina —see Cyst, retina

Pseudoelephantiasis neuroarthritica Q82.0

Pseudoexfoliation, capsule (lens) —see Cataract, specified NEC

Pseudofolliculitis barbae L73.1

Pseudoglioma H44.89

Pseudohemophilia (Bernuth's) (hereditary) (type B) —see Disease, von Willebrand
  Type A D69.8
  vascular D69.8

Pseudohermaphroditism Q56.3
  adrenal E25.8
  female (see also Disorder, adrenogenital) Q56.2
    with adrenocortical disorder E25.8
    without adrenocortical disorder Q56.2
    adrenal (congenital) E25.0
  male (see also Disorder, adrenogenital) Q56.1
    with
      adrenocortical disorder E25.8
      androgen resistance E34.51
      cleft scrotum Q56.1
      feminizing testis E34.51
      5-alpha-reductase deficiency E29.1
    without gonadal disorder Q56.1
    adrenal E25.8

Pseudo-Hurler's polydystrophy E77.0

Pseudohydrocephalus G93.2

Pseudohypertrophic muscular dystrophy (Erb's) G71.02

Pseudohypertrophy, muscle (see also Dystrophy, muscular, by type, if applicable) G71.09

Pseudohypoparathyroidism E20.1

Pseudoinsomnia F51.03

Pseudoleukemia, infantile D64.89

Pseudomembranous —see condition

Pseudomenses (newborn) P54.6

Pseudomenstruation (newborn) P54.6

Pseudomeningocele (cerebral) (infective) (post-traumatic) G96.198
  postprocedural (spinal) G97.82

Pseudomonas
  aeruginosa, as cause of disease classified elsewhere B96.5
  mallei infection A24.0
    as cause of disease classified elsewhere B96.5
  pseudomallei, as cause of disease classified elsewhere B96.5

Pseudomyotonia G71.19

Pseudomyxoma peritonei C78.6

Pseudoneuritis, optic (nerve) (disc) (papilla), congenital Q14.2

Pseudo-obstruction intestine (acute) (chronic) (idiopathic) (intermittent secondary) (primary) K59.89
  colonic K59.81

Pseudopapilledema H47.33-
  congenital Q14.2

Pseudoparalysis
  arm or leg R29.818
  atonic, congenital P94.2

Pseudopelade L66.0

Pseudophakia Z96.1

Pseudopolyarthritis, rhizomelic M35.3

Pseudopolycythemia D75.1

Pseudopseudohypoparathyroidism E20.1

Pseudopterygium H11.81-

Pseudoptosis (eyelid) —see Blepharochalasis

Pseudopuberty, precocious
  female heterosexual E25.8
  male isosexual E25.8

Pseudorickets (renal) N25.0

Pseudorubella B08.20

Pseudosclerema, newborn P83.88

Pseudosclerosis (brain)
  of Westphal (Strümpell) E83.01
  Jakob's —see Creutzfeldt-Jakob disease or syndrome
  spastic —see Creutzfeldt-Jakob disease or syndrome

Pseudotetanus —see Convulsions

Pseudotetany R29.0
  hysterical F44.5

Pseudotruncus arteriosus Q25.49

Pseudotuberculosis A28.2
  enterocolitis A04.8
  pasteurella (infection) A28.0

Pseudotumor G93.2
  cerebri G93.2
  orbital H05.11-

Pseudoxanthoma elasticum Q82.8

Psilosis (sprue) (tropical) K90.1
  nontropical K90.0

Psittacosis A70

Psoitis M60.88

Psoriasis L40.9
  arthropathic L40.50
    arthritis mutilans L40.52
    distal interphalangeal L40.51
    juvenile L40.54
    other specified L40.59
    spondylitis L40.53
  buccal K13.29
  flexural L40.8
  guttate L40.4
  mouth K13.29
  nummular L40.0
  plaque L40.0
  psychogenic F54
  pustular (generalized) L40.1
    palmaris et plantaris L40.3
  specified NEC L40.8
  vulgaris L40.0

Psychasthenia F48.8

Psychiatric disorder or problem F99

Psychogenic —see also condition
  factors associated with physical conditions F54

Psychological and behavioral factors affecting medical condition F59

Psychoneurosis, psychoneurotic —see also Neurosis
  anxiety (state) F41.1
  depersonalization F48.1
  hypochondriacal F45.21
  hysteria F44.9
  neurasthenic F48.8
  personality NEC F60.89

Psychopathy, psychopathic
  affectionless F94.2
  autistic F84.5
  constitution, post-traumatic F07.81
  personality —see Disorder, personality
  sexual —see Deviation, sexual
  state F60.2

Psychosexual identity disorder of childhood F64.2

Psychosis, psychotic F29
  acute (transient) F23
    hysterical F44.9
  affective —see Disorder, mood
  alcoholic F10.959
    with
      abuse F10.159
      anxiety disorder F10.980
        with
          abuse F10.180
          dependence F10.280
      delirium tremens F10.231
      delusions F10.950
        with
          abuse F10.150
          dependence F10.250
      dementia F10.97
        with dependence F10.27
      dependence F10.259
      hallucinosis F10.951
        with
          abuse F10.151
          dependence F10.251
      mood disorder F10.94
        with
          abuse F10.14
          dependence F10.24
      paranoia F10.950
        with
          abuse F10.150
          dependence F10.250
      persisting amnesia F10.96
        with dependence F10.26
      amnestic confabulatory F10.96
        with dependence F10.26
      delirium tremens F10.231
      Korsakoff's, Korsakov's, Korsakow's F10.26
      paranoid type F10.950
        with
          abuse F10.150
          dependence F10.250
  anergastic —see Psychosis, organic
  arteriosclerotic (simple type) (uncomplicated) (see also Dementia, vascular) F01.50
    with behavioral disturbance —see Dementia, vascular
  childhood F84.0
    atypical F84.8
  climacteric —see Psychosis, involutional
  confusional F29
    acute or subacute F05
    reactive F23
  cycloid F23
  depressive —see Disorder, depressive
  disintegrative (childhood) F84.3
  drug-induced —see F11-F19 with .x59
    paranoid and hallucinatory states —see F11-F19 with .x50 or .x51
  due to or associated with
    addiction, drug —see F11-F19 with .x59
    dependence
      alcohol F10.259
      drug —see F11-F19 with .x59
    epilepsy F06.8
    Huntington's chorea F06.8
    ischemia, cerebrovascular (generalized) F06.8
    multiple sclerosis F06.8
    physical disease F06.8
    presenile dementia F03
    senile dementia F03

Psychosis, psychotic *(continued)*
  due to or associated with *(continued)*
    vascular disease (arteriosclerotic) (cerebral) *(see also* Dementia, vascular) F01.50
      with behavioral disturbance — *see* Dementia, vascular
  epileptic F06.8
  episode F23
    due to or associated with physical condition F06.8
  exhaustive F43.0
  hallucinatory, chronic F28
  hypomanic F30.8
  hysterical (acute) F44.9
  induced F24
  infantile F84.0
    atypical F84.8
  infective (acute) (subacute) F05
  involutional F28
    depressive —*see* Disorder, depressive
    melancholic —*see* Disorder, depressive
    paranoid (state) F22
  Korsakoff's, Korsakov's, Korsakow's (nonalcoholic) F04
    alcoholic F10.96
      in dependence F10.26
    induced by other psychoactive substance —*see* categories F11-F19 with .x5x
  mania, manic (single episode) F30.2
    recurrent type F31.89
  manic-depressive —*see* Disorder, bipolar
  menopausal —*see* Psychosis, involutional
  mixed schizophrenic and affective F25.8
  multi-infarct (cerebrovascular) *(see also* Dementia, vascular) F01.50
    with behavioral disturbance — *see* Dementia, vascular
  nonorganic F29
    specified NEC F28
  organic F09
    due to or associated with
      arteriosclerosis (cerebral) —*see* Psychosis, arteriosclerotic
      cerebrovascular disease, arteriosclerotic —*see* Psychosis, arteriosclerotic
      childbirth —*see* Psychosis, puerperal
      Creutzfeldt-Jakob disease or syndrome —*see* Creutzfeldt-Jakob disease or syndrome
      dependence, alcohol F10.259
      disease
        alcoholic liver F10.259
        brain, arteriosclerotic —*see* Psychosis, arteriosclerotic
        cerebrovascular *(see also* Dementia, vascular) F01.50
          with behavioral disturbance —*see* Dementia, vascular
        Creutzfeldt-Jakob —*see* Creutzfeldt-Jakob disease or syndrome
        endocrine or metabolic F06.8
          acute or subacute F05
        liver, alcoholic F10.259
      epilepsy transient (acute) F05

Psychosis, psychotic *(continued)*
  organic *(continued)*
    due to or associated with *(continued)*
      infection
        brain (intracranial) F06.8
          acute or subacute F05
      intoxication
        alcoholic (acute) F10.259
        drug F11-F19 with .x59
      ischemia, cerebrovascular (generalized) —*see* Psychosis, arteriosclerotic
      puerperium —*see* Psychosis, puerperal
      trauma, brain (birth) (from electric current) (surgical) F06.8
        acute or subacute F05
    infective F06.8
      acute or subacute F05
    post-traumatic F06.8
      acute or subacute F05
  paranoiac F22
  paranoid (climacteric) (involutional) (menopausal) F22
    psychogenic (acute) F23
    schizophrenic F20.0
    senile F03
  postpartum (NOS) F53.1
  presbyophrenic (type) F03
  presenile F03
  psychogenic (paranoid) F23
    depressive (NOS) F32.3
  puerperal F53
    specified type —*see* Psychosis, by type
  reactive (brief) (transient) (emotional stress) (psychological trauma) F23
    depressive F32.3
      recurrent F33.3
    excitative type F30.8
  schizoaffective F25.9
    depressive type F25.1
    manic type F25.0
  schizophrenia, schizophrenic —*see* Schizophrenia
  schizophrenia-like, in epilepsy F06.2
  schizophreniform F20.81
    affective type F25.9
    brief F23
    confusional type F23
    mixed type F25.0
  senile NEC F03
    depressed or paranoid type F03
    simple deterioration F03
    specified type - code to condition
  shared F24
  situational (reactive) F23
  symbiotic (childhood) F84.3
  symptomatic F09

Psychosomatic —*see* Disorder, psychosomatic

Psychosyndrome, organic F07.9

Psychotic episode due to or associated with physical condition F06.8

Pterygium (eye) H11.00-
  amyloid H11.01-
  central H11.02-
  colli Q18.3
  double H11.03-
  peripheral
    progressive H11.05-
    stationary H11.04-
  recurrent H11.06-

Ptilosis (eyelid) —*see* Madarosis

Ptomaine (poisoning) —*see* Poisoning, food

Ptosis —*see also* Blepharoptosis
  adiposa (false) —*see* Blepharoptosis
  breast N64.81
  brow H57.81-
  cecum K63.4
  colon K63.4
  congenital (eyelid) Q10.0
    specified site NEC —*see* Anomaly, by site
  eyebrow H57.81-
  eyelid —*see* Blepharoptosis
    congenital Q10.0
  gastric K31.89
  intestine K63.4
  kidney N28.83
  liver K76.89
  renal N28.83
  splanchnic K63.4
  spleen D73.89
  stomach K31.89
  viscera K63.4

PTP D69.51

Ptyalism (periodic) K11.7
  hysterical F45.8
  pregnancy —*see* Pregnancy, complicated by, specified pregnancy-related condition NEC
  psychogenic F45.8

Ptyalolithiasis K11.5

Pubarche, precocious E30.1

Pubertas praecox E30.1

Puberty (development state) Z00.3
  bleeding (excessive) N92.2
  delayed E30.0
  precocious (constitutional) (cryptogenic) (idiopathic) E30.1
    central E22.8
    due to
      ovarian hyperfunction E28.1
        estrogen E28.0
      testicular hyperfunction E29.0
  premature E30.1
    due to
      adrenal cortical hyperfunction E25.8
      pineal tumor E34.8
      pituitary (anterior) hyperfunction E22.8

Puckering, macula —*see* Degeneration, macula, puckering

Pudenda, pudendum —*see* condition

Puente's disease (simple glandular cheilitis) K13.0

Puerperal, puerperium (complicated by, complications)
  abnormal glucose (tolerance test) O99.815
  abscess
    areola O91.02
      associated with lactation O91.03
    Bartholin's gland O86.19
    breast O91.12
      associated with lactation O91.13
    cervix (uteri) O86.11
    genital organ NEC O86.19
    kidney O86.21
    mammary O91.12
      associated with lactation O91.13
    nipple O91.02
      associated with lactation O91.03
    peritoneum O85

Puerperal, puerperium *(continued)*
  abscess *(continued)*
    subareolar O91.12
      associated with lactation O91.13
    urinary tract —*see* Puerperal, infection, urinary
    uterus O86.12
    vagina (wall) O86.13
    vaginorectal O86.13
    vulvovaginal gland O86.13
  adnexitis O86.19
  afibrinogenemia, or other coagulation defect O72.3
  albuminuria (acute) (subacute) —*see* Proteinuria, gestational
  alcohol use O99.315
  anemia O90.81
    pre-existing (pre-pregnancy) O99.03
  anesthetic death O89.8
  apoplexy O99.43
  bariatric surgery status O99.845
  blood disorder NEC O99.13
  blood dyscrasia O72.3
  cardiomyopathy O90.3
  cerebrovascular disorder (conditions in I60-I69) O99.43
  cervicitis O86.11
  circulatory system disorder O99.43
  coagulopathy (any) O99.13
    with hemorrhage O72.3
  complications O90.9
    specified NEC O90.89
  convulsions —*see* Eclampsia
  cystitis O86.22
  cystopyelitis O86.29
  delirium NEC F05
  diabetes O24.93
    gestational —*see* Puerperal, gestational diabetes
    pre-existing O24.33
      specified NEC O24.83
      type 1 O24.03
      type 2 O24.13
  digestive system disorder O99.63
  disease O90.9
    breast NEC O92.29
    cerebrovascular (acute) O99.43
    nonobstetric NEC O99.893
    tubo-ovarian O86.19
    Valsuani's O99.03
  disorder O90.9
    biliary tract O26.63
    lactation O92.70
    liver O26.63
    nonobstetric NEC O99.893
  disruption
    cesarean wound O90.0
    episiotomy wound O90.1
    perineal laceration wound O90.1
  drug use O99.325
  eclampsia (with pre-existing hypertension) O15.2
  embolism (pulmonary) (blood clot) —*see* Embolism, obstetric, puerperal
  endocrine, nutritional or metabolic disease NEC O99.285
  endophlebitis —*see* Puerperal, phlebitis
  endotrachelitis O86.11
  failure
    lactation (complete) O92.3
      partial O92.4
    renal, acute O90.49
  fever (of unknown origin) O86.4
    septic O85
  fissure, nipple O92.12
    associated with lactation O92.13

281

Puerperal, puerperium (continued)
  fistula
    breast (due to mastitis) O91.12
      associated with lactation O91.13
    nipple O91.02
      associated with lactation O91.03
  galactophoritis O91.22
    associated with lactation O91.23
  galactorrhea O92.6
  gastric banding status O99.845
  gastric bypass status O99.845
  gastrointestinal disease NEC O99.63
  gestational
    diabetes O24.439
      diet controlled O24.430
      insulin (and diet) controlled O24.434
      oral drug controlled (antidiabetic) (hypoglycemic) O24.435
    edema O12.05
      with proteinuria O12.25
    proteinuria O12.15
  gonorrhea O98.23
  hematoma, subdural O99.43
  hemiplegia, cerebral O99.355
    due to cerbrovascular disorder O99.43
  hemorrhage O72.1
    brain O99.43
    bulbar O99.43
    cerebellar O99.43
    cerebral O99.43
    cortical O99.43
    delayed or secondary O72.2
    extradural O99.43
    internal capsule O99.43
    intracranial O99.43
    intrapontine O99.43
    meningeal O99.43
    pontine O99.43
    retained placenta O72.0
    subarachnoid O99.43
    subcortical O99.43
    subdural O99.43
    third stage O72.0
    uterine, delayed O72.2
    ventricular O99.43
  hemorrhoids O87.2
  hepatorenal syndrome O90.41
  hypertension —*see* Hypertension, complicating, puerperium
  hypertrophy, breast O92.29
  induration breast (fibrous) O92.29
  infection O86.4
    cervix O86.11
    generalized O85
    genital tract NEC O86.19
      obstetric surgical wound O86.09
    kidney (bacillus coli) O86.21
    maternal O98.93
      carrier state NEC O99.835
      gonorrhea O98.23
      human immunodeficiency virus (HIV) O98.73
      protozoal O98.63
      sexually transmitted NEC O98.33
      specified NEC O98.83
      streptococcus group B (GBS) carrier state O99.825
      syphilis O98.13
      tuberculosis O98.03
      viral hepatitis O98.43
      viral NEC O98.53
    nipple O91.02
      associated with lactation O91.03

Puerperal, puerperium (continued)
  infection (continued)
    peritoneum O85
    renal O86.21
    specified NEC O86.89
    urinary (asymptomatic) (tract) NEC O86.20
      bladder O86.22
      kidney O86.21
      specified site NEC O86.29
      urethra O86.22
    vagina O86.13
    vein —*see* Puerperal, phlebitis
  ischemia, cerebral O99.43
  lymphangitis O86.89
    breast O91.22
      associated with lactation O91.23
  malignancy O9A.13
  malnutrition O25.3
  mammillitis O91.02
    associated with lactation O91.03
  mammitis O91.22
    associated with lactation O91.23
  mania F30.8
  mastitis O91.22
    associated with lactation O91.23
    purulent O91.12
      associated with lactation O91.13
  melancholia —*see* Disorder, depressive
  mental disorder NEC O99.345
  metroperitonitis O85
  metrorrhagia —*see* Hemorrhage, postpartum
  metrosalpingitis O86.19
  metrovaginitis O86.13
  milk leg O87.1
  monoplegia, cerebral O99.43
  mood disturbance O90.6
  necrosis, liver (acute) (subacute) (conditions in subcategory K72.0) O26.63
    with renal failure O90.49
  nervous system disorder O99.355
  neuritis O90.89
  obesity (pre-existing prior to pregnancy) O99.215
  obesity surgery status O99.845
  occlusion, precerebral artery O99.43
  paralysis
    bladder (sphincter) O90.89
    cerebral O99.43
  paralytic stroke O99.43
  parametritis O85
  paravaginitis O86.13
  pelviperitonitis O85
  perimetritis O86.12
  perimetrosalpingitis O86.19
  perinephritis O86.21
  periphlebitis —*see* Puerperal, phlebitis
  peritoneal infection O85
  peritonitis (pelvic) O85
  perivaginitis O86.13
  phlebitis O87.0
    deep O87.1
    pelvic O87.1
    superficial O87.0
  phlebothrombosis, deep O87.1
  phlegmasia alba dolens O87.1
  placental polyp O90.89
  pneumonia, embolic —*see* Embolism, obstetric, puerperal
  pre-eclampsia (NOS) —*see* Pre-eclampsia
  psychosis F53.1
  pyelitis O86.21
  pyelocystitis O86.29
  pyelonephritis O86.21

Puerperal, puerperium (continued)
  pyelonephrosis O86.21
  pyemia O85
  pyocystitis O86.29
  pyohemia O85
  pyometra O86.12
  pyonephritis O86.21
  pyosalpingitis O86.19
  pyrexia (of unknown origin) O86.4
  renal
    disease NEC O90.89
    failure O90.49
  respiratory disease NEC O99.53
  retention
    decidua —*see* Retention, decidua
    placenta O72.0
    secundines —*see* Retention, secundines
  retrated nipple O92.02
  salpingo-ovaritis O86.19
  salpingoperitonitis O85
  secondary perineal tear O90.1
  sepsis (pelvic) O85
  sepsis O85
  septic thrombophlebitis O86.81
  skin disorder NEC O99.73
  specified condition NEC O99.893
  stroke O99.43
  subinvolution (uterus) O90.89
  subluxation of symphysis (pubis) O26.73
  suppuration —*see* Puerperal, abscess
  tetanus A34
  thelitis O91.02
    associated with lactation O91.03
  thrombocytopenia O72.3
  thrombophlebitis (superficial) O87.0
    deep O87.1
    pelvic O87.1
    septic O86.81
  thrombosis (venous) —*see* Thrombosis, puerperal
  thyroiditis O90.5
  toxemia (eclamptic) (pre-eclamptic) (with convulsions) O15.2
  trauma, non-obstetric O9A.23
    caused by abuse (physical) (suspected) O9A.33
      confirmed O9A.33
    psychological (suspected) O9A.53
      confirmed O9A.53
    sexual (suspected) O9A.43
      confirmed O9A.43
  uremia (due to renal failure) O90.49
  urethritis O86.22
  vaginitis O86.13
  varicose veins (legs) O87.4
    vulva or perineum O87.8
  venous O87.9
  vulvitis O86.19
  vulvovaginitis O86.13
  white leg O87.1

Puerperium —*see* Puerperal

Pulmolithiasis J98.4

Pulmonary —*see* condition

Pulpitis (acute) (anachoretic) (chronic) (hyperplastic) (putrescent) (suppurative) (ulcerative) K04.01
  irreversible K04.02
  reversible K04.01

Pulpless tooth K04.99

Pulse
  alternating R00.8
  bigeminal R00.8
  fast R00.0
  feeble, rapid due to shock following injury T79.4
  rapid R00.0
  weak R09.89

Pulsus alternans or trigeminus R00.8

Punch drunk F07.81

Punctum lacrimale occlusion —*see* Obstruction, lacrimal

Puncture
  abdomen, abdominal
    wall S31.139
      with
        foreign body S31.149
        penetration into peritoneal cavity S31.639
          with foreign body S31.649
    wall S31.139
      epigastric region S31.132
        with
          foreign body S31.142
          penetration into peritoneal cavity S31.632
            with foreign body S31.642
      left
        lower quadrant S31.134
          with
            foreign body S31.144
            penetration into peritoneal cavity S31.634
              with foreign body S31.644
        upper quadrant S31.131
          with
            foreign body S31.141
            penetration into peritoneal cavity S31.631
              with foreign body S31.641
      periumbilic region S31.135
        with
          foreign body S31.145
          penetration into peritoneal cavity S31.635
            with foreign body S31.645
      right
        lower quadrant S31.133
          with
            foreign body S31.143
            penetration into peritoneal cavity S31.633
              with foreign body S31.643
        upper quadrant S31.130
          with
            foreign body S31.140
            penetration into peritoneal cavity S31.630
              with foreign body S31.640
  accidental, complicating surgery —*see* Complication, accidental puncture or laceration
  alveolar (process) —*see* Puncture, oral cavity
  ankle S91.039
    with
      foreign body S91.049

Puncture (continued)
  ankle (continued)
    left S91.032
      with
        foreign body S91.042
    right S91.031
      with
        foreign body S91.041
  anus S31.833
    with foreign body S31.834
  arm (upper) S41.139
    with foreign body S41.149
    left S41.132
      with foreign body S41.142
    lower —see Puncture, forearm
    right S41.131
      with foreign body S41.141
  auditory canal (external) (meatus) —see Puncture, ear
  auricle, ear —see Puncture, ear
  axilla —see Puncture, arm
  back —see also Puncture, thorax, back
    lower S31.030
      with
        foreign body S31.040
          with penetration into retroperitoneal space S31.041
        penetration into retroperitoneal space S31.031
  bladder (traumatic) S37.29
    nontraumatic N32.89
  breast S21.039
    with foreign body S21.049
    left S21.032
      with foreign body S21.042
    right S21.031
      with foreign body S21.041
  buttock S31.803
    with foreign body S31.804
    left S31.823
      with foreign body S31.824
    right S31.813
      with foreign body S31.814
  by
    device, implant or graft —see Complications, by site and type, mechanical
    foreign body left accidentally in operative wound T81.539
    instrument (any) during a procedure, accidental —see Puncture, accidental complicating surgery
  calf —see Puncture, leg
  canaliculus lacrimalis —see Puncture, eyelid
  canthus, eye —see Puncture, eyelid
  cervical esophagus S11.23
    with foreign body S11.24
  cheek (external) S01.439
    with foreign body S01.449
    left S01.432
      with foreign body S01.442
    right S01.431
      with foreign body S01.441
    internal —see Puncture, oral cavity
  chest wall —see Puncture, thorax
  chin —see Puncture, head, specified site NEC
  clitoris —see Puncture, vulva
  costal region —see Puncture, thorax
  digit(s)
    hand —see Puncture, finger
    foot —see Puncture, toe
  ear (canal) (external) S01.339
    with foreign body S01.349

Puncture (continued)
  ear (continued)
    left S01.332
      with foreign body S01.342
    right S01.331
      with foreign body S01.341
    drum S09.2-
  elbow S51.039
    with
      foreign body S51.049
    left S51.032
      with
        foreign body S51.042
    right S51.031
      with
        foreign body S51.041
  epididymis —see Puncture, testis
  epigastric region —see Puncture, abdomen, wall, epigastric
  epiglottis S11.83
    with foreign body S11.84
  esophagus
    cervical S11.23
      with foreign body S11.24
    thoracic S27.818
  eyeball S05.6-
    with foreign body S05.5-
  eyebrow —see Puncture, eyelid
  eyelid S01.13-
    with foreign body S01.14-
    left S01.132
      with foreign body S01.142
    right S01.131
      with foreign body S01.141
  face NEC —see Puncture, head, specified site NEC
  finger(s) S61.239
    with
      damage to nail S61.339
        with
          foreign body S61.349
      foreign body S61.249
    index S61.238
      with
        damage to nail S61.338
          with
            foreign body S61.348
        foreign body S61.248
      left S61.231
        with
          damage to nail S61.331
            with
              foreign body S61.341
          foreign body S61.241
      right S61.230
        with
          damage to nail S61.330
            with
              foreign body S61.340
          foreign body S61.240
    little S61.238
      with
        damage to nail S61.338
          with
            foreign body S61.348
        foreign body S61.248
      left S61.237
        with
          damage to nail S61.337
            with
              foreign body S61.347
          foreign body S61.247
      right S61.236
        with
          damage to nail S61.336
            with
              foreign body S61.346
          foreign body S61.246

Puncture (continued)
  finger(s) (continued)
    middle S61.238
      with
        damage to nail S61.338
          with
            foreign body S61.348
        foreign body S61.248
      left S61.233
        with
          damage to nail S61.333
            with
              foreign body S61.343
          foreign body S61.243
      right S61.232
        with
          damage to nail S61.332
            with
              foreign body S61.342
          foreign body S61.242
    ring S61.238
      with
        damage to nail S61.338
          with
            foreign body S61.348
        foreign body S61.248
      left S61.235
        with
          damage to nail S61.335
            with
              foreign body S61.345
          foreign body S61.245
      right S61.234
        with
          damage to nail S61.334
            with
              foreign body S61.344
          foreign body S61.244
  flank S31.139
    with foreign body S31.149
  foot (except toe(s) alone) S91.339
    with foreign body S91.349
    left S91.332
      with foreign body S91.342
    right S91.331
      with foreign body S91.341
    toe —see Puncture, toe
  forearm S51.839
    with
      foreign body S51.849
    elbow only —see Puncture, elbow
    left S51.832
      with
        foreign body S51.842
    right S51.831
      with
        foreign body S51.841
  forehead —see Puncture, head, specified site NEC
  genital organs, external
    female S31.532
      with foreign body S31.542
      vagina —see Puncture, vagina
      vulva —see Puncture, vulva
    male S31.531
      with foreign body S31.541
      penis —see Puncture, penis
      scrotum —see Puncture, scrotum
      testis —see Puncture, testis
  groin —see Puncture, abdomen, wall
  gum —see Puncture, oral cavity
  hand S61.439
    with
      foreign body S61.449

Puncture (continued)
  hand (continued)
    finger —see Puncture, finger
    left S61.432
      with
        foreign body S61.442
    right S61.431
      with
        foreign body S61.441
    thumb —see Puncture, thumb
  head S01.93
    with foreign body S01.94
    cheek —see Puncture, cheek
    ear —see Puncture, ear
    eyelid —see Puncture, eyelid
    lip —see Puncture, oral cavity
    nose —see Puncture, nose
    oral cavity —see Puncture, oral cavity
    scalp S01.03
      with foreign body S01.04
    specified site NEC S01.83
      with foreign body S01.84
    temporomandibular area —see Puncture, cheek
  heart S26.99
    with hemopericardium S26.09
    without hemopericardium S26.19
  heel —see Puncture, foot
  hip S71.039
    with foreign body S71.049
    left S71.032
      with foreign body S71.042
    right S71.031
      with foreign body S71.041
  hymen —see Puncture, vagina
  hypochondrium —see Puncture, abdomen, wall
  hypogastric region —see Puncture, abdomen, wall
  inguinal region —see Puncture, abdomen, wall
  instep —see Puncture, foot
  internal organs —see Injury, by site
  interscapular region —see Puncture, thorax, back
  intestine
    large
      colon S36.599
        ascending S36.590
        descending S36.592
        sigmoid S36.593
        specified site NEC S36.598
        transverse S36.591
      rectum S36.69
    small S36.499
      duodenum S36.490
      specified site NEC S36.498
  intra-abdominal organ S36.99
    gallbladder S36.128
    intestine —see Puncture, intestine
    liver S36.118
    pancreas —see Puncture, pancreas
    peritoneum S36.81
    specified site NEC S36.898
    spleen S36.09
    stomach S36.39
  jaw —see Puncture, head, specified site NEC
  knee S81.039
    with foreign body S81.049
    left S81.032
      with foreign body S81.042
    right S81.031
      with foreign body S81.041
  labium (majus) (minus) —see Puncture, vulva

Puncture *(continued)*
  lacrimal duct —*see* Puncture, eyelid
  larynx S11.013
    with foreign body S11.014
  leg (lower) S81.839
    with foreign body S81.849
    foot —*see* Puncture, foot
    knee —*see* Puncture, knee
    left S81.832
      with foreign body S81.842
    right S81.831
      with foreign body S81.841
    upper —*see* Puncture, thigh
  lip S01.531
    with foreign body S01.541
  loin —*see* Puncture, abdomen, wall
  lower back —*see* Puncture, back, lower
  lumbar region —*see* Puncture, back, lower
  malar region —*see* Puncture, head, specified site NEC
  mammary —*see* Puncture, breast
  mastoid region —*see* Puncture, head, specified site NEC
  mouth —*see* Puncture, oral cavity
  nail
    finger —*see* Puncture, finger, with damage to nail
    toe —*see* Puncture, toe, with damage to nail
  nasal (septum) (sinus) —*see* Puncture, nose
  nasopharynx —*see* Puncture, head, specified site NEC
  neck S11.93
    with foreign body S11.94
    involving
      cervical esophagus —*see* Puncture, cervical esophagus
      larynx —*see* Puncture, larynx
      pharynx —*see* Puncture, pharynx
      thyroid gland —*see* Puncture, thyroid gland
      trachea —*see* Puncture, trachea
    specified site NEC S11.83
      with foreign body S11.84
  nose (septum) (sinus) S01.23
    with foreign body S01.24
  ocular —*see* Puncture, eyeball
  oral cavity S01.532
    with foreign body S01.542
  orbit S05.4-
  palate —*see* Puncture, oral cavity
  palm —*see* Puncture, hand
  pancreas S36.299
    body S36.291
    head S36.290
    tail S36.292
  pelvis —*see* Puncture, back, lower
  penis S31.23
    with foreign body S31.24
  perineum
    female S31.43
      with foreign body S31.44
    male S31.139
      with foreign body S31.149
  periocular area (with or without lacrimal passages) —*see* Puncture, eyelid
  phalanges
    finger —*see* Puncture, finger
    toe —*see* Puncture, toe
  pharynx S11.23
    with foreign body S11.24
  pinna —*see* Puncture, ear
  popliteal space —*see* Puncture, knee

Puncture *(continued)*
  prepuce —*see* Puncture, penis
  pubic region S31.139
    with foreign body S31.149
  pudendum —*see* Puncture, genital organs, external
  rectovaginal septum —*see* Puncture, vagina
  sacral region —*see* Puncture, back, lower
  sacroiliac region —*see* Puncture, back, lower
  salivary gland —*see* Puncture, oral cavity
  scalp S01.03
    with foreign body S01.04
  scapular region —*see* Puncture, shoulder
  scrotum S31.33
    with foreign body S31.34
  shin —*see* Puncture, leg
  shoulder S41.039
    with foreign body S41.049
    left S41.032
      with foreign body S41.042
    right S41.031
      with foreign body S41.041
  spermatic cord —*see* Puncture, testis
  sternal region —*see* Puncture, thorax, front
  submaxillary region —*see* Puncture, head, specified site NEC
  submental region —*see* Puncture, head, specified site NEC
  subungual
    finger(s) —*see* Puncture, finger, with damage to nail
    toe —*see* Puncture, toe, with damage to nail
  supraclavicular fossa —*see* Puncture, neck, specified site NEC
  temple, temporal region —*see* Puncture, head, specified site NEC
  temporomandibular area —*see* Puncture, cheek
  testis S31.33
    with foreign body S31.34
  thigh S71.139
    with foreign body S71.149
    left S71.132
      with foreign body S71.142
    right S71.131
      with foreign body S71.141
  thorax, thoracic (wall) S21.93
    with foreign body S21.94
    back S21.23-
      with
        foreign body S21.24-
          with penetration S21.44
        penetration S21.43
    breast —*see* Puncture, breast
    front S21.13-
      with
        foreign body S21.14-
          with penetration S21.34
        penetration S21.33
  throat —*see* Puncture, neck
  thumb S61.039
    with
      damage to nail S61.139
        with
          foreign body S61.149
      foreign body S61.049
    left S61.032
      with
        damage to nail S61.132
          with
            foreign body S61.142
        foreign body S61.042

Puncture *(continued)*
  thumb *(continued)*
    left *(continued)*
    right S61.031
      with
        damage to nail S61.131
          with
            foreign body S61.141
        foreign body S61.041
  thyroid gland S11.13
    with foreign body S11.14
  toe(s) S91.139
    with
      damage to nail S91.239
        with
          foreign body S91.249
      foreign body S91.149
    great S91.133
      with
        damage to nail S91.233
          with
            foreign body S91.243
        foreign body S91.143
      left S91.132
        with
          damage to nail S91.232
            with
              foreign body S91.242
          foreign body S91.142
      right S91.131
        with
          damage to nail S91.231
            with
              foreign body S91.241
          foreign body S91.141
    lesser S91.136
      with
        damage to nail S91.236
          with
            foreign body S91.246
        foreign body S91.146
      left S91.135
        with
          damage to nail S91.235
            with
              foreign body S91.245
          foreign body S91.145
      right S91.134
        with
          damage to nail S91.234
            with
              foreign body S91.244
          foreign body S91.144
  tongue —*see* Puncture, oral cavity
  trachea S11.023
    with foreign body S11.024
  tunica vaginalis —*see* Puncture, testis
  tympanum, tympanic membrane S09.2-
  umbilical region S31.135
    with foreign body S31.145
  uvula —*see* Puncture, oral cavity
  vagina S31.43
    with foreign body S31.44
  vocal cords S11.033
    with foreign body S11.034
  vulva S31.43
    with foreign body S31.44
  wrist S61.539
    with
      foreign body S61.549
    left S61.532
      with
        foreign body S61.542
    right S61.531
      with
        foreign body S61.541

PUO (pyrexia of unknown origin) R50.9

Pupillary membrane (persistent) Q13.89

Pupillotonia —*see* Anomaly, pupil, function, tonic pupil

Purpura D69.2
  abdominal D69.0
  allergic D69.0
  anaphylactoid D69.0
  annularis telangiectodes L81.7
  arthritic D69.0
  autoerythrocyte sensitization D69.2
  autoimmune D69.0
  bacterial D69.0
  Bateman's (senile) D69.2
  capillary fragility (hereditary) (idiopathic) D69.8
  cryoglobulinemic D89.1
  Devil's pinches D69.2
  fibrinolytic —*see* Fibrinolysis
  fulminans, fulminous D65
  gangrenous D65
  hemorrhagic, hemorrhagica D69.3
    not due to thrombocytopenia D69.0
  Henoch (-Schönlein) (allergic) D69.0
  hypergammaglobulinemic (benign) (Waldenström) D89.0
  idiopathic (thrombocytopenic) D69.3
    nonthrombocytopenic D69.0
  immune thrombocytopenic D69.3
  infectious D69.0
  malignant D69.0
  neonatorum P54.5
  nervosa D69.0
  newborn P54.5
  nonthrombocytopenic D69.2
    hemorrhagic D69.0
    idiopathic D69.0
  nonthrombopenic D69.2
  peliosis rheumatica D69.0
  posttransfusion (post-transfusion) (from (fresh) whole blood or blood products) D69.51
  primary D69.49
  red cell membrane sensitivity D69.2
  rheumatica D69.0
  Schönlein (-Henoch) (allergic) D69.0
  scorbutic E54 *[D77]*
  senile D69.2
  simplex D69.2
  symptomatica D69.0
  telangiectasia annularis L81.7
  thrombocytopenic D69.49
    congenital D69.42
    hemorrhagic D69.3
    hereditary D69.42
    idiopathic D69.3
    immune D69.3
    neonatal, transitory P61.0
    thrombotic M31.19
  thrombohemolytic —*see* Fibrinolysis
  thrombolytic —*see* Fibrinolysis
  thrombopenic D69.49
  thrombotic, thrombocytopenic M31.19
  toxic D69.0
  vascular D69.0
  visceral symptoms D69.0

Purpuric spots R23.3

Purulent —*see* condition

Pus
  in
    stool R19.5
    urine N39.0
  tube (rupture) —see Salpingo-oophoritis
Pustular rash L08.0
Pustule (nonmalignant) L08.9
  malignant A22.0
Pustulosis palmaris et plantaris L40.3
Putnam (-Dana) disease or syndrome —see Degeneration, combined
Putrescent pulp (dental) K04.1
Pyarthritis, pyarthrosis —see Arthritis, pyogenic or pyemic
  tuberculous —see Tuberculosis, joint
Pyelectasis —see Hydronephrosis
Pyelitis (congenital) (uremic) —see also Pyelonephritis
  with
    calculus —see category N20
      with hydronephrosis N13.6
      contracted kidney N11.9
    acute N10
    chronic N11.9
      with calculus —see category N20
        with hydronephrosis N13.6
    cystica N28.84
    puerperal (postpartum) O86.21
    tuberculous A18.11
Pyelocystitis —see Pyelonephritis
Pyelonephritis —see also Nephritis, tubulo-interstitial
  with
    calculus —see category N20
      with hydronephrosis N13.6
      contracted kidney N11.9
    acute N10
    calculous —see category N20
      with hydronephrosis N13.6
    chronic N11.9
      with calculus —see category N20
        with hydronephrosis N13.6
      associated with ureteral obstruction or stricture N11.1
      nonobstructive N11.8
        with reflux (vesicoureteral) N11.0
      obstructive N11.1
      specified NEC N11.8
    in (due to)
      brucellosis A23.9 [N16]
      cryoglobulinemia (mixed) D89.1 [N16]
      cystinosis E72.04
      diphtheria A36.84
      glycogen storage disease E74.09 [N16]
      leukemia NEC C95.9- [N16]
      lymphoma NEC C85.90 [N16]
      multiple myeloma C90.0- [N16]
      obstruction N11.1
      Salmonella infection A02.25
      sarcoidosis D86.84
      sepsis A41.9 [N16]
      Sjögren's disease M35.04
      toxoplasmosis B58.83
      transplant rejection T86.91 [N16]
      Wilson's disease E83.01 [N16]
    nonobstructive N12
      with reflux (vesicoureteral) N11.0
      chronic N11.8
    syphilitic A52.75

Pyelonephrosis (obstructive) N11.1
  chronic N11.9
Pyelophlebitis I80.8
Pyeloureteritis cystica N28.85
Pyemia, pyemic (fever) (infection) (purulent) —see also Sepsis
  joint —see Arthritis, pyogenic or pyemic
  liver K75.1
  pneumococcal A40.3
  portal K75.1
  postvaccinal T88.0
  puerperal, postpartum, childbirth O85
  specified organism NEC A41.89
  tuberculous —see Tuberculosis, miliary
Pygopagus Q89.4
Pyknoepilepsy (idiopathic) —see Pyknolepsy
Pyknolepsy G40.A09
  intractable G40.A19
    with status epilepticus G40.A11
    without status epilepticus G40.A19
  not intractable G40.A09
    with status epilepticus G40.A01
    without status epilepticus G40.A09
Pylephlebitis K75.1
Pyle's syndrome Q78.5
Pylethrombophlebitis K75.1
Pylethrombosis K75.1
Pyloritis K29.90
  with bleeding K29.91
Pylorospasm (reflex) NEC K31.3
  congenital or infantile Q40.0
  newborn Q40.0
  neurotic F45.8
  psychogenic F45.8
Pylorus, pyloric —see condition
Pyoarthrosis —see Arthritis, pyogenic or pyemic
Pyocele
  mastoid —see Mastoiditis, acute
  sinus (accessory) —see Sinusitis
  turbinate (bone) J32.9
  urethra (see also Urethritis) N34.0
Pyocolpos —see Vaginitis
Pyocystitis N30.80
  with hematuria N30.81
Pyoderma, pyodermia L08.0
  gangrenosum L88
  newborn P39.4
  phagedenic L88
  vegetans L08.81
Pyodermatitis L08.0
  vegetans L08.81
Pyogenic —see condition
Pyohydronephrosis N13.6
Pyometra, pyometrium, pyometritis —see Endometritis
Pyomyositis (tropical) —see Myositis, infective
Pyonephritis N12
Pyonephrosis N13.6
  tuberculous A18.11
Pyo-oophoritis —see Salpingo-oophoritis
Pyo-ovarium —see Salpingo-oophoritis

Pyopericarditis, pyopericardium I30.1
Pyophlebitis —see Phlebitis
Pyopneumopericardium I30.1
Pyopneumothorax (infective) J86.9
  with fistula J86.0
  tuberculous NEC A15.6
Pyosalpinx, pyosalpingitis —see also Salpingo-oophoritis
Pyothorax J86.9
  with fistula J86.0
  tuberculous NEC A15.6
Pyoureter N28.89
  tuberculous A18.11
Pyramidopallidonigral syndrome G20.C
Pyrexia (of unknown origin) R50.9
  atmospheric T67.01
  during labor NEC O75.2
  heat T67.01
  newborn P81.9
    environmentally-induced P81.0
  persistent R50.9
  puerperal O86.4
Pyroglobulinemia NEC E88.09
Pyromania F63.1
Pyrosis R12
Pyuria (bacterial) (sterile) R82.81

Q

Q fever A78
  with pneumonia A78
Quadricuspid aortic valve Q23.8
Quadrilateral fever A78
Quadriparesis —see Quadriplegia
  meaning muscle weakness M62.81
Quadriplegia G82.50
  complete
    C1-C4 level G82.51
    C5-C7 level G82.53
  congenital (cerebral) (spinal) G80.8
    spastic G80.0
  embolic (current episode) I63.4-
  functional R53.2
  incomplete
    C1-C4 level G82.52
    C5-C7 level G82.54
  thrombotic (current episode) I63.3-
  traumatic -- code to injury with seventh character S
    current episode —see Injury, spinal (cord), cervical
Quadruplet, pregnancy —see Pregnancy, quadruplet
Quarrelsomeness F60.3
Queensland fever A77.3
Quervain's disease M65.4
  thyroid E06.1
Queyrat's erythroplasia D07.4
  penis D07.4
  specified site —see Neoplasm, skin, in situ
  unspecified site D07.4
Quincke's disease or edema T78.3
  hereditary D84.1
Quinsy (gangrenous) J36
Quintan fever A79.0
Quintuplet, pregnancy —see Pregnancy, quintuplet

R

Rabbit fever —see Tularemia
Rabies A82.9
  contact Z20.3
  exposure to Z20.3
  inoculation reaction —see Complications, vaccination
  sylvatic A82.0
  urban A82.1
Rachischisis —see Spina bifida
Rachitic —see also condition
  deformities of spine (late effect) (sequelae) E64.3
  pelvis (late effect) (sequelae) E64.3
    with disproportion (fetopelvic) O33.0
      causing obstructed labor O65.0
Rachitis, rachitism (acute) (tarda) —see also Rickets
  renalis N25.0
  sequelae E64.3
Radial nerve —see condition
Radiation
  burn —see Burn
  effects NOS T66
  sickness NOS T66
  therapy, encounter for Z51.0
Radiculitis (pressure) (vertebrogenic) —see Radiculopathy
Radiculomyelitis —see also Encephalitis
  toxic, due to
    Clostridium tetani A35
    Corynebacterium diphtheriae A36.82
Radiculopathy M54.10
  cervical region M54.12
  cervicothoracic region M54.13
  due to
    disc disorder
      C3 M50.11
      C4 M50.11
      C5 M50.121
      C6 M50.122
      C7 M50.123
      C8 M50.13
    displacement of intervertebral disc —see Disorder, disc, with, radiculopathy
  leg M54.1-
  lumbar region M54.16
  lumbosacral region M54.17
  occipito-atlanto-axial region M54.11
  postherpetic B02.29
  sacrococcygeal region M54.18
  syphilitic A52.11
  thoracic region (with visceral pain) M54.14
  thoracolumbar region M54.15
Radiodermal burns (acute, chronic, or occupational) —see Burn
Radiodermatitis L58.9
  acute L58.0
  chronic L58.1
Radiotherapy session Z51.0
RAEB (refractory anemia with excess blasts) D46.2-
Rage, meaning rabies —see Rabies
Ragpicker's disease A22.1
Ragsorter's disease A22.1
Raillietiniasis B71.8
Railroad neurosis F48.8

285

Railway spine F48.8

Raised —see also Elevated
  antibody titer R76.0

Rake teeth, tooth M26.39

Rales R09.89

Ramifying renal pelvis Q63.8

Ramsay-Hunt disease or syndrome
  (see also Hunt's, disease) B02.21
  meaning dyssynergia cerebellaris
    myoclonica G11.19

Ranula K11.6
  congenital Q38.4

Rape
  adult
    confirmed T74.21
    suspected T76.21
    alleged, observation or
      examination, ruled out
        adult Z04.41
        child Z04.42
  child
    confirmed T74.22
    suspected T76.22

Rapid
  feeble pulse, due to shock,
    following injury T79.4
  heart (beat) R00.0
    psychogenic F45.8
  second stage (delivery) O62.3
  time-zone change syndrome G47.25

Rarefaction, bone —see Disorder,
  bone, density and structure,
  specified NEC

Rash (toxic) R21
  canker A38.9
  diaper L22
  drug (internal use) L27.0
    contact (see also Dermatitis, due
      to, drugs, external) L25.1
  following immunization T88.1
  food —see Dermatitis, due to, food
  heat L74.0
  napkin (psoriasiform) L22
  nettle —see Urticaria
  pustular L08.0
  rose R21
    epidemic B06.9
  scarlet A38.9
  serum (see also Reaction, serum)
    T80.69
  wandering tongue K14.1

Rasmussen aneurysm —see
  Tuberculosis, pulmonary

Rasmussen encephalitis G04.81

Rat-bite fever A25.9
  due to Streptobacillus moniliformis
    A25.1
  spirochetal (morsus muris) A25.0

Rathke's pouch tumor D44.3

Raymond (-Céstan) **syndrome** I65.8

Raynaud's disease, phenomenon or
  syndrome (secondary) I73.00
  with gangrene (symmetric) I73.01

RDS (newborn) (type I) P22.0
  type II P22.1

Reaction —see also Disorder
  adaptation —see Disorder,
    adjustment
  adjustment (anxiety) (conduct
    disorder) (depressiveness) (distress)
    —see Disorder, adjustment
  with
    mutism, elective (child)
      (adolescent) F94.0

Reaction (continued)
  adverse
    food (any) (ingested) NEC T78.1
      anaphylactic —see Shock,
        anaphylactic, due to food
  affective —see Disorder, mood
  allergic —see Allergy
  anaphylactic —see Shock,
    anaphylactic
  anaphylactoid —see Shock,
    anaphylactic
  anesthesia —see Anesthesia,
    complication
  antitoxin (prophylactic)
    (therapeutic) —see
    Complications, vaccination
  anxiety F41.1
  Arthus —see Arthus' phenomenon
  asthenic F48.8
  combat and operational stress F43.0
  compulsive F42.8
  conversion F44.9
  crisis, acute F43.0
  deoxyribonuclease (DNA) (DNase)
    hypersensitivity D69.2
  depressive (single episode) F32.9
    affective (single episode) F31.4
      recurrent episode F33.9
    neurotic F34.1
    psychoneurotic F34.1
    psychotic F32.3
    recurrent —see Disorder,
      depressive, recurrent
  dissociative F44.9
  drug NEC T88.7
    addictive —see Dependence,
      drug
    transmitted via placenta
      or breast milk —see
        Absorption, drug, addictive,
        through placenta
    allergic —see Allergy, drug
    lichenoid L43.2
    newborn P93.8
      gray baby syndrome P93.0
    overdose or poisoning (by
      accident) —see Table of
      Drugs and Chemicals, by
      drug, poisoning
    photoallergic L56.1
    phototoxic L56.0
    withdrawal —see Dependence,
      by drug, with, withdrawal
      infant of dependent mother
        P96.1
      newborn P96.1
    wrong substance given or taken
      (by accident) —see Table
      of Drugs and Chemicals, by
      drug, poisoning
  fear F40.9
    child (abnormal) F93.8
  febrile nonhemolytic transfusion
    (FNHTR) R50.84
  fluid loss, cerebrospinal G97.1
  foreign
    body NEC —see Granuloma,
      foreign body
    in operative wound
      (inadvertently left) —see
        Foreign body, accidentally
        left during a procedure
  substance accidentally left
    during a procedure (chemical)
    (powder) (talc) T81.60
  aseptic peritonitis T81.61
  body or object (instrument)
    (sponge) (swab) —see
      Foreign body, accidentally
      left during a procedure
  specified reaction NEC T81.69

Reaction (continued)
  grief —see Disorder, adjustment
  Herxheimer's R68.89
  hyperkinetic —see Hyperkinesia
  hypochondriacal F45.20
  hypoglycemic, due to insulin E16.0
    with coma (diabetic) —see
      Diabetes, coma
      nondiabetic E15
    therapeutic misadventure —see
      subcategory T38.3
  hypomanic F30.8
  hysterical F44.9
  immunization —see Complications,
    vaccination
  incompatibility
    ABO blood group (infusion)
      (transfusion) —see
        Complication(s), transfusion,
        incompatibility reaction,
        ABO
      delayed serologic T80.39
    minor blood group (Duffy) (E)
      (K) (Kell) (Kidd) (Lewis) (M)
      (N) (P) (S) T80.89
    Rh (factor) (infusion)
      (transfusion) —see
        Complication(s), transfusion,
        incompatibility reaction, Rh
        (factor)
  inflammatory —see Infection
  infusion —see Complications,
    infusion
  inoculation (immune serum) —see
    Complications, vaccination
  insulin T38.3-
  involutional psychotic —see
    Disorder, depressive
  leukemoid D72.823
    basophilic D72.823
    lymphocytic D72.823
    monocytic D72.823
    myelocytic D72.823
    neutrophilic D72.823
  LSD (acute)
    due to drug abuse —see Abuse,
      drug, hallucinogen
    due to drug dependence —see
      Dependence, drug,
      hallucinogen
  lumbar puncture G97.1
  manic-depressive —see Disorder,
    bipolar
  neurasthenic F48.8
  neurogenic —see Neurosis
  neurotic F48.9
  neurotic-depressive F34.1
  nitritoid —see Crisis, nitritoid
  nonspecific
    to
      cell mediated immunity
        measurement of gamma
        interferon antigen response
        without active tuberculosis
        R76.12
      QuantiFERON-TB test (QFT)
        without active tuberculosis
        R76.12
      tuberculin test (see also
        Reaction, tuberculin skin
        test) R76.11
  obsessive-compulsive F42.8
  organic, acute or subacute —see
    Delirium
  paranoid (acute) F23
    chronic F22
    senile F03
  passive dependency F60.7
  phobic F40.9
  post-traumatic stress,
    uncomplicated Z73.3

Reaction (continued)
  psychogenic F99
  psychoneurotic —see also Neurosis
    compulsive F42.8
    depersonalization F48.1
    depressive F34.1
    hypochondriacal F45.20
    neurasthenic F48.8
    obsessive F42.8
  psychophysiologic —see Disorder,
    somatoform
  psychosomatic —see Disorder,
    somatoform
  psychotic —see Psychosis
  scarlet fever toxin —see
    Complications, vaccination
  schizophrenic F23
    acute (brief) (undifferentiated)
      F23
    latent F21
    undifferentiated (acute) (brief)
      F23
  serological for syphilis —see
    Serology for syphilis
  serum T80.69
    anaphylactic (immediate) —see
      also Shock, anaphylactic T80.59
    specified reaction NEC
      due to
        administration of blood and
          blood products T80.61
        immunization T80.62
        serum specified NEC
          T80.69
        vaccination T80.62
  situational —see Disorder, adjustment
  somatization —see Disorder,
    somatoform
  spinal puncture G97.1
    dural G97.1
  stress (severe) F43.9
    acute (agitation) ("daze")
      (disorientation) (disturbance
      of consciousness) (flight
      reaction) (fugue) F43.0
    specified NEC F43.89
  surgical procedure —see
    Complications, surgical
    procedure
  tetanus antitoxin —see
    Complications, vaccination
  toxic, to local anesthesia
    T88.59
    in labor and delivery O74.4
    in pregnancy O29.3X-
    postpartum, puerperal O89.3
  toxin-antitoxin —see
    Complications, vaccination
  transfusion (blood) (bone marrow)
    (lymphocytes) (allergic) —see
    Complications, transfusion
  tuberculin skin test, abnormal R76.11
  vaccination (any) —see
    Complications, vaccination
  withdrawing, child or adolescent
    F93.8

Reactive airway disease —see
  Asthma

Reactive depression —see Reaction,
  depressive

Rearrangement
  chromosomal
    balanced (in) Q95.9
      abnormal individual
        (autosomal) Q95.2
      non-sex (autosomal)
        chromosomes Q95.2
      sex/non-sex chromosomes
        Q95.3
      specified NEC Q95.8

Recalcitrant patient —*see* Noncompliance

Recanalization, thrombus —*see* Thrombosis

Recession, receding
chamber angle (eye) H21.55-
chin M26.09
gingival (postinfective) (postoperative)
generalized K06.020
minimal K06.021
moderate K06.022
severe K06.023
localized K06.010
minimal K06.011
moderate K06.012
severe K06.013

Recklinghausen disease Q85.01
bones E21.0

Reclus' disease (cystic) —*see* Mastopathy, cystic

Recrudescence
deficit
cerebral infarction —*see* Sequelae, infarction, cerebral
stroke —*see* Sequelae, infarction, cerebral
sequelae
cerebral infarction —*see* Sequelae, infarction, cerebral
stroke —*see* Sequelae, infarction, cerebral

Recrudescent typhus (fever) A75.1

Recruitment, auditory H93.21-

Rectalgia K62.89

Rectitis K62.89

Rectocele
female (without uterine prolapse) N81.6
with uterine prolapse N81.4
complete N81.3
incomplete N81.2
in pregnancy —*see* Pregnancy, complicated by, abnormal, pelvic organs or tissues NEC
male K62.3

Rectosigmoid junction —*see* condition

Rectosigmoiditis K63.89
ulcerative (chronic) K51.30
with
complication K51.319
abscess K51.314
fistula K51.313
obstruction K51.312
rectal bleeding K51.311
specified NEC K51.318

Rectourethral —*see* condition

Rectovaginal —*see* condition

Rectovesical —*see* condition

Rectum, rectal —*see* condition

Recurrent —*see* condition
pregnancy loss —*see* Loss (of), pregnancy, recurrent

Red bugs B88.0

Red-cedar lung or pneumonitis J67.8

Red tide (*see also* Table of Drugs and Chemicals) T65.82-

Reduced
mobility Z74.09
ventilatory or vital capacity R94.2

Redundant, redundancy
anus (congenital) Q43.8
clitoris N90.89
colon (congenital) Q43.8
foreskin (congenital) N47.8
intestine (congenital) Q43.8
labia N90.69
organ or site, congenital NEC —*see* Accessory
panniculus (abdominal) E65
prepuce (congenital) N47.8
pylorus K31.89
rectum (congenital) Q43.8
scrotum N50.89
sigmoid (congenital) Q43.8
skin L98.7
and subcutaneous tissue L98.7
of face L57.4
eyelids —*see* Blepharochalasis
stomach K31.89

Reduplication —*see* Duplication

Reflex R29.2
hyperactive gag J39.2
pupillary, abnormal —*see* Anomaly, pupil, function
vasoconstriction I73.9
vasovagal R55

Reflux K21.9
acid K21.9
esophageal K21.9
with esophagitis (without bleeding) K21.00
with bleeding K21.01
newborn P78.83
gastroesophageal K21.9
with esophagitis (without bleeding) K21.00
with bleeding K21.01
mitral —*see* Insufficiency, mitral
ureteral —*see* Reflux, vesicoureteral
vesicoureteral (with scarring) N13.70
with
nephropathy N13.729
with hydroureter N13.739
bilateral N13.732
unilateral N13.731
bilateral N13.722
unilateral N13.721
without hydroureter N13.729
bilateral N13.722
unilateral N13.721
pyelonephritis (chronic) N11.0
congenital Q62.7
without nephropathy N13.71

Reforming, artificial openings —*see* Attention to, artificial, opening

Refractive error —*see* Disorder, refraction

Refsum's disease or syndrome G60.1

Refusal of
food, psychogenic F50.89
treatment (because of) Z53.20
left against medical advice (AMA) Z53.29
left without being seen Z53.21
patient's decision NEC Z53.29
reasons of belief or group pressure Z53.9

Regional —*see* condition

Regurgitation R11.10
aortic (valve) —*see* Insufficiency, aortic
food —*see also* Vomiting
with reswallowing —*see* Rumination
newborn P92.1

Regurgitation (*continued*)
gastric contents —*see* Vomiting
heart —*see* Endocarditis
mitral (valve) —*see* Insufficiency, mitral
congenital Q23.3
myocardial —*see* Endocarditis
pulmonary (valve) (heart) I37.1
congenital Q22.2
syphilitic A52.03
tricuspid —*see* Insufficiency, tricuspid
valve, valvular —*see* Endocarditis
congenital Q24.8
vesicoureteral —*see* Reflux, vesicoureteral

Reifenstein syndrome E34.52

Reinsertion
implantable subdermal contraceptive Z30.46
intrauterine contraceptive device Z30.433

Reiter's disease, syndrome, or urethritis M02.30
ankle M02.37-
elbow M02.32-
foot joint M02.37-
hand joint M02.34-
hip M02.35-
knee M02.36-
multiple site M02.39
shoulder M02.31-
vertebra M02.38
wrist M02.33-

Reichmann's disease or syndrome K31.89

Rejection
food, psychogenic F50.89
transplant T86.91
bone T86.830
marrow T86.01
cornea T86.840-
heart T86.21
with lung(s) T86.31
intestine T86.850
kidney T86.11
liver T86.41
lung(s) T86.810
with heart T86.31
organ (immune or nonimmune cause) T86.91
pancreas T86.890
skin (allograft) (autograft) T86.820
specified NEC T86.890
stem cell (peripheral blood) (umbilical cord) T86.5

Relapsing fever A68.9
Carter's (Asiatic) A68.1
Dutton's (West African) A68.1
Koch's A68.9
louse-borne (epidemic) A68.0
Novy's (American) A68.1
Obermeyers's (European) A68.0
Spirillum A68.9
tick-borne (endemic) A68.1

Relationship
occlusal
open anterior M26.220
open posterior M26.221

Relaxation
anus (sphincter) K62.89
psychogenic F45.8
arch (foot) —*see also* Deformity, limb, flat foot
back ligaments —*see* Instability, joint, spine
bladder (sphincter) N31.2
cardioesophageal K21.9

Relaxation (*continued*)
cervix —*see* Incompetency, cervix
diaphragm J98.6
joint (capsule) (ligament) (paralytic) —*see* Flail, joint
congenital NEC Q74.8
lumbosacral (joint) —*see* subcategory M53.2
pelvic floor N81.89
perineum N81.89
posture R29.3
rectum (sphincter) K62.89
sacroiliac (joint) —*see* subcategory M53.2
scrotum N50.89
urethra (sphincter) N36.44
vesical N31.2

Release from prison, anxiety concerning Z65.2

Remains
canal of Cloquet Q14.0
capsule (opaque) Q14.8

Remittent fever (malarial) B54

Remnant
canal of Cloquet Q14.0
capsule (opaque) Q14.8
cervix, cervical stump (acquired) (postoperative) N88.8
cystic duct, postcholecystectomy K91.5
fingernail L60.8
congenital Q84.6
meniscus, knee —*see* Derangement, knee, meniscus, specified NEC
thyroglossal duct Q89.2
tonsil J35.8
infected (chronic) J35.01
urachus Q64.4

Removal (from) (of)
artificial
arm Z44.00-
complete Z44.01-
partial Z44.02-
eye Z44.2-
leg Z44.10-
complete Z44.11-
partial Z44.12-
breast implant Z45.81
cardiac pulse generator (battery) (end-of-life) Z45.010
catheter (urinary) (indwelling) Z46.6
from artificial opening —*see* Attention to, artificial, opening
non-vascular Z46.82
vascular NEC Z45.2
drains Z48.03
device Z46.9
contraceptive Z30.432
implantable subdermal Z30.46
implanted NEC Z45.89
specified NEC Z46.89
dressing (nonsurgical) Z48.00
surgical Z48.01
external
fixation device - code to fracture with seventh character D
prosthesis, prosthetic device Z44.9
breast Z44.3-
specified NEC Z44.8
home in childhood (to foster home or institution) Z62.29
ileostomy Z43.2
insulin pump Z46.81
myringotomy device (stent) (tube) Z45.82

Removal *(continued)*
  nervous system device NEC Z46.2
    brain neuropacemaker Z46.2
    visual substitution device Z46.2
      implanted Z45.31
  non-vascular catheter Z46.82
  orthodontic device Z46.4
  organ, prophylactic (for neoplasia management) —*see* Prophylactic, organ removal
  staples Z48.02
  stent
    ureteral Z46.6
  suture Z48.02
  urinary device Z46.6
  vascular access device or catheter Z45.2

Ren
  arcuatus Q63.1
  mobile, mobilis N28.89
    congenital Q63.8
  unguliformis Q63.1

Renal —*see* condition

Rendu-Osler-Weber disease or syndrome I78.0

Reninoma D41.0-

Renon-Delille syndrome E23.3

Reovirus, as cause of disease classified elsewhere B97.5

Repeated falls NEC R29.6

Replaced chromosome by dicentric ring Q93.2

Replacement by artificial or mechanical device or prosthesis of
  bladder Z96.0
  blood vessel NEC Z95.828
  bone NEC Z96.7
  cochlea Z96.21
  coronary artery Z95.5
  eustachian tube Z96.29
  eye globe Z97.0
  heart Z95.812
    valve Z95.2
      prosthetic Z95.2
      specified NEC Z95.4
      xenogenic Z95.3
  intestine Z96.89
  joint Z96.60
    hip —*see* Presence, hip joint implant
    knee —*see* Presence, knee joint implant
    specified site NEC Z96.698
  larynx Z96.3
  lens Z96.1
  limb(s) —*see* Presence, artificial, limb
  mandible NEC (for tooth root implant(s)) Z96.5
  organ NEC Z96.89
  peripheral vessel NEC Z95.828
  stapes Z96.29
  teeth Z97.2
  tendon Z96.7
  tissue NEC Z96.89
  tooth root(s) Z96.5
  vessel NEC Z95.828
    coronary (artery) Z95.5

Request for expert evidence Z04.89

Reserve, decreased or low
  cardiac —*see* Disease, heart
  kidney N28.89

Residing
  in place not meant for human habitation (abandoned building) (car) (park) (sidewalk) Z59.02
    on the street Z59.02

Residual —*see also* condition
  ovary syndrome N99.83
  state, schizophrenic F20.5
  urine R39.198

Resistance, resistant (to)
  activated protein C D68.51
  insulin E88.819
    complicating pregnancy O26.89-
    specified type NEC E88.818
  organism(s)
    to
      drug Z16.30
        aminoglycosides Z16.29
        amoxicillin Z16.11
        ampicillin Z16.11
        antibiotic(s) Z16.20
          multiple Z16.24
          specified NEC Z16.29
        antifungal Z16.32
        antimicrobial (single) Z16.30
          multiple Z16.35
          specified NEC Z16.39
        antimycobacterial (single) Z16.341
          multiple Z16.342
        antiparasitic Z16.31
        antiviral Z16.33
        beta lactam antibiotics Z16.10
          specified NEC Z16.19
        carbapenem Z16.13
        cephalosporins Z16.19
        extended beta lactamase (ESBL) Z16.12
        fluoroquinolones Z16.23
        macrolides Z16.29
        methicillin —*see* MRSA
        multiple drugs (MDRO)
          antibiotics Z16.24
          antimicrobial Z16.35
          antimycobacterials Z16.342
        penicillins Z16.11
        quinine (and related compounds) Z16.31
        quinolones Z16.23
        sulfonamides Z16.29
        tetracyclines Z16.29
        tuberculostatics (single) Z16.341
          multiple Z16.342
        vancomycin Z16.21
          related antibiotics Z16.22
  thyroid hormone E07.89

Resorption
  dental (roots) K03.3
    alveoli M26.79
  teeth (external) (internal) (pathological) (roots) K03.3

Respiration
  Cheyne-Stokes R06.3
  decreased due to shock, following injury T79.4
  disorder of, psychogenic F45.8
  insufficient, or poor R06.89
    newborn P28.5
  painful R07.1
  sighing, psychogenic F45.8

Respiratory —*see also* condition
  distress syndrome (newborn) (type I) P22.0
    type II P22.1

Respiratory *(continued)*
  syncytial virus, as cause of disease classified elsewhere (*see also* Virus, respiratory syncytial (RSV)) B97.4

Respite care Z75.5

Response (drug)
  photoallergic L56.1
  phototoxic L56.0

Restenosis
  stent
    vascular
      end stent
        adjacent to stent —*see* Arteriosclerosis
        within the stent
          coronary T82.855
          peripheral T82.856
      in stent
        coronary vessel T82.855
        peripheral vessel T82.856

Restless legs (syndrome) G25.81

Restlessness R45.1

Restriction of housing space Z59.19

Restoration (of)
  dental
    aesthetically inadequate or displeasing K08.56
    defective K08.50
      specified NEC K08.59
    failure of marginal integrity K08.51
    failure of periodontal anatomical intergrity K08.54
  organ continuity from previous sterilization (tuboplasty) (vasoplasty) Z31.0
    aftercare Z31.42
  tooth (existing)
    contours biologically incompatible with oral health K08.54
    open margins K08.51
    overhanging K08.52
    poor aesthetic K08.56
    poor gingival margins K08.51
  unsatisfactory, of tooth K08.50
    specified NEC K08.59

Restorative material (dental)
  allergy to K08.55
  fractured K08.539
    with loss of material K08.531
    without loss of material K08.530
  unrepairable overhanging of K08.52

Rests, ovarian, in fallopian tube Q50.6

Restzustand (schizophrenic) F20.5

Retained —*see also* Retention
  cholelithiasis following cholecystectomy K91.86
  foreign body fragments (type of) Z18.9
    acrylics Z18.2
    animal quill(s) or spines Z18.31
    cement Z18.83
    concrete Z18.83
    crystalline Z18.83
    depleted isotope Z18.09
    depleted uranium Z18.01
    diethylhexyl phthalates Z18.2
    glass Z18.81
    isocyanate Z18.2
    magnetic metal Z18.11
    metal Z18.10
    nonmagnectic metal Z18.12
    nontherapeutic radioactive Z18.09

Retained *(continued)*
  foreign body fragments *(continued)*
    organic NEC Z18.39
    plastic Z18.2
    quill(s) (animal) Z18.31
    radioactive (nontherapeutic) NEC Z18.09
    specified NEC Z18.89
    spine(s) (animal) Z18.31
    stone Z18.83
    tooth (teeth) Z18.32
    wood Z18.33
  fragments (type of) Z18.9
    acrylics Z18.2
    animal quill(s) or spines Z18.31
    cement Z18.83
    concrete Z18.83
    crystalline Z18.83
    depleted isotope Z18.09
    depleted uranium Z18.01
    diethylhexyl phthalates Z18.2
    glass Z18.81
    isocyanate Z18.2
    magnetic metal Z18.11
    metal Z18.10
    nonmagnectic metal Z18.12
    nontherapeutic radioactive Z18.09
    organic NEC Z18.39
    plastic Z18.2
    quill(s) (animal) Z18.31
    radioactive (nontherapeutic) NEC Z18.09
    specified NEC Z18.89
    spine(s) (animal) Z18.31
    stone Z18.83
    tooth (teeth) Z18.32
    wood Z18.33
  gallstones, following cholecystectomy K91.86

Retardation
  development, developmental, specific —*see* Disorder, developmental
  endochondral bone growth —*see* Disorder, bone, development or growth
  growth R62.50
    due to malnutrition E45
  mental —*see* Disability, intellectual
  motor function, specific F82
  physical (child) R62.52
    due to malnutrition E45
  reading (specific) F81.0
  spelling (specific) (without reading disorder) F81.81

Retching —*see* Vomiting

Retention —*see also* Retained
  bladder —*see* Retention, urine
  carbon dioxide E87.29
  cholelithiasis following cholecystectomy K91.86
  cyst —*see* Cyst
  dead
    fetus (at or near term) (mother) O36.4
      early fetal death O02.1
    ovum O02.0
  decidua (fragments) (following delivery) (with hemorrhage) O72.2
    without hemorrhage O73.1
  deciduous tooth K00.6
  dental root K08.3
  fecal —*see* Constipation
  fetus
    dead O36.4
      early O02.1

Retention (continued)
  fluid R60.9
  foreign body —see also Foreign
      body, retained
      current trauma - code as Foreign
          body, by site or type
  gallstones, following
      cholecystectomy K91.86
  gastric K31.89
  intrauterine contraceptive device,
      in pregnancy —see Pregnancy,
      complicated by, retention,
      intrauterine device
  membranes (complicating delivery)
      (with hemorrhage) O72.2
      with abortion —see Abortion,
          by type
      without hemorrhage O73.1
  meniscus —see Derangement,
      meniscus
  menses N94.89
  milk (puerperal, postpartum) O92.79
  nitrogen, extrarenal R39.2
  ovary syndrome N99.83
  placenta (total) (with hemorrhage)
      O72.0
      without hemorrhage O73.0
      portions or fragments (with
          hemorrhage) O72.2
          without hemorrhage O73.1
  products of conception
      early pregnancy (dead fetus)
          O02.1
      following
          delivery (with hemorrhage)
              O72.2
              without hemorrhage O73.1
  secundines (following delivery)
      (with hemorrhage) O72.0
      without hemorrhage O73.0
      complicating puerperium
          (delayed hemorrhage) O72.2
      partial O72.2
          without hemorrhage O73.1
  smegma, clitoris N90.89
  urine R33.9
      due to hyperplasia (hypertrophy)
          of prostate —see Hyperplasia,
          prostate
      drug-induced R33.0
      organic R33.8
          drug-induced R33.0
      psychogenic F45.8
      specified NEC R33.8
  water (in tissues) —see Edema

Reticular erythematous mucinosis
  L98.5

Reticulation, dust —see
  Pneumoconiosis

Reticulocytosis R70.1

Reticuloendotheliosis
  acute infantile C96.0
  leukemic C91.4-
  nonlipid C96.0

Reticulohistiocytoma (giant-cell)
  D76.3

Reticuloid, actinic L57.1

Reticulosis (skin)
  acute of infancy C96.0
  hemophagocytic, familial D76.1
  histiocytic medullary C96.A
  lipomelanotic I89.8
  malignant (midline) C86.0
  polymorphic C86.0
  Sézary —see Sézary disease

Retina, retinal —see also condition
  dark area D49.81

Retinitis —see also Inflammation,
  chorioretinal
  albuminurica N18.9 *[H32]*
  diabetic —see Diabetes, retinitis
  disciformis —see Degeneration,
      macula
  focal —see Inflammation,
      chorioretinal, focal
  gravidarum —see Pregnancy,
      complicated by, specified
      pregnancy-related condition NEC
  juxtapapillaris —see Inflammation,
      chorioretinal, focal,
      juxtapapillary
  luetic —see Retinitis, syphilitic
  pigmentosa H35.52
  proliferans —see Disorder, globe,
      degenerative, specified type NEC
  proliferating —see Disorder, globe,
      degenerative, specified type NEC
  renal N18.9 *[H32]*
  syphilitic (early) (secondary) A51.43
      central, recurrent A52.71
      congenital (early) A50.01 *[H32]*
      late A52.71
  tuberculous A18.53

Retinoblastoma C69.2-
  differentiated C69.2-
  undifferentiated C69.2-

Retinochoroiditis —see also
  Inflammation, chorioretinal
  disseminated —see Inflammation,
      chorioretinal, disseminated
      syphilitic A52.71
  focal —see Inflammation,
      chorioretinal
  juxtapapillaris —see Inflammation,
      chorioretinal, focal,
      juxtapapillary

Retinopathy (background) H35.00
  arteriosclerotic I70.8 *[H35.0-]*
  atherosclerotic I70.8 *[H35.0-]*
  central serous —see
      Chorioretinopathy, central serous
  Coats H35.02-
  diabetic —see Diabetes,
      retinopathy
  exudative H35.02-
  hypertensive H35.03-
  in (due to)
      diabetes —see Diabetes,
          retinopathy
      sickle-cell disorders
          nonproliferative D57.-
              [H36.81-]
          proliferative D57.- *[H36.82-]*
  of prematurity H35.10-
      stage 0 H35.11-
      stage 1 H35.12-
      stage 2 H35.13-
      stage 3 H35.14-
      stage 4 H35.15-
      stage 5 H35.16-
  pigmentary, congenital —see
      Dystrophy, retina
  proliferative NEC H35.2-
      diabetic —see Diabetes,
          retinopathy, proliferative
      sickle-cell D57.- *[H36.82-]*
  thaslassemia H35.2
  solar H31.02-

Retinoschisis H33.10-
  congenital Q14.1
  specified type NEC H33.19-

Retortamoniasis A07.8

Retractile testis Q55.22

Retraction
  cervix —see Retroversion, uterus

Retraction (continued)
  drum (membrane) —see Disorder,
      tympanic membrane, specified
      NEC
  finger —see Deformity, finger
  lid H02.539
      left H02.536
          lower H02.535
          upper H02.534
      right H02.533
          lower H02.532
          upper H02.531
  lung J98.4
  mediastinum J98.59
  nipple N64.53
      associated with
          lactation O92.03
          pregnancy O92.01-
          puerperium O92.02
      congenital Q83.8
  palmar fascia M72.0
  pleura —see Pleurisy
  ring, uterus (Bandl's) (pathological)
      O62.4
  sternum (congenital) Q76.7
      acquired M95.4
  uterus —see Retroversion, uterus
  valve (heart) —see Endocarditis

Retrobulbar —see condition

Retrocecal —see condition

Retrocession —see Retroversion

Retrodisplacement —see
  Retroversion

Retroflection, retroflexion —see
  Retroversion

Retrognathia, retrognathism
  (mandibular) (maxillary) M26.19

Retrograde menstruation N92.5

Retroperineal —see condition

Retroperitoneal —see condition

Retroperitonitis K68.9

Retropharyngeal —see condition

Retroplacental —see condition

Retroposition —see Retroversion

Retroprosthetic membrane
  T85.398

Retrosternal thyroid (congenital)
  Q89.2

Retroversion, retroverted
  cervix —see Retroversion, uterus
  female NEC —see Retroversion,
      uterus
  iris H21.89
  testis (congenital) Q55.29
  uterus (acquired) (acute) (any
      degree) (asymptomatic) (cervix)
      (postinfectional) (postpartal, old)
      N85.4
      congenital Q51.818
      in pregnancy O34.53-

**Retrovirus, as cause of disease
  classified elsewhere** B97.30
  human
      immunodeficiency, type 2 (HIV
          2) B97.35
      T-cell lymphotropic
          type I (HTLV-I) B97.33
          type II (HTLV-II) B97.34
  lentivirus B97.31
  oncovirus B97.32
  specified NEC B97.39

Retrusion, premaxilla
  (developmental) M26.09

Rett's disease or syndrome F84.2

Reverse peristalsis R19.2

Reye's syndrome G93.7

Rh (factor)
  hemolytic disease (newborn) P55.0
  incompatibility, immunization or
      sensitization
      affecting management of
          pregnancy NEC O36.09-
              anti-D antibody O36.01-
          newborn P55.0
      transfusion reaction —see
          Complication(s), transfusion,
          incompatibility reaction, Rh
          (factor)
  negative mother affecting newborn
      P55.0
  titer elevated —see
      Complication(s), transfusion,
      incompatibility reaction, Rh
      (factor)
  transfusion reaction —see
      Complication(s), transfusion,
      incompatibility reaction, Rh
      (factor)

Rhabdomyolysis (idiopathic) **NEC**
  M62.82
  traumatic T79.6

Rhabdomyoma —see also
  Neoplasm, connective tissue,
  benign
  adult —see Neoplasm, connective
      tissue, benign
  fetal —see Neoplasm, connective
      tissue, benign
  glycogenic —see Neoplasm,
      connective tissue, benign

Rhabdomyosarcoma (any type)
  —see Neoplasm, connective tissue,
  malignant

Rhabdosarcoma —see
  Rhabdomyosarcoma

Rhesus (factor) **incompatibility**
  —see Rh, incompatibility

Rheumatic (acute) (subacute)
  adherent pericardium I09.2
  chronic I09.89
  coronary arteritis I01.8
  degeneration, myocardium I09.0
  fever (acute) —see Fever,
      rheumatic
  heart —see Disease, heart,
      rheumatic
  myocardial degeneration —see
      Degeneration, myocardium
  myocarditis (chronic) (inactive)
      (with chorea) I09.0
      active or acute I01.2
          with chorea (acute) (rheumatic)
              (Sydenham's) I02.0
  pancarditis, acute I01.8
      with chorea (acute) (rheumatic)
          Sydenham's) I02.0
  pericarditis (active) (acute) (with
      effusion) (with pneumonia) I01.0
      with chorea (acute) (rheumatic)
          (Sydenham's) I02.0
      chronic or inactive I09.2
  pneumonia I00 *[J17]*
  torticollis M43.6
  typhoid fever A01.09

Rheumatism (articular) (neuralgic)
  (nonarticular) M79.0
  gout —see Arthritis, rheumatoid
  intercostal, meaning Tietze's
      disease M94.0
  palindromic (any site) M12.30
      ankle M12.37-

Rheumatism *(continued)*
  palindromic *(continued)*
    elbow M12.32-
    foot joint M12.37-
    hand joint M12.34-
    hip M12.35-
    knee M12.36-
    multiple site M12.39
    shoulder M12.31-
    specified joint NEC M12.38
    vertebrae M12.38
    wrist M12.33-
  sciatic M54.4-
Rheumatoid —see also condition
  arthritis —see also Arthritis, rheumatoid
    with involvement of organs NEC M05.60
      ankle M05.67-
      elbow M05.62-
      foot joint M05.67-
      hand joint M05.64-
      hip M05.65-
      knee M05.66-
      multiple site M05.69
      shoulder M05.61-
      vertebra —see Spondylitis, ankylosing
      wrist M05.63-
    seronegative —see Arthritis, rheumatoid, seronegative
    seropositive —see Arthritis, rheumatoid, seropositive
  carditis M05.30
    ankle M05.37-
    elbow M05.32-
    foot joint M05.37-
    hand joint M05.34-
    hip M05.35-
    knee M05.36-
    multiple site M05.39
    shoulder M05.31-
    vertebra —see Spondylitis, ankylosing
    wrist M05.33-
  endocarditis —see Rheumatoid, carditis
  lung (disease) M05.10
    ankle M05.17-
    elbow M05.12-
    foot joint M05.17-
    hand joint M05.14-
    hip M05.15-
    knee M05.16-
    multiple site M05.19
    shoulder M05.11-
    vertebra —see Spondylitis, ankylosing
    wrist M05.13-
  myocarditis —see Rheumatoid, carditis
  myopathy M05.40
    ankle M05.47-
    elbow M05.42-
    foot joint M05.47-
    hand joint M05.44-
    hip M05.45-
    knee M05.46-
    multiple site M05.49
    shoulder M05.41-
    vertebra —see Spondylitis, ankylosing
    wrist M05.43-
  pericarditis —see Rheumatoid, carditis
  polyarthritis —see Arthritis, rheumatoid
  polyneuropathy M05.50
    ankle M05.57-
    elbow M05.52-
    foot joint M05.57-

Rheumatoid *(continued)*
  polyneuropathy *(continued)*
    hand joint M05.54-
    hip M05.55-
    knee M05.56-
    multiple site M05.59
    shoulder M05.51-
    vertebra —see Spondylitis, ankylosing
    wrist M05.53-
  vasculitis M05.20
    ankle M05.27-
    elbow M05.22-
    foot joint M05.27-
    hand joint M05.24-
    hip M05.25-
    knee M05.26-
    multiple site M05.29
    shoulder M05.21-
    vertebra —see Spondylitis, ankylosing
    wrist M05.23-
Rhinitis (atrophic) (catarrhal) (chronic) (croupous) (fibrinous) (granulomatous) (hyperplastic) (hypertrophic) (membranous) (obstructive) (purulent) (suppurative) (ulcerative) J31.0
  with
    sore throat —see Nasopharyngitis
  acute J00
  allergic J30.9
    with asthma J45.909
      with
        exacerbation (acute) J45.901
        status asthmaticus J45.902
    due to
      food J30.5
      pollen J30.1
    nonseasonal J30.89
    perennial J30.89
    seasonal NEC J30.2
    specified NEC J30.89
  infective J00
  pneumococcal J00
  syphilitic A52.73
    congenital A50.05 *[J99]*
  tuberculous A15.8
  vasomotor J30.0
Rhinoantritis (chronic) —see Sinusitis, maxillary
Rhinodacryolith —see Dacryolith
Rhinolith (nasal sinus) J34.89
Rhinomegaly J34.89
Rhinopharyngitis (acute) (subacute) —see also Nasopharyngitis
  chronic J31.1
  destructive ulcerating A66.5
  mutilans A66.5
Rhinophyma L71.1
Rhinorrhea J34.89
  cerebrospinal (fluid) G96.01
    postoperative G96.08
    specified NEC G96.08
    spontaneous G96.01
    traumatic G96.08
  paroxysmal —see Rhinitis, allergic
  spasmodic —see Rhinitis, allergic
Rhinosalpingitis —see Salpingitis, eustachian
Rhinoscleroma A48.8
Rhinosinusitis —see Sinusitis
Rhinosporidiosis B48.1
Rhinovirus infection NEC B34.8

Rhizomelic chondrodysplasia punctata E71.540
Rhythm
  atrioventricular nodal I49.8
  disorder I49.9
    coronary sinus I49.8
    ectopic I49.8
    nodal I49.8
  escape I49.9
  heart, abnormal I49.9
  idioventricular I44.2
  nodal I49.8
  sleep, inversion G47.2-
    nonorganic origin —see Disorder, sleep, circadian rhythm, psychogenic
Rhytidosis facialis L98.8
Rib —see also condition
  cervical Q76.5
Riboflavin deficiency E53.0
Rice bodies —see also Loose, body, joint
  knee M23.4-
Richter syndrome —see Leukemia, chronic lymphocytic, B-cell type
Richter's hernia —see Hernia, abdomen, with obstruction
Ricinism —see Poisoning, food, noxious, plant
Rickets (active) (acute) (adolescent) (chest wall) (congenital) (current) (infantile) (intestinal) E55.0
  adult —see Osteomalacia
  celiac K90.0
  hypophosphatemic with nephrotic-glycosuric dwarfism E72.09
  inactive E64.3
  kidney N25.0
  renal N25.0
  sequelae, any E64.3
  vitamin-D-resistant E83.31 *[M90.80]*
Rickettsia 364D/R. philipii (Pacific Coast tick fever) A77.8
Rickettsial disease A79.9
  specified type NEC A79.89
Rickettsialpox (Rickettsia akari) A79.1
Rickettsiosis A79.9
  due to
    Ehrlichia sennetsu A79.81
    Neorickettsia sennetsu A79.81
    Rickettsia akari (rickettsialpox) A79.1
  specified type NEC A79.89
  tick-borne A77.9
  vesicular A79.1
Rider's bone —see Ossification, muscle, specified NEC
Ridge, alveolus —see also condition
  flabby K06.8
Ridged ear, congenital Q17.3
Riedel's
  lobe, liver Q44.79
  struma, thyroiditis or disease E06.5
Rieger's anomaly or syndrome Q13.81
Riehl's melanosis L81.4
Rietti-Greppi-Micheli anemia D56.9
Rieux's hernia —see Hernia, abdomen, specified site NEC
Riga (-Fede) disease K14.0

Riggs' disease —see Periodontitis
Right aortic arch Q25.47
Right middle lobe syndrome J98.11
Rigid, rigidity —see also condition
  abdominal R19.30
    with severe abdominal pain R10.0
    epigastric R19.36
    generalized R19.37
    left lower quadrant R19.34
    left upper quadrant R19.32
    periumbilic R19.35
    right lower quadrant R19.33
    right upper quadrant R19.31
  articular, multiple, congenital Q68.8
  cervix (uteri) in pregnancy —see Pregnancy, complicated by, abnormal, cervix
  hymen (acquired) (congenital) N89.6
  nuchal R29.1
  pelvic floor in pregnancy —see Pregnancy, complicated by, abnormal, pelvic organs or tissues NEC
  perineum or vulva in pregnancy —see Pregnancy, complicated by, abnormal, vulva
  spine —see Dorsopathy, specified NEC
  vagina in pregnancy —see Pregnancy, complicated by, abnormal, vagina
Rigors R68.89
  with fever R50.9
Riley-Day syndrome G90.1
RIND (reversible ischemic neurologic deficit) I63.9
Ring(s)
  aorta (vascular) Q25.45
  Bandl's O62.4
  contraction, complicating delivery O62.4
  esophageal, lower (muscular) K22.2
  Fleischer's (cornea) H18.04-
  hymenal, tight (acquired) (congenital) N89.6
  Kayser-Fleischer (cornea) H18.04-
  retraction, uterus, pathological O62.4
  Schatzki's (esophagus) (lower) K22.2
    congenital Q39.3
  Soemmerring's —see Cataract, secondary
  vascular (congenital) Q25.8
    aorta Q25.45
Ringed hair (congenital) Q84.1
Ringworm B35.9
  beard B35.0
  black dot B35.0
  body B35.4
  Burmese B35.5
  corporeal B35.4
  foot B35.3
  groin B35.6
  hand B35.2
  honeycomb B35.0
  nails B35.1
  perianal (area) B35.6
  scalp B35.0
  specified NEC B35.8
  Tokelau B35.5
Rise, venous pressure I87.8
Rising, PSA following treatment for malignant neoplasm of prostate R97.21

Risk
for
dental caries Z91.849
high Z91.843
low Z91.841
moderate Z91.842
homelessness, imminent Z59.811
suffocation (smothering) under another while sleeping Z72.823
suicidal
meaning personal history of attempted suicide Z91.51
meaning suicidal ideation —see Ideation, suicidal

Ritter's disease L00
Rivalry, sibling Z62.891
Rivalta's disease A42.2
River blindness B73.01
Robert's pelvis Q74.2
with disproportion (fetopelvic) O33.0
causing obstructed labor O65.0
Robin (-Pierre) **syndrome** Q87.0
Robinow-Silvermann-Smith syndrome Q87.19
Robinson's (hidrotic) **ectodermal dysplasia or syndrome** Q82.4
Robles' disease B73.01
Rocky Mountain (spotted) **fever** A77.0
Roetheln —see Rubella
Roger's disease Q21.0
Rokitansky-Aschoff sinuses (gallbladder) K82.8
Rolando's fracture (displaced) S62.22-
nondisplaced S62.22-
Romano-Ward (prolonged QT interval) **syndrome** I45.81
Romberg's disease or syndrome G51.8
Roof, mouth —see condition
Rosacea L71.9
acne L71.9
keratitis L71.8
specified NEC L71.8
Rosary, rachitic E55.0
Rose
cold J30.1
fever J30.1
rash R21
epidemic B06.9
Rosenbach's erysipeloid A26.0
Rosenthal's disease or syndrome D68.1
Roseola B09
infantum B08.20
due to human herpesvirus 6 B08.21
due to human herpesvirus 7 B08.22
Rossbach's disease K31.89
psychogenic F45.8
Ross River disease or fever B33.1
Rostan's asthma (cardiac) —see Failure, ventricular, left
Rotation
anomalous, incomplete or insufficient, intestine Q43.3
cecum (congenital) Q43.3
colon (congenital) Q43.3

Rotation (continued)
spine, incomplete or insufficient —see Dorsopathy, deforming, specified NEC
tooth, teeth, fully erupted M26.35
vertebra, incomplete or insufficient —see Dorsopathy, deforming, specified NEC
Rotes Quérol disease or syndrome —see Hyperostosis, ankylosing
Roth (-Bernhardt) **disease or syndrome** —see Meralgia paraesthetica
Rothmund (-Thomson) **syndrome** Q82.8
Rotor's disease or syndrome E80.6
Round
back (with wedging of vertebrae) —see Kyphosis
sequelae (late effect) of rickets E64.3
worms (large) (infestation) NEC B82.0
Ascariasis (see also Ascariasis) B77.9
Roussy-Lévy syndrome G60.0
Rubella (German measles) B06.9
complication NEC B06.09
neurological B06.00
congenital P35.0
contact Z20.4
exposure to Z20.4
maternal
manifest rubella in infant P35.0
care for (suspected) damage to fetus O35.3
suspected damage to fetus affecting management of pregnancy O35.3
specified complications NEC B06.89
Rubeola (meaning measles) —see Measles
meaning rubella —see Rubella
Rubeosis, iris —see Disorder, iris, vascular
Rubinstein-Taybi syndrome Q87.2
Rudimentary (congenital) —see also Agenesis
arm —see Defect, reduction, upper limb
bone Q79.9
cervix uteri Q51.828
eye Q11.2
lobule of ear Q17.3
patella Q74.1
respiratory organs in thoracopagus Q89.4
tracheal bronchus Q32.4
uterus Q51.818
in male Q56.1
vagina Q52.0
Ruled out condition —see Observation, suspected
Rumination R11.10
with nausea R11.2
disorder of infancy F98.21
neurotic F42.8
newborn P92.1
obsessional F42.8
psychogenic F42.8
Runaway [from current living environment] Z62.892
Runeberg's disease D51.0
Running out of money Z59.86
Runny nose R09.89

Rupia (syphilitic) A51.39
congenital A50.06
tertiary A52.79
Rupture, ruptured
abscess (spontaneous) - code by site under Abscess
aneurysm —see Aneurysm
anus (sphincter) —see Laceration, anus
aorta, aortic I71.8
abdominal I71.30
infrarenal I71.33
juxtarenal I71.32
pararenal I71.31
arch I71.12
ascending I71.11
descending I71.8
abdominal I71.30
thoracic I71.13
syphilitic A52.01
thoracoabdominal I71.50
paravisceral I71.52
supraceliac I71.51
thorax, thoracic I71.10
transverse I71.12
traumatic —see Injury, aorta, laceration, major
valve or cusp (see also Endocarditis, aortic) I35.8
appendix (with peritonitis) (see also Appendicitis) K35.32
with localized peritonitis (see also Appendicitis) K35.32
arteriovenous fistula, brain —see Fistula, arteriovenous, brain, ruptured
artery I77.2
brain —see Hemorrhage, intracranial, intracerebral
coronary —see Infarct, myocardium
heart —see Infarct, myocardium
pulmonary I28.8
traumatic (complication) —see Injury, blood vessel
bile duct (common) (hepatic) K83.2
cystic K82.2
bladder (sphincter) (nontraumatic) (spontaneous) N32.89
following ectopic or molar pregnancy O08.6
obstetrical trauma O71.5
traumatic S37.29
blood vessel —see also Hemorrhage
brain —see Hemorrhage, intracranial, intracerebral
heart —see Infarct, myocardium
traumatic (complication) — see Injury, blood vessel, laceration, major, by site
bone —see Fracture
bowel (nontraumatic) K63.1
brain
aneurysm (congenital) —see also Hemorrhage, intracranial, subarachnoid
syphilitic A52.05
hemorrhagic —see Hemorrhage, intracranial, intracerebral
capillaries I78.8
cardiac (auricle) (ventricle) (wall) I23.3
with hemopericardium I23.0
infectional I40.9
traumatic —see Injury, heart
cartilage (articular) (current) —see also Sprain
knee S83.3-
semilunar —see Tear, meniscus

Rupture, ruptured (continued)
cecum (with peritonitis) K65.0
with peritoneal abscess K35.33
traumatic S36.598
celiac artery, traumatic —see Injury, blood vessel, celiac artery, laceration, major
cerebral aneurysm (congenital) (see Hemorrhage, intracranial, subarachnoid)
cervix (uteri)
with ectopic or molar pregnancy O08.6
following ectopic or molar pregnancy O08.6
obstetrical trauma O71.3
traumatic S37.69
chordae tendineae NEC I51.1
concurrent with acute myocardial infarction —see Infarct, myocardium
following acute myocardial infarction (current complication) I23.4
choroid (direct) (indirect) (traumatic) H31.32-
circle of Willis I60.6
colon (nontraumatic) K63.1
traumatic —see Injury, intestine, large
cornea (traumatic) —see Injury, eye, laceration
coronary (artery) (thrombotic) —see Infarct, myocardium
corpus luteum (infected) (ovary) N83.1-
cyst —see Cyst
cystic duct K82.2
Descemet's membrane —see Change, corneal membrane, Descemet's, rupture
traumatic —see Injury, eye, laceration
diaphragm, traumatic —see Injury, intrathoracic, diaphragm
disc —see Rupture, intervertebral disc
diverticulum (intestine) K57.80
with bleeding K57.81
bladder N32.3
large intestine K57.20
with
bleeding K57.21
small intestine K57.40
with bleeding K57.41
small intestine K57.00
with
bleeding K57.01
large intestine K57.40
with bleeding K57.41
duodenal stump K31.89
ear drum (nontraumatic) —see also Perforation, tympanum
traumatic S09.2-
due to blast injury —see Injury, blast, ear
esophagus K22.3
eye (without prolapse or loss of intraocular tissue) —see Injury, eye, laceration
fallopian tube NEC (nonobstetric) (nontraumatic) N83.8
due to pregnancy O00.10-
with intrauterine pregnancy O00.11-
fontanel P13.1
gallbladder K82.2
traumatic S36.128
gastric —see also Rupture, stomach
vessel K92.2

Rupture, ruptured (*continued*)
  globe (eye) (traumatic) —*see*
    Injury, eye, laceration
  graafian follicle (hematoma) N83.0-
  heart —*see* Rupture, cardiac
  hymen (nontraumatic)
    (nonintentional) N89.8
  internal organ, traumatic —*see*
    Injury, by site
  intervertebral disc —*see*
    Displacement, intervertebral disc
    traumatic —*see* Rupture,
      traumatic, intervertebral disc
  intestine NEC (nontraumatic) K63.1
    traumatic —*see* Injury, intestine
  iris —*see also* Abnormality, pupillary
    traumatic —*see* Injury, eye,
      laceration
  joint capsule, traumatic —*see* Sprain
  kidney (traumatic) S37.06-
    birth injury P15.8
    nontraumatic N28.89
  lacrimal duct (traumatic) —*see*
    Injury, eye, specified site NEC
  lens (cataract) (traumatic) —*see*
    Cataract, traumatic
  ligament, traumatic —*see* Rupture,
    traumatic, ligament, by site
  liver S36.116
    birth injury P15.0
  lymphatic vessel I89.8
  marginal sinus (placental) (with
    hemorrhage) —*see* Hemorrhage,
    antepartum, specified cause NEC
  membrana tympani (nontraumatic)
    —*see* Perforation, tympanum
  membranes (spontaneous)
    artificial
      delayed delivery following
        O75.5
    delayed delivery following
      —*see* Pregnancy, complicated
      by, premature rupture of
      membranes
  meningeal artery I60.8
  meniscus (knee) —*see also* Tear,
    meniscus
    old —*see* Derangement, meniscus
    site other than knee - code as Sprain
  mesenteric artery, traumatic —*see*
    Injury, mesenteric, artery,
    laceration, major
  mesentery (nontraumatic) K66.8
    traumatic —*see* Injury, intra-
      abdominal, specified, site NEC
  mitral (valve) I34.89
  muscle (traumatic) —*see also* Strain
    diastasis —*see* Diastasis, muscle
    nontraumatic M62.10
      ankle M62.17-
      foot M62.17-
      forearm M62.13-
      hand M62.14-
      lower leg M62.16-
      pelvic region M62.15-
      shoulder region M62.11-
      specified site NEC M62.18
      thigh M62.15-
      upper arm M62.12-
    traumatic —*see* Strain, by site
  musculotendinous junction NEC,
    nontraumatic —*see* Rupture,
    tendon, spontaneous
  mycotic aneurysm causing cerebral
    hemorrhage —*see* Hemorrhage,
    intracranial, subarachnoid
  myocardium, myocardial —*see*
    Rupture, cardiac
    traumatic —*see* Injury, heart
  nontraumatic, meaning hernia
    —*see* Hernia

Rupture, ruptured (*continued*)
  obstructed —*see* Hernia, by site,
    obstructed
  operation wound —*see* Disruption,
    wound, operation
  ovary, ovarian N83.8
    corpus luteum cyst N83.1-
    follicle (graafian) N83.0-
  oviduct (nonobstetric)
    (nontraumatic) N83.8
    due to pregnancy O00.10-
      with intrauterine pregnancy
        O00.11-
  pancreas (nontraumatic) K86.89
    traumatic S36.299
  papillary muscle NEC I51.2
    following acute myocardial
      infarction (current
      complication) I23.5
  pelvic
    floor, complicating delivery O70.1
    organ NEC, obstetrical trauma
      O71.5
  perineum (nonobstetric)
    (nontraumatic) N90.89
    complicating delivery —*see*
      Delivery, complicated, by,
      laceration, anus (sphincter)
  postoperative wound —*see*
    Disruption, wound, operation
  prostate (traumatic) S37.828
  pulmonary
    artery I28.8
    valve (heart) I37.8
    vein I28.8
    vessel I28.8
  pus tube —*see* Salpingitis
  pyosalpinx —*see* Salpingitis
  rectum (nontraumatic) K63.1
    traumatic S36.69
  retina, retinal (traumatic) (without
    detachment) —*see also* Break,
    retina
    with detachment —*see*
      Detachment, retina, with
      retinal, break
  rotator cuff (nontraumatic)
    M75.10-
    complete M75.12-
    incomplete M75.11-
  sclera —*see* Injury, eye, laceration
  sigmoid (nontraumatic) K63.1
    traumatic S36.593
  spinal cord —*see also* Injury, spinal
    cord, by region
    due to injury at birth P11.5
    newborn (birth injury) P11.5
  spleen (traumatic) S36.09
    birth injury P15.1
    congenital (birth injury) P15.1
    due to P. vivax malaria B51.0
    nontraumatic D73.5
    spontaneous D73.5
  splenic vein R58
    traumatic —*see* Injury, blood
      vessel, splenic vein
  stomach (nontraumatic)
    (spontaneous) K31.89
    traumatic S36.39
  supraspinatus (complete)
    (incomplete) (nontraumatic)
    —*see* Tear, rotator cuff
  symphysis pubis
    obstetric O71.6
    traumatic S33.4
  synovium (cyst) M66.10
    ankle M66.17-
    elbow M66.12-
    finger M66.14-
    foot M66.17-
    forearm M66.13-

Rupture, ruptured (*continued*)
  synovium (cyst) (*continued*)
    hand M66.14-
    pelvic region M66.15-
    shoulder region M66.11-
    specified site NEC M66.18
    thigh M66.15-
    toe M66.17-
    upper arm M66.12-
    wrist M66.13-
  tendon (traumatic) —*see* Strain
    nontraumatic (spontaneous)
      M66.9
      ankle M66.87-
      extensor M66.20
        ankle M66.27-
        foot M66.27-
        forearm M66.23-
        hand M66.24-
        lower leg M66.26-
        multiple sites M66.29
        pelvic region M66.25-
        shoulder region M66.21-
        specified site NEC M66.28
        thigh M66.25-
        upper arm M66.22-
      flexor M66.30
        ankle M66.37-
        foot M66.37-
        forearm M66.33-
        hand M66.34-
        lower leg M66.36-
        multiple sites M66.39
        pelvic region M66.35-
        shoulder region M66.31-
        specified site NEC M66.38
        thigh M66.35-
        upper arm M66.32-
      foot M66.87-
      forearm M66.83-
      hand M66.84-
      lower leg M66.86-
      multiple sites M66.89
      pelvic region M66.85-
      shoulder region M66.81-
      specified
        site NEC M66.88
        tendon M66.80
      thigh M66.85-
      upper arm M66.82-
  thoracic duct I89.8
  tonsil J35.8
  traumatic
    aorta —*see* Injury, aorta,
      laceration, major
    diaphragm —*see* Injury,
      intrathoracic, diaphragm
    external site —*see* Wound, open,
      by site
    eye —*see* Injury, eye, laceration
    internal organ —*see* Injury, by
      site
    intervertebral disc
      cervical S13.0
      lumbar S33.0
      thoracic S23.0
    kidney S37.06-
    ligament —*see also* Sprain
      ankle —*see* Sprain, ankle
      carpus —*see* Rupture,
        traumatic, ligament, wrist
      collateral (hand) —*see*
        Rupture, traumatic,
        ligament, finger, collateral
      finger (metacarpophalangeal)
        (interphalangeal) S63.40-
        collateral S63.41-
          index S63.41-
          little S63.41-
          middle S63.41-
          ring S63.41-

Rupture, ruptured (*continued*)
  traumatic (*continued*)
    ligament (*continued*)
      finger (*continued*)
        index S63.40-
        little S63.40-
        middle S63.40-
        palmar S63.42-
          index S63.42-
          little S63.42-
          middle S63.42-
          ring S63.42-
        ring S63.40-
        specified site NEC S63.499
          index S63.49-
          little S63.49-
          middle S63.49-
          ring S63.49-
        volar plate S63.43-
          index S63.43-
          little S63.43-
          middle S63.43-
          ring S63.43-
      foot —*see* Sprain, foot
      radial collateral S53.2-
      radiocarpal —*see* Rupture,
        traumatic, ligament, wrist,
        radiocarpal
      ulnar collateral S53.3-
      ulnocarpal —*see* Rupture,
        traumatic, ligament, wrist,
        ulnocarpal
      wrist S63.30-
        collateral S63.31-
        radiocarpal S63.32-
        specified site NEC S63.39-
        ulnocarpal (palmar) S63.33-
    liver S36.116
    membrana tympani —*see*
      Rupture, ear drum,
      traumatic
    muscle or tendon —*see* Strain
    myocardium —*see* Injury, heart
    pancreas S36.299
    rectum S36.69
    sigmoid S36.593
    spleen S36.09
    stomach S36.39
    symphysis pubis S33.4
    tympanum, tympanic
      (membrane) —*see* Rupture,
      ear drum, traumatic
    ureter S37.19
    uterus S37.69
    vagina —*see* Injury, vagina
    vena cava —*see* Injury, vena
      cava, laceration, major
  tricuspid (heart) (valve) I07.8
  tube, tubal (nonobstetric)
    (nontraumatic) N83.8
    abscess —*see* Salpingitis
    due to pregnancy O00.10-
      with intrauterine pregnancy
        O00.11-
  tympanum, tympanic (membrane)
    (nontraumatic) (*see also*
    Perforation, tympanic
    membrane) H72.9-
    traumatic —*see* Rupture, ear
      drum, traumatic
  umbilical cord, complicating
    delivery O69.89
  ureter (traumatic) S37.19
    nontraumatic N28.89
  urethra (nontraumatic) N36.8
    with ectopic or molar pregnancy
      O08.6
    following ectopic or molar
      pregnancy O08.6
    obstetrical trauma O71.5
    traumatic S37.39

Rupture, ruptured *(continued)*
  uterosacral ligament (nonobstetric) (nontraumatic) N83.8
  uterus (traumatic) S37.69
    before labor O71.0-
    during or after labor O71.1
    nonpuerperal, nontraumatic N85.8
    pregnant (during labor) O71.1
      before labor O71.0-
  vagina —*see* Injury, vagina
  valve, valvular (heart) —*see* Endocarditis
  varicose vein —*see* Varix
  varix —*see* Varix
  vena cava R58
    traumatic —*see* Injury, vena cava, laceration, major
  vesical (urinary) N32.89
  vessel (blood) R58
    pulmonary I28.8
    traumatic —*see* Injury, blood vessel
  viscus R19.8
  vulva complicating delivery O70.0
Russell-Silver syndrome Q87.19
Russian spring-summer type encephalitis A84.0
Rust's disease (tuberculous cervical spondylitis) A18.01
Ruvalcaba-Myhre-Smith syndrome E71.440
Rytand-Lipsitch syndrome I44.2

S

Saber, sabre shin or tibia (syphilitic) A50.56 *[M90.8-]*
Sac lacrimal —*see* condition
Saccharomyces infection B37.9
Saccharopinuria E72.3
Saccular —*see* condition
Sacculation
  aorta (nonsyphilitic) —*see* Aneurysm, aorta
  bladder N32.3
  intralaryngeal (congenital) (ventricular) Q31.3
  larynx (congenital) (ventricular) Q31.3
  organ or site, congenital —*see* Distortion
  pregnant uterus —*see* Pregnancy, complicated by, abnormal, uterus
  ureter N28.89
  urethra N36.1
  vesical N32.3
Sachs' amaurotic familial idiocy or disease E75.02
Sachs-Tay disease E75.02
Sacks-Libman disease M32.11
Sacralgia M53.3
Sacralization Q76.49
Sacrodynia M53.3
Sacroiliac joint —*see* condition
Sacroiliitis NEC M46.1
Sacrum —*see* condition
Saddle
  back —*see* Lordosis
  embolus
    abdominal aorta I74.01
    pulmonary artery I26.92
      with acute cor pulmonale I26.02

Saddle *(continued)*
  injury - code to condition
  nose M95.0
    due to syphilis A50.57
Sadism (sexual) F65.52
Sadness, postpartal O90.6
Sadomasochism F65.50
Saemisch's ulcer (cornea) —*see* Ulcer, cornea, central
Sagging
  skin and subcutaneous tissue (following bariatric surgery weight loss) (following dietary weight loss) L98.7
Sahib disease B55.0
Sailors' skin L57.8
Saint
  Anthony's fire —*see* Erysipelas
  triad —*see* Hernia, diaphragm
  Vitus' dance —*see* Chorea, Sydenham's
Salaam
  attack(s) —*see* Epilepsy, spasms
  tic R25.8
Salicylism
  abuse F55.8
  overdose or wrong substance given —*see* Table of Drugs and Chemicals, by drug, poisoning
Salivary duct or gland —*see* condition
Salivation, excessive K11.7
Salmonella —*see* Infection, Salmonella
Salmonellosis A02.0
Salpingitis (catarrhal) (fallopian tube) (nodular) (pseudofollicular) (purulent) (septic) N70.91
  with oophoritis N70.93
  acute N70.01
    with oophoritis N70.03
  chlamydial A56.11
  chronic N70.11
    with oophoritis N70.13
  complicating abortion —*see* Abortion, by type, complicated by, salpingitis
  ear —*see* Salpingitis, eustachian
  eustachian (tube) H68.00-
    acute H68.01-
    chronic H68.02-
  follicularis N70.11
    with oophoritis N70.13
  gonococcal (acute) (chronic) A54.24
  interstitial, chronic N70.11
    with oophoritis N70.13
  isthmica nodosa N70.11
    with oophoritis N70.13
  specific (gonococcal) (acute) (chronic) A54.24
  tuberculous (acute) (chronic) A18.17
  venereal (gonococcal) (acute) (chronic) A54.24
Salpingocele N83.4-
Salpingo-oophoritis (catarrhal) (purulent) (ruptured) (septic) (suppurative) N70.93
  acute N70.03
    with ectopic or molar pregnancy O08.0
    following ectopic or molar pregnancy O08.0
    gonococcal A54.24

Salpingo-oophoritis *(continued)*
  chronic N70.13
    following ectopic or molar pregnancy O08.0
  gonococcal (acute) (chronic) A54.24
  puerperal O86.19
  specific (gonococcal) (acute) (chronic) A54.24
  subacute N70.03
  tuberculous (acute) (chronic) A18.17
  venereal (gonococcal) (acute) (chronic) A54.24
Salpingo-ovaritis —*see* Salpingo-oophoritis
Salpingoperitonitis —*see* Salpingo-oophoritis
Salzmann's nodular dystrophy —*see* Degeneration, cornea, nodular
Sampson's cyst or tumor N80.10-
San Joaquin (Valley) **fever** B38.0
Sandblaster's asthma, lung or pneumoconiosis J62.8
Sander's disease (paranoia) F22
Sandfly fever A93.1
Sandhoff's disease E75.01
Sanfilippo (Type B) (Type C) (Type D) **syndrome** E76.22
Sanger-Brown ataxia G11.2
Sao Paulo fever or typhus A77.0
Saponification, mesenteric K65.8
Sarcocele (benign)
  syphilitic A52.76
    congenital A50.59
Sarcocystosis A07.8
Sarcoepiplocele —*see* Hernia
Sarcoepiplomphalocele Q79.2
Sarcoglycanopathy G71.0340
  alpha G71.0341
  beta G71.0342
  delta G71.0349
  gamma G71.0349
Sarcoid —*see also* Sarcoidosis
  arthropathy D86.86
  Boeck's D86.9
  Darier-Roussy D86.3
  iridocyclitis D86.83
  meningitis D86.81
  myocarditis D86.85
  myositis D86.87
  pyelonephritis D86.84
  Spiegler-Fendt L08.89
Sarcoidosis D86.9
  with
    cranial nerve palsies D86.82
    hepatic granuloma D86.89
    polyarthritis D86.86
    tubulo-interstitial nephropathy D86.84
  combined sites NEC D86.89
  lung D86.0
    and lymph nodes D86.2
  lymph nodes D86.1
    and lung D86.2
  meninges D86.81
  skin D86.3
  specified type NEC D86.89
Sarcoma (of) —*see also* Neoplasm, connective tissue, malignant
  alveolar soft part —*see* Neoplasm, connective tissue, malignant
  ameloblastic C41.1
    upper jaw (bone) C41.0

Sarcoma *(continued)*
  botryoid —*see* Neoplasm, connective tissue, malignant
  botryoides —*see* Neoplasm, connective tissue, malignant
  cerebellar C71.6
    circumscribed (arachnoidal) C71.6
  circumscribed (arachnoidal) cerebellar C71.6
  clear cell —*see also* Neoplasm, connective tissue, malignant
    kidney C64.-
  dendritic cells (accessory cells) C96.4
  embryonal —*see* Neoplasm, connective tissue, malignant
  endometrial (stromal) C54.1
    isthmus C54.0
  epithelioid (cell) —*see* Neoplasm, connective tissue, malignant
  Ewing's —*see* Neoplasm, bone, malignant
  follicular dendritic cell C96.4
  germinoblastic (diffuse) —*see* Lymphoma, diffuse large cell
  follicular —*see* Lymphoma, follicular, specified NEC
  giant cell (except of bone) —*see also* Neoplasm, connective tissue, malignant
    bone —*see* Neoplasm, bone, malignant
  glomoid —*see* Neoplasm, connective tissue, malignant
  granulocytic C92.3-
  hemangioendothelial —*see* Neoplasm, connective tissue, malignant
  hemorrhagic, multiple —*see* Sarcoma, Kaposi's
  histiocytic C96.A
  Hodgkin —*see* Lymphoma, Hodgkin
  immunoblastic (diffuse) —*see* Lymphoma, diffuse large cell
  interdigitating dendritic cell C96.4
  Kaposi's
    colon C46.4
    connective tissue C46.1
    gastrointestinal organ C46.4
    lung C46.5-
    lymph node(s) C46.3
    palate (hard) (soft) C46.2
    rectum C46.4
    skin C46.0
    specified site NEC C46.7
    stomach C46.4
    unspecified site C46.9
  Kupffer cell C22.3
  Langerhans cell C96.4
  leptomeningeal —*see* Neoplasm, meninges, malignant
  liver NEC C22.4
  lymphangioendothelial —*see* Neoplasm, connective tissue, malignant
  lymphoblastic —*see* Lymphoma, lymphoblastic (diffuse)
  lymphocytic —*see* Lymphoma, small cell B-cell
  mast cell C96.22
  melanotic —*see* Melanoma
  meningeal —*see* Neoplasm, meninges, malignant
  meningothelial —*see* Neoplasm, meninges, malignant

293

Sarcoma (continued)
  mesenchymal —see also
    Neoplasm, connective tissue,
    malignant
    mixed —see Neoplasm,
      connective tissue, malignant
  mesothelial —see Mesothelioma
  monstrocellular
    specified site —see Neoplasm,
      malignant, by site
    unspecified site C71.9
  myeloid C92.8-
  neurogenic —see Neoplasm, nerve,
    malignant
  odontogenic C41.1
    upper jaw (bone) C41.0
  osteoblastic —see Neoplasm, bone,
    malignant
  osteogenic —see also Neoplasm,
    bone, malignant
    juxtacortical —see Neoplasm,
      bone, malignant
    periosteal —see Neoplasm,
      bone, malignant
  periosteal —see also Neoplasm,
    bone, malignant
    osteogenic —see Neoplasm,
      bone, malignant
  pleomorphic cell —see Neoplasm,
    connective tissue, malignant
  reticulum cell (diffuse) —see
    Lymphoma, diffuse large cell
    nodular —see Lymphoma,
      follicular
    pleomorphic cell type —see
      Lymphoma, diffuse large cell
  rhabdoid —see Neoplasm,
    malignant, by site
  round cell —see Neoplasm,
    connective tissue, malignant
  small cell —see Neoplasm,
    connective tissue, malignant
  soft tissue —see Neoplasm,
    connective tissue, malignant
  spindle cell —see Neoplasm,
    connective tissue, malignant
  stromal (endometrial) C54.1
    isthmus C54.0
  synovial —see also Neoplasm,
    connective tissue, malignant
    biphasic —see Neoplasm,
      connective tissue, malignant
    epithelioid cell —see Neoplasm,
      connective tissue, malignant
    spindle cell —see Neoplasm,
      connective tissue, malignant

Sarcomatosis
  meningeal —see Neoplasm,
    meninges, malignant
  specified site NEC —see Neoplasm,
    connective tissue, malignant
  unspecified site C80.1

Sarcopenia (age-related) M62.84
Sarcosinemia E72.59
Sarcosporidiosis (intestinal) A07.8
SARS-CoV-2 —see also COVID-19
  sequelae (post acute) U09.9
Satiety, early R68.81
Saturnine —see condition
Saturnism
  overdose or wrong substance
    given or taken —see Table of
    Drugs and Chemicals, by drug,
    poisoning
Satyriasis F52.8
Sauriasis —see Ichthyosis

SBE (subacute bacterial endocarditis)
  I33.0
Scabs R23.4
Scabies (any site) B86
Scaglietti-Dagnini syndrome E22.0
Scald —see Burn
Scalenus anticus (anterior)
  syndrome G54.0
Scales R23.4
Scaling, skin R23.4
Scalp —see condition
Scapegoating affecting child Z62.3
Scaphocephaly, non-deformational
  Q75.01
Scapulalgia M89.8X1
Scapulohumeral myopathy
  G71.02
Scar, scarring (see also Cicatrix)
  L90.5
  adherent L90.5
  atrophic L90.5
  cervix
    in pregnancy or childbirth —see
      Pregnancy, complicated by,
      abnormal cervix
  cheloid L91.0
  chorioretinal H31.00-
    posterior pole macula H31.01-
    postsurgical H59.81-
    solar retinopathy H31.02-
    specified type NEC H31.09-
  choroid —see Scar, chorioretinal
  conjunctiva H11.24-
  cornea H17.9
    xerophthalmic —see also
      Opacity, cornea
      vitamin A deficiency E50.6
  defect (isthmocele) O34.22
  duodenum, obstructive K31.5
  hypertrophic L91.0
  keloid L91.0
  labia N90.89
  lung (base) J98.4
  macula —see Scar, chorioretinal,
    posterior pole
  muscle M62.89
  myocardium, myocardial I25.2
  painful L90.5
  posterior pole (eye) —see Scar,
    chorioretinal, posterior pole
  retina —see Scar, chorioretinal
  trachea J39.8
  transmural uterine, in pregnancy
    O34.29
  uterus N85.8
    in pregnancy O34.29
  vagina N89.8
    postoperative N99.2
  vulva N90.89
Scarabiasis B88.2
Scarlatina (anginosa) (maligna)
  A38.9
  myocarditis (acute) A38.1
  old —see Myocarditis
  otitis media A38.0
  ulcerosa A38.8
Scarlet fever (albuminuria) (angina)
  A38.9
Schamberg's disease (progressive
  pigmentary dermatosis) L81.7
Schatzki's ring (acquired)
  (esophagus) (lower) K22.2
  congenital Q39.3
Schaufenster krankheit I20.89

Schaumann's
  benign lymphogranulomatosis D86.1
  disease or syndrome —see
    Sarcoidosis
Scheie's syndrome E76.03
Schenck's disease B42.1
**Scheuermann's disease or
  osteochondrosis** —see
  Osteochondrosis, juvenile, spine
Schilder (-Flatau) **disease** G37.0
Schilling-type monocytic leukemia
  C93.0-
**Schimmelbusch's disease, cystic
  mastitis, or hyperplasia** —see
  Mastopathy, cystic
Schistosoma infestation —see
  Infestation, Schistosoma
Schistosomiasis B65.9
  with muscle disorder B65.9 [M63.80]
    ankle B65.9 [M63.87-]
    foot B65.9 [M63.87-]
    forearm B65.9 [M63.83-]
    hand B65.9 [M63.84-]
    lower leg B65.9 [M63.86-]
    multiple sites B65.9 [M63.89]
    pelvic region B65.9 [M63.85-]
    shoulder region B65.9 [M63.81-]
    specified site NEC B65.9 [M63.88]
    thigh B65.9 [M63.85-]
    upper arm B65.9 [M63.82-]
  Asiatic B65.2
  bladder B65.0
  chestermani B65.8
  colon B65.1
  cutaneous B65.3
  due to
    S. haematobium B65.0
    S. japonicum B65.2
    S. mansoni B65.1
    S. mattheii B65.8
  Eastern B65.2
  genitourinary tract B65.0
  intestinal B65.1
  lung NEC B65.9 [J99]
    pneumonia B65.9 [J17]
  Manson's (intestinal) B65.1
  oriental B65.2
  pulmonary NEC B65.9 [J99]
    pneumonia B65.9
  Schistosoma
    haematobium B65.0
    japonicum B65.2
    mansoni B65.1
  specified type NEC B65.8
  urinary B65.0
  vesical B65.0
Schizencephaly Q04.6
Schizoaffective psychosis F25.9
Schizodontia K00.2
Schizoid personality F60.1
Schizophrenia, schizophrenic F20.9
  acute (brief) (undifferentiated) F23
  atypical (form) F20.3
  borderline F21
  catalepsy F20.2
  catatonic (type) (excited)
    (withdrawn) F20.2
  cenesthopathic, cenesthesiopathic
    F20.89
  childhood type F20.9
  chronic undifferentiated F20.9
  cyclic F25.0
  disorganized (type) F20.1
  flexibilitas cerea F20.2
  hebephrenic (type) F20.1
  incipient F21

Schizophrenia, schizophrenic
  (continued)
  latent F21
  negative type F20.5
  paranoid (type) F20.0
  paraphrenic F20.0
  post-psychotic depression F32.89
  prepsychotic F21
  prodromal F21
  pseudoneurotic F21
  pseudopsychopathic F21
  reaction F23
  residual (state) (type) F20.5
  restzustand F20.5
  schizoaffective (type) —see
    Psychosis, schizoaffective
  simple (type) F20.89
  simplex F20.89
  specified type NEC F20.89
  spectrum and other psychotic
    disorder F29
    specified NEC F28
  stupor F20.2
  syndrome of childhood F84.5
  undifferentiated (type) F20.3
    chronic F20.5
Schizothymia (persistent) F60.1
**Schlatter-Osgood disease or
  osteochondrosis** M92.52-
Schlatter's tibia —see
  Osteochondrosis, juvenile, tibia
Schmidt's syndrome (polyglandular,
  autoimmune) E31.0
Schmincke's carcinoma or tumor
  —see Neoplasm, nasopharynx,
  malignant
Schmitz (-Stutzer) **dysentery**
  A03.0
Schmorl's disease or nodes
  lumbar region M51.46
  lumbosacral region M51.47
  sacrococcygeal region M53.3
  thoracic region M51.44
  thoracolumbar region M51.45
Schneiderian
  papilloma —see Neoplasm,
    nasopharynx, benign
    specified site —see Neoplasm,
      benign, by site
    unspecified site D14.0
  specified site —see Neoplasm,
    malignant, by site
  unspecified site C30.0
Scholte's syndrome (malignant
  carcinoid) E34.0
Scholz (-Bielchowsky-Henneberg)
  disease or syndrome E75.25
Schönlein (-Henoch) **disease or
  purpura** (primary) (rheumatic)
  D69.0
Schottmuller's disease A01.4
Schroeder's syndrome (endocrine
  hypertensive) E27.0
**Schüller-Christian disease or
  syndrome** C96.5
**Schultze's type acroparesthesia,
  simple** I73.89
Schultz's disease or syndrome —see
  Agranulocytosis
**Schwalbe-Ziehen-Oppenheim
  disease** G24.1
Schwannoma —see also Neoplasm,
  nerve, benign
  malignant —see also Neoplasm,
    nerve, malignant

Schwannoma (continued)
  malignant (continued)
    with rhabdomyoblastic differentiation —see Neoplasm, nerve, malignant
  melanocytic —see Neoplasm, nerve, benign
  pigmented —see Neoplasm, nerve, benign
Schwannomatosis Q85.03
Schwartz (-Jampel) **syndrome** G71.13
Schwartz-Bartter syndrome E22.2
Schweniger-Buzzi anetoderma L90.1
Sciatic —see condition
Sciatica (infective) M54.3-
  with lumbago M54.4-
    due to intervertebral disc disorder —see Disorder, disc, with, radiculopathy
  due to displacement of intervertebral disc (with lumbago) —see Disorder, disc, with, radiculopathy
  wallet M54.3-
Scimitar syndrome Q26.8
Sclera —see condition
Sclerectasia H15.84-
Scleredema
  adultorum —see Sclerosis, systemic
  Buschke's —see Sclerosis, systemic
  newborn P83.0
Sclerema (adiposum) (edematosum) (neonatorum) (newborn) P83.0
  adultorum —see Sclerosis, systemic
Scleriasis —see Scleroderma
Scleritis H15.00-
  with corneal involvement H15.04-
  anterior H15.01-
  brawny H15.02-
  in (due to) zoster B02.34
  posterior H15.03-
  specified type NEC H15.09-
  syphilitic A52.71
  tuberculous (nodular) A18.51
Sclerochoroiditis H31.8
Scleroconjunctivitis —see Scleritis
Sclerocystic ovary syndrome E28.2
Sclerodactyly, sclerodactylia L94.3
Scleroderma, sclerodermia
  (acrosclerotic) (diffuse) (generalized) (progressive) (pulmonary) (see also Sclerosis, systemic) M34.9-
  circumscribed L94.0
  linear L94.1
  localized L94.0
  newborn P83.88
  systemic M34.9
Sclerokeratitis H16.8
  tuberculous A18.52
Scleroma nasi A48.8
Scleromalacia (perforans) H15.05-
Scleromyxedema L98.5
Sclérose en plaques G35
Sclerosis, sclerotic
  adrenal (gland) E27.8
  Alzheimer's —see Disease, Alzheimer's
  amyotrophic (lateral) G12.21
  aorta, aortic I70.0
    valve —see Endocarditis, aortic

Sclerosis, sclerotic (continued)
  artery, arterial, arteriolar, arteriovascular —see Arteriosclerosis
  ascending multiple G35
  brain (generalized) (lobular) G37.9
    artery, arterial I67.2
    diffuse G37.0
    disseminated G35
    insular G35
    Krabbe's E75.23
    miliary G35
    multiple G35
    presenile (Alzheimer's) —see Disease, Alzheimer's, early onset
    senile (arteriosclerotic) I67.2
    stem, multiple G35
    tuberous Q85.1
  bulbar, multiple G35
  bundle of His I44.39
  cardiac —see Disease, heart, ischemic, atherosclerotic
  cardiorenal —see Hypertension, cardiorenal
  cardiovascular —see also Disease, cardiovascular
    renal —see Hypertension, cardiorenal
  cerebellar —see Sclerosis, brain
  cerebral —see Sclerosis, brain
  cerebrospinal (disseminated) (multiple) G35
  cerebrovascular I67.2
  choroid —see Degeneration, choroid
  combined (spinal cord) —see also Degeneration, combined
    multiple G35
  concentric (Balo) G37.5
  cornea —see Opacity, cornea
  coronary (artery) I25.10
    with angina pectoris —see Arteriosclerosis, coronary (artery),
  corpus cavernosum
    female N90.89
    male N48.6
  diffuse (brain) (spinal cord) G37.0
  disseminated G35
  dorsal G35
  dorsolateral (spinal cord) —see Degeneration, combined
  endometrium N85.5
  extrapyramidal G25.9
  eye, nuclear (senile) —see Cataract, senile, nuclear
  focal and segmental (glomerular) (see also N00-N07 with fourth character .1) N05.1
  Friedreich's (spinal cord) G11.11
  funicular (spermatic cord) N50.89
  general (vascular) —see Arteriosclerosis
  gland (lymphatic) I89.8
  hepatic K74.1
    alcoholic K70.2
  hereditary
    cerebellar G11.9
    spinal (Friedreich's ataxia) G11.11
  hippocampal G93.81
  insular G35
  kidney —see Sclerosis, renal
  larynx J38.7
  lateral (amyotrophic) (descending) (spinal) G12.21
    primary G12.23
  lens, senile nuclear —see Cataract, senile, nuclear
  liver K74.1
    with fibrosis K74.2
      alcoholic K70.2

Sclerosis, sclerotic (continued)
  liver (continued)
    alcoholic K70.2
    cardiac K76.1
  lung —see Fibrosis, lung
  mastoid —see Mastoiditis, chronic
  mesial temporal G93.81
  mitral I05.8
  Mönckeberg's (medial) —see Arteriosclerosis, extremities
  multiple (brain stem) (cerebral) (generalized) (spinal cord) G35
  myocardium, myocardial —see Disease, heart, ischemic, atherosclerotic
  nuclear (senile), eye —see Cataract, senile, nuclear
  ovary N83.8
  pancreas K86.89
  penis N48.6
  peripheral arteries —see Arteriosclerosis, extremities
  plaques G35
  pluriglandular E31.8
  polyglandular E31.8
  posterolateral (spinal cord) —see Degeneration, combined
  presenile (Alzheimer's) —see Disease, Alzheimer's, early onset
  primary, lateral G12.23
  progressive, systemic M34.0
  pulmonary —see Fibrosis, lung
    artery I27.0
    valve (heart) —see Endocarditis, pulmonary
  renal N26.9
    with
      cystine storage disease E72.09
      hypertensive heart disease (conditions in I11) —see Hypertension, cardiorenal
    arteriolar (hyaline) (hyperplastic) —see Hypertension, kidney
  retina (senile) (vascular) H35.00
  senile (vascular) —see Arteriosclerosis
  spinal (cord) (progressive) G95.89
    ascending G61.0
    combined —see also Degeneration, combined
      multiple G35
      syphilitic A52.11
    disseminated G35
    dorsolateral —see Degeneration, combined
    hereditary (Friedreich's) (mixed form) G11.11
    lateral (amyotrophic) G12.21
    progressive G12.23
    multiple G35
    posterior (syphilitic) A52.11
  stomach K31.89
  subendocardial, congenital I42.4
  systemic M34.9
    with
      lung involvement M34.81
      myopathy M34.82
      polyneuropathy M34.83
    drug-induced M34.2
    due to chemicals NEC M34.2
    progressive M34.0
    specified NEC M34.89
  temporal (mesial) G93.81
  tricuspid (heart) (valve) I07.8
  tuberous (brain) Q85.1
  tympanic membrane —see Disorder, tympanic membrane, specified NEC
  valve, valvular (heart) —see Endocarditis

Sclerosis, sclerotic (continued)
  vascular —see Arteriosclerosis
  vein I87.8
Scoliosis (acquired) (postural) M41.9
  adolescent (idiopathic) —see Scoliosis, idiopathic, adolescent
  congenital Q67.5
    due to bony malformation Q76.3
    failure of segmentation (hemivertebra) Q76.3
    hemivertebra fusion Q76.3
  postural Q67.5
  degenerative M41.5-
  idiopathic M41.20
    adolescent M41.129
      cervical region M41.122
      cervicothoracic region M41.123
      lumbar region M41.126
      lumbosacral region M41.127
      thoracic region M41.124
      thoracolumbar region M41.125
    cervical region M41.22
    cervicothoracic region M41.23
    infantile M41.00
      cervical region M41.02
      cervicothoracic region M41.03
      lumbar region M41.06
      lumbosacral region M41.07
      sacrococcygeal region M41.08
      thoracic region M41.04
      thoracolumbar region M41.05
    juvenile M41.119
      cervical region M41.112
      cervicothoracic region M41.113
      lumbar region M41.116
      lumbosacral region M41.117
      thoracic region M41.114
      thoracolumbar region M41.115
    lumbar region M41.26
    lumbosacral region M41.27
    thoracic region M41.24
    thoracolumbar region M41.25
  infantile —see Scoliosis, idiopathic, infantile
  neuromuscular M41.40
    cervical region M41.42
    cervicothoracic region M41.43
    lumbar region M41.46
    lumbosacral region M41.47
    occipito-atlanto-axial region M41.41
    thoracic region M41.44
    thoracolumbar region M41.45
  paralytic —see Scoliosis, neuromuscular
  postprocedural M96.89
  postradiation therapy M96.5
  rachitic (late effect or sequelae) E64.3 [M49.80]
    cervical region E64.3 [M49.82]
    cervicothoracic region E64.3 [M49.83]
    lumbar region E64.3 [M49.86]
    lumbosacral region E64.3 [M49.87]
    multiple sites E64.3 [M49.89]
    occipito-atlanto-axial region E64.3 [M49.81]
    sacrococcygeal region E64.3 [M49.88]
    thoracic region E64.3 [M49.84]
    thoracolumbar region E64.3 [M49.85]
  sciatic M54.4-
  secondary (to) NEC M41.50
    cerebral palsy, Friedreich's ataxia, poliomyelitis, neuromuscular disorders —see Scoliosis, neuromuscular
    cervical region M41.52

Scoliosis (continued)
　secondary (continued)
　　cervicothoracic region M41.53
　　lumbar region M41.56
　　lumbosacral region M41.57
　　thoracic region M41.54
　　thoracolumbar region M41.55
　　specified form NEC M41.80
　　　cervical region M41.82
　　　cervicothoracic region M41.83
　　　lumbar region M41.86
　　　lumbosacral region M41.87
　　　thoracic region M41.84
　　　thoracolumbar region M41.85
　　thoracogenic M41.30
　　　thoracic region M41.34
　　　thoracolumbar region M41.35
　　tuberculous A18.01

Scoliotic pelvis
　with disproportion (fetopelvic) O33.0
　　causing obstructed labor O65.0

Scorbutus, scorbutic —see also Scurvy
　anemia D53.2

Score, NIHSS (National Institutes of Health Stoke Scale) R29.7-

Scotoma (arcuate) (Bjerrum) (central) (ring) —see also Defect, visual field, localized, scotoma
　scintillating H53.12-

Scratch —see Abrasion

Scratchy throat R09.89

Screening (for) Z13.9
　alcoholism Z13.39
　anemia Z13.0
　anomaly, congenital Z13.89
　antenatal, of mother (see also Encounter, antenatal screening) Z36.9
　arterial hypertension Z13.6
　arthropod-borne viral disease NEC Z11.59
　autism Z13.41
　bacteriuria, asymptomatic Z13.89
　behavioral disorder Z13.30
　　specified NEC Z13.39
　brain injury, traumatic Z13.850
　bronchitis, chronic Z13.83
　brucellosis Z11.2
　cardiovascular disorder Z13.6
　cataract Z13.5
　chlamydial diseases Z11.8
　cholera Z11.0
　chromosomal abnormalities (nonprocreative) NEC Z13.79
　colonoscopy Z12.11
　congenital
　　dislocation of hip Z13.89
　　eye disorder Z13.5
　　malformation or deformation Z13.89
　contamination NEC Z13.88
　coronavirus (disease) (novel) 2019 Z11.52
　COVID-19 Z11.52
　cystic fibrosis Z13.228
　dengue fever Z11.59
　dental disorder Z13.84
　depression (adult) (adolescent) (child) Z13.31
　　maternal Z13.32
　　perinatal Z13.32
　developmental
　　delays Z13.40
　　　global (milestones) Z13.42
　　　specified NEC Z13.49
　　handicap Z13.42
　　　in early childhood Z13.42

Screening (continued)
　diabetes mellitus Z13.1
　diphtheria Z11.2
　disability, intellectual Z13.39
　disease or disorder Z13.9
　　bacterial NEC Z11.2
　　　intestinal infectious Z11.0
　　　respiratory tuberculosis Z11.1
　　behavioral Z13.30
　　　specified NEC Z13.39
　　blood or blood-forming organ Z13.0
　　cardiovascular Z13.6
　　Chagas' Z11.6
　　chlamydial Z11.8
　　coronavirus (disease) (novel) 2019 Z11.52
　　　COVID-19 Z11.52
　　dental Z13.89
　　developmental delays Z13.40
　　　global (milestones) Z13.42
　　　specified NEC Z13.49
　　digestive tract NEC Z13.818
　　　lower GI Z13.811
　　　upper GI Z13.810
　　ear Z13.5
　　endocrine Z13.29
　　eye Z13.5
　　genitourinary Z13.89
　　heart Z13.6
　　human immunodeficiency virus (HIV) infection Z11.4
　　immunity Z13.0
　　infection
　　　intestinal Z11.0
　　　　specified NEC Z11.6
　　infectious Z11.9
　　mental health and behavioral Z13.30
　　　specified NEC Z13.39
　　metabolic Z13.228
　　neurological Z13.89
　　nutritional Z13.21
　　　metabolic Z13.228
　　　　lipoid disorders Z13.220
　　protozoal Z11.6
　　　intestinal Z11.0
　　respiratory Z13.83
　　rheumatic Z13.828
　　rickettsial Z11.8
　　sexually-transmitted NEC Z11.3
　　　human immunodeficiency virus (HIV) Z11.4
　　sickle-cell (trait) Z13.0
　　skin Z13.89
　　specified NEC Z13.89
　　spirochetal Z11.8
　　thyroid Z13.29
　　vascular Z13.6
　　venereal Z11.3
　　viral NEC Z11.59
　　　human immunodeficiency virus (HIV) Z11.4
　　　intestinal Z11.0
　　　coronavirus (disease) (novel) 2019 Z11.52
　　　　COVID-19 Z11.52
　　　　SARS-CoV-2 Z11.52
　elevated titer Z13.89
　emphysema Z13.83
　encephalitis, viral (mosquito- or tick-borne) Z11.59
　exposure to contaminants (toxic) Z13.88
　fever
　　dengue Z11.59
　　hemorrhagic Z11.59
　　yellow Z11.59
　filariasis Z11.6
　galactosemia Z13.228
　gastrointestinal condition Z13.818

Screening (continued)
　genetic (nonprocreative) - for procreative management —see Testing, genetic, for procreative management
　　disease carrier status (nonprocreative) Z13.71
　　specified NEC (nonprocreative) Z13.79
　genitourinary condition Z13.89
　glaucoma Z13.5
　gonorrhea Z11.3
　gout Z13.89
　helminthiasis (intestinal) Z11.6
　hematopoietic malignancy Z12.89
　hemoglobinopathies NEC Z13.0
　hemorrhagic fever Z11.59
　Hodgkin disease Z12.89
　human immunodeficiency virus (HIV) Z11.4
　human papillomavirus Z11.51
　hypertension Z13.6
　immunity disorders Z13.0
　infant or child (over 28 days old) Z00.129
　　with abnormal findings Z00.121
　infection
　　mycotic Z11.8
　　parasitic Z11.8
　ingestion of radioactive substance Z13.88
　intellectual disability Z13.39
　intestinal
　　helminthiasis Z11.6
　　infectious disease Z11.0
　leishmaniasis Z11.6
　leprosy Z11.2
　leptospirosis Z11.8
　leukemia Z12.89
　lymphoma Z12.89
　malaria Z11.6
　malnutrition Z13.29
　　metabolic Z13.228
　　nutritional Z13.21
　measles Z11.59
　mental health disorder Z13.30
　　specified NEC Z13.39
　metabolic errors, inborn Z13.228
　multiphasic Z13.89
　musculoskeletal disorder Z13.828
　　osteoporosis Z13.820
　mycoses Z11.8
　myocardial infarction (acute) Z13.6
　neoplasm (malignant) (of) Z12.9
　　bladder Z12.6
　　blood Z12.89
　　breast Z12.39
　　　routine mammogram Z12.31
　　cervix Z12.4
　　colon Z12.11
　　genitourinary organs NEC Z12.79
　　　bladder Z12.6
　　　cervix Z12.4
　　　ovary Z12.73
　　　prostate Z12.5
　　　testis Z12.71
　　　vagina Z12.72
　　hematopoietic system Z12.89
　　intestinal tract Z12.10
　　　colon Z12.11
　　　rectum Z12.12
　　　small intestine Z12.13
　　lung Z12.2
　　lymph (glands) Z12.89
　　nervous system Z12.82
　　oral cavity Z12.81
　　prostate Z12.5
　　rectum Z12.12
　　respiratory organs Z12.2
　　skin Z12.83

Screening (continued)
　neoplasm (continued)
　　small intestine Z12.13
　　specified site NEC Z12.89
　　stomach Z12.0
　nephropathy Z13.89
　nervous system disorders NEC Z13.858
　neurological condition Z13.89
　osteoporosis Z13.820
　parasitic infestation Z11.9
　　specified NEC Z11.8
　phenylketonuria Z13.228
　plague Z11.2
　poisoning (chemical) (heavy metal) Z13.88
　poliomyelitis Z11.59
　postnatal, chromosomal abnormalities Z13.89
　prenatal, of mother (see also Encounter, antenatal screening) Z36.9
　protozoal disease Z11.6
　　intestinal Z11.0
　pulmonary tuberculosis Z11.1
　radiation exposure Z13.88
　respiratory condition Z13.83
　respiratory tuberculosis Z11.1
　rheumatoid arthritis Z13.828
　rubella Z11.59
　SARS-CoV-2 Z11.52
　schistosomiasis Z11.6
　sexually-transmitted disease NEC Z11.3
　　human immunodeficiency virus (HIV) Z11.4
　sickle-cell disease or trait Z13.0
　skin condition Z13.89
　sleeping sickness Z11.6
　special Z13.9
　　specified NEC Z13.89
　syphilis Z11.3
　tetanus Z11.2
　trachoma Z11.8
　traumatic brain injury Z13.850
　trypanosomiasis Z11.6
　tuberculosis, respiratory Z11.1
　　active Z11.1
　　latent Z11.7
　venereal disease Z11.3
　viral encephalitis (mosquito- or tick-borne) Z11.59
　whooping cough Z11.2
　worms, intestinal Z11.6
　yaws Z11.8
　yellow fever Z11.59

Scrofula, scrofulosis (tuberculosis of cervical lymph glands) A18.2

Scrofulide (primary) (tuberculous) A18.4

Scrofuloderma, scrofulodermia (any site) (primary) A18.4

Scrofulosus lichen (primary) (tuberculous) A18.4

Scrofulous —see condition

Scrotal tongue K14.5

Scrotum —see condition

Scurvy, scorbutic E54
　anemia D53.2
　gum E54
　infantile E54
　rickets E55.0 [M90.80]

Sealpox B08.62

Seasickness T75.3

Seatworm (infection) (infestation) B80

Sebaceous —see also condition
　cyst —see Cyst, sebaceous

Seborrhea, seborrheic L21.9
- capillitii R23.8
- capitis L21.0
- dermatitis L21.9
  - infantile L21.1
- eczema L21.9
  - infantile L21.1
- sicca L21.0

Seckel's syndrome Q87.19

Seclusion, pupil —*see* Membrane, pupillary

Second hand tobacco smoke exposure (acute) (chronic) Z77.22
- in the perinatal period P96.81

Secondary
- dentin (in pulp) K04.3
- neoplasm, secondaries —*see* Table of Neoplasms, secondary

Secretion
- antidiuretic hormone, inappropriate E22.2
- catecholamine, by pheochromocytoma E27.5
- hormone
  - antidiuretic, inappropriate (syndrome) E22.2
  - by
    - carcinoid tumor E34.0
    - pheochromocytoma E27.5
  - ectopic NEC E34.2
- urinary
  - excessive R35.89
  - suppression R34

Section
- nerve, traumatic —*see* Injury, nerve

Sedative, hypnotic, or anxiolytic-induced
- anxiety disorder F13.980
- bipolar and related disorder F13.94
- delirium F13.921
- depressive disorder F13.94
- major neurocognitive disorder F13.97
- mild neurocognitive disorder F13.988
- psychotic disorder F13.959
- sexual dysfunction F13.981
- sleep disorder F13.982

Segmentation, incomplete (congenital) —*see also* Fusion
- bone NEC Q78.8
- lumbosacral (joint) (vertebra) Q76.49

SEID (systemic exertion intolerance disease) G93.32

Seitelberger's syndrome (infantile neuraxonal dystrophy) G31.89

Seizure(s) (*see also* Convulsions) R56.9
- absence G40.A-
- akinetic —*see* Epilepsy, generalized, specified NEC
- atonic —*see* Epilepsy, generalized, specified NEC
- autonomic (hysterical) F44.5
- convulsive —*see* Convulsions
- cortical (focal) (motor) —*see* Epilepsy, localization-related, symptomatic, with simple partial seizures
- disorder (*see also* Epilepsy) G40.909
- due to stroke —*see* Sequelae (of), disease, cerebrovascular, by type, specified NEC
- epileptic —*see* Epilepsy

Seizure(s) *(continued)*
- febrile (simple) R56.00
  - with status epilepticus G40.901
  - complex (atypical) (complicated) R56.01
    - with status epilepticus G40.901
- grand mal G40.409
  - intractable G40.419
    - with status epilepticus G40.411
    - without status epilepticus G40.419
  - not intractable G40.409
    - with status epilepticus G40.401
    - without status epilepticus G40.409
- heart —*see* Disease, heart
- hysterical F44.5
- intractable G40.919
  - with status epilepticus G40.911
- Jacksonian (focal) (motor type) (sensory type) —*see* Epilepsy, localization-related, symptomatic, with simple partial seizures
- newborn P90
- nonspecific epileptic
  - atonic —*see* Epilepsy, generalized, specified NEC
  - clonic —*see* Epilepsy, generalized, specified NEC
  - myoclonic —*see* Epilepsy, generalized, specified NEC
  - tonic —*see* Epilepsy, generalized, specified NEC
  - tonic-clonic —*see* Epilepsy, generalized, specified NEC
- partial, developing into secondarily generalized seizures
  - complex —*see* Epilepsy, localization-related, symptomatic, with complex partial seizures
  - simple —*see* Epilepsy, localization-related, symptomatic, with simple partial seizures
- petit mal G40.A-
  - intractable G40.A1-
    - with status epilepticus G40.A11
    - without status epilepticus G40.A19
  - not intractable G40.A0-
    - with status epilepticus G40.A01
    - without status epilepticus G40.A09
- post traumatic R56.1
- recurrent G40.909
- specified NEC G40.89
- uncinate —*see* Epilepsy, localization-related, symptomatic, with complex partial seizures

Selenium deficiency, dietary E59

Self-damaging behavior (life-style) Z72.89

Self-harm (attempted)
- history (personal)
  - in family Z81.8
    - nonsuicidal Z91.52
    - suicidal Z91.51
  - nonsuicidal R45.88

Self-injury, nonsuicidal R45.88
- personal history Z91.52

Self-mutilation (attempted)
- history (personal)
  - in family Z81.8
    - nonsuicidal Z91.52
    - suicidal Z91.51
  - nonsuicidal R45.88

Self-poisoning
- history (personal) Z91.51
  - in family Z81.8
- observation following (alleged) attempt Z03.6

Semicoma R40.1

Seminal vesiculitis N49.0

Seminoma C62.9-
- specified site —*see* Neoplasm, malignant, by site

Senear-Usher disease or syndrome L10.4

Senectus R54

Senescence (without mention of psychosis) R54

Senile, senility (*see also* condition) R41.81
- with
  - acute confusional state F05
  - mental changes NOS F03
  - psychosis NEC —*see* Psychosis, senile
- asthenia R54
- cervix (atrophic) N88.8
- debility R54
- endometrium (atrophic) N85.8
- fallopian tube (atrophic) —*see* Atrophy, fallopian tube
- heart (failure) R54
- ovary (atrophic) —*see* Atrophy, ovary
- premature E34.8
- vagina, vaginitis (atrophic) N95.2
- wart L82.1

Sensation
- burning (skin) R20.8
  - tongue K14.6
- foreign body R09.A0
  - eye H57.8A-
  - globus R09.A2
  - nose R09.A1
  - specified site NEC R09.A9
  - throat R09.A2
- loss of R20.8
- prickling (skin) R20.2
- tingling (skin) R20.2

Sense loss
- smell —*see* Disturbance, sensation, smell
- taste —*see* Disturbance, sensation, taste
- touch R20.8

Sensibility disturbance (cortical) (deep) (vibratory) R20.9

Sensitive, sensitivity —*see also* Allergy
- carotid sinus G90.01
- child (excessive) F93.8
- cold, autoimmune D59.12
- dentin K03.89
- gluten (non-celiac) K90.41
- latex Z91.040
- methemoglobin D74.8
- tuberculin, without clinical or radiological symptoms R76.11
- visual
  - glare H53.71
  - impaired contrast H53.72

Sensitiver Beziehungswahn F22

Sensitization, auto-erythrocytic D69.2

Separation
- anxiety, abnormal (of childhood) F93.0
- apophysis, traumatic - code as Fracture, by site

Separation *(continued)*
- choroid —*see* Detachment, choroid
- epiphysis, epiphyseal
  - nontraumatic —*see also* Osteochondropathy, specified type NEC
    - upper femoral —*see* Slipped, epiphysis, upper femoral
  - traumatic - code as Fracture, by site
- fracture —*see* Fracture
- infundibulum cardiac from right ventricle by a partition Q24.3
- joint (traumatic) (current) - code by site under Dislocation
- muscle (nontraumatic) —*see* Diastasis, muscle
- pubic bone, obstetrical trauma O71.6
- retina, retinal —*see* Detachment, retina
- symphysis pubis, obstetrical trauma O71.6
- tracheal ring, incomplete, congenital Q32.1

Sepsis (generalized) (unspecified organism) A41.9
- with
  - organ dysfunction (acute) (multiple) R65.20
    - with septic shock R65.21
- Acinetobacter baumannii A41.54
- actinomycotic A42.7
- adrenal hemorrhage syndrome (meningococcal) A39.1
- anaerobic A41.4
- Bacillus anthracis A22.7
- Brucella —*see also* Brucellosis A23.9
- candidal B37.7
- Cronobacter A41.59
- cryptogenic A41.9
- due to device, implant or graft T85.79
  - arterial graft NEC T82.7
  - breast (implant) T85.79
  - catheter NEC T85.79
    - dialysis (renal) T82.7
      - intraperitoneal T85.71
    - infusion NEC T82.7
      - spinal (cranial) (epidural) (intrathecal) (spinal) (subarachnoid) (subdural) T85.735
    - urethral (indwelling) T83.511
    - urinary T83.518
  - ectopic or molar pregnancy O08.82
  - electronic (electrode) (pulse generator) (stimulator)
    - bone T84.7
    - cardiac T82.7
    - nervous system T85.738
      - brain T85.731
      - neurostimulator generator T85.734
      - peripheral nerve T85.732
      - spinal cord T85.733
    - urinary T83.590
  - fixation, internal (orthopedic) —*see* Complication, fixation device, infection
  - gastrointestinal (bile duct) (esophagus) T85.79
    - neurostimulator electrode (lead) T85.732
  - genital T83.69
  - heart NEC T82.7
    - valve (prosthesis) T82.6
      - graft T82.7

Sepsis (continued)
  due to device, implant or graft (continued)
    joint prosthesis —see Complication, joint prosthesis, infection
    ocular (corneal graft) (orbital implant) T85.79
    orthopedic NEC T84.7
      fixation device, internal —see Complication, fixation device, infection
    specified NEC T85.79
    vascular T82.7
    ventricular intracranial (communicating) shunt T85.730
  during labor O75.3
  Enterococcus A41.81
  Erysipelothrix (rhusiopathiae) (erysipeloid) A26.7
  Escherichia coli (E. coli) A41.51
  extraintestinal yersiniosis A28.2
  following
    abortion (subsequent episode) O08.0
      current episode —see Abortion
    ectopic or molar pregnancy O08.82
    immunization T88.0
    infusion, therapeutic injection or transfusion NEC T80.29
    obstetrical procedure O86.04
  gangrenous A41.9
  gonococcal A54.86
  Gram-negative (organism) A41.50
    anaerobic A41.4
  Haemophilus influenzae A41.3
  herpesviral B00.7
  intra-abdominal K65.1
  intraocular —see Endophthalmitis, purulent
  Listeria monocytogenes A32.7
  localized - code to specific localized infection
    in operation wound T81.49
    skin —see Abscess
  malleus A24.0
  melioidosis A24.1
  meningeal —see Meningitis
  meningococcal A39.4
    acute A39.2
    chronic A39.3
  MRSA (Methicillin resistant Staphylococcus aureus) A41.02
  MSSA (Methicillin susceptible Staphylococcus aureus) A41.01
  newborn P36.9
    due to
      anaerobes NEC P36.5
      Escherichia coli P36.4
      Staphylococcus P36.30
        aureus P36.2
        specified NEC P36.39
      Streptococcus P36.10
        group B P36.0
        specified NEC P36.19
      specified NEC P36.8
  other gram-negative A41.59
  Pasteurella multocida A28.0
  pelvic, puerperal, postpartum, childbirth O85
  postprocedural T81.44
  pneumococcal A40.3
  puerperal, postpartum, childbirth (pelvic) O85
  Pseudomonas (pseudomonas aeruginosa) A41.52

Sepsis (continued)
  Salmonella (arizonae) (choleraesuis) (enteritidis) (typhimurium) A02.1
  Serratia A41.53
  severe R65.20
    with septic shock R65.21
  skin, localized —see Abscess
  Shigella (see also Dysentery, bacillary) A03.9
  specified organism NEC A41.89
  Staphylococcus, staphylococcal A41.2
    aureus (methicillin susceptible) (MSSA) A41.01
      methicillin resistant (MRSA) A41.02
    coagulase-negative A41.1
    specified NEC A41.1
  Streptococcus, streptococcal A40.9
    agalactiae A40.1
    group
      A A40.0
      B A40.1
      D A41.81
    neonatal P36.10
      group B P36.0
      specified NEC P36.19
    pneumoniae A40.3
    pyogenes A40.0
    specified NEC A40.8
  tracheostomy stoma J95.02
  tularemic A21.7
  umbilical, umbilical cord (newborn) —see Sepsis, newborn
  Yersinia pestis A20.7

Septate —see Septum

Septic —see condition
  arm —see Cellulitis, upper limb
    with lymphangitis —see Lymphangitis, acute, upper limb
  embolus —see Embolism
  finger —see Cellulitis, digit
    with lymphangitis —see Lymphangitis, acute, digit
  foot —see Cellulitis, lower limb
    with lymphangitis —see Lymphangitis, acute, lower limb
  gallbladder (acute) K81.0
  hand —see Cellulitis, upper limb
    with lymphangitis —see Lymphangitis, acute, upper limb
  joint —see Arthritis, pyogenic or pyemic
  leg —see Cellulitis, lower limb
    with lymphangitis —see Lymphangitis, acute, lower limb
  nail —see also Cellulitis, digit
    with lymphangitis —see Lymphangitis, acute, digit
  sore —see also Abscess
    throat J02.0
      streptococcal J02.0
  spleen (acute) D73.89
  teeth, tooth (pulpal origin) K04.4
  throat —see Pharyngitis
  thrombus —see Thrombosis
  toe —see Cellulitis, digit
    with lymphangitis —see Lymphangitis, acute, digit
  tonsils, chronic J35.01
    with adenoiditis J35.03
  uterus —see Endometritis

Septicemia A41.9
  meaning sepsis —see Sepsis

Septum, septate (congenital) —see also Anomaly, by site
  anal Q42.3
    with fistula Q42.2
  aqueduct of Sylvius Q03.0
    with spina bifida —see Spina bifida, by site, with hydrocephalus
  uterus Q51.28
    complete Q51.21
    partial Q51.22
    specified NEC Q51.28
  vagina Q52.10
    in pregnancy —see Pregnancy, complicated by, abnormal vagina
      causing obstructed labor O65.5
    longitudinal Q52.129
      microperforate
        left side Q52.124
        right side Q52.123
      nonobstruction Q52.120
      obstructing Q52.129
        left side Q52.122
        right side Q52.1221
    transverse Q52.11

Sequelae (of) —see also condition
  abscess, intracranial or intraspinal (conditions in G06) G09
  amputation -- code to injury with seventh character S
  burn and corrosion -- code to injury with seventh character S
  calcium deficiency E64.8
  cerebrovascular disease —see Sequelae, disease, cerebrovascular
  childbirth O94
  contusion -- code to injury with seventh character S
  corrosion —see Sequelae, burn and corrosion
  COVID-19 (post acute) U09.9
  crushing injury -- code to injury with seventh character S
  disease
    cerebrovascular I69.90
      alteration of sensation I69.998
      aphasia I69.920
      apraxia I69.990
      ataxia I69.993
      cognitive deficits I69.91
      disturbance of vision I69.998
      dysarthria I69.922
      dysphagia I69.991
      dysphasia I69.921
      facial droop I69.992
      facial weakness I69.992
      fluency disorder I69.923
      hemiplegia I69.95-
      hemorrhage
        intracerebral —see Sequelae, hemorrhage, intracerebral
        intracranial, nontraumatic NEC —see Sequelae, hemorrhage, intracranial, nontraumatic
        subarachnoid —see Sequelae, hemorrhage, subarachnoid
      language deficit I69.928
      monoplegia
        lower limb I69.94-
        upper limb I69.93-
      paralytic syndrome I69.96-
      specified effect NEC I69.998
      specified type NEC I69.80
        alteration of sensation I69.898
        aphasia I69.820
        apraxia I69.890

Sequelae (continued)
  disease (continued)
    cerebrovascular (continued)
      specified type (continued)
        ataxia I69.893
        cognitive deficits I69.81
        disturbance of vision I69.898
        dysarthria I69.822
        dysphagia I69.891
        dysphasia I69.821
        facial droop I69.892
        facial weakness I69.892
        fluency disorder I69.823
        hemiplegia I69.85-
        language deficit I69.828
        monoplegia
          lower limb I69.84-
          upper limb I69.83-
        paralytic syndrome I69.86-
        specified effect NEC I69.898
      speech deficit I69.928
        speech deficit I69.828
      stroke NOS —see Sequelae, stroke NOS
  dislocation -- code to injury with seventh character S
  encephalitis or encephalomyelitis (conditions in G04) G09
    in infectious disease NEC B94.8
    viral B94.1
  external cause -- code to injury with seventh character S
  foreign body entering natural orifice -- code to injury with seventh character S
  fracture -- code to injury with seventh character S
  frostbite -- code to injury with seventh character S
  Hansen's disease B92
  hemorrhage
    intracerebral I69.10
      alteration of sensation I69.198
      aphasia I69.120
      apraxia I69.190
      ataxia I69.193
      cognitive deficits I69.11
      disturbance of vision I69.198
      dysarthria I69.122
      dysphagia I69.191
      dysphasia I69.121
      facial droop I69.192
      facial weakness I69.192
      fluency disorder I69.123
      hemiplegia I69.15-
      language deficit NEC I69.128
      monoplegia
        lower limb I69.14-
        upper limb I69.13-
      paralytic syndrome I69.16-
      specified effect NEC I69.198
      speech deficit NEC I69.128
    intracranial, nontraumatic NEC I69.20
      alteration of sensation I69.298
      aphasia I69.220
      apraxia I69.290
      ataxia I69.293
      cognitive deficits I69.21
      disturbance of vision I69.298
      dysarthria I69.222
      dysphagia I69.291
      dysphasia I69.221
      facial droop I69.292
      facial weakness I69.292
      fluency disorder I69.223
      hemiplegia I69.25-
      language deficit NEC I69.228
      monoplegia
        lower limb I69.24-
        upper limb I69.23-

Sequelae (continued)
  hemorrhage (continued)
    intracranial, nontraumatic (continued)
      paralytic syndrome I69.26-
      specified effect NEC I69.298
      speech deficit NEC I69.228
    subarachnoid I69.00
      alteration of sensation I69.098
      aphasia I69.020
      apraxia I69.090
      ataxia I69.093
      cognitive deficits —see subcategory I69.01-
      disturbance of vision I69.098
      dysarthria I69.022
      dysphagia I69.091
      dysphasia I69.021
      facial droop I69.092
      facial weakness I69.092
      fluency disorder I69.023
      hemiplegia I69.05-
      language deficit NEC I69.028
      monoplegia
        lower limb I69.04-
        upper limb I69.03-
      paralytic syndrome I69.06-
      specified effect NEC I69.098
      speech deficit NEC I69.028
  hepatitis, viral B94.2
  hyperalimentation E68
  infarction
    cerebral I69.30
      alteration of sensation I69.398
      aphasia I69.320
      apraxia I69.390
      ataxia I69.393
      cognitive deficits I69.31
      disturbance of vision I69.398
      dysarthria I69.322
      dysphagia I69.391
      dysphasia I69.321
      facial droop I69.392
      facial weakness I69.392
      fluency disorder I69.323
      hemiplegia I69.35-
      language deficit NEC I69.328
      monoplegia
        lower limb I69.34-
        upper limb I69.33-
      paralytic syndrome I69.36-
      specified effect NEC I69.398
      speech deficit NEC I69.328
  infection, pyogenic, intracranial or intraspinal G09
  infectious disease B94.9
    specified NEC B94.8
  injury -- code to injury with seventh character S
  leprosy B92
  meningitis
    bacterial (conditions in G00) G09
    other or unspecified cause (conditions in G03) G09
  muscle (and tendon) injury - code to injury with seventh character S
  myelitis —see Sequelae, encephalitis
  niacin deficiency E64.8
  nutritional deficiency E64.9
    specified NEC E64.8
  obstetrical condition O94
  parasitic disease B94.9
  phlebitis or thrombophlebitis of intracranial or intraspinal venous sinuses and veins (conditions in G08) G09

Sequelae (continued)
  poisoning -- code to poisoning with seventh character S
    nonmedicinal substance —see Sequelae, toxic effect, nonmedicinal substance
  poliomyelitis (acute) B91
  pregnancy O94
  protein-energy malnutrition E64.0
  puerperium O94
  rickets E64.3
  SARS-CoV-2 (post acute) U09.9
  selenium deficiency E64.8
  sprain and strain - code to injury with seventh character S
  stroke NOS I69.30
    alteration in sensation I69.398
    aphasia I69.320
    apraxia I69.390
    ataxia I69.393
    cognitive deficits I69.31
    disturbance of vision I69.398
    dysarthria I69.322
    dysphagia I69.391
    dysphasia I69.321
    facial droop I69.392
    facial weakness I69.392
    hemiplegia I69.35-
    language deficit NEC I69.328
    monoplegia
      lower limb I69.34-
      upper limb I69.33-
    paralytic syndrome I69.36-
    specified effect NEC I69.398
    speech deficit NEC I69.328
  tendon and muscle injury - code to injury with seventh character S
  thiamine deficiency E64.8
  trachoma B94.0
  tuberculosis B90.9
    bones and joints B90.2
    central nervous system B90.0
    genitourinary B90.1
    pulmonary (respiratory) B90.9
    specified organs NEC B90.8
  viral
    encephalitis B94.1
    hepatitis B94.2
  vitamin deficiency NEC E64.8
    A E64.1
    B E64.8
    C E64.2
  wound, open - code to injury with seventh character S

Sequestration —see also Sequestrum
  disc —see Displacement, intervertebral disc
  lung, congenital Q33.2

Sequestrum
  bone —see Osteomyelitis, chronic
  dental M27.2
  jaw bone M27.2
  orbit —see Osteomyelitis, orbit
  sinus (accessory) (nasal) —see Sinusitis

Sequoiosis lung or pneumonitis J67.8

Serology for syphilis
  doubtful
    with signs or symptoms - code by site and stage under Syphilis
    follow-up of latent syphilis —see Syphilis, latent
  negative, with signs or symptoms - code by site and stage under Syphilis

Serology for syphilis (continued)
  positive A53.0
    with signs or symptoms - code by site and stage under Syphilis
  reactivated A53.0

Seroma —see also Hematoma
  postprocedural —see Complication, postprocedural, seroma
  traumatic, secondary and recurrent T79.2

Seropurulent —see condition

Serositis, multiple K65.8
  pericardial I31.1
  peritoneal K65.8

Serous —see condition

Sertoli cell
  adenoma
    specified site —see Neoplasm, benign, by site
    unspecified site
      female D27.9
      male D29.20
  carcinoma
    specified site —see Neoplasm, malignant, by site
    unspecified site (male) C62.9-
    female C56.9
  tumor
    with lipid storage
      specified site —see Neoplasm, benign, by site
      unspecified site
        female D27.9
        male D29.20
    specified site —see Neoplasm, benign, by site
    unspecified site
      female D27.9
      male D29.20

Sertoli-Leydig cell tumor —see Neoplasm, benign, by site
  specified site —see Neoplasm, benign, by site
  unspecified site
    female D27.9
    male D29.20

Serum
  allergy, allergic reaction (see also Reaction, serum) T80.69
    shock (see also Shock, anaphylactic) T80.59
  arthritis (see also Reaction, serum) T80.69
  complication or reaction NEC (see also Reaction, serum) T80.69
  disease NEC (see also Reaction, serum) T80.69
  hepatitis —see also Hepatitis, viral, type B
    carrier (suspected) of B18.1
  intoxication (see also Reaction, serum) T80.69
  neuritis (see also Reaction, serum) T80.69
  neuropathy G61.1
  poisoning NEC (see also Reaction, serum) T80.69
  rash NEC (see also Reaction, serum) T80.69
  reaction NEC (see also Reaction, serum) T80.69
  sickness NEC (see also Reaction, serum) T80.69
  urticaria (see also Reaction, serum) T80.69

Sesamoiditis M25.8-

Sever's disease or osteochondrosis —see Osteochondrosis, juvenile, tarsus

Severe sepsis R65.20
  with septic shock R65.21

Sex
  chromosome mosaics Q97.8
    lines with various numbers of X chromosomes Q97.2
  education Z70.8
  reassignment surgery status Z87.890

Sextuplet pregnancy —see Pregnancy, sextuplet

Sexual
  function, disorder of (psychogenic) F52.9
  immaturity (female) (male) E30.0
  impotence (psychogenic) organic origin NEC —see Dysfunction, sexual, male
  precocity (constitutional) (cryptogenic) (female) (idiopathic) (male) E30.1

Sexuality, pathologic —see Deviation, sexual

Sézary disease C84.1-

Shadow, lung R91.8

Shaking palsy or paralysis —see Parkinsonism

Shallowness, acetabulum —see Derangement, joint, specified type NEC, hip

Shaver's disease J63.1

Sheath (tendon) —see condition

Sheathing, retinal vessels H35.01-

Shedding
  nail L60.8
  premature, primary (deciduous) teeth K00.6

Sheehan's disease or syndrome E23.0

Shelf, rectal K62.89

Shell teeth K00.5

Shellshock (current) F43.0
  lasting state —see Disorder, post-traumatic stress

Shield kidney Q63.1

Shift
  auditory threshold (temporary) H93.24-
  mediastinal R93.89

Shifting sleep-work schedule (affecting sleep) G47.26

Shiga (-Kruse) **dysentery** A03.0

Shiga's bacillus A03.0

Shigella (dysentery) —see Dysentery, bacillary

Shigellosis A03.9
  Group A A03.0
  Group B A03.1
  Group C A03.2
  Group D A03.3

Shin splints S86.89

Shingles —see Herpes, zoster

Shipyard disease or eye B30.0

Shirodkar suture, in pregnancy —see Pregnancy, complicated by, incompetent cervix

Shock R57.9
- with ectopic or molar pregnancy O08.3
- adrenal (cortical) (Addisonian) E27.2
- adverse food reaction (anaphylactic) —*see* Shock, anaphylactic, due to food
- allergic —*see* Shock, anaphylactic
- anaphylactic T78.2
  - chemical —*see* Table of Drugs and Chemicals
  - due to drug or medicinal substance
    - correct substance properly administered T88.6
    - overdose or wrong substance given or taken (by accident) —*see* Table of Drugs and Chemicals, by drug, poisoning
  - due to food (nonpoisonous) T78.00
    - additives T78.06
    - dairy products T78.07
    - eggs T78.08
    - fish T78.03
      - shellfish T78.02
    - fruit T78.04
    - milk T78.07
    - nuts T78.05
      - multiple types T78.05
      - peanuts T78.01
    - peanuts T78.01
    - seeds T78.05
    - specified type NEC T78.09
    - vegetable T78.04
  - following sting(s) —*see* Venom
  - immunization T80.52
  - serum T80.59
    - blood and blood products T80.51
    - immunization T80.52
    - specified NEC T80.59
    - vaccination T80.52
- anaphylactoid —*see* Shock, anaphylactic
- anesthetic
  - correct substance properly administered T88.2
  - overdose or wrong substance given or taken —*see* Table of Drugs and Chemicals, by drug, poisoning
  - specified anesthetic —*see* Table of Drugs and Chemicals, by drug, poisoning
- cardiogenic R57.0
- chemical substance —*see* Table of Drugs and Chemicals
- complicating ectopic or molar pregnancy O08.3
- culture —*see* Disorder, adjustment
- drug
  - due to correct substance properly administered T88.6
  - overdose or wrong substance given or taken (by accident) —*see* Table of Drugs and Chemicals, by drug, poisoning
- during or after labor and delivery O75.1
- electric T75.4
  - (taser) T75.4
- endotoxic R65.21
  - postprocedural (resulting from a procedure, not elsewhere classified) T81.12

Shock *(continued)*
- following
  - ectopic or molar pregnancy O08.3
  - injury (immediate) (delayed) T79.4
  - labor and delivery O75.1
- food (anaphylactic) —*see* Shock, anaphylactic, due to food
- from electroshock gun (taser) T75.4
- gram-negative R65.21
  - postprocedural (resulting from a procedure, not elsewhere classified) T81.12
- hematologic R57.8
- hemorrhagic R57.8
  - surgery (intraoperative) (postoperative) T81.19
  - trauma T79.4
- hypovolemic R57.1
  - surgical T81.19
  - traumatic T79.4
- insulin E15
  - therapeutic misadventure —*see* subcategory T38.3
- kidney N17.0
  - traumatic (following crushing) T79.5
- lightning T75.01
- liver K72.00
- lung J80
- obstetric O75.1
  - with ectopic or molar pregnancy O08.3
  - following ectopic or molar pregnancy O08.3
- pleural (surgical) T81.19
  - due to trauma T79.4
- postprocedural (postoperative) T81.10
  - with ectopic or molar pregnancy O08.3
  - cardiogenic T81.11
  - endotoxic T81.12
  - following ectopic or molar pregnancy O08.3
  - gram-negative T81.12
  - hypovolemic T81.19
  - septic T81.12
  - specified type NEC T81.19
- psychic F43.0
- septic (due to severe sepsis) R65.21
- specified NEC R57.8
- surgical T81.10
- taser gun (taser) T75.4
- therapeutic misadventure NEC T81.10
- thyroxin
  - overdose or wrong substance given or taken —*see* Table of Drugs and Chemicals, by drug, poisoning
- toxic, syndrome A48.3
- transfusion —*see* Complications, transfusion
- traumatic (immediate) (delayed) T79.4

Shoemaker's chest M95.4

Short, shortening, shortness
- arm (acquired) —*see also* Deformity, limb, unequal length
  - congenital Q71.81-
  - forearm —*see* Deformity, limb, unequal length
- bowel syndrome K91.2
- breath R06.02
- cervical (complicating pregnancy) O26.87-
  - non-gravid uterus N88.3

Short, shortening, shortness *(continued)*
- common bile duct, congenital Q44.5
- cord (umbilical), complicating delivery O69.3
- cystic duct, congenital Q44.5
- esophagus (congenital) Q39.8
- femur (acquired) —*see* Deformity, limb, unequal length, femur
  - congenital —*see* Defect, reduction, lower limb, longitudinal, femur
- frenum, frenulum, linguae (congenital) Q38.1
- hip (acquired) —*see also* Deformity, limb, unequal length
  - congenital Q65.89
- leg (acquired) —*see also* Deformity, limb, unequal length
  - congenital Q72.81-
  - lower leg —*see also* Deformity, limb, unequal length
- limbed stature, with immunodeficiency D82.2
- lower limb (acquired) —*see also* Deformity, limb, unequal length
  - congenital Q72.81-
- organ or site, congenital NEC —*see* Distortion
- palate, congenital Q38.5
- radius (acquired) —*see also* Deformity, limb, unequal length
  - congenital —*see* Defect, reduction, upper limb, longitudinal, radius
- rib syndrome Q77.2
- stature (child) (hereditary) (idiopathic) NEC R62.52
  - constitutional E34.31
  - due to
    - endocrine disorder E34.30
      - specified type NEC, due to endocrine disorder E34.39
    - genetic causes E34.329
      - ACAN gene variant E34.328
      - acid-labile subunit gene (IGFALS) defect E34.321
      - aggrecan deficiency E34.328
      - genetic syndrome with resistance to insulin-like growth factor-1 E34.322
      - growth hormone gene 1 (GH1) defect with growth hormone neutralizing antibodies E34.321
      - growth hormone insensitivity syndrome (GHIS) E34.321
      - insulin-like growth factor 1 gene (IGF1) defect E34.321
      - insulin-like growth factor-1 receptor (IGF-1R) defect E34.322
      - insulin-like growth factor-1 (IGF-1) resistance E34.322
      - NPR-2 gene variant E34.328
      - post-insulin-like growth factor-1 receptor signaling defect E34.322
      - primary insulin-like growth factor-1 (IGF-1) deficiency E34.321
      - severe primary insulin-like growth factor-1 deficiency (SPIGFD) E34.321

Short, shortening, shortness *(continued)*
- stature *(continued)*
  - due to *(continued)*
    - genetic causes *(continued)*
      - signal transducer and activator of transcription 5B gene (STAT5b) defect E34.321
      - specified genetic cause NEC E34.328
    - Laron-type E34.321
- tendon —*see also* Contraction, tendon
  - with contracture of joint —*see* Contraction, joint
  - Achilles (acquired) M67.0-
    - congenital Q66.89
  - congenital Q79.8
- thigh (acquired) —*see also* Deformity, limb, unequal length, femur
  - congenital —*sese* Defect, reduction, lower limb, longitudinal, femur
- tibialis anterior (tendon) —*see* Contraction, tendon
- umbilical cord
  - complicating delivery O69.3
- upper limb, congenital —*see* Defect, reduction, upper limb, specified type NEC
- urethra N36.8
- uvula, congenital Q38.5
- vagina (congenital) Q52.4

Shortsightedness —*see* Myopia

Shoshin (acute fulminating beriberi) E51.11

Shoulder —*see* condition

Shovel-shaped incisors K00.2

Shower, thromboembolic —*see* Embolism

Shunt
- arterial-venous (dialysis) Z99.2
- arteriovenous, pulmonary (acquired) I28.0
  - congenital Q25.72
- cerebral ventricle (communicating) in situ Z98.2
- surgical, prosthetic, with complications —*see* Complications, cardiovascular, device or implant

Shutdown, renal N28.9

Shy-Drager syndrome G90.3

Sialadenitis, sialadenosis (any gland) (chronic) (periodic) (suppurative) —*see* Sialoadenitis

Sialectasia K11.8

Sialidosis E77.1

Sialitis, silitis (any gland) (chronic) (suppurative) —*see* Sialoadenitis

Sialoadenitis (any gland) (periodic) (suppurative) K11.20
- acute K11.21
  - recurrent K11.22
- chronic K11.23

Sialoadenopathy K11.9

Sialoangitis —*see* Sialoadenitis

Sialodochitis (fibrinosa) —*see* Sialoadenitis

Sialodocholithiasis K11.5

Sialolithiasis K11.5

Sialometaplasia, necrotizing K11.8

Sialorrhea —see also Ptyalism
  periodic —see Sialoadenitis
Sialosis K11.7
Siamese twin Q89.4
Sibling rivalry Z62.891
Sicard's syndrome G52.7
Sicca syndrome —see Syndrome, Sjögren
Sick R69
  or handicapped person in family Z63.79
    needing care at home Z63.6
  sinus (syndrome) I49.5
Sick-euthyroid syndrome E07.81
Sickle-cell
  anemia —see Disease, sickle-cell
  beta plus —see Disease, sickle-cell, thalassemia, beta plus
  beta zero —see Disease, sickle-cell, thalassemia, beta zero
  trait D57.3
Sicklemia —see also Disease, sickle-cell
  trait D57.3
Sickness
  air (travel) T75.3
  airplane T75.3
  alpine T70.29
  altitude T70.20
  Andes T70.29
  aviator's T70.29
  balloon T70.29
  car T75.3
  compressed air T70.3
  decompression T70.3
  green D50.8
  milk —see Poisoning, food, noxious
  motion T75.3
  mountain T70.29
    acute D75.1
  protein (see also Reaction, serum) T80.69
  radiation T66
  roundabout (motion) T75.3
  sea T75.3
  serum NEC (see also Reaction, serum) T80.69
  sleeping (African) B56.9
    by Trypanosoma B56.9
      brucei
        gambiense B56.0
        rhodesiense B56.1
    East African B56.1
    Gambian B56.0
    Rhodesian B56.1
    West African B56.0
  swing (motion) T75.3
  train (railway) (travel) T75.3
  travel (any vehicle) T75.3
Sideropenia —see Anemia, iron deficiency
Siderosilicosis J62.8
Siderosis (lung) J63.4
  brain G93.89
  eye (globe) —see Disorder, globe, degenerative, siderosis
Siemens' syndrome (ectodermal dysplasia) Q82.8
Sighing R06.89
  psychogenic F45.8
Sigmoid —see also condition
  flexure —see condition
  kidney Q63.1

Sigmoiditis (see also Enteritis) K52.9
  infectious A09
  noninfectious K52.9
Silfverskiöld's syndrome Q78.9
Silicosiderosis J62.8
Silicosis, silicotic (simple) (complicated) J62.8
  with tuberculosis J65
Silicotuberculosis J65
Silo-fillers' disease J68.8
  bronchitis J68.0
  pneumonitis J68.0
  pulmonary edema J68.1
Silver's syndrome Q87.19
Simian malaria B53.1
Simmonds' cachexia or disease E23.0
Simons' disease or syndrome (progressive lipodystrophy) E88.1
Simple, simplex —see condition
Simulation, conscious (of illness) Z76.5
Simultanagnosia (asimultagnosia) R48.3
Sin Nombre virus disease (Hantavirus) (cardio)-**pulmonary syndrome**) B33.4
Sinding-Larsen disease or osteochondrosis —see Osteochondrosis, juvenile, patella
Singapore hemorrhagic fever A91
Singer's node or nodule J38.2
Single
  atrium Q21.20
  coronary artery Q24.5
  umbilical artery Q27.0
  ventricle Q20.4
Singultus R06.6
  epidemicus B33.0
Sinus —see also Fistula
  abdominal K63.89
  arrest I45.5
  arrhythmia I49.8
  bradycardia R00.1
  branchial cleft (internal) (external) Q18.0
  coccygeal —see Sinus, pilonidal
  dental K04.6
  dermal (congenital) Q06.8
    with abscess Q06.8
      coccygeal, pilonidal —see Sinus, coccygeal
  infected, skin NEC L08.89
  marginal, ruptured or bleeding — see Hemorrhage, antepartum, specified cause NEC
  medial, face and neck Q18.8
  pause I45.5
  pericranii Q01.9
  pilonidal (infected) (rectum) L05.92
    with abscess L05.02
  preauricular Q18.1
  rectovaginal N82.3
  Rokitansky-Aschoff (gallbladder) K82.8
  sacrococcygeal (dermoid) (infected) —see Sinus, pilonidal
  tachycardia R00.0
    paroxysmal I47.19
  tarsi syndrome M25.57-
  testis N50.89
  tract (postinfective) —see Fistula
  urachus Q64.4

Sinusitis (accessory) (chronic) (hyperplastic) (nasal) (nonpurulent) (purulent) J32.9
  acute J01.90
    ethmoidal J01.20
      recurrent J01.21
    frontal J01.10
      recurrent J01.11
    involving more than one sinus, other than pansinusitis J01.80
      recurrent J01.81
    maxillary J01.00
      recurrent J01.01
    pansinusitis J01.40
      recurrent J01.41
    recurrent J01.91
    specified NEC J01.80
      recurrent J01.81
    sphenoidal J01.30
      recurrent J01.31
  allergic —see Rhinitis, allergic
  due to high altitude T70.1
  ethmoidal J32.2
    acute J01.20
      recurrent J01.21
  frontal J32.1
    acute J01.10
      recurrent J01.11
  influenzal —see Influenza, with, respiratory manifestations NEC
  involving more than one sinus but not pansinusitis J32.8
    acute J01.80
      recurrent J01.81
  maxillary J32.0
    acute J01.00
      recurrent J01.01
  sphenoidal J32.3
    acute J01.30
      recurrent J01.31
  tuberculous, any sinus A15.8
Sinusitis-bronchiectasis-situs inversus (syndrome) (triad) Q89.3
Sipple's syndrome E31.22
Sirenomelia (syndrome) Q87.2
Siriasis T67.01
Sirkari's disease B55.0
Siti A65
Situation, psychiatric F99
Situational
  disturbance (transient) —see Disorder, adjustment
    acute F43.0
  maladjustment —see Disorder, adjustment
  reaction —see Disorder, adjustment
    acute F43.0
Situs inversus or transversus (abdominalis) (thoracis) Q89.3
Sixth disease B08.20
  due to human herpesvirus 6 B08.21
  due to human herpesvirus 7 B08.22
Sjögren-Larsson syndrome Q87.19
Sjögren's syndrome or disease — see Syndrome, Sjögren
Skeletal —see condition
Skene's gland —see condition
Skenitis —see Urethritis
Skerljevo A65
Skevas-Zerfus disease —see Toxicity, venom, marine animal, sea anemone
Skin —see also condition
  clammy R23.1
  donor —see Donor, skin

Skin *(continued)*
  dry L85.3
  hidebound M35.9
Slate-dressers' or slate-miners' lung J62.8
Sleep
  apnea —see Apnea, sleep
  deprivation Z72.820
  disorder or disturbance G47.9
    child F51.9
      nonorganic origin F51.9
      specified NEC G47.8
  disturbance G47.9
    nonorganic origin F51.9
  drunkenness F51.9
  rhythm inversion G47.2-
  terrors F51.4
  walking F51.3
    hysterical F44.89
Sleep hygiene
  abuse Z72.821
  inadequate Z72.821
  poor Z72.821
Sleeping sickness —see Sickness, sleeping
Sleeplessness —see Insomnia
  menopausal N95.1
Sleep-wake schedule disorder G47.20
Slim disease (in HIV infection) B20
Slipped, slipping
  epiphysis (traumatic) —see also Osteochondropathy, specified type NEC
    capital femoral (traumatic) [SCFE]
      acute (on chronic) S79.01-
      nontraumatic M93.00-
    current traumatic - code as Fracture, by site
    upper femoral (nontraumatic) [SUFE] M93.00-
      acute M93.01-
        on chronic M93.03-
      chronic M93.02-
  intervertebral disc —see Displacement, intervertebral disc
  ligature, umbilical P51.8
  patella —see Disorder, patella, derangement NEC
  rib M89.8X8
  sacroiliac joint —see subcategory M53.2
  tendon —see Disorder, tendon
  ulnar nerve, nontraumatic —see Lesion, nerve, ulnar
  vertebra NEC —see Spondylolisthesis
Slocumb's syndrome E27.0
Sloughing (multiple) (phagedena) (skin) —see also Gangrene
  abscess —see Abscess
  appendix K38.8
  sfascia —see Disorder, soft tissue, specified type NEC
  scrotum N50.89
  tendon —see Disorder, tendon
  transplanted organ —see Rejection, transplant
  ulcer —see Ulcer, skin
Slow
  feeding, newborn P92.2
  flow syndrome, coronary I20.89
  heart (beat) R00.1
Slowing, urinary stream R39.198
Sluder's neuralgia (syndrome) G44.89

Slurred, slurring speech R47.81
Small (ness)
  for gestational age —see Small for dates
  introitus, vagina N89.6
  kidney (unknown cause) N27.9
    bilateral N27.1
    unilateral N27.0
  ovary (congenital) Q50.39
  pelvis
    with disproportion (fetopelvic) O33.1
      causing obstructed labor O65.1
  uterus N85.8
  white kidney N03.9
Small-and-light-for-dates —see Small for dates
Small-for-dates (infant) P05.10
  with weight of
    499 grams or less P05.11
    500-749 grams P05.12
    750-999 grams P05.13
    1000-1249 grams P05.14
    1250-1499 grams P05.15
    1500-1749 grams P05.16
    1750-1999 grams P05.17
    2000-2499 grams P05.18
    2500 grams and over P05.19
  specified NEC P05.19
Smallpox B03
Smearing, fecal R15.1
SMEI (severe myoclonic epilepsy in infancy) G40.83-
Smith-Lemli-Opitz syndrome E78.72
Smith's fracture S52.54-
Smoker —see Dependence, drug, nicotine
Smoker's
  bronchitis J41.0
  cough J41.0
  palate K13.24
  throat J31.2
  tongue K13.24
Smoking
  passive Z77.22
Smothering spells R06.81
Snaggle teeth, tooth M26.39
Snapping
  finger —see Trigger finger
  hip —see Derangement, joint, specified type NEC, hip
    involving the iliotibial band M76.3-
  knee —see Derangement, knee
    involving the iliotibial band M76.3-
Sneddon-Wilkinson disease or syndrome (sub-corneal pustular dermatosis) L13.1
Sneezing (intractable) R06.7
Sniffing
  cocaine
    abuse —see Abuse, drug, cocaine
    dependence —see Dependence, drug, cocaine
  gasoline
    abuse —see Abuse, drug, inhalant
    dependence —see Dependence, drug, inhalant
  glue (airplane)
    abuse —see Abuse, drug, inhalant
    drug dependence —see Dependence, drug, inhalant

Sniffles
  newborn P28.89
Snoring R06.83
Snow blindness —see Photokeratitis
Snuffles (non-syphilitic) R06.5
  newborn P28.89
  syphilitic (infant) A50.05 [J99]
Social
  exclusion Z60.4
    due to discrimination or persecution (perceived) Z60.5
  migrant Z59.00
    acculturation difficulty Z60.3
  rejection Z60.4
    due to discrimination or persecution Z60.5
  role conflict NEC Z73.5
  skills inadequacy NEC Z73.4
  transplantation Z60.3
Sodoku A25.0
Soemmerring's ring —see Cataract, secondary
Soft —see also condition
  nails L60.3
Softening
  bone —see Osteomalacia
  brain (necrotic) (progressive) G93.89
    congenital Q04.8
    embolic I63.4-
    hemorrhagic —see Hemorrhage, intracranial, intracerebral
    occlusive I63.5-
    thrombotic I63.3-
  cartilage M94.2-
    patella M22.4-
  cerebellar —see Softening, brain
  cerebral —see Softening, brain
  cerebrospinal —see Softening, brain
  myocardial, heart —see Degeneration, myocardial
  spinal cord G95.89
  stomach K31.89
Soldier's
  heart F45.8
  patches I31.0
Solitary
  cyst, kidney N28.1
  kidney, congenital Q60.0
Solvent abuse —see Abuse, drug, inhalant
  dependence —see Dependence, drug, inhalant
Somatization reaction, somatic reaction —see Disorder, somatoform
Somnambulism F51.3
  hysterical F44.89
Somnolence R40.0
  nonorganic origin F51.11
Sonne dysentery A03.3
Soor B37.0
Sore
  bed —see Ulcer, pressure, by site
  chiclero B55.1
  Delhi B55.1
  desert —see Ulcer, skin
  eye H57.1-
  Lahore B55.1
  mouth K13.79
    canker K12.0
  muscle M79.10
  Naga —see Ulcer, skin

Sore (continued)
  of skin —see Ulcer, skin
  oriental B55.1
  pressure —see Ulcer, pressure, by site
  skin L98.9
  soft A57
  throat (acute) —see also Pharyngitis
    with influenza, flu, or grippe —see Influenza, with, respiratory manifestations NEC
    chronic J31.2
    coxsackie (virus) B08.5
    diphtheritic A36.0
    herpesviral B00.2
    influenzal —see Influenza, with, respiratory manifestations NEC
    septic J02.0
    streptococcal (ulcerative) J02.0
    viral NEC J02.8
      coxsackie B08.5
  tropical —see Ulcer, skin
  veldt —see Ulcer, skin
Soto's syndrome (cerebral gigantism) Q87.3
South African cardiomyopathy syndrome I42.8
Southeast Asian hemorrhagic fever A91
Spacing
  abnormal, tooth, teeth, fully erupted M26.30
  excessive, tooth, fully erupted M26.32
Spade-like hand (congenital) Q68.1
Spading nail L60.8
  congenital Q84.6
Spanish collar N47.1
Sparganosis B70.1
Spasm(s), spastic, spasticity (see also condition) R25.2
  accommodation —see Spasm, of accommodation
  ampulla of Vater K83.4
  anus, ani (sphincter) (reflex) K59.4
    psychogenic F45.8
  artery I73.9
    cerebral G45.9
  Bell's G51.3-
  bladder (sphincter, external or internal) N32.89
    psychogenic F45.8
  bronchus, bronchiole J98.01
  cardia K22.0
  cardiac I20.1
  carpopedal —see Tetany
  cerebral (arteries) (vascular) G45.9
  cervix, complicating delivery O62.4
  ciliary body (of accommodation) —see Spasm, of accommodation
  colon (see also Irritable, bowel) K58.9
    with diarrhea K58.0
    psychogenic F45.8
  common duct K83.8
  compulsive —see Tic
  conjugate H51.8
  coronary (artery) I20.1
  diaphragm (reflex) R06.6
    epidemic B33.0
    psychogenic F45.8
  duodenum K59.89
  epidemic diaphragmatic (transient) B33.0
  esophagus (diffuse) K22.4
    psychogenic F45.8
  facial G51.3-

Spasm(s), spastic, spasticity (continued)
  fallopian tube N83.8
  gastrointestinal (tract) K31.89
    psychogenic F45.8
  glottis J38.5
    hysterical F44.4
    psychogenic F45.8
      conversion reaction F44.4
    reflex through recurrent laryngeal nerve J38.5
  habit —see Tic
  heart I20.1
  hemifacial (clonic) G51.3-
  hourglass —see Contraction, hourglass
  hysterical F44.4
  infantile —see Epilepsy, spasms
  inferior oblique, eye H51.8
  intestinal (see also Syndrome, irritable bowel) K58.9
    psychogenic F45.8
  larynx, laryngeal J38.5
    hysterical F44.4
    psychogenic F45.8
      conversion reaction F44.4
  levator palpebrae superioris —see Disorder, eyelid function
  muscle NEC M62.838
    back M62.830
  nerve, trigeminal G51.0
  nervous F45.8
  nodding F98.4
  occupational F48.8
  oculogyric H51.8
    psychogenic F45.8
  of accommodation H52.53-
  ophthalmic artery —see Occlusion, artery, retina
  perineal, female N94.89
  peroneo-extensor —see also Deformity, limb, flat foot
  pharynx (reflex) J39.2
    hysterical F45.8
    psychogenic F45.8
  psychogenic F45.8
  pylorus NEC K31.3
    adult hypertrophic K31.89
    congenital or infantile Q40.0
    psychogenic F45.8
  rectum (sphincter) K59.4
    psychogenic F45.8
  retinal (artery) —see Occlusion, artery, retina
  sigmoid (see also Syndrome, irritable bowel) K58.9
    psychogenic F45.8
  sphincter of Oddi K83.4
  stomach K31.89
    neurotic F45.8
  throat J39.2
    hysterical F45.8
    psychogenic F45.8
  tic F95.9
    chronic F95.1
    transient of childhood F95.0
  tongue K14.8
  torsion (progressive) G24.1
  trigeminal nerve —see Neuralgia, trigeminal
  ureter N13.5
  urethra (sphincter) N35.919
  uterus N85.8
    complicating labor O62.4
  vagina N94.2
    psychogenic F52.5
  vascular I73.9
  vasomotor I73.9
  vein NEC I87.8
  viscera —see Pain, abdominal

Spasmodic —see condition
Spasmophilia —see Tetany
Spasmus nutans F98.4
Spastic, spasticity —see also Spasm
 child (cerebral) (congenital) (paralysis) G80.1
Speaker's throat R49.8
Specific, specified —see condition
Speech
 defect, disorder, disturbance, impediment —see Disorder, speech R47.9
 psychogenic, in childhood and adolescence F98.8
 slurring R47.81
 specified NEC R47.89
Spells, transient oxygen desaturation of newborn (see also Apnea, newborn) P28.40
 during sleep (see also Apnea, newborn, sleep, primary) P28.30
Spencer's disease A08.19
Spens' syndrome (syncope with heart block) I45.9
Sperm counts (fertility testing) Z31.41
 postvasectomy Z30.8
 reversal Z31.42
Spermatic cord —see condition
Spermatocele N43.40
 congenital Q55.4
 multiple N43.42
 single N43.41
Spermatocystitis N49.0
Spermatocytoma C62.9-
 specified site —see Neoplasm, malignant, by site
Spermatorrhea N50.89
Sphacelus —see Gangrene
Sphenoidal —see condition
Sphenoiditis (chronic) —see Sinusitis, sphenoidal
Sphenopalatine ganglion neuralgia G90.09
Sphericity, increased, lens (congenital) Q12.4
Spherocytosis (congenital) (familial) (hereditary) D58.0
 hemoglobin disease D58.0
 sickle-cell (disease) D57.8-
Spherophakia Q12.4
Sphincter —see condition
Sphincteritis, sphincter of Oddi —see Cholangitis
Sphingolipidosis E75.3
 specified NEC E75.29
Sphingomyelinosis E75.3
Spicule tooth K00.2
Spider
 bite —see Toxicity, venom, spider
 nonvenomous —see Bite, by site, superficial, insect
 fingers —see Syndrome, Marfan
 nevus I78.1
 toes —see Syndrome, Marfan
 vascular I78.1
Spiegler-Fendt
 benign lymphocytoma L98.8
 sarcoid L08.89
Spielmeyer-Vogt disease E75.4

Spina bifida (aperta) Q05.9
 with hydrocephalus NEC Q05.4
 cervical Q05.5
  with hydrocephalus Q05.0
 dorsal Q05.6
  with hydrocephalus Q05.1
 lumbar Q05.7
  with hydrocephalus Q05.2
 lumbosacral Q05.7
  with hydrocephalus Q05.2
 occulta Q76.0
 sacral Q05.8
  with hydrocephalus Q05.3
 thoracic Q05.6
  with hydrocephalus Q05.1
 thoracolumbar Q05.6
  with hydrocephalus Q05.1
Spindle, Krukenberg's —see Pigmentation, cornea, posterior
Spine, spinal —see condition
Spiradenoma (eccrine) —see Neoplasm, skin, benign
Spirillosis A25.0
Spirillum
 minus A25.0
 obermeieri infection A68.0
Spirochetal —see condition
Spirochetosis A69.9
 arthritic, arthritica A69.9
 bronchopulmonary A69.8
 icterohemorrhagic A27.0
 lung A69.8
Spirometrosis B70.1
Spitting blood —see Hemoptysis
Splanchnoptosis K63.4
Spleen, splenic —see condition
Splenectasis —see Splenomegaly
Splenitis (interstitial) (malignant) (nonspecific) D73.89
 malarial (see also Malaria) B54 [D77]
 tuberculous A18.85
Splenocele D73.89
Splenomegaly, splenomegalia (Bengal) (cryptogenic) (idiopathic) (tropical) R16.1
 with hepatomegaly R16.2
 cirrhotic D73.2
 congenital Q89.09
 congestive, chronic D73.2
 Egyptian B65.1
 Gaucher's E75.22
 malarial (see also Malaria) B54 [D77]
 neutropenic D73.81
 Niemann-Pick —see Niemann-Pick disease or syndrome
 siderotic D73.2
 syphilitic A52.79
  congenital (early) A50.08 [D77]
Splenopathy D73.9
Splenoptosis D73.89
Splenosis D73.89
Splinter —see Foreign body, superficial, by site
Split, splitting
 foot Q72.7-
 hand Q71.6
 heart sounds R01.2
 lip, congenital —see Cleft, lip
 nails L60.3
 urinary stream R39.13
Spondylarthrosis —see Spondylosis

Spondylitis (chronic) —see also Spondylopathy, inflammatory
 ankylopoietica —see Spondylitis, ankylosing
 ankylosing (chronic) M45.9
  with lung involvement M45.9 [J99]
  cervical region M45.2
  cervicothoracic region M45.3
  juvenile M08.1
  lumbar region M45.6
  lumbosacral region M45.7
  multiple sites M45.0
  occipito-atlanto-axial region M45.1
  sacrococcygeal region M45.8
  thoracic region M45.4
  thoracolumbar region M45.5
 atrophic (ligamentous) —see Spondylitis, ankylosing
 deformans (chronic) —see Spondylosis
 gonococcal A54.41
 gouty (see also Gout, by type, vertebrae) M10.08
 in (due to)
  brucellosis A23.9 [M49.80]
   cervical region A23.9 [M49.82]
   cervicothoracic region A23.9 [M49.83]
   lumbar region A23.9 [M49.86]
   lumbosacral region A23.9 [M49.87]
   multiple sites A23.9 [M49.89]
   occipito-atlanto-axial region A23.9 [M49.81]
   sacrococcygeal region A23.9 [M49.88]
   thoracic region A23.9 [M49.84]
   thoracolumbar region A23.9 [M49.85]
  enterobacteria (see also subcategory M49.8) A04.9
  tuberculosis A18.01
 infectious NEC —see Spondylopathy, infective
 juvenile ankylosing (chronic) M08.1
 Kümmell's —see Spondylopathy, traumatic
 Marie-Strümpell —see Spondylitis, ankylosing
 muscularis —see Spondylopathy, specified NEC
 psoriatic L40.53
 rheumatoid —see Spondylitis, ankylosing
 rhizomelica —see Spondylitis, ankylosing
 sacroiliac NEC M46.1
 senescent, senile —see Spondylosis
 traumatic (chronic) or post-traumatic —see Spondylopathy, traumatic
 tuberculosa A18.01
 typhosa A01.05
Spondyloarthritis
 axial —see also Spondylitis, ankylosing
  non-radiographic M45.A0
   cervical M45.A2
   cervicothoracic M45.A3
   lumbar M45.A6
   lumbosacral M45.A7
   multiple sites M45.AB
   occipito-atlanto-axial region M45.A1
   sacral and sacrococcygeal M45.A8
   thoracic M45.A4
   thoracolumbar M45.A5

Spondylolisthesis (acquired) (degenerative) M43.10
 with disproportion (fetopelvic) O33.0
  causing obstructed labor O65.0
 cervical region M43.12
 cervicothoracic region M43.13
 congenital Q76.2
 lumbar region M43.16
 lumbosacral region M43.17
 multiple sites M43.19
 occipito-atlanto-axial region M43.11
 sacrococcygeal region M43.18
 thoracic region M43.14
 thoracolumbar region M43.15
 traumatic (old) M43.10
  acute
   fifth cervical (displaced) S12.430
    nondisplaced S12.431
    specified type NEC (displaced) S12.450
    nondisplaced S12.451
    type III S12.44
   fourth cervical (displaced) S12.330
    nondisplaced S12.331
    specified type NEC (displaced) S12.350
    nondisplaced S12.351
    type III S12.34
   second cervical (displaced) S12.130
    nondisplaced S12.131
    specified type NEC (displaced) S12.150
    nondisplaced S12.151
    type III S12.14
   seventh cervical (displaced) S12.630
    nondisplaced S12.631
    specified type NEC (displaced) S12.650
    nondisplaced S12.651
    type III S12.64
   sixth cervical (displaced) S12.530
    nondisplaced S12.531
    specified type NEC (displaced) S12.550
    nondisplaced S12.551
    type III S12.54
   third cervical (displaced) S12.230
    nondisplaced S12.231
    specified type NEC (displaced) S12.250
    nondisplaced S12.251
    type III S12.24
Spondylolysis (acquired) M43.00
 cervical region M43.02
 cervicothoracic region M43.03
 congenital Q76.2
 lumbar region M43.06
 lumbosacral region M43.07
  with disproportion (fetopelvic) O33.0
   causing obstructed labor O65.8
 multiple sites M43.09
 occipito-atlanto-axial region M43.01
 sacrococcygeal region M43.08
 thoracic region M43.04
 thoracolumbar region M43.05
Spondylopathy M48.9
 infective NEC M46.50
  cervical region M46.52
  cervicothoracic region M46.53
  lumbar region M46.56
  lumbosacral region M46.57
  multiple sites M46.59

Spondylopathy *(continued)*
  infective *(continued)*
    occipito-atlanto-axial region M46.51
    sacrococcygeal region M46.58
    thoracic region M46.54
    thoracolumbar region M46.55
  inflammatory M46.90
    cervical region M46.92
    cervicothoracic region M46.93
    lumbar region M46.96
    lumbosacral region M46.97
    multiple sites M46.99
    occipito-atlanto-axial region M46.91
    sacrococcygeal region M46.98
    specified type NEC M46.80
      cervical region M46.82
      cervicothoracic region M46.83
      lumbar region M46.86
      lumbosacral region M46.87
      multiple sites M46.89
      occipito-atlanto-axial region M46.81
      sacrococcygeal region M46.88
      thoracic region M46.84
      thoracolumbar region M46.85
    thoracic region M46.94
    thoracolumbar region M46.95
  neuropathic, in
    syringomyelia and syringobulbia G95.0
    tabes dorsalis A52.11
  specified NEC M48.8
  traumatic M48.30
    cervical region M48.32
    cervicothoracic region M48.33
    lumbar region M48.36
    lumbosacral region M48.37
    occipito-atlanto-axial region M48.31
    sacrococcygeal region M48.38
    thoracic region M48.34
    thoracolumbar region M48.35
Spondylosis M47.9
  with
    disproportion (fetopelvic) O33.0
      causing obstructed labor O65.0
    myelopathy NEC M47.10
      cervical region M47.12
      cervicothoracic region M47.13
      lumbar region M47.16
      occipito-atlanto-axial region M47.11
      thoracic region M47.14
      thoracolumbar region M47.15
    radiculopathy M47.20
      cervical region M47.22
      cervicothoracic region M47.23
      lumbar region M47.26
      lumbosacral region M47.27
      occipito-atlanto-axial region M47.21
      sacrococcygeal region M47.28
      thoracic region M47.24
      thoracolumbar region M47.25
  specified NEC M47.899
    cervical region M47.892
    cervicothoracic region M47.893
    facet joint M47.819
    lumbar region M47.896
    lumbosacral region M47.897
    occipito-atlanto-axial region M47.891
    sacrococcygeal region M47.898
    thoracic region M47.894
    thoracolumbar region M47.895
  traumatic —*see* Spondylopathy, traumatic

Spondylosis *(continued)*
  without myelopathy or radiculopathy M47.819
    cervical region M47.812
    cervicothoracic region M47.813
    lumbar region M47.816
    lumbosacral region M47.817
    occipito-atlanto-axial region M47.811
    sacrococcygeal region M47.818
    thoracic region M47.814
    thoracolumbar region M47.815
Sponge
  inadvertently left in operation wound —*see* Foreign body, accidentally left during a procedure
  kidney (medullary) Q61.5
Sponge-diver's disease —*see* Toxicity, venom, marine animal, sea anemone
Spongioblastoma (any type) —*see* Neoplasm, malignant, by site
  specified site —*see* Neoplasm, malignant, by site
  unspecified site C71.9
Spongioneuroblastoma —*see* Neoplasm, malignant, by site
Spontaneous —*see also* condition
  fracture (cause unknown) —*see* Fracture, pathological
Spoon nail L60.3
  congenital Q84.6
Sporadic —*see* condition
Sporothrix schenckii infection —*see* Sporotrichosis
Sporotrichosis B42.9
  arthritis B42.82
  disseminated B42.7
  generalized B42.7
  lymphocutaneous (fixed) (progressive) B42.1
  pulmonary B42.0
  specified NEC B42.89
Spots, spotting (in) (of)
  Bitot's —*see also* Pigmentation, conjunctiva
    in the young child E50.1
    vitamin A deficiency E50.1
  café, au lait L81.3
  Cayenne pepper I78.1
  cotton wool, retina —*see* Occlusion, artery, retina
  de Morgan's (senile angiomas) I78.1
  Fuchs' black (myopic) (*see also* Myopia, degenerative) H44.2-
  intermenstrual (regular) N92.0
    irregular N92.1
  Koplik's B05.9
  liver L81.4
  pregnancy O26.85-
  purpuric R23.3
  ruby I78.1
Spotted fever —*see* Fever, spotted A77.9
Sprain (joint) (ligament)
  acromioclavicular joint or ligament S43.5-
  ankle S93.40-
    calcaneofibular ligament S93.41-
    deltoid ligament S93.42-
    internal collateral ligament —*see* Sprain, ankle, specified ligament NEC
    specified ligament NEC S93.49-

Sprain *(continued)*
  ankle *(continued)*
    talofibular ligament —*see* Sprain, ankle, specified ligament NEC
    tibiofibular ligament S93.43-
  anterior longitudinal, cervical S13.4
  atlas, atlanto-axial, atlanto-occipital S13.4
  breast bone —*see* Sprain, sternum
  calcaneofibular —*see* Sprain, ankle
  carpal —*see* Sprain, wrist
  carpometacarpal —*see* Sprain, hand, specified site NEC
  cartilage
    costal S23.41
    semilunar (knee) —*see* Sprain, knee, specified site NEC
      with current tear —*see* Tear, meniscus
    thyroid region S13.5
    xiphoid —*see* Sprain, sternum
  cervical, cervicodorsal, cervicothoracic S13.4
  chondrosternal S23.421
  coracoclavicular S43.8-
  coracohumeral S43.41-
  coronary, knee —*see* Sprain, knee, specified site NEC
  costal cartilage S23.41
  cricoarytenoid articulation or ligament S13.5
  cricothyroid articulation S13.5
  cruciate, knee —*see* Sprain, knee, cruciate
  deltoid, ankle —*see* Sprain, ankle
  dorsal (spine) S23.3
  elbow S53.40-
    radial collateral ligament S53.43-
    radiohumeral S53.41-
    rupture
      radial collateral ligament —*see* Rupture, traumatic, ligament, radial collateral
      ulnar collateral ligament —*see* Rupture, traumatic, ligament, ulnar collateral
    specified type NEC S53.49-
    ulnar collateral ligament S53.44-
    ulnohumeral S53.42-
  femur, head —*see* Sprain, hip
  fibular collateral, knee —*see* Sprain, knee, collateral
  fibulocalcaneal —*see* Sprain, ankle
  finger(s) S63.61-
    index S63.61-
    interphalangeal (joint) S63.63-
      index S63.63-
      little S63.63-
      middle S63.63-
      ring S63.63-
    little S63.61-
    middle S63.61-
    ring S63.61-
    metacarpophalangeal (joint) S63.65-
    specified site NEC S63.69-
      index S63.69-
      little S63.69-
      middle S63.69-
      ring S63.69-
  foot S93.60-
    specified ligament NEC S93.69-
    tarsal ligament S93.61-
    tarsometatarsal ligament S93.62-
    toe —*see* Sprain, toe
  hand S63.9-
    finger —*see* Sprain, finger
    specified site NEC S63.8
    thumb —*see* Sprain, thumb

Sprain *(continued)*
  head S03.9
  hip S73.10-
    iliofemoral ligament S73.11-
    ischiocapsular (ligament) S73.12-
    specified NEC S73.19-
  iliofemoral —*see* Sprain, hip
  innominate
    acetabulum —*see* Sprain, hip
    sacral junction S33.6
  internal
    collateral, ankle —*see* Sprain, ankle
    semilunar cartilage —*see* Sprain, knee, specified site NEC
  interphalangeal
    finger —*see* Sprain, finger, interphalangeal (joint)
    toe —*see* Sprain, toe, interphalangeal joint
  ischiocapsular —*see* Sprain, hip
  ischiofemoral —*see* Sprain, hip
  jaw (articular disc) (cartilage) (meniscus) S03.4-
    old M26.69
  knee S83.9-
    collateral ligament S83.40-
      lateral (fibular) S83.42-
      medial (tibial) S83.41-
    cruciate ligament S83.50-
      anterior S83.51-
      posterior S83.52-
    lateral (fibular) collateral ligament S83.42-
    medial (tibial) collateral ligament S83.41-
    patellar ligament S76.11-
    specified site NEC S83.8X-
    superior tibiofibular joint (ligament) S83.6-
  lateral collateral, knee —*see* Sprain, knee, collateral
  lumbar (spine) S33.5
  lumbosacral S33.9
  mandible (articular disc) S03.4-
    old M26.69
  medial collateral, knee —*see* Sprain, knee, collateral
  meniscus
    jaw S03.4-
      old M26.69
    knee —*see* Sprain, knee, specified site NEC
      with current tear —*see* Tear, meniscus
      old —*see* Derangement, knee, meniscus, due to old tear
    mandible S03.4-
      old M26.69
  metacarpal (distal) (proximal) —*see* Sprain, hand, specified site NEC
  metacarpophalangeal —*see* Sprain, finger, metacarpophalangeal (joint)
  metatarsophalangeal —*see* Sprain, toe, metatarsophalangeal joint
  midcarpal —*see* Sprain, hand, specified site NEC
  midtarsal —*see* Sprain, foot, specified site NEC
  neck S13.9
    anterior longitudinal cervical ligament S13.4
    atlanto-axial joint S13.4
    atlanto-occipital joint S13.4
    cervical spine S13.4
    cricoarytenoid ligament S13.5
    cricothyroid ligament S13.5
    specified site NEC S13.8
    thyroid region (cartilage) S13.5

Sprain (continued)
nose S03.8
orbicular, hip —see Sprain, hip
patella —see Sprain, knee, specified site NEC
patellar ligament S76.11-
pelvis NEC S33.8
phalanx
  finger —see Sprain, finger
  toe —see Sprain, toe
pubofemoral —see Sprain, hip
radiocarpal —see Sprain, wrist
radiohumeral —see Sprain, elbow
radius, collateral —see Rupture, traumatic, ligament, radial collateral
rib (cage) S23.41
rotator cuff (capsule) S43.42-
sacroiliac (region)
  chronic or old —see subcategory M53.2
  joint S33.6
scaphoid (hand) —see Sprain, hand, specified site NEC
scapula (r) —see Sprain, shoulder girdle, specified site NEC
semilunar cartilage (knee) —see Sprain, knee, specified site NEC
  with current tear —see Tear, meniscus
    old —see Derangement, knee, meniscus, due to old tear
shoulder joint S43.40-
  acromioclavicular joint (ligament) —see Sprain, acromioclavicular joint
  blade —see Sprain, shoulder, girdle, specified site NEC
  coracoclavicular joint (ligament) —see Sprain, coracoclavicular joint
  coracohumeral ligament —see Sprain, coracohumeral joint
  girdle S43.9-
    specified site NEC S43.8-
  rotator cuff —see Sprain, rotator cuff
  specified site NEC S43.49-
  sternoclavicular joint (ligament) —see Sprain, sternoclavicular joint
spine
  cervical S13.4
  lumbar S33.5
  thoracic S23.3
sternoclavicular joint S43.6-
sternum S23.429
  chondrosternal joint S23.421
  specified site NEC S23.428
  sternoclavicular (joint) (ligament) S23.420
symphysis
  jaw S03.4-
    old M26.69
  mandibular S03.4-
    old M26.69
talofibular —see Sprain, ankle
tarsal —see Sprain, foot, specified site NEC
tarsometatarsal —see Sprain, foot, specified site NEC
temporomandibular S03.4-
  old M26.69
thorax S23.9
  ribs S23.41
  specified site NEC S23.8
  spine S23.3
  sternum —see Sprain, sternum

Sprain (continued)
thumb S63.60-
  interphalangeal (joint) S63.62-
  metacarpophalangeal (joint) S63.64-
  specified site NEC S63.68-
thyroid cartilage or region S13.5
tibia (proximal end) —see Sprain, knee, specified site NEC
tibial collateral, knee —see Sprain, knee, collateral
tibiofibular
  distal —see Sprain, ankle
  superior —see Sprain, knee, specified site NEC
toe(s) S93.50-
  great S93.50-
    interphalangeal joint S93.51-
      great S93.51-
      lesser S93.51-
  lesser S93.50-
  metatarsophalangeal joint S93.52-
    great S93.52-
    lesser S93.52-
ulna, collateral —see Rupture, traumatic, ligament, ulnar collateral
ulnohumeral —see Sprain, elbow
wrist S63.50-
  carpal S63.51-
  radiocarpal S63.52-
  specified site NEC S63.59-
xiphoid cartilage —see Sprain, sternum

Sprengel's deformity (congenital) Q74.0

Sprue (tropical) K90.1
celiac K90.0
idiopathic K90.49
meaning thrush B37.0
nontropical K90.0

Spur, bone —see also Enthesopathy
calcaneal M77.3-
iliac crest M76.2-
nose (septum) J34.89

Spurway's syndrome Q78.0

Sputum
abnormal (amount) (color) (odor) (purulent) R09.3
blood-stained R04.2
excessive (cause unknown) R09.3

Squamous —see also condition
epithelium in
  cervical canal (congenital) Q51.828
  uterine mucosa (congenital) Q51.818

Squashed nose M95.0
congenital Q67.4

Squeeze, diver's T70.3

Squint —see also Strabismus
accommodative —see Strabismus, convergent concomitant

SSADHD (succinic semialdehyde dehydrogenase deficiency) E72.81

St. Hubert's disease A82.9

Stab —see also Laceration
internal organs —see Injury, by site

Stafne's cyst or cavity M27.0

Staggering gait R26.0
hysterical F44.4

Staghorn calculus —see Calculus, kidney

Stähli's line (cornea) (pigment) —see Pigmentation, cornea, anterior

Stain, staining
meconium (newborn) P96.83
port wine Q82.5
tooth, teeth (hard tissues) (extrinsic) K03.6
  due to
    accretions K03.6
    deposits (betel) (black) (green) (materia alba) (orange) (soft) (tobacco) K03.6
    metals (copper) (silver) K03.7
    nicotine K03.6
    pulpal bleeding K03.7
    tobacco K03.6
  intrinsic K00.8

Stammering (see also Disorder, fluency) F80.81

Standstill
auricular I45.5
cardiac —see Arrest, cardiac
sinoatrial I45.5
ventricular —see Arrest, cardiac

Stannosis J63.5

Stanton's disease —see Melioidosis

Staphylitis (acute) (catarrhal) (chronic) (gangrenous) (membranous) (suppurative) (ulcerative) K12.2

Staphylococcal scalded skin syndrome L00

Staphylococcemia A41.2

Staphylococcus, staphylococcal
—see also condition
as cause of disease classified elsewhere B95.8
  aureus (methicillin susceptible) (MSSA) B95.61
    methicillin resistant (MRSA) B95.62
  specified NEC, as cause of disease classified elsewhere B95.7

Staphyloma (sclera)
cornea H18.72-
equatorial H15.81-
localized (anterior) H15.82-
posticum H15.83-
ring H15.85-

Stargardt's disease —see Dystrophy, retina

Starvation (inanition) (due to lack of food) T73.0
edema —see Malnutrition, severe

Stasis
bile (noncalculous) K83.1
bronchus J98.09
  with infection —see Bronchitis
cardiac —see Failure, heart, congestive
cecum K59.89
colon K59.89
dermatitis I87.2
  with
    varicose ulcer —see Varix, leg, with ulcer, with inflammation
    varicose veins —see Varix, leg, with inflammation
  due to postthrombotic syndrome —see Syndrome, postthrombotic
duodenal K31.5
eczema —see Varix, leg, with, inflammation
edema —see Hypertension, venous (chronic), idiopathic
foot T69.0-
ileocecal coil K59.89

Stasis (continued)
ileum K59.89
intestinal K59.89
jejunum K59.89
kidney N19
liver (cirrhotic) K76.1
lymphatic I89.8
pneumonia J18.2
pulmonary —see Edema, lung
rectal K59.89
renal N19
  tubular N17.0
ulcer —see Varix, leg, with, ulcer
  without varicose veins (see also Ulcer, by site) I87.2
urine —see Retention, urine
venous I87.8

State (of)
affective and paranoid, mixed, organic psychotic F06.8
agitated R45.1
  acute reaction to stress F43.0
anxiety (neurotic) F41.1
apprehension F41.1
burn-out Z73.0
climacteric, female Z78.0
  symptomatic N95.1
compulsive F42.8
  mixed with obsessional thoughts F42.2
confusional (psychogenic) F44.89
  acute —see also Delirium
    with
      arteriosclerotic dementia (see also Dementia, vascular) F01.50
        with behavioral disturbance —see Dementia, vascular
      senility or dementia F05
        alcoholic F10.231
      epileptic F05
      reactive (from emotional stress, psychological trauma) F44.89
  subacute —see Delirium
convulsive —see Convulsions
crisis F43.0
depressive F32.A
  neurotic F34.1
dissociative F44.9
emotional shock (stress) R45.7
hypercoagulation —see Hypercoagulable
locked-in G83.5
menopausal Z78.0
  symptomatic N95.1
neurotic F48.9
  with depersonalization F48.1
obsessional F42.8
oneiroid (schizophrenia-like) F23
organic
  hallucinatory (nonalcoholic) F06.0
  paranoid (-hallucinatory) F06.2
panic F41.0
paranoid F22
  climacteric F22
  involutional F22
  menopausal F22
  organic F06.2
  senile F03
  simple F22
persistent vegetative R40.3
phobic F40.9
postleukotomy F07.0
pregnant
  gestational carrier Z33.3
  incidental Z33.1
psychogenic, twilight F44.89
psychopathic (constitutional) F60.2

State (continued)
  psychotic, organic —see also
      Psychosis, organic
    mixed paranoid and affective
        F06.8
    senile or presenile F03
    transient NEC F06.8
      with
        hallucinations F06.0
        depression F06.31
  residual schizophrenic F20.5
  restlessness R45.1
  stress (emotional) R45.7
  tension (mental) F48.9
    specified NEC F48.8
  transient organic psychotic NEC
      F06.8
    depressive type F06.31
    hallucinatory type F06.0
  twilight
    epileptic F05
    psychogenic F44.89
  vegetative, persistent R40.3
  vital exhaustion Z73.0
  withdrawal, —see Withdrawal,
      state

Status (post) —see also Presence (of)
  absence, epileptic —see Epilepsy,
      by type, with status epilepticus
  administration of tPA (rtPA) in a
      different facility within the last
      24 hours prior to admission to
      current facility Z92.82
  adrenalectomy (unilateral)
      (bilateral) E89.6
  anastomosis Z98.0
  angioplasty (peripheral) Z98.62
    with implant Z95.820
    coronary artery Z98.61
      with implant Z95.5
  anginosus I20.9
  aortocoronary bypass Z95.1
  arthrodesis Z98.1
  artificial opening (of) Z93.9
    gastrointestinal tract Z93.4
    specified NEC Z93.8
    urinary tract Z93.6
    vagina Z93.8
  asthmaticus —see Asthma, by type,
      with status asthmaticus
  awaiting organ transplant
      Z76.82
  bariatric surgery Z98.84
  bed confinement Z74.01
  bleb, filtering (vitreous), after
      glaucoma surgery Z98.83
  breast implant Z98.82
    removal Z98.86
  cataract extraction Z98.4-
  cholecystectomy Z90.49
  clitorectomy N90.811
    with excision of labia minora
        N90.812
  colectomy (complete) (partial)
      Z90.49
  colonization —see Carrier
      (suspected) of
  colostomy Z93.3
  convulsivus idiopathicus —see
      Epilepsy, by type, with status
      epilepticus
  coronary artery angioplasty —see
      Status, angioplasty, coronary
      artery
  coronary artery bypass graft Z95.1
  cystectomy (urinary bladder) Z90.6
  cystostomy Z93.50
    appendico-vesicostomy Z93.52
    cutaneous Z93.51
    specified NEC Z93.59
  delinquent immunization Z28.39

Status (continued)
  dental Z98.818
    crown Z98.811
    fillings Z98.811
    restoration Z98.811
    sealant Z98.810
    specified NEC Z98.818
  deployment (current) (military)
      Z56.82
  dialysis (hemodialysis) (peritoneal)
      Z99.2
  do not resuscitate (DNR) Z66
  donor —see Donor
  embedded fragments —see
      Retained, foreign body
      fragments (type of)
  embedded splinter —see Retained,
      foreign body fragments (type of)
  enterostomy Z93.4
  epileptic, epilepticus (see also
      Epilepsy, by type, with status
      epilepticus) G40.901
  estrogen receptor
    negative Z17.1
    positive Z17.0
  female genital cutting —see
      Female genital mutilation status
  female genital mutilation —see
      Female genital mutilation status
  filtering (vitreous) bleb after
      glaucoma surgery Z98.83
  gastrectomy (complete) (partial)
      Z90.3
  gastric banding Z98.84
  gastric bypass for obesity Z98.84
  gastrostomy Z93.1
  human immunodeficiency virus
      (HIV) infection, asymptomatic
      Z21
  hysterectomy (complete) (total)
      Z90.710
    partial (with remaining cervial
        stump) Z90.711
  ileostomy Z93.2
  implant
    breast Z98.82
  infibulation N90.813
  intestinal bypass Z98.0
  jejunostomy Z93.4
  laryngectomy Z90.02
  lapsed immunization schedule
      Z28.39
  lymphaticus E32.8
  malignancy
    castrate resistant prostate Z19.2
    hormone resistant Z19.2
    hormone sensitive Z19.1
  marmoratus G80.3
  mastectomy (unilateral) (bilateral)
      Z90.1-
  military deployment status
      (current) Z56.82
    in theater or in support of
        military war, peacekeeping
        and humanitarian operations
        Z56.82
  nephrectomy (unilateral) (bilateral)
      Z90.5
  nephrostomy Z93.6
  obesity surgery Z98.84
  oophorectomy
    bilateral Z90.722
    unilateral Z90.721
  organ replacement
    by artificial or mechanical device
        or prosthesis of
      artery Z95.828
      bladder Z96.0
      blood vessel Z95.828
      breast Z97.8
      eye globe Z97.0

Status (continued)
  organ replacement (continued)
    by artificial or mechanical device
        or prosthesis of (continued)
      heart Z95.812
        valve Z95.2
      intestine Z97.8
      joint Z96.60
        hip —see Presence, hip
            joint implant
        knee —see Presence, knee
            joint implant
        specified site NEC Z96.698
      kidney Z97.8
      larynx Z96.3
      lens Z96.1
      limbs —see Presence,
          artificial, limb
      liver Z97.8
      lung Z97.8
      pancreas Z97.8
    by organ transplant
        (heterologous)(homologous)
        —see Transplant
  pacemaker
    brain Z96.89
    cardiac Z95.0
    specified NEC Z96.89
  pancreatectomy Z90.410
    complete Z90.410
    partial Z90.411
    total Z90.410
  physical restraint Z78.1
  pneumonectomy (complete)
      (partial) Z90.2
  pneumothorax, therapeutic Z98.3
  postcommotio cerebri F07.81
  postoperative (postprocedural)
      NEC Z98.890
    breast implant Z98.82
    dental Z98.818
      crown Z98.811
      fillings Z98.811
      restoration Z98.811
      sealant Z98.810
      specified NEC Z98.818
    pneumothorax, therapeutic Z98.3
    uterine scar Z98.891
  postpartum (routine follow-up)
      Z39.2
    care immediately after delivery
        Z39.0
  postsurgical (postprocedural) NEC
      Z98.890
    pneumothorax, therapeutic Z98.3
  pregnancy, incidental Z33.1
  prosthesis coronary angioplasty
      Z95.5
  pseudophakia Z96.1
  renal dialysis (hemodialysis)
      (peritoneal) Z99.2
  retained foreign body —see
      Retained, foreign body
      fragments (type of)
  reversed jejunal transposition (for
      bypass) Z98.0
  salpingo-oophorectomy
    bilateral Z90.722
    unilateral Z90.721
  sex reassignment surgery status
      Z87.890
  shunt
    arteriovenous (for dialysis) Z99.2
    cerebrospinal fluid Z98.2
    ventricular (communicating)
        (for drainage) Z98.2
  splenectomy Z90.81
  thymicolymphaticus E32.8
  thymicus E32.8
  thymolymphaticus E32.8

Status (continued)
  thyroidectomy (hypothyroidism)
      E89.0
  tooth (teeth) extraction (see also
      Absence, teeth, acquired)
      K08.409
  tPA (rtPA) administration in a
      different facility within the last
      24 hours prior to admission to
      current facility Z92.82
  tracheostomy Z93.0
  transplant —see Transplant
    organ removed Z98.85
  tubal ligation Z98.51
  underimmunization Z28.39
    COVID-19 Z28.31-
      partially vaccinated (for)
          Z28.311
      unvaccinated (for) Z28.310
  ureterostomy Z93.6
  urethrostomy Z93.6
  vagina, artificial Z93.8
  vasectomy Z98.52
  wheelchair confinement Z99.3

Stealing
  child problem F91.8
    in company with others
        Z72.810
  pathological (compulsive)
      F63.2

Steam burn —see Burn

Steatocystoma multiplex L72.2

Steatohepatitis (nonalcoholic)
    (NASH) K75.81

Steatoma L72.3
  eyelid (cystic) —see Dermatosis,
      eyelid
  infected —see Hordeolum

Steatorrhea (chronic) K90.4
  with lacteal obstruction K90.2
  idiopathic (adult) (infantile)
      K90.9
  pancreatic K90.3
  primary K90.0
  tropical K90.1

Steatosis E88.89
  heart —see Degeneration,
      myocardial
  kidney N28.89
  liver NEC K76.0

**Steele-Richardson-Olszewski
disease or syndrome** G23.1

Steinbrocker's syndrome G90.8

Steinert's disease G71.11

Stein-Leventhal syndrome E28.2

Stein's syndrome E28.2

STEMI (see also Infarct,
    myocardium ST elevation) I21.3

Stenocardia I20.89

Stenocephaly Q75.8

Stenosis, stenotic (cicatricial) —see
    also Stricture
  ampulla of Vater K83.1
  anus, anal (canal) (sphincter)
      K62.4
    and rectum K62.4
    congenital Q42.3
      with fistula Q42.2
  aorta (ascending) (supraventricular)
      (congenital) Q25.1
    arteriosclerotic I70.0
    calcified I70.0
    supravalvular Q25.3
  aortic (valve) I35.0
    with insufficiency I35.2
    congenital Q23.0

Stenosis, stenotic (*continued*)
- aortic (*continued*)
  - rheumatic I06.0
    - with
      - incompetency, insufficiency or regurgitation I06.2
        - with mitral (valve) disease I08.0
          - with tricuspid (valve) disease I08.3
      - mitral (valve) disease I08.0
        - with tricuspid (valve) disease I08.3
      - tricuspid (valve) disease I08.2
        - with mitral (valve) disease I08.3
  - specified cause NEC I35.0
  - syphilitic A52.03
- aqueduct of Sylvius (congenital) Q03.0
  - with spina bifida —*see* Spina bifida, by site, with hydrocephalus
  - acquired G91.1
- artery NEC (*see also* Arteriosclerosis) I77.1
  - celiac I77.4
  - cerebral —*see* Occlusion, artery, cerebral
  - extremities —*see* Arteriosclerosis, extremities
  - precerebral —*see* Occlusion, artery, precerebral
  - pulmonary (congenital) Q25.6
    - acquired I28.8
  - renal I70.1
  - stent
    - coronary T82.855
    - peripheral T82.856
- bile duct (common) (hepatic) K83.1
  - congenital Q44.3
- bladder-neck (acquired) N32.0
  - congenital Q64.31
- brain G93.89
- bronchus J98.09
  - congenital Q32.3
  - syphilitic A52.72
- cardia (stomach) K22.2
  - congenital Q39.3
- cardiovascular —*see* Disease, cardiovascular
- caudal M48.08
- cervix, cervical (canal) N88.2
  - congenital Q51.828
  - in pregnancy or childbirth —*see* Pregnancy, complicated by, abnormal cervix
- colon —*see also* Obstruction, intestine
  - congenital Q42.9
    - specified NEC Q42.8
- colostomy K94.03
- common (bile) duct K83.1
  - congenital Q44.3
- coronary (artery) —*see* Disease, heart, ischemic, atherosclerotic
- cystic duct —*see* Obstruction, gallbladder
- due to presence of device, implant or graft (*see also* Complications, by site and type, specified NEC) T85.858
  - arterial graft NEC T82.858
  - breast (implant) T85.858
  - catheter T85.858
    - dialysis (renal) T82.858
      - intraperitoneal T85.858
    - infusion NEC T82.858
      - spinal (epidural) (subdural) T85.850
    - urinary (indwelling) T83.85

Stenosis, stenotic (*continued*)
- due to presence of device, implant or graft (*continued*)
  - fixation, internal (orthopedic) NEC T84.85
  - gastrointestinal (bile duct) (esophagus) T85.858
  - genital NEC T83.85
  - heart NEC T82.857
  - joint prosthesis T84.85
  - ocular (corneal graft) (orbital implant) NEC T85.858
  - orthopedic NEC T84.85
  - specified NEC T85.858
  - urinary NEC T83.85
  - vascular NEC T82.858
  - ventricular intracranial shunt T85.850
- duodenum K31.5
  - congenital Q41.0
- ejaculatory duct NEC N50.89
- endocervical os —*see* Stenosis, cervix
- enterostomy K94.13
- esophagus K22.2
  - congenital Q39.3
  - syphilitic A52.79
    - congenital A50.59 [K23]
- eustachian tube —*see* Obstruction, eustachian tube
- external ear canal (acquired) H61.30-
  - congenital Q16.1
  - due to
    - inflammation H61.32-
    - trauma H61.31-
  - postprocedural H95.81-
  - specified cause NEC H61.39-
- gallbladder —*see* Obstruction, gallbladder
- glottis J38.6
- heart valve (*see also* Endocarditis) I38
  - aortic —*see* Stenosis, aortic
  - congenital Q24.8
  - mitral —*see* Stenosis, mitral
  - pulmonary —*see* Stenosis, pulmonary, valve
  - tricuspid —*see* Stenosis, tricuspid Q22.4
- hepatic duct K83.1
- hymen N89.6
- hypertrophic subaortic (idiopathic) I42.1
- ileum (*see also* Obstruction, intestine, specified NEC) K56.699
  - congenital Q41.2
- infundibulum cardia Q24.3
- intervertebral foramina —*see also* Lesion, biomechanical, specified NEC
  - connective tissue M99.79
    - abdomen M99.79
    - cervical region M99.71
    - cervicothoracic M99.71
    - head region M99.70
    - lumbar region M99.73
    - lumbosacral M99.73
    - occipitocervical M99.70
    - sacral region M99.74
    - sacrococcygeal M99.74
    - sacroiliac M99.74
    - specified NEC M99.79
    - thoracic region M99.72
    - thoracolumbar M99.72
  - disc M99.79
    - abdomen M99.79
    - cervical region M99.71
    - cervicothoracic M99.71
    - head region M99.70
    - lower extremity M99.76

Stenosis, stenotic (*continued*)
- intervertebral foramina (*continued*)
  - disc (*continued*)
    - lumbar region M99.73
    - lumbosacral M99.73
    - occipitocervical M99.70
    - pelvic M99.75
    - rib cage M99.78
    - sacral region M99.74
    - sacrococcygeal M99.74
    - sacroiliac M99.74
    - specified NEC M99.79
    - thoracic region M99.72
    - thoracolumbar M99.72
    - upper extremity M99.77
  - osseous M99.69
    - abdomen M99.69
    - cervical region M99.61
    - cervicothoracic M99.61
    - head region M99.60
    - lower extremity M99.66
    - lumbar region M99.63
    - lumbosacral M99.63
    - occipitocervical M99.60
    - pelvic M99.65
    - rib cage M99.68
    - sacral region M99.64
    - sacrococcygeal M99.64
    - sacroiliac M99.64
    - specified NEC M99.69
    - thoracic region M99.62
    - thoracolumbar M99.62
    - upper extremity M99.67
  - subluxation —*see* Stenosis, intervertebral foramina, Vosseous
- intestine —*see also* Obstruction, intestine
  - congenital (small) Q41.9
    - large Q42.9
      - specified NEC Q42.8
    - specified NEC Q41.8
- jejunum (*see also* Obstruction, intestine, specified NEC) K56.699
  - congenital Q41.1
- lacrimal (passage)
  - canaliculi H04.54-
  - congenital Q10.5
  - duct H04.55-
  - punctum H04.56-
  - sac H04.57-
- lacrimonasal duct —*see* Stenosis, lacrimal, duct
  - congenital Q10.5
- larynx J38.6
  - congenital NEC Q31.8
    - subglottic Q31.1
  - syphilitic A52.73
    - congenital A50.59 [J99]
- mitral (chronic) (inactive) (valve) I05.0
  - with
    - aortic valve disease I08.0
    - incompetency, insufficiency or regurgitation I05.2
  - active or acute I01.1
    - with rheumatic or Sydenham's chorea I02.0
  - congenital Q23.2
  - specified cause, except rheumatic I34.2
  - syphilitic A52.03
- myocardium, myocardial —*see also* Degeneration, myocardial
  - hypertrophic subaortic (idiopathic) I42.1
- nares (anterior) (posterior) J34.89
  - congenital Q30.0
- nasal duct —*see also* Stenosis, lacrimal, duct
  - congenital Q10.5

Stenosis, stenotic (*continued*)
- nasolacrimal duct —*see also* Stenosis, lacrimal, duct
  - congenital Q10.5
- neural canal —*see also* Lesion, biomechanical, specified NEC
  - connective tissue M99.49
    - abdomen M99.49
    - cervical region M99.41
    - cervicothoracic M99.41
    - head region M99.40
    - lower extremity M99.46
    - lumbar region M99.43
    - lumbosacral M99.43
    - occipitocervical M99.40
    - pelvic M99.45
    - rib cage M99.48
    - sacral region M99.44
    - sacrococcygeal M99.44
    - sacroiliac M99.44
    - specified NEC M99.49
    - thoracic region M99.42
    - thoracolumbar M99.42
    - upper extremity M99.47
  - intervertebral disc M99.59
    - abdomen M99.59
    - cervical region M99.51
    - cervicothoracic M99.51
    - head region M99.50
    - lower extremity M99.56
    - lumbar region M99.53
    - lumbosacral M99.53
    - occipitocervical M99.50
    - pelvic M99.55
    - rib cage M99.58
    - sacral region M99.54
    - sacrococcygeal M99.54
    - sacroiliac M99.54
    - specified NEC M99.59
    - thoracic region M99.52
    - thoracolumbar M99.52
    - upper extremity M99.57
  - osseous M99.39
    - abdomen M99.39
    - cervical region M99.31
    - cervicothoracic M99.31
    - head region M99.30
    - lower extremity M99.36
    - lumbar region M99.33
    - lumbosacral M99.33
    - pelvic M99.35
    - rib cage M99.38
    - occipitocervical M99.30
    - sacral region M99.34
    - sacrococcygeal M99.34
    - sacroiliac M99.34
    - specified NEC M99.39
    - thoracic region M99.32
    - thoracolumbar M99.32
    - upper extremity M99.37
  - subluxation M99.29
    - cervical region M99.21
    - cervicothoracic M99.21
    - head region M99.20
    - lower extremity M99.26
    - lumbar region M99.23
    - lumbosacral M99.23
    - occipitocervical M99.20
    - pelvic M99.25
    - rib cage M99.28
    - sacral region M99.24
    - sacrococcygeal M99.24
    - sacroiliac M99.24
    - specified NEC M99.29
    - thoracic region M99.22
    - thoracolumbar M99.22
    - upper extremity M99.27
- organ or site, congenital NEC —*see* Atresia, by site
- papilla of Vater K83.1

Stenosis, stenotic *(continued)*
  pulmonary (artery) (congenital) Q25.6
    with ventricular septal defect, transposition of aorta, and hypertrophy of right ventricle Q21.3
    acquired I28.8
    in tetralogy of Fallot Q21.3
    infundibular Q24.3
    subvalvular Q24.3
    supravalvular Q25.6
    valve I37.0
      with insufficiency I37.2
      congenital Q22.1
      rheumatic I09.89
        with aortic, mitral or tricuspid (valve) disease I08.8
    vein, acquired I28.8
    vessel NEC I28.8
  pulmonic (congenital) Q22.1
    infundibular Q24.3
    subvalvular Q24.3
  pylorus (hypertrophic) (acquired) K31.1
    adult K31.1
    congenital Q40.0
    infantile Q40.0
  rectum (sphincter) —*see* Stricture, rectum
  renal artery I70.1
    congenital Q27.1
  salivary duct (any) K11.8
  sphincter of Oddi K83.1
  spinal M48.00
    cervical region M48.02
    cervicothoracic region M48.03
    lumbar region (NOS) (without neurogenic claudication) M48.061
      with neurogenic claudication M48.062
    lumbosacral region M48.07
    occipito-atlanto-axial region M48.01
    sacrococcygeal region M48.08
    thoracic region M48.04
    thoracolumbar region M48.05
  stent
    vascular
      end stent
        adjacent to stent —*see* Arteriosclerosis
        within the stent
          coronary T82.855
          peripheral T82.856
      in stent
        coronary vessel T82.855
        peripheral vessel T82.856
  stomach, hourglass K31.2
  subaortic (congenital) Q24.4
    hypertrophic (idiopathic) I42.1
  subglottic J38.6
    congenital Q31.1
    postprocedural J95.5
  trachea J39.8
    congenital Q32.1
    syphilitic A52.73
    tuberculous NEC A15.5
  tracheostomy J95.03
  tricuspid (valve) I07.0
    with
      aortic (valve) disease I08.2
      incompetency, insufficiency or regurgitation I07.2
        with aortic (valve) disease I08.2
          with mitral (valve) disease I08.3
        mitral (valve) disease I08.1
          with aortic (valve) disease I08.3

Stenosis, stenotic *(continued)*
  tricuspid *(continued)*
    congenital Q22.4
    nonrheumatic I36.0
      with insufficiency I36.2
  tubal N97.1
  ureter —*see* Atresia, ureter
  ureteropelvic junction, congenital Q62.11
  ureterovesical orifice, congenital Q62.12
  urethra (valve) —*see also* Stricture, urethra
    congenital Q64.32
  urinary meatus, congenital Q64.33
  vagina N89.5
    congenital Q52.4
    in pregnancy —*see* Pregnancy, complicated by, abnormal vagina
      causing obstructed labor O65.5
  valve (cardiac) (heart) (*see also* Endocarditis) I38
    congenital Q24.8
      aortic Q23.0
      mitral Q23.2
      pulmonary Q22.1
      tricuspid Q22.4
  vena cava (inferior) (superior) I87.1
    congenital Q26.0
  vesicourethral orifice Q64.31
  vulva N90.5
Stent jail T82.897
Stercolith (impaction) K56.41
  appendix K38.1
Stercoraceous, stercoral ulcer K63.3
  anus or rectum K62.6
Stereotypies NEC F98.4
Sterility —*see* Infertility
Sterilization —*see* Encounter (for), sterilization
Sternalgia —*see* Angina
Sternopagus Q89.4
Sternum bifidum Q76.7
Steroid
  effects (adverse) (adrenocortical) (iatrogenic)
    cushingoid E24.2
      correct substance properly administered —*see* Table of Drugs and Chemicals, by drug, adverse effect
      overdose or wrong substance given or taken —*see* Table of Drugs and Chemicals, by drug, poisoning
    diabetes —*see* category E09
      correct substance properly administered —*see* Table of Drugs and Chemicals, by drug, adverse effect
      overdose or wrong substance given or taken —*see* Table of Drugs and Chemicals, by drug, poisoning
    fever R50.2
    insufficiency E27.3
      correct substance properly administered —*see* Table of Drugs and Chemicals, by drug, adverse effect
      overdose or wrong substance given or taken —*see* Table of Drugs and Chemicals, by drug, poisoning
  responder H40.04-

Stevens-Johnson disease or syndrome L51.1
  toxic epidermal necrolysis overlap L51.3
Stewart-Morel syndrome M85.2
Sticker's disease B08.3
Sticky eye —*see* Conjunctivitis, acute, mucopurulent
Stieda's disease —*see* Bursitis, tibial collateral
Stiff neck —*see* Torticollis
Stiff-man syndrome G25.82
Stiffness, joint NEC M25.60-
  ankle M25.67-
  ankylosis —*see* Ankylosis, joint
  contracture —*see* Contraction, joint
  elbow M25.62-
  foot M25.67-
  hand M25.64-
  hip M25.65-
  knee M25.66-
  shoulder M25.61-
  specified site NEC M25.69
  wrist M25.63-
Stigmata congenital syphilis A50.59
Stillbirth P95
Still-Felty syndrome —*see* Felty's syndrome
Still's disease or syndrome (juvenile) M08.20
  adult-onset M06.1
  ankle M08.27-
  elbow M08.22-
  foot joint M08.27-
  hand joint M08.24-
  hip M08.25-
  knee M08.26-
  multiple site M08.29
  shoulder M08.21-
  specified site NEC M08.2A
  vertebra M08.28
  wrist M08.23-
Stimulation, ovary E28.1
Sting (venomous) (with allergic or anaphylactic shock) —*see* Table of Drugs and Chemicals, by animal or substance, poisoning
Stippled epiphyses Q78.8
Stitch
  abscess T81.41
  burst (in operation wound) —*see* Disruption, wound, operation
Stokes-Adams disease or syndrome I45.9
Stokes' disease E05.00
  with thyroid storm E05.01
Stokvis (-Talma) disease D74.8
Stoma malfunction
  colostomy K94.03
  enterostomy K94.13
  gastrostomy K94.23
  ileostomy K94.13
  tracheostomy J95.03
Stomach —*see* condition
Stomatitis (denture) (ulcerative) K12.1
  angular K13.0
    due to dietary or vitamin deficiency E53.0
  aphthous K12.0
  bovine B08.61
  candidal B37.0
  catarrhal K12.1

Stomatitis *(continued)*
  diphtheritic A36.89
  due to
    dietary deficiency E53.0
    thrush B37.0
    vitamin deficiency
      B group NEC E53.9
      B2(riboflavin) E53.0
  epidemic B08.8
  epizootic B08.8
  follicular K12.1
  gangrenous A69.0
  Geotrichum B48.3
  herpesviral, herpetic B00.2
  herpetiformis K12.0
  malignant K12.1
  membranous acute K12.1
  monilial B37.0
  mycotic B37.0
  necrotizing ulcerative A69.0
  parasitic B37.0
  septic K12.1
  spirochetal A69.1
  suppurative (acute) K12.2
  ulceromembranous A69.1
  vesicular K12.1
    with exanthem (enteroviral) B08.4
    virus disease A93.8
  Vincent's A69.1
Stomatocytosis D58.8
Stomatomycosis B37.0
Stomatorrhagia K13.79
Stone(s) —*see also* Calculus
  bladder (diverticulum) N21.0
  cystine E72.09
  heart syndrome I50.1
  kidney N20.0
  prostate N42.0
  pulpal (dental) K04.2
  renal N20.0
  salivary gland or duct (any) K11.5
  urethra (impacted) N21.1
  urinary (duct) (impacted) (passage) N20.9
    bladder (diverticulum) N21.0
    lower tract N21.9
    specified NEC N21.8
  xanthine E79.82 *[N22]*
Stonecutter's lung J62.8
Stonemason's asthma, disease, lung or pneumoconiosis J62.8
Stoppage
  heart —*see* Arrest, cardiac
  urine —*see* Retention, urine
Storm, thyroid —*see* Thyrotoxicosis
Strabismus (congenital) (nonparalytic) H50.9
  concomitant H50.40
    convergent —*see* Strabismus, convergent concomitant
    divergent —*see* Strabismus, divergent concomitant
  convergent concomitant H50.00
    accommodative component H50.43
    alternating H50.05
      with
        A pattern H50.06
        specified nonconcomitances NEC H50.08
        V pattern H50.07
    monocular H50.01-
      with
        A pattern H50.02-
        specified nonconcomitances NEC H50.04-
        V pattern H50.03-
    intermittent H50.31-
      alternating H50.32

Strabismus *(continued)*
  cyclotropia H50.41
  divergent concomitant H50.10
    alternating H50.15
      with
        A pattern H50.16
        specified noncomitances
          NEC H50.18
        V pattern H50.17
    monocular H50.11-
      with
        A pattern H50.12-
        specified noncomitances
          NEC H50.14-
        V pattern H50.13-
      intermittent H50.33
        alternating H50.34
  Duane's syndrome H50.81-
  due to adhesions, scars H50.69
  heterophoria H50.50
    alternating H50.55
    cyclophoria H50.54
    esophoria H50.51
    exophoria H50.52
    vertical H50.53
  heterotropia H50.40
    intermittent H50.30
  hypertropia H50.2-
  hypotropia —*see* Hypertropia
  latent H50.50
  mechanical H50.60
    Brown's sheath syndrome H50.61-
    specified type NEC H50.69
  monofixation syndrome H50.42
  paralytic H49.9
    abducens nerve H49.2-
    fourth nerve H49.1-
    Kearns-Sayre syndrome H49.81-
    ophthalmoplegia (external)
      progressive H49.4-
        with pigmentary retinopathy
          H49.81-
      total H49.3-
    sixth nerve H49.2-
    specified type NEC H49.88-
    third nerve H49.0-
    trochlear nerve H49.1-
  specified type NEC H50.89
  vertical H50.2-

Strain
  back S39.012
  cervical S16.1
  eye NEC —*see* Disturbance,
    vision, subjective
  heart —*see* Disease, heart
  low back S39.012
  mental NOS Z73.3
    work-related Z56.6
  muscle (tendon) —*see* Injury,
    muscle, by site, strain
  neck S16.1
  postural —*see also* Disorder, soft
    tissue, due to use
  physical NOS Z73.3
    work-related Z56.6
  psychological NEC Z73.3
  tendon —*see* Injury, muscle, by
    site, strain

Straining, on urination R39.16

Strand, vitreous —*see* Opacity,
  vitreous, membranes and strands

Strangulation, strangulated
  —*see also* Asphyxia, traumatic
  appendix K38.8
  bladder-neck N32.0
  bowel or colon K56.2
  food or foreign body —*see* Foreign
    body, by site

Strangulation, strangulated
(continued)
  hemorrhoids —*see* Hemorrhoids,
    with complication
  hernia —*see also* Hernia, by site,
    with obstruction
    with gangrene —*see* Hernia, by
      site, with gangrene
  intestine (large) (small) K56.2
    with hernia —*see also* Hernia,
      by site, with obstruction
      with gangrene —*see* Hernia,
        by site, with gangrene
  mesentery K56.2
  mucus —*see* Asphyxia, mucus
  omentum K56.2
  organ or site, congenital NEC
    —*see* Atresia, by site
  ovary —*see* Torsion, ovary
  penis N48.89
    foreign body T19.4
  rupture —*see* Hernia, by site, with
    obstruction
  stomach due to hernia —*see also*
    Hernia, by site, with obstruction
    with gangrene —*see* Hernia, by
      site, with gangrene
  vesicourethral orifice N32.0

Strangury R30.0

Straw itch B88.0

Strawberry
  gallbladder K82.4
  mark Q82.5
  tongue (red) (white) K14.3

Streak(s)
  macula, angioid H35.33
  ovarian Q50.32

Strephosymbolia F81.0
  secondary to organic lesion R48.8

Streptobacillary fever A25.1

Streptobacillosis A25.1

Streptobacillus moniliformis A25.1

Streptococcus, streptococcal —*see
also* condition
  as cause of disease classified
    elsewhere B95.5
  group
    A, as cause of disease classified
      elsewhere B95.0
    B, as cause of disease classified
      elsewhere B95.1
    D, as cause of disease classified
      elsewhere B95.2
  pneumoniae, as cause of disease
    classified elsewhere B95.3
  specified NEC, as cause of
    disease classified elsewhere
    B95.4

Streptomycosis B47.1

Streptotrichosis A48.8

Stress F43.9
  family —*see* Disruption, family
  fetal P84
    complicating pregnancy O77.9
    due to drug administration
      O77.1
  mental NEC Z73.3
    work-related Z56.6
  physical NEC Z73.3
    work-related Z56.6
  polycythemia D75.1
  reaction (*see also* Reaction, stress)
    F43.9
  work schedule Z56.3

Stretching, nerve —*see* Injury, nerve

**Striae albicantes, atrophicae or
distensae** (cutis) L90.6

Stricture —*see also* Stenosis
  ampulla of Vater K83.1
  anus (sphincter) K62.4
    congenital Q42.3
      with fistula Q42.2
    infantile Q42.3
      with fistula Q42.2
  aorta (ascending) (congenital) Q25.1
    arteriosclerotic I70.0
    calcified I70.0
    supravalvular, congenital Q25.3
  aortic (valve) —*see* Stenosis, aortic
  aqueduct of Sylvius (congenital)
    Q03.0
    with spina bifida —*see*
      Spina bifida, by site, with
      hydrocephalus
    acquired G91.1
  artery I77.1
    basilar —*see* Occlusion, artery,
      basilar
    carotid —*see* Occlusion, artery,
      carotid
    celiac I77.4
    congenital (peripheral) Q27.8
      cerebral Q28.3
      coronary Q24.5
      digestive system Q27.8
      lower limb Q27.8
      retinal Q14.1
      specified site NEC Q27.8
      umbilical Q27.0
      upper limb Q27.8
    coronary —*see* Disease, heart,
      ischemic, atherosclerotic
      congenital Q24.5
    precerebral —*see* Occlusion,
      artery, precerebral
    pulmonary (congenital)
      Q25.6
      acquired I28.8
    renal I70.1
    vertebral —*see* Occlusion,
      artery, vertebral
  auditory canal (external)
    (congenital)
    acquired —*see* Stenosis, external
      ear canal
  bile duct (common) (hepatic) K83.1
    congenital Q44.3
    postoperative K91.89
  bladder N32.89
    neck N32.0
  bowel —*see* Obstruction, intestine
  brain G93.89
  bronchus J98.09
    congenital Q32.3
    syphilitic A52.72
  cardia (stomach) K22.2
    congenital Q39.3
  cardiac —*see also* Disease, heart
    orifice (stomach) K22.2
  cecum —*see* Obstruction, intestine
  cervix, cervical (canal) N88.2
    congenital Q51.828
    in pregnancy —*see* Pregnancy,
      complicated by, abnormal
      cervix
      causing obstructed labor
        O65.5
  colon —*see also* Obstruction,
    intestine
    congenital Q42.9
      specified NEC Q42.8
  colostomy K94.03
  common (bile) duct K83.1
  coronary (artery) —*see* Disease,
    heart, ischemic, atherosclerotic

Stricture *(continued)*
  cystic duct —*see* Obstruction,
    gallbladder
  digestive organs NEC, congenital
    Q45.8
  duodenum K31.5
    congenital Q41.0
  ear canal (external) (congenital)
    Q16.1
    acquired —*see* Stricture,
      auditory canal, acquired
  ejaculatory duct N50.89
  enterostomy K94.13
  esophagus K22.2
    congenital Q39.3
    syphilitic A52.79
      congenital A50.59 *[K23]*
  eustachian tube —*see also*
    Obstruction, eustachian tube
    congenital Q17.8
  fallopian tube N97.1
    gonococcal A54.24
    tuberculous A18.17
  gallbladder —*see* Obstruction,
    gallbladder
  glottis J38.6
  heart —*see also* Disease, heart
    valve (*see also* Endocarditis) I38
      aortic Q23.0
      mitral Q23.2
      pulmonary Q22.1
      tricuspid Q22.4
  hepatic duct K83.1
  hourglass, of stomach K31.2
  hymen N89.6
  hypopharynx J39.2
  ileum (*see also* Obstruction, intestine,
    specified NEC) K56.699
    congenital Q41.2
  intestine —*see also* Obstruction,
    intestine
    congenital (small) Q41.9
      large Q42.9
        specified NEC Q42.8
      specified NEC Q41.8
    ischemic K55.1
  jejunum (*see also* Obstruction,
    intestine, specified NEC)
    K56.699
    congenital Q41.1
  lacrimal passages —*see also*
    Stenosis, lacrimal
    congenital Q10.5
  larynx J38.6
    congenital NEC Q31.8
      subglottic Q31.1
    syphilitic A52.73
      congenital A50.59 *[J99]*
  meatus
    ear (congenital) Q16.1
      acquired —*see* Stricture,
        auditory canal, acquired
    osseous (ear) (congenital) Q16.1
      acquired —*see* Stricture,
        auditory canal, acquired
    urinarius —*see also* Stricture,
      urethra
      congenital Q64.33
  mitral (valve) —*see* Stenosis,
    mitral
  myocardium, myocardial I51.5
    hypertrophic subaortic
      (idiopathic) I42.1
  nares (anterior) (posterior) J34.89
    congenital Q30.0
  nasal duct —*see also* Stenosis,
    lacrimal, duct
    congenital Q10.5
  nasolacrimal duct —*see also*
    Stenosis, lacrimal, duct
    congenital Q10.5

Stricture (continued)
  nasopharynx J39.2
    syphilitic A52.73
  nose J34.89
    congenital Q30.0
  nostril (anterior) (posterior) J34.89
    congenital Q30.0
    syphilitic A52.73
      congenital A50.59 [J99]
  organ or site, congenital NEC
    —see Atresia, by site
  os uteri —see Stricture, cervix
  osseous meatus (ear) (congenital)
    Q16.1
    acquired —see Stricture,
      auditory canal, acquired
  oviduct —see Stricture, fallopian
    tube
  pelviureteric junction (congenital)
    Q62.11
    acquired, with hydronephrosis
      N13.0
  penis, by foreign body T19.4
  pharynx J39.2
  prostate N42.89
  pulmonary, pulmonic
    artery (congenital) Q25.6
      acquired I28.8
      noncongenital I28.8
    infundibulum (congenital) Q24.3
    valve I37.0
      congenital Q22.1
    vein, acquired I28.8
    vessel NEC I28.8
  punctum lacrimale —see also
    Stenosis, lacrimal, punctum
    congenital Q10.5
  pylorus (hypertrophic) K31.1
    adult K31.1
    congenital Q40.0
    infantile Q40.0
  rectosigmoid (see also Obstruction,
    intestine, specified NEC)
    K56.699
  rectum (sphincter) K62.4
    congenital Q42.1
      with fistula Q42.0
    due to
      chlamydial lymphogranuloma
        A55
      irradiation K91.89
      lymphogranuloma venereum
        A55
    gonococcal A54.6
    inflammatory (chlamydial) A55
    syphilitic A52.74
    tuberculous A18.32
  renal artery I70.1
    congenital Q27.1
  salivary duct or gland (any) K11.8
  sigmoid (flexure) —see
    Obstruction, intestine
  spermatic cord N50.89
  stoma (following) (of)
    colostomy K94.03
    enterostomy K94.13
    gastrostomy K94.23
    ileostomy K94.13
    tracheostomy J95.03
  stomach K31.89
    congenital Q40.2
    hourglass K31.2
  subaortic Q24.4
    hypertrophic (acquired)
      (idiopathic) I42.1
  subglottic J38.6
  syphilitic NEC A52.79
  trachea J39.8
    congenital Q32.1
    syphilitic A52.73
    tuberculous NEC A15.5

Stricture (continued)
  tracheostomy J95.03
  tricuspid (valve) —see Stenosis,
    tricuspid
  tunica vaginalis N50.89
  ureter (postoperative) N13.5
    with
      hydronephrosis N13.1
        with infection N13.6
      pyelonephritis (chronic)
        N11.1
    congenital —see Atresia, ureter
    tuberculous A18.11
  ureteropelvic junction (congenital)
    Q62.11
    acquired, with hydronephrosis
      N13.0
  ureterovesical orifice N13.5
    with infection N13.6
  urethra (organic) (spasmodic) (see
    also Stricture, urethra, male)
    N35.919
    associated with schistosomiasis
      B65.0 [N37]
    congenital Q64.39
      valvular (posterior) Q64.2
    due to
      infection —see Stricture,
        urethra, postinfective
      trauma —see Stricture,
        urethra, post-traumatic
    female N35.92
    gonococcal, gonorrheal
      A54.01
    infective NEC —see Stricture,
      urethra, postinfective
    late effect (sequelae) of injury
      —see Stricture, urethra, post-
      traumatic
    male N35.919
      anterior urethra N35.914
      bulbous urethra N35.912
      meatal N35.911
      membranous urethra N35.913
      overlapping site N35.916
    postcatheterization —see Stricture,
      urethra, postprocedural
    postinfective NEC
      female N35.12
      male N35.119
        anterior urethra N35.114
        bulbous urethra N35.112
        meatal N35.111
        membranous urethra
          N35.113
        overlapping sites N35.116
    postobstetric N35.021
    postoperative —see Stricture,
      urethra, postprocedural
    postprocedural
      female N99.12
      male N99.114
        anterior bulbous urethra
          N99.113
        bulbous urethra N99.111
        fossa navicularis N99.115
        meatal N99.110
        membranous urethra
          N99.112
        overlapping sites N99.116
    post-traumatic
      female N35.028
        due to childbirth N35.021
      male N35.014
        anterior urethra N35.013
        bulbous urethra N35.011
        meatal N35.010
        membranous urethra
          N35.012
        overlapping sites N35.016

Stricture (continued)
  urethra (continued)
    sequela (late effect) of
      childbirth N35.021
      injury —see Stricture, urethra,
        post-traumatic
    specified cause NEC
      female N35.82
      male N35.819
        anterior urethra N35.814
        bulbous urethra N35.812
        meatal N35.811
        membranous urethra N35.813
        overlapping site N35.816
    syphilitic A52.76
    traumatic —see Stricture,
      urethra, post-traumatic
    valvular (posterior), congenital
      Q64.2
  urinary meatus —see Stricture,
    urethra
  uterus, uterine (synechiae) N85.6
    os (external) (internal) —see
      Stricture, cervix
  vagina (outlet) —see Stenosis, vagina
  valve (cardiac) (heart) —see also
    Endocarditis
    congenital
      aortic Q23.0
      mitral Q23.2
      pulmonary Q22.1
      tricuspid Q22.4
  vas deferens N50.89
    congenital Q55.4
  vein I87.1
  vena cava (inferior) (superior) NEC
    I87.1
    congenital Q26.0
  vesicourethral orifice N32.0
    congenital Q64.31
  vulva (acquired) N90.5
Stridor R06.1
  congenital (larynx) P28.89
Stridulous —see condition
Stroke (apoplectic) (brain) (ischemic)
  (paralytic) I63.9
  cerebral, perinatal P91.82-
  cerebrovascular (ischemic) I63.9
    chronic (old) (remote) (imaging)
      (without sequelae) Z86.73
      with residual defects
        —see Sequelae, disease,
        cerebrovascular
  embolic I63.-
  thrombolic I63.-
  cryptogenic (see also Infarction,
    cerebral) I63.9
  epileptic —see Epilepsy
  heat T67.01
    exertional T67.02
    specified NEC T67.09
  in evolution I63.9
  intraoperative
    during cardiac surgery I97.810
    during other surgery I97.811
  ischemic, perinatal arterial P91.82-
  lightning —see Lightning
  meaning
    cerebral hemorrhage - code to
      Hemorrhage, intracranial
    cerebral infarction - code to
      Infarction, cerebral
  neonatal P91.82-
  postprocedural
    following cardiac surgery I97.820
    following other surgery I97.821
  sun T67.01
    specified NEC T67.09
  unspecified (NOS) I63.9

Stromatosis, endometrial D39.0
Strongyloidiasis, strongyloidosis
  B78.9
  cutaneous B78.1
  disseminated B78.7
  intestinal B78.0
Strophulus pruriginosus L28.2
Struck by lightning —see Lightning
Struma —see also Goiter
  Hashimoto E06.3
  lymphomatosa E06.3
  nodosa (simplex) E04.9
    endemic E01.2
      multinodular E01.1
    multinodular E04.2
      iodine-deficiency related
        E01.1
    toxic or with hyperthyroidism
      E05.20
      with thyroid storm E05.21
      multinodular E05.20
        with thyroid storm E05.21
      uninodular E05.10
        with thyroid storm E05.11
    toxicosa E05.20
      with thyroid storm E05.21
      multinodular E05.20
        with thyroid storm E05.21
      uninodular E05.10
        with thyroid storm E05.11
    uninodular E04.1
  ovarii D27.-
  Riedel's E06.5
Strumipriva cachexia E03.4
Strümpell-Marie spine —see
  Spondylitis, ankylosing
Strümpell-Westphal pseudosclerosis
  E83.01
Stuart deficiency disease (factor X)
  D68.2
Stuart-Prower factor deficiency
  (factor X) D68.2
Student's elbow —see Bursitis,
  elbow, olecranon
Stump —see Amputation
Stunting, nutritional E45
Stupor (catatonic) R40.1
  depressive (single episode) F32.89
    recurrent episode F33.8
  dissociative F44.2
  manic F30.2
  manic-depressive F31.89
  psychogenic (anergic) F44.2
  reaction to exceptional stress
    (transient) F43.0
Sturge (-Weber) (-Dimitri) (-Kalischer)
  disease or syndrome Q85.89
Stuttering F80.81
  adult onset F98.5
  childhood onset F80.81
  following cerebrovascular
    disease —see Disorder, fluency.
  following cerebrovascular disease
  in conditions classified elsewhere
    R47.82
Sty, stye (external) (internal)
  (meibomian) (zeisian) —see
  Hordeolum
Subacidity, gastric K31.89
  psychogenic F45.8
Subacute —see condition
Subarachnoid —see condition
Subcortical —see condition

Subcostal syndrome, nerve compression —*see* Mononeuropathy, upper limb, specified site NEC
Subcutaneous, subcuticular —*see* condition
Subdural —*see* condition
Subendocardium —*see* condition
Subependymoma
  specified site —*see* Neoplasm, uncertain behavior, by site
  unspecified site D43.2
Suberosis J67.3
Subglossitis —*see* Glossitis
Subhemophilia D66
Subinvolution
  breast (postlactational) (postpuerperal) N64.89
  puerperal O90.89
  uterus (chronic) (nonpuerperal) N85.3
  puerperal O90.89
Sublingual —*see* condition
Sublinguitis —*see* Sialoadenitis
Subluxatable hip Q65.6
Subluxation —*see also* Dislocation
  acromioclavicular S43.11-
  ankle S93.0-
  atlantoaxial, recurrent M43.4
    with myelopathy M43.3
  carpometacarpal (joint) NEC S63.05-
    thumb S63.04-
  complex, vertebral —*see* Complex, subluxation
  congenital —*see also* Malposition, congenital
    hip —*see* Dislocation, hip, congenital, partial
    joint (excluding hip)
      lower limb Q68.8
      shoulder Q68.8
      upper limb Q68.8
  elbow (traumatic) S53.10-
    anterior S53.11-
    lateral S53.14-
    medial S53.13-
    posterior S53.12-
    specified type NEC S53.19-
  finger S63.20-
    index S63.20-
    interphalangeal S63.22-
      distal S63.24-
        index S63.24-
        little S63.24-
        middle S63.24-
        ring S63.24-
      index S63.22-
      little S63.22-
      middle S63.22-
      proximal S63.23-
        index S63.23-
        little S63.23-
        middle S63.23-
        ring S63.23-
      ring S63.22-
    little S63.20-
    metacarpophalangeal S63.21-
      index S63.21-
      little S63.21-
      middle S63.21-
      ring S63.21-
    middle S63.20-
    ring S63.20-
  foot S93.30-
    specified site NEC S93.33-
    tarsal joint S93.31-

Subluxation (*continued*)
  foot (*continued*)
    tarsometatarsal joint S93.32-
    toe —*see* Subluxation, toe
  hip S73.00-
    anterior S73.03-
      obturator S73.02-
    central S73.04-
    posterior S73.01-
  interphalangeal (joint)
    finger S63.22-
      distal joint S63.24-
        index S63.24-
        little S63.24-
        middle S63.24-
        ring S63.24-
      index S63.22-
      little S63.22-
      middle S63.22-
      proximal joint S63.23-
        index S63.23-
        little S63.23-
        middle S63.23-
        ring S63.23-
      ring S63.22-
    thumb S63.12-
    toe S93.13-
      great S93.13-
      lesser S93.13-
  joint prosthesis —*see* Complications, joint prosthesis, mechanical, displacement, by site
  knee S83.10-
    cap —*see* Subluxation, patella
    patella —*see* Subluxation, patella
    proximal tibia
      anteriorly S83.11-
      laterally S83.14-
      medially S83.13-
      posteriorly S83.12-
    specified type NEC S83.19-
  lens —*see* Dislocation, lens, partial
  ligament, traumatic —*see* Sprain, by site
  metacarpal (bone)
    proximal end S63.06-
  metacarpophalangeal (joint)
    finger S63.21-
      index S63.21-
      little S63.21-
      middle S63.21-
      ring S63.21-
    thumb S63.11-
  metatarsophalangeal joint S93.14-
    great toe S93.14-
    lesser toe S93.14-
  midcarpal (joint) S63.03-
  patella S83.00-
    lateral S83.01-
    recurrent (nontraumatic) —*see* Dislocation, patella, recurrent, incomplete
    specified type NEC S83.09-
  pathological —*see* Dislocation, pathological
  radial head S53.00-
    anterior S53.01-
    nursemaid's elbow S53.03-
    posterior S53.02-
    specified type NEC S53.09-
  radiocarpal (joint) S63.02-
  radioulnar (joint)
    distal S63.01-
    proximal —*see* Subluxation, elbow
  shoulder
    congenital Q68.8
    girdle S43.30-
      scapula S43.31-
      specified site NEC S43.39-

Subluxation (*continued*)
  shoulder (*continued*)
    traumatic S43.00-
      anterior S43.01-
      inferior S43.03-
      posterior S43.02-
      specified type NEC S43.08-
  sternoclavicular (joint) S43.20-
    anterior S43.21-
    posterior S43.22-
  symphysis (pubis) —*see also* Dislocation, symphysis pubis
  thumb S63.103
    interphalangeal joint —*see* Subluxation, interphalangeal (joint), thumb
    metacarpophalangeal joint —*see* Subluxation, metacarpophalangeal (joint), thumb
  toe(s) S93.10-
    great S93.10-
      interphalangeal joint S93.13-
      metatarsophalangeal joint S93.14-
    interphalangeal joint S93.13-
    lesser S93.10-
      interphalangeal joint S93.13-
      metatarsophalangeal joint S93.14-
    metatarsophalangeal joint S93.149
  ulna
    distal end S63.07-
    proximal end —*see* Subluxation, elbow
  ulnohumeral joint —*see* Subluxation, elbow
  vertebral
    recurrent NEC —*see* subcategory M43.5
    traumatic
      cervical S13.100
        atlantoaxial joint S13.120
        atlantooccipital joint S13.110
        atloidooccipital joint S13.110
        joint between
          C0 and C1 S13.110
          C1 and C2 S13.120
          C2 and C3 S13.130
          C3 and C4 S13.140
          C4 and C5 S13.150
          C5 and C6 S13.160
          C6 and C7 S13.170
          C7 and T1 S13.180
        occipitoatloid joint S13.110
      lumbar S33.100
        joint between
          L1 and L2 S33.110
          L2 and L3 S33.120
          L3 and L4 S33.130
          L4 and L5 S33.140
      thoracic S23.100
        joint between
          T1 and T2 S23.110
          T2 and T3 S23.120
          T3 and T4 S23.122
          T4 and T5 S23.130
          T5 and T6 S23.132
          T6 and T7 S23.140
          T7 and T8 S23.142
          T8 and T9 S23.150
          T9 and T10 S23.152
          T10 and T11 S23.160
          T11 and T12 S23.162
          T12 and L1 S23.170

Subluxation (*continued*)
  wrist (carpal bone) S63.00-
    carpometacarpal joint —*see* Subluxation, carpometacarpal (joint)
    distal radioulnar joint —*see* Subluxation, radioulnar (joint), distal
    metacarpal bone, proximal —*see* Subluxation, metacarpal (bone), proximal end
    midcarpal —*see* Subluxation, midcarpal (joint)
    radiocarpal joint —*see* Subluxation, radiocarpal (joint)
    recurrent —*see* Dislocation, recurrent, wrist
    specified site NEC S63.09-
    ulna —*see* Subluxation, ulna, distal end
Submaxillary —*see* condition
Submersion (fatal) (nonfatal) T75.1
Submucous —*see* condition
Subnormal, subnormality
  accommodation (old age) H52.4
  mental —*see* Disability, intellectual
  temperature (accidental) T68
Subphrenic —*see* condition
Subscapular nerve —*see* condition
Subseptus uterus Q51.28
Subsiding appendicitis K36
Substance (other psychoactive) -induced
  anxiety disorder F19.980
  bipolar and related disorder F19.94
  delirium F19.921
  depressive disorder F19.94
  major neurocognitive disorder F19.97
  mild neurocognitive disorder F19.988
  obsessive-compulsive and related disorder F19.988
  psychotic disorder F19.959
  sexual dysfunction F19.981
  sleep disorder F19.982
Substernal thyroid E04.9
  congenital Q89.2
Substitution disorder F44.9
Subtentorial —*see* condition
Subthyroidism (acquired) —*see also* Hypothyroidism
  congenital E03.1
Succenturiate placenta O43.19-
Sucking thumb, child (excessive) F98.8
Sudamen, sudamina L74.1
Sudanese kala-azar B55.0
Sudden
  heart failure —*see* Failure, heart
  hearing loss —*see* Deafness, sudden
Sudeck's atrophy, disease, or syndrome —*see* Algoneurodystrophy
Suffocation —*see* Asphyxia, traumatic
Sugar
  blood
    high (transient) R73.9
    low (transient) E16.2
  in urine R81

Suicide, suicidal (attempted) T14.91
- by poisoning —see Table of Drugs and Chemicals
- history of (personal) Z91.51
  - in family Z81.8
- ideation —see Ideation, suicidal
- risk
  - meaning personal history of attempted suicide Z91.51
  - meaning suicidal ideation —see Ideation, suicidal
- tendencies
  - meaning personal history of attempted suicide Z91.51
  - meaning suicidal ideation —see Ideation, suicidal
- trauma —see nature of injury by site

Suipestifer infection —see Infection, salmonella

Sulfhemoglobinemia, sulphemoglobinemia (acquired) (with methemoglobinemia) D74.8

Sumatran mite fever A75.3

Summer —see condition

Sunburn L55.9
- due to
  - tanning bed (acute) L56.8
    - chronic L57.8
  - ultraviolet radiation (acute) L56.8
    - chronic L57.8
- first degree L55.0
- second degree L55.1
- third degree L55.2

SUNCT (short lasting unilateral neuralgiform headache with conjunctival injection and tearing) G44.059
- intractable G44.051
- not intractable G44.059

Sundowning F05

Sunken acetabulum —see Derangement, joint, specified type NEC, hip

Sunstroke T67.01
- specified NEC T67.09

Superfecundation —see Pregnancy, multiple

Superfetation —see Pregnancy, multiple

Superinvolution (uterus) N85.8

Supernumerary (congenital)
- aortic cusps Q23.8
- auditory ossicles Q16.3
- bone Q79.8
- breast Q83.1
- carpal bones Q74.0
- cusps, heart valve NEC Q24.8
  - aortic Q23.8
  - mitral Q23.2
  - pulmonary Q22.3
- digit(s) Q69.9
- ear (lobule) Q17.0
- fallopian tube Q50.6
- finger Q69.0
- hymen Q52.4
- kidney Q63.0
- lacrimonasal duct Q10.6
- lobule (ear) Q17.0
- mitral cusps Q23.2
- muscle Q79.8
- nipple(s) Q83.3
- organ or site not listed —see Accessory
- ossicles, auditory Q16.3
- ovary Q50.31

Supernumerary (continued)
- oviduct Q50.6
- pulmonary, pulmonic cusps Q22.3
- rib Q76.6
  - cervical or first (syndrome) Q76.5
- roots (of teeth) K00.2
- spleen Q89.09
- tarsal bones Q74.2
- teeth K00.1
- testis Q55.29
- thumb Q69.1
- toe Q69.2
- uterus Q51.28
- vagina Q52.1
- vertebra Q76.49

Supervision (of)
- contraceptive —see Prescription, contraceptives
- dietary (for) Z71.3
  - allergy (food) Z71.3
  - colitis Z71.3
  - diabetes mellitus Z71.3
  - food allergy or intolerance Z71.3
  - gastritis Z71.3
  - hypercholesterolemia Z71.3
  - hypoglycemia Z71.3
  - intolerance (food) Z71.3
  - obesity Z71.3
  - specified NEC Z71.3
- healthy infant or child Z76.2
  - foundling Z76.1
- high-risk pregnancy —see Pregnancy, supervision of, high, risk
- lactation Z39.1
- pregnancy —see Pregnancy, supervision of

Supplemental teeth K00.1

Suppression
- binocular vision H53.34
- lactation O92.5
- menstruation N94.89
- ovarian secretion E28.39
- renal N28.9
- urine, urinary secretion R34

Suppuration, suppurative —see also condition
- accessory sinus (chronic) —see Sinusitis
- adrenal gland
- antrum (chronic) —see Sinusitis, maxillary
- bladder —see Cystitis
- brain G06.0
  - sequelae G09
- breast N61.1
  - puerperal, postpartum or gestational —see Mastitis, obstetric, purulent
- dental periosteum M27.3
- ear (middle) —see also Otitis, media
  - external NEC —see Otitis, externa, infective
  - internal —see subcategory H83.0
- ethmoidal (chronic) (sinus) —see Sinusitis, ethmoidal
- fallopian tube —see Salpingo-oophoritis
- frontal (chronic) (sinus) —see Sinusitis, frontal
- gallbladder (acute) K81.0
- gum K05.20
  - generalized —see Periodontitis, aggressive, generalized
  - localized —see Periodontitis, aggressive, localized
- intracranial G06.0
- joint —see Arthritis, pyogenic or pyemic
- labyrinthine —see subcategory H83.0

Suppuration, suppurative (continued)
- lung —see Abscess, lung
- mammary gland N61.1
  - puerperal, postpartum O91.12
  - associated with lactation O91.13
- maxilla, maxillary M27.2
  - sinus (chronic) —see Sinusitis, maxillary
- muscle —see Myositis, infective
- nasal sinus (chronic) —see Sinusitis
- pancreas, acute (see also Pancreatitis, acute) K85.80
- parotid gland —see Sialoadenitis
- pelvis, pelvic
  - female —see Disease, pelvis, inflammatory
  - male K65.0
- pericranial —see Osteomyelitis
- salivary duct or gland (any) —see Sialoadenitis
- sinus (accessory) (chronic) (nasal) —see Sinusitis
- sphenoidal sinus (chronic) —see Sinusitis, sphenoidal
- thymus (gland) E32.1
- thyroid (gland) E06.0
- tonsil —see Tonsillitis
- uterus —see Endometritis

Supraeruption of tooth (teeth) M26.34

Supraglottitis J04.30
- with obstruction J04.31

Suprarenal (gland) —see condition

Suprascapular nerve —see condition

Suprasellar —see condition

Surfer's knots or nodules S89.8-

Surgical
- emphysema T81.82
- procedures, complication or misadventure —see Complications, surgical procedures
- shock T81.10

Surveillance (of) (for) —see also Observation
- alcohol abuse Z71.41
- contraceptive —see Prescription, contraceptives
- dietary Z71.3
- drug abuse Z71.51

Susceptibility to disease, genetic Z15.89
- malignant neoplasm Z15.09
  - breast Z15.01
  - endometrium Z15.04
  - ovary Z15.02
  - prostate Z15.03
  - specified NEC Z15.09
- multiple endocrine neoplasia Z15.81

Suspected condition, ruled out —see also Observation, suspected
- amniotic cavity and membrane Z03.71
- cervical shortening Z03.75
- fetal anomaly Z03.73
- fetal growth Z03.74
- maternal and fetal conditions NEC Z03.79
- newborn (see also Observation, newborn, suspected condition ruled out) Z05.9
- oligohydramnios Z03.71
- placental problem Z03.72
- polyhydramnios Z03.71

Suspended uterus
- in pregnancy or childbirth —see Pregnancy, complicated by, abnormal uterus

Sutton's nevus D22.9

Suture
- burst (in operation wound) T81.31
  - external operation wound T81.31
  - internal operation wound T81.32
- inadvertently left in operation wound —see Foreign body, accidentally left during a procedure
- removal Z48.02

Swab inadvertently left in operation wound —see Foreign body, accidentally left during a procedure

Swallowed, swallowing
- difficulty —see Dysphagia
- foreign body —see Foreign body, alimentary tract

Swan-neck deformity (finger) —see Deformity, finger, swan-neck

Swearing, compulsive F42.8
- in Gilles de la Tourette's syndrome F95.2

Sweat, sweats
- fetid L75.0
- night R61

Sweating, excessive R61

Sweeley-Klionsky disease E75.21

Sweet's disease or dermatosis L98.2

Swelling (of) R60.9
- abdomen, abdominal (not referable to any particular organ) —see Mass, abdominal
- ankle —see Effusion, joint, ankle
- arm M79.89
  - forearm M79.89
- breast (see also Lump, breast) N63.0
- Calabar B74.3
- cervical gland R59.0
- chest, localized R22.2
- ear H93.8-
- extremity (lower) (upper) —see Disorder, soft tissue, specified type NEC
- finger M79.89
- foot M79.89
- glands R59.9
  - generalized R59.1
  - localized R59.0
- hand M79.89
- head (localized) R22.0
- inflammatory —see Inflammation
- intra-abdominal —see Mass, abdominal
- joint —see Effusion, joint
- leg M79.89
  - lower M79.89
- limb —see Disorder, soft tissue, specified type NEC
- localized (skin) R22.9
  - chest R22.2
  - head R22.0
  - limb
    - lower —see Mass, localized, limb, lower
    - upper —see Mass, localized, limb, upper
  - neck R22.1
  - trunk R22.2
- neck (localized) R22.1
- pelvic —see Mass, abdominal
- scrotum N50.89
- splenic —see Splenomegaly

Swelling *(continued)*
    testis N50.89
    toe M79.89
    umbilical R19.09
    wandering, due to Gnathostoma (spinigerum) B83.1
    white —*see* Tuberculosis, arthritis
Swift (-Feer) disease
    overdose or wrong substance given or taken —*see* Table of Drugs and Chemicals, by drug, poisoning
Swimmer's
    cramp T75.1
    ear H60.33-
    itch B65.3
Swimming in the head R42
Swollen —*see* Swelling
Swyer syndrome Q99.1
Sycosis L73.8
    barbae (not parasitic) L73.8
    contagiosa (mycotic) B35.0
    lupoides L73.8
    mycotic B35.0
    parasitic B35.0
    vulgaris L73.8
Sydenham's chorea —*see* Chorea, Sydenham's
Sylvatic yellow fever A95.0
Sylvest's disease B33.0
Symblepharon H11.23-
    congenital Q10.3
Symond's syndrome G93.2
Sympathetic —*see* condition
Sympatheticotonia G90.8
Sympathicoblastoma
    specified site —*see* Neoplasm, malignant, by site
    unspecified site C74.90
Sympathogonioma —*see* Sympathicoblastoma
Symphalangy (fingers) (toes) Q70.9
Symptoms NEC R68.89
    breast NEC N64.59
    cold J00
    development NEC R63.8
    factitious, self-induced —*see* Disorder, factitious
    genital organs, female R10.2
    involving
        abdomen NEC R19.8
        appearance NEC R46.89
        awareness R41.9
            altered mental status R41.82
            amnesia —*see* Amnesia
            borderline intellectual functioning R41.83
            coma —*see* Coma
            disorientation R41.0
            neurologic neglect syndrome R41.4
            senile cognitive decline R41.81
            specified symptom NEC R41.89
        behavior NEC R46.89
        cardiovascular system NEC R09.89
        chest NEC R09.89
        circulatory system NEC R09.89
        cognitive functions R41.9
            altered mental status R41.82
            amnesia —*see* Amnesia
            borderline intellectual functioning R41.83
            coma —*see* Coma

Symptoms NEC *(continued)*
    involving *(continued)*
        cognitive functions *(continued)*
            disorientation R41.0
            neurologic neglect syndrome R41.4
            senile cognitive decline R41.81
            specified symptom NEC R41.89
        development NEC R62.50
        digestive system NEC R19.8
        emotional state NEC R45.89
            emotional lability R45.86
        food and fluid intake R63.8
        general perceptions and sensations R44.9
            specified NEC R44.8
        musculoskeletal system R29.91
            specified NEC R29.898
        nervous system R29.90
            specified NEC R29.818
        pelvis NEC R19.8
        respiratory system NEC R09.89
        skin and integument R23.9
        urinary system R39.9
    menopausal N95.1
    metabolism NEC R63.8
    neurotic F48.8
    of infancy R68.19
    pelvis NEC, female R10.2
    skin and integument NEC R23.9
    subcutaneous tissue NEC R23.9
    viral cold J00
Sympus Q74.2
Syncephalus Q89.4
Synchondrosis
    abnormal (congenital) Q78.8
    ischiopubic M91.0
Synchysis (scintillans) (senile) (vitreous body) H43.89
Syncope (near) (pre-) R55
    anginosa I20.89
    bradycardia R00.1
    cardiac R55
    carotid sinus G90.01
    due to spinal (lumbar) puncture G97.1
    heart R55
    heat T67.1
    laryngeal R05.4
    psychogenic F48.8
    tussive R05.8
    vasoconstriction R55
    vasodepressor R55
    vasomotor R55
    vasovagal R55
Syndactylism, syndactyly Q70.9
    complex (with synostosis)
        fingers Q70.0-
        toes Q70.2-
    simple (without synostosis)
        fingers Q70.1-
        toes Q70.3-
Syndrome —*see also* Disease
    4H G11.5
    5q minus NOS D46.C
    22q13.3 deletion Q93.52
    48, XXXX Q97.1
    49, XXXXX Q97.1
    abdominal
        acute R10.0
        muscle deficiency Q79.4
        abnormal innervation H02.519
            left H02.516
                lower H02.515
                upper H02.514
            right H02.513
                lower H02.512
                upper H02.511

Syndrome *(continued)*
    abstinence, neonatal P96.1
    acid pulmonary aspiration, obstetric O74.0
    acquired immunodeficiency —*see* Human, immunodeficiency virus (HIV) disease
    activated phosphoinositide 3-kinase delta syndrome [APDS] D81.82
    acute abdominal R10.0
    acute respiratory distress (adult) (child) J80
        idiopathic J84.114
    Adair-Dighton Q78.0
    Adams-Stokes (-Morgagni) I45.9
    adiposogenital E23.6
    adrenal
        hemorrhage (meningococcal) A39.1
        meningococcic A39.1
    adrenocortical —*see* Cushing's, syndrome
    adrenogenital E25.9
        congenital, associated with enzyme deficiency E25.0
    afferent loop NEC K91.89
    Aicardi-Goutières E79.81
    Alagille (-Watson) Q44.71
    alcohol withdrawal (without convulsions) —*see* Dependence, alcohol, with, withdrawal
    Alder's D72.0
    Aldrich (-Wiskott) D82.0
    alien hand R41.4
    Alport Q87.81
    alveolar hypoventilation E66.2
    alveolocapillary block J84.10
    amnesic, amnestic (confabulatory) (due to) —*see* Disorder, amnesic
    amyostatic (Wilson's disease) E83.01
    androgen insensitivity E34.50
        complete E34.51
        partial E34.52
    androgen resistance (*see also* Syndrome, androgen insensitivity) E34.50
    Angelman Q93.51
    anginal —*see* Angina
    ankyloglossia superior Q38.1
    anterior
        chest wall R07.89
        cord G83.82
        spinal artery G95.19
            compression M47.019
                cervical region M47.012
                cervicothoracic region M47.013
                lumbar region M47.016
                occipito-atlanto-axial region M47.011
                thoracic region M47.014
                thoracolumbar region M47.015
        tibial M76.81-
    antibody deficiency D80.9
        agammaglobulinemic D80.1
            hereditary D80.0
            congenital D80.0
        hypogammaglobulinemic D80.1
            hereditary D80.0
    anticardiolipin (-antibody) D68.61
    antidepressant discontinuation T43.205
    antiphospholipid (-antibody) D68.61
    aortic
        arch M31.4
        bifurcation I74.09
    aortomesenteric duodenum occlusion K31.5
    apical ballooning (transient left ventricular) I51.81

Syndrome *(continued)*
    arcuate ligament I77.4
    argentaffin, argintaffinoma E34.0
    Arnold-Chiari —*see* Arnold-Chiari disease
    Arrillaga-Ayerza I27.0
    arterial tortuosity Q87.82
    arteriovenous steal T82.898-
    Asherman's N85.6
    aspiration, of newborn —*see* Aspiration, by substance, with pneumonia
        meconium P24.01
    ataxia-telangiectasia G11.3
    auriculotemporal G50.8
    autoerythrocyte sensitization (Gardner-Diamond) D69.2
    autoimmune polyglandular E31.0
    autoimmune lymphoproliferative [ALPS] D89.82
    autoinflammatory M04.9
        specified type NEC M04.8
    autosomal —*see* Abnormal, autosomes
    Avellis' G46.8
    Ayerza (-Arrillaga) I27.0
    Babinski-Nageotte G83.89
    Bakwin-Krida Q78.5
    Bardet-Biedl Q87.83
    bare lymphocyte D81.6
    Barré-Guillain G61.0
    Barré-Liéou M53.0
    Barrett's —*see* Barrett's, esophagus
    Barsony-Polgar K22.4
    Barsony-Teschendorf K22.4
    Barth E78.71
    Bartter's E26.81
    basal cell nevus Q87.89
    Basedow's E05.00
        with thyroid storm E05.01
    basilar artery G45.0
    Batten-Steinert G71.11
    battered
        baby or child —*see* Maltreatment, child, physical abuse
        spouse —*see* Maltreatment, adult, physical abuse
    Beals Q87.40
    Beau's I51.5
    Beck's I65.8
    Benedikt's G46.3
    Béquez César (-Steinbrinck-Chédiak-Higashi) E70.330
    Bernhardt-Roth —*see* Meralgia paresthetica
    Bernheim's —*see* Failure, heart, right
    big spleen D73.1
    bilateral polycystic ovarian E28.2
    Bing-Horton's —*see* Horton's headache
    Birt-Hogg-Dube syndrome Q87.89
    Björck (-Thorsen) E34.0
    black
        lung J60
        widow spider bite —*see* Toxicity, venom, spider, black widow
    Blackfan-Diamond D61.01
    Blau M04.8
    blind loop K90.2
        congenital Q43.8
        postsurgical K91.2
    blue sclera Q78.0
    blue toe I75.02-
    Boder-Sedgewick G11.3
    Boerhaave's K22.3
    Borjeson Forssman Lehmann Q89.8
    Bouillaud's I01.9
    Bourneville (-Pringle) Q85.1

Syndrome (continued)
  Bouveret (-Hoffman) I47.9
  brachial plexus G54.0
  bradycardia-tachycardia I49.5
  brain (nonpsychotic) F09
    with psychosis, psychotic reaction F09
    acute or subacute —see Delirium
    congenital —see Disability, intellectual
    organic F09
      post-traumatic (nonpsychotic) F07.81
        psychotic F09
      personality change F07.0
      postcontusional F07.81
      post-traumatic, nonpsychotic F07.81
      psycho-organic F09
      psychotic F06.8
  brain stem stroke G46.3
  Brandt's (acrodermatitis enteropathica) E83.2
  broad ligament laceration N83.8
  Brock's J98.11
  bronchiolitis obliterans (see also Bronchiolitis, obliterative) J44.81
  bronze baby P83.88
  Brown-Sequard G83.81
  Brugada I49.8
  bubbly lung P27.0
  Buchem's M85.2
  Budd-Chiari I82.0
  bulbar (progressive) G12.22
  Bürger-Grütz E78.3
  Burke's K86.89
  Burnett's (milk-alkali) E83.52
  burning feet E53.9
  Bywaters' T79.5
  Call-Fleming I67.841
  carbohydrate-deficient glycoprotein (CDGS) E77.8
  carcinogenic thrombophlebitis I82.1
  carcinoid E34.0
  cardiac asthma I50.1
  cardiacos negros I27.0
  cardiofaciocutaneous Q87.89
  cardiopulmonary-obesity E66.2
  cardiorenal —see Hypertension, cardiorenal
  cardiorespiratory distress (idiopathic), newborn P22.0
  cardiovascular renal —see Hypertension, cardiorenal
  carotid
    artery (hemispheric) (internal) G45.1
    body G90.01
    sinus G90.01
  carpal tunnel G56.0-
  Cassidy (-Scholte) E34.0
  cat cry Q93.4
  cat eye Q92.8
  cauda equina G83.4
  causalgia —see Causalgia
  celiac K90.0
    artery compression I77.4
    axis I77.4
  central pain G89.0
  cerebellar
    hereditary G11.9
    stroke G46.4
  cerebellomedullary malformation —see Spina bifida
  cerebral
    artery
      anterior G46.1
      middle G46.0
      posterior G46.2
      gigantism E22.0

Syndrome (continued)
  cervical (root) M53.1
    disc —see Disorder, disc, cervical, with neuritis
    fusion Q76.1
    posterior, sympathicus M53.0
    rib Q76.5
    sympathetic paralysis G90.2
  cervicobrachial (diffuse) M53.1
  cervicocranial M53.0
  cervicodorsal outlet G54.2
  cervicothoracic outlet G54.0
  Céstan (-Raymond) I65.8
  Charcot's (angina cruris) (intermittent claudication) I73.9
  Charcot-Weiss-Baker G90.09
  CHARGE Q89.8
  Chédiak-Higashi (-Steinbrinck) E70.330
  chest wall R07.1
  Chiari's (hepatic vein thrombosis) I82.0
  Chilaiditi's Q43.3
  child maltreatment —see Maltreatment, child
  chondrocostal junction M94.0
  chondroectodermal dysplasia Q77.6
  chromosome 4 short arm deletion Q93.3
  chromosome 5 short arm deletion Q93.4
  chronic
    infantile neurological, cutaneous and articular (CINCA) M04.2
    pain G89.4
      personality F68.8
  Churg-Strauss M30.1
  Clarke-Hadfield K86.89
  Clerambault's automatism G93.89
  Clouston's (hidrotic ectodermal dysplasia) Q82.4
  clumsiness, clumsy child F82
  cluster headache G44.009
    intractable G44.001
    not intractable G44.009
  Coffin-Lowry Q89.8
  cold injury (newborn) P80.0
  combined immunity deficiency D81.9
  compartment (deep) (posterior) (traumatic) T79.A0
    abdomen T79.A3
    lower extremity (hip, buttock, thigh, leg, foot, toes) T79.A2
    nontraumatic
      abdomen M79.A3
      lower extremity (hip, buttock, thigh, leg, foot, toes) M79.A2-
      specified site NEC M79.A9
      upper extremity (shoulder, arm, forearm, wrist, hand, fingers) M79.A1-
    postprocedural —see Syndrome, compartment, nontraumatic
    specified site NEC T79.A9
    upper extremity (shoulder, arm, forearm, wrist, hand, fingers) T79.A1
  complex regional pain —see Syndrome, pain, complex regional
  compression T79.5
    anterior spinal —see Syndrome, anterior, spinal artery, compression
    cauda equina G83.4
    celiac artery I77.4
    vertebral artery M47.029
      occipito-atlanto-axial region M47.021
      cervical region M47.022

Syndrome (continued)
  concussion F07.81
  congenital
    affecting multiple systems NEC Q87.89
    central alveolar hypoventilation G47.35
    facial diplegia Q87.0
    muscular hypertrophy-cerebral Q87.89
    oculo-auriculovertebral Q87.0
    oculofacial diplegia (Moebius) Q87.0
    rubella (manifest) P35.0
  congestion-fibrosis (pelvic), female N94.89
  congestive dysmenorrhea N94.6
  Conn's E26.01
  connective tissue M35.9
    overlap NEC M35.1
  conus medullaris G95.81
  cord
    anterior G83.82
    posterior G83.83
  coronary
    acute NEC I24.9
    insufficiency or intermediate I20.0
    slow flow I20.89
  Costen's (complex) M26.69
  costochondral junction M94.0
  costoclavicular G54.0
  costovertebral E22.0
  Cowden
    PTEN related Q85.81
    specified NEC Q85.82
  craniovertebral M53.0
  Creutzfeldt-Jakob —see Creutzfeldt-Jakob disease or syndrome
  cri-du-chat Q93.4
  crib death R99
  cricopharyngeal —see Dysphagia
  croup J05.0
  CRPS I —see Syndrome, pain, complex regional I
  crush T79.5
  cryopyrin-associated periodic M04.2
  cryptophthalmos Q87.0
  cubital tunnel —see Lesion, nerve, ulnar
  Curschmann (-Batten) (-Steinert) G71.11
  Cushing's E24.9
    alcohol-induced E24.4
    due to
      alcohol
        drugs E24.2
        ectopic ACTH E24.3
        overproduction of pituitary ACTH E24.0
    drug-induced E24.2
    overdose or wrong substance given or taken —see Table of Drugs and Chemicals, by drug, poisoning
    pituitary-dependent E24.0
    specified type NEC E24.8
  cystic duct stump K91.5
  cytokine release D89.839
    grade 1 D89.831
    grade 2 D89.832
    grade 3 D89.833
    grade 4 D89.834
    grade 5 D89.835
  Dana-Putnam D51.0
  Danbolt (-Cross) (acrodermatitis enteropathica) E83.2
  Dandy-Walker Q03.1
    with spina bifida Q07.01
  Danlos' (see also Syndrome, Ehlers-Danlos) Q79.60

Syndrome (continued)
  defibrination —see also Fibrinolysis
    with
      antepartum hemorrhage —see Hemorrhage, antepartum, with coagulation defect
      intrapartum hemorrhage —see Hemorrhage, complicating, delivery
    newborn P60
    postpartum O72.3
  Degos' I77.89
  Déjérine-Roussy G89.0
  delayed sleep phase G47.21
  demyelinating G37.9
  dependence —see F10-F19 with fourth character .2
  depersonalization (-derealization) F48.1
  De Quervain E34.51
  de Toni-Fanconi (-Debré) E72.09
    with cystinosis E72.04
  diabetes mellitus-hypertension-nephrosis —see Diabetes, nephrosis
  de Vivo syndrome E74.810
  diabetes mellitus in newborn infant P70.2
  diabetes-nephrosis —see Diabetes, nephrosis
  diabetic amyotrophy —see Diabetes, amyotrophy
  dialysis associated steal T82.898-
  Diamond-Blackfan D61.01
  Diamond-Gardner D69.2
  DIC (diffuse or disseminated intravascular coagulopathy) D65
  di George's D82.1
  Dighton's Q78.0
  disequilibrium E87.8
  Döhle body-panmyelopathic D72.0
  dorsolateral medullary G46.4
  double athetosis G80.3
  Down (see also Down syndrome) Q90.9
  Dravet (intractable) G40.834
    with status epilepticus G40.833
    without status epilepticus G40.834
  DRESS (drug rash with eosinophilia and systemic symptoms) D72.12
  Dresbach's (elliptocytosis) D58.1
  Dressler's (postmyocardial infarction) I24.1
    postcardiotomy I97.0
  drug rash with eosinophilia and systemic symptoms (DRESS) D72.12
  drug withdrawal, infant of dependent mother P96.1
  dry eye H04.12-
  due to abnormality
    chromosomal Q99.9
    sex
      female phenotype Q97.9
      male phenotype Q98.9
      specified NEC Q99.8
  dumping (postgastrectomy) K91.1
    nonsurgical K31.89
  Dupré's (meningism) R29.1
  dysmetabolic X E88.810
  dyspraxia, developmental F82
  Eagle-Barrett Q79.4
  Eaton-Lambert —see Syndrome, Lambert-Eaton
  Ebstein's Q22.5
  ectopic ACTH E24.3
  eczema-thrombocytopenia D82.0
  Eddowes' Q78.0

Syndrome (*continued*)
 effort (psychogenic) F45.8
 Eisenmenger's I27.83
 Ehlers-Danlos Q79.60
  classical (cEDS) (classical EDS) Q79.61
  hypermobile (hEDS) (hypermobile EDS) Q79.62
  specified NEC Q79.69
  vascular (vascular EDS) (vEDS) Q79.63
 Ekman's Q78.0
 electric feet E53.8
 Ellis-van Creveld Q77.6
 empty nest Z60.0
 endocrine-hypertensive E27.0
 entrapment —*see* Neuropathy, entrapment
 eosinophilia-myalgia M35.89
 epileptic —*see also* Epilepsy, by type
  absence G40.A09
   intractable G40.A19
    with status epilepticus G40.A11
    without status epilepticus G40.A19
   not intractable G40.A09
    with status epilepticus G40.A01
    without status epilepticus G40.A09
 Erdheim-Chester (ECD) E88.89
 Erdheim's E22.0
 erythrocyte fragmentation D59.4
 Evans D69.41
 exhaustion F48.8
 extrapyramidal G25.9
  specified NEC G25.89
 eye retraction —*see* Strabismus
 eyelid-malar-mandible Q87.0
 Faber's D50.9
 facet M47.89-
 facet joint (*see also* Spondylosis) M47.819
 facial pain, paroxysmal G50.0
 Fallot's Q21.3
 familial cold autoinflammatory M04.2
 familial eczema-thrombocytopenia (Wiskott-Aldrich) D82.0
 Fanconi (-de Toni) (-Debré) E72.09
  with cystinosis E72.04
 Fanconi's (anemia) (congenital pancytopenia) D61.09
 fatigue
  chronic G93.32
  postviral G93.31
  psychogenic F48.8
 faulty bowel habit K59.39
 Feil-Klippel (brevicollis) Q76.1
 Felty's —*see* Felty's syndrome
 fertile eunuch E23.0
 fetal
  alcohol (dysmorphic) Q86.0
  hydantoin Q86.1
 Fiedler's I40.1
 first arch Q87.0
 fish odor E72.89
 Fisher's G61.0
 Fitzhugh-Curtis
  due to
   Chlamydia trachomatis A74.81
   Neisseria gonorrhorea (gonococcal peritonitis) A54.85
 Fitz's (*see also* Pancreatitis, acute) K85.80
 Flajani (-Basedow) E05.00
  with thyroid storm E05.01
 flatback —*see* Flatback syndrome

Syndrome (*continued*)
 floppy
  baby P94.2
  iris (intraoeprative) (IFIS) H21.81
  mitral valve I34.1
 flush E34.0
 Foix-Alajouanine G95.19
 Fong's Q87.2
 food protein-induced enterocolitis (FPIES) K52.21
 foramen magnum G93.5
 Foster-Kennedy H47.14-
 Foville's (peduncular) G46.3
 fragile X Q99.2
 Franceschetti Q75.4
 Frey's
  auriculotemporal G50.8
  hyperhidrosis L74.52
 Friderichsen-Waterhouse A39.1
 Froin's G95.89
 frontal lobe F07.0
 Fukuhara E88.49
 functional
  bowel K59.9
  prepubertal castrate E29.1
 Gaisböck's D75.1
 ganglion (basal ganglia brain) G25.9
  geniculi G51.1
 Gardner-Diamond D69.2
 gastroesophageal
  junction K22.0
  laceration-hemorrhage K22.6
 gastrojejunal loop obstruction K91.89
 Gee-Herter-Heubner K90.0
 Gelineau's G47.419
  with cataplexy G47.411
 genito-anorectal A55
 Gerstmann-Sträussler-Scheinker (GSS) A81.82
 Gianotti-Crosti L44.4
 giant platelet (Bernard-Soulier) D69.1
 Gilles de la Tourette's F95.2
 Glass Q87.89
 Gleich's D72.118
 goiter-deafness E07.1
 Goldberg Q89.8
 Goldberg-Maxwell E34.51
 Good's D83.8
 Gopalan' (burning feet) E53.8
 Gorlin's Q87.89
 Gougerot-Blum L81.7
 Gouley's I31.1
 Gower's R55
 gray or grey (newborn) P93.0
  platelet D69.1
 Gubler-Millard G46.3
 Guillain-Barré (-Strohl) G61.0
 gustatory sweating G50.8
 Hadfield-Clarke K86.89
 hair tourniquet —*see* Constriction, external, by site
 Hamman's J98.19
 hand-foot L27.1
 hand-shoulder G90.8
 hantavirus (cardio)-pulmonary (HPS) (HCPS) B33.4
 happy puppet Q93.51
 Harada's H30.81-
 Hayem-Faber D50.9
 headache NEC G44.89
  complicated NEC G44.59
 Heberden's I20.89
 Hedinger's E34.0
 Hegglin's D72.
 HELLP (hemolysis, elevated liver enzymes and low platelet count) O14.2-
  complicating
   childbirth O14.24
   puerperium O14.25

Syndrome (*continued*)
 hemolytic-uremic D59.30
  atypical D59.39
   genetic D59.32
   hereditary D59.32
   infection-associated D59.31
   secondary D59.39
   specified NEC D59.39
  due to genetic disorder D59.32
  familial D59.32
  hereditary D59.32
  infection-associated D59.31
  secondary D59.39
  Shiga toxin-producing E. coli [STEC] related D59.31
  specified NEC D59.39
  typical D59.31
 hemophagocytic, infection-associated D76.2
 Henoch-Schönlein D69.0
 hepatic flexure K59.89
 hepatopulmonary K76.81
 hepatorenal K76.7
  following delivery O90.41
  postoperative or postprocedural K91.83
  postpartum, puerperal O90.41
 hepatourologic K76.7
 hereditary alpha tryptasemia D89.44
 Herter (-Gee) (nontropical sprue) K90.0
 Heubner-Herter K90.0
 Heyd's K76.7
 Hilger's G90.09
 histamine-like (fish poisoning) —*see* Poisoning, fish
 histiocytic D76.3
 histiocytosis NEC D76.3
 HIV infection, acute B20
 Hoffmann-Werdnig G12.0
 Hollander-Simons E88.1
 Hoppe-Goldflam G70.00
  with exacerbation (acute) G70.01
  in crisis G70.01
 Horner's G90.2
 hungry bone E83.81
 hunterian glossitis D51.0
 Hunt's (herpetic geniculate ganglionitis) (neuralgia) B02.21
  dyssynergia cerebellaris myoclonica G11.19
 Hutchinson's triad A50.53
 hyperabduction G54.0
 hyperammonemia-hyperornithinemia-homocitrullinemia E72.4
 hypereosinophilic (HES) D72.119
  idiopathic (IHES) D72.110
  lymphocytic variant (LHES) D72.111
  myeloid D72.118
  specified NEC D72.118
 hyperimmunoglobulin D M04.1
 hyperimmunoglobulin E (IgE) D82.4
 hyperkalemic E87.5
 hyperkinetic —*see* Hyperkinesia
 hypermobility M35.7
 hypernatremia E87.0
 hyperosmolarity (*see also*, Diabetes, by type, with hyperosmolarity) E87.0
 hyperperfusion G97.82
 hypersplenic D73.1
 hypertransfusion, newborn P61.1
 hyperventilation F45.8
 hyperviscosity (of serum)
  polycythemic D75.1
  sclerothymic D58.8
 hypoglycemic (familial) (neonatal) E16.2
 hypokalemic E87.6

Syndrome (*continued*)
 hyponatremic E87.1
 hypopituitarism E23.0
 hypoplastic left-heart Q23.4
 hypopotassemia E87.6
 hyposmolality E87.1
 hypotension, maternal O26.5-
 hypothenar hammer I73.89
 hypoventilation, obesity (OHS) E66.2
 ICF (intravascular coagulation-fibrinolysis) D65
 idiopathic
  cardiorespiratory distress, newborn P22.0
  nephrotic (infantile) N04.9
 iliotibial band M76.3-
 immobility, immobilization (paraplegic) M62.3
 immune effector cell-associated neurotoxicity (ICANS) G92.00
  grade
   1 G92.01
   2 G92.02
   3 G92.03
   4 G92.04
   5 G92.05
  unspecified G92.00
 immune reconstitution D89.3
 immune reconstitution inflammatory [IRIS] D89.3
 immunity deficiency, combined D81.9
 immunodeficiency
  acquired —*see* Human, immunodeficiency virus (HIV) disease
  combined D81.9
 impending coronary I20.0
 impingement, shoulder M75.4-
 inappropriate secretion of antidiuretic hormone E22.2
 infant
  of diabetic mother P70.1
  gestational diabetes P70.0
 infantilism (pituitary) E23.0
 inferior vena cava I87.1
 inspissated bile (newborn) P59.1
 institutional (childhood) F94.2
 insufficient sleep F51.12
 insulin resistance
  type A E88.811
  type B E88.818
 intermediate coronary (artery) I20.0
 interspinous ligament —*see* Spondylopathy, specified NEC
 intestinal
  carcinoid E34.0
  knot K56.2
 intravascular coagulation-fibrinolysis (ICF) D65
 iodine-deficiency, congenital E00.9
  type
   mixed E00.2
   myxedematous E00.1
   neurological E00.0
 IRDS (idiopathic respiratory distress, newborn) P22.0
 irritable
  bowel K58.9
   with
    constipation K58.1
    diarrhea K58.0
   mixed K58.2
   psychogenic F45.8
   specified NEC K58.8
  heart (psychogenic) F45.8
  weakness F48.8
 ischemic
  bowel (transient) K55.9
  chronic K55.1

Syndrome (continued)
ischemic (continued)
due to mesenteric artery insufficiency K55.1
steal T82.898
IVC (intravascular coagulopathy) D65
Ivemark's Q89.01
Jaccoud's —see Arthropathy, postrheumatic, chronic
Jackson's G83.89
Jakob-Creutzfeldt —see Creutzfeldt-Jakob disease or syndrome
jaw-winking Q07.8
Jervell-Lange-Nielsen I45.81
jet lag G47.25
Job's D71
Joseph-Diamond-Blackfan D61.01
jugular foramen G52.7
Kabuki Q89.8
Kanner's (autism) F84.0
Kartagener's Q89.3
Kelly's D50.1
Kimmelstiel-Wilson —see Diabetes, specified type, with Kimmelstiel-Wilson disease
Klein (e)-Levine G47.13
Klippel-Feil (brevicollis) Q76.1
Köhler-Pellegrini-Steida —see Bursitis, tibial collateral
König's K59.89
Korsakoff (-Wernicke) (nonalcoholic) F04
alcoholic F10.26
Kostmann's D70.0
Krabbe's congenital muscle hypoplasia Q79.8
labyrinthine H83.2
lacunar NEC G46.7
Lambert-Eaton G70.80
in
neoplastic disease G73.1
specified disease NEC G70.81
Landau-Kleffner —see Epilepsy, specified NEC
Larsen's Q74.8
lateral
cutaneous nerve of thigh G57.1-
medullary G46.4
Launois' E22.0
Laurence-Moon Q87.84
lazy
leukocyte D70.8
posture M62.3
Lemiere I80.8
Lennox-Gastaut G40.812
intractable G40.814
with status epilepticus G40.813
without status epilepticus G40.814
not intractable G40.812
with status epilepticus G40.811
without status epilepticus G40.812
lenticular, progressive E83.01
Leopold-Levi's E05.90
Lev's I44.2
Li-Fraumeni Z15.01
Lichtheim's D51.0
Lightwood's N25.89
Lignac (de Toni) (-Fanconi) (-Debré) E72.09
with cystinosis E72.04
Likoff's I20.89
limbic epilepsy personality F07.0
liver-kidney K76.7
lobotomy F07.0
Loffler's J82.89
long arm 18 or 21 deletion Q93.89
long QT I45.81
Louis-Barré G11.3

Syndrome (continued)
low
atmospheric pressure T70.29
back M54.50
output (cardiac) I50.9
lower radicular, newborn (birth injury) P14.8
Luetscher's (dehydration) E86.0
Lupus anticoagulant D68.62
Lutembacher's Q21.19
macrophage activation D76.1
due to infection D76.2
magnesium-deficiency R29.0
Majeed M04.8
Mal de Debarquement R42
malabsorption K90.9
postsurgical K91.2
malformation, congenital, due to
alcohol Q86.0
exogenous cause NEC Q86.8
hydantoin Q86.1
warfarin Q86.2
malignant
carcinoid E34.0
neuroleptic G21.0
Mallory-Weiss K22.6
mandibulofacial dysostosis Q75.4
manic-depressive —see Disorder, bipolar
maple-syrup-urine E71.0
Marable's I77.4
Marfan Q87.40
with
cardiovascular manifestations Q87.418
aortic dilation Q87.410
ocular manifestations Q87.42
skeletal manifestations Q87.43
Marie's (acromegaly) E22.0
mast cell activation —see Activation, mast cell
maternal hypotension —see Syndrome, hypotension, maternal
May (-Hegglin) D72.0
McArdle (-Schmidt) (-Pearson) E74.04
McQuarrie's E16.2
meconium plug (newborn) P76.0
MED13L (mediator complex subunit 13L) Q87.85
median arcuate ligament I77.4
mediator complex subunit 13L (MED13L) Q87.85
Meekeren-Ehlers-Danlos Q79.6
megavitamin-B6 E67.2
Meige G24.4
MELAS E88.41
Mendelson's O74.0
MERRF (myoclonic epilepsy associated with ragged-red fibers) E88.42
mesenteric
artery (superior) K55.1
vascular insufficiency K55.1
metabolic E88.810
metastatic carcinoid E34.0
micrognathia-glossoptosis Q87.0
midbrain NEC G93.89
middle lobe (lung) J98.19
middle radicular G54.0
migraine (see also Migraine) G43.909-
Mikulicz' K11.8
milk-alkali E83.52
Millard-Gubler G46.3
Miller-Dieker Q93.88
Miller-Fisher G61.0
Minkowski-Chauffard D58.0
Mirizzi's K83.1
MNGIE (Mitochondrial Neurogastrointestinal Encephalopathy) E88.49

Syndrome (continued)
Möbius, ophthalmoplegic migraine —see Migraine, ophthalmoplegic
monofixation H50.42
Morel-Moore M85.2
Morel-Morgagni M85.2
Morgagni (-Morel) (-Stewart) M85.2
Morgagni-Adams-Stokes I45.9
Mounier-Kuhn Q32.4
with bronchiectasis J47.9
with
exacerbation (acute) J47.1
lower respiratory infection J47.0
acquired J98.09
with bronchiectasis J47.9
with
exacerbation (acute) J47.1
lower respiratory infection J47.0
Muckle-Wells M04.2
mucocutaneous lymph node (acute febrile) (MCLS) M30.3
multiple endocrine neoplasia (MEN) —see Neoplasia, endocrine, multiple (MEN)
multiple operations —see Disorder, factitious
multisystem inflammatory (in adults) (in children) M35.81
myasthenic G70.9
in
diabetes mellitus —see Diabetes, amyotrophy
endocrine disease NEC E34.9 [G73.3]
neoplastic disease (see also Neoplasm) D49.9 [G73.3]
thyrotoxicosis (hyperthyroidism) E05.90 [G73.3]
with thyroid storm E05.91 [G73.3]
myelodysplastic D46.9
with
5q deletion D46.C
isolated del (5q) chromosomal abnormality D46.C
multilineage dysplasia D46.A
with ringed sideroblasts D46.B
lesions, low grade D46.20
specified NEC D46.Z
myeloid hypereosinophilic D72.118
myelopathic pain G89.0
myeloproliferative (chronic) D47.1
myofascial pain M79.18
Naffziger's G54.0
nail patella Q87.2
NARP (Neuropathy, Ataxia and Retinitis pigmentosa) E88.49
neonatal abstinence P96.1
nephritic —see also Nephritis
with edema —see Nephrosis
acute N00.9
chronic N03.9
rapidly progressive N01.9
nephrotic (congenital) (see also Nephrosis) N04.9
with
C3
glomerulonephritis N04.A
glomerulopathy N04.A
with dense deposit disease N04.6
dense deposit disease N04.6
diffuse
crescentic glomerulonephritis N04.7
endocapillary proliferative glomerulonephritis N04.4

Syndrome (continued)
nephrotic (continued)
with (continued)
diffuse (continued)
membranous glomerulonephritis N04.20
mesangial proliferative glomerulonephritis N04.3
mesangiocapillary glomerulonephritis N04.5
focal and segmental glomerular lesions N04.1
minor glomerular abnormality N04.0
specified morphological changes NEC N04.8
specified type NEC with diffuse membranous glomerulonephritis N04.29
diabetic —see Diabetes, nephrosis
neurologic neglect R41.4
Nezelof's D81.4
Nonne-Milroy-Meige Q82.0
Nothnagel's vasomotor acroparesthesia I73.89
obesity hypoventilation (OHS) E66.2
obliterans
bronchiolitis (see also Bronchiolitis, obliterative) J44.81
oculomotor H51.9
Ogilvie K59.81
Oliver-McFarlane Q87.89
ophthalmoplegia-cerebellar ataxia —see Strabismus, paralytic, third nerve
oral allergy T78.1
oral-facial-digital Q87.0
organic
affective F06.30
amnesic (not alcohol- or drug-induced) F04
brain F09
depressive F06.31
hallucinosis F06.0
personality F07.0
Ormond's N13.5
oro-facial-digital Q87.0
os trigonum Q68.8
Osler-Weber-Rendu I78.0
osteoporosis-osteomalacia M83.8
Osterreicher-Turner Q87.2
otolith —see subcategory H81.8
oto-palatal-digital Q87.0
outlet (thoracic) G54.0
ovary
polycystic E28.2
resistant E28.39
sclerocystic E28.2
Owren's D68.2
Paget-Schroetter I82.890
pain —see also Pain
complex regional I G90.50
lower limb G90.52-
specified site NEC G90.59
upper limb G90.51-
complex regional II —see Causalgia
painful
bruising D69.2
feet E53.8
prostate N42.81
paralysis agitans —see Parkinsonism
paralytic G83.9
specified NEC G83.89
Parinaud's H51.0
parkinsonian —see Parkinsonism
Parkinson's —see Parkinsonism

Syndrome *(continued)*
paroxysmal facial pain G50.0
Parry's E05.00
  with thyroid storm E05.01
Parsonage (-Aldren)-Turner G54.5
patella clunk M25.86-
Paterson (-Brown) (-Kelly) D50.1
pectoral girdle I77.89
pectoralis minor I77.89
pediatric autoimmune
   neuropsychiatric disorders
   associated with streptococcal
   infections (PANDAS) D89.89
Pelger-Huet D72.0
pellagra-cerebellar ataxia-renal
   aminoaciduria E72.02
pellagroid E52
Pellegrini-Stieda —see Bursitis,
   tibial collateral
pelvic congestion-fibrosis, female
   N94.89
penta X Q97.1
peptic ulcer —see Ulcer, peptic
perabduction I77.89
periodic fever M04.1
periodic fever, aphthous stomatitis,
   pharyngitis, and adenopathy
   [PFAPA] M04.8
periodic headache, in adults and
   children —see Headache, periodic
   syndromes in adults and children
periurethral fibrosis N13.5
Peutz-Jeghers Q85.89
phantom limb (without pain) G54.7
   with pain G54.6
pharyngeal pouch D82.1
Phelan-McDermid Q93.52
Pick's see Disease, Pick's
Pickwickian E66.2
PIE (pulmonary infiltration
   with eosinophilia) (see also
   Eosinophilia, pulmonary) J82.89
pigmentary pallidal degeneration
   (progressive) G23.0
pineal E34.8
pituitary E22.0
plantar fascia M72.2
placental transfusion —see
   Pregnancy, complicated by,
   placental transfusion syndromes
plateau iris (post-iridectomy)
   (postprocedural) H21.82
Plummer-Vinson D50.1
pluricarential of infancy E40
plurideficiency E40
pluriglandular (compensatory) E31.8
   autoimmune E31.0
pneumatic hammer T75.21
polyangiitis overlap M30.8
polycarential of infancy E40
polyglandular E31.8
   autoimmune E31.0
polysplenia Q89.09
pontine NEC G93.89
popliteal
   artery entrapment I77.89
   web Q87.89
postbacterial fatigue G93.39
postcardiac injury
   postcardiotomy I97.0
   postmyocardial infarction I24.1
postcardiotomy I97.0
post chemoembolization - code to
   associated conditions
postcholecystectomy K91.5
postcommissurotomy I97.0
postconcussional F07.81
postcontusional F07.81
post-COVID (-19) U09.9
postencephalitic F07.89
post endometrial ablation N99.85

Syndrome *(continued)*
posterior
   cervical sympathetic M53.0
   cord G83.83
   fossa compression G93.5
   reversible encephalopathy
      (PRES) I67.83
postgastrectomy (dumping) K91.1
postgastric surgery K91.1
postinfarction I24.1
postinfectious fatigue G93.39
postlaminectomy NEC M96.1
postleukotomy F07.0
postmastectomy lymphedema I97.2
postmyocardial infarction I24.1
postoperative NEC T81.9
   blind loop K90.2
postpartum panhypopituitary
   (Sheehan) E23.0
postpolio (myelitic) G14
postthrombotic I87.009
   with
      inflammation I87.02-
         with ulcer I87.03-
      specified complication NEC
         I87.09-
      ulcer I87.01-
         with inflammation I87.03-
   asymptomatic I87.00-
postural
   orthostatic tachycardia [POTS]
      G90.A
   tachycardia G90.A
postvagotomy K91.1
postvalvulotomy I97.0
postviral NEC G93.31
   fatigue G93.31
Potain's K31.0
potassium intoxication E87.5
Prader-Willi Q87.11
Prader-Willi-like Q87.19
precerebral artery (multiple)
   (bilateral) G45.2
preinfarction I20.0
preleukemic D46.9
premature senility E34.8
premenstrual dysphoric F32.81
premenstrual tension N94.3
Prinzmetal-Massumi R07.1
prune belly Q79.4
pseudocarpal tunnel (sublimis)
   —see Syndrome, carpal tunnel
pseudoparalytica G70.00
   with exacerbation (acute) G70.01
   in crisis G70.01
pseudo -Turner's Q87.19
psycho-organic (nonpsychotic
   severity) F07.9
   acute or subacute F05
   depressive type F06.31
   hallucinatory type F06.0
   nonpsychotic severity F07.0
   specified NEC F07.89
PTEN (hamartoma) tumor Q85.81
pulmonary
   arteriosclerosis I27.0
   dysmaturity (Wilson-Mikity)
      P27.0
   hypoperfusion (idiopathic) P22.0
   renal (hemorrhagic)
      (Goodpasture's) M31.0
pure
   motor lacunar G46.5
   sensory lacunar G46.6
Putnam-Dana D51.0
pyogenic arthritis, pyoderma
   gangrenosum, and acne [PAPA]
   M04.8
pyramidopallidonigral G20.C
pyriformis —see Lesion, nerve,
   sciatic

Syndrome *(continued)*
QT interval prolongation I45.81
radicular NEC —see
   Radiculopathy
   upper limbs, newborn (birth
      injury) P14.3
rapid time-zone change G47.25
Rasmussen G04.81
Raymond (-Céstan) I65.8
Raynaud's I73.00
   with gangrene I73.01
RDS (respiratory distress
   syndrome, newborn) P22.0
reactive airways dysfunction J68.3
Refsum's G60.1
Reifenstein E34.52
renal glomerulohyalinosis-diabetic
   —see Diabetes, nephrosis
Rendu-Osler-Weber I78.0
residual ovary N99.83
resistant ovary E28.39
respiratory
   distress
      acute J80
      adult J80
      child J80
      idiopathic J84.114
      newborn (idiopathic) (type I)
         P22.0
      type II P22.1
restless legs G25.81
restrictive allograft J4A.0
retinoblastoma (familial) C69.2
retroperitoneal fibrosis K68.2
retroviral seroconversion (acute) Z21
Reye's G93.7
Richter —see Leukemia, chronic
   lymphocytic, B-cell type
Ridley's I50.1
right
   heart, hypoplastic Q22.6
   ventricular obstruction —see
      Failure, heart, right
Romano-Ward (prolonged QT
   interval) I45.81
rotator cuff, shoulder (see also
   Tear, rotator cuff) M75.10-
Rotes Quérol —see Hyperostosis,
   ankylosing
Roth —see Meralgia paresthetica
rubella (congenital) P35.0
Ruvalcaba-Myhre-Smith E71.440
Rytand-Lipsitch I44.2
salt
   depletion E87.1
      due to heat NEC T67.8
         causing heat exhaustion or
            prostration T67.4
   low E87.1
salt-losing N28.89
SATB2-associated Q87.89
Scaglietti-Dagnini E22.0
scalenus anticus (anterior) G54.0
scapulocostal —see
   Mononeuropathy, upper limb,
   specified site NEC
scapuloperoneal G71.09
schizophrenic, of childhood NEC
   F20.9
Schnitzler D47.2
Scholte's E34.0
Schroeder's E27.0
Schüller-Christian C96.5
Schwachman (-Diamond) D61.02
Schwartz (-Jampel) G71.13
Schwartz-Bartter E22.2
scimitar Q26.8
sclerocystic ovary E28.2
Seitelberger's G31.89
septicemic adrenal hemorrhage A39.1
seroconversion, retroviral (acute) Z21

Syndrome *(continued)*
serous meningitis G93.2
severe acute respiratory (SARS)
   J12.81
   coronavirus 2019 (see also
      COVID-19) U07.1
   pneumonia J12.82
shaken infant T74.4
shock (traumatic) T79.4
   kidney N17.0
      following crush injury T79.5
   toxic A48.3
shock-lung J80
Shone's — code to specific
   anomalies
short
   bowel K90.829
      with
         colon in continuity K90.821
         ileocolonic anastomosis
            K90.821
         without colon in continuity
            K90.822
   gut —see Syndrome, short,
      bowel
   rib Q77.2
shoulder-hand —see
   Algoneurodystrophy
Shwachman (-Diamond) D61.02
sicca —see Syndrome, Sjögren
sick
   cell E87.1
   sinus I49.5
sick-euthyroid E07.81
sideropenic D50.1
Siemens' ectodermal dysplasia Q82.4
Silfverskiöld's Q78.9
Simons' E88.1
sinus tarsi M25.57-
sinusitis-bronchiectasis-situs
   inversus Q89.3
Sipple's E31.22
sirenomelia Q87.2
Sjögren M35.00
   with
      central nervous system
         involvement M35.07
      dental involvement M35.0C
      gastrointestinal involvement
         M35.08
      glomerular disease M35.0A
      inflammatory arthritis M35.05
      keratoconjunctivitis M35.01
      lung involvement M35.02
      myopathy M35.03
      peripheral nervous system
         involvement M35.06
      renal tubular acidosis M35.04
      specified organ involvement,
         NEC M35.09
      tubulo-interstitial nephropathy
         M35.04
      vasculitis M35.0B
Slocumb's E27.0
slow flow, coronary I20.89
Sluder's G44.89
Smith-Magenis Q93.88
Sneddon-Wilkinson L13.1
Snyder-Robinson Q87.89
Sotos' Q87.3
South African cardiomyopathy
   I42.8
spasmodic
   upward movement, eyes H51.8
   winking F95.8
Spen's I45.9
splenic
   agenesis Q89.01
   flexure K59.89
   neutropenia D73.81
Spurway's Q78.0

317

Syndrome (continued)
staphylococcal scalded skin L00
steal
arteriovenous T82.898-
ischemic T82.898-
subclavian G45.8
Stein-Leventhal E28.2
Stein's E28.2
Stevens-Johnson syndrome L51.1
toxic epidermal necrolysis overlap L51.3
Stewart-Morel M85.2
Stickler Q89.8
stiff baby Q89.8
stiff man G25.82
Still-Felty —*see* Felty's syndrome
Stokes (-Adams) I45.9
stone heart I50.1
straight back, congenital Q76.49
Sturge-Weber (-Dimitri) Q85.89
subclavian steal G45.8
subcoracoid-pectoralis minor G54.0
subcostal nerve compression I77.89
subphrenic interposition Q43.3
superior
cerebellar artery I63.89
mesenteric artery K55.1
semi-circular canal dehiscence H83.8X-
vena cava I87.1
supine hypotensive (maternal) —*see* Syndrome, hypotension, maternal
suprarenal cortical E27.0
supraspinatus (*see also* Tear, rotator cuff) M75.10-
Susac G93.49
swallowed blood P78.2
sweat retention L74.0
Swyer Q99.1
Symond's G93.2
sympathetic
cervical paralysis G90.2
pelvic, female N94.89
systemic inflammatory response (SIRS), of non-infective origin (without organ dysfunction) R65.10
with acute organ dysfunction R65.11
tachycardia-bradycardia I49.5
takotsubo I51.81
TAR (thrombocytopenia with absent radius) Q87.2
tarsal tunnel G57.5-
teething K00.7
tegmental G93.89
telangiectasic-pigmentation-cataract Q82.8
temporal pyramidal apex —*see* Otitis, media, suppurative, acute
temporomandibular joint-pain-dysfunction M26.62-
Terry's (*see also* Myopia, degenerative) H44.2-
testicular feminization (*see also* Syndrome, androgen insensitivity) E34.51
thalamic pain (hyperesthetic) G89.0
thoracic outlet (compression) G54.0
Thorson-Björck E34.0
thrombocytopenia with absent radius (TAR) Q87.2
thrombosis with thrombocytopenia D75.84
thyroid-adrenocortical insufficiency E31.0
tibial
anterior M76.81-
posterior M76.82-

Syndrome (continued)
Tietze's M94.0
time-zone (rapid) G47.25
Toni-Fanconi E72.09
with cystinosis E72.04
Touraine's Q79.8
tourniquet —*see* Constriction, external, by site
toxic shock A48.3
transient left ventricular apical ballooning I51.81
traumatic vasospastic T75.22
Treacher Collins Q75.4
triple X, female Q97.0
trisomy Q92.9
13 Q91.7
meiotic nondisjunction Q91.4
mitotic nondisjunction Q91.5
mosaicism Q91.5
translocation Q91.6
18 Q91.3
meiotic nondisjunction Q91.0
mitotic nondisjunction Q91.1
mosaicism Q91.1
translocation Q91.2
20 (q)(p) Q92.8
21 Q90.9
meiotic nondisjunction Q90.0
mitotic nondisjunction Q90.1
mosaicism Q90.1
translocation Q90.2
22 Q92.8
tropical wet feet T69.0-
Trousseau's I82.1
tumor lysis (following antineoplastic chemotherapy) (spontaneous) NEC E88.3
tumor necrosis factor receptor associated periodic (TRAPS) M04.1
Twiddler's (due to)
automatic implantable defibrillator T82.198
cardiac pacemaker T82.198
Unverricht (-Lundborg) —*see* Epilepsy, generalized, idiopathic
upward gaze H51.8
uremia, chronic (*see also* Disease, kidney, chronic) N18.9
urethral N34.3
urethro-oculo-articular —*see* Reiter's disease
urohepatic K76.7
vago-hypoglossal G52.7
vascular NEC in cerebrovascular disease G46.8
vasoconstriction, reversible cerebrovascular I67.841
vasomotor I73.9
vasospastic (traumatic) T75.22
vasovagal R55
van Buchem's M85.2
van der Hoeve's Q78.0
VATER Q87.2
velo-cardio-facial Q93.81
vena cava (inferior) (superior) (obstruction) I87.1
vertebral
artery G45.0
compression —*see* Syndrome, anterior, spinal artery, compression
steal G45.0
vertebro-basilar artery G45.0
vertebrogenic (pain) (*see also,* Pain, vertebrogenic) M54.89
vertiginous —*see* Disorder, vestibular function
Vinson-Plummer D50.1
virus B34.9
visceral larva migrans B83.0

Syndrome (continued)
visual disorientation H53.8
vitamin B6 deficiency E53.1
vitreal corneal H59.01-
vitreous (touch) H59.01-
Vogt-Koyanagi H20.82-
Volkmann's T79.6
von Hippel-Lindau Q85.83
von Schroetter's I82.890
von Willebrand (-Jürgen) —*see* Disease, von Willebrand
acquired (*see also* Disease, von Willebrand) D68.04
Waldenström-Kjellberg D50.1
Wallenberg's G46.3
wasting (syndrome) due to underlying condition E88.A
water retention E87.79
Waterhouse (-Friderichsen) A39.1
Weber-Gubler G46.3
Weber-Leyden G46.3
Weber's G46.3
Wegener's M31.30
with
kidney involvement M31.31
lung involvement M31.30
with kidney involvement M31.31
Weingarten's (tropical eosinophilia) J82.89
Weiss-Baker G90.09
Werdnig-Hoffman G12.0
Wermer's E31.21
Werner's E34.8
Wernicke-Korsakoff (nonalcoholic) F04
alcoholic F10.26
West's —*see* Epilepsy, spasms
Westphal-Strümpell E83.01
wet
feet (maceration) (tropical) T69.0-
lung, newborn P22.1
whiplash S13.4
whistling face Q87.0
Wilkie's K55.1
Wilkinson-Sneddon L13.1
Willebrand (-Jürgens) —*see* Disease, von Willebrand
Williams Q93.82
Wilson's (hepatolenticular degeneration) E83.01
Wiskott-Aldrich D82.0
withdrawal —*see* Withdrawal, state drug
infant of dependent mother P96.1
therapeutic use, newborn P96.2
Woakes' (ethmoiditis) J33.1
Wright's (hyperabduction) G54.0
X I20.9
XXXX Q97.1
XXXXX Q97.1
XXXXY Q98.1
XXY Q98.0
Yao M04.8
yellow nail L60.5
Zahorsky's B08.5
Zellweger syndrome E71.510
Zellweger-like syndrome E71.541

Synechia (anterior) (iris) (posterior) (pupil) —*see also* Adhesions, iris
intra-uterine (traumatic) N85.6

Synesthesia R20.8

Syngamiasis, syngamosis B83.3

Synodontia K00.2

Synorchidism, synorchism Q55.1

Synostosis (congenital) Q78.8
astragalo-scaphoid Q74.2
radioulnar Q74.0

Synovial sarcoma —*see* Neoplasm, connective tissue, malignant

Synovioma (malignant) —*see also* Neoplasm, connective tissue, malignant
benign —*see* Neoplasm, connective tissue, benign

Synoviosarcoma —*see* Neoplasm, connective tissue, malignant

Synovitis (*see also* Tenosynovitis) M65.9
crepitant
hand M70.0-
wrist M70.03-
gonococcal A54.49
gouty —*see* Gout,
in (due to)
crystals M65.8-
gonorrhea A54.49
syphilis (late) A52.78
use, overuse, pressure —*see* Disorder, soft tissue, due to use
infective NEC —*see* Tenosynovitis, infective NEC
specified NEC —*see* Tenosynovitis, specified type NEC
syphilitic A52.78
congenital (early) A50.02
toxic —*see* Synovitis, transient
transient M67.3-
ankle M67.37-
elbow M67.32-
foot joint M67.37-
hand joint M67.34-
hip M67.35-
knee M67.36-
multiple site M67.39
pelvic region M67.35-
shoulder M67.31-
specified joint NEC M67.38
wrist M67.33-
traumatic, current —*see* Sprain
tuberculous —*see* Tuberculosis, synovitis
villonodular (pigmented) M12.2-
ankle M12.27-
elbow M12.22-
foot joint M12.27-
hand joint M12.24-
hip M12.25-
knee M12.26-
multiple site M12.29
pelvic region M12.25-
shoulder M12.21-
specified joint NEC M12.28
vertebrae M12.28
wrist M12.23-

Syphilid A51.39
congenital A50.06
newborn A50.06
tubercular (late) A52.79

Syphilis, syphilitic (acquired) A53.9
abdomen (late) A52.79
acoustic nerve A52.15
adenopathy (secondary) A51.49
adrenal (gland) (with cortical hypofunction) A52.79
age under 2 years NOS —*see also* Syphilis, congenital, early acquired A51.9
alopecia (secondary) A51.32
anemia (late) A52.79 *[D63.8]*
aneurysm (aorta) (ruptured) A52.01
central nervous system A52.05
congenital A50.54 *[I79.0]*
anus (late) A52.74
primary A51.1
secondary A51.39

Syphilis, syphilitic *(continued)*
  aorta (arch) (abdominal) (thoracic) A52.02
    aneurysm A52.01
  aortic (insufficiency) (regurgitation) (stenosis) A52.03
    aneurysm A52.01
  arachnoid (adhesive) (cerebral) (spinal) A52.13
  asymptomatic —see Syphilis, latent
  ataxia (locomotor) A52.11
  atrophoderma maculatum A51.39
  auricular fibrillation A52.06
  bladder (late) A52.76
  bone A52.77
    secondary A51.46
  brain A52.17
  breast (late) A52.79
  bronchus (late) A52.72
  bubo (primary) A51.0
  bulbar palsy A52.19
  bursa (late) A52.78
  cardiac decompensation A52.06
  cardiovascular A52.00
  central nervous system (late) (recurrent) (relapse) (tertiary) A52.3
    with
      ataxia A52.11
      general paralysis A52.17
        juvenile A50.45
      paresis (general) A52.17
        juvenile A50.45
      tabes (dorsalis) A52.11
        juvenile A50.45
      taboparesis A52.17
        juvenile A50.45
    aneurysm A52.05
    congenital A50.40
    juvenile A50.40
    remission in (sustained) A52.3
    serology doubtful, negative, or positive A52.3
    specified nature or site NEC A52.19
    vascular A52.05
  cerebral A52.17
    meningovascular A52.13
    nerves (multiple palsies) A52.15
    sclerosis A52.17
    thrombosis A52.05
  cerebrospinal (tabetic type) A52.12
  cerebrovascular A52.05
  cervix (late) A52.76
  chancre (multiple) A51.0
    extragenital A51.2
    Rollet's A51.0
  Charcot's joint A52.16
  chorioretinitis A51.43
    congenital A50.01
    late A52.71
    prenatal A50.01
  choroiditis —see Syphilitic chorioretinitis
  choroidoretinitis —see Syphilitic chorioretinitis
  ciliary body (secondary) A51.43
    late A52.71
  colon (late) A52.74
  combined spinal sclerosis A52.11
  condyloma (latum) A51.31
  congenital A50.9
    with
      paresis (general) A50.45
      tabes (dorsalis) A50.45
      taboparesis A50.45
    chorioretinitis, choroiditis A50.01 *[H32]*

Syphilis, syphilitic *(continued)*
  congenital *(continued)*
    early, or less than 2 years after birth NEC A50.2
      with manifestations —see Syphilis, congenital, early, symptomatic
      latent (without manifestations) A50.1
        negative spinal fluid test A50.1
        serology positive A50.1
      symptomatic A50.09
        cutaneous A50.06
        mucocutaneous A50.07
        oculopathy A50.01
        osteochondropathy A50.02
        pharyngitis A50.03
        pneumonia A50.04
        rhinitis A50.05
        visceral A50.08
    interstitial keratitis A50.31
    juvenile neurosyphilis A50.45
    late, or 2 years or more after birth NEC A50.7
      chorioretinitis, choroiditis A50.32
      interstitial keratitis A50.31
      juvenile neurosyphilis A50.45
      latent (without manifestations) A50.6
        negative spinal fluid test A50.6
        serology positive A50.6
      symptomatic or with manifestations NEC A50.59
        arthropathy A50.55
        cardiovascular A50.54
        Clutton's joints A50.51
        Hutchinson's teeth A50.52
        Hutchinson's triad A50.53
        osteochondropathy A50.56
        saddle nose A50.57
  conjugal A53.9
    tabes A52.11
  conjunctiva (late) A52.71
  contact Z20.2
  cord bladder A52.19
  cornea, late A52.71
  coronary (artery) (sclerosis) A52.06
  coryza, congenital A50.05
  cranial nerve A52.15
    multiple palsies A52.15
  cutaneous —see Syphilis, skin
  dacryocystitis (late) A52.71
  degeneration, spinal cord A52.12
  dementia paralytica A52.17
    juvenilis A50.45
  destruction of bone A52.77
  dilatation, aorta A52.01
  due to blood transfusion A53.9
  dura mater A52.13
  ear A52.79
    inner A52.79
    nerve (eighth) A52.15
    neurorecurrence A52.15
  early A51.9
    cardiovascular A52.00
    central nervous system A52.3
    latent (without manifestations) (less than 2 years after infection) A51.5
      negative spinal fluid test A51.5
      serological relapse after treatment A51.5
      serology positive A51.5
    relapse (treated, untreated) A51.9
    skin A51.39
    symptomatic A51.9
      extragenital chancre A51.2

Syphilis, syphilitic *(continued)*
  early *(continued)*
    symptomatic *(continued)*
      primary, except extragenital chancre A51.0
      secondary (see also Syphilis, secondary) A51.39
        relapse (treated, untreated) A51.49
      ulcer A51.39
  eighth nerve (neuritis) A52.15
  endemic A65
  endocarditis A52.03
    aortic A52.03
    pulmonary A52.03
  epididymis (late) A52.76
  epiglottis (late) A52.73
  epiphysitis (congenital) (early) A50.02
  episcleritis (late) A52.71
  esophagus A52.79
  eustachian tube A52.73
  exposure to Z20.2
  eye A52.71
  eyelid (late) (with gumma) A52.71
  fallopian tube (late) A52.76
  fracture A52.77
  gallbladder (late) A52.74
  gastric (polyposis) (late) A52.74
  general A53.9
    paralysis A52.17
      juvenile A50.45
  genital (primary) A51.0
  glaucoma A52.71
  gumma NEC A52.79
    cardiovascular system A52.00
    central nervous system A52.3
    congenital A50.59
  heart (block) (decompensation) (disease) (failure) A52.06 *[I52]*
    valve NEC A52.03
  hemianesthesia A52.19
  hemianopsia A52.71
  hemiparesis A52.17
  hemiplegia A52.17
  hepatic artery A52.09
  hepatis A52.74
  hepatomegaly, congenital A50.08
  hereditaria tarda —see Syphilis, congenital, late
  hereditary —see Syphilis, congenital
  Hutchinson's teeth A50.52
  hyalitis A52.71
  inactive —see Syphilis, latent
  infantum —see Syphilis, congenital
  inherited —see Syphilis, congenital
  internal ear A52.79
  intestine (late) A52.74
  iris, iritis (secondary) A51.43
    late A52.71
  joint (late) A52.77
  keratitis (congenital) (interstitial) (late) A50.31
  kidney (late) A52.75
  lacrimal passages (late) A52.71
  larynx (late) A52.73
  late A52.9
    cardiovascular A52.00
    central nervous system A52.3
    kidney A52.75
    latent or 2 years or more after infection (without manifestations) A52.8
      negative spinal fluid test A52.8
      serology positive A52.8
    paresis A52.17
    specified site NEC A52.79
    symptomatic or with manifestations A52.79
    tabes A52.11

Syphilis, syphilitic *(continued)*
  latent A53.0
    with signs or symptoms - code by site and stage under Syphilis
    central nervous system A52.2
    date of infection unspecified A53.0
    early, or less than 2 years after infection A51.5
    follow-up of latent syphilis A53.0
      date of infection unspecified A53.0
      late, or 2 years or more after infection A52.8
    late, or 2 years or more after infection A52.8
    positive serology (only finding) A53.0
      date of infection unspecified A53.0
      early, or less than 2 years after infection A51.5
      late, or 2 years or more after infection A52.8
  lens (late) A52.71
  leukoderma A51.39
    late A52.79
  lienitis A52.79
  lip A51.39
    chancre (primary) A51.2
    late A52.79
  Lissauer's paralysis A52.17
  liver A52.74
  locomotor ataxia A52.11
  lung A52.72
  lymph gland (early) (secondary) A51.49
    late A52.79
  lymphadenitis (secondary) A51.49
  macular atrophy of skin A51.39
    striated A52.79
  mediastinum (late) A52.73
  meninges (adhesive) (brain) (spinal cord) A52.13
  meningitis A52.13
    acute (secondary) A51.41
    congenital A50.41
  meningoencephalitis A52.14
  meningovascular A52.13
    congenital A50.41
  mesarteritis A52.09
    brain A52.04
  middle ear A52.77
  mitral stenosis A52.03
  monoplegia A52.17
  mouth (secondary) A51.39
    late A52.79
  mucocutaneous (secondary) A51.39
    late A52.79
  mucous
    membrane (secondary) A51.39
      late A52.79
    patches A51.39
      congenital A50.07
  mulberry molars A50.52
  muscle A52.78
  myocardium A52.06
  nasal sinus (late) A52.73
  neonatorum —see Syphilis, congenital
  nephrotic syndrome (secondary) A51.44
  nerve palsy (any cranial nerve) A52.15
    multiple A52.15
  nervous system, central A52.3
  neuritis A52.15
    acoustic A52.15
  neurorecidive of retina A52.19

Syphilis, syphilitic (continued)
  neuroretinitis A52.19
  newborn —see Syphilis, congenital
  nodular superficial (late) A52.79
  nonvenereal A65
  nose (late) A52.73
    saddle back deformity A50.57
  occlusive arterial disease A52.09
  oculopathy A52.71
  ophthalmic (late) A52.71
  optic nerve (atrophy) (neuritis) (papilla) A52.15
  orbit (late) A52.71
  organic A53.9
  osseous (late) A52.77
  osteochondritis (congenital) (early) A50.02 [M90.80]
  osteoporosis A52.77
  ovary (late) A52.76
  oviduct (late) A52.76
  palate (late) A52.79
  pancreas (late) A52.74
  paralysis A52.17
    general A52.17
      juvenile A50.45
  paresis (general) A52.17
    juvenile A50.45
  paresthesia A52.19
  Parkinson's disease or syndrome A52.19
  paroxysmal tachycardia A52.06
  pemphigus (congenital) A50.06
  penis (chancre) A51.0
    late A52.76
  pericardium A52.06
  perichondritis, larynx (late) A52.73
  periosteum (late) A52.77
    congenital (early) A50.02 [M90.80]
    early (secondary) A51.46
  peripheral nerve A52.79
  petrous bone (late) A52.77
  pharynx (late) A52.73
    secondary A51.39
  pituitary (gland) A52.79
  pleura (late) A52.73
  pneumonia, white A50.04
  pontine lesion A52.17
  portal vein A52.09
  primary A51.0
    anal A51.1
    and secondary —see Syphilis, secondary
    central nervous system A52.3
    extragenital chancre NEC A51.2
    fingers A51.2
    genital A51.0
    lip A51.2
    specified site NEC A51.2
    tonsils A51.2
  prostate (late) A52.76
  ptosis (eyelid) A52.71
  pulmonary (late) A52.72
    artery A52.09
  pyelonephritis (late) A52.75
  recently acquired, symptomatic A51.9
  rectum (late) A52.74
  respiratory tract (late) A52.73
  retina, late A52.71
  retrobulbar neuritis A52.15
  salpingitis A52.76
  sclera (late) A52.71
  sclerosis
    cerebral A52.17
    coronary A52.06
    multiple A52.11
  scotoma (central) A52.71
  scrotum (late) A52.76
  secondary (and primary) A51.49
    adenopathy A51.49
    anus A51.39

Syphilis, syphilitic (continued)
  secondary (continued)
    bone A51.46
    chorioretinitis, choroiditis A51.43
    hepatitis A51.45
    liver A51.45
    lymphadenitis A51.49
    meningitis (acute) A51.41
    mouth A51.39
    mucous membranes A51.39
    periosteum, periostitis A51.46
    pharynx A51.39
    relapse (treated, untreated) A51.49
    skin A51.39
    specified form NEC A51.49
    tonsil A51.39
    ulcer A51.39
    viscera NEC A51.49
    vulva A51.39
  seminal vesicle (late) A52.76
  seronegative with signs or symptoms - code by site and stage under Syphilis
  seropositive
    with signs or symptoms - code by site and stage under Syphilis
    follow-up of latent syphilis —see Syphilis, latent
    only finding —see Syphilis, latent
  seventh nerve (paralysis) A52.15
  sinus, sinusitis (late) A52.73
  skeletal system A52.77
  skin (with ulceration) (early) (secondary) A51.39
    late or tertiary A52.79
  small intestine A52.74
  spastic spinal paralysis A52.17
  spermatic cord (late) A52.76
  spinal (cord) A52.12
  spleen A52.79
  splenomegaly A52.79
  spondylitis A52.77
  staphyloma A52.71
  stigmata (congenital) A50.59
  stomach A52.74
  synovium A52.78
  tabes dorsalis (late) A52.11
    juvenile A50.45
  tabetic type A52.11
    juvenile A50.45
  taboparesis A52.17
    juvenile A50.45
  tachycardia A52.06
  tendon (late) A52.78
  tertiary A52.9
    with symptoms NEC A52.79
    cardiovascular A52.00
    central nervous system A52.3
    multiple NEC A52.79
    specified site NEC A52.79
  testis A52.76
  thorax A52.73
  throat A52.73
  thymus (gland) (late) A52.79
  thyroid (late) A52.79
  tongue (late) A52.79
  tonsil (lingual) (late) A52.73
    primary A51.2
    secondary A51.39
  trachea (late) A52.73
  tunica vaginalis (late) A52.76
  ulcer (any site) (early) (secondary) A51.39
    late A52.79
    perforating A52.79
      foot A52.11
  urethra (late) A52.76

Syphilis, syphilitic (continued)
  urogenital (late) A52.76
  uterus (late) A52.76
  uveal tract (secondary) A51.43
    late A52.71
  uveitis (secondary) A51.43
    late A52.71
  uvula (late) (perforated) A52.79
  vagina A51.0
    late A52.76
  valvulitis NEC A52.03
  vascular A52.00
    brain (cerebral) A52.05
  ventriculi A52.74
  vesicae urinariae (late) A52.76
  viscera (abdominal) (late) A52.74
    secondary A51.49
  vitreous (opacities) (late) A52.71
    hemorrhage A52.71
  vulva A51.0
    late A52.76
    secondary A51.39
Syphiloma A52.79
  cardiovascular system A52.00
  central nervous system A52.3
  circulatory system A52.00
  congenital A50.59
Syphilophobia F45.29
Syringadenoma —see also Neoplasm, skin, benign
  papillary —see Neoplasm, skin, benign
Syringobulbia G95.0
Syringocystadenoma —see Neoplasm, skin, benign
  papillary —see Neoplasm, skin, benign
Syringoma —see also Neoplasm, skin, benign
  chondroid —see Neoplasm, skin, benign
Syringomyelia G95.0
Syringomyelitis —see Encephalitis
Syringomyelocele —see Spina bifida
Syringopontia G95.0
System, systemic —see also condition
  disease, combined —see Degeneration, combined
  inflammatory response syndrome (SIRS) of non-infectious origin (without organ dysfunction) R65.10
    with acute organ dysfunction R65.11
  lupus erythematosus M32.9
    inhibitor present D68.62
Systemic exertion intolerance disease [SEID] G93.32

T

Tabacism, tabacosis, tabagism —see also Poisoning, tobacco
  meaning dependence (without remission) F17.200
    with
      disorder F17.299
        in remission F17.211
        specified disorder NEC F17.298
        withdrawal F17.203
Tabardillo A75.9
  flea-borne A75.2
  louse-borne A75.0

Tabes, tabetic A52.10
  with
    central nervous system syphilis A52.10
    Charcot's joint A52.16
    cord bladder A52.19
    crisis, viscera (any) A52.19
    paralysis, general A52.17
    paresis (general) A52.17
    perforating ulcer (foot) A52.19
  arthropathy (Charcot) A52.16
  bladder A52.19
  bone A52.11
  cerebrospinal A52.12
  congenital A50.45
  conjugal A52.10
  dorsalis A52.11
    juvenile A50.49
  juvenile A50.49
  latent A52.19
  mesenterica A18.39
  paralysis, insane, general A52.17
  spasmodic A52.17
  syphilis (cerebrospinal) A52.12
Taboparalysis A52.17
Taboparesis (remission) A52.17
  juvenile A50.45
TAC (trigeminal autonomic cephalgia) NEC G44.099
  intractable G44.091
  not intractable G44.099
Tache noir S60.22-
Tachyalimentation K91.2
Tachyarrhythmia, tachyrhythmia —see Tachycardia
Tachycardia R00.0
  atrial (paroxysmal) I47.19
  auricular I47.19
  AV nodal re-entry (re-entrant) I47.19
  junctional (paroxysmal) I47.19
  newborn P29.11
  nodal (paroxysmal) I47.19
  non-paroxysmal AV nodal I45.89
  paroxysmal (sustained) (nonsustained) I47.9
    with sinus bradycardia I49.5
    atrial (PAT) I47.19
    atrioventricular (AV) (re-entrant) I47.19
      psychogenic F54
    junctional I47.19
      ectopic I47.19
    nodal I47.19
    psychogenic (atrial) (supraventricular) (ventricular) F54
    supraventricular (sustained) I47.10
      psychogenic F54
    ventricular I47.20
      psychogenic F54
      specified type NEC I47.29
  psychogenic F45.8
  sick sinus I49.5
  sinoauricular NOS R00.0
    paroxysmal I47.19
  sinus [sinusal] NOS R00.0
    inappropriate, so stated (IST) I47.11
    paroxysmal I47.19
  supraventricular I47.10
  ventricular (paroxysmal) (sustained) I47.20
    psychogenic F54
    specified type NEC I47.29
Tachygastria K31.89

Tachypnea R06.82
 hysterical F45.8
 newborn (idiopathic) (transitory) P22.1
 psychogenic F45.8
 transitory, of newborn P22.1
TAD (transfusion-associated dyspnea) J95.87
Taenia (infection) (infestation) B68.9
 diminuta B71.0
 echinococcal infestation B67.90
 mediocanellata B68.1
 nana B71.0
 saginata B68.1
 solium (intestinal form) B68.0
  larval form —*see* Cysticercosis
Taeniasis (intestine) —*see* Taenia
TACO (transfusion associated circulatory overload) E87.71
Tag (hypertrophied skin) (infected) L91.8
 adenoid J35.8
 anus K64.4
 hemorrhoidal K64.4
 hymen N89.8
 perineal N90.89
 preauricular Q17.0
 sentinel K64.4
 skin L91.8
  accessory (congenital) Q82.8
  anus K64.4
  congenital Q82.8
  preauricular Q17.0
 tonsil J35.8
 urethra, urethral N36.8
 vulva N90.89
Tahyna fever B33.8
Takahara's disease E80.3
Takayasu's disease or syndrome M31.4
Talaromycosis B48.4
Talcosis (pulmonary) J62.0
Talipes (congenital) Q66.89
 acquired, planus —*see* Deformity, limb, flat foot
 asymmetric Q66.89
 calcaneovalgus Q66.4-
 calcaneovarus Q66.1-
 calcaneus Q66.89
 cavus Q66.7-
 equinovalgus Q66.6
 equinovarus Q66.0-
 equinus Q66.89
 percavus Q66.7-
 planovalgus Q66.6
 planus (acquired) (any degree) —*see also* Deformity, limb, flat foot
  congenital Q66.5-
  due to rickets (sequelae) E64.3
 valgus Q66.6
 varus Q66.3-
Tall stature, constitutional E34.4
Talma's disease M62.89
Talon noir S90.3-
 hand S60.22-
 heel S90.3-
 toe S90.1-
Tamponade, heart I31.4
Tanapox (virus disease) B08.71
Tangier disease E78.6
Tantrum, child problem F91.8
Tapeworm (infection) (infestation) —*see* Infestation, tapeworm
Tapia's syndrome G52.7

TAR (thrombocytopenia with absent radius) **syndrome** Q87.2
Tarral-Besnier disease L44.0
Tarsal tunnel syndrome —*see* Syndrome, tarsal tunnel
Tarsalgia —*see* Pain, limb, lower
Tarsitis (eyelid) H01.8
 syphilitic A52.71
 tuberculous A18.4
Tartar (teeth) (dental calculus) K03.6
Tattoo (mark) L81.8
Tauri's disease E74.09
Taurodontism K00.2
Taussig-Bing syndrome Q20.1
Taybi's syndrome Q87.2
Tay-Sachs amaurotic familial idiocy or disease E75.02
TBI (traumatic brain injury) S06.9
Teacher's node or nodule J38.2
Tear, torn (traumatic) —*see also* Laceration
 with abortion —*see* Abortion
 annular fibrosis M51.35
 anus, anal (sphincter) S31.831
  complicating delivery
   with third degree perineal laceration (*see also* Delivery, complicated, by, laceration, perineum, third degree) O70.20
    with mucosa O70.3
   without third degree perineal laceration O70.4
  nontraumatic (healed) (old) K62.81
 articular cartilage, old —*see* Derangement, joint, articular cartilage, by site
 bladder
  with ectopic or molar pregnancy O08.6
  following ectopic or molar pregnancy O08.6
  obstetrical O71.5
  traumatic —*see* Injury, bladder
 bowel
  with ectopic or molar pregnancy O08.6
  following ectopic or molar pregnancy O08.6
  obstetrical trauma O71.5
 broad ligament
  with ectopic or molar pregnancy O08.6
 broad ligament
  following ectopic or molar pregnancy O08.6
  obstetrical trauma O71.6
 bucket handle (knee) (meniscus) —*see* Tear, meniscus
 capsule, joint —*see* Sprain
 cartilage —*see also* Sprain
  articular, old —*see* Derangement, joint, articular cartilage, by site
 cervix
  with ectopic or molar pregnancy O08.6
  following ectopic or molar pregnancy O08.6
  obstetrical trauma (current) O71.3
  old N88.1
  traumatic —*see* Injury, uterus
 dural G97.41
  nontraumatic G96.11

Tear, torn (*continued*)
 internal organ —*see* Injury, by site
 knee cartilage
  articular (current) S83.3-
  old —*see* Derangement, knee, meniscus, due to old tear
 ligament —*see* Sprain
 meniscus (knee) (current injury) S83.209
  bucket-handle S83.20-
  lateral
   bucket-handle S83.25-
   complex S83.27-
   peripheral S83.26-
   specified type NEC S83.28-
  medial
   bucket-handle S83.21-
   complex S83.23-
   peripheral S83.22-
   specified type NEC S83.24-
  old —*see* Derangement, knee, meniscus, due to old tear
  site other than knee - code as Sprain
  specified type NEC S83.20-
 muscle —*see* Strain
 pelvic
  floor, complicating delivery O70.1
  organ NEC, obstetrical trauma O71.5
   with ectopic or molar pregnancy O08.6
   following ectopic or molar pregnancy O08.6
 perineal, secondary O90.1
 periurethral tissue, obstetrical trauma O71.82
  with ectopic or molar pregnancy O08.6
  following ectopic or molar pregnancy O08.6
 rectovaginal septum —*see* Laceration, vagina
 retina, retinal (without detachment) (horseshoe) —*see also* Break, retina, horseshoe
  with detachment —*see* Detachment, retina, with retinal, break
 rotator cuff (nontraumatic) M75.10-
  complete M75.12-
  incomplete M75.11-
  traumatic S46.01-
   capsule S43.42-
 semilunar cartilage, knee —*see* Tear, meniscus
 supraspinatus (complete) (incomplete) (nontraumatic) (*see also* Tear, rotator cuff) M75.10-
 tendon —*see* Strain
 tentorial, at birth P10.4
 umbilical cord
  complicating delivery O69.89
 urethra
  with ectopic or molar pregnancy O08.6
  following ectopic or molar pregnancy O08.6
  obstetrical trauma O71.5
 uterus —*see* Injury, uterus
 vagina —*see* Laceration, vagina
 vessel, from catheter —*see* Puncture, accidental complicating surgery
 vulva, complicating delivery O70.0
Tear-stone —*see* Dacryolith

Teeth —*see also* condition
 grinding
  psychogenic F45.8
  sleep related G47.63
Teething (syndrome) K00.7
Telangiectasia, telangiectasis (verrucous) I78.1
 ataxic (cerebellar) (Louis-Bar) G11.3
 familial I78.0
 hemorrhagic, hereditary (congenital) (senile) I78.0
 hereditary, hemorrhagic (congenital) (senile) I78.0
 juxtafoveal H35.07-
 macular H35.07-
 macularis eruptiva perstans D47.01
 parafoveal H35.07-
 retinal (idiopathic) (juxtafoveal) (macular) (parafoveal) H35.07-
 spider I78.1
Telephone scatologia F65.89
Telescoped bowel or intestine K56.1
 congenital Q43.8
Temperature
 body, high (of unknown origin) R50.9
 cold, trauma from T69.9
  newborn P80.0
  specified effect NEC T69.8
Temple —*see* condition
Temporal —*see* condition
Temporomandibular joint pain-dysfunction syndrome M26.62-
Temporosphenoidal —*see* condition
Tendency
 bleeding —*see* Defect, coagulation
 suicide
  meaning personal history of attempted suicide Z91.51
  meaning suicidal ideation —*see* Ideation, suicidal
 to fall R29.6
Tenderness, abdominal R10.819
 epigastric R10.816
 generalized R10.817
 left lower quadrant R10.814
 left upper quadrant R10.812
 periumbilic R10.815
 right lower quadrant R10.813
 right upper quadrant R10.811
 rebound R10.829
  epigastric R10.826
  generalized R10.827
  left lower quadrant R10.824
  left upper quadrant R10.822
  periumbilic R10.825
  right lower quadrant R10.823
  right upper quadrant R10.821
Tendinitis, tendonitis —*see also* Enthesopathy
 Achilles M76.6-
 adhesive —*see* Tenosynovitis, specified type NEC
  shoulder —*see* Capsulitis, adhesive
 bicipital M75.2-
 calcific M65.2-
  ankle M65.27-
  foot M65.27-
  forearm M65.23-
  hand M65.24-
  lower leg M65.26-
  multiple sites M65.29
  pelvic region M65.25-
  shoulder M75.3-

Tendinitis, tendonitis *(continued)*
  calcific *(continued)*
    specified site NEC M65.28
      thigh M65.25-
      upper arm M65.22-
  due to use, overuse, pressure —*see also* Disorder, soft tissue, due to use
    specified NEC —*see* Disorder, soft tissue, due to use, specified NEC
  gluteal M76.0-
  patellar M76.5-
  peroneal M76.7-
  psoas M76.1-
  tibial (posterior) M76.82-
    anterior M76.81-
  trochanteric —*see* Bursitis, hip, trochanteric

Tendon —*see* condition

Tendosynovitis —*see* Tenosynovitis

Tenesmus (rectal) R19.8
  vesical R30.1

Tennis elbow —*see* Epicondylitis, lateral

Tenonitis —*see also* Tenosynovitis
  eye (capsule) H05.04-

Tenontosynovitis —*see* Tenosynovitis

Tenontothecitis —*see* Tenosynovitis

Tenophyte —*see* Disorder, synovium, specified type NEC

Tenosynovitis (*see also* Synovitis) M65.9
  adhesive —*see* Tenosynovitis, specified type NEC
    shoulder —*see* Capsulitis, adhesive
  bicipital (calcifying) —*see* Tendinitis, bicipital
  gonococcal A54.49
  in (due to)
    crystals M65.8-
    gonorrhea A54.49
    syphilis (late) A52.78
    use, overuse, pressure —*see also* Disorder, soft tissue, due to use
      specified NEC —*see* Disorder, soft tissue, due to use, specified NEC
  infective NEC M65.1-
    ankle M65.17-
    foot M65.17-
    forearm M65.13-
    hand M65.14-
    lower leg M65.16-
    multiple sites M65.19
    pelvic region M65.15-
    shoulder region M65.11-
    specified site NEC M65.18
    thigh M65.15-
    upper arm M65.12-
  radial styloid M65.4
  shoulder region M65.81-
    adhesive —*see* Capsulitis, adhesive
  specified type NEC M65.88
    ankle M65.87-
    foot M65.87-
    forearm M65.83-
    hand M65.84-
    lower leg M65.86-
    multiple sites M65.89
    pelvic region M65.85-
    shoulder region M65.81-

Tenosynovitis *(continued)*
  specified type *(continued)*
    specified site NEC M65.88
      thigh M65.85-
      upper arm M65.82-
  tuberculous —*see* Tuberculosis, tenosynovitis

Tenovaginitis —*see* Tenosynovitis

Tension
  arterial, high —*see also* Hypertension
    without diagnosis of hypertension R03.0
  headache G44.209
    intractable G44.201
    not intractable G44.209
  nervous R45.0
  pneumothorax J93.0
  premenstrual N94.3
  state (mental) F48.9

Tentorium —*see* condition

Teratencephalus Q89.8

Teratism Q89.7

Teratoblastoma (malignant) —*see* Neoplasm, malignant, by site

Teratocarcinoma —*see also* Neoplasm, malignant, by site
  liver C22.7

Teratoma (solid) —*see also* Neoplasm, uncertain behavior, by site
  with embryonal carcinoma, mixed —*see* Neoplasm, malignant, by site
  with malignant transformation —*see* Neoplasm, malignant, by site
  adult (cystic) —*see* Neoplasm, benign, by site
  benign —*see* Neoplasm, benign, by site
  combined with choriocarcinoma —*see* Neoplasm, malignant, by site
  cystic (adult) —*see* Neoplasm, benign, by site
  differentiated —*see* Neoplasm, benign, by site
  embryonal —*see also* Neoplasm, malignant, by site
    liver C22.7
  immature —*see* Neoplasm, malignant, by site
  liver C22.7
    adult, benign, cystic, differentiated type or mature D13.4
  malignant —*see also* Neoplasm, malignant, by site
    anaplastic —*see* Neoplasm, malignant, by site
    intermediate —*see* Neoplasm, malignant, by site
    specified site —*see* Neoplasm, malignant, by site
    unspecified site C62.90
    undifferentiated —*see* Neoplasm, malignant, by site
  mature —*see* Neoplasm, uncertain behavior, by site
  malignant —*see* Neoplasm, by site, malignant, by site
  ovary D27.-
    embryonal, immature or malignant C56-

Teratoma *(continued)*
  solid —*see* Neoplasm, uncertain behavior, by site
  testis C62.9-
    adult, benign, cystic, differentiated type or mature D29.2-
    scrotal C62.1-
    undescended C62.0-

Termination
  anomalous —*see also* Malposition, congenital
    right pulmonary vein Q26.3
  pregnancy, elective Z33.2

Ternidens diminutus infestation B81.8

Ternidensiasis B81.8

Terror(s) **night** (child) F51.4

Terrorism, victim of Z65.4

Terry's syndrome (*see also* Myopia, degenerative) H44.2-

Tertiary —*see* condition

Test, tests, testing (for)
  adequacy (for dialysis)
    hemodialysis Z49.31
    peritoneal Z49.32
  blood-alcohol Z02.83
    positive —*see* Findings, abnormal, in blood
  blood-drug Z02.83
    positive —*see* Findings, abnormal, in blood
  blood pressure Z01.30
    abnormal reading —*see* Blood, pressure
  blood typing Z01.83
    Rh typing Z01.83
  cardiac pulse generator (battery) Z45.010
  fertility Z31.41
  genetic
    disease carrier status for procreative management
      female Z31.430
      male Z31.440
    male partner of patient with recurrent pregnancy loss Z31.441
    procreative management NEC
      female Z31.438
      male Z31.448
  hearing Z01.10
    with abnormal findings NEC Z01.118
    infant or child (over 28 days old) Z00.129
      with abnormal findings Z00.121
  HIV (human immunodeficiency virus)
    nonconclusive (in infants) R75
    positive Z21
    seropositive Z21
  immunity status Z01.84
  intelligence NEC Z01.89
  laboratory (as part of a general medical examination) Z00.00
    with abnormal finding Z00.01
  for medicolegal reason NEC Z04.89
  male partner of patient with recurrent pregnancy loss Z31.441
  Mantoux (for tuberculosis) Z11.1
    abnormal result R76.11

Test, tests, testing *(continued)*
  pregnancy, positive first pregnancy —*see* Pregnancy, normal, first
  procreative Z31.49
    fertility Z31.41
  skin, diagnostic
    allergy Z01.82
      special screening examination —*see* Screening, by name of disease
    Mantoux Z11.1
    tuberculin Z11.1
  specified NEC Z01.89
  tuberculin Z11.1
    abnormal result R76.11
  vision Z01.00
    with abnormal findings Z01.01
    following failed vision screening Z01.020
      with abnormal findings Z01.021
    infant or child (over 28 days old) Z00.129
      with abnormal findings Z00.121
  Wassermann Z11.3
    positive —*see* Serology for syphilis, positive

Testicle, testicular, testis —*see also* condition
  feminization syndrome (*see also* Syndrome, androgen insensitivity) E34.51
  migrans Q55.29

Tetanus, tetanic (cephalic) (convulsions) A35
  with
    abortion A34
    ectopic or molar pregnancy O08.0
    following ectopic or molar pregnancy O08.0
  inoculation reaction (due to serum) —*see* Complications, vaccination
  neonatorum A33
  obstetrical A34
  puerperal, postpartum, childbirth A34

Tetany (due to) R29.0
  alkalosis E87.3
  associated with rickets E55.0
  convulsions R29.0
    hysterical F44.5
  functional (hysterical) F44.5
  hyperkinetic R29.0
    hysterical F44.5
  hyperpnea R06.4
    hysterical F44.5
    psychogenic F45.8
  hyperventilation (*see also* Hyperventilation) R06.4
    hysterical F44.5
  neonatal (without calcium or magnesium deficiency) P71.3
  parathyroid (gland) E20.9
  parathyroprival E89.2
  post- (para)thyroidectomy E89.2
  postoperative E89.2
  pseudotetany R29.0
  psychogenic (conversion reaction) F44.5

Tetralogy of Fallot Q21.3

Tetraplegia (chronic) (*see also* Quadriplegia) G82.50

Thailand hemorrhagic fever A91

Thalassanemia —*see* Thalassemia

Thalassemia (anemia) (disease) D56.9
 with other hemoglobinopathy D56.8
 alpha (major) (severe) (triple gene defect) D56.0
  minor D56.3
  silent carrier D56.3
  trait D56.3
 beta (severe) D56.1
  homozygous D56.1
  major D56.1
  minor D56.3
  trait D56.3
 delta-beta (homozygous) D56.2
  minor D56.3
  trait D56.3
 dominant D56.8
 hemoglobin
  C D56.8
  E-beta D56.5
 intermedia D56.1
 major D56.1
 minor D56.3
 mixed D56.8
 sickle-cell —see Disease, sickle-cell, thalassemia
 specified type NEC D56.8
 trait D56.3
 variants D56.8

Thanatophoric dwarfism or short stature Q77.1

Thaysen-Gee disease (nontropical sprue) K90.0

Thaysen's disease K90.0

Thecoma D27-
 luteinized D27-
 malignant C56-

Thelarche, premature E30.8

Thelaziasis B83.8

Thelitis N61.0
 puerperal, postpartum or gestational —see Infection, nipple

Therapeutic —see condition

Therapy
 drug, long-term (current) (prophylactic)
  agents affecting estrogen receptors and estrogen levels NEC Z79.818
  anastrozole (Arimidex) Z79.811
  antibiotics Z79.2
   short-term use - omit code
  anticoagulants Z79.01
  anti-inflammatory Z79.1
  antiplatelet Z79.02
  antithrombotics Z79.02
  aromatase inhibitors Z79.811
  aspirin Z79.82
  birth control pill or patch Z79.3
  bisphosphonates Z79.83
  contraceptive, oral Z79.3
  drug, specified NEC Z79.899
  estrogen receptor downregulators Z79.818
  Evista Z79.810
  exemestane (Aromasin) Z79.811
  Fareston Z79.810
  fulvestrant (Faslodex) Z79.818
  gonadotropin-releasing hormone (GnRH) agonist Z79.818
  goserelin acetate (Zoladex) Z79.818
  hormone replacement Z79.890
  insulin Z79.4
  letrozole (Femara) Z79.811

Therapy (continued)
 drug, long-term (continued)
  leuprolide acetate (leuprorelin) (Lupron) Z79.818
  megestrol acetate (Megace) Z79.818
  methadone
   for pain management Z79.891
   maintenance therapy F11.20
  Nolvadex Z79.810
  oral antidiabetic Z79.84
  opiate analgesic Z79.891
  oral contraceptive Z79.3
  oral hypoglycemic Z79.84
  raloxifene (Evista) Z79.810
  selective estrogen receptor modulators (SERMs) Z79.810
  short term - omit code
  steroids
   inhaled Z79.51
   systemic Z79.52
  tamoxifen (Nolvadex) Z79.810
  toremifene (Fareston) Z79.810

Thermic —see condition

Thermography (abnormal) (see also Abnormal, diagnostic imaging) R93.89
 breast R92.8

Thermoplegia T67.01

Thesaurismosis, glycogen —see Disease, glycogen storage

Thiamin deficiency E51.9
 specified NEC E51.8

Thiaminic deficiency with beriberi E51.11

Thibierge-Weissenbach syndrome —see Sclerosis, systemic

Thickening
 bone —see Hypertrophy, bone
 breast N64.59
 endometrium R93.89
 epidermal L85.9
  specified NEC L85.8
 hymen N89.6
 larynx J38.7
 nail L60.2
  congenital Q84.5
 periosteal —see Hypertrophy, bone
 pleura J92.9
  with asbestos J92.0
 skin R23.4
 subepiglottic J38.7
 tongue K14.8
 valve, heart —see Endocarditis

Thigh —see condition

Thinning vertebra —see Spondylopathy, specified NEC

Thirst, excessive R63.1
 due to deprivation of water T73.1

Thomsen disease G71.12

Thoracic —see also condition
 kidney Q63.2
 outlet syndrome G54.0

Thoracogastroschisis (congenital) Q79.8

Thoracopagus Q89.4

Thorax —see condition

Thorn's syndrome N28.89

Thorson-Björck syndrome E34.0

Threadworm (infection) (infestation) B80

Threatened
 abortion O20.0
  with subsequent abortion O03.9

Threatened (continued)
 abuse (harm) —see Maltreatment
 job loss, anxiety concerning Z56.2
 labor (without delivery) O47.9
  at or after 37 completed weeks of gestation O47.1
  before 37 completed weeks of gestation O47.0-
 loss of job, anxiety concerning Z56.2
 miscarriage O20.0
 unemployment, anxiety concerning Z56.2

Three-day fever A93.1

Threshers' lung J67.0

Thrix annulata (congenital) Q84.1

Throat —see condition

Thrombasthenia (Glanzmann) (hemorrhagic) (hereditary) D69.1

Thromboangiitis I73.1
 obliterans (general) I73.1
  cerebral I67.89
  vessels
   brain I67.89
   spinal cord I67.89

Thromboarteritis —see Arteritis

Thromboasthenia (Glanzmann) (hemorrhagic) (hereditary) D69.1

Thrombocytasthenia (Glanzmann) D69.1

Thrombocythemia (hemorrhagic) (see also Thrombocytosis) D75.839
 essential D47.3
 idiopathic D47.3
 primary D47.3

Thrombocytopathy (dystrophic) (granulopenic) D69.1

Thrombocytopenia, thrombocytopenic D69.6
 with absent radius (TAR) Q87.2
 congenital D69.42
 dilutional D69.59
 due to
  drugs D69.59
  extracorporeal circulation of blood D69.59
  (massive) blood transfusion D69.59
  platelet alloimmunization D69.59
 essential D69.3
 heparin-associated D75.821
 heparin induced (HIT) D75.829
  delayed-onset D75.828
  immune-mediated D75.822
  non-immune D75.821
  persisting D75.828
  syndrome
   autoimmune D75.828
   specified NEC D75.828
   spontaneous (without heparin exposure) D75.84
  type 1 D75.821
  type 2 D75.822
 hereditary D69.42
 idiopathic D69.3
 neonatal, transitory P61.0
  due to
   exchange transfusion P61.0
   idiopathic maternal thrombocytopenia P61.0
   isoimmunization P61.0
 primary NEC D69.49
  idiopathic D69.3
 puerperal, postpartum O72.3
 secondary D69.59
 transient neonatal P61.0
 vaccine-induced thrombotic D75.84

Thrombocytosis D75.839
 essential D47.3
 idiopathic D47.3
 primary D47.3
 reactive D75.838
 secondary D75.838
 specified NEC D75.838

Thromboembolism —see Embolism

Thrombopathy (Bernard-Soulier) D69.1
 constitutional —see Disease, von Willebrand
 Willebrand-Jurgens —see Disease, von Willebrand

Thrombopenia —see Thrombocytopenia

Thrombophilia D68.59
 primary NEC D68.59
 secondary NEC D68.69
 specified NEC D68.69

Thrombophlebitis I80.9
 antepartum O22.2-
  deep O22.3-
  superficial O22.2-
 calf muscular vein (NOS) I80.25-
 cavernous (venous) sinus G08
  complicating pregnancy O22.5-
  nonpyogenic I67.6
 cerebral (sinus) (vein) G08
  nonpyogenic I67.6
  sequelae G09
 due to implanted device —see Complications, by site and type, specified NEC
 during or resulting from a procedure NEC T81.72
 femoral vein (superficial) I80.1-
 femoropopliteal vein I80.0-
 gastrocnemial vein I80.25
 hepatic (vein) I80.8
 idiopathic, recurrent I82.1
 iliac vein (common) (external) (internal) I80.21-
 iliofemoral I80.1-
 intracranial venous sinus (any) G08
  nonpyogenic I67.6
  sequelae G09
 intraspinal venous sinuses and veins G08
  nonpyogenic G95.19
 lateral (venous) sinus G08
  nonpyogenic I67.6
 leg I80.3
  superficial I80.0-
 longitudinal (venous) sinus G08
  nonpyogenic I67.6
 lower extremity I80.299
 migrans, migrating I82.1
 pelvic
  with ectopic or molar pregnancy O08.0
  following ectopic or molar pregnancy O08.0
  puerperal O87.1
 peroneal vein I80.24-
 popliteal vein —see Phlebitis, leg, deep, popliteal
 portal (vein) K75.1
 postoperative T81.72
 pregnancy —see Thrombophlebitis, antepartum
 puerperal, postpartum, childbirth O87.0
  deep O87.1
  pelvic O87.1
  septic O86.81
  superficial O87.0
 saphenous (greater) (lesser) I80.0-

Thrombophlebitis (continued)
  sinus (intracranial) G08
    nonpyogenic I67.6
  soleal vein I80.25-
  specified site NEC I80.8
  tibial vein (anterior) (posterior) I80.23-

Thrombosis, thrombotic (bland) (multiple) (progressive) (silent) (vessel) I82.90
  anal K64.5
  antepartum —see Thrombophlebitis, antepartum
  aorta, aortic I74.10
    abdominal I74.09
      saddle I74.01
    bifurcation I74.09
    saddle I74.01
    specified site NEC I74.19
    terminal I74.09
    thoracic I74.11
    valve —see Endocarditis, aortic
  apoplexy I63.3-
  artery, arteries (postinfectional) I74.9
    auditory, internal —see Occlusion, artery, precerebral, specified NEC
    basilar —see Occlusion, artery, basilar
    carotid (common) (internal) —see Occlusion, artery, carotid
    cerebellar (anterior inferior) (posterior inferior) (superior) —see Occlusion, artery, cerebellar
    cerebral —see Occlusion, artery, cerebral
    choroidal (anterior) —see Occlusion, artery, precerebral, specified NEC
    communicating, posterior —see Occlusion, artery, precerebral, specified NEC
    coronary —see also Infarct, myocardium
      not resulting in infarction I24.0
    hepatic I74.8
    hypophyseal —see Occlusion, artery, precerebral, specified NEC
    iliac I74.5
    limb I74.4
      lower I74.3
      upper I74.2
    meningeal, anterior or posterior —see Occlusion, artery, cerebral, specified NEC
    mesenteric (with gangrene) (see also Infarct, intestine) K55.069
    ophthalmic —see Occlusion, artery, retina
    pontine —see Occlusion, artery, precerebral, specified NEC
    precerebral —see Occlusion, artery, precerebral
    pulmonary (iatrogenic) —see Embolism, pulmonary
    renal N28.0
    retinal —see Occlusion, artery, retina
    spinal, anterior or posterior G95.11
    traumatic NEC T14.8
    vertebral —see Occlusion, artery, vertebral
  atrium, auricular —see also Infarct, myocardium
    following acute myocardial infarction (current complication) I23.6
    not resulting in infarction I51.3
    old I51.3

Thrombosis, thrombotic (continued)
  basilar (artery) —see Occlusion, artery, basilar
  brain (artery) (stem) —see also Occlusion, artery, cerebral
    due to syphilis A52.05
    puerperal O99.43
    sinus —see Thrombosis, intracranial venous sinus
  capillary I78.8
  cardiac —see also Infarct, myocardium
    not resulting in infarction I51.3
    old I51.3
    valve —see Endocarditis
  carotid (artery) (common) (internal) —see Occlusion, artery, carotid
  cavernous (venous) sinus —see Thrombosis, intracranial venous sinus
  cerebellar artery (anterior inferior) (posterior inferior) (superior) I66.3
  cerebral (artery) —see Occlusion, artery, cerebral
  cerebrovenous sinus —see also Thrombosis, intracranial venous sinus
    puerperium O87.3
  chronic I82.91
  coronary (artery) (vein) —see also Infarct, myocardium
    not resulting in infarction I24.0
  corpus cavernosum N48.89
  cortical I66.9
  deep —see Embolism, vein, lower extremity
  due to device, implant or graft (see also Complications, by site and type, specified NEC) T85.868
    arterial graft NEC T82.868
    breast (implant) T85.868
    catheter NEC T85.868
      dialysis (renal) T82.868
        intraperitoneal T85.868
      infusion NEC T82.868
        spinal (epidural) (subdural) T85.860
      urinary (indwelling) T83.86
    electronic (electrode) (pulse generator) (stimulator)
      bone T84.86
      cardiac T82.867
      nervous system (brain) (peripheral nerve) (spinal) T85.860
      urinary T83.86
    fixation, internal (orthopedic) NEC T84.86
    gastrointestinal (bile duct) (esophagus) T85.868
    genital NEC T83.86
    heart T82.867
    joint prosthesis T84.86
    ocular (corneal graft) (orbital implant) NEC T85.868
    orthopedic NEC T84.86
    specified NEC T85.868
    urinary NEC T83.86
    vascular NEC T82.868
    ventricular intracranial shunt T85.860
  during the puerperium —see Thrombosis, puerperal
  endocardial —see also Infarct, myocardium
    not resulting in infarction I51.3

Thrombosis, thrombotic (continued)
  eye —see Occlusion, retina
  genital organ
    female NEC N94.89
      pregnancy —see Thrombophlebitis, antepartum
    male N50.1
  gestational —see Phlebopathy, gestational
  heart (chamber) —see also Infarct, myocardium
    not resulting in infarction I51.3
    old I51.3
  hepatic (vein) I82.0
    artery I74.8
  history (of) Z86.718
  intestine (with gangrene (see also Infarct, intestine)) K55.069
  intracardiac NEC (apical) (atrial) (auricular) (ventricular) (old) I51.3
  intracranial (arterial) I66.9
    venous sinus (any) G08
      nonpyogenic origin I67.6
      puerperium O87.3
  intramural —see also Infarct, myocardium
    not resulting in infarction I51.3
    old I51.3
  intraspinal venous sinuses and veins G08
    nonpyogenic G95.19
  kidney (artery) N28.0
  lateral (venous) sinus —see Thrombosis, intracranial venous sinus
  leg —see Thrombosis, vein, lower extremity
    arterial I74.3
  liver (venous) I82.0
    artery I74.8
    portal vein I81
  longitudinal (venous) sinus —see Thrombosis, intracranial venous sinus
  lower limb —see Thrombosis, vein, lower extremity
  lung (iatrogenic) (postoperative) —see Embolism, pulmonary
  meninges (brain) (arterial) I66.8
  mesenteric (artery) (with gangrene) (see also Infarct, intestine) K55.069
    vein (inferior) (superior) K55.0-
  mitral I34.89
  mural —see also Infarct, myocardium
    due to syphilis A52.06
    not resulting in infarction I51.3
    old I51.3
  omentum (with gangrene) (see also Infarct, intestine) K55.069
  ophthalmic —see Occlusion, retina
  pampiniform plexus (male) N50.1
  parietal —see also Infarct, myocardium
    not resulting in infarction I24.0
  penis, superficial vein N48.81
  perianal venous K64.5
  peripheral arteries I74.4
    upper I74.2
  personal history (of) Z86.718
  portal I81
    due to syphilis A52.09
  precerebral artery —see Occlusion, artery, precerebral
  puerperal, postpartum O87.0
    brain (artery) O99.43
      venous (sinus) O87.3
    cardiac O99.43

Thrombosis, thrombotic (continued)
  puerperal, postpartum (continued)
    cerebral (artery) O99.43
      venous (sinus) O87.3
      superficial O87.0
    pulmonary (artery) (iatrogenic) (postoperative) (vein) —see Embolism, pulmonary
    renal (artery) N28.0
      vein I82.3
  resulting from presence of device, implant or graft —see Complications, by site and type, specified NEC
  retina, retinal —see Occlusion, retina
  scrotum N50.1
  seminal vesicle N50.1
  sigmoid (venous) sinus —see Thrombosis, intracranial venous sinus
  sinus, intracranial (any) —see Thrombosis, intracranial venous sinus
  specified site NEC I82.890
    chronic I82.891
  spermatic cord N50.1
  spinal cord (arterial) G95.11
    due to syphilis A52.09
    pyogenic origin G06.1
  spleen, splenic D73.5
    artery I74.8
  testis N50.1
  tumor —see Neoplasm, unspecified behavior, by site
  traumatic NEC T14.8
  tricuspid I07.8
  tunica vaginalis N50.1
  umbilical cord (vessels), complicating delivery O69.5
  vas deferens N50.1
  vein (acute) I82.90
    antecubital I82.61-
      chronic I82.71-
    axillary I82.A1-
      chronic I82.A2-
    basilic I82.61-
      chronic I82.71-
    brachial I82.62-
      chronic I82.72-
    brachiocephalic (innominate) I82.290
      chronic I82.291
    calf muscular I82.46-
      chronic I82.56-
    cerebral, nonpyogenic I67.6
    cephalic I82.61-
      chronic I82.71-
    chronic I82.91
    deep (DVT) I82.40-
      calf I82.4Z-
        chronic I82.5Z-
      lower leg I82.4Z-
        chronic I82.5Z-
      thigh I82.4Y-
        chronic I82.5Y-
      upper leg I82.4Y-
        chronic I82.5Y-
    femoral I82.41-
      chronic I82.51-
    iliac (iliofemoral) I82.42-
      chronic I82.52-
    innominate I82.290
      chronic I82.291
    internal jugular I82.C1-
      chronic I82.C2-
    lower extremity
      deep I82.40-
        chronic I82.50-
        specified NEC I82.49-
          chronic NEC I82.59-

Thrombosis, thrombotic *(continued)*
  vein *(continued)*
    lower extremity *(continued)*
      distal
        deep I82.4Z-
        proximal
          deep I82.4Y-
            chronic I82.5Y-
        superficial I82.81-
      perianal K64.5
      peroneal I82.45-
        chronic I82.55-
      popliteal I82.43-
        chronic I82.53-
      radial I82.62-
        chronic I82.72-
      renal I82.3
      saphenous (greater) (lesser) I82.81-
      specified NEC I82.890
        chronic NEC I82.891
      subclavian I82.B1-
        chronic I82.B2-
      thoracic NEC I82.290
        chronic I82.291
      tibial I82.44-
        chronic I82.54-
      ulnar I82.62-
        chronic I82.72-
      upper extremity I82.60-
        chronic I82.70-
        deep I82.62-
          chronic I82.72-
        superficial I82.61-
          chronic I82.71-
    vena cava
      inferior I82.220
        chronic I82.221
      superior I82.210
        chronic I82.211
    venous, perianal K64.5
    ventricle —*see also* Infarct,
        myocardium
      following acute myocardial
          infarction (current
          complication) I23.6
      not resulting in infarction I24.0
      old I51.3

Thrombus —*see* Thrombosis

Thrush —*see also* Candidiasis
  oral B37.0
  newborn P37.5
  vaginal (acute) B37.31
    chronic (recurrent) B37.32

Thumb —*see also* condition
  sucking (child problem) F98.8

Thymitis E32.8

Thymoma —*see also* Neoplasm,
    thymus, by type
  malignant C37
  metaplastic C37
  microscopic D15.0
  sclerosing C37
  type A C37
  type AB C37
  type B1 C37
  type B2 C37
  type B3 C37

Thymus, thymic (gland) —*see*
    condition

Thyrocele —*see* Goiter

Thyroglossal —*see also* condition
  cyst Q89.2
  duct, persistent Q89.2

Thyroid (gland) (body) —*see also*
    condition
  hormone resistance E07.89
  lingual Q89.2
  nodule (cystic) (nontoxic) (single)
      E04.1

Thyroiditis E06.9
  acute (nonsuppurative) (pyogenic)
      (suppurative) E06.0
  autoimmune E06.3
  chronic (nonspecific) (sclerosing)
      E06.5
    with thyrotoxicosis, transient
        E06.2
    fibrous E06.5
    lymphadenoid E06.3
    lymphocytic E06.3
    lymphoid E06.3
  de Quervain's E06.1
  drug-induced E06.4
  fibrous (chronic) E06.5
  giant-cell (follicular) E06.1
  granulomatous (de Quervain)
      (subacute) E06.1
  Hashimoto's (struma
      lymphomatosa) E06.3
  iatrogenic E06.4
  ligneous E06.5
  lymphocytic (chronic) E06.3
  lymphoid E06.3
  lymphomatous E06.3
  nonsuppurative E06.1
  postpartum, puerperal O90.5
  pseudotuberculous E06.1
  pyogenic E06.0
  radiation E06.4
  Riedel's E06.5
  subacute (granulomatous) E06.1
  suppurative E06.0
  tuberculous A18.81
  viral E06.1
  woody E06.5

Thyrolingual duct, persistent Q89.2

Thyromegaly E01.0

Thyrotoxic
  crisis —*see* Thyrotoxicosis
  heart disease or failure (*see also*
      Thyrotoxicosis) E05.90 [I43]
    with thyroid storm E05.91 [I43]
  storm —*see* Thyrotoxicosis

Thyrotoxicosis (recurrent) E05.90
  with
    goiter (diffuse) E05.00
      with thyroid storm E05.01
      adenomatous uninodular E05.10
        with thyroid storm E05.11
      multinodular E05.20
        with thyroid storm E05.21
      nodular E05.20
        with thyroid storm E05.21
      uninodular E05.10
        with thyroid storm E05.11
    infiltrative
      dermopathy E05.00
        with thyroid storm E05.01
      ophthalmopathy E05.00
        with thyroid storm E05.01
    single thyroid nodule E05.10
      with thyroid storm E05.11
    thyroid storm E05.91
  due to
    ectopic thyroid nodule or tissue
        E05.30
      with thyroid storm E05.31
    ingestion of (excessive) thyroid
        material E05.40
      with thyroid storm E05.41
    overproduction of thyroid-
        stimulating hormone E05.80
      with thyroid storm E05.81
    specified cause NEC E05.80
      with thyroid storm E05.81
  factitia E05.40
    with thyroid storm E05.41

Thyrotoxicosis *(continued)*
  heart (*see also* Failure, heart, high-
      output) E05.90 [I43]
    with thyroid storm (*see also*
        Failure, heart, high-output)
        E05.91 [I43]
    failure (*see also* Failure, heart,
        high-output) E05.90 [I43]
  neonatal (transient) P72.1
  transient with chronic thyroiditis
      E06.2

Tibia vara M92.51-

Tic (disorder) F95.9
  breathing F95.8
  child problem F95.0
  compulsive F95.1
  de la Tourette F95.2
  degenerative (generalized)
      (localized) G25.69
    facial G25.69
  disorder
    chronic
      motor F95.1
      vocal F95.1
    combined vocal and multiple
        motor F95.2
    transient F95.0
  douloureux G50.0
    atypical G50.1
    postherpetic, postzoster
        B02.22
  drug-induced G25.61
  eyelid F95.8
  habit F95.9
    chronic F95.1
    transient of childhood F95.0
  lid, transient of childhood F95.0
  motor-verbal F95.2
  occupational F48.8
  orbicularis F95.8
    transient of childhood F95.0
  organic origin G25.69
  postchoreic G25.69
  provisional F95.0
  psychogenic, compulsive F95.1
  salaam R25.8
  spasm (motor or vocal) F95.9
    chronic F95.1
    transient of childhood F95.0
  specified NEC F95.8

Tick-borne —*see* condition

Tietze's disease or syndrome M94.0

Tight, tightness
  anus K62.89
  chest R07.89
  fascia (lata) M62.89
  foreskin (congenital) N47.1
  hymen, hymenal ring N89.6
  introitus (acquired) (congenital)
      N89.6
  rectal sphincter K62.89
  tendon —*see* Short, tendon
  urethral sphincter N35.919

Tilting vertebra —*see* Dorsopathy,
    deforming, specified NEC

Timidity, child F93.8

Tin-miner's lung J63.5

Tinea (intersecta) (tarsi) B35.9
  amiantacea L44.8
  asbestina B35.0
  barbae B35.0
  beard B35.0
  black dot B35.0
  blanca B36.2
  capitis B35.0
  corporis B35.4
  cruris B35.6

Tinea *(continued)*
  flava B36.0
  foot B35.3
  furfuracea B36.0
  imbricata (Tokelau) B35.5
  kerion B35.0
  manuum B35.2
  microsporic —*see* Dermatophytosis
  nigra B36.1
  nodosa —*see* Piedra
  pedis B35.3
  scalp B35.0
  specified NEC B35.8
  sycosis B35.0
  tonsurans B35.0
  trichophytic —*see*
      Dermatophytosis
  unguium B35.1
  versicolor B36.0

Tingling sensation (skin) R20.2

Tinnitus NOS H93.1-
  audible H93.1-
  aurium H93.1-
  pulsatile H93.A-
  subjective H93.1-

Tipped tooth (teeth) M26.33

Tipping
  pelvis M95.5
    with disproportion (fetopelvic)
        O33.0
      causing obstructed labor
          O65.0
  tooth (teeth), fully erupted
      M26.33

Tiredness R53.83

Tissue —*see* condition

Tobacco (nicotine)
  abuse, —*see* Tobacco, use
  dependence —*see* Dependence,
      drug, nicotine
  harmful use Z72.0
  heart —*see* Tobacco, toxic
      effect
  maternal use, affecting newborn
      P04.2
  toxic effect —*see* Table of Drugs
      and Chemicals, by substance,
      poisoning
    chewing tobacco —*see* Table
        of Drugs and Chemicals, by
        substance, poisoning
    cigarettes —*see* Table of Drugs
        and Chemicals, by substance,
        poisoning
  use Z72.0
    complicating
      childbirth O99.334
      pregnancy O99.33-
      puerperium O99.335
    counseling and surveillance
        Z71.6
    history Z87.891
    withdrawal state (*see also*
        Dependence, drug, nicotine)
        F17.203

Tocopherol deficiency E56.0

Todd's
  cirrhosis K74.3
  paralysis (postepileptic) (transitory)
      G83.84

Toe —*see* condition

Toilet, artificial opening —*see*
    Attention to, artificial, opening

Tokelau (ringworm) B35.5

Tollwut —*see* Rabies

Tommaselli's disease R31.9
  correct substance properly administered —*see* Table of Drugs and Chemicals, by drug, adverse effect
  overdose or wrong substance given or taken —*see* Table of Drugs and Chemicals, by drug, poisoning

Tongue —*see also* condition
  tie Q38.1

Tonic pupil —*see* Anomaly, pupil, function, tonic pupil

Toni-Fanconi syndrome (cystinosis) E72.09
  with cystinosis E72.04

Tonsil —*see* condition

Tonsillitis (acute) (catarrhal) (croupous) (follicular) (gangrenous) (infective) (lacunar) (lingual) (malignant) (membranous) (parenchymatous) (phlegmonous) (pseudomembranous) (purulent) (septic) (subacute) (suppurative) (toxic) (ulcerative) (vesicular) (viral) J03.90
  chronic J35.01
    with adenoiditis J35.03
  diphtheritic A36.0
  hypertrophic J35.01
    with adenoiditis J35.03
  recurrent J03.91
  specified organism NEC J03.80
    recurrent J03.81
  staphylococcal J03.80
    recurrent J03.81
  streptococcal J03.00
    recurrent J03.01
  tuberculous A15.8
  Vincent's A69.1

Tooth, teeth —*see* condition

Toothache K08.89

Topagnosis R20.8

Tophi —*see* Gout, chronic

TORCH infection —*see* Infection, congenital
  without active infection P00.2

Torn —*see* Tear

Tornwaldt's cyst or disease J39.2

Torsades de pointes I47.21

Torsion
  accessory tube —*see* Torsion, fallopian tube
  adnexa (female) —*see* Torsion, fallopian tube
  aorta, acquired I77.1
  appendix epididymis N44.04
  appendix testis N44.03
  bile duct (common) (hepatic) K83.8
    congenital Q44.5
  bowel, colon or intestine K56.2
  cervix —*see* Malposition, uterus
  cystic duct K82.8
  dystonia —*see* Dystonia, torsion
  epididymis (appendix) N44.04
  fallopian tube N83.52-
    with ovary N83.53
  gallbladder K82.8
    congenital Q44.1
  hydatid of Morgagni
    female N83.52-
    male N44.03
  kidney (pedicle) (leading to infarction) N28.0

Torsion (continued)
  Meckel's diverticulum (congenital) Q43.0
    malignant —*see* Table of Neoplasms, small intestine, malignant
  mesentery K56.2
  omentum K56.2
  organ or site, congenital NEC —*see* Anomaly, by site
  ovary (pedicle) N83.51-
    with fallopian tube N83.53
    congenital Q50.2
  oviduct —*see* Torsion, fallopian tube
  penis (acquired) N48.82
    congenital Q55.63
  spasm —*see* Dystonia, torsion
  spermatic cord N44.02
    extravaginal N44.01
    intravaginal N44.02
  spleen D73.5
  testis, testicle N44.00
    appendix N44.03
  tibia —*see* Deformity, limb, specified type NEC, lower leg
  uterus —*see* Malposition, uterus

Torticollis (intermittent) (spastic) M43.6
  congenital (sternomastoid) Q68.0
  due to birth injury P15.8
  hysterical F44.4
  ocular R29.891
  psychogenic F45.8
    conversion reaction F44.4
  rheumatic M43.6
  rheumatoid M06.88
  spasmodic G24.3
  traumatic, current S13.4

Tortipelvis G24.1

Tortuous
  aortic arch Q25.46
  artery I77.1
  organ or site, congenital NEC —*see* Distortion
  retinal vessel, congenital Q14.1
  ureter N13.8
  urethra N36.8
  vein —*see* Varix

Torture, victim of Z65.4

Torula, torular (histolytica) (infection) —*see* Cryptococcosis

Torulosis —*see* Cryptococcosis

Torus (mandibularis) (palatinus) M27.0
  fracture —*see* Fracture, by site, torus

Touraine's syndrome Q79.8

Tourette's syndrome F95.2

Tourniquet syndrome —*see* Constriction, external, by site

Tower skull Q75.009
  with exophthalmos Q87.0

Toxemia R68.89
  bacterial —*see* Sepsis
  burn —*see* Burn
  eclamptic (with pre-existing hypertension) —*see* Eclampsia
  erysipelatous —*see* Erysipelas
  fatigue R68.89
  food —*see* Poisoning, food
  gastrointestinal K52.1
  intestinal K52.1
  kidney —*see* Uremia
  malarial —*see* Malaria
  myocardial —*see* Myocarditis, toxic

Toxemia (continued)
  of pregnancy —*see* Pre-eclampsia
  pre-eclamptic —*see* Pre-eclampsia
  small intestine K52.1
  staphylococcal, due to food A05.0
  stasis R68.89
  uremic —*see* Uremia
  urinary —*see* Uremia

Toxemica cerebropathia psychica (nonalcoholic) F04
  alcoholic —*see* Alcohol, amnestic disorder

Toxic (poisoning) (*see also* condition) T65.91
  effect —*see* Table of Drugs and Chemicals, by substance, poisoning
  shock syndrome A48.3
  thyroid (gland) —*see* Thyrotoxicosis

Toxicemia —*see* Toxemia

Toxicity —*see* Table of Drugs and Chemicals, by substance, poisoning
  fava bean D55.0
  food, noxious —*see* Poisoning, food
  from drug or nonmedicinal substance —*see* Table of Drugs and Chemicals, by drug

Toxicosis —*see also* Toxemia
  capillary, hemorrhagic D69.0

Toxinfection, gastrointestinal K52.1

Toxocariasis B83.0

Toxoplasma, toxoplasmosis (acquired) B58.9
  with
    hepatitis B58.1
    meningoencephalitis B58.2
    ocular involvement B58.00
    other organ involvement B58.89
    pneumonia, pneumonitis B58.3
  congenital (acute) (subacute) (chronic) P37.1
  maternal, manifest toxoplasmosis in infant (acute) (subacute) (chronic) P37.1

tPA (rtPA) administration in a different facility within the last 24 hours prior to admission to current facility Z92.82

Trabeculation, bladder N32.89

Trachea —*see* condition

Tracheitis (catarrhal) (infantile) (membranous) (plastic) (septal) (suppurative) (viral) J04.10
  with
    bronchitis (15 years of age and above) J40
      acute or subacute —*see* Bronchitis, acute
      chronic J42
      tuberculous NEC A15.5
      under 15 years of age J20.9
    laryngitis (acute) J04.2
      chronic J37.1
      tuberculous NEC A15.5
  acute J04.10
    with obstruction J04.11
  chronic J42
    with
      bronchitis (chronic) J42
      laryngitis (chronic) J37.1
  diphtheritic (membranous) A36.89

Tracheitis (continued)
  due to external agent —*see* Inflammation, respiratory, upper, due to
  syphilitic A52.73
  tuberculous A15.5

Trachelitis (nonvenereal) —*see* Cervicitis

Tracheobronchial —*see* condition

Tracheobronchitis (15 years of age and above) —*see also* Bronchitis
  due to
    Bordetella bronchiseptica A37.80
      with pneumonia A37.81
    Francisella tularensis A21.8

Tracheobronchomegaly Q32.4
  with bronchiectasis J47.9
    with
      exacerbation (acute) J47.1
      lower respiratory infection J47.0
  acquired J98.09
    with bronchiectasis J47.9
      with
        exacerbation (acute) J47.1
        lower respiratory infection J47.0

Tracheobronchopneumonitis —*see* Pneumonia, broncho-

Tracheocele (external) (internal) J39.8
  congenital Q32.1

Tracheomalacia J39.8
  congenital Q32.0

Tracheopharyngitis (acute) J06.9
  chronic J42
  due to external agent —*see* Inflammation, respiratory, upper, due to

Tracheostenosis J39.8

Tracheostomy
  complication —*see* Complication, tracheostomy
  status Z93.0
    attention to Z43.0
    malfunctioning J95.03

Trachoma, trachomatous A71.9
  active (stage) A71.1
  contraction of conjunctiva A71.1
  dubium A71.0
  initial (stage) A71.0
  healed or sequelae B94.0
  pannus A71.1
  Türck's J37.0

Traction, vitreomacular H43.82-

Train sickness T75.3

Trait(s)
  Hb-S D57.3
  hemoglobin
    abnormal NEC D58.2
      with thalassemia D56.3
    C —*see* Disease, hemoglobin C
    S (Hb-S) D57.3
  Lepore D56.3
  personality, accentuated Z73.1
  sickle-cell D57.3
    with elliptocytosis or spherocytosis D57.3
  type A personality Z73.1

Tramp Z59.00

Trance R41.89
  hysterical F44.89

Transaminasemia R74.01

Transection
 abdomen (partial) S38.3
 aorta (incomplete) —see also
   Injury, aorta
   complete —see Injury, aorta,
     laceration, major
 carotid artery (incomplete) —see
   also Injury, blood vessel, carotid,
   laceration
   complete —see Injury, blood
     vessel, carotid, laceration,
     major
 celiac artery (incomplete) S35.211
   branch (incomplete) S35.291
     complete S35.292
   complete S35.212
 innominate
   artery (incomplete) —see also
     Injury, blood vessel, thoracic,
     innominate, artery, laceration
     complete —see Injury, blood
       vessel, thoracic, innominate,
       artery, laceration, major
   vein (incomplete) —see also
     Injury, blood vessel, thoracic,
     innominate, vein, laceration
     complete —see Injury, blood
       vessel, thoracic, innominate,
       vein, laceration, major
 jugular vein (external) (incomplete)
   —see also Injury, blood vessel,
   jugular vein, laceration
   complete —see Injury,
     blood vessel, jugular vein,
     laceration, major
   internal (incomplete) —see
     also Injury, blood vessel,
     jugular vein, internal,
     laceration
     complete —see Injury,
       blood vessel, jugular vein,
       internal, laceration, major
 mesenteric artery (incomplete)
   —see also Injury, mesenteric,
   artery, laceration
   complete —see Injury,
     mesenteric artery, laceration,
     major
 pulmonary vessel (incomplete)
   —see also Injury, blood
   vessel, thoracic, pulmonary,
   laceration
   complete —see Injury, blood
     vessel, thoracic, pulmonary,
     laceration, major
 subclavian —see Transection,
   innominate
 vena cava (incomplete) —see also
   Injury, vena cava
   complete —see Injury, vena
     cava, laceration, major
 vertebral artery (incomplete)
   —see also Injury, blood vessel,
   vertebral, laceration
   complete —see Injury, blood
     vessel, vertebral, laceration,
     major

Transfusion
 associated (red blood cell)
   hemochromatosis E83.111
 blood
   ABO incompatible —see
     Complication(s), transfusion,
     incompatibility reaction,
     ABO
   minor blood group (Duffy)
     (E) (K) (Kell) (Kidd) (Lewis)
     (M) (N) (P) (S) T80.89
   reaction or complication —see
     Complications, transfusion

Transfusion (continued)
 fetomaternal (mother) —see
   Pregnancy, complicated
   by, placenta, transfusion
   syndrome
 maternofetal (mother) —see
   Pregnancy, complicated by,
   placenta, transfusion syndrome
 placental (syndrome) (mother)
   —see Pregnancy, complicated
   by, placenta, transfusion
   syndrome
 reaction (adverse) —see
   Complications, transfusion
 related acute lung injury (TRALI)
   J95.84
 twin-to-twin —see Pregnancy,
   complicated by, placenta,
   transfusion syndrome, fetus to
   fetus

Transgender F64.0

Transient (meaning homeless) —see
 also condition Z59.00

Translocation
 balanced autosomal Q95.9
   in normal individual Q95.0
 chromosomes NEC Q99.8
   balanced and insertion in normal
     individual Q95.0
 Down syndrome Q90.2
 trisomy
   13 Q91.6
   18 Q91.2
   21 Q90.2

Translucency, iris —see
 Degeneration, iris

**Transmission of chemical
 substances through the placenta**
 —see Absorption, chemical,
 through placenta

Transparency, lung, unilateral
 J43.0

Transplant (ed) (status) Z94.9
 awaiting organ Z76.82
 bone Z94.6
   marrow Z94.81
 candidate Z76.82
 complication —see Complication,
   transplant
 cornea Z94.7
 heart Z94.1
   and lung(s) Z94.3
   valve Z95.2
     prosthetic Z95.2
     specified NEC Z95.4
     xenogenic Z95.3
 intestine Z94.82
 kidney Z94.0
 liver Z94.4
 lung(s) Z94.2
   and heart Z94.3
 organ (failure) (infection)
   (rejection) Z94.9
   removal status Z98.85
 pancreas Z94.83
 skin Z94.5
 social Z60.3
 specified organ or tissue NEC
   Z94.89
 stem cells Z94.84
 tissue Z94.9

Transplants, ovarian, endometrial
 N80.10-

Transposed —see Transposition

Transposition (congenital) —see
 also Malposition, congenital
 abdominal viscera Q89.3

Transposition (continued)
 aorta (dextra) Q20.3
 appendix Q43.8
 colon Q43.8
 corrected Q20.5
 great vessels (complete) (partial)
   Q20.3
 heart Q24.0
   with complete transposition of
     viscera Q89.3
 intestine (large) (small) Q43.8
 reversed jejunal (for bypass)
   (status) Z98.0
 scrotum Q55.23
 stomach Q40.2
   with general transposition of
     viscera Q89.3
 tooth, teeth, fully erupted M26.30
 vessels, great (complete) (partial)
   Q20.3
 viscera (abdominal) (thoracic) Q89.3

Transsexualism F64.0

Transverse —see also condition
 arrest (deep), in labor O64.0
 lie (mother) O32.2
   causing obstructed labor O64.8

Transvestism, transvestitism (dual-
 role) F64.1
 fetihistic F65.1

Trapped placenta (with hemorrhage)
 O72.0
 without hemorrhage O73.0

**TRAPS (tumor necrosis factor
 receptor associated periodic
 syndrome)** M04.1

Trauma, traumatism —see also
 Injury
 acoustic —see subcategory H83.3
 birth —see Birth, injury
 complicating ectopic or molar
   pregnancy O08.6
 during delivery O71.9
 following ectopic or molar
   pregnancy O08.6
 non-accidental —see Abuse,
   physical
 obstetric O71.9
   specified NEC O71.89
 occlusal
   primary K08.81
   secondary K08.82

Traumatic —see also condition
 brain injury S06.9

Treacher Collins syndrome Q75.4

Treitz's hernia —see Hernia,
 abdomen, specified site NEC

Trematode infestation —see
 Infestation, fluke

Trematodiasis —see Infestation, fluke

Trembling paralysis —see
 Parkinsonism

Tremor(s) R25.1
 drug induced G25.1
 essential (benign) G25.0
 familial G25.0
 hereditary G25.0
 hysterical F44.4
 intention G25.2
 medication induced postural G25.1
 mercurial —see subcategory T56.1
 Parkinson's —see Parkinsonism
 psychogenic (conversion reaction)
   F44.4
 senilis R54
 specified type NEC G25.2

Trench
 fever A79.0
 foot —see Immersion, foot
 mouth A69.1

Treponema pallidum infection
 —see Syphilis

Treponematosis
 due to
   T. pallidum —see Syphilis
   T. pertenue —see Yaws

Triad
 Hutchinson's (congenital syphilis)
   A50.53
 Kartagener's Q89.3
 Saint's —see Hernia, diaphragm

Trichiasis (eyelid) H02.059
 with entropion —see Entropion
 left H02.056
   lower H02.055
   upper H02.054
 right H02.053
   lower H02.052
   upper H02.051

Trichinella spiralis (infection)
 (infestation) B75

**Trichinellosis, trichiniasis,
 trichinelliasis, trichinosis** B75
 with muscle disorder B75 [M63.80]
   ankle B75 [M63.87-]
   foot B75 [M63.87-]
   forearm B75 [M63.83-]
   hand B75 [M63.84-]
   lower leg B75 [M63.86-]
   multiple sites B75 [M63.89]
   pelvic region B75 [M63.85-]
   shoulder region B75 [M63.81-]
   specified site NEC B75 [M63.88]
   thigh B75 [M63.85-]
   upper arm B75 [M63.82-]

Trichobezoar T18.9
 intestine T18.3
 stomach T18.2

Trichocephaliasis, trichocephalosis
 B79

Trichocephalus infestation B79

Trichoclasis L67.8

Trichoepithelioma —see also
 Neoplasm, skin, benign
 malignant —see Neoplasm, skin,
   malignant

Trichofolliculoma —see Neoplasm,
 skin, benign

Tricholemmoma —see Neoplasm,
 skin, benign

Trichomoniasis A59.9
 bladder A59.03
 cervix A59.09
 intestinal A07.8
 prostate A59.02
 seminal vesicles A59.09
 specified site NEC A59.8
 urethra A59.03
 urogenitalis A59.00
 vagina A59.01
 vulva A59.01

Trichomycosis
 axillaris A48.8
 nodosa, nodularis B36.8

Trichonodosis L67.8

**Trichophytid, trichophyton
 infection** —see Dermatophytosis

Trichophytobezoar T18.9
 intestine T18.3
 stomach T18.2

327

Trichophytosis —*see* Dermatophytosis
Trichoptilosis L67.8
Trichorrhexis (nodosa) (invaginata) L67.0
Trichosis axillaris A48.8
Trichosporosis nodosa B36.2
Trichostasis spinulosa (congenital) Q84.1
Trichostrongyliasis, trichostrongylosis (small intestine) B81.2
Trichostrongylus infection B81.2
Trichotillomania F63.3
Trichromat, trichromatopsia, anomalous (congenital) H53.55
Trichuriasis B79
Trichuris trichiura (infection) (infestation) (any site) B79
Tricuspid (valve) —*see* condition
Trifid —*see also* Accessory
  kidney (pelvis) Q63.8
  tongue Q38.3
Trigeminal neuralgia —*see* Neuralgia, trigeminal
Trigeminy R00.8
Trigger finger (acquired) M65.30
  congenital Q74.0
  index finger M65.32
  little finger M65.35-
  middle finger M65.33-
  ring finger M65.34-
  thumb M65.31-
Trigonitis (bladder) (chronic) (pseudomembranous) N30.30
  with hematuria N30.31
Trigonocephaly Q75.03
Trilocular heart —*see* Cor triloculare
Trimethylaminuria E72.52
Tripartite placenta O43.19-
Triphalangeal thumb Q74.0
Triple —*see also* Accessory
  kidneys Q63.0
  uteri Q51.818
  X, female Q97.0
Triple I O41.12-
Triplegia G83.89
  congenital G80.8
Triplet (newborn) —*see also* Newborn, triplet
  complicating pregnancy —*see* Pregnancy, triplet
Triplication —*see* Accessory
Triploidy Q92.7
Trismus R25.2
  neonatorum A33
  newborn A33
Trisomy (syndrome) Q92.9
  autosomes Q92.9
  chromosome specified NEC Q92.8
    partial Q92.2
      due to unbalanced translocation Q92.5
  whole (nonsex chromosome)
    meiotic nondisjunction Q92.0
    mitotic nondisjunction Q92.1
    mosaicism Q92.1
    specified NEC Q92.8

Trisomy (continued)
  due to
    dicentrics —*see* Extra, marker chromosomes
    extra rings —*see* Extra, marker chromosomes
    isochromosomes —*see* Extra, marker chromosomes
  specified NEC Q92.8
  whole chromosome Q92.9
    meiotic nondisjunction Q92.0
    mitotic nondisjunction Q92.1
    mosaicism Q92.1
    partial Q92.9
    specified NEC Q92.8
  13 (partial) Q91.7
    meiotic nondisjunction Q91.4
    mitotic nondisjunction Q91.5
    mosaicism Q91.5
    translocation Q91.6
  18 (partial) Q91.3
    meiotic nondisjunction Q91.0
    mitotic nondisjunction Q91.1
    mosaicism Q91.1
    translocation Q91.2
  20 Q92.8
  21 (partial) Q90.9
    meiotic nondisjunction Q90.0
    mitotic nondisjunction Q90.1
    mosaicism Q90.1
    translocation Q90.2
  22 Q92.8
Tritanomaly, tritanopia H53.55
Trombiculosis, trombiculiasis, trombidiosis B88.0
Trophedema (congenital) (hereditary) Q82.0
Trophoblastic disease (*see also* Mole, hydatidiform) O01.9
Tropholymphedema Q82.0
Trophoneurosis NEC G96.89
  disseminated M34.9
Tropical —*see* condition
Trouble —*see also* Disease
  heart —*see* Disease, heart
  kidney —*see* Disease, renal
  nervous R45.0
  sinus —*see* Sinusitis
Trousseau's syndrome (thrombophlebitis migrans) I82.1
Truancy, childhood
  from school Z72.810
Truncus
  arteriosus (persistent) Q20.0
  communis Q20.0
Trunk —*see* condition
Trypanosomiasis
  African B56.9
    by Trypanosoma brucei
      gambiense B56.0
      rhodesiense B56.1
  American —*see* Chagas' disease
  Brazilian —*see* Chagas' disease
  by Trypanosoma
    brucei gambiense B56.0
    brucei rhodesiense B56.1
    cruzi —*see* Chagas' disease
  gambiensis, Gambian B56.0
  rhodesiensis, Rhodesian B56.1
  South American —*see* Chagas' disease
  where
    African trypanosomiasis is prevalent B56.9
    Chagas' disease is prevalent B57.2

Tryptasemia, hereditary alpha D89.44
T-shaped incisors K00.2
Tsutsugamushi (disease) (fever) A75.3
Tube, tubal, tubular —*see* condition
Tubercle —*see also* Tuberculosis
  brain, solitary A17.81
  Darwin's Q17.8
  Ghon, primary infection A15.7
Tuberculid, tuberculide (indurating, subcutaneous) (lichenoid) (miliary) (papulonecrotic) (primary) (skin) A18.4
Tuberculoma —*see also* Tuberculosis
  brain A17.81
  meninges (cerebral) (spinal) A17.1
  spinal cord A17.81
Tuberculosis, tubercular, tuberculous (calcification) (calcified) (caseous) (chromogenic acid-fast bacilli) (degeneration) (fibrocaseous) (fistula) (interstitial) (isolated circumscribed lesions) (necrosis) (parenchymatous) (ulcerative) A15.9
  with pneumoconiosis (any condition in J60-J64) J65
  abdomen (lymph gland) A18.39
  abscess (respiratory) A15.9
    bone A18.03
      hip A18.02
      knee A18.02
      sacrum A18.01
      specified site NEC A18.03
      spinal A18.01
      vertebra A18.01
    brain A17.81
    breast A18.89
    Cowper's gland A18.15
    dura (mater) (cerebral) (spinal) A17.81
    epidural (cerebral) (spinal) A17.81
    female pelvis A18.17
    frontal sinus A15.8
    genital organs NEC A18.10
    genitourinary A18.10
    gland (lymphatic) —*see* Tuberculosis, lymph gland
    hip A18.02
    intestine A18.32
    ischiorectal A18.32
    joint NEC A18.02
      hip A18.02
      knee A18.02
      specified NEC A18.02
      vertebral A18.01
    kidney A18.11
    knee A18.02
    latent Z22.7
    lumbar (spine) A18.01
    lung —*see* Tuberculosis, pulmonary
    meninges (cerebral) (spinal) A17.0
    muscle A18.09
    perianal (fistula) A18.32
    perinephritic A18.11
    perirectal A18.32
    rectum A18.32
    retropharyngeal A15.8
    sacrum A18.01
    scrofulous A18.2
    scrotum A18.15
    skin (primary) A18.4
    spinal cord A17.81
    spine or vertebra (column) A18.01
    subdiaphragmatic A18.31

Tuberculosis, tubercular, tuberculous (continued)
  abscess (continued)
    testis A18.15
    urinary A18.13
    uterus A18.17
  accessory sinus —*see* Tuberculosis, sinus
  Addison's disease A18.7
  adenitis —*see* Tuberculosis, lymph gland
  adenoids A15.8
  adenopathy —*see* Tuberculosis, lymph gland
  adherent pericardium A18.84
  adnexa (uteri) A18.17
  adrenal (capsule) (gland) A18.7
  alimentary canal A18.32
  anemia A18.89
  ankle (joint) (bone) A18.02
  anus A18.32
  apex, apical —*see* Tuberculosis, pulmonary
  appendicitis, appendix A18.32
  arachnoid A17.0
  artery, arteritis A18.89
    cerebral A18.89
  arthritis (chronic) (synovial) A18.02
    spine or vertebra (column) A18.01
  articular —*see* Tuberculosis, joint
  ascites A18.31
  asthma —*see* Tuberculosis, pulmonary
  axilla, axillary (gland) A18.2
  bladder A18.12
  bone A18.03
    hip A18.02
    knee A18.02
    limb NEC A18.03
    sacrum A18.01
    spine or vertebral column A18.01
  bowel (miliary) A18.32
  brain A17.81
  breast A18.89
  broad ligament A18.17
  bronchi, bronchial, bronchus A15.5
    ectasia, ectasis (bronchiectasis) —*see* Tuberculosis, pulmonary
    fistula A15.5
      primary (progressive) A15.7
    gland or node A15.4
      primary (progressive) A15.7
    lymph gland or node A15.4
      primary (progressive) A15.7
  bronchiectasis —*see* Tuberculosis, pulmonary
  bronchitis A15.5
  bronchopleural A15.6
  bronchopneumonia, bronchopneumonic —*see* Tuberculosis, pulmonary
  bronchorrhagia A15.5
  bronchotracheal A15.5
  bronze disease A18.7
  buccal cavity A18.83
  bulbourethral gland A18.15
  bursa A18.09
  cachexia A15.9
  cardiomyopathy A18.84
  caries —*see* Tuberculosis, bone
  cartilage A18.02
    intervertebral A18.01
  catarrhal —*see* Tuberculosis, respiratory
  cecum A18.32
  cellulitis (primary) A18.4
  cerebellum A17.81

Tuberculosis, tubercular, tuberculous (continued)
cerebral, cerebrum A17.81
cerebrospinal A17.81
 meninges A17.0
cervical (lymph gland or node) A18.2
cervicitis, cervix (uteri) A18.16
chest —see Tuberculosis, respiratory
chorioretinitis A18.53
choroid, choroiditis A18.53
ciliary body A18.54
colitis A18.32
collier's J65
colliquativa (primary) A18.4
colon A18.32
complex, primary A15.7
congenital P37.0
conjunctiva A18.59
connective tissue (systemic) A18.89
contact Z20.1
cornea (ulcer) A18.52
Cowper's gland A18.15
coxae A18.02
coxalgia A18.02
cul-de-sac of Douglas A18.17
curvature, spine A18.01
cutis (colliquativa) (primary) A18.4
cyst, ovary A18.18
cystitis A18.12
dactylitis A18.03
diarrhea A18.32
diffuse —see Tuberculosis, miliary
digestive tract A18.32
disseminated —see Tuberculosis, miliary
duodenum A18.32
dura (mater) (cerebral) (spinal) A17.0
 abscess (cerebral) (spinal) A17.81
dysentery A18.32
ear (inner) (middle) A18.6
 bone A18.03
 external (primary) A18.4
 skin (primary) A18.4
elbow A18.02
emphysema —see Tuberculosis, pulmonary
empyema A15.6
encephalitis A17.82
endarteritis A18.89
endocarditis A18.84
 aortic A18.84
 mitral A18.84
 pulmonary A18.84
 tricuspid A18.84
endocrine glands NEC A18.82
endometrium A18.17
enteric, enterica, enteritis A18.32
enterocolitis A18.32
epididymis, epididymitis A18.15
epidural abscess (cerebral) (spinal) A17.81
epiglottis A15.5
episcleritis A18.51
erythema (induratum) (nodosum) (primary) A18.4
esophagus A18.83
eustachian tube A18.6
exposure (to) Z20.1
exudative —see Tuberculosis, pulmonary
eye A18.50
eyelid (primary) (lupus) A18.4
fallopian tube (acute) (chronic) A18.17
fascia A18.09
fauces A15.8

Tuberculosis, tubercular, tuberculous (continued)
female pelvic inflammatory disease A18.17
finger A18.03
first infection A15.7
gallbladder A18.83
ganglion A18.09
gastritis A18.83
gastrocolic fistula A18.32
gastroenteritis A18.32
gastrointestinal tract A18.32
general, generalized —see Tuberculosis, miliary
genital organs A18.10
genitourinary A18.10
genu A18.02
glandula suprarenalis A18.7
glandular, general A18.2
glottis A15.5
grinder's J65
gum A18.83
hand A18.03
heart A18.84
hematogenous —see Tuberculosis, miliary
hemoptysis —see Tuberculosis, pulmonary
hemorrhage NEC —see Tuberculosis, pulmonary
hemothorax A15.6
hepatitis A18.83
hilar lymph nodes A15.4
 primary (progressive) A15.7
hip (joint) (disease) (bone) A18.02
hydropneumothorax A15.6
hydrothorax A15.6
hypoadrenalism A18.7
hypopharynx A15.8
ileocecal (hyperplastic) A18.32
ileocolitis A18.32
ileum A18.32
iliac spine (superior) A18.03
immunological findings only A15.7
indurativa (primary) A18.4
infantile A15.7
infection A15.9
 without clinical manifestations A15.7
infraclavicular gland A18.2
inguinal gland A18.2
inguinalis A18.2
intestine (any part) A18.32
iridocyclitis A18.54
iris, iritis A18.54
ischiorectal A18.32
jaw A18.03
jejunum A18.32
joint A18.02
 vertebral A18.01
keratitis (interstitial) A18.52
keratoconjunctivitis A18.52
kidney A18.11
knee (joint) A18.02
kyphosis, kyphoscoliosis A18.01
laryngitis A15.5
larynx A15.5
latent Z22.7
leptomeninges, leptomeningitis (cerebral) (spinal) A17.0
lichenoides (primary) A18.4
linguae A18.83
lip A18.83
liver A18.83
lordosis A18.01
lung —see Tuberculosis, pulmonary
lupus vulgaris A18.4

Tuberculosis, tubercular, tuberculous (continued)
lymph gland or node (peripheral) A18.2
 abdomen A18.39
 bronchial A15.4
  primary (progressive) A15.7
 cervical A18.2
 hilar A15.4
  primary (progressive) A15.7
 intrathoracic A15.4
  primary (progressive) A15.7
 mediastinal A15.4
  primary (progressive) A15.7
 mesenteric A18.39
 retroperitoneal A18.39
 tracheobronchial A15.4
  primary (progressive) A15.7
lymphadenitis —see Tuberculosis, lymph gland
lymphangitis —see Tuberculosis, lymph gland
lymphatic (gland) (vessel) —see Tuberculosis, lymph gland
mammary gland A18.89
marasmus A15.9
mastoiditis A18.03
mediastinal lymph gland or node A15.4
 primary (progressive) A15.7
mediastinitis A15.8
 primary (progressive) A15.7
mediastinum A15.8
 primary (progressive) A15.7
medulla A17.81
melanosis, Addisonian A18.7
meninges, meningitis (basilar) (cerebral) (cerebrospinal) (spinal) A17.0
meningoencephalitis A17.82
mesentery, mesenteric (gland or node) A18.39
miliary A19.9
 acute A19.2
  multiple sites A19.1
  single specified site A19.0
 chronic A19.8
 specified NEC A19.8
millstone makers' J65
miner's J65
molder's J65
mouth A18.83
multiple A19.9
 acute A19.1
 chronic A19.8
muscle A18.09
myelitis A17.82
myocardium, myocarditis A18.84
nasal (passage) (sinus) A15.8
nasopharynx A15.8
neck gland A18.2
nephritis A18.11
nerve (mononeuropathy) A17.83
nervous system A17.9
nose (septum) A15.8
ocular A18.50
omentum A18.31
oophoritis (acute) (chronic) A18.17
optic (nerve trunk) (papilla) A18.59
orbit A18.59
orchitis A18.15
organ, specified NEC A18.89
osseous —see Tuberculosis, bone
osteitis —see Tuberculosis, bone
osteomyelitis —see Tuberculosis, bone
otitis media A18.6
ovary, ovaritis (acute) (chronic) A18.17
oviduct (acute) (chronic) A18.17
pachymeningitis A17.0

Tuberculosis, tubercular, tuberculous (continued)
palate (soft) A18.83
pancreas A18.83
papulonecrotic (a) (primary) A18.4
parathyroid glands A18.82
paronychia (primary) A18.4
parotid gland or region A18.83
pelvis (bony) A18.03
penis A18.15
peribronchitis A15.5
pericardium, pericarditis A18.84
perichondritis, larynx A15.5
periostitis —see Tuberculosis, bone
perirectal fistula A18.32
peritoneum NEC A18.31
peritonitis A18.31
pharynx, pharyngitis A15.8
phlyctenulosis (keratoconjunctivitis) A18.52
phthisis NEC —see Tuberculosis, pulmonary
pituitary gland A18.82
pleura, pleural, pleurisy, pleuritis (fibrinous) (obliterative) (purulent) (simple plastic) (with effusion) A15.6
 primary (progressive) A15.7
pneumonia, pneumonic —see Tuberculosis, pulmonary
pneumothorax (spontaneous) (tense valvular) —see Tuberculosis, pulmonary
polyneuropathy A17.89
polyserositis A19.9
 acute A19.1
 chronic A19.8
potter's J65
prepuce A18.15
primary (complex) A15.7
proctitis A18.32
prostate, prostatitis A18.14
pulmonalis —see Tuberculosis, pulmonary
pulmonary (cavitated) (fibrotic) (infiltrative) (nodular) A15.0
 childhood type or first infection A15.7
 primary (complex) A15.7
pyelitis A18.11
pyelonephritis A18.11
pyemia —see Tuberculosis, miliary
pyonephrosis A18.11
pyopneumothorax A15.6
pyothorax A15.6
rectum (fistula) (with abscess) A18.32
reinfection stage —see Tuberculosis, pulmonary
renal A18.11
renis A18.11
respiratory A15.9
 primary A15.7
 specified site NEC A15.8
retina, retinitis A18.53
retroperitoneal (lymph gland or node) A18.39
rheumatism NEC A18.09
rhinitis A15.8
sacroiliac (joint) A18.01
sacrum A18.01
salivary gland A18.83
salpingitis (acute) (chronic) A18.17
sandblaster's J65
sclera A18.51
scoliosis A18.01
scrofulous A18.2
scrotum A18.15
seminal tract or vesicle A18.15

329

Tuberculosis, tubercular, tuberculous *(continued)*
 senile A15.9
 septic —*see* Tuberculosis, miliary
 shoulder (joint) A18.02
  blade A18.03
 sigmoid A18.32
 sinus (any nasal) A15.8
  bone A18.03
  epididymis A18.15
 skeletal NEC A18.03
 skin (any site) (primary) A18.4
 small intestine A18.32
 soft palate A18.83
 spermatic cord A18.15
 spine, spinal (column) A18.01
  cord A17.81
  medulla A17.81
  membrane A17.0
  meninges A17.0
 spleen, splenitis A18.85
 spondylitis A18.01
 sternoclavicular joint A18.02
 stomach A18.83
 stonemason's J65
 subcutaneous tissue (cellular) (primary) A18.4
 subcutis (primary) A18.4
 subdeltoid bursa A18.83
 submaxillary (region) A18.83
 supraclavicular gland A18.2
 suprarenal (capsule) (gland) A18.7
 swelling, joint (*see also* category M01) (*see also* Tuberculosis, joint) A18.02
 symphysis pubis A18.02
 synovitis A18.09
  articular A18.02
  spine or vertebra A18.01
 systemic —*see* Tuberculosis, miliary
 tarsitis A18.4
 tendon (sheath) —*see* Tuberculosis, tenosynovitis
 tenosynovitis A18.09
  spine or vertebra A18.01
 testis A18.15
 throat A15.8
 thymus gland A18.82
 thyroid gland A18.81
 tongue A18.83
 tonsil, tonsillitis A15.8
 trachea, tracheal A15.5
  lymph gland or node A15.4
   primary (progressive) A15.7
 tracheobronchial A15.5
  lymph gland or node A15.4
   primary (progressive) A15.7
 tubal (acute) (chronic) A18.17
 tunica vaginalis A18.15
 ulcer (skin) (primary) A18.4
  bowel or intestine A18.32
  specified NEC - code under Tuberculosis, by site
 unspecified site A15.9
 ureter A18.11
 urethra, urethral (gland) A18.13
 urinary organ or tract A18.13
 uterus A18.17
 uveal tract A18.54
 uvula A18.83
 vagina A18.18
 vas deferens A18.15
 verruca, verrucosa (cutis) (primary) A18.4
 vertebra (column) A18.01
 vesiculitis A18.15
 vulva A18.18
 wrist (joint) A18.02

Tuberculum
 Carabelli —*see* Note at K00.2
 occlusal —*see* Note at K00.2
 paramolare K00.2

Tuberosity, enitre maxillary M26.07

Tuberous sclerosis (brain) Q85.1

Tubo-ovarian —*see* condition

Tuboplasty, after previous sterilization Z31.0
 aftercare Z31.42

Tubotympanitis, catarrhal (chronic) —*see* Otitis, media, nonsuppurative, chronic, serous

Tularemia A21.9
 with
  conjunctivitis A21.1
  pneumonia A21.2
 abdominal A21.3
 bronchopneumonic A21.2
 conjunctivitis A21.1
 cryptogenic A21.3
 enteric A21.3
 gastrointestinal A21.3
 generalized A21.7
 ingestion A21.3
 intestinal A21.3
 oculoglandular A21.1
 ophthalmic A21.1
 pneumonia (any), pneumonic A21.2
 pulmonary A21.2
 sepsis A21.7
 specified NEC A21.8
 typhoidal A21.7
 ulceroglandular A21.0

Tularensis conjunctivitis A21.1

Tumefaction —*see also* Swelling
 liver —*see* Hypertrophy, liver

Tumor —*see also* Neoplasm, unspecified behavior, by site
 acinar cell —*see* Neoplasm, uncertain behavior, by site
 acinic cell —*see* Neoplasm, uncertain behavior, by site
 adenocarcinoid —*see* Neoplasm, malignant, by site
 adenomatoid —*see also* Neoplasm, benign, by site
  odontogenic —*see* Cyst, calcifying odontogenic
 adnexal (skin) —*see* Neoplasm, skin, benign, by site
 adrenal
  cortical (benign) D35.0-
   malignant C74.0-
  rest —*see* Neoplasm, benign, by site
 alpha-cell
  malignant
   pancreas C25.4
   specified site NEC —*see* Neoplasm, malignant, by site
   unspecified site C25.4
  pancreas D13.7
  specified site NEC —*see* Neoplasm, benign, by site
  unspecified site D13.7
 aneurysmal —*see* Aneurysm
 aortic body D44.7
  malignant C75.5
 Askin's —*see* Neoplasm, connective tissue, malignant
 basal cell (*see also* Neoplasm, skin, uncertain behavior) D48.5
 Bednar —*see* Neoplasm, skin, malignant

Tumor *(continued)*
 benign (unclassified) —*see* Neoplasm, benign, by site
 beta-cell
  malignant
   pancreas C25.4
   specified site NEC —*see* Neoplasm, malignant, by site
   unspecified site C25.4
  pancreas D13.7
  specified site NEC —*see* Neoplasm, benign, by site
  unspecified site D13.7
 Brenner D27.9
  borderline malignancy D39.1-
  malignant C56-
  proliferating D39.1-
 bronchial alveolar, intravascular D38.1
 Brooke's —*see* Neoplasm, skin, benign
 brown fat —*see* Lipoma
 Burkitt —*see* Lymphoma, Burkitt
 calcifying epithelial odontogenic —*see* Cyst, calcifying
 odontogenic
 carcinoid D3A.00
  benign D3A.00
   appendix D3A.020
   ascending colon D3A.022
   bronchus (lung) D3A.090
   cecum D3A.021
   colon D3A.029
   descending colon D3A.024
   duodenum D3A.010
   foregut NOS D3A.094
   hindgut NOS D3A.096
   ileum D3A.012
   jejunum D3A.011
   kidney D3A.093
   large intestine D3A.029
   lung (bronchus) D3A.090
   midgut NOS D3A.095
   rectum D3A.026
   sigmoid colon D3A.025
   small intestine D3A.019
   specified NEC D3A.098
   stomach D3A.092
   thymus D3A.091
   transverse colon D3A.023
  malignant C7A.00
   appendix C7A.020
   ascending colon C7A.022
   bronchus (lung) C7A.090
   cecum C7A.021
   colon C7A.029
   descending colon C7A.024
   duodenum C7A.010
   foregut NOS C7A.094
   hindgut NOS C7A.096
   ileum C7A.012
   jejunum C7A.011
   kidney C7A.093
   large intestine C7A.029
   lung (bronchus) C7A.090
   midgut NOS C7A.095
   rectum C7A.026
   sigmoid colon C7A.025
   small intestine C7A.019
   specified NEC C7A.098
   stomach C7A.092
   thymus C7A.091
   transverse colon C7A.023
  mesentary metastasis C7B.04
  secondary C7B.00
   bone C7B.03
   distant lymph nodes C7B.01
   liver C7B.02
   peritoneum C7B.04
   specified NEC C7B.09

Tumor *(continued)*
 carotid body D44.6
  malignant C75.4
 cells —*see also* Neoplasm, unspecified behavior, by site
  benign —*see* Neoplasm, benign, by site
  malignant —*see* Neoplasm, malignant, by site
  uncertain whether benign or malignant —*see* Neoplasm, uncertain behavior, by site
 cervix, in pregnancy or childbirth —*see* Pregnancy, complicated by, tumor, cervix
 chondromatous giant cell —*see* Neoplasm, bone, benign
 chromaffin —*see also* Neoplasm, benign, by site
  malignant —*see* Neoplasm, malignant, by site
 Cock's peculiar L72.3
 Codman's —*see* Neoplasm, bone, benign
 dentigerous, mixed —*see* Cyst, calcifying odontogenic
 dermoid —*see* Neoplasm, benign, by site
  with malignant transformation C56-
 desmoid (extra-abdominal) —*see also* Neoplasm, connective tissue, uncertain behavior
  abdominal —*see* Neoplasm, connective tissue, uncertain behavior
 embolus —*see* Neoplasm, secondary, by site
 embryonal (mixed) —*see also* Neoplasm, uncertain behavior, by site
  liver C22.7
 endodermal sinus
  specified site —*see* Neoplasm, malignant, by site
  unspecified site
   female C56.-
   male C62.90
 epithelial
  benign —*see* Neoplasm, benign, by site
  malignant —*see* Neoplasm, malignant, by site
 Ewing's —*see* Neoplasm, bone, malignant, by site
 fatty —*see* Lipoma
 fibroid —*see* Leiomyoma
 G cell
  malignant
   pancreas C25.4
   specified site NEC —*see* Neoplasm, malignant, by site
   unspecified site C25.4
  specified site —*see* Neoplasm, uncertain behavior, by site
  unspecified site D37.8
 germ cell —*see also* Neoplasm, malignant, by site
  mixed —*see* Neoplasm, malignant, by site
 ghost cell, odontogenic —*see* Cyst, calcifying odontogenic
 giant cell —*see also* Neoplasm, uncertain behavior, by site
  bone D48.0
   malignant —*see* Neoplasm, bone, malignant
  chondromatous —*see* Neoplasm, bone, benign
  malignant —*see* Neoplasm, malignant, by site

Tumor *(continued)*
- giant cell *(continued)*
  - soft parts —*see* Neoplasm, connective tissue, uncertain behavior
    - malignant —*see* Neoplasm, connective tissue, malignant
- glomus D18.00
  - intra-abdominal D18.03
  - intracranial D18.02
  - jugulare D44.7
    - malignant C75.5
  - skin D18.01
  - specified site NEC D18.09
- gonadal stromal —*see* Neoplasm, uncertain behavior, by site
- granular cell —*see also* Neoplasm, connective tissue, benign
  - malignant —*see* Neoplasm, connective tissue, malignant
- granulosa cell D39.1-
  - juvenile D39.1-
  - malignant C56-
- granulosa cell-theca cell D39.1-
  - malignant C56-
- Grawitz's C64-
- hemorrhoidal —*see* Hemorrhoids
- hilar cell D27-
- hilus cell D27-
- Hurthle cell (benign) D34
  - malignant C73
- hydatid —*see* Echinococcus
- hypernephroid —*see also* Neoplasm, uncertain behavior, by site
- interstitial cell —*see also* Neoplasm, uncertain behavior, by site
  - benign —*see* Neoplasm, benign, by site
  - malignant —*see* Neoplasm, malignant, by site
- intravascular bronchial alveolar D38.1
- islet cell —*see* Neoplasm, benign, by site
  - malignant —*see* Neoplasm, malignant, by site
    - pancreas C25.4
    - specified site NEC —*see* Neoplasm, malignant, by site
    - unspecified site C25.4
  - pancreas D13.7
  - specified site NEC —*see* Neoplasm, benign, by site
  - unspecified site D13.7
- juxtaglomerular D41.0-
- Klatskin's C24.0
- Krukenberg's C79.6-
- Leydig cell —*see* Neoplasm, uncertain behavior, by site
  - benign —*see* Neoplasm, benign, by site
    - specified site —*see* Neoplasm, benign, by site
    - unspecified site
      - female D27.9
      - male D29.20
  - malignant —*see* Neoplasm, malignant, by site
    - specified site —*see* Neoplasm, malignant, by site
    - unspecified site
      - female C56.9
      - male C62.90
  - specified site —*see* Neoplasm, uncertain behavior, by site
  - unspecified site
    - female D39.10
    - male D40.10

Tumor *(continued)*
- lipid cell, ovary D27-
- lipoid cell, ovary D27-
- malignant *(see also* Neoplasm, malignant, by site) C80.1
  - fusiform cell (type) C80.1
  - giant cell (type) C80.1
  - localized, plasma cell —*see* Plasmacytoma, solitary
  - mixed NEC C80.1
  - small cell (type) C80.1
  - spindle cell (type) C80.1
  - unclassified C80.1
- mast cell D47.09
- melanotic, neuroectodermal —*see* Neoplasm, benign, by site
- Merkel cell —*see* Carcinoma, Merkel cell
- mesenchymal
  - malignant —*see* Neoplasm, connective tissue, malignant
  - mixed —*see* Neoplasm, connective tissue, uncertain behavior
- mesodermal, mixed —*see also* Neoplasm, malignant, by site
  - liver C22.4
- mesonephric —*see also* Neoplasm, uncertain behavior, by site
  - malignant —*see* Neoplasm, malignant, by site
- metastatic
  - from specified site —*see* Neoplasm, malignant, by site
  - of specified site —*see* Neoplasm, malignant, by site
  - to specified site —*see* Neoplasm, secondary, by site
- mixed NEC —*see also* Neoplasm, benign, by site
  - malignant —*see* Neoplasm, malignant, by site
- mucinous of low malignant potential
  - specified site —*see* Neoplasm, malignant, by site
  - unspecified site C56.9
- mucocarcinoid
  - specified site —*see* Neoplasm, malignant, by site
  - unspecified site C18.1
- mucoepidermoid —*see* Neoplasm, uncertain behavior, by site
- Müllerian, mixed
  - specified site —*see* Neoplasm, malignant, by site
  - unspecified site C54.9
- myoepithelial —*see* Neoplasm, benign, by site
- neuroectodermal (peripheral) —*see* Neoplasm, malignant, by site
  - primitive
    - specified site —*see* Neoplasm, malignant, by site
    - unspecified site C71.9
- neuroendocrine D3A.8
  - malignant poorly differentiated C7A.1
  - secondary NEC C7B.8
  - specified NEC C7A.8
- neurogenic olfactory C30.0
- nonencapsulated sclerosing C73
- odontogenic (adenomatoid) (benign) (calcifying epithelial) (keratocystic) (squamous) —*see* Cyst, calcifying odontogenic
  - malignant C41.1
    - upper jaw (bone) C41.0
- ovarian stromal D39.1-
- ovary, in pregnancy —*see* Pregnancy, complicated by

Tumor *(continued)*
- pacinian —*see* Neoplasm, skin, benign
- Pancoast's —*see* Pancoast's syndrome
- papillary —*see also* Papilloma
  - cystic D37.9
  - mucinous of low malignant potential C56-
    - specified site —*see* Neoplasm, malignant, by site
    - unspecified site C56.9
  - serous of low malignant potential
    - specified site —*see* Neoplasm, malignant, by site
    - unspecified site C56.9
- pelvic, in pregnancy or childbirth —*see* Pregnancy, complicated by
- phantom F45.8
- phyllodes D48.6-
  - benign D24-
  - malignant —*see* Neoplasm, breast, malignant
- Pindborg —*see* Cyst, calcifying odontogenic
- placental site trophoblastic D39.2
- plasma cell (malignant) (localized) —*see* Plasmacytoma, solitary
- polyvesicular vitelline
  - specified site —*see* Neoplasm, malignant, by site
  - unspecified site
    - female C56.9
    - male C62.90
- Pott's puffy —*see* Osteomyelitis, specified NEC
- Rathke's pouch D44.3
- retinal anlage —*see* Neoplasm, benign, by site
- salivary gland type, mixed —*see* Neoplasm, salivary gland, benign
  - malignant —*see* Neoplasm, salivary gland, malignant
- Sampson's N80.10-
- Schmincke's —*see* Neoplasm, nasopharynx, malignant
- sclerosing stromal D27-
- sebaceous —*see* Cyst, sebaceous
- secondary —*see* Neoplasm, secondary, by site
  - carcinoid C7B.00
    - bone C7B.03
    - distant lymph nodes C7B.01
    - liver C7B.02
    - peritoneum C7B.04
    - specified NEC C7B.09
  - neuroendocrine NEC C7B.8
- serous of low malignant potential
  - specified site —*see* Neoplasm, malignant, by site
  - unspecified site C56.9
- Sertoli cell —*see* Neoplasm, benign, by site
  - with lipid storage
    - specified site —*see* Neoplasm, benign, by site
    - unspecified site
      - female D27.9
      - male D29.20
  - specified site —*see* Neoplasm, benign, by site
  - unspecified site
    - female D27.9
    - male D29.20
- Sertoli-Leydig cell —*see* Neoplasm, benign, by site
  - specified site —*see* Neoplasm, benign, by site

Tumor *(continued)*
- Sertoli-Leydig cell *(continued)*
  - unspecified site
    - female D27.9
    - male D29.20
- sex cord (-stromal) —*see* Neoplasm, uncertain behavior, by site
  - with annular tubules D39.1-
- skin appendage —*see* Neoplasm, skin, benign
- smooth muscle —*see* Neoplasm, connective tissue, uncertain behavior
- soft tissue
  - benign —*see* Neoplasm, connective tissue, benign
  - malignant —*see* Neoplasm, connective tissue, malignant
- sternomastoid (congenital) Q68.0
- stromal
  - endometrial D39.0
  - gastric D48.19
    - benign D21.4
    - malignant C16.9
    - uncertain behavior D48.19
  - gastrointestinal C49.A-
    - benign D21.4
    - esophagus C49.A1
    - malignant C49.A0
      - colon C49.A4
      - duodenum C49.A3
      - esophagus C49.A1
      - ileum C49.A3
      - jejunum C49.A3
      - Meckel diverticulum C49.A3
      - large intestine C49.A4
      - omentum C49.A9
      - peritoneum C49.A9
      - rectum C49.A5
      - small intestine C49.A3
      - specified site NEC C49.A9
      - stomach C49.A2
    - rectum C49.A5
    - small intestine C49.A3
    - specified site NEC C49.A9
    - stomach C49.A2
    - uncertain behavior D48.19
  - intestine
    - benign D21.4
    - malignant
      - large C49.A4
      - small C49.A3
    - uncertain behavior D48.19
  - ovarian D39.1-
  - stomach C49.A2
    - benign D21.4
    - malignant C49.A2
    - uncertain behavior D48.19
- testicular D40.10
- sweat gland —*see also* Neoplasm, skin, uncertain behavior
  - benign —*see* Neoplasm, skin, benign
  - malignant —*see* Neoplasm, skin, malignant
- syphilitic, brain A52.17
- testicular stromal D40.1-
- theca cell D27.-
- theca cell-granulosa cell D39.1-
- Triton, malignant —*see* Neoplasm, nerve, malignant
- trophoblastic, placental site D39.2
- turban D23.4
- uterus (body), in pregnancy or childbirth —*see* Pregnancy, complicated by, tumor, uterus

Tumor (continued)
vagina, in pregnancy or childbirth —*see* Pregnancy, complicated by
varicose —*see* Varix
von Recklinghausen's —*see* Neurofibromatosis
vulva or perineum, in pregnancy or childbirth —*see* Pregnancy, complicated by causing obstructed labor O65.5
Warthin's —*see* Neoplasm, salivary gland, benign
Wilms' C64-
yolk sac —*see* Neoplasm, malignant, by site
specified site —*see* Neoplasm, malignant, by site
unspecified site
female C56.9
male C62.90

Tumor lysis syndrome (following antineoplastic chemotherapy) (spontaneous) **NEC** E88.3

Tumorlet —*see* Neoplasm, uncertain behavior, by site

Tungiasis B88.1

Tunica vasculosa lentis Q12.2

Turban tumor D23.4

Türck's trachoma J37.0

Turner-Kieser syndrome Q87.2

Turner-like syndrome Q87.19

Turner's
hypoplasia (tooth) K00.4
syndrome Q96.9
specified NEC Q96.8
tooth K00.4

Turner-Ullrich syndrome Q96.9

Tussis convulsiva —*see* Whooping cough

Twiddler's syndrome (due to)
automatic implantable defibrillator T82.198
cardiac pacemaker T82.198

Twilight state
epileptic F05
psychogenic F44.89

Twin (newborn) —*see also* Newborn, twin
conjoined Q89.4
pregnancy —*see* Pregnancy, twin

Twinning, teeth K00.2

Twist, twisted
bowel, colon or intestine K56.2
hair (congenital) Q84.1
mesentery K56.2
omentum K56.2
organ or site, congenital NEC —*see* Anomaly, by site
ovarian pedicle —*see* Torsion, ovary

Twitching R25.3

Tylosis (acquired) L84
buccalis K13.29
linguae K13.29
palmaris et plantaris (congenital) (inherited) Q82.8
acquired L85.1

Tympanism R14.0

Tympanites (abdominal) (intestinal) R14.0

Tympanitis —*see* Myringitis

Tympanosclerosis —*see* subcategory H74.0

Tympanum —*see* condition

Tympany
abdomen R14.0
chest R09.89

Type A behavior pattern Z73.1

Typhlitis —*see* Cecitis

Typhoenteritis —*see* Typhoid

Typhoid (abortive) (ambulant) (any site) (clinical) (fever) (hemorrhagic) (infection) (intermittent) (malignant) (rheumatic) (Widal negative) A01.00
with pneumonia A01.03
abdominal A01.09
arthritis A01.04
carrier (suspected) of Z22.0
cholecystitis (current) A01.09
endocarditis A01.02
heart involvement A01.02
inoculation reaction —*see* Complications, vaccination
meningitis A01.01
mesenteric lymph nodes A01.09
myocarditis A01.02
osteomyelitis A01.05
perichondritis, larynx A01.09
pneumonia A01.03
spine A01.05
specified NEC A01.09
ulcer (perforating) A01.09

Typhomalaria (fever) —*see* Malaria

Typhomania A01.00

Typhoperitonitis A01.09

Typhus (fever) A75.9
abdominal, abdominalis —*see* Typhoid
African tick A77.1
amarillic A95.9
brain A75.9 *[G94]*
cerebral A75.9 *[G94]*
classical A75.0
due to Rickettsia
prowazekii A75.0
recrudescent A75.1
tsutsugamushi A75.3
typhi A75.2
endemic (flea-borne) A75.2
epidemic (louse-borne) A75.0
exanthematic NEC A75.0
exanthematicus SAI A75.0
brillii SAI A75.1
mexicanus SAI A75.2
typhus murinus A75.2
flea-borne A75.2
India tick A77.1
Kenya (tick) A77.1
louse-borne A75.0
Mexican A75.2
mite-borne A75.3
murine A75.2
North Asian tick-borne A77.2
Orientia Tsutsugamushi (scrub typhus) A75.3
petechial A75.9
Queensland tick A77.3
rat A75.2
recrudescent A75.1
recurrens —*see* Fever, relapsing
Sao Paulo A77.0
scrub (China) (India) (Malaysia) (New Guinea) A75.3
shop (of Malaysia) A75.2
Siberian tick A77.2
tick-borne A77.9
tropical (mite-borne) A75.3

Tyrosinemia E70.21
newborn, transitory P74.5

Tyrosinosis E70.21

Tyrosinuria E70.29

U

Uhl's anomaly or disease Q24.8

Ulcer, ulcerated, ulcerating, ulceration, ulcerative
alveolar process M27.3
amebic (intestine) A06.1
skin A06.7
anastomotic —*see* Ulcer, gastrojejunal
anorectal K62.6
antral —*see* Ulcer, stomach
anus (sphincter) (solitary) K62.6
aorta —*see* Aneurysm
aphthous (oral) (recurrent) K12.0
genital organ(s)
female N76.6
male N50.89
artery I77.2
atrophic —*see* Ulcer, skin
decubitus —*see* Ulcer, pressure, by site
back L98.429
with
bone involvement without evidence of necrosis L98.426
bone necrosis L98.424
exposed fat layer L98.422
muscle involvement without evidence of necrosis L98.425
muscle necrosis L98.423
skin breakdown only L98.421
specified severity NEC L98.428
Barrett's (esophagus) K22.10
with bleeding K22.11
bile duct (common) (hepatic) K83.8
bladder (solitary) (sphincter) NEC N32.89
bilharzial B65.9 *[N33]*
in schistosomiasis (bilharzial) B65.9 *[N33]*
submucosal —*see* Cystitis, interstitial
tuberculous A18.12
bleeding K27.4
bone —*see* Osteomyelitis, specified type NEC
bowel —*see* Ulcer, intestine
breast N61.1
bronchus J98.09
buccal (cavity) (traumatic) K12.1
Buruli A31.1
buttock L98.419
with
bone involvement without evidence of necrosis L98.416
bone necrosis L98.414
exposed fat layer L98.412
muscle involvement without evidence of necrosis L98.415
muscle necrosis L98.413
skin breakdown only L98.411
specified severity NEC L98.418
cameron —*see* Ulcer, stomach
cancerous —*see* Neoplasm, malignant, by site
cardia K22.10
with bleeding K22.11
cardioesophageal (peptic) K22.10
with bleeding K22.11

Ulcer, ulcerated, ulcerating, ulceration, ulcerative
(continued)
cecum —*see* Ulcer, intestine
cervix (uteri) (decubitus) (trophic) N86
with cervicitis N72
chancroidal A57
chiclero B55.1
chronic (cause unknown) —*see* Ulcer, skin
Cochin-China B55.1
colon —*see* Ulcer, intestine
conjunctiva H10.89
cornea H16.00-
with hypopyon H16.03-
central H16.01-
dendritic (herpes simplex) B00.52
marginal H16.04-
Mooren's H16.05-
mycotic H16.06-
perforated H16.07-
ring H16.02-
tuberculous (phlyctenular) A18.52
corpus cavernosum (chronic) N48.5
crural —*see* Ulcer, lower limb
Curling's —*see* Ulcer, peptic, acute
Cushing's —*see* Ulcer, peptic, acute
cystic duct K82.8
cystitis (interstitial) —*see* Cystitis, interstitial
decubitus —*see* Ulcer, pressure, by site
dendritic, cornea (herpes simplex) B00.52
diabetes, diabetic —*see* Diabetes, ulcer
Dieulafoy's K25.0
due to
infection NEC —*see* Ulcer, skin
radiation NEC L59.8
trophic disturbance (any region) —*see* Ulcer, skin
X-ray L58.1
duodenum, duodenal (eroded) (peptic) K26.9
with
hemorrhage K26.4
and perforation K26.6
perforation K26.5
acute K26.3
with
hemorrhage K26.0
and perforation K26.2
perforation K26.1
chronic (erosive) K26.7
with
hemorrhage K26.4
and perforation K26.6
perforation K26.5
dysenteric A09
elusive —*see* Cystitis, interstitial
endocarditis (acute) (chronic) (subacute) I28.8
epiglottis J38.7
esophagus (peptic) K22.10
with bleeding K22.11
due to
aspirin K22.10
with bleeding K22.11
gastrointestinal reflux disease (without bleeding) K21.00
with bleeding K21.01
ingestion of chemical or medicament K22.10
with bleeding K22.11
fungal K22.10
with bleeding K22.11

Ulcer, ulcerated, ulcerating, ulceration, ulcerative *(continued)*
  esophagus *(continued)*
    infective K22.10
      with bleeding K22.11
    varicose —*see* Varix, esophagus
  eyelid (region) H01.8
  fauces J39.2
  Fenwick (-Hunner) (solitary) —*see* Cystitis, interstitial
  fistulous —*see* Ulcer, skin
  foot (indolent) (trophic) —*see* Ulcer, lower limb
  frambesial, initial A66.0
  frenum (tongue) K14.0
  gallbladder or duct K82.8
  gangrenous —*see* Gangrene
  gastric —*see* Ulcer, stomach
  gastrocolic —*see* Ulcer, gastrojejunal
  gastroduodenal —*see* Ulcer, peptic
  gastroesophageal —*see* Ulcer, stomach
  gastrointestinal —*see* Ulcer, gastrojejunal
  gastrojejunal (peptic) K28.9
    with
      hemorrhage K28.4
        and perforation K28.6
      perforation K28.5
    acute K28.3
      with
        hemorrhage K28.0
          and perforation K28.2
        perforation K28.1
    chronic K28.7
      with
        hemorrhage K28.4
          and perforation K28.6
        perforation K28.5
  gastrojejunocolic —*see* Ulcer, gastrojejunal
  gingiva K06.8
  gingivitis K05.10
    nonplaque induced K05.11
    plaque induced K05.10
  glottis J38.7
  granuloma of pudenda A58
  gum K06.8
  gumma, due to yaws A66.4
  heel —*see* Ulcer, lower limb
  hemorrhoid (*see also* Hemorrhoids, by degree) K64.8
  Hunner's —*see* Cystitis, interstitial
  hypopharynx J39.2
  hypopyon (chronic) (subacute) —*see* Ulcer, cornea, with hypopyon
  hypostaticum —*see* Ulcer, varicose
  ileum —*see* Ulcer, intestine
  intestine, intestinal K63.3
    with perforation K63.1
    amebic A06.1
    duodenal —*see* Ulcer, duodenum
    granulocytopenic (with hemorrhage) —*see* Neutropenia
    marginal —*see* Ulcer, gastrojejunal
    perforating K63.1
      newborn P78.0
    primary, small intestine K63.3
    rectum K62.6
    stercoraceous, stercoral K63.3
    tuberculous A18.32
    typhoid (fever) —*see* Typhoid
    varicose I86.8
  jejunum, jejunal —*see* Ulcer, gastrojejunal
  keratitis —*see* Ulcer, cornea
  knee —*see* Ulcer, lower limb

Ulcer, ulcerated, ulcerating, ulceration, ulcerative *(continued)*
  labium (majus) (minus) N76.6
  laryngitis —*see* Laryngitis
  larynx (aphthous) (contact) J38.7
    diphtheritic A36.2
  leg —*see* Ulcer, lower limb
  lip K13.0
  Lipschütz's N76.6
  lower limb (atrophic) (chronic) (neurogenic) (perforating) (pyogenic) (trophic) (tropical) L97.909
    with
      bone involvement without evidence of necrosis L97.906
      bone necrosis L97.904
      exposed fat layer L97.902
      muscle involvement without evidence of necrosis L97.905
      muscle necrosis L97.903
      skin breakdown only L97.901
      specified severity NEC L97.908
    ankle L97.309
      with
        bone involvement without evidence of necrosis L97.306
        bone necrosis L97.304
        exposed fat layer L97.302
        muscle involvement without evidence of necrosis L97.305
        muscle necrosis L97.303
        skin breakdown only L97.301
        specified severity NEC L97.308
      left L97.329
        with
          bone involvement without evidence of necrosis L97.326
          bone necrosis L97.324
          exposed fat layer L97.322
          muscle involvement without evidence of necrosis L97.325
          muscle necrosis L97.323
          skin breakdown only L97.321
          specified severity NEC L97.328
      right L97.319
        with
          bone involvement without evidence of necrosis L97.316
          bone necrosis L97.314
          exposed fat layer L97.312
          muscle involvement without evidence of necrosis L97.315
          muscle necrosis L97.313
          skin breakdown only L97.311
          specified severity NEC L97.318
    calf L97.209
      with
        bone involvement without evidence of necrosis L97.206
        bone necrosis L97.204
        exposed fat layer L97.202
        muscle involvement without evidence of necrosis L97.205
        muscle necrosis L97.203

Ulcer, ulcerated, ulcerating, ulceration, ulcerative *(continued)*
  lower limb *(continued)*
    calf *(continued)*
      with *(continued)*
        skin breakdown only L97.201
        specified severity NEC L97.208
      left L97.229
        with
          bone involvement without evidence of necrosis L97.226
          bone necrosis L97.224
          exposed fat layer L97.222
          muscle involvement without evidence of necrosis L97.225
          muscle necrosis L97.223
          skin breakdown only L97.221
          specified severity NEC L97.228
      right L97.219
        with
          bone involvement without evidence of necrosis L97.216
          bone necrosis L97.214
          exposed fat layer L97.212
          muscle involvement without evidence of necrosis L97.215
          muscle necrosis L97.213
          skin breakdown only L97.211
          specified severity NEC L97.218
    decubitus —*see* Ulcer, pressure, by site
    foot specified NEC L97.509
      with
        bone involvement without evidence of necrosis L97.506
        bone necrosis L97.504
        exposed fat layer L97.502
        muscle involvement without evidence of necrosis L97.505
        muscle necrosis L97.503
        skin breakdown only L97.501
        specified severity NEC L97.508
      left L97.529
        with
          bone involvement without evidence of necrosis L97.526
          bone necrosis L97.524
          exposed fat layer L97.522
          muscle involvement without evidence of necrosis L97.525
          muscle necrosis L97.523
          skin breakdown only L97.521
          specified severity NEC L97.528
      right L97.519
        with
          bone involvement without evidence of necrosis L97.516

Ulcer, ulcerated, ulcerating, ulceration, ulcerative *(continued)*
  lower limb *(continued)*
    foot specified NEC *(continued)*
      right *(continued)*
        with *(continued)*
          bone necrosis L97.514
          exposed fat layer L97.512
          muscle involvement without evidence of necrosis L97.515
          muscle necrosis L97.513
          skin breakdown only L97.511
          specified severity NEC L97.518
    heel L97.409
      with
        bone involvement without evidence of necrosis L97.406
        bone necrosis L97.404
        exposed fat layer L97.402
        muscle involvement without evidence of necrosis L97.405
        muscle necrosis L97.403
        skin breakdown only L97.401
        specified severity NEC L97.408
      left L97.429
        with
          bone involvement without evidence of necrosis L97.426
          bone necrosis L97.424
          exposed fat layer L97.422
          muscle involvement without evidence of necrosis L97.425
          muscle necrosis L97.423
          skin breakdown only L97.421
          specified severity NEC L97.428
      right L97.419
        with
          bone involvement without evidence of necrosis L97.416
          bone necrosis L97.414
          exposed fat layer L97.412
          muscle involvement without evidence of necrosis L97.415
          muscle necrosis L97.413
          skin breakdown only L97.411
          specified severity NEC L97.418
    left L97.929
      with
        bone involvement without evidence of necrosis L97.926
        bone necrosis L97.924
        exposed fat layer L97.922
        muscle involvement without evidence of necrosis L97.925
        muscle necrosis L97.923
        skin breakdown only L97.921
        specified severity NEC L97.928

Ulcer, ulcerated, ulcerating, ulceration, ulcerative *(continued)*
- lower limb *(continued)*
  - lower leg NOS L97.909
    - with
      - bone involvement without evidence of necrosis L97.906
      - bone necrosis L97.904
      - exposed fat layer L97.902
      - muscle involvement without evidence of necrosis L97.905
      - muscle necrosis L97.903
      - skin breakdown only L97.901
      - specified severity NEC L97.908
    - left L97.929
      - with
        - bone involvement without evidence of necrosis L97.926
        - bone necrosis L97.924
        - exposed fat layer L97.922
        - muscle involvement without evidence of necrosis L97.925
        - muscle necrosis L97.923
        - skin breakdown only L97.921
        - specified severity NEC L97.928
    - right L97.919
      - with
        - bone involvement without evidence of necrosis L97.916
        - bone necrosis L97.914
        - exposed fat layer L97.912
        - muscle involvement without evidence of necrosis L97.915
        - muscle necrosis L97.913
        - skin breakdown only L97.911
        - specified severity NEC L97.918
    - specified site NEC L97.809
      - with
        - bone involvement without evidence of necrosis L97.806
        - bone necrosis L97.804
        - exposed fat layer L97.802
        - muscle involvement without evidence of necrosis L97.805
        - muscle necrosis L97.803
        - skin breakdown only L97.801
        - specified severity NEC L97.808
      - left L97.829
        - with
          - bone involvement without evidence of necrosis L97.826
          - bone necrosis L97.824
          - exposed fat layer L97.822
          - muscle involvement without evidence of necrosis L97.825
          - muscle necrosis L97.823
          - skin breakdown only L97.821
          - specified severity NEC L97.828
        - right L97.819
          - with
            - bone involvement without evidence of necrosis L97.816
            - bone necrosis L97.814
            - exposed fat layer L97.812
            - muscle involvement without evidence of necrosis L97.815
            - muscle necrosis L97.813
            - skin breakdown only L97.811
            - specified severity NEC L97.818
  - midfoot L97.409
    - with
      - bone involvement without evidence of necrosis L97.406
      - bone necrosis L97.404
      - exposed fat layer L97.402
      - muscle involvement without evidence of necrosis L97.405
      - muscle necrosis L97.403
      - skin breakdown only L97.401
      - specified severity NEC L97.408
    - left L97.429
      - with
        - bone involvement without evidence of necrosis L97.426
        - bone necrosis L97.424
        - exposed fat layer L97.422
        - muscle involvement without evidence of necrosis L97.425
        - muscle necrosis L97.423
        - skin breakdown only L97.421
        - specified severity NEC L97.428
    - right L97.419
      - with
        - bone involvement without evidence of necrosis L97.416
        - bone necrosis L97.414
        - exposed fat layer L97.412
        - muscle involvement without evidence of necrosis L97.415
        - muscle necrosis L97.413
        - skin breakdown only L97.411
        - specified severity NEC L97.418
    - right L97.919
      - with
        - bone involvement without evidence of necrosis L97.916
        - bone necrosis L97.914
        - exposed fat layer L97.912
        - muscle involvement without evidence of necrosis L97.915
        - muscle necrosis L97.913
        - skin breakdown only L97.911
        - specified severity NEC L97.918
  - thigh L97.109
    - with
      - bone involvement without evidence of necrosis L97.106
      - bone necrosis L97.104
      - exposed fat layer L97.102
      - muscle involvement without evidence of necrosis L97.105
      - muscle necrosis L97.103
      - skin breakdown only L97.101
      - specified severity NEC L97.108
    - left L97.129
      - with
        - bone involvement without evidence of necrosis L97.126
        - bone necrosis L97.124
        - exposed fat layer L97.122
        - muscle involvement without evidence of necrosis L97.125
        - muscle necrosis L97.123
        - skin breakdown only L97.121
        - specified severity NEC L97.128
    - right L97.119
      - with
        - bone involvement without evidence of necrosis L97.116
        - bone necrosis L97.114
        - exposed fat layer L97.112
        - muscle involvement without evidence of necrosis L97.115
        - muscle necrosis L97.113
        - skin breakdown only L97.111
        - specified severity NEC L97.118
  - toe L97.509
    - with
      - bone involvement without evidence of necrosis L97.506
      - bone necrosis L97.504
      - exposed fat layer L97.502
      - muscle involvement without evidence of necrosis L97.505
      - muscle necrosis L97.503
      - skin breakdown only L97.501
      - specified severity NEC L97.508
    - left L97.529
      - with
        - bone involvement without evidence of necrosis L97.526
        - bone necrosis L97.524
        - exposed fat layer L97.522
        - muscle involvement without evidence of necrosis L97.525
        - muscle necrosis L97.523
        - skin breakdown only L97.521
        - specified severity NEC L97.528
    - right L97.519
      - with
        - bone involvement without evidence of necrosis L97.516
        - bone necrosis L97.514
        - exposed fat layer L97.512
        - muscle involvement without evidence of necrosis L97.515
        - muscle necrosis L97.513
        - skin breakdown only L97.511
        - specified severity NEC L97.518
- leprous A30.1
- syphilitic A52.19
- varicose —*see* Varix, leg, with, ulcer
- luetic —*see* Ulcer, syphilitic
- lung J98.4
  - tuberculous —*see* Tuberculosis, pulmonary
- malignant —*see* Neoplasm, malignant, by site
- marginal NEC —*see* Ulcer, gastrojejunal
- meatus (urinarius) N34.2
- Meckel's diverticulum Q43.0
  - malignant —*see* Table of Neoplasms, small intestine, malignant
- Meleney's (chronic undermining) —*see* Ulcer, skin
- Mooren's (cornea) —*see* Ulcer, cornea, Mooren's
- mycobacterial (skin) A31.1
- nasopharynx J39.2
- neck, uterus N86
- neurogenic NEC —*see* Ulcer, skin
- nose, nasal (passage) (infective) (septum) J34.0
  - skin —*see* Ulcer, skin
  - spirochetal A69.8
  - varicose (bleeding) I86.8
- oral mucosa (traumatic) K12.1

Ulcer, ulcerated, ulcerating, ulceration, ulcerative
(continued)
- palate (soft) K12.1
- penis (chronic) N48.5
- peptic (site unspecified) K27.9
  - with
    - hemorrhage K27.4
      - and perforation K27.6
    - perforation K27.5
  - acute K27.3
    - with
      - hemorrhage K27.0
        - and perforation K27.2
      - perforation K27.1
  - chronic K27.7
    - with
      - hemorrhage K27.4
        - and perforation K27.6
      - perforation K27.5
  - esophagus K22.10
    - with bleeding K22.11
  - newborn P78.82
  - perforating K27.5
  - skin —*see* Ulcer, skin
- peritonsillar J35.8
- phagedenic (tropical) —*see* Ulcer, skin
- pharynx J39.2
- phlebitis —*see* Phlebitis
- plaster —*see* Ulcer, pressure, by site
- popliteal space —*see* Ulcer, lower limb
- postpyloric —*see* Ulcer, duodenum
- prepuce N47.7
- prepyloric —*see* Ulcer, stomach
- pressure (pressure area) L89.9-
  - ankle L89.5-
  - back L89.1-
  - buttock L89.3-
  - coccyx L89.15-
  - contiguous site of back, buttock, hip L89.4-
  - elbow L89.0-
  - face L89.81-
  - head L89.81-
  - heel L89.6-
  - hip L89.2-
  - sacral region (tailbone) L89.15-
  - specified site NEC L89.89-
  - stage 1 (healing) (pre-ulcer skin changes limited to persistent focal edema)
    - ankle L89.5-
    - back L89.1-
    - buttock L89.3-
    - coccyx L89.15-
    - contiguous site of back, buttock, hip L89.4-
    - elbow L89.0-
    - face L89.81-
    - head L89.81-
    - heel L89.6-
    - hip L89.2-
    - sacral region (tailbone) L89.15-
    - specified site NEC L89.89-
  - stage 2 (healing) (abrasion, blister, partial thickness skin loss involving epidermis and/or dermis)
    - ankle L89.5-
    - back L89.1-
    - buttock L89.3-
    - coccyx L89.15-
    - contiguous site of back, buttock, hip L89.4-
    - elbow L89.0-
    - face L89.81-

Ulcer, ulcerated, ulcerating, ulceration, ulcerative
(continued)
- pressure *(continued)*
  - stage 2 *(continued)*
    - head L89.81-
    - heel L89.6-
    - hip L89.2-
    - sacral region (tailbone) L89.15-
    - specified site NEC L89.89-
  - stage 3 (healing) (full thickness skin loss involving damage or necrosis of subcutaneous tissue)
    - ankle L89.5-
    - back L89.1-
    - buttock L89.3-
    - coccyx L89.15-
    - contiguous site of back, buttock, hip L89.4-
    - elbow L89.0-
    - face L89.81-
    - head L89.81-
    - heel L89.6-
    - hip L89.2-
    - sacral region (tailbone) L89.15-
    - specified site NEC L89.89-
  - stage 4 (healing) (necrosis of soft tissues through to underlying muscle, tendon, or bone)
    - ankle L89.5-
    - back L89.1-
    - buttock L89.3-
    - coccyx L89.15-
    - contiguous site of back, buttock, hip L89.4-
    - elbow L89.0-
    - face L89.81-
    - head L89.81-
    - heel L89.6-
    - hip L89.2-
    - sacral region (tailbone) L89.15-
    - specified site NEC L89.89-
  - unspecified stage
    - ankle L89.5-
    - back L89.1-
    - buttock L89.3-
    - coccyx L89.15-
    - contiguous site of back, buttock, hip L89.4-
    - elbow L89.0-
    - face L89.81-
    - head L89.81-
    - heel L89.6-
    - hip L89.2-
    - sacral region (tailbone) L89.15-
    - specified site NEC L89.89-
  - unstageable
    - ankle L89.5-
    - back L89.1-
    - buttock L89.3-
    - coccyx L89.15-
    - contiguous site of back, buttock, hip L89.4-
    - elbow L89.0-
    - face L89.81-
    - head L89.81-
    - heel L89.6-
    - hip L89.2-
    - sacral region (tailbone) L89.15-
    - specified site NEC L89.89-
- primary of intestine K63.3
  - with perforation K63.1
- prostate N41.9

Ulcer, ulcerated, ulcerating, ulceration, ulcerative
(continued)
- pyloric —*see* Ulcer, stomach
- rectosigmoid K63.3
  - with perforation K63.1
- rectum (sphincter) (solitary) K62.6
  - stercoraceous, stercoral K62.6
- retina —*see* Inflammation, chorioretinal
- rodent —*see also* Neoplasm, skin, malignant
- sclera —*see* Scleritis
- scrofulous (tuberculous) A18.2
- scrotum N50.89
  - tuberculous A18.15
  - varicose I86.1
- seminal vesicle N50.89
- sigmoid —*see* Ulcer, intestine
- skin (atrophic) (chronic) (neurogenic) (non-healing) (perforating) (pyogenic) (trophic) (tropical) L98.499
  - with gangrene —*see* Gangrene
  - amebic A06.7
  - back —*see* Ulcer, back
  - buttock —*see* Ulcer, buttock
  - decubitus —*see* Ulcer, pressure
  - lower limb —*see* Ulcer, lower limb
  - mycobacterial A31.1
  - specified site NEC L98.499
    - with
      - bone involvement without evidence of necrosis L98.496
      - bone necrosis L98.494
      - exposed fat layer L98.492
      - muscle involvement without evidence of necrosis L98.495
      - muscle necrosis L98.493
      - skin breakdown only L98.491
      - specified severity NEC L98.498
  - tuberculous (primary) A18.4
  - varicose —*see* Ulcer, varicose
- sloughing —*see* Ulcer, skin
- solitary, anus or rectum (sphincter) K62.6
- sore throat J02.9
  - streptococcal J02.0
- spermatic cord N50.89
- spine (tuberculous) A18.01
- stasis (venous) —*see* Varix, leg, with, ulcer
  - without varicose veins (*see also* Ulcer, by site) I87.2
- stercoraceous, stercoral K63.3
  - with perforation K63.1
  - anus or rectum K62.6
- stoma, stomal —*see* Ulcer, gastrojejunal
- stomach (eroded) (peptic) (round) K25.9
  - with
    - hemorrhage K25.4
      - and perforation K25.6
    - perforation K25.5
  - acute K25.3
    - with
      - hemorrhage K25.0
        - and perforation K25.2
      - perforation K25.1
  - chronic K25.7
    - with
      - hemorrhage K25.4
        - and perforation K25.6
      - perforation K25.5
- stomal —*see* Ulcer, gastrojejunal

Ulcer, ulcerated, ulcerating, ulceration, ulcerative
(continued)
- stomatitis K12.1
- stress —*see* Ulcer, peptic
- strumous (tuberculous) A18.2
- submucosal, bladder —*see* Cystitis, interstitial
- syphilitic (any site) (early) (secondary) A51.39
  - late A52.79
  - perforating A52.79
    - foot A52.11
- testis N50.89
- thigh —*see* Ulcer, lower limb
- throat J39.2
  - diphtheritic A36.0
- toe —*see* Ulcer, lower limb
- tongue (traumatic) K14.0
- tonsil J35.8
  - diphtheritic A36.0
- trachea J39.8
- trophic —*see* Ulcer, skin
- tropical —*see* Ulcer, skin
- tuberculous —*see* Tuberculosis, ulcer
- tunica vaginalis N50.89
- turbinate J34.89
- typhoid (perforating) —*see* Typhoid
- unspecified site —*see* Ulcer, skin
- urethra (meatus) —*see* Urethritis
- uterus N85.8
  - cervix N86
    - with cervicitis N72
  - neck N86
    - with cervicitis N72
- vagina N76.5
  - in Behçet's disease M35.2 [N77.0]
  - pessary N89.8
- valve, heart I33.0
- varicose (lower limb, any part) —*see also* Varix, leg, with, ulcer
  - broad ligament I86.2
  - esophagus —*see* Varix, esophagus
  - inflamed or infected —*see* Varix, leg, with ulcer, with inflammation
  - nasal septum I86.8
  - perineum I86.3
  - scrotum I86.1
  - specified site NEC I86.8
  - sublingual I86.0
  - vulva I86.3
- vas deferens N50.89
- vulva (acute) (infectional) N76.6
  - in (due to)
    - Behçet's disease M35.2 [N77.0]
    - herpesviral (herpes simplex) infection A60.04
    - tuberculosis A18.18
- vulvobuccal, recurring N76.6
- X-ray L58.1
- yaws A66.4

Ulcerosa scarlatina A38.8

Ulcus —*see also* Ulcer
- cutis tuberculosum A18.4
- duodeni —*see* Ulcer, duodenum
- durum (syphilitic) A51.0
  - extragenital A51.2
- gastrojejunale —*see* Ulcer, gastrojejunal
- hypostaticum —*see* Ulcer, varicose
- molle (cutis) (skin) A57
- serpens corneae —*see* Ulcer, cornea, central
- ventriculi —*see* Ulcer, stomach

Ulegyria Q04.8
Ulerythema
  ophryogenes, congenital Q84.2
  sycosiforme L73.8
Ullrich (-Bonnevie) (-Turner)
  syndrome (see also Turner's
  syndrome) Q87.19
Ullrich-Feichtiger syndrome Q87.0
Ulnar —see condition
Ulorrhagia, ulorrhea K06.8
Umbilicus, umbilical —see condition
Unable to
  make ends meet Z59.86
  obtain
    adequate
      childcare due to limited
        financial resources,
        specified NEC Z59.87
      clothing due to limited
        financial resources,
        specified NEC Z59.87
      internet services, due to
        unavailability in geographic
        area Z58.81
      telephone services, due to
        unavailability in geographic
        area Z58.81
      utilities, due to inadequate
        physical environment Z58.81
      utilities due to limited
        financial resources,
        specified NEC Z59.87
    basic
      needs due to limited financial
        resources, specified NEC
        Z59.87
      services in physical
        environment Z58.81
Unacceptable
  contours of tooth K08.54
  morphology of tooth K08.54
Unaffordable transportation Z59.82
Unavailability (of)
  bed at medical facility Z75.1
  health service-related agencies Z75.4
  medical facilities (at) Z75.3
    due to
      investigation by social service
        agency Z75.2
      lack of services at home Z75.0
      remoteness from facility Z75.3
      waiting list Z75.1
    home Z75.0
    outpatient clinic Z75.3
  schooling Z55.1
  social service agencies Z75.4
Uncinaria americana infestation
  B76.1
Uncinariasis B76.9
Uncongenial work Z56.5
Unconscious (ness) —see Coma
Under observation —see Observation
Underachievement in school Z55.3
Underdevelopment —see also
  Undeveloped
  nose Q30.1
  sexual E30.0
Underdosing (see also Tables of
  Drugs and Chemicals, categories
  T36-T50, with final character 6)
  Z91.14
  intentional NEC Z91.128
    due to financial hardship of
      patient Z91.120

Underdosing (continued)
  unintentional NEC Z91.138
    due to patient's age related
      debility Z91.130
Underfeeding, newborn P92.3
Underfill, endodontic M27.53
Underimmunization status Z28.39
  COVID-19 Z28.31-
    partially vaccinated (for) Z28.311
    unvaccinated (for) Z28.310
Undernourishment —see Malnutrition
Undernutrition —see Malnutrition
Underweight R63.6
  for gestational age —see Light for
    dates
Underwood's disease P83.0
Undescended —see also
  Malposition, congenital
  cecum Q43.3
  colon Q43.3
  testicle —see Cryptorchid
Undeveloped, undevelopment
  —see also Hypoplasia
  brain (congenital) Q02
  cerebral (congenital) Q02
  heart Q24.8
  lung Q33.6
  testis E29.1
  uterus E30.0
Undiagnosed (disease) R69
Undulant fever —see Brucellosis
Unemployment, anxiety concerning
  Z56.0
  threatened Z56.2
Unequal length (acquired) (limb)
  —see also Deformity, limb,
  unequal length
  leg —see also Deformity, limb,
    unequal length
    congenital Q72.9-
Unextracted dental root K08.3
Unguis incarnatus L60.0
Unhappiness R45.2
Unicornate uterus Q51.4
  in pregnancy or childbirth O34.00
Unilateral —see also condition
  development, breast N64.89
  organ or site, congenital NEC
    —see Agenesis, by site
Unilocular heart Q20.8
Unimmunized —see also
  Underimmunization status
  for COVID-19 Z28.310
Union, abnormal —see also Fusion
  larynx and trachea Q34.8
Universal mesentery Q43.3
Unreliable transportation Z59.82
Unrepairable overhanging of dental
  restorative materials K08.52
Unroofed coronary sinus Q21.13
Unsafe transportation Z59.82
Unsatisfactory
  restoration of tooth K08.50
    specified NEC K08.59
  sample of cytologic smear
    anus R85.615
    cervix R87.615
    vagina R87.625
  surroundings Z59.19
  work Z56.5
Unsoundness of mind —see Psychosis

Unstable
  back NEC —see Instability, joint,
    spine
  hip (congenital) Q65.6
    acquired —see Derangement,
      joint, specified type NEC, hip
  joint —see Instability, joint
    secondary to removal of joint
      prosthesis M96.89
  lie (mother) O32.0
  lumbosacral joint (congenital)
    —see subcategory M53.2
  sacroiliac —see subcategory M53.2
  spine NEC —see Instability, joint,
    spine
Unsteadiness on feet R26.81
Untruthfulness, child problem F91.8
Unvaccinated —see also
  Underimmunization status
  for COVID-19 Z28.310
Unverricht (-Lundborg) **disease**
  or epilepsy —see Epilepsy,
  generalized, idiopathic
Unwanted
  multiple moves in the last
    12 months Z59.81-
  pregnancy Z64.0
Upbringing, institutional Z62.22
  away from parents NEC Z62.29
  in care of non-parental family
    member Z62.21
  in foster care Z62.21
  in orphanage or group home
    Z62.22
  in welfare custody Z62.21
Upper respiratory —see condition
Upset
  gastric K30
  gastrointestinal K30
    psychogenic F45.8
  intestinal (large) (small) K59.9
    psychogenic F45.8
  menstruation N93.9
  mental F48.9
  stomach K30
    psychogenic F45.8
Urachus —see also condition
  patent or persistent Q64.4
Urbach-Oppenheim disease
  (necrobiosis lipoidica diabeticorum)
  —see E08-E13 with .620
Urbach's lipoid proteinosis E78.89
Urbach-Wiethe disease E78.89
Urban yellow fever A95.1
Urea
  blood, high —see Uremia
  cycle metabolism disorder —see
    Disorder, urea cycle metabolism
Uremia, uremic N19
  with
    ectopic or molar pregnancy
      O08.4
    polyneuropathy N18.9 [G63]
  chronic NOS (see also Disease,
    kidney, chronic) N18.9
    due to hypertension —see
      Hypertensive, kidney
  complicating
    ectopic or molar pregnancy O08.4
  congenital P96.0
  extrarenal R39.2
  following ectopic or molar
    pregnancy O08.4
  newborn P96.0
  prerenal R39.2

Ureter, ureteral —see condition
Ureteralgia N23
Ureterectasis —see Hydroureter
Ureteritis N28.89
  cystica N28.86
  due to calculus N20.1
    with calculus, kidney N20.2
      with hydronephrosis N13.2
  gonococcal (acute) (chronic)
    A54.21
  nonspecific N28.89
Ureterocele N28.89
  congenital (orthotopic) Q62.31
  ectopic Q62.32
Ureterolith, ureterolithiasis —see
  Calculus, ureter
Ureterostomy
  attention to Z43.6
  status Z93.6
Urethra, urethral —see condition
Urethralgia R39.89
Urethritis (anterior) (posterior) N34.2
  calculous N21.1
  candidal B37.41
  chlamydial A56.01
  diplococcal (gonococcal) A54.01
    with abscess (accessory gland)
      (periurethral) A54.1
  gonococcal A54.01
    with abscess (accessory gland)
      (periurethral) A54.1
  nongonococcal N34.1
    Reiter's —see Reiter's disease
  nonspecific N34.1
  nonvenereal N34.1
  postmenopausal N34.2
  puerperal O86.22
  Reiter's —see Reiter's disease
  specified NEC N34.2
  trichomonal or due to Trichomonas
    (vaginalis) A59.03
Urethrocele N81.0
  with
    cystocele —see Cystocele
    prolapse of uterus —see
      Prolapse, uterus
Urethrolithiasis (with colic or
  infection) N21.1
Urethrorectal —see condition
Urethrorrhagia N36.8
Urethrorrhea R36.9
Urethrostomy
  attention to Z43.6
  status Z93.6
Urethrotrigonitis —see Trigonitis
Urethrovaginal —see condition
Urgency
  fecal R15.2
  hypertensive —see Hypertension
  urinary R39.15
Urhidrosis, uridrosis L74.8
Uric acid in blood (increased) E79.0
Uricacidemia (asymptomatic) E79.0
Uricemia (asymptomatic) E79.0
Uricosuria R82.998
Urinary —see condition
Urination
  frequent R35.0
  painful R30.9
Urine
  blood in —see Hematuria
  discharge, excessive R35.89
  enuresis, nonorganic origin F98.0
  extravasation R39.0

Urine (continued)
  frequency R35.0
  incontinence R32
    nonorganic origin F98.0
  intermittent stream R39.198
  pus in N39.0
  retention or stasis R33.9
    organic R33.8
      drug-induced R33.0
    psychogenic F45.8
  secretion
    deficient R34
    excessive R35.89
    frequency R35.0
  stream
    intermittent R39.198
    slowing R39.198
    splitting R39.13
    weak R39.12

Urinemia —*see* Uremia

Urinoma, urethra N36.8

Uroarthritis, infectious (Reiter's) —*see* Reiter's disease

Urodialysis R34

Urolithiasis —*see* Calculus, urinary

Uronephrosis —*see* Hydronephrosis

Uropathy N39.9
  obstructive N13.9
    specified NEC N13.8
  reflux N13.9
    specified NEC N13.8
  vesicoureteral reflux-associated —*see* Reflux, vesicoureteral

Urosepsis - code to condition

Urticaria L50.9
  with angioneurotic edema T78.3
    hereditary D84.1
  allergic L50.0
  cholinergic L50.5
  chronic L50.8
  cold, familial L50.2
  contact L50.6
  dermatographic L50.3
  due to
    cold or heat L50.2
    drugs L50.0
    food L50.0
    inhalants L50.0
    plants L50.6
    serum (*see also* Reaction, serum) T80.69
  factitial L50.3
  familial cold M04.2
  giant T78.3
    hereditary D84.1
  gigantea T78.3
  idiopathic L50.1
  larynx T78.3
    hereditary D84.1
  neonatorum P83.88
  nonallergic L50.1
  papulosa (Hebra) L28.2
  pigmentosa D47.01
    congenital Q82.2
      of neonatal onset Q82.2
      of newborn onset Q82.2
    recurrent periodic L50.8
    serum (*see also* Reaction, serum) T80.69
  solar L56.3
  specified type NEC L50.8
  thermal (cold) (heat) L50.2
  vibratory L50.4
  xanthelasmoidea —*see* Urticaria pigmentosa

Use (of)
  alcohol F10.90

Use (continued)
  alcohol (continued)
    with
      intoxication F10.929
      sleep disorder F10.982
      sleep disorder (continued)
        withdrawal F10.939
          with
            perceptual disturbance F10.932
          delirium F10.931
          uncomplicated F10.930
    harmful —*see* Abuse, alcohol
    in remission F10.91
  amphetamines —*see* Use, stimulant NEC
  caffeine —*see* Use, stimulant NEC
  cannabis F12.90
    with
      anxiety disorder F12.980
      intoxication F12.929
        with
          delirium F12.921
          perceptual disturbance F12.922
          uncomplicated F12.920
      other specified disorder F12.988
      psychosis F12.959
        delusions F12.950
        hallucinations F12.951
      unspecified disorder F12.99
      withdrawal F12.93
    in remission F12.91
  cocaine F14.90
    with
      anxiety disorder F14.980
      intoxication F14.929
        with
          delirium F14.921
          perceptual disturbance F14.922
          uncomplicated F14.920
      other specified disorder F14.988
      psychosis F14.959
        delusions F14.950
        hallucinations F14.951
      sexual dysfunction F14.981
      sleep disorder F14.982
      unspecified disorder F14.99
      withdrawal F14.93
    harmful —*see* Abuse, drug, cocaine
    in remission F14.91
  drug(s) NEC F19.90
    with sleep disorder F19.982
    harmful —*see* Abuse, drug, by type
  hallucinogen NEC F16.90
    with
      anxiety disorder F16.980
      intoxication F16.929
        with
          delirium F16.921
          uncomplicated F16.920
      mood disorder F16.94
      other specified disorder F16.988
      perception disorder (flashbacks) F16.983
      psychosis F16.959
        delusions F16.950
        hallucinations F16.951
      unspecified disorder F16.99
    harmful —*see* Abuse, drug, hallucinogen NEC
    in remission F16.91
  inhalants F18.90
    with
      anxiety disorder F18.980

Use (continued)
  inhalants (continued)
    with (continued)
      intoxication F18.929
        with delirium F18.921
        uncomplicated F18.920
      mood disorder F18.94
      other specified disorder F18.988
      persisting dementia F18.97
      psychosis F18.959
        delusions F18.950
        hallucinations F18.951
      unspecified disorder F18.99
    harmful —*see* Abuse, drug, inhalant
    in remission F18.91
  methadone —*see* Use, opioid
  nonprescribed drugs F19.90
    harmful —*see* Abuse, non-psychoactive substance
  opioid F11.90
    with
      disorder F11.99
        mood F11.94
        sleep F11.982
        specified type NEC F11.988
      intoxication F11.929
        with
          delirium F11.921
          perceptual disturbance F11.922
          uncomplicated F11.920
      opioid-associated amnestic syndrome F11.988
      withdrawal F11.93
    harmful —*see* Abuse, drug, opioid
    in remission F11.91
  patent medicines F19.90
    harmful —*see* Abuse, non-psychoactive substance
  psychoactive drug NEC F19.90
    with
      anxiety disorder F19.980
      intoxication F19.929
        with
          delirium F19.921
          perceptual disturbance F19.922
          uncomplicated F19.920
      mood disorder F19.94
      other specified disorder F19.988
      persisting
        amnestic disorder F19.96
        dementia F19.97
      psychosis F19.959
        delusions F19.950
        hallucinations F19.951
      sexual dysfunction F19.981
      sleep disorder F19.982
      unspecified disorder F19.99
      withdrawal F19.939
        with
          delirium F19.931
          perceptual disturbance F19.932
          uncomplicated F19.930
    harmful —*see* Abuse, drug NEC, psychoactive NEC
    in remission F19.91
  sedative, hypnotic, or anxiolytic F13.90
    with
      anxiety disorder F13.980
      intoxication F13.929
        with
          delirium F13.921
          uncomplicated F13.920
      other specified disorder F13.988
      persisting
        amnestic disorder F13.96
        dementia F13.97

Use (continued)
  sedative, hypnotic, or anxiolytic (continued)
    with (continued)
      psychosis F13.959
        delusions F13.950
        hallucinations F13.951
      sexual dysfunction F13.981
      sleep disorder F13.982
      unspecified disorder F13.99
    harmful —*see* Abuse, drug, sedative, hypnotic, or anxiolytic
    in remission F13.91
  stimulant NEC F15.90
    with
      anxiety disorder F15.980
      intoxication F15.929
        with
          delirium F15.921
          perceptual disturbance F15.922
          uncomplicated F15.920
      mood disorder F15.94
      other specified disorder F15.988
      psychosis F15.959
        delusions F15.950
        hallucinations F15.951
      sexual dysfunction F15.981
      sleep disorder F15.982
      unspecified disorder F15.99
      withdrawal F15.93
    harmful —*see* Abuse, drug, stimulant NEC
    in remission F15.91
  volatile solvents (*see also* Use, inhalant) F18.90
    harmful —*see* Abuse, drug, inhalant
  tobacco Z72.0
    with dependence —*see* Dependence, drug, nicotine

Usher-Senear disease or syndrome L10.4

Uta B55.1

Uteromegaly N85.2

Uterovaginal —*see* condition

Uterovesical —*see* condition

Uveal —*see* condition

Uveitis (anterior) —*see also* Iridocyclitis
  acute —*see* Iridocyclitis, acute
  chronic —*see* Iridocyclitis, chronic
  due to toxoplasmosis (acquired) B58.09
    congenital P37.1
  granulomatous —*see* Iridocyclitis, chronic
  heterochromic —*see* Cyclitis, Fuchs' heterochromic
  lens-induced —*see* Iridocyclitis, lens-induced
  posterior —*see* Chorioretinitis
  sympathetic H44.13-
  syphilitic (secondary) A51.43
    congenital (early) A50.01
    late A52.71
  tuberculous A18.54

Uveoencephalitis —*see* Inflammation, chorioretinal

Uveokeratitis —*see* Iridocyclitis

Uveoparotitis D86.89

Uvula —*see* condition

Uvulitis (acute) (catarrhal) (chronic) (membranous) (suppurative) (ulcerative) K12.2

V

Vaccination (prophylactic)
- complication or reaction —*see* Complications, vaccination
- delayed Z28.9
- encounter for Z23
- not done —*see* Immunization, not done, because (of)
- partial —*see also* Underimmunization status
- for COVID-19 Z28.311

Vaccinia (generalized) (localized) T88.1
- congenital P35.8
- without vaccination B08.011

Vacuum, in sinus (accessory) (nasal) J34.89

Vagabond, vagabondage Z59.00

Vagabond's disease B85.1

Vagina, vaginal —*see* condition

Vaginalitis (tunica) (testis) N49.1

Vaginismus (reflex) N94.2
- functional F52.5
- nonorganic F52.5
- psychogenic F52.5
- secondary N94.2

Vaginitis (acute) (circumscribed) (diffuse) (emphysematous) (nonvenereal) (ulcerative) N76.0
- with ectopic or molar pregnancy O08.0
- amebic A06.82
- atrophic, postmenopausal N95.2
- bacterial N76.0
- blennorrhagic (gonococcal) A54.02
- candidal (acute) B37.31
  - chronic (recurrent) B37.32
- chlamydial A56.02
- chronic N76.1
- due to Trichomonas (vaginalis) A59.01
- following ectopic or molar pregnancy O08.0
- gonococcal A54.02
  - with abscess (accessory gland) (periurethral) A54.1
- granuloma A58
- in (due to)
  - candidiasis (acute) B37.31
    - chronic (recurrent) B37.32
  - herpesviral (herpes simplex) infection A60.04
  - pinworm infection B80 [N77.1]
- monilial (acute) B37.31
  - chronic (recurrent) B37.32
- mycotic (candidal) (acute) B37.31
  - chronic (recurrent) B37.32
- postmenopausal atrophic N95.2
- puerperal (postpartum) O86.13
- senile (atrophic) N95.2
- subacute or chronic N76.1
- syphilitic (early) A51.0
  - late A52.76
- trichomonal A59.01
- tuberculous A18.18

Vaginosis —*see* Vaginitis

Vagotonia G52.2

Vagrancy Z59.00

VAIN —*see* Neoplasia, intraepithelial, vagina

Vallecula —*see* condition

Valley fever B38.0

Valsuani's disease —*see* Anemia, obstetric

Valve, valvular (formation) —*see also* condition
- cerebral ventricle (communicating) in situ Z98.2
- cervix, internal os Q51.828
- congenital NEC —*see* Atresia, by site
- ureter (pelvic junction) (vesical orifice) Q62.39
- urethra (congenital) (posterior) Q64.2

Valvulitis (chronic) —*see* Endocarditis

Valvulopathy —*see* Endocarditis

Van Bogaert's leukoencephalopathy (sclerosing) (subacute) A81.1

Van Bogaert-Scherer-Epstein disease or syndrome E75.5

Van Buchem's syndrome M85.2

Van Creveld-von Gierke disease E74.01

Van der Hoeve (-de Kleyn) **syndrome** Q78.0

Van der Woude's syndrome Q38.0

Van Neck's disease or osteochondrosis M91.0

Vanishing lung J44.89

Vapor asphyxia or suffocation T59.9
- specified agent —*see* Table of Drugs and Chemicals

Variance, lethal ball, prosthetic heart valve T82.09

Variants, thalassemic D56.8

Variations in hair color L67.1

Varicella B01.9
- with
  - complications NEC B01.89
  - encephalitis B01.11
  - encephalomyelitis B01.11
  - meningitis B01.0
  - myelitis B01.12
  - pneumonia B01.2
- congenital P35.8

Varices —*see* Varix

Varicocele (scrotum) (thrombosed) I86.1
- ovary I86.2
- perineum I86.3
- spermatic cord (ulcerated) I86.1

Varicose
- aneurysm (ruptured) I77.0
- dermatitis —*see* Varix, leg, with, inflammation
- eczema —*see* Varix, leg, with, inflammation
- phlebitis —*see* Varix, with, inflammation
- tumor —*see* Varix
- ulcer (lower limb, any part) —*see also* Varix, leg, with, ulcer
  - anus (*see also* Hemorrhoids) K64.8
  - esophagus —*see* Varix, esophagus
  - inflamed or infected —*see* Varix, leg, with ulcer, with inflammation
  - nasal septum I86.8

Varicose (*continued*)
- ulcer (*continued*)
  - perineum I86.3
  - scrotum I86.1
  - specified site NEC I86.8
- vein —*see* Varix
- vessel —*see* Varix, leg

Varicosis, varicosities, varicosity —*see* Varix

Variola (major) (minor) B03

Varioloid B03

Varix (lower limb) (ruptured) I83.90
- with
  - bleeding I83.899
  - edema I83.899
  - inflammation I83.10
    - with ulcer (venous) I83.209
  - pain I83.819
  - rupture I83.899
  - specified complication NEC I83.899
  - stasis dermatitis I83.10
    - with ulcer (venous) I83.209
  - swelling I83.899
  - ulcer I83.0-
    - with inflammation I83.2-
- aneurysmal I77.0
- asymptomatic I83.9-
- bladder I86.2
- broad ligament I86.2
- complicating
  - childbirth (lower extremity) O87.4
    - anus or rectum O87.2
    - genital (vagina, vulva or perineum) O87.8
  - pregnancy (lower extremity) O22.0-
    - anus or rectum O22.4-
    - genital (vagina, vulva or perineum) O22.1-
  - puerperium (lower extremity) O87.4
    - anus or rectum O87.2
    - genital (vagina, vulva, perineum) O87.8
- congenital (any site) Q27.8
- esophagus (idiopathic) (primary) (ulcerated) I85.00
  - bleeding I85.01
  - congenital Q27.8
  - in (due to)
    - alcoholic liver disease I85.10
      - bleeding I85.11
    - cirrhosis of liver I85.10
      - bleeding I85.11
    - portal hypertension I85.10
      - bleeding I85.11
    - schistosomiasis I85.10
      - bleeding I85.11
    - toxic liver disease I85.10
      - bleeding I85.11
  - secondary I85.10
    - bleeding I85.11
- gastric I86.4
- inflamed or infected I83.10
  - ulcerated I83.209
- labia (majora) I86.3
- leg (asymptomatic) I83.9-
  - with
    - edema I83.899
    - inflammation I83.10
      - with ulcer —*see* Varix, leg, with, ulcer, with inflammation by site
    - pain I83.819
    - specified complication NEC I83.899

Varix (*continued*)
- leg (*continued*)
  - with (*continued*)
    - swelling I83.899
    - ulcer I83.0-
      - with inflammation I83.2-
      - ankle I83.003
        - with inflammation I83.203
      - calf I83.002
        - with inflammation I83.202
      - foot NEC I83.005
        - with inflammation I83.205
      - heel I83.004
        - with inflammation I83.204
      - lower leg NEC I83.008
        - with inflammation I83.208
      - midfoot I83.004
        - with inflammation I83.204
      - thigh I83.001
        - with inflammation I83.201
  - bilateral (asymptomatic) I83.93
    - with
      - edema I83.893
      - pain I83.813
      - specified complication NEC I83.893
      - swelling I83.893
      - ulcer I83.0-
        - with inflammation I83.209
  - left (asymptomatic) I83.92
    - with
      - edema I83.892
      - pain I83.812
      - specified complication NEC I83.892
      - swelling I83.892
      - inflammation I83.12
        - with ulcer —*see* Varix, leg, with, ulcer, with inflammation by site
      - ulcer I83.029
        - with inflammation I83.229
      - ankle I83.023
        - with inflammation I83.223
      - calf I83.022
        - with inflammation I83.222
      - foot NEC I83.025
        - with inflammation I83.225
      - heel I83.024
        - with inflammation I83.224
      - lower leg NEC I83.028
        - with inflammation I83.228
      - midfoot I83.024
        - with inflammation I83.224
      - thigh I83.021
        - with inflammation I83.221
  - right (asymptomatic) I83.91
    - with
      - edema I83.891
      - pain I83.811
      - specified complication NEC I83.891
      - swelling I83.891

Varix *(continued)*
  leg *(continued)*
    right *(continued)*
      with *(continued)*
        inflammation I83.11
          with ulcer —*see* Varix, leg, with, ulcer, with inflammation by site
        ulcer I83.019
          with inflammation I83.219
          ankle I83.013
            with inflammation I83.213
          calf I83.012
            with inflammation I83.212
          foot NEC I83.015
            with inflammation I83.215
          heel I83.014
            with inflammation I83.214
          lower leg NEC I83.018
            with inflammation I83.218
          midfoot I83.014
            with inflammation I83.214
          thigh I83.011
            with inflammation I83.211
  nasal septum I86.8
  orbit I86.8
    congenital Q27.8
  ovary I86.2
  papillary I78.1
  pelvis I86.2
  perineum I86.3
  pharynx I86.8
  placenta O43.89-
  renal papilla I86.8
  retina H35.09
  scrotum (ulcerated) I86.1
  sigmoid colon I86.8
  specified site NEC I86.8
  spinal (cord) (vessels) I86.8
  spleen, splenic (vein) (with phlebolith) I86.8
  stomach I86.4
  sublingual I86.0
  ulcerated I83.009
    inflamed or infected I83.209
  uterine ligament I86.2
  vagina I86.8
  vocal cord I86.8
  vulva I86.3
Vas deferens —*see* condition
Vas deferentitis N49.1
Vasa previa O69.4
  hemorrhage from, affecting newborn P50.0
Vascular —*see also* condition
  loop on optic papilla Q14.2
  spasm I73.9
  spider I78.1
Vascularization, cornea —*see* Neovascularization, cornea
Vasculitis I77.6
  allergic D69.0
  ANCA (antineutrophilic cytoplasmic antibody) associated I77.82
  ANCA (antineutrophilic cytoplasmic antibody) positive I77.82
  antineutrophilic cytoplasmic antibody [ANCA] I77.82
  cryoglobulinemic D89.1

Vasculitis *(continued)*
  disseminated I77.6
  hypocomplementemic M31.8
  kidney I77.89
  leukocytoclastic M31.0
  livedoid L95.0
  nodular L95.8
  retina H35.06-
  rheumatic —*see* Fever, rheumatic
  rheumatoid —*see* Rheumatoid, vasculitis
  skin (limited to) L95.9
    specified NEC L95.8
  systemic M31.8
Vasculopathy, necrotizing M31.9
  cardiac allograft T86.290
  specified NEC M31.8
Vasitis (nodosa) N49.1
  tuberculous A18.15
Vasodilation I73.9
Vasomotor —*see* condition
Vasoplasty, after previous sterilization Z31.0
  aftercare Z31.42
Vasospasm (vasoconstriction) (*see also* Angiospasm) I73.9
  cerebral (cerebrovascular) (artery) I67.848
    reversible I67.841
  coronary I20.1
  nerve
    arm —*see* Mononeuropathy, upper limb
    brachial plexus G54.0
    cervical plexus G54.2
    leg —*see* Mononeuropathy, lower limb
  peripheral NOS I73.9
  retina (artery) —*see* Occlusion, artery, retina
Vasospastic —*see* condition
Vasovagal attack (paroxysmal) R55
  psychogenic F45.8
VATER syndrome Q87.2
Vater's ampulla —*see* condition
Vegetation, vegetative
  adenoid (nasal fossa) J35.8
  endocarditis (acute) (any valve) (subacute) I33.0
  heart (mycotic) (valve) I33.0
Veil
  Jackson's Q43.3
Vein, venous —*see* condition
Veldt sore —*see* Ulcer, skin
Velpeau's hernia —*see* Hernia, femoral
Venereal
  bubo A55
  disease A64
  granuloma inguinale A58
  lymphogranuloma (Durand-Nicolas-Favre) A55
Venofibrosis I87.8
Venom, venomous —*see* Table of Drugs and Chemicals, by animal or substance, poisoning
Venous —*see* condition
Ventilator lung, newborn P27.8
Ventral —*see* condition
Ventricle, ventricular —*see also* condition
  escape I49.3
  inversion Q20.5

Ventriculitis (cerebral) (*see also* Encephalitis) G04.90
Ventriculostomy status Z98.2
Vernet's syndrome G52.7
Verneuil's disease (syphilitic bursitis) A52.78
Verruca (due to HPV) (filiformis) (simplex) (viral) (vulgaris) B07.9
  acuminata A63.0
  necrogenica (primary) (tuberculosa) A18.4
  plana B07.8
  plantaris B07.0
  seborrheica L82.1
    inflamed L82.0
  senile (seborrheic) L82.1
    inflamed L82.0
  tuberculosa (primary) A18.4
  venereal A63.0
Verrucosities —*see* Verruca
Verruga peruana, peruviana A44.1
Version
  cervix —*see* Malposition, uterus
  uterus (postinfectional) (postpartal, old) —*see* Malposition, uterus
Vertebra, vertebral —*see* condition
Vertical talus (congenital) Q66.80
  left foot Q66.82
  right foot Q66.81
Vertigo R42
  auditory —*see* Vertigo, aural
  aural H81.31-
  benign paroxysmal (positional) H81.1-
  central (origin) H81.4
  cerebral H81.4
  Dix and Hallpike (epidemic) —*see* Neuronitis, vestibular
  due to infrasound T75.23
  epidemic A88.1
    Dix and Hallpike —*see* Neuronitis, vestibular
    Pedersen's —*see* Neuronitis, vestibular
    vestibular neuronitis —*see* Neuronitis, vestibular
  hysterical F44.89
  infrasound —*see* subcategory T75.23
  labyrinthine H81.0
  laryngeal R05.4
  malignant positional H81.4
  Ménière's —*see* subcategory H81.0
  menopausal N95.1
  otogenic —*see* Vertigo, aural
  paroxysmal positional, benign —*see* Vertigo, benign paroxysmal
  Pedersen's (epidemic) —*see* Neuronitis, vestibular
  peripheral NEC H81.39-
  positional
    benign paroxysmal —*see* Vertigo, benign paroxysmal
  malignant H81.4
Very-low-density-lipoprotein-type (VLDL) hyperlipoproteinemia E78.1
Vesania —*see* Psychosis
Vesical —*see* condition
Vesicle
  cutaneous R23.8
  seminal —*see* condition
  skin R23.8
Vesicocolic —*see* condition

Vesicoperineal —*see* condition
Vesicorectal —*see* condition
Vesicourethrorectal —*see* condition
Vesicovaginal —*see* condition
Vesicular —*see* condition
Vesiculitis (seminal) N49.0
  amebic A06.82
  gonorrheal (acute) (chronic) A54.23
  trichomonal A59.09
  tuberculous A18.15
Vestibulitis (ear) —*see also* subcategory H83.0
  nose (external) J34.89
  vulvar N94.810
Vestibulopathy, acute peripheral (recurrent) —*see* Neuronitis, vestibular
Vestige, vestigial —*see also* Persistence
  branchial Q18.0
  structures in vitreous Q14.0
Vibration
  adverse effects T75.20
    pneumatic hammer syndrome T75.21
    specified effect NEC T75.29
    vasospastic syndrome T75.22
    vertigo from infrasound T75.23
  exposure (occupational) Z57.7
  vertigo T75.23
Vibriosis A28.9
Victim (of)
  crime Z65.4
  disaster Z65.5
  terrorism Z65.4
  torture Z65.4
  war Z65.5
Vidal's disease L28.0
Villaret's syndrome G52.7
Villous —*see* condition
VIN —*see* Neoplasia, intraepithelial, vulva
Vincent's infection (angina) (gingivitis) A69.1
  stomatitis NEC A69.1
Vinson-Plummer syndrome D50.1
Violence, physical R45.6
Viosterol deficiency —*see* Deficiency, calciferol
Vipoma —*see* Neoplasm, malignant, by site
Viremia B34.9
Virilism (adrenal) E25.9
  congenital E25.0
Virilization (female) (suprarenal) E25.9
  congenital E25.0
  isosexual E28.2
Virulent bubo A57
Virus, viral —*see also* condition
  as cause of disease classified elsewhere B97.89
    respiratory syncytial virus (RSV) —*see* Virus, respiratory syncytial (RSV)
  cytomegalovirus B25.9
  human immunodeficiency (HIV) —*see* Human, immunodeficiency virus (HIV) disease

Virus, viral *(continued)*
  infection —*see* Infection, virus
  respiratory syncytial (RSV)
    as cause of disease classified elsewhere B97.4
    bronchiolitis J21.0
    bronchitis J20.5
    bronchopneumonia J12.1
    otitis media H65- *[B97.4]*
    pneumonia J12.1
    upper respiratory infection J06.9 *[B97.4]*
  specified NEC B34.8
  swine influenza (viruses that normally cause infections in pigs) (*see also* Influenza, due to, identified novel influenza A virus) J09.X2
  West Nile (fever) A92.30
    with
      complications NEC A92.39
      cranial nerve disorders A92.32
      encephalitis A92.31
      encephalomyelitis A92.31
      neurologic manifestation NEC A92.32
      optic neuritis A92.32
      polyradiculitis A92.32
Viscera, visceral —*see* condition
Visceroptosis K63.4
Visible peristalsis R19.2
Vision, visual
  binocular, suppression H53.34
  blurred, blurring H53.8
    hysterical F44.6
  defect, defective NEC H54.7
  disorientation (syndrome) H53.8
  disturbance H53.9
    hysterical F44.6
  double H53.2
  examination Z01.00
    following failed vision screening Z01.020
      with abnormal findings Z01.021
    with abnormal findings Z01.01
  field, limitation (defect) —*see* Defect, visual field
  hallucinations R44.1
  halos H53.19
  loss —*see* Loss, vision
    sudden —*see* Disturbance, vision, subjective, loss, sudden
  low (both eyes) —*see* Low, vision
  perception, simultaneous without fusion H53.33
Vitality, lack or want of R53.83
  newborn P96.89
Vitamin deficiency —*see* Deficiency, vitamin
Vitelline duct, persistent Q43.0
Vitiligo L80
  eyelid H02.739
    left H02.736
      lower H02.735
      upper H02.734
    right H02.733
      lower H02.732
      upper H02.731
  pinta A67.2
  vulva N90.89

Vitreal corneal syndrome H59.01-
Vitreoretinopathy, proliferative —*see also* Retinopathy, proliferative
  with retinal detachment —*see* Detachment, retina, traction
Vitreous —*see also* condition
  touch syndrome —*see* Complication, postprocedural, following cataract surgery
Vocal cord —*see* condition
Vogt-Koyanagi syndrome H20.82-
Vogt's disease or syndrome G80.3
Vogt-Spielmeyer amaurotic idiocy or disease E75.4
Voice
  change R49.9
    specified NEC R49.8
  loss —*see* Aphonia
Volhynian fever A79.0
Volkmann's ischemic contracture or paralysis (complicating trauma) T79.6
Volvulus (bowel) (colon) (intestine) K56.2
  with perforation K56.2
  congenital Q43.8
  duodenum K31.5
  fallopian tube —*see* Torsion, fallopian tube
  oviduct —*see* Torsion, fallopian tube
  stomach (due to absence of gastrocolic ligament) K31.89
Vomiting R11.10
  with nausea R11.2
  asphyxia —*see* Foreign body, by site, causing asphyxia, gastric contents
  bilious (cause unknown) R11.14
    in newborn P92.01
    following gastro-intestinal surgery K91.0
  blood —*see* Hematemesis
  causing asphyxia, choking, or suffocation —*see* Foreign body, by site
  cyclical, in migraine, G43.A0
    with refractory migraine G43.A1
    intractable G43.A1
    not intractable G43.A0
    psychogenic F50.89
    without refractory migraine G43.A0
  cyclical syndrome NOS (unrelated to migraine) R11.15
  fecal matter R11.13AB
  following gastrointestinal surgery K91.0
    psychogenic F50.89
  functional K31.89
  hysterical F50.89
  nervous F50.89
  neurotic F50.89
  newborn NEC P92.09
    bilious P92.01
  periodic R11.10
    psychogenic F50.89
  persistent R11.15
  projectile R11.12
  psychogenic F50.89
  uremic —*see* Uremia
  without nausea R11.11
Vomito negro —*see* Fever, yellow

Von Bezold's abscess —*see* Mastoiditis, acute
Von Economo-Cruchet disease A85.8
Von Eulenburg's disease G71.19
Von Gierke's disease E74.01
Von Hippel (-Lindau) **disease or syndrome** Q85.83
Von Jaksch's anemia or disease D64.89
Von Recklinghausen
  disease (neurofibromatosis) Q85.01
  bones E21.0
Von Schroetter's syndrome I82.890
Von Willebrand (-Jurgens) (-Minot) **disease or syndrome** —*see* Disease, von Willebrand
Von Zumbusch's disease L40.1
Voyeurism F65.3
Vrolik's disease Q78.0
Vulva —*see* condition
Vulvismus N94.2
Vulvitis (acute) (allergic) (atrophic) (hypertrophic) (intertriginous) (senile) N76.2
  with ectopic or molar pregnancy O08.0
  adhesive, congenital Q52.79
  blennorrhagic (gonococcal) A54.02
  candidal (acute) B37.31
    chronic (recurrent) B37.32
  chlamydial A56.02
  due to Haemophilus ducreyi A57
  following ectopic or molar pregnancy O08.0
  gonococcal A54.02
    with abscess (accessory gland) (periurethral) A54.1
  herpesviral A60.04
  leukoplakic N90.4
  monilial (acute) B37.31
    chronic (recurrent) B37.32
  puerperal (postpartum) O86.19
  subacute or chronic N76.3
  syphilitic (early) A51.0
    late A52.76
  trichomonal A59.01
  tuberculous A18.18
Vulvodynia N94.819
  specified NEC N94.818
Vulvorectal —*see* condition
Vulvovaginitis (acute) —*see* Vaginitis

W

Waiting list, person on Z75.1
  for organ transplant Z76.82
  undergoing social agency investigation Z75.2
Waldenström-Kjellberg syndrome D50.1
Waldenström
  hypergammaglobulinemia D89.0
  syndrome or macroglobulinemia C88.0
Walking
  difficulty R26.2
    psychogenic F44.4
  sleep F51.3
    hysterical F44.89
Wall, abdominal —*see* condition
Wallenberg's disease or syndrome G46.3

Wallgren's disease I87.8
Wandering
  gallbladder, congenital Q44.1
  in diseases classified elsewhere Z91.83
  kidney, congenital Q63.8
  organ or site, congenital NEC —*see* Malposition, congenital, by site
  pacemaker (heart) I49.8
  spleen D73.89
War neurosis F48.8
Wart (due to HPV) (filiform) (infectious) (viral) B07.9
  anogenital region (venereal) A63.0
  common B07.8
  external genital organs (venereal) A63.0
  flat B07.8
  Hassal-Henle's (of cornea) H18.49
  Peruvian A44.1
  plantar B07.0
  prosector (tuberculous) A18.4
  seborrheic L82.1
    inflamed L82.0
  senile (seborrheic) L82.1
    inflamed L82.0
  tuberculous A18.4
  venereal A63.0
Warthin's tumor —*see* Neoplasm, salivary gland, benign
Wassilieff's disease A27.0
Wasting
  disease (syndrome) E88.A
    due to
      malnutrition E43
        with marasmus E41
      underlying condition E88.A
  extreme (due to malnutrition) E43
    with marasmus E41
  muscle NEC —*see* Atrophy, muscle
Water
  clefts (senile cataract) —*see* Cataract, senile, incipient
  deprivation of T73.1
  intoxication E87.79
  itch B76.9
  lack of T73.1
    safe drinking Z58.6
  loading E87.70
  on
    brain —*see* Hydrocephalus
    chest J94.8
  poisoning E87.79
Waterbrash R12
Waterhouse (-Friderichsen) **syndrome or disease** (meningococcal) A39.1
Water-losing nephritis N25.89
Watermelon stomach K31.819
  with hemorrhage K31.811
  without hemorrhage K31.819
Watsoniasis B66.8
Wax in ear —*see* Impaction, cerumen
Weak, weakening, weakness (generalized) R53.1
  arches (acquired) —*see also* Deformity, limb, flat foot
  bladder (sphincter) R32
  facial R29.810
    following
      cerebrovascular disease I69.992
      cerebral infarction I69.392
      intracerebral hemorrhage I69.192

Weak, weakening, weakness (continued)
- nontraumatic intracranial hemorrhage NEC I69.292
- specified disease NEC I69.892
- stroke I69.392
- subarachnoid hemorrhage I69.092
- foot (double) —see also Weak, arches
- heart, cardiac —see Failure, heart
- mind F70
- muscle M62.81
- myocardium —see Failure, heart
- newborn P96.89
- pelvic fundus N81.89
- pubocervical tissue N81.82
- senile R54
- rectovaginal tissue N81.83
- urinary stream R39.12
- valvular —see Endocarditis

Wear, worn (with normal or routine use)
- articular bearing surface of internal joint prosthesis —see Complications, joint prosthesis, mechanical, wear of articular bearing surfaces, by site
- device, implant or graft —see Complications, by site, mechanical complication
- tooth, teeth (approximal) (hard tissues) (interproximal) (occlusal) K03.0

Weather, weathered
- effects of
  - cold T69.9
    - specified effect NEC T69.8
  - hot —see Heat
- skin L57.8

Weaver's syndrome Q87.3

Web, webbed (congenital)
- duodenal Q43.8
- esophagus Q39.4
- fingers Q70.1-
- larynx (glottic) (subglottic) Q31.0
- neck (pterygium colli) Q18.3
- Paterson-Kelly D50.1
- popliteal syndrome Q87.89
- toes Q70.3-

Weber-Christian disease M35.6

Weber-Cockayne syndrome (epidermolysis bullosa) Q81.8

Weber-Gubler syndrome G46.3

Weber-Leyden syndrome G46.3

Weber-Osler syndrome I78.0

Weber's paralysis or syndrome G46.3

Wedge-shaped or wedging vertebra —see Collapse, vertebra NEC

Wegener's granulomatosis or syndrome M31.30
- with
  - kidney involvement M31.31
  - lung involvement M31.30
    - with kidney involvement M31.31

Wegner's disease A50.02

Weight
- 1000-2499 grams at birth (low) —see Low, birthweight
- 999 grams or less at birth (extremely low) —see Low, birthweight, extreme

Weight (continued)
- and length below 10th percentile for gestational age P05.1-
- below but length above 10th percentile for gestational age P05.0-
- gain (abnormal) (excessive) R63.5
  - in pregnancy —see Pregnancy, complicated by, excessive weight gain
  - low —see Pregnancy, complicated by, insufficient, weight gain
- loss (abnormal) (cause unknown) R63.4

Weightlessness (effect of) T75.82

Weil (I)-Marchesani syndrome Q87.19

Weil's disease A27.0

Weingarten's syndrome J82.89

Weir Mitchell's disease I73.81

Weiss-Baker syndrome G90.09

Wells' disease L98.3

Wen —see Cyst, sebaceous

Wenckebach's block or phenomenon I44.1

Werdnig-Hoffmann syndrome (muscular atrophy) G12.0

Werlhof's disease D69.3

Wermer's disease or syndrome E31.21

Werner-His disease A79.0

Werner's disease or syndrome E34.8

Wernicke-Korsakoff's syndrome or psychosis (alcoholic) F10.96
- with dependence F10.26
- drug-induced
  - due to drug abuse —see Abuse, drug, by type, with amnestic disorder
  - due to drug dependence —see Dependence, drug, by type, with amnestic disorder
- nonalcoholic F04

Wernicke-Posadas disease B38.9

Wernicke's
- developmental aphasia F80.2
- disease or syndrome E51.2
- encephalopathy E51.2
- polioencephalitis, superior E51.2

West African fever B50.8

Westphal-Strümpell syndrome E83.01

West's syndrome —see Epilepsy, spasms

Wet
- feet, tropical (maceration) (syndrome) —see Immersion, foot
- lung (syndrome), newborn P22.1

Wharton's duct —see condition

Wheal —see Urticaria

Wheezing R06.2

Whiplash injury S13.4

Whipple's disease (see also subcategory M14.8-) K90.81

Whipworm (disease) (infection) (infestation) B79

Whistling face Q87.0

White —see also condition
- kidney, small N03.9
- leg, puerperal, postpartum, childbirth O87.1
- mouth B37.0
- patches of mouth K13.29
- spot lesions, teeth
  - chewing surface K02.51
  - pit and fissure surface K02.51
  - smooth surface K02.61

Whitehead L70.0

Whitlow —see also Cellulitis, digit
- with lymphangitis —see Lymphangitis, acute, digit
- herpesviral B00.89

Whitmore's disease or fever —see Melioidosis

Whooping cough A37.90
- with pneumonia A37.91
- due to Bordetella
  - bronchiseptica A37.81
  - parapertussis A37.11
  - pertussis A37.01
  - specified organism NEC A37.81
- due to
  - Bordetella
    - bronchiseptica A37.80
      - with pneumonia A37.81
    - parapertussis A37.10
      - with pneumonia A37.11
    - pertussis A37.00
      - with pneumonia A37.01
  - specified NEC A37.80
    - with pneumonia A37.81

Wichman's asthma J38.5

Wide cranial sutures, newborn P96.3

Widening aorta —see Ectasia, aorta
- with aneurysm —see Aneurysm, aorta

Wilkie's disease or syndrome K55.1

Wilkinson-Sneddon disease or syndrome L13.1

Willebrand (-Jürgens) **thrombopathy** —see Disease, von Willebrand

Willige-Hunt disease or syndrome G23.1

Williams syndrome Q93.82

Wilms' tumor C64-

Wilson-Mikity syndrome P27.0

Wilson's
- disease or syndrome E83.01
- hepatolenticular degeneration E83.01
- lichen ruber L43.9

Window —see also Imperfect, closure
- aorticopulmonary Q21.4

Winter —see condition

Wiskott-Aldrich syndrome D82.0

Withdrawal state —see also Dependence, drug by type, with withdrawal
- alcohol
  - with perceptual disturbances F10.232
    - due to alcohol abuse F10.132
    - due to alcohol use F10.932
    - abuse —see Abuse, alcohol, with, withdrawal
    - dependence —see Dependence, alcohol, with, withdrawal

Withdrawal state (continued)
- alcohol (continued)
  - use —see Use, alcohol, with, withdrawal
  - without perceptual disturbances F10.239
    - due to alcohol abuse F10.139
    - due to alcohol use F10.939
- caffeine F15.93
- cannabis F12.23
- newborn
  - correct therapeutic substance properly administered P96.2
  - infant of dependent mother P96.1
- therapeutic substance, neonatal P96.2

Witts' anemia D50.8

Witzelsucht F07.0

Woakes' ethmoiditis or syndrome J33.1

Wolff-Hirschorn syndrome Q93.3

Wolff-Parkinson-White syndrome I45.6

Wolhynian fever A79.0

Wolman's disease E75.5

Wood lung or pneumonitis J67.8

Woolly, wooly hair (congenital) (nevus) Q84.1

Woolsorter's disease A22.1

Word
- blindness (congenital) (developmental) F81.0
- deafness (congenital) (developmental) H93.25

Worm(s) (infection) (infestation) —see also Infestation, helminth
- guinea B72
- in intestine NEC B82.0

Worm-eaten soles A66.3

Worn out —see Exhaustion
- cardiac
  - defibrillator (with synchronous cardiac pacemaker) Z45.02
  - pacemaker
    - battery Z45.010
    - lead Z45.018
  - device, implant or graft —see Complications, by site, mechanical

Worried well Z71.1

Worries R45.82

Wound check Z48.0-
- due to injury - code to Injury, by site, using appropriate seventh character for subsequent encounter
- postoperative —see Aftercare

Wound, open T14.8-
- abdomen, abdominal
  - wall S31.109
    - with penetration into peritoneal cavity S31.609
    - bite —see Bite, abdomen, wall
    - epigastric region S31.102
      - with penetration into peritoneal cavity S31.602
      - bite —see Bite, abdomen, wall, epigastric region
      - laceration —see Laceration, abdomen, wall, epigastric region
      - puncture —see Puncture, abdomen, wall, epigastric region

Wound, open (continued)
  abdomen, abdominal (continued)
    wall (continued)
      laceration —see Laceration, abdomen, wall
      left
        lower quadrant S31.104
          with penetration into peritoneal cavity S31.604
          bite —see Bite, abdomen, wall, left, lower quadrant
          laceration —see Laceration, abdomen, wall, left, lower quadrant
          puncture —see Puncture, abdomen, wall, left, lower quadrant
        upper quadrant S31.101
          with penetration into peritoneal cavity S31.601
          bite —see Bite, abdomen, wall, left, upper quadrant
          laceration —see Laceration, abdomen, wall, left, upper quadrant
          puncture —see Puncture, abdomen, wall, left, upper quadrant
      periumbilic region S31.105
        with penetration into peritoneal cavity S31.605
        bite —see Bite, abdomen, wall, periumbilic region
        laceration —see Laceration, abdomen, wall, periumbilic region
        puncture —see Puncture, abdomen, wall, periumbilic region
      puncture —see Puncture, abdomen, wall
      right
        lower quadrant S31.103
          with penetration into peritoneal cavity S31.603
          bite —see Bite, abdomen, wall, right, lower quadrant
          laceration —see Laceration, abdomen, wall, right, lower quadrant
          puncture —see Puncture, abdomen, wall, right, lower quadrant
        upper quadrant S31.100
          with penetration into peritoneal cavity S31.600
          bite —see Bite, abdomen, wall, right, upper quadrant
          laceration —see Laceration, abdomen, wall, right, upper quadrant
          puncture —see Puncture, abdomen, wall, right, upper quadrant
  alveolar (process) —see Wound, open, oral cavity

Wound, open (continued)
  ankle S91.00-
    bite —see Bite, ankle
    laceration —see Laceration, ankle
    puncture —see Puncture, ankle
  antecubital space —see Wound, open, elbow
  anterior chamber, eye —see Wound, open, ocular
  anus S31.839
    bite S31.835
    laceration —see Laceration, anus
    puncture —see Puncture, anus
  arm (upper) S41.10-
    with amputation —see Amputation, traumatic, arm
    bite —see Bite, arm
    forearm —see Wound, open, forearm
    laceration —see Laceration, arm
    puncture —see Puncture, arm
  auditory canal (external) (meatus) —see Wound, open, ear
  auricle, ear —see Wound, open, ear
  axilla —see Wound, open, arm
  back —see also Wound, open, thorax, back
    lower S31.000
      with penetration into retroperitoneal space S31.001
      bite —see Bite, back, lower
      laceration —see Laceration, back, lower
      puncture —see Puncture, back, lower
    bite —see Bite
  blood vessel —see Injury, blood vessel
  breast S21.00-
    with amputation —see Amputation, traumatic, breast
    bite —see Bite, breast
    laceration —see Laceration, breast
    puncture —see Puncture, breast
  buttock S31.809
    bite —see Bite, buttock
    laceration —see Laceration, buttock
    left S31.829
    puncture —see Puncture, buttock
    right S31.819
  calf —see Wound, open, leg
  canaliculus lacrimalis —see Wound, open, eyelid
  canthus, eye —see Wound, open, eyelid
  cervical esophagus S11.20
    bite S11.25
    laceration —see Laceration, esophagus, traumatic, cervical
    puncture —see Puncture, cervical esophagus
  cheek (external) S01.40-
    bite —see Bite, cheek
    laceration —see Laceration, cheek
    puncture —see Puncture, cheek
    internal —see Wound, open, oral cavity
  chest wall —see Wound, open, thorax
  chin —see Wound, open, head, specified site NEC
  choroid —see Wound, open, ocular
  ciliary body (eye) —see Wound, open, ocular

Wound, open (continued)
  clitoris S31.40
    with amputation —see Amputation, traumatic, clitoris
    bite S31.45
    laceration —see Laceration, vulva
    puncture —see Puncture, vulva
  conjunctiva —see Wound, open, ocular
  cornea —see Wound, open, ocular
  costal region —see Wound, open, thorax
  Descemet's membrane —see Wound, open, ocular
  digit(s)
    foot —see Wound, open, toe
    hand —see Wound, open, finger
  ear (canal) (external) S01.30-
    with amputation —see Amputation, traumatic, ear
    bite —see Bite, ear
    laceration —see Laceration, ear
    puncture —see Puncture, ear
    drum S09.2-
  elbow S51.00-
    bite —see Bite, elbow
    laceration —see Laceration, elbow
    puncture —see Puncture, elbow
  epididymis —see Wound, open, testis
  epigastric region S31.102
    with penetration into peritoneal cavity S31.602
    bite —see Bite, abdomen, wall, epigastric region
    laceration —see Laceration, abdomen, wall, epigastric region
    puncture —see Puncture, abdomen, wall, epigastric region
  epiglottis —see Wound, open, neck, specified site NEC
  esophagus (thoracic) S27.819
    cervical —see Wound, open, cervical esophagus
    laceration S27.813
    specified type NEC S27.818
  eye —see Wound, open, ocular
  eyeball —see Wound, open, ocular
  eyebrow —see Wound, open, eyelid
  eyelid S01.10-
    bite —see Bite, eyelid
    laceration —see Laceration, eyelid
    puncture —see Puncture, eyelid
  face NEC —see Wound, open, head, specified site NEC
  finger(s) S61.209
    with
      amputation —see Amputation, traumatic, finger
      damage to nail S61.309
    bite —see Bite, finger
    index S61.208
      with
        damage to nail S61.308
      left S61.201
        with
          damage to nail S61.301
      right S61.200
        with
          damage to nail S61.300

Wound, open (continued)
  finger(s) (continued)
    laceration —see Laceration, finger
    little S61.208
      with
        damage to nail S61.308
      left S61.207
        with damage to nail S61.307
      right S61.206
        with damage to nail S61.306
    middle S61.208
      with
        damage to nail S61.308
      left S61.203
        with damage to nail S61.303
      right S61.202
        with damage to nail S61.302
    puncture —see Puncture, finger
    ring S61.208
      with
        damage to nail S61.308
      left S61.205
        with damage to nail S61.305
      right S61.204
        with damage to nail S61.304
  flank —see Wound, open, abdomen, wall
  foot (except toe(s) alone) S91.30-
    with amputation —see Amputation, traumatic, foot
    bite —see Bite, foot
    laceration —see Laceration, foot
    puncture —see Puncture, foot
    toe —see Wound, open, toe
  forearm S51.80-
    with
      amputation —see Amputation, traumatic, forearm
    bite —see Bite, forearm
    elbow only —see Wound, open, elbow
    laceration —see Laceration, forearm
    puncture —see Puncture, forearm
  forehead —see Wound, open, head, specified site NEC
  genital organs, external
    with amputation —see Amputation, traumatic, genital organs
    bite —see Bite, genital organ
    female S31.502
      vagina S31.40
      vulva S31.40
    laceration —see Laceration, genital organ
    male S31.501
      penis S31.20
      scrotum S31.30
      testes S31.30
    puncture —see Puncture, genital organ
  globe (eye) —see Wound, open, ocular
  groin —see Wound, open, abdomen, wall
  gum —see Wound, open, oral cavity
  hand S61.40-
    with
      amputation —see Amputation, traumatic, hand

Wound, open *(continued)*
  hand *(continued)*
    bite —*see* Bite, hand
    finger(s) —*see* Wound, open, finger
    laceration —*see* Laceration, hand
    puncture —*see* Puncture, hand
    thumb —*see* Wound, open, thumb
  head S01.90
    bite —*see* Bite, head
    cheek —*see* Wound, open, cheek
    ear —*see* Wound, open, ear
    eyelid —*see* Wound, open, eyelid
    laceration —*see* Laceration, head
    lip —*see* Wound, open, lip
    nose S01.20
    oral cavity —*see* Wound, open, oral cavity
    puncture —*see* Puncture, head
    scalp —*see* Wound, open, scalp
    specified site NEC S01.80
    temporomandibular area —*see* Wound, open, cheek
  heel —*see* Wound, open, foot
  hip S71.00-
    with amputation —*see* Amputation, traumatic, hip
    bite —*see* Bite, hip
    laceration —*see* Laceration, hip
    puncture —*see* Puncture, hip
  hymen S31.40
    bite —*see* Bite, vulva
    laceration —*see* Laceration, vagina
    puncture —*see* Puncture, vagina
  hypochondrium S31.109
    bite —*see* Bite, hypochondrium
    laceration —*see* Laceration, hypochondrium
    puncture —*see* Puncture, hypochondrium
  hypogastric region S31.109
    bite —*see* Bite, hypogastric region
    laceration —*see* Laceration, hypogastric region
    puncture —*see* Puncture, hypogastric region
  iliac (region) —*see* Wound, open, inguinal region
  inguinal region S31.109
    bite —*see* Bite, abdomen, wall, lower quadrant
    laceration —*see* Laceration, inguinal region
    puncture —*see* Puncture, inguinal region
  instep —*see* Wound, open, foot
  interscapular region —*see* Wound, open, thorax, back
  intraocular —*see* Wound, open, ocular
  iris —*see* Wound, open, ocular
  jaw —*see* Wound, open, head, specified site NEC
  knee S81.00-
    bite —*see* Bite, knee
    laceration —*see* Laceration, knee
    puncture —*see* Puncture, knee
  labium (majus) (minus) —*see* Wound, open, vulva
  laceration —*see* Laceration, by site

Wound, open *(continued)*
  lacrimal duct —*see* Wound, open, eyelid
  larynx S11.019
    bite —*see* Bite, larynx
    laceration —*see* Laceration, larynx
    puncture —*see* Puncture, larynx
  left
    lower quadrant S31.104
      with penetration into peritoneal cavity S31.604
      bite —*see* Bite, abdomen, wall, left, lower quadrant
      laceration —*see* Laceration, abdomen, wall, left, lower quadrant
      puncture —*see* Puncture, abdomen, wall, left, lower quadrant
    upper quadrant S31.101
      with penetration into peritoneal cavity S31.601
      bite —*see* Bite, abdomen, wall, left, upper quadrant
      laceration —*see* Laceration, abdomen, wall, left, upper quadrant
      puncture —*see* Puncture, abdomen, wall, left, upper quadrant
  leg (lower) S81.80-
    with amputation —*see* Amputation, traumatic, leg
    ankle —*see* Wound, open, ankle
    bite —*see* Bite, leg
    foot —*see* Wound, open, foot
    knee —*see* Wound, open, knee
    laceration —*see* Laceration, leg
    puncture —*see* Puncture, leg
    toe —*see* Wound, open, toe
    upper —*see* Wound, open, thigh
  lip S01.501
    bite —*see* Bite, lip
    laceration —*see* Laceration, lip
    puncture —*see* Puncture, lip
  loin S31.109
    bite —*see* Bite, abdomen wall
    laceration —*see* Laceration, loin
    puncture —*see* Puncture, loin
  lower back —*see* Wound, open, back, lower
  lumbar region —*see* Wound, open, back, lower
  malar region —*see* Wound, open, head, specified site NEC
  mammary —*see* Wound, open, breast
  mastoid region —*see* Wound, open, head, specified site NEC
  mouth —*see* Wound, open, oral cavity
  nail
    finger —*see* Wound, open, finger, with damage to nail
    toe —*see* Wound, open, toe, with damage to nail
  nape (neck) —*see* Wound, open, neck
  nasal (septum) (sinus) —*see* Wound, open, nose
  nasopharynx —*see* Wound, open, head, specified site NEC

Wound, open *(continued)*
  neck S11.90
    bite —*see* Bite, neck
    involving
      cervical esophagus S11.20
      larynx —*see* Wound, open, larynx
      pharynx S11.20
      thyroid S11.10
      trachea (cervical) S11.029
        bite —*see* Bite, trachea
        laceration S11.021
          with foreign body S11.022
        puncture S11.023
          with foreign body S11.024
    laceration —*see* Laceration, neck
    puncture —*see* Puncture, neck
    specified site NEC S11.80
    specified type NEC S11.89
  nose (septum) (sinus) S01.20
    with amputation —*see* Amputation, traumatic, nose
    bite —*see* Bite, nose
    laceration —*see* Laceration, nose
    puncture —*see* Puncture, nose
  ocular S05.90
    avulsion (traumatic enucleation) S05.7-
    eyeball S05.6-
      with foreign body S05.5-
    eyelid —*see* Wound, open, eyelid
    laceration and rupture S05.3-
      with prolapse or loss of intraocular tissue S05.2-
    orbit (penetrating) (with or without foreign body) S05.4-
    periocular area —*see* Wound, open, eyelid
    specified NEC S05.8X-
  oral cavity S01.502
    bite S01.552
    laceration —*see* Laceration, oral cavity
    puncture —*see* Puncture, oral cavity
  orbit —*see* Wound, open, ocular, orbit
  palate —*see* Wound, open, oral cavity
  palm —*see* Wound, open, hand
  pelvis, pelvic —*see also* Wound, open, back, lower
    girdle —*see* Wound, open, hip
  penetrating —*see* Puncture, by site
  penis S31.20
    with amputation —*see* Amputation, traumatic, penis
    bite S31.25
    laceration —*see* Laceration, penis
    puncture —*see* Puncture, penis
  perineum
    bite —*see* Bite, perineum
    female S31.502
    laceration —*see* Laceration, perineum
    male S31.501
    puncture —*see* Puncture, perineum
  periocular area (with or without lacrimal passages) —*see* Wound, open, eyelid

Wound, open *(continued)*
  periumbilic region S31.105
    with penetration into peritoneal cavity S31.605
    bite —*see* Bite, abdomen, wall, periumbilic region
    laceration —*see* Laceration, abdomen, wall, periumbilic region
    puncture —*see* Puncture, abdomen, wall, periumbilic region
  phalanges
    finger —*see* Wound, open, finger
    toe —*see* Wound, open, toe
  pharynx S11.20
  pinna —*see* Wound, open, ear
  popliteal space —*see* Wound, open, knee
  prepuce —*see* Wound, open, penis
  pubic region —*see* Wound, open, back, lower
  pudendum —*see* Wound, open, genital organs, external
  puncture wound —*see* Puncture
  rectovaginal septum —*see* Wound, open, vagina
  right
    lower quadrant S31.103
      with penetration into peritoneal cavity S31.603
      bite —*see* Bite, abdomen, wall, right, lower quadrant
      laceration —*see* Laceration, abdomen, wall, right, lower quadrant
      puncture —*see* Puncture, abdomen, wall, right, lower quadrant
    upper quadrant S31.100
      with penetration into peritoneal cavity S31.600
      bite —*see* Bite, abdomen, wall, right, upper quadrant
      laceration —*see* Laceration, abdomen, wall, right, upper quadrant
      puncture —*see* Puncture, abdomen, wall, right, upper quadrant
  sacral region —*see* Wound, open, back, lower
  sacroiliac region —*see* Wound, open, back, lower
  salivary gland —*see* Wound, open, oral cavity
  scalp S01.00
    bite S01.05
    laceration —*see* Laceration, scalp
    puncture —*see* Puncture, scalp
  scalpel, newborn (birth injury) P15.8
  scapular region —*see* Wound, open, shoulder
  sclera —*see* Wound, open, ocular
  scrotum S31.30
    with amputation —*see* Amputation, traumatic, scrotum
    bite S31.35
    laceration —*see* Laceration, scrotum
    puncture —*see* Puncture, scrotum
  shin —*see* Wound, open, leg

343

Wound, open *(continued)*
  shoulder S41.00-
    with amputation —see
      Amputation, traumatic, arm
    bite —see Bite, shoulder
    laceration —see Laceration,
      shoulder
    puncture —see Puncture,
      shoulder
  skin NOS T14.8
  spermatic cord —see Wound, open,
    testis
  sternal region —see Wound, open,
    thorax, front wall
  submaxillary region —see
    Wound, open, head, specified
    site NEC
  submental region —see
    Wound, open, head, specified
    site NEC
  subungual
    finger(s) —see Wound, open,
      finger
    toe(s) —see Wound, open, toe
  supraclavicular region —see
    Wound, open, neck, specified
    site NEC
  temple, temporal region —see
    Wound, open, head, specified
    site NEC
  temporomandibular area —see
    Wound, open, cheek
  testis S31.30
    with amputation —see
      Amputation, traumatic, testes
    bite S31.35
    laceration —see Laceration,
      testis
    puncture —see Puncture, testis
  thigh S71.10-
    with amputation —see
      Amputation, traumatic, hip
    bite —see Bite, thigh
    laceration —see Laceration,
      thigh
    puncture —see Puncture, thigh
  thorax, thoracic (wall) S21.90
    back S21.20-
      with penetration S21.40
    bite —see Bite, thorax
    breast —see Wound, open,
      breast
    front S21.10-
      with penetration S21.30
    laceration —see Laceration,
      thorax
    puncture —see Puncture, thorax
  throat —see Wound, open, neck
  thumb S61.009
    with
      amputation —see Amputation,
        traumatic, thumb
      damage to nail S61.109
    bite —see Bite, thumb
    laceration —see Laceration,
      thumb
    left S61.002
      with
        damage to nail S61.102
    puncture —see Puncture, thumb
    right S61.001
      with
        damage to nail S61.101
  thyroid (gland) —see Wound, open,
    neck, thyroid
  toe(s) S91.109
    with
      amputation —see Amputation,
        traumatic, toe
      damage to nail S91.209

Wound, open *(continued)*
  toe(s) *(continued)*
    bite —see Bite, toe
    great S91.103
      with
        damage to nail S91.203
      left S91.102
        with
          damage to nail S91.202
      right S91.101
        with
          damage to nail S91.201
    laceration —see Laceration, toe
    lesser S91.106
      with
        damage to nail S91.206
      left S91.105
        with
          damage to nail S91.205
      right S91.104
        with
          damage to nail S91.204
    puncture —see Puncture, toe
  tongue —see Wound, open, oral
    cavity
  trachea (cervical region) —see
    Wound, open, neck, trachea
  tunica vaginalis —see Wound,
    open, testis
  tympanum, tympanic membrane
    S09.2-
    laceration —see Laceration, ear,
      drum
    puncture —see Puncture,
      tympanum
  umbilical region —see Wound,
    open, abdomen, wall,
    periumbilic region
  uvula —see Wound, open, oral
    cavity
  vagina S31.40
    bite S31.45
    laceration —see Laceration,
      vagina
    puncture —see Puncture,
      vagina
  vocal cord S11.039
    bite —see Bite, vocal cord
    laceration S11.031
      with foreign body S11.032
    puncture S11.033
      with foreign body S11.034
  vitreous (humor) —see Wound,
    open, ocular
  vulva S31.40
    with amputation —see
      Amputation, traumatic, vulva
    bite S31.45
    laceration —see Laceration,
      vulva
    puncture —see Puncture, vulva
  wrist S61.50-
    bite —see Bite, wrist
    laceration —see Laceration,
      wrist
    puncture —see Puncture, wrist
Wound, superficial —see Injury —
  see also specified injury type
Wright's syndrome G54.0
Wrist —see condition
Wrong drug (by accident) (given in
  error) —see Table of Drugs and
  Chemicals, by drug, poisoning
Wry neck —see Torticollis
Wuchereria (bancrofti) **infestation**
  B74.0
Wuchereriasis B74.0
Wuchernde Struma Langhans C73

X

Xanthelasma (eyelid) (palpebrarum)
  H02.60
  left H02.66
    lower H02.65
    upper H02.64
  right H02.63
    lower H02.62
    upper H02.61
Xanthelasmatosis (essential)
  E78.2
Xanthinuria, hereditary E79.82
Xanthoastrocytoma
  specified site —see Neoplasm,
    malignant, by site
  unspecified site C71.9
Xanthofibroma —see Neoplasm,
  connective tissue, benign
Xanthogranuloma D76.3
Xanthoma(s), xanthomatosis (primary)
  (familial) (hereditary) E75.5
  with
    hyperlipoproteinemia
      Type I E78.3
      Type III E78.2
      Type IV E78.1
      Type V E78.3
  bone (generalisata) C96.5
  cerebrotendinous E75.5
  cutaneotendinous E75.5
  disseminatum (skin) E78.2
  eruptive E78.2
  hypercholesterinemic E78.00
  hypercholesterolemic E78.00
  hyperlipidemic E78.5
  joint E75.5
  multiple (skin) E78.2
  tendon (sheath) E75.5
  tubo-eruptive E78.2
  tuberosum E78.2
  tuberous E78.2
  verrucous, oral mucosa
    K13.4
Xanthosis R23.8
Xenophobia F40.10
Xeroderma —see also Ichthyosis
  acquired L85.0
  eyelid H01.149
    left H01.146
      lower H01.145
      upper H01.144
    right H01.143
      lower H01.142
      upper H01.141
  pigmentosum Q82.1
  vitamin A deficiency E50.8
Xerophthalmia (vitamin A
  deficiency) E50.7
  unrelated to vitamin A deficiency
    —see Keratoconjunctivitis
Xerosis
  conjunctiva H11.14-
    with Bitot's spots —see also
      Pigmentation, conjunctiva
      vitamin A deficiency E50.1
    vitamin A deficiency E50.0
  cornea H18.89-
    with ulceration —see Ulcer,
      cornea
    vitamin A deficiency
      E50.3
    vitamin A deficiency E50.2
  cutis (dry skin) L85.3
  skin L85.3
Xerostomia K11.7

Xiphopagus Q89.4
XO syndrome Q96.9
X-ray (of)
  abnormal findings —see Abnormal,
    diagnostic imaging
  breast (mammogram) (routine)
    Z12.31
  chest
    routine (as part of a general
      medical examination)
      Z00.00
      with abnormal findings
        Z00.01
    routine (as part of a general
      medical examination) Z00.00
      with abnormal findings
        Z00.01
XXXXY syndrome Q98.1
XXY syndrome Q98.0

Y

Yaba pox (virus disease)
  B08.72
Yatapoxvirus B08.70
  specified NEC B08.79
Yawning R06.89
  psychogenic F45.8
Yaws A66.9
  bone lesions A66.6
  butter A66.1
  chancre A66.0
  cutaneous, less than five years after
    infection A66.2
  early (cutaneous) (macular)
    (maculopapular) (micropapular)
    (papular) A66.2
    frambeside A66.2
    skin lesions NEC A66.2
  eyelid A66.2
  ganglion A66.6
  gangosis, gangosa A66.5
  gumma, gummata A66.4
    bone A66.6
  gummatous
    frambeside A66.4
    osteitis A66.6
    periostitis A66.6
  hydrarthrosis (see also subcategory
    M14.8-) A66.6
  hyperkeratosis (early) (late)
    A66.3
  initial lesions A66.0
  joint lesions (see also subcategory
    M14.8-) A66.6
  juxta-articular nodules A66.7
  late nodular (ulcerated) A66.4
  latent (without clinical
    manifestations) (with positive
    serology) A66.8
  mother A66.0
  mucosal A66.7
  multiple papillomata A66.1
  nodular, late (ulcerated) A66.4
  osteitis A66.6
  papilloma, plantar or palmar
    A66.1
  periostitis (hypertrophic) A66.6
  specified NEC A66.7
  ulcers A66.4
  wet crab A66.1
Yeast infection (see also Candidiasis)
  B37.9
Yellow
  atrophy (liver) —see Failure,
    hepatic
  fever —see Fever, yellow

Yellow *(continued)*
  jack —*see* Fever, yellow
  jaundice —*see* Jaundice
  nail syndrome L60.5
Yersiniosis —*see also* Infection, Yersinia
  extraintestinal A28.2
  intestinal A04.6

Z

Zahorsky's syndrome (herpangina) B08.5
Zellweger's syndrome E71.510
Zenker's diverticulum (esophagus) K22.5

Ziehen-Oppenheim disease G24.1
Zieve's syndrome K70.0
Zika NOS A92.5
  congenital P35.4
Zinc
  deficiency, dietary E60
  metabolism disorder E83.2

Zollinger-Ellison syndrome E16.4
Zona —*see* Herpes, zoster
Zoophobia F40.218
Zoster (herpes) —*see* Herpes, zoster
Zygomycosis B46.9
  specified NEC B46.8
Zymotic —*see* condition

Neoplasm Table Guidance

The Neoplasm Table gives the code numbers for neoplasms by anatomical site. For each site there are six possible code numbers according to whether the neoplasm in question is malignant, benign, in situ, of uncertain behavior, or of unspecified nature. The description of the neoplasm will often indicate which of the six columns is appropriate; e.g., malignant melanoma of skin, benign fibroadenoma of breast, carcinoma in situ of cervix uteri.

Where such descriptors are not present, the remainder of the Index should be consulted where guidance is given to the appropriate column for each morphological (histological) variety listed; e.g., Mesonephroma—see Neoplasm, malignant; Embryoma—see also Neoplasm, uncertain behavior; Disease, Bowen's—see Neoplasm, skin, in situ. However, the guidance in the Index can be overridden if one of the descriptors mentioned above is present; e.g., malignant adenoma of colon is coded to C18.9 and not to D12.6 as the adjective "malignant" overrides the Index entry "Adenoma—see also Neoplasm, benign."

Codes listed with a dash -, following the code have a required additional character for laterality. The tabular must be reviewed for the complete code.

Table of Neoplasms

	Malignant Primary	Malignant Secondary	Ca in situ	Benign	Uncertain Behavior	Unspecified Behavior
Neoplasm, neoplastic	C80.1	C79.9	D09.9	D36.9	D48.9	D49.9
A						
abdomen, abdominal	C76.2	C79.8-	D09.8	D36.7	D48.7	D49.89
cavity	C76.2	C79.8-	D09.8	D36.7	D48.7	D49.89
organ	C76.2	C79.8-	D09.8	D36.7	D48.7	D49.89
viscera	C76.2	C79.8-	D09.8	D36.7	D48.7	D49.89
wall—see also Neoplasm, abdomen, wall, skin	C44.509	C79.2	D04.5	D23.5	D48.5	D49.2
connective tissue	C49.4	C79.8-	-	D21.4	D48.1	D49.2
skin	C44.509					
basal cell carcinoma	C44.519	-	-	-	-	-
specified type NEC	C44.599	-	-	-	-	-
squamous cell carcinoma	C44.529	-	-	-	-	-
abdominopelvic	C76.8	C79.8-	-	D36.7	D48.7	D49.89
accessory sinus—see Neoplasm, sinus						
acoustic nerve	C72.4-	C79.49	-	D33.3	D43.3	D49.7
adenoid (pharynx) (tissue)	C11.1	C79.89	D00.08	D10.6	D37.05	D49.0
adipose tissue —see also Neoplasm, connective tissue	C49.4	C79.89	-	D21.9	D48.1	D49.2
adnexa (uterine)	C57.4	C79.89	D07.39	D28.7	D39.8	D49.59
adrenal	C74.9-	C79.7-	D09.3	D35.0-	D44.1-	D49.7
capsule	C74.9-	C79.7-	D09.3	D35.0-	D44.1-	D49.7
cortex	C74.0-	C79.7-	D09.3	D35.0-	D44.1-	D49.7
gland	C74.9-	C79.7-	D09.3	D35.0-	D44.1-	D49.7
medulla	C74.1-	C79.7-	D09.3	D35.0-	D44.1-	D49.7
ala nasi (external)—see also Neoplasm, skin, nose	C44.301	C79.2	D04.39	D23.39	D48.5	D49.2
alimentary canal or tract NEC	C26.9	C78.80	D01.9	D13.99	D37.9	D49.0
alveolar	C03.9	C79.89	D00.03	D10.39	D37.09	D49.0
mucosa	C03.9	C79.89	D00.03	D10.39	D37.09	D49.0
lower	C03.1	C79.89	D00.03	D10.39	D37.09	D49.0
upper	C03.0	C79.89	D00.03	D10.39	D37.09	D49.0
ridge or process	C41.1	C79.51	-	D16.5	D48.0	D49.2
carcinoma	C03.9	C79.8-	-	-	-	-
lower	C03.1	C79.8-	-	-	-	-
upper	C03.0	C79.8-	-	-	-	-
lower	C41.1	C79.51	-	D16.5-	D48.0	D49.2
mucosa	C03.9	C79.89	D00.03	D10.39	D37.09	D49.0
lower	C03.1	C79.89	D00.03	D10.39	D37.09	D49.0
upper	C03.0	C79.89	D00.03	D10.39	D37.09	D49.0
upper	C41.0	C79.51	-	D16.4-	D48.0	D49.2
sulcus	C06.1	C79.89	D00.02	D10.39	D37.09	D49.0
alveolus	C03.9	C79.89	D00.03	D10.39	D37.09	D49.0
lower	C03.1	C79.89	D00.03	D10.39	D37.09	D49.0
upper	C03.0	C79.89	D00.03	D10.39	D37.09	D49.0
ampulla of Vater	C24.1	C78.89	D01.5	D13.5	D37.6	D49.0
ankle NEC	C76.5-	C79.89	D04.7-	D36.7	D48.7	D49.89

	Malignant Primary	Malignant Secondary	Ca in situ	Benign	Uncertain Behavior	Unspecified Behavior
anorectum, anorectal (junction)	C21.8	C78.5	D01.3	D12.9	D37.8	D49.0
antecubital fossa or space	C76.4-	C79.89	D04.6-	D36.7	D48.7	D49.89
antrum (Highmore) (maxillary)	C31.0	C78.39	D02.3	D14.0	D38.5	D49.1
pyloric	C16.3	C78.89	D00.2	D13.1	D37.1	D49.0
tympanicum	C30.1	C78.39	D02.3	D14.0	D38.5	D49.1
anus, anal	C21.0	C78.5	D01.3	D12.9	D37.8	D49.0
canal	C21.1	C78.5	D01.3	D12.9	D37.8	D49.0
cloacogenic zone	C21.2	C78.5	D01.3	D12.9	D37.8	D49.0
margin—see also Neoplasm, anus, skin	C44.500	C79.2	D04.5	D23.5	D48.5	D49.2
overlapping lesion with rectosigmoid junction or rectum	C21.8	-	-	-	-	-
skin	C44.500	C79.2	D04.5	D23.5	D48.5	D49.2
basal cell carcinoma	C44.510	-	-	-	-	-
specified type NEC	C44.590	-	-	-	-	-
squamous cell carcinoma	C44.520	-	-	-	-	-
sphincter	C21.1	C78.5	D01.3	D12.9	D37.8	D49.0
aorta (thoracic)	C49.3	C79.89	-	D21.3	D48.1	D49.2
abdominal	C49.4	C79.89	-	D21.4	D48.1	D49.2
aortic body	C75.5	C79.89	-	D35.6	D44.7	D49.7
aponeurosis	C49.9	C79.89	-	D21.9	D48.1	D49.2
palmar	C49.1-	C79.89	-	D21.1-	D48.1	D49.2
plantar	C49.2-	C79.89	-	D21.2-	D48.1	D49.2
appendix	C18.1	C78.5	D01.0	D12.1	D37.3	D49.0
arachnoid	C70.9	C79.49	-	D32.9	D42.9	D49.7
cerebral	C70.0	C79.32	-	D32.0	D42.0	D49.7
spinal	C70.1	C79.49	-	D32.1	D42.1	D49.7
areola	C50.0-	C79.81	D05.-	D24.-	D48.6-	D49.3
arm NEC	C76.4-	C79.89	D04.6-	D36.7	D48.7	D49.89
artery—see Neoplasm, connective tissue						
aryepiglottic fold	C13.1	C79.89	D00.08	D10.7	D37.05	D49.0
hypopharyngeal aspect	C13.1	C79.89	D00.08	D10.7	D37.05	D49.0
laryngeal aspect	C32.1	C78.39	D02.0	D14.1	D38.0	D49.1
marginal zone	C13.1	C79.89	D00.08	D10.7	D37.05	D49.0
arytenoid (cartilage)	C32.3	C78.39	D02.0	D14.1	D38.0	D49.1
fold—see Neoplasm, aryepiglottic						
associated with transplanted organ	C80.2	-	-	-	-	-
atlas	C41.2	C79.51	-	D16.6	D48.0	D49.2
atrium, cardiac	C38.0	C79.89	-	D15.1	D48.7	D49.89
auditory						
canal (external) (skin)	C44.20-	C79.2	D04.2-	D23.2-	D48.5	D49.2
internal	C30.1	C78.39	D02.3	D14.0	D38.5	D49.1
nerve	C72.4-	C79.49	-	D33.3	D43.3	D49.7
tube	C30.1	C78.39	D02.3	D14.0	D38.5	D49.1
opening	C11.2	C79.89	D00.08	D10.6	D37.05	D49.0

347

Table of Neoplasms

	Malignant Primary	Malignant Secondary	Ca in situ	Benign	Uncertain Behavior	Unspecified Behavior
auricle, ear—see also Neoplasm, skin, ear	C44.20-	C79.2	D04.2-	D23.2-	D48.5	D49.2
auricular canal (external)—see also Neoplasm, skin, ear	C44.20-	C79.2	D04.2-	D23.2-	D48.5	D49.2
internal	C30.1	C78.39	D02.3	D14.0	D38.5	D49.2
autonomic nerve or nervous system NEC (see Neoplasm, nerve, peripheral)						
axilla, axillary	C76.1	C79.89	D09.8	D36.7	D48.7	D49.89
fold—see also Neoplasm, skin, trunk	C44.509	C79.2	D04.5	D23.5	D48.5	D49.2
B						
back NEC	C76.8	C79.89	D04.5	D36.7	D48.7	D49.89
Bartholin's gland	C51.0	C79.82	D07.1	D28.0	D39.8	D49.59
basal ganglia	C71.0	C79.31	-	D33.0	D43.0	D49.6
basis pedunculi	C71.7	C79.31	-	D33.1	D43.1	D49.6
bile or biliary (tract)	C24.9	C78.89	D01.5	D13.5	D37.6	D49.0
canaliculi (biliferi) (intrahepatic)	C22.1	C78.7	D01.5	D13.4	D37.6	D49.0
canals, interlobular	C22.1	C78.89	D01.5	D13.4	D37.6	D49.0
duct or passage (common) (cystic) (extrahepatic)	C24.0	C78.89	D01.5	D13.5	D37.6	D49.0
interlobular	C22.1	C78.89	D01.5	D13.4	D37.6	D49.0
intrahepatic	C22.1	C78.7	D01.5	D13.4	D37.6	D49.0
and extrahepatic	C24.8	C78.89	D01.5	D13.5	D37.6	D49.0
bladder (urinary)	C67.9	C79.11	D09.0	D30.3	D41.4	D49.4
dome	C67.1	C79.11	D09.0	D30.3	D41.4	D49.4
neck	C67.5	C79.11	D09.0	D30.3	D41.4	D49.4
orifice	C67.9	C79.11	D09.0	D30.3	D41.4	D49.4
ureteric	C67.6	C79.11	D09.0	D30.3	D41.4	D49.4
urethral	C67.5	C79.11	D09.0	D30.3	D41.4	D49.4
overlapping lesion	C67.8	-	-	-	-	-
sphincter	C67.8	C79.11	D09.0	D30.3	D41.4	D49.4
trigone	C67.0	C79.11	D09.0	D30.3	D41.4	D49.4
urachus	C67.7	C79.11	D09.0	D30.3	D41.4	D49.4
wall	C67.9	C79.11	D09.0	D30.3	D41.4	D49.4
anterior	C67.3	C79.11	D09.0	D30.3	D41.4	D49.4
lateral	C67.2	C79.11	D09.0	D30.3	D41.4	D49.4
posterior	C67.4	C79.11	D09.0	D30.3	D41.4	D49.4
blood vessel—see Neoplasm, connective tissue						
bone (periosteum)	C41.9	C79.51	-	D16.9	D48.0	D49.2
acetabulum	C41.4	C79.51	-	D16.8	D48.0	D49.2
ankle	C40.3-	C79.51	-	D16.3-	-	-
arm NEC	C40.0-	C79.51	-	D16.0-	-	-
astragalus	C40.3-	C79.51	-	D16.3-	-	-
atlas	C41.2	C79.51	-	D16.6	D48.0	D49.2
axis	C41.2	C79.51	-	D16.6	D48.0	D49.2
back NEC	C41.2	C79.51	-	D16.6	D48.0	D49.2
calcaneus	C40.3-	C79.51	-	D16.3-	-	-
calvarium	C41.0	C79.51	-	D16.4	D48.0	D49.2
carpus (any)	C40.1-	C79.51	-	D16.1-	-	-
cartilage NEC	C41.9	C79.51	-	D16.9	D48.0	D49.2

	Malignant Primary	Malignant Secondary	Ca in situ	Benign	Uncertain Behavior	Unspecified Behavior
bone — continued						
clavicle	C41.3	C79.51	-	D16.7	D48.0	D49.2
clivus	C41.0	C79.51	-	D16.4	D48.0	D49.2
coccygeal vertebra	C41.4	C79.51	-	D16.8	D48.0	D49.2
coccyx	C41.4	C79.51	-	D16.8	D48.0	D49.2
costal cartilage	C41.3	C79.51	-	D16.7	D48.0	D49.2
costovertebral joint	C41.3	C79.51	-	D16.7	D48.0	D49.2
cranial	C41.0	C79.51	-	D16.4	D48.0	D49.2
cuboid	C40.3-	C79.51	-	D16.3-	-	-
cuneiform	C41.9	C79.51	-	D16.9	D48.0	D49.2
elbow	C40.0-	C79.51	-	D16.0-	-	-
ethmoid (labyrinth)	C41.0	C79.51	-	D16.4	D48.0	D49.2
face	C41.0	C79.51	-	D16.4	D48.0	D49.2
femur (any part)	C40.2-	C79.51	-	D16.2-	-	-
fibula (any part)	C40.2-	C79.51	-	D16.2-	-	-
finger (any)	C40.1-	C79.51	-	D16.1-	-	-
foot	C40.3-	C79.51	-	D16.3-	-	-
forearm	C40.0-	C79.51	-	D16.0-	-	-
frontal	C41.0	C79.51	-	D16.4	D48.0	D49.2
hand	C40.1-	C79.51	-	D16.1-	-	-
heel	C40.3-	C79.51	-	D16.3-	-	-
hip	C41.4	C79.51	-	D16.8	D48.0	D49.2
humerus (any part)	C40.0-	C79.51	-	D16.0-	-	-
hyoid	C41.0	C79.51	-	D16.4	D48.0	D49.2
ilium	C41.4	C79.51	-	D16.8	D48.0	D49.2
innominate	C41.4	C79.51	-	D16.8	D48.0	D49.2
intervertebral cartilage or disc	C41.2	C79.51	-	D16.6	D48.0	D49.2
ischium	C41.4	C79.51	-	D16.8	D48.0	D49.2
jaw (lower)	C41.1	C79.51	-	D16.5	D48.0	D49.2
knee	C40.2-	C79.51	-	D16.2-	-	-
leg NEC	C40.2-	C79.51	-	D16.2-	-	-
limb NEC	C40.9-	C79.51	-	D16.9	-	-
lower (long bones)	C40.2-	C79.51	-	D16.2-	-	-
short bones	C40.3-	C79.51	-	D16.3-	-	-
upper (long bones)	C40.0-	C79.51	-	D16.0-	-	-
short bones	C40.1-	C79.51	-	D16.1-	-	-
malar	C41.0	C79.51	-	D16.4	D48.0	D49.2
mandible	C41.1	C79.51	-	D16.5	D48.0	D49.2
marrow NEC (any bone)	C96.9	C79.52	-	-	D47.9	D49.89
mastoid	C41.0	C79.51	-	D16.4	D48.0	D49.2
maxilla, maxillary (superior)	C41.0	C79.51	-	D16.4	D48.0	D49.2
inferior	C41.1	C79.51	-	D16.4	D48.0	D49.2
metacarpus (any)	C40.1-	C79.51	-	D16.1-	-	-
metatarsus (any)	C40.3-	C79.51	-	D16.3-	-	-
navicular						
ankle	C40.3-	C79.51	-	-	-	-
hand	C40.1-	C79.51	-	-	-	-
nose, nasal	C41.0	C79.51	-	D16.4	D48.0	D49.2
occipital	C41.0	C79.51	-	D16.4	D48.0	D49.2
orbit	C41.0	C79.51	-	D16.4	D48.0	D49.2

	Malignant Primary	Malignant Secondary	Ca in situ	Benign	Uncertain Behavior	Unspecified Behavior
bone — *continued*						
overlapping sites	C40.8-	-	-	-	-	-
parietal	C41.0	C79.51	-	D16.4	D48.0	D49.2
patella	C40.2-	C79.51	-	-	-	-
pelvic	C41.4	C79.51	-	D16.8	D48.0	D49.2
phalanges						
foot	C40.3-	C79.51	-	-	-	-
hand	C40.1-	C79.51	-	-	-	-
pubic	C41.4	C79.51	-	D16.8	D48.0	D49.2
radius (any part)	C40.0-	C79.51	-	D16.0-	-	-
rib	C41.3	C79.51	-	D16.7	D48.0	D49.2
sacral vertebra	C41.4	C79.51	-	D16.8	D48.0	D49.2
sacrum	C41.4	C79.51	-	D16.8	D48.0	D49.2
scaphoid	-	-	-	-	-	-
of ankle	C40.3-	C79.51	-	-	-	-
of hand	C40.1-	C79.51	-	-	-	-
scapula (any part)	C40.0-	C79.51	-	D16.0-	-	-
sella turcica	C41.0	C79.51	-	D16.4	D48.0	D49.2
shoulder	C40.0-	C79.51	-	D16.0-	-	-
skull	C41.0	C79.51	-	D16.4	D48.0	D49.2
sphenoid	C41.0	C79.51	-	D16.4	D48.0	D49.2
spine, spinal (column)	C41.2	C79.51	-	D16.6	D48.0	D49.2
coccyx	C41.4	C79.51	-	D16.8	D48.0	D49.2
sacrum	C41.4	C79.51	-	D16.8	D48.0	D49.2
sternum	C41.3	C79.51	-	D16.7	D48.0	D49.2
tarsus (any)	C40.3-	C79.51	-	-	-	-
temporal	C41.0	C79.51	-	D16.4	D48.0	D49.2
thumb	C40.1-	C79.51	-	-	-	-
tibia (any part)	C40.2-	C79.51	-	-	-	-
toe (any)	C40.3-	C79.51	-	-	-	-
trapezium	C40.1-	C79.51	-	-	-	-
trapezoid	C40.1-	C79.51	-	-	-	-
turbinate	C41.0	C79.51	-	D16.4	D48.0	D49.2
ulna (any part)	C40.0-	C79.51	-	D16.0-	-	-
unciform	C40.1-	C79.51	-	-	-	-
vertebra (column)	C41.2	C79.51	-	D16.6	D48.0	D49.2
coccyx	C41.4	C79.51	-	D16.8	D48.0	D49.2
sacrum	C41.4	C79.51	-	D16.8	D48.0	D49.2
vomer	C41.0	C79.51	-	D16.4	D48.0	D49.2
wrist	C40.1-	C79.51	-	-	-	-
xiphoid process	C41.3	C79.51	-	D16.7	D48.0	D49.2
zygomatic	C41.0	C79.51	-	D16.4	D48.0	D49.2
book-leaf (mouth)	C06.89	C79.89	D00.00	D10.39	D37.09	D49.0
bowel — see Neoplasm, intestine						
brachial plexus	C47.1-	C79.89	-	D36.12	D48.2	D49.2
brain NEC	C71.9	C79.31	-	D33.2	D43.2	D49.6
basal ganglia	C71.0	C79.31	-	D33.0	D43.0	D49.6
cerebellopontine angle	C71.6	C79.31	-	D33.1	D43.1	D49.6
cerebellum NOS	C71.6	C79.31	-	D33.1	D43.1	D49.6
cerebrum	C71.0	C79.31	-	D33.0	D43.0	D49.6
choroid plexus	C71.7	C79.31	-	D33.1	D43.1	D49.6
corpus callosum	C71.8	C79.31	-	D33.2	D43.2	D49.6

	Malignant Primary	Malignant Secondary	Ca in situ	Benign	Uncertain Behavior	Unspecified Behavior
brain NEC — *continued*						
corpus striatum	C71.0	C79.31	-	D33.0	D43.0	D49.6
cortex (cerebral)	C71.0	C79.31	-	D33.0	D43.0	D49.6
frontal lobe	C71.1	C79.31	-	D33.0	D43.0	D49.6
globus pallidus	C71.0	C79.31	-	D33.0	D43.0	D49.6
hippocampus	C71.2	C79.31	-	D33.0	D43.0	D49.6
hypothalamus	C71.0	C79.31	-	D33.0	D43.0	D49.6
internal capsule	C71.0	C79.31	-	D33.0	D43.0	D49.6
medulla oblongata	C71.7	C79.31	-	D33.1	D43.1	D49.6
meninges	C70.0	C79.32	-	D32.0	D42.0	D49.7
midbrain	C71.7	C79.31	-	D33.1	D43.1	D49.6
occipital lobe	C71.4	C79.31	-	D33.0	D43.0	D49.6
overlapping lesion	C71.8	C79.31	-	-	-	-
parietal lobe	C71.3	C79.31	-	D33.0	D43.0	D49.6
peduncle	C71.7	C79.31	-	D33.1	D43.1	D49.6
pons	C71.7	C79.31	-	D33.1	D43.1	D49.6
stem	C71.7	C79.31	-	D33.1	D43.1	D49.6
tapetum	C71.8	C79.31	-	D33.2	D43.2	D49.6
temporal lobe	C71.2	C79.31	-	D33.0	D43.0	D49.6
thalamus	C71.0	C79.31	-	D33.0	D43.0	D49.6
uncus	C71.2	C79.31	-	D33.0	D43.0	D49.6
ventricle (floor)	C71.5	C79.31	-	D33.0	D43.0	D49.6
fourth	C71.7	C79.31	-	D33.1	D43.1	D49.6
branchial (cleft) (cyst) (vestiges)	C10.4	C79.89	D00.08	D10.5	D37.05	D49.0
breast (connective tissue) (glandular tissue) (soft parts)	C50.9-	C79.81	D05.-	D24.-	D48.6-	D49.3
areola	C50.0-	C79.81	D05.-	D24.-	D48.6-	D49.3
axillary tail	C50.6-	C79.81	D05.-	D24.-	D48.6-	D49.3
central portion	C50.1-	C79.81	D05.-	D24.-	D48.6-	D49.3
inner	C50.8-	C79.81	D05.-	D24.-	D48.6-	D49.3
lower	C50.8-	C79.81	D05.-	D24.-	D48.6-	D49.3
lower-inner quadrant	C50.3-	C79.81	D05.-	D24.-	D48.6-	D49.3
lower-outer quadrant	C50.5-	C79.81	D05.-	D24.-	D48.6-	D49.3
mastectomy site (skin)— see also Neoplasm, breast, skin	C44.501	C79.2	-	-	-	-
specified as breast tissue	C50.8-	C79.81	-	-	-	-
midline	C50.8-	C79.81	D05.-	D24.-	D48.6-	D49.3
nipple	C50.0-	C79.81	D05.-	D24.-	D48.6-	D49.3
outer	C50.8-	C79.81	D05.-	D24.-	D48.6-	D49.3
overlapping lesion	C50.8-	-	-	-	-	-
skin	C44.501	C79.2	D04.5	D23.5	D48.5	D49.2
basal cell carcinoma	C44.511	-	-	-	-	-
specified type NEC	C44.591	-	-	-	-	-
squamous cell carcinoma	C44.521	-	-	-	-	-
tail (axillary)	C50.6-	C79.81	D05.-	D24.-	D48.6-	D49.3
upper	C50.8-	C79.81	D05.-	D24.-	D48.6-	D49.3
upper-inner quadrant	C50.2-	C79.81	D05.-	D24.-	D48.6-	D49.3
upper-outer quadrant	C50.4-	C79.81	D05.-	D24.-	D48.6-	D49.3
broad ligament	C57.1-	C79.82	D07.39	D28.2	D39.8	D49.59

Table of Neoplasms

	Malignant Primary	Malignant Secondary	Ca in situ	Benign	Uncertain Behavior	Unspecified Behavior
bronchiogenic, bronchogenic (lung)	C34.9-	C78.0-	D02.2-	D14.3-	D38.1	D49.1
bronchiole	C34.9-	C78.0-	D02.2-	D14.3-	D38.1	D49.1
bronchus	C34.9-	C78.0-	D02.2-	D14.3-	D38.1	D49.1
carina	C34.0-	C78.0-	D02.2-	D14.3-	D38.1	D49.1
lower lobe of lung	C34.3-	C78.0-	D02.2-	D14.3-	D38.1	D49.1
main	C34.0-	C78.0-	D02.2-	D14.3-	D38.1	D49.1
middle lobe of lung	C34.2	C78.0-	D02.21	D14.31	D38.1	D49.1
overlapping lesion	C34.8-	-	-	-	-	-
upper lobe of lung	C34.1-	C78.0-	D02.2-	D14.3-	D38.1	D49.1
brow	C44.309	C79.2	D04.39	D23.39	D48.5	D49.2
basal cell carcinoma	C44.319	-	-	-	-	-
specified type NEC	C44.399	-	-	-	-	-
squamous cell carcinoma	C44.329	-	-	-	-	-
buccal (cavity)	C06.9	C79.89	D00.00	D10.39	D37.09	D49.0
commissure	C06.0	C79.89	D00.02	D10.39	D37.09	D49.0
groove (lower) (upper)	C06.1	C79.89	D00.02	D10.39	D37.09	D49.0
mucosa	C06.0	C79.89	D00.02	D10.39	D37.09	D49.0
sulcus (lower) (upper)	C06.1	C79.89	D00.02	D10.39	D37.09	D49.0
bulbourethral gland	C68.0	C79.19	D09.19	D30.4	D41.3	D49.59
bursa—see Neoplasm, connective tissue						
buttock NEC	C76.3	C79.89	D04.5	D36.7	D48.7	D49.89

C

	Malignant Primary	Malignant Secondary	Ca in situ	Benign	Uncertain Behavior	Unspecified Behavior
calf	C76.5-	C79.89	D04.7-	D36.7	D48.7	D49.89
calvarium	C41.0	C79.51	-	D16.4	D48.0	D49.2
calyx, renal	C65.-	C79.0-	D09.19	D30.1-	D41.1-	D49.51-
canal						
anal	C21.1	C78.5	D01.3	D12.9	D37.8	D49.0
auditory (external)—see also Neoplasm, skin, ear	C44.20-	C79.2	D04.2-	D23.2-	D48.5	D49.2
auricular (external)—see also Neoplasm, skin, ear	C44.20-	C79.2	D04.2-	D23.2-	D48.5	D49.2
canaliculi, biliary (biliferi) (intrahepatic)	C22.1	C78.7	D01.5	D13.4	D37.6	D49.0
canthus (eye) (inner) (outer)	C44.10-	C79.2	D04.1-	D23.1-	D48.5	D49.2
basal cell carcinoma	C44.11-	-	-	-	-	-
sebaceous cell	C44.13-	-	-	-	-	-
specified type NEC	C44.19-	-	-	-	-	-
squamous cell carcinoma	C44.12-	-	-	-	-	-
capillary—see Neoplasm, connective tissue						
caput coli	C18.0	C78.5	D01.0	D12.0	D37.4	D49.0
carcinoid—see Tumor, carcinoid						
cardia (gastric)	C16.0	C78.89	D00.2	D13.1	D37.1	D49.0
cardiac orifice (stomach)	C16.0	C78.89	D00.2	D13.1	D37.1	D49.0
cardio-esophageal junction	C16.0	C78.89	D00.2	D13.1	D37.1	D49.0
cardio-esophagus	C16.0	C78.89	D00.2	D13.1	D37.1	D49.0
carina (bronchus)	C34.0-	C78.0-	D02.2-	D14.3-	D38.1	D49.1
carotid (artery)	C49.0	C79.89	-	D21.0	D48.1	D49.2
body	C75.4	C79.89	-	D35.5	D44.6	D49.7
carpus (any bone)	C40.1-	C79.51	-	D16.1-	-	-
cartilage (articular) (joint) NEC—see also Neoplasm, bone	C41.9	C79.51	-	D16.9	D48.0	D49.2
arytenoid	C32.3	C78.39	D02.0	D14.1	D38.0	D49.1

	Malignant Primary	Malignant Secondary	Ca in situ	Benign	Uncertain Behavior	Unspecified Behavior
cartilage NEC — continued						
auricular	C49.0	C79.89	-	D21.0	D48.1	D49.2
bronchi	C34.0-	C78.39	-	D14.3-	D38.1	D49.1
costal	C41.3	C79.51	-	D16.7	D48.0	D49.2
cricoid	C32.3	C78.39	D02.0	D14.1	D38.0	D49.1
cuneiform	C32.3	C78.39	D02.0	D14.1	D38.0	D49.1
ear (external)	C49.0	C79.89	-	D21.0	D48.1	D49.2
ensiform	C41.3	C79.51	-	D16.7	D48.0	D49.2
epiglottis	C32.1	C78.39	D02.0	D14.1	D38.0	D49.1
anterior surface	C10.1	C79.89	D00.08	D10.5	D37.05	D49.0
eyelid	C49.0	C79.89	-	D21.0	D48.1	D49.2
intervertebral	C41.2	C79.51	-	D16.6	D48.0	D49.2
larynx, laryngeal	C32.3	C78.39	D02.0	D14.1	D38.0	D49.1
nose, nasal	C30.0	C78.39	D02.3	D14.0	D38.5	D49.1
pinna	C49.0	C79.89	-	D21.0	D48.1	D49.2
rib	C41.3	C79.51	-	D16.7	D48.0	D49.2
semilunar (knee)	C40.2-	C79.51	-	D16.2-	D48.0	D49.2
thyroid	C32.3	C78.39	D02.0	D14.1	D38.0	D49.1
trachea	C33	C78.39	D02.1	D14.2	D38.1	D49.1
cauda equina	C72.1	C79.49	-	D33.4	D43.4	D49.7
cavity						
buccal	C06.9	C79.89	D00.00	D10.30	D37.09	D49.0
nasal	C30.0	C78.39	D02.3	D14.0	D38.5	D49.1
oral	C06.9	C79.89	D00.00	D10.30	D37.09	D49.0
peritoneal	C48.2	C78.6	-	D20.1	D48.4	D49.0
tympanic	C30.1	C78.39	D02.3	D14.0	D38.5	D49.1
cecum	C18.0	C78.5	D01.0	D12.0	D37.4	D49.0
central nervous system	C72.9	C79.40	-	-	-	-
cerebellopontine (angle)	C71.6	C79.31	-	D33.1	D43.1	D49.6
cerebellum, cerebellar	C71.6	C79.31	-	D33.1	D43.1	D49.6
cerebrum, cerebral (cortex) (hemisphere) (white matter)	C71.0	C79.31	-	D33.0	D43.0	D49.6
meninges	C70.0	C79.32	-	D32.0	D42.0	D49.7
peduncle	C71.7	C79.31	-	D33.1	D43.1	D49.6
ventricle	C71.5	C79.31	-	D33.0	D43.0	D49.6
fourth	C71.7	C79.31	-	D33.1	D43.1	D49.6
cervical region	C76.0	C79.89	D09.8	D36.7	D48.7	D49.89
cervix (cervical) (uteri) (uterus)	C53.9	C79.82	D06.9	D26.0	D39.0	D49.59
canal	C53.0	C79.82	D06.0	D26.0	D39.0	D49.59
endocervix (canal) (gland)	C53.0	C79.82	D06.0	D26.0	D39.0	D49.59
exocervix	C53.1	C79.82	D06.1	D26.0	D39.0	D49.59
external os	C53.1	C79.82	D06.1	D26.0	D39.0	D49.59
internal os	C53.0	C79.82	D06.0	D26.0	D39.0	D49.59
nabothian gland	C53.0	C79.82	D06.0	D26.0	D39.0	D49.59
overlapping lesion	C53.8	-	-	-	-	-
squamocolumnar junction	C53.8	C79.82	D06.7	D26.0	D39.0	D49.59
stump	C53.8	C79.82	D06.7	D26.0	D39.0	D49.59
cheek	C76.0	C79.89	D09.8	D36.7	D48.7	D49.89
external	C44.309	C79.2	D04.39	D23.39	D48.5	D49.2
basal cell carcinoma	C44.319	-	-	-	-	-
specified type NEC	C44.399	-	-	-	-	-
squamous cell carcinoma	C44.329	-	-	-	-	-

	Malignant Primary	Malignant Secondary	Ca in situ	Benign	Uncertain Behavior	Unspecified Behavior
cheek — *continued*						
inner aspect	C06.0	C79.89	D00.02	D10.39	D37.09	D49.0
internal	C06.0	C79.89	D00.02	D10.39	D37.09	D49.0
mucosa	C06.0	C79.89	D00.02	D10.39	D37.09	D49.0
chest (wall) NEC	C76.1	C79.89	D09.8	D36.7	D48.7	D49.89
chiasma opticum	C72.3-	C79.49	-	D33.3	D43.3	D49.7
chin	C44.309	C79.2	D04.39	D23.39	D48.5	D49.2
basal cell carcinoma	C44.319	-	-	-	-	-
specified type NEC	C44.399	-	-	-	-	-
squamous cell carcinoma	C44.329	-	-	-	-	-
choana	C11.3	C79.89	D00.08	D10.6	D37.05	D49.0
cholangiole	C22.1	C78.89	D01.5	D13.4	D37.6	D49.0
choledochal duct	C24.0	C78.89	D01.5	D13.5	D37.6	D49.0
choroid	C69.3-	C79.49	D09.2-	D31.3-	D48.7	D49.81
plexus	C71.5	C79.31	-	D33.0	D43.0	D49.6
ciliary body	C69.4-	C79.49	D09.2-	D31.4-	D48.7	D49.89
clavicle	C41.3	C79.51	-	D16.7	D48.0	D49.2
clitoris	C51.2	C79.82	D07.1	D28.0	D39.8	D49.59
clivus	C41.0	C79.51	-	D16.4-	D48.0	D49.2
cloacogenic zone	C21.2	C78.5	D01.3	D12.9	D37.8	D49.0
coccygeal						
body or glomus	C49.5	C79.89	-	D21.5	D48.1	D49.2
vertebra	C41.4	C79.51	-	D16.8	D48.0	D49.2
coccyx	C41.4	C79.51	-	D16.8	D48.0	D49.2
colon—see also Neoplasm, intestine, large	C18.9	C78.5	-	-	-	-
with rectum	C19	C78.5	D01.1	D12.7	D37.5	D49.0
column, spinal—see Neoplasm, spine						
columnella—see also Neoplasm, skin, face	C44.390	C79.2	D04.39	D23.39	D48.5	D49.2
commissure						
labial, lip	C00.6	C79.89	D00.01	D10.39	D37.01	D49.0
laryngeal	C32.0	C78.39	D02.0	D14.1	D38.0	D49.1
common (bile) duct	C24.0	C78.89	D01.5	D13.5	D37.6	D49.0
concha—see also Neoplasm, skin, ear	C44.20-	C79.2	D04.2-	D23.2-	D48.5	D49.2
nose	C30.0	C78.39	D02.3	D14.0	D38.5	D49.1
conjunctiva	C69.0-	C79.49	D09.2-	D31.0-	D48.7	D49.89
connective tissue NEC	C49.9	C79.89	-	D21.9	D48.1	D49.2

Note: For neoplasms of connective tissue (blood vessel, bursa, fascia, ligament, muscle, peripheral nerves, sympathetic and parasympathetic nerves and ganglia, synovia, tendon, etc.) or of morphological types that indicate connective tissue, code according to the list under "Neoplasm, connective tissue". For sites that do not appear in this list, code to neoplasm of that site; e.g., fibrosarcoma, pancreas (C25.9)

	Malignant Primary	Malignant Secondary	Ca in situ	Benign	Uncertain Behavior	Unspecified Behavior
connective tissue NEC — *continued*						
Note: Morphological types that indicate connective tissue appear in their proper place in the alphabetic index with the instruction "see Neoplasm, connective tissue ...."						
abdomen	C49.4	C79.89	-	D21.4	D48.1	D49.2
abdominal wall	C49.4	C79.89	-	D21.4	D48.1	D49.2
ankle	C49.2-	C79.89	-	D21.2-	D48.1	D49.2
antecubital fossa or space	C49.1-	C79.89	-	D21.1-	D48.1	D49.2
arm	C49.1-	C79.89	-	D21.1-	D48.1	D49.2
auricle (ear)	C49.0	C79.89	-	D21.0	D48.1	D49.2
axilla	C49.3	C79.89	-	D21.3	D48.1	D49.2
back	C49.6	C79.89	-	D21.6	D48.1	D49.2
breast—see Neoplasm, breast						
buttock	C49.5	C79.89	-	D21.5	D48.1	D49.2
calf	C49.2-	C79.89	-	D21.2-	D48.1	D49.2
cervical region	C49.0	C79.89	-	D21.0	D48.1	D49.2
cheek	C49.0	C79.89	-	D21.0	D48.1	D49.2
chest (wall)	C49.3	C79.89	-	D21.3	D48.1	D49.2
chin	C49.0	C79.89	-	D21.0	D48.1	D49.2
diaphragm	C49.3	C79.89	-	D21.3	D48.1	D49.2
ear (external)	C49.0	C79.89	-	D21.0	D48.1	D49.2
elbow	C49.1-	C79.89	-	D21.1-	D48.1	D49.2
extrarectal	C49.5	C79.89	-	D21.5	D48.1	D49.2
extremity	C49.9	C79.89	-	D21.9	D48.1	D49.2
lower	C49.2-	C79.89	-	D21.2-	D48.1	D49.2
upper	C49.1-	C79.89	-	D21.1-	D48.1	D49.2
eyelid	C49.0	C79.89	-	D21.0	D48.1	D49.2
face	C49.0	C79.89	-	D21.0	D48.1	D49.2
finger	C49.1-	C79.89	-	D21.1-	D48.1	D49.2
flank	C49.6	C79.89	-	D21.6	D48.1	D49.2
foot	C49.2-	C79.89	-	D21.2-	D48.1	D49.2
forearm	C49.1-	C79.89	-	D21.1-	D48.1	D49.2
forehead	C49.0	C79.89	-	D21.0	D48.1	D49.2
gastric	C49.4	C79.89	-	D21.4	D48.1	D49.2
gastrointestinal	C49.4	C79.89	-	D21.4	D48.1	D49.2
gluteal region	C49.5	C79.89	-	D21.5	D48.1	D49.2
great vessels NEC	C49.3	C79.89	-	D21.3	D48.1	D49.2
groin	C49.5	C79.89	-	D21.5	D48.1	D49.2
hand	C49.1-	C79.89	-	D21.1-	D48.1	D49.2
head	C49.0	C79.89	-	D21.0	D48.1	D49.2
heel	C49.2-	C79.89	-	D21.2-	D48.1	D49.2
hip	C49.2-	C79.89	-	D21.2-	D48.1	D49.2
hypochondrium	C49.4	C79.89	-	D21.4	D48.1	D49.2
iliopsoas muscle	C49.5	C79.89	-	D21.5	D48.1	D49.2
infraclavicular region	C49.3	C79.89	-	D21.3	D48.1	D49.2
inguinal (canal) (region)	C49.5	C79.89	-	D21.5	D48.1	D49.2
intestinal	C49.4	C79.89	-	D21.4	D48.1	D49.2
intrathoracic	C49.3	C79.89	-	D21.3	D48.1	D49.2
ischiorectal fossa	C49.5	C79.89	-	D21.5	D48.1	D49.2

Table of Neoplasms

	Malignant Primary	Malignant Secondary	Ca in situ	Benign	Uncertain Behavior	Unspecified Behavior
connective tissue NEC — *continued*						
jaw	C03.9	C79.89	D00.03	D10.39	D48.1	D49.0
knee	C49.2-	C79.89	-	D21.2-	D48.1	D49.2
leg	C49.2-	C79.89	-	D21.2-	D48.1	D49.2
limb NEC	C49.9	C79.89	-	D21.9	D48.1	D49.2
lower	C49.2-	C79.89	-	D21.2-	D48.1	D49.2
upper	C49.1-	C79.89	-	D21.1-	D48.1	D49.2
nates	C49.5	C79.89	-	D21.5	D48.1	D49.2
neck	C49.0	C79.89	-	D21.0	D48.1	D49.2
orbit	C69.6-	C79.49	D09.2-	D31.6-	D48.1	D49.89
overlapping lesion	C49.8	-	-	-	-	-
pararectal	C49.5	C79.89	-	D21.5	D48.1	D49.2
para-urethral	C49.5	C79.89	-	D21.5	D48.1	D49.2
paravaginal	C49.5	C79.89	-	D21.5	D48.1	D49.2
pelvis (floor)	C49.5	C79.89	-	D21.5	D48.1	D49.2
pelvo-abdominal	C49.8	C79.89	-	D21.6	D48.1	D49.2
perineum	C49.5	C79.89	-	D21.5	D48.1	D49.2
perirectal (tissue)	C49.5	C79.89	-	D21.5	D48.1	D49.2
periurethral (tissue)	C49.5	C79.89	-	D21.5	D48.1	D49.2
popliteal fossa or space	C49.2-	C79.89	-	D21.2-	D48.1	D49.2
presacral	C49.5	C79.89	-	D21.5	D48.1	D49.2
psoas muscle	C49.4	C79.89	-	D21.4	D48.1	D49.2
pterygoid fossa	C49.0	C79.89	-	D21.0	D48.1	D49.2
rectovaginal septum or wall	C49.5	C79.89	-	D21.5	D48.1	D49.2
rectovesical	C49.5	C79.89	-	D21.5	D48.1	D49.2
retroperitoneum	C48.0	C78.6	-	D20.0	D48.3	D49.0
sacrococcygeal region	C49.5	C79.89	-	D21.5	D48.1	D49.2
scalp	C49.0	C79.89	-	D21.0	D48.1	D49.2
scapular region	C49.3	C79.89	-	D21.3	D48.1	D49.2
shoulder	C49.1-	C79.89	-	D21.1-	D48.1	D49.2
skin (dermis) NEC—see also Neoplasm, skin, by site	C44.90	C79.2	D04.9	D23.9	D48.5	D49.2
stomach	C49.4	C79.89	-	D21.4	D48.1	D49.2
submental	C49.0	C79.89	-	D21.0	D48.1	D49.2
supraclavicular region	C49.0	C79.89	-	D21.0	D48.1	D49.2
temple	C49.0	C79.89	-	D21.0	D48.1	D49.2
temporal region	C49.0	C79.89	-	D21.0	D48.1	D49.2
thigh	C49.2-	C79.89	-	D21.2-	D48.1	D49.2
thoracic (duct) (wall)	C49.3	C79.89	-	D21.3	D48.1	D49.2
thorax	C49.3	C79.89	-	D21.3	D48.1	D49.2
thumb	C49.1-	C79.89	-	D21.1-	D48.1	D49.2
toe	C49.2-	C79.89	-	D21.2-	D48.1	D49.2
trunk	C49.6	C79.89	-	D21.6	D48.1	D49.2
umbilicus	C49.4	C79.89	-	D21.4	D48.1	D49.2
vesicorectal	C49.5	C79.89	-	D21.5	D48.1	D49.2
wrist	C49.1-	C79.89	-	D21.1-	D48.1	D49.2
conus medullaris	C72.0	C79.49	-	D33.4	D43.4	D49.7
cord (true) (vocal)	C32.0	C78.39	D02.0	D14.1	D38.0	D49.1
false	C32.1	C78.39	D02.0	D14.1	D38.0	D49.1
spermatic	C63.1-	C79.82	D07.69	D29.8	D40.8	D49.59

	Malignant Primary	Malignant Secondary	Ca in situ	Benign	Uncertain Behavior	Unspecified Behavior
cord (true) (vocal) — *continued*						
spinal (cervical) (lumbar) (thoracic)	C72.0	C79.49	-	D33.4	D43.4	D49.7
cornea (limbus)	C69.1-	C79.49	D09.2-	D31.1-	D48.7	D49.89
corpus						
albicans	C56.-	C79.6-	D07.39	D27.-	D39.1-	D49.59
callosum, brain	C71.0	C79.31	-	D33.2	D43.2	D49.6
cavernosum	C60.2	C79.82	D07.4	D29.0	D40.8	D49.59
gastric	C16.2	C78.89	D00.2	D13.1	D37.1	D49.0
overlapping sites	C54.8	-	-	-	-	-
penis	C60.2	C79.82	D07.4	D29.0	D40.8	D49.59
striatum, cerebrum	C71.0	C79.31	-	D33.0	D43.0	D49.6
uteri	C54.9	C79.82	D07.0	D26.1	D39.0	D49.59
isthmus	C54.0	C79.82	D07.0	D26.1	D39.0	D49.59
cortex						
adrenal	C74.0-	C79.7-	D09.3	D35.0-	D44.1-	D49.7
cerebral	C71.0	C79.31	-	D33.0	D43.0	D49.6
costal cartilage	C41.3	C79.51	-	D16.7	D48.0	D49.2
costovertebral joint	C41.3	C79.51	-	D16.7	D48.0	D49.2
Cowper's gland	C68.0	C79.19	D09.19	D30.4	D41.3	D49.59
cranial (fossa, any)	C71.9	C79.31	-	D33.2	D43.2	D49.6
meninges	C70.0	C79.32	-	D32.0	D42.0	D49.7
nerve	C72.50	C79.49	-	D33.3	D43.3	D49.7
specified NEC	C72.59	C79.49	-	D33.3	D43.3	D49.7
craniobuccal pouch	C75.2	C79.89	D09.3	D35.2	D44.3	D49.7
craniopharyngeal (duct) (pouch)	C75.2	C79.89	D09.3	D35.3	D44.4	D49.7
cricoid	C13.0	C79.89	D00.08	D10.7	D37.05	D49.0
cartilage	C32.3	C78.39	D02.0	D14.1	D38.0	D49.1
cricopharynx	C13.0	C79.89	D00.08	D10.7	D37.05	D49.0
crypt of Morgagni	C21.8	C78.5	D01.3	D12.9	D37.8	D49.0
crystalline lens	C69.4-	C79.49	D09.2-	D31.4-	D48.7	D49.89
cul-de-sac (Douglas')	C48.1	C78.6	-	D20.1	D48.4	D49.0
cuneiform cartilage	C32.3	C78.39	D02.0	D14.1	D38.0	D49.1
cutaneous—see Neoplasm, skin						
cutis—see Neoplasm, skin						
cystic (bile) duct (common)	C24.0	C78.89	D01.5	D13.5	D37.6	D49.0
D						
dermis—see Neoplasm, skin						
diaphragm	C49.3	C79.89	-	D21.3	D48.1	D49.2
digestive organs, system, tube, or tract NEC	C26.9	C78.89	D01.9	D13.99	D37.9	D49.0
disc, intervertebral	C41.2	C79.51	-	D16.6	D48.0	D49.2
disease, generalized	C80.0	-	-	-	-	-
disseminated	C80.0	-	-	-	-	-
Douglas' cul-de-sac or pouch	C48.1	C78.6	-	D20.1	D48.4	D49.0
duodenojejunal junction	C17.8	C78.4	D01.49	D13.39	D37.2	D49.0
duodenum	C17.0	C78.4	D01.49	D13.2	D37.2	D49.0
dura (cranial) (mater)	C70.9	C79.49	-	D32.9	D42.9	D49.7
cerebral	C70.0	C79.32	-	D32.0	D42.0	D49.7
spinal	C70.1	C79.49	-	D32.1	D42.1	D49.7

	Malignant Primary	Malignant Secondary	Ca in situ	Benign	Uncertain Behavior	Unspecified Behavior
E							
ear (external)—see also Neoplasm, skin, ear	C44.20-	C79.2	D04.2-	D23.2-	D48.5	D49.2
auricle or auris—see also Neoplasm, skin, ear	C44.20-	C79.2	D04.2-	D23.2-	D48.5	D49.2
canal, external—see also Neoplasm, skin, ear	C44.20-	C79.2	D04.2-	D23.2-	D48.5	D49.2
cartilage	C49.0	C79.89	-	D21.0	D48.1	D49.2
external meatus—see also Neoplasm, skin, ear	C44.20-	C79.2	D04.2-	D23.2-	D48.5	D49.2
inner	C30.1	C78.39	D02.3	D14.0	D38.5	D49.1
lobule—see also Neoplasm, skin, ear	C44.20-	C79.2	D04.2-	D23.2-	D48.5	D49.2
middle	C30.1	C78.39	D02.3	D14.0	D38.5	D49.1
overlapping lesion with accessory sinuses	C31.8	-	-	-	-	-
skin	C44.20-	C79.2	D04.2-	D23.2-	D48.5	D49.2
basal cell carcinoma	C44.21-	-	-	-	-	-
specified type NEC	C44.29-	-	-	-	-	-
squamous cell carcinoma	C44.22-	-	-	-	-	-
earlobe	C44.20-	C79.2	D04.2-	D23.2-	D48.5	D49.2
basal cell carcinoma	C44.21-	-	-	-	-	-
specified type NEC	C44.29-	-	-	-	-	-
squamous cell carcinoma	C44.22-	-	-	-	-	-
ejaculatory duct	C63.7	C79.82	D07.69	D29.8	D40.8	D49.59
elbow NEC	C76.4-	C79.89	D04.6-	D36.7	D48.7	D49.89
endocardium	C38.0	C79.89	-	D15.1	D48.7	D49.89
endocervix (canal) (gland)	C53.0	C79.82	D06.0	D26.0	D39.0	D49.59
endocrine gland NEC	C75.9	C79.89	D09.3	D35.9	D44.9	D49.7
pluriglandular	C75.8	C79.89	D09.3	D35.7	D44.9	D49.7
endometrium (gland) (stroma)	C54.1	C79.82	D07.0	D26.1	D39.0	D49.59
ensiform cartilage	C41.3	C79.51	-	D16.7	D48.0	D49.2
enteric—see Neoplasm, intestine							
ependyma (brain)	C71.5	C79.31	-	D33.0	D43.0	D49.6
fourth ventricle	C71.7	C79.31	-	D33.1	D43.1	D49.6
epicardium	C38.0	C79.89	-	D15.1	D48.7	D49.89
epididymis	C63.0-	C79.82	D07.69	D29.3-	D40.8	D49.59
epidural	C72.9	C79.49	-	D33.9	D43.9	D49.7
epiglottis	C32.1	C78.39	D02.0	D14.1	D38.0	D49.1
anterior aspect or surface	C10.1	C79.89	D00.08	D10.5	D37.05	D49.0
cartilage	C32.3	C78.39	D02.0	D14.1	D38.0	D49.1
free border (margin)	C10.1	C79.89	D00.08	D10.5	D37.05	D49.0
junctional region	C10.8	C79.89	D00.08	D10.5	D37.05	D49.0
posterior (laryngeal) surface	C32.1	C78.39	D02.0	D14.1	D38.0	D49.1
suprahyoid portion	C32.1	C78.39	D02.0	D14.1	D38.0	D49.1
esophagogastric junction	C16.0	C78.89	D00.2	D13.1	D37.1	D49.0
esophagus	C15.9	C78.89	D00.1	D13.0	D37.8	D49.0
abdominal	C15.5	C78.89	D00.1	D13.0	D37.8	D49.0
cervical	C15.3	C78.89	D00.1	D13.0	D37.8	D49.0
distal (third)	C15.5	C78.89	D00.1	D13.0	D37.8	D49.0
lower (third)	C15.5	C78.89	D00.1	D13.0	D37.8	D49.0

	Malignant Primary	Malignant Secondary	Ca in situ	Benign	Uncertain Behavior	Unspecified Behavior
esophagus — continued							
middle (third)	C15.4	C78.89	D00.1	D13.0	D37.8	D49.0
overlapping lesion	C15.8	-	-	-	-	-
proximal (third)	C15.3	C78.89	D00.1	D13.0	D37.8	D49.0
thoracic	C15.4	C78.89	D00.1	D13.0	D37.8	D49.0
upper (third)	C15.3	C78.89	D00.1	D13.0	D37.8	D49.0
ethmoid (sinus)	C31.1	C78.39	D02.3	D14.0	D38.5	D49.1
bone or labyrinth	C41.0	C79.51	-	D16.4-	D48.0	D49.2
eustachian tube	C30.1	C78.39	D02.3	D14.0	D38.5	D49.1
exocervix	C53.1	C79.82	D06.1	D26.0	D39.0	D49.59
external							
meatus (ear)—see also Neoplasm, skin, ear	C44.20-	C79.2	D04.2-	D23.2-	D48.5	D49.2
os, cervix uteri	C53.1	C79.82	D06.1	D26.0	D39.0	D49.59
extradural	C72.9	C79.49	-	D33.9	D43.9	D49.7
extrahepatic (bile) duct	C24.0	C78.89	D01.5	D13.5	D37.6	D49.0
overlapping lesion with gallbladder	C24.8	-	-	-	-	-
extraocular muscle	C69.6-	C79.49	D09.2-	D31.6-	D48.7	D49.89
extrarectal	C76.3	C79.89	D09.8	D36.7	D48.7	D49.89
extremity	C76.8	C79.89	D04.8	D36.7	D48.7	D49.89
lower	C76.5-	C79.89	D04.7-	D36.7	D48.7	D49.89
upper	C76.4-	C79.89	D04.6-	D36.7	D48.7	D49.89
eye NEC	C69.9-	C79.49	D09.2-	D31.9	D48.7	D49.89
overlapping sites	C69.8-	-	-	-	-	-
eyeball	C69.9-	C79.49	D09.2-	D31.9-	D48.7	D49.89
eyebrow	C44.309	C79.2	D04.39	D23.39	D48.5	D49.2
basal cell carcinoma	C44.319	-	-	-	-	-
specified type NEC	C44.399	-	-	-	-	-
squamous cell carcinoma	C44.329	-	-	-	-	-
eyelid (lower) (skin) (upper)	C44.10-	-	-	-	-	-
basal cell carcinoma	C44.11-	-	-	-	-	-
sebaceous cell	C44.13-	-	-	-	-	-
specified type NEC	C44.19-	-	-	-	-	-
squamous cell carcinoma	C44.12-	-	-	-	-	-
cartilage	C49.0	C79.89	-	D21.0	D48.1	D49.2
F							
face NEC	C76.0	C79.89	D04.39	D36.7	D48.7	D49.89
fallopian tube (accessory)	C57.0-	C79.82	D07.39	D28.2	D39.8	D49.59
falx (cerebella) (cerebri)	C70.0	C79.32	-	D32.0	D42.0	D49.7
fascia—see also Neoplasm, connective tissue							
palmar	C49.1-	C79.89	-	D21.1-	D48.1	D49.2
plantar	C49.2-	C79.89	-	D21.2-	D48.1	D49.2
fatty tissue—see Neoplasm, connective tissue							
fauces, faucial NEC	C10.9	C79.89	D00.08	D10.5	D37.05	D49.0
pillars	C09.1	C79.89	D00.08	D10.5	D37.05	D49.0
tonsil	C09.9	C79.89	D00.08	D10.4	D37.05	D49.0
femur (any part)	C40.2-	-	-	D16.2-	-	-
fetal membrane	C58	C79.82	D07.0	D26.7	D39.2	D49.59
fibrous tissue—see Neoplasm, connective tissue							

353

	Malignant Primary	Malignant Secondary	Ca in situ	Benign	Uncertain Behavior	Unspecified Behavior
fibula (any part)	C40.2-	C79.51	-	D16.2-	-	-
filum terminale	C72.0	C79.49	-	D33.4	D43.4	D49.7
finger NEC	C76.4-	C79.89	D04.6-	D36.7	D48.7	D49.89
flank NEC	C76.8	C79.89	D04.5	D36.7	D48.7	D49.89
follicle, nabothian	C53.0	C79.82	D06.0	D26.0	D39.0	D49.59
foot NEC	C76.5-	C79.89	D04.7-	D36.7	D48.7	D49.89
forearm NEC	C76.4-	C79.89	D04.6-	D36.7	D48.7	D49.89
forehead (skin)	C44.309	C79.2	D04.39	D23.39	D48.5	D49.2
basal cell carcinoma	C44.319	-	-	-	-	-
specified type NEC	C44.399	-	-	-	-	-
squamous cell carcinoma	C44.329	-	-	-	-	-
foreskin	C60.0	C79.82	D07.4	D29.0	D40.8	D49.59
fornix						
pharyngeal	C11.3	C79.89	D00.08	D10.6	D37.05	D49.0
vagina	C52	C79.82	D07.2	D28.1	D39.8	D49.59
fossa (of)						
anterior (cranial)	C71.9	C79.31	-	D33.2	D43.2	D49.6
cranial	C71.9	C79.31	-	D33.2	D43.2	D49.6
ischiorectal	C76.3	C79.89	D09.8	D36.7	D48.7	D49.89
middle (cranial)	C71.9	C79.31	-	D33.2	D43.2	D49.6
piriform	C12	C79.89	D00.08	D10.7	D37.05	D49.0
pituitary	C75.1	C79.89	D09.3	D35.2	D44.3	D49.7
posterior (cranial)	C71.9	C79.31	-	D33.2	D43.2	D49.6
pterygoid	C49.0	C79.89	-	D21.0	D48.1	D49.2
pyriform	C12	C79.89	D00.08	D10.7	D37.05	D49.0
Rosenmuller	C11.2	C79.89	D00.08	D10.6	D37.05	D49.0
tonsillar	C09.0	C79.89	D00.08	D10.5	D37.05	D49.0
fourchette	C51.9	C79.82	D07.1	D28.0	D39.8	D49.59
frenulum						
labii—see Neoplasm, lip, internal						
linguae	C02.2	C79.89	D00.07	D10.1	D37.02	D49.0
frontal						
bone	C41.0	C79.51	-	D16.4	D48.0	D49.2
lobe, brain	C71.1	C79.31	-	D33.0	D43.0	D49.6
pole	C71.1	C79.31	-	D33.0	D43.0	D49.6
sinus	C31.2	C78.39	D02.3	D14.0	D38.5	D49.1
fundus						
stomach	C16.1	C78.89	D00.2	D13.1	D37.1	D49.0
uterus	C54.3	C79.82	D07.0	D26.1	D39.0	D49.59
G						
gall duct (extrahepatic)	C24.0	C78.89	D01.5	D13.5	D37.6	D49.0
intrahepatic	C22.1	C78.7	D01.5	D13.4	D37.6	D49.0
gallbladder	C23	C78.89	D01.5	D13.5	D37.6	D49.0
overlapping lesion with extrahepatic bile ducts	C24.8	-	-	-	-	-
ganglia—see also Neoplasm, nerve, peripheral	C47.9	C79.89	-	D36.10	D48.2	D49.2
basal	C71.0	C79.31	-	D33.0	D43.0	D49.6
cranial nerve	C72.50	C79.49	-	D33.3	D43.3	D49.7
Gartner's duct	C52	C79.82	D07.2	D28.1	D39.8	D49.59
gastric—see Neoplasm, stomach						
gastrocolic	C26.9	C78.89	D01.9	D13.99	D37.9	D49.0

	Malignant Primary	Malignant Secondary	Ca in situ	Benign	Uncertain Behavior	Unspecified Behavior
gastroesophageal junction	C16.0	C78.89	D00.2	D13.1	D37.1	D49.0
gastrointestinal (tract) NEC	C26.9	C78.89	D01.9	D13.99	D37.9	D49.0
generalized	C80.0	-	-	-	-	-
genital organ or tract						
female NEC	C57.9	C79.82	D07.30	D28.9	D39.9	D49.59
overlapping lesion	C57.8	-	-	-	-	-
specified site NEC	C57.7	C79.82	D07.39	D28.7	D39.8	D49.59
male NEC	C63.9	C79.82	D07.60	D29.9	D40.9	D49.59
overlapping lesion	C63.8	-	-	-	-	-
specified site NEC	C63.7	C79.82	D07.69	D29.8	D40.8	D49.59
genitourinary tract						
female	C57.9	C79.82	D07.30	D28.9	D39.9	D49.59
male	C63.9	C79.82	D07.60	D29.9	D40.9	D49.59
gingiva (alveolar) (marginal)	C03.9	C79.89	D00.03	D10.39	D37.09	D49.0
lower	C03.1	C79.89	D00.03	D10.39	D37.09	D49.0
mandibular	C03.1	C79.89	D00.03	D10.39	D37.09	D49.0
maxillary	C03.0	C79.89	D00.03	D10.39	D37.09	D49.0
upper	C03.0	C79.89	D00.03	D10.39	D37.09	D49.0
gland, glandular (lymphatic) (system)—see also Neoplasm, lymph gland						
endocrine NEC	C75.9	C79.89	D09.3	D35.9	D44.9	D49.7
salivary—see Neoplasm, salivary gland						
glans penis	C60.1	C79.82	D07.4	D29.0	D40.8	D49.59
globus pallidus	C71.0	C79.31	-	D33.0	D43.0	D49.6
glomus						
coccygeal	C49.5	C79.89	-	D21.5	D48.1	D49.2
jugularis	C75.5	C79.89	-	D35.6	D44.7	D49.7
glosso-epiglottic fold(s)	C10.1	C79.89	D00.08	D10.5	D37.05	D49.0
glossopalatine fold	C09.1	C79.89	D00.08	D10.5	D37.05	D49.0
glossopharyngeal sulcus	C09.0	C79.89	D00.08	D10.5	D37.05	D49.0
glottis	C32.0	C78.39	D02.0	D14.1	D38.0	D49.1
gluteal region	C76.3	C79.89	D04.5	D36.7	D48.7	D49.89
great vessels NEC	C49.3	C79.89	-	D21.3	D48.1	D49.2
groin NEC	C76.3	C79.89	D04.5	D36.7	D48.7	D49.89
gum	C03.9	C79.89	D00.03	D10.39	D37.09	D49.0
lower	C03.1	C79.89	D00.03	D10.39	D37.09	D49.0
upper	C03.0	C79.89	D00.03	D10.39	D37.09	D49.0
H						
hand NEC	C76.4-	C79.89	D04.6-	D36.7	D48.7	D49.89
head NEC	C76.0	C79.89	D04.4	D36.7	D48.7	D49.89
heart	C38.0	C79.89	-	D15.1	D48.7	D49.89
heel NEC	C76.5-	C79.89	D04.7-	D36.7	D48.7	D49.89
helix—see also Neoplasm, skin, ear	C44.20-	C79.2	D04.2-	D23.2-	D48.5	D49.2
hematopoietic, hemopoietic tissue NEC	C96.9	-	-	-	-	-
specified NEC	C96.Z	-	-	-	-	-
hemisphere, cerebral	C71.0	C79.31	-	D33.0	D43.0	D49.6
hemorrhoidal zone	C21.1	C78.5	D01.3	D12.9	D37.8	D49.0
hepatic—see also Index to disease, by histology	C22.9	C78.7	D01.5	D13.4	D37.6	D49.0

	Malignant Primary	Malignant Secondary	Ca in situ	Benign	Uncertain Behavior	Unspecified Behavior
hepatic — *continued*						
duct (bile)	C24.0	C78.89	D01.5	D13.5	D37.6	D49.0
flexure (colon)	C18.3	C78.5	D01.0	D12.3	D37.4	D49.0
primary	C22.8	C78.7	D01.5	D13.4	D37.6	D49.0
hepatobiliary	C24.9	C78.89	D01.5	D13.5	D37.6	D49.0
hepatoblastoma	C22.2	C78.7	D01.5	D13.4	D37.6	D49.0
hepatoma	C22.0	C78.7	D01.5	D13.4	D37.6	D49.0
hilus of lung	C34.0-	C78.0-	D02.2-	D14.3-	D38.1	D49.1
hip NEC	C76.5-	C79.89	D04.7-	D36.7	D48.7	D49.89
hippocampus, brain	C71.2	C79.31	-	D33.0	D43.0	D49.6
humerus (any part)	C40.0-	C79.51	-	D16.0-	-	-
hymen	C52	C79.82	D07.2	D28.1	D39.8	D49.59
hypopharynx, hypopharyngeal NEC	C13.9	C79.89	D00.08	D10.7	D37.05	D49.0
overlapping lesion	C13.8	-	-	-	-	-
postcricoid region	C13.0	C79.89	D00.08	D10.7	D37.05	D49.0
posterior wall	C13.2	C79.89	D00.08	D10.7	D37.05	D49.0
pyriform fossa (sinus)	C12	C79.89	D00.08	D10.7	D37.05	D49.0
hypophysis	C75.1	C79.89	D09.3	D35.2	D44.3	D49.7
hypothalamus	C71.0	C79.31	-	D33.0	D43.0	D49.6
I						
ileocecum, ileocecal (coil) (junction) (valve)	C18.0	C78.5	D01.0	D12.0	D37.4	D49.0
ileum	C17.2	C78.4	D01.49	D13.39	D37.2	D49.0
ilium	C41.4	C79.51	-	D16.8	D48.0	D49.2
immunoproliferative NEC	C88.9	-	-	-	-	-
infraclavicular (region)	C76.1	C79.89	D04.5	D36.7	D48.7	D49.89
inguinal (region)	C76.3	C79.89	D04.5	D36.7	D48.7	D49.89
insula	C71.0	C79.31	-	D33.0	D43.0	D49.6
insular tissue (pancreas)	C25.4	C78.89	D01.7	D13.7	D37.8	D49.0
brain	C71.0	C79.31	-	D33.0	D43.0	D49.6
interarytenoid fold	C13.1	C79.89	D00.08	D10.7	D37.05	D49.0
hypopharyngeal aspect	C13.1	C79.89	D00.08	D10.7	D37.05	D49.0
laryngeal aspect	C32.1	C78.39	D02.0	D14.1	D38.0	D49.1
marginal zone	C13.1	C79.89	D00.08	D10.7	D37.05	D49.0
interdental papillae	C03.9	C79.89	D00.03	D10.39	D37.09	D49.0
lower	C03.1	C79.89	D00.03	D10.39	D37.09	D49.0
upper	C03.0	C79.89	D00.03	D10.39	D37.09	D49.0
internal						
capsule	C71.0	C79.31	-	D33.0	D43.0	D49.6
os (cervix)	C53.0	C79.82	D06.0	D26.0	D39.0	D49.59
intervertebral cartilage or disc	C41.2	C79.51	-	D16.6	D48.0	D49.2
intestine, intestinal	C26.0	C78.80	D01.40	D13.99	D37.8	D49.0
large	C18.9	C78.5	D01.0	D12.6	D37.4	D49.0
appendix	C18.1	C78.5	D01.0	D12.1	D37.3	D49.0
caput coli	C18.0	C78.5	D01.0	D12.0	D37.4	D49.0
cecum	C18.0	C78.5	D01.0	D12.0	D37.4	D49.0
colon	C18.9	C78.5	D01.0	D12.6	D37.4	D49.0
and rectum	C19	C78.5	D01.1	D12.7	D37.5	D49.0
ascending	C18.2	C78.5	D01.0	D12.2	D37.4	D49.0
caput	C18.0	C78.5	D01.0	D12.0	D37.4	D49.0

	Malignant Primary	Malignant Secondary	Ca in situ	Benign	Uncertain Behavior	Unspecified Behavior
intestine, intestinal, large, colon — *continued*						
descending	C18.6	C78.5	D01.0	D12.4	D37.4	D49.0
distal	C18.6	C78.5	D01.0	D12.4	D37.4	D49.0
left	C18.6	C78.5	D01.0	D12.4	D37.4	D49.0
overlapping lesion	C18.8	-	-	-	-	-
pelvic	C18.7	C78.5	D01.0	D12.5	D37.4	D49.0
right	C18.2	C78.5	D01.0	D12.2	D37.4	D49.0
sigmoid (flexure)	C18.7	C78.5	D01.0	D12.5	D37.4	D49.0
transverse	C18.4	C78.5	D01.0	D12.3	D37.4	D49.0
hepatic flexure	C18.3	C78.5	D01.0	D12.3	D37.4	D49.0
ileocecum, ileocecal (coil) (valve)	C18.0	C78.5	D01.0	D12.0	D37.4	D49.0
overlapping lesion	C18.8	-	-	-	-	-
sigmoid flexure (lower) (upper)	C18.7	C78.5	D01.0	D12.5	D37.4	D49.0
splenic flexure	C18.5	C78.5	D01.0	D12.3	D37.4	D49.0
small	C17.9	C78.4	D01.40	D13.30	D37.2	D49.0
duodenum	C17.0	C78.4	D01.49	D13.2	D37.2	D49.0
ileum	C17.2	C78.4	D01.49	D13.39	D37.2	D49.0
jejunum	C17.1	C78.4	D01.49	D13.39	D37.2	D49.0
overlapping lesion	C17.8	-	-	-	-	-
tract NEC	C26.0	C78.89	D01.40	D13.99	D37.8	D49.0
intra-abdominal	C76.2	C79.89	D09.8	D36.7	D48.7	D49.89
intracranial NEC	C71.9	C79.31	-	D33.2	D43.2	D49.6
intrahepatic (bile) duct	C22.1	C78.7	D01.5	D13.4	D37.6	D49.0
intraocular	C69.9-	C79.49	D09.2-	D31.9-	D48.7	D49.89
intraorbital	C69.6-	C79.49	D09.2-	D31.6-	D48.7	D49.89
intrasellar	C75.1	C79.89	D09.3	D35.2	D44.3	D49.7
intrathoracic (cavity) (organs)	C76.1	C79.89	D09.8	D15.9	D48.7	D49.89
specified NEC	C76.1	C79.89	D09.8	D15.7	-	-
iris	C69.4-	C79.49	D09.2-	D31.4-	D48.7	D49.89
ischiorectal (fossa)	C76.3	C79.89	D09.8	D36.7	D48.7	D49.89
ischium	C41.4	C79.51	-	D16.8	D48.0	D49.2
island of Reil	C71.0	C79.31	-	D33.0	D43.0	D49.6
islands or islets of Langerhans	C25.4	C78.89	D01.7	D13.7	D37.8	D49.0
isthmus uteri	C54.0	C79.82	D07.0	D26.1	D39.0	D49.59
J						
jaw	C76.0	C79.89	D09.8	D36.7	D48.7	D49.89
bone	C41.1	C79.51	-	D16.5	D48.0	D49.2
lower	C41.1	C79.51	-	D16.5	-	-
upper	C41.0	C79.51	-	D16.4	-	-
carcinoma (any type) (lower) (upper)	C76.0	C79.89	-	-	-	-
skin—see also Neoplasm, skin, face	C44.309	C79.2	D04.39	D23.39	D48.5	D49.2
soft tissues	C03.9	C79.89	D00.03	D10.39	D37.09	D49.0
lower	C03.1	C79.89	D00.03	D10.39	D37.09	D49.0
upper	C03.0	C79.89	D00.03	D10.39	D37.09	D49.0
jejunum	C17.1	C78.4	D01.49	D13.39	D37.2	D49.0
joint NEC—see also Neoplasm, bone	C41.9	C79.51	-	D16.9	D48.0	D49.2

Table of Neoplasms

	Malignant Primary	Malignant Secondary	Ca in situ	Benign	Uncertain Behavior	Unspecified Behavior
joint NEC — *continued*						
acromioclavicular	C40.0-	C79.51	-	D16.0-	-	-
bursa or synovial membrane—see Neoplasm, connective tissue						
costovertebral	C41.3	C79.51	-	D16.7	D48.0	D49.2
sternocostal	C41.3	C79.51	-	D16.7	D48.0	D49.2
temporomandibular	C41.1	C79.51	-	D16.5	D48.0	D49.2
junction						
anorectal	C21.8	C78.5	D01.3	D12.9	D37.8	D49.0
cardioesophageal	C16.0	C78.89	D00.2	D13.1	D37.1	D49.0
esophagogastric	C16.0	C78.89	D00.2	D13.1	D37.1	D49.0
gastroesophageal	C16.0	C78.89	D00.2	D13.1	D37.1	D49.0
hard and soft palate	C05.9	C79.89	D00.00	D10.39	D37.09	D49.0
ileocecal	C18.0	C78.5	D01.0	D12.0	D37.4	D49.0
pelvirectal	C19	C78.5	D01.1	D12.7	D37.5	D49.0
pelviureteric	C65.-	C79.0-	D09.19	D30.1-	D41.1-	D49.59
rectosigmoid	C19	C78.5	D01.1	D12.7	D37.5	D49.0
squamocolumnar, of cervix	C53.8	C79.82	D06.7	D26.0	D39.0	D49.59
K						
Kaposi's sarcoma—see Kaposi's, sarcoma						
kidney (parenchymal)	C64.-	C79.0-	D09.19	D30.0-	D41.0-	D49.51-
calyx	C65.-	C79.0-	D09.19	D30.1-	D41.1-	D49.51-
hilus	C65.-	C79.0-	D09.19	D30.1-	D41.1-	D49.51-
pelvis	C65.-	C79.0-	D09.19	D30.1-	D41.1-	D49.51-
knee NEC	C76.5-	C79.89	D04.7-	D36.7	D48.7	D49.89
L						
labia (skin)	C51.9	C79.82	D07.1	D28.0	D39.8	D49.59
majora	C51.0	C79.82	D07.1	D28.0	D39.8	D49.59
minora	C51.1	C79.82	D07.1	D28.0	D39.8	D49.59
labial—see also Neoplasm, lip	C00.9	C79.89	D00.01	D10.0	D37.01	D49.0
sulcus (lower) (upper)	C06.1	C79.89	D00.02	D10.39	D37.09	D49.0
labium (skin)	C51.9	C79.82	D07.1	D28.0	D39.8	D49.59
majus	C51.0	C79.82	D07.1	D28.0	D39.8	D49.59
minus	C51.1	C79.82	D07.1	D28.0	D39.8	D49.59
lacrimal						
canaliculi	C69.5-	C79.49	D09.2-	D31.5-	D48.7	D49.89
duct (nasal)	C69.5-	C79.49	D09.2-	D31.5-	D48.7	D49.89
gland	C69.5-	C79.49	D09.2-	D31.5-	D48.7	D49.89
punctum	C69.5-	C79.49	D09.2-	D31.5-	D48.7	D49.89
sac	C69.5-	C79.49	D09.2-	D31.5-	D48.7	D49.89
Langerhans, islands or islets	C25.4	C78.89	D01.7	D13.7	D37.8	D49.0
laryngopharynx	C13.9	C79.89	D00.08	D10.7	D37.05	D49.0
larynx, laryngeal NEC	C32.9	C78.39	D02.0	D14.1	D38.0	D49.1
aryepiglottic fold	C32.1	C78.39	D02.0	D14.1	D38.0	D49.1
cartilage (arytenoid) (cricoid) (cuneiform) (thyroid)	C32.3	C78.39	D02.0	D14.1	D38.0	D49.1
commissure (anterior) (posterior)	C32.0	C78.39	D02.0	D14.1	D38.0	D49.1

	Malignant Primary	Malignant Secondary	Ca in situ	Benign	Uncertain Behavior	Unspecified Behavior
larynx, laryngeal NEC — *continued*						
extrinsic NEC	C32.1	C78.39	D02.0	D14.1	D38.0	D49.1
meaning hypopharynx	C13.9	C79.89	D00.08	D10.7	D37.05	D49.0
interarytenoid fold	C32.1	C78.39	D02.0	D14.1	D38.0	D49.1
intrinsic	C32.0	C78.39	D02.0	D14.1	D38.0	D49.1
overlapping lesion	C32.8	-	-	-	-	-
ventricular band	C32.1	C78.39	D02.0	D14.1	D38.0	D49.1
leg NEC	C76.5-	C79.89	D04.7-	D36.7	D48.7	D49.89
lens, crystalline	C69.4-	C79.49	D09.2-	D31.4-	D48.7	D49.89
lid (lower) (upper)	C44.10-	C79.2	D04.1-	D23.1-	D48.5	D49.2
basal cell carcinoma	C44.11-	-	-	-	-	-
sebaceous cell	C44.13-	-	-	-	-	-
specified type NEC	C44.19-	-	-	-	-	-
squamous cell carcinoma	C44.12-	-	-	-	-	-
ligament—see also Neoplasm, connective tissue						
broad	C57.1-	C79.82	D07.39	D28.2	D39.8	D49.59
Mackenrodt's	C57.7	C79.82	D07.39	D28.7	D39.8	D49.59
non-uterine—see Neoplasm, connective tissue						
round	C57.2-	C79.82	-	D28.2	D39.8	D49.59
sacro-uterine	C57.3	C79.82	-	D28.2	D39.8	D49.59
uterine	C57.3	C79.82	-	D28.2	D39.8	D49.59
utero-ovarian	C57.7	C79.82	D07.39	D28.2	D39.8	D49.59
uterosacral	C57.3	C79.82	-	D28.2	D39.8	D49.59
limb	C76.8	C79.89	D04.8	D36.7	D48.7	D49.89
lower	C76.5-	C79.89	D04.7-	D36.7	D48.7	D49.89
upper	C76.4-	C79.89	D04.6-	D36.7	D48.7	D49.89
limbus of cornea	C69.1-	C79.49	D09.2-	D31.1-	D48.7	D49.89
lingual NEC—see also Neoplasm, tongue	C02.9	C79.89	D00.07	D10.1	D37.02	D49.0
lingula, lung	C34.1-	C78.0-	D02.2-	D14.3-	D38.1	D49.1
lip	C00.9	C79.89	D00.01	D10.0	D37.01	D49.0
buccal aspect—see Neoplasm, lip, internal						
commissure	C00.6	C79.89	D00.01	D10.0	D37.01	D49.0
external	C00.2	C79.89	D00.01	D10.0	D37.01	D49.0
lower	C00.1	C79.89	D00.01	D10.0	D37.01	D49.0
upper	C00.0	C79.89	D00.01	D10.0	D37.01	D49.0
frenulum—see Neoplasm, lip, internal						
inner aspect—see Neoplasm, lip, internal						
internal	C00.5	C79.89	D00.01	D10.0	D37.01	D49.0
lower	C00.4	C79.89	D00.01	D10.0	D37.01	D49.0
upper	C00.3	C79.89	D00.01	D10.0	D37.01	D49.0
lipstick area	C00.2	C79.89	D00.01	D10.0	D37.01	D49.0
lower	C00.1	C79.89	D00.01	D10.0	D37.01	D49.0
upper	C00.0	C79.89	D00.01	D10.0	D37.01	D49.0
lower	C00.1	C79.89	D00.01	D10.0	D37.01	D49.0
internal	C00.4	C79.89	D00.01	D10.0	D37.01	D49.0

	Malignant Primary	Malignant Secondary	Ca in situ	Benign	Uncertain Behavior	Unspecified Behavior
lip — *continued*						
mucosa—see Neoplasm, lip, intervnal						
oral aspect—see Neoplasm, lip, internal						
overlapping lesion	C00.8	-	-	-	-	-
with oral cavity or pharynx	C14.8	-	-	-	-	-
skin (commissure) (lower) (upper)	C44.00	C79.2	D04.0	D23.0	D48.5	D49.2
basal cell carcinoma	C44.01	-	-	-	-	-
specified type NEC	C44.09	-	-	-	-	-
squamous cell carcinoma	C44.02	-	-	-	-	-
upper	C00.0	C79.89	D00.01	D10.0	D37.01	D49.0
internal	C00.3	C79.89	D00.01	D10.0	D37.01	D49.0
vermilion border	C00.2	C79.89	D00.01	D10.0	D37.01	D49.0
lower	C00.1	C79.89	D00.01	D10.0	D37.01	D49.0
upper	C00.0	C79.89	D00.01	D10.0	D37.01	D49.0
lipomatous—see Lipoma, by site						
liver—see also Index to disease, by histology	C22.9	C78.7	D01.5	D13.4	D37.6	D49.0
primary	C22.8	C78.7	D01.5	D13.4	D37.6	D49.0
lumbosacral plexus	C47.5	C79.89	-	D36.16	D48.2	D49.2
lung	C34.9-	C78.0-	D02.2-	D14.3-	D38.1	D49.1
azygos lobe	C34.1-	C78.0-	D02.2-	D14.3-	D38.1	D49.1
carina	C34.0-	C78.0-	D02.2-	D14.3-	D38.1	D49.1
hilus	C34.0-	C78.0-	D02.2-	D14.3-	D38.1	D49.1
linqula	C34.1-	C78.0-	D02.2-	D14.3-	D38.1	D49.1
lobe NEC	C34.9-	C78.0-	D02.2-	D14.3-	D38.1	D49.1
lower lobe	C34.3-	C78.0-	D02.2-	D14.3-	D38.1	D49.1
main bronchus	C34.0-	C78.0-	D02.2-	D14.3-	D38.1	D49.1
mesothelioma—see Mesothelioma						
middle lobe	C34.2	C78.0-	D02.21	D14.31	D38.1	D49.1
overlapping lesion	C34.8-	-	-	-	-	-
upper lobe	C34.1-	C78.0-	D02.2-	D14.3-	D38.1	D49.1
lymph, lymphatic channel NEC	C49.9	C79.89	-	D21.9	D48.1	D49.2
gland (secondary)	-	C77.9	-	D36.0	D48.7	D49.89
abdominal	-	C77.2	-	D36.0	D48.7	D49.89
aortic	-	C77.2	-	D36.0	D48.7	D49.89
arm	-	C77.3	-	D36.0	D48.7	D49.89
auricular (anterior) (posterior)	-	C77.0	-	D36.0	D48.7	D49.89
axilla, axillary	-	C77.3	-	D36.0	D48.7	D49.89
brachial	-	C77.3	-	D36.0	D48.7	D49.89
bronchial	-	C77.1	-	D36.0	D48.7	D49.89
bronchopulmonary	-	C77.1	-	D36.0	D48.7	D49.89
celiac	-	C77.2	-	D36.0	D48.7	D49.89
cervical	-	C77.0	-	D36.0	D48.7	D49.89
cervicofacial	-	C77.0	-	D36.0	D48.7	D49.89
Cloquet	-	C77.4	-	D36.0	D48.7	D49.89
colic	-	C77.2	-	D36.0	D48.7	D49.89
common duct	-	C77.2	-	D36.0	D48.7	D49.89

	Malignant Primary	Malignant Secondary	Ca in situ	Benign	Uncertain Behavior	Unspecified Behavior
lymph, lymphatic channel NEC, gland — *continued*						
cubital	-	C77.3	-	D36.0	D48.7	D49.89
diaphragmatic	-	C77.1	-	D36.0	D48.7	D49.89
epigastric, inferior	-	C77.1	-	D36.0	D48.7	D49.89
epitrochlear	-	C77.3	-	D36.0	D48.7	D49.89
esophageal	-	C77.1	-	D36.0	D48.7	D49.89
face	-	C77.0	-	D36.0	D48.7	D49.89
femoral	-	C77.4	-	D36.0	D48.7	D49.89
gastric	-	C77.2	-	D36.0	D48.7	D49.89
groin	-	C77.4	-	D36.0	D48.7	D49.89
head	-	C77.0	-	D36.0	D48.7	D49.89
hepatic	-	C77.2	-	D36.0	D48.7	D49.89
hilar (pulmonary)	-	C77.1	-	D36.0	D48.7	D49.89
splenic	-	C77.2	-	D36.0	D48.7	D49.89
hypogastric	-	C77.5	-	D36.0	D48.7	D49.89
ileocolic	-	C77.2	-	D36.0	D48.7	D49.89
iliac	-	C77.5	-	D36.0	D48.7	D49.89
infraclavicular	-	C77.3	-	D36.0	D48.7	D49.89
inguina, inguinal	-	C77.4	-	D36.0	D48.7	D49.89
innominate	-	C77.1	-	D36.0	D48.7	D49.89
intercostal	-	C77.1	-	D36.0	D48.7	D49.89
intestinal	-	C77.2	-	D36.0	D48.7	D49.89
intrabdominal	-	C77.2	-	D36.0	D48.7	D49.89
intrapelvic	-	C77.5	-	D36.0	D48.7	D49.89
intrathoracic	-	C77.1	-	D36.0	D48.7	D49.89
jugular	-	C77.0	-	D36.0	D48.7	D49.89
leg	-	C77.4	-	D36.0	D48.7	D49.89
limb						
lower	-	C77.4	-	D36.0	D48.7	D49.89
upper	-	C77.3	-	D36.0	D48.7	D49.89
lower limb	-	C77.4	-	D36.0	D48.7	D49.89
lumbar	-	C77.2	-	D36.0	D48.7	D49.89
mandibular	-	C77.0	-	D36.0	D48.7	D49.89
mediastinal	-	C77.1	-	D36.0	D48.7	D49.89
mesenteric (inferior) (superior)	-	C77.2	-	D36.0	D48.7	D49.89
midcolic	-	C77.2	-	D36.0	D48.7	D49.89
multiple sites in categories C77.0 - C77.5	-	C77.8	-	D36.0	D48.7	D49.89
neck	-	C77.0	-	D36.0	D48.7	D49.89
obturator	-	C77.5	-	D36.0	D48.7	D49.89
occipital	-	C77.0	-	D36.0	D48.7	D49.89
pancreatic	-	C77.2	-	D36.0	D48.7	D49.89
para-aortic	-	C77.2	-	D36.0	D48.7	D49.89
paracervical	-	C77.5	-	D36.0	D48.7	D49.89
parametrial	-	C77.5	-	D36.0	D48.7	D49.89
parasternal	-	C77.1	-	D36.0	D48.7	D49.89
parotid	-	C77.0	-	D36.0	D48.7	D49.89
pectoral	-	C77.3	-	D36.0	D48.7	D49.89
pelvic	-	C77.5	-	D36.0	D48.7	D49.89
peri-aortic	-	C77.2	-	D36.0	D48.7	D49.89
peripancreatic	-	C77.2	-	D36.0	D48.7	D49.89

Table of Neoplasms

	Malignant Primary	Malignant Secondary	Ca in situ	Benign	Uncertain Behavior	Unspecified Behavior
lymph, lymphatic channel NEC, gland — *continued*						
popliteal	-	C77.4	-	D36.0	D48.7	D49.89
porta hepatis	-	C77.2	-	D36.0	D48.7	D49.89
portal	-	C77.2	-	D36.0	D48.7	D49.89
preauricular	-	C77.0	-	D36.0	D48.7	D49.89
prelaryngeal	-	C77.0	-	D36.0	D48.7	D49.89
presymphysial	-	C77.5	-	D36.0	D48.7	D49.89
pretracheal	-	C77.0	-	D36.0	D48.7	D49.89
primary (any site) NEC	C96.9	-	-	-	-	-
pulmonary (hiler)	-	C77.1	-	D36.0	D48.7	D49.89
pyloric	-	C77.2	-	D36.0	D48.7	D49.89
retroperitoneal	-	C77.2	-	D36.0	D48.7	D49.89
retropharyngeal	-	C77.0	-	D36.0	D48.7	D49.89
Rosenmuller's	-	C77.4	-	D36.0	D48.7	D49.89
sacral	-	C77.5	-	D36.0	D48.7	D49.89
scalene	-	C77.0	-	D36.0	D48.7	D49.89
site NEC	-	C77.9	-	D36.0	D48.7	D49.89
splenic (hilar)	-	C77.2	-	D36.0	D48.7	D49.89
subclavicular	-	C77.3	-	D36.0	D48.7	D49.89
subinguinal	-	C77.4	-	D36.0	D48.7	D49.89
sublingual	-	C77.0	-	D36.0	D48.7	D49.89
submandibular	-	C77.0	-	D36.0	D48.7	D49.89
submaxillary	-	C77.0	-	D36.0	D48.7	D49.89
submental	-	C77.0	-	D36.0	D48.7	D49.89
subscapular	-	C77.3	-	D36.0	D48.7	D49.89
supraclavicular	-	C77.0	-	D36.0	D48.7	D49.89
thoracic	-	C77.1	-	D36.0	D48.7	D49.89
tibial	-	C77.4	-	D36.0	D48.7	D49.89
tracheal	-	C77.1	-	D36.0	D48.7	D49.89
tracheobronchial	-	C77.1	-	D36.0	D48.7	D49.89
upper limb	-	C77.3	-	D36.0	D48.7	D49.89
Virchow's	-	C77.0	-	D36.0	D48.7	D49.89
node—see also Neoplasm, lymph gland						
primary NEC	C96.9	-	-	-	-	-
vessel—see also Neoplasm, connective tissue	C49.9	C79.89	-	D21.9	D48.1	D49.2
M						
Mackenrodt's ligament	C57.7	C79.82	D07.39	D28.7	D39.8	D49.59
malar	C41.0	C79.51	-	D16.4	D48.0	D49.2
region—see Neoplasm, cheek						
mammary gland—see Neoplasm, breast						
mandible	C41.1	C79.51	-	D16.5	D48.0	D49.2
alveolar						
mucosa (carcinoma)	C03.1	C79.89	D00.03	D10.39	D37.09	D49.0
ridge or process	C41.1	C79.51	-	D16.5	D48.0	D49.2
marrow (bone) NEC	C96.9	C79.52	-	-	D47.9	D49.89
mastectomy site (skin)—see also Neoplasm, breast, skin	C44.501	C79.2	-	-	-	-
specified as breast tissue	C50.8-	C79.81	-	-	-	-
mastoid (air cells) (antrum) (cavity)	C30.1	C78.39	D02.3	D14.0	D38.5	D49.1
bone or process	C41.0	C79.51	-	D16.4	D48.0	D49.2
maxilla, maxillary (superior)	C41.0	C79.51	-	D16.4	D48.0	D49.2
alveolar						
mucosa	C03.0	C79.89	D00.03	D10.39	D37.09	D49.0
ridge or process (carcinoma)	C41.0	C79.51	-	D16.4	D48.0	D49.2
antrum	C31.0	C78.39	D02.3	D14.0	D38.5	D49.1
carcinoma	C03.0	C79.51	-	-	-	-
inferior—see Neoplasm, mandible						
sinus	C31.0	C78.39	D02.3	D14.0	D38.5	D49.1
meatus external (ear)—see also Neoplasm, skin, ear	C44.20-	C79.2	D04.2-	D23.2-	D48.5	D49.2
Meckel diverticulum, malignant	C17.3	C78.4	D01.49	D13.39	D37.2	D49.0
mediastinum, mediastinal	C38.3	C78.1	-	D15.2	D38.3	D49.89
anterior	C38.1	C78.1	-	D15.2	D38.3	D49.89
posterior	C38.2	C78.1	-	D15.2	D38.3	D49.89
medulla						
adrenal	C74.1-	C79.7-	D09.3	D35.0-	D44.1-	D49.7
oblongata	C71.7	C79.31	-	D33.1	D43.1	D49.6
meibomian gland	C44.10-	C79.2	D04.1-	D23.1-	D48.5	D49.2
basal cell carcinoma	C44.11-	-	-	-	-	-
sebaceous cell	C44.13-	-	-	-	-	-
specified type NEC	C44.19-	-	-	-	-	-
squamous cell carcinoma	C44.12-	-	-	-	-	-
melanoma—see Melanoma						
meninges	C70.9	C79.49	-	D32.9	D42.9	D49.7
brain	C70.0	C79.32	-	D32.0	D42.0	D49.7
cerebral	C70.0	C79.32	-	D32.0	D42.0	D49.7
crainial	C70.0	C79.32	-	D32.0	D42.0	D49.7
intracranial	C70.0	C79.32	-	D32.0	D42.0	D49.7
spinal (cord)	C70.1	C79.49	-	D32.1	D42.1	D49.7
meniscus, knee joint (lateral) (medial)	C40.2-	C79.51	-	D16.2-	D48.0	D49.2
Merkel cell—see Carcinoma, Merkel cell						
mesentery, mesenteric	C48.1	C78.6	-	D20.1	D48.4	D49.0
mesoappendix	C48.1	C78.6	-	D20.1	D48.4	D49.0
mesocolon	C48.1	C78.6	-	D20.1	D48.4	D49.0
mesopharynx—see Neoplasm, oropharynx						
mesosalpinx	C57.1-	C79.82	D07.39	D28.2	D39.8	D49.59
mesothelial tissue—see Mesothelioma						
mesothelioma—see Mesothelioma						
mesovarium	C57.1-	C79.82	D07.39	D28.2	D39.8	D49.59
metacarpus (any bone)	C40.1-	C79.51	-	D16.1-	-	-
metastatic NEC—see also Neoplasm, by site, secondary	-	C79.9	-	-	-	-
metatarsus (any bone)	C40.3-	C79.51	-	D16.3-	-	-
midbrain	C71.7	C79.31	-	D33.1	D43.1	D49.6

	Malignant Primary	Malignant Secondary	Ca in situ	Benign	Uncertain Behavior	Unspecified Behavior
milk duct—see Neoplasm, breast						
mons						
pubis	C51.9	C79.82	D07.1	D28.0	D39.8	D49.59
veneris	C51.9	C79.82	D07.1	D28.0	D39.8	D49.59
motor tract	C72.9	C79.49	-	D33.9	D43.9	D49.7
brain	C71.9	C79.31	-	D33.2	D43.2	D49.6
cauda equina	C72.1	C79.49	-	D33.4	D43.4	D49.7
spinal	C72.0	C79.49	-	D33.4	D43.4	D49.7
mouth	C06.9	C79.89	D00.00	D10.30	D37.09	D49.0
book-leaf	C06.89	C79.89	-	-	-	-
floor	C04.9	C79.89	D00.06	D10.2	D37.09	D49.0
anterior portion	C04.0	C79.89	D00.06	D10.2	D37.09	D49.0
lateral portion	C04.1	C79.89	D00.06	D10.2	D37.09	D49.0
overlapping lesion	C04.8	-	-	-	-	-
overlapping NEC	C06.80	-	-	-	-	-
roof	C05.9	C79.89	D00.00	D10.39	D37.09	D49.0
specified part NEC	C06.89	C79.89	D00.00	D10.39	D37.09	D49.0
vestibule	C06.1	C79.89	D00.00	D10.39	D37.09	D49.0
mucosa						
alveolar (ridge or process)	C03.9	C79.89	D00.03	D10.39	D37.09	D49.0
lower	C03.1	C79.89	D00.03	D10.39	D37.09	D49.0
upper	C03.0	C79.89	D00.03	D10.39	D37.09	D49.0
buccal	C06.0	C79.89	D00.02	D10.39	D37.09	D49.0
cheek	C06.0	C79.89	D00.02	D10.39	D37.09	D49.0
lip—see Neoplasm, lip, internal						
nasal	C30.0	C78.39	D02.3	D14.0	D38.5	D49.1
oral	C06.0	C79.89	D00.02	D10.39	D37.09	D49.0
Mullerian duct						
female	C57.7	C79.82	D07.39	D28.7	D39.8	D49.59
male	C63.7	C79.82	D07.69	D29.8	D40.8	D49.59
muscle—see also Neoplasm, connective tissue						
extraocular	C69.6-	C79.49	D09.2-	D31.6-	D48.7	D49.89
myocardium	C38.0	C79.89	-	D15.1	D48.7	D49.89
myometrium	C54.2	C79.82	D07.0	D26.1	D39.0	D49.59
myopericardium	C38.0	C79.89	-	D15.1	D48.7	D49.89
N						
nabothian gland (follicle)	C53.0	C79.82	D06.0	D26.0	D39.0	D49.59
nail—see also Neoplasm, skin, limb	C44.90	C79.2	D04.9	D23.9	D48.5	D49.2
finger—see also Neoplasm, skin, limb, upper	C44.60-	C79.2	D04.6-	D23.6-	D48.5	D49.2
toe—see also Neoplasm, skin, limb, lower	C44.70-	C79.2	D04.7-	D23.7-	D48.5	D49.2
nares, naris (anterior) (posterior)	C30.0	C78.39	D02.3	D14.0	D38.5	D49.1
nasal—see Neoplasm, nose						
nasolabial groove—see also Neoplasm, skin, face	C44.309	C79.2	D04.39	D23.39	D48.5	D49.2
nasolacrimal duct	C69.5-	C79.49	D09.2-	D31.5-	D48.7	D49.89

	Malignant Primary	Malignant Secondary	Ca in situ	Benign	Uncertain Behavior	Unspecified Behavior
nasopharynx, nasopharyngeal	C11.9	C79.89	D00.08	D10.6	D37.05	D49.0
floor	C11.3	C79.89	D00.08	D10.6	D37.05	D49.0
overlapping lesion	C11.8	-	-	-	-	-
roof	C11.0	C79.89	D00.08	D10.6	D37.05	D49.0
wall	C11.9	C79.89	D00.08	D10.6	D37.05	D49.0
anterior	C11.3	C79.89	D00.08	D10.6	D37.05	D49.0
lateral	C11.2	C79.89	D00.08	D10.6	D37.05	D49.0
posterior	C11.1	C79.89	D00.08	D10.6	D37.05	D49.0
superior	C11.0	C79.89	D00.08	D10.6	D37.05	D49.0
nates—see also Neoplasm, skin, trunk	C44.509	C79.2	D04.5	D23.5	D48.5	D49.2
neck NEC	C76.0	C79.89	D09.8	D36.7	D48.7	D49.89
skin	C44.40	-	-	-	-	-
basal cell carcinoma	C44.41	-	-	-	-	-
specified type NEC	C44.49	-	-	-	-	-
squamous cell carcinoma	C44.42	-	-	-	-	-
nerve (ganglion)	C47.9	C79.89	-	D36.10	D48.2	D49.2
abducens	C72.59	C79.49	-	D33.3	D43.3	D49.7
accessory (spinal)	C72.59	C79.49	-	D33.3	D43.3	D49.7
acoustic	C72.4-	C79.49	-	D33.3	D43.3	D49.7
auditory	C72.4-	C79.49	-	D33.3	D43.3	D49.7
autonomic NEC—see also Neoplasm, nerve, peripheral	C47.9	C79.89	-	D36.10	D48.2	D49.2
brachial	C47.1-	C79.89	-	D36.12	D48.2	D49.2
cranial	C72.50	C79.49	-	D33.3	D43.3	D49.7
specified NEC	C72.59	C79.49	-	D33.3	D43.3	D49.7
facial	C72.59	C79.49	-	D33.3	D43.3	D49.7
femoral	C47.2-	C79.89	-	D36.13	D48.2	D49.2
ganglion NEC—see also Neoplasm, nerve, peripheral	C47.9	C79.89	-	D36.10	D48.2	D49.2
glossopharyngeal	C72.59	C79.49	-	D33.3	D43.3	D49.7
hypoglossal	C72.59	C79.49	-	D33.3	D43.3	D49.7
intercostal	C47.3	C79.89	-	D36.14	D48.2	D49.2
lumbar	C47.6	C79.89	-	D36.17	D48.2	D49.2
median	C47.1-	C79.89	-	D36.12	D48.2	D49.2
obturator	C47.2-	C79.89	-	D36.13	D48.2	D49.2
oculomotor	C72.59	C79.49	-	D33.3	D43.3	D49.7
olfactory	C47.2-	C79.49	-	D33.3	D43.3	D49.7
optic	C72.3-	C79.49	-	D33.3	D43.3	D49.7
parasympathetic NEC	C47.9	C79.89	-	D36.10	D48.2	D49.2
peripheral NEC	C47.9	C79.89	-	D36.10	D48.2	D49.2
abdomen	C47.4	C79.89	-	D36.15	D48.2	D49.2
abdominal wall	C47.4	C79.89	-	D36.15	D48.2	D49.2
ankle	C47.2-	C79.89	-	D36.13	D48.2	D49.2
antecubital fossa or space	C47.1-	C79.89	-	D36.12	D48.2	D49.2
arm	C47.1-	C79.89	-	D36.12	D48.2	D49.2
auricle (ear)	C47.0	C79.89	-	D36.11	D48.2	D49.2
axilla	C47.3	C79.89	-	D36.12	D48.2	D49.2
back	C47.6	C79.89	-	D36.17	D48.2	D49.2
buttock	C47.5	C79.89	-	D36.16	D48.2	D49.2

Table of Neoplasms

	Malignant Primary	Malignant Secondary	Ca in situ	Benign	Uncertain Behavior	Unspecified Behavior
nerve (ganglion), peripheral NEC — *continued*						
calf	C47.2-	C79.89	-	D36.13	D48.2	D49.2
cervical region	C47.0	C79.89	-	D36.11	D48.2	D49.2
cheek	C47.0	C79.89	-	D36.11	D48.2	D49.2
chest (wall)	C47.3	C79.89	-	D36.14	D48.2	D49.2
chin	C47.0	C79.89	-	D36.11	D48.2	D49.2
ear (external)	C47.0	C79.89	-	D36.11	D48.2	D49.2
elbow	C47.1-	C79.89	-	D36.12	D48.2	D49.2
extrarectal	C47.5	C79.89	-	D36.16	D48.2	D49.2
extremity	C47.9	C79.89	-	D36.10	D48.2	D49.2
lower	C47.2-	C79.89	-	D36.13	D48.2	D49.2
upper	C47.1-	C79.89	-	D36.12	D48.2	D49.2
eyelid	C47.0	C79.89	-	D36.11	D48.2	D49.2
face	C47.0	C79.89	-	D36.11	D48.2	D49.2
finger	C47.1-	C79.89	-	D36.12	D48.2	D49.2
flank	C47.6	C79.89	-	D36.17	D48.2	D49.2
foot	C47.2-	C79.89	-	D36.13	D48.2	D49.2
forearm	C47.1-	C79.89	-	D36.12	D48.2	D49.2
forehead	C47.0	C79.89	-	D36.11	D48.2	D49.2
gluteal region	C47.5	C79.89	-	D36.16	D48.2	D49.2
groin	C47.5	C79.89	-	D36.16	D48.2	D49.2
hand	C47.1-	C79.89	-	D36.12	D48.2	D49.2
head	C47.0	C79.89	-	D36.11	D48.2	D49.2
heel	C47.2-	C79.89	-	D36.13	D48.2	D49.2
hip	C47.2-	C79.89	-	D36.13	D48.2	D49.2
infraclavicular region	C47.3	C79.89	-	D36.14	D48.2	D49.2
inguinal (canal) (region)	C47.5	C79.89	-	D36.16	D48.2	D49.2
intrathoracic	C47.3	C79.89	-	D36.14	D48.2	D49.2
ischiorectal fossa	C47.5	C79.89	-	D36.16	D48.2	D49.2
knee	C47.2-	C79.89	-	D36.13	D48.2	D49.2
leg	C47.2-	C79.89	-	D36.13	D48.2	D49.2
limb NEC	C47.9	C79.89	-	D36.10	D48.2	D49.2
lower	C47.2-	C79.89	-	D36.13	D48.2	D49.2
upper	C47.1-	C79.89	-	D36.12	D48.2	D49.2
nates	C47.5	C79.89	-	D36.16	D48.2	D49.2
neck	C47.0	C79.89	-	D36.11	D48.2	D49.2
orbit	C69.6-	C79.49	-	D31.6-	D48.7	D49.2
pararectal	C47.5	C79.89	-	D36.16	D48.2	D49.2
paraurethral	C47.5	C79.89	-	D36.16	D48.2	D49.2
paravaginal	C47.5	C79.89	-	D36.16	D48.2	D49.2
pelvis (floor)	C47.5	C79.89	-	D36.16	D48.2	D49.2
pelvoabdominal	C47.8	C79.89	-	D36.17	D48.2	D49.2
perineum	C47.5	C79.89	-	D36.16	D48.2	D49.2
perirectal (tissue)	C47.5	C79.89	-	D36.16	D48.2	D49.2
periurethral (tissue)	C47.5	C79.89	-	D36.16	D48.2	D49.2
popliteal fossa or space	C47.2-	C79.89	-	D36.13	D48.2	D49.2
presacral	C47.5	C79.89	-	D36.16	D48.2	D49.2
pterygoid fossa	C47.0	C79.89	-	D36.11	D48.2	D49.2
rectovaginal septum or wall	C47.5	C79.89	-	D36.16	D48.2	D49.2
rectovesical	C47.5	C79.89	-	D36.16	D48.2	D49.2
sacrococcygeal region	C47.5	C79.89	-	D36.16	D48.2	D49.2

	Malignant Primary	Malignant Secondary	Ca in situ	Benign	Uncertain Behavior	Unspecified Behavior
nerve (ganglion), peripheral NEC — *continued*						
scalp	C47.0	C79.89	-	D36.11	D48.2	D49.2
scapular region	C47.3	C79.89	-	D36.14	D48.2	D49.2
shoulder	C47.1-	C79.89	-	D36.12	D48.2	D49.2
submental	C47.0	C79.89	-	D36.11	D48.2	D49.2
supraclavicular region	C47.0	C79.89	-	D36.11	D48.2	D49.2
temple	C47.0	C79.89	-	D36.11	D48.2	D49.2
temporal region	C47.0	C79.89	-	D36.11	D48.2	D49.2
thigh	C47.2-	C79.89	-	D36.13	D48.2	D49.2
thoracic (duct) (wall)	C47.3	C79.89	-	D36.14	D48.2	D49.2
thorax	C47.3	C79.89	-	D36.14	D48.2	D49.2
thumb	C47.1-	C79.89	-	D36.12	D48.2	D49.2
toe	C47.2-	C79.89	-	D36.13	D48.2	D49.2
trunk	C47.6	C79.89	-	D36.17	D48.2	D49.2
umbilicus	C47.4	C79.89	-	D36.15	D48.2	D49.2
vesicorectal	C47.5	C79.89	-	D36.16	D48.2	D49.2
wrist	C47.1-	C79.89	-	D36.12	D48.2	D49.2
radial	C47.1-	C79.89	-	D36.12	D48.2	D49.2
sacral	C47.5	C79.89	-	D36.16	D48.2	D49.2
sciatic	C47.2-	C79.89	-	D36.13	D48.2	D49.2
spinal NEC	C47.9	C79.89	-	D36.10	D48.2	D49.2
accessory	C72.59	C79.49	-	D33.3	D43.3	D49.7
sympathetic NEC—see also Neoplasm, nerve, peripheral	C47.9	C79.89	-	D36.10	D48.2	D49.2
trigeminal	C72.59	C79.49	-	D33.3	D43.3	D49.7
trochlear	C72.59	C79.49	-	D33.3	D43.3	D49.7
ulnar	C47.1-	C79.89	-	D36.12	D48.2	D49.2
vagus	C72.59	C79.49	-	D33.3	D43.3	D49.7
nervous system (central)	C72.9	C79.40	-	D33.9	D43.9	D49.7
autonomic—see Neoplasm, nerve, peripheral						
parasympathetic—see Neoplasm, nerve, peripheral						
specified site NEC	-	C79.49	-	D33.7	D43.8	-
sympathetic—see Neoplasm, nerve, peripheral						
nevus—see Nevus						
nipple	C50.0-	C79.81	D05.-	D24.-	-	-
nose, nasal	C76.0	C79.89	D09.8	D36.7	D48.7	D49.89
ala (external) (nasi)—see also Neoplasm, nose, skin	C44.301	C79.2	D04.39	D23.39	D48.5	D49.2
bone	C41.0	C79.51	-	D16.4	D48.0	D49.2
cartilage	C30.0	C78.39	D02.3	D14.0	D38.5	D49.1
cavity	C30.0	C78.39	D02.3	D14.0	D38.5	D49.1
choana	C11.3	C79.89	D00.08	D10.6	D37.05	D49.0
external (skin)—see also Neoplasm, nose, skin	C44.301	C79.2	D04.39	D23.39	D48.5	D49.2
fossa	C30.0	C78.39	D02.3	D14.0	D38.5	D49.1
internal	C30.0	C78.39	D02.3	D14.0	D38.5	D49.1
mucosa	C30.0	C78.39	D02.3	D14.0	D38.5	D49.1
septum	C30.0	C78.39	D02.3	D14.0	D38.5	D49.1

360

	Malignant Primary	Malignant Secondary	Ca in situ	Benign	Uncertain Behavior	Unspecified Behavior
nose, nasal, septum — *continued*						
posterior margin	C11.3	C79.89	D00.08	D10.6	D37.05	D49.0
sinus—see Neoplasm, sinus						
skin	C44.301	C79.2	D04.39	D23.39	D48.5	D49.2
basal cell carcinoma	C44.311	-	-	-	-	-
specified type NEC	C44.391	-	-	-	-	-
squamous cell carcinoma	C44.321	-	-	-	-	-
turbinate (mucosa)	C30.0	C78.39	D02.3	D14.0	D38.5	D49.1
bone	C41.0	C79.51	-	D16.4	D48.0	D49.2
vestibule	C30.0	C78.39	D02.3	D14.0	D38.5	D49.1
nostril	C30.0	C78.39	D02.3	D14.0	D38.5	D49.1
nucleus pulposus	C41.2	C79.51	-	D16.6	D48.0	D49.2
O						
occipital						
bone	C41.0	C79.51	-	D16.4	D48.0	D49.2
lobe or pole, brain	C71.4	C79.31	-	D33.0	D43.0	D49.6
odontogenic—see Neoplasm, jaw bone						
olfactory nerve or bulb	C72.2-	C79.49	-	D33.3	D43.3	D49.7
olive (brain)	C71.7	C79.31	-	D33.1	D43.1	D49.6
omentum	C48.1	C78.6	-	D20.1	D48.4	D49.0
operculum (brain)	C71.0	C79.31	-	D33.0	D43.0	D49.6
optic nerve, chiasm, or tract	C72.3-	C79.49	-	D33.3	D43.3	D49.7
oral (cavity)	C06.9	C79.89	D00.00	D10.30	D37.09	D49.0
ill-defined	C14.8	C79.89	D00.00	D10.30	D37.09	D49.0
mucosa	C06.0	C79.89	D00.02	D10.39	D37.09	D49.0
orbit	C69.6-	C79.49	D09.2-	D31.6-	D48.7	D49.89
autonomic nerve	C69.6-	C79.49	-	D31.6-	D48.7	D49.2
bone	C41.0	C79.51	-	D16.4	D48.0	D49.2
eye	C69.6-	C79.49	D09.2-	D31.6-	D48.7	D49.89
peripheral nerves	C69.6-	C79.49	-	D31.6-	D48.7	D49.2
soft parts	C69.6-	C79.49	D09.2-	D31.6-	D48.7	D49.89
organ of Zuckerkandl	C75.5	C79.89	-	D35.6	D44.7	D49.7
oropharynx	C10.9	C79.89	D00.08	D10.5	D37.05	D49.0
branchial cleft (vestige)	C10.4	C79.89	D00.08	D10.5	D37.05	D49.0
junctional region	C10.8	C79.89	D00.08	D10.5	D37.05	D49.0
lateral wall	C10.2	C79.89	D00.08	D10.5	D37.05	D49.0
overlapping lesion	C10.8	-	-	-	-	-
pillars or fauces	C09.1	C79.89	D00.08	D10.5	D37.05	D49.0
posterior wall	C10.3	C79.89	D00.08	D10.5	D37.05	D49.0
vallecula	C10.0	C79.89	D00.08	D10.5	D37.05	D49.0
os						
external	C53.1	C79.82	D06.1	D26.0	D39.0	D49.59
internal	C53.0	C79.82	D06.0	D26.0	D39.0	D49.59
ovary	C56.-	C79.6-	D07.39	D27.-	D39.1-	D49.59
oviduct	C57.0-	C79.82	D07.39	D28.2	D39.8	D49.59
P						
palate	C05.9	C79.89	D00.00	D10.39	D37.09	D49.0
hard	C05.0	C79.89	D00.05	D10.39	D37.09	D49.0
junction of hard and soft palate	C05.9	C79.89	D00.00	D10.39	D37.09	D49.0

	Malignant Primary	Malignant Secondary	Ca in situ	Benign	Uncertain Behavior	Unspecified Behavior
palate — *continued*						
overlapping lesions	C05.8	-	-	-	-	-
soft	C05.1	C79.89	D00.04	D10.39	D37.09	D49.0
nasopharyngeal surface	C11.3	C79.89	D00.08	D10.6	D37.05	D49.0
posterior surface	C11.3	C79.89	D00.08	D10.6	D37.05	D49.0
superior surface	C11.3	C79.89	D00.08	D10.6	D37.05	D49.0
palatoglossal arch	C09.1	C79.89	D00.00	D10.5	D37.09	D49.0
palatopharyngeal arch	C09.1	C79.89	D00.00	D10.5	D37.09	D49.0
pallium	C71.0	C79.31	-	D33.0	D43.0	D49.6
palpebra	C44.10-	C79.2	D04.1-	D23.1-	D48.5	D49.2
basal cell carcinoma	C44.11-	-	-	-	-	-
sebaceous cell	C44.13-	-	-	-	-	-
specified type NEC	C44.19-	-	-	-	-	-
squamous cell carcinoma	C44.12-	-	-	-	-	-
pancreas	C25.9	C78.89	D01.7	D13.6	D37.8	D49.0
body	C25.1	C78.89	D01.7	D13.6	D37.8	D49.0
duct (of Santorini) (of Wirsung)	C25.3	C78.89	D01.7	D13.6	D37.8	D49.0
ectopic tissue	C25.7	C78.89	-	D13.6	D37.8	D49.0
head	C25.0	C78.89	D01.7	D13.6	D37.8	D49.0
islet cells	C25.4	C78.89	D01.7	D13.7	D37.8	D49.0
neck	C25.7	C78.89	D01.7	D13.6	D37.8	D49.0
overlapping lesion	C25.8	-	-	-	-	-
tail	C25.2	C78.89	D01.7	D13.6	D37.8	D49.0
para-aortic body	C75.5	C79.89	-	D35.6	D44.7	D49.7
paraganglion NEC	C75.5	C79.89	-	D35.6	D44.7	D49.7
parametrium	C57.3	C79.82	-	D28.2	D39.8	D49.59
paranephric	C48.0	C78.6	-	D20.0	D48.3	D49.0
pararectal	C76.3	C79.89	-	D36.7	D48.7	D49.89
parasagittal (region)	C76.0	C79.89	D09.8	D36.7	D48.7	D49.89
parasellar	C72.9	C79.49	-	D33.9	D43.8	D49.7
parathyroid (gland)	C75.0	C79.89	D09.3	D35.1	D44.2	D49.7
paraurethral	C76.3	C79.89	-	D36.7	D48.7	D49.89
gland	C68.1	C79.19	D09.19	D30.8	D41.8	D49.59
paravaginal	C76.3	C79.89	-	D36.7	D48.7	D49.89
parenchyma, kidney	C64.-	C79.0-	D09.19	D30.0-	D41.0-	D49.51-
parietal						
bone	C41.0	C79.51	-	D16.4	D48.0	D49.2
lobe, brain	C71.3	C79.31	-	D33.0	D43.0	D49.6
paroophoron	C57.1-	C79.82	D07.39	D28.2	D39.8	D49.59
parotid (duct) (gland)	C07	C79.89	D00.00	D11.0	D37.030	D49.0
parovarium	C57.1-	C79.82	D07.39	D28.2	D39.8	D49.59
patella	C40.20	C79.51	-	-	-	-
peduncle, cerebral	C71.7	C79.31	-	D33.1	D43.1	D49.6
pelvirectal junction	C19	C78.5	D01.1	D12.7	D37.5	D49.0
pelvis, pelvic	C76.3	C79.89	D09.8	D36.7	D48.7	D49.89
bone	C41.4	C79.51	-	D16.8	D48.0	D49.2
floor	C76.3	C79.89	D09.8	D36.7	D48.7	D49.89
renal	C65.-	C79.0-	D09.19	D30.1-	D41.1-	D49.51-
viscera	C76.3	C79.89	D09.8	D36.7	D48.7	D49.89
wall	C76.3	C79.89	D09.8	D36.7	D48.7	D49.89
pelvo-abdominal	C76.8	C79.89	D09.8	D36.7	D48.7	D49.89

361

Table of Neoplasms

	Malignant Primary	Malignant Secondary	Ca in situ	Benign	Uncertain Behavior	Unspecified Behavior
penis	C60.9	C79.82	D07.4	D29.0	D40.8	D49.59
body	C60.2	C79.82	D07.4	D29.0	D40.8	D49.59
corpus (cavernosum)	C60.2	C79.82	D07.4	D29.0	D40.8	D49.59
glans	C60.1	C79.82	D07.4	D29.0	D40.8	D49.59
overlapping sites	C60.8	-	-	-	-	-
skin NEC	C60.9	C79.82	D07.4	D29.0	D40.8	D49.59
periadrenal (tissue)	C48.0	C78.6	-	D20.0	D48.3	D49.0
perianal (skin)—see also Neoplasm, anus, skin	C44.500	C79.2	D04.5	D23.5	D48.5	D49.2
pericardium	C38.0	C79.89	-	D15.1	D48.7	D49.89
perinephric	C48.0	C78.6	-	D20.0	D48.3	D49.0
perineum	C76.3	C79.89	D09.8	D36.7	D48.7	D49.89
periodontal tissue NEC	C03.9	C79.89	D00.03	D10.39	D37.09	D49.0
periosteum—see Neoplasm, bone						
peripancreatic	C48.0	C78.6	-	D20.0	D48.3	D49.0
peripheral nerve NEC	C47.9	C79.89	-	D36.10	D48.2	D49.2
perirectal (tissue)	C76.3	C79.89	-	D36.7	D48.7	D49.89
perirenal (tissue)	C48.0	C78.6	-	D20.0	D48.3	D49.0
peritoneum, peritoneal (cavity)	C48.2	C78.6	-	D20.1	D48.4	D49.0
benign mesothelial tissue—see Mesothelioma, benign						
overlapping lesion	C48.8	-	-	-	-	-
with digestive organs	C26.9	-	-	-	-	-
parietal	C48.1	C78.6	-	D20.1	D48.4	D49.0
pelvic	C48.1	C78.6	-	D20.1	D48.4	D49.0
specified part NEC	C48.1	C78.6	-	D20.1	D48.4	D49.0
peritonsillar (tissue)	C76.0	C79.89	D09.8	D36.7	D48.7	D49.89
periurethral tissue	C76.3	C79.89	-	D36.7	D48.7	D49.89
phalanges						
foot	C40.3-	C79.51	-	D16.3-	-	-
hand	C40.1-	C79.51	-	D16.1-	-	-
pharynx, pharyngeal	C14.0	C79.89	D00.08	D10.9	D37.05	D49.0
bursa	C11.1	C79.89	D00.08	D10.6	D37.05	D49.0
fornix	C11.3	C79.89	D00.08	D10.6	D37.05	D49.0
recess	C11.2	C79.89	D00.08	D10.6	D37.05	D49.0
region	C14.0	C79.89	D00.08	D10.9	D37.05	D49.0
tonsil	C11.1	C79.89	D00.08	D10.6	D37.05	D49.0
wall (lateral) (posterior)	C14.0	C79.89	D00.08	D10.9	D37.05	D49.0
pia mater	C70.9	C79.40	-	D32.9	D42.9	D49.7
cerebral	C70.0	C79.32	-	D32.0	D42.0	D49.7
cranial	C70.0	C79.32	-	D32.0	D42.0	D49.7
spinal	C70.1	C79.49	-	D32.1	D42.1	D49.7
pillars of fauces	C09.1	C79.89	D00.08	D10.5	D37.05	D49.0
pineal (body) (gland)	C75.3	C79.89	D09.3	D35.4	D44.5	D49.7
pinna (ear) NEC—see also Neoplasm, skin, ear	C44.20-	C79.2	D04.2-	D23.2-	D48.5	D49.2
piriform fossa or sinus	C12	C79.89	D00.08	D10.7	D37.05	D49.0
pituitary (body) (fossa) (gland) (lobe)	C75.1	C79.89	D09.3	D35.2	D44.3	D49.7
placenta	C58	C79.82	D07.0	D26.7	D39.2	D49.59

	Malignant Primary	Malignant Secondary	Ca in situ	Benign	Uncertain Behavior	Unspecified Behavior
pleura, pleural (cavity)	C38.4	C78.2	-	D19.0	D38.2	D49.1
overlapping lesion with heart or mediastinum	C38.8	-	-	-	-	-
parietal	C38.4	C78.2	-	D19.0	D38.2	D49.1
visceral	C38.4	C78.2	-	D19.0	D38.2	D49.1
plexus						
brachial	C47.1-	C79.89	-	D36.12	D48.2	D49.2
cervical	C47.0	C79.89	-	D36.11	D48.2	D49.2
choroid	C71.5	C79.31	-	D33.0	D43.0	D49.6
lumbosacral	C47.5	C79.89	-	D36.16	D48.2	D49.2
sacral	C47.5	C79.89	-	D36.16	D48.2	D49.2
pluriendocrine	C75.8	C79.89	D09.3	D35.7	D44.9	D49.7
pole						
frontal	C71.1	C79.31	-	D33.0	D43.0	D49.6
occipital	C71.4	C79.31	-	D33.0	D43.0	D49.6
pons (varolii)	C71.7	C79.31	-	D33.1	D43.1	D49.6
popliteal fossa or space	C76.5-	C79.89	D04.7-	D36.7	D48.7	D49.89
postcricoid (region)	C13.0	C79.89	D00.08	D10.7	D37.05	D49.0
posterior fossa (cranial)	C71.9	C79.31	-	D33.2	D43.2	D49.6
postnasal space	C11.9	C79.89	D00.08	D10.6	D37.05	D49.0
prepuce	C60.0	C79.82	D07.4	D29.0	D40.8	D49.59
prepylorus	C16.4	C78.89	D00.2	D13.1	D37.1	D49.0
presacral (region)	C76.3	C79.89	-	D36.7	D48.7	D49.89
prostate (gland)	C61	C79.82	D07.5	D29.1	D40.0	D49.59
utricle	C68.0	C79.19	D09.19	D30.4	D41.3	D49.59
pterygoid fossa	C49.0	C79.89	-	D21.0	D48.1	D49.2
pubic bone	C41.4	C79.51	-	D16.8	D48.0	D49.2
pudenda, pudendum (female)	C51.9	C79.82	D07.1	D28.0	D39.8	D49.59
pulmonary—see also Neoplasm, lung	C34.9-	C78.0-	D02.2-	D14.3-	D38.1	D49.1
putamen	C71.0	C79.31	-	D33.0	D43.0	D49.6
pyloric						
antrum	C16.3	C78.89	D00.2	D13.1	D37.1	D49.0
canal	C16.4	C78.89	D00.2	D13.1	D37.1	D49.0
pylorus	C16.4	C78.89	D00.2	D13.1	D37.1	D49.0
pyramid (brain)	C71.7	C79.31	-	D33.1	D43.1	D49.6
pyriform fossa or sinus	C12	C79.89	D00.08	D10.7	D37.05	D49.0
R						
radius (any part)	C40.0-	C79.51	-	D16.0-	-	-
Rathke's pouch	C75.1	C79.89	D09.3	D35.2	D44.3	D49.7
rectosigmoid (junction)	C19	C78.5	D01.1	D12.7	D37.5	D49.0
overlapping lesion with anus or rectum	C21.8	-	-	-	-	-
rectouterine pouch	C48.1	C78.6	-	D20.1	D48.4	D49.0
rectovaginal septum or wall	C76.3	C79.89	D09.8	D36.7	D48.7	D49.89
rectovesical septum	C76.3	C79.89	D09.8	D36.7	D48.7	D49.89
rectum (ampulla)	C20	C78.5	D01.2	D12.8	D37.5	D49.0
and colon	C19	C78.5	D01.1	D12.7	D37.5	D49.0
overlapping lesion with anus or rectosigmoid junction	C21.8	-	-	-	-	-

	Malignant Primary	Malignant Secondary	Ca in situ	Benign	Uncertain Behavior	Unspecified Behavior
renal	C64.-	C79.0-	D09.19	D30.0-	D41.0-	D49.51-
calyx	C65.-	C79.0-	D09.19	D30.1-	D41.1-	D49.51-
hilus	C65.-	C79.0-	D09.19	D30.1-	D41.1-	D49.51-
parenchyma	C64.-	C79.0-	D09.19	D30.0-	D41.0-	D49.51-
pelvis	C65.-	C79.0-	D09.19	D30.1-	D41.1-	D49.51-
respiratory						
organs or system NEC	C39.9	C78.30	D02.4	D14.4	D38.6	D49.1
tract NEC	C39.9	C78.30	D02.4	D14.4	D38.5	D49.1
upper	C39.0	C78.30	D02.4	D14.4	D38.5	D49.1
retina	C69.2-	C79.49	D09.2-	D31.2-	D48.7	D49.81
retrobulbar	C69.6-	C79.49	-	D31.6-	D48.7	D49.89
retrocecal	C48.0	C78.6	-	D20.0	D48.3	D49.0
retromolar (area) (triangle) (trigone)	C06.2	C79.89	D00.00	D10.39	D37.09	D49.0
retro-orbital	C76.0	C79.89	D09.8	D36.7	D48.7	D49.89
retroperitoneal (space) (tissue)	C48.0	C78.6	-	D20.0	D48.3	D49.0
retroperitoneum	C48.0	C78.6	-	D20.0	D48.3	D49.0
retropharyngeal	C14.0	C79.89	D00.08	D10.9	D37.05	D49.0
retrovesical (septum)	C76.3	C79.89	D09.8	D36.7	D48.7	D49.89
rhinencephalon	C71.0	C79.31	-	D33.0	D43.0	D49.6
rib	C41.3	C79.51	-	D16.7	D48.0	D49.2
Rosenmuller's fossa	C11.2	C79.89	D00.08	D10.6	D37.05	D49.0
round ligament	C57.2-	C79.82	-	D28.2	D39.8	D49.59
S						
sacrococcyx, sacrococcygeal	C41.4	C79.51		D16.8	D48.0	D49.2
region	C76.3	C79.89	D09.8	D36.7	D48.7	D49.89
sacrouterine ligament	C57.3	C79.82	-	D28.2	D39.8	D49.59
sacrum, sacral (vertebra)	C41.4	C79.51	-	D16.8	D48.0	D49.2
salivary gland or duct (major)	C08.9	C79.89	D00.00	D11.9	D37.039	D49.0
minor NEC	C06.9	C79.89	D00.00	D10.39	D37.04	D49.0
overlapping lesion	C08.9	-	-	-	-	-
parotid	C07	C79.89	D00.00	D11.0	D37.030	D49.0
pluriglandular	C08.9	C79.89	D00.00	D11.9	D37.039	D49.0
sublingual	C08.1	C79.89	D00.00	D11.7	D37.031	D49.0
submandibular	C08.0	C79.89	D00.00	D11.7	D37.032	D49.0
submaxillary	C08.0	C79.89	D00.00	D11.7	D37.032	D49.0
salpinx (uterine)	C57.0-	C79.82	D07.39	D28.2	D39.8	D49.59
Santorini's duct	C25.3	C78.89	D01.7	D13.6	D37.8	D49.0
scalp	C44.40	C79.2	D04.4	D23.4	D48.5	D49.2
basal cell carcinoma	C44.41	-	-	-	-	-
specified type NEC	C44.49	-	-	-	-	-
squamous cell carcinoma	C44.42	-	-	-	-	-
scapula (any part)	C40.0-	C79.51	-	D16.0-	-	-
scapular region	C76.1	C79.89	D09.8	D36.7	D48.7	D49.89
scar NEC—see also Neoplasm, skin, by site	C44.90	C79.2	D04.9	D23.9	D48.5	D49.2
sciatic nerve	C47.2-	C79.89		D36.13	D48.2	D49.2
sclera	C69.4-	C79.49	D09.2-	D31.4-	D48.7	D49.89
scrotum (skin)	C63.2	C79.82	D07.61	D29.4	D40.8	D49.59
sebaceous gland—see Neoplasm, skin						

	Malignant Primary	Malignant Secondary	Ca in situ	Benign	Uncertain Behavior	Unspecified Behavior
sella turcica	C75.1	C79.89	D09.3	D35.2	D44.3	D49.7
bone	C41.0	C79.51	-	D16.4	D48.0	D49.2
semilunar cartilage (knee)	C40.2-	C79.51	-	D16.2-	D48.0	D49.2
seminal vesicle	C63.7	C79.82	D07.69	D29.8	D40.8	D49.59
septum						
nasal	C30.0	C78.39	D02.3	D14.0	D38.5	D49.1
posterior margin	C11.3	C79.89	D00.08	D10.6	D37.05	D49.0
rectovaginal	C76.3	C79.89	D09.8	D36.7	D48.7	D49.89
rectovesical	C76.3	C79.89	D09.8	D36.7	D48.7	D49.89
urethrovaginal	C57.9	C79.82	D07.30	D28.9	D39.9	D49.59
vesicovaginal	C57.9	C79.82	D07.30	D28.9	D39.9	D49.59
shoulder NEC	C76.4-	C79.89	D04.6-	D36.7	D48.7	D49.89
sigmoid flexure (lower) (upper)	C18.7	C78.5	D01.0	D12.5	D37.4	D49.0
sinus (accessory)	C31.9	C78.39	D02.3	D14.0	D38.5	D49.1
bone (any)	C41.0	C79.51	-	D16.4	D48.0	D49.2
ethmoidal	C31.1	C78.39	D02.3	D14.0	D38.5	D49.1
frontal	C31.2	C78.39	D02.3	D14.0	D38.5	D49.1
maxillary	C31.0	C78.39	D02.3	D14.0	D38.5	D49.1
nasal, paranasal NEC	C31.9	C78.39	D02.3	D14.0	D38.5	D49.1
overlapping lesion	C31.8	-	-	-	-	-
pyriform	C12	C79.89	D00.08	D10.7	D37.05	D49.0
sphenoid	C31.3	C78.39	D02.3	D14.0	D38.5	D49.1
skeleton, skeletal NEC	C41.9	C79.51	-	D16.9	D48.0	D49.2
Skene's gland	C68.1	C79.19	D09.19	D30.8	D41.8	D49.59
skin NOS	C44.90	C79.2	D04.9	D23.9	D48.5	D49.2
abdominal wall	C44.509	C79.2	D04.5	D23.5	D48.5	D49.2
basal cell carcinoma	C44.519	-	-	-	-	-
specified type NEC	C44.599	-	-	-	-	-
squamous cell carcinoma	C44.529	-	-	-	-	-
ala nasi—see also Neoplasm, nose, skin	C44.301	C79.2	D04.39	D23.39	D48.5	D49.2
ankle—see also Neoplasm, skin, limb, lower	C44.70-	C79.2	D04.7-	D23.7-	D48.5	D49.2
antecubital space—see also Neoplasm, skin, limb, upper	C44.60-	C79.2	D04.6-	D23.6-	D48.5	D49.2
anus	C44.500	C79.2	D04.5	D23.5	D48.5	D49.2
basal cell carcinoma	C44.510	-	-	-	-	-
specified type NEC	C44.590	-	-	-	-	-
squamous cell carcinoma	C44.520	-	-	-	-	-
arm—see also Neoplasm, skin, limb, upper	C44.60-	C79.2	D04.6-	D23.6-	D48.5	D49.2
auditory canal (external)—see also Neoplasm, skin, ear	C44.20-	C79.2	D04.2-	D23.2-	D48.5	D49.2
auricle (ear)—see also Neoplasm, skin, ear	C44.20-	C79.2	D04.2-	D23.2-	D48.5	D49.2
auricular canal (external)—see also Neoplasm, skin, ear	C44.20-	C79.2	D04.2-	D23.2-	D48.5	D49.2
axilla, axillary fold—see also Neoplasm, skin, trunk	C44.509	C79.2	D04.5	D23.5	D48.5	D49.2

Table of Neoplasms

	Malignant Primary	Malignant Secondary	Ca in situ	Benign	Uncertain Behavior	Unspecified Behavior
skin NOS — *continued*						
back—see also Neoplasm, skin, trunk	C44.509	C79.2	D04.5	D23.5	D48.5	D49.2
basal cell carcinoma	C44.91					
breast	C44.501	C79.2	D04.5	D23.5	D48.5	D49.2
basal cell carcinoma	C44.511	-	-	-	-	-
specified type NEC	C44.591	-	-	-	-	-
squamous cell carcinoma	C44.521	-	-	-	-	-
brow—see also Neoplasm, skin, face	C44.309	C79.2	D04.39	D23.39	D48.5	D49.2
buttock—see also Neoplasm, skin, trunk	C44.509	C79.2	D04.5	D23.5	D48.5	D49.2
calf—see also Neoplasm, skin, limb, lower	C44.70-	C79.2	D04.7-	D23.7-	D48.5	D49.2
canthus (eye) (inner) (outer)	C44.10-	C79.2	D04.1-	D23.1-	D48.5	D49.2
basal cell carcinoma	C44.11-	-	-	-	-	-
sebaceous cell	C44.13-	-	-	-	-	-
specified type NEC	C44.19-	-	-	-	-	-
squamous cell carcinoma	C44.12-	-	-	-	-	-
cervical region—see also Neoplasm, skin, neck	C44.40	C79.2	D04.4	D23.4	D48.5	D49.2
cheek (external) —see also Neoplasm, skin, face	C44.309	C79.2	D04.39	D23.39	D48.5	D49.2
chest (wall)—see also Neoplasm, skin, trunk	C44.509	C79.2	D04.5	D23.5	D48.5	D49.2
chin—see also Neoplasm, skin, face	C44.309	C79.2	D04.39	D23.39	D48.5	D49.2
clavicular area—see also Neoplasm, skin, trunk	C44.509	C79.2	D04.5	D23.5	D48.5	D49.2
clitoris	C51.2	C79.82	D07.1	D28.0	D39.8	D49.59
columnella—see also Neoplasm, skin, face	C44.309	C79.2	D04.39	D23.39	D48.5	D49.2
concha—see also Neoplasm, skin, ear	C44.20-	C79.2	D04.2-	D23.2-	D48.5	D49.2
ear (external)	C44.20-	C79.2	D04.2-	D23.2-	D48.5	D49.2
basal cell carcinoma	C44.21-	-	-	-	-	-
specified type NEC	C44.29-	-	-	-	-	-
squamous cell carcinoma	C44.22-	-	-	-	-	-
elbow—see also Neoplasm, skin, limb, upper	C44.60-	C79.2	D04.6-	D23.6-	D48.5	D49.2
eyebrow—see also Neoplasm, skin, face	C44.309	C79.2	D04.39	D23.39	D48.5	D49.2
eyelid	C44.10-	C79.2	D04.1-	D23.1-	D48.5	D49.2
basal cell carcinoma	C44.11-	-	-	-	-	-
sebaceous cell	C44.13-	-	-	-	-	-
specified type NEC	C44.19-	-	-	-	-	-
squamous cell carcinoma	C44.12-	-	-	-	-	-
face NOS	C44.300	C79.2	D04.30	D23.30	D48.5	D49.2
basal cell carcinoma	C44.310	-	-	-	-	-
specified type NEC	C44.390	-	-	-	-	-

	Malignant Primary	Malignant Secondary	Ca in situ	Benign	Uncertain Behavior	Unspecified Behavior
skin NOS, face NOS — *continued*						
squamous cell carcinoma	C44.320	-	-	-	-	-
female genital organs (external)	C51.9	C79.82	D07.1	D28.0	D39.8	D49.59
clitoris	C51.2	C79.82	D07.1	D28.0	D39.8	D49.59
labium NEC	C51.9	C79.82	D07.1	D28.0	D39.8	D49.59
majus	C51.0	C79.82	D07.1	D28.0	D39.8	D49.59
minus	C51.1	C79.82	D07.1	D28.0	D39.8	D49.59
pudendum	C51.9	C79.82	D07.1	D28.0	D39.8	D49.59
vulva	C51.9	C79.82	D07.1	D28.0	D39.8	D49.59
finger—see also Neoplasm, skin, limb, upper	C44.60-	C79.2	D04.6-	D23.6-	D48.5	D49.2
flank—see also Neoplasm, skin, trunk	C44.509	C79.2	D04.5	D23.5	D48.5	D49.2
foot—see also Neoplasm, skin, limb, lower	C44.70-	C79.2	D04.7-	D23.7-	D48.5	D49.2
forearm—see also Neoplasm, skin, limb, upper	C44.60-	C79.2	D04.6-	D23.6-	D48.5	D49.2
forehead—see also *Neoplasm, skin, face*	C44.309	C79.2	D04.39	D23.39	D48.5	D49.2
glabella—see also Neoplasm, skin, face	C44.309	C79.2	D04.39	D23.39	D48.5	D49.2
gluteal region—see also Neoplasm, skin, trunk	C44.509	C79.2	D04.5	D23.5	D48.5	D49.2
groin—see also Neoplasm, skin, trunk	C44.509	C79.2	D04.5	D23.5	D48.5	D49.2
hand—see also Neoplasm, skin, limb, upper	C44.60-	C79.2	D04.6-	D23.6-	D48.5	D49.2
head NEC—see also Neoplasm, skin, scalp	C44.40	C79.2	D04.4	D23.4	D48.5	D49.2
heel—see also Neoplasm, skin, limb, lower	C44.70-	C79.2	D04.7-	D23.7-	D48.5	D49.2
helix—see also Neoplasm, skin, ear	C44.20-	C79.2	D04.2-	D23.2-	D48.5	D49.2
hip—see also Neoplasm, skin, limb, lower	C44.70-	C79.2	D04.7-	D23.7-	D48.5	D49.2
infraclavicular region— see also Neoplasm, skin, trunk	C44.509	C79.2	D04.5	D23.5	D48.5	D49.2
inguinal region—see also Neoplasm, skin, trunk	C44.509	C79.2	D04.5	D23.5	D48.5	D49.2
jaw—see also Neoplasm, skin, face	C44.309	C79.2	D04.39	D23.39	D48.5	D49.2
Kaposi's sarcoma —see Kaposi's, sarcoma, skin						
knee—see also Neoplasm, skin, limb, lower	C44.70-	C79.2	D04.7-	D23.7-	D48.5	D49.2
labia						
majora	C51.0	C79.82	D07.1	D28.0	D39.8	D49.59
minora	C51.1	C79.82	D07.1	D28.0	D39.8	D49.59
leg—see also Neoplasm, skin, limb, lower	C44.70-	C79.2	D04.7-	D23.7-	D48.5	D49.2
lid (lower) (upper)	C44.10-	C79.2	D04.1-	D23.1-	D48.5	D49.2
basal cell carcinoma	C44.11-	-	-	-	-	-

	Malignant Primary	Malignant Secondary	Ca in situ	Benign	Uncertain Behavior	Unspecified Behavior
skin NOS, lid (lower) (upper) — *continued*						
sebaceous cell	C44.13-	-	-	-	-	-
specified type NEC	C44.19-	-	-	-	-	-
squamous cell carcinoma	C44.12-	-	-	-	-	-
limb NEC	C44.90	C79.2	D04.9	D23.9	D48.5	D49.2
basal cell carcinoma	C44.91					
lower	C44.70-	C79.2	D04.7-	D23.7-	D48.5	D49.2
basal cell carcinoma	C44.71-	-	-	-	-	-
specified type NEC	C44.79-	-	-	-	-	-
squamous cell carcinoma	C44.72-	-	-	-	-	-
upper	C44.60-	C79.2	D04.6-	D23.6-	D48.5	D49.2
basal cell carcinoma	C44.61-	-	-	-	-	-
specified type NEC	C44.69-	-	-	-	-	-
squamous cell carcinoma	C44.62-	-	-	-	-	-
lip (lower) (upper)	C44.00	C79.2	D04.0	D23.0	D48.5	D49.2
basal cell carcinoma	C44.01					
specified type NEC	C44.09	-	-	-	-	-
squamous cell carcinoma	C44.02	-	-	-	-	-
male genital organs	C63.9	C79.82	D07.60	D29.9	D40.8	D49.59
penis	C60.9	C79.82	D07.4	D29.0	D40.8	D49.59
prepuce	C60.0	C79.82	D07.4	D29.0	D40.8	D49.59
scrotum	C63.2	C79.82	D07.61	D29.4	D40.8	D49.59
mastectomy site (skin)— see also Neoplasm, skin, breast	C44.501	C79.2				
specified as breast tissue	C50.8-	C79.81	-	-	-	-
meatus, acoustic (external)—see also Neoplasm, skin, ear	C44.20-	C79.2	D04.2-	D23.2-	D48.5	D49.2
melanotic—see Melanoma						
Merkel cell—see Carcinoma, Merkel cell						
nates—see also Neoplasm, skin, trunk	C44.509	C79.2	D04.5	D23.5	D48.5	D49.2
neck	C44.40	C79.2	D04.4	D23.4	D48.5	D49.2
basal cell carcinoma	C44.41	-	-	-	-	-
specified type NEC	C44.49	-	-	-	-	-
squamous cell carcinoma	C44.42	-	-	-	-	-
nevus—see Nevus, skin						
nose (external)—see also Neoplasm, nose, skin	C44.301	C79.2	D04.39	D23.39	D48.5	D49.2
overlapping lesion	C44.80	-	-	-	-	-
basal cell carcinoma	C44.81	-	-	-	-	-
specified type NEC	C44.89	-	-	-	-	-
squamous cell carcinoma	C44.82	-	-	-	-	-
palm—see also Neoplasm, skin, limb, upper	C44.60-	C79.2	D04.6-	D23.6-	D48.5	D49.2
palpebra	C44.10-	C79.2	D04.1-	D23.1-	D48.5	D49.2
basal cell carcinoma	C44.11-	-	-	-	-	-
sebaceous cell	C44.13-	-	-	-	-	-

	Malignant Primary	Malignant Secondary	Ca in situ	Benign	Uncertain Behavior	Unspecified Behavior
skin NOS, palpebra — *continued*						
specified type NEC	C44.19-	-	-	-	-	-
squamous cell carcinoma	C44.12-	-	-	-	-	-
penis NEC	C60.9	C79.82	D07.4	D29.0	D40.8	D49.59
perianal—see also Neoplasm, skin, anus	C44.500	C79.2	D04.5	D23.5	D48.5	D49.2
perineum—see also Neoplasm, skin, anus	C44.500	C79.2	D04.5	D23.5	D48.5	D49.2
pinna—see also Neoplasm, skin, ear	C44.20-	C79.2	D04.2-	D23.2-	D48.5	D49.2
plantar—see also Neoplasm, skin, limb, lower	C44.70-	C79.2	D04.7-	D23.7-	D48.5	D49.2
popliteal fossa or space—see also Neoplasm, skin, limb, lower	C44.70-	C79.2	D04.7-	D23.7-	D48.5	D49.2
prepuce	C60.0	C79.82	D07.4	D29.0	D40.8	D49.59
pubes—see also Neoplasm, skin, trunk	C44.509	C79.2	D04.5	D23.5	D48.5	D49.2
sacrococcygeal region—see also Neoplasm, skin, trunk	C44.509	C79.2	D04.5	D23.5	D48.5	D49.2
scalp	C44.40	C79.2	D04.4	D23.4	D48.5	D49.2
basal cell carcinoma	C44.41	-	-	-	-	-
specified type NEC	C44.49	-	-	-	-	-
squamous cell carcinoma	C44.42	-	-	-	-	-
scapular region—see also Neoplasm, skin, trunk	C44.509	C79.2	D04.5	D23.5	D48.5	D49.2
scrotum	C63.2	C79.82	D07.61	D29.4	D40.8	D49.59
shoulder—see also Neoplasm, skin, limb, upper	C44.60-	C79.2	D04.6-	D23.6-	D48.5	D49.2
sole (foot)—see also Neoplasm, skin, limb, lower	C44.70-	C79.2	D04.7-	D23.7-	D48.5	D49.2
specified sites NEC	C44.80	C79.2	D04.8	D23.9	D48.5	D49.2
basal cell carcinoma	C44.81	-	-	-	-	-
specified type NEC	C44.89	-	-	-	-	-
squamous cell carcinoma	C44.82	-	-	-	-	-
specified type NEC	C44.99	-	-	-	-	-
squamous cell carcinoma	C44.92					
submammary fold—see also Neoplasm, skin, trunk	C44.509	C79.2	D04.5	D23.5	D48.5	D49.2
supraclavicular region—see also Neoplasm, skin, neck	C44.40	C79.2	D04.4	D23.4	D48.5	D49.2
temple—see also Neoplasm, skin, face	C44.309	C79.2	D04.39	D23.39	D48.5	D49.2
thigh—see also Neoplasm, skin, limb, lower	C44.70-	C79.2	D04.7-	D23.7-	D48.5	D49.2
thoracic wall—see also Neoplasm, skin, trunk	C44.509	C79.2	D04.5	D23.5	D48.5	D49.2
thumb—see also Neoplasm, skin, limb, upper	C44.60-	C79.2	D04.6-	D23.6-	D48.5	D49.2

	Malignant Primary	Malignant Secondary	Ca in situ	Benign	Uncertain Behavior	Unspecified Behavior
skin NOS — *continued*						
toe—see also Neoplasm, skin, limb, lower	C44.70-	C79.2	D04.7-	D23.7-	D48.5	D49.2
tragus—see also Neoplasm, skin, ear	C44.20-	C79.2	D04.2-	D23.2-	D48.5	D49.2
trunk	C44.509	C79.2	D04.5	D23.5	D48.5	D49.2
basal cell carcinoma	C44.519	-	-	-	-	-
specified type NEC	C44.599	-	-	-	-	-
squamous cell carcinoma	C44.529	-	-	-	-	-
umbilicus—see also Neoplasm, skin, trunk	C44.509	C79.2	D04.5	D23.5	D48.5	D49.2
vulva	C51.9	C79.82	D07.1	D28.0	D39.8	D49.59
overlapping lesion	C51.8	-	-	-	-	-
wrist—see also Neoplasm, skin, limb, upper	C44.60-	C79.2	D04.6-	D23.6-	D48.5	D49.2
skull	C41.0	C79.51	-	D16.4	D48.0	D49.2
soft parts or tissues—see Neoplasm, connective tissue						
specified site NEC	C76.8	C79.89	D09.8	D36.7	D48.7	D49.89
spermatic cord	C63.1-	C79.82	D07.69	D29.8	D40.8	D49.59
sphenoid	C31.3	C78.39	D02.3	D14.0	D38.5	D49.1
bone	C41.0	C79.51	-	D16.4	D48.0	D49.2
sinus	C31.3	C78.39	D02.3	D14.0	D38.5	D49.1
sphincter						
anal	C21.1	C78.5	D01.3	D12.9	D37.8	D49.0
of Oddi	C24.0	C78.89	D01.5	D13.5	D37.6	D49.0
spine, spinal (column)	C41.2	C79.51	-	D16.6	D48.0	D49.2
bulb	C71.7	C79.31	-	D33.1	D43.1	D49.6
coccyx	C41.4	C79.51	-	D16.8	D48.0	D49.2
cord (cervical) (lumbar) (sacral) (thoracic)	C72.0	C79.49	-	D33.4	D43.4	D49.7
dura mater	C70.1	C79.49	-	D32.1	D42.1	D49.7
lumbosacral	C41.2	C79.51	-	D16.6	D48.0	D49.2
marrow NEC	C96.9	C79.52	-	-	D47.9	D49.89
membrane	C70.1	C79.49	-	D32.1	D42.1	D49.7
meninges	C70.1	C79.49	-	D32.1	D42.1	D49.7
nerve (root)	C47.9	C79.89	-	D36.10	D48.2	D49.2
pia mater	C70.1	C79.49	-	D32.1	D42.1	D49.7
root	C47.9	C79.89	-	D36.10	D48.2	D49.2
sacrum	C41.4	C79.51	-	D16.8	D48.0	D49.2
spleen, splenic NEC	C26.1	C78.89	D01.7	D13.99	D37.8	D49.0
flexure (colon)	C18.5	C78.5	D01.0	D12.3	D37.4	D49.0
stem, brain	C71.7	C79.31	-	D33.1	D43.1	D49.6
Stensen's duct	C07	C79.89	D00.00	D11.0	D37.030	D49.0
sternum	C41.3	C79.51	-	D16.7	D48.0	D49.2
stomach	C16.9	C78.89	D00.2	D13.1	D37.1	D49.0
antrum (pyloric)	C16.3	C78.89	D00.2	D13.1	D37.1	D49.0
body	C16.2	C78.89	D00.2	D13.1	D37.1	D49.0
cardia	C16.0	C78.89	D00.2	D13.1	D37.1	D49.0
cardiac orifice	C16.0	C78.89	D00.2	D13.1	D37.1	D49.0
corpus	C16.2	C78.89	D00.2	D13.1	D37.1	D49.0
fundus	C16.1	C78.89	D00.2	D13.1	D37.1	D49.0

	Malignant Primary	Malignant Secondary	Ca in situ	Benign	Uncertain Behavior	Unspecified Behavior
stomach — *continued*						
greater curvature NEC	C16.6	C78.89	D00.2	D13.1	D37.1	D49.0
lesser curvature NEC	C16.5	C78.89	D00.2	D13.1	D37.1	D49.0
overlapping lesion	C16.8	-	-	-	-	-
prepylorus	C16.4	C78.89	D00.2	D13.1	D37.1	D49.0
pylorus	C16.4	C78.89	D00.2	D13.1	D37.1	D49.0
wall NEC	C16.9	C78.89	D00.2	D13.1	D37.1	D49.0
anterior NEC	C16.8	C78.89	D00.2	D13.1	D37.1	D49.0
posterior NEC	C16.8	C78.89	D00.2	D13.1	D37.1	D49.0
stroma, endometrial	C54.1	C79.82	D07.0	D26.1	D39.0	D49.59
stump, cervical	C53.8	C79.82	D06.7	D26.0	D39.0	D49.59
subcutaneous (nodule) (tissue) NEC—see Neoplasm, connective tissue						
subdural	C70.9	C79.32	-	D32.9	D42.9	D49.7
subglottis, subglottic	C32.2	C78.39	D02.0	D14.1	D38.0	D49.1
sublingual	C04.9	C79.89	D00.06	D10.2	D37.09	D49.0
gland or duct	C08.1	C79.89	D00.00	D11.7	D37.031	D49.0
submandibular gland	C08.0	C79.89	D00.00	D11.7	D37.032	D49.0
submaxillary gland or duct	C08.0	C79.89	D00.00	D11.7	D37.032	D49.0
submental	C76.0	C79.89	D09.8	D36.7	D48.7	D49.89
subpleural	C34.9-	C78.0-	D02.2-	D14.3-	D38.1	D49.1
substernal	C38.1	C78.1	-	D15.2	D38.3	D49.89
sudoriferous, sudoriparous gland, site unspecified	C44.90	C79.2	D04.9	D23.9	D48.5	D49.2
specified site—see Neoplasm, skin						
supraclavicular region	C76.0	C79.89	D09.8	D36.7	D48.7	D49.89
supraglottis	C32.1	C78.39	D02.0	D14.1	D38.0	D49.1
suprarenal	C74.9-	C79.7-	D09.3	D35.0-	D44.1-	D49.7
capsule	C74.9-	C79.7-	D09.3	D35.0-	D44.1-	D49.7
cortex	C74.0-	C79.7-	D09.3	D35.0-	D44.1-	D49.7
gland	C74.9-	C79.7-	D09.3	D35.0-	D44.1-	D49.7
medulla	C74.1-	C79.7-	D09.3	D35.0-	D44.1-	D49.7
suprasellar (region)	C71.9	C79.31	-	D33.2	D43.2	D49.6
supratentorial (brain) NEC	C71.0	C79.31	-	D33.0	D43.0	D49.6
sweat gland (apocrine) (eccrine), site unspecified	C44.90	C79.2	D04.9	D23.9	D48.5	D49.2
specified site—see Neoplasm, skin						
sympathetic nerve or nervous system NEC	C47.9	C79.89	-	D36.10	D48.2	D49.2
symphysis pubis	C41.4	C79.51	-	D16.8	D48.0	D49.2
synovial membrane—see Neoplasm, connective tissue						
T						
tapetum, brain	C71.8	C79.31	-	D33.2	D43.2	D49.6
tarsus (any bone)	C40.3-	C79.51	-	D16.3-	-	-
temple (skin)—see also Neoplasm, skin, face	C44.309	C79.2	D04.39	D23.39	D48.5	D49.2
temporal						
bone	C41.0	C79.51	-	D16.4	D48.0	D49.2

	Malignant Primary	Malignant Secondary	Ca in situ	Benign	Uncertain Behavior	Unspecified Behavior
temporal — *continued*						
lobe or pole	C71.2	C79.31	-	D33.0	D43.0	D49.6
region	C76.0	C79.89	D09.8	D36.7	D48.7	D49.89
skin—see also Neoplasm, skin, face	C44.309	C79.2	D04.39	D23.39	D48.5	D49.2
tendon (sheath)—see Neoplasm, connective tissue						
tentorium (cerebelli)	C70.0	C79.32	-	D32.0	D42.0	D49.7
testis, testes	C62.9-	C79.82	D07.69	D29.2-	D40.1-	D49.59
descended	C62.1-	C79.82	D07.69	D29.2-	D40.1-	D49.59
ectopic	C62.0-	C79.82	D07.69	D29.2-	D40.1-	D49.59
retained	C62.0-	C79.82	D07.69	D29.2-	D40.1-	D49.59
scrotal	C62.1-	C79.82	D07.69	D29.2-	D40.1-	D49.59
undescended	C62.0-	C79.82	D07.69	D29.2-	D40.1-	D49.59
unspecified whether descended or undescended	C62.9-	C79.82	D07.69	D29.2-	D40.1-	D49.59
thalamus	C71.0	C79.31	-	D33.0	D43.0	D49.6
thigh NEC	C76.5-	C79.89	D04.7-	D36.7	D48.7	D49.89
thorax, thoracic (cavity) (organs NEC)	C76.1	C79.89	D09.8	D36.7	D48.7	D49.89
duct	C49.3	C79.89	-	D21.3	D48.1	D49.2
wall NEC	C76.1	C79.89	D09.8	D36.7	D48.7	D49.89
throat	C14.0	C79.89	D00.08	D10.9	D37.05	D49.0
thumb NEC	C76.4-	C79.89	D04.6-	D36.7	D48.7	D49.89
thymus (gland)	C37	C79.89	D09.3	D15.0	D38.4	D49.89
thyroglossal duct	C73	C79.89	D09.3	D34	D44.0	D49.7
thyroid (gland)	C73	C79.89	D09.3	D34	D44.0	D49.7
cartilage	C32.3	C78.39	D02.0	D14.1	D38.0	D49.1
tibia (any part)	C40.2-	C79.51	-	D16.2-	-	-
toe NEC	C76.5-	C79.89	D04.7-	D36.7	D48.7	D49.89
tongue	C02.9	C79.89	D00.07	D10.1	D37.02	D49.0
anterior (two-thirds) NEC	C02.3	C79.89	D00.07	D10.1	D37.02	D49.0
dorsal surface	C02.0	C79.89	D00.07	D10.1	D37.02	D49.0
ventral surface	C02.2	C79.89	D00.07	D10.1	D37.02	D49.0
base (dorsal surface)	C01	C79.89	D00.07	D10.1	D37.02	D49.0
border (lateral)	C02.1	C79.89	D00.07	D10.1	D37.02	D49.0
dorsal surface NEC	C02.0	C79.89	D00.07	D10.1	D37.02	D49.0
fixed part NEC	C01	C79.89	D00.07	D10.1	D37.02	D49.0
foreamen cecum	C02.0	C79.89	D00.07	D10.1	D37.02	D49.0
frenulum linguae	C02.2	C79.89	D00.07	D10.1	D37.02	D49.0
junctional zone	C02.8	C79.89	D00.07	D10.1	D37.02	D49.0
margin (lateral)	C02.1	C79.89	D00.07	D10.1	D37.02	D49.0
midline NEC	C02.0	C79.89	D00.07	D10.1	D37.02	D49.0
mobile part NEC	C02.3	C79.89	D00.07	D10.1	D37.02	D49.0
overlapping lesion	C02.8	-	-	-	-	-
posterior (third)	C01	C79.89	D00.07	D10.1	D37.02	D49.0
root	C01	C79.89	D00.07	D10.1	D37.02	D49.0
surface (dorsal)	C02.0	C79.89	D00.07	D10.1	D37.02	D49.0
base	C01	C79.89	D00.07	D10.1	D37.02	D49.0
ventral	C02.2	C79.89	D00.07	D10.1	D37.02	D49.0
tip	C02.1	C79.89	D00.07	D10.1	D37.02	D49.0
tonsil	C02.4	C79.89	D00.07	D10.1	D37.02	D49.0

	Malignant Primary	Malignant Secondary	Ca in situ	Benign	Uncertain Behavior	Unspecified Behavior
tonsil	C09.9	C79.89	D00.08	D10.4	D37.05	D49.0
fauces, faucial	C09.9	C79.89	D00.08	D10.4	D37.05	D49.0
lingual	C02.4	C79.89	D00.07	D10.1	D37.02	D49.0
overlapping sites	C09.8	-	-	-	-	-
palatine	C09.9	C79.89	D00.08	D10.4	D37.05	D49.0
pharyngeal	C11.1	C79.89	D00.08	D10.6	D37.05	D49.0
pillar (anterior) (posterior)	C09.1	C79.89	D00.08	D10.5	D37.05	D49.0
tonsillar fossa	C09.0	C79.89	D00.08	D10.5	D37.05	D49.0
tooth socket NEC	C03.9	C79.89	D00.03	D10.39	D37.09	D49.0
trachea (cartilage) (mucosa)	C33	C78.39	D02.1	D14.2	D38.1	D49.1
overlapping lesion with bronchus or lung	C34.8-	-	-	-	-	-
tracheobronchial	C34.8-	C78.39	D02.1	D14.2	D38.1	D49.1
overlapping lesion with lung	C34.8-	-	-	-	-	-
tragus—see also Neoplasm, skin, ear	C44.20-	C79.2	D04.2-	D23.2-	D48.5	D49.2
trunk NEC	C76.8	C79.89	D04.5	D36.7	D48.7	D49.89
tubo-ovarian	C57.8	C79.82	D07.39	D28.7	D39.8	D49.59
tunica vaginalis	C63.7	C79.82	D07.69	D29.8	D40.8	D49.59
turbinate (bone)	C41.0	C79.51	-	D16.4	D48.0	D49.2
nasal	C30.0	C78.39	D02.3	D14.0	D38.5	D49.1
tympanic cavity	C30.1	C78.39	D02.3	D14.0	D38.5	D49.1
U						
ulna (any part)	C40.0-	C79.51	-	D16.0-	-	-
umbilicus, umbilical—see also Neoplasm, skin, trunk	C44.509	C79.2	D04.5	D23.5	D48.5	D49.2
uncus, brain	C71.2	C79.31	-	D33.0	D43.0	D49.6
unknown site or unspecified	C80.1	C79.9	D09.9	D36.9	D48.9	D49.9
urachus	C67.7	C79.11	D09.0	D30.3	D41.4	D49.4
ureter, ureteral	C66.-	C79.19	D09.19	D30.2-	D41.2-	D49.59
orifice (bladder)	C67.6	C79.11	D09.0	D30.3	D41.4	D49.4
ureter-bladder (junction)	C67.6	C79.11	D09.0	D30.3	D41.4	D49.4
urethra, urethral (gland)	C68.0	C79.19	D09.19	D30.4	D41.3	D49.59
orifice, internal	C67.5	C79.11	D09.0	D30.3	D41.4	D49.4
urethrovaginal (septum)	C57.9	C79.82	D07.30	D28.9	D39.8	D49.59
urinary organ or system	C68.9	C79.10	D09.10	D30.9	D41.9	D49.59
bladder—see Neoplasm, bladder						
overlapping lesion	C68.8	-	-	-	-	-
specified sites NEC	C68.8	C79.19	D09.19	D30.8	D41.8	D49.59
utero-ovarian	C57.8	C79.82	D07.39	D28.7	D39.8	D49.59
ligament	C57.1	C79.82	D07.39	D28.2	D39.8	D49.59
uterosacral ligament	C57.3	C79.82	-	D28.2	D39.8	D49.59
uterus, uteri, uterine	C55	C79.82	D07.0	D26.9	D39.0	D49.59
adnexa NEC	C57.4	C79.82	D07.39	D28.7	D39.8	D49.59
body	C54.9	C79.82	D07.0	D26.1	D39.0	D49.59
cervix	C53.9	C79.82	D06.9	D26.0	D39.0	D49.59
cornu	C54.9	C79.82	D07.0	D26.1	D39.0	D49.59
corpus	C54.9	C79.82	D07.0	D26.1	D39.0	D49.59
endocervix (canal) (gland)	C53.0	C79.82	D06.0	D26.0	D39.0	D49.59
endometrium	C54.1	C79.82	D07.0	D26.1	D39.0	D49.59
exocervix	C53.1	C79.82	D06.1	D26.0	D39.0	D49.59

Table of Neoplasms

	Malignant Primary	Malignant Secondary	Ca in situ	Benign	Uncertain Behavior	Unspecified Behavior
uterus, uteri, uterine — *continued*						
external os	C53.1	C79.82	D06.1	D26.0	D39.0	D49.59
fundus	C54.3	C79.82	D07.0	D26.1	D39.0	D49.59
internal os	C53.0	C79.82	D06.0	D26.0	D39.0	D49.59
isthmus	C54.0	C79.82	D07.0	D26.1	D39.0	D49.59
ligament	C57.3	C79.82	-	D28.2	D39.8	D49.59
broad	C57.1	C79.82	D07.39	D28.2	D39.8	D49.59
round	C57.2	C79.82	-	D28.2	D39.8	D49.59
lower segment	C54.0	C79.82	D07.0	D26.1	D39.0	D49.59
myometrium	C54.2	C79.82	D07.0	D26.1	D39.0	D49.59
overlapping sites	C54.8	-	-	-	-	-
squamocolumnar junction	C53.8	C79.82	D06.7	D26.0	D39.0	D49.59
tube	C57.0-	C79.82	D07.39	D28.2	D39.8	D49.59
utricle, prostatic	C68.0	C79.19	D09.19	D30.4	D41.3	D49.59
uveal tract	C69.4-	C79.49	D09.2-	D31.4-	D48.7	D49.89
uvula	C05.2	C79.89	D00.04	D10.39	D37.09	D49.0
V						
vagina, vaginal (fornix) (vault) (wall)	C52	C79.82	D07.2	D28.1	D39.8	D49.59
vaginovesical	C57.9	C79.82	D07.30	D28.9	D39.9	D49.59
septum	C57.9	C79.82	D07.30	D28.9	D39.9	D49.59
vallecula (epiglottis)	C10.0	C79.89	D00.08	D10.5	D37.05	D49.0
vas deferens	C63.1-	C79.82	D07.69	D29.8	D40.8	D49.59
vascular—see Neoplasm, connective tissue						
Vater's ampulla	C24.1	C78.89	D01.5	D13.5	D37.6	D49.0
vein, venous—see Neoplasm, connective tissue						
vena cava (abdominal) (inferior)	C49.4	C79.89	-	D21.4	D48.1	D49.2
superior	C49.3	C79.89	-	D21.3	D48.1	D49.2
ventricle (cerebral) (floor) (lateral) (third)	C71.5	C79.31	-	D33.0	D43.0	D49.6
cardiac (left) (right)	C38.0	C79.89	-	D15.1	D48.7	D49.89
fourth	C71.7	C79.31	-	D33.1	D43.1	D49.6
ventricular band of larynx	C32.1	C78.39	D02.0	D14.1	D38.0	D49.1
ventriculus—see Neoplasm, stomach						
vermillion border—see Neoplasm, lip						
vermis, cerebellum	C71.6	C79.31	-	D33.1	D43.1	D49.6
vertebra (column)	C41.2	C79.51	-	D16.6	D48.0	D49.2
coccyx	C41.4	C79.51	-	D16.8	D48.0	D49.2
marrow NEC	C96.9	C79.52	-	-	D47.9	D49.89
sacrum	C41.4	C79.51	-	D16.8	D48.0	D49.2
vesical—see Neoplasm, bladder						
vesicle, seminal	C63.7	C79.82	D07.69	D29.8	D40.8	D49.59
vesicocervical tissue	C57.9	C79.82	D07.30	D28.9	D39.9	D49.59
vesicorectal	C76.3	C79.82	D09.8	D36.7	D48.7	D49.89
vesicovaginal	C57.9	C79.82	D07.30	D28.9	D39.9	D49.59
septum	C57.9	C79.82	D07.30	D28.9	D39.8	D49.59
vessel (blood)—see Neoplasm, connective tissue						
vestibular gland, greater	C51.0	C79.82	D07.1	D28.0	D39.8	D49.59
vestibule						
mouth	C06.1	C79.89	D00.00	D10.39	D37.09	D49.0
nose	C30.0	C78.39	D02.3	D14.0	D38.5	D49.1
Virchow's gland	C77.0	C77.0	-	D36.0	D48.7	D49.89
viscera NEC	C76.8	C79.89	D09.8	D36.7	D48.7	D49.89
vocal cords (true)	C32.0	C78.39	D02.0	D14.1	D38.0	D49.1
false	C32.1	C78.39	D02.0	D14.1	D38.0	D49.1
vomer	C41.0	C79.51	-	D16.4	D48.0	D49.2
vulva	C51.9	C79.82	D07.1	D28.0	D39.8	D49.59
vulvovaginal gland	C51.0	C79.82	D07.1	D28.0	D39.8	D49.59
W						
Waldeyer's ring	C14.2	C79.89	D00.08	D10.9	D37.05	D49.0
Wharton's duct	C08.0	C79.89	D00.00	D11.7	D37.032	D49.0
white matter (central) (cerebral)	C71.0	C79.31	-	D33.0	D43.0	D49.6
windpipe	C33	C78.39	D02.1	D14.2	D38.1	D49.1
Wirsung's duct	C25.3	C78.89	D01.7	D13.6	D37.8	D49.0
wolffian (body) (duct)						
female	C57.7	C79.82	D07.39	D28.7	D39.8	D49.59
male	C63.7	C79.82	D07.69	D29.8	D40.8	D49.59
womb—see Neoplasm, uterus						
wrist NEC	C76.4-	C79.89	D04.6-	D36.7	D48.7	D49.89
X						
xiphoid process	C41.3	C79.51	-	D16.7	D48.0	D49.2
Z						
Zuckerkandl organ	C75.5	C79.89	-	D35.6	D44.7	D49.7

Table of Drugs and Chemicals

Substance	Poisoning, Accidental (unintentional)	Poisoning, Intentional self-harm	Poisoning, Assault	Poisoning, Undetermined	Adverse effect	Underdosing
1-propanol	T51.3X1	T51.3X2	T51.3X3	T51.3X4	—	—
2-propanol	T51.2X1	T51.2X2	T51.2X3	T51.2X4	—	—
2,4-D (dichlorophen-oxyacetic acid)	T60.3X1	T60.3X2	T60.3X3	T60.3X4	—	—
2,4-toluene diisocyanate	T65.0X1	T65.0X2	T65.0X3	T65.0X4	—	—
2,4,5-T (trichloro-phenoxyacetic acid)	T60.1X1	T60.1X2	T60.1X3	T60.1X4	—	—
3,4-methylenedioxy-methamphetamine	T43.641	T43.642	T43.643	T43.644	—	—
14-hydroxydihydro-morphinone	T40.2X1	T40.2X2	T40.2X3	T40.2X4	T40.2X5	T40.2X6
A						
ABOB	T37.5X1	T37.5X2	T37.5X3	T37.5X4	T37.5X5	T37.5X6
Abrine	T62.2X1	T62.2X2	T62.2X3	T62.2X4	—	—
Abrus (seed)	T62.2X1	T62.2X2	T62.2X3	T62.2X4	—	—
Absinthe	T51.0X1	T51.0X2	T51.0X3	T51.0X4	—	—
beverage	T51.0X1	T51.0X2	T51.0X3	T51.0X4	—	—
Acaricide	T60.8X1	T60.8X2	T60.8X3	T60.8X4	—	—
Acebutolol	T44.7X1	T44.7X2	T44.7X3	T44.7X4	T44.7X5	T44.7X6
Acecarbromal	T42.6X1	T42.6X2	T42.6X3	T42.6X4	T42.6X5	T42.6X6
Aceclidine	T44.1X1	T44.1X2	T44.1X3	T44.1X4	T44.1X5	T44.1X6
Acedapsone	T37.0X1	T37.0X2	T37.0X3	T37.0X4	T37.0X5	T37.0X6
Acefylline piperazine	T48.6X1	T48.6X2	T48.6X3	T48.6X4	T48.6X5	T48.6X6
Acemorphan	T40.2X1	T40.2X2	T40.2X3	T40.2X4	T40.2X5	T40.2X6
Acenocoumarin	T45.511	T45.512	T45.513	T45.514	T45.515	T45.516
Acenocoumarol	T45.511	T45.512	T45.513	T45.514	T45.515	T45.516
Acepifylline	T48.6X1	T48.6X2	T48.6X3	T48.6X4	T48.6X5	T48.6X6
Acepromazine	T43.3X1	T43.3X2	T43.3X3	T43.3X4	T43.3X5	T43.3X6
Acesulfamethoxy-pyridazine	T37.0X1	T37.0X2	T37.0X3	T37.0X4	T37.0X5	T37.0X6
Acetal	T52.8X1	T52.8X2	T52.8X3	T52.8X4	—	—
Acetaldehyde (vapor)	T52.8X1	T52.8X2	T52.8X3	T52.8X4	—	—
liquid	T65.891	T65.892	T65.893	T65.894	—	—
P-Acetamidophenol	T39.1X1	T39.1X2	T39.1X3	T39.1X4	T39.1X5	T39.1X6
Acetaminophen	T39.1X1	T39.1X2	T39.1X3	T39.1X4	T39.1X5	T39.1X6
Acetaminosalol	T39.1X1	T39.1X2	T39.1X3	T39.1X4	T39.1X5	T39.1X6
Acetanilide	T39.1X1	T39.1X2	T39.1X3	T39.1X4	T39.1X5	T39.1X6
Acetarsol	T37.3X1	T37.3X2	T37.3X3	T37.3X4	T37.3X5	T37.3X6
Acetazolamide	T50.2X1	T50.2X2	T50.2X3	T50.2X4	T50.2X5	T50.2X6
Acetiamine	T45.2X1	T45.2X2	T45.2X3	T45.2X4	T45.2X5	T45.2X6
Acetic						
acid	T54.2X1	T54.2X2	T54.2X3	T54.2X4	—	—
with sodium acetate (ointment)	T49.3X1	T49.3X2	T49.3X3	T49.3X4	T49.3X5	T49.3X6
ester (solvent) (vapor)	T52.8X1	T52.8X2	T52.8X3	T52.8X4	—	—
irrigating solution	T50.3X1	T50.3X2	T50.3X3	T50.3X4	T50.3X5	T50.3X6
medicinal (lotion)	T49.2X1	T49.2X2	T49.2X3	T49.2X4	T49.2X5	T49.2X6
anhydride	T65.891	T65.892	T65.893	T65.894	—	—
ether (vapor)	T52.8X1	T52.8X2	T52.8X3	T52.8X4	—	—

Substance	Poisoning, Accidental (unintentional)	Poisoning, Intentional self-harm	Poisoning, Assault	Poisoning, Undetermined	Adverse effect	Underdosing
Acetohexamide	T38.3X1	T38.3X2	T38.3X3	T38.3X4	T38.3X5	T38.3X6
Acetohydroxamic acid	T50.991	T50.992	T50.993	T50.994	T50.995	T50.996
Acetomenaphthone	T45.7X1	T45.7X2	T45.7X3	T45.7X4	T45.7X5	T45.7X6
Acetomorphine	T40.1X1	T40.1X2	T40.1X3	T40.1X4	—	—
Acetone (oils)	T52.4X1	T52.4X2	T52.4X3	T52.4X4	—	—
chlorinated	T52.4X1	T52.4X2	T52.4X3	T52.4X4	—	—
vapor	T52.4X1	T52.4X2	T52.4X3	T52.4X4	—	—
Acetonitrile	T52.8X1	T52.8X2	T52.8X3	T52.8X4	—	—
Acetophenazine	T43.3X1	T43.3X2	T43.3X3	T43.3X4	T43.3X5	T43.3X6
Acetophenetedin	T39.1X1	T39.1X2	T39.1X3	T39.1X4	T39.1X5	T39.1X6
Acetophenone	T52.4X1	T52.4X2	T52.4X3	T52.4X4	—	—
Acetorphine	T40.2X1	T40.2X2	T40.2X3	T40.2X4	—	—
Acetosulfone (sodium)	T37.1X1	T37.1X2	T37.1X3	T37.1X4	T37.1X5	T37.1X6
Acetrizoate (sodium)	T50.8X1	T50.8X2	T50.8X3	T50.8X4	T50.8X5	T50.8X6
Acetrizoic acid	T50.8X1	T50.8X2	T50.8X3	T50.8X4	T50.8X5	T50.8X6
Acetyl						
bromide	T53.6X1	T53.6X2	T53.6X3	T53.6X4	—	—
chloride	T53.6X1	T53.6X2	T53.6X3	T53.6X4	—	—
Acetylcarbromal	T42.6X1	T42.6X2	T42.6X3	T42.6X4	T42.6X5	T42.6X6
Acetylcholine						
chloride	T44.1X1	T44.1X2	T44.1X3	T44.1X4	T44.1X5	T44.1X6
derivative	T44.1X1	T44.1X2	T44.1X3	T44.1X4	T44.1X5	T44.1X6
Acetylcysteine	T48.4X1	T48.4X2	T48.4X3	T48.4X4	T48.4X5	T48.4X6
Acetyldigitoxin	T46.0X1	T46.0X2	T46.0X3	T46.0X4	T46.0X5	T46.0X6
Acetyldigoxin	T46.0X1	T46.0X2	T46.0X3	T46.0X4	T46.0X5	T46.0X6
Acetyldihydrocodeine	T40.2X1	T40.2X2	T40.2X3	T40.2X4	—	—
Acetyldihydroco-deinone	T40.2X1	T40.2X2	T40.2X3	T40.2X4	—	—
Acetylene (gas)	T59.891	T59.892	T59.893	T59.894		
dichloride	T53.6X1	T53.6X2	T53.6X3	T53.6X4	—	—
incomplete combustion of	T58.11	T58.12	T58.13	T58.14		
industrial	T59.891	T59.892	T59.893	T59.894		
tetrachloride	T53.6X1	T53.6X2	T53.6X3	T53.6X4	—	—
vapor	T53.6X1	T53.6X2	T53.6X3	T53.6X4	—	—
Acetylpheneturide	T42.6X1	T42.6X2	T42.6X3	T42.6X4	T42.6X5	T42.6X6
Acetylphenylhydra-zine	T39.8X1	T39.8X2	T39.8X3	T39.8X4	T39.8X5	T39.8X6
Acetylsalicylic acid (salts)	T39.011	T39.012	T39.013	T39.014	T39.015	T39.016
enteric coated	T39.011	T39.012	T39.013	T39.014	T39.015	T39.016
Acetylsulfamethoxy-pyridazine	T37.0X1	T37.0X2	T37.0X3	T37.0X4	T37.0X5	T37.0X6
Achromycin	T36.4X1	T36.4X2	T36.4X3	T36.4X4	T36.4X5	T36.4X6
ophthalmic preparation	T49.5X1	T49.5X2	T49.5X3	T49.5X4	T49.5X5	T49.5X6
topical NEC	T49.0X1	T49.0X2	T49.0X3	T49.0X4	T49.0X5	T49.0X6
Aciclovir	T37.5X1	T37.5X2	T37.5X3	T37.5X4	T37.5X5	T37.5X6
Acid (corrosive) NEC	T54.2X1	T54.2X2	T54.2X3	T54.2X4	—	—
Acidifying agent NEC	T50.901	T50.902	T50.903	T50.904	T50.905	T50.906

Substance	Poisoning, Accidental (unintentional)	Poisoning, Intentional self-harm	Poisoning, Assault	Poisoning, Undetermined	Adverse effect	Underdosing
Acipimox	T46.6X1	T46.6X2	T46.6X3	T46.6X4	T46.6X5	T46.6X6
Acitretin	T50.991	T50.992	T50.993	T50.994	T50.995	T50.996
Aclarubicin	T45.1X1	T45.1X2	T45.1X3	T45.1X4	T45.1X5	T45.1X6
Aclatonium napadisilate	T48.1X1	T48.1X2	T48.1X3	T48.1X4	T48.1X5	T48.1X6
Aconite (wild)	T46.991	T46.992	T46.993	T46.994	T46.995	T46.996
Aconitine	T46.991	T46.992	T46.993	T46.994	T46.995	T46.996
Aconitum ferox	T46.991	T46.992	T46.993	T46.994	T46.995	T46.996
Acridine	T65.6X1	T65.6X2	T65.6X3	T65.6X4	—	—
vapor	T59.891	T59.892	T59.893	T59.894	—	—
Acriflavine	T37.91	T37.92	T37.93	T37.94	T37.95	T37.96
Acriflavinium chloride	T49.0X1	T49.0X2	T49.0X3	T49.0X4	T49.0X5	T49.0X6
Acrinol	T49.0X1	T49.0X2	T49.0X3	T49.0X4	T49.0X5	T49.0X6
Acrisorcin	T49.0X1	T49.0X2	T49.0X3	T49.0X4	T49.0X5	T49.0X6
Acrivastine	T45.0X1	T45.0X2	T45.0X3	T45.0X4	T45.0X5	T45.0X6
Acrolein (gas)	T59.891	T59.892	T59.893	T59.894	—	—
liquid	T54.1X1	T54.1X2	T54.1X3	T54.1X4	—	—
Acrylamide	T65.891	T65.892	T65.893	T65.894	—	—
Acrylic resin	T49.3X1	T49.3X2	T49.3X3	T49.3X4	T49.3X5	T49.3X6
Acrylonitrile	T65.891	T65.892	T65.893	T65.894	—	—
Actaea spicata	T62.2X1	T62.2X2	T62.2X3	T62.2X4	—	—
berry	T62.1X1	T62.1X2	T62.1X3	T62.1X4	—	—
Acterol	T37.3X1	T37.3X2	T37.3X3	T37.3X4	T37.3X5	T37.3X6
ACTH	T38.811	T38.812	T38.813	T38.814	T38.815	T38.816
Actinomycin C	T45.1X1	T45.1X2	T45.1X3	T45.1X4	T45.1X5	T45.1X6
Actinomycin D	T45.1X1	T45.1X2	T45.1X3	T45.1X4	T45.1X5	T45.1X6
Activated charcoal—see also Charcoal, medicinal	T47.6X1	T47.6X2	T47.6X3	T47.6X4	T47.6X5	T47.6X6
Acyclovir	T37.5X1	T37.5X2	T37.5X3	T37.5X4	T37.5X5	T37.5X6
Adenine	T45.2X1	T45.2X2	T45.2X3	T45.2X4	T45.2X5	T45.2X6
arabinoside	T37.5X1	T37.5X2	T37.5X3	T37.5X4	T37.5X5	T37.5X6
Adenosine (phosphate)	T46.2X1	T46.2X2	T46.2X3	T46.2X4	T46.2X5	T46.2X6
ADH	T38.891	T38.892	T38.893	T38.894	T38.895	T38.896
Adhesive NEC	T65.891	T65.892	T65.893	T65.894	—	—
Adicillin	T36.0X1	T36.0X2	T36.0X3	T36.0X4	T36.0X5	T36.0X6
Adiphenine	T44.3X1	T44.3X2	T44.3X3	T44.3X4	T44.3X5	T44.3X6
Adipiodone	T50.8X1	T50.8X2	T50.8X3	T50.8X4	T50.8X5	T50.8X6
Adjunct, pharmaceutical	T50.901	T50.902	T50.903	T50.904	T50.905	T50.906
Adrenal (extract, cortex or medulla) (glucocorticoids) (hormones) (mineralocorticoids)	T38.0X1	T38.0X2	T38.0X3	T38.0X4	T38.0X5	T38.0X6
ENT agent	T49.6X1	T49.6X2	T49.6X3	T49.6X4	T49.6X5	T49.6X6
ophthalmic preparation	T49.5X1	T49.5X2	T49.5X3	T49.5X4	T49.5X5	T49.5X6
topical NEC	T49.0X1	T49.0X2	T49.0X3	T49.0X4	T49.0X5	T49.0X6
Adrenaline	T44.5X1	T44.5X2	T44.5X3	T44.5X4	T44.5X5	T44.5X6
Adrenalin—see Adrenaline						
Adrenergic NEC	T44.901	T44.902	T44.903	T44.904	T44.905	T44.906
blocking agent NEC	T44.8X1	T44.8X2	T44.8X3	T44.8X4	T44.8X5	T44.8X6
beta, heart	T44.7X1	T44.7X2	T44.7X3	T44.7X4	T44.7X5	T44.7X6
specified NEC	T44.991	T44.992	T44.993	T44.994	T44.995	T44.996

Substance	Poisoning, Accidental (unintentional)	Poisoning, Intentional self-harm	Poisoning, Assault	Poisoning, Undetermined	Adverse effect	Underdosing
Adrenochrome						
(mono) semicarbazone	T46.991	T46.992	T46.993	T46.994	T46.995	T46.996
derivative	T46.991	T46.992	T46.993	T46.994	T46.995	T46.996
Adrenocorticotrophic hormone	T38.811	T38.812	T38.813	T38.814	T38.815	T38.816
Adrenocorticotro-phin	T38.811	T38.812	T38.813	T38.814	T38.815	T38.816
Adriamycin	T45.1X1	T45.1X2	T45.1X3	T45.1X4	T45.1X5	T45.1X6
Aerosol spray NEC	T65.91	T65.92	T65.93	T65.94	—	—
Aerosporin	T36.8X1	T36.8X2	T36.8X3	T36.8X4	T36.8X5	T36.8X6
ENT agent	T49.6X1	T49.6X2	T49.6X3	T49.6X4	T49.6X5	T49.6X6
ophthalmic preparation	T49.5X1	T49.5X2	T49.5X3	T49.5X4	T49.5X5	T49.5X6
topical NEC	T49.0X1	T49.0X2	T49.0X3	T49.0X4	T49.0X5	T49.0X6
Aethusa cynapium	T62.2X1	T62.2X2	T62.2X3	T62.2X4	—	—
Afghanistan black	T40.711	T40.712	T40.713	T40.714	T40.715	T40.716
Aflatoxin	T64.01	T64.02	T64.03	T64.04	—	—
Afloqualone	T42.8X1	T42.8X2	T42.8X3	T42.8X4	T42.8X5	T42.8X6
African boxwood	T62.2X1	T62.2X2	T62.2X3	T62.2X4	—	—
Agar	T47.4X1	T47.4X2	T47.4X3	T47.4X4	T47.4X5	T47.4X6
Agonist						
predominantly						
alpha-adrenoreceptor	T44.4X1	T44.4X2	T44.4X3	T44.4X4	T44.4X5	T44.4X6
beta-adrenoreceptor	T44.5X1	T44.5X2	T44.5X3	T44.5X4	T44.5X5	T44.5X6
Agricultural agent NEC	T65.91	T65.92	T65.93	T65.94	—	—
Agrypnal	T42.3X1	T42.3X2	T42.3X3	T42.3X4	T42.3X5	T42.3X6
AHLG	T50.Z11	T50.Z12	T50.Z13	T50.Z14	T50.Z15	T50.Z16
Air contaminant (s), source/type NOS	T65.91	T65.92	T65.93	T65.94	—	—
Ajmaline	T46.2X1	T46.2X2	T46.2X3	T46.2X4	T46.2X5	T46.2X6
Akee	T62.1X1	T62.1X2	T62.1X3	T62.1X4	—	—
Akrinol	T49.0X1	T49.0X2	T49.0X3	T49.0X4	T49.0X5	T49.0X6
Akritoin	T37.8X1	T37.8X2	T37.8X3	T37.8X4	T37.8X5	T37.8X6
Alacepril	T46.4X1	T46.4X2	T46.4X3	T46.4X4	T46.4X5	T46.4X6
Alantolactone	T37.4X1	T37.4X2	T37.4X3	T37.4X4	T37.4X5	T37.4X6
Albamycin	T36.8X1	T36.8X2	T36.8X3	T36.8X4	T36.8X5	T36.8X6
Albendazole	T37.4X1	T37.4X2	T37.4X3	T37.4X4	T37.4X5	T37.4X6
Albumin						
bovine	T45.8X1	T45.8X2	T45.8X3	T45.8X4	T45.8X5	T45.8X6
human serum	T45.8X1	T45.8X2	T45.8X3	T45.8X4	T45.8X5	T45.8X6
salt-poor	T45.8X1	T45.8X2	T45.8X3	T45.8X4	T45.8X5	T45.8X6
normal human serum	T45.8X1	T45.8X2	T45.8X3	T45.8X4	T45.8X5	T45.8X6
Albuterol	T48.6X1	T48.6X2	T48.6X3	T48.6X4	T48.6X5	T48.6X6
Albutoin	T42.0X1	T42.0X2	T42.0X3	T42.0X4	T42.0X5	T42.0X6
Alclometasone	T49.0X1	T49.0X2	T49.0X3	T49.0X4	T49.0X5	T49.0X6
Alcohol	T51.91	T51.92	T51.93	T51.94	—	—
absolute	T51.0X1	T51.0X2	T51.0X3	T51.0X4	—	—
beverage	T51.0X1	T51.0X2	T51.0X3	T51.0X4	—	—
allyl	T51.8X1	T51.8X2	T51.8X3	T51.8X4	—	—
amyl	T51.3X1	T51.3X2	T51.3X3	T51.3X4	—	—
antifreeze	T51.1X1	T51.1X2	T51.1X3	T51.1X4	—	—
beverage	T51.0X1	T51.0X2	T51.0X3	T51.0X4	—	—
butyl	T51.3X1	T51.3X2	T51.3X3	T51.3X4	—	—

Substance	Poisoning, Accidental (unintentional)	Poisoning, Intentional self-harm	Poisoning, Assault	Poisoning, Undetermined	Adverse effect	Underdosing
Alcohol — Continued						
dehydrated	T51.0X1	T51.0X2	T51.0X3	T51.0X4	—	—
beverage	T51.0X1	T51.0X2	T51.0X3	T51.0X4	—	—
denatured	T51.0X1	T51.0X2	T51.0X3	T51.0X4	—	—
deterrent NEC	T50.6X1	T50.6X2	T50.6X3	T50.6X4	T50.6X5	T50.6X6
diagnostic (gastric function)	T50.8X1	T50.8X2	T50.8X3	T50.8X4	T50.8X5	T50.8X6
ethyl	T51.0X1	T51.0X2	T51.0X3	T51.0X4	—	—
beverage	T51.0X1	T51.0X2	T51.0X3	T51.0X4	—	—
grain	T51.0X1	T51.0X2	T51.0X3	T51.0X4	—	—
beverage	T51.0X1	T51.0X2	T51.0X3	T51.0X4	—	—
industrial	T51.0X1	T51.0X2	T51.0X3	T51.0X4	—	—
isopropyl	T51.2X1	T51.2X2	T51.2X3	T51.2X4	—	—
methyl	T51.1X1	T51.1X2	T51.1X3	T51.1X4	—	—
preparation for consumption	T51.0X1	T51.0X2	T51.0X3	T51.0X4	—	—
propyl	T51.3X1	T51.3X2	T51.3X3	T51.3X4	—	—
secondary	T51.2X1	T51.2X2	T51.2X3	T51.2X4	—	—
radiator	T51.1X1	T51.1X2	T51.1X3	T51.1X4	—	—
rubbing	T51.2X1	T51.2X2	T51.2X3	T51.2X4	—	—
specified type NEC	T51.8X1	T51.8X2	T51.8X3	T51.8X4	—	—
surgical	T51.0X1	T51.0X2	T51.0X3	T51.0X4	—	—
vapor (from any type of Alcohol)	T59.891	T59.892	T59.893	T59.894	—	—
wood	T51.1X1	T51.1X2	T51.1X3	T51.1X4	—	—
Alcuronium (chloride)	T48.1X1	T48.1X2	T48.1X3	T48.1X4	T48.1X5	T48.1X6
Aldactone	T50.0X1	T50.0X2	T50.0X3	T50.0X4	T50.0X5	T50.0X6
Aldesulfone sodium	T37.1X1	T37.1X2	T37.1X3	T37.1X4	T37.1X5	T37.1X6
Aldicarb	T60.0X1	T60.0X2	T60.0X3	T60.0X4	—	—
Aldomet	T46.5X1	T46.5X2	T46.5X3	T46.5X4	T46.5X5	T46.5X6
Aldosterone	T50.0X1	T50.0X2	T50.0X3	T50.0X4	T50.0X5	T50.0X6
Aldrin (dust)	T60.1X1	T60.1X2	T60.1X3	T60.1X4	—	—
Aleve—see Naproxen						
Alexitol sodium	T47.1X1	T47.1X2	T47.1X3	T47.1X4	T47.1X5	T47.1X6
Alfacalcidol	T45.2X1	T45.2X2	T45.2X3	T45.2X4	T45.2X5	T45.2X6
Alfadolone	T41.1X1	T41.1X2	T41.1X3	T41.1X4	T41.1X5	T41.1X6
Alfaxalone	T41.1X1	T41.1X2	T41.1X3	T41.1X4	T41.1X5	T41.1X6
Alfentanil	T40.411	T40.412	T40.413	T40.414	T40.415	T40.416
Alfuzosin (hydrochloride)	T44.8X1	T44.8X2	T44.8X3	T44.8X4	T44.8X5	T44.8X6
Algae (harmful) (toxin)	T65.821	T65.822	T65.823	T65.824	—	—
Algeldrate	T47.1X1	T47.1X2	T47.1X3	T47.1X4	T47.1X5	T47.1X6
Algin	T47.8X1	T47.8X2	T47.8X3	T47.8X4	T47.8X5	T47.8X6
Alglucerase	T45.3X1	T45.3X2	T45.3X3	T45.3X4	T45.3X5	T45.3X6
Alidase	T45.3X1	T45.3X2	T45.3X3	T45.3X4	T45.3X5	T45.3X6
Alimemazine	T43.3X1	T43.3X2	T43.3X3	T43.3X4	T43.3X5	T43.3X6
Aliphatic thiocyanates	T65.0X1	T65.0X2	T65.0X3	T65.0X4	—	—
Alizapride	T45.0X1	T45.0X2	T45.0X3	T45.0X4	T45.0X5	T45.0X6
Alkali (caustic)	T54.3X1	T54.3X2	T54.3X3	T54.3X4	—	—
Alkaline antiseptic solution (aromatic)	T49.6X1	T49.6X2	T49.6X3	T49.6X4	T49.6X5	T49.6X6
Alkalinizing agents (medicinal)	T50.901	T50.902	T50.903	T50.904	T50.905	T50.906
Alkalizing agent NEC	T50.901	T50.902	T50.903	T50.904	T50.905	T50.906
Alka-seltzer	T39.011	T39.012	T39.013	T39.014	T39.015	T39.016
Alkavervir	T46.5X1	T46.5X2	T46.5X3	T46.5X4	T46.5X5	T46.5X6
Alkonium (bromide)	T49.0X1	T49.0X2	T49.0X3	T49.0X4	T49.0X5	T49.0X6
Alkylating drug NEC	T45.1X1	T45.1X2	T45.1X3	T45.1X4	T45.1X5	T45.1X6
antimyeloprolifera-tive	T45.1X1	T45.1X2	T45.1X3	T45.1X4	T45.1X5	T45.1X6
lymphatic	T45.1X1	T45.1X2	T45.1X3	T45.1X4	T45.1X5	T45.1X6
Alkylisocyanate	T65.0X1	T65.0X2	T65.0X3	T65.0X4	—	—
Allantoin	T49.4X1	T49.4X2	T49.4X3	T49.4X4	T49.4X5	T49.4X6
Allegron	T43.011	T43.012	T43.013	T43.014	T43.015	T43.016
Allethrin	T49.0X1	T49.0X2	T49.0X3	T49.0X4	T49.0X5	T49.0X6
Allobarbital	T42.3X1	T42.3X2	T42.3X3	T42.3X4	T42.3X5	T42.3X6
Allopurinol	T50.4X1	T50.4X2	T50.4X3	T50.4X4	T50.4X5	T50.4X6
Allyl						
Alcohol	T51.8X1	T51.8X2	T51.8X3	T51.8X4	—	—
disulfide	T46.6X1	T46.6X2	T46.6X3	T46.6X4	T46.6X5	T46.6X6
Allylestrenol	T38.5X1	T38.5X2	T38.5X3	T38.5X4	T38.5X5	T38.5X6
Allylisopropyl-acetylurea	T42.6X1	T42.6X2	T42.6X3	T42.6X4	T42.6X5	T42.6X6
Allylisopropyl-malonylurea	T42.3X1	T42.3X2	T42.3X3	T42.3X4	T42.3X5	T42.3X6
Allylthiourea	T49.3X1	T49.3X2	T49.3X3	T49.3X4	T49.3X5	T49.3X6
Allyltribromide	T42.6X1	T42.6X2	T42.6X3	T42.6X4	T42.6X5	T42.6X6
Allypropymal	T42.3X1	T42.3X2	T42.3X3	T42.3X4	T42.3X5	T42.3X6
Almagate	T47.1X1	T47.1X2	T47.1X3	T47.1X4	T47.1X5	T47.1X6
Almasilate	T47.1X1	T47.1X2	T47.1X3	T47.1X4	T47.1X5	T47.1X6
Almitrine	T50.7X1	T50.7X2	T50.7X3	T50.7X4	T50.7X5	T50.7X6
Aloes	T47.2X1	T47.2X2	T47.2X3	T47.2X4	T47.2X5	T47.2X6
Aloglutamol	T47.1X1	T47.1X2	T47.1X3	T47.1X4	T47.1X5	T47.1X6
Aloin	T47.2X1	T47.2X2	T47.2X3	T47.2X4	T47.2X5	T47.2X6
Aloxidone	T42.2X1	T42.2X2	T42.2X3	T42.2X4	T42.2X5	T42.2X6
Alpha						
acetyldigoxin	T46.0X1	T46.0X2	T46.0X3	T46.0X4	T46.0X5	T46.0X6
adrenergic blocking drug	T44.6X1	T44.6X2	T44.6X3	T44.6X4	T44.6X5	T44.6X6
amylase	T45.3X1	T45.3X2	T45.3X3	T45.3X4	T45.3X5	T45.3X6
tocoferol (acetate)	T45.2X1	T45.2X2	T45.2X3	T45.2X4	T45.2X5	T45.2X6
tocopherol	T45.2X1	T45.2X2	T45.2X3	T45.2X4	T45.2X5	T45.2X6
Alphadolone	T41.1X1	T41.1X2	T41.1X3	T41.1X4	T41.1X5	T41.1X6
Alphaprodine	T40.491	T40.492	T40.493	T40.494	T40.495	T40.496
Alphaxalone	T41.1X1	T41.1X2	T41.1X3	T41.1X4	T41.1X5	T41.1X6
Alprazolam	T42.4X1	T42.4X2	T42.4X3	T42.4X4	T42.4X5	T42.4X6
Alprenolol	T44.7X1	T44.7X2	T44.7X3	T44.7X4	T44.7X5	T44.7X6
Alprostadil	T46.7X1	T46.7X2	T46.7X3	T46.7X4	T46.7X5	T46.7X6
Alsactide	T38.811	T38.812	T38.813	T38.814	T38.815	T38.816
Alseroxylon	T46.5X1	T46.5X2	T46.5X3	T46.5X4	T46.5X5	T46.5X6
Alteplase	T45.611	T45.612	T45.613	T45.614	T45.615	T45.616
Altizide	T50.2X1	T50.2X2	T50.2X3	T50.2X4	T50.2X5	T50.2X6

Substance	Poisoning, Accidental (unintentional)	Poisoning, Intentional self-harm	Poisoning, Assault	Poisoning, Undetermined	Adverse effect	Underdosing
Altretamine	T45.1X1	T45.1X2	T45.1X3	T45.1X4	T45.1X5	T45.1X6
Alum (medicinal)	T49.4X1	T49.4X2	T49.4X3	T49.4X4	T49.4X5	T49.4X6
nonmedicinal (ammonium) (potassium)	T56.891	T56.892	T56.893	T56.894	—	—
Aluminium, aluminum						
acetate	T49.2X1	T49.2X2	T49.2X3	T49.2X4	T49.2X5	T49.2X6
solution	T49.0X1	T49.0X2	T49.0X3	T49.0X4	T49.0X5	T49.0X6
aspirin	T39.011	T39.012	T39.013	T39.014	T39.015	T39.016
bis (acetylsalicylate)	T39.011	T39.012	T39.013	T39.014	T39.015	T39.016
carbonate (gel, basic)	T47.1X1	T47.1X2	T47.1X3	T47.1X4	T47.1X5	T47.1X6
chlorhydroxide-complex	T47.1X1	T47.1X2	T47.1X3	T47.1X4	T47.1X5	T47.1X6
chloride	T49.2X1	T49.2X2	T49.2X3	T49.2X4	T49.2X5	T49.2X6
clofibrate	T46.6X1	T46.6X2	T46.6X3	T46.6X4	T46.6X5	T46.6X6
diacetate	T49.2X1	T49.2X2	T49.2X3	T49.2X4	T49.2X5	T49.2X6
glycinate	T47.1X1	T47.1X2	T47.1X3	T47.1X4	T47.1X5	T47.1X6
hydroxide (gel)	T47.1X1	T47.1X2	T47.1X3	T47.1X4	T47.1X5	T47.1X6
hydroxide-magnesium carb. gel	T47.1X1	T47.1X2	T47.1X3	T47.1X4	T47.1X5	T47.1X6
magnesium silicate	T47.1X1	T47.1X2	T47.1X3	T47.1X4	T47.1X5	T47.1X6
nicotinate	T46.7X1	T46.7X2	T46.7X3	T46.7X4	T46.7X5	T46.7X6
ointment (surgical) (topical)	T49.3X1	T49.3X2	T49.3X3	T49.3X4	T49.3X5	T49.3X6
phosphate	T47.1X1	T47.1X2	T47.1X3	T47.1X4	T47.1X5	T47.1X6
salicylate	T39.091	T39.092	T39.093	T39.094	T39.095	T39.096
silicate	T47.1X1	T47.1X2	T47.1X3	T47.1X4	T47.1X5	T47.1X6
sodium silicate	T47.1X1	T47.1X2	T47.1X3	T47.1X4	T47.1X5	T47.1X6
subacetate	T49.2X1	T49.2X2	T49.2X3	T49.2X4	T49.2X5	T49.2X6
sulfate	T49.0X1	T49.0X2	T49.0X3	T49.0X4	T49.0X5	T49.0X6
tannate	T47.6X1	T47.6X2	T47.6X3	T47.6X4	T47.6X5	T47.6X6
topical NEC	T49.3X1	T49.3X2	T49.3X3	T49.3X4	T49.3X5	T49.3X6
Alurate	T42.3X1	T42.3X2	T42.3X3	T42.3X4	T42.3X5	T42.3X6
Alverine	T44.3X1	T44.3X2	T44.3X3	T44.3X4	T44.3X5	T44.3X6
Alvodine	T40.2X1	T40.2X2	T40.2X3	T40.2X4	T40.2X5	T40.2X6
Amanita phalloides	T62.0X1	T62.0X2	T62.0X3	T62.0X4	—	—
Amanitine	T62.0X1	T62.0X2	T62.0X3	T62.0X4	—	—
Amantadine	T42.8X1	T42.8X2	T42.8X3	T42.8X4	T42.8X5	T42.8X6
Ambazone	T49.6X1	T49.6X2	T49.6X3	T49.6X4	T49.6X5	T49.6X6
Ambenonium (chloride)	T44.0X1	T44.0X2	T44.0X3	T44.0X4	T44.0X5	T44.0X6
Ambroxol	T48.4X1	T48.4X2	T48.4X3	T48.4X4	T48.4X5	T48.4X6
Ambuphylline	T48.6X1	T48.6X2	T48.6X3	T48.6X4	T48.6X5	T48.6X6
Ambutonium bromide	T44.3X1	T44.3X2	T44.3X3	T44.3X4	T44.3X5	T44.3X6
Amcinonide	T49.0X1	T49.0X2	T49.0X3	T49.0X4	T49.0X5	T49.0X6
Amdinocillin	T36.0X1	T36.0X2	T36.0X3	T36.0X4	T36.0X5	T36.0X6
Ametazole	T50.8X1	T50.8X2	T50.8X3	T50.8X4	T50.8X5	T50.8X6
Amethocaine	T41.3X1	T41.3X2	T41.3X3	T41.3X4	T41.3X5	T41.3X6
regional	T41.3X1	T41.3X2	T41.3X3	T41.3X4	T41.3X5	T41.3X6
spinal	T41.3X1	T41.3X2	T41.3X3	T41.3X4	T41.3X5	T41.3X6
Amethopterin	T45.1X1	T45.1X2	T45.1X3	T45.1X4	T45.1X5	T45.1X6
Amezinium metilsulfate	T44.991	T44.992	T44.993	T44.994	T44.995	T44.996

Substance	Poisoning, Accidental (unintentional)	Poisoning, Intentional self-harm	Poisoning, Assault	Poisoning, Undetermined	Adverse effect	Underdosing
Amfebutamone	T43.291	T43.292	T43.293	T43.294	T43.295	T43.296
Amfepramone	T50.5X1	T50.5X2	T50.5X3	T50.5X4	T50.5X5	T50.5X6
Amfetamine	T43.621	T43.622	T43.623	T43.624	T43.625	T43.626
Amfetaminil	T43.621	T43.622	T43.623	T43.624	T43.625	T43.626
Amfomycin	T36.8X1	T36.8X2	T36.8X3	T36.8X4	T36.8X5	T36.8X6
Amidefrine mesilate	T48.5X1	T48.5X2	T48.5X3	T48.5X4	T48.5X5	T48.5X6
Amidone	T40.3X1	T40.3X2	T40.3X3	T40.3X4	T40.3X5	T40.3X6
Amidopyrine	T39.2X1	T39.2X2	T39.2X3	T39.2X4	T39.2X5	T39.2X6
Amidotrizoate	T50.8X1	T50.8X2	T50.8X3	T50.8X4	T50.8X5	T50.8X6
Amiflamine	T43.1X1	T43.1X2	T43.1X3	T43.1X4	T43.1X5	T43.1X6
Amikacin	T36.5X1	T36.5X2	T36.5X3	T36.5X4	T36.5X5	T36.5X6
Amikhelline	T46.3X1	T46.3X2	T46.3X3	T46.3X4	T46.3X5	T46.3X6
Amiloride	T50.2X1	T50.2X2	T50.2X3	T50.2X4	T50.2X5	T50.2X6
Aminacrine	T49.0X1	T49.0X2	T49.0X3	T49.0X4	T49.0X5	T49.0X6
Amineptine	T43.011	T43.012	T43.013	T43.014	T43.015	T43.016
Aminitrozole	T37.3X1	T37.3X2	T37.3X3	T37.3X4	T37.3X5	T37.3X6
Amino acids	T50.3X1	T50.3X2	T50.3X3	T50.3X4	T50.3X5	T50.3X6
Aminoacetic acid (derivatives)	T50.3X1	T50.3X2	T50.3X3	T50.3X4	T50.3X5	T50.3X6
Aminoacridine	T49.0X1	T49.0X2	T49.0X3	T49.0X4	T49.0X5	T49.0X6
Aminobenzoic acid(-p)	T49.3X1	T49.3X2	T49.3X3	T49.3X4	T49.3X5	T49.3X6
4-Aminobutyric acid	T43.8X1	T43.8X2	T43.8X3	T43.8X4	T43.8X5	T43.8X6
Aminocaproic acid	T45.621	T45.622	T45.623	T45.624	T45.625	T45.626
Aminoethyl-isothiourium	T45.8X1	T45.8X2	T45.8X3	T45.8X4	T45.8X5	T45.8X6
Aminofenazone	T39.2X1	T39.2X2	T39.2X3	T39.2X4	T39.2X5	T39.2X6
Aminoglutethimide	T45.1X1	T45.1X2	T45.1X3	T45.1X4	T45.1X5	T45.1X6
Aminohippuric acid	T50.8X1	T50.8X2	T50.8X3	T50.8X4	T50.8X5	T50.8X6
Aminomethylbenzoic acid	T45.691	T45.692	T45.693	T45.694	T45.695	T45.696
Aminometradine	T50.2X1	T50.2X2	T50.2X3	T50.2X4	T50.2X5	T50.2X6
Aminopentamide	T44.3X1	T44.3X2	T44.3X3	T44.3X4	T44.3X5	T44.3X6
Aminophenazone	T39.2X1	T39.2X2	T39.2X3	T39.2X4	T39.2X5	T39.2X6
Aminophenol	T54.0X1	T54.0X2	T54.0X3	T54.0X4	—	—
4-Aminophenol derivatives	T39.1X1	T39.1X2	T39.1X3	T39.1X4	T39.1X5	T39.1X6
Aminophenylpyri-done	T43.591	T43.592	T43.593	T43.594	T43.595	T43.596
Aminophylline	T48.6X1	T48.6X2	T48.6X3	T48.6X4	T48.6X5	T48.6X6
Aminopterin sodium	T45.1X1	T45.1X2	T45.1X3	T45.1X4	T45.1X5	T45.1X6
Aminopyrine	T39.2X1	T39.2X2	T39.2X3	T39.2X4	T39.2X5	T39.2X6
8-Aminoquinoline drugs	T37.2X1	T37.2X2	T37.2X3	T37.2X4	T37.2X5	T37.2X6
Aminorex	T50.5X1	T50.5X2	T50.5X3	T50.5X4	T50.5X5	T50.5X6
Aminosalicylic acid	T37.1X1	T37.1X2	T37.1X3	T37.1X4	T37.1X5	T37.1X6
Aminosalylum	T37.1X1	T37.1X2	T37.1X3	T37.1X4	T37.1X5	T37.1X6
Amiodarone	T46.2X1	T46.2X2	T46.2X3	T46.2X4	T46.2X5	T46.2X6
Amiphenazole	T50.7X1	T50.7X2	T50.7X3	T50.7X4	T50.7X5	T50.7X6
Amiquinsin	T46.5X1	T46.5X2	T46.5X3	T46.5X4	T46.5X5	T46.5X6
Amisometradine	T50.2X1	T50.2X2	T50.2X3	T50.2X4	T50.2X5	T50.2X6
Amisulpride	T43.591	T43.592	T43.593	T43.594	T43.595	T43.596
Amitriptyline	T43.011	T43.012	T43.013	T43.014	T43.015	T43.016
Amitriptylinoxide	T43.011	T43.012	T43.013	T43.014	T43.015	T43.016

Substance	Poisoning, Accidental (unintentional)	Poisoning, Intentional self-harm	Poisoning, Assault	Poisoning, Undetermined	Adverse effect	Underdosing
Amlexanox	T48.6X1	T48.6X2	T48.6X3	T48.6X4	T48.6X5	T48.6X6
Ammonia (fumes) (gas) (vapor)	T59.891	T59.892	T59.893	T59.894	—	—
aromatic spirit	T48.991	T48.992	T48.993	T48.994	T48.995	T48.996
liquid (household)	T54.3X1	T54.3X2	T54.3X3	T54.3X4	—	—
Ammoniated mercury	T49.0X1	T49.0X2	T49.0X3	T49.0X4	T49.0X5	T49.0X6
Ammonium						
acid tartrate	T49.5X1	T49.5X2	T49.5X3	T49.5X4	T49.5X5	T49.5X6
bromide	T42.6X1	T42.6X2	T42.6X3	T42.6X4	T42.6X5	T42.6X6
carbonate	T54.3X1	T54.3X2	T54.3X3	T54.3X4	—	—
chloride	T50.991	T50.992	T50.993	T50.994	T50.995	T50.996
expectorant	T48.4X1	T48.4X2	T48.4X3	T48.4X4	T48.4X5	T48.4X6
compounds (household) NEC	T54.3X1	T54.3X2	T54.3X3	T54.3X4	—	—
fumes (any usage)	T59.891	T59.892	T59.893	T59.894	—	—
industrial	T54.3X1	T54.3X2	T54.3X3	T54.3X4	—	—
ichthyosulronate	T49.4X1	T49.4X2	T49.4X3	T49.4X4	T49.4X5	T49.4X6
mandelate	T37.91	T37.92	T37.93	T37.94	T37.95	T37.96
sulfamate	T60.3X1	T60.3X2	T60.3X3	T60.3X4	—	—
sulfonate resin	T47.8X1	T47.8X2	T47.8X3	T47.8X4	T47.8X5	T47.8X6
Amobarbital (sodium)	T42.3X1	T42.3X2	T42.3X3	T42.3X4	T42.3X5	T42.3X6
Amodiaquine	T37.2X1	T37.2X2	T37.2X3	T37.2X4	T37.2X5	T37.2X6
Amopyroquin(e)	T37.2X1	T37.2X2	T37.2X3	T37.2X4	T37.2X5	T37.2X6
Amoxapine	T43.011	T43.012	T43.013	T43.014	T43.015	T43.016
Amoxicillin	T36.0X1	T36.0X2	T36.0X3	T36.0X4	T36.0X5	T36.0X6
Amperozide	T43.591	T43.592	T43.593	T43.594	T43.595	T43.596
Amphenidone	T43.591	T43.592	T43.593	T43.594	T43.595	T43.596
Amphetamine NEC	T43.621	T43.622	T43.623	T43.624	T43.625	T43.626
Amphomycin	T36.8X1	T36.8X2	T36.8X3	T36.8X4	T36.8X5	T36.8X6
Amphotalide	T37.4X1	T37.4X2	T37.4X3	T37.4X4	T37.4X5	T37.4X6
Amphotericin B	T36.7X1	T36.7X2	T36.7X3	T36.7X4	T36.7X5	T36.7X6
topical	T49.0X1	T49.0X2	T49.0X3	T49.0X4	T49.0X5	T49.0X6
Ampicillin	T36.0X1	T36.0X2	T36.0X3	T36.0X4	T36.0X5	T36.0X6
Amprotropine	T44.3X1	T44.3X2	T44.3X3	T44.3X4	T44.3X5	T44.3X6
Amsacrine	T45.1X1	T45.1X2	T45.1X3	T45.1X4	T45.1X5	T45.1X6
Amygdaline	T62.2X1	T62.2X2	T62.2X3	T62.2X4	—	—
Amyl						
acetate	T52.8X1	T52.8X2	T52.8X3	T52.8X4	—	—
vapor	T59.891	T59.892	T59.893	T59.894	—	—
alcohol	T51.3X1	T51.3X2	T51.3X3	T51.3X4	—	—
chloride	T53.6X1	T53.6X2	T53.6X3	T53.6X4	—	—
formate	T52.8X1	T52.8X2	T52.8X3	T52.8X4	—	—
nitrite	T46.3X1	T46.3X2	T46.3X3	T46.3X4	T46.3X5	T46.3X6
propionate	T65.891	T65.892	T65.893	T65.894	—	—
Amylase	T47.5X1	T47.5X2	T47.5X3	T47.5X4	T47.5X5	T47.5X6
Amyleine, regional	T41.3X1	T41.3X2	T41.3X3	T41.3X4	T41.3X5	T41.3X6
Amylene						
dichloride	T53.6X1	T53.6X2	T53.6X3	T53.6X4	—	—
hydrate	T51.3X1	T51.3X2	T51.3X3	T51.3X4	—	—
Amylmetacresol	T49.6X1	T49.6X2	T49.6X3	T49.6X4	T49.6X5	T49.6X6
Amylobarbitone	T42.3X1	T42.3X2	T42.3X3	T42.3X4	T42.3X5	T42.3X6

Substance	Poisoning, Accidental (unintentional)	Poisoning, Intentional self-harm	Poisoning, Assault	Poisoning, Undetermined	Adverse effect	Underdosing
Amylocaine, regional	T41.3X1	T41.3X2	T41.3X3	T41.3X4	T41.3X5	T41.3X6
infiltration (subcutaneous)	T41.3X1	T41.3X2	T41.3X3	T41.3X4	T41.3X5	T41.3X6
nerve block (peripheral) (plexus)	T41.3X1	T41.3X2	T41.3X3	T41.3X4	T41.3X5	T41.3X6
spinal	T41.3X1	T41.3X2	T41.3X3	T41.3X4	T41.3X5	T41.3X6
topical (surface)	T41.3X1	T41.3X2	T41.3X3	T41.3X4	T41.3X5	T41.3X6
Amylopectin	T47.6X1	T47.6X2	T47.6X3	T47.6X4	T47.6X5	T47.6X6
Amytal (sodium)	T42.3X1	T42.3X2	T42.3X3	T42.3X4	T42.3X5	T42.3X6
Anabolic steroid	T38.7X1	T38.7X2	T38.7X3	T38.7X4	T38.7X5	T38.7X6
Analeptic NEC	T50.7X1	T50.7X2	T50.7X3	T50.7X4	T50.7X5	T50.7X6
Analgesic	T39.91	T39.92	T39.93	T39.94	T39.95	T39.96
anti-inflammatory NEC	T39.91	T39.92	T39.93	T39.94	T39.95	T39.96
propionic acid derivative	T39.311	T39.312	T39.313	T39.314	T39.315	T39.316
antirheumatic NEC	T39.4X1	T39.4X2	T39.4X3	T39.4X4	T39.4X5	T39.4X6
aromatic NEC	T39.1X1	T39.1X2	T39.1X3	T39.1X4	T39.1X5	T39.1X6
narcotic NEC	T40.601	T40.602	T40.603	T40.604	T40.605	T40.606
combination	T40.601	T40.602	T40.603	T40.604	T40.605	T40.606
obstetric	T40.601	T40.602	T40.603	T40.604	T40.605	T40.606
non-narcotic NEC	T39.91	T39.92	T39.93	T39.94	T39.95	T39.96
combination	T39.91	T39.92	T39.93	T39.94	T39.95	T39.96
pyrazole	T39.2X1	T39.2X2	T39.2X3	T39.2X4	T39.2X5	T39.2X6
specified NEC	T39.8X1	T39.8X2	T39.8X3	T39.8X4	T39.8X5	T39.8X6
Analgin	T39.2X1	T39.2X2	T39.2X3	T39.2X4	T39.2X5	T39.2X6
Anamirta cocculus	T62.1X1	T62.1X2	T62.1X3	T62.1X4	—	—
Ancillin	T36.0X1	T36.0X2	T36.0X3	T36.0X4	T36.0X5	T36.0X6
Ancrod	T45.691	T45.692	T45.693	T45.694	T45.695	T45.696
Androgen	T38.7X1	T38.7X2	T38.7X3	T38.7X4	T38.7X5	T38.7X6
Androgen-estrogen mixture	T38.7X1	T38.7X2	T38.7X3	T38.7X4	T38.7X5	T38.7X6
Androstalone	T38.7X1	T38.7X2	T38.7X3	T38.7X4	T38.7X5	T38.7X6
Androstanolone	T38.7X1	T38.7X2	T38.7X3	T38.7X4	T38.7X5	T38.7X6
Androsterone	T38.7X1	T38.7X2	T38.7X3	T38.7X4	T38.7X5	T38.7X6
Anemone pulsatilla	T62.2X1	T62.2X2	T62.2X3	T62.2X4	—	—
Anesthesia						
caudal	T41.3X1	T41.3X2	T41.3X3	T41.3X4	T41.3X5	T41.3X6
endotracheal	T41.0X1	T41.0X2	T41.0X3	T41.0X4	T41.0X5	T41.0X6
epidural	T41.3X1	T41.3X2	T41.3X3	T41.3X4	T41.3X5	T41.3X6
inhalation	T41.0X1	T41.0X2	T41.0X3	T41.0X4	T41.0X5	T41.0X6
local	T41.3X1	T41.3X2	T41.3X3	T41.3X4	T41.3X5	T41.3X6
mucosal	T41.3X1	T41.3X2	T41.3X3	T41.3X4	T41.3X5	T41.3X6
muscle relaxation	T48.1X1	T48.1X2	T48.1X3	T48.1X4	T48.1X5	T48.1X6
nerve blocking	T41.3X1	T41.3X2	T41.3X3	T41.3X4	T41.3X5	T41.3X6
plexus blocking	T41.3X1	T41.3X2	T41.3X3	T41.3X4	T41.3X5	T41.3X6
potentiated	T41.201	T41.202	T41.203	T41.204	T41.205	T41.206
rectal	T41.201	T41.202	T41.203	T41.204	T41.205	T41.206
general	T41.201	T41.202	T41.203	T41.204	T41.205	T41.206
local	T41.3X1	T41.3X2	T41.3X3	T41.3X4	T41.3X5	T41.3X6
regional	T41.3X1	T41.3X2	T41.3X3	T41.3X4	T41.3X5	T41.3X6
surface	T41.3X1	T41.3X2	T41.3X3	T41.3X4	T41.3X5	T41.3X6

Substance	Poisoning, Accidental (unintentional)	Poisoning, Intentional self-harm	Poisoning, Assault	Poisoning, Undetermined	Adverse effect	Underdosing
Anesthetic NEC —see also Anesthesia	T41.41	T41.42	T41.43	T41.44	T41.45	T41.46
with muscle relaxant	T41.201	T41.202	T41.203	T41.204	T41.205	T41.206
general	T41.201	T41.202	T41.203	T41.204	T41.205	T41.206
local	T41.3X1	T41.3X2	T41.3X3	T41.3X4	T41.3X5	T41.3X6
gaseous NEC	T41.0X1	T41.0X2	T41.0X3	T41.0X4	T41.0X5	T41.0X6
general NEC	T41.201	T41.202	T41.203	T41.204	T41.205	T41.206
halogenated hydrocarbon derivatives NEC	T41.0X1	T41.0X2	T41.0X3	T41.0X4	T41.0X5	T41.0X6
infiltration NEC	T41.3X1	T41.3X2	T41.3X3	T41.3X4	T41.3X5	T41.3X6
intravenous NEC	T41.1X1	T41.1X2	T41.1X3	T41.1X4	T41.1X5	T41.1X6
local NEC	T41.3X1	T41.3X2	T41.3X3	T41.3X4	T41.3X5	T41.3X6
rectal	T41.201	T41.202	T41.203	T41.204	T41.205	T41.206
general	T41.201	T41.202	T41.203	T41.204	T41.205	T41.206
local	T41.3X1	T41.3X2	T41.3X3	T41.3X4	T41.3X5	T41.3X6
regional NEC	T41.3X1	T41.3X2	T41.3X3	T41.3X4	T41.3X5	T41.3X6
spinal NEC	T41.3X1	T41.3X2	T41.3X3	T41.3X4	T41.3X5	T41.3X6
thiobarbiturate	T41.1X1	T41.1X2	T41.1X3	T41.1X4	T41.1X5	T41.1X6
topical	T41.3X1	T41.3X2	T41.3X3	T41.3X4	T41.3X5	T41.3X6
Aneurine	T45.2X1	T45.2X2	T45.2X3	T45.2X4	T45.2X5	T45.2X6
Angio-Conray	T50.8X1	T50.8X2	T50.8X3	T50.8X4	T50.8X5	T50.8X6
Angiotensin	T44.5X1	T44.5X2	T44.5X3	T44.5X4	T44.5X5	T44.5X6
Angiotensinamide	T44.991	T44.992	T44.993	T44.994	T44.995	T44.996
Anhydrohydroxy-progesterone	T38.5X1	T38.5X2	T38.5X3	T38.5X4	T38.5X5	T38.5X6
Anhydron	T50.2X1	T50.2X2	T50.2X3	T50.2X4	T50.2X5	T50.2X6
Anileridine	T40.491	T40.492	T40.493	T40.494	T40.495	T40.496
Aniline (dye) (liquid)	T65.3X1	T65.3X2	T65.3X3	T65.3X4	—	—
analgesic	T39.1X1	T39.1X2	T39.1X3	T39.1X4	T39.1X5	T39.1X6
derivatives, therapeutic NEC	T39.1X1	T39.1X2	T39.1X3	T39.1X4	T39.1X5	T39.1X6
vapor	T65.3X1	T65.3X2	T65.3X3	T65.3X4	—	—
Aniscoropine	T44.3X1	T44.3X2	T44.3X3	T44.3X4	T44.3X5	T44.3X6
Anise oil	T47.5X1	T47.5X2	T47.5X3	T47.5X4	T47.5X5	T47.5X6
Anisidine	T65.3X1	T65.3X2	T65.3X3	T65.3X4	—	—
Anisindione	T45.511	T45.512	T45.513	T45.514	T45.515	T45.516
Anisotropine methyl-bromide	T44.3X1	T44.3X2	T44.3X3	T44.3X4	T44.3X5	T44.3X6
Anistreplase	T45.611	T45.612	T45.613	T45.614	T45.615	T45.616
Anorexiant (central)	T50.5X1	T50.5X2	T50.5X3	T50.5X4	T50.5X5	T50.5X6
Anorexic agents	T50.5X1	T50.5X2	T50.5X3	T50.5X4	T50.5X5	T50.5X6
Ansamycin	T36.6X1	T36.6X2	T36.6X3	T36.6X4	T36.6X5	T36.6X6
Ant (bite) (sting)	T63.421	T63.422	T63.423	T63.424	—	—
Ant poison—see Insecticide						
Antabuse	T50.6X1	T50.6X2	T50.6X3	T50.6X4	T50.6X5	T50.6X6
Antacid NEC	T47.1X1	T47.1X2	T47.1X3	T47.1X4	T47.1X5	T47.1X6
Antagonist						
Aldosterone	T50.0X1	T50.0X2	T50.0X3	T50.0X4	T50.0X5	T50.0X6
alpha-adrenoreceptor	T44.6X1	T44.6X2	T44.6X3	T44.6X4	T44.6X5	T44.6X6
anticoagulant	T45.7X1	T45.7X2	T45.7X3	T45.7X4	T45.7X5	T45.7X6

Substance	Poisoning, Accidental (unintentional)	Poisoning, Intentional self-harm	Poisoning, Assault	Poisoning, Undetermined	Adverse effect	Underdosing
Antagonist — Continued						
beta-adrenoreceptor	T44.7X1	T44.7X2	T44.7X3	T44.7X4	T44.7X5	T44.7X6
extrapyramidal NEC	T44.3X1	T44.3X2	T44.3X3	T44.3X4	T44.3X5	T44.3X6
folic acid	T45.1X1	T45.1X2	T45.1X3	T45.1X4	T45.1X5	T45.1X6
H2 receptor	T47.0X1	T47.0X2	T47.0X3	T47.0X4	T47.0X5	T47.0X6
heavy metal	T45.8X1	T45.8X2	T45.8X3	T45.8X4	T45.8X5	T45.8X6
narcotic analgesic	T50.7X1	T50.7X2	T50.7X3	T50.7X4	T50.7X5	T50.7X6
opiate	T50.7X1	T50.7X2	T50.7X3	T50.7X4	T50.7X5	T50.7X6
pyrimidine	T45.1X1	T45.1X2	T45.1X3	T45.1X4	T45.1X5	T45.1X6
serotonin	T46.5X1	T46.5X2	T46.5X3	T46.5X4	T46.5X5	T46.5X6
Antazolin(e)	T45.0X1	T45.0X2	T45.0X3	T45.0X4	T45.0X5	T45.0X6
Anterior pituitary hormone NEC	T38.811	T38.812	T38.813	T38.814	T38.815	T38.816
Anthelmintic NEC	T37.4X1	T37.4X2	T37.4X3	T37.4X4	T37.4X5	T37.4X6
Anthiolimine	T37.4X1	T37.4X2	T37.4X3	T37.4X4	T37.4X5	T37.4X6
Anthralin	T49.4X1	T49.4X2	T49.4X3	T49.4X4	T49.4X5	T49.4X6
Anthramycin	T45.1X1	T45.1X2	T45.1X3	T45.1X4	T45.1X5	T45.1X6
Antiadrenergic NEC	T44.8X1	T44.8X2	T44.8X3	T44.8X4	T44.8X5	T44.8X6
Antiallergic NEC	T45.0X1	T45.0X2	T45.0X3	T45.0X4	T45.0X5	T45.0X6
Anti-anemic (drug) (preparation)	T45.8X1	T45.8X2	T45.8X3	T45.8X4	T45.8X5	T45.8X6
Antiandrogen NEC	T38.6X1	T38.6X2	T38.6X3	T38.6X4	T38.6X5	T38.6X6
Antianxiety drug NEC	T43.501	T43.502	T43.503	T43.504	T43.505	T43.506
Antiaris toxicaria	T65.891	T65.892	T65.893	T65.894	—	—
Antiarteriosclerotic drug	T46.6X1	T46.6X2	T46.6X3	T46.6X4	T46.6X5	T46.6X6
Antiasthmatic drug NEC	T48.6X1	T48.6X2	T48.6X3	T48.6X4	T48.6X5	T48.6X6
Antibiotic NEC	T36.91	T36.92	T36.93	T36.94	T36.95	T36.96
aminoglycoside	T36.5X1	T36.5X2	T36.5X3	T36.5X4	T36.5X5	T36.5X6
anticancer	T45.1X1	T45.1X2	T45.1X3	T45.1X4	T45.1X5	T45.1X6
antifungal	T36.7X1	T36.7X2	T36.7X3	T36.7X4	T36.7X5	T36.7X6
antimycobacterial	T36.5X1	T36.5X2	T36.5X3	T36.5X4	T36.5X5	T36.5X6
antineoplastic	T45.1X1	T45.1X2	T45.1X3	T45.1X4	T45.1X5	T45.1X6
cephalosporin (group)	T36.1X1	T36.1X2	T36.1X3	T36.1X4	T36.1X5	T36.1X6
chloramphenicol (group)	T36.2X1	T36.2X2	T36.2X3	T36.2X4	T36.2X5	T36.2X6
ENT	T49.6X1	T49.6X2	T49.6X3	T49.6X4	T49.6X5	T49.6X6
eye	T49.5X1	T49.5X2	T49.5X3	T49.5X4	T49.5X5	T49.5X6
fungicidal (local)	T49.0X1	T49.0X2	T49.0X3	T49.0X4	T49.0X5	T49.0X6
intestinal	T36.8X1	T36.8X2	T36.8X3	T36.8X4	T36.8X5	T36.8X6
b-lactam NEC	T36.1X1	T36.1X2	T36.1X3	T36.1X4	T36.1X5	T36.1X6
local	T49.0X1	T49.0X2	T49.0X3	T49.0X4	T49.0X5	T49.0X6
macrolides	T36.3X1	T36.3X2	T36.3X3	T36.3X4	T36.3X5	T36.3X6
polypeptide	T36.8X1	T36.8X2	T36.8X3	T36.8X4	T36.8X5	T36.8X6
specified NEC	T36.8X1	T36.8X2	T36.8X3	T36.8X4	T36.8X5	T36.8X6
tetracycline (group)	T36.4X1	T36.4X2	T36.4X3	T36.4X4	T36.4X5	T36.4X6
throat	T49.6X1	T49.6X2	T49.6X3	T49.6X4	T49.6X5	T49.6X6
Anticancer agents NEC	T45.1X1	T45.1X2	T45.1X3	T45.1X4	T45.1X5	T45.1X6
Anticholesterolemic drug NEC	T46.6X1	T46.6X2	T46.6X3	T46.6X4	T46.6X5	T46.6X6
Anticholinergic NEC	T44.3X1	T44.3X2	T44.3X3	T44.3X4	T44.3X5	T44.3X6

Substance	Poisoning, Accidental (unintentional)	Poisoning, Intentional self-harm	Poisoning, Assault	Poisoning, Undetermined	Adverse effect	Underdosing
Anticholinesterase	T44.0X1	T44.0X2	T44.0X3	T44.0X4	T44.0X5	T44.0X6
organophosphorus	T44.0X1	T44.0X2	T44.0X3	T44.0X4	T44.0X5	T44.0X6
insecticide	T60.0X1	T60.0X2	T60.0X3	T60.0X4	—	—
nerve gas	T59.891	T59.892	T59.893	T59.894	—	—
reversible	T44.0X1	T44.0X2	T44.0X3	T44.0X4	T44.0X5	T44.0X6
ophthalmological	T49.5X1	T49.5X2	T49.5X3	T49.5X4	T49.5X5	T49.5X6
Anticoagulant NEC	T45.511	T45.512	T45.513	T45.514	T45.515	T45.516
Antagonist	T45.7X1	T45.7X2	T45.7X3	T45.7X4	T45.7X5	T45.7X6
Anti-common-cold drug NEC	T48.5X1	T48.5X2	T48.5X3	T48.5X4	T48.5X5	T48.5X6
Anticonvulsant	T42.71	T42.72	T42.73	T42.74	T42.75	T42.76
barbiturate	T42.3X1	T42.3X2	T42.3X3	T42.3X4	T42.3X5	T42.3X6
combination (with barbiturate)	T42.3X1	T42.3X2	T42.3X3	T42.3X4	T42.3X5	T42.3X6
hydantoin	T42.0X1	T42.0X2	T42.0X3	T42.0X4	T42.0X5	T42.0X6
hypnotic NEC	T42.6X1	T42.6X2	T42.6X3	T42.6X4	T42.6X5	T42.6X6
oxazolidinedione	T42.2X1	T42.2X2	T42.2X3	T42.2X4	T42.2X5	T42.2X6
pyrimidinedione	T42.6X1	T42.6X2	T42.6X3	T42.6X4	T42.6X5	T42.6X6
specified NEC	T42.6X1	T42.6X2	T42.6X3	T42.6X4	T42.6X5	T42.6X6
succinimide	T42.2X1	T42.2X2	T42.2X3	T42.2X4	T42.2X5	T42.2X6
Anti-D immuno-globulin (human)	T50.Z11	T50.Z12	T50.Z13	T50.Z14	T50.Z15	T50.Z16
Antidepressant	T43.201	T43.202	T43.203	T43.204	T43.205	T43.206
monoamine oxidase inhibitor	T43.1X1	T43.1X2	T43.1X3	T43.1X4	T43.1X5	T43.1X6
selective serotonin norepinephrine reuptake inhibitor	T43.211	T43.212	T43.213	T43.214	T43.215	T43.216
selective serotonin reuptake inhibitor	T43.221	T43.222	T43.223	T43.224	T43.225	T43.226
specified NEC	T43.291	T43.292	T43.293	T43.294	T43.295	T43.296
tetracyclic	T43.021	T43.022	T43.023	T43.024	T43.025	T43.026
triazolopyridine	T43.211	T43.212	T43.213	T43.214	T43.215	T43.216
tricyclic	T43.011	T43.012	T43.013	T43.014	T43.015	T43.016
Antidiabetic NEC	T38.3X1	T38.3X2	T38.3X3	T38.3X4	T38.3X5	T38.3X6
biguanide	T38.3X1	T38.3X2	T38.3X3	T38.3X4	T38.3X5	T38.3X6
and sulfonyl combined	T38.3X1	T38.3X2	T38.3X3	T38.3X4	T38.3X5	T38.3X6
combined	T38.3X1	T38.3X2	T38.3X3	T38.3X4	T38.3X5	T38.3X6
sulfonylurea	T38.3X1	T38.3X2	T38.3X3	T38.3X4	T38.3X5	T38.3X6
Antidiarrheal drug NEC	T47.6X1	T47.6X2	T47.6X3	T47.6X4	T47.6X5	T47.6X6
absorbent	T47.6X1	T47.6X2	T47.6X3	T47.6X4	T47.6X5	T47.6X6
Antidiphtheria serum	T50.Z11	T50.Z12	T50.Z13	T50.Z14	T50.Z15	T50.Z16
Antidiuretic hormone	T38.891	T38.892	T38.893	T38.894	T38.895	T38.896
Antidote NEC	T50.6X1	T50.6X2	T50.6X3	T50.6X4	T50.6X5	T50.6X6
heavy metal	T45.8X1	T45.8X2	T45.8X3	T45.8X4	T45.8X5	T45.8X6
Antidysrhythmic NEC	T46.2X1	T46.2X2	T46.2X3	T46.2X4	T46.2X5	T46.2X6
Antiemetic drug	T45.0X1	T45.0X2	T45.0X3	T45.0X4	T45.0X5	T45.0X6
Antiepilepsy agent	T42.71	T42.72	T42.73	T42.74	T42.75	T42.76
combination	T42.5X1	T42.5X2	T42.5X3	T42.5X4	T42.5X5	T42.5X6
mixed	T42.5X1	T42.5X2	T42.5X3	T42.5X4	T42.5X5	T42.5X6
specified, NEC	T42.6X1	T42.6X2	T42.6X3	T42.6X4	T42.6X5	T42.6X6

Substance	Poisoning, Accidental (unintentional)	Poisoning, Intentional self-harm	Poisoning, Assault	Poisoning, Undetermined	Adverse effect	Underdosing
Antiestrogen NEC	T38.6X1	T38.6X2	T38.6X3	T38.6X4	T38.6X5	T38.6X6
Antifertility pill	T38.4X1	T38.4X2	T38.4X3	T38.4X4	T38.4X5	T38.4X6
Antifibrinolytic drug	T45.621	T45.622	T45.623	T45.624	T45.625	T45.626
Antifilarial drug	T37.4X1	T37.4X2	T37.4X3	T37.4X4	T37.4X5	T37.4X6
Antiflatulent	T47.5X1	T47.5X2	T47.5X3	T47.5X4	T47.5X5	T47.5X6
Antifreeze	T65.91	T65.92	T65.93	T65.94	—	—
alcohol	T51.1X1	T51.1X2	T51.1X3	T51.1X4	—	—
ethylene glycol	T51.8X1	T51.8X2	T51.8X3	T51.8X4	—	—
Antifungal						
antibiotic (systemic)	T36.7X1	T36.7X2	T36.7X3	T36.7X4	T36.7X5	T36.7X6
anti-infective NEC	T37.91	T37.92	T37.93	T37.94	T37.95	T37.96
disinfectant, local	T49.0X1	T49.0X2	T49.0X3	T49.0X4	T49.0X5	T49.0X6
nonmedicinal (spray)	T60.3X1	T60.3X2	T60.3X3	T60.3X4	—	—
topical	T49.0X1	T49.0X2	T49.0X3	T49.0X4	T49.0X5	T49.0X6
Anti-gastric-secretion drug NEC	T47.1X1	T47.1X2	T47.1X3	T47.1X4	T47.1X5	T47.1X6
Antigonadotrophin NEC	T38.6X1	T38.6X2	T38.6X3	T38.6X4	T38.6X5	T38.6X6
Antihallucinogen	T43.501	T43.502	T43.503	T43.504	T43.505	T43.506
Antihelmintics	T37.4X1	T37.4X2	T37.4X3	T37.4X4	T37.4X5	T37.4X6
Antihemophilic						
factor	T45.8X1	T45.8X2	T45.8X3	T45.8X4	T45.8X5	T45.8X6
fraction	T45.8X1	T45.8X2	T45.8X3	T45.8X4	T45.8X5	T45.8X6
globulin concentrate	T45.7X1	T45.7X2	T45.7X3	T45.7X4	T45.7X5	T45.7X6
human plasma	T45.8X1	T45.8X2	T45.8X3	T45.8X4	T45.8X5	T45.8X6
plasma, dried	T45.7X1	T45.7X2	T45.7X3	T45.7X4	T45.7X5	T45.7X6
Antihemorrhoidal preparation	T49.2X1	T49.2X2	T49.2X3	T49.2X4	T49.2X5	T49.2X6
Antiheparin drug	T45.7X1	T45.7X2	T45.7X3	T45.7X4	T45.7X5	T45.7X6
Antihistamine	T45.0X1	T45.0X2	T45.0X3	T45.0X4	T45.0X5	T45.0X6
Antihookworm drug	T37.4X1	T37.4X2	T37.4X3	T37.4X4	T37.4X5	T37.4X6
Anti-human lymphocytic globulin	T50.Z11	T50.Z12	T50.Z13	T50.Z14	T50.Z15	T50.Z16
Antihyperlipidemic drug	T46.6X1	T46.6X2	T46.6X3	T46.6X4	T46.6X5	T46.6X6
Antihypertensive drug NEC	T46.5X1	T46.5X2	T46.5X3	T46.5X4	T46.5X5	T46.5X6
Anti-infective NEC	T37.91	T37.92	T37.93	T37.94	T37.95	T37.96
anthelmintic	T37.4X1	T37.4X2	T37.4X3	T37.4X4	T37.4X5	T37.4X6
antibiotics	T36.91	T36.92	T36.93	T36.94	T36.95	T36.96
specified NEC	T36.8X1	T36.8X2	T36.8X3	T36.8X4	T36.8X5	T36.8X6
antimalarial	T37.2X1	T37.2X2	T37.2X3	T37.2X4	T37.2X5	T37.2X6
antimycobacterial NEC	T37.1X1	T37.1X2	T37.1X3	T37.1X4	T37.1X5	T37.1X6
antibiotics	T36.5X1	T36.5X2	T36.5X3	T36.5X4	T36.5X5	T36.5X6
antiprotozoal NEC	T37.3X1	T37.3X2	T37.3X3	T37.3X4	T37.3X5	T37.3X6
blood	T37.2X1	T37.2X2	T37.2X3	T37.2X4	T37.2X5	T37.2X6
antiviral	T37.5X1	T37.5X2	T37.5X3	T37.5X4	T37.5X5	T37.5X6
arsenical	T37.8X1	T37.8X2	T37.8X3	T37.8X4	T37.8X5	T37.8X6
bismuth, local	T49.0X1	T49.0X2	T49.0X3	T49.0X4	T49.0X5	T49.0X6
ENT	T49.6X1	T49.6X2	T49.6X3	T49.6X4	T49.6X5	T49.6X6
eye NEC	T49.5X1	T49.5X2	T49.5X3	T49.5X4	T49.5X5	T49.5X6
heavy metals NEC	T37.8X1	T37.8X2	T37.8X3	T37.8X4	T37.8X5	T37.8X6

Substance	Poisoning, Accidental (unintentional)	Poisoning, Intentional self-harm	Poisoning, Assault	Poisoning, Undetermined	Adverse effect	Underdosing
Anti-infective NEC — *Continued*						
local NEC	T49.0X1	T49.0X2	T49.0X3	T49.0X4	T49.0X5	T49.0X6
specified NEC	T49.0X1	T49.0X2	T49.0X3	T49.0X4	T49.0X5	T49.0X6
mixed	T37.91	T37.92	T37.93	T37.94	T37.95	T37.96
ophthalmic preparation	T49.5X1	T49.5X2	T49.5X3	T49.5X4	T49.5X5	T49.5X6
topical NEC	T49.0X1	T49.0X2	T49.0X3	T49.0X4	T49.0X5	T49.0X6
Anti-inflammatory drug NEC	T39.391	T39.392	T39.393	T39.394	T39.395	T39.396
local	T49.0X1	T49.0X2	T49.0X3	T49.0X4	T49.0X5	T49.0X6
nonsteroidal NEC	T39.391	T39.392	T39.393	T39.394	T39.395	T39.396
propionic acid derivative	T39.311	T39.312	T39.313	T39.314	T39.315	T39.316
specified NEC	T39.391	T39.392	T39.393	T39.394	T39.395	T39.396
Antikaluretic	T50.3X1	T50.3X2	T50.3X3	T50.3X4	T50.3X5	T50.3X6
Antiknock (tetraethyl lead)	T56.0X1	T56.0X2	T56.0X3	T56.0X4	—	—
Antilipemic drug NEC	T46.6X1	T46.6X2	T46.6X3	T46.6X4	T46.6X5	T46.6X6
Antimalarial	T37.2X1	T37.2X2	T37.2X3	T37.2X4	T37.2X5	T37.2X6
prophylactic NEC	T37.2X1	T37.2X2	T37.2X3	T37.2X4	T37.2X5	T37.2X6
pyrimidine derivative	T37.2X1	T37.2X2	T37.2X3	T37.2X4	T37.2X5	T37.2X6
Antimetabolite	T45.1X1	T45.1X2	T45.1X3	T45.1X4	T45.1X5	T45.1X6
Antimitotic agent	T45.1X1	T45.1X2	T45.1X3	T45.1X4	T45.1X5	T45.1X6
Antimony (compounds) (vapor)NEC	T56.891	T56.892	T56.893	T56.894	—	—
anti-infectives	T37.8X1	T37.8X2	T37.8X3	T37.8X4	T37.8X5	T37.8X6
dimercaptosuccinate	T37.3X1	T37.3X2	T37.3X3	T37.3X4	T37.3X5	T37.3X6
hydride	T56.891	T56.892	T56.893	T56.894	—	—
pesticide (vapor)	T60.8X1	T60.8X2	T60.8X3	T60.8X4	—	—
potassium (sodium) tartrate	T37.8X1	T37.8X2	T37.8X3	T37.8X4	T37.8X5	T37.8X6
sodium dimercaptosuccinate	T37.3X1	T37.3X2	T37.3X3	T37.3X4	T37.3X5	T37.3X6
tartrated	T37.8X1	T37.8X2	T37.8X3	T37.8X4	T37.8X5	T37.8X6
Antimuscarinic NEC	T44.3X1	T44.3X2	T44.3X3	T44.3X4	T44.3X5	T44.3X6
Antimycobacterial drug NEC	T37.1X1	T37.1X2	T37.1X3	T37.1X4	T37.1X5	T37.1X6
antibiotics	T36.5X1	T36.5X2	T36.5X3	T36.5X4	T36.5X5	T36.5X6
combination	T37.1X1	T37.1X2	T37.1X3	T37.1X4	T37.1X5	T37.1X6
Antinausea drug	T45.0X1	T45.0X2	T45.0X3	T45.0X4	T45.0X5	T45.0X6
Antinematode drug	T37.4X1	T37.4X2	T37.4X3	T37.4X4	T37.4X5	T37.4X6
Antineoplastic NEC	T45.1X1	T45.1X2	T45.1X3	T45.1X4	T45.1X5	T45.1X6
alkaloidal	T45.1X1	T45.1X2	T45.1X3	T45.1X4	T45.1X5	T45.1X6
antibiotics	T45.1X1	T45.1X2	T45.1X3	T45.1X4	T45.1X5	T45.1X6
combination	T45.1X1	T45.1X2	T45.1X3	T45.1X4	T45.1X5	T45.1X6
estrogen	T38.5X1	T38.5X2	T38.5X3	T38.5X4	T38.5X5	T38.5X6
steroid	T38.7X1	T38.7X2	T38.7X3	T38.7X4	T38.7X5	T38.7X6
Antiparasitic drug (systemic)	T37.91	T37.92	T37.93	T37.94	T37.95	T37.96
local	T49.0X1	T49.0X2	T49.0X3	T49.0X4	T49.0X5	T49.0X6
specified NEC	T37.8X1	T37.8X2	T37.8X3	T37.8X4	T37.8X5	T37.8X6
Antiparkinsonism drug NEC	T42.8X1	T42.8X2	T42.8X3	T42.8X4	T42.8X5	T42.8X6
Antiperspirant NEC	T49.2X1	T49.2X2	T49.2X3	T49.2X4	T49.2X5	T49.2X6
Antiphlogistic NEC	T39.4X1	T39.4X2	T39.4X3	T39.4X4	T39.4X5	T39.4X6
Antiplatyhelmintic drug	T37.4X1	T37.4X2	T37.4X3	T37.4X4	T37.4X5	T37.4X6
Antiprotozoal drug NEC	T37.3X1	T37.3X2	T37.3X3	T37.3X4	T37.3X5	T37.3X6
blood	T37.2X1	T37.2X2	T37.2X3	T37.2X4	T37.2X5	T37.2X6
local	T49.0X1	T49.0X2	T49.0X3	T49.0X4	T49.0X5	T49.0X6
Antipruritic drug NEC	T49.1X1	T49.1X2	T49.1X3	T49.1X4	T49.1X5	T49.1X6
Antipsychotic drug	T43.501	T43.502	T43.503	T43.504	T43.505	T43.506
specified NEC	T43.591	T43.592	T43.593	T43.594	T43.595	T43.596
Antipyretic	T39.91	T39.92	T39.93	T39.94	T39.95	T39.96
specified NEC	T39.8X1	T39.8X2	T39.8X3	T39.8X4	T39.8X5	T39.8X6
Antipyrine	T39.2X1	T39.2X2	T39.2X3	T39.2X4	T39.2X5	T39.2X6
Antirabies hyperimmune serum	T50.Z11	T50.Z12	T50.Z13	T50.Z14	T50.Z15	T50.Z16
Antirheumatic NEC	T39.4X1	T39.4X2	T39.4X3	T39.4X4	T39.4X5	T39.4X6
Antirigidity drug NEC	T42.8X1	T42.8X2	T42.8X3	T42.8X4	T42.8X5	T42.8X6
Antischistosomal drug	T37.4X1	T37.4X2	T37.4X3	T37.4X4	T37.4X5	T37.4X6
Antiscorpion sera	T50.Z11	T50.Z12	T50.Z13	T50.Z14	T50.Z15	T50.Z16
Antiseborrheics	T49.4X1	T49.4X2	T49.4X3	T49.4X4	T49.4X5	T49.4X6
Antiseptics (external) (medicinal)	T49.0X1	T49.0X2	T49.0X3	T49.0X4	T49.0X5	T49.0X6
Antistine	T45.0X1	T45.0X2	T45.0X3	T45.0X4	T45.0X5	T45.0X6
Antitapeworm drug	T37.4X1	T37.4X2	T37.4X3	T37.4X4	T37.4X5	T37.4X6
Antitetanus immunoglobulin	T50.Z11	T50.Z12	T50.Z13	T50.Z14	T50.Z15	T50.Z16
Antithrombotic	T45.521	T45.522	T45.523	T45.524	T45.525	T45.526
Antithyroid drug NEC	T38.2X1	T38.2X2	T38.2X3	T38.2X4	T38.2X5	T38.2X6
Antitoxin	T50.Z11	T50.Z12	T50.Z13	T50.Z14	T50.Z15	T50.Z16
diphtheria	T50.Z11	T50.Z12	T50.Z13	T50.Z14	T50.Z15	T50.Z16
gas gangrene	T50.Z11	T50.Z12	T50.Z13	T50.Z14	T50.Z15	T50.Z16
tetanus	T50.Z11	T50.Z12	T50.Z13	T50.Z14	T50.Z15	T50.Z16
Antitrichomonal drug	T37.3X1	T37.3X2	T37.3X3	T37.3X4	T37.3X5	T37.3X6
Antituberculars	T37.1X1	T37.1X2	T37.1X3	T37.1X4	T37.1X5	T37.1X6
antibiotics	T36.5X1	T36.5X2	T36.5X3	T36.5X4	T36.5X5	T36.5X6
Antitussive NEC	T48.3X1	T48.3X2	T48.3X3	T48.3X4	T48.3X5	T48.3X6
codeine mixture	T40.2X1	T40.2X2	T40.2X3	T40.2X4	T40.2X5	T40.2X6
opiate	T40.2X1	T40.2X2	T40.2X3	T40.2X4	T40.2X5	T40.2X6
Antivaricose drug	T46.8X1	T46.8X2	T46.8X3	T46.8X4	T46.8X5	T46.8X6
Antivenin, antivenom (sera)	T50.Z11	T50.Z12	T50.Z13	T50.Z14	T50.Z15	T50.Z16
crotaline	T50.Z11	T50.Z12	T50.Z13	T50.Z14	T50.Z15	T50.Z16
spider bite	T50.Z11	T50.Z12	T50.Z13	T50.Z14	T50.Z15	T50.Z16
Antivertigo drug	T45.0X1	T45.0X2	T45.0X3	T45.0X4	T45.0X5	T45.0X6
Antiviral drug NEC	T37.5X1	T37.5X2	T37.5X3	T37.5X4	T37.5X5	T37.5X6
eye	T49.5X1	T49.5X2	T49.5X3	T49.5X4	T49.5X5	T49.5X6
Antiwhipworm drug	T37.4X1	T37.4X2	T37.4X3	T37.4X4	T37.4X5	T37.4X6
Antrol—see also by specific chemical substance	T60.91	T60.92	T60.93	T60.94	—	—
fungicide	T60.91	T60.92	T60.93	T60.94	—	—
ANTU (alpha naphthylthiourea)	T60.4X1	T60.4X2	T60.4X3	T60.4X4	—	—
Apalcillin	T36.0X1	T36.0X2	T36.0X3	T36.0X4	T36.0X5	T36.0X6

Substance	Poisoning, Accidental (unintentional)	Poisoning, Intentional self-harm	Poisoning, Assault	Poisoning, Undetermined	Adverse effect	Underdosing
APC	T48.5X1	T48.5X2	T48.5X3	T48.5X4	T48.5X5	T48.5X6
Aplonidine	T44.4X1	T44.4X2	T44.4X3	T44.4X4	T44.4X5	T44.4X6
Apomorphine	T47.7X1	T47.7X2	T47.7X3	T47.7X4	T47.7X5	T47.7X6
Appetite depressants, central	T50.5X1	T50.5X2	T50.5X3	T50.5X4	T50.5X5	T50.5X6
Apraclonidine (hydrochloride)	T44.4X1	T44.4X2	T44.4X3	T44.4X4	T44.4X5	T44.4X6
Apresoline	T46.5X1	T46.5X2	T46.5X3	T46.5X4	T46.5X5	T46.5X6
Aprindine	T46.2X1	T46.2X2	T46.2X3	T46.2X4	T46.2X5	T46.2X6
Aprobarbital	T42.3X1	T42.3X2	T42.3X3	T42.3X4	T42.3X5	T42.3X6
Apronalide	T42.6X1	T42.6X2	T42.6X3	T42.6X4	T42.6X5	T42.6X6
Aprotinin	T45.621	T45.622	T45.623	T45.624	T45.625	T45.626
Aptocaine	T41.3X1	T41.3X2	T41.3X3	T41.3X4	T41.3X5	T41.3X6
Aqua fortis	T54.2X1	T54.2X2	T54.2X3	T54.2X4	—	—
Ara-A	T37.5X1	T37.5X2	T37.5X3	T37.5X4	T37.5X5	T37.5X6
Ara-C	T45.1X1	T45.1X2	T45.1X3	T45.1X4	T45.1X5	T45.1X6
Arachis oil	T49.3X1	T49.3X2	T49.3X3	T49.3X4	T49.3X5	T49.3X6
cathartic	T47.4X1	T47.4X2	T47.4X3	T47.4X4	T47.4X5	T47.4X6
Aralen	T37.2X1	T37.2X2	T37.2X3	T37.2X4	T37.2X5	T37.2X6
Arecoline	T44.1X1	T44.1X2	T44.1X3	T44.1X4	T44.1X5	T44.1X6
Arginine	T50.991	T50.992	T50.993	T50.994	T50.995	T50.996
glutamate	T50.991	T50.992	T50.993	T50.994	T50.995	T50.996
Argyrol	T49.0X1	T49.0X2	T49.0X3	T49.0X4	T49.0X5	T49.0X6
ENT agent	T49.6X1	T49.6X2	T49.6X3	T49.6X4	T49.6X5	T49.6X6
ophthalmic preparation	T49.5X1	T49.5X2	T49.5X3	T49.5X4	T49.5X5	T49.5X6
Aristocort	T38.0X1	T38.0X2	T38.0X3	T38.0X4	T38.0X5	T38.0X6
ENT agent	T49.6X1	T49.6X2	T49.6X3	T49.6X4	T49.6X5	T49.6X6
ophthalmic preparation	T49.5X1	T49.5X2	T49.5X3	T49.5X4	T49.5X5	T49.5X6
topical NEC	T49.0X1	T49.0X2	T49.0X3	T49.0X4	T49.0X5	T49.0X6
Aromatics, corrosive	T54.1X1	T54.1X2	T54.1X3	T54.1X4	—	—
disinfectants	T54.1X1	T54.1X2	T54.1X3	T54.1X4	—	—
Arsenate of lead	T57.0X1	T57.0X2	T57.0X3	T57.0X4	—	—
herbicide	T57.0X1	T57.0X2	T57.0X3	T57.0X4	—	—
Arsenic, arsenicals (compounds) (dust) (vapor) NEC	T57.0X1	T57.0X2	T57.0X3	T57.0X4	—	—
anti-infectives	T37.8X1	T37.8X2	T37.8X3	T37.8X4	T37.8X5	T37.8X6
pesticide (dust) (fumes)	T57.0X1	T57.0X2	T57.0X3	T57.0X4	—	—
Arsine (gas)	T57.0X1	T57.0X2	T57.0X3	T57.0X4	—	—
Arsphenamine (silver)	T37.8X1	T37.8X2	T37.8X3	T37.8X4	T37.8X5	T37.8X6
Arsthinol	T37.3X1	T37.3X2	T37.3X3	T37.3X4	T37.3X5	T37.3X6
Artane	T44.3X1	T44.3X2	T44.3X3	T44.3X4	T44.3X5	T44.3X6
Arthropod (venomous) NEC	T63.481	T63.482	T63.483	T63.484	—	—
Articaine	T41.3X1	T41.3X2	T41.3X3	T41.3X4	T41.3X5	T41.3X6
Asbestos	T57.8X1	T57.8X2	T57.8X3	T57.8X4	—	—
Ascaridole	T37.4X1	T37.4X2	T37.4X3	T37.4X4	T37.4X5	T37.4X6
Ascorbic acid	T45.2X1	T45.2X2	T45.2X3	T45.2X4	T45.2X5	T45.2X6
Asiaticoside	T49.0X1	T49.0X2	T49.0X3	T49.0X4	T49.0X5	T49.0X6
Asparaginase	T45.1X1	T45.1X2	T45.1X3	T45.1X4	T45.1X5	T45.1X6
Aspidium (oleoresin)	T37.4X1	T37.4X2	T37.4X3	T37.4X4	T37.4X5	T37.4X6

Substance	Poisoning, Accidental (unintentional)	Poisoning, Intentional self-harm	Poisoning, Assault	Poisoning, Undetermined	Adverse effect	Underdosing
Aspirin (aluminum) (soluble)	T39.011	T39.012	T39.013	T39.014	T39.015	T39.016
Aspoxicillin	T36.0X1	T36.0X2	T36.0X3	T36.0X4	T36.0X5	T36.0X6
Astemizole	T45.0X1	T45.0X2	T45.0X3	T45.0X4	T45.0X5	T45.0X6
Astringent (local)	T49.2X1	T49.2X2	T49.2X3	T49.2X4	T49.2X5	T49.2X6
specified NEC	T49.2X1	T49.2X2	T49.2X3	T49.2X4	T49.2X5	T49.2X6
Astromicin	T36.5X1	T36.5X2	T36.5X3	T36.5X4	T36.5X5	T36.5X6
Ataractic drug NEC	T43.501	T43.502	T43.503	T43.504	T43.505	T43.506
Atenolol	T44.7X1	T44.7X2	T44.7X3	T44.7X4	T44.7X5	T44.7X6
Atonia drug, intestinal	T47.4X1	T47.4X2	T47.4X3	T47.4X4	T47.4X5	T47.4X6
Atophan	T50.4X1	T50.4X2	T50.4X3	T50.4X4	T50.4X5	T50.4X6
Atracurium besilate	T48.1X1	T48.1X2	T48.1X3	T48.1X4	T48.1X5	T48.1X6
Atropine	T44.3X1	T44.3X2	T44.3X3	T44.3X4	T44.3X5	T44.3X6
derivative	T44.3X1	T44.3X2	T44.3X3	T44.3X4	T44.3X5	T44.3X6
methonitrate	T44.3X1	T44.3X2	T44.3X3	T44.3X4	T44.3X5	T44.3X6
Attapulgite	T47.6X1	T47.6X2	T47.6X3	T47.6X4	T47.6X5	T47.6X6
Auramine	T65.891	T65.892	T65.893	T65.894	—	—
dye	T65.6X1	T65.6X2	T65.6X3	T65.6X4	—	—
fungicide	T60.3X1	T60.3X2	T60.3X3	T60.3X4	—	—
Auranofin	T39.4X1	T39.4X2	T39.4X3	T39.4X4	T39.4X5	T39.4X6
Aurantiin	T46.991	T46.992	T46.993	T46.994	T46.995	T46.996
Aureomycin	T36.4X1	T36.4X2	T36.4X3	T36.4X4	T36.4X5	T36.4X6
ophthalmic preparation	T49.5X1	T49.5X2	T49.5X3	T49.5X4	T49.5X5	T49.5X6
topical NEC	T49.0X1	T49.0X2	T49.0X3	T49.0X4	T49.0X5	T49.0X6
Aurothioglucose	T39.4X1	T39.4X2	T39.4X3	T39.4X4	T39.4X5	T39.4X6
Aurothioglycanide	T39.4X1	T39.4X2	T39.4X3	T39.4X4	T39.4X5	T39.4X6
Aurothiomalate sodium	T39.4X1	T39.4X2	T39.4X3	T39.4X4	T39.4X5	T39.4X6
Aurotioprol	T39.4X1	T39.4X2	T39.4X3	T39.4X4	T39.4X5	T39.4X6
Automobile fuel	T52.0X1	T52.0X2	T52.0X3	T52.0X4	—	—
Autonomic nervous system agent NEC	T44.901	T44.902	T44.903	T44.904	T44.905	T44.906
Avlosulfon	T37.1X1	T37.1X2	T37.1X3	T37.1X4	T37.1X5	T37.1X6
Avomine	T42.6X1	T42.6X2	T42.6X3	T42.6X4	T42.6X5	T42.6X6
Axerophthol	T45.2X1	T45.2X2	T45.2X3	T45.2X4	T45.2X5	T45.2X6
Azacitidine	T45.1X1	T45.1X2	T45.1X3	T45.1X4	T45.1X5	T45.1X6
Azacyclonol	T43.591	T43.592	T43.593	T43.594	T43.595	T43.596
Azadirachta	T60.2X1	T60.2X2	T60.2X3	T60.2X4	—	—
Azanidazole	T37.3X1	T37.3X2	T37.3X3	T37.3X4	T37.3X5	T37.3X6
Azapetine	T46.7X1	T46.7X2	T46.7X3	T46.7X4	T46.7X5	T46.7X6
Azapropazone	T39.2X1	T39.2X2	T39.2X3	T39.2X4	T39.2X5	T39.2X6
Azaribine	T45.1X1	T45.1X2	T45.1X3	T45.1X4	T45.1X5	T45.1X6
Azaserine	T45.1X1	T45.1X2	T45.1X3	T45.1X4	T45.1X5	T45.1X6
Azatadine	T45.0X1	T45.0X2	T45.0X3	T45.0X4	T45.0X5	T45.0X6
Azatepa	T45.1X1	T45.1X2	T45.1X3	T45.1X4	T45.1X5	T45.1X6
Azathioprine	T45.1X1	T45.1X2	T45.1X3	T45.1X4	T45.1X5	T45.1X6
Azelaic acid	T49.0X1	T49.0X2	T49.0X3	T49.0X4	T49.0X5	T49.0X6
Azelastine	T45.0X1	T45.0X2	T45.0X3	T45.0X4	T45.0X5	T45.0X6
Azidocillin	T36.0X1	T36.0X2	T36.0X3	T36.0X4	T36.0X5	T36.0X6
Azidothymidine	T37.5X1	T37.5X2	T37.5X3	T37.5X4	T37.5X5	T37.5X6

Substance	Poisoning, Accidental (unintentional)	Poisoning, Intentional self-harm	Poisoning, Assault	Poisoning, Undetermined	Adverse effect	Underdosing
Azinphos (ethyl) (methyl)	T60.0X1	T60.0X2	T60.0X3	T60.0X4	—	—
Aziridine (chelating)	T54.1X1	T54.1X2	T54.1X3	T54.1X4	—	—
Azithromycin	T36.3X1	T36.3X2	T36.3X3	T36.3X4	T36.3X5	T36.3X6
Azlocillin	T36.0X1	T36.0X2	T36.0X3	T36.0X4	T36.0X5	T36.0X6
Azobenzene smoke	T65.3X1	T65.3X2	T65.3X3	T65.3X4	—	—
acaricide	T60.8X1	T60.8X2	T60.8X3	T60.8X4	—	—
Azosulfamide	T37.0X1	T37.0X2	T37.0X3	T37.0X4	T37.0X5	T37.0X6
AZT	T37.5X1	T37.5X2	T37.5X3	T37.5X4	T37.5X5	T37.5X6
Aztreonam	T36.1X1	T36.1X2	T36.1X3	T36.1X4	T36.1X5	T36.1X6
Azulfidine	T37.0X1	T37.0X2	T37.0X3	T37.0X4	T37.0X5	T37.0X6
Azuresin	T50.8X1	T50.8X2	T50.8X3	T50.8X4	T50.8X5	T50.8X6
B						
Bacampicillin	T36.0X1	T36.0X2	T36.0X3	T36.0X4	T36.0X5	T36.0X6
Bacillus						
lactobacillus	T47.8X1	T47.8X2	T47.8X3	T47.8X4	T47.8X5	T47.8X6
subtilis	T47.6X1	T47.6X2	T47.6X3	T47.6X4	T47.6X5	T47.6X6
Bacimycin	T49.0X1	T49.0X2	T49.0X3	T49.0X4	T49.0X5	T49.0X6
ophthalmic preparation	T49.5X1	T49.5X2	T49.5X3	T49.5X4	T49.5X5	T49.5X6
Bacitracin zinc	T49.0X1	T49.0X2	T49.0X3	T49.0X4	T49.0X5	T49.0X6
with neomycin	T49.0X1	T49.0X2	T49.0X3	T49.0X4	T49.0X5	T49.0X6
ENT agent	T49.6X1	T49.6X2	T49.6X3	T49.6X4	T49.6X5	T49.6X6
ophthalmic preparation	T49.5X1	T49.5X2	T49.5X3	T49.5X4	T49.5X5	T49.5X6
topical NEC	T49.0X1	T49.0X2	T49.0X3	T49.0X4	T49.0X5	T49.0X6
Baclofen	T42.8X1	T42.8X2	T42.8X3	T42.8X4	T42.8X5	T42.8X6
Baking soda	T50.991	T50.992	T50.993	T50.994	T50.995	T50.996
BAL	T45.8X1	T45.8X2	T45.8X3	T45.8X4	T45.8X5	T45.8X6
Bambuterol	T48.6X1	T48.6X2	T48.6X3	T48.6X4	T48.6X5	T48.6X6
Bamethan (sulfate)	T46.7X1	T46.7X2	T46.7X3	T46.7X4	T46.7X5	T46.7X6
Bamifylline	T48.6X1	T48.6X2	T48.6X3	T48.6X4	T48.6X5	T48.6X6
Bamipine	T45.0X1	T45.0X2	T45.0X3	T45.0X4	T45.0X5	T45.0X6
Baneberry—see Actauseea spicata						
Banewort—see Belladonna						
Barbenyl	T42.3X1	T42.3X2	T42.3X3	T42.3X4	T42.3X5	T42.3X6
Barbexaclone	T42.6X1	T42.6X2	T42.6X3	T42.6X4	T42.6X5	T42.6X6
Barbital	T42.3X1	T42.3X2	T42.3X3	T42.3X4	T42.3X5	T42.3X6
sodium	T42.3X1	T42.3X2	T42.3X3	T42.3X4	T42.3X5	T42.3X6
Barbitone	T42.3X1	T42.3X2	T42.3X3	T42.3X4	T42.3X5	T42.3X6
Barbiturate NEC	T42.3X1	T42.3X2	T42.3X3	T42.3X4	T42.3X5	T42.3X6
with tranquilizer	T42.3X1	T42.3X2	T42.3X3	T42.3X4	T42.3X5	T42.3X6
anesthetic (intravenous)	T41.1X1	T41.1X2	T41.1X3	T41.1X4	T41.1X5	T41.1X6
Barium (carbonate) (chloride) (sulfite)	T57.8X1	T57.8X2	T57.8X3	T57.8X4	—	—
diagnostic agent	T50.8X1	T50.8X2	T50.8X3	T50.8X4	T50.8X5	T50.8X6
pesticide	T60.4X1	T60.4X2	T60.4X3	T60.4X4	—	—
rodenticide	T60.4X1	T60.4X2	T60.4X3	T60.4X4	—	—
sulfate (medicinal)	T50.8X1	T50.8X2	T50.8X3	T50.8X4	T50.8X5	T50.8X6
Barrier cream	T49.3X1	T49.3X2	T49.3X3	T49.3X4	T49.3X5	T49.3X6
Basic fuchsin	T49.0X1	T49.0X2	T49.0X3	T49.0X4	T49.0X5	T49.0X6

Substance	Poisoning, Accidental (unintentional)	Poisoning, Intentional self-harm	Poisoning, Assault	Poisoning, Undetermined	Adverse effect	Underdosing
Battery acid or fluid	T54.2X1	T54.2X2	T54.2X3	T54.2X4	—	—
Bay rum	T51.8X1	T51.8X2	T51.8X3	T51.8X4	—	—
BCG (vaccine)	T50.A91	T50.A92	T50.A93	T50.A94	T50.A95	T50.A96
BCNU	T45.1X1	T45.1X2	T45.1X3	T45.1X4	T45.1X5	T45.1X6
Bearsfoot	T62.2X1	T62.2X2	T62.2X3	T62.2X4	—	—
Beclamide	T42.6X1	T42.6X2	T42.6X3	T42.6X4	T42.6X5	T42.6X6
Beclomethasone	T44.5X1	T44.5X2	T44.5X3	T44.5X4	T44.5X5	T44.5X6
Bee (sting) (venom)	T63.441	T63.442	T63.443	T63.444	—	—
Befunolol	T49.5X1	T49.5X2	T49.5X3	T49.5X4	T49.5X5	T49.5X6
Bekanamycin	T36.5X1	T36.5X2	T36.5X3	T36.5X4	T36.5X5	T36.5X6
Belladonna—see also Nightshade						
alkaloids	T44.3X1	T44.3X2	T44.3X3	T44.3X4	T44.3X5	T44.3X6
extract	T44.3X1	T44.3X2	T44.3X3	T44.3X4	T44.3X5	T44.3X6
herb	T44.3X1	T44.3X2	T44.3X3	T44.3X4	T44.3X5	T44.3X6
Bemegride	T50.7X1	T50.7X2	T50.7X3	T50.7X4	T50.7X5	T50.7X6
Benactyzine	T44.3X1	T44.3X2	T44.3X3	T44.3X4	T44.3X5	T44.3X6
Benadryl	T45.0X1	T45.0X2	T45.0X3	T45.0X4	T45.0X5	T45.0X6
Benaprizine	T44.3X1	T44.3X2	T44.3X3	T44.3X4	T44.3X5	T44.3X6
Benazepril	T46.4X1	T46.4X2	T46.4X3	T46.4X4	T46.4X5	T46.4X6
Bencyclane	T46.7X1	T46.7X2	T46.7X3	T46.7X4	T46.7X5	T46.7X6
Bendazol	T46.3X1	T46.3X2	T46.3X3	T46.3X4	T46.3X5	T46.3X6
Bendrofluazide	T50.2X1	T50.2X2	T50.2X3	T50.2X4	T50.2X5	T50.2X6
Bendroflumethiazide	T50.2X1	T50.2X2	T50.2X3	T50.2X4	T50.2X5	T50.2X6
Benemid	T50.4X1	T50.4X2	T50.4X3	T50.4X4	T50.4X5	T50.4X6
Benethamine penicillin	T36.0X1	T36.0X2	T36.0X3	T36.0X4	T36.0X5	T36.0X6
Benexate	T47.1X1	T47.1X2	T47.1X3	T47.1X4	T47.1X5	T47.1X6
Benfluorex	T46.6X1	T46.6X2	T46.6X3	T46.6X4	T46.6X5	T46.6X6
Benfotiamine	T45.2X1	T45.2X2	T45.2X3	T45.2X4	T45.2X5	T45.2X6
Benisone	T49.0X1	T49.0X2	T49.0X3	T49.0X4	T49.0X5	T49.0X6
Benomyl	T60.0X1	T60.0X2	T60.0X3	T60.0X4	—	—
Benoquin	T49.8X1	T49.8X2	T49.8X3	T49.8X4	T49.8X5	T49.8X6
Benoxinate	T41.3X1	T41.3X2	T41.3X3	T41.3X4	T41.3X5	T41.3X6
Benperidol	T43.4X1	T43.4X2	T43.4X3	T43.4X4	T43.4X5	T43.4X6
Benproperine	T48.3X1	T48.3X2	T48.3X3	T48.3X4	T48.3X5	T48.3X6
Benserazide	T42.8X1	T42.8X2	T42.8X3	T42.8X4	T42.8X5	T42.8X6
Bentazepam	T42.4X1	T42.4X2	T42.4X3	T42.4X4	T42.4X5	T42.4X6
Bentiromide	T50.8X1	T50.8X2	T50.8X3	T50.8X4	T50.8X5	T50.8X6
Bentonite	T49.3X1	T49.3X2	T49.3X3	T49.3X4	T49.3X5	T49.3X6
Benzalbutyramide	T46.6X1	T46.6X2	T46.6X3	T46.6X4	T46.6X5	T46.6X6
Benzalkonium (chloride)	T49.0X1	T49.0X2	T49.0X3	T49.0X4	T49.0X5	T49.0X6
ophthalmic preparation	T49.5X1	T49.5X2	T49.5X3	T49.5X4	T49.5X5	T49.5X6
Benzamidosali cylate (calcium)	T37.1X1	T37.1X2	T37.1X3	T37.1X4	T37.1X5	T37.1X6
Benzamine	T41.3X1	T41.3X2	T41.3X3	T41.3X4	T41.3X5	T41.3X6
lactate	T49.1X1	T49.1X2	T49.1X3	T49.1X4	T49.1X5	T49.1X6
Benzamphetamine	T50.5X1	T50.5X2	T50.5X3	T50.5X4	T50.5X5	T50.5X6
Benzapril hydrochloride	T46.5X1	T46.5X2	T46.5X3	T46.5X4	T46.5X5	T46.5X6
Benzathine benzylpenicillin	T36.0X1	T36.0X2	T36.0X3	T36.0X4	T36.0X5	T36.0X6
Benzathine penicillin	T36.0X1	T36.0X2	T36.0X3	T36.0X4	T36.0X5	T36.0X6

Table of Drugs and Chemicals

Substance	Poisoning, Accidental (unintentional)	Poisoning, Intentional self-harm	Poisoning, Assault	Poisoning, Undetermined	Adverse effect	Underdosing
Benzatropine	T42.8X1	T42.8X2	T42.8X3	T42.8X4	T42.8X5	T42.8X6
Benzbromarone	T50.4X1	T50.4X2	T50.4X3	T50.4X4	T50.4X5	T50.4X6
Benzcarbimine	T45.1X1	T45.1X2	T45.1X3	T45.1X4	T45.1X5	T45.1X6
Benzedrex	T44.991	T44.992	T44.993	T44.994	T44.995	T44.996
Benzedrine (amphetamine)	T43.621	T43.622	T43.623	T43.624	T43.625	T43.626
Benzenamine	T65.3X1	T65.3X2	T65.3X3	T65.3X4	—	—
Benzene	T52.1X1	T52.1X2	T52.1X3	T52.1X4		
homologues (acetyl) (dimethyl) (methyl) (solvent)	T52.2X1	T52.2X2	T52.2X3	T52.2X4	—	—
Benzethonium (chloride)	T49.0X1	T49.0X2	T49.0X3	T49.0X4	T49.0X5	T49.0X6
Benzfetamine	T50.5X1	T50.5X2	T50.5X3	T50.5X4	T50.5X5	T50.5X6
Benzhexol	T44.3X1	T44.3X2	T44.3X3	T44.3X4	T44.3X5	T44.3X6
Benzhydramine (chloride)	T45.0X1	T45.0X2	T45.0X3	T45.0X4	T45.0X5	T45.0X6
Benzidine	T65.891	T65.892	T65.893	T65.894	—	—
Benzilonium bromide	T44.3X1	T44.3X2	T44.3X3	T44.3X4	T44.3X5	T44.3X6
Benzimidazole	T60.3X1	T60.3X2	T60.3X3	T60.3X4	—	—
Benzin(e)—see Ligroin						
Benziodarone	T46.3X1	T46.3X2	T46.3X3	T46.3X4	T46.3X5	T46.3X6
Benznidazole	T37.3X1	T37.3X2	T37.3X3	T37.3X4	T37.3X5	T37.3X6
Benzocaine	T41.3X1	T41.3X2	T41.3X3	T41.3X4	T41.3X5	T41.3X6
Benzodiapin	T42.4X1	T42.4X2	T42.4X3	T42.4X4	T42.4X5	T42.4X6
Benzodiazepine NEC	T42.4X1	T42.4X2	T42.4X3	T42.4X4	T42.4X5	T42.4X6
Benzoic acid	T49.0X1	T49.0X2	T49.0X3	T49.0X4	T49.0X5	T49.0X6
with salicylic acid	T49.0X1	T49.0X2	T49.0X3	T49.0X4	T49.0X5	T49.0X6
Benzoin (tincture)	T48.5X1	T48.5X2	T48.5X3	T48.5X4	T48.5X5	T48.5X6
Benzol (benzene)	T52.1X1	T52.1X2	T52.1X3	T52.1X4	—	—
vapor	T52.0X1	T52.0X2	T52.0X3	T52.0X4	—	—
Benzomorphan	T40.2X1	T40.2X2	T40.2X3	T40.2X4	T40.2X5	T40.2X6
Benzonatate	T48.3X1	T48.3X2	T48.3X3	T48.3X4	T48.3X5	T48.3X6
Benzophenones	T49.3X1	T49.3X2	T49.3X3	T49.3X4	T49.3X5	T49.3X6
Benzopyrone	T46.991	T46.992	T46.993	T46.994	T46.995	T46.996
Benzothiadiazides	T50.2X1	T50.2X2	T50.2X3	T50.2X4	T50.2X5	T50.2X6
Benzoxonium chloride	T49.0X1	T49.0X2	T49.0X3	T49.0X4	T49.0X5	T49.0X6
Benzoyl peroxide	T49.0X1	T49.0X2	T49.0X3	T49.0X4	T49.0X5	T49.0X6
Benzoylpas calcium	T37.1X1	T37.1X2	T37.1X3	T37.1X4	T37.1X5	T37.1X6
Benzperidin	T43.591	T43.592	T43.593	T43.594	T43.595	T43.596
Benzperidol	T43.591	T43.592	T43.593	T43.594	T43.595	T43.596
Benzphetamine	T50.5X1	T50.5X2	T50.5X3	T50.5X4	T50.5X5	T50.5X6
Benzpyrinium bromide	T44.1X1	T44.1X2	T44.1X3	T44.1X4	T44.1X5	T44.1X6
Benzquinamide	T45.0X1	T45.0X2	T45.0X3	T45.0X4	T45.0X5	T45.0X6
Benzthiazide	T50.2X1	T50.2X2	T50.2X3	T50.2X4	T50.2X5	T50.2X6
Benztropine						
anticholinergic	T44.3X1	T44.3X2	T44.3X3	T44.3X4	T44.3X5	T44.3X6
antiparkinson	T42.8X1	T42.8X2	T42.8X3	T42.8X4	T42.8X5	T42.8X6
Benzydamine	T49.0X1	T49.0X2	T49.0X3	T49.0X4	T49.0X5	T49.0X6
Benzyl						
acetate	T52.8X1	T52.8X2	T52.8X3	T52.8X4	—	—
alcohol	T49.0X1	T49.0X2	T49.0X3	T49.0X4	T49.0X5	T49.0X6

Substance	Poisoning, Accidental (unintentional)	Poisoning, Intentional self-harm	Poisoning, Assault	Poisoning, Undetermined	Adverse effect	Underdosing
Benzyl — Continued						
benzoate	T49.0X1	T49.0X2	T49.0X3	T49.0X4	T49.0X5	T49.0X6
Benzoic acid	T49.0X1	T49.0X2	T49.0X3	T49.0X4	T49.0X5	T49.0X6
morphine	T40.2X1	T40.2X2	T40.2X3	T40.2X4	—	—
nicotinate	T46.6X1	T46.6X2	T46.6X3	T46.6X4	T46.6X5	T46.6X6
penicillin	T36.0X1	T36.0X2	T36.0X3	T36.0X4	T36.0X5	T36.0X6
Benzylhydrochl-orthia-zide	T50.2X1	T50.2X2	T50.2X3	T50.2X4	T50.2X5	T50.2X6
Benzylpenicillin	T36.0X1	T36.0X2	T36.0X3	T36.0X4	T36.0X5	T36.0X6
Benzylthiouracil	T38.2X1	T38.2X2	T38.2X3	T38.2X4	T38.2X5	T38.2X6
Bephenium hydroxy-naphthoate	T37.4X1	T37.4X2	T37.4X3	T37.4X4	T37.4X5	T37.4X6
Bepridil	T46.1X1	T46.1X2	T46.1X3	T46.1X4	T46.1X5	T46.1X6
Bergamot oil	T65.891	T65.892	T65.893	T65.894	—	—
Bergapten	T50.991	T50.992	T50.993	T50.994	T50.995	T50.996
Berries, poisonous	T62.1X1	T62.1X2	T62.1X3	T62.1X4	—	—
Beryllium (compounds)	T56.7X1	T56.7X2	T56.7X3	T56.7X4	—	—
b-acetyldigoxin	T46.0X1	T46.0X2	T46.0X3	T46.0X4	T46.0X5	T46.0X6
beta adrenergic blocking agent, heart	T44.7X1	T44.7X2	T44.7X3	T44.7X4	T44.7X5	T44.7X6
b-benzalbutyramide	T46.6X1	T46.6X2	T46.6X3	T46.6X4	T46.6X5	T46.6X6
Betacarotene	T45.2X1	T45.2X2	T45.2X3	T45.2X4	T45.2X5	T45.2X6
b-eucaine	T49.1X1	T49.1X2	T49.1X3	T49.1X4	T49.1X5	T49.1X6
Beta-Chlor	T42.6X1	T42.6X2	T42.6X3	T42.6X4	T42.6X5	T42.6X6
b-galactosidase	T47.5X1	T47.5X2	T47.5X3	T47.5X4	T47.5X5	T47.5X6
Betahistine	T46.7X1	T46.7X2	T46.7X3	T46.7X4	T46.7X5	T46.7X6
Betaine	T47.5X1	T47.5X2	T47.5X3	T47.5X4	T47.5X5	T47.5X6
Betamethasone	T49.0X1	T49.0X2	T49.0X3	T49.0X4	T49.0X5	T49.0X6
topical	T49.0X1	T49.0X2	T49.0X3	T49.0X4	T49.0X5	T49.0X6
Betamicin	T36.8X1	T36.8X2	T36.8X3	T36.8X4	T36.8X5	T36.8X6
Betanidine	T46.5X1	T46.5X2	T46.5X3	T46.5X4	T46.5X5	T46.5X6
b-sitosterol(s)	T46.6X1	T46.6X2	T46.6X3	T46.6X4	T46.6X5	T46.6X6
Betaxolol	T44.7X1	T44.7X2	T44.7X3	T44.7X4	T44.7X5	T44.7X6
Betazole	T50.8X1	T50.8X2	T50.8X3	T50.8X4	T50.8X5	T50.8X6
Bethanechol	T44.1X1	T44.1X2	T44.1X3	T44.1X4	T44.1X5	T44.1X6
chloride	T44.1X1	T44.1X2	T44.1X3	T44.1X4	T44.1X5	T44.1X6
Bethanidine	T46.5X1	T46.5X2	T46.5X3	T46.5X4	T46.5X5	T46.5X6
Betoxycaine	T41.3X1	T41.3X2	T41.3X3	T41.3X4	T41.3X5	T41.3X6
Betula oil	T49.3X1	T49.3X2	T49.3X3	T49.3X4	T49.3X5	T49.3X6
Bevantolol	T44.7X1	T44.7X2	T44.7X3	T44.7X4	T44.7X5	T44.7X6
Bevonium metilsulfate	T44.3X1	T44.3X2	T44.3X3	T44.3X4	T44.3X5	T44.3X6
Bezafibrate	T46.6X1	T46.6X2	T46.6X3	T46.6X4	T46.6X5	T46.6X6
Bezitramide	T40.491	T40.492	T40.493	T40.494	T40.495	T40.496
BHA	T50.991	T50.992	T50.993	T50.994	T50.995	T50.996
Bhang	T40.711	T40.712	T40.713	T40.714	T40.715	T40.716
BHC (medicinal)	T49.0X1	T49.0X2	T49.0X3	T49.0X4	T49.0X5	T49.0X6
nonmedicinal (vapor)	T53.6X1	T53.6X2	T53.6X3	T53.6X4	—	—
Bialamicol	T37.3X1	T37.3X2	T37.3X3	T37.3X4	T37.3X5	T37.3X6
Bibenzonium bromide	T48.3X1	T48.3X2	T48.3X3	T48.3X4	T48.3X5	T48.3X6
Bibrocathol	T49.5X1	T49.5X2	T49.5X3	T49.5X4	T49.5X5	T49.5X6
Bichloride of mercury— see Mercury, chloride						

Table of Drugs and Chemicals

Bichromates–Brass

Substance	Poisoning, Accidental (unintentional)	Poisoning, Intentional self-harm	Poisoning, Assault	Poisoning, Undetermined	Adverse effect	Underdosing
Bichromates (calcium) (potassium) (sodium) (crystals)	T57.8X1	T57.8X2	T57.8X3	T57.8X4	—	—
fumes	T56.2X1	T56.2X2	T56.2X3	T56.2X4	—	—
Biclotymol	T49.6X1	T49.6X2	T49.6X3	T49.6X4	T49.6X5	T49.6X6
Bicuculline	T50.7X1	T50.7X2	T50.7X3	T50.7X4	T50.7X5	T50.7X6
Bifemelane	T43.291	T43.292	T43.293	T43.294	T43.295	T43.296
Biguanide derivatives, oral	T38.3X1	T38.3X2	T38.3X3	T38.3X4	T38.3X5	T38.3X6
Bile salts	T47.5X1	T47.5X2	T47.5X3	T47.5X4	T47.5X5	T47.5X6
Biligrafin	T50.8X1	T50.8X2	T50.8X3	T50.8X4	T50.8X5	T50.8X6
Bilopaque	T50.8X1	T50.8X2	T50.8X3	T50.8X4	T50.8X5	T50.8X6
Binifibrate	T46.6X1	T46.6X2	T46.6X3	T46.6X4	T46.6X5	T46.6X6
Binitrobenzol	T65.3X1	T65.3X2	T65.3X3	T65.3X4	—	—
Bioflavonoid(s)	T46.991	T46.992	T46.993	T46.994	T46.995	T46.996
Biological substance NEC	T50.901	T50.902	T50.903	T50.904	T50.905	T50.906
Biotin	T45.2X1	T45.2X2	T45.2X3	T45.2X4	T45.2X5	T45.2X6
Biperiden	T44.3X1	T44.3X2	T44.3X3	T44.3X4	T44.3X5	T44.3X6
Bisacodyl	T47.2X1	T47.2X2	T47.2X3	T47.2X4	T47.2X5	T47.2X6
Bisbentiamine	T45.2X1	T45.2X2	T45.2X3	T45.2X4	T45.2X5	T45.2X6
Bisbutiamine	T45.2X1	T45.2X2	T45.2X3	T45.2X4	T45.2X5	T45.2X6
Bisdequalinium (salts) (diacetate)	T49.6X1	T49.6X2	T49.6X3	T49.6X4	T49.6X5	T49.6X6
Bishydroxycoumarin	T45.511	T45.512	T45.513	T45.514	T45.515	T45.516
Bismarsen	T37.8X1	T37.8X2	T37.8X3	T37.8X4	T37.8X5	T37.8X6
Bismuth salts	T47.6X1	T47.6X2	T47.6X3	T47.6X4	T47.6X5	T47.6X6
aluminate	T47.1X1	T47.1X2	T47.1X3	T47.1X4	T47.1X5	T47.1X6
anti-infectives	T37.8X1	T37.8X2	T37.8X3	T37.8X4	T37.8X5	T37.8X6
formic iodide	T49.0X1	T49.0X2	T49.0X3	T49.0X4	T49.0X5	T49.0X6
glycolylarsenate	T49.0X1	T49.0X2	T49.0X3	T49.0X4	T49.0X5	T49.0X6
nonmedicinal (compounds) NEC	T65.91	T65.92	T65.93	T65.94	—	—
subcarbonate	T47.6X1	T47.6X2	T47.6X3	T47.6X4	T47.6X5	T47.6X6
subsalicylate	T37.8X1	T37.8X2	T37.8X3	T37.8X4	T37.8X5	T37.8X6
sulfarsphenamine	T37.8X1	T37.8X2	T37.8X3	T37.8X4	T37.8X5	T37.8X6
Bisoprolol	T44.7X1	T44.7X2	T44.7X3	T44.7X4	T44.7X5	T44.7X6
Bisoxatin	T47.2X1	T47.2X2	T47.2X3	T47.2X4	T47.2X5	T47.2X6
Bisulepin (hydrochloride)	T45.0X1	T45.0X2	T45.0X3	T45.0X4	T45.0X5	T45.0X6
Bithionol	T37.8X1	T37.8X2	T37.8X3	T37.8X4	T37.8X5	T37.8X6
anthelminthic	T37.4X1	T37.4X2	T37.4X3	T37.4X4	T37.4X5	T37.4X6
Bitolterol	T48.6X1	T48.6X2	T48.6X3	T48.6X4	T48.6X5	T48.6X6
Bitoscanate	T37.4X1	T37.4X2	T37.4X3	T37.4X4	T37.4X5	T37.4X6
Bitter almond oil	T62.8X1	T62.8X2	T62.8X3	T62.8X4	—	—
Bittersweet	T62.2X1	T62.2X2	T62.2X3	T62.2X4	—	—
Black						
flag	T60.91	T60.92	T60.93	T60.94	—	—
henbane	T62.2X1	T62.2X2	T62.2X3	T62.2X4	—	—
leaf (40)	T60.91	T60.92	T60.93	T60.94	—	—
widow spider (bite)	T63.311	T63.312	T63.313	T63.314	—	—
antivenin	T50.Z11	T50.Z12	T50.Z13	T50.Z14	T50.Z15	T50.Z16

Substance	Poisoning, Accidental (unintentional)	Poisoning, Intentional self-harm	Poisoning, Assault	Poisoning, Undetermined	Adverse effect	Underdosing
Blast furnace gas (carbon monoxide from)	T58.8X1	T58.8X2	T58.8X3	T58.8X4	—	—
Bleach	T54.91	T54.92	T54.93	T54.94	—	—
Bleaching agent (medicinal)	T49.4X1	T49.4X2	T49.4X3	T49.4X4	T49.4X5	T49.4X6
Bleomycin	T45.1X1	T45.1X2	T45.1X3	T45.1X4	T45.1X5	T45.1X6
Blockain	T41.3X1	T41.3X2	T41.3X3	T41.3X4	T41.3X5	T41.3X6
infiltration (subcutaneous)	T41.3X1	T41.3X2	T41.3X3	T41.3X4	T41.3X5	T41.3X6
nerve block (peripheral) (plexus)	T41.3X1	T41.3X2	T41.3X3	T41.3X4	T41.3X5	T41.3X6
topical (surface)	T41.3X1	T41.3X2	T41.3X3	T41.3X4	T41.3X5	T41.3X6
Blockers, calcium channel	T46.1X1	T46.1X2	T46.1X3	T46.1X4	T46.1X5	T46.1X6
Blood (derivatives) (natural) (plasma) (whole)	T45.8X1	T45.8X2	T45.8X3	T45.8X4	T45.8X5	T45.8X6
dried	T45.8X1	T45.8X2	T45.8X3	T45.8X4	T45.8X5	T45.8X6
drug affecting NEC	T45.91	T45.92	T45.93	T45.94	T45.95	T45.96
expander NEC	T45.8X1	T45.8X2	T45.8X3	T45.8X4	T45.8X5	T45.8X6
fraction NEC	T45.8X1	T45.8X2	T45.8X3	T45.8X4	T45.8X5	T45.8X6
substitute (macromolecular)	T45.8X1	T45.8X2	T45.8X3	T45.8X4	T45.8X5	T45.8X6
Blue velvet	T40.2X1	T40.2X2	T40.2X3	T40.2X4	—	—
Bone meal	T62.8X1	T62.8X2	T62.8X3	T62.8X4	—	—
Bonine	T45.0X1	T45.0X2	T45.0X3	T45.0X4	T45.0X5	T45.0X6
Bopindolol	T44.7X1	T44.7X2	T44.7X3	T44.7X4	T44.7X5	T44.7X6
Boracic acid	T49.0X1	T49.0X2	T49.0X3	T49.0X4	T49.0X5	T49.0X6
ENT agent	T49.6X1	T49.6X2	T49.6X3	T49.6X4	T49.6X5	T49.6X6
ophthalmic preparation	T49.5X1	T49.5X2	T49.5X3	T49.5X4	T49.5X5	T49.5X6
Borane complex	T57.8X1	T57.8X2	T57.8X3	T57.8X4	—	—
Borate (s)	T57.8X1	T57.8X2	T57.8X3	T57.8X4	—	—
buffer	T50.991	T50.992	T50.993	T50.994	T50.995	T50.996
cleanser	T54.91	T54.92	T54.93	T54.94	—	—
sodium	T57.8X1	T57.8X2	T57.8X3	T57.8X4	—	—
Borax (cleanser)	T54.91	T54.92	T54.93	T54.94	—	—
Bordeaux mixture	T60.3X1	T60.3X2	T60.3X3	T60.3X4	—	—
Boric acid	T49.0X1	T49.0X2	T49.0X3	T49.0X4	T49.0X5	T49.0X6
ENT agent	T49.6X1	T49.6X2	T49.6X3	T49.6X4	T49.6X5	T49.6X6
ophthalmic preparation	T49.5X1	T49.5X2	T49.5X3	T49.5X4	T49.5X5	T49.5X6
Bornaprine	T44.3X1	T44.3X2	T44.3X3	T44.3X4	T44.3X5	T44.3X6
Boron	T57.8X1	T57.8X2	T57.8X3	T57.8X4	—	—
hydride NEC	T57.8X1	T57.8X2	T57.8X3	T57.8X4	—	—
fumes or gas	T57.8X1	T57.8X2	T57.8X3	T57.8X4	—	—
trifluoride	T59.891	T59.892	T59.893	T59.894	—	—
Botox	T48.291	T48.292	T48.293	T48.294	T48.295	T48.296
Botulinus anti-toxin (type A, B)	T50.Z11	T50.Z12	T50.Z13	T50.Z14	T50.Z15	T50.Z16
Brake fluid vapor	T59.891	T59.892	T59.893	T59.894	—	—
Brallobarbital	T42.3X1	T42.3X2	T42.3X3	T42.3X4	T42.3X5	T42.3X6
Bran (wheat)	T47.4X1	T47.4X2	T47.4X3	T47.4X4	T47.4X5	T47.4X6
Brass (fumes)	T56.891	T56.892	T56.893	T56.894	—	—

Substance	Poisoning, Accidental (unintentional)	Poisoning, Intentional self-harm	Poisoning, Assault	Poisoning, Undetermined	Adverse effect	Underdosing
Brasso	T52.0X1	T52.0X2	T52.0X3	T52.0X4	—	—
Bretylium tosilate	T46.2X1	T46.2X2	T46.2X3	T46.2X4	T46.2X5	T46.2X6
Brevital (sodium)	T41.1X1	T41.1X2	T41.1X3	T41.1X4	T41.1X5	T41.1X6
Brinase	T45.3X1	T45.3X2	T45.3X3	T45.3X4	T45.3X5	T45.3X6
British antilewisite	T45.8X1	T45.8X2	T45.8X3	T45.8X4	T45.8X5	T45.8X6
Brodifacoum	T60.4X1	T60.4X2	T60.4X3	T60.4X4	—	—
Bromal (hydrate)	T42.6X1	T42.6X2	T42.6X3	T42.6X4	T42.6X5	T42.6X6
Bromazepam	T42.4X1	T42.4X2	T42.4X3	T42.4X4	T42.4X5	T42.4X6
Bromazine	T45.0X1	T45.0X2	T45.0X3	T45.0X4	T45.0X5	T45.0X6
Brombenzylcyanide	T59.3X1	T59.3X2	T59.3X3	T59.3X4	—	—
Bromelains	T45.3X1	T45.3X2	T45.3X3	T45.3X4	T45.3X5	T45.3X6
Bromethalin	T60.4X1	T60.4X2	T60.4X3	T60.4X4	—	—
Bromhexine	T48.4X1	T48.4X2	T48.4X3	T48.4X4	T48.4X5	T48.4X6
Bromide salts	T42.6X1	T42.6X2	T42.6X3	T42.6X4	T42.6X5	T42.6X6
Bromindione	T45.511	T45.512	T45.513	T45.514	T45.515	T45.516
Bromine						
compounds (medicinal)	T42.6X1	T42.6X2	T42.6X3	T42.6X4	T42.6X5	T42.6X6
sedative	T42.6X1	T42.6X2	T42.6X3	T42.6X4	T42.6X5	T42.6X6
vapor	T59.891	T59.892	T59.893	T59.894	—	—
Bromisoval	T42.6X1	T42.6X2	T42.6X3	T42.6X4	T42.6X5	T42.6X6
Bromisovalum	T42.6X1	T42.6X2	T42.6X3	T42.6X4	T42.6X5	T42.6X6
Bromobenzylcyanide	T59.3X1	T59.3X2	T59.3X3	T59.3X4	—	—
Bromochloro-salicylanilide	T49.0X1	T49.0X2	T49.0X3	T49.0X4	T49.0X5	T49.0X6
Bromocriptine	T42.8X1	T42.8X2	T42.8X3	T42.8X4	T42.8X5	T42.8X6
Bromodiphenhydramine	T45.0X1	T45.0X2	T45.0X3	T45.0X4	T45.0X5	T45.0X6
Bromoform	T42.6X1	T42.6X2	T42.6X3	T42.6X4	T42.6X5	T42.6X6
Bromophenol blue reagent	T50.991	T50.992	T50.993	T50.994	T50.995	T50.996
Bromopride	T47.8X1	T47.8X2	T47.8X3	T47.8X4	T47.8X5	T47.8X6
Bromosalicyl chloranitide	T49.0X1	T49.0X2	T49.0X3	T49.0X4	T49.0X5	T49.0X6
Bromosalicyl hydroxamic acid	T37.1X1	T37.1X2	T37.1X3	T37.1X4	T37.1X5	T37.1X6
Bromo-seltzer	T39.1X1	T39.1X2	T39.1X3	T39.1X4	T39.1X5	T39.1X6
Bromoxynil	T60.3X1	T60.3X2	T60.3X3	T60.3X4	—	—
Bromperidol	T43.4X1	T43.4X2	T43.4X3	T43.4X4	T43.4X5	T43.4X6
Brompheniramine	T45.0X1	T45.0X2	T45.0X3	T45.0X4	T45.0X5	T45.0X6
Bromsulphthalein	T50.8X1	T50.8X2	T50.8X3	T50.8X4	T50.8X5	T50.8X6
Bromural	T42.6X1	T42.6X2	T42.6X3	T42.6X4	T42.6X5	T42.6X6
Bromvaletone	T42.6X1	T42.6X2	T42.6X3	T42.6X4	T42.6X5	T42.6X6
Bronchodilator NEC	T48.6X1	T48.6X2	T48.6X3	T48.6X4	T48.6X5	T48.6X6
Brotizolam	T42.4X1	T42.4X2	T42.4X3	T42.4X4	T42.4X5	T42.4X6
Brovincamine	T46.7X1	T46.7X2	T46.7X3	T46.7X4	T46.7X5	T46.7X6
Brown recluse spider (bite) (venom)	T63.331	T63.332	T63.333	T63.334	—	—
Brown spider (bite) (venom)	T63.391	T63.392	T63.393	T63.394	—	—
Broxaterol	T48.6X1	T48.6X2	T48.6X3	T48.6X4	T48.6X5	T48.6X6
Broxuridine	T45.1X1	T45.1X2	T45.1X3	T45.1X4	T45.1X5	T45.1X6

Substance	Poisoning, Accidental (unintentional)	Poisoning, Intentional self-harm	Poisoning, Assault	Poisoning, Undetermined	Adverse effect	Underdosing
Broxyquinoline	T37.8X1	T37.8X2	T37.8X3	T37.8X4	T37.8X5	T37.8X6
Bruceine	T48.291	T48.292	T48.293	T48.294	T48.295	T48.296
Brucia	T62.2X1	T62.2X2	T62.2X3	T62.2X4	—	—
Brucine	T65.1X1	T65.1X2	T65.1X3	T65.1X4	—	—
Brunswick green—see Copper						
Bruten—see Ibuprofen						
Bryonia	T47.2X1	T47.2X2	T47.2X3	T47.2X4	T47.2X5	T47.2X6
Buclizine	T45.0X1	T45.0X2	T45.0X3	T45.0X4	T45.0X5	T45.0X6
Buclosamide	T49.0X1	T49.0X2	T49.0X3	T49.0X4	T49.0X5	T49.0X6
Budesonide	T44.5X1	T44.5X2	T44.5X3	T44.5X4	T44.5X5	T44.5X6
Budralazine	T46.5X1	T46.5X2	T46.5X3	T46.5X4	T46.5X5	T46.5X6
Bufferin	T39.011	T39.012	T39.013	T39.014	T39.015	T39.016
Buflomedil	T46.7X1	T46.7X2	T46.7X3	T46.7X4	T46.7X5	T46.7X6
Buformin	T38.3X1	T38.3X2	T38.3X3	T38.3X4	T38.3X5	T38.3X6
Bufotenine	T40.991	T40.992	T40.993	T40.994	—	—
Bufrolin	T48.6X1	T48.6X2	T48.6X3	T48.6X4	T48.6X5	T48.6X6
Bufylline	T48.6X1	T48.6X2	T48.6X3	T48.6X4	T48.6X5	T48.6X6
Bulk filler	T50.5X1	T50.5X2	T50.5X3	T50.5X4	T50.5X5	T50.5X6
cathartic	T47.4X1	T47.4X2	T47.4X3	T47.4X4	T47.4X5	T47.4X6
Bumetanide	T50.1X1	T50.1X2	T50.1X3	T50.1X4	T50.1X5	T50.1X6
Bunaftine	T46.2X1	T46.2X2	T46.2X3	T46.2X4	T46.2X5	T46.2X6
Bunamiodyl	T50.8X1	T50.8X2	T50.8X3	T50.8X4	T50.8X5	T50.8X6
Bunazosin	T44.6X1	T44.6X2	T44.6X3	T44.6X4	T44.6X5	T44.6X6
Bunitrolol	T44.7X1	T44.7X2	T44.7X3	T44.7X4	T44.7X5	T44.7X6
Buphenine	T46.7X1	T46.7X2	T46.7X3	T46.7X4	T46.7X5	T46.7X6
Bupivacaine	T41.3X1	T41.3X2	T41.3X3	T41.3X4	T41.3X5	T41.3X6
infiltration (subcutaneous)	T41.3X1	T41.3X2	T41.3X3	T41.3X4	T41.3X5	T41.3X6
nerve block (peripheral) (plexus)	T41.3X1	T41.3X2	T41.3X3	T41.3X4	T41.3X5	T41.3X6
spinal	T41.3X1	T41.3X2	T41.3X3	T41.3X4	T41.3X5	T41.3X6
Bupranolol	T44.7X1	T44.7X2	T44.7X3	T44.7X4	T44.7X5	T44.7X6
Buprenorphine	T40.491	T40.492	T40.493	T40.494	T40.495	T40.496
Bupropion	T43.291	T43.292	T43.293	T43.294	T43.295	T43.296
Burimamide	T47.1X1	T47.1X2	T47.1X3	T47.1X4	T47.1X5	T47.1X6
Buserelin	T38.891	T38.892	T38.893	T38.894	T38.895	T38.896
Buspirone	T43.591	T43.592	T43.593	T43.594	T43.595	T43.596
Busulfan, busulphan	T45.1X1	T45.1X2	T45.1X3	T45.1X4	T45.1X5	T45.1X6
Butabarbital (sodium)	T42.3X1	T42.3X2	T42.3X3	T42.3X4	T42.3X5	T42.3X6
Butabarbitone	T42.3X1	T42.3X2	T42.3X3	T42.3X4	T42.3X5	T42.3X6
Butabarpal	T42.3X1	T42.3X2	T42.3X3	T42.3X4	T42.3X5	T42.3X6
Butacaine	T41.3X1	T41.3X2	T41.3X3	T41.3X4	T41.3X5	T41.3X6
Butalamine	T46.7X1	T46.7X2	T46.7X3	T46.7X4	T46.7X5	T46.7X6
Butalbital	T42.3X1	T42.3X2	T42.3X3	T42.3X4	T42.3X5	T42.3X6
Butallylonal	T42.3X1	T42.3X2	T42.3X3	T42.3X4	T42.3X5	T42.3X6
Butamben	T41.3X1	T41.3X2	T41.3X3	T41.3X4	T41.3X5	T41.3X6
Butamirate	T48.3X1	T48.3X2	T48.3X3	T48.3X4	T48.3X5	T48.3X6

Substance	Poisoning, Accidental (unintentional)	Poisoning, Intentional self-harm	Poisoning, Assault	Poisoning, Undetermined	Adverse effect	Underdosing
Butane (distributed in mobile container)	T59.891	T59.892	T59.893	T59.894	—	—
distributed through pipes	T59.891	T59.892	T59.893	T59.894	—	—
incomplete combustion	T58.11	T58.12	T58.13	T58.14	—	—
Butanilicaine	T41.3X1	T41.3X2	T41.3X3	T41.3X4	T41.3X5	T41.3X6
Butanol	T51.3X1	T51.3X2	T51.3X3	T51.3X4		
Butanone, 2-butanone	T52.4X1	T52.4X2	T52.4X3	T52.4X4		
Butantrone	T49.4X1	T49.4X2	T49.4X3	T49.4X4	T49.4X5	T49.4X6
Butaperazine	T43.3X1	T43.3X2	T43.3X3	T43.3X4	T43.3X5	T43.3X6
Butazolidin	T39.2X1	T39.2X2	T39.2X3	T39.2X4	T39.2X5	T39.2X6
Butetamate	T48.6X1	T48.6X2	T48.6X3	T48.6X4	T48.6X5	T48.6X6
Butethal	T42.3X1	T42.3X2	T42.3X3	T42.3X4	T42.3X5	T42.3X6
Butethamate	T44.3X1	T44.3X2	T44.3X3	T44.3X4	T44.3X5	T44.3X6
Buthalitone (sodium)	T41.1X1	T41.1X2	T41.1X3	T41.1X4	T41.1X5	T41.1X6
Butisol (sodium)	T42.3X1	T42.3X2	T42.3X3	T42.3X4	T42.3X5	T42.3X6
Butizide	T50.2X1	T50.2X2	T50.2X3	T50.2X4	T50.2X5	T50.2X6
Butobarbital	T42.3X1	T42.3X2	T42.3X3	T42.3X4	T42.3X5	T42.3X6
sodium	T42.3X1	T42.3X2	T42.3X3	T42.3X4	T42.3X5	T42.3X6
Butobarbitone	T42.3X1	T42.3X2	T42.3X3	T42.3X4	T42.3X5	T42.3X6
Butoconazole (nitrate)	T49.0X1	T49.0X2	T49.0X3	T49.0X4	T49.0X5	T49.0X6
Butorphanol	T40.491	T40.492	T40.493	T40.494	T40.495	T40.496
Butriptyline	T43.011	T43.012	T43.013	T43.014	T43.015	T43.016
Butropium bromide	T44.3X1	T44.3X2	T44.3X3	T44.3X4	T44.3X5	T44.3X6
Butter of antimony—see Antimony						
Buttercups	T62.2X1	T62.2X2	T62.2X3	T62.2X4	—	—
Butyl						
acetate (secondary)	T52.8X1	T52.8X2	T52.8X3	T52.8X4	—	—
alcohol	T51.3X1	T51.3X2	T51.3X3	T51.3X4	—	—
aminobenzoate	T41.3X1	T41.3X2	T41.3X3	T41.3X4	T41.3X5	T41.3X6
butyrate	T52.8X1	T52.8X2	T52.8X3	T52.8X4	—	—
carbinol	T51.3X1	T51.3X2	T51.3X3	T51.3X4	—	—
carbitol	T52.3X1	T52.3X2	T52.3X3	T52.3X4	—	—
cellosolve	T52.3X1	T52.3X2	T52.3X3	T52.3X4	—	—
chloral (hydrate)	T42.6X1	T42.6X2	T42.6X3	T42.6X4	T42.6X5	T42.6X6
formate	T52.8X1	T52.8X2	T52.8X3	T52.8X4	—	—
lactate	T52.8X1	T52.8X2	T52.8X3	T52.8X4	—	—
propionate	T52.8X1	T52.8X2	T52.8X3	T52.8X4	—	—
scopolamine bromide	T44.3X1	T44.3X2	T44.3X3	T44.3X4	T44.3X5	T44.3X6
thiobarbital sodium	T41.1X1	T41.1X2	T41.1X3	T41.1X4	T41.1X5	T41.1X6
Butylated hydroxy-anisole	T50.991	T50.992	T50.993	T50.994	T50.995	T50.996
Butylchloral hydrate	T42.6X1	T42.6X2	T42.6X3	T42.6X4	T42.6X5	T42.6X6
Butyltoluene	T52.2X1	T52.2X2	T52.2X3	T52.2X4	—	—
Butyn	T41.3X1	T41.3X2	T41.3X3	T41.3X4	T41.3X5	T41.3X6
Butyrophenone (-based tranquilizers)	T43.4X1	T43.4X2	T43.4X3	T43.4X4	T43.4X5	T43.4X6

C

Substance	Poisoning, Accidental (unintentional)	Poisoning, Intentional self-harm	Poisoning, Assault	Poisoning, Undetermined	Adverse effect	Underdosing
Cabergoline	T42.8X1	T42.8X2	T42.8X3	T42.8X4	T42.8X5	T42.8X6
Cacodyl, cacodylic acid	T57.0X1	T57.0X2	T57.0X3	T57.0X4	—	—
Cactinomycin	T45.1X1	T45.1X2	T45.1X3	T45.1X4	T45.1X5	T45.1X6
Cade oil	T49.4X1	T49.4X2	T49.4X3	T49.4X4	T49.4X5	T49.4X6
Cadexomer iodine	T49.0X1	T49.0X2	T49.0X3	T49.0X4	T49.0X5	T49.0X6
Cadmium (chloride) (fumes) (oxide)	T56.3X1	T56.3X2	T56.3X3	T56.3X4	—	—
sulfide (medicinal) NEC	T49.4X1	T49.4X2	T49.4X3	T49.4X4	T49.4X5	T49.4X6
Cadralazine	T46.5X1	T46.5X2	T46.5X3	T46.5X4	T46.5X5	T46.5X6
Caffeine	T43.611	T43.612	T43.613	T43.614	T43.615	T43.616
Calabar bean	T62.2X1	T62.2X2	T62.2X3	T62.2X4	—	—
Caladium seguinum	T62.2X1	T62.2X2	T62.2X3	T62.2X4	—	—
Calamine (lotion)	T49.3X1	T49.3X2	T49.3X3	T49.3X4	T49.3X5	T49.3X6
Calcifediol	T45.2X1	T45.2X2	T45.2X3	T45.2X4	T45.2X5	T45.2X6
Calciferol	T45.2X1	T45.2X2	T45.2X3	T45.2X4	T45.2X5	T45.2X6
Calcitonin	T50.991	T50.992	T50.993	T50.994	T50.995	T50.996
Calcitriol	T45.2X1	T45.2X2	T45.2X3	T45.2X4	T45.2X5	T45.2X6
Calcium	T50.3X1	T50.3X2	T50.3X3	T50.3X4	T50.3X5	T50.3X6
actylsalicylate	T39.011	T39.012	T39.013	T39.014	T39.015	T39.016
benzamidosalicylate	T37.1X1	T37.1X2	T37.1X3	T37.1X4	T37.1X5	T37.1X6
bromide	T42.6X1	T42.6X2	T42.6X3	T42.6X4	T42.6X5	T42.6X6
bromolactobionate	T42.6X1	T42.6X2	T42.6X3	T42.6X4	T42.6X5	T42.6X6
carbaspirin	T39.011	T39.012	T39.013	T39.014	T39.015	T39.016
carbimide	T50.6X1	T50.6X2	T50.6X3	T50.6X4	T50.6X5	T50.6X6
carbonate	T47.1X1	T47.1X2	T47.1X3	T47.1X4	T47.1X5	T47.1X6
chloride	T50.991	T50.992	T50.993	T50.994	T50.995	T50.996
anhydrous	T50.991	T50.992	T50.993	T50.994	T50.995	T50.996
cyanide	T57.8X1	T57.8X2	T57.8X3	T57.8X4	—	—
dioctyl sulfosuccinate	T47.4X1	T47.4X2	T47.4X3	T47.4X4	T47.4X5	T47.4X6
disodium edathamil	T45.8X1	T45.8X2	T45.8X3	T45.8X4	T45.8X5	T45.8X6
disodium edetate	T45.8X1	T45.8X2	T45.8X3	T45.8X4	T45.8X5	T45.8X6
dobesilate	T46.991	T46.992	T46.993	T46.994	T46.995	T46.996
EDTA	T45.8X1	T45.8X2	T45.8X3	T45.8X4	T45.8X5	T45.8X6
ferrous citrate	T45.4X1	T45.4X2	T45.4X3	T45.4X4	T45.4X5	T45.4X6
folinate	T45.8X1	T45.8X2	T45.8X3	T45.8X4	T45.8X5	T45.8X6
glubionate	T50.3X1	T50.3X2	T50.3X3	T50.3X4	T50.3X5	T50.3X6
gluconate	T50.3X1	T50.3X2	T50.3X3	T50.3X4	T50.3X5	T50.3X6
gluconogalactogluconate	T50.3X1	T50.3X2	T50.3X3	T50.3X4	T50.3X5	T50.3X6
hydrate, hydroxide	T54.3X1	T54.3X2	T54.3X3	T54.3X4	—	—
hypochlorite	T54.3X1	T54.3X2	T54.3X3	T54.3X4	—	—
iodide	T48.4X1	T48.4X2	T48.4X3	T48.4X4	T48.4X5	T48.4X6
ipodate	T50.8X1	T50.8X2	T50.8X3	T50.8X4	T50.8X5	T50.8X6
lactate	T50.3X1	T50.3X2	T50.3X3	T50.3X4	T50.3X5	T50.3X6
leucovorin	T45.8X1	T45.8X2	T45.8X3	T45.8X4	T45.8X5	T45.8X6
mandelate	T37.91	T37.92	T37.93	T37.94	T37.95	T37.96
oxide	T54.3X1	T54.3X2	T54.3X3	T54.3X4	—	—
pantothenate	T45.2X1	T45.2X2	T45.2X3	T45.2X4	T45.2X5	T45.2X6
phosphate	T50.3X1	T50.3X2	T50.3X3	T50.3X4	T50.3X5	T50.3X6
salicylate	T39.091	T39.092	T39.093	T39.094	T39.095	T39.096
salts	T50.3X1	T50.3X2	T50.3X3	T50.3X4	T50.3X5	T50.3X6
Calculus-dissolving drug	T50.991	T50.992	T50.993	T50.994	T50.995	T50.996
Calomel	T49.0X1	T49.0X2	T49.0X3	T49.0X4	T49.0X5	T49.0X6
Caloric agent	T50.3X1	T50.3X2	T50.3X3	T50.3X4	T50.3X5	T50.3X6

Substance	Poisoning, Accidental (unintentional)	Poisoning, Intentional self-harm	Poisoning, Assault	Poisoning, Undetermined	Adverse effect	Underdosing
Calusterone	T38.7X1	T38.7X2	T38.7X3	T38.7X4	T38.7X5	T38.7X6
Camazepam	T42.4X1	T42.4X2	T42.4X3	T42.4X4	T42.4X5	T42.4X6
Camomile	T49.0X1	T49.0X2	T49.0X3	T49.0X4	T49.0X5	T49.0X6
Camoquin	T37.2X1	T37.2X2	T37.2X3	T37.2X4	T37.2X5	T37.2X6
Camphor						
insecticide	T60.2X1	T60.2X2	T60.2X3	T60.2X4	—	—
medicinal	T49.8X1	T49.8X2	T49.8X3	T49.8X4	T49.8X5	T49.8X6
Camylofin	T44.3X1	T44.3X2	T44.3X3	T44.3X4	T44.3X5	T44.3X6
Cancer chemotherapy drug regimen	T45.1X1	T45.1X2	T45.1X3	T45.1X4	T45.1X5	T45.1X6
Candeptin	T49.0X1	T49.0X2	T49.0X3	T49.0X4	T49.0X5	T49.0X6
Candicidin	T49.0X1	T49.0X2	T49.0X3	T49.0X4	T49.0X5	T49.0X6
Cannabinoids, synthetic	T40.721	T40.722	T40.723	T40.724	T40.725	T40.726
Cannabinol	T40.711	T40.712	T40.713	T40.714	T40.715	T40.716
Cannabis (derivatives)	T40.711	T40.712	T40.713	T40.714	T40.715	T40.716
Canned heat	T51.1X1	T51.1X2	T51.1X3	T51.1X4	—	—
Canrenoic acid	T50.0X1	T50.0X2	T50.0X3	T50.0X4	T50.0X5	T50.0X6
Canrenone	T50.0X1	T50.0X2	T50.0X3	T50.0X4	T50.0X5	T50.0X6
Cantharides, cantharidin, cantharis	T49.8X1	T49.8X2	T49.8X3	T49.8X4	T49.8X5	T49.8X6
Canthaxanthin	T50.991	T50.992	T50.993	T50.994	T50.995	T50.996
Capillary-active drug NEC	T46.901	T46.902	T46.903	T46.904	T46.905	T46.906
Capreomycin	T36.8X1	T36.8X2	T36.8X3	T36.8X4	T36.8X5	T36.8X6
Capsicum	T49.4X1	T49.4X2	T49.4X3	T49.4X4	T49.4X5	T49.4X6
Captafol	T60.3X1	T60.3X2	T60.3X3	T60.3X4	—	—
Captan	T60.3X1	T60.3X2	T60.3X3	T60.3X4	—	—
Captodiame, captodiamine	T43.591	T43.592	T43.593	T43.594	T43.595	T43.596
Captopril	T46.4X1	T46.4X2	T46.4X3	T46.4X4	T46.4X5	T46.4X6
Caramiphen	T44.3X1	T44.3X2	T44.3X3	T44.3X4	T44.3X5	T44.3X6
Carazolol	T44.7X1	T44.7X2	T44.7X3	T44.7X4	T44.7X5	T44.7X6
Carbachol	T44.1X1	T44.1X2	T44.1X3	T44.1X4	T44.1X5	T44.1X6
Carbacrylamine (resin)	T50.3X1	T50.3X2	T50.3X3	T50.3X4	T50.3X5	T50.3X6
Carbamate (insecticide)	T60.0X1	T60.0X2	T60.0X3	T60.0X4	—	—
Carbamate (sedative)	T42.6X1	T42.6X2	T42.6X3	T42.6X4	T42.6X5	T42.6X6
herbicide	T60.0X1	T60.0X2	T60.0X3	T60.0X4	—	—
insecticide	T60.0X1	T60.0X2	T60.0X3	T60.0X4	—	—
Carbamazepine	T42.1X1	T42.1X2	T42.1X3	T42.1X4	T42.1X5	T42.1X6
Carbamide	T47.3X1	T47.3X2	T47.3X3	T47.3X4	T47.3X5	T47.3X6
peroxide	T49.0X1	T49.0X2	T49.0X3	T49.0X4	T49.0X5	T49.0X6
topical	T49.8X1	T49.8X2	T49.8X3	T49.8X4	T49.8X5	T49.8X6
Carbamylcholine chloride	T44.1X1	T44.1X2	T44.1X3	T44.1X4	T44.1X5	T44.1X6
Carbaril	T60.0X1	T60.0X2	T60.0X3	T60.0X4	—	—
Carbarsone	T37.3X1	T37.3X2	T37.3X3	T37.3X4	T37.3X5	T37.3X6
Carbaryl	T60.0X1	T60.0X2	T60.0X3	T60.0X4	—	—
Carbaspirin	T39.011	T39.012	T39.013	T39.014	T39.015	T39.016
Carbazochrome (salicylate) (sodium sulfonate)	T49.4X1	T49.4X2	T49.4X3	T49.4X4	T49.4X5	T49.4X6
Carbenicillin	T36.0X1	T36.0X2	T36.0X3	T36.0X4	T36.0X5	T36.0X6

Substance	Poisoning, Accidental (unintentional)	Poisoning, Intentional self-harm	Poisoning, Assault	Poisoning, Undetermined	Adverse effect	Underdosing
Carbenoxolone	T47.1X1	T47.1X2	T47.1X3	T47.1X4	T47.1X5	T47.1X6
Carbetapentane	T48.3X1	T48.3X2	T48.3X3	T48.3X4	T48.3X5	T48.3X6
Carbethyl salicylate	T39.091	T39.092	T39.093	T39.094	T39.095	T39.096
Carbidopa (with levodopa)	T42.8X1	T42.8X2	T42.8X3	T42.8X4	T42.8X5	T42.8X6
Carbimazole	T38.2X1	T38.2X2	T38.2X3	T38.2X4	T38.2X5	T38.2X6
Carbinol	T51.1X1	T51.1X2	T51.1X3	T51.1X4	—	—
Carbinoxamine	T45.0X1	T45.0X2	T45.0X3	T45.0X4	T45.0X5	T45.0X6
Carbiphene	T39.8X1	T39.8X2	T39.8X3	T39.8X4	T39.8X5	T39.8X6
Carbitol	T52.3X1	T52.3X2	T52.3X3	T52.3X4	—	—
Carbo medicinalis	T47.6X1	T47.6X2	T47.6X3	T47.6X4	T47.6X5	T47.6X6
Carbocaine	T41.3X1	T41.3X2	T41.3X3	T41.3X4	T41.3X5	T41.3X6
infiltration (subcutaneous)	T41.3X1	T41.3X2	T41.3X3	T41.3X4	T41.3X5	T41.3X6
nerve block (peripheral) (plexus)	T41.3X1	T41.3X2	T41.3X3	T41.3X4	T41.3X5	T41.3X6
topical (surface)	T41.3X1	T41.3X2	T41.3X3	T41.3X4	T41.3X5	T41.3X6
Carbocisteine	T48.4X1	T48.4X2	T48.4X3	T48.4X4	T48.4X5	T48.4X6
Carbocromen	T46.3X1	T46.3X2	T46.3X3	T46.3X4	T46.3X5	T46.3X6
Carbol fuchsin	T49.0X1	T49.0X2	T49.0X3	T49.0X4	T49.0X5	T49.0X6
Carbolic acid—see also Phenol	T54.0X1	T54.0X2	T54.0X3	T54.0X4	—	—
Carbolonium (bromide)	T48.1X1	T48.1X2	T48.1X3	T48.1X4	T48.1X5	T48.1X6
Carbomycin	T36.8X1	T36.8X2	T36.8X3	T36.8X4	T36.8X5	T36.8X6
Carbon						
bisulfide (liquid)	T65.4X1	T65.4X2	T65.4X3	T65.4X4	—	—
vapor	T65.4X1	T65.4X2	T65.4X3	T65.4X4	—	—
dioxide (gas)	T59.7X1	T59.7X2	T59.7X3	T59.7X4	—	—
medicinal	T41.5X1	T41.5X2	T41.5X3	T41.5X4	T41.5X5	T41.5X6
nonmedicinal	T59.7X1	T59.7X2	T59.7X3	T59.7X4	—	—
snow	T49.4X1	T49.4X2	T49.4X3	T49.4X4	T49.4X5	T49.4X6
disulfide (liquid)	T65.4X1	T65.4X2	T65.4X3	T65.4X4	—	—
vapor	T65.4X1	T65.4X2	T65.4X3	T65.4X4	—	—
monoxide (from incomplete combustion)	T58.91	T58.92	T58.93	T58.94	—	—
blast furnace gas	T58.8X1	T58.8X2	T58.8X3	T58.8X4	—	—
butane (distributed in mobile container)	T58.11	T58.12	T58.13	T58.14	—	—
distributed through pipes	T58.11	T58.12	T58.13	T58.14	—	—
charcoal fumes	T58.2X1	T58.2X2	T58.2X3	T58.2X4	—	—
coal	T58.2X1	T58.2X2	T58.2X3	T58.2X4	—	—
coke (in domestic stoves, fireplaces)	T58.2X1	T58.2X2	T58.2X3	T58.2X4	—	—
gas (piped)	T58.11	T58.12	T58.13	T58.14	—	—
solid (in domestic stoves, fireplaces)	T58.2X1	T58.2X2	T58.2X3	T58.2X4	—	—
exhaust gas (motor) not in transit	T58.01	T58.02	T58.03	T58.04	—	—
combustion engine, any not in watercraft	T58.01	T58.02	T58.03	T58.04	—	—
farm tractor, not in transit	T58.01	T58.02	T58.03	T58.04	—	—

Table of Drugs and Chemicals

Carbon–Cathomycin

Substance	Poisoning, Accidental (unintentional)	Poisoning, Intentional self-harm	Poisoning, Assault	Poisoning, Undetermined	Adverse effect	Underdosing
Carbon — Continued						
gas engine	T58.01	T58.02	T58.03	T58.04	—	—
motor pump	T58.01	T58.02	T58.03	T58.04	—	—
motor vehicle, not in transit	T58.01	T58.02	T58.03	T58.04	—	—
fuel (in domestic use)	T58.2X1	T58.2X2	T58.2X3	T58.2X4	—	—
gas (piped)	T58.11	T58.12	T58.13	T58.14	—	—
in mobile container	T58.11	T58.12	T58.13	T58.14	—	—
piped (natural)	T58.11	T58.12	T58.13	T58.14	—	—
utility	T58.11	T58.12	T58.13	T58.14	—	—
in mobile container	T58.11	T58.12	T58.13	T58.14	—	—
illuminating gas	T58.11	T58.12	T58.13	T58.14	—	—
industrial fuels or gases, any	T58.8X1	T58.8X2	T58.8X3	T58.8X4	—	—
kerosene (in domestic stoves, fireplaces)	T58.2X1	T58.2X2	T58.2X3	T58.2X4	—	—
kiln gas or vapor	T58.8X1	T58.8X2	T58.8X3	T58.8X4	—	—
motor exhaust gas, not in transit	T58.01	T58.02	T58.03	T58.04	—	—
piped gas (manufactured) (natural)	T58.11	T58.12	T58.13	T58.14	—	—
producer gas	T58.8X1	T58.8X2	T58.8X3	T58.8X4	—	—
propane (distributed in mobile container)	T58.11	T58.12	T58.13	T58.14	—	—
distributed through pipes	T58.11	T58.12	T58.13	T58.14	—	—
specified source NEC	T58.8X1	T58.8X2	T58.8X3	T58.8X4	—	—
stove gas	T58.11	T58.12	T58.13	T58.14	—	—
piped	T58.11	T58.12	T58.13	T58.14	—	—
utility gas	T58.11	T58.12	T58.13	T58.14	—	—
piped	T58.11	T58.12	T58.13	T58.14	—	—
water gas	T58.11	T58.12	T58.13	T58.14	—	—
wood (in domestic stoves, fireplaces)	T58.2X1	T58.2X2	T58.2X3	T58.2X4	—	—
tetrachloride (vapor) NEC	T53.0X1	T53.0X2	T53.0X3	T53.0X4	—	—
liquid (cleansing agent) NEC	T53.0X1	T53.0X2	T53.0X3	T53.0X4	—	—
solvent	T53.0X1	T53.0X2	T53.0X3	T53.0X4	—	—
Carbonic acid gas	T59.7X1	T59.7X2	T59.7X3	T59.7X4	—	—
anhydrase inhibitor NEC	T50.2X1	T50.2X2	T50.2X3	T50.2X4	T50.2X5	T50.2X6
Carbophenothion	T60.0X1	T60.0X2	T60.0X3	T60.0X4	—	—
Carboplatin	T45.1X1	T45.1X2	T45.1X3	T45.1X4	T45.1X5	T45.1X6
Carboprost	T48.0X1	T48.0X2	T48.0X3	T48.0X4	T48.0X5	T48.0X6
Carboquone	T45.1X1	T45.1X2	T45.1X3	T45.1X4	T45.1X5	T45.1X6
Carbowax	T49.3X1	T49.3X2	T49.3X3	T49.3X4	T49.3X5	T49.3X6
Carboxymethyl-cellulose	T47.4X1	T47.4X2	T47.4X3	T47.4X4	T47.4X5	T47.4X6
S-Carboxymethyl-cysteine	T48.4X1	T48.4X2	T48.4X3	T48.4X4	T48.4X5	T48.4X6
Carbrital	T42.3X1	T42.3X2	T42.3X3	T42.3X4	T42.3X5	T42.3X6

Substance	Poisoning, Accidental (unintentional)	Poisoning, Intentional self-harm	Poisoning, Assault	Poisoning, Undetermined	Adverse effect	Underdosing
Carbromal	T42.6X1	T42.6X2	T42.6X3	T42.6X4	T42.6X5	T42.6X6
Carbutamide	T38.3X1	T38.3X2	T38.3X3	T38.3X4	T38.3X5	T38.3X6
Carbuterol	T48.6X1	T48.6X2	T48.6X3	T48.6X4	T48.6X5	T48.6X6
Cardiac						
depressants	T46.2X1	T46.2X2	T46.2X3	T46.2X4	T46.2X5	T46.2X6
rhythm regulator	T46.2X1	T46.2X2	T46.2X3	T46.2X4	T46.2X5	T46.2X6
specified NEC	T46.2X1	T46.2X2	T46.2X3	T46.2X4	T46.2X5	T46.2X6
Cardiografin	T50.8X1	T50.8X2	T50.8X3	T50.8X4	T50.8X5	T50.8X6
Cardio-green	T50.8X1	T50.8X2	T50.8X3	T50.8X4	T50.8X5	T50.8X6
Cardiotonic (glycoside)NEC	T46.0X1	T46.0X2	T46.0X3	T46.0X4	T46.0X5	T46.0X6
Cardiovascular drug NEC	T46.901	T46.902	T46.903	T46.904	T46.905	T46.906
Cardrase	T50.2X1	T50.2X2	T50.2X3	T50.2X4	T50.2X5	T50.2X6
Carfecillin	T36.0X1	T36.0X2	T36.0X3	T36.0X4	T36.0X5	T36.0X6
Carfenazine	T43.3X1	T43.3X2	T43.3X3	T43.3X4	T43.3X5	T43.3X6
Carfusin	T49.0X1	T49.0X2	T49.0X3	T49.0X4	T49.0X5	T49.0X6
Carindacillin	T36.0X1	T36.0X2	T36.0X3	T36.0X4	T36.0X5	T36.0X6
Carisoprodol	T42.8X1	T42.8X2	T42.8X3	T42.8X4	T42.8X5	T42.8X6
Carmellose	T47.4X1	T47.4X2	T47.4X3	T47.4X4	T47.4X5	T47.4X6
Carminative	T47.5X1	T47.5X2	T47.5X3	T47.5X4	T47.5X5	T47.5X6
Carmofur	T45.1X1	T45.1X2	T45.1X3	T45.1X4	T45.1X5	T45.1X6
Carmustine	T45.1X1	T45.1X2	T45.1X3	T45.1X4	T45.1X5	T45.1X6
Carotene	T45.2X1	T45.2X2	T45.2X3	T45.2X4	T45.2X5	T45.2X6
Carphenazine	T43.3X1	T43.3X2	T43.3X3	T43.3X4	T43.3X5	T43.3X6
Carpipramine	T42.4X1	T42.4X2	T42.4X3	T42.4X4	T42.4X5	T42.4X6
Carprofen	T39.311	T39.312	T39.313	T39.314	T39.315	T39.316
Carpronium chloride	T44.3X1	T44.3X2	T44.3X3	T44.3X4	T44.3X5	T44.3X6
Carrageenan	T47.8X1	T47.8X2	T47.8X3	T47.8X4	T47.8X5	T47.8X6
Carteolol	T44.7X1	T44.7X2	T44.7X3	T44.7X4	T44.7X5	T44.7X6
Carter's Little Pills	T47.2X1	T47.2X2	T47.2X3	T47.2X4	T47.2X5	T47.2X6
Cascara (sagrada)	T47.2X1	T47.2X2	T47.2X3	T47.2X4	T47.2X5	T47.2X6
Cassava	T62.2X1	T62.2X2	T62.2X3	T62.2X4	—	—
Castellani's paint	T49.0X1	T49.0X2	T49.0X3	T49.0X4	T49.0X5	T49.0X6
Castor						
bean	T62.2X1	T62.2X2	T62.2X3	T62.2X4	—	—
oil	T47.2X1	T47.2X2	T47.2X3	T47.2X4	T47.2X5	T47.2X6
Catalase	T45.3X1	T45.3X2	T45.3X3	T45.3X4	T45.3X5	T45.3X6
Caterpillar (sting)	T63.431	T63.432	T63.433	T63.434	—	—
Catha (edulis) (tea)	T43.691	T43.692	T43.693	T43.694	—	—
Cathartic NEC	T47.4X1	T47.4X2	T47.4X3	T47.4X4	T47.4X5	T47.4X6
anthacene derivative	T47.2X1	T47.2X2	T47.2X3	T47.2X4	T47.2X5	T47.2X6
bulk	T47.4X1	T47.4X2	T47.4X3	T47.4X4	T47.4X5	T47.4X6
contact	T47.2X1	T47.2X2	T47.2X3	T47.2X4	T47.2X5	T47.2X6
emollient NEC	T47.4X1	T47.4X2	T47.4X3	T47.4X4	T47.4X5	T47.4X6
irritant NEC	T47.2X1	T47.2X2	T47.2X3	T47.2X4	T47.2X5	T47.2X6
mucilage	T47.4X1	T47.4X2	T47.4X3	T47.4X4	T47.4X5	T47.4X6
saline	T47.3X1	T47.3X2	T47.3X3	T47.3X4	T47.3X5	T47.3X6
vegetable	T47.2X1	T47.2X2	T47.2X3	T47.2X4	T47.2X5	T47.2X6
Cathine	T50.5X1	T50.5X2	T50.5X3	T50.5X4	T50.5X5	T50.5X6
Cathomycin	T36.8X1	T36.8X2	T36.8X3	T36.8X4	T36.8X5	T36.8X6

Substance	Poisoning, Accidental (unintentional)	Poisoning, Intentional self-harm	Poisoning, Assault	Poisoning, Undetermined	Adverse effect	Underdosing
Cation exchange resin	T50.3X1	T50.3X2	T50.3X3	T50.3X4	T50.3X5	T50.3X6
Caustic(s) NEC	T54.91	T54.92	T54.93	T54.94	—	—
alkali	T54.3X1	T54.3X2	T54.3X3	T54.3X4	—	—
hydroxide	T54.3X1	T54.3X2	T54.3X3	T54.3X4	—	—
potash	T54.3X1	T54.3X2	T54.3X3	T54.3X4	—	—
soda	T54.3X1	T54.3X2	T54.3X3	T54.3X4	—	—
specified NEC	T54.91	T54.92	T54.93	T54.94	—	—
Ceepryn	T49.0X1	T49.0X2	T49.0X3	T49.0X4	T49.0X5	T49.0X6
ENT agent	T49.6X1	T49.6X2	T49.6X3	T49.6X4	T49.6X5	T49.6X6
lozenges	T49.6X1	T49.6X2	T49.6X3	T49.6X4	T49.6X5	T49.6X6
Cefacetrile	T36.1X1	T36.1X2	T36.1X3	T36.1X4	T36.1X5	T36.1X6
Cefaclor	T36.1X1	T36.1X2	T36.1X3	T36.1X4	T36.1X5	T36.1X6
Cefadroxil	T36.1X1	T36.1X2	T36.1X3	T36.1X4	T36.1X5	T36.1X6
Cefalexin	T36.1X1	T36.1X2	T36.1X3	T36.1X4	T36.1X5	T36.1X6
Cefaloglycin	T36.1X1	T36.1X2	T36.1X3	T36.1X4	T36.1X5	T36.1X6
Cefaloridine	T36.1X1	T36.1X2	T36.1X3	T36.1X4	T36.1X5	T36.1X6
Cefalosporins	T36.1X1	T36.1X2	T36.1X3	T36.1X4	T36.1X5	T36.1X6
Cefalotin	T36.1X1	T36.1X2	T36.1X3	T36.1X4	T36.1X5	T36.1X6
Cefamandole	T36.1X1	T36.1X2	T36.1X3	T36.1X4	T36.1X5	T36.1X6
Cefamycin antibiotic	T36.1X1	T36.1X2	T36.1X3	T36.1X4	T36.1X5	T36.1X6
Cefapirin	T36.1X1	T36.1X2	T36.1X3	T36.1X4	T36.1X5	T36.1X6
Cefatrizine	T36.1X1	T36.1X2	T36.1X3	T36.1X4	T36.1X5	T36.1X6
Cefazedone	T36.1X1	T36.1X2	T36.1X3	T36.1X4	T36.1X5	T36.1X6
Cefazolin	T36.1X1	T36.1X2	T36.1X3	T36.1X4	T36.1X5	T36.1X6
Cefbuperazone	T36.1X1	T36.1X2	T36.1X3	T36.1X4	T36.1X5	T36.1X6
Cefetamet	T36.1X1	T36.1X2	T36.1X3	T36.1X4	T36.1X5	T36.1X6
Cefixime	T36.1X1	T36.1X2	T36.1X3	T36.1X4	T36.1X5	T36.1X6
Cefmenoxime	T36.1X1	T36.1X2	T36.1X3	T36.1X4	T36.1X5	T36.1X6
Cefmetazole	T36.1X1	T36.1X2	T36.1X3	T36.1X4	T36.1X5	T36.1X6
Cefminox	T36.1X1	T36.1X2	T36.1X3	T36.1X4	T36.1X5	T36.1X6
Cefonicid	T36.1X1	T36.1X2	T36.1X3	T36.1X4	T36.1X5	T36.1X6
Cefoperazone	T36.1X1	T36.1X2	T36.1X3	T36.1X4	T36.1X5	T36.1X6
Ceforanide	T36.1X1	T36.1X2	T36.1X3	T36.1X4	T36.1X5	T36.1X6
Cefotaxime	T36.1X1	T36.1X2	T36.1X3	T36.1X4	T36.1X5	T36.1X6
Cefotetan	T36.1X1	T36.1X2	T36.1X3	T36.1X4	T36.1X5	T36.1X6
Cefotiam	T36.1X1	T36.1X2	T36.1X3	T36.1X4	T36.1X5	T36.1X6
Cefoxitin	T36.1X1	T36.1X2	T36.1X3	T36.1X4	T36.1X5	T36.1X6
Cefpimizole	T36.1X1	T36.1X2	T36.1X3	T36.1X4	T36.1X5	T36.1X6
Cefpiramide	T36.1X1	T36.1X2	T36.1X3	T36.1X4	T36.1X5	T36.1X6
Cefradine	T36.1X1	T36.1X2	T36.1X3	T36.1X4	T36.1X5	T36.1X6
Cefroxadine	T36.1X1	T36.1X2	T36.1X3	T36.1X4	T36.1X5	T36.1X6
Cefsulodin	T36.1X1	T36.1X2	T36.1X3	T36.1X4	T36.1X5	T36.1X6
Ceftazidime	T36.1X1	T36.1X2	T36.1X3	T36.1X4	T36.1X5	T36.1X6
Cefteram	T36.1X1	T36.1X2	T36.1X3	T36.1X4	T36.1X5	T36.1X6
Ceftezole	T36.1X1	T36.1X2	T36.1X3	T36.1X4	T36.1X5	T36.1X6
Ceftizoxime	T36.1X1	T36.1X2	T36.1X3	T36.1X4	T36.1X5	T36.1X6
Ceftriaxone	T36.1X1	T36.1X2	T36.1X3	T36.1X4	T36.1X5	T36.1X6
Cefuroxime	T36.1X1	T36.1X2	T36.1X3	T36.1X4	T36.1X5	T36.1X6
Cefuzonam	T36.1X1	T36.1X2	T36.1X3	T36.1X4	T36.1X5	T36.1X6
Celestone	T38.0X1	T38.0X2	T38.0X3	T38.0X4	T38.0X5	T38.0X6
topical	T49.0X1	T49.0X2	T49.0X3	T49.0X4	T49.0X5	T49.0X6

Substance	Poisoning, Accidental (unintentional)	Poisoning, Intentional self-harm	Poisoning, Assault	Poisoning, Undetermined	Adverse effect	Underdosing
Celiprolol	T44.7X1	T44.7X2	T44.7X3	T44.7X4	T44.7X5	T44.7X6
Cell stimulants and proliferants	T49.8X1	T49.8X2	T49.8X3	T49.8X4	T49.8X5	T49.8X6
Cellosolve	T52.91	T52.92	T52.93	T52.94	—	—
Cellulose						
cathartic	T47.4X1	T47.4X2	T47.4X3	T47.4X4	T47.4X5	T47.4X6
hydroxyethyl	T47.4X1	T47.4X2	T47.4X3	T47.4X4	T47.4X5	T47.4X6
nitrates (topical)	T49.3X1	T49.3X2	T49.3X3	T49.3X4	T49.3X5	T49.3X6
oxidized	T49.4X1	T49.4X2	T49.4X3	T49.4X4	T49.4X5	T49.4X6
Centipede (bite)	T63.411	T63.412	T63.413	T63.414	—	—
Central nervous system						
depressants	T42.71	T42.72	T42.73	T42.74	T42.75	T42.76
anesthetic (general) NEC	T41.201	T41.202	T41.203	T41.204	T41.205	T41.206
gases NEC	T41.0X1	T41.0X2	T41.0X3	T41.0X4	T41.0X5	T41.0X6
intravenous	T41.1X1	T41.1X2	T41.1X3	T41.1X4	T41.1X5	T41.1X6
barbiturates	T42.3X1	T42.3X2	T42.3X3	T42.3X4	T42.3X5	T42.3X6
benzodiazepines	T42.4X1	T42.4X2	T42.4X3	T42.4X4	T42.4X5	T42.4X6
bromides	T42.6X1	T42.6X2	T42.6X3	T42.6X4	T42.6X5	T42.6X6
cannabis sativa	T40.711	T40.712	T40.713	T40.714	T40.715	T40.716
chloral hydrate	T42.6X1	T42.6X2	T42.6X3	T42.6X4	T42.6X5	T42.6X6
ethanol	T51.0X1	T51.0X2	T51.0X3	T51.0X4	—	—
hallucinogenics	T40.901	T40.902	T40.903	T40.904	T40.905	T40.906
hypnotics	T42.71	T42.72	T42.73	T42.74	T42.75	T42.76
specified NEC	T42.6X1	T42.6X2	T42.6X3	T42.6X4	T42.6X5	T42.6X6
muscle relaxants	T42.8X1	T42.8X2	T42.8X3	T42.8X4	T42.8X5	T42.8X6
paraldehyde	T42.6X1	T42.6X2	T42.6X3	T42.6X4	T42.6X5	T42.6X6
sedatives; sedative-hypnotics	T42.71	T42.72	T42.73	T42.74	T42.75	T42.76
mixed NEC	T42.6X1	T42.6X2	T42.6X3	T42.6X4	T42.6X5	T42.6X6
specified NEC	T42.6X1	T42.6X2	T42.6X3	T42.6X4	T42.6X5	T42.6X6
muscle-tone depressants	T42.8X1	T42.8X2	T42.8X3	T42.8X4	T42.8X5	T42.8X6
stimulants	T43.601	T43.602	T43.603	T43.604	T43.605	T43.606
amphetamines	T43.621	T43.622	T43.623	T43.624	T43.625	T43.626
analeptics	T50.7X1	T50.7X2	T50.7X3	T50.7X4	T50.7X5	T50.7X6
antidepressants	T43.201	T43.202	T43.203	T43.204	T43.205	T43.206
opiate antagonists	T50.7X1	T50.7X2	T50.7X3	T50.7X4	T50.7X5	T50.7X6
specified NEC	T43.691	T43.692	T43.693	T43.694	T43.695	T43.696
Cephalexin	T36.1X1	T36.1X2	T36.1X3	T36.1X4	T36.1X5	T36.1X6
Cephaloglycin	T36.1X1	T36.1X2	T36.1X3	T36.1X4	T36.1X5	T36.1X6
Cephaloridine	T36.1X1	T36.1X2	T36.1X3	T36.1X4	T36.1X5	T36.1X6
Cephalosporins	T36.1X1	T36.1X2	T36.1X3	T36.1X4	T36.1X5	T36.1X6
N(adicillin)	T36.0X1	T36.0X2	T36.0X3	T36.0X4	T36.0X5	T36.0X6
Cephalothin	T36.1X1	T36.1X2	T36.1X3	T36.1X4	T36.1X5	T36.1X6
Cephalotin	T36.1X1	T36.1X2	T36.1X3	T36.1X4	T36.1X5	T36.1X6
Cephradine	T36.1X1	T36.1X2	T36.1X3	T36.1X4	T36.1X5	T36.1X6
Cerbera (odallam)	T62.2X1	T62.2X2	T62.2X3	T62.2X4	—	—
Cerberin	T46.0X1	T46.0X2	T46.0X3	T46.0X4	T46.0X5	T46.0X6
Cerebral stimulants	T43.601	T43.602	T43.603	T43.604	T43.605	T43.606
psychotherapeutic	T43.601	T43.602	T43.603	T43.604	T43.605	T43.606
specified NEC	T43.691	T43.692	T43.693	T43.694	T43.695	T43.696

Substance	Poisoning, Accidental (unintentional)	Poisoning, Intentional self-harm	Poisoning, Assault	Poisoning, Undetermined	Adverse effect	Underdosing
Cerium oxalate	T45.0X1	T45.0X2	T45.0X3	T45.0X4	T45.0X5	T45.0X6
Cerous oxalate	T45.0X1	T45.0X2	T45.0X3	T45.0X4	T45.0X5	T45.0X6
Ceruletide	T50.8X1	T50.8X2	T50.8X3	T50.8X4	T50.8X5	T50.8X6
Cetalkonium (chloride)	T49.0X1	T49.0X2	T49.0X3	T49.0X4	T49.0X5	T49.0X6
Cethexonium chloride	T49.0X1	T49.0X2	T49.0X3	T49.0X4	T49.0X5	T49.0X6
Cetiedil	T46.7X1	T46.7X2	T46.7X3	T46.7X4	T46.7X5	T46.7X6
Cetirizine	T45.0X1	T45.0X2	T45.0X3	T45.0X4	T45.0X5	T45.0X6
Cetomacrogol	T50.991	T50.992	T50.993	T50.994	T50.995	T50.996
Cetotiamine	T45.2X1	T45.2X2	T45.2X3	T45.2X4	T45.2X5	T45.2X6
Cetoxime	T45.0X1	T45.0X2	T45.0X3	T45.0X4	T45.0X5	T45.0X6
Cetraxate	T47.1X1	T47.1X2	T47.1X3	T47.1X4	T47.1X5	T47.1X6
Cetrimide	T49.0X1	T49.0X2	T49.0X3	T49.0X4	T49.0X5	T49.0X6
Cetrimonium (bromide)	T49.0X1	T49.0X2	T49.0X3	T49.0X4	T49.0X5	T49.0X6
Cetylpyridinium chloride	T49.0X1	T49.0X2	T49.0X3	T49.0X4	T49.0X5	T49.0X6
ENT agent	T49.6X1	T49.6X2	T49.6X3	T49.6X4	T49.6X5	T49.6X6
lozenges	T49.6X1	T49.6X2	T49.6X3	T49.6X4	T49.6X5	T49.6X6
Cevadilla—see Sabadilla						
Cevitamic acid	T45.2X1	T45.2X2	T45.2X3	T45.2X4	T45.2X5	T45.2X6
Chalk, precipitated	T47.1X1	T47.1X2	T47.1X3	T47.1X4	T47.1X5	T47.1X6
Chamomile	T49.0X1	T49.0X2	T49.0X3	T49.0X4	T49.0X5	T49.0X6
Ch'an su	T46.0X1	T46.0X2	T46.0X3	T46.0X4	T46.0X5	T46.0X6
Charcoal	T47.6X1	T47.6X2	T47.6X3	T47.6X4	T47.6X5	T47.6X6
activated—see also Charcoal, medicinal	T47.6X1	T47.6X2	T47.6X3	T47.6X4	T47.6X5	T47.6X6
fumes (Carbon monoxide)	T58.2X1	T58.2X2	T58.2X3	T58.2X4	—	—
industrial	T58.8X1	T58.8X2	T58.8X3	T58.8X4	—	—
medicinal (activated)	T47.6X1	T47.6X2	T47.6X3	T47.6X4	T47.6X5	T47.6X6
antidiarrheal	T47.6X1	T47.6X2	T47.6X3	T47.6X4	T47.6X5	T47.6X6
poison control	T47.8X1	T47.8X2	T47.8X3	T47.8X4	T47.8X5	T47.8X6
specified use other than for diarrhea	T47.8X1	T47.8X2	T47.8X3	T47.8X4	T47.8X5	T47.8X6
topical	T49.8X1	T49.8X2	T49.8X3	T49.8X4	T49.8X5	T49.8X6
Chaulmosulfone	T37.1X1	T37.1X2	T37.1X3	T37.1X4	T37.1X5	T37.1X6
Chelating agent NEC	T50.6X1	T50.6X2	T50.6X3	T50.6X4	T50.6X5	T50.6X6
Chelidonium majus	T62.2X1	T62.2X2	T62.2X3	T62.2X4	—	—
Chemical substance NEC	T65.91	T65.92	T65.93	T65.94	—	—
Chenodeoxycholic acid	T47.5X1	T47.5X2	T47.5X3	T47.5X4	T47.5X5	T47.5X6
Chenodiol	T47.5X1	T47.5X2	T47.5X3	T47.5X4	T47.5X5	T47.5X6
Chenopodium	T37.4X1	T37.4X2	T37.4X3	T37.4X4	T37.4X5	T37.4X6
Cherry laurel	T62.2X1	T62.2X2	T62.2X3	T62.2X4	—	—
Chinidin(e)	T46.2X1	T46.2X2	T46.2X3	T46.2X4	T46.2X5	T46.2X6
Chiniofon	T37.8X1	T37.8X2	T37.8X3	T37.8X4	T37.8X5	T37.8X6
Chlophedianol	T48.3X1	T48.3X2	T48.3X3	T48.3X4	T48.3X5	T48.3X6
Chloral	T42.6X1	T42.6X2	T42.6X3	T42.6X4	T42.6X5	T42.6X6
derivative	T42.6X1	T42.6X2	T42.6X3	T42.6X4	T42.6X5	T42.6X6
hydrate	T42.6X1	T42.6X2	T42.6X3	T42.6X4	T42.6X5	T42.6X6
Chloralamide	T42.6X1	T42.6X2	T42.6X3	T42.6X4	T42.6X5	T42.6X6
Chloralodol	T42.6X1	T42.6X2	T42.6X3	T42.6X4	T42.6X5	T42.6X6
Chloralose	T60.4X1	T60.4X2	T60.4X3	T60.4X4	—	—

Substance	Poisoning, Accidental (unintentional)	Poisoning, Intentional self-harm	Poisoning, Assault	Poisoning, Undetermined	Adverse effect	Underdosing
Chlorambucil	T45.1X1	T45.1X2	T45.1X3	T45.1X4	T45.1X5	T45.1X6
Chloramine	T57.8X1	T57.8X2	T57.8X3	T57.8X4	—	—
T	T49.0X1	T49.0X2	T49.0X3	T49.0X4	T49.0X5	T49.0X6
topical	T49.0X1	T49.0X2	T49.0X3	T49.0X4	T49.0X5	T49.0X6
Chloramphenicol	T36.2X1	T36.2X2	T36.2X3	T36.2X4	T36.2X5	T36.2X6
ENT agent	T49.6X1	T49.6X2	T49.6X3	T49.6X4	T49.6X5	T49.6X6
ophthalmic preparation	T49.5X1	T49.5X2	T49.5X3	T49.5X4	T49.5X5	T49.5X6
topical NEC	T49.0X1	T49.0X2	T49.0X3	T49.0X4	T49.0X5	T49.0X6
Chlorate (potassium) (sodium) NEC	T60.3X1	T60.3X2	T60.3X3	T60.3X4	—	—
herbicide	T60.3X1	T60.3X2	T60.3X3	T60.3X4	—	—
Chlorazanil	T50.2X1	T50.2X2	T50.2X3	T50.2X4	T50.2X5	T50.2X6
Chlorbenzene, chlorbenzol	T53.7X1	T53.7X2	T53.7X3	T53.7X4	—	—
Chlorbenzoxamine	T44.3X1	T44.3X2	T44.3X3	T44.3X4	T44.3X5	T44.3X6
Chlorbutol	T42.6X1	T42.6X2	T42.6X3	T42.6X4	T42.6X5	T42.6X6
Chlorcyclizine	T45.0X1	T45.0X2	T45.0X3	T45.0X4	T45.0X5	T45.0X6
Chlordan(e) (dust)	T60.1X1	T60.1X2	T60.1X3	T60.1X4	—	—
Chlordantoin	T49.0X1	T49.0X2	T49.0X3	T49.0X4	T49.0X5	T49.0X6
Chlordiazepoxide	T42.4X1	T42.4X2	T42.4X3	T42.4X4	T42.4X5	T42.4X6
Chlordiethyl benzamide	T49.3X1	T49.3X2	T49.3X3	T49.3X4	T49.3X5	T49.3X6
Chloresium	T49.8X1	T49.8X2	T49.8X3	T49.8X4	T49.8X5	T49.8X6
Chlorethiazol	T42.6X1	T42.6X2	T42.6X3	T42.6X4	T42.6X5	T42.6X6
Chlorethyl—see Ethyl, chloride						
Chloretone	T42.6X1	T42.6X2	T42.6X3	T42.6X4	T42.6X5	T42.6X6
Chlorex	T53.6X1	T53.6X2	T53.6X3	T53.6X4	—	—
insecticide	T60.1X1	T60.1X2	T60.1X3	T60.1X4	—	—
Chlorfenvinphos	T60.0X1	T60.0X2	T60.0X3	T60.0X4	—	—
Chlorhexadol	T42.6X1	T42.6X2	T42.6X3	T42.6X4	T42.6X5	T42.6X6
Chlorhexamide	T45.1X1	T45.1X2	T45.1X3	T45.1X4	T45.1X5	T45.1X6
Chlorhexidine	T49.0X1	T49.0X2	T49.0X3	T49.0X4	T49.0X5	T49.0X6
Chlorhydro-xyquinolin	T49.0X1	T49.0X2	T49.0X3	T49.0X4	T49.0X5	T49.0X6
Chloride of lime (bleach)	T54.3X1	T54.3X2	T54.3X3	T54.3X4	—	—
Chlorimipramine	T43.011	T43.012	T43.013	T43.014	T43.015	T43.016
Chlorinated						
camphene	T53.6X1	T53.6X2	T53.6X3	T53.6X4	—	—
diphenyl	T53.7X1	T53.7X2	T53.7X3	T53.7X4	—	—
hydrocarbons NEC	T53.91	T53.92	T53.93	T53.94	—	—
solvents	T53.91	T53.92	T53.93	T53.94	—	—
lime (bleach)	T54.3X1	T54.3X2	T54.3X3	T54.3X4	—	—
and boric acid solution	T49.0X1	T49.0X2	T49.0X3	T49.0X4	T49.0X5	T49.0X6
naphthalene (insecticide)	T60.1X1	T60.1X2	T60.1X3	T60.1X4	—	—
industrial (non-pesticide)	T53.7X1	T53.7X2	T53.7X3	T53.7X4	—	—
pesticide NEC	T60.8X1	T60.8X2	T60.8X3	T60.8X4	—	—
soda—see also sodium hypochlorite						
solution	T49.0X1	T49.0X2	T49.0X3	T49.0X4	T49.0X5	T49.0X6

Substance	Poisoning, Accidental (unintentional)	Poisoning, Intentional self-harm	Poisoning, Assault	Poisoning, Undetermined	Adverse effect	Underdosing
Chlorine (fumes) (gas)	T59.4X1	T59.4X2	T59.4X3	T59.4X4	—	—
bleach	T54.3X1	T54.3X2	T54.3X3	T54.3X4	—	—
compound gas NEC	T59.4X1	T59.4X2	T59.4X3	T59.4X4	—	—
disinfectant	T59.4X1	T59.4X2	T59.4X3	T59.4X4	—	—
releasing agents NEC	T59.4X1	T59.4X2	T59.4X3	T59.4X4	—	—
Chlorisondamine chloride	T46.991	T46.992	T46.993	T46.994	T46.995	T46.996
Chlormadinone	T38.5X1	T38.5X2	T38.5X3	T38.5X4	T38.5X5	T38.5X6
Chlormephos	T60.0X1	T60.0X2	T60.0X3	T60.0X4	—	—
Chlormerodrin	T50.2X1	T50.2X2	T50.2X3	T50.2X4	T50.2X5	T50.2X6
Chlormethiazole	T42.6X1	T42.6X2	T42.6X3	T42.6X4	T42.6X5	T42.6X6
Chlormethine	T45.1X1	T45.1X2	T45.1X3	T45.1X4	T45.1X5	T45.1X6
Chlormethyle-necycline	T36.4X1	T36.4X2	T36.4X3	T36.4X4	T36.4X5	T36.4X6
Chlormezanone	T42.6X1	T42.6X2	T42.6X3	T42.6X4	T42.6X5	T42.6X6
Chloroacetic acid	T60.3X1	T60.3X2	T60.3X3	T60.3X4	—	—
Chloroacetone	T59.3X1	T59.3X2	T59.3X3	T59.3X4	—	—
Chloroacetophenone	T59.3X1	T59.3X2	T59.3X3	T59.3X4	—	—
Chloroaniline	T53.7X1	T53.7X2	T53.7X3	T53.7X4	—	—
Chlorobenzene, chlorobenzol	T53.7X1	T53.7X2	T53.7X3	T53.7X4	—	—
Chlorobromo methane (fire extinguisher)	T53.6X1	T53.6X2	T53.6X3	T53.6X4	—	—
Chlorobutanol	T49.0X1	T49.0X2	T49.0X3	T49.0X4	T49.0X5	T49.0X6
Chlorocresol	T49.0X1	T49.0X2	T49.0X3	T49.0X4	T49.0X5	T49.0X6
Chlorodehydro-methyltestosterone	T38.7X1	T38.7X2	T38.7X3	T38.7X4	T38.7X5	T38.7X6
Chlorodinitro-benzene	T53.7X1	T53.7X2	T53.7X3	T53.7X4	—	—
dust or vapor	T53.7X1	T53.7X2	T53.7X3	T53.7X4	—	—
Chlorodiphenyl	T53.7X1	T53.7X2	T53.7X3	T53.7X4	—	—
Chloroethane—see Ethyl, chloride						
Chloroethylene	T53.6X1	T53.6X2	T53.6X3	T53.6X4	—	—
Chlorofluorocarbons	T53.5X1	T53.5X2	T53.5X3	T53.5X4	—	—
Chloroform (fumes) (vapor)	T53.1X1	T53.1X2	T53.1X3	T53.1X4	—	—
anesthetic	T41.0X1	T41.0X2	T41.0X3	T41.0X4	T41.0X5	T41.0X6
solvent	T53.1X1	T53.1X2	T53.1X3	T53.1X4	—	—
water, concentrated	T41.0X1	T41.0X2	T41.0X3	T41.0X4	T41.0X5	T41.0X6
Chloroguanide	T37.2X1	T37.2X2	T37.2X3	T37.2X4	T37.2X5	T37.2X6
Chloromycetin	T36.2X1	T36.2X2	T36.2X3	T36.2X4	T36.2X5	T36.2X6
ENT agent	T49.6X1	T49.6X2	T49.6X3	T49.6X4	T49.6X5	T49.6X6
ophthalmic preparation	T49.5X1	T49.5X2	T49.5X3	T49.5X4	T49.5X5	T49.5X6
otic solution	T49.6X1	T49.6X2	T49.6X3	T49.6X4	T49.6X5	T49.6X6
topical NEC	T49.0X1	T49.0X2	T49.0X3	T49.0X4	T49.0X5	T49.0X6
Chloronitrobenzene	T53.7X1	T53.7X2	T53.7X3	T53.7X4	—	—
dust or vapor	T53.7X1	T53.7X2	T53.7X3	T53.7X4	—	—
Chlorophacinone	T60.4X1	T60.4X2	T60.4X3	T60.4X4	—	—
Chlorophenol	T53.7X1	T53.7X2	T53.7X3	T53.7X4	—	—
Chlorophenothane	T60.1X1	T60.1X2	T60.1X3	T60.1X4	—	—
Chlorophyll	T50.991	T50.992	T50.993	T50.994	T50.995	T50.996
Chloropicrin (fumes)	T53.6X1	T53.6X2	T53.6X3	T53.6X4	—	—
fumigant	T60.8X1	T60.8X2	T60.8X3	T60.8X4	—	—

Substance	Poisoning, Accidental (unintentional)	Poisoning, Intentional self-harm	Poisoning, Assault	Poisoning, Undetermined	Adverse effect	Underdosing
Chloropicrin — Continued						
fungicide	T60.3X1	T60.3X2	T60.3X3	T60.3X4	—	—
pesticide	T60.8X1	T60.8X2	T60.8X3	T60.8X4	—	—
Chloroprocaine	T41.3X1	T41.3X2	T41.3X3	T41.3X4	T41.3X5	T41.3X6
infiltration (subcutaneous)	T41.3X1	T41.3X2	T41.3X3	T41.3X4	T41.3X5	T41.3X6
nerve block (peripheral) (plexus)	T41.3X1	T41.3X2	T41.3X3	T41.3X4	T41.3X5	T41.3X6
spinal	T41.3X1	T41.3X2	T41.3X3	T41.3X4	T41.3X5	T41.3X6
Chloroptic	T49.5X1	T49.5X2	T49.5X3	T49.5X4	T49.5X5	T49.5X6
Chloropurine	T45.1X1	T45.1X2	T45.1X3	T45.1X4	T45.1X5	T45.1X6
Chloropyramine	T45.0X1	T45.0X2	T45.0X3	T45.0X4	T45.0X5	T45.0X6
Chloropyrifos	T60.0X1	T60.0X2	T60.0X3	T60.0X4	—	—
Chloropyrilene	T45.0X1	T45.0X2	T45.0X3	T45.0X4	T45.0X5	T45.0X6
Chloroquine	T37.2X1	T37.2X2	T37.2X3	T37.2X4	T37.2X5	T37.2X6
Chlorothalonil	T60.3X1	T60.3X2	T60.3X3	T60.3X4	—	—
Chlorothen	T45.0X1	T45.0X2	T45.0X3	T45.0X4	T45.0X5	T45.0X6
Chlorothiazide	T50.2X1	T50.2X2	T50.2X3	T50.2X4	T50.2X5	T50.2X6
Chlorothymol	T49.4X1	T49.4X2	T49.4X3	T49.4X4	T49.4X5	T49.4X6
Chlorotrianisene	T38.5X1	T38.5X2	T38.5X3	T38.5X4	T38.5X5	T38.5X6
Chlorovinyldichloro-arsine, not in war	T57.0X1	T57.0X2	T57.0X3	T57.0X4	—	—
Chloroxine	T49.4X1	T49.4X2	T49.4X3	T49.4X4	T49.4X5	T49.4X6
Chloroxylenol	T49.0X1	T49.0X2	T49.0X3	T49.0X4	T49.0X5	T49.0X6
Chlorphenamine	T45.0X1	T45.0X2	T45.0X3	T45.0X4	T45.0X5	T45.0X6
Chlorphenesin	T42.8X1	T42.8X2	T42.8X3	T42.8X4	T42.8X5	T42.8X6
topical (antifungal)	T49.0X1	T49.0X2	T49.0X3	T49.0X4	T49.0X5	T49.0X6
Chlorpheniramine	T45.0X1	T45.0X2	T45.0X3	T45.0X4	T45.0X5	T45.0X6
Chlorphenoxamine	T45.0X1	T45.0X2	T45.0X3	T45.0X4	T45.0X5	T45.0X6
Chlorphentermine	T50.5X1	T50.5X2	T50.5X3	T50.5X4	T50.5X5	T50.5X6
Chlorprocaine—see Chloroprocaine						
Chlorproguanil	T37.2X1	T37.2X2	T37.2X3	T37.2X4	T37.2X5	T37.2X6
Chlorpromazine	T43.3X1	T43.3X2	T43.3X3	T43.3X4	T43.3X5	T43.3X6
Chlorpropamide	T38.3X1	T38.3X2	T38.3X3	T38.3X4	T38.3X5	T38.3X6
Chlorprothixene	T43.4X1	T43.4X2	T43.4X3	T43.4X4	T43.4X5	T43.4X6
Chlorquinaldol	T49.0X1	T49.0X2	T49.0X3	T49.0X4	T49.0X5	T49.0X6
Chlorquinol	T49.0X1	T49.0X2	T49.0X3	T49.0X4	T49.0X5	T49.0X6
Chlortalidone	T50.2X1	T50.2X2	T50.2X3	T50.2X4	T50.2X5	T50.2X6
Chlortetracycline	T36.4X1	T36.4X2	T36.4X3	T36.4X4	T36.4X5	T36.4X6
Chlorthalidone	T50.2X1	T50.2X2	T50.2X3	T50.2X4	T50.2X5	T50.2X6
Chlorthiophos	T60.0X1	T60.0X2	T60.0X3	T60.0X4	—	—
Chlortrianisene	T38.5X1	T38.5X2	T38.5X3	T38.5X4	T38.5X5	T38.5X6
Chlor-Trimeton	T45.0X1	T45.0X2	T45.0X3	T45.0X4	T45.0X5	T45.0X6
Chlorthion	T60.0X1	T60.0X2	T60.0X3	T60.0X4	—	—
Chlorzoxazone	T42.8X1	T42.8X2	T42.8X3	T42.8X4	T42.8X5	T42.8X6
Choke damp	T59.7X1	T59.7X2	T59.7X3	T59.7X4	—	—
Cholagogues	T47.5X1	T47.5X2	T47.5X3	T47.5X4	T47.5X5	T47.5X6
Cholebrine	T50.8X1	T50.8X2	T50.8X3	T50.8X4	T50.8X5	T50.8X6
Cholecalciferol	T45.2X1	T45.2X2	T45.2X3	T45.2X4	T45.2X5	T45.2X6

Substance	Poisoning, Accidental (unintentional)	Poisoning, Intentional self-harm	Poisoning, Assault	Poisoning, Undetermined	Adverse effect	Underdosing
Cholecystokinin	T50.8X1	T50.8X2	T50.8X3	T50.8X4	T50.8X5	T50.8X6
Cholera vaccine	T50.A91	T50.A92	T50.A93	T50.A94	T50.A95	T50.A96
Choleretic	T47.5X1	T47.5X2	T47.5X3	T47.5X4	T47.5X5	T47.5X6
Cholesterol-lowering agents	T46.6X1	T46.6X2	T46.6X3	T46.6X4	T46.6X5	T46.6X6
Cholestyramine (resin)	T46.6X1	T46.6X2	T46.6X3	T46.6X4	T46.6X5	T46.6X6
Cholic acid	T47.5X1	T47.5X2	T47.5X3	T47.5X4	T47.5X5	T47.5X6
Choline	T48.6X1	T48.6X2	T48.6X3	T48.6X4	T48.6X5	T48.6X6
chloride	T50.991	T50.992	T50.993	T50.994	T50.995	T50.996
dihydrogen citrate	T50.991	T50.992	T50.993	T50.994	T50.995	T50.996
salicylate	T39.091	T39.092	T39.093	T39.094	T39.095	T39.096
theophyllinate	T48.6X1	T48.6X2	T48.6X3	T48.6X4	T48.6X5	T48.6X6
Cholinergic (drug) NEC	T44.1X1	T44.1X2	T44.1X3	T44.1X4	T44.1X5	T44.1X6
muscle tone enhancer	T44.1X1	T44.1X2	T44.1X3	T44.1X4	T44.1X5	T44.1X6
organophosphorus	T44.0X1	T44.0X2	T44.0X3	T44.0X4	T44.0X5	T44.0X6
insecticide	T60.0X1	T60.0X2	T60.0X3	T60.0X4	—	—
nerve gas	T59.891	T59.892	T59.893	T59.894	—	—
trimethyl ammonium propanediol	T44.1X1	T44.1X2	T44.1X3	T44.1X4	T44.1X5	T44.1X6
Cholinesterase reactivator	T50.6X1	T50.6X2	T50.6X3	T50.6X4	T50.6X5	T50.6X6
Cholografin	T50.8X1	T50.8X2	T50.8X3	T50.8X4	T50.8X5	T50.8X6
Chorionic gonadotropin	T38.891	T38.892	T38.893	T38.894	T38.895	T38.896
Chromate	T56.2X1	T56.2X2	T56.2X3	T56.2X4	—	—
dust or mist	T56.2X1	T56.2X2	T56.2X3	T56.2X4	—	—
lead—see also lead	T56.0X1	T56.0X2	T56.0X3	T56.0X4	—	—
paint	T56.0X1	T56.0X2	T56.0X3	T56.0X4	—	—
Chromic						
acid	T56.2X1	T56.2X2	T56.2X3	T56.2X4	—	—
dust or mist	T56.2X1	T56.2X2	T56.2X3	T56.2X4	—	—
phosphate 32P	T45.1X1	T45.1X2	T45.1X3	T45.1X4	T45.1X5	T45.1X6
Chromium	T56.2X1	T56.2X2	T56.2X3	T56.2X4	—	—
compounds—see Chromate						
sesquioxide	T50.8X1	T50.8X2	T50.8X3	T50.8X4	T50.8X5	T50.8X6
Chromomycin A3	T45.1X1	T45.1X2	T45.1X3	T45.1X4	T45.1X5	T45.1X6
Chromonar	T46.3X1	T46.3X2	T46.3X3	T46.3X4	T46.3X5	T46.3X6
Chromyl chloride	T56.2X1	T56.2X2	T56.2X3	T56.2X4	—	—
Chrysarobin	T49.4X1	T49.4X2	T49.4X3	T49.4X4	T49.4X5	T49.4X6
Chrysazin	T47.2X1	T47.2X2	T47.2X3	T47.2X4	T47.2X5	T47.2X6
Chymar	T45.3X1	T45.3X2	T45.3X3	T45.3X4	T45.3X5	T45.3X6
ophthalmic preparation	T49.5X1	T49.5X2	T49.5X3	T49.5X4	T49.5X5	T49.5X6
Chymopapain	T45.3X1	T45.3X2	T45.3X3	T45.3X4	T45.3X5	T45.3X6
Chymotrypsin	T45.3X1	T45.3X2	T45.3X3	T45.3X4	T45.3X5	T45.3X6
ophthalmic preparation	T49.5X1	T49.5X2	T49.5X3	T49.5X4	T49.5X5	T49.5X6
Cianidanol	T50.991	T50.992	T50.993	T50.994	T50.995	T50.996
Cianopramine	T43.011	T43.012	T43.013	T43.014	T43.015	T43.016
Cibenzoline	T46.2X1	T46.2X2	T46.2X3	T46.2X4	T46.2X5	T46.2X6
Ciclacillin	T36.0X1	T36.0X2	T36.0X3	T36.0X4	T36.0X5	T36.0X6
Ciclobarbital—see Hexobarbital						

Substance	Poisoning, Accidental (unintentional)	Poisoning, Intentional self-harm	Poisoning, Assault	Poisoning, Undetermined	Adverse effect	Underdosing
Ciclonicate	T46.7X1	T46.7X2	T46.7X3	T46.7X4	T46.7X5	T46.7X6
Ciclopirox (olamine)	T49.0X1	T49.0X2	T49.0X3	T49.0X4	T49.0X5	T49.0X6
Ciclosporin	T45.1X1	T45.1X2	T45.1X3	T45.1X4	T45.1X5	T45.1X6
Cicuta maculata or virosa	T62.2X1	T62.2X2	T62.2X3	T62.2X4	—	—
Cicutoxin	T62.2X1	T62.2X2	T62.2X3	T62.2X4	—	—
Cigarette lighter fluid	T52.0X1	T52.0X2	T52.0X3	T52.0X4	—	—
Cigarettes (tobacco)	T65.221	T65.222	T65.223	T65.224	—	—
Ciguatoxin	T61.01	T61.02	T61.03	T61.04	—	—
Cilazapril	T46.4X1	T46.4X2	T46.4X3	T46.4X4	T46.4X5	T46.4X6
Cimetidine	T47.0X1	T47.0X2	T47.0X3	T47.0X4	T47.0X5	T47.0X6
Cimetropium bromide	T44.3X1	T44.3X2	T44.3X3	T44.3X4	T44.3X5	T44.3X6
Cinchocaine	T41.3X1	T41.3X2	T41.3X3	T41.3X4	T41.3X5	T41.3X6
topical (surface)	T41.3X1	T41.3X2	T41.3X3	T41.3X4	T41.3X5	T41.3X6
Cinchona	T37.2X1	T37.2X2	T37.2X3	T37.2X4	T37.2X5	T37.2X6
Cinchonine alkaloids	T37.2X1	T37.2X2	T37.2X3	T37.2X4	T37.2X5	T37.2X6
Cinchophen	T50.4X1	T50.4X2	T50.4X3	T50.4X4	T50.4X5	T50.4X6
Cinepazide	T46.7X1	T46.7X2	T46.7X3	T46.7X4	T46.7X5	T46.7X6
Cinnamedrine	T48.5X1	T48.5X2	T48.5X3	T48.5X4	T48.5X5	T48.5X6
Cinnarizine	T45.0X1	T45.0X2	T45.0X3	T45.0X4	T45.0X5	T45.0X6
Cinoxacin	T37.8X1	T37.8X2	T37.8X3	T37.8X4	T37.8X5	T37.8X6
Ciprofibrate	T46.6X1	T46.6X2	T46.6X3	T46.6X4	T46.6X5	T46.6X6
Ciprofloxacin	T36.8X1	T36.8X2	T36.8X3	T36.8X4	T36.8X5	T36.8X6
Cisapride	T47.8X1	T47.8X2	T47.8X3	T47.8X4	T47.8X5	T47.8X6
Cisplatin	T45.1X1	T45.1X2	T45.1X3	T45.1X4	T45.1X5	T45.1X6
Citalopram	T43.221	T43.222	T43.223	T43.224	T43.225	T43.226
Citanest						
infiltration (subcutaneous)	T41.3X1	T41.3X2	T41.3X3	T41.3X4	T41.3X5	T41.3X6
nerve block (peripheral) (plexus)	T41.3X1	T41.3X2	T41.3X3	T41.3X4	T41.3X5	T41.3X6
Citric acid	T47.5X1	T47.5X2	T47.5X3	T47.5X4	T47.5X5	T47.5X6
Citrovorum (factor)	T45.8X1	T45.8X2	T45.8X3	T45.8X4	T45.8X5	T45.8X6
Claviceps purpurea	T62.2X1	T62.2X2	T62.2X3	T62.2X4	—	—
Clavulanic acid	T36.1X1	T36.1X2	T36.1X3	T36.1X4	T36.1X5	T36.1X6
Cleaner, cleansing agent, type not specified	T65.891	T65.892	T65.893	T65.894		
of paint or varnish	T52.91	T52.92	T52.93	T52.94	—	—
specified type NEC	T65.891	T65.892	T65.893	T65.894	—	—
Clebopride	T47.8X1	T47.8X2	T47.8X3	T47.8X4	T47.8X5	T47.8X6
Clefamide	T37.3X1	T37.3X2	T37.3X3	T37.3X4	T37.3X5	T37.3X6
Clemastine	T45.0X1	T45.0X2	T45.0X3	T45.0X4	T45.0X5	T45.0X6
Clematis vitalba	T62.2X1	T62.2X2	T62.2X3	T62.2X4	—	—
Clemizole	T45.0X1	T45.0X2	T45.0X3	T45.0X4	T45.0X5	T45.0X6
penicillin	T36.0X1	T36.0X2	T36.0X3	T36.0X4	T36.0X5	T36.0X6
Clenbuterol	T48.6X1	T48.6X2	T48.6X3	T48.6X4	T48.6X5	T48.6X6
Clidinium bromide	T44.3X1	T44.3X2	T44.3X3	T44.3X4	T44.3X5	T44.3X6
Clindamycin	T36.8X1	T36.8X2	T36.8X3	T36.8X4	T36.8X5	T36.8X6
Clinofibrate	T46.6X1	T46.6X2	T46.6X3	T46.6X4	T46.6X5	T46.6X6
Clioquinol	T37.8X1	T37.8X2	T37.8X3	T37.8X4	T37.8X5	T37.8X6
Cliradon	T40.2X1	T40.2X2	T40.2X3	T40.2X4	—	—

Substance	Poisoning, Accidental (unintentional)	Poisoning, Intentional self-harm	Poisoning, Assault	Poisoning, Undetermined	Adverse effect	Underdosing
Clobazam	T42.4X1	T42.4X2	T42.4X3	T42.4X4	T42.4X5	T42.4X6
Clobenzorex	T50.5X1	T50.5X2	T50.5X3	T50.5X4	T50.5X5	T50.5X6
Clobetasol	T49.0X1	T49.0X2	T49.0X3	T49.0X4	T49.0X5	T49.0X6
Clobetasone	T49.0X1	T49.0X2	T49.0X3	T49.0X4	T49.0X5	T49.0X6
Clobutinol	T48.3X1	T48.3X2	T48.3X3	T48.3X4	T48.3X5	T48.3X6
Clocortolone	T38.0X1	T38.0X2	T38.0X3	T38.0X4	T38.0X5	T38.0X6
Clodantoin	T49.0X1	T49.0X2	T49.0X3	T49.0X4	T49.0X5	T49.0X6
Clodronic acid	T50.991	T50.992	T50.993	T50.994	T50.995	T50.996
Clofazimine	T37.1X1	T37.1X2	T37.1X3	T37.1X4	T37.1X5	T37.1X6
Clofedanol	T48.3X1	T48.3X2	T48.3X3	T48.3X4	T48.3X5	T48.3X6
Clofenamide	T50.2X1	T50.2X2	T50.2X3	T50.2X4	T50.2X5	T50.2X6
Clofenotane	T49.0X1	T49.0X2	T49.0X3	T49.0X4	T49.0X5	T49.0X6
Clofezone	T39.2X1	T39.2X2	T39.2X3	T39.2X4	T39.2X5	T39.2X6
Clofibrate	T46.6X1	T46.6X2	T46.6X3	T46.6X4	T46.6X5	T46.6X6
Clofibride	T46.6X1	T46.6X2	T46.6X3	T46.6X4	T46.6X5	T46.6X6
Cloforex	T50.5X1	T50.5X2	T50.5X3	T50.5X4	T50.5X5	T50.5X6
Clomethiazole	T42.6X1	T42.6X2	T42.6X3	T42.6X4	T42.6X5	T42.6X6
Clometocillin	T36.0X1	T36.0X2	T36.0X3	T36.0X4	T36.0X5	T36.0X6
Clomifene	T38.5X1	T38.5X2	T38.5X3	T38.5X4	T38.5X5	T38.5X6
Clomiphene	T38.5X1	T38.5X2	T38.5X3	T38.5X4	T38.5X5	T38.5X6
Clomipramine	T43.011	T43.012	T43.013	T43.014	T43.015	T43.016
Clomocycline	T36.4X1	T36.4X2	T36.4X3	T36.4X4	T36.4X5	T36.4X6
Clonazepam	T42.4X1	T42.4X2	T42.4X3	T42.4X4	T42.4X5	T42.4X6
Clonidine	T46.5X1	T46.5X2	T46.5X3	T46.5X4	T46.5X5	T46.5X6
Clonixin	T39.8X1	T39.8X2	T39.8X3	T39.8X4	T39.8X5	T39.8X6
Clopamide	T50.2X1	T50.2X2	T50.2X3	T50.2X4	T50.2X5	T50.2X6
Clopenthixol	T43.4X1	T43.4X2	T43.4X3	T43.4X4	T43.4X5	T43.4X6
Cloperastine	T48.3X1	T48.3X2	T48.3X3	T48.3X4	T48.3X5	T48.3X6
Clophedianol	T48.3X1	T48.3X2	T48.3X3	T48.3X4	T48.3X5	T48.3X6
Cloponone	T36.2X1	T36.2X2	T36.2X3	T36.2X4	T36.2X5	T36.2X6
Cloprednol	T38.0X1	T38.0X2	T38.0X3	T38.0X4	T38.0X5	T38.0X6
Cloral betaine	T42.6X1	T42.6X2	T42.6X3	T42.6X4	T42.6X5	T42.6X6
Cloramfenicol	T36.2X1	T36.2X2	T36.2X3	T36.2X4	T36.2X5	T36.2X6
Clorazepate (dipotassium)	T42.4X1	T42.4X2	T42.4X3	T42.4X4	T42.4X5	T42.4X6
Clorexolone	T50.2X1	T50.2X2	T50.2X3	T50.2X4	T50.2X5	T50.2X6
Clorfenamine	T45.0X1	T45.0X2	T45.0X3	T45.0X4	T45.0X5	T45.0X6
Clorgiline	T43.1X1	T43.1X2	T43.1X3	T43.1X4	T43.1X5	T43.1X6
Clorotepine	T44.3X1	T44.3X2	T44.3X3	T44.3X4	T44.3X5	T44.3X6
Clorox (bleach)	T54.91	T54.92	T54.93	T54.94	—	—
Clorprenaline	T48.6X1	T48.6X2	T48.6X3	T48.6X4	T48.6X5	T48.6X6
Clortermine	T50.5X1	T50.5X2	T50.5X3	T50.5X4	T50.5X5	T50.5X6
Clotiapine	T43.591	T43.592	T43.593	T43.594	T43.595	T43.596
Clotiazepam	T42.4X1	T42.4X2	T42.4X3	T42.4X4	T42.4X5	T42.4X6
Clotibric acid	T46.6X1	T46.6X2	T46.6X3	T46.6X4	T46.6X5	T46.6X6
Clotrimazole	T49.0X1	T49.0X2	T49.0X3	T49.0X4	T49.0X5	T49.0X6
Cloxacillin	T36.0X1	T36.0X2	T36.0X3	T36.0X4	T36.0X5	T36.0X6
Cloxazolam	T42.4X1	T42.4X2	T42.4X3	T42.4X4	T42.4X5	T42.4X6
Cloxiquine	T49.0X1	T49.0X2	T49.0X3	T49.0X4	T49.0X5	T49.0X6
Clozapine	T42.4X1	T42.4X2	T42.4X3	T42.4X4	T42.4X5	T42.4X6

Substance	Poisoning, Accidental (unintentional)	Poisoning, Intentional self-harm	Poisoning, Assault	Poisoning, Undetermined	Adverse effect	Underdosing
Coagulant NEC	T45.7X1	T45.7X2	T45.7X3	T45.7X4	T45.7X5	T45.7X6
Coal (carbon monoxide from)—see also Carbon, monoxide, coal	T58.2X1	T58.2X2	T58.2X3	T58.2X4	—	—
oil—see Kerosene						
tar	T49.1X1	T49.1X2	T49.1X3	T49.1X4	T49.1X5	T49.1X6
fumes	T59.891	T59.892	T59.893	T59.894	—	—
medicinal (ointment)	T49.4X1	T49.4X2	T49.4X3	T49.4X4	T49.4X5	T49.4X6
analgesics NEC	T39.2X1	T39.2X2	T39.2X3	T39.2X4	T39.2X5	T39.2X6
naphtha (solvent)	T52.0X1	T52.0X2	T52.0X3	T52.0X4	—	—
Cobalamine	T45.2X1	T45.2X2	T45.2X3	T45.2X4	T45.2X5	T45.2X6
Cobalt (nonmedicinal) (fumes) (industrial)	T56.891	T56.892	T56.893	T56.894	—	—
medicinal (trace) (chloride)	T45.8X1	T45.8X2	T45.8X3	T45.8X4	T45.8X5	T45.8X6
Cobra (venom)	T63.041	T63.042	T63.043	T63.044	—	—
Coca (leaf)	T40.5X1	T40.5X2	T40.5X3	T40.5X4	T40.5X5	T40.5X6
Cocaine	T40.5X1	T40.5X2	T40.5X3	T40.5X4	T40.5X5	T40.5X6
topical anesthetic	T41.3X1	T41.3X2	T41.3X3	T41.3X4	T41.3X5	T41.3X6
Cocarboxylase	T45.3X1	T45.3X2	T45.3X3	T45.3X4	T45.3X5	T45.3X6
Coccidioidin	T50.8X1	T50.8X2	T50.8X3	T50.8X4	T50.8X5	T50.8X6
Cocculus indicus	T62.1X1	T62.1X2	T62.1X3	T62.1X4	—	—
Cochineal	T65.6X1	T65.6X2	T65.6X3	T65.6X4	—	—
medicinal products	T50.991	T50.992	T50.993	T50.994	T50.995	T50.996
Codeine	T40.2X1	T40.2X2	T40.2X3	T40.2X4	T40.2X5	T40.2X6
Cod-liver oil	T45.2X1	T45.2X2	T45.2X3	T45.2X4	T45.2X5	T45.2X6
Coenzyme A	T50.991	T50.992	T50.993	T50.994	T50.995	T50.996
Coffee	T62.8X1	T62.8X2	T62.8X3	T62.8X4	—	—
Cogalactoiso-merase	T50.991	T50.992	T50.993	T50.994	T50.995	T50.996
Cogentin	T44.3X1	T44.3X2	T44.3X3	T44.3X4	T44.3X5	T44.3X6
Coke fumes or gas (carbon monoxide)	T58.2X1	T58.2X2	T58.2X3	T58.2X4	—	—
industrial use	T58.8X1	T58.8X2	T58.8X3	T58.8X4	—	—
Colace	T47.4X1	T47.4X2	T47.4X3	T47.4X4	T47.4X5	T47.4X6
Colaspase	T45.1X1	T45.1X2	T45.1X3	T45.1X4	T45.1X5	T45.1X6
Colchicine	T50.4X1	T50.4X2	T50.4X3	T50.4X4	T50.4X5	T50.4X6
Colchicum	T62.2X1	T62.2X2	T62.2X3	T62.2X4	—	—
Cold cream	T49.3X1	T49.3X2	T49.3X3	T49.3X4	T49.3X5	T49.3X6
Colecalciferol	T45.2X1	T45.2X2	T45.2X3	T45.2X4	T45.2X5	T45.2X6
Colestipol	T46.6X1	T46.6X2	T46.6X3	T46.6X4	T46.6X5	T46.6X6
Colestyramine	T46.6X1	T46.6X2	T46.6X3	T46.6X4	T46.6X5	T46.6X6
Colimycin	T36.8X1	T36.8X2	T36.8X3	T36.8X4	T36.8X5	T36.8X6
Colistimethate	T36.8X1	T36.8X2	T36.8X3	T36.8X4	T36.8X5	T36.8X6
Colistin	T36.8X1	T36.8X2	T36.8X3	T36.8X4	T36.8X5	T36.8X6
sulfate (eye preparation)	T49.5X1	T49.5X2	T49.5X3	T49.5X4	T49.5X5	T49.5X6
Collagen	T50.991	T50.992	T50.993	T50.994	T50.995	T50.996
Collagenase	T49.4X1	T49.4X2	T49.4X3	T49.4X4	T49.4X5	T49.4X6
Collodion	T49.3X1	T49.3X2	T49.3X3	T49.3X4	T49.3X5	T49.3X6
Colocynth	T47.2X1	T47.2X2	T47.2X3	T47.2X4	T47.2X5	T47.2X6
Colophony adhesive	T49.3X1	T49.3X2	T49.3X3	T49.3X4	T49.3X5	T49.3X6
Colorant—see also Dye	T50.991	T50.992	T50.993	T50.994	T50.995	T50.996

Substance	Poisoning, Accidental (unintentional)	Poisoning, Intentional self-harm	Poisoning, Assault	Poisoning, Undetermined	Adverse effect	Underdosing
Coloring matter—see Dye(s)						
Combustion gas (after combustion)—see Carbon, monoxide						
prior to combustion	T59.891	T59.892	T59.893	T59.894	—	—
Compazine	T43.3X1	T43.3X2	T43.3X3	T43.3X4	T43.3X5	T43.3X6
Compound						
42 (warfarin)	T60.4X1	T60.4X2	T60.4X3	T60.4X4	—	—
269 (endrin)	T60.1X1	T60.1X2	T60.1X3	T60.1X4	—	—
497 (dieldrin)	T60.1X1	T60.1X2	T60.1X3	T60.1X4	—	—
1080 (sodium fluoroacetate)	T60.4X1	T60.4X2	T60.4X3	T60.4X4	—	—
3422 (parathion)	T60.0X1	T60.0X2	T60.0X3	T60.0X4	—	—
3911 (phorate)	T60.0X1	T60.0X2	T60.0X3	T60.0X4	—	—
3956 (toxaphene)	T60.1X1	T60.1X2	T60.1X3	T60.1X4	—	—
4049 (malathion)	T60.0X1	T60.0X2	T60.0X3	T60.0X4	—	—
4069 (malathion)	T60.0X1	T60.0X2	T60.0X3	T60.0X4	—	—
4124 (dicapthon)	T60.0X1	T60.0X2	T60.0X3	T60.0X4	—	—
E (cortisone)	T38.0X1	T38.0X2	T38.0X3	T38.0X4	T38.0X5	T38.0X6
F (hydrocortisone)	T38.0X1	T38.0X2	T38.0X3	T38.0X4	T38.0X5	T38.0X6
Congener, avnnabolic	T38.7X1	T38.7X2	T38.7X3	T38.7X4	T38.7X5	T38.7X6
Congo red	T50.8X1	T50.8X2	T50.8X3	T50.8X4	T50.8X5	T50.8X6
Coniine, conine	T62.2X1	T62.2X2	T62.2X3	T62.2X4	—	—
Conium (maculatum)	T62.2X1	T62.2X2	T62.2X3	T62.2X4	—	—
Conjugated estrogenic substances	T38.5X1	T38.5X2	T38.5X3	T38.5X4	T38.5X5	T38.5X6
Contac	T48.5X1	T48.5X2	T48.5X3	T48.5X4	T48.5X5	T48.5X6
Contact lens solution	T49.5X1	T49.5X2	T49.5X3	T49.5X4	T49.5X5	T49.5X6
Contraceptive (oral)	T38.4X1	T38.4X2	T38.4X3	T38.4X4	T38.4X5	T38.4X6
vaginal	T49.8X1	T49.8X2	T49.8X3	T49.8X4	T49.8X5	T49.8X6
Contrast medium, radiography	T50.8X1	T50.8X2	T50.8X3	T50.8X4	T50.8X5	T50.8X6
Convallaria glycosides	T46.0X1	T46.0X2	T46.0X3	T46.0X4	T46.0X5	T46.0X6
Convallaria majalis	T62.2X1	T62.2X2	T62.2X3	T62.2X4	—	—
berry	T62.1X1	T62.1X2	T62.1X3	T62.1X4	—	—
Copper (dust) (fumes) (nonmedicinal) NEC	T56.4X1	T56.4X2	T56.4X3	T56.4X4	—	—
arsenate, arsenite	T57.0X1	T57.0X2	T57.0X3	T57.0X4	—	—
insecticide	T60.2X1	T60.2X2	T60.2X3	T60.2X4	—	—
emetic	T47.7X1	T47.7X2	T47.7X3	T47.7X4	T47.7X5	T47.7X6
fungicide	T60.3X1	T60.3X2	T60.3X3	T60.3X4	—	—
gluconate	T49.0X1	T49.0X2	T49.0X3	T49.0X4	T49.0X5	T49.0X6
insecticide	T60.2X1	T60.2X2	T60.2X3	T60.2X4	—	—
medicinal (trace)	T45.8X1	T45.8X2	T45.8X3	T45.8X4	T45.8X5	T45.8X6
oleate	T49.0X1	T49.0X2	T49.0X3	T49.0X4	T49.0X5	T49.0X6
sulfate	T56.4X1	T56.4X2	T56.4X3	T56.4X4	—	—
cupric	T56.4X1	T56.4X2	T56.4X3	T56.4X4	—	—
fungicide	T60.3X1	T60.3X2	T60.3X3	T60.3X4	—	—
medicinal						
ear	T49.6X1	T49.6X2	T49.6X3	T49.6X4	T49.6X5	T49.6X6
emetic	T47.7X1	T47.7X2	T47.7X3	T47.7X4	T47.7X5	T47.7X6

Substance	Poisoning, Accidental (unintentional)	Poisoning, Intentional self-harm	Poisoning, Assault	Poisoning, Undetermined	Adverse effect	Underdosing
Copper NEC — Continued						
eye	T49.5X1	T49.5X2	T49.5X3	T49.5X4	T49.5X5	T49.5X6
cuprous	T56.4X1	T56.4X2	T56.4X3	T56.4X4	—	—
fungicide	T60.3X1	T60.3X2	T60.3X3	T60.3X4	—	—
medicinal						
ear	T49.6X1	T49.6X2	T49.6X3	T49.6X4	T49.6X5	T49.6X6
emetic	T47.7X1	T47.7X2	T47.7X3	T47.7X4	T47.7X5	T47.7X6
eye	T49.5X1	T49.5X2	T49.5X3	T49.5X4	T49.5X5	T49.5X6
Copperhead snake (bite) (venom)	T63.061	T63.062	T63.063	T63.064	—	—
Coral (sting)	T63.691	T63.692	T63.693	T63.694	—	—
snake (bite) (venom)	T63.021	T63.022	T63.023	T63.024	—	—
Corbadrine	T49.6X1	T49.6X2	T49.6X3	T49.6X4	T49.6X5	T49.6X6
Cordite	T65.891	T65.892	T65.893	T65.894	—	—
vapor	T59.891	T59.892	T59.893	T59.894	—	—
Cordran	T49.0X1	T49.0X2	T49.0X3	T49.0X4	T49.0X5	T49.0X6
Corn cures	T49.4X1	T49.4X2	T49.4X3	T49.4X4	T49.4X5	T49.4X6
Corn starch	T49.3X1	T49.3X2	T49.3X3	T49.3X4	T49.3X5	T49.3X6
Cornhusker's lotion	T49.3X1	T49.3X2	T49.3X3	T49.3X4	T49.3X5	T49.3X6
Coronary vasodilator NEC	T46.3X1	T46.3X2	T46.3X3	T46.3X4	T46.3X5	T46.3X6
Corrosive NEC	T54.91	T54.92	T54.93	T54.94	—	—
acid NEC	T54.2X1	T54.2X2	T54.2X3	T54.2X4	—	—
aromatics	T54.1X1	T54.1X2	T54.1X3	T54.1X4	—	—
disinfectant	T54.1X1	T54.1X2	T54.1X3	T54.1X4	—	—
fumes NEC	T54.91	T54.92	T54.93	T54.94	—	—
specified NEC	T54.91	T54.92	T54.93	T54.94	—	—
sublimate	T56.1X1	T56.1X2	T56.1X3	T56.1X4	—	—
Cortate	T38.0X1	T38.0X2	T38.0X3	T38.0X4	T38.0X5	T38.0X6
Cort-Dome	T38.0X1	T38.0X2	T38.0X3	T38.0X4	T38.0X5	T38.0X6
ENT agent	T49.6X1	T49.6X2	T49.6X3	T49.6X4	T49.6X5	T49.6X6
ophthalmic preparation	T49.5X1	T49.5X2	T49.5X3	T49.5X4	T49.5X5	T49.5X6
topical NEC	T49.0X1	T49.0X2	T49.0X3	T49.0X4	T49.0X5	T49.0X6
Cortef	T38.0X1	T38.0X2	T38.0X3	T38.0X4	T38.0X5	T38.0X6
ENT agent	T49.6X1	T49.6X2	T49.6X3	T49.6X4	T49.6X5	T49.6X6
ophthalmic preparation	T49.5X1	T49.5X2	T49.5X3	T49.5X4	T49.5X5	T49.5X6
topical NEC	T49.0X1	T49.0X2	T49.0X3	T49.0X4	T49.0X5	T49.0X6
Corticosteroid	T38.0X1	T38.0X2	T38.0X3	T38.0X4	T38.0X5	T38.0X6
ENT agent	T49.6X1	T49.6X2	T49.6X3	T49.6X4	T49.6X5	T49.6X6
mineral	T50.0X1	T50.0X2	T50.0X3	T50.0X4	T50.0X5	T50.0X6
ophthalmic	T49.5X1	T49.5X2	T49.5X3	T49.5X4	T49.5X5	T49.5X6
topical NEC	T49.0X1	T49.0X2	T49.0X3	T49.0X4	T49.0X5	T49.0X6
Corticotropin	T38.811	T38.812	T38.813	T38.814	T38.815	T38.816
Cortisol	T49.0X1	T49.0X2	T49.0X3	T49.0X4	T49.0X5	T49.0X6
ENT agent	T49.6X1	T49.6X2	T49.6X3	T49.6X4	T49.6X5	T49.6X6
ophthalmic preparation	T49.5X1	T49.5X2	T49.5X3	T49.5X4	T49.5X5	T49.5X6
topical NEC	T49.0X1	T49.0X2	T49.0X3	T49.0X4	T49.0X5	T49.0X6
Cortisone (acetate)	T38.0X1	T38.0X2	T38.0X3	T38.0X4	T38.0X5	T38.0X6
ENT agent	T49.6X1	T49.6X2	T49.6X3	T49.6X4	T49.6X5	T49.6X6

Substance	Poisoning, Accidental (unintentional)	Poisoning, Intentional self-harm	Poisoning, Assault	Poisoning, Undetermined	Adverse effect	Underdosing
Cortisone — *Continued*						
ophthalmic preparation	T49.5X1	T49.5X2	T49.5X3	T49.5X4	T49.5X5	T49.5X6
topical NEC	T49.0X1	T49.0X2	T49.0X3	T49.0X4	T49.0X5	T49.0X6
Cortivazol	T38.0X1	T38.0X2	T38.0X3	T38.0X4	T38.0X5	T38.0X6
Cortogen	T38.0X1	T38.0X2	T38.0X3	T38.0X4	T38.0X5	T38.0X6
ENT agent	T49.6X1	T49.6X2	T49.6X3	T49.6X4	T49.6X5	T49.6X6
ophthalmic preparation	T49.5X1	T49.5X2	T49.5X3	T49.5X4	T49.5X5	T49.5X6
Cortone	T38.0X1	T38.0X2	T38.0X3	T38.0X4	T38.0X5	T38.0X6
ENT agent	T49.6X1	T49.6X2	T49.6X3	T49.6X4	T49.6X5	T49.6X6
ophthalmic preparation	T49.5X1	T49.5X2	T49.5X3	T49.5X4	T49.5X5	T49.5X6
Cortril	T38.0X1	T38.0X2	T38.0X3	T38.0X4	T38.0X5	T38.0X6
ENT agent	T49.6X1	T49.6X2	T49.6X3	T49.6X4	T49.6X5	T49.6X6
ophthalmic preparation	T49.5X1	T49.5X2	T49.5X3	T49.5X4	T49.5X5	T49.5X6
topical NEC	T49.0X1	T49.0X2	T49.0X3	T49.0X4	T49.0X5	T49.0X6
Corynebacterium parvum	T45.1X1	T45.1X2	T45.1X3	T45.1X4	T45.1X5	T45.1X6
Cosmetic preparation	T49.8X1	T49.8X2	T49.8X3	T49.8X4	T49.8X5	T49.8X6
Cosmetics	T49.8X1	T49.8X2	T49.8X3	T49.8X4	T49.8X5	T49.8X6
Cosyntropin	T38.811	T38.812	T38.813	T38.814	T38.815	T38.816
Cotarnine	T45.7X1	T45.7X2	T45.7X3	T45.7X4	T45.7X5	T45.7X6
Co-trimoxazole	T36.8X1	T36.8X2	T36.8X3	T36.8X4	T36.8X5	T36.8X6
Cottonseed oil	T49.3X1	T49.3X2	T49.3X3	T49.3X4	T49.3X5	T49.3X6
Cough mixture (syrup)	T48.4X1	T48.4X2	T48.4X3	T48.4X4	T48.4X5	T48.4X6
containing opiates	T40.2X1	T40.2X2	T40.2X3	T40.2X4	T40.2X5	T40.2X6
expectorants	T48.4X1	T48.4X2	T48.4X3	T48.4X4	T48.4X5	T48.4X6
Coumadin	T45.511	T45.512	T45.513	T45.514	T45.515	T45.516
rodenticide	T60.4X1	T60.4X2	T60.4X3	T60.4X4	—	—
Coumaphos	T60.0X1	T60.0X2	T60.0X3	T60.0X4	—	—
Coumarin	T45.511	T45.512	T45.513	T45.514	T45.515	T45.516
Coumetarol	T45.511	T45.512	T45.513	T45.514	T45.515	T45.516
Cowbane	T62.2X1	T62.2X2	T62.2X3	T62.2X4	—	—
Cozyme	T45.2X1	T45.2X2	T45.2X3	T45.2X4	T45.2X5	T45.2X6
Crack	T40.5X1	T40.5X2	T40.5X3	T40.5X4		
Crataegus extract	T46.0X1	T46.0X2	T46.0X3	T46.0X4	T46.0X5	T46.0X6
Creolin	T54.1X1	T54.1X2	T54.1X3	T54.1X4	—	—
disinfectant	T54.1X1	T54.1X2	T54.1X3	T54.1X4	—	—
Creosol (compound)	T49.0X1	T49.0X2	T49.0X3	T49.0X4	T49.0X5	T49.0X6
Creosote (coal tar) (beechwood)	T49.0X1	T49.0X2	T49.0X3	T49.0X4	T49.0X5	T49.0X6
medicinal (expectorant)	T48.4X1	T48.4X2	T48.4X3	T48.4X4	T48.4X5	T48.4X6
syrup	T48.4X1	T48.4X2	T48.4X3	T48.4X4	T48.4X5	T48.4X6
Cresol(s)	T49.0X1	T49.0X2	T49.0X3	T49.0X4	T49.0X5	T49.0X6
and soap solution	T49.0X1	T49.0X2	T49.0X3	T49.0X4	T49.0X5	T49.0X6
Cresyl acetate	T49.0X1	T49.0X2	T49.0X3	T49.0X4	T49.0X5	T49.0X6
Cresylic acid	T49.0X1	T49.0X2	T49.0X3	T49.0X4	T49.0X5	T49.0X6
Crimidine	T60.4X1	T60.4X2	T60.4X3	T60.4X4	—	—
Croconazole	T37.8X1	T37.8X2	T37.8X3	T37.8X4	T37.8X5	T37.8X6
Cromoglicic acid	T48.6X1	T48.6X2	T48.6X3	T48.6X4	T48.6X5	T48.6X6
Cromolyn	T48.6X1	T48.6X2	T48.6X3	T48.6X4	T48.6X5	T48.6X6
Cromonar	T46.3X1	T46.3X2	T46.3X3	T46.3X4	T46.3X5	T46.3X6
Cropropamide	T39.8X1	T39.8X2	T39.8X3	T39.8X4	T39.8X5	T39.8X6

Substance	Poisoning, Accidental (unintentional)	Poisoning, Intentional self-harm	Poisoning, Assault	Poisoning, Undetermined	Adverse effect	Underdosing
Cropropamide — *Continued*						
with crotethamide	T50.7X1	T50.7X2	T50.7X3	T50.7X4	T50.7X5	T50.7X6
Crotamiton	T49.0X1	T49.0X2	T49.0X3	T49.0X4	T49.0X5	T49.0X6
Crotethamide	T39.8X1	T39.8X2	T39.8X3	T39.8X4	T39.8X5	T39.8X6
with cropropamide	T50.7X1	T50.7X2	T50.7X3	T50.7X4	T50.7X5	T50.7X6
Croton (oil)	T47.2X1	T47.2X2	T47.2X3	T47.2X4	T47.2X5	T47.2X6
chloral	T42.6X1	T42.6X2	T42.6X3	T42.6X4	T42.6X5	T42.6X6
Crude oil	T52.0X1	T52.0X2	T52.0X3	T52.0X4	—	—
Cryogenine	T39.8X1	T39.8X2	T39.8X3	T39.8X4	T39.8X5	T39.8X6
Cryolite (vapor)	T60.1X1	T60.1X2	T60.1X3	T60.1X4	—	—
insecticide	T60.1X1	T60.1X2	T60.1X3	T60.1X4		
Cryptenamine (tannates)	T46.5X1	T46.5X2	T46.5X3	T46.5X4	T46.5X5	T46.5X6
Crystal violet	T49.0X1	T49.0X2	T49.0X3	T49.0X4	T49.0X5	T49.0X6
Cuckoopint	T62.2X1	T62.2X2	T62.2X3	T62.2X4	—	—
Cumetharol	T45.511	T45.512	T45.513	T45.514	T45.515	T45.516
Cupric						
acetate	T60.3X1	T60.3X2	T60.3X3	T60.3X4		
acetoarsenite	T57.0X1	T57.0X2	T57.0X3	T57.0X4	—	—
arsenate	T57.0X1	T57.0X2	T57.0X3	T57.0X4	—	—
gluconate	T49.0X1	T49.0X2	T49.0X3	T49.0X4	T49.0X5	T49.0X6
oleate	T49.0X1	T49.0X2	T49.0X3	T49.0X4	T49.0X5	T49.0X6
sulfate	T56.4X1	T56.4X2	T56.4X3	T56.4X4		
Cuprous sulfate—see also *Copper, sulfate*	T56.4X1	T56.4X2	T56.4X3	T56.4X4		
Curare, curarine	T48.1X1	T48.1X2	T48.1X3	T48.1X4	T48.1X5	T48.1X6
Cyamemazine	T43.3X1	T43.3X2	T43.3X3	T43.3X4	T43.3X5	T43.3X6
Cyamopsis tetragono-loba	T46.6X1	T46.6X2	T46.6X3	T46.6X4	T46.6X5	T46.6X6
Cyanacetyl hydrazide	T37.1X1	T37.1X2	T37.1X3	T37.1X4	T37.1X5	T37.1X6
Cyanic acid (gas)	T59.891	T59.892	T59.893	T59.894		
Cyanide(s) (compounds) (potassium) (sodium) NEC	T65.0X1	T65.0X2	T65.0X3	T65.0X4		
dust or gas (inhalation) NEC	T57.3X1	T57.3X2	T57.3X3	T57.3X4	—	—
fumigant	T65.0X1	T65.0X2	T65.0X3	T65.0X4		
hydrogen	T57.3X1	T57.3X2	T57.3X3	T57.3X4		
mercuric—see *Mercury*						
pesticide (dust) (fumes)	T65.0X1	T65.0X2	T65.0X3	T65.0X4		
Cyanoacrylate adhesive	T49.3X1	T49.3X2	T49.3X3	T49.3X4	T49.3X5	T49.3X6
Cyanocobalamin	T45.8X1	T45.8X2	T45.8X3	T45.8X4	T45.8X5	T45.8X6
Cyanogen (chloride) (gas) NEC	T59.891	T59.892	T59.893	T59.894	—	—
Cyclacillin	T36.0X1	T36.0X2	T36.0X3	T36.0X4	T36.0X5	T36.0X6
Cyclaine	T41.3X1	T41.3X2	T41.3X3	T41.3X4	T41.3X5	T41.3X6
Cyclamate	T50.991	T50.992	T50.993	T50.994	T50.995	T50.996
Cyclamen europaeum	T62.2X1	T62.2X2	T62.2X3	T62.2X4	—	—
Cyclandelate	T46.7X1	T46.7X2	T46.7X3	T46.7X4	T46.7X5	T46.7X6
Cyclazocine	T50.7X1	T50.7X2	T50.7X3	T50.7X4	T50.7X5	T50.7X6
Cyclizine	T45.0X1	T45.0X2	T45.0X3	T45.0X4	T45.0X5	T45.0X6
Cyclobarbital	T42.3X1	T42.3X2	T42.3X3	T42.3X4	T42.3X5	T42.3X6

391

Substance	Poisoning, Accidental (unintentional)	Poisoning, Intentional self-harm	Poisoning, Assault	Poisoning, Undetermined	Adverse effect	Underdosing
Cyclobarbitone	T42.3X1	T42.3X2	T42.3X3	T42.3X4	T42.3X5	T42.3X6
Cyclobenzaprine	T48.1X1	T48.1X2	T48.1X3	T48.1X4	T48.1X5	T48.1X6
Cyclodrine	T44.3X1	T44.3X2	T44.3X3	T44.3X4	T44.3X5	T44.3X6
Cycloguanil embonate	T37.2X1	T37.2X2	T37.2X3	T37.2X4	T37.2X5	T37.2X6
Cyclohexane	T52.8X1	T52.8X2	T52.8X3	T52.8X4	—	—
Cyclohexanol	T51.8X1	T51.8X2	T51.8X3	T51.8X4	—	—
Cyclohexanone	T52.4X1	T52.4X2	T52.4X3	T52.4X4	—	—
Cycloheximide	T60.3X1	T60.3X2	T60.3X3	T60.3X4	—	—
Cyclohexyl acetate	T52.8X1	T52.8X2	T52.8X3	T52.8X4	—	—
Cycloleucin	T45.1X1	T45.1X2	T45.1X3	T45.1X4	T45.1X5	T45.1X6
Cyclomethycaine	T41.3X1	T41.3X2	T41.3X3	T41.3X4	T41.3X5	T41.3X6
Cyclopentamine	T44.4X1	T44.4X2	T44.4X3	T44.4X4	T44.4X5	T44.4X6
Cyclopenthiazide	T50.2X1	T50.2X2	T50.2X3	T50.2X4	T50.2X5	T50.2X6
Cyclopentolate	T44.3X1	T44.3X2	T44.3X3	T44.3X4	T44.3X5	T44.3X6
Cyclophosphamide	T45.1X1	T45.1X2	T45.1X3	T45.1X4	T45.1X5	T45.1X6
Cycloplegic drug	T49.5X1	T49.5X2	T49.5X3	T49.5X4	T49.5X5	T49.5X6
Cyclopropane	T41.291	T41.292	T41.293	T41.294	T41.295	T41.296
Cyclopyrabital	T39.8X1	T39.8X2	T39.8X3	T39.8X4	T39.8X5	T39.8X6
Cycloserine	T37.1X1	T37.1X2	T37.1X3	T37.1X4	T37.1X5	T37.1X6
Cyclosporin	T45.1X1	T45.1X2	T45.1X3	T45.1X4	T45.1X5	T45.1X6
Cyclothiazide	T50.2X1	T50.2X2	T50.2X3	T50.2X4	T50.2X5	T50.2X6
Cycrimine	T44.3X1	T44.3X2	T44.3X3	T44.3X4	T44.3X5	T44.3X6
Cyhalothrin	T60.1X1	T60.1X2	T60.1X3	T60.1X4	—	—
Cymarin	T46.0X1	T46.0X2	T46.0X3	T46.0X4	T46.0X5	T46.0X6
Cypermethrin	T60.1X1	T60.1X2	T60.1X3	T60.1X4	—	—
Cyphenothrin	T60.2X1	T60.2X2	T60.2X3	T60.2X4	—	—
Cyproheptadine	T45.0X1	T45.0X2	T45.0X3	T45.0X4	T45.0X5	T45.0X6
Cyproterone	T38.6X1	T38.6X2	T38.6X3	T38.6X4	T38.6X5	T38.6X6
Cysteamine	T50.6X1	T50.6X2	T50.6X3	T50.6X4	T50.6X5	T50.6X6
Cytarabine	T45.1X1	T45.1X2	T45.1X3	T45.1X4	T45.1X5	T45.1X6
Cytisus						
laburnum	T62.2X1	T62.2X2	T62.2X3	T62.2X4	—	—
scoparius	T62.2X1	T62.2X2	T62.2X3	T62.2X4	—	—
Cytochrome C	T47.5X1	T47.5X2	T47.5X3	T47.5X4	T47.5X5	T47.5X6
Cytomel	T38.1X1	T38.1X2	T38.1X3	T38.1X4	T38.1X5	T38.1X6
Cytosine arabinoside	T45.1X1	T45.1X2	T45.1X3	T45.1X4	T45.1X5	T45.1X6
Cytoxan	T45.1X1	T45.1X2	T45.1X3	T45.1X4	T45.1X5	T45.1X6
Cytozyme	T45.7X1	T45.7X2	T45.7X3	T45.7X4	T45.7X5	T45.7X6
2,4-D	T60.3X1	T60.3X2	T60.3X3	T60.3X4	—	—
D						
Dacarbazine	T45.1X1	T45.1X2	T45.1X3	T45.1X4	T45.1X5	T45.1X6
Dactinomycin	T45.1X1	T45.1X2	T45.1X3	T45.1X4	T45.1X5	T45.1X6
DADPS	T37.1X1	T37.1X2	T37.1X3	T37.1X4	T37.1X5	T37.1X6
Dakin's solution	T49.0X1	T49.0X2	T49.0X3	T49.0X4	T49.0X5	T49.0X6
Dalapon (sodium)	T60.3X1	T60.3X2	T60.3X3	T60.3X4	—	—
Dalmane	T42.4X1	T42.4X2	T42.4X3	T42.4X4	T42.4X5	T42.4X6
Danazol	T38.6X1	T38.6X2	T38.6X3	T38.6X4	T38.6X5	T38.6X6
Danilone	T45.511	T45.512	T45.513	T45.514	T45.515	T45.516
Danthron	T47.2X1	T47.2X2	T47.2X3	T47.2X4	T47.2X5	T47.2X6
Dantrolene	T42.8X1	T42.8X2	T42.8X3	T42.8X4	T42.8X5	T42.8X6

Substance	Poisoning, Accidental (unintentional)	Poisoning, Intentional self-harm	Poisoning, Assault	Poisoning, Undetermined	Adverse effect	Underdosing
Dantron	T47.2X1	T47.2X2	T47.2X3	T47.2X4	T47.2X5	T47.2X6
Daphne (gnidium) (mezereum)	T62.2X1	T62.2X2	T62.2X3	T62.2X4	—	—
berry	T62.1X1	T62.1X2	T62.1X3	T62.1X4	—	—
Dapsone	T37.1X1	T37.1X2	T37.1X3	T37.1X4	T37.1X5	T37.1X6
Daraprim	T37.2X1	T37.2X2	T37.2X3	T37.2X4	T37.2X5	T37.2X6
Darnel	T62.2X1	T62.2X2	T62.2X3	T62.2X4	—	—
Darvon	T39.8X1	T39.8X2	T39.8X3	T39.8X4	T39.8X5	T39.8X6
Daunomycin	T45.1X1	T45.1X2	T45.1X3	T45.1X4	T45.1X5	T45.1X6
Daunorubicin	T45.1X1	T45.1X2	T45.1X3	T45.1X4	T45.1X5	T45.1X6
DBI	T38.3X1	T38.3X2	T38.3X3	T38.3X4	T38.3X5	T38.3X6
D-Con	T60.91	T60.92	T60.93	T60.94	—	—
insecticide	T60.2X1	T60.2X2	T60.2X3	T60.2X4		
rodenticide	T60.4X1	T60.4X2	T60.4X3	T60.4X4		
DDAVP	T38.891	T38.892	T38.893	T38.894	T38.895	T38.896
DDE (bis (chlorophenyl)-dichloroethylene)	T60.2X1	T60.2X2	T60.2X3	T60.2X4	—	—
DDS	T37.1X1	T37.1X2	T37.1X3	T37.1X4	T37.1X5	T37.1X6
DDT (dust)	T60.1X1	T60.1X2	T60.1X3	T60.1X4	—	—
Deadly nightshade—see also Belladonna	T62.2X1	T62.2X2	T62.2X3	T62.2X4	—	—
berry	T62.1X1	T62.1X2	T62.1X3	T62.1X4		
Deamino-D-arginine vasopressin	T38.891	T38.892	T38.893	T38.894	T38.895	T38.896
Deanol (aceglumate)	T50.991	T50.992	T50.993	T50.994	T50.995	T50.996
Debrisoquine	T46.5X1	T46.5X2	T46.5X3	T46.5X4	T46.5X5	T46.5X6
Decaborane	T57.8X1	T57.8X2	T57.8X3	T57.8X4	—	—
fumes	T59.891	T59.892	T59.893	T59.894		
Decadron	T38.0X1	T38.0X2	T38.0X3	T38.0X4	T38.0X5	T38.0X6
ENT agent	T49.6X1	T49.6X2	T49.6X3	T49.6X4	T49.6X5	T49.6X6
ophthalmic preparation	T49.5X1	T49.5X2	T49.5X3	T49.5X4	T49.5X5	T49.5X6
topical NEC	T49.0X1	T49.0X2	T49.0X3	T49.0X4	T49.0X5	T49.0X6
Decahydro-naphthalene	T52.8X1	T52.8X2	T52.8X3	T52.8X4	—	—
Decalin	T52.8X1	T52.8X2	T52.8X3	T52.8X4	—	—
Decamethonium (bromide)	T48.1X1	T48.1X2	T48.1X3	T48.1X4	T48.1X5	T48.1X6
Decholin	T47.5X1	T47.5X2	T47.5X3	T47.5X4	T47.5X5	T47.5X6
Declomycin	T36.4X1	T36.4X2	T36.4X3	T36.4X4	T36.4X5	T36.4X6
Decongestant, nasal (mucosa)	T48.5X1	T48.5X2	T48.5X3	T48.5X4	T48.5X5	T48.5X6
combination	T48.5X1	T48.5X2	T48.5X3	T48.5X4	T48.5X5	T48.5X6
Deet	T60.8X1	T60.8X2	T60.8X3	T60.8X4	—	—
Deferoxamine	T45.8X1	T45.8X2	T45.8X3	T45.8X4	T45.8X5	T45.8X6
Deflazacort	T38.0X1	T38.0X2	T38.0X3	T38.0X4	T38.0X5	T38.0X6
Deglycyrrhizinized extract of licorice	T48.4X1	T48.4X2	T48.4X3	T48.4X4	T48.4X5	T48.4X6
Dehydrocholic acid	T47.5X1	T47.5X2	T47.5X3	T47.5X4	T47.5X5	T47.5X6
Dehydroemetine	T37.3X1	T37.3X2	T37.3X3	T37.3X4	T37.3X5	T37.3X6
Dekalin	T52.8X1	T52.8X2	T52.8X3	T52.8X4	—	—
Delalutin	T38.5X1	T38.5X2	T38.5X3	T38.5X4	T38.5X5	T38.5X6
Delorazepam	T42.4X1	T42.4X2	T42.4X3	T42.4X4	T42.4X5	T42.4X6
Delphinium	T62.2X1	T62.2X2	T62.2X3	T62.2X4	—	—

Substance	Poisoning, Accidental (unintentional)	Poisoning, Intentional self-harm	Poisoning, Assault	Poisoning, Undetermined	Adverse effect	Underdosing
Deltamethrin	T60.1X1	T60.1X2	T60.1X3	T60.1X4	—	—
Deltasone	T38.0X1	T38.0X2	T38.0X3	T38.0X4	T38.0X5	T38.0X6
Deltra	T38.0X1	T38.0X2	T38.0X3	T38.0X4	T38.0X5	T38.0X6
Delvinal	T42.3X1	T42.3X2	T42.3X3	T42.3X4	T42.3X5	T42.3X6
Demecarium (bromide)	T49.5X1	T49.5X2	T49.5X3	T49.5X4	T49.5X5	T49.5X6
Demeclocycline	T36.4X1	T36.4X2	T36.4X3	T36.4X4	T36.4X5	T36.4X6
Demecolcine	T45.1X1	T45.1X2	T45.1X3	T45.1X4	T45.1X5	T45.1X6
Demegestone	T38.5X1	T38.5X2	T38.5X3	T38.5X4	T38.5X5	T38.5X6
Demelanizing agents	T49.8X1	T49.8X2	T49.8X3	T49.8X4	T49.8X5	T49.8X6
Demephion -O and -S	T60.0X1	T60.0X2	T60.0X3	T60.0X4	—	—
Demerol	T40.2X1	T40.2X2	T40.2X3	T40.2X4	T40.2X5	T40.2X6
Demethylchlor-tetracycline	T36.4X1	T36.4X2	T36.4X3	T36.4X4	T36.4X5	T36.4X6
Demethyltetracycline	T36.4X1	T36.4X2	T36.4X3	T36.4X4	T36.4X5	T36.4X6
Demeton -O and -S	T60.0X1	T60.0X2	T60.0X3	T60.0X4	—	—
Demulcent (external)	T49.3X1	T49.3X2	T49.3X3	T49.3X4	T49.3X5	T49.3X6
specified NEC	T49.3X1	T49.3X2	T49.3X3	T49.3X4	T49.3X5	T49.3X6
Demulen	T38.4X1	T38.4X2	T38.4X3	T38.4X4	T38.4X5	T38.4X6
Denatured alcohol	T51.0X1	T51.0X2	T51.0X3	T51.0X4	—	—
Dendrid	T49.5X1	T49.5X2	T49.5X3	T49.5X4	T49.5X5	T49.5X6
Dental drug, topical application NEC	T49.7X1	T49.7X2	T49.7X3	T49.7X4	T49.7X5	T49.7X6
Dentifrice	T49.7X1	T49.7X2	T49.7X3	T49.7X4	T49.7X5	T49.7X6
Deodorant spray (feminine hygiene)	T49.8X1	T49.8X2	T49.8X3	T49.8X4	T49.8X5	T49.8X6
Deoxycortone	T50.0X1	T50.0X2	T50.0X3	T50.0X4	T50.0X5	T50.0X6
2-Deoxy-5-fluorouridine	T45.1X1	T45.1X2	T45.1X3	T45.1X4	T45.1X5	T45.1X6
5-Deoxy-5-fluorouridine	T45.1X1	T45.1X2	T45.1X3	T45.1X4	T45.1X5	T45.1X6
Deoxyribonuclease (pancreatic)	T45.3X1	T45.3X2	T45.3X3	T45.3X4	T45.3X5	T45.3X6
Depilatory	T49.4X1	T49.4X2	T49.4X3	T49.4X4	T49.4X5	T49.4X6
Deprenalin	T42.8X1	T42.8X2	T42.8X3	T42.8X4	T42.8X5	T42.8X6
Deprenyl	T42.8X1	T42.8X2	T42.8X3	T42.8X4	T42.8X5	T42.8X6
Depressant, appetite	T50.5X1	T50.5X2	T50.5X3	T50.5X4	T50.5X5	T50.5X6
Depressant						
appetite (central)	T50.5X1	T50.5X2	T50.5X3	T50.5X4	T50.5X5	T50.5X6
cardiac	T46.2X1	T46.2X2	T46.2X3	T46.2X4	T46.2X5	T46.2X6
central nervous system (anesthetic)—see also Central nervous system, depressants	T42.71	T42.72	T42.73	T42.74	T42.75	T42.76
general anesthetic	T41.201	T41.202	T41.203	T41.204	T41.205	T41.206
muscle tone	T42.8X1	T42.8X2	T42.8X3	T42.8X4	T42.8X5	T42.8X6
muscle tone, central	T42.8X1	T42.8X2	T42.8X3	T42.8X4	T42.8X5	T42.8X6
psychotherapeutic	T43.501	T43.502	T43.503	T43.504	T43.505	T43.506
Deptropine	T45.0X1	T45.0X2	T45.0X3	T45.0X4	T45.0X5	T45.0X6
Dequalinium (chloride)	T49.0X1	T49.0X2	T49.0X3	T49.0X4	T49.0X5	T49.0X6
Derris root	T60.2X1	T60.2X2	T60.2X3	T60.2X4	—	—
Deserpidine	T46.5X1	T46.5X2	T46.5X3	T46.5X4	T46.5X5	T46.5X6
Desferrioxamine	T45.8X1	T45.8X2	T45.8X3	T45.8X4	T45.8X5	T45.8X6
Desipramine	T43.011	T43.012	T43.013	T43.014	T43.015	T43.016
Deslanoside	T46.0X1	T46.0X2	T46.0X3	T46.0X4	T46.0X5	T46.0X6

Substance	Poisoning, Accidental (unintentional)	Poisoning, Intentional self-harm	Poisoning, Assault	Poisoning, Undetermined	Adverse effect	Underdosing
Desloughing agent	T49.4X1	T49.4X2	T49.4X3	T49.4X4	T49.4X5	T49.4X6
Desmethy-limipramine	T43.011	T43.012	T43.013	T43.014	T43.015	T43.016
Desmopressin	T38.891	T38.892	T38.893	T38.894	T38.895	T38.896
Desocodeine	T40.2X1	T40.2X2	T40.2X3	T40.2X4	T40.2X5	T40.2X6
Desogestrel	T38.5X1	T38.5X2	T38.5X3	T38.5X4	T38.5X5	T38.5X6
Desomorphine	T40.2X1	T40.2X2	T40.2X3	T40.2X4	—	—
Desonide	T49.0X1	T49.0X2	T49.0X3	T49.0X4	T49.0X5	T49.0X6
Desoximetasone	T49.0X1	T49.0X2	T49.0X3	T49.0X4	T49.0X5	T49.0X6
Desoxycorticosteroid	T50.0X1	T50.0X2	T50.0X3	T50.0X4	T50.0X5	T50.0X6
Desoxycortone	T50.0X1	T50.0X2	T50.0X3	T50.0X4	T50.0X5	T50.0X6
Desoxyephedrine	T43.651	T43.652	T43.653	T43.654	T43.655	T43.656
Detaxtran	T46.6X1	T46.6X2	T46.6X3	T46.6X4	T46.6X5	T46.6X6
Detergent	T49.2X1	T49.2X2	T49.2X3	T49.2X4	T49.2X5	T49.2X6
external medication	T49.2X1	T49.2X2	T49.2X3	T49.2X4	T49.2X5	T49.2X6
local	T49.2X1	T49.2X2	T49.2X3	T49.2X4	T49.2X5	T49.2X6
medicinal	T49.2X1	T49.2X2	T49.2X3	T49.2X4	T49.2X5	T49.2X6
nonmedicinal	T55.1X1	T55.1X2	T55.1X3	T55.1X4	—	—
specified NEC	T55.1X1	T55.1X2	T55.1X3	T55.1X4	—	—
Deterrent, alcohol	T50.6X1	T50.6X2	T50.6X3	T50.6X4	T50.6X5	T50.6X6
Detoxifying agent	T50.6X1	T50.6X2	T50.6X3	T50.6X4	T50.6X5	T50.6X6
Detrothyronine	T38.1X1	T38.1X2	T38.1X3	T38.1X4	T38.1X5	T38.1X6
Dettol (external medication)	T49.0X1	T49.0X2	T49.0X3	T49.0X4	T49.0X5	T49.0X6
Dexamethasone	T38.0X1	T38.0X2	T38.0X3	T38.0X4	T38.0X5	T38.0X6
ENT agent	T49.6X1	T49.6X2	T49.6X3	T49.6X4	T49.6X5	T49.6X6
ophthalmic preparation	T49.5X1	T49.5X2	T49.5X3	T49.5X4	T49.5X5	T49.5X6
topical NEC	T49.0X1	T49.0X2	T49.0X3	T49.0X4	T49.0X5	T49.0X6
Dexamfetamine	T43.621	T43.622	T43.623	T43.624	T43.625	T43.626
Dexamphetamine	T43.621	T43.622	T43.623	T43.624	T43.625	T43.626
Dexbrom-pheniramine	T45.0X1	T45.0X2	T45.0X3	T45.0X4	T45.0X5	T45.0X6
Dexchlorpheniramine	T45.0X1	T45.0X2	T45.0X3	T45.0X4	T45.0X5	T45.0X6
Dexedrine	T43.621	T43.622	T43.623	T43.624	T43.625	T43.626
Dexetimide	T44.3X1	T44.3X2	T44.3X3	T44.3X4	T44.3X5	T44.3X6
Dexfenfluramine	T50.5X1	T50.5X2	T50.5X3	T50.5X4	T50.5X5	T50.5X6
Dexpanthenol	T45.2X1	T45.2X2	T45.2X3	T45.2X4	T45.2X5	T45.2X6
Dextran (40) (70) (150)	T45.8X1	T45.8X2	T45.8X3	T45.8X4	T45.8X5	T45.8X6
Dextriferron	T45.4X1	T45.4X2	T45.4X3	T45.4X4	T45.4X5	T45.4X6
Dextro calcium pantothenate	T45.2X1	T45.2X2	T45.2X3	T45.2X4	T45.2X5	T45.2X6
Dextro pantothenyl alcohol	T45.2X1	T45.2X2	T45.2X3	T45.2X4	T45.2X5	T45.2X6
Dextroamphetamine	T43.621	T43.622	T43.623	T43.624	T43.625	T43.626
Dextromethorphan	T48.3X1	T48.3X2	T48.3X3	T48.3X4	T48.3X5	T48.3X6
Dextromoramide	T40.491	T40.492	T40.493	T40.494	—	—
topical	T49.8X1	T49.8X2	T49.8X3	T49.8X4	T49.8X5	T49.8X6
Dextropropoxyphene	T40.491	T40.492	T40.493	T40.494	T40.495	T40.496
Dextrorphan	T40.2X1	T40.2X2	T40.2X3	T40.2X4	T40.2X5	T40.2X6
Dextrose	T50.3X1	T50.3X2	T50.3X3	T50.3X4	T50.3X5	T50.3X6
concentrated solution, intravenous	T46.8X1	T46.8X2	T46.8X3	T46.8X4	T46.8X5	T46.8X6
Dextrothyroxin	T38.1X1	T38.1X2	T38.1X3	T38.1X4	T38.1X5	T38.1X6

393

Substance	Poisoning, Accidental (unintentional)	Poisoning, Intentional self-harm	Poisoning, Assault	Poisoning, Undetermined	Adverse effect	Underdosing
Dextrothyroxine sodium	T38.1X1	T38.1X2	T38.1X3	T38.1X4	T38.1X5	T38.1X6
DFP	T44.0X1	T44.0X2	T44.0X3	T44.0X4	T44.0X5	T44.0X6
DHE	T37.3X1	T37.3X2	T37.3X3	T37.3X4	T37.3X5	T37.3X6
45	T46.5X1	T46.5X2	T46.5X3	T46.5X4	T46.5X5	T46.5X6
Diabinese	T38.3X1	T38.3X2	T38.3X3	T38.3X4	T38.3X5	T38.3X6
Diacetone alcohol	T52.4X1	T52.4X2	T52.4X3	T52.4X4	—	—
Diacetyl monoxime	T50.991	T50.992	T50.993	T50.994	—	—
Diacetylmorphine	T40.1X1	T40.1X2	T40.1X3	T40.1X4	—	—
Diachylon plaster	T49.4X1	T49.4X2	T49.4X3	T49.4X4	T49.4X5	T49.4X6
Diaethylst-ilboestrolum	T38.5X1	T38.5X2	T38.5X3	T38.5X4	T38.5X5	T38.5X6
Diagnostic agent NEC	T50.8X1	T50.8X2	T50.8X3	T50.8X4	T50.8X5	T50.8X6
Dial (soap)	T49.2X1	T49.2X2	T49.2X3	T49.2X4	T49.2X5	T49.2X6
sedative	T42.3X1	T42.3X2	T42.3X3	T42.3X4	T42.3X5	T42.3X6
Dialkyl carbonate	T52.91	T52.92	T52.93	T52.94	—	—
Diallylbarbituric acid	T42.3X1	T42.3X2	T42.3X3	T42.3X4	T42.3X5	T42.3X6
Diallymal	T42.3X1	T42.3X2	T42.3X3	T42.3X4	T42.3X5	T42.3X6
Dialysis solution (intraperitoneal)	T50.3X1	T50.3X2	T50.3X3	T50.3X4	T50.3X5	T50.3X6
Diaminodi-phenylsulfone	T37.1X1	T37.1X2	T37.1X3	T37.1X4	T37.1X5	T37.1X6
Diamorphine	T40.1X1	T40.1X2	T40.1X3	T40.1X4	—	—
Diamox	T50.2X1	T50.2X2	T50.2X3	T50.2X4	T50.2X5	T50.2X6
Diamthazole	T49.0X1	T49.0X2	T49.0X3	T49.0X4	T49.0X5	T49.0X6
Dianthone	T47.2X1	T47.2X2	T47.2X3	T47.2X4	T47.2X5	T47.2X6
Diaphenylsulfone	T37.0X1	T37.0X2	T37.0X3	T37.0X4	T37.0X5	T37.0X6
Diasone (sodium)	T37.1X1	T37.1X2	T37.1X3	T37.1X4	T37.1X5	T37.1X6
Diastase	T47.5X1	T47.5X2	T47.5X3	T47.5X4	T47.5X5	T47.5X6
Diatrizoate	T50.8X1	T50.8X2	T50.8X3	T50.8X4	T50.8X5	T50.8X6
Diazepam	T42.4X1	T42.4X2	T42.4X3	T42.4X4	T42.4X5	T42.4X6
Diazinon	T60.0X1	T60.0X2	T60.0X3	T60.0X4	—	—
Diazomethane (gas)	T59.891	T59.892	T59.893	T59.894	—	—
Diazoxide	T46.5X1	T46.5X2	T46.5X3	T46.5X4	T46.5X5	T46.5X6
Dibekacin	T36.5X1	T36.5X2	T36.5X3	T36.5X4	T36.5X5	T36.5X6
Dibenamine	T44.6X1	T44.6X2	T44.6X3	T44.6X4	T44.6X5	T44.6X6
Dibenzepin	T43.011	T43.012	T43.013	T43.014	T43.015	T43.016
Dibenzheptropine	T45.0X1	T45.0X2	T45.0X3	T45.0X4	T45.0X5	T45.0X6
Dibenzyline	T44.6X1	T44.6X2	T44.6X3	T44.6X4	T44.6X5	T44.6X6
Diborane (gas)	T59.891	T59.892	T59.893	T59.894	—	—
Dibromoch-loropropane	T60.8X1	T60.8X2	T60.8X3	T60.8X4	—	—
Dibromodulcitol	T45.1X1	T45.1X2	T45.1X3	T45.1X4	T45.1X5	T45.1X6
Dibromoethane	T53.6X1	T53.6X2	T53.6X3	T53.6X4	—	—
Dibromomannitol	T45.1X1	T45.1X2	T45.1X3	T45.1X4	T45.1X5	T45.1X6
Dibromopropamidine isethionate	T49.0X1	T49.0X2	T49.0X3	T49.0X4	T49.0X5	T49.0X6
Dibrompropamidine	T49.0X1	T49.0X2	T49.0X3	T49.0X4	T49.0X5	T49.0X6
Dibucaine	T41.3X1	T41.3X2	T41.3X3	T41.3X4	T41.3X5	T41.3X6
topical (surface)	T41.3X1	T41.3X2	T41.3X3	T41.3X4	T41.3X5	T41.3X6
Dibunate sodium	T48.3X1	T48.3X2	T48.3X3	T48.3X4	T48.3X5	T48.3X6
Dibutoline sulfate	T44.3X1	T44.3X2	T44.3X3	T44.3X4	T44.3X5	T44.3X6
Dicamba	T60.3X1	T60.3X2	T60.3X3	T60.3X4	—	—
Dicapthon	T60.0X1	T60.0X2	T60.0X3	T60.0X4	—	—

Substance	Poisoning, Accidental (unintentional)	Poisoning, Intentional self-harm	Poisoning, Assault	Poisoning, Undetermined	Adverse effect	Underdosing
Dichlobenil	T60.3X1	T60.3X2	T60.3X3	T60.3X4	—	—
Dichlone	T60.3X1	T60.3X2	T60.3X3	T60.3X4	—	—
Dichloralphenozone	T42.6X1	T42.6X2	T42.6X3	T42.6X4	T42.6X5	T42.6X6
Dichlorbenzidine	T65.3X1	T65.3X2	T65.3X3	T65.3X4	—	—
Dichlorhydrin	T52.8X1	T52.8X2	T52.8X3	T52.8X4	—	—
Dichlorhydroxy-quinoline	T37.8X1	T37.8X2	T37.8X3	T37.8X4	T37.8X5	T37.8X6
Dichlorobenzene	T53.7X1	T53.7X2	T53.7X3	T53.7X4	—	—
Dichlorobenzyl alcohol	T49.6X1	T49.6X2	T49.6X3	T49.6X4	T49.6X5	T49.6X6
Dichlorodifluoro-methane	T53.5X1	T53.5X2	T53.5X3	T53.5X4	—	—
Dichloroethane	T52.8X1	T52.8X2	T52.8X3	T52.8X4	—	—
Sym-Dichloroethyl ether	T53.6X1	T53.6X2	T53.6X3	T53.6X4	—	—
Dichloroethyl sulfide, not in war	T59.891	T59.892	T59.893	T59.894	—	—
Dichloroethylene	T53.6X1	T53.6X2	T53.6X3	T53.6X4	—	—
Dichloroformoxine, not in war	T59.891	T59.892	T59.893	T59.894	—	—
Dichlorohydrin, alpha-dichlorohydrin	T52.8X1	T52.8X2	T52.8X3	T52.8X4	—	—
Dichloromethane (solvent)	T53.4X1	T53.4X2	T53.4X3	T53.4X4	—	—
vapor	T53.4X1	T53.4X2	T53.4X3	T53.4X4	—	—
Dichloronaphtho-quinone	T60.3X1	T60.3X2	T60.3X3	T60.3X4	—	—
Dichlorophen	T37.4X1	T37.4X2	T37.4X3	T37.4X4	T37.4X5	T37.4X6
2,4-Dichlorophenoxy-acetic acid	T60.3X1	T60.3X2	T60.3X3	T60.3X4	—	—
Dichloropropene	T60.3X1	T60.3X2	T60.3X3	T60.3X4	—	—
Dichloropropionic acid	T60.3X1	T60.3X2	T60.3X3	T60.3X4	—	—
Dichlorphenamide	T50.2X1	T50.2X2	T50.2X3	T50.2X4	T50.2X5	T50.2X6
Dichlorvos	T60.0X1	T60.0X2	T60.0X3	T60.0X4	—	—
Diclofenac	T39.391	T39.392	T39.393	T39.394	T39.395	T39.396
Diclofenamide	T50.2X1	T50.2X2	T50.2X3	T50.2X4	T50.2X5	T50.2X6
Diclofensine	T43.291	T43.292	T43.293	T43.294	T43.295	T43.296
Diclonixine	T39.8X1	T39.8X2	T39.8X3	T39.8X4	T39.8X5	T39.8X6
Dicloxacillin	T36.0X1	T36.0X2	T36.0X3	T36.0X4	T36.0X5	T36.0X6
Dicophane	T49.0X1	T49.0X2	T49.0X3	T49.0X4	T49.0X5	T49.0X6
Dicoumarol, dicoumarin, dicumarol	T45.511	T45.512	T45.513	T45.514	T45.515	T45.516
Dicrotophos	T60.0X1	T60.0X2	T60.0X3	T60.0X4	—	—
Dicyanogen (gas)	T65.0X1	T65.0X2	T65.0X3	T65.0X4	—	—
Dicyclomine	T44.3X1	T44.3X2	T44.3X3	T44.3X4	T44.3X5	T44.3X6
Dicycloverine	T44.3X1	T44.3X2	T44.3X3	T44.3X4	T44.3X5	T44.3X6
Dideoxycytidine	T37.5X1	T37.5X2	T37.5X3	T37.5X4	T37.5X5	T37.5X6
Dideoxyinosine	T37.5X1	T37.5X2	T37.5X3	T37.5X4	T37.5X5	T37.5X6
Dieldrin (vapor)	T60.1X1	T60.1X2	T60.1X3	T60.1X4	—	—
Diemal	T42.3X1	T42.3X2	T42.3X3	T42.3X4	T42.3X5	T42.3X6
Dienestrol	T38.5X1	T38.5X2	T38.5X3	T38.5X4	T38.5X5	T38.5X6
Dienoestrol	T38.5X1	T38.5X2	T38.5X3	T38.5X4	T38.5X5	T38.5X6
Dietetic drug NEC	T50.901	T50.902	T50.903	T50.904	T50.905	T50.906
Diethazine	T42.8X1	T42.8X2	T42.8X3	T42.8X4	T42.8X5	T42.8X6

Substance	Poisoning, Accidental (unintentional)	Poisoning, Intentional self-harm	Poisoning, Assault	Poisoning, Undetermined	Adverse effect	Underdosing
Diethyl						
barbituric acid	T42.3X1	T42.3X2	T42.3X3	T42.3X4	T42.3X5	T42.3X6
carbamazine	T37.4X1	T37.4X2	T37.4X3	T37.4X4	T37.4X5	T37.4X6
carbinol	T51.3X1	T51.3X2	T51.3X3	T51.3X4	—	—
carbonate	T52.8X1	T52.8X2	T52.8X3	T52.8X4	—	—
ether (vapor)—see also ether	T41.0X1	T41.0X2	T41.0X3	T41.0X4	T41.0X5	T41.0X6
oxide	T52.8X1	T52.8X2	T52.8X3	T52.8X4	—	—
propion	T50.5X1	T50.5X2	T50.5X3	T50.5X4	T50.5X5	T50.5X6
stilbestrol	T38.5X1	T38.5X2	T38.5X3	T38.5X4	T38.5X5	T38.5X6
toluamide (nonmedicinal)	T60.8X1	T60.8X2	T60.8X3	T60.8X4	—	—
medicinal	T49.3X1	T49.3X2	T49.3X3	T49.3X4	T49.3X5	T49.3X6
Diethylcarbamazine	T37.4X1	T37.4X2	T37.4X3	T37.4X4	T37.4X5	T37.4X6
Diethylene						
dioxide	T52.8X1	T52.8X2	T52.8X3	T52.8X4	—	—
glycol (monoacetate) (monobutyl ether) (monoethyl ether)	T52.3X1	T52.3X2	T52.3X3	T52.3X4	—	—
Diethylhexy-lphthalate	T65.891	T65.892	T65.893	T65.894	—	—
Diethylpropion	T50.5X1	T50.5X2	T50.5X3	T50.5X4	T50.5X5	T50.5X6
Diethylstilbestrol	T38.5X1	T38.5X2	T38.5X3	T38.5X4	T38.5X5	T38.5X6
Diethylstilboestrol	T38.5X1	T38.5X2	T38.5X3	T38.5X4	T38.5X5	T38.5X6
Diethylsulfone-diethylmethane	T42.6X1	T42.6X2	T42.6X3	T42.6X4	T42.6X5	T42.6X6
Diethyltoluamide	T49.0X1	T49.0X2	T49.0X3	T49.0X4	T49.0X5	T49.0X6
Diethyltryptamine (DET)	T40.991	T40.992	T40.993	T40.994		
Difebarbamate	T42.3X1	T42.3X2	T42.3X3	T42.3X4	T42.3X5	T42.3X6
Difencloxazine	T40.2X1	T40.2X2	T40.2X3	T40.2X4	T40.2X5	T40.2X6
Difenidol	T45.0X1	T45.0X2	T45.0X3	T45.0X4	T45.0X5	T45.0X6
Difenoxin	T47.6X1	T47.6X2	T47.6X3	T47.6X4	T47.6X5	T47.6X6
Difetarsone	T37.3X1	T37.3X2	T37.3X3	T37.3X4	T37.3X5	T37.3X6
Diffusin	T45.3X1	T45.3X2	T45.3X3	T45.3X4	T45.3X5	T45.3X6
Diflorasone	T49.0X1	T49.0X2	T49.0X3	T49.0X4	T49.0X5	T49.0X6
Diflos	T44.0X1	T44.0X2	T44.0X3	T44.0X4	T44.0X5	T44.0X6
Diflubenzuron	T60.1X1	T60.1X2	T60.1X3	T60.1X4	—	—
Diflucortolone	T49.0X1	T49.0X2	T49.0X3	T49.0X4	T49.0X5	T49.0X6
Diflunisal	T39.091	T39.092	T39.093	T39.094	T39.095	T39.096
Difluoromethyldopa	T42.8X1	T42.8X2	T42.8X3	T42.8X4	T42.8X5	T42.8X6
Difluorophate	T44.0X1	T44.0X2	T44.0X3	T44.0X4	T44.0X5	T44.0X6
Digestant NEC	T47.5X1	T47.5X2	T47.5X3	T47.5X4	T47.5X5	T47.5X6
Digitalin(e)	T46.0X1	T46.0X2	T46.0X3	T46.0X4	T46.0X5	T46.0X6
Digitalis (leaf) (glycoside)	T46.0X1	T46.0X2	T46.0X3	T46.0X4	T46.0X5	T46.0X6
lanata	T46.0X1	T46.0X2	T46.0X3	T46.0X4	T46.0X5	T46.0X6
purpurea	T46.0X1	T46.0X2	T46.0X3	T46.0X4	T46.0X5	T46.0X6
Digitoxin	T46.0X1	T46.0X2	T46.0X3	T46.0X4	T46.0X5	T46.0X6
Digitoxose	T46.0X1	T46.0X2	T46.0X3	T46.0X4	T46.0X5	T46.0X6
Digoxin	T46.0X1	T46.0X2	T46.0X3	T46.0X4	T46.0X5	T46.0X6
Digoxine	T46.0X1	T46.0X2	T46.0X3	T46.0X4	T46.0X5	T46.0X6
Dihydralazine	T46.5X1	T46.5X2	T46.5X3	T46.5X4	T46.5X5	T46.5X6
Dihydrazine	T46.5X1	T46.5X2	T46.5X3	T46.5X4	T46.5X5	T46.5X6

Substance	Poisoning, Accidental (unintentional)	Poisoning, Intentional self-harm	Poisoning, Assault	Poisoning, Undetermined	Adverse effect	Underdosing
Dihydrocodeine	T40.2X1	T40.2X2	T40.2X3	T40.2X4	T40.2X5	T40.2X6
Dihydrocodeinone	T40.2X1	T40.2X2	T40.2X3	T40.2X4	T40.2X5	T40.2X6
Dihydroergocornine	T46.7X1	T46.7X2	T46.7X3	T46.7X4	T46.7X5	T46.7X6
Dihydroergocristine (mesilate)	T46.7X1	T46.7X2	T46.7X3	T46.7X4	T46.7X5	T46.7X6
Dihydroergokryptine	T46.7X1	T46.7X2	T46.7X3	T46.7X4	T46.7X5	T46.7X6
Dihydroergotamine	T46.5X1	T46.5X2	T46.5X3	T46.5X4	T46.5X5	T46.5X6
Dihydroergotoxine	T46.7X1	T46.7X2	T46.7X3	T46.7X4	T46.7X5	T46.7X6
mesilate	T46.7X1	T46.7X2	T46.7X3	T46.7X4	T46.7X5	T46.7X6
Dihydrohydroxy-codeinone	T40.2X1	T40.2X2	T40.2X3	T40.2X4	T40.2X5	T40.2X6
Dihydrohydroxy-morphinone	T40.2X1	T40.2X2	T40.2X3	T40.2X4	T40.2X5	T40.2X6
Dihydroisocodeine	T40.2X1	T40.2X2	T40.2X3	T40.2X4	T40.2X5	T40.2X6
Dihydromorphine	T40.2X1	T40.2X2	T40.2X3	T40.2X4	—	—
Dihydromorphinone	T40.2X1	T40.2X2	T40.2X3	T40.2X4	T40.2X5	T40.2X6
Dihydrostreptomycin	T36.5X1	T36.5X2	T36.5X3	T36.5X4	T36.5X5	T36.5X6
Dihydrotachysterol	T45.2X1	T45.2X2	T45.2X3	T45.2X4	T45.2X5	T45.2X6
Dihydroxyaluminum aminoacetate	T47.1X1	T47.1X2	T47.1X3	T47.1X4	T47.1X5	T47.1X6
Dihydroxyaluminum sodium carbonate	T47.1X1	T47.1X2	T47.1X3	T47.1X4	T47.1X5	T47.1X6
Dihydroxyanthra-quinone	T47.2X1	T47.2X2	T47.2X3	T47.2X4	T47.2X5	T47.2X6
Dihydroxycodeinone	T40.2X1	T40.2X2	T40.2X3	T40.2X4	T40.2X5	T40.2X6
Dihydroxypropyl theophylline	T50.2X1	T50.2X2	T50.2X3	T50.2X4	T50.2X5	T50.2X6
Diiodohydroxyquin	T37.8X1	T37.8X2	T37.8X3	T37.8X4	T37.8X5	T37.8X6
topical	T49.0X1	T49.0X2	T49.0X3	T49.0X4	T49.0X5	T49.0X6
Diiodo-hydroxyquinoline	T37.8X1	T37.8X2	T37.8X3	T37.8X4	T37.8X5	T37.8X6
Diiodotyrosine	T38.2X1	T38.2X2	T38.2X3	T38.2X4	T38.2X5	T38.2X6
Diisopromine	T44.3X1	T44.3X2	T44.3X3	T44.3X4	T44.3X5	T44.3X6
Diisopropylamine	T46.3X1	T46.3X2	T46.3X3	T46.3X4	T46.3X5	T46.3X6
Diisopropyl-fluorophos-phonate	T44.0X1	T44.0X2	T44.0X3	T44.0X4	T44.0X5	T44.0X6
Dilantin	T42.0X1	T42.0X2	T42.0X3	T42.0X4	T42.0X5	T42.0X6
Dilaudid	T40.2X1	T40.2X2	T40.2X3	T40.2X4	T40.2X5	T40.2X6
Dilazep	T46.3X1	T46.3X2	T46.3X3	T46.3X4	T46.3X5	T46.3X6
Dill	T47.5X1	T47.5X2	T47.5X3	T47.5X4	T47.5X5	T47.5X6
Diloxanide	T37.3X1	T37.3X2	T37.3X3	T37.3X4	T37.3X5	T37.3X6
Diltiazem	T46.1X1	T46.1X2	T46.1X3	T46.1X4	T46.1X5	T46.1X6
Dimazole	T49.0X1	T49.0X2	T49.0X3	T49.0X4	T49.0X5	T49.0X6
Dimefline	T50.7X1	T50.7X2	T50.7X3	T50.7X4	T50.7X5	T50.7X6
Dimefox	T60.0X1	T60.0X2	T60.0X3	T60.0X4	—	—
Dimemorfan	T48.3X1	T48.3X2	T48.3X3	T48.3X4	T48.3X5	T48.3X6
Dimenhydrinate	T45.0X1	T45.0X2	T45.0X3	T45.0X4	T45.0X5	T45.0X6
Dimercaprol (British anti-lewisite)	T45.8X1	T45.8X2	T45.8X3	T45.8X4	T45.8X5	T45.8X6
Dimercaptopropanol	T45.8X1	T45.8X2	T45.8X3	T45.8X4	T45.8X5	T45.8X6
Dimestrol	T38.5X1	T38.5X2	T38.5X3	T38.5X4	T38.5X5	T38.5X6
Dimetane	T45.0X1	T45.0X2	T45.0X3	T45.0X4	T45.0X5	T45.0X6
Dimethicone	T47.1X1	T47.1X2	T47.1X3	T47.1X4	T47.1X5	T47.1X6
Dimethindene	T45.0X1	T45.0X2	T45.0X3	T45.0X4	T45.0X5	T45.0X6

395

Substance	Poisoning, Accidental (unintentional)	Poisoning, Intentional self-harm	Poisoning, Assault	Poisoning, Undetermined	Adverse effect	Underdosing
Dimethisoquin	T49.1X1	T49.1X2	T49.1X3	T49.1X4	T49.1X5	T49.1X6
Dimethisterone	T38.5X1	T38.5X2	T38.5X3	T38.5X4	T38.5X5	T38.5X6
Dimethoate	T60.0X1	T60.0X2	T60.0X3	T60.0X4	—	—
Dimethocaine	T41.3X1	T41.3X2	T41.3X3	T41.3X4	T41.3X5	T41.3X6
Dimethoxanate	T48.3X1	T48.3X2	T48.3X3	T48.3X4	T48.3X5	T48.3X6
Dimethyl						
arsine, arsinic acid	T57.0X1	T57.0X2	T57.0X3	T57.0X4	—	—
carbinol	T51.2X1	T51.2X2	T51.2X3	T51.2X4	—	—
carbonate	T52.8X1	T52.8X2	T52.8X3	T52.8X4	—	—
diguanide	T38.3X1	T38.3X2	T38.3X3	T38.3X4	T38.3X5	T38.3X6
ketone	T52.4X1	T52.4X2	T52.4X3	T52.4X4	—	—
vapor	T52.4X1	T52.4X2	T52.4X3	T52.4X4	—	—
meperidine	T40.2X1	T40.2X2	T40.2X3	T40.2X4	T40.2X5	T40.2X6
parathion	T60.0X1	T60.0X2	T60.0X3	T60.0X4	—	—
phthlate	T49.3X1	T49.3X2	T49.3X3	T49.3X4	T49.3X5	T49.3X6
polysiloxane	T47.8X1	T47.8X2	T47.8X3	T47.8X4	T47.8X5	T47.8X6
sulfate (fumes)	T59.891	T59.892	T59.893	T59.894	—	—
liquid	T65.891	T65.892	T65.893	T65.894	—	—
sulfoxide (nonmedicinal)	T52.8X1	T52.8X2	T52.8X3	T52.8X4	—	—
medicinal	T49.4X1	T49.4X2	T49.4X3	T49.4X4	T49.4X5	T49.4X6
tryptamine	T40.991	T40.992	T40.993	T40.994	—	—
tubocurarine	T48.1X1	T48.1X2	T48.1X3	T48.1X4	T48.1X5	T48.1X6
Dimethylamine sulfate	T49.4X1	T49.4X2	T49.4X3	T49.4X4	T49.4X5	T49.4X6
Dimethylformamide	T52.8X1	T52.8X2	T52.8X3	T52.8X4	—	—
Dimethyltubocurarinium chloride	T48.1X1	T48.1X2	T48.1X3	T48.1X4	T48.1X5	T48.1X6
Dimeticone	T47.1X1	T47.1X2	T47.1X3	T47.1X4	T47.1X5	T47.1X6
Dimetilan	T60.0X1	T60.0X2	T60.0X3	T60.0X4	—	—
Dimetindene	T45.0X1	T45.0X2	T45.0X3	T45.0X4	T45.0X5	T45.0X6
Dimetotiazine	T43.3X1	T43.3X2	T43.3X3	T43.3X4	T43.3X5	T43.3X6
Dimorpholamine	T50.7X1	T50.7X2	T50.7X3	T50.7X4	T50.7X5	T50.7X6
Dimoxyline	T46.3X1	T46.3X2	T46.3X3	T46.3X4	T46.3X5	T46.3X6
Dinitrobenzene	T65.3X1	T65.3X2	T65.3X3	T65.3X4	—	—
vapor	T59.891	T59.892	T59.893	T59.894	—	—
Dinitrobenzol	T65.3X1	T65.3X2	T65.3X3	T65.3X4	—	—
vapor	T59.891	T59.892	T59.893	T59.894	—	—
Dinitrobutylphenol	T65.3X1	T65.3X2	T65.3X3	T65.3X4	—	—
Dinitro (-ortho-)cresol (pesticide) (spray)	T65.3X1	T65.3X2	T65.3X3	T65.3X4	—	—
Dinitro-cyclohexylphenol	T65.3X1	T65.3X2	T65.3X3	T65.3X4	—	—
Dinitrophenol	T65.3X1	T65.3X2	T65.3X3	T65.3X4	—	—
Dinoprost	T48.0X1	T48.0X2	T48.0X3	T48.0X4	T48.0X5	T48.0X6
Dinoprostone	T48.0X1	T48.0X2	T48.0X3	T48.0X4	T48.0X5	T48.0X6
Dinoseb	T60.3X1	T60.3X2	T60.3X3	T60.3X4	—	—
Dioctyl sulfosuccinate (calcium) (sodium)	T47.4X1	T47.4X2	T47.4X3	T47.4X4	T47.4X5	T47.4X6
Diodone	T50.8X1	T50.8X2	T50.8X3	T50.8X4	T50.8X5	T50.8X6
Diodoquin	T37.8X1	T37.8X2	T37.8X3	T37.8X4	T37.8X5	T37.8X6
Dionin	T40.2X1	T40.2X2	T40.2X3	T40.2X4	T40.2X5	T40.2X6
Diosmin	T46.991	T46.992	T46.993	T46.994	T46.995	T46.996

Substance	Poisoning, Accidental (unintentional)	Poisoning, Intentional self-harm	Poisoning, Assault	Poisoning, Undetermined	Adverse effect	Underdosing
Dioxane	T52.8X1	T52.8X2	T52.8X3	T52.8X4	—	—
Dioxathion	T60.0X1	T60.0X2	T60.0X3	T60.0X4	—	—
Dioxin	T53.7X1	T53.7X2	T53.7X3	T53.7X4	—	—
Dioxopromethazine	T43.3X1	T43.3X2	T43.3X3	T43.3X4	T43.3X5	T43.3X6
Dioxyline	T46.3X1	T46.3X2	T46.3X3	T46.3X4	T46.3X5	T46.3X6
Dipentene	T52.8X1	T52.8X2	T52.8X3	T52.8X4	—	—
Diperodon	T41.3X1	T41.3X2	T41.3X3	T41.3X4	T41.3X5	T41.3X6
Diphacinone	T60.4X1	T60.4X2	T60.4X3	T60.4X4	—	—
Diphemanil	T44.3X1	T44.3X2	T44.3X3	T44.3X4	T44.3X5	T44.3X6
metilsulfate	T44.3X1	T44.3X2	T44.3X3	T44.3X4	T44.3X5	T44.3X6
Diphenadione	T45.511	T45.512	T45.513	T45.514	T45.515	T45.516
rodenticide	T60.4X1	T60.4X2	T60.4X3	T60.4X4	—	—
Diphenhydramine	T45.0X1	T45.0X2	T45.0X3	T45.0X4	T45.0X5	T45.0X6
Diphenidol	T45.0X1	T45.0X2	T45.0X3	T45.0X4	T45.0X5	T45.0X6
Diphenoxylate	T47.6X1	T47.6X2	T47.6X3	T47.6X4	T47.6X5	T47.6X6
Diphenylamine	T65.3X1	T65.3X2	T65.3X3	T65.3X4	—	—
Diphenylbutazone	T39.2X1	T39.2X2	T39.2X3	T39.2X4	T39.2X5	T39.2X6
Diphenyl-chloroarsine, not in war	T57.0X1	T57.0X2	T57.0X3	T57.0X4	—	—
Diphenylhydantoin	T42.0X1	T42.0X2	T42.0X3	T42.0X4	T42.0X5	T42.0X6
Diphenylmethane dye	T52.1X1	T52.1X2	T52.1X3	T52.1X4	—	—
Diphenylpyraline	T45.0X1	T45.0X2	T45.0X3	T45.0X4	T45.0X5	T45.0X6
Diphtheria						
antitoxin	T50.Z11	T50.Z12	T50.Z13	T50.Z14	T50.Z15	T50.Z16
toxoid	T50.A91	T50.A92	T50.A93	T50.A94	T50.A95	T50.A96
with tetanus toxoid	T50.A21	T50.A22	T50.A23	T50.A24	T50.A25	T50.A26
with pertussis component	T50.A11	T50.A12	T50.A13	T50.A14	T50.A15	T50.A16
vaccine	T50.A91	T50.A92	T50.A93	T50.A94	T50.A95	T50.A96
combination						
including pertussis	T50.A11	T50.A12	T50.A13	T50.A14	T50.A15	T50.A16
without pertussis	T50.A21	T50.A22	T50.A23	T50.A24	T50.A25	T50.A26
Diphylline	T50.2X1	T50.2X2	T50.2X3	T50.2X4	T50.2X5	T50.2X6
Dipipanone	T40.491	T40.492	T40.493	T40.494	—	—
Dipivefrine	T49.5X1	T49.5X2	T49.5X3	T49.5X4	T49.5X5	T49.5X6
Diplovax	T50.B91	T50.B92	T50.B93	T50.B94	T50.B95	T50.B96
Diprophylline	T50.2X1	T50.2X2	T50.2X3	T50.2X4	T50.2X5	T50.2X6
Dipropyline	T48.291	T48.292	T48.293	T48.294	T48.295	T48.296
Dipyridamole	T46.3X1	T46.3X2	T46.3X3	T46.3X4	T46.3X5	T46.3X6
Dipyrone	T39.2X1	T39.2X2	T39.2X3	T39.2X4	T39.2X5	T39.2X6
Diquat (dibromide)	T60.3X1	T60.3X2	T60.3X3	T60.3X4	—	—
Disinfectant	T65.891	T65.892	T65.893	T65.894	—	—
alkaline	T54.3X1	T54.3X2	T54.3X3	T54.3X4	—	—
aromatic	T54.1X1	T54.1X2	T54.1X3	T54.1X4	—	—
intestinal	T37.8X1	T37.8X2	T37.8X3	T37.8X4	T37.8X5	T37.8X6
Disipal	T42.8X1	T42.8X2	T42.8X3	T42.8X4	T42.8X5	T42.8X6
Disodium edetate	T50.6X1	T50.6X2	T50.6X3	T50.6X4	T50.6X5	T50.6X6
Disoprofol	T41.291	T41.292	T41.293	T41.294	T41.295	T41.296
Disopyramide	T46.2X1	T46.2X2	T46.2X3	T46.2X4	T46.2X5	T46.2X6
Distigmine (bromide)	T44.0X1	T44.0X2	T44.0X3	T44.0X4	T44.0X5	T44.0X6
Disulfamide	T50.2X1	T50.2X2	T50.2X3	T50.2X4	T50.2X5	T50.2X6

Substance	Poisoning, Accidental (unintentional)	Poisoning, Intentional self-harm	Poisoning, Assault	Poisoning, Undetermined	Adverse effect	Underdosing
Disulfanilamide	T37.0X1	T37.0X2	T37.0X3	T37.0X4	T37.0X5	T37.0X6
Disulfiram	T50.6X1	T50.6X2	T50.6X3	T50.6X4	T50.6X5	T50.6X6
Disulfoton	T60.0X1	T60.0X2	T60.0X3	T60.0X4	—	—
Dithiazanine iodide	T37.4X1	T37.4X2	T37.4X3	T37.4X4	T37.4X5	T37.4X6
Dithiocarbamate	T60.0X1	T60.0X2	T60.0X3	T60.0X4	—	—
Dithranol	T49.4X1	T49.4X2	T49.4X3	T49.4X4	T49.4X5	T49.4X6
Diucardin	T50.2X1	T50.2X2	T50.2X3	T50.2X4	T50.2X5	T50.2X6
Diupres	T50.2X1	T50.2X2	T50.2X3	T50.2X4	T50.2X5	T50.2X6
Diuretic NEC	T50.2X1	T50.2X2	T50.2X3	T50.2X4	T50.2X5	T50.2X6
benzothiadiazine	T50.2X1	T50.2X2	T50.2X3	T50.2X4	T50.2X5	T50.2X6
carbonic acid anhydrase inhibitors	T50.2X1	T50.2X2	T50.2X3	T50.2X4	T50.2X5	T50.2X6
furfuryl NEC	T50.2X1	T50.2X2	T50.2X3	T50.2X4	T50.2X5	T50.2X6
loop (high-ceiling)	T50.1X1	T50.1X2	T50.1X3	T50.1X4	T50.1X5	T50.1X6
mercurial NEC	T50.2X1	T50.2X2	T50.2X3	T50.2X4	T50.2X5	T50.2X6
osmotic	T50.2X1	T50.2X2	T50.2X3	T50.2X4	T50.2X5	T50.2X6
purine NEC	T50.2X1	T50.2X2	T50.2X3	T50.2X4	T50.2X5	T50.2X6
saluretic NEC	T50.2X1	T50.2X2	T50.2X3	T50.2X4	T50.2X5	T50.2X6
sulfonamide	T50.2X1	T50.2X2	T50.2X3	T50.2X4	T50.2X5	T50.2X6
thiazide NEC	T50.2X1	T50.2X2	T50.2X3	T50.2X4	T50.2X5	T50.2X6
xanthine	T50.2X1	T50.2X2	T50.2X3	T50.2X4	T50.2X5	T50.2X6
Diurgin	T50.2X1	T50.2X2	T50.2X3	T50.2X4	T50.2X5	T50.2X6
Diuril	T50.2X1	T50.2X2	T50.2X3	T50.2X4	T50.2X5	T50.2X6
Diuron	T60.3X1	T60.3X2	T60.3X3	T60.3X4	—	—
Divalproex	T42.6X1	T42.6X2	T42.6X3	T42.6X4	T42.6X5	T42.6X6
Divinyl ether	T41.0X1	T41.0X2	T41.0X3	T41.0X4	T41.0X5	T41.0X6
Dixanthogen	T49.0X1	T49.0X2	T49.0X3	T49.0X4	T49.0X5	T49.0X6
Dixyrazine	T43.3X1	T43.3X2	T43.3X3	T43.3X4	T43.3X5	T43.3X6
D-lysergic acid diethylamide	T40.8X1	T40.8X2	T40.8X3	T40.8X4	—	—
DMCT	T36.4X1	T36.4X2	T36.4X3	T36.4X4	T36.4X5	T36.4X6
DMSO—see Dimethyl, sulfoxide						
DNBP	T60.3X1	T60.3X2	T60.3X3	T60.3X4	—	—
DNOC	T65.3X1	T65.3X2	T65.3X3	T65.3X4	—	—
Dobutamine	T44.5X1	T44.5X2	T44.5X3	T44.5X4	T44.5X5	T44.5X6
DOCA	T38.0X1	T38.0X2	T38.0X3	T38.0X4	T38.0X5	T38.0X6
Docusate sodium	T47.4X1	T47.4X2	T47.4X3	T47.4X4	T47.4X5	T47.4X6
Dodicin	T49.0X1	T49.0X2	T49.0X3	T49.0X4	T49.0X5	T49.0X6
Dofamium chloride	T49.0X1	T49.0X2	T49.0X3	T49.0X4	T49.0X5	T49.0X6
Dolophine	T40.3X1	T40.3X2	T40.3X3	T40.3X4	T40.3X5	T40.3X6
Doloxene	T39.8X1	T39.8X2	T39.8X3	T39.8X4	T39.8X5	T39.8X6
Domestic gas (after combustion)—see Gas, utility						
prior to combustion	T59.891	T59.892	T59.893	T59.894	—	—
Domiodol	T48.4X1	T48.4X2	T48.4X3	T48.4X4	T48.4X5	T48.4X6
Domiphen (bromide)	T49.0X1	T49.0X2	T49.0X3	T49.0X4	T49.0X5	T49.0X6
Domperidone	T45.0X1	T45.0X2	T45.0X3	T45.0X4	T45.0X5	T45.0X6
Dopa	T42.8X1	T42.8X2	T42.8X3	T42.8X4	T42.8X5	T42.8X6
Dopamine	T44.991	T44.992	T44.993	T44.994	T44.995	T44.996
Doriden	T42.6X1	T42.6X2	T42.6X3	T42.6X4	T42.6X5	T42.6X6
Dormiral	T42.3X1	T42.3X2	T42.3X3	T42.3X4	T42.3X5	T42.3X6
Dormison	T42.6X1	T42.6X2	T42.6X3	T42.6X4	T42.6X5	T42.6X6
Dornase	T48.4X1	T48.4X2	T48.4X3	T48.4X4	T48.4X5	T48.4X6
Dorsacaine	T41.3X1	T41.3X2	T41.3X3	T41.3X4	T41.3X5	T41.3X6
Dosulepin	T43.011	T43.012	T43.013	T43.014	T43.015	T43.016
Dothiepin	T43.011	T43.012	T43.013	T43.014	T43.015	T43.016
Doxantrazole	T48.6X1	T48.6X2	T48.6X3	T48.6X4	T48.6X5	T48.6X6
Doxapram	T50.7X1	T50.7X2	T50.7X3	T50.7X4	T50.7X5	T50.7X6
Doxazosin	T44.6X1	T44.6X2	T44.6X3	T44.6X4	T44.6X5	T44.6X6
Doxepin	T43.011	T43.012	T43.013	T43.014	T43.015	T43.016
Doxifluridine	T45.1X1	T45.1X2	T45.1X3	T45.1X4	T45.1X5	T45.1X6
Doxorubicin	T45.1X1	T45.1X2	T45.1X3	T45.1X4	T45.1X5	T45.1X6
Doxycycline	T36.4X1	T36.4X2	T36.4X3	T36.4X4	T36.4X5	T36.4X6
Doxylamine	T45.0X1	T45.0X2	T45.0X3	T45.0X4	T45.0X5	T45.0X6
Dramamine	T45.0X1	T45.0X2	T45.0X3	T45.0X4	T45.0X5	T45.0X6
Drano (drain cleaner)	T54.3X1	T54.3X2	T54.3X3	T54.3X4	—	—
Dressing, live pulp	T49.7X1	T49.7X2	T49.7X3	T49.7X4	T49.7X5	T49.7X6
Drocode	T40.2X1	T40.2X2	T40.2X3	T40.2X4	T40.2X5	T40.2X6
Dromoran	T40.2X1	T40.2X2	T40.2X3	T40.2X4	T40.2X5	T40.2X6
Dromostanolone	T38.7X1	T38.7X2	T38.7X3	T38.7X4	T38.7X5	T38.7X6
Dronabinol	T40.711	T40.712	T40.713	T40.714	T40.715	T40.716
Droperidol	T43.591	T43.592	T43.593	T43.594	T43.595	T43.596
Dropropizine	T48.3X1	T48.3X2	T48.3X3	T48.3X4	T48.3X5	T48.3X6
Drostanolone	T38.7X1	T38.7X2	T38.7X3	T38.7X4	T38.7X5	T38.7X6
Drotaverine	T44.3X1	T44.3X2	T44.3X3	T44.3X4	T44.3X5	T44.3X6
Drotrecogin alfa	T45.511	T45.512	T45.513	T45.514	T45.515	T45.516
Drug NEC	T50.901	T50.902	T50.903	T50.904	T50.905	T50.906
specified NEC	T50.991	T50.992	T50.993	T50.994	T50.995	T50.996
DTIC	T45.1X1	T45.1X2	T45.1X3	T45.1X4	T45.1X5	T45.1X6
Duboisine	T44.3X1	T44.3X2	T44.3X3	T44.3X4	T44.3X5	T44.3X6
Dulcolax	T47.2X1	T47.2X2	T47.2X3	T47.2X4	T47.2X5	T47.2X6
Duponol (C) (EP)	T49.2X1	T49.2X2	T49.2X3	T49.2X4	T49.2X5	T49.2X6
Durabolin	T38.7X1	T38.7X2	T38.7X3	T38.7X4	T38.7X5	T38.7X6
Dyclone	T41.3X1	T41.3X2	T41.3X3	T41.3X4	T41.3X5	T41.3X6
Dyclonine	T41.3X1	T41.3X2	T41.3X3	T41.3X4	T41.3X5	T41.3X6
Dydrogesterone	T38.5X1	T38.5X2	T38.5X3	T38.5X4	T38.5X5	T38.5X6
Dye NEC	T65.6X1	T65.6X2	T65.6X3	T65.6X4	—	—
antiseptic	T49.0X1	T49.0X2	T49.0X3	T49.0X4	T49.0X5	T49.0X6
diagnostic agents	T50.8X1	T50.8X2	T50.8X3	T50.8X4	T50.8X5	T50.8X6
pharmaceutical NEC	T50.901	T50.902	T50.903	T50.904	T50.905	T50.906
Dyflos	T44.0X1	T44.0X2	T44.0X3	T44.0X4	T44.0X5	T44.0X6
Dymelor	T38.3X1	T38.3X2	T38.3X3	T38.3X4	T38.3X5	T38.3X6
Dynamite	T65.3X1	T65.3X2	T65.3X3	T65.3X4	—	—
fumes	T59.891	T59.892	T59.893	T59.894	—	—
Dyphylline	T44.3X1	T44.3X2	T44.3X3	T44.3X4	T44.3X5	T44.3X6
E						
Ear drug NEC	T49.6X1	T49.6X2	T49.6X3	T49.6X4	T49.6X5	T49.6X6
Ear preparations	T49.6X1	T49.6X2	T49.6X3	T49.6X4	T49.6X5	T49.6X6
Echothiophate, echothiopate, ecothiopate	T49.5X1	T49.5X2	T49.5X3	T49.5X4	T49.5X5	T49.5X6

Substance	Poisoning, Accidental (unintentional)	Poisoning, Intentional self-harm	Poisoning, Assault	Poisoning, Undetermined	Adverse effect	Underdosing
Econazole	T49.0X1	T49.0X2	T49.0X3	T49.0X4	T49.0X5	T49.0X6
Ecothiopate iodide	T49.5X1	T49.5X2	T49.5X3	T49.5X4	T49.5X5	T49.5X6
Ecstasy	T43.641	T43.642	T43.643	T43.644	—	—
Ectylurea	T42.6X1	T42.6X2	T42.6X3	T42.6X4	T42.6X5	T42.6X6
Edathamil disodium	T45.8X1	T45.8X2	T45.8X3	T45.8X4	T45.8X5	T45.8X6
Edecrin	T50.1X1	T50.1X2	T50.1X3	T50.1X4	T50.1X5	T50.1X6
Edetate, disodium (calcium)	T45.8X1	T45.8X2	T45.8X3	T45.8X4	T45.8X5	T45.8X6
Edoxudine	T49.5X1	T49.5X2	T49.5X3	T49.5X4	T49.5X5	T49.5X6
Edrophonium	T44.0X1	T44.0X2	T44.0X3	T44.0X4	T44.0X5	T44.0X6
chloride	T44.0X1	T44.0X2	T44.0X3	T44.0X4	T44.0X5	T44.0X6
EDTA	T50.6X1	T50.6X2	T50.6X3	T50.6X4	T50.6X5	T50.6X6
Eflornithine	T37.2X1	T37.2X2	T37.2X3	T37.2X4	T37.2X5	T37.2X6
Efloxate	T46.3X1	T46.3X2	T46.3X3	T46.3X4	T46.3X5	T46.3X6
Elase	T49.8X1	T49.8X2	T49.8X3	T49.8X4	T49.8X5	T49.8X6
Elastase	T47.5X1	T47.5X2	T47.5X3	T47.5X4	T47.5X5	T47.5X6
Elaterium	T47.2X1	T47.2X2	T47.2X3	T47.2X4	T47.2X5	T47.2X6
Elcatonin	T50.991	T50.992	T50.993	T50.994	T50.995	T50.996
Elder	T62.2X1	T62.2X2	T62.2X3	T62.2X4	—	—
berry, (unripe)	T62.1X1	T62.1X2	T62.1X3	T62.1X4	—	—
Electrolyte balance drug	T50.3X1	T50.3X2	T50.3X3	T50.3X4	T50.3X5	T50.3X6
Electrolytes NEC	T50.3X1	T50.3X2	T50.3X3	T50.3X4	T50.3X5	T50.3X6
Electrolytic agent NEC	T50.3X1	T50.3X2	T50.3X3	T50.3X4	T50.3X5	T50.3X6
Elemental diet	T50.901	T50.902	T50.903	T50.904	T50.905	T50.906
Elliptinium acetate	T45.1X1	T45.1X2	T45.1X3	T45.1X4	T45.1X5	T45.1X6
Embramine	T45.0X1	T45.0X2	T45.0X3	T45.0X4	T45.0X5	T45.0X6
Emepronium (salts)	T44.3X1	T44.3X2	T44.3X3	T44.3X4	T44.3X5	T44.3X6
bromide	T44.3X1	T44.3X2	T44.3X3	T44.3X4	T44.3X5	T44.3X6
Emetic NEC	T47.7X1	T47.7X2	T47.7X3	T47.7X4	T47.7X5	T47.7X6
Emetine	T37.3X1	T37.3X2	T37.3X3	T37.3X4	T37.3X5	T37.3X6
Emollient NEC	T49.3X1	T49.3X2	T49.3X3	T49.3X4	T49.3X5	T49.3X6
Emorfazone	T39.8X1	T39.8X2	T39.8X3	T39.8X4	T39.8X5	T39.8X6
Emylcamate	T43.591	T43.592	T43.593	T43.594	T43.595	T43.596
Enalapril	T46.4X1	T46.4X2	T46.4X3	T46.4X4	T46.4X5	T46.4X6
Enalaprilat	T46.4X1	T46.4X2	T46.4X3	T46.4X4	T46.4X5	T46.4X6
Encainide	T46.2X1	T46.2X2	T46.2X3	T46.2X4	T46.2X5	T46.2X6
Endocaine	T41.3X1	T41.3X2	T41.3X3	T41.3X4	T41.3X5	T41.3X6
Endosulfan	T60.2X1	T60.2X2	T60.2X3	T60.2X4	—	—
Endothall	T60.3X1	T60.3X2	T60.3X3	T60.3X4	—	—
Endralazine	T46.5X1	T46.5X2	T46.5X3	T46.5X4	T46.5X5	T46.5X6
Endrin	T60.1X1	T60.1X2	T60.1X3	T60.1X4	—	—
Enflurane	T41.0X1	T41.0X2	T41.0X3	T41.0X4	T41.0X5	T41.0X6
Enhexymal	T42.3X1	T42.3X2	T42.3X3	T42.3X4	T42.3X5	T42.3X6
Enocitabine	T45.1X1	T45.1X2	T45.1X3	T45.1X4	T45.1X5	T45.1X6
Enovid	T38.4X1	T38.4X2	T38.4X3	T38.4X4	T38.4X5	T38.4X6
Enoxacin	T36.8X1	T36.8X2	T36.8X3	T36.8X4	T36.8X5	T36.8X6
Enoxaparin (sodium)	T45.511	T45.512	T45.513	T45.514	T45.515	T45.516
Enpiprazole	T43.591	T43.592	T43.593	T43.594	T43.595	T43.596
Enprofylline	T48.6X1	T48.6X2	T48.6X3	T48.6X4	T48.6X5	T48.6X6
Enprostil	T47.1X1	T47.1X2	T47.1X3	T47.1X4	T47.1X5	T47.1X6

Substance	Poisoning, Accidental (unintentional)	Poisoning, Intentional self-harm	Poisoning, Assault	Poisoning, Undetermined	Adverse effect	Underdosing
ENT preparations (anti-infectives)	T49.6X1	T49.6X2	T49.6X3	T49.6X4	T49.6X5	T49.6X6
Enterogastrone	T38.891	T38.892	T38.893	T38.894	T38.895	T38.896
Enviomycin	T36.8X1	T36.8X2	T36.8X3	T36.8X4	T36.8X5	T36.8X6
Enzodase	T45.3X1	T45.3X2	T45.3X3	T45.3X4	T45.3X5	T45.3X6
Enzyme NEC	T45.3X1	T45.3X2	T45.3X3	T45.3X4	T45.3X5	T45.3X6
depolymerizing	T49.8X1	T49.8X2	T49.8X3	T49.8X4	T49.8X5	T49.8X6
fibrolytic	T45.3X1	T45.3X2	T45.3X3	T45.3X4	T45.3X5	T45.3X6
gastric	T47.5X1	T47.5X2	T47.5X3	T47.5X4	T47.5X5	T47.5X6
intestinal	T47.5X1	T47.5X2	T47.5X3	T47.5X4	T47.5X5	T47.5X6
local action	T49.4X1	T49.4X2	T49.4X3	T49.4X4	T49.4X5	T49.4X6
proteolytic	T49.4X1	T49.4X2	T49.4X3	T49.4X4	T49.4X5	T49.4X6
thrombolytic	T45.3X1	T45.3X2	T45.3X3	T45.3X4	T45.3X5	T45.3X6
EPAB	T41.3X1	T41.3X2	T41.3X3	T41.3X4	T41.3X5	T41.3X6
Epanutin	T42.0X1	T42.0X2	T42.0X3	T42.0X4	T42.0X5	T42.0X6
Ephedra	T44.991	T44.992	T44.993	T44.994	T44.995	T44.996
Ephedrine	T44.991	T44.992	T44.993	T44.994	T44.995	T44.996
Epichlorhydrin, epichlorohydrin	T52.8X1	T52.8X2	T52.8X3	T52.8X4	—	—
Epicillin	T36.0X1	T36.0X2	T36.0X3	T36.0X4	T36.0X5	T36.0X6
Epiestriol	T38.5X1	T38.5X2	T38.5X3	T38.5X4	T38.5X5	T38.5X6
Epilim—see Sodium, valproate						
Epimestrol	T38.5X1	T38.5X2	T38.5X3	T38.5X4	T38.5X5	T38.5X6
Epinephrine	T44.5X1	T44.5X2	T44.5X3	T44.5X4	T44.5X5	T44.5X6
Epirubicin	T45.1X1	T45.1X2	T45.1X3	T45.1X4	T45.1X5	T45.1X6
Epitiostanol	T38.7X1	T38.7X2	T38.7X3	T38.7X4	T38.7X5	T38.7X6
Epitizide	T50.2X1	T50.2X2	T50.2X3	T50.2X4	T50.2X5	T50.2X6
EPN	T60.0X1	T60.0X2	T60.0X3	T60.0X4	—	—
EPO	T45.8X1	T45.8X2	T45.8X3	T45.8X4	T45.8X5	T45.8X6
Epoetin alpha	T45.8X1	T45.8X2	T45.8X3	T45.8X4	T45.8X5	T45.8X6
Epomediol	T50.991	T50.992	T50.993	T50.994	T50.995	T50.996
Epoprostenol	T45.521	T45.522	T45.523	T45.524	T45.525	T45.526
Epoxy resin	T65.891	T65.892	T65.893	T65.894	—	—
Eprazinone	T48.4X1	T48.4X2	T48.4X3	T48.4X4	T48.4X5	T48.4X6
Epsilon amino-caproic acid	T45.621	T45.622	T45.623	T45.624	T45.625	T45.626
Epsom salt	T47.3X1	T47.3X2	T47.3X3	T47.3X4	T47.3X5	T47.3X6
Eptazocine	T40.491	T40.492	T40.493	T40.494	T40.495	T40.496
Equanil	T43.591	T43.592	T43.593	T43.594	T43.595	T43.596
Equisetum	T62.2X1	T62.2X2	T62.2X3	T62.2X4	—	—
diuretic	T50.2X1	T50.2X2	T50.2X3	T50.2X4	T50.2X5	T50.2X6
Ergobasine	T48.0X1	T48.0X2	T48.0X3	T48.0X4	T48.0X5	T48.0X6
Ergocalciferol	T45.2X1	T45.2X2	T45.2X3	T45.2X4	T45.2X5	T45.2X6
Ergoloid mesylates	T46.7X1	T46.7X2	T46.7X3	T46.7X4	T46.7X5	T46.7X6
Ergometrine	T48.0X1	T48.0X2	T48.0X3	T48.0X4	T48.0X5	T48.0X6
Ergonovine	T48.0X1	T48.0X2	T48.0X3	T48.0X4	T48.0X5	T48.0X6
Ergot NEC	T64.81	T64.82	T64.83	T64.84	—	—
derivative	T48.0X1	T48.0X2	T48.0X3	T48.0X4	T48.0X5	T48.0X6
medicinal (alkaloids)	T48.0X1	T48.0X2	T48.0X3	T48.0X4	T48.0X5	T48.0X6
prepared	T48.0X1	T48.0X2	T48.0X3	T48.0X4	T48.0X5	T48.0X6

Substance	Poisoning, Accidental (unintentional)	Poisoning, Intentional self-harm	Poisoning, Assault	Poisoning, Undetermined	Adverse effect	Underdosing
Ergotamine	T46.5X1	T46.5X2	T46.5X3	T46.5X4	T46.5X5	T46.5X6
Ergotocine	T48.0X1	T48.0X2	T48.0X3	T48.0X4	T48.0X5	T48.0X6
Ergotrate	T48.0X1	T48.0X2	T48.0X3	T48.0X4	T48.0X5	T48.0X6
Eritrityl tetranitrate	T46.3X1	T46.3X2	T46.3X3	T46.3X4	T46.3X5	T46.3X6
Erythrityl tetranitrate	T46.3X1	T46.3X2	T46.3X3	T46.3X4	T46.3X5	T46.3X6
Erythrol tetranitrate	T46.3X1	T46.3X2	T46.3X3	T46.3X4	T46.3X5	T46.3X6
Erythromycin (salts)	T36.3X1	T36.3X2	T36.3X3	T36.3X4	T36.3X5	T36.3X6
ophthalmic preparation	T49.5X1	T49.5X2	T49.5X3	T49.5X4	T49.5X5	T49.5X6
topical NEC	T49.0X1	T49.0X2	T49.0X3	T49.0X4	T49.0X5	T49.0X6
Erythropoietin	T45.8X1	T45.8X2	T45.8X3	T45.8X4	T45.8X5	T45.8X6
human	T45.8X1	T45.8X2	T45.8X3	T45.8X4	T45.8X5	T45.8X6
Escin	T46.991	T46.992	T46.993	T46.994	T46.995	T46.996
Esculin	T45.2X1	T45.2X2	T45.2X3	T45.2X4	T45.2X5	T45.2X6
Esculoside	T45.2X1	T45.2X2	T45.2X3	T45.2X4	T45.2X5	T45.2X6
ESDT (ether-soluble tar distillate)	T49.1X1	T49.1X2	T49.1X3	T49.1X4	T49.1X5	T49.1X6
Eserine	T49.5X1	T49.5X2	T49.5X3	T49.5X4	T49.5X5	T49.5X6
Esflurbiprofen	T39.311	T39.312	T39.313	T39.314	T39.315	T39.316
Eskabarb	T42.3X1	T42.3X2	T42.3X3	T42.3X4	T42.3X5	T42.3X6
Eskalith	T43.8X1	T43.8X2	T43.8X3	T43.8X4	T43.8X5	T43.8X6
Esmolol	T44.7X1	T44.7X2	T44.7X3	T44.7X4	T44.7X5	T44.7X6
Estanozolol	T38.7X1	T38.7X2	T38.7X3	T38.7X4	T38.7X5	T38.7X6
Estazolam	T42.4X1	T42.4X2	T42.4X3	T42.4X4	T42.4X5	T42.4X6
Estradiol	T38.5X1	T38.5X2	T38.5X3	T38.5X4	T38.5X5	T38.5X6
with testosterone	T38.7X1	T38.7X2	T38.7X3	T38.7X4	T38.7X5	T38.7X6
benzoate	T38.5X1	T38.5X2	T38.5X3	T38.5X4	T38.5X5	T38.5X6
Estramustine	T45.1X1	T45.1X2	T45.1X3	T45.1X4	T45.1X5	T45.1X6
Estriol	T38.5X1	T38.5X2	T38.5X3	T38.5X4	T38.5X5	T38.5X6
Estrogen	T38.5X1	T38.5X2	T38.5X3	T38.5X4	T38.5X5	T38.5X6
with progesterone	T38.5X1	T38.5X2	T38.5X3	T38.5X4	T38.5X5	T38.5X6
conjugated	T38.5X1	T38.5X2	T38.5X3	T38.5X4	T38.5X5	T38.5X6
Estrone	T38.5X1	T38.5X2	T38.5X3	T38.5X4	T38.5X5	T38.5X6
Estropipate	T38.5X1	T38.5X2	T38.5X3	T38.5X4	T38.5X5	T38.5X6
Etacrynate sodium	T50.1X1	T50.1X2	T50.1X3	T50.1X4	T50.1X5	T50.1X6
Etacrynic acid	T50.1X1	T50.1X2	T50.1X3	T50.1X4	T50.1X5	T50.1X6
Etafedrine	T48.6X1	T48.6X2	T48.6X3	T48.6X4	T48.6X5	T48.6X6
Etafenone	T46.3X1	T46.3X2	T46.3X3	T46.3X4	T46.3X5	T46.3X6
Etambutol	T37.1X1	T37.1X2	T37.1X3	T37.1X4	T37.1X5	T37.1X6
Etamiphyllin	T48.6X1	T48.6X2	T48.6X3	T48.6X4	T48.6X5	T48.6X6
Etamivan	T50.7X1	T50.7X2	T50.7X3	T50.7X4	T50.7X5	T50.7X6
Etamsylate	T45.7X1	T45.7X2	T45.7X3	T45.7X4	T45.7X5	T45.7X6
Etebenecid	T50.4X1	T50.4X2	T50.4X3	T50.4X4	T50.4X5	T50.4X6
Ethacridine	T49.0X1	T49.0X2	T49.0X3	T49.0X4	T49.0X5	T49.0X6
Ethacrynic acid	T50.1X1	T50.1X2	T50.1X3	T50.1X4	T50.1X5	T50.1X6
Ethadione	T42.2X1	T42.2X2	T42.2X3	T42.2X4	T42.2X5	T42.2X6
Ethambutol	T37.1X1	T37.1X2	T37.1X3	T37.1X4	T37.1X5	T37.1X6
Ethamide	T50.2X1	T50.2X2	T50.2X3	T50.2X4	T50.2X5	T50.2X6
Ethamivan	T50.7X1	T50.7X2	T50.7X3	T50.7X4	T50.7X5	T50.7X6
Ethamsylate	T45.7X1	T45.7X2	T45.7X3	T45.7X4	T45.7X5	T45.7X6

Substance	Poisoning, Accidental (unintentional)	Poisoning, Intentional self-harm	Poisoning, Assault	Poisoning, Undetermined	Adverse effect	Underdosing
Ethanol	T51.0X1	T51.0X2	T51.0X3	T51.0X4	—	—
beverage	T51.0X1	T51.0X2	T51.0X3	T51.0X4	—	—
Ethanolamine oleate	T46.8X1	T46.8X2	T46.8X3	T46.8X4	T46.8X5	T46.8X6
Ethaverine	T44.3X1	T44.3X2	T44.3X3	T44.3X4	T44.3X5	T44.3X6
Ethchlorvynol	T42.6X1	T42.6X2	T42.6X3	T42.6X4	T42.6X5	T42.6X6
Ethebenecid	T50.4X1	T50.4X2	T50.4X3	T50.4X4	T50.4X5	T50.4X6
Ether (vapor)	T41.0X1	T41.0X2	T41.0X3	T41.0X4	T41.0X5	T41.0X6
anesthetic	T41.0X1	T41.0X2	T41.0X3	T41.0X4	T41.0X5	T41.0X6
divinyl	T41.0X1	T41.0X2	T41.0X3	T41.0X4	T41.0X5	T41.0X6
ethyl (medicinal)	T41.0X1	T41.0X2	T41.0X3	T41.0X4	T41.0X5	T41.0X6
nonmedicinal	T52.8X1	T52.8X2	T52.8X3	T52.8X4	—	—
petroleum—see Ligroin						
solvent	T52.8X1	T52.8X2	T52.8X3	T52.8X4	—	—
Ethiazide	T50.2X1	T50.2X2	T50.2X3	T50.2X4	T50.2X5	T50.2X6
Ethidium chloride (vapor)	T59.891	T59.892	T59.893	T59.894	—	—
Ethinamate	T42.6X1	T42.6X2	T42.6X3	T42.6X4	T42.6X5	T42.6X6
Ethinylestradiol, ethinyloestradiol	T38.5X1	T38.5X2	T38.5X3	T38.5X4	T38.5X5	T38.5X6
with						
levonorgestrel	T38.4X1	T38.4X2	T38.4X3	T38.4X4	T38.4X5	T38.4X6
norethisterone	T38.4X1	T38.4X2	T38.4X3	T38.4X4	T38.4X5	T38.4X6
Ethiodized oil (131 I)	T50.8X1	T50.8X2	T50.8X3	T50.8X4	T50.8X5	T50.8X6
Ethion	T60.0X1	T60.0X2	T60.0X3	T60.0X4	—	—
Ethionamide	T37.1X1	T37.1X2	T37.1X3	T37.1X4	T37.1X5	T37.1X6
Ethioniamide	T37.1X1	T37.1X2	T37.1X3	T37.1X4	T37.1X5	T37.1X6
Ethisterone	T38.5X1	T38.5X2	T38.5X3	T38.5X4	T38.5X5	T38.5X6
Ethobral	T42.3X1	T42.3X2	T42.3X3	T42.3X4	T42.3X5	T42.3X6
Ethocaine (infiltration) (topical)	T41.3X1	T41.3X2	T41.3X3	T41.3X4	T41.3X5	T41.3X6
nerve block (peripheral) (plexus)	T41.3X1	T41.3X2	T41.3X3	T41.3X4	T41.3X5	T41.3X6
spinal	T41.3X1	T41.3X2	T41.3X3	T41.3X4	T41.3X5	T41.3X6
Ethoheptazine	T40.491	T40.492	T40.493	T40.494	T40.495	T40.496
Ethopropazine	T44.3X1	T44.3X2	T44.3X3	T44.3X4	T44.3X5	T44.3X6
Ethosuximide	T42.2X1	T42.2X2	T42.2X3	T42.2X4	T42.2X5	T42.2X6
Ethotoin	T42.0X1	T42.0X2	T42.0X3	T42.0X4	T42.0X5	T42.0X6
Ethoxazene	T37.91	T37.92	T37.93	T37.94	T37.95	T37.96
Ethoxazorutoside	T46.991	T46.992	T46.993	T46.994	T46.995	T46.996
2-Ethoxyethanol	T52.3X1	T52.3X2	T52.3X3	T52.3X4	—	—
Ethoxzolamide	T50.2X1	T50.2X2	T50.2X3	T50.2X4	T50.2X5	T50.2X6
Ethyl						
acetate	T52.8X1	T52.8X2	T52.8X3	T52.8X4	—	—
alcohol	T51.0X1	T51.0X2	T51.0X3	T51.0X4	—	—
beverage	T51.0X1	T51.0X2	T51.0X3	T51.0X4	—	—
aldehyde (vapor)	T59.891	T59.892	T59.893	T59.894	—	—
liquid	T52.8X1	T52.8X2	T52.8X3	T52.8X4	—	—
aminobenzoate	T41.3X1	T41.3X2	T41.3X3	T41.3X4	T41.3X5	T41.3X6
aminophenthiazine	T43.3X1	T43.3X2	T43.3X3	T43.3X4	T43.3X5	T43.3X6
benzoate	T52.8X1	T52.8X2	T52.8X3	T52.8X4	—	—

Substance	Poisoning, Accidental (unintentional)	Poisoning, Intentional self-harm	Poisoning, Assault	Poisoning, Undetermined	Adverse effect	Underdosing
Ethyl — *Continued*						
biscoumacetate	T45.511	T45.512	T45.513	T45.514	T45.515	T45.516
bromide (anesthetic)	T41.0X1	T41.0X2	T41.0X3	T41.0X4	T41.0X5	T41.0X6
carbamate	T45.1X1	T45.1X2	T45.1X3	T45.1X4	T45.1X5	T45.1X6
carbinol	T51.3X1	T51.3X2	T51.3X3	T51.3X4	—	—
carbonate	T52.8X1	T52.8X2	T52.8X3	T52.8X4	—	—
chaulmoograte	T37.1X1	T37.1X2	T37.1X3	T37.1X4	T37.1X5	T37.1X6
chloride (anesthetic)	T41.0X1	T41.0X2	T41.0X3	T41.0X4	T41.0X5	T41.0X6
anesthetic (local)	T41.3X1	T41.3X2	T41.3X3	T41.3X4	T41.3X5	T41.3X6
inhaled	T41.0X1	T41.0X2	T41.0X3	T41.0X4	T41.0X5	T41.0X6
local	T49.4X1	T49.4X2	T49.4X3	T49.4X4	T49.4X5	T49.4X6
solvent	T53.6X1	T53.6X2	T53.6X3	T53.6X4	—	—
dibunate	T48.3X1	T48.3X2	T48.3X3	T48.3X4	T48.3X5	T48.3X6
dichloroarsine (vapor)	T57.0X1	T57.0X2	T57.0X3	T57.0X4	—	—
estranol	T38.7X1	T38.7X2	T38.7X3	T38.7X4	T38.7X5	T38.7X6
ether—see also ether	T52.8X1	T52.8X2	T52.8X3	T52.8X4	—	—
formate NEC (solvent)	T52.0X1	T52.0X2	T52.0X3	T52.0X4	—	—
fumarate	T49.4X1	T49.4X2	T49.4X3	T49.4X4	T49.4X5	T49.4X6
hydroxyisobutyrate NEC (solvent)	T52.8X1	T52.8X2	T52.8X3	T52.8X4	—	—
iodoacetate	T59.3X1	T59.3X2	T59.3X3	T59.3X4	—	—
lactate NEC (solvent)	T52.8X1	T52.8X2	T52.8X3	T52.8X4	—	—
loflazepate	T42.4X1	T42.4X2	T42.4X3	T42.4X4	T42.4X5	T42.4X6
mercuric chloride	T56.1X1	T56.1X2	T56.1X3	T56.1X4	—	—
methylcarbinol	T51.8X1	T51.8X2	T51.8X3	T51.8X4	—	—
morphine	T40.2X1	T40.2X2	T40.2X3	T40.2X4	T40.2X5	T40.2X6
noradrenaline	T48.6X1	T48.6X2	T48.6X3	T48.6X4	T48.6X5	T48.6X6
oxybutyrate NEC (solvent)	T52.8X1	T52.8X2	T52.8X3	T52.8X4	—	—
Ethylene (gas)	T59.891	T59.892	T59.893	T59.894	—	—
anesthetic (general)	T41.0X1	T41.0X2	T41.0X3	T41.0X4	T41.0X5	T41.0X6
chlorohydrin	T52.8X1	T52.8X2	T52.8X3	T52.8X4	—	—
vapor	T53.6X1	T53.6X2	T53.6X3	T53.6X4	—	—
dichloride	T52.8X1	T52.8X2	T52.8X3	T52.8X4	—	—
vapor	T53.6X1	T53.6X2	T53.6X3	T53.6X4	—	—
dinitrate	T52.3X1	T52.3X2	T52.3X3	T52.3X4	—	—
glycol(s)	T52.8X1	T52.8X2	T52.8X3	T52.8X4	—	—
dinitrate	T52.3X1	T52.3X2	T52.3X3	T52.3X4	—	—
monobutyl ether	T52.3X1	T52.3X2	T52.3X3	T52.3X4	—	—
imine	T54.1X1	T54.1X2	T54.1X3	T54.1X4	—	—
oxide (fumigant) (nonmedicinal)	T59.891	T59.892	T59.893	T59.894	—	—
medicinal	T49.0X1	T49.0X2	T49.0X3	T49.0X4	T49.0X5	T49.0X6
Ethylenediamine theophylline	T48.6X1	T48.6X2	T48.6X3	T48.6X4	T48.6X5	T48.6X6
Ethylenediaminetetra-acetic acid	T50.6X1	T50.6X2	T50.6X3	T50.6X4	T50.6X5	T50.6X6
Ethylen-edinitrilotetra-acetate	T50.6X1	T50.6X2	T50.6X3	T50.6X4	T50.6X5	T50.6X6
Ethylestrenol	T38.7X1	T38.7X2	T38.7X3	T38.7X4	T38.7X5	T38.7X6
Ethylhydro-xycellulose	T47.4X1	T47.4X2	T47.4X3	T47.4X4	T47.4X5	T47.4X6

Substance	Poisoning, Accidental (unintentional)	Poisoning, Intentional self-harm	Poisoning, Assault	Poisoning, Undetermined	Adverse effect	Underdosing
Ethylidene						
chloride NEC	T53.6X1	T53.6X2	T53.6X3	T53.6X4	—	—
diacetate	T60.3X1	T60.3X2	T60.3X3	T60.3X4	—	—
dicoumarin	T45.511	T45.512	T45.513	T45.514	T45.515	T45.516
dicoumarol	T45.511	T45.512	T45.513	T45.514	T45.515	T45.516
diethyl ether	T52.0X1	T52.0X2	T52.0X3	T52.0X4	—	—
Ethylmorphine	T40.2X1	T40.2X2	T40.2X3	T40.2X4	T40.2X5	T40.2X6
Ethylnorepinephrine	T48.6X1	T48.6X2	T48.6X3	T48.6X4	T48.6X5	T48.6X6
Ethylparachloro-phenoxyisobutyrate	T46.6X1	T46.6X2	T46.6X3	T46.6X4	T46.6X5	T46.6X6
Ethynodiol	T38.4X1	T38.4X2	T38.4X3	T38.4X4	T38.4X5	T38.4X6
with mestranol diacetate	T38.4X1	T38.4X2	T38.4X3	T38.4X4	T38.4X5	T38.4X6
Etidocaine	T41.3X1	T41.3X2	T41.3X3	T41.3X4	T41.3X5	T41.3X6
infiltration (subcutaneous)	T41.3X1	T41.3X2	T41.3X3	T41.3X4	T41.3X5	T41.3X6
nerve (peripheral) (plexus)	T41.3X1	T41.3X2	T41.3X3	T41.3X4	T41.3X5	T41.3X6
Etidronate	T50.991	T50.992	T50.993	T50.994	T50.995	T50.996
Etidronic acid (disodium salt)	T50.991	T50.992	T50.993	T50.994	T50.995	T50.996
Etifoxine	T42.6X1	T42.6X2	T42.6X3	T42.6X4	T42.6X5	T42.6X6
Etilefrine	T44.4X1	T44.4X2	T44.4X3	T44.4X4	T44.4X5	T44.4X6
Etilfen	T42.3X1	T42.3X2	T42.3X3	T42.3X4	T42.3X5	T42.3X6
Etinodiol	T38.4X1	T38.4X2	T38.4X3	T38.4X4	T38.4X5	T38.4X6
Etiroxate	T46.6X1	T46.6X2	T46.6X3	T46.6X4	T46.6X5	T46.6X6
Etizolam	T42.4X1	T42.4X2	T42.4X3	T42.4X4	T42.4X5	T42.4X6
Etodolac	T39.391	T39.392	T39.393	T39.394	T39.395	T39.396
Etofamide	T37.3X1	T37.3X2	T37.3X3	T37.3X4	T37.3X5	T37.3X6
Etofibrate	T46.6X1	T46.6X2	T46.6X3	T46.6X4	T46.6X5	T46.6X6
Etofylline	T46.7X1	T46.7X2	T46.7X3	T46.7X4	T46.7X5	T46.7X6
clofibrate	T46.6X1	T46.6X2	T46.6X3	T46.6X4	T46.6X5	T46.6X6
Etoglucid	T45.1X1	T45.1X2	T45.1X3	T45.1X4	T45.1X5	T45.1X6
Etomidate	T41.1X1	T41.1X2	T41.1X3	T41.1X4	T41.1X5	T41.1X6
Etomide	T39.8X1	T39.8X2	T39.8X3	T39.8X4	T39.8X5	T39.8X6
Etomidoline	T44.3X1	T44.3X2	T44.3X3	T44.3X4	T44.3X5	T44.3X6
Etoposide	T45.1X1	T45.1X2	T45.1X3	T45.1X4	T45.1X5	T45.1X6
Etorphine	T40.2X1	T40.2X2	T40.2X3	T40.2X4	T40.2X5	T40.2X6
Etoval	T42.3X1	T42.3X2	T42.3X3	T42.3X4	T42.3X5	T42.3X6
Etozolin	T50.1X1	T50.1X2	T50.1X3	T50.1X4	T50.1X5	T50.1X6
Etretinate	T50.991	T50.992	T50.993	T50.994	T50.995	T50.996
Etryptamine	T43.691	T43.692	T43.693	T43.694	T43.695	T43.696
Etybenzatropine	T44.3X1	T44.3X2	T44.3X3	T44.3X4	T44.3X5	T44.3X6
Etynodiol	T38.4X1	T38.4X2	T38.4X3	T38.4X4	T38.4X5	T38.4X6
Eucaine	T41.3X1	T41.3X2	T41.3X3	T41.3X4	T41.3X5	T41.3X6
Eucalyptus oil	T49.7X1	T49.7X2	T49.7X3	T49.7X4	T49.7X5	T49.7X6
Eucatropine	T49.5X1	T49.5X2	T49.5X3	T49.5X4	T49.5X5	T49.5X6
Eucodal	T40.2X1	T40.2X2	T40.2X3	T40.2X4	T40.2X5	T40.2X6
Euneryl	T42.3X1	T42.3X2	T42.3X3	T42.3X4	T42.3X5	T42.3X6
Euphthalmine	T44.3X1	T44.3X2	T44.3X3	T44.3X4	T44.3X5	T44.3X6

Table of Drugs and Chemicals

Substance	Poisoning, Accidental (unintentional)	Poisoning, Intentional self-harm	Poisoning, Assault	Poisoning, Undetermined	Adverse effect	Underdosing
Eurax	T49.0X1	T49.0X2	T49.0X3	T49.0X4	T49.0X5	T49.0X6
Euresol	T49.4X1	T49.4X2	T49.4X3	T49.4X4	T49.4X5	T49.4X6
Euthroid	T38.1X1	T38.1X2	T38.1X3	T38.1X4	T38.1X5	T38.1X6
Evans blue	T50.8X1	T50.8X2	T50.8X3	T50.8X4	T50.8X5	T50.8X6
Evipal	T42.3X1	T42.3X2	T42.3X3	T42.3X4	T42.3X5	T42.3X6
sodium	T41.1X1	T41.1X2	T41.1X3	T41.1X4	T41.1X5	T41.1X6
Evipan	T42.3X1	T42.3X2	T42.3X3	T42.3X4	T42.3X5	T42.3X6
sodium	T41.1X1	T41.1X2	T41.1X3	T41.1X4	T41.1X5	T41.1X6
Exalamide	T49.0X1	T49.0X2	T49.0X3	T49.0X4	T49.0X5	T49.0X6
Exalgin	T39.1X1	T39.1X2	T39.1X3	T39.1X4	T39.1X5	T39.1X6
Excipients, pharmaceutical	T50.901	T50.902	T50.903	T50.904	T50.905	T50.906
Exhaust gas (engine) (motor vehicle)	T58.01	T58.02	T58.03	T58.04	—	—
Ex-Lax (phenolphthalein)	T47.2X1	T47.2X2	T47.2X3	T47.2X4	T47.2X5	T47.2X6
Expectorant NEC	T48.4X1	T48.4X2	T48.4X3	T48.4X4	T48.4X5	T48.4X6
Extended insulin zinc suspension	T38.3X1	T38.3X2	T38.3X3	T38.3X4	T38.3X5	T38.3X6
External medications (skin) (mucous membrane)	T49.91	T49.92	T49.93	T49.94	T49.95	T49.96
dental agent	T49.7X1	T49.7X2	T49.7X3	T49.7X4	T49.7X5	T49.7X6
ENT agent	T49.6X1	T49.6X2	T49.6X3	T49.6X4	T49.6X5	T49.6X6
ophthalmic preparation	T49.5X1	T49.5X2	T49.5X3	T49.5X4	T49.5X5	T49.5X6
specified NEC	T49.8X1	T49.8X2	T49.8X3	T49.8X4	T49.8X5	T49.8X6
Extrapyramidal antagonist NEC	T44.3X1	T44.3X2	T44.3X3	T44.3X4	T44.3X5	T44.3X6
Eye agents (anti-infective)	T49.5X1	T49.5X2	T49.5X3	T49.5X4	T49.5X5	T49.5X6
Eye drug NEC	T49.5X1	T49.5X2	T49.5X3	T49.5X4	T49.5X5	T49.5X6

F

Substance	Poisoning, Accidental (unintentional)	Poisoning, Intentional self-harm	Poisoning, Assault	Poisoning, Undetermined	Adverse effect	Underdosing
FAC (fluorouracil + doxorubicin + cyclophosphamide)	T45.1X1	T45.1X2	T45.1X3	T45.1X4	T45.1X5	T45.1X6
Factor						
I (fibrinogen)	T45.8X1	T45.8X2	T45.8X3	T45.8X4	T45.8X5	T45.8X6
III (thromboplastin)	T45.8X1	T45.8X2	T45.8X3	T45.8X4	T45.8X5	T45.8X6
VIII (antihemophilic Factor) (concentrate)	T45.8X1	T45.8X2	T45.8X3	T45.8X4	T45.8X5	T45.8X6
IX complex	T45.7X1	T45.7X2	T45.7X3	T45.7X4	T45.7X5	T45.7X6
human	T45.8X1	T45.8X2	T45.8X3	T45.8X4	T45.8X5	T45.8X6
Famotidine	T47.0X1	T47.0X2	T47.0X3	T47.0X4	T47.0X5	T47.0X6
Fat suspension, intravenous	T50.991	T50.992	T50.993	T50.994	T50.995	T50.996
Fazadinium bromide	T48.1X1	T48.1X2	T48.1X3	T48.1X4	T48.1X5	T48.1X6
Febarbamate	T42.3X1	T42.3X2	T42.3X3	T42.3X4	T42.3X5	T42.3X6
Fecal softener	T47.4X1	T47.4X2	T47.4X3	T47.4X4	T47.4X5	T47.4X6
Fedrilate	T48.3X1	T48.3X2	T48.3X3	T48.3X4	T48.3X5	T48.3X6
Felodipine	T46.1X1	T46.1X2	T46.1X3	T46.1X4	T46.1X5	T46.1X6
Felypressin	T38.891	T38.892	T38.893	T38.894	T38.895	T38.896
Femoxetine	T43.221	T43.222	T43.223	T43.224	T43.225	T43.226
Fenalcomine	T46.3X1	T46.3X2	T46.3X3	T46.3X4	T46.3X5	T46.3X6
Fenamisal	T37.1X1	T37.1X2	T37.1X3	T37.1X4	T37.1X5	T37.1X6
Fenazone	T39.2X1	T39.2X2	T39.2X3	T39.2X4	T39.2X5	T39.2X6
Fenbendazole	T37.4X1	T37.4X2	T37.4X3	T37.4X4	T37.4X5	T37.4X6
Fenbutrazate	T50.5X1	T50.5X2	T50.5X3	T50.5X4	T50.5X5	T50.5X6
Fencamfamine	T43.691	T43.692	T43.693	T43.694	T43.695	T43.696
Fendiline	T46.1X1	T46.1X2	T46.1X3	T46.1X4	T46.1X5	T46.1X6
Fenetylline	T43.691	T43.692	T43.693	T43.694	T43.695	T43.696
Fenflumizole	T39.391	T39.392	T39.393	T39.394	T39.395	T39.396
Fenfluramine	T50.5X1	T50.5X2	T50.5X3	T50.5X4	T50.5X5	T50.5X6
Fenobarbital	T42.3X1	T42.3X2	T42.3X3	T42.3X4	T42.3X5	T42.3X6
Fenofibrate	T46.6X1	T46.6X2	T46.6X3	T46.6X4	T46.6X5	T46.6X6
Fenoprofen	T39.311	T39.312	T39.313	T39.314	T39.315	T39.316
Fenoterol	T48.6X1	T48.6X2	T48.6X3	T48.6X4	T48.6X5	T48.6X6
Fenoverine	T44.3X1	T44.3X2	T44.3X3	T44.3X4	T44.3X5	T44.3X6
Fenoxazoline	T48.5X1	T48.5X2	T48.5X3	T48.5X4	T48.5X5	T48.5X6
Fenproporex	T50.5X1	T50.5X2	T50.5X3	T50.5X4	T50.5X5	T50.5X6
Fenquizone	T50.2X1	T50.2X2	T50.2X3	T50.2X4	T50.2X5	T50.2X6
Fentanyl (analogs)	T40.411	T40.412	T40.413	T40.414	T40.415	T40.416
Fentazin	T43.3X1	T43.3X2	T43.3X3	T43.3X4	T43.3X5	T43.3X6
Fenthion	T60.0X1	T60.0X2	T60.0X3	T60.0X4	—	—
Fenticlor	T49.0X1	T49.0X2	T49.0X3	T49.0X4	T49.0X5	T49.0X6
Fenylbutazone	T39.2X1	T39.2X2	T39.2X3	T39.2X4	T39.2X5	T39.2X6
Feprazone	T39.2X1	T39.2X2	T39.2X3	T39.2X4	T39.2X5	T39.2X6
Fer de lance (bite) (venom)	T63.061	T63.062	T63.063	T63.064	—	—
Ferric—see also Iron						
chloride	T45.4X1	T45.4X2	T45.4X3	T45.4X4	T45.4X5	T45.4X6
citrate	T45.4X1	T45.4X2	T45.4X3	T45.4X4	T45.4X5	T45.4X6
hydroxide						
colloidal	T45.4X1	T45.4X2	T45.4X3	T45.4X4	T45.4X5	T45.4X6
polymaltose	T45.4X1	T45.4X2	T45.4X3	T45.4X4	T45.4X5	T45.4X6
pyrophosphate	T45.4X1	T45.4X2	T45.4X3	T45.4X4	T45.4X5	T45.4X6
Ferritin	T45.4X1	T45.4X2	T45.4X3	T45.4X4	T45.4X5	T45.4X6
Ferrocholinate	T45.4X1	T45.4X2	T45.4X3	T45.4X4	T45.4X5	T45.4X6
Ferrodextrane	T45.4X1	T45.4X2	T45.4X3	T45.4X4	T45.4X5	T45.4X6
Ferropolimaler	T45.4X1	T45.4X2	T45.4X3	T45.4X4	T45.4X5	T45.4X6
Ferrous—see also Iron						
phosphate	T45.4X1	T45.4X2	T45.4X3	T45.4X4	T45.4X5	T45.4X6
salt	T45.4X1	T45.4X2	T45.4X3	T45.4X4	T45.4X5	T45.4X6
with folic acid	T45.4X1	T45.4X2	T45.4X3	T45.4X4	T45.4X5	T45.4X6
Ferrous fumarate, gluconate, lactate, salt NEC, sulfate (medicinal)	T45.4X1	T45.4X2	T45.4X3	T45.4X4	T45.4X5	T45.4X6
Ferrovanadium (fumes)	T59.891	T59.892	T59.893	T59.894	—	—
Ferrum—see Iron						
Fertilizers NEC	T65.891	T65.892	T65.893	T65.894	—	—
with herbicide mixture	T60.3X1	T60.3X2	T60.3X3	T60.3X4	—	—
Fetoxilate	T47.6X1	T47.6X2	T47.6X3	T47.6X4	T47.6X5	T47.6X6
Fiber, dietary	T47.4X1	T47.4X2	T47.4X3	T47.4X4	T47.4X5	T47.4X6
Fiberglass	T65.831	T65.832	T65.833	T65.834	—	—
Fibrinogen (human)	T45.8X1	T45.8X2	T45.8X3	T45.8X4	T45.8X5	T45.8X6
Fibrinolysin (human)	T45.691	T45.692	T45.693	T45.694	T45.695	T45.696

Substance	Poisoning, Accidental (unintentional)	Poisoning, Intentional self-harm	Poisoning, Assault	Poisoning, Undetermined	Adverse effect	Underdosing
Fibrinolysis						
affecting drug	T45.601	T45.602	T45.603	T45.604	T45.605	T45.606
inhibitor NEC	T45.621	T45.622	T45.623	T45.624	T45.625	T45.626
Fibrinolytic drug	T45.611	T45.612	T45.613	T45.614	T45.615	T45.616
Filix mas	T37.4X1	T37.4X2	T37.4X3	T37.4X4	T37.4X5	T37.4X6
Filtering cream	T49.3X1	T49.3X2	T49.3X3	T49.3X4	T49.3X5	T49.3X6
Fiorinal	T39.011	T39.012	T39.013	T39.014	T39.015	T39.016
Firedamp	T59.891	T59.892	T59.893	T59.894	—	—
Fish, noxious, nonbacterial	T61.91	T61.92	T61.93	T61.94	—	—
ciguatera	T61.01	T61.02	T61.03	T61.04	—	—
scombroid	T61.11	T61.12	T61.13	T61.14	—	—
shell	T61.781	T61.782	T61.783	T61.784	—	—
specified NEC	T61.771	T61.772	T61.773	T61.774	—	—
Flagyl	T37.3X1	T37.3X2	T37.3X3	T37.3X4	T37.3X5	T37.3X6
Flavine adenine dinucleotide	T45.2X1	T45.2X2	T45.2X3	T45.2X4	T45.2X5	T45.2X6
Flavodic acid	T46.991	T46.992	T46.993	T46.994	T46.995	T46.996
Flavoxate	T44.3X1	T44.3X2	T44.3X3	T44.3X4	T44.3X5	T44.3X6
Flaxedil	T48.1X1	T48.1X2	T48.1X3	T48.1X4	T48.1X5	T48.1X6
Flaxseed (medicinal)	T49.3X1	T49.3X2	T49.3X3	T49.3X4	T49.3X5	T49.3X6
Flecainide	T46.2X1	T46.2X2	T46.2X3	T46.2X4	T46.2X5	T46.2X6
Fleroxacin	T36.8X1	T36.8X2	T36.8X3	T36.8X4	T36.8X5	T36.8X6
Floctafenine	T39.8X1	T39.8X2	T39.8X3	T39.8X4	T39.8X5	T39.8X6
Flomax	T44.6X1	T44.6X2	T44.6X3	T44.6X4	T44.6X5	T44.6X6
Flomoxef	T36.1X1	T36.1X2	T36.1X3	T36.1X4	T36.1X5	T36.1X6
Flopropione	T44.3X1	T44.3X2	T44.3X3	T44.3X4	T44.3X5	T44.3X6
Florantyrone	T47.5X1	T47.5X2	T47.5X3	T47.5X4	T47.5X5	T47.5X6
Floraquin	T37.8X1	T37.8X2	T37.8X3	T37.8X4	T37.8X5	T37.8X6
Florinef	T38.0X1	T38.0X2	T38.0X3	T38.0X4	T38.0X5	T38.0X6
ENT agent	T49.6X1	T49.6X2	T49.6X3	T49.6X4	T49.6X5	T49.6X6
ophthalmic preparation	T49.5X1	T49.5X2	T49.5X3	T49.5X4	T49.5X5	T49.5X6
topical NEC	T49.0X1	T49.0X2	T49.0X3	T49.0X4	T49.0X5	T49.0X6
Flowers of sulfur	T49.4X1	T49.4X2	T49.4X3	T49.4X4	T49.4X5	T49.4X6
Floxuridine	T45.1X1	T45.1X2	T45.1X3	T45.1X4	T45.1X5	T45.1X6
Fluanisone	T43.4X1	T43.4X2	T43.4X3	T43.4X4	T43.4X5	T43.4X6
Flubendazole	T37.4X1	T37.4X2	T37.4X3	T37.4X4	T37.4X5	T37.4X6
Fluclorolone acetonide	T49.0X1	T49.0X2	T49.0X3	T49.0X4	T49.0X5	T49.0X6
Flucloxacillin	T36.0X1	T36.0X2	T36.0X3	T36.0X4	T36.0X5	T36.0X6
Fluconazole	T37.8X1	T37.8X2	T37.8X3	T37.8X4	T37.8X5	T37.8X6
Flucytosine	T37.8X1	T37.8X2	T37.8X3	T37.8X4	T37.8X5	T37.8X6
Fludeoxyglucose (18F)	T50.8X1	T50.8X2	T50.8X3	T50.8X4	T50.8X5	T50.8X6
Fludiazepam	T42.4X1	T42.4X2	T42.4X3	T42.4X4	T42.4X5	T42.4X6
Fludrocortisone	T50.0X1	T50.0X2	T50.0X3	T50.0X4	T50.0X5	T50.0X6
ENT agent	T49.6X1	T49.6X2	T49.6X3	T49.6X4	T49.6X5	T49.6X6
ophthalmic preparation	T49.5X1	T49.5X2	T49.5X3	T49.5X4	T49.5X5	T49.5X6
topical NEC	T49.0X1	T49.0X2	T49.0X3	T49.0X4	T49.0X5	T49.0X6
Fludroxycortide	T49.0X1	T49.0X2	T49.0X3	T49.0X4	T49.0X5	T49.0X6
Flufenamic acid	T39.391	T39.392	T39.393	T39.394	T39.395	T39.396
Fluindione	T45.511	T45.512	T45.513	T45.514	T45.515	T45.516
Flumequine	T37.8X1	T37.8X2	T37.8X3	T37.8X4	T37.8X5	T37.8X6

Substance	Poisoning, Accidental (unintentional)	Poisoning, Intentional self-harm	Poisoning, Assault	Poisoning, Undetermined	Adverse effect	Underdosing
Flumethasone	T49.0X1	T49.0X2	T49.0X3	T49.0X4	T49.0X5	T49.0X6
Flumethiazide	T50.2X1	T50.2X2	T50.2X3	T50.2X4	T50.2X5	T50.2X6
Flumidin	T37.5X1	T37.5X2	T37.5X3	T37.5X4	T37.5X5	T37.5X6
Flunarizine	T46.7X1	T46.7X2	T46.7X3	T46.7X4	T46.7X5	T46.7X6
Flunidazole	T37.8X1	T37.8X2	T37.8X3	T37.8X4	T37.8X5	T37.8X6
Flunisolide	T48.6X1	T48.6X2	T48.6X3	T48.6X4	T48.6X5	T48.6X6
Flunitrazepam	T42.4X1	T42.4X2	T42.4X3	T42.4X4	T42.4X5	T42.4X6
Fluocinolone (acetonide)	T49.0X1	T49.0X2	T49.0X3	T49.0X4	T49.0X5	T49.0X6
Fluocinonide	T49.0X1	T49.0X2	T49.0X3	T49.0X4	T49.0X5	T49.0X6
Fluocortin (butyl)	T49.0X1	T49.0X2	T49.0X3	T49.0X4	T49.0X5	T49.0X6
Fluocortolone	T49.0X1	T49.0X2	T49.0X3	T49.0X4	T49.0X5	T49.0X6
Fluohydrocortisone	T38.0X1	T38.0X2	T38.0X3	T38.0X4	T38.0X5	T38.0X6
ENT agent	T49.6X1	T49.6X2	T49.6X3	T49.6X4	T49.6X5	T49.6X6
ophthalmic preparation	T49.5X1	T49.5X2	T49.5X3	T49.5X4	T49.5X5	T49.5X6
topical NEC	T49.0X1	T49.0X2	T49.0X3	T49.0X4	T49.0X5	T49.0X6
Fluonid	T49.0X1	T49.0X2	T49.0X3	T49.0X4	T49.0X5	T49.0X6
Fluopromazine	T43.3X1	T43.3X2	T43.3X3	T43.3X4	T43.3X5	T43.3X6
Fluoracetate	T60.8X1	T60.8X2	T60.8X3	T60.8X4	—	—
Fluorescein	T50.8X1	T50.8X2	T50.8X3	T50.8X4	T50.8X5	T50.8X6
Fluorhydrocortisone	T50.0X1	T50.0X2	T50.0X3	T50.0X4	T50.0X5	T50.0X6
Fluoride (nonmedicinal)(pesticide) (sodium) NEC	T60.8X1	T60.8X2	T60.8X3	T60.8X4	—	—
hydrogen—see Hydrofluoric acid						
medicinal NEC	T50.991	T50.992	T50.993	T50.994	T50.995	T50.996
dental use	T49.7X1	T49.7X2	T49.7X3	T49.7X4	T49.7X5	T49.7X6
not pesticide NEC	T54.91	T54.92	T54.93	T54.94	—	—
stannous	T49.7X1	T49.7X2	T49.7X3	T49.7X4	T49.7X5	T49.7X6
Fluorinated corticosteroids	T38.0X1	T38.0X2	T38.0X3	T38.0X4	T38.0X5	T38.0X6
Fluorine (gas)	T59.5X1	T59.5X2	T59.5X3	T59.5X4	—	—
salt—see Fluoride(s)						
Fluoristan	T49.7X1	T49.7X2	T49.7X3	T49.7X4	T49.7X5	T49.7X6
Fluormetholone	T49.0X1	T49.0X2	T49.0X3	T49.0X4	T49.0X5	T49.0X6
Fluoroacetate	T60.8X1	T60.8X2	T60.8X3	T60.8X4	—	—
Fluorocarbon monomer	T53.6X1	T53.6X2	T53.6X3	T53.6X4	—	—
Fluorocytosine	T37.8X1	T37.8X2	T37.8X3	T37.8X4	T37.8X5	T37.8X6
Fluorodeoxyuridine	T45.1X1	T45.1X2	T45.1X3	T45.1X4	T45.1X5	T45.1X6
Fluorometholone	T49.0X1	T49.0X2	T49.0X3	T49.0X4	T49.0X5	T49.0X6
ophthalmic preparation	T49.5X1	T49.5X2	T49.5X3	T49.5X4	T49.5X5	T49.5X6
Fluorophosphate insecticide	T60.0X1	T60.0X2	T60.0X3	T60.0X4	—	—
Fluorosol	T46.3X1	T46.3X2	T46.3X3	T46.3X4	T46.3X5	T46.3X6
Fluorouracil	T45.1X1	T45.1X2	T45.1X3	T45.1X4	T45.1X5	T45.1X6
Fluorphenylalanine	T49.5X1	T49.5X2	T49.5X3	T49.5X4	T49.5X5	T49.5X6
Fluothane	T41.0X1	T41.0X2	T41.0X3	T41.0X4	T41.0X5	T41.0X6
Fluoxetine	T43.221	T43.222	T43.223	T43.224	T43.225	T43.226
Fluoxymesterone	T38.7X1	T38.7X2	T38.7X3	T38.7X4	T38.7X5	T38.7X6
Flupenthixol	T43.4X1	T43.4X2	T43.4X3	T43.4X4	T43.4X5	T43.4X6
Flupentixol	T43.4X1	T43.4X2	T43.4X3	T43.4X4	T43.4X5	T43.4X6

Substance	Poisoning, Accidental (unintentional)	Poisoning, Intentional self-harm	Poisoning, Assault	Poisoning, Undetermined	Adverse effect	Underdosing
Fluphenazine	T43.3X1	T43.3X2	T43.3X3	T43.3X4	T43.3X5	T43.3X6
Fluprednidene	T49.0X1	T49.0X2	T49.0X3	T49.0X4	T49.0X5	T49.0X6
Fluprednisolone	T38.0X1	T38.0X2	T38.0X3	T38.0X4	T38.0X5	T38.0X6
Fluradoline	T39.8X1	T39.8X2	T39.8X3	T39.8X4	T39.8X5	T39.8X6
Flurandrenolide	T49.0X1	T49.0X2	T49.0X3	T49.0X4	T49.0X5	T49.0X6
Flurandrenolone	T49.0X1	T49.0X2	T49.0X3	T49.0X4	T49.0X5	T49.0X6
Flurazepam	T42.4X1	T42.4X2	T42.4X3	T42.4X4	T42.4X5	T42.4X6
Flurbiprofen	T39.311	T39.312	T39.313	T39.314	T39.315	T39.316
Flurobate	T49.0X1	T49.0X2	T49.0X3	T49.0X4	T49.0X5	T49.0X6
Fluroxene	T41.0X1	T41.0X2	T41.0X3	T41.0X4	T41.0X5	T41.0X6
Fluspirilene	T43.591	T43.592	T43.593	T43.594	T43.595	T43.596
Flutamide	T38.6X1	T38.6X2	T38.6X3	T38.6X4	T38.6X5	T38.6X6
Flutazolam	T42.4X1	T42.4X2	T42.4X3	T42.4X4	T42.4X5	T42.4X6
Fluticasone propionate	T38.0X1	T38.0X2	T38.0X3	T38.0X4	T38.0X5	T38.0X6
Flutoprazepam	T42.4X1	T42.4X2	T42.4X3	T42.4X4	T42.4X5	T42.4X6
Flutropium bromide	T48.6X1	T48.6X2	T48.6X3	T48.6X4	T48.6X5	T48.6X6
Fluvoxamine	T43.221	T43.222	T43.223	T43.224	T43.225	T43.226
Folacin	T45.8X1	T45.8X2	T45.8X3	T45.8X4	T45.8X5	T45.8X6
Folic acid	T45.8X1	T45.8X2	T45.8X3	T45.8X4	T45.8X5	T45.8X6
with ferrous salt	T45.2X1	T45.2X2	T45.2X3	T45.2X4	T45.2X5	T45.2X6
antagonist	T45.1X1	T45.1X2	T45.1X3	T45.1X4	T45.1X5	T45.1X6
Folinic acid	T45.8X1	T45.8X2	T45.8X3	T45.8X4	T45.8X5	T45.8X6
Folium stramoniae	T48.6X1	T48.6X2	T48.6X3	T48.6X4	T48.6X5	T48.6X6
Follicle-stimulating hormone, human	T38.811	T38.812	T38.813	T38.814	T38.815	T38.816
Folpet	T60.3X1	T60.3X2	T60.3X3	T60.3X4	—	—
Fominoben	T48.3X1	T48.3X2	T48.3X3	T48.3X4	T48.3X5	T48.3X6
Food, foodstuffs, noxious, nonbacterial, NEC	T62.91	T62.92	T62.93	T62.94	—	—
berries	T62.1X1	T62.1X2	T62.1X3	T62.1X4	—	—
fish—see also Fish	T61.91	T61.92	T61.93	T61.94	—	—
mushrooms	T62.0X1	T62.0X2	T62.0X3	T62.0X4	—	—
plants	T62.2X1	T62.2X2	T62.2X3	T62.2X4	—	—
seafood	T61.91	T61.92	T61.93	T61.94	—	—
specified NEC	T61.8X1	T61.8X2	T61.8X3	T61.8X4	—	—
seeds	T62.2X1	T62.2X2	T62.2X3	T62.2X4	—	—
shellfish	T61.781	T61.782	T61.783	T61.784	—	—
specified NEC	T62.8X1	T62.8X2	T62.8X3	T62.8X4	—	—
Fool's parsley	T62.2X1	T62.2X2	T62.2X3	T62.2X4	—	—
Formaldehyde (solution), gas or vapor	T59.2X1	T59.2X2	T59.2X3	T59.2X4	—	—
fungicide	T60.3X1	T60.3X2	T60.3X3	T60.3X4	—	—
Formalin	T59.2X1	T59.2X2	T59.2X3	T59.2X4	—	—
fungicide	T60.3X1	T60.3X2	T60.3X3	T60.3X4	—	—
vapor	T59.2X1	T59.2X2	T59.2X3	T59.2X4	—	—
Formic acid	T54.2X1	T54.2X2	T54.2X3	T54.2X4	—	—
vapor	T59.891	T59.892	T59.893	T59.894	—	—
Foscarnet sodium	T37.5X1	T37.5X2	T37.5X3	T37.5X4	T37.5X5	T37.5X6
Fosfestrol	T38.5X1	T38.5X2	T38.5X3	T38.5X4	T38.5X5	T38.5X6
Fosfomycin	T36.8X1	T36.8X2	T36.8X3	T36.8X4	T36.8X5	T36.8X6
Fosfonet sodium	T37.5X1	T37.5X2	T37.5X3	T37.5X4	T37.5X5	T37.5X6

Substance	Poisoning, Accidental (unintentional)	Poisoning, Intentional self-harm	Poisoning, Assault	Poisoning, Undetermined	Adverse effect	Underdosing
Fosinopril	T46.4X1	T46.4X2	T46.4X3	T46.4X4	T46.4X5	T46.4X6
sodium	T46.4X1	T46.4X2	T46.4X3	T46.4X4	T46.4X5	T46.4X6
Fowler's solution	T57.0X1	T57.0X2	T57.0X3	T57.0X4	—	—
Foxglove	T62.2X1	T62.2X2	T62.2X3	T62.2X4	—	—
Framycetin	T36.5X1	T36.5X2	T36.5X3	T36.5X4	T36.5X5	T36.5X6
Frangula	T47.2X1	T47.2X2	T47.2X3	T47.2X4	T47.2X5	T47.2X6
extract	T47.2X1	T47.2X2	T47.2X3	T47.2X4	T47.2X5	T47.2X6
Frei antigen	T50.8X1	T50.8X2	T50.8X3	T50.8X4	T50.8X5	T50.8X6
Freon	T53.5X1	T53.5X2	T53.5X3	T53.5X4	—	—
Fructose	T50.3X1	T50.3X2	T50.3X3	T50.3X4	T50.3X5	T50.3X6
Frusemide	T50.1X1	T50.1X2	T50.1X3	T50.1X4	T50.1X5	T50.1X6
FSH	T38.811	T38.812	T38.813	T38.814	T38.815	T38.816
Ftorafur	T45.1X1	T45.1X2	T45.1X3	T45.1X4	T45.1X5	T45.1X6
Fuel						
automobile	T52.0X1	T52.0X2	T52.0X3	T52.0X4	—	—
exhaust gas, not in transit	T58.01	T58.02	T58.03	T58.04	—	—
vapor NEC	T52.0X1	T52.0X2	T52.0X3	T52.0X4	—	—
gas (domestic use)—see also Carbon, monoxide, fuel, utility	T59.891	T59.892	T59.893	T59.894	—	—
utility	T59.891	T59.892	T59.893	T59.894	—	—
in mobile container	T59.891	T59.892	T59.893	T59.894	—	—
incomplete combustion of—see Carbon, monoxide, fuel, utility						
piped (natural)	T59.891	T59.892	T59.893	T59.894	—	—
industrial, incomplete combustion	T58.8X1	T58.8X2	T58.8X3	T58.8X4	—	—
Fugillin	T36.8X1	T36.8X2	T36.8X3	T36.8X4	T36.8X5	T36.8X6
Fulminate of mercury	T56.1X1	T56.1X2	T56.1X3	T56.1X4	—	—
Fulvicin	T36.7X1	T36.7X2	T36.7X3	T36.7X4	T36.7X5	T36.7X6
Fumadil	T36.8X1	T36.8X2	T36.8X3	T36.8X4	T36.8X5	T36.8X6
Fumagillin	T36.8X1	T36.8X2	T36.8X3	T36.8X4	T36.8X5	T36.8X6
Fumaric acid	T49.4X1	T49.4X2	T49.4X3	T49.4X4	T49.4X5	T49.4X6
Fumes (from)	T59.91	T59.92	T59.93	T59.94	—	—
carbon monoxide—see Carbon, monoxide						
charcoal (domestic use)—see Charcoal, fumes						
chloroform—see Chloroform						
coke (in domestic stoves, fireplaces)—see Coke fumes						
corrosive NEC	T54.91	T54.92	T54.93	T54.94	—	—
ether—see ether						
freons	T53.5X1	T53.5X2	T53.5X3	T53.5X4	—	—
hydrocarbons	T59.891	T59.892	T59.893	T59.894	—	—
petroleum (liquefied)	T59.891	T59.892	T59.893	T59.894	—	—
distributed through pipes (pure or mixed with air)	T59.891	T59.892	T59.893	T59.894	—	—

Substance	Poisoning, Accidental (unintentional)	Poisoning, Intentional self-harm	Poisoning, Assault	Poisoning, Undetermined	Adverse effect	Underdosing
Fumes — *Continued*						
lead—see lead						
metal—see Metals, or the specified metal						
nitrogen dioxide	T59.0X1	T59.0X2	T59.0X3	T59.0X4	—	—
pesticides—see Pesticide						
petroleum (liquefied)	T59.891	T59.892	T59.893	T59.894	—	—
distributed through pipes (pure or mixed with air)	T59.891	T59.892	T59.893	T59.894	—	—
polyester	T59.891	T59.892	T59.893	T59.894	—	—
specified source NEC— see also substance specified	T59.891	T59.892	T59.893	T59.894	—	—
sulfur dioxide	T59.1X1	T59.1X2	T59.1X3	T59.1X4	—	—
Fumigant NEC	T60.91	T60.92	T60.93	T60.94	—	—
Fungi, noxious, used as food	T62.0X1	T62.0X2	T62.0X3	T62.0X4	—	—
Fungicide NEC (nonmedicinal)	T60.3X1	T60.3X2	T60.3X3	T60.3X4	—	—
Fungizone	T36.7X1	T36.7X2	T36.7X3	T36.7X4	T36.7X5	T36.7X6
topical	T49.0X1	T49.0X2	T49.0X3	T49.0X4	T49.0X5	T49.0X6
Furacin	T49.0X1	T49.0X2	T49.0X3	T49.0X4	T49.0X5	T49.0X6
Furadantin	T37.91	T37.92	T37.93	T37.94	T37.95	T37.96
Furazolidone	T37.8X1	T37.8X2	T37.8X3	T37.8X4	T37.8X5	T37.8X6
Furazolium chloride	T49.0X1	T49.0X2	T49.0X3	T49.0X4	T49.0X5	T49.0X6
Furfural	T52.8X1	T52.8X2	T52.8X3	T52.8X4	—	—
Furnace (coal burning) (domestic), gas from	T58.2X1	T58.2X2	T58.2X3	T58.2X4	—	—
industrial	T58.8X1	T58.8X2	T58.8X3	T58.8X4	—	—
Furniture polish	T65.891	T65.892	T65.893	T65.894	—	—
Furosemide	T50.1X1	T50.1X2	T50.1X3	T50.1X4	T50.1X5	T50.1X6
Furoxone	T37.91	T37.92	T37.93	T37.94	T37.95	T37.96
Fursultiamine	T45.2X1	T45.2X2	T45.2X3	T45.2X4	T45.2X5	T45.2X6
Fusafungine	T36.8X1	T36.8X2	T36.8X3	T36.8X4	T36.8X5	T36.8X6
Fusel oil (any) (amyl) (butyl) (propyl), vapor	T51.3X1	T51.3X2	T51.3X3	T51.3X4	—	—
Fusidate (ethanolamine) (sodium)	T36.8X1	T36.8X2	T36.8X3	T36.8X4	T36.8X5	T36.8X6
Fusidic acid	T36.8X1	T36.8X2	T36.8X3	T36.8X4	T36.8X5	T36.8X6
Fytic acid, nonasodium	T50.6X1	T50.6X2	T50.6X3	T50.6X4	T50.6X5	T50.6X6
G						
GABA	T43.8X1	T43.8X2	T43.8X3	T43.8X4	T43.8X5	T43.8X6
Gadolinium	T56.821	T56.822	T56.823	T56.824	—	—
Gadopentetic acid	T50.8X1	T50.8X2	T50.8X3	T50.8X4	T50.8X5	T50.8X6
Galactose	T50.3X1	T50.3X2	T50.3X3	T50.3X4	T50.3X5	T50.3X6
b-Galactosidase	T47.5X1	T47.5X2	T47.5X3	T47.5X4	T47.5X5	T47.5X6
Galantamine	T44.0X1	T44.0X2	T44.0X3	T44.0X4	T44.0X5	T44.0X6
Gallamine (triethiodide)	T48.1X1	T48.1X2	T48.1X3	T48.1X4	T48.1X5	T48.1X6
Gallium citrate	T50.991	T50.992	T50.993	T50.994	T50.995	T50.996
Gallopamil	T46.1X1	T46.1X2	T46.1X3	T46.1X4	T46.1X5	T46.1X6
Gamboge	T47.2X1	T47.2X2	T47.2X3	T47.2X4	T47.2X5	T47.2X6

Substance	Poisoning, Accidental (unintentional)	Poisoning, Intentional self-harm	Poisoning, Assault	Poisoning, Undetermined	Adverse effect	Underdosing
Gamimune	T50.Z11	T50.Z12	T50.Z13	T50.Z14	T50.Z15	T50.Z16
Gamma globulin	T50.Z11	T50.Z12	T50.Z13	T50.Z14	T50.Z15	T50.Z16
Gamma-aminobutyric acid	T43.8X1	T43.8X2	T43.8X3	T43.8X4	T43.8X5	T43.8X6
Gamma-benzene hexachloride (medicinal)	T49.0X1	T49.0X2	T49.0X3	T49.0X4	T49.0X5	T49.0X6
nonmedicinal, vapor	T53.6X1	T53.6X2	T53.6X3	T53.6X4	—	—
Gamma-BHC (medicinal)—see also **Gamma-benzene hexachloride**	T49.0X1	T49.0X2	T49.0X3	T49.0X4	T49.0X5	T49.0X6
Gamulin	T50.Z11	T50.Z12	T50.Z13	T50.Z14	T50.Z15	T50.Z16
Ganciclovir (sodium)	T37.5X1	T37.5X2	T37.5X3	T37.5X4	T37.5X5	T37.5X6
Ganglionic blocking drug NEC	T44.2X1	T44.2X2	T44.2X3	T44.2X4	T44.2X5	T44.2X6
specified NEC	T44.2X1	T44.2X2	T44.2X3	T44.2X4	T44.2X5	T44.2X6
Ganja	T40.711	T40.712	T40.713	T40.714	T40.715	T40.716
Garamycin	T36.5X1	T36.5X2	T36.5X3	T36.5X4	T36.5X5	T36.5X6
ophthalmic preparation	T49.5X1	T49.5X2	T49.5X3	T49.5X4	T49.5X5	T49.5X6
topical NEC	T49.0X1	T49.0X2	T49.0X3	T49.0X4	T49.0X5	T49.0X6
Gardenal	T42.3X1	T42.3X2	T42.3X3	T42.3X4	T42.3X5	T42.3X6
Gardepanyl	T42.3X1	T42.3X2	T42.3X3	T42.3X4	T42.3X5	T42.3X6
Gas NEC	T59.91	T59.92	T59.93	T59.94	—	—
acetylene	T59.891	T59.892	T59.893	T59.894	—	—
incomplete combustion of	T58.11	T58.12	T58.13	T58.14	—	—
air contaminants, source or type not specified	T59.91	T59.92	T59.93	T59.94	—	—
anesthetic	T41.0X1	T41.0X2	T41.0X3	T41.0X4	T41.0X5	T41.0X6
blast furnace	T58.8X1	T58.8X2	T58.8X3	T58.8X4	—	—
butane—see butane						
carbon monoxide—see Carbon, monoxide						
chlorine	T59.4X1	T59.4X2	T59.4X3	T59.4X4	—	—
coal	T58.2X1	T58.2X2	T58.2X3	T58.2X4	—	—
cyanide	T57.3X1	T57.3X2	T57.3X3	T57.3X4	—	—
dicyanogen	T65.0X1	T65.0X2	T65.0X3	T65.0X4	—	—
domestic—see Domestic gas						
exhaust	T58.01	T58.02	T58.03	T58.04	—	—
from utility (for cooking, heating, or lighting) (after combustion)—see Carbon, monoxide, fuel, utility						
prior to combustion	T59.891	T59.892	T59.893	T59.894	—	—
from wood- or coal-burning stove or fireplace	T58.2X1	T58.2X2	T58.2X3	T58.2X4	—	—
fuel (domestic use) (after combustion)—see also Carbon, monoxide, fuel						

404

Substance	Poisoning, Accidental (unintentional)	Poisoning, Intentional self-harm	Poisoning, Assault	Poisoning, Undetermined	Adverse effect	Underdosing
Gas NEC — *Continued*						
industrial use	T58.8X1	T58.8X2	T58.8X3	T58.8X4	—	—
prior to combustion	T59.891	T59.892	T59.893	T59.894	—	—
utility	T59.891	T59.892	T59.893	T59.894	—	—
in mobile container	T59.891	T59.892	T59.893	T59.894	—	—
incomplete combustion of—see Carbon, monoxide, fuel, utility						
piped (natural)	T59.891	T59.892	T59.893	T59.894	—	—
garage	T58.01	T58.02	T58.03	T58.04	—	—
hydrocarbon NEC	T59.891	T59.892	T59.893	T59.894	—	—
incomplete combustion of—see Carbon, monoxide, fuel, utility						
liquefied—see butane						
piped	T59.891	T59.892	T59.893	T59.894	—	—
hydrocyanic acid	T65.0X1	T65.0X2	T65.0X3	T65.0X4	—	—
illuminating (after combustion)	T58.11	T58.12	T58.13	T58.14	—	—
prior to combustion	T59.891	T59.892	T59.893	T59.894	—	—
incomplete combustion, any—see Carbon, monoxide						
kiln	T58.8X1	T58.8X2	T58.8X3	T58.8X4	—	—
lacrimogenic	T59.3X1	T59.3X2	T59.3X3	T59.3X4	—	—
liquefied petroleum—see butane						
marsh	T59.891	T59.892	T59.893	T59.894	—	—
motor exhaust, not in transit	T58.01	T58.02	T58.03	T58.04	—	—
mustard, not in war	T59.891	T59.892	T59.893	T59.894	—	—
natural	T59.891	T59.892	T59.893	T59.894	—	—
nerve, not in war	T59.91	T59.92	T59.93	T59.94	—	—
oil	T52.0X1	T52.0X2	T52.0X3	T52.0X4	—	—
petroleum (liquefied) (distributed in mobile containers)	T59.891	T59.892	T59.893	T59.894	—	—
piped (pure or mixed with air)	T59.891	T59.892	T59.893	T59.894	—	—
piped (manufactured) (natural) NEC	T59.891	T59.892	T59.893	T59.894	—	—
producer	T58.8X1	T58.8X2	T58.8X3	T58.8X4	—	—
propane—see propane						
refrigerant (chlorofluoro-carbon)	T53.5X1	T53.5X2	T53.5X3	T53.5X4	—	—
not chlorofluoro-carbon	T59.891	T59.892	T59.893	T59.894	—	—
sewer	T59.91	T59.92	T59.93	T59.94	—	—
specified source NEC	T59.91	T59.92	T59.93	T59.94	—	—
stove (after combustion)	T58.11	T58.12	T58.13	T58.14	—	—
prior to combustion	T59.891	T59.892	T59.893	T59.894	—	—
tear	T59.3X1	T59.3X2	T59.3X3	T59.3X4	—	—
therapeutic	T41.5X1	T41.5X2	T41.5X3	T41.5X4	T41.5X5	T41.5X6

Substance	Poisoning, Accidental (unintentional)	Poisoning, Intentional self-harm	Poisoning, Assault	Poisoning, Undetermined	Adverse effect	Underdosing
Gas NEC — *Continued*						
utility (for cooking, heating, or lighting) (piped) NEC	T59.891	T59.892	T59.893	T59.894	—	—
in mobile container	T59.891	T59.892	T59.893	T59.894	—	—
incomplete combustion of—see Carbon, monoxide, fuel, utilty						
piped (natural)	T59.891	T59.892	T59.893	T59.894	—	—
water	T58.11	T58.12	T58.13	T58.14	—	—
incomplete combustion of—see Carbon, monoxide, fuel, utility						
Gaseous substance—see Gas						
Gasoline	T52.0X1	T52.0X2	T52.0X3	T52.0X4	—	—
vapor	T52.0X1	T52.0X2	T52.0X3	T52.0X4	—	—
Gastric enzymes	T47.5X1	T47.5X2	T47.5X3	T47.5X4	T47.5X5	T47.5X6
Gastrografin	T50.8X1	T50.8X2	T50.8X3	T50.8X4	T50.8X5	T50.8X6
Gastrointestinal drug	T47.91	T47.92	T47.93	T47.94	T47.95	T47.96
biological	T47.8X1	T47.8X2	T47.8X3	T47.8X4	T47.8X5	T47.8X6
specified NEC	T47.8X1	T47.8X2	T47.8X3	T47.8X4	T47.8X5	T47.8X6
Gaultheria procumbens	T62.2X1	T62.2X2	T62.2X3	T62.2X4	—	—
Gefarnate	T44.3X1	T44.3X2	T44.3X3	T44.3X4	T44.3X5	T44.3X6
Gelatin (intravenous)	T45.8X1	T45.8X2	T45.8X3	T45.8X4	T45.8X5	T45.8X6
absorbable (sponge)	T45.7X1	T45.7X2	T45.7X3	T45.7X4	T45.7X5	T45.7X6
Gelfilm	T49.8X1	T49.8X2	T49.8X3	T49.8X4	T49.8X5	T49.8X6
Gelfoam	T45.7X1	T45.7X2	T45.7X3	T45.7X4	T45.7X5	T45.7X6
Gelsemine	T50.991	T50.992	T50.993	T50.994	T50.995	T50.996
Gelsemium (sempervirens)	T62.2X1	T62.2X2	T62.2X3	T62.2X4	—	—
Gemeprost	T48.0X1	T48.0X2	T48.0X3	T48.0X4	T48.0X5	T48.0X6
Gemfibrozil	T46.6X1	T46.6X2	T46.6X3	T46.6X4	T46.6X5	T46.6X6
Gemonil	T42.3X1	T42.3X2	T42.3X3	T42.3X4	T42.3X5	T42.3X6
Gentamicin	T36.5X1	T36.5X2	T36.5X3	T36.5X4	T36.5X5	T36.5X6
ophthalmic preparation	T49.5X1	T49.5X2	T49.5X3	T49.5X4	T49.5X5	T49.5X6
topical NEC	T49.0X1	T49.0X2	T49.0X3	T49.0X4	T49.0X5	T49.0X6
Gentian	T47.5X1	T47.5X2	T47.5X3	T47.5X4	T47.5X5	T47.5X6
violet	T49.0X1	T49.0X2	T49.0X3	T49.0X4	T49.0X5	T49.0X6
Gepefrine	T44.4X1	T44.4X2	T44.4X3	T44.4X4	T44.4X5	T44.4X6
Gestonorone caproate	T38.5X1	T38.5X2	T38.5X3	T38.5X4	T38.5X5	T38.5X6
Gexane	T49.0X1	T49.0X2	T49.0X3	T49.0X4	T49.0X5	T49.0X6
Gila monster (venom)	T63.111	T63.112	T63.113	T63.114	—	—
Ginger	T47.5X1	T47.5X2	T47.5X3	T47.5X4	T47.5X5	T47.5X6
Jamaica—see Jamaica, ginger						
Gitalin	T46.0X1	T46.0X2	T46.0X3	T46.0X4	T46.0X5	T46.0X6
amorphous	T46.0X1	T46.0X2	T46.0X3	T46.0X4	T46.0X5	T46.0X6
Gitaloxin	T46.0X1	T46.0X2	T46.0X3	T46.0X4	T46.0X5	T46.0X6
Gitoxin	T46.0X1	T46.0X2	T46.0X3	T46.0X4	T46.0X5	T46.0X6
Glafenine	T39.8X1	T39.8X2	T39.8X3	T39.8X4	T39.8X5	T39.8X6

Table of Drugs and Chemicals

Glandular extract–Guano

Substance	Poisoning, Accidental (unintentional)	Poisoning, Intentional self-harm	Poisoning, Assault	Poisoning, Undetermined	Adverse effect	Underdosing
Glandular extract (medicinal) NEC	T50.Z91	T50.Z92	T50.Z93	T50.Z94	T50.Z95	T50.Z96
Glaucarubin	T37.3X1	T37.3X2	T37.3X3	T37.3X4	T37.3X5	T37.3X6
Glibenclamide	T38.3X1	T38.3X2	T38.3X3	T38.3X4	T38.3X5	T38.3X6
Glibornuride	T38.3X1	T38.3X2	T38.3X3	T38.3X4	T38.3X5	T38.3X6
Gliclazide	T38.3X1	T38.3X2	T38.3X3	T38.3X4	T38.3X5	T38.3X6
Glimidine	T38.3X1	T38.3X2	T38.3X3	T38.3X4	T38.3X5	T38.3X6
Glipizide	T38.3X1	T38.3X2	T38.3X3	T38.3X4	T38.3X5	T38.3X6
Gliquidone	T38.3X1	T38.3X2	T38.3X3	T38.3X4	T38.3X5	T38.3X6
Glisolamide	T38.3X1	T38.3X2	T38.3X3	T38.3X4	T38.3X5	T38.3X6
Glisoxepide	T38.3X1	T38.3X2	T38.3X3	T38.3X4	T38.3X5	T38.3X6
Globin zinc insulin	T38.3X1	T38.3X2	T38.3X3	T38.3X4	T38.3X5	T38.3X6
Globulin						
antilymphocytic	T50.Z11	T50.Z12	T50.Z13	T50.Z14	T50.Z15	T50.Z16
antirhesus	T50.Z11	T50.Z12	T50.Z13	T50.Z14	T50.Z15	T50.Z16
antivenin	T50.Z11	T50.Z12	T50.Z13	T50.Z14	T50.Z15	T50.Z16
antiviral	T50.Z11	T50.Z12	T50.Z13	T50.Z14	T50.Z15	T50.Z16
Glucagon	T38.3X1	T38.3X2	T38.3X3	T38.3X4	T38.3X5	T38.3X6
Glucocorticoids	T38.0X1	T38.0X2	T38.0X3	T38.0X4	T38.0X5	T38.0X6
Glucocorticosteroid	T38.0X1	T38.0X2	T38.0X3	T38.0X4	T38.0X5	T38.0X6
Gluconic acid	T50.991	T50.992	T50.993	T50.994	T50.995	T50.996
Glucosamine sulfate	T39.4X1	T39.4X2	T39.4X3	T39.4X4	T39.4X5	T39.4X6
Glucose	T50.3X1	T50.3X2	T50.3X3	T50.3X4	T50.3X5	T50.3X6
with sodium chloride	T50.3X1	T50.3X2	T50.3X3	T50.3X4	T50.3X5	T50.3X6
Glucosulfone sodium	T37.1X1	T37.1X2	T37.1X3	T37.1X4	T37.1X5	T37.1X6
Glucurolactone	T47.8X1	T47.8X2	T47.8X3	T47.8X4	T47.8X5	T47.8X6
Glue NEC	T52.8X1	T52.8X2	T52.8X3	T52.8X4	—	—
Glutamic acid	T47.5X1	T47.5X2	T47.5X3	T47.5X4	T47.5X5	T47.5X6
Glutaral (medicinal)	T49.0X1	T49.0X2	T49.0X3	T49.0X4	T49.0X5	T49.0X6
nonmedicinal	T65.891	T65.892	T65.893	T65.894	—	—
Glutaraldehyde (nonmedicinal)	T65.891	T65.892	T65.893	T65.894		
medicinal	T49.0X1	T49.0X2	T49.0X3	T49.0X4	T49.0X5	T49.0X6
Glutathione	T50.6X1	T50.6X2	T50.6X3	T50.6X4	T50.6X5	T50.6X6
Glutethimide	T42.6X1	T42.6X2	T42.6X3	T42.6X4	T42.6X5	T42.6X6
Glyburide	T38.3X1	T38.3X2	T38.3X3	T38.3X4	T38.3X5	T38.3X6
Glycerin	T47.4X1	T47.4X2	T47.4X3	T47.4X4	T47.4X5	T47.4X6
Glycerol	T47.4X1	T47.4X2	T47.4X3	T47.4X4	T47.4X5	T47.4X6
borax	T49.6X1	T49.6X2	T49.6X3	T49.6X4	T49.6X5	T49.6X6
intravenous	T50.3X1	T50.3X2	T50.3X3	T50.3X4	T50.3X5	T50.3X6
iodinated	T48.4X1	T48.4X2	T48.4X3	T48.4X4	T48.4X5	T48.4X6
Glycerophosphate	T50.991	T50.992	T50.993	T50.994	T50.995	T50.996
Glyceryl						
gualacolate	T48.4X1	T48.4X2	T48.4X3	T48.4X4	T48.4X5	T48.4X6
nitrate	T46.3X1	T46.3X2	T46.3X3	T46.3X4	T46.3X5	T46.3X6
triacetate (topical)	T49.0X1	T49.0X2	T49.0X3	T49.0X4	T49.0X5	T49.0X6
trinitrate	T46.3X1	T46.3X2	T46.3X3	T46.3X4	T46.3X5	T46.3X6
Glycine	T50.3X1	T50.3X2	T50.3X3	T50.3X4	T50.3X5	T50.3X6
Glyclopyramide	T38.3X1	T38.3X2	T38.3X3	T38.3X4	T38.3X5	T38.3X6
Glycobiarsol	T37.3X1	T37.3X2	T37.3X3	T37.3X4	T37.3X5	T37.3X6
Glycols (ether)	T52.3X1	T52.3X2	T52.3X3	T52.3X4	—	—
Glyconiazide	T37.1X1	T37.1X2	T37.1X3	T37.1X4	T37.1X5	T37.1X6
Glycopyrrolate	T44.3X1	T44.3X2	T44.3X3	T44.3X4	T44.3X5	T44.3X6
Glycopyrronium	T44.3X1	T44.3X2	T44.3X3	T44.3X4	T44.3X5	T44.3X6
bromide	T44.3X1	T44.3X2	T44.3X3	T44.3X4	T44.3X5	T44.3X6
Glycoside, cardiac (stimulant)	T46.0X1	T46.0X2	T46.0X3	T46.0X4	T46.0X5	T46.0X6
Glycyclamide	T38.3X1	T38.3X2	T38.3X3	T38.3X4	T38.3X5	T38.3X6
Glycyrrhiza extract	T48.4X1	T48.4X2	T48.4X3	T48.4X4	T48.4X5	T48.4X6
Glycyrrhizic acid	T48.4X1	T48.4X2	T48.4X3	T48.4X4	T48.4X5	T48.4X6
Glycyrrhizinate potassium	T48.4X1	T48.4X2	T48.4X3	T48.4X4	T48.4X5	T48.4X6
Glymidine sodium	T38.3X1	T38.3X2	T38.3X3	T38.3X4	T38.3X5	T38.3X6
Glyphosate	T60.3X1	T60.3X2	T60.3X3	T60.3X4	—	—
Glyphylline	T48.6X1	T48.6X2	T48.6X3	T48.6X4	T48.6X5	T48.6X6
Gold						
colloidal (198Au)	T45.1X1	T45.1X2	T45.1X3	T45.1X4	T45.1X5	T45.1X6
salts	T39.4X1	T39.4X2	T39.4X3	T39.4X4	T39.4X5	T39.4X6
Golden sulfide of antimony	T56.891	T56.892	T56.893	T56.894	—	—
Goldylocks	T62.2X1	T62.2X2	T62.2X3	T62.2X4	—	—
Gonadal tissue extract	T38.901	T38.902	T38.903	T38.904	T38.905	T38.906
female	T38.5X1	T38.5X2	T38.5X3	T38.5X4	T38.5X5	T38.5X6
male	T38.7X1	T38.7X2	T38.7X3	T38.7X4	T38.7X5	T38.7X6
Gonadorelin	T38.891	T38.892	T38.893	T38.894	T38.895	T38.896
Gonadotropin	T38.891	T38.892	T38.893	T38.894	T38.895	T38.896
chorionic	T38.891	T38.892	T38.893	T38.894	T38.895	T38.896
pituitary	T38.811	T38.812	T38.813	T38.814	T38.815	T38.816
Goserelin	T45.1X1	T45.1X2	T45.1X3	T45.1X4	T45.1X5	T45.1X6
Grain alcohol	T51.0X1	T51.0X2	T51.0X3	T51.0X4	—	—
Gramicidin	T49.0X1	T49.0X2	T49.0X3	T49.0X4	T49.0X5	T49.0X6
Granisetron	T45.0X1	T45.0X2	T45.0X3	T45.0X4	T45.0X5	T45.0X6
Gratiola officinalis	T62.2X1	T62.2X2	T62.2X3	T62.2X4	—	—
Grease	T65.891	T65.892	T65.893	T65.894	—	—
Green hellebore	T62.2X1	T62.2X2	T62.2X3	T62.2X4	—	—
Green soap	T49.2X1	T49.2X2	T49.2X3	T49.2X4	T49.2X5	T49.2X6
Grifulvin	T36.7X1	T36.7X2	T36.7X3	T36.7X4	T36.7X5	T36.7X6
Griseofulvin	T36.7X1	T36.7X2	T36.7X3	T36.7X4	T36.7X5	T36.7X6
Growth hormone	T38.811	T38.812	T38.813	T38.814	T38.815	T38.816
Guaiac reagent	T50.991	T50.992	T50.993	T50.994	T50.995	T50.996
Guaiacol derivatives	T48.4X1	T48.4X2	T48.4X3	T48.4X4	T48.4X5	T48.4X6
Guaifenesin	T48.4X1	T48.4X2	T48.4X3	T48.4X4	T48.4X5	T48.4X6
Guaimesal	T48.4X1	T48.4X2	T48.4X3	T48.4X4	T48.4X5	T48.4X6
Guaiphenesin	T48.4X1	T48.4X2	T48.4X3	T48.4X4	T48.4X5	T48.4X6
Guamecycline	T36.4X1	T36.4X2	T36.4X3	T36.4X4	T36.4X5	T36.4X6
Guanabenz	T46.5X1	T46.5X2	T46.5X3	T46.5X4	T46.5X5	T46.5X6
Guanacline	T46.5X1	T46.5X2	T46.5X3	T46.5X4	T46.5X5	T46.5X6
Guanadrel	T46.5X1	T46.5X2	T46.5X3	T46.5X4	T46.5X5	T46.5X6
Guanatol	T37.2X1	T37.2X2	T37.2X3	T37.2X4	T37.2X5	T37.2X6
Guanethidine	T46.5X1	T46.5X2	T46.5X3	T46.5X4	T46.5X5	T46.5X6
Guanfacine	T46.5X1	T46.5X2	T46.5X3	T46.5X4	T46.5X5	T46.5X6
Guano	T65.891	T65.892	T65.893	T65.894	—	—

Substance	Poisoning, Accidental (unintentional)	Poisoning, Intentional self-harm	Poisoning, Assault	Poisoning, Undetermined	Adverse effect	Underdosing
Guanochlor	T46.5X1	T46.5X2	T46.5X3	T46.5X4	T46.5X5	T46.5X6
Guanoclor	T46.5X1	T46.5X2	T46.5X3	T46.5X4	T46.5X5	T46.5X6
Guanoctine	T46.5X1	T46.5X2	T46.5X3	T46.5X4	T46.5X5	T46.5X6
Guanoxabenz	T46.5X1	T46.5X2	T46.5X3	T46.5X4	T46.5X5	T46.5X6
Guanoxan	T46.5X1	T46.5X2	T46.5X3	T46.5X4	T46.5X5	T46.5X6
Guar gum (medicinal)	T46.6X1	T46.6X2	T46.6X3	T46.6X4	T46.6X5	T46.6X6
H						
Hachimycin	T36.7X1	T36.7X2	T36.7X3	T36.7X4	T36.7X5	T36.7X6
Hair						
dye	T49.4X1	T49.4X2	T49.4X3	T49.4X4	T49.4X5	T49.4X6
preparation NEC	T49.4X1	T49.4X2	T49.4X3	T49.4X4	T49.4X5	T49.4X6
Halazepam	T42.4X1	T42.4X2	T42.4X3	T42.4X4	T42.4X5	T42.4X6
Halcinolone	T49.0X1	T49.0X2	T49.0X3	T49.0X4	T49.0X5	T49.0X6
Halcinonide	T49.0X1	T49.0X2	T49.0X3	T49.0X4	T49.0X5	T49.0X6
Halethazole	T49.0X1	T49.0X2	T49.0X3	T49.0X4	T49.0X5	T49.0X6
Hallucinogen NOS	T40.901	T40.902	T40.903	T40.904	T40.905	T40.906
specified NEC	T40.991	T40.992	T40.993	T40.994	T40.995	T40.996
Halofantrine	T37.2X1	T37.2X2	T37.2X3	T37.2X4	T37.2X5	T37.2X6
Halofenate	T46.6X1	T46.6X2	T46.6X3	T46.6X4	T46.6X5	T46.6X6
Halometasone	T49.0X1	T49.0X2	T49.0X3	T49.0X4	T49.0X5	T49.0X6
Haloperidol	T43.4X1	T43.4X2	T43.4X3	T43.4X4	T43.4X5	T43.4X6
Haloprogin	T49.0X1	T49.0X2	T49.0X3	T49.0X4	T49.0X5	T49.0X6
Halotex	T49.0X1	T49.0X2	T49.0X3	T49.0X4	T49.0X5	T49.0X6
Halothane	T41.0X1	T41.0X2	T41.0X3	T41.0X4	T41.0X5	T41.0X6
Haloxazolam	T42.4X1	T42.4X2	T42.4X3	T42.4X4	T42.4X5	T42.4X6
Halquinols	T49.0X1	T49.0X2	T49.0X3	T49.0X4	T49.0X5	T49.0X6
Hamamelis	T49.2X1	T49.2X2	T49.2X3	T49.2X4	T49.2X5	T49.2X6
Haptendextran	T45.8X1	T45.8X2	T45.8X3	T45.8X4	T45.8X5	T45.8X6
Harmonyl	T46.5X1	T46.5X2	T46.5X3	T46.5X4	T46.5X5	T46.5X6
Hartmann's solution	T50.3X1	T50.3X2	T50.3X3	T50.3X4	T50.3X5	T50.3X6
Hashish	T40.711	T40.712	T40.713	T40.714	T40.715	T40.716
Hawaiian Woodrose seeds	T40.991	T40.992	T40.993	T40.994	—	—
HCB	T60.3X1	T60.3X2	T60.3X3	T60.3X4	—	—
HCH	T53.6X1	T53.6X2	T53.6X3	T53.6X4	—	—
medicinal	T49.0X1	T49.0X2	T49.0X3	T49.0X4	T49.0X5	T49.0X6
HCN	T57.3X1	T57.3X2	T57.3X3	T57.3X4	—	—
Headache cures, drugs, powders NEC	T50.901	T50.902	T50.903	T50.904	T50.905	T50.906
Heavenly Blue (morning glory)	T40.991	T40.992	T40.993	T40.994	—	—
Heavy metal antidote	T45.8X1	T45.8X2	T45.8X3	T45.8X4	T45.8X5	T45.8X6
Hedaquinium	T49.0X1	T49.0X2	T49.0X3	T49.0X4	T49.0X5	T49.0X6
Hedge hyssop	T62.2X1	T62.2X2	T62.2X3	T62.2X4	—	—
Heet	T49.8X1	T49.8X2	T49.8X3	T49.8X4	T49.8X5	T49.8X6
Helenin	T37.4X1	T37.4X2	T37.4X3	T37.4X4	T37.4X5	T37.4X6
Helium (nonmedicinal) NEC	T59.891	T59.892	T59.893	T59.894	—	—
medicinal	T48.991	T48.992	T48.993	T48.994	T48.995	T48.996
Hellebore (black) (green) (white)	T62.2X1	T62.2X2	T62.2X3	T62.2X4	—	—
Hematin	T45.8X1	T45.8X2	T45.8X3	T45.8X4	T45.8X5	T45.8X6
Hematinic preparation	T45.8X1	T45.8X2	T45.8X3	T45.8X4	T45.8X5	T45.8X6
Hematological agent	T45.91	T45.92	T45.93	T45.94	T45.95	T45.96
specified NEC	T45.8X1	T45.8X2	T45.8X3	T45.8X4	T45.8X5	T45.8X6
Hemlock	T62.2X1	T62.2X2	T62.2X3	T62.2X4	—	—
Hemostatic	T45.621	T45.622	T45.623	T45.624	T45.625	T45.626
drug, systemic	T45.621	T45.622	T45.623	T45.624	T45.625	T45.626
Hemostyptic	T49.4X1	T49.4X2	T49.4X3	T49.4X4	T49.4X5	T49.4X6
Henbane	T62.2X1	T62.2X2	T62.2X3	T62.2X4	—	—
Heparin (sodium)	T45.511	T45.512	T45.513	T45.514	T45.515	T45.516
action reverser	T45.7X1	T45.7X2	T45.7X3	T45.7X4	T45.7X5	T45.7X6
Heparin-fraction	T45.511	T45.512	T45.513	T45.514	T45.515	T45.516
Heparinoid (systemic)	T45.511	T45.512	T45.513	T45.514	T45.515	T45.516
Hepatic secretion stimulant	T47.8X1	T47.8X2	T47.8X3	T47.8X4	T47.8X5	T47.8X6
Hepatitis B						
immune globulin	T50.Z11	T50.Z12	T50.Z13	T50.Z14	T50.Z15	T50.Z16
vaccine	T50.B91	T50.B92	T50.B93	T50.B94	T50.B95	T50.B96
Hepronicate	T46.7X1	T46.7X2	T46.7X3	T46.7X4	T46.7X5	T46.7X6
Heptabarb	T42.3X1	T42.3X2	T42.3X3	T42.3X4	T42.3X5	T42.3X6
Heptabarbital	T42.3X1	T42.3X2	T42.3X3	T42.3X4	T42.3X5	T42.3X6
Heptabarbitone	T42.3X1	T42.3X2	T42.3X3	T42.3X4	T42.3X5	T42.3X6
Heptachlor	T60.1X1	T60.1X2	T60.1X3	T60.1X4	—	—
Heptalgin	T40.2X1	T40.2X2	T40.2X3	T40.2X4	T40.2X5	T40.2X6
Heptaminol	T46.3X1	T46.3X2	T46.3X3	T46.3X4	T46.3X5	T46.3X6
Herbicide NEC	T60.3X1	T60.3X2	T60.3X3	T60.3X4	—	—
Heroin	T40.1X1	T40.1X2	T40.1X3	T40.1X4	—	—
Herplex	T49.5X1	T49.5X2	T49.5X3	T49.5X4	T49.5X5	T49.5X6
HES	T45.8X1	T45.8X2	T45.8X3	T45.8X4	T45.8X5	T45.8X6
Hesperidin	T46.991	T46.992	T46.993	T46.994	T46.995	T46.996
Hetacillin	T36.0X1	T36.0X2	T36.0X3	T36.0X4	T36.0X5	T36.0X6
Hetastarch	T45.8X1	T45.8X2	T45.8X3	T45.8X4	T45.8X5	T45.8X6
HETP	T60.0X1	T60.0X2	T60.0X3	T60.0X4	—	—
Hexachlorobenzene (vapor)	T60.3X1	T60.3X2	T60.3X3	T60.3X4	—	—
Hexachlorocyclohexane	T53.6X1	T53.6X2	T53.6X3	T53.6X4	—	—
Hexachlorophene	T49.0X1	T49.0X2	T49.0X3	T49.0X4	T49.0X5	T49.0X6
Hexadiline	T46.3X1	T46.3X2	T46.3X3	T46.3X4	T46.3X5	T46.3X6
Hexadimethrine (bromide)	T45.7X1	T45.7X2	T45.7X3	T45.7X4	T45.7X5	T45.7X6
Hexadylamine	T46.3X1	T46.3X2	T46.3X3	T46.3X4	T46.3X5	T46.3X6
Hexaethyl tetraphosphate	T60.0X1	T60.0X2	T60.0X3	T60.0X4	—	—
Hexafluorenium bromide	T48.1X1	T48.1X2	T48.1X3	T48.1X4	T48.1X5	T48.1X6
Hexafluronium (bromide)	T48.1X1	T48.1X2	T48.1X3	T48.1X4	T48.1X5	T48.1X6
Hexa-germ	T49.2X1	T49.2X2	T49.2X3	T49.2X4	T49.2X5	T49.2X6
Hexahydrobenzol	T52.8X1	T52.8X2	T52.8X3	T52.8X4	—	—
Hexahydrocresol(s)	T51.8X1	T51.8X2	T51.8X3	T51.8X4	—	—
arsenide	T57.0X1	T57.0X2	T57.0X3	T57.0X4	—	—
arseniurated	T57.0X1	T57.0X2	T57.0X3	T57.0X4	—	—
cyanide	T57.3X1	T57.3X2	T57.3X3	T57.3X4	—	—

407

Substance	Poisoning, Accidental (unintentional)	Poisoning, Intentional self-harm	Poisoning, Assault	Poisoning, Undetermined	Adverse effect	Underdosing
Hexahydrocresol(s) — *Continued*						
gas	T59.891	T59.892	T59.893	T59.894	—	—
Fluoride (liquid)	T57.8X1	T57.8X2	T57.8X3	T57.8X4	—	—
vapor	T59.891	T59.892	T59.893	T59.894	—	—
phophorated	T60.0X1	T60.0X2	T60.0X3	T60.0X4	—	—
sulfate	T57.8X1	T57.8X2	T57.8X3	T57.8X4	—	—
sulfide (gas)	T59.6X1	T59.6X2	T59.6X3	T59.6X4	—	—
arseniurated	T57.0X1	T57.0X2	T57.0X3	T57.0X4	—	—
sulfurated	T57.8X1	T57.8X2	T57.8X3	T57.8X4	—	—
Hexahydrophenol	T51.8X1	T51.8X2	T51.8X3	T51.8X4	—	—
Hexalen	T51.8X1	T51.8X2	T51.8X3	T51.8X4	—	—
Hexamethonium bromide	T44.2X1	T44.2X2	T44.2X3	T44.2X4	T44.2X5	T44.2X6
Hexamethylene	T52.8X1	T52.8X2	T52.8X3	T52.8X4	—	—
Hexamethylmelamine	T45.1X1	T45.1X2	T45.1X3	T45.1X4	T45.1X5	T45.1X6
Hexamidine	T49.0X1	T49.0X2	T49.0X3	T49.0X4	T49.0X5	T49.0X6
Hexamine (mandelate)	T37.8X1	T37.8X2	T37.8X3	T37.8X4	T37.8X5	T37.8X6
Hexanone, 2-hexanone	T52.4X1	T52.4X2	T52.4X3	T52.4X4	—	—
Hexanuorenium	T48.1X1	T48.1X2	T48.1X3	T48.1X4	T48.1X5	T48.1X6
Hexapropymate	T42.6X1	T42.6X2	T42.6X3	T42.6X4	T42.6X5	T42.6X6
Hexasonium iodide	T44.3X1	T44.3X2	T44.3X3	T44.3X4	T44.3X5	T44.3X6
Hexcarbacholine bromide	T48.1X1	T48.1X2	T48.1X3	T48.1X4	T48.1X5	T48.1X6
Hexemal	T42.3X1	T42.3X2	T42.3X3	T42.3X4	T42.3X5	T42.3X6
Hexestrol	T38.5X1	T38.5X2	T38.5X3	T38.5X4	T38.5X5	T38.5X6
Hexethal (sodium)	T42.3X1	T42.3X2	T42.3X3	T42.3X4	T42.3X5	T42.3X6
Hexetidine	T37.8X1	T37.8X2	T37.8X3	T37.8X4	T37.8X5	T37.8X6
Hexobarbital	T42.3X1	T42.3X2	T42.3X3	T42.3X4	T42.3X5	T42.3X6
rectal	T41.291	T41.292	T41.293	T41.294	T41.295	T41.296
sodium	T41.1X1	T41.1X2	T41.1X3	T41.1X4	T41.1X5	T41.1X6
Hexobendine	T46.3X1	T46.3X2	T46.3X3	T46.3X4	T46.3X5	T46.3X6
Hexocyclium	T44.3X1	T44.3X2	T44.3X3	T44.3X4	T44.3X5	T44.3X6
metilsulfate	T44.3X1	T44.3X2	T44.3X3	T44.3X4	T44.3X5	T44.3X6
Hexoestrol	T38.5X1	T38.5X2	T38.5X3	T38.5X4	T38.5X5	T38.5X6
Hexone	T52.4X1	T52.4X2	T52.4X3	T52.4X4	—	—
Hexoprenaline	T48.6X1	T48.6X2	T48.6X3	T48.6X4	T48.6X5	T48.6X6
Hexylcaine	T41.3X1	T41.3X2	T41.3X3	T41.3X4	T41.3X5	T41.3X6
Hexylresorcinol	T52.2X1	T52.2X2	T52.2X3	T52.2X4	—	—
HGH (human growth hormone)	T38.811	T38.812	T38.813	T38.814	T38.815	T38.816
Hinkle's pills	T47.2X1	T47.2X2	T47.2X3	T47.2X4	T47.2X5	T47.2X6
Histalog	T50.8X1	T50.8X2	T50.8X3	T50.8X4	T50.8X5	T50.8X6
Histamine (phosphate)	T50.8X1	T50.8X2	T50.8X3	T50.8X4	T50.8X5	T50.8X6
Histoplasmin	T50.8X1	T50.8X2	T50.8X3	T50.8X4	T50.8X5	T50.8X6
Holly berries	T62.2X1	T62.2X2	T62.2X3	T62.2X4	—	—
Homatropine	T44.3X1	T44.3X2	T44.3X3	T44.3X4	T44.3X5	T44.3X6
methylbromide	T44.3X1	T44.3X2	T44.3X3	T44.3X4	T44.3X5	T44.3X6
Homochlorcyclizine	T45.0X1	T45.0X2	T45.0X3	T45.0X4	T45.0X5	T45.0X6
Homosalate	T49.3X1	T49.3X2	T49.3X3	T49.3X4	T49.3X5	T49.3X6
Homo-tet	T50.Z11	T50.Z12	T50.Z13	T50.Z14	T50.Z15	T50.Z16

Substance	Poisoning, Accidental (unintentional)	Poisoning, Intentional self-harm	Poisoning, Assault	Poisoning, Undetermined	Adverse effect	Underdosing
Hormone	T38.801	T38.802	T38.803	T38.804	T38.805	T38.806
adrenal cortical steroids	T38.0X1	T38.0X2	T38.0X3	T38.0X4	T38.0X5	T38.0X6
androgenic	T38.7X1	T38.7X2	T38.7X3	T38.7X4	T38.7X5	T38.7X6
anterior pituitary NEC	T38.811	T38.812	T38.813	T38.814	T38.815	T38.816
antidiabetic agents	T38.3X1	T38.3X2	T38.3X3	T38.3X4	T38.3X5	T38.3X6
antidiuretic	T38.891	T38.892	T38.893	T38.894	T38.895	T38.896
cancer therapy	T45.1X1	T45.1X2	T45.1X3	T45.1X4	T45.1X5	T45.1X6
follicle stimulating	T38.811	T38.812	T38.813	T38.814	T38.815	T38.816
gonadotropic	T38.891	T38.892	T38.893	T38.894	T38.895	T38.896
pituitary	T38.811	T38.812	T38.813	T38.814	T38.815	T38.816
growth	T38.811	T38.812	T38.813	T38.814	T38.815	T38.816
luteinizing	T38.811	T38.812	T38.813	T38.814	T38.815	T38.816
ovarian	T38.5X1	T38.5X2	T38.5X3	T38.5X4	T38.5X5	T38.5X6
oxytocic	T48.0X1	T48.0X2	T48.0X3	T48.0X4	T48.0X5	T48.0X6
parathyroid (derivatives)	T50.991	T50.992	T50.993	T50.994	T50.995	T50.996
pituitary (posterior) NEC	T38.891	T38.892	T38.893	T38.894	T38.895	T38.896
anterior	T38.811	T38.812	T38.813	T38.814	T38.815	T38.816
specified, NEC	T38.891	T38.892	T38.893	T38.894	T38.895	T38.896
thyroid	T38.1X1	T38.1X2	T38.1X3	T38.1X4	T38.1X5	T38.1X6
Hornet (sting)	T63.451	T63.452	T63.453	T63.454	—	—
Horse anti-human lymphocytic serum	T50.Z11	T50.Z12	T50.Z13	T50.Z14	T50.Z15	T50.Z16
Horticulture agent NEC	T65.91	T65.92	T65.93	T65.94	—	—
with pesticide	T60.91	T60.92	T60.93	T60.94	—	—
Human						
albumin	T45.8X1	T45.8X2	T45.8X3	T45.8X4	T45.8X5	T45.8X6
growth hormone (HGH)	T38.811	T38.812	T38.813	T38.814	T38.815	T38.816
immune serum	T50.Z11	T50.Z12	T50.Z13	T50.Z14	T50.Z15	T50.Z16
Hyaluronidase	T45.3X1	T45.3X2	T45.3X3	T45.3X4	T45.3X5	T45.3X6
Hyazyme	T45.3X1	T45.3X2	T45.3X3	T45.3X4	T45.3X5	T45.3X6
Hycodan	T40.2X1	T40.2X2	T40.2X3	T40.2X4	T40.2X5	T40.2X6
Hydantoin derivative NEC	T42.0X1	T42.0X2	T42.0X3	T42.0X4	T42.0X5	T42.0X6
Hydeltra	T38.0X1	T38.0X2	T38.0X3	T38.0X4	T38.0X5	T38.0X6
Hydergine	T44.6X1	T44.6X2	T44.6X3	T44.6X4	T44.6X5	T44.6X6
Hydrabamine penicillin	T36.0X1	T36.0X2	T36.0X3	T36.0X4	T36.0X5	T36.0X6
Hydralazine	T46.5X1	T46.5X2	T46.5X3	T46.5X4	T46.5X5	T46.5X6
Hydrargaphen	T49.0X1	T49.0X2	T49.0X3	T49.0X4	T49.0X5	T49.0X6
Hydrargyri amino-chloridum	T49.0X1	T49.0X2	T49.0X3	T49.0X4	T49.0X5	T49.0X6
Hydrastine	T48.291	T48.292	T48.293	T48.294	T48.295	T48.296
Hydrazine	T54.1X1	T54.1X2	T54.1X3	T54.1X4	—	—
monoamine oxidase inhibitors	T43.1X1	T43.1X2	T43.1X3	T43.1X4	T43.1X5	T43.1X6
Hydrazoic acid, azides	T54.2X1	T54.2X2	T54.2X3	T54.2X4	—	—
Hydriodic acid	T48.4X1	T48.4X2	T48.4X3	T48.4X4	T48.4X5	T48.4X6
Hydrocarbon gas	T59.891	T59.892	T59.893	T59.894	—	—
incomplete combustion of—see Carbon, monoxide, fuel, utility						

Substance	Poisoning, Accidental (unintentional)	Poisoning, Intentional self-harm	Poisoning, Assault	Poisoning, Undetermined	Adverse effect	Underdosing
Hydrocarbon gas — *Continued*						
liquefied (mobile container)	T59.891	T59.892	T59.893	T59.894	—	—
piped (natural)	T59.891	T59.892	T59.893	T59.894	—	—
Hydrochloric acid (liquid)	T54.2X1	T54.2X2	T54.2X3	T54.2X4	—	—
medicinal (digestant)	T47.5X1	T47.5X2	T47.5X3	T47.5X4	T47.5X5	T47.5X6
vapor	T59.891	T59.892	T59.893	T59.894	—	—
Hydrochlorothiazide	T50.2X1	T50.2X2	T50.2X3	T50.2X4	T50.2X5	T50.2X6
Hydrocodone	T40.2X1	T40.2X2	T40.2X3	T40.2X4	T40.2X5	T40.2X6
Hydrocortisone (derivatives)	T38.0X1	T38.0X2	T38.0X3	T38.0X4	T38.0X5	T38.0X6
aceponate	T49.0X1	T49.0X2	T49.0X3	T49.0X4	T49.0X5	T49.0X6
ENT agent	T49.6X1	T49.6X2	T49.6X3	T49.6X4	T49.6X5	T49.6X6
ophthalmic preparation	T49.5X1	T49.5X2	T49.5X3	T49.5X4	T49.5X5	T49.5X6
topical NEC	T49.0X1	T49.0X2	T49.0X3	T49.0X4	T49.0X5	T49.0X6
Hydrocortone	T38.0X1	T38.0X2	T38.0X3	T38.0X4	T38.0X5	T38.0X6
ENT agent	T49.6X1	T49.6X2	T49.6X3	T49.6X4	T49.6X5	T49.6X6
ophthalmic preparation	T49.5X1	T49.5X2	T49.5X3	T49.5X4	T49.5X5	T49.5X6
topical NEC	T49.0X1	T49.0X2	T49.0X3	T49.0X4	T49.0X5	T49.0X6
Hydrocyanic acid (liquid)	T57.3X1	T57.3X2	T57.3X3	T57.3X4	—	—
gas	T65.0X1	T65.0X2	T65.0X3	T65.0X4	—	—
Hydroflumethiazide	T50.2X1	T50.2X2	T50.2X3	T50.2X4	T50.2X5	T50.2X6
Hydrofluoric acid (liquid)	T54.2X1	T54.2X2	T54.2X3	T54.2X4	—	—
vapor	T59.891	T59.892	T59.893	T59.894	—	—
Hydrogen	T59.891	T59.892	T59.893	T59.894	—	—
arsenide	T57.0X1	T57.0X2	T57.0X3	T57.0X4	—	—
arseniureted	T57.0X1	T57.0X2	T57.0X3	T57.0X4	—	—
chloride	T57.8X1	T57.8X2	T57.8X3	T57.8X4	—	—
cyanide (salts)	T57.3X1	T57.3X2	T57.3X3	T57.3X4	—	—
gas	T57.3X1	T57.3X2	T57.3X3	T57.3X4	—	—
Fluoride	T59.5X1	T59.5X2	T59.5X3	T59.5X4	—	—
vapor	T59.5X1	T59.5X2	T59.5X3	T59.5X4	—	—
peroxide	T49.0X1	T49.0X2	T49.0X3	T49.0X4	T49.0X5	T49.0X6
phosphureted	T57.1X1	T57.1X2	T57.1X3	T57.1X4	—	—
sulfide	T59.6X1	T59.6X2	T59.6X3	T59.6X4	—	—
arseniureted	T57.0X1	T57.0X2	T57.0X3	T57.0X4	—	—
sulfureted	T59.6X1	T59.6X2	T59.6X3	T59.6X4	—	—
Hydromethylpyridine	T46.7X1	T46.7X2	T46.7X3	T46.7X4	T46.7X5	T46.7X6
Hydromorphinol	T40.2X1	T40.2X2	T40.2X3	T40.2X4	—	—
Hydromorphinone	T40.2X1	T40.2X2	T40.2X3	T40.2X4	T40.2X5	T40.2X6
Hydromorphone	T40.2X1	T40.2X2	T40.2X3	T40.2X4	T40.2X5	T40.2X6
Hydromox	T50.2X1	T50.2X2	T50.2X3	T50.2X4	T50.2X5	T50.2X6
Hydrophilic lotion	T49.3X1	T49.3X2	T49.3X3	T49.3X4	T49.3X5	T49.3X6
Hydroquinidine	T46.2X1	T46.2X2	T46.2X3	T46.2X4	T46.2X5	T46.2X6
Hydroquinone	T52.2X1	T52.2X2	T52.2X3	T52.2X4	—	—
vapor	T59.891	T59.892	T59.893	T59.894	—	—
Hydrosulfuric acid (gas)	T59.6X1	T59.6X2	T59.6X3	T59.6X4	—	—

Substance	Poisoning, Accidental (unintentional)	Poisoning, Intentional self-harm	Poisoning, Assault	Poisoning, Undetermined	Adverse effect	Underdosing
Hydrotalcite	T47.1X1	T47.1X2	T47.1X3	T47.1X4	T47.1X5	T47.1X6
Hydrous wool fat	T49.3X1	T49.3X2	T49.3X3	T49.3X4	T49.3X5	T49.3X6
Hydroxide, caustic	T54.3X1	T54.3X2	T54.3X3	T54.3X4	—	—
Hydroxocobalamin	T45.8X1	T45.8X2	T45.8X3	T45.8X4	T45.8X5	T45.8X6
Hydroxyamp-hetamine	T49.5X1	T49.5X2	T49.5X3	T49.5X4	T49.5X5	T49.5X6
Hydroxycarbamide	T45.1X1	T45.1X2	T45.1X3	T45.1X4	T45.1X5	T45.1X6
Hydroxychloroquine	T37.8X1	T37.8X2	T37.8X3	T37.8X4	T37.8X5	T37.8X6
Hydroxydihydro-codeinone	T40.2X1	T40.2X2	T40.2X3	T40.2X4	T40.2X5	T40.2X6
Hydroxyestrone	T38.5X1	T38.5X2	T38.5X3	T38.5X4	T38.5X5	T38.5X6
Hydroxyethyl starch	T45.8X1	T45.8X2	T45.8X3	T45.8X4	T45.8X5	T45.8X6
Hydroxyme-thylpentanone	T52.4X1	T52.4X2	T52.4X3	T52.4X4	—	—
Hydroxyphenamate	T43.591	T43.592	T43.593	T43.594	T43.595	T43.596
Hydroxypheny-lbutazone	T39.2X1	T39.2X2	T39.2X3	T39.2X4	T39.2X5	T39.2X6
Hydroxyprogesterone	T38.5X1	T38.5X2	T38.5X3	T38.5X4	T38.5X5	T38.5X6
caproate	T38.5X1	T38.5X2	T38.5X3	T38.5X4	T38.5X5	T38.5X6
Hydroxyquinoline (derivatives) NEC	T37.8X1	T37.8X2	T37.8X3	T37.8X4	T37.8X5	T37.8X6
Hydroxystilbamidine	T37.3X1	T37.3X2	T37.3X3	T37.3X4	T37.3X5	T37.3X6
Hydroxytoluene (nonmedicinal)	T54.0X1	T54.0X2	T54.0X3	T54.0X4	—	—
medicinal	T49.0X1	T49.0X2	T49.0X3	T49.0X4	T49.0X5	T49.0X6
Hydroxyurea	T45.1X1	T45.1X2	T45.1X3	T45.1X4	T45.1X5	T45.1X6
Hydroxyzine	T43.591	T43.592	T43.593	T43.594	T43.595	T43.596
Hyoscine	T44.3X1	T44.3X2	T44.3X3	T44.3X4	T44.3X5	T44.3X6
Hyoscyamine	T44.3X1	T44.3X2	T44.3X3	T44.3X4	T44.3X5	T44.3X6
Hyoscyamus	T44.3X1	T44.3X2	T44.3X3	T44.3X4	T44.3X5	T44.3X6
dry extract	T44.3X1	T44.3X2	T44.3X3	T44.3X4	T44.3X5	T44.3X6
Hypaque	T50.8X1	T50.8X2	T50.8X3	T50.8X4	T50.8X5	T50.8X6
Hypertussis	T50.Z11	T50.Z12	T50.Z13	T50.Z14	T50.Z15	T50.Z16
Hypnotic	T42.71	T42.72	T42.73	T42.74	T42.75	T42.76
anticonvulsant	T42.71	T42.72	T42.73	T42.74	T42.75	T42.76
specified NEC	T42.6X1	T42.6X2	T42.6X3	T42.6X4	T42.6X5	T42.6X6
Hypochlorite	T49.0X1	T49.0X2	T49.0X3	T49.0X4	T49.0X5	T49.0X6
Hypophysis, posterior	T38.891	T38.892	T38.893	T38.894	T38.895	T38.896
Hypotensive NEC	T46.5X1	T46.5X2	T46.5X3	T46.5X4	T46.5X5	T46.5X6
Hypromellose	T49.5X1	T49.5X2	T49.5X3	T49.5X4	T49.5X5	T49.5X6
I						
Ibacitabine	T37.5X1	T37.5X2	T37.5X3	T37.5X4	T37.5X5	T37.5X6
Ibopamine	T44.991	T44.992	T44.993	T44.994	T44.995	T44.996
Ibufenac	T39.311	T39.312	T39.313	T39.314	T39.315	T39.316
Ibuprofen	T39.311	T39.312	T39.313	T39.314	T39.315	T39.316
Ibuproxam	T39.311	T39.312	T39.313	T39.314	T39.315	T39.316
Ibuterol	T48.6X1	T48.6X2	T48.6X3	T48.6X4	T48.6X5	T48.6X6
Ichthammol	T49.0X1	T49.0X2	T49.0X3	T49.0X4	T49.0X5	T49.0X6
Ichthyol	T49.4X1	T49.4X2	T49.4X3	T49.4X4	T49.4X5	T49.4X6
Idarubicin	T45.1X1	T45.1X2	T45.1X3	T45.1X4	T45.1X5	T45.1X6
Idrocilamide	T42.8X1	T42.8X2	T42.8X3	T42.8X4	T42.8X5	T42.8X6
Ifenprodil	T46.7X1	T46.7X2	T46.7X3	T46.7X4	T46.7X5	T46.7X6

Substance	Poisoning, Accidental (unintentional)	Poisoning, Intentional self-harm	Poisoning, Assault	Poisoning, Undetermined	Adverse effect	Underdosing
Ifosfamide	T45.1X1	T45.1X2	T45.1X3	T45.1X4	T45.1X5	T45.1X6
Iletin	T38.3X1	T38.3X2	T38.3X3	T38.3X4	T38.3X5	T38.3X6
Ilex	T62.2X1	T62.2X2	T62.2X3	T62.2X4	—	—
Illuminating gas (after combustion)	T58.11	T58.12	T58.13	T58.14	—	—
prior to combustion	T59.891	T59.892	T59.893	T59.894	—	—
Ilopan	T45.2X1	T45.2X2	T45.2X3	T45.2X4	T45.2X5	T45.2X6
Iloprost	T46.7X1	T46.7X2	T46.7X3	T46.7X4	T46.7X5	T46.7X6
Ilotycin	T36.3X1	T36.3X2	T36.3X3	T36.3X4	T36.3X5	T36.3X6
ophthalmic preparation	T49.5X1	T49.5X2	T49.5X3	T49.5X4	T49.5X5	T49.5X6
topical NEC	T49.0X1	T49.0X2	T49.0X3	T49.0X4	T49.0X5	T49.0X6
Imidazole-4-carboxamide	T45.1X1	T45.1X2	T45.1X3	T45.1X4	T45.1X5	T45.1X6
Imipenem	T36.0X1	T36.0X2	T36.0X3	T36.0X4	T36.0X5	T36.0X6
Imipramine	T43.011	T43.012	T43.013	T43.014	T43.015	T43.016
Iminostilbene	T42.1X1	T42.1X2	T42.1X3	T42.1X4	T42.1X5	T42.1X6
Immu-G	T50.Z11	T50.Z12	T50.Z13	T50.Z14	T50.Z15	T50.Z16
Immuglobin	T50.Z11	T50.Z12	T50.Z13	T50.Z14	T50.Z15	T50.Z16
Immune						
globulin	T50.Z11	T50.Z12	T50.Z13	T50.Z14	T50.Z15	T50.Z16
serum globulin	T50.Z11	T50.Z12	T50.Z13	T50.Z14	T50.Z15	T50.Z16
Immunoglobin human (intravenous) (normal)	T50.Z11	T50.Z12	T50.Z13	T50.Z14	T50.Z15	T50.Z16
unmodified	T50.Z11	T50.Z12	T50.Z13	T50.Z14	T50.Z15	T50.Z16
Immunosuppressive drug	T45.1X1	T45.1X2	T45.1X3	T45.1X4	T45.1X5	T45.1X6
Immu-tetanus	T50.Z11	T50.Z12	T50.Z13	T50.Z14	T50.Z15	T50.Z16
Indalpine	T43.221	T43.222	T43.223	T43.224	T43.225	T43.226
Indanazoline	T48.5X1	T48.5X2	T48.5X3	T48.5X4	T48.5X5	T48.5X6
Indandione (derivatives)	T45.511	T45.512	T45.513	T45.514	T45.515	T45.516
Indapamide	T46.5X1	T46.5X2	T46.5X3	T46.5X4	T46.5X5	T46.5X6
Indendione (derivatives)	T45.511	T45.512	T45.513	T45.514	T45.515	T45.516
Indenolol	T44.7X1	T44.7X2	T44.7X3	T44.7X4	T44.7X5	T44.7X6
Inderal	T44.7X1	T44.7X2	T44.7X3	T44.7X4	T44.7X5	T44.7X6
Indian						
hemp	T40.711	T40.712	T40.713	T40.714	T40.715	T40.716
tobacco	T62.2X1	T62.2X2	T62.2X3	T62.2X4	—	—
Indigo carmine	T50.8X1	T50.8X2	T50.8X3	T50.8X4	T50.8X5	T50.8X6
Indobufen	T45.521	T45.522	T45.523	T45.524	T45.525	T45.526
Indocin	T39.2X1	T39.2X2	T39.2X3	T39.2X4	T39.2X5	T39.2X6
Indocyanine green	T50.8X1	T50.8X2	T50.8X3	T50.8X4	T50.8X5	T50.8X6
Indometacin	T39.391	T39.392	T39.393	T39.394	T39.395	T39.396
Indomethacin	T39.391	T39.392	T39.393	T39.394	T39.395	T39.396
farnesil	T39.4X1	T39.4X2	T39.4X3	T39.4X4	T39.4X5	T39.4X6
Indoramin	T44.6X1	T44.6X2	T44.6X3	T44.6X4	T44.6X5	T44.6X6
Industrial						
alcohol	T51.0X1	T51.0X2	T51.0X3	T51.0X4	—	—
fumes	T59.891	T59.892	T59.893	T59.894	—	—
solvents (fumes) (vapors)	T52.91	T52.92	T52.93	T52.94	—	—
Influenza vaccine	T50.B91	T50.B92	T50.B93	T50.B94	T50.B95	T50.B96
Ingested substance NEC	T65.91	T65.92	T65.93	T65.94	—	—

Substance	Poisoning, Accidental (unintentional)	Poisoning, Intentional self-harm	Poisoning, Assault	Poisoning, Undetermined	Adverse effect	Underdosing
INH	T37.1X1	T37.1X2	T37.1X3	T37.1X4	T37.1X5	T37.1X6
Inhalation, gas (noxious)—see Gas						
Inhibitor						
angiotensin-converting enzyme	T46.4X1	T46.4X2	T46.4X3	T46.4X4	T46.4X5	T46.4X6
carbonic anhydrase	T50.2X1	T50.2X2	T50.2X3	T50.2X4	T50.2X5	T50.2X6
fibrinolysis	T45.621	T45.622	T45.623	T45.624	T45.625	T45.626
monoamine oxidase NEC	T43.1X1	T43.1X2	T43.1X3	T43.1X4	T43.1X5	T43.1X6
hydrazine	T43.1X1	T43.1X2	T43.1X3	T43.1X4	T43.1X5	T43.1X6
postsynaptic	T43.8X1	T43.8X2	T43.8X3	T43.8X4	T43.8X5	T43.8X6
prothrombin synthesis	T45.511	T45.512	T45.513	T45.514	T45.515	T45.516
Ink	T65.891	T65.892	T65.893	T65.894	—	—
Inorganic substance NEC	T57.91	T57.92	T57.93	T57.94	—	—
Inosine pranobex	T37.5X1	T37.5X2	T37.5X3	T37.5X4	T37.5X5	T37.5X6
Inositol	T50.991	T50.992	T50.993	T50.994	T50.995	T50.996
nicotinate	T46.7X1	T46.7X2	T46.7X3	T46.7X4	T46.7X5	T46.7X6
Inproquone	T45.1X1	T45.1X2	T45.1X3	T45.1X4	T45.1X5	T45.1X6
Insect (sting), venomous	T63.481	T63.482	T63.483	T63.484	—	—
ant	T63.421	T63.422	T63.423	T63.424	—	—
bee	T63.441	T63.442	T63.443	T63.444	—	—
caterpillar	T63.431	T63.432	T63.433	T63.434	—	—
hornet	T63.451	T63.452	T63.453	T63.454	—	—
wasp	T63.461	T63.462	T63.463	T63.464	—	—
Insecticide NEC	T60.91	T60.92	T60.93	T60.94		
carbamate	T60.0X1	T60.0X2	T60.0X3	T60.0X4		
chlorinated	T60.1X1	T60.1X2	T60.1X3	T60.1X4		
mixed	T60.91	T60.92	T60.93	T60.94		
organochlorine	T60.1X1	T60.1X2	T60.1X3	T60.1X4		
organophosphorus	T60.0X1	T60.0X2	T60.0X3	T60.0X4		
Insular tissue extract	T38.3X1	T38.3X2	T38.3X3	T38.3X4	T38.3X5	T38.3X6
Insulin (amorphous) (globin) (isophane) (Lente) (NPH) (Semilente) (Ultralente)	T38.3X1	T38.3X2	T38.3X3	T38.3X4	T38.3X5	T38.3X6
defalan	T38.3X1	T38.3X2	T38.3X3	T38.3X4	T38.3X5	T38.3X6
human	T38.3X1	T38.3X2	T38.3X3	T38.3X4	T38.3X5	T38.3X6
injection, soluble	T38.3X1	T38.3X2	T38.3X3	T38.3X4	T38.3X5	T38.3X6
biphasic	T38.3X1	T38.3X2	T38.3X3	T38.3X4	T38.3X5	T38.3X6
intermediate acting	T38.3X1	T38.3X2	T38.3X3	T38.3X4	T38.3X5	T38.3X6
protamine zinc	T38.3X1	T38.3X2	T38.3X3	T38.3X4	T38.3X5	T38.3X6
slow acting	T38.3X1	T38.3X2	T38.3X3	T38.3X4	T38.3X5	T38.3X6
zinc						
protamine injection	T38.3X1	T38.3X2	T38.3X3	T38.3X4	T38.3X5	T38.3X6
suspension (amorphous) (crystalline)	T38.3X1	T38.3X2	T38.3X3	T38.3X4	T38.3X5	T38.3X6
Interferon (alpha) (beta) (gamma)	T37.5X1	T37.5X2	T37.5X3	T37.5X4	T37.5X5	T37.5X6
Intestinal motility control drug	T47.6X1	T47.6X2	T47.6X3	T47.6X4	T47.6X5	T47.6X6
biological	T47.8X1	T47.8X2	T47.8X3	T47.8X4	T47.8X5	T47.8X6

Substance	Poisoning, Accidental (unintentional)	Poisoning, Intentional self-harm	Poisoning, Assault	Poisoning, Undetermined	Adverse effect	Underdosing
Intranarcon	T41.1X1	T41.1X2	T41.1X3	T41.1X4	T41.1X5	T41.1X6
Intravenous						
amino acids	T50.991	T50.992	T50.993	T50.994	T50.995	T50.996
fat suspension	T50.991	T50.992	T50.993	T50.994	T50.995	T50.996
Inulin	T50.8X1	T50.8X2	T50.8X3	T50.8X4	T50.8X5	T50.8X6
Invert sugar	T50.3X1	T50.3X2	T50.3X3	T50.3X4	T50.3X5	T50.3X6
Inza—see Naproxen						
Iobenzamic acid	T50.8X1	T50.8X2	T50.8X3	T50.8X4	T50.8X5	T50.8X6
Iocarmic acid	T50.8X1	T50.8X2	T50.8X3	T50.8X4	T50.8X5	T50.8X6
Iocetamic acid	T50.8X1	T50.8X2	T50.8X3	T50.8X4	T50.8X5	T50.8X6
Iodamide	T50.8X1	T50.8X2	T50.8X3	T50.8X4	T50.8X5	T50.8X6
Iodide NEC—see also Iodine	T49.0X1	T49.0X2	T49.0X3	T49.0X4	T49.0X5	T49.0X6
mercury (ointment)	T49.0X1	T49.0X2	T49.0X3	T49.0X4	T49.0X5	T49.0X6
methylate	T49.0X1	T49.0X2	T49.0X3	T49.0X4	T49.0X5	T49.0X6
potassium (expectorant) NEC	T48.4X1	T48.4X2	T48.4X3	T48.4X4	T48.4X5	T48.4X6
Iodinated						
contrast medium	T50.8X1	T50.8X2	T50.8X3	T50.8X4	T50.8X5	T50.8X6
glycerol	T48.4X1	T48.4X2	T48.4X3	T48.4X4	T48.4X5	T48.4X6
human serum albumin (131I)	T50.8X1	T50.8X2	T50.8X3	T50.8X4	T50.8X5	T50.8X6
Iodine (antiseptic, external) (tincture) NEC	T49.0X1	T49.0X2	T49.0X3	T49.0X4	T49.0X5	T49.0X6
125—see also Radiation sickness, and exposure to radioactive isotopes	T50.8X1	T50.8X2	T50.8X3	T50.8X4	T50.8X5	T50.8X6
therapeutic	T50.991	T50.992	T50.993	T50.994	T50.995	T50.996
131—see also Radiation sickness, and exposure to radioactive isotopes	T50.8X1	T50.8X2	T50.8X3	T50.8X4	T50.8X5	T50.8X6
therapeutic	T38.2X1	T38.2X2	T38.2X3	T38.2X4	T38.2X5	T38.2X6
diagnostic	T50.8X1	T50.8X2	T50.8X3	T50.8X4	T50.8X5	T50.8X6
for thyroid conditions (antithyroid)	T38.2X1	T38.2X2	T38.2X3	T38.2X4	T38.2X5	T38.2X6
solution	T49.0X1	T49.0X2	T49.0X3	T49.0X4	T49.0X5	T49.0X6
vapor	T59.891	T59.892	T59.893	T59.894	—	—
Iodipamide	T50.8X1	T50.8X2	T50.8X3	T50.8X4	T50.8X5	T50.8X6
Iodized (poppy seed) oil	T50.8X1	T50.8X2	T50.8X3	T50.8X4	T50.8X5	T50.8X6
Iodobismitol	T37.8X1	T37.8X2	T37.8X3	T37.8X4	T37.8X5	T37.8X6
Iodochlorhyd-roxyquin	T37.8X1	T37.8X2	T37.8X3	T37.8X4	T37.8X5	T37.8X6
topical	T49.0X1	T49.0X2	T49.0X3	T49.0X4	T49.0X5	T49.0X6
Iodochlorhydroxy-quinoline	T37.8X1	T37.8X2	T37.8X3	T37.8X4	T37.8X5	T37.8X6
Iodocholesterol (131I)	T50.8X1	T50.8X2	T50.8X3	T50.8X4	T50.8X5	T50.8X6
Iodoform	T49.0X1	T49.0X2	T49.0X3	T49.0X4	T49.0X5	T49.0X6
Iodohippuric acid	T50.8X1	T50.8X2	T50.8X3	T50.8X4	T50.8X5	T50.8X6
Iodopanoic acid	T50.8X1	T50.8X2	T50.8X3	T50.8X4	T50.8X5	T50.8X6
Iodophthalein (sodium)	T50.8X1	T50.8X2	T50.8X3	T50.8X4	T50.8X5	T50.8X6
Iodopyracet	T50.8X1	T50.8X2	T50.8X3	T50.8X4	T50.8X5	T50.8X6
Iodoquinol	T37.8X1	T37.8X2	T37.8X3	T37.8X4	T37.8X5	T37.8X6
Iodoxamic acid	T50.8X1	T50.8X2	T50.8X3	T50.8X4	T50.8X5	T50.8X6
Iofendylate	T50.8X1	T50.8X2	T50.8X3	T50.8X4	T50.8X5	T50.8X6
Ioglycamic acid	T50.8X1	T50.8X2	T50.8X3	T50.8X4	T50.8X5	T50.8X6

Substance	Poisoning, Accidental (unintentional)	Poisoning, Intentional self-harm	Poisoning, Assault	Poisoning, Undetermined	Adverse effect	Underdosing
Iohexol	T50.8X1	T50.8X2	T50.8X3	T50.8X4	T50.8X5	T50.8X6
Ion exchange resin						
anion	T47.8X1	T47.8X2	T47.8X3	T47.8X4	T47.8X5	T47.8X6
cation	T50.3X1	T50.3X2	T50.3X3	T50.3X4	T50.3X5	T50.3X6
cholestyramine	T46.6X1	T46.6X2	T46.6X3	T46.6X4	T46.6X5	T46.6X6
intestinal	T47.8X1	T47.8X2	T47.8X3	T47.8X4	T47.8X5	T47.8X6
Iopamidol	T50.8X1	T50.8X2	T50.8X3	T50.8X4	T50.8X5	T50.8X6
Iopanoic acid	T50.8X1	T50.8X2	T50.8X3	T50.8X4	T50.8X5	T50.8X6
Iophenoic acid	T50.8X1	T50.8X2	T50.8X3	T50.8X4	T50.8X5	T50.8X6
Iopodate, sodium	T50.8X1	T50.8X2	T50.8X3	T50.8X4	T50.8X5	T50.8X6
Iopodic acid	T50.8X1	T50.8X2	T50.8X3	T50.8X4	T50.8X5	T50.8X6
Iopromide	T50.8X1	T50.8X2	T50.8X3	T50.8X4	T50.8X5	T50.8X6
Iopydol	T50.8X1	T50.8X2	T50.8X3	T50.8X4	T50.8X5	T50.8X6
Iotalamic acid	T50.8X1	T50.8X2	T50.8X3	T50.8X4	T50.8X5	T50.8X6
Iothalamate	T50.8X1	T50.8X2	T50.8X3	T50.8X4	T50.8X5	T50.8X6
Iothiouracil	T38.2X1	T38.2X2	T38.2X3	T38.2X4	T38.2X5	T38.2X6
Iotrol	T50.8X1	T50.8X2	T50.8X3	T50.8X4	T50.8X5	T50.8X6
Iotrolan	T50.8X1	T50.8X2	T50.8X3	T50.8X4	T50.8X5	T50.8X6
Iotroxate	T50.8X1	T50.8X2	T50.8X3	T50.8X4	T50.8X5	T50.8X6
Iotroxic acid	T50.8X1	T50.8X2	T50.8X3	T50.8X4	T50.8X5	T50.8X6
Ioversol	T50.8X1	T50.8X2	T50.8X3	T50.8X4	T50.8X5	T50.8X6
Ioxaglate	T50.8X1	T50.8X2	T50.8X3	T50.8X4	T50.8X5	T50.8X6
Ioxaglic acid	T50.8X1	T50.8X2	T50.8X3	T50.8X4	T50.8X5	T50.8X6
Ioxitalamic acid	T50.8X1	T50.8X2	T50.8X3	T50.8X4	T50.8X5	T50.8X6
Ipecac	T47.7X1	T47.7X2	T47.7X3	T47.7X4	T47.7X5	T47.7X6
Ipecacuanha	T48.4X1	T48.4X2	T48.4X3	T48.4X4	T48.4X5	T48.4X6
Ipodate, calcium	T50.8X1	T50.8X2	T50.8X3	T50.8X4	T50.8X5	T50.8X6
Ipral	T42.3X1	T42.3X2	T42.3X3	T42.3X4	T42.3X5	T42.3X6
Ipratropium (bromide)	T48.6X1	T48.6X2	T48.6X3	T48.6X4	T48.6X5	T48.6X6
Ipriflavone	T46.3X1	T46.3X2	T46.3X3	T46.3X4	T46.3X5	T46.3X6
Iprindole	T43.011	T43.012	T43.013	T43.014	T43.015	T43.016
Iproclozide	T43.1X1	T43.1X2	T43.1X3	T43.1X4	T43.1X5	T43.1X6
Iprofenin	T50.8X1	T50.8X2	T50.8X3	T50.8X4	T50.8X5	T50.8X6
Iproheptine	T49.2X1	T49.2X2	T49.2X3	T49.2X4	T49.2X5	T49.2X6
Iproniazid	T43.1X1	T43.1X2	T43.1X3	T43.1X4	T43.1X5	T43.1X6
Iproplatin	T45.1X1	T45.1X2	T45.1X3	T45.1X4	T45.1X5	T45.1X6
Iproveratril	T46.1X1	T46.1X2	T46.1X3	T46.1X4	T46.1X5	T46.1X6
Iron (compounds) (medicinal) NEC	T45.4X1	T45.4X2	T45.4X3	T45.4X4	T45.4X5	T45.4X6
ammonium	T45.4X1	T45.4X2	T45.4X3	T45.4X4	T45.4X5	T45.4X6
dextran injection	T45.4X1	T45.4X2	T45.4X3	T45.4X4	T45.4X5	T45.4X6
nonmedicinal	T56.891	T56.892	T56.893	T56.894	—	—
salts	T45.4X1	T45.4X2	T45.4X3	T45.4X4	T45.4X5	T45.4X6
sorbitex	T45.4X1	T45.4X2	T45.4X3	T45.4X4	T45.4X5	T45.4X6
sorbitol citric acid complex	T45.4X1	T45.4X2	T45.4X3	T45.4X4	T45.4X5	T45.4X6
Irrigating fluid (vaginal)	T49.8X1	T49.8X2	T49.8X3	T49.8X4	T49.8X5	T49.8X6
eye	T49.5X1	T49.5X2	T49.5X3	T49.5X4	T49.5X5	T49.5X6
Isepamicin	T36.5X1	T36.5X2	T36.5X3	T36.5X4	T36.5X5	T36.5X6
Isoaminile (citrate)	T48.3X1	T48.3X2	T48.3X3	T48.3X4	T48.3X5	T48.3X6
Isoamyl nitrite	T46.3X1	T46.3X2	T46.3X3	T46.3X4	T46.3X5	T46.3X6
Isobenzan	T60.1X1	T60.1X2	T60.1X3	T60.1X4	—	—

Substance	Poisoning, Accidental (unintentional)	Poisoning, Intentional self-harm	Poisoning, Assault	Poisoning, Undetermined	Adverse effect	Underdosing
Isobutyl acetate	T52.8X1	T52.8X2	T52.8X3	T52.8X4	—	—
Isocarboxazid	T43.1X1	T43.1X2	T43.1X3	T43.1X4	T43.1X5	T43.1X6
Isoconazole	T49.0X1	T49.0X2	T49.0X3	T49.0X4	T49.0X5	T49.0X6
Isocyanate	T65.0X1	T65.0X2	T65.0X3	T65.0X4	—	—
Isoephedrine	T44.991	T44.992	T44.993	T44.994	T44.995	T44.996
Isoetarine	T48.6X1	T48.6X2	T48.6X3	T48.6X4	T48.6X5	T48.6X6
Isoethadione	T42.2X1	T42.2X2	T42.2X3	T42.2X4	T42.2X5	T42.2X6
Isoetharine	T44.5X1	T44.5X2	T44.5X3	T44.5X4	T44.5X5	T44.5X6
Isoflurane	T41.0X1	T41.0X2	T41.0X3	T41.0X4	T41.0X5	T41.0X6
Isoflurophate	T44.0X1	T44.0X2	T44.0X3	T44.0X4	T44.0X5	T44.0X6
Isomaltose, ferric complex	T45.4X1	T45.4X2	T45.4X3	T45.4X4	T45.4X5	T45.4X6
Isometheptene	T44.3X1	T44.3X2	T44.3X3	T44.3X4	T44.3X5	T44.3X6
Isoniazid	T37.1X1	T37.1X2	T37.1X3	T37.1X4	T37.1X5	T37.1X6
with						
rifampicin	T36.6X1	T36.6X2	T36.6X3	T36.6X4	T36.6X5	T36.6X6
thioacetazone	T37.1X1	T37.1X2	T37.1X3	T37.1X4	T37.1X5	T37.1X6
Isonicotinic acid hydrazide	T37.1X1	T37.1X2	T37.1X3	T37.1X4	T37.1X5	T37.1X6
Isonipecaine	T40.491	T40.492	T40.493	T40.494	T40.495	T40.496
Isopentaquine	T37.2X1	T37.2X2	T37.2X3	T37.2X4	T37.2X5	T37.2X6
Isophane insulin	T38.3X1	T38.3X2	T38.3X3	T38.3X4	T38.3X5	T38.3X6
Isophorone	T65.891	T65.892	T65.893	T65.894	—	—
Isophosphamide	T45.1X1	T45.1X2	T45.1X3	T45.1X4	T45.1X5	T45.1X6
Isopregnenone	T38.5X1	T38.5X2	T38.5X3	T38.5X4	T38.5X5	T38.5X6
Isoprenaline	T48.6X1	T48.6X2	T48.6X3	T48.6X4	T48.6X5	T48.6X6
Isopromethazine	T43.3X1	T43.3X2	T43.3X3	T43.3X4	T43.3X5	T43.3X6
Isopropamide	T44.3X1	T44.3X2	T44.3X3	T44.3X4	T44.3X5	T44.3X6
iodide	T44.3X1	T44.3X2	T44.3X3	T44.3X4	T44.3X5	T44.3X6
Isopropanol	T51.2X1	T51.2X2	T51.2X3	T51.2X4	—	—
Isopropyl						
acetate	T52.8X1	T52.8X2	T52.8X3	T52.8X4	—	—
alcohol	T51.2X1	T51.2X2	T51.2X3	T51.2X4	—	—
medicinal	T49.4X1	T49.4X2	T49.4X3	T49.4X4	T49.4X5	T49.4X6
ether	T52.8X1	T52.8X2	T52.8X3	T52.8X4	—	—
Isopropylamino-phenazone	T39.2X1	T39.2X2	T39.2X3	T39.2X4	T39.2X5	T39.2X6
Isoproterenol	T48.6X1	T48.6X2	T48.6X3	T48.6X4	T48.6X5	T48.6X6
Isosorbide dinitrate	T46.3X1	T46.3X2	T46.3X3	T46.3X4	T46.3X5	T46.3X6
Isothipendyl	T45.0X1	T45.0X2	T45.0X3	T45.0X4	T45.0X5	T45.0X6
Isotretinoin	T50.991	T50.992	T50.993	T50.994	T50.995	T50.996
Isoxazolyl penicillin	T36.0X1	T36.0X2	T36.0X3	T36.0X4	T36.0X5	T36.0X6
Isoxicam	T39.391	T39.392	T39.393	T39.394	T39.395	T39.396
Isoxsuprine	T46.7X1	T46.7X2	T46.7X3	T46.7X4	T46.7X5	T46.7X6
Ispagula	T47.4X1	T47.4X2	T47.4X3	T47.4X4	T47.4X5	T47.4X6
husk	T47.4X1	T47.4X2	T47.4X3	T47.4X4	T47.4X5	T47.4X6
Isradipine	T46.1X1	T46.1X2	T46.1X3	T46.1X4	T46.1X5	T46.1X6
I-thyroxine sodium	T38.1X1	T38.1X2	T38.1X3	T38.1X4	T38.1X5	T38.1X6
Itraconazole	T37.8X1	T37.8X2	T37.8X3	T37.8X4	T37.8X5	T37.8X6
Itramin tosilate	T46.3X1	T46.3X2	T46.3X3	T46.3X4	T46.3X5	T46.3X6
Ivermectin	T37.4X1	T37.4X2	T37.4X3	T37.4X4	T37.4X5	T37.4X6
Izoniazid	T37.1X1	T37.1X2	T37.1X3	T37.1X4	T37.1X5	T37.1X6
with thioacetazone	T37.1X1	T37.1X2	T37.1X3	T37.1X4	T37.1X5	T37.1X6

Substance	Poisoning, Accidental (unintentional)	Poisoning, Intentional self-harm	Poisoning, Assault	Poisoning, Undetermined	Adverse effect	Underdosing
J						
Jalap	T47.2X1	T47.2X2	T47.2X3	T47.2X4	T47.2X5	T47.2X6
Jamaica						
dogwood (bark)	T39.8X1	T39.8X2	T39.8X3	T39.8X4	T39.8X5	T39.8X6
ginger	T65.891	T65.892	T65.893	T65.894	—	—
root	T62.2X1	T62.2X2	T62.2X3	T62.2X4	—	—
Jatropha	T62.2X1	T62.2X2	T62.2X3	T62.2X4	—	—
curcas	T62.2X1	T62.2X2	T62.2X3	T62.2X4	—	—
Jectofer	T45.4X1	T45.4X2	T45.4X3	T45.4X4	T45.4X5	T45.4X6
Jellyfish (sting)	T63.621	T63.622	T63.623	T63.624	—	—
Jequirity (bean)	T62.2X1	T62.2X2	T62.2X3	T62.2X4	—	—
Jimson weed (stramonium)	T62.2X1	T62.2X2	T62.2X3	T62.2X4	—	—
seeds	T62.2X1	T62.2X2	T62.2X3	T62.2X4	—	—
Josamycin	T36.3X1	T36.3X2	T36.3X3	T36.3X4	T36.3X5	T36.3X6
Juniper tar	T49.1X1	T49.1X2	T49.1X3	T49.1X4	T49.1X5	T49.1X6
K						
Kallidinogenase	T46.7X1	T46.7X2	T46.7X3	T46.7X4	T46.7X5	T46.7X6
Kallikrein	T46.7X1	T46.7X2	T46.7X3	T46.7X4	T46.7X5	T46.7X6
Kanamycin	T36.5X1	T36.5X2	T36.5X3	T36.5X4	T36.5X5	T36.5X6
Kantrex	T36.5X1	T36.5X2	T36.5X3	T36.5X4	T36.5X5	T36.5X6
Kaolin	T47.6X1	T47.6X2	T47.6X3	T47.6X4	T47.6X5	T47.6X6
light	T47.6X1	T47.6X2	T47.6X3	T47.6X4	T47.6X5	T47.6X6
Karaya (gum)	T47.4X1	T47.4X2	T47.4X3	T47.4X4	T47.4X5	T47.4X6
Kebuzone	T39.2X1	T39.2X2	T39.2X3	T39.2X4	T39.2X5	T39.2X6
Kelevan	T60.1X1	T60.1X2	T60.1X3	T60.1X4	—	—
Kemithal	T41.1X1	T41.1X2	T41.1X3	T41.1X4	T41.1X5	T41.1X6
Kenacort	T38.0X1	T38.0X2	T38.0X3	T38.0X4	T38.0X5	T38.0X6
Keratolytic drug NEC	T49.4X1	T49.4X2	T49.4X3	T49.4X4	T49.4X5	T49.4X6
anthracene	T49.4X1	T49.4X2	T49.4X3	T49.4X4	T49.4X5	T49.4X6
Keratoplastic NEC	T49.4X1	T49.4X2	T49.4X3	T49.4X4	T49.4X5	T49.4X6
Kerosene, kerosine (fuel) (solvent) NEC	T52.0X1	T52.0X2	T52.0X3	T52.0X4	—	—
insecticide	T52.0X1	T52.0X2	T52.0X3	T52.0X4	—	—
vapor	T52.0X1	T52.0X2	T52.0X3	T52.0X4	—	—
Ketamine	T41.291	T41.292	T41.293	T41.294	T41.295	T41.296
Ketazolam	T42.4X1	T42.4X2	T42.4X3	T42.4X4	T42.4X5	T42.4X6
Ketazon	T39.2X1	T39.2X2	T39.2X3	T39.2X4	T39.2X5	T39.2X6
Ketobemidone	T40.491	T40.492	T40.493	T40.494	—	—
Ketoconazole	T49.0X1	T49.0X2	T49.0X3	T49.0X4	T49.0X5	T49.0X6
Ketols	T52.4X1	T52.4X2	T52.4X3	T52.4X4	—	—
Ketone oils	T52.4X1	T52.4X2	T52.4X3	T52.4X4	—	—
Ketoprofen	T39.311	T39.312	T39.313	T39.314	T39.315	T39.316
Ketorolac	T39.8X1	T39.8X2	T39.8X3	T39.8X4	T39.8X5	T39.8X6
Ketotifen	T45.0X1	T45.0X2	T45.0X3	T45.0X4	T45.0X5	T45.0X6
Khat	T43.691	T43.692	T43.693	T43.694	—	—
Khellin	T46.3X1	T46.3X2	T46.3X3	T46.3X4	T46.3X5	T46.3X6
Khelloside	T46.3X1	T46.3X2	T46.3X3	T46.3X4	T46.3X5	T46.3X6
Kiln gas or vapor (carbon monoxide)	T58.8X1	T58.8X2	T58.8X3	T58.8X4	—	—
Kitasamycin	T36.3X1	T36.3X2	T36.3X3	T36.3X4	T36.3X5	T36.3X6
Konsyl	T47.4X1	T47.4X2	T47.4X3	T47.4X4	T47.4X5	T47.4X6

Substance	Poisoning, Accidental (unintentional)	Poisoning, Intentional self-harm	Poisoning, Assault	Poisoning, Undetermined	Adverse effect	Underdosing
Kosam seed	T62.2X1	T62.2X2	T62.2X3	T62.2X4	—	—
Krait (venom)	T63.091	T63.092	T63.093	T63.094	—	—
Kwell (insecticide)	T60.1X1	T60.1X2	T60.1X3	T60.1X4	—	—
anti-infective (topical)	T49.0X1	T49.0X2	T49.0X3	T49.0X4	T49.0X5	T49.0X6
L						
Labetalol	T44.8X1	T44.8X2	T44.8X3	T44.8X4	T44.8X5	T44.8X6
Laburnum (seeds)	T62.2X1	T62.2X2	T62.2X3	T62.2X4	—	—
leaves	T62.2X1	T62.2X2	T62.2X3	T62.2X4	—	—
Lachesine	T49.5X1	T49.5X2	T49.5X3	T49.5X4	T49.5X5	T49.5X6
Lacidipine	T46.5X1	T46.5X2	T46.5X3	T46.5X4	T46.5X5	T46.5X6
Lacquer	T65.6X1	T65.6X2	T65.6X3	T65.6X4	—	—
Lacrimogenic gas	T59.3X1	T59.3X2	T59.3X3	T59.3X4	—	—
Lactated potassic saline	T50.3X1	T50.3X2	T50.3X3	T50.3X4	T50.3X5	T50.3X6
Lactic acid	T49.8X1	T49.8X2	T49.8X3	T49.8X4	T49.8X5	T49.8X6
Lactobacillus						
acidophilus	T47.6X1	T47.6X2	T47.6X3	T47.6X4	T47.6X5	T47.6X6
compound	T47.6X1	T47.6X2	T47.6X3	T47.6X4	T47.6X5	T47.6X6
bifidus, lyophilized	T47.6X1	T47.6X2	T47.6X3	T47.6X4	T47.6X5	T47.6X6
bulgaricus	T47.6X1	T47.6X2	T47.6X3	T47.6X4	T47.6X5	T47.6X6
sporogenes	T47.6X1	T47.6X2	T47.6X3	T47.6X4	T47.6X5	T47.6X6
Lactoflavin	T45.2X1	T45.2X2	T45.2X3	T45.2X4	T45.2X5	T45.2X6
Lactose (as excipient)	T50.901	T50.902	T50.903	T50.904	T50.905	T50.906
Lactuca (virosa) (extract)	T42.6X1	T42.6X2	T42.6X3	T42.6X4	T42.6X5	T42.6X6
Lactucarium	T42.6X1	T42.6X2	T42.6X3	T42.6X4	T42.6X5	T42.6X6
Lactulose	T47.3X1	T47.3X2	T47.3X3	T47.3X4	T47.3X5	T47.3X6
Laevo—see Levo-						
Lanatosides	T46.0X1	T46.0X2	T46.0X3	T46.0X4	T46.0X5	T46.0X6
Lanolin	T49.3X1	T49.3X2	T49.3X3	T49.3X4	T49.3X5	T49.3X6
Largactil	T43.3X1	T43.3X2	T43.3X3	T43.3X4	T43.3X5	T43.3X6
Larkspur	T62.2X1	T62.2X2	T62.2X3	T62.2X4	—	—
Laroxyl	T43.011	T43.012	T43.013	T43.014	T43.015	T43.016
Lasix	T50.1X1	T50.1X2	T50.1X3	T50.1X4	T50.1X5	T50.1X6
Lassar's paste	T49.4X1	T49.4X2	T49.4X3	T49.4X4	T49.4X5	T49.4X6
Latamoxef	T36.1X1	T36.1X2	T36.1X3	T36.1X4	T36.1X5	T36.1X6
Latex	T65.811	T65.812	T65.813	T65.814	—	—
Lathyrus (seed)	T62.2X1	T62.2X2	T62.2X3	T62.2X4	—	—
Laudanum	T40.0X1	T40.0X2	T40.0X3	T40.0X4	T40.0X5	T40.0X6
Laudexium	T48.1X1	T48.1X2	T48.1X3	T48.1X4	T48.1X5	T48.1X6
Laughing gas	T41.0X1	T41.0X2	T41.0X3	T41.0X4	T41.0X5	T41.0X6
Laurel, black or cherry	T62.2X1	T62.2X2	T62.2X3	T62.2X4	—	—
Laurolinium	T49.0X1	T49.0X2	T49.0X3	T49.0X4	T49.0X5	T49.0X6
Lauryl sulfoacetate	T49.2X1	T49.2X2	T49.2X3	T49.2X4	T49.2X5	T49.2X6
Laxative NEC	T47.4X1	T47.4X2	T47.4X3	T47.4X4	T47.4X5	T47.4X6
osmotic	T47.3X1	T47.3X2	T47.3X3	T47.3X4	T47.3X5	T47.3X6
saline	T47.3X1	T47.3X2	T47.3X3	T47.3X4	T47.3X5	T47.3X6
stimulant	T47.2X1	T47.2X2	T47.2X3	T47.2X4	T47.2X5	T47.2X6
L-dopa	T42.8X1	T42.8X2	T42.8X3	T42.8X4	T42.8X5	T42.8X6
Lead (dust) (fumes) (vapor) NEC	T56.0X1	T56.0X2	T56.0X3	T56.0X4	—	—
acetate	T49.2X1	T49.2X2	T49.2X3	T49.2X4	T49.2X5	T49.2X6

Substance	Poisoning, Accidental (unintentional)	Poisoning, Intentional self-harm	Poisoning, Assault	Poisoning, Undetermined	Adverse effect	Underdosing
Lead NEC — *Continued*						
alkyl (fuel additive)	T56.0X1	T56.0X2	T56.0X3	T56.0X4	—	—
anti-infectives	T37.8X1	T37.8X2	T37.8X3	T37.8X4	T37.8X5	T37.8X6
antiknock compound (tetraethyl)	T56.0X1	T56.0X2	T56.0X3	T56.0X4	—	—
arsenate, arsenite (dust) (herbicide) (insecticide) (vapor)	T57.0X1	T57.0X2	T57.0X3	T57.0X4	—	—
carbonate	T56.0X1	T56.0X2	T56.0X3	T56.0X4	—	—
paint	T56.0X1	T56.0X2	T56.0X3	T56.0X4	—	—
chromate	T56.0X1	T56.0X2	T56.0X3	T56.0X4	—	—
paint	T56.0X1	T56.0X2	T56.0X3	T56.0X4	—	—
dioxide	T56.0X1	T56.0X2	T56.0X3	T56.0X4	—	—
inorganic	T56.0X1	T56.0X2	T56.0X3	T56.0X4	—	—
iodide	T56.0X1	T56.0X2	T56.0X3	T56.0X4	—	—
pigment (paint)	T56.0X1	T56.0X2	T56.0X3	T56.0X4	—	—
monoxide (dust)	T56.0X1	T56.0X2	T56.0X3	T56.0X4	—	—
paint	T56.0X1	T56.0X2	T56.0X3	T56.0X4	—	—
organic	T56.0X1	T56.0X2	T56.0X3	T56.0X4	—	—
oxide	T56.0X1	T56.0X2	T56.0X3	T56.0X4	—	—
paint	T56.0X1	T56.0X2	T56.0X3	T56.0X4	—	—
paint	T56.0X1	T56.0X2	T56.0X3	T56.0X4	—	—
salts	T56.0X1	T56.0X2	T56.0X3	T56.0X4	—	—
specified compound NEC	T56.0X1	T56.0X2	T56.0X3	T56.0X4	—	—
tetra-ethyl	T56.0X1	T56.0X2	T56.0X3	T56.0X4	—	—
Lebanese red	T40.711	T40.712	T40.713	T40.714	T40.715	T40.716
Lefetamine	T39.8X1	T39.8X2	T39.8X3	T39.8X4	T39.8X5	T39.8X6
Lenperone	T43.4X1	T43.4X2	T43.4X3	T43.4X4	T43.4X5	T43.4X6
Lente lietin (insulin)	T38.3X1	T38.3X2	T38.3X3	T38.3X4	T38.3X5	T38.3X6
Leptazol	T50.7X1	T50.7X2	T50.7X3	T50.7X4	T50.7X5	T50.7X6
Leptophos	T60.0X1	T60.0X2	T60.0X3	T60.0X4	—	—
Leritine	T40.2X1	T40.2X2	T40.2X3	T40.2X4	T40.2X5	T40.2X6
Letosteine	T48.4X1	T48.4X2	T48.4X3	T48.4X4	T48.4X5	T48.4X6
Letter	T38.1X1	T38.1X2	T38.1X3	T38.1X4	T38.1X5	T38.1X6
Lettuce opium	T42.6X1	T42.6X2	T42.6X3	T42.6X4	T42.6X5	T42.6X6
Leucinocaine	T41.3X1	T41.3X2	T41.3X3	T41.3X4	T41.3X5	T41.3X6
Leucocianidol	T46.991	T46.992	T46.993	T46.994	T46.995	T46.996
Leucovorin (factor)	T45.8X1	T45.8X2	T45.8X3	T45.8X4	T45.8X5	T45.8X6
Leukeran	T45.1X1	T45.1X2	T45.1X3	T45.1X4	T45.1X5	T45.1X6
Leuprolide	T38.891	T38.892	T38.893	T38.894	T38.895	T38.896
Levalbuterol	T48.6X1	T48.6X2	T48.6X3	T48.6X4	T48.6X5	T48.6X6
Levallorphan	T50.7X1	T50.7X2	T50.7X3	T50.7X4	T50.7X5	T50.7X6
Levamisole	T37.4X1	T37.4X2	T37.4X3	T37.4X4	T37.4X5	T37.4X6
Levanil	T42.6X1	T42.6X2	T42.6X3	T42.6X4	T42.6X5	T42.6X6
Levarterenol	T44.4X1	T44.4X2	T44.4X3	T44.4X4	T44.4X5	T44.4X6
Levdropropizine	T48.3X1	T48.3X2	T48.3X3	T48.3X4	T48.3X5	T48.3X6
Levobunolol	T49.5X1	T49.5X2	T49.5X3	T49.5X4	T49.5X5	T49.5X6
Levocabastine (hydrochloride)	T45.0X1	T45.0X2	T45.0X3	T45.0X4	T45.0X5	T45.0X6
Levocarnitine	T50.991	T50.992	T50.993	T50.994	T50.995	T50.996

413

Substance	Poisoning, Accidental (unintentional)	Poisoning, Intentional self-harm	Poisoning, Assault	Poisoning, Undetermined	Adverse effect	Underdosing
Levodopa	T42.8X1	T42.8X2	T42.8X3	T42.8X4	T42.8X5	T42.8X6
with carbidopa	T42.8X1	T42.8X2	T42.8X3	T42.8X4	T42.8X5	T42.8X6
Levo-dromoran	T40.2X1	T40.2X2	T40.2X3	T40.2X4	T40.2X5	T40.2X6
Levoglutamide	T50.991	T50.992	T50.993	T50.994	T50.995	T50.996
Levoid	T38.1X1	T38.1X2	T38.1X3	T38.1X4	T38.1X5	T38.1X6
Levo-iso-methadone	T40.3X1	T40.3X2	T40.3X3	T40.3X4	T40.3X5	T40.3X6
Levomepromazine	T43.3X1	T43.3X2	T43.3X3	T43.3X4	T43.3X5	T43.3X6
Levonordefrin	T49.6X1	T49.6X2	T49.6X3	T49.6X4	T49.6X5	T49.6X6
Levonorgestrel	T38.4X1	T38.4X2	T38.4X3	T38.4X4	T38.4X5	T38.4X6
with ethinylestradiol	T38.5X1	T38.5X2	T38.5X3	T38.5X4	T38.5X5	T38.5X6
Levopromazine	T43.3X1	T43.3X2	T43.3X3	T43.3X4	T43.3X5	T43.3X6
Levoprome	T42.6X1	T42.6X2	T42.6X3	T42.6X4	T42.6X5	T42.6X6
Levopropoxyphene	T40.491	T40.492	T40.493	T40.494	T40.495	T40.496
Levopropylhexedrine	T50.5X1	T50.5X2	T50.5X3	T50.5X4	T50.5X5	T50.5X6
Levoproxyphylline	T48.6X1	T48.6X2	T48.6X3	T48.6X4	T48.6X5	T48.6X6
Levorphanol	T40.491	T40.492	T40.493	T40.494	T40.495	T40.496
Levothyroxine	T38.1X1	T38.1X2	T38.1X3	T38.1X4	T38.1X5	T38.1X6
sodium	T38.1X1	T38.1X2	T38.1X3	T38.1X4	T38.1X5	T38.1X6
Levsin	T44.3X1	T44.3X2	T44.3X3	T44.3X4	T44.3X5	T44.3X6
Levulose	T50.3X1	T50.3X2	T50.3X3	T50.3X4	T50.3X5	T50.3X6
Lewisite (gas), not in war	T57.0X1	T57.0X2	T57.0X3	T57.0X4	—	—
Librium	T42.4X1	T42.4X2	T42.4X3	T42.4X4	T42.4X5	T42.4X6
Lidex	T49.0X1	T49.0X2	T49.0X3	T49.0X4	T49.0X5	T49.0X6
Lidocaine	T41.3X1	T41.3X2	T41.3X3	T41.3X4	T41.3X5	T41.3X6
regional	T41.3X1	T41.3X2	T41.3X3	T41.3X4	T41.3X5	T41.3X6
spinal	T41.3X1	T41.3X2	T41.3X3	T41.3X4	T41.3X5	T41.3X6
Lidofenin	T50.8X1	T50.8X2	T50.8X3	T50.8X4	T50.8X5	T50.8X6
Lidoflazine	T46.1X1	T46.1X2	T46.1X3	T46.1X4	T46.1X5	T46.1X6
Lighter fluid	T52.0X1	T52.0X2	T52.0X3	T52.0X4	—	—
Lignin hemicellulose	T47.6X1	T47.6X2	T47.6X3	T47.6X4	T47.6X5	T47.6X6
Lignocaine	T41.3X1	T41.3X2	T41.3X3	T41.3X4	T41.3X5	T41.3X6
regional	T41.3X1	T41.3X2	T41.3X3	T41.3X4	T41.3X5	T41.3X6
spinal	T41.3X1	T41.3X2	T41.3X3	T41.3X4	T41.3X5	T41.3X6
Ligroin(e) (solvent)	T52.0X1	T52.0X2	T52.0X3	T52.0X4	—	—
vapor	T59.891	T59.892	T59.893	T59.894	—	—
Ligustrum vulgare	T62.2X1	T62.2X2	T62.2X3	T62.2X4	—	—
Lily of the valley	T62.2X1	T62.2X2	T62.2X3	T62.2X4	—	—
Lime (chloride)	T54.3X1	T54.3X2	T54.3X3	T54.3X4	—	—
Limonene	T52.8X1	T52.8X2	T52.8X3	T52.8X4	—	—
Lincomycin	T36.8X1	T36.8X2	T36.8X3	T36.8X4	T36.8X5	T36.8X6
Lindane (insecticide) (nonmedicinal) (vapor)	T53.6X1	T53.6X2	T53.6X3	T53.6X4	—	—
medicinal	T49.0X1	T49.0X2	T49.0X3	T49.0X4	T49.0X5	T49.0X6
Liniments NEC	T49.91	T49.92	T49.93	T49.94	T49.95	T49.96
Linoleic acid	T46.6X1	T46.6X2	T46.6X3	T46.6X4	T46.6X5	T46.6X6
Linolenic acid	T46.6X1	T46.6X2	T46.6X3	T46.6X4	T46.6X5	T46.6X6
Linseed	T47.4X1	T47.4X2	T47.4X3	T47.4X4	T47.4X5	T47.4X6
Liothyronine	T38.1X1	T38.1X2	T38.1X3	T38.1X4	T38.1X5	T38.1X6
Liotrix	T38.1X1	T38.1X2	T38.1X3	T38.1X4	T38.1X5	T38.1X6
Lipancreatin	T47.5X1	T47.5X2	T47.5X3	T47.5X4	T47.5X5	T47.5X6

Substance	Poisoning, Accidental (unintentional)	Poisoning, Intentional self-harm	Poisoning, Assault	Poisoning, Undetermined	Adverse effect	Underdosing
Lipo-alprostadil	T46.7X1	T46.7X2	T46.7X3	T46.7X4	T46.7X5	T46.7X6
Lipo-Lutin	T38.5X1	T38.5X2	T38.5X3	T38.5X4	T38.5X5	T38.5X6
Lipotropic drug NEC	T50.901	T50.902	T50.903	T50.904	T50.905	T50.906
Liquefied petroleum gases	T59.891	T59.892	T59.893	T59.894	—	—
piped (pure or mixed with air)	T59.891	T59.892	T59.893	T59.894	—	—
Liquid						
paraffin	T47.4X1	T47.4X2	T47.4X3	T47.4X4	T47.4X5	T47.4X6
petrolatum	T47.4X1	T47.4X2	T47.4X3	T47.4X4	T47.4X5	T47.4X6
topical	T49.3X1	T49.3X2	T49.3X3	T49.3X4	T49.3X5	T49.3X6
specified NEC	T65.891	T65.892	T65.893	T65.894		
substance	T65.91	T65.92	T65.93	T65.94	—	—
Liquor creosolis compositus	T65.891	T65.892	T65.893	T65.894		
Liquorice	T48.4X1	T48.4X2	T48.4X3	T48.4X4	T48.4X5	T48.4X6
extract	T47.8X1	T47.8X2	T47.8X3	T47.8X4	T47.8X5	T47.8X6
Lisinopril	T46.4X1	T46.4X2	T46.4X3	T46.4X4	T46.4X5	T46.4X6
Lisuride	T42.8X1	T42.8X2	T42.8X3	T42.8X4	T42.8X5	T42.8X6
Lithane	T43.8X1	T43.8X2	T43.8X3	T43.8X4	T43.8X5	T43.8X6
Lithium	T56.891	T56.892	T56.893	T56.894	—	—
gluconate	T43.591	T43.592	T43.593	T43.594	T43.595	T43.596
salts (carbonate)	T43.591	T43.592	T43.593	T43.594	T43.595	T43.596
Lithonate	T43.8X1	T43.8X2	T43.8X3	T43.8X4	T43.8X5	T43.8X6
Liver						
extract	T45.8X1	T45.8X2	T45.8X3	T45.8X4	T45.8X5	T45.8X6
for parenteral use	T45.8X1	T45.8X2	T45.8X3	T45.8X4	T45.8X5	T45.8X6
fraction 1	T45.8X1	T45.8X2	T45.8X3	T45.8X4	T45.8X5	T45.8X6
hydrolysate	T45.8X1	T45.8X2	T45.8X3	T45.8X4	T45.8X5	T45.8X6
Lizard (bite) (venom)	T63.121	T63.122	T63.123	T63.124	—	—
LMD	T45.8X1	T45.8X2	T45.8X3	T45.8X4	T45.8X5	T45.8X6
Lobelia	T62.2X1	T62.2X2	T62.2X3	T62.2X4	—	—
Lobeline	T50.7X1	T50.7X2	T50.7X3	T50.7X4	T50.7X5	T50.7X6
Local action drug NEC	T49.8X1	T49.8X2	T49.8X3	T49.8X4	T49.8X5	T49.8X6
Locorten	T49.0X1	T49.0X2	T49.0X3	T49.0X4	T49.0X5	T49.0X6
Lofepramine	T43.011	T43.012	T43.013	T43.014	T43.015	T43.016
Lolium temulentum	T62.2X1	T62.2X2	T62.2X3	T62.2X4	—	—
Lomotil	T47.6X1	T47.6X2	T47.6X3	T47.6X4	T47.6X5	T47.6X6
Lomustine	T45.1X1	T45.1X2	T45.1X3	T45.1X4	T45.1X5	T45.1X6
Lonidamine	T45.1X1	T45.1X2	T45.1X3	T45.1X4	T45.1X5	T45.1X6
Loperamide	T47.6X1	T47.6X2	T47.6X3	T47.6X4	T47.6X5	T47.6X6
Loprazolam	T42.4X1	T42.4X2	T42.4X3	T42.4X4	T42.4X5	T42.4X6
Lorajmine	T46.2X1	T46.2X2	T46.2X3	T46.2X4	T46.2X5	T46.2X6
Loratidine	T45.0X1	T45.0X2	T45.0X3	T45.0X4	T45.0X5	T45.0X6
Lorazepam	T42.4X1	T42.4X2	T42.4X3	T42.4X4	T42.4X5	T42.4X6
Lorcainide	T46.2X1	T46.2X2	T46.2X3	T46.2X4	T46.2X5	T46.2X6
Lormetazepam	T42.4X1	T42.4X2	T42.4X3	T42.4X4	T42.4X5	T42.4X6
Lotions NEC	T49.91	T49.92	T49.93	T49.94	T49.95	T49.96
Lotusate	T42.3X1	T42.3X2	T42.3X3	T42.3X4	T42.3X5	T42.3X6
Lovastatin	T46.6X1	T46.6X2	T46.6X3	T46.6X4	T46.6X5	T46.6X6
Lowila	T49.2X1	T49.2X2	T49.2X3	T49.2X4	T49.2X5	T49.2X6

Substance	Poisoning, Accidental (unintentional)	Poisoning, Intentional self-harm	Poisoning, Assault	Poisoning, Undetermined	Adverse effect	Underdosing
Loxapine	T43.591	T43.592	T43.593	T43.594	T43.595	T43.596
Lozenges (throat)	T49.6X1	T49.6X2	T49.6X3	T49.6X4	T49.6X5	T49.6X6
LSD	T40.8X1	T40.8X2	T40.8X3	T40.8X4	—	—
L-Tryptophan—see amino acid						
Lubricant, eye	T49.5X1	T49.5X2	T49.5X3	T49.5X4	T49.5X5	T49.5X6
Lubricating oil NEC	T52.0X1	T52.0X2	T52.0X3	T52.0X4	—	—
Lucanthone	T37.4X1	T37.4X2	T37.4X3	T37.4X4	T37.4X5	T37.4X6
Luminal	T42.3X1	T42.3X2	T42.3X3	T42.3X4	T42.3X5	T42.3X6
Lung irritant (gas) NEC	T59.91	T59.92	T59.93	T59.94	—	—
Luteinizing hormone	T38.811	T38.812	T38.813	T38.814	T38.815	T38.816
Lutocylol	T38.5X1	T38.5X2	T38.5X3	T38.5X4	T38.5X5	T38.5X6
Lutromone	T38.5X1	T38.5X2	T38.5X3	T38.5X4	T38.5X5	T38.5X6
Lututrin	T48.291	T48.292	T48.293	T48.294	T48.295	T48.296
Lye (concentrated)	T54.3X1	T54.3X2	T54.3X3	T54.3X4	—	—
Lygranum (skin test)	T50.8X1	T50.8X2	T50.8X3	T50.8X4	T50.8X5	T50.8X6
Lymecycline	T36.4X1	T36.4X2	T36.4X3	T36.4X4	T36.4X5	T36.4X6
Lymphogranuloma venereum antigen	T50.8X1	T50.8X2	T50.8X3	T50.8X4	T50.8X5	T50.8X6
Lynestrenol	T38.4X1	T38.4X2	T38.4X3	T38.4X4	T38.4X5	T38.4X6
Lyovac Sodium Edecrin	T50.1X1	T50.1X2	T50.1X3	T50.1X4	T50.1X5	T50.1X6
Lypressin	T38.891	T38.892	T38.893	T38.894	T38.895	T38.896
Lysergic acid diethylamide	T40.8X1	T40.8X2	T40.8X3	T40.8X4	—	—
Lysergide	T40.8X1	T40.8X2	T40.8X3	T40.8X4	—	—
Lysine vasopressin	T38.891	T38.892	T38.893	T38.894	T38.895	T38.896
Lysol	T54.1X1	T54.1X2	T54.1X3	T54.1X4	—	—
Lysozyme	T49.0X1	T49.0X2	T49.0X3	T49.0X4	T49.0X5	T49.0X6
Lytta (vitatta)	T49.8X1	T49.8X2	T49.8X3	T49.8X4	T49.8X5	T49.8X6
M						
Mace	T59.3X1	T59.3X2	T59.3X3	T59.3X4	—	—
Macrogol	T50.991	T50.992	T50.993	T50.994	T50.995	T50.996
Macrolide						
anabolic drug	T38.7X1	T38.7X2	T38.7X3	T38.7X4	T38.7X5	T38.7X6
antibiotic	T36.3X1	T36.3X2	T36.3X3	T36.3X4	T36.3X5	T36.3X6
Mafenide	T49.0X1	T49.0X2	T49.0X3	T49.0X4	T49.0X5	T49.0X6
Magaldrate	T47.1X1	T47.1X2	T47.1X3	T47.1X4	T47.1X5	T47.1X6
Magic mushroom	T40.991	T40.992	T40.993	T40.994	—	—
Magnamycin	T36.8X1	T36.8X2	T36.8X3	T36.8X4	T36.8X5	T36.8X6
Magnesia magma	T47.1X1	T47.1X2	T47.1X3	T47.1X4	T47.1X5	T47.1X6
Magnesium NEC	T56.891	T56.892	T56.893	T56.894	—	—
carbonate	T47.1X1	T47.1X2	T47.1X3	T47.1X4	T47.1X5	T47.1X6
citrate	T47.4X1	T47.4X2	T47.4X3	T47.4X4	T47.4X5	T47.4X6
hydroxide	T47.1X1	T47.1X2	T47.1X3	T47.1X4	T47.1X5	T47.1X6
oxide	T47.1X1	T47.1X2	T47.1X3	T47.1X4	T47.1X5	T47.1X6
peroxide	T49.0X1	T49.0X2	T49.0X3	T49.0X4	T49.0X5	T49.0X6
salicylate	T39.091	T39.092	T39.093	T39.094	T39.095	T39.096
silicofluoride	T50.3X1	T50.3X2	T50.3X3	T50.3X4	T50.3X5	T50.3X6
sulfate	T47.4X1	T47.4X2	T47.4X3	T47.4X4	T47.4X5	T47.4X6
thiosulfate	T45.0X1	T45.0X2	T45.0X3	T45.0X4	T45.0X5	T45.0X6
trisilicate	T47.1X1	T47.1X2	T47.1X3	T47.1X4	T47.1X5	T47.1X6

Substance	Poisoning, Accidental (unintentional)	Poisoning, Intentional self-harm	Poisoning, Assault	Poisoning, Undetermined	Adverse effect	Underdosing
Malathion (medicinal)	T49.0X1	T49.0X2	T49.0X3	T49.0X4	T49.0X5	T49.0X6
insecticide	T60.0X1	T60.0X2	T60.0X3	T60.0X4	—	—
Male fern extract	T37.4X1	T37.4X2	T37.4X3	T37.4X4	T37.4X5	T37.4X6
M-AMSA	T45.1X1	T45.1X2	T45.1X3	T45.1X4	T45.1X5	T45.1X6
Mandelic acid	T37.8X1	T37.8X2	T37.8X3	T37.8X4	T37.8X5	T37.8X6
Manganese (dioxide) (salts)	T57.2X1	T57.2X2	T57.2X3	T57.2X4	—	—
medicinal	T50.991	T50.992	T50.993	T50.994	T50.995	T50.996
Mannitol	T47.3X1	T47.3X2	T47.3X3	T47.3X4	T47.3X5	T47.3X6
hexanitrate	T46.3X1	T46.3X2	T46.3X3	T46.3X4	T46.3X5	T46.3X6
Mannomustine	T45.1X1	T45.1X2	T45.1X3	T45.1X4	T45.1X5	T45.1X6
MAO inhibitors	T43.1X1	T43.1X2	T43.1X3	T43.1X4	T43.1X5	T43.1X6
Mapharsen	T37.8X1	T37.8X2	T37.8X3	T37.8X4	T37.8X5	T37.8X6
Maphenide	T49.0X1	T49.0X2	T49.0X3	T49.0X4	T49.0X5	T49.0X6
Maprotiline	T43.021	T43.022	T43.023	T43.024	T43.025	T43.026
Marcaine	T41.3X1	T41.3X2	T41.3X3	T41.3X4	T41.3X5	T41.3X6
infiltration (subcutaneous)	T41.3X1	T41.3X2	T41.3X3	T41.3X4	T41.3X5	T41.3X6
nerve block (peripheral) (plexus)	T41.3X1	T41.3X2	T41.3X3	T41.3X4	T41.3X5	T41.3X6
Marezine	T45.0X1	T45.0X2	T45.0X3	T45.0X4	T45.0X5	T45.0X6
Marihuana	T40.711	T40.712	T40.713	T40.714	T40.715	T40.716
Marijuana	T40.711	T40.712	T40.713	T40.714	T40.715	T40.716
Marine (sting)	T63.691	T63.692	T63.693	T63.694	—	—
animals (sting)	T63.691	T63.692	T63.693	T63.694	—	—
plants (sting)	T63.711	T63.712	T63.713	T63.714	—	—
Marplan	T43.1X1	T43.1X2	T43.1X3	T43.1X4	T43.1X5	T43.1X6
Marsh gas	T59.891	T59.892	T59.893	T59.894	—	—
Marsilid	T43.1X1	T43.1X2	T43.1X3	T43.1X4	T43.1X5	T43.1X6
Matulane	T45.1X1	T45.1X2	T45.1X3	T45.1X4	T45.1X5	T45.1X6
Mazindol	T50.5X1	T50.5X2	T50.5X3	T50.5X4	T50.5X5	T50.5X6
MCPA	T60.3X1	T60.3X2	T60.3X3	T60.3X4	—	—
MDMA	T43.641	T43.642	T43.643	T43.644	—	—
Meadow saffron	T62.2X1	T62.2X2	T62.2X3	T62.2X4	—	—
Measles virus vaccine (attenuated)	T50.B91	T50.B92	T50.B93	T50.B94	T50.B95	T50.B96
Meat, noxious	T62.8X1	T62.8X2	T62.8X3	T62.8X4	—	—
Meballymal	T42.3X1	T42.3X2	T42.3X3	T42.3X4	T42.3X5	T42.3X6
Mebanazine	T43.1X1	T43.1X2	T43.1X3	T43.1X4	T43.1X5	T43.1X6
Mebaral	T42.3X1	T42.3X2	T42.3X3	T42.3X4	T42.3X5	T42.3X6
Mebendazole	T37.4X1	T37.4X2	T37.4X3	T37.4X4	T37.4X5	T37.4X6
Mebeverine	T44.3X1	T44.3X2	T44.3X3	T44.3X4	T44.3X5	T44.3X6
Mebhydrolin	T45.0X1	T45.0X2	T45.0X3	T45.0X4	T45.0X5	T45.0X6
Mebumal	T42.3X1	T42.3X2	T42.3X3	T42.3X4	T42.3X5	T42.3X6
Mebutamate	T43.591	T43.592	T43.593	T43.594	T43.595	T43.596
Mecamylamine	T44.2X1	T44.2X2	T44.2X3	T44.2X4	T44.2X5	T44.2X6
Mechlorethamine	T45.1X1	T45.1X2	T45.1X3	T45.1X4	T45.1X5	T45.1X6
Mecillinam	T36.0X1	T36.0X2	T36.0X3	T36.0X4	T36.0X5	T36.0X6
Meclizine (hydrochloride)	T45.0X1	T45.0X2	T45.0X3	T45.0X4	T45.0X5	T45.0X6
Meclocycline	T36.4X1	T36.4X2	T36.4X3	T36.4X4	T36.4X5	T36.4X6

Table of Drugs and Chemicals

Meclofenamate–Mercurophylline

Substance	Poisoning, Accidental (unintentional)	Poisoning, Intentional self-harm	Poisoning, Assault	Poisoning, Undetermined	Adverse effect	Underdosing
Meclofenamate	T39.391	T39.392	T39.393	T39.394	T39.395	T39.396
Meclofenamic acid	T39.391	T39.392	T39.393	T39.394	T39.395	T39.396
Meclofenoxate	T43.691	T43.692	T43.693	T43.694	T43.695	T43.696
Meclozine	T45.0X1	T45.0X2	T45.0X3	T45.0X4	T45.0X5	T45.0X6
Mecobalamin	T45.8X1	T45.8X2	T45.8X3	T45.8X4	T45.8X5	T45.8X6
Mecoprop	T60.3X1	T60.3X2	T60.3X3	T60.3X4	—	—
Mecrilate	T49.3X1	T49.3X2	T49.3X3	T49.3X4	T49.3X5	T49.3X6
Mecysteine	T48.4X1	T48.4X2	T48.4X3	T48.4X4	T48.4X5	T48.4X6
Medazepam	T42.4X1	T42.4X2	T42.4X3	T42.4X4	T42.4X5	T42.4X6
Medicament NEC	T50.901	T50.902	T50.903	T50.904	T50.905	T50.906
Medinal	T42.3X1	T42.3X2	T42.3X3	T42.3X4	T42.3X5	T42.3X6
Medomin	T42.3X1	T42.3X2	T42.3X3	T42.3X4	T42.3X5	T42.3X6
Medrogestone	T38.5X1	T38.5X2	T38.5X3	T38.5X4	T38.5X5	T38.5X6
Medroxalol	T44.8X1	T44.8X2	T44.8X3	T44.8X4	T44.8X5	T44.8X6
Medroxyprogesteron eacetate (depot)	T38.5X1	T38.5X2	T38.5X3	T38.5X4	T38.5X5	T38.5X6
Medrysone	T49.0X1	T49.0X2	T49.0X3	T49.0X4	T49.0X5	T49.0X6
Mefenamic acid	T39.391	T39.392	T39.393	T39.394	T39.395	T39.396
Mefenorex	T50.5X1	T50.5X2	T50.5X3	T50.5X4	T50.5X5	T50.5X6
Mefloquine	T37.2X1	T37.2X2	T37.2X3	T37.2X4	T37.2X5	T37.2X6
Mefruside	T50.2X1	T50.2X2	T50.2X3	T50.2X4	T50.2X5	T50.2X6
Megahallucinogen	T40.901	T40.902	T40.903	T40.904	T40.905	T40.906
Megestrol	T38.5X1	T38.5X2	T38.5X3	T38.5X4	T38.5X5	T38.5X6
Meglumine						
antimoniate	T37.8X1	T37.8X2	T37.8X3	T37.8X4	T37.8X5	T37.8X6
diatrizoate	T50.8X1	T50.8X2	T50.8X3	T50.8X4	T50.8X5	T50.8X6
iodipamide	T50.8X1	T50.8X2	T50.8X3	T50.8X4	T50.8X5	T50.8X6
iotroxate	T50.8X1	T50.8X2	T50.8X3	T50.8X4	T50.8X5	T50.8X6
MEK (methyl ethyl ketone)	T52.4X1	T52.4X2	T52.4X3	T52.4X4	—	—
Meladinin	T49.3X1	T49.3X2	T49.3X3	T49.3X4	T49.3X5	T49.3X6
Meladrazine	T44.3X1	T44.3X2	T44.3X3	T44.3X4	T44.3X5	T44.3X6
Melaleuca alternifolia oil	T49.0X1	T49.0X2	T49.0X3	T49.0X4	T49.0X5	T49.0X6
Melanizing agents	T49.3X1	T49.3X2	T49.3X3	T49.3X4	T49.3X5	T49.3X6
Melanocyte-stimulating hormone	T38.891	T38.892	T38.893	T38.894	T38.895	T38.896
Melarsonyl potassium	T37.3X1	T37.3X2	T37.3X3	T37.3X4	T37.3X5	T37.3X6
Melarsoprol	T37.3X1	T37.3X2	T37.3X3	T37.3X4	T37.3X5	T37.3X6
Melia azedarach	T62.2X1	T62.2X2	T62.2X3	T62.2X4	—	—
Melitracen	T43.011	T43.012	T43.013	T43.014	T43.015	T43.016
Mellaril	T43.3X1	T43.3X2	T43.3X3	T43.3X4	T43.3X5	T43.3X6
Meloxine	T49.3X1	T49.3X2	T49.3X3	T49.3X4	T49.3X5	T49.3X6
Melperone	T43.4X1	T43.4X2	T43.4X3	T43.4X4	T43.4X5	T43.4X6
Melphalan	T45.1X1	T45.1X2	T45.1X3	T45.1X4	T45.1X5	T45.1X6
Memantine	T43.8X1	T43.8X2	T43.8X3	T43.8X4	T43.8X5	T43.8X6
Menadiol	T45.7X1	T45.7X2	T45.7X3	T45.7X4	T45.7X5	T45.7X6
sodium sulfate	T45.7X1	T45.7X2	T45.7X3	T45.7X4	T45.7X5	T45.7X6
Menadione	T45.7X1	T45.7X2	T45.7X3	T45.7X4	T45.7X5	T45.7X6
sodium bisulfite	T45.7X1	T45.7X2	T45.7X3	T45.7X4	T45.7X5	T45.7X6
Menaphthone	T45.7X1	T45.7X2	T45.7X3	T45.7X4	T45.7X5	T45.7X6
Menaquinone	T45.7X1	T45.7X2	T45.7X3	T45.7X4	T45.7X5	T45.7X6
Menatetrenone	T45.7X1	T45.7X2	T45.7X3	T45.7X4	T45.7X5	T45.7X6
Meningococcal vaccine	T50.A91	T50.A92	T50.A93	T50.A94	T50.A95	T50.A96
Menningovax (-AC) (-C)	T50.A91	T50.A92	T50.A93	T50.A94	T50.A95	T50.A96
Menotropins	T38.811	T38.812	T38.813	T38.814	T38.815	T38.816
Menthol	T48.5X1	T48.5X2	T48.5X3	T48.5X4	T48.5X5	T48.5X6
Mepacrine	T37.2X1	T37.2X2	T37.2X3	T37.2X4	T37.2X5	T37.2X6
Meparfynol	T42.6X1	T42.6X2	T42.6X3	T42.6X4	T42.6X5	T42.6X6
Mepartricin	T36.7X1	T36.7X2	T36.7X3	T36.7X4	T36.7X5	T36.7X6
Mepazine	T43.3X1	T43.3X2	T43.3X3	T43.3X4	T43.3X5	T43.3X6
Mepenzolate	T44.3X1	T44.3X2	T44.3X3	T44.3X4	T44.3X5	T44.3X6
bromide	T44.3X1	T44.3X2	T44.3X3	T44.3X4	T44.3X5	T44.3X6
Meperidine	T40.491	T40.492	T40.493	T40.494	T40.495	T40.496
Mephebarbital	T42.3X1	T42.3X2	T42.3X3	T42.3X4	T42.3X5	T42.3X6
Mephenamin (e)	T42.8X1	T42.8X2	T42.8X3	T42.8X4	T42.8X5	T42.8X6
Mephenesin	T42.8X1	T42.8X2	T42.8X3	T42.8X4	T42.8X5	T42.8X6
Mephenhydramine	T45.0X1	T45.0X2	T45.0X3	T45.0X4	T45.0X5	T45.0X6
Mephenoxalone	T42.8X1	T42.8X2	T42.8X3	T42.8X4	T42.8X5	T42.8X6
Mephentermine	T44.991	T44.992	T44.993	T44.994	T44.995	T44.996
Mephenytoin	T42.0X1	T42.0X2	T42.0X3	T42.0X4	T42.0X5	T42.0X6
with phenobarbital	T42.3X1	T42.3X2	T42.3X3	T42.3X4	T42.3X5	T42.3X6
Mephobarbital	T42.3X1	T42.3X2	T42.3X3	T42.3X4	T42.3X5	T42.3X6
Mephosfolan	T60.0X1	T60.0X2	T60.0X3	T60.0X4	—	—
Mepindolol	T44.7X1	T44.7X2	T44.7X3	T44.7X4	T44.7X5	T44.7X6
Mepiperphenidol	T44.3X1	T44.3X2	T44.3X3	T44.3X4	T44.3X5	T44.3X6
Mepitiostane	T38.7X1	T38.7X2	T38.7X3	T38.7X4	T38.7X5	T38.7X6
Mepivacaine	T41.3X1	T41.3X2	T41.3X3	T41.3X4	T41.3X5	T41.3X6
epidural	T41.3X1	T41.3X2	T41.3X3	T41.3X4	T41.3X5	T41.3X6
Meprednisone	T38.0X1	T38.0X2	T38.0X3	T38.0X4	T38.0X5	T38.0X6
Meprobam	T43.591	T43.592	T43.593	T43.594	T43.595	T43.596
Meprobamate	T43.591	T43.592	T43.593	T43.594	T43.595	T43.596
Meproscillarin	T46.0X1	T46.0X2	T46.0X3	T46.0X4	T46.0X5	T46.0X6
Meprylcaine	T41.3X1	T41.3X2	T41.3X3	T41.3X4	T41.3X5	T41.3X6
Meptazinol	T39.8X1	T39.8X2	T39.8X3	T39.8X4	T39.8X5	T39.8X6
Mepyramine	T45.0X1	T45.0X2	T45.0X3	T45.0X4	T45.0X5	T45.0X6
Mequitazine	T43.3X1	T43.3X2	T43.3X3	T43.3X4	T43.3X5	T43.3X6
Meralluride	T50.2X1	T50.2X2	T50.2X3	T50.2X4	T50.2X5	T50.2X6
Merbaphen	T50.2X1	T50.2X2	T50.2X3	T50.2X4	T50.2X5	T50.2X6
Merbromin	T49.0X1	T49.0X2	T49.0X3	T49.0X4	T49.0X5	T49.0X6
Mercaptoben-zothiazole salts	T49.0X1	T49.0X2	T49.0X3	T49.0X4	T49.0X5	T49.0X6
Mercaptomerin	T50.2X1	T50.2X2	T50.2X3	T50.2X4	T50.2X5	T50.2X6
Mercaptopurine	T45.1X1	T45.1X2	T45.1X3	T45.1X4	T45.1X5	T45.1X6
Mercumatilin	T50.2X1	T50.2X2	T50.2X3	T50.2X4	T50.2X5	T50.2X6
Mercuramide	T50.2X1	T50.2X2	T50.2X3	T50.2X4	T50.2X5	T50.2X6
Mercurochrome	T49.0X1	T49.0X2	T49.0X3	T49.0X4	T49.0X5	T49.0X6
Mercurophylline	T50.2X1	T50.2X2	T50.2X3	T50.2X4	T50.2X5	T50.2X6

Substance	Poisoning, Accidental (unintentional)	Poisoning, Intentional self-harm	Poisoning, Assault	Poisoning, Undetermined	Adverse effect	Underdosing
Mercury, mercurial, mercuric, mercurous (compounds) (cyanide) (fumes) (nonmedicinal) (vapor) NEC	T56.1X1	T56.1X2	T56.1X3	T56.1X4	—	—
ammoniated	T49.0X1	T49.0X2	T49.0X3	T49.0X4	T49.0X5	T49.0X6
anti-infective						
local	T49.0X1	T49.0X2	T49.0X3	T49.0X4	T49.0X5	T49.0X6
systemic	T37.8X1	T37.8X2	T37.8X3	T37.8X4	T37.8X5	T37.8X6
topical	T49.0X1	T49.0X2	T49.0X3	T49.0X4	T49.0X5	T49.0X6
chloride (ammoniated)	T49.0X1	T49.0X2	T49.0X3	T49.0X4	T49.0X5	T49.0X6
fungicide	T56.1X1	T56.1X2	T56.1X3	T56.1X4	—	—
diuretic NEC	T50.2X1	T50.2X2	T50.2X3	T50.2X4	T50.2X5	T50.2X6
fungicide	T56.1X1	T56.1X2	T56.1X3	T56.1X4	—	—
organic (fungicide)	T56.1X1	T56.1X2	T56.1X3	T56.1X4	—	—
oxide, yellow	T49.0X1	T49.0X2	T49.0X3	T49.0X4	T49.0X5	T49.0X6
Mersalyl	T50.2X1	T50.2X2	T50.2X3	T50.2X4	T50.2X5	T50.2X6
Merthiolate	T49.0X1	T49.0X2	T49.0X3	T49.0X4	T49.0X5	T49.0X6
ophthalmic preparation	T49.5X1	T49.5X2	T49.5X3	T49.5X4	T49.5X5	T49.5X6
Meruvax	T50.B91	T50.B92	T50.B93	T50.B94	T50.B95	T50.B96
Mesalazine	T47.8X1	T47.8X2	T47.8X3	T47.8X4	T47.8X5	T47.8X6
Mescal buttons	T40.991	T40.992	T40.993	T40.994	—	—
Mescaline	T40.991	T40.992	T40.993	T40.994	—	—
Mesna	T48.4X1	T48.4X2	T48.4X3	T48.4X4	T48.4X5	T48.4X6
Mesoglycan	T46.6X1	T46.6X2	T46.6X3	T46.6X4	T46.6X5	T46.6X6
Mesoridazine	T43.3X1	T43.3X2	T43.3X3	T43.3X4	T43.3X5	T43.3X6
Mestanolone	T38.7X1	T38.7X2	T38.7X3	T38.7X4	T38.7X5	T38.7X6
Mesterolone	T38.7X1	T38.7X2	T38.7X3	T38.7X4	T38.7X5	T38.7X6
Mestranol	T38.5X1	T38.5X2	T38.5X3	T38.5X4	T38.5X5	T38.5X6
Mesulergine	T42.8X1	T42.8X2	T42.8X3	T42.8X4	T42.8X5	T42.8X6
Mesulfen	T49.0X1	T49.0X2	T49.0X3	T49.0X4	T49.0X5	T49.0X6
Mesuximide	T42.2X1	T42.2X2	T42.2X3	T42.2X4	T42.2X5	T42.2X6
Metabutethamine	T41.3X1	T41.3X2	T41.3X3	T41.3X4	T41.3X5	T41.3X6
Metactesylacetate	T49.0X1	T49.0X2	T49.0X3	T49.0X4	T49.0X5	T49.0X6
Metacycline	T36.4X1	T36.4X2	T36.4X3	T36.4X4	T36.4X5	T36.4X6
Metaldehyde (snail killer) NEC	T60.8X1	T60.8X2	T60.8X3	T60.8X4	—	—
Metals (heavy) (nonmedicinal)	T56.91	T56.92	T56.93	T56.94	—	—
dust, fumes, or vapor NEC	T56.91	T56.92	T56.93	T56.94	—	—
gadolinium	T56.821	T56.822	T56.823	T56.824	—	—
light NEC	T56.91	T56.92	T56.93	T56.94	—	—
dust, fumes, or vapor NEC	T56.91	T56.92	T56.93	T56.94	—	—
specified NEC	T56.891	T56.892	T56.893	T56.894	—	—
thallium	T56.811	T56.812	T56.813	T56.814	—	—
Metamfetamine	T43.651	T43.652	T43.653	T43.654	T43.655	T43.656
Metamizole sodium	T39.2X1	T39.2X2	T39.2X3	T39.2X4	T39.2X5	T39.2X6
Metampicillin	T36.0X1	T36.0X2	T36.0X3	T36.0X4	T36.0X5	T36.0X6
Metamucil	T47.4X1	T47.4X2	T47.4X3	T47.4X4	T47.4X5	T47.4X6
Metandienone	T38.7X1	T38.7X2	T38.7X3	T38.7X4	T38.7X5	T38.7X6
Metandrostenolone	T38.7X1	T38.7X2	T38.7X3	T38.7X4	T38.7X5	T38.7X6

Substance	Poisoning, Accidental (unintentional)	Poisoning, Intentional self-harm	Poisoning, Assault	Poisoning, Undetermined	Adverse effect	Underdosing
Metaphen	T49.0X1	T49.0X2	T49.0X3	T49.0X4	T49.0X5	T49.0X6
Metaphos	T60.0X1	T60.0X2	T60.0X3	T60.0X4	—	—
Metapramine	T43.011	T43.012	T43.013	T43.014	T43.015	T43.016
Metaproterenol	T48.291	T48.292	T48.293	T48.294	T48.295	T48.296
Metaraminol	T44.4X1	T44.4X2	T44.4X3	T44.4X4	T44.4X5	T44.4X6
Metaxalone	T42.8X1	T42.8X2	T42.8X3	T42.8X4	T42.8X5	T42.8X6
Metenolone	T38.7X1	T38.7X2	T38.7X3	T38.7X4	T38.7X5	T38.7X6
Metergoline	T42.8X1	T42.8X2	T42.8X3	T42.8X4	T42.8X5	T42.8X6
Metescufylline	T46.991	T46.992	T46.993	T46.994	T46.995	T46.996
Metetoin	T42.0X1	T42.0X2	T42.0X3	T42.0X4	T42.0X5	T42.0X6
Metformin	T38.3X1	T38.3X2	T38.3X3	T38.3X4	T38.3X5	T38.3X6
Methacholine	T44.1X1	T44.1X2	T44.1X3	T44.1X4	T44.1X5	T44.1X6
Methacycline	T36.4X1	T36.4X2	T36.4X3	T36.4X4	T36.4X5	T36.4X6
Methadone	T40.3X1	T40.3X2	T40.3X3	T40.3X4	T40.3X5	T40.3X6
Methallenestril	T38.5X1	T38.5X2	T38.5X3	T38.5X4	T38.5X5	T38.5X6
Methallenoestril	T38.5X1	T38.5X2	T38.5X3	T38.5X4	T38.5X5	T38.5X6
Methamphetamine	T43.651	T43.652	T43.653	T43.654	T43.655	T43.656
Methampyrone	T39.2X1	T39.2X2	T39.2X3	T39.2X4	T39.2X5	T39.2X6
Methandienone	T38.7X1	T38.7X2	T38.7X3	T38.7X4	T38.7X5	T38.7X6
Methandriol	T38.7X1	T38.7X2	T38.7X3	T38.7X4	T38.7X5	T38.7X6
Methandrostenolone	T38.7X1	T38.7X2	T38.7X3	T38.7X4	T38.7X5	T38.7X6
Methane	T59.891	T59.892	T59.893	T59.894	—	—
Methanethiol	T59.891	T59.892	T59.893	T59.894	—	—
Methaniazide	T37.1X1	T37.1X2	T37.1X3	T37.1X4	T37.1X5	T37.1X6
Methanol (vapor)	T51.1X1	T51.1X2	T51.1X3	T51.1X4	—	—
Methantheline	T44.3X1	T44.3X2	T44.3X3	T44.3X4	T44.3X5	T44.3X6
Methanthelinium bromide	T44.3X1	T44.3X2	T44.3X3	T44.3X4	T44.3X5	T44.3X6
Methaphenilene	T45.0X1	T45.0X2	T45.0X3	T45.0X4	T45.0X5	T45.0X6
Methapyrilene	T45.0X1	T45.0X2	T45.0X3	T45.0X4	T45.0X5	T45.0X6
Methaqualone (compound)	T42.6X1	T42.6X2	T42.6X3	T42.6X4	T42.6X5	T42.6X6
Metharbital	T42.3X1	T42.3X2	T42.3X3	T42.3X4	T42.3X5	T42.3X6
Methazolamide	T50.2X1	T50.2X2	T50.2X3	T50.2X4	T50.2X5	T50.2X6
Methdilazine	T43.3X1	T43.3X2	T43.3X3	T43.3X4	T43.3X5	T43.3X6
Methedrine	T43.651	T43.652	T43.653	T43.654	T43.655	T43.656
Methenamine (mandelate)	T37.8X1	T37.8X2	T37.8X3	T37.8X4	T37.8X5	T37.8X6
Methenolone	T38.7X1	T38.7X2	T38.7X3	T38.7X4	T38.7X5	T38.7X6
Methergine	T48.0X1	T48.0X2	T48.0X3	T48.0X4	T48.0X5	T48.0X6
Methetoin	T42.0X1	T42.0X2	T42.0X3	T42.0X4	T42.0X5	T42.0X6
Methiacil	T38.2X1	T38.2X2	T38.2X3	T38.2X4	T38.2X5	T38.2X6
Methicillin	T36.0X1	T36.0X2	T36.0X3	T36.0X4	T36.0X5	T36.0X6
Methimazole	T38.2X1	T38.2X2	T38.2X3	T38.2X4	T38.2X5	T38.2X6
Methiodal sodium	T50.8X1	T50.8X2	T50.8X3	T50.8X4	T50.8X5	T50.8X6
Methionine	T50.991	T50.992	T50.993	T50.994	T50.995	T50.996
Methisazone	T37.5X1	T37.5X2	T37.5X3	T37.5X4	T37.5X5	T37.5X6
Methisoprinol	T37.5X1	T37.5X2	T37.5X3	T37.5X4	T37.5X5	T37.5X6
Methitural	T42.3X1	T42.3X2	T42.3X3	T42.3X4	T42.3X5	T42.3X6
Methixene	T44.3X1	T44.3X2	T44.3X3	T44.3X4	T44.3X5	T44.3X6
Methobarbital, methobarbitone	T42.3X1	T42.3X2	T42.3X3	T42.3X4	T42.3X5	T42.3X6

Substance	Poisoning, Accidental (unintentional)	Poisoning, Intentional self-harm	Poisoning, Assault	Poisoning, Undetermined	Adverse effect	Underdosing
Methocarbamol	T42.8X1	T42.8X2	T42.8X3	T42.8X4	T42.8X5	T42.8X6
skeletal muscle relaxant	T48.1X1	T48.1X2	T48.1X3	T48.1X4	T48.1X5	T48.1X6
Methohexital	T41.1X1	T41.1X2	T41.1X3	T41.1X4	T41.1X5	T41.1X6
Methohexitone	T41.1X1	T41.1X2	T41.1X3	T41.1X4	T41.1X5	T41.1X6
Methoin	T42.0X1	T42.0X2	T42.0X3	T42.0X4	T42.0X5	T42.0X6
Methopholine	T39.8X1	T39.8X2	T39.8X3	T39.8X4	T39.8X5	T39.8X6
Methopromazine	T43.3X1	T43.3X2	T43.3X3	T43.3X4	T43.3X5	T43.3X6
Methorate	T48.3X1	T48.3X2	T48.3X3	T48.3X4	T48.3X5	T48.3X6
Methoserpidine	T46.5X1	T46.5X2	T46.5X3	T46.5X4	T46.5X5	T46.5X6
Methotrexate	T45.1X1	T45.1X2	T45.1X3	T45.1X4	T45.1X5	T45.1X6
Methotrimeprazine	T43.3X1	T43.3X2	T43.3X3	T43.3X4	T43.3X5	T43.3X6
Methoxa-Dome	T49.3X1	T49.3X2	T49.3X3	T49.3X4	T49.3X5	T49.3X6
Methoxamine	T44.4X1	T44.4X2	T44.4X3	T44.4X4	T44.4X5	T44.4X6
Methoxsalen	T50.991	T50.992	T50.993	T50.994	T50.995	T50.996
Methoxyaniline	T65.3X1	T65.3X2	T65.3X3	T65.3X4	—	—
Methoxybenzyl penicillin	T36.0X1	T36.0X2	T36.0X3	T36.0X4	T36.0X5	T36.0X6
Methoxychlor	T53.7X1	T53.7X2	T53.7X3	T53.7X4	—	—
Methoxy-DDT	T53.7X1	T53.7X2	T53.7X3	T53.7X4	—	—
2-Methoxyethanol	T52.3X1	T52.3X2	T52.3X3	T52.3X4	—	—
Methoxyflurane	T41.0X1	T41.0X2	T41.0X3	T41.0X4	T41.0X5	T41.0X6
Methoxyphenamine	T48.6X1	T48.6X2	T48.6X3	T48.6X4	T48.6X5	T48.6X6
Methoxypromazine	T43.3X1	T43.3X2	T43.3X3	T43.3X4	T43.3X5	T43.3X6
5-Methoxypsoralen (5-MOP)	T50.991	T50.992	T50.993	T50.994	T50.995	T50.996
8-Methoxypsoralen (8-MOP)	T50.991	T50.992	T50.993	T50.994	T50.995	T50.996
Methscopolamine bromide	T44.3X1	T44.3X2	T44.3X3	T44.3X4	T44.3X5	T44.3X6
Methsuximide	T42.2X1	T42.2X2	T42.2X3	T42.2X4	T42.2X5	T42.2X6
Methyclothiazide	T50.2X1	T50.2X2	T50.2X3	T50.2X4	T50.2X5	T50.2X6
Methyl						
acetate	T52.4X1	T52.4X2	T52.4X3	T52.4X4	—	—
acetone	T52.4X1	T52.4X2	T52.4X3	T52.4X4	—	—
acrylate	T65.891	T65.892	T65.893	T65.894	—	—
alcohol	T51.1X1	T51.1X2	T51.1X3	T51.1X4	—	—
aminophenol	T65.3X1	T65.3X2	T65.3X3	T65.3X4	—	—
amphetamine	T43.651	T43.652	T43.653	T43.654	T43.655	T43.656
androstanolone	T38.7X1	T38.7X2	T38.7X3	T38.7X4	T38.7X5	T38.7X6
atropine	T44.3X1	T44.3X2	T44.3X3	T44.3X4	T44.3X5	T44.3X6
benzene	T52.2X1	T52.2X2	T52.2X3	T52.2X4	—	—
benzoate	T52.8X1	T52.8X2	T52.8X3	T52.8X4	—	—
benzol	T52.2X1	T52.2X2	T52.2X3	T52.2X4	—	—
bromide (gas)	T59.891	T59.892	T59.893	T59.894	—	—
fumigant	T60.8X1	T60.8X2	T60.8X3	T60.8X4	—	—
butanol	T51.3X1	T51.3X2	T51.3X3	T51.3X4	—	—
carbinol	T51.1X1	T51.1X2	T51.1X3	T51.1X4	—	—
carbonate	T52.8X1	T52.8X2	T52.8X3	T52.8X4	—	—
CCNU	T45.1X1	T45.1X2	T45.1X3	T45.1X4	T45.1X5	T45.1X6
cellosolve	T52.91	T52.92	T52.93	T52.94	—	—
cellulose	T47.4X1	T47.4X2	T47.4X3	T47.4X4	T47.4X5	T47.4X6

Substance	Poisoning, Accidental (unintentional)	Poisoning, Intentional self-harm	Poisoning, Assault	Poisoning, Undetermined	Adverse effect	Underdosing
Methyl — Continued						
chloride (gas)	T59.891	T59.892	T59.893	T59.894	—	—
chloroformate	T59.3X1	T59.3X2	T59.3X3	T59.3X4	—	—
cyclohexane	T52.8X1	T52.8X2	T52.8X3	T52.8X4	—	—
cyclohexanol	T51.8X1	T51.8X2	T51.8X3	T51.8X4	—	—
cyclohexanone	T52.8X1	T52.8X2	T52.8X3	T52.8X4	—	—
cyclohexyl acetate	T52.8X1	T52.8X2	T52.8X3	T52.8X4	—	—
demeton	T60.0X1	T60.0X2	T60.0X3	T60.0X4	—	—
dihydromorphinone	T40.2X1	T40.2X2	T40.2X3	T40.2X4	T40.2X5	T40.2X6
ergometrine	T48.0X1	T48.0X2	T48.0X3	T48.0X4	T48.0X5	T48.0X6
ergonovine	T48.0X1	T48.0X2	T48.0X3	T48.0X4	T48.0X5	T48.0X6
ethyl ketone	T52.4X1	T52.4X2	T52.4X3	T52.4X4	—	—
glucamine antimonate	T37.8X1	T37.8X2	T37.8X3	T37.8X4	T37.8X5	T37.8X6
hydrazine	T65.891	T65.892	T65.893	T65.894	—	—
iodide	T65.891	T65.892	T65.893	T65.894	—	—
isobutyl ketone	T52.4X1	T52.4X2	T52.4X3	T52.4X4	—	—
isothiocyanate	T60.3X1	T60.3X2	T60.3X3	T60.3X4	—	—
mercaptan	T59.891	T59.892	T59.893	T59.894	—	—
morphine NEC	T40.2X1	T40.2X2	T40.2X3	T40.2X4	T40.2X5	T40.2X6
nicotinate	T49.4X1	T49.4X2	T49.4X3	T49.4X4	T49.4X5	T49.4X6
paraben	T49.0X1	T49.0X2	T49.0X3	T49.0X4	T49.0X5	T49.0X6
parafynol	T42.6X1	T42.6X2	T42.6X3	T42.6X4	T42.6X5	T42.6X6
parathion	T60.0X1	T60.0X2	T60.0X3	T60.0X4	—	—
peridol	T43.4X1	T43.4X2	T43.4X3	T43.4X4	T43.4X5	T43.4X6
phenidate	T43.631	T43.632	T43.633	T43.634	T43.635	T43.636
prednisolone	T38.0X1	T38.0X2	T38.0X3	T38.0X4	T38.0X5	T38.0X6
ENT agent	T49.6X1	T49.6X2	T49.6X3	T49.6X4	T49.6X5	T49.6X6
ophthalmic preparation	T49.5X1	T49.5X2	T49.5X3	T49.5X4	T49.5X5	T49.5X6
topical NEC	T49.0X1	T49.0X2	T49.0X3	T49.0X4	T49.0X5	T49.0X6
propylcarbinol	T51.3X1	T51.3X2	T51.3X3	T51.3X4	—	—
rosaniline NEC	T49.0X1	T49.0X2	T49.0X3	T49.0X4	T49.0X5	T49.0X6
salicylate	T49.2X1	T49.2X2	T49.2X3	T49.2X4	T49.2X5	T49.2X6
sulfate (fumes)	T59.891	T59.892	T59.893	T59.894	—	—
liquid	T52.8X1	T52.8X2	T52.8X3	T52.8X4	—	—
sulfonal	T42.6X1	T42.6X2	T42.6X3	T42.6X4	T42.6X5	T42.6X6
testosterone	T38.7X1	T38.7X2	T38.7X3	T38.7X4	T38.7X5	T38.7X6
thiouracil	T38.2X1	T38.2X2	T38.2X3	T38.2X4	T38.2X5	T38.2X6
Methylamphetamine	T43.651	T43.652	T43.653	T43.654	T43.655	T43.656
Methylated spirit	T51.1X1	T51.1X2	T51.1X3	T51.1X4	—	—
Methylatropine nitrate	T44.3X1	T44.3X2	T44.3X3	T44.3X4	T44.3X5	T44.3X6
Methylbenactyzium bromide	T44.3X1	T44.3X2	T44.3X3	T44.3X4	T44.3X5	T44.3X6
Methylbenzethonium chloride	T49.0X1	T49.0X2	T49.0X3	T49.0X4	T49.0X5	T49.0X6
Methylcellulose	T47.4X1	T47.4X2	T47.4X3	T47.4X4	T47.4X5	T47.4X6
laxative	T47.4X1	T47.4X2	T47.4X3	T47.4X4	T47.4X5	T47.4X6
Methylchlorophenoxy-acetic acid	T60.3X1	T60.3X2	T60.3X3	T60.3X4	—	—
Methyldopa	T46.5X1	T46.5X2	T46.5X3	T46.5X4	T46.5X5	T46.5X6
Methyldopate	T46.5X1	T46.5X2	T46.5X3	T46.5X4	T46.5X5	T46.5X6

Substance	Poisoning, Accidental (unintentional)	Poisoning, Intentional self-harm	Poisoning, Assault	Poisoning, Undetermined	Adverse effect	Underdosing
Methylene						
blue	T50.6X1	T50.6X2	T50.6X3	T50.6X4	T50.6X5	T50.6X6
chloride or dichloride (solvent) NEC	T53.4X1	T53.4X2	T53.4X3	T53.4X4	—	—
Methylenedioxy-amphetamine	T43.621	T43.622	T43.623	T43.624	T43.625	T43.626
Methylenedioxy-methamphetamine	T43.641	T43.642	T43.643	T43.644	—	—
Methylergometrine	T48.0X1	T48.0X2	T48.0X3	T48.0X4	T48.0X5	T48.0X6
Methylergonovine	T48.0X1	T48.0X2	T48.0X3	T48.0X4	T48.0X5	T48.0X6
Methylestrenolone	T38.5X1	T38.5X2	T38.5X3	T38.5X4	T38.5X5	T38.5X6
Methylethyl cellulose	T50.991	T50.992	T50.993	T50.994	T50.995	T50.996
Methylhexabital	T42.3X1	T42.3X2	T42.3X3	T42.3X4	T42.3X5	T42.3X6
Methylmorphine	T40.2X1	T40.2X2	T40.2X3	T40.2X4	T40.2X5	T40.2X6
Methylparaben (ophthalmic)	T49.5X1	T49.5X2	T49.5X3	T49.5X4	T49.5X5	T49.5X6
Methylparafynol	T42.6X1	T42.6X2	T42.6X3	T42.6X4	T42.6X5	T42.6X6
Methylpentynol, methylpenthynol	T42.6X1	T42.6X2	T42.6X3	T42.6X4	T42.6X5	T42.6X6
Methylphenidate	T43.631	T43.632	T43.633	T43.634	T43.635	T43.636
Methylphenobarbital	T42.3X1	T42.3X2	T42.3X3	T42.3X4	T42.3X5	T42.3X6
Methylpolysiloxane	T47.1X1	T47.1X2	T47.1X3	T47.1X4	T47.1X5	T47.1X6
Methylprednisolone— see Methyl, prednisolone						
Methylrosaniline	T49.0X1	T49.0X2	T49.0X3	T49.0X4	T49.0X5	T49.0X6
Methylrosanilinium chloride	T49.0X1	T49.0X2	T49.0X3	T49.0X4	T49.0X5	T49.0X6
Methyltestosterone	T38.7X1	T38.7X2	T38.7X3	T38.7X4	T38.7X5	T38.7X6
Methylthionine chloride	T50.6X1	T50.6X2	T50.6X3	T50.6X4	T50.6X5	T50.6X6
Methylthioninium chloride	T50.6X1	T50.6X2	T50.6X3	T50.6X4	T50.6X5	T50.6X6
Methylthiouracil	T38.2X1	T38.2X2	T38.2X3	T38.2X4	T38.2X5	T38.2X6
Methyprylon	T42.6X1	T42.6X2	T42.6X3	T42.6X4	T42.6X5	T42.6X6
Methysergide	T46.5X1	T46.5X2	T46.5X3	T46.5X4	T46.5X5	T46.5X6
Metiamide	T47.1X1	T47.1X2	T47.1X3	T47.1X4	T47.1X5	T47.1X6
Meticillin	T36.0X1	T36.0X2	T36.0X3	T36.0X4	T36.0X5	T36.0X6
Meticrane	T50.2X1	T50.2X2	T50.2X3	T50.2X4	T50.2X5	T50.2X6
Metildigoxin	T46.0X1	T46.0X2	T46.0X3	T46.0X4	T46.0X5	T46.0X6
Metipranolol	T49.5X1	T49.5X2	T49.5X3	T49.5X4	T49.5X5	T49.5X6
Metirosine	T46.5X1	T46.5X2	T46.5X3	T46.5X4	T46.5X5	T46.5X6
Metisazone	T37.5X1	T37.5X2	T37.5X3	T37.5X4	T37.5X5	T37.5X6
Metixene	T44.3X1	T44.3X2	T44.3X3	T44.3X4	T44.3X5	T44.3X6
Metizoline	T48.5X1	T48.5X2	T48.5X3	T48.5X4	T48.5X5	T48.5X6
Metoclopramide	T45.0X1	T45.0X2	T45.0X3	T45.0X4	T45.0X5	T45.0X6
Metofenazate	T43.3X1	T43.3X2	T43.3X3	T43.3X4	T43.3X5	T43.3X6
Metofoline	T39.8X1	T39.8X2	T39.8X3	T39.8X4	T39.8X5	T39.8X6
Metolazone	T50.2X1	T50.2X2	T50.2X3	T50.2X4	T50.2X5	T50.2X6
Metopon	T40.2X1	T40.2X2	T40.2X3	T40.2X4	T40.2X5	T40.2X6
Metoprine	T45.1X1	T45.1X2	T45.1X3	T45.1X4	T45.1X5	T45.1X6
Metoprolol	T44.7X1	T44.7X2	T44.7X3	T44.7X4	T44.7X5	T44.7X6
Metrifonate	T60.0X1	T60.0X2	T60.0X3	T60.0X4	—	—
Metrizamide	T50.8X1	T50.8X2	T50.8X3	T50.8X4	T50.8X5	T50.8X6
Metrizoic acid	T50.8X1	T50.8X2	T50.8X3	T50.8X4	T50.8X5	T50.8X6

Substance	Poisoning, Accidental (unintentional)	Poisoning, Intentional self-harm	Poisoning, Assault	Poisoning, Undetermined	Adverse effect	Underdosing
Metronidazole	T37.8X1	T37.8X2	T37.8X3	T37.8X4	T37.8X5	T37.8X6
Metycaine	T41.3X1	T41.3X2	T41.3X3	T41.3X4	T41.3X5	T41.3X6
infiltration (subcutaneous)	T41.3X1	T41.3X2	T41.3X3	T41.3X4	T41.3X5	T41.3X6
nerve block (peripheral) (plexus)	T41.3X1	T41.3X2	T41.3X3	T41.3X4	T41.3X5	T41.3X6
topical (surface)	T41.3X1	T41.3X2	T41.3X3	T41.3X4	T41.3X5	T41.3X6
Metyrapone	T50.8X1	T50.8X2	T50.8X3	T50.8X4	T50.8X5	T50.8X6
Mevinphos	T60.0X1	T60.0X2	T60.0X3	T60.0X4	—	—
Mexazolam	T42.4X1	T42.4X2	T42.4X3	T42.4X4	T42.4X5	T42.4X6
Mexenone	T49.3X1	T49.3X2	T49.3X3	T49.3X4	T49.3X5	T49.3X6
Mexiletine	T46.2X1	T46.2X2	T46.2X3	T46.2X4	T46.2X5	T46.2X6
Mezereon	T62.2X1	T62.2X2	T62.2X3	T62.2X4		
berries	T62.1X1	T62.1X2	T62.1X3	T62.1X4		
Mezlocillin	T36.0X1	T36.0X2	T36.0X3	T36.0X4	T36.0X5	T36.0X6
Mianserin	T43.021	T43.022	T43.023	T43.024	T43.025	T43.026
Micatin	T49.0X1	T49.0X2	T49.0X3	T49.0X4	T49.0X5	T49.0X6
Miconazole	T49.0X1	T49.0X2	T49.0X3	T49.0X4	T49.0X5	T49.0X6
Micronomicin	T36.5X1	T36.5X2	T36.5X3	T36.5X4	T36.5X5	T36.5X6
Midazolam	T42.4X1	T42.4X2	T42.4X3	T42.4X4	T42.4X5	T42.4X6
Midecamycin	T36.3X1	T36.3X2	T36.3X3	T36.3X4	T36.3X5	T36.3X6
Mifepristone	T38.6X1	T38.6X2	T38.6X3	T38.6X4	T38.6X5	T38.6X6
Milk of magnesia	T47.1X1	T47.1X2	T47.1X3	T47.1X4	T47.1X5	T47.1X6
Millipede (tropical) (venomous)	T63.411	T63.412	T63.413	T63.414	—	—
Miltown	T43.591	T43.592	T43.593	T43.594	T43.595	T43.596
Milverine	T44.3X1	T44.3X2	T44.3X3	T44.3X4	T44.3X5	T44.3X6
Minaprine	T43.291	T43.292	T43.293	T43.294	T43.295	T43.296
Minaxolone	T41.291	T41.292	T41.293	T41.294	T41.295	T41.296
Mineral						
acids	T54.2X1	T54.2X2	T54.2X3	T54.2X4	—	—
oil (laxative) (medicinal)	T47.4X1	T47.4X2	T47.4X3	T47.4X4	T47.4X5	T47.4X6
emulsion	T47.2X1	T47.2X2	T47.2X3	T47.2X4	T47.2X5	T47.2X6
nonmedicinal	T52.0X1	T52.0X2	T52.0X3	T52.0X4	—	—
topical	T49.3X1	T49.3X2	T49.3X3	T49.3X4	T49.3X5	T49.3X6
salt NEC	T50.3X1	T50.3X2	T50.3X3	T50.3X4	T50.3X5	T50.3X6
spirits	T52.0X1	T52.0X2	T52.0X3	T52.0X4	—	—
Mineralocorticosteroid	T50.0X1	T50.0X2	T50.0X3	T50.0X4	T50.0X5	T50.0X6
Minocycline	T36.4X1	T36.4X2	T36.4X3	T36.4X4	T36.4X5	T36.4X6
Minoxidil	T46.7X1	T46.7X2	T46.7X3	T46.7X4	T46.7X5	T46.7X6
Miokamycin	T36.3X1	T36.3X2	T36.3X3	T36.3X4	T36.3X5	T36.3X6
Miotic drug	T49.5X1	T49.5X2	T49.5X3	T49.5X4	T49.5X5	T49.5X6
Mipafox	T60.0X1	T60.0X2	T60.0X3	T60.0X4		
Mirex	T60.1X1	T60.1X2	T60.1X3	T60.1X4	—	—
Mirtazapine	T43.021	T43.022	T43.023	T43.024	T43.025	T43.026
Misonidazole	T37.3X1	T37.3X2	T37.3X3	T37.3X4	T37.3X5	T37.3X6
Misoprostol	T47.1X1	T47.1X2	T47.1X3	T47.1X4	T47.1X5	T47.1X6
Mithramycin	T45.1X1	T45.1X2	T45.1X3	T45.1X4	T45.1X5	T45.1X6
Mitobronitol	T45.1X1	T45.1X2	T45.1X3	T45.1X4	T45.1X5	T45.1X6
Mitoguazone	T45.1X1	T45.1X2	T45.1X3	T45.1X4	T45.1X5	T45.1X6

Substance	Poisoning, Accidental (unintentional)	Poisoning, Intentional self-harm	Poisoning, Assault	Poisoning, Undetermined	Adverse effect	Underdosing
Mitolactol	T45.1X1	T45.1X2	T45.1X3	T45.1X4	T45.1X5	T45.1X6
Mitomycin	T45.1X1	T45.1X2	T45.1X3	T45.1X4	T45.1X5	T45.1X6
Mitopodozide	T45.1X1	T45.1X2	T45.1X3	T45.1X4	T45.1X5	T45.1X6
Mitotane	T45.1X1	T45.1X2	T45.1X3	T45.1X4	T45.1X5	T45.1X6
Mitoxantrone	T45.1X1	T45.1X2	T45.1X3	T45.1X4	T45.1X5	T45.1X6
Mivacurium chloride	T48.1X1	T48.1X2	T48.1X3	T48.1X4	T48.1X5	T48.1X6
Miyari bacteria	T47.6X1	T47.6X2	T47.6X3	T47.6X4	T47.6X5	T47.6X6
Moclobemide	T43.1X1	T43.1X2	T43.1X3	T43.1X4	T43.1X5	T43.1X6
Moderil	T46.5X1	T46.5X2	T46.5X3	T46.5X4	T46.5X5	T46.5X6
Mofebutazone	T39.2X1	T39.2X2	T39.2X3	T39.2X4	T39.2X5	T39.2X6
Mogadon—see Nitrazepam						
Molindone	T43.591	T43.592	T43.593	T43.594	T43.595	T43.596
Molsidomine	T46.3X1	T46.3X2	T46.3X3	T46.3X4	T46.3X5	T46.3X6
Mometasone	T49.0X1	T49.0X2	T49.0X3	T49.0X4	T49.0X5	T49.0X6
Monistat	T49.0X1	T49.0X2	T49.0X3	T49.0X4	T49.0X5	T49.0X6
Monkshood	T62.2X1	T62.2X2	T62.2X3	T62.2X4	—	—
Monoamine oxidase inhibitor NEC	T43.1X1	T43.1X2	T43.1X3	T43.1X4	T43.1X5	T43.1X6
hydrazine	T43.1X1	T43.1X2	T43.1X3	T43.1X4	T43.1X5	T43.1X6
Monobenzone	T49.4X1	T49.4X2	T49.4X3	T49.4X4	T49.4X5	T49.4X6
Monochloroacetic acid	T60.3X1	T60.3X2	T60.3X3	T60.3X4	—	—
Monochlorobenzene	T53.7X1	T53.7X2	T53.7X3	T53.7X4	—	—
Monoethanolamine	T46.8X1	T46.8X2	T46.8X3	T46.8X4	T46.8X5	T46.8X6
oleate	T46.8X1	T46.8X2	T46.8X3	T46.8X4	T46.8X5	T46.8X6
Monooctanoin	T50.991	T50.992	T50.993	T50.994	T50.995	T50.996
Monophenylbutazone	T39.2X1	T39.2X2	T39.2X3	T39.2X4	T39.2X5	T39.2X6
Monosodium glutamate	T65.891	T65.892	T65.893	T65.894	—	—
Monosulfiram	T49.0X1	T49.0X2	T49.0X3	T49.0X4	T49.0X5	T49.0X6
Monoxide, carbon—see Carbon, monoxide						
Monoxidine hydrochloride	T46.1X1	T46.1X2	T46.1X3	T46.1X4	T46.1X5	T46.1X6
Monuron	T60.3X1	T60.3X2	T60.3X3	T60.3X4	—	—
Moperone	T43.4X1	T43.4X2	T43.4X3	T43.4X4	T43.4X5	T43.4X6
Mopidamol	T45.1X1	T45.1X2	T45.1X3	T45.1X4	T45.1X5	T45.1X6
MOPP (mechlorethamine + vincristine + prednisone + procarbazine)	T45.1X1	T45.1X2	T45.1X3	T45.1X4	T45.1X5	T45.1X6
Morfin	T40.2X1	T40.2X2	T40.2X3	T40.2X4	T40.2X5	T40.2X6
Morinamide	T37.1X1	T37.1X2	T37.1X3	T37.1X4	T37.1X5	T37.1X6
Morning glory seeds	T40.991	T40.992	T40.993	T40.994	—	—
Moroxydine	T37.5X1	T37.5X2	T37.5X3	T37.5X4	T37.5X5	T37.5X6
Morphazinamide	T37.1X1	T37.1X2	T37.1X3	T37.1X4	T37.1X5	T37.1X6
Morphine	T40.2X1	T40.2X2	T40.2X3	T40.2X4	T40.2X5	T40.2X6
antagonist	T50.7X1	T50.7X2	T50.7X3	T50.7X4	T50.7X5	T50.7X6
Morpholinylethylmorphine	T40.2X1	T40.2X2	T40.2X3	T40.2X4	—	—
Morsuximide	T42.2X1	T42.2X2	T42.2X3	T42.2X4	T42.2X5	T42.2X6
Mosapramine	T43.591	T43.592	T43.593	T43.594	T43.595	T43.596

Substance	Poisoning, Accidental (unintentional)	Poisoning, Intentional self-harm	Poisoning, Assault	Poisoning, Undetermined	Adverse effect	Underdosing
Moth balls—see also Pesticide	T60.2X1	T60.2X2	T60.2X3	T60.2X4	—	—
naphthalene	T60.2X1	T60.2X2	T60.2X3	T60.2X4	—	—
paradichlorobenzene	T60.1X1	T60.1X2	T60.1X3	T60.1X4	—	—
Motor exhaust gas	T58.01	T58.02	T58.03	T58.04	—	—
Mouthwash (antiseptic) (zincchloride)	T49.6X1	T49.6X2	T49.6X3	T49.6X4	T49.6X5	T49.6X6
Moxastine	T45.0X1	T45.0X2	T45.0X3	T45.0X4	T45.0X5	T45.0X6
Moxaverine	T44.3X1	T44.3X2	T44.3X3	T44.3X4	T44.3X5	T44.3X6
Moxisylyte	T46.7X1	T46.7X2	T46.7X3	T46.7X4	T46.7X5	T46.7X6
Mucilage, plant	T47.4X1	T47.4X2	T47.4X3	T47.4X4	T47.4X5	T47.4X6
Mucolytic drug	T48.4X1	T48.4X2	T48.4X3	T48.4X4	T48.4X5	T48.4X6
Mucomyst	T48.4X1	T48.4X2	T48.4X3	T48.4X4	T48.4X5	T48.4X6
Mucous membrane agents (external)	T49.91	T49.92	T49.93	T49.94	T49.95	T49.96
specified NEC	T49.8X1	T49.8X2	T49.8X3	T49.8X4	T49.8X5	T49.8X6
Multiple unspecified drugs, medicaments and biological substances	T50.911	T50.912	T50.913	T50.914	T50.915	T50.916
Mumps						
immune globulin (human)	T50.Z11	T50.Z12	T50.Z13	T50.Z14	T50.Z15	T50.Z16
skin test antigen	T50.8X1	T50.8X2	T50.8X3	T50.8X4	T50.8X5	T50.8X6
vaccine	T50.B91	T50.B92	T50.B93	T50.B94	T50.B95	T50.B96
Mumpsvax	T50.B91	T50.B92	T50.B93	T50.B94	T50.B95	T50.B96
Mupirocin	T49.0X1	T49.0X2	T49.0X3	T49.0X4	T49.0X5	T49.0X6
Muriatic acid—see Hydrochloric acid						
Muromonab-CD3	T45.1X1	T45.1X2	T45.1X3	T45.1X4	T45.1X5	T45.1X6
Muscle-action drug NEC	T48.201	T48.202	T48.203	T48.204	T48.205	T48.206
Muscle affecting agents NEC	T48.201	T48.202	T48.203	T48.204	T48.205	T48.206
oxytocic	T48.0X1	T48.0X2	T48.0X3	T48.0X4	T48.0X5	T48.0X6
relaxants	T48.201	T48.202	T48.203	T48.204	T48.205	T48.206
central nervous system	T42.8X1	T42.8X2	T42.8X3	T42.8X4	T42.8X5	T42.8X6
skeletal	T48.1X1	T48.1X2	T48.1X3	T48.1X4	T48.1X5	T48.1X6
smooth	T44.3X1	T44.3X2	T44.3X3	T44.3X4	T44.3X5	T44.3X6
Muscle relaxant—see Relaxant, muscle						
Muscle-tone depressant, central NEC	T42.8X1	T42.8X2	T42.8X3	T42.8X4	T42.8X5	T42.8X6
specified NEC	T42.8X1	T42.8X2	T42.8X3	T42.8X4	T42.8X5	T42.8X6
Mushroom, noxious	T62.0X1	T62.0X2	T62.0X3	T62.0X4	—	—
Mussel, noxious	T61.781	T61.782	T61.783	T61.784	—	—
Mustard (emetic)	T47.7X1	T47.7X2	T47.7X3	T47.7X4	T47.7X5	T47.7X6
black	T47.7X1	T47.7X2	T47.7X3	T47.7X4	T47.7X5	T47.7X6
gas, not in war	T59.91	T59.92	T59.93	T59.94	—	—
nitrogen	T45.1X1	T45.1X2	T45.1X3	T45.1X4	T45.1X5	T45.1X6
Mustine	T45.1X1	T45.1X2	T45.1X3	T45.1X4	T45.1X5	T45.1X6
M-vac	T45.1X1	T45.1X2	T45.1X3	T45.1X4	T45.1X5	T45.1X6
Mycifradin	T36.5X1	T36.5X2	T36.5X3	T36.5X4	T36.5X5	T36.5X6
topical	T49.0X1	T49.0X2	T49.0X3	T49.0X4	T49.0X5	T49.0X6

Substance	Poisoning, Accidental (unintentional)	Poisoning, Intentional self-harm	Poisoning, Assault	Poisoning, Undetermined	Adverse effect	Underdosing
Mycitracin	T36.8X1	T36.8X2	T36.8X3	T36.8X4	T36.8X5	T36.8X6
ophthalmic preparation	T49.5X1	T49.5X2	T49.5X3	T49.5X4	T49.5X5	T49.5X6
Mycostatin	T36.7X1	T36.7X2	T36.7X3	T36.7X4	T36.7X5	T36.7X6
topical	T49.0X1	T49.0X2	T49.0X3	T49.0X4	T49.0X5	T49.0X6
Mycotoxins	T64.81	T64.82	T64.83	T64.84	—	—
aflatoxin	T64.01	T64.02	T64.03	T64.04	—	—
specified NEC	T64.81	T64.82	T64.83	T64.84	—	—
Mydriacyl	T44.3X1	T44.3X2	T44.3X3	T44.3X4	T44.3X5	T44.3X6
Mydriatic drug	T49.5X1	T49.5X2	T49.5X3	T49.5X4	T49.5X5	T49.5X6
Myelobromal	T45.1X1	T45.1X2	T45.1X3	T45.1X4	T45.1X5	T45.1X6
Myleran	T45.1X1	T45.1X2	T45.1X3	T45.1X4	T45.1X5	T45.1X6
Myochrysin(e)	T39.2X1	T39.2X2	T39.2X3	T39.2X4	T39.2X5	T39.2X6
Myoneural blocking agents	T48.1X1	T48.1X2	T48.1X3	T48.1X4	T48.1X5	T48.1X6
Myralact	T49.0X1	T49.0X2	T49.0X3	T49.0X4	T49.0X5	T49.0X6
Myristica fragrans	T62.2X1	T62.2X2	T62.2X3	T62.2X4	—	—
Myristicin	T65.891	T65.892	T65.893	T65.894	—	—
Mysoline	T42.3X1	T42.3X2	T42.3X3	T42.3X4	T42.3X5	T42.3X6
N						
Nabilone	T40.711	T40.712	T40.713	T40.714	T40.715	T40.716
Nabumetone	T39.391	T39.392	T39.393	T39.394	T39.395	T39.396
Nadolol	T44.7X1	T44.7X2	T44.7X3	T44.7X4	T44.7X5	T44.7X6
Nafcillin	T36.0X1	T36.0X2	T36.0X3	T36.0X4	T36.0X5	T36.0X6
Nafoxidine	T38.6X1	T38.6X2	T38.6X3	T38.6X4	T38.6X5	T38.6X6
Naftazone	T46.991	T46.992	T46.993	T46.994	T46.995	T46.996
Naftidrofuryl (oxalate)	T46.7X1	T46.7X2	T46.7X3	T46.7X4	T46.7X5	T46.7X6
Naftifine	T49.0X1	T49.0X2	T49.0X3	T49.0X4	T49.0X5	T49.0X6
Nail polish remover	T52.91	T52.92	T52.93	T52.94	—	—
Nalbuphine	T40.491	T40.492	T40.493	T40.494	T40.495	T40.496
Naled	T60.0X1	T60.0X2	T60.0X3	T60.0X4	—	—
Nalidixic acid	T37.8X1	T37.8X2	T37.8X3	T37.8X4	T37.8X5	T37.8X6
Nalorphine	T50.7X1	T50.7X2	T50.7X3	T50.7X4	T50.7X5	T50.7X6
Naloxone	T50.7X1	T50.7X2	T50.7X3	T50.7X4	T50.7X5	T50.7X6
Naltrexone	T50.7X1	T50.7X2	T50.7X3	T50.7X4	T50.7X5	T50.7X6
Namenda	T43.8X1	T43.8X2	T43.8X3	T43.8X4	T43.8X5	T43.8X6
Nandrolone	T38.7X1	T38.7X2	T38.7X3	T38.7X4	T38.7X5	T38.7X6
Naphazoline	T48.5X1	T48.5X2	T48.5X3	T48.5X4	T48.5X5	T48.5X6
Naphtha (painters') (petroleum)	T52.0X1	T52.0X2	T52.0X3	T52.0X4	—	—
solvent	T52.0X1	T52.0X2	T52.0X3	T52.0X4	—	—
vapor	T52.0X1	T52.0X2	T52.0X3	T52.0X4	—	—
Naphthalene (non-chlorinated)	T60.2X1	T60.2X2	T60.2X3	T60.2X4	—	—
chlorinated	T60.1X1	T60.1X2	T60.1X3	T60.1X4	—	—
vapor	T60.1X1	T60.1X2	T60.1X3	T60.1X4	—	—
insecticide or moth repellent	T60.2X1	T60.2X2	T60.2X3	T60.2X4	—	—
chlorinated	T60.1X1	T60.1X2	T60.1X3	T60.1X4	—	—
vapor	T60.2X1	T60.2X2	T60.2X3	T60.2X4	—	—
chlorinated	T60.1X1	T60.1X2	T60.1X3	T60.1X4	—	—
Naphthol	T65.891	T65.892	T65.893	T65.894	—	—

Substance	Poisoning, Accidental (unintentional)	Poisoning, Intentional self-harm	Poisoning, Assault	Poisoning, Undetermined	Adverse effect	Underdosing
Naphthylamine	T65.891	T65.892	T65.893	T65.894	—	—
Naphthylthiourea (ANTU)	T60.4X1	T60.4X2	T60.4X3	T60.4X4	—	—
Naprosyn—see Naproxen						
Naproxen	T39.311	T39.312	T39.313	T39.314	T39.315	T39.316
Narcotic (drug)	T40.601	T40.602	T40.603	T40.604	T40.605	T40.606
analgesic NEC	T40.601	T40.602	T40.603	T40.604	T40.605	T40.606
antagonist	T50.7X1	T50.7X2	T50.7X3	T50.7X4	T50.7X5	T50.7X6
specified NEC	T40.691	T40.692	T40.693	T40.694	T40.695	T40.696
synthetic	T40.491	T40.492	T40.493	T40.494	T40.495	T40.496
Narcotine	T48.3X1	T48.3X2	T48.3X3	T48.3X4	T48.3X5	T48.3X6
Nardil	T43.1X1	T43.1X2	T43.1X3	T43.1X4	T43.1X5	T43.1X6
Nasal drug NEC	T49.6X1	T49.6X2	T49.6X3	T49.6X4	T49.6X5	T49.6X6
Natamycin	T49.0X1	T49.0X2	T49.0X3	T49.0X4	T49.0X5	T49.0X6
Natrium cyanide—see Cyanide (s)						
Natural						
blood (product)	T45.8X1	T45.8X2	T45.8X3	T45.8X4	T45.8X5	T45.8X6
gas (piped)	T59.891	T59.892	T59.893	T59.894	—	—
incomplete combustion	T58.11	T58.12	T58.13	T58.14	—	—
Nealbarbital	T42.3X1	T42.3X2	T42.3X3	T42.3X4	T42.3X5	T42.3X6
Nectadon	T48.3X1	T48.3X2	T48.3X3	T48.3X4	T48.3X5	T48.3X6
Nedocromil	T48.6X1	T48.6X2	T48.6X3	T48.6X4	T48.6X5	T48.6X6
Nefopam	T39.8X1	T39.8X2	T39.8X3	T39.8X4	T39.8X5	T39.8X6
Nematocyst (sting)	T63.691	T63.692	T63.693	T63.694	—	—
Nembutal	T42.3X1	T42.3X2	T42.3X3	T42.3X4	T42.3X5	T42.3X6
Nemonapride	T43.591	T43.592	T43.593	T43.594	T43.595	T43.596
Neoarsphenamine	T37.8X1	T37.8X2	T37.8X3	T37.8X4	T37.8X5	T37.8X6
Neocinchophen	T50.4X1	T50.4X2	T50.4X3	T50.4X4	T50.4X5	T50.4X6
Neomycin (derivatives)	T36.5X1	T36.5X2	T36.5X3	T36.5X4	T36.5X5	T36.5X6
with						
bacitracin	T49.0X1	T49.0X2	T49.0X3	T49.0X4	T49.0X5	T49.0X6
neostigmine	T44.0X1	T44.0X2	T44.0X3	T44.0X4	T44.0X5	T44.0X6
ENT agent	T49.6X1	T49.6X2	T49.6X3	T49.6X4	T49.6X5	T49.6X6
ophthalmic preparation	T49.5X1	T49.5X2	T49.5X3	T49.5X4	T49.5X5	T49.5X6
topical NEC	T49.0X1	T49.0X2	T49.0X3	T49.0X4	T49.0X5	T49.0X6
Neonal	T42.3X1	T42.3X2	T42.3X3	T42.3X4	T42.3X5	T42.3X6
Neoprontosil	T37.0X1	T37.0X2	T37.0X3	T37.0X4	T37.0X5	T37.0X6
Neosalvarsan	T37.8X1	T37.8X2	T37.8X3	T37.8X4	T37.8X5	T37.8X6
Neosilversalvarsan	T37.8X1	T37.8X2	T37.8X3	T37.8X4	T37.8X5	T37.8X6
Neosporin	T36.8X1	T36.8X2	T36.8X3	T36.8X4	T36.8X5	T36.8X6
ENT agent	T49.6X1	T49.6X2	T49.6X3	T49.6X4	T49.6X5	T49.6X6
opthalmic preparation	T49.5X1	T49.5X2	T49.5X3	T49.5X4	T49.5X5	T49.5X6
topical NEC	T49.0X1	T49.0X2	T49.0X3	T49.0X4	T49.0X5	T49.0X6
Neostigmine bromide	T44.0X1	T44.0X2	T44.0X3	T44.0X4	T44.0X5	T44.0X6
Neraval	T42.3X1	T42.3X2	T42.3X3	T42.3X4	T42.3X5	T42.3X6
Neravan	T42.3X1	T42.3X2	T42.3X3	T42.3X4	T42.3X5	T42.3X6
Nerium oleander	T62.2X1	T62.2X2	T62.2X3	T62.2X4	—	—
Nerve gas, not in war	T59.91	T59.92	T59.93	T59.94	—	—

Substance	Poisoning, Accidental (unintentional)	Poisoning, Intentional self-harm	Poisoning, Assault	Poisoning, Undetermined	Adverse effect	Underdosing
Nesacaine	T41.3X1	T41.3X2	T41.3X3	T41.3X4	T41.3X5	T41.3X6
infiltration (subcutaneous)	T41.3X1	T41.3X2	T41.3X3	T41.3X4	T41.3X5	T41.3X6
nerve block (peripheral) (plexus)	T41.3X1	T41.3X2	T41.3X3	T41.3X4	T41.3X5	T41.3X6
Netilmicin	T36.5X1	T36.5X2	T36.5X3	T36.5X4	T36.5X5	T36.5X6
Neurobarb	T42.3X1	T42.3X2	T42.3X3	T42.3X4	T42.3X5	T42.3X6
Neuroleptic drug NEC	T43.501	T43.502	T43.503	T43.504	T43.505	T43.506
Neuromuscular blocking drug	T48.1X1	T48.1X2	T48.1X3	T48.1X4	T48.1X5	T48.1X6
Neutral insulin injection	T38.3X1	T38.3X2	T38.3X3	T38.3X4	T38.3X5	T38.3X6
Neutral spirits	T51.0X1	T51.0X2	T51.0X3	T51.0X4	—	—
beverage	T51.0X1	T51.0X2	T51.0X3	T51.0X4	—	—
Niacin	T46.7X1	T46.7X2	T46.7X3	T46.7X4	T46.7X5	T46.7X6
Niacinamide	T45.2X1	T45.2X2	T45.2X3	T45.2X4	T45.2X5	T45.2X6
Nialamide	T43.1X1	T43.1X2	T43.1X3	T43.1X4	T43.1X5	T43.1X6
Niaprazine	T42.6X1	T42.6X2	T42.6X3	T42.6X4	T42.6X5	T42.6X6
Nicametate	T46.7X1	T46.7X2	T46.7X3	T46.7X4	T46.7X5	T46.7X6
Nicardipine	T46.1X1	T46.1X2	T46.1X3	T46.1X4	T46.1X5	T46.1X6
Nicergoline	T46.7X1	T46.7X2	T46.7X3	T46.7X4	T46.7X5	T46.7X6
Nickel (carbonyl) (tetra-carbonyl) (fumes) (vapor)	T56.891	T56.892	T56.893	T56.894	—	—
Nickelocene	T56.891	T56.892	T56.893	T56.894	—	—
Niclosamide	T37.4X1	T37.4X2	T37.4X3	T37.4X4	T37.4X5	T37.4X6
Nicofuranose	T46.7X1	T46.7X2	T46.7X3	T46.7X4	T46.7X5	T46.7X6
Nicomorphine	T40.2X1	T40.2X2	T40.2X3	T40.2X4	—	—
Nicorandil	T46.3X1	T46.3X2	T46.3X3	T46.3X4	T46.3X5	T46.3X6
Nicotiana (plant)	T62.2X1	T62.2X2	T62.2X3	T62.2X4	—	—
Nicotinamide	T45.2X1	T45.2X2	T45.2X3	T45.2X4	T45.2X5	T45.2X6
Nicotine (insecticide) (spray) (sulfate) NEC	T60.2X1	T60.2X2	T60.2X3	T60.2X4	—	—
from tobacco	T65.291	T65.292	T65.293	T65.294	—	—
cigarettes	T65.221	T65.222	T65.223	T65.224	—	—
not insecticide	T65.291	T65.292	T65.293	T65.294	—	—
Nicotinic acid	T46.7X1	T46.7X2	T46.7X3	T46.7X4	T46.7X5	T46.7X6
Nicotinyl alcohol	T46.7X1	T46.7X2	T46.7X3	T46.7X4	T46.7X5	T46.7X6
Nicoumalone	T45.511	T45.512	T45.513	T45.514	T45.515	T45.516
Nifedipine	T46.1X1	T46.1X2	T46.1X3	T46.1X4	T46.1X5	T46.1X6
Nifenazone	T39.2X1	T39.2X2	T39.2X3	T39.2X4	T39.2X5	T39.2X6
Nifuraldezone	T37.91	T37.92	T37.93	T37.94	T37.95	T37.96
Nifuratel	T37.8X1	T37.8X2	T37.8X3	T37.8X4	T37.8X5	T37.8X6
Nifurtimox	T37.3X1	T37.3X2	T37.3X3	T37.3X4	T37.3X5	T37.3X6
Nifurtoinol	T37.8X1	T37.8X2	T37.8X3	T37.8X4	T37.8X5	T37.8X6
Nightshade, deadly (solanum)—see also Belladonna	T62.2X1	T62.2X2	T62.2X3	T62.2X4	—	—
berry	T62.1X1	T62.1X2	T62.1X3	T62.1X4	—	—
Nikethamide	T50.7X1	T50.7X2	T50.7X3	T50.7X4	T50.7X5	T50.7X6
Nilstat	T36.7X1	T36.7X2	T36.7X3	T36.7X4	T36.7X5	T36.7X6
topical	T49.0X1	T49.0X2	T49.0X3	T49.0X4	T49.0X5	T49.0X6
Nilutamide	T38.6X1	T38.6X2	T38.6X3	T38.6X4	T38.6X5	T38.6X6
Nimesulide	T39.391	T39.392	T39.393	T39.394	T39.395	T39.396
Nimetazepam	T42.4X1	T42.4X2	T42.4X3	T42.4X4	T42.4X5	T42.4X6
Nimodipine	T46.1X1	T46.1X2	T46.1X3	T46.1X4	T46.1X5	T46.1X6
Nimorazole	T37.3X1	T37.3X2	T37.3X3	T37.3X4	T37.3X5	T37.3X6
Nimustine	T45.1X1	T45.1X2	T45.1X3	T45.1X4	T45.1X5	T45.1X6
Niridazole	T37.4X1	T37.4X2	T37.4X3	T37.4X4	T37.4X5	T37.4X6
Nisentil	T40.2X1	T40.2X2	T40.2X3	T40.2X4	T40.2X5	T40.2X6
Nisoldipine	T46.1X1	T46.1X2	T46.1X3	T46.1X4	T46.1X5	T46.1X6
Nitramine	T65.3X1	T65.3X2	T65.3X3	T65.3X4	—	—
Nitrate, organic	T46.3X1	T46.3X2	T46.3X3	T46.3X4	T46.3X5	T46.3X6
Nitrazepam	T42.4X1	T42.4X2	T42.4X3	T42.4X4	T42.4X5	T42.4X6
Nitrefazole	T50.6X1	T50.6X2	T50.6X3	T50.6X4	T50.6X5	T50.6X6
Nitrendipine	T46.1X1	T46.1X2	T46.1X3	T46.1X4	T46.1X5	T46.1X6
Nitric						
acid (liquid)	T54.2X1	T54.2X2	T54.2X3	T54.2X4	—	—
vapor	T59.891	T59.892	T59.893	T59.894	—	—
oxide (gas)	T59.0X1	T59.0X2	T59.0X3	T59.0X4	—	—
Nitrimidazine	T37.3X1	T37.3X2	T37.3X3	T37.3X4	T37.3X5	T37.3X6
Nitrite, amyl (medicinal) (vapor)	T46.3X1	T46.3X2	T46.3X3	T46.3X4	T46.3X5	T46.3X6
Nitroaniline	T65.3X1	T65.3X2	T65.3X3	T65.3X4	—	—
vapor	T59.891	T59.892	T59.893	T59.894	—	—
Nitrobenzene, nitrobenzol	T65.3X1	T65.3X2	T65.3X3	T65.3X4	—	—
vapor	T65.3X1	T65.3X2	T65.3X3	T65.3X4	—	—
Nitrocellulose	T65.891	T65.892	T65.893	T65.894	—	—
lacquer	T65.891	T65.892	T65.893	T65.894	—	—
Nitrodiphenyl	T65.3X1	T65.3X2	T65.3X3	T65.3X4	—	—
Nitrofural	T49.0X1	T49.0X2	T49.0X3	T49.0X4	T49.0X5	T49.0X6
Nitrofurantoin	T37.8X1	T37.8X2	T37.8X3	T37.8X4	T37.8X5	T37.8X6
Nitrofurazone	T49.0X1	T49.0X2	T49.0X3	T49.0X4	T49.0X5	T49.0X6
Nitrogen	T59.0X1	T59.0X2	T59.0X3	T59.0X4	—	—
mustard	T45.1X1	T45.1X2	T45.1X3	T45.1X4	T45.1X5	T45.1X6
Nitroglycerin, nitro-glycerol (medicinal)	T46.3X1	T46.3X2	T46.3X3	T46.3X4	T46.3X5	T46.3X6
nonmedicinal	T65.5X1	T65.5X2	T65.5X3	T65.5X4	—	—
fumes	T65.5X1	T65.5X2	T65.5X3	T65.5X4	—	—
Nitroglycol	T52.3X1	T52.3X2	T52.3X3	T52.3X4	—	—
Nitrohydrochloric acid	T54.2X1	T54.2X2	T54.2X3	T54.2X4	—	—
Nitromersol	T49.0X1	T49.0X2	T49.0X3	T49.0X4	T49.0X5	T49.0X6
Nitronaphthalene	T65.891	T65.892	T65.893	T65.894	—	—
Nitrophenol	T54.0X1	T54.0X2	T54.0X3	T54.0X4	—	—
Nitropropane	T52.8X1	T52.8X2	T52.8X3	T52.8X4	—	—
Nitroprusside	T46.5X1	T46.5X2	T46.5X3	T46.5X4	T46.5X5	T46.5X6
Nitrosodimethylamine	T65.3X1	T65.3X2	T65.3X3	T65.3X4	—	—
Nitrothiazol	T37.4X1	T37.4X2	T37.4X3	T37.4X4	T37.4X5	T37.4X6
Nitrotoluene, nitrotoluol	T65.3X1	T65.3X2	T65.3X3	T65.3X4	—	—
vapor	T65.3X1	T65.3X2	T65.3X3	T65.3X4	—	—
Nitrous						
acid (liquid)	T54.2X1	T54.2X2	T54.2X3	T54.2X4	—	—
fumes	T59.891	T59.892	T59.893	T59.894	—	—

Substance	Poisoning, Accidental (unintentional)	Poisoning, Intentional self-harm	Poisoning, Assault	Poisoning, Undetermined	Adverse effect	Underdosing
Nitrous — *Continued*						
ether spirit	T46.3X1	T46.3X2	T46.3X3	T46.3X4	T46.3X5	T46.3X6
oxide	T41.0X1	T41.0X2	T41.0X3	T41.0X4	T41.0X5	T41.0X6
Nitroxoline	T37.8X1	T37.8X2	T37.8X3	T37.8X4	T37.8X5	T37.8X6
Nitrozone	T49.0X1	T49.0X2	T49.0X3	T49.0X4	T49.0X5	T49.0X6
Nizatidine	T47.0X1	T47.0X2	T47.0X3	T47.0X4	T47.0X5	T47.0X6
Nizofenone	T43.8X1	T43.8X2	T43.8X3	T43.8X4	T43.8X5	T43.8X6
Noctec	T42.6X1	T42.6X2	T42.6X3	T42.6X4	T42.6X5	T42.6X6
Noludar	T42.6X1	T42.6X2	T42.6X3	T42.6X4	T42.6X5	T42.6X6
Nomegestrol	T38.5X1	T38.5X2	T38.5X3	T38.5X4	T38.5X5	T38.5X6
Nomifensine	T43.291	T43.292	T43.293	T43.294	T43.295	T43.296
Nonoxinol	T49.8X1	T49.8X2	T49.8X3	T49.8X4	T49.8X5	T49.8X6
Nonylphenoxy (polyethoxy-ethanol)	T49.8X1	T49.8X2	T49.8X3	T49.8X4	T49.8X5	T49.8X6
Noptil	T42.3X1	T42.3X2	T42.3X3	T42.3X4	T42.3X5	T42.3X6
Noradrenaline	T44.4X1	T44.4X2	T44.4X3	T44.4X4	T44.4X5	T44.4X6
Noramidopyrine	T39.2X1	T39.2X2	T39.2X3	T39.2X4	T39.2X5	T39.2X6
methanesulfonate sodium	T39.2X1	T39.2X2	T39.2X3	T39.2X4	T39.2X5	T39.2X6
Norbormide	T60.4X1	T60.4X2	T60.4X3	T60.4X4	—	—
Nordazepam	T42.4X1	T42.4X2	T42.4X3	T42.4X4	T42.4X5	T42.4X6
Norepinephrine	T44.4X1	T44.4X2	T44.4X3	T44.4X4	T44.4X5	T44.4X6
Norethandrolone	T38.7X1	T38.7X2	T38.7X3	T38.7X4	T38.7X5	T38.7X6
Norethindrone	T38.4X1	T38.4X2	T38.4X3	T38.4X4	T38.4X5	T38.4X6
Norethisterone (acetate) (enantate)	T38.4X1	T38.4X2	T38.4X3	T38.4X4	T38.4X5	T38.4X6
with ethinylestradiol	T38.5X1	T38.5X2	T38.5X3	T38.5X4	T38.5X5	T38.5X6
Noretynodrel	T38.5X1	T38.5X2	T38.5X3	T38.5X4	T38.5X5	T38.5X6
Norfenefrine	T44.4X1	T44.4X2	T44.4X3	T44.4X4	T44.4X5	T44.4X6
Norfloxacin	T36.8X1	T36.8X2	T36.8X3	T36.8X4	T36.8X5	T36.8X6
Norgestrel	T38.4X1	T38.4X2	T38.4X3	T38.4X4	T38.4X5	T38.4X6
Norgestrienone	T38.4X1	T38.4X2	T38.4X3	T38.4X4	T38.4X5	T38.4X6
Norlestrin	T38.4X1	T38.4X2	T38.4X3	T38.4X4	T38.4X5	T38.4X6
Norlutin	T38.4X1	T38.4X2	T38.4X3	T38.4X4	T38.4X5	T38.4X6
Normal serum albumin (human), salt-poor	T45.8X1	T45.8X2	T45.8X3	T45.8X4	T45.8X5	T45.8X6
Normethandrone	T38.5X1	T38.5X2	T38.5X3	T38.5X4	T38.5X5	T38.5X6
Normison—see Benzodiazepines						
Normorphine	T40.2X1	T40.2X2	T40.2X3	T40.2X4	—	—
Norpseudoephedrine	T50.5X1	T50.5X2	T50.5X3	T50.5X4	T50.5X5	T50.5X6
Nortestosterone (furanpro pionate)	T38.7X1	T38.7X2	T38.7X3	T38.7X4	T38.7X5	T38.7X6
Nortriptyline	T43.011	T43.012	T43.013	T43.014	T43.015	T43.016
Noscapine	T48.3X1	T48.3X2	T48.3X3	T48.3X4	T48.3X5	T48.3X6
Nose preparations	T49.6X1	T49.6X2	T49.6X3	T49.6X4	T49.6X5	T49.6X6
Novobiocin	T36.5X1	T36.5X2	T36.5X3	T36.5X4	T36.5X5	T36.5X6
Novocain (infiltration) (topical)	T41.3X1	T41.3X2	T41.3X3	T41.3X4	T41.3X5	T41.3X6
nerve block (peripheral) (plexus)	T41.3X1	T41.3X2	T41.3X3	T41.3X4	T41.3X5	T41.3X6
spinal	T41.3X1	T41.3X2	T41.3X3	T41.3X4	T41.3X5	T41.3X6

Substance	Poisoning, Accidental (unintentional)	Poisoning, Intentional self-harm	Poisoning, Assault	Poisoning, Undetermined	Adverse effect	Underdosing
Noxious foodstuff	T62.91	T62.92	T62.93	T62.94	—	—
specified NEC	T62.8X1	T62.8X2	T62.8X3	T62.8X4	—	—
Noxiptiline	T43.011	T43.012	T43.013	T43.014	T43.015	T43.016
Noxytiolin	T49.0X1	T49.0X2	T49.0X3	T49.0X4	T49.0X5	T49.0X6
NPH Iletin (insulin)	T38.3X1	T38.3X2	T38.3X3	T38.3X4	T38.3X5	T38.3X6
Numorphan	T40.2X1	T40.2X2	T40.2X3	T40.2X4	T40.2X5	T40.2X6
Nunol	T42.3X1	T42.3X2	T42.3X3	T42.3X4	T42.3X5	T42.3X6
Nupercaine (spinal anesthetic)	T41.3X1	T41.3X2	T41.3X3	T41.3X4	T41.3X5	T41.3X6
topical (surface)	T41.3X1	T41.3X2	T41.3X3	T41.3X4	T41.3X5	T41.3X6
Nutmeg oil (liniment)	T49.3X1	T49.3X2	T49.3X3	T49.3X4	T49.3X5	T49.3X6
Nutritional supplement	T50.901	T50.902	T50.903	T50.904	T50.905	T50.906
Nux vomica	T65.1X1	T65.1X2	T65.1X3	T65.1X4	—	—
Nydrazid	T37.1X1	T37.1X2	T37.1X3	T37.1X4	T37.1X5	T37.1X6
Nylidrin	T46.7X1	T46.7X2	T46.7X3	T46.7X4	T46.7X5	T46.7X6
Nystatin	T36.7X1	T36.7X2	T36.7X3	T36.7X4	T36.7X5	T36.7X6
topical	T49.0X1	T49.0X2	T49.0X3	T49.0X4	T49.0X5	T49.0X6
Nytol	T45.0X1	T45.0X2	T45.0X3	T45.0X4	T45.0X5	T45.0X6
O						
Obidoxime chloride	T50.6X1	T50.6X2	T50.6X3	T50.6X4	T50.6X5	T50.6X6
Octafonium (chloride)	T49.3X1	T49.3X2	T49.3X3	T49.3X4	T49.3X5	T49.3X6
Octamethyl pyrophosphoramide	T60.0X1	T60.0X2	T60.0X3	T60.0X4	—	—
Octanoin	T50.991	T50.992	T50.993	T50.994	T50.995	T50.996
Octatropine methyl-bromide	T44.3X1	T44.3X2	T44.3X3	T44.3X4	T44.3X5	T44.3X6
Octotiamine	T45.2X1	T45.2X2	T45.2X3	T45.2X4	T45.2X5	T45.2X6
Octoxinol (9)	T49.8X1	T49.8X2	T49.8X3	T49.8X4	T49.8X5	T49.8X6
Octreotide	T38.991	T38.992	T38.993	T38.994	T38.995	T38.996
Octyl nitrite	T46.3X1	T46.3X2	T46.3X3	T46.3X4	T46.3X5	T46.3X6
Oestradiol	T38.5X1	T38.5X2	T38.5X3	T38.5X4	T38.5X5	T38.5X6
Oestriol	T38.5X1	T38.5X2	T38.5X3	T38.5X4	T38.5X5	T38.5X6
Oestrogen	T38.5X1	T38.5X2	T38.5X3	T38.5X4	T38.5X5	T38.5X6
Oestrone	T38.5X1	T38.5X2	T38.5X3	T38.5X4	T38.5X5	T38.5X6
Ofloxacin	T36.8X1	T36.8X2	T36.8X3	T36.8X4	T36.8X5	T36.8X6
Oil (of)	T65.891	T65.892	T65.893	T65.894	—	—
bitter almond	T62.8X1	T62.8X2	T62.8X3	T62.8X4	—	—
cloves	T49.7X1	T49.7X2	T49.7X3	T49.7X4	T49.7X5	T49.7X6
colors	T65.6X1	T65.6X2	T65.6X3	T65.6X4	—	—
fumes	T59.891	T59.892	T59.893	T59.894	—	—
lubricating	T52.0X1	T52.0X2	T52.0X3	T52.0X4	—	—
Niobe	T52.8X1	T52.8X2	T52.8X3	T52.8X4	—	—
vitriol (liquid)	T54.2X1	T54.2X2	T54.2X3	T54.2X4	—	—
fumes	T54.2X1	T54.2X2	T54.2X3	T54.2X4	—	—
wintergreen (bitter) NEC	T49.3X1	T49.3X2	T49.3X3	T49.3X4	T49.3X5	T49.3X6
Oily preparation (for skin)	T49.3X1	T49.3X2	T49.3X3	T49.3X4	T49.3X5	T49.3X6
Ointment NEC	T49.3X1	T49.3X2	T49.3X3	T49.3X4	T49.3X5	T49.3X6
Olanzapine	T43.591	T43.592	T43.593	T43.594	T43.595	T43.596
Oleander	T62.2X1	T62.2X2	T62.2X3	T62.2X4	—	—
Oleandomycin	T36.3X1	T36.3X2	T36.3X3	T36.3X4	T36.3X5	T36.3X6

Substance	Poisoning, Accidental (unintentional)	Poisoning, Intentional self-harm	Poisoning, Assault	Poisoning, Undetermined	Adverse effect	Underdosing
Oleandrin	T46.0X1	T46.0X2	T46.0X3	T46.0X4	T46.0X5	T46.0X6
Oleic acid	T46.6X1	T46.6X2	T46.6X3	T46.6X4	T46.6X5	T46.6X6
Oleovitamin A	T45.2X1	T45.2X2	T45.2X3	T45.2X4	T45.2X5	T45.2X6
Oleum ricini	T47.2X1	T47.2X2	T47.2X3	T47.2X4	T47.2X5	T47.2X6
Olive oil (medicinal) NEC	T47.4X1	T47.4X2	T47.4X3	T47.4X4	T47.4X5	T47.4X6
Olivomycin	T45.1X1	T45.1X2	T45.1X3	T45.1X4	T45.1X5	T45.1X6
Olsalazine	T47.8X1	T47.8X2	T47.8X3	T47.8X4	T47.8X5	T47.8X6
Omeprazole	T47.1X1	T47.1X2	T47.1X3	T47.1X4	T47.1X5	T47.1X6
OMPA	T60.0X1	T60.0X2	T60.0X3	T60.0X4	—	—
Oncovin	T45.1X1	T45.1X2	T45.1X3	T45.1X4	T45.1X5	T45.1X6
Ondansetron	T45.0X1	T45.0X2	T45.0X3	T45.0X4	T45.0X5	T45.0X6
Ophthaine	T41.3X1	T41.3X2	T41.3X3	T41.3X4	T41.3X5	T41.3X6
Ophthetic	T41.3X1	T41.3X2	T41.3X3	T41.3X4	T41.3X5	T41.3X6
Opiate NEC	T40.601	T40.602	T40.603	T40.604	T40.605	T40.606
antagonists	T50.7X1	T50.7X2	T50.7X3	T50.7X4	T50.7X5	T50.7X6
Opioid NEC	T40.2X1	T40.2X2	T40.2X3	T40.2X4	T40.2X5	T40.2X6
Opipramol	T43.011	T43.012	T43.013	T43.014	T43.015	T43.016
Opium alkaloids (total)	T40.0X1	T40.0X2	T40.0X3	T40.0X4	T40.0X5	T40.0X6
standardized powdered	T40.0X1	T40.0X2	T40.0X3	T40.0X4	T40.0X5	T40.0X6
tincture (camphorated)	T40.0X1	T40.0X2	T40.0X3	T40.0X4	T40.0X5	T40.0X6
Oracon	T38.4X1	T38.4X2	T38.4X3	T38.4X4	T38.4X5	T38.4X6
Oragrafin	T50.8X1	T50.8X2	T50.8X3	T50.8X4	T50.8X5	T50.8X6
Oral contraceptives	T38.4X1	T38.4X2	T38.4X3	T38.4X4	T38.4X5	T38.4X6
Oral rehydration salts	T50.3X1	T50.3X2	T50.3X3	T50.3X4	T50.3X5	T50.3X6
Orazamide	T50.991	T50.992	T50.993	T50.994	T50.995	T50.996
Orciprenaline	T48.291	T48.292	T48.293	T48.294	T48.295	T48.296
Organidin	T48.4X1	T48.4X2	T48.4X3	T48.4X4	T48.4X5	T48.4X6
Organonitrate NEC	T46.3X1	T46.3X2	T46.3X3	T46.3X4	T46.3X5	T46.3X6
Organophosphates	T60.0X1	T60.0X2	T60.0X3	T60.0X4	—	—
Orimune	T50.B91	T50.B92	T50.B93	T50.B94	T50.B95	T50.B96
Orinase	T38.3X1	T38.3X2	T38.3X3	T38.3X4	T38.3X5	T38.3X6
Ormeloxifene	T38.6X1	T38.6X2	T38.6X3	T38.6X4	T38.6X5	T38.6X6
Ornidazole	T37.3X1	T37.3X2	T37.3X3	T37.3X4	T37.3X5	T37.3X6
Ornithine aspartate	T50.991	T50.992	T50.993	T50.994	T50.995	T50.996
Ornoprostil	T47.1X1	T47.1X2	T47.1X3	T47.1X4	T47.1X5	T47.1X6
Orphenadrine (hydrochloride)	T42.8X1	T42.8X2	T42.8X3	T42.8X4	T42.8X5	T42.8X6
Ortal (sodium)	T42.3X1	T42.3X2	T42.3X3	T42.3X4	T42.3X5	T42.3X6
Orthoboric acid	T49.0X1	T49.0X2	T49.0X3	T49.0X4	T49.0X5	T49.0X6
ENT agent	T49.6X1	T49.6X2	T49.6X3	T49.6X4	T49.6X5	T49.6X6
ophthalmic preparation	T49.5X1	T49.5X2	T49.5X3	T49.5X4	T49.5X5	T49.5X6
Orthocaine	T41.3X1	T41.3X2	T41.3X3	T41.3X4	T41.3X5	T41.3X6
Orthodichlorobenzene	T53.7X1	T53.7X2	T53.7X3	T53.7X4	—	—
Ortho-Novum	T38.4X1	T38.4X2	T38.4X3	T38.4X4	T38.4X5	T38.4X6
Orthotolidine (reagent)	T54.2X1	T54.2X2	T54.2X3	T54.2X4	—	—
Osmic acid (liquid)	T54.2X1	T54.2X2	T54.2X3	T54.2X4	—	—
fumes	T54.2X1	T54.2X2	T54.2X3	T54.2X4	—	—
Osmotic diuretics	T50.2X1	T50.2X2	T50.2X3	T50.2X4	T50.2X5	T50.2X6
Otilonium bromide	T44.3X1	T44.3X2	T44.3X3	T44.3X4	T44.3X5	T44.3X6

Substance	Poisoning, Accidental (unintentional)	Poisoning, Intentional self-harm	Poisoning, Assault	Poisoning, Undetermined	Adverse effect	Underdosing
Otorhinolaryngological drug NEC	T49.6X1	T49.6X2	T49.6X3	T49.6X4	T49.6X5	T49.6X6
Ouabain(e)	T46.0X1	T46.0X2	T46.0X3	T46.0X4	T46.0X5	T46.0X6
Ovarian						
hormone	T38.5X1	T38.5X2	T38.5X3	T38.5X4	T38.5X5	T38.5X6
stimulant	T38.5X1	T38.5X2	T38.5X3	T38.5X4	T38.5X5	T38.5X6
Ovral	T38.4X1	T38.4X2	T38.4X3	T38.4X4	T38.4X5	T38.4X6
Ovulen	T38.4X1	T38.4X2	T38.4X3	T38.4X4	T38.4X5	T38.4X6
Oxacillin	T36.0X1	T36.0X2	T36.0X3	T36.0X4	T36.0X5	T36.0X6
Oxalic acid	T54.2X1	T54.2X2	T54.2X3	T54.2X4	—	—
ammonium salt	T50.991	T50.992	T50.993	T50.994	T50.995	T50.996
Oxamniquine	T37.4X1	T37.4X2	T37.4X3	T37.4X4	T37.4X5	T37.4X6
Oxanamide	T43.591	T43.592	T43.593	T43.594	T43.595	T43.596
Oxandrolone	T38.7X1	T38.7X2	T38.7X3	T38.7X4	T38.7X5	T38.7X6
Oxantel	T37.4X1	T37.4X2	T37.4X3	T37.4X4	T37.4X5	T37.4X6
Oxapium iodide	T44.3X1	T44.3X2	T44.3X3	T44.3X4	T44.3X5	T44.3X6
Oxaprotiline	T43.021	T43.022	T43.023	T43.024	T43.025	T43.026
Oxaprozin	T39.311	T39.312	T39.313	T39.314	T39.315	T39.316
Oxatomide	T45.0X1	T45.0X2	T45.0X3	T45.0X4	T45.0X5	T45.0X6
Oxazepam	T42.4X1	T42.4X2	T42.4X3	T42.4X4	T42.4X5	T42.4X6
Oxazimedrine	T50.5X1	T50.5X2	T50.5X3	T50.5X4	T50.5X5	T50.5X6
Oxazolam	T42.4X1	T42.4X2	T42.4X3	T42.4X4	T42.4X5	T42.4X6
Oxazolidine derivatives	T42.2X1	T42.2X2	T42.2X3	T42.2X4	T42.2X5	T42.2X6
Oxazolidinedione (derivative)	T42.2X1	T42.2X2	T42.2X3	T42.2X4	T42.2X5	T42.2X6
Ox bile extract	T47.5X1	T47.5X2	T47.5X3	T47.5X4	T47.5X5	T47.5X6
Oxcarbazepine	T42.1X1	T42.1X2	T42.1X3	T42.1X4	T42.1X5	T42.1X6
Oxedrine	T44.4X1	T44.4X2	T44.4X3	T44.4X4	T44.4X5	T44.4X6
Oxeladin (citrate)	T48.3X1	T48.3X2	T48.3X3	T48.3X4	T48.3X5	T48.3X6
Oxendolone	T38.5X1	T38.5X2	T38.5X3	T38.5X4	T38.5X5	T38.5X6
Oxetacaine	T41.3X1	T41.3X2	T41.3X3	T41.3X4	T41.3X5	T41.3X6
Oxethazine	T41.3X1	T41.3X2	T41.3X3	T41.3X4	T41.3X5	T41.3X6
Oxetorone	T39.8X1	T39.8X2	T39.8X3	T39.8X4	T39.8X5	T39.8X6
Oxiconazole	T49.0X1	T49.0X2	T49.0X3	T49.0X4	T49.0X5	T49.0X6
Oxidizing agent NEC	T54.91	T54.92	T54.93	T54.94	—	—
Oxipurinol	T50.4X1	T50.4X2	T50.4X3	T50.4X4	T50.4X5	T50.4X6
Oxitriptan	T43.291	T43.292	T43.293	T43.294	T43.295	T43.296
Oxitropium bromide	T48.6X1	T48.6X2	T48.6X3	T48.6X4	T48.6X5	T48.6X6
Oxodipine	T46.1X1	T46.1X2	T46.1X3	T46.1X4	T46.1X5	T46.1X6
Oxolamine	T48.3X1	T48.3X2	T48.3X3	T48.3X4	T48.3X5	T48.3X6
Oxolinic acid	T37.8X1	T37.8X2	T37.8X3	T37.8X4	T37.8X5	T37.8X6
Oxomemazine	T43.3X1	T43.3X2	T43.3X3	T43.3X4	T43.3X5	T43.3X6
Oxophenarsine	T37.3X1	T37.3X2	T37.3X3	T37.3X4	T37.3X5	T37.3X6
Oxprenolol	T44.7X1	T44.7X2	T44.7X3	T44.7X4	T44.7X5	T44.7X6
Oxsoralen	T49.3X1	T49.3X2	T49.3X3	T49.3X4	T49.3X5	T49.3X6
Oxtriphylline	T48.6X1	T48.6X2	T48.6X3	T48.6X4	T48.6X5	T48.6X6
Oxybate sodium	T41.291	T41.292	T41.293	T41.294	T41.295	T41.296
Oxybuprocaine	T41.3X1	T41.3X2	T41.3X3	T41.3X4	T41.3X5	T41.3X6
Oxybutynin	T44.3X1	T44.3X2	T44.3X3	T44.3X4	T44.3X5	T44.3X6
Oxychlorosene	T49.0X1	T49.0X2	T49.0X3	T49.0X4	T49.0X5	T49.0X6

Substance	Poisoning, Accidental (unintentional)	Poisoning, Intentional self-harm	Poisoning, Assault	Poisoning, Undetermined	Adverse effect	Underdosing
Oxycodone	T40.2X1	T40.2X2	T40.2X3	T40.2X4	T40.2X5	T40.2X6
Oxyfedrine	T46.3X1	T46.3X2	T46.3X3	T46.3X4	T46.3X5	T46.3X6
Oxygen	T41.5X1	T41.5X2	T41.5X3	T41.5X4	T41.5X5	T41.5X6
Oxylone	T49.0X1	T49.0X2	T49.0X3	T49.0X4	T49.0X5	T49.0X6
ophthalmic preparation	T49.5X1	T49.5X2	T49.5X3	T49.5X4	T49.5X5	T49.5X6
Oxymesterone	T38.7X1	T38.7X2	T38.7X3	T38.7X4	T38.7X5	T38.7X6
Oxymetazoline	T48.5X1	T48.5X2	T48.5X3	T48.5X4	T48.5X5	T48.5X6
Oxymetholone	T38.7X1	T38.7X2	T38.7X3	T38.7X4	T38.7X5	T38.7X6
Oxymorphone	T40.2X1	T40.2X2	T40.2X3	T40.2X4	T40.2X5	T40.2X6
Oxypertine	T43.591	T43.592	T43.593	T43.594	T43.595	T43.596
Oxyphenbutazone	T39.2X1	T39.2X2	T39.2X3	T39.2X4	T39.2X5	T39.2X6
Oxyphencyclimine	T44.3X1	T44.3X2	T44.3X3	T44.3X4	T44.3X5	T44.3X6
Oxyphenisatine	T47.2X1	T47.2X2	T47.2X3	T47.2X4	T47.2X5	T47.2X6
Oxyphenonium bromide	T44.3X1	T44.3X2	T44.3X3	T44.3X4	T44.3X5	T44.3X6
Oxypolygelatin	T45.8X1	T45.8X2	T45.8X3	T45.8X4	T45.8X5	T45.8X6
Oxyquinoline (derivatives)	T37.8X1	T37.8X2	T37.8X3	T37.8X4	T37.8X5	T37.8X6
Oxytetracycline	T36.4X1	T36.4X2	T36.4X3	T36.4X4	T36.4X5	T36.4X6
Oxytocic drug NEC	T48.0X1	T48.0X2	T48.0X3	T48.0X4	T48.0X5	T48.0X6
Oxytocin (synthetic)	T48.0X1	T48.0X2	T48.0X3	T48.0X4	T48.0X5	T48.0X6
Ozone	T59.891	T59.892	T59.893	T59.894	—	—
P						
PABA	T49.3X1	T49.3X2	T49.3X3	T49.3X4	T49.3X5	T49.3X6
Packed red cells	T45.8X1	T45.8X2	T45.8X3	T45.8X4	T45.8X5	T45.8X6
Padimate	T49.3X1	T49.3X2	T49.3X3	T49.3X4	T49.3X5	T49.3X6
Paint NEC	T65.6X1	T65.6X2	T65.6X3	T65.6X4	—	—
cleaner	T52.91	T52.92	T52.93	T52.94	—	—
fumes NEC	T59.891	T59.892	T59.893	T59.894	—	—
lead (fumes)	T56.0X1	T56.0X2	T56.0X3	T56.0X4	—	—
solvent NEC	T52.8X1	T52.8X2	T52.8X3	T52.8X4	—	—
stripper	T52.8X1	T52.8X2	T52.8X3	T52.8X4	—	—
Palfium	T40.2X1	T40.2X2	T40.2X3	T40.2X4	—	—
Palm kernel oil	T50.991	T50.992	T50.993	T50.994	T50.995	T50.996
Paludrine	T37.2X1	T37.2X2	T37.2X3	T37.2X4	T37.2X5	T37.2X6
PAM (pralidoxime)	T50.6X1	T50.6X2	T50.6X3	T50.6X4	T50.6X5	T50.6X6
Pamaquine (naphthoute)	T37.2X1	T37.2X2	T37.2X3	T37.2X4	T37.2X5	T37.2X6
Panadol	T39.1X1	T39.1X2	T39.1X3	T39.1X4	T39.1X5	T39.1X6
Pancreatic						
digestive secretion stimulant	T47.8X1	T47.8X2	T47.8X3	T47.8X4	T47.8X5	T47.8X6
dornase	T45.3X1	T45.3X2	T45.3X3	T45.3X4	T45.3X5	T45.3X6
Pancreatin	T47.5X1	T47.5X2	T47.5X3	T47.5X4	T47.5X5	T47.5X6
Pancrelipase	T47.5X1	T47.5X2	T47.5X3	T47.5X4	T47.5X5	T47.5X6
Pancuronium (bromide)	T48.1X1	T48.1X2	T48.1X3	T48.1X4	T48.1X5	T48.1X6
Pangamic acid	T45.2X1	T45.2X2	T45.2X3	T45.2X4	T45.2X5	T45.2X6
Panthenol	T45.2X1	T45.2X2	T45.2X3	T45.2X4	T45.2X5	T45.2X6
topical	T49.8X1	T49.8X2	T49.8X3	T49.8X4	T49.8X5	T49.8X6
Pantopon	T40.0X1	T40.0X2	T40.0X3	T40.0X4	T40.0X5	T40.0X6
Pantothenic acid	T45.2X1	T45.2X2	T45.2X3	T45.2X4	T45.2X5	T45.2X6
Panwarfin	T45.511	T45.512	T45.513	T45.514	T45.515	T45.516

Substance	Poisoning, Accidental (unintentional)	Poisoning, Intentional self-harm	Poisoning, Assault	Poisoning, Undetermined	Adverse effect	Underdosing
Papain	T47.5X1	T47.5X2	T47.5X3	T47.5X4	T47.5X5	T47.5X6
digestant	T47.5X1	T47.5X2	T47.5X3	T47.5X4	T47.5X5	T47.5X6
Papaveretum	T40.0X1	T40.0X2	T40.0X3	T40.0X4	T40.0X5	T40.0X6
Papaverine	T44.3X1	T44.3X2	T44.3X3	T44.3X4	T44.3X5	T44.3X6
Para-acetamidophenol	T39.1X1	T39.1X2	T39.1X3	T39.1X4	T39.1X5	T39.1X6
Para-aminobenzoic acid	T49.3X1	T49.3X2	T49.3X3	T49.3X4	T49.3X5	T49.3X6
Para-aminophenol derivatives	T39.1X1	T39.1X2	T39.1X3	T39.1X4	T39.1X5	T39.1X6
Para-aminosalicylic acid	T37.1X1	T37.1X2	T37.1X3	T37.1X4	T37.1X5	T37.1X6
Paracetaldehyde	T42.6X1	T42.6X2	T42.6X3	T42.6X4	T42.6X5	T42.6X6
Paracetamol	T39.1X1	T39.1X2	T39.1X3	T39.1X4	T39.1X5	T39.1X6
Parachlorophenol (camphorated)	T49.0X1	T49.0X2	T49.0X3	T49.0X4	T49.0X5	T49.0X6
Paracodin	T40.2X1	T40.2X2	T40.2X3	T40.2X4	T40.2X5	T40.2X6
Paradione	T42.2X1	T42.2X2	T42.2X3	T42.2X4	T42.2X5	T42.2X6
Paraffin(s) (wax)	T52.0X1	T52.0X2	T52.0X3	T52.0X4	—	—
liquid (medicinal)	T47.4X1	T47.4X2	T47.4X3	T47.4X4	T47.4X5	T47.4X6
nonmedicinal	T52.0X1	T52.0X2	T52.0X3	T52.0X4	—	—
Paraformaldehyde	T60.3X1	T60.3X2	T60.3X3	T60.3X4	—	—
Paraldehyde	T42.6X1	T42.6X2	T42.6X3	T42.6X4	T42.6X5	T42.6X6
Paramethadione	T42.2X1	T42.2X2	T42.2X3	T42.2X4	T42.2X5	T42.2X6
Paramethasone	T38.0X1	T38.0X2	T38.0X3	T38.0X4	T38.0X5	T38.0X6
acetate	T49.0X1	T49.0X2	T49.0X3	T49.0X4	T49.0X5	T49.0X6
Paraoxon	T60.0X1	T60.0X2	T60.0X3	T60.0X4	—	—
Paraquat	T60.3X1	T60.3X2	T60.3X3	T60.3X4	—	—
Parasympatholytic NEC	T44.3X1	T44.3X2	T44.3X3	T44.3X4	T44.3X5	T44.3X6
Parasympathomimetic drug NEC	T44.1X1	T44.1X2	T44.1X3	T44.1X4	T44.1X5	T44.1X6
Parathion	T60.0X1	T60.0X2	T60.0X3	T60.0X4	—	—
Parathormone	T50.991	T50.992	T50.993	T50.994	T50.995	T50.996
Parathyroid extract	T50.991	T50.992	T50.993	T50.994	T50.995	T50.996
Paratyphoid vaccine	T50.A91	T50.A92	T50.A93	T50.A94	T50.A95	T50.A96
Paredrine	T44.4X1	T44.4X2	T44.4X3	T44.4X4	T44.4X5	T44.4X6
Paregoric	T40.0X1	T40.0X2	T40.0X3	T40.0X4	T40.0X5	T40.0X6
Pargyline	T46.5X1	T46.5X2	T46.5X3	T46.5X4	T46.5X5	T46.5X6
Paris green	T57.0X1	T57.0X2	T57.0X3	T57.0X4	—	—
insecticide	T57.0X1	T57.0X2	T57.0X3	T57.0X4	—	—
Parnate	T43.1X1	T43.1X2	T43.1X3	T43.1X4	T43.1X5	T43.1X6
Paromomycin	T36.5X1	T36.5X2	T36.5X3	T36.5X4	T36.5X5	T36.5X6
Paroxypropione	T45.1X1	T45.1X2	T45.1X3	T45.1X4	T45.1X5	T45.1X6
Parzone	T40.2X1	T40.2X2	T40.2X3	T40.2X4	T40.2X5	T40.2X6
PAS	T37.1X1	T37.1X2	T37.1X3	T37.1X4	T37.1X5	T37.1X6
Pasiniazid	T37.1X1	T37.1X2	T37.1X3	T37.1X4	T37.1X5	T37.1X6
PBB (polybrominated biphenyls)	T65.891	T65.892	T65.893	T65.894	—	—
PCB	T65.891	T65.892	T65.893	T65.894	—	—
PCP						
meaning pentachlorophenol	T60.1X1	T60.1X2	T60.1X3	T60.1X4	—	—
fungicide	T60.3X1	T60.3X2	T60.3X3	T60.3X4	—	—
herbicide	T60.3X1	T60.3X2	T60.3X3	T60.3X4	—	—
insecticide	T60.1X1	T60.1X2	T60.1X3	T60.1X4	—	—
meaning phencyclidine	T40.991	T40.992	T40.993	T40.994	—	—

Table of Drugs and Chemicals

Peach kernel oil–Pertofrane

Substance	Poisoning, Accidental (unintentional)	Poisoning, Intentional self-harm	Poisoning, Assault	Poisoning, Undetermined	Adverse effect	Underdosing
Peach kernel oil (emulsion)	T47.4X1	T47.4X2	T47.4X3	T47.4X4	T47.4X5	T47.4X6
Peanut oil (emulsion) NEC	T47.4X1	T47.4X2	T47.4X3	T47.4X4	T47.4X5	T47.4X6
topical	T49.3X1	T49.3X2	T49.3X3	T49.3X4	T49.3X5	T49.3X6
Pearly Gates (morning glory seeds)	T40.991	T40.992	T40.993	T40.994	—	—
Pecazine	T43.3X1	T43.3X2	T43.3X3	T43.3X4	T43.3X5	T43.3X6
Pectin	T47.6X1	T47.6X2	T47.6X3	T47.6X4	T47.6X5	T47.6X6
Pefloxacin	T37.8X1	T37.8X2	T37.8X3	T37.8X4	T37.8X5	T37.8X6
Pegademase, bovine	T50.Z91	T50.Z92	T50.Z93	T50.Z94	T50.Z95	T50.Z96
Pelletierine tannate	T37.4X1	T37.4X2	T37.4X3	T37.4X4	T37.4X5	T37.4X6
Pemirolast (potassium)	T48.6X1	T48.6X2	T48.6X3	T48.6X4	T48.6X5	T48.6X6
Pemoline	T50.7X1	T50.7X2	T50.7X3	T50.7X4	T50.7X5	T50.7X6
Pempidine	T44.2X1	T44.2X2	T44.2X3	T44.2X4	T44.2X5	T44.2X6
Penamecillin	T36.0X1	T36.0X2	T36.0X3	T36.0X4	T36.0X5	T36.0X6
Penbutolol	T44.7X1	T44.7X2	T44.7X3	T44.7X4	T44.7X5	T44.7X6
Penethamate	T36.0X1	T36.0X2	T36.0X3	T36.0X4	T36.0X5	T36.0X6
Penfluridol	T43.591	T43.592	T43.593	T43.594	T43.595	T43.596
Penflutizide	T50.2X1	T50.2X2	T50.2X3	T50.2X4	T50.2X5	T50.2X6
Pengitoxin	T46.0X1	T46.0X2	T46.0X3	T46.0X4	T46.0X5	T46.0X6
Penicillamine	T50.6X1	T50.6X2	T50.6X3	T50.6X4	T50.6X5	T50.6X6
Penicillin (any)	T36.0X1	T36.0X2	T36.0X3	T36.0X4	T36.0X5	T36.0X6
Penicillinase	T45.3X1	T45.3X2	T45.3X3	T45.3X4	T45.3X5	T45.3X6
Penicilloyl polylysine	T50.8X1	T50.8X2	T50.8X3	T50.8X4	T50.8X5	T50.8X6
Penimepicycline	T36.4X1	T36.4X2	T36.4X3	T36.4X4	T36.4X5	T36.4X6
Pentachloroethane	T53.6X1	T53.6X2	T53.6X3	T53.6X4	—	—
Pentachloronaphthalene	T53.7X1	T53.7X2	T53.7X3	T53.7X4	—	—
Pentachlorophenol (pesticide)	T60.1X1	T60.1X2	T60.1X3	T60.1X4	—	—
fungicide	T60.3X1	T60.3X2	T60.3X3	T60.3X4	—	—
herbicide	T60.3X1	T60.3X2	T60.3X3	T60.3X4	—	—
insecticide	T60.1X1	T60.1X2	T60.1X3	T60.1X4	—	—
Pentaerythritol	T46.3X1	T46.3X2	T46.3X3	T46.3X4	T46.3X5	T46.3X6
chloral	T42.6X1	T42.6X2	T42.6X3	T42.6X4	T42.6X5	T42.6X6
tetranitrate NEC	T46.3X1	T46.3X2	T46.3X3	T46.3X4	T46.3X5	T46.3X6
Pentaerythrityl tetranitrate	T46.3X1	T46.3X2	T46.3X3	T46.3X4	T46.3X5	T46.3X6
Pentagastrin	T50.8X1	T50.8X2	T50.8X3	T50.8X4	T50.8X5	T50.8X6
Pentalin	T53.6X1	T53.6X2	T53.6X3	T53.6X4	—	—
Pentamethonium bromide	T44.2X1	T44.2X2	T44.2X3	T44.2X4	T44.2X5	T44.2X6
Pentamidine	T37.3X1	T37.3X2	T37.3X3	T37.3X4	T37.3X5	T37.3X6
Pentanol	T51.3X1	T51.3X2	T51.3X3	T51.3X4	—	—
Pentapyrrolinium (bitartrate)	T44.2X1	T44.2X2	T44.2X3	T44.2X4	T44.2X5	T44.2X6
Pentaquine	T37.2X1	T37.2X2	T37.2X3	T37.2X4	T37.2X5	T37.2X6
Pentazocine	T40.491	T40.492	T40.493	T40.494	T40.495	T40.496
Pentetrazole	T50.7X1	T50.7X2	T50.7X3	T50.7X4	T50.7X5	T50.7X6
Penthienate bromide	T44.3X1	T44.3X2	T44.3X3	T44.3X4	T44.3X5	T44.3X6
Pentifylline	T46.7X1	T46.7X2	T46.7X3	T46.7X4	T46.7X5	T46.7X6

Substance	Poisoning, Accidental (unintentional)	Poisoning, Intentional self-harm	Poisoning, Assault	Poisoning, Undetermined	Adverse effect	Underdosing
Pentobarbital	T42.3X1	T42.3X2	T42.3X3	T42.3X4	T42.3X5	T42.3X6
sodium	T42.3X1	T42.3X2	T42.3X3	T42.3X4	T42.3X5	T42.3X6
Pentobarbitone	T42.3X1	T42.3X2	T42.3X3	T42.3X4	T42.3X5	T42.3X6
Pentolonium tartrate	T44.2X1	T44.2X2	T44.2X3	T44.2X4	T44.2X5	T44.2X6
Pentosan polysulfate (sodium)	T39.8X1	T39.8X2	T39.8X3	T39.8X4	T39.8X5	T39.8X6
Pentostatin	T45.1X1	T45.1X2	T45.1X3	T45.1X4	T45.1X5	T45.1X6
Pentothal	T41.1X1	T41.1X2	T41.1X3	T41.1X4	T41.1X5	T41.1X6
Pentoxifylline	T46.7X1	T46.7X2	T46.7X3	T46.7X4	T46.7X5	T46.7X6
Pentoxyverine	T48.3X1	T48.3X2	T48.3X3	T48.3X4	T48.3X5	T48.3X6
Pentrinat	T46.3X1	T46.3X2	T46.3X3	T46.3X4	T46.3X5	T46.3X6
Pentylenetetrazole	T50.7X1	T50.7X2	T50.7X3	T50.7X4	T50.7X5	T50.7X6
Pentylsalicylamide	T37.1X1	T37.1X2	T37.1X3	T37.1X4	T37.1X5	T37.1X6
Pentymal	T42.3X1	T42.3X2	T42.3X3	T42.3X4	T42.3X5	T42.3X6
Peplomycin	T45.1X1	T45.1X2	T45.1X3	T45.1X4	T45.1X5	T45.1X6
Peppermint (oil)	T47.5X1	T47.5X2	T47.5X3	T47.5X4	T47.5X5	T47.5X6
Pepsin	T47.5X1	T47.5X2	T47.5X3	T47.5X4	T47.5X5	T47.5X6
digestant	T47.5X1	T47.5X2	T47.5X3	T47.5X4	T47.5X5	T47.5X6
Pepstatin	T47.1X1	T47.1X2	T47.1X3	T47.1X4	T47.1X5	T47.1X6
Peptavlon	T50.8X1	T50.8X2	T50.8X3	T50.8X4	T50.8X5	T50.8X6
Perazine	T43.3X1	T43.3X2	T43.3X3	T43.3X4	T43.3X5	T43.3X6
Percaine (spinal)	T41.3X1	T41.3X2	T41.3X3	T41.3X4	T41.3X5	T41.3X6
topical (surface)	T41.3X1	T41.3X2	T41.3X3	T41.3X4	T41.3X5	T41.3X6
Perchloroethylene	T53.3X1	T53.3X2	T53.3X3	T53.3X4	—	—
medicinal	T37.4X1	T37.4X2	T37.4X3	T37.4X4	T37.4X5	T37.4X6
vapor	T53.3X1	T53.3X2	T53.3X3	T53.3X4	—	—
Percodan	T40.2X1	T40.2X2	T40.2X3	T40.2X4	T40.2X5	T40.2X6
Percogesic—see also acetaminophen	T45.0X1	T45.0X2	T45.0X3	T45.0X4	T45.0X5	T45.0X6
Percorten	T38.0X1	T38.0X2	T38.0X3	T38.0X4	T38.0X5	T38.0X6
Pergolide	T42.8X1	T42.8X2	T42.8X3	T42.8X4	T42.8X5	T42.8X6
Pergonal	T38.811	T38.812	T38.813	T38.814	T38.815	T38.816
Perhexilene	T46.3X1	T46.3X2	T46.3X3	T46.3X4	T46.3X5	T46.3X6
Perhexiline (maleate)	T46.3X1	T46.3X2	T46.3X3	T46.3X4	T46.3X5	T46.3X6
Periactin	T45.0X1	T45.0X2	T45.0X3	T45.0X4	T45.0X5	T45.0X6
Periciazine	T43.3X1	T43.3X2	T43.3X3	T43.3X4	T43.3X5	T43.3X6
Periclor	T42.6X1	T42.6X2	T42.6X3	T42.6X4	T42.6X5	T42.6X6
Perindopril	T46.4X1	T46.4X2	T46.4X3	T46.4X4	T46.4X5	T46.4X6
Perisoxal	T39.8X1	T39.8X2	T39.8X3	T39.8X4	T39.8X5	T39.8X6
Peritoneal dialysis solution	T50.3X1	T50.3X2	T50.3X3	T50.3X4	T50.3X5	T50.3X6
Peritrate	T46.3X1	T46.3X2	T46.3X3	T46.3X4	T46.3X5	T46.3X6
Perlapine	T42.4X1	T42.4X2	T42.4X3	T42.4X4	T42.4X5	T42.4X6
Permanganate	T65.891	T65.892	T65.893	T65.894	—	—
Permethrin	T60.1X1	T60.1X2	T60.1X3	T60.1X4	—	—
Pernocton	T42.3X1	T42.3X2	T42.3X3	T42.3X4	T42.3X5	T42.3X6
Pernoston	T42.3X1	T42.3X2	T42.3X3	T42.3X4	T42.3X5	T42.3X6
Peronine	T40.2X1	T40.2X2	T40.2X3	T40.2X4	—	—
Perphenazine	T43.3X1	T43.3X2	T43.3X3	T43.3X4	T43.3X5	T43.3X6
Pertofrane	T43.011	T43.012	T43.013	T43.014	T43.015	T43.016

Substance	Poisoning, Accidental (unintentional)	Poisoning, Intentional self-harm	Poisoning, Assault	Poisoning, Undetermined	Adverse effect	Underdosing
Pertussis						
immune serum (human)	T50.Z11	T50.Z12	T50.Z13	T50.Z14	T50.Z15	T50.Z16
vaccine (with diphtheria toxoid) (with tetanus toxoid)	T50.A11	T50.A12	T50.A13	T50.A14	T50.A15	T50.A16
Peruvian balsam	T49.0X1	T49.0X2	T49.0X3	T49.0X4	T49.0X5	T49.0X6
Peruvoside	T46.0X1	T46.0X2	T46.0X3	T46.0X4	T46.0X5	T46.0X6
Pesticide (dust) (fumes) (vapor) NEC	T60.91	T60.92	T60.93	T60.94	—	—
arsenic	T57.0X1	T57.0X2	T57.0X3	T57.0X4		
chlorinated	T60.1X1	T60.1X2	T60.1X3	T60.1X4		
cyanide	T65.0X1	T65.0X2	T65.0X3	T65.0X4		
kerosene	T52.0X1	T52.0X2	T52.0X3	T52.0X4		
mixture (of compounds)	T60.91	T60.92	T60.93	T60.94		
naphthalene	T60.2X1	T60.2X2	T60.2X3	T60.2X4		
organochlorine (compounds)	T60.1X1	T60.1X2	T60.1X3	T60.1X4		
petroleum (distillate) (products) NEC	T60.8X1	T60.8X2	T60.8X3	T60.8X4		
specified ingredient NEC	T60.8X1	T60.8X2	T60.8X3	T60.8X4		
strychnine	T65.1X1	T65.1X2	T65.1X3	T65.1X4		
thallium	T60.4X1	T60.4X2	T60.4X3	T60.4X4		
Pethidine	T40.491	T40.492	T40.493	T40.494	T40.495	T40.496
Petrichloral	T42.6X1	T42.6X2	T42.6X3	T42.6X4	T42.6X5	T42.6X6
Petrol	T52.0X1	T52.0X2	T52.0X3	T52.0X4		
vapor	T52.0X1	T52.0X2	T52.0X3	T52.0X4	—	—
Petrolatum	T49.3X1	T49.3X2	T49.3X3	T49.3X4	T49.3X5	T49.3X6
hydrophilic	T49.3X1	T49.3X2	T49.3X3	T49.3X4	T49.3X5	T49.3X6
liquid	T47.4X1	T47.4X2	T47.4X3	T47.4X4	T47.4X5	T47.4X6
topical	T49.3X1	T49.3X2	T49.3X3	T49.3X4	T49.3X5	T49.3X6
nonmedicinal	T52.0X1	T52.0X2	T52.0X3	T52.0X4	—	—
red veterinary	T49.3X1	T49.3X2	T49.3X3	T49.3X4	T49.3X5	T49.3X6
white	T49.3X1	T49.3X2	T49.3X3	T49.3X4	T49.3X5	T49.3X6
Petroleum (products) NEC	T52.0X1	T52.0X2	T52.0X3	T52.0X4	—	—
benzine(s)—see Ligroin						
ether—see Ligroin						
jelly—see Petrolatum						
naphtha—see Ligroin						
pesticide	T60.8X1	T60.8X2	T60.8X3	T60.8X4	—	—
solids	T52.0X1	T52.0X2	T52.0X3	T52.0X4		
solvents	T52.0X1	T52.0X2	T52.0X3	T52.0X4		
vapor	T52.0X1	T52.0X2	T52.0X3	T52.0X4		
Peyote	T40.991	T40.992	T40.993	T40.994	—	—
Phanodorm, phanodorn	T42.3X1	T42.3X2	T42.3X3	T42.3X4	T42.3X5	T42.3X6
Phanquinone	T37.3X1	T37.3X2	T37.3X3	T37.3X4	T37.3X5	T37.3X6
Phanquone	T37.3X1	T37.3X2	T37.3X3	T37.3X4	T37.3X5	T37.3X6
Pharmaceutical						
adjunct NEC	T50.901	T50.902	T50.903	T50.904	T50.905	T50.906
excipient NEC	T50.901	T50.902	T50.903	T50.904	T50.905	T50.906
sweetener	T50.901	T50.902	T50.903	T50.904	T50.905	T50.906
viscous agent	T50.901	T50.902	T50.903	T50.904	T50.905	T50.906

Substance	Poisoning, Accidental (unintentional)	Poisoning, Intentional self-harm	Poisoning, Assault	Poisoning, Undetermined	Adverse effect	Underdosing
Phemitone	T42.3X1	T42.3X2	T42.3X3	T42.3X4	T42.3X5	T42.3X6
Phenacaine	T41.3X1	T41.3X2	T41.3X3	T41.3X4	T41.3X5	T41.3X6
Phenacemide	T42.6X1	T42.6X2	T42.6X3	T42.6X4	T42.6X5	T42.6X6
Phenacetin	T39.1X1	T39.1X2	T39.1X3	T39.1X4	T39.1X5	T39.1X6
Phenadoxone	T40.2X1	T40.2X2	T40.2X3	T40.2X4	—	—
Phenaglycodol	T43.591	T43.592	T43.593	T43.594	T43.595	T43.596
Phenantoin	T42.0X1	T42.0X2	T42.0X3	T42.0X4	T42.0X5	T42.0X6
Phenaphthazine reagent	T50.991	T50.992	T50.993	T50.994	T50.995	T50.996
Phenazocine	T40.491	T40.492	T40.493	T40.494	T40.495	T40.496
Phenazone	T39.2X1	T39.2X2	T39.2X3	T39.2X4	T39.2X5	T39.2X6
Phenazopyridine	T39.8X1	T39.8X2	T39.8X3	T39.8X4	T39.8X5	T39.8X6
Phenbenicillin	T36.0X1	T36.0X2	T36.0X3	T36.0X4	T36.0X5	T36.0X6
Phenbutrazate	T50.5X1	T50.5X2	T50.5X3	T50.5X4	T50.5X5	T50.5X6
Phencyclidine	T40.991	T40.992	T40.993	T40.994	T40.995	T40.996
Phendimetrazine	T50.5X1	T50.5X2	T50.5X3	T50.5X4	T50.5X5	T50.5X6
Phenelzine	T43.1X1	T43.1X2	T43.1X3	T43.1X4	T43.1X5	T43.1X6
Phenemal	T42.3X1	T42.3X2	T42.3X3	T42.3X4	T42.3X5	T42.3X6
Phenergan	T42.6X1	T42.6X2	T42.6X3	T42.6X4	T42.6X5	T42.6X6
Pheneticillin	T36.0X1	T36.0X2	T36.0X3	T36.0X4	T36.0X5	T36.0X6
Pheneturide	T42.6X1	T42.6X2	T42.6X3	T42.6X4	T42.6X5	T42.6X6
Phenformin	T38.3X1	T38.3X2	T38.3X3	T38.3X4	T38.3X5	T38.3X6
Phenglutarimide	T44.3X1	T44.3X2	T44.3X3	T44.3X4	T44.3X5	T44.3X6
Phenicarbazide	T39.8X1	T39.8X2	T39.8X3	T39.8X4	T39.8X5	T39.8X6
Phenindamine	T45.0X1	T45.0X2	T45.0X3	T45.0X4	T45.0X5	T45.0X6
Phenindione	T45.511	T45.512	T45.513	T45.514	T45.515	T45.516
Pheniprazine	T43.1X1	T43.1X2	T43.1X3	T43.1X4	T43.1X5	T43.1X6
Pheniramine	T45.0X1	T45.0X2	T45.0X3	T45.0X4	T45.0X5	T45.0X6
Phenisatin	T47.2X1	T47.2X2	T47.2X3	T47.2X4	T47.2X5	T47.2X6
Phenmetrazine	T50.5X1	T50.5X2	T50.5X3	T50.5X4	T50.5X5	T50.5X6
Phenobal	T42.3X1	T42.3X2	T42.3X3	T42.3X4	T42.3X5	T42.3X6
Phenobarbital	T42.3X1	T42.3X2	T42.3X3	T42.3X4	T42.3X5	T42.3X6
with						
mephenytoin	T42.3X1	T42.3X2	T42.3X3	T42.3X4	T42.3X5	T42.3X6
phenytoin	T42.3X1	T42.3X2	T42.3X3	T42.3X4	T42.3X5	T42.3X6
sodium	T42.3X1	T42.3X2	T42.3X3	T42.3X4	T42.3X5	T42.3X6
Phenobarbitone	T42.3X1	T42.3X2	T42.3X3	T42.3X4	T42.3X5	T42.3X6
Phenobutiodil	T50.8X1	T50.8X2	T50.8X3	T50.8X4	T50.8X5	T50.8X6
Phenoctide	T49.0X1	T49.0X2	T49.0X3	T49.0X4	T49.0X5	T49.0X6
Phenol	T49.0X1	T49.0X2	T49.0X3	T49.0X4	T49.0X5	T49.0X6
disinfectant	T54.0X1	T54.0X2	T54.0X3	T54.0X4	—	—
in oil injection	T46.8X1	T46.8X2	T46.8X3	T46.8X4	T46.8X5	T46.8X6
medicinal	T49.1X1	T49.1X2	T49.1X3	T49.1X4	T49.1X5	T49.1X6
nonmedicinal NEC	T54.0X1	T54.0X2	T54.0X3	T54.0X4	—	—
pesticide	T60.8X1	T60.8X2	T60.8X3	T60.8X4	—	—
red	T50.8X1	T50.8X2	T50.8X3	T50.8X4	T50.8X5	T50.8X6
Phenolic preparation	T49.1X1	T49.1X2	T49.1X3	T49.1X4	T49.1X5	T49.1X6
Phenolphthalein	T47.2X1	T47.2X2	T47.2X3	T47.2X4	T47.2X5	T47.2X6
Phenolsulfonphthalein	T50.8X1	T50.8X2	T50.8X3	T50.8X4	T50.8X5	T50.8X6
Phenomorphan	T40.2X1	T40.2X2	T40.2X3	T40.2X4	—	—
Phenonyl	T42.3X1	T42.3X2	T42.3X3	T42.3X4	T42.3X5	T42.3X6

Substance	Poisoning, Accidental (unintentional)	Poisoning, Intentional self-harm	Poisoning, Assault	Poisoning, Undetermined	Adverse effect	Underdosing
Phenoperidine	T40.491	T40.492	T40.493	T40.494	—	—
Phenopyrazone	T46.991	T46.992	T46.993	T46.994	T46.995	T46.996
Phenoquin	T50.4X1	T50.4X2	T50.4X3	T50.4X4	T50.4X5	T50.4X6
Phenothiazine (psychotropic) NEC	T43.3X1	T43.3X2	T43.3X3	T43.3X4	T43.3X5	T43.3X6
insecticide	T60.2X1	T60.2X2	T60.2X3	T60.2X4	—	—
Phenothrin	T49.0X1	T49.0X2	T49.0X3	T49.0X4	T49.0X5	T49.0X6
Phenoxybenzamine	T46.7X1	T46.7X2	T46.7X3	T46.7X4	T46.7X5	T46.7X6
Phenoxyethanol	T49.0X1	T49.0X2	T49.0X3	T49.0X4	T49.0X5	T49.0X6
Phenoxymethyl penicillin	T36.0X1	T36.0X2	T36.0X3	T36.0X4	T36.0X5	T36.0X6
Phenprobamate	T42.8X1	T42.8X2	T42.8X3	T42.8X4	T42.8X5	T42.8X6
Phenprocoumon	T45.511	T45.512	T45.513	T45.514	T45.515	T45.516
Phensuximide	T42.2X1	T42.2X2	T42.2X3	T42.2X4	T42.2X5	T42.2X6
Phentermine	T50.5X1	T50.5X2	T50.5X3	T50.5X4	T50.5X5	T50.5X6
Phenthicillin	T36.0X1	T36.0X2	T36.0X3	T36.0X4	T36.0X5	T36.0X6
Phentolamine	T46.7X1	T46.7X2	T46.7X3	T46.7X4	T46.7X5	T46.7X6
Phenyl						
butazone	T39.2X1	T39.2X2	T39.2X3	T39.2X4	T39.2X5	T39.2X6
enediamine	T65.3X1	T65.3X2	T65.3X3	T65.3X4	—	—
hydrazine	T65.3X1	T65.3X2	T65.3X3	T65.3X4	—	—
antineoplastic	T45.1X1	T45.1X2	T45.1X3	T45.1X4	T45.1X5	T45.1X6
mercuric compounds— see Mercury						
salicylate	T49.3X1	T49.3X2	T49.3X3	T49.3X4	T49.3X5	T49.3X6
Phenylalanine mustard	T45.1X1	T45.1X2	T45.1X3	T45.1X4	T45.1X5	T45.1X6
Phenylbutazone	T39.2X1	T39.2X2	T39.2X3	T39.2X4	T39.2X5	T39.2X6
Phenylenediamine	T65.3X1	T65.3X2	T65.3X3	T65.3X4	—	—
Phenylephrine	T44.4X1	T44.4X2	T44.4X3	T44.4X4	T44.4X5	T44.4X6
Phenylethylbiguanide	T38.3X1	T38.3X2	T38.3X3	T38.3X4	T38.3X5	T38.3X6
Phenylmercuric						
acetate	T49.0X1	T49.0X2	T49.0X3	T49.0X4	T49.0X5	T49.0X6
borate	T49.0X1	T49.0X2	T49.0X3	T49.0X4	T49.0X5	T49.0X6
nitrate	T49.0X1	T49.0X2	T49.0X3	T49.0X4	T49.0X5	T49.0X6
Phenylmethylbarbitone	T42.3X1	T42.3X2	T42.3X3	T42.3X4	T42.3X5	T42.3X6
Phenylpropanol	T47.5X1	T47.5X2	T47.5X3	T47.5X4	T47.5X5	T47.5X6
Phenylpropanolamine	T44.991	T44.992	T44.993	T44.994	T44.995	T44.996
Phenylsulfthion	T60.0X1	T60.0X2	T60.0X3	T60.0X4	—	—
Phenyltoloxamine	T45.0X1	T45.0X2	T45.0X3	T45.0X4	T45.0X5	T45.0X6
Phenyramidol, phenyramidon	T39.8X1	T39.8X2	T39.8X3	T39.8X4	T39.8X5	T39.8X6
Phenytoin	T42.0X1	T42.0X2	T42.0X3	T42.0X4	T42.0X5	T42.0X6
with Phenobarbital	T42.3X1	T42.3X2	T42.3X3	T42.3X4	T42.3X5	T42.3X6
pHisoHex	T49.2X1	T49.2X2	T49.2X3	T49.2X4	T49.2X5	T49.2X6
Pholcodine	T48.3X1	T48.3X2	T48.3X3	T48.3X4	T48.3X5	T48.3X6
Pholedrine	T46.991	T46.992	T46.993	T46.994	T46.995	T46.996
Phorate	T60.0X1	T60.0X2	T60.0X3	T60.0X4	—	—
Phosdrin	T60.0X1	T60.0X2	T60.0X3	T60.0X4	—	—
Phosfolan	T60.0X1	T60.0X2	T60.0X3	T60.0X4	—	—
Phosgene (gas)	T59.891	T59.892	T59.893	T59.894	—	—
Phosphamidon	T60.0X1	T60.0X2	T60.0X3	T60.0X4	—	—

Substance	Poisoning, Accidental (unintentional)	Poisoning, Intentional self-harm	Poisoning, Assault	Poisoning, Undetermined	Adverse effect	Underdosing
Phosphate	T65.891	T65.892	T65.893	T65.894	—	—
laxative	T47.4X1	T47.4X2	T47.4X3	T47.4X4	T47.4X5	T47.4X6
organic	T60.0X1	T60.0X2	T60.0X3	T60.0X4	—	—
solvent	T52.91	T52.92	T52.93	T52.94	—	—
tricresyl	T65.891	T65.892	T65.893	T65.894	—	—
Phosphine	T57.1X1	T57.1X2	T57.1X3	T57.1X4	—	—
fumigant	T57.1X1	T57.1X2	T57.1X3	T57.1X4	—	—
Phospholine	T49.5X1	T49.5X2	T49.5X3	T49.5X4	T49.5X5	T49.5X6
Phosphoric acid	T54.2X1	T54.2X2	T54.2X3	T54.2X4	—	—
Phosphorus (compound) NEC	T57.1X1	T57.1X2	T57.1X3	T57.1X4	—	—
pesticide	T60.0X1	T60.0X2	T60.0X3	T60.0X4	—	—
Phthalates	T65.891	T65.892	T65.893	T65.894	—	—
Phthalic anhydride	T65.891	T65.892	T65.893	T65.894	—	—
Phthalimidoglutarimide	T42.6X1	T42.6X2	T42.6X3	T42.6X4	T42.6X5	T42.6X6
Phthalylsulfathiazole	T37.0X1	T37.0X2	T37.0X3	T37.0X4	T37.0X5	T37.0X6
Phylloquinone	T45.7X1	T45.7X2	T45.7X3	T45.7X4	T45.7X5	T45.7X6
Physeptone	T40.3X1	T40.3X2	T40.3X3	T40.3X4	T40.3X5	T40.3X6
Physostigma venenosum	T62.2X1	T62.2X2	T62.2X3	T62.2X4	—	—
Physostigmine	T49.5X1	T49.5X2	T49.5X3	T49.5X4	T49.5X5	T49.5X6
Phytolacca decandra	T62.2X1	T62.2X2	T62.2X3	T62.2X4	—	—
berries	T62.1X1	T62.1X2	T62.1X3	T62.1X4	—	—
Phytomenadione	T45.7X1	T45.7X2	T45.7X3	T45.7X4	T45.7X5	T45.7X6
Phytonadione	T45.7X1	T45.7X2	T45.7X3	T45.7X4	T45.7X5	T45.7X6
Picoperine	T48.3X1	T48.3X2	T48.3X3	T48.3X4	T48.3X5	T48.3X6
Picosulfate (sodium)	T47.2X1	T47.2X2	T47.2X3	T47.2X4	T47.2X5	T47.2X6
Picric (acid)	T54.2X1	T54.2X2	T54.2X3	T54.2X4	—	—
Picrotoxin	T50.7X1	T50.7X2	T50.7X3	T50.7X4	T50.7X5	T50.7X6
Piketoprofen	T49.0X1	T49.0X2	T49.0X3	T49.0X4	T49.0X5	T49.0X6
Pilocarpine	T44.1X1	T44.1X2	T44.1X3	T44.1X4	T44.1X5	T44.1X6
Pilocarpus (jaborandi) extract	T44.1X1	T44.1X2	T44.1X3	T44.1X4	T44.1X5	T44.1X6
Pilsicainide (hydrochloride)	T46.2X1	T46.2X2	T46.2X3	T46.2X4	T46.2X5	T46.2X6
Pimaricin	T36.7X1	T36.7X2	T36.7X3	T36.7X4	T36.7X5	T36.7X6
Pimeclone	T50.7X1	T50.7X2	T50.7X3	T50.7X4	T50.7X5	T50.7X6
Pimelic ketone	T52.8X1	T52.8X2	T52.8X3	T52.8X4	—	—
Pimethixene	T45.0X1	T45.0X2	T45.0X3	T45.0X4	T45.0X5	T45.0X6
Piminodine	T40.2X1	T40.2X2	T40.2X3	T40.2X4	T40.2X5	T40.2X6
Pimozide	T43.591	T43.592	T43.593	T43.594	T43.595	T43.596
Pinacidil	T46.5X1	T46.5X2	T46.5X3	T46.5X4	T46.5X5	T46.5X6
Pinaverium bromide	T44.3X1	T44.3X2	T44.3X3	T44.3X4	T44.3X5	T44.3X6
Pinazepam	T42.4X1	T42.4X2	T42.4X3	T42.4X4	T42.4X5	T42.4X6
Pindolol	T44.7X1	T44.7X2	T44.7X3	T44.7X4	T44.7X5	T44.7X6
Pindone	T60.4X1	T60.4X2	T60.4X3	T60.4X4	—	—
Pine oil (disinfectant)	T65.891	T65.892	T65.893	T65.894	—	—
Pinkroot	T37.4X1	T37.4X2	T37.4X3	T37.4X4	T37.4X5	T37.4X6
Pipadone	T40.2X1	T40.2X2	T40.2X3	T40.2X4	—	—
Pipamazine	T45.0X1	T45.0X2	T45.0X3	T45.0X4	T45.0X5	T45.0X6
Pipamperone	T43.4X1	T43.4X2	T43.4X3	T43.4X4	T43.4X5	T43.4X6
Pipazetate	T48.3X1	T48.3X2	T48.3X3	T48.3X4	T48.3X5	T48.3X6

Substance	Poisoning, Accidental (unintentional)	Poisoning, Intentional self-harm	Poisoning, Assault	Poisoning, Undetermined	Adverse effect	Underdosing
Pipemidic acid	T37.8X1	T37.8X2	T37.8X3	T37.8X4	T37.8X5	T37.8X6
Pipenzolate bromide	T44.3X1	T44.3X2	T44.3X3	T44.3X4	T44.3X5	T44.3X6
Piperacetazine	T43.3X1	T43.3X2	T43.3X3	T43.3X4	T43.3X5	T43.3X6
Piperacillin	T36.0X1	T36.0X2	T36.0X3	T36.0X4	T36.0X5	T36.0X6
Piperazine	T37.4X1	T37.4X2	T37.4X3	T37.4X4	T37.4X5	T37.4X6
estrone sulfate	T38.5X1	T38.5X2	T38.5X3	T38.5X4	T38.5X5	T38.5X6
Piper cubeba	T62.2X1	T62.2X2	T62.2X3	T62.2X4	—	—
Piperidione	T48.3X1	T48.3X2	T48.3X3	T48.3X4	T48.3X5	T48.3X6
Piperidolate	T44.3X1	T44.3X2	T44.3X3	T44.3X4	T44.3X5	T44.3X6
Piperocaine	T41.3X1	T41.3X2	T41.3X3	T41.3X4	T41.3X5	T41.3X6
infiltration (subcutaneous)	T41.3X1	T41.3X2	T41.3X3	T41.3X4	T41.3X5	T41.3X6
nerve block (peripheral) (plexus)	T41.3X1	T41.3X2	T41.3X3	T41.3X4	T41.3X5	T41.3X6
topical (surface)	T41.3X1	T41.3X2	T41.3X3	T41.3X4	T41.3X5	T41.3X6
Piperonyl butoxide	T60.8X1	T60.8X2	T60.8X3	T60.8X4	—	—
Pipethanate	T44.3X1	T44.3X2	T44.3X3	T44.3X4	T44.3X5	T44.3X6
Pipobroman	T45.1X1	T45.1X2	T45.1X3	T45.1X4	T45.1X5	T45.1X6
Pipotiazine	T43.3X1	T43.3X2	T43.3X3	T43.3X4	T43.3X5	T43.3X6
Pipoxizine	T45.0X1	T45.0X2	T45.0X3	T45.0X4	T45.0X5	T45.0X6
Pipradrol	T43.691	T43.692	T43.693	T43.694	T43.695	T43.696
Piprinhydrinate	T45.0X1	T45.0X2	T45.0X3	T45.0X4	T45.0X5	T45.0X6
Pirarubicin	T45.1X1	T45.1X2	T45.1X3	T45.1X4	T45.1X5	T45.1X6
Pirazinamide	T37.1X1	T37.1X2	T37.1X3	T37.1X4	T37.1X5	T37.1X6
Pirbuterol	T48.6X1	T48.6X2	T48.6X3	T48.6X4	T48.6X5	T48.6X6
Pirenzepine	T47.1X1	T47.1X2	T47.1X3	T47.1X4	T47.1X5	T47.1X6
Piretanide	T50.1X1	T50.1X2	T50.1X3	T50.1X4	T50.1X5	T50.1X6
Piribedil	T42.8X1	T42.8X2	T42.8X3	T42.8X4	T42.8X5	T42.8X6
Piridoxilate	T46.3X1	T46.3X2	T46.3X3	T46.3X4	T46.3X5	T46.3X6
Piritramide	T40.491	T40.492	T40.493	T40.494	—	—
Piromidic acid	T37.8X1	T37.8X2	T37.8X3	T37.8X4	T37.8X5	T37.8X6
Piroxicam	T39.391	T39.392	T39.393	T39.394	T39.395	T39.396
beta-cyclodextrin complex	T39.8X1	T39.8X2	T39.8X3	T39.8X4	T39.8X5	T39.8X6
Pirozadil	T46.6X1	T46.6X2	T46.6X3	T46.6X4	T46.6X5	T46.6X6
Piscidia (bark) (erythrina)	T39.8X1	T39.8X2	T39.8X3	T39.8X4	T39.8X5	T39.8X6
Pitch	T65.891	T65.892	T65.893	T65.894	—	—
Pitkin's solution	T41.3X1	T41.3X2	T41.3X3	T41.3X4	T41.3X5	T41.3X6
Pitocin	T48.0X1	T48.0X2	T48.0X3	T48.0X4	T48.0X5	T48.0X6
Pitressin (tannate)	T38.891	T38.892	T38.893	T38.894	T38.895	T38.896
Pituitary extracts (posterior)	T38.891	T38.892	T38.893	T38.894	T38.895	T38.896
anterior	T38.811	T38.812	T38.813	T38.814	T38.815	T38.816
Pituitrin	T38.891	T38.892	T38.893	T38.894	T38.895	T38.896
Pivampicillin	T36.0X1	T36.0X2	T36.0X3	T36.0X4	T36.0X5	T36.0X6
Pivmecillinam	T36.0X1	T36.0X2	T36.0X3	T36.0X4	T36.0X5	T36.0X6
Placental hormone	T38.891	T38.892	T38.893	T38.894	T38.895	T38.896
Placidyl	T42.6X1	T42.6X2	T42.6X3	T42.6X4	T42.6X5	T42.6X6
Plague vaccine	T50.A91	T50.A92	T50.A93	T50.A94	T50.A95	T50.A96

Substance	Poisoning, Accidental (unintentional)	Poisoning, Intentional self-harm	Poisoning, Assault	Poisoning, Undetermined	Adverse effect	Underdosing
Plant						
food or fertilizer NEC	T65.891	T65.892	T65.893	T65.894	—	—
containing herbicide	T60.3X1	T60.3X2	T60.3X3	T60.3X4	—	—
noxious, used as food	T62.2X1	T62.2X2	T62.2X3	T62.2X4	—	—
berries	T62.1X1	T62.1X2	T62.1X3	T62.1X4	—	—
seeds	T62.2X1	T62.2X2	T62.2X3	T62.2X4	—	—
specified type NEC	T62.2X1	T62.2X2	T62.2X3	T62.2X4	—	—
Plasma	T45.8X1	T45.8X2	T45.8X3	T45.8X4	T45.8X5	T45.8X6
expander NEC	T45.8X1	T45.8X2	T45.8X3	T45.8X4	T45.8X5	T45.8X6
protein fraction (human)	T45.8X1	T45.8X2	T45.8X3	T45.8X4	T45.8X5	T45.8X6
Plasmanate	T45.8X1	T45.8X2	T45.8X3	T45.8X4	T45.8X5	T45.8X6
Plasminogen (tissue) activator	T45.611	T45.612	T45.613	T45.614	T45.615	T45.616
Plaster dressing	T49.3X1	T49.3X2	T49.3X3	T49.3X4	T49.3X5	T49.3X6
Plastic dressing	T49.3X1	T49.3X2	T49.3X3	T49.3X4	T49.3X5	T49.3X6
Plegicil	T43.3X1	T43.3X2	T43.3X3	T43.3X4	T43.3X5	T43.3X6
Plicamycin	T45.1X1	T45.1X2	T45.1X3	T45.1X4	T45.1X5	T45.1X6
Podophyllotoxin	T49.8X1	T49.8X2	T49.8X3	T49.8X4	T49.8X5	T49.8X6
Podophyllum (resin)	T49.4X1	T49.4X2	T49.4X3	T49.4X4	T49.4X5	T49.4X6
Poison NEC	T65.91	T65.92	T65.93	T65.94	—	—
Poisonous berries	T62.1X1	T62.1X2	T62.1X3	T62.1X4	—	—
Pokeweed (any part)	T62.2X1	T62.2X2	T62.2X3	T62.2X4	—	—
Poldine metilsulfate	T44.3X1	T44.3X2	T44.3X3	T44.3X4	T44.3X5	T44.3X6
Polidexide (sulfate)	T46.6X1	T46.6X2	T46.6X3	T46.6X4	T46.6X5	T46.6X6
Polidocanol	T46.8X1	T46.8X2	T46.8X3	T46.8X4	T46.8X5	T46.8X6
Poliomyelitis vaccine	T50.B91	T50.B92	T50.B93	T50.B94	T50.B95	T50.B96
Polish (car) (floor) (furniture) (metal) (porcelain) (silver)	T65.891	T65.892	T65.893	T65.894	—	—
abrasive	T65.891	T65.892	T65.893	T65.894	—	—
porcelain	T65.891	T65.892	T65.893	T65.894	—	—
Poloxalkol	T47.4X1	T47.4X2	T47.4X3	T47.4X4	T47.4X5	T47.4X6
Poloxamer	T47.4X1	T47.4X2	T47.4X3	T47.4X4	T47.4X5	T47.4X6
Polyaminostyrene resins	T50.3X1	T50.3X2	T50.3X3	T50.3X4	T50.3X5	T50.3X6
Polycarbophil	T47.4X1	T47.4X2	T47.4X3	T47.4X4	T47.4X5	T47.4X6
Polychlorinated biphenyl	T65.891	T65.892	T65.893	T65.894	—	—
Polycycline	T36.4X1	T36.4X2	T36.4X3	T36.4X4	T36.4X5	T36.4X6
Polyester fumes	T59.891	T59.892	T59.893	T59.894	—	—
Polyester resin hardener	T52.91	T52.92	T52.93	T52.94	—	—
fumes	T59.891	T59.892	T59.893	T59.894	—	—
Polyestradiol phosphate	T38.5X1	T38.5X2	T38.5X3	T38.5X4	T38.5X5	T38.5X6
Polyethanolamine alkyl sulfate	T49.2X1	T49.2X2	T49.2X3	T49.2X4	T49.2X5	T49.2X6
Polyethylene adhesive	T49.3X1	T49.3X2	T49.3X3	T49.3X4	T49.3X5	T49.3X6
Polyferose	T45.4X1	T45.4X2	T45.4X3	T45.4X4	T45.4X5	T45.4X6
Polygeline	T45.8X1	T45.8X2	T45.8X3	T45.8X4	T45.8X5	T45.8X6
Polymyxin	T36.8X1	T36.8X2	T36.8X3	T36.8X4	T36.8X5	T36.8X6
B	T36.8X1	T36.8X2	T36.8X3	T36.8X4	T36.8X5	T36.8X6
ENT agent	T49.6X1	T49.6X2	T49.6X3	T49.6X4	T49.6X5	T49.6X6

Substance	Poisoning, Accidental (unintentional)	Poisoning, Intentional self-harm	Poisoning, Assault	Poisoning, Undetermined	Adverse effect	Underdosing
Polymyxin — *Continued*						
ophthalmic preparation	T49.5X1	T49.5X2	T49.5X3	T49.5X4	T49.5X5	T49.5X6
topical NEC	T49.0X1	T49.0X2	T49.0X3	T49.0X4	T49.0X5	T49.0X6
E sulfate (eye preparation)	T49.5X1	T49.5X2	T49.5X3	T49.5X4	T49.5X5	T49.5X6
Polynoxylin	T49.0X1	T49.0X2	T49.0X3	T49.0X4	T49.0X5	T49.0X6
Polyoestradiol phosphate	T38.5X1	T38.5X2	T38.5X3	T38.5X4	T38.5X5	T38.5X6
Polyoxymethyleneurea	T49.0X1	T49.0X2	T49.0X3	T49.0X4	T49.0X5	T49.0X6
Polysilane	T47.8X1	T47.8X2	T47.8X3	T47.8X4	T47.8X5	T47.8X6
Polytetrafluoroethylene (inhaled)	T59.891	T59.892	T59.893	T59.894	—	—
Polythiazide	T50.2X1	T50.2X2	T50.2X3	T50.2X4	T50.2X5	T50.2X6
Polyvidone	T45.8X1	T45.8X2	T45.8X3	T45.8X4	T45.8X5	T45.8X6
Polyvinylpyrrolidone	T45.8X1	T45.8X2	T45.8X3	T45.8X4	T45.8X5	T45.8X6
Pontocaine (hydrochloride) (infiltration) (topical)	T41.3X1	T41.3X2	T41.3X3	T41.3X4	T41.3X5	T41.3X6
nerve block (peripheral) (plexus)	T41.3X1	T41.3X2	T41.3X3	T41.3X4	T41.3X5	T41.3X6
spinal	T41.3X1	T41.3X2	T41.3X3	T41.3X4	T41.3X5	T41.3X6
Porfiromycin	T45.1X1	T45.1X2	T45.1X3	T45.1X4	T45.1X5	T45.1X6
Posterior pituitary hormone NEC	T38.891	T38.892	T38.893	T38.894	T38.895	T38.896
Pot	T40.711	T40.712	T40.713	T40.714	T40.715	T40.716
Potash (caustic)	T54.3X1	T54.3X2	T54.3X3	T54.3X4	—	—
Potassic saline injection (lactated)	T50.3X1	T50.3X2	T50.3X3	T50.3X4	T50.3X5	T50.3X6
Potassium (salts) NEC	T50.3X1	T50.3X2	T50.3X3	T50.3X4	T50.3X5	T50.3X6
aminobenzoate	T45.8X1	T45.8X2	T45.8X3	T45.8X4	T45.8X5	T45.8X6
aminosalicylate	T37.1X1	T37.1X2	T37.1X3	T37.1X4	T37.1X5	T37.1X6
antimony 'tartrate'	T37.8X1	T37.8X2	T37.8X3	T37.8X4	T37.8X5	T37.8X6
arsenite (solution)	T57.0X1	T57.0X2	T57.0X3	T57.0X4	—	—
bichromate	T56.2X1	T56.2X2	T56.2X3	T56.2X4	—	—
bisulfate	T47.3X1	T47.3X2	T47.3X3	T47.3X4	T47.3X5	T47.3X6
bromide	T42.6X1	T42.6X2	T42.6X3	T42.6X4	T42.6X5	T42.6X6
canrenoate	T50.0X1	T50.0X2	T50.0X3	T50.0X4	T50.0X5	T50.0X6
carbonate	T54.3X1	T54.3X2	T54.3X3	T54.3X4	—	—
chlorate NEC	T65.891	T65.892	T65.893	T65.894	—	—
chloride	T50.3X1	T50.3X2	T50.3X3	T50.3X4	T50.3X5	T50.3X6
citrate	T50.991	T50.992	T50.993	T50.994	T50.995	T50.996
cyanide	T65.0X1	T65.0X2	T65.0X3	T65.0X4	—	—
ferric hexacyano-ferrate (medicinal)	T50.6X1	T50.6X2	T50.6X3	T50.6X4	T50.6X5	T50.6X6
nonmedicinal	T65.891	T65.892	T65.893	T65.894	—	—
Fluoride	T57.8X1	T57.8X2	T57.8X3	T57.8X4	—	—
glucaldrate	T47.1X1	T47.1X2	T47.1X3	T47.1X4	T47.1X5	T47.1X6
hydroxide	T54.3X1	T54.3X2	T54.3X3	T54.3X4	—	—
iodate	T49.0X1	T49.0X2	T49.0X3	T49.0X4	T49.0X5	T49.0X6
iodide	T48.4X1	T48.4X2	T48.4X3	T48.4X4	T48.4X5	T48.4X6
nitrate	T57.8X1	T57.8X2	T57.8X3	T57.8X4	—	—
oxalate	T65.891	T65.892	T65.893	T65.894	—	—

Substance	Poisoning, Accidental (unintentional)	Poisoning, Intentional self-harm	Poisoning, Assault	Poisoning, Undetermined	Adverse effect	Underdosing
Potassium — *Continued*						
perchlorate (nonmedicinal) NEC	T65.891	T65.892	T65.893	T65.894	—	—
antithyroid	T38.2X1	T38.2X2	T38.2X3	T38.2X4	T38.2X5	T38.2X6
medicinal	T38.2X1	T38.2X2	T38.2X3	T38.2X4	T38.2X5	T38.2X6
Permanganate (nonmedicinal)	T65.891	T65.892	T65.893	T65.894	—	—
medicinal	T49.0X1	T49.0X2	T49.0X3	T49.0X4	T49.0X5	T49.0X6
sulfate	T47.2X1	T47.2X2	T47.2X3	T47.2X4	T47.2X5	T47.2X6
Potassium-removing resin	T50.3X1	T50.3X2	T50.3X3	T50.3X4	T50.3X5	T50.3X6
Potassium-retaining drug	T50.3X1	T50.3X2	T50.3X3	T50.3X4	T50.3X5	T50.3X6
Povidone	T45.8X1	T45.8X2	T45.8X3	T45.8X4	T45.8X5	T45.8X6
iodine	T49.0X1	T49.0X2	T49.0X3	T49.0X4	T49.0X5	T49.0X6
Practolol	T44.7X1	T44.7X2	T44.7X3	T44.7X4	T44.7X5	T44.7X6
Prajmalium bitartrate	T46.2X1	T46.2X2	T46.2X3	T46.2X4	T46.2X5	T46.2X6
Pralidoxime (iodide)	T50.6X1	T50.6X2	T50.6X3	T50.6X4	T50.6X5	T50.6X6
chloride	T50.6X1	T50.6X2	T50.6X3	T50.6X4	T50.6X5	T50.6X6
Pramiverine	T44.3X1	T44.3X2	T44.3X3	T44.3X4	T44.3X5	T44.3X6
Pramocaine	T49.1X1	T49.1X2	T49.1X3	T49.1X4	T49.1X5	T49.1X6
Pramoxine	T49.1X1	T49.1X2	T49.1X3	T49.1X4	T49.1X5	T49.1X6
Prasterone	T38.7X1	T38.7X2	T38.7X3	T38.7X4	T38.7X5	T38.7X6
Pravastatin	T46.6X1	T46.6X2	T46.6X3	T46.6X4	T46.6X5	T46.6X6
Prazepam	T42.4X1	T42.4X2	T42.4X3	T42.4X4	T42.4X5	T42.4X6
Praziquantel	T37.4X1	T37.4X2	T37.4X3	T37.4X4	T37.4X5	T37.4X6
Prazitone	T43.291	T43.292	T43.293	T43.294	T43.295	T43.296
Prazosin	T44.6X1	T44.6X2	T44.6X3	T44.6X4	T44.6X5	T44.6X6
Prednicarbate	T49.0X1	T49.0X2	T49.0X3	T49.0X4	T49.0X5	T49.0X6
Prednimustine	T45.1X1	T45.1X2	T45.1X3	T45.1X4	T45.1X5	T45.1X6
Prednisolone	T38.0X1	T38.0X2	T38.0X3	T38.0X4	T38.0X5	T38.0X6
ENT agent	T49.6X1	T49.6X2	T49.6X3	T49.6X4	T49.6X5	T49.6X6
ophthalmic preparation	T49.5X1	T49.5X2	T49.5X3	T49.5X4	T49.5X5	T49.5X6
steaglate	T49.0X1	T49.0X2	T49.0X3	T49.0X4	T49.0X5	T49.0X6
topical NEC	T49.0X1	T49.0X2	T49.0X3	T49.0X4	T49.0X5	T49.0X6
Prednisone	T38.0X1	T38.0X2	T38.0X3	T38.0X4	T38.0X5	T38.0X6
Prednylidene	T38.0X1	T38.0X2	T38.0X3	T38.0X4	T38.0X5	T38.0X6
Pregnandiol	T38.5X1	T38.5X2	T38.5X3	T38.5X4	T38.5X5	T38.5X6
Pregneninolone	T38.5X1	T38.5X2	T38.5X3	T38.5X4	T38.5X5	T38.5X6
Preludin	T43.691	T43.692	T43.693	T43.694	T43.695	T43.696
Premarin	T38.5X1	T38.5X2	T38.5X3	T38.5X4	T38.5X5	T38.5X6
Premedication anesthetic	T41.201	T41.202	T41.203	T41.204	T41.205	T41.206
Prenalterol	T44.5X1	T44.5X2	T44.5X3	T44.5X4	T44.5X5	T44.5X6
Prenoxdiazine	T48.3X1	T48.3X2	T48.3X3	T48.3X4	T48.3X5	T48.3X6
Prenylamine	T46.3X1	T46.3X2	T46.3X3	T46.3X4	T46.3X5	T46.3X6
Preparation H	T49.8X1	T49.8X2	T49.8X3	T49.8X4	T49.8X5	T49.8X6
Preparation, local	T49.4X1	T49.4X2	T49.4X3	T49.4X4	T49.4X5	T49.4X6
Preservative (nonmedicinal)	T65.891	T65.892	T65.893	T65.894	—	—
medicinal	T50.901	T50.902	T50.903	T50.904	T50.905	T50.906
wood	T60.91	T60.92	T60.93	T60.94	—	—

Substance	Poisoning, Accidental (unintentional)	Poisoning, Intentional self-harm	Poisoning, Assault	Poisoning, Undetermined	Adverse effect	Underdosing
Prethcamide	T50.7X1	T50.7X2	T50.7X3	T50.7X4	T50.7X5	T50.7X6
Pride of China	T62.2X1	T62.2X2	T62.2X3	T62.2X4	—	—
Pridinol	T44.3X1	T44.3X2	T44.3X3	T44.3X4	T44.3X5	T44.3X6
Prifinium bromide	T44.3X1	T44.3X2	T44.3X3	T44.3X4	T44.3X5	T44.3X6
Prilocaine	T41.3X1	T41.3X2	T41.3X3	T41.3X4	T41.3X5	T41.3X6
infiltration (subcutaneous)	T41.3X1	T41.3X2	T41.3X3	T41.3X4	T41.3X5	T41.3X6
nerve block (peripheral) (plexus)	T41.3X1	T41.3X2	T41.3X3	T41.3X4	T41.3X5	T41.3X6
regional	T41.3X1	T41.3X2	T41.3X3	T41.3X4	T41.3X5	T41.3X6
Primaquine	T37.2X1	T37.2X2	T37.2X3	T37.2X4	T37.2X5	T37.2X6
Primidone	T42.6X1	T42.6X2	T42.6X3	T42.6X4	T42.6X5	T42.6X6
Primula (veris)	T62.2X1	T62.2X2	T62.2X3	T62.2X4	—	—
Prinadol	T40.2X1	T40.2X2	T40.2X3	T40.2X4	T40.2X5	T40.2X6
Priscol, Priscoline	T44.6X1	T44.6X2	T44.6X3	T44.6X4	T44.6X5	T44.6X6
Pristinamycin	T36.3X1	T36.3X2	T36.3X3	T36.3X4	T36.3X5	T36.3X6
Privet	T62.2X1	T62.2X2	T62.2X3	T62.2X4	—	—
berries	T62.1X1	T62.1X2	T62.1X3	T62.1X4	—	—
Privine	T44.4X1	T44.4X2	T44.4X3	T44.4X4	T44.4X5	T44.4X6
Pro-Banthine	T44.3X1	T44.3X2	T44.3X3	T44.3X4	T44.3X5	T44.3X6
Probarbital	T42.3X1	T42.3X2	T42.3X3	T42.3X4	T42.3X5	T42.3X6
Probenecid	T50.4X1	T50.4X2	T50.4X3	T50.4X4	T50.4X5	T50.4X6
Probucol	T46.6X1	T46.6X2	T46.6X3	T46.6X4	T46.6X5	T46.6X6
Procainamide	T46.2X1	T46.2X2	T46.2X3	T46.2X4	T46.2X5	T46.2X6
Procaine	T41.3X1	T41.3X2	T41.3X3	T41.3X4	T41.3X5	T41.3X6
benzylpenicillin	T36.0X1	T36.0X2	T36.0X3	T36.0X4	T36.0X5	T36.0X6
nerve block (peripheral) (plexus)	T41.3X1	T41.3X2	T41.3X3	T41.3X4	T41.3X5	T41.3X6
penicillin G	T36.0X1	T36.0X2	T36.0X3	T36.0X4	T36.0X5	T36.0X6
regional	T41.3X1	T41.3X2	T41.3X3	T41.3X4	T41.3X5	T41.3X6
spinal	T41.3X1	T41.3X2	T41.3X3	T41.3X4	T41.3X5	T41.3X6
Procalmidol	T43.591	T43.592	T43.593	T43.594	T43.595	T43.596
Procarbazine	T45.1X1	T45.1X2	T45.1X3	T45.1X4	T45.1X5	T45.1X6
Procaterol	T44.5X1	T44.5X2	T44.5X3	T44.5X4	T44.5X5	T44.5X6
Prochlorperazine	T43.3X1	T43.3X2	T43.3X3	T43.3X4	T43.3X5	T43.3X6
Procyclidine	T44.3X1	T44.3X2	T44.3X3	T44.3X4	T44.3X5	T44.3X6
Producer gas	T58.8X1	T58.8X2	T58.8X3	T58.8X4	—	—
Profadol	T40.491	T40.492	T40.493	T40.494	T40.495	T40.496
Profenamine	T44.3X1	T44.3X2	T44.3X3	T44.3X4	T44.3X5	T44.3X6
Profenil	T44.3X1	T44.3X2	T44.3X3	T44.3X4	T44.3X5	T44.3X6
Proflavine	T49.0X1	T49.0X2	T49.0X3	T49.0X4	T49.0X5	T49.0X6
Progabide	T42.6X1	T42.6X2	T42.6X3	T42.6X4	T42.6X5	T42.6X6
Progesterone	T38.5X1	T38.5X2	T38.5X3	T38.5X4	T38.5X5	T38.5X6
Progestin	T38.5X1	T38.5X2	T38.5X3	T38.5X4	T38.5X5	T38.5X6
oral contraceptive	T38.4X1	T38.4X2	T38.4X3	T38.4X4	T38.4X5	T38.4X6
Progestogen NEC	T38.5X1	T38.5X2	T38.5X3	T38.5X4	T38.5X5	T38.5X6
Progestone	T38.5X1	T38.5X2	T38.5X3	T38.5X4	T38.5X5	T38.5X6
Proglumide	T47.1X1	T47.1X2	T47.1X3	T47.1X4	T47.1X5	T47.1X6
Proguanil	T37.2X1	T37.2X2	T37.2X3	T37.2X4	T37.2X5	T37.2X6
Prolactin	T38.811	T38.812	T38.813	T38.814	T38.815	T38.816

Substance	Poisoning, Accidental (unintentional)	Poisoning, Intentional self-harm	Poisoning, Assault	Poisoning, Undetermined	Adverse effect	Underdosing
Prolintane	T43.691	T43.692	T43.693	T43.694	T43.695	T43.696
Proloid	T38.1X1	T38.1X2	T38.1X3	T38.1X4	T38.1X5	T38.1X6
Proluton	T38.5X1	T38.5X2	T38.5X3	T38.5X4	T38.5X5	T38.5X6
Promacetin	T37.1X1	T37.1X2	T37.1X3	T37.1X4	T37.1X5	T37.1X6
Promazine	T43.3X1	T43.3X2	T43.3X3	T43.3X4	T43.3X5	T43.3X6
Promedol	T40.2X1	T40.2X2	T40.2X3	T40.2X4	—	—
Promegestone	T38.5X1	T38.5X2	T38.5X3	T38.5X4	T38.5X5	T38.5X6
Promethazine (teoclate)	T43.3X1	T43.3X2	T43.3X3	T43.3X4	T43.3X5	T43.3X6
Promin	T37.1X1	T37.1X2	T37.1X3	T37.1X4	T37.1X5	T37.1X6
Pronase	T45.3X1	T45.3X2	T45.3X3	T45.3X4	T45.3X5	T45.3X6
Pronestyl (hydrochloride)	T46.2X1	T46.2X2	T46.2X3	T46.2X4	T46.2X5	T46.2X6
Pronetalol	T44.7X1	T44.7X2	T44.7X3	T44.7X4	T44.7X5	T44.7X6
Prontosil	T37.0X1	T37.0X2	T37.0X3	T37.0X4	T37.0X5	T37.0X6
Propachlor	T60.3X1	T60.3X2	T60.3X3	T60.3X4	—	—
Propafenone	T46.2X1	T46.2X2	T46.2X3	T46.2X4	T46.2X5	T46.2X6
Propallylonal	T42.3X1	T42.3X2	T42.3X3	T42.3X4	T42.3X5	T42.3X6
Propamidine	T49.0X1	T49.0X2	T49.0X3	T49.0X4	T49.0X5	T49.0X6
Propane (distributed in mobile container)	T59.891	T59.892	T59.893	T59.894	—	—
distributed through pipes	T59.891	T59.892	T59.893	T59.894	—	—
incomplete combustion	T58.11	T58.12	T58.13	T58.14	—	—
Propanidid	T41.291	T41.292	T41.293	T41.294	T41.295	T41.296
Propanil	T60.3X1	T60.3X2	T60.3X3	T60.3X4	—	—
1-Propanol	T51.3X1	T51.3X2	T51.3X3	T51.3X4	—	—
2-Propanol	T51.2X1	T51.2X2	T51.2X3	T51.2X4	—	—
Propantheline	T44.3X1	T44.3X2	T44.3X3	T44.3X4	T44.3X5	T44.3X6
bromide	T44.3X1	T44.3X2	T44.3X3	T44.3X4	T44.3X5	T44.3X6
Proparacaine	T41.3X1	T41.3X2	T41.3X3	T41.3X4	T41.3X5	T41.3X6
Propatylnitrate	T46.3X1	T46.3X2	T46.3X3	T46.3X4	T46.3X5	T46.3X6
Propicillin	T36.0X1	T36.0X2	T36.0X3	T36.0X4	T36.0X5	T36.0X6
Propiolactone	T49.0X1	T49.0X2	T49.0X3	T49.0X4	T49.0X5	T49.0X6
Propiomazine	T45.0X1	T45.0X2	T45.0X3	T45.0X4	T45.0X5	T45.0X6
Propionaldehyde (medicinal)	T42.6X1	T42.6X2	T42.6X3	T42.6X4	T42.6X5	T42.6X6
Propionate (calcium) (sodium)	T49.0X1	T49.0X2	T49.0X3	T49.0X4	T49.0X5	T49.0X6
Propion gel	T49.0X1	T49.0X2	T49.0X3	T49.0X4	T49.0X5	T49.0X6
Propitocaine	T41.3X1	T41.3X2	T41.3X3	T41.3X4	T41.3X5	T41.3X6
infiltration (subcutaneous)	T41.3X1	T41.3X2	T41.3X3	T41.3X4	T41.3X5	T41.3X6
nerve block (peripheral) (plexus)	T41.3X1	T41.3X2	T41.3X3	T41.3X4	T41.3X5	T41.3X6
Propofol	T41.291	T41.292	T41.293	T41.294	T41.295	T41.296
Propoxur	T60.0X1	T60.0X2	T60.0X3	T60.0X4	—	—
Propoxycaine	T41.3X1	T41.3X2	T41.3X3	T41.3X4	T41.3X5	T41.3X6
infiltration (subcutaneous)	T41.3X1	T41.3X2	T41.3X3	T41.3X4	T41.3X5	T41.3X6
nerve block (peripheral) (plexus)	T41.3X1	T41.3X2	T41.3X3	T41.3X4	T41.3X5	T41.3X6
topical (surface)	T41.3X1	T41.3X2	T41.3X3	T41.3X4	T41.3X5	T41.3X6

Substance	Poisoning, Accidental (unintentional)	Poisoning, Intentional self-harm	Poisoning, Assault	Poisoning, Undetermined	Adverse effect	Underdosing
Propoxyphene	T40.491	T40.492	T40.493	T40.494	T40.495	T40.496
Propranolol	T44.7X1	T44.7X2	T44.7X4	T44.7X4	T44.7X5	T44.7X6
Propyl						
alcohol	T51.3X1	T51.3X2	T51.3X3	T51.3X4	—	—
carbinol	T51.3X1	T51.3X2	T51.3X3	T51.3X4	—	—
hexadrine	T44.4X1	T44.4X2	T44.4X3	T44.4X4	T44.4X5	T44.4X6
iodone	T50.8X1	T50.8X2	T50.8X3	T50.8X4	T50.8X5	T50.8X6
thiouracil	T38.2X1	T38.2X2	T38.2X3	T38.2X4	T38.2X5	T38.2X6
Propylaminophenothiazine	T43.3X1	T43.3X2	T43.3X3	T43.3X4	T43.3X5	T43.3X6
Propylene	T59.891	T59.892	T59.893	T59.894	—	—
Propylhexedrine	T48.5X1	T48.5X2	T48.5X3	T48.5X4	T48.5X5	T48.5X6
Propyliodone	T50.8X1	T50.8X2	T50.8X3	T50.8X4	T50.8X5	T50.8X6
Propylparaben (ophthalmic)	T49.5X1	T49.5X2	T49.5X3	T49.5X4	T49.5X5	T49.5X6
Propylthiouracil	T38.2X1	T38.2X2	T38.2X3	T38.2X4	T38.2X5	T38.2X6
Propyphenazone	T39.2X1	T39.2X2	T39.2X3	T39.2X4	T39.2X5	T39.2X6
Proquazone	T39.391	T39.392	T39.393	T39.394	T39.395	T39.396
Proscillaridin	T46.0X1	T46.0X2	T46.0X3	T46.0X4	T46.0X5	T46.0X6
Prostacyclin	T45.521	T45.522	T45.523	T45.524	T45.525	T45.526
Prostaglandin (I2)	T45.521	T45.522	T45.523	T45.524	T45.525	T45.526
E1	T46.7X1	T46.7X2	T46.7X3	T46.7X4	T46.7X5	T46.7X6
E2	T48.0X1	T48.0X2	T48.0X3	T48.0X4	T48.0X5	T48.0X6
F2 alpha	T48.0X1	T48.0X2	T48.0X3	T48.0X4	T48.0X5	T48.0X6
Prostigmin	T44.0X1	T44.0X2	T44.0X3	T44.0X4	T44.0X5	T44.0X6
Prosultiamine	T45.2X1	T45.2X2	T45.2X3	T45.2X4	T45.2X5	T45.2X6
Protamine sulfate	T45.7X1	T45.7X2	T45.7X3	T45.7X4	T45.7X5	T45.7X6
zinc insulin	T38.3X1	T38.3X2	T38.3X3	T38.3X4	T38.3X5	T38.3X6
Protease	T47.5X1	T47.5X2	T47.5X3	T47.5X4	T47.5X5	T47.5X6
Protectant, skin NEC	T49.3X1	T49.3X2	T49.3X3	T49.3X4	T49.3X5	T49.3X6
Protein hydrolysate	T50.991	T50.992	T50.993	T50.994	T50.995	T50.996
Prothiaden—see Dothiepin hydrochloride						
Prothionamide	T37.1X1	T37.1X2	T37.1X3	T37.1X4	T37.1X5	T37.1X6
Prothipendyl	T43.591	T43.592	T43.593	T43.594	T43.595	T43.596
Prothoate	T60.0X1	T60.0X2	T60.0X3	T60.0X4	—	—
Prothrombin						
activator	T45.7X1	T45.7X2	T45.7X3	T45.7X4	T45.7X5	T45.7X6
synthesis inhibitor	T45.511	T45.512	T45.513	T45.514	T45.515	T45.516
Protionamide	T37.1X1	T37.1X2	T37.1X3	T37.1X4	T37.1X5	T37.1X6
Protirelin	T38.891	T38.892	T38.893	T38.894	T38.895	T38.896
Protokylol	T48.6X1	T48.6X2	T48.6X3	T48.6X4	T48.6X5	T48.6X6
Protopam	T50.6X1	T50.6X2	T50.6X3	T50.6X4	T50.6X5	T50.6X6
Protoveratrine (s) (A) (B)	T46.5X1	T46.5X2	T46.5X3	T46.5X4	T46.5X5	T46.5X6
Protriptyline	T43.011	T43.012	T43.013	T43.014	T43.015	T43.016
Provera	T38.5X1	T38.5X2	T38.5X3	T38.5X4	T38.5X5	T38.5X6
Provitamin A	T45.2X1	T45.2X2	T45.2X3	T45.2X4	T45.2X5	T45.2X6
Proxibarbal	T42.3X1	T42.3X2	T42.3X3	T42.3X4	T42.3X5	T42.3X6
Proxymetacaine	T41.3X1	T41.3X2	T41.3X3	T41.3X4	T41.3X5	T41.3X6
Proxyphylline	T48.6X1	T48.6X2	T48.6X3	T48.6X4	T48.6X5	T48.6X6

Substance	Poisoning, Accidental (unintentional)	Poisoning, Intentional self-harm	Poisoning, Assault	Poisoning, Undetermined	Adverse effect	Underdosing
Prozac—see Fluoxetine hydrochloride						
Prunus						
laurocerasus	T62.2X1	T62.2X2	T62.2X3	T62.2X4	—	—
virginiana	T62.2X1	T62.2X2	T62.2X3	T62.2X4	—	—
Prussian blue						
commercial	T65.891	T65.892	T65.893	T65.894	—	—
therapeutic	T50.6X1	T50.6X2	T50.6X3	T50.6X4	T50.6X5	T50.6X6
Prussic acid	T65.0X1	T65.0X2	T65.0X3	T65.0X4	—	—
vapor	T57.3X1	T57.3X2	T57.3X3	T57.3X4	—	—
Pseudoephedrine	T44.991	T44.992	T44.993	T44.994	T44.995	T44.996
Psilocin	T40.991	T40.992	T40.993	T40.994	—	—
Psilocybin	T40.991	T40.992	T40.993	T40.994	—	—
Psilocybine	T40.991	T40.992	T40.993	T40.994	—	—
Psoralene (nonmedicinal)	T65.891	T65.892	T65.893	T65.894	—	—
Psoralens (medicinal)	T50.991	T50.992	T50.993	T50.994	T50.995	T50.996
PSP (phenolsulfonphthalein)	T50.8X1	T50.8X2	T50.8X3	T50.8X4	T50.8X5	T50.8X6
Psychodysleptic drug NOS	T40.901	T40.902	T40.903	T40.904	T40.905	T40.906
specified NEC	T40.991	T40.992	T40.993	T40.994	T40.995	T40.996
Psychostimulant	T43.601	T43.602	T43.603	T43.604	T43.605	T43.606
amphetamine	T43.621	T43.622	T43.623	T43.624	T43.625	T43.626
caffeine	T43.611	T43.612	T43.613	T43.614	T43.615	T43.616
methylphenidate	T43.631	T43.632	T43.633	T43.634	T43.635	T43.636
specified NEC	T43.691	T43.692	T43.693	T43.694	T43.695	T43.696
Psychotherapeutic drug NEC	T43.91	T43.92	T43.93	T43.94	T43.95	T43.96
antidepressants—see also Antidepressant	T43.201	T43.202	T43.203	T43.204	T43.205	T43.206
specified NEC	T43.8X1	T43.8X2	T43.8X3	T43.8X4	T43.8X5	T43.8X6
tranquilizers NEC	T43.501	T43.502	T43.503	T43.504	T43.505	T43.506
Psychotomimetic agents	T40.901	T40.902	T40.903	T40.904	T40.905	T40.906
Psychotropic drug NEC	T43.91	T43.92	T43.93	T43.94	T43.95	T43.96
specified NEC	T43.8X1	T43.8X2	T43.8X3	T43.8X4	T43.8X5	T43.8X6
Psyllium hydrophilic mucilloid	T47.4X1	T47.4X2	T47.4X3	T47.4X4	T47.4X5	T47.4X6
Pteroylglutamic acid	T45.8X1	T45.8X2	T45.8X3	T45.8X4	T45.8X5	T45.8X6
Pteroyltriglutamate	T45.1X1	T45.1X2	T45.1X3	T45.1X4	T45.1X5	T45.1X6
PTFE—see Polytetrafluoroethylene						
Pulp						
devitalizing paste	T49.7X1	T49.7X2	T49.7X3	T49.7X4	T49.7X5	T49.7X6
dressing	T49.7X1	T49.7X2	T49.7X3	T49.7X4	T49.7X5	T49.7X6
Pulsatilla	T62.2X1	T62.2X2	T62.2X3	T62.2X4	—	—
Pumpkin seed extract	T37.4X1	T37.4X2	T37.4X3	T37.4X4	T37.4X5	T37.4X6
Purex (bleach)	T54.91	T54.92	T54.93	T54.94	—	—
Purgative NEC—also Cathartic	T47.4X1	T47.4X2	T47.4X3	T47.4X4	T47.4X5	T47.4X6
Purine analogue (antineoplastic)	T45.1X1	T45.1X2	T45.1X3	T45.1X4	T45.1X5	T45.1X6

Substance	Poisoning, Accidental (unintentional)	Poisoning, Intentional self-harm	Poisoning, Assault	Poisoning, Undetermined	Adverse effect	Underdosing
Purine diuretics	T50.2X1	T50.2X2	T50.2X3	T50.2X4	T50.2X5	T50.2X6
Purinethol	T45.1X1	T45.1X2	T45.1X3	T45.1X4	T45.1X5	T45.1X6
PVP	T45.8X1	T45.8X2	T45.8X3	T45.8X4	T45.8X5	T45.8X6
Pyrabital	T39.8X1	T39.8X2	T39.8X3	T39.8X4	T39.8X5	T39.8X6
Pyramidon	T39.2X1	T39.2X2	T39.2X3	T39.2X4	T39.2X5	T39.2X6
Pyrantel	T37.4X1	T37.4X2	T37.4X3	T37.4X4	T37.4X5	T37.4X6
Pyrathiazine	T45.0X1	T45.0X2	T45.0X3	T45.0X4	T45.0X5	T45.0X6
Pyrazinamide	T37.1X1	T37.1X2	T37.1X3	T37.1X4	T37.1X5	T37.1X6
Pyrazinoic acid (amide)	T37.1X1	T37.1X2	T37.1X3	T37.1X4	T37.1X5	T37.1X6
Pyrazole (derivatives)	T39.2X1	T39.2X2	T39.2X3	T39.2X4	T39.2X5	T39.2X6
Pyrazolone analgesic NEC	T39.2X1	T39.2X2	T39.2X3	T39.2X4	T39.2X5	T39.2X6
Pyrethrin, pyrethrum (nonmedicinal)	T60.2X1	T60.2X2	T60.2X3	T60.2X4	—	—
Pyrethrum extract	T49.0X1	T49.0X2	T49.0X3	T49.0X4	T49.0X5	T49.0X6
Pyribenzamine	T45.0X1	T45.0X2	T45.0X3	T45.0X4	T45.0X5	T45.0X6
Pyridine	T52.8X1	T52.8X2	T52.8X3	T52.8X4	—	—
aldoxime methiodide	T50.6X1	T50.6X2	T50.6X3	T50.6X4	T50.6X5	T50.6X6
aldoxime methyl chloride	T50.6X1	T50.6X2	T50.6X3	T50.6X4	T50.6X5	T50.6X6
vapor	T59.891	T59.892	T59.893	T59.894	—	—
Pyridium	T39.8X1	T39.8X2	T39.8X3	T39.8X4	T39.8X5	T39.8X6
Pyridostigmine bromide	T44.0X1	T44.0X2	T44.0X3	T44.0X4	T44.0X5	T44.0X6
Pyridoxal phosphate	T45.2X1	T45.2X2	T45.2X3	T45.2X4	T45.2X5	T45.2X6
Pyridoxine	T45.2X1	T45.2X2	T45.2X3	T45.2X4	T45.2X5	T45.2X6
Pyrilamine	T45.0X1	T45.0X2	T45.0X3	T45.0X4	T45.0X5	T45.0X6
Pyrimethamine	T37.2X1	T37.2X2	T37.2X3	T37.2X4	T37.2X5	T37.2X6
with sulfadoxine	T37.2X1	T37.2X2	T37.2X3	T37.2X4	T37.2X5	T37.2X6
Pyrimidine antagonist	T45.1X1	T45.1X2	T45.1X3	T45.1X4	T45.1X5	T45.1X6
Pyriminil	T60.4X1	T60.4X2	T60.4X3	T60.4X4	—	—
Pyrithione zinc	T49.4X1	T49.4X2	T49.4X3	T49.4X4	T49.4X5	T49.4X6
Pyrithyldione	T42.6X1	T42.6X2	T42.6X3	T42.6X4	T42.6X5	T42.6X6
Pyrogallic acid	T49.0X1	T49.0X2	T49.0X3	T49.0X4	T49.0X5	T49.0X6
Pyrogallol	T49.0X1	T49.0X2	T49.0X3	T49.0X4	T49.0X5	T49.0X6
Pyroxylin	T49.3X1	T49.3X2	T49.3X3	T49.3X4	T49.3X5	T49.3X6
Pyrrobutamine	T45.0X1	T45.0X2	T45.0X3	T45.0X4	T45.0X5	T45.0X6
Pyrrolizidine alkaloids	T62.8X1	T62.8X2	T62.8X3	T62.8X4	—	—
Pyrvinium chloride	T37.4X1	T37.4X2	T37.4X3	T37.4X4	T37.4X5	T37.4X6
PZI	T38.3X1	T38.3X2	T38.3X3	T38.3X4	T38.3X5	T38.3X6
Q						
Quaalude	T42.6X1	T42.6X2	T42.6X3	T42.6X4	T42.6X5	T42.6X6
Quarternary ammonium						
anti-infective	T49.0X1	T49.0X2	T49.0X3	T49.0X4	T49.0X5	T49.0X6
ganglion blocking	T44.2X1	T44.2X2	T44.2X3	T44.2X4	T44.2X5	T44.2X6
parasympatholytic	T44.3X1	T44.3X2	T44.3X3	T44.3X4	T44.3X5	T44.3X6
Quazepam	T42.4X1	T42.4X2	T42.4X3	T42.4X4	T42.4X5	T42.4X6
Quicklime	T54.3X1	T54.3X2	T54.3X3	T54.3X4	—	—
Quillaja extract	T48.4X1	T48.4X2	T48.4X3	T48.4X4	T48.4X5	T48.4X6
Quinacrine	T37.2X1	T37.2X2	T37.2X3	T37.2X4	T37.2X5	T37.2X6
Quinaglute	T46.2X1	T46.2X2	T46.2X3	T46.2X4	T46.2X5	T46.2X6
Quinalbarbital	T42.3X1	T42.3X2	T42.3X3	T42.3X4	T42.3X5	T42.3X6

Substance	Poisoning, Accidental (unintentional)	Poisoning, Intentional self-harm	Poisoning, Assault	Poisoning, Undetermined	Adverse effect	Underdosing
Quinalbarbitone sodium	T42.3X1	T42.3X2	T42.3X3	T42.3X4	T42.3X5	T42.3X6
Quinalphos	T60.0X1	T60.0X2	T60.0X3	T60.0X4	—	—
Quinapril	T46.4X1	T46.4X2	T46.4X3	T46.4X4	T46.4X5	T46.4X6
Quinestradiol	T38.5X1	T38.5X2	T38.5X3	T38.5X4	T38.5X5	T38.5X6
Quinestradol	T38.5X1	T38.5X2	T38.5X3	T38.5X4	T38.5X5	T38.5X6
Quinestrol	T38.5X1	T38.5X2	T38.5X3	T38.5X4	T38.5X5	T38.5X6
Quinethazone	T50.2X1	T50.2X2	T50.2X3	T50.2X4	T50.2X5	T50.2X6
Quingestanol	T38.4X1	T38.4X2	T38.4X3	T38.4X4	T38.4X5	T38.4X6
Quinidine	T46.2X1	T46.2X2	T46.2X3	T46.2X4	T46.2X5	T46.2X6
Quinine	T37.2X1	T37.2X2	T37.2X3	T37.2X4	T37.2X5	T37.2X6
Quiniobine	T37.8X1	T37.8X2	T37.8X3	T37.8X4	T37.8X5	T37.8X6
Quinisocaine	T49.1X1	T49.1X2	T49.1X3	T49.1X4	T49.1X5	T49.1X6
Quinocide	T37.2X1	T37.2X2	T37.2X3	T37.2X4	T37.2X5	T37.2X6
Quinoline (derivatives) NEC	T37.8X1	T37.8X2	T37.8X3	T37.8X4	T37.8X5	T37.8X6
Quinupramine	T43.011	T43.012	T43.013	T43.014	T43.015	T43.016
Quotane	T41.3X1	T41.3X2	T41.3X3	T41.3X4	T41.3X5	T41.3X6
R						
Rabies						
immune globulin (human)	T50.Z11	T50.Z12	T50.Z13	T50.Z14	T50.Z15	T50.Z16
vaccine	T50.B91	T50.B92	T50.B93	T50.B94	T50.B95	T50.B96
Racemoramide	T40.2X1	T40.2X2	T40.2X3	T40.2X4	—	—
Racemorphan	T40.2X1	T40.2X2	T40.2X3	T40.2X4	T40.2X5	T40.2X6
Racepinefrin	T44.5X1	T44.5X2	T44.5X3	T44.5X4	T44.5X5	T44.5X6
Raclopride	T43.591	T43.592	T43.593	T43.594	T43.595	T43.596
Radiator alcohol	T51.1X1	T51.1X2	T51.1X3	T51.1X4	—	—
Radioactive drug NEC	T50.8X1	T50.8X2	T50.8X3	T50.8X4	T50.8X5	T50.8X6
Radio-opaque (drugs) (materials)	T50.8X1	T50.8X2	T50.8X3	T50.8X4	T50.8X5	T50.8X6
Ramifenazone	T39.2X1	T39.2X2	T39.2X3	T39.2X4	T39.2X5	T39.2X6
Ramipril	T46.4X1	T46.4X2	T46.4X3	T46.4X4	T46.4X5	T46.4X6
Ranitidine	T47.0X1	T47.0X2	T47.0X3	T47.0X4	T47.0X5	T47.0X6
Ranunculus	T62.2X1	T62.2X2	T62.2X3	T62.2X4		
Rat poison NEC	T60.4X1	T60.4X2	T60.4X3	T60.4X4		
Rattlesnake (venom)	T63.011	T63.012	T63.013	T63.014	—	—
Raubasine	T46.7X1	T46.7X2	T46.7X3	T46.7X4	T46.7X5	T46.7X6
Raudixin	T46.5X1	T46.5X2	T46.5X3	T46.5X4	T46.5X5	T46.5X6
Rautensin	T46.5X1	T46.5X2	T46.5X3	T46.5X4	T46.5X5	T46.5X6
Rautina	T46.5X1	T46.5X2	T46.5X3	T46.5X4	T46.5X5	T46.5X6
Rautotal	T46.5X1	T46.5X2	T46.5X3	T46.5X4	T46.5X5	T46.5X6
Rauwiloid	T46.5X1	T46.5X2	T46.5X3	T46.5X4	T46.5X5	T46.5X6
Rauwoldin	T46.5X1	T46.5X2	T46.5X3	T46.5X4	T46.5X5	T46.5X6
Rauwolfia (alkaloids)	T46.5X1	T46.5X2	T46.5X3	T46.5X4	T46.5X5	T46.5X6
Razoxane	T45.1X1	T45.1X2	T45.1X3	T45.1X4	T45.1X5	T45.1X6
Realgar	T57.0X1	T57.0X2	T57.0X3	T57.0X4	—	—
Recombinant(R)—see specific protein						
Red blood cells, packed	T45.8X1	T45.8X2	T45.8X3	T45.8X4	T45.8X5	T45.8X6
Red squill (scilliroside)	T60.4X1	T60.4X2	T60.4X3	T60.4X4		
Reducing agent, industrial NEC	T65.891	T65.892	T65.893	T65.894	—	—

Substance	Poisoning, Accidental (unintentional)	Poisoning, Intentional self-harm	Poisoning, Assault	Poisoning, Undetermined	Adverse effect	Underdosing
Refrigerant gas (chlorofluoro-carbon)	T53.5X1	T53.5X2	T53.5X3	T53.5X4	—	—
not chlorofluoro-carbon	T59.891	T59.892	T59.893	T59.894	—	—
Regroton	T50.2X1	T50.2X2	T50.2X3	T50.2X4	T50.2X5	T50.2X6
Rehydration salts (oral)	T50.3X1	T50.3X2	T50.3X3	T50.3X4	T50.3X5	T50.3X6
Rela	T42.8X1	T42.8X2	T42.8X3	T42.8X4	T42.8X5	T42.8X6
Relaxant, muscle						
anesthetic	T48.1X1	T48.1X2	T48.1X3	T48.1X4	T48.1X5	T48.1X6
central nervous system	T42.8X1	T42.8X2	T42.8X3	T42.8X4	T42.8X5	T42.8X6
skeletal NEC	T48.1X1	T48.1X2	T48.1X3	T48.1X4	T48.1X5	T48.1X6
smooth NEC	T44.3X1	T44.3X2	T44.3X3	T44.3X4	T44.3X5	T44.3X6
Remoxipride	T43.591	T43.592	T43.593	T43.594	T43.595	T43.596
Renese	T50.2X1	T50.2X2	T50.2X3	T50.2X4	T50.2X5	T50.2X6
Renografin	T50.8X1	T50.8X2	T50.8X3	T50.8X4	T50.8X5	T50.8X6
Replacement solution	T50.3X1	T50.3X2	T50.3X3	T50.3X4	T50.3X5	T50.3X6
Reproterol	T48.6X1	T48.6X2	T48.6X3	T48.6X4	T48.6X5	T48.6X6
Rescinnamine	T46.5X1	T46.5X2	T46.5X3	T46.5X4	T46.5X5	T46.5X6
Reserpin(e)	T46.5X1	T46.5X2	T46.5X3	T46.5X4	T46.5X5	T46.5X6
Resorcin, resorcinol (nonmedicinal)	T65.891	T65.892	T65.893	T65.894	—	—
medicinal	T49.4X1	T49.4X2	T49.4X3	T49.4X4	T49.4X5	T49.4X6
Respaire	T48.4X1	T48.4X2	T48.4X3	T48.4X4	T48.4X5	T48.4X6
Respiratory drug NEC	T48.901	T48.902	T48.903	T48.904	T48.905	T48.906
antiasthmatic NEC	T48.6X1	T48.6X2	T48.6X3	T48.6X4	T48.6X5	T48.6X6
anti-common-cold NEC	T48.5X1	T48.5X2	T48.5X3	T48.5X4	T48.5X5	T48.5X6
expectorant NEC	T48.4X1	T48.4X2	T48.4X3	T48.4X4	T48.4X5	T48.4X6
stimulant	T48.901	T48.902	T48.903	T48.904	T48.905	T48.906
Retinoic acid	T49.0X1	T49.0X2	T49.0X3	T49.0X4	T49.0X5	T49.0X6
Retinol	T45.2X1	T45.2X2	T45.2X3	T45.2X4	T45.2X5	T45.2X6
Rh(D) immune globulin (human)	T50.Z11	T50.Z12	T50.Z13	T50.Z14	T50.Z15	T50.Z16
Rhodine	T39.011	T39.012	T39.013	T39.014	T39.015	T39.016
RhoGAM	T50.Z11	T50.Z12	T50.Z13	T50.Z14	T50.Z15	T50.Z16
Rhubarb						
dry extract	T47.2X1	T47.2X2	T47.2X3	T47.2X4	T47.2X5	T47.2X6
tincture, compound	T47.2X1	T47.2X2	T47.2X3	T47.2X4	T47.2X5	T47.2X6
Ribavirin	T37.5X1	T37.5X2	T37.5X3	T37.5X4	T37.5X5	T37.5X6
Riboflavin	T45.2X1	T45.2X2	T45.2X3	T45.2X4	T45.2X5	T45.2X6
Ribostamycin	T36.5X1	T36.5X2	T36.5X3	T36.5X4	T36.5X5	T36.5X6
Ricin	T62.2X1	T62.2X2	T62.2X3	T62.2X4	—	—
Ricinus communis	T62.2X1	T62.2X2	T62.2X3	T62.2X4	—	—
Rickettsial vaccine NEC	T50.A91	T50.A92	T50.A93	T50.A94	T50.A95	T50.A96
Rifabutin	T36.6X1	T36.6X2	T36.6X3	T36.6X4	T36.6X5	T36.6X6
Rifamide	T36.6X1	T36.6X2	T36.6X3	T36.6X4	T36.6X5	T36.6X6
Rifampicin	T36.6X1	T36.6X2	T36.6X3	T36.6X4	T36.6X5	T36.6X6
with isoniazid	T37.1X1	T37.1X2	T37.1X3	T37.1X4	T37.1X5	T37.1X6
Rifampin	T36.6X1	T36.6X2	T36.6X3	T36.6X4	T36.6X5	T36.6X6
Rifamycin	T36.6X1	T36.6X2	T36.6X3	T36.6X4	T36.6X5	T36.6X6
Rifaximin	T36.6X1	T36.6X2	T36.6X3	T36.6X4	T36.6X5	T36.6X6

Substance	Poisoning, Accidental (unintentional)	Poisoning, Intentional self-harm	Poisoning, Assault	Poisoning, Undetermined	Adverse effect	Underdosing
Rimantadine	T37.5X1	T37.5X2	T37.5X3	T37.5X4	T37.5X5	T37.5X6
Rimazolium metilsulfate	T39.8X1	T39.8X2	T39.8X3	T39.8X4	T39.8X5	T39.8X6
Rimifon	T37.1X1	T37.1X2	T37.1X3	T37.1X4	T37.1X5	T37.1X6
Rimiterol	T48.6X1	T48.6X2	T48.6X3	T48.6X4	T48.6X5	T48.6X6
Ringer (lactate) solution	T50.3X1	T50.3X2	T50.3X3	T50.3X4	T50.3X5	T50.3X6
Ristocetin	T36.8X1	T36.8X2	T36.8X3	T36.8X4	T36.8X5	T36.8X6
Ritalin	T43.631	T43.632	T43.633	T43.634	T43.635	T43.636
Ritodrine	T44.5X1	T44.5X2	T44.5X3	T44.5X4	T44.5X5	T44.5X6
Roach killer—see Insecticide						
Rociverine	T44.3X1	T44.3X2	T44.3X3	T44.3X4	T44.3X5	T44.3X6
Rocky Mountain spotted fever vaccine	T50.A91	T50.A92	T50.A93	T50.A94	T50.A95	T50.A96
Rodenticide NEC	T60.4X1	T60.4X2	T60.4X3	T60.4X4	—	—
Rohypnol	T42.4X1	T42.4X2	T42.4X3	T42.4X4	T42.4X5	T42.4X6
Rokitamycin	T36.3X1	T36.3X2	T36.3X3	T36.3X4	T36.3X5	T36.3X6
Rolaids	T47.1X1	T47.1X2	T47.1X3	T47.1X4	T47.1X5	T47.1X6
Rolitetracycline	T36.4X1	T36.4X2	T36.4X3	T36.4X4	T36.4X5	T36.4X6
Romilar	T48.3X1	T48.3X2	T48.3X3	T48.3X4	T48.3X5	T48.3X6
Ronifibrate	T46.6X1	T46.6X2	T46.6X3	T46.6X4	T46.6X5	T46.6X6
Rosaprostol	T47.1X1	T47.1X2	T47.1X3	T47.1X4	T47.1X5	T47.1X6
Rose bengal sodium (131I)	T50.8X1	T50.8X2	T50.8X3	T50.8X4	T50.8X5	T50.8X6
Rose water ointment	T49.3X1	T49.3X2	T49.3X3	T49.3X4	T49.3X5	T49.3X6
Rosoxacin	T37.8X1	T37.8X2	T37.8X3	T37.8X4	T37.8X5	T37.8X6
Rotenone	T60.2X1	T60.2X2	T60.2X3	T60.2X4	—	—
Rotoxamine	T45.0X1	T45.0X2	T45.0X3	T45.0X4	T45.0X5	T45.0X6
Rough-on-rats	T60.4X1	T60.4X2	T60.4X3	T60.4X4	—	—
Roxatidine	T47.0X1	T47.0X2	T47.0X3	T47.0X4	T47.0X5	T47.0X6
Roxithromycin	T36.3X1	T36.3X2	T36.3X3	T36.3X4	T36.3X5	T36.3X6
Rt-PA	T45.611	T45.612	T45.613	T45.614	T45.615	T45.616
Rubbing alcohol	T51.2X1	T51.2X2	T51.2X3	T51.2X4	—	—
Rubefacient	T49.4X1	T49.4X2	T49.4X3	T49.4X4	T49.4X5	T49.4X6
Rubella vaccine	T50.B91	T50.B92	T50.B93	T50.B94	T50.B95	T50.B96
Rubeola vaccine	T50.B91	T50.B92	T50.B93	T50.B94	T50.B95	T50.B96
Rubidium chloride Rb82	T50.8X1	T50.8X2	T50.8X3	T50.8X4	T50.8X5	T50.8X6
Rubidomycin	T45.1X1	T45.1X2	T45.1X3	T45.1X4	T45.1X5	T45.1X6
Rue	T62.2X1	T62.2X2	T62.2X3	T62.2X4	—	—
Rufocromomycin	T45.1X1	T45.1X2	T45.1X3	T45.1X4	T45.1X5	T45.1X6
Russel's viper venin	T45.7X1	T45.7X2	T45.7X3	T45.7X4	T45.7X5	T45.7X6
Ruta (graveolens)	T62.2X1	T62.2X2	T62.2X3	T62.2X4	—	—
Rutinum	T46.991	T46.992	T46.993	T46.994	T46.995	T46.996
Rutoside	T46.991	T46.992	T46.993	T46.994	T46.995	T46.996
S						
Sabadilla (plant)	T62.2X1	T62.2X2	T62.2X3	T62.2X4	—	—
pesticide	T60.2X1	T60.2X2	T60.2X3	T60.2X4	—	—
Saccharated iron oxide	T45.8X1	T45.8X2	T45.8X3	T45.8X4	T45.8X5	T45.8X6
Saccharin	T50.901	T50.902	T50.903	T50.904	T50.905	T50.906
Saccharomyces boulardii	T47.6X1	T47.6X2	T47.6X3	T47.6X4	T47.6X5	T47.6X6
Safflower oil	T46.6X1	T46.6X2	T46.6X3	T46.6X4	T46.6X5	T46.6X6
Safrazine	T43.1X1	T43.1X2	T43.1X3	T43.1X4	T43.1X5	T43.1X6

Substance	Poisoning, Accidental (unintentional)	Poisoning, Intentional self-harm	Poisoning, Assault	Poisoning, Undetermined	Adverse effect	Underdosing
Salazosulfapyridine	T37.0X1	T37.0X2	T37.0X3	T37.0X4	T37.0X5	T37.0X6
Salbutamol	T48.6X1	T48.6X2	T48.6X3	T48.6X4	T48.6X5	T48.6X6
Salicylamide	T39.091	T39.092	T39.093	T39.094	T39.095	T39.096
Salicylate NEC	T39.091	T39.092	T39.093	T39.094	T39.095	T39.096
methyl	T49.3X1	T49.3X2	T49.3X3	T49.3X4	T49.3X5	T49.3X6
theobromine calcium	T50.2X1	T50.2X2	T50.2X3	T50.2X4	T50.2X5	T50.2X6
Salicylazosulfapyridine	T37.0X1	T37.0X2	T37.0X3	T37.0X4	T37.0X5	T37.0X6
Salicylhydroxamic acid	T49.0X1	T49.0X2	T49.0X3	T49.0X4	T49.0X5	T49.0X6
Salicylic acid	T49.4X1	T49.4X2	T49.4X3	T49.4X4	T49.4X5	T49.4X6
with benzoic acid	T49.4X1	T49.4X2	T49.4X3	T49.4X4	T49.4X5	T49.4X6
congeners	T39.091	T39.092	T39.093	T39.094	T39.095	T39.096
derivative	T39.091	T39.092	T39.093	T39.094	T39.095	T39.096
salts	T39.091	T39.092	T39.093	T39.094	T39.095	T39.096
Salinazid	T37.1X1	T37.1X2	T37.1X3	T37.1X4	T37.1X5	T37.1X6
Salmeterol	T48.6X1	T48.6X2	T48.6X3	T48.6X4	T48.6X5	T48.6X6
Salol	T49.3X1	T49.3X2	T49.3X3	T49.3X4	T49.3X5	T49.3X6
Salsalate	T39.091	T39.092	T39.093	T39.094	T39.095	T39.096
Salt substitute	T50.901	T50.902	T50.903	T50.904	T50.905	T50.906
Salt-replacing drug	T50.901	T50.902	T50.903	T50.904	T50.905	T50.906
Salt-retaining mineralocorticoid	T50.0X1	T50.0X2	T50.0X3	T50.0X4	T50.0X5	T50.0X6
Saluretic NEC	T50.2X1	T50.2X2	T50.2X3	T50.2X4	T50.2X5	T50.2X6
Saluron	T50.2X1	T50.2X2	T50.2X3	T50.2X4	T50.2X5	T50.2X6
Salvarsan 606 (neosilver) (silver)	T37.8X1	T37.8X2	T37.8X3	T37.8X4	T37.8X5	T37.8X6
Sambucus canadensis	T62.2X1	T62.2X2	T62.2X3	T62.2X4	—	—
berry	T62.1X1	T62.1X2	T62.1X3	T62.1X4	—	—
Sandril	T46.5X1	T46.5X2	T46.5X3	T46.5X4	T46.5X5	T46.5X6
Sanguinaria canadensis	T62.2X1	T62.2X2	T62.2X3	T62.2X4	—	—
Saniflush (cleaner)	T54.2X1	T54.2X2	T54.2X3	T54.2X4	—	—
Santonin	T37.4X1	T37.4X2	T37.4X3	T37.4X4	T37.4X5	T37.4X6
Santyl	T49.8X1	T49.8X2	T49.8X3	T49.8X4	T49.8X5	T49.8X6
Saralasin	T46.5X1	T46.5X2	T46.5X3	T46.5X4	T46.5X5	T46.5X6
Sarcolysin	T45.1X1	T45.1X2	T45.1X3	T45.1X4	T45.1X5	T45.1X6
Sarkomycin	T45.1X1	T45.1X2	T45.1X3	T45.1X4	T45.1X5	T45.1X6
Saroten	T43.011	T43.012	T43.013	T43.014	T43.015	T43.016
Saturnine—see Lead						
Savin (oil)	T49.4X1	T49.4X2	T49.4X3	T49.4X4	T49.4X5	T49.4X6
Scammony	T47.2X1	T47.2X2	T47.2X3	T47.2X4	T47.2X5	T47.2X6
Scarlet red	T49.8X1	T49.8X2	T49.8X3	T49.8X4	T49.8X5	T49.8X6
Scheele's green	T57.0X1	T57.0X2	T57.0X3	T57.0X4	—	—
insecticide	T57.0X1	T57.0X2	T57.0X3	T57.0X4	—	—
Schizontozide (blood) (tissue)	T37.2X1	T37.2X2	T37.2X3	T37.2X4	T37.2X5	T37.2X6
Schradan	T60.0X1	T60.0X2	T60.0X3	T60.0X4	—	—
Schweinfurth green	T57.0X1	T57.0X2	T57.0X3	T57.0X4	—	—
insecticide	T57.0X1	T57.0X2	T57.0X3	T57.0X4	—	—
Scilla, rat poison	T60.4X1	T60.4X2	T60.4X3	T60.4X4	—	—
Scillaren	T60.4X1	T60.4X2	T60.4X3	T60.4X4	—	—
Sclerosing agent	T46.8X1	T46.8X2	T46.8X3	T46.8X4	T46.8X5	T46.8X6
Scombrotoxin	T61.11	T61.12	T61.13	T61.14	—	—

Substance	Poisoning, Accidental (unintentional)	Poisoning, Intentional self-harm	Poisoning, Assault	Poisoning, Undetermined	Adverse effect	Underdosing
Scopolamine	T44.3X1	T44.3X2	T44.3X3	T44.3X4	T44.3X5	T44.3X6
Scopolia extract	T44.3X1	T44.3X2	T44.3X3	T44.3X4	T44.3X5	T44.3X6
Scouring powder	T65.891	T65.892	T65.893	T65.894	—	—
Sea						
anemone (sting)	T63.631	T63.632	T63.633	T63.634		
cucumber (sting)	T63.691	T63.692	T63.693	T63.694		
snake (bite) (venom)	T63.091	T63.092	T63.093	T63.094		
urchin spine (puncture)	T63.691	T63.692	T63.693	T63.694		
Seafood	T61.91	T61.92	T61.93	T61.94		
specified NEC	T61.8X1	T61.8X2	T61.8X3	T61.8X4		
Secbutabarbital	T42.3X1	T42.3X2	T42.3X3	T42.3X4	T42.3X5	T42.3X6
Secbutabarbitone	T42.3X1	T42.3X2	T42.3X3	T42.3X4	T42.3X5	T42.3X6
Secnidazole	T37.3X1	T37.3X2	T37.3X3	T37.3X4	T37.3X5	T37.3X6
Secobarbital	T42.3X1	T42.3X2	T42.3X3	T42.3X4	T42.3X5	T42.3X6
Seconal	T42.3X1	T42.3X2	T42.3X3	T42.3X4	T42.3X5	T42.3X6
Secretin	T50.8X1	T50.8X2	T50.8X3	T50.8X4	T50.8X5	T50.8X6
Sedative NEC	T42.71	T42.72	T42.73	T42.74	T42.75	T42.76
mixed NEC	T42.6X1	T42.6X2	T42.6X3	T42.6X4	T42.6X5	T42.6X6
Sedormid	T42.6X1	T42.6X2	T42.6X3	T42.6X4	T42.6X5	T42.6X6
Seed disinfectant or dressing	T60.8X1	T60.8X2	T60.8X3	T60.8X4	—	—
Seeds (poisonous)	T62.2X1	T62.2X2	T62.2X3	T62.2X4	—	—
Selegiline	T42.8X1	T42.8X2	T42.8X3	T42.8X4	T42.8X5	T42.8X6
Selenium NEC	T56.891	T56.892	T56.893	T56.894	—	—
disulfide or sulfide	T49.4X1	T49.4X2	T49.4X3	T49.4X4	T49.4X5	T49.4X6
fumes	T59.891	T59.892	T59.893	T59.894	—	—
sulfide	T49.4X1	T49.4X2	T49.4X3	T49.4X4	T49.4X5	T49.4X6
Selenomethionine (75Se)	T50.8X1	T50.8X2	T50.8X3	T50.8X4	T50.8X5	T50.8X6
Selsun	T49.4X1	T49.4X2	T49.4X3	T49.4X4	T49.4X5	T49.4X6
Semustine	T45.1X1	T45.1X2	T45.1X3	T45.1X4	T45.1X5	T45.1X6
Senega syrup	T48.4X1	T48.4X2	T48.4X3	T48.4X4	T48.4X5	T48.4X6
Senna	T47.2X1	T47.2X2	T47.2X3	T47.2X4	T47.2X5	T47.2X6
Sennoside A+B	T47.2X1	T47.2X2	T47.2X3	T47.2X4	T47.2X5	T47.2X6
Septisol	T49.2X1	T49.2X2	T49.2X3	T49.2X4	T49.2X5	T49.2X6
Seractide	T38.811	T38.812	T38.813	T38.814	T38.815	T38.816
Serax	T42.4X1	T42.4X2	T42.4X3	T42.4X4	T42.4X5	T42.4X6
Serenesil	T42.6X1	T42.6X2	T42.6X3	T42.6X4	T42.6X5	T42.6X6
Serenium (hydrochloride)	T37.91	T37.92	T37.93	T37.94	T37.95	T37.96
Serepax—see Oxazepam						
Sermorelin	T38.891	T38.892	T38.893	T38.894	T38.895	T38.896
Sernyl	T41.1X1	T41.1X2	T41.1X3	T41.1X4	T41.1X5	T41.1X6
Serotonin	T50.991	T50.992	T50.993	T50.994	T50.995	T50.996
Serpasil	T46.5X1	T46.5X2	T46.5X3	T46.5X4	T46.5X5	T46.5X6
Serrapeptase	T45.3X1	T45.3X2	T45.3X3	T45.3X4	T45.3X5	T45.3X6
Serum						
antibotulinus	T50.Z11	T50.Z12	T50.Z13	T50.Z14	T50.Z15	T50.Z16
anticytotoxic	T50.Z11	T50.Z12	T50.Z13	T50.Z14	T50.Z15	T50.Z16
antidiphtheria	T50.Z11	T50.Z12	T50.Z13	T50.Z14	T50.Z15	T50.Z16
antimeningococcus	T50.Z11	T50.Z12	T50.Z13	T50.Z14	T50.Z15	T50.Z16
anti-Rh	T50.Z11	T50.Z12	T50.Z13	T50.Z14	T50.Z15	T50.Z16

Substance	Poisoning, Accidental (unintentional)	Poisoning, Intentional self-harm	Poisoning, Assault	Poisoning, Undetermined	Adverse effect	Underdosing
Serum — *Continued*						
anti-snake-bite	T50.Z11	T50.Z12	T50.Z13	T50.Z14	T50.Z15	T50.Z16
antitetanic	T50.Z11	T50.Z12	T50.Z13	T50.Z14	T50.Z15	T50.Z16
antitoxic	T50.Z11	T50.Z12	T50.Z13	T50.Z14	T50.Z15	T50.Z16
complement (inhibitor)	T45.8X1	T45.8X2	T45.8X3	T45.8X4	T45.8X5	T45.8X6
convalescent	T50.Z11	T50.Z12	T50.Z13	T50.Z14	T50.Z15	T50.Z16
hemolytic complement	T45.8X1	T45.8X2	T45.8X3	T45.8X4	T45.8X5	T45.8X6
immune (human)	T50.Z11	T50.Z12	T50.Z13	T50.Z14	T50.Z15	T50.Z16
protective NEC	T50.Z11	T50.Z12	T50.Z13	T50.Z14	T50.Z15	T50.Z16
Setastine	T45.0X1	T45.0X2	T45.0X3	T45.0X4	T45.0X5	T45.0X6
Setoperone	T43.591	T43.592	T43.593	T43.594	T43.595	T43.596
Sewer gas	T59.91	T59.92	T59.93	T59.94	—	—
Shampoo	T55.0X1	T55.0X2	T55.0X3	T55.0X4	—	—
Shellfish, noxious, nonbacterial	T61.781	T61.782	T61.783	T61.784	—	—
Sildenafil	T46.7X1	T46.7X2	T46.7X3	T46.7X4	T46.7X5	T46.7X6
Silibinin	T50.991	T50.992	T50.993	T50.994	T50.995	T50.996
Silicone NEC	T65.891	T65.892	T65.893	T65.894	—	—
medicinal	T49.3X1	T49.3X2	T49.3X3	T49.3X4	T49.3X5	T49.3X6
Silvadene	T49.0X1	T49.0X2	T49.0X3	T49.0X4	T49.0X5	T49.0X6
Silver	T49.0X1	T49.0X2	T49.0X3	T49.0X4	T49.0X5	T49.0X6
anti-infectives	T49.0X1	T49.0X2	T49.0X3	T49.0X4	T49.0X5	T49.0X6
arsphenamine	T37.8X1	T37.8X2	T37.8X3	T37.8X4	T37.8X5	T37.8X6
colloidal	T49.0X1	T49.0X2	T49.0X3	T49.0X4	T49.0X5	T49.0X6
nitrate	T49.0X1	T49.0X2	T49.0X3	T49.0X4	T49.0X5	T49.0X6
ophthalmic preparation	T49.5X1	T49.5X2	T49.5X3	T49.5X4	T49.5X5	T49.5X6
toughened (keratolytic)	T49.4X1	T49.4X2	T49.4X3	T49.4X4	T49.4X5	T49.4X6
nonmedicinal (dust)	T56.891	T56.892	T56.893	T56.894	—	—
protein	T49.5X1	T49.5X2	T49.5X3	T49.5X4	T49.5X5	T49.5X6
salvarsan	T37.8X1	T37.8X2	T37.8X3	T37.8X4	T37.8X5	T37.8X6
sulfadiazine	T49.4X1	T49.4X2	T49.4X3	T49.4X4	T49.4X5	T49.4X6
Silymarin	T50.991	T50.992	T50.993	T50.994	T50.995	T50.996
Simaldrate	T47.1X1	T47.1X2	T47.1X3	T47.1X4	T47.1X5	T47.1X6
Simazine	T60.3X1	T60.3X2	T60.3X3	T60.3X4	—	—
Simethicone	T47.1X1	T47.1X2	T47.1X3	T47.1X4	T47.1X5	T47.1X6
Simfibrate	T46.6X1	T46.6X2	T46.6X3	T46.6X4	T46.6X5	T46.6X6
Simvastatin	T46.6X1	T46.6X2	T46.6X3	T46.6X4	T46.6X5	T46.6X6
Sincalide	T50.8X1	T50.8X2	T50.8X3	T50.8X4	T50.8X5	T50.8X6
Sinequan	T43.011	T43.012	T43.013	T43.014	T43.015	T43.016
Singoserp	T46.5X1	T46.5X2	T46.5X3	T46.5X4	T46.5X5	T46.5X6
Sintrom	T45.511	T45.512	T45.513	T45.514	T45.515	T45.516
Sisomicin	T36.5X1	T36.5X2	T36.5X3	T36.5X4	T36.5X5	T36.5X6
Sitosterols	T46.6X1	T46.6X2	T46.6X3	T46.6X4	T46.6X5	T46.6X6
Skeletal muscle relaxants	T48.1X1	T48.1X2	T48.1X3	T48.1X4	T48.1X5	T48.1X6
Skin						
agents (external)	T49.91	T49.92	T49.93	T49.94	T49.95	T49.96
specified NEC	T49.8X1	T49.8X2	T49.8X3	T49.8X4	T49.8X5	T49.8X6
test antigen	T50.8X1	T50.8X2	T50.8X3	T50.8X4	T50.8X5	T50.8X6

Substance	Poisoning, Accidental (unintentional)	Poisoning, Intentional self-harm	Poisoning, Assault	Poisoning, Undetermined	Adverse effect	Underdosing
Sleep-eze	T45.0X1	T45.0X2	T45.0X3	T45.0X4	T45.0X5	T45.0X6
Sleeping draught, pill	T42.71	T42.72	T42.73	T42.74	T42.75	T42.76
Smallpox vaccine	T50.B11	T50.B12	T50.B13	T50.B14	T50.B15	T50.B16
Smelter fumes NEC	T56.91	T56.92	T56.93	T56.94	—	—
Smog	T59.1X1	T59.1X2	T59.1X3	T59.1X4	—	—
Smoke NEC	T59.811	T59.812	T59.813	T59.814	—	—
Smooth muscle relaxant	T44.3X1	T44.3X2	T44.3X3	T44.3X4	T44.3X5	T44.3X6
Snail killer NEC	T60.8X1	T60.8X2	T60.8X3	T60.8X4	—	—
Snake venom or bite	T63.001	T63.002	T63.003	T63.004		
hemocoagulase	T45.7X1	T45.7X2	T45.7X3	T45.7X4	T45.7X5	T45.7X6
Snuff	T65.211	T65.212	T65.213	T65.214	—	—
Soap (powder) (product)	T55.0X1	T55.0X2	T55.0X3	T55.0X4		
enema	T47.4X1	T47.4X2	T47.4X3	T47.4X4	T47.4X5	T47.4X6
medicinal, soft	T49.2X1	T49.2X2	T49.2X3	T49.2X4	T49.2X5	T49.2X6
superfatted	T49.2X1	T49.2X2	T49.2X3	T49.2X4	T49.2X5	T49.2X6
Sobrerol	T48.4X1	T48.4X2	T48.4X3	T48.4X4	T48.4X5	T48.4X6
Soda (caustic)	T54.3X1	T54.3X2	T54.3X3	T54.3X4	—	—
bicarb	T47.1X1	T47.1X2	T47.1X3	T47.1X4	T47.1X5	T47.1X6
chlorinated—see Sodium, hypochlorite						
Sodium						
acetosulfone	T37.1X1	T37.1X2	T37.1X3	T37.1X4	T37.1X5	T37.1X6
acetrizoate	T50.8X1	T50.8X2	T50.8X3	T50.8X4	T50.8X5	T50.8X6
acid phosphate	T50.3X1	T50.3X2	T50.3X3	T50.3X4	T50.3X5	T50.3X6
alginate	T47.8X1	T47.8X2	T47.8X3	T47.8X4	T47.8X5	T47.8X6
amidotrizoate	T50.8X1	T50.8X2	T50.8X3	T50.8X4	T50.8X5	T50.8X6
aminopterin	T45.1X1	T45.1X2	T45.1X3	T45.1X4	T45.1X5	T45.1X6
amylosulfate	T47.8X1	T47.8X2	T47.8X3	T47.8X4	T47.8X5	T47.8X6
amytal	T42.3X1	T42.3X2	T42.3X3	T42.3X4	T42.3X5	T42.3X6
antimony gluconate	T37.3X1	T37.3X2	T37.3X3	T37.3X4	T37.3X5	T37.3X6
arsenate	T57.0X1	T57.0X2	T57.0X3	T57.0X4	—	—
aurothiomalate	T39.4X1	T39.4X2	T39.4X3	T39.4X4	T39.4X5	T39.4X6
aurothiosulfate	T39.4X1	T39.4X2	T39.4X3	T39.4X4	T39.4X5	T39.4X6
barbiturate	T42.3X1	T42.3X2	T42.3X3	T42.3X4	T42.3X5	T42.3X6
basic phosphate	T47.4X1	T47.4X2	T47.4X3	T47.4X4	T47.4X5	T47.4X6
bicarbonate	T47.1X1	T47.1X2	T47.1X3	T47.1X4	T47.1X5	T47.1X6
bichromate	T57.8X1	T57.8X2	T57.8X3	T57.8X4	—	—
biphosphate	T50.3X1	T50.3X2	T50.3X3	T50.3X4	T50.3X5	T50.3X6
bisulfate	T65.891	T65.892	T65.893	T65.894	—	—
borate						
cleanser	T57.8X1	T57.8X2	T57.8X3	T57.8X4	—	—
eye	T49.5X1	T49.5X2	T49.5X3	T49.5X4	T49.5X5	T49.5X6
therapeutic	T49.8X1	T49.8X2	T49.8X3	T49.8X4	T49.8X5	T49.8X6
bromide	T42.6X1	T42.6X2	T42.6X3	T42.6X4	T42.6X5	T42.6X6
cacodylate (nonmedicinal) NEC	T50.8X1	T50.8X2	T50.8X3	T50.8X4	T50.8X5	T50.8X6
anti-infective	T37.8X1	T37.8X2	T37.8X3	T37.8X4	T37.8X5	T37.8X6
herbicide	T60.3X1	T60.3X2	T60.3X3	T60.3X4	—	—
calcium edetate	T45.8X1	T45.8X2	T45.8X3	T45.8X4	T45.8X5	T45.8X6
carbonate NEC	T54.3X1	T54.3X2	T54.3X3	T54.3X4	—	—
chlorate NEC	T65.891	T65.892	T65.893	T65.894	—	—

Substance	Poisoning, Accidental (unintentional)	Poisoning, Intentional self-harm	Poisoning, Assault	Poisoning, Undetermined	Adverse effect	Underdosing
Sodium — *Continued*						
herbicide	T54.91	T54.92	T54.93	T54.94	—	—
chloride	T50.3X1	T50.3X2	T50.3X3	T50.3X4	T50.3X5	T50.3X6
with glucose	T50.3X1	T50.3X2	T50.3X3	T50.3X4	T50.3X5	T50.3X6
chromate	T65.891	T65.892	T65.893	T65.894	—	—
citrate	T50.991	T50.992	T50.993	T50.994	T50.995	T50.996
cromoglicate	T48.6X1	T48.6X2	T48.6X3	T48.6X4	T48.6X5	T48.6X6
cyanide	T65.0X1	T65.0X2	T65.0X3	T65.0X4	—	—
cyclamate	T50.3X1	T50.3X2	T50.3X3	T50.3X4	T50.3X5	T50.3X6
dehydrocholate	T45.8X1	T45.8X2	T45.8X3	T45.8X4	T45.8X5	T45.8X6
diatrizoate	T50.8X1	T50.8X2	T50.8X3	T50.8X4	T50.8X5	T50.8X6
dibunate	T48.4X1	T48.4X2	T48.4X3	T48.4X4	T48.4X5	T48.4X6
dioctyl sulfosuccinate	T47.4X1	T47.4X2	T47.4X3	T47.4X4	T47.4X5	T47.4X6
dipantoyl ferrate	T45.8X1	T45.8X2	T45.8X3	T45.8X4	T45.8X5	T45.8X6
edetate	T45.8X1	T45.8X2	T45.8X3	T45.8X4	T45.8X5	T45.8X6
ethacrynate	T50.1X1	T50.1X2	T50.1X3	T50.1X4	T50.1X5	T50.1X6
feredetate	T45.8X1	T45.8X2	T45.8X3	T45.8X4	T45.8X5	T45.8X6
Fluoride—see Fluoride						
fluoroacetate (dust) (pesticide)	T60.4X1	T60.4X2	T60.4X3	T60.4X4	—	—
free salt	T50.3X1	T50.3X2	T50.3X3	T50.3X4	T50.3X5	T50.3X6
fusidate	T36.8X1	T36.8X2	T36.8X3	T36.8X4	T36.8X5	T36.8X6
glucaldrate	T47.1X1	T47.1X2	T47.1X3	T47.1X4	T47.1X5	T47.1X6
glucosulfone	T37.1X1	T37.1X2	T37.1X3	T37.1X4	T37.1X5	T37.1X6
glutamate	T45.8X1	T45.8X2	T45.8X3	T45.8X4	T45.8X5	T45.8X6
hydrogen carbonate	T50.3X1	T50.3X2	T50.3X3	T50.3X4	T50.3X5	T50.3X6
hydroxide	T54.3X1	T54.3X2	T54.3X3	T54.3X4	—	—
hypochlorite (bleach) NEC	T54.3X1	T54.3X2	T54.3X3	T54.3X4	—	—
disinfectant	T54.3X1	T54.3X2	T54.3X3	T54.3X4	—	—
medicinal (anti-infective) (external)	T49.0X1	T49.0X2	T49.0X3	T49.0X4	T49.0X5	T49.0X6
vapor	T54.3X1	T54.3X2	T54.3X3	T54.3X4	—	—
hyposulfite	T49.0X1	T49.0X2	T49.0X3	T49.0X4	T49.0X5	T49.0X6
indigotin disulfonate	T50.8X1	T50.8X2	T50.8X3	T50.8X4	T50.8X5	T50.8X6
iodide	T50.991	T50.992	T50.993	T50.994	T50.995	T50.996
I-131	T50.8X1	T50.8X2	T50.8X3	T50.8X4	T50.8X5	T50.8X6
therapeutic	T38.2X1	T38.2X2	T38.2X3	T38.2X4	T38.2X5	T38.2X6
iodohippurate (131I)	T50.8X1	T50.8X2	T50.8X3	T50.8X4	T50.8X5	T50.8X6
iopodate	T50.8X1	T50.8X2	T50.8X3	T50.8X4	T50.8X5	T50.8X6
iothalamate	T50.8X1	T50.8X2	T50.8X3	T50.8X4	T50.8X5	T50.8X6
iron edetate	T45.4X1	T45.4X2	T45.4X3	T45.4X4	T45.4X5	T45.4X6
lactate (compound solution)	T45.8X1	T45.8X2	T45.8X3	T45.8X4	T45.8X5	T45.8X6
lauryl (sulfate)	T49.2X1	T49.2X2	T49.2X3	T49.2X4	T49.2X5	T49.2X6
L-triiodothyronine	T38.1X1	T38.1X2	T38.1X3	T38.1X4	T38.1X5	T38.1X6
magnesium citrate	T50.991	T50.992	T50.993	T50.994	T50.995	T50.996
mersalate	T50.2X1	T50.2X2	T50.2X3	T50.2X4	T50.2X5	T50.2X6
metasilicate	T65.891	T65.892	T65.893	T65.894	—	—
metrizoate	T50.8X1	T50.8X2	T50.8X3	T50.8X4	T50.8X5	T50.8X6
monofluoroacetate (pesticide)	T60.1X1	T60.1X2	T60.1X3	T60.1X4	—	—

Substance	Poisoning, Accidental (unintentional)	Poisoning, Intentional self-harm	Poisoning, Assault	Poisoning, Undetermined	Adverse effect	Underdosing
Sodium — *Continued*						
morrhuate	T46.8X1	T46.8X2	T46.8X3	T46.8X4	T46.8X5	T46.8X6
nafcillin	T36.0X1	T36.0X2	T36.0X3	T36.0X4	T36.0X5	T36.0X6
nitrate (oxidizing agent)	T65.891	T65.892	T65.893	T65.894	—	—
nitrite	T50.6X1	T50.6X2	T50.6X3	T50.6X4	T50.6X5	T50.6X6
nitroferricyanide	T46.5X1	T46.5X2	T46.5X3	T46.5X4	T46.5X5	T46.5X6
nitroprusside	T46.5X1	T46.5X2	T46.5X3	T46.5X4	T46.5X5	T46.5X6
oxalate	T65.891	T65.892	T65.893	T65.894	—	—
oxide/peroxide	T65.891	T65.892	T65.893	T65.894	—	—
oxybate	T41.291	T41.292	T41.293	T41.294	T41.295	T41.296
para-aminohippurate	T50.8X1	T50.8X2	T50.8X3	T50.8X4	T50.8X5	T50.8X6
perborate (nonmedicinal) NEC	T65.891	T65.892	T65.893	T65.894	—	—
medicinal	T49.0X1	T49.0X2	T49.0X3	T49.0X4	T49.0X5	T49.0X6
soap	T55.0X1	T55.0X2	T55.0X3	T55.0X4	—	—
percarbonate—see Sodium, perborate						
pertechnetate Tc99m	T50.8X1	T50.8X2	T50.8X3	T50.8X4	T50.8X5	T50.8X6
phosphate						
cellulose	T45.8X1	T45.8X2	T45.8X3	T45.8X4	T45.8X5	T45.8X6
dibasic	T47.2X1	T47.2X2	T47.2X3	T47.2X4	T47.2X5	T47.2X6
monobasic	T47.2X1	T47.2X2	T47.2X3	T47.2X4	T47.2X5	T47.2X6
phytate	T50.6X1	T50.6X2	T50.6X3	T50.6X4	T50.6X5	T50.6X6
picosulfate	T47.2X1	T47.2X2	T47.2X3	T47.2X4	T47.2X5	T47.2X6
polyhydroxyaluminium monocarbonate	T47.1X1	T47.1X2	T47.1X3	T47.1X4	T47.1X5	T47.1X6
polystyrene sulfonate	T50.3X1	T50.3X2	T50.3X3	T50.3X4	T50.3X5	T50.3X6
propionate	T49.0X1	T49.0X2	T49.0X3	T49.0X4	T49.0X5	T49.0X6
propyl hydroxybenzoate	T50.991	T50.992	T50.993	T50.994	T50.995	T50.996
psylliate	T46.8X1	T46.8X2	T46.8X3	T46.8X4	T46.8X5	T46.8X6
removing resins	T50.3X1	T50.3X2	T50.3X3	T50.3X4	T50.3X5	T50.3X6
salicylate	T39.091	T39.092	T39.093	T39.094	T39.095	T39.096
salt NEC	T50.3X1	T50.3X2	T50.3X3	T50.3X4	T50.3X5	T50.3X6
selenate	T60.2X1	T60.2X2	T60.2X3	T60.2X4	—	—
stibogluconate	T37.3X1	T37.3X2	T37.3X3	T37.3X4	T37.3X5	T37.3X6
sulfate	T47.4X1	T47.4X2	T47.4X3	T47.4X4	T47.4X5	T47.4X6
sulfoxone	T37.1X1	T37.1X2	T37.1X3	T37.1X4	T37.1X5	T37.1X6
tetradecyl sulfate	T46.8X1	T46.8X2	T46.8X3	T46.8X4	T46.8X5	T46.8X6
thiopental	T41.1X1	T41.1X2	T41.1X3	T41.1X4	T41.1X5	T41.1X6
thiosalicylate	T39.091	T39.092	T39.093	T39.094	T39.095	T39.096
thiosulfate	T50.6X1	T50.6X2	T50.6X3	T50.6X4	T50.6X5	T50.6X6
tolbutamide	T38.3X1	T38.3X2	T38.3X3	T38.3X4	T38.3X5	T38.3X6
(L)-triiodothyronine	T38.1X1	T38.1X2	T38.1X3	T38.1X4	T38.1X5	T38.1X6
tyropanoate	T50.8X1	T50.8X2	T50.8X3	T50.8X4	T50.8X5	T50.8X6
valproate	T42.6X1	T42.6X2	T42.6X3	T42.6X4	T42.6X5	T42.6X6
versenate	T50.6X1	T50.6X2	T50.6X3	T50.6X4	T50.6X5	T50.6X6
Sodium-free salt	T50.901	T50.902	T50.903	T50.904	T50.905	T50.906
Sodium-removing resin	T50.3X1	T50.3X2	T50.3X3	T50.3X4	T50.3X5	T50.3X6
Soft soap	T55.0X1	T55.0X2	T55.0X3	T55.0X4	—	—
Solanine	T62.2X1	T62.2X2	T62.2X3	T62.2X4	—	—
berries	T62.1X1	T62.1X2	T62.1X3	T62.1X4	—	—

Substance	Poisoning, Accidental (unintentional)	Poisoning, Intentional self-harm	Poisoning, Assault	Poisoning, Undetermined	Adverse effect	Underdosing
Solanum dulcamara	T62.2X1	T62.2X2	T62.2X3	T62.2X4	—	—
berries	T62.1X1	T62.1X2	T62.1X3	T62.1X4	—	—
Solapsone	T37.1X1	T37.1X2	T37.1X3	T37.1X4	T37.1X5	T37.1X6
Solar lotion	T49.3X1	T49.3X2	T49.3X3	T49.3X4	T49.3X5	T49.3X6
Solasulfone	T37.1X1	T37.1X2	T37.1X3	T37.1X4	T37.1X5	T37.1X6
Soldering fluid	T65.891	T65.892	T65.893	T65.894	—	—
Solid substance	T65.91	T65.92	T65.93	T65.94	—	—
specified NEC	T65.891	T65.892	T65.893	T65.894	—	—
Solvent, industrial NEC	T52.91	T52.92	T52.93	T52.94	—	—
naphtha	T52.0X1	T52.0X2	T52.0X3	T52.0X4	—	—
petroleum	T52.0X1	T52.0X2	T52.0X3	T52.0X4	—	—
specified NEC	T52.8X1	T52.8X2	T52.8X3	T52.8X4	—	—
Soma	T42.8X1	T42.8X2	T42.8X3	T42.8X4	T42.8X5	T42.8X6
Somatorelin	T38.891	T38.892	T38.893	T38.894	T38.895	T38.896
Somatostatin	T38.991	T38.992	T38.993	T38.994	T38.995	T38.996
Somatotropin	T38.811	T38.812	T38.813	T38.814	T38.815	T38.816
Somatrem	T38.811	T38.812	T38.813	T38.814	T38.815	T38.816
Somatropin	T38.811	T38.812	T38.813	T38.814	T38.815	T38.816
Sominex	T45.0X1	T45.0X2	T45.0X3	T45.0X4	T45.0X5	T45.0X6
Somnos	T42.6X1	T42.6X2	T42.6X3	T42.6X4	T42.6X5	T42.6X6
Somonal	T42.3X1	T42.3X2	T42.3X3	T42.3X4	T42.3X5	T42.3X6
Soneryl	T42.3X1	T42.3X2	T42.3X3	T42.3X4	T42.3X5	T42.3X6
Soothing syrup	T50.901	T50.902	T50.903	T50.904	T50.905	T50.906
Sopor	T42.6X1	T42.6X2	T42.6X3	T42.6X4	T42.6X5	T42.6X6
Soporific	T42.71	T42.72	T42.73	T42.74	T42.75	T42.76
Soporific drug	T42.71	T42.72	T42.73	T42.74	T42.75	T42.76
specified type NEC	T42.6X1	T42.6X2	T42.6X3	T42.6X4	T42.6X5	T42.6X6
Sorbide nitrate	T46.3X1	T46.3X2	T46.3X3	T46.3X4	T46.3X5	T46.3X6
Sorbitol	T47.4X1	T47.4X2	T47.4X3	T47.4X4	T47.4X5	T47.4X6
Sotalol	T44.7X1	T44.7X2	T44.7X3	T44.7X4	T44.7X5	T44.7X6
Sotradecol	T46.8X1	T46.8X2	T46.8X3	T46.8X4	T46.8X5	T46.8X6
Soysterol	T46.6X1	T46.6X2	T46.6X3	T46.6X4	T46.6X5	T46.6X6
Spacoline	T44.3X1	T44.3X2	T44.3X3	T44.3X4	T44.3X5	T44.3X6
Spanish fly	T49.8X1	T49.8X2	T49.8X3	T49.8X4	T49.8X5	T49.8X6
Sparine	T43.3X1	T43.3X2	T43.3X3	T43.3X4	T43.3X5	T43.3X6
Sparteine	T48.0X1	T48.0X2	T48.0X3	T48.0X4	T48.0X5	T48.0X6
Spasmolytic						
anticholinergics	T44.3X1	T44.3X2	T44.3X3	T44.3X4	T44.3X5	T44.3X6
autonomic	T44.3X1	T44.3X2	T44.3X3	T44.3X4	T44.3X5	T44.3X6
bronchial NEC	T48.6X1	T48.6X2	T48.6X3	T48.6X4	T48.6X5	T48.6X6
quaternary ammonium	T44.3X1	T44.3X2	T44.3X3	T44.3X4	T44.3X5	T44.3X6
skeletal muscle NEC	T48.1X1	T48.1X2	T48.1X3	T48.1X4	T48.1X5	T48.1X6
Spectinomycin	T36.5X1	T36.5X2	T36.5X3	T36.5X4	T36.5X5	T36.5X6
Speed	T43.651	T43.652	T43.653	T43.654	T43.655	T43.656
Spermicide	T49.8X1	T49.8X2	T49.8X3	T49.8X4	T49.8X5	T49.8X6
Spider (bite) (venom)	T63.391	T63.392	T63.393	T63.394	—	—
antivenin	T50.Z11	T50.Z12	T50.Z13	T50.Z14	T50.Z15	T50.Z16
Spigelia (root)	T37.4X1	T37.4X2	T37.4X3	T37.4X4	T37.4X5	T37.4X6
Spindle inactivator	T50.4X1	T50.4X2	T50.4X3	T50.4X4	T50.4X5	T50.4X6
Spiperone	T43.4X1	T43.4X2	T43.4X3	T43.4X4	T43.4X5	T43.4X6

Substance	Poisoning, Accidental (unintentional)	Poisoning, Intentional self-harm	Poisoning, Assault	Poisoning, Undetermined	Adverse effect	Underdosing
Spiramycin	T36.3X1	T36.3X2	T36.3X3	T36.3X4	T36.3X5	T36.3X6
Spirapril	T46.4X1	T46.4X2	T46.4X3	T46.4X4	T46.4X5	T46.4X6
Spirilene	T43.591	T43.592	T43.593	T43.594	T43.595	T43.596
Spirit(s) (neutral) NEC	T51.0X1	T51.0X2	T51.0X3	T51.0X4	—	—
beverage	T51.0X1	T51.0X2	T51.0X3	T51.0X4	—	—
industrial	T51.0X1	T51.0X2	T51.0X3	T51.0X4	—	—
mineral	T52.0X1	T52.0X2	T52.0X3	T52.0X4	—	—
of salt—see Hydrochloric acid						
surgical	T51.0X1	T51.0X2	T51.0X3	T51.0X4	—	—
Spironolactone	T50.0X1	T50.0X2	T50.0X3	T50.0X4	T50.0X5	T50.0X6
Spiroperidol	T43.4X1	T43.4X2	T43.4X3	T43.4X4	T43.4X5	T43.4X6
Sponge, absorbable (gelatin)	T45.7X1	T45.7X2	T45.7X3	T45.7X4	T45.7X5	T45.7X6
Sporostacin	T49.0X1	T49.0X2	T49.0X3	T49.0X4	T49.0X5	T49.0X6
Spray (aerosol)	T65.91	T65.92	T65.93	T65.94	—	—
cosmetic	T65.891	T65.892	T65.893	T65.894	—	—
medicinal NEC	T50.901	T50.902	T50.903	T50.904	T50.905	T50.906
pesticides—see Pesticide						
specified content—see specific substance						
Spurge flax	T62.2X1	T62.2X2	T62.2X3	T62.2X4	—	—
Spurges	T62.2X1	T62.2X2	T62.2X3	T62.2X4	—	—
Sputum viscosity-lowering drug	T48.4X1	T48.4X2	T48.4X3	T48.4X4	T48.4X5	T48.4X6
Squill	T46.0X1	T46.0X2	T46.0X3	T46.0X4	T46.0X5	T46.0X6
rat poison	T60.4X1	T60.4X2	T60.4X3	T60.4X4	—	—
Squirting cucumber (cathartic)	T47.2X1	T47.2X2	T47.2X3	T47.2X4	T47.2X5	T47.2X6
Stains	T65.6X1	T65.6X2	T65.6X3	T65.6X4	—	—
Stannous fluoride	T49.7X1	T49.7X2	T49.7X3	T49.7X4	T49.7X5	T49.7X6
Stanolone	T38.7X1	T38.7X2	T38.7X3	T38.7X4	T38.7X5	T38.7X6
Stanozolol	T38.7X1	T38.7X2	T38.7X3	T38.7X4	T38.7X5	T38.7X6
Staphisagria or stavesacre (pediculicide)	T49.0X1	T49.0X2	T49.0X3	T49.0X4	T49.0X5	T49.0X6
Starch	T50.901	T50.902	T50.903	T50.904	T50.905	T50.906
Stelazine	T43.3X1	T43.3X2	T43.3X3	T43.3X4	T43.3X5	T43.3X6
Stemetil	T43.3X1	T43.3X2	T43.3X3	T43.3X4	T43.3X5	T43.3X6
Stepronin	T48.4X1	T48.4X2	T48.4X3	T48.4X4	T48.4X5	T48.4X6
Sterculia	T47.4X1	T47.4X2	T47.4X3	T47.4X4	T47.4X5	T47.4X6
Sternutator gas	T59.891	T59.892	T59.893	T59.894	—	—
Steroid	T38.0X1	T38.0X2	T38.0X3	T38.0X4	T38.0X5	T38.0X6
anabolic	T38.7X1	T38.7X2	T38.7X3	T38.7X4	T38.7X5	T38.7X6
androgenic	T38.7X1	T38.7X2	T38.7X3	T38.7X4	T38.7X5	T38.7X6
antineoplastic, hormone	T38.7X1	T38.7X2	T38.7X3	T38.7X4	T38.7X5	T38.7X6
estrogen	T38.5X1	T38.5X2	T38.5X3	T38.5X4	T38.5X5	T38.5X6
ENT agent	T49.6X1	T49.6X2	T49.6X3	T49.6X4	T49.6X5	T49.6X6
ophthalmic preparation	T49.5X1	T49.5X2	T49.5X3	T49.5X4	T49.5X5	T49.5X6
topical NEC	T49.0X1	T49.0X2	T49.0X3	T49.0X4	T49.0X5	T49.0X6
Stibine	T56.891	T56.892	T56.893	T56.894	—	—
Stibogluconate	T37.3X1	T37.3X2	T37.3X3	T37.3X4	T37.3X5	T37.3X6

Substance	Poisoning, Accidental (unintentional)	Poisoning, Intentional self-harm	Poisoning, Assault	Poisoning, Undetermined	Adverse effect	Underdosing
Stibophen	T37.4X1	T37.4X2	T37.4X3	T37.4X4	T37.4X5	T37.4X6
Stilbamidine (isetionate)	T37.3X1	T37.3X2	T37.3X3	T37.3X4	T37.3X5	T37.3X6
Stilbestrol	T38.5X1	T38.5X2	T38.5X3	T38.5X4	T38.5X5	T38.5X6
Stilboestrol	T38.5X1	T38.5X2	T38.5X3	T38.5X4	T38.5X5	T38.5X6
Stimulant						
central nervous system—see also Psychostimulant	T43.601	T43.602	T43.603	T43.604	T43.605	T43.606
analeptics	T50.7X1	T50.7X2	T50.7X3	T50.7X4	T50.7X5	T50.7X6
opiate antagonist	T50.7X1	T50.7X2	T50.7X3	T50.7X4	T50.7X5	T50.7X6
psychotherapeutic NEC—see also Psychotherapeutic drug	T43.601	T43.602	T43.603	T43.604	T43.605	T43.606
specified NEC	T43.691	T43.692	T43.693	T43.694	T43.695	T43.696
respiratory	T48.901	T48.902	T48.903	T48.904	T48.905	T48.906
Stone-dissolving drug	T50.901	T50.902	T50.903	T50.904	T50.905	T50.906
Storage battery (cells) (acid)	T54.2X1	T54.2X2	T54.2X3	T54.2X4	—	—
Stovaine	T41.3X1	T41.3X2	T41.3X3	T41.3X4	T41.3X5	T41.3X6
infiltration (subcutaneous)	T41.3X1	T41.3X2	T41.3X3	T41.3X4	T41.3X5	T41.3X6
nerve block (peripheral) (plexus)	T41.3X1	T41.3X2	T41.3X3	T41.3X4	T41.3X5	T41.3X6
spinal	T41.3X1	T41.3X2	T41.3X3	T41.3X4	T41.3X5	T41.3X6
topical (surface)	T41.3X1	T41.3X2	T41.3X3	T41.3X4	T41.3X5	T41.3X6
Stovarsal	T37.8X1	T37.8X2	T37.8X3	T37.8X4	T37.8X5	T37.8X6
Stove gas—see Gas, stove						
Stoxil	T49.5X1	T49.5X2	T49.5X3	T49.5X4	T49.5X5	T49.5X6
Stramonium	T48.6X1	T48.6X2	T48.6X3	T48.6X4	T48.6X5	T48.6X6
natural state	T62.2X1	T62.2X2	T62.2X3	T62.2X4	—	—
Streptodornase	T45.3X1	T45.3X2	T45.3X3	T45.3X4	T45.3X5	T45.3X6
Streptoduocin	T36.5X1	T36.5X2	T36.5X3	T36.5X4	T36.5X5	T36.5X6
Streptokinase	T45.611	T45.612	T45.613	T45.614	T45.615	T45.616
Streptomycin (derivative)	T36.5X1	T36.5X2	T36.5X3	T36.5X4	T36.5X5	T36.5X6
Streptonivicin	T36.5X1	T36.5X2	T36.5X3	T36.5X4	T36.5X5	T36.5X6
Streptovarycin	T36.5X1	T36.5X2	T36.5X3	T36.5X4	T36.5X5	T36.5X6
Streptozocin	T45.1X1	T45.1X2	T45.1X3	T45.1X4	T45.1X5	T45.1X6
Streptozotocin	T45.1X1	T45.1X2	T45.1X3	T45.1X4	T45.1X5	T45.1X6
Stripper (paint) (solvent)	T52.8X1	T52.8X2	T52.8X3	T52.8X4	—	—
Strobane	T60.1X1	T60.1X2	T60.1X3	T60.1X4	—	—
Strofantina	T46.0X1	T46.0X2	T46.0X3	T46.0X4	T46.0X5	T46.0X6
Strophanthin (g) (k)	T46.0X1	T46.0X2	T46.0X3	T46.0X4	T46.0X5	T46.0X6
Strophanthus	T46.0X1	T46.0X2	T46.0X3	T46.0X4	T46.0X5	T46.0X6
Strophantin	T46.0X1	T46.0X2	T46.0X3	T46.0X4	T46.0X5	T46.0X6
Strophantin-g	T46.0X1	T46.0X2	T46.0X3	T46.0X4	T46.0X5	T46.0X6
Strychnine (nonmedicinal) (pesticide) (salts)	T65.1X1	T65.1X2	T65.1X3	T65.1X4	—	—
medicinal	T48.291	T48.292	T48.293	T48.294	T48.295	T48.296
Strychnos (ignatii)—see Strychnine						

Substance	Poisoning, Accidental (unintentional)	Poisoning, Intentional self-harm	Poisoning, Assault	Poisoning, Undetermined	Adverse effect	Underdosing
Styramate	T42.8X1	T42.8X2	T42.8X3	T42.8X4	T42.8X5	T42.8X6
Styrene	T65.891	T65.892	T65.893	T65.894	—	—
Succinimide, antiepileptic or anticonvulsant	T42.2X1	T42.2X2	T42.2X3	T42.2X4	T42.2X5	T42.2X6
mercuric—see Mercury						
Succinylcholine	T48.1X1	T48.1X2	T48.1X3	T48.1X4	T48.1X5	T48.1X6
Succinylsulfathiazole	T37.0X1	T37.0X2	T37.0X3	T37.0X4	T37.0X5	T37.0X6
Sucralfate	T47.1X1	T47.1X2	T47.1X3	T47.1X4	T47.1X5	T47.1X6
Sucrose	T50.3X1	T50.3X2	T50.3X3	T50.3X4	T50.3X5	T50.3X6
Sufentanil	T40.411	T40.412	T40.413	T40.414	T40.415	T40.416
Sulbactam	T36.0X1	T36.0X2	T36.0X3	T36.0X4	T36.0X5	T36.0X6
Sulbenicillin	T36.0X1	T36.0X2	T36.0X3	T36.0X4	T36.0X5	T36.0X6
Sulbentine	T49.0X1	T49.0X2	T49.0X3	T49.0X4	T49.0X5	T49.0X6
Sulfacetamide	T49.0X1	T49.0X2	T49.0X3	T49.0X4	T49.0X5	T49.0X6
ophthalmic preparation	T49.5X1	T49.5X2	T49.5X3	T49.5X4	T49.5X5	T49.5X6
Sulfachlorpyridazine	T37.0X1	T37.0X2	T37.0X3	T37.0X4	T37.0X5	T37.0X6
Sulfacitine	T37.0X1	T37.0X2	T37.0X3	T37.0X4	T37.0X5	T37.0X6
Sulfadiasulfone sodium	T37.0X1	T37.0X2	T37.0X3	T37.0X4	T37.0X5	T37.0X6
Sulfadiazine	T37.0X1	T37.0X2	T37.0X3	T37.0X4	T37.0X5	T37.0X6
silver (topical)	T49.0X1	T49.0X2	T49.0X3	T49.0X4	T49.0X5	T49.0X6
Sulfadimethoxine	T37.0X1	T37.0X2	T37.0X3	T37.0X4	T37.0X5	T37.0X6
Sulfadimidine	T37.0X1	T37.0X2	T37.0X3	T37.0X4	T37.0X5	T37.0X6
Sulfadoxine	T37.0X1	T37.0X2	T37.0X3	T37.0X4	T37.0X5	T37.0X6
with pyrimethamine	T37.2X1	T37.2X2	T37.2X3	T37.2X4	T37.2X5	T37.2X6
Sulfaethidole	T37.0X1	T37.0X2	T37.0X3	T37.0X4	T37.0X5	T37.0X6
Sulfafurazole	T37.0X1	T37.0X2	T37.0X3	T37.0X4	T37.0X5	T37.0X6
Sulfaguanidine	T37.0X1	T37.0X2	T37.0X3	T37.0X4	T37.0X5	T37.0X6
Sulfalene	T37.0X1	T37.0X2	T37.0X3	T37.0X4	T37.0X5	T37.0X6
Sulfaloxate	T37.0X1	T37.0X2	T37.0X3	T37.0X4	T37.0X5	T37.0X6
Sulfaloxic acid	T37.0X1	T37.0X2	T37.0X3	T37.0X4	T37.0X5	T37.0X6
Sulfamazone	T39.2X1	T39.2X2	T39.2X3	T39.2X4	T39.2X5	T39.2X6
Sulfamerazine	T37.0X1	T37.0X2	T37.0X3	T37.0X4	T37.0X5	T37.0X6
Sulfameter	T37.0X1	T37.0X2	T37.0X3	T37.0X4	T37.0X5	T37.0X6
Sulfamethazine	T37.0X1	T37.0X2	T37.0X3	T37.0X4	T37.0X5	T37.0X6
Sulfamethizole	T37.0X1	T37.0X2	T37.0X3	T37.0X4	T37.0X5	T37.0X6
Sulfamethoxazole	T37.0X1	T37.0X2	T37.0X3	T37.0X4	T37.0X5	T37.0X6
with trimethoprim	T36.8X1	T36.8X2	T36.8X3	T36.8X4	T36.8X5	T36.8X6
Sulfamethoxydiazine	T37.0X1	T37.0X2	T37.0X3	T37.0X4	T37.0X5	T37.0X6
Sulfamethoxypyridazine	T37.0X1	T37.0X2	T37.0X3	T37.0X4	T37.0X5	T37.0X6
Sulfamethylthiazole	T37.0X1	T37.0X2	T37.0X3	T37.0X4	T37.0X5	T37.0X6
Sulfametoxydiazine	T37.0X1	T37.0X2	T37.0X3	T37.0X4	T37.0X5	T37.0X6
Sulfamidopyrine	T39.2X1	T39.2X2	T39.2X3	T39.2X4	T39.2X5	T39.2X6
Sulfamonomethoxine	T37.0X1	T37.0X2	T37.0X3	T37.0X4	T37.0X5	T37.0X6
Sulfamoxole	T37.0X1	T37.0X2	T37.0X3	T37.0X4	T37.0X5	T37.0X6
Sulfamylon	T49.0X1	T49.0X2	T49.0X3	T49.0X4	T49.0X5	T49.0X6
Sulfan blue (diagnostic dye)	T50.8X1	T50.8X2	T50.8X3	T50.8X4	T50.8X5	T50.8X6
Sulfanilamide	T37.0X1	T37.0X2	T37.0X3	T37.0X4	T37.0X5	T37.0X6
Sulfanilylguanidine	T37.0X1	T37.0X2	T37.0X3	T37.0X4	T37.0X5	T37.0X6
Sulfaperin	T37.0X1	T37.0X2	T37.0X3	T37.0X4	T37.0X5	T37.0X6

Substance	Poisoning, Accidental (unintentional)	Poisoning, Intentional self-harm	Poisoning, Assault	Poisoning, Undetermined	Adverse effect	Underdosing
Sulfaphenazole	T37.0X1	T37.0X2	T37.0X3	T37.0X4	T37.0X5	T37.0X6
Sulfaphenylthiazole	T37.0X1	T37.0X2	T37.0X3	T37.0X4	T37.0X5	T37.0X6
Sulfaproxyline	T37.0X1	T37.0X2	T37.0X3	T37.0X4	T37.0X5	T37.0X6
Sulfapyridine	T37.0X1	T37.0X2	T37.0X3	T37.0X4	T37.0X5	T37.0X6
Sulfapyrimidine	T37.0X1	T37.0X2	T37.0X3	T37.0X4	T37.0X5	T37.0X6
Sulfarsphenamine	T37.8X1	T37.8X2	T37.8X3	T37.8X4	T37.8X5	T37.8X6
Sulfasalazine	T37.0X1	T37.0X2	T37.0X3	T37.0X4	T37.0X5	T37.0X6
Sulfasuxidine	T37.0X1	T37.0X2	T37.0X3	T37.0X4	T37.0X5	T37.0X6
Sulfasymazine	T37.0X1	T37.0X2	T37.0X3	T37.0X4	T37.0X5	T37.0X6
Sulfated amylopectin	T47.8X1	T47.8X2	T47.8X3	T47.8X4	T47.8X5	T47.8X6
Sulfathiazole	T37.0X1	T37.0X2	T37.0X3	T37.0X4	T37.0X5	T37.0X6
Sulfatostearate	T49.2X1	T49.2X2	T49.2X3	T49.2X4	T49.2X5	T49.2X6
Sulfinpyrazone	T50.4X1	T50.4X2	T50.4X3	T50.4X4	T50.4X5	T50.4X6
Sulfiram	T49.0X1	T49.0X2	T49.0X3	T49.0X4	T49.0X5	T49.0X6
Sulfisomidine	T37.0X1	T37.0X2	T37.0X3	T37.0X4	T37.0X5	T37.0X6
Sulfisoxazole	T37.0X1	T37.0X2	T37.0X3	T37.0X4	T37.0X5	T37.0X6
ophthalmic preparation	T49.5X1	T49.5X2	T49.5X3	T49.5X4	T49.5X5	T49.5X6
Sulfobromophthalein (sodium)	T50.8X1	T50.8X2	T50.8X3	T50.8X4	T50.8X5	T50.8X6
Sulfobromphthalein	T50.8X1	T50.8X2	T50.8X3	T50.8X4	T50.8X5	T50.8X6
Sulfogaiacol	T48.4X1	T48.4X2	T48.4X3	T48.4X4	T48.4X5	T48.4X6
Sulfomyxin	T36.8X1	T36.8X2	T36.8X3	T36.8X4	T36.8X5	T36.8X6
Sulfonal	T42.6X1	T42.6X2	T42.6X3	T42.6X4	T42.6X5	T42.6X6
Sulfonamide NEC	T37.0X1	T37.0X2	T37.0X3	T37.0X4	T37.0X5	T37.0X6
eye	T49.5X1	T49.5X2	T49.5X3	T49.5X4	T49.5X5	T49.5X6
Sulfonazide	T37.1X1	T37.1X2	T37.1X3	T37.1X4	T37.1X5	T37.1X6
Sulfones	T37.1X1	T37.1X2	T37.1X3	T37.1X4	T37.1X5	T37.1X6
Sulfonethylmethane	T42.6X1	T42.6X2	T42.6X3	T42.6X4	T42.6X5	T42.6X6
Sulfonmethane	T42.6X1	T42.6X2	T42.6X3	T42.6X4	T42.6X5	T42.6X6
Sulfonphthal, sulfonphthol	T50.8X1	T50.8X2	T50.8X3	T50.8X4	T50.8X5	T50.8X6
Sulfonylurea derivatives, oral	T38.3X1	T38.3X2	T38.3X3	T38.3X4	T38.3X5	T38.3X6
Sulforidazine	T43.3X1	T43.3X2	T43.3X3	T43.3X4	T43.3X5	T43.3X6
Sulfoxone	T37.1X1	T37.1X2	T37.1X3	T37.1X4	T37.1X5	T37.1X6
Sulfur, sulfurated, sulfuric, sulfurous, sulfuryl (compounds NEC) (medicinal)	T49.4X1	T49.4X2	T49.4X3	T49.4X4	T49.4X5	T49.4X6
acid	T54.2X1	T54.2X2	T54.2X3	T54.2X4	—	—
dioxide (gas)	T59.1X1	T59.1X2	T59.1X3	T59.1X4	—	—
ether—see Ether(s)						
hydrogen	T59.6X1	T59.6X2	T59.6X3	T59.6X4	—	—
medicinal (keratolytic) (ointment) NEC	T49.4X1	T49.4X2	T49.4X3	T49.4X4	T49.4X5	T49.4X6
ointment	T49.0X1	T49.0X2	T49.0X3	T49.0X4	T49.0X5	T49.0X6
pesticide (vapor)	T60.91	T60.92	T60.93	T60.94	—	—
vapor NEC	T59.891	T59.892	T59.893	T59.894	—	—
Sulfuric acid	T54.2X1	T54.2X2	T54.2X3	T54.2X4	—	—
Sulglicotide	T47.1X1	T47.1X2	T47.1X3	T47.1X4	T47.1X5	T47.1X6
Sulindac	T39.391	T39.392	T39.393	T39.394	T39.395	T39.396
Sulisatin	T47.2X1	T47.2X2	T47.2X3	T47.2X4	T47.2X5	T47.2X6

Substance	Poisoning, Accidental (unintentional)	Poisoning, Intentional self-harm	Poisoning, Assault	Poisoning, Undetermined	Adverse effect	Underdosing
Sulisobenzone	T49.3X1	T49.3X2	T49.3X3	T49.3X4	T49.3X5	T49.3X6
Sulkowitch's reagent	T50.8X1	T50.8X2	T50.8X3	T50.8X4	T50.8X5	T50.8X6
Sulmetozine	T44.3X1	T44.3X2	T44.3X3	T44.3X4	T44.3X5	T44.3X6
Suloctidil	T46.7X1	T46.7X2	T46.7X3	T46.7X4	T46.7X5	T46.7X6
Sulph——see also Sulf-						
Sulphadiazine	T37.0X1	T37.0X2	T37.0X3	T37.0X4	T37.0X5	T37.0X6
Sulphadimethoxine	T37.0X1	T37.0X2	T37.0X3	T37.0X4	T37.0X5	T37.0X6
Sulphadimidine	T37.0X1	T37.0X2	T37.0X3	T37.0X4	T37.0X5	T37.0X6
Sulphadione	T37.1X1	T37.1X2	T37.1X3	T37.1X4	T37.1X5	T37.1X6
Sulphafurazole	T37.0X1	T37.0X2	T37.0X3	T37.0X4	T37.0X5	T37.0X6
Sulphamethizole	T37.0X1	T37.0X2	T37.0X3	T37.0X4	T37.0X5	T37.0X6
Sulphamethoxazole	T37.0X1	T37.0X2	T37.0X3	T37.0X4	T37.0X5	T37.0X6
Sulphan blue	T50.8X1	T50.8X2	T50.8X3	T50.8X4	T50.8X5	T50.8X6
Sulphaphenazole	T37.0X1	T37.0X2	T37.0X3	T37.0X4	T37.0X5	T37.0X6
Sulphapyridine	T37.0X1	T37.0X2	T37.0X3	T37.0X4	T37.0X5	T37.0X6
Sulphasalazine	T37.0X1	T37.0X2	T37.0X3	T37.0X4	T37.0X5	T37.0X6
Sulphinpyrazone	T50.4X1	T50.4X2	T50.4X3	T50.4X4	T50.4X5	T50.4X6
Sulpiride	T43.591	T43.592	T43.593	T43.594	T43.595	T43.596
Sulprostone	T48.0X1	T48.0X2	T48.0X3	T48.0X4	T48.0X5	T48.0X6
Sulpyrine	T39.2X1	T39.2X2	T39.2X3	T39.2X4	T39.2X5	T39.2X6
Sultamicillin	T36.0X1	T36.0X2	T36.0X3	T36.0X4	T36.0X5	T36.0X6
Sulthiame	T42.6X1	T42.6X2	T42.6X3	T42.6X4	T42.6X5	T42.6X6
Sultiame	T42.6X1	T42.6X2	T42.6X3	T42.6X4	T42.6X5	T42.6X6
Sultopride	T43.591	T43.592	T43.593	T43.594	T43.595	T43.596
Sumatriptan	T39.8X1	T39.8X2	T39.8X3	T39.8X4	T39.8X5	T39.8X6
Sunflower seed oil	T46.6X1	T46.6X2	T46.6X3	T46.6X4	T46.6X5	T46.6X6
Superinone	T48.4X1	T48.4X2	T48.4X3	T48.4X4	T48.4X5	T48.4X6
Suprofen	T39.311	T39.312	T39.313	T39.314	T39.315	T39.316
Suramin (sodium)	T37.4X1	T37.4X2	T37.4X3	T37.4X4	T37.4X5	T37.4X6
Surfacaine	T41.3X1	T41.3X2	T41.3X3	T41.3X4	T41.3X5	T41.3X6
Surital	T41.1X1	T41.1X2	T41.1X3	T41.1X4	T41.1X5	T41.1X6
Sutilains	T45.3X1	T45.3X2	T45.3X3	T45.3X4	T45.3X5	T45.3X6
Suxamethonium (chloride)	T48.1X1	T48.1X2	T48.1X3	T48.1X4	T48.1X5	T48.1X6
Suxethonium (chloride)	T48.1X1	T48.1X2	T48.1X3	T48.1X4	T48.1X5	T48.1X6
Suxibuzone	T39.2X1	T39.2X2	T39.2X3	T39.2X4	T39.2X5	T39.2X6
Sweet niter spirit	T46.3X1	T46.3X2	T46.3X3	T46.3X4	T46.3X5	T46.3X6
Sweet oil (birch)	T49.3X1	T49.3X2	T49.3X3	T49.3X4	T49.3X5	T49.3X6
Sweetener	T50.901	T50.902	T50.903	T50.904	T50.905	T50.906
Sym-dichloroethyl ether	T53.6X1	T53.6X2	T53.6X3	T53.6X4	—	—
Sympatholytic NEC	T44.8X1	T44.8X2	T44.8X3	T44.8X4	T44.8X5	T44.8X6
haloalkylamine	T44.8X1	T44.8X2	T44.8X3	T44.8X4	T44.8X5	T44.8X6
Sympathomimetic NEC	T44.901	T44.902	T44.903	T44.904	T44.905	T44.906
anti-common-cold	T48.5X1	T48.5X2	T48.5X3	T48.5X4	T48.5X5	T48.5X6
bronchodilator	T48.6X1	T48.6X2	T48.6X3	T48.6X4	T48.6X5	T48.6X6
specified NEC	T44.991	T44.992	T44.993	T44.994	T44.995	T44.996
Synagis	T50.B91	T50.B92	T50.B93	T50.B94	T50.B95	T50.B96
Synalar	T49.0X1	T49.0X2	T49.0X3	T49.0X4	T49.0X5	T49.0X6
Synthetic cannabinoids	T40.721	T40.722	T40.723	T40.724	T40.725	T40.726
Synthroid	T38.1X1	T38.1X2	T38.1X3	T38.1X4	T38.1X5	T38.1X6
Syntocinon	T48.0X1	T48.0X2	T48.0X3	T48.0X4	T48.0X5	T48.0X6

Substance	Poisoning, Accidental (unintentional)	Poisoning, Intentional self-harm	Poisoning, Assault	Poisoning, Undetermined	Adverse effect	Underdosing
Syrosingopine	T46.5X1	T46.5X2	T46.5X3	T46.5X4	T46.5X5	T46.5X6
Systemic drug	T45.91	T45.92	T45.93	T45.94	T45.95	T45.96
specified NEC	T45.8X1	T45.8X2	T45.8X3	T45.8X4	T45.8X5	T45.8X6
2,4,5-T	T60.3X1	T60.3X2	T60.3X3	T60.3X4	—	—

T

Substance	Poisoning, Accidental (unintentional)	Poisoning, Intentional self-harm	Poisoning, Assault	Poisoning, Undetermined	Adverse effect	Underdosing
Tablets—see also specified substance	T50.901	T50.902	T50.903	T50.904	T50.905	T50.906
Tace	T38.5X1	T38.5X2	T38.5X3	T38.5X4	T38.5X5	T38.5X6
Tacrine	T44.0X1	T44.0X2	T44.0X3	T44.0X4	T44.0X5	T44.0X6
Tadalafil	T46.7X1	T46.7X2	T46.7X3	T46.7X4	T46.7X5	T46.7X6
Talampicillin	T36.0X1	T36.0X2	T36.0X3	T36.0X4	T36.0X5	T36.0X6
Talbutal	T42.3X1	T42.3X2	T42.3X3	T42.3X4	T42.3X5	T42.3X6
Talc powder	T49.3X1	T49.3X2	T49.3X3	T49.3X4	T49.3X5	T49.3X6
Talcum	T49.3X1	T49.3X2	T49.3X3	T49.3X4	T49.3X5	T49.3X6
Taleranol	T38.6X1	T38.6X2	T38.6X3	T38.6X4	T38.6X5	T38.6X6
Tamoxifen	T38.6X1	T38.6X2	T38.6X3	T38.6X4	T38.6X5	T38.6X6
Tamsulosin	T44.6X1	T44.6X2	T44.6X3	T44.6X4	T44.6X5	T44.6X6
Tandearil, tanderil	T39.2X1	T39.2X2	T39.2X3	T39.2X4	T39.2X5	T39.2X6
Tannic acid	T49.2X1	T49.2X2	T49.2X3	T49.2X4	T49.2X5	T49.2X6
medicinal (astringent)	T49.2X1	T49.2X2	T49.2X3	T49.2X4	T49.2X5	T49.2X6
Tannin—see Tannic acid						
Tansy	T62.2X1	T62.2X2	T62.2X3	T62.2X4	—	—
TAO	T36.3X1	T36.3X2	T36.3X3	T36.3X4	T36.3X5	T36.3X6
Tapazole	T38.2X1	T38.2X2	T38.2X3	T38.2X4	T38.2X5	T38.2X6
Tar NEC	T52.0X1	T52.0X2	T52.0X3	T52.0X4	—	—
camphor	T60.1X1	T60.1X2	T60.1X3	T60.1X4	—	—
distillate	T49.1X1	T49.1X2	T49.1X3	T49.1X4	T49.1X5	T49.1X6
fumes	T59.891	T59.892	T59.893	T59.894	—	—
medicinal	T49.1X1	T49.1X2	T49.1X3	T49.1X4	T49.1X5	T49.1X6
ointment	T49.1X1	T49.1X2	T49.1X3	T49.1X4	T49.1X5	T49.1X6
Taractan	T43.591	T43.592	T43.593	T43.594	T43.595	T43.596
Tarantula (venomous)	T63.321	T63.322	T63.323	T63.324	—	—
Tartar emetic	T37.8X1	T37.8X2	T37.8X3	T37.8X4	T37.8X5	T37.8X6
Tartaric acid	T65.891	T65.892	T65.893	T65.894	—	—
Tartrate, laxative	T47.4X1	T47.4X2	T47.4X3	T47.4X4	T47.4X5	T47.4X6
Tartrated antimony (anti-infective)	T37.8X1	T37.8X2	T37.8X3	T37.8X4	T37.8X5	T37.8X6
Tauromustine	T45.1X1	T45.1X2	T45.1X3	T45.1X4	T45.1X5	T45.1X6
TCA—see Trichloroacetic acid						
TCDD	T53.7X1	T53.7X2	T53.7X3	T53.7X4	—	—
TDI (vapor)	T65.0X1	T65.0X2	T65.0X3	T65.0X4	—	—
Tear						
gas	T59.3X1	T59.3X2	T59.3X3	T59.3X4	—	—
solution	T49.5X1	T49.5X2	T49.5X3	T49.5X4	T49.5X5	T49.5X6
Teclothiazide	T50.2X1	T50.2X2	T50.2X3	T50.2X4	T50.2X5	T50.2X6
Teclozan	T37.3X1	T37.3X2	T37.3X3	T37.3X4	T37.3X5	T37.3X6
Tegafur	T45.1X1	T45.1X2	T45.1X3	T45.1X4	T45.1X5	T45.1X6
Tegretol	T42.1X1	T42.1X2	T42.1X3	T42.1X4	T42.1X5	T42.1X6
Teicoplanin	T36.8X1	T36.8X2	T36.8X3	T36.8X4	T36.8X5	T36.8X6
Telepaque	T50.8X1	T50.8X2	T50.8X3	T50.8X4	T50.8X5	T50.8X6

Substance	Poisoning, Accidental (unintentional)	Poisoning, Intentional self-harm	Poisoning, Assault	Poisoning, Undetermined	Adverse effect	Underdosing
Tellurium	T56.891	T56.892	T56.893	T56.894	—	—
fumes	T56.891	T56.892	T56.893	T56.894	—	—
TEM	T45.1X1	T45.1X2	T45.1X3	T45.1X4	T45.1X5	T45.1X6
Temazepam	T42.4X1	T42.4X2	T42.4X3	T42.4X4	T42.4X5	T42.4X6
Temocillin	T36.0X1	T36.0X2	T36.0X3	T36.0X4	T36.0X5	T36.0X6
Tenamfetamine	T43.621	T43.622	T43.623	T43.624	T43.625	T43.626
Teniposide	T45.1X1	T45.1X2	T45.1X3	T45.1X4	T45.1X5	T45.1X6
Tenitramine	T46.3X1	T46.3X2	T46.3X3	T46.3X4	T46.3X5	T46.3X6
Tenoglicin	T48.4X1	T48.4X2	T48.4X3	T48.4X4	T48.4X5	T48.4X6
Tenonitrozole	T37.3X1	T37.3X2	T37.3X3	T37.3X4	T37.3X5	T37.3X6
Tenoxicam	T39.391	T39.392	T39.393	T39.394	T39.395	T39.396
TEPA	T45.1X1	T45.1X2	T45.1X3	T45.1X4	T45.1X5	T45.1X6
TEPP	T60.0X1	T60.0X2	T60.0X3	T60.0X4	—	—
Teprotide	T46.5X1	T46.5X2	T46.5X3	T46.5X4	T46.5X5	T46.5X6
Terazosin	T44.6X1	T44.6X2	T44.6X3	T44.6X4	T44.6X5	T44.6X6
Terbufos	T60.0X1	T60.0X2	T60.0X3	T60.0X4	—	—
Terbutaline	T48.6X1	T48.6X2	T48.6X3	T48.6X4	T48.6X5	T48.6X6
Terconazole	T49.0X1	T49.0X2	T49.0X3	T49.0X4	T49.0X5	T49.0X6
Terfenadine	T45.0X1	T45.0X2	T45.0X3	T45.0X4	T45.0X5	T45.0X6
Teriparatide (acetate)	T50.991	T50.992	T50.993	T50.994	T50.995	T50.996
Terizidone	T37.1X1	T37.1X2	T37.1X3	T37.1X4	T37.1X5	T37.1X6
Terlipressin	T38.891	T38.892	T38.893	T38.894	T38.895	T38.896
Terodiline	T46.3X1	T46.3X2	T46.3X3	T46.3X4	T46.3X5	T46.3X6
Teroxalene	T37.4X1	T37.4X2	T37.4X3	T37.4X4	T37.4X5	T37.4X6
Terpin(cis) hydrate	T48.4X1	T48.4X2	T48.4X3	T48.4X4	T48.4X5	T48.4X6
Terramycin	T36.4X1	T36.4X2	T36.4X3	T36.4X4	T36.4X5	T36.4X6
Tertatolol	T44.7X1	T44.7X2	T44.7X3	T44.7X4	T44.7X5	T44.7X6
Tessalon	T48.3X1	T48.3X2	T48.3X3	T48.3X4	T48.3X5	T48.3X6
Testolactone	T38.7X1	T38.7X2	T38.7X3	T38.7X4	T38.7X5	T38.7X6
Testosterone	T38.7X1	T38.7X2	T38.7X3	T38.7X4	T38.7X5	T38.7X6
Tetanus toxoid or vaccine	T50.A91	T50.A92	T50.A93	T50.A94	T50.A95	T50.A96
antitoxin	T50.Z11	T50.Z12	T50.Z13	T50.Z14	T50.Z15	T50.Z16
immune globulin (human)	T50.Z11	T50.Z12	T50.Z13	T50.Z14	T50.Z15	T50.Z16
toxoid	T50.A91	T50.A92	T50.A93	T50.A94	T50.A95	T50.A96
with diphtheria toxoid	T50.A21	T50.A22	T50.A23	T50.A24	T50.A25	T50.A26
with pertussis	T50.A11	T50.A12	T50.A13	T50.A14	T50.A15	T50.A16
Tetrabenazine	T43.591	T43.592	T43.593	T43.594	T43.595	T43.596
Tetracaine	T41.3X1	T41.3X2	T41.3X3	T41.3X4	T41.3X5	T41.3X6
nerve block (peripheral) (plexus)	T41.3X1	T41.3X2	T41.3X3	T41.3X4	T41.3X5	T41.3X6
regional	T41.3X1	T41.3X2	T41.3X3	T41.3X4	T41.3X5	T41.3X6
spinal	T41.3X1	T41.3X2	T41.3X3	T41.3X4	T41.3X5	T41.3X6
Tetrachlorethylene—see Tetrachloroethylene						
Tetrachlormethiazide	T50.2X1	T50.2X2	T50.2X3	T50.2X4	T50.2X5	T50.2X6
2,3,7,8-Tetrachlorodi-benzo-p-dioxin	T53.7X1	T53.7X2	T53.7X3	T53.7X4	—	—
Tetrachloroethane	T53.6X1	T53.6X2	T53.6X3	T53.6X4	—	—
vapor	T53.6X1	T53.6X2	T53.6X3	T53.6X4	—	—

Substance	Poisoning, Accidental (unintentional)	Poisoning, Intentional self-harm	Poisoning, Assault	Poisoning, Undetermined	Adverse effect	Underdosing
Tetrachloroethane — *Continued*						
paint or varnish	T53.6X1	T53.6X2	T53.6X3	T53.6X4	—	—
Tetrachloroethylene (liquid)	T53.3X1	T53.3X2	T53.3X3	T53.3X4		
medicinal	T37.4X1	T37.4X2	T37.4X3	T37.4X4	T37.4X5	T37.4X6
vapor	T53.3X1	T53.3X2	T53.3X3	T53.3X4		
Tetrachloromethane— see Carbon tetrachloride						
Tetracosactide	T38.811	T38.812	T38.813	T38.814	T38.815	T38.816
Tetracosactrin	T38.811	T38.812	T38.813	T38.814	T38.815	T38.816
Tetracycline	T36.4X1	T36.4X2	T36.4X3	T36.4X4	T36.4X5	T36.4X6
ophthalmic preparation	T49.5X1	T49.5X2	T49.5X3	T49.5X4	T49.5X5	T49.5X6
topical NEC	T49.0X1	T49.0X2	T49.0X3	T49.0X4	T49.0X5	T49.0X6
Tetradifon	T60.8X1	T60.8X2	T60.8X3	T60.8X4	—	—
Tetradotoxin	T61.771	T61.772	T61.773	T61.774	—	—
Tetraethyl						
lead	T56.0X1	T56.0X2	T56.0X3	T56.0X4		
pyrophosphate	T60.0X1	T60.0X2	T60.0X3	T60.0X4		
Tetraethylammonium chloride	T44.2X1	T44.2X2	T44.2X3	T44.2X4	T44.2X5	T44.2X6
Tetraethylthiuram disulfide	T50.6X1	T50.6X2	T50.6X3	T50.6X4	T50.6X5	T50.6X6
Tetrahydroamino-acridine	T44.0X1	T44.0X2	T44.0X3	T44.0X4	T44.0X5	T44.0X6
Tetrahydrocannabinol	T40.711	T40.712	T40.713	T40.714	T40.715	T40.716
Tetrahydrofuran	T52.8X1	T52.8X2	T52.8X3	T52.8X4	—	—
Tetrahydronaphthalene	T52.8X1	T52.8X2	T52.8X3	T52.8X4		
Tetrahydrozoline	T49.5X1	T49.5X2	T49.5X3	T49.5X4	T49.5X5	T49.5X6
Tetralin	T52.8X1	T52.8X2	T52.8X3	T52.8X4		
Tetramethrin	T60.2X1	T60.2X2	T60.2X3	T60.2X4		
Tetramethylthiuram (disulfide) NEC	T60.3X1	T60.3X2	T60.3X3	T60.3X4		
medicinal	T49.0X1	T49.0X2	T49.0X3	T49.0X4	T49.0X5	T49.0X6
Tetramisole	T37.4X1	T37.4X2	T37.4X3	T37.4X4	T37.4X5	T37.4X6
Tetranicotinoyl fructose	T46.7X1	T46.7X2	T46.7X3	T46.7X4	T46.7X5	T46.7X6
Tetrazepam	T42.4X1	T42.4X2	T42.4X3	T42.4X4	T42.4X5	T42.4X6
Tetronal	T42.6X1	T42.6X2	T42.6X3	T42.6X4	T42.6X5	T42.6X6
Tetryl	T65.3X1	T65.3X2	T65.3X3	T65.3X4	—	—
Tetrylammonium chloride	T44.2X1	T44.2X2	T44.2X3	T44.2X4	T44.2X5	T44.2X6
Tetryzoline	T49.5X1	T49.5X2	T49.5X3	T49.5X4	T49.5X5	T49.5X6
Thalidomide	T45.1X1	T45.1X2	T45.1X3	T45.1X4	T45.1X5	T45.1X6
Thallium (compounds) (dust) NEC	T56.811	T56.812	T56.813	T56.814	—	—
pesticide	T60.4X1	T60.4X2	T60.4X3	T60.4X4		
THC	T40.711	T40.712	T40.713	T40.714	T40.715	T40.716
Thebacon	T48.3X1	T48.3X2	T48.3X3	T48.3X4	T48.3X5	T48.3X6
Thebaine	T40.2X1	T40.2X2	T40.2X3	T40.2X4	T40.2X5	T40.2X6
Thenoic acid	T49.6X1	T49.6X2	T49.6X3	T49.6X4	T49.6X5	T49.6X6
Thenyldiamine	T45.0X1	T45.0X2	T45.0X3	T45.0X4	T45.0X5	T45.0X6

Substance	Poisoning, Accidental (unintentional)	Poisoning, Intentional self-harm	Poisoning, Assault	Poisoning, Undetermined	Adverse effect	Underdosing
Theobromine (calcium salicylate)	T48.6X1	T48.6X2	T48.6X3	T48.6X4	T48.6X5	T48.6X6
sodium salicylate	T48.6X1	T48.6X2	T48.6X3	T48.6X4	T48.6X5	T48.6X6
Theophyllamine	T48.6X1	T48.6X2	T48.6X3	T48.6X4	T48.6X5	T48.6X6
Theophylline	T48.6X1	T48.6X2	T48.6X3	T48.6X4	T48.6X5	T48.6X6
aminobenzoic acid	T48.6X1	T48.6X2	T48.6X3	T48.6X4	T48.6X5	T48.6X6
ethylenediamine	T48.6X1	T48.6X2	T48.6X3	T48.6X4	T48.6X5	T48.6X6
piperazine p-amino-benzoate	T48.6X1	T48.6X2	T48.6X3	T48.6X4	T48.6X5	T48.6X6
Thiabendazole	T37.4X1	T37.4X2	T37.4X3	T37.4X4	T37.4X5	T37.4X6
Thialbarbital	T41.1X1	T41.1X2	T41.1X3	T41.1X4	T41.1X5	T41.1X6
Thiamazole	T38.2X1	T38.2X2	T38.2X3	T38.2X4	T38.2X5	T38.2X6
Thiambutosine	T37.1X1	T37.1X2	T37.1X3	T37.1X4	T37.1X5	T37.1X6
Thiamine	T45.2X1	T45.2X2	T45.2X3	T45.2X4	T45.2X5	T45.2X6
Thiamphenicol	T36.2X1	T36.2X2	T36.2X3	T36.2X4	T36.2X5	T36.2X6
Thiamylal	T41.1X1	T41.1X2	T41.1X3	T41.1X4	T41.1X5	T41.1X6
sodium	T41.1X1	T41.1X2	T41.1X3	T41.1X4	T41.1X5	T41.1X6
Thiazesim	T43.291	T43.292	T43.293	T43.294	T43.295	T43.296
Thiazides (diuretics)	T50.2X1	T50.2X2	T50.2X3	T50.2X4	T50.2X5	T50.2X6
Thiazinamium metilsulfate	T43.3X1	T43.3X2	T43.3X3	T43.3X4	T43.3X5	T43.3X6
Thiethylperazine	T43.3X1	T43.3X2	T43.3X3	T43.3X4	T43.3X5	T43.3X6
Thimerosal	T49.0X1	T49.0X2	T49.0X3	T49.0X4	T49.0X5	T49.0X6
ophthalmic preparation	T49.5X1	T49.5X2	T49.5X3	T49.5X4	T49.5X5	T49.5X6
Thioacetazone	T37.1X1	T37.1X2	T37.1X3	T37.1X4	T37.1X5	T37.1X6
with isoniazid	T37.1X1	T37.1X2	T37.1X3	T37.1X4	T37.1X5	T37.1X6
Thiobarbital sodium	T41.1X1	T41.1X2	T41.1X3	T41.1X4	T41.1X5	T41.1X6
Thiobarbiturate anesthetic	T41.1X1	T41.1X2	T41.1X3	T41.1X4	T41.1X5	T41.1X6
Thiobismol	T37.8X1	T37.8X2	T37.8X3	T37.8X4	T37.8X5	T37.8X6
Thiobutabarbital sodium	T41.1X1	T41.1X2	T41.1X3	T41.1X4	T41.1X5	T41.1X6
Thiocarbamate (insecticide)	T60.0X1	T60.0X2	T60.0X3	T60.0X4	—	—
Thiocarbamide	T38.2X1	T38.2X2	T38.2X3	T38.2X4	T38.2X5	T38.2X6
Thiocarbarsone	T37.8X1	T37.8X2	T37.8X3	T37.8X4	T37.8X5	T37.8X6
Thiocarlide	T37.1X1	T37.1X2	T37.1X3	T37.1X4	T37.1X5	T37.1X6
Thioctamide	T50.991	T50.992	T50.993	T50.994	T50.995	T50.996
Thioctic acid	T50.991	T50.992	T50.993	T50.994	T50.995	T50.996
Thiofos	T60.0X1	T60.0X2	T60.0X3	T60.0X4		
Thioglycolate	T49.4X1	T49.4X2	T49.4X3	T49.4X4	T49.4X5	T49.4X6
Thioglycolic acid	T65.891	T65.892	T65.893	T65.894	—	—
Thioguanine	T45.1X1	T45.1X2	T45.1X3	T45.1X4	T45.1X5	T45.1X6
Thiomercaptomerin	T50.2X1	T50.2X2	T50.2X3	T50.2X4	T50.2X5	T50.2X6
Thiomerin	T50.2X1	T50.2X2	T50.2X3	T50.2X4	T50.2X5	T50.2X6
Thiomersal	T49.0X1	T49.0X2	T49.0X3	T49.0X4	T49.0X5	T49.0X6
Thionazin	T60.0X1	T60.0X2	T60.0X3	T60.0X4	—	—
Thiopental (sodium)	T41.1X1	T41.1X2	T41.1X3	T41.1X4	T41.1X5	T41.1X6
Thiopentone (sodium)	T41.1X1	T41.1X2	T41.1X3	T41.1X4	T41.1X5	T41.1X6
Thiopropazate	T43.3X1	T43.3X2	T43.3X3	T43.3X4	T43.3X5	T43.3X6
Thioproperazine	T43.3X1	T43.3X2	T43.3X3	T43.3X4	T43.3X5	T43.3X6

Substance	Poisoning, Accidental (unintentional)	Poisoning, Intentional self-harm	Poisoning, Assault	Poisoning, Undetermined	Adverse effect	Underdosing
Thioridazine	T43.3X1	T43.3X2	T43.3X3	T43.3X4	T43.3X5	T43.3X6
Thiosinamine	T49.3X1	T49.3X2	T49.3X3	T49.3X4	T49.3X5	T49.3X6
Thiotepa	T45.1X1	T45.1X2	T45.1X3	T45.1X4	T45.1X5	T45.1X6
Thiothixene	T43.4X1	T43.4X2	T43.4X3	T43.4X4	T43.4X5	T43.4X6
Thiouracil (benzyl) (methyl) (propyl)	T38.2X1	T38.2X2	T38.2X3	T38.2X4	T38.2X5	T38.2X6
Thiourea	T38.2X1	T38.2X2	T38.2X3	T38.2X4	T38.2X5	T38.2X6
Thiphenamil	T44.3X1	T44.3X2	T44.3X3	T44.3X4	T44.3X5	T44.3X6
Thiram	T60.3X1	T60.3X2	T60.3X3	T60.3X4	—	—
medicinal	T49.2X1	T49.2X2	T49.2X3	T49.2X4	T49.2X5	T49.2X6
Thonzylamine (systemic)	T45.0X1	T45.0X2	T45.0X3	T45.0X4	T45.0X5	T45.0X6
mucosal decongestant	T48.5X1	T48.5X2	T48.5X3	T48.5X4	T48.5X5	T48.5X6
Thorazine	T43.3X1	T43.3X2	T43.3X3	T43.3X4	T43.3X5	T43.3X6
Thorium dioxide suspension	T50.8X1	T50.8X2	T50.8X3	T50.8X4	T50.8X5	T50.8X6
Thornapple	T62.2X1	T62.2X2	T62.2X3	T62.2X4	—	—
Throat drug NEC	T49.6X1	T49.6X2	T49.6X3	T49.6X4	T49.6X5	T49.6X6
Thrombin	T45.7X1	T45.7X2	T45.7X3	T45.7X4	T45.7X5	T45.7X6
Thrombolysin	T45.611	T45.612	T45.613	T45.614	T45.615	T45.616
Thromboplastin	T45.7X1	T45.7X2	T45.7X3	T45.7X4	T45.7X5	T45.7X6
Thurfyl nicotinate	T46.7X1	T46.7X2	T46.7X3	T46.7X4	T46.7X5	T46.7X6
Thymol	T49.0X1	T49.0X2	T49.0X3	T49.0X4	T49.0X5	T49.0X6
Thymopentin	T37.5X1	T37.5X2	T37.5X3	T37.5X4	T37.5X5	T37.5X6
Thymoxamine	T46.7X1	T46.7X2	T46.7X3	T46.7X4	T46.7X5	T46.7X6
Thymus extract	T38.891	T38.892	T38.893	T38.894	T38.895	T38.896
Thyreotrophic hormone	T38.811	T38.812	T38.813	T38.814	T38.815	T38.816
Thyroglobulin	T38.1X1	T38.1X2	T38.1X3	T38.1X4	T38.1X5	T38.1X6
Thyroid (hormone)	T38.1X1	T38.1X2	T38.1X3	T38.1X4	T38.1X5	T38.1X6
Thyrolar	T38.1X1	T38.1X2	T38.1X3	T38.1X4	T38.1X5	T38.1X6
Thyrotrophin	T38.811	T38.812	T38.813	T38.814	T38.815	T38.816
Thyrotropic hormone	T38.811	T38.812	T38.813	T38.814	T38.815	T38.816
Thyroxine	T38.1X1	T38.1X2	T38.1X3	T38.1X4	T38.1X5	T38.1X6
Tiabendazole	T37.4X1	T37.4X2	T37.4X3	T37.4X4	T37.4X5	T37.4X6
Tiamizide	T50.2X1	T50.2X2	T50.2X3	T50.2X4	T50.2X5	T50.2X6
Tianeptine	T43.291	T43.292	T43.293	T43.294	T43.295	T43.296
Tiapamil	T46.1X1	T46.1X2	T46.1X3	T46.1X4	T46.1X5	T46.1X6
Tiapride	T43.591	T43.592	T43.593	T43.594	T43.595	T43.596
Tiaprofenic acid	T39.311	T39.312	T39.313	T39.314	T39.315	T39.316
Tiaramide	T39.8X1	T39.8X2	T39.8X3	T39.8X4	T39.8X5	T39.8X6
Ticarcillin	T36.0X1	T36.0X2	T36.0X3	T36.0X4	T36.0X5	T36.0X6
Ticlatone	T49.0X1	T49.0X2	T49.0X3	T49.0X4	T49.0X5	T49.0X6
Ticlopidine	T45.521	T45.522	T45.523	T45.524	T45.525	T45.526
Ticrynafen	T50.1X1	T50.1X2	T50.1X3	T50.1X4	T50.1X5	T50.1X6
Tidiacic	T50.991	T50.992	T50.993	T50.994	T50.995	T50.996
Tiemonium	T44.3X1	T44.3X2	T44.3X3	T44.3X4	T44.3X5	T44.3X6
iodide	T44.3X1	T44.3X2	T44.3X3	T44.3X4	T44.3X5	T44.3X6
Tienilic acid	T50.1X1	T50.1X2	T50.1X3	T50.1X4	T50.1X5	T50.1X6
Tifenamil	T44.3X1	T44.3X2	T44.3X3	T44.3X4	T44.3X5	T44.3X6
Tigan	T45.0X1	T45.0X2	T45.0X3	T45.0X4	T45.0X5	T45.0X6
Tigloidine	T44.3X1	T44.3X2	T44.3X3	T44.3X4	T44.3X5	T44.3X6

Substance	Poisoning, Accidental (unintentional)	Poisoning, Intentional self-harm	Poisoning, Assault	Poisoning, Undetermined	Adverse effect	Underdosing
Tilactase	T47.5X1	T47.5X2	T47.5X3	T47.5X4	T47.5X5	T47.5X6
Tiletamine	T41.291	T41.292	T41.293	T41.294	T41.295	T41.296
Tilidine	T40.491	T40.492	T40.493	T40.494	—	—
Timepidium bromide	T44.3X1	T44.3X2	T44.3X3	T44.3X4	T44.3X5	T44.3X6
Timiperone	T43.4X1	T43.4X2	T43.4X3	T43.4X4	T43.4X5	T43.4X6
Timolol	T44.7X1	T44.7X2	T44.7X3	T44.7X4	T44.7X5	T44.7X6
Tin (chloride) (dust) (oxide) NEC	T56.6X1	T56.6X2	T56.6X3	T56.6X4	—	—
anti-infectives	T37.8X1	T37.8X2	T37.8X3	T37.8X4	T37.8X5	T37.8X6
Tincture, iodine—see Iodine						
Tindal	T43.3X1	T43.3X2	T43.3X3	T43.3X4	T43.3X5	T43.3X6
Tinidazole	T37.3X1	T37.3X2	T37.3X3	T37.3X4	T37.3X5	T37.3X6
Tinoridine	T39.8X1	T39.8X2	T39.8X3	T39.8X4	T39.8X5	T39.8X6
Tiocarlide	T37.1X1	T37.1X2	T37.1X3	T37.1X4	T37.1X5	T37.1X6
Tioclomarol	T45.511	T45.512	T45.513	T45.514	T45.515	T45.516
Tioconazole	T49.0X1	T49.0X2	T49.0X3	T49.0X4	T49.0X5	T49.0X6
Tioguanine	T45.1X1	T45.1X2	T45.1X3	T45.1X4	T45.1X5	T45.1X6
Tiopronin	T50.991	T50.992	T50.993	T50.994	T50.995	T50.996
Tiotixene	T43.4X1	T43.4X2	T43.4X3	T43.4X4	T43.4X5	T43.4X6
Tioxolone	T49.4X1	T49.4X2	T49.4X3	T49.4X4	T49.4X5	T49.4X6
Tipepidine	T48.3X1	T48.3X2	T48.3X3	T48.3X4	T48.3X5	T48.3X6
Tiquizium bromide	T44.3X1	T44.3X2	T44.3X3	T44.3X4	T44.3X5	T44.3X6
Tiratricol	T38.1X1	T38.1X2	T38.1X3	T38.1X4	T38.1X5	T38.1X6
Tisopurine	T50.4X1	T50.4X2	T50.4X3	T50.4X4	T50.4X5	T50.4X6
Titanium (compounds) (vapor)	T56.891	T56.892	T56.893	T56.894	—	—
dioxide	T49.3X1	T49.3X2	T49.3X3	T49.3X4	T49.3X5	T49.3X6
ointment	T49.3X1	T49.3X2	T49.3X3	T49.3X4	T49.3X5	T49.3X6
oxide	T49.3X1	T49.3X2	T49.3X3	T49.3X4	T49.3X5	T49.3X6
tetrachloride	T56.891	T56.892	T56.893	T56.894	—	—
Titanocene	T56.891	T56.892	T56.893	T56.894	—	—
Titroid	T38.1X1	T38.1X2	T38.1X3	T38.1X4	T38.1X5	T38.1X6
Tizanidine	T42.8X1	T42.8X2	T42.8X3	T42.8X4	T42.8X5	T42.8X6
TMTD	T60.3X1	T60.3X2	T60.3X3	T60.3X4	—	—
TNT (fumes)	T65.3X1	T65.3X2	T65.3X3	T65.3X4	—	—
Toadstool	T62.0X1	T62.0X2	T62.0X3	T62.0X4	—	—
Tobacco NEC	T65.291	T65.292	T65.293	T65.294	—	—
cigarettes	T65.221	T65.222	T65.223	T65.224	—	—
Indian	T62.2X1	T62.2X2	T62.2X3	T62.2X4	—	—
smoke, second-hand	T65.221	T65.222	T65.223	T65.224	—	—
Tobramycin	T36.5X1	T36.5X2	T36.5X3	T36.5X4	T36.5X5	T36.5X6
Tocainide	T46.2X1	T46.2X2	T46.2X3	T46.2X4	T46.2X5	T46.2X6
Tocoferol	T45.2X1	T45.2X2	T45.2X3	T45.2X4	T45.2X5	T45.2X6
Tocopherol	T45.2X1	T45.2X2	T45.2X3	T45.2X4	T45.2X5	T45.2X6
acetate	T45.2X1	T45.2X2	T45.2X3	T45.2X4	T45.2X5	T45.2X6
Tocosamine	T48.0X1	T48.0X2	T48.0X3	T48.0X4	T48.0X5	T48.0X6
Todralazine	T46.5X1	T46.5X2	T46.5X3	T46.5X4	T46.5X5	T46.5X6
Tofisopam	T42.4X1	T42.4X2	T42.4X3	T42.4X4	T42.4X5	T42.4X6
Tofranil	T43.011	T43.012	T43.013	T43.014	T43.015	T43.016
Toilet deodorizer	T65.891	T65.892	T65.893	T65.894	—	—

Substance	Poisoning, Accidental (unintentional)	Poisoning, Intentional self-harm	Poisoning, Assault	Poisoning, Undetermined	Adverse effect	Underdosing
Tolamolol	T44.7X1	T44.7X2	T44.7X3	T44.7X4	T44.7X5	T44.7X6
Tolazamide	T38.3X1	T38.3X2	T38.3X3	T38.3X4	T38.3X5	T38.3X6
Tolazoline	T46.7X1	T46.7X2	T46.7X3	T46.7X4	T46.7X5	T46.7X6
Tolbutamide (sodium)	T38.3X1	T38.3X2	T38.3X3	T38.3X4	T38.3X5	T38.3X6
Tolciclate	T49.0X1	T49.0X2	T49.0X3	T49.0X4	T49.0X5	T49.0X6
Tolmetin	T39.391	T39.392	T39.393	T39.394	T39.395	T39.396
Tolnaftate	T49.0X1	T49.0X2	T49.0X3	T49.0X4	T49.0X5	T49.0X6
Tolonidine	T46.5X1	T46.5X2	T46.5X3	T46.5X4	T46.5X5	T46.5X6
Toloxatone	T42.6X1	T42.6X2	T42.6X3	T42.6X4	T42.6X5	T42.6X6
Tolperisone	T44.3X1	T44.3X2	T44.3X3	T44.3X4	T44.3X5	T44.3X6
Tolserol	T42.8X1	T42.8X2	T42.8X3	T42.8X4	T42.8X5	T42.8X6
Toluene (liquid)	T52.2X1	T52.2X2	T52.2X3	T52.2X4	—	—
diisocyanate	T65.0X1	T65.0X2	T65.0X3	T65.0X4	—	—
Toluidine	T65.891	T65.892	T65.893	T65.894	—	—
vapor	T59.891	T59.892	T59.893	T59.894	—	—
Toluol (liquid)	T52.2X1	T52.2X2	T52.2X3	T52.2X4	—	—
vapor	T52.2X1	T52.2X2	T52.2X3	T52.2X4	—	—
Toluylenediamine	T65.3X1	T65.3X2	T65.3X3	T65.3X4	—	—
Tolylene-2,4-diisocyanate	T65.0X1	T65.0X2	T65.0X3	T65.0X4	—	—
Tonic NEC	T50.901	T50.902	T50.903	T50.904	T50.905	T50.906
Topical action drug NEC	T49.91	T49.92	T49.93	T49.94	T49.95	T49.96
ear, nose or throat	T49.6X1	T49.6X2	T49.6X3	T49.6X4	T49.6X5	T49.6X6
eye	T49.5X1	T49.5X2	T49.5X3	T49.5X4	T49.5X5	T49.5X6
skin	T49.91	T49.92	T49.93	T49.94	T49.95	T49.96
specified NEC	T49.8X1	T49.8X2	T49.8X3	T49.8X4	T49.8X5	T49.8X6
Toquizine	T44.3X1	T44.3X2	T44.3X3	T44.3X4	T44.3X5	T44.3X6
Toremifene	T38.6X1	T38.6X2	T38.6X3	T38.6X4	T38.6X5	T38.6X6
Tosylchloramide sodium	T49.8X1	T49.8X2	T49.8X3	T49.8X4	T49.8X5	T49.8X6
Toxaphene (dust) (spray)	T60.1X1	T60.1X2	T60.1X3	T60.1X4	—	—
Toxin, diphtheria (Schick Test)	T50.8X1	T50.8X2	T50.8X3	T50.8X4	T50.8X5	T50.8X6
Toxoid						
combined	T50.A21	T50.A22	T50.A23	T50.A24	T50.A25	T50.A26
diphtheria	T50.A91	T50.A92	T50.A93	T50.A94	T50.A95	T50.A96
tetanus	T50.A91	T50.A92	T50.A93	T50.A94	T50.A95	T50.A96
Trace element NEC	T45.8X1	T45.8X2	T45.8X3	T45.8X4	T45.8X5	T45.8X6
Tractor fuel NEC	T52.0X1	T52.0X2	T52.0X3	T52.0X4	—	—
Tragacanth	T50.991	T50.992	T50.993	T50.994	T50.995	T50.996
Tramadol	T40.421	T40.422	T40.423	T40.424	T40.425	T40.426
Tramazoline	T48.5X1	T48.5X2	T48.5X3	T48.5X4	T48.5X5	T48.5X6
Tranexamic acid	T45.621	T45.622	T45.623	T45.624	T45.625	T45.626
Tranilast	T45.0X1	T45.0X2	T45.0X3	T45.0X4	T45.0X5	T45.0X6
Tranquilizer NEC	T43.501	T43.502	T43.503	T43.504	T43.505	T43.506
with hypnotic or sedative	T42.6X1	T42.6X2	T42.6X3	T42.6X4	T42.6X5	T42.6X6
benzodiazepine NEC	T42.4X1	T42.4X2	T42.4X3	T42.4X4	T42.4X5	T42.4X6
butyrophenone NEC	T43.4X1	T43.4X2	T43.4X3	T43.4X4	T43.4X5	T43.4X6
carbamate	T43.591	T43.592	T43.593	T43.594	T43.595	T43.596
dimethylamine	T43.3X1	T43.3X2	T43.3X3	T43.3X4	T43.3X5	T43.3X6
ethylamine	T43.3X1	T43.3X2	T43.3X3	T43.3X4	T43.3X5	T43.3X6

Substance	Poisoning, Accidental (unintentional)	Poisoning, Intentional self-harm	Poisoning, Assault	Poisoning, Undetermined	Adverse effect	Underdosing
Tranquilizer NEC — Continued						
hydroxyzine	T43.591	T43.592	T43.593	T43.594	T43.595	T43.596
major NEC	T43.501	T43.502	T43.503	T43.504	T43.505	T43.506
penothiazine NEC	T43.3X1	T43.3X2	T43.3X3	T43.3X4	T43.3X5	T43.3X6
phenothiazine-based	T43.3X1	T43.3X2	T43.3X3	T43.3X4	T43.3X5	T43.3X6
piperazine NEC	T43.3X1	T43.3X2	T43.3X3	T43.3X4	T43.3X5	T43.3X6
piperidine	T43.3X1	T43.3X2	T43.3X3	T43.3X4	T43.3X5	T43.3X6
propylamine	T43.3X1	T43.3X2	T43.3X3	T43.3X4	T43.3X5	T43.3X6
specified NEC	T43.591	T43.592	T43.593	T43.594	T43.595	T43.596
thioxanthene NEC	T43.591	T43.592	T43.593	T43.594	T43.595	T43.596
Tranxene	T42.4X1	T42.4X2	T42.4X3	T42.4X4	T42.4X5	T42.4X6
Tranylcypromine	T43.1X1	T43.1X2	T43.1X3	T43.1X4	T43.1X5	T43.1X6
Trapidil	T46.3X1	T46.3X2	T46.3X3	T46.3X4	T46.3X5	T46.3X6
Trasentine	T44.3X1	T44.3X2	T44.3X3	T44.3X4	T44.3X5	T44.3X6
Travert	T50.3X1	T50.3X2	T50.3X3	T50.3X4	T50.3X5	T50.3X6
Trazodone	T43.211	T43.212	T43.213	T43.214	T43.215	T43.216
Trecator	T37.1X1	T37.1X2	T37.1X3	T37.1X4	T37.1X5	T37.1X6
Treosulfan	T45.1X1	T45.1X2	T45.1X3	T45.1X4	T45.1X5	T45.1X6
Tretamine	T45.1X1	T45.1X2	T45.1X3	T45.1X4	T45.1X5	T45.1X6
Tretinoin	T49.0X1	T49.0X2	T49.0X3	T49.0X4	T49.0X5	T49.0X6
Tretoquinol	T48.6X1	T48.6X2	T48.6X3	T48.6X4	T48.6X5	T48.6X6
Triacetin	T49.0X1	T49.0X2	T49.0X3	T49.0X4	T49.0X5	T49.0X6
Triacetoxyanthracene	T49.4X1	T49.4X2	T49.4X3	T49.4X4	T49.4X5	T49.4X6
Triacetyloleandomycin	T36.3X1	T36.3X2	T36.3X3	T36.3X4	T36.3X5	T36.3X6
Triamcinolone	T38.0X1	T38.0X2	T38.0X3	T38.0X4	T38.0X5	T38.0X6
ENT agent	T49.6X1	T49.6X2	T49.6X3	T49.6X4	T49.6X5	T49.6X6
hexacetonide	T49.0X1	T49.0X2	T49.0X3	T49.0X4	T49.0X5	T49.0X6
ophthalmic preparation	T49.5X1	T49.5X2	T49.5X3	T49.5X4	T49.5X5	T49.5X6
topical NEC	T49.0X1	T49.0X2	T49.0X3	T49.0X4	T49.0X5	T49.0X6
Triampyzine	T44.3X1	T44.3X2	T44.3X3	T44.3X4	T44.3X5	T44.3X6
Triamterene	T50.2X1	T50.2X2	T50.2X3	T50.2X4	T50.2X5	T50.2X6
Triazine (herbicide)	T60.3X1	T60.3X2	T60.3X3	T60.3X4	—	—
Triaziquone	T45.1X1	T45.1X2	T45.1X3	T45.1X4	T45.1X5	T45.1X6
Triazolam	T42.4X1	T42.4X2	T42.4X3	T42.4X4	T42.4X5	T42.4X6
Triazole (herbicide)	T60.3X1	T60.3X2	T60.3X3	T60.3X4	—	—
Tribenoside	T46.991	T46.992	T46.993	T46.994	T46.995	T46.996
Tribromacetaldehyde	T42.6X1	T42.6X2	T42.6X3	T42.6X4	T42.6X5	T42.6X6
Tribromoethanol, rectal	T41.291	T41.292	T41.293	T41.294	T41.295	T41.296
Tribromomethane	T42.6X1	T42.6X2	T42.6X3	T42.6X4	T42.6X5	T42.6X6
Trichlorethane	T53.2X1	T53.2X2	T53.2X3	T53.2X4	—	—
Trichlorethylene	T53.2X1	T53.2X2	T53.2X3	T53.2X4	—	—
Trichlorfon	T60.0X1	T60.0X2	T60.0X3	T60.0X4	—	—
Trichlormethiazide	T50.2X1	T50.2X2	T50.2X3	T50.2X4	T50.2X5	T50.2X6
Trichlormethine	T45.1X1	T45.1X2	T45.1X3	T45.1X4	T45.1X5	T45.1X6
Trichloroacetic acid, Trichloracetic acid	T54.2X1	T54.2X2	T54.2X3	T54.2X4	—	—
medicinal	T49.4X1	T49.4X2	T49.4X3	T49.4X4	T49.4X5	T49.4X6
Trichloroethane	T53.2X1	T53.2X2	T53.2X3	T53.2X4	—	—
Trichloroethanol	T42.6X1	T42.6X2	T42.6X3	T42.6X4	T42.6X5	T42.6X6

Substance	Poisoning, Accidental (unintentional)	Poisoning, Intentional self-harm	Poisoning, Assault	Poisoning, Undetermined	Adverse effect	Underdosing
Trichloroethyl phosphate	T42.6X1	T42.6X2	T42.6X3	T42.6X4	T42.6X5	T42.6X6
Trichloroethylene (liquid) (vapor)	T53.2X1	T53.2X2	T53.2X3	T53.2X4	—	—
anesthetic (gas)	T41.0X1	T41.0X2	T41.0X3	T41.0X4	T41.0X5	T41.0X6
vapor NEC	T53.2X1	T53.2X2	T53.2X3	T53.2X4	—	—
Trichlorofluoromethane NEC	T53.5X1	T53.5X2	T53.5X3	T53.5X4	—	—
Trichloronate	T60.0X1	T60.0X2	T60.0X3	T60.0X4	—	—
2,4,5-Trichlorophen-oxyacetic acid	T60.3X1	T60.3X2	T60.3X3	T60.3X4	—	—
Trichloropropane	T53.6X1	T53.6X2	T53.6X3	T53.6X4	—	—
Trichlorotriethylamine	T45.1X1	T45.1X2	T45.1X3	T45.1X4	T45.1X5	T45.1X6
Trichomonacides NEC	T37.3X1	T37.3X2	T37.3X3	T37.3X4	T37.3X5	T37.3X6
Trichomycin	T36.7X1	T36.7X2	T36.7X3	T36.7X4	T36.7X5	T36.7X6
Triclobisonium chloride	T49.0X1	T49.0X2	T49.0X3	T49.0X4	T49.0X5	T49.0X6
Triclocarban	T49.0X1	T49.0X2	T49.0X3	T49.0X4	T49.0X5	T49.0X6
Triclofos	T42.6X1	T42.6X2	T42.6X3	T42.6X4	T42.6X5	T42.6X6
Triclosan	T49.0X1	T49.0X2	T49.0X3	T49.0X4	T49.0X5	T49.0X6
Tricresyl phosphate	T65.891	T65.892	T65.893	T65.894	—	—
solvent	T52.91	T52.92	T52.93	T52.94	—	—
Tricyclamol chloride	T44.3X1	T44.3X2	T44.3X3	T44.3X4	T44.3X5	T44.3X6
Tridesilon	T49.0X1	T49.0X2	T49.0X3	T49.0X4	T49.0X5	T49.0X6
Tridihexethyl iodide	T44.3X1	T44.3X2	T44.3X3	T44.3X4	T44.3X5	T44.3X6
Tridione	T42.2X1	T42.2X2	T42.2X3	T42.2X4	T42.2X5	T42.2X6
Trientine	T45.8X1	T45.8X2	T45.8X3	T45.8X4	T45.8X5	T45.8X6
Triethanolamine NEC	T54.3X1	T54.3X2	T54.3X3	T54.3X4	—	—
detergent	T54.3X1	T54.3X2	T54.3X3	T54.3X4	—	—
trinitrate (biphosphate)	T46.3X1	T46.3X2	T46.3X3	T46.3X4	T46.3X5	T46.3X6
Triethanomelamine	T45.1X1	T45.1X2	T45.1X3	T45.1X4	T45.1X5	T45.1X6
Triethylenemelamine	T45.1X1	T45.1X2	T45.1X3	T45.1X4	T45.1X5	T45.1X6
Triethylenephos-phoramide	T45.1X1	T45.1X2	T45.1X3	T45.1X4	T45.1X5	T45.1X6
Triethylenethiophos-phoramide	T45.1X1	T45.1X2	T45.1X3	T45.1X4	T45.1X5	T45.1X6
Trifluoperazine	T43.3X1	T43.3X2	T43.3X3	T43.3X4	T43.3X5	T43.3X6
Trifluoroethyl vinyl ether	T41.0X1	T41.0X2	T41.0X3	T41.0X4	T41.0X5	T41.0X6
Trifluperidol	T43.4X1	T43.4X2	T43.4X3	T43.4X4	T43.4X5	T43.4X6
Triflupromazine	T43.3X1	T43.3X2	T43.3X3	T43.3X4	T43.3X5	T43.3X6
Trifluridine	T37.5X1	T37.5X2	T37.5X3	T37.5X4	T37.5X5	T37.5X6
Triflusal	T45.521	T45.522	T45.523	T45.524	T45.525	T45.526
Trihexyphenidyl	T44.3X1	T44.3X2	T44.3X3	T44.3X4	T44.3X5	T44.3X6
Triiodothyronine	T38.1X1	T38.1X2	T38.1X3	T38.1X4	T38.1X5	T38.1X6
Trilene	T41.0X1	T41.0X2	T41.0X3	T41.0X4	T41.0X5	T41.0X6
Trilostane	T38.991	T38.992	T38.993	T38.994	T38.995	T38.996
Trimebutine	T44.3X1	T44.3X2	T44.3X3	T44.3X4	T44.3X5	T44.3X6
Trimecaine	T41.3X1	T41.3X2	T41.3X3	T41.3X4	T41.3X5	T41.3X6
Trimeprazine (tartrate)	T44.3X1	T44.3X2	T44.3X3	T44.3X4	T44.3X5	T44.3X6
Trimetaphan camsilate	T44.2X1	T44.2X2	T44.2X3	T44.2X4	T44.2X5	T44.2X6
Trimetazidine	T46.7X1	T46.7X2	T46.7X3	T46.7X4	T46.7X5	T46.7X6
Trimethadione	T42.2X1	T42.2X2	T42.2X3	T42.2X4	T42.2X5	T42.2X6
Trimethaphan	T44.2X1	T44.2X2	T44.2X3	T44.2X4	T44.2X5	T44.2X6
Trimethidinium	T44.2X1	T44.2X2	T44.2X3	T44.2X4	T44.2X5	T44.2X6
Trimethobenzamide	T45.0X1	T45.0X2	T45.0X3	T45.0X4	T45.0X5	T45.0X6
Trimethoprim	T37.8X1	T37.8X2	T37.8X3	T37.8X4	T37.8X5	T37.8X6
with sulfamethoxazole	T36.8X1	T36.8X2	T36.8X3	T36.8X4	T36.8X5	T36.8X6
Trimethylcarbinol	T51.3X1	T51.3X2	T51.3X3	T51.3X4	—	—
Trimethylpsoralen	T49.3X1	T49.3X2	T49.3X3	T49.3X4	T49.3X5	T49.3X6
Trimeton	T45.0X1	T45.0X2	T45.0X3	T45.0X4	T45.0X5	T45.0X6
Trimetrexate	T45.1X1	T45.1X2	T45.1X3	T45.1X4	T45.1X5	T45.1X6
Trimipramine	T43.011	T43.012	T43.013	T43.014	T43.015	T43.016
Trimustine	T45.1X1	T45.1X2	T45.1X3	T45.1X4	T45.1X5	T45.1X6
Trinitrine	T46.3X1	T46.3X2	T46.3X3	T46.3X4	T46.3X5	T46.3X6
Trinitrobenzol	T65.3X1	T65.3X2	T65.3X3	T65.3X4	—	—
Trinitrophenol	T65.3X1	T65.3X2	T65.3X3	T65.3X4	—	—
Trinitrotoluene (fumes)	T65.3X1	T65.3X2	T65.3X3	T65.3X4	—	—
Trional	T42.6X1	T42.6X2	T42.6X3	T42.6X4	T42.6X5	T42.6X6
Triorthocresyl phosphate	T65.891	T65.892	T65.893	T65.894	—	—
Trioxide of arsenic	T57.0X1	T57.0X2	T57.0X3	T57.0X4	—	—
Trioxysalen	T49.4X1	T49.4X2	T49.4X3	T49.4X4	T49.4X5	T49.4X6
Tripamide	T50.2X1	T50.2X2	T50.2X3	T50.2X4	T50.2X5	T50.2X6
Triparanol	T46.6X1	T46.6X2	T46.6X3	T46.6X4	T46.6X5	T46.6X6
Tripelennamine	T45.0X1	T45.0X2	T45.0X3	T45.0X4	T45.0X5	T45.0X6
Triperiden	T44.3X1	T44.3X2	T44.3X3	T44.3X4	T44.3X5	T44.3X6
Triperidol	T43.4X1	T43.4X2	T43.4X3	T43.4X4	T43.4X5	T43.4X6
Triphenylphosphate	T65.891	T65.892	T65.893	T65.894	—	—
Triple						
bromides	T42.6X1	T42.6X2	T42.6X3	T42.6X4	T42.6X5	T42.6X6
carbonate	T47.1X1	T47.1X2	T47.1X3	T47.1X4	T47.1X5	T47.1X6
vaccine						
DPT	T50.A11	T50.A12	T50.A13	T50.A14	T50.A15	T50.A16
including pertussis	T50.A11	T50.A12	T50.A13	T50.A14	T50.A15	T50.A16
MMR	T50.B91	T50.B92	T50.B93	T50.B94	T50.B95	T50.B96
Triprolidine	T45.0X1	T45.0X2	T45.0X3	T45.0X4	T45.0X5	T45.0X6
Trisodium hydrogen edetate	T50.6X1	T50.6X2	T50.6X3	T50.6X4	T50.6X5	T50.6X6
Trisoralen	T49.3X1	T49.3X2	T49.3X3	T49.3X4	T49.3X5	T49.3X6
Trisulfapyrimidines	T37.0X1	T37.0X2	T37.0X3	T37.0X4	T37.0X5	T37.0X6
Trithiozine	T44.3X1	T44.3X2	T44.3X3	T44.3X4	T44.3X5	T44.3X6
Tritiozine	T44.3X1	T44.3X2	T44.3X3	T44.3X4	T44.3X5	T44.3X6
Tritoqualine	T45.0X1	T45.0X2	T45.0X3	T45.0X4	T45.0X5	T45.0X6
Trofosfamide	T45.1X1	T45.1X2	T45.1X3	T45.1X4	T45.1X5	T45.1X6
Troleandomycin	T36.3X1	T36.3X2	T36.3X3	T36.3X4	T36.3X5	T36.3X6
Trolnitrate (phosphate)	T46.3X1	T46.3X2	T46.3X3	T46.3X4	T46.3X5	T46.3X6
Tromantadine	T37.5X1	T37.5X2	T37.5X3	T37.5X4	T37.5X5	T37.5X6
Trometamol	T50.2X1	T50.2X2	T50.2X3	T50.2X4	T50.2X5	T50.2X6
Tromethamine	T50.2X1	T50.2X2	T50.2X3	T50.2X4	T50.2X5	T50.2X6
Tronothane	T41.3X1	T41.3X2	T41.3X3	T41.3X4	T41.3X5	T41.3X6
Tropacine	T44.3X1	T44.3X2	T44.3X3	T44.3X4	T44.3X5	T44.3X6
Tropatepine	T44.3X1	T44.3X2	T44.3X3	T44.3X4	T44.3X5	T44.3X6

Substance	Poisoning, Accidental (unintentional)	Poisoning, Intentional self-harm	Poisoning, Assault	Poisoning, Undetermined	Adverse effect	Underdosing
Tropicamide	T44.3X1	T44.3X2	T44.3X3	T44.3X4	T44.3X5	T44.3X6
Trospium chloride	T44.3X1	T44.3X2	T44.3X3	T44.3X4	T44.3X5	T44.3X6
Troxerutin	T46.991	T46.992	T46.993	T46.994	T46.995	T46.996
Troxidone	T42.2X1	T42.2X2	T42.2X3	T42.2X4	T42.2X5	T42.2X6
Tryparsamide	T37.3X1	T37.3X2	T37.3X3	T37.3X4	T37.3X5	T37.3X6
Trypsin	T45.3X1	T45.3X2	T45.3X3	T45.3X4	T45.3X5	T45.3X6
Tryptizol	T43.011	T43.012	T43.013	T43.014	T43.015	T43.016
TSH	T38.811	T38.812	T38.813	T38.814	T38.815	T38.816
Tuaminoheptane	T48.5X1	T48.5X2	T48.5X3	T48.5X4	T48.5X5	T48.5X6
Tuberculin, purified protein derivative (PPD)	T50.8X1	T50.8X2	T50.8X3	T50.8X4	T50.8X5	T50.8X6
Tubocurare	T48.1X1	T48.1X2	T48.1X3	T48.1X4	T48.1X5	T48.1X6
Tubocurarine (chloride)	T48.1X1	T48.1X2	T48.1X3	T48.1X4	T48.1X5	T48.1X6
Tulobuterol	T48.6X1	T48.6X2	T48.6X3	T48.6X4	T48.6X5	T48.6X6
Turpentine (spirits of)	T52.8X1	T52.8X2	T52.8X3	T52.8X4	—	—
vapor	T52.8X1	T52.8X2	T52.8X3	T52.8X4	—	—
Tybamate	T43.591	T43.592	T43.593	T43.594	T43.595	T43.596
Tyloxapol	T48.4X1	T48.4X2	T48.4X3	T48.4X4	T48.4X5	T48.4X6
Tymazoline	T48.5X1	T48.5X2	T48.5X3	T48.5X4	T48.5X5	T48.5X6
Typhoid-paratyphoid vaccine	T50.A91	T50.A92	T50.A93	T50.A94	T50.A95	T50.A96
Typhus vaccine	T50.A91	T50.A92	T50.A93	T50.A94	T50.A95	T50.A96
Tyropanoate	T50.8X1	T50.8X2	T50.8X3	T50.8X4	T50.8X5	T50.8X6
Tyrothricin	T49.6X1	T49.6X2	T49.6X3	T49.6X4	T49.6X5	T49.6X6
ENT agent	T49.6X1	T49.6X2	T49.6X3	T49.6X4	T49.6X5	T49.6X6
ophthalmic preparation	T49.5X1	T49.5X2	T49.5X3	T49.5X4	T49.5X5	T49.5X6

U

Substance	Poisoning, Accidental (unintentional)	Poisoning, Intentional self-harm	Poisoning, Assault	Poisoning, Undetermined	Adverse effect	Underdosing
Ufenamate	T39.391	T39.392	T39.393	T39.394	T39.395	T39.396
Ultraviolet light protectant	T49.3X1	T49.3X2	T49.3X3	T49.3X4	T49.3X5	T49.3X6
Undecenoic acid	T49.0X1	T49.0X2	T49.0X3	T49.0X4	T49.0X5	T49.0X6
Undecoylium	T49.0X1	T49.0X2	T49.0X3	T49.0X4	T49.0X5	T49.0X6
Undecylenic acid (derivatives)	T49.0X1	T49.0X2	T49.0X3	T49.0X4	T49.0X5	T49.0X6
Unna's boot	T49.3X1	T49.3X2	T49.3X3	T49.3X4	T49.3X5	T49.3X6
Unsaturated fatty acid	T46.6X1	T46.6X2	T46.6X3	T46.6X4	T46.6X5	T46.6X6
Uracil mustard	T45.1X1	T45.1X2	T45.1X3	T45.1X4	T45.1X5	T45.1X6
Uramustine	T45.1X1	T45.1X2	T45.1X3	T45.1X4	T45.1X5	T45.1X6
Urapidil	T46.5X1	T46.5X2	T46.5X3	T46.5X4	T46.5X5	T46.5X6
Urari	T48.1X1	T48.1X2	T48.1X3	T48.1X4	T48.1X5	T48.1X6
Urate oxidase	T50.4X1	T50.4X2	T50.4X3	T50.4X4	T50.4X5	T50.4X6
Urea	T47.3X1	T47.3X2	T47.3X3	T47.3X4	T47.3X5	T47.3X6
peroxide	T49.0X1	T49.0X2	T49.0X3	T49.0X4	T49.0X5	T49.0X6
stibamine	T37.4X1	T37.4X2	T37.4X3	T37.4X4	T37.4X5	T37.4X6
topical	T49.8X1	T49.8X2	T49.8X3	T49.8X4	T49.8X5	T49.8X6
Urethane	T45.1X1	T45.1X2	T45.1X3	T45.1X4	T45.1X5	T45.1X6
Urginea (maritima) (scilla)—see Squill						
Uric acid metabolism drug NEC	T50.4X1	T50.4X2	T50.4X3	T50.4X4	T50.4X5	T50.4X6
Uricosuric agent	T50.4X1	T50.4X2	T50.4X3	T50.4X4	T50.4X5	T50.4X6
Urinary anti-infective	T37.8X1	T37.8X2	T37.8X3	T37.8X4	T37.8X5	T37.8X6
Urofollitropin	T38.811	T38.812	T38.813	T38.814	T38.815	T38.816
Urokinase	T45.611	T45.612	T45.613	T45.614	T45.615	T45.616
Urokon	T50.8X1	T50.8X2	T50.8X3	T50.8X4	T50.8X5	T50.8X6
Ursodeoxycholic acid	T50.991	T50.992	T50.993	T50.994	T50.995	T50.996
Ursodiol	T50.991	T50.992	T50.993	T50.994	T50.995	T50.996
Urtica	T62.2X1	T62.2X2	T62.2X3	T62.2X4	—	—
Utility gas—see Gas, utility						

V

Substance	Poisoning, Accidental (unintentional)	Poisoning, Intentional self-harm	Poisoning, Assault	Poisoning, Undetermined	Adverse effect	Underdosing
Vaccine NEC	T50.Z91	T50.Z92	T50.Z93	T50.Z94	T50.Z95	T50.Z96
antineoplastic	T50.Z91	T50.Z92	T50.Z93	T50.Z94	T50.Z95	T50.Z96
bacterial NEC	T50.A91	T50.A92	T50.A93	T50.A94	T50.A95	T50.A96
with						
other bacterial component	T50.A21	T50.A22	T50.A23	T50.A24	T50.A25	T50.A26
pertussis component	T50.A11	T50.A12	T50.A13	T50.A14	T50.A15	T50.A16
viral-rickettsial component	T50.A21	T50.A22	T50.A23	T50.A24	T50.A25	T50.A26
mixed NEC	T50.A21	T50.A22	T50.A23	T50.A24	T50.A25	T50.A26
BCG	T50.A91	T50.A92	T50.A93	T50.A94	T50.A95	T50.A96
cholera	T50.A91	T50.A92	T50.A93	T50.A94	T50.A95	T50.A96
diphtheria	T50.A91	T50.A92	T50.A93	T50.A94	T50.A95	T50.A96
with tetanus	T50.A21	T50.A22	T50.A23	T50.A24	T50.A25	T50.A26
and pertussis	T50.A11	T50.A12	T50.A13	T50.A14	T50.A15	T50.A16
influenza	T50.B91	T50.B92	T50.B93	T50.B94	T50.B95	T50.B96
measles	T50.B91	T50.B92	T50.B93	T50.B94	T50.B95	T50.B96
with mumps and rubella	T50.B91	T50.B92	T50.B93	T50.B94	T50.B95	T50.B96
meningococcal	T50.A91	T50.A92	T50.A93	T50.A94	T50.A95	T50.A96
mumps	T50.B91	T50.B92	T50.B93	T50.B94	T50.B95	T50.B96
paratyphoid	T50.A91	T50.A92	T50.A93	T50.A94	T50.A95	T50.A96
pertussis	T50.A11	T50.A12	T50.A13	T50.A14	T50.A15	T50.A16
with diphtheria	T50.A11	T50.A12	T50.A13	T50.A14	T50.A15	T50.A16
and tetanus	T50.A11	T50.A12	T50.A13	T50.A14	T50.A15	T50.A16
with other component	T50.A11	T50.A12	T50.A13	T50.A14	T50.A15	T50.A16
plague	T50.A91	T50.A92	T50.A93	T50.A94	T50.A95	T50.A96
poliomyelitis	T50.B91	T50.B92	T50.B93	T50.B94	T50.B95	T50.B96
poliovirus	T50.B91	T50.B92	T50.B93	T50.B94	T50.B95	T50.B96
rabies	T50.B91	T50.B92	T50.B93	T50.B94	T50.B95	T50.B96
respiratory syncytial virus	T50.B91	T50.B92	T50.B93	T50.B94	T50.B95	T50.B96
rickettsial NEC	T50.A91	T50.A92	T50.A93	T50.A94	T50.A95	T50.A96
with						
bacterial component	T50.A21	T50.A22	T50.A23	T50.A24	T50.A25	T50.A26
Rocky Mountain spotted fever	T50.A91	T50.A92	T50.A93	T50.A94	T50.A95	T50.A96
rubella	T50.B91	T50.B92	T50.B93	T50.B94	T50.B95	T50.B96
sabin oral	T50.B91	T50.B92	T50.B93	T50.B94	T50.B95	T50.B96
smallpox	T50.B11	T50.B12	T50.B13	T50.B14	T50.B15	T50.B16
TAB	T50.A91	T50.A92	T50.A93	T50.A94	T50.A95	T50.A96
tetanus	T50.A91	T50.A92	T50.A93	T50.A94	T50.A95	T50.A96

Substance	Poisoning, Accidental (unintentional)	Poisoning, Intentional self-harm	Poisoning, Assault	Poisoning, Undetermined	Adverse effect	Underdosing
Vaccine NEC — *Continued*						
typhoid	T50.A91	T50.A92	T50.A93	T50.A94	T50.A95	T50.A96
typhus	T50.A91	T50.A92	T50.A93	T50.A94	T50.A95	T50.A96
viral NEC	T50.B91	T50.B92	T50.B93	T50.B94	T50.B95	T50.B96
yellow fever	T50.B91	T50.B92	T50.B93	T50.B94	T50.B95	T50.B96
Vaccinia immune globulin	T50.Z11	T50.Z12	T50.Z13	T50.Z14	T50.Z15	T50.Z16
Vaginal contraceptives	T49.8X1	T49.8X2	T49.8X3	T49.8X4	T49.8X5	T49.8X6
Valerian						
root	T42.6X1	T42.6X2	T42.6X3	T42.6X4	T42.6X5	T42.6X6
tincture	T42.6X1	T42.6X2	T42.6X3	T42.6X4	T42.6X5	T42.6X6
Valethamate bromide	T44.3X1	T44.3X2	T44.3X3	T44.3X4	T44.3X5	T44.3X6
Valisone	T49.0X1	T49.0X2	T49.0X3	T49.0X4	T49.0X5	T49.0X6
Valium	T42.4X1	T42.4X2	T42.4X3	T42.4X4	T42.4X5	T42.4X6
Valmid	T42.6X1	T42.6X2	T42.6X3	T42.6X4	T42.6X5	T42.6X6
Valnoctamide	T42.6X1	T42.6X2	T42.6X3	T42.6X4	T42.6X5	T42.6X6
Valproate (sodium)	T42.6X1	T42.6X2	T42.6X3	T42.6X4	T42.6X5	T42.6X6
Valproic acid	T42.6X1	T42.6X2	T42.6X3	T42.6X4	T42.6X5	T42.6X6
Valpromide	T42.6X1	T42.6X2	T42.6X3	T42.6X4	T42.6X5	T42.6X6
Vanadium	T56.891	T56.892	T56.893	T56.894	—	—
Vancomycin	T36.8X1	T36.8X2	T36.8X3	T36.8X4	T36.8X5	T36.8X6
Vapor—see also Gas	T59.91	T59.92	T59.93	T59.94	—	—
kiln (carbon monoxide)	T58.8X1	T58.8X2	T58.8X3	T58.8X4	—	—
lead—see lead						
specified source NEC	T59.891	T59.892	T59.893	T59.894	—	—
Vardenafil	T46.7X1	T46.7X2	T46.7X3	T46.7X4	T46.7X5	T46.7X6
Varicose reduction drug	T46.8X1	T46.8X2	T46.8X3	T46.8X4	T46.8X5	T46.8X6
Varnish	T65.4X1	T65.4X2	T65.4X3	T65.4X4	—	—
cleaner	T52.91	T52.92	T52.93	T52.94	—	—
Vaseline	T49.3X1	T49.3X2	T49.3X3	T49.3X4	T49.3X5	T49.3X6
Vasodilan	T46.7X1	T46.7X2	T46.7X3	T46.7X4	T46.7X5	T46.7X6
Vasodilator						
coronary NEC	T46.3X1	T46.3X2	T46.3X3	T46.3X4	T46.3X5	T46.3X6
peripheral NEC	T46.7X1	T46.7X2	T46.7X3	T46.7X4	T46.7X5	T46.7X6
Vasopressin	T38.891	T38.892	T38.893	T38.894	T38.895	T38.896
Vasopressor drugs	T38.891	T38.892	T38.893	T38.894	T38.895	T38.896
Vecuronium bromide	T48.1X1	T48.1X2	T48.1X3	T48.1X4	T48.1X5	T48.1X6
Vegetable extract, astringent	T49.2X1	T49.2X2	T49.2X3	T49.2X4	T49.2X5	T49.2X6
Venlafaxine	T43.211	T43.212	T43.213	T43.214	T43.215	T43.216
Venom, venomous (bite) (sting)	T63.91	T63.92	T63.93	T63.94	—	—
amphibian NEC	T63.831	T63.832	T63.833	T63.834	—	—
animal NEC	T63.891	T63.892	T63.893	T63.894	—	—
ant	T63.421	T63.422	T63.423	T63.424	—	—
arthropod NEC	T63.481	T63.482	T63.483	T63.484	—	—
bee	T63.441	T63.442	T63.443	T63.444	—	—
centipede	T63.411	T63.412	T63.413	T63.414	—	—
fish	T63.591	T63.592	T63.593	T63.594	—	—
frog	T63.811	T63.812	T63.813	T63.814	—	—

Substance	Poisoning, Accidental (unintentional)	Poisoning, Intentional self-harm	Poisoning, Assault	Poisoning, Undetermined	Adverse effect	Underdosing
Venom, venomous — *Continued*						
hornet	T63.451	T63.452	T63.453	T63.454	—	—
insect NEC	T63.481	T63.482	T63.483	T63.484	—	—
lizard	T63.121	T63.122	T63.123	T63.124	—	—
marine						
animals	T63.691	T63.692	T63.693	T63.694	—	—
bluebottle	T63.611	T63.612	T63.613	T63.614	—	—
jellyfish NEC	T63.621	T63.622	T63.623	T63.624	—	—
Portuguese Man-o-war	T63.611	T63.612	T63.613	T63.614	—	—
sea anemone	T63.631	T63.632	T63.633	T63.634	—	—
specified NEC	T63.691	T63.692	T63.693	T63.694	—	—
fish	T63.591	T63.592	T63.593	T63.594	—	—
plants	T63.711	T63.712	T63.713	T63.714	—	—
sting ray	T63.511	T63.512	T63.513	T63.514	—	—
millipede (tropical)	T63.411	T63.412	T63.413	T63.414	—	—
plant NEC	T63.791	T63.792	T63.793	T63.794	—	—
marine	T63.711	T63.712	T63.713	T63.714	—	—
reptile	T63.191	T63.192	T63.193	T63.194	—	—
gila monster	T63.111	T63.112	T63.113	T63.114	—	—
lizard NEC	T63.121	T63.122	T63.123	T63.124	—	—
scorpion	T63.2X1	T63.2X2	T63.2X3	T63.2X4	—	—
snake	T63.001	T63.002	T63.003	T63.004	—	—
African NEC	T63.081	T63.082	T63.083	T63.084	—	—
American (North) (South) NEC	T63.061	T63.062	T63.063	T63.064	—	—
Asian	T63.081	T63.082	T63.083	T63.084	—	—
Australian	T63.071	T63.072	T63.073	T63.074	—	—
cobra	T63.041	T63.042	T63.043	T63.044	—	—
coral snake	T63.021	T63.022	T63.023	T63.024	—	—
rattlesnake	T63.011	T63.012	T63.013	T63.014	—	—
specified NEC	T63.091	T63.092	T63.093	T63.094	—	—
taipan	T63.031	T63.032	T63.033	T63.034	—	—
specified NEC	T63.891	T63.892	T63.893	T63.894	—	—
spider	T63.301	T63.302	T63.303	T63.304	—	—
black widow	T63.311	T63.312	T63.313	T63.314	—	—
brown recluse	T63.331	T63.332	T63.333	T63.334	—	—
specified NEC	T63.391	T63.392	T63.393	T63.394	—	—
tarantula	T63.321	T63.322	T63.323	T63.324	—	—
sting ray	T63.511	T63.512	T63.513	T63.514	—	—
toad	T63.821	T63.822	T63.823	T63.824	—	—
wasp	T63.461	T63.462	T63.463	T63.464	—	—
Venous sclerosing drug NEC	T46.8X1	T46.8X2	T46.8X3	T46.8X4	T46.8X5	T46.8X6
Ventolin—see Albuterol						
Veramon	T42.3X1	T42.3X2	T42.3X3	T42.3X4	T42.3X5	T42.3X6
Verapamil	T46.1X1	T46.1X2	T46.1X3	T46.1X4	T46.1X5	T46.1X6
Veratrine	T46.5X1	T46.5X2	T46.5X3	T46.5X4	T46.5X5	T46.5X6
Veratrum						
album	T62.2X1	T62.2X2	T62.2X3	T62.2X4	—	—
alkaloids	T46.5X1	T46.5X2	T46.5X3	T46.5X4	T46.5X5	T46.5X6

Substance	Poisoning, Accidental (unintentional)	Poisoning, Intentional self-harm	Poisoning, Assault	Poisoning, Undetermined	Adverse effect	Underdosing
Veratrum — *Continued*						
viride	T62.2X1	T62.2X2	T62.2X3	T62.2X4	—	—
Verdigris	T60.3X1	T60.3X2	T60.3X3	T60.3X4	—	—
Veronal	T42.3X1	T42.3X2	T42.3X3	T42.3X4	T42.3X5	T42.3X6
Veroxil	T37.4X1	T37.4X2	T37.4X3	T37.4X4	T37.4X5	T37.4X6
Versenate	T50.6X1	T50.6X2	T50.6X3	T50.6X4	T50.6X5	T50.6X6
Versidyne	T39.8X1	T39.8X2	T39.8X3	T39.8X4	T39.8X5	T39.8X6
Vetrabutine	T48.0X1	T48.0X2	T48.0X3	T48.0X4	T48.0X5	T48.0X6
Vidarabine	T37.5X1	T37.5X2	T37.5X3	T37.5X4	T37.5X5	T37.5X6
Vienna						
green	T57.0X1	T57.0X2	T57.0X3	T57.0X4		
insecticide	T60.2X1	T60.2X2	T60.2X3	T60.2X4	—	—
red	T57.0X1	T57.0X2	T57.0X3	T57.0X4	—	—
pharmaceutical dye	T50.991	T50.992	T50.993	T50.994	T50.995	T50.996
Vigabatrin	T42.6X1	T42.6X2	T42.6X3	T42.6X4	T42.6X5	T42.6X6
Viloxazine	T43.291	T43.292	T43.293	T43.294	T43.295	T43.296
Viminol	T39.8X1	T39.8X2	T39.8X3	T39.8X4	T39.8X5	T39.8X6
Vinbarbital, vinbarbitone	T42.3X1	T42.3X2	T42.3X3	T42.3X4	T42.3X5	T42.3X6
Vinblastine	T45.1X1	T45.1X2	T45.1X3	T45.1X4	T45.1X5	T45.1X6
Vinburnine	T46.7X1	T46.7X2	T46.7X3	T46.7X4	T46.7X5	T46.7X6
Vincamine	T45.1X1	T45.1X2	T45.1X3	T45.1X4	T45.1X5	T45.1X6
Vincristine	T45.1X1	T45.1X2	T45.1X3	T45.1X4	T45.1X5	T45.1X6
Vindesine	T45.1X1	T45.1X2	T45.1X3	T45.1X4	T45.1X5	T45.1X6
Vinesthene, vinethene	T41.0X1	T41.0X2	T41.0X3	T41.0X4	T41.0X5	T41.0X6
Vinorelbine tartrate	T45.1X1	T45.1X2	T45.1X3	T45.1X4	T45.1X5	T45.1X6
Vinpocetine	T46.7X1	T46.7X2	T46.7X3	T46.7X4	T46.7X5	T46.7X6
Vinyl						
acetate	T65.891	T65.892	T65.893	T65.894	—	—
bital	T42.3X1	T42.3X2	T42.3X3	T42.3X4	T42.3X5	T42.3X6
bromide	T65.891	T65.892	T65.893	T65.894	—	—
chloride	T59.891	T59.892	T59.893	T59.894	—	—
ether	T41.0X1	T41.0X2	T41.0X3	T41.0X4	T41.0X5	T41.0X6
Vinylbital	T42.3X1	T42.3X2	T42.3X3	T42.3X4	T42.3X5	T42.3X6
Vinylidene chloride	T65.891	T65.892	T65.893	T65.894	—	—
Vioform	T37.8X1	T37.8X2	T37.8X3	T37.8X4	T37.8X5	T37.8X6
topical	T49.0X1	T49.0X2	T49.0X3	T49.0X4	T49.0X5	T49.0X6
Viomycin	T36.8X1	T36.8X2	T36.8X3	T36.8X4	T36.8X5	T36.8X6
Viosterol	T45.2X1	T45.2X2	T45.2X3	T45.2X4	T45.2X5	T45.2X6
Viper (venom)	T63.091	T63.092	T63.093	T63.094	—	—
Viprynium	T37.4X1	T37.4X2	T37.4X3	T37.4X4	T37.4X5	T37.4X6
Viquidil	T46.7X1	T46.7X2	T46.7X3	T46.7X4	T46.7X5	T46.7X6
Viral vaccine NEC	T50.B91	T50.B92	T50.B93	T50.B94	T50.B95	T50.B96
Virginiamycin	T36.8X1	T36.8X2	T36.8X3	T36.8X4	T36.8X5	T36.8X6
Virugon	T37.5X1	T37.5X2	T37.5X3	T37.5X4	T37.5X5	T37.5X6
Viscous agent	T50.901	T50.902	T50.903	T50.904	T50.905	T50.906
Visine	T49.5X1	T49.5X2	T49.5X3	T49.5X4	T49.5X5	T49.5X6
Visnadine	T46.3X1	T46.3X2	T46.3X3	T46.3X4	T46.3X5	T46.3X6
Vitamin NEC	T45.2X1	T45.2X2	T45.2X3	T45.2X4	T45.2X5	T45.2X6
A	T45.2X1	T45.2X2	T45.2X3	T45.2X4	T45.2X5	T45.2X6
B NEC	T45.2X1	T45.2X2	T45.2X3	T45.2X4	T45.2X5	T45.2X6

Substance	Poisoning, Accidental (unintentional)	Poisoning, Intentional self-harm	Poisoning, Assault	Poisoning, Undetermined	Adverse effect	Underdosing
Vitamin NEC — *Continued*						
nicotinic acid	T46.7X1	T46.7X2	T46.7X3	T46.7X4	T46.7X5	T46.7X6
B1	T45.2X1	T45.2X2	T45.2X3	T45.2X4	T45.2X5	T45.2X6
B2	T45.2X1	T45.2X2	T45.2X3	T45.2X4	T45.2X5	T45.2X6
B6	T45.2X1	T45.2X2	T45.2X3	T45.2X4	T45.2X5	T45.2X6
B12	T45.2X1	T45.2X2	T45.2X3	T45.2X4	T45.2X5	T45.2X6
B15	T45.2X1	T45.2X2	T45.2X3	T45.2X4	T45.2X5	T45.2X6
C	T45.2X1	T45.2X2	T45.2X3	T45.2X4	T45.2X5	T45.2X6
D	T45.2X1	T45.2X2	T45.2X3	T45.2X4	T45.2X5	T45.2X6
D2	T45.2X1	T45.2X2	T45.2X3	T45.2X4	T45.2X5	T45.2X6
D3	T45.2X1	T45.2X2	T45.2X3	T45.2X4	T45.2X5	T45.2X6
E	T45.2X1	T45.2X2	T45.2X3	T45.2X4	T45.2X5	T45.2X6
E acetate	T45.2X1	T45.2X2	T45.2X3	T45.2X4	T45.2X5	T45.2X6
hematopoietic	T45.8X1	T45.8X2	T45.8X3	T45.8X4	T45.8X5	T45.8X6
K NEC	T45.7X1	T45.7X2	T45.7X3	T45.7X4	T45.7X5	T45.7X6
K1	T45.7X1	T45.7X2	T45.7X3	T45.7X4	T45.7X5	T45.7X6
K2	T45.7X1	T45.7X2	T45.7X3	T45.7X4	T45.7X5	T45.7X6
PP	T45.2X1	T45.2X2	T45.2X3	T45.2X4	T45.2X5	T45.2X6
ulceroprotectant	T47.1X1	T47.1X2	T47.1X3	T47.1X4	T47.1X5	T47.1X6
Vleminckx's solution	T49.4X1	T49.4X2	T49.4X3	T49.4X4	T49.4X5	T49.4X6
Voltaren—see Diclofenac sodium						
W						
Warfarin	T45.511	T45.512	T45.513	T45.514	T45.515	T45.516
rodenticide	T60.4X1	T60.4X2	T60.4X3	T60.4X4	—	—
sodium	T45.511	T45.512	T45.513	T45.514	T45.515	T45.516
Wasp (sting)	T63.461	T63.462	T63.463	T63.464		
Water						
balance drug	T50.3X1	T50.3X2	T50.3X3	T50.3X4	T50.3X5	T50.3X6
distilled	T50.3X1	T50.3X2	T50.3X3	T50.3X4	T50.3X5	T50.3X6
gas—see Gas, water						
incomplete combustion of—see Carbon, monoxide, fuel, utility						
hemlock	T62.2X1	T62.2X2	T62.2X3	T62.2X4	—	—
moccasin (venom)	T63.061	T63.062	T63.063	T63.064		
purified	T50.3X1	T50.3X2	T50.3X3	T50.3X4	T50.3X5	T50.3X6
Wax (paraffin) (petroleum)	T52.0X1	T52.0X2	T52.0X3	T52.0X4		
automobile	T65.891	T65.892	T65.893	T65.894	—	—
floor	T52.0X1	T52.0X2	T52.0X3	T52.0X4		
Weed killers NEC	T60.3X1	T60.3X2	T60.3X3	T60.3X4	—	—
Welldorm	T42.6X1	T42.6X2	T42.6X3	T42.6X4	T42.6X5	T42.6X6
White						
arsenic	T57.0X1	T57.0X2	T57.0X3	T57.0X4	—	—
hellebore	T62.2X1	T62.2X2	T62.2X3	T62.2X4		
lotion (keratolytic)	T49.4X1	T49.4X2	T49.4X3	T49.4X4	T49.4X5	T49.4X6
spirit	T52.0X1	T52.0X2	T52.0X3	T52.0X4		
Whitewash	T65.891	T65.892	T65.893	T65.894	—	—
Whole blood (human)	T45.8X1	T45.8X2	T45.8X3	T45.8X4	T45.8X5	T45.8X6

Substance	Poisoning, Accidental (unintentional)	Poisoning, Intentional self-harm	Poisoning, Assault	Poisoning, Undetermined	Adverse effect	Underdosing
Wild						
black cherry	T62.2X1	T62.2X2	T62.2X3	T62.2X4	—	—
poisonous plants NEC	T62.2X1	T62.2X2	T62.2X3	T62.2X4	—	—
Window cleaning fluid	T65.891	T65.892	T65.893	T65.894	—	—
Wintergreen (oil)	T49.3X1	T49.3X2	T49.3X3	T49.3X4	T49.3X5	T49.3X6
Wisterine	T62.2X1	T62.2X2	T62.2X3	T62.2X4	—	—
Witch hazel	T49.2X1	T49.2X2	T49.2X3	T49.2X4	T49.2X5	T49.2X6
Wood alcohol or spirit	T51.1X1	T51.1X2	T51.1X3	T51.1X4	—	—
Wool fat (hydrous)	T49.3X1	T49.3X2	T49.3X3	T49.3X4	T49.3X5	T49.3X6
Woorali	T48.1X1	T48.1X2	T48.1X3	T48.1X4	T48.1X5	T48.1X6
Wormseed, American	T37.4X1	T37.4X2	T37.4X3	T37.4X4	T37.4X5	T37.4X6
X						
Xamoterol	T44.5X1	T44.5X2	T44.5X3	T44.5X4	T44.5X5	T44.5X6
Xanthine diuretics	T50.2X1	T50.2X2	T50.2X3	T50.2X4	T50.2X5	T50.2X6
Xanthinol nicotinate	T46.7X1	T46.7X2	T46.7X3	T46.7X4	T46.7X5	T46.7X6
Xanthotoxin	T49.3X1	T49.3X2	T49.3X3	T49.3X4	T49.3X5	T49.3X6
Xantinol nicotinate	T46.7X1	T46.7X2	T46.7X3	T46.7X4	T46.7X5	T46.7X6
Xantocillin	T36.0X1	T36.0X2	T36.0X3	T36.0X4	T36.0X5	T36.0X6
Xenon (127Xe) (133Xe)	T50.8X1	T50.8X2	T50.8X3	T50.8X4	T50.8X5	T50.8X6
Xenysalate	T49.4X1	T49.4X2	T49.4X3	T49.4X4	T49.4X5	T49.4X6
Xibornol	T37.8X1	T37.8X2	T37.8X3	T37.8X4	T37.8X5	T37.8X6
Xigris	T45.511	T45.512	T45.513	T45.514	T45.515	T45.516
Xipamide	T50.2X1	T50.2X2	T50.2X3	T50.2X4	T50.2X5	T50.2X6
Xylene (vapor)	T52.2X1	T52.2X2	T52.2X3	T52.2X4	—	—
Xylocaine (infiltration) (topical)	T41.3X1	T41.3X2	T41.3X3	T41.3X4	T41.3X5	T41.3X6
nerve block (peripheral) (plexus)	T41.3X1	T41.3X2	T41.3X3	T41.3X4	T41.3X5	T41.3X6
spinal	T41.3X1	T41.3X2	T41.3X3	T41.3X4	T41.3X5	T41.3X6
Xylol (vapor)	T52.2X1	T52.2X2	T52.2X3	T52.2X4	—	—
Xylometazoline	T48.5X1	T48.5X2	T48.5X3	T48.5X4	T48.5X5	T48.5X6
Y						
Yeast	T45.2X1	T45.2X2	T45.2X3	T45.2X4	T45.2X5	T45.2X6
dried	T45.2X1	T45.2X2	T45.2X3	T45.2X4	T45.2X5	T45.2X6
Yellow						
fever vaccine	T50.B91	T50.B92	T50.B93	T50.B94	T50.B95	T50.B96
jasmine	T62.2X1	T62.2X2	T62.2X3	T62.2X4	—	—
phenolphthalein	T47.2X1	T47.2X2	T47.2X3	T47.2X4	T47.2X5	T47.2X6
Yew	T62.2X1	T62.2X2	T62.2X3	T62.2X4	—	—
Yohimbic acid	T40.991	T40.992	T40.993	T40.994	T40.995	T40.996
Z						
Zactane	T39.8X1	T39.8X2	T39.8X3	T39.8X4	T39.8X5	T39.8X6

Substance	Poisoning, Accidental (unintentional)	Poisoning, Intentional self-harm	Poisoning, Assault	Poisoning, Undetermined	Adverse effect	Underdosing
Zalcitabine	T37.5X1	T37.5X2	T37.5X3	T37.5X4	T37.5X5	T37.5X6
Zaroxolyn	T50.2X1	T50.2X2	T50.2X3	T50.2X4	T50.2X5	T50.2X6
Zephiran (topical)	T49.0X1	T49.0X2	T49.0X3	T49.0X4	T49.0X5	T49.0X6
ophthalmic preparation	T49.5X1	T49.5X2	T49.5X3	T49.5X4	T49.5X5	T49.5X6
Zeranol	T38.7X1	T38.7X2	T38.7X3	T38.7X4	T38.7X5	T38.7X6
Zerone	T51.1X1	T51.1X2	T51.1X3	T51.1X4	—	—
Zidovudine	T37.5X1	T37.5X2	T37.5X3	T37.5X4	T37.5X5	T37.5X6
Zimeldine	T43.221	T43.222	T43.223	T43.224	T43.225	T43.226
Zinc (compounds) (fumes) (vapor) NEC	T56.5X1	T56.5X2	T56.5X3	T56.5X4	—	—
anti-infectives	T49.0X1	T49.0X2	T49.0X3	T49.0X4	T49.0X5	T49.0X6
antivaricose	T46.8X1	T46.8X2	T46.8X3	T46.8X4	T46.8X5	T46.8X6
bacitracin	T49.0X1	T49.0X2	T49.0X3	T49.0X4	T49.0X5	T49.0X6
chloride (mouthwash)	T49.6X1	T49.6X2	T49.6X3	T49.6X4	T49.6X5	T49.6X6
chromate	T56.5X1	T56.5X2	T56.5X3	T56.5X4	—	—
gelatin	T49.3X1	T49.3X2	T49.3X3	T49.3X4	T49.3X5	T49.3X6
oxide	T49.3X1	T49.3X2	T49.3X3	T49.3X4	T49.3X5	T49.3X6
plaster	T49.3X1	T49.3X2	T49.3X3	T49.3X4	T49.3X5	T49.3X6
peroxide	T49.0X1	T49.0X2	T49.0X3	T49.0X4	T49.0X5	T49.0X6
pesticides	T56.5X1	T56.5X2	T56.5X3	T56.5X4	—	—
phosphide	T60.4X1	T60.4X2	T60.4X3	T60.4X4	—	—
pyrithionate	T49.4X1	T49.4X2	T49.4X3	T49.4X4	T49.4X5	T49.4X6
stearate	T49.3X1	T49.3X2	T49.3X3	T49.3X4	T49.3X5	T49.3X6
sulfate	T49.5X1	T49.5X2	T49.5X3	T49.5X4	T49.5X5	T49.5X6
ENT agent	T49.6X1	T49.6X2	T49.6X3	T49.6X4	T49.6X5	T49.6X6
ophthalmic solution	T49.5X1	T49.5X2	T49.5X3	T49.5X4	T49.5X5	T49.5X6
topical NEC	T49.0X1	T49.0X2	T49.0X3	T49.0X4	T49.0X5	T49.0X6
undecylenate	T49.0X1	T49.0X2	T49.0X3	T49.0X4	T49.0X5	T49.0X6
Zineb	T60.0X1	T60.0X2	T60.0X3	T60.0X4	—	—
Zinostatin	T45.1X1	T45.1X2	T45.1X3	T45.1X4	T45.1X5	T45.1X6
Zipeprol	T48.3X1	T48.3X2	T48.3X3	T48.3X4	T48.3X5	T48.3X6
Zofenopril	T46.4X1	T46.4X2	T46.4X3	T46.4X4	T46.4X5	T46.4X6
Zolpidem	T42.6X1	T42.6X2	T42.6X3	T42.6X4	T42.6X5	T42.6X6
Zomepirac	T39.391	T39.392	T39.393	T39.394	T39.395	T39.396
Zopiclone	T42.6X1	T42.6X2	T42.6X3	T42.6X4	T42.6X5	T42.6X6
Zorubicin	T45.1X1	T45.1X2	T45.1X3	T45.1X4	T45.1X5	T45.1X6
Zotepine	T43.591	T43.592	T43.593	T43.594	T43.595	T43.596
Zovant	T45.511	T45.512	T45.513	T45.514	T45.515	T45.516
Zoxazolamine	T42.8X1	T42.8X2	T42.8X3	T42.8X4	T42.8X5	T42.8X6
Zuclopenthixol	T43.4X1	T43.4X2	T43.4X3	T43.4X4	T43.4X5	T43.4X6
Zygadenus (venenosus)	T62.2X1	T62.2X2	T62.2X3	T62.2X4	—	—
Zyprexa	T43.591	T43.592	T43.593	T43.594	T43.595	T43.596

External Cause of Injuries Index

A

Abandonment (causing exposure to weather conditions) (with intent to injure or kill) NEC X58

Abuse (adult) (child) (mental) (physical) (sexual) X58

Accident (to) X58
  aircraft (in transit) (powered) —*see also* Accident, transport, aircraft
    due to, caused by cataclysm — *see* Forces of nature, by type
  animal-drawn vehicle —*see* Accident, transport, animal-drawn vehicle occupant
  animal-rider —*see* Accident, transport, animal-rider
  automobile —*see* Accident, transport, car occupant
  bare foot water skiier V94.4
  boat, boating —*see also* Accident, watercraft
    striking swimmer
      powered V94.11
      unpowered V94.12
  bus —*see* Accident, transport, bus occupant
  cable car, not on rails V98.0
    on rails —*see* Accident, transport, streetcar occupant
  car —*see* Accident, transport, car occupant
  caused by, due to
    animal NEC W64
    chain hoist W24.0
    cold (excessive) —*see* Exposure, cold
    corrosive liquid, substance —*see* Table of Drugs and Chemicals
    cutting or piercing instrument —*see* Contact, with, by type of instrument
    drive belt W24.0
    electric
      current —*see* Exposure, electric current
      motor —*see also* Contact, with, by type of machine W31.3
        current (of) W86.8
    environmental factor NEC X58
    explosive material —*see* Explosion
    fire, flames —*see* Exposure, fire
    firearm missile —*see* Discharge, firearm by type
    heat (excessive) —*see* Heat
    hot —*see* Contact, with, hot
    ignition —*see* Ignition
    lifting device W24.0
    lightning —*see* subcategory T75.0
      causing fire —*see* Exposure, fire
    machine, machinery —*see* Contact, with, by type of machine
    natural factor NEC X58
    pulley (block) W24.0
    radiation —*see* Radiation
    steam X13.1
      inhalation X13.0
      pipe X16

Accident (continued)
  caused by, due to (continued)
    thunderbolt —*see* subcategory T75.0
      causing fire —*see* Exposure, fire
    transmission device W24.1
  coach —*see* Accident, transport, bus occupant
  coal car —*see* Accident, transport, industrial vehicle occupant
  diving —*see also* Fall, into, water with
    drowning or submersion —*see* Drowning
  forklift —*see* Accident, transport, industrial vehicle occupant
  heavy transport vehicle NOS — *see* Accident, transport, truck occupant
  ice yacht V98.2
  in
    medical, surgical procedure
      as, or due to misadventure —*see* Misadventure
      causing an abnormal reaction or later complication without mention of misadventure —*see also* Complication of or following, by type of procedure Y84.9
  land yacht V98.1
  late effect of —*see* W00-X58 with 7th character S
  logging car —*see* Accident, transport, industrial vehicle occupant
  machine, machinery —*see also* Contact, with, by type of machine
    on board watercraft V93.69
      explosion —*see* Explosion, in, watercraft
      fire —*see* Burn, on board watercraft
      powered craft V93.63
        ferry boat V93.61
        fishing boat V93.62
        jetskis V93.63
        liner V93.61
        merchant ship V93.60
        passenger ship V93.61
        sailboat V93.64
  mine tram —*see* Accident, transport, industrial vehicle occupant
  mobility scooter (motorized) —*see* Accident, transport, pedestrian, conveyance, specified type NEC
  motor scooter —*see* Accident, transport, motorcycle
  motor vehicle NOS (traffic) —*see also* Accident, transport V89.2
    nontraffic V89.0
    three-wheeled NOS —*see* Accident, transport, three-wheeled motor vehicle occupant
  motorcycle NOS —*see* Accident, transport, motorcycle
  nonmotor vehicle NOS (nontraffic) —*see also* Accident, transport V89.1
    traffic NOS V89.3
  nontraffic (victim's mode of transport NOS) V88.9

Accident (continued)
  nontraffic (continued)
    collision (between) V88.7
      bus and truck V88.5
      car and:
        bus V88.3
        pickup V88.2
        three-wheeled motor vehicle V88.0
        train V88.6
        truck V88.4
        two-wheeled motor vehicle V88.0
        van V88.2
      specified vehicle NEC and:
        three-wheeled motor vehicle V88.1
        two-wheeled motor vehicle V88.1
      known mode of transport —*see* Accident, transport, by type of vehicle
    noncollision V88.8
  on board watercraft V93.89
    powered craft V93.83
      ferry boat V93.81
      fishing boat V93.82
      jetskis V93.83
      liner V93.81
      merchant ship V93.80
      passenger ship V93.81
    unpowered craft V93.88
      canoe V93.85
      inflatable V93.86
        in tow
          recreational V94.31
          specified NEC V94.32
      kayak V93.85
      sailboat V93.84
      surf-board V93.88
      water skis V93.87
      windsurfer V93.88
  parachutist V97.29
    entangled in object V97.21
    injured on landing V97.22
  pedal cycle —*see* Accident, transport, pedal cyclist
  pedestrian (on foot)
    with
      another pedestrian W51
        with fall W03
          due to ice or snow W00.0
          on pedestrian conveyance NEC V00.09
      rider of
        hoverboard V00.038
        Segway V00.038
        standing
          electric scooter V00.031
          micro-mobility pedestrian conveyance NEC V00.038
        roller skater (in-line) V00.01
        skate boarder V00.02
      transport vehicle —*see* Accident, transport, pedestrian, conveyance
  pick-up truck or van —*see* Accident, transport, pickup truck occupant
  quarry truck —*see* Accident, transport, industrial vehicle occupant

Accident (continued)
  railway vehicle (any) (in motion) — *see* Accident, transport, railway vehicle occupant
    due to cataclysm —*see* Forces of nature, by type
  scooter (non-motorized) —*see* Accident, transport, pedestrian, conveyance, scooter
  sequelae of —*see* W00-X58 with 7th character S
  skateboard —*see* Accident, transport, pedestrian, conveyance, skateboard
  ski (ing) —*see* Accident, transport, pedestrian, conveyance
    lift V98.3
  specified cause NEC X58
  streetcar —*see* Accident, transport, streetcar occupant
  traffic (victim's mode of transport NOS) V87.9
    collision (between) V87.7
      bus and truck V87.5
      car and:
        bus V87.3
        pickup V87.2
        three-wheeled motor vehicle V87.0
        train V87.6
        truck V87.4
        two-wheeled motor vehicle V87.0
        van V87.2
      specified vehicle NEC V86.39
        and
          three-wheeled motor vehicle V87.1
          two-wheeled motor vehicle V87.1
        driver V86.09
        person on outside V86.29
        passenger V86.19
        while boarding or alighting V86.49
      known mode of transport —*see* Accident, transport, by type of vehicle
    noncollision V87.8
  transport (involving injury to) V99
    18 wheeler —*see* Accident, transport, truck occupant
    agricultural vehicle occupant (nontraffic) V84.9
      driver V84.5
      hanger-on V84.7
      passenger V84.6
      traffic V84.3
        driver V84.0
        hanger-on V84.2
        passenger V84.1
      while boarding or alighting V84.4
    aircraft NEC V97.89
      military NEC V97.818
        with civilian aircraft V97.810
        civilian injured by V97.811
      occupant injured (in)
        nonpowered craft accident V96.9
          balloon V96.00
            collision V96.03
            crash V96.01
            explosion V96.05

Accident (continued)
transport (continued)
  aircraft NEC (continued)
    occupant injured (continued)
      nonpowered craft accident (continued)
        balloon (continued)
          fire V96.04
          forced landing V96.02
          specified type NEC V96.09
        glider V96.20
          collision V96.23
          crash V96.21
          explosion V96.25
          fire V96.24
          forced landing V96.22
          specified type NEC V96.29
        hang glider V96.10
          collision V96.13
          crash V96.11
          explosion V96.15
          fire V96.14
          forced landing V96.12
          specified type NEC V96.19
        specified craft NEC V96.8
      powered craft accident V95.9
        fixed wing NEC
          commercial V95.30
            collision V95.33
            crash V95.31
            explosion V95.35
            fire V95.34
            forced landing V95.32
            specified type NEC V95.39
          private V95.20
            collision V95.23
            crash V95.21
            explosion V95.25
            fire V95.24
            forced landing V95.22
            specified type NEC V95.29
        glider V95.10
          collision V95.13
          crash V95.11
          explosion V95.15
          fire V95.14
          forced landing V95.12
          specified type NEC V95.19
        helicopter V95.00
          collision V95.03
          crash V95.01
          explosion V95.05
          fire V95.04
          forced landing V95.02
          specified type NEC V95.09
        spacecraft V95.40
          collision V95.43
          crash V95.41
          explosion V95.45
          fire V95.44
          forced landing V95.42
          specified type NEC V95.49
        specified craft NEC V95.8
        ultralight V95.10
          collision V95.13
          crash V95.11
          explosion V95.15
          fire V95.14
          forced landing V95.12
          specified type NEC V95.19

Accident (continued)
transport (continued)
  aircraft NEC (continued)
    occupant injured (continued)
      specified accident NEC V97.0
      while boarding or alighting V97.1
      person (injured by)
        falling from, in or on aircraft V97.0
        machinery on aircraft V97.89
        on ground with aircraft involvement V97.39
        rotating propeller V97.32
        struck by object falling from aircraft V97.31
        sucked into aircraft jet V97.33
        while boarding or alighting aircraft V97.1
  airport (battery-powered) passenger vehicle —see Accident, transport, industrial vehicle occupant
  all-terrain vehicle occupant (nontraffic) V86.95
    driver V86.55
    dune buggy —see Accident, transport, dune buggy occupant
    hanger-on V86.75
    passenger V86.65
    snowmobile —see Accident, transport, snowmobile occupant
    specified type NEC V86.99
      driver V86.59
      passenger V86.69
      person on outside V86.79
      traffic V86.35
        driver V86.05
        hanger-on V86.25
        passenger V86.15
      while boarding or alighting V86.45
  ambulance occupant (traffic) V86.31
    driver V86.01
    hanger-on V86.21
    nontraffic V86.91
      driver V86.51
      hanger-on V86.71
      passenger V86.61
    passenger V86.11
    while boarding or alighting V86.41
  animal-drawn vehicle occupant (in) V80.929
    collision (with)
      animal V80.12
        being ridden V80.711
      animal-drawn vehicle V80.721
      bus V80.42
      car V80.42
      fixed or stationary object V80.82
      military vehicle V80.920
      nonmotor vehicle V80.791
      pedal cycle V80.22
      pedestrian V80.12
      pickup V80.42
      railway train or vehicle V80.62
      specified motor vehicle NEC V80.52
      streetcar V80.731
      truck V80.42
      two- or three-wheeled motor vehicle V80.32
      van V80.42

Accident (continued)
transport (continued)
  animal-drawn vehicle occupant (continued)
    noncollision V80.02
    specified circumstance NEC V80.928
  animal-rider V80.919
    collision (with)
      animal V80.11
        being ridden V80.710
      animal-drawn vehicle V80.720
      bus V80.41
      car V80.41
      fixed or stationary object V80.81
      military vehicle V80.910
      nonmotor vehicle V80.790
      pedal cycle V80.21
      pedestrian V80.11
      pickup V80.41
      railway train or vehicle V80.61
      specified motor vehicle NEC V80.51
      streetcar V80.730
      truck V80.41
      two- or three-wheeled motor vehicle V80.31
      van V80.41
    noncollision V80.018
      specified as horse rider V80.010
    specified circumstance NEC V80.918
  armored car —see Accident, transport, truck occupant
  battery-powered truck (baggage) (mail) —see Accident, transport, industrial vehicle occupant
  bus occupant V79.9
    collision (with)
      animal (traffic) V70.9
        being ridden (traffic) V76.9
          nontraffic V76.3
          while boarding or alighting V76.4
        nontraffic V70.3
        while boarding or alighting V70.4
      animal-drawn vehicle (traffic) V76.9
        nontraffic V76.3
        while boarding or alighting V76.4
      bus (traffic) V74.9
        nontraffic V74.3
        while boarding or alighting V74.4
      car (traffic) V73.9
        nontraffic V73.3
        while boarding or alighting V73.4
      motor vehicle NOS (traffic) V79.60
        nontraffic V79.20
        specified type NEC (traffic) V79.69
          nontraffic V79.29
      pedal cycle (traffic) V71.9
        nontraffic V71.3
        while boarding or alighting V71.4
      pickup truck (traffic) V73.9
        nontraffic V73.3
        while boarding or alighting V73.4
      railway vehicle (traffic) V75.9
        nontraffic V75.3
        while boarding or alighting V75.4

Accident (continued)
transport (continued)
  bus occupant (continued)
    collision (continued)
      specified vehicle NEC (traffic) V76.9
        nontraffic V76.3
        while boarding or alighting V76.4
      stationary object (traffic) V77.9
        nontraffic V77.3
        while boarding or alighting V77.4
      streetcar (traffic) V76.9
        nontraffic V76.3
        while boarding or alighting V76.4
      three wheeled motor vehicle (traffic) V72.9
        nontraffic V72.3
        while boarding or alighting V72.4
      truck (traffic) V74.9
        nontraffic V74.3
        while boarding or alighting V74.4
      two wheeled motor vehicle (traffic) V72.9
        nontraffic V72.3
        while boarding or alighting V72.4
      van (traffic) V73.9
        nontraffic V73.3
        while boarding or alighting V73.4
    driver
      collision (with)
        animal (traffic) V70.5
          being ridden (traffic) V76.5
            nontraffic V76.0
          nontraffic V70.0
        animal-drawn vehicle (traffic) V76.5
          nontraffic V76.0
        bus (traffic) V74.5
          nontraffic V74.0
        car (traffic) V73.5
          nontraffic V73.0
        motor vehicle NOS (traffic) V79.40
          nontraffic V79.00
          specified type NEC (traffic) V79.49
            nontraffic V79.09
        pedal cycle (traffic) V71.5
          nontraffic V71.0
        pickup truck (traffic) V73.5
          nontraffic V73.0
        railway vehicle (traffic) V75.5
          nontraffic V75.0
        specified vehicle NEC (traffic) V76.5
          nontraffic V76.0
        stationary object (traffic) V77.5
          nontraffic V77.0
        streetcar (traffic) V76.5
          nontraffic V76.0
        three wheeled motor vehicle (traffic) V72.5
          nontraffic V72.0
        truck (traffic) V74.5
          nontraffic V74.0
        two wheeled motor vehicle (traffic) V72.5
          nontraffic V72.0

451

Accident (continued)
  transport (continued)
    bus occupant (continued)
      driver (continued)
        collision (continued)
          van (traffic) V73.5
            nontraffic V73.0
        noncollision accident
          (traffic) V78.5
          nontraffic V78.0
      noncollision accident (traffic)
        V78.9
        nontraffic V78.3
        while boarding or alighting
          V78.4
      nontraffic V79.3
      hanger-on
        collision (with)
          animal (traffic) V70.7
            being ridden (traffic)
              V76.7
              nontraffic V76.2
            nontraffic V70.2
          animal-drawn vehicle
            (traffic) V76.7
            nontraffic V76.2
          bus (traffic) V74.7
            nontraffic V74.2
          car (traffic) V73.7
            nontraffic V73.2
          pedal cycle (traffic) V71.7
            nontraffic V71.2
          pickup truck (traffic) V73.7
            nontraffic V73.2
          railway vehicle (traffic)
            V75.7
            nontraffic V75.2
          specified vehicle NEC
            (traffic) V76.7
            nontraffic V76.2
          stationary object (traffic)
            V77.7
            nontraffic V77.2
          streetcar (traffic) V76.7
            nontraffic V76.2
          three wheeled motor
            vehicle (traffic) V72.7
            nontraffic V72.2
          truck (traffic) V74.7
            nontraffic V74.2
          two wheeled motor
            vehicle (traffic) V72.7
            nontraffic V72.2
          van (traffic) V73.7
            nontraffic V73.2
        noncollision accident
          (traffic) V78.7
          nontraffic V78.2
      passenger
        collision (with)
          animal (traffic) V70.6
            being ridden (traffic)
              V76.6
              nontraffic V76.1
            nontraffic V70.1
          animal-drawn vehicle
            (traffic) V76.6
            nontraffic V76.1
          bus (traffic) V74.6
            nontraffic V74.1
          car (traffic) V73.6
            nontraffic V73.1
          motor vehicle NOS
            (traffic) V79.50
            nontraffic V79.10
            specified type NEC
              (traffic) V79.59
              nontraffic V79.19
          pedal cycle (traffic)
            V71.6
            nontraffic V71.1

Accident (continued)
  transport (continued)
    bus occupant (continued)
      passenger (continued)
        collision (continued)
          pickup truck (traffic) V73.6
            nontraffic V73.1
          railway vehicle (traffic)
            V75.6
            nontraffic V75.1
          specified vehicle NEC
            (traffic) V76.6
            nontraffic V76.1
          stationary object (traffic)
            V77.6
            nontraffic V77.1
          streetcar (traffic) V76.6
            nontraffic V76.1
          three wheeled motor
            vehicle (traffic) V72.6
            nontraffic V72.1
          truck (traffic) V74.6
            nontraffic V74.1
          two wheeled motor
            vehicle (traffic) V72.6
            nontraffic V72.1
          van (traffic) V73.6
            nontraffic V73.1
        noncollision accident
          (traffic) V78.6
          nontraffic V78.1
      specified type NEC V79.88
      military vehicle V79.81
    cable car, not on rails V98.0
    on rails —*see* Accident,
      transport, streetcar occupant
    car occupant V49.9
      ambulance occupant —*see*
        Accident, transport,
        ambulance occupant
      collision (with)
        animal (traffic) V40.9
          being ridden (traffic)
            V46.9
            nontraffic V46.3
            while boarding or
              alighting V46.4
          nontraffic V40.3
          while boarding or
            alighting V40.4
        animal-drawn vehicle
          (traffic) V46.9
          nontraffic V46.3
          while boarding or
            alighting V46.4
        bus (traffic) V44.9
          nontraffic V44.3
          while boarding or
            alighting V44.4
        car (traffic) V43.92
          nontraffic V43.32
          while boarding or
            alighting V43.42
        motor vehicle NOS (traffic)
          V49.60
          nontraffic V49.20
          specified type NEC
            (traffic) V49.69
            nontraffic V49.29
        pedal cycle (traffic)
          V41.9
          nontraffic V41.3
          while boarding or
            alighting V41.4
        pickup truck (traffic)
          V43.93
          nontraffic V43.33
          while boarding or
            alighting V43.43
        railway vehicle (traffic)
          V45.9

Accident (continued)
  transport (continued)
    car occupant (continued)
      collision (continued)
        railway vehicle
          (continued)
          nontraffic V45.3
          while boarding or
            alighting V45.4
        specified vehicle NEC
          (traffic) V46.9
          nontraffic V46.3
          while boarding or
            alighting V46.4
        sport utility vehicle (traffic)
          V43.91
          nontraffic V43.31
          while boarding or
            alighting V43.41
        stationary object (traffic)
          V47.9
          nontraffic V47.3
          while boarding or
            alighting V47.4
        streetcar (traffic) V46.9
          nontraffic V46.3
          while boarding or
            alighting V46.4
        three wheeled motor vehicle
          (traffic) V42.9
          nontraffic V42.3
          while boarding or
            alighting V42.4
        truck (traffic) V44.9
          nontraffic V44.3
          while boarding or
            alighting V44.4
        two wheeled motor vehicle
          (traffic) V42.9
          nontraffic V42.3
          while boarding or
            alighting V42.4
        van (traffic) V43.94
          nontraffic V43.34
          while boarding or
            alighting V43.44
      driver
        collision (with)
          animal (traffic) V40.5
            being ridden (traffic)
              V46.5
              nontraffic V46.0
            nontraffic V40.0
          animal-drawn vehicle
            (traffic) V46.5
            nontraffic V46.0
          bus (traffic) V44.5
            nontraffic V44.0
          car (traffic) V43.52
            nontraffic V43.02
          motor vehicle NOS
            (traffic) V49.40
            nontraffic V49.00
            specified type NEC
              (traffic) V49.49
              nontraffic
                V49.09
          pedal cycle (traffic)
            V41.5
            nontraffic V41.0
          pickup truck (traffic)
            V43.53
            nontraffic V43.03
          railway vehicle (traffic)
            V45.5
            nontraffic V45.0
          specified vehicle NEC
            (traffic) V46.5
            nontraffic V46.0
          sport utility vehicle
            (traffic) V43.51

Accident (continued)
  transport (continued)
    car occupant (continued)
      driver (continued)
        collision (continued)
          sport utility vehicle
            (continued)
            nontraffic V43.01
          stationary object (traffic)
            V47.5
            nontraffic V47.0
          streetcar (traffic) V46.5
            nontraffic V46.0
          three wheeled motor
            vehicle (traffic) V42.5
            nontraffic V42.0
          truck (traffic) V44.5
            nontraffic V44.0
          two wheeled motor
            vehicle (traffic) V42.5
            nontraffic V42.0
          van (traffic) V43.54
            nontraffic V43.04
        noncollision accident
          (traffic) V48.5
          nontraffic V48.0
          noncollision accident (traffic)
            V48.9
            nontraffic V48.3
            while boarding or alighting
              V48.4
      nontraffic V49.3
      hanger-on
        collision (with)
          animal (traffic) V40.7
            being ridden (traffic)
              V46.7
              nontraffic V46.2
            nontraffic V40.2
          animal-drawn vehicle
            (traffic) V46.7
            nontraffic V46.2
          bus (traffic) V44.7
            nontraffic V44.2
          car (traffic) V43.72
            nontraffic V43.22
          pedal cycle (traffic)
            V41.7
            nontraffic V41.2
          pickup truck (traffic)
            V43.73
            nontraffic V43.23
          railway vehicle (traffic)
            V45.7
            nontraffic V45.2
          specified vehicle NEC
            (traffic) V46.7
            nontraffic V46.2
          sport utility vehicle
            (traffic) V43.71
            nontraffic V43.21
          stationary object (traffic)
            V47.7
            nontraffic V47.2
          streetcar (traffic) V46.7
            nontraffic V46.2
          three wheeled motor
            vehicle (traffic)
            V42.7
            nontraffic V42.2
          truck (traffic) V44.7
            nontraffic V44.2
          two wheeled motor
            vehicle (traffic)
            V42.7
            nontraffic V42.2
          van (traffic) V43.74
            nontraffic V43.24
        noncollision accident
          (traffic) V48.7
          nontraffic V48.2

Accident *(continued)*
transport *(continued)*
  car occupant *(continued)*
    passenger
      collision (with)
        animal (traffic) V40.6
          being ridden (traffic)
            V46.6
            nontraffic V46.1
          nontraffic V40.1
        animal-drawn vehicle
          (traffic) V46.6
          nontraffic V46.1
        bus (traffic) V44.6
          nontraffic V44.1
        car (traffic) V43.62
          nontraffic V43.12
        motor vehicle NOS
          (traffic) V49.50
          nontraffic V49.10
          specified type NEC
            (traffic) V49.59
            nontraffic V49.19
        pedal cycle (traffic)
          V41.6
          nontraffic V41.1
        pickup truck (traffic)
          V43.63
          nontraffic V43.13
        railway vehicle (traffic)
          V45.6
          nontraffic V45.1
        specified vehicle NEC
          (traffic) V46.6
          nontraffic V46.1
        sport utility vehicle
          (traffic) V43.61
          nontraffic V43.11
        stationary object (traffic)
          V47.6
          nontraffic V47.1
        streetcar (traffic) V46.6
          nontraffic V46.1
        three wheeled motor
          vehicle (traffic) V42.6
          nontraffic V42.1
        truck (traffic) V44.6
          nontraffic V44.1
        two wheeled motor vehicle
          (traffic) V42.6
          nontraffic V42.1
        van (traffic) V43.64
          nontraffic V43.14
      noncollision accident
        (traffic) V48.6
        nontraffic V48.1
      specified type NEC V49.88
      military vehicle V49.81
  coal car —*see* Accident,
    transport, industrial vehicle
    occupant
  construction vehicle occupant
    (nontraffic) V85.9
    driver V85.5
    hanger-on V85.7
    passenger V85.6
    traffic V85.3
      driver V85.0
      hanger-on V85.2
      passenger V85.1
    while boarding or alighting
      V85.4
  dirt bike rider (nontraffic)
    V86.96
    driver V86.56
    hanger-on V86.76
    passenger V86.66
    traffic V86.36
      driver V86.06
      hanger-on V86.26
      passenger V86.16

Accident *(continued)*
transport *(continued)*
  dirt bike rider *(continued)*
    while boarding or alighting
      V86.46
  due to cataclysm —*see* Forces of
    nature, by type
  dune buggy occupant (nontraffic)
    V86.93
    driver V86.53
    hanger-on V86.73
    passenger V86.63
    traffic V86.33
      driver V86.03
      hanger-on V86.23
      passenger V86.13
    while boarding or alighting
      V86.43
  e-bicycle —*see* Accident,
    transport, electric (assisted)
    bicyclist
  e-bike —*see* Accident, transport,
    electric (assisted) bicyclist
  electric (assisted) bicyclist
    V29.91
    collision (with)
      animal (traffic) V20.91
        being ridden (traffic)
          V26.91
          nontraffic V26.21
          while boarding or
            alighting V26.31
        nontraffic V20.21
        while boarding or
          alighting V20.31
      animal-drawn vehicle
        (traffic) V26.91
        nontraffic V26.21
        while boarding or
          alighting V26.31
      bus (traffic) V24.91
        nontraffic V24.21
        while boarding or
          alighting V24.31
      car (traffic) V23.91
        nontraffic V23.21
        while boarding or
          alighting V23.31
      motor vehicle NOS (traffic)
        V29.601
        nontraffic V29.201
        specified type NEC
          (traffic) V29.691
          nontraffic V29.291
      pedal cycle (traffic) V21.91
        nontraffic V21.21
        while boarding or
          alighting V21.31
      pedestrian V20.91
        nontraffic V20.01
        while boarding or
          alighting V20.31
      pickup truck (traffic) V23.91
        nontraffic V23.21
        while boarding or
          alighting V23.31
      railway vehicle (traffic)
        V25.91
        nontraffic V25.21
        while boarding or
          alighting V25.31
      specified vehicle NEC
        (traffic) V26.91
        nontraffic V26.21
        while boarding or
          alighting V26.31
      stationary object (traffic)
        V27.91
        nontraffic V27.21
        while boarding or
          alighting V27.31

Accident *(continued)*
transport *(continued)*
  electric (assisted) bicyclist
    (continued)
    collision (with) *(continued)*
      streetcar (traffic) V26.91
        nontraffic V26.21
        while boarding or
          alighting V26.31
      three wheeled motor vehicle
        (traffic) V22.91
        nontraffic V22.21
        while boarding or
          alighting V22.31
      truck (traffic) V24.91
        nontraffic V24.21
        while boarding or
          alighting V24.31
      two wheeled motor vehicle
        (traffic) V22.91
        nontraffic V22.21
        while boarding or
          alighting V22.31
      van (traffic) V23.91
        nontraffic V23.21
        while boarding or
          alighting V23.31
    driver
      collision (with)
        animal (traffic) V20.41
          being ridden (traffic)
            V26.41
            nontraffic V26.01
          nontraffic V20.01
        animal-drawn vehicle
          (traffic) V26.41
          nontraffic V26.01
        bus (traffic) V24.41
          nontraffic V24.01
        car (traffic) V23.41
          nontraffic V23.01
        motor vehicle NOS
          (traffic) V29.401
          nontraffic V29.001
          specified type NEC
            (traffic) V29.491
            nontraffic V29.091
        pedal cycle (traffic)
          V21.41
          nontraffic V21.01
        pedestrian
          nontraffic V20.01
          traffic V20.41
        pickup truck (traffic)
          V23.41
          nontraffic V23.01
        railway vehicle (traffic)
          V25.41
          nontraffic V25.01
        specified vehicle NEC
          (traffic) V26.41
          nontraffic V26.01
        stationary object (traffic)
          V27.41
          nontraffic V27.01
        streetcar (traffic) V26.41
          nontraffic V26.01
        three wheeled motor
          vehicle (traffic) V22.41
          nontraffic V22.01
        truck (traffic) V24.41
          nontraffic V24.01
        two wheeled motor
          vehicle (traffic)
          V22.41
          nontraffic V22.01
        van (traffic) V23.41
          nontraffic V23.01
      noncollision accident
        (traffic) V28.41
        nontraffic V28.01

Accident *(continued)*
transport *(continued)*
  electric (assisted) bicyclist
    (continued)
    noncollision accident (traffic)
      V28.91
      nontraffic V28.21
      while boarding or alighting
        V28.31
    nontraffic V29.31
    passenger
      collision (with)
        animal (traffic) V20.51
          being ridden (traffic)
            V26.51
            nontraffic V26.11
          nontraffic V20.11
        animal-drawn vehicle
          (traffic) V26.51
          nontraffic V26.11
        bus (traffic) V24.51
          nontraffic V24.11
        car (traffic) V23.51
          nontraffic V23.11
        motor vehicle NOS
          (traffic) V29.501
          nontraffic V29.101
          specified type NEC
            (traffic) V29.591
            nontraffic V29.191
        pedal cycle (traffic)
          V21.51
          nontraffic V21.11
        pedestrian
          nontraffic V20.11
          traffic V20.51
        pickup truck (traffic)
          V23.51
          nontraffic V23.11
        railway vehicle (traffic)
          V25.51
          nontraffic 25.11
        specified vehicle NEC
          (traffic) V26.51
          nontraffic V26.11
        stationary object (traffic)
          V27.51
          nontraffic V27.11
        streetcar (traffic) V26.51
          nontraffic V26.11
        three wheeled motor
          vehicle (traffic) V22.51
          nontraffic V22.11
        truck (traffic) V24.51
          nontraffic V24.11
        two wheeled motor
          vehicle (traffic) V22.51
          nontraffic V22.11
        van (traffic) V23.51
          nontraffic V23.11
      noncollision accident
        (traffic) V28.51
        nontraffic V28.11
    specified type NEC V29.881
    military vehicle V29.811
  forklift —*see* Accident, transport,
    industrial vehicle occupant
  go cart —*see* Accident, transport,
    all-terrain vehicle occupant
  golf cart —*see* Accident,
    transport, all-terrain vehicle
    occupant
  heavy transport vehicle
    occupant —*see* Accident,
    transport, truck occupant
  hoverboard V00.848
  ice yacht V98.2
  industrial vehicle occupant
    (nontraffic) V83.9
    driver V83.5
    hanger-on V83.7

Accident (*continued*)
 transport (*continued*)
  industrial vehicle occupant
   (nontraffic) (*continued*)
   passenger V83.6
   traffic V83.3
    driver V83.0
    hanger-on V83.2
    passenger V83.1
   while boarding or alighting
    V83.4
  interurban electric car —*see*
   Accident, transport, streetcar
  land yacht V98.1
  logging car —*see* Accident,
   transport, industrial vehicle
   occupant
  military vehicle occupant
   (traffic) V86.34
   driver V86.04
   hanger-on V86.24
   nontraffic V86.94
    driver V86.54
    hanger-on V86.74
    passenger V86.64
   passenger V86.14
   while boarding or alighting
    V86.44
  mine tram —*see* Accident,
   transport, industrial vehicle
   occupant
  motorcoach —*see* Accident,
   transport, bus occupant
  motorcycle V29.99
   collision (with)
    animal (traffic) V20.99
     being ridden (traffic)
      V26.99
      nontraffic V26.29
      while boarding
       or alighting V26.39
     nontraffic V20.29
     while boarding or
      alighting V20.39
    animal-drawn vehicle
     (traffic) V26.99
     nontraffic V26.29
     while boarding
      or alighting V26.39
    bus (traffic) V24.99
     nontraffic V24.29
     while boarding
      or alighting V24.39
    car (traffic) V23.99
     nontraffic V23.29
     while boarding or
      alighting V23.39
    motor vehicle NOS (traffic)
     V29.608
     nontraffic V29.208
     specified type NEC
      (traffic) V29.698
      nontraffic V29.298
    pedal cycle (traffic) V21.99
     nontraffic V21.29
     while boarding or
      alighting V21.39
    pickup truck (traffic) V23.99
     nontraffic V23.29
     while boarding or
      alighting V23.39
    railway vehicle (traffic)
     V25.99
     nontraffic V25.29
     while boarding or
      alighting V25.39
    specified vehicle NEC
     (traffic) V26.99
     nontraffic V26.29
     while boarding or
      alighting V26.39

Accident (*continued*)
 transport (*continued*)
  motorcycle (*continued*)
   collision (*continued*)
    stationary object (traffic)
     V27.99
     nontraffic V27.29
     while boarding or
      alighting V27.39
    streetcar (traffic) V26.99
     nontraffic V26.29
     while boarding or
      alighting V26.39
    three wheeled motor vehicle
     (traffic) V22.99
     nontraffic V22.29
     while boarding or
      alighting V22.39
    truck (traffic) V24.99
     nontraffic V24.29
     while boarding or
      alighting V24.39
    two wheeled motor vehicle
     (traffic) V22.99
     nontraffic V22.29
     while boarding or
      alighting V22.39
    van (traffic) V23.99
     nontraffic V23.29
     while boarding or
      alighting V23.39
   driver
    collision (with)
     animal (traffic) V20.49
      being ridden (traffic)
       V26.49
       nontraffic V26.09
      nontraffic V20.09
     animal-drawn vehicle
      (traffic) V26.49
      nontraffic V26.09
     bus (traffic) V24.49
      nontraffic V24.09
     car (traffic) V23.49
      nontraffic V23.09
     motor vehicle NOS
      (traffic) V29.408
      nontraffic V29.008
      specified type NEC
       (traffic) V29.498
       nontraffic V29.098
     pedal cycle (traffic)
      V21.49
      nontraffic V21.09
     pedestrian
      nontraffic V20.09
      traffic V20.49
     pickup truck (traffic)
      V23.49
      nontraffic V23.09
     railway vehicle (traffic)
      V25.49
      nontraffic V25.09
     specified vehicle NEC
      (traffic) V26.49
      nontraffic V26.09
     stationary object (traffic)
      V27.49
      nontraffic V27.09
     streetcar (traffic) V26.49
      nontraffic V26.09
     three wheeled motor
      vehicle (traffic)
      V22.49
      nontraffic V22.09
     truck (traffic) V24.49
      nontraffic V24.09
     two wheeled motor
      vehicle (traffic)
      V22.49
      nontraffic V22.09

Accident (*continued*)
 transport (*continued*)
  driver (*continued*)
   collision (*continued*)
    van (traffic) V23.49
    nontraffic V23.09
   noncollision accident
    (traffic) V28.49
    nontraffic V28.09
   noncollision accident (traffic)
    V28.99
    nontraffic V28.29
   while boarding or alighting
    V28.39
   nontraffic V29.39
   passenger
    collision (with)
     animal (traffic) V20.59
      being ridden (traffic)
       V26.59
       nontraffic V26.19
      nontraffic V20.19
     animal-drawn vehicle
      (traffic) V26.59
      nontraffic V26.19
     bus (traffic) V24.59
      nontraffic V24.19
     car (traffic) V23.59
      nontraffic V23.19
     motor vehicle NOS (traffic)
      V29.508
      nontraffic V29.108
      specified type NEC
       (traffic) V29.598
       nontraffic V29.198
     pedal cycle (traffic)
      V21.59
      nontraffic V21.19
     pedestrian
      nontraffic V20.19
      traffic V20.59
     pickup truck (traffic)
      V23.59
      nontraffic V23.19
     railway vehicle (traffic)
      V25.59
      nontraffic V25.19
     specified vehicle NEC
      (traffic) V26.59
      nontraffic V26.19
     stationary object (traffic)
      V27.59
      nontraffic V27.19
     streetcar (traffic) V26.59
      nontraffic V26.19
     three wheeled motor vehicle
      (traffic) V22.59
      nontraffic V22.19
     truck (traffic) V24.59
      nontraffic V24.19
     two wheeled motor vehicle
      (traffic) V22.59
      nontraffic V22.19
     van (traffic) V23.59
      nontraffic V23.19
    noncollision accident (traffic)
     V28.59
     nontraffic V28.19
   specified type NEC V29.888
   military vehicle V29.818
  motor vehicle NEC occupant
   (traffic) V89.2
  occupant (of)
   aircraft (powered) V95.9
    fixed wing
     commercial
      —*see* Accident,
      transport, aircraft,
      occupant, powered,
      fixed wing,
      commercial

Accident (*continued*)
 transport (*continued*)
  occupant (*continued*)
   aircraft (powered)
    (*continued*)
    fixed wing (*continued*)
     private —*see* Accident,
      transport, aircraft,
      occupant, powered,
      fixed wing, private
   nonpowered V96.9
   specified NEC V95.8
  airport battery-powered
   vehicle —*see* Accident,
   transport, industrial vehicle
   occupant
  all-terrain vehicle (ATV)
   —*see* Accident, transport,
   all-terrain vehicle
   occupant
  animal-drawn vehicle —
   see Accident, transport,
   animal-drawn vehicle
   occupant
  automobile —*see* Accident,
   transport, car occupant
  balloon V96.00
  battery-powered vehicle
   —*see* Accident, transport,
   industrial vehicle occupant
  bicycle —*see* Accident,
   transport, pedal cyclist
   motorized —*see* Accident,
    transport, motorcycle
    rider
  boat NEC —*see* Accident,
   watercraft
  bulldozer —*see* Accident,
   transport, construction
   vehicle occupant
  bus —*see* Accident, transport,
   bus occupant
  cable car (on rails)
   —*see also* Accident,
   transport, streetcar
   occupant
   not on rails V98.0
  car —*see also* Accident,
   transport, car occupant
   cable (on rails) —*see also*
    Accident, transport,
    streetcar occupant
    not on rails V98.0
  coach —*see* Accident,
   transport, bus occupant
  coal-car —*see* Accident,
   transport, industrial vehicle
   occupant
  digger —*see* Accident,
   transport, construction
   vehicle occupant
  dump truck —*see* Accident,
   transport, construction
   vehicle occupant
  earth-leveler —*see* Accident,
   transport, construction
   vehicle occupant
  farm machinery (self-
   propelled) —*see* Accident,
   transport, agricultural
   vehicle occupant
  forklift —*see* Accident,
   transport, industrial vehicle
   occupant
  glider (unpowered) V96.20
   hang V96.10
   powered (microlight)
    (ultralight) —*see*
    Accident, transport,
    aircraft, occupant,
    powered, glider

Accident *(continued)*
  transport *(continued)*
    occupant *(continued)*
      glider (unpowered) NEC V96.20
      hang-glider V96.10
      harvester —*see* Accident, transport, agricultural vehicle occupant
      heavy (transport) vehicle —*see* Accident, transport, truck occupant
      helicopter —*see* Accident, transport, aircraft, occupant, helicopter
      ice-yacht V98.2
      kite (carrying person) V96.8
      land-yacht V98.1
      logging car —*see* Accident, transport, industrial vehicle occupant
      mechanical shovel —*see* Accident, transport, construction vehicle occupant
      microlight —*see* Accident, transport, aircraft, occupant, powered, glider
      minibus —*see* Accident, transport, pickup truck occupant
      minivan —*see* Accident, transport, pickup truck occupant
      moped —*see* Accident, transport, motorcycle
      motor scooter —*see* Accident, transport, motorcycle
      motorcycle (with sidecar) —*see* Accident, transport, motorcycle
      off-road motor-vehicle (*see also* Accident, transport, all-terrain vehicle occupant) V86.99
      pedal cycle —*see also* Accident, transport, pedal cyclist
      pick-up (truck) —*see* Accident, transport, pickup truck occupant
      railway (train) (vehicle) (subterranean) (elevated) —*see* Accident, transport, railway vehicle occupant
      rickshaw —*see* Accident, transport, pedal cycle
      motorized —*see* Accident, transport, three-wheeled motor vehicle
      pedal driven —*see* Accident, transport, pedal cyclist
      road-roller —*see* Accident, transport, construction vehicle occupant
      ship NOS V94.9
      ski-lift (chair) (gondola) V98.3
      snowmobile —*see* Accident, transport, snowmobile occupant
      spacecraft, spaceship —*see* Accident, transport, aircraft, occupant, spacecraft

Accident *(continued)*
  transport *(continued)*
    occupant *(continued)*
      sport utility vehicle —*see* Accident, transport, pickup truck occupant
      streetcar (interurban) (operating on public street or highway) —*see* Accident, transport, streetcar occupant
      SUV —*see* Accident, transport, pickup truck occupant
      téléférique V98.0
      three-wheeled vehicle (motorized) —*see also* Accident, transport, three-wheeled motor vehicle occupant
      nonmotorized —*see* Accident, transport, pedal cycle
      tractor (farm) (and trailer) —*see* Accident, transport, agricultural vehicle occupant
      train —*see* Accident, transport, railway vehicle occupant
      tram —*see* Accident, transport, streetcar occupant
      in mine or quarry —*see* Accident, transport, industrial vehicle occupant
      tricycle —*see* Accident, transport, pedal cycle
      motorized —*see* Accident, transport, three-wheeled motor vehicle
      trolley —*see* Accident, transport, streetcar occupant
      in mine or quarry —*see* Accident, transport, industrial vehicle occupant
      tub, in mine or quarry —*see* Accident, transport, industrial vehicle occupant
      ultralight —*see* Accident, transport, aircraft, occupant, powered, glider
      van —*see* Accident, transport, van occupant
      vehicle NEC V89.9
        heavy transport —*see* Accident, transport, truck occupant
        motor (traffic) NEC V89.2
        nontraffic NEC V89.0
      watercraft NOS V94.9
        causing drowning —*see* Drowning, resulting from accident to boat
      off-road motor-vehicle (*see also* Accident, transport, all-terrain occupant) V86.99
      parachutist V97.29
        after accident to aircraft —*see* Accident, transport, aircraft
        entangled in object V97.21
        injured on landing V97.22
    pedal cyclist V19.9
      collision (with)
        animal (traffic) V10.9

Accident *(continued)*
  transport *(continued)*
    pedal cyclist *(continued)*
      collision *(continued)*
        animal (traffic) *(continued)*
          being ridden (traffic) V16.9
          nontraffic V16.2
          while boarding or alighting V16.3
        nontraffic V10.2
        while boarding or alighting V10.3
        animal-drawn vehicle (traffic) V16.9
          nontraffic V16.2
          while boarding or alighting V16.3
        bus (traffic) V14.9
          nontraffic V14.2
          while boarding or alighting V14.3
        car (traffic) V13.9
          nontraffic V13.2
          while boarding or alighting V13.3
        motor vehicle NOS (traffic) V19.60
          nontraffic V19.20
          specified type NEC (traffic) V19.69
          nontraffic V19.29
        pedal cycle (traffic) V11.9
          nontraffic V11.2
          while boarding or alighting V11.3
        pickup truck (traffic) V13.9
          nontraffic V13.2
          while boarding or alighting V13.3
        railway vehicle (traffic) V15.9
          nontraffic V15.2
          while boarding or alighting V15.3
        specified vehicle NEC (traffic) V16.9
          nontraffic V16.2
          while boarding or alighting V16.3
        stationary object (traffic) V17.9
          nontraffic V17.2
          while boarding or alighting V17.3
        streetcar (traffic) V16.9
          nontraffic V16.2
          while boarding or alighting V16.3
        three wheeled motor vehicle (traffic) V12.9
          nontraffic V12.2
          while boarding or alighting V12.3
        truck (traffic) V14.9
          nontraffic V14.2
          while boarding or alighting V14.3
        two wheeled motor vehicle (traffic) V12.9
          nontraffic V12.2
          while boarding or alighting V12.3
        van (traffic) V13.9
          nontraffic V13.2
          while boarding or alighting V13.3
      driver
        collision (with)
          animal (traffic) V10.4

Accident *(continued)*
  transport *(continued)*
    pedal cyclist *(continued)*
      driver *(continued)*
        collision *(continued)*
          animal (traffic) *(continued)*
            being ridden (traffic) V16.4
            nontraffic V16.0
          nontraffic V10.0
          animal-drawn vehicle (traffic) V16.4
            nontraffic V16.0
          bus (traffic) V14.4
            nontraffic V14.0
          car (traffic) V13.4
            nontraffic V13.0
          motor vehicle NOS (traffic) V19.40
            nontraffic V19.00
            specified type NEC (traffic) V19.49
            nontraffic V19.09
          pedal cycle (traffic) V11.4
            nontraffic V11.0
          pickup truck (traffic) tV13.4
            nontraffic V13.0
          railway vehicle (traffic) V15.4
            nontraffic V15.0
          specified vehicle NEC (traffic) V16.4
            nontraffic V16.0
          stationary object (traffic) V17.4
            nontraffic V17.0
          streetcar (traffic) V16.4
            nontraffic V16.0
          three wheeled motor vehicle (traffic) V12.4
            nontraffic V12.0
          truck (traffic) V14.4
            nontraffic V14.0
          two wheeled motor vehicle (traffic) V12.4
            nontraffic V12.0
          van (traffic) V13.4
            nontraffic V13.0
        noncollision accident (traffic) V18.4
          nontraffic V18.0
      noncollision accident (traffic) V18.9
        nontraffic V18.2
        while boarding or alighting V18.3
      nontraffic V19.3
      passenger
        collision (with)
          animal (traffic) V10.5
            being ridden (traffic) V16.5
            nontraffic V16.1
          nontraffic V10.1
          animal-drawn vehicle (traffic) V16.5
            nontraffic V16.1
          bus (traffic) V14.5
            nontraffic V14.1
          car (traffic) V13.5
            nontraffic V13.1
          motor vehicle NOS (traffic) V19.50
            nontraffic V19.10
            specified type NEC (traffic) V19.59
            nontraffic V19.19
          pedal cycle (traffic) V11.5

455

Accident (continued)
  transport (continued)
    pedal cyclist (continued)
      passenger (continued)
        collision (continued)
          pedal cycle (traffic)
          (continued)
            nontraffic V11.1
          pickup truck (traffic)
            V13.5
            nontraffic V13.1
          railway vehicle (traffic)
            V15.5
            nontraffic V15.1
          specified vehicle NEC
            (traffic) V16.5
            nontraffic V16.1
          stationary object (traffic)
            V17.5
            nontraffic V17.1
          streetcar (traffic) V16.5
            nontraffic V16.1
          three wheeled motor
            vehicle (traffic) V12.5
            nontraffic V12.1
          truck (traffic) V14.5
            nontraffic V14.1
          two wheeled motor
            vehicle (traffic) V12.5
            nontraffic V12.1
          van (traffic) V13.5
            nontraffic V13.1
        noncollision accident
          (traffic) V18.5
          nontraffic V18.1
        specified type NEC V19.88
        military vehicle V19.81
    pedestrian
      conveyance (occupant) V09.9
        baby stroller V00.828
          collision (with) V09.9
            animal being
              ridden or animal
              drawn vehicle
              V06.99
              nontraffic V06.09
              traffic V06.19
            bus or heavy transport
              V04.99
              nontraffic V04.09
              traffic V04.19
            car V03.99
              nontraffic V03.09
              traffic V03.19
            pedal cycle V01.99
              nontraffic V01.09
              traffic V01.19
            pick-up truck or van
              V03.99
              nontraffic V03.09
              traffic V03.19
            railway (train)
              (vehicle) V05.99
              nontraffic V05.09
              traffic V05.19
            streetcar V06.99
              nontraffic V06.09
              traffic V06.19
            stationary object
              V00.822
            two- or three-wheeled
              motor vehicle
              V02.99
              nontraffic V02.09
              traffic V02.19
            vehicle V09.9
              animal-drawn
                V06.99
                nontraffic
                  V06.09
                traffic V06.19

Accident (continued)
  transport (continued)
    pedestrian (continued)
      conveyance (continued)
        baby stroller (continued)
          collision (continued)
            vehicle (continued)
              motor
                nontraffic V09.00
                traffic V09.20
          fall V00.821
          nontraffic V09.1
            involving motor
              vehicle NEC
              V09.00
          traffic V09.3
            involving motor
              vehicle NEC
              V09.20
        flat-bottomed NEC
          V00.388
          collision (with) V09.9
            animal being ridden or
              animal drawn
              vehicle V06.99
              nontraffic V06.09
              traffic V06.19
            bus or heavy transport
              V04.99
              nontraffic V04.09
              traffic V04.19
            car V03.99
              nontraffic V03.09
              traffic V03.19
            pedal cycle V01.99
              nontraffic V01.09
              traffic V01.19
            pick-up truck or van
              V03.99
              nontraffic V03.09
              traffic V03.19
            railway (train)
              (vehicle) V05.99
              nontraffic V05.09
              traffic V05.19
            stationary object
              V00.382
            streetcar V06.99
              nontraffic V06.09
              traffic V06.19
            two- or three-wheeled
              motor vehicle
              V02.99
              nontraffic V02.09
              traffic V02.19
            vehicle V09.9
              animal-drawn
                V06.99
                nontraffic V06.09
                traffic V06.19
              motor
                nontraffic V09.00
                traffic V09.20
          fall V00.381
          nontraffic V09.1
            involving motor
              vehicle NEC
              V09.00
          snow
            board —see Accident,
              transport, pedestrian,
              conveyance, snow
              board
            ski —see Accident,
              transport, pedestrian,
              conveyance, skis
              (snow)
          traffic V09.3
            involving motor
              vehicle NEC
              V09.20

Accident (continued)
  transport (continued)
    pedestrian (continued)
      conveyance (continued)
        flat-bottomed NEC
          (continued)
          gliding type NEC V00.288
          collision (with) V09.9
            animal being ridden
              or animal drawn
              vehicle V06.99
              nontraffic V06.09
              traffic V06.19
            bus or heavy transport
              V04.99
              nontraffic V04.09
              traffic V04.19
            car V03.99
              nontraffic V03.09
              traffic V03.19
            pedal cycle V01.99
              nontraffic V01.09
              traffic V01.19
            pick-up truck or van
              V03.99
              nontraffic V03.09
              traffic V03.19
            railway (train)
              (vehicle) V05.99
              nontraffic V05.09
              traffic V05.19
            stationary object
              V00.282
            streetcar V06.99
              nontraffic V06.09
              traffic V06.19
            two- or three-wheeled
              motor vehicle V02.99
              nontraffic V02.09
              traffic V02.19
            vehicle V09.9
              animal-drawn
                V06.99
                nontraffic V06.09
                traffic V06.19
              motor
                nontraffic V09.00
                traffic V09.20
          fall V00.281
          heelies —see Accident,
            transport, pedestrian,
            conveyance, heelies
          ice skate —see Accident,
            transport, pedestrian,
            conveyance, ice skate
          nontraffic V09.1
            involving motor
              vehicle NEC V09.00
          sled —see Accident,
            transport, pedestrian,
            conveyance, sled
          traffic V09.3
            involving motor
              vehicle NEC V09.20
          wheelies —see
            Accident, transport,
            pedestrian,
            conveyance, heelies
        heelies V00.158
          colliding with stationary
            object V00.152
          fall V00.151
        hoverboard
          collision with
            animal being ridden
              or animal drawn
              vehicle V06.938
              nontraffic V06.038
              traffic V06.138
            bus or heavy transport
              V04.938

Accident (continued)
  transport (continued)
    pedestrian (continued)
      conveyance (continued)
        hoverboard (continued)
          collision (continued)
            bus or heavy transport
            (continued)
              nontraffic V04.038
              traffic V04.138
            car V03.938
              nontraffic V03.038
              traffic V03.138
            pedal cycle V01.938
              nontraffic V01.038
              traffic V01.138
            pick-up or van
              V03.938
              nontraffic
                V03.038
              traffic V03.138
            railway (train)
              (vehicle) V05.938
              nontraffic
                V05.038
              traffic V05.138
            streetcar V06.938
              nontraffic
                V06.038
              traffic V06.138
            three-wheeled motor
              vehicle V02.938
              nontraffic V02.038
              traffic V02.138
            two-wheeled motor
              vehicle V02.938
              nontraffic
                V02.038
              traffic V02.138
            vehicle, nonmotor,
              specified NEC
              V06.938
              nontraffic
                V06.038
              traffic V06.138
          fall V00.838
        ice skates V00.218
          collision (with) V09.9
            animal being ridden
              or animal drawn
              vehicle V06.99
              nontraffic V06.09
              traffic V06.19
            bus or heavy transport
              V04.99
              nontraffic V04.09
              traffic V04.19
            car V03.99
              nontraffic V03.09
              traffic V03.19
            pedal cycle V01.99
              nontraffic V01.09
              traffic V01.19
            pick-up truck or van
              V03.99
              nontraffic V03.09
              traffic V03.19
            railway (train)
              (vehicle) V05.99
              nontraffic V05.09
              traffic V05.19
            streetcar V06.99
              nontraffic V06.09
              traffic V06.19
            stationary object
              V00.212
            two- or three-
              wheeled motor
              vehicle V02.99
              nontraffic V02.09
              traffic V02.19

Accident *(continued)*
transport *(continued)*
pedestrian *(continued)*
conveyance *(continued)*
ice skates *(continued)*
collision *(continued)*
vehicle V09.9
animal-drawn
V06.99
nontraffic V06.09
traffic V06.19
motor
nontraffic V09.00
traffic V09.20
fall V00.211
nontraffic V09.1
involving motor
vehicle NEC
V09.00
traffic V09.3
involving motor
vehicle NEC
V09.20
motorized mobility scooter
V00.838
collision with stationary
object V00.832
fall from V00.831
nontraffic V09.1
involving motor vehicle
V09.00
military V09.01
specified type NEC
V09.09
roller skates (non in-line)
V00.128
collision (with) V09.9
animal being ridden
or animal drawn
vehicle V06.91
nontraffic V06.01
traffic V06.11
bus or heavy transport
V04.91
nontraffic V04.01
traffic V04.11
car V03.91
nontraffic V03.01
traffic V03.11
pedal cycle V01.91
nontraffic V01.01
traffic V01.11
pick-up truck or van
V03.91
nontraffic V03.01
traffic V03.11
railway (train)
(vehicle) V05.91
nontraffic V05.01
traffic V05.11
streetcar V06.91
nontraffic V06.01
traffic V06.11
stationary object
V00.122
two- or three-wheeled
motor vehicle
V02.91
nontraffic V02.01
traffic V02.11
vehicle V09.9
animal-drawn
V06.91
nontraffic
V06.01
traffic V06.11
motor
nontraffic
V09.00
traffic V09.20
fall V00.121

Accident *(continued)*
transport *(continued)*
pedestrian *(continued)*
conveyance *(continued)*
roller skates *(continued)*
in-line V00.118
collision —*see also*
Accident, transport,
pedestrian,
conveyance
occupant, roller
skates, collision
with stationary
object V00.112
fall V00.111
nontraffic V09.1
involving motor
vehicle NEC V09.00
traffic V09.3
involving motor
vehicle NEC V09.20
rolling shoes V00.158
colliding with stationary
object V00.152
fall V00.151
rolling type NEC V00.188
collision (with) V09.9
animal being ridden
or animal drawn
vehicle V06.99
nontraffic V06.09
traffic V06.19
bus or heavy transport
V04.99
nontraffic V04.09
traffic V04.19
car V03.99
nontraffic V03.09
traffic V03.19
pedal cycle V01.99
nontraffic V01.09
traffic V01.19
pick-up truck or van
V03.99
nontraffic V03.09
traffic V03.19
railway (train)
(vehicle) V05.99
nontraffic V05.09
traffic V05.19
stationary object
V00.182
streetcar V06.99
nontraffic V06.09
traffic V06.19
two- or three-wheeled
motor vehicle V02.99
nontraffic V02.09
traffic V02.19
vehicle V09.9
animal-drawn
V06.99
nontraffic V06.09
traffic V06.19
motor
nontraffic V09.00
traffic V09.20
fall V00.181
in-line roller skate
—*see* Accident,
transport, pedestrian,
conveyance, roller
skate, in-line
nontraffic V09.1
involving motor
vehicle NEC
V09.00
roller skate —*see*
Accident, transport,
pedestrian, conveyance,
roller skate

Accident *(continued)*
transport *(continued)*
pedestrian *(continued)*
conveyance *(continued)*
rolling type NEC
(continued)
scooter (non-motorized)
—*see* Accident,
transport, pedestrian,
conveyance, scooter
skateboard —*see*
Accident, transport,
pedestrian, conveyance,
skateboard
traffic V09.3
involving motor
vehicle NEC V09.20
scooter (non-motorized)
V00.148
collision (with) V09.9
animal being ridden
or animal drawn
vehicle V06.99
nontraffic V06.09
traffic V06.19
bus or heavy transport
V04.99
nontraffic V04.09
traffic V04.19
car V03.99
nontraffic V03.09
traffic V03.19
pedal cycle V01.99
nontraffic V01.09
traffic V01.19
pick-up truck or van
V03.99
nontraffic V03.09
traffic V03.19
railway (train)
(vehicle) V05.99
nontraffic V05.09
traffic V05.19
streetcar V06.99
nontraffic V06.09
traffic V06.19
stationary object
V00.142
two- or three-wheeled
motor vehicle
V02.99
nontraffic V02.09
traffic V02.19
vehicle V09.9
animal-drawn V06.99
nontraffic V06.09
traffic V06.19
motor
nontraffic V09.00
traffic V09.20
fall V00.141
nontraffic V09.1
involving motor
vehicle NEC V09.00
traffic V09.3
involving motor
vehicle NEC V09.20
Segway
collision with
animal being ridden
or animal drawn
vehicle V06.938
nontraffic V06.038
traffic V06.138
bus or heavy transport
V04.938
nontraffic V04.038
traffic V04.138
car V03.938
nontraffic V03.038
traffic V03.138

Accident *(continued)*
transport *(continued)*
pedestrian *(continued)*
conveyance *(continued)*
Segway *(continued)*
collision *(continued)*
pedal cycle V01.938
nontraffic V01.038
traffic V01.138
pick-up or van
V03.938
nontraffic V03.038
traffic V03.138
railway (train)
(vehicle) V05.938
nontraffic V05.038
traffic V05.138
streetcar V06.938
nontraffic V06.038
traffic V06.138
three-wheeled motor
vehicle V02.938
nontraffic V02.038
traffic V02.138
two-wheeled motor
vehicle V02.938
nontraffic V02.038
traffic V02.138
vehicle, nonmotor,
specified NEC
V06.938
nontraffic V06.038
traffic V06.138
fall V00.848
skateboard V00.138
collision (with) V09.9
animal being
ridden or animal
drawn vehicle
V06.92
nontraffic V06.02
traffic V06.12
bus or heavy transport
V04.92
nontraffic V04.02
traffic V04.12
car V03.92
nontraffic V03.02
traffic V03.12
pedal cycle V01.92
nontraffic V01.02
traffic V01.12
pick-up truck or van
V03.92
nontraffic V03.02
traffic V03.12
railway (train)
(vehicle) V05.92
nontraffic V05.02
traffic V05.12
streetcar V06.92
nontraffic V06.02
traffic V06.12
stationary object
V00.132
two- or three-wheeled
motor vehicle
V02.92
nontraffic V02.02
traffic V02.12
vehicle V09.9
animal-drawn
V06.92
nontraffic
V06.02
traffic V06.12
motor
nontraffic
V09.00
traffic V09.20
fall V00.131

Accident (continued)
  transport (continued)
    pedestrian (continued)
      conveyance (continued)
        skateboard (continued)
          nontraffic V09.1
            involving motor
              vehicle NEC V09.00
          traffic V09.3
            involving motor
              vehicle NEC V09.20
        sled V00.228
          collision (with) V09.9
            animal being ridden or
              animal drawn
              vehicle V06.99
                nontraffic V06.09
                traffic V06.19
            bus or heavy transport
              V04.99
              nontraffic V04.09
              traffic V04.19
            car V03.99
              nontraffic V03.09
              traffic V03.19
            pedal cycle V01.99
              nontraffic V01.09
              traffic V01.19
            pick-up truck or van
              V03.99
              nontraffic V03.09
              traffic V03.19
            railway (train)
              (vehicle) V05.99
              nontraffic V05.09
              traffic V05.19
            streetcar V06.99
              nontraffic V06.09
              traffic V06.19
            stationary object
              V00.222
            two- or three-wheeled
              motor vehicle
              V02.99
              nontraffic
                V02.09
              traffic V02.19
            vehicle V09.9
              animal-drawn
                V06.99
                nontraffic V06.09
                traffic V06.19
              motor
                nontraffic V09.00
                traffic V09.20
          fall V00.221
          nontraffic V09.1
            involving motor
              vehicle NEC
              V09.00
          traffic V09.3
            involving motor
              vehicle NEC
              V09.20
        skis (snow) V00.328
          collision (with) V09.9
            animal being ridden
              or animal drawn
              vehicle V06.99
                nontraffic V06.09
                traffic V06.19
            bus or heavy transport
              V04.99
              nontraffic V04.09
              traffic V04.19
            car V03.99
              nontraffic V03.09
              traffic V03.19
            pedal cycle V01.99
              nontraffic V01.09
              traffic V01.19

Accident (continued)
  transport (continued)
    pedestrian (continued)
      conveyance (continued)
        skis (continued)
          collision (continued)
            pick-up truck or van
              V03.99
              nontraffic V03.09
              traffic V03.19
            railway (train)
              (vehicle) V05.99
              nontraffic V05.09
              traffic V05.19
            streetcar V06.99
              nontraffic V06.09
              traffic V06.19
            stationary object
              V00.322
            two- or three-wheeled
              motor vehicle
              V02.99
              nontraffic V02.09
              traffic V02.19
            vehicle V09.9
              animal-drawn
                V06.99
                nontraffic V06.09
                traffic V06.19
              motor
                nontraffic V09.00
                traffic V09.20
          fall V00.321
          nontraffic V09.1
            involving motor
              vehicle NEC V09.00
          traffic V09.3
            involving motor
              vehicle NEC
              V09.20
        snow board V00.318
          collision (with) V09.9
            animal being ridden
              or animal drawn
              vehicle V06.99
                nontraffic V06.09
                traffic V06.19
            bus or heavy transport
              V04.99
              nontraffic V04.09
              traffic V04.19
            car V03.99
              nontraffic V03.09
              traffic V03.19
            pedal cycle V01.99
              nontraffic V01.09
              traffic V01.19
            pick-up truck or van
              V03.99
              nontraffic V03.09
              traffic V03.19
            railway (train)
              (vehicle) V05.99
              nontraffic V05.09
              traffic V05.19
            streetcar V06.99
              nontraffic
                V06.09
              traffic V06.19
            stationary object
              V00.312
            two- or three-wheeled
              motor vehicle
              V02.99
              nontraffic V02.09
              traffic V02.19
            vehicle V09.9
              animal-drawn
                V06.99
                nontraffic V06.09
                traffic V06.19

Accident (continued)
  transport (continued)
    pedestrian (continued)
      conveyance (continued)
        snow board (continued)
          collision (continued)
            vehicle (continued)
              motor
                nontraffic V09.00
                traffic V09.20
          fall V00.311
          nontraffic V09.1
            involving motor
              vehicle NEC V09.00
          traffic V09.3
            involving motor
              vehicle NEC V09.20
        specified type NEC
          V00.898
          collision (with) V09.9
            animal being ridden
              or animal drawn
              vehicle V06.99
                nontraffic V06.09
                traffic V06.19
            bus or heavy transport
              V04.99
              nontraffic V04.09
              traffic V04.19
            car V03.99
              nontraffic V03.09
              traffic V03.19
            pedal cycle V01.99
              nontraffic V01.09
              traffic V01.19
            pick-up truck or van
              V03.99
              nontraffic V03.09
              traffic V03.19
            railway (train)
              (vehicle) V05.99
              nontraffic V05.09
              traffic V05.19
            streetcar V06.99
              nontraffic V06.09
              traffic V06.19
            stationary object
              V00.892
            two- or three-wheeled
              motor vehicle
              V02.99
              nontraffic V02.09
              traffic V02.19
            vehicle V09.9
              animal-drawn
                V06.99
                nontraffic V06.09
                traffic V06.19
              motor
                nontraffic V09.00
                traffic V09.20
          fall V00.891
          nontraffic V09.1
            involving motor
              vehicle NEC V09.00
          traffic V09.3
            involving motor
              vehicle NEC V09.20
        Standing
          electric scooter
            collision with
              animal being ridden
                or animal drawn
                vehicle V06.931
                  nontraffic V06.031
                  traffic V06.131
              bus or heavy
                transport V04.931
                nontraffic
                  V04.031
                traffic V04.131

Accident (continued)
  transport (continued)
    pedestrian (continued)
      conveyance (continued)
        Standing (continued)
          electric scooter
          (continued)
            collision with
            (continued)
              car V03.931
                nontraffic
                  V03.031
                traffic V03.131
              pedal cycle V01.931
                nontraffic V01.031
                traffic V01.131
              pick-up or
                vanV03.931
                nontraffic
                  V03.031
                traffic V03.131
              railway (train)
                (vehicle)V05.931
                nontraffic
                  V05.031
                traffic V05.131
              streetcar V06.931
                nontraffic
                  V06.031
                traffic V06.131
              three-wheeled motor
                vehicle V02.931
                nontraffic
                  V02.031
                traffic V02.131
              two-wheeled motor
                vehicle V02.931
                nontraffic
                  V02.031
                traffic V02.131
              vehicle, nonmotor,
                specified NEC
                V06.931
                nontraffic
                  V06.031
                traffic V06.131
          fall V00.841
          micro-mobility
          pedestrian conveyance
          collision with
            animal being ridden
              or animal drawn
              vehicle V06.938
              nontraffic
                V06.038
              traffic V06.138
            bus or heavy
              transport V04.938
              nontraffic
                V04.038
              traffic V04.138
            car V03.938
              nontraffic
                V03.038
              traffic V03.138
            pedal cycle V01.938
              nontraffic
                V01.038
              traffic V01.138
            pick-up or
              vanV03.938
              nontraffic
                V03.038
              traffic V03.138
            railway (train)
              (vehicle)V05.938
              nontraffic
                V05.038
              traffic V05.138
            stationary object
              V00.842

Accident (continued)
 transport (continued)
  pedestrian (continued)
   conveyance (continued)
    Standing (continued)
     micro-mobility
      (continued)
      collision with
       (continued)
       streetcar V06.938
        nontraffic V06.038
        traffic V06.138
       three-wheeled motor
        vehicle V02.938
        nontraffic
         V02.038
        traffic V02.138
       two-wheeled motor
        vehicle V02.938
        nontraffic
         V02.038
        traffic V02.138
       vehicle, nonmotor,
        specified NEC
        V06.938
        nontraffic
         V06.038
        traffic V06.138
      fall V00.848
     traffic V09.3
      involving motor vehicle
       V09.20
       military V09.21
       specified type NEC
        V09.29
     wheelchair (powered)
      V00.818
      collision (with) V09.9
       animal being ridden
        or animal drawn
        vehicle V06.99
        nontraffic V06.09
        traffic V06.19
       bus or heavy transport
        V04.99
        nontraffic V04.09
        traffic V04.19
       car V03.99
        nontraffic V03.09
        traffic V03.19
       pedal cycle V01.99
        nontraffic V01.09
        traffic V01.19
       pick-up truck or van
        V03.99
        nontraffic V03.09
        traffic V03.19
       railway (train)
        (vehicle) V05.99
        nontraffic V05.09
        traffic V05.19
       streetcar V06.99
        nontraffic V06.09
        traffic V06.19
       stationary object
        V00.812
       two- or three-wheeled
        motor vehicle V02.99
        nontraffic V02.09
        traffic V02.19
       vehicle V09.9
        animal-drawn V06.99
         nontraffic V06.09
         traffic V06.19
        motor
         nontraffic V09.00
         traffic V09.20
      fall V00.811
      nontraffic V09.1
       involving motor
        vehicle NEC V09.00

Accident (continued)
 transport (continued)
  pedestrian (continued)
   conveyance (continued)
    wheelchair (continued)
     nontraffic (continued)
      traffic V09.3
       involving motor
        vehicle NEC
        V09.20
     wheeled shoe V00.158
      colliding with
       stationary object
       V00.152
      fall V00.151
  on foot —see also Accident,
   pedestrian
   collision (with)
    animal being ridden or
     animal drawn vehicle
     V06.90
     nontraffic V06.00
     traffic V06.10
    bus or heavy transport
     V04.90
     nontraffic V04.00
     traffic V04.10
    car V03.90
     nontraffic V03.00
     traffic V03.10
    pedal cycle V01.90
     nontraffic V01.00
     traffic V01.10
    pick-up truck or van
     V03.90
     nontraffic V03.00
     traffic V03.10
    railway (train) (vehicle)
     V05.90
     nontraffic V05.00
     traffic V05.10
    streetcar V06.90
     nontraffic V06.00
     traffic V06.10
    two- or three-wheeled
     motor vehicle V02.90
     nontraffic V02.00
     traffic V02.10
    vehicle V09.9
     animal-drawn V06.90
      nontraffic V06.00
      traffic V06.10
     motor
      nontraffic V09.00
      traffic V09.20
     nontraffic V09.1
      involving motor vehicle
       V09.00
       military V09.01
       specified type NEC
        V09.09
     traffic V09.3
      involving motor vehicle
       V09.20
       military V09.21
       specified type NEC
        V09.29
  person NEC (unknown way or
   transportation) V99
   collision (between)
    bus (with)
     heavy transport vehicle
      (traffic) V87.5
      nontraffic V88.5
    car (with)
     nontraffic V88.5
     bus (traffic) V87.3
      nontraffic V88.3
     heavy transport vehicle
      (traffic) V87.4
      nontraffic V88.4

Accident (continued)
 transport (continued)
  person NEC (continued)
   collision (continued)
    car (continued)
     pick-up truck or van
      (traffic) V87.2
      nontraffic V88.2
     train or railway vehicle
      (traffic) V87.6
      nontraffic V88.6
     two- or three-wheeled
      motor vehicle (traffic)
      V87.0
      nontraffic V88.0
    motor vehicle (traffic) NEC
     V87.7
     nontraffic V88.7
    two-or three-wheeled
     vehicle (with) (traffic)
     motor vehicle NEC
     V87.1
     nontraffic V88.1
    nonmotor vehicle (collision)
     (noncollision) (traffic) V87.9
     nontraffic V88.9
  pickup truck occupant V59.9
   collision (with)
    animal (traffic) V50.9
     being ridden (traffic)
      V56.9
      nontraffic V56.3
      while boarding or
       alighting V56.4
     nontraffic V50.3
     while boarding or
      alighting V50.4
    animal-drawn vehicle
     (traffic) V56.9
     nontraffic V56.3
     while boarding or
      alighting V56.4
    bus (traffic) V54.9
     nontraffic V54.3
     while boarding or
      alighting V54.4
    car (traffic) V53.9
     nontraffic V53.3
     while boarding or
      alighting V53.4
    motor vehicle NOS (traffic)
     V59.60
     nontraffic V59.20
     specified type NEC
      (traffic) V59.69
      nontraffic V59.29
    pedal cycle (traffic)
     V51.9
     nontraffic V51.3
     while boarding or
      alighting V51.4
    pickup truck (traffic)
     V53.9
     nontraffic V53.3
     while boarding or
      alighting V53.4
    railway vehicle (traffic)
     V55.9
     nontraffic V55.3
     while boarding or
      alighting V55.4
    specified vehicle NEC
     (traffic) V56.9
     nontraffic V56.3
     while boarding or
      alighting V56.4
    stationary object (traffic)
     V57.9
     nontraffic V57.3
     while boarding or
      alighting V57.4

Accident (continued)
 transport (continued)
  pickup truck occupant (continued)
   collision (continued)
    streetcar (traffic) V56.9
     nontraffic V56.3
     while boarding or
      alighting V56.4
    three wheeled motor
     vehicle (traffic) V52.9
     nontraffic V52.3
     while boarding or
      alighting V52.4
    truck (traffic) V54.9
     nontraffic V54.3
     while boarding or
      alighting V54.4
    two wheeled motor vehicle
     (traffic) V52.9
     nontraffic V52.3
     while boarding or
      alighting V52.4
    van (traffic) V53.9
     nontraffic V53.3
     while boarding or
      alighting V53.4
   driver
    collision (with)
     animal (traffic) V50.5
      being ridden (traffic)
       V56.5
       nontraffic V56.0
      nontraffic V50.0
     animal-drawn vehicle
      (traffic) V56.5
      nontraffic V56.0
     bus (traffic) V54.5
      nontraffic V54.0
     car (traffic) V53.5
      nontraffic V53.0
     motor vehicle NOS
      (traffic) V59.40
      nontraffic V59.00
      specified type NEC
       (traffic) V59.49
       nontraffic V59.09
     pedal cycle (traffic) V51.5
      nontraffic V51.0
     pickup truck (traffic)
      V53.5
      nontraffic V53.0
     railway vehicle (traffic)
      V55.5
      nontraffic V55.0
     specified vehicle NEC
      (traffic) V56.5
      nontraffic V56.0
     stationary object (traffic)
      V57.5
      nontraffic V57.0
     streetcar (traffic) V56.5
      nontraffic V56.0
     three wheeled motor
      vehicle (traffic) V52.5
      nontraffic V52.0
     truck (traffic) V54.5
      nontraffic V54.0
     two wheeled motor
      vehicle (traffic) V52.5
      nontraffic V52.0
     van (traffic) V53.5
      nontraffic V53.0
    noncollision accident
     (traffic) V58.5
     nontraffic V58.0
    noncollision accident (traffic)
     V58.9
     nontraffic V58.3
     while boarding or alighting
      V58.4
   nontraffic V59.3

459

Accident (*continued*)
 transport (*continued*)
  pickup truck occupant (*continued*)
   hanger-on
    collision (with)
     animal (traffic) V50.7
      being ridden (traffic) V56.7
       nontraffic V56.2
      nontraffic V50.2
     animal-drawn vehicle (traffic) V56.7
      nontraffic V56.2
     bus (traffic) V54.7
      nontraffic V54.2
     car (traffic) V53.7
      nontraffic V53.2
     pedal cycle (traffic) V51.7
      nontraffic V51.2
     pickup truck (traffic) V53.7
      nontraffic V53.2
     railway vehicle (traffic) V55.7
      nontraffic V55.2
     specified vehicle NEC (traffic) V56.7
      nontraffic V56.2
     stationary object (traffic) V57.7
      nontraffic V57.2
     streetcar (traffic) V56.7
      nontraffic V56.2
     three wheeled motor vehicle (traffic) V52.7
      nontraffic V52.2
     truck (traffic) V54.7
      nontraffic V54.2
     two wheeled motor vehicle (traffic) V52.7
      nontraffic V52.2
     van (traffic) V53.7
      nontraffic V53.2
    noncollision accident (traffic) V58.7
     nontraffic V58.2
   passenger
    collision (with)
     animal (traffic) V50.6
      being ridden (traffic) V56.6
       nontraffic V56.1
      nontraffic V50.1
     animal-drawn vehicle (traffic) V56.6
      nontraffic V56.1
     bus (traffic) V54.6
      nontraffic V54.1
     car (traffic) V53.6
      nontraffic V53.1
     motor vehicle NOS (traffic) V59.50
      nontraffic V59.10
     specified type NEC (traffic) V59.59
      nontraffic V59.19
     pedal cycle (traffic) V51.6
      nontraffic V51.1
     pickup truck (traffic) V53.6
      nontraffic V53.1
     railway vehicle (traffic) V55.6
      nontraffic V55.1
     specified vehicle NEC (traffic) V56.6
      nontraffic V56.1
     stationary object (traffic) V57.6
      nontraffic V57.1

Accident (*continued*)
 transport (*continued*)
  pickup truck occupant (*continued*)
   passenger
    collision (with)
     streetcar (traffic) V56.6
      nontraffic V56.1
     three wheeled motor vehicle (traffic) V52.6
      nontraffic V52.1
     truck (traffic) V54.6
      nontraffic V54.1
     two wheeled motor vehicle (traffic) V52.6
      nontraffic V52.1
     van (traffic) V53.6
      nontraffic V53.1
    noncollision accident (traffic) V58.6
     nontraffic V58.1
   specified type NEC V59.88
   military vehicle V59.81
  quarry truck —*see* Accident, transport, industrial vehicle occupant
  race car —*see* Accident, transport, motor vehicle NEC occupant
  railway vehicle occupant V81.9
   collision (with) V81.3
    motor vehicle (non-military) (traffic) V81.1
    military V81.83
    nontraffic V81.0
    rolling stock V81.2
    specified object NEC V81.3
   during derailment V81.7
    with antecedent collision
     —*see* Accident, transport, railway vehicle occupant, collision
   explosion V81.81
   fall (in railway vehicle) V81.5
    during derailment V81.7
     with antecedent collision
      —*see* Accident, transport, railway vehicle occupant, collision
    from railway vehicle V81.6
     during derailment V81.7
      with antecedent collision —*see* Accident, transport, railway vehicle occupant, collision
    while boarding or alighting V81.4
   fire V81.81
   object falling onto train V81.82
   specified type NEC V81.89
   while boarding or alighting V81.4
  Segway V00.848
  ski lift V98.3
  snowmobile occupant (nontraffic) V86.92
   driver V86.52
   hanger-on V86.72
   passenger V86.62
   traffic V86.32
    driver V86.02
    hanger-on V86.22
    passenger V86.12
   while boarding or alighting V86.42
  specified NEC V98.8
  sport utility vehicle occupant
   —*see also* Accident, transport, pickup truck occupant

Accident (*continued*)
 transport (*continued*)
  streetcar occupant V82.9
   collision (with) V82.3
    motor vehicle (traffic) V82.1
     nontraffic V82.0
    rolling stock V82.2
   during derailment V82.7
    with antecedent collision
     —*see* Accident, transport, streetcar occupant, collision
   fall (in streetcar) V82.5
    during derailment V82.7
     with antecedent collision —*see* Accident, transport, streetcar occupant, collision
    from streetcar V82.6
     during derailment V82.7
      with antecedent collision —*see* Accident, transport, streetcar occupant, collision
    while boarding or alighting V82.4
   while boarding or alighting V82.4
   specified type NEC V82.8
   while boarding or alighting V82.4
  three-wheeled motor vehicle occupant V39.9
   collision (with)
    animal (traffic) V30.9
     being ridden (traffic) V36.9
      nontraffic V36.3
      while boarding or alighting V36.4
     nontraffic V30.3
     while boarding or alighting V30.4
    animal-drawn vehicle (traffic) V36.9
     nontraffic V36.3
     while boarding or alighting V36.4
    bus (traffic) V34.9
     nontraffic V34.3
     while boarding or alighting V34.4
    car (traffic) V33.9
     nontraffic V33.3
     while boarding or alighting V33.4
    motor vehicle NOS (traffic) V39.60
     nontraffic V39.20
     specified type NEC (traffic) V39.69
      nontraffic V39.29
    pedal cycle (traffic) V31.9
     nontraffic V31.3
     while boarding or alighting V31.4
    pickup truck (traffic) V33.9
     nontraffic V33.3
     while boarding or alighting V33.4
    railway vehicle (traffic) V35.9
     nontraffic V35.3
     while boarding or alighting V35.4
    specified vehicle NEC (traffic) V36.9
     nontraffic V36.3
     while boarding or alighting V36.4

Accident (*continued*)
 transport (*continued*)
  three-wheeled motor vehicle occupant (*continued*)
   collision (*continued*)
    stationary object (traffic) V37.9
     nontraffic V37.3
     while boarding or alighting V37.4
    streetcar (traffic) V36.9
     nontraffic V36.3
     while boarding or alighting V36.4
    three wheeled motor vehicle (traffic) V32.9
     nontraffic V32.3
     while boarding or alighting V32.4
    truck (traffic) V34.9
     nontraffic V34.3
     while boarding or alighting V34.4
    two wheeled motor vehicle (traffic) V32.9
     nontraffic V32.3
     while boarding or alighting V32.4
    van (traffic) V33.9
     nontraffic V33.3
     while boarding or alighting V33.4
   driver
    collision (with)
     animal (traffic) V30.5
      being ridden (traffic) V36.5
       nontraffic V36.0
      nontraffic V30.0
     animal-drawn vehicle (traffic) V36.5
      nontraffic V36.0
     bus (traffic) V34.5
      nontraffic V34.0
     car (traffic) V33.5
      nontraffic V33.0
     motor vehicle NOS (traffic) V39.40
      nontraffic V39.00
     specified type NEC (traffic) V39.49
      nontraffic V39.09
     pedal cycle (traffic) V31.5
      nontraffic V31.0
     pickup truck (traffic) V33.5
      nontraffic V33.0
     railway vehicle (traffic) V35.5
      nontraffic V35.0
     specified vehicle NEC (traffic) V36.5
      nontraffic V36.0
     stationary object (traffic) V37.5
      nontraffic V37.0
     streetcar (traffic) V36.5
      nontraffic V36.0
     three wheeled motor vehicle (traffic) V32.5
      nontraffic V32.0
     truck (traffic) V34.5
      nontraffic V34.0
     two wheeled motor vehicle (traffic) V32.5
      nontraffic V32.0
     van (traffic) V33.5
      nontraffic V33.0
    noncollision accident (traffic) V38.5
     nontraffic V38.0

Accident (continued)
  transport (continued)
    three-wheeled motor vehicle
      occupant (continued)
        noncollision accident (traffic)
          V38.9
          nontraffic V38.3
          while boarding or alighting
            V38.4
          nontraffic V39.3
        hanger-on
          collision (with)
            animal (traffic) V30.7
              being ridden (traffic)
                V36.7
                nontraffic V36.2
              nontraffic V30.2
            animal-drawn vehicle
              (traffic) V36.7
              nontraffic V36.2
            bus (traffic) V34.7
              nontraffic V34.2
            car (traffic) V33.7
              nontraffic V33.2
            pedal cycle (traffic) V31.7
              nontraffic V31.2
            pickup truck (traffic) V33.7
              nontraffic V33.2
            railway vehicle (traffic)
              V35.7
              nontraffic V35.2
            specified vehicle NEC
              (traffic) V36.7
              nontraffic V36.2
            stationary object (traffic)
              V37.7
              nontraffic V37.2
            streetcar (traffic) V36.7
              nontraffic V36.2
            three wheeled motor
              vehicle (traffic)
                V32.7
                nontraffic V32.2
            truck (traffic) V34.7
              nontraffic V34.2
            two wheeled motor
              vehicle (traffic)
                V32.7
                nontraffic V32.2
            van (traffic) V33.7
              nontraffic V33.2
          noncollision accident
            (traffic) V38.7
            nontraffic V38.2
        passenger
          collision (with)
            animal (traffic) V30.6
              being ridden (traffic)
                V36.6
                nontraffic V36.1
              nontraffic V30.1
            animal-drawn vehicle
              (traffic) V36.6
              nontraffic V36.1
            bus (traffic) V34.6
              nontraffic V34.1
            car (traffic) V33.6
              nontraffic V33.1
            motor vehicle NOS
              (traffic) V39.50
              nontraffic V39.10
            specified type NEC
              (traffic) V39.59
              nontraffic V39.19
            pedal cycle (traffic) V31.6
              nontraffic V31.1
            pickup truck (traffic) V33.6
              nontraffic V33.1
            railway vehicle (traffic)
              V35.6
              nontraffic V35.1

Accident (continued)
  transport (continued)
    three-wheeled motor vehicle
      occupant (continued)
        passenger (continued)
          collision (continued)
            specified vehicle NEC
              (traffic) V36.6
              nontraffic V36.1
            stationary object (traffic)
              V37.6
              nontraffic V37.1
            streetcar (traffic) V36.6
              nontraffic V36.1
            three wheeled motor
              vehicle (traffic) V32.6
              nontraffic V32.1
            truck (traffic) V34.6
              nontraffic V34.1
            two wheeled motor
              vehicle (traffic) V32.6
              nontraffic V32.1
            van (traffic) V33.6
              nontraffic V33.1
          noncollision accident
            (traffic) V38.6
            nontraffic V38.1
        specified type NEC V39.89
        military vehicle V39.81
    tractor (farm) (and trailer)
      —see Accident, transport,
      agricultural vehicle occupant
    tram —see Accident, transport,
      streetcar
      in mine or quarry —see
        Accident, transport,
        industrial vehicle occupant
    trolley —see Accident, transport,
      streetcar
      in mine or quarry
        —see Accident, transport,
        industrial vehicle occupant
    truck occupant V69.9
      collision (with)
        animal (traffic) V60.9
          being ridden (traffic)
            V66.9
            nontraffic V66.3
            while boarding or
              alighting V66.4
          nontraffic V60.3
          while boarding or
            alighting V60.4
        animal-drawn vehicle
          (traffic) V66.9
          nontraffic V66.3
          while boarding or
            alighting V66.4
        bus (traffic) V64.9
          nontraffic V64.3
          while boarding or
            alighting V64.4
        car (traffic) V63.9
          nontraffic V63.3
          while boarding or
            alighting V63.4
        motor vehicle NOS (traffic)
          V69.60
          nontraffic V69.20
          specified type NEC
            (traffic) V69.69
            nontraffic V69.29
        pedal cycle (traffic) V61.9
          nontraffic V61.3
          while boarding or
            alighting V61.4
        pickup truck (traffic)
          V63.9
          nontraffic V63.3
          while boarding or
            alighting V63.4

Accident (continued)
  transport (continued)
    truck occupant (continued)
      collision (continued)
        railway vehicle (traffic) V65.9
          nontraffic V65.3
          while boarding or
            alighting V65.4
        specified vehicle NEC
          (traffic) V66.9
          nontraffic V66.3
          while boarding or
            alighting V66.4
        stationary object (traffic)
          V67.9
          nontraffic V67.3
          while boarding or
            alighting V67.4
        streetcar (traffic) V66.9
          nontraffic V66.3
          while boarding or
            alighting V66.4
        three wheeled motor vehicle
          (traffic) V62.9
          nontraffic V62.3
          while boarding or
            alighting V62.4
        truck (traffic) V64.9
          nontraffic V64.3
          while boarding or
            alighting V64.4
        two wheeled motor vehicle
          (traffic) V62.9
          nontraffic V62.3
          while boarding or
            alighting V62.4
        van (traffic) V63.9
          nontraffic V63.3
          while boarding or
            alighting V63.4
      driver
        collision (with)
          animal (traffic) V60.5
            being ridden (traffic)
              V66.5
              nontraffic V66.0
            nontraffic V60.0
          animal-drawn vehicle
            (traffic) V66.5
            nontraffic V66.0
          bus (traffic) V64.5
            nontraffic V64.0
          car (traffic) V63.5
            nontraffic V63.0
          motor vehicle NOS
            (traffic) V69.40
            nontraffic V69.00
            specified type NEC
              (traffic) V69.49
              nontraffic V69.09
          pedal cycle (traffic)
            V61.5
            nontraffic V61.0
          pickup truck (traffic) V63.5
            nontraffic V63.0
          railway vehicle (traffic)
            V65.5
            nontraffic V65.0
          specified vehicle NEC
            (traffic) V66.5
            nontraffic V66.0
          stationary object (traffic)
            V67.5
            nontraffic V67.0
          streetcar (traffic) V66.5
            nontraffic V66.0
          three wheeled motor
            vehicle (traffic) V62.5
            nontraffic V62.0
          truck (traffic) V64.5
            nontraffic V64.0

Accident (continued)
  transport (continued)
    truck occupant (continued)
      driver (continued)
        collision (continued)
          two wheeled motor
            vehicle (traffic) V62.5
            nontraffic V62.0
          van (traffic) V63.5
            nontraffic V63.0
        noncollision accident
          (traffic) V68.5
          nontraffic V68.0
      dump —see Accident,
        transport, construction
        vehicle occupant
      hanger-on
        collision (with)
          animal (traffic) V60.7
            being ridden (traffic)
              V66.7
              nontraffic V66.2
            nontraffic V60.2
          animal-drawn vehicle
            (traffic) V66.7
            nontraffic V66.2
          bus (traffic) V64.7
            nontraffic V64.2
          car (traffic) V63.7
            nontraffic V63.2
          pedal cycle (traffic)
            V61.7
            nontraffic V61.2
          pickup truck (traffic)
            V63.7
            nontraffic V63.2
          railway vehicle (traffic)
            V65.7
            nontraffic V65.2
          specified vehicle NEC
            (traffic) V66.7
            nontraffic V66.2
          stationary object (traffic)
            V67.7
            nontraffic V67.2
          streetcar (traffic) V66.7
            nontraffic V66.2
          three wheeled motor
            vehicle (traffic)
              V62.7
              nontraffic V62.2
          truck (traffic) V64.7
            nontraffic V64.2
          two wheeled motor
            vehicle (traffic) V62.7
            nontraffic V62.2
          van (traffic) V63.7
            nontraffic V63.2
        noncollision accident
          (traffic) V68.7
          nontraffic V68.2
      noncollision accident (traffic)
        V68.9
        nontraffic V68.3
        while boarding or alighting
          V68.4
      nontraffic V69.3
      passenger
        collision (with)
          animal (traffic) V60.6
            being ridden (traffic)
              V66.6
              nontraffic V66.1
            nontraffic V60.1
          animal-drawn vehicle
            (traffic) V66.6
            nontraffic V66.1
          bus (traffic) V64.6
            nontraffic V64.1
          car (traffic) V63.6
            nontraffic V63.1

Accident (continued)
  transport (continued)
    truck occupant (continued)
      passenger (continued)
        collision (continued)
          motor vehicle NOS
            (traffic) V69.50
            nontraffic V69.10
            specified type NEC
              (traffic) V69.59
              nontraffic V69.19
          pedal cycle (traffic) V61.6
            nontraffic V61.1
          pickup truck (traffic)
            V63.6
            nontraffic V63.1
          railway vehicle (traffic)
            V65.6
            nontraffic V65.1
          specified vehicle NEC
            (traffic) V66.6
            nontraffic V66.1
          stationary object (traffic)
            V67.6
            nontraffic V67.1
          streetcar (traffic) V66.6
            nontraffic V66.1
          three wheeled motor
            vehicle (traffic) V62.6
            nontraffic V62.1
          truck (traffic) V64.6
            nontraffic V64.1
          two wheeled motor
            vehicle (traffic)
            V62.6
            nontraffic V62.1
          van (traffic) V63.6
            nontraffic V63.1
        noncollision accident
          (traffic) V68.6
        nontraffic V68.1
      pickup —see Accident,
        transport, pickup truck
        occupant
      specified type NEC V69.88
      military vehicle V69.81
    van occupant V59.9
      collision (with)
        animal (traffic) V50.9
          being ridden (traffic)
            V56.9
            nontraffic V56.3
            while boarding or
              alighting V56.4
          nontraffic V50.3
          while boarding or
            alighting V50.4
        animal-drawn vehicle
          (traffic) V56.9
          nontraffic V56.3
          while boarding or
            alighting V56.4
        bus (traffic) V54.9
          nontraffic V54.3
          while boarding or
            alighting V54.4
        car (traffic) V53.9
          nontraffic V53.3
          while boarding or
            alighting V53.4
        motor vehicle NOS (traffic)
          V59.60
          nontraffic V59.20
          specified type NEC
            (traffic) V59.69
            nontraffic V59.29
        pedal cycle (traffic)
          V51.9
          nontraffic V51.3
          while boarding or
            alighting V51.4

Accident (continued)
  transport (continued)
    van occupant (continued)
      collision (continued)
        pickup truck (traffic) V53.9
          nontraffic V53.3
          while boarding or
            alighting V53.4
        railway vehicle (traffic) V55.9
          nontraffic V55.3
          while boarding or
            alighting V55.4
        specified vehicle NEC
          (traffic) V56.9
          nontraffic V56.3
          while boarding or
            alighting V56.4
        stationary object (traffic)
          V57.9
          nontraffic V57.3
          while boarding or
            alighting V57.4
        streetcar (traffic) V56.9
          nontraffic V56.3
          while boarding or
            alighting V56.4
        three wheeled motor vehicle
          (traffic) V52.9
          nontraffic V52.3
          while boarding or
            alighting V52.4
        truck (traffic) V54.9
          nontraffic V54.3
          while boarding or
            alighting V54.4
        two wheeled motor vehicle
          (traffic) V52.9
          nontraffic V52.3
          while boarding or
            alighting V52.4
        van (traffic) V53.9
          nontraffic V53.3
          while boarding or
            alighting V53.4
      driver
        collision (with)
          animal (traffic) V50.5
            being ridden (traffic)
              V56.5
              nontraffic V56.0
            nontraffic V50.0
          animal-drawn vehicle
            (traffic) V56.5
            nontraffic V56.0
          bus (traffic) V54.5
            nontraffic V54.0
          car (traffic) V53.5
            nontraffic V53.0
          motor vehicle NOS
            (traffic) V59.40
            nontraffic V59.00
            specified type NEC
              (traffic) V59.49
              nontraffic V59.09
          pedal cycle (traffic)
            V51.5
            nontraffic V51.0
          pickup truck (traffic)
            V53.5
            nontraffic V53.0
          railway vehicle (traffic)
            V55.5
            nontraffic V55.0
          specified vehicle NEC
            (traffic) V56.5
            nontraffic V56.0
          stationary object (traffic)
            V57.5
            nontraffic V57.0
          streetcar (traffic) V56.5
            nontraffic V56.0

Accident (continued)
  transport (continued)
    van occupant (continued)
      driver (continued)
        collision (continued)
          three wheeled motor
            vehicle (traffic) V52.5
            nontraffic V52.0
          truck (traffic) V54.5
            nontraffic V54.0
          two wheeled motor
            vehicle (traffic)V52.5
            nontraffic V52.0
          van (traffic) V53.5
            nontraffic V53.0
        noncollision accident
          (traffic) V58.5
          nontraffic V58.0
      noncollision accident (traffic)
        V58.9
        nontraffic V58.3
        while boarding or alighting
          V58.4
      nontraffic V59.3
      hanger-on
        collision (with)
          animal (traffic) V50.7
            being ridden (traffic)
              V56.7
              nontraffic V56.2
            nontraffic V50.2
          animal-drawn vehicle
            (traffic) V56.7
            nontraffic V56.2
          bus (traffic) V54.7
            nontraffic V54.2
          car (traffic) V53.7
            nontraffic V53.2
          pedal cycle (traffic) V51.7
            nontraffic V51.2
          pickup truck (traffic)
            V53.7
            nontraffic V53.2
          railway vehicle (traffic)
            V55.7
            nontraffic V55.2
          specified vehicle NEC
            (traffic) V56.7
            nontraffic V56.2
          stationary object (traffic)
            V57.7
            nontraffic V57.2
          streetcar (traffic) V56.7
            nontraffic V56.2
          three wheeled motor
            vehicle (traffic) V52.7
            nontraffic V52.2
          truck (traffic) V54.7
            nontraffic V54.2
          two wheeled motor
            vehicle (traffic) V52.7
            nontraffic V52.2
          van (traffic) V53.7
            nontraffic V53.2
        noncollision accident
          (traffic) V58.7
          nontraffic V58.2
      passenger
        collision (with)
          animal (traffic) V50.6
            being ridden (traffic)
              V56.6
              nontraffic V56.1
            nontraffic V50.1
          animal-drawn vehicle
            (traffic) V56.6
            nontraffic V56.1
          bus (traffic) V54.6
            nontraffic V54.1
          car (traffic) V53.6
            nontraffic V53.1

Accident (continued)
  transport (continued)
    van occupant (continued)
      passenger (continued)
        collision (with)
          motor vehicle NOS
            (traffic) V59.50
            nontraffic V59.10
            specified type NEC
              (traffic) V59.59
              nontraffic V59.19
          pedal cycle (traffic) V51.6
            nontraffic V51.1
          pickup truck (traffic)
            V53.6
            nontraffic V53.1
          railway vehicle (traffic)
            V55.6
            nontraffic V55.1
          specified vehicle NEC
            (traffic) V56.6
            nontraffic V56.1
          stationary object (traffic)
            V57.6
            nontraffic V57.1
          streetcar (traffic) V56.6
            nontraffic V56.1
          three wheeled motor
            vehicle (traffic) V52.6
            nontraffic V52.1
          truck (traffic) V54.6
            nontraffic V54.1
          two wheeled motor
            vehicle (traffic) V52.6
            nontraffic V52.1
          van (traffic) V53.6
            nontraffic V53.1
        noncollision accident
          (traffic) V58.6
          nontraffic V58.1
      specified type NEC V59.88
      military vehicle V59.81
    watercraft occupant
      —see Accident, watercraft
  vehicle NEC V89.9
    animal-drawn NEC —see
      Accident, transport, animal-
      drawn vehicle occupant
    special
      agricultural —see Accident,
        transport, agricultural
        vehicle occupant
      construction —see Accident,
        transport, construction
        vehicle occupant
      industrial —see Accident,
        transport, industrial vehicle
        occupant
    three-wheeled NEC (motorized)
      —see Accident, transport,
      three-wheeled motor vehicle
      occupant
  watercraft V94.9
    causing
      drowning —see Drowning,
        due to, accident to,
        watercraft
      injury NEC V91.89
        crushed between craft and
          object V91.19
        powered craft V91.13
          ferry boat V91.11
          fishing boat V91.12
          jetskis V91.13
          liner V91.11
          merchant ship V91.10
          passenger ship V91.11
        unpowered craft V91.18
          canoe V91.15
          inflatable V91.16
          kayak V91.15

Accident (continued)
 watercraft (continued)
  causing (continued)
   injury NEC (continued)
    crushed between craft and object (continued)
     unpowered craft (continued)
      sailboat V91.14
      surf-board V91.18
      windsurfer V91.18
    fall on board V91.29
     powered craft V91.23
      ferry boat V91.21
      fishing boat V91.22
      jetskis V91.23
      liner V91.21
      merchant ship V91.20
      passenger ship V91.21
     unpowered craft
      canoe V91.25
      inflatable V91.26
      kayak V91.25
      sailboat V91.24
    fire on board causing burn V91.09
     powered craft V91.03
      ferry boat V91.01
      fishing boat V91.02
      jetskis V91.03
      liner V91.01
      merchant ship V91.00
      passenger ship V91.01
     unpowered craft V91.08
      canoe V91.05
      inflatable V91.06
      kayak V91.05
      sailboat V91.04
      surf-board V91.08
      water skis V91.07
      windsurfer V91.08
    hit by falling object V91.39
     powered craft V91.33
      ferry boat V91.31
      fishing boat V91.32
      jetskis V91.33
      liner V91.31
      merchant ship V91.30
      passenger ship V91.31
     unpowered craft V91.38
      canoe V91.35
      inflatable V91.36
      kayak V91.35
      sailboat V91.34
      surf-board V91.38
      water skis V91.37
      windsurfer V91.38
    specified type NEC V91.89
     powered craft V91.83
      ferry boat V91.81
      fishing boat V91.82
      jetskis V91.83
      liner V91.81
      merchant ship V91.80
      passenger ship V91.81
     unpowered craft V91.88
      canoe V91.85
      inflatable V91.86
      kayak V91.85
      sailboat V91.84
      surf-board V91.88
      water skis V91.87
      windsurfer V91.88
   due to, caused by cataclysm — see Forces of nature, by type
  military NEC V94.818
   with civilian watercraft V94.810
    civilian in water injured by V94.811

Accident (continued)
 watercraft (continued)
  nonpowered, struck by
   nonpowered vessel V94.22
   powered vessel V94.21
  specified type NEC V94.89
  striking swimmer
   powered V94.11
   unpowered V94.12

Acid throwing (assault) Y08.89

Activity (involving) (of victim at time of event) Y93.9
 aerobic and step exercise (class) Y93.A3
 alpine skiing Y93.23
 animal care NEC Y93.K9
 arts and handcrafts NEC Y93.D9
 athletics NEC Y93.79
 athletics played as a team or group NEC Y93.69
 athletics played individually NEC Y93.59
 baking Y93.G3
 ballet Y93.41
 barbells Y93.B3
 BASE (Building, Antenna, Span, Earth) jumping Y93.33
 baseball Y93.64
 basketball Y93.67
 bathing (personal) Y93.E1
 beach volleyball Y93.68
 bike riding Y93.55
 blackout game Y93.85
 boogie boarding Y93.18
 bowling Y93.54
 boxing Y93.71
 brass instrument playing Y93.J4
 building construction Y93.H3
 bungee jumping Y93.34
 calisthenics Y93.A2
 canoeing (in calm and turbulent water) Y93.16
 capture the flag Y93.6A
 cardiorespiratory exercise NEC Y93.A9
 caregiving (providing) NEC Y93 F9
  bathing Y93.F1
  lifting Y93.F2
 cellular
  communication device Y93.C2
  telephone Y93.C2
 challenge course Y93.A5
 cheerleading Y93.45
 choking game Y93.85
 circuit training Y93.A4
 cleaning
  floor Y93.E5
 climbing NEC Y93.39
  mountain Y93.31
  rock Y93.31
  wall Y93.31
 clothing care and maintenance NEC Y93.E9
 combatives Y93.75
 computer
  keyboarding Y93.C1
  technology NEC Y93.C9
 confidence course Y93.A5
 construction (building) Y93.H3
 cooking and baking Y93.G3
 cool down exercises Y93.A2
 cricket Y93.69
 crocheting Y93.D1
 cross country skiing Y93.24
 dancing (all types) Y93.41
 digging
  dirt Y93.H1
 dirt digging Y93.H1
 dishwashing Y93.G1

Activity (continued)
 diving (platform) (springboard) Y93.12
  underwater Y93.15
 dodge ball Y93.6A
 downhill skiing Y93.23
 drum playing Y93.J2
 dumbbells Y93.B3
 electronic
  devices NEC Y93.C9
   hand held interactive Y93.C2
  game playing (using) (with)
   interactive device Y93.C2
   keyboard or other stationary device Y93.C1
 elliptical machine Y93.A1
 exercise(s)
  machines ((primarily) for)
   cardiorespiratory conditioning Y93.A1
   muscle strengthening Y93.B1
  muscle strengthening (non-machine) NEC Y93.B9
 external motion NEC Y93.I9
  rollercoaster Y93.I1
 fainting game Y93.85
 field hockey Y93.65
 figure skating (pairs) (singles) Y93.21
 flag football Y93.62
 floor mopping and cleaning Y93.E5
 food preparation and clean up Y93.G1
 football (American) NOS Y93.61
  flag Y93.62
  tackle Y93.61
  touch Y93.62
 four square Y93.6A
 free weights Y93.B3
 frisbee (ultimate) Y93.74
 furniture
  building Y93.D3
  finishing Y93.D3
  repair Y93.D3
 game playing (electronic)
  using keyboard or other stationary device Y93.C1
  using interactive device Y93.C2
 gardening Y93.H2
 golf Y93.53
 grass drills Y93.A6
 grilling and smoking food Y93.G2
 grooming and shearing an animal Y93.K3
 guerilla drills Y93.A6
 gymnastics (rhythmic) Y93.43
 handball Y93.73
 handcrafts NEC Y93.D9
 hand held interactive electronic device Y93.C2
 hang gliding Y93.35
 hiking (on level or elevated terrain) Y93.01
 hockey (ice) Y93.22
  field Y93.65
 horseback riding Y93.52
 household (interior) maintenance NEC Y93.E9
 ice NEC Y93.29
  dancing Y93.21
  hockey Y93.22
  skating Y93.21
 inline roller skating Y93.51
 ironing Y93.E4
 judo Y93.75
 jumping (off) NEC Y93.39
  BASE (Building, Antenna, Span, Earth) Y93.33
  bungee Y93.34
  jacks Y93.A2
  rope Y93.56
 jumping jacks Y93.A2

Activity (continued)
 jumping rope Y93.56
 karate Y93.75
 kayaking (in calm and turbulent water) Y93.16
 keyboarding (computer) Y93.C1
 kickball Y93.6A
 knitting Y93.D1
 lacrosse Y93.65
 land maintenance NEC Y93.H9
 landscaping Y93.H2
 laundry Y93.E2
 machines (exercise)
  primarily for cardiorespiratory conditioning Y93.A1
  primarily for muscle strengthening Y93.B1
 maintenance
  exterior building NEC Y93.H9
  household (interior) NEC Y93.E9
  land Y93.H9
  property Y93.H9
 marching (on level or elevated terrain) Y93.01
 martial arts Y93.75
 microwave oven Y93.G3
 milking an animal Y93.K2
 mopping (floor) Y93.E5
 mountain climbing Y93.31
 muscle strengthening
  exercises (non-machine) NEC Y93.B9
  machines Y93.B1
 musical keyboard (electronic) playing Y93.J1
 nordic skiing Y93.24
 obstacle course Y93.A5
 oven (microwave) Y93.G3
 packing up and unpacking in moving to a new residence Y93.E6
 parasailing Y93.19
 pass out game Y93.85
 percussion instrument playing NEC Y93.J2
 personal
  bathing and showering Y93.E1
  hygiene NEC Y93.E8
  showering Y93.E1
 physical games generally associated with school recess, summer camp and children Y93.6A
 physical training NEC Y93.A9
 piano playing Y93.J1
 pilates Y93.B4
 platform diving Y93.12
 playing musical instrument
  brass instrument Y93.J4
  drum Y93.J2
  musical keyboard (electronic) Y93.J1
  percussion instrument NEC Y93.J2
  piano Y93.J1
  string instrument Y93.J3
  winds instrument Y93.J4
 property maintenance
  exterior NEC Y93.H9
  interior NEC Y93.E9
 pruning (garden and lawn) Y93.H2
 pull-ups Y93.B2
 push-ups Y93.B2
 racquetball Y93.73
 rafting (in calm and turbulent water) Y93.16
 raking (leaves) Y93.H1
 rappelling Y93.32
 refereeing a sports activity Y93.81
 residential relocation Y93.E6
 rhythmic gymnastics Y93.43
 rhythmic movement NEC Y93.49
 riding
  horseback Y93.52
  rollercoaster Y93.I1

463

Activity (continued)
rock climbing Y93.31
rollercoaster riding Y93.I1
roller skating (inline) Y93.51
rough housing and horseplay Y93.83
rowing (in calm and turbulent water) Y93.16
rugby Y93.63
running Y93.02
SCUBA diving Y93.15
sewing Y93.D2
shoveling Y93.H1
   dirt Y93.H1
   snow Y93.H1
showering (personal) Y93.E1
sit-ups Y93.B2
skateboarding Y93.51
skating (ice) Y93.21
   roller Y93.51
skiing (alpine) (downhill) Y93.23
   cross country Y93.24
   nordic Y93.24
   water Y93.17
sledding (snow) Y93.23
sleeping (sleep) Y93.84
smoking and grilling food Y93.G2
snorkeling Y93.15
snow NEC Y93.29
   boarding Y93.23
   shoveling Y93.H1
   sledding Y93.23
   tubing Y93.23
soccer Y93.66
softball Y93.64
specified NEC Y93.89
spectator at an event Y93.82
sports NEC Y93.79
   sports played as a team or group NEC Y93.69
   sports played individually NEC Y93.59
springboard diving Y93.12
squash Y93.73
stationary bike Y93.A1
step (stepping) exercise (class) Y93.A3
stepper machine Y93.A1
stove Y93.G3
string instrument playing Y93.J3
surfing Y93.18
   wind Y93.18
swimming Y93.11
tackle football Y93.61
tap dancing Y93.41
tennis Y93.73
tobogganing Y93.23
touch football Y93.62
track and field events (non-running) Y93.57
   running Y93.02
trampoline Y93.44
treadmill Y93.A1
trimming shrubs Y93.H2
tubing (in calm and turbulent water) Y93.16
   snow Y93.23
ultimate frisbee Y93.74
underwater diving Y93.15
unpacking in moving to a new residence Y93.E6
use of stove, oven and microwave oven Y93.G3
vacuuming Y93.E3
volleyball (beach) (court) Y93.68
wake boarding Y93.17
walking an animal Y93.K1
walking (on level or elevated terrain) Y93.01
   an animal Y93.K1
wall climbing Y93.31
warm up and cool down exercises Y93.A2

Activity (continued)
water NEC Y93.19
   aerobics Y93.14
   craft NEC Y93.19
   exercise Y93.14
   polo Y93.13
   skiing Y93.17
   sliding Y93.18
   survival training and testing Y93.19
weeding (garden and lawn) Y93.H2
wind instrument playing Y93.J4
windsurfing Y93.18
wrestling Y93.72
yoga Y93.42

Adverse effect of drugs —see Table of Drugs and Chemicals

Aerosinusitis —see Air, pressure

After-effect, late —see Sequelae

Air
blast in war operations —see War operations, air blast
pressure
   change, rapid
     during
         ascent W94.29
         while (in) (surfacing from)
            aircraft W94.23
            deep water diving W94.21
            underground W94.22
         descent W94.39
         in
            aircraft W94.31
            water W94.32
   high, prolonged W94.0
   low, prolonged W94.12
     due to residence or long visit at high altitude W94.11

Alpine sickness W94.11

Altitude sickness W94.11

Anaphylactic shock, anaphylaxis —see Table of Drugs and Chemicals

Andes disease W94.11

Arachnidism, arachnoidism X58

Arson (with intent to injure or kill) X97

Asphyxia, asphyxiation
by
   food (bone) (seed) —see categories T17 and T18
   gas —see also Table of Drugs and Chemicals
     legal
        execution —see Legal, intervention, gas
        intervention —see Legal, intervention, gas
from
   fire —see also Exposure, fire
     in war operations —see War operations, fire
   ignition —see Ignition
   vomitus T17.81
in war operations —see War operations, restriction of airway

Aspiration
food (any type) (into respiratory tract) (with asphyxia, obstruction respiratory tract, suffocation) —see categories T17 and T18
foreign body —see Foreign body, aspiration
vomitus (with asphyxia, obstruction respiratory tract, suffocation) T17.81

Assassination (attempt) —see Assault

Assault (homicidal) (by) (in) Y09
arson X97
bite (of human being) Y04.1
bodily force Y04.8
   bite Y04.1
   bumping into Y04.2
   sexual —see subcategories T74.0, T76.0
   unarmed fight Y04.0
bomb X96.9
   antipersonnel X96.0
   fertilizer X96.3
   gasoline X96.1
   letter X96.2
   petrol X96.1
   pipe X96.3
   specified NEC X96.8
brawl (hand) (fists) (foot) (unarmed) Y04.0
burning, burns (by fire) NEC X97
   acid Y08.89
   caustic, corrosive substance Y08.89
   chemical from swallowing caustic, corrosive substance —see Table of Drugs and Chemicals
   cigarette(s) X97
   hot object X98.9
     fluid NEC X98.2
     household appliance X98.3
     specified NEC X98.8
     steam X98.0
     tap water X98.1
     vapors X98.0
   scalding —see Assault, burning
   steam X98.0
   vitriol Y08.89
caustic, corrosive substance (gas) Y08.89
crashing of
   aircraft Y08.81
   motor vehicle Y03.8
     pushed in front of Y02.0
     run over Y03.0
     specified NEC Y03.8
cutting or piercing instrument X99.9
   dagger X99.2
   glass X99.0
   knife X99.1
   specified NEC X99.8
   sword X99.2
dagger X99.2
drowning (in) X92.9
   bathtub X92.0
   natural water X92.3
   specified NEC X92.8
   swimming pool X92.1
     following fall X92.2
dynamite X96.8
explosive(s) (material) X96.9
fight (hand) (fists) (foot) (unarmed) Y04.0
   with weapon —see Assault, by type of weapon
fire X97
firearm X95.9
   airgun X95.01
   handgun X93
   hunting rifle X94.1
   larger X94.9
     specified NEC X94.8
   machine gun X94.2
   shotgun X94.0
   specified NEC X95.8

Assault (continued)
gunshot (wound) NEC —see Assault, firearm, by type
incendiary device X97
injury Y09
   to child due to criminal abortion attempt NEC Y08.89
knife X99.1
late effect of —see X92-Y08 with 7th character S
placing before moving object NEC Y02.8
   motor vehicle Y02.0
poisoning —see categories T36-T65 with 7th character S
puncture, any part of body —see Assault, cutting or piercing instrument
pushing
   before moving object NEC Y02.8
     motor vehicle Y02.0
     subway train Y02.1
     train Y02.1
   from high place Y01
rape T74.2-
scalding —see Assault, burning
sequelae of —see X92-Y08 with 7th character S
sexual (by bodily force) T74.2-
shooting —see Assault, firearm
specified means NEC Y08.89
stab, any part of body —see Assault, cutting or piercing instrument
steam X98.0
striking against
   other person Y04.2
   sports equipment Y08.09
     baseball bat Y08.02
     hockey stick Y08.01
struck by
   sports equipment Y08.09
     baseball bat Y08.02
     hockey stick Y08.01
submersion —see Assault, drowning
violence Y09
weapon Y09
   blunt Y00
   cutting or piercing —see Assault, cutting or piercing instrument
   firearm —see Assault, firearm
wound Y09
   cutting —see Assault, cutting or piercing instrument
   gunshot —see Assault, firearm
   knife X99.1
   piercing —see Assault, cutting or piercing instrument
   puncture —see Assault, cutting or piercing instrument
   stab —see Assault, cutting or piercing instrument

Attack by mammals NEC W55.89

Avalanche —see Landslide

Aviator's disease —see Air, pressure

B

Barotitis, barodontalgia, barosinusitis, barotrauma (otitic) (sinus) —see Air, pressure

Battered (baby) (child) (person) (syndrome) X58

Bayonet wound W26.1
in

Bayonet wound (continued)
in (continued)
legal intervention —see Legal, intervention, sharp object, bayonet
war operations —see War operations, combat
stated as undetermined whether accidental or intentional Y28.8
suicide (attempt) X78.2

Bean in nose —see categories T17 and T18

Bed set on fire NEC
—see Exposure, fire, uncontrolled, building, bed

Beheading (by guillotine)
homicide X99.9
legal execution —see Legal, intervention

Bending, injury in (prolonged) (static) X50.1

Bends —see Air, pressure, change

Bite, bitten by
alligator W58.01
arthropod (nonvenomous) NEC W57
bull W55.21
cat W55.01
cow W55.21
crocodile W58.11
dog W54.0
goat W55.31
hoof stock NEC W55.31
horse W55.11
human being (accidentally) W50.3
with intent to injure or kill Y04.1
as, or caused by, a crowd or human stampede (with fall) W52
assault Y04.1
homicide (attempt) Y04.1
in
fight Y04.1
insect (nonvenomous) W57
lizard (nonvenomous) W59.01
mammal NEC W55.81
marine W56.31
marine animal (nonvenomous) W56.81
millipede W57
moray eel W56.51
mouse W53.01
person(s) (accidentally) W50.3
with intent to injure or kill Y04.1
as, or caused by, a crowd or human stampede (with fall) W52
assault Y04.1
homicide (attempt) Y04.1
in
fight Y04.1
pig W55.41
raccoon W55.51
rat W53.11
reptile W59.81
lizard W59.01
snake W59.11
turtle W59.21
terrestrial W59.81
rodent W53.81
mouse W53.01
rat W53.11
specified NEC W53.81
squirrel W53.21
shark W56.41
sheep W55.31
snake (nonvenomous) W59.11
spider (nonvenomous) W57
squirrel W53.21

Blast (air) **in war operations**
—see War operations, blast

Blizzard X37.2

Blood alcohol level Y90.9
less than 20mg/100ml Y90.0
presence in blood, level not specified Y90.9
20-39mg/100ml Y90.1
40-59mg/100ml Y90.2
60-79mg/100ml Y90.3
80-99mg/100ml Y90.4
100-119mg/100ml Y90.5
120-199mg/100ml Y90.6
200-239mg/100ml Y90.7

Blow X58
by law-enforcing agent, police (on duty) —see Legal, intervention, manhandling
blunt object —see Legal, intervention, blunt object

Blowing up —see Explosion

Brawl (hand) (fists) (foot) Y04.0

Breakage (accidental) (part of)
ladder (causing fall) W11
scaffolding (causing fall) W12

Broken
glass, contact with —see Contact, with, glass
power line (causing electric shock) W85

Bumping against, into (accidentally)
object NEC W22.8
with fall —see Fall, due to, bumping against, object
caused by crowd or human stampede (with fall) W52
sports equipment W21.9
person(s) W51
with fall W03
due to ice or snow W00.0
assault Y04.2
caused by, a crowd or human stampede (with fall) W52
homicide (attempt) Y04.2
sports equipment W21.9

Burn, burned, burning (accidental) (by) (from) (on)
acid NEC —see Table of Drugs and Chemicals
bed linen —see Exposure, fire, uncontrolled, in building, bed
blowtorch X08.8
with ignition of clothing NEC X06.2
nightwear X05
bonfire, campfire (controlled) —see also Exposure, fire, controlled, not in building
uncontrolled —see Exposure, fire, uncontrolled, not in building
candle X08.8
with ignition of clothing NEC X06.2
nightwear X05
caustic liquid, substance (external) (internal) NEC —see Table of Drugs and Chemicals
chemical (external) (internal) —see also Table of Drugs and Chemicals
in war operations —see War operations, fire
cigar(s) or cigarette(s) X08.8
with ignition of clothing NEC X06.2
nightwear X05
clothes, clothing NEC (from controlled fire) X06.2
with conflagration —see Exposure, fire, uncontrolled, building

Burn, burned, burning (continued)
clothes, clothing NEC (continued)
with conflagration (continued)
not in building or structure —see Exposure, fire, uncontrolled, not in building
cooker (hot) X15.8
stated as undetermined whether accidental or intentional Y27.3
suicide (attempt) X77.3
electric blanket X16
engine (hot) X17
fire, flames —see Exposure, fire
flare, Very pistol —see Discharge, firearm NEC
heat
from appliance (electrical) (household) X15.8
cooker X15.8
hotplate X15.2
kettle X15.8
light bulb X15.8
saucepan X15.3
skillet X15.3
stove X15.0
stated as undetermined whether accidental or intentional Y27.3
suicide (attempt) X77.3
toaster X15.1
in local application or packing during medical or surgical procedure Y63.5
heating
appliance, radiator or pipe X16
homicide (attempt) —see Assault, burning
hot
air X14.1
cooker X15.8
drink X10.0
engine X17
fat X10.2
fluid NEC X12
food X10.1
gases X14.1
heating appliance X16
household appliance NEC X15.8
kettle X15.8
liquid NEC X12
machinery X17
metal (molten) (liquid) NEC X18
object (not producing fire or flames) NEC X19
oil (cooking) X10.2
pipe(s) X16
radiator X16
saucepan (glass) (metal) X15.3
stove (kitchen) X15.0
substance NEC X19
caustic or corrosive NEC —see Table of Drugs and Chemicals
toaster X15.1
tool X17
vapor X13.1
water (tap) —see Contact, with, hot, tap water
hotplate X15.2
suicide (attempt) X77.3
ignition —see Ignition
in war operations —see War operations, fire
inflicted by other person X97
by hot objects, hot vapor, and steam —see Assault, burning, hot object

Burn, burned, burning (continued)
internal, from swallowed caustic, corrosive liquid, substance —see Table of Drugs and Chemicals
iron (hot) X15.8
stated as undetermined whether accidental or intentional Y27.3
suicide (attempt) X77.3
kettle (hot) X15.8
stated as undetermined whether accidental or intentional Y27.3
suicide (attempt) X77.3
lamp (flame) X08.8
with ignition of clothing NEC X06.2
nightwear X05
lighter (cigar) (cigarette) X08.8
with ignition of clothing NEC X06.2
nightwear X05
lightning —see subcategory T75.0
causing fire —see Exposure, fire
liquid (boiling) (hot) NEC X12
stated as undetermined whether accidental or intentional Y27.2
suicide (attempt) X77.2
local application of externally applied substance in medical or surgical care Y63.5
machinery (hot) X17
matches X08.8
with ignition of clothing NEC X06.2
nightwear X05
mattress —see Exposure, fire, uncontrolled, building, bed
medicament, externally applied Y63.5
metal (hot) (liquid) (molten) NEC X18
nightwear (nightclothes, nightdress, gown, pajamas, robe) X05
object (hot) NEC X19
on board watercraft
due to
accident to watercraft V91.09
powered craft V91.03
ferry boat V91.01
fishing boat V91.02
jetskis V91.03
liner V91.01
merchant ship V91.00
passenger ship V91.01
unpowered craft V91.08
canoe V91.05
inflatable V91.06
kayak V91.05
sailboat V91.04
surf-board V91.08
water skis V91.07
windsurfer V91.08
fire on board V93.09
ferry boat V93.01
fishing boat V93.02
jetskis V93.03
liner V93.01
merchant ship V93.00
passenger ship V93.01
powered craft NEC V93.03
sailboat V93.04
specified heat source NEC on board V93.19
ferry boat V93.11
fishing boat V93.12
jetskis V93.13
liner V93.11
merchant ship V93.10
passenger ship V93.11
powered craft NEC V93.13
sailboat V93.14

465

Burn, burned, burning (continued)
  pipe (hot) X16
    smoking X08.8
      with ignition of clothing NEC X06.2
        nightwear X05
  powder —see Powder burn
  radiator (hot) X16
  saucepan (hot) (glass) (metal) X15.3
    stated as undetermined whether accidental or intentional Y27.3
    suicide (attempt) X77.3
  self-inflicted X76
    stated as undetermined whether accidental or intentional Y26
  steam X13.1
    pipe X16
    stated as undetermined whether accidental or intentional Y27.8
  stated as undetermined whether accidental or intentional Y27.0
  suicide (attempt) X77.0
  stove (hot) (kitchen) X15.0
    stated as undetermined whether accidental or intentional Y27.3
    suicide (attempt) X77.3
  substance (hot) NEC X19
    boiling X12
      stated as undetermined whether accidental or intentional Y27.2
      suicide (attempt) X77.2
    molten (metal) X18
  suicide (attempt) NEC X76
    hot
      household appliance X77.3
      object X77.9
  therapeutic misadventure
    heat in local application or packing during medical or surgical procedure Y63.5
    overdose of radiation Y63.2
  toaster (hot) X15.1
    stated as undetermined whether accidental or intentional Y27.3
    suicide (attempt) X77.3
  tool (hot) X17
  torch, welding X08.8
    with ignition of clothing NEC X06.2
      nightwear X05
  trash fire (controlled)
    —see Exposure, fire, controlled, not in building
    uncontrolled —see Exposure, fire, uncontrolled, not in building
  vapor (hot) X13.1
    stated as undetermined whether accidental or intentional Y27.0
    suicide (attempt) X77.0
  Very pistol —see Discharge, firearm NEC

Butted by animal W55.82
  bull W55.22
  cow W55.22
  goat W55.32
  horse W55.12
  pig W55.42
  sheep W55.32

C

Caisson disease —see Air, pressure, change
Campfire (exposure to) (controlled)
  —see also Exposure, fire, controlled, not in building

Camfire (continued)
  uncontrolled —see Exposure, fire, uncontrolled, not in building
Capital punishment (any means) —see Legal, intervention
Car sickness T75.3
Casualty (not due to war) NEC X58
  war —see War operations
Cat
  bite W55.01
  scratch W55.03
Cataclysm, cataclysmic (any injury) NEC —see Forces of nature
Catching fire —see Exposure, fire
Caught
  between
    folding object W23.0
    objects (moving) W23.0
      and
        machinery —see Contact, with, by type of machine
        stationary W23.2
      stationary W23.1
        and moving W23.2
    sliding door and door frame W23.0
  by, in
    machinery (moving parts of) —see Contact, with, by type of machine
    washing-machine wringer W23.0
  under packing crate (due to losing grip) W23.1
Cave-in caused by cataclysmic earth surface movement or eruption —see Landslide
Change(s) in air pressure —see Air, pressure, change
Choked, choking (on) (any object except food or vomitus)
  food (bone) (seed) —see categories T17 and T18
  vomitus T17.81-
Civil insurrection —see War operations
Cloudburst (any injury) X37.8
Cold, exposure to (accidental) (excessive) (extreme) (natural) (place) NEC —see Exposure, cold
Collapse
  building W20.1
    burning (uncontrolled fire) X00.2
  dam or man-made structure (causing earth movement) X36.0
  machinery —see Contact, with, by type of machine
  structure W20.1
    burning (uncontrolled fire) X00.2
Collision (accidental) NEC —see also Accident, transport V89.9
  pedestrian W51
    with fall W03
    due to ice or snow W00.0
      involving pedestrian conveyance —see Accident, transport, pedestrian, conveyance
    and
      crowd or human stampede (with fall) W52
      object W22.8
        with fall —see Fall, due to, bumping against, object
  person(s) —see Collision, pedestrian
  transport vehicle NEC V89.9

Collision (continued)
  transport vehicle NEC (continued)
    and
      avalanche, fallen or not moving —see Accident, transport
        falling or moving —see Landslide
      landslide, fallen or not moving —see Accident, transport
        falling or moving —see Landslide
    due to cataclysm —see Forces of nature, by type
    intentional, purposeful suicide (attempt) —see Suicide, collision
Combustion, spontaneous —see Ignition
Complication (delayed) of or following (medical or surgical procedure) Y84.9
  with misadventure —see Misadventure
  amputation of limb(s) Y83.5
  anastomosis (arteriovenous) (blood vessel) (gastrojejunal) (tendon) (natural or artificial material) Y83.2
  aspiration (of fluid) Y84.4
    tissue Y84.8
  biopsy Y84.8
  blood
    sampling Y84.7
    transfusion
      procedure Y84.8
  bypass Y83.2
  catheterization (urinary) Y84.6
    cardiac Y84.0
  colostomy Y83.3
  cystostomy Y83.3
  dialysis (kidney) Y84.1
  drug —see Table of Drugs and Chemicals
  due to misadventure —see Misadventure
  duodenostomy Y83.3
  electroshock therapy Y84.3
  external stoma, creation of Y83.3
  formation of external stoma Y83.3
  gastrostomy Y83.3
  graft Y83.2
  hypothermia (medically-induced) Y84.8
  implant, implantation (of)
    artificial
      internal device (cardiac pacemaker) (electrodes in brain) (heart valve prosthesis) (orthopedic) Y83.1
      material or tissue (for anastomosis or bypass) Y83.2
    with creation of external stoma Y83.3
    natural tissues (for anastomosis or bypass) Y83.2
      with creation of external stoma Y83.3
  infusion
    procedure Y84.8
  injection —see Table of Drugs and Chemicals
    procedure Y84.8
  insertion of gastric or duodenal sound Y84.5
  insulin-shock therapy Y84.3
  paracentesis (abdominal) (thoracic) (aspirative) Y84.4

Complication (continued)
  procedures other than surgical operation —see Complication of or following, by type of procedure
  radiological procedure or therapy Y84.2
  removal of organ (partial) (total) NEC Y83.6
  sampling
    blood Y84.7
    fluid NEC Y84.4
    tissue Y84.8
  shock therapy Y84.3
  surgical operation NEC —see also Complication of or following, by type of operation Y83.9
    reconstructive NEC Y83.4
      with
        anastomosis, bypass or graft Y83.2
        formation of external stoma Y83.3
    specified NEC Y83.8
  transfusion —see also Table of Drugs and Chemicals
    procedure Y84.8
  transplant, transplantation (heart) (kidney) (liver) (whole organ, any) Y83.0
    partial organ Y83.4
  ureterostomy Y83.3
  vaccination —see also Table of Drugs and Chemicals
    procedure Y84.8
Compression
  divers' squeeze —see Air, pressure, change
  trachea by
    food (lodged in esophagus) —see categories T17 and T18
    vomitus (lodged in esophagus) T17.81-
Conflagration —see Exposure, fire, uncontrolled
Constriction (external)
  hair W49.01
  jewelry W49.04
  ring W49.04
  rubber band W49.03
  specified item NEC W49.09
  string W49.02
  thread W49.02
Contact (accidental)
  with
    abrasive wheel (metalworking) W31.1
    alligator W58.09
      bite W58.01
      crushing W58.03
      strike W58.02
    amphibian W62.9
      frog W62.0
      toad W62.1
    animal (nonvenomous) NEC W64
      marine W56.89
        bite W56.81
        dolphin —see Contact, with, dolphin
        fish NEC —see Contact, with, fish
        mammal —see Contact, with, mammal, marine
        orca —see Contact, with, orca
        sea lion —see Contact, with, sea lion

Contact (continued)
  with (continued)
    animal (continued)
      marine (continued)
        shark —see Contact, with, shark
        strike W56.82
      animate mechanical force NEC W64
    arrow W21.89
      not thrown, projected or falling W45.8
    arthropods (nonvenomous) W57
    axe W27.0
    band-saw (industrial) W31.2
    bayonet —see Bayonet wound
    bee(s) X58
    bench-saw (industrial) W31.2
    bird W61.99
      bite W61.91
      chicken —see Contact, with, chicken
      duck —see Contact, with, duck
      goose —see Contact, with, goose
      macaw —see Contact, with, macaw
      parrot —see Contact, with, parrot
      psittacine —see Contact, with, psittacine
      strike W61.92
      turkey —see Contact, with, turkey
    blender W29.0
    boiling water X12
      stated as undetermined whether accidental or intentional Y27.2
      suicide (attempt) X77.2
    bore, earth-drilling or mining (land) (seabed) W31.0
    buffalo —see Contact, with, hoof stock NEC
    bull W55.29
      bite W55.21
      gored W55.22
      strike W55.22
    bumper cars W31.81
    camel —see Contact, with, hoof stock NEC
    can
      lid W26.8
      opener W27.4
        powered W29.0
    cat W55.09
      bite W55.01
      scratch W55.03
    caterpillar (venomous) X58
    centipede (venomous) X58
    chain
      hoist W24.0
        agricultural operations W30.89
      saw W29.3
    chicken W61.39
      peck W61.33
      strike W61.32
    chisel W27.0
    circular saw W31.2
    cobra X58
    combine (harvester) W30.0
    conveyer belt W24.1
    cooker (hot) X15.8
      stated as undetermined whether accidental or intentional Y27.3
      suicide (attempt) X77.3
    coral X58

Contact (continued)
  with (continued)
    cotton gin W31.82
    cow W55.29
      bite W55.21
      strike W55.22
    crane W24.0
      agricultural operations W30.89
    crocodile W58.19
      bite W58.11
      crushing W58.13
      strike W58.12
    dagger W26.1
      stated as undetermined whether accidental or intentional Y28.2
      suicide (attempt) X78.2
    dairy equipment W31.82
    dart W21.89
      not thrown, projected or falling W45.8
    deer —see Contact, with, hoof stock NEC
    derrick W24.0
      agricultural operations W30.89
      hay W30.2
    dog W54.8
      bite W54.0
      strike W54.1
    dolphin W56.09
      bite W56.01
      strike W56.02
    donkey —see Contact, with, hoof stock NEC
    drill (powered) W29.8
      earth (land) (seabed) W31.0
      nonpowered W27.8
    drive belt W24.0
      agricultural operations W30.89
    dry ice —see Exposure, cold, man-made
    dryer (clothes) (powered) (spin) W29.2
    duck W61.69
      bite W61.61
      strike W61.62
    earth (-)
      drilling machine (industrial) W31.0
      scraping machine in stationary use W31.83
    edge of stiff paper W26.2
    electric
      beater W29.0
      blanket X16
      fan W29.2
        commercial W31.82
      knife W29.1
      mixer W29.0
    elevator (building) W24.0
      agricultural operations W30.89
      grain W30.3
    engine(s), hot NEC X17
    excavating machine W31.0
    farm machine W30.9
    feces —see Contact, with, by type of animal
    fer de lance X58
    fish W56.59
      bite W56.51
      shark —see Contact, with, shark
      strike W56.52
    flying horses W31.81
    forging (metalworking) machine W31.1
    fork W27.4
    forklift (truck) W24.0

Contact (continued)
  with (continued)
    forklift (continued)
      agricultural operations W30.89
    frog W62.0
    garden
      cultivator (powered) W29.3
        riding W30.89
      fork W27.1
    gas turbine W31.3
    Gila monster X58
    giraffe —see Contact, with, hoof stock NEC
    glass (sharp) (broken) W25
      with subsequent fall W18.02
      assault X99.0
      due to fall —see Fall, by type
      stated as undetermined whether accidental or intentional Y28.0
      suicide (attempt) X78.0
    goat W55.39
      bite W55.31
      strike W55.32
    goose W61.59
      bite W61.51
      strike W61.52
    hand
      saw W27.0
      tool (not powered) NEC W27.8
        powered W29.8
    harvester W30.0
    hay-derrick W30.2
    heat NEC X19
      from appliance (electrical) (household) —see Contact, with, hot, household appliance
      heating appliance X16
    heating
      appliance (hot) X16
      pad (electric) X16
    hedge-trimmer (powered) W29.3
    hoe W27.1
    hoist (chain) (shaft) NEC W24.0
      agricultural W30.89
    hoof stock NEC W55.39
      bite W55.31
      strike W55.32
    hornet(s) X58
    horse W55.19
      bite W55.11
      strike W55.12
    hot
      air X14.1
        inhalation X14.0
      cooker X15.8
      cooking
        pan X15.3
        pot X15.3
      drinks X10.0
      engine X17
      fats X10.2
      fluids NEC X12
        assault X98.2
        suicide (attempt) X77.2
        undetermined whether accidental or intentional Y27.2
      food X10.1
      gases X14.1
        inhalation X14.0
      heating appliance X16
      household appliance X15.8
        assault X98.3
        cooker X15.8
        hotplate X15.2
        kettle X15.8
        light bulb X15.8
        object NEC X19
          assault X98.8

Contact (continued)
  with (continued)
    hot (continued)
      household appliance (continued)
        object NEC (continued)
          stated as undetermined whether accidental or intentional Y27.9
          suicide (attempt) X77.8
        saucepan X15.3
        skillet X15.3
        stove X15.0
        stated as undetermined whether accidental or intentional Y27.3
        suicide (attempt) X77.3
        toaster X15.1
      kettle X15.8
      light bulb X15.8
      liquid NEC (see also Burn) X12
        drinks X10.0
        stated as undetermined whether accidental or intentional Y27.2
        suicide (attempt) X77.2
        tap water X11.8
          stated as undetermined whether accidental or intentional Y27.1
          suicide (attempt) X77.1
      machinery X17
      metal (molten) (liquid) NEC X18
      object (not producing fire or flames) NEC X19
      oil (cooking) X10.2
      pipe X16
      plate X15.2
      radiator X16
      saucepan (glass) (metal) X15.3
      skillet X15.3
      stove (kitchen) X15.0
      substance NEC X19
      tap-water X11.8
        assault X98.1
        heated on stove X12
          stated as undetermined whether accidental or intentional Y27.2
          suicide (attempt) X77.2
        in bathtub X11.0
          running X11.1
        stated as undetermined whether accidental or intentional Y27.1
        suicide (attempt) X77.1
      toaster X15.1
      tool X17
      vapors X13.1
        inhalation X13.0
      water (tap) X11.8
        boiling X12
          stated as undetermined whether accidental or intentional Y27.2
          suicide (attempt) X77.2
          heated on stove X12
            stated as undetermined whether accidental or intentional Y27.2
            suicide (attempt) X77.2
        in bathtub X11.0
          running X11.1
        stated as undetermined whether accidental or intentional Y27.1
        suicide (attempt) X77.1
    hotplate X15.2
    ice-pick W27.4
    insect (nonvenomous) NEC W57
    kettle (hot) X15.8

467

Contact (continued)
  with (continued)
    knife W26.0
      assault X99.1
      electric W29.1
      stated as undetermined whether accidental or intentional Y28.1
      suicide (attempt) X78.1
    lathe (metalworking) W31.1
      turnings W45.8
      woodworking W31.2
    lawnmower (powered) (ridden) W28
      causing electrocution W86.8
        suicide (attempt) X83.1
      unpowered W27.1
    lift, lifting (devices) W24.0
      agricultural operations W30.89
      shaft W24.0
    liquefied gas —see Exposure, cold, man-made
    liquid air, hydrogen, nitrogen —see Exposure, cold, man-made
    lizard (nonvenomous) W59.09
      bite W59.01
      strike W59.02
    llama —see Contact, with, hoof stock NEC
    macaw W61.19
      bite W61.11
      strike W61.12
    machine, machinery W31.9
      abrasive wheel W31.1
      agricultural including animal-powered W30.9
        combine harvester W30.0
        grain storage elevator W30.3
        hay derrick W30.2
        power take-off device W30.1
        reaper W30.0
        specified NEC W30.89
        thresher W30.0
        transport vehicle, stationary W30.81
      band saw W31.2
      bench saw W31.2
      circular saw W31.2
      commercial NEC W31.82
      drilling, metal (industrial) W31.1
      earth-drilling W31.0
      earthmoving or scraping W31.89
      excavating W31.89
      forging machine W31.1
      gas turbine W31.3
      hot X17
      internal combustion engine W31.3
      land drill W31.0
      lathe W31.1
      lifting (devices) W24.0
      metal drill W31.1
      metalworking (industrial) W31.1
      milling, metal W31.1
      mining W31.0
      molding W31.2
      overhead plane W31.2
      power press, metal W31.1
      prime mover W31.3
      printing W31.89
      radial saw W31.2
      recreational W31.81
      roller-coaster W31.81
      rolling mill, metal W31.1

Contact (continued)
  with (continued)
    machine, machinery (continued)
      sander W31.2
      seabed drill W31.0
      shaft
        hoist W31.0
        lift W31.0
        specified NEC W31.89
      spinning W31.89
      steam engine W31.3
      transmission W24.1
      undercutter W31.0
      water driven turbine W31.3
      weaving W31.89
      woodworking or forming (industrial) W31.2
    mammal (feces) (urine) W55.89
      bull —see Contact, with, bull
      cat —see Contact, with, cat
      cow —see Contact, with, cow
      goat —see Contact, with, goat
      hoof stock —see Contact, with, hoof stock
      horse —see Contact, with, horse
      marine W56.39
        dolphin —see Contact, with, dolphin
        orca —see Contact, with, orca
        sea lion —see Contact, with, sea lion
        specified NEC W56.39
          bite W56.31
          strike W56.32
      pig —see Contact, with, pig
      raccoon —see Contact, with, raccoon
      rodent —see Contact, with, rodent
      sheep —see Contact, with, sheep
      specified NEC W55.89
        bite W55.81
        strike W55.82
    marine
      animal W56.89
        bite W56.81
        dolphin —see Contact, with, dolphin
        fish NEC —see Contact, with, fish
        mammal —see Contact, with, mammal, marine
        orca —see Contact, with, orca
        sea lion —see Contact, with, sea lion
        shark —see Contact, with, shark
        strike W56.82
    meat
      grinder (domestic) W29.0
        industrial W31.82
        nonpowered W27.4
      slicer (domestic) W29.0
        industrial W31.82
    merry go round W31.81
    metal, hot (liquid) (molten) NEC X18
    millipede W57
    nail W45.0
      gun W29.4
    needle (sewing) W27.3
      hypodermic W46.0
        contaminated W46.1
    object (blunt) NEC
      hot NEC X19

Contact (continued)
  with (continued)
    object (continued)
      legal intervention —see Legal, intervention, blunt object
      sharp NEC W45.8
        inflicted by other person NEC W45.8
          stated as intentional homicide (attempt) —see Assault, cutting or piercing instrument
        legal intervention —see Legal, intervention, sharp object
        self-inflicted X78.9
    orca W56.29
      bite W56.21
      strike W56.22
    overhead plane W31.2
    paper (as sharp object) W26.2
    paper-cutter W27.5
    parrot W61.09
      bite W61.01
      strike W61.02
    pig W55.49
      bite W55.41
      strike W55.42
    pipe, hot X16
    pitchfork W27.1
    plane (metal) (wood) W27.0
      overhead W31.2
    plant thorns, spines, sharp leaves or other mechanisms W60
    powered
      garden cultivator W29.3
      household appliance, implement, or machine W29.8
      saw (industrial) W31.2
      hand W29.8
    printing machine W31.89
    psittacine bird W61.29
      bite W61.21
      macaw —see Contact, with, macaw
      parrot —see Contact, with, parrot
      strike W61.22
    pulley (block) (transmission) W24.0
      agricultural operations W30.89
    raccoon W55.59
      bite W55.51
      strike W55.52
    radial-saw (industrial) W31.2
    radiator (hot) X16
    rake W27.1
    rattlesnake X58
    reaper W30.0
    reptile W59.89
      lizard —see Contact, with, lizard
      snake —see Contact, with, snake
      specified NEC W59.89
        bite W59.81
        crushing W59.83
        strike W59.82
      turtle —see Contact, with, turtle
    rivet gun (powered) W29.4
    road scraper —see Accident, transport, construction vehicle
    rodent (feces) (urine) W53.89
      bite W53.81
      mouse W53.09
        bite W53.01
      rat W53.19
        bite W53.11

Contact (continued)
  with (continued)
    rodent (continued)
      specified NEC W53.89
        bite W53.81
      squirrel W53.29
        bite W53.21
    roller coaster W31.81
    rope NEC W24.0
      agricultural operations W30.89
    saliva —see Contact, with, by type of animal
    sander W29.8
      industrial W31.2
    saucepan (hot) (glass) (metal) X15.3
    saw W27.0
      band (industrial) W31.2
      bench (industrial) W31.2
      chain W29.3
      hand W27.0
    sawing machine, metal W31.1
    scissors W27.2
    scorpion X58
    screwdriver W27.0
      powered W29.8
    sea
      anemone, cucumber or urchin (spine) X58
      lion W56.19
        bite W56.11
        strike W56.12
    serpent —see Contact, with, snake, by type
    sewing-machine (electric) (powered) W29.2
      not powered W27.8
    shaft (hoist) (lift) (transmission) NEC W24.0
      agricultural W30.89
    shark W56.49
      bite W56.41
      strike W56.42
    sharp object(s) W26.9
      specified NEC W26.8
    shears (hand) W27.2
      powered (industrial) W31.1
        domestic W29.2
    sheep W55.39
      bite W55.31
      strike W55.32
    shovel W27.8
      steam —see Accident, transport, construction vehicle
    snake (nonvenomous) W59.19
      bite W59.11
      crushing W59.13
      strike W59.12
    spade W27.1
    spider (venomous) X58
    spin-drier W29.2
    spinning machine W31.89
    splinter W45.8
    sports equipment W21.9
    staple gun (powered) W29.8
    steam X13.1
      engine W31.3
      inhalation X13.0
      pipe X16
      shovel W31.89
    stove (hot) (kitchen) X15.0
    substance, hot NEC X19
      molten (metal) X18
    sword W26.1
      assault X99.2
      stated as undetermined whether accidental or intentional Y28.2
      suicide (attempt) X78.2

Contact (continued)
  with (continued)
    tarantula X58
    thresher W30.0
    tin can lid W26.8
    toad W62.1
    toaster (hot) X15.1
    tool W27.8
      hand (not powered) W27.8
        auger W27.8
        axe W27.0
        can opener W27.4
        chisel W27.0
        fork W27.4
        garden W27.1
        handsaw W27.0
        hoe W27.1
        ice-pick W27.4
        kitchen utensil W27.4
        manual
          lawn mower W27.1
          sewing machine W27.8
        meat grinder W27.4
        needle (sewing) W27.3
          hypodermic W46.0
            contaminated W46.1
        paper cutter W27.5
        pitchfork W27.1
        rake W27.1
        scissors W27.2
        screwdriver W27.0
        specified NEC W27.8
        workbench W27.0
    hot X17
    powered W29.8
      blender W29.0
        commercial W31.82
      can opener W29.0
        commercial W31.82
      chainsaw W29.3
      clothes dryer W29.2
        commercial W31.82
      dishwasher W29.2
        commercial W31.82
      edger W29.3
      electric fan W29.2
        commercial W31.82
      electric knife W29.1
      food processor W29.0
        commercial W31.82
      garbage disposal W29.0
        commercial W31.82
      garden tool W29.3
      hedge trimmer W29.3
      ice maker W29.0
        commercial W31.82
      kitchen appliance
        W29.0
        commercial W31.82
      lawn mower W28
      meat grinder W29.0
        commercial W31.82
      mixer W29.0
        commercial W31.82
      rototiller W29.3
      sewing machine W29.2
        commercial W31.82
      washing machine W29.2
        commercial W31.82
    transmission device (belt, cable, chain, gear, pinion, shaft) W24.1
      agricultural operations W30.89
    turbine (gas) (water-driven) W31.3
    turkey W61.49
      peck W61.43
      strike W61.42
    turtle (nonvenomous) W59.29
      bite W59.21

Contact (continued)
  with (continued)
    turtle (continued)
      strike W59.22
      terrestrial W59.89
        bite W59.81
        crushing W59.83
        strike W59.82
    under-cutter W31.0
    urine —see Contact, with, by type of animal
    vehicle
      agricultural use (transport)
        —see Accident, transport, agricultural vehicle
        not on public highway W30.81
      industrial use (transport)
        —see Accident, transport, industrial vehicle
        not on public highway W31.83
      off-road use (transport)
        —see Accident, transport, all-terrain or off-road vehicle
        not on public highway W31.83
    special construction use (transport)
      —see Accident, transport, construction vehicle
      not on public highway W31.83
    venomous
      animal X58
      arthropods X58
      lizard X58
      marine animal NEC X58
      marine plant NEC X58
      millipedes (tropical) X58
      plant(s) X58
      snake X58
      spider X58
    viper X58
    washing-machine (powered) W29.2
    wasp X58
    weaving-machine W31.89
    winch W24.0
      agricultural operations W30.89
    wire NEC W24.0
      agricultural operations W30.89
    wood slivers W45.8
    yellow jacket X58
    zebra —see Contact, with, hoof stock NEC
  pressure X50.9
  stress X50.9

Coup de soleil X32

Crash
  aircraft (in transit) (powered) V95.9
    balloon V96.01
    fixed wing NEC (private) V95.21
      commercial V95.31
    glider V96.21
      hang V96.11
      powered V95.11
    helicopter V95.01
    in war operations —see War operations, destruction of aircraft
    microlight V95.11
    nonpowered V96.9
      specified NEC V96.8
    powered NEC V95.8
    stated as
      homicide (attempt) Y08.81
      suicide (attempt) X83.0

Crush (continued)
  aircraft (continued)
    ultralight V95.11
  spacecraft V95.41
  transport vehicle NEC —see also Accident, transport V89.9
    homicide (attempt) Y03.8
    motor NEC (traffic) V89.2
      homicide (attempt) Y03.8
      suicide (attempt)
        —see Suicide, collision

Cruelty (mental) (physical) (sexual) X58

Crushed (accidentally) X58
  between objects (moving) (stationary and moving) W23.0
    stationary W23.1
  by
    alligator W58.03
    avalanche NEC —see Landslide
    cave-in W20.0
      caused by cataclysmic earth surface movement —see Landslide
    crocodile W58.13
    crowd or human stampede W52
    falling
      aircraft V97.39
        in war operations —see War operations, destruction of aircraft
      earth, material W20.0
        caused by cataclysmic earth surface movement —see Landslide
      object NEC W20.8
    landslide NEC —see Landslide
    lizard (nonvenomous) W59.09
    machinery —see Contact, with, by type of machine
    reptile NEC W59.89
    snake (nonvenomous) W59.13
  in
    machinery —see Contact, with, by type of machine

Cut, cutting (any part of body) (accidental) —see also Contact, with, by object or machine
  during medical or surgical treatment as misadventure —see Index to Diseases and Injuries, Complications
  homicide (attempt) —see Assault, cutting or piercing instrument
  inflicted by other person —see Assault, cutting or piercing instrument
  legal
    execution —see Legal, intervention
    intervention —see Legal, intervention, sharp object
  machine NEC —see also Contact, with, by type of machine W31.9
  self-inflicted —see Suicide, cutting or piercing instrument
  suicide (attempt) —see Suicide, cutting or piercing instrument

Cyclone (any injury) X37.1

D

Decapitation (accidental circumstances) NEC X58
  homicide X99.9
  legal execution —see Legal, intervention

Dehydration from lack of water X58

Deprivation X58

Derailment (accidental)
  railway (rolling stock) (train) (vehicle) (without antecedent collision) V81.7
    with antecedent collision —see Accident, transport, railway vehicle occupant
  streetcar (without antecedent collision) V82.7
    with antecedent collision —see Accident, transport, streetcar occupant

Descent
  parachute (voluntary) (without accident to aircraft) V97.29
    due to accident to aircraft —see Accident, transport, aircraft

Desertion X58

Destitution X58

Disability, late effect or sequela of injury —see Sequelae

Discharge (accidental)
  airgun W34.010
    assault X95.01
    homicide (attempt) X95.01
    stated as undetermined whether accidental or intentional Y24.0
    suicide (attempt) X74.01
  BB gun —see Discharge, airgun
  firearm (accidental) W34.00
    assault X95.9
    handgun (pistol) (revolver) W32.0
      assault X93
      homicide (attempt) X93
      legal intervention —see Legal, intervention, firearm, handgun
      stated as undetermined whether accidental or intentional Y22
      suicide (attempt) X72
    homicide (attempt) X95.9
    hunting rifle W33.02
      assault X94.1
      homicide (attempt) X94.1
      legal intervention
        injuring
          bystander Y35.032
          law enforcement personnel Y35.031
          suspect Y35.033
          unspecified person Y35.039
      stated as undetermined whether accidental or intentional Y23.1
      suicide (attempt) X73.1
    larger W33.00
      assault X94.9
      homicide (attempt) X94.9
      hunting rifle —see Discharge, firearm, hunting rifle
      legal intervention —see Legal, intervention, firearm by type of firearm
      machine gun —see Discharge, firearm, machine gun
      shotgun —see Discharge, firearm, shotgun
      specified NEC W33.09
        assault X94.8
        homicide (attempt) X94.8
        legal intervention
          injuring
            bystander Y35.092
            law enforcement personnel Y35.091

Discharge (continued)
  firearm (continued)
    larger (continued)
      specified NEC (continued)
        legal intervention (continued)
          injuring (continued)
            suspect Y35.093
            unspecified person Y35.099
        stated as undetermined whether accidental or intentional Y23.8
      specified NEC W33.09
        suicide (attempt) X73.8
      stated as undetermined whether accidental or intentional Y23.9
      suicide (attempt) X73.9
    legal intervention
      injuring
        bystander Y35.002
        law enforcement personnel Y35.001
        suspect Y35.03
        unspecified person Y35.049
      using rubber bullet
        injuring
          bystander Y35.042
          law enforcement personnel Y35.041
          suspect Y35.043
          unspecified person Y35.049
    machine gun W33.03
      assault X94.2
      homicide (attempt) X94.2
      legal intervention —see Legal, intervention, firearm, machine gun
      stated as undetermined whether accidental or intentional Y23.3
      suicide (attempt) X73.2
    pellet gun —see Discharge, airgun
    shotgun W33.01
      assault X94.0
      homicide (attempt) X94.0
      legal intervention —see Legal, intervention, firearm, specified NEC
      stated as undetermined whether accidental or intentional Y23.0
      suicide (attempt) X73.0
    specified NEC W34.09
      assault X95.8
      homicide (attempt) X95.8
      legal intervention —see Legal, intervention, firearm, specified NEC
      stated as undetermined whether accidental or intentional Y24.8
      suicide (attempt) X74.8
    stated as undetermined whether accidental or intentional Y24.9
    suicide (attempt) X74.9
    Very pistol W34.09
      assault X95.8
      homicide (attempt) X95.8
      stated as undetermined whether accidental or intentional Y24.8
      suicide (attempt) X74.8
  firework(s) W39
    stated as undetermined whether accidental or intentional Y25
  gas-operated gun NEC W34.018

Discharge (continued)
  gas-operated gun NEC (continued)
    airgun —see Discharge, airgun
    assault X95.09
    homicide (attempt) X95.09
    paintball gun —see Discharge, paintball gun
    stated as undetermined whether accidental or intentional Y24.8
    suicide (attempt) X74.09
  gun NEC —see also Discharge, firearm NEC
    air —see Discharge, airgun
    BB —see Discharge, airgun
    for single hand use —see Discharge, firearm, handgun
    hand —see Discharge, firearm, handgun
    machine —see Discharge, firearm, machine gun
    other specified —see Discharge, firearm NEC
    paintball —see Discharge, paintball gun
    pellet —see Discharge, airgun
  handgun —see Discharge, firearm, handgun
  machine gun —see Discharge, firearm, machine gun
  paintball gun W34.011
    assault X95.02
    homicide (attempt) X95.02
    stated as undetermined whether accidental or intentional Y24.8
    suicide (attempt) X74.02
  pistol —see Discharge, firearm, handgun
  flare —see Discharge, firearm, Very pistol
  pellet —see Discharge, airgun
  Very —see Discharge, firearm, Very pistol
  revolver —see Discharge, firearm, handgun
  rifle (hunting) —see Discharge, firearm, hunting rifle
  shotgun —see Discharge, firearm, shotgun
  spring-operated gun NEC W34.018
    assault X95.09
    homicide (attempt) X95.09
    stated as undetermined whether accidental or intentional Y24.8
    suicide (attempt) X74.09

Disease
  Andes W94.11
  aviator's —see Air, pressure
  range W94.11

Diver's disease, palsy, paralysis, squeeze —see Air, pressure

Diving (into water) —see Accident, diving

Dog bite W54.0

Dragged by transport vehicle NEC —see also Accident, transport V09.9

Drinking poison (accidental) —see Table of Drugs and Chemicals

Dropped (accidentally) while being carried or supported by other person W04

Drowning (accidental) W74
  assault X92.9
  due to
    accident (to)
      machinery —see Contact, with, by type of machine
      watercraft V90.89

Drowning (continued)
  due to (continued)
    accident (continued)
      watercraft (continued)
        burning V90.29
          powered V90.23
            fishing boat V90.22
            jetskis V90.23
            merchant ship V90.20
            passenger ship V90.21
          unpowered V90.28
            canoe V90.25
            inflatable V90.26
            kayak V90.25
            sailboat V90.24
            water skis V90.27
        crushed V90.39
          powered V90.33
            fishing boat V90.32
            jetskis V90.33
            merchant ship V90.30
            passenger ship V90.31
          unpowered V90.38
            canoe V90.35
            inflatable V90.36
            kayak V90.35
            sailboat V90.34
            water skis V90.37
        overturning V90.09
          powered V90.03
            fishing boat V90.02
            jetskis V90.03
            merchant ship V90.00
            passenger ship V90.01
          unpowered V90.08
            canoe V90.05
            inflatable V90.06
            kayak V90.05
            sailboat V90.04
        sinking V90.19
          powered V90.13
            fishing boat V90.12
            jetskis V90.13
            merchant ship V90.10
            passenger ship V90.11
          unpowered V90.18
            canoe V90.15
            inflatable V90.16
            kayak V90.15
            sailboat V90.14
        specified type NEC V90.89
          powered V90.83
            fishing boat V90.82
            jetskis V90.83
            merchant ship V90.80
            passenger ship V90.81
          unpowered V90.88
            canoe V90.85
            inflatable V90.86
            kayak V90.85
            sailboat V90.84
            water skis V90.87
    avalanche —see Landslide
    cataclysmic
      earth surface movement NEC —see Forces of nature, earth movement
      storm —see Forces of nature, cataclysmic storm
    cloudburst X37.8
    cyclone X37.1
    fall overboard (from) V92.09
      powered craft V92.03
        ferry boat V92.01
        fishing boat V92.02
        jetskis V92.03
        liner V92.01
        merchant ship V92.00
        passenger ship V92.01
      unpowered craft V92.08

Drowning (continued)
  due to (continued)
    fall overboard (continued)
      unpowered craft (continued)
        canoe V92.05
        inflatable V92.06
        kayak V92.05
        sailboat V92.04
        surf-board V92.08
        water skis V92.07
        windsurfer V92.08
    resulting from
      accident to watercraft —see Drowning, due to, accident to, watercraft
      being washed overboard (from) V92.29
        powered craft V92.23
          ferry boat V92.21
          fishing boat V92.22
          jetskis V92.23
          liner V92.21
          merchant ship V92.20
          passenger ship V92.21
        unpowered craft V92.28
          canoe V92.25
          inflatable V92.26
          kayak V92.25
          sailboat V92.24
          surf-board V92.28
          water skis V92.27
          windsurfer V92.28
      motion of watercraft V92.19
        powered craft V92.13
          ferry boat V92.11
          fishing boat V92.12
          jetskis V92.13
          liner V92.11
          merchant ship V92.10
          passenger ship V92.11
        unpowered craft
          canoe V92.15
          inflatable V92.16
          kayak V92.15
          sailboat V92.14
    hurricane X37.0
    jumping into water from watercraft (involved in accident) —see also Drowning, due to, accident to, watercraft without accident to or on watercraft W16.711
    tidal wave NEC —see Forces of nature, tidal wave
    torrential rain X37.8
  following
    fall
      into
        bathtub W16.211
        bucket W16.221
        fountain —see Drowning, following, fall, into, water, specified NEC
        quarry —see Drowning, following, fall, into, water, specified NEC
        reservoir —see Drowning, following, fall, into, water, specified NEC
        swimming-pool W16.011
          striking
            bottom W16.021
            wall W16.031
          stated as undetermined whether accidental or intentional Y21.3
          suicide (attempt) X71.2
        water NOS W16.41
          natural (lake) (open sea) (river) (stream) (pond) W16.111

Drowning (continued)
 following (continued)
  fall (continued)
   into (continued)
    water NOS (continued)
     natural (continued)
      striking
       bottom W16.121
       side W16.131
      specified NEC W16.311
       striking
        bottom W16.321
        wall W16.331
    overboard NEC
     —see Drowning, due to, fall overboard
   jump or dive
    from boat W16.711
     striking bottom W16.721
    into
     fountain —see Drowning, following, jump or dive, into, water, specified NEC
     quarry —see Drowning, following, jump or dive, into, water, specified NEC
     reservoir —see Drowning, following, jump or dive, into, water, specified NEC
     swimming-pool W16.511
      striking
       bottom W16.521
       wall W16.531
      suicide (attempt) X71.2
     water NOS W16.91
      natural (lake) (open sea) (river) (stream) (pond) W16.611
      specified NEC W16.811
       striking
        bottom W16.821
        wall W16.831
      striking bottom W16.621
 homicide (attempt) X92.9
 in
  bathtub (accidental) W65
   assault X92.0
   following fall W16.211
    stated as undetermined whether accidental or intentional Y21.1
   stated as undetermined whether accidental or intentional Y21.0
   suicide (attempt) X71.0
  lake —see Drowning, in, natural water
  natural water (lake) (open sea) (river) (stream) (pond) W69
   assault X92.3
   following
    dive or jump W16.611
     striking bottom W16.621
    fall W16.111
     striking
      bottom W16.121
      side W16.131
   stated as undetermined whether accidental or intentional Y21.4
   suicide (attempt) X71.3
  quarry —see Drowning, in, specified place NEC
  quenching tank —see Drowning, in, specified place NEC
  reservoir —see Drowning, in, specified place NEC

Drowning (continued)
 in (continued)
  river —see Drowning, in, natural water
  sea —see Drowning, in, natural water
  specified place NEC W73
   assault X92.8
   following
    dive or jump W16.811
     striking
      bottom W16.821
      wall W16.831
    fall W16.311
     striking
      bottom W16.321
      wall W16.331
   stated as undetermined whether accidental or intentional Y21.8
   suicide (attempt) X71.8
  stream —see Drowning, in, natural water
  swimming-pool W67
   assault X92.1
    following fall X92.2
   following
    dive or jump W16.511
     striking
      bottom W16.521
      wall W16.531
    fall W16.011
     striking
      bottom W16.021
      wall W16.031
   stated as undetermined whether accidental or intentional Y21.2
    following fall Y21.3
   suicide (attempt) X71.1
    following fall X71.2
  war operations —see War operations, restriction of airway
 resulting from accident to watercraft see Drowning, due to, accident, watercraft
 self-inflicted X71.9
  stated as undetermined whether accidental or intentional Y21.9
  suicide (attempt) X71.9

E

Earth (surface) movement NEC
 —see Forces of nature, earth movement
Earth falling (on) W20.0
 caused by cataclysmic earth surface movement or eruption —see Landslide
Earthquake (any injury) X34
Effect(s) (adverse) of
 air pressure (any)- —see Air, pressure
 cold, excessive (exposure to) —see Exposure, cold
 heat (excessive) —see Heat
 hot place (weather) —see Heat
 insolation X30
 late —see Sequelae
 motion —see Motion
 nuclear explosion or weapon in war operations —see War operations, nuclear weapon
 radiation —see Radiation
 travel —see Travel
Electric shock (accidental) (by) (in) —see Exposure, electric current

Electrocution (accidental)
 —see Exposure, electric current
Endotracheal tube wrongly placed during anesthetic procedure
Entanglement
 in
  bed linen, causing suffocation —see categories T71
  wheel of pedal cycle V19.88
Entry of foreign body or material —see Foreign body
Environmental pollution related condition —see Z57
Execution, legal (any method) —see Legal, intervention
Exhaustion
 cold —see Exposure, cold
 due to excessive exertion (see also Overexertion) X50.9
 heat —see Heat
Explosion (accidental) (of) (with secondary fire) W40.9
 acetylene W40.1
 aerosol can W36.1
 air tank (compressed) (in machinery) W36.2
 aircraft (in transit) (powered) NEC V95.9
  balloon V96.05
  fixed wing NEC (private) V95.25
   commercial V95.35
  glider V96.25
   hang V96.15
  helicopter V95.05
  in war operations —see War operations, destruction of aircraft
  microlight V95.15
  nonpowered V96.9
   specified NEC V96.8
  powered NEC V95.8
  stated as
   homicide (attempt) Y03.8
   suicide (attempt) X83.0
  ultralight V95.15
 anesthetic gas in operating room W40.1
 antipersonnel bomb W40.8
  assault X96.0
  homicide (attempt) X96.0
  suicide (attempt) X75
 assault X96.9
 bicycle tire W37.0
 blasting (cap) (materials) W40.0
 boiler (machinery), not on transport vehicle W35
  on watercraft —see Explosion, in, watercraft
 butane W40.1
 caused by other person X96.9
 coal gas W40.1
 detonator W40.0
 dump (munitions) W40.8
 dynamite W40.0
  in
   assault X96.8
   homicide (attempt) X96.8
   legal intervention
    injuring
     bystander Y35.112
     law enforcement personnel Y35.111
     unspecified person Y35.119
     suspect Y35.113
    unspecified person Y35.119
   suicide (attempt) X75

Explosion (continued)
 explosive (material) W40.9
  gas W40.1
  in blasting operation W40.0
  specified NEC W40.8
   in
    assault X96.8
    homicide (attempt) X96.8
    legal intervention
     injuring
      bystander Y35.192
      law enforcement personnel Y35.191
      suspect Y35.193
      unspecified person Y35.199
    suicide (attempt) X75
 factory (munitions) W40.8
 fertilizer bomb W40.8
  assault X96.3
  homicide (attempt) X96.3
  suicide (attempt) X75
 firearm (parts) NEC W34.19
  airgun W34.110
  BB gun W34.110
  gas, air or spring-operated gun NEC W34.118
  handgun W32.1
  hunting rifle W33.12
  larger firearm W33.10
   specified NEC W33.19
  machine gun W33.13
  paintball gun W34.111
  pellet gun W34.110
  shotgun W33.11
  Very pistol [flare] W34.19
 fire-damp W40.1
 fireworks W39
 gas (coal) (explosive) W40.1
  cylinder W36.9
   aerosol can W36.1
   air tank W36.2
   pressurized W36.3
   specified NEC W36.8
 gasoline (fumes) (tank) not in moving motor vehicle W40.1
  bomb W40.8
   assault X96.1
   homicide (attempt) X96.1
   suicide (attempt) X75
  in motor vehicle —see Accident, transport, by type of vehicle
 grain store W40.8
 grenade W40.8
  in
   assault X96.8
   homicide (attempt) X96.8
   legal intervention
    injuring
     bystander Y35.192
     law enforcement personnel Y35.191
     suspect Y35.193
     unspecified person Y35.199
    suicide (attempt) X75
 handgun (parts) —see Explosion, firearm, hangun (parts)
 homicide (attempt) X96.9
  antipersonnel bomb —see Explosion, antipersonnel bomb
  fertilizer bomb —see Explosion, fertilizer bomb
  gasoline bomb —see Explosion, gasoline bomb
  letter bomb —see Explosion, letter bomb
  pipe bomb —see Explosion, pipe bomb

471

Explosion *(continued)*
  homicide *(continued)*
    specified NEC X96.8
  hose, pressurized W37.8
  hot water heater, tank (in machinery) W35
    on watercraft —*see* Explosion, in, watercraft
  in, on
    dump W40.8
    factory W40.8
    mine (of explosive gases) NEC W40.1
    watercraft V93.59
      powered craft V93.53
        ferry boat V93.51
        fishing boat V93.52
        jetskis V93.53
        liner V93.51
        merchant ship V93.50
        passenger ship V93.51
        sailboat V93.54
  letter bomb W40.8
    assault X96.2
    homicide (attempt) X96.2
    suicide (attempt) X75
  machinery —*see also* Contact, with, by type of machine
    on board watercraft —*see* Explosion, in, watercraft
    pressure vessel —*see* Explosion, by type of vessel
  methane W40.1
  mine W40.1
  missile NEC W40.8
  mortar bomb W40.8
    in
      assault X96.8
      homicide (attempt) X96.8
      legal intervention
        injuring
          bystander Y35.192
          law enforcement personnel Y35.191
          suspect Y35.193
          unspecified person Y35.199
      suicide (attempt) X75
  munitions (dump) (factory) W40.8
  pipe, pressurized W37.8
    bomb W40.8
      assault X96.4
      homicide (attempt) X96.4
      suicide (attempt) X75
  pressure, pressurized
    cooker W38
    gas tank (in machinery) W36.3
    hose W37.8
    pipe W37.8
    specified device NEC W38
    tire W37.8
      bicycle W37.0
    vessel (in machinery) W38
  propane W40.1
  self-inflicted X75
  shell (artillery) NEC W40.8
    during war operations —*see* War operations, explosion
    in
      legal intervention
        injuring
          bystander Y35.122
          law enforcement personnel Y35.121
          suspect Y35.123
          unspecified person Y35.129
    war —*see* War operations, explosion
  spacecraft V95.45

Explosion *(continued)*
  stated as undetermined whether accidental or intentional Y25
  steam or water lines (in machinery) W37.8
  stove W40.9
  suicide (attempt) X75
  tire, pressurized W37.8
    bicycle W37.0
  undetermined whether accidental or intentional Y25
  vehicle tire NEC W37.8
    bicycle W37.0
  war operations —*see* War operations, explosion

Exposure (to) X58
  air pressure change —*see* Air, pressure
  cold (accidental) (excessive) (extreme) (natural) (place) X31
    assault Y08.89
    due to
      man-made conditions W93.8
        dry ice (contact) W93.01
          inhalation W93.02
        liquid air (contact) (hydrogen) (nitrogen) W93.11
          inhalation W93.12
        refrigeration unit (deep freeze) W93.2
        suicide (attempt) X83.2
      weather (conditions) X31
    homicide (attempt) Y08.89
    self-inflicted X83.2
  due to abandonment or neglect X58
  electric current W86.8
    appliance (faulty) W86.8
      domestic W86.0
    caused by other person Y08.89
    conductor (faulty) W86.1
    control apparatus (faulty) W86.1
    electric power generating plant, distribution station W86.1
    electroshock gun —*see* Exposure, electric current, taser
    high-voltage cable W85
    homicide (attempt) Y08.89
    legal execution —*see* Legal, intervention, specified means NEC
    lightning —*see* subcategory T75.0
    live rail W86.8
    misadventure in medical or surgical procedure in electroshock therapy Y63.4
    motor (electric) (faulty) W86.8
      domestic W86.0
    self-inflicted X83.1
    specified NEC W86.8
      domestic W86.0
    stun gun —*see* Exposure, electric current, taser
    suicide (attempt) X83.1
    taser W86.8
      assault Y08.89
      legal intervention —*see* categories Y35
      self-harm (intentional) X83.8
      undetermined intent Y33
    third rail W86.8
    transformer (faulty) W86.1
    transmission lines W85
  environmental tobacco smoke X58
  excessive
    cold —*see* Exposure, cold
    heat (natural) NEC X30
      man-made W92

Exposure *(continued)*
  factor(s) NOS X58
    environmental NEC X58
      man-made NEC W99
      natural NEC —*see* Forces of nature
    specified NEC X58
  fire, flames (accidental) X08.8
    assault X97
    campfire —*see* Exposure, fire, controlled, not in building
    controlled (in)
      with ignition (of) clothing —*see also* Ignition, clothes X06.2
        nightwear X05
      bonfire —*see* Exposure, fire, controlled, not in building
      brazier (in building or structure) —*see also* Exposure, fire, controlled, building
        not in building or structure —*see* Exposure, fire, controlled, not in building
      building or structure X02.0
        with
          fall from building X02.3
          injury due to building collapse X02.2
          from building X02.5
          smoke inhalation X02.1
          hit by object from building X02.4
          specified mode of injury NEC X02.8
      fireplace, furnace or stove —*see* Exposure, fire, controlled, building
      not in building or structure X03.0
        with
          fall X03.3
          smoke inhalation X03.1
          hit by object X03.4
          specified mode of injury NEC X03.8
      trash —*see* Exposure, fire, controlled, not in building
    fireplace —*see* Exposure, fire, controlled, building
    fittings or furniture (in building or structure) (uncontrolled) —*see* Exposure, fire, uncontrolled, building
    forest (uncontrolled) —*see* Exposure, fire, uncontrolled, not in building
    grass (uncontrolled) —*see* Exposure, fire, uncontrolled, not in building
    hay (uncontrolled) —*see* Exposure, fire, uncontrolled, not in building
    homicide (attempt) X97
    ignition of highly flammable material X04
    in, of, on, starting in
      machinery —*see* Contact, with, by type of machine
      motor vehicle (in motion) —*see also* Accident, transport, occupant by type of vehicle V87.8
        with collision —*see* Collision
      railway rolling stock, train, vehicle V81.81
        with collision —*see* Accident, transport, railway vehicle occupant

Exposure *(continued)*
  fire, flames *(continued)*
    in *(continued)*
      street car (in motion) V82.8
        with collision —*see* Accident, transport, streetcar occupant
      transport vehicle NEC —*see also* Accident, transport with collision —*see* Collision
    war operations —*see also* War operations, fire
      from nuclear explosion —*see* War operations, nuclear weapons
    watercraft (in transit) (not in transit) V91.09
      localized —*see* Burn, on board watercraft, due to, fire on board
      powered craft V91.03
        ferry boat V91.01
        fishing boat V91.02
        jet skis V91.03
        liner V91.01
        merchant ship V91.00
        passenger ship V91.01
      unpowered craft V91.08
        canoe V91.05
        inflatable V91.06
        kayak V91.05
        sailboat V91.04
        surf-board V91.08
        waterskis V91.07
        windsurfer V91.08
    lumber (uncontrolled) —*see* Exposure, fire, uncontrolled, not in building
    mine (uncontrolled) —*see* Exposure, fire, uncontrolled, not in building
    prairie (uncontrolled) —*see* Exposure, fire, uncontrolled, not in building
    resulting from
      explosion —*see* Explosion
      lightning X08.8
    self-inflicted X76
    specified NEC X08.8
    started by other person X97
    stated as undetermined whether accidental or intentional Y26
    stove —*see* Exposure, fire, controlled, building
    suicide (attempt) X76
    tunnel (uncontrolled) —*see* Exposure, fire, uncontrolled, not in building
    uncontrolled
      in building or structure X00.0
        with
          fall from building X00.3
          injury due to building collapse X00.2
          jump from building X00.5
          smoke inhalation X00.1
        bed X08.00
          due to
            cigarette X08.01
            specified material NEC X08.09
        furniture NEC X08.20
          due to
            cigarette X08.21
            specified material NEC X08.29
        hit by object from building X00.4
        sofa X08.10

Exposure *(continued)*
  fire, flames *(continued)*
    uncontrolled *(continued)*
      in building or structure *(continued)*
        sofa *(continued)*
          due to
            cigarette X08.11
            specified material NEC X08.19
        specified mode of injury NEC X00.8
      not in building or structure (any) X01.0
        with
          fall X01.3
          smoke inhalation X01.1
          hit by object X01.4
          specified mode of injury NEC X01.8
      undetermined whether accidental or intentional Y26
  forces of nature NEC —*see* Forces of nature
  G-forces (abnormal) W49.9
  gravitational forces (abnormal) W49.9
  heat (natural) NEC —*see* Heat
  high-pressure jet (hydraulic) (pneumatic) W49.9
  hydraulic jet W49.9
  inanimate mechanical force W49.9
  jet, high-pressure (hydraulic) (pneumatic) W49.9
  lightning —*see* subcategory T75.0
    causing fire —*see* Exposure, fire
  mechanical forces NEC W49.9
    animate NEC W64
    inanimate NEC W49.9
  noise W42.9
    supersonic W42.0
  noxious substance —*see* Table of Drugs and Chemical
  pneumatic jet W49.9
  prolonged in deep-freeze unit or refrigerator W93.2
  radiation —*see* Radiation
  smoke —*see also* Exposure, fire
    tobacco, second hand Z77.22
  specified factors NEC X58
  sunlight X32
    man-made (sun lamp) W89.8
      tanning bed W89.1
  supersonic waves W42.0
  transmission line(s), electric W85
  vibration W49.9
  waves
    infrasound W49.9
    sound W42.9
    supersonic W42.0
  weather NEC —*see* Forces of nature

External cause status Y99.9
  child assisting in compensated work for family Y99.8
  civilian activity done for financial or other compensation Y99.0
  civilian activity done for income or pay Y99.0
  family member assisting in compensated work for other family member Y99.8
  hobby not done for income Y99.8
  leisure activity Y99.8
  military activity Y99.1
  off-duty activity of military personnel Y99.8
  recreation or sport not for income or while a student Y99.8
  specified NEC Y99.8
  student activity Y99.8
  volunteer activity Y99.2

F

Factors, supplemental
  alcohol
    blood level
      less than 20mg/100ml Y90.0
      presence in blood, level not specified Y90.9
      20-39mg/100ml Y90.1
      40-59mg/100ml Y90.2
      60-79mg/100ml Y90.3
      80-99mg/100ml Y90.4
      100-119mg/100ml Y90.5
      120-199mg/100ml Y90.6
      200-239mg/100ml Y90.7
      240mg/100ml or more Y90.8
    presence in blood, but level not specified Y90.9
  environmental-pollution-related condition- *see* Z57
  nosocomial condition Y95
  work-related condition Y99.0

Failure
  in suture or ligature during surgical procedure Y65.2
  mechanical, of instrument or apparatus (any) (during any medical or surgical procedure) Y65.8
  sterile precautions (during medical and surgical care) —*see* Misadventure, failure, sterile precautions, by type of procedure
  to
    introduce tube or instrument Y65.4
      endotracheal tube during anesthesia Y65.3
    make curve (transport vehicle) NEC —*see* Accident, transport
    remove tube or instrument Y65.4

Fall, falling *(accidental)* W19
  building W20.1
    burning (uncontrolled fire) X00.3
  down
    embankment W17.81
    escalator W10.0
    hill W17.81
    ladder W11
    ramp W10.2
    stairs, steps W10.9
  due to
    bumping against
      object W18.00
        sharp glass W18.02
        specified NEC W18.09
        sports equipment W18.01
      person W03
        due to ice or snow W00.0
        on pedestrian conveyance —*see* Accident, transport, pedestrian, conveyance
    collision with another person W03
      due to ice or snow W00.0
      involving pedestrian conveyance —*see* Accident, transport, pedestrian, conveyance
    grocery cart tipping over W17.82
    ice or snow W00.9
      from one level to another W00.2
      on stairs or steps W00.1
      involving pedestrian conveyance —*see* Accident, transport, pedestrian, conveyance
      on same level W00.0

Fall, falling *(continued)*
  due to *(continued)*
    slipping (on moving sidewalk) W01.0
      with subsequent striking against object W01.10
        furniture W01.190
        sharp object W01.119
          glass W01.110
        power tool or machine W01.111
        specified NEC W01.118
      specified NEC W01.198
    striking against
      object W18.00
        sharp glass W18.02
        specified NEC W18.09
        sports equipment W18.01
      person W03
        due to ice or snow W00.0
        on pedestrian conveyance —*see* Accident, transport, pedestrian, conveyance
  earth (with asphyxia or suffocation (by pressure)) —*see* Earth, falling
  from, off, out of
    aircraft NEC (with accident to aircraft NEC) V97.0
      while boarding or alighting V97.1
    balcony W13.0
    bed W06
    boat, ship, watercraft NEC (with drowning or submersion) —*see* Drowning, due to, fall overboard
      with hitting bottom or object V94.0
    bridge W13.1
    building W13.9
      burning (uncontrolled fire) X00.3
    cavity W17.2
    chair W07
    cherry picker W17.89
    cliff W15
    dock W17.4
    embankment W17.81
    escalator W10.0
    flagpole W13.8
    furniture NEC W08
    grocery cart W17.82
    haystack W17.89
    high place NEC W17.89
      stated as undetermined whether accidental or intentional Y30
    hole W17.2
    incline W10.2
    ladder W11
    lifting device W17.89
    machine, machinery —*see also* Contact, with, by type of machine
      not in operation W17.89
    manhole W17.1
    mobile elevated work platform [MEWP] W17.89
    motorized mobility scooter W05.2
    one level to another NEC W17.89
      intentional, purposeful, suicide (attempt) X80
      stated as undetermined whether accidental or intentional Y30
    pit W17.2
    playground equipment W09.8
      jungle gym W09.2
      slide W09.0

Fall, falling *(continued)*
  from, off, out of *(continued)*
    playground equipment *(continued)*
      swing W09.1
    quarry W17.89
    railing W13.9
    ramp W10.2
    roof W13.2
    scaffolding W12
    scooter (nonmotorized) W05.1
      motorized mobility W05.2
    sky lift W17.89
    stairs, steps W10.9
      curb W10.1
      due to ice or snow W00.1
      escalator W10.0
      incline W10.2
      ramp W10.2
      sidewalk curb W10.1
      specified NEC W10.8
      standing
        electric scooter V00.841
        micro-mobility pedestrian conveyance V00.848
    stepladder W11
    stool W08
    storm drain W17.1
    streetcar NEC V82.6
      with antecedent collision —*see* Accident, transport, streetcar occupant
      while boarding or alighting V82.4
    structure NEC W13.8
      burning (uncontrolled fire) X00.3
    table W08
    toilet W18.11
      with subsequent striking against object W18.12
    train NEC V81.6
      during derailment (without antecedent collision) V81.7
      with antecedent collision —*see* Accident, transport, railway vehicle occupant
      while boarding or alighting V81.4
    transport vehicle after collision —*see* Accident, transport, by type of vehicle, collision
    tree W14
    vehicle (in motion) NEC —*see also* Accident, transport V89.9
      motor NEC —*see also* Accident, transport, occupant, by type of vehicle V87.8
      stationary W17.89
      while boarding or alighting —*see* Accident, transport, by type of vehicle, while boarding or alighting
    viaduct W13.8
    wall W13.8
    watercraft —*see also* Drowning, due to, fall overboard
      with hitting bottom or object V94.0
    well W17.0
    wheelchair, non-moving W05.0
      powered —*see* Accident, transport, pedestrian, conveyance occupant, specified type NEC
    window W13.4
  in, on
    aircraft NEC V97.0
      with accident to aircraft V97.0
      while boarding or alighting V97.1

473

Fall, falling (continued)
  in, on (continued)
    bathtub (empty) W18.2
      filled W16.212
        causing drowning W16.211
    escalator W10.0
    incline W10.2
    ladder W11
    machine, machinery
      —*see* Contact, with, by type of machine
    object, edged, pointed or sharp (with cut) —*see* Fall, by type
    playground equipment W09.8
      jungle gym W09.2
      slide W09.0
      swing W09.1
    ramp W10.2
    scaffolding W12
    shower W18.2
      causing drowning W16.211
    staircase, stairs, steps W10.9
      curb W10.1
      due to ice or snow W00.1
      escalator W10.0
      incline W10.2
      specified NEC W10.8
    streetcar (without antecedent collision) V82.5
      with antecedent collision
        —*see* Accident, transport, streetcar occupant
      while boarding or alighting V82.4
    train (without antecedent collision) V81.5
      with antecedent collision
        —*see* Accident, transport, railway vehicle occupant
      during derailment (without antecedent collision) V81.7
        with antecedent collision
          —*see* Accident, transport, railway vehicle occupant
      while boarding or alighting V81.4
    transport vehicle after collision —*see* Accident, transport, by type of vehicle, collision
    watercraft V93.39
      due to
        accident to craft V91.29
          powered craft V91.23
            ferry boat V91.21
            fishing boat V91.22
            jetskis V91.23
            liner V91.21
            merchant ship V91.20
            passenger ship V91.21
          unpowered craft
            canoe V91.25
            inflatable V91.26
            kayak V91.25
            sailboat V91.24
      powered craft V93.33
        ferry boat V93.31
        fishing boat V93.32
        jetskis V93.33
        liner V93.31
        merchant ship V93.30
        passenger ship V93.31
      unpowered craft V93.38
        canoe V93.35
        inflatable V93.36
        kayak V93.35
        sailboat V93.34
        surf-board V93.38
        windsurfer V93.38
  into
    cavity W17.2
    dock W17.4

Fall, falling (continued)
  into (continued)
    fire —*see* Exposure, fire, by type
    haystack W17.89
    hole W17.2
    manhole W17.1
    moving part of machinery —*see* Contact, with, by type of machine
    ocean —*see* Fall, into, water
    opening in surface NEC W17.89
    pit W17.2
    pond —*see* Fall, into, water
    quarry W17.89
    river —*see* Fall, into, water
    shaft W17.89
    storm drain W17.1
    stream —*see* Fall, into, water
    swimming pool —*see also* Fall, into, water, in, swimming pool
      empty W17.3
    tank W17.89
    water W16.42
      causing drowning W16.41
      from watercraft —*see* Drowning, due to, fall overboard
      hitting diving board W21.4
      in
        bathtub W16.212
          causing drowning W16.211
        bucket W16.222
          causing drowning W16.221
        natural body of water W16.112
          causing drowning W16.111
          striking
            bottom W16.122
              causing drowning W16.121
            side W16.132
              causing drowning W16.131
        specified water NEC W16.312
          causing drowning W16.311
          striking
            bottom W16.322
              causing drowning W16.321
            wall W16.332
              causing drowning W16.331
        swimming pool W16.012
          causing drowning W16.011
          striking
            bottom W16.022
              causing drowning W16.021
            wall W16.032
              causing drowning W16.031
        utility bucket W16.222
          causing drowning W16.221
    well W17.0
  involving
    bed W06
    chair W07
    furniture NEC W08
    glass —*see* Fall, by type
    playground equipment W09.8
      jungle gym W09.2
      slide W09.0
      swing W09.1

Fall, falling (continued)
  involvin (continued)
    roller blades —*see* Accident, transport, pedestrian, conveyance
    skateboard(s) —*see* Accident, transport, pedestrian, conveyance
    skates (ice) (in line) (roller) —*see* Accident, transport, pedestrian, conveyance
    skis —*see* Accident, transport, pedestrian, conveyance
    table W08
    wheelchair, non-moving W05.0
      powered —*see* Accident, transport, pedestrian, conveyance, specified type NEC
  object —*see* Struck by, object, falling
  off
    toilet W18.11
      with subsequent striking against object W18.12
  on same level W18.30
    due to
      specified NEC W18.39
      stepping on an object W18.31
  out of
    bed W06
    building NEC W13.8
    chair W07
    furniture NEC W08
    wheelchair, non-moving W05.0
      powered —*see* Accident, transport, pedestrian, conveyance, specified type NEC
    window W13.4
  over
    animal W01.0
    cliff W15
    embankment W17.81
    small object W01.0
  rock W20.8
  same level W18.30
    from
      being crushed, pushed, or stepped on by a crowd or human stampede W52
      collision, pushing, shoving, by or with other person W03
      slipping, stumbling, tripping W01.0
    involving ice or snow W00.0
      involving skates (ice) (roller), skateboard, skis —*see* Accident, transport, pedestrian, conveyance
  snowslide (avalanche) —*see* Landslide
  stone W20.8
  structure W20.1
    burning (uncontrolled fire) X00.3
  through
    bridge W13.1
    floor W13.3
    roof W13.2
    wall W13.8
    window W13.4
  timber W20.8
  tree (caused by lightning) W20.8
  while being carried or supported by other person(s) W04

Fallen on by
  animal (not being ridden) NEC W55.89

Felo-de-se —*see* Suicide

Fight (hand) (fists) (foot)
  —*see* Assault, fight

Fire (accidental) —*see* Exposure, fire

Firearm discharge
  —*see* Discharge, firearm

Fireball effects from nuclear explosion in war operations —*see* War operations, nuclear weapons

Fireworks (explosion) W39

Flash burns from explosion
  —*see* Explosion

Flood (any injury) (caused by) X38
  collapse of man-made structure causing earth movement X36.0
  tidal wave —*see* Forces of nature, tidal wave

Food (any type) in
  air passages (with asphyxia, obstruction, or suffocation) —*see* categories T17 and T18
  alimentary tract causing asphyxia (due to compression of trachea) —*see* categories T17 and T18

Forces of nature X39.8
  avalanche X36.1
    causing transport accident —*see* Accident, transport, by type of vehicle
  blizzard X37.2
  cataclysmic storm X37.9
    with flood X38
    blizzard X37.2
    cloudburst X37.8
    cyclone X37.1
    dust storm X37.3
    hurricane X37.0
    specified storm NEC X37.8
    storm surge X37.0
    tornado X37.1
    twister X37.1
    typhoon X37.0
  cloudburst X37.8
  cold (natural) X31
  cyclone X37.1
  dam collapse causing earth movement X36.0
  dust storm X37.3
  earth movement X36.1
    earthquake X34
    caused by dam or structure collapse X36.0
  earthquake X34
  flood (caused by) X38
    dam collapse X36.0
    tidal wave —*see* Forces of nature, tidal wave
  heat (natural) X30
  hurricane X37.0
  landslide X36.1
    causing transport accident —*see* Accident, transport, by type of vehicle
  lightning —*see subcategory* T75.0
    causing fire —*see* Exposure, fire
  mudslide X36.1
    causing transport accident —*see* Accident, transport, by type of vehicle
  radiation (natural) X39.08
    radon X39.01
  radon X39.01
  specified force NEC X39.8
  storm surge X37.0

Forces of nature *(continued)*
structure collapse causing earth movement X36.0
sunlight X32
tidal wave X37.41
  due to
    earthquake X37.41
    landslide X37.43
    storm X37.42
    volcanic eruption X37.41
tornado X37.1
tsunami X37.41
twister X37.1
typhoon X37.0
volcanic eruption X35

Foreign body
aspiration —*see* Index to Diseases and Injuries, Foreign body, respiratory tract
embedded in skin W45.-
entering through
  natural orifice W44.9
    audio device W44.G1
    battery W44.A0
      button W44.A1
      cylindrical W44.A9
      other specified NEC W44.A9
    bezoar W44.F1
    bottle cap W44.E9
    can lid W44.E9
      combination metal and plastic
      jewelry W44.G3
      toy and toy part W44.G2
    dagger W44.H2
    dart W44.H1
    ear buds W44.G1
    food W44.F3
    glass W44.C0
      intact W44.C2
        bottle W44.C2
      shard W44.C1
      sharp W44.C1
    hearing aids W44.G1
    insect W44.F4
    knife W44.H2
    magnetic metal W44.D0
      bead W44.D1
      coin W44.D2
      jewelry W44.D4
      object specified NEC W44.D9
      toy W44.D3
    needle (hypodermic) (sewing) W44.H1
    non-magnetic metal W44.E0
      bead W44.E1
      coin W44.E2
      jewelry W44.E4
      object specified NEC W44.E9
      toy W44.E3
    objects of natural or organic material W44.F0
      specified NEC W44.F9
    other
      non-organic objects W44.G0
        specified NEC W44.G9
      sharp object unspecified W44.H0
    plastic
      bead W44.B1
      bottle W44.B5
      coin W44.B2
      jewelry W44.B4
      object W44.B0
        specified NEC W44.B9
      toy and toy part W44.B3

entering *(continued)*
natural orifice *(continued)*
    pull tab W44.E9
    rubber band W44.F2
    safety pin W44.H1
    specified NEC W44.8
    sword W44.H2
  skin W45.8
    can lid W26.8
    nail W45.0
    paper W26.2
    specified NEC W45.8
    splinter W45.8

Forest fire (exposure to) —*see* Exposure, fire, uncontrolled, not in building

Found injured X58
from exposure (to) —*see* Exposure
on
  highway, road (way), street V89.9
  railway right of way V81.9

Fracture (circumstances unknown or unspecified) X58
due to specified cause NEC X58

Freezing —*see* Exposure, cold

Frostbite X31
due to man-made conditions —*see* Exposure, cold, man-made

Frozen —*see* Exposure, cold

G

Gored by bull W55.22
Gunshot wound W34.00

H

Hailstones, injured by X39.8
Hanged herself or himself —*see* Hanging, self-inflicted
Hanging (accidental) —*see also* category T71
legal execution —*see* Legal, intervention, specified means NEC
Heat (effects of) (excessive) X30
  due to
    man-made conditions W92
      on board watercraft V93.29
        fishing boat V93.22
        merchant ship V93.20
        passenger ship V93.21
        sailboat V93.24
        specified powered craft NEC V93.23
    weather (conditions) X30
  from
    electric heating apparatus causing burning X16
    nuclear explosion in war operations —*see* War operations, nuclear weapons
    inappropriate in local application or packing in medical or surgical procedure Y63.5

Hemorrhage
delayed following medical or surgical treatment without mention of misadventure —*see* Index to Diseases and Injuries, Complication(s)
during medical or surgical treatment as misadventure —*see* Index to Diseases and Injuries, Complication(s)

High
altitude (effects) —*see* Air, pressure, low
level of radioactivity, effects —*see* Radiation
pressure (effects) —*see* Air, pressure, high
temperature, effects —*see* Heat

Hit, hitting (accidental) by —*see* Struck by

Hitting against —*see* Striking against

Homicide (attempt) (justifiable) —*see* Assault

Hot
place, effects —*see also* Heat
weather, effects X30

House fire (uncontrolled) —*see* Exposure, fire, uncontrolled, building

Humidity, causing problem X39.8

Hunger X58

Hurricane (any injury) X37.0

Hypobarism, hypobaropathy —*see* Air, pressure, low

I

Ictus
caloris —*see also* Heat
solaris X30

Ignition (accidental) —*see also* Exposure, fire X08.8
anesthetic gas in operating room W40.1
apparel X06.2
  from highly flammable material X04
  nightwear X05
bed linen (sheets) (spreads) (pillows) (mattress) —*see* Exposure, fire, uncontrolled, building, bed
benzine X04
clothes, clothing NEC (from controlled fire) X06.2
  from
    highly flammable material X04
ether X04
  in operating room W40.1
explosive material —*see* Explosion
gasoline X04
jewelry (plastic) (any) X06.0
kerosene X04
material
  explosive —*see* Explosion
  highly flammable with secondary explosion X04
nightwear X05
paraffin X04
petrol X04

Immersion (accidental) —*see also* Drowning
hand or foot due to cold (excessive) X31

Implantation of quills of porcupine W55.89

Inanition (from) (hunger) X58
thirst X58

Inappropriate operation performed
correct operation on wrong side or body part (wrong side) (wrong site) Y65.53
operation intended for another patient done on wrong patient Y65.52
wrong operation performed on correct patient Y65.51

Inattention after, at birth (homicidal intent) (infanticidal intent) X58

Incident, adverse
device
  anesthesiology Y70.8
    accessory Y70.2
    diagnostic Y70.0
    miscellaneous Y70.8
    monitoring Y70.0
    prosthetic Y70.2
    rehabilitative Y70.1
    surgical Y70.3
    therapeutic Y70.1
  cardiovascular Y71.8
    accessory Y71.2
    diagnostic Y71.0
    miscellaneous Y71.8
    monitoring Y71.0
    prosthetic Y71.2
    rehabilitative Y71.1
    surgical Y71.3
    therapeutic Y71.1
  gastroenterology Y73.8
    accessory Y73.2
    diagnostic Y73.0
    miscellaneous Y73.8
    monitoring Y73.0
    prosthetic Y73.2
    rehabilitative Y73.1
    surgical Y73.3
    therapeutic Y73.1
  general
    hospital Y74.8
      accessory Y74.2
      diagnostic Y74.0
      miscellaneous Y74.8
      monitoring Y74.0
      prosthetic Y74.2
      rehabilitative Y74.1
      surgical Y74.3
      therapeutic Y74.1
    surgical Y81.8
      accessory Y81.2
      diagnostic Y81.0
      miscellaneous Y81.8
      monitoring Y81.0
      prosthetic Y81.2
      rehabilitative Y81.1
      surgical Y81.3
      therapeutic Y81.1
  gynecological Y76.8
    accessory Y76.2
    diagnostic Y76.0
    miscellaneous Y76.8
    monitoring Y76.0
    prosthetic Y76.2
    rehabilitative Y76.1
    surgical Y76.3
    therapeutic Y76.1
  medical Y82.9
    specified type NEC Y82.8
  neurological Y75.8
    accessory Y75.2
    diagnostic Y75.0
    miscellaneous Y75.8
    monitoring Y75.0
    prosthetic Y75.2
    rehabilitative Y75.1
    surgical Y75.3
    therapeutic Y75.1

Incident, adverse (continued)
  device (continued)
    obstetrical Y76.8
      accessory Y76.2
      diagnostic Y76.0
      miscellaneous Y76.8
      monitoring Y76.0
      prosthetic Y76.2
      rehabilitative Y76.1
      surgical Y76.3
      therapeutic Y76.1
    ophthalmic Y77.8
      accessory Y77.2
      contact lens (rigid gas permeable) (soft (hydrophilic)) Y77.11
      diagnostic Y77.0
      miscellaneous Y77.8
      monitoring Y77.0
      prosthetic Y77.2
      rehabilitative Y77.19
      surgical Y77.3
      therapeutic Y77.19
    orthopedic Y79.8
      accessory Y79.2
      diagnostic Y79.0
      miscellaneous Y79.8
      monitoring Y79.0
      prosthetic Y79.2
      rehabilitative Y79.1
      surgical Y79.3
      therapeutic Y79.1
    otorhinolaryngological Y72.8
      accessory Y72.2
      diagnostic Y72.0
      miscellaneous Y72.8
      monitoring Y72.0
      prosthetic Y72.2
      rehabilitative Y72.1
      surgical Y72.3
      therapeutic Y72.1
    personal use Y74.8
      accessory Y74.2
      diagnostic Y74.0
      miscellaneous Y74.8
      monitoring Y74.0
      prosthetic Y74.2
      rehabilitative Y74.1
      surgical Y74.3
      therapeutic Y74.1
    physical medicine Y80.8
      accessory Y80.2
      diagnostic Y80.0
      miscellaneous Y80.8
      monitoring Y80.0
      prosthetic Y80.2
      rehabilitative Y80.1
      surgical Y80.3
      therapeutic Y80.1
    plastic surgical Y81.8
      accessory Y81.2
      diagnostic Y81.0
      miscellaneous Y81.8
      monitoring Y81.0
      prosthetic Y81.2
      rehabilitative Y81.1
      surgical Y81.3
      therapeutic Y81.1
    radiological Y78.8
      accessory Y78.2
      diagnostic Y78.0
      miscellaneous Y78.8
      monitoring Y78.0
      prosthetic Y78.2
      rehabilitative Y78.1
      surgical Y78.3
      therapeutic Y78.1
    urology Y73.8
      accessory Y73.2
      diagnostic Y73.0

Incident, adverse (continued)
  device (continued)
    urology (continued)
      miscellaneous Y73.8
      monitoring Y73.0
      prosthetic Y73.2
      rehabilitative Y73.1
      surgical Y73.3
      therapeutic Y73.1

Incineration (accidental) —see Exposure, fire

Infanticide —see Assault

Infrasound waves (causing injury) W49.9

Ingestion
  foreign body (causing injury) (with obstruction) —see Foreign body, alimentary canal
  poisonous
    plant(s) X58
    substance NEC —see Table of Drugs and Chemicals

Inhalation
  excessively cold substance, man-made —see Exposure, cold, man-made
  food (any type) (into respiratory tract) (with asphyxia, obstruction respiratory tract, suffocation) —see categories T17 and T18
  foreign body —see Foreign body, aspiration
  gastric contents (with asphyxia, obstruction respiratory passage, suffocation) T17.81-
  hot air or gases X14.0
  liquid air, hydrogen, nitrogen W93.12
    suicide (attempt) X83.2
  steam X13.0
    assault X98.0
    stated as undetermined whether accidental or intentional Y27.0
    suicide (attempt) X77.0
  toxic gas —see Table of Drugs and Chemicals
  vomitus (with asphyxia, obstruction respiratory passage, suffocation) T17.81-

Injury, injured (accidental(ly)) NOS X58
  by, caused by, from
    assault —see Assault
    law-enforcing agent, police, in course of legal intervention —see Legal intervention
    suicide (attempt) X83.8
  due to, in
    civil insurrection —see War operations
    fight —see also Assault, fight Y04.0
    war operations —see War operations
  homicide —see also Assault Y09
  inflicted (by)
    in course of arrest (attempted), suppression of disturbance, maintenance of order, by law-enforcing agents —see Legal intervention

Injury (continued)
  inflicted (continued)
    other person
      stated as
        accidental X58
        intentional, homicide (attempt) —see Assault
        undetermined whether accidental or intentional Y33
    purposely (inflicted) by other person(s) —see Assault
    self-inflicted X83.8
      stated as accidental X58
    specified cause NEC X58
    undetermined whether accidental or intentional Y33

Insolation, effects X30

Insufficient nourishment X58

Interruption of respiration (by)
  food (lodged in esophagus) —see categories T17 and T18
  vomitus (lodged in esophagus) T17.81-

Intervention, legal —see Legal intervention

Intoxication
  drug —see Table of Drugs and Chemicals
  poison —see Table of Drugs and Chemicals

J

Jammed (accidentally)
  between objects (moving) (stationary and moving) W23.0
    stationary W23.1

Jumped, jumping
  before moving object NEC X81.8
    motor vehicle X81.0
    subway train X81.1
    train X81.1
    undetermined whether accidental or intentional Y31
  from
    boat (into water) voluntarily, without accident (to or on boat) W16.712
      with
        accident to or on boat —see Accident, watercraft
        drowning or submersion W16.711
          suicide (attempt) X71.3
      striking bottom W16.722
        causing drowning W16.721
    building —see also Jumped, from, high place W13.9
      burning (uncontrolled fire) X00.5
    high place NEC W17.89
      suicide (attempt) X80
      undetermined whether accidental or intentional Y30
    structure —see also Jumped, from, high place W13.9
      burning (uncontrolled fire) X00.5
  into water W16.92
    causing drowning W16.91
    from, off watercraft —see Jumped, from, boat
    in
      natural body W16.612
        causing drowning W16.611
        striking bottom W16.622
          causing drowning W16.621

Jumped (continued)
  into water (continued)
    in (continued)
      specified place NEC W16.812
        causing drowning W16.811
        striking
          bottom W16.822
            causing drowning W16.821
          wall W16.832
            causing drowning W16.831
      swimming pool W16.512
        causing drowning W16.511
        striking
          bottom W16.522
            causing drowning W16.521
          wall W16.532
            causing drowning W16.531
    suicide (attempt) X71.3

K

Kicked by
  animal NEC W55.82
  person(s) (accidentally) W50.1
    with intent to injure or kill Y04.0
    as, or caused by, a crowd or human stampede (with fall) W52
    assault Y04.0
    homicide (attempt) Y04.0
    in
      fight Y04.0
      legal intervention
        injuring
          bystander Y35.812
          law enforcement personnel Y35.811
          suspect Y35.813
          unspecified person Y35.819

Kicking
  against
    object W22.8
      sports equipment W21.9
    stationary W22.09
      sports equipment W21.89
    person —see Striking against, person
    sports equipment W21.9
  carpet stretcher with knee X50.3

Killed, killing (accidentally)
  NOS —see also Injury X58
  in action —see War operations
  brawl, fight (hand) (fists) (foot) Y04.0
  by weapon —see also Assault
    cutting, piercing —see Assault, cutting or piercing instrument
    firearm —see Discharge, firearm, by type, homicide
  self
    stated as
      accident NOS X58
      suicide —see Suicide
      undetermined whether accidental or intentional Y33

Kneeling (prolonged) (static) X50.1

Knocked down (accidentally) (by) NOS X58
  animal (not being ridden) NEC —see also Struck by, by type of animal

Knocked down (continued)
  crowd or human stampede W52
  person W51
    in brawl, fight Y04.0
  transport vehicle NEC —*see also* Accident, transport V09.9

L

Laceration NEC —*see* Injury
Lack of
  care (helpless person) (infant) (newborn) X58
  food except as result of abandonment or neglect X58
    due to abandonment or neglect X58
  water except as result of transport accident X58
    due to transport accident —*see* Accident, transport, by type
  helpless person, infant, newborn X58
Landslide (falling on transport vehicle) X36.1
  caused by collapse of man-made structure X36.0
Late effect —*see* Sequelae
Legal
  execution (any method) —*see* Legal, intervention
  intervention (by)
    baton —*see* Legal, intervention, blunt object, baton
    bayonet —*see* Legal, intervention, sharp object, bayonet
    blow —*see* Legal, intervention, manhandling
    blunt object
      baton
        injuring
          bystander Y35.312
          law enforcement personnel Y35.311
          suspect Y35.313
          unspecified person Y35.319
        injuring
          bystander Y35.302
          law enforcement personnel Y35.301
          suspect Y35.303
          unspecified person Y35.309
        specified NEC
          injuring
            bystander Y35.392
            law enforcement personnel Y35.391
            suspect Y35.393
            unspecified person Y35.399
        stave
          injuring
            bystander Y35.392
            law enforcement personnel Y35.391
            suspect Y35.393
            unspecified person Y35.399
    bomb —*see* Legal, intervention, explosive
    conducted energy device
      injuring
        bystander Y35.832
        law enforcement personnel Y35.831
        suspect Y35.833
        unspecified person Y35.839
    cutting or piercing instrument —*see* Legal, intervention, sharp object

Legal (continued)
  intervention (continued)
    dynamite —*see* Legal, intervention, explosive, dynamite
    electroshock device (taser)
      injuring
        bystander Y35.832
        law enforcement personnel Y35.831
        suspect Y35.833
        unspecified person Y35.839
    explosive(s)
      dynamite
        injuring
          bystander Y35.112
          law enforcement personnel Y35.111
          suspect Y35.113
          unspecified person Y35.119
      grenade
        injuring
          bystander Y35.192
          law enforcement personnel Y35.191
          suspect Y35.193
          unspecified person Y35.199
      injuring
        bystander Y35.102
        law enforcement personnel Y35.101
        suspect Y35.103
        unspecified person Y35.109
      mortar bomb
        injuring
          bystander Y35.192
          law enforcement personnel Y35.191
          suspect Y35.193
          unspecified person Y35.199
      shell
        injuring
          bystander Y35.122
          law enforcement personnel Y35.121
          suspect Y35.123
          unspecified person Y35.129
      specified NEC
        injuring
          bystander Y35.192
          law enforcement personnel Y35.191
          suspect Y35.193
          unspecified person Y35.199
    firearm(s) (discharge)
      handgun
        injuring
          bystander Y35.022
          law enforcement personnel Y35.021
          suspect Y35.023
          unspecified person Y35.029
      injuring
        bystander Y35.002
        law enforcement personnel Y35.001
        suspect Y35.003
        unspecified person Y35.009
      machine gun
        injuring
          bystander Y35.012
          law enforcement personnel Y35.011
          suspect Y35.013
          unspecified person Y35.019

Legal (continued)
  intervention (continued)
    firearm (continued)
      rifle pellet
        injuring
          bystander Y35.032
          law enforcement personnel Y35.031
          suspect Y35.033
          unspecified person Y35.039
      rubber bullet
        injuring
          bystander Y35.042
          law enforcement personnel Y35.041
          suspect Y35.043
          unspecified person Y35.049
      shotgun —*see* Legal, intervention, firearm, specified NEC
      specified NEC
        injuring
          bystander Y35.092
          law enforcement personnel Y35.091
          suspect Y35.093
          unspecified person Y35.099
    gas (asphyxiation) (poisoning)
      injuring
        bystander Y35.202
        law enforcement personnel Y35.201
        suspect Y35.203
        unspecified person Y35.209
      specified NEC
        injuring
          bystander Y35.292
          law enforcement personnel Y35.291
          suspect Y35.293
          unspecified person Y35.299
      tear gas
        injuring
          bystander Y35.212
          law enforcement personnel Y35.211
          suspect Y35.213
          unspecified person Y35.219
    grenade —*see* Legal, intervention, explosive, grenade
    injuring
      bystander Y35.92
      law enforcement personnel Y35.91
      suspect Y35.93
      unspecified person Y35.99
    late effect (of) —*see* with 7th character S Y35
    manhandling
      injuring
        bystander Y35.812
        law enforcement personnel Y35.811
        suspect Y35.813
        unspecified person Y35.819
    sequelae (of) —*see* with 7th character S Y35
    sharp objects
      bayonet
        injuring
          bystander Y35.412
          law enforcement personnel Y35.411
          suspect Y35.413
          unspecified person Y35.419

Legal (continued)
  intervention (continued)
    sharp object (continued)
      injuring
        bystander Y35.402
        law enforcement personnel Y35.401
        suspect Y35.403
        unspecified person Y35.409
      specified NEC
        injuring
          bystander Y35.492
          law enforcement personnel Y35.491
          suspect Y35.493
          unspecified person Y35.499
    specified means NEC
      injuring
        bystander Y35.892
        law enforcement personnel Y35.891
        suspect Y35.893
        unspecified person Y35.899
    stabbing —*see* Legal, intervention, sharp object
    stave —*see* Legal, intervention, blunt object, stave
    stun gun
      injuring
        bystander Y35.832
        law enforcement personnel Y35.831
        suspect Y35.833
        unspecified person Y35.839
    taser
      injuring
        bystander Y35.832
        law enforcement personnel Y35.831
        suspect Y35.833
        unspecified person Y35.839
    tear gas —*see* Legal, intervention, gas, tear gas
    truncheon —*see* Legal, intervention, blunt object, stave
Lifting - *see also* Overexertion
  heavy objects X50.0
  weights X50.0
Lightning (shock) (stroke) (struck by) —*see* subcategory T75.0
  causing fire —*see* Exposure, fire
Loss of control (transport vehicle) NEC —*see* Accident, transport
Lost at sea NOS —*see* Drowning, due to, fall overboard
Low
  pressure (effects) —*see* Air, pressure, low
  temperature (effects) —*see* Exposure, cold
Lying before train, vehicle or other moving object X81.8
  subway train X81.1
  train X81.1
  undetermined whether accidental or intentional Y31
Lynching —*see* Assault

M

Malfunction (mechanism or component) (of)
  firearm W34.10
    airgun W34.110
    BB gun W34.110
    gas, air or spring-operated gun NEC W34.118
    handgun W32.1

477

Malfunction (continued)
  firearm (continued)
    hunting rifle W33.12
    larger firearm W33.10
      specified NEC W33.19
    machine gun W33.13
    paintball gun W34.111
    pellet gun W34.110
    shotgun W33.11
    specified NEC W34.19
    Very pistol [flare] W34.19
  handgun —see Malfunction, firearm, handgun

Maltreatment —see Perpetrator

Mangled (accidentally) NOS X58

Manhandling (in brawl, fight) Y04.0
  legal intervention —see Legal, intervention, manhandling

Manslaughter (nonaccidental) —see Assault

Mauled by animal NEC W55.89

Medical procedure, complication
  of (delayed or as an abnormal reaction without mention of misadventure) —see Complication of or following, by specified type of procedure
  due to or as a result of misadventure —see Misadventure

Melting (due to fire) —see also Exposure, fire
  apparel NEC X06.3
  clothes, clothing NEC X06.3
    nightwear X05
  fittings or furniture (burning building) (uncontrolled fire) X00.8
  nightwear X05
  plastic jewelry X06.1

Mental cruelty X58

Military operations (injuries to military and civilians occuring during peacetime on military property and during routine military exercises and operations) (by) (from) (involving) Y37.90-
  air blast Y37.20-
  aircraft
    destruction —see Military operations, destruction of aircraft
    airway restriction —see Military operations, restriction of airways
    asphyxiation —see Military operations, restriction of airways
  biological weapons Y37.6X-
  blast Y37.20-
  blast fragments Y37.20-
  blast wave Y37.20-
  blast wind Y37.20-
  bomb Y37.20-
    dirty Y37.50-
    gasoline Y37.31-
    incendiary Y37.31-
    petrol Y37.31-
  bullet Y37.43-
    incendiary Y37.32-
    rubber Y37.41-
  chemical weapons Y37.7X-
  combat
    hand to hand (unarmed) combat Y37.44-
    using blunt or piercing object Y37.45-

Military operations (continued)
  conflagration —see Military operations, fire
  conventional warfare NEC Y37.49-
  depth-charge Y37.01-
  destruction of aircraft Y37.10-
    due to
      air to air missile Y37.11-
      collision with other aircraft Y37.12-
      detonation (accidental) of onboard munitions and explosives Y37.14-
      enemy fire or explosives Y37.11-
      explosive placed on aircraft Y37.11-
      onboard fire Y37.13-
      rocket propelled grenade [RPG] Y37.11-
      small arms fire Y37.11-
      surface to air missile Y37.11-
    specified NEC Y37.19-
  detonation (accidental) of onboard marine weapons Y37.05-
  own munitions or munitions launch device Y37.24-
  dirty bomb Y37.50-
  explosion (of) Y37.20-
    aerial bomb Y37.21-
    bomb NOS —see also Military operations, bomb(s) Y37.20-
    fragments Y37.20-
    grenade Y37.29-
    guided missile Y37.22-
    improvised explosive device [IED] (person-borne) (roadside) (vehicle-borne) Y37.23-
    land mine Y37.29-
    marine mine (at sea) (in harbor) Y37.02-
    marine weapon Y37.00-
      specified NEC Y37.09-
    own munitions or munitions launch device (accidental) Y37.24-
    sea-based artillery shell Y37.03-
    specified NEC Y37.29-
    torpedo Y37.04-
  fire Y37.30-
    specified NEC Y37.39-
  firearms
    discharge Y37.43-
    pellets Y37.42-
  flamethrower Y37.33-
  fragments (from) (of)
    improvised explosive device [IED] (person-borne) (roadside) (vehicle-borne) Y37.26-
    munitions Y37.25-
    specified NEC Y37.29-
    weapons Y37.27-
  friendly fire Y37.92-
  hand to hand (unarmed) combat Y37.44-
  hot substances —see Military operations, fire
  incendiary bullet Y37.32-
  nuclear weapon (effects of) Y37.50-
    acute radiation exposure Y37.54-
    blast pressure Y37.51-
    direct blast Y37.51-
    direct heat Y37.53-

Military operations (continued)
  nuclear weapon (continued)
    fallout exposure Y37.54-
    fireball Y37.53-
    indirect blast (struck or crushed by blast debris) (being thrown by blast) Y37.52-
    ionizing radiation (immediate exposure) Y37.54-
    nuclear radiation Y37.54-
    radiation
      ionizing (immediate exposure) Y37.54-
      nuclear Y37.54-
      thermal Y37.53-
    specified NEC Y37.59-
    secondary effects Y37.54-
    thermal radiation Y37.53-
  restriction of air (airway)
    intentional Y37.46-
    unintentional Y37.47-
  rubber bullets Y37.41-
  shrapnel NOS Y37.29-
  suffocation —see Military operations, restriction of airways
  unconventional warfare NEC Y37.7X-
  underwater blast NOS Y37.00-
  warfare
    conventional NEC Y37.49-
    unconventional NEC Y37.7X-
  weapons
    biological weapons Y37.6X-
    chemical Y37.7X-
    nuclear (effects of) Y37.50-
      acute radiation exposure Y37.54-
      blast pressure Y37.51-
      direct blast Y37.51-
      direct heat Y37.53-
      fallout exposure Y37.54-
      fireball Y37.53-
      radiation
        ionizing (immediate exposure) Y37.54-
        nuclear Y37.54-
        thermal Y37.53-
      secondary effects Y37.54-
      specified NEC Y37.59-
    of mass destruction [WMD] Y37.91-
  weapon of mass destruction [WMD] Y37.91-

Misadventure(s) to patient(s) during surgical or medical care Y69
  contaminated medical or biological substance (blood, drug, fluid) Y64.9
    administered (by) NEC Y64.9
      immunization Y64.1
      infusion Y64.0
      injection Y64.1
      specified means NEC Y64.8
      transfusion Y64.0
      vaccination Y64.1
  excessive amount of blood or other fluid during transfusion or infusion Y63.0
  failure
    in dosage Y63.9
      electroshock therapy Y63.4
      inappropriate temperature (too hot or too cold) in local application and packing Y63.5

Misadventure(s) to patient(s) during surgical or medical care (continued)
  failure (continued)
    in dosage (continued)
      infusion
        excessive amount of fluid Y63.0
        incorrect dilution of fluid Y63.1
      insulin-shock therapy Y63.4
      nonadministration of necessary drug or biological substance Y63.6
      overdose —see Table of Drugs and Chemicals
      radiation, in therapy Y63.2
    radiation
      overdose Y63.2
      specified procedure NEC Y63.8
    transfusion
      excessive amount of blood Y63.0
    mechanical, of instrument or apparatus (any) (during any procedure) Y65.8
    sterile precautions (during procedure) Y62.9
      aspiration of fluid or tissue (by puncture or catheterization, except heart) Y62.6
      biopsy (except needle aspiration) Y62.8
        needle (aspirating) Y62.6
      blood sampling Y62.6
      catheterization Y62.6
        heart Y62.5
      dialysis (kidney) Y62.2
      endoscopic examination Y62.4
      enema Y62.8
      immunization Y62.3
      infusion Y62.1
      injection Y62.3
      needle biopsy Y62.6
      paracentesis (abdominal) (thoracic) Y62.6
      perfusion Y62.2
      puncture (lumbar) Y62.6
      removal of catheter or packing Y62.8
      specified procedure NEC Y62.8
      surgical operation Y62.0
      transfusion Y62.1
      vaccination Y62.3
    suture or ligature during surgical procedure Y65.2
    to introduce or to remove tube or instrument —see Failure, to
  hemorrhage —see Index to Diseases and Injuries, Complication(s)
  inadvertent exposure of patient to radiation Y63.3
  inappropriate
    operation performed —see Inappropriate operation performed
    temperature (too hot or too cold) in local application or packing Y63.5
  infusion —see also Misadventure, by type, infusion Y69
    excessive amount of fluid Y63.0

Misadventure(s) to patient(s) during surgical or medical care (*continued*)
  infusion (*continued*)
    incorrect dilution of fluid Y63.1
    wrong fluid Y65.1
  mismatched blood in transfusion Y65.0
  nonadministration of necessary drug or biological substance Y63.6
  overdose —*see* Table of Drugs and Chemicals
  radiation (in therapy) Y63.2
  perforation —*see* Index to Diseases and Injuries, Complication(s)
  performance of inappropriate operation —*see* Inappropriate operation performed
  puncture —*see* Index to Diseases and Injuries, Complication(s)
  specified type NEC Y65.8
    failure
      suture or ligature during surgical operation Y65.2
      to introduce or to remove tube or instrument —*see* Failure, to
    infusion of wrong fluid Y65.1
    performance of inappropriate operation —*see* Inappropriate operation performed
    transfusion of mismatched blood Y65.0
    wrong
      drug given in error —*see* Table of Drugs and Chemicals
      fluid in infusion Y65.1
      placement of endotracheal tube during anesthetic procedure Y65.3
  transfusion —*see* Misadventure, by type, transfusion
    excessive amount of blood Y63.0
    mismatched blood Y65.0
  wrong
    drug given in error —*see* Table of Drugs and Chemicals
    fluid in infusion Y65.1
    placement of endotracheal tube during anesthetic procedure Y65.3

Mismatched blood in transfusion Y65.0

Motion sickness T75.3

Mountain sickness W94.11

Mudslide (of cataclysmic nature) —*see* Landslide

Murder (attempt) —*see* Assault

N

Nail
  contact with W45.0
    gun W29.4
  embedded in skin W45.0

Neglect (criminal) (homicidal intent) X58

Noise (causing injury) (pollution) W42.9
  supersonic W42.0

Nonadministration (of)
  drug or biological substance (necessary) Y63.6
  surgical and medical care Y66

Nosocomial condition Y95

O

Object
  falling
    from, in, on, hitting
      machinery —*see* Contact, with, by type of machine
  set in motion by
    accidental explosion or rupture of pressure vessel W38
    firearm —*see* Discharge, firearm, by type
    machine (ry) —*see* Contact, with, by type of machine

Overdose (drug) —*see* Table of Drugs and Chemicals
  radiation Y63.2

Overexertion X50.9
  from
    prolonged static or awkward postures X50.1
    repetitive movements X50.3
    specified strenuous movements or postures NEC X50.9
    strenuous movement or load X50.0

Overexposure (accidental) (to)
  cold —*see also* Exposure, cold X31
    due to man-made conditions —*see* Exposure, cold, man-made
  heat —*see also* Heat X30
  radiation —*see* Radiation
  radioactivity W88.0
  sun (sunburn) X32
  weather NEC —*see* Forces of nature
  wind NEC —*see* Forces of nature

Overheated —*see* Heat

Overturning (accidental)
  machinery —*see* Contact, with, by type of machine
  transport vehicle NEC —*see also* Accident, transport V89.9
  watercraft (causing drowning, submersion) —*see also* Drowning, due to, accident to, watercraft, overturning
    causing injury except drowning or submersion —*see* Accident, watercraft, causing, injury NEC

P

Parachute descent (voluntary) (without accident to aircraft) V97.29
  due to accident to aircraft —*see* Accident, transport, aircraft

Pecked by bird W61.99

Perforation during medical or surgical treatment as misadventure —*see* Index to Diseases and Injuries, Complication(s)

Perpetrator, perpetration, of assault, maltreatment and neglect (by) Y07.9
  acquaintance Y07.54
  aunt Y07.47
  boyfriend
    current Y07.030
    former Y07.031
  brother Y07.410
    stepbrother Y07.435
  child (adopted) (biological) (foster) (in-law) (step) Y07.44
  coach Y07.53
  cousin
    female Y07.491
    male Y07.490
  daughter (adopted) (biological) (foster) (in-law) (step) Y07.44
  daycare provider Y07.519
    at-home
      adult care Y07.512
      childcare Y07.510
    care center
      adult care Y07.513
      childcare Y07.511
  family member NEC Y07.499
  father Y07.11
    adoptive Y07.13
    foster Y07.420
    stepfather Y07.430
  foster father Y07.420
  foster mother Y07.421
  friend Y07.54
  girl friend Y07.04
    current Y07.040
    former Y07.041
  grandchild (adopted) (biological) (foster) (in-law) (step) Y07.45
  granddaughter (adopted) (biological) (foster) (in-law) (step) Y07.45
  grandfather Y07.46
  grandmother Y07.46
  grandparent Y07.46
  grandson (adopted) (biological) (foster) (in-law) (step) Y07.45
  healthcare provider Y07.529
    mental health Y07.521
    specified NEC Y07.528
  husband Y07.01
    current Y07.010
    former Y07.011
  instructor Y07.53
  mother Y07.12
    adoptive Y07.14
    foster Y07.421
    stepmother Y07.433
  multiple perpetrators Y07.6
  non-binary
    child (adopted) (biological) (foster) (in-law) (step) Y07.44
    grandchild (adopted) (biological) (foster) (in-law) (step) Y07.45
    grandparent Y07.46
    parental sibling Y07.47
  nonfamily member Y07.50
    specified NEC Y07.59
  nurse Y07.528
  occupational therapist Y07.528
  parental sibling Y07.47
  partner
    female (dating) (intimate)
      current Y07.040
      former Y07.041
      gender non-conforming
        current Y07.050
        former Y07.051

Perpetrator, perpetration, of assault, maltreatment and neglect (*continued*)
  partner (*continued*)
    male (dating) (intimate)
      current Y07.030
      former Y07.031
    non-binary
      current Y07.050
      former Y07.051
    of parent
      female Y07.434
      male Y07.432
  physical therapist Y07.528
  sister Y07.411
  son (adopted) (biological) (foster) (in-law) (step) Y07.44
  speech therapist Y07.528
  stepbrother Y07.435
  stepfather Y07.430
  stepmother Y07.433
  stepsister Y07.436
  teacher Y07.53
  uncle Y07.47
  wife
    current Y07.020
    former Y07.021

Piercing —*see* Contact, with, by type of object or machine

Pinched
  between objects (moving) (stationary and moving) W23.0
  stationary W23.1

Pinned under machine (ry) —*see* Contact, with, by type of machine

Place of occurrence Y92.9
  abandoned house Y92.89
  airplane Y92.813
  airport Y92.520
  ambulatory health services establishment NEC Y92.538
  ambulatory surgery center Y92.530
  amusement park Y92.831
  apartment (co-op) —*see* Place of occurrence, residence, apartment
  assembly hall Y92.29
  bank Y92.510
  bar Y92.59
  barn Y92.71
  baseball field Y92.320
  basketball court Y92.310
  beach Y92.832
  boarding house —*see* Place of occurrence, residence, boarding house
  boat Y92.814
  bowling alley Y92.39
  bridge Y92.89
  building under construction Y92.61
  bus Y92.811
    station Y92.521
  cafe Y92.511
  campsite Y92.833
  campus —*see* Place of occurrence, school
  canal Y92.89
  car Y92.810
  casino Y92.59
  children's home —*see* Place of occurrence, residence, institutional, orphanage
  church Y92.22
  cinema Y92.26
  clubhouse Y92.29
  coal pit Y92.64
  college (community) Y92.214

Place of occurrence (*continued*)
- condominium —*see* Place of occurrence, residence, apartment
- construction area —*see* Place of occurrence, industrial and construction area
- convalescent home —*see* Place of occurrence, residence, institutional, nursing home
- court-house Y92.240
- cricket ground Y92.328
- cultural building Y92.258
  - art gallery Y92.250
  - museum Y92.251
  - music hall Y92.252
  - opera house Y92.253
  - specified NEC Y92.258
  - theater Y92.254
- dancehall Y92.252
- day nursery Y92.210
- dentist office Y92.531
- derelict house Y92.89
- desert Y92.820
- dock NOS Y92.89
- dockyard Y92.62
- doctor's office Y92.531
- dormitory —*see* Place of occurrence, residence, institutional, school dormitory
- dry dock Y92.62
- factory (building) (premises) Y92.63
- farm (land under cultivation) (outbuildings) Y92.79
  - barn Y92.71
  - chicken coop Y92.72
  - field Y92.73
  - hen house Y92.72
  - house —*see* Place of occurrence, residence, house
  - orchard Y92.74
  - specified NEC Y92.79
- football field Y92.321
- forest Y92.821
- freeway Y92.411
- gallery Y92.250
- garage (commercial) Y92.59
  - boarding house Y92.044
  - military base Y92.135
  - mobile home Y92.025
  - nursing home Y92.124
  - orphanage Y92.114
  - private house Y92.015
  - reform school Y92.155
- gas station Y92.524
- gasworks Y92.69
- golf course Y92.39
- gravel pit Y92.64
- grocery Y92.512
- gymnasium Y92.39
- handball court Y92.318
- harbor Y92.89
- harness racing course Y92.39
- healthcare provider office Y92.531
- highway Y92.410
  - interstate Y92.411
- hill Y92.828
- hockey rink Y92.330
- home —*see* Place of occurrence, residence
- hospice —*see* Place of occurrence, residence, institutional, nursing home
- hospital Y92.239
  - cafeteria Y92.233
  - corridor Y92.232
  - operating room Y92.234
  - patient
    - bathroom Y92.231
    - room Y92.230
  - specified NEC Y92.238

Place of occurrence (*continued*)
- hotel Y92.59
- house —*see also* Place of occurrence, residence
  - abandoned Y92.89
  - under construction Y92.61
- industrial and construction area (yard) Y92.69
  - building under construction Y92.61
  - dock Y92.62
  - dry dock Y92.62
  - factory Y92.63
  - gasworks Y92.69
  - mine Y92.64
  - oil rig Y92.65
  - pit Y92.64
  - power station Y92.69
  - shipyard Y92.62
  - specified NEC Y92.69
  - tunnel under construction Y92.69
  - workshop Y92.69
- interstate Y92.411
- kindergarten Y92.211
- lacrosse field Y92.328
- lake Y92.838
  - wilderness Y92.828
- library Y92.241
- mall Y92.59
- market Y92.512
- marsh Y92.828
- military
  - base —*see* Place of occurrence, residence, institutional, military base
  - training ground Y92.84
- mine Y92.64
- mosque Y92.22
- motel Y92.59
- motorway (interstate) Y92.411
- mountain Y92.828
- movie-house Y92.26
- museum Y92.251
- music-hall Y92.252
- not applicable Y92.9
- nuclear power station Y92.69
- nursing home —*see* Place of occurrence, residence, institutional, nursing home
- office building Y92.59
- offshore installation Y92.65
- oil rig Y92.65
- old people's home —*see* Place of occurrence, residence, institutional, specified NEC
- opera-house Y92.253
- orphanage —*see* Place of occurrence, residence, institutional, orphanage
- outpatient surgery center Y92.530
- park (public) Y92.830
  - amusement Y92.831
- parking garage Y92.89
  - lot Y92.481
- pavement Y92.480
- physician office Y92.531
- polo field Y92.328
- pond Y92.828
- post office Y92.242
- power station Y92.69
- prairie Y92.828
- prison —*see* Place of occurrence, residence, institutional, prison
- public
  - administration building Y92.248
    - city hall Y92.243
    - courthouse Y92.240
    - library Y92.241
    - post office Y92.242
    - specified NEC Y92.248
  - building NEC Y92.29
  - hall Y92.29

Place of occurrence (*continued*)
- public (*continued*)
  - place NOS Y92.89
- race course Y92.39
- radio station Y92.59
- railway line (bridge) Y92.85
- ranch (outbuildings) —*see* Place of occurrence, farm
- recreation area Y92.838
  - amusement park Y92.831
  - beach Y92.832
  - campsite Y92.833
  - park (public) Y92.830
  - seashore Y92.832
  - specified NEC Y92.838
- religious institution Y92.22
- reform school —*see* Place of occurrence, residence, institutional, reform school
- residence (non-institutional) (private) Y92.009
  - apartment Y92.039
    - bathroom Y92.031
    - bedroom Y92.032
    - kitchen Y92.030
    - specified NEC Y92.038
  - bathroom Y92.002
  - bedroom Y92.003
  - boarding house Y92.049
    - bathroom Y92.041
    - bedroom Y92.042
    - driveway Y92.043
    - garage Y92.044
    - garden Y92.046
    - kitchen Y92.040
    - specified NEC Y92.048
    - swimming pool Y92.045
    - yard Y92.046
  - dining room Y92.001
  - garden Y92.007
  - home Y92.009
  - house, single family Y92.019
    - bathroom Y92.012
    - bedroom Y92.013
    - dining room Y92.011
    - driveway Y92.014
    - garage Y92.015
    - garden Y92.017
    - kitchen Y92.010
    - specified NEC Y92.018
    - swimming pool Y92.016
    - yard Y92.017
  - institutional Y92.10
    - children's home —*see* Place of occurrence, residence, institutional, orphanage
    - hospice —*see* Place of occurrence, residence, institutional, nursing home
    - military base Y92.139
      - barracks Y92.133
      - garage Y92.135
      - garden Y92.137
      - kitchen Y92.130
      - mess hall Y92.131
      - specified NEC Y92.138
      - swimming pool Y92.136
      - yard Y92.137
    - nursing home Y92.129
      - bathroom Y92.121
      - bedroom Y92.122
      - driveway Y92.123
      - garage Y92.124
      - garden Y92.126
      - kitchen Y92.120
      - specified NEC Y92.128
      - swimming pool Y92.125
      - yard Y92.126
    - orphanage Y92.119
      - bathroom Y92.111

Place of occurrence (*continued*)
- residence (*continued*)
  - institutional (*continued*)
    - orphanage (*continued*)
      - bedroom Y92.112
      - driveway Y92.113
      - garage Y92.114
      - garden Y92.116
      - kitchen Y92.110
      - specified NEC Y92.118
      - swimming pool Y92.115
      - yard Y92.116
    - prison Y92.149
      - bathroom Y92.142
      - cell Y92.143
      - courtyard Y92.147
      - dining room Y92.141
      - kitchen Y92.140
      - specified NEC Y92.148
      - swimming pool Y92.146
    - reform school Y92.159
      - bathroom Y92.152
      - bedroom Y92.153
      - dining room Y92.151
      - driveway Y92.154
      - garage Y92.155
      - garden Y92.157
      - kitchen Y92.150
      - specified NEC Y92.158
      - swimming pool Y92.156
      - yard Y92.157
    - school dormitory Y92.169
      - bathroom Y92.162
      - bedroom Y92.163
      - dining room Y92.161
      - kitchen Y92.160
      - specified NEC Y92.168
    - specified NEC Y92.199
      - bathroom Y92.192
      - bedroom Y92.193
      - dining room Y92.191
      - driveway Y92.194
      - garage Y92.195
      - garden Y92.197
      - kitchen Y92.190
      - specified NEC Y92.198
      - swimming pool Y92.196
      - yard Y92.197
  - kitchen Y92.000
  - mobile home Y92.029
    - bathroom Y92.022
    - bedroom Y92.023
    - dining room Y92.021
    - driveway Y92.024
    - garage Y92.025
    - garden Y92.027
    - kitchen Y92.020
    - specified NEC Y92.028
    - swimming pool Y92.026
    - yard Y92.027
  - specified place in residence NEC Y92.008
  - specified residence type NEC Y92.099
    - bathroom Y92.091
    - bedroom Y92.092
    - driveway Y92.093
    - garage Y92.094
    - garden Y92.096
    - kitchen Y92.090
    - specified NEC Y92.098
    - swimming pool Y92.095
    - yard Y92.096
- restaurant Y92.511
- riding school Y92.39
- river Y92.828
- road Y92.410
- rodeo ring Y92.39
- rugby field Y92.328
- same day surgery center Y92.530
- sand pit Y92.64

Place of occurrence (continued)
school (private) (public) (state) Y92.219
  college Y92.214
  daycare center Y92.210
  elementary school Y92.211
  high school Y92.213
  kindergarten Y92.211
  middle school Y92.212
  specified NEC Y92.218
  trace school Y92.215
  university Y92.214
  vocational school Y92.215
sea (shore) Y92.832
senior citizen center Y92.29
service area
  airport Y92.520
  bus station Y92.521
  gas station Y92.524
  highway rest stop Y92.523
  railway station Y92.522
shipyard Y92.62
shop (commercial) Y92.513
sidewalk Y92.480
silo Y92.79
skating rink (roller) Y92.331
  ice Y92.330
slaughter house Y92.86
soccer field Y92.322
specified place NEC Y92.89
sports area Y92.39
  athletic
    court Y92.318
      basketball Y92.310
      specified NEC Y92.318
      squash Y92.311
      tennis Y92.312
    field Y92.328
      baseball Y92.320
      cricket ground Y92.328
      football Y92.321
      hockey Y92.328
      soccer Y92.322
      specified NEC Y92.328
  golf course Y92.39
  gymnasium Y92.39
  riding school Y92.39
  skating rink (roller) Y92.331
    ice Y92.330
  stadium Y92.39
  swimming pool Y92.34
squash court Y92.311
stadium Y92.39
steeplechasing course Y92.39
store Y92.512
stream Y92.828
street and highway Y92.410
  bike path Y92.482
  freeway Y92.411
  highway ramp Y92.415
  interstate highway Y92.411
  local residential or business street Y92.414
  motorway Y92.411
  parkway Y92.412
  parking lot Y92.481
  sidewalk Y92.480
  specified NEC Y92.488
  state road Y92.413
subway car Y92.816
supermarket Y92.512
swamp Y92.828
swimming pool (public) Y92.34
  private (at) Y92.095
    boarding house Y92.045
    military base Y92.136
    mobile home Y92.026
    nursing home Y92.125
    orphanage Y92.115
    prison Y92.146
    reform school Y92.156

Place of occurrence (continued)
swimming pool (continued)
  private (continued)
    single family residence Y92.016
synagogue Y92.22
tavern Y92.59
television station Y92.59
tennis court Y92.312
theater Y92.254
trade area Y92.59
  bank Y92.510
  cafe Y92.511
  casino Y92.59
  garage Y92.59
  hotel Y92.59
  market Y92.512
  office building Y92.59
  radio station Y92.59
  restaurant Y92.511
  shop Y92.513
  shopping mall Y92.59
  store Y92.512
  supermarket Y92.512
  television station Y92.59
  warehouse Y92.59
trailer park, residential —see Place of occurrence, residence, mobile home
trailer site NOS Y92.89
train Y92.815
  station Y92.522
truck Y92.812
tunnel under construction Y92.69
urgent (health) care center Y92.532
university Y92.214
vehicle (transport) Y92.818
  airplane Y92.813
  boat Y92.814
  bus Y92.811
  car Y92.810
  specified NEC Y92.818
  subway car Y92.816
  train Y92.815
  truck Y92.812
warehouse Y92.59
water reservoir Y92.89
wilderness area Y92.828
  desert Y92.820
  forest Y92.821
  marsh Y92.828
  mountain Y92.828
  prairie Y92.828
  specified NEC Y92.828
  swamp Y92.828
workshop Y92.69
yard, private Y92.096
  boarding house Y92.046
  single family house Y92.017
  mobile home Y92.027
youth center Y92.29
zoo (zoological garden) Y92.834

Plumbism —see Table of Drugs and Chemicals, lead

Poisoning (accidental) (by)
—see also Table of Drugs and Chemicals
  by plant, thorns, spines, sharp leaves or other mechanisms NEC X58
  carbon monoxide
    generated by
      motor vehicle —see Accident, transport
      watercraft (in transit) (not in transit) V93.89
        ferry boat V93.81
        fishing boat V93.82
        jet skis V93.83
        liner V93.81

Poisoning (continued)
carbon monoxide (continued)
  generated by (continued)
    watercraft (continued)
      merchant ship V93.80
      passenger ship V93.81
      powered craft NEC V93.83
caused by injection of poisons into skin by plant thorns, spines, sharp leaves X58
marine or sea plants (venomous) X58
exhaust gas
  generated by
    motor vehicle —see Accident, transport
    watercraft (in transit) (not in transit) V93.89
      ferry boat V93.81
      fishing boat V93.82
      jet skis V93.83
      liner V93.81
      merchant ship V93.80
      passenger ship V93.81
      powered craft NEC V93.83
fumes or smoke due to
  explosion —see also Explosion W40.9
  fire —see Exposure, fire
  ignition —see Ignition gas
  in legal intervention —see Legal, intervention, gas
  legal execution —see Legal, intervention, gas
in war operations —see War operations

Powder burn (by) (from)
airgun W34.110
BB gun W34.110
firearm NEC W34.19
gas, air or spring-operated gun NEC W34.118
handgun W32.1
hunting rifle W33.12
larger firearm W33.10
  specified NEC W33.19
machine gun W33.13
paintball gun W34.111
pellet gun W34.110
shotgun W33.11
Very pistol [flare] W34.19

Premature cessation (of) surgical and medical care Y66

Privation (food) (water) X58

Procedure (operation)
correct, on wrong side or body part (wrong side) (wrong site) Y65.53
intended for another patient done on wrong patient Y65.52
performed on patient not scheduled for surgery Y65.52
performed on wrong patient Y65.52
wrong, performed on correct patient Y65.51

Prolonged
sitting in transport vehicle —see Sitting
stay in
  high altitude as cause of anoxia, barodontalgia, barotitis or hypoxia W94.11
  weightless environment X52

Pulling, excessive (see also Overexertion) X50.9

Puncture, puncturing —see also Contact, with, by type of object or machine
by
  plant thorns, spines, sharp leaves or other mechanisms NEC W60
during medical or surgical treatment as misadventure —see Index to Diseases and Injuries, Complication(s)

Pushed, pushing (accidental) (injury in)
by other person(s) (accidental) W51
  with fall W03
    due to ice or snow W00.0
  as, or caused by, a crowd or human stampede (with fall) W52
  before moving object NEC Y02.8
    motor vehicle Y02.0
    subway train Y02.1
    train Y02.1
  from
    high place NEC
      in accidental circumstances W17.89
      stated as
        intentional, homicide (attempt) Y01
        undetermined whether accidental or intentional Y30
    transport vehicle NEC —see also Accident, transport V89.9
      stated as
        intentional, homicide (attempt) Y08.89
overexertion X50.9

R

Radiation (exposure to)
arc lamps W89.0
atomic power plant (malfunction) NEC W88.1
complication of or abnormal reaction to medical radiotherapy Y84.2
electromagnetic, ionizing W88.0
gamma rays W88.1
in
  war operations (from or following nuclear explosion) —see War operations
inadvertent exposure of patient (receiving test or therapy) Y63.3
infrared (heaters and lamps) W90.1
excessive heat from W92
ionized, ionizing (particles, artificially accelerated)
  radioisotopes W88.1
  specified NEC W88.8
  x-rays W88.0
isotopes, radioactive —see Radiation, radioactive isotopes
laser(s) W90.2
  in war operations —see War operations
  misadventure in medical care Y63.2
light sources (man-made visible and ultraviolet) W89.9
  natural X32
  specified NEC W89.8
  tanning bed W89.1
  welding light W89.0

Radiation (continued)
- man-made visible light W89.9
  - specified NEC W89.8
  - tanning bed W89.1
  - welding light W89.0
- microwave W90.8
- misadventure in medical or surgical procedure Y63.2
- natural NEC X39.08
  - radon X39.01
- overdose (in medical or surgical procedure) Y63.2
- radar W90.0
- radioactive isotopes (any) W88.1
  - atomic power plant malfunction W88.1
  - misadventure in medical or surgical treatment Y63.2
- radiofrequency W90.0
- radium NEC W88.1
- sun X32
- ultraviolet (light) (man-made) W89.9
  - natural X32
  - specified NEC W89.8
  - tanning bed W89.1
  - welding light W89.0
- welding arc, torch, or light W89.0
  - excessive heat from W92
- x-rays (hard) (soft) W88.0

Range disease W94.11

Rape (attempted) T74.2-

Rat bite W53.11

Reaching (prolonged) (static) X50.1

Reaction, abnormal to medical procedure —*see also* Complication of or following, by type of procedure Y84.9
- with misadventure —*see* Misadventure
- biologicals —*see* Table of Drugs and Chemicals
- drugs —*see* Table of Drugs and Chemicals
- vaccine —*see* Table of Drugs and Chemicals

Recoil
- airgun W34.110
- BB gun W34.110
- firearm NEC W34.19
- gas, air or spring-operated gun NEC W34.118
- handgun W32.1
- hunting rifle W33.12
- larger firearm W33.10
  - specified NEC W33.19
- machine gun W33.13
- paintball gun W34.111
- pellet W34.110
- shotgun W33.11
- Very pistol [flare] W34.19

Reduction in
- atmospheric pressure —*see* Air, pressure, change

Rock falling on or hitting (accidentally) (person) W20.8
- in cave-in W20.0

Run over (accidentally) (by)
- animal (not being ridden) NEC W55.89
- machinery —*see* Contact, with, by specified type of machine
- transport vehicle NEC —*see also* Accident, transport V09.9
  - intentional homicide (attempt) Y03.0
  - motor NEC V09.20
    - intentional homicide (attempt) Y03.0

Running
- before moving object X81.8
- motor vehicle X81.0

Running off, away
- animal (being ridden) —*see also* Accident, transport V80.918
  - not being ridden W55.89
- animal-drawn vehicle NEC —*see also* Accident, transport V80.928
- highway, road (way), street transport vehicle NEC —*see also* Accident, transport V89.9

Rupture pressurized devices —*see* Explosion, by type of device

S

Saturnism —*see* Table of Drugs and Chemicals, lead

Scald, scalding (accidental) (by) (from) (in) X19
- air (hot) X14.1
- gases (hot) X14.1
- homicide (attempt) —*see* Assault, burning, hot object
- inflicted by other person
  - stated as intentional, homicide (attempt) —*see* Assault, burning, hot object
- liquid (boiling) (hot) NEC X12
  - stated as undetermined whether accidental or intentional Y27.2
  - suicide (attempt) X77.2
- local application of externally applied substance in medical or surgical care Y63.5
- metal (molten) (liquid) (hot) NEC X18
- self-inflicted X77.9
  - stated as undetermined whether accidental or intentional Y27.8
- steam X13.1
  - assault X98.0
  - stated as undetermined whether accidental or intentional Y27.0
  - suicide (attempt) X77.0
- suicide (attempt) X77.9
- vapor (hot) X13.1
  - assault X98.0
  - stated as undetermined whether accidental or intentional Y27.0
  - suicide (attempt) X77.0

Scratched by
- cat W55.03
- person(s) (accidentally) W50.4
  - with intent to injure or kill Y04.0
  - as, or caused by, a crowd or human stampede (with fall) W52
  - assault Y04.0
  - homicide (attempt) Y04.0
  - in
    - fight Y04.0
    - legal intervention
      - injuring
        - bystander Y35.892
        - law enforcement personnel Y35.891
        - suspect Y35.893
        - unspecified person Y35.899

Seasickness T75.3

Self-harm NEC —*see also* External cause by type, undetermined whether accidental or intentional
- intentional —*see* Suicide
- poisoning NEC —*see* Table of drugs and biologicals, accident

Self-inflicted (injury) NEC —*see also* External cause by type, undetermined whether accidental or intentional —*see* Suicide
- poisoning NEC —*see* Table of drugs and biologicals, accident

Sequelae (of)
- accident NEC —*see* W00-X58 with 7th character S
- assault (homicidal) (any means) —*see* X92-Y08 with 7th character S
- homicide, attempt (any means) —*see* X92-Y08 with 7th character S
- injury undetermined whether accidentally or purposely inflicted —*see* Y21-Y33 with 7th character S
- intentional self-harm (classifiable to X71-X83) —*see* X71-X83 with 7th character S
- legal intervention —*see* with 7th character S Y35
- motor vehicle accident —*see* V00-V99 with 7th character S
- suicide, attempt (any means) —*see* X71-X83 with 7th character S
- transport accident —*see* V00-V99 with 7th character S
- war operations —*see* War operations

Shock
- electric —*see* Exposure, electric current
- from electric appliance (any) (faulty) W86.8
  - domestic W86.0
  - suicide (attempt) X83.1

Shooting, shot (accidental(ly)) —*see also* Discharge, firearm, by type
- herself or himself —*see* Discharge, firearm by type, self-inflicted
- homicide (attempt) —*see* Discharge, firearm by type, homicide
- in war operations —*see* War operations
- inflicted by other person —*see* Discharge, firearm by type, homicide
  - accidental —*see* Discharge, firearm, by type of firearm
  - legal
    - execution —*see* Legal, intervention, firearm
    - intervention —*see* Legal, intervention, firearm
  - self-inflicted —*see* Discharge, firearm by type, suicide
  - accidental —*see* Discharge, firearm, by type of firearm
  - suicide (attempt) —*see* Discharge, firearm by type, suicide

Shoving (accidentally) by other person —*see* Pushed, by other person

Sickness
- alpine W94.11
- motion —*see* Motion
- mountain W94.11

Sinking (accidental)
- watercraft (causing drowning, submersion) —*see also* Drowning, due to, accident to, watercraft, sinking
- causing injury except drowning or submersion —*see* Accident, watercraft, causing, injury NEC

Siriasis X32

Sitting (prolonged) (static) X50.1

Slashed wrists —*see* Cut, self-inflicted

Slipping (accidental) (on same level) (with fall) W01.0
- on
  - ice W00.0
    - with skates —*see* Accident, transport, pedestrian, conveyance
  - mud W01.0
  - oil W01.0
  - snow W00.0
    - with skis —*see* Accident, transport, pedestrian, conveyance
  - surface (slippery) (wet) NEC W01.0
- without fall W18.40
  - due to
    - specified NEC W18.49
    - stepping from one level to another W18.43
    - stepping into hole or opening W18.42
    - stepping on object W18.41

Sliver, wood, contact with W45.8

Smoldering (due to fire) —*see* Exposure, fire

Sodomy (attempted) by force T74.2-

Sound waves (causing injury) W42.9
- supersonic W42.0

Splinter, contact with W45.8

Stab, stabbing —*see* Cut

Standing (prolonged) (static) X50.1

Starvation X58

Status of external cause Y99.9
- child assisting in compensated work for family Y99.8
- civilian activity done for financial or other compensation Y99.0
- civilian activity done for income or pay Y99.0
- family member assisting in compensated work for other family member Y99.8
- hobby not done for income Y99.8
- leisure activity Y99.8
- military activity Y99.1
- off-duty activity of military personnel Y99.8
- recreation or sport not for income or while a student Y99.8
- specified NEC Y99.8
- student activity Y99.8
- volunteer activity Y99.2

Stepped on
- by
  - animal (not being ridden) NEC W55.89
  - crowd or human stampede W52
  - person W50.0

Stepping on
- object W22.8
  - with fall W18.31
  - sports equipment W21.9
  - stationary W22.09
    - sports equipment W21.89
- person W51
  - by crowd or human stampede W52
- sports equipment W21.9

Sting
- arthropod, nonvenomous W57
- insect, nonvenomous W57

Storm (cataclysmic) —see Forces of nature, cataclysmic storm
Straining, excessive —(see also Overexertion) X50.9
Strangling —see Strangulation
Strangulation (accidental) —see categories T71
Strenuous movements (see also Overexertion) X50.9
Striking against
- airbag (automobile) W22.10
  - driver side W22.11
  - front passenger side W22.12
  - specified NEC W22.19
- bottom when
  - diving or jumping into water (in) W16.822
    - causing drowning W16.821
    - from boat W16.722
      - causing drowning W16.721
    - natural body W16.622
      - causing drowning W16.821
    - swimming pool W16.522
      - causing drowning W16.521
  - falling into water (in) W16.322
    - causing drowning W16.321
    - fountain —see Striking against, bottom when, falling into water, specified NEC
    - natural body W16.122
      - causing drowning W16.121
    - reservoir —see Striking against, bottom when, falling into water, specified NEC
    - specified NEC W16.322
      - causing drowning W16.321
    - swimming pool W16.022
      - causing drowning W16.021
- diving board (swimming-pool) W21.4
- object W22.8
  - with
    - drowning or submersion —see Drowning
    - fall —see Fall, due to, bumping against, object
  - caused by crowd or human stampede (with fall) W52
  - furniture W22.03
  - lamppost W22.02
  - sports equipment W21.9
  - stationary W22.09
    - sports equipment W21.89
  - wall W22.01
- person(s) W51
  - with fall W03
    - due to ice or snow W00.0
  - as, or caused by, a crowd or human stampede (with fall) W52
  - assault Y04.2
  - homicide (attempt) Y04.2
- sports equipment W21.9
- wall (when) W22.01
  - diving or jumping into water (in) W16.832
    - causing drowning W16.831
    - swimming pool W16.532
      - causing drowning W16.531
  - falling into water (in) W16.332
    - causing drowning W16.331
    - fountain —see Striking against, wall when, falling into water, specified NEC
    - natural body W16.132
      - causing drowning W16.131

Striking against (continued)
- wall (continued)
  - falling into water (continued)
    - reservoir —see Striking against, wall when, falling into water, specified NEC
    - specified NEC W16.332
      - causing drowning W16.331
    - swimming pool W16.032
      - causing drowning W16.031
  - swimming pool (when) W22.042
    - causing drowning W22.041
    - diving or jumping into water W16.532
      - causing drowning W16.531
    - falling into water W16.032
      - causing drowning W16.031

Struck (accidentally) by
- airbag (automobile) W22.10
  - driver side W22.11
  - front passenger side W22.12
  - specified NEC W22.19
- alligator W58.02
- animal (not being ridden) NEC W55.89
- avalanche —see Landslide
- ball (hit) (thrown) W21.00
  - assault Y08.09
  - baseball W21.03
  - basketball W21.05
  - golf ball W21.04
  - football W21.01
  - soccer W21.02
  - softball W21.07
  - specified NEC W21.09
  - volleyball W21.06
- bat or racquet
  - baseball bat W21.11
    - assault Y08.02
  - golf club W21.13
    - assault Y08.09
  - specified NEC W21.19
    - assault Y08.09
  - tennis racquet W21.12
    - assault Y08.09
- bullet —see also Discharge, firearm by type
  - in war operations —see War operations
- crocodile W58.12
- dog W54.1
- flare, Very pistol —see Discharge, firearm NEC
- hailstones X39.8
- hockey (ice)
  - field
    - puck W21.221
    - stick W21.211
  - puck W21.220
  - stick W21.210
  - assault Y08.01
- landslide —see Landslide
- law-enforcement agent (on duty) —see Legal, intervention, manhandling
  - with blunt object —see Legal, intervention, blunt object
- lightning —see subcategory T75.0
  - causing fire —see Exposure, fire
- machine —see Contact, with, by type of machine
- mammal NEC W55.89
  - marine W56.32
- marine animal W56.82
- missile
  - firearm —see Discharge, firearm by type
  - in war operations —see War operations, missile
- object W22.8
  - blunt W22.8

Struck (continued)
- object (continued)
  - blunt (continued)
    - assault Y00
    - suicide (attempt) X79
    - undetermined whether accidental or intentional Y29
  - falling W20.8
    - from, in, on
      - building W20.1
        - burning (uncontrolled fire) X00.4
      - cataclysmic
        - earth surface movement NEC —see Landslide
        - storm —see Forces of nature, cataclysmic storm
      - cave-in W20.0
      - earthquake X34
      - machine (in operation) —see Contact, with, by type of machine
      - structure W20.1
        - burning X00.4
      - transport vehicle (in motion) —see Accident, transport, by type of vehicle
      - watercraft V93.49
        - due to
          - accident to craft V91.39
            - powered craft V91.33
              - ferry boat V91.31
              - fishing boat V91.32
              - jetskis V91.33
              - liner V91.31
              - merchant ship V91.30
              - passenger ship V91.31
            - unpowered craft V91.38
              - canoe V91.35
              - inflatable V91.36
              - kayak V91.35
              - sailboat V91.34
              - surf-board V91.38
              - windsurfer V91.38
          - powered craft V93.43
            - ferry boat V93.41
            - fishing boat V93.42
            - jetskis V93.43
            - liner V93.41
            - merchant ship V93.40
            - passenger ship V93.41
          - unpowered craft V93.48
            - sailboat V93.44
            - surf-board V93.48
            - windsurfer V93.48
  - moving NEC W20.8
  - projected W20.8
    - assault Y00
    - in sports W21.9
      - assault Y08.09
      - ball W21.00
        - baseball W21.03
        - basketball W21.05
        - football W21.01
        - golf ball W21.04
        - soccer W21.02
        - softball W21.07
        - specified NEC W21.09
        - volleyball W21.06
      - bat or racquet
        - baseball bat W21.11

Struck (continued)
- object (continued)
  - projected (continued)
    - in sports (continued)
      - bat or racquet (continued)
        - baseball bat (continued)
          - assault Y08.02
        - golf club W21.13
          - assault Y08.09
        - specified NEC W21.19
          - assault Y08.09
        - tennis racquet W21.12
          - assault Y08.09
      - hockey (ice)
        - field
          - puck W21.221
          - stick W21.211
        - puck W21.220
        - stick W21.210
        - assault Y08.01
      - specified NEC W21.89
    - set in motion by explosion —see Explosion
  - thrown W20.8
    - assault Y00
    - in sports W21.9
      - assault Y08.09
      - ball W21.00
        - baseball W21.03
        - basketball W21.05
        - football W21.01
        - golf ball W21.04
        - soccer W21.02
        - soft ball W21.07
        - specified NEC W21.09
        - volleyball W21.06
      - bat or racquet
        - baseball bat W21.11
          - assault Y08.02
        - golf club W21.13
          - assault Y08.09
        - specified NEC W21.19
          - assault Y08.09
        - tennis racquet W21.12
          - assault Y08.09
      - hockey (ice)
        - field
          - puck W21.221
          - stick W21.211
        - puck W21.220
        - stick W21.210
        - assault Y08.01
      - specified NEC W21.89
- other person(s) W50.0
  - with
    - blunt object W22.8
      - intentional, homicide (attempt) Y00
      - sports equipment W21.9
      - undetermined whether accidental or intentional Y29
    - fall W03
      - due to ice or snow W00.0
    - as, or caused by, a crowd or human stampede (with fall) W52
  - assault Y04.2
  - homicide (attempt) Y04.2
  - in legal intervention
    - injuring
      - bystander Y35.812
      - law enforcement personnel Y35.811
      - suspect Y35.813
      - unspecified person Y35.819
  - sports equipment W21.9
- police (on duty) —see Legal, intervention, manhandling
  - with blunt object —see Legal, intervention, blunt object
- sports equipment W21.9

483

Struck (continued)
   sports equipment (continued)
      assault Y08.09
      ball W21.00
         baseball W21.03
         basketball W21.05
         football W21.01
         golf ball W21.04
         soccer W21.02
         soft ball W21.07
         specified NEC W21.09
         volleyball W21.06
      bat or racquet
         baseball bat W21.11
            assault Y08.02
         golf club W21.13
            assault Y08.09
         specified NEC W21.19
         tennis racquet W21.12
            assault Y08.09
      cleats (shoe) W21.31
      foot wear NEC W21.39
      football helmet W21.81
      hockey (ice)
         field
            puck W21.221
            stick W21.211
         puck W21.220
         stick W21.210
            assault Y08.01
      skate blades W21.32
      specified NEC W21.89
         assault Y08.09
   thunderbolt —see subcategory T75.0
      causing fire —see Exposure, fire
   transport vehicle NEC —see
      also Accident, transport V09.9
      intentional, homicide (attempt)
         Y03.0
      motor NEC —see also Accident,
         transport V09.20
         homicide Y03.0
   vehicle (transport) NEC
      —see Accident, transport, by
      type of vehicle
      stationary (falling from jack,
         hydraulic lift, ramp) W20.8

Stumbling
   over
      animal NEC W01.0
         with fall W18.09
      carpet, rug or (small) object
         W22.8
         with fall W18.09
      person W51
         with fall W03
            due to ice or snow W00.0
   without fall W18.40
      due to
         specified NEC W18.49
         stepping from one level to
            another W18.43
         stepping into hole or opening
            W18.42
         stepping on object W18.41

Submersion (accidental)
   —see Drowning

Suffocation (accidental) (by external means) (by pressure) (mechanical)
   —see also category T71
   due to, by
      avalanche —see Landslide
      explosion —see Explosion
      fire —see Exposure, fire
      food, any type (aspiration)
         (ingestion) (inhalation)
            —see categories T17 and T18
      ignition —see Ignition
      landslide —see Landslide

Suffocation (continued)
   due to, by (continued)
      machine (ry) —see Contact, with, by type of machine
      vomitus (aspiration) (inhalation) T17.81-
   in
      burning building X00.8

Suicide, suicidal (attempted) (by) X83.8
   blunt object X79
   burning, burns X76
      hot object X77.9
         fluid NEC X77.2
         household appliance X77.3
         specified NEC X77.8
         steam X77.0
         tap water X77.1
         vapors X77.0
   caustic substance —see Table of Drugs and Chemicals
   cold, extreme X83.2
   collision of motor vehicle with
      motor vehicle X82.0
      specified NEC X82.8
      train X82.1
      tree X82.2
   crashing of aircraft X83.0
   cut (any part of body) X78.9
   cutting or piercing instrument X78.9
      dagger X78.2
      glass X78.0
      knife X78.1
      specified NEC X78.8
      sword X78.2
   drowning (in) X71.9
      bathtub X71.0
      natural water X71.3
      specified NEC X71.8
      swimming pool X71.1
         following fall X71.2
   electrocution X83.1
   explosive(s) (material) X75
   fire, flames X76
   firearm X74.9
      airgun X74.01
      handgun X72
      hunting rifle X73.1
      larger X73.9
         specified NEC X73.8
      machine gun X73.2
      shotgun X73.0
      specified NEC X74.8
   hanging X83.8
   hot object —see Suicide, burning, hot object
   jumping
      before moving object X81.8
         motor vehicle X81.0
         subway train X81.1
         train X81.1
      from high place X80
   late effect of attempt
      —see X71-X83 with 7th character S
   lying before moving object, train, vehicle X81.8
   poisoning —see Table of Drugs and Chemicals
   puncture (any part of body)
      —see Suicide, cutting or piercing instrument
   scald —see Suicide, burning, hot object
   sequelae of attempt —see X71-X83 with 7th character S
   sharp object (any) —see Suicide, cutting or piercing instrument

Suicide, suicidal (continued)
   shooting —see Suicide, firearm
   specified means NEC X83.8
   stab (any part of body)
      —see Suicide, cutting or piercing instrument
   steam, hot vapors X77.0
   strangulation X83.8
   submersion —see Suicide, drowning
   suffocation X83.8
   wound NEC X83.8

Sunstroke X32

Supersonic waves (causing injury) W42.0

Surgical procedure, complication of (delayed or as an abnormal reaction without mention of misadventure) —see also Complication of or following, by type of procedure
   due to or as a result of
      misadventure —see Misadventure

Swallowed, swallowing
   foreign body —see Foreign body, alimentary canal
   poison —see Table of Drugs and Chemicals
   substance
      caustic or corrosive —see Table of Drugs and Chemicals
      poisonous —see Table of Drugs and Chemicals

T

Tackle in sport W03

Terrorism (involving) Y38.80
   biological weapons Y38.6X-
   chemical weapons Y38.7X-
   conflagration Y38.3X-
   drowning and submersion Y38.89-
   explosion Y38.2X-
      destruction of aircraft Y38.1X-
      marine weapons Y38.0X-
   fire Y38.3X-
   firearms Y38.4X-
   hot substances Y38.3X-
   lasers Y38.89-
   nuclear weapons Y38.3X-
   piercing or stabbing instruments Y38.89-
   secondary effects Y38.9X-
   specified method NEC Y38.89-
   suicide bomber Y38.81-

Thirst X58

Threat to breathing
   aspiration —see Aspiration
   due to cave-in, falling earth or substance NEC —see categories T71

Thrown (accidentally)
   against part (any) of or object in transport vehicle (in motion) NEC —see also Accident, transport
   from
      high place, homicide (attempt) Y01
      machinery —see Contact, with, by type of machine
      transport vehicle NEC —see also Accident, transport V89.9
   off —see Thrown, from

Thunderbolt —see subcategory T75.0
   causing fire —see Exposure, fire

Tidal wave (any injury) NEC —see Forces of nature, tidal wave

Took
   overdose (drug) —see Table of Drugs and Chemicals
   poison —see Table of Drugs and Chemicals

Tornado (any injury) X37.1

Torrential rain (any injury) X37.8

Torture X58

Trampled by animal NEC W55.89

Trapped (accidentally)
   between objects (moving) (stationary and moving) —see Caught
   by part (any) of
      electric (assisted) bicycle V29.881
      motorcycle V29.888
      pedal cycle V19.88
      transport vehicle NEC —see also Accident, transport V89.9

Travel (effects) (sickness) T75.3

Tree falling on or hitting (accidentally) (person) W20.8

Tripping
   over
      animal W01.0
         with fall W01.0
      carpet, rug or (small) object W22.8
         with fall W18.09
      person W51
         with fall W03
            due to ice or snow W00.0
   without fall W18.40
      due to
         specified NEC W18.49
         stepping from one level to another W18.43
         stepping into hole or opening W18.42
         stepping on object W18.41

Twisted by person(s) (accidentally) W50.2
   with intent to injure or kill Y04.0
   as, or caused by, a crowd or human stampede (with fall) W52
   assault Y04.0
   homicide (attempt) Y04.0
   in
      fight Y04.0
      legal intervention —see Legal, intervention, manhandling

Twisting (prolonged) (static) X50.1

U

Underdosing of necessary drugs, medicaments or biological substances Y63.6

Undetermined intent (contact) (exposure)
   automobile collision Y32
   blunt object Y29
   drowning (submersion) (in) Y21.9
      bathtub Y21.0
         after fall Y21.1
      natural water (lake) (ocean) (pond) (river) (stream) Y21.4
      specified place NEC Y21.8
      swimming pool Y21.2
         after fall Y21.3
   explosive material Y25

Undetermined intent (continued)
fall, jump or push from high place Y30
falling, lying or running before moving object Y31
fire Y26
firearm discharge Y24.9
  airgun (BB) (pellet) Y24.0
  handgun (pistol) (revolver) Y22
  hunting rifle Y23.1
  larger Y23.9
    hunting rifle Y23.1
    machine gun Y23.3
    military Y23.2
    shotgun Y23.0
    specified type NEC Y23.8
  machine gun Y23.3
  military Y23.2
  shotgun Y23.0
  specified type NEC Y24.8
  Very pistol Y24.8
hot object Y27.9
  fluid NEC Y27.2
  household appliance Y27.3
  specified object NEC Y27.8
  steam Y27.0
  tap water Y27.1
  vapor Y27.0
jump, fall or push from high place Y30
lying, falling or running before moving object Y31
motor vehicle crash Y32
push, fall or jump from high place Y30
running, falling or lying before moving object Y31
sharp object Y28.9
  dagger Y28.2
  glass Y28.0
  knife Y28.1
  specified object NEC Y28.8
  sword Y28.2
smoke Y26
specified event NEC Y33

Use of hand as hammer X50.3

V

Vibration (causing injury) W49.9
Victim (of)
  avalanche —*see* Landslide
  earth movements NEC —*see* Forces of nature, earth movement
  earthquake X34
  flood —*see* Flood
  landslide —*see* Landslide
  lightning —*see subcategory* T75.0
  causing fire —*see* Exposure, fire
  storm (cataclysmic) NEC —*see* Forces of nature, cataclysmic storm
  volcanic eruption X35
Volcanic eruption (any injury) X35
Vomitus, gastric contents in air passages (with asphyxia, obstruction or suffocation) T17.81-

W

Walked into stationary object (any) W22.09
  furniture W22.03
  lamppost W22.02
  wall W22.01
War operations (injuries to military personnel and civilians during war, civil insurrection and peacekeeping missions) (by) (from) (involving) Y36.90
  after cessation of hostilities Y36.89-
    explosion (of)
      bomb placed during war operations Y36.82-
      mine placed during war operations Y36.81-
      specified NEC Y36.88-
  air blast Y36.20-
  aircraft
    destruction —*see* War operations, destruction of aircraft
  airway restriction —*see* War operations, restriction of airways
  asphyxiation —*see* War operations, restriction of airways
  biological weapons Y36.6X-
  blast Y36.20-
  blast fragments Y36.20-
  blast wave Y36.20-
  blast wind Y36.20-
  bomb Y36.20-
    dirty Y36.50-
    gasoline Y36.31-
    incendiary Y36.31-
    petrol Y36.31-
  bullet Y36.43-
    incendiary Y36.32-
    rubber Y36.41-
  chemical weapons Y36.7X-
  combat
    hand to hand (unarmed) combat Y36.44-
    using blunt or piercing object Y36.45-
  conflagration —*see* War operations, fire
  conventional warfare NEC Y36.49-
  depth-charge Y36.01-
  destruction of aircraft Y36.10-
    due to
      air to air missile Y36.11-
      collision with other aircraft Y36.12-
      detonation (accidental) of onboard munitions and explosives Y36.14-
      enemy fire or explosives Y36.11-
      explosive placed on aircraft Y36.11-
      onboard fire Y36.13-
      rocket propelled grenade [RPG] Y36.11-
      small arms fire Y36.11-
      surface to air missile Y36.11-
      specified NEC Y36.19-
  detonation (accidental) of onboard marine weapons Y36.05-

War operations (continued)
detonation (continued)
  own munitions or munitions launch device Y36.24-
dirty bomb Y36.50-
explosion (of) Y36.20-
  after cessation of hostilities
    bomb placed during war operations Y36.82-
    mine placed during war operations Y36.81-
  aerial bomb Y36.21-
  bomb NOS —*see also* War operations, bomb(s) Y36.20-
  own munitions or munitions launch device (accidental) Y36.24-
  fragments Y36.20-
  grenade Y36.29-
  guided missile Y36.22-
  improvised explosive device [IED] (person-borne) (roadside) (vehicle-borne) Y36.23-
  land mine Y36.29-
  marine mine (at sea) (in harbor) Y36.02-
  marine weapon Y36.00-
    specified NEC Y36.09-
  sea-based artillery shell Y36.03-
  specified NEC Y36.29-
  torpedo Y36.04-
fire Y36.30-
  specified NEC Y36.39-
firearms
  discharge Y36.43-
  pellets Y36.42-
flamethrower Y36.33-
fragments (from) (of)
  improvised explosive device [IED] (person-borne) (roadside) (vehicle-borne) Y36.26-
  munitions Y36.25-
  specified NEC Y36.29-
  weapons Y36.27-
friendly fire Y36.92
hand to hand (unarmed) combat Y36.44-
hot substances —*see* War operations, fire
incendiary bullet Y36.32-
nuclear weapon (effects of) Y36.50-
  acute radiation exposure Y36.54-
  blast pressure Y36.51-
  direct blast Y36.51-
  direct heat Y36.53-
  fallout exposure Y36.54-
  fireball Y36.53-
  indirect blast (struck or crushed by blast debris) (being thrown by blast) Y36.52-
  ionizing radiation (immediate exposure) Y36.54-
  nuclear radiation Y36.54-
  radiation
    ionizing (immediate exposure) Y36.54-
    nuclear Y36.54-
    thermal Y36.53-

War operations (continued)
nuclear weapon (continued)
  specified NEC Y36.59-
  secondary effects Y36.54-
  thermal radiation Y36.53-
restriction of air (airway)
  intentional Y36.46-
  unintentional Y36.47-
rubber bullets Y36.41-
shrapnel NOS Y36.29-
suffocation —*see* War operations, restriction of airways
unconventional warfare NEC Y36.7X-
underwater blast NOS Y36.00-
warfare
  conventional NEC Y36.49-
  unconventional NEC Y36.7X-
weapons
  biological weapons Y36.6X-
  chemical Y36.7X-
  nuclear (effects of) Y36.50-
    acute radiation exposure Y36.54-
    blast pressure Y36.51-
    direct blast Y36.51-
    direct heat Y36.53-
    fallout exposure Y36.54-
    fireball Y36.53-
    radiation
      ionizing (immediate exposure) Y36.54-
      nuclear Y36.54-
      thermal Y36.53-
    secondary effects Y36.54-
    specified NEC Y36.59-
  of mass destruction [WMD] Y36.91
weapon of mass destruction [WMD] Y36.91

Washed
  away by flood —*see* Flood
  off road by storm (transport vehicle) —*see* Forces of nature, cataclysmic storm

Weather exposure NEC
  —*see* Forces of nature

Weightlessness (causing injury) (effects of) (in spacecraft, real or simulated) X52

Work related condition Y99.0

Wound (accidental) NEC
  —*see also* Injury X58
  battle —*see also* War operations Y36.90
  gunshot —*see* Discharge, firearm by type

Wreck transport vehicle NEC
  —*see also* Accident, transport V89.9

Wrong
  device implanted into correct surgical site Y65.51
  fluid in infusion Y65.1
  procedure (operation) on correct patient Y65.51
  patient, procedure performed on Y65.52

Tabular List of Diseases and Injuries

Table of Contents

1. Certain infectious and parasitic diseases (A00-B99)
2. Neoplasms (C00-D49)
3. Diseases of the blood and blood-forming organs and certain disorders involving the immune mechanism (D50-D89)
4. Endocrine, nutritional and metabolic diseases (E00-E89)
5. Mental, Behavioral and Neurodevelopmental disorders (F01-F99)
6. Diseases of the nervous system (G00-G99)
7. Diseases of the eye and adnexa (H00-H59)
8. Diseases of the ear and mastoid process (H60-H95)
9. Diseases of the circulatory system (I00-I99)
10. Diseases of the respiratory system (J00-J99)
11. Diseases of the digestive system (K00-K95)
12. Diseases of the skin and subcutaneous tissue (L00-L99)
13. Diseases of the musculoskeletal system and connective tissue (M00-M99)
14. Diseases of the genitourinary system (N00-N99)
15. Pregnancy, childbirth and the puerperium (O00-O9A)
16. Certain conditions originating in the perinatal period (P00-P96)
17. Congenital malformations, deformations and chromosomal abnormalities (Q00-Q99)
18. Symptoms, signs and abnormal clinical and laboratory findings, not elsewhere classified (R00-R99)
19. Injury, poisoning and certain other consequences of external causes (S00-T88)
20. External causes of morbidity (V00-Y99)
21. Factors influencing health status and contact with health services (Z00-Z99)
22. Codes for Special Purposes (U00-U85)

Instructional Notations

Includes:
The word 'Includes' appears immediately under certain categories to further define, or give examples of, the content of the category.

Excludes Notes
The ICD-10-CM has two types of excludes notes. Each note has a different definition for use but they are both similar in that they indicate that codes excluded from each other are independent of each other.

Excludes1
A type 1 Excludes note is a pure excludes. It means 'NOT CODED HERE!' An Excludes1 note indicates that the code excluded should never be used at the same time as the code above the Excludes1 note. An Excludes1 is used when two conditions cannot occur together, such as a congenital form versus an acquired form of the same condition.

Excludes2
A type 2 excludes note represents 'Not included here'. An Excludes2 note indicates that the condition excluded is not part of the condition it is excluded from but a patient may have both conditions at the same time. When an Excludes2 note appears under a code it is acceptable to use both the code and the excluded code together.

Code First/Use Additional Code notes (etiology/manifestation paired codes)
Certain conditions have both an underlying etiology and multiple body system manifestations due to the underlying etiology. For such conditions the ICD-10-CM has a coding convention that requires the underlying condition be sequenced first followed by the manifestation. Wherever such a combination exists there is a 'use additional code' note at the etiology code, and a 'code first' note at the manifestation code. These instructional notes indicate the proper sequencing order of the codes, etiology followed by manifestation.

In most cases the manifestation codes will have in the code title, 'in diseases classified elsewhere.' Codes with this title are a component of the etiology/manifestation convention. The code title indicates that it is a manifestation code. 'In diseases classified elsewhere' codes are never permitted to be used as first listed or principal diagnosis codes. They must be used in conjunction with an underlying condition code and they must be listed following the underlying condition.

Code Also
A "code also" note instructs that two codes may be required to fully describe a condition, but this note does not provide sequencing direction. **The sequencing depends on the circumstances of the encounter.**

7th characters and placeholder X
Certain ICD-10-CM categories have applicable 7th characters. The applicable 7th character is required for all codes within the category, or as the notes in the Tabular List instruct. The 7th character must always be the 7th character in the data field. If a code that requires a 7th character is not 6 characters, a placeholder X must be used to fill in the empty characters.

486   +, +7th, X + 7th   ● Newborn   ● Pediatric   ● Maternity   ● Adult   ♀ Female    Male   Manifestation   Unacceptable PDX   HCC   CC   MCC   HAC

Chapter 1: Certain Infectious and Parasitic Diseases (A00-B99)

Includes: diseases generally recognized as communicable or transmissible

Use additional code to identify resistance to antimicrobial drugs (Z16-)

Excludes1: certain localized infections - see body system-related chapters

Excludes2: carrier or suspected carrier of infectious disease (Z22.-)
infectious and parasitic diseases specific to the perinatal period (P35-P39)
infectious and parasitic diseases complicating pregnancy, childbirth and the puerperium (O98.-)
influenza and other acute respiratory infections (J00-J22)

This chapter contains the following category blocks:

A00-A09	Intestinal infectious diseases
A15-A19	Tuberculosis
A20-A28	Certain zoonotic bacterial diseases
A30-A49	Other bacterial diseases
A50-A64	Infections with a predominantly sexual mode of transmission
A65-A69	Other spirochetal diseases
A70-A74	Other diseases caused by chlamydiae
A75-A79	Rickettsioses
A80-A89	Viral and prion infections of the central nervous system
A90-A99	Arthropod-borne viral fevers and viral hemorrhagic fevers
B00-B09	Viral infections characterized by skin and mucous membrane lesions
B10	Other human herpesviruses
B15-B19	Viral hepatitis
B20	Human immunodeficiency virus [HIV] disease
B25-B34	Other viral diseases
B35-B49	Mycoses
B50-B64	Protozoal diseases
B65-B83	Helminthiases
B85-B89	Pediculosis, acariasis and other infestations
B90-B94	Sequelae of infectious and parasitic diseases
B95-B97	Bacterial and viral infectious agents
B99	Other infectious diseases

C. Chapter-Specific Coding Guidelines

In addition to general coding guidelines, there are guidelines for specific diagnoses and/or conditions in the classification. Unless otherwise indicated, these guidelines apply to all health care settings. Please refer to Section II for guidelines on the selection of principal diagnosis.

1. **Chapter 1: Certain Infectious and Parasitic Diseases (A00-B99)**, *U07.1*

    a. **Human Immunodeficiency Virus (HIV) Infections**

    1) **Code only confirmed cases**

    Code only confirmed cases of HIV infection/illness. This is an exception to the hospital inpatient guideline Section II, H.

    In this context, "confirmation" does not require documentation of positive serology or culture for HIV; the provider's diagnostic statement that the patient is HIV positive, or has an HIV-related illness is sufficient.

    2) **Selection and sequencing of HIV codes**

    (a) **Patient admitted for HIV-related condition**

    If a patient is admitted for an HIV-related condition, the principal diagnosis should be B20, Human immunodeficiency virus [HIV] disease followed by additional diagnosis codes for all reported HIV-related conditions.
    An exception to this guideline is if the reason for admission is hemolytic-uremic syndrome associated with HIV disease. Assign code D59.31, Infection-associated hemolytic-uremic syndrome, followed by code B20, Human immunodeficiency virus [HIV] disease.

    (b) **Patient with HIV disease admitted for unrelated condition**

    If a patient with HIV disease is admitted for an unrelated condition (such as a traumatic injury), the code for the unrelated condition (e.g., the nature of injury code) should be the principal diagnosis. Other diagnoses would be B20 followed by additional diagnosis codes for all reported HIV-related conditions.

    (c) **Whether the patient is newly diagnosed**

    Whether the patient is newly diagnosed or has had previous admissions/encounters for HIV conditions is irrelevant to the sequencing decision.

    (d) **Asymptomatic human immunodeficiency virus**

    Z21, Asymptomatic human immunodeficiency virus [HIV] infection status, is to be applied when the patient without any documentation of symptoms is listed as being "HIV positive," "known HIV," "HIV test positive," or similar terminology. Do not use this code if the term "AIDS" is used or if the patient is treated for any HIV-related illness or is described as having any condition(s) resulting from his/her HIV positive status; use B20 in these cases.

    (e) **Patients with inconclusive HIV serology**

    Patients with inconclusive HIV serology, but no definitive diagnosis or manifestations of the illness, may be assigned code R75, Inconclusive laboratory evidence of human immunodeficiency virus [HIV].

    (f) **Previously diagnosed HIV-related illness**

    Patients with any known prior diagnosis of an HIV-related illness should be coded to B20. Once a patient has developed an HIV-related illness, the patient should always be assigned code B20 on every subsequent admission/encounter. Patients previously diagnosed with any HIV illness (B20) should never be assigned to R75 or Z21, Asymptomatic human immunodeficiency virus [HIV] infection status.

    (g) **HIV Infection in Pregnancy, Childbirth and the Puerperium**

    During pregnancy, childbirth or the puerperium, a patient admitted (or presenting for a health care encounter) because of an HIV-related illness should receive a principal diagnosis code of O98.7-, Human immunodeficiency [HIV] disease complicating pregnancy, childbirth and the puerperium, followed by B20 and the code(s) for the HIV-related illness(es). Codes from Chapter 15 always take sequencing priority. Patients with asymptomatic HIV infection status admitted (or presenting for a health care encounter) during pregnancy, childbirth, or the puerperium should receive codes of O98.7- and Z21.

    (h) **Encounters for testing for HIV**

    If a patient is being seen to determine his/her HIV status, use code Z11.4, Encounter for screening for human immunodeficiency virus [HIV]. Use additional codes for any associated high risk behavior.

    If a patient with signs or symptoms is being seen for HIV testing, code the signs and symptoms. An additional counseling code Z71.7, Human immunodeficiency virus [HIV] counseling, may be used if counseling is provided during the encounter for the test.

    When a patient returns to be informed of his/her HIV test results and the test result is negative, use code Z71.7, Human immunodeficiency virus [HIV] counseling.

    If the results are positive, see previous guidelines and assign codes as appropriate.

    (i) **HIV managed by antiretroviral medication**

    If a patient with documented history of HIV disease, HIV-related illness or AIDS is currently managed on antiretroviral medications, assign code B20, Human immunodeficiency virus [HIV] disease. Code Z79.899, Other long term (current) drug therapy, may be assigned as an additional code to identify the long-term (current) use of antiretroviral medications.

    (j) **Encounter for HIV Prophylaxis Measures**

    When a patient is seen for administration of pre-exposure prophylaxis medication for HIV, assign code Z29.81, Encounter for HIV pre-exposure prophylaxis. Pre-exposure prophylaxis (PrEP) is intended to prevent infection in people who are at risk for getting HIV through sex or injection drug use. Any risk factors for HIV should also be coded.

    b. **Infectious agents as the cause of diseases classified to other chapters**

    Certain infections are classified in chapters other than Chapter 1 and no organism is identified as part of the infection code. In these instances, it is necessary to use an additional code from Chapter 1 to identify the organism. A code from category B95, Streptococcus, Staphylococcus, and Enterococcus as the cause of diseases classified to other chapters, B96, Other bacterial agents as the cause of diseases classified to other chapters, or B97, Viral agents as the cause of diseases classified to other chapters, is to be used as an additional code to identify the organism. An instructional note will be found at the infection code advising that an additional organism code is required.

    c. **Infections resistant to antibiotics**

    Many bacterial infections are resistant to current antibiotics. It is necessary to identify all infections documented as antibiotic resistant. Assign a code from category Z16, Resistance to antimicrobial drugs, following the infection code only if the infection code does not identify drug resistance.

    d. **Sepsis, Severe Sepsis, and Septic Shock**

    1) **Coding of Sepsis and Severe Sepsis**

    (a) **Sepsis**

    For a diagnosis of sepsis, assign the appropriate code for the underlying systemic infection. If the type of infection or causal organism is not further specified, assign code A41.9, Sepsis, unspecified organism.

    A code from subcategory R65.2, Severe sepsis, should not be assigned unless severe sepsis or an associated acute organ dysfunction is documented.

(i) Negative or inconclusive blood cultures and sepsis

Negative or inconclusive blood cultures do not preclude a diagnosis of sepsis in patients with clinical evidence of the condition, however, the provider should be queried.

(ii) Urosepsis

The term urosepsis is a nonspecific term. It is not to be considered synonymous with sepsis. It has no default code in the Alphabetic Index. Should a provider use this term, he/she must be queried for clarification.

(iii) Sepsis with organ dysfunction

If a patient has sepsis and associated acute organ dysfunction or multiple organ dysfunction (MOD), follow the instructions for coding severe sepsis.

(iv) Acute organ dysfunction that is not clearly associated with the sepsis

If a patient has sepsis and an acute organ dysfunction, but the medical record documentation indicates that the acute organ dysfunction is related to a medical condition other than the sepsis, do not assign a code from subcategory R65.2, Severe sepsis. An acute organ dysfunction must be associated with the sepsis in order to assign the severe sepsis code. If the documentation is not clear as to whether an acute organ dysfunction is related to the sepsis or another medical condition, query the provider.

(b) Severe sepsis

The coding of severe sepsis requires a minimum of 2 codes: first a code for the underlying systemic infection, followed by a code from subcategory R65.2, Severe sepsis. If the causal organism is not documented, assign code A41.9, Sepsis, unspecified organism, for the infection. Additional code(s) for the associated acute organ dysfunction are also required.

Due to the complex nature of severe sepsis, some cases may require querying the provider prior to assignment of the codes.

2) Septic shock

Septic shock generally refers to circulatory failure associated with severe sepsis, and therefore, it represents a type of acute organ dysfunction.

For cases of septic shock, the code for the systemic infection should be sequenced first, followed by code R65.21, Severe sepsis with septic shock or code T81.12, Postprocedural septic shock. Any additional codes for the other acute organ dysfunctions should also be assigned. As noted in the sequencing instructions in the Tabular List, the code for septic shock cannot be assigned as a principal diagnosis.

3) Sequencing of severe sepsis

If severe sepsis is present on admission, and meets the definition of principal diagnosis, the underlying systemic infection should be assigned as principal diagnosis followed by the appropriate code from subcategory R65.2 as required by the sequencing rules in the Tabular List. A code from subcategory R65.2 can never be assigned as a principal diagnosis.

When severe sepsis develops during an encounter (it was not present on admission) the underlying systemic infection and the appropriate code from subcategory R65.2 should be assigned as secondary diagnoses.

Severe sepsis may be present on admission but the diagnosis may not be confirmed until sometime after admission. If the documentation is not clear whether severe sepsis was present on admission, the provider should be queried.

For infection-associated hemolytic-uremic syndrome with severe sepsis, see guideline I.C.1.d.9.

4) Sepsis or severe sepsis with a localized infection

If the reason for admission is both sepsis or severe sepsis and a localized infection, such as pneumonia or cellulitis, a code(s) for the underlying systemic infection should be assigned first and the code for the localized infection should be assigned as a secondary diagnosis. If the patient has severe sepsis, a code from subcategory R65.2 should also be assigned as a secondary diagnosis. If the patient is admitted with a localized infection, such as pneumonia, and sepsis/severe sepsis doesn't develop until after admission, the localized infection should be assigned first, followed by the appropriate sepsis/severe sepsis codes.

For hemolytic-uremic syndrome associated with sepsis, see guideline I.C.1.d.9.

5) Sepsis due to a postprocedural infection

(a) Documentation of causal relationship

As with all postprocedural complications, code assignment is based on the provider's documentation of the relationship between the infection and the procedure.

(b) Sepsis due to a postprocedural infection

For **sepsis** following a **postprocedural wound (surgical site) infection**, a code from T81.41, to T81.43, Infection following a procedure, or a code from O86.00 to O86.03, Infection of obstetric surgical wound, that identifies the site of the infection should be **sequenced** first, if known. Assign an additional code for sepsis following a procedure (T81.44) or sepsis following an obstetrical procedure (O86.04). Use an additional code to identify the infectious agent. If the patient has severe sepsis the appropriate code from subcategory R65.2 should also be assigned with the additional code(s) for any acute organ dysfunction.

For infections following infusion, transfusion, therapeutic injection, or immunization, a code from subcategory T80.2, Infections following infusion, transfusion, and therapeutic injection, or code T88.0-, Infection following immunization, should be coded first, followed by the code for the specific infection. If the patient has severe sepsis, the appropriate code from subcategory R65.2 should also be assigned, with the additional code(s) for any acute organ dysfunction.

(c) Postprocedural infection and postprocedural septic shock

If a postprocedural infection has resulted in postprocedural septic shock, assign the codes indicated above for sepsis due to a postprocedural infection, followed by code T81.12-, Postprocedural septic shock. Do not assign code R65.21, Severe sepsis with septic shock. Additional code(s) should be assigned for any acute organ dysfunction.

6) Sepsis and severe sepsis associated with a noninfectious process (condition)

In some cases a noninfectious process (condition), such as trauma, may lead to an infection which can result in sepsis or severe sepsis. If sepsis or severe sepsis is documented as associated with a noninfectious condition, such as a burn or serious injury, and this condition meets the definition for principal diagnosis, the code for the noninfectious condition should be sequenced first, followed by the code for the resulting infection. If severe sepsis, is present a code from subcategory R65.2 should also be assigned with any associated organ dysfunction(s) codes. It is not necessary to assign a code from subcategory R65.1, Systemic inflammatory response syndrome (SIRS) of non-infectious origin, for these cases.

If the infection meets the definition of principal diagnosis it should be sequenced before the non-infectious condition. When both the associated non-infectious condition and the infection meet the definition of principal diagnosis either may be assigned as principal diagnosis.

Only one code from category R65, Symptoms and signs specifically associated with systemic inflammation and infection, should be assigned. Therefore, when a non-infectious condition leads to an infection resulting in severe sepsis, assign the appropriate code from subcategory R65.2, Severe sepsis. Do not additionally assign a code from subcategory R65.1, Systemic inflammatory response syndrome (SIRS) of non-infectious origin.

See Section I.C.18. SIRS due to non-infectious process

7) Sepsis and septic shock complicating abortion, pregnancy, childbirth, and the puerperium

See Section I.C.15. Sepsis and septic shock complicating abortion, pregnancy, childbirth and the puerperium

8) Newborn sepsis

See Section I.C.16. f. Bacterial sepsis of Newborn

9) Hemolytic-uremic syndrome associated with sepsis

If the reason for admission is hemolytic-uremic syndrome that is associated with sepsis, assign code D59.31, Infection-associated hemolytic-uremic syndrome, as the principal diagnosis. Codes for the underlying systemic infection and any other conditions (such as severe sepsis) should be assigned as secondary diagnoses.

e. Methicillin Resistant *Staphylococcus aureus* (MRSA) Conditions

1) Selection and sequencing of MRSA codes

(a) Combination codes for MRSA infection

When a patient is diagnosed with an infection that is due to methicillin resistant Staphylococcus aureus (MRSA), and that infection has a combination code that includes the causal organism (e.g., sepsis, pneumonia) assign the appropriate combination code for the condition (e.g., code A41.02, Sepsis due to Methicillin resistant Staphylococcus aureus or code J15.212, Pneumonia due to Methicillin resistant Staphylococcus aureus). Do not assign code B95.62, Methicillin resistant Staphylococcus aureus infection as the cause of diseases classified elsewhere, as an additional code because the combination code includes the type of infection and the MRSA organism. Do not assign a code from subcategory Z16.11, Resistance to penicillins, as an additional diagnosis.

See Section C.1. for instructions on coding and sequencing of sepsis and severe sepsis.

(b) Other codes for MRSA infection

When there is documentation of a current infection (e.g., wound infection, stitch abscess, urinary tract infection) due to MRSA, and that infection does not have a combination code that includes the causal organism, assign the appropriate code to identify the condition along with code B95.62, Methicillin resistant Staphylococcus aureus infection as the cause of diseases classified elsewhere for the MRSA infection. Do not assign a code from subcategory Z16.11, Resistance to penicillins.

(c) Methicillin susceptible Staphylococcus aureus (MSSA) and MRSA colonization

The condition or state of being colonized or carrying MSSA or MRSA is called colonization or carriage, while an individual person is described as being colonized or being a carrier. Colonization means that MSSA or MSRA is present on or in the body without necessarily causing illness. A positive MRSA colonization test might be documented by the provider as "MRSA screen positive" or "MRSA nasal swab positive".

Assign code Z22.322, Carrier or suspected carrier of Methicillin resistant Staphylococcus aureus, for patients documented as having MRSA colonization. Assign code Z22.321, Carrier or suspected carrier of Methicillin susceptible Staphylococcus aureus, for patient documented as having MSSA colonization. Colonization is not necessarily indicative of a disease process or as the cause of a specific condition the patient may have unless documented as such by the provider.

(d) MRSA colonization and infection

If a patient is documented as having both MRSA colonization and infection during a hospital admission, code Z22.322, Carrier or suspected carrier of Methicillin resistant Staphylococcus aureus, and a code for the MRSA infection may both be assigned.

f. Zika virus infections

1) Code only confirmed cases

Code only a confirmed diagnosis of Zika virus (A92.5, Zika virus disease) as documented by the provider. This is an exception to the hospital inpatient guideline Section II, H. In this context, "confirmation" does not require documentation of the type of test performed; the provider's diagnostic statement that the condition is confirmed is sufficient. This code should be assigned regardless of the stated mode of transmission.

If the provider documents "suspected", "possible" or "provable" Zika, do not assign code A92.5. Assign a code(s) explaining the reason for encounter (such as fever, rash, or joint pain) or Z20.821, Contact with and (suspected) exposure to Zika virus.

g. Coronavirus infections

1) COVID-19 infection (infection due to SARS-CoV-2)

(a) Code only confirmed cases

Code only a confirmed diagnosis of the 2019 novel coronavirus disease (COVID-19) as documented by the provider or documentation of a positive COVID-19 test result. For a confirmed diagnosis, assign code U07.1, COVID-19. This is an exception to the hospital inpatient guideline Section II, H. In this context, "confirmation" does not require documentation of a positive test result for COVID-19; the provider's documentation that the individual has COVID-19 is sufficient.

If the provider documents "suspected," "possible," "probable," or "inconclusive" COVID-19, do not assign code U07.1. Instead, code the signs and symptoms reported.

See guideline I.C.1.g.1.g.

(b) Sequencing of codes

When COVID-19 meets the definition of principle diagnosis, code U07.1, COVID-19, should be sequenced first, followed by the appropriate codes for associated manifestations, except when another guideline requires that certain codes be sequenced first, such as obstetrics, sepsis, or transplant complications.

For a COVID-19 infection that progresses to sepsis, see Section I.C.1.d Sepsis, Severe Sepsis, and Septic Shock

See Section I.C.15.s. for COVID-19 infection in pregnancy, childbirth, and the puerperium

See Section I.C.16.h. for COVID-19 infection in newborn

For a COVID-19 infection in a lung transplant patient, see Section I.C.19.g.3.a. Transplant complications other than kidney

(c) Acute respiratory manifestations of COVID-19

When the reason for the encounter/admission is a respiratory manifestation of COVID-19, assign code U07.1, COVID-19, as the principal/first-listed diagnosis and assign code(s) for the respiratory manifestation(s) as additional diagnoses.

The following conditions are examples of common respiratory manifestations of COVID-19.

(i) Pneumonia

For a patient with pneumonia confirmed as due to COVID-19, assign codes U07.1, COVID-19, and J12.82, Pneumonia due to coronavirus disease 2019.

(ii) Acute bronchitis

For a patient with acute bronchitis confirmed as due to COVID-19, assign codes U07.1, and J20.8, Acute bronchitis due to other specified organisms.

Bronchitis not otherwise specified (NOS) due to COVID-19 should be coded using code U07.1 and J40, Bronchitis, not specified as acute or chronic.

(iii) Lower respiratory infection

If the COVID-19 is documented as being associated with lower respiratory infection, not otherwise specified (NOS), or an acute respiratory infection, NOS, codes U07.1 and J22, Unspecified acute lower respiratory infection, should be assigned.

If the COVID-19 is documented as being associated with a respiratory infection, NOS, codes U07.1 and J98.8, Other specified respiratory disorders, should be assigned.

(iv) Acute respiratory distress syndrome

For acute respiratory distress syndrome (ARDS) due to COVID-19, assign codes U07.1 and J80, Acute respiratory distress syndrome.

(v) Acute respiratory failure

For acute respiratory failure due to COVID-19, assign code U07.1 and code J96.0-, Acute respiratory failure.

(d) Non-respiratory manifestations of COVID-19

When the reason for the encounter/admission is a non-respiratory manifestation (e.g., viral enteritis) of COVID-19, assign code U07.1, COVID-19, as the principal/first-listed diagnosis and assign code(s) for the manifestation(s) as additional diagnoses.

(e) Exposure to COVID-19

For asymptomatic individuals with actual or suspected exposure to COVID-19, assign code Z20.822, Contact with and (suspected) exposure to COVID-19.

For symptomatic individuals with actual or suspected exposure to COVID-19 and the infection has been ruled out, or test results are inconclusive or unknown, assign code Z20.822, Contact with and (suspected) exposure to COVID-19.

See guidelines I.C.21.c.1, Contact/Exposure, for additional guidance regarding the use of category Z20 codes.

If COVID-19 is confirmed, see guidelines I.C.1.g.1.a.

(f) Screening for COVID-19

For screening for COVID-19, including preoperative testing, assign code Z11.52, Encounter for screening for COVID-19.

(g) Signs and symptoms without definitive diagnosis of COVID-19

For patient presenting with any signs/symptoms associated with COVID-19 (such as fever, etc.) but a definitive diagnosis has not been established, assign the appropriate code(s) for each of the presenting signs and symptoms such as:

- R05.1, Acute cough, or R05.9, Cough, unspecified
- R06.02 Shortness of breath
- R50.9 Fever, unspecified

If a patient with signs/symptoms associated with COVID-19 also has an actual or suspected contact with or exposure to COVID-19, assign Z20.828, Contact with and (suspected) exposure to other viral communicable diseases, as an additional code.

(h) Asymptomatic individuals who test positive for COVID-19

For asymptomatic individuals who test positive for COVID-19, *see guideline I.C.1.g.1.a.* Although the individual is asymptomatic, the individual has tested positive and is considered to have a COVID-19 infection.

(i) Personal history of COVID-19

For patients with a history of COVID-19, assign code Z86.16, Personal history of COVID-19.

(j) Follow-up visits after COVID-19 infection has resolved

For individuals who previously had COVID-19, without residual symptom(s) or condition(s) and are being seen for follow-up evaluation, and COVID-19 test results are negative, assign codes Z09, Encounter for follow-up examination after completed treatment for conditions other than malignant neoplasm, and Z86.16, Personal history of COVID-19.

For follow-up visits for individuals with symptom(s) or condition(s) related to a previous COVID-19 infection, see guideline I.C.1.g.1.m.

See Section I.C.21.c.8, Factors influencing health states and contact with health services, Follow-up.

(k) Encounter for antibody testing

For an encounter for antibody testing that is not being performed to confirm a current COVID-19 infection, nor is a follow-up test after resolution of COVID-19, assign Z01.84, Encounter for antibody response examination.

Follow the applicable guidelines above if the individual is being tested to confirm a current COVID-19 infection.

For follow-up testing after a COVID-19 infection, see guideline I.C.1.g.1.j

(l) Multisystem Inflammatory Syndrome

For individuals with multisystem inflammatory syndrome (MIS) and COVID-19, assign code U07.1, COVID-19, as the principal/first-listed diagnosis and assign code M35.81, Multisystem inflammatory syndrome, as an additional diagnosis.

If an individual with a history of COVID-19 develops MIS, assign codes M35.81, Multisystem inflammatory syndrome, and U09.9, Post COVID-19 condition, unspecified.

If an individual with a known or suspected exposure to COVID-19, and no current COVID-19 infection or history of COVID-19, develops MIS, assign codes M35.81, Muyltisystem Inflammatory Syndrome, and Z20.822, Contact with and (suspected) exposure to COVID-19.

Additional codes should be assigned for any associated complications of MIS.

(m) Post COVID-19 Condition

For sequela of COVID-19, or associated symptoms or conditions that develop following a previous COVID-19 infection, assign a code(s) for the specific symptom(s) or condition(s) related to the previous COVID-19 infection, if known, and code U09.9, Post COVID-19 condition, unspecified.

Code U09.9 should not be assigned for manifestations of an active (current) COVID-19 infection.

If a patient has a condition(s) associated with a previous COVID-19 infection and develops a new active (current) COVID-19 infection, code U09.9 may be assigned in conjunction with code U07.1, COVID-19, to identify that the patient also has a condition(s) associated with a previous COVID-19 infection. Code(s) for the specific condition(s) associated with the previous COVID-19 infection and code(s) for manifestation(s) of the new active (current) COVID-19 infection should also be assigned.

(n) Underimmunization for COVID-19 Status

Code Z28.310, Unvaccinated for COVID-19, may be assigned when the patient has not received a COVID-19 vaccine of any type. Code Z28.311, Partially vaccinated for COVID-19, may be assigned when the patient has been partially vaccinated for COVID-19 as per the recommendations of the Centers for Disease Control and Prevention (CDC) in place at the time of the encounter. For information, visit the CDC's website https://www.cdc.gov/coronavirus/2019-ncov/vaccines/.

See Section I.B.14. for underimmunization documentation by clinicians other than patient's provider.

Intestinal infectious diseases (A00-A09)

A00 Cholera
- **CC A00.0** Cholera due to Vibrio cholerae 01, biovar cholerae
  - Classical cholera
- **CC A00.1** Cholera due to Vibrio cholerae 01, biovar eltor
  - Cholera eltor
- **CC A00.9** Cholera, unspecified

A01 Typhoid and paratyphoid fevers
- **+ A01.0** Typhoid fever
  - Infection due to Salmonella typhi
  - **CC A01.00** Typhoid fever, unspecified
  - **CC A01.01** Typhoid meningitis
  - **CC A01.02** Typhoid fever with heart involvement
    - Typhoid endocarditis
    - Typhoid myocarditis
  - **CC A01.03** Typhoid pneumonia
  - **CC A01.04** Typhoid arthritis
  - **CC A01.05** Typhoid osteomyelitis
  - **CC A01.09** Typhoid fever with other complications
- **CC A01.1** Paratyphoid fever A
- **CC A01.2** Paratyphoid fever B
- **CC A01.3** Paratyphoid fever C
- **CC A01.4** Paratyphoid fever, unspecified
  - Infection due to Salmonella paratyphi NOS

A02 Other salmonella infections
Includes: infection or foodborne intoxication due to any Salmonella species other than S. typhi and S. paratyphi
- **CC A02.0** Salmonella enteritis
  - Salmonellosis
- **MCC A02.1** Salmonella sepsis
  - **Review coding guideline C.1.d**
- **+ A02.2** Localized salmonella infections
  - **A02.20** Localized salmonella infection, unspecified
  - **MCC A02.21** Salmonella meningitis
  - **MCC A02.22** Salmonella pneumonia
  - **CC A02.23** Salmonella arthritis
  - **CC A02.24** Salmonella osteomyelitis
  - **CC A02.25** Salmonella pyelonephritis
    - Salmonella tubulo-interstitial nephropathy
  - **CC A02.29** Salmonella with other localized infection
- **CC A02.8** Other specified salmonella infections
- **CC A02.9** Salmonella infection, unspecified

A03 Shigellosis
- **CC A03.0** Shigellosis due to Shigella dysenteriae
  - Group A shigellosis [Shiga-Kruse dysentery]
- **A03.1** Shigellosis due to Shigella flexneri
  - Group B shigellosis
- **A03.2** Shigellosis due to Shigella boydii
  - Group C shigellosis
- **A03.3** Shigellosis due to Shigella sonnei
  - Group D shigellosis
- **A03.8** Other shigellosis
- **A03.9** Shigellosis, unspecified
  - Bacillary dysentery NOS

A04 Other bacterial intestinal infections
Excludes1: bacterial foodborne intoxications, NEC (A05.-)
tuberculous enteritis (A18.32)
- **CC A04.0** Enteropathogenic Escherichia coli infection
- **CC A04.1** Enterotoxigenic Escherichia coli infection
- **CC A04.2** Enteroinvasive Escherichia coli infection
- **CC A04.3** Enterohemorrhagic Escherichia coli infection
- **CC A04.4** Other intestinal Escherichia coli infections
  - Escherichia coli enteritis NOS
- **CC A04.5** Campylobacter enteritis
- **CC A04.6** Enteritis due to Yersinia enterocolitica
  - **Excludes1:** extraintestinal yersiniosis (A28.2)
- **+ A04.7** Enterocolitis due to Clostridium difficile
  - Foodborne intoxication by Clostridium difficile
  - Pseudomembraneous colitis
  - *AHA CC: 4Q, 2017, 4*
  - **CC A04.71** Enterocolitis due to clostridium difficile, recurrent
    - *AHA CC: 1Q, 2020, 18*
  - **CC A04.72** Enterocolitis due to clostridium difficile, not specified as recurrent
- **CC A04.8** Other specified bacterial intestinal infections
- **CC A04.9** Bacterial intestinal infection, unspecified
  - Bacterial enteritis NOS

A05 Other bacterial foodborne intoxications, not elsewhere classified

> **Excludes1:** *Clostridium difficile foodborne intoxication and infection (A04.7-)*
> *Escherichia coli infection (A04.0-A04.4)*
> *listeriosis (A32.-)*
> *salmonella foodborne intoxication and infection (A02.-)*
> *toxic effect of noxious foodstuffs (T61-T62)*

- **CC A05.0** Foodborne staphylococcal intoxication
- **CC A05.1** Botulism food poisoning
  - Botulism NOS
  - Classical foodborne intoxication due to Clostridium botulinum
  - **Excludes1:** *infant botulism (A48.51)*
    wound botulism (A48.52)
- **CC A05.2** Foodborne Clostridium perfringens [Clostridium welchii] intoxication
  - Enteritis necroticans
  - Pig-bel
- **CC A05.3** Foodborne Vibrio parahaemolyticus intoxication
- **CC A05.4** Foodborne Bacillus cereus intoxication
- **CC A05.5** Foodborne Vibrio vulnificus intoxication
- **CC A05.8** Other specified bacterial foodborne intoxications
- **A05.9** Bacterial foodborne intoxication, unspecified

A06 Amebiasis

> **Includes:** infection due to Entamoeba histolytica
> **Excludes1:** *other protozoal intestinal diseases (A07.-)*
> **Excludes2:** *acanthamebiasis (B60.1-)*
> *Naegleriasis (B60.2)*

- **CC A06.0** Acute amebic dysentery
  - Acute amebiasis
  - Intestinal amebiasis NOS
- **CC A06.1** Chronic intestinal amebiasis
- **CC A06.2** Amebic nondysenteric colitis
- **CC A06.3** Ameboma of intestine
  - Ameboma NOS
- **MCC A06.4** Amebic liver abscess
  - Hepatic amebiasis
- **MCC A06.5** Amebic lung abscess
  - Amebic abscess of lung (and liver)
- **MCC A06.6** Amebic brain abscess
  - Amebic abscess of brain (and liver) (and lung)
- **A06.7** Cutaneous amebiasis
- **+ A06.8** Amebic infection of other sites
  - **CC A06.81** Amebic cystitis
  - **CC A06.82** Other amebic genitourinary infections
    - Amebic balanitis
    - Amebic vesiculitis
    - Amebic vulvovaginitis
  - **CC A06.89** Other amebic infections
    - Amebic appendicitis
    - Amebic splenic abscess
- **A06.9** Amebiasis, unspecified

A07 Other protozoal intestinal diseases

- **A07.0** Balantidiasis
  - Balantidial dysentery
- **CC A07.1** Giardiasis [lambliasis]
- **CC A07.2** Cryptosporidiosis
- **CC A07.3** Isosporiasis
  - Infection due to Isospora belli and Isospora hominis
  - Intestinal coccidiosis
  - Isosporosis
- **CC A07.4** Cyclosporiasis
- **CC A07.8** Other specified protozoal intestinal diseases
  - Intestinal microsporidiosis
  - Intestinal trichomoniasis
  - Sarcocystosis
  - Sarcosporidiosis
- **CC A07.9** Protozoal intestinal disease, unspecified
  - Flagellate diarrhea
  - Protozoal colitis
  - Protozoal diarrhea
  - Protozoal dysentery

A08 Viral and other specified intestinal infections

> **Excludes1:** *influenza with involvement of gastrointestinal tract (J09.X3, J10.2, J11.2)*

- **CC A08.0** Rotaviral enteritis
- **+ A08.1** Acute gastroenteropathy due to Norwalk agent and other small round viruses
  - **CC A08.11** Acute gastroenteropathy due to Norwalk agent
    - Acute gastroenteropathy due to Norovirus
    - Acute gastroenteropathy due to Norwalk-like agent
  - **CC A08.19** Acute gastroenteropathy due to other small round viruses
    - Acute gastroenteropathy due to small round virus [SRV] NOS
- **CC A08.2** Adenoviral enteritis
- **+ A08.3** Other viral enteritis
  - **CC A08.31** Calicivirus enteritis
  - **CC A08.32** Astrovirus enteritis
  - **CC A08.39** Other viral enteritis
    - Coxsackie virus enteritis
    - Echovirus enteritis
    - Enterovirus enteritis NEC
    - Torovirus enteritis
- **A08.4** Viral intestinal infection, unspecified
  - Viral enteritis NOS
  - Viral gastroenteritis NOS
  - Viral gastroenteropathy NOS
  - *AHA CC: 3Q, 2016, 12*
- **A08.8** Other specified intestinal infections

- **CC A09** Infectious gastroenteritis and colitis, unspecified
  - Infectious colitis NOS
  - Infectious enteritis NOS
  - Infectious gastroenteritis NOS
  - **Excludes1:** *colitis NOS (K52.9)*
    diarrhea NOS (R19.7)
    enteritis NOS (K52.9)
    gastroenteritis NOS (K52.9)
    noninfective gastroenteritis and colitis, unspecified (K52.9)
  - **Valid 3-character code, no further characters required**

Tuberculosis (A15-A19)

> **Includes:** infections due to Mycobacterium tuberculosis and Mycobacterium bovis
> **Excludes1:** *congenital tuberculosis (P37.0)*
> *nonspecific reaction to test for tuberculosis without active tuberculosis (R76.1-)*
> *pneumoconiosis associated with tuberculosis, any type in A15 (J65)*
> *positive PPD (R76.11)*
> *positive tuberculin skin test without active tuberculosis (R76.11)*
> *sequelae of tuberculosis (B90.-)*
> *silicotuberculosis (J65)*

A15 Respiratory tuberculosis

- **CC A15.0** Tuberculosis of lung
  - Tuberculous bronchiectasis
  - Tuberculous fibrosis of lung
  - Tuberculous pneumonia
  - Tuberculous pneumothorax
- **CC A15.4** Tuberculosis of intrathoracic lymph nodes
  - Tuberculosis of hilar lymph nodes
  - Tuberculosis of mediastinal lymph nodes
  - Tuberculosis of tracheobronchial lymph nodes
  - **Excludes1:** *tuberculosis specified as primary (A15.7)*
- **CC A15.5** Tuberculosis of larynx, trachea and bronchus
  - Tuberculosis of bronchus
  - Tuberculosis of glottis
  - Tuberculosis of larynx
  - Tuberculosis of trachea
- **CC A15.6** Tuberculous pleurisy
  - Tuberculosis of pleura Tuberculous empyema
  - **Excludes1:** *primary respiratory tuberculosis (A15.7)*
- **CC A15.7** Primary respiratory tuberculosis
- **CC A15.8** Other respiratory tuberculosis
  - Mediastinal tuberculosis
  - Nasopharyngeal tuberculosis
  - Tuberculosis of nose
  - Tuberculosis of sinus [any nasal]
- **CC A15.9** Respiratory tuberculosis unspecified

A17 Tuberculosis of nervous system

- **MCC A17.0** Tuberculous meningitis
  - Tuberculosis of meninges (cerebral)(spinal)
  - Tuberculous leptomeningitis
  - **Excludes1:** *tuberculous meningoencephalitis (A17.82)*

A17.1–A21.9 — Chapter 1: Certain Infectious and Parasitic Diseases

> MCC **A17.1** **Meningeal tuberculoma**
> Tuberculoma of meninges (cerebral) (spinal)
> **Excludes2:** *tuberculoma of brain and spinal cord (A17.81)*
>
> + **A17.8** **Other tuberculosis of nervous system**
> MCC **A17.81** **Tuberculoma of brain and spinal cord**
> Tuberculous abscess of brain and spinal cord
> MCC **A17.82** **Tuberculous meningoencephalitis**
> Tuberculous myelitis
> MCC **A17.83** **Tuberculous neuritis**
> Tuberculous mononeuropathy
> MCC **A17.89** **Other tuberculosis of nervous system**
> Tuberculous polyneuropathy
> CC **A17.9** **Tuberculosis of nervous system, unspecified**

A18 Tuberculosis of other organs

> + **A18.0** **Tuberculosis of bones and joints**
> CC **A18.01** **Tuberculosis of spine**
> Pott's disease or curvature of spine
> Tuberculous arthritis
> Tuberculous osteomyelitis of spine
> Tuberculous spondylitis
> CC **A18.02** **Tuberculous arthritis of other joints**
> Tuberculosis of hip (joint)
> Tuberculosis of knee (joint)
> CC **A18.03** **Tuberculosis of other bones**
> Tuberculous mastoiditis
> Tuberculous osteomyelitis
> CC **A18.09** **Other musculoskeletal tuberculosis**
> Tuberculous myositis
> Tuberculous synovitis
> Tuberculous tenosynovitis
>
> + **A18.1** **Tuberculosis of genitourinary system**
> CC **A18.10** **Tuberculosis of genitourinary system, unspecified**
> CC **A18.11** **Tuberculosis of kidney and ureter**
> CC **A18.12** **Tuberculosis of bladder**
> CC **A18.13** **Tuberculosis of other urinary organs**
> Tuberculous urethritis
> ● ♂ CC **A18.14** **Tuberculosis of prostate**
> ♂ CC **A18.15** **Tuberculosis of other male genital organs**
> ♀ CC **A18.16** **Tuberculosis of cervix**
> ♀ CC **A18.17** **Tuberculous female pelvic inflammatory disease**
> Tuberculous endometritis
> Tuberculous oophoritis and salpingitis
> ♀ CC **A18.18** **Tuberculosis of other female genital organs**
> Tuberculous ulceration of vulva
>
> CC **A18.2** **Tuberculous peripheral lymphadenopathy**
> Tuberculous adenitis
> **Excludes2:** *tuberculosis of bronchial and mediastinal lymph nodes (A15.4)*
> *tuberculosis of mesenteric and retroperitoneal lymph nodes (A18.39)*
> *tuberculous tracheobronchial adenopathy (A15.4)*
>
> + **A18.3** **Tuberculosis of intestines, peritoneum and mesenteric glands**
> MCC **A18.31** **Tuberculous peritonitis**
> Tuberculous ascites
> CC **A18.32** **Tuberculous enteritis**
> Tuberculosis of anus and rectum
> Tuberculosis of intestine (large) (small)
> CC **A18.39** **Retroperitoneal tuberculosis**
> Tuberculosis of mesenteric glands
> Tuberculosis of retroperitoneal (lymph glands)
>
> CC **A18.4** **Tuberculosis of skin and subcutaneous tissue**
> Erythema induratum, tuberculous
> Lupus excedens
> Lupus vulgaris NOS
> Lupus vulgaris of eyelid
> Scrofuloderma
> Tuberculosis of external ear
> **Excludes2:** *lupus erythematosus (L93.-)*
> *systemic lupus erythematosus (M32.-)*
>
> + **A18.5** **Tuberculosis of eye**
> **Excludes2:** *lupus vulgaris of eyelid (A18.4)*
> CC **A18.50** **Tuberculosis of eye, unspecified**
> CC **A18.51** **Tuberculous episcleritis**
> CC **A18.52** **Tuberculous keratitis**
> Tuberculous interstitial keratitis
> Tuberculous keratoconjunctivitis (interstitial) (phlyctenular)
> CC **A18.53** **Tuberculous chorioretinitis**
> CC **A18.54** **Tuberculous iridocyclitis**
> CC **A18.59** **Other tuberculosis of eye**
> Tuberculous conjunctivitis
>
> CC **A18.6** **Tuberculosis of (inner) (middle) ear**
> Tuberculous otitis media
> **Excludes2:** *tuberculosis of external ear (A18.4)*
> *tuberculous mastoiditis (A18.03)*
>
> CC **A18.7** **Tuberculosis of adrenal glands**
> Tuberculous Addison's disease
>
> + **A18.8** **Tuberculosis of other specified organs**
> CC **A18.81** **Tuberculosis of thyroid gland**
> CC **A18.82** **Tuberculosis of other endocrine glands**
> Tuberculosis of pituitary gland
> Tuberculosis of thymus gland
> CC **A18.83** **Tuberculosis of digestive tract organs, not elsewhere classified**
> **Excludes1:** *tuberculosis of intestine (A18.32)*
> CC **A18.84** **Tuberculosis of heart**
> Tuberculous cardiomyopathy
> Tuberculous endocarditis
> Tuberculous myocarditis
> Tuberculous pericarditis
> CC **A18.85** **Tuberculosis of spleen**
> CC **A18.89** **Tuberculosis of other sites**
> Tuberculosis of muscle
> Tuberculous cerebral arteritis

A19 Miliary tuberculosis

> **Includes:** disseminated tuberculosis
> generalized tuberculosis
> tuberculous polyserositis
> MCC **A19.0** **Acute miliary tuberculosis of a single specified site**
> MCC **A19.1** **Acute miliary tuberculosis of multiple sites**
> MCC **A19.2** **Acute miliary tuberculosis, unspecified**
> MCC **A19.8** **Other miliary tuberculosis**
> MCC **A19.9** **Miliary tuberculosis, unspecified**

Certain zoonotic bacterial diseases (A20-A28)

A20 Plague

> **Includes:** infection due to Yersinia pestis
> MCC **A20.0** **Bubonic plague**
> MCC **A20.1** **Cellulocutaneous plague**
> MCC **A20.2** **Pneumonic plague**
> MCC **A20.3** **Plague meningitis**
> MCC **A20.7** **Septicemic plague**
> *Review coding guideline C.1.d*
> MCC **A20.8** **Other forms of plague**
> Abortive plague
> Asymptomatic plague
> Pestis minor
> MCC **A20.9** **Plague, unspecified**

A21 Tularemia

> **Includes:** deer-fly fever
> infection due to Francisella tularensis
> rabbit fever
> CC **A21.0** **Ulceroglandular tularemia**
> CC **A21.1** **Oculoglandular tularemia**
> Ophthalmic tularemia
> CC **A21.2** **Pulmonary tularemia**
> CC **A21.3** **Gastrointestinal tularemia**
> Abdominal tularemia
> CC **A21.7** **Generalized tularemia**
> *Review coding guideline C.1.d*
> CC **A21.8** **Other forms of tularemia**
> CC **A21.9** **Tularemia, unspecified**

A22 Anthrax
    Includes: infection due to Bacillus anthracis
  CC **A22.0 Cutaneous anthrax**
      Malignant carbuncle
      Malignant pustule
  MCC **A22.1 Pulmonary anthrax**
      Inhalation anthrax
      Ragpicker's disease
      Woolsorter's disease
  CC **A22.2 Gastrointestinal anthrax**
  MCC **A22.7 Anthrax sepsis**
      Review coding guideline C.1.d
  CC **A22.8 Other forms of anthrax**
      Anthrax meningitis
  CC **A22.9 Anthrax, unspecified**

A23 Brucellosis
    Includes: Malta fever
           Mediterranean fever
           undulant fever
  A23.0 Brucellosis due to Brucella melitensis
  A23.1 Brucellosis due to Brucella abortus
  A23.2 Brucellosis due to Brucella suis
  A23.3 Brucellosis due to Brucella canis
  CC **A23.8 Other brucellosis**
  CC **A23.9 Brucellosis, unspecified**
      Review coding guideline C.1.d

A24 Glanders and melioidosis
  CC **A24.0 Glanders**
      Infection due to Pseudomonas mallei
      Malleus
      Review coding guideline C.1.d
  CC **A24.1 Acute and fulminating melioidosis**
      Melioidosis pneumonia
      Melioidosis sepsis
      Review coding guideline C.1.d
  CC **A24.2 Subacute and chronic melioidosis**
  CC **A24.3 Other melioidosis**
  CC **A24.9 Melioidosis, unspecified**
      Infection due to Pseudomonas pseudomallei NOS
      Whitmore's disease

A25 Rat-bite fevers
  CC **A25.0 Spirillosis**
      Sodoku
  CC **A25.1 Streptobacillosis**
      Epidemic arthritic erythema
      Haverhill fever
      Streptobacillary rat-bite fever
  CC **A25.9 Rat-bite fever, unspecified**

A26 Erysipeloid
  A26.0 Cutaneous erysipeloid
      Erythema migrans
  MCC **A26.7 Erysipelothrix sepsis**
      Review coding guideline C.1.d
  A26.8 Other forms of erysipeloid
  A26.9 Erysipeloid, unspecified

A27 Leptospirosis
  CC **A27.0 Leptospirosis icterohemorrhagica**
      Leptospiral or spirochetal jaundice (hemorrhagic)
      Weil's disease
  + **A27.8 Other forms of leptospirosis**
    MCC **A27.81 Aseptic meningitis in leptospirosis**
    CC **A27.89 Other forms of leptospirosis**
  CC **A27.9 Leptospirosis, unspecified**

A28 Other zoonotic bacterial diseases, not elsewhere classified
  CC **A28.0 Pasteurellosis**
      Review coding guideline C.1.d
  CC **A28.1 Cat-scratch disease**
      Cat-scratch fever
  CC **A28.2 Extraintestinal yersiniosis**
      Excludes1: enteritis due to Yersinia enterocolitica (A04.6)
                plague (A20.-)
      Review coding guideline C.1.d
  CC **A28.8 Other specified zoonotic bacterial diseases, not elsewhere classified**
  CC **A28.9 Zoonotic bacterial disease, unspecified**

Other bacterial diseases (A30-A49)

A30 Leprosy [Hansen's disease]
    Includes: infection due to Mycobacterium leprae
    Excludes1: sequelae of leprosy (B92)
  CC **A30.0 Indeterminate leprosy**
      I leprosy
  CC **A30.1 Tuberculoid leprosy**
      TT leprosy
  CC **A30.2 Borderline tuberculoid leprosy**
      BT leprosy
  CC **A30.3 Borderline leprosy**
      BB leprosy
  CC **A30.4 Borderline lepromatous leprosy**
      BL leprosy
  CC **A30.5 Lepromatous leprosy**
      LL leprosy
  CC **A30.8 Other forms of leprosy**
  CC **A30.9 Leprosy, unspecified**

A31 Infection due to other mycobacteria
    Excludes2: leprosy (A30.-)
              tuberculosis (A15-A19)
  CC **A31.0 Pulmonary mycobacterial infection**
      Infection due to Mycobacterium avium
      Infection due to Mycobacterium intracellulare [Battey bacillus]
      Infection due to Mycobacterium kansasii
  CC **A31.1 Cutaneous mycobacterial infection**
      Buruli ulcer
      Infection due to Mycobacterium marinum
      Infection due to Mycobacterium ulcerans
  CC **A31.2 Disseminated mycobacterium avium-intracellulare complex (DMAC)**
      MAC sepsis
  CC **A31.8 Other mycobacterial infections**
  CC **A31.9 Mycobacterial infection, unspecified**
      Atypical mycobacterial infection NOS
      Mycobacteriosis NOS

A32 Listeriosis
    Includes: listerial foodborne infection
    Excludes1: neonatal (disseminated) listeriosis (P37.2)
  CC **A32.0 Cutaneous listeriosis**
  + **A32.1 Listerial meningitis and meningoencephalitis**
    CC **A32.11 Listerial meningitis**
    CC **A32.12 Listerial meningoencephalitis**
  MCC **A32.7 Listerial sepsis**
      Review coding guideline C.1.d
  + **A32.8 Other forms of listeriosis**
    CC **A32.81 Oculoglandular listeriosis**
    CC **A32.82 Listerial endocarditis**
    CC **A32.89 Other forms of listeriosis**
        Listerial cerebral arteritis
  CC **A32.9 Listeriosis, unspecified**

A33 Tetanus neonatorum
MCC
  Valid 3-character code, no further characters required

A34 Obstetrical tetanus
♀ CC
  Valid 3-character code, no further characters required

A35 Other tetanus
MCC
  Tetanus NOS
    Excludes1: obstetrical tetanus (A34)
                tetanus neonatorum (A33)
  Valid 3-character code, no further characters required

A36 Diphtheria
  CC **A36.0 Pharyngeal diphtheria**
      Diphtheritic membranous angina
      Tonsillar diphtheria
  CC **A36.1 Nasopharyngeal diphtheria**
  CC **A36.2 Laryngeal diphtheria**
      Diphtheritic laryngotracheitis
  CC **A36.3 Cutaneous diphtheria**
      Excludes2: erythrasma (L08.1)
  + **A36.8 Other diphtheria**
    CC **A36.81 Diphtheritic cardiomyopathy**
        Diphtheritic myocarditis
    CC **A36.82 Diphtheritic radiculomyelitis**
    CC **A36.83 Diphtheritic polyneuritis**
    CC **A36.84 Diphtheritic tubulo-interstitial nephropathy**

CC A36.85	Diphtheritic cystitis
CC A36.86	Diphtheritic conjunctivitis
CC A36.89	Other diphtheritic complications
	Diphtheritic peritonitis
CC A36.9	Diphtheria, unspecified

A37 Whooping cough

- **A37.0** Whooping cough due to Bordetella pertussis
  - CC **A37.00** Whooping cough due to Bordetella pertussis without pneumonia
    - Paroxysmal cough due to Bordetella pertussis without pneumonia
  - MCC **A37.01** Whooping cough due to Bordetella pertussis with pneumonia
    - Paroxysmal cough due to Bordetella pertussis with pneumonia
- **A37.1** Whooping cough due to Bordetella parapertussis
  - CC **A37.10** Whooping cough due to Bordetella parapertussis without pneumonia
  - MCC **A37.11** Whooping cough due to Bordetella parapertussis with pneumonia
- **A37.8** Whooping cough due to other Bordetella species
  - CC **A37.80** Whooping cough due to other Bordetella species without pneumonia
  - MCC **A37.81** Whooping cough due to other Bordetella species with pneumonia
- **A37.9** Whooping cough, unspecified species
  - CC **A37.90** Whooping cough, unspecified species without pneumonia
  - MCC **A37.91** Whooping cough, unspecified species with pneumonia

A38 Scarlet fever

Includes: scarlatina
Excludes2: streptococcal sore throat (J02.0)

CC A38.0	Scarlet fever with otitis media
CC A38.1	Scarlet fever with myocarditis
CC A38.8	Scarlet fever with other complications
CC A38.9	Scarlet fever, uncomplicated
	Scarlet fever, NOS

A39 Meningococcal infection

MCC A39.0	Meningococcal meningitis
MCC A39.1	Waterhouse-Friderichsen syndrome
	Meningococcal hemorrhagic adrenalitis
	Meningococcic adrenal syndrome
	Review coding guideline C.1.d
MCC A39.2	Acute meningococcemia
	Review coding guideline C.1.d
MCC A39.3	Chronic meningococcemia
	Review coding guideline C.1.d
MCC A39.4	Meningococcemia, unspecified
	Review coding guideline C.1.d

- **A39.5** Meningococcal heart disease
  - MCC **A39.50** Meningococcal carditis, unspecified
  - MCC **A39.51** Meningococcal endocarditis
  - MCC **A39.52** Meningococcal myocarditis
  - MCC **A39.53** Meningococcal pericarditis
- **A39.8** Other meningococcal infections
  - MCC **A39.81** Meningococcal encephalitis
  - CC **A39.82** Meningococcal retrobulbar neuritis
  - CC **A39.83** Meningococcal arthritis
  - CC **A39.84** Postmeningococcal arthritis
  - CC **A39.89** Other meningococcal infections
    - Meningococcal conjunctivitis

CC **A39.9** Meningococcal infection, unspecified
  Meningococcal disease NOS

A40 Streptococcal sepsis

Code first, if applicable, postprocedural sepsis (T81.44-)
  sepsis due to central venous catheter (T80.211-)
  streptococcal sepsis during labor (O75.3)
  streptococcal sepsis following abortion or ectopic or molar pregnancy (O03.37, O03.87, O04.87, O07.37, O08.82)
  streptococcal sepsis following immunization (T88.0-)
  streptococcal sepsis following infusion, transfusion or therapeutic injection (T80.22-, T80.29-)

Excludes1: neonatal (P36.0-P36.1)
  puerperal sepsis (O85)
  sepsis due to Streptococcus, group D (A41.81)

Review coding guideline C.1.d

MCC A40.0	Sepsis due to streptococcus, group A
MCC A40.1	Sepsis due to streptococcus, group B
	AHA CC: 4Q, 2018, 89; 1Q, 2019, 14
MCC A40.3	Sepsis due to Streptococcus pneumoniae
	Pneumococcal sepsis
MCC A40.8	Other streptococcal sepsis
MCC A40.9	Streptococcal sepsis, unspecified

A41 Other sepsis

Code first, if applicable, postprocedural sepsis (T81.44-)
  sepsis due to central venous catheter (T80.211-)
  sepsis during labor (O75.3)
  sepsis following abortion, ectopic or molar pregnancy (O03.37, O03.87, O04.87, O07.37, O08.82)
  sepsis following immunization (T88.0-)
  sepsis following infusion, transfusion or therapeutic injection (T80.22-, T80.29-)

Excludes1: bacteremia NOS (R78.81)
  neonatal (P36.-)
  puerperal sepsis (O85)
  streptococcal sepsis (A40.-)

Excludes2: sepsis (due to) (in) actinomycotic (A42.7)
  sepsis (due to) (in) anthrax (A22.7)
  sepsis (due to) (in) candidal (B37.7)
  sepsis (due to) (in) Erysipelothrix (A26.7)
  sepsis (due to) (in) extraintestinal yersiniosis (A28.2)
  sepsis (due to) (in) gonococcal (A54.86)
  sepsis (due to) (in) herpesviral (B00.7)
  sepsis (due to) (in) listerial (A32.7)
  sepsis (due to) (in) melioidosis (A24.1)
  sepsis (due to) (in) meningococcal (A39.2-A39.4)
  sepsis (due to) (in) plague (A20.7)
  sepsis (due to) (in) tularemia (A21.7)
  toxic shock syndrome (A48.3)

Review coding guideline C.1.d

- **A41.0** Sepsis due to Staphylococcus aureus
  - MCC **A41.01** Sepsis due to Methicillin susceptible Staphylococcus aureus
    - MSSA sepsis
    - Staphylococcus aureus sepsis NOS
    - *AHA CC: 2Q, 2020, 17-18*
  - MCC **A41.02** Sepsis due to Methicillin resistant Staphylococcus aureus
    - **Review coding guideline C.1.e.1.a**

MCC A41.1	Sepsis due to other specified staphylococcus
	Coagulase negative staphylococcus sepsis
MCC A41.2	Sepsis due to unspecified staphylococcus
MCC A41.3	Sepsis due to Hemophilus influenzae
MCC A41.4	Sepsis due to anaerobes
	Excludes1: gas gangrene (A48.0)

- **A41.5** Sepsis due to other Gram-negative organisms
  - MCC **A41.50** Gram-negative sepsis, unspecified
    - Gram-negative sepsis NOS
    - *AHA CC: 2Q, 2020, 29*
  - MCC **A41.51** Sepsis due to Escherichia coli [E. coli]
    - *AHA CC: 1Q, 2018, 16; 2Q, 2020, 17-18*
  - MCC **A41.52** Sepsis due to Pseudomonas
    - Pseudomonas aeruginosa
  - MCC **A41.53** Sepsis due to Serratia
  - MCC **A41.54** Sepsis due to Acinetobacter baumannii
  - MCC **A41.59** Other Gram-negative sepsis
    - *AHA CC: 1Q, 2019, 13*
- **A41.8** Other specified sepsis
  - MCC **A41.81** Sepsis due to Enterococcus
  - MCC **A41.89** Other specified sepsis
    - *AHA CC: 3Q, 2016, 9-14; 2Q, 2020, 8; 1Q, 2021, 33*

MCC **A41.9** Sepsis, unspecified organism
  Septicemia NOS
  AHA CC: 4Q, 2018, 18; 2Q, 2020, 28; 1Q, 2022, 35; 2Q, 2022, 5

A42 Actinomycosis

Excludes1: actinomycetoma (B47.1)

CC A42.0	Pulmonary actinomycosis
CC A42.1	Abdominal actinomycosis
CC A42.2	Cervicofacial actinomycosis
MCC A42.7	Actinomycotic sepsis
	Review coding guideline C.1.d

- **A42.8** Other forms of actinomycosis
  - CC **A42.81** Actinomycotic meningitis
  - CC **A42.82** Actinomycotic encephalitis
  - CC **A42.89** Other forms of actinomycosis

CC **A42.9** Actinomycosis, unspecified

A43 Nocardiosis
  CC **A43.0** Pulmonary nocardiosis
  CC **A43.1** Cutaneous nocardiosis
  CC **A43.8** Other forms of nocardiosis
  CC **A43.9** Nocardiosis, unspecified

A44 Bartonellosis
  CC **A44.0** Systemic bartonellosis
        Oroya fever
  CC **A44.1** Cutaneous and mucocutaneous bartonellosis
        Verruga peruana
  CC **A44.8** Other forms of bartonellosis
  CC **A44.9** Bartonellosis, unspecified

A46 Erysipelas
  Excludes1: postpartum or puerperal erysipelas (O86.89)
  Valid 3-character code, no further characters required

A48 Other bacterial diseases, not elsewhere classified
  Excludes1: actinomycetoma (B47.1)
  MCC **A48.0** Gas gangrene
        Clostridial cellulitis
        Clostridial myonecrosis
        AHA CC: 4Q, 2017, 102
  MCC **A48.1** Legionnaires' disease
      A48.2 Nonpneumonic Legionnaires' disease [Pontiac fever]
  MCC **A48.3** Toxic shock syndrome
        Use additional code to identify the organism (B95, B96)
        Excludes1: endotoxic shock NOS (R57.8)
                sepsis NOS (A41.9)
        AHA CC: 1Q, 2022, 35
      A48.4 Brazilian purpuric fever
        Systemic Hemophilus aegyptius infection
  + **A48.5** Other specified botulism
        Non-foodborne intoxication due to toxins of Clostridium botulinum [C. botulinum]
        Excludes1: food poisoning due to toxins of Clostridium botulinum (A05.1)
    • CC **A48.51** Infant botulism
      CC **A48.52** Wound botulism
        Non-foodborne botulism NOS
        Use additional code for associated wound
      A48.8 Other specified bacterial diseases

A49 Bacterial infection of unspecified site
  Excludes1: bacterial agents as the cause of diseases classified elsewhere (B95-B96)
          chlamydial infection NOS (A74.9)
          meningococcal infection NOS (A39.9)
          rickettsial infection NOS (A79.9)
          spirochetal infection NOS (A69.9)
  + **A49.0** Staphylococcal infection, unspecified
      A49.01 Methicillin susceptible Staphylococcus aureus infection, unspecified site
        Methicillin susceptible Staphylococcus aureus (MSSA) infection
        Staphylococcus aureus infection NOS
      A49.02 Methicillin resistant Staphylococcus aureus infection, unspecified site
        Methicillin resistant Staphylococcus aureus (MRSA) infection
    A49.1 Streptococcal infection, unspecified site
    A49.2 Hemophilus influenzae infection, unspecified site
    A49.3 Mycoplasma infection, unspecified site
    A49.8 Other bacterial infections of unspecified site
    A49.9 Bacterial infection, unspecified
        Excludes1: bacteremia NOS (R78.81)

Infections with a predominantly sexual mode of transmission (A50-A64)

Excludes1: nonspecific and nongonococcal urethritis (N34.1)
         Reiter's disease (M02.3-)
Excludes2: human immunodeficiency virus [HIV] disease (B20)

A50 Congenital syphilis
  + **A50.0** Early congenital syphilis, symptomatic
        Any congenital syphilitic condition specified as early or manifest less than two years after birth.
    CC **A50.01** Early congenital syphilitic oculopathy
    CC **A50.02** Early congenital syphilitic osteochondropathy
    CC **A50.03** Early congenital syphilitic pharyngitis
        Early congenital syphilitic laryngitis
    CC **A50.04** Early congenital syphilitic pneumonia
    CC **A50.05** Early congenital syphilitic rhinitis
    CC **A50.06** Early cutaneous congenital syphilis
    CC **A50.07** Early mucocutaneous congenital syphilis
    CC **A50.08** Early visceral congenital syphilis
    CC **A50.09** Other early congenital syphilis, symptomatic
    A50.1 Early congenital syphilis, latent
        Congenital syphilis without clinical manifestations, with positive serological reaction and negative spinal fluid test, less than two years after birth.
  CC **A50.2** Early congenital syphilis, unspecified
        Congenital syphilis NOS less than two years after birth.
  + **A50.3** Late congenital syphilitic oculopathy
        Excludes1: Hutchinson's triad (A50.53)
    CC **A50.30** Late congenital syphilitic oculopathy, unspecified
    CC **A50.31** Late congenital syphilitic interstitial keratitis
    CC **A50.32** Late congenital syphilitic chorioretinitis
    CC **A50.39** Other late congenital syphilitic oculopathy
  + **A50.4** Late congenital neurosyphilis [juvenile neurosyphilis]
        Use additional code to identify any associated mental disorder
        Excludes1: Hutchinson's triad (A50.53)
    CC **A50.40** Late congenital neurosyphilis, unspecified
        Juvenile neurosyphilis NOS
    MCC **A50.41** Late congenital syphilitic meningitis
    MCC **A50.42** Late congenital syphilitic encephalitis
    CC **A50.43** Late congenital syphilitic polyneuropathy
    CC **A50.44** Late congenital syphilitic optic nerve atrophy
    CC **A50.45** Juvenile general paresis
        Dementia paralytica juvenilis
        Juvenile tabetoparetic neurosyphilis
    CC **A50.49** Other late congenital neurosyphilis
        Juvenile tabes dorsalis
  + **A50.5** Other late congenital syphilis, symptomatic
        Any congenital syphilitic condition specified as late or manifest two years or more after birth.
    CC **A50.51** Clutton's joints
    CC **A50.52** Hutchinson's teeth
    CC **A50.53** Hutchinson's triad
    CC **A50.54** Late congenital cardiovascular syphilis
    CC **A50.55** Late congenital syphilitic arthropathy
    CC **A50.56** Late congenital syphilitic osteochondropathy
    CC **A50.57** Syphilitic saddle nose
    CC **A50.59** Other late congenital syphilis, symptomatic
    A50.6 Late congenital syphilis, latent
        Congenital syphilis without clinical manifestations, with positive serological reaction and negative spinal fluid test, two years or more after birth.
    A50.7 Late congenital syphilis, unspecified
        Congenital syphilis NOS two years or more after birth.
    A50.9 Congenital syphilis, unspecified

A51 Early syphilis
  A51.0 Primary genital syphilis
        Syphilitic chancre NOS
  A51.1 Primary anal syphilis
  A51.2 Primary syphilis of other sites
  + **A51.3** Secondary syphilis of skin and mucous membranes
    CC **A51.31** Condyloma latum
    CC **A51.32** Syphilitic alopecia
    CC **A51.39** Other secondary syphilis of skin
        Syphilitic leukoderma
        Syphilitic mucous patch
        Excludes1: late syphilitic leukoderma (A52.79)
  + **A51.4** Other secondary syphilis
    MCC **A51.41** Secondary syphilitic meningitis
    ♀ CC **A51.42** Secondary syphilitic female pelvic disease
    CC **A51.43** Secondary syphilitic oculopathy
        Secondary syphilitic chorioretinitis
        Secondary syphilitic iridocyclitis, iritis
        Secondary syphilitic uveitis
    CC **A51.44** Secondary syphilitic nephritis
    CC **A51.45** Secondary syphilitic hepatitis
    CC **A51.46** Secondary syphilitic osteopathy
    CC **A51.49** Other secondary syphilitic conditions
        Secondary syphilitic lymphadenopathy
        Secondary syphilitic myositis

A51.5 Early syphilis, latent
Syphilis (acquired) without clinical manifestations, with positive serological reaction and negative spinal fluid test, less than two years after infection.
A51.9 Early syphilis, unspecified

A52 Late syphilis
+ **A52.0** Cardiovascular and cerebrovascular syphilis
  - CC **A52.00** Cardiovascular syphilis, unspecified
  - CC **A52.01** Syphilitic aneurysm of aorta
  - CC **A52.02** Syphilitic aortitis
  - CC **A52.03** Syphilitic endocarditis
    Syphilitic aortic valve incompetence or stenosis
    Syphilitic mitral valve stenosis
    Syphilitic pulmonary valve regurgitation
  - CC **A52.04** Syphilitic cerebral arteritis
  - CC **A52.05** Other cerebrovascular syphilis
    Syphilitic cerebral aneurysm (ruptured) (non-ruptured)
    Syphilitic cerebral thrombosis
  - CC **A52.06** Other syphilitic heart involvement
    Syphilitic coronary artery disease
    Syphilitic myocarditis
    Syphilitic pericarditis
  - CC **A52.09** Other cardiovascular syphilis
+ **A52.1** Symptomatic neurosyphilis
  - CC **A52.10** Symptomatic neurosyphilis, unspecified
  - CC **A52.11** Tabes dorsalis
    Locomotor ataxia (progressive)
    Tabetic neurosyphilis
  - CC **A52.12** Other cerebrospinal syphilis
  - MCC **A52.13** Late syphilitic meningitis
  - MCC **A52.14** Late syphilitic encephalitis
  - CC **A52.15** Late syphilitic neuropathy
    Late syphilitic acoustic neuritis
    Late syphilitic optic (nerve) atrophy
    Late syphilitic polyneuropathy
    Late syphilitic retrobulbar neuritis
  - CC **A52.16** Charcôt's arthropathy (tabetic)
  - CC **A52.17** General paresis
    Dementia paralytica
  - CC **A52.19** Other symptomatic neurosyphilis
    Syphilitic parkinsonism
- CC **A52.2** Asymptomatic neurosyphilis
- CC **A52.3** Neurosyphilis, unspecified
    Gumma (syphilitic)
    Syphilis (late)
    Syphiloma
    AHA CC: 2Q, 2021, 6
+ **A52.7** Other symptomatic late syphilis
  - CC **A52.71** Late syphilitic oculopathy
    Late syphilitic chorioretinitis
    Late syphilitic episcleritis
  - **A52.72** Syphilis of lung and bronchus
  - CC **A52.73** Symptomatic late syphilis of other respiratory organs
  - CC **A52.74** Syphilis of liver and other viscera
    Late syphilitic peritonitis
  - CC **A52.75** Syphilis of kidney and ureter
    Syphilitic glomerular disease
  - CC **A52.76** Other genitourinary symptomatic late syphilis
    Late syphilitic female pelvic inflammatory disease
  - CC **A52.77** Syphilis of bone and joint
  - CC **A52.78** Syphilis of other musculoskeletal tissue
    Late syphilitic bursitis
    Syphilis [stage unspecified] of bursa
    Syphilis [stage unspecified] of muscle
    Syphilis [stage unspecified] of synovium
    Syphilis [stage unspecified] of tendon
  - CC **A52.79** Other symptomatic late syphilis
    Late syphilitic leukoderma
    Syphilis of adrenal gland
    Syphilis of pituitary gland
    Syphilis of thyroid gland
    Syphilitic splenomegaly
    Excludes1: syphilitic leukoderma (secondary) (A51.39)
- **A52.8** Late syphilis, latent
    Syphilis (acquired) without clinical manifestations, with positive serological reaction and negative spinal fluid test, two years or more after infection.
- **A52.9** Late syphilis, unspecified

A53 Other and unspecified syphilis
- **A53.0** Latent syphilis, unspecified as early or late
    Latent syphilis NOS
    Positive serological reaction for syphilis
- **A53.9** Syphilis, unspecified
    Infection due to Treponema pallidum NOS
    Syphilis (acquired) NOS
    Excludes1: syphilis NOS under two years of age (A50.2)

A54 Gonococcal infection
+ **A54.0** Gonococcal infection of lower genitourinary tract without periurethral or accessory gland abscess
    Excludes1: gonococcal infection with genitourinary gland abscess (A54.1)
    gonococcal infection with periurethral abscess (A54.1)
  - CC **A54.00** Gonococcal infection of lower genitourinary tract, unspecified
  - CC **A54.01** Gonococcal cystitis and urethritis, unspecified
  - ♀ CC **A54.02** Gonococcal vulvovaginitis, unspecified
  - ♀ CC **A54.03** Gonococcal cervicitis, unspecified
  - CC **A54.09** Other gonococcal infection of lower genitourinary tract
- CC **A54.1** Gonococcal infection of lower genitourinary tract with periurethral and accessory gland abscess
    Gonococcal Bartholin's gland abscess
+ **A54.2** Gonococcal pelviperitonitis and other gonococcal genitourinary infection
  - CC **A54.21** Gonococcal infection of kidney and ureter
  - ♂ CC **A54.22** Gonococcal prostatitis
  - ♂ CC **A54.23** Gonococcal infection of other male genital organs
    Gonococcal epididymitis
    Gonococcal orchitis
  - ♀ CC **A54.24** Gonococcal female pelvic inflammatory disease
    Gonococcal pelviperitonitis
    Excludes1: gonococcal peritonitis (A54.85)
  - CC **A54.29** Other gonococcal genitourinary infections
+ **A54.3** Gonococcal infection of eye
  - CC **A54.30** Gonococcal infection of eye, unspecified
  - CC **A54.31** Gonococcal conjunctivitis
    Ophthalmia neonatorum due to gonococcus
  - CC **A54.32** Gonococcal iridocyclitis
  - CC **A54.33** Gonococcal keratitis
  - CC **A54.39** Other gonococcal eye infection
    Gonococcal endophthalmia
+ **A54.4** Gonococcal infection of musculoskeletal system
  - CC **A54.40** Gonococcal infection of musculoskeletal system, unspecified
  - CC **A54.41** Gonococcal spondylopathy
  - CC **A54.42** Gonococcal arthritis
    Excludes2: gonococcal infection of spine (A54.41)
  - CC **A54.43** Gonococcal osteomyelitis
    Excludes2: gonococcal infection of spine (A54.41)
  - CC **A54.49** Gonococcal infection of other musculoskeletal tissue
    Gonococcal bursitis
    Gonococcal myositis
    Gonococcal synovitis
    Gonococcal tenosynovitis
- **A54.5** Gonococcal pharyngitis
- **A54.6** Gonococcal infection of anus and rectum
+ **A54.8** Other gonococcal infections
  - MCC **A54.81** Gonococcal meningitis
  - CC **A54.82** Gonococcal brain abscess
  - CC **A54.83** Gonococcal heart infection
    Gonococcal endocarditis
    Gonococcal myocarditis
    Gonococcal pericarditis
  - CC **A54.84** Gonococcal pneumonia
  - CC **A54.85** Gonococcal peritonitis
    Excludes1: gonococcal pelviperitonitis (A54.24)
  - MCC **A54.86** Gonococcal sepsis
    Review coding guideline C.1.d
  - CC **A54.89** Other gonococcal infections
    Gonococcal keratoderma
    Gonococcal lymphadenitis
- CC **A54.9** Gonococcal infection, unspecified

A55 Chlamydial lymphogranuloma (venereum)
    Climatic or tropical bubo
    Durand-Nicolas-Favre disease
    Esthiomene
    Lymphogranuloma inguinale
    Valid 3-character code, no further characters required

A56 Other sexually transmitted chlamydial diseases
    Includes: sexually transmitted diseases due to Chlamydia trachomatis
    Excludes1: neonatal chlamydial conjunctivitis (P39.1)
        neonatal chlamydial pneumonia (P23.1)
    Excludes2: chlamydial lymphogranuloma (A55)
        conditions classified to A74.-
  + **A56.0 Chlamydial infection of lower genitourinary tract**
      A56.00 Chlamydial infection of lower genitourinary tract, unspecified
      A56.01 Chlamydial cystitis and urethritis
    ♀ **A56.02 Chlamydial vulvovaginitis**
      A56.09 Other chlamydial infection of lower genitourinary tract
        Chlamydial cervicitis
  + **A56.1 Chlamydial infection of pelviperitoneum and other genitourinary organs**
    ♀ **A56.11 Chlamydial female pelvic inflammatory disease**
      A56.19 Other chlamydial genitourinary infection
        Chlamydial epididymitis
        Chlamydial orchitis
  A56.2 Chlamydial infection of genitourinary tract, unspecified
  A56.3 Chlamydial infection of anus and rectum
  A56.4 Chlamydial infection of pharynx
  A56.8 Sexually transmitted chlamydial infection of other sites

A57 Chancroid
    Ulcus molle
    Valid 3-character code, no further characters required

A58 Granuloma inguinale
    Donovanosis
    Valid 3-character code, no further characters required

A59 Trichomoniasis
    Excludes2: *intestinal trichomoniasis (A07.8)*
  + **A59.0 Urogenital trichomoniasis**
      A59.00 Urogenital trichomoniasis, unspecified
        Fluor (vaginalis) due to Trichomonas
        Leukorrhea (vaginalis) due to Trichomonas
    ♀ **A59.01 Trichomonal vulvovaginitis**
    ♂ **A59.02 Trichomonal prostatitis**
      A59.03 Trichomonal cystitis and urethritis
      A59.09 Other urogenital trichomoniasis
        Trichomonas cervicitis
  A59.8 Trichomoniasis of other sites
  A59.9 Trichomoniasis, unspecified

A60 Anogenital herpesviral [herpes simplex] infections
  + **A60.0 Herpesviral infection of genitalia and urogenital tract**
      A60.00 Herpesviral infection of urogenital system, unspecified
    ♂ **A60.01 Herpesviral infection of penis**
    ♂ **A60.02 Herpesviral infection of other male genital organs**
    ♀ **A60.03 Herpesviral cervicitis**
    ♀ **A60.04 Herpesviral vulvovaginitis**
        Herpesviral [herpes simplex] ulceration
        Herpesviral [herpes simplex] vaginitis
        Herpesviral [herpes simplex] vulvitis
      A60.09 Herpesviral infection of other urogenital tract
  A60.1 Herpesviral infection of perianal skin and rectum
  A60.9 Anogenital herpesviral infection, unspecified
    AHA CC: 1Q, 2020, 20

A63 Other predominantly sexually transmitted diseases, not elsewhere classified
    Excludes2: *molluscum contagiosum (B08.1)*
        papilloma of cervix (D26.0)
  A63.0 Anogenital (venereal) warts
    Anogenital warts due to (human) papillomavirus [HPV]
    Condyloma acuminatum
  A63.8 Other specified predominantly sexually transmitted diseases

A64 Unspecified sexually transmitted disease
    Valid 3-character code, no further characters required

Other spirochetal diseases (A65-A69)
Excludes2: *leptospirosis (A27.-)*
    syphilis (A50-A53)

A65 Nonvenereal syphilis
    Bejel
    Endemic syphilis
    Njovera
    Valid 3-character code, no further characters required

A66 Yaws
    Includes: bouba
        frambesia (tropica)
        pian
  A66.0 Initial lesions of yaws
    Chancre of yaws
    Frambesia, initial or primary
    Initial frambesial ulcer
    Mother yaw
  A66.1 Multiple papillomata and wet crab yaws
    Frambesioma
    Pianoma
    Plantar or palmar papilloma of yaws
  A66.2 Other early skin lesions of yaws
    Cutaneous yaws, less than five years after infection
    Early yaws (cutaneous)(macular)(maculopapular) (micropapular)(papular)
    Frambeside of early yaws
  A66.3 Hyperkeratosis of yaws
    Ghoul hand
    Hyperkeratosis, palmar or plantar (early) (late) due to yaws
    Worm-eaten soles
  A66.4 Gummata and ulcers of yaws
    Gummatous frambeside
    Nodular late yaws (ulcerated)
  A66.5 Gangosa
    Rhinopharyngitis mutilans
  A66.6 Bone and joint lesions of yaws
    Yaws ganglion
    Yaws goundou
    Yaws gumma, bone
    Yaws gummatous osteitis or periostitis
    Yaws hydrarthrosis
    Yaws osteitis
    Yaws periostitis (hypertrophic)
  A66.7 Other manifestations of yaws
    Juxta-articular nodules of yaws
    Mucosal yaws
  A66.8 Latent yaws
    Yaws without clinical manifestations, with positive serology
  A66.9 Yaws, unspecified

A67 Pinta [carate]
  A67.0 Primary lesions of pinta
    Chancre (primary) of pinta
    Papule (primary) of pinta
  A67.1 Intermediate lesions of pinta
    Erythematous plaques of pinta
    Hyperchromic lesions of pinta
    Hyperkeratosis of pinta
    Pintids
  A67.2 Late lesions of pinta
    Achromic skin lesions of pinta
    Cicatricial skin lesions of pinta
    Dyschromic skin lesions of pinta
  A67.3 Mixed lesions of pinta
    Achromic with hyperchromic skin lesions of pinta [carate]
  A67.9 Pinta, unspecified

A68 Relapsing fevers
    Includes: recurrent fever
    Excludes2: *Lyme disease (A69.2-)*
  CC **A68.0 Louse-borne relapsing fever**
    Relapsing fever due to Borrelia recurrentis
  CC **A68.1 Tick-borne relapsing fever**
    Relapsing fever due to any Borrelia species other than Borrelia recurrentis
  CC **A68.9 Relapsing fever, unspecified**

A69 Other spirochetal infections
- **A69.0** Necrotizing ulcerative stomatitis
  - Cancrum oris
  - Fusospirochetal gangrene
  - Noma
  - Stomatitis gangrenosa
- CC **A69.1** Other Vincent's infections
  - Fusospirochetal pharyngitis
  - Necrotizing ulcerative (acute) gingivitis
  - Necrotizing ulcerative (acute) gingivostomatitis
  - Spirochetal stomatitis
  - Trench mouth
  - Vincent's angina
  - Vincent's gingivitis
- + **A69.2** Lyme disease
  - Erythema chronicum migrans due to Borrelia burgdorferi
  - CC **A69.20** Lyme disease, unspecified
    - *AHA CC: 4Q, 2021, 4-5*
  - CC **A69.21** Meningitis due to Lyme disease
  - CC **A69.22** Other neurologic disorders in Lyme disease
    - Cranial neuritis
    - Meningoencephalitis
    - Polyneuropathy
  - CC **A69.23** Arthritis due to Lyme disease
  - CC **A69.29** Other conditions associated with Lyme disease
    - Myopericarditis due to Lyme disease
    - *AHA CC: 3Q, 2016, 12*
- **A69.8** Other specified spirochetal infections
- **A69.9** Spirochetal infection, unspecified

Other diseases caused by chlamydiae (A70-A74)

Excludes1: *sexually transmitted chlamydial diseases (A55-A56)*

CC A70 Chlamydia psittaci infections
- Ornithosis
- Parrot fever
- Psittacosis
- **Valid 3-character code, no further characters required**

A71 Trachoma
Excludes1: *sequelae of trachoma (B94.0)*
- **A71.0** Initial stage of trachoma
  - Trachoma dubium
- **A71.1** Active stage of trachoma
  - Granular conjunctivitis (trachomatous)
  - Trachomatous follicular conjunctivitis
  - Trachomatous pannus
- **A71.9** Trachoma, unspecified

A74 Other diseases caused by chlamydiae
Excludes1: *neonatal chlamydial conjunctivitis (P39.1)*
neonatal chlamydial pneumonia (P23.1)
Reiter's disease (M02.3-)
sexually transmitted chlamydial diseases (A55-A56)
Excludes2: *chlamydial pneumonia (J16.0)*
- **A74.0** Chlamydial conjunctivitis
  - Paratrachoma
- + **A74.8** Other chlamydial diseases
  - **A74.81** Chlamydial peritonitis
  - **A74.89** Other chlamydial diseases
- **A74.9** Chlamydial infection, unspecified
  - Chlamydiosis NOS

Rickettsioses (A75-A79)

A75 Typhus fever
Excludes1: *rickettsiosis due to Ehrlichia sennetsu (A79.81)*
- CC **A75.0** Epidemic louse-borne typhus fever due to Rickettsia prowazekii
  - Classical typhus (fever)
  - Epidemic (louse-borne) typhus
- CC **A75.1** Recrudescent typhus [Brill's disease]
  - Brill-Zinsser disease
- CC **A75.2** Typhus fever due to Rickettsia typhi
  - Murine (flea-borne) typhus
- CC **A75.3** Typhus fever due to Rickettsia tsutsugamushi
  - Scrub (mite-borne) typhus
  - Typhus fever due to Orientia Tsutsugamushi (scrub typhus)
  - Tsutsugamushi fever
- CC **A75.9** Typhus fever, unspecified
  - Typhus (fever) NOS

A77 Spotted fever [tick-borne rickettsioses]
- CC **A77.0** Spotted fever due to Rickettsia rickettsii
  - Rocky Mountain spotted fever
  - Sao Paulo fever
- CC **A77.1** Spotted fever due to Rickettsia conorii
  - African tick typhus
  - Boutonneuse fever
  - India tick typhus
  - Kenya tick typhus
  - Marseilles fever
  - Mediterranean tick fever
- CC **A77.2** Spotted fever due to Rickettsia siberica
  - North Asian tick fever
  - Siberian tick typhus
- CC **A77.3** Spotted fever due to Rickettsia australis
  - Queensland tick typhus
- + **A77.4** Ehrlichiosis
  - **Excludes1:** *anaplasmosis [A. phagocytophilum] (A79.82)*
  rickettsiosis due to Ehrlichia sennetsu (A79.81)
  AHA CC: 4Q, 2021, 4-5
  - CC **A77.40** Ehrlichiosis, unspecified
  - CC **A77.41** Ehrlichiosis chafeensis [E. chafeensis]
  - CC **A77.49** Other ehrlichiosis
    - Ehrlichiosis due to E. ewingii
    - Ehrlichiosis due to E. muris euclairensis
- CC **A77.8** Other spotted fevers
  - Rickettsia 364D/R. philipii (Pacific Coast tick fever)
  - Spotted fever due to Rickettsia africae (African tick bite fever)
  - Spotted fever due to Rickettsia parkeri
- CC **A77.9** Spotted fever, unspecified
  - Tick-borne typhus NOS

CC A78 Q fever
- Infection due to Coxiella burnetii
- Nine Mile fever
- Quadrilateral fever
- **Valid 3-character code, no further characters required**

A79 Other rickettsioses
- CC **A79.0** Trench fever
  - Quintan fever
  - Wolhynian fever
- CC **A79.1** Rickettsialpox due to Rickettsia akari
  - Kew Garden fever
  - Vesicular rickettsiosis
- + **A79.8** Other specified rickettsioses
  - CC **A79.81** Rickettsiosis due to Ehrlichia sennetsu
    - Rickettsiosis due to Neorickettsia sennetsu
    - **Excludes1:** *rickettsiosis due to Ehrlichia sennetsu (A79.81)*
  - CC **A79.82** Anaplasmosis [A. phagocytophilum]
    - Transfusion transmitted A. phagocytophilum
    - *AHA CC: 4Q, 2021, 4-5*
  - CC **A79.89** Other specified rickettsioses
- CC **A79.9** Rickettsiosis, unspecified
  - Rickettsial infection NOS

Viral and prion infections of the central nervous system (A80-A89)

Excludes1: *postpolio syndrome (G14)*
sequelae of poliomyelitis (B91)
sequelae of viral encephalitis (B94.1)

A80 Acute poliomyelitis
Excludes1: *acute flaccid myelitis (G04.82)*
- MCC **A80.0** Acute paralytic poliomyelitis, vaccine-associated
- MCC **A80.1** Acute paralytic poliomyelitis, wild virus, imported
- MCC **A80.2** Acute paralytic poliomyelitis, wild virus, indigenous
- + **A80.3** Acute paralytic poliomyelitis, other and unspecified
  - MCC **A80.30** Acute paralytic poliomyelitis, unspecified
  - MCC **A80.39** Other acute paralytic poliomyelitis
- **A80.4** Acute nonparalytic poliomyelitis
- **A80.9** Acute poliomyelitis, unspecified

A81 Atypical virus infections of central nervous system

Includes: diseases of the central nervous system caused by prions

Use additional code, if applicable, to identify:
dementia with anxiety (F02.84, F02.A4, F02.B4, F02.C4)
dementia with behavioral disturbance (F02.81-, F02.A1-, F02.B1-, F02.C1-)
dementia with mood disturbance (F02.83, F02.A3, F02.B3, F02.C3)
dementia with psychotic disturbance (F02.82, F02.A2, F02.B2, F02.C2)
dementia without behavioral disturbance (F02.80, F02.A0, F02.B0, F02.C0)
mild neurocognitive disorder due to known physiological condition (F06.7-)

- **+ A81.0 Creutzfeldt-Jakob disease**
  - **CC A81.00** Creutzfeldt-Jakob disease, unspecified
    Jakob-Creutzfeldt disease, unspecified
  - **CC A81.01** Variant Creutzfeldt-Jakob disease
    CJD
  - **CC A81.09** Other Creutzfeldt-Jakob disease
    CJD
    Familial Creutzfeldt-Jakob disease
    Iatrogenic Creutzfeldt-Jakob disease
    Sporadic Creutzfeldt-Jakob disease
    Subacute spongiform encephalopathy (with dementia)
- **CC A81.1 Subacute sclerosing panencephalitis**
  Dawson's inclusion body encephalitis
  Van Bogaert's sclerosing leukoencephalopathy
- **CC A81.2 Progressive multifocal leukoencephalopathy**
  Multifocal leukoencephalopathy NOS
- **+ A81.8 Other atypical virus infections of central nervous system**
  - **CC A81.81** Kuru
  - **CC A81.82** Gerstmann-Sträussler-Scheinker syndrome
    GSS syndrome
  - **CC A81.83** Fatal familial insomnia
    FFI
  - **CC A81.89** Other atypical virus infections of central nervous system
- **CC A81.9 Atypical virus infection of central nervous system, unspecified**
  Prion diseases of the central nervous system NOS

A82 Rabies

- **CC A82.0** Sylvatic rabies
- **CC A82.1** Urban rabies
- **CC A82.9** Rabies, unspecified

A83 Mosquito-borne viral encephalitis

Includes: mosquito-borne viral meningoencephalitis
Excludes2: Venezuelan equine encephalitis (A92.2)
West Nile fever (A92.3-)
West Nile virus (A92.3-)

- **MCC A83.0** Japanese encephalitis
- **MCC A83.1** Western equine encephalitis
- **MCC A83.2** Eastern equine encephalitis
- **MCC A83.3** St Louis encephalitis
- **MCC A83.4** Australian encephalitis
  Kunjin virus disease
- **MCC A83.5** California encephalitis
  California meningoencephalitis
  La Crosse encephalitis
- **MCC A83.6** Rocio virus disease
- **MCC A83.8** Other mosquito-borne viral encephalitis
- **MCC A83.9** Mosquito-borne viral encephalitis, unspecified

A84 Tick-borne viral encephalitis

Includes: tick-borne viral meningoencephalitis

- **MCC A84.0** Far Eastern tick-borne encephalitis [Russian spring-summer encephalitis]
- **MCC A84.1** Central European tick-borne encephalitis
- **+ A84.8 Other tick-borne viral encephalitis**
  - **MCC A84.81** Powassan virus disease
    AHA CC: 4Q, 2020, 4-5
  - **MCC A84.89** Other tick-borne viral encephalitis
    Louping ill
    Code first, if applicable, transfusion related infection (T80.22-)
- **MCC A84.9** Tick-borne viral encephalitis, unspecified

A85 Other viral encephalitis, not elsewhere classified

Includes: specified viral encephalomyelitis NEC
specified viral meningoencephalitis NEC
Excludes1: encephalitis due to cytomegalovirus (B25.8)
encephalitis due to herpesvirus NEC (B10.0-)
encephalitis due to herpesvirus [herpes simplex] (B00.4)
encephalitis due to measles virus (B05.0)
encephalitis due to mumps virus (B26.2)
encephalitis due to poliomyelitis virus (A80.-)
encephalitis due to zoster (B02.0)
lymphocytic choriomeningitis (A87.2)
myalgic encephalomyelitis (G93.32)

- **CC A85.0** Enteroviral encephalitis
  Enteroviral encephalomyelitis
- **CC A85.1** Adenoviral encephalitis
  Adenoviral meningoencephalitis
- **MCC A85.2** Arthropod-borne viral encephalitis, unspecified
  Excludes1: West nile virus with encephalitis (A92.31)
- **CC A85.8** Other specified viral encephalitis
  Encephalitis lethargica
  Von Economo-Cruchet disease

CC A86 Unspecified viral encephalitis

Viral encephalomyelitis NOS
Viral meningoencephalitis NOS
Valid 3-character code, no further characters required

A87 Viral meningitis

Excludes1: meningitis due to herpesvirus [herpes simplex] (B00.3)
meningitis due to herpesvirus [herpes simplex] (B00.3)
meningitis due to measles virus (B05.1)
meningitis due to mumps virus (B26.1)
meningitis due to poliomyelitis virus (A80.-)
meningitis due to zoster (B02.1)

- **CC A87.0** Enteroviral meningitis
  Coxsackievirus meningitis
  Echovirus meningitis
- **CC A87.1** Adenoviral meningitis
- **CC A87.2** Lymphocytic choriomeningitis
  Lymphocytic meningoencephalitis
- **CC A87.8** Other viral meningitis
- **CC A87.9** Viral meningitis, unspecified

A88 Other viral infections of central nervous system, not elsewhere classified

Excludes1: viral encephalitis NOS (A86)
viral meningitis NOS (A87.9)

- **CC A88.0** Enteroviral exanthematous fever [Boston exanthem]
- **A88.1** Epidemic vertigo
- **CC A88.8** Other specified viral infections of central nervous system

CC A89 Unspecified viral infection of central nervous system

Valid 3-character code, no further characters required

Arthropod-borne viral fevers and viral hemorrhagic fevers (A90-A99)

CC A90 Dengue fever [classical dengue]

Excludes1: dengue hemorrhagic fever (A91)
AHA CC: 3Q, 2016, 13
Valid 3-character code, no further characters required

CC A91 Dengue hemorrhagic fever

Valid 3-character code, no further characters required

A92 Other mosquito-borne viral fevers

Excludes1: Ross River disease (B33.1)

- **CC A92.0** Chikungunya virus disease
  Chikungunya (hemorrhagic) fever
- **CC A92.1** O'nyong-nyong fever
- **CC A92.2** Venezuelan equine fever
  Venezuelan equine encephalitis
  Venezuelan equine encephalomyelitis virus disease
- **+ A92.3 West Nile virus infection**
  West Nile fever
  - **MCC A92.30** West Nile virus infection, unspecified
    West Nile fever NOS
    West Nile fever without complications
    West Nile virus NOS

MCC A92.31 West Nile virus infection with encephalitis
    West Nile encephalitis
    West Nile encephalomyelitis
    AHA CC: 3Q, 2016, 12-13
MCC A92.32 West Nile virus infection with other neurologic manifestation
    Use additional code to specify the neurologic manifestation
MCC A92.39 West Nile virus infection with other complications
    Use additional code to specify the other conditions
CC A92.4 Rift Valley fever
CC A92.5 Zika virus disease
    Zika virus fever
    Zika virus infection
    Zika NOS
    Excludes1: congenital Zika virus disease (P35.4)
    Review coding guideline C.1.f
    AHA CC: 4Q, 2016, 4-7
CC A92.8 Other specified mosquito-borne viral fevers
CC A92.9 Mosquito-borne viral fever, unspecified

A93 Other arthropod-borne viral fevers, not elsewhere classified
CC A93.0 Oropouche virus disease
    Oropouche fever
CC A93.1 Sandfly fever
    Pappataci fever
    Phlebotomus fever
CC A93.2 Colorado tick fever
CC A93.8 Other specified arthropod-borne viral fevers
    Piry virus disease
    Vesicular stomatitis virus disease [Indiana fever]

CC A94 Unspecified arthropod-borne viral fever
    Arboviral fever NOS
    Arbovirus infection NOS
    Valid 3-character code, no further characters required

A95 Yellow fever
CC A95.0 Sylvatic yellow fever
    Jungle yellow fever
CC A95.1 Urban yellow fever
CC A95.9 Yellow fever, unspecified

A96 Arenaviral hemorrhagic fever
CC A96.0 Junin hemorrhagic fever
    Argentinian hemorrhagic fever
CC A96.1 Machupo hemorrhagic fever
    Bolivian hemorrhagic fever
A96.2 Lassa fever
CC A96.8 Other arenaviral hemorrhagic fevers
CC A96.9 Arenaviral hemorrhagic fever, unspecified

A98 Other viral hemorrhagic fevers, not elsewhere classified
    Excludes1: chikungunya hemorrhagic fever (A92.0)
        dengue hemorrhagic fever (A91)
CC A98.0 Crimean-Congo hemorrhagic fever
    Central Asian hemorrhagic fever
CC A98.1 Omsk hemorrhagic fever
CC A98.2 Kyasanur Forest disease
A98.3 Marburg virus disease
A98.4 Ebola virus disease
CC A98.5 Hemorrhagic fever with renal syndrome
    Epidemic hemorrhagic fever
    Korean hemorrhagic fever
    Russian hemorrhagic fever
    Hantaan virus disease
    Hantavirus disease with renal manifestations
    Nephropathia epidemica
    Songo fever
    Excludes1: hantavirus (cardio)-pulmonary syndrome (B33.4)
CC A98.8 Other specified viral hemorrhagic fevers

CC A99 Unspecified viral hemorrhagic fever
    Valid 3-character code, no further characters

Viral infections characterized by skin and mucous membrane lesions (B00-B09)

B00 Herpesviral [herpes simplex] infections
    Excludes1: congenital herpesviral infections (P35.2)
    Excludes2: anogenital herpesviral infection (A60.-)
        gammaherpesviral mononucleosis (B27.0-)
        herpangina (B08.5)
    B00.0 Eczema herpeticum
        Kaposi's varicelliform eruption
    B00.1 Herpesviral vesicular dermatitis
        Herpes simplex facialis
        Herpes simplex labialis
        Herpes simplex otitis externa
        Vesicular dermatitis of ear
        Vesicular dermatitis of lip
    CC B00.2 Herpesviral gingivostomatitis and pharyngotonsillitis
        Herpesviral pharyngitis
    MCC B00.3 Herpesviral meningitis
    MCC B00.4 Herpesviral encephalitis
        Herpesviral meningoencephalitis
        Simian B disease
        Excludes1: herpesviral encephalitis due to herpesvirus 6 and 7 (B10.01, B10.09)
            non-simplex herpesviral encephalitis (B10.0-)
    + **B00.5** Herpesviral ocular disease
        CC B00.50 Herpesviral ocular disease, unspecified
        CC B00.51 Herpesviral iridocyclitis
            Herpesviral iritis
            Herpesviral uveitis, anterior
        CC B00.52 Herpesviral keratitis
            Herpesviral keratoconjunctivitis
        CC B00.53 Herpesviral conjunctivitis
        CC B00.59 Other herpesviral disease of eye
            Herpesviral dermatitis of eyelid
    MCC B00.7 Disseminated herpesviral disease
        Herpesviral sepsis
        Review coding guideline C.1.d
    + **B00.8** Other forms of herpesviral infections
        CC B00.81 Herpesviral hepatitis
        MCC B00.82 Herpes simplex myelitis
        CC B00.89 Other herpesviral infection
            Herpesviral whitlow
    B00.9 Herpesviral infection, unspecified
        Herpes simplex infection NOS

B01 Varicella [chickenpox]
    CC B01.0 Varicella meningitis
    + **B01.1** Varicella encephalitis, myelitis and encephalomyelitis
        Postchickenpox encephalitis, myelitis and encephalomyelitis
        MCC B01.11 Varicella encephalitis and encephalomyelitis
            Postchickenpox encephalitis and encephalomyelitis
        MCC B01.12 Varicella myelitis
            Postchickenpox myelitis
    MCC B01.2 Varicella pneumonia
    + **B01.8** Varicella with other complications
        CC B01.81 Varicella keratitis
        CC B01.89 Other varicella complications
    CC B01.9 Varicella without complication
        Varicella NOS

B02 Zoster [herpes zoster]
    Includes: shingles
        zona
    CC B02.0 Zoster encephalitis
        Zoster meningoencephalitis
    MCC B02.1 Zoster meningitis
        AHA CC: 1Q, 2019, 18
    + **B02.2** Zoster with other nervous system involvement
        CC B02.21 Postherpetic geniculate ganglionitis
        CC B02.22 Postherpetic trigeminal neuralgia
        CC B02.23 Postherpetic polyneuropathy
        MCC B02.24 Postherpetic myelitis
            Herpes zoster myelitis
        CC B02.29 Other postherpetic nervous system involvement
            Postherpetic radiculopathy
    + **B02.3** Zoster ocular disease
        CC B02.30 Zoster ocular disease, unspecified
        CC B02.31 Zoster conjunctivitis
        CC B02.32 Zoster iridocyclitis
        CC B02.33 Zoster keratitis
            Herpes zoster keratoconjunctivitis

CC B02.34 Zoster scleritis
CC B02.39 Other herpes zoster eye disease
Zoster blepharitis
CC B02.7 Disseminated zoster
CC B02.8 Zoster with other complications
Herpes zoster otitis externa
B02.9 Zoster without complications
Zoster NOS

CC **B03 Smallpox**
NOTE In 1980 the 33rd World Health Assembly declared that smallpox had been eradicated. The classification is maintained for surveillance purposes.
Valid 3-character code, no further characters required

CC **B04 Monkeypox**
AHA CC: 3Q, 2022, 3
Valid 3-character code, no further characters required

B05 Measles
Includes: morbilli
Excludes1: subacute sclerosing panencephalitis (A81.1)
MCC B05.0 Measles complicated by encephalitis
Postmeasles encephalitis
CC B05.1 Measles complicated by meningitis
Postmeasles meningitis
MCC B05.2 Measles complicated by pneumonia
Postmeasles pneumonia
B05.3 Measles complicated by otitis media
Postmeasles otitis media
CC B05.4 Measles with intestinal complications
+ B05.8 Measles with other complications
CC B05.81 Measles keratitis and keratoconjunctivitis
CC B05.89 Other measles complications
B05.9 Measles without complication
Measles NOS

B06 Rubella [German measles]
Excludes1: congenital rubella (P35.0)
+ B06.0 Rubella with neurological complications
CC B06.00 Rubella with neurological complication, unspecified
MCC B06.01 Rubella encephalitis
Rubella meningoencephalitis
CC B06.02 Rubella meningitis
CC B06.09 Other neurological complications of rubella
+ B06.8 Rubella with other complications
CC B06.81 Rubella pneumonia
CC B06.82 Rubella arthritis
CC B06.89 Other rubella complications
B06.9 Rubella without complication
Rubella NOS

B07 Viral warts
Includes: verruca simplex
verruca vulgaris
viral warts due to human papillomavirus
Excludes2: anogenital (venereal) warts (A63.0)
papilloma of bladder (D41.4)
papilloma of cervix (D26.0)
papilloma of larynx (D14.1)
B07.0 Plantar wart
Verruca plantaris
B07.8 Other viral warts
Common wart
Flat wart
Verruca plana
B07.9 Viral wart, unspecified

B08 Other viral infections characterized by skin and mucous membrane lesions, not elsewhere classified
Excludes1: vesicular stomatitis virus disease (A93.8)
B08.0 Other orthopoxvirus infections
Excludes2: monkeypox (B04)
+ B08.01 Cowpox and vaccinia not from vaccine
B08.010 Cowpox
B08.011 Vaccinia not from vaccine
Excludes1: vaccinia (from vaccination) (generalized) (T88.1)
B08.02 Orf virus disease
Contagious pustular dermatitis
Ecthyma contagiosum
B08.03 Pseudocowpox [milker's node]
B08.04 Paravaccinia, unspecified
B08.09 Other orthopoxvirus infections
Orthopoxvirus infection NOS
B08.1 Molluscum contagiosum
+ B08.2 Exanthema subitum [sixth disease]
Roseola infantum
• B08.20 Exanthema subitum [sixth disease], unspecified
Roseola infantum, unspecified
• B08.21 Exanthema subitum [sixth disease] due to human herpesvirus 6
Roseola infantum due to human herpesvirus 6
• B08.22 Exanthema subitum [sixth disease] due to human herpesvirus 7
Roseola infantum due to human herpesvirus 7
CC B08.3 Erythema infectiosum [fifth disease]
B08.4 Enteroviral vesicular stomatitis with exanthem
Hand, foot and mouth disease
B08.5 Enteroviral vesicular pharyngitis
Herpangina
+ B08.6 Parapoxvirus infections
B08.60 Parapoxvirus infection, unspecified
B08.61 Bovine stomatitis
B08.62 Sealpox
B08.69 Other parapoxvirus infections
+ B08.7 Yatapoxvirus infections
B08.70 Yatapoxvirus infection, unspecified
CC B08.71 Tanapox virus disease
B08.72 Yaba pox virus disease
Yaba monkey tumor disease
B08.79 Other yatapoxvirus infections
B08.8 Other specified viral infections characterized by skin and mucous membrane lesions
Enteroviral lymphonodular pharyngitis
Foot-and-mouth disease
Poxvirus NEC

B09 Unspecified viral infection characterized by skin and mucous membrane lesions
Viral enanthema NOS
Viral exanthema NOS
Valid 3-character code, no further characters required

Other human herpesviruses (B10)
B10 Other human herpesviruses
Excludes2: cytomegalovirus (B25.9)
Epstein-Barr virus (B27.0-)
herpes NOS (B00.9)
herpes simplex (B00.-)
herpes zoster (B02.-)
human herpesvirus NOS (B00.-)
human herpesvirus 1 and 2 (B00.-)
human herpesvirus 3 (B01.-, B02.-)
human herpesvirus 4 (B27.0-)
human herpesvirus 5 (B25.-)
varicella (B01.-)
zoster (B02.-)
+ B10.0 Other human herpesvirus encephalitis
Excludes2: herpes encephalitis NOS (B00.4)
herpes simplex encephalitis (B00.4)
human herpesvirus encephalitis (B00.4)
simian B herpes virus encephalitis (B00.4)
MCC B10.01 Human herpesvirus 6 encephalitis
MCC B10.09 Other human herpesvirus encephalitis
Human herpesvirus 7 encephalitis
+ B10.8 Other human herpesvirus infection
B10.81 Human herpesvirus 6 infection
B10.82 Human herpesvirus 7 infection
B10.89 Other human herpesvirus infection
Human herpesvirus 8 infection
Kaposi's sarcoma-associated herpesvirus infection

Viral hepatitis (B15-B19)
Excludes1: sequelae of viral hepatitis (B94.2)
Excludes2: cytomegaloviral hepatitis (B25.1)
herpesviral [herpes simplex] hepatitis (B00.81)

B15 Acute hepatitis A
MCC B15.0 Hepatitis A with hepatic coma
CC B15.9 Hepatitis A without hepatic coma
Hepatitis A (acute)(viral) NOS

B16 Acute hepatitis B
- MCC **B16.0** Acute hepatitis B with delta-agent with hepatic coma
- CC **B16.1** Acute hepatitis B with delta-agent without hepatic coma
- MCC **B16.2** Acute hepatitis B without delta-agent with hepatic coma
- CC **B16.9** Acute hepatitis B without delta-agent and without hepatic coma
  Hepatitis B (acute) (viral) NOS
  AHA CC: 3Q, 2016, 13

B17 Other acute viral hepatitis
- CC **B17.0** Acute delta-(super) infection of hepatitis B carrier
- + **B17.1** Acute hepatitis C
  - CC **B17.10** Acute hepatitis C without hepatic coma
    Acute hepatitis C NOS
  - MCC **B17.11** Acute hepatitis C with hepatic coma
- CC **B17.2** Acute hepatitis E
- CC **B17.8** Other specified acute viral hepatitis
  Hepatitis non-A non-B (acute) (viral) NEC
- CC **B17.9** Acute viral hepatitis, unspecified
  Acute hepatitis NOS
  Acute infectious hepatitis NOS

B18 Chronic viral hepatitis
Includes: Carrier of viral hepatitis
- CC **B18.0** Chronic viral hepatitis B with delta-agent
- CC **B18.1** Chronic viral hepatitis B without delta-agent
  Carrier of viral hepatitis B
  Chronic (viral) hepatitis B
- **B18.2** Chronic viral hepatitis C
  Carrier of viral hepatitis C
  AHA CC: 1Q, 2017, 41; 1Q, 2018, 4-5
- CC **B18.8** Other chronic viral hepatitis
  Carrier of other viral hepatitis
- CC **B18.9** Chronic viral hepatitis, unspecified
  Carrier of unspecified viral hepatitis

B19 Unspecified viral hepatitis
- MCC **B19.0** Unspecified viral hepatitis with hepatic coma
- + **B19.1** Unspecified viral hepatitis B
  - CC **B19.10** Unspecified viral hepatitis B without hepatic coma
    Unspecified viral hepatitis B NOS
  - MCC **B19.11** Unspecified viral hepatitis B with hepatic coma
- + **B19.2** Unspecified viral hepatitis C
  - **B19.20** Unspecified viral hepatitis C without hepatic coma
    Viral hepatitis C NOS
  - MCC **B19.21** Unspecified viral hepatitis C with hepatic coma
- CC **B19.9** Unspecified viral hepatitis without hepatic coma
  Viral hepatitis NOS

Human immunodeficiency virus [HIV] disease (B20)

CC B20 Human immunodeficiency virus [HIV] disease
Includes: acquired immune deficiency syndrome [AIDS]
AIDS-related complex [ARC]
HIV infection, symptomatic

Code first Human immunodeficiency virus [HIV] disease complicating pregnancy, childbirth and the puerperium, if applicable (O98.7-)

Use additional code(s) to identify all manifestations of HIV infection
Excludes1: asymptomatic human immunodeficiency virus [HIV] infection status (Z21)
exposure to HIV virus (Z20.6)
inconclusive serologic evidence of HIV (R75)
Review coding guideline C.1.a
AHA CC: 1Q, 2019, 8-11; 4Q, 2020, 97-98; 1Q, 2021, 52; 2Q, 2021, 6; 1Q, 2022, 36-37
Valid 3-character code, no further characters required

Other viral diseases (B25-B34)

B25 Cytomegaloviral disease
Excludes1: congenital cytomegalovirus infection (P35.1)
cytomegaloviral mononucleosis (B27.1-)
- MCC **B25.0** Cytomegaloviral pneumonitis
- CC **B25.1** Cytomegaloviral hepatitis
- MCC **B25.2** Cytomegaloviral pancreatitis
- CC **B25.8** Other cytomegaloviral diseases
  Cytomegaloviral encephalitis
- CC **B25.9** Cytomegaloviral disease, unspecified

B26 Mumps
Includes: epidemic parotitis
infectious parotitis
- ♂ CC **B26.0** Mumps orchitis
- MCC **B26.1** Mumps meningitis
- MCC **B26.2** Mumps encephalitis
- CC **B26.3** Mumps pancreatitis
- + **B26.8** Mumps with other complications
  - CC **B26.81** Mumps hepatitis
  - CC **B26.82** Mumps myocarditis
  - CC **B26.83** Mumps nephritis
  - CC **B26.84** Mumps polyneuropathy
  - CC **B26.85** Mumps arthritis
  - CC **B26.89** Other mumps complications
- **B26.9** Mumps without complication
  Mumps NOS
  Mumps parotitis NOS

B27 Infectious mononucleosis
Includes: glandular fever
monocytic angina
- + **B27.0** Gammaherpesviral mononucleosis
  Mononucleosis due to Epstein-Barr virus
  - **B27.00** Gammaherpesviral mononucleosis without complication
  - **B27.01** Gammaherpesviral mononucleosis with polyneuropathy
  - **B27.02** Gammaherpesviral mononucleosis with meningitis
  - **B27.09** Gammaherpesviral mononucleosis with other complications
    Hepatomegaly in gammaherpesviral mononucleosis
- + **B27.1** Cytomegaloviral mononucleosis
  - **B27.10** Cytomegaloviral mononucleosis without complications
  - **B27.11** Cytomegaloviral mononucleosis with polyneuropathy
  - **B27.12** Cytomegaloviral mononucleosis with meningitis
  - **B27.19** Cytomegaloviral mononucleosis with other complication
    Hepatomegaly in cytomegaloviral mononucleosis
- + **B27.8** Other infectious mononucleosis
  - **B27.80** Other infectious mononucleosis without complication
  - **B27.81** Other infectious mononucleosis with polyneuropathy
  - **B27.82** Other infectious mononucleosis with meningitis
  - **B27.89** Other infectious mononucleosis with other complication
    Hepatomegaly in other infectious mononucleosis
- + **B27.9** Infectious mononucleosis, unspecified
  - **B27.90** Infectious mononucleosis, unspecified without complication
  - **B27.91** Infectious mononucleosis, unspecified with polyneuropathy
  - **B27.92** Infectious mononucleosis, unspecified with meningitis
  - **B27.99** Infectious mononucleosis, unspecified with other complication
    Hepatomegaly in unspecified infectious mononucleosis

B30 Viral conjunctivitis
Excludes1: herpesviral [herpes simplex] ocular disease (B00.5)
ocular zoster (B02.3)
- **B30.0** Keratoconjunctivitis due to adenovirus
  Epidemic keratoconjunctivitis
  Shipyard eye
- **B30.1** Conjunctivitis due to adenovirus
  Acute adenoviral follicular conjunctivitis
  Swimming-pool conjunctivitis
- **B30.2** Viral pharyngoconjunctivitis
- **B30.3** Acute epidemic hemorrhagic conjunctivitis (enteroviral)
  Conjunctivitis due to coxsackievirus 24
  Conjunctivitis due to enterovirus 70
  Hemorrhagic conjunctivitis (acute)(epidemic)
- **B30.8** Other viral conjunctivitis
  Newcastle conjunctivitis
- **B30.9** Viral conjunctivitis, unspecified

B33 Other viral diseases, not elsewhere classified
- **B33.0** Epidemic myalgia
  Bornholm disease

CC	B33.1	Ross River disease
		Epidemic polyarthritis and exanthema
		Ross River fever
+	B33.2	Viral carditis
		Coxsackie (virus) carditis
CC	B33.20	Viral carditis, unspecified
CC	B33.21	Viral endocarditis
CC	B33.22	Viral myocarditis
CC	B33.23	Viral pericarditis
	B33.24	Viral cardiomyopathy
	B33.3	Retrovirus infections, not elsewhere classified
		Retrovirus infection NOS
CC	B33.4	Hantavirus (cardio)-pulmonary syndrome [HPS] [HCPS]
		Hantavirus disease with pulmonary manifestations
		Sin nombre virus disease

Use additional code to identify any associated acute kidney failure (N17.9)

Excludes1: hantavirus disease with renal manifestations (A98.5)
hemorrhagic fever with renal manifestations (A98.5)

B33.8 Other specified viral diseases

Excludes1: anogenital human papillomavirus infection (A63.0)
viral warts due to human papillomavirus infection (B07)

B34 Viral infection of unspecified site

Excludes1: anogenital human papillomavirus infection (A63.0)
cytomegaloviral disease NOS (B25.9)
herpesvirus [herpes simplex] infection NOS (B00.9)
retrovirus infection NOS (B33.3)
viral agents as the cause of diseases classified elsewhere (B97.-)
viral warts due to human papillomavirus infection (B07)

- B34.0 Adenovirus infection, unspecified
- B34.1 Enterovirus infection, unspecified
  - Coxsackievirus infection NOS
  - Echovirus infection NOS
- B34.2 Coronavirus infection, unspecified
  - **Excludes1:** COVID-19 (U07.1)
    pneumonia due to SARS associated coronavirus (J12.81)
  - AHA CC: 1Q, 2020, 34-36
- CC B34.3 Parvovirus infection, unspecified
- B34.4 Papovavirus infection, unspecified
- B34.8 Other viral infections of unspecified site
- B34.9 Viral infection, unspecified
  - Viremia NOS
  - AHA CC: 3Q, 2016, 10

Mycoses (B35-B49)

Excludes2: hypersensitivity pneumonitis due to organic dust (J67.-)
mycosis fungoides (C84.0-)

B35 Dermatophytosis

Includes: favus
infections due to species of Epidermophyton, Micro-sporum and Trichophyton
tinea, any type except those in B36.-

- B35.0 Tinea barbae and tinea capitis
  - Beard ringworm
  - Kerion
  - Scalp ringworm
  - Sycosis, mycotic
- B35.1 Tinea unguium
  - Dermatophytic onychia
  - Dermatophytosis of nail
  - Onychomycosis
  - Ringworm of nails
- B35.2 Tinea manuum
  - Dermatophytosis of hand
  - Hand ringworm
- B35.3 Tinea pedis
  - Athlete's foot
  - Dermatophytosis of foot
  - Foot ringworm
- B35.4 Tinea corporis
  - Ringworm of the body
- B35.5 Tinea imbricata
  - Tokelau
- B35.6 Tinea cruris
  - Dhobi itch
  - Groin ringworm
  - Jock itch
- B35.8 Other dermatophytoses
  - Disseminated dermatophytosis
  - Granulomatous dermatophytosis
- B35.9 Dermatophytosis, unspecified
  - Ringworm NOS

B36 Other superficial mycoses

- B36.0 Pityriasis versicolor
  - Tinea flava
  - Tinea versicolor
- B36.1 Tinea nigra
  - Keratomycosis nigricans palmaris
  - Microsporosis nigra
  - Pityriasis nigra
- B36.2 White piedra
  - Tinea blanca
- B36.3 Black piedra
- B36.8 Other specified superficial mycoses
- B36.9 Superficial mycosis, unspecified

B37 Candidiasis

Includes: candidosis
moniliasis

Excludes1: neonatal candidiasis (P37.5)

- CC B37.0 Candidal stomatitis
  - Oral thrush
- MCC B37.1 Pulmonary candidiasis
  - Candidal bronchitis
  - Candidal pneumonia
- B37.2 Candidiasis of skin and nail
  - Candidal onychia
  - Candidal paronychia
  - **Excludes2:** diaper dermatitis (L22)
- + B37.3 Candidiasis of vulva and vagina
  - Candidal vulvovaginitis
  - Monilial vulvovaginitis
  - Vaginal thrush
  - ♀ B37.31 Acute candidiasis of vulva and vagina
    - Candidiasis of vulva and vagina NOS
    - AHA CC: 4Q, 2022, 4-5
  - ♀ B37.32 Chronic candidiasis of vulva and vagina
    - Recurrent candidiasis of vulva and vagina
    - AHA CC: 4Q, 2022, 4-5
- + B37.4 Candidiasis of other urogenital sites
  - CC B37.41 Candidal cystitis and urethritis
    - HAC see Appendix B for HAC conditional logic
  - ♂ B37.42 Candidal balanitis
  - CC B37.49 Other urogenital candidiasis
    - Candidal pyelonephritis
    - HAC see Appendix B for HAC conditional logic
- MCC B37.5 Candidal meningitis
- MCC B37.6 Candidal endocarditis
- MCC B37.7 Candidal sepsis
  - Disseminated candidiasis
  - Systemic candidiasis
  - Review coding guideline C.1.d
  - AHA CC: 4Q, 2014, 46
- + B37.8 Candidiasis of other sites
  - CC B37.81 Candidal esophagitis
  - CC B37.82 Candidal enteritis
    - Candidal proctitis
  - CC B37.83 Candidal cheilitis
  - CC B37.84 Candidal otitis externa
  - CC B37.89 Other sites of candidiasis
    - Candidal osteomyelitis
- B37.9 Candidiasis, unspecified
  - Thrush NOS

B38 Coccidioidomycosis

- CC B38.0 Acute pulmonary coccidioidomycosis
- CC B38.1 Chronic pulmonary coccidioidomycosis
- CC B38.2 Pulmonary coccidioidomycosis, unspecified
- CC B38.3 Cutaneous coccidioidomycosis
- MCC B38.4 Coccidioidomycosis meningitis
- CC B38.7 Disseminated coccidioidomycosis
  - Generalized coccidioidomycosis
- + B38.8 Other forms of coccidioidomycosis
  - ♂ CC B38.81 Prostatic coccidioidomycosis
  - CC B38.89 Other forms of coccidioidomycosis
- CC B38.9 Coccidioidomycosis, unspecified

B39 Histoplasmosis
Code first associated AIDS (B20)
Use additional code for any associated manifestations, such as:
endocarditis (I39)
meningitis (G02)
pericarditis (I32)
retinitis (H32)
- MCC **B39.0** Acute pulmonary histoplasmosis capsulati
- MCC **B39.1** Chronic pulmonary histoplasmosis capsulati
- MCC **B39.2** Pulmonary histoplasmosis capsulati, unspecified
- CC **B39.3** Disseminated histoplasmosis capsulati
  Generalized histoplasmosis capsulati
- **B39.4** Histoplasmosis capsulati, unspecified
  American histoplasmosis
- **B39.5** Histoplasmosis duboisii
  African histoplasmosis
- **B39.9** Histoplasmosis, unspecified

B40 Blastomycosis
Excludes1: Brazilian blastomycosis (B41.-)
keloidal blastomycosis (B48.0)
- CC **B40.0** Acute pulmonary blastomycosis
- CC **B40.1** Chronic pulmonary blastomycosis
- CC **B40.2** Pulmonary blastomycosis, unspecified
- CC **B40.3** Cutaneous blastomycosis
- CC **B40.7** Disseminated blastomycosis
  Generalized blastomycosis
- + **B40.8** Other forms of blastomycosis
  - CC **B40.81** Blastomycotic meningoencephalitis
    Meningomyelitis due to blastomycosis
  - CC **B40.89** Other forms of blastomycosis
- CC **B40.9** Blastomycosis, unspecified

B41 Paracoccidioidomycosis
Includes: Brazilian blastomycosis
Lutz' disease
- CC **B41.0** Pulmonary paracoccidioidomycosis
- CC **B41.7** Disseminated paracoccidioidomycosis
  Generalized paracoccidioidomycosis
- CC **B41.8** Other forms of paracoccidioidomycosis
- CC **B41.9** Paracoccidioidomycosis, unspecified

B42 Sporotrichosis
- **B42.0** Pulmonary sporotrichosis
- **B42.1** Lymphocutaneous sporotrichosis
- **B42.7** Disseminated sporotrichosis
  Generalized sporotrichosis
- + **B42.8** Other forms of sporotrichosis
  - **B42.81** Cerebral sporotrichosis
    Meningitis due to sporotrichosis
  - **B42.82** Sporotrichosis arthritis
  - **B42.89** Other forms of sporotrichosis
- **B42.9** Sporotrichosis, unspecified

B43 Chromomycosis and pheomycotic abscess
- **B43.0** Cutaneous chromomycosis
  Dermatitis verrucosa
- **B43.1** Pheomycotic brain abscess
  Cerebral chromomycosis
- **B43.2** Subcutaneous pheomycotic abscess and cyst
- **B43.8** Other forms of chromomycosis
- **B43.9** Chromomycosis, unspecified

B44 Aspergillosis
Includes: aspergilloma
- MCC **B44.0** Invasive pulmonary aspergillosis
- CC **B44.1** Other pulmonary aspergillosis
- CC **B44.2** Tonsillar aspergillosis
- CC **B44.7** Disseminated aspergillosis
  Generalized aspergillosis
- + **B44.8** Other forms of aspergillosis
  - CC **B44.81** Allergic bronchopulmonary aspergillosis
  - CC **B44.89** Other forms of aspergillosis
- CC **B44.9** Aspergillosis, unspecified

B45 Cryptococcosis
- CC **B45.0** Pulmonary cryptococcosis
- MCC **B45.1** Cerebral cryptococcosis
  Cryptococcal meningitis
  Cryptococcosis meningocerebralis
- CC **B45.2** Cutaneous cryptococcosis
- CC **B45.3** Osseous cryptococcosis
- CC **B45.7** Disseminated cryptococcosis
  Generalized cryptococcosis
- CC **B45.8** Other forms of cryptococcosis
- CC **B45.9** Cryptococcosis, unspecified

B46 Zygomycosis
- MCC **B46.0** Pulmonary mucormycosis
- MCC **B46.1** Rhinocerebral mucormycosis
- MCC **B46.2** Gastrointestinal mucormycosis
- MCC **B46.3** Cutaneous mucormycosis
  Subcutaneous mucormycosis
- MCC **B46.4** Disseminated mucormycosis
  Generalized mucormycosis
- MCC **B46.5** Mucormycosis, unspecified
- MCC **B46.8** Other zygomycoses
  Entomophthoromycosis
- MCC **B46.9** Zygomycosis, unspecified
  Phycomycosis NOS

B47 Mycetoma
- CC **B47.0** Eumycetoma
  Madura foot, mycotic
  Maduromycosis
- CC **B47.1** Actinomycetoma
- CC **B47.9** Mycetoma, unspecified
  Madura foot NOS

B48 Other mycoses, not elsewhere classified
- **B48.0** Lobomycosis
  Keloidal blastomycosis
  Lobo's disease
- **B48.1** Rhinosporidiosis
- **B48.2** Allescheriasis
  Infection due to Pseudallescheria boydii
  Excludes1: eumycetoma (B47.0)
- CC **B48.3** Geotrichosis
  Geotrichum stomatitis
- CC **B48.4** Penicillosis
  Talaromycosis
- CC **B48.8** Other specified mycoses
  Adiaspiromycosis
  Infection of tissue and organs by Alternaria
  Infection of tissue and organs by Drechslera
  Infection of tissue and organs by Fusarium
  Infection of tissue and organs by saprophytic fungi NEC
  AHA CC: 2Q, 2014, 13; 4Q, 2014, 46

- CC **B49** Unspecified mycosis
  Fungemia NOS
  Valid 3-character code, no further characters required

Protozoal diseases (B50-B64)

Excludes1: amebiasis (A06.-)
other protozoal intestinal diseases (A07.-)

B50 Plasmodium falciparum malaria
Includes: mixed infections of Plasmodium falciparum with any other Plasmodium species
- CC **B50.0** Plasmodium falciparum malaria with cerebral complications
  Cerebral malaria NOS
- CC **B50.8** Other severe and complicated Plasmodium falciparum malaria
  Severe or complicated Plasmodium falciparum malaria NOS
- MCC **B50.9** Plasmodium falciparum malaria, unspecified

B51 Plasmodium vivax malaria
Includes: mixed infections of Plasmodium vivax with other Plasmodium species, except Plasmodium falciparum
Excludes1: plasmodium vivax with Plasmodium falciparum (B50.-)
- CC **B51.0** Plasmodium vivax malaria with rupture of spleen
- CC **B51.8** Plasmodium vivax malaria with other complications
- CC **B51.9** Plasmodium vivax malaria without complication
  Plasmodium vivax malaria NOS

B52 Plasmodium malariae malaria
Includes: mixed infections of Plasmodium malariae with other Plasmodium species, except Plasmodium falciparum and Plasmodium vivax
Excludes1: Plasmodium falciparum (B50.-)
Plasmodium vivax (B51.-)
- CC **B52.0** Plasmodium malariae malaria with nephropathy

CC B52.8 Plasmodium malariae malaria with other complications
CC B52.9 Plasmodium malariae malaria without complication
    Plasmodium malariae malaria NOS

B53 Other specified malaria
  CC B53.0 Plasmodium ovale malaria
    Excludes1: Plasmodium ovale with Plasmodium falciparum (B50.-)
               Plasmodium ovale with Plasmodium malariae (B52.-)
               Plasmodium ovale with Plasmodium vivax (B51.-)
  CC B53.1 Malaria due to simian plasmodia
    Excludes1: Malaria due to simian plasmodia with Plasmodium falciparum (B50.-)
               Malaria due to simian plasmodia with Plasmodium malariae (B52.-)
               Malaria due to simian plasmodia with Plasmodium ovale (B53.0)
               Malaria due to simian plasmodia with Plasmodium vivax (B51.-)
  CC B53.8 Other malaria, not elsewhere classified

CC **B54** Unspecified malaria
    Valid 3-character code, no further characters required

B55 Leishmaniasis
  CC B55.0 Visceral leishmaniasis
    Kala-azar
    Post-kala-azar dermal leishmaniasis
  CC B55.1 Cutaneous leishmaniasis
  CC B55.2 Mucocutaneous leishmaniasis
  CC B55.9 Leishmaniasis, unspecified

B56 African trypanosomiasis
  CC B56.0 Gambiense trypanosomiasis
    Infection due to Trypanosoma brucei gambiense
    West African sleeping sickness
  CC B56.1 Rhodesiense trypanosomiasis
    East African sleeping sickness
    Infection due to Trypanosoma brucei rhodesiense
  CC B56.9 African trypanosomiasis, unspecified
    Sleeping sickness NOS

B57 Chagas' disease
    Includes: American trypanosomiasis
             infection due to Trypanosoma cruzi
  CC B57.0 Acute Chagas' disease with heart involvement
    Acute Chagas' disease with myocarditis
  CC B57.1 Acute Chagas' disease without heart involvement
    Acute Chagas' disease NOS
  CC B57.2 Chagas' disease (chronic) with heart involvement
    American trypanosomiasis NOS
    Chagas' disease (chronic) NOS
    Chagas' disease (chronic) with myocarditis
    Trypanosomiasis NOS
  + B57.3 Chagas' disease (chronic) with digestive system involvement
    CC B57.30 Chagas' disease with digestive system involvement, unspecified
    CC B57.31 Megaesophagus in Chagas' disease
    CC B57.32 Megacolon in Chagas' disease
    CC B57.39 Other digestive system involvement in Chagas' disease
  + B57.4 Chagas' disease (chronic) with nervous system involvement
    CC B57.40 Chagas' disease with nervous system involvement, unspecified
    CC B57.41 Meningitis in Chagas' disease
    CC B57.42 Meningoencephalitis in Chagas' disease
    CC B57.49 Other nervous system involvement in Chagas' disease
  CC B57.5 Chagas' disease (chronic) with other organ involvement

B58 Toxoplasmosis
    Includes: infection due to Toxoplasma gondii
    Excludes1: congenital toxoplasmosis (P37.1)
  + B58.0 Toxoplasma oculopathy
    CC B58.00 Toxoplasma oculopathy, unspecified
    CC B58.01 Toxoplasma chorioretinitis
    CC B58.09 Other toxoplasma oculopathy
      Toxoplasma uveitis
  CC B58.1 Toxoplasma hepatitis
  MCC B58.2 Toxoplasma meningoencephalitis
  MCC B58.3 Pulmonary toxoplasmosis
  + B58.8 Toxoplasmosis with other organ involvement
    MCC B58.81 Toxoplasma myocarditis
    CC B58.82 Toxoplasma myositis
    CC B58.83 Toxoplasma tubulo-interstitial nephropathy
      Toxoplasma pyelonephritis
    CC B58.89 Toxoplasmosis with other organ involvement
  CC B58.9 Toxoplasmosis, unspecified

B59 Pneumocystosis
  MCC Pneumonia due to Pneumocystis carinii
       Pneumonia due to Pneumocystis jiroveci
    Valid 3-character code, no further characters required

B60 Other protozoal diseases, not elsewhere classified
    Excludes1: cryptosporidiosis (A07.2)
               intestinal microsporidiosis (A07.8)
               isosporiasis (A07.3)
  + B60.0 Babesiosis
    AHA CC: 4Q, 2020, 5-6
    CC B60.00 Babesiosis, unspecified
      Babesiosis due to unspecified Babesia species
      Piroplasmosis, unspecified
    CC B60.01 Babesiosis due to Babesia microti
      Infection due to B. microti
    CC B60.02 Babesiosis due to Babesia duncani
      Infection due to B. duncani and B. duncani-type species
    CC B60.03 Babesiosis due to Babesia divergens
      Babesiosis due to Babesia MO-1
      Infection due to B. divergens and B. divergens-like strains
    CC B60.09 Other babesiosis
      Babesiosis due to Babesia KO-1
      Babesiosis due to Babesia venatorum
      Infection due to other Babesia species
      Infection due to other protozoa of the order Piroplasmida
      Other piroplasmosis
  + B60.1 Acanthamebiasis
    CC B60.10 Acanthamebiasis, unspecified
    B60.11 Meningoencephalitis due to Acanthamoeba (culbertsoni)
    B60.12 Conjunctivitis due to Acanthamoeba
    B60.13 Keratoconjunctivitis due to Acanthamoeba
    CC B60.19 Other acanthamebic disease
  CC B60.2 Naegleriasis
    Primary amebic meningoencephalitis
  B60.8 Other specified protozoal diseases
    Microsporidiosis

B64 Unspecified protozoal disease
    Valid 3-character code, no further characters required

Helminthiases (B65-B83)

B65 Schistosomiasis [bilharziasis]
    Includes: snail fever
  CC B65.0 Schistosomiasis due to Schistosoma haematobium [urinary schistosomiasis]
  CC B65.1 Schistosomiasis due to Schistosoma mansoni [intestinal schistosomiasis]
  CC B65.2 Schistosomiasis due to Schistosoma japonicum
    Asiatic schistosomiasis
  CC B65.3 Cercarial dermatitis
    Swimmer's itch
  CC B65.8 Other schistosomiasis
    Infection due to Schistosoma intercalatum
    Infection due to Schistosoma mattheei
    Infection due to Schistosoma mekongi
  CC B65.9 Schistosomiasis, unspecified

B66 Other fluke infections
  CC B66.0 Opisthorchiasis
    Infection due to cat liver fluke
    Infection due to Opisthorchis (felineus)(viverrini)
  CC B66.1 Clonorchiasis
    Chinese liver fluke disease
    Infection due to Clonorchis sinensis
    Oriental liver fluke disease
  CC B66.2 Dicroceliasis
    Infection due to Dicrocoelium dendriticum
    Lancet fluke infection

Chapter 1: Certain Infectious and Parasitic Diseases

B66.3–B81

- CC **B66.3** Fascioliasis
  - Infection due to Fasciola gigantica
  - Infection due to Fasciola hepatica
  - Infection due to Fasciola indica
  - Sheep liver fluke disease
- CC **B66.4** Paragonimiasis
  - Infection due to Paragonimus species
  - Lung fluke disease
  - Pulmonary distomiasis
- CC **B66.5** Fasciolopsiasis
  - Infection due to Fasciolopsis buski
  - Intestinal distomiasis
- CC **B66.8** Other specified fluke infections
  - Echinostomiasis
  - Heterophyiasis
  - Metagonimiasis
  - Nanophyetiasis
  - Watsoniasis
- **B66.9** Fluke infection, unspecified

B67 Echinococcosis
Includes: hydatidosis
- CC **B67.0** Echinococcus granulosus infection of liver
- CC **B67.1** Echinococcus granulosus infection of lung
- CC **B67.2** Echinococcus granulosus infection of bone
- + **B67.3** Echinococcus granulosus infection, other and multiple sites
  - CC **B67.31** Echinococcus granulosus infection, thyroid gland
  - CC **B67.32** Echinococcus granulosus infection, multiple sites
  - CC **B67.39** Echinococcus granulosus infection, other sites
- CC **B67.4** Echinococcus granulosus infection, unspecified
  - Dog tapeworm (infection)
- CC **B67.5** Echinococcus multilocularis infection of liver
- + **B67.6** Echinococcus multilocularis infection, other and multiple sites
  - CC **B67.61** Echinococcus multilocularis infection, multiple sites
  - CC **B67.69** Echinococcus multilocularis infection, other sites
- CC **B67.7** Echinococcus multilocularis infection, unspecified
- CC **B67.8** Echinococcosis, unspecified, of liver
- + **B67.9** Echinococcosis, other and unspecified
  - CC **B67.90** Echinococcosis, unspecified
    - Echinococcosis NOS
  - CC **B67.99** Other echinococcosis

B68 Taeniasis
Excludes1: cysticercosis (B69.-)
- CC **B68.0** Taenia solium taeniasis
  - Pork tapeworm (infection)
- CC **B68.1** Taenia saginata taeniasis
  - Beef tapeworm (infection)
  - Infection due to adult tapeworm Taenia saginata
- CC **B68.9** Taeniasis, unspecified

B69 Cysticercosis
Includes: cysticerciasis infection due to larval form of Taenia solium
- CC **B69.0** Cysticercosis of central nervous system
- CC **B69.1** Cysticercosis of eye
- + **B69.8** Cysticercosis of other sites
  - CC **B69.81** Myositis in cysticercosis
  - CC **B69.89** Cysticercosis of other sites
- CC **B69.9** Cysticercosis, unspecified

B70 Diphyllobothriasis and sparganosis
- CC **B70.0** Diphyllobothriasis
  - Diphyllobothrium (adult) (latum) (pacificum) infection
  - Fish tapeworm (infection)
  - **Excludes2:** larval diphyllobothriasis (B70.1)
- CC **B70.1** Sparganosis
  - Infection due to Sparganum (mansoni) (proliferum)
  - Infection due to Spirometra larva
  - Larval diphyllobothriasis
  - Spirometrosis

B71 Other cestode infections
- CC **B71.0** Hymenolepiasis
  - Dwarf tapeworm infection
  - Rat tapeworm (infection)
- CC **B71.1** Dipylidiasis
- CC **B71.8** Other specified cestode infections
  - Coenurosis
- **B71.9** Cestode infection, unspecified
  - Tapeworm (infection) NOS

CC B72 Dracunculiasis
Includes: guinea worm infection
infection due to Dracunculus medinensis
Valid 3-character code, no further characters required

B73 Onchocerciasis
Includes: onchocerca volvulus infection
onchocercosis
river blindness
- + **B73.0** Onchocerciasis with eye disease
  - CC **B73.00** Onchocerciasis with eye involvement, unspecified
  - CC **B73.01** Onchocerciasis with endophthalmitis
  - CC **B73.02** Onchocerciasis with glaucoma
  - CC **B73.09** Onchocerciasis with other eye involvement
    - Infestation of eyelid due to onchocerciasis
- CC **B73.1** Onchocerciasis without eye disease

B74 Filariasis
Excludes2: onchocerciasis (B73)
tropical (pulmonary) eosinophilia NOS (J82.89)
- CC **B74.0** Filariasis due to Wuchereria bancrofti
  - Bancroftian elephantiasis
  - Bancroftian filariasis
- CC **B74.1** Filariasis due to Brugia malayi
- CC **B74.2** Filariasis due to Brugia timori
- CC **B74.3** Loiasis
  - Calabar swelling
  - Eyeworm disease of Africa
  - Loa loa infection
- CC **B74.4** Mansonelliasis
  - Infection due to Mansonella ozzardi
  - Infection due to Mansonella perstans
  - Infection due to Mansonella streptocerca
- CC **B74.8** Other filariases
  - Dirofilariasis
- CC **B74.9** Filariasis, unspecified

CC B75 Trichinellosis
Includes: infection due to Trichinella species
trichiniasis
Valid 3-character code, no further characters required

B76 Hookworm diseases
Includes: uncinariasis
- CC **B76.0** Ancylostomiasis
  - Infection due to Ancylostoma species
- CC **B76.1** Necatoriasis
  - Infection due to Necator americanus
- CC **B76.8** Other hookworm diseases
- CC **B76.9** Hookworm disease, unspecified
  - Cutaneous larva migrans NOS

B77 Ascariasis
Includes: ascaridiasis
roundworm infection
- CC **B77.0** Ascariasis with intestinal complications
- + **B77.8** Ascariasis with other complications
  - MCC **B77.81** Ascariasis pneumonia
  - CC **B77.89** Ascariasis with other complications
- CC **B77.9** Ascariasis, unspecified

B78 Strongyloidiasis
Excludes1: trichostrongyliasis (B81.2)
- CC **B78.0** Intestinal strongyloidiasis
- **B78.1** Cutaneous strongyloidiasis
- CC **B78.7** Disseminated strongyloidiasis
- CC **B78.9** Strongyloidiasis, unspecified

CC B79 Trichuriasis
Includes: trichocephaliasis
whipworm (disease)(infection)
Valid 3-character code, no further characters required

CC B80 Enterobiasis
Includes: oxyuriasis
pinworm infection
threadworm infection
Valid 3-character code, no further characters required

B81 Other intestinal helminthiases, not elsewhere classified
Excludes1: angiostrongyliasis due to:
Angiostrongylus cantonensis (B83.2)
Parastrongylus cantonensis (B83.2)

CC **B81.0** **Anisakiasis**
  Infection due to Anisakis larva
CC **B81.1** **Intestinal capillariasis**
  Capillariasis NOS
  Infection due to Capillaria philippinensis
  Excludes2: *hepatic capillariasis (B83.8)*
CC **B81.2** **Trichostrongyliasis**
CC **B81.3** **Intestinal angiostrongyliasis**
  Angiostrongyliasis due to:
    Angiostrongylus costaricensis
    Parastrongylus cantonensis
CC **B81.4** **Mixed intestinal helminthiases**
  Infection due to intestinal helminths classified to more than one of the categories B65.0-B81.3 and B81.8
  Mixed helminthiasis NOS
CC **B81.8** **Other specified intestinal helminthiases**
  Infection due to Oesophagostomum species [esophagostomiasis]
  Infection due to Ternidens diminutus [ternidensiasis]

B82 Unspecified intestinal parasitism
  CC **B82.0** **Intestinal helminthiasis, unspecified**
  B82.9 **Intestinal parasitism, unspecified**

B83 Other helminthiases
  Excludes1: *capillariasis NOS (B81.1)*
  Excludes2: *intestinal capillariasis (B81.1)*
  B83.0 **Visceral larva migrans**
    Toxocariasis
  B83.1 **Gnathostomiasis**
    Wandering swelling
  B83.2 **Angiostrongyliasis due to Parastrongylus cantonensis**
    Eosinophilic meningoencephalitis due to Parastrongylus cantonensis
    Excludes2: *intestinal angiostrongyliasis (B81.3)*
  B83.3 **Syngamiasis**
    Syngamosis
  B83.4 **Internal hirudiniasis**
    Excludes2: *external hirudiniasis (B88.3)*
  B83.8 **Other specified helminthiases**
    Acanthocephaliasis
    Gongylonemiasis
    Hepatic capillariasis
    Metastrongyliasis
    Thelaziasis
  B83.9 **Helminthiasis, unspecified**
    Worms NOS
    Excludes1: *intestinal helminthiasis NOS (B82.0)*

Pediculosis, acariasis and other infestations (B85-B89)

B85 Pediculosis and phthiriasis
  B85.0 **Pediculosis due to Pediculus humanus capitis**
    Head-louse infestation
  B85.1 **Pediculosis due to Pediculus humanus corporis**
    Body-louse infestation
  B85.2 **Pediculosis, unspecified**
  B85.3 **Phthiriasis**
    Infestation by crab-louse
    Infestation by Phthirus pubis
  B85.4 **Mixed pediculosis and phthiriasis**
    Infestation classifiable to more than one of the categories B85.0-B85.3

B86 Scabies
  Sarcoptic itch
  Valid 3-character code, no further characters required

B87 Myiasis
  Includes: infestation by larva of flies
  B87.0 **Cutaneous myiasis**
    Creeping myiasis
  B87.1 **Wound myiasis**
    Traumatic myiasis
  B87.2 **Ocular myiasis**
  B87.3 **Nasopharyngeal myiasis**
    Laryngeal myiasis
  B87.4 **Aural myiasis**
  + B87.8 **Myiasis of other sites**
    B87.81 **Genitourinary myiasis**
    B87.82 **Intestinal myiasis**
    B87.89 **Myiasis of other sites**
  B87.9 **Myiasis, unspecified**

B88 Other infestations
  B88.0 **Other acariasis**
    Acarine dermatitis
    Dermatitis due to Demodex species
    Dermatitis due to Dermanyssus gallinae
    Dermatitis due to Liponyssoides sanguineus
    Trombiculosis
    Excludes2: *scabies (B86)*
  B88.1 **Tungiasis [sandflea infestation]**
  B88.2 **Other arthropod infestations**
    Scarabiasis
  B88.3 **External hirudiniasis**
    Leech infestation NOS
    Excludes2: *internal hirudiniasis (B83.4)*
  B88.8 **Other specified infestations**
    Ichthyoparasitism due to Vandellia cirrhosa
    Linguatulosis
    Porocephaliasis
  B88.9 **Infestation, unspecified**
    Infestation (skin) NOS
    Infestation by mites NOS
    Skin parasites NOS

B89 Unspecified parasitic disease
  Valid 3-character code, no further characters required

Sequelae of infectious and parasitic diseases (B90-B94)

NOTE Categories B90-B94 are to be used to indicate conditions in categories A00-B89 as the cause of sequelae, which are themselves classified elsewhere. The 'sequelae' include conditions specified as such; they also include residuals of diseases classifiable to the above categories if there is evidence that the disease itself is no longer present. Codes from these categories are not to be used for chronic infections. Code chronic current infections to active infectious disease as appropriate.

Code first condition resulting from (sequela) the infectious or parasitic disease

B90 Sequelae of tuberculosis
  B90.0 **Sequelae of central nervous system tuberculosis**
  B90.1 **Sequelae of genitourinary tuberculosis**
  B90.2 **Sequelae of tuberculosis of bones and joints**
  B90.8 **Sequelae of tuberculosis of other organs**
    Excludes2: *sequelae of respiratory tuberculosis (B90.9)*
  B90.9 **Sequelae of respiratory and unspecified tuberculosis**
    Sequelae of tuberculosis NOS

B91 Sequelae of poliomyelitis
  Excludes1: *postpolio syndrome (G14)*
  Valid 3-character code, no further characters required

B92 Sequelae of leprosy
  Valid 3-character code, no further characters required

B94 Sequelae of other and unspecified infectious and parasitic diseases
  B94.0 **Sequelae of trachoma**
  B94.1 **Sequelae of viral encephalitis**
  B94.2 **Sequelae of viral hepatitis**
  B94.8 **Sequelae of other specified infectious and parasitic diseases**
    AHA CC: 4Q, 2017, 109; 3Q, 2020, 10-14; 1Q, 2021, 35, 44-46, 48; 4Q, 2021, 102-103
  B94.9 **Sequelae of unspecified infectious and parasitic disease**
    Excludes2: *post COVID-19 condition (U09.9)*

Bacterial and viral infectious agents (B95-B97)

NOTE These categories are provided for use as supplementary or additional codes to identify the infectious agent(s) in diseases classified elsewhere.

B95 Streptococcus, Staphylococcus, and Enterococcus as the cause of diseases classified elsewhere
  Review coding guideline C.1.b
  B95.0 **Streptococcus, group A, as the cause of diseases classified elsewhere**
  B95.1 **Streptococcus, group B, as the cause of diseases classified elsewhere**
    AHA CC: 4Q, 2018, 23; 2Q, 2019, 9-10; 1Q, 2020, 10
  B95.2 **Enterococcus as the cause of diseases classified elsewhere**
  B95.3 **Streptococcus pneumoniae as the cause of diseases classified elsewhere**
  B95.4 **Other streptococcus as the cause of diseases classified elsewhere**
  B95.5 **Unspecified streptococcus as the cause of diseases classified elsewhere**

- **+ B95.6** Staphylococcus aureus as the cause of diseases classified elsewhere
  - **B95.61** Methicillin susceptible Staphylococcus aureus infection as the cause of diseases classified elsewhere
    - Methicillin susceptible Staphylococcus aureus (MSSA) infection as the cause of diseases classified elsewhere
    - Staphylococcus aureus infection NOS as the cause of diseases classified elsewhere
  - **B95.62** Methicillin resistant Staphylococcus aureus infection as the cause of diseases classified elsewhere
    - Methicillin resistant staphylococcus aureus (MRSA) infection as the cause of diseases classified elsewhere
    - *Review coding guidelines C.1.e.1.a and C.1.e.1.b*
    - *AHA CC: 1Q, 2016, 12-13*
- **B95.7** Other staphylococcus as the cause of diseases classified elsewhere
- **B95.8** Unspecified staphylococcus as the cause of diseases classified elsewhere

B96 Other bacterial agents as the cause of diseases classified elsewhere
Review coding guideline C.1.b
- **B96.0** Mycoplasma pneumoniae [M. pneumoniae] as the cause of diseases classified elsewhere
  - Pleuro-pneumonia-like-organism [PPLO]
- **B96.1** Klebsiella pneumoniae [K. pneumoniae] as the cause of diseases classified elsewhere
- **+ B96.2** Escherichia coli [E. coli] as the cause of diseases classified elsewhere
  - **B96.20** Unspecified Escherichia coli [E. coli] as the cause of diseases classified elsewhere
    - Escherichia coli [E. coli] NOS
    - *AHA CC: 1Q, 2018, 16; 4Q, 2018, 34; 1Q, 2022, 31*
  - **B96.21** Shiga toxin-producing Escherichia coli [E. coli] [STEC] O157 as the cause of diseases classified elsewhere
    - E. coli O157:H- (nonmotile) with confirmation of Shiga toxin
    - E. coli O157 with confirmation of Shiga toxin when H antigen is unknown, or is not H7
    - O157:H7 Escherichia coli [E.coli] with or without confirmation of Shiga toxin-production
    - Shiga toxin-producing Escherichia coli [E.coli] O157:H7 with or without confirmation of Shiga toxin-production
    - STEC O157:H7 with or without confirmation of Shiga toxin-production
  - **B96.22** Other specified Shiga toxin-producing Escherichia coli [E. coli] [STEC] as the cause of diseases classified elsewhere
    - Non-O157 Shiga toxin-producing Escherichia coli [E.coli]
    - Non-O157 Shiga toxin-producing Escherichia coli [E.coli] with known O group
  - **B96.23** Unspecified Shiga toxin-producing Escherichia coli [E. coli] [STEC] as the cause of diseases classified elsewhere
    - Shiga toxin-producing Escherichia coli [E. coli] with unspecified O group
    - STEC NOS
  - **B96.29** Other Escherichia coli [E. coli] as the cause of diseases classified elsewhere
    - Non-Shiga toxin-producing E. coli
- **B96.3** Hemophilus influenzae [H. influenzae] as the cause of diseases classified elsewhere
- **B96.4** Proteus (mirabilis) (morganii) as the cause of diseases classified elsewhere
- **B96.5** Pseudomonas (aeruginosa) (mallei) (pseudomallei) as the cause of diseases classified elsewhere
  - *AHA CC: 1Q, 2015, 18-19*
- **B96.6** Bacteroides fragilis [B. fragilis] as the cause of diseases classified elsewhere
- **B96.7** Clostridium perfringens [C. perfringens] as the cause of diseases classified elsewhere

- **+ B96.8** Other specified bacterial agents as the cause of diseases classified elsewhere
  - **B96.81** Helicobacter pylori [H. pylori] as the cause of diseases classified elsewhere
  - **B96.82** Vibrio vulnificus as the cause of diseases classified elsewhere
  - **B96.83** Acinetobacter baumannii as the cause of diseases classified elsewhere
  - **B96.89** Other specified bacterial agents as the cause of diseases classified elsewhere

B97 Viral agents as the cause of diseases classified elsewhere
Review coding guideline C.1.b
- **B97.0** Adenovirus as the cause of diseases classified elsewhere
- **+ B97.1** Enterovirus as the cause of diseases classified elsewhere
  - **B97.10** Unspecified enterovirus as the cause of diseases classified elsewhere
  - **B97.11** Coxsackievirus as the cause of diseases classified elsewhere
  - **B97.12** Echovirus as the cause of diseases classified elsewhere
  - **B97.19** Other enterovirus as the cause of diseases classified elsewhere
- **+ B97.2** Coronavirus as the cause of diseases classified elsewhere
  - **CC B97.21** SARS-associated coronavirus as the cause of diseases classified elsewhere
    - **Excludes1:** pneumonia due to SARS-associated coronavirus (J12.81)
  - **B97.29** Other coronavirus as the cause of diseases classified elsewhere
    - *AHA CC: 1Q, 2020, 34-36*
- **+ B97.3** Retrovirus as the cause of diseases classified elsewhere
  - **Excludes1:** Human immunodeficiency virus [HIV] disease (B20)
  - **B97.30** Unspecified retrovirus as the cause of diseases classified elsewhere
  - **B97.31** Lentivirus as the cause of diseases classified elsewhere
  - **B97.32** Oncovirus as the cause of diseases classified elsewhere
  - **CC B97.33** Human T-cell lymphotrophic virus, type I [HTLV-I] as the cause of diseases classified elsewhere
  - **CC B97.34** Human T-cell lymphotrophic virus, type II [HTLV-II] as the cause of diseases classified elsewhere
  - **CC B97.35** Human immunodeficiency virus, type 2 [HIV 2] as the cause of diseases classified elsewhere
  - **B97.39** Other retrovirus as the cause of diseases classified elsewhere
- **B97.4** Respiratory syncytial virus as the cause of diseases classified elsewhere
  - RSV as the cause of diseases classified elsewhere
  - Code first related disorders, such as:
    - otitis media (H65.-)
    - upper respiratory infection (J06.9)
  - **Excludes1:** acute bronchiolitis due to respiratory syncytial virus (RSV) (J21.0)
    - acute bronchitis due to respiratory syncytial virus (RSV) (J20.5)
    - respiratory syncytial virus (RSV) pneumonia (J12.1)
- **B97.5** Reovirus as the cause of diseases classified elsewhere
- **B97.6** Parvovirus as the cause of diseases classified elsewhere
- **B97.7** Papillomavirus as the cause of diseases classified elsewhere
- **+ B97.8** Other viral agents as the cause of diseases classified elsewhere
  - **B97.81** Human metapneumovirus as the cause of diseases classified elsewhere
  - **B97.89** Other viral agents as the cause of diseases classified elsewhere
    - *AHA CC: 3Q, 2016, 9-14*

Other infectious diseases (B99)

B99 Other and unspecified infectious diseases
- **B99.8** Other infectious disease
- **B99.9** Unspecified infectious disease

Chapter 2: Neoplasms (C00-D49)

NOTE **Functional activity**
All neoplasms are classified in this chapter, whether they are functionally active or not. An additional code from Chapter 4 may be used, to identify functional activity associated with any neoplasm.

Morphology [Histology]
Chapter 2 classifies neoplasms primarily by site (topography), with broad groupings for behavior, malignant, in situ, benign, etc. The Table of Neoplasms should be used to identify the correct topography code. In a few cases, such as for malignant melanoma and certain neuroendocrine tumors, the morphology (histologic type) is included in the category and codes.

Primary malignant neoplasms overlapping site boundaries
A primary malignant neoplasm that overlaps two or more contiguous (next to each other) sites should be classified to the subcategory/code .8 ('overlapping lesion'), unless the combination is specifically indexed elsewhere. For multiple neoplasms of the same site that are not contiguous, such as tumors in different quadrants of the same breast, codes for each site should be assigned.

Malignant neoplasm of ectopic tissue
Malignant neoplasms of ectopic tissue are to be coded to the site mentioned, e.g., ectopic pancreatic malignant neoplasms are coded to pancreas, unspecified (C25.9).

This chapter contains the following category blocks:

C00-C14	Malignant neoplasms of lip, oral cavity and pharynx
C15-C26	Malignant neoplasms of digestive organs
C30-C39	Malignant neoplasms of respiratory and intrathoracic organs
C40-C41	Malignant neoplasms of bone and articular cartilage
C43-C44	Melanoma and other malignant neoplasms of skin
C45-C49	Malignant neoplasms of mesothelial and soft tissue
C50	Malignant neoplasms of breast
C51-C58	Malignant neoplasms of female genital organs
C60-C63	Malignant neoplasms of male genital organs
C64-C68	Malignant neoplasms of urinary tract
C69-C72	Malignant neoplasms of eye, brain and other parts of central nervous system
C73-C75	Malignant neoplasms of thyroid and other endocrine glands
C7A	Malignant neuroendocrine tumors
C7B	Secondary neuroendocrine tumors
C76-C80	Malignant neoplasms of ill-defined, other secondary and unspecified sites
C81-C96	Malignant neoplasms of lymphoid, hematopoietic and related tissue
D00-D09	In situ neoplasms
D10-D36	Benign neoplasms, except benign neuroendocrine tumors
D3A	Benign neuroendocrine tumors
D37-D48	Neoplasms of uncertain behavior, polycythemia vera and myelodysplastic syndromes
D49	Neoplasms of unspecified behavior

C. Chapter-Specific Coding Guidelines

In addition to general coding guidelines, there are guidelines for specific diagnoses and/or conditions in the classification. Unless otherwise indicated, these guidelines apply to all health care settings. Please refer to Section II for guidelines on the selection of principal diagnosis.

2. Chapter 2: Neoplasms (C00-D49)

General guidelines

Chapter 2 of the ICD-10-CM contains the codes for most benign and all malignant neoplasms. Certain benign neoplasms, such as prostatic adenomas, may be found in the specific body system chapters. To properly code a neoplasm it is necessary to determine from the record if the neoplasm is benign, in-situ, malignant, or of uncertain histologic behavior. If malignant, any secondary (metastatic) sites should also be determined.

Primary malignant neoplasms overlapping site boundaries

A primary malignant neoplasm that overlaps two or more contiguous (next to each other) sites should be classified to the subcategory/code .8 ('overlapping lesion'), unless the combination is specifically indexed elsewhere. For multiple neoplasms of the same site that are not contiguous such as tumors in different quadrants of the same breast, codes for each site should be assigned.

Malignant neoplasm of ectopic tissue

Malignant neoplasms of ectopic tissue are to be coded to the site of origin mentioned, e.g., ectopic pancreatic malignant neoplasms involving the stomach are coded to malignant neoplasm of pancreas, unspecified (C25.9).

The neoplasm table in the Alphabetic Index should be referenced first. However, if the histological term is documented, that term should be referenced first, rather than going immediately to the Neoplasm Table, in order to determine which column in the Neoplasm Table is appropriate. For example, if the documentation indicates "adenoma," refer to the term in the Alphabetic Index to review the entries under this term and the instructional note to "see also neoplasm, by site, benign." The table provides the proper code based on the type of neoplasm and the site. It is important to select the proper column in the table that corresponds to the type of neoplasm. The Tabular List should then be referenced to verify that the correct code has been selected from the table and that a more specific site code does not exist.

See Section I.C.21. Factors influencing health status and contact with health services, Status, for information regarding Z15.0, codes for genetic susceptibility to cancer.

a. **Admission/Encounter for treatment of primary site**

If the malignancy is chiefly responsible for occasioning the patient admission/encounter and treatment is directed at the primary site, designate the primary malignancy as the principal/first-listed diagnosis.

The only exception to this guideline is if the administration of chemotherapy, immunotherapy or external beam radiation therapy is chiefly responsible for occasioning the admission/encounter. In that case, assign the appropriate Z51.-- code as the first-listed or principal diagnosis, and the underlying diagnosis or problem for which the service is being performed as a secondary diagnosis.

b. **Admission/Encounter for treatment of secondary site**

When a patient is admitted because of a primary neoplasm with metastasis and treatment is directed toward the secondary site only, the secondary neoplasm is designated as the principal diagnosis even though the primary malignancy is still present.

c. **Coding and sequencing of complications**

Coding and sequencing of complications associated with the malignancies or with the therapy thereof are subject to the following guidelines:

1) **Anemia associated with malignancy**

When admission/encounter is for management of an anemia associated with the malignancy, and the treatment is only for anemia, the appropriate code for the malignancy is sequenced as the principal or first-listed diagnosis followed by the appropriate code for the anemia (such as code D63.0, Anemia in neoplastic disease).

2) **Anemia associated with chemotherapy, immunotherapy and radiation therapy**

When the admission/encounter is for management of an anemia associated with an adverse effect of the administration of chemotherapy or immunotherapy and the only treatment is for the anemia, the anemia code is sequenced first followed by the appropriate codes for the neoplasm and the adverse effect (T45.1X5-, Adverse effect of antineoplastic and immunosuppressive drugs).

When the admission/encounter is for management of an anemia associated with an adverse effect of radiotherapy, the anemia code should be sequenced first, followed by the appropriate neoplasm code and code Y84.2, Radiological procedure and radiotherapy as the cause of abnormal reaction of the patient, or of later complication, without mention of misadventure at the time of the procedure.

3) **Management of dehydration due to the malignancy**

When the admission/encounter is for management of dehydration due to the malignancy and only the dehydration is being treated (intravenous rehydration), the dehydration is sequenced first, followed by the code(s) for the malignancy.

4) **Treatment of a complication resulting from a surgical procedure**

When the admission/encounter is for treatment of a complication resulting from a surgical procedure, designate the complication as the principal or first-listed diagnosis if treatment is directed at resolving the complication.

d. **Primary malignancy previously excised**

When a primary malignancy has been previously excised or eradicated from its site and there is no further treatment directed to that site and there is no evidence of any existing primary malignancy at that site, a code from category Z85, Personal history of malignant neoplasm, should be used to indicate the former site of the malignancy. Any mention of extension, invasion, or metastasis to another site is coded as a secondary malignant neoplasm to that site. The secondary site may be the principal or first-listed diagnosis with the Z85 code used as a secondary code.

See section I.C.2.t. Secondary malignant neoplasm of lymphoid tissue.

e. **Admissions/Encounters involving chemotherapy, immunotherapy and radiation therapy**

1) **Episode of care involves surgical removal of neoplasm**

When an episode of care involves the surgical removal of a neoplasm, primary or secondary site, followed by adjunct chemotherapy or

509

radiation treatment during the same episode of care, the code for the neoplasm should be assigned as principal or first-listed diagnosis.

2) **Patient admission/encounter chiefly for administration of chemotherapy, immunotherapy and radiation therapy**

If a patient admission/encounter is **chiefly** for the administration of chemotherapy, immunotherapy or external beam radiation therapy assign code Z51.0, Encounter for antineoplastic radiation therapy, or Z51.11, Encounter for antineoplastic chemotherapy, or Z51.12, Encounter for antineoplastic immunotherapy as the first-listed or principal diagnosis. If a patient receives more than one of these therapies during the same admission more than one of these codes may be assigned, in any sequence.

The malignancy for which the therapy is being administered should be assigned as a secondary diagnosis.

If a patient admission/encounter is for the insertion or implantation of radioactive elements (e.g., brachytherapy) the appropriate code for the malignancy is sequenced as the principal or first-listed diagnosis. Code Z51.0 should not be assigned.

3) **Patient admitted for radiation therapy, chemotherapy or immunotherapy and develops complications**

When a patient is admitted for the purpose of external beam radiotherapy, immunotherapy or chemotherapy and develops complications such as uncontrolled nausea and vomiting or dehydration, the principal or first-listed diagnosis is Z51.0, Encounter for antineoplastic radiation therapy, or Z51.11, Encounter for antineoplastic chemotherapy, or Z51.12, Encounter for antineoplastic immunotherapy followed by any codes for the complications.

When a patient is admitted for the purpose of insertion or implantation of radioactive elements (e.g., brachytherapy) and develops complications such as uncontrolled nausea and vomiting or dehydration, the principal or first-listed diagnosis is the appropriate code for the malignancy followed by any codes for the complications.

f. **Admission/encounter to determine extent of malignancy**

When the reason for admission/encounter is to determine the extent of the malignancy, or for a procedure such as paracentesis or thoracentesis, the primary malignancy or appropriate metastatic site is designated as the principal or first-listed diagnosis, even though chemotherapy or radiotherapy is administered.

g. **Symptoms, signs, and abnormal findings listed in Chapter 18 associated with neoplasms**

Symptoms, signs, and ill-defined conditions listed in Chapter 18 characteristic of, or associated with, an existing primary or secondary site malignancy cannot be used to replace the malignancy as principal or first-listed diagnosis, regardless of the number of admissions or encounters for treatment and care of the neoplasm.

See section I.C.21. Factors influencing health status and contact with health services, Encounter for prophylactic organ removal.

h. **Admission/encounter for pain control/management**

See Section I.C.6. for information on coding admission/encounter for pain control/management.

i. **Malignancy in two or more noncontiguous sites**

A patient may have more than one malignant tumor in the same organ. These tumors may represent different primaries or metastatic disease, depending on the site. Should the documentation be unclear, the provider should be queried as to the status of each tumor so that the correct codes can be assigned.

j. **Disseminated malignant neoplasm, unspecified**

Code C80.0, Disseminated malignant neoplasm, unspecified, is for use only in those cases where the patient has advanced metastatic disease and no known primary or secondary sites are specified. It should not be used in place of assigning codes for the primary site and all known secondary sites.

k. **Malignant neoplasm without specification of site**

Code C80.1, Malignant (primary) neoplasm, unspecified, equates to Cancer, unspecified. This code should only be used when no determination can be made as to the primary site of a malignancy. This code should rarely be used in the inpatient setting.

l. **Sequencing of neoplasm codes**

1) **Encounter for treatment of primary malignancy**

If the reason for the encounter is for treatment of a primary malignancy, assign the malignancy as the principal/first-listed diagnosis. The primary site is to be sequenced first, followed by any metastatic sites.

2) **Encounter for treatment of secondary malignancy**

When an encounter is for a primary malignancy with metastasis and treatment is directed toward the metastatic (secondary) site(s) only, the metastatic site(s) is designated as the principal/first-listed diagnosis. The primary malignancy is coded as an additional code.

3) **Malignant neoplasm in a pregnant patient**

When a pregnant woman has a malignant neoplasm, a code from subcategory O9A.1-, Malignant neoplasm complicating pregnancy, childbirth, and the puerperium, should be sequenced first, followed by the appropriate code from Chapter 2 to indicate the type of neoplasm.

4) **Encounter for complication associated with a neoplasm**

When an encounter is for management of a complication associated with a neoplasm, such as dehydration, and the treatment is only for the complication, the complication is coded first, followed by the appropriate code(s) for the neoplasm.

The exception to this guideline is anemia. When the admission/encounter is for management of an anemia associated with the malignancy, and the treatment is only for anemia, the appropriate code for the malignancy is sequenced as the principal or first-listed diagnosis followed by code D63.0, Anemia in neoplastic disease.

5) **Complication from surgical procedure for treatment of a neoplasm**

When an encounter is for treatment of a complication resulting from a surgical procedure performed for the treatment of the neoplasm, designate the complication as the principal/first-listed diagnosis. See the guideline regarding the coding of a current malignancy versus personal history to determine if the code for the neoplasm should also be assigned.

6) **Pathologic fracture due to a neoplasm**

When an encounter is for a pathological fracture due to a neoplasm, and the focus of treatment is the fracture, a code from subcategory M84.5, Pathological fracture in neoplastic disease, should be sequenced first, followed by the code for the neoplasm.

If the focus of treatment is the neoplasm with an associated pathological fracture, the neoplasm code should be sequenced first, followed by a code from M84.5 for the pathological fracture.

m. **Current malignancy versus personal history of malignancy**

When a primary malignancy has been excised but further treatment, such as an additional surgery for the malignancy, radiation therapy or chemotherapy is directed to that site, the primary malignancy code should be used until treatment is completed.

When a primary malignancy has been previously excised or eradicated from its site, there is no further treatment (of the malignancy) directed to that site, and there is no evidence of any existing primary malignancy at that site, a code from category Z85, Personal history of malignant neoplasm, should be used to indicate the former site of the malignancy.

Subcategories Z85.0 - Z85.7 should only be assigned for the former site of a primary malignancy, not the site of a secondary malignancy. Codes from subcategory Z85.8-, may be assigned for the former site(s) of either a primary or secondary malignancy included in this subcategory.

See Section I.C.21. Factors influencing health status and contact with health services, History (of)

n. **Leukemia, Multiple Myeloma, and Malignant Plasma Cell Neoplasms in remission versus personal history**

The categories for leukemia, and category C90, Multiple myeloma and malignant plasma cell neoplasms, have codes indicating whether or not the leukemia has achieved remission. There are also codes Z85.6, Personal history of leukemia, and Z85.79, Personal history of other malignant neoplasms of lymphoid, hematopoietic and related tissues. If the documentation is unclear, as to whether the leukemia has achieved remission, the provider should be queried.

See Section I.C.21. Factors influencing health status and contact with health services, History (of)

o. **Aftercare following surgery for neoplasm**

See Section I.C.21. Factors influencing health status and contact with health services, Aftercare

p. **Follow-up care for completed treatment of a malignancy**

See Section I.C.21. Factors influencing health status and contact with health services, Follow-up

q. **Prophylactic organ removal for prevention of malignancy**

See Section I.C. 21, Factors influencing health status and contact with health services, Prophylactic organ removal

r. **Malignant neoplasm associated with transplanted organ**

A malignant neoplasm of a transplanted organ should be coded as a transplant complication. Assign first the appropriate code from category T86.-, Complications of transplanted organs and tissue, followed by code

C80.2, Malignant neoplasm associated with transplanted organ. Use an additional code for the specific malignancy.

- **s. Breast Implant Associated Anaplastic Large Cell Lymphoma**
  Breast implant associated anaplastic large cell lymphoma (BIA-ALCL) is a type of lymphoma that can develop around breast implants. Assign code C84.7A, Anaplastic large cell lymphoma, ALK-negative, breast, for BIA-ALCL. Do not assign a complication code from chapter 19.

- **t. Secondary malignant neoplasm of lymphoid tissue**
  When a malignant neoplasm of lymphoid tissue metastasizes beyond the lymph nodes, a code from categories C81-C85 with a final character "9" should be assigned identifying "extranodal and solid organ sites" rather than a code for the secondary neoplasm of the affected solid organ. For example, for metastasis of **diffuse large** B-cell lymphoma to the lung, brain and left adrenal gland, assign code C83.39, Diffuse large B-cell lymphoma, extranodal and solid organ sites.

Malignant neoplasms (C00-C96)

Malignant neoplasms, stated or presumed to be primary (of specified sites), and certain specified histologies, except neuroendocrine, and of lymphoid, hematopoietic and related tissue (C00-C75)

Malignant neoplasms of lip, oral cavity and pharynx (C00-C14)

C00 Malignant neoplasm of lip
   Use additional code to identify:
   alcohol abuse and dependence (F10.-)
   history of tobacco dependence (Z87.891)
   tobacco dependence (F17.-)
   tobacco use (Z72.0)
   Excludes1: malignant melanoma of lip (C43.0)
   Merkel cell carcinoma of lip (C4A.0)
   other and unspecified malignant neoplasm of skin of lip (C44.0-)

   C00.0 Malignant neoplasm of external upper lip
   Malignant neoplasm of lipstick area of upper lip
   Malignant neoplasm of upper lip NOS
   Malignant neoplasm of vermilion border of upper lip

   C00.1 Malignant neoplasm of external lower lip
   Malignant neoplasm of lower lip NOS
   Malignant neoplasm of lipstick area of lower lip
   Malignant neoplasm of vermilion border of lower lip

   C00.2 Malignant neoplasm of external lip, unspecified
   Malignant neoplasm of vermilion border of lip NOS

   C00.3 Malignant neoplasm of upper lip, inner aspect
   Malignant neoplasm of buccal aspect of upper lip
   Malignant neoplasm of frenulum of upper lip
   Malignant neoplasm of mucosa of upper lip
   Malignant neoplasm of oral aspect of upper lip

   C00.4 Malignant neoplasm of lower lip, inner aspect
   Malignant neoplasm of buccal aspect of lower lip
   Malignant neoplasm of frenulum of lower lip
   Malignant neoplasm of mucosa of lower lip
   Malignant neoplasm of oral aspect of lower lip

   C00.5 Malignant neoplasm of lip, unspecified, inner aspect
   Malignant neoplasm of buccal aspect of lip, unspecified
   Malignant neoplasm of frenulum of lip, unspecified
   Malignant neoplasm of mucosa of lip, unspecified
   Malignant neoplasm of oral aspect of lip, unspecified

   C00.6 Malignant neoplasm of commissure of lip, unspecified
   C00.8 Malignant neoplasm of overlapping sites of lip
   C00.9 Malignant neoplasm of lip, unspecified

C01 Malignant neoplasm of base of tongue
   Malignant neoplasm of dorsal surface of base of tongue
   Malignant neoplasm of fixed part of tongue NOS
   Malignant neoplasm of posterior third of tongue
   Use additional code to identify:
   alcohol abuse and dependence (F10.-)
   history of tobacco dependence (Z87.891)
   tobacco dependence (F17.-)
   tobacco use (Z72.0)
   Valid 3-character code, no further characters required

C02 Malignant neoplasm of other and unspecified parts of tongue
   Use additional code to identify:
   alcohol abuse and dependence (F10.-)
   history of tobacco dependence (Z87.891)
   tobacco dependence (F17.-)
   tobacco use (Z72.0)

   C02.0 Malignant neoplasm of dorsal surface of tongue
   Malignant neoplasm of anterior two-thirds of tongue, dorsal surface
   Excludes2: malignant neoplasm of dorsal surface of base of tongue (C01)

   C02.1 Malignant neoplasm of border of tongue
   Malignant neoplasm of tip of tongue

   C02.2 Malignant neoplasm of ventral surface of tongue
   Malignant neoplasm of anterior two-thirds of tongue, ventral surface
   Malignant neoplasm of frenulum linguae

   C02.3 Malignant neoplasm of anterior two-thirds of tongue, part unspecified
   Malignant neoplasm of middle third of tongue NOS
   Malignant neoplasm of mobile part of tongue NOS

   C02.4 Malignant neoplasm of lingual tonsil
   Excludes2: malignant neoplasm of tonsil NOS (C09.9)

   C02.8 Malignant neoplasm of overlapping sites of tongue
   Malignant neoplasm of two or more contiguous sites of tongue

   C02.9 Malignant neoplasm of tongue, unspecified

C03 Malignant neoplasm of gum
   Includes: malignant neoplasm of alveolar (ridge) mucosa
   malignant neoplasm of gingiva
   Use additional code to identify:
   alcohol abuse and dependence (F10.-)
   history of tobacco dependence (Z87.891)
   tobacco dependence (F17.-)
   tobacco use (Z72.0)
   Excludes2: malignant odontogenic neoplasms (C41.0-C41.1)

   C03.0 Malignant neoplasm of upper gum
   C03.1 Malignant neoplasm of lower gum
   C03.9 Malignant neoplasm of gum, unspecified

C04 Malignant neoplasm of floor of mouth
   Use additional code to identify:
   alcohol abuse and dependence (F10.-)
   history of tobacco dependence (Z87.891)
   tobacco dependence (F17.-)
   tobacco use (Z72.0)

   C04.0 Malignant neoplasm of anterior floor of mouth
   Malignant neoplasm of anterior to the premolar-canine junction

   C04.1 Malignant neoplasm of lateral floor of mouth
   C04.8 Malignant neoplasm of overlapping sites of floor of mouth
   C04.9 Malignant neoplasm of floor of mouth, unspecified

C05 Malignant neoplasm of palate
   Use additional code to identify:
   alcohol abuse and dependence (F10.-)
   history of tobacco dependence (Z87.891)
   tobacco dependence (F17.-)
   tobacco use (Z72.0)
   Excludes1: Kaposi's sarcoma of palate (C46.2)

   C05.0 Malignant neoplasm of hard palate
   C05.1 Malignant neoplasm of soft palate
   Excludes2: malignant neoplasm of nasopharyngeal surface of soft palate (C11.3)

   C05.2 Malignant neoplasm of uvula
   C05.8 Malignant neoplasm of overlapping sites of palate
   C05.9 Malignant neoplasm of palate, unspecified
   Malignant neoplasm of roof of mouth

C06 Malignant neoplasm of other and unspecified parts of mouth
   Use additional code to identify:
   alcohol abuse and dependence (F10.-)
   history of tobacco dependence (Z87.891)
   tobacco dependence (F17.-)
   tobacco use (Z72.0)

   C06.0 Malignant neoplasm of cheek mucosa
   Malignant neoplasm of buccal mucosa NOS
   Malignant neoplasm of internal cheek

   C06.1 Malignant neoplasm of vestibule of mouth
   Malignant neoplasm of buccal sulcus (upper) (lower)
   Malignant neoplasm of labial sulcus (upper) (lower)

   C06.2 Malignant neoplasm of retromolar area

Tumor Biology and Chemotherapy

Tumor heterogeneity

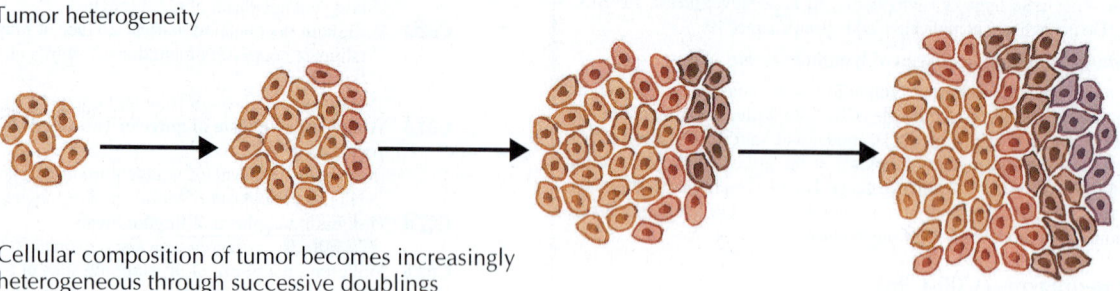

Cellular composition of tumor becomes increasingly heterogeneous through successive doublings

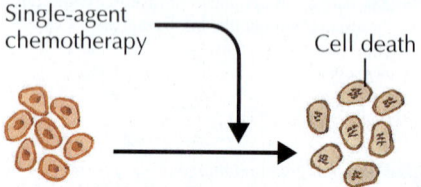

Single-agent chemotherapy may be successful in susceptible homogeneous tumors

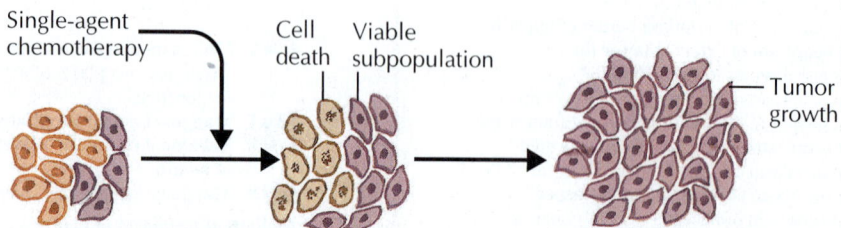

Single-agent chemotherapy for heterogeneous tumors may result only in death of susceptible cell line, selecting nonresponsive cells for growth and spread

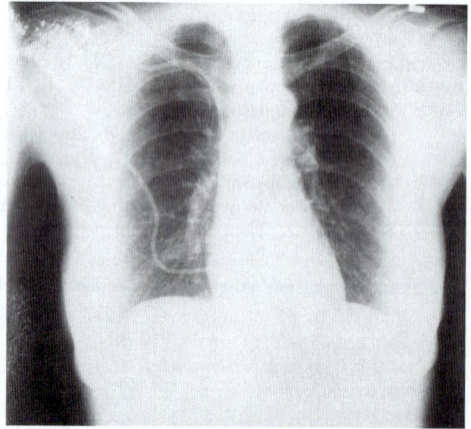

Radiograph of lungs after multiple-agent chemotherapy

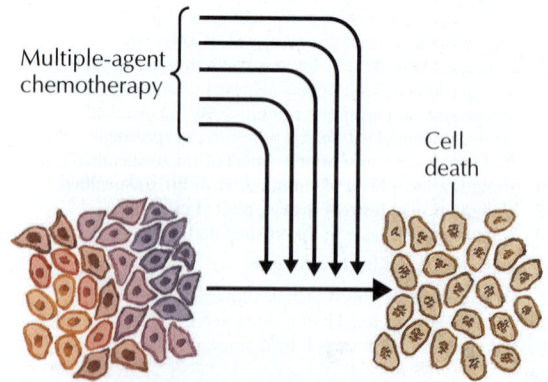

Multiple-agent chemotherapy affects subpopulations of heterogeneous tumors

© Elsevier Inc. All rights reserved. www.netterimages.com

+ C06.8 Malignant neoplasm of overlapping sites of other and unspecified parts of mouth
- **C06.80** Malignant neoplasm of overlapping sites of unspecified parts of mouth
- **C06.89** Malignant neoplasm of overlapping sites of other parts of mouth
  - 'book leaf' neoplasm [ventral surface of tongue and floor of mouth]

C06.9 Malignant neoplasm of mouth, unspecified
- Malignant neoplasm of minor salivary gland, unspecified site
- Malignant neoplasm of oral cavity NOS

C07 Malignant neoplasm of parotid gland
Use additional code to identify:
- alcohol abuse and dependence (F10.-)
- exposure to environmental tobacco smoke (Z77.22)
- exposure to tobacco smoke in the perinatal period (P96.81)
- history of tobacco dependence (Z87.891)
- occupational exposure to environmental tobacco smoke (Z57.31)
- tobacco dependence (F17.-)
- tobacco use (Z72.0)

Valid 3-character code, no further characters required

C08 Malignant neoplasm of other and unspecified major salivary glands
Includes: malignant neoplasm of salivary ducts
Use additional code to identify:
- alcohol abuse and dependence (F10.-)
- exposure to environmental tobacco smoke (Z77.22)
- exposure to tobacco smoke in the perinatal period (P96.81)
- history of tobacco dependence (Z87.891)
- occupational exposure to environmental tobacco smoke (Z57.31)
- tobacco dependence (F17.-)
- tobacco use (Z72.0)

Excludes1: malignant neoplasms of specified minor salivary glands which are classified according to their anatomical location

Excludes2: malignant neoplasms of minor salivary glands NOS (C06.9)
malignant neoplasm of parotid gland (C07)

- **C08.0** Malignant neoplasm of submandibular gland
  - Malignant neoplasm of submaxillary gland
- **C08.1** Malignant neoplasm of sublingual gland
- **C08.9** Malignant neoplasm of major salivary gland, unspecified
  - Malignant neoplasm of salivary gland (major) NOS

C09 Malignant neoplasm of tonsil
Use additional code to identify:
- alcohol abuse and dependence (F10.-)
- exposure to environmental tobacco smoke (Z77.22)
- exposure to tobacco smoke in the perinatal period (P96.81)
- history of tobacco dependence (Z87.891)
- occupational exposure to environmental tobacco smoke (Z57.31)
- tobacco dependence (F17.-)
- tobacco use (Z72.0)

Excludes2: malignant neoplasm of lingual tonsil (C02.4)
malignant neoplasm of pharyngeal tonsil (C11.1)

- **C09.0** Malignant neoplasm of tonsillar fossa
- **C09.1** Malignant neoplasm of tonsillar pillar (anterior) (posterior)
- **C09.8** Malignant neoplasm of overlapping sites of tonsil
- **C09.9** Malignant neoplasm of tonsil, unspecified
  - Malignant neoplasm of tonsil NOS
  - Malignant neoplasm of faucial tonsils
  - Malignant neoplasm of palatine tonsils

C10 Malignant neoplasm of oropharynx
Use additional code to identify:
- alcohol abuse and dependence (F10.-)
- exposure to environmental tobacco smoke (Z77.22)
- exposure to tobacco smoke in the perinatal period (P96.81)
- history of tobacco dependence (Z87.891)
- occupational exposure to environmental tobacco smoke (Z57.31)
- tobacco dependence (F17.-)
- tobacco use (Z72.0)

Excludes2: malignant neoplasm of tonsil (C09.-)

- **C10.0** Malignant neoplasm of vallecula
- **C10.1** Malignant neoplasm of anterior surface of epiglottis
  - Malignant neoplasm of epiglottis, free border [margin]
  - Malignant neoplasm of glossoepiglottic fold(s)
  - **Excludes2:** malignant neoplasm of epiglottis (suprahyoid portion) NOS (C32.1)
- **C10.2** Malignant neoplasm of lateral wall of oropharynx
- **C10.3** Malignant neoplasm of posterior wall of oropharynx
- **C10.4** Malignant neoplasm of branchial cleft
  - Malignant neoplasm of branchial cyst [site of neoplasm]
- **C10.8** Malignant neoplasm of overlapping sites of oropharynx
  - Malignant neoplasm of junctional region of oropharynx
- **C10.9** Malignant neoplasm of oropharynx, unspecified

C11 Malignant neoplasm of nasopharynx
Use additional code to identify:
- exposure to environmental tobacco smoke (Z77.22)
- exposure to tobacco smoke in the perinatal period (P96.81)
- history of tobacco dependence (Z87.891)
- occupational exposure to environmental tobacco smoke (Z57.31)
- tobacco dependence (F17.-)
- tobacco use (Z72.0)

- **C11.0** Malignant neoplasm of superior wall of nasopharynx
  - Malignant neoplasm of roof of nasopharynx
- **C11.1** Malignant neoplasm of posterior wall of nasopharynx
  - Malignant neoplasm of adenoid
  - Malignant neoplasm of pharyngeal tonsil
- **C11.2** Malignant neoplasm of lateral wall of nasopharynx
  - Malignant neoplasm of fossa of Rosenmüller
  - Malignant neoplasm of opening of auditory tube
  - Malignant neoplasm of pharyngeal recess
- **C11.3** Malignant neoplasm of anterior wall of nasopharynx
  - Malignant neoplasm of floor of nasopharynx
  - Malignant neoplasm of nasopharyngeal (anterior) (posterior) surface of soft palate
  - Malignant neoplasm of posterior margin of nasal choana
  - Malignant neoplasm of posterior margin of nasal septum
- **C11.8** Malignant neoplasm of overlapping sites of nasopharynx
- **C11.9** Malignant neoplasm of nasopharynx, unspecified
  - Malignant neoplasm of nasopharyngeal wall NOS

C12 Malignant neoplasm of pyriform sinus
Malignant neoplasm of pyriform fossa
Use additional code to identify:
- exposure to environmental tobacco smoke (Z77.22)
- exposure to tobacco smoke in the perinatal period (P96.81)
- history of tobacco dependence (Z87.891)
- occupational exposure to environmental tobacco smoke (Z57.31)
- tobacco dependence (F17.-)
- tobacco use (Z72.0)

Valid 3-character code, no further characters required

C13 Malignant neoplasm of hypopharynx
Use additional code to identify:
- exposure to environmental tobacco smoke (Z77.22)
- exposure to tobacco smoke in the perinatal period (P96.81)
- history of tobacco dependence (Z87.891)
- occupational exposure to environmental tobacco smoke (Z57.31)
- tobacco dependence (F17.-)
- tobacco use (Z72.0)

Excludes2: malignant neoplasm of pyriform sinus (C12)

- **C13.0** Malignant neoplasm of postcricoid region
- **C13.1** Malignant neoplasm of aryepiglottic fold, hypopharyngeal aspect
  - Malignant neoplasm of aryepiglottic fold NOS
  - Malignant neoplasm of interarytenoid fold NOS
  - Malignant neoplasm of aryepiglottic fold, marginal zone
  - Malignant neoplasm of interarytenoid fold, marginal zone
  - **Excludes2:** malignant neoplasm of aryepiglottic fold or interarytenoid fold, laryngeal aspect (C32.1)
- **C13.2** Malignant neoplasm of posterior wall of hypopharynx
- **C13.8** Malignant neoplasm of overlapping sites of hypopharynx
- **C13.9** Malignant neoplasm of hypopharynx, unspecified
  - Malignant neoplasm of hypopharyngeal wall NOS

C14 Malignant neoplasm of other and ill-defined sites in the lip, oral cavity and pharynx
Use additional code to identify:
- alcohol abuse and dependence (F10.-)
- exposure to environmental tobacco smoke (Z77.22)
- exposure to tobacco smoke in the perinatal period (P96.81)
- history of tobacco dependence (Z87.891)
- occupational exposure to environmental tobacco smoke (Z57.31)
- tobacco dependence (F17.-)
- tobacco use (Z72.0)

Excludes1: malignant neoplasm of oral cavity NOS (C06.9)

- **C14.0** Malignant neoplasm of pharynx, unspecified
- **C14.2** Malignant neoplasm of Waldeyer's ring

C14.8 Malignant neoplasm of overlapping sites of lip, oral cavity and pharynx
Primary malignant neoplasm of two or more contiguous sites of lip, oral cavity and pharynx
Excludes1: 'book leaf' neoplasm [ventral surface of tongue and floor of mouth] (C06.89)

Malignant neoplasms of digestive organs (C15-C26)

Excludes1: Kaposi's sarcoma of gastrointestinal sites (C46.4)
Excludes2: gastrointestinal stromal tumors (C49.A-)

C15 Malignant neoplasm of esophagus
Use additional code to identify:
alcohol abuse and dependence (F10.-)
- CC **C15.3** Malignant neoplasm of upper third of esophagus
- CC **C15.4** Malignant neoplasm of middle third of esophagus
- CC **C15.5** Malignant neoplasm of lower third of esophagus
  Excludes1: malignant neoplasm of cardio-esophageal junction (C16.0)
  AHA CC: 3Q, 2022, 10
- CC **C15.8** Malignant neoplasm of overlapping sites of esophagus
- CC **C15.9** Malignant neoplasm of esophagus, unspecified

C16 Malignant neoplasm of stomach
Use additional code to identify:
alcohol abuse and dependence (F10.-)
Excludes2: malignant carcinoid tumor of the stomach (C7A.092)
- CC **C16.0** Malignant neoplasm of cardia
  Malignant neoplasm of cardiac orifice
  Malignant neoplasm of cardio-esophageal junction
  Malignant neoplasm of esophagus and stomach
  Malignant neoplasm of gastro-esophageal junction
- CC **C16.1** Malignant neoplasm of fundus of stomach
- CC **C16.2** Malignant neoplasm of body of stomach
- CC **C16.3** Malignant neoplasm of pyloric antrum
  Malignant neoplasm of gastric antrum
- CC **C16.4** Malignant neoplasm of pylorus
  Malignant neoplasm of prepylorus
  Malignant neoplasm of pyloric canal
- CC **C16.5** Malignant neoplasm of lesser curvature of stomach, unspecified
  Malignant neoplasm of lesser curvature of stomach, not classifiable to C16.1-C16.4
- CC **C16.6** Malignant neoplasm of greater curvature of stomach, unspecified
  Malignant neoplasm of greater curvature of stomach, not classifiable to C16.0-C16.4
- CC **C16.8** Malignant neoplasm of overlapping sites of stomach
- CC **C16.9** Malignant neoplasm of stomach, unspecified
  Gastric cancer NOS

C17 Malignant neoplasm of small intestine
Excludes1: malignant carcinoid tumors of the small intestine (C7A.01)
- CC **C17.0** Malignant neoplasm of duodenum
- CC **C17.1** Malignant neoplasm of jejunum
- CC **C17.2** Malignant neoplasm of ileum
  Excludes1: malignant neoplasm of ileocecal valve (C18.0)
- CC **C17.3** Meckel's diverticulum, malignant
  Excludes1: Meckel's diverticulum, congenital (Q43.0)
- CC **C17.8** Malignant neoplasm of overlapping sites of small intestine
- CC **C17.9** Malignant neoplasm of small intestine, unspecified

C18 Malignant neoplasm of colon
Excludes1: malignant carcinoid tumors of the colon (C7A.02-)
- CC **C18.0** Malignant neoplasm of cecum
  Malignant neoplasm of ileocecal valve
- CC **C18.1** Malignant neoplasm of appendix
- CC **C18.2** Malignant neoplasm of ascending colon
- CC **C18.3** Malignant neoplasm of hepatic flexure
- CC **C18.4** Malignant neoplasm of transverse colon
- CC **C18.5** Malignant neoplasm of splenic flexure
- CC **C18.6** Malignant neoplasm of descending colon
- CC **C18.7** Malignant neoplasm of sigmoid colon
  Malignant neoplasm of sigmoid (flexure)
  Excludes1: malignant neoplasm of rectosigmoid junction (C19)
- CC **C18.8** Malignant neoplasm of overlapping sites of colon
- CC **C18.9** Malignant neoplasm of colon, unspecified
  Malignant neoplasm of large intestine NOS

CC **C19** Malignant neoplasm of rectosigmoid junction
Malignant neoplasm of colon with rectum
Malignant neoplasm of rectosigmoid (colon)
Excludes1: malignant carcinoid tumors of the colon (C7A.02-)
Valid 3-character code, no further characters required

CC **C20** Malignant neoplasm of rectum
Malignant neoplasm of rectal ampulla
Excludes1: malignant carcinoid tumor of the rectum (C7A.026)
Valid 3-character code, no further characters required

CC **C21** Malignant neoplasm of anus and anal canal
Excludes2: malignant carcinoid tumors of the colon (C7A.02-)
malignant melanoma of anal margin (C43.51)
malignant melanoma of anal skin (C43.51)
malignant melanoma of perianal skin (C43.51)
other and unspecified malignant neoplasm of anal margin (C44.500, C44.510, C44.520, C44.590)
other and unspecified malignant neoplasm of anal skin (C44.500, C44.510, C44.520, C44.590)
other and unspecified malignant neoplasm of perianal skin (C44.500, C44.510, C44.520, C44.590)
- CC **C21.0** Malignant neoplasm of anus, unspecified
- CC **C21.1** Malignant neoplasm of anal canal
  Malignant neoplasm of anal sphincter
- CC **C21.2** Malignant neoplasm of cloacogenic zone
- CC **C21.8** Malignant neoplasm of overlapping sites of rectum, anus and anal canal
  Malignant neoplasm of anorectal junction
  Malignant neoplasm of anorectum
  Primary malignant neoplasm of two or more contiguous sites of rectum, anus and anal canal

C22 Malignant neoplasm of liver and intrahepatic bile ducts
Excludes1: malignant neoplasm of biliary tract NOS (C24.9)
secondary malignant neoplasm of liver and intrahepatic bile duct (C78.7)
Use additional code to identify:
alcohol abuse and dependence (F10.-)
hepatitis B (B16.-, B18.0-B18.1)
hepatitis C (B17.1-, B18.2)
- CC **C22.0** Liver cell carcinoma
  Hepatocellular carcinoma
  Hepatoma
  AHA CC: 1Q, 2016, 18-19
- CC **C22.1** Intrahepatic bile duct carcinoma
  Cholangiocarcinoma
  Excludes1: malignant neoplasm of hepatic duct (C24.0)
  AHA CC: 1Q, 2023, 24-25
- CC **C22.2** Hepatoblastoma
- CC **C22.3** Angiosarcoma of liver
  Kupffer cell sarcoma
- CC **C22.4** Other sarcomas of liver
- CC **C22.7** Other specified carcinomas of liver
- CC **C22.8** Malignant neoplasm of liver, primary, unspecified as to type
- CC **C22.9** Malignant neoplasm of liver, not specified as primary or secondary

CC **C23** Malignant neoplasm of gallbladder
Valid 3-character code, no further characters required

C24 Malignant neoplasm of other and unspecified parts of biliary tract
Excludes1: malignant neoplasm of intrahepatic bile duct (C22.1)
- CC **C24.0** Malignant neoplasm of extrahepatic bile duct
  Malignant neoplasm of biliary duct or passage NOS
  Malignant neoplasm of common bile duct
  Malignant neoplasm of cystic duct
  Malignant neoplasm of hepatic duct
- CC **C24.1** Malignant neoplasm of ampulla of Vater
- CC **C24.8** Malignant neoplasm of overlapping sites of biliary tract
  Malignant neoplasm involving both intrahepatic and extrahepatic bile ducts
  Primary malignant neoplasm of two or more contiguous sites of biliary tract
- CC **C24.9** Malignant neoplasm of biliary tract, unspecified

C25 Malignant neoplasm of pancreas
Code also, if applicable, exocrine pancreatic insufficiency (K86.81)
Use additional code to identify:
alcohol abuse and dependence (F10.-)
- CC **C25.0** Malignant neoplasm of head of pancreas
- CC **C25.1** Malignant neoplasm of body of pancreas
  AHA CC: 4Q, 2018, 40

Clinical Manifestations of Colorectal Cancer

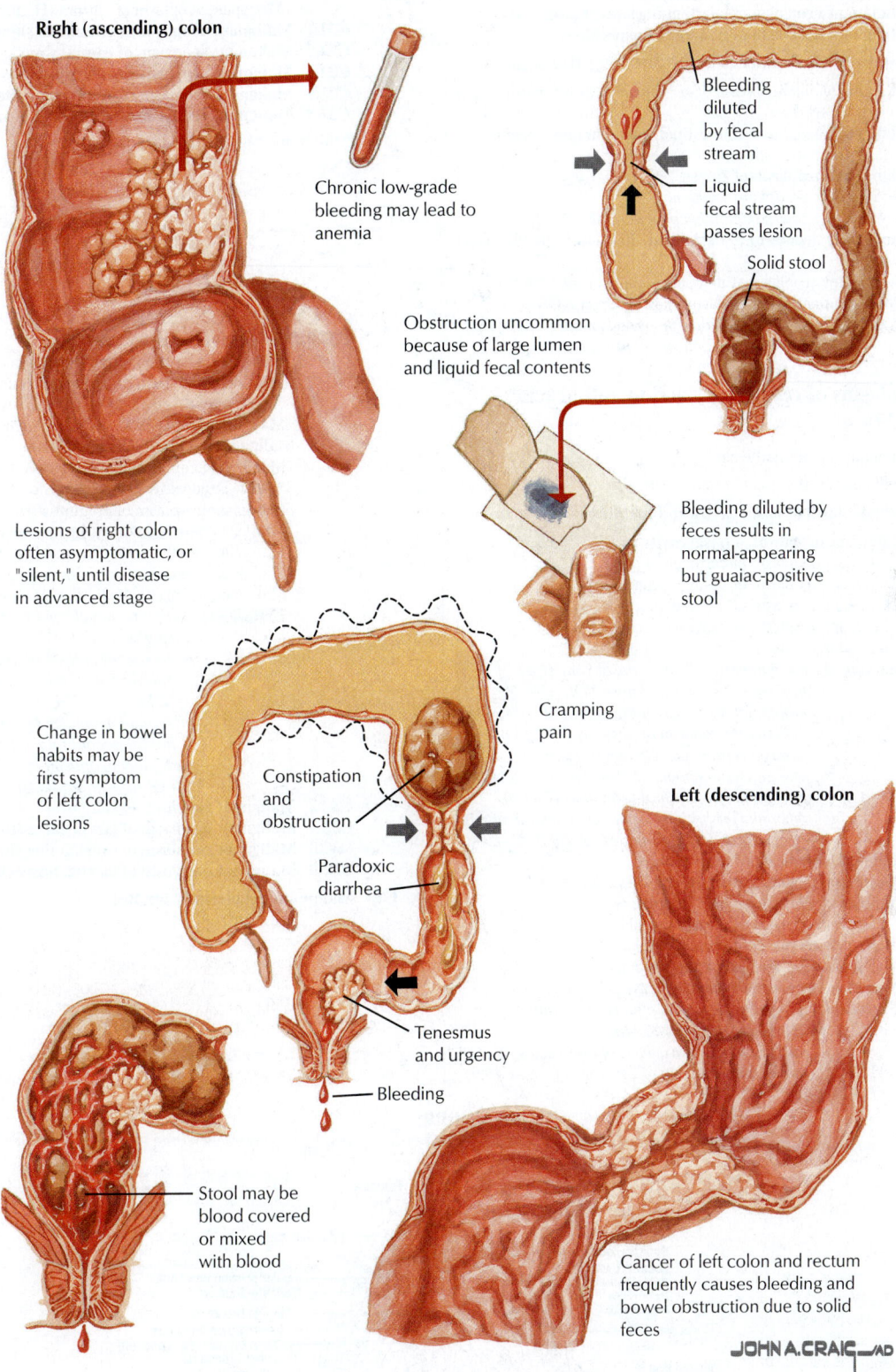

Chapter 2: Neoplasms

515

CC **C25.2** Malignant neoplasm of tail of pancreas
CC **C25.3** Malignant neoplasm of pancreatic duct
CC **C25.4** Malignant neoplasm of endocrine pancreas
Malignant neoplasm of islets of Langerhans
Use additional code to identify any functional activity.
CC **C25.7** Malignant neoplasm of other parts of pancreas
Malignant neoplasm of neck of pancreas
CC **C25.8** Malignant neoplasm of overlapping sites of pancreas
CC **C25.9** Malignant neoplasm of pancreas, unspecified

C26 Malignant neoplasm of other and ill-defined digestive organs
Excludes1: malignant neoplasm of peritoneum and retroperitoneum (C48.-)
C26.0 Malignant neoplasm of intestinal tract, part unspecified
Malignant neoplasm of intestine NOS
C26.1 Malignant neoplasm of spleen
Excludes1: Hodgkin lymphoma (C81.-)
non-Hodgkin lymphoma (C82-C85)
C26.9 Malignant neoplasm of ill-defined sites within the digestive system
Malignant neoplasm of alimentary canal or tract NOS
Malignant neoplasm of gastrointestinal tract NOS
Excludes1: malignant neoplasm of abdominal NOS (C76.2)
malignant neoplasm of intra-abdominal NOS (C76.2)

Malignant neoplasms of respiratory and intrathoracic organs (C30-C39)

Includes: malignant neoplasm of middle ear
Excludes1: mesothelioma (C45.-)

C30 Malignant neoplasm of nasal cavity and middle ear
C30.0 Malignant neoplasm of nasal cavity
Malignant neoplasm of cartilage of nose
Malignant neoplasm of nasal concha
Malignant neoplasm of internal nose
Malignant neoplasm of septum of nose
Malignant neoplasm of vestibule of nose
Excludes1: malignant neoplasm of nasal bone (C41.0)
malignant neoplasm of nose NOS (C76.0)
malignant neoplasm of olfactory bulb (C72.2-)
malignant neoplasm of posterior margin of nasal septum and choana (C11.3)
malignant melanoma of skin of nose (C43.31)
malignant neoplasm of turbinates (C41.0)
other and unspecified malignant neoplasm of skin of nose (C44.301, C44.311, C44.321, C44.391)
C30.1 Malignant neoplasm of middle ear
Malignant neoplasm of antrum tympanicum
Malignant neoplasm of auditory tube
Malignant neoplasm of eustachian tube
Malignant neoplasm of inner ear
Malignant neoplasm of mastoid air cells
Malignant neoplasm of tympanic cavity
Excludes1: malignant neoplasm of auricular canal (external) (C43.2-,C44.2-)
malignant neoplasm of bone of ear (meatus) (C41.0)
malignant neoplasm of cartilage of ear (C49.0)
malignant melanoma of skin of (external) ear (C43.2-)
other and unspecified malignant neoplasm of skin of (external) ear (C44.2-)

C31 Malignant neoplasm of accessory sinuses
C31.0 Malignant neoplasm of maxillary sinus
Malignant neoplasm of antrum (Highmore) (maxillary)
C31.1 Malignant neoplasm of ethmoidal sinus
C31.2 Malignant neoplasm of frontal sinus
C31.3 Malignant neoplasm of sphenoid sinus
C31.8 Malignant neoplasm of overlapping sites of accessory sinuses
C31.9 Malignant neoplasm of accessory sinus, unspecified

C32 Malignant neoplasm of larynx
Use additional code to identify:
alcohol abuse and dependence (F10.-)
exposure to environmental tobacco smoke (Z77.22)
exposure to tobacco smoke in the perinatal period (P96.81)
history of tobacco dependence (Z87.891)
occupational exposure to environmental tobacco smoke (Z57.31)
tobacco dependence (F17.-)
tobacco use (Z72.0)
C32.0 Malignant neoplasm of glottis
Malignant neoplasm of intrinsic larynx
Malignant neoplasm of laryngeal commissure (anterior) (posterior)
Malignant neoplasm of vocal cord (true) NOS
C32.1 Malignant neoplasm of supraglottis
Malignant neoplasm of aryepiglottic fold or interarytenoid fold, laryngeal aspect
Malignant neoplasm of epiglottis (suprahyoid portion) NOS
Malignant neoplasm of extrinsic larynx
Malignant neoplasm of false vocal cord
Malignant neoplasm of posterior (laryngeal) surface of epiglottis
Malignant neoplasm of ventricular bands
Excludes2: malignant neoplasm of anterior surface of epiglottis (C10.1)
malignant neoplasm of aryepiglottic fold or interarytenoid fold, hypopharyngeal aspect (C13.1)
malignant neoplasm of aryepiglottic fold or interarytenoid fold, marginal zone (C13.1)
malignant neoplasm of aryepiglottic fold or interarytenoid fold NOS (C13.1)
C32.2 Malignant neoplasm of subglottis
C32.3 Malignant neoplasm of laryngeal cartilage
C32.8 Malignant neoplasm of overlapping sites of larynx
C32.9 Malignant neoplasm of larynx, unspecified

CC **C33** Malignant neoplasm of trachea
Use additional code to identify:
exposure to environmental tobacco smoke (Z77.22)
exposure to tobacco smoke in the perinatal period (P96.81)
history of tobacco dependence (Z87.891)
occupational exposure to environmental tobacco smoke (Z57.31)
tobacco dependence (F17.-)
tobacco use (Z72.0)
Valid 3-character code, no further characters required

Lungs

Right — Left

Labels: Trachea, Apex, Superior lobe, Lobar bronchus: Right superior, Right middle, Right inferior, Horizontal fissure, Oblique fissure, Middle lobe, Inferior lobe, Diaphragm, Superior Lobe, Lingular division bronchus, Carina of trachea, Lingula bronchus, Intermediate bronchus, Main bronchi (right and left), Lobar bronchus: Left superior, Left inferior, Oblique fissure, Cardiac notch, Lingula of lung, Inferior lobe

©AHIMA

C34 Malignant neoplasm of bronchus and lung

Use additional code to identify:
exposure to environmental tobacco smoke (Z77.22)
exposure to tobacco smoke in the perinatal period (P96.81)
history of tobacco dependence (Z87.891)
occupational exposure to environmental tobacco smoke (Z57.31)
tobacco dependence (F17.-)
tobacco use (Z72.0)

Excludes1: Kaposi's sarcoma of lung (C46.5-)
malignant carcinoid tumor of the bronchus and lung (C7A.090)

- C34.0 **Malignant neoplasm of main bronchus**
  Malignant neoplasm of carina
  Malignant neoplasm of hilus (of lung)
  - CC C34.00 Malignant neoplasm of unspecified main bronchus
  - CC C34.01 Malignant neoplasm of right main bronchus
  - CC C34.02 Malignant neoplasm of left main bronchus
- C34.1 **Malignant neoplasm of upper lobe, bronchus or lung**
  - CC C34.10 Malignant neoplasm of upper lobe, unspecified bronchus or lung
  - CC C34.11 Malignant neoplasm of upper lobe, right bronchus or lung
  - CC C34.12 Malignant neoplasm of upper lobe, left bronchus or lung
- CC C34.2 **Malignant neoplasm of middle lobe, bronchus or lung**
- C34.3 **Malignant neoplasm of lower lobe, bronchus or lung**
  - CC C34.30 Malignant neoplasm of lower lobe, unspecified bronchus or lung
  - CC C34.31 Malignant neoplasm of lower lobe, right bronchus or lung
  - CC C34.32 Malignant neoplasm of lower lobe, left bronchus or lung
- C34.8 **Malignant neoplasm of overlapping sites of bronchus and lung**
  - CC C34.80 Malignant neoplasm of overlapping sites of unspecified bronchus and lung
  - CC C34.81 Malignant neoplasm of overlapping sites of right bronchus and lung
  - CC C34.82 Malignant neoplasm of overlapping sites of left bronchus and lung
- C34.9 **Malignant neoplasm of unspecified part of bronchus or lung**
  - CC C34.90 Malignant neoplasm of unspecified part of unspecified bronchus or lung
    Lung cancer NOS
    AHA CC: 2Q, 2014, 10; 4Q, 2022, 22-23
  - CC C34.91 Malignant neoplasm of unspecified part of right bronchus or lung
  - CC C34.92 Malignant neoplasm of unspecified part of left bronchus or lung

CC C37 Malignant neoplasm of thymus

Excludes1: malignant carcinoid tumor of the thymus (C7A.091)
Valid 3-character code, no further characters required

C38 Malignant neoplasm of heart, mediastinum and pleura

Excludes1: mesothelioma (C45.-)
- CC C38.0 **Malignant neoplasm of heart**
  Malignant neoplasm of pericardium
  Excludes1: malignant neoplasm of great vessels (C49.3)
- CC C38.1 Malignant neoplasm of anterior mediastinum
- CC C38.2 Malignant neoplasm of posterior mediastinum
- CC C38.3 Malignant neoplasm of mediastinum, part unspecified
- CC C38.4 Malignant neoplasm of pleura
- CC C38.8 Malignant neoplasm of overlapping sites of heart, mediastinum and pleura

C39 Malignant neoplasm of other and ill-defined sites in the respiratory system and intrathoracic organs

Use additional code to identify:
exposure to environmental tobacco smoke (Z77.22)
exposure to tobacco smoke in the perinatal period (P96.81)
history of tobacco dependence (Z87.891)
occupational exposure to environmental tobacco smoke (Z57.31)
tobacco dependence (F17.-)
tobacco use (Z72.0)

Excludes1: intrathoracic malignant neoplasm NOS (C76.1)
thoracic malignant neoplasm NOS (C76.1)

- C39.0 **Malignant neoplasm of upper respiratory tract, part unspecified**
- C39.9 **Malignant neoplasm of lower respiratory tract, part unspecified**
  Malignant neoplasm of respiratory tract NOS

Malignant neoplasms of bone and articular cartilage (C40-C41)

Includes: malignant neoplasm of cartilage (articular) (joint)
malignant neoplasm of periosteum

Excludes1: malignant neoplasm of bone marrow NOS (C96.9)
malignant neoplasm of synovia (C49.-)

C40 Malignant neoplasm of bone and articular cartilage of limbs

Use additional code to identify major osseous defect, if applicable (M89.7-)

- C40.0 **Malignant neoplasm of scapula and long bones of upper limb**
  - CC C40.00 Malignant neoplasm of scapula and long bones of unspecified upper limb
  - CC C40.01 Malignant neoplasm of scapula and long bones of right upper limb
  - CC C40.02 Malignant neoplasm of scapula and long bones of left upper limb
- C40.1 **Malignant neoplasm of short bones of upper limb**
  - CC C40.10 Malignant neoplasm of short bones of unspecified upper limb
  - CC C40.11 Malignant neoplasm of short bones of right upper limb
  - CC C40.12 Malignant neoplasm of short bones of left upper limb
- C40.2 **Malignant neoplasm of long bones of lower limb**
  - CC C40.20 Malignant neoplasm of long bones of unspecified lower limb
  - CC C40.21 Malignant neoplasm of long bones of right lower limb
  - CC C40.22 Malignant neoplasm of long bones of left lower limb
- C40.3 **Malignant neoplasm of short bones of lower limb**
  - CC C40.30 Malignant neoplasm of short bones of unspecified lower limb
  - CC C40.31 Malignant neoplasm of short bones of right lower limb
  - CC C40.32 Malignant neoplasm of short bones of left lower limb
- C40.8 **Malignant neoplasm of overlapping sites of bone and articular cartilage of limb**
  - CC C40.80 Malignant neoplasm of overlapping sites of bone and articular cartilage of unspecified limb
  - CC C40.81 Malignant neoplasm of overlapping sites of bone and articular cartilage of right limb
  - CC C40.82 Malignant neoplasm of overlapping sites of bone and articular cartilage of left limb
- C40.9 **Malignant neoplasm of unspecified bones and articular cartilage of limb**
  - CC C40.90 Malignant neoplasm of unspecified bones and articular cartilage of unspecified limb
  - CC C40.91 Malignant neoplasm of unspecified bones and articular cartilage of right limb
  - CC C40.92 Malignant neoplasm of unspecified bones and articular cartilage of left limb

C41 Malignant neoplasm of bone and articular cartilage of other and unspecified sites

Excludes1: malignant neoplasm of bones of limbs (C40.-)
malignant neoplasm of cartilage of ear (C49.0)
malignant neoplasm of cartilage of eyelid (C49.0)
malignant neoplasm of cartilage of larynx (C32.3)
malignant neoplasm of cartilage of limbs (C40.-)
malignant neoplasm of cartilage of nose (C30.0)

- CC C41.0 **Malignant neoplasm of bones of skull and face**
  Malignant neoplasm of maxilla (superior)
  Malignant neoplasm of orbital bone
  Excludes2: carcinoma, any type except intraosseous or odontogenic of:
  maxillary sinus (C31.0)
  upper jaw (C03.0)
  malignant neoplasm of jaw bone (lower) (C41.1)
- CC C41.1 **Malignant neoplasm of mandible**
  Malignant neoplasm of inferior maxilla
  Malignant neoplasm of lower jaw bone
  Excludes2: carcinoma, any type except intraosseous or odontogenic of:
  jaw NOS (C03.9)
  lower (C03.1)
  malignant neoplasm of upper jaw bone (C41.0)

CC **C41.2** Malignant neoplasm of vertebral column
Excludes1: malignant neoplasm of sacrum and coccyx (C41.4)
CC **C41.3** Malignant neoplasm of ribs, sternum and clavicle
CC **C41.4** Malignant neoplasm of pelvic bones, sacrum and coccyx
CC **C41.9** Malignant neoplasm of bone and articular cartilage, unspecified

Melanoma and other malignant neoplasms of skin (C43-C44)

C43 Malignant melanoma of skin
Excludes1: melanoma in situ (D03.-)
Excludes2: malignant melanoma of skin of genital organs (C51-C52, C60.-, C63.-)
Merkel cell carcinoma (C4A.-)
sites other than skin-code to malignant neoplasm of the site

C43.0 Malignant melanoma of lip
Excludes1: malignant neoplasm of vermilion border of lip (C00.0-C00.2)

+ **C43.1** Malignant melanoma of eyelid, including canthus
C43.10 Malignant melanoma of unspecified eyelid, including canthus
+ **C43.11** Malignant melanoma of right eyelid, including canthus
C43.111 Malignant melanoma of right upper eyelid, including canthus
C43.112 Malignant melanoma of right lower eyelid, including canthus
+ **C43.12** Malignant melanoma of left eyelid, including canthus
C43.121 Malignant melanoma of left upper eyelid, including canthus
C43.122 Malignant melanoma of left lower eyelid, including canthus

+ **C43.2** Malignant melanoma of ear and external auricular canal
C43.20 Malignant melanoma of unspecified ear and external auricular canal
C43.21 Malignant melanoma of right ear and external auricular canal
C43.22 Malignant melanoma of left ear and external auricular canal

+ **C43.3** Malignant melanoma of other and unspecified parts of face
C43.30 Malignant melanoma of unspecified part of face
C43.31 Malignant melanoma of nose
C43.39 Malignant melanoma of other parts of face

C43.4 Malignant melanoma of scalp and neck
+ **C43.5** Malignant melanoma of trunk
Excludes2: malignant neoplasm of anus NOS (C21.0)
malignant neoplasm of scrotum (C63.2)
C43.51 Malignant melanoma of anal skin
Malignant melanoma of anal margin
Malignant melanoma of perianal skin
C43.52 Malignant melanoma of skin of breast
C43.59 Malignant melanoma of other part of trunk

+ **C43.6** Malignant melanoma of upper limb, including shoulder
C43.60 Malignant melanoma of unspecified upper limb, including shoulder
C43.61 Malignant melanoma of right upper limb, including shoulder
C43.62 Malignant melanoma of left upper limb, including shoulder

+ **C43.7** Malignant melanoma of lower limb, including hip
C43.70 Malignant melanoma of unspecified lower limb, including hip
C43.71 Malignant melanoma of right lower limb, including hip
C43.72 Malignant melanoma of left lower limb, including hip

C43.8 Malignant melanoma of overlapping sites of skin
C43.9 Malignant melanoma of skin, unspecified
Malignant melanoma of unspecified site of skin
Melanoma (malignant) NOS

C4A Merkel cell carcinoma
C4A.0 Merkel cell carcinoma of lip
Excludes1: malignant neoplasm of vermilion border of lip (C00.0-C00.2)

+ **C4A.1** Merkel cell carcinoma of eyelid, including canthus
C4A.10 Merkel cell carcinoma of unspecified eyelid, including canthus
+ **C4A.11** Merkel cell carcinoma of right eyelid, including canthus
C4A.111 Merkel cell carcinoma of right upper eyelid, including canthus
C4A.112 Merkel cell carcinoma of right lower eyelid, including canthus
+ **C4A.12** Merkel cell carcinoma of left eyelid, including canthus
C4A.121 Merkel cell carcinoma of left upper eyelid, including canthus
C4A.122 Merkel cell carcinoma of left lower eyelid, including canthus

+ **C4A.2** Merkel cell carcinoma of ear and external auricular canal
C4A.20 Merkel cell carcinoma of unspecified ear and external auricular canal
C4A.21 Merkel cell carcinoma of right ear and external auricular canal
C4A.22 Merkel cell carcinoma of left ear and external auricular canal

+ **C4A.3** Merkel cell carcinoma of other and unspecified parts of face
C4A.30 Merkel cell carcinoma of unspecified part of face
C4A.31 Merkel cell carcinoma of nose
C4A.39 Merkel cell carcinoma of other parts of face

C4A.4 Merkel cell carcinoma of scalp and neck
+ **C4A.5** Merkel cell carcinoma of trunk
Excludes2: malignant neoplasm of anus NOS (C21.0)
malignant neoplasm of scrotum (C63.2)
C4A.51 Merkel cell carcinoma of anal skin
Merkel cell carcinoma of anal margin
Merkel cell carcinoma of perianal skin
C4A.52 Merkel cell carcinoma of skin of breast
C4A.59 Merkel cell carcinoma of other part of trunk

+ **C4A.6** Merkel cell carcinoma of upper limb, including shoulder
C4A.60 Merkel cell carcinoma of unspecified upper limb, including shoulder
C4A.61 Merkel cell carcinoma of right upper limb, including shoulder
C4A.62 Merkel cell carcinoma of left upper limb, including shoulder

+ **C4A.7** Merkel cell carcinoma of lower limb, including hip
C4A.70 Merkel cell carcinoma of unspecified lower limb, including hip
C4A.71 Merkel cell carcinoma of right lower limb, including hip
C4A.72 Merkel cell carcinoma of left lower limb, including hip

C4A.8 Merkel cell carcinoma of overlapping sites
C4A.9 Merkel cell carcinoma, unspecified
Merkel cell carcinoma of unspecified site
Merkel cell carcinoma NOS

C44 Other and unspecified malignant neoplasm of skin
Includes: malignant neoplasm of sebaceous glands
malignant neoplasm of sweat glands
Excludes1: Kaposi's sarcoma of skin (C46.0)
malignant melanoma of skin (C43.-)
malignant neoplasm of skin of genital organs (C51-C52, C60.-, C63.2)
Merkel cell carcinoma (C4A.-)

+ **C44.0** Other and unspecified malignant neoplasm of skin of lip
Excludes1: malignant neoplasm of lip (C00.-)
C44.00 Unspecified malignant neoplasm of skin of lip
C44.01 Basal cell carcinoma of skin of lip
C44.02 Squamous cell carcinoma of skin of lip
C44.09 Other specified malignant neoplasm of skin of lip

- **C44.1** Other and unspecified malignant neoplasm of skin of eyelid, including canthus
  Excludes1: connective tissue of eyelid (C49.0)
  - **C44.10** Unspecified malignant neoplasm of skin of eyelid, including canthus
    - C44.101 Unspecified malignant neoplasm of skin of unspecified eyelid, including canthus
    - C44.102 Unspecified malignant neoplasm of skin of right eyelid, including canthus
      - C44.1021 Unspecified malignant neoplasm of skin of right upper eyelid, including canthus
      - C44.1022 Unspecified malignant neoplasm of skin of right lower eyelid, including canthus
    - C44.109 Unspecified malignant neoplasm of skin of left eyelid, including canthus
      - C44.1091 Unspecified malignant neoplasm of skin of left upper eyelid, including canthus
      - C44.1092 Unspecified malignant neoplasm of skin of left lower eyelid, including canthus
  - **C44.11** Basal cell carcinoma of skin of eyelid, including canthus
    - C44.111 Basal cell carcinoma of skin of unspecified eyelid, including canthus
    - C44.112 Basal cell carcinoma of skin of right eyelid, including canthus
      - C44.1121 Basal cell carcinoma of skin of right upper eyelid, including canthus
      - C44.1122 Basal cell carcinoma of skin of right lower eyelid, including canthus
    - C44.119 Basal cell carcinoma of skin of left eyelid, including canthus
      - C44.1191 Basal cell carcinoma of skin of left upper eyelid, including canthus
      - C44.1192 Basal cell carcinoma of skin of left lower eyelid, including canthus
  - **C44.12** Squamous cell carcinoma of skin of eyelid, including canthus
    - C44.121 Squamous cell carcinoma of skin of unspecified eyelid, including canthus
    - C44.122 Squamous cell carcinoma of skin of right eyelid, including canthus
      - C44.1221 Squamous cell carcinoma of skin of right upper eyelid, including canthus
      - C44.1222 Squamous cell carcinoma of skin of right lower eyelid, including canthus
    - C44.129 Squamous cell carcinoma of skin of left eyelid, including canthus
      - C44.1291 Squamous cell carcinoma of skin of left upper eyelid, including canthus
      - C44.1292 Squamous cell carcinoma of skin of left lower eyelid, including canthus
  - **C44.13** Sebaceous cell carcinoma of skin of eyelid, including canthus
    - C44.131 Sebaceous cell carcinoma of skin of unspecified eyelid, including canthus
    - C44.132 Sebaceous cell carcinoma of skin of right eyelid, including canthus
      - C44.1321 Sebaceous cell carcinoma of skin of right upper eyelid, including canthus
      - C44.1322 Sebaceous cell carcinoma of skin of right lower eyelid, including canthus
    - C44.139 Sebaceous cell carcinoma of skin of left eyelid, including canthus
      - C44.1391 Sebaceous cell carcinoma of skin of left upper eyelid, including canthus
      - C44.1392 Sebaceous cell carcinoma of skin of left lower eyelid, including canthus
  - **C44.19** Other specified malignant neoplasm of skin of eyelid, including canthus
    - C44.191 Other specified malignant neoplasm of skin of unspecified eyelid, including canthus
    - C44.192 Other specified malignant neoplasm of skin of right eyelid, including canthus
      - C44.1921 Other specified malignant neoplasm of skin of right upper eyelid, including canthus
      - C44.1922 Other specified malignant neoplasm of skin of right lower eyelid, including canthus
    - C44.199 Other specified malignant neoplasm of skin of left eyelid, including canthus
      - C44.1991 Other specified malignant neoplasm of skin of left upper eyelid, including canthus
      - C44.1992 Other specified malignant neoplasm of skin of left lower eyelid, including canthus
- **C44.2** Other and unspecified malignant neoplasm of skin of ear and external auricular canal
  Excludes1: connective tissue of ear (C49.0)
  - **C44.20** Unspecified malignant neoplasm of skin of ear and external auricular canal
    - C44.201 Unspecified malignant neoplasm of skin of unspecified ear and external auricular canal
    - C44.202 Unspecified malignant neoplasm of skin of right ear and external auricular canal
    - C44.209 Unspecified malignant neoplasm of skin of left ear and external auricular canal
  - **C44.21** Basal cell carcinoma of skin of ear and external auricular canal
    - C44.211 Basal cell carcinoma of skin of unspecified ear and external auricular canal
    - C44.212 Basal cell carcinoma of skin of right ear and external auricular canal
    - C44.219 Basal cell carcinoma of skin of left ear and external auricular canal
  - **C44.22** Squamous cell carcinoma of skin of ear and external auricular canal
    - C44.221 Squamous cell carcinoma of skin of unspecified ear and external auricular canal
    - C44.222 Squamous cell carcinoma of skin of right ear and external auricular canal
    - C44.229 Squamous cell carcinoma of skin of left ear and external auricular canal

- **C44.29** Other specified malignant neoplasm of skin of ear and external auricular canal
  - C44.291 Other specified malignant neoplasm of skin of unspecified ear and external auricular canal
  - C44.292 Other specified malignant neoplasm of skin of right ear and external auricular canal
  - C44.299 Other specified malignant neoplasm of skin of left ear and external auricular canal
- **C44.3** Other and unspecified malignant neoplasm of skin of other and unspecified parts of face
  - **C44.30** Unspecified malignant neoplasm of skin of other and unspecified parts of face
    - C44.300 Unspecified malignant neoplasm of skin of unspecified part of face
    - C44.301 Unspecified malignant neoplasm of skin of nose
    - C44.309 Unspecified malignant neoplasm of skin of other parts of face
  - **C44.31** Basal cell carcinoma of skin of other and unspecified parts of face
    - C44.310 Basal cell carcinoma of skin of unspecified parts of face
    - C44.311 Basal cell carcinoma of skin of nose
    - C44.319 Basal cell carcinoma of skin of other parts of face
      - *AHA CC: 1Q, 2017, 4*
  - **C44.32** Squamous cell carcinoma of skin of other and unspecified parts of face
    - C44.320 Squamous cell carcinoma of skin of unspecified parts of face
    - C44.321 Squamous cell carcinoma of skin of nose
    - C44.329 Squamous cell carcinoma of skin of other parts of face
  - **C44.39** Other specified malignant neoplasm of skin of other and unspecified parts of face
    - C44.390 Other specified malignant neoplasm of skin of unspecified parts of face
    - C44.391 Other specified malignant neoplasm of skin of nose
    - C44.399 Other specified malignant neoplasm of skin of other parts of face
- **C44.4** Other and unspecified malignant neoplasm of skin of scalp and neck
  - C44.40 Unspecified malignant neoplasm of skin of scalp and neck
  - C44.41 Basal cell carcinoma of skin of scalp and neck
  - C44.42 Squamous cell carcinoma of skin of scalp and neck
  - C44.49 Other specified malignant neoplasm of skin of scalp and neck
- **C44.5** Other and unspecified malignant neoplasm of skin of trunk
  - **Excludes1:** anus NOS (C21.0)
    scrotum (C63.2)
  - **C44.50** Unspecified malignant neoplasm of skin of trunk
    - C44.500 Unspecified malignant neoplasm of anal skin
      Unspecified malignant neoplasm of anal margin
      Unspecified malignant neoplasm of perianal skin
    - C44.501 Unspecified malignant neoplasm of skin of breast
    - C44.509 Unspecified malignant neoplasm of skin of other part of trunk
  - **C44.51** Basal cell carcinoma of skin of trunk
    - C44.510 Basal cell carcinoma of anal skin
      Basal cell carcinoma of anal margin
      Basal cell carcinoma of perianal skin
    - C44.511 Basal cell carcinoma of skin of breast
    - C44.519 Basal cell carcinoma of skin of other part of trunk
  - **C44.52** Squamous cell carcinoma of skin of trunk
    - C44.520 Squamous cell carcinoma of anal skin
      Squamous cell carcinoma of anal margin
      Squamous cell carcinoma of perianal skin
    - C44.521 Squamous cell carcinoma of skin of breast
    - C44.529 Squamous cell carcinoma of skin of other part of trunk
  - **C44.59** Other specified malignant neoplasm of skin of trunk
    - C44.590 Other specified malignant neoplasm of anal skin
      Other specified malignant neoplasm of anal margin
      Other specified malignant neoplasm of perianal skin
    - C44.591 Other specified malignant neoplasm of skin of breast
    - C44.599 Other specified malignant neoplasm of skin of other part of trunk
- **C44.6** Other and unspecified malignant neoplasm of skin of upper limb, including shoulder
  - **C44.60** Unspecified malignant neoplasm of skin of upper limb, including shoulder
    - C44.601 Unspecified malignant neoplasm of skin of unspecified upper limb, including shoulder
    - C44.602 Unspecified malignant neoplasm of skin of right upper limb, including shoulder
    - C44.609 Unspecified malignant neoplasm of skin of left upper limb, including shoulder
  - **C44.61** Basal cell carcinoma of skin of upper limb, including shoulder
    - C44.611 Basal cell carcinoma of skin of unspecified upper limb, including shoulder
    - C44.612 Basal cell carcinoma of skin of right upper limb, including shoulder
    - C44.619 Basal cell carcinoma of skin of left upper limb, including shoulder
  - **C44.62** Squamous cell carcinoma of skin of upper limb, including shoulder
    - C44.621 Squamous cell carcinoma of skin of unspecified upper limb, including shoulder
    - C44.622 Squamous cell carcinoma of skin of right upper limb, including shoulder
    - C44.629 Squamous cell carcinoma of skin of left upper limb, including shoulder
  - **C44.69** Other specified malignant neoplasm of skin of upper limb, including shoulder
    - C44.691 Other specified malignant neoplasm of skin of unspecified upper limb, including shoulder
    - C44.692 Other specified malignant neoplasm of skin of right upper limb, including shoulder
    - C44.699 Other specified malignant neoplasm of skin of left upper limb, including shoulder
- **C44.7** Other and unspecified malignant neoplasm of skin of lower limb, including hip
  - **C44.70** Unspecified malignant neoplasm of skin of lower limb, including hip
    - C44.701 Unspecified malignant neoplasm of skin of unspecified lower limb, including hip
    - C44.702 Unspecified malignant neoplasm of skin of right lower limb, including hip
    - C44.709 Unspecified malignant neoplasm of skin of left lower limb, including hip
  - **C44.71** Basal cell carcinoma of skin of lower limb, including hip
    - C44.711 Basal cell carcinoma of skin of unspecified lower limb, including hip
    - C44.712 Basal cell carcinoma of skin of right lower limb, including hip
    - C44.719 Basal cell carcinoma of skin of left lower limb, including hip

- **+ C44.72** Squamous cell carcinoma of skin of lower limb, including hip
  - **C44.721** Squamous cell carcinoma of skin of unspecified lower limb, including hip
  - **C44.722** Squamous cell carcinoma of skin of right lower limb, including hip
  - **C44.729** Squamous cell carcinoma of skin of left lower limb, including hip
- **+ C44.79** Other specified malignant neoplasm of skin of lower limb, including hip
  - **C44.791** Other specified malignant neoplasm of skin of unspecified lower limb, including hip
  - **C44.792** Other specified malignant neoplasm of skin of right lower limb, including hip
  - **C44.799** Other specified malignant neoplasm of skin of left lower limb, including hip
- **+ C44.8** Other and unspecified malignant neoplasm of overlapping sites of skin
  - **C44.80** Unspecified malignant neoplasm of overlapping sites of skin
  - **C44.81** Basal cell carcinoma of overlapping sites of skin
  - **C44.82** Squamous cell carcinoma of overlapping sites of skin
  - **C44.89** Other specified malignant neoplasm of overlapping sites of skin
- **+ C44.9** Other and unspecified malignant neoplasm of skin, unspecified
  - **C44.90** Unspecified malignant neoplasm of skin, unspecified
    - Malignant neoplasm of unspecified site of skin
  - **C44.91** Basal cell carcinoma of skin, unspecified
  - **C44.92** Squamous cell carcinoma of skin, unspecified
  - **C44.99** Other specified malignant neoplasm of skin, unspecified

Malignant neoplasms of mesothelial and soft tissue (C45-C49)

C45 Mesothelioma
- CC **C45.0** Mesothelioma of pleura
  - *Excludes1:* other malignant neoplasm of pleura (C38.4)
  - AHA CC: 2Q, 2017, 11
- CC **C45.1** Mesothelioma of peritoneum
  - Mesothelioma of cul-de-sac
  - Mesothelioma of mesentery
  - Mesothelioma of mesocolon
  - Mesothelioma of omentum
  - Mesothelioma of peritoneum (parietal) (pelvic)
  - *Excludes1:* other malignant neoplasm of soft tissue of peritoneum (C48.-)
- CC **C45.2** Mesothelioma of pericardium
  - *Excludes1:* other malignant neoplasm of pericardium (C38.0)
- **C45.7** Mesothelioma of other sites
- **C45.9** Mesothelioma, unspecified

C46 Kaposi's sarcoma
- Code first any human immunodeficiency virus [HIV] disease (B20)
- CC **C46.0** Kaposi's sarcoma of skin
- CC **C46.1** Kaposi's sarcoma of soft tissue
  - Kaposi's sarcoma of blood vessel
  - Kaposi's sarcoma of connective tissue
  - Kaposi's sarcoma of fascia
  - Kaposi's sarcoma of ligament
  - Kaposi's sarcoma of lymphatic(s) NEC
  - Kaposi's sarcoma of muscle
  - *Excludes2:* Kaposi's sarcoma of lymph glands and nodes (C46.3)
- CC **C46.2** Kaposi's sarcoma of palate
- CC **C46.3** Kaposi's sarcoma of lymph nodes
- CC **C46.4** Kaposi's sarcoma of gastrointestinal sites
- **+ C46.5** Kaposi's sarcoma of lung
  - CC **C46.50** Kaposi's sarcoma of unspecified lung
  - CC **C46.51** Kaposi's sarcoma of right lung
  - CC **C46.52** Kaposi's sarcoma of left lung
- CC **C46.7** Kaposi's sarcoma of other sites
- CC **C46.9** Kaposi's sarcoma, unspecified
  - Kaposi's sarcoma of unspecified site

C47 Malignant neoplasm of peripheral nerves and autonomic nervous system
- *Includes:* malignant neoplasm of sympathetic and parasympathetic nerves and ganglia
- *Excludes1:* Kaposi's sarcoma of soft tissue (C46.1)
- CC **C47.0** Malignant neoplasm of peripheral nerves of head, face and neck
  - *Excludes1:* malignant neoplasm of peripheral nerves of orbit (C69.6-)
- **+ C47.1** Malignant neoplasm of peripheral nerves of upper limb, including shoulder
  - CC **C47.10** Malignant neoplasm of peripheral nerves of unspecified upper limb, including shoulder
  - CC **C47.11** Malignant neoplasm of peripheral nerves of right upper limb, including shoulder
  - CC **C47.12** Malignant neoplasm of peripheral nerves of left upper limb, including shoulder
- **+ C47.2** Malignant neoplasm of peripheral nerves of lower limb, including hip
  - CC **C47.20** Malignant neoplasm of peripheral nerves of unspecified lower limb, including hip
  - CC **C47.21** Malignant neoplasm of peripheral nerves of right lower limb, including hip
  - CC **C47.22** Malignant neoplasm of peripheral nerves of left lower limb, including hip
- CC **C47.3** Malignant neoplasm of peripheral nerves of thorax
- CC **C47.4** Malignant neoplasm of peripheral nerves of abdomen
- CC **C47.5** Malignant neoplasm of peripheral nerves of pelvis
- CC **C47.6** Malignant neoplasm of peripheral nerves of trunk, unspecified
  - Malignant neoplasm of peripheral nerves of unspecified part of trunk
- CC **C47.8** Malignant neoplasm of overlapping sites of peripheral nerves and autonomic nervous system
- CC **C47.9** Malignant neoplasm of peripheral nerves and autonomic nervous system, unspecified
  - Malignant neoplasm of unspecified site of peripheral nerves and autonomic nervous system

C48 Malignant neoplasm of retroperitoneum and peritoneum
- *Excludes1:* Kaposi's sarcoma of connective tissue (C46.1)
  - mesothelioma (C45.-)
- CC **C48.0** Malignant neoplasm of retroperitoneum
- CC **C48.1** Malignant neoplasm of specified parts of peritoneum
  - Malignant neoplasm of cul-de-sac
  - Malignant neoplasm of mesentery
  - Malignant neoplasm of mesocolon
  - Malignant neoplasm of omentum
  - Malignant neoplasm of parietal peritoneum
  - Malignant neoplasm of pelvic peritoneum
- CC **C48.2** Malignant neoplasm of peritoneum, unspecified
- CC **C48.8** Malignant neoplasm of overlapping sites of retroperitoneum and peritoneum

C49 Malignant neoplasm of other connective and soft tissue
- *Includes:* malignant neoplasm of blood vessel
  - malignant neoplasm of bursa
  - malignant neoplasm of cartilage
  - malignant neoplasm of fascia
  - malignant neoplasm of fat
  - malignant neoplasm of ligament, except uterine
  - malignant neoplasm of lymphatic vessel
  - malignant neoplasm of muscle
  - malignant neoplasm of synovia
  - malignant neoplasm of tendon (sheath)
- *Excludes1:* malignant neoplasm of cartilage (of):
  - articular (C40-C41)
  - larynx (C32.3)
  - nose (C30.0)
  - malignant neoplasm of connective tissue of breast (C50.-)
- *Excludes2:* Kaposi's sarcoma of soft tissue (C46.1)
  - malignant neoplasm of heart (C38.0)
  - malignant neoplasm of peripheral nerves and autonomic nervous system (C47.-)
  - malignant neoplasm of peritoneum (C48.2)
  - malignant neoplasm of retroperitoneum (C48.0)
  - malignant neoplasm of uterine ligament (C57.3)
  - mesothelioma (C45.-)

CC C49.0 Malignant neoplasm of connective and soft tissue of head, face and neck
    Malignant neoplasm of connective tissue of ear
    Malignant neoplasm of connective tissue of eyelid
    Excludes1: connective tissue of orbit (C69.6-)

+ **C49.1** Malignant neoplasm of connective and soft tissue of upper limb, including shoulder
    CC C49.10 Malignant neoplasm of connective and soft tissue of unspecified upper limb, including shoulder
    CC C49.11 Malignant neoplasm of connective and soft tissue of right upper limb, including shoulder
    CC C49.12 Malignant neoplasm of connective and soft tissue of left upper limb, including shoulder

+ **C49.2** Malignant neoplasm of connective and soft tissue of lower limb, including hip
    CC C49.20 Malignant neoplasm of connective and soft tissue of unspecified lower limb, including hip
    CC C49.21 Malignant neoplasm of connective and soft tissue of right lower limb, including hip
    CC C49.22 Malignant neoplasm of connective and soft tissue of left lower limb, including hip

CC C49.3 Malignant neoplasm of connective and soft tissue of thorax
    Malignant neoplasm of axilla
    Malignant neoplasm of diaphragm
    Malignant neoplasm of great vessels
    Excludes1: malignant neoplasm of breast (C50.-)
        malignant neoplasm of heart (C38.0)
        malignant neoplasm of mediastinum (C38.1-C38.3)
        malignant neoplasm of thymus (C37)
    AHA CC: 3Q, 2015, 19-20

CC C49.4 Malignant neoplasm of connective and soft tissue of abdomen
    Malignant neoplasm of abdominal wall
    Malignant neoplasm of hypochondrium

CC C49.5 Malignant neoplasm of connective and soft tissue of pelvis
    Malignant neoplasm of buttock
    Malignant neoplasm of groin
    Malignant neoplasm of perineum

CC C49.6 Malignant neoplasm of connective and soft tissue of trunk, unspecified
    Malignant neoplasm of back NOS

CC C49.8 Malignant neoplasm of overlapping sites of connective and soft tissue
    Primary malignant neoplasm of two or more contiguous sites of connective and soft tissue

CC C49.9 Malignant neoplasm of connective and soft tissue, unspecified

+ **C49.A** Gastrointestinal stromal tumor
    AHA CC: 4Q, 2016, 8
    CC C49.A0 Gastrointestinal stromal tumor, unspecified site
    CC C49.A1 Gastrointestinal stromal tumor of esophagus
    CC C49.A2 Gastrointestinal stromal tumor of stomach
    CC C49.A3 Gastrointestinal stromal tumor of small intestine
    CC C49.A4 Gastrointestinal stromal tumor of large intestine
    CC C49.A5 Gastrointestinal stromal tumor of rectum
    CC C49.A9 Gastrointestinal stromal tumor of other sites

Malignant neoplasms of breast (C50)

C50 Malignant neoplasm of breast
    Includes: connective tissue of breast
        Paget's disease of breast
        Paget's disease of nipple
    Use additional code to identify estrogen receptor status (Z17.0, Z17.1)
    Excludes1: skin of breast (C44.501, C44.511, C44.521, C44.591)

+ **C50.0** Malignant neoplasm of nipple and areola
    + **C50.01** Malignant neoplasm of nipple and areola, female
        ♀ **C50.011** Malignant neoplasm of nipple and areola, right female breast
        ♀ **C50.012** Malignant neoplasm of nipple and areola, left female breast
        ♀ **C50.019** Malignant neoplasm of nipple and areola, unspecified female breast
    + **C50.02** Malignant neoplasm of nipple and areola, male
        ♂ **C50.021** Malignant neoplasm of nipple and areola, right male breast
        ♂ **C50.022** Malignant neoplasm of nipple and areola, left male breast
        ♂ **C50.029** Malignant neoplasm of nipple and areola, unspecified male breast

+ **C50.1** Malignant neoplasm of central portion of breast
    + **C50.11** Malignant neoplasm of central portion of breast, female
        ♀ **C50.111** Malignant neoplasm of central portion of right female breast
        ♀ **C50.112** Malignant neoplasm of central portion of left female breast
        ♀ **C50.119** Malignant neoplasm of central portion of unspecified female breast
    + **C50.12** Malignant neoplasm of central portion of breast, male
        ♂ **C50.121** Malignant neoplasm of central portion of right male breast
        ♂ **C50.122** Malignant neoplasm of central portion of left male breast
        ♂ **C50.129** Malignant neoplasm of central portion of unspecified male breast

+ **C50.2** Malignant neoplasm of upper-inner quadrant of breast
    + **C50.21** Malignant neoplasm of upper-inner quadrant of breast, female
        ♀ **C50.211** Malignant neoplasm of upper-inner quadrant of right female breast
        ♀ **C50.212** Malignant neoplasm of upper-inner quadrant of left female breast
        ♀ **C50.219** Malignant neoplasm of upper-inner quadrant of unspecified female breast
    + **C50.22** Malignant neoplasm of upper-inner quadrant of breast, male
        ♂ **C50.221** Malignant neoplasm of upper-inner quadrant of right male breast
        ♂ **C50.222** Malignant neoplasm of upper-inner quadrant of left male breast
        ♂ **C50.229** Malignant neoplasm of upper-inner quadrant of unspecified male breast

+ **C50.3** Malignant neoplasm of lower-inner quadrant of breast
    + **C50.31** Malignant neoplasm of lower-inner quadrant of breast, female
        ♀ **C50.311** Malignant neoplasm of lower-inner quadrant of right female breast
        ♀ **C50.312** Malignant neoplasm of lower-inner quadrant of left female breast
        ♀ **C50.319** Malignant neoplasm of lower-inner quadrant of unspecified female breast
    + **C50.32** Malignant neoplasm of lower-inner quadrant of breast, male
        ♂ **C50.321** Malignant neoplasm of lower-inner quadrant of right male breast
        ♂ **C50.322** Malignant neoplasm of lower-inner quadrant of left male breast
        ♂ **C50.329** Malignant neoplasm of lower-inner quadrant of unspecified male breast

+ **C50.4** Malignant neoplasm of upper-outer quadrant of breast
    + **C50.41** Malignant neoplasm of upper-outer quadrant of breast, female
        ♀ **C50.411** Malignant neoplasm of upper-outer quadrant of right female breast
        ♀ **C50.412** Malignant neoplasm of upper-outer quadrant of left female breast
        ♀ **C50.419** Malignant neoplasm of upper-outer quadrant of unspecified female breast
    + **C50.42** Malignant neoplasm of upper-outer quadrant of breast, male
        ♂ **C50.421** Malignant neoplasm of upper-outer quadrant of right male breast
        ♂ **C50.422** Malignant neoplasm of upper-outer quadrant of left male breast
        ♂ **C50.429** Malignant neoplasm of upper-outer quadrant of unspecified male breast

- **C50.5 Malignant neoplasm of lower-outer quadrant of breast**
  - **C50.51 Malignant neoplasm of lower-outer quadrant of breast, female**
    - ♀ **C50.511** Malignant neoplasm of lower-outer quadrant of right female breast
    - ♀ **C50.512** Malignant neoplasm of lower-outer quadrant of left female breast
    - ♀ **C50.519** Malignant neoplasm of lower-outer quadrant of unspecified female breast
  - **C50.52 Malignant neoplasm of lower-outer quadrant of breast, male**
    - ♂ **C50.521** Malignant neoplasm of lower-outer quadrant of right male breast
    - ♂ **C50.522** Malignant neoplasm of lower-outer quadrant of left male breast
    - ♂ **C50.529** Malignant neoplasm of lower-outer quadrant of unspecified male breast
- **C50.6 Malignant neoplasm of axillary tail of breast**
  - **C50.61 Malignant neoplasm of axillary tail of breast, female**
    - ♀ **C50.611** Malignant neoplasm of axillary tail of right female breast
    - ♀ **C50.612** Malignant neoplasm of axillary tail of left female breast
    - ♀ **C50.619** Malignant neoplasm of axillary tail of unspecified female breast
  - **C50.62 Malignant neoplasm of axillary tail of breast, male**
    - ♂ **C50.621** Malignant neoplasm of axillary tail of right male breast
    - ♂ **C50.622** Malignant neoplasm of axillary tail of left male breast
    - ♂ **C50.629** Malignant neoplasm of axillary tail of unspecified male breast
- **C50.8 Malignant neoplasm of overlapping sites of breast**
  - **C50.81 Malignant neoplasm of overlapping sites of breast, female**
    - ♀ **C50.811** Malignant neoplasm of overlapping sites of right female breast
    - ♀ **C50.812** Malignant neoplasm of overlapping sites of left female breast
    - ♀ **C50.819** Malignant neoplasm of overlapping sites of unspecified female breast
  - **C50.82 Malignant neoplasm of overlapping sites of breast, male**
    - ♂ **C50.821** Malignant neoplasm of overlapping sites of right male breast
    - ♂ **C50.822** Malignant neoplasm of overlapping sites of left male breast
    - ♂ **C50.829** Malignant neoplasm of overlapping sites of unspecified male breast
- **C50.9 Malignant neoplasm of breast of unspecified site**
  - **C50.91 Malignant neoplasm of breast of unspecified site, female**
    - ♀ **C50.911** Malignant neoplasm of unspecified site of right female breast
    - ♀ **C50.912** Malignant neoplasm of unspecified site of left female breast
      AHA CC: 3Q, 2022, 11, 14-15
    - ♀ **C50.919** Malignant neoplasm of unspecified site of unspecified female breast
  - **C50.92 Malignant neoplasm of breast of unspecified site, male**
    - ♂ **C50.921** Malignant neoplasm of unspecified site of right male breast
    - ♂ **C50.922** Malignant neoplasm of unspecified site of left male breast
    - ♂ **C50.929** Malignant neoplasm of unspecified site of unspecified male breast

Malignant neoplasms of female genital organs (C51-C58)

Includes: malignant neoplasm of skin of female genital organs

C51 Malignant neoplasm of vulva
Excludes1: carcinoma in situ of vulva (D07.1)
- ♀ **C51.0** Malignant neoplasm of labium majus
  Malignant neoplasm of Bartholin's [greater vestibular] gland
- ♀ **C51.1** Malignant neoplasm of labium minus
- ♀ **C51.2** Malignant neoplasm of clitoris
- ♀ **C51.8** Malignant neoplasm of overlapping sites of vulva
- ♀ **C51.9** Malignant neoplasm of vulva, unspecified
  Malignant neoplasm of external female genitalia NOS
  Malignant neoplasm of pudendum

♀ C52 Malignant neoplasm of vagina
Excludes1: carcinoma in situ of vagina (D07.2)
Valid 3-character code, no further characters required

C53 Malignant neoplasm of cervix uteri
Excludes1: carcinoma in situ of cervix uteri (D06.-)
- ♀ **C53.0** Malignant neoplasm of endocervix
- ♀ **C53.1** Malignant neoplasm of exocervix
- ♀ **C53.8** Malignant neoplasm of overlapping sites of cervix uteri
- ♀ **C53.9** Malignant neoplasm of cervix uteri, unspecified
  AHA CC: 4Q, 2017, 103-104

C54 Malignant neoplasm of corpus uteri
- ♀ **C54.0** Malignant neoplasm of isthmus uteri
  Malignant neoplasm of lower uterine segment
- ♀ **C54.1** Malignant neoplasm of endometrium
- ♀ **C54.2** Malignant neoplasm of myometrium
- ♀ **C54.3** Malignant neoplasm of fundus uteri
- ♀ **C54.8** Malignant neoplasm of overlapping sites of corpus uteri
- ♀ **C54.9** Malignant neoplasm of corpus uteri, unspecified

♀ C55 Malignant neoplasm of uterus, part unspecified
Valid 3-character code, no further characters required

C56 Malignant neoplasm of ovary
Use additional code to identify any functional activity
- ♀ CC **C56.1** Malignant neoplasm of right ovary
- ♀ CC **C56.2** Malignant neoplasm of left ovary
- ♀ CC **C56.3** Malignant neoplasm of bilateral ovaries
  AHA CC: 4Q, 2021, 6
- ♀ CC **C56.9** Malignant neoplasm of unspecified ovary

C57 Malignant neoplasm of other and unspecified female genital organs
- **C57.0 Malignant neoplasm of fallopian tube**
  Malignant neoplasm of oviduct
  Malignant neoplasm of uterine tube
  - ♀ **C57.00** Malignant neoplasm of unspecified fallopian tube
  - ♀ **C57.01** Malignant neoplasm of right fallopian tube
  - ♀ **C57.02** Malignant neoplasm of left fallopian tube
- **C57.1 Malignant neoplasm of broad ligament**
  - ♀ **C57.10** Malignant neoplasm of unspecified broad ligament
  - ♀ **C57.11** Malignant neoplasm of right broad ligament
  - ♀ **C57.12** Malignant neoplasm of left broad ligament
- **C57.2 Malignant neoplasm of round ligament**
  - ♀ **C57.20** Malignant neoplasm of unspecified round ligament
  - ♀ **C57.21** Malignant neoplasm of right round ligament
  - ♀ **C57.22** Malignant neoplasm of left round ligament
- ♀ **C57.3** Malignant neoplasm of parametrium
  Malignant neoplasm of uterine ligament NOS
- ♀ **C57.4** Malignant neoplasm of uterine adnexa, unspecified
- ♀ **C57.7** Malignant neoplasm of other specified female genital organs
  Malignant neoplasm of wolffian body or duct
- ♀ **C57.8** Malignant neoplasm of overlapping sites of female genital organs
  Primary malignant neoplasm of two or more contiguous sites of the female genital organs whose point of origin cannot be determined
  Primary tubo-ovarian malignant neoplasm whose point of origin cannot be determined
  Primary utero-ovarian malignant neoplasm whose point of origin cannot be determined
- ♀ **C57.9** Malignant neoplasm of female genital organ, unspecified
  Malignant neoplasm of female genitourinary tract NOS

♀ C58 Malignant neoplasm of placenta
Includes: choriocarcinoma NOS
chorionepithelioma NOS
Excludes1: chorioadenoma (destruens) (D39.2)
hydatidiform mole NOS (O01.9)
invasive hydatidiform mole (D39.2)
male choriocarcinoma NOS (C62.9-)
malignant hydatidiform mole (D39.2)
Valid 3-character code, no further characters required

Malignant neoplasms of male genital organs (C60-C63)

Includes: malignant neoplasm of skin of male genital organs

C60 Malignant neoplasm of penis
- ♂ **C60.0** Malignant neoplasm of prepuce
  - Malignant neoplasm of foreskin
- ♂ **C60.1** Malignant neoplasm of glans penis
- ♂ **C60.2** Malignant neoplasm of body of penis
  - Malignant neoplasm of corpus cavernosum
- ♂ **C60.8** Malignant neoplasm of overlapping sites of penis
- ♂ **C60.9** Malignant neoplasm of penis, unspecified
  - Malignant neoplasm of skin of penis NOS

♂ C61 Malignant neoplasm of prostate
Use additional code, if applicable, to identify:
  hormone sensitivity status (Z19.1-Z19.2)
  rising PSA following treatment for malignant neoplasm of prostate (R97.21)
Excludes1: malignant neoplasm of seminal vesicle (C63.7)
AHA CC: 1Q, 2017, 17-18
Valid 3-character code, no further characters required

C62 Malignant neoplasm of testis
Use additional code to identify any functional activity
- + **C62.0** Malignant neoplasm of undescended testis
  - Malignant neoplasm of ectopic testis
  - Malignant neoplasm of retained testis
  - ♂ **C62.00** Malignant neoplasm of unspecified undescended testis
  - ♂ **C62.01** Malignant neoplasm of undescended right testis
  - ♂ **C62.02** Malignant neoplasm of undescended left testis
- + **C62.1** Malignant neoplasm of descended testis
  - Malignant neoplasm of scrotal testis
  - ♂ **C62.10** Malignant neoplasm of unspecified descended testis
  - ♂ **C62.11** Malignant neoplasm of descended right testis
  - ♂ **C62.12** Malignant neoplasm of descended left testis
- + **C62.9** Malignant neoplasm of testis, unspecified whether descended or undescended
  - ♂ **C62.90** Malignant neoplasm of unspecified testis, unspecified whether descended or undescended
    - Malignant neoplasm of testis NOS
  - ♂ **C62.91** Malignant neoplasm of right testis, unspecified whether descended or undescended
  - ♂ **C62.92** Malignant neoplasm of left testis, unspecified whether descended or undescended

C63 Malignant neoplasm of other and unspecified male genital organs
- + **C63.0** Malignant neoplasm of epididymis
  - ♂ **C63.00** Malignant neoplasm of unspecified epididymis
  - ♂ **C63.01** Malignant neoplasm of right epididymis
  - ♂ **C63.02** Malignant neoplasm of left epididymis
- + **C63.1** Malignant neoplasm of spermatic cord
  - ♂ **C63.10** Malignant neoplasm of unspecified spermatic cord
  - ♂ **C63.11** Malignant neoplasm of right spermatic cord
  - ♂ **C63.12** Malignant neoplasm of left spermatic cord
- ♂ **C63.2** Malignant neoplasm of scrotum
  - Malignant neoplasm of skin of scrotum
- ♂ **C63.7** Malignant neoplasm of other specified male genital organs
  - Malignant neoplasm of seminal vesicle
  - Malignant neoplasm of tunica vaginalis
- ♂ **C63.8** Malignant neoplasm of overlapping sites of male genital organs
  - Primary malignant neoplasm of two or more contiguous sites of male genital organs whose point of origin cannot be determined
- ♂ **C63.9** Malignant neoplasm of male genital organ, unspecified
  - Malignant neoplasm of male genitourinary tract NOS

Malignant neoplasms of urinary tract (C64-C68)

C64 Malignant neoplasm of kidney, except renal pelvis
Excludes1: malignant carcinoid tumor of the kidney (C7A.093)
  malignant neoplasm of renal calyces (C65.-)
  malignant neoplasm of renal pelvis (C65.-)
- CC **C64.1** Malignant neoplasm of right kidney, except renal pelvis
- CC **C64.2** Malignant neoplasm of left kidney, except renal pelvis
- CC **C64.9** Malignant neoplasm of unspecified kidney, except renal pelvis

C65 Malignant neoplasm of renal pelvis
Includes: malignant neoplasm of pelviureteric junction
  malignant neoplasm of renal calyces
- CC **C65.1** Malignant neoplasm of right renal pelvis
- CC **C65.2** Malignant neoplasm of left renal pelvis
- CC **C65.9** Malignant neoplasm of unspecified renal pelvis

C66 Malignant neoplasm of ureter
Excludes1: malignant neoplasm of ureteric orifice of bladder (C67.6)
- CC **C66.1** Malignant neoplasm of right ureter
- CC **C66.2** Malignant neoplasm of left ureter
- CC **C66.9** Malignant neoplasm of unspecified ureter

C67 Malignant neoplasm of bladder
- **C67.0** Malignant neoplasm of trigone of bladder
- **C67.1** Malignant neoplasm of dome of bladder
- **C67.2** Malignant neoplasm of lateral wall of bladder
- **C67.3** Malignant neoplasm of anterior wall of bladder
- **C67.4** Malignant neoplasm of posterior wall of bladder
- **C67.5** Malignant neoplasm of bladder neck
  - Malignant neoplasm of internal urethral orifice
- **C67.6** Malignant neoplasm of ureteric orifice
- **C67.7** Malignant neoplasm of urachus
- **C67.8** Malignant neoplasm of overlapping sites of bladder
- **C67.9** Malignant neoplasm of bladder, unspecified
AHA CC: 1Q, 2016, 19; 1Q, 2017, 6

C68 Malignant neoplasm of other and unspecified urinary organs
Excludes1: malignant neoplasm of female genitourinary tract NOS (C57.9)
  malignant neoplasm of male genitourinary tract NOS (C63.9)
- CC **C68.0** Malignant neoplasm of urethra
  Excludes1: malignant neoplasm of urethral orifice of bladder (C67.5)
- CC **C68.1** Malignant neoplasm of paraurethral glands
- CC **C68.8** Malignant neoplasm of overlapping sites of urinary organs
  - Primary malignant neoplasm of two or more contiguous sites of urinary organs whose point of origin cannot be determined
- CC **C68.9** Malignant neoplasm of urinary organ, unspecified
  - Malignant neoplasm of urinary system NOS

Malignant neoplasms of eye, brain and other parts of central nervous system (C69-C72)

C69 Malignant neoplasm of eye and adnexa
Excludes1: malignant neoplasm of connective tissue of eyelid (C49.0)
  malignant neoplasm of eyelid (skin) (C43.1-, C44.1-)
  malignant neoplasm of optic nerve (C72.3-)
- + **C69.0** Malignant neoplasm of conjunctiva
  - **C69.00** Malignant neoplasm of unspecified conjunctiva
  - **C69.01** Malignant neoplasm of right conjunctiva
  - **C69.02** Malignant neoplasm of left conjunctiva
- + **C69.1** Malignant neoplasm of cornea
  - **C69.10** Malignant neoplasm of unspecified cornea
  - **C69.11** Malignant neoplasm of right cornea
  - **C69.12** Malignant neoplasm of left cornea
- + **C69.2** Malignant neoplasm of retina
  Excludes1: dark area on retina (D49.81)
    neoplasm of unspecified behavior of retina and choroid (D49.81)
    retinal freckle (D49.81)
  - **C69.20** Malignant neoplasm of unspecified retina
  - **C69.21** Malignant neoplasm of right retina
  - **C69.22** Malignant neoplasm of left retina
- + **C69.3** Malignant neoplasm of choroid
  - **C69.30** Malignant neoplasm of unspecified choroid
  - **C69.31** Malignant neoplasm of right choroid
  - **C69.32** Malignant neoplasm of left choroid
- + **C69.4** Malignant neoplasm of ciliary body
  - **C69.40** Malignant neoplasm of unspecified ciliary body
  - **C69.41** Malignant neoplasm of right ciliary body
  - **C69.42** Malignant neoplasm of left ciliary body
- + **C69.5** Malignant neoplasm of lacrimal gland and duct
  - Malignant neoplasm of lacrimal sac
  - Malignant neoplasm of nasolacrimal duct

- **C69.50** Malignant neoplasm of unspecified lacrimal gland and duct
- **C69.51** Malignant neoplasm of right lacrimal gland and duct
- **C69.52** Malignant neoplasm of left lacrimal gland and duct
- **+ C69.6** Malignant neoplasm of orbit
  - Malignant neoplasm of connective tissue of orbit
  - Malignant neoplasm of extraocular muscle
  - Malignant neoplasm of peripheral nerves of orbit
  - Malignant neoplasm of retrobulbar tissue
  - Malignant neoplasm of retro-ocular tissue
  - **Excludes1:** malignant neoplasm of orbital bone (C41.0)
  - **C69.60** Malignant neoplasm of unspecified orbit
  - **C69.61** Malignant neoplasm of right orbit
  - **C69.62** Malignant neoplasm of left orbit
- **+ C69.8** Malignant neoplasm of overlapping sites of eye and adnexa
  - **C69.80** Malignant neoplasm of overlapping sites of unspecified eye and adnexa
  - **C69.81** Malignant neoplasm of overlapping sites of right eye and adnexa
  - **C69.82** Malignant neoplasm of overlapping sites of left eye and adnexa
- **+ C69.9** Malignant neoplasm of unspecified site of eye
  - Malignant neoplasm of eyeball
  - **C69.90** Malignant neoplasm of unspecified site of unspecified eye
  - **C69.91** Malignant neoplasm of unspecified site of right eye
  - **C69.92** Malignant neoplasm of unspecified site of left eye

C70 Malignant neoplasm of meninges
- CC **C70.0** Malignant neoplasm of cerebral meninges
- CC **C70.1** Malignant neoplasm of spinal meninges
- CC **C70.9** Malignant neoplasm of meninges, unspecified

C71 Malignant neoplasm of brain
Excludes1: malignant neoplasm of cranial nerves (C72.2-C72.5)
retrobulbar malignant neoplasm (C69.6-)
- CC **C71.0** Malignant neoplasm of cerebrum, except lobes and ventricles
  - Malignant neoplasm of supratentorial NOS
- CC **C71.1** Malignant neoplasm of frontal lobe
- CC **C71.2** Malignant neoplasm of temporal lobe
- CC **C71.3** Malignant neoplasm of parietal lobe
- CC **C71.4** Malignant neoplasm of occipital lobe
- CC **C71.5** Malignant neoplasm of cerebral ventricle
  - **Excludes1:** malignant neoplasm of fourth cerebral ventricle (C71.7)
- CC **C71.6** Malignant neoplasm of cerebellum
- CC **C71.7** Malignant neoplasm of brain stem
  - Malignant neoplasm of fourth cerebral ventricle
  - Infratentorial malignant neoplasm NOS
- CC **C71.8** Malignant neoplasm of overlapping sites of brain
- CC **C71.9** Malignant neoplasm of brain, unspecified
  - *AHA CC: 3Q, 2014, 3-4*

C72 Malignant neoplasm of spinal cord, cranial nerves and other parts of central nervous system
Excludes1: malignant neoplasm of meninges (C70.-)
malignant neoplasm of peripheral nerves and autonomic nervous system (C47.-)
- CC **C72.0** Malignant neoplasm of spinal cord
- CC **C72.1** Malignant neoplasm of cauda equina
- **+ C72.2** Malignant neoplasm of olfactory nerve
  - Malignant neoplasm of olfactory bulb
  - CC **C72.20** Malignant neoplasm of unspecified olfactory nerve
  - CC **C72.21** Malignant neoplasm of right olfactory nerve
  - CC **C72.22** Malignant neoplasm of left olfactory nerve
- **+ C72.3** Malignant neoplasm of optic nerve
  - CC **C72.30** Malignant neoplasm of unspecified optic nerve
  - CC **C72.31** Malignant neoplasm of right optic nerve
  - CC **C72.32** Malignant neoplasm of left optic nerve
- **+ C72.4** Malignant neoplasm of acoustic nerve
  - CC **C72.40** Malignant neoplasm of unspecified acoustic nerve
  - CC **C72.41** Malignant neoplasm of right acoustic nerve
  - CC **C72.42** Malignant neoplasm of left acoustic nerve
- **+ C72.5** Malignant neoplasm of other and unspecified cranial nerves
  - CC **C72.50** Malignant neoplasm of unspecified cranial nerve
    - Malignant neoplasm of cranial nerve NOS
  - CC **C72.59** Malignant neoplasm of other cranial nerves
- CC **C72.9** Malignant neoplasm of central nervous system, unspecified
  - Malignant neoplasm of unspecified site of central nervous system
  - Malignant neoplasm of nervous system NOS

Malignant neoplasms of thyroid and other endocrine glands (C73-C75)

C73 Malignant neoplasm of thyroid gland
Use additional code to identify any functional activity
Valid 3-character code, no further characters required

C74 Malignant neoplasm of adrenal gland
- **+ C74.0** Malignant neoplasm of cortex of adrenal gland
  - CC **C74.00** Malignant neoplasm of cortex of unspecified adrenal gland
  - CC **C74.01** Malignant neoplasm of cortex of right adrenal gland
  - CC **C74.02** Malignant neoplasm of cortex of left adrenal gland
- **+ C74.1** Malignant neoplasm of medulla of adrenal gland
  - CC **C74.10** Malignant neoplasm of medulla of unspecified adrenal gland
  - CC **C74.11** Malignant neoplasm of medulla of right adrenal gland
  - CC **C74.12** Malignant neoplasm of medulla of left adrenal gland
- **+ C74.9** Malignant neoplasm of unspecified part of adrenal gland
  - CC **C74.90** Malignant neoplasm of unspecified part of unspecified adrenal gland
  - CC **C74.91** Malignant neoplasm of unspecified part of right adrenal gland
  - CC **C74.92** Malignant neoplasm of unspecified part of left adrenal gland

C75 Malignant neoplasm of other endocrine glands and related structures
Excludes1: malignant carcinoid tumors (C7A.0-)
malignant neoplasm of adrenal gland (C74.-)
malignant neoplasm of endocrine pancreas (C25.4)
malignant neoplasm of islets of Langerhans (C25.4)
malignant neoplasm of ovary (C56.-)
malignant neoplasm of testis (C62.-)
malignant neoplasm of thymus (C37)
malignant neoplasm of thyroid gland (C73)
malignant neuroendocrine tumors (C7A.-)
- CC **C75.0** Malignant neoplasm of parathyroid gland
- CC **C75.1** Malignant neoplasm of pituitary gland
- CC **C75.2** Malignant neoplasm of craniopharyngeal duct
- CC **C75.3** Malignant neoplasm of pineal gland
- CC **C75.4** Malignant neoplasm of carotid body
- CC **C75.5** Malignant neoplasm of aortic body and other paraganglia
- CC **C75.8** Malignant neoplasm with pluriglandular involvement, unspecified
- CC **C75.9** Malignant neoplasm of endocrine gland, unspecified

Malignant neuroendocrine tumors (C7A)

C7A Malignant neuroendocrine tumors
Code also any associated multiple endocrine neoplasia [MEN] syndromes (E31.2-)
Use additional code to identify any associated endocrine syndrome, such as:
carcinoid syndrome (E34.0)
Excludes2: malignant pancreatic islet cell tumors (C25.4)
Merkel cell carcinoma (C4A.-)
- **+ C7A.0** Malignant carcinoid tumors
  - CC **C7A.00** Malignant carcinoid tumor of unspecified site
  - **+ C7A.01** Malignant carcinoid tumors of the small intestine
    - CC **C7A.010** Malignant carcinoid tumor of the duodenum
    - CC **C7A.011** Malignant carcinoid tumor of the jejunum
    - CC **C7A.012** Malignant carcinoid tumor of the ileum
    - CC **C7A.019** Malignant carcinoid tumor of the small intestine, unspecified portion
  - **+ C7A.02** Malignant carcinoid tumors of the appendix, large intestine, and rectum
    - CC **C7A.020** Malignant carcinoid tumor of the appendix
    - CC **C7A.021** Malignant carcinoid tumor of the cecum
    - CC **C7A.022** Malignant carcinoid tumor of the ascending colon
    - CC **C7A.023** Malignant carcinoid tumor of the transverse colon
    - CC **C7A.024** Malignant carcinoid tumor of the descending colon

CC **C7A.025** Malignant carcinoid tumor of the sigmoid colon
CC **C7A.026** Malignant carcinoid tumor of the rectum
CC **C7A.029** Malignant carcinoid tumor of the large intestine, unspecified portion
   Malignant carcinoid tumor of the colon NOS
+ **C7A.09** Malignant carcinoid tumors of other sites
   CC **C7A.090** Malignant carcinoid tumor of the bronchus and lung
   CC **C7A.091** Malignant carcinoid tumor of the thymus
   CC **C7A.092** Malignant carcinoid tumor of the stomach
   CC **C7A.093** Malignant carcinoid tumor of the kidney
   CC **C7A.094** Malignant carcinoid tumor of the foregut, unspecified
   CC **C7A.095** Malignant carcinoid tumor of the midgut, unspecified
   CC **C7A.096** Malignant carcinoid tumor of the hindgut, unspecified
   CC **C7A.098** Malignant carcinoid tumors of other sites
CC **C7A.1** Malignant poorly differentiated neuroendocrine tumors
   Malignant poorly differentiated neuroendocrine tumor NOS
   Malignant poorly differentiated neuroendocrine carcinoma, any site
   High grade neuroendocrine carcinoma, any site
   AHA CC: 1Q, 2023, 20-22
CC **C7A.8** Other malignant neuroendocrine tumors
   AHA CC: 3Q, 2019, 7-8

Secondary neuroendocrine tumors (C7B)

C7B Secondary neuroendocrine tumors
   Use additional code to identify any functional activity
+ **C7B.0** Secondary carcinoid tumors
   C7B.00 Secondary carcinoid tumors, unspecified site
   CC **C7B.01** Secondary carcinoid tumors of distant lymph nodes
   CC **C7B.02** Secondary carcinoid tumors of liver
   CC **C7B.03** Secondary carcinoid tumors of bone
   CC **C7B.04** Secondary carcinoid tumors of peritoneum
      Mesentary metastasis of carcinoid tumor
   CC **C7B.09** Secondary carcinoid tumors of other sites
C7B.1 Secondary Merkel cell carcinoma
   Merkel cell carcinoma nodal presentation
   Merkel cell carcinoma visceral metastatic presentation
CC **C7B.8** Other secondary neuroendocrine tumors
   AHA CC: 3Q, 2019, 7-8; 1Q, 2023, 20-22

Malignant neoplasms of ill-defined, other secondary and unspecified sites (C76-C80)

Review coding guidelines C.2.b and C.2.l.2

C76 Malignant neoplasm of other and ill-defined sites
   Excludes1: malignant neoplasm of female genitourinary tract NOS (C57.9)
   malignant neoplasm of male genitourinary tract NOS (C63.9)
   malignant neoplasm of lymphoid, hematopoietic and related tissue (C81-C96)
   malignant neoplasm of skin (C44.-)
   malignant neoplasm of unspecified site NOS (C80.1)
   C76.0 Malignant neoplasm of head, face and neck
      Malignant neoplasm of cheek NOS
      Malignant neoplasm of nose NOS
   C76.1 Malignant neoplasm of thorax
      Intrathoracic malignant neoplasm NOS
      Malignant neoplasm of axilla NOS
      Thoracic malignant neoplasm NOS
   C76.2 Malignant neoplasm of abdomen
   C76.3 Malignant neoplasm of pelvis
      Malignant neoplasm of groin NOS
      Malignant neoplasm of sites overlapping systems within the pelvis
      Rectovaginal (septum) malignant neoplasm
      Rectovesical (septum) malignant neoplasm
+ **C76.4** Malignant neoplasm of upper limb
   C76.40 Malignant neoplasm of unspecified upper limb
   C76.41 Malignant neoplasm of right upper limb
   C76.42 Malignant neoplasm of left upper limb
+ **C76.5** Malignant neoplasm of lower limb
   C76.50 Malignant neoplasm of unspecified lower limb
   C76.51 Malignant neoplasm of right lower limb
   C76.52 Malignant neoplasm of left lower limb
C76.8 Malignant neoplasm of other specified ill-defined sites
   Malignant neoplasm of overlapping ill-defined sites
+ **C77** Secondary and unspecified malignant neoplasm of lymph nodes
   Excludes1: malignant neoplasm of lymph nodes, specified as primary (C81-C86, C88, C96.-)
   mesentary metastasis of carcinoid tumor (C7B.04)
   secondary carcinoid tumors of distant lymph nodes (C7B.01)
CC **C77.0** Secondary and unspecified malignant neoplasm of lymph nodes of head, face and neck
   Secondary and unspecified malignant neoplasm of supraclavicular lymph nodes
   AHA CC: 3Q, 2022, 14-15
CC **C77.1** Secondary and unspecified malignant neoplasm of intrathoracic lymph nodes
CC **C77.2** Secondary and unspecified malignant neoplasm of intra-abdominal lymph nodes
CC **C77.3** Secondary and unspecified malignant neoplasm of axilla and upper limb lymph nodes
   Secondary and unspecified malignant neoplasm of pectoral lymph nodes
CC **C77.4** Secondary and unspecified malignant neoplasm of inguinal and lower limb lymph nodes
CC **C77.5** Secondary and unspecified malignant neoplasm of intrapelvic lymph nodes
CC **C77.8** Secondary and unspecified malignant neoplasm of lymph nodes of multiple regions
CC **C77.9** Secondary and unspecified malignant neoplasm of lymph node, unspecified

C78 Secondary malignant neoplasm of respiratory and digestive organs
   Excludes1: secondary carcinoid tumors of liver (C7B.02)
   secondary carcinoid tumors of peritoneum (C7B.04)
   Excludes2: lymph node metastases (C77.0)
+ **C78.0** Secondary malignant neoplasm of lung
   CC **C78.00** Secondary malignant neoplasm of unspecified lung
      AHA CC: 3Q, 2022, 9
   CC **C78.01** Secondary malignant neoplasm of right lung
   CC **C78.02** Secondary malignant neoplasm of left lung
CC **C78.1** Secondary malignant neoplasm of mediastinum
CC **C78.2** Secondary malignant neoplasm of pleura
+ **C78.3** Secondary malignant neoplasm of other and unspecified respiratory organs
   CC **C78.30** Secondary malignant neoplasm of unspecified respiratory organ
   CC **C78.39** Secondary malignant neoplasm of other respiratory organs
CC **C78.4** Secondary malignant neoplasm of small intestine
CC **C78.5** Secondary malignant neoplasm of large intestine and rectum
CC **C78.6** Secondary malignant neoplasm of retroperitoneum and peritoneum
   AHA CC: 2Q, 2017, 12
CC **C78.7** Secondary malignant neoplasm of liver and intrahepatic bile duct
   AHA CC: 3Q, 2022, 14-15
+ **C78.8** Secondary malignant neoplasm of other and unspecified digestive organs
   CC **C78.80** Secondary malignant neoplasm of unspecified digestive organ
   CC **C78.89** Secondary malignant neoplasm of other digestive organs
      Code also exocrine pancreatic insufficiency (K86.81)

C79 Secondary malignant neoplasm of other and unspecified sites
   Excludes1: secondary carcinoid tumors (C7B.-)
   secondary neuroendocrine tumors (C7B.-)
+ **C79.0** Secondary malignant neoplasm of kidney and renal pelvis
   CC **C79.00** Secondary malignant neoplasm of unspecified kidney and renal pelvis
   CC **C79.01** Secondary malignant neoplasm of right kidney and renal pelvis
   CC **C79.02** Secondary malignant neoplasm of left kidney and renal pelvis

- **C79.1** Secondary malignant neoplasm of bladder and other and unspecified urinary organs
  - CC **C79.10** Secondary malignant neoplasm of unspecified urinary organs
  - CC **C79.11** Secondary malignant neoplasm of bladder
    - *Excludes2:* lymph node metastases (C77.0)
  - CC **C79.19** Secondary malignant neoplasm of other urinary organs
- CC **C79.2** Secondary malignant neoplasm of skin
  - *Excludes1:* secondary Merkel cell carcinoma (C7B.1)
- **C79.3** Secondary malignant neoplasm of brain and cerebral meninges
  - CC **C79.31** Secondary malignant neoplasm of brain
    - *AHA CC: 3Q, 2022, 9-11*
  - CC **C79.32** Secondary malignant neoplasm of cerebral meninges
    - *AHA CC: 1Q, 2020, 13-14*
- **C79.4** Secondary malignant neoplasm of other and unspecified parts of nervous system
  - CC **C79.40** Secondary malignant neoplasm of unspecified part of nervous system
  - CC **C79.49** Secondary malignant neoplasm of other parts of nervous system
- **C79.5** Secondary malignant neoplasm of bone and bone marrow
  - *Excludes1:* secondary carcinoid tumors of bone (C7B.03)
  - CC **C79.51** Secondary malignant neoplasm of bone
    - *AHA CC: 3Q, 2022, 14-15*
  - CC **C79.52** Secondary malignant neoplasm of bone marrow
- **C79.6** Secondary malignant neoplasm of ovary
  - ♀ CC **C79.60** Secondary malignant neoplasm of unspecified ovary
  - ♀ CC **C79.61** Secondary malignant neoplasm of right ovary
  - ♀ CC **C79.62** Secondary malignant neoplasm of left ovary
  - ♀ CC **C79.63** Secondary malignant neoplasm of bilateral ovaries
    - *AHA CC: 4Q, 2021, 6*
- **C79.7** Secondary malignant neoplasm of adrenal gland
  - CC **C79.70** Secondary malignant neoplasm of unspecified adrenal gland
  - CC **C79.71** Secondary malignant neoplasm of right adrenal gland
  - CC **C79.72** Secondary malignant neoplasm of left adrenal gland
- **C79.8** Secondary malignant neoplasm of other specified sites
  - CC **C79.81** Secondary malignant neoplasm of breast
  - CC **C79.82** Secondary malignant neoplasm of genital organs
  - CC **C79.89** Secondary malignant neoplasm of other specified sites
    - *AHA CC: 2Q, 2017, 11*
- CC **C79.9** Secondary malignant neoplasm of unspecified site
  - Metastatic cancer NOS
  - Metastatic disease NOS
  - *Excludes1:* carcinomatosis NOS (C80.0)
    - generalized cancer NOS (C80.0)
    - malignant (primary) neoplasm of unspecified site (C80.1)
  - *AHA CC: 2Q, 2023, 5-6*

C80 Malignant neoplasm without specification of site
- *Excludes1:* malignant carcinoid tumor of unspecified site (C7A.00)
  - malignant neoplasm of specified multiple sites- code to each site
- CC **C80.0** Disseminated malignant neoplasm, unspecified
  - Carcinomatosis NOS
  - Generalized cancer, unspecified site (primary) (secondary)
  - Generalized malignancy, unspecified site (primary) (secondary)
  - *Review coding guideline C.2.j*
- **C80.1** Malignant (primary) neoplasm, unspecified
  - Cancer NOS
  - Cancer unspecified site (primary)
  - Carcinoma unspecified site (primary)
  - Malignancy unspecified site (primary)
  - *Excludes1:* secondary malignant neoplasm of unspecified site (C79.9)
  - *Review coding guideline C.2.k*
- CC **C80.2** Malignant neoplasm associated with transplanted organ
  - Code first complication of transplanted organ (T86.-)
  - Use additional code to identify the specific malignancy
  - *Review coding guideline C.2.r*

Malignant neoplasms of lymphoid, hematopoietic and related tissue (C81-C96)

Excludes2: Kaposi's sarcoma of lymph nodes (C46.3)
secondary and unspecified neoplasm of lymph nodes (C77.-)
secondary neoplasm of bone marrow (C79.52)
secondary neoplasm of spleen (C78.89)

C81 Hodgkin lymphoma
- *Excludes1:* personal history of Hodgkin lymphoma (Z85.71)
- **C81.0** Nodular lymphocyte predominant Hodgkin lymphoma
  - CC **C81.00** Nodular lymphocyte predominant Hodgkin lymphoma, unspecified site
  - CC **C81.01** Nodular lymphocyte predominant Hodgkin lymphoma, lymph nodes of head, face, and neck
  - CC **C81.02** Nodular lymphocyte predominant Hodgkin lymphoma, intrathoracic lymph nodes
  - CC **C81.03** Nodular lymphocyte predominant Hodgkin lymphoma, intra-abdominal lymph nodes
  - CC **C81.04** Nodular lymphocyte predominant Hodgkin lymphoma, lymph nodes of axilla and upper limb
  - CC **C81.05** Nodular lymphocyte predominant Hodgkin lymphoma, lymph nodes of inguinal region and lower limb
  - CC **C81.06** Nodular lymphocyte predominant Hodgkin lymphoma, intrapelvic lymph nodes
  - CC **C81.07** Nodular lymphocyte predominant Hodgkin lymphoma, spleen
  - CC **C81.08** Nodular lymphocyte predominant Hodgkin lymphoma, lymph nodes of multiple sites
  - CC **C81.09** Nodular lymphocyte predominant Hodgkin lymphoma, extranodal and solid organ sites
- **C81.1** Nodular sclerosis Hodgkin lymphoma
  - Nodular sclerosis classical Hodgkin lymphoma
  - CC **C81.10** Nodular sclerosis Hodgkin lymphoma, unspecified site
  - CC **C81.11** Nodular sclerosis Hodgkin lymphoma, lymph nodes of head, face, and neck
  - CC **C81.12** Nodular sclerosis Hodgkin lymphoma, intrathoracic lymph nodes
  - CC **C81.13** Nodular sclerosis Hodgkin lymphoma, intra-abdominal lymph nodes
  - CC **C81.14** Nodular sclerosis Hodgkin lymphoma, lymph nodes of axilla and upper limb
  - CC **C81.15** Nodular sclerosis Hodgkin lymphoma, lymph nodes of inguinal region and lower limb
  - CC **C81.16** Nodular sclerosis Hodgkin lymphoma, intrapelvic lymph nodes
  - CC **C81.17** Nodular sclerosis Hodgkin lymphoma, spleen
  - CC **C81.18** Nodular sclerosis Hodgkin lymphoma, lymph nodes of multiple sites
  - CC **C81.19** Nodular sclerosis Hodgkin lymphoma, extranodal and solid organ sites
- **C81.2** Mixed cellularity Hodgkin lymphoma
  - Mixed cellularity classical Hodgkin lymphoma
  - CC **C81.20** Mixed cellularity Hodgkin lymphoma, unspecified site
  - CC **C81.21** Mixed cellularity Hodgkin lymphoma, lymph nodes of head, face, and neck
  - CC **C81.22** Mixed cellularity Hodgkin lymphoma, intrathoracic lymph nodes
  - CC **C81.23** Mixed cellularity Hodgkin lymphoma, intra-abdominal lymph nodes
  - CC **C81.24** Mixed cellularity Hodgkin lymphoma, lymph nodes of axilla and upper limb
  - CC **C81.25** Mixed cellularity Hodgkin lymphoma, lymph nodes of inguinal region and lower limb
  - CC **C81.26** Mixed cellularity Hodgkin lymphoma, intrapelvic lymph nodes
  - CC **C81.27** Mixed cellularity Hodgkin lymphoma, spleen
  - CC **C81.28** Mixed cellularity Hodgkin lymphoma, lymph nodes of multiple sites
  - CC **C81.29** Mixed cellularity Hodgkin lymphoma, extranodal and solid organ sites

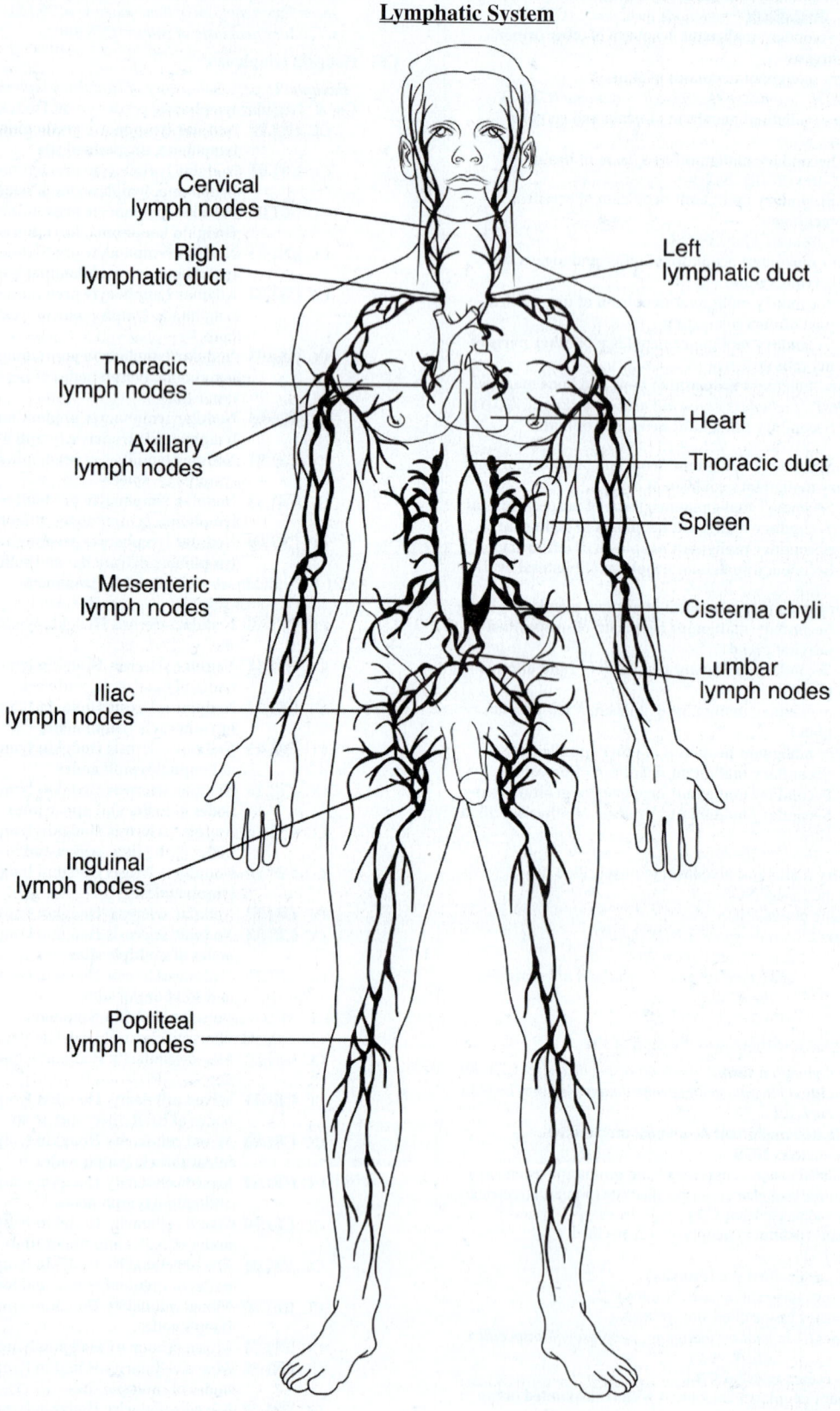

- **C81.3 Lymphocyte depleted Hodgkin lymphoma**
  Lymphocyte depleted classical Hodgkin lymphoma
  - CC **C81.30** Lymphocyte depleted Hodgkin lymphoma, unspecified site
  - CC **C81.31** Lymphocyte depleted Hodgkin lymphoma, lymph nodes of head, face, and neck
  - CC **C81.32** Lymphocyte depleted Hodgkin lymphoma, intrathoracic lymph nodes
  - CC **C81.33** Lymphocyte depleted Hodgkin lymphoma, intra-abdominal lymph nodes
  - CC **C81.34** Lymphocyte depleted Hodgkin lymphoma, lymph nodes of axilla and upper limb
  - CC **C81.35** Lymphocyte depleted Hodgkin lymphoma, lymph nodes of inguinal region and lower limb
  - CC **C81.36** Lymphocyte depleted Hodgkin lymphoma, intrapelvic lymph nodes
  - CC **C81.37** Lymphocyte depleted Hodgkin lymphoma, spleen
  - CC **C81.38** Lymphocyte depleted Hodgkin lymphoma, lymph nodes of multiple sites
  - CC **C81.39** Lymphocyte depleted Hodgkin lymphoma, extranodal and solid organ sites
- **C81.4 Lymphocyte-rich Hodgkin lymphoma**
  Lymphocyte-rich classical Hodgkin lymphoma
  Excludes1: *nodular lymphocyte predominant Hodgkin lymphoma (C81.0-)*
  - CC **C81.40** Lymphocyte-rich Hodgkin lymphoma, unspecified site
  - CC **C81.41** Lymphocyte-rich Hodgkin lymphoma, lymph nodes of head, face, and neck
  - CC **C81.42** Lymphocyte-rich Hodgkin lymphoma, intrathoracic lymph nodes
  - CC **C81.43** Lymphocyte-rich Hodgkin lymphoma, intra-abdominal lymph nodes
  - CC **C81.44** Lymphocyte-rich Hodgkin lymphoma, lymph nodes of axilla and upper limb
  - CC **C81.45** Lymphocyte-rich Hodgkin lymphoma, lymph nodes of inguinal region and lower limb
  - CC **C81.46** Lymphocyte-rich Hodgkin lymphoma, intrapelvic lymph nodes
  - CC **C81.47** Lymphocyte-rich Hodgkin lymphoma, spleen
  - CC **C81.48** Lymphocyte-rich Hodgkin lymphoma, lymph nodes of multiple sites
  - CC **C81.49** Lymphocyte-rich Hodgkin lymphoma, extranodal and solid organ sites
- **C81.7 Other Hodgkin lymphoma**
  Classical Hodgkin lymphoma NOS
  Other classical Hodgkin lymphoma
  - CC **C81.70** Other Hodgkin lymphoma, unspecified site
  - CC **C81.71** Other Hodgkin lymphoma, lymph nodes of head, face, and neck
  - CC **C81.72** Other Hodgkin lymphoma, intrathoracic lymph nodes
  - CC **C81.73** Other Hodgkin lymphoma, intra-abdominal lymph nodes
  - CC **C81.74** Other Hodgkin lymphoma, lymph nodes of axilla and upper limb
  - CC **C81.75** Other Hodgkin lymphoma, lymph nodes of inguinal region and lower limb
  - CC **C81.76** Other Hodgkin lymphoma, intrapelvic lymph nodes
  - CC **C81.77** Other Hodgkin lymphoma, spleen
  - CC **C81.78** Other Hodgkin lymphoma, lymph nodes of multiple sites
  - CC **C81.79** Other Hodgkin lymphoma, extranodal and solid organ sites
- **C81.9 Hodgkin lymphoma, unspecified**
  - CC **C81.90** Hodgkin lymphoma, unspecified, unspecified site
  - CC **C81.91** Hodgkin lymphoma, unspecified, lymph nodes of head, face, and neck
  - CC **C81.92** Hodgkin lymphoma, unspecified, intrathoracic lymph nodes
  - CC **C81.93** Hodgkin lymphoma, unspecified, intra-abdominal lymph nodes
  - CC **C81.94** Hodgkin lymphoma, unspecified, lymph nodes of axilla and upper limb
  - CC **C81.95** Hodgkin lymphoma, unspecified, lymph nodes of inguinal region and lower limb
  - CC **C81.96** Hodgkin lymphoma, unspecified, intrapelvic lymph nodes
  - CC **C81.97** Hodgkin lymphoma, unspecified, spleen
  - CC **C81.98** Hodgkin lymphoma, unspecified, lymph nodes of multiple sites
  - CC **C81.99** Hodgkin lymphoma, unspecified, extranodal and solid organ sites

C82 Follicular lymphoma
  Includes: follicular lymphoma with or without diffuse areas
  Excludes1: *mature T/NK-cell lymphomas (C84.-)*
  personal history of non-Hodgkin lymphoma (Z85.72)
- **C82.0 Follicular lymphoma grade I**
  - CC **C82.00** Follicular lymphoma grade I, unspecified site
  - CC **C82.01** Follicular lymphoma grade I, lymph nodes of head, face, and neck
  - CC **C82.02** Follicular lymphoma grade I, intrathoracic lymph nodes
  - CC **C82.03** Follicular lymphoma grade I, intra-abdominal lymph nodes
  - CC **C82.04** Follicular lymphoma grade I, lymph nodes of axilla and upper limb
  - CC **C82.05** Follicular lymphoma grade I, lymph nodes of inguinal region and lower limb
  - CC **C82.06** Follicular lymphoma grade I, intrapelvic lymph nodes
  - CC **C82.07** Follicular lymphoma grade I, spleen
  - CC **C82.08** Follicular lymphoma grade I, lymph nodes of multiple sites
  - CC **C82.09** Follicular lymphoma grade I, extranodal and solid organ sites
- **C82.1 Follicular lymphoma grade II**
  - CC **C82.10** Follicular lymphoma grade II, unspecified site
  - CC **C82.11** Follicular lymphoma grade II, lymph nodes of head, face, and neck
  - CC **C82.12** Follicular lymphoma grade II, intrathoracic lymph nodes
  - CC **C82.13** Follicular lymphoma grade II, intra-abdominal lymph nodes
  - CC **C82.14** Follicular lymphoma grade II, lymph nodes of axilla and upper limb
  - CC **C82.15** Follicular lymphoma grade II, lymph nodes of inguinal region and lower limb
  - CC **C82.16** Follicular lymphoma grade II, intrapelvic lymph nodes
  - CC **C82.17** Follicular lymphoma grade II, spleen
  - CC **C82.18** Follicular lymphoma grade II, lymph nodes of multiple sites
  - CC **C82.19** Follicular lymphoma grade II, extranodal and solid organ sites
- **C82.2 Follicular lymphoma grade III, unspecified**
  - CC **C82.20** Follicular lymphoma grade III, unspecified, unspecified site
  - CC **C82.21** Follicular lymphoma grade III, unspecified, lymph nodes of head, face, and neck
  - CC **C82.22** Follicular lymphoma grade III, unspecified, intrathoracic lymph nodes
  - CC **C82.23** Follicular lymphoma grade III, unspecified, intra-abdominal lymph nodes
  - CC **C82.24** Follicular lymphoma grade III, unspecified, lymph nodes of axilla and upper limb
  - CC **C82.25** Follicular lymphoma grade III, unspecified, lymph nodes of inguinal region and lower limb
  - CC **C82.26** Follicular lymphoma grade III, unspecified, intrapelvic lymph nodes
  - CC **C82.27** Follicular lymphoma grade III, unspecified, spleen
  - CC **C82.28** Follicular lymphoma grade III, unspecified, lymph nodes of multiple sites
  - CC **C82.29** Follicular lymphoma grade III, unspecified, extranodal and solid organ sites
- **C82.3 Follicular lymphoma grade IIIa**
  - CC **C82.30** Follicular lymphoma grade IIIa, unspecified site
  - CC **C82.31** Follicular lymphoma grade IIIa, lymph nodes of head, face, and neck
  - CC **C82.32** Follicular lymphoma grade IIIa, intrathoracic lymph nodes
  - CC **C82.33** Follicular lymphoma grade IIIa, intra-abdominal lymph nodes
  - CC **C82.34** Follicular lymphoma grade IIIa, lymph nodes of axilla and upper limb
  - CC **C82.35** Follicular lymphoma grade IIIa, lymph nodes of inguinal region and lower limb

- CC **C82.36** Follicular lymphoma grade IIIa, intrapelvic lymph nodes
- CC **C82.37** Follicular lymphoma grade IIIa, spleen
- CC **C82.38** Follicular lymphoma grade IIIa, lymph nodes of multiple sites
- CC **C82.39** Follicular lymphoma grade IIIa, extranodal and solid organ sites

+ **C82.4** Follicular lymphoma grade IIIb
- CC **C82.40** Follicular lymphoma grade IIIb, unspecified site
- CC **C82.41** Follicular lymphoma grade IIIb, lymph nodes of head, face, and neck
- CC **C82.42** Follicular lymphoma grade IIIb, intrathoracic lymph nodes
- CC **C82.43** Follicular lymphoma grade IIIb, intra-abdominal lymph nodes
- CC **C82.44** Follicular lymphoma grade IIIb, lymph nodes of axilla and upper limb
- CC **C82.45** Follicular lymphoma grade IIIb, lymph nodes of inguinal region and lower limb
- CC **C82.46** Follicular lymphoma grade IIIb, intrapelvic lymph nodes
- CC **C82.47** Follicular lymphoma grade IIIb, spleen
- CC **C82.48** Follicular lymphoma grade IIIb, lymph nodes of multiple sites
- CC **C82.49** Follicular lymphoma grade IIIb, extranodal and solid organ sites

+ **C82.5** Diffuse follicle center lymphoma
- CC **C82.50** Diffuse follicle center lymphoma, unspecified site
- CC **C82.51** Diffuse follicle center lymphoma, lymph nodes of head, face, and neck
- CC **C82.52** Diffuse follicle center lymphoma, intrathoracic lymph nodes
- CC **C82.53** Diffuse follicle center lymphoma, intra-abdominal lymph nodes
- CC **C82.54** Diffuse follicle center lymphoma, lymph nodes of axilla and upper limb
- CC **C82.55** Diffuse follicle center lymphoma, lymph nodes of inguinal region and lower limb
- CC **C82.56** Diffuse follicle center lymphoma, intrapelvic lymph nodes
- CC **C82.57** Diffuse follicle center lymphoma, spleen
- CC **C82.58** Diffuse follicle center lymphoma, lymph nodes of multiple sites
- CC **C82.59** Diffuse follicle center lymphoma, extranodal and solid organ sites

+ **C82.6** Cutaneous follicle center lymphoma
- CC **C82.60** Cutaneous follicle center lymphoma, unspecified site
- CC **C82.61** Cutaneous follicle center lymphoma, lymph nodes of head, face, and neck
- CC **C82.62** Cutaneous follicle center lymphoma, intrathoracic lymph nodes
- CC **C82.63** Cutaneous follicle center lymphoma, intra-abdominal lymph nodes
- CC **C82.64** Cutaneous follicle center lymphoma, lymph nodes of axilla and upper limb
- CC **C82.65** Cutaneous follicle center lymphoma, lymph nodes of inguinal region and lower limb
- CC **C82.66** Cutaneous follicle center lymphoma, intrapelvic lymph nodes
- CC **C82.67** Cutaneous follicle center lymphoma, spleen
- CC **C82.68** Cutaneous follicle center lymphoma, lymph nodes of multiple sites
- CC **C82.69** Cutaneous follicle center lymphoma, extranodal and solid organ sites

+ **C82.8** Other types of follicular lymphoma
- CC **C82.80** Other types of follicular lymphoma, unspecified site
- CC **C82.81** Other types of follicular lymphoma, lymph nodes of head, face, and neck
- CC **C82.82** Other types of follicular lymphoma, intrathoracic lymph nodes
- CC **C82.83** Other types of follicular lymphoma, intra-abdominal lymph nodes
- CC **C82.84** Other types of follicular lymphoma, lymph nodes of axilla and upper limb
- CC **C82.85** Other types of follicular lymphoma, lymph nodes of inguinal region and lower limb
- CC **C82.86** Other types of follicular lymphoma, intrapelvic lymph nodes
- CC **C82.87** Other types of follicular lymphoma, spleen
- CC **C82.88** Other types of follicular lymphoma, lymph nodes of multiple sites
- CC **C82.89** Other types of follicular lymphoma, extranodal and solid organ sites

+ **C82.9** Follicular lymphoma, unspecified
- CC **C82.90** Follicular lymphoma, unspecified, unspecified site
- CC **C82.91** Follicular lymphoma, unspecified, lymph nodes of head, face, and neck
- CC **C82.92** Follicular lymphoma, unspecified, intrathoracic lymph nodes
- CC **C82.93** Follicular lymphoma, unspecified, intra-abdominal lymph nodes
- CC **C82.94** Follicular lymphoma, unspecified, lymph nodes of axilla and upper limb
- CC **C82.95** Follicular lymphoma, unspecified, lymph nodes of inguinal region and lower limb
- CC **C82.96** Follicular lymphoma, unspecified, intrapelvic lymph nodes
- CC **C82.97** Follicular lymphoma, unspecified, spleen
- CC **C82.98** Follicular lymphoma, unspecified, lymph nodes of multiple sites
- CC **C82.99** Follicular lymphoma, unspecified, extranodal and solid organ sites

C83 Non-follicular lymphoma

Excludes1: personal history of non-Hodgkin lymphoma (Z85.72)

+ **C83.0** Small cell B-cell lymphoma
  Lymphoplasmacytic lymphoma
  Nodal marginal zone lymphoma
  Non-leukemic variant of B-CLL
  Splenic marginal zone lymphoma
  Excludes1: chronic lymphocytic leukemia (C91.1)
  mature T/NK-cell lymphomas (C84.-)
  Waldenström macroglobulinemia (C88.0)
  AHA CC: 1Q, 2023, 18-19
- CC **C83.00** Small cell B-cell lymphoma, unspecified site
- CC **C83.01** Small cell B-cell lymphoma, lymph nodes of head, face, and neck
- CC **C83.02** Small cell B-cell lymphoma, intrathoracic lymph nodes
- CC **C83.03** Small cell B-cell lymphoma, intra-abdominal lymph nodes
- CC **C83.04** Small cell B-cell lymphoma, lymph nodes of axilla and upper limb
- CC **C83.05** Small cell B-cell lymphoma, lymph nodes of inguinal region and lower limb
- CC **C83.06** Small cell B-cell lymphoma, intrapelvic lymph nodes
- CC **C83.07** Small cell B-cell lymphoma, spleen
- CC **C83.08** Small cell B-cell lymphoma, lymph nodes of multiple sites
- CC **C83.09** Small cell B-cell lymphoma, extranodal and solid organ sites

+ **C83.1** Mantle cell lymphoma
  Centrocytic lymphoma
  Malignant lymphomatous polyposis
- CC **C83.10** Mantle cell lymphoma, unspecified site
- CC **C83.11** Mantle cell lymphoma, lymph nodes of head, face, and neck
- CC **C83.12** Mantle cell lymphoma, intrathoracic lymph nodes
- CC **C83.13** Mantle cell lymphoma, intra-abdominal lymph nodes
- CC **C83.14** Mantle cell lymphoma, lymph nodes of axilla and upper limb
- CC **C83.15** Mantle cell lymphoma, lymph nodes of inguinal region and lower limb
- CC **C83.16** Mantle cell lymphoma, intrapelvic lymph nodes
- CC **C83.17** Mantle cell lymphoma, spleen
- CC **C83.18** Mantle cell lymphoma, lymph nodes of multiple sites
- CC **C83.19** Mantle cell lymphoma, extranodal and solid organ sites

+ C83.3 Diffuse large B-cell lymphoma
  Anaplastic diffuse large B-cell lymphoma
  CD30-positive diffuse large B-cell lymphoma
  Centroblastic diffuse large B-cell lymphoma
  Diffuse large B-cell lymphoma, subtype not specified
  Immunoblastic diffuse large B-cell lymphoma
  Plasmablastic diffuse large B-cell lymphoma
  Diffuse large B-cell lymphoma, subtype not specified
  T-cell rich diffuse large B-cell lymphoma
  Excludes1: mediastinal (thymic) large B-cell lymphoma (C85.2-)
      mature T/NK-cell lymphomas (C84.-)
  - CC **C83.30** Diffuse large B-cell lymphoma, unspecified site
  - CC **C83.31** Diffuse large B-cell lymphoma, lymph nodes of head, face, and neck
  - CC **C83.32** Diffuse large B-cell lymphoma, intrathoracic lymph nodes
  - CC **C83.33** Diffuse large B-cell lymphoma, intra-abdominal lymph nodes
  - CC **C83.34** Diffuse large B-cell lymphoma, lymph nodes of axilla and upper limb
  - CC **C83.35** Diffuse large B-cell lymphoma, lymph nodes of inguinal region and lower limb
  - CC **C83.36** Diffuse large B-cell lymphoma, intrapelvic lymph nodes
  - CC **C83.37** Diffuse large B-cell lymphoma, spleen
  - CC **C83.38** Diffuse large B-cell lymphoma, lymph nodes of multiple sites
    AHA CC: 1Q, 2023, 22-23
  - CC **C83.39** Diffuse large B-cell lymphoma, extranodal and solid organ sites
    AHA CC: 1Q, 2023, 22-23

+ C83.5 Lymphoblastic (diffuse) lymphoma
  B-precursor lymphoma
  Lymphoblastic B-cell lymphoma
  Lymphoblastic lymphoma NOS
  Lymphoblastic T-cell lymphoma
  T-precursor lymphoma
  - CC **C83.50** Lymphoblastic (diffuse) lymphoma, unspecified site
  - CC **C83.51** Lymphoblastic (diffuse) lymphoma, lymph nodes of head, face, and neck
  - CC **C83.52** Lymphoblastic (diffuse) lymphoma, intrathoracic lymph nodes
  - CC **C83.53** Lymphoblastic (diffuse) lymphoma, intra-abdominal lymph nodes
  - CC **C83.54** Lymphoblastic (diffuse) lymphoma, lymph nodes of axilla and upper limb
  - CC **C83.55** Lymphoblastic (diffuse) lymphoma, lymph nodes of inguinal region and lower limb
  - CC **C83.56** Lymphoblastic (diffuse) lymphoma, intrapelvic lymph nodes
  - CC **C83.57** Lymphoblastic (diffuse) lymphoma, spleen
  - CC **C83.58** Lymphoblastic (diffuse) lymphoma, lymph nodes of multiple sites
  - CC **C83.59** Lymphoblastic (diffuse) lymphoma, extranodal and solid organ sites

+ C83.7 Burkitt lymphoma
  Atypical Burkitt lymphoma
  Burkitt-like lymphoma
  Excludes1: mature B-cell leukemia Burkitt type (C91.A-)
  - CC **C83.70** Burkitt lymphoma, unspecified site
  - CC **C83.71** Burkitt lymphoma, lymph nodes of head, face, and neck
  - CC **C83.72** Burkitt lymphoma, intrathoracic lymph nodes
  - CC **C83.73** Burkitt lymphoma, intra-abdominal lymph nodes
  - CC **C83.74** Burkitt lymphoma, lymph nodes of axilla and upper limb
  - CC **C83.75** Burkitt lymphoma, lymph nodes of inguinal region and lower limb
  - CC **C83.76** Burkitt lymphoma, intrapelvic lymph nodes
  - CC **C83.77** Burkitt lymphoma, spleen
  - CC **C83.78** Burkitt lymphoma, lymph nodes of multiple sites
  - CC **C83.79** Burkitt lymphoma, extranodal and solid organ sites

+ C83.8 Other non-follicular lymphoma
  Intravascular large B-cell lymphoma
  Lymphoid granulomatosis
  Primary effusion B-cell lymphoma
  Excludes1: mediastinal (thymic) large B-cell lymphoma (C85.2-)
      T-cell rich B-cell lymphoma (C83.3-)
  - CC **C83.80** Other non-follicular lymphoma, unspecified site
  - CC **C83.81** Other non-follicular lymphoma, lymph nodes of head, face, and neck
  - CC **C83.82** Other non-follicular lymphoma, intrathoracic lymph nodes
  - CC **C83.83** Other non-follicular lymphoma, intra-abdominal lymph nodes
  - CC **C83.84** Other non-follicular lymphoma, lymph nodes of axilla and upper limb
  - CC **C83.85** Other non-follicular lymphoma, lymph nodes of inguinal region and lower limb
  - CC **C83.86** Other non-follicular lymphoma, intrapelvic lymph nodes
  - CC **C83.87** Other non-follicular lymphoma, spleen
  - CC **C83.88** Other non-follicular lymphoma, lymph nodes of multiple sites
  - CC **C83.89** Other non-follicular lymphoma, extranodal and solid organ sites

+ C83.9 Non-follicular (diffuse) lymphoma, unspecified
  - CC **C83.90** Non-follicular (diffuse) lymphoma, unspecified, unspecified site
  - CC **C83.91** Non-follicular (diffuse) lymphoma, unspecified, lymph nodes of head, face, and neck
  - CC **C83.92** Non-follicular (diffuse) lymphoma, unspecified, intrathoracic lymph nodes
  - CC **C83.93** Non-follicular (diffuse) lymphoma, unspecified, intra-abdominal lymph nodes
  - CC **C83.94** Non-follicular (diffuse) lymphoma, unspecified, lymph nodes of axilla and upper limb
  - CC **C83.95** Non-follicular (diffuse) lymphoma, unspecified, lymph nodes of inguinal region and lower limb
  - CC **C83.96** Non-follicular (diffuse) lymphoma, unspecified, intrapelvic lymph nodes
  - CC **C83.97** Non-follicular (diffuse) lymphoma, unspecified, spleen
  - CC **C83.98** Non-follicular (diffuse) lymphoma, unspecified, lymph nodes of multiple sites
  - CC **C83.99** Non-follicular (diffuse) lymphoma, unspecified, extranodal and solid organ sites

C84 Mature T/NK-cell lymphomas
  Excludes1: personal history of non-Hodgkin lymphoma (Z85.72)

+ C84.0 Mycosis fungoides
  Excludes1: peripheral T-cell lymphoma, not elsewhere classified (C84.4-)
  - CC **C84.00** Mycosis fungoides, unspecified site
  - CC **C84.01** Mycosis fungoides, lymph nodes of head, face, and neck
  - CC **C84.02** Mycosis fungoides, intrathoracic lymph nodes
  - CC **C84.03** Mycosis fungoides, intra-abdominal lymph nodes
  - CC **C84.04** Mycosis fungoides, lymph nodes of axilla and upper limb
  - CC **C84.05** Mycosis fungoides, lymph nodes of inguinal region and lower limb
  - CC **C84.06** Mycosis fungoides, intrapelvic lymph nodes
  - CC **C84.07** Mycosis fungoides, spleen
  - CC **C84.08** Mycosis fungoides, lymph nodes of multiple sites
  - CC **C84.09** Mycosis fungoides, extranodal and solid organ sites

+ C84.1 Sézary disease
  - CC **C84.10** Sézary disease, unspecified site
  - CC **C84.11** Sézary disease, lymph nodes of head, face, and neck
  - CC **C84.12** Sézary disease, intrathoracic lymph nodes
  - CC **C84.13** Sézary disease, intra-abdominal lymph nodes
  - CC **C84.14** Sézary disease, lymph nodes of axilla and upper limb
  - CC **C84.15** Sézary disease, lymph nodes of inguinal region and lower limb
  - CC **C84.16** Sézary disease, intrapelvic lymph nodes
  - CC **C84.17** Sézary disease, spleen
  - CC **C84.18** Sézary disease, lymph nodes of multiple sites
  - CC **C84.19** Sézary disease, extranodal and solid organ sites

+ C84.4 Peripheral T-cell lymphoma, not elsewhere classified
  Lennert's lymphoma
  Lymphoepithelioid lymphoma
  Mature T-cell lymphoma, not elsewhere classified
  - CC **C84.40** Peripheral T-cell lymphoma, not elsewhere classified, unspecified site
  - CC **C84.41** Peripheral T-cell lymphoma, not elsewhere classified, lymph nodes of head, face, and neck
  - CC **C84.42** Peripheral T-cell lymphoma, not elsewhere classified, intrathoracic lymph nodes
  - CC **C84.43** Peripheral T-cell lymphoma, not elsewhere classified, intra-abdominal lymph nodes

- CC **C84.44** Peripheral T-cell lymphoma, not elsewhere classified, lymph nodes of axilla and upper limb
- CC **C84.45** Peripheral T-cell lymphoma, not elsewhere classified, lymph nodes of inguinal region and lower limb
- CC **C84.46** Peripheral T-cell lymphoma, not elsewhere classified, intrapelvic lymph nodes
- CC **C84.47** Peripheral T-cell lymphoma, not elsewhere classified, spleen
- CC **C84.48** Peripheral T-cell lymphoma, not elsewhere classified, lymph nodes of multiple sites
- CC **C84.49** Peripheral T-cell lymphoma, not elsewhere classified, extranodal and solid organ sites

+ **C84.6** Anaplastic large cell lymphoma, ALK-positive
  Anaplastic large cell lymphoma, CD30-positive
  - CC **C84.60** Anaplastic large cell lymphoma, ALK-positive, unspecified site
  - CC **C84.61** Anaplastic large cell lymphoma, ALK-positive, lymph nodes of head, face, and neck
  - CC **C84.62** Anaplastic large cell lymphoma, ALK-positive, intrathoracic lymph nodes
  - CC **C84.63** Anaplastic large cell lymphoma, ALK-positive, intra-abdominal lymph nodes
  - CC **C84.64** Anaplastic large cell lymphoma, ALK-positive, lymph nodes of axilla and upper limb
  - CC **C84.65** Anaplastic large cell lymphoma, ALK-positive, lymph nodes of inguinal region and lower limb
  - CC **C84.66** Anaplastic large cell lymphoma, ALK-positive, intrapelvic lymph nodes
  - CC **C84.67** Anaplastic large cell lymphoma, ALK-positive, spleen
  - CC **C84.68** Anaplastic large cell lymphoma, ALK-positive, lymph nodes of multiple sites
  - CC **C84.69** Anaplastic large cell lymphoma, ALK-positive, extranodal and solid organ sites

+ **C84.7** Anaplastic large cell lymphoma, ALK-negative
  Excludes1: *primary cutaneous CD30-positive T-cell proliferations (C86.6-)*
  - CC **C84.70** Anaplastic large cell lymphoma, ALK-negative, unspecified site
  - CC **C84.71** Anaplastic large cell lymphoma, ALK-negative, lymph nodes of head, face, and neck
  - CC **C84.72** Anaplastic large cell lymphoma, ALK-negative, intrathoracic lymph nodes
  - CC **C84.73** Anaplastic large cell lymphoma, ALK-negative, intra-abdominal lymph nodes
  - CC **C84.74** Anaplastic large cell lymphoma, ALK-negative, lymph nodes of axilla and upper limb
  - CC **C84.75** Anaplastic large cell lymphoma, ALK-negative, lymph nodes of inguinal region and lower limb
  - CC **C84.76** Anaplastic large cell lymphoma, ALK-negative, intrapelvic lymph nodes
  - CC **C84.77** Anaplastic large cell lymphoma, ALK-negative, spleen
  - CC **C84.78** Anaplastic large cell lymphoma, ALK-negative, lymph nodes of multiple sites
  - CC **C84.79** Anaplastic large cell lymphoma, ALK-negative, extranodal and solid organ sites
  - CC **C84.7A** Anaplastic large cell lymphoma, ALK-negative, breast
    Breast implant associated anaplastic large cell lymphoma (BIA-ALCL)
    Use additional code to identify:
    breast implant status (Z98.82)
    personal history of breast implant removal (Z98.86)
    AHA CC: 4Q, 2021, 6

+ **C84.A** Cutaneous T-cell lymphoma, unspecified
  - CC **C84.A0** Cutaneous T-cell lymphoma, unspecified, unspecified site
  - CC **C84.A1** Cutaneous T-cell lymphoma, unspecified lymph nodes of head, face, and neck
  - CC **C84.A2** Cutaneous T-cell lymphoma, unspecified, intrathoracic lymph nodes
  - CC **C84.A3** Cutaneous T-cell lymphoma, unspecified, intra-abdominal lymph nodes
  - CC **C84.A4** Cutaneous T-cell lymphoma, unspecified, lymph nodes of axilla and upper limb
  - CC **C84.A5** Cutaneous T-cell lymphoma, unspecified, lymph nodes of inguinal region and lower limb
  - CC **C84.A6** Cutaneous T-cell lymphoma, unspecified, intrapelvic lymph nodes
  - CC **C84.A7** Cutaneous T-cell lymphoma, unspecified, spleen
    AHA CC: 2Q, 2021, 6-7
  - CC **C84.A8** Cutaneous T-cell lymphoma, unspecified, lymph nodes of multiple sites
    AHA CC: 2Q, 2021, 6-7
  - CC **C84.A9** Cutaneous T-cell lymphoma, unspecified, extranodal and solid organ sites

+ **C84.Z** Other mature T/NK-cell lymphomas
  NOTE If T-cell lineage or involvement is mentioned in conjunction with a specific lymphoma, code to the more specific description.
  Excludes1: *angioimmunoblastic T-cell lymphoma (C86.5)*
  blastic NK-cell lymphoma (C86.4)
  enteropathy-type T-cell lymphoma (C86.2)
  extranodal NK-cell lymphoma, nasal type (C86.0)
  hepatosplenic T-cell lymphoma (C86.1)
  primary cutaneous CD30-positive T-cell proliferations (C86.6)
  subcutaneous panniculitis-like T-cell lymphoma (C86.3)
  T-cell leukemia (C91.1-)
  - CC **C84.Z0** Other mature T/NK-cell lymphomas, unspecified site
  - CC **C84.Z1** Other mature T/NK-cell lymphomas, lymph nodes of head, face, and neck
  - CC **C84.Z2** Other mature T/NK-cell lymphomas, intrathoracic lymph nodes
  - CC **C84.Z3** Other mature T/NK-cell lymphomas, intra-abdominal lymph nodes
  - CC **C84.Z4** Other mature T/NK-cell lymphomas, lymph nodes of axilla and upper limb
  - CC **C84.Z5** Other mature T/NK-cell lymphomas, lymph nodes of inguinal region and lower limb
  - CC **C84.Z6** Other mature T/NK-cell lymphomas, intrapelvic lymph nodes
  - CC **C84.Z7** Other mature T/NK-cell lymphomas, spleen
  - CC **C84.Z8** Other mature T/NK-cell lymphomas, lymph nodes of multiple sites
  - CC **C84.Z9** Other mature T/NK-cell lymphomas, extranodal and solid organ sites

+ **C84.9** Mature T/NK-cell lymphomas, unspecified
  NK/T cell lymphoma NOS
  Excludes1: *mature T-cell lymphoma, not elsewhere classified (C84.4-)*
  - CC **C84.90** Mature T/NK-cell lymphomas, unspecified, unspecified site
  - CC **C84.91** Mature T/NK-cell lymphomas, unspecified, lymph nodes of head, face, and neck
  - CC **C84.92** Mature T/NK-cell lymphomas, unspecified, intrathoracic lymph nodes
  - CC **C84.93** Mature T/NK-cell lymphomas, unspecified, intra-abdominal lymph nodes
  - CC **C84.94** Mature T/NK-cell lymphomas, unspecified, lymph nodes of axilla and upper limb
  - CC **C84.95** Mature T/NK-cell lymphomas, unspecified, lymph nodes of inguinal region and lower limb
  - CC **C84.96** Mature T/NK-cell lymphomas, unspecified, intrapelvic lymph nodes
  - CC **C84.97** Mature T/NK-cell lymphomas, unspecified, spleen
  - CC **C84.98** Mature T/NK-cell lymphomas, unspecified, lymph nodes of multiple sites
  - CC **C84.99** Mature T/NK-cell lymphomas, unspecified, extranodal and solid organ sites

C85 Other specified and unspecified types of non-Hodgkin lymphoma
  Excludes1: *other specified types of T/NK-cell lymphoma (C86.-)*
  personal history of non-Hodgkin lymphoma (Z85.72)

+ **C85.1** Unspecified B-cell lymphoma
  NOTE If B-cell lineage or involvement is mentioned in conjunction with a specific lymphoma, code to the more specific description.
  - CC **C85.10** Unspecified B-cell lymphoma, unspecified site
  - CC **C85.11** Unspecified B-cell lymphoma, lymph nodes of head, face, and neck
  - CC **C85.12** Unspecified B-cell lymphoma, intrathoracic lymph nodes
  - CC **C85.13** Unspecified B-cell lymphoma, intra-abdominal lymph nodes

- CC **C85.14** Unspecified B-cell lymphoma, lymph nodes of axilla and upper limb
- CC **C85.15** Unspecified B-cell lymphoma, lymph nodes of inguinal region and lower limb
- CC **C85.16** Unspecified B-cell lymphoma, intrapelvic lymph nodes
- CC **C85.17** Unspecified B-cell lymphoma, spleen
- CC **C85.18** Unspecified B-cell lymphoma, lymph nodes of multiple sites
- CC **C85.19** Unspecified B-cell lymphoma, extranodal and solid organ sites

+ **C85.2** Mediastinal (thymic) large B-cell lymphoma
- CC **C85.20** Mediastinal (thymic) large B-cell lymphoma, unspecified site
- CC **C85.21** Mediastinal (thymic) large B-cell lymphoma, lymph nodes of head, face, and neck
- CC **C85.22** Mediastinal (thymic) large B-cell lymphoma, intrathoracic lymph nodes
- CC **C85.23** Mediastinal (thymic) large B-cell lymphoma, intra-abdominal lymph nodes
- CC **C85.24** Mediastinal (thymic) large B-cell lymphoma, lymph nodes of axilla and upper limb
- CC **C85.25** Mediastinal (thymic) large B-cell lymphoma, lymph nodes of inguinal region and lower limb
- CC **C85.26** Mediastinal (thymic) large B-cell lymphoma, intrapelvic lymph nodes
- CC **C85.27** Mediastinal (thymic) large B-cell lymphoma, spleen
- CC **C85.28** Mediastinal (thymic) large B-cell lymphoma, lymph nodes of multiple sites
- CC **C85.29** Mediastinal (thymic) large B-cell lymphoma, extranodal and solid organ sites

+ **C85.8** Other specified types of non-Hodgkin lymphoma
- CC **C85.80** Other specified types of non-Hodgkin lymphoma, unspecified site
- CC **C85.81** Other specified types of non-Hodgkin lymphoma, lymph nodes of head, face, and neck
- CC **C85.82** Other specified types of non-Hodgkin lymphoma, intrathoracic lymph nodes
- CC **C85.83** Other specified types of non-Hodgkin lymphoma, intra-abdominal lymph nodes
- CC **C85.84** Other specified types of non-Hodgkin lymphoma, lymph nodes of axilla and upper limb
- CC **C85.85** Other specified types of non-Hodgkin lymphoma, lymph nodes of inguinal region and lower limb
- CC **C85.86** Other specified types of non-Hodgkin lymphoma, intrapelvic lymph nodes
- CC **C85.87** Other specified types of non-Hodgkin lymphoma, spleen
- CC **C85.88** Other specified types of non-Hodgkin lymphoma, lymph nodes of multiple sites
- CC **C85.89** Other specified types of non-Hodgkin lymphoma, extranodal and solid organ sites

+ **C85.9** Non-Hodgkin lymphoma, unspecified
  Lymphoma NOS
  Malignant lymphoma NOS
  Non-Hodgkin lymphoma NOS
- CC **C85.90** Non-Hodgkin lymphoma, unspecified, unspecified site
- CC **C85.91** Non-Hodgkin lymphoma, unspecified, lymph nodes of head, face, and neck
- CC **C85.92** Non-Hodgkin lymphoma, unspecified, intrathoracic lymph nodes
- CC **C85.93** Non-Hodgkin lymphoma, unspecified, intra-abdominal lymph nodes
- CC **C85.94** Non-Hodgkin lymphoma, unspecified, lymph nodes of axilla and upper limb
- CC **C85.95** Non-Hodgkin lymphoma, unspecified, lymph nodes of inguinal region and lower limb
- CC **C85.96** Non-Hodgkin lymphoma, unspecified, intrapelvic lymph nodes
- CC **C85.97** Non-Hodgkin lymphoma, unspecified, spleen
- CC **C85.98** Non-Hodgkin lymphoma, unspecified, lymph nodes of multiple sites
- CC **C85.99** Non-Hodgkin lymphoma, unspecified, extranodal and solid organ sites

C86 Other specified types of T/NK-cell lymphoma

Excludes1: anaplastic large cell lymphoma, ALK negative (C84.7-)
anaplastic large cell lymphoma, ALK positive (C84.6-)
mature T/NK-cell lymphomas (C84.-)
other specified types of non-Hodgkin lymphoma (C85.8-)

- CC **C86.0** Extranodal NK/T-cell lymphoma, nasal type
- CC **C86.1** Hepatosplenic T-cell lymphoma
  Alpha-beta and gamma delta types
- CC **C86.2** Enteropathy-type (intestinal) T-cell lymphoma
  Enteropathy associated T-cell lymphoma
- CC **C86.3** Subcutaneous panniculitis-like T-cell lymphoma
- CC **C86.4** Blastic NK-cell lymphoma
  Blastic plasmacytoid dendritic cell neoplasm (BPDCN)
- CC **C86.5** Angioimmunoblastic T-cell lymphoma
  Angioimmunoblastic lymphadenopathy with dysproteinemia (AILD)
- CC **C86.6** Primary cutaneous CD30-positive T-cell proliferations
  Lymphomatoid papulosis
  Primary cutaneous anaplastic large cell lymphoma
  Primary cutaneous CD30-positive large T-cell lymphoma

C88 Malignant immunoproliferative diseases and certain other B-cell lymphomas

Excludes1: B-cell lymphoma, unspecified (C85.1-)
personal history of other malignant neoplasms of lymphoid, hematopoietic and related tissues (Z85.79)

- **C88.0** Waldenström macroglobulinemia
  Lymphoplasmacytic lymphoma with IgM-production
  Macroglobulinemia (idiopathic) (primary)
  Excludes1: small cell B-cell lymphoma (C83.0)
- CC **C88.2** Heavy chain disease
  Franklin disease
  Gamma heavy chain disease
  Mu heavy chain disease
- CC **C88.3** Immunoproliferative small intestinal disease
  Alpha heavy chain disease
  Mediterranean lymphoma
- CC **C88.4** Extranodal marginal zone B-cell lymphoma of mucosa-associated lymphoid tissue [MALT-lymphoma]
  Lymphoma of skin-associated lymphoid tissue [SALT-lymphoma]
  Lymphoma of bronchial-associated lymphoid tissue [BALT-lymphoma]
  Excludes1: high malignant (diffuse large B-cell) lymphoma (C83.3-)
- CC **C88.8** Other malignant immunoproliferative diseases
- CC **C88.9** Malignant immunoproliferative disease, unspecified
  Immunoproliferative disease NOS

C90 Multiple myeloma and malignant plasma cell neoplasms

Excludes1: personal history of other malignant neoplasms of lymphoid, hematopoietic and related tissues (Z85.79)

+ **C90.0** Multiple myeloma
  Kahler's disease
  Medullary plasmacytoma
  Myelomatosis
  Plasma cell myeloma
  Excludes1: solitary myeloma (C90.3-)
  solitary plasmactyoma (C90.3-)
- CC **C90.00** Multiple myeloma not having achieved remission
  Multiple myeloma with failed remission
  Multiple myeloma NOS
  AHA CC: 4Q, 2020, 11-12, 14
- CC **C90.01** Multiple myeloma in remission
- CC **C90.02** Multiple myeloma in relapse

+ **C90.1** Plasma cell leukemia
  Plasmacytic leukemia
- CC **C90.10** Plasma cell leukemia not having achieved remission
  Plasma cell leukemia with failed remission
  Plasma cell leukemia NOS
  AHA CC: 2Q, 2019, 30
- CC **C90.11** Plasma cell leukemia in remission
- CC **C90.12** Plasma cell leukemia in relapse

- **C90.2 Extramedullary plasmacytoma**
  - CC **C90.20 Extramedullary plasmacytoma not having achieved remission**
    - Extramedullary plasmacytoma with failed remission
    - Extramedullary plasmacytoma NOS
  - CC **C90.21 Extramedullary plasmacytoma in remission**
  - CC **C90.22 Extramedullary plasmacytoma in relapse**
- **C90.3 Solitary plasmacytoma**
  - Localized malignant plasma cell tumor NOS
  - Plasmacytoma NOS
  - Solitary myeloma
  - CC **C90.30 Solitary plasmacytoma not having achieved remission**
    - Solitary plasmacytoma with failed remission
    - Solitary plasmacytoma NOS
  - CC **C90.31 Solitary plasmacytoma in remission**
  - CC **C90.32 Solitary plasmacytoma in relapse**

C91 Lymphoid leukemia

Excludes1: personal history of leukemia (Z85.6)

- **C91.0 Acute lymphoblastic leukemia [ALL]**
  - NOTE: Codes in subcategory C91.0- should only be used for T-cell and B-cell precursor leukemia
  - CC **C91.00 Acute lymphoblastic leukemia not having achieved remission**
    - Acute lymphoblastic leukemia with failed remission
    - Acute lymphoblastic leukemia NOS
    - AHA CC: 4Q, 2020, 14-15; 1Q, 2022, 16-17
  - CC **C91.01 Acute lymphoblastic leukemia, in remission**
  - CC **C91.02 Acute lymphoblastic leukemia, in relapse**
- **C91.1 Chronic lymphocytic leukemia of B-cell type**
  - Lymphoplasmacytic leukemia
  - Richter syndrome
  - *Excludes1:* lymphoplasmacytic lymphoma (C83.0-)
  - CC **C91.10 Chronic lymphocytic leukemia of B-cell type not having achieved remission**
    - Chronic lymphocytic leukemia of B-cell type with failed remission
    - Chronic lymphocytic leukemia of B-cell type NOS
  - CC **C91.11 Chronic lymphocytic leukemia of B-cell type in remission**
  - CC **C91.12 Chronic lymphocytic leukemia of B-cell type in relapse**
    - AHA CC: 1Q, 2023, 18-19
- **C91.3 Prolymphocytic leukemia of B-cell type**
  - CC **C91.30 Prolymphocytic leukemia of B-cell type not having achieved remission**
    - Prolymphocytic leukemia of B-cell type with failed remission
    - Prolymphocytic leukemia of B-cell type NOS
  - CC **C91.31 Prolymphocytic leukemia of B-cell type, in remission**
  - CC **C91.32 Prolymphocytic leukemia of B-cell type, in relapse**
- **C91.4 Hairy cell leukemia**
  - Leukemic reticuloendotheliosis
  - CC **C91.40 Hairy cell leukemia not having achieved remission**
    - Hairy cell leukemia with failed remission
    - Hairy cell leukemia NOS
  - CC **C91.41 Hairy cell leukemia, in remission**
  - CC **C91.42 Hairy cell leukemia, in relapse**
- **C91.5 Adult T-cell lymphoma/leukemia (HTLV-1-associated)**
  - Acute variant of adult T-cell lymphoma/leukemia (HTLV-1-associated)
  - Chronic variant of adult T-cell lymphoma/leukemia (HTLV-1-associated)
  - Lymphomatoid variant of adult T-cell lymphoma/leukemia (HTLV-1-associated)
  - Smouldering variant of adult T-cell lymphoma/leukemia (HTLV-1-associated)
  - • CC **C91.50 Adult T-cell lymphoma/leukemia (HTLV-1-associated) not having achieved remission**
    - Adult T-cell lymphoma/leukemia (HTLV-1-associated) with failed remission
    - Adult T-cell lymphoma/leukemia (HTLV-1-associated) NOS
  - • CC **C91.51 Adult T-cell lymphoma/leukemia (HTLV-1-associated), in remission**
  - • CC **C91.52 Adult T-cell lymphoma/leukemia (HTLV-1-associated), in relapse**
- **C91.6 Prolymphocytic leukemia of T-cell type**
  - CC **C91.60 Prolymphocytic leukemia of T-cell type not having achieved remission**
    - Prolymphocytic leukemia of T-cell type with failed remission
    - Prolymphocytic leukemia of T-cell type NOS
  - CC **C91.61 Prolymphocytic leukemia of T-cell type, in remission**
  - CC **C91.62 Prolymphocytic leukemia of T-cell type, in relapse**
- **C91.A Mature B-cell leukemia Burkitt-type**
  - *Excludes1:* Burkitt lymphoma (C83.7-)
  - CC **C91.A0 Mature B-cell leukemia Burkitt-type not having achieved remission**
    - Mature B-cell leukemia Burkitt-type with failed remission
    - Mature B-cell leukemia Burkitt-type NOS
  - CC **C91.A1 Mature B-cell leukemia Burkitt-type, in remission**
  - CC **C91.A2 Mature B-cell leukemia Burkitt-type, in relapse**
- **C91.Z Other lymphoid leukemia**
  - T-cell large granular lymphocytic leukemia (associated with rheumatoid arthritis)
  - CC **C91.Z0 Other lymphoid leukemia not having achieved remission**
    - Other lymphoid leukemia with failed remission
    - Other lymphoid leukemia NOS
    - AHA CC: 2Q, 2019, 24-26
  - CC **C91.Z1 Other lymphoid leukemia, in remission**
  - CC **C91.Z2 Other lymphoid leukemia, in relapse**
- **C91.9 Lymphoid leukemia, unspecified**
  - CC **C91.90 Lymphoid leukemia, unspecified not having achieved remission**
    - Lymphoid leukemia with failed remission
    - Lymphoid leukemia NOS
  - CC **C91.91 Lymphoid leukemia, unspecified, in remission**
  - CC **C91.92 Lymphoid leukemia, unspecified, in relapse**

C92 Myeloid leukemia

Code also, if applicable, pancytopenia (acquired) (D61.818)
Includes: granulocytic leukemia
myelogenous leukemia
Excludes1: personal history of leukemia (Z85.6)
AHA CC: 1Q, 2019, 16-17

- **C92.0 Acute myeloblastic leukemia**
  - Acute myeloblastic leukemia, minimal differentiation
  - Acute myeloblastic leukemia (with maturation)
  - Acute myeloblastic leukemia 1/ETO
  - Acute myeloblastic leukemia M0
  - Acute myeloblastic leukemia M1
  - Acute myeloblastic leukemia M2
  - Acute myeloblastic leukemia with t(8;21)
  - Acute myeloblastic leukemia (without a FAB classification) NOS
  - Refractory anemia with excess blasts in transformation [RAEB T]
  - *Excludes1:* acute exacerbation of chronic myeloid leukemia (C92.10)
    refractory anemia with excess of blasts not in transformation (D46.2-)
  - AHA CC: 4Q, 2018, 87
  - CC **C92.00 Acute myeloblastic leukemia, not having achieved remission**
    - Acute myeloblastic leukemia with failed remission
    - Acute myeloblastic leukemia NOS
  - CC **C92.01 Acute myeloblastic leukemia, in remission**
    - AHA CC: 3Q, 2021, 4
  - CC **C92.02 Acute myeloblastic leukemia, in relapse**
    - AHA CC: 1Q, 2023, 23

- **C92.1 Chronic myeloid leukemia, BCR/ABL-positive**
  Chronic myelogenous leukemia, Philadelphia chromosome (Ph1) positive
  Chronic myelogenous leukemia, t(9;22) (q34;q11)
  Chronic myelogenous leukemia with crisis of blast cells
  Excludes1: atypical chronic myeloid leukemia BCR/ABL-negative (C92.2-)
   chronic myelomonocytic leukemia (C93.1-)
   chronic myeloproliferative disease (D47.1)
  - CC **C92.10 Chronic myeloid leukemia, BCR/ABL-positive, not having achieved remission**
    Chronic myeloid leukemia, BCR/ABL-positive with failed remission
    Chronic myeloid leukemia, BCR/ABL-positive NOS
    AHA CC: 1Q, 2017, 7
  - CC **C92.11 Chronic myeloid leukemia, BCR/ABL-positive, in remission**
  - CC **C92.12 Chronic myeloid leukemia, BCR/ABL-positive, in relapse**
- **C92.2 Atypical chronic myeloid leukemia, BCR/ABL-negative**
  - CC **C92.20 Atypical chronic myeloid leukemia, BCR/ABL-negative, not having achieved remission**
    Atypical chronic myeloid leukemia, BCR/ABL-negative with failed remission
    Atypical chronic myeloid leukemia, BCR/ABL-negative NOS
  - CC **C92.21 Atypical chronic myeloid leukemia, BCR/ABL-negative, in remission**
  - CC **C92.22 Atypical chronic myeloid leukemia, BCR/ABL-negative, in relapse**
- **C92.3 Myeloid sarcoma**
  A malignant tumor of immature myeloid cells
  Chloroma
  Granulocytic sarcoma
  - CC **C92.30 Myeloid sarcoma, not having achieved remission**
    Myeloid sarcoma with failed remission
    Myeloid sarcoma NOS
  - CC **C92.31 Myeloid sarcoma, in remission**
  - CC **C92.32 Myeloid sarcoma, in relapse**
- **C92.4 Acute promyelocytic leukemia**
  AML M3
  AML Me with t(15;17) and variants
  - CC **C92.40 Acute promyelocytic leukemia, not having achieved remission**
    Acute promyelocytic leukemia with failed remission
    Acute promyelocytic leukemia NOS
  - CC **C92.41 Acute promyelocytic leukemia, in remission**
  - CC **C92.42 Acute promyelocytic leukemia, in relapse**
- **C92.5 Acute myelomonocytic leukemia**
  AML M4
  AML M4 Eo with inv(16) or t(16;16)
  - CC **C92.50 Acute myelomonocytic leukemia, not having achieved remission**
    Acute myelomonocytic leukemia with failed remission
    Acute myelomonocytic leukemia NOS
  - CC **C92.51 Acute myelomonocytic leukemia, in remission**
  - CC **C92.52 Acute myelomonocytic leukemia, in relapse**
- **C92.6 Acute myeloid leukemia with 11q23-abnormality**
  Acute myeloid leukemia with variation of MLL-gene
  - CC **C92.60 Acute myeloid leukemia with 11q23-abnormality not having achieved remission**
    Acute myeloid leukemia with 11q23-abnormality with failed remission
    Acute myeloid leukemia with 11q23-abnormality NOS
  - CC **C92.61 Acute myeloid leukemia with 11q23-abnormality in remission**
  - CC **C92.62 Acute myeloid leukemia with 11q23-abnormality in relapse**
- **C92.A Acute myeloid leukemia with multilineage dysplasia**
  Acute myeloid leukemia with dysplasia of remaining hematopoesis and/or myelodysplastic disease in its history
  - CC **C92.A0 Acute myeloid leukemia with multilineage dysplasia, not having achieved remission**
    Acute myeloid leukemia with multilineage dysplasia with failed remission
    Acute myeloid leukemia with multilineage dysplasia NOS
  - CC **C92.A1 Acute myeloid leukemia with multilineage dysplasia, in remission**
  - CC **C92.A2 Acute myeloid leukemia with multilineage dysplasia, in relapse**
- **C92.Z Other myeloid leukemia**
  - CC **C92.Z0 Other myeloid leukemia not having achieved remission**
    Myeloid leukemia NEC with failed remission
    Myeloid leukemia NEC
  - CC **C92.Z1 Other myeloid leukemia, in remission**
  - CC **C92.Z2 Other myeloid leukemia, in relapse**
- **C92.9 Myeloid leukemia, unspecified**
  - CC **C92.90 Myeloid leukemia, unspecified, not having achieved remission**
    Myeloid leukemia, unspecified with failed remission
    Myeloid leukemia, unspecified NOS
  - CC **C92.91 Myeloid leukemia, unspecified in remission**
  - CC **C92.92 Myeloid leukemia, unspecified in relapse**

C93 Monocytic leukemia
Includes: monocytoid leukemia
Excludes1: personal history of leukemia (Z85.6)

- **C93.0 Acute monoblastic/monocytic leukemia**
  AML M5
  AML M5a
  AML M5b
  - CC **C93.00 Acute monoblastic/monocytic leukemia, not having achieved remission**
    Acute monoblastic/monocytic leukemia with failed remission
    Acute monoblastic/monocytic leukemia NOS
  - CC **C93.01 Acute monoblastic/monocytic leukemia, in remission**
  - CC **C93.02 Acute monoblastic/monocytic leukemia, in relapse**
- **C93.1 Chronic myelomonocytic leukemia**
  Chronic monocytic leukemia
  CMML-1
  CMML-2
  CMML with eosinophilia
  Code also, if applicable, eosinophilia (D72.18)
  - CC **C93.10 Chronic myelomonocytic leukemia not having achieved remission**
    Chronic myelomonocytic leukemia with failed remission
    Chronic myelomonocytic leukemia NOS
  - CC **C93.11 Chronic myelomonocytic leukemia, in remission**
  - CC **C93.12 Chronic myelomonocytic leukemia, in relapse**
- **C93.3 Juvenile myelomonocytic leukemia**
  - CC **C93.30 Juvenile myelomonocytic leukemia, not having achieved remission**
    Juvenile myelomonocytic leukemia with failed remission
    Juvenile myelomonocytic leukemia NOS
  - CC **C93.31 Juvenile myelomonocytic leukemia, in remission**
  - CC **C93.32 Juvenile myelomonocytic leukemia, in relapse**
- **C93.Z Other monocytic leukemia**
  - CC **C93.Z0 Other monocytic leukemia, not having achieved remission**
    Other monocytic leukemia NOS
  - CC **C93.Z1 Other monocytic leukemia, in remission**
  - CC **C93.Z2 Other monocytic leukemia, in relapse**
- **C93.9 Monocytic leukemia, unspecified**
  - CC **C93.90 Monocytic leukemia, unspecified, not having achieved remission**
    Monocytic leukemia, unspecified with failed remission
    Monocytic leukemia, unspecified NOS
  - CC **C93.91 Monocytic leukemia, unspecified in remission**
  - CC **C93.92 Monocytic leukemia, unspecified in relapse**

C94 Other leukemias of specified cell type

Excludes1: leukemic reticuloendotheliosis (C91.4-)
myelodysplastic syndromes (D46.-)
personal history of leukemia (Z85.6)
plasma cell leukemia (C90.1-)

- **C94.0 Acute erythroid leukemia**
  Acute myeloid leukemia M6(a)(b)
  Erythroleukemia
  - **CC C94.00 Acute erythroid leukemia, not having achieved remission**
    Acute erythroid leukemia with failed remission
    Acute erythroid leukemia NOS
  - **CC C94.01 Acute erythroid leukemia, in remission**
  - **CC C94.02 Acute erythroid leukemia, in relapse**

- **C94.2 Acute megakaryoblastic leukemia**
  Acute myeloid leukemia M7
  Acute megakaryocytic leukemia
  - **CC C94.20 Acute megakaryoblastic leukemia not having achieved remission**
    Acute megakaryoblastic leukemia with failed remission
    Acute megakaryoblastic leukemia NOS
  - **CC C94.21 Acute megakaryoblastic leukemia, in remission**
  - **CC C94.22 Acute megakaryoblastic leukemia, in relapse**

- **C94.3 Mast cell leukemia**
  AHA CC: 4Q, 2017, 5
  - **CC C94.30 Mast cell leukemia not having achieved remission**
    Mast cell leukemia with failed remission
    Mast cell leukemia NOS
  - **CC C94.31 Mast cell leukemia, in remission**
  - **CC C94.32 Mast cell leukemia, in relapse**

- **C94.4 Acute panmyelosis with myelofibrosis**
  Acute myelofibrosis
  Excludes1: myelofibrosis NOS (D75.81)
  secondary myelofibrosis NOS (D75.81)
  - **CC C94.40 Acute panmyelosis with myelofibrosis not having achieved remission**
    Acute myelofibrosis NOS
    Acute panmyelosis with myelofibrosis with failed remission
    Acute panmyelosis NOS
  - **CC C94.41 Acute panmyelosis with myelofibrosis, in remission**
  - **CC C94.42 Acute panmyelosis with myelofibrosis, in relapse**

- **CC C94.6 Myelodysplastic disease, not elsewhere classified**
  Myelodysplastic/myeloproliferative neoplasm, unclassifiable
  Myeloproliferative disease, not elsewhere classified

- **C94.8 Other specified leukemias**
  Aggressive NK-cell leukemia
  Acute basophilic leukemia
  Code also, if applicable, eosinophilia (D72.18)
  - **CC C94.80 Other specified leukemias not having achieved remission**
    Other specified leukemia with failed remission
    Other specified leukemias NOS
  - **CC C94.81 Other specified leukemias, in remission**
  - **CC C94.82 Other specified leukemias, in relapse**

C95 Leukemia of unspecified cell type

Excludes1: personal history of leukemia (Z85.6)

- **C95.0 Acute leukemia of unspecified cell type**
  Acute bilineal leukemia
  Acute mixed lineage leukemia
  Biphenotypic acute leukemia
  Stem cell leukemia of unclear lineage
  Excludes1: acute exacerbation of unspecified chronic leukemia (C95.10)
  - **CC C95.00 Acute leukemia of unspecified cell type not having achieved remission**
    Acute leukemia of unspecified cell type with failed remission
    Acute leukemia NOS
  - **CC C95.01 Acute leukemia of unspecified cell type, in remission**
  - **CC C95.02 Acute leukemia of unspecified cell type, in relapse**

- **C95.1 Chronic leukemia of unspecified cell type**
  - **CC C95.10 Chronic leukemia of unspecified cell type not having achieved remission**
    Chronic leukemia of unspecified cell type with failed remission
    Chronic leukemia NOS
  - **CC C95.11 Chronic leukemia of unspecified cell type, in remission**
  - **CC C95.12 Chronic leukemia of unspecified cell type, in relapse**

- **C95.9 Leukemia, unspecified**
  - **CC C95.90 Leukemia, unspecified not having achieved remission**
    Leukemia, unspecified with failed remission
    Leukemia NOS
  - **CC C95.91 Leukemia, unspecified, in remission**
  - **CC C95.92 Leukemia, unspecified, in relapse**

C96 Other and unspecified malignant neoplasms of lymphoid, hematopoietic and related tissue

Excludes1: personal history of other malignant neoplasms of lymphoid, hematopoietic and related tissues (Z85.79)

- **CC C96.0 Multifocal and multisystemic (disseminated) Langerhans-cell histiocytosis**
  Histiocytosis X, multisystemic
  Letterer-Siwe disease
  Excludes1: adult pulmonary Langerhans cell histiocytosis (J84.82)
  multifocal and unisystemic Langerhans-cell histiocytosis (C96.5)
  unifocal Langerhans-cell histiocytosis (C96.6)

- **C96.2 Malignant mast cell neoplasm**
  Excludes1: indolent mastocytosis (D47.02)
  mast cell leukemia (C94.30)
  mastocytosis (congenital) (cutaneous) (Q82.2)
  AHA CC: 4Q, 2017, 5
  - **CC C96.20 Malignant mast cell neoplasm, unspecified**
  - **CC C96.21 Aggressive systemic mastocytosis**
  - **CC C96.22 Mast cell sarcoma**
  - **CC C96.29 Other malignant mast cell neoplasm**

- **CC C96.4 Sarcoma of dendritic cells (accessory cells)**
  Follicular dendritic cell sarcoma
  Interdigitating dendritic cell sarcoma
  Langerhans cell sarcoma

- **CC C96.5 Multifocal and unisystemic Langerhans-cell histiocytosis**
  Hand-Schüller-Christian disease
  Histiocytosis X, multifocal
  Excludes1: multifocal and multisystemic (disseminated) Langerhans-cell histiocytosis (C96.0)
  unifocal Langerhans-cell histiocytosis (C96.6)

- **CC C96.6 Unifocal Langerhans-cell histiocytosis**
  Eosinophilic granuloma
  Histiocytosis X, unifocal
  Histiocytosis X NOS
  Langerhans-cell histiocytosis NOS
  Excludes1: multifocal and multisysemic (disseminated) Langerhans-cell histiocytosis (C96.0)
  multifocal and unisystemic Langerhans-cell histiocytosis (C96.5)

- **CC C96.A Histiocytic sarcoma**
  Malignant histiocytosis

- **CC C96.Z Other specified malignant neoplasms of lymphoid, hematopoietic and related tissue**

- **CC C96.9 Malignant neoplasm of lymphoid, hematopoietic and related tissue, unspecified**

In situ neoplasms (D00-D09)

Includes: Bowen's disease
erythroplasia
grade III intraepithelial neoplasia
Queyrat's erythroplasia

D00 Carcinoma in situ of oral cavity, esophagus and stomach

Excludes1: melanoma in situ (D03.-)

- **D00.0 Carcinoma in situ of lip, oral cavity and pharynx**
  Use additional code to identify:
  exposure to environmental tobacco smoke (Z77.22)
  exposure to tobacco smoke in the perinatal period (P96.81)
  history of tobacco dependence (Z87.891)
  occupational exposure to environmental tobacco smoke (Z57.31)
  tobacco dependence (F17.-)
  tobacco use (Z72.0)
  Excludes1: carcinoma in situ of aryepiglottic fold or interarytenoid fold, laryngeal aspect (D02.0)
  carcinoma in situ of epiglottis NOS (D02.0)
  carcinoma in situ of epiglottis suprahyoid portion (D02.0)
  carcinoma in situ of skin of lip (D03.0, D04.0)

  - **D00.00** Carcinoma in situ of oral cavity, unspecified site
  - **D00.01** Carcinoma in situ of labial mucosa and vermilion border
  - **D00.02** Carcinoma in situ of buccal mucosa
  - **D00.03** Carcinoma in situ of gingiva and edentulous alveolar ridge
  - **D00.04** Carcinoma in situ of soft palate
  - **D00.05** Carcinoma in situ of hard palate
  - **D00.06** Carcinoma in situ of floor of mouth
  - **D00.07** Carcinoma in situ of tongue
  - **D00.08** Carcinoma in situ of pharynx
    Carcinoma in situ of aryepiglottic fold NOS
    Carcinoma in situ of hypopharyngeal aspect of aryepiglottic fold
    Carcinoma in situ of marginal zone of aryepiglottic fold

- **D00.1** Carcinoma in situ of esophagus
- **D00.2** Carcinoma in situ of stomach

D01 Carcinoma in situ of other and unspecified digestive organs

Excludes1: melanoma in situ (D03.-)

- **D01.0 Carcinoma in situ of colon**
  Excludes1: carcinoma in situ of rectosigmoid junction (D01.1)
- **D01.1** Carcinoma in situ of rectosigmoid junction
- **D01.2** Carcinoma in situ of rectum
- **D01.3** Carcinoma in situ of anus and anal canal
  Anal intraepithelial neoplasia III [AIN III]
  Severe dysplasia of anus
  Excludes1: anal intraepithelial neoplasia I and II [AIN I and AIN II] (K62.82)
  carcinoma in situ of anal margin (D04.5)
  carcinoma in situ of anal skin (D04.5)
  carcinoma in situ of perianal skin (D04.5)
- **D01.4 Carcinoma in situ of other and unspecified parts of intestine**
  Excludes1: carcinoma in situ of ampulla of Vater (D01.5)
  - **D01.40** Carcinoma in situ of unspecified part of intestine
  - **D01.49** Carcinoma in situ of other parts of intestine
- **D01.5** Carcinoma in situ of liver, gallbladder and bile ducts
  Carcinoma in situ of ampulla of Vater
- **D01.7** Carcinoma in situ of other specified digestive organs
  Carcinoma in situ of pancreas
- **D01.9** Carcinoma in situ of digestive organ, unspecified

D02 Carcinoma in situ of middle ear and respiratory system

Use additional code to identify:
exposure to environmental tobacco smoke (Z77.22)
exposure to tobacco smoke in the perinatal period (P96.81)
history of tobacco dependence (Z87.891)
occupational exposure to environmental tobacco smoke (Z57.31)
tobacco dependence (F17.-)
tobacco use (Z72.0)
Excludes1: melanoma in situ (D03.-)

- **D02.0** Carcinoma in situ of larynx
  Carcinoma in situ of aryepiglottic fold or interarytenoid fold, laryngeal aspect
  Carcinoma in situ of epiglottis (suprahyoid portion)
  Excludes1: carcinoma in situ of aryepiglottic fold or interarytenoid fold NOS (D00.08)
  carcinoma in situ of hypopharyngeal aspect (D00.08)
  carcinoma in situ of marginal zone (D00.08)
- **D02.1** Carcinoma in situ of trachea
- **D02.2 Carcinoma in situ of bronchus and lung**
  - **D02.20** Carcinoma in situ of unspecified bronchus and lung
  - **D02.21** Carcinoma in situ of right bronchus and lung
  - **D02.22** Carcinoma in situ of left bronchus and lung
- **D02.3** Carcinoma in situ of other parts of respiratory system
  Carcinoma in situ of accessory sinuses
  Carcinoma in situ of middle ear
  Carcinoma in situ of nasal cavities
  Excludes1: carcinoma in situ of ear (external) (skin) (D04.2-)
  carcinoma in situ of nose NOS (D09.8)
  carcinoma in situ of skin of nose (D04.3)
- **D02.4** Carcinoma in situ of respiratory system, unspecified

D03 Melanoma in situ

- **D03.0** Melanoma in situ of lip
- **D03.1 Melanoma in situ of eyelid, including canthus**
  - **D03.10** Melanoma in situ of unspecified eyelid, including canthus
  - **D03.11 Melanoma in situ of right eyelid, including canthus**
    - **D03.111** Melanoma in situ of right upper eyelid, including canthus
    - **D03.112** Melanoma in situ of right lower eyelid, including canthus
  - **D03.12 Melanoma in situ of left eyelid, including canthus**
    - **D03.121** Melanoma in situ of left upper eyelid, including canthus
    - **D03.122** Melanoma in situ of left lower eyelid, including canthus
- **D03.2 Melanoma in situ of ear and external auricular canal**
  - **D03.20** Melanoma in situ of unspecified ear and external auricular canal
  - **D03.21** Melanoma in situ of right ear and external auricular canal
  - **D03.22** Melanoma in situ of left ear and external auricular canal
- **D03.3 Melanoma in situ of other and unspecified parts of face**
  - **D03.30** Melanoma in situ of unspecified part of face
  - **D03.39** Melanoma in situ of other parts of face
- **D03.4** Melanoma in situ of scalp and neck
- **D03.5 Melanoma in situ of trunk**
  - **D03.51** Melanoma in situ of anal skin
    Melanoma in situ of anal margin
    Melanoma in situ of perianal skin
  - **D03.52** Melanoma in situ of breast (skin) (soft tissue)
  - **D03.59** Melanoma in situ of other part of trunk
- **D03.6 Melanoma in situ of upper limb, including shoulder**
  - **D03.60** Melanoma in situ of unspecified upper limb, including shoulder
  - **D03.61** Melanoma in situ of right upper limb, including shoulder
  - **D03.62** Melanoma in situ of left upper limb, including shoulder
- **D03.7 Melanoma in situ of lower limb, including hip**
  - **D03.70** Melanoma in situ of unspecified lower limb, including hip
  - **D03.71** Melanoma in situ of right lower limb, including hip
  - **D03.72** Melanoma in situ of left lower limb, including hip

D03.8 Melanoma in situ of other sites
　　Melanoma in situ of scrotum
　　Excludes1: carcinoma in situ of scrotum (D07.61)
D03.9 Melanoma in situ, unspecified

D04　Carcinoma in situ of skin
Excludes1: erythroplasia of Queyrat (penis) NOS (D07.4)
　　melanoma in situ (D03.-)

D04.0 Carcinoma in situ of skin of lip
　　Excludes2: carcinoma in situ of vermilion border of lip (D00.01)
+ **D04.1** Carcinoma in situ of skin of eyelid, including canthus
　　D04.10 Carcinoma in situ of skin of unspecified eyelid, including canthus
　+ **D04.11** Carcinoma in situ of skin of right eyelid, including canthus
　　　D04.111 Carcinoma in situ of skin of right upper eyelid, including canthus
　　　D04.112 Carcinoma in situ of skin of right lower eyelid, including canthus
　+ **D04.12** Carcinoma in situ of skin of left eyelid, including canthus
　　　D04.121 Carcinoma in situ of skin of left upper eyelid, including canthus
　　　D04.122 Carcinoma in situ of skin of left lower eyelid, including canthus
+ **D04.2** Carcinoma in situ of skin of ear and external auricular canal
　　D04.20 Carcinoma in situ of skin of unspecified ear and external auricular canal
　　D04.21 Carcinoma in situ of skin of right ear and external auricular canal
　　D04.22 Carcinoma in situ of skin of left ear and external auricular canal
+ **D04.3** Carcinoma in situ of skin of other and unspecified parts of face
　　D04.30 Carcinoma in situ of skin of unspecified part of face
　　D04.39 Carcinoma in situ of skin of other parts of face
D04.4 Carcinoma in situ of skin of scalp and neck
D04.5 Carcinoma in situ of skin of trunk
　　Carcinoma in situ of anal margin
　　Carcinoma in situ of anal skin
　　Carcinoma in situ of perianal skin
　　Carcinoma in situ of skin of breast
　　Excludes1: carcinoma in situ of anus NOS (D01.3)
　　　　carcinoma in situ of scrotum (D07.61)
　　　　carcinoma in situ of skin of genital organs (D07.-)
+ **D04.6** Carcinoma in situ of skin of upper limb, including shoulder
　　D04.60 Carcinoma in situ of skin of unspecified upper limb, including shoulder
　　D04.61 Carcinoma in situ of skin of right upper limb, including shoulder
　　D04.62 Carcinoma in situ of skin of left upper limb, including shoulder
+ **D04.7** Carcinoma in situ of skin of lower limb, including hip
　　D04.70 Carcinoma in situ of skin of unspecified lower limb, including hip
　　D04.71 Carcinoma in situ of skin of right lower limb, including hip
　　D04.72 Carcinoma in situ of skin of left lower limb, including hip
D04.8 Carcinoma in situ of skin of other sites
D04.9 Carcinoma in situ of skin, unspecified

D05　Carcinoma in situ of breast
Excludes1: carcinoma in situ of skin of breast (D04.5)
　　melanoma in situ of breast (skin) (D03.5)
　　Paget's disease of breast or nipple (C50.-)
+ **D05.0** Lobular carcinoma in situ of breast
　　D05.00 Lobular carcinoma in situ of unspecified breast
　　D05.01 Lobular carcinoma in situ of right breast
　　D05.02 Lobular carcinoma in situ of left breast
+ **D05.1** Intraductal carcinoma in situ of breast
　　D05.10 Intraductal carcinoma in situ of unspecified breast
　　D05.11 Intraductal carcinoma in situ of right breast
　　D05.12 Intraductal carcinoma in situ of left breast
+ **D05.8** Other specified type of carcinoma in situ of breast
　　D05.80 Other specified type of carcinoma in situ of unspecified breast
　　D05.81 Other specified type of carcinoma in situ of right breast
　　D05.82 Other specified type of carcinoma in situ of left breast
+ **D05.9** Unspecified type of carcinoma in situ of breast
　　D05.90 Unspecified type of carcinoma in situ of unspecified breast
　　D05.91 Unspecified type of carcinoma in situ of right breast
　　D05.92 Unspecified type of carcinoma in situ of left breast

D06　Carcinoma in situ of cervix uteri
Includes: cervical adenocarcinoma in situ
　　cervical intraepithelial glandular neoplasia
　　cervical intraepithelial neoplasia III [CIN III]
　　severe dysplasia of cervix uteri
Excludes1: cervical intraepithelial neoplasia II [CIN II] (N87.1)
　　cytologic evidence of malignancy of cervix without histologic confirmation (R87.614)
　　high grade squamous intraepithelial lesion (HGSIL) of cervix (R87.613)
　　melanoma in situ of cervix (D03.5)
　　moderate cervical dysplasia (N87.1)
♀ **D06.0** Carcinoma in situ of endocervix
♀ **D06.1** Carcinoma in situ of exocervix
♀ **D06.7** Carcinoma in situ of other parts of cervix
♀ **D06.9** Carcinoma in situ of cervix, unspecified

D07　Carcinoma in situ of other and unspecified genital organs
Excludes1: melanoma in situ of trunk (D03.5)
♀ **D07.0** Carcinoma in situ of endometrium
♀ **D07.1** Carcinoma in situ of vulva
　　Severe dysplasia of vulva
　　Vulvar intraepithelial neoplasia III [VIN III]
　　Excludes1: moderate dysplasia of vulva (N90.1)
　　　　vulvar intraepithelial neoplasia II [VIN II] (N90.1)
♀ **D07.2** Carcinoma in situ of vagina
　　Severe dysplasia of vagina
　　Vaginal intraepithelial neoplasia III [VAIN III]
　　Excludes1: moderate dysplasia of vagina (N89.1)
　　　　vaginal intraepithelial neoplasia II [VIN II] (N89.1)
+ **D07.3** Carcinoma in situ of other and unspecified female genital organs
　♀ **D07.30** Carcinoma in situ of unspecified female genital organs
　♀ **D07.39** Carcinoma in situ of other female genital organs
♂ **D07.4** Carcinoma in situ of penis
　　Erythroplasia of Queyrat NOS
♂ **D07.5** Carcinoma in situ of prostate
　　Prostatic intraepithelial neoplasia III (PIN III)
　　Severe dysplasia of prostate
　　Excludes1: dysplasia (mild) (moderate) of prostate (N42.3-)
　　　　prostatic intraepithelial neoplasia II [PIN II] (N42.3-)
+ **D07.6** Carcinoma in situ of other and unspecified male genital organs
　♂ **D07.60** Carcinoma in situ of unspecified male genital organs
　♂ **D07.61** Carcinoma in situ of scrotum
　♂ **D07.69** Carcinoma in situ of other male genital organs

D09　Carcinoma in situ of other and unspecified sites
Excludes1: melanoma in situ (D03.-)
D09.0 Carcinoma in situ of bladder
+ **D09.1** Carcinoma in situ of other and unspecified urinary organs
　　D09.10 Carcinoma in situ of unspecified urinary organ
　　D09.19 Carcinoma in situ of other urinary organs
+ **D09.2** Carcinoma in situ of eye
　　Excludes1: carcinoma in situ of skin of eyelid (D04.1-)
　　D09.20 Carcinoma in situ of unspecified eye
　　D09.21 Carcinoma in situ of right eye
　　D09.22 Carcinoma in situ of left eye
D09.3 Carcinoma in situ of thyroid and other endocrine glands
　　Excludes1: carcinoma in situ of endocrine pancreas (D01.7)
　　　　carcinoma in situ of ovary (D07.39)
　　　　carcinoma in situ of testis (D07.69)
D09.8 Carcinoma in situ of other specified sites
D09.9 Carcinoma in situ, unspecified

Benign neoplasms, except benign neuroendocrine tumors (D10-D36)

D10 Benign neoplasm of mouth and pharynx

- **D10.0** Benign neoplasm of lip
  Benign neoplasm of lip (frenulum) (inner aspect) (mucosa) (vermilion border)
  Excludes1: benign neoplasm of skin of lip (D22.0, D23.0)
- **D10.1** Benign neoplasm of tongue
  Benign neoplasm of lingual tonsil
- **D10.2** Benign neoplasm of floor of mouth
- + **D10.3** Benign neoplasm of other and unspecified parts of mouth
  - **D10.30** Benign neoplasm of unspecified part of mouth
  - **D10.39** Benign neoplasm of other parts of mouth
    Benign neoplasm of minor salivary gland NOS
    Excludes1: benign odontogenic neoplasms (D16.4-D16.5)
    benign neoplasm of mucosa of lip (D10.0)
    benign neoplasm of nasopharyngeal surface of soft palate (D10.6)
- **D10.4** Benign neoplasm of tonsil
  Benign neoplasm of tonsil (faucial) (palatine)
  Excludes1: benign neoplasm of lingual tonsil (D10.1)
  benign neoplasm of pharyngeal tonsil (D10.6)
  benign neoplasm of tonsillar fossa (D10.5)
  benign neoplasm of tonsillar pillars (D10.5)
- **D10.5** Benign neoplasm of other parts of oropharynx
  Benign neoplasm of epiglottis, anterior aspect
  Benign neoplasm of tonsillar fossa
  Benign neoplasm of tonsillar pillars
  Benign neoplasm of vallecula
  Excludes1: benign neoplasm of epiglottis NOS (D14.1)
  benign neoplasm of epiglottis, suprahyoid portion (D14.1)
- **D10.6** Benign neoplasm of nasopharynx
  Benign neoplasm of pharyngeal tonsil
  Benign neoplasm of posterior margin of septum and choanae
- **D10.7** Benign neoplasm of hypopharynx
- **D10.9** Benign neoplasm of pharynx, unspecified

D11 Benign neoplasm of major salivary glands

Excludes1: benign neoplasms of specified minor salivary glands which are classified according to their anatomical location
benign neoplasms of minor salivary glands NOS (D10.39)

- **D11.0** Benign neoplasm of parotid gland
- **D11.7** Benign neoplasm of other major salivary glands
  Benign neoplasm of sublingual salivary gland
  Benign neoplasm of submandibular salivary gland
- **D11.9** Benign neoplasm of major salivary gland, unspecified

D12 Benign neoplasm of colon, rectum, anus and anal canal

Excludes2: benign carcinoid tumors of the large intestine, and rectum (D3A.02-)
polyp of colon NOS (K63.5)

- **D12.0** Benign neoplasm of cecum
  Benign neoplasm of ileocecal valve
  AHA CC: 3Q, 2018, 22
- **D12.1** Benign neoplasm of appendix
  Excludes1: benign carcinoid tumor of the appendix (D3A.020)
- **D12.2** Benign neoplasm of ascending colon
  AHA CC: 2Q, 2018, 14
- **D12.3** Benign neoplasm of transverse colon
  Benign neoplasm of hepatic flexure
  Benign neoplasm of splenic flexure
- **D12.4** Benign neoplasm of descending colon
- **D12.5** Benign neoplasm of sigmoid colon
- **D12.6** Benign neoplasm of colon, unspecified
  Adenomatosis of colon
  Benign neoplasm of large intestine NOS
  Polyposis (hereditary) of colon
  Excludes1: inflammatory polyp of colon (K51.4-)
  AHA CC: 1Q, 2017, 8-9
- **D12.7** Benign neoplasm of rectosigmoid junction
- **D12.8** Benign neoplasm of rectum
  Excludes1: benign carcinoid tumor of the rectum (D3A.026)
  AHA CC: 1Q, 2018, 6-7
- **D12.9** Benign neoplasm of anus and anal canal
  Benign neoplasm of anus NOS
  Excludes1: benign neoplasm of anal margin (D22.5, D23.5)
  benign neoplasm of anal skin (D22.5, D23.5)
  benign neoplasm of perianal skin (D22.5, D23.5)

D13 Benign neoplasm of other and ill-defined parts of digestive system

Excludes1: benign stromal tumors of digestive system (D21.4)

- **D13.0** Benign neoplasm of esophagus
- **D13.1** Benign neoplasm of stomach
  Excludes1: benign carcinoid tumor of the stomach (D3A.092)
- **D13.2** Benign neoplasm of duodenum
  Excludes1: benign carcinoid tumor of the duodenum (D3A.010)
- + **D13.3** Benign neoplasm of other and unspecified parts of small intestine
  Excludes1: benign carcinoid tumors of the small intestine (D3A.01-)
  benign neoplasm of ileocecal valve (D12.0)
  - **D13.30** Benign neoplasm of unspecified part of small intestine
  - **D13.39** Benign neoplasm of other parts of small intestine
- **D13.4** Benign neoplasm of liver
  Benign neoplasm of intrahepatic bile ducts
- **D13.5** Benign neoplasm of extrahepatic bile ducts
- **D13.6** Benign neoplasm of pancreas
  Excludes1: benign neoplasm of endocrine pancreas (D13.7)
- **D13.7** Benign neoplasm of endocrine pancreas
  Islet cell tumor
  Benign neoplasm of islets of Langerhans
  Use additional code to identify any functional activity.
- + **D13.9** Benign neoplasm of ill-defined sites within the digestive system
  - **D13.91** Familial adenomatous polyposis
    Code also associated conditions, such as:
    benign neoplasm of colon (D12.6)
    malignant neoplasm of colon (C18.-)
  - **D13.99** Benign neoplasm of ill-defined sites within the digestive system
    Benign neoplasm of digestive system NOS
    Benign neoplasm of intestine NOS
    Benign neoplasm of spleen

D14 Benign neoplasm of middle ear and respiratory system

- **D14.0** Benign neoplasm of middle ear, nasal cavity and accessory sinuses
  Benign neoplasm of cartilage of nose
  Excludes1: benign neoplasm of auricular canal (external) (D22.2-, D23.2-)
  benign neoplasm of bone of ear (D16.4)
  benign neoplasm of bone of nose (D16.4)
  benign neoplasm of cartilage of ear (D21.0)
  benign neoplasm of ear (external)(skin) (D22.2-, D23.2-)
  benign neoplasm of nose NOS (D36.7)
  benign neoplasm of skin of nose (D22.39, D23.39)
  benign neoplasm of olfactory bulb (D33.3)
  benign neoplasm of posterior margin of septum and choanae (D10.6)
  polyp of accessory sinus (J33.8)
  polyp of ear (middle) (H74.4)
  polyp of nasal (cavity) (J33.-)
- **D14.1** Benign neoplasm of larynx
  Adenomatous polyp of larynx
  Benign neoplasm of epiglottis (suprahyoid portion)
  Excludes1: benign neoplasm of epiglottis, anterior aspect (D10.5)
  polyp (nonadenomatous) of vocal cord or larynx (J38.1)
- **D14.2** Benign neoplasm of trachea

- **+ D14.3** Benign neoplasm of bronchus and lung
  - *Excludes1:* benign carcinoid tumor of the bronchus and lung (D3A.090)
  - **D14.30** Benign neoplasm of unspecified bronchus and lung
  - **D14.31** Benign neoplasm of right bronchus and lung
  - **D14.32** Benign neoplasm of left bronchus and lung
- **D14.4** Benign neoplasm of respiratory system, unspecified

D15 Benign neoplasm of other and unspecified intrathoracic organs
Excludes1: benign neoplasm of mesothelial tissue (D19.-)
- **D15.0** Benign neoplasm of thymus
  - *Excludes1:* benign carcinoid tumor of the thymus (D3A.091)
- **D15.1** Benign neoplasm of heart
  - *Excludes1:* benign neoplasm of great vessels (D21.3)
- **D15.2** Benign neoplasm of mediastinum
- **D15.7** Benign neoplasm of other specified intrathoracic organs
- **D15.9** Benign neoplasm of intrathoracic organ, unspecified

D16 Benign neoplasm of bone and articular cartilage
Excludes1: benign neoplasm of connective tissue of ear (D21.0)
benign neoplasm of connective tissue of eyelid (D21.0)
benign neoplasm of connective tissue of larynx (D14.1)
benign neoplasm of connective tissue of nose (D14.0)
benign neoplasm of synovia (D21.-)
- **+ D16.0** Benign neoplasm of scapula and long bones of upper limb
  - **D16.00** Benign neoplasm of scapula and long bones of unspecified upper limb
  - **D16.01** Benign neoplasm of scapula and long bones of right upper limb
  - **D16.02** Benign neoplasm of scapula and long bones of left upper limb
- **+ D16.1** Benign neoplasm of short bones of upper limb
  - **D16.10** Benign neoplasm of short bones of unspecified upper limb
  - **D16.11** Benign neoplasm of short bones of right upper limb
  - **D16.12** Benign neoplasm of short bones of left upper limb
- **+ D16.2** Benign neoplasm of long bones of lower limb
  - **D16.20** Benign neoplasm of long bones of unspecified lower limb
  - **D16.21** Benign neoplasm of long bones of right lower limb
  - **D16.22** Benign neoplasm of long bones of left lower limb
- **+ D16.3** Benign neoplasm of short bones of lower limb
  - **D16.30** Benign neoplasm of short bones of unspecified lower limb
  - **D16.31** Benign neoplasm of short bones of right lower limb
  - **D16.32** Benign neoplasm of short bones of left lower limb
- **D16.4** Benign neoplasm of bones of skull and face
  - Benign neoplasm of maxilla (superior)
  - Benign neoplasm of orbital bone
  - Keratocyst of maxilla
  - Keratocystic odontogenic tumor of maxilla
  - *Excludes2:* benign neoplasm of lower jaw bone (D16.5)
- **D16.5** Benign neoplasm of lower jaw bone
  - Keratocyst of mandible
  - Keratocystic odontogenic tumor of mandible
- **D16.6** Benign neoplasm of vertebral column
  - *Excludes1:* benign neoplasm of sacrum and coccyx (D16.8)
- **D16.7** Benign neoplasm of ribs, sternum and clavicle
- **D16.8** Benign neoplasm of pelvic bones, sacrum and coccyx
- **D16.9** Benign neoplasm of bone and articular cartilage, unspecified

D17 Benign lipomatous neoplasm
- **D17.0** Benign lipomatous neoplasm of skin and subcutaneous tissue of head, face and neck
- **D17.1** Benign lipomatous neoplasm of skin and subcutaneous tissue of trunk
- **+ D17.2** Benign lipomatous neoplasm of skin and subcutaneous tissue of limb
  - **D17.20** Benign lipomatous neoplasm of skin and subcutaneous tissue of unspecified limb
  - **D17.21** Benign lipomatous neoplasm of skin and subcutaneous tissue of right arm
  - **D17.22** Benign lipomatous neoplasm of skin and subcutaneous tissue of left arm
  - **D17.23** Benign lipomatous neoplasm of skin and subcutaneous tissue of right leg
  - **D17.24** Benign lipomatous neoplasm of skin and subcutaneous tissue of left leg
- **+ D17.3** Benign lipomatous neoplasm of skin and subcutaneous tissue of other and unspecified sites
  - **D17.30** Benign lipomatous neoplasm of skin and subcutaneous tissue of unspecified sites
  - **D17.39** Benign lipomatous neoplasm of skin and subcutaneous tissue of other sites
- **D17.4** Benign lipomatous neoplasm of intrathoracic organs
- **D17.5** Benign lipomatous neoplasm of intra-abdominal organs
  - *Excludes1:* benign lipomatous neoplasm of peritoneum and retroperitoneum (D17.79)
- ♂ **D17.6** Benign lipomatous neoplasm of spermatic cord
- **+ D17.7** Benign lipomatous neoplasm of other sites
  - **D17.71** Benign lipomatous neoplasm of kidney
  - **D17.72** Benign lipomatous neoplasm of other genitourinary organ
  - **D17.79** Benign lipomatous neoplasm of other sites
    - Benign lipomatous neoplasm of peritoneum
    - Benign lipomatous neoplasm of retroperitoneum
- **D17.9** Benign lipomatous neoplasm, unspecified
  - Lipoma NOS

D18 Hemangioma and lymphangioma, any site
Excludes1: benign neoplasm of glomus jugulare (D35.6)
blue or pigmented nevus (D22.-)
nevus NOS (D22.-)
vascular nevus (Q82.5)
- **+ D18.0** Hemangioma
  - Angioma NOS
  - Cavernous nevus
  - **D18.00** Hemangioma unspecified site
  - **D18.01** Hemangioma of skin and subcutaneous tissue
  - **D18.02** Hemangioma of intracranial structures
  - **D18.03** Hemangioma of intra-abdominal structures
  - **D18.09** Hemangioma of other sites
- **D18.1** Lymphangioma, any site
  - AHA CC: 2Q, 2018, 13; 3Q, 2018, 31

D19 Benign neoplasm of mesothelial tissue
- **D19.0** Benign neoplasm of mesothelial tissue of pleura
- **D19.1** Benign neoplasm of mesothelial tissue of peritoneum
- **D19.7** Benign neoplasm of mesothelial tissue of other sites
- **D19.9** Benign neoplasm of mesothelial tissue, unspecified
  - Benign mesothelioma NOS

D20 Benign neoplasm of soft tissue of retroperitoneum and peritoneum
Excludes1: benign lipomatous neoplasm of peritoneum and retroperitoneum (D17.79)
benign neoplasm of mesothelial tissue (D19.-)
- **D20.0** Benign neoplasm of soft tissue of retroperitoneum
- **D20.1** Benign neoplasm of soft tissue of peritoneum

D21 Other benign neoplasms of connective and other soft tissue

Includes: benign neoplasm of blood vessel
benign neoplasm of bursa
benign neoplasm of cartilage
benign neoplasm of fascia
benign neoplasm of fat
benign neoplasm of ligament, except uterine
benign neoplasm of lymphatic channel
benign neoplasm of muscle
benign neoplasm of synovia
benign neoplasm of tendon (sheath)
benign stromal tumors

Excludes1: benign neoplasm of articular cartilage (D16.-)
benign neoplasm of cartilage of larynx (D14.1)
benign neoplasm of cartilage of nose (D14.0)
benign neoplasm of connective tissue of breast (D24.-)
benign neoplasm of peripheral nerves and autonomic nervous system (D36.1-)
benign neoplasm of peritoneum (D20.1)
benign neoplasm of retroperitoneum (D20.0)
benign neoplasm of uterine ligament, any (D28.2)
benign neoplasm of vascular tissue (D18.-)
hemangioma (D18.0-)
lipomatous neoplasm (D17.-)
lymphangioma (D18.1)
uterine leiomyoma (D25.-)

- **D21.0** Benign neoplasm of connective and other soft tissue of head, face and neck
    Benign neoplasm of connective tissue of ear
    Benign neoplasm of connective tissue of eyelid
    Excludes1: benign neoplasm of connective tissue of orbit (D31.6-)
- **+ D21.1** Benign neoplasm of connective and other soft tissue of upper limb, including shoulder
    - **D21.10** Benign neoplasm of connective and other soft tissue of unspecified upper limb, including shoulder
    - **D21.11** Benign neoplasm of connective and other soft tissue of right upper limb, including shoulder
    - **D21.12** Benign neoplasm of connective and other soft tissue of left upper limb, including shoulder
- **+ D21.2** Benign neoplasm of connective and other soft tissue of lower limb, including hip
    - **D21.20** Benign neoplasm of connective and other soft tissue of unspecified lower limb, including hip
    - **D21.21** Benign neoplasm of connective and other soft tissue of right lower limb, including hip
    - **D21.22** Benign neoplasm of connective and other soft tissue of left lower limb, including hip
- **D21.3** Benign neoplasm of connective and other soft tissue of thorax
    Benign neoplasm of axilla
    Benign neoplasm of diaphragm
    Benign neoplasm of great vessels
    Excludes1: benign neoplasm of heart (D15.1)
    benign neoplasm of mediastinum (D15.2)
    benign neoplasm of thymus (D15.0)
- **D21.4** Benign neoplasm of connective and other soft tissue of abdomen
    Benign stromal tumors of abdomen
- **D21.5** Benign neoplasm of connective and other soft tissue of pelvis
    Excludes1: benign neoplasm of any uterine ligament (D28.2)
    uterine leiomyoma (D25.-)
- **D21.6** Benign neoplasm of connective and other soft tissue of trunk, unspecified
    Benign neoplasm of connective and other soft tissue of back NOS
- **D21.9** Benign neoplasm of connective and other soft tissue, unspecified

D22 Melanocytic nevi

Includes: atypical nevus
blue hairy pigmented nevus
nevus NOS

- **D22.0** Melanocytic nevi of lip
- **+ D22.1** Melanocytic nevi of eyelid, including canthus
    - **D22.10** Melanocytic nevi of unspecified eyelid, including canthus
    - **+ D22.11** Melanocytic nevi of right eyelid, including canthus
        - **D22.111** Melanocytic nevi of right upper eyelid, including canthus
        - **D22.112** Melanocytic nevi of right lower eyelid, including canthus
    - **+ D22.12** Melanocytic nevi of left eyelid, including canthus
        - **D22.121** Melanocytic nevi of left upper eyelid, including canthus
        - **D22.122** Melanocytic nevi of left lower eyelid, including canthus
- **+ D22.2** Melanocytic nevi of ear and external auricular canal
    - **D22.20** Melanocytic nevi of unspecified ear and external auricular canal
    - **D22.21** Melanocytic nevi of right ear and external auricular canal
    - **D22.22** Melanocytic nevi of left ear and external auricular canal
- **+ D22.3** Melanocytic nevi of other and unspecified parts of face
    - **D22.30** Melanocytic nevi of unspecified part of face
    - **D22.39** Melanocytic nevi of other parts of face
- **D22.4** Melanocytic nevi of scalp and neck
- **D22.5** Melanocytic nevi of trunk
    Melanocytic nevi of anal margin
    Melanocytic nevi of anal skin
    Melanocytic nevi of perianal skin
    Melanocytic nevi of skin of breast
- **+ D22.6** Melanocytic nevi of upper limb, including shoulder
    - **D22.60** Melanocytic nevi of unspecified upper limb, including shoulder
    - **D22.61** Melanocytic nevi of right upper limb, including shoulder
    - **D22.62** Melanocytic nevi of left upper limb, including shoulder
- **+ D22.7** Melanocytic nevi of lower limb, including hip
    - **D22.70** Melanocytic nevi of unspecified lower limb, including hip
    - **D22.71** Melanocytic nevi of right lower limb, including hip
    - **D22.72** Melanocytic nevi of left lower limb, including hip
- **D22.9** Melanocytic nevi, unspecified

D23 Other benign neoplasms of skin

Includes: benign neoplasm of hair follicles
benign neoplasm of sebaceous glands
benign neoplasm of sweat glands

Excludes1: benign lipomatous neoplasms of skin (D17.0-D17.3)
Excludes2: melanocytic nevi (D22.-)

- **D23.0** Other benign neoplasm of skin of lip
    Excludes1: benign neoplasm of vermilion border of lip (D10.0)
- **+ D23.1** Other benign neoplasm of skin of eyelid, including canthus
    - **D23.10** Other benign neoplasm of skin of unspecified eyelid, including canthus
    - **+ D23.11** Other benign neoplasm of skin of right eyelid, including canthus
        - **D23.111** Other benign neoplasm of skin of right upper eyelid, including canthus
        - **D23.112** Other benign neoplasm of skin of right lower eyelid, including canthus
    - **+ D23.12** Other benign neoplasm of skin of left eyelid, including canthus
        - **D23.121** Other benign neoplasm of skin of left upper eyelid, including canthus
        - **D23.122** Other benign neoplasm of skin of left lower eyelid, including canthus

- **+ D23.2** Other benign neoplasm of skin of ear and external auricular canal
  - **D23.20** Other benign neoplasm of skin of unspecified ear and external auricular canal
  - **D23.21** Other benign neoplasm of skin of right ear and external auricular canal
  - **D23.22** Other benign neoplasm of skin of left ear and external auricular canal
- **+ D23.3** Other benign neoplasm of skin of other and unspecified parts of face
  - **D23.30** Other benign neoplasm of skin of unspecified part of face
  - **D23.39** Other benign neoplasm of skin of other parts of face
- **D23.4** Other benign neoplasm of skin of scalp and neck
- **D23.5** Other benign neoplasm of skin of trunk
  - Other benign neoplasm of anal margin
  - Other benign neoplasm of anal skin
  - Other benign neoplasm of perianal skin
  - Other benign neoplasm of skin of breast
  - **Excludes1:** benign neoplasm of anus NOS (D12.9)
- **+ D23.6** Other benign neoplasm of skin of upper limb, including shoulder
  - **D23.60** Other benign neoplasm of skin of unspecified upper limb, including shoulder
  - **D23.61** Other benign neoplasm of skin of right upper limb, including shoulder
  - **D23.62** Other benign neoplasm of skin of left upper limb, including shoulder
- **+ D23.7** Other benign neoplasm of skin of lower limb, including hip
  - **D23.70** Other benign neoplasm of skin of unspecified lower limb, including hip
  - **D23.71** Other benign neoplasm of skin of right lower limb, including hip
  - **D23.72** Other benign neoplasm of skin of left lower limb, including hip
- **D23.9** Other benign neoplasm of skin, unspecified

D24 Benign neoplasm of breast
Includes: benign neoplasm of connective tissue of breast
benign neoplasm of soft parts of breast
fibroadenoma of breast
Excludes2: adenofibrosis of breast (N60.2)
benign cyst of breast (N60.-)
benign mammary dysplasia (N60.-)
benign neoplasm of skin of breast (D22.5, D23.5)
fibrocystic disease of breast (N60.-)
- **D24.1** Benign neoplasm of right breast
  - *AHA CC: 1Q, 2017, 5-6*
- **D24.2** Benign neoplasm of left breast
- **D24.9** Benign neoplasm of unspecified breast

D25 Leiomyoma of uterus
Includes: uterine fibroid
uterine fibromyoma
uterine myoma
- ♀ **D25.0** Submucous leiomyoma of uterus
- ♀ **D25.1** Intramural leiomyoma of uterus
  - Interstitial leiomyoma of uterus
- ♀ **D25.2** Subserosal leiomyoma of uterus
  - Subperitoneal leiomyoma of uterus
- ♀ **D25.9** Leiomyoma of uterus, unspecified

D26 Other benign neoplasms of uterus
- ♀ **D26.0** Other benign neoplasm of cervix uteri
- ♀ **D26.1** Other benign neoplasm of corpus uteri
- ♀ **D26.7** Other benign neoplasm of other parts of uterus
- ♀ **D26.9** Other benign neoplasm of uterus, unspecified

D27 Benign neoplasm of ovary
Use additional code to identify any functional activity.
Excludes2: corpus albicans cyst (N83.2-)
corpus luteum cyst (N83.1-)
endometrial cyst (N80.1-)
follicular (atretic) cyst (N83.0-)
graafian follicle cyst (N83.0-)
ovarian cyst NEC (N83.2-)
ovarian retention cyst (N83.2-)
- ♀ **D27.0** Benign neoplasm of right ovary
- ♀ **D27.1** Benign neoplasm of left ovary
- ♀ **D27.9** Benign neoplasm of unspecified ovary

D28 Benign neoplasm of other and unspecified female genital organs
Includes: adenomatous polyp
benign neoplasm of skin of female genital organs
benign teratoma
Excludes1: epoophoron cyst (Q50.5)
fimbrial cyst (Q50.4)
Gartner's duct cyst (Q52.4)
parovarian cyst (Q50.5)
- ♀ **D28.0** Benign neoplasm of vulva
- ♀ **D28.1** Benign neoplasm of vagina
- ♀ **D28.2** Benign neoplasm of uterine tubes and ligaments
  - Benign neoplasm of fallopian tube
  - Benign neoplasm of uterine ligament (broad) (round)
- ♀ **D28.7** Benign neoplasm of other specified female genital organs
- ♀ **D28.9** Benign neoplasm of female genital organ, unspecified

D29 Benign neoplasm of male genital organs
Includes: benign neoplasm of skin of male genital organs
- ♂ **D29.0** Benign neoplasm of penis
- ♂ **D29.1** Benign neoplasm of prostate
  - **Excludes1:** enlarged prostate (N40.-)
- **+ D29.2** Benign neoplasm of testis
  - Use additional code to identify any functional activity.
  - ♂ **D29.20** Benign neoplasm of unspecified testis
  - ♂ **D29.21** Benign neoplasm of right testis
  - ♂ **D29.22** Benign neoplasm of left testis
- **+ D29.3** Benign neoplasm of epididymis
  - ♂ **D29.30** Benign neoplasm of unspecified epididymis
  - ♂ **D29.31** Benign neoplasm of right epididymis
  - ♂ **D29.32** Benign neoplasm of left epididymis
- ♂ **D29.4** Benign neoplasm of scrotum
  - Benign neoplasm of skin of scrotum
- ♂ **D29.8** Benign neoplasm of other specified male genital organs
  - Benign neoplasm of seminal vesicle
  - Benign neoplasm of spermatic cord
  - Benign neoplasm of tunica vaginalis
- ♂ **D29.9** Benign neoplasm of male genital organ, unspecified

D30 Benign neoplasm of urinary organs
- **+ D30.0** Benign neoplasm of kidney
  - **Excludes1:** benign carcinoid tumor of the kidney (D3A.093)
  - benign neoplasm of renal calyces (D30.1-)
  - benign neoplasm of renal pelvis (D30.1-)
  - **D30.00** Benign neoplasm of unspecified kidney
  - **D30.01** Benign neoplasm of right kidney
  - **D30.02** Benign neoplasm of left kidney
- **+ D30.1** Benign neoplasm of renal pelvis
  - **D30.10** Benign neoplasm of unspecified renal pelvis
  - **D30.11** Benign neoplasm of right renal pelvis
  - **D30.12** Benign neoplasm of left renal pelvis
- **+ D30.2** Benign neoplasm of ureter
  - **Excludes1:** benign neoplasm of ureteric orifice of bladder (D30.3)
  - **D30.20** Benign neoplasm of unspecified ureter
  - **D30.21** Benign neoplasm of right ureter
  - **D30.22** Benign neoplasm of left ureter
- **D30.3** Benign neoplasm of bladder
  - Benign neoplasm of ureteric orifice of bladder
  - Benign neoplasm of urethral orifice of bladder
- **D30.4** Benign neoplasm of urethra
  - **Excludes1:** benign neoplasm of urethral orifice of bladder (D30.3)
- **D30.8** Benign neoplasm of other specified urinary organs
  - Benign neoplasm of paraurethral glands
- **D30.9** Benign neoplasm of urinary organ, unspecified
  - Benign neoplasm of urinary system NOS

D31 Benign neoplasm of eye and adnexa
Excludes1: benign neoplasm of connective tissue of eyelid (D21.0)
benign neoplasm of optic nerve (D33.3)
benign neoplasm of skin of eyelid (D22.1-, D23.1-)
- **+ D31.0** Benign neoplasm of conjunctiva
  - **D31.00** Benign neoplasm of unspecified conjunctiva
  - **D31.01** Benign neoplasm of right conjunctiva
  - **D31.02** Benign neoplasm of left conjunctiva
- **+ D31.1** Benign neoplasm of cornea
  - **D31.10** Benign neoplasm of unspecified cornea
  - **D31.11** Benign neoplasm of right cornea
  - **D31.12** Benign neoplasm of left cornea

- **D31.2** Benign neoplasm of retina
  - *Excludes1:* dark area on retina (D49.81)
    hemangioma of retina (D49.81)
    neoplasm of unspecified behavior of retina and choroid (D49.81)
    retinal freckle (D49.81)
  - D31.20 Benign neoplasm of unspecified retina
  - D31.21 Benign neoplasm of right retina
  - D31.22 Benign neoplasm of left retina
- **D31.3** Benign neoplasm of choroid
  - D31.30 Benign neoplasm of unspecified choroid
  - D31.31 Benign neoplasm of right choroid
  - D31.32 Benign neoplasm of left choroid
- **D31.4** Benign neoplasm of ciliary body
  - D31.40 Benign neoplasm of unspecified ciliary body
  - D31.41 Benign neoplasm of right ciliary body
  - D31.42 Benign neoplasm of left ciliary body
- **D31.5** Benign neoplasm of lacrimal gland and duct
  Benign neoplasm of lacrimal sac
  Benign neoplasm of nasolacrimal duct
  - D31.50 Benign neoplasm of unspecified lacrimal gland and duct
  - D31.51 Benign neoplasm of right lacrimal gland and duct
  - D31.52 Benign neoplasm of left lacrimal gland and duct
- **D31.6** Benign neoplasm of unspecified site of orbit
  Benign neoplasm of connective tissue of orbit
  Benign neoplasm of extraocular muscle
  Benign neoplasm of peripheral nerves of orbit
  Benign neoplasm of retrobulbar tissue
  Benign neoplasm of retro-ocular tissue
  - *Excludes1:* benign neoplasm of orbital bone (D16.4-)
  - D31.60 Benign neoplasm of unspecified site of unspecified orbit
  - D31.61 Benign neoplasm of unspecified site of right orbit
  - D31.62 Benign neoplasm of unspecified site of left orbit
- **D31.9** Benign neoplasm of unspecified part of eye
  Benign neoplasm of eyeball
  - D31.90 Benign neoplasm of unspecified part of unspecified eye
  - D31.91 Benign neoplasm of unspecified part of right eye
  - D31.92 Benign neoplasm of unspecified part of left eye

D32 Benign neoplasm of meninges
- **D32.0** Benign neoplasm of cerebral meninges
- **D32.1** Benign neoplasm of spinal meninges
- **D32.9** Benign neoplasm of meninges, unspecified
  Meningioma NOS

D33 Benign neoplasm of brain and other parts of central nervous system
Excludes1: angioma (D18.0-)
  benign neoplasm of meninges (D32.-)
  benign neoplasm of peripheral nerves and autonomic nervous system (D36.1-)
  hemangioma (D18.0-)
  neurofibromatosis (Q85.0-)
  retro-ocular benign neoplasm (D31.6-)
- **D33.0** Benign neoplasm of brain, supratentorial
  Benign neoplasm of cerebral ventricle
  Benign neoplasm of cerebrum
  Benign neoplasm of frontal lobe
  Benign neoplasm of occipital lobe
  Benign neoplasm of parietal lobe
  Benign neoplasm of temporal lobe
  - *Excludes1:* benign neoplasm of fourth ventricle (D33.1)
- **D33.1** Benign neoplasm of brain, infratentorial
  Benign neoplasm of brain stem
  Benign neoplasm of cerebellum
  Benign neoplasm of fourth ventricle
- **D33.2** Benign neoplasm of brain, unspecified
- **D33.3** Benign neoplasm of cranial nerves
  Benign neoplasm of olfactory bulb
- **D33.4** Benign neoplasm of spinal cord
- **D33.7** Benign neoplasm of other specified parts of central nervous system
- **D33.9** Benign neoplasm of central nervous system, unspecified
  Benign neoplasm of nervous system (central) NOS

D34 Benign neoplasm of thyroid gland
Use additional code to identify any functional activity
Valid 3-character code, no further characters required

D35 Benign neoplasm of other and unspecified endocrine glands
Use additional code to identify any functional activity
Excludes1: benign neoplasm of endocrine pancreas (D13.7)
  benign neoplasm of ovary (D27.-)
  benign neoplasm of testis (D29.2.-)
  benign neoplasm of thymus (D15.0)
- **D35.0** Benign neoplasm of adrenal gland
  - D35.00 Benign neoplasm of unspecified adrenal gland
  - D35.01 Benign neoplasm of right adrenal gland
  - D35.02 Benign neoplasm of left adrenal gland
- **D35.1** Benign neoplasm of parathyroid gland
- **D35.2** Benign neoplasm of pituitary gland
  AHA CC: 3Q, 2014, 22-23
- **D35.3** Benign neoplasm of craniopharyngeal duct
- **D35.4** Benign neoplasm of pineal gland
- **D35.5** Benign neoplasm of carotid body
- **D35.6** Benign neoplasm of aortic body and other paraganglia
  Benign tumor of glomus jugulare
- **D35.7** Benign neoplasm of other specified endocrine glands
- **D35.9** Benign neoplasm of endocrine gland, unspecified
  Benign neoplasm of unspecified endocrine gland

D36 Benign neoplasm of other and unspecified sites
- **D36.0** Benign neoplasm of lymph nodes
  - *Excludes1:* lymphangioma (D18.1)
- **D36.1** Benign neoplasm of peripheral nerves and autonomic nervous system
  - *Excludes1:* benign neoplasm of peripheral nerves of orbit (D31.6-)
    neurofibromatosis (Q85.0-)
  - D36.10 Benign neoplasm of peripheral nerves and autonomic nervous system, unspecified
  - D36.11 Benign neoplasm of peripheral nerves and autonomic nervous system of face, head, and neck
  - D36.12 Benign neoplasm of peripheral nerves and autonomic nervous system, upper limb, including shoulder
  - D36.13 Benign neoplasm of peripheral nerves and autonomic nervous system of lower limb, including hip
  - D36.14 Benign neoplasm of peripheral nerves and autonomic nervous system of thorax
  - D36.15 Benign neoplasm of peripheral nerves and autonomic nervous system of abdomen
  - D36.16 Benign neoplasm of peripheral nerves and autonomic nervous system of pelvis
  - D36.17 Benign neoplasm of peripheral nerves and autonomic nervous system of trunk, unspecified
- **D36.7** Benign neoplasm of other specified sites
  Benign neoplasm of nose NOS
  Benign neoplasm of back NOS
- **D36.9** Benign neoplasm, unspecified site

Benign neuroendocrine tumors (D3A)

D3A Benign neuroendocrine tumors
Code also any associated multiple endocrine neoplasia [MEN] syndromes (E31.2-)

Use additional code to identify any associated endocrine syndrome, such as:
carotid syndrome (E34.0)
Excludes2: benign pancreatic islet cell tumors (D13.7)
- **D3A.0** Benign carcinoid tumors
  - D3A.00 Benign carcinoid tumor of unspecified site
    Carcinoid tumor NOS
  - **D3A.01** Benign carcinoid tumors of the small intestine
    - D3A.010 Benign carcinoid tumor of the duodenum
    - D3A.011 Benign carcinoid tumor of the jejunum
    - D3A.012 Benign carcinoid tumor of the ileum
    - D3A.019 Benign carcinoid tumor of the small intestine, unspecified portion

- **+ D3A.02 Benign carcinoid tumors of the appendix, large intestine, and rectum**
  - D3A.020 Benign carcinoid tumor of the appendix
  - D3A.021 Benign carcinoid tumor of the cecum
  - D3A.022 Benign carcinoid tumor of the ascending colon
  - D3A.023 Benign carcinoid tumor of the transverse colon
  - D3A.024 Benign carcinoid tumor of the descending colon
  - D3A.025 Benign carcinoid tumor of the sigmoid colon
  - D3A.026 Benign carcinoid tumor of the rectum
  - D3A.029 Benign carcinoid tumor of the large intestine, unspecified portion
    - Benign carcinoid tumor of the colon NOS
- **+ D3A.09 Benign carcinoid tumors of other sites**
  - D3A.090 Benign carcinoid tumor of the bronchus and lung
  - D3A.091 Benign carcinoid tumor of the thymus
  - D3A.092 Benign carcinoid tumor of the stomach
  - D3A.093 Benign carcinoid tumor of the kidney
  - D3A.094 Benign carcinoid tumor of the foregut, unspecified
  - D3A.095 Benign carcinoid tumor of the midgut, unspecified
  - D3A.096 Benign carcinoid tumor of the hindgut, unspecified
  - D3A.098 Benign carcinoid tumors of other sites
- **D3A.8 Other benign neuroendocrine tumors**
  - Neuroendocrine tumor NOS

Neoplasms of uncertain behavior, polycythemia vera and myelodysplastic syndromes (D37-D48)

NOTE Categories D37-D44, and D48 classify by site neoplasms of uncertain behavior, i.e., histologic confirmation whether the neoplasm is malignant or benign cannot be made.

Excludes1: neoplasms of unspecified behavior (D49.-)

D37 Neoplasm of uncertain behavior of oral cavity and digestive organs

Excludes1: stromal tumors of uncertain behavior of digestive system (D48.1-)

- **+ D37.0 Neoplasm of uncertain behavior of lip, oral cavity and pharynx**

  Excludes1: neoplasm of uncertain behavior of aryepiglottic fold or interarytenoid fold, laryngeal aspect (D38.0)
  neoplasm of uncertain behavior of epiglottis NOS (D38.0)
  neoplasm of uncertain behavior of skin of lip (D48.5)
  neoplasm of uncertain behavior of suprahyoid portion of epiglottis (D38.0)

  - D37.01 Neoplasm of uncertain behavior of lip
    - Neoplasm of uncertain behavior of vermilion border of lip
  - D37.02 Neoplasm of uncertain behavior of tongue
  - **+ D37.03 Neoplasm of uncertain behavior of the major salivary glands**
    - D37.030 Neoplasm of uncertain behavior of the parotid salivary glands
    - D37.031 Neoplasm of uncertain behavior of the sublingual salivary glands
    - D37.032 Neoplasm of uncertain behavior of the submandibular salivary glands
    - D37.039 Neoplasm of uncertain behavior of the major salivary glands, unspecified
  - D37.04 Neoplasm of uncertain behavior of the minor salivary glands
    - Neoplasm of uncertain behavior of submucosal salivary glands of lip
    - Neoplasm of uncertain behavior of submucosal salivary glands of cheek
    - Neoplasm of uncertain behavior of submucosal salivary glands of hard palate
    - Neoplasm of uncertain behavior of submucosal salivary glands of soft palate
  - D37.05 Neoplasm of uncertain behavior of pharynx
    - Neoplasm of uncertain behavior of aryepiglottic fold of pharynx NOS
    - Neoplasm of uncertain behavior of hypopharyngeal aspect of aryepiglottic fold of pharynx
    - Neoplasm of uncertain behavior of marginal zone of aryepiglottic fold of pharynx
  - D37.09 Neoplasm of uncertain behavior of other specified sites of the oral cavity
- D37.1 Neoplasm of uncertain behavior of stomach
- D37.2 Neoplasm of uncertain behavior of small intestine
- D37.3 Neoplasm of uncertain behavior of appendix
- D37.4 Neoplasm of uncertain behavior of colon
- D37.5 Neoplasm of uncertain behavior of rectum
  - Neoplasm of uncertain behavior of rectosigmoid junction
- D37.6 Neoplasm of uncertain behavior of liver, gallbladder and bile ducts
  - Neoplasm of uncertain behavior of ampulla of Vater
- D37.8 Neoplasm of uncertain behavior of other specified digestive organs
  - Neoplasm of uncertain behavior of anal canal
  - Neoplasm of uncertain behavior of anal sphincter
  - Neoplasm of uncertain behavior of anus NOS
  - Neoplasm of uncertain behavior of esophagus
  - Neoplasm of uncertain behavior of intestine NOS
  - Neoplasm of uncertain behavior of pancreas

  Excludes1: neoplasm of uncertain behavior of anal margin (D48.5)
  neoplasm of uncertain behavior of anal skin (D48.5)
  neoplasm of uncertain behavior of perianal skin (D48.5)
- D37.9 Neoplasm of uncertain behavior of digestive organ, unspecified

D38 Neoplasm of uncertain behavior of middle ear and respiratory and intrathoracic organs

Excludes1: neoplasm of uncertain behavior of heart (D48.7)

- D38.0 Neoplasm of uncertain behavior of larynx
  - Neoplasm of uncertain behavior of aryepiglottic fold or interarytenoid fold, laryngeal aspect
  - Neoplasm of uncertain behavior of epiglottis (suprahyoid portion)

  Excludes1: neoplasm of uncertain behavior of aryepiglottic fold or interarytenoid fold NOS (D37.05)
  neoplasm of uncertain behavior of hypopharyngeal aspect of aryepiglottic fold (D37.05)
  neoplasm of uncertain behavior of marginal zone of aryepiglottic fold (D37.05)
- D38.1 Neoplasm of uncertain behavior of trachea, bronchus and lung
- D38.2 Neoplasm of uncertain behavior of pleura
- D38.3 Neoplasm of uncertain behavior of mediastinum
- D38.4 Neoplasm of uncertain behavior of thymus
- D38.5 Neoplasm of uncertain behavior of other respiratory organs
  - Neoplasm of uncertain behavior of accessory sinuses
  - Neoplasm of uncertain behavior of cartilage of nose
  - Neoplasm of uncertain behavior of middle ear
  - Neoplasm of uncertain behavior of nasal cavities

  Excludes1: neoplasm of uncertain behavior of ear (external) (skin) (D48.5)
  neoplasm of uncertain behavior of nose NOS (D48.7)
  neoplasm of uncertain behavior of skin of nose (D48.5)
- D38.6 Neoplasm of uncertain behavior of respiratory organ, unspecified

D39 Neoplasm of uncertain behavior of female genital organs
- ♀ **D39.0** Neoplasm of uncertain behavior of uterus
- + **D39.1** Neoplasm of uncertain behavior of ovary
  Use additional code to identify any functional activity.
  - ♀ **D39.10** Neoplasm of uncertain behavior of unspecified ovary
  - ♀ **D39.11** Neoplasm of uncertain behavior of right ovary
  - ♀ **D39.12** Neoplasm of uncertain behavior of left ovary
- ♀ **D39.2** Neoplasm of uncertain behavior of placenta
  Chorioadenoma destruens
  Invasive hydatidiform mole
  Malignant hydatidiform mole
  Excludes1: hydatidiform mole NOS (O01.9)
- ♀ **D39.8** Neoplasm of uncertain behavior of other specified female genital organs
  Neoplasm of uncertain behavior of skin of female genital organs
- ♀ **D39.9** Neoplasm of uncertain behavior of female genital organ, unspecified

D40 Neoplasm of uncertain behavior of male genital organs
- ♂ **D40.0** Neoplasm of uncertain behavior of prostate
- + **D40.1** Neoplasm of uncertain behavior of testis
  - ♂ **D40.10** Neoplasm of uncertain behavior of unspecified testis
  - ♂ **D40.11** Neoplasm of uncertain behavior of right testis
  - ♂ **D40.12** Neoplasm of uncertain behavior of left testis
- ♂ **D40.8** Neoplasm of uncertain behavior of other specified male genital organs
  Neoplasm of uncertain behavior of skin of male genital organs
- ♂ **D40.9** Neoplasm of uncertain behavior of male genital organ, unspecified

D41 Neoplasm of uncertain behavior of urinary organs
- + **D41.0** Neoplasm of uncertain behavior of kidney
  Excludes1: neoplasm of uncertain behavior of renal pelvis (D41.1-)
  - **D41.00** Neoplasm of uncertain behavior of unspecified kidney
  - **D41.01** Neoplasm of uncertain behavior of right kidney
  - **D41.02** Neoplasm of uncertain behavior of left kidney
- + **D41.1** Neoplasm of uncertain behavior of renal pelvis
  - **D41.10** Neoplasm of uncertain behavior of unspecified renal pelvis
  - **D41.11** Neoplasm of uncertain behavior of right renal pelvis
  - **D41.12** Neoplasm of uncertain behavior of left renal pelvis
- + **D41.2** Neoplasm of uncertain behavior of ureter
  - **D41.20** Neoplasm of uncertain behavior of unspecified ureter
  - **D41.21** Neoplasm of uncertain behavior of right ureter
  - **D41.22** Neoplasm of uncertain behavior of left ureter
- **D41.3** Neoplasm of uncertain behavior of urethra
- **D41.4** Neoplasm of uncertain behavior of bladder
- **D41.8** Neoplasm of uncertain behavior of other specified urinary organs
- **D41.9** Neoplasm of uncertain behavior of unspecified urinary organ

D42 Neoplasm of uncertain behavior of meninges
- **D42.0** Neoplasm of uncertain behavior of cerebral meninges
- **D42.1** Neoplasm of uncertain behavior of spinal meninges
- **D42.9** Neoplasm of uncertain behavior of meninges, unspecified

D43 Neoplasm of uncertain behavior of brain and central nervous system
Excludes1: neoplasm of uncertain behavior of peripheral nerves and autonomic nervous system (D48.2)
- **D43.0** Neoplasm of uncertain behavior of brain, supratentorial
  Neoplasm of uncertain behavior of cerebral ventricle
  Neoplasm of uncertain behavior of cerebrum
  Neoplasm of uncertain behavior of frontal lobe
  Neoplasm of uncertain behavior of occipital lobe
  Neoplasm of uncertain behavior of parietal lobe
  Neoplasm of uncertain behavior of temporal lobe
  Excludes1: neoplasm of uncertain behavior of fourth ventricle (D43.1)
- **D43.1** Neoplasm of uncertain behavior of brain, infratentorial
  Neoplasm of uncertain behavior of brain stem
  Neoplasm of uncertain behavior of cerebellum
  Neoplasm of uncertain behavior of fourth ventricle
  AHA CC: 2Q, 2023, 16
- **D43.2** Neoplasm of uncertain behavior of brain, unspecified
- **D43.3** Neoplasm of uncertain behavior of cranial nerves
- **D43.4** Neoplasm of uncertain behavior of spinal cord
- **D43.8** Neoplasm of uncertain behavior of other specified parts of central nervous system
- **D43.9** Neoplasm of uncertain behavior of central nervous system, unspecified
  Neoplasm of uncertain behavior of nervous system (central) NOS

D44 Neoplasm of uncertain behavior of endocrine glands
Excludes1: multiple endocrine adenomatosis (E31.2-)
multiple endocrine neoplasia (E31.2-)
neoplasm of uncertain behavior of endocrine pancreas (D37.8)
neoplasm of uncertain behavior of ovary (D39.1-)
neoplasm of uncertain behavior of testis (D40.1-)
neoplasm of uncertain behavior of thymus (D38.4)
- **D44.0** Neoplasm of uncertain behavior of thyroid gland
- + **D44.1** Neoplasm of uncertain behavior of adrenal gland
  Use additional code to identify any functional activity.
  - **D44.10** Neoplasm of uncertain behavior of unspecified adrenal gland
  - **D44.11** Neoplasm of uncertain behavior of right adrenal gland
  - **D44.12** Neoplasm of uncertain behavior of left adrenal gland
- **D44.2** Neoplasm of uncertain behavior of parathyroid gland
- **D44.3** Neoplasm of uncertain behavior of pituitary gland
  Use additional code to identify any functional activity.
- **D44.4** Neoplasm of uncertain behavior of craniopharyngeal duct
- **D44.5** Neoplasm of uncertain behavior of pineal gland
- **D44.6** Neoplasm of uncertain behavior of carotid body
- **D44.7** Neoplasm of uncertain behavior of aortic body and other paraganglia
  AHA CC: 4Q, 2016, 26; 2Q, 2021, 7
- **D44.9** Neoplasm of uncertain behavior of unspecified endocrine gland

D45 Polycythemia vera
Excludes1: familial polycythemia (D75.0)
secondary polycythemia (D75.1)
Valid 3-character code, no further characters required

D46 Myelodysplastic syndromes
Use additional code for adverse effect, if applicable, to identify drug (T36-T50 with fifth or sixth character 5)
Excludes2: drug-induced aplastic anemia (D61.1)
- **D46.0** Refractory anemia without ring sideroblasts, so stated
  Refractory anemia without sideroblasts, without excess of blasts
- **D46.1** Refractory anemia with ring sideroblasts
  RARS
- + **D46.2** Refractory anemia with excess of blasts [RAEB]
  - **D46.20** Refractory anemia with excess of blasts, unspecified
    RAEB NOS
  - **D46.21** Refractory anemia with excess of blasts 1
    RAEB 1
  - CC **D46.22** Refractory anemia with excess of blasts 2
    RAEB 2
- **D46.A** Refractory cytopenia with multilineage dysplasia
- **D46.B** Refractory cytopenia with multilineage dysplasia and ring sideroblasts
  RCMD RS
- CC **D46.C** Myelodysplastic syndrome with isolated del(5q) chromosomal abnormality
  Myelodysplastic syndrome with 5q deletion
  5q minus syndrome NOS
- **D46.4** Refractory anemia, unspecified
- **D46.Z** Other myelodysplastic syndromes
  Excludes1: chronic myelomonocytic leukemia (C93.1-)
- **D46.9** Myelodysplastic syndrome, unspecified
  Myelodysplasia NOS

D47 Other neoplasms of uncertain behavior of lymphoid, hematopoietic and related tissue

D47.0 Mast cell neoplasms of uncertain behavior
Excludes1: congenital cutaneous mastocytosis (Q82.2)
histiocytic neoplasms of uncertain behavior (D47.Z9)
malignant mast cell neoplasm (C96.2-)
AHA CC: 4Q, 2017, 5

CC D47.01 Cutaneous mastocytosis
Diffuse cutaneous mastocytosis
Maculopapular cutaneous mastocytosis
Solitary mastocytoma
Telangiectasia macularis eruptiva perstans
Urticaria pigmentosa
Excludes1: congenital (diffuse) (maculopapular) cutaneous mastocytosis (Q82.2)
congenital urticaria pigmentosa (Q82.2)
extracutaneous mastocytoma (D47.09)

CC D47.02 Systemic mastocytosis
Indolent systemic mastocytosis
Isolated bone marrow mastocytosis
Smoldering systemic mastocytosis
Systemic mastocytosis, with an associated hematological non-mast cell lineage disease (SM-AHNMD)
Code also, if applicable, any associated hematological non-mast cell lineage disease, such as:
acute myeloid leukemia (C92.6-, C92.A-)
chronic myelomonocytic leukemia (C93.1-)
essential thrombocytosis (D47.3)
hypereosinophilic syndrome (D72.1)
myelodysplastic syndrome (D46.9)
myeloproliferative syndrome (D47.1)
non-Hodgkin lymphoma (C82-C85)
plasma cell myeloma (C90.0-)
polycythemia vera (D45)
Excludes1: aggressive systemic mastocytosis (C96.21)
mast cell leukemia (C94.3-)

CC D47.09 Other mast cell neoplasms of uncertain behavior
Extracutaneous mastocytoma
Mast cell tumor NOS
Mastocytoma NOS
Mastocytosis NOS
Excludes1: malignant mast cell tumor (C96.2)
mastocytosis (congenital) (cutaneous) (Q82.2)

CC D47.1 Chronic myeloproliferative disease
Chronic neutrophilic leukemia
Myeloproliferative disease, unspecified
Excludes1: atypical chronic myeloid leukemia BCR/ABL-negative (C92.2-)
chronic myeloid leukemia BCR/ABL-positive (C92.1-)
myelofibrosis NOS (D75.81)
myelophthisic anemia (D61.82)
myelophthisis (D61.82)
secondary myelofibrosis NOS (D75.81)

D47.2 Monoclonal gammopathy
Monoclonal gammopathy of undetermined significance [MGUS]
AHA CC: 3Q, 2021, 5

D47.3 Essential (hemorrhagic) thrombocythemia
Essential thrombocytosis
Idiopathic hemorrhagic thrombocythemia
Primary thrombocytosis
Excludes2: reactive thrombocytosis (D75.838)
secondary thrombocytosis (D75.838)
thrombocythemia NOS (D75.839)
thrombocytosis NOS (D75.839)

D47.4 Osteomyelofibrosis
Chronic idiopathic myelofibrosis
Myelofibrosis (idiopathic) (with myeloid metaplasia)
Myelosclerosis (megakaryocytic) with myeloid metaplasia
Secondary myelofibrosis in myeloproliferative disease
Excludes1: acute myelofibrosis (C94.4-)

+ D47.Z Other specified neoplasms of uncertain behavior of lymphoid, hematopoietic and related tissue

CC D47.Z1 Post-transplant lymphoproliferative disorder (PTLD)
Code first complications of transplanted organs and tissue (T86.-)

CC D47.Z2 Castleman disease
Code also, if applicable, human herpesvirus 8 infection (B10.89)
Excludes2: Kaposi's sarcoma (C46.-)
AHA CC: 4Q, 2016, 8

CC D47.Z9 Other specified neoplasms of uncertain behavior of lymphoid, hematopoietic and related tissue
Histiocytic tumors of uncertain behavior

CC D47.9 Neoplasm of uncertain behavior of lymphoid, hematopoietic and related tissue, unspecified
Lymphoproliferative disease NOS

D48 Neoplasm of uncertain behavior of other and unspecified sites
Excludes1: neurofibromatosis (nonmalignant) (Q85.0-)

D48.0 Neoplasm of uncertain behavior of bone and articular cartilage
Excludes1: neoplasm of uncertain behavior of cartilage of ear (D48.1-)
neoplasm of uncertain behavior of cartilage of larynx (D38.0)
neoplasm of uncertain behavior of cartilage of nose (D38.5)
neoplasm of uncertain behavior of connective tissue of eyelid (D48.1-)
neoplasm of uncertain behavior of synovia (D48.1-)

+ D48.1 Neoplasm of uncertain behavior of connective and other soft tissue
Neoplasm of uncertain behavior of connective tissue of ear
Neoplasm of uncertain behavior of connective tissue of eyelid
Stromal tumors of uncertain behavior of digestive system
Excludes1: neoplasm of uncertain behavior of articular cartilage (D48.0)
neoplasm of uncertain behavior of cartilage of larynx (D38.0)
neoplasm of uncertain behavior of cartilage of nose (D38.5)
neoplasm of uncertain behavior of connective tissue of breast (D48.6-)

+ D48.11 Desmoid tumor
- D48.110 Desmoid tumor of head and neck
- D48.111 Desmoid tumor of chest wall
- D48.112 Desmoid tumor, intrathoracic
- D48.113 Desmoid tumor of abdominal wall
- D48.114 Desmoid tumor, intraabdominal
  Desmoid tumor of pelvic cavity
  Desmoid tumor, peritoneal, retroperitoneal
- D48.115 Desmoid tumor of upper extremity and shoulder girdle
- D48.116 Desmoid tumor of lower extremity and pelvic girdle
  Desmoid tumor of buttock
- D48.117 Desmoid tumor of back
- D48.118 Desmoid tumor of other site
- D48.119 Desmoid tumor of unspecified site

D48.19 Other specified neoplasm of uncertain behavior of connective and other soft tissue

D48.2 Neoplasm of uncertain behavior of peripheral nerves and autonomic nervous system
Excludes1: neoplasm of uncertain behavior of peripheral nerves of orbit (D48.7)

D48.3 Neoplasm of uncertain behavior of retroperitoneum
D48.4 Neoplasm of uncertain behavior of peritoneum
D48.5 Neoplasm of uncertain behavior of skin
Neoplasm of uncertain behavior of anal margin
Neoplasm of uncertain behavior of anal skin
Neoplasm of uncertain behavior of perianal skin
Neoplasm of uncertain behavior of skin of breast
Excludes1: neoplasm of uncertain behavior of anus NOS (D37.8)
neoplasm of uncertain behavior of skin of genital organs (D39.8, D40.8)
neoplasm of uncertain behavior of vermilion border of lip (D37.0)

+ **D48.6** **Neoplasm of uncertain behavior of breast**
Neoplasm of uncertain behavior of connective tissue of breast
Cystosarcoma phyllodes
Excludes1: *neoplasm of uncertain behavior of skin of breast (D48.5)*

- **D48.60** Neoplasm of uncertain behavior of unspecified breast
- **D48.61** Neoplasm of uncertain behavior of right breast
- **D48.62** Neoplasm of uncertain behavior of left breast

D48.7 **Neoplasm of uncertain behavior of other specified sites**
Neoplasm of uncertain behavior of eye
Neoplasm of uncertain behavior of heart
Neoplasm of uncertain behavior of peripheral nerves of orbit
Excludes1: *neoplasm of uncertain behavior of connective tissue (D48.1-)*
neoplasm of uncertain behavior of skin of eyelid (D48.5)

D48.9 **Neoplasm of uncertain behavior, unspecified**

Neoplasms of unspecified behavior (D49)

D49 **Neoplasms of unspecified behavior**

NOTE Category D49 classifies by site neoplasms of unspecified morphology and behavior. The term 'mass', unless otherwise stated, is not to be regarded as a neoplastic growth.

Includes: 'growth' NOS
neoplasm NOS
new growth NOS
tumor NOS

Excludes1: *neoplasms of uncertain behavior (D37-D44, D48)*

D49.0 **Neoplasm of unspecified behavior of digestive system**
Excludes1: *neoplasm of unspecified behavior of margin of anus (D49.2)*
neoplasm of unspecified behavior of perianal skin (D49.2)
neoplasm of unspecified behavior of skin of anus (D49.2)

D49.1 **Neoplasm of unspecified behavior of respiratory system**

D49.2 **Neoplasm of unspecified behavior of bone, soft tissue, and skin**
Excludes1: *neoplasm of unspecified behavior of anal canal (D49.0)*
neoplasm of unspecified behavior of anus NOS (D49.0)
neoplasm of unspecified behavior of bone marrow (D49.89)
neoplasm of unspecified behavior of cartilage of larynx (D49.1)
neoplasm of unspecified behavior of cartilage of nose (D49.1)
neoplasm of unspecified behavior of connective tissue of breast (D49.3)
neoplasm of unspecified behavior of skin of genital organs (D49.59)
neoplasm of unspecified behavior of vermilion border of lip (D49.0)

D49.3 **Neoplasm of unspecified behavior of breast**
Excludes1: *neoplasm of unspecified behavior of skin of breast (D49.2)*

D49.4 **Neoplasm of unspecified behavior of bladder**

+ **D49.5** **Neoplasm of unspecified behavior of other genitourinary organs**
AHA CC: 4Q, 2016, 9

+ **D49.51** Neoplasm of unspecified behavior of kidney
- **D49.511** Neoplasm of unspecified behavior of right kidney
- **D49.512** Neoplasm of unspecified behavior of left kidney
- **D49.519** Neoplasm of unspecified behavior of unspecified kidney

D49.59 Neoplasm unspecified behavior of other genitourinary organ

D49.6 **Neoplasm of unspecified behavior of brain**
Excludes1: *neoplasm of unspecified behavior of cerebral meninges (D49.7)*
neoplasm of unspecified behavior of cranial nerves (D49.7)

D49.7 **Neoplasm of unspecified behavior of endocrine glands and other parts of nervous system**
Excludes1: *neoplasm of unspecified behavior of peripheral, sympathetic, and parasympathetic nerves and ganglia (D49.2)*

+ **D49.8** **Neoplasm of unspecified behavior of other specified sites**
Excludes1: *neoplasm of unspecified behavior of eyelid (skin) (D49.2)*
neoplasm of unspecified behavior of eyelid cartilage (D49.2)
neoplasm of unspecified behavior of great vessels (D49.2)
neoplasm of unspecified behavior of optic nerve (D49.7)

D49.81 Neoplasm of unspecified behavior of retina and choroid
Dark area on retina
Retinal freckle

D49.89 Neoplasm of unspecified behavior of other specified sites

D49.9 **Neoplasm of unspecified behavior of unspecified site**

Chapter 3: Diseases of the Blood and Blood-Forming Organs and Certain Disorders Involving the Immune Mechanism (D50-D89)

Excludes2: autoimmune disease (systemic) NOS (M35.9)
certain conditions originating in the perinatal period (P00-P96)
complications of pregnancy, childbirth and the puerperium (O00-O9A)
congenital malformations, deformations and chromosomal abnormalities (Q00-Q99)
endocrine, nutritional and metabolic diseases (E00-E88)
human immunodeficiency virus [HIV] disease (B20)
injury, poisoning and certain other consequences of external causes (S00-T88)
neoplasms (C00-D49)
symptoms, signs and abnormal clinical and laboratory findings, not elsewhere classified (R00-R94)

This chapter contains the following category blocks:
- D50-D53 Nutritional anemias
- D55-D59 Hemolytic anemias
- D60-D64 Aplastic and other anemias and other bone marrow failure syndromes
- D65-D69 Coagulation defects, purpura and other hemorrhagic conditions
- D70-D77 Other disorders of blood and blood-forming organs
- D78 Intraoperative and postprocedural complications of the spleen
- D80-D89 Certain disorders involving the immune mechanism

C. Chapter-Specific Coding Guidelines

In addition to general coding guidelines, there are guidelines for specific diagnoses and/or conditions in the classification. Unless otherwise indicated, these guidelines apply to all health care settings. Please refer to Section II for guidelines on the selection of principal diagnosis.

3. Chapter 3: Diseases of the Blood and Blood-Forming Organs and Certain Disorders Involving the Immune Mechanism (D50-D89)

Reserved for future guideline expansion

Nutritional anemias (D50-D53)

D50 Iron deficiency anemia
  Includes: asiderotic anemia
  hypochromic anemia
  D50.0 Iron deficiency anemia secondary to blood loss (chronic)
    Posthemorrhagic anemia (chronic)
    Excludes1: acute posthemorrhagic anemia (D62)
    congenital anemia from fetal blood loss (P61.3)
  D50.1 Sideropenic dysphagia
    Kelly-Paterson syndrome
    Plummer-Vinson syndrome
  D50.8 Other iron deficiency anemias
    Iron deficiency anemia due to inadequate dietary iron intake
  D50.9 Iron deficiency anemia, unspecified

D51 Vitamin B12 deficiency anemia
  Excludes1: vitamin B12 deficiency (E53.8)
  D51.0 Vitamin B12 deficiency anemia due to intrinsic factor deficiency
    Addison anemia
    Biermer anemia
    Pernicious (congenital) anemia
    Congenital intrinsic factor deficiency
  D51.1 Vitamin B12 deficiency anemia due to selective vitamin B12 malabsorption with proteinuria
    Imerslund (Gräsbeck) syndrome
    Megaloblastic hereditary anemia
  D51.2 Transcobalamin II deficiency
  D51.3 Other dietary vitamin B12 deficiency anemia
    Vegan anemia
  D51.8 Other vitamin B12 deficiency anemias
  D51.9 Vitamin B12 deficiency anemia, unspecified

D52 Folate deficiency anemia
  Excludes1: folate deficiency without anemia (E53.8)
  D52.0 Dietary folate deficiency anemia
    Nutritional megaloblastic anemia
  D52.1 Drug-induced folate deficiency anemia
    Use additional code for adverse effect, if applicable, to identify drug (T36-T50 with fifth or sixth character 5)
  D52.8 Other folate deficiency anemias
  D52.9 Folate deficiency anemia, unspecified
    Folic acid deficiency anemia NOS

D53 Other nutritional anemias
  Includes: megaloblastic anemia unresponsive to vitamin B12 or folate therapy
  D53.0 Protein deficiency anemia
    Amino-acid deficiency anemia
    Orotaciduric anemia
    Excludes1: Lesch-Nyhan syndrome (E79.1)
  D53.1 Other megaloblastic anemias, not elsewhere classified
    Megaloblastic anemia NOS
    Excludes1: Di Guglielmo's disease (C94.0)
  D53.2 Scorbutic anemia
    Excludes1: scurvy (E54)
  D53.8 Other specified nutritional anemias
    Anemia associated with deficiency of copper
    Anemia associated with deficiency of molybdenum
    Anemia associated with deficiency of zinc
    Excludes1: nutritional deficiencies without anemia, such as:
      copper deficiency NOS (E61.0)
      molybdenum deficiency NOS (E61.5)
      zinc deficiency NOS (E60)
  D53.9 Nutritional anemia, unspecified
    Simple chronic anemia
    Excludes1: anemia NOS (D64.9)
    AHA CC: 4Q, 2018, 88

Hemolytic anemias (D55-D59)

D55 Anemia due to enzyme disorders
  Excludes1: drug-induced enzyme deficiency anemia (D59.2)
  D55.0 Anemia due to glucose-6-phosphate dehydrogenase [G6PD] deficiency
    Favism
    G6PD deficiency anemia
    Excludes1: glucose-6-phosphate dehydrogenase (G6PD) deficiency without anemia (D75.A)
  D55.1 Anemia due to other disorders of glutathione metabolism
    Anemia (due to) enzyme deficiencies, except G6PD, related to the hexose monophosphate [HMP] shunt pathway
    Anemia (due to) hemolytic nonspherocytic (hereditary), type I
  + **D55.2 Anemia due to disorders of glycolytic enzymes**
    Excludes1: disorders of glycolysis not associated with anemia (E74.81-)
    D55.21 Anemia due to pyruvate kinase deficiency
      PK deficiency anemia
      Pyruvate kinase deficiency anemia
      AHA CC: 4Q, 2021, 6-7
    D55.29 Anemia due to other disorders of glycolytic enzymes
      Hexokinase deficiency anemia
      Triose-phosphate isomerase deficiency anemia
      AHA CC: 4Q, 2021, 6-7
  D55.3 Anemia due to disorders of nucleotide metabolism
  D55.8 Other anemias due to enzyme disorders
  D55.9 Anemia due to enzyme disorder, unspecified

D56 Thalassemia
  Excludes1: sickle-cell thalassemia (D57.4-)
  D56.0 Alpha thalassemia
    Alpha thalassemia major
    Hemoglobin H Constant Spring
    Hemoglobin H disease
    Hydrops fetalis due to alpha thalassemia
    Severe alpha thalassemia
    Triple gene defect alpha thalassemia
    Use additional code, if applicable, for hydrops fetalis due to alpha thalassemia (P56.99)
    Excludes1: alpha thalassemia trait or minor (D56.3)
      asymptomatic alpha thalassemia (D56.3)
      hydrops fetalis due to isoimmunization (P56.0)
      hydrops fetalis not due to immune hemolysis (P83.2)
  D56.1 Beta thalassemia
    Beta thalassemia major
    Cooley's anemia
    Homozygous beta thalassemia
    Severe beta thalassemia
    Thalassemia intermedia
    Thalassemia major
    Excludes1: beta thalassemia minor (D56.3)
      beta thalassemia trait (D56.3)
      delta-beta thalassemia (D56.2)
      hemoglobin E-beta thalassemia (D56.5)
      sickle-cell beta thalassemia (D57.4-)

D56.2 **Delta-beta thalassemia**
Homozygous delta-beta thalassemia
Excludes1: *delta-beta thalassemia minor (D56.3)*
delta-beta thalassemia trait (D56.3)

D56.3 **Thalassemia minor**
Alpha thalassemia minor
Alpha thalassemia silent carrier
Alpha thalassemia trait
Beta thalassemia minor
Beta thalassemia trait
Delta-beta thalassemia minor
Delta-beta thalassemia trait
Thalassemia trait NOS
Excludes1: *alpha thalassemia (D56.0)*
beta thalassemia (D56.1)
delta-beta thalassemia (D56.2)
hemoglobin E-beta thalassemia (D56.5)
sickle-cell trait (D57.3)

D56.4 **Hereditary persistence of fetal hemoglobin [HPFH]**

D56.5 **Hemoglobin E-beta thalassemia**
Excludes1: *beta thalassemia (D56.1)*
beta thalassemia minor (D56.3)
beta thalassemia trait (D56.3)
delta-beta thalassemia (D56.2)
delta-beta thalassemia trait (D56.3)
hemoglobin E disease (D58.2)
other hemoglobinopathies (D58.2)
sickle-cell beta thalassemia (D57.4-)

D56.8 **Other thalassemias**
Dominant thalassemia
Hemoglobin C thalassemia
Mixed thalassemia
Thalassemia with other hemoglobinopathy
Excludes1: *hemoglobin C disease (D58.2)*
hemoglobin E disease (D58.2)
other hemoglobinopathies (D58.2)
sickle-cell anemia (D57.-)
sickle-cell thalassemia (D57.4-)

D56.9 **Thalassemia, unspecified**
Mediterranean anemia (with other hemoglobinopathy)

D57 **Sickle-cell disorders**
Use additional code for any associated fever (R50.81)
Excludes1: *other hemoglobinopathies (D58.-)*
AHA CC: 4Q, 2020, 6-7; 2Q, 2022, 28-29

+ **D57.0** **Hb-SS disease with crisis**
Sickle-cell disease with crisis
Hb-SS disease with (vaso-occlusive) pain
MCC **D57.00** **Hb-SS disease with crisis, unspecified**
Hb-SS disease with (painful) crisis NOS
Hb-SS disease with (vaso-occlusive) pain NOS
MCC **D57.01** **Hb-SS disease with acute chest syndrome**
MCC **D57.02** **Hb-SS disease with splenic sequestration**
MCC **D57.03** **Hb-SS disease with cerebral vascular involvement**
Code also, if applicable, cerebral infarction (I63.-)
MCC **D57.04** **Hb-SS disease with dactylitis**
MCC **D57.09** **Hb-SS disease with crisis with other specified complication**
Use additional code to identify complications, such as:
cholelithiasis (K80.-)
priapism (N48.32)

D57.1 **Sickle-cell disease without crisis**
Hb-SS disease without crisis
Sickle-cell anemia NOS
Sickle-cell disease NOS
Sickle-cell disorder NOS

+ **D57.2** **Sickle-cell/Hb-C disease**
Hb-SC disease
Hb-S/Hb-C disease
D57.20 **Sickle-cell/Hb-C disease without crisis**
+ **D57.21** **Sickle-cell/Hb-C disease with crisis**
MCC **D57.211** **Sickle-cell/Hb-C disease with acute chest syndrome**
MCC **D57.212** **Sickle-cell/Hb-C disease with splenic sequestration**
MCC **D57.213** **Sickle-cell/Hb-C disease with cerebral vascular involvement**
Code also, if applicable, cerebral infarction (I63.-)
MCC **D57.214** **Sickle-cell/Hb-C disease with dactylitis**
MCC **D57.218** **Sickle-cell/Hb-C disease with crisis with other specified complication**
Use additional code to identify complications, such as:
cholelithiasis (K80.-)
priapism (N48.32)
MCC **D57.219** **Sickle-cell/Hb-C disease with crisis, unspecified**
Sickle-cell/Hb-C disease with crisis NOS
Sickle-cell/Hb-C disease with (vaso-occlusive) pain NOS

D57.3 **Sickle-cell trait**
Hb-S trait
Heterozygous hemoglobin S

+ **D57.4** **Sickle-cell thalassemia**
Sickle-cell beta thalassemia
Thalassemia Hb-S disease
D57.40 **Sickle-cell thalassemia without crisis**
Microdrepanocytosis
Sickle-cell thalassemia NOS
+ **D57.41** **Sickle-cell thalassemia, unspecified, with crisis**
Sickle-cell thalassemia with (painful) crisis NOS
Sickle-cell thalassemia with (vaso-occlusive) pain NOS
MCC **D57.411** **Sickle-cell thalassemia, unspecified, with acute chest syndrome**
MCC **D57.412** **Sickle-cell thalassemia, unspecified, with splenic sequestration**
MCC **D57.413** **Sickle-cell thalassemia, unspecified, with cerebral vascular involvement**
Code also, if applicable, cerebral infarction (I63.-)
MCC **D57.414** **Sickle-cell thalassemia, unspecified, with dactylitis**
MCC **D57.418** **Sickle-cell thalassemia, unspecified, with crisis with other specified complication**
Use additional code to identify complications, such as:
cholelithiasis (K80.-)
priapism (N48.32)
MCC **D57.419** **Sickle-cell thalassemia, unspecified, with crisis**
Sickle-cell thalassemia with (painful) crisis NOS
Sickle-cell thalassemia with (vaso-occlusive) pain NOS
D57.42 **Sickle-cell thalassemia beta zero without crisis**
HbS-beta zero without crisis
Sickle-cell beta zero without crisis
+ **D57.43** **Sickle-cell thalassemia beta zero with crisis**
HbS-beta zero with crisis
Sickle-cell beta zero with crisis
MCC **D57.431** **Sickle-cell thalassemia beta zero with acute chest syndrome**
HbS-beta zero with acute chest syndrome
Sickle-cell beta zero with acute chest syndrome
MCC **D57.432** **Sickle-cell thalassemia beta zero with splenic sequestration**
HbS-beta zero with splenic sequestration
Sickle-cell beta zero with splenic sequestration
MCC **D57.433** **Sickle-cell thalassemia beta zero with cerebral vascular involvement**
HbS-beta zero with cerebral vascular involvement
Sickle-cell beta zero with cerebral vascular involvement
Code also, if applicable, cerebral infarction (I63.-)
MCC **D57.434** **Sickle-cell thalassemia beta zero with dactylitis**

MCC D57.438 Sickle-cell thalassemia beta zero with crisis with other specified complication
    HbS-beta zero with other specified complication
    Sickle-cell beta zero with other specified complication
    Use additional code to identify complications, such as:
      cholelithiasis (K80.-)
      priapism (N48.32)

MCC D57.439 Sickle-cell thalassemia beta zero with crisis, unspecified
    HbS-beta zero with other specified complication
    Sickle-cell beta zero with crisis unspecified
    Sickle-cell thalassemia beta zero with (painful) crisis NOS
    Sickle-cell thalassemia beta zero with (vaso-occlusive) pain NOS

D57.44 Sickle-cell thalassemia beta plus without crisis
    HbS-beta plus without crisis
    Sickle-cell beta plus without crisis

+ D57.45 Sickle-cell thalassemia beta plus with crisis
    HbS-beta plus with crisis
    Sickle-cell beta plus with crisis

MCC D57.451 Sickle-cell thalassemia beta plus with acute chest syndrome
    HbS-beta plus with acute chest syndrome
    Sickle-cell beta plus with acute chest syndrome

MCC D57.452 Sickle-cell thalassemia beta plus with splenic sequestration
    HbS-beta plus with splenic sequestration
    Sickle-cell beta plus with splenic sequestration

MCC D57.453 Sickle-cell thalassemia beta plus with cerebral vascular involvement
    HbS-beta plus with cerebral vascular involvement
    Sickle-cell beta plus with cerebral vascular involvement
    Code also, if applicable, cerebral infarction (I63.-)

MCC D57.454 Sickle-cell thalassemia beta plus with dactylitis

MCC D57.458 Sickle-cell thalassemia beta plus with crisis with other specified complication
    HbS-beta plus with crisis with other specified complication
    Sickle-cell beta plus with crisis with other specified complication
    Use additional code to identify complications, such as:
      cholelithiasis (K80.-)
      priapism (N48.32)

MCC D57.459 Sickle-cell thalassemia beta plus with crisis, unspecified
    HbS-beta plus with crisis with unspecified complication
    Sickle-cell beta plus with crisis with unspecified complication
    Sickle-cell thalassemia beta plus with (painful) crisis NOS
    Sickle-cell thalassemia beta plus with (vaso-occlusive) pain NOS

+ D57.8 Other sickle-cell disorders
    Hb-SD disease
    Hb-SE disease

D57.80 Other sickle-cell disorders without crisis

+ D57.81 Other sickle-cell disorders with crisis

MCC D57.811 Other sickle-cell disorders with acute chest syndrome

MCC D57.812 Other sickle-cell disorders with splenic sequestration

MCC D57.813 Other sickle-cell disorders with cerebral vascular involvement
    Code also, if applicable, cerebral infarction (I63.-)

MCC D57.814 Other sickle-cell disorders with dactylitis

MCC D57.818 Other sickle-cell disorders with crisis with other specified complication
    Use additional code to identify complications, such as:
      cholelithiasis (K80.-)
      priapism (N48.32)

MCC D57.819 Other sickle-cell disorders with crisis, unspecified
    Other sickle-cell disorders with crisis NOS
    Other sickle-cell disorders with (vaso-occlusive) pain NOS

D58 Other hereditary hemolytic anemias

Excludes1: hemolytic anemia of the newborn (P55.-)

D58.0 Hereditary spherocytosis
    Acholuric (familial) jaundice
    Congenital (spherocytic) hemolytic icterus
    Minkowski-Chauffard syndrome

D58.1 Hereditary elliptocytosis
    Elliptocytosis (congenital)
    Ovalocytosis (congenital) (hereditary)

D58.2 Other hemoglobinopathies
    Abnormal hemoglobin NOS
    Congenital Heinz body anemia
    Hb-C disease
    Hb-D disease
    Hb-E disease
    Hemoglobinopathy NOS
    Unstable hemoglobin hemolytic disease
    Excludes1: familial polycythemia (D75.0)
      Hb-M disease (D74.0)
      hemoglobin E-beta thalassemia (D56.5)
      hereditary persistence of fetal hemoglobin [HPFH] (D56.4)
      high-altitude polycythemia (D75.1)
      methemoglobinemia (D74.-)
      other hemoglobinopathies with thalassemia (D56.8)

CC D58.8 Other specified hereditary hemolytic anemias
    Stomatocytosis

CC D58.9 Hereditary hemolytic anemia, unspecified

D59 Acquired hemolytic anemia

CC D59.0 Drug-induced autoimmune hemolytic anemia
    Use additional code for adverse effect, if applicable, to identify drug (T36-T50 with fifth or sixth character 5)

+ D59.1 Other autoimmune hemolytic anemias
    Excludes2: Evans syndrome (D69.41)
      hemolytic disease of newborn (P55.-)
      paroxysmal cold hemoglobinuria (D59.6)
    AHA CC: 4Q, 2020, 7-8

CC D59.10 Autoimmune hemolytic anemia, unspecified

CC D59.11 Warm autoimmune hemolytic anemia
    Warm type (primary) (secondary) (symptomatic) autoimmune hemolytic anemia
    Warm type autoimmune hemolytic disease

CC D59.12 Cold autoimmune hemolytic anemia
    Chronic cold hemagglutinin disease
    Cold agglutinin disease
    Cold agglutinin hemoglobinuria
    Cold type (primary) (secondary) (symptomatic) autoimmune hemolytic anemia
    Cold type autoimmune hemolytic disease

CC D59.13 Mixed type autoimmune hemolytic anemia
    Mixed type autoimmune hemolytic disease
    Mixed type, cold and warm, (primary) (secondary) (symptomatic) autoimmune hemolytic anemia

CC D59.19 Other autoimmune hemolytic anemia

CC D59.2 Drug-induced nonautoimmune hemolytic anemia
    Drug-induced enzyme deficiency anemia
    Use additional code for adverse effect, if applicable, to identify drug (T36-T50 with fifth or sixth character 5)

+ D59.3 Hemolytic-uremic syndrome
    Code also, if applicable, any associated:
      acute kidney failure (N17.-)
      chronic kidney disease (N18.-)
    AHA CC: 4Q, 2022, 5-6
    Review coding guideline C.1.a.2.a

MCC D59.30 Hemolytic-uremic syndrome, unspecified
    Hemolytic-uremic syndrome NOS

MCC **D59.31** **Infection-associated hemolytic-uremic syndrome**
  Shiga toxin-producing E. coli [STEC] related hemolytic uremic syndrome
  Typical hemolytic uremic syndrome
  Use additional code to identify associated infection, such as:
    E. coli infection (B96.2-)
    Human immunodeficiency virus [HIV] disease (B20)
    Pneumococcal meningitis (G00.1)
    Pneumococcal pneumonia (J13)
    Sepsis due to Streptococcus pneumoniae (A40.3)
    Shigella dysenteriae (A03.9)
    Streptococcus pneumoniae as the cause of diseases classified elsewhere (B95.3)

MCC **D59.32** **Hereditary hemolytic-uremic syndrome**
  Atypical hemolytic uremic syndrome with an identified genetic cause
  Code also, if applicable:
    defects in the complement system (D84.1)
    methylmalonic acidemia (E71.120)

MCC **D59.39** **Other hemolytic-uremic syndrome**
  Atypical (nongenetic) hemolytic uremic syndrome
  Secondary hemolytic-uremic syndrome
  Code first, if applicable, any associated:
    COVID-19 (U07.1)
    complications of kidney transplant (T86.1-)
    complications of heart transplant (T86.2-)
    complications of liver transplant (T86.4-)

  Code also, if applicable, any associated condition, such as:
    hypertensive emergency (I16.1)
    malignant neoplasm (C00-C96)
    systemic lupus erythematosus (M32.-)

  Use additional code, if applicable, for adverse effect to identify drug (T36-T50 with fifth or sixth character 5)
  AHA CC: 4Q, 2022, 5-6

CC **D59.4** **Other nonautoimmune hemolytic anemias**
  Mechanical hemolytic anemia
  Microangiopathic hemolytic anemia
  Toxic hemolytic anemia

D59.5 **Paroxysmal nocturnal hemoglobinuria [Marchiafava-Micheli]**
  Excludes1: hemoglobinuria NOS (R82.3)

D59.6 **Hemoglobinuria due to hemolysis from other external causes**
  Hemoglobinuria from exertion
  March hemoglobinuria
  Paroxysmal cold hemoglobinuria
  Use additional code (Chapter 20) to identify external cause
  Excludes1: hemoglobinuria NOS (R82.3)

D59.8 **Other acquired hemolytic anemias**
CC **D59.9** **Acquired hemolytic anemia, unspecified**
  Idiopathic hemolytic anemia, chronic

Aplastic and other anemias and other bone marrow failure syndromes (D60-D64)

D60 **Acquired pure red cell aplasia [erythroblastopenia]**
  Includes: red cell aplasia (acquired) (adult) (with thymoma)
  Excludes1: congenital red cell aplasia (D61.01)
MCC **D60.0** Chronic acquired pure red cell aplasia
MCC **D60.1** Transient acquired pure red cell aplasia
MCC **D60.8** Other acquired pure red cell aplasias
MCC **D60.9** Acquired pure red cell aplasia, unspecified

D61 **Other aplastic anemias and other bone marrow failure syndromes**
  Excludes2: neutropenia (D70.-)
  + **D61.0** **Constitutional aplastic anemia**
    CC **D61.01** **Constitutional (pure) red blood cell aplasia**
      Blackfan-Diamond syndrome
      Congenital (pure) red cell aplasia
      Familial hypoplastic anemia
      Primary (pure) red cell aplasia
      Red cell (pure) aplasia of infants
      Excludes1: acquired red cell aplasia (D60.9)

CC **D61.02** **Shwachman-Diamond syndrome**
  Code also, if applicable, associated conditions such as:
    acute myeloblastic leukemia (C92.0-)
    exocrine pancreatic insufficiency (K86.81)
    myelodysplastic syndrome (D46.-)
  Use Additional code, if applicable, for genetic susceptibility to other malignant neoplasm (Z15.09)

CC **D61.09** **Other constitutional aplastic anemia**
  Fanconi's anemia
  Pancytopenia with malformations

MCC **D61.1** **Drug-induced aplastic anemia**
  Use additional code for adverse effect, if applicable, to identify drug (T36-T50 with fifth or sixth character 5)

MCC **D61.2** **Aplastic anemia due to other external agents**
  Code first, if applicable, toxic effects of substances chiefly nonmedicinal as to source (T51-T65)

MCC **D61.3** **Idiopathic aplastic anemia**
  + **D61.8** **Other specified aplastic anemias and other bone marrow failure syndromes**
    + **D61.81** **Pancytopenia**
      Excludes1: pancytopenia (due to) (with) aplastic anemia (D61.9)
        pancytopenia (due to) (with) bone marrow infiltration (D61.82)
        pancytopenia (due to) (with) congenital (pure) red cell aplasia (D61.01)
        pancytopenia (due to) (with) hairy cell leukemia (C91.4-)
        pancytopenia (due to) (with) human immunodeficiency virus disease (B20.-)
        pancytopenia (due to) (with) leukoerythroblastic anemia (D61.82)
        pancytopenia (due to) (with) myeloproliferative disease (D47.1)
      Excludes2: pancytopenia (due to) (with) myelodysplastic syndromes (D46.-)

      MCC **D61.810** **Antineoplastic chemotherapy induced pancytopenia**
        Excludes2: aplastic anemia due to antineoplastic chemotherapy (D61.1)
        AHA CC: 3Q, 2020, 22-23
      MCC **D61.811** **Other drug-induced pancytopenia**
        Excludes2: aplastic anemia due to drugs (D61.1)
      CC **D61.818** **Other pancytopenia**
        AHA CC: 1Q, 2019, 16-17; 1Q, 2023, 23

    CC **D61.82** **Myelophthisis**
      Leukoerythroblastic anemia
      Myelophthisic anemia
      Panmyelophthisis
      Code also the underlying disorder, such as:
        malignant neoplasm of breast (C50.-)
        tuberculosis (A15.-)
      Excludes1: idiopathic myelofibrosis (D47.1)
        myelofibrosis NOS (D75.81)
        myelofibrosis with myeloid metaplasia (D47.4)
        primary myelofibrosis (D47.1)
        secondary myelofibrosis (D75.81)

    MCC **D61.89** **Other specified aplastic anemias and other bone marrow failure syndromes**

CC **D61.9** **Aplastic anemia, unspecified**
  Hypoplastic anemia NOS
  Medullary hypoplasia

CC **D62** **Acute posthemorrhagic anemia**
  Excludes1: anemia due to chronic blood loss (D50.0)
    blood loss anemia NOS (D50.0)
    congenital anemia from fetal blood loss (P61.3)
  AHA CC: 3Q, 2019, 11-12, 17
  Valid 3-character code, no further characters required

D63 Anemia in chronic diseases classified elsewhere

D63.0 Anemia in neoplastic disease
Code first neoplasm (C00-D49)
Excludes1: aplastic anemia due to antineoplastic chemotherapy (D61.1)
Excludes2: anemia due to antineoplastic chemotherapy (D64.81)
Review coding guidelines C.2.c.1, C.2.c.2 and C.2.l.4

D63.1 Anemia in chronic kidney disease
Erythropoietin resistant anemia (EPO resistant anemia)
Code first underlying chronic kidney disease (CKD) (N18.-)

D63.8 Anemia in other chronic diseases classified elsewhere
Code first underlying disease, such as:
diphyllobothriasis (B70.0)
hookworm disease (B76.0-B76.9)
hypothyroidism (E00.0-E03.9)
malaria (B50.0-B54)
symptomatic late syphilis (A52.79)
tuberculosis (A18.89)

D64 Other anemias
Excludes1: refractory anemia (D46.-)
refractory anemia with excess blasts in transformation [RAEB T] (C92.0-)

D64.0 Hereditary sideroblastic anemia
Sex-linked hypochromic sideroblastic anemia

D64.1 Secondary sideroblastic anemia due to disease
Code first underlying disease

D64.2 Secondary sideroblastic anemia due to drugs and toxins
Code first poisoning due to drug or toxin, if applicable (T36-T65 with fifth or sixth character 1-4)
Use additional code for adverse effect, if applicable, to identify drug (T36-T50 with fifth or sixth character 5)

D64.3 Other sideroblastic anemias
Sideroblastic anemia NOS
Pyridoxine-responsive sideroblastic anemia NEC

D64.4 Congenital dyserythropoietic anemia
Dyshematopoietic anemia (congenital)
Excludes1: Blackfan-Diamond syndrome (D61.01)
Di Guglielmo's disease (C94.0)

+ D64.8 Other specified anemias
D64.81 Anemia due to antineoplastic chemotherapy
Antineoplastic chemotherapy induced anemia
Excludes2: anemia in neoplastic disease (D63.0)
aplastic anemia due to antineoplastic chemotherapy (D61.1)
AHA CC: 4Q, 2014, 22-23; 3Q, 2021, 4

D64.89 Other specified anemias
Infantile pseudoleukemia

D64.9 Anemia, unspecified
AHA CC: 4Q, 2018, 88

Coagulation defects, purpura and other hemorrhagic conditions (D65-D69)

MCC D65 Disseminated intravascular coagulation [defibrination syndrome]
Afibrinogenemia, acquired
Consumption coagulopathy
COVID-19 associated diffuse or disseminated intravascular coagulopathy
Diffuse or disseminated intravascular coagulation [DIC]
Fibrinolytic hemorrhage, acquired
Fibrinolytic purpura
Purpura fulminans
Code also, if applicable, associated condition
Excludes1: disseminated intravascular coagulation (complicating):
abortion or ectopic or molar pregnancy (O00-O07, O08.1)
in newborn (P60)
pregnancy, childbirth and the puerperium (O45.0, O46.0, O67.0, O72.3)
AHA CC: 1Q, 2021, 39
Valid 3-character code, no further characters required

MCC D66 Hereditary factor VIII deficiency
Classical hemophilia
Deficiency factor VIII (with functional defect)
Hemophilia NOS
Hemophilia A
Excludes1: factor VIII deficiency with vascular defect (D68.0-)
Valid 3-character code, no further characters required

MCC D67 Hereditary factor IX deficiency
Christmas disease
Factor IX deficiency (with functional defect)
Hemophilia B
Plasma thromboplastin component [PTC] deficiency
Valid 3-character code, no further characters required

D68 Other coagulation defects
Excludes1: abnormal coagulation profile NOS (R79.1)
Excludes2: coagulation defects complicating abortion or ectopic or molar pregnancy (O00-O07, O08.1)
coagulation defects complicating pregnancy, childbirth and the puerperium (O45.0, O46.0, O67.0, O72.3)

+ D68.0 Von Willebrand's disease
Excludes1: capillary fragility (hereditary) (D69.8)
factor VIII deficiency NOS (D66)
factor VIII deficiency with functional defect (D66)
AHA CC: 4Q, 2022, 7-9

CC D68.00 Von Willebrand disease, unspecified
CC D68.01 Von Willebrand disease, type 1
Partial quantitative deficiency of von Willebrand factor
Type 1C von Willebrand disease
AHA CC: 4Q, 2022, 9

+ D68.02 Von Willebrand disease, type 2
Qualitative defects of von Willebrand factor

CC D68.020 Von Willebrand disease, type 2A
Qualitative defects of von Willebrand factor with decreased platelet adhesion and selective deficiency of high-molecular-weight multimers

CC D68.021 Von Willebrand disease, type 2B
Qualitative defects of von Willebrand factor with high-molecular-weight von Willebrand factor loss
Qualitative defects of von Willebrand factor with hyper-adhesive forms
Qualitative defects of von Willebrand factor with increased affinity for platelet glycoprotein Ib

CC D68.022 Von Willebrand disease, type 2M
Qualitative defects of von Willebrand factor with defective platelet adhesion with a normal size distribution of von Willebrand factor multimers

CC D68.023 Von Willebrand disease, type 2N
Qualitative defects of von Willebrand factor with defective von Willebrand factor to factor VIII binding
Qualitative defects of von Willebrand factor with markedly decreased affinity for factor VIII

CC D68.029 Von Willebrand disease, type 2, unspecified
Qualitative defect in von Willebrand factor function, with no further subtyping

CC D68.03 Von Willebrand disease, type 3
(Near) complete absence of von Willebrand factor
Total quantitative deficiency of von Willebrand factor

CC D68.04 Acquired von Willebrand disease
Acquired von Willebrand syndrome

CC D68.09 Other von Willebrand disease
Platelet-type von Willebrand disease
Pseudo-von Willebrand disease
Code also, if applicable, qualitative platelet defects (D69.1)

CC D68.1 Hereditary factor XI deficiency
Hemophilia C
Plasma thromboplastin antecedent [PTA] deficiency
Rosenthal's disease

CC **D68.2** **Hereditary deficiency of other clotting factors**
    AC globulin deficiency
    Congenital afibrinogenemia
    Deficiency of factor I [fibrinogen]
    Deficiency of factor II [prothrombin]
    Deficiency of factor V [labile]
    Deficiency of factor VII [stable]
    Deficiency of factor X [Stuart-Prower]
    Deficiency of factor XII [Hageman]
    Deficiency of factor XIII [fibrin stabilizing]
    Dysfibrinogenemia (congenital)
    Hypoproconvertinemia
    Owren's disease
    Proaccelerin deficiency

+ **D68.3** **Hemorrhagic disorder due to circulating anticoagulants**
  + **D68.31** **Hemorrhagic disorder due to intrinsic circulating anticoagulants, antibodies, or inhibitors**
    CC **D68.311** **Acquired hemophilia**
        Autoimmune hemophilia
        Autoimmune inhibitors to clotting factors
        Secondary hemophilia
    CC **D68.312** **Antiphospholipid antibody with hemorrhagic disorder**
        Lupus anticoagulant (LAC) with hemorrhagic disorder
        Systemic lupus erythematosus [SLE] inhibitor with hemorrhagic disorder
        Excludes1: *antiphospholipid antibody, finding without diagnosis (R76.0)*
            antiphospholipid antibody syndrome (D68.61)
            antiphospholipid antibody with hypercoagulable state (D68.61)
            lupus anticoagulant (LAC) finding without diagnosis (R76.0)
            lupus anticoagulant (LAC) with hypercoagulable state (D68.62)
            systemic lupus erythematosus [SLE] inhibitor finding without diagnosis (R76.0)
            systemic lupus erythematosus [SLE] inhibitor with hypercoagulable state (D68.62)
    CC **D68.318** **Other hemorrhagic disorder due to intrinsic circulating anticoagulants, antibodies, or inhibitors**
        Antithromboplastinemia
        Antithromboplastinogenemia
        Hemorrhagic disorder due to intrinsic increase in antithrombin
        Hemorrhagic disorder due to intrinsic increase in anti-VIIIa
        Hemorrhagic disorder due to intrinsic increase in anti-IXa
        Hemorrhagic disorder due to intrinsic increase in anti-XIa
  CC **D68.32** **Hemorrhagic disorder due to extrinsic circulating anticoagulants**
    Drug-induced hemorrhagic disorder
    Hemorrhagic disorder due to increase in anti-IIa
    Hemorrhagic disorder due to increase in anti-Xa
    Hyperheparinemia
    Use additional code for adverse effect, if applicable, to identify drug (T45.515, T45.525)
    AHA CC: 1Q, 2016, 14-15; 1Q, 2021, 4-5

CC **D68.4** **Acquired coagulation factor deficiency**
    Deficiency of coagulation factor due to liver disease
    Deficiency of coagulation factor due to vitamin K deficiency
    Excludes1: *vitamin K deficiency of newborn (P53)*

+ **D68.5** **Primary thrombophilia**
    Primary hypercoagulable states
    Excludes1: *antiphospholipid syndrome (D68.61)*
        lupus anticoagulant (D68.62)
        secondary activated protein C resistance (D68.69)
        secondary antiphospholipid antibody syndrome (D68.69)
        secondary lupus anticoagulant with hypercoagulable state (D68.69)
        secondary systemic lupus erythematosus [SLE] inhibitor with hypercoagulable state (D68.69)
        systemic lupus erythematosus [SLE] inhibitor finding without diagnosis (R76.0)
        systemic lupus erythematosus [SLE] inhibitor with hemorrhagic disorder (D68.312)
        thrombotic thrombocytopenic purpura (M31.19)
  CC **D68.51** **Activated protein C resistance**
    Factor V Leiden mutation
  CC **D68.52** **Prothrombin gene mutation**
  CC **D68.59** **Other primary thrombophilia**
    Antithrombin III deficiency
    Hypercoagulable state NOS
    Primary hypercoagulable state NEC
    Primary thrombophilia NEC
    Protein C deficiency
    Protein S deficiency
    Thrombophilia NOS
    AHA CC: 2Q, 2021, 8-9

+ **D68.6** **Other thrombophilia**
    Other hypercoagulable states
    Excludes1: *diffuse or disseminated intravascular coagulation [DIC] (D65)*
        heparin induced thrombocytopenia (HIT) (D75.82-)
        hyperhomocysteinemia (E72.11)
  CC **D68.61** **Antiphospholipid syndrome**
    Anticardiolipin syndrome
    Antiphospholipid antibody syndrome
    Excludes1: *anti-phospholipid antibody, finding without diagnosis (R76.0)*
        anti-phospholipid antibody with hemorrhagic disorder (D68.312)
        lupus anticoagulant syndrome (D68.62)
  CC **D68.62** **Lupus anticoagulant syndrome**
    Lupus anticoagulant
    Presence of systemic lupus erythematosus [SLE] inhibitor
    Excludes1: *anticardiolipin syndrome (D68.61)*
        antiphospholipid syndrome (D68.61)
        lupus anticoagulant (LAC) finding without diagnosis (R76.0)
        lupus anticoagulant (LAC) with hemorrhagic disorder (D68.312)
  CC **D68.69** **Other thrombophilia**
    COVID-19 associated hypercoagulability
    Hypercoagulable states NEC
    Secondary hypercoagulable state NOS
    Code also, if applicable, associated condition
    AHA CC: 2Q, 2021, 8

CC **D68.8** **Other specified coagulation defects**
    COVID-19 associated coagulopathy
    Code also, if applicable, associated condition
    Excludes1: *hemorrhagic disease of newborn (P53)*
    AHA CC: 1Q, 2021, 39-40

CC **D68.9** **Coagulation defect, unspecified**

D69 Purpura and other hemorrhagic conditions

Excludes1: benign hypergammaglobulinemic purpura (D89.0)
cryoglobulinemic purpura (D89.1)
essential (hemorrhagic) thrombocythemia (D47.3)
hemorrhagic thrombocythemia (D47.3)
purpura fulminans (D65)
thrombotic thrombocytopenic purpura (M31.19)
Waldenström hypergammaglobulinemic purpura (D89.0)

CC D69.0 Allergic purpura
Allergic vasculitis
Nonthrombocytopenic hemorrhagic purpura
Nonthrombocytopenic idiopathic purpura
Purpura anaphylactoid
Purpura Henoch(-Schönlein)
Purpura rheumatica
Vascular purpura
Excludes1: thrombocytopenic hemorrhagic purpura (D69.3)
AHA CC: 3Q, 2020, 26-27

CC D69.1 Qualitative platelet defects
Bernard-Soulier [giant platelet] syndrome
Glanzmann's disease
Grey platelet syndrome
Thromboasthenia (hemorrhagic) (hereditary)
Thrombocytopathy
Excludes1: hemolytic-uremic syndrome (D59.3-)
Excludes2: von Willebrand disease (D68.0-)

D69.2 Other nonthrombocytopenic purpura
Purpura NOS
Purpura simplex
Senile purpura

CC D69.3 Immune thrombocytopenic purpura
Hemorrhagic (thrombocytopenic) purpura
Idiopathic thrombocytopenic purpura
Tidal platelet dysgenesis

+ D69.4 Other primary thrombocytopenia
Excludes1: transient neonatal thrombocytopenia (P61.0)
Wiskott-Aldrich syndrome (D82.0)

CC D69.41 Evans syndrome
CC D69.42 Congenital and hereditary thrombocytopenia purpura
Congenital thrombocytopenia
Hereditary thrombocytopenia
Code first congenital or hereditary disorder, such as:
thrombocytopenia with absent radius (TAR syndrome) (Q87.2)

D69.49 Other primary thrombocytopenia
Megakaryocytic hypoplasia
Primary thrombocytopenia NOS

+ D69.5 Secondary thrombocytopenia
Excludes1: heparin induced thrombocytopenia (HIT) (D75.82-)
transient thrombocytopenia of newborn (P61.0)

D69.51 Posttransfusion purpura
Posttransfusion purpura from whole blood (fresh) or blood products PTP

D69.59 Other secondary thrombocytopenia
AHA CC: 4Q, 2014, 22-23

D69.6 Thrombocytopenia, unspecified
D69.8 Other specified hemorrhagic conditions
Capillary fragility (hereditary)
Vascular pseudohemophilia
D69.9 Hemorrhagic condition, unspecified

Other disorders of blood and blood-forming organs (D70-D77)

D70 Neutropenia
Includes: agranulocytosis
decreased absolute neurophile count (ANC)
Use additional code for any associated:
fever (R50.81)
Code also, if applicable, mucositis (J34.81, K12.3-, K92.81, N76.81)
Excludes1: neutropenic splenomegaly (D73.81)
transient neonatal neutropenia (P61.5)

D70.0 Congenital agranulocytosis
Congenital neutropenia
Infantile genetic agranulocytosis
Kostmann's disease

D70.1 Agranulocytosis secondary to cancer chemotherapy
Use additional code for adverse effect, if applicable, to identify drug (T45.1X5)

Code also underlying neoplasm
AHA CC: 4Q, 2014, 22-23

D70.2 Other drug-induced agranulocytosis
Use additional code for adverse effect, if applicable, to identify drug (T36-T50 with fifth or sixth character 5)

D70.3 Neutropenia due to infection
D70.4 Cyclic neutropenia
Cyclic hematopoiesis
Periodic neutropenia

D70.8 Other neutropenia
D70.9 Neutropenia, unspecified
AHA CC: 2Q, 2019, 24-26

D71 Functional disorders of polymorphonuclear neutrophils
Cell membrane receptor complex [CR3] defect
Chronic (childhood) granulomatous disease
Congenital dysphagocytosis
Progressive septic granulomatosis
Valid 3-character code, no further characters required

D72 Other disorders of white blood cells
Excludes1: basophilia (D72.824)
immunity disorders (D80-D89)
neutropenia (D70)
preleukemia (syndrome) (D46.9)

D72.0 Genetic anomalies of leukocytes
Alder (granulation) (granulocyte) anomaly
Alder syndrome
Hereditary leukocytic hypersegmentation
Hereditary leukocytic hyposegmentation
Hereditary leukomelanopathy
May-Hegglin (granulation) (granulocyte) anomaly
May-Hegglin syndrome
Pelger-Huët (granulation) (granulocyte) anomaly
Pelger-Huët syndrome
Excludes1: Chédiak (-Steinbrinck)-Higashi syndrome (E70.330)

+ D72.1 Eosinophilia
Excludes2: Löffler's syndrome (J82.89)
pulmonary eosinophilia (J82.-)
AHA CC: 4Q, 2020, 8-10

D72.10 Eosinophilia, unspecified
+ D72.11 Hypereosinophilic syndrome [HES]

D72.110 Idiopathic hypereosinophilic syndrome [IHES]

D72.111 Lymphocytic Variant Hypereosinophilic Syndrome [LHES]
Lymphocyte variant hypereosinophilia
Code also, if applicable, any associated lymphocytic neoplastic disorder
AHA CC: 4Q, 2020, 10

D72.118 Other hypereosinophilic syndrome
Episodic angioendema with eosinophilia
Gleich's syndrome

D72.119 Hypereosinophilic syndrome [HES], unspecified

D72.12 Drug rash with eosinophilia and systemic symptoms syndrome
  DRESS syndrome
  Use additional code for adverse effect, if applicable, to identify drug (T36-T50 with fifth or sixth character 5)

D72.18 Eosinophilia in diseases classified elsewhere
  Code first underlying disease, such as: chronic myelomonocytic leukemia (C93.1-)

D72.19 Other eosinophilia
  Familial eosinophilia
  Hereditary eosinophilia

+ **D72.8** Other specified disorders of white blood cells
  Excludes1: *leukemia (C91-C95)*

+ **D72.81** Decreased white blood cell count
  Excludes1: *neutropenia (D70.-)*

  D72.810 Lymphocytopenia
    Decreased lymphocytes

  D72.818 Other decreased white blood cell count
    Basophilic leukopenia
    Eosinophilic leukopenia
    Monocytopenia
    Other decreased leukocytes
    Plasmacytopenia

  D72.819 Decreased white blood cell count, unspecified
    Decreased leukocytes, unspecified
    Leukocytopenia, unspecified
    Leukopenia
    Excludes1: *malignant leukopenia (D70.9)*

+ **D72.82** Elevated white blood cell count
  Excludes1: *eosinophilia (D72.1)*

  D72.820 Lymphocytosis (symptomatic)
    Elevated lymphocytes

  D72.821 Monocytosis (symptomatic)
    Excludes1: *infectious mononucleosis (B27.-)*

  D72.822 Plasmacytosis

  D72.823 Leukemoid reaction
    Basophilic leukemoid reaction
    Leukemoid reaction NOS
    Lymphocytic leukemoid reaction
    Monocytic leukemoid reaction
    Myelocytic leukemoid reaction
    Neutrophilic leukemoid reaction

  D72.824 Basophilia

  D72.825 Bandemia
    Bandemia without diagnosis of specific infection
    Excludes1: *confirmed infection - code to infection*
      leukemia (C91.-, C92.-, C93.-, C94.-, C95.-)

  D72.828 Other elevated white blood cell count

  D72.829 Elevated white blood cell count, unspecified
    Elevated leukocytes, unspecified
    Leukocytosis, unspecified

D72.89 Other specified disorders of white blood cells
  Abnormality of white blood cells NEC

D72.9 Disorder of white blood cells, unspecified
  Abnormal leukocyte differential NOS

D73 **Diseases of spleen**

D73.0 Hyposplenism
  Atrophy of spleen
  Excludes1: *asplenia (congenital) (Q89.01)*
    postsurgical absence of spleen (Z90.81)

D73.1 Hypersplenism
  Excludes1: *neutropenic splenomegaly (D73.81)*
    primary splenic neutropenia (D73.81)
    splenitis, splenomegaly in late syphilis (A52.79)
    splenitis, splenomegaly in tuberculosis (A18.85)
    splenomegaly NOS (R16.1)
    splenomegaly congenital (Q89.0)

D73.2 Chronic congestive splenomegaly

D73.3 Abscess of spleen

D73.4 Cyst of spleen

D73.5 Infarction of spleen
  Splenic rupture, nontraumatic
  Torsion of spleen
  Excludes1: *rupture of spleen due to Plasmodium vivax malaria (B51.0)*
    traumatic rupture of spleen (S36.03-)

+ **D73.8** Other diseases of spleen

  D73.81 Neutropenic splenomegaly
    Werner-Schultz disease

  D73.89 Other diseases of spleen
    Fibrosis of spleen NOS
    Perisplenitis
    Splenitis NOS

D73.9 Disease of spleen, unspecified

D74 **Methemoglobinemia**

CC **D74.0** Congenital methemoglobinemia
  Congenital NADH-methemoglobin reductase deficiency
  Hemoglobin-M [Hb-M] disease
  Methemoglobinemia, hereditary

CC **D74.8** Other methemoglobinemias
  Acquired methemoglobinemia (with sulfhemoglobinemia)
  Toxic methemoglobinemia

CC **D74.9** Methemoglobinemia, unspecified

D75 **Other and unspecified diseases of blood and blood-forming organs**
  Excludes2: *acute lymphadenitis (L04.-)*
    chronic lymphadenitis (I88.1)
    enlarged lymph nodes (R59.-)
    hypergammaglobulinemia NOS (D89.2)
    lymphadenitis NOS (I88.9)
    mesenteric lymphadenitis (acute) (chronic) (I88.0)

D75.0 Familial erythrocytosis
  Benign polycythemia
  Familial polycythemia
  Excludes1: *hereditary ovalocytosis (D58.1)*

D75.1 Secondary polycythemia
  Acquired polycythemia
  Emotional polycythemia
  Erythrocytosis NOS
  Hypoxemic polycythemia
  Nephrogenous polycythemia
  Polycythemia due to erythropoietin
  Polycythemia due to fall in plasma volume
  Polycythemia due to high altitude
  Polycythemia due to stress
  Polycythemia NOS
  Relative polycythemia
  Excludes1: *polycythemia neonatorum (P61.1)*
    polycythemia vera (D45)

+ **D75.8** Other specified diseases of blood and blood-forming organs

CC **D75.81** Myelofibrosis
    Myelofibrosis NOS
    Secondary myelofibrosis NOS
    Code first the underlying disorder, such as: malignant neoplasm of breast (C50.-)
    Use additional code, if applicable, for associated therapy-related myelodysplastic syndrome (D46.-)
    Use additional code for adverse effect, if applicable, to identify drug (T45.1X5)
    Excludes1: *acute myelofibrosis (C94.4-)*
      idiopathic myelofibrosis (D47.1)
      leukoerythroblastic anemia (D61.82)
      myelofibrosis with myeloid metaplasia (D47.4)
      myelophthisic anemia (D61.82)
      myelophthisis (D61.82)
      primary myelofibrosis (D47.1)

- **D75.82** Heparin induced thrombocytopenia (HIT)
  Use additional code, if applicable, for adverse effect of heparin (T45.515-)
  AHA CC: 4Q, 2022, 9-10
  - **D75.821** Non-immune heparin-induced thrombocytopenia
    Non-immune HIT
    Type 1 heparin-induced thrombocytopenia
  - **D75.822** Immune-mediated heparin-induced thrombocytopenia
    Immune-mediated HIT
    Type 2 heparin-induced thrombocytopenia
  - **D75.828** Other heparin-induced thrombocytopenia syndrome
    Autoimmune heparin-induced thrombocytopenia syndrome
    Delayed-onset heparin-induced thrombocytopenia
    Persisting heparin-induced thrombocytopenia
  - **D75.829** Heparin-induced thrombocytopenia, unspecified
- **D75.83** Thrombocytosis
  Excludes2: essential thrombocythemia (D47.3)
  AHA CC: 4Q, 2021, 7-8
  - **D75.838** Other thrombocytosis
    Reactive thrombocytosis
    Secondary thrombocytosis
    Code also underlying condition, if known and applicable
  - **D75.839** Thrombocytosis, unspecified
    Thrombocythemia NOS
    Thrombocytosis NOS
- **D75.84** Other platelet-activating anti-PF4 disorders
  Spontaneous heparin-induced thrombocytopenia syndrome (without heparin exposure)
  Thrombosis with thrombocytopenia syndrome
  Vaccine-induced thrombotic thrombocytopenia
  Use additional code, if applicable, for adverse effect of other viral vaccine (T50.B95-)
- **D75.89** Other specified diseases of blood and blood-forming organs
- **D75.9** Disease of blood and blood-forming organs, unspecified
- **D75.A** Glucose-6-phosphate dehydrogenase (G6PD) deficiency without anemia
  Excludes1: glucose-6-phosphate dehydrogenase (G6PD) deficiency with anemia (D55.0)
  AHA CC: 4Q, 2019, 4-5

D76 Other specified diseases with participation of lymphoreticular and reticulohistiocytic tissue
Excludes1: (Abt-) Letterer-Siwe disease (C96.0)
eosinophilic granuloma (C96.6)
Hand-Schüller-Christian disease (C96.5)
histiocytic medullary reticulosis (C96.9)
histiocytic sarcoma (C96.A)
histiocytosis X, multifocal (C96.5)
histiocytosis X, unifocal (C96.6)
Langerhans-cell histiocytosis, multifocal (C96.5)
Langerhans-cell histiocytosis NOS (C96.6)
Langerhans-cell histiocytosis, unifocal (C96.6)
leukemic reticuloendotheliosis (C91.4-)
lipomelanotic reticulosis (I89.8)
malignant histiocytosis (C96.A)
malignant reticulosis (C86.0)
nonlipid reticuloendotheliosis (C96.0)
- CC **D76.1** Hemophagocytic lymphohistiocytosis
  Familial hemophagocytic reticulosis
  Histiocytoses of mononuclear phagocytes
- CC **D76.2** Hemophagocytic syndrome, infection-associated
  Use additional code to identify infectious agent or disease.
- CC **D76.3** Other histiocytosis syndromes
  Reticulohistiocytoma (giant-cell)
  Sinus histiocytosis with massive lymphadenopathy
  Xanthogranuloma

D77 Other disorders of blood and blood-forming organs in diseases classified elsewhere
Code first underlying disease, such as:
amyloidosis (E85.-)
congenital early syphilis (A50.0-)
echinococcosis (B67.0-B67.9)
malaria (B50.0-B54)
schistosomiasis [bilharziasis] (B65.0-B65.9)
vitamin C deficiency (E54)
Excludes1: rupture of spleen due to Plasmodium vivax malaria (B51.0)
splenitis, splenomegaly in late syphilis (A52.79)
splenitis, splenomegaly in tuberculosis (A18.85)
Valid 3-character code, no further characters required

Intraoperative and postprocedural complications of the spleen (D78)

D78 Intraoperative and postprocedural complications of the spleen
AHA CC: 4Q, 2016, 9-10
- **D78.0** Intraoperative hemorrhage and hematoma of the spleen complicating a procedure
  Excludes1: intraoperative hemorrhage and hematoma of the spleen due to accidental puncture or laceration during a procedure (D78.1-)
  - CC **D78.01** Intraoperative hemorrhage and hematoma of the spleen complicating a procedure on the spleen
  - CC **D78.02** Intraoperative hemorrhage and hematoma of the spleen complicating other procedure
- **D78.1** Accidental puncture and laceration of the spleen during a procedure
  - CC **D78.11** Accidental puncture and laceration of the spleen during a procedure on the spleen
  - CC **D78.12** Accidental puncture and laceration of the spleen during other procedure
    AHA CC: 1Q, 2022, 22-23
- **D78.2** Postprocedural hemorrhage of the spleen following a procedure
  - CC **D78.21** Postprocedural hemorrhage of the spleen following a procedure on the spleen
  - CC **D78.22** Postprocedural hemorrhage of the spleen following other procedure
- **D78.3** Postprocedural hematoma and seroma of the spleen following a procedure
  - CC **D78.31** Postprocedural hematoma of the spleen following a procedure on the spleen
  - CC **D78.32** Postprocedural hematoma of the spleen following other procedure
  - CC **D78.33** Postprocedural seroma of the spleen following a procedure on the spleen
  - CC **D78.34** Postprocedural seroma of the spleen following other procedure
- **D78.8** Other intraoperative and postprocedural complications of the spleen
  Use additional code, if applicable, to further specify disorder
  - CC **D78.81** Other intraoperative complications of the spleen
  - CC **D78.89** Other postprocedural complications of the spleen

Certain disorders involving the immune mechanism (D80-D89)

Includes: defects in the complement system
immunodeficiency disorders, except human immunodeficiency virus [HIV] disease sarcoidosis

Excludes1: autoimmune disease (systemic) NOS (M35.9)
functional disorders of polymorphonuclear neutrophils (D71)
human immunodeficiency virus [HIV] disease (B20)

D80 Immunodeficiency with predominantly antibody defects
- CC **D80.0** Hereditary hypogammaglobulinemia
  Autosomal recessive agammaglobulinemia (Swiss type)
  X-linked agammaglobulinemia [Bruton] (with growth hormone deficiency)
- CC **D80.1** Nonfamilial hypogammaglobulinemia
  Agammaglobulinemia with immunoglobulin-bearing B-lymphocytes
  Common variable agammaglobulinemia [CVAgamma]
  Hypogammaglobulinemia NOS
- CC **D80.2** Selective deficiency of immunoglobulin A [IgA]
- CC **D80.3** Selective deficiency of immunoglobulin G [IgG] subclasses
- CC **D80.4** Selective deficiency of immunoglobulin M [IgM]

Pathways of Immune Response

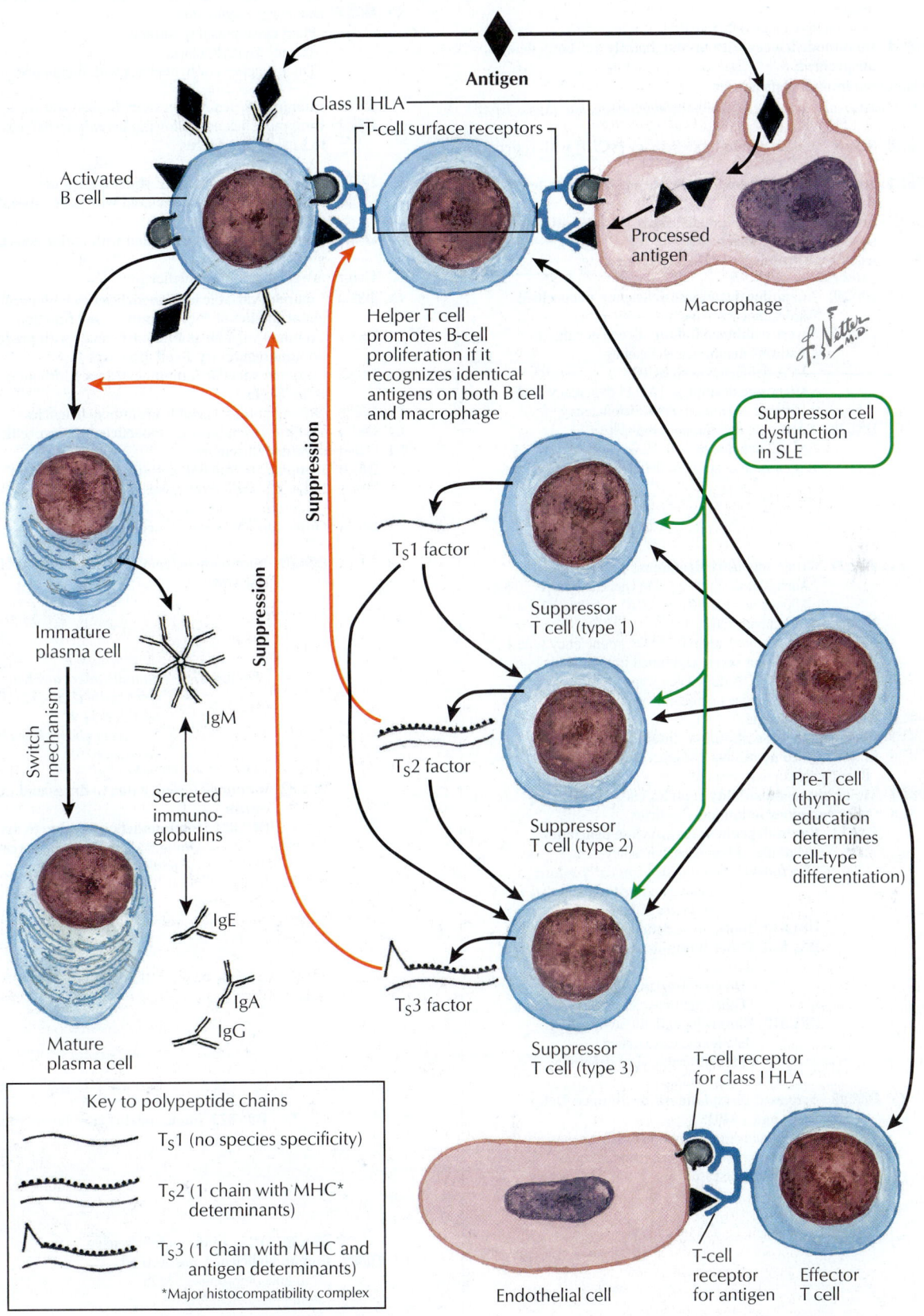

CC D80.5 Immunodeficiency with increased immunoglobulin M [IgM]
CC D80.6 Antibody deficiency with near-normal immunoglobulins or with hyperimmunoglobulinemia
CC D80.7 Transient hypogammaglobulinemia of infancy
+ D80.8 Other immunodeficiencies with predominantly antibody defects
    Kappa light chain deficiency
CC D80.9 Immunodeficiency with predominantly antibody defects, unspecified

D81 Combined immunodeficiencies
   Excludes1: autosomal recessive agammaglobulinemia (Swiss type) (D80.0)
CC D81.0 Severe combined immunodeficiency [SCID] with reticular dysgenesis
CC D81.1 Severe combined immunodeficiency [SCID] with low T- and B-cell numbers
CC D81.2 Severe combined immunodeficiency [SCID] with low or normal B-cell numbers
+ D81.3 Adenosine deaminase [ADA] deficiency
    AHA CC: 4Q, 2019, 5-6
  CC D81.30 Adenosine deaminase deficiency, unspecified
    ADA deficiency NOS
  CC D81.31 Severe combined immunodeficiency due to adenosine deaminase deficiency
    ADA deficiency with SCID
    Adenosine deaminase [ADA] deficiency with severe combined immunodeficiency
  CC D81.32 Adenosine deaminase 2 deficiency
    ADA2 deficiency
    Adenosine deaminase deficiency type 2
    Code also, if applicable, any associated manifestations, such as:
      polyarteritis nodosa (M30.0)
      stroke (I63.-)
  CC D81.39 Other adenosine deaminase deficiency
    Adenosine deaminase [ADA] deficiency type 1, NOS
    Adenosine deaminase [ADA] deficiency type 1, without SCID
    Adenosine deaminase [ADA] deficiency type 1, without severe combined immunodeficiency
    Partial ADA deficiency (type 1)
    Partial adenosine deaminase deficiency (type 1)
CC D81.4 Nezelof's syndrome
CC D81.5 Purine nucleoside phosphorylase [PNP] deficiency
CC D81.6 Major histocompatibility complex class I deficiency
    Bare lymphocyte syndrome
CC D81.7 Major histocompatibility complex class II deficiency
+ D81.8 Other combined immunodeficiencies
  + D81.81 Biotin-dependent carboxylase deficiency
    Multiple carboxylase deficiency
   Excludes1: biotin-dependent carboxylase deficiency due to dietary deficiency of biotin (E53.8)
    D81.810 Biotinidase deficiency
    D81.818 Other biotin-dependent carboxylase deficiency
      Holocarboxylase synthetase deficiency
      Other multiple carboxylase deficiency
    D81.819 Biotin-dependent carboxylase deficiency, unspecified
      Multiple carboxylase deficiency, unspecified
  CC D81.82 Activated Phosphoinositide 3-kinase Delta Syndrome [APDS]
    p110d-activating mutation causing senescent T cells, lymphadenopathy, and immunodeficiency [PASLI] disease
    Code also, if applicable, any associated manifestations, such as:
      bronchiectasis (J47.-)
      herpes virus infections (B00.-)
      other acute respiratory tract infections (J00-J06; J20-J22)
      other infections (A00-B99)
      pneumonia (J12-J18)
    AHA CC: 4Q, 2022, 11
  CC D81.89 Other combined immunodeficiencies

CC D81.9 Combined immunodeficiency, unspecified
    Severe combined immunodeficiency disorder [SCID]NOS

D82 Immunodeficiency associated with other major defects
   Excludes1: ataxia telangiectasia [Louis-Bar] (G11.3)
CC D82.0 Wiskott-Aldrich syndrome
    Immunodeficiency with thrombocytopenia and eczema
CC D82.1 Di George's syndrome
    Pharyngeal pouch syndrome
    Thymic alymphoplasia
    Thymic aplasia or hypoplasia with immunodeficiency
    AHA CC: 3Q, 2019, 14-15
D82.2 Immunodeficiency with short-limbed stature
D82.3 Immunodeficiency following hereditary defective response to Epstein-Barr virus
    X-linked lymphoproliferative disease
D82.4 Hyperimmunoglobulin E [IgE] syndrome
D82.8 Immunodeficiency associated with other specified major defects
D82.9 Immunodeficiency associated with major defect, unspecified

D83 Common variable immunodeficiency
CC D83.0 Common variable immunodeficiency with predominant abnormalities of B-cell numbers and function
CC D83.1 Common variable immunodeficiency with predominant immunoregulatory T-cell disorders
CC D83.2 Common variable immunodeficiency with autoantibodies to B- or T-cells
CC D83.8 Other common variable immunodeficiencies
CC D83.9 Common variable immunodeficiency, unspecified

D84 Other immunodeficiencies
D84.0 Lymphocyte function antigen-1 [LFA-1] defect
D84.1 Defects in the complement system
    C1 esterase inhibitor [C1-INH] deficiency
+ D84.8 Other specified immunodeficiencies
    AHA CC: 4Q, 2020, 10-11
  CC D84.81 Immunodeficiency due to conditions classified elsewhere
    Code first underlying condition, such as:
      chromosomal abnormalities (Q90-Q99)
      diabetes mellitus (E08-E13)
      malignant neoplasms (C00-C96)
   Excludes1: certain disorders involving the immune mechanism (D80-D83, D84.0, D84.1, D84.9)
      human immunodeficiency virus [HIV] disease (B20)
    AHA CC: 1Q, 2021, 52
  + D84.82 Immunodeficiency due to drugs and external causes
    CC D84.821 Immunodeficiency due to drugs
      Immunodeficiency due to (current or past) medication
      Use additional code for adverse effect if applicable, to identify adverse effect of drug (T36-T50 with fifth or sixth character 5)
      Use additional code, if applicable, for associated long term (current) drug therapy drug or medication such as:
        long term (current) drug therapy systemic steroids (Z79.52)
        other long term (current) drug therapy (Z79.899)
    AHA CC: 4Q, 2020, 11-12
    CC D84.822 Immunodeficiency due to external causes
      Code also, if applicable, radiological procedure and radiotherapy (Y84.2)
      Use additional code for external cause such as:
        exposure to ionizing radiation (W88)
  CC D84.89 Other immunodeficiencies
CC D84.9 Immunodeficiency, unspecified
    Immunocompromised NOS
    Immunodeficient NOS
    Immunosuppressed NOS

D86 Sarcoidosis
D86.0 Sarcoidosis of lung
D86.1 Sarcoidosis of lymph nodes
D86.2 Sarcoidosis of lung with sarcoidosis of lymph nodes
D86.3 Sarcoidosis of skin

- **D86.8** Sarcoidosis of other sites
  - **D86.81** Sarcoid meningitis
  - **D86.82** Multiple cranial nerve palsies in sarcoidosis
  - **D86.83** Sarcoid iridocyclitis
  - **D86.84** Sarcoid pyelonephritis
    Tubulo-interstitial nephropathy in sarcoidosis
  - **D86.85** Sarcoid myocarditis
  - **D86.86** Sarcoid arthropathy
    Polyarthritis in sarcoidosis
  - **D86.87** Sarcoid myositis
  - **D86.89** Sarcoidosis of other sites
    Hepatic granuloma
    Uveoparotid fever [Heerfordt]
- **D86.9** Sarcoidosis, unspecified

D89 Other disorders involving the immune mechanism, not elsewhere classified

Excludes1: hyperglobulinemia NOS (R77.1)
monoclonal gammopathy (of undetermined significance) (D47.2)

Excludes2: transplant failure and rejection (T86.-)

- **D89.0** Polyclonal hypergammaglobulinemia
  Benign hypergammaglobulinemic purpura
  Polyclonal gammopathy NOS
- **D89.1** Cryoglobulinemia
  Cryoglobulinemic purpura
  Cryoglobulinemic vasculitis
  Essential cryoglobulinemia
  Idiopathic cryoglobulinemia
  Mixed cryoglobulinemia
  Primary cryoglobulinemia
  Secondary cryoglobulinemia
- **D89.2** Hypergammaglobulinemia, unspecified
- **D89.3** Immune reconstitution syndrome
  Immune reconstitution inflammatory syndrome [IRIS]
  Use additional code for adverse effect, if applicable, to identify drug (T36-T50 with fifth or sixth character 5)
  Add the following new codes after D89.3.
- **D89.4** Mast cell activation syndrome and related disorders

  Excludes1: aggressive systemic mastocytosis (C96.21)
  congenital cutaneous mastocytosis (Q82.2)
  (indolent) systemic mastocytosis (D47.02)
  malignant mast cell neoplasm (C96.2-)
  malignant mastocytoma (C96.29)
  mast cell sarcoma (C96.22)
  mastocytoma NOS (D47.09)
  (non-congenital) cutaneous mastocytosis (D47.01)
  other mast cell neoplasms of uncertain behavior (D47.09)
  systemic mastocytosis associated with a clonal hematologic non-mast cell lineage disease (SM-AHNMD) (D47.02)

  AHA CC: 4Q, 2016, 11

  - **D89.40** Mast cell activation, unspecified
    Mast cell activation disorder, unspecified
    Mast cell activation syndrome, NOS
  - **D89.41** Monoclonal mast cell activation syndrome
  - **D89.42** Idiopathic mast cell activation syndrome
  - **D89.43** Secondary mast cell activation
    Secondary mast cell activation syndrome
    Code also underlying etiology, if known
  - **D89.44** Hereditary alpha tryptasemia
    Use additional code, if applicable, for:
      allergy status, other than to drugs and biological substances (Z91.0-)
      personal history of anaphylaxis (Z87.892)
    AHA CC: 4Q, 2021, 8
  - **D89.49** Other mast cell activation disorder
    Other mast cell activation syndrome
- **D89.8** Other specified disorders involving the immune mechanism, not elsewhere classified
  - **D89.81** Graft-versus-host disease
    Code first underlying cause, such as:
      complications of transplanted organs and tissues (T86.-)
      complications of blood transfusion (T80.89)
    Use additional code to identify associated manifestations, such as:
      desquamative dermatitis (L30.8)
      diarrhea (R19.7)
      elevated bilirubin (R17)
      hair loss (L65.9)
    - **D89.810** Acute graft-versus-host disease
    - **D89.811** Chronic graft-versus-host disease
    - **D89.812** Acute on chronic graft-versus-host disease
    - **D89.813** Graft-versus-host disease, unspecified
  - **D89.82** Autoimmune lymphoproliferative syndrome [ALPS]
  - **D89.83** Cytokine release syndrome
    Code first underlying cause, such as:
      complications following infusion, transfusion and therapeutic injection (T80.89-)
      complications of transplanted organs and tissues (T86.-)
    Use additional code to identify associated manifestations
    AHA CC: 4Q, 2020, 12-13
    - **D89.831** Cytokine release syndrome, grade 1
    - **D89.832** Cytokine release syndrome, grade 2
      AHA CC: 4Q, 2020, 14-15
    - **D89.833** Cytokine release syndrome, grade 3
      AHA CC: 4Q, 2020, 14
    - **D89.834** Cytokine release syndrome, grade 4
    - **D89.835** Cytokine release syndrome, grade 5
    - **D89.839** Cytokine release syndrome, grade unspecified
  - **D89.84** IgG4-related disease
    Immunoglobulin G4-related disease
  - **D89.89** Other specified disorders involving the immune mechanism, not elsewhere classified
    Excludes1: human immunodeficiency virus disease (B20)
    AHA CC: 4Q, 2017, 109
- **D89.9** Disorder involving the immune mechanism, unspecified
  Immune disease NOS
  AHA CC: 3Q, 2015, 22

Chapter 4: Endocrine, Nutritional and Metabolic Disease (E00-E89)

NOTE All neoplasms, whether functionally active or not, are classified in Chapter 2. Appropriate codes in this chapter (i.e. E05.8, E07.0, E16-E31, E34.-) may be used as additional codes to indicate either functional activity by neoplasms and ectopic endocrine tissue or hyperfunction and hypofunction of endocrine glands associated with neoplasms and other conditions classified elsewhere.

Excludes1: transitory endocrine and metabolic disorders specific to newborn (P70-P74)

This chapter contains the following category blocks:
- E00-E07 Disorders of thyroid gland
- E08-E13 Diabetes mellitus
- E15-E16 Other disorders of glucose regulation and pancreatic internal secretion
- E20-E35 Disorders of other endocrine glands
- E36 Intraoperative complications of endocrine system
- E40-E46 Malnutrition
- E50-E64 Other nutritional deficiencies
- E65-E68 Overweight, obesity and other hyperalimentation
- E70-E88 Metabolic disorders
- E89 Postprocedural endocrine and metabolic complications and disorders, not elsewhere classified

C. Chapter-Specific Coding Guidelines

In addition to general coding guidelines, there are guidelines for specific diagnoses and/or conditions in the classification. Unless otherwise indicated, these guidelines apply to all health care settings. Please refer to Section II for guidelines on the selection of principal diagnosis.

4. Chapter 4: Endocrine, Nutritional and Metabolic Diseases (E00-E89)

a. Diabetes mellitus

The diabetes mellitus codes are combination codes that include the type of diabetes mellitus, the body system affected, and the complications affecting that body system. As many codes within a particular category as are necessary to describe all of the complications of the disease may be used. They should be sequenced based on the reason for a particular encounter. Assign as many codes from categories E08 – E13 as needed to identify all of the associated conditions that the patient has.

1) Type of diabetes

The age of a patient is not the sole determining factor, though most type 1 diabetics develop the condition before reaching puberty. For this reason type 1 diabetes mellitus is also referred to as juvenile diabetes.

2) Type of diabetes mellitus not documented

If the type of diabetes mellitus is not documented in the medical record the default is E11.-, Type 2 diabetes mellitus.

3) Diabetes mellitus and the use of insulin and oral hypoglycemics

If the documentation in a medical record does not indicate the type of diabetes but does indicate that the patient uses insulin, code E11-, Type 2 diabetes mellitus, should be assigned. Additional code(s) should be assigned from category Z79 to identify the long-term (current) use of insulin, oral hypoglycemic drugs, or injectable non-insulin antidiabetic, as follows:

If the patient is treated with both oral hypoglycemic drugs and insulin, both code Z79.4, Long term (current) use of insulin, and code Z79.84, Long term (current) use of oral hypoglycemic drugs, should be assigned. If the patient is treated with both insulin and an injectable non-insulin antidiabetic drug, assign codes Z79.4, Long-term (current) use of insulin, and Z79.85, Long-term (current) use of injectable non-insulin antidiabetic drugs. If the patient is treated with both oral hypoglycemic drugs and an injectable non-insulin antidiabetic drug, assign codes Z79.84, Long-term (current) use of oral hypoglycemic drugs, and Z79.85, Long-term (current) use of injectable non-insulin antidiabetic drugs. Code Z79.4 should not be assigned if insulin is given temporarily to bring a type 2 patient's blood sugar under control during an encounter.

4) Diabetes mellitus in pregnancy and gestational diabetes

See Section I.C.15. Diabetes mellitus in pregnancy.
See Section I.C.15. Gestational (pregnancy induced) diabetes.

5) Complications due to insulin pump malfunction

(a) Underdose of insulin due to insulin pump failure

An underdose of insulin due to an insulin pump failure should be assigned to a code from subcategory T85.6, Mechanical complication of other specified internal and external prosthetic devices, implants and grafts, that specifies the type of pump malfunction, as the principal or first-listed code, followed by code T38.3x6-, Underdosing of insulin and oral hypoglycemic [antidiabetic] drugs. Additional codes for the type of diabetes mellitus and any associated complications due to the underdosing should also be assigned.

(b) Overdose of insulin due to insulin pump failure

The principal or first-listed code for an encounter due to an insulin pump malfunction resulting in an overdose of insulin, should also be T85.6-, Mechanical complication of other specified internal and external prosthetic devices, implants and grafts, followed by code T38.3x1-, Poisoning by insulin and oral hypoglycemic [antidiabetic] drugs, accidental (unintentional).

6) Secondary diabetes mellitus

Codes under categories E08, Diabetes mellitus due to underlying condition, E09, Drug or chemical induced diabetes mellitus, and E13, Other specified diabetes mellitus, identify complications/manifestations associated with secondary diabetes mellitus. Secondary diabetes is always caused by another condition or event (e.g., cystic fibrosis, malignant neoplasm of pancreas, pancreatectomy, adverse effect of drug, or poisoning).

(a) Secondary diabetes mellitus and the use of insulin or oral hypoglycemic drugs

For patients with secondary diabetes mellitus who routinely use insulin or oral hypoglycemic drugs, or injectable non-insulin drugs, an additional code(s) from category Z79 should be assigned to identify the long-term (current) use of insulin, oral hypoglycemic drugs or non-injectable non-insulin drugs as follows: If the patient is treated with both oral hypoglycemic drugs and insulin, both code Z79.4, Long term (current) use of insulin, and code Z79.84, Long term (current) use of oral hypoglycemic drugs, should be assigned. If the patient is treated with both insulin and an injectable non-insulin antidiabetic drug, assign codes Z79.4, Long-term (current) use of insulin, and Z79.85, Long-term (current) use of injectable non-insulin antidiabetic drugs. If the patient is treated with both oral hypoglycemic drugs and an injectable non-insulin antidiabetic drug, assign codes Z79.84, Long-term (current) use of oral hypoglycemic drugs, and Z79.85, Long-term (current) use of injectable non-insulin antidiabetic drugs. Code Z79.4 should not be assigned if insulin is given temporarily to bring a secondary diabetic patient's blood sugar under control during an encounter.

(b) Assigning and sequencing secondary diabetes codes and its causes

The sequencing of the secondary diabetes codes in relationship to codes for the cause of the diabetes is based on the Tabular List instructions for categories E08, E09 and E13.

(i) Secondary diabetes mellitus due to pancreatectomy

For postpancreatectomy diabetes mellitus (lack of insulin due to the surgical removal of all or part of the pancreas), assign code E89.1, Postprocedural hypoinsulinemia. Assign a code from category E13 and a code from subcategory Z90.41-, Acquired absence of pancreas, as additional codes.

(ii) Secondary diabetes due to drugs

Secondary diabetes may be caused by an adverse effect of correctly administered medications, poisoning or sequela of poisoning.

See section I.C.19.e for coding of adverse effects and poisoning, and section I.C.20 for external cause code reporting.

Disorders of thyroid gland (E00-E07)

E00 Congenital iodine-deficiency syndrome

Use additional code (F70-F79) to identify associated intellectual disabilities.

Excludes1: subclinical iodine-deficiency hypothyroidism (E02)

- **E00.0 Congenital iodine-deficiency syndrome, neurological type**
  Endemic cretinism, neurological type
- **E00.1 Congenital iodine-deficiency syndrome, myxedematous type**
  Endemic hypothyroid cretinism
  Endemic cretinism, myxedematous type
- **E00.2 Congenital iodine-deficiency syndrome, mixed type**
  Endemic cretinism, mixed type
- **E00.9 Congenital iodine-deficiency syndrome, unspecified**
  Congenital iodine-deficiency hypothyroidism NOS
  Endemic cretinism NOS

E01 Iodine-deficiency related thyroid disorders and allied conditions

Excludes1: congenital iodine-deficiency syndrome (E00.-)
subclinical iodine-deficiency hypothyroidism (E02)

- **E01.0 Iodine-deficiency related diffuse (endemic) goiter**
- **E01.1 Iodine-deficiency related multinodular (endemic) goiter**
  Iodine-deficiency related nodular goiter
- **E01.2 Iodine-deficiency related (endemic) goiter, unspecified**
  Endemic goiter NOS
- **E01.8 Other iodine-deficiency related thyroid disorders and allied conditions**
  Acquired iodine-deficiency hypothyroidism NOS

Endocrine System

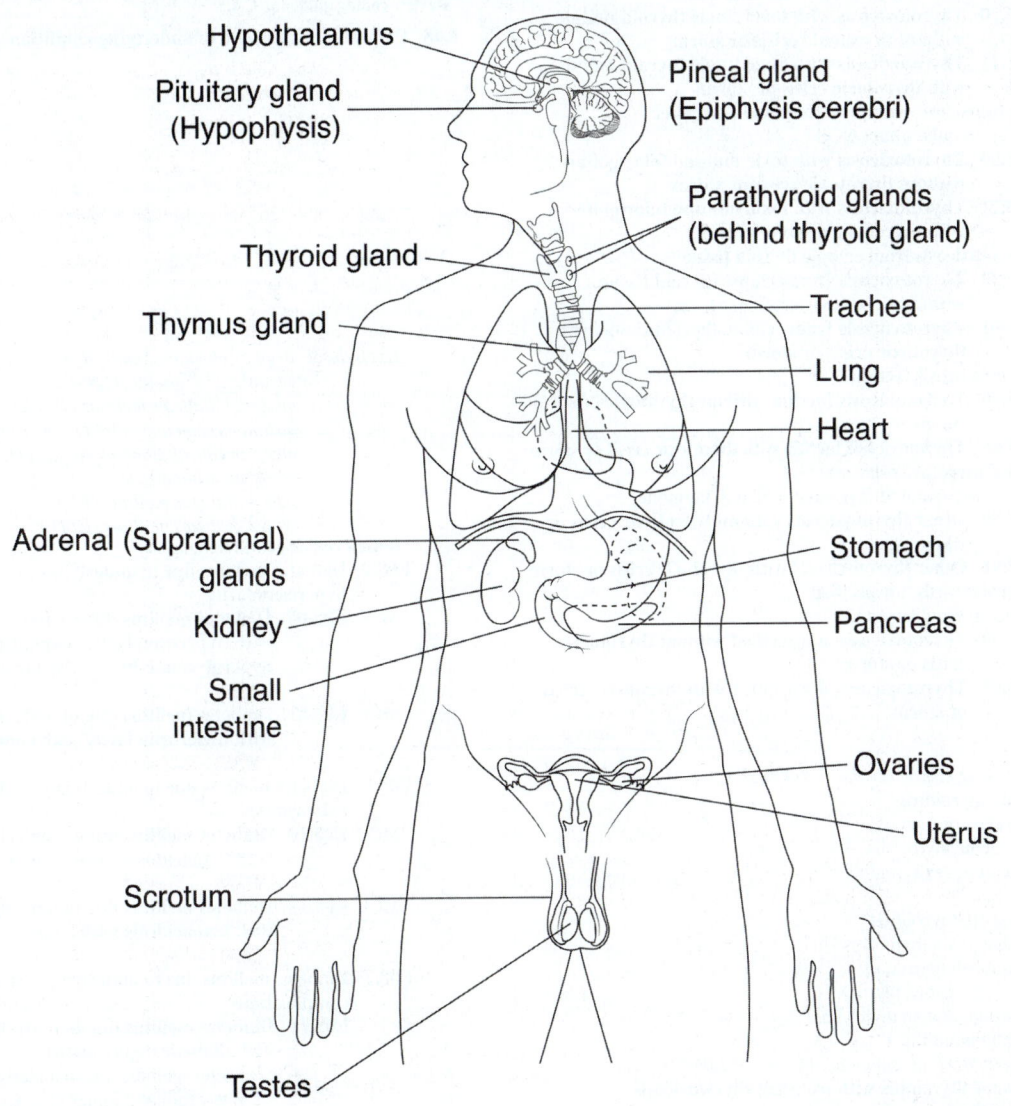

©AHIMA

E02 Subclinical iodine-deficiency hypothyroidism
   AHA CC: 1Q, 2021, 8-9
   Valid 3-character code, no further characters required

E03 Other hypothyroidism
   Excludes1: *iodine-deficiency related hypothyroidism (E00-E02)*
      postprocedural hypothyroidism (E89.0)
   E03.0 Congenital hypothyroidism with diffuse goiter
      Congenital parenchymatous goiter (nontoxic)
      Congenital goiter (nontoxic) NOS
      Excludes1: *transitory congenital goiter with normal function (P72.0)*
   E03.1 Congenital hypothyroidism without goiter
      Aplasia of thyroid (with myxedema)
      Congenital atrophy of thyroid
      Congenital hypothyroidism NOS
   E03.2 Hypothyroidism due to medicaments and other exogenous substances
      Code first poisoning due to drug or toxin, if applicable (T36-T65 with fifth or sixth character 1-4)
      Use additional code for adverse effect, if applicable, to identify drug (T36-T50 with fifth or sixth character 5)
   E03.3 Postinfectious hypothyroidism
   E03.4 Atrophy of thyroid (acquired)
      Excludes1: *congenital atrophy of thyroid (E03.1)*
   MCC **E03.5 Myxedema coma**
   E03.8 Other specified hypothyroidism
      AHA CC: 1Q, 2021, 8-9
   E03.9 Hypothyroidism, unspecified
      Myxedema NOS

E04 Other nontoxic goiter
   Excludes1: *congenital goiter (NOS) (diffuse) (parenchymatous) (E03.0)*
      iodine-deficiency related goiter (E00-E02)
   E04.0 Nontoxic diffuse goiter
      Diffuse (colloid) nontoxic goiter
      Simple nontoxic goiter
   E04.1 Nontoxic single thyroid nodule
      Colloid nodule (cystic) (thyroid)
      Nontoxic uninodular goiter
      Thyroid (cystic) nodule NOS
   E04.2 Nontoxic multinodular goiter
      Cystic goiter NOS
      Multinodular (cystic) goiter NOS
   E04.8 Other specified nontoxic goiter
   E04.9 Nontoxic goiter, unspecified
      Goiter NOS
      Nodular goiter (nontoxic) NOS

E05 Thyrotoxicosis [hyperthyroidism]
   Excludes1: *chronic thyroiditis with transient thyrotoxicosis (E06.2)*
      neonatal thyrotoxicosis (P72.1)
   + **E05.0 Thyrotoxicosis with diffuse goiter**
      Exophthalmic or toxic goiter NOS
      Graves' disease
      Toxic diffuse goiter
      E05.00 Thyrotoxicosis with diffuse goiter without thyrotoxic crisis or storm
   MCC **E05.01 Thyrotoxicosis with diffuse goiter with thyrotoxic crisis or storm**

- **+ E05.1** Thyrotoxicosis with toxic single thyroid nodule
  Thyrotoxicosis with toxic uninodular goiter
  - **E05.10** Thyrotoxicosis with toxic single thyroid nodule without thyrotoxic crisis or storm
  - **MCC E05.11** Thyrotoxicosis with toxic single thyroid nodule with thyrotoxic crisis or storm
- **+ E05.2** Thyrotoxicosis with toxic multinodular goiter
  Toxic nodular goiter NOS
  - **E05.20** Thyrotoxicosis with toxic multinodular goiter without thyrotoxic crisis or storm
  - **MCC E05.21** Thyrotoxicosis with toxic multinodular goiter with thyrotoxic crisis or storm
- **+ E05.3** Thyrotoxicosis from ectopic thyroid tissue
  - **E05.30** Thyrotoxicosis from ectopic thyroid tissue without thyrotoxic crisis or storm
  - **MCC E05.31** Thyrotoxicosis from ectopic thyroid tissue with thyrotoxic crisis or storm
- **+ E05.4** Thyrotoxicosis factitia
  - **E05.40** Thyrotoxicosis factitia without thyrotoxic crisis or storm
  - **MCC E05.41** Thyrotoxicosis factitia with thyrotoxic crisis or storm
- **+ E05.8** Other thyrotoxicosis
  Overproduction of thyroid-stimulating hormone
  - **E05.80** Other thyrotoxicosis without thyrotoxic crisis or storm
  - **MCC E05.81** Other thyrotoxicosis with thyrotoxic crisis or storm
- **+ E05.9** Thyrotoxicosis, unspecified
  Hyperthyroidism NOS
  - **E05.90** Thyrotoxicosis, unspecified without thyrotoxic crisis or storm
  - **MCC E05.91** Thyrotoxicosis, unspecified with thyrotoxic crisis or storm

E06 Thyroiditis
Excludes1: postpartum thyroiditis (O90.5)
- **CC E06.0** Acute thyroiditis
  Abscess of thyroid
  Pyogenic thyroiditis
  Suppurative thyroiditis
  Use additional code (B95-B97) to identify infectious agent.
- **E06.1** Subacute thyroiditis
  de Quervain thyroiditis
  Giant-cell thyroiditis
  Granulomatous thyroiditis
  Nonsuppurative thyroiditis
  Viral thyroiditis
  Excludes1: autoimmune thyroiditis (E06.3)
- **E06.2** Chronic thyroiditis with transient thyrotoxicosis
  Excludes1: autoimmune thyroiditis (E06.3)
- **E06.3** Autoimmune thyroiditis
  Hashimoto's thyroiditis
  Hashitoxicosis (transient)
  Lymphadenoid goiter
  Lymphocytic thyroiditis
  Struma lymphomatosa
- **E06.4** Drug-induced thyroiditis
  Use additional code for adverse effect, if applicable, to identify drug (T36-T50 with fifth or sixth character 5)
- **E06.5** Other chronic thyroiditis
  Chronic fibrous thyroiditis
  Chronic thyroiditis NOS
  Ligneous thyroiditis
  Riedel thyroiditis
- **E06.9** Thyroiditis, unspecified

E07 Other disorders of thyroid
- **E07.0** Hypersecretion of calcitonin
  C-cell hyperplasia of thyroid
  Hypersecretion of thyrocalcitonin
- **E07.1** Dyshormogenetic goiter
  Familial dyshormogenetic goiter
  Pendred's syndrome
  Excludes1: transitory congenital goiter with normal function (P72.0)
- **+ E07.8** Other specified disorders of thyroid
  - **E07.81** Sick-euthyroid syndrome
    Euthyroid sick-syndrome
  - **E07.89** Other specified disorders of thyroid
    Abnormality of thyroid-binding globulin
    Hemorrhage of thyroid
    Infarction of thyroid
- **E07.9** Disorder of thyroid, unspecified

Diabetes mellitus (E08-E13)
Review coding guideline C.4.a

E08 Diabetes mellitus due to underlying condition
Code first the underlying condition, such as:
congenital rubella (P35.0)
Cushing's syndrome (E24.-)
cystic fibrosis (E84.-)
malignant neoplasm (C00-C96)
malnutrition (E40-E46)
pancreatitis and other diseases of the pancreas (K85-K86.-)

Use additional code to identify control using:
insulin (Z79.4)
oral antidiabetic drugs (Z79.84)
oral hypoglycemic drugs (Z79.84)

Excludes1: drug or chemical induced diabetes mellitus (E09.-)
gestational diabetes (O24.4-)
neonatal diabetes mellitus (P70.2)
postpancreatectomy diabetes mellitus (E13.-)
postprocedural diabetes mellitus (E13.-)
secondary diabetes mellitus NEC (E13.-)
type 1 diabetes mellitus (E10.-)
type 2 diabetes mellitus (E11.-)

Review coding guideline C.4.a.6.a
- **+ E08.0** Diabetes mellitus due to underlying condition with hyperosmolarity
  - **MCC E08.00** Diabetes mellitus due to underlying condition with hyperosmolarity without nonketotic hyperglycemic-hyperosmolar coma (NKHHC)
    HAC see Appendix B for HAC conditional logic
  - **MCC E08.01** Diabetes mellitus due to underlying condition with hyperosmolarity with coma
    HAC see Appendix B for HAC conditional logic
- **+ E08.1** Diabetes mellitus due to underlying condition with ketoacidosis
  - **MCC E08.10** Diabetes mellitus due to underlying condition with ketoacidosis without coma
    HAC see Appendix B for HAC conditional logic
  - **MCC E08.11** Diabetes mellitus due to underlying condition with ketoacidosis with coma
    HAC see Appendix B for HAC conditional logic
- **+ E08.2** Diabetes mellitus due to underlying condition with kidney complications
  - **E08.21** Diabetes mellitus due to underlying condition with diabetic nephropathy
    Diabetes mellitus due to underlying condition with intercapillary glomerulosclerosis
    Diabetes mellitus due to underlying condition with intracapillary glomerulonephrosis
    Diabetes mellitus due to underlying condition with Kimmelstiel-Wilson disease
  - **E08.22** Diabetes mellitus due to underlying condition with diabetic chronic kidney disease
    Use additional code to identify stage of chronic kidney disease (N18.1-N18.6)
  - **E08.29** Diabetes mellitus due to underlying condition with other diabetic kidney complication
    Renal tubular degeneration in diabetes mellitus due to underlying condition
- **+ E08.3** Diabetes mellitus due to underlying condition with ophthalmic complications
  AHA CC: 4Q, 2016, 11-13
  - **+ E08.31** Diabetes mellitus due to underlying condition with unspecified diabetic retinopathy
    - **E08.311** Diabetes mellitus due to underlying condition with unspecified diabetic retinopathy with macular edema
    - **E08.319** Diabetes mellitus due to underlying condition with unspecified diabetic retinopathy without macular edema

+ **E08.32** Diabetes mellitus due to underlying condition with mild nonproliferative diabetic retinopathy
Diabetes mellitus due to underlying condition with nonproliferative diabetic retinopathy NOS

> One of the following 7th characters is to be assigned to codes in subcategory **E08.32** to designate laterality of the disease:
> 1 right eye
> 2 left eye
> 3 bilateral
> 9 unspecified eye

+7th **E08.321** Diabetes mellitus due to underlying condition with mild nonproliferative diabetic retinopathy with macular edema

+7th **E08.329** Diabetes mellitus due to underlying condition with mild nonproliferative diabetic retinopathy without macular edema

+ **E08.33** Diabetes mellitus due to underlying condition with moderate nonproliferative diabetic retinopathy

> One of the following 7th characters is to be assigned to codes in subcategory **E08.33** to designate laterality of the disease:
> 1 right eye
> 2 left eye
> 3 bilateral
> 9 unspecified eye

+7th **E08.331** Diabetes mellitus due to underlying condition with moderate nonproliferative diabetic retinopathy with macular edema

+7th **E08.339** Diabetes mellitus due to underlying condition with moderate nonproliferative diabetic retinopathy without macular edema

+ **E08.34** Diabetes mellitus due to underlying condition with severe nonproliferative diabetic retinopathy

> One of the following 7th characters is to be assigned to codes in subcategory **E08.34** to designate laterality of the disease:
> 1 right eye
> 2 left eye
> 3 bilateral
> 9 unspecified eye

+7th **E08.341** Diabetes mellitus due to underlying condition with severe nonproliferative diabetic retinopathy with macular edema

+7th **E08.349** Diabetes mellitus due to underlying condition with severe nonproliferative diabetic retinopathy without macular edema

+ **E08.35** Diabetes mellitus due to underlying condition with proliferative diabetic retinopathy

> One of the following 7th characters is to be assigned to codes in subcategory **E08.35** to designate laterality of the disease:
> 1 right eye
> 2 left eye
> 3 bilateral
> 9 unspecified eye

+7th **E08.351** Diabetes mellitus due to underlying condition with proliferative diabetic retinopathy with macular edema

+7th **E08.352** Diabetes mellitus due to underlying condition with proliferative diabetic retinopathy with traction retinal detachment involving the macula

+7th **E08.353** Diabetes mellitus due to underlying condition with proliferative diabetic retinopathy with traction retinal detachment not involving the macula

+7th **E08.354** Diabetes mellitus due to underlying condition with proliferative diabetic retinopathy with combined traction retinal detachment and rhegmatogenous retinal detachment

+7th **E08.355** Diabetes mellitus due to underlying condition with stable proliferative diabetic retinopathy

+7th **E08.359** Diabetes mellitus due to underlying condition with proliferative diabetic retinopathy without macular edema

E08.36 Diabetes mellitus due to underlying condition with diabetic cataract

X+7th **E08.37** Diabetes mellitus due to underlying condition with diabetic macular edema, resolved following treatment

> One of the following 7th characters is to be assigned to codes in subcategory **E08.37** to designate laterality of the disease:
> 1 right eye
> 2 left eye
> 3 bilateral
> 9 unspecified eye

E08.39 Diabetes mellitus due to underlying condition with other diabetic ophthalmic complication
Use additional code to identify manifestation, such as:
diabetic glaucoma (H40-H42)

+ **E08.4** Diabetes mellitus due to underlying condition with neurological complications

E08.40 Diabetes mellitus due to underlying condition with diabetic neuropathy, unspecified

E08.41 Diabetes mellitus due to underlying condition with diabetic mononeuropathy

E08.42 Diabetes mellitus due to underlying condition with diabetic polyneuropathy
Diabetes mellitus due to underlying condition with diabetic neuralgia

E08.43 Diabetes mellitus due to underlying condition with diabetic autonomic (poly)neuropathy
Diabetes mellitus due to underlying condition with diabetic gastroparesis
AHA CC: 3Q, 2013, 114-115

E08.44 Diabetes mellitus due to underlying condition with diabetic amyotrophy

E08.49 Diabetes mellitus due to underlying condition with other diabetic neurological complication

+ **E08.5** Diabetes mellitus due to underlying condition with circulatory complications

E08.51 Diabetes mellitus due to underlying condition with diabetic peripheral angiopathy without gangrene

CC **E08.52** Diabetes mellitus due to underlying condition with diabetic peripheral angiopathy with gangrene
Diabetes mellitus due to underlying condition with diabetic gangrene

E08.59 Diabetes mellitus due to underlying condition with other circulatory complications

+ **E08.6** Diabetes mellitus due to underlying condition with other specified complications

+ **E08.61** Diabetes mellitus due to underlying condition with diabetic arthropathy

E08.610 Diabetes mellitus due to underlying condition with diabetic neuropathic arthropathy
Diabetes mellitus due to underlying condition with Charcôt's joints

E08.618 Diabetes mellitus due to underlying condition with other diabetic arthropathy

- **E08.62** Diabetes mellitus due to underlying condition with skin complications
  - **E08.620** Diabetes mellitus due to underlying condition with diabetic dermatitis
    - Diabetes mellitus due to underlying condition with diabetic necrobiosis lipoidica
  - **E08.621** Diabetes mellitus due to underlying condition with foot ulcer
    - Use additional code to identify site of ulcer (L97.4-, L97.5-)
  - **E08.622** Diabetes mellitus due to underlying condition with other skin ulcer
    - Use additional code to identify site of ulcer (L97.1-L97.9, L98.41-L98.49)
  - **E08.628** Diabetes mellitus due to underlying condition with other skin complications
- **E08.63** Diabetes mellitus due to underlying condition with oral complications
  - **E08.630** Diabetes mellitus due to underlying condition with periodontal disease
  - **E08.638** Diabetes mellitus due to underlying condition with other oral complications
- **E08.64** Diabetes mellitus due to underlying condition with hypoglycemia
  - MCC **E08.641** Diabetes mellitus due to underlying condition with hypoglycemia with coma
  - **E08.649** Diabetes mellitus due to underlying condition with hypoglycemia without coma
- **E08.65** Diabetes mellitus due to underlying condition with hyperglycemia
- **E08.69** Diabetes mellitus due to underlying condition with other specified complication
  - Use additional code to identify complication
- **E08.8** Diabetes mellitus due to underlying condition with unspecified complications
- **E08.9** Diabetes mellitus due to underlying condition without complications

E09 Drug or chemical induced diabetes mellitus

Code first poisoning due to drug or toxin, if applicable (T36-T65 with fifth or sixth character 1-4)

Use additional code for adverse effect, if applicable, to identify drug (T36-T50 with fifth or sixth character 5)

Use additional code to identify control using:
- insulin (Z79.4)
- oral antidiabetic drugs (Z79.84)
- oral hypoglycemic drugs (Z79.84)

Excludes1: diabetes mellitus due to underlying condition (E08.-)
gestational diabetes (O24.4-)
neonatal diabetes mellitus (P70.2)
postpancreatectomy diabetes mellitus (E13.-)
postprocedural diabetes mellitus (E13.-)
secondary diabetes mellitus NEC (E13.-)
type 1 diabetes mellitus (E10.-)
type 2 diabetes mellitus (E11.-)

Review coding guideline C.4.a.6.a

- **E09.0** Drug or chemical induced diabetes mellitus with hyperosmolarity
  - MCC **E09.00** Drug or chemical induced diabetes mellitus with hyperosmolarity without nonketotic hyperglycemic-hyperosmolar coma (NKHHC)
    - HAC see Appendix B for HAC conditional logic
  - MCC **E09.01** Drug or chemical induced diabetes mellitus with hyperosmolarity with coma
    - HAC see Appendix B for HAC conditional logic
- **E09.1** Drug or chemical induced diabetes mellitus with ketoacidosis
  - MCC **E09.10** Drug or chemical induced diabetes mellitus with ketoacidosis without coma
    - HAC see Appendix B for HAC conditional logic
  - MCC **E09.11** Drug or chemical induced diabetes mellitus with ketoacidosis with coma
    - HAC see Appendix B for HAC conditional logic
- **E09.2** Drug or chemical induced diabetes mellitus with kidney complications
  - **E09.21** Drug or chemical induced diabetes mellitus with diabetic nephropathy
    - Drug or chemical induced diabetes mellitus with intercapillary glomerulosclerosis
    - Drug or chemical induced diabetes mellitus with intracapillary glomerulonephrosis
    - Drug or chemical induced diabetes mellitus with Kimmelstiel-Wilson disease
  - **E09.22** Drug or chemical induced diabetes mellitus with diabetic chronic kidney disease
    - Use additional code to identify stage of chronic kidney disease (N18.1-N18.6)
  - **E09.29** Drug or chemical induced diabetes mellitus with other diabetic kidney complication
    - Drug or chemical induced diabetes mellitus with renal tubular degeneration
- **E09.3** Drug or chemical induced diabetes mellitus with ophthalmic complications
  - AHA CC: 4Q, 2016, 11-13
  - **E09.31** Drug or chemical induced diabetes mellitus with unspecified diabetic retinopathy
    - **E09.311** Drug or chemical induced diabetes mellitus with unspecified diabetic retinopathy with macular edema
    - **E09.319** Drug or chemical induced diabetes mellitus with unspecified diabetic retinopathy without macular edema
  - **E09.32** Drug or chemical induced diabetes mellitus with mild nonproliferative diabetic retinopathy
    - Drug or chemical induced diabetes mellitus with nonproliferative diabetic retinopathy NOS

    One of the following 7th characters is to be assigned to codes in subcategory **E09.32** to designate laterality of the disease:
    1 right eye
    2 left eye
    3 bilateral
    9 unspecified eye

    - +7th **E09.321** Drug or chemical induced diabetes mellitus with mild nonproliferative diabetic retinopathy with macular edema
    - +7th **E09.329** Drug or chemical induced diabetes mellitus with mild nonproliferative diabetic retinopathy without macular edema
  - +7th **E09.33** Drug or chemical induced diabetes mellitus with moderate nonproliferative diabetic retinopathy

    One of the following 7th characters is to be assigned to codes in subcategory **E09.33** to designate laterality of the disease:
    1 right eye
    2 left eye
    3 bilateral
    9 unspecified eye

    - +7th **E09.331** Drug or chemical induced diabetes mellitus with moderate nonproliferative diabetic retinopathy with macular edema
    - +7th **E09.339** Drug or chemical induced diabetes mellitus with moderate nonproliferative diabetic retinopathy without macular edema
  - **E09.34** Drug or chemical induced diabetes mellitus with severe nonproliferative diabetic retinopathy

    One of the following 7th characters is to be assigned to codes in subcategory **E09.34** to designate laterality of the disease:
    1 right eye
    2 left eye
    3 bilateral
    9 unspecified eye

+7th E09.341 Drug or chemical induced diabetes mellitus with severe nonproliferative diabetic retinopathy with macular edema

+7th E09.349 Drug or chemical induced diabetes mellitus with severe nonproliferative diabetic retinopathy without macular edema

+ E09.35 Drug or chemical induced diabetes mellitus with proliferative diabetic retinopathy

> One of the following 7th characters is to be assigned to codes in subcategory **E09.35** to designate laterality of the disease:
> 1 right eye
> 2 left eye
> 3 bilateral
> 9 unspecified eye

+7th E09.351 Drug or chemical induced diabetes mellitus with proliferative diabetic retinopathy with macular edema

+7th E09.352 Drug or chemical induced diabetes mellitus with proliferative diabetic retinopathy with traction retinal detachment involving the macula

+7th E09.353 Drug or chemical induced diabetes mellitus with proliferative diabetic retinopathy with traction retinal detachment not involving the macula

+7th E09.354 Drug or chemical induced diabetes mellitus with proliferative diabetic retinopathy with combined traction retinal detachment and rhegmatogenous retinal detachment

+7th E09.355 Drug or chemical induced diabetes mellitus with stable proliferative diabetic retinopathy

+7th E09.359 Drug or chemical induced diabetes mellitus with proliferative diabetic retinopathy without macular edema

E09.36 Drug or chemical induced diabetes mellitus with diabetic cataract

X+7th E09.37 Drug or chemical induced diabetes mellitus with diabetic macular edema, resolved following treatment

> One of the following 7th characters is to be assigned to codes in subcategory **E09.37** to designate laterality of the disease:
> 1 right eye
> 2 left eye
> 3 bilateral
> 9 unspecified eye

E09.39 Drug or chemical induced diabetes mellitus with other diabetic ophthalmic complication
Use additional code to identify manifestation, such as: diabetic glaucoma (H40-H42)

+ E09.4 Drug or chemical induced diabetes mellitus with neurological complications

E09.40 Drug or chemical induced diabetes mellitus with neurological complications with diabetic neuropathy, unspecified

E09.41 Drug or chemical induced diabetes mellitus with neurological complications with diabetic mononeuropathy

E09.42 Drug or chemical induced diabetes mellitus with neurological complications with diabetic polyneuropathy
Drug or chemical induced diabetes mellitus with diabetic neuralgia

E09.43 Drug or chemical induced diabetes mellitus with neurological complications with diabetic autonomic (poly)neuropathy
Drug or chemical induced diabetes mellitus with diabetic gastroparesis
AHA CC: 3Q, 2013, 114-115

E09.44 Drug or chemical induced diabetes mellitus with neurological complications with diabetic amyotrophy

E09.49 Drug or chemical induced diabetes mellitus with neurological complications with other diabetic neurological complication

+ E09.5 Drug or chemical induced diabetes mellitus with circulatory complications

E09.51 Drug or chemical induced diabetes mellitus with diabetic peripheral angiopathy without gangrene

CC E09.52 Drug or chemical induced diabetes mellitus with diabetic peripheral angiopathy with gangrene
Drug or chemical induced diabetes mellitus with diabetic gangrene

E09.59 Drug or chemical induced diabetes mellitus with other circulatory complications

+ E09.6 Drug or chemical induced diabetes mellitus with other specified complications

+ E09.61 Drug or chemical induced diabetes mellitus with diabetic arthropathy

E09.610 Drug or chemical induced diabetes mellitus with diabetic neuropathic arthropathy
Drug or chemical induced diabetes mellitus with Charcôt's joints

E09.618 Drug or chemical induced diabetes mellitus with other diabetic arthropathy

+ E09.62 Drug or chemical induced diabetes mellitus with skin complications

E09.620 Drug or chemical induced diabetes mellitus with diabetic dermatitis
Drug or chemical induced diabetes mellitus with diabetic necrobiosis lipoidica

E09.621 Drug or chemical induced diabetes mellitus with foot ulcer
Use additional code to identify site of ulcer (L97.4-, L97.5-)

E09.622 Drug or chemical induced diabetes mellitus with other skin ulcer
Use additional code to identify site of ulcer (L97.1-L97.9, L98.41-L98.49)

E09.628 Drug or chemical induced diabetes mellitus with other skin complications

+ E09.63 Drug or chemical induced diabetes mellitus with oral complications

E09.630 Drug or chemical induced diabetes mellitus with periodontal disease

E09.638 Drug or chemical induced diabetes mellitus with other oral complications

+ E09.64 Drug or chemical induced diabetes mellitus with hypoglycemia

MCC E09.641 Drug or chemical induced diabetes mellitus with hypoglycemia with coma

E09.649 Drug or chemical induced diabetes mellitus with hypoglycemia without coma

CC E09.65 Drug or chemical induced diabetes mellitus with hyperglycemia

CC E09.69 Drug or chemical induced diabetes mellitus with other specified complication
Use additional code to identify complication

CC E09.8 Drug or chemical induced diabetes mellitus with unspecified complications

CC E09.9 Drug or chemical induced diabetes mellitus without complications

E10 Type 1 diabetes mellitus

Includes: brittle diabetes (mellitus)
diabetes (mellitus) due to autoimmune process
diabetes (mellitus) due to immune mediated pancreatic islet beta-cell destruction
idiopathic diabetes (mellitus)
juvenile onset diabetes (mellitus)
ketosis-prone diabetes (mellitus)

Excludes1: diabetes mellitus due to underlying condition (E08.-)
drug or chemical induced diabetes mellitus (E09.-)
gestational diabetes (O24.4-)
hyperglycemia NOS (R73.9)
neonatal diabetes mellitus (P70.2)
postpancreatectomy diabetes mellitus (E13.-)
postprocedural diabetes mellitus (E13.-)
secondary diabetes mellitus NEC (E13.-)
type 2 diabetes mellitus (E11.-)

Diabetes Mellitus and Its Complications: Micro and Macrovascular Complications

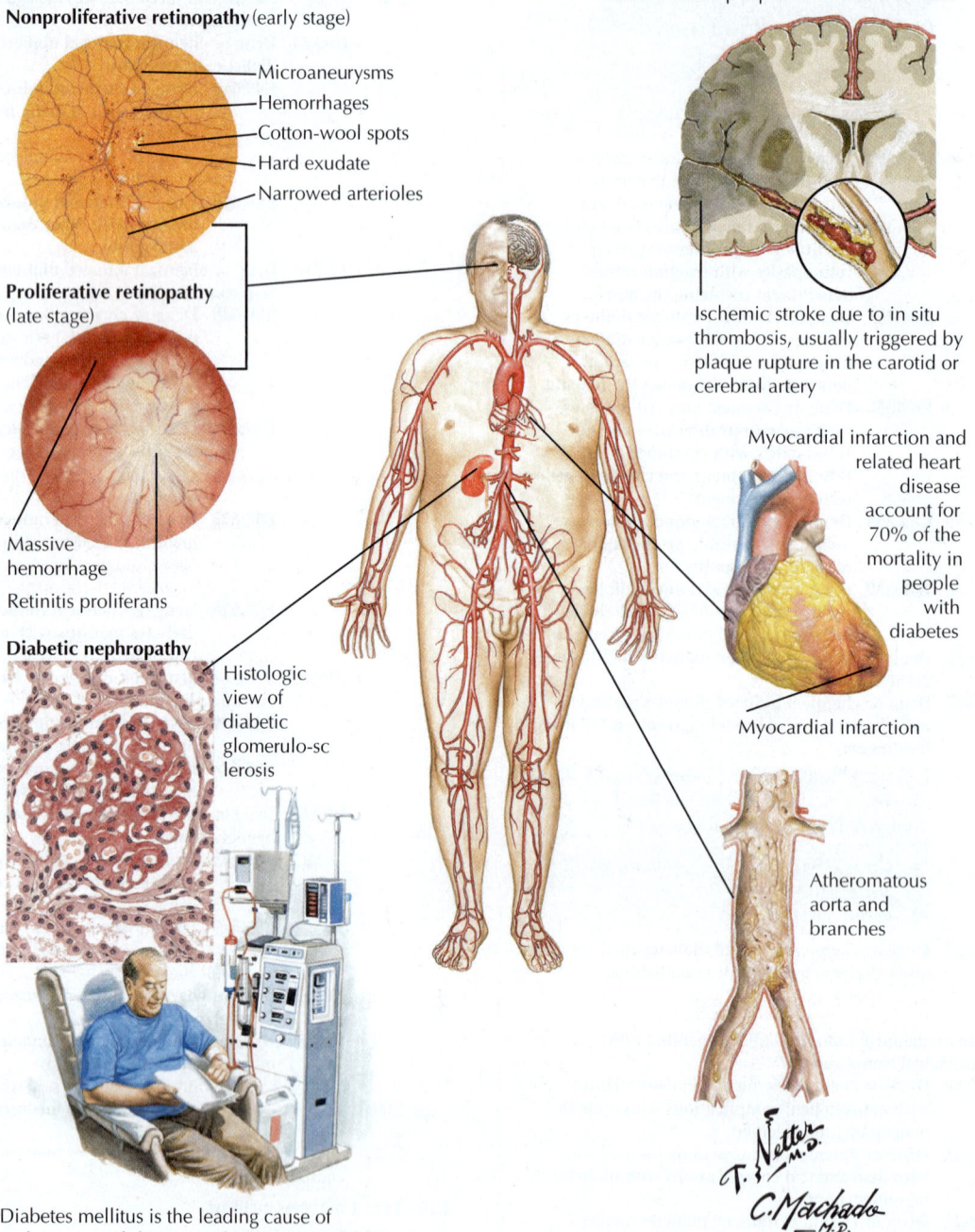

- **E10.1** Type 1 diabetes mellitus with ketoacidosis
  - MCC **E10.10** Type 1 diabetes mellitus with ketoacidosis without coma
    - HAC see Appendix B for HAC conditional logic
    - *AHA CC: 3Q, 2013, 20*
  - MCC **E10.11** Type 1 diabetes mellitus with ketoacidosis with coma
    - HAC see Appendix B for HAC conditional logic
- **E10.2** Type 1 diabetes mellitus with kidney complications
  - **E10.21** Type 1 diabetes mellitus with diabetic nephropathy
    - Type 1 diabetes mellitus with intercapillary glomerulosclerosis
    - Type 1 diabetes mellitus with intracapillary glomerulonephrosis
    - Type 1 diabetes mellitus with Kimmelstiel-Wilson disease
  - **E10.22** Type 1 diabetes mellitus with diabetic chronic kidney disease
    - *Use additional code to identify stage of chronic kidney disease (N18.1-N18.6)*
  - **E10.29** Type 1 diabetes mellitus with other diabetic kidney complication
    - Type 1 diabetes mellitus with renal tubular degeneration
- **E10.3** Type 1 diabetes mellitus with ophthalmic complications
  - *AHA CC: 4Q, 2016, 11-13*
  - **E10.31** Type 1 diabetes mellitus with unspecified diabetic retinopathy
    - **E10.311** Type 1 diabetes mellitus with unspecified diabetic retinopathy with macular edema
    - **E10.319** Type 1 diabetes mellitus with unspecified diabetic retinopathy without macular edema
  - **E10.32** Type 1 diabetes mellitus with mild nonproliferative diabetic retinopathy
    - Type 1 diabetes mellitus with nonproliferative diabetic retinopathy NOS

    One of the following 7th characters is to be assigned to codes in subcategory **E10.32** to designate laterality of the disease:
    1 right eye
    2 left eye
    3 bilateral
    9 unspecified eye

    - +7th **E10.321** Type 1 diabetes mellitus with mild nonproliferative diabetic retinopathy with macular edema
    - +7th **E10.329** Type 1 diabetes mellitus with mild nonproliferative diabetic retinopathy without macular edema
  - **E10.33** Type 1 diabetes mellitus with moderate nonproliferative diabetic retinopathy

    One of the following 7th characters is to be assigned to codes in subcategory **E10.33** to designate laterality of the disease:
    1 right eye
    2 left eye
    3 bilateral
    9 unspecified eye

    - +7th **E10.331** Type 1 diabetes mellitus with moderate nonproliferative diabetic retinopathy with macular edema
    - +7th **E10.339** Type 1 diabetes mellitus with moderate nonproliferative diabetic retinopathy without macular edema
  - **E10.34** Type 1 diabetes mellitus with severe nonproliferative diabetic retinopathy

    One of the following 7th characters is to be assigned to codes in subcategory **E10.34** to designate laterality of the disease:
    1 right eye
    2 left eye
    3 bilateral
    9 unspecified eye

    - +7th **E10.341** Type 1 diabetes mellitus with severe nonproliferative diabetic retinopathy with macular edema
    - +7th **E10.349** Type 1 diabetes mellitus with severe nonproliferative diabetic retinopathy without macular edema
  - **E10.35** Type 1 diabetes mellitus with proliferative diabetic retinopathy

    One of the following 7th characters is to be assigned to codes in subcategory **E10.35** to designate laterality of the disease:
    1 right eye
    2 left eye
    3 bilateral
    9 unspecified eye

    - +7th **E10.351** Type 1 diabetes mellitus with proliferative diabetic retinopathy with macular edema
    - +7th **E10.352** Type 1 diabetes mellitus with proliferative diabetic retinopathy with traction retinal detachment involving the macula
    - +7th **E10.353** Type 1 diabetes mellitus with proliferative diabetic retinopathy with traction retinal detachment not involving the macula
    - +7th **E10.354** Type 1 diabetes mellitus with proliferative diabetic retinopathy with combined traction retinal detachment and rhegmatogenous retinal detachment
    - +7th **E10.355** Type 1 diabetes mellitus with stable proliferative diabetic retinopathy
    - +7th **E10.359** Type 1 diabetes mellitus with proliferative diabetic retinopathy without macular edema
  - **E10.36** Type 1 diabetes mellitus with diabetic cataract
  - X+7th **E10.37** Type 1 diabetes mellitus with diabetic macular edema, resolved following treatment

    One of the following 7th characters is to be assigned to codes in subcategory **E10.37** to designate laterality of the disease:
    1 right eye
    2 left eye
    3 bilateral
    9 unspecified eye

  - **E10.39** Type 1 diabetes mellitus with other diabetic ophthalmic complication
    - *Use additional code to identify manifestation, such as: diabetic glaucoma (H40-H42)*
- **E10.4** Type 1 diabetes mellitus with neurological complications
  - **E10.40** Type 1 diabetes mellitus with diabetic neuropathy, unspecified
  - **E10.41** Type 1 diabetes mellitus with diabetic mononeuropathy
  - **E10.42** Type 1 diabetes mellitus with diabetic polyneuropathy
    - Type 1 diabetes mellitus with diabetic neuralgia
  - **E10.43** Type 1 diabetes mellitus with diabetic autonomic (poly)neuropathy
    - Type 1 diabetes mellitus with diabetic gastroparesis
    - *AHA CC: 3Q, 2013, 114-115*
  - **E10.44** Type 1 diabetes mellitus with diabetic amyotrophy
  - **E10.49** Type 1 diabetes mellitus with other diabetic neurological complication
- **E10.5** Type 1 diabetes mellitus with circulatory complications
  - **E10.51** Type 1 diabetes mellitus with diabetic peripheral angiopathy without gangrene
  - CC **E10.52** Type 1 diabetes mellitus with diabetic peripheral angiopathy with gangrene
    - Type 1 diabetes mellitus with diabetic gangrene
  - **E10.59** Type 1 diabetes mellitus with other circulatory complications

- **E10.6** Type 1 diabetes mellitus with other specified complications
  - **E10.61** Type 1 diabetes mellitus with diabetic arthropathy
    - **E10.610** Type 1 diabetes mellitus with diabetic neuropathic arthropathy
      Type 1 diabetes mellitus with Charcôt's joints
    - **E10.618** Type 1 diabetes mellitus with other diabetic arthropathy
  - **E10.62** Type 1 diabetes mellitus with skin complications
    - **E10.620** Type 1 diabetes mellitus with diabetic dermatitis
      Type 1 diabetes mellitus with diabetic necrobiosis lipoidica
    - **E10.621** Type 1 diabetes mellitus with foot ulcer
      Use additional code to identify site of ulcer (L97.4-, L97.5-)
    - **E10.622** Type 1 diabetes mellitus with other skin ulcer
      Use additional code to identify site of ulcer (L97.1-L97.9, L98.41-L98.49)
    - **E10.628** Type 1 diabetes mellitus with other skin complications
  - **E10.63** Type 1 diabetes mellitus with oral complications
    - **E10.630** Type 1 diabetes mellitus with periodontal disease
    - **E10.638** Type 1 diabetes mellitus with other oral complications
  - **E10.64** Type 1 diabetes mellitus with hypoglycemia
    - MCC **E10.641** Type 1 diabetes mellitus with hypoglycemia with coma
    - **E10.649** Type 1 diabetes mellitus with hypoglycemia without coma
      AHA CC: 1Q, 2016, 13
  - **E10.65** Type 1 diabetes mellitus with hyperglycemia
    AHA CC: 1Q, 2022, 28-29
  - **E10.69** Type 1 diabetes mellitus with other specified complication
    Use additional code to identify complication
    AHA CC: 1Q, 2022, 28-29
- **E10.8** Type 1 diabetes mellitus with unspecified complications
- **E10.9** Type 1 diabetes mellitus without complications

E11 Type 2 diabetes mellitus

Includes: diabetes (mellitus) due to insulin secretory defect
diabetes NOS
insulin resistant diabetes (mellitus)

Use additional code to identify control using:
  insulin (Z79.4)
  oral antidiabetic drugs (Z79.84)
  oral hypoglycemic drugs (Z79.84)

Excludes1: diabetes mellitus due to underlying condition (E08.-)
  drug or chemical induced diabetes mellitus (E09.-)
  gestational diabetes (O24.4-)
  neonatal diabetes mellitus (P70.2)
  postpancreatectomy diabetes mellitus (E13.-)
  postprocedural diabetes mellitus (E13.-)
  secondary diabetes mellitus NEC (E13.-)
  type 1 diabetes mellitus (E10.-)

Review coding guidelines C.4.a.2 and C.4.a.3

- **E11.0** Type 2 diabetes mellitus with hyperosmolarity
  AHA CC: 4Q, 2017, 6
  - MCC **E11.00** Type 2 diabetes mellitus with hyperosmolarity without nonketotic hyperglycemic-hyperosmolar coma (NKHHC)
    AHA CC: 1Q, 2022, 28
    HAC see Appendix B for HAC conditional logic
  - MCC **E11.01** Type 2 diabetes mellitus with hyperosmolarity with coma
    HAC see Appendix B for HAC conditional logic
- **E11.1** Type 2 diabetes mellitus with ketoacidosis
  - MCC **E11.10** Type 2 diabetes mellitus with ketoacidosis without coma
    HAC see Appendix B for HAC conditional logic
  - MCC **E11.11** Type 2 diabetes mellitus with ketoacidosis with coma
    AHA CC: 4Q, 2017, 6
    HAC see Appendix B for HAC conditional logic

- **E11.2** Type 2 diabetes mellitus with kidney complications
  - **E11.21** Type 2 diabetes mellitus with diabetic nephropathy
    Type 2 diabetes mellitus with intercapillary glomerulosclerosis
    Type 2 diabetes mellitus with intracapillary glomerulonephrosis
    Type 2 diabetes mellitus with Kimmelstiel-Wilson disease
  - **E11.22** Type 2 diabetes mellitus with diabetic chronic kidney disease
    Use additional code to identify stage of chronic kidney disease (N18.1-N18.6)
    AHA CC: 4Q, 2018, 88-89; 3Q, 2019, 3; 3Q, 2022, 15-16
  - **E11.29** Type 2 diabetes mellitus with other diabetic kidney complication
    Type 2 diabetes mellitus with renal tubular degeneration
- **E11.3** Type 2 diabetes mellitus with ophthalmic complications
  AHA CC: 4Q, 2016, 11-13
  - **E11.31** Type 2 diabetes mellitus with unspecified diabetic retinopathy
    - **E11.311** Type 2 diabetes mellitus with unspecified diabetic retinopathy with macular edema
    - **E11.319** Type 2 diabetes mellitus with unspecified diabetic retinopathy without macular edema
      AHA CC: 3Q, 2013, 20
  - **E11.32** Type 2 diabetes mellitus with mild nonproliferative diabetic retinopathy
    Type 2 diabetes mellitus with nonproliferative diabetic retinopathy NOS

    > One of the following 7th characters is to be assigned to codes in subcategory **E11.32** to designate laterality of the disease:
    > 1 right eye
    > 2 left eye
    > 3 bilateral
    > 9 unspecified eye

    - +7th **E11.321** Type 2 diabetes mellitus with mild nonproliferative diabetic retinopathy with macular edema
    - +7th **E11.329** Type 2 diabetes mellitus with mild nonproliferative diabetic retinopathy without macular edema
  - **E11.33** Type 2 diabetes mellitus with moderate nonproliferative diabetic retinopathy

    > One of the following 7th characters is to be assigned to codes in subcategory **E11.33** to designate laterality of the disease:
    > 1 right eye
    > 2 left eye
    > 3 bilateral
    > 9 unspecified eye

    - +7th **E11.331** Type 2 diabetes mellitus with moderate nonproliferative diabetic retinopathy with macular edema
    - +7th **E11.339** Type 2 diabetes mellitus with moderate nonproliferative diabetic retinopathy without macular edema
  - **E11.34** Type 2 diabetes mellitus with severe nonproliferative diabetic retinopathy

    > One of the following 7th characters is to be assigned to codes in subcategory **E11.34** to designate laterality of the disease:
    > 1 right eye
    > 2 left eye
    > 3 bilateral
    > 9 unspecified eye

    - +7th **E11.341** Type 2 diabetes mellitus with severe nonproliferative diabetic retinopathy with macular edema
    - +7th **E11.349** Type 2 diabetes mellitus with severe nonproliferative diabetic retinopathy without macular edema

+ **E11.35** Type 2 diabetes mellitus with proliferative diabetic retinopathy

> One of the following 7th characters is to be assigned to codes in subcategory **E11.35** to designate laterality of the disease:
> 1 right eye
> 2 left eye
> 3 bilateral
> 9 unspecified eye

+7th **E11.351** Type 2 diabetes mellitus with proliferative diabetic retinopathy with macular edema

+7th **E11.352** Type 2 diabetes mellitus with proliferative diabetic retinopathy with traction retinal detachment involving the macula

+7th **E11.353** Type 2 diabetes mellitus with proliferative diabetic retinopathy with traction retinal detachment not involving the macula

+7th **E11.354** Type 2 diabetes mellitus with proliferative diabetic retinopathy with combined traction retinal detachment and rhegmatogenous retinal detachment

+7th **E11.355** Type 2 diabetes mellitus with stable proliferative diabetic retinopathy

+7th **E11.359** Type 2 diabetes mellitus with proliferative diabetic retinopathy without macular edema

E11.36 Type 2 diabetes mellitus with diabetic cataract
AHA CC: 2Q, 2019, 30-31

X+7th **E11.37** Type 2 diabetes mellitus with diabetic macular edema, resolved following treatment

> One of the following 7th characters is to be assigned to codes in subcategory **E11.37** to designate laterality of the disease:
> 1 right eye
> 2 left eye
> 3 bilateral
> 9 unspecified eye

E11.39 Type 2 diabetes mellitus with other diabetic ophthalmic complication
Use additional code to identify manifestation, such as:
diabetic glaucoma (H40-H42)

+ **E11.4** Type 2 diabetes mellitus with neurological complications
AHA CC: 3Q, 2022, 15-16

E11.40 Type 2 diabetes mellitus with diabetic neuropathy, unspecified
AHA CC: 4Q, 2013, 129; 3Q, 2018, 3-4

E11.41 Type 2 diabetes mellitus with diabetic mononeuropathy

E11.42 Type 2 diabetes mellitus with diabetic polyneuropathy
Type 2 diabetes mellitus with diabetic neuralgia
AHA CC: 1Q, 2020, 12

E11.43 Type 2 diabetes mellitus with diabetic autonomic (poly)neuropathy
Type 2 diabetes mellitus with diabetic gastroparesis
AHA CC: 4Q, 2013, 114-115; 2Q, 2023, 8-9

E11.44 Type 2 diabetes mellitus with diabetic amyotrophy

E11.49 Type 2 diabetes mellitus with other diabetic neurological complication

+ **E11.5** Type 2 diabetes mellitus with circulatory complications

E11.51 Type 2 diabetes mellitus with diabetic peripheral angiopathy without gangrene
AHA CC: 3Q, 2018, 3-4

CC **E11.52** Type 2 diabetes mellitus with diabetic peripheral angiopathy with gangrene
Type 2 diabetes mellitus with diabetic gangrene
AHA CC: 4Q, 2017, 102

E11.59 Type 2 diabetes mellitus with other circulatory complications

+ **E11.6** Type 2 diabetes mellitus with other specified complications

+ **E11.61** Type 2 diabetes mellitus with diabetic arthropathy

E11.610 Type 2 diabetes mellitus with diabetic neuropathic arthropathy

Type 2 diabetes mellitus with Charcôt's joints

E11.618 Type 2 diabetes mellitus with other diabetic arthropathy

+ **E11.62** Type 2 diabetes mellitus with skin complications

E11.620 Type 2 diabetes mellitus with diabetic dermatitis
Type 2 diabetes mellitus with diabetic necrobiosis lipoidica

E11.621 Type 2 diabetes mellitus with foot ulcer
Use additional code to identify site of ulcer (L97.4-, L97.5-)
AHA CC: 1Q, 2016, 12-13; 1Q, 2020, 12; 2Q, 2020, 19

E11.622 Type 2 diabetes mellitus with other skin ulcer
Use additional code to identify site of ulcer (L97.1-L97.9, L98.41-L98.49)
AHA CC: 4Q, 2017, 17; 1Q, 2021, 7-8

E11.628 Type 2 diabetes mellitus with other skin complications

+ **E11.63** Type 2 diabetes mellitus with oral complications

E11.630 Type 2 diabetes mellitus with periodontal disease

E11.638 Type 2 diabetes mellitus with other oral complications

+ **E11.64** Type 2 diabetes mellitus with hypoglycemia

MCC **E11.641** Type 2 diabetes mellitus with hypoglycemia with coma

E11.649 Type 2 diabetes mellitus with hypoglycemia without coma
AHA CC: 3Q, 2015, 21; 3Q, 2016, 42

E11.65 Type 2 diabetes mellitus with hyperglycemia
AHA CC: 3Q, 2013, 20; 1Q, 2022, 28-29; 2Q, 2023, 10

E11.69 Type 2 diabetes mellitus with other specified complication
Use additional code to identify complication
AHA CC: 4Q, 2016, 141-142; 1Q, 2020, 12

E11.8 Type 2 diabetes mellitus with unspecified complications

E11.9 Type 2 diabetes mellitus without complications
AHA CC: 4Q, 2013, 128; 2Q, 2020, 18

E13 **Other specified diabetes mellitus**

Includes: diabetes mellitus due to genetic defects of beta-cell function diabetes mellitus due to genetic defects in insulin action postpancreatectomy diabetes mellitus postprocedural diabetes mellitus secondary diabetes mellitus NEC

Use additional code to identify control using:
insulin (Z79.4)
oral antidiabetic drugs (Z79.84)
oral hypoglycemic drugs (Z79.84)

Excludes1: diabetes (mellitus) due to autoimmune process (E10.-)
diabetes (mellitus) due to immune mediated pancreatic islet beta-cell destruction (E10.-)
diabetes mellitus due to underlying condition (E08.-)
drug or chemical induced diabetes mellitus (E09.-)
gestational diabetes (O24.4-)
neonatal diabetes mellitus (P70.2)
type 1 diabetes mellitus (E10.-)

AHA CC: 3Q, 2018, 4-5
Review coding guidelines C.4.a.6.a and C.4.a.6.b.i

+ **E13.0** Other specified diabetes mellitus with hyperosmolarity

MCC **E13.00** Other specified diabetes mellitus with hyperosmolarity without nonketotic hyperglycemic-hyperosmolar coma (NKHHC)
HAC see Appendix B for HAC conditional logic

MCC **E13.01** Other specified diabetes mellitus with hyperosmolarity with coma
HAC see Appendix B for HAC conditional logic

+ **E13.1** Other specified diabetes mellitus with ketoacidosis

MCC **E13.10** Other specified diabetes mellitus with ketoacidosis without coma
HAC see Appendix B for HAC conditional logic
AHA CC: 1Q, 2013, 26-27; 2Q, 2016, 10

MCC **E13.11** Other specified diabetes mellitus with ketoacidosis with coma
HAC see Appendix B for HAC conditional logic

+ E13.2 Other specified diabetes mellitus with kidney complications
- **E13.21** Other specified diabetes mellitus with diabetic nephropathy
  - Other specified diabetes mellitus with intercapillary glomerulosclerosis
  - Other specified diabetes mellitus with intracapillary glomerulonephrosis
  - Other specified diabetes mellitus with Kimmelstiel-Wilson disease
- **E13.22** Other specified diabetes mellitus with diabetic chronic kidney disease
  - *Use additional code to identify stage of chronic kidney disease (N18.1-N18.6)*
- **E13.29** Other specified diabetes mellitus with other diabetic kidney complication
  - Other specified diabetes mellitus with renal tubular degeneration

+ E13.3 Other specified diabetes mellitus with ophthalmic complications
AHA CC: 4Q, 2016, 11-13
- **+ E13.31** Other specified diabetes mellitus with unspecified diabetic retinopathy
  - **E13.311** Other specified diabetes mellitus with unspecified diabetic retinopathy with macular edema
  - **E13.319** Other specified diabetes mellitus with unspecified diabetic retinopathy without macular edema
- **+ E13.32** Other specified diabetes mellitus with mild nonproliferative diabetic retinopathy
  - Other specified diabetes mellitus with nonproliferative diabetic retinopathy NOS

  One of the following 7th characters is to be assigned to codes in subcategory **E13.32** to designate laterality of the disease:
  1 right eye
  2 left eye
  3 bilateral
  9 unspecified eye

  - **+7th E13.321** Other specified diabetes mellitus with mild nonproliferative diabetic retinopathy with macular edema
  - **+7th E13.329** Other specified diabetes mellitus with mild nonproliferative diabetic retinopathy without macular edema
- **+ E13.33** Other specified diabetes mellitus with moderate nonproliferative diabetic retinopathy

  One of the following 7th characters is to be assigned to codes in subcategory **E13.33** to designate laterality of the disease:
  1 right eye
  2 left eye
  3 bilateral
  9 unspecified eye

  - **+7th E13.331** Other specified diabetes mellitus with moderate nonproliferative diabetic retinopathy with macular edema
  - **+7th E13.339** Other specified diabetes mellitus with moderate nonproliferative diabetic retinopathy without macular edema
- **+ E13.34** Other specified diabetes mellitus with severe nonproliferative diabetic retinopathy

  One of the following 7th characters is to be assigned to codes in subcategory **E13.34** to designate laterality of the disease:
  1 right eye
  2 left eye
  3 bilateral
  9 unspecified eye

  - **+7th E13.341** Other specified diabetes mellitus with severe nonproliferative diabetic retinopathy with macular edema
  - **+7th E13.349** Other specified diabetes mellitus with severe nonproliferative diabetic retinopathy without macular edema

+ E13.35 Other specified diabetes mellitus with proliferative diabetic retinopathy

One of the following 7th characters is to be assigned to codes in subcategory **E13.35** to designate laterality of the disease:
1 right eye
2 left eye
3 bilateral
9 unspecified eye

- **+7th E13.351** Other specified diabetes mellitus with proliferative diabetic retinopathy with macular edema
- **+7th E13.352** Other specified diabetes mellitus with proliferative diabetic retinopathy with traction retinal detachment involving the macula
- **+7th E13.353** Other specified diabetes mellitus with proliferative diabetic retinopathy with traction retinal detachment not involving the macula
- **+7th E13.354** Other specified diabetes mellitus with proliferative diabetic retinopathy with combined traction retinal detachment and rhegmatogenous retinal detachment
- **+7th E13.355** Other specified diabetes mellitus with stable proliferative diabetic retinopathy
- **+7th E13.359** Other specified diabetes mellitus with proliferative diabetic retinopathy without macular edema

- **E13.36** Other specified diabetes mellitus with diabetic cataract
- **X+7th E13.37** Other specified diabetes mellitus with diabetic macular edema, resolved following treatment

  One of the following 7th characters is to be assigned to codes in subcategory **E13.37** to designate laterality of the disease:
  1 right eye
  2 left eye
  3 bilateral
  9 unspecified eye

- **E13.39** Other specified diabetes mellitus with other diabetic ophthalmic complication
  - *Use additional code to identify manifestation, such as: diabetic glaucoma (H40-H42)*

+ E13.4 Other specified diabetes mellitus with neurological complications
- **E13.40** Other specified diabetes mellitus with diabetic neuropathy, unspecified
  - *AHA CC: 4Q, 2013, 129*
- **E13.41** Other specified diabetes mellitus with diabetic mononeuropathy
- **E13.42** Other specified diabetes mellitus with diabetic polyneuropathy
  - Other specified diabetes mellitus with diabetic neuralgia
- **E13.43** Other specified diabetes mellitus with diabetic autonomic (poly)neuropathy
  - Other specified diabetes mellitus with diabetic gastroparesis
  - *AHA CC: 4Q, 2013, 114-115*
- **E13.44** Other specified diabetes mellitus with diabetic amyotrophy
- **E13.49** Other specified diabetes mellitus with other diabetic neurological complication

+ E13.5 Other specified diabetes mellitus with circulatory complications
- **E13.51** Other specified diabetes mellitus with diabetic peripheral angiopathy without gangrene
- **CC E13.52** Other specified diabetes mellitus with diabetic peripheral angiopathy with gangrene
  - Other specified diabetes mellitus with diabetic gangrene
- **E13.59** Other specified diabetes mellitus with other circulatory complications

+ **E13.6** Other specified diabetes mellitus with other specified complications
  + **E13.61** Other specified diabetes mellitus with diabetic arthropathy
      E13.610 Other specified diabetes mellitus with diabetic neuropathic arthropathy
        Other specified diabetes mellitus with Charcôt's joints
      E13.618 Other specified diabetes mellitus with other diabetic arthropathy
  + **E13.62** Other specified diabetes mellitus with skin complications
      E13.620 Other specified diabetes mellitus with diabetic dermatitis
        Other specified diabetes mellitus with diabetic necrobiosis lipoidica
      E13.621 Other specified diabetes mellitus with foot ulcer
        Use additional code to identify site of ulcer (L97.4-, L97.5-)
      E13.622 Other specified diabetes mellitus with other skin ulcer
        Use additional code to identify site of ulcer (L97.1-L97.9, L98.41-L98.49)
      E13.628 Other specified diabetes mellitus with other skin complications
  + **E13.63** Other specified diabetes mellitus with oral complications
      E13.630 Other specified diabetes mellitus with periodontal disease
      E13.638 Other specified diabetes mellitus with other oral complications
  + **E13.64** Other specified diabetes mellitus with hypoglycemia
      MCC **E13.641** Other specified diabetes mellitus with hypoglycemia with coma
      E13.649 Other specified diabetes mellitus with hypoglycemia without coma
    E13.65 Other specified diabetes mellitus with hyperglycemia
        AHA CC: 3Q, 2018, 4-5
    E13.69 Other specified diabetes mellitus with other specified complication
        Use additional code to identify complication
  E13.8 Other specified diabetes mellitus with unspecified complications
  E13.9 Other specified diabetes mellitus without complications

Other disorders of glucose regulation and pancreatic internal secretion (E15-E16)

CC **E15** Nondiabetic hypoglycemic coma
  Includes: drug-induced insulin coma in nondiabetic
      hyperinsulinism with hypoglycemic coma
      hypoglycemic coma NOS
    HAC see Appendix B for HAC conditional logic
    Valid 3-character code, no further characters required

E16 Other disorders of pancreatic internal secretion
  E16.0 Drug-induced hypoglycemia without coma
      Use additional code for adverse effect, if applicable, to identify drug (T36-T50 with fifth or sixth character 5)
      Excludes1: diabetes with hypoglycemia without coma (E09.649)
  E16.1 Other hypoglycemia
      Functional hyperinsulinism
      Functional nonhyperinsulinemic hypoglycemia
      Hyperinsulinism NOS
      Hyperplasia of pancreatic islet beta cells NOS
      Excludes1: diabetes with hypoglycemia (E08.649, E10.649, E11.649, E13.649)
        hypoglycemia in infant of diabetic mother (P70.1)
        neonatal hypoglycemia (P70.4)
  E16.2 Hypoglycemia, unspecified
      Excludes1: diabetes with hypoglycemia (E08.649, E10.649, E11.649, E13.649)
  E16.3 Increased secretion of glucagon
      Hyperplasia of pancreatic endocrine cells with glucagon excess
  E16.4 Increased secretion of gastrin
      Hypergastrinemia
      Hyperplasia of pancreatic endocrine cells with gastrin excess
      Zollinger-Ellison syndrome
  E16.8 Other specified disorders of pancreatic internal secretion
      Increased secretion from endocrine pancreas of growth hormone-releasing hormone
      Increased secretion from endocrine pancreas of pancreatic polypeptide
      Increased secretion from endocrine pancreas of somatostatin
      Increased secretion from endocrine pancreas of vasoactive-intestinal polypeptide
  E16.9 Disorder of pancreatic internal secretion, unspecified
      Islet-cell hyperplasia NOS
      Pancreatic endocrine cell hyperplasia NOS

Disorders of other endocrine glands (E20-E35)

  Excludes1: galactorrhea (N64.3)
      gynecomastia (N62)

E20 Hypoparathyroidism
  Excludes1: Di George's syndrome (D82.1)
      postprocedural hypoparathyroidism (E89.2)
      tetany NOS (R29.0)
      transitory neonatal hypoparathyroidism (P71.4)
  E20.0 Idiopathic hypoparathyroidism
  E20.1 Pseudohypoparathyroidism
+ **E20.8** Other hypoparathyroidism
  + **E20.81** Hypoparathyroidism due to impaired parathyroid hormone secretion
      E20.810 Autosomal dominant hypocalcemia
        Autosomal dominant hypocalcemia type 1 (ADH1)
        Autosomal dominant hypocalcemia type 2 (ADH2)
        Code also, if applicable, any associated conditions, such as:
          calculus of kidney (N20.0)
          chronic kidney disease (N18.-)
          respiratory distress (J80, R06.-)
          seizure disorder (G40.-, R56.9)
      E20.811 Secondary hypoparathyroidism in diseases classified elsewhere
        Code first underlying condition, if known
      E20.812 Autoimmune hypoparathyroidism
        Code first, if applicable, underlying condition such as:
          autoimmune polyglandular failure (E31.0)
          Schmidt's syndrome (E31.0)
      E20.818 Other specified hypoparathyroidism due to impaired parathyroid hormonesecretion
        Familial isolated hypoparathyroidism
      E20.819 Hypoparathyroidism due to impaired parathyroid hormone secretion, unspecified
    E20.89 Other specified hypoparathyroidism
      Familial hypoparathyroidism
  E20.9 Hypoparathyroidism, unspecified
      Parathyroid tetany

E21 Hyperparathyroidism and other disorders of parathyroid gland
  Excludes1: adult osteomalacia (M83.-)
      ectopic hyperparathyroidism (E34.2)
      hungry bone syndrome (E83.81)
      infantile and juvenile osteomalacia (E55.0)
  Excludes2: familial hypocalciuric hypercalcemia (E83.52)
  E21.0 Primary hyperparathyroidism
      Hyperplasia of parathyroid
      Osteitis fibrosa cystica generalisata [von Recklinghausen's disease of bone]
  E21.1 Secondary hyperparathyroidism, not elsewhere classified
      Excludes1: secondary hyperparathyroidism of renal origin (N25.81)

- **E21.2** Other hyperparathyroidism
  Tertiary hyperparathyroidism
  Excludes1: familial hypocalciuric hypercalcemia (E83.52)
- **E21.3** Hyperparathyroidism, unspecified
- **E21.4** Other specified disorders of parathyroid gland
- **E21.5** Disorder of parathyroid gland, unspecified

E22 Hyperfunction of pituitary gland
Excludes1: Cushing's syndrome (E24.-)
Nelson's syndrome (E24.1)
overproduction of ACTH not associated with Cushing's disease (E27.0)
overproduction of pituitary ACTH (E24.0)
overproduction of thyroid-stimulating hormone (E05.8-)

- **E22.0** Acromegaly and pituitary gigantism
  Overproduction of growth hormone
  Excludes1: constitutional gigantism (E34.4)
  constitutional tall stature (E34.4)
  increased secretion from endocrine pancreas of growth hormone-releasing hormone (E16.8)
- CC **E22.1** Hyperprolactinemia
  Use additional code for adverse effect, if applicable, to identify drug (T36-T50 with fifth or sixth character 5)
- CC **E22.2** Syndrome of inappropriate secretion of antidiuretic hormone
- CC **E22.8** Other hyperfunction of pituitary gland
  Central precocious puberty
- CC **E22.9** Hyperfunction of pituitary gland, unspecified

E23 Hypofunction and other disorders of the pituitary gland
Includes: the listed conditions whether the disorder is in the pituitary or the hypothalamus
Excludes1: postprocedural hypopituitarism (E89.3)
short stature due to endocrine disorder (E34.3-)

- CC **E23.0** Hypopituitarism
  Fertile eunuch syndrome
  Hypogonadotropic hypogonadism
  Idiopathic growth hormone deficiency
  Isolated deficiency of gonadotropin
  Isolated deficiency of growth hormone
  Isolated deficiency of pituitary hormone
  Kallmann's syndrome
  Lorain-Levi short stature
  Necrosis of pituitary gland (postpartum)
  Panhypopituitarism
  Pituitary cachexia
  Pituitary insufficiency NOS
  Pituitary short stature
  Sheehan's syndrome
  Simmonds' disease
- **E23.1** Drug-induced hypopituitarism
  Use additional code for adverse effect, if applicable, to identify drug (T36-T50 with fifth or sixth character 5)
- CC **E23.2** Diabetes insipidus
  Excludes1: nephrogenic diabetes insipidus (N25.1)
- **E23.3** Hypothalamic dysfunction, not elsewhere classified
  Excludes1: Prader-Willi syndrome (Q87.11)
  Russell-Silver syndrome (Q87.19)
- **E23.6** Other disorders of pituitary gland
  Abscess of pituitary
  Adiposogenital dystrophy
- **E23.7** Disorder of pituitary gland, unspecified

E24 Cushing's syndrome
Excludes1: congenital adrenal hyperplasia (E25.0)
- CC **E24.0** Pituitary-dependent Cushing's disease
  Overproduction of pituitary ACTH
  Pituitary-dependent hypercorticalism
- **E24.1** Nelson's syndrome
- CC **E24.2** Drug-induced Cushing's syndrome
  Use additional code for adverse effect, if applicable, to identify drug (T36-T50 with fifth or sixth character 5)
- CC **E24.3** Ectopic ACTH syndrome
- CC **E24.4** Alcohol-induced pseudo-Cushing's syndrome
- CC **E24.8** Other Cushing's syndrome
- CC **E24.9** Cushing's syndrome, unspecified

E25 Adrenogenital disorders
Includes: adrenogenital syndromes, virilizing or feminizing, whether acquired or due to adrenal hyperplasia consequent on inborn enzyme defects in hormone synthesis
Female adrenal pseudohermaphroditism
Female heterosexual precocious pseudopuberty
Male isosexual precocious pseudopuberty
Male macrogenitosomia praecox
Male sexual precocity with adrenal hyperplasia
Male virilization (female)
Excludes1: indeterminate sex and pseudohermaphroditism (Q56)
chromosomal abnormalities (Q90-Q99)

- CC **E25.0** Congenital adrenogenital disorders associated with enzyme deficiency
  Congenital adrenal hyperplasia
  21-Hydroxylase deficiency
  Salt-losing congenital adrenal hyperplasia
- **E25.8** Other adrenogenital disorders
  Idiopathic adrenogenital disorder
  Use additional code for adverse effect, if applicable, to identify drug (T36-T50 with fifth or sixth character 5)
- **E25.9** Adrenogenital disorder, unspecified
  Adrenogenital syndrome NOS

E26 Hyperaldosteronism
- + **E26.0** Primary hyperaldosteronism
  - **E26.01** Conn's syndrome
    Code also adrenal adenoma (D35.0-)
  - **E26.02** Glucocorticoid-remediable aldosteronism
    Familial aldosteronism type I
  - **E26.09** Other primary hyperaldosteronism
    Primary aldosteronism due to adrenal hyperplasia (bilateral)
- **E26.1** Secondary hyperaldosteronism
- + **E26.8** Other hyperaldosteronism
  - **E26.81** Bartter's syndrome
  - **E26.89** Other hyperaldosteronism
- **E26.9** Hyperaldosteronism, unspecified
  Aldosteronism NOS
  Hyperaldosteronism NOS

E27 Other disorders of adrenal gland
- CC **E27.0** Other adrenocortical overactivity
  Overproduction of ACTH, not associated with Cushing's disease
  Premature adrenarche
  Excludes1: Cushing's syndrome (E24.-)
- **E27.1** Primary adrenocortical insufficiency
  Addison's disease
  Autoimmune adrenalitis
  Excludes1: Addison only phenotype adrenoleukodystrophy (E71.528)
  amyloidosis (E85.-)
  tuberculous Addison's disease (A18.7)
  Waterhouse-Friderichsen syndrome (A39.1)
- CC **E27.2** Addisonian crisis
  Adrenal crisis
  Adrenocortical crisis
- CC **E27.3** Drug-induced adrenocortical insufficiency
  Use additional code for adverse effect, if applicable, to identify drug (T36-T50 with fifth or sixth character 5)
- + **E27.4** Other and unspecified adrenocortical insufficiency
  Excludes1: adrenoleukodystrophy [Addison-Schilder] (E71.528)
  Waterhouse-Friderichsen syndrome (A39.1)
  - CC **E27.40** Unspecified adrenocortical insufficiency
    Adrenocortical insufficiency NOS
    Hypoaldosteronism
  - CC **E27.49** Other adrenocortical insufficiency
    Adrenal hemorrhage
    Adrenal infarction
- CC **E27.5** Adrenomedullary hyperfunction
  Adrenomedullary hyperplasia
  Catecholamine hypersecretion
- **E27.8** Other specified disorders of adrenal gland
  Abnormality of cortisol-binding globulin
- **E27.9** Disorder of adrenal gland, unspecified

E28 Ovarian dysfunction
  Excludes1: isolated gonadotropin deficiency (E23.0)
    postprocedural ovarian failure (E89.4-)
  ♀ **E28.0 Estrogen excess**
    Use additional code for adverse effect, if applicable, to identify drug (T36-T50 with fifth or sixth character 5)
  ♀ **E28.1 Androgen excess**
    Hypersecretion of ovarian androgens
    Use additional code for adverse effect, if applicable, to identify drug (T36-T50 with fifth or sixth character 5)
  ♀ **E28.2 Polycystic ovarian syndrome**
    Sclerocystic ovary syndrome
    Stein-Leventhal syndrome
  + **E28.3 Primary ovarian failure**
    Excludes1: pure gonadal dysgenesis (Q99.1)
      Turner's syndrome (Q96.-)
    + **E28.31 Premature menopause**
      • ♀ **E28.310 Symptomatic premature menopause**
        Symptoms such as flushing, sleeplessness, headache, lack of concentration, associated with premature menopause
      • ♀ **E28.319 Asymptomatic premature menopause**
        Premature menopause NOS
    ♀ **E28.39 Other primary ovarian failure**
      Decreased estrogen
      Resistant ovary syndrome
  ♀ **E28.8 Other ovarian dysfunction**
    Ovarian hyperfunction NOS
    Excludes1: postprocedural ovarian failure (E89.4-)
  ♀ **E28.9 Ovarian dysfunction, unspecified**

E29 Testicular dysfunction
  Excludes1: androgen insensitivity syndrome (E34.5-)
    azoospermia or oligospermia NOS (N46.0-N46.1)
    isolated gonadotropin deficiency (E23.0)
    Klinefelter's syndrome (Q98.0-Q98.1, Q98.4)
  ♂ **E29.0 Testicular hyperfunction**
    Hypersecretion of testicular hormones
  ♂ **E29.1 Testicular hypofunction**
    Defective biosynthesis of testicular androgen NOS
    5-delta-Reductase deficiency (with male pseudohermaphroditism)
    Testicular hypogonadism NOS
    Use additional code for adverse effect, if applicable, to identify drug (T36-T50 with fifth or sixth character 5)
    Excludes1: postprocedural testicular hypofunction (E89.5)
  ♂ **E29.8 Other testicular dysfunction**
  ♂ **E29.9 Testicular dysfunction, unspecified**

E30 Disorders of puberty, not elsewhere classified
  E30.0 Delayed puberty
    Constitutional delay of puberty
    Delayed sexual development
  • **E30.1 Precocious puberty**
    Precocious menstruation
    Excludes1: Albright (-McCune) (-Sternberg) syndrome (Q78.1)
      central precocious puberty (E22.8)
      congenital adrenal hyperplasia (E25.0)
      female heterosexual precocious pseudopuberty (E25.-)
      male isosexual precocious pseudopuberty (E25.-)
  • **E30.8 Other disorders of puberty**
    Premature thelarche
  E30.9 Disorder of puberty, unspecified

E31 Polyglandular dysfunction
  Excludes1: ataxia telangiectasia [Louis-Bar] (G11.3)
    dystrophia myotonica [Steinert] (G71.11)
    pseudohypoparathyroidism (E20.1)
  E31.0 Autoimmune polyglandular failure
    Schmidt's syndrome
  E31.1 Polyglandular hyperfunction
    Excludes1: multiple endocrine adenomatosis (E31.2-)
      multiple endocrine neoplasia (E31.2-)
  + **E31.2 Multiple endocrine neoplasia [MEN] syndromes**
    Multiple endocrine adenomatosis
    Code also any associated malignancies and other conditions associated with the syndromes
    E31.20 Multiple endocrine neoplasia [MEN] syndrome, unspecified
      Multiple endocrine adenomatosis NOS
      Multiple endocrine neoplasia [MEN] syndrome NOS
    E31.21 Multiple endocrine neoplasia [MEN] type I
      Wermer's syndrome
    E31.22 Multiple endocrine neoplasia [MEN] type IIA
      Sipple's syndrome
    E31.23 Multiple endocrine neoplasia [MEN] type IIB
  E31.8 Other polyglandular dysfunction
  E31.9 Polyglandular dysfunction, unspecified

E32 Diseases of thymus
  Excludes1: aplasia or hypoplasia of thymus with immunodeficiency (D82.1)
    myasthenia gravis (G70.0)
  E32.0 Persistent hyperplasia of thymus
    Hypertrophy of thymus
  CC **E32.1 Abscess of thymus**
  E32.8 Other diseases of thymus
    Excludes1: aplasia or hypoplasia with immunodeficiency (D82.1)
      thymoma (D15.0)
  E32.9 Disease of thymus, unspecified

E34 Other endocrine disorders
  Excludes1: pseudohypoparathyroidism (E20.1)
  CC **E34.0 Carcinoid syndrome**
    NOTE May be used as an additional code to identify functional activity associated with a carcinoid tumor.
  E34.1 Other hypersecretion of intestinal hormones
  E34.2 Ectopic hormone secretion, not elsewhere classified
    Excludes1: ectopic ACTH syndrome (E24.3)
  + **E34.3 Short stature due to endocrine disorder**
    Excludes1: achondroplastic short stature (Q77.4)
      hypochondroplastic short stature (Q77.4)
      nutritional short stature (E45)
      pituitary short stature (E23.0)
      progeria (E34.8)
      renal short stature (N25.0)
      Russell-Silver syndrome (Q87.19)
      short-limbed stature with immunodeficiency (D82.2)
      short stature in specific dysmorphic syndromes - code to syndrome - see Alphabetical Index
      short stature (child) (R62.52)
      short stature NOS (R62.52)
    AHA CC: 4Q, 2022, 11-13
    E34.30 Short stature due to endocrine disorder, unspecified
    E34.31 Constitutional short stature
      Constitutional delay of growth, puberty, or maturation
    + **E34.32 Genetic causes of short stature**
      E34.321 Primary insulin-like growth factor-1 (IGF-1) deficiency
        Acid-labile subunit gene (IGFALS) defect
        Growth hormone gene 1 (GH1) defect with growth hormone neutralizing antibodies
        Growth hormone insensitivity syndrome (GHIS)
        Insulin-like growth factor 1 gene (IGF1) defect
        Laron type short stature
        Severe primary insulin-like growth factor-1 deficiency (SPIGFD)
        Signal transducer and activator of transcription 5B gene (STAT5b) defect

E34.322 **Insulin-like growth factor-1 (IGF-1) resistance**
Genetic syndrome with resistance to insulin-like growth factor-1
Insulin-like growth factor-1 receptor (IGF-1R) defect
Post-insulin-like growth factor-1 receptor signaling defect
E34.328 **Other genetic causes of short stature**
Short stature due to ACAN gene variant
Short stature due to aggrecan deficiency
Short stature due to NPR-2 gene variant
E34.329 **Unspecified genetic causes of short stature**
E34.39 **Other short stature due to endocrine disorder**
E34.4 **Constitutional tall stature**
Constitutional gigantism
+ E34.5 **Androgen insensitivity syndrome**
E34.50 **Androgen insensitivity syndrome, unspecified**
Androgen insensitivity NOS
E34.51 **Complete androgen insensitivity syndrome**
Complete androgen insensitivity
de Quervain syndrome
Goldberg-Maxwell syndrome
E34.52 **Partial androgen insensitivity syndrome**
Partial androgen insensitivity
Reifenstein syndrome
E34.8 **Other specified endocrine disorders**
Pineal gland dysfunction
Progeria
Excludes2: *pseudohypoparathyroidism (E20.1)*
E34.9 **Endocrine disorder, unspecified**
Endocrine disturbance NOS
Hormone disturbance NOS

E35 Disorders of endocrine glands in diseases classified elsewhere

Code first underlying disease, such as:
late congenital syphilis of thymus gland [Dubois disease] (A50.59)

Use additional code, if applicable, to identify:
sequelae of tuberculosis of other organs (B90.8)
Excludes1: *Echinococcus granulosus infection of thyroid gland (B67.3)*
meningococcal hemorrhagic adrenalitis (A39.1)
syphilis of endocrine gland (A52.79)
tuberculosis of adrenal gland, except calcification (A18.7)
tuberculosis of endocrine gland NEC (A18.82)
tuberculosis of thyroid gland (A18.81)
Waterhouse-Friderichsen syndrome (A39.1)
Valid 3-character code, no further characters required

Intraoperative complications of endocrine system (E36)

E36 Intraoperative complications of endocrine system
Excludes2: *postprocedural endocrine and metabolic complications and disorders, not elsewhere classified (E89.-)*
+ E36.0 **Intraoperative hemorrhage and hematoma of an endocrine system organ or structure complicating a procedure**
Excludes1: *intraoperative hemorrhage and hematoma of an endocrine system organ or structure due to accidental puncture or laceration during a procedure (E36.1-)*
CC E36.01 **Intraoperative hemorrhage and hematoma of an endocrine system organ or structure complicating an endocrine system procedure**
AHA CC: 1Q, 2020, 19
CC E36.02 **Intraoperative hemorrhage and hematoma of an endocrine system organ or structure complicating other procedure**
+ E36.1 **Accidental puncture and laceration of an endocrine system organ or structure during a procedure**
CC E36.11 **Accidental puncture and laceration of an endocrine system organ or structure during an endocrine system procedure**
CC E36.12 **Accidental puncture and laceration of an endocrine system organ or structure during other procedure**
E36.8 **Other intraoperative complications of endocrine system**
Use additional code, if applicable, to further specify disorder

Malnutrition (E40-E46)

Excludes1: *intestinal malabsorption (K90.-)*
sequelae of protein-calorie malnutrition (E64.0)
Excludes2: *nutritional anemias (D50-D53)*
starvation (T73.0)

MCC **E40 Kwashiorkor**
Severe malnutrition with nutritional edema with dyspigmentation of skin and hair
Excludes1: *marasmic kwashiorkor (E42)*
AHA CC: 3Q, 2017, 25-26
Valid 3-character code, no further characters required

MCC **E41 Nutritional marasmus**
Severe malnutrition with marasmus
Excludes1: *marasmic kwashiorkor (E42)*
AHA CC: 3Q, 2017, 24-25
Valid 3-character code, no further characters required

MCC **E42 Marasmic kwashiorkor**
Intermediate form severe protein-calorie malnutrition
Severe protein-calorie malnutrition with signs of both kwashiorkor and marasmus
AHA CC: 3Q, 2017, 25-26
Valid 3-character code, no further characters required

MCC **E43 Unspecified severe protein-calorie malnutrition**
Starvation edema
AHA CC: 3Q, 2017, 25-26; 4Q, 2017, 108-109; 1Q, 2020, 4-7; 1Q, 2022, 13-14
Valid 3-character code, no further characters required

E44 Protein-calorie malnutrition of moderate and mild degree
CC E44.0 **Moderate protein-calorie malnutrition**
CC E44.1 **Mild protein-calorie malnutrition**

CC **E45 Retarded development following protein-calorie malnutrition**
Nutritional short stature
Nutritional stunting
Physical retardation due to malnutrition
Valid 3-character code, no further characters required

CC **E46 Unspecified protein-calorie malnutrition**
Malnutrition NOS
Protein-calorie imbalance NOS
Excludes1: *nutritional deficiency NOS (E63.9)*
Valid 3-character code, no further characters required

Other nutritional deficiencies (E50-E64)

Excludes2: *nutritional anemias (D50-D53)*

E50 Vitamin A deficiency
Excludes1: *sequelae of vitamin A deficiency (E64.1)*
E50.0 **Vitamin A deficiency with conjunctival xerosis**
E50.1 **Vitamin A deficiency with Bitot's spot and conjunctival xerosis**
Bitot's spot in the young child
E50.2 **Vitamin A deficiency with corneal xerosis**
E50.3 **Vitamin A deficiency with corneal ulceration and xerosis**
E50.4 **Vitamin A deficiency with keratomalacia**
E50.5 **Vitamin A deficiency with night blindness**
E50.6 **Vitamin A deficiency with xerophthalmic scars of cornea**
E50.7 **Other ocular manifestations of vitamin A deficiency**
Xerophthalmia NOS
E50.8 **Other manifestations of vitamin A deficiency**
Follicular keratosis
Xeroderma
E50.9 **Vitamin A deficiency, unspecified**
Hypovitaminosis A NOS

E51 Thiamine deficiency
Excludes1: *sequelae of thiamine deficiency (E64.8)*
+ E51.1 **Beriberi**
CC E51.11 **Dry beriberi**
Beriberi NOS
Beriberi with polyneuropathy
CC E51.12 **Wet beriberi**
Beriberi with cardiovascular manifestations
Cardiovascular beriberi
Shoshin disease
CC E51.2 **Wernicke's encephalopathy**
CC E51.8 **Other manifestations of thiamine deficiency**
CC E51.9 **Thiamine deficiency, unspecified**

E52 Niacin deficiency [pellagra]
Niacin (-tryptophan) deficiency
Nicotinamide deficiency
Pellagra (alcoholic)
Excludes1: *sequelae of niacin deficiency (E64.8)*
Valid 3-character code, no further characters required

E53 Deficiency of other B group vitamins
Excludes1: *sequelae of vitamin B deficiency (E64.8)*

CC **E53.0 Riboflavin deficiency**
Ariboflavinosis
Vitamin B2 deficiency

E53.1 Pyridoxine deficiency
Vitamin B6 deficiency
Excludes1: *pyridoxine-responsive sideroblastic anemia (D64.3)*

E53.8 Deficiency of other specified B group vitamins
Biotin deficiency
Cyanocobalamin deficiency
Folate deficiency
Folic acid deficiency
Pantothenic acid deficiency
Vitamin B12 deficiency
Excludes1: *folate deficiency anemia (D52.-)*
vitamin B12 deficiency anemia (D51.-)

E53.9 Vitamin B deficiency, unspecified

E54 Ascorbic acid deficiency
Deficiency of vitamin C
Scurvy
Excludes1: *scorbutic anemia (D53.2)*
sequelae of vitamin C deficiency (E64.2)
Valid 3-character code, no further characters required

E55 Vitamin D deficiency
Excludes1: *adult osteomalacia (M83.-)*
osteoporosis (M80.-)
sequelae of rickets (E64.3)

CC **E55.0 Rickets, active**
Infantile osteomalacia
Juvenile osteomalacia
Excludes1: *celiac rickets (K90.0)*
Crohn's rickets (K50.-)
hereditary vitamin D-dependent rickets (E83.32)
inactive rickets (E64.3)
renal rickets (N25.0)
sequelae of rickets (E64.3)
vitamin D-resistant rickets (E83.31)

E55.9 Vitamin D deficiency, unspecified
Avitaminosis D

E56 Other vitamin deficiencies
Excludes1: *sequelae of other vitamin deficiencies (E64.8)*

E56.0 Deficiency of vitamin E
E56.1 Deficiency of vitamin K
Excludes1: *deficiency of coagulation factor due to vitamin K deficiency (D68.4)*
vitamin K deficiency of newborn (P53)

E56.8 Deficiency of other vitamins
E56.9 Vitamin deficiency, unspecified

E58 Dietary calcium deficiency
Excludes1: *disorders of calcium metabolism (E83.5-)*
sequelae of calcium deficiency (E64.8)
Valid 3-character code, no further characters required

E59 Dietary selenium deficiency
Keshan disease
Excludes1: *sequelae of selenium deficiency (E64.8)*
Valid 3-character code, no further characters required

E60 Dietary zinc deficiency
Valid 3-character code, no further characters required

E61 Deficiency of other nutrient elements
Use additional code for adverse effect, if applicable, to identify drug (T36-T50 with fifth or sixth character 5)
Excludes1: *disorders of mineral metabolism (E83.-)*
iodine deficiency related thyroid disorders (E00-E02)
sequelae of malnutrition and other nutritional deficiencies (E64.-)

E61.0 Copper deficiency
E61.1 Iron deficiency
Excludes1: *iron deficiency anemia (D50.-)*
E61.2 Magnesium deficiency
E61.3 Manganese deficiency
E61.4 Chromium deficiency
E61.5 Molybdenum deficiency
E61.6 Vanadium deficiency
E61.7 Deficiency of multiple nutrient elements
E61.8 Deficiency of other specified nutrient elements
E61.9 Deficiency of nutrient element, unspecified

E63 Other nutritional deficiencies
Excludes2: *dehydration (E86.0)*
failure to thrive, adult (R62.7)
failure to thrive, child (R62.51)
feeding problems in newborn (P92.-)
sequelae of malnutrition and other nutritional deficiencies (E64.-)

E63.0 Essential fatty acid [EFA] deficiency
E63.1 Imbalance of constituents of food intake
E63.8 Other specified nutritional deficiencies
E63.9 Nutritional deficiency, unspecified

E64 Sequelae of malnutrition and other nutritional deficiencies
NOTE This category is to be used to indicate conditions in categories E43, E44, E46, E50-E63 as the cause of sequelae, which are themselves classified elsewhere. The 'sequelae' include conditions specified as such; they also include the late effects of diseases classifiable to the above categories if the disease itself is no longer present
Code first condition resulting from (sequela) of malnutrition and other nutritional deficiencies

CC **E64.0 Sequelae of protein-calorie malnutrition**
Excludes2: *retarded development following protein-calorie malnutrition (E45)*

E64.1 Sequelae of vitamin A deficiency
E64.2 Sequelae of vitamin C deficiency
E64.3 Sequelae of rickets
E64.8 Sequelae of other nutritional deficiencies
E64.9 Sequelae of unspecified nutritional deficiency

Overweight, obesity and other hyperalimentation (E65-E68)

E65 Localized adiposity
Fat pad
Valid 3-character code, no further characters required

E66 Overweight and obesity
Code first obesity complicating pregnancy, childbirth and the puerperium, if applicable (O99.21-)

Use additional code to identify body mass index (BMI), if known (Z68.-)
Excludes1: *adiposogenital dystrophy (E23.6)*
lipomatosis NOS (E88.2)
lipomatosis dolorosa [Dercum] (E88.2)
Prader-Willi syndrome (Q87.11)
AHA CC: 4Q, 2018, 80

+ **E66.0 Obesity due to excess calories**
E66.01 Morbid (severe) obesity due to excess calories
Excludes1: *morbid (severe) obesity with alveolar hypoventilation (E66.2)*
AHA CC: 4Q, 2018, 79; 2Q, 2022, 9; 3Q, 2022, 6-7
HAC see Appendix B for HAC conditional logic
E66.09 Other obesity due to excess calories

E66.1 Drug-induced obesity
Use additional code for adverse effect, if applicable, to identify drug (T36-T50 with fifth or sixth character 5)

CC **E66.2 Morbid (severe) obesity with alveolar hypoventilation**
Obesity hypoventilation syndrome (OHS)
Pickwickian syndrome

E66.3 Overweight
E66.8 Other obesity
E66.9 Obesity, unspecified
Obesity NOS
AHA CC: 4Q, 2013, 129; 2Q, 2021, 10-11

E67 Other hyperalimentation
  Excludes1: hyperalimentation NOS (R63.2)
  sequelae of hyperalimentation (E68)
  E67.0 Hypervitaminosis A
  E67.1 Hypercarotenemia
  E67.2 Megavitamin-B6 syndrome
  E67.3 Hypervitaminosis D
  E67.8 Other specified hyperalimentation

E68 Sequelae of hyperalimentation
  Code first condition resulting from (sequela) of hyperalimentation
  Valid 3-character code, no further characters required

Metabolic disorders (E70-E88)

Excludes1: androgen insensitivity syndrome (E34.5-)
  congenital adrenal hyperplasia (E25.0)
  hemolytic anemias attributable to enzyme disorders (D55.-)
  Marfan syndrome (Q87.4-)
  5-alpha-reductase deficiency (E29.1)
Excludes2: Ehlers-Danlos syndromes (Q79.6-)

E70 Disorders of aromatic amino-acid metabolism
  CC E70.0 Classical phenylketonuria
  CC E70.1 Other hyperphenylalaninemias
  + E70.2 Disorders of tyrosine metabolism
    Excludes1: transitory tyrosinemia of newborn (P74.5)
    CC E70.20 Disorder of tyrosine metabolism, unspecified
    CC E70.21 Tyrosinemia
      Hypertyrosinemia
    CC E70.29 Other disorders of tyrosine metabolism
      Alkaptonuria
      Ochronosis
  + E70.3 Albinism
    CC E70.30 Albinism, unspecified
    + E70.31 Ocular albinism
      CC E70.310 X-linked ocular albinism
      CC E70.311 Autosomal recessive ocular albinism
      CC E70.318 Other ocular albinism
      CC E70.319 Ocular albinism, unspecified
    + E70.32 Oculocutaneous albinism
      Excludes1: Chediak-Higashi syndrome (E70.330)
        Hermansky-Pudlak syndrome (E70.331)
      CC E70.320 Tyrosinase negative oculocutaneous albinism
        Albinism I
        Oculocutaneous albinism ty-neg
      CC E70.321 Tyrosinase positive oculocutaneous albinism
        Albinism II
        Oculocutaneous albinism ty-pos
      CC E70.328 Other oculocutaneous albinism
        Cross syndrome
      CC E70.329 Oculocutaneous albinism, unspecified
    + E70.33 Albinism with hematologic abnormality
      CC E70.330 Chediak-Higashi syndrome
      CC E70.331 Hermansky-Pudlak syndrome
      CC E70.338 Other albinism with hematologic abnormality
      CC E70.339 Albinism with hematologic abnormality, unspecified
    CC E70.39 Other specified albinism
      Piebaldism
  + E70.4 Disorders of histidine metabolism
    CC E70.40 Disorders of histidine metabolism, unspecified
    CC E70.41 Histidinemia
    CC E70.49 Other disorders of histidine metabolism
  CC E70.5 Disorders of tryptophan metabolism
  + E70.8 Other disorders of aromatic amino-acid metabolism
    CC E70.81 Aromatic L-amino acid decarboxylase deficiency
      AADC deficiency
      AHA CC: 4Q, 2020, 15-16
    CC E70.89 Other disorders of aromatic amino-acid metabolism
  + E70.9 Disorder of aromatic amino-acid metabolism, unspecified

E71 Disorders of branched-chain amino-acid metabolism and fatty-acid metabolism
  CC E71.0 Maple-syrup-urine disease
  + E71.1 Other disorders of branched-chain amino-acid metabolism
    + E71.11 Branched-chain organic acidurias
      CC E71.110 Isovaleric acidemia
      CC E71.111 3-methylglutaconic aciduria
      CC E71.118 Other branched-chain organic acidurias
    + E71.12 Disorders of propionate metabolism
      CC E71.120 Methylmalonic acidemia
      CC E71.121 Propionic acidemia
      CC E71.128 Other disorders of propionate metabolism
    CC E71.19 Other disorders of branched-chain amino-acid metabolism
      Hyperleucine-isoleucinemia
      Hypervalinemia
  CC E71.2 Disorder of branched-chain amino-acid metabolism, unspecified
  + E71.3 Disorders of fatty-acid metabolism
    Excludes1: peroxisomal disorders (E71.5)
      Refsum's disease (G60.1)
      Schilder's disease (G37.0)
    Excludes2: carnitine deficiency due to inborn error of metabolism (E71.42)
    E71.30 Disorder of fatty-acid metabolism, unspecified
    + E71.31 Disorders of fatty-acid oxidation
      CC E71.310 Long chain/very long chain acyl CoA dehydrogenase deficiency
        LCAD deficiency
        VLCAD deficiency
      CC E71.311 Medium chain acyl CoA dehydrogenase deficiency
        MCAD deficiency
      CC E71.312 Short chain acyl CoA dehydrogenase deficiency
        SCAD deficiency
      CC E71.313 Glutaric aciduria type II
        Glutaric aciduria type II A
        Glutaric aciduria type II B
        Glutaric aciduria type II C
        Excludes1: glutaric aciduria (type 1) NOS (E72.3)
      CC E71.314 Muscle carnitine palmitoyltransferase deficiency
      CC E71.318 Other disorders of fatty-acid oxidation
    CC E71.32 Disorders of ketone metabolism
    CC E71.39 Other disorders of fatty-acid metabolism
  + E71.4 Disorders of carnitine metabolism
    Excludes1: Muscle carnitine palmitoyltransferase deficiency (E71.314)
    E71.40 Disorder of carnitine metabolism, unspecified
    E71.41 Primary carnitine deficiency
    E71.42 Carnitine deficiency due to inborn errors of metabolism
      Code also associated inborn error or metabolism
    E71.43 Iatrogenic carnitine deficiency
      Carnitine deficiency due to hemodialysis
      Carnitine deficiency due to Valproic acid therapy
    + E71.44 Other secondary carnitine deficiency
      E71.440 Ruvalcaba-Myhre-Smith syndrome
      E71.448 Other secondary carnitine deficiency
  + E71.5 Peroxisomal disorders
    Excludes1: Schilder's disease (G37.0)
    CC E71.50 Peroxisomal disorder, unspecified
    + E71.51 Disorders of peroxisome biogenesis
      Group 1 peroxisomal disorders
      Excludes1: Refsum's disease (G60.1)
      CC E71.510 Zellweger syndrome
      CC E71.511 Neonatal adrenoleukodystrophy
        Excludes1: X-linked adrenoleukodystrophy (E71.42-)
      CC E71.518 Other disorders of peroxisome biogenesis
    + E71.52 X-linked adrenoleukodystrophy
      CC E71.520 Childhood cerebral X-linked adrenoleukodystrophy
      CC E71.521 Adolescent X-linked adrenoleukodystrophy
      CC E71.522 Adrenomyeloneuropathy

CC **E71.528** Other X-linked adrenoleukodystrophy
Addison only phenotype adrenoleukodystrophy
Addison-Schilder adrenoleukodystrophy
CC **E71.529** X-linked adrenoleukodystrophy, unspecified type
CC **E71.53** Other group 2 peroxisomal disorders
+ **E71.54** Other peroxisomal disorders
CC **E71.540** Rhizomelic chondrodysplasia punctata
Excludes1: *chondrodysplasia punctata NOS (Q77.3)*
CC **E71.541** Zellweger-like syndrome
CC **E71.542** Other group 3 peroxisomal disorders
CC **E71.548** Other peroxisomal disorders

E72 Other disorders of amino-acid metabolism
Excludes1: disorders of:
aromatic amino-acid metabolism (E70.-)
branched-chain amino-acid metabolism (E71.0-E71.2)
fatty-acid metabolism (E71.3)
purine and pyrimidine metabolism (E79.-)
gout (M1A.-, M10.-)

+ **E72.0** Disorders of amino-acid transport
Excludes1: *disorders of tryptophan metabolism (E70.5)*
CC **E72.00** Disorders of amino-acid transport, unspecified
CC **E72.01** Cystinuria
CC **E72.02** Hartnup's disease
CC **E72.03** Lowe's syndrome
Use additional code for associated glaucoma (H42)
CC **E72.04** Cystinosis
Fanconi (-de Toni) (-Debré) syndrome with cystinosis
Excludes1: *Fanconi (-de Toni) (-Debré) syndrome without cystinosis (E72.09)*
CC **E72.09** Other disorders of amino-acid transport
Fanconi (-de Toni) (-Debré) syndrome, unspecified

+ **E72.1** Disorders of sulfur-bearing amino-acid metabolism
Excludes1: cystinosis (E72.04)
cystinuria (E72.01)
transcobalamin II deficiency (D51.2)
CC **E72.10** Disorders of sulfur-bearing amino-acid metabolism, unspecified
CC **E72.11** Homocystinuria
Cystathionine synthase deficiency
CC **E72.12** Methylenetetrahydrofolate reductase deficiency
CC **E72.19** Other disorders of sulfur-bearing amino-acid metabolism
Cystathioninuria
Methioninemia
Sulfite oxidase deficiency

+ **E72.2** Disorders of urea cycle metabolism
Excludes1: *disorders of ornithine metabolism (E72.4)*
CC **E72.20** Disorder of urea cycle metabolism, unspecified
Hyperammonemia
Excludes1: hyperammonemia-hyperornithinemia-homocitrullinemia syndrome E72.4
transient hyperammonemia of newborn (P74.6)
CC **E72.21** Argininemia
CC **E72.22** Arginosuccinic aciduria
CC **E72.23** Citrullinemia
CC **E72.29** Other disorders of urea cycle metabolism

CC **E72.3** Disorders of lysine and hydroxylysine metabolism
Glutaric aciduria NOS
Glutaric aciduria (type I)
Hydroxylysinemia
Hyperlysinemia
Excludes1: glutaric aciduria type II (E71.313)
Refsum's disease (G60.1)
Zellweger syndrome (E71.510)

CC **E72.4** Disorders of ornithine metabolism
Hyperammonemia-Hyperornithinemia-Homocitrullinemia syndrome
Ornithinemia (types I, II)
Ornithine transcarbamylase deficiency
Excludes1: *hereditary choroidal dystrophy (H31.2-)*

+ **E72.5** Disorders of glycine metabolism
CC **E72.50** Disorder of glycine metabolism, unspecified
CC **E72.51** Non-ketotic hyperglycinemia
CC **E72.52** Trimethylaminuria
CC **E72.53** Primary hyperoxaluria
Oxalosis
Oxaluria
AHA CC: 4Q, 2018, 29
CC **E72.59** Other disorders of glycine metabolism
D-glycericacidemia
Hyperhydroxyprolinemia
Hyperprolinemia (types I, II)
Sarcosinemia

+ **E72.8** Other specified disorders of amino-acid metabolism
CC **E72.81** Disorders of gamma aminobutyric acid metabolism
4-hydroxybutyric aciduria
Disorders of GABA metabolism
GABA metabolic defect
GABA transaminase deficiency
GABA-T deficiency
Gamma-hydroxybutyric aciduria
SSADHA
Succinic semialdehyde dehydrogenase deficiency
AHA CC: 4Q, 2018, 5
CC **E72.89** Other specified disorders of amino-acid metabolism
Disorders of beta-amino-acid metabolism
Disorders of gamma-glutamyl cycle

CC **E72.9** Disorder of amino-acid metabolism, unspecified

E73 Lactose intolerance
E73.0 Congenital lactase deficiency
E73.1 Secondary lactase deficiency
E73.8 Other lactose intolerance
E73.9 Lactose intolerance, unspecified

E74 Other disorders of carbohydrate metabolism
Excludes1: diabetes mellitus (E08-E13)
NOS (E16.2)
increased secretion of glucagon (E16.3)
mucopolysaccharidosis (E76.0-E76.3)

+ **E74.0** Glycogen storage disease
CC **E74.00** Glycogen storage disease, unspecified
CC **E74.01** von Gierke disease
Type I glycogen storage disease
CC **E74.02** Pompe disease
Cardiac glycogenosis
Type II glycogen storage disease
CC **E74.03** Cori disease
Forbes disease
Type III glycogen storage disease
CC **E74.04** McArdle disease
Type V glycogen storage disease
CC **E74.05** Lysosome-associated membrane protein 2 [LAMP2] deficiency
Danon disease
Code also, if applicable, associated manifestations such as:
dilated cardiomyopathy (I42.0)
obstructive hypertrophic cardiomyopathy (I42.1)
CC **E74.09** Other glycogen storage disease
Andersen disease
Glycogen storage disease, types 0, IV, VI-XI
Hers disease
Liver phosphorylase deficiency
Muscle phosphofructokinase deficiency
Tauri disease

+ **E74.1** Disorders of fructose metabolism
Excludes1: *muscle phosphofructokinase deficiency (E74.09)*
E74.10 Disorder of fructose metabolism, unspecified
E74.11 Essential fructosuria
Fructokinase deficiency
E74.12 Hereditary fructose intolerance
Fructosemia
E74.19 Other disorders of fructose metabolism
Fructose-1, 6-diphosphatase deficiency

- **E74.2 Disorders of galactose metabolism**
  - CC **E74.20** Disorders of galactose metabolism, unspecified
  - CC **E74.21** Galactosemia
  - CC **E74.29** Other disorders of galactose metabolism
    - Galactokinase deficiency
- **E74.3 Other disorders of intestinal carbohydrate absorption**
  - *Excludes2:* lactose intolerance (E73.-)
  - **E74.31** Sucrase-isomaltase deficiency
  - **E74.39** Other disorders of intestinal carbohydrate absorption
    - Disorder of intestinal carbohydrate absorption NOS
    - Glucose-galactose malabsorption
    - Sucrase deficiency
- CC **E74.4 Disorders of pyruvate metabolism and gluconeogenesis**
  - Deficiency of phosphoenolpyruvate carboxykinase
  - Deficiency of pyruvate carboxylase
  - Deficiency of pyruvate dehydrogenase
  - *Excludes1:* disorders of pyruvate metabolism and gluconeogenesis with anemia (D55.-)
    - Leigh's syndrome (G31.82)
- **E74.8 Other specified disorders of carbohydrate metabolism**
  - **E74.81 Disorders of glucose transport, not elsewhere classified**
    - *AHA CC: 4Q, 2020, 16*
    - CC **E74.810** Glucose transporter protein type 1 deficiency
      - De Vivo syndrome
      - Glucose transport defect, blood-brain barrier
      - Glut1 deficiency
      - GLUT1 deficiency syndrome 1, infantile onset
      - GLUT1 deficiency syndrome 2, childhood onset
    - CC **E74.818** Other disorders of glucose transport
      - (Familial) renal glycosuria
    - CC **E74.819** Disorders of glucose transport, unspecified
  - CC **E74.89** Other specified disorders of carbohydrate metabolism
    - Essential pentosuria
- **E74.9** Disorder of carbohydrate metabolism, unspecified

- **E75 Disorders of sphingolipid metabolism and other lipid storage disorders**
  - *Excludes1:* mucolipidosis, types I-III (E77.0-E77.1)
    - Refsum's disease (G60.1)
  - **E75.0 GM2 gangliosidosis**
    - CC **E75.00** GM2 gangliosidosis, unspecified
    - CC **E75.01** Sandhoff disease
    - CC **E75.02** Tay-Sachs disease
    - CC **E75.09** Other GM2 gangliosidosis
      - Adult GM2 gangliosidosis
      - Juvenile GM2 gangliosidosis
  - **E75.1 Other and unspecified gangliosidosis**
    - CC **E75.10** Unspecified gangliosidosis
      - Gangliosidosis NOS
    - CC **E75.11** Mucolipidosis IV
    - CC **E75.19** Other gangliosidosis
      - GM1 gangliosidosis
      - GM3 gangliosidosis
  - **E75.2 Other sphingolipidosis**
    - *Excludes1:* adrenoleukodystrophy [Addison-Schilder] (E71.528)
    - **E75.21** Fabry (-Anderson) disease
    - **E75.22** Gaucher disease
    - CC **E75.23** Krabbe disease
    - **E75.24 Niemann-Pick disease**
      - *AHA CC: 4Q, 2021, 8-9*
      - Acid sphingomyelinase deficiency (ASMD)
      - **E75.240** Niemann-Pick disease type A
        - Acid sphingomyelinase deficiency type A (ASMD type A)
        - Infantile neurovisceral acid sphingomyelinase deficiency
      - **E75.241** Niemann-Pick disease type B
        - Acid sphingomyelinase deficiency type B (ASMD type B)
        - Chronic visceral acid sphingomyelinase deficiency
      - **E75.242** Niemann-Pick disease type C
      - **E75.243** Niemann-Pick disease type D
      - **E75.244** Niemann-Pick disease type A/B
        - Acid sphingomyelinase deficiency type A/B (ASMD type A/B)
        - Chronic neurovisceral acid sphingomyelinase deficiency
      - **E75.248** Other Niemann-Pick disease
      - **E75.249** Niemann-Pick disease, unspecified
        - Acid sphingomyelinase deficiency (ASMD) NOS
    - CC **E75.25** Metachromatic leukodystrophy
    - CC **E75.26** Sulfatase deficiency
      - Multiple sulfatase deficiency (MSD)
      - *AHA CC: 4Q, 2018, 5-6*
    - CC **E75.27** Pelizaeus-Merzbacher disease
    - CC **E75.28** Canavan disease
    - CC **E75.29** Other sphingolipidosis
      - Farber's syndrome
      - Sulfatide lipidosis
  - **E75.3** Sphingolipidosis, unspecified
  - CC **E75.4** Neuronal ceroid lipofuscinosis
    - Batten disease
    - Bielschowsky-Jansky disease
    - Kufs disease
    - Spielmeyer-Vogt disease
  - **E75.5** Other lipid storage disorders
    - Cerebrotendinous cholesterosis [van Bogaert-Scherer-Epstein]
    - Wolman's disease
  - **E75.6** Lipid storage disorder, unspecified

- **E76 Disorders of glycosaminoglycan metabolism**
  - **E76.0 Mucopolysaccharidosis, type I**
    - CC **E76.01** Hurler's syndrome
    - CC **E76.02** Hurler-Scheie syndrome
    - CC **E76.03** Scheie's syndrome
  - CC **E76.1 Mucopolysaccharidosis, type II**
    - Hunter's syndrome
  - **E76.2 Other mucopolysaccharidoses**
    - **E76.21 Morquio mucopolysaccharidoses**
      - CC **E76.210** Morquio A mucopolysaccharidoses
        - Classic Morquio syndrome
        - Morquio syndrome A
        - Mucopolysaccharidosis, type IVA
      - CC **E76.211** Morquio B mucopolysaccharidoses
        - Morquio-like mucopolysaccharidoses
        - Morquio-like syndrome
        - Morquio syndrome B
        - Mucopolysaccharidosis, type IVB
      - CC **E76.219** Morquio mucopolysaccharidoses, unspecified
        - Morquio syndrome
        - Mucopolysaccharidosis, type IV
    - CC **E76.22** Sanfilippo mucopolysaccharidoses
      - Mucopolysaccharidosis, type III (A) (B) (C) (D)
      - Sanfilippo A syndrome
      - Sanfilippo B syndrome
      - Sanfilippo C syndrome
      - Sanfilippo D syndrome
    - CC **E76.29** Other mucopolysaccharidoses
      - beta-Glucuronidase deficiency
      - Maroteaux-Lamy (mild) (severe) syndrome
      - Mucopolysaccharidosis, types VI, VII
  - CC **E76.3** Mucopolysaccharidosis, unspecified
  - CC **E76.8** Other disorders of glucosaminoglycan metabolism
  - CC **E76.9** Glucosaminoglycan metabolism disorder, unspecified

- **E77 Disorders of glycoprotein metabolism**
  - **E77.0** Defects in post-translational modification of lysosomal enzymes
    - Mucolipidosis II [I-cell disease]
    - Mucolipidosis III [pseudo-Hurler polydystrophy]
  - **E77.1** Defects in glycoprotein degradation
    - Aspartylglucosaminuria
    - Fucosidosis
    - Mannosidosis
    - Sialidosis [mucolipidosis I]
  - **E77.8** Other disorders of glycoprotein metabolism
  - **E77.9** Disorder of glycoprotein metabolism, unspecified

E78 Disorders of lipoprotein metabolism and other lipidemias
    Excludes1: sphingolipidosis (E75.0-E75.3)
- **E78.0 Pure hypercholesterolemia**
  - **E78.00 Pure hypercholesterolemia, unspecified**
    Fedrickson's hyperlipoproteinemia, type IIa
    Hyperbetalipoproteinemia
    Low-density-lipoprotein-type [LDL] hyperlipoproteinemia
    (Pure) hypercholesterolemia, NOS
    AHA CC: 4Q, 2016, 13-14; 2Q, 2022, 5-7; 2Q, 2023, 9-10
  - **E78.01 Familial hypercholesterolemia**
- **E78.1 Pure hyperglyceridemia**
  Elevated fasting triglycerides
  Endogenous hyperglyceridemia
  Fredrickson's hyperlipoproteinemia, type IV
  Hyperlipidemia, group B
  Hyperprebetalipoproteinemia
  Very-low-density-lipoprotein-type [VLDL] hyperlipoproteinemia
- **E78.2 Mixed hyperlipidemia**
  Broad- or floating-betalipoproteinemia
  Combined hyperlipidemia NOS
  Elevated cholesterol with elevated triglycerides NEC
  Fredrickson's hyperlipoproteinemia, type IIb or III
  Hyperbetalipoproteinemia with prebetalipoproteinemia
  Hypercholesteremia with endogenous hyperglyceridemia
  Hyperlipidemia, group C
  Tubo-eruptive xanthoma
  Xanthoma tuberosum
     Excludes1: cerebrotendinous cholesterosis [van Bogaert-Scherer-Epstein] (E75.5)
              familial combined hyperlipidemia (E78.49)
  AHA CC: 2Q, 2022, 6-7; 2Q, 2023, 9-10
- **E78.3 Hyperchylomicronemia**
  Chylomicron retention disease
  Fredrickson's hyperlipoproteinemia, type I or V
  Hyperlipidemia, group D
  Mixed hyperglyceridemia
- **E78.4 Other hyperlipidemia**
  AHA CC: 4Q, 2018, 6
  - **E78.41 Elevated Lipoprotein(a)**
    Elevated Lp(a)
  - **E78.49 Other hyperlipidemia**
    Familial combined hyperlipidemia
- **E78.5 Hyperlipidemia, unspecified**
  AHA CC: 2Q, 2022, 5-6
- **E78.6 Lipoprotein deficiency**
  Abetalipoproteinemia
  Depressed HDL cholesterol
  High-density lipoprotein deficiency
  Hypoalphalipoproteinemia
  Hypobetalipoproteinemia (familial)
  Lecithin cholesterol acyltransferase deficiency
  Tangier disease
- **E78.7 Disorders of bile acid and cholesterol metabolism**
     Excludes1: Niemann-Pick disease type C (E75.242)
  - **E78.70 Disorder of bile acid and cholesterol metabolism, unspecified**
  - **CC E78.71 Barth syndrome**
  - **CC E78.72 Smith-Lemli-Opitz syndrome**
  - **E78.79 Other disorders of bile acid and cholesterol metabolism**
    AHA CC: 1Q, 2023, 27
- **E78.8 Other disorders of lipoprotein metabolism**
  - **E78.81 Lipoid dermatoarthritis**
  - **E78.89 Other lipoprotein metabolism disorders**
- **E78.9 Disorder of lipoprotein metabolism, unspecified**

E79 Disorders of purine and pyrimidine metabolism
    Excludes1: Ataxia-telangiectasia (Q87.19)
              Bloom's syndrome (Q82.8)
              Cockayne's syndrome (Q87.19)
              calculus of kidney (N20.0)
              combined immunodeficiency disorders (D81.-)
              Fanconi's anemia (D61.09)
              gout (M1A.-, M10.-)
              orotaciduric anemia (D53.0)
              progeria (E34.8)
              Werner's syndrome (E34.8)
              xeroderma pigmentosum (Q82.1)
- **E79.0 Hyperuricemia without signs of inflammatory arthritis and tophaceous disease**
  Asymptomatic hyperuricemia
- **CC E79.1 Lesch-Nyhan syndrome**
  HGPRT deficiency
- **CC E79.2 Myoadenylate deaminase deficiency**
- **E79.8 Other disorders of purine and pyrimidine metabolism**
  - **CC E79.81 Aicardi-Goutières syndrome**
  - **CC E79.82 Hereditary xanthinuria**
  - **CC E79.89 Other specified disorders of purine and pyrimidine metabolism**
- **CC E79.9 Disorder of purine and pyrimidine metabolism, unspecified**

E80 Disorders of porphyrin and bilirubin metabolism
   Includes: defects of catalase and peroxidase
- **CC E80.0 Hereditary erythropoietic porphyria**
  Congenital erythropoietic porphyria
  Erythropoietic protoporphyria
- **CC E80.1 Porphyria cutanea tarda**
- **E80.2 Other and unspecified porphyria**
  - **CC E80.20 Unspecified porphyria**
    Porphyria NOS
  - **CC E80.21 Acute intermittent (hepatic) porphyria**
  - **CC E80.29 Other porphyria**
    Hereditary coproporphyria
- **CC E80.3 Defects of catalase and peroxidase**
  Acatalasia [Takahara]
- **E80.4 Gilbert syndrome**
- **E80.5 Crigler-Najjar syndrome**
- **E80.6 Other disorders of bilirubin metabolism**
  Dubin-Johnson syndrome
  Rotor's syndrome
  AHA CC: 3Q, 2022, 7
- **E80.7 Disorder of bilirubin metabolism, unspecified**

E83 Disorders of mineral metabolism
   Excludes1: dietary mineral deficiency (E58-E61)
           parathyroid disorders (E20-E21)
           vitamin D deficiency (E55.-)
- **E83.0 Disorders of copper metabolism**
  - **E83.00 Disorder of copper metabolism, unspecified**
  - **E83.01 Wilson's disease**
    Code also associated Kayser Fleischer ring (H18.04-)
  - **E83.09 Other disorders of copper metabolism**
    Menkes' (kinky hair) (steely hair) disease
- **E83.1 Disorders of iron metabolism**
     Excludes1: iron deficiency anemia (D50.-)
             sideroblastic anemia (D64.0-D64.3)
  - **E83.10 Disorder of iron metabolism, unspecified**
  - **E83.11 Hemochromatosis**
       Excludes1: GALD (P78.84)
               Gestational alloimmune liver disease (P78.84)
               Neonatal hemochromatosis (P78.84)
    - **E83.110 Hereditary hemochromatosis**
      Bronzed diabetes
      Pigmentary cirrhosis (of liver)
      Primary (hereditary) hemochromatosis

- **E83.111** Hemochromatosis due to repeated red blood cell transfusions
  - Iron overload due to repeated red blood cell transfusions
  - Transfusion (red blood cell) associated hemochromatosis
- **E83.118** Other hemochromatosis
- **E83.119** Hemochromatosis, unspecified
- **E83.19** Other disorders of iron metabolism
  - Use additional code, if applicable, for idiopathic pulmonary hemosiderosis (J84.03)
- **E83.2** Disorders of zinc metabolism
  - Acrodermatitis enteropathica
- **+ E83.3** Disorders of phosphorus metabolism and phosphatases
  - **Excludes1:** adult osteomalacia (M83.-)
    - osteoporosis (M80.-)
  - **E83.30** Disorder of phosphorus metabolism, unspecified
  - **E83.31** Familial hypophosphatemia
    - Vitamin D-resistant osteomalacia
    - Vitamin D-resistant rickets
    - **Excludes1:** vitamin D-deficiency rickets (E55.0)
  - **E83.32** Hereditary vitamin D-dependent rickets (type 1) (type 2)
    - 25-hydroxyvitamin D 1-alpha-hydroxylase deficiency
    - Pseudovitamin D deficiency
    - Vitamin D receptor defect
  - **E83.39** Other disorders of phosphorus metabolism
    - Acid phosphatase deficiency
    - Hypophosphatasia
- **+ E83.4** Disorders of magnesium metabolism
  - **E83.40** Disorders of magnesium metabolism, unspecified
  - **E83.41** Hypermagnesemia
    - *AHA CC: 4Q, 2016, 54-55*
  - **E83.42** Hypomagnesemia
  - **E83.49** Other disorders of magnesium metabolism
- **+ E83.5** Disorders of calcium metabolism
  - **Excludes1:** autoimmune hypoparathyroidism (E20.812)
    - autosomal dominant hypocalcemia (E20.810)
    - chondrocalcinosis (M11.1-M11.2)
    - hungry bone syndrome (E83.81)
    - hyperparathyroidism (E21.0-E21.3)
    - secondary hypoparathyroidism in diseases classified elsewhere (E20.811)
  - **E83.50** Unspecified disorder of calcium metabolism
  - **E83.51** Hypocalcemia
  - **E83.52** Hypercalcemia
    - Familial hypocalciuric hypercalcemia
  - **E83.59** Other disorders of calcium metabolism
- **+ E83.8** Other disorders of mineral metabolism
  - **E83.81** Hungry bone syndrome
  - **E83.89** Other disorders of mineral metabolism
- **E83.9** Disorder of mineral metabolism, unspecified

E84 Cystic fibrosis
Code also exocrine pancreatic insufficiency (K86.81)
Includes: mucoviscidosis
- **MCC E84.0** Cystic fibrosis with pulmonary manifestations
  - Use additional code to identify any infectious organism present, such as:
    - Pseudomonas (B96.5)
  - *AHA CC: 1Q, 2021, 23-24*
- **+ E84.1** Cystic fibrosis with intestinal manifestations
  - **● MCC E84.11** Meconium ileus in cystic fibrosis
    - **Excludes1:** meconium ileus not due to cystic fibrosis (P76.0)
  - **CC E84.19** Cystic fibrosis with other intestinal manifestations
    - Distal intestinal obstruction syndrome
- **CC E84.8** Cystic fibrosis with other manifestations
- **CC E84.9** Cystic fibrosis, unspecified

E85 Amyloidosis
Excludes2: Alzheimer's disease (G30.0-)
- **CC E85.0** Non-neuropathic heredofamilial amyloidosis
  - Hereditary amyloid nephropathy
  - Code also associated disorders, such as:
    - autoinflammatory syndromes (M04.-)
  - **Excludes2:** Transthyretin-related (ATTR) familial amyloid cardiomyopathy (E85.4)
- **CC E85.1** Neuropathic heredofamilial amyloidosis
  - Amyloid polyneuropathy (Portuguese)
  - Transthyretin-related (ATTR) familial amyloid polyneuropathy
  - *AHA CC: 4Q, 2012, 99-101*
- **CC E85.2** Heredofamilial amyloidosis, unspecified
- **CC E85.3** Secondary systemic amyloidosis
  - Hemodialysis-associated amyloidosis
- **CC E85.4** Organ-limited amyloidosis
  - Localized amyloidosis
  - Transthyretin-related (ATTR) familial amyloid cardiomyopathy
- **+ E85.8** Other amyloidosis
  - *AHA CC: 4Q, 2017, 7*
  - **CC E85.81** Light chain (AL) amyloidosis
  - **CC E85.82** Wild-type transthyretin-related (ATTR) amyloidosis
    - Senile systemic amyloidosis (SSA)
  - **CC E85.89** Other amyloidosis
- **CC E85.9** Amyloidosis, unspecified

E86 Volume depletion
Use Additional code(s) for any associated disorders of electrolyte and acid-base balance (E87.-)
Excludes1: dehydration of newborn (P74.1)
- postprocedural hypovolemic shock (T81.19)
- traumatic hypovolemic shock (T79.4)
Excludes2: hypovolemic shock NOS (R57.1)
- **E86.0** Dehydration
  - Review coding guidelines C.2.c.3
  - *AHA CC: 1Q, 2014, 7; 2Q, 2019, 7-8*
- **E86.1** Hypovolemia
  - Depletion of volume of plasma
- **E86.9** Volume depletion, unspecified
  - *AHA CC: 2Q, 2019, 7-8*

E87 Other disorders of fluid, electrolyte and acid-base balance
Excludes1: diabetes insipidus (E23.2)
- electrolyte imbalance associated with hyperemesis gravidarum (O21.1)
- electrolyte imbalance following ectopic or molar pregnancy (O08.5)
- familial periodic paralysis (G72.3)
- metabolic acidemia in newborn, unspecified (P19.9)
- **CC E87.0** Hyperosmolality and hypernatremia
  - Sodium [Na] excess
  - Sodium [Na] overload
  - **Excludes1:** diabetes with hyperosmolarity (E08, E09, E11, E13 with final characters .00 or .01)
  - *AHA CC: 1Q, 2014, 7; 1Q, 2022, 28-29*
- **CC E87.1** Hypo-osmolality and hyponatremia
  - Sodium [Na] deficiency
  - **Excludes1:** syndrome of inappropriate secretion of antidiuretic hormone (E22.2)
  - *AHA CC: 1Q, 2014, 7*
- **+ E87.2** Acidosis
  - **Excludes1:** diabetic acidosis - see categories E08-E10, E11, E13 with ketoacidosis
  - *AHA CC: 3Q, 2020, 30-31; 4Q, 2022, 13-14*
  - **CC E87.20** Acidosis, unspecified
    - Lactic acidosis NOS
    - Metabolic acidosis NOS
    - Code also, if applicable, respiratory failure with hypercapnia (J96. with 5th character 2)
  - **CC E87.21** Acute metabolic acidosis
    - Acute lactic acidosis
  - **CC E87.22** Chronic metabolic acidosis
    - Chronic lactic acidosis
    - Code first underlying etiology, if applicable
    - *AHA CC: 4Q, 2022, 14*
  - **CC E87.29** Other acidosis
    - Respiratory acidosis NOS
    - **Excludes2:** acute respiratory acidosis (J96.02)
      - chronic respiratory acidosis (J96.12)
- **CC E87.3** Alkalosis
  - Alkalosis NOS
  - Metabolic alkalosis
  - Respiratory alkalosis
- **CC E87.4** Mixed disorder of acid-base balance

- **E87.5 Hyperkalemia**
  - Potassium [K] excess
  - Potassium [K] overload
- **E87.6 Hypokalemia**
  - Potassium [K] deficiency
- + **E87.7 Fluid overload**
  - *Excludes1:* edema NOS (R60.9)
    - fluid retention (R60.9)
  - **E87.70 Fluid overload, unspecified**
    - *AHA CC: 1Q, 2023, 19-20*
  - **E87.71 Transfusion associated circulatory overload**
    - Fluid overload due to transfusion (blood) (blood components)
    - TACO
  - **E87.79 Other fluid overload**
- **E87.8 Other disorders of electrolyte and fluid balance, not elsewhere classified**
  - Electrolyte imbalance NOS
  - Hyperchloremia
  - Hypochloremia

E88 Other and unspecified metabolic disorders

Use additional codes for associated conditions
Excludes1: histiocytosis X (chronic) (C96.6)

- + **E88.0 Disorders of plasma-protein metabolism, not elsewhere classified**
  - *Excludes1:* monoclonal gammopathy (of undetermined significance) (D47.2)
    - polyclonal hypergammaglobulinemia (D89.0)
    - Waldenström macroglobulinemia (C88.0)
  - *Excludes2:* disorder of lipoprotein metabolism (E78.-)
  - **E88.01 Alpha-1-antitrypsin deficiency**
    - AAT deficiency
  - CC **E88.02 Plasminogen deficiency**
    - Dysplasminogenemia
    - Hypoplasminogenemia
    - Type 1 plasminogen deficiency
    - Type 2 plasminogen deficiency
    - Code also, if applicable, ligneous conjunctivitis (H10.51)
    - Use additional code for associated findings, such as:
      - hydrocephalus (G91.4)
      - otitis media (H67.-)
      - respiratory disorder related to plasminogen deficiency (J99)
    - *AHA CC: 4Q, 2018, 6-7*
  - **E88.09 Other disorders of plasma-protein metabolism, not elsewhere classified**
    - Bisalbuminemia
- **E88.1 Lipodystrophy, not elsewhere classified**
  - Lipodystrophy NOS
  - *Excludes1:* Whipple's disease (K90.81)
- **E88.2 Lipomatosis, not elsewhere classified**
  - Lipomatosis NOS
  - Lipomatosis (Check) dolorosa [Dercum]
- MCC **E88.3 Tumor lysis syndrome**
  - Tumor lysis syndrome (spontaneous)
  - Tumor lysis syndrome following antineoplastic drug chemotherapy
  - Use additional code for adverse effect, if applicable, to identify drug (T45.1X5)
  - *AHA CC: 2Q, 2019, 24-26*
- + **E88.4 Mitochondrial metabolism disorders**
  - *Excludes1:* disorders of pyruvate metabolism (E74.4)
    - Kearns-Sayre syndrome (H49.81)
    - Leber's disease (H47.22)
    - Leigh's encephalopathy (G31.82)
    - Mitochondrial myopathy, NEC (G71.3)
    - Reye's syndrome (G93.7)
  - CC **E88.40 Mitochondrial metabolism disorder, unspecified**
  - CC **E88.41 MELAS syndrome**
    - Mitochondrial myopathy, encephalopathy, lactic acidosis and stroke-like episodes
  - CC **E88.42 MERRF syndrome**
    - Myoclonic epilepsy associated with ragged-red fibers
    - Code also progressive myoclonic epilepsy (G40.3-)
  - CC **E88.43 Disorders of mitochondrial tRNA synthetases**
  - CC **E88.49 Other mitochondrial metabolism disorders**
- + **E88.8 Other specified metabolic disorders**
  - + **E88.81 Metabolic syndrome and other insulin resistance**
    - Use additional codes for associated manifestations, such as:
      - obesity (E66.-)
    - *AHA CC: 3Q, 2022, 6-7*
    - **E88.810 Metabolic syndrome**
      - Dysmetabolic syndrome
    - **E88.811 Insulin resistance syndrome, Type A**
    - **E88.818 Other insulin resistance**
      - Insulin resistance syndrome, Type B
    - **E88.819 Insulin resistance, unspecified**
  - **E88.89 Other specified metabolic disorders**
    - Launois-Bensaude adenolipomatosis
    - *Excludes1:* adult pulmonary Langerhans cell histiocytosis (J84.82)
- **E88.9 Metabolic disorder, unspecified**
- **E88.A Wasting disease (syndrome) due to underlying condition**
  - Cachexia due to underlying condition
  - Code first underlying condition
  - *Excludes1:* cachexia NOS (R64)
    - nutritional marasmus (E41)
  - *Excludes2:* failure to thrive (R62.51, R62.7)

Postprocedural endocrine and metabolic complications and disorders, not elsewhere classified (E89)

- **E89 Postprocedural endocrine and metabolic complications and disorders, not elsewhere classified**
  - *Excludes2:* intraoperative complications of endocrine system organ or structure (E36.0-, E36.1-, E36.8)
- **E89.0 Postprocedural hypothyroidism**
  - Postirradiation hypothyroidism
  - Postsurgical hypothyroidism
- CC **E89.1 Postprocedural hypoinsulinemia**
  - Postpancreatectomy hyperglycemia
  - Postsurgical hypoinsulinemia
  - Use additional code, if applicable, to identify:
    - acquired absence of pancreas (Z90.41-)
    - diabetes mellitus (postpancreatectomy) (postprocedural) (E13.-)
    - insulin use (Z79.4)
  - *Excludes1:* transient postprocedural hyperglycemia (R73.9)
    - transient postprocedural hypoglycemia (E16.2)
  - Review coding guideline C.4.a.6.b.i
- **E89.2 Postprocedural hypoparathyroidism**
  - Parathyroprival tetany
- **E89.3 Postprocedural hypopituitarism**
  - Postirradiation hypopituitarism
- + **E89.4 Postprocedural ovarian failure**
  - ♀ **E89.40 Asymptomatic postprocedural ovarian failure**
    - Postprocedural ovarian failure NOS
  - ♀ **E89.41 Symptomatic postprocedural ovarian failure**
    - Symptoms such as flushing, sleeplessness, headache, lack of concentration, associated with postprocedural menopause
- ♂ **E89.5 Postprocedural testicular hypofunction**
- CC **E89.6 Postprocedural adrenocortical (-medullary) hypofunction**
- + **E89.8 Other postprocedural endocrine and metabolic complications and disorders**
  - *AHA CC: 4Q, 2016, 9-10*
  - + **E89.81 Postprocedural hemorrhage of an endocrine system organ or structure following a procedure**
    - CC **E89.810 Postprocedural hemorrhage of an endocrine system organ or structure following an endocrine system procedure**
    - CC **E89.811 Postprocedural hemorrhage of an endocrine system organ or structure following other procedure**

+ E89.82 Postprocedural hematoma and seroma of an endocrine system organ or structre

CC **E89.820** Postprocedural hematoma of an endocrine system organ or structure following an endocrine system procedure

CC **E89.821** Postprocedural hematoma of an endocrine system organ or structure following other procedure

CC **E89.822** Postprocedural seroma of an endocrine system organ or structure following an endocrine system procedure

CC **E89.823** Postprocedural seroma of an endocrine system organ or structure following other procedure

CC **E89.89** Other postprocedural endocrine and metabolic complications and disorders

Use additional code, if applicable, to further specify disorder

Chapter 5: Mental, Behavioral and Neurodevelopmental Disorders (F01-F99)

Includes: disorders of psychological development

Excludes2: symptoms, signs and abnormal clinical laboratory findings, not elsewhere classified (R00-R99)

This chapter contains the following category blocks:

F01-F09	Mental disorders due to known physiological conditions
F10-F19	Mental and behavioral disorders due to psychoactive substance use
F20-F29	Schizophrenia, schizotypal, delusional, and other non-mood psychotic disorders
F30-F39	Mood [affective] disorders
F40-F48	Anxiety, dissociative, stress-related, somatoform and other nonpsychotic mental disorders
F50-F59	Behavioral syndromes associated with physiological disturbances and physical factors
F60-F69	Disorders of adult personality and behavior
F70-F79	Intellectual disabilities
F80-F89	Pervasive and specific developmental disorders
F90-F98	Behavioral and emotional disorders with onset usually occurring in childhood and adolescence
F99	Unspecified mental disorder

C. Chapter-Specific Coding Guidelines

In addition to general coding guidelines, there are guidelines for specific diagnoses and/or conditions in the classification. Unless otherwise indicated, these guidelines apply to all health care settings. Please refer to Section II for guidelines on the selection of principal diagnosis.

5. Chapter 5: Mental, Behavioral and Neurodevelopmental Disorders (F01-F99)

a. Pain disorders related to psychological factors

Assign code F45.41, for pain that is exclusively related to psychological disorders. As indicated by the Excludes 1 note under category G89, a code from category G89 should not be assigned with code F45.41

Code F45.42, Pain disorders with related psychological factors, should be used with a code from category G89, Pain, not elsewhere classified, if there is documentation of a psychological component for a patient with acute or chronic pain.

See Section I.C.6. Pain

b. Mental and behavioral disorders due to psychoactive substance use

1) In Remission

Selection of codes describing "in remission" for categories F10-F19, Mental and behavioral disorders due to psychoactive substance use (categories F10-F19 with -.11, -.21, -91) requires the provider's clinical judgment and are assigned only on the basis of provider documentation (as defined in the Official Guidelines for Coding and Reporting), unless otherwise instructed by the classification.

Mild substance use disorders in early or sustained remission are classified to the appropriate codes for substance abuse in remission, and moderate or severe substance use disorders in early or sustained remission are classified to the appropriate codes for substance dependence in remission.

2) Psychoactive Substance Use, Abuse And Dependence

When the provider documentation refers to use, abuse and dependence of the same substance (e.g. alcohol, opioid, cannabis, etc.), only one code should be assigned to identify the pattern of use based on the following hierarchy:

- If both use and abuse are documented, assign only the code for abuse
- If both abuse and dependence are documented, assign only the code for dependence
- If use, abuse and dependence are all documented, assign only the code for dependence
- If both use and dependence are documented, assign only the code for dependence.

3) Psychoactive Substance Use Unspecified

As with all other unspecified diagnoses, the codes for unspecified psychoactive substance use disorders (F10.9-, F11.9-, F12.9-, F13.9-, F14.9-, F15.9-, F16.9-, F18.9-, F19.9-) should only be assigned based on provider documentation and when they meet the definition of a reportable diagnosis (see Section III, Reporting Additional Diagnoses). These codes are to be used only when the psychoactive substance use is associated with a substance related disorder (chapter 5 disorders such as sexual dysfunction, sleep disorder, or a mental or behavioral disorder) or medical condition, and such a relationship is documented by the provider.

4) Medical Conditions Due to Psychoactive Substance Use, Abuse and Dependence

Medical conditions due to substance use, abuse, and dependence are not classified as substance-induced disorders. Assign the diagnosis code for the medical condition as directed by the Alphabetical Index along with the appropriate psychoactive substance use, abuse or dependence code. For example, for alcoholic pancreatitis due to alcohol dependence, assign the appropriate code from subcategory K85.2, Alcohol induced acute pancreatitis, and the appropriate code from subcategory F10.2, such as code F10.20, Alcohol dependence, uncomplicated. It would not be appropriate to assign code F10.288, Alcohol dependence with other alcohol-induced disorder.

5) Blood Alcohol Level

A code from category Y90, Evidence of alcohol involvement determined by blood alcohol level, may be assigned when this information is documented and the patient's provider has documented a condition classifiable to category F10, Alcohol related disorders. The blood alcohol level does not need to be documented by the patient's provider in order for it to be coded.

See Section I.B.14. for blood alcohol level documentation by clinicians other than patient's provider.

c. Factitious Disorder

Factitious disorder imposed on self or Munchausen's syndrome is a disorder in which a person falsely reports or causes his or her own physical or psychological signs or symptoms. For patients with documented factitious disorder on self or Munchausen's syndrome, assign the appropriate code from subcategory F68.1-, Factitious disorder imposed on self.

Munchausen's syndrome by proxy (MSBP) is a disorder in which a caregiver (perpetrator) falsely reports or causes an illness or injury in another person (victim) under his or her care, such as a child, an elderly adult, or a person who has a disability. The conditions is also referred to as "factitious disorder imposed on another" or "factitious disorder by proxy." The perpetrator, not the victim, receives this diagnosis. Assign code F68.A, Factitious disorder imposed on another, to the perpetrator's record. For the victim of a patient suffering from MSBP, assign the appropriate code from categories T74, Adult and child abuse, neglect and other maltreatment, confirmed, or T76, Adult and child abuse, neglect and other maltreatment, suspected.

See Section I.C.19.f. Adult and child abuse, neglect and other maltreatment

d. Dementia

The ICD-10-CM classifies dementia (categories F01, F02, and F03) on the basis of the etiology and severity (unspecified, mild, moderate or severe). Selection of the appropriate severity level requires the provider's clinical judgment and codes should be assigned only on the basis of provider documentation (as defined in the *Official Guidelines for Coding and Reporting*), unless otherwise instructed by the classification. If the documentation does not provide information about the severity of the dementia, assign the appropriate code for unspecified severity.

If a patient is admitted to an inpatient acute care hospital or other inpatient facility setting with dementia at one severity level and it progresses to a higher severity level, assign one code for the highest severity level reported during the stay.

Mental disorders due to known physiological conditions (F01-F09)

NOTE This block comprises a range of mental disorders grouped together on the basis of their having in common a demonstrable etiology in cerebral disease, brain injury, or other insult leading to cerebral dysfunction. The dysfunction may be primary, as in diseases, injuries, and insults that affect the brain directly and selectively; or secondary, as in systemic diseases and disorders that attack the brain only as one of the multiple organs or systems of the body that are involved.

F01 Vascular dementia

Vascular dementia as a result of infarction of the brain due to vascular disease, including hypertensive cerebrovascular disease.

Includes: arteriosclerotic dementia
major neurocognitive disorder due to vascular disease
multi-infarct dementia

Code first the underlying physiological condition or sequelae of cerebrovascular disease.
AHA CC: 4Q, 2022, 14-15
Review coding guideline C.5.d

- **+ F01.5 Vascular dementia, unspecified severity**
  - **F01.50 Vascular dementia, unspecified severity, without behavioral disturbance psychotic disturbance, mood disturbance, and anxiety**
    Major neurocognitive disorder due to vascular disease NOS
    Vascular dementia NOS
    AHA CC: 2Q, 2021, 4

- **+ F01.51 Vascular dementia, unspecified severity, with behavioral disturbance**
  - **CC F01.511 Vascular dementia, unspecified severity, with agitation**
    - Major neurocognitive disorder due to vascular disease, unspecified severity, with aberrant motor behavior such as restlessness, rocking, pacing, or exit-seeking
    - Major neurocognitive disorder due to vascular disease, unspecified severity, with verbal or physical behaviors such as profanity, shouting, threatening, anger, aggression, combativeness, or violence
    - Vascular dementia, unspecified severity, with aberrant motor behavior such as restlessness, rocking, pacing, or exit-seeking
    - Vascular dementia, unspecified severity, with verbal or physical behaviors such as profanity, shouting, threatening, anger, aggression, combativeness, or violence
  - **CC F01.518 Vascular dementia, unspecified severity, with other behavioral disturbance**
    - Major neurocognitive disorder due to vascular disease, unspecified severity, with behavioral disturbances such as sleep disturbance, social disinhibition, or sexual disinhibition
    - Vascular dementia, unspecified severity, with behavioral disturbances such as sleep disturbance, social disinhibition, or sexual disinhibition
    - Use additional code, if applicable, to identify wandering in vascular dementia (Z91.83)
- **CC F01.52 Vascular dementia, unspecified severity, with psychotic disturbance**
  - Major neurocognitive disorder due to vascular disease, unspecified severity, with psychotic disturbance such as hallucinations, paranoia, suspiciousness, or delusional state
  - Vascular dementia, unspecified severity, with psychotic disturbance such as hallucinations, paranoia, suspiciousness, or delusional state
- **CC F01.53 Vascular dementia, unspecified severity, with mood disturbance**
  - Major neurocognitive disorder due to vascular disease, unspecified severity, with mood disturbance such as depression, apathy, or anhedonia
  - Vascular dementia, unspecified severity, with mood disturbance such as depression, apathy, or anhedonia
- **CC F01.54 Vascular dementia, unspecified severity, with anxiety**
  - Major neurocognitive disorder due to vascular disease, unspecified severity, with anxiety
- **+ F01.A Vascular dementia, mild**
  - **Excludes1:** *mild neurocognitive disorder due to known physiological condition with or without behavioral disturbance (F06.7-)*
  - **F01.A0 Vascular dementia, mild, without behavioral disturbance, psychotic disturbance, mood disturbance, and anxiety**
    - Major neurocognitive disorder due to vascular disease, mild, NOS
    - Vascular dementia, mild, NOS
  - **+ F01.A1 Vascular dementia, mild, with behavioral disturbance**
    - **CC F01.A11 Vascular dementia, mild, with agitation**
      - Major neurocognitive disorder due to vascular disease, mild, with aberrant motor behavior such as restlessness, rocking, pacing, or exit-seeking
      - Major neurocognitive disorder due to vascular disease, mild, with verbal or physical behaviors such as profanity, shouting, threatening, anger, aggression, combativeness, or violence
      - Vascular dementia, mild, with aberrant motor behavior such as restlessness, rocking, pacing, or exit-seeking
      - Vascular dementia, mild, with verbal or physical behaviors such as profanity, shouting, threatening, anger, aggression, combativeness, or violence
    - **CC F01.A18 Vascular dementia, mild, with other behavioral disturbance**
      - Major neurocognitive disorder due to vascular disease, mild, with behavioral disturbances such as sleep disturbance, social disinhibition, or sexual disinhibition
      - Vascular dementia, mild, with behavioral disturbances such as sleep disturbance, social disinhibition, or sexual disinhibition
      - Use additional code, if applicable, to identify wandering in vascular dementia (Z91.83)
  - **CC F01.A2 Vascular dementia, mild, with psychotic disturbance**
    - Major neurocognitive disorder due to vascular disease, mild, with psychotic disturbance such as hallucinations, paranoia, suspiciousness, or delusional state
    - Vascular dementia, mild, with psychotic disturbance such as hallucinations, paranoia, suspiciousness, or delusional state
  - **CC F01.A3 Vascular dementia, mild, with mood disturbance**
    - Major neurocognitive disorder due to vascular disease, mild, with mood disturbance such as depression, apathy, or anhedonia
    - Vascular dementia, mild, with mood disturbance such as depression, apathy, or anhedonia
  - **CC F01.A4 Vascular dementia, mild, with anxiety**
    - Major neurocognitive disorder due to vascular disease, mild, with anxiety
- **+ F01.B Vascular dementia, moderate**
  - **F01.B0 Vascular dementia, moderate, without behavioral disturbance, psychotic disturbance, mood disturbance, and anxiety**
    - Major neurocognitive disorder due to vascular disease, moderate, NOS
    - Vascular dementia, moderate, NOS
  - **+ F01.B1 Vascular dementia, moderate, with behavioral disturbance**
    - **CC F01.B11 Vascular dementia, moderate, with agitation**
      - Major neurocognitive disorder due to vascular disease, moderate, with aberrant motor behavior such as restlessness, rocking, pacing, or exit-seeking
      - Major neurocognitive disorder due to vascular disease, moderate, with verbal or physical behaviors such as profanity, shouting, threatening, anger, aggression, combativeness, or violence
      - Vascular dementia, moderate, with aberrant motor behavior such as restlessness, rocking, pacing, or exit-seeking
      - Vascular dementia, moderate, with verbal or physical behaviors such as profanity, shouting, threatening, anger, aggression, combativeness, or violence

- **CC F01.B18 Vascular dementia, moderate, with other behavioral disturbance**
  Major neurocognitive disorder due to vascular disease, moderate, with behavioral disturbances such as sleep disturbance, social disinhibition, or sexual disinhibition
  Vascular dementia, moderate, with behavioral disturbances such as sleep disturbance, social disinhibition, or sexual disinhibition
  Use additional code, if applicable, to identify wandering in vascular dementia (Z91.83)

- **CC F01.B2 Vascular dementia, moderate, with psychotic disturbance**
  Major neurocognitive disorder due to vascular disease, moderate, with psychotic disturbance such as hallucinations, paranoia, suspiciousness, or delusional state
  Vascular dementia, moderate, with psychotic disturbance such as hallucinations, paranoia, suspiciousness, or delusional state

- **CC F01.B3 Vascular dementia, moderate, with mood disturbance**
  Major neurocognitive disorder due to vascular disease, moderate, with mood disturbance such as depression, apathy, or anhedonia
  Vascular dementia, moderate, with mood disturbance such as depression, apathy, or anhedonia

- **CC F01.B4 Vascular dementia, moderate, with anxiety**
  Major neurocognitive disorder due to vascular disease, moderate, with anxiety

+ **F01.C Vascular dementia, severe**

  - **F01.C0 Vascular dementia, severe, without behavioral disturbance, psychotic disturbance, mood disturbance, and anxiety**
    Major neurocognitive disorder due to vascular disease, severe, NOS
    Vascular dementia, severe, NOS

  + **F01.C1 Vascular dementia, severe, with behavioral disturbance**

    - **CC F01.C11 Vascular dementia, severe, with agitation**
      Major neurocognitive disorder due to vascular disease, severe, with aberrant motor behavior such as restlessness, rocking, pacing, or exit-seeking
      Major neurocognitive disorder due to vascular disease, severe, with verbal or physical behaviors such as profanity, shouting, threatening, anger, aggression, combativeness, or violence
      Vascular dementia, severe, with aberrant motor behavior such as restlessness, rocking, pacing, or exit-seeking
      Vascular dementia, severe, with verbal or physical behaviors such as profanity, shouting, threatening, anger, aggression, combativeness, or violence

    - **CC F01.C18 Vascular dementia, severe, with other behavioral disturbance**
      Major neurocognitive disorder due to vascular disease, severe, with behavioral disturbances such as sleep disturbance, social disinhibition, or sexual disinhibition
      Vascular dementia, severe, with behavioral disturbances such as sleep disturbance, social disinhibition, or sexual disinhibition
      Use additional code, if applicable, to identify wandering in vascular dementia (Z91.83)

- **CC F01.C2 Vascular dementia, severe, with psychotic disturbance**
  Major neurocognitive disorder due to vascular disease, severe, with psychotic disturbance such as hallucinations, paranoia, suspiciousness, or delusional state
  Vascular dementia, severe, with psychotic disturbance such as hallucinations, paranoia, suspiciousness, or delusional state

- **CC F01.C3 Vascular dementia, severe, with mood disturbance**
  Major neurocognitive disorder due to vascular disease, severe, with mood disturbance such as depression, apathy, or anhedonia
  Vascular dementia, severe, with mood disturbance such as depression, apathy, or anhedonia

- **CC F01.C4 Vascular dementia, severe, with anxiety**
  Major neurocognitive disorder due to vascular disease, severe, with anxiety

F02 Dementia in other diseases classified elsewhere

Includes: Major neurocognitive disorder in other diseases classified elsewhere

Code first the underlying physiological condition, such as:
  Alzheimer's (G30.-)
  cerebral lipidosis (E75.4)
  Creutzfeldt-Jakob disease (A81.0-)
  dementia with Lewy bodies (G31.83)
  dementia with Parkinsonism (G31.83)
  epilepsy and recurrent seizures (G40.-)
  frontotemporal dementia (G31.09)
  hepatolenticular degeneration (E83.01)
  human immunodeficiency virus [HIV] disease (B20)
  Huntington's disease (G10)
  hypercalcemia (E83.52)
  hypothyroidism, acquired (E00-E03.-)
  intoxications (T36-T65)
  Jakob-Creutzfeldt disease (A81.0-)
  multiple sclerosis (G35)
  neurosyphilis (A52.17)
  niacin deficiency [pellagra] (E52)
  Parkinson's disease (G20.-)
  Pick's disease (G31.01)
  polyarteritis nodosa (M30.0)
  prion disease (A81.9)
  systemic lupus erythematosus (M32.-)
  traumatic brain injury (S06.-)
  trypanosomiasis (B56.-, B57.-)
  vitamin B deficiency (E53.8)

Excludes1: mild neurocognitive disorder due to known physiological condition with or without behavioral disturbance (F06.7-)

Excludes2: dementia in alcohol and psychoactive substance disorders (F10-F19, with .17, .27, .97)
  vascular dementia (F01.5-, F01.A-, F01.B-, F01.C-)

AHA CC: 4Q, 2022, 14-15
Review coding guideline C.5.d

+ **F02.8 Dementia in other diseases classified elsewhere, unspecified severity**

  F02.80 Dementia in other diseases classified elsewhere, unspecified severity, without behavioral disturbance, psychotic disturbance, mood disturbance, and anxiety
    Dementia in other diseases classified elsewhere NOS
    Major neurocognitive disorder in other diseases classified elsewhere NOS
    AHA CC: 2Q, 2016, 6; 4Q, 2016, 141; 1Q, 2017, 43-44; 1Q, 2022, 25

  + **F02.81 Dementia in other diseases classified elsewhere, unspecified severity, with behavioral disturbance**
    AHA CC: 2Q, 2017, 7-8

- **CC** **F02.811** **Dementia in other diseases classified elsewhere, unspecified severity, with agitation**
  - Dementia in other diseases classified elsewhere, unspecified severity, with aberrant motor behavior such as restlessness, rocking, pacing, or exit-seeking
  - Dementia in other diseases classified elsewhere, unspecified severity, with verbal or physical behaviors such as profanity, shouting, threatening, anger, aggression, combativeness, or violence
  - Major neurocognitive disorder in other diseases classified elsewhere, unspecified severity, with aberrant motor behavior such as restlessness, rocking, pacing, or exit-seeking
  - Major neurocognitive disorder in other diseases classified elsewhere, unspecified severity, with verbal or physical behaviors such as profanity, shouting, threatening, anger, aggression, combativeness, or violence
- **CC** **F02.818** **Dementia in other diseases classified elsewhere, unspecified severity, with other behavioral disturbance**
  - Dementia in other diseases classified elsewhere with sleep disturbance, social disinhibition, or sexual disinhibition
  - Major neurocognitive disorder in other diseases classified elsewhere with sleep disturbance, social disinhibition, or sexual disinhibition
  - Use additional code, if applicable, to identify wandering in dementia in conditions classified elsewhere (Z91.83)
- **CC** **F02.82** **Dementia in other diseases classified elsewhere, unspecified severity, with psychotic disturbance**
  - Dementia in other diseases classified elsewhere, unspecified severity, with psychotic disturbance such as hallucinations, paranoia, suspiciousness, or delusional state
  - Major neurocognitive disorder in other diseases classified elsewhere, unspecified, with psychotic disturbance such as hallucinations, paranoia, suspiciousness, or delusional state
- **CC** **F02.83** **Dementia in other diseases classified elsewhere, unspecified severity, with mood disturbance**
  - Dementia in other diseases classified elsewhere, unspecified severity, with mood disturbance such as depression, apathy, or anhedonia
  - Major neurocognitive disorder in other diseases classified elsewhere unspecified severity, with mood disturbance such as with depression, apathy, or anhedonia
- **CC** **F02.84** **Dementia in other diseases classified elsewhere, unspecified severity, with anxiety**
  - Major neurocognitive disorder in other diseases classified elsewhere unspecified severity, with anxiety
- **+** **F02.A** **Dementia in other diseases classified elsewhere, mild**
  - *Excludes1:* mild neurocognitive disorder due to known physiological condition with or without behavioral disturbance (F06.7-)
  - **F02.A0** **Dementia in other diseases classified elsewhere, mild, without behavioral disturbance, psychotic disturbance, mood disturbance, and anxiety**
    - Dementia in other diseases classified elsewhere, mild, NOS
    - Major neurocognitive disorder in other diseases classified elsewhere, mild, NOS
- **+** **F02.A1** **Dementia in other diseases classified elsewhere, mild, with behavioral disturbance**
  - **CC** **F02.A11** **Dementia in other diseases classified elsewhere, mild, with agitation**
    - Dementia in other diseases classified elsewhere, mild, with aberrant motor behavior such as restlessness, rocking, pacing, or exit-seeking
    - Dementia in other diseases classified elsewhere, mild, with verbal or physical behaviors such as profanity, shouting, threatening, anger, aggression, combativeness, or violence
    - Major neurocognitive disorder in other diseases classified elsewhere, mild, with aberrant motor behavior such as restlessness, rocking, pacing, or exit-seeking
    - Major neurocognitive disorder in other diseases classified elsewhere, mild, with verbal or physical behaviors such as profanity, shouting, threatening, anger, aggression, combativeness, or violence
  - **CC** **F02.A18** **Dementia in other diseases classified elsewhere, mild, with other behavioral disturbance**
    - Dementia in other diseases classified elsewhere, mild, with behavioral disturbances such as sleep disturbance, social disinhibition, or sexual disinhibition
    - Major neurocognitive disorder in other diseases classified elsewhere, mild, with behavioral disturbances such as sleep disturbance, social disinhibition, or sexual disinhibition
    - Use additional code, if applicable, to identify wandering in dementia in conditions classified elsewhere (Z91.83)
- **CC** **F02.A2** **Dementia in other diseases classified elsewhere, mild, with psychotic disturbance**
  - Dementia in other diseases classified elsewhere, mild, with psychotic disturbance such as hallucinations, paranoia, suspiciousness, or delusional state
  - Major neurocognitive disorder in other diseases classified elsewhere, mild, with psychotic disturbance such as hallucinations, paranoia, suspiciousness, or delusional state
- **CC** **F02.A3** **Dementia in other diseases classified elsewhere, mild, with mood disturbance**
  - Dementia in other diseases classified elsewhere, mild, with mood disturbance such as depression, apathy, or anhedonia
  - Major neurocognitive disorder in other diseases classified elsewhere, mild, with mood disturbance such as depression, apathy, or anhedonia
- **CC** **F02.A4** **Dementia in other diseases classified elsewhere, mild, with anxiety**
  - Major neurocognitive disorder in other diseases classified elsewhere, mild, with anxiety
- **+** **F02.B** **Dementia in other diseases classified elsewhere, moderate**
  - **F02.B0** **Dementia in other diseases classified elsewhere, moderate, without behavioral disturbance, psychotic disturbance, mood disturbance, and anxiety**
    - Dementia in other diseases classified elsewhere, moderate, NOS
    - Major neurocognitive disorder in other diseases classified elsewhere, moderate, NOS

+ F02.B1 Dementia in other diseases classified elsewhere, moderate, with behavioral disturbance

    CC F02.B11 Dementia in other diseases classified elsewhere, moderate, with agitation

        Dementia in other diseases classified elsewhere, moderate, with aberrant motor behavior such as restlessness, rocking, pacing, or exit-seeking

        Dementia in other diseases classified elsewhere, moderate, with verbal or physical behaviors such as profanity, shouting, threatening, anger, aggression, combativeness, or violence

        Major neurocognitive disorder in other diseases classified elsewhere, moderate, with aberrant motor behavior such as restlessness, rocking, pacing, or exit-seeking

        Major neurocognitive disorder in other diseases classified elsewhere, moderate, with verbal or physical behaviors such as profanity, shouting, threatening, anger, aggression, combativeness, or violence

    CC F02.B18 Dementia in other diseases classified elsewhere, moderate, with other behavioral disturbance

        Dementia in other diseases classified elsewhere, moderate, with behavioral disturbances such as sleep disturbance, social disinhibition, or sexual disinhibition

        Major neurocognitive disorder in other diseases classified elsewhere, moderate, with behavioral disturbance such as sleep disturbance, social disinhibition, or sexual disinhibition

        Use additional code, if applicable, to identify wandering in dementia in conditions classified elsewhere (Z91.83)

    CC F02.B2 Dementia in other diseases classified elsewhere, moderate, with psychotic disturbance

        Dementia in other diseases classified elsewhere, moderate, with psychotic disturbance such as hallucinations, paranoia, suspiciousness, or delusional state

        Major neurocognitive disorder in other diseases classified elsewhere, moderate, with psychotic disturbance such as hallucinations, paranoia, suspiciousness, or delusional state

    CC F02.B3 Dementia in other diseases classified elsewhere, moderate, with mood disturbance

        Dementia in other diseases classified elsewhere, moderate, with mood disturbance such as depression, apathy, or anhedonia

        Major neurocognitive disorder in other diseases classified elsewhere, moderate, with mood disturbance such as depression, apathy, or anhedonia

    CC F02.B4 Dementia in other diseases classified elsewhere, moderate, with anxiety

        Major neurocognitive disorder in other diseases classified elsewhere, moderate, with anxiety

+ F02.C Dementia in other diseases classified elsewhere, severe

    F02.C0 Dementia in other diseases classified elsewhere, severe, without behavioral disturbance, psychotic disturbance, mood disturbance, and anxiety

        Dementia in other diseases classified elsewhere, severe, NOS

        Major neurocognitive disorder in other diseases classified elsewhere, severe, NOS

+ F02.C1 Dementia in other diseases classified elsewhere, severe, with behavioral disturbance

    CC F02.C11 Dementia in other diseases classified elsewhere, severe, with agitation

        Dementia in other diseases classified elsewhere, severe, with aberrant motor behavior such as restlessness, rocking, pacing, or exit-seeking

        Dementia in other diseases classified elsewhere, severe, with verbal or physical behaviors such as profanity, shouting, threatening, anger, aggression, combativeness, or violence

        Major neurocognitive disorder in other diseases classified elsewhere, severe, with aberrant motor behavior such as restlessness, rocking, pacing, or exit-seeking

        Major neurocognitive disorder in other diseases classified elsewhere, severe, with verbal or physical behaviors such as profanity, shouting, threatening, anger, aggression, combativeness, or violence

        AHA CC: 4Q, 2022, 15

    CC F02.C18 Dementia in other diseases classified elsewhere, severe, with other behavioral disturbance

        Dementia in other diseases classified elsewhere, severe, with behavioral disturbances such as sleep disturbance, social disinhibition, or sexual disinhibition

        Major neurocognitive disorder in other diseases classified elsewhere, severe, with behavioral disturbances such as sleep disturbance, social disinhibition, or sexual disinhibition

        Use additional code, if applicable, to identify wandering in dementia in conditions classified elsewhere (Z91.83)

    CC F02.C2 Dementia in other diseases classified elsewhere, severe, with psychotic disturbance

        Dementia in other diseases classified elsewhere, severe, with psychotic disturbance such as hallucinations, paranoia, suspiciousness, or delusional state

        Major neurocognitive disorder in other diseases classified elsewhere, severe, with psychotic disturbance such as hallucinations, paranoia, suspiciousness, or delusional state

    CC F02.C3 Dementia in other diseases classified elsewhere, severe, with mood disturbance

        Dementia in other diseases classified elsewhere, severe, with mood disturbance such as depression, apathy, or anhedonia

        Major neurocognitive disorder in other diseases classified elsewhere, severe, with mood disturbance such as depression, apathy, or anhedonia

    CC F02.C4 Dementia in other diseases classified elsewhere, severe, with anxiety

        Major neurocognitive disorder in other diseases classified elsewhere, severe, with anxiety

F03 Unspecified dementia

    Major neurocognitive disorder NOS
    Presenile dementia NOS
    Presenile psychosis NOS
    Primary degenerative dementia NOS
    Senile dementia NOS
    Senile dementia depressed or paranoid type
    Senile psychosis NOS

    Excludes1: senility NOS (R41.81)
    Excludes2: mild memory disturbance due to known physiological condition (F06.8)
        senile dementia with delirium or acute confusional state (F05)

    AHA CC: 4Q, 2022, 14-15
    Review coding guideline C.5.d

- **+ F03.9 Unspecified dementia, unspecified severity**
  - **• F03.90** Unspecified dementia, unspecified severity, without behavioral disturbance, psychotic disturbance, mood disturbance, and anxiety
    Dementia NOS
    AHA CC: 4Q, 2012, 92-93; 2Q, 2021, 4
  - **• + F03.91** Unspecified dementia, unspecified severity, with behavioral disturbance
    - CC **F03.911** Unspecified dementia, unspecified severity, with agitation
      Unspecified dementia, unspecified severity, with aberrant motor behavior such as restlessness, rocking, pacing, or exit-seeking
      Unspecified dementia, unspecified severity, with verbal or physical behaviors such as profanity, shouting, threatening, anger, aggression, combativeness, or violence
    - CC **F03.918** Unspecified dementia, unspecified severity, with other behavioral disturbance
      Unspecified dementia, unspecified severity, with behavioral disturbances such as sleep disturbance, social disinhibition, or sexual disinhibition
      Use additional code, if applicable, to identify wandering in unspecified dementia(Z91.83)
  - CC **F03.92** Unspecified dementia, unspecified severity, with psychotic disturbance
    Unspecified dementia, unspecified severity, with psychotic disturbance such as hallucinations, paranoia, suspiciousness, or delusional state
  - CC **F03.93** Unspecified dementia, unspecified severity, with mood disturbance
    Unspecified dementia, unspecified severity, with mood disturbance such as depression, apathy, or anhedonia
  - CC **F03.94** Unspecified dementia, unspecified severity, with anxiety
- **+ F03.A Unspecified dementia, mild**
  Excludes1: mild neurocognitive disorder due to known physiological condition with or without behavioral disturbance (F06.7-)
  - **F03.A0** Unspecified dementia, mild, without behavioral disturbance, psychotic disturbance, mood disturbance, and anxiety
    Dementia, mild, NOS
  - **+ F03.A1** Unspecified dementia, mild, with behavioral disturbance
    - CC **F03.A11** Unspecified dementia, mild, with agitation
      Unspecified dementia, mild, with aberrant motor behavior such as restlessness, rocking, pacing, or exit-seeking
      Unspecified dementia, mild, with verbal or physical behaviors such as profanity, shouting, threatening, anger, aggression, combativeness, or violence
    - CC **F03.A18** Unspecified dementia, mild, with other behavioral disturbance
      Unspecified dementia, mild, with behavioral disturbances such as sleep disturbance, social disinhibition, or sexual disinhibition
      Use additional code, if applicable, to identify wandering in unspecified dementia(Z91.83)
  - CC **F03.A2** Unspecified dementia, mild, with psychotic disturbance
    Unspecified dementia, mild, with psychotic disturbance such as hallucinations, paranoia, suspiciousness, or delusional state
  - CC **F03.A3** Unspecified dementia, mild, with mood disturbance
    Unspecified dementia, mild, with mood disturbance such as depression, apathy, or anhedonia
  - CC **F03.A4** Unspecified dementia, mild, with anxiety

- **+ F03.B Unspecified dementia, moderate**
  - **F03.B0** Unspecified dementia, moderate, without behavioral disturbance, psychotic disturbance, mood disturbance, and anxiety
    Dementia, moderate, NOS
  - **+ F03.B1** Unspecified dementia, moderate, with behavioral disturbance
    - CC **F03.B11** Unspecified dementia, moderate, with agitation
      Unspecified dementia, moderate, with aberrant motor behavior such as restlessness, rocking, pacing, or exit-seeking
      Unspecified dementia, moderate, with verbal or physical behaviors such as profanity, shouting, threatening, anger, aggression, combativeness, or violence
    - CC **F03.B18** Unspecified dementia, moderate, with other behavioral disturbance
      Unspecified dementia, moderate, with behavioral disturbances such as sleep disturbance, social disinhibition, or sexual disinhibition
      Use additional code, if applicable, to identify wandering in unspecified dementia(Z91.83)
  - CC **F03.B2** Unspecified dementia, moderate, with psychotic disturbance
    Unspecified dementia, moderate, with psychotic disturbance such as hallucinations, paranoia, suspiciousness, or delusional state
  - CC **F03.B3** Unspecified dementia, moderate, with mood disturbance
    Unspecified dementia, moderate, with mood disturbance such as depression, apathy, or anhedonia
  - CC **F03.B4** Unspecified dementia, moderate, with anxiety
- **+ F03.C Unspecified dementia, severe**
  - **F03.C0** Unspecified dementia, severe, without behavioral disturbance, psychotic disturbance, mood disturbance, and anxiety
    Dementia, severe, NOS
  - **+ F03.C1** Unspecified dementia, severe, with behavioral disturbance
    - CC **F03.C11** Unspecified dementia, severe, with agitation
      Unspecified dementia, severe, with aberrant motor behavior such as restlessness, rocking, pacing, or exit-seeking
      Unspecified dementia, severe, with verbal or physical behaviors such as profanity, shouting, threatening, anger, aggression, combativeness, or violence
    - CC **F03.C18** Unspecified dementia, severe, with other behavioral disturbance
      Unspecified dementia, severe, with behavioral disturbances such as sleep disturbance, social disinhibition, or sexual disinhibition
      Use additional code, if applicable, to identify wandering in unspecified dementia(Z91.83)
  - CC **F03.C2** Unspecified dementia, severe, with psychotic disturbance
    Unspecified dementia, severe, with psychotic disturbance such as hallucinations, paranoia, suspiciousness, or delusional state
  - CC **F03.C3** Unspecified dementia, severe, with mood disturbance
    Unspecified dementia, severe, with mood disturbance such as depression, apathy, or anhedonia
  - CC **F03.C4** Unspecified dementia, severe, with anxiety

F04 **Amnestic disorder due to known physiological condition**
   Korsakov's psychosis or syndrome, nonalcoholic
   Code first the underlying physiological condition
   Excludes1: amnesia NOS (R41.3)
      anterograde amnesia (R41.1)
      dissociative amnesia (F44.0)
      retrograde amnesia (R41.2)
   Excludes2: alcohol-induced or unspecified Korsakov's syndrome (F10.26, F10.96)
      Korsakov's syndrome induced by other psychoactive substances (F13.26, F13.96, F19.16, F19.26, F19.96)
   Valid 3-character code, no further characters required

CC **F05** **Delirium due to known physiological condition**
   Acute or subacute brain syndrome
   Acute or subacute confusional state (nonalcoholic)
   Acute or subacute infective psychosis
   Acute or subacute organic reaction
   Acute or subacute psycho-organic syndrome
   Delirium of mixed etiology
   Delirium superimposed on dementia
   Sundowning
   Code first the underlying physiological condition, such as: dementia (F03.9-)
   Excludes1: delirium NOS (R41.0)
   Excludes2: delirium tremens alcohol-induced or unspecified (F10.231, F10.921)
   AHA CC: 2Q, 2019, 34
   Valid 3-character code, no further characters required

F06 **Other mental disorders due to known physiological condition**
   Includes: mental disorders due to endocrine disorder
      mental disorders due to exogenous hormone
      mental disorders due to exogenous toxic substance
      mental disorders due to primary cerebral disease
      mental disorders due to somatic illness
      mental disorders due to systemic disease affecting the brain
   Code first the underlying physiological condition
   Excludes1: unspecified dementia (F03)
   Excludes2: delirium due to known physiological condition (F05)
      dementia as classified in F01-F02
      other mental disorders associated with alcohol and other psychoactive substances (F10-F19)

CC **F06.0** **Psychotic disorder with hallucinations due to known physiological condition**
   Organic hallucinatory state (nonalcoholic)
   Excludes2: hallucinations and perceptual disturbance induced by alcohol and other psychoactive substances (F10-F19 with .151, .251, .951)
      schizophrenia (F20.-)

F06.1 **Catatonic disorder due to known physiological condition**
   Catatonia associated with another mental disorder
   Catatonia NOS
   Excludes1: catatonic stupor (R40.1)
      stupor NOS (R40.1)
   Excludes2: catatonic schizophrenia (F20.2)
      dissociative stupor (F44.2)

CC **F06.2** **Psychotic disorder with delusions due to known physiological condition**
   Paranoid and paranoid-hallucinatory organic states
   Schizophrenia-like psychosis in epilepsy
   Excludes2: alcohol and drug-induced psychotic disorder (F10-F19 with .150, .250, .950)
      brief psychotic disorder (F23)
      delusional disorder (F22)
      schizophrenia (F20.-)

+ **F06.3** **Mood disorder due to known physiological condition**
   Excludes2: mood disorders due to alcohol and other psychoactive substances (F10-F19 with .14, .24, .94)
      mood disorders, not due to known physiological condition or unspecified (F30-F39)

   F06.30 Mood disorder due to known physiological condition, unspecified
   F06.31 Mood disorder due to known physiological condition with depressive features
      Depressive disorder due to known physiological condition, with depressive features
   F06.32 Mood disorder due to known physiological condition with major depressive-like episode
      Depressive disorder due to known physiological condition, with major depressive-like episode
   F06.33 Mood disorder due to known physiological condition with manic features
      Bipolar and related disorder due to a known physiological condition, with manic features
      Bipolar and related disorder due to known physiological condition, with manic- or hypomanic-like episodes
   F06.34 Mood disorder due to known physiological condition with mixed features
      Bipolar and related disorder due to known physiological condition, with mixed features
      Depressive disorder due to known physiological condition, with mixed features

F06.4 **Anxiety disorder due to known physiological condition**
   Excludes2: anxiety disorders due to alcohol and other psychoactive substances (F10-F19 with .180, .280, .980)
      anxiety disorders, not due to known physiological condition or unspecified (F40.-, F41.-)

+ **F06.7** **Mild neurocognitive disorder due to known physiological condition**
   Mild neurocognitive impairment due to a known physiological condition
   Code first the underlying physiological condition, such as:
      Alzheimer's disease (G30.-)
      frontotemporal neurocognitive disorder (G31.09)
      human immunodeficiency virus [HIV] disease (B20)
      Huntington's disease (G10)
      Neurocognitive disorder with Lewy bodies (G31.83)
      Parkinson's disease (G20.-)
      systemic lupus erythematosus (M32.-)
      traumatic brain injury (S06.-)
      vitamin B deficiency (E53.-)
   Excludes1: age related cognitive decline (R41.81)
      altered mental status (R41.82)
      cerebral degeneration (G31.9)
      change in mental status (R41.82)
      cognitive deficits following (sequelae of) cerebral hemorrhage or infarction (I69.01-I69.11-, I69.21-I69.31-, I69.81-I69.91-)
      dementia (F01.-, F02.-, F03)
      mild cognitive impairment due to unknown or unspecified etiology (G31.84)
      neurologic neglect syndrome (R41.4)
      personality change, nonpsychotic (F68.8)
   AHA CC: 4Q, 2022, 16

   F06.70 Mild neurocognitive disorder due to known physiological condition without behavioral disturbance
      Mild neurocognitive disorder due to known physiological condition, NOS
   CC **F06.71** Mild neurocognitive disorder due to known physiological condition with behavioral disturbance

F06.8 **Other specified mental disorders due to known physiological condition**
   Epileptic psychosis NOS
   Obsessive-compulsive and related disorder due to a known physiological condition
   Organic dissociative disorder
   Organic emotionally labile [asthenic] disorder

F07 **Personality and behavioral disorders due to known physiological condition**
   Code first the underlying physiological condition

   F07.0 **Personality change due to known physiological condition**
      Frontal lobe syndrome
      Limbic epilepsy personality syndrome
      Lobotomy syndrome
      Organic personality disorder
      Organic pseudopsychopathic personality
      Organic pseudoretarded personality
      Postleucotomy syndrome
      Excludes1: mild cognitive impairment (G31.84)
         postconcussional syndrome (F07.81)
         postencephalitic syndrome (F07.89)
         signs and symptoms involving emotional state (R45.-)
      Excludes2: specific personality disorder (F60.-)

- **F07.8** Other personality and behavioral disorders due to known physiological condition
  - **F07.81** Postconcussional syndrome
    Postcontusional syndrome (encephalopathy)
    Post-traumatic brain syndrome, nonpsychotic
    Use additional code to identify associated post-traumatic headache, if applicable (G44.3-)
    Excludes1: current concussion (brain) (S06.0-)
    postencephalitic syndrome (F07.89)
  - **F07.89** Other personality and behavioral disorders due to known physiological condition
    Postencephalitic syndrome
    Right hemispheric organic affective disorder
- **F07.9** Unspecified personality and behavioral disorder due to known physiological condition
  Organic psychosyndrome

F09 Unspecified mental disorder due to known physiological condition
  Mental disorder NOS due to known physiological condition
  Organic brain syndrome NOS
  Organic mental disorder NOS
  Organic psychosis NOS
  Symptomatic psychosis NOS
  Code first the underlying physiological condition
  Excludes1: mild neurocognitive disorder due to known physiological condition (F06.7-)
  psychosis NOS (F29)
  Valid 3-character code, no further characters required

Mental and behavioral disorders due to psychoactive substance use (F10-F19)
Review coding guideline C.5.b
AHA CC: 4Q, 2017, 8; 1Q, 2020, 9; 1Q, 2022, 33-34; 4Q, 2022, 16-17

F10 Alcohol related disorders
Use additional code for blood alcohol level, if applicable (Y90.-)
- **F10.1** Alcohol abuse
  Excludes1: alcohol dependence (F10.2-)
  alcohol use, unspecified (F10.9-)
  - **F10.10** Alcohol abuse, uncomplicated
    Alcohol use disorder, mild
  - **F10.11** Alcohol abuse, in remission
    Alcohol use disorder, mild, in early remission
    Alcohol use disorder, mild, in sustained remission
    AHA CC: 1Q, 2022, 25
  - **F10.12** Alcohol abuse with intoxication
    - **F10.120** Alcohol abuse with intoxication, uncomplicated
    - CC **F10.121** Alcohol abuse with intoxication delirium
    - **F10.129** Alcohol abuse with intoxication, unspecified
  - **F10.13** Alcohol abuse, with withdrawal
    AHA CC: 4Q, 2020, 16-17
    - CC **F10.130** Alcohol abuse with withdrawal, uncomplicated
    - CC **F10.131** Alcohol abuse with withdrawal delirium
    - CC **F10.132** Alcohol abuse with withdrawal with perceptual disturbance
    - CC **F10.139** Alcohol abuse with withdrawal, unspecified
  - CC **F10.14** Alcohol abuse with alcohol-induced mood disorder
    Alcohol use disorder, mild, with alcohol-induced bipolar or related disorder
    Alcohol use disorder, mild, with alcohol-induced depressive disorder
  - **F10.15** Alcohol abuse with alcohol-induced psychotic disorder
    - **F10.150** Alcohol abuse with alcohol-induced psychotic disorder with delusions
    - CC **F10.151** Alcohol abuse with alcohol-induced psychotic disorder with hallucinations
    - CC **F10.159** Alcohol abuse with alcohol-induced psychotic disorder, unspecified
  - **F10.18** Alcohol abuse with other alcohol-induced disorders
    AHA CC: 1Q, 2022, 33-34
    - CC **F10.180** Alcohol abuse with alcohol-induced anxiety disorder
    - CC **F10.181** Alcohol abuse with alcohol-induced sexual dysfunction
    - **F10.182** Alcohol abuse with alcohol-induced sleep disorder
    - CC **F10.188** Alcohol abuse with other alcohol-induced disorder
    AHA CC: 1Q, 2022, 25
  - CC **F10.19** Alcohol abuse with unspecified alcohol-induced disorder
- **F10.2** Alcohol dependence
  Excludes1: alcohol abuse (F10.1-)
  alcohol use, unspecified (F10.9-)
  Excludes2: toxic effect of alcohol (T51.0-)
  - **F10.20** Alcohol dependence, uncomplicated
    Alcohol use disorder, moderate
    Alcohol use disorder, severe
    AHA CC: 1Q, 2020, 9
  - **F10.21** Alcohol dependence, in remission
    Alcohol use disorder, moderate, in early remission
    Alcohol use disorder, moderate, in sustained remission
    Alcohol use disorder, severe, in early remission
    Alcohol use disorder, severe, in sustained remission
  - **F10.22** Alcohol dependence with intoxication
    Acute drunkenness (in alcoholism)
    Excludes2: alcohol dependence with withdrawal (F10.23-)
    - **F10.220** Alcohol dependence with intoxication, uncomplicated
    - CC **F10.221** Alcohol dependence with intoxication delirium
    - **F10.229** Alcohol dependence with intoxication, unspecified
  - **F10.23** Alcohol dependence with withdrawal
    Excludes2: Alcohol dependence with intoxication (F10.22-)
    - CC **F10.230** Alcohol dependence with withdrawal, uncomplicated
    - CC **F10.231** Alcohol dependence with withdrawal delirium
    - CC **F10.232** Alcohol dependence with withdrawal with perceptual disturbance
    - CC **F10.239** Alcohol dependence with withdrawal, unspecified
  - CC **F10.24** Alcohol dependence with alcohol-induced mood disorder
    Alcohol use disorder, moderate, with alcohol-induced bipolar or related disorder
    Alcohol use disorder, moderate, with alcohol-induced depressive disorder
    Alcohol use disorder, severe, with alcohol-induced bipolar or related disorder
    Alcohol use disorder, severe, with alcohol-induced depressive disorder
  - **F10.25** Alcohol dependence with alcohol-induced psychotic disorder
    - **F10.250** Alcohol dependence with alcohol-induced psychotic disorder with delusions
    - CC **F10.251** Alcohol dependence with alcohol-induced psychotic disorder with hallucinations
    - CC **F10.259** Alcohol dependence with alcohol-induced psychotic disorder, unspecified
  - **F10.26** Alcohol dependence with alcohol-induced persisting amnestic disorder
    Alcohol use disorder, moderate, with alcohol-induced major neurocognitive disorder, amnestic-confabulatory type
    Alcohol use disorder, severe, with alcohol-induced major neurocognitive disorder, amnestic-confabulatory type
  - CC **F10.27** Alcohol dependence with alcohol-induced persisting dementia
    Alcohol use disorder, moderate, with alcohol-induced major neurocognitive disorder, nonamnestic-confabulatory type
    Alcohol use disorder, severe, with alcohol-induced major neurocognitive disorder, nonamnestic-confabulatory type

- **+ F10.28** Alcohol dependence with other alcohol-induced disorders
  - CC **F10.280** Alcohol dependence with alcohol-induced anxiety disorder
  - CC **F10.281** Alcohol dependence with alcohol-induced sexual dysfunction
  - **F10.282** Alcohol dependence with alcohol-induced sleep disorder
  - CC **F10.288** Alcohol dependence with other alcohol-induced disorder
    - Alcohol use disorder, moderate, with alcohol-induced mild neurocognitive disorder
    - Alcohol use disorder, severe, with alcohol-induced mild neurocognitive disorder
  - CC **F10.29** Alcohol dependence with unspecified alcohol-induced disorder
- **+ F10.9** Alcohol use, unspecified
  - *Excludes1:* alcohol abuse (F10.1-)
  - alcohol dependence (F10.2-)
  - **F10.90** Alcohol use, unspecified, uncomplicated
  - **F10.91** Alcohol use, unspecified, in remission
  - **+ F10.92** Alcohol use, unspecified with intoxication
    - **F10.920** Alcohol use, unspecified with intoxication, uncomplicated
    - CC **F10.921** Alcohol use, unspecified with intoxication delirium
    - **F10.929** Alcohol use, unspecified with intoxication, unspecified
  - **+ F10.93** Alcohol use, unspecified with withdrawal
    - *AHA CC: 4Q, 2020, 16-17*
    - CC **F10.930** Alcohol use, unspecified with withdrawal, uncomplicated
    - CC **F10.931** Alcohol use, unspecified with withdrawal delirium
    - CC **F10.932** Alcohol use, unspecified with withdrawal with perceptual disturbance
    - CC **F10.939** Alcohol use, unspecified with withdrawal, unspecified
  - CC **F10.94** Alcohol use, unspecified with alcohol-induced mood disorder
    - Alcohol-induced bipolar or related disorder, without use disorder
    - Alcohol-induced depressive disorder, without use disorder
  - **+ F10.95** Alcohol use, unspecified with alcohol-induced psychotic disorder
    - **F10.950** Alcohol use, unspecified with alcohol-induced psychotic disorder with delusions
    - CC **F10.951** Alcohol use, unspecified with alcohol-induced psychotic disorder with hallucinations
    - CC **F10.959** Alcohol use, unspecified with alcohol-induced psychotic disorder, unspecified
      - Alcohol-induced psychotic disorder without use disorder
  - **F10.96** Alcohol use, unspecified with alcohol-induced persisting amnestic disorder
    - Alcohol-induced major neurocognitive disorder, amnestic-confabulatory type, without use disorder
  - **F10.97** Alcohol use, unspecified with alcohol-induced persisting dementia
    - Alcohol-induced major neurocognitive disorder, nonamnestic-confabulatory type, without use disorder
  - **+ F10.98** Alcohol use, unspecified with other alcohol-induced disorders
    - CC **F10.980** Alcohol use, unspecified with alcohol-induced anxiety disorder
      - Alcohol-induced anxiety disorder, without use disorder
    - CC **F10.981** Alcohol use, unspecified with alcohol-induced sexual dysfunction
      - Alcohol-induced sexual dysfunction, without use disorder
    - **F10.982** Alcohol use, unspecified with alcohol-induced sleep disorder
      - Alcohol-induced sleep disorder, without use disorder
    - CC **F10.988** Alcohol use, unspecified with other alcohol-induced disorder
      - Alcohol-induced mild neurocognitive disorder, without use disorder
      - *AHA CC: 3Q, 2019, 8*
    - CC **F10.99** Alcohol use, unspecified with unspecified alcohol-induced disorder

F11 Opioid related disorders

- **+ F11.1** Opioid abuse
  - *Excludes1:* opioid dependence (F11.2-)
  - opioid use, unspecified (F11.9-)
  - **F11.10** Opioid abuse, uncomplicated
    - Opioid use disorder, mild
  - **F11.11** Opioid abuse, in remission
    - Opioid use disorder, mild, in early remission
    - Opioid use disorder, mild, in sustained remission
  - **+ F11.12** Opioid abuse with intoxication
    - **F11.120** Opioid abuse with intoxication, uncomplicated
    - CC **F11.121** Opioid abuse with intoxication delirium
    - **F11.122** Opioid abuse with intoxication with perceptual disturbance
    - **F11.129** Opioid abuse with intoxication, unspecified
  - CC **F11.13** Opioid abuse with withdrawal
    - *AHA CC: 4Q, 2020, 16-17*
  - **F11.14** Opioid abuse with opioid-induced mood disorder
    - Opioid use disorder, mild, with opioid-induced depressive disorder
  - **+ F11.15** Opioid abuse with opioid-induced psychotic disorder
    - CC **F11.150** Opioid abuse with opioid-induced psychotic disorder with delusions
    - CC **F11.151** Opioid abuse with opioid-induced psychotic disorder with hallucinations
    - **F11.159** Opioid abuse with opioid-induced psychotic disorder, unspecified
  - **+ F11.18** Opioid abuse with other opioid-induced disorder
    - **F11.181** Opioid abuse with opioid-induced sexual dysfunction
    - **F11.182** Opioid abuse with opioid-induced sleep disorder
    - **F11.188** Opioid abuse with other opioid-induced disorder
      - Opioid-associated amnestic syndrome with opioid abuse
  - **F11.19** Opioid abuse with unspecified opioid-induced disorder
- **+ F11.2** Opioid dependence
  - *Excludes1:* opioid abuse (F11.1-)
  - opioid use, unspecified (F11.9-)
  - *Excludes2:* opioid poisoning (T40.0-T40.2-)
  - CC **F11.20** Opioid dependence, uncomplicated
    - Opioid use disorder, moderate
    - Opioid use disorder, severe
  - **F11.21** Opioid dependence, in remission
    - Opioid use disorder, moderate, in early remission
    - Opioid use disorder, moderate, in sustained remission
    - Opioid use disorder, severe, in early remission
    - Opioid use disorder, severe, in sustained remission
  - **+ F11.22** Opioid dependence with intoxication
    - *Excludes1:* opioid dependence with withdrawal (F11.23)
    - **F11.220** Opioid dependence with intoxication, uncomplicated
    - CC **F11.221** Opioid dependence with intoxication delirium
    - CC **F11.222** Opioid dependence with intoxication with perceptual disturbance
    - **F11.229** Opioid dependence with intoxication, unspecified
  - CC **F11.23** Opioid dependence with withdrawal
    - *Excludes1:* opioid dependence with intoxication (F11.22-)
  - **F11.24** Opioid dependence with opioid-induced mood disorder
    - Opioid use disorder, moderate, with opioid-induced depressive disorder

- **+ F11.25** Opioid dependence with opioid-induced psychotic disorder
  - CC **F11.250** Opioid dependence with opioid-induced psychotic disorder with delusions
  - CC **F11.251** Opioid dependence with opioid-induced psychotic disorder with hallucinations
  - CC **F11.259** Opioid dependence with opioid-induced psychotic disorder, unspecified
- **+ F11.28** Opioid dependence with other opioid-induced disorder
  - CC **F11.281** Opioid dependence with opioid-induced sexual dysfunction
  - CC **F11.282** Opioid dependence with opioid-induced sleep disorder
  - CC **F11.288** Opioid dependence with other opioid-induced disorder
    - Opioid-associated amnestic syndrome with opioid dependence
- **F11.29** Opioid dependence with unspecified opioid-induced disorder
- **+ F11.9** Opioid use, unspecified
  - **Excludes1:** opioid abuse (F11.1-)
    - opioid dependence (F11.2-)
  - **F11.90** Opioid use, unspecified, uncomplicated
  - **F11.91** Opioid use, unspecified, in remission
  - **+ F11.92** Opioid use, unspecified with intoxication
    - **Excludes1:** opioid use, unspecified with withdrawal (F11.93)
    - **F11.920** Opioid use, unspecified with intoxication, uncomplicated
    - CC **F11.921** Opioid use, unspecified with intoxication delirium
      - Opioid use delirium
    - **F11.922** Opioid use, unspecified with intoxication with perceptual disturbance
    - **F11.929** Opioid use, unspecified with intoxication, unspecified
  - CC **F11.93** Opioid use, unspecified with withdrawal
    - **Excludes1:** opioid use, unspecified with intoxication (F11.92-)
  - **F11.94** Opioid use, unspecified with opioid-induced mood disorder
    - Opioid-induced depressive disorder, without use disorder
  - **+ F11.95** Opioid use, unspecified with opioid-induced psychotic disorder
    - CC **F11.950** Opioid use, unspecified with opioid-induced psychotic disorder with delusions
    - CC **F11.951** Opioid use, unspecified with opioid-induced psychotic disorder with hallucinations
    - **F11.959** Opioid use, unspecified with opioid-induced psychotic disorder, unspecified
  - **+ F11.98** Opioid use, unspecified with other specified opioid-induced disorder
    - **F11.981** Opioid use, unspecified with opioid-induced sexual dysfunction
      - Opioid-induced sexual dysfunction, without use disorder
    - **F11.982** Opioid use, unspecified with opioid-induced sleep disorder
      - Opioid-induced sleep disorder, without use disorder
    - **F11.988** Opioid use, unspecified with other opioid-induced disorder
      - Opioid-associated amnestic syndrome without use disorder
      - Opioid-induced anxiety disorder, without use disorder
  - **F11.99** Opioid use, unspecified with unspecified opioid-induced disorder

F12 Cannabis related disorders
Includes: marijuana
AHA CC: 1Q, 2020, 8

- **+ F12.1** Cannabis abuse
  - **Excludes1:** cannabis dependence (F12.2-)
    - cannabis use, unspecified (F12.9-)
  - **F12.10** Cannabis abuse, uncomplicated
    - Cannabis use disorder, mild
  - **F12.11** Cannabis abuse, in remission
    - Cannabis use disorder, mild, in early remission
    - Cannabis use disorder, mild, in sustained remission
  - **+ F12.12** Cannabis abuse with intoxication
    - **F12.120** Cannabis abuse with intoxication, uncomplicated
    - CC **F12.121** Cannabis abuse with intoxication delirium
    - **F12.122** Cannabis abuse with intoxication with perceptual disturbance
    - **F12.129** Cannabis abuse with intoxication, unspecified
  - CC **F12.13** Cannabis abuse with withdrawal
    - *AHA CC: 4Q, 2020, 16-17*
  - **+ F12.15** Cannabis abuse with psychotic disorder
    - CC **F12.150** Cannabis abuse with psychotic disorder with delusions
    - CC **F12.151** Cannabis abuse with psychotic disorder with hallucinations
    - **F12.159** Cannabis abuse with psychotic disorder, unspecified
  - **+ F12.18** Cannabis abuse with other cannabis-induced disorder
    - **F12.180** Cannabis abuse with cannabis-induced anxiety disorder
    - **F12.188** Cannabis abuse with other cannabis-induced disorder
      - Cannabis use disorder, mild, with cannabis-induced sleep disorder
  - **F12.19** Cannabis abuse with unspecified cannabis-induced disorder
- **+ F12.2** Cannabis dependence
  - **Excludes1:** cannabis abuse (F12.1-)
    - cannabis use, unspecified (F12.9-)
  - **Excludes2:** cannabis poisoning (T40.7-)
  - **F12.20** Cannabis dependence, uncomplicated
    - Cannabis use disorder, moderate
    - Cannabis use disorder, severe
  - **F12.21** Cannabis dependence, in remission
    - Cannabis use disorder, moderate, in early remission
    - Cannabis use disorder, moderate, in sustained remission
    - Cannabis use disorder, severe, in early remission
    - Cannabis use disorder, severe, in sustained remission
  - **+ F12.22** Cannabis dependence with intoxication
    - **F12.220** Cannabis dependence with intoxication, uncomplicated
    - CC **F12.221** Cannabis dependence with intoxication delirium
    - **F12.222** Cannabis dependence with intoxication with perceptual disturbance
    - **F12.229** Cannabis dependence with intoxication, unspecified
  - **F12.23** Cannabis dependence with withdrawal
    - *AHA CC: 4Q, 2018, 7*
  - **+ F12.25** Cannabis dependence with psychotic disorder
    - CC **F12.250** Cannabis dependence with psychotic disorder with delusions
    - CC **F12.251** Cannabis dependence with psychotic disorder with hallucinations
    - **F12.259** Cannabis dependence with psychotic disorder, unspecified
  - **+ F12.28** Cannabis dependence with other cannabis-induced disorder
    - **F12.280** Cannabis dependence with cannabis-induced anxiety disorder
    - **F12.288** Cannabis dependence with other cannabis-induced disorder
      - Cannabis use disorder, moderate, with cannabis-induced sleep disorder
      - Cannabis use disorder, severe, with cannabis-induced sleep disorder
  - **F12.29** Cannabis dependence with unspecified cannabis-induced disorder
- **+ F12.9** Cannabis use, unspecified
  - **Excludes1:** cannabis abuse (F12.1-)
    - cannabis dependence (F12.2-)
  - **F12.90** Cannabis use, unspecified, uncomplicated
  - **F12.91** Cannabis use, unspecified, in remission

- **+ F12.92** Cannabis use, unspecified with intoxication
  - **F12.920** Cannabis use, unspecified with intoxication, uncomplicated
  - CC **F12.921** Cannabis use, unspecified with intoxication delirium
  - **F12.922** Cannabis use, unspecified with intoxication with perceptual disturbance
  - **F12.929** Cannabis use, unspecified with intoxication, unspecified
- **F12.93** Cannabis use, unspecified with withdrawal
  - *AHA CC: 4Q, 2018, 7*
- **+ F12.95** Cannabis use, unspecified with psychotic disorder
  - CC **F12.950** Cannabis use, unspecified with psychotic disorder with delusions
  - CC **F12.951** Cannabis use, unspecified with psychotic disorder with hallucinations
  - **F12.959** Cannabis use, unspecified with psychotic disorder, unspecified
    - Cannabis-induced psychotic disorder, without use disorder
- **+ F12.98** Cannabis use, unspecified with other cannabis-induced disorder
  - **F12.980** Cannabis use, unspecified with anxiety disorder
    - Cannabis-induced anxiety disorder, without use disorder
  - **F12.988** Cannabis use, unspecified with other cannabis-induced disorder
    - Cannabis-induced sleep disorder, without use disorder
- **F12.99** Cannabis use, unspecified with unspecified cannabis-induced disorder

F13 Sedative, hypnotic, or anxiolytic related disorders

- **+ F13.1** Sedative, hypnotic or anxiolytic-related abuse
  - **Excludes1:** *sedative, hypnotic or anxiolytic-related dependence (F13.2-)*
    sedative, hypnotic, or anxiolytic use, unspecified (F13.9-)
  - **F13.10** Sedative, hypnotic or anxiolytic abuse, uncomplicated
    - Sedative, hypnotic, or anxiolytic use disorder, mild
  - **F13.11** Sedative, hypnotic or anxiolytic abuse, in remission
    - Sedative, hypnotic or anxiolytic use disorder, mild, in early remission
    - Sedative, hypnotic or anxiolytic use disorder, mild, in sustained remission
  - **+ F13.12** Sedative, hypnotic or anxiolytic abuse with intoxication
    - **F13.120** Sedative, hypnotic or anxiolytic abuse with intoxication, uncomplicated
    - CC **F13.121** Sedative, hypnotic or anxiolytic abuse with intoxication delirium
    - **F13.129** Sedative, hypnotic or anxiolytic abuse with intoxication, unspecified
  - **+ F13.13** Sedative, hypnotic or anxiolytic abuse with withdrawal
    - *AHA CC: 4Q, 2020, 16-17*
    - CC **F13.130** Sedative, hypnotic or anxiolytic abuse with withdrawal, uncomplicated
    - CC **F13.131** Sedative, hypnotic or anxiolytic abuse with withdrawal delirium
    - CC **F13.132** Sedative, hypnotic or anxiolytic abuse with withdrawal with perceptual disturbance
    - CC **F13.139** Sedative, hypnotic or anxiolytic abuse with withdrawal, unspecified
  - **F13.14** Sedative, hypnotic or anxiolytic abuse with sedative, hypnotic or anxiolytic-induced mood disorder
    - Sedative, hypnotic, or anxiolytic use disorder, mild, with sedative, hypnotic, or anxiolytic-induced bipolar or related disorder
    - Sedative, hypnotic, or anxiolytic use disorder, mild, with sedative, hypnotic, or anxiolytic-induced depressive disorder
  - **+ F13.15** Sedative, hypnotic or anxiolytic abuse with sedative, hypnotic or anxiolytic-induced psychotic disorder
    - CC **F13.150** Sedative, hypnotic or anxiolytic abuse with sedative, hypnotic or anxiolytic-induced psychotic disorder with delusions
    - CC **F13.151** Sedative, hypnotic or anxiolytic abuse with sedative, hypnotic or anxiolytic-induced psychotic disorder with hallucinations
    - **F13.159** Sedative, hypnotic or anxiolytic abuse with sedative, hypnotic or anxiolytic-induced psychotic disorder, unspecified
  - **+ F13.18** Sedative, hypnotic or anxiolytic abuse with other sedative, hypnotic or anxiolytic-induced disorders
    - **F13.180** Sedative, hypnotic or anxiolytic abuse with sedative, hypnotic or anxiolytic-induced anxiety disorder
    - **F13.181** Sedative, hypnotic or anxiolytic abuse with sedative, hypnotic or anxiolytic-induced sexual dysfunction
    - **F13.182** Sedative, hypnotic or anxiolytic abuse with sedative, hypnotic or anxiolytic-induced sleep disorder
    - **F13.188** Sedative, hypnotic or anxiolytic abuse with other sedative, hypnotic or anxiolytic-induced disorder
  - **F13.19** Sedative, hypnotic or anxiolytic abuse with unspecified sedative, hypnotic or anxiolytic-induced disorder
- **+ F13.2** Sedative, hypnotic or anxiolytic-related dependence
  - **Excludes1:** *sedative, hypnotic or anxiolytic-related abuse (F13.1-)*
    sedative, hypnotic, or anxiolytic use, unspecified (F13.9-)
  - **Excludes2:** *sedative, hypnotic, or anxiolytic poisoning (T42.-)*
  - CC **F13.20** Sedative, hypnotic or anxiolytic dependence, uncomplicated
  - **F13.21** Sedative, hypnotic or anxiolytic dependence, in remission
    - Sedative, hypnotic or anxiolytic use disorder, moderate, in early remission
    - Sedative, hypnotic or anxiolytic use disorder, moderate, in sustained remission
    - Sedative, hypnotic or anxiolytic use disorder, severe, in early remission
    - Sedative, hypnotic or anxiolytic use disorder, severe, in sustained remission
  - **+ F13.22** Sedative, hypnotic or anxiolytic dependence with intoxication
    - **Excludes1:** *sedative, hypnotic or anxiolytic dependence with withdrawal (F13.23-)*
    - **F13.220** Sedative, hypnotic or anxiolytic dependence with intoxication, uncomplicated
    - CC **F13.221** Sedative, hypnotic or anxiolytic dependence with intoxication delirium
    - **F13.229** Sedative, hypnotic or anxiolytic dependence with intoxication, unspecified
  - **+ F13.23** Sedative, hypnotic or anxiolytic dependence with withdrawal
    - Sedative, hypnotic, or anxiolytic use disorder, moderate
    - Sedative, hypnotic, or anxiolytic use disorder, severe
    - **Excludes1:** *sedative, hypnotic or anxiolytic dependence with intoxication (F13.22-)*
    - CC **F13.230** Sedative, hypnotic or anxiolytic dependence with withdrawal, uncomplicated
    - CC **F13.231** Sedative, hypnotic or anxiolytic dependence with withdrawal delirium
    - CC **F13.232** Sedative, hypnotic or anxiolytic dependence with withdrawal with perceptual disturbance
      - Sedative, hypnotic, or anxiolytic withdrawal with perceptual disturbances
    - CC **F13.239** Sedative, hypnotic or anxiolytic dependence with withdrawal, unspecified
      - Sedative, hypnotic, or anxiolytic withdrawal without perceptual disturbances

F13.24 Sedative, hypnotic or anxiolytic dependence with sedative, hypnotic or anxiolytic-induced mood disorder
- Sedative, hypnotic, or anxiolytic use disorder, moderate, with sedative, hypnotic, or anxiolytic-induced bipolar or related disorder
- Sedative, hypnotic, or anxiolytic use disorder, moderate, with sedative, hypnotic, or anxiolytic-induced depressive disorder
- Sedative, hypnotic, or anxiolytic use disorder, severe, with sedative, hypnotic, or anxiolytic-induced bipolar or related disorder
- Sedative, hypnotic, or anxiolytic use disorder, severe, with sedative, hypnotic, or anxiolytic-induced depressive disorder

+ **F13.25** Sedative, hypnotic or anxiolytic dependence with sedative, hypnotic or anxiolytic-induced psychotic disorder
- CC **F13.250** Sedative, hypnotic or anxiolytic dependence with sedative, hypnotic or anxiolytic-induced psychotic disorder with delusions
- CC **F13.251** Sedative, hypnotic or anxiolytic dependence with sedative, hypnotic or anxiolytic-induced psychotic disorder with hallucinations
- CC **F13.259** Sedative, hypnotic or anxiolytic dependence with sedative, hypnotic or anxiolytic-induced psychotic disorder, unspecified

CC **F13.26** Sedative, hypnotic or anxiolytic dependence with sedative, hypnotic or anxiolytic-induced persisting amnestic disorder

CC **F13.27** Sedative, hypnotic or anxiolytic dependence with sedative, hypnotic or anxiolytic-induced persisting dementia
- Sedative, hypnotic, or anxiolytic use disorder, moderate, with sedative, hypnotic, or anxiolytic-induced major neurocognitive disorder
- Sedative, hypnotic, or anxiolytic use disorder, severe, with sedative, hypnotic, or anxiolytic-induced major neurocognitive disorder

+ **F13.28** Sedative, hypnotic or anxiolytic dependence with other sedative, hypnotic or anxiolytic-induced disorders
- CC **F13.280** Sedative, hypnotic or anxiolytic dependence with sedative, hypnotic or anxiolytic-induced anxiety disorder
- CC **F13.281** Sedative, hypnotic or anxiolytic dependence with sedative, hypnotic or anxiolytic-induced sexual dysfunction
- CC **F13.282** Sedative, hypnotic or anxiolytic dependence with sedative, hypnotic or anxiolytic-induced sleep disorder
- CC **F13.288** Sedative, hypnotic or anxiolytic dependence with other sedative, hypnotic or anxiolytic-induced disorder
  - Sedative, hypnotic, or anxiolytic use disorder, moderate, with sedative, hypnotic, or anxiolytic-induced mild neurocognitive disorder
  - Sedative, hypnotic, or anxiolytic use disorder, severe, with sedative, hypnotic, or anxiolytic-induced mild neurocognitive disorder

F13.29 Sedative, hypnotic or anxiolytic dependence with unspecified sedative, hypnotic or anxiolytic-induced disorder

+ **F13.9** Sedative, hypnotic or anxiolytic-related use, unspecified
  Excludes1: sedative, hypnotic or anxiolytic-related abuse (F13.1-)
  sedative, hypnotic or anxiolytic-related dependence (F13.2-)
  Review coding guideline C.5.b.3

F13.90 Sedative, hypnotic, or anxiolytic use, unspecified, uncomplicated

F13.91 Sedative, hypnotic or anxiolytic use, unspecified, in remission

+ **F13.92** Sedative, hypnotic or anxiolytic use, unspecified with intoxication
  Excludes1: sedative, hypnotic or anxiolytic use, unspecified with withdrawal (F13.93-)
- **F13.920** Sedative, hypnotic or anxiolytic use, unspecified with intoxication, uncomplicated
- CC **F13.921** Sedative, hypnotic or anxiolytic use, unspecified with intoxication delirium
  - Sedative, hypnotic, or anxiolytic-induced delirium
- **F13.929** Sedative, hypnotic or anxiolytic use, unspecified with intoxication, unspecified

+ **F13.93** Sedative, hypnotic or anxiolytic use, unspecified with withdrawal
  Excludes1: sedative, hypnotic or anxiolytic use, unspecified with intoxication (F13.92-)
- CC **F13.930** Sedative, hypnotic or anxiolytic use, unspecified with withdrawal, uncomplicated
- CC **F13.931** Sedative, hypnotic or anxiolytic use, unspecified with withdrawal delirium
- CC **F13.932** Sedative, hypnotic or anxiolytic use, unspecified with withdrawal with perceptual disturbances
- CC **F13.939** Sedative, hypnotic or anxiolytic use, unspecified with withdrawal, unspecified

F13.94 Sedative, hypnotic or anxiolytic use, unspecified with sedative, hypnotic or anxiolytic-induced mood disorder
- Sedative, hypnotic, or anxiolytic-induced bipolar or related disorder, without use disorder
- Sedative, hypnotic, or anxiolytic-induced depressive disorder, without use disorder

+ **F13.95** Sedative, hypnotic or anxiolytic use, unspecified with sedative, hypnotic or anxiolytic-induced psychotic disorder
- CC **F13.950** Sedative, hypnotic or anxiolytic use, unspecified with sedative, hypnotic or anxiolytic-induced psychotic disorder with delusions
- CC **F13.951** Sedative, hypnotic or anxiolytic use, unspecified with sedative, hypnotic or anxiolytic-induced psychotic disorder with hallucinations
- **F13.959** Sedative, hypnotic or anxiolytic use, unspecified with sedative, hypnotic or anxiolytic-induced psychotic disorder, unspecified
  - Sedative, hypnotic, or anxiolytic-induced psychotic disorder, without use disorder

F13.96 Sedative, hypnotic or anxiolytic use, unspecified with sedative, hypnotic or anxiolytic-induced persisting amnestic disorder

CC **F13.97** Sedative, hypnotic or anxiolytic use, unspecified with sedative, hypnotic or anxiolytic-induced persisting dementia
- Sedative, hypnotic, or anxiolytic-induced major neurocognitive disorder, without use disorder

+ **F13.98** Sedative, hypnotic or anxiolytic use, unspecified with other sedative, hypnotic or anxiolytic-induced disorders
- **F13.980** Sedative, hypnotic or anxiolytic use, unspecified with sedative, hypnotic or anxiolytic-induced anxiety disorder
  - Sedative, hypnotic, or anxiolytic-induced anxiety disorder, without use disorder
- **F13.981** Sedative, hypnotic or anxiolytic use, unspecified with sedative, hypnotic or anxiolytic-induced sexual dysfunction
  - Sedative, hypnotic, or anxiolytic-induced sexual dysfunction, without use disorder
- **F13.982** Sedative, hypnotic or anxiolytic use, unspecified with sedative, hypnotic or anxiolytic-induced sleep disorder
  - Sedative, hypnotic, or anxiolytic-induced sleep, without use disorder

F13.988 Sedative, hypnotic or anxiolytic use, unspecified with other sedative, hypnotic or anxiolytic-induced disorder
    Sedative, hypnotic, or anxiolytic-induced mild neurocognitive disorder

F13.99 Sedative, hypnotic or anxiolytic use, unspecified with unspecified sedative, hypnotic or anxiolytic-induced disorder

F14 Cocaine related disorders
Excludes2: other stimulant-related disorders (F15.-)

+ **F14.1** Cocaine abuse
    Excludes1: cocaine dependence (F14.2-)
               cocaine use, unspecified (F14.9-)

  F14.10 Cocaine abuse, uncomplicated
    Cocaine use disorder, mild

  F14.11 Cocaine abuse, in remission
    Cocaine use disorder, mild, in early remission
    Cocaine use disorder, mild, in sustained remission

+ **F14.12** Cocaine abuse with intoxication
  F14.120 Cocaine abuse with intoxication, uncomplicated
  CC F14.121 Cocaine abuse with intoxication with delirium
  F14.122 Cocaine abuse with intoxication with perceptual disturbance
  F14.129 Cocaine abuse with intoxication, unspecified

CC F14.13 Cocaine abuse, unspecified with withdrawal
    AHA CC: 4Q, 2020, 16-17

F14.14 Cocaine abuse with cocaine-induced mood disorder
    Cocaine use disorder, mild, with cocaine-induced bipolar or related disorder
    Cocaine use disorder, mild, with cocaine-induced depressive disorder

+ **F14.15** Cocaine abuse with cocaine-induced psychotic disorder
  CC F14.150 Cocaine abuse with cocaine-induced psychotic disorder with delusions
  CC F14.151 Cocaine abuse with cocaine-induced psychotic disorder with hallucinations
  F14.159 Cocaine abuse with cocaine-induced psychotic disorder, unspecified

+ **F14.18** Cocaine abuse with other cocaine-induced disorder
  F14.180 Cocaine abuse with cocaine-induced anxiety disorder
  F14.181 Cocaine abuse with cocaine-induced sexual dysfunction
  F14.182 Cocaine abuse with cocaine-induced sleep disorder
  F14.188 Cocaine abuse with other cocaine-induced disorder
    Cocaine use disorder, mild, with cocaine-induced obsessive compulsive or related disorder

F14.19 Cocaine abuse with unspecified cocaine-induced disorder

+ **F14.2** Cocaine dependence
    Excludes1: cocaine abuse (F14.1-)
               cocaine use, unspecified (F14.9-)
    Excludes2: cocaine poisoning (T40.5-)

CC F14.20 Cocaine dependence, uncomplicated
    Cocaine use disorder, moderate
    Cocaine use disorder, severe

F14.21 Cocaine dependence, in remission
    Cocaine use disorder, moderate, in early remission
    Cocaine use disorder, moderate, in sustained remission
    Cocaine use disorder, severe, in early remission
    Cocaine use disorder, severe, in sustained remission
    AHA CC: 2Q, 2017, 26-28

+ **F14.22** Cocaine dependence with intoxication
    Excludes1: cocaine dependence with withdrawal (F14.23)
  F14.220 Cocaine dependence with intoxication, uncomplicated
  CC F14.221 Cocaine dependence with intoxication delirium
  F14.222 Cocaine dependence with intoxication with perceptual disturbance
  CC F14.229 Cocaine dependence with intoxication, unspecified

CC F14.23 Cocaine dependence with withdrawal
    Excludes1: cocaine dependence with intoxication (F14.22-)

F14.24 Cocaine dependence with cocaine-induced mood disorder
    Cocaine use disorder, moderate, with cocaine-induced bipolar or related disorder
    Cocaine use disorder, moderate, with cocaine-induced depressive disorder
    Cocaine use disorder, severe, with cocaine-induced bipolar or related disorder
    Cocaine use disorder, severe, with cocaine-induced depressive disorder

+ **F14.25** Cocaine dependence with cocaine-induced psychotic disorder
  CC F14.250 Cocaine dependence with cocaine-induced psychotic disorder with delusions
  CC F14.251 Cocaine dependence with cocaine-induced psychotic disorder with hallucinations
  CC F14.259 Cocaine dependence with cocaine-induced psychotic disorder, unspecified

+ **F14.28** Cocaine dependence with other cocaine-induced disorder
  CC F14.280 Cocaine dependence with cocaine-induced anxiety disorder
  CC F14.281 Cocaine dependence with cocaine-induced sexual dysfunction
  CC F14.282 Cocaine dependence with cocaine-induced sleep disorder
  CC F14.288 Cocaine dependence with other cocaine-induced disorder
    Cocaine use disorder, moderate, with cocaine-induced obsessive compulsive or related disorder
    Cocaine use disorder, severe, with cocaine-induced obsessive compulsive or related disorder

F14.29 Cocaine dependence with unspecified cocaine-induced disorder

+ **F14.9** Cocaine use, unspecified
    Excludes1: cocaine abuse (F14.1-)
               cocaine dependence (F14.2-)
    Review coding guideline C.5.b.3

F14.90 Cocaine use, unspecified, uncomplicated
    AHA CC: 2Q, 2018, 10-11

F14.91 Cocaine use, unspecified, in remission

+ **F14.92** Cocaine use, unspecified with intoxication
  F14.920 Cocaine use, unspecified with intoxication, uncomplicated
  CC F14.921 Cocaine use, unspecified with intoxication delirium
  F14.922 Cocaine use, unspecified with intoxication with perceptual disturbance
  F14.929 Cocaine use, unspecified with intoxication, unspecified

CC F14.93 Cocaine use, unspecified with withdrawal
    AHA CC: 4Q, 2020, 16-17

F14.94 Cocaine use, unspecified with cocaine-induced mood disorder
    Cocaine-induced bipolar or related disorder, without use disorder
    Cocaine-induced depressive disorder, without use disorder

+ **F14.95** Cocaine use, unspecified with cocaine-induced psychotic disorder
  CC F14.950 Cocaine use, unspecified with cocaine-induced psychotic disorder with delusions
  CC F14.951 Cocaine use, unspecified with cocaine-induced psychotic disorder with hallucinations
  F14.959 Cocaine use, unspecified with cocaine-induced psychotic disorder, unspecified
    Cocaine-induced psychotic disorder, without use disorder

+ **F14.98** Cocaine use, unspecified with other specified cocaine-induced disorder
  F14.980 Cocaine use, unspecified with cocaine-induced anxiety disorder
    Cocaine-induced anxiety disorder, without use disorder

F14.981 Cocaine use, unspecified with cocaine-induced sexual dysfunction
Cocaine-induced sexual dysfunction, without use disorder
F14.982 Cocaine use, unspecified with cocaine-induced sleep disorder
Cocaine-induced sleep disorder, without use disorder
F14.988 Cocaine use, unspecified with other cocaine-induced disorder
Cocaine-induced obsessive compulsive or related disorder
F14.99 Cocaine use, unspecified with unspecified cocaine-induced disorder

F15 Other stimulant related disorders
Includes: amphetamine-related disorders
caffeine
Excludes2: cocaine-related disorders (F14.-)

+ **F15.1 Other stimulant abuse**
Excludes1: other stimulant dependence (F15.2-)
other stimulant use, unspecified (F15.9-)
- **F15.10** Other stimulant abuse, uncomplicated
Amphetamine type substance use disorder, mild
Other or unspecified stimulant use disorder, mild
- **F15.11** Other stimulant abuse, in remission
Amphetamine type substance use disorder, mild, in early remission
Amphetamine type substance use disorder, mild, in sustained remission
Other or unspecified stimulant use disorder, mild, in early remission
Other or unspecified stimulant use disorder, mild, in sustained remission
AHA CC: 3Q, 2021, 8
+ **F15.12 Other stimulant abuse with intoxication**
- **F15.120** Other stimulant abuse with intoxication, uncomplicated
- CC **F15.121** Other stimulant abuse with intoxication delirium
- **F15.122** Other stimulant abuse with intoxication with perceptual disturbance
Amphetamine or other stimulant use disorder, mild, with amphetamine or other stimulant intoxication, with perceptual disturbances
- **F15.129** Other stimulant abuse with intoxication, unspecified
Amphetamine or other stimulant use disorder, mild, with amphetamine or other stimulant intoxication, without perceptual disturbances
- CC **F15.13** Other stimulant abuse with withdrawal
AHA CC: 4Q, 2020, 16-17
- **F15.14** Other stimulant abuse with stimulant-induced mood disorder
Amphetamine or other stimulant use disorder, mild, with amphetamine or other stimulant-induced bipolar or related disorder
Amphetamine or other stimulant use disorder, mild, with amphetamine or other stimulant-induced depressive disorder
+ **F15.15 Other stimulant abuse with stimulant-induced psychotic disorder**
- CC **F15.150** Other stimulant abuse with stimulant-induced psychotic disorder with delusions
- CC **F15.151** Other stimulant abuse with stimulant-induced psychotic disorder with hallucinations
- **F15.159** Other stimulant abuse with stimulant-induced psychotic disorder, unspecified
+ **F15.18 Other stimulant abuse with other stimulant-induced disorder**
- **F15.180** Other stimulant abuse with stimulant-induced anxiety disorder
- **F15.181** Other stimulant abuse with stimulant-induced sexual dysfunction
- **F15.182** Other stimulant abuse with stimulant-induced sleep disorder
- **F15.188** Other stimulant abuse with other stimulant-induced disorder
Amphetamine or other stimulant use disorder, mild, with amphetamine or other stimulant-induced obsessive-compulsive or related disorder
- **F15.19** Other stimulant abuse with unspecified stimulant-induced disorder

+ **F15.2 Other stimulant dependence**
Excludes1: other stimulant abuse (F15.1-)
other stimulant use, unspecified (F15.9-)
- CC **F15.20** Other stimulant dependence, uncomplicated
Amphetamine type substance use disorder, moderate
Amphetamine type substance use disorder, severe
Other or unspecified stimulant use disorder, moderate
Other or unspecified stimulant use disorder, severe
- **F15.21** Other stimulant dependence, in remission
Amphetamine type substance use disorder, moderate, in early remission
Amphetamine type substance use disorder, moderate, in sustained remission
Amphetamine type substance use disorder, severe, in early remission
Amphetamine type substance use disorder, severe, in sustained remission
Other or unspecified stimulant use disorder, moderate, in early remission
Other or unspecified stimulant use disorder, moderate, in sustained remission
Other or unspecified stimulant use disorder, severe, in early remission
Other or unspecified stimulant use disorder, severe, in sustained remission
+ **F15.22 Other stimulant dependence with intoxication**
Excludes1: other stimulant dependence with withdrawal (F15.23)
- **F15.220** Other stimulant dependence with intoxication, uncomplicated
- CC **F15.221** Other stimulant dependence with intoxication delirium
- CC **F15.222** Other stimulant dependence with intoxication with perceptual disturbance
Amphetamine or other stimulant use disorder, moderate, with amphetamine or other stimulant intoxication, with perceptual disturbances
Amphetamine or other stimulant use disorder, severe, with amphetamine or other stimulant intoxication, with perceptual disturbances
- **F15.229** Other stimulant dependence with intoxication, unspecified
Amphetamine or other stimulant use disorder, moderate, with amphetamine or other stimulant intoxication, without perceptual disturbances
Amphetamine or other stimulant use disorder, severe, with amphetamine or other stimulant intoxication, without perceptual disturbances
- CC **F15.23** Other stimulant dependence with withdrawal
Amphetamine or other stimulant withdrawal
Excludes1: other stimulant dependence with intoxication (F15.22-)
- **F15.24** Other stimulant dependence with stimulant-induced mood disorder
Amphetamine or other stimulant use disorder, moderate, with amphetamine or other stimulant-induced bipolar or related disorder
Amphetamine or other stimulant use disorder, moderate, with amphetamine or other stimulant-induced depressive disorder
Amphetamine or other stimulant use disorder, severe, with amphetamine or other stimulant-induced bipolar or related disorder
Amphetamine or other stimulant use disorder, severe, with amphetamine or other stimulant-induced depressive disorder

- **+ F15.25** Other stimulant dependence with stimulant-induced psychotic disorder
  - **CC F15.250** Other stimulant dependence with stimulant-induced psychotic disorder with delusions
  - **CC F15.251** Other stimulant dependence with stimulant-induced psychotic disorder with hallucinations
  - **CC F15.259** Other stimulant dependence with stimulant-induced psychotic disorder, unspecified
- **+ F15.28** Other stimulant dependence with other stimulant-induced disorder
  - **CC F15.280** Other stimulant dependence with stimulant-induced anxiety disorder
  - **CC F15.281** Other stimulant dependence with stimulant-induced sexual dysfunction
  - **CC F15.282** Other stimulant dependence with stimulant-induced sleep disorder
  - **CC F15.288** Other stimulant dependence with other stimulant-induced disorder
    - Amphetamine or other stimulant use disorder, moderate, with amphetamine or other stimulant-induced obsessive-compulsive or related disorder
    - Amphetamine or other stimulant use disorder, severe, with amphetamine or other stimulant-induced obsessive-compulsive or related disorder
- **F15.29** Other stimulant dependence with unspecified stimulant-induced disorder
- **+ F15.9** Other stimulant use, unspecified
  - **Excludes1:** other stimulant abuse (F15.1-)
    other stimulant dependence (F15.2-)
  - Review coding guideline C.5.b.3
  - **F15.90** Other stimulant use, unspecified, uncomplicated
    - AHA CC: 4Q, 2022, 46
  - **F15.91** Other stimulant use, unspecified, in remission
  - **+ F15.92** Other stimulant use, unspecified with intoxication
    - **Excludes1:** other stimulant use, unspecified with withdrawal (F15.93)
    - **F15.920** Other stimulant use, unspecified with intoxication, uncomplicated
    - **CC F15.921** Other stimulant use, unspecified with intoxication delirium
      - Amphetamine or other stimulant-induced delirium
    - **F15.922** Other stimulant use, unspecified with intoxication with perceptual disturbance
    - **F15.929** Other stimulant use, unspecified with intoxication, unspecified
      - Caffeine intoxication
  - **CC F15.93** Other stimulant use, unspecified with withdrawal
    - Caffeine withdrawal
    - **Excludes1:** other stimulant use, unspecified with intoxication (F15.92-)
  - **F15.94** Other stimulant use, unspecified with stimulant-induced mood disorder
    - Amphetamine or other stimulant-induced bipolar or related disorder, without use disorder
    - Amphetamine or other stimulant-induced depressive disorder, without use disorder
  - **+ F15.95** Other stimulant use, unspecified with stimulant-induced psychotic disorder
    - **CC F15.950** Other stimulant use, unspecified with stimulant-induced psychotic disorder with delusions
    - **CC F15.951** Other stimulant use, unspecified with stimulant-induced psychotic disorder with hallucinations
    - **F15.959** Other stimulant use, unspecified with stimulant-induced psychotic disorder, unspecified
      - Amphetamine or other stimulant-induced psychotic disorder, without use disorder
  - **+ F15.98** Other stimulant use, unspecified with other stimulant-induced disorder
    - **F15.980** Other stimulant use, unspecified with stimulant-induced anxiety disorder
      - Amphetamine or other stimulant-induced anxiety disorder, without use disorder
      - Caffeine induced anxiety disorder, without use disorder
    - **F15.981** Other stimulant use, unspecified with stimulant-induced sexual dysfunction
      - Amphetamine or other stimulant-induced sexual dysfunction, without use disorder
    - **F15.982** Other stimulant use, unspecified with stimulant-induced sleep disorder
      - Amphetamine or other stimulant-induced sleep disorder, without use disorder
      - Caffeine induced sleep disorder, without use disorder
    - **F15.988** Other stimulant use, unspecified with other stimulant-induced disorder
      - Amphetamine or other stimulant-induced obsessive-compulsive or related disorder, without use disorder
  - **F15.99** Other stimulant use, unspecified with unspecified stimulant-induced disorder

F16 Hallucinogen related disorders
Includes: ecstasy
PCP
phencyclidine

- **+ F16.1** Hallucinogen abuse
  - **Excludes1:** hallucinogen dependence (F16.2-)
    hallucinogen use, unspecified (F16.9-)
  - **F16.10** Hallucinogen abuse, uncomplicated
    - Other hallucinogen use disorder, mild
    - Phencyclidine use disorder, mild
    - AHA CC: 4Q, 2018, 31
  - **F16.11** Hallucinogen abuse, in remission
    - Other hallucinogen use disorder, mild, in early remission
    - Other hallucinogen use disorder, mild, in sustained remission
    - Phencyclidine use disorder, mild, in early remission
    - Phencyclidine use disorder, mild, in sustained remission
  - **+ F16.12** Hallucinogen abuse with intoxication
    - **F16.120** Hallucinogen abuse with intoxication, uncomplicated
    - **CC F16.121** Hallucinogen abuse with intoxication with delirium
    - **F16.122** Hallucinogen abuse with intoxication with perceptual disturbance
    - **F16.129** Hallucinogen abuse with intoxication, unspecified
  - **F16.14** Hallucinogen abuse with hallucinogen-induced mood disorder
    - Other hallucinogen use disorder, mild, with other hallucinogen-induced bipolar or related disorder
    - Other hallucinogen use disorder, mild, with other hallucinogen-induced depressive disorder
    - Phencyclidine use disorder, mild, with other hallucinogen-induced bipolar or related disorder
    - Phencyclidine use disorder, mild, with other hallucinogen-induced depressive disorder
  - **+ F16.15** Hallucinogen abuse with hallucinogen-induced psychotic disorder
    - **CC F16.150** Hallucinogen abuse with hallucinogen-induced psychotic disorder with delusions
    - **CC F16.151** Hallucinogen abuse with hallucinogen-induced psychotic disorder with hallucinations
    - **F16.159** Hallucinogen abuse with hallucinogen-induced psychotic disorder, unspecified
  - **+ F16.18** Hallucinogen abuse with other hallucinogen-induced disorder
    - **F16.180** Hallucinogen abuse with hallucinogen-induced anxiety disorder
    - **F16.183** Hallucinogen abuse with hallucinogen persisting perception disorder (flashbacks)
    - **F16.188** Hallucinogen abuse with other hallucinogen-induced disorder

F16.19 Hallucinogen abuse with unspecified hallucinogen-induced disorder
+ **F16.2 Hallucinogen dependence**
Excludes1: *hallucinogen abuse (F16.1-)*
hallucinogen use, unspecified (F16.9-)
CC F16.20 Hallucinogen dependence, uncomplicated
  Other hallucinogen use disorder, moderate
  Other hallucinogen use disorder, severe
  Phencyclidine use disorder, moderate
  Phencyclidine use disorder, severe
F16.21 Hallucinogen dependence, in remission
  Other hallucinogen use disorder, moderate, in early remission
  Other hallucinogen use disorder, moderate, in sustained remission
  Other hallucinogen use disorder, severe, in early remission
  Other hallucinogen use disorder, severe, in sustained remission
  Phencyclidine use disorder, moderate, in early remission
  Phencyclidine use disorder, moderate, in sustained remission
  Phencyclidine use disorder, severe, in early remission
  Phencyclidine use disorder, severe, in sustained remission
+ F16.22 Hallucinogen dependence with intoxication
  F16.220 Hallucinogen dependence with intoxication, uncomplicated
  CC F16.221 Hallucinogen dependence with intoxication with delirium
  F16.229 Hallucinogen dependence with intoxication, unspecified
F16.24 Hallucinogen dependence with hallucinogen-induced mood disorder
  Other hallucinogen use disorder, moderate, with other hallucinogen-induced bipolar or related disorder
  Other hallucinogen use disorder, moderate, with other hallucinogen-induced depressive disorder
  Other hallucinogen use disorder, severe, with other hallucinogen-induced bipolar or related disorder
  Other hallucinogen use disorder, severe, with other hallucinogen-induced depressive disorder
  Phencyclidine use disorder, moderate, with other phencyclidine-induced bipolar or related disorder
  Phencyclidine use disorder, moderate, with other phencyclidine-induced depressive disorder
  Phencyclidine use disorder, severe, with other phencyclidine-induced bipolar or related disorder
  Phencyclidine use disorder, severe, with other phencyclidine-induced depressive disorder
+ F16.25 Hallucinogen dependence with hallucinogen-induced psychotic disorder
  CC F16.250 Hallucinogen dependence with hallucinogen-induced psychotic disorder with delusions
  CC F16.251 Hallucinogen dependence with hallucinogen-induced psychotic disorder with hallucinations
  CC F16.259 Hallucinogen dependence with hallucinogen-induced psychotic disorder, unspecified
+ F16.28 Hallucinogen dependence with other hallucinogen-induced disorder
  CC F16.280 Hallucinogen dependence with hallucinogen-induced anxiety disorder
  CC F16.283 Hallucinogen dependence with hallucinogen persisting perception disorder (flashbacks)
  CC F16.288 Hallucinogen dependence with other hallucinogen-induced disorder
  F16.29 Hallucinogen dependence with unspecified hallucinogen-induced disorder
+ **F16.9 Hallucinogen use, unspecified**
Excludes1: *hallucinogen abuse (F16.1-)*
hallucinogen dependence (F16.2-)
Review coding guideline C.5.b.3
F16.90 Hallucinogen use, unspecified, uncomplicated
F16.91 Hallucinogen use, unspecified, in remission
+ F16.92 Hallucinogen use, unspecified with intoxication
  F16.920 Hallucinogen use, unspecified with intoxication, uncomplicated
  CC F16.921 Hallucinogen use, unspecified with intoxication with delirium
    Other hallucinogen intoxication delirium
  F16.929 Hallucinogen use, unspecified with intoxication, unspecified
F16.94 Hallucinogen use, unspecified with hallucinogen-induced mood disorder
  Other hallucinogen-induced bipolar or related disorder, without use disorder
  Other hallucinogen-induced depressive disorder, without use disorder
  Phencyclidine-induced bipolar or related disorder, without use disorder
  Phencyclidine-induced depressive disorder, without use disorder
+ F16.95 Hallucinogen use, unspecified with hallucinogen-induced psychotic disorder
  CC F16.950 Hallucinogen use, unspecified with hallucinogen-induced psychotic disorder with delusions
  CC F16.951 Hallucinogen use, unspecified with hallucinogen-induced psychotic disorder with hallucinations
  F16.959 Hallucinogen use, unspecified with hallucinogen-induced psychotic disorder, unspecified
    Other hallucinogen-induced psychotic disorder, without use disorder
    Phencyclidine-induced psychotic disorder, without use disorder
+ F16.98 Hallucinogen use, unspecified with other specified hallucinogen-induced disorder
  F16.980 Hallucinogen use, unspecified with hallucinogen-induced anxiety disorder
    Other hallucinogen-induced anxiety disorder, without use disorder
    Phencyclidine-induced anxiety disorder, without use disorder
  F16.983 Hallucinogen use, unspecified with hallucinogen persisting perception disorder (flashbacks)
  F16.988 Hallucinogen use, unspecified with other hallucinogen-induced disorder
  F16.99 Hallucinogen use, unspecified with unspecified hallucinogen-induced disorder

F17 Nicotine dependence
Excludes1: *history of tobacco dependence (Z87.891)*
tobacco use NOS (Z72.0)
Excludes2: *tobacco use (smoking) during pregnancy, childbirth and the puerperium (O99.33-)*
toxic effect of nicotine (T65.2-)
Review coding guideline C.15.1.2
+ **F17.2 Nicotine dependence**
+ F17.20 Nicotine dependence, unspecified
  F17.200 Nicotine dependence, unspecified, uncomplicated
    Tobacco use disorder, mild
    Tobacco use disorder, moderate
    Tobacco use disorder, severe
    AHA CC: 4Q, 2013, 108; 1Q, 2016, 36-37
  F17.201 Nicotine dependence, unspecified, in remission
    Tobacco use disorder, mild, in early remission
    Tobacco use disorder, mild, in sustained remission
    Tobacco use disorder, moderate, in early remission
    Tobacco use disorder, moderate, in sustained remission
    Tobacco use disorder, severe, in early remission
    Tobacco use disorder, severe, in sustained remission
  CC F17.203 Nicotine dependence unspecified, with withdrawal
    Tobacco withdrawal

F17.208 Nicotine dependence, unspecified, with other nicotine-induced disorders
F17.209 Nicotine dependence, unspecified, with unspecified nicotine-induced disorders

+ **F17.21** Nicotine dependence, cigarettes
  F17.210 Nicotine dependence, cigarettes, uncomplicated
  AHA CC: 4Q, 2013, 109; 2Q, 2017, 28-29
  F17.211 Nicotine dependence, cigarettes, in remission
  Tobacco use disorder, cigarettes, mild, in early remission
  Tobacco use disorder, cigarettes, mild, in sustained remission
  Tobacco use disorder, cigarettes, moderate, in early remission
  Tobacco use disorder, cigarettes, moderate, in sustained remission
  Tobacco use disorder, cigarettes, severe, in early remission
  Tobacco use disorder, cigarettes, severe, in sustained remission
  CC **F17.213** Nicotine dependence, cigarettes, with withdrawal
  F17.218 Nicotine dependence, cigarettes, with other nicotine-induced disorders
  F17.219 Nicotine dependence, cigarettes, with unspecified nicotine-induced disorders

+ **F17.22** Nicotine dependence, chewing tobacco
  F17.220 Nicotine dependence, chewing tobacco, uncomplicated
  F17.221 Nicotine dependence, chewing tobacco, in remission
  Tobacco use disorder, chewing tobacco, mild, in early remission
  Tobacco use disorder, chewing tobacco, mild, in sustained remission
  Tobacco use disorder, chewing tobacco, moderate, in early remission
  Tobacco use disorder, chewing tobacco, moderate, in sustained remission
  Tobacco use disorder, chewing tobacco, severe, in early remission
  Tobacco use disorder, chewing tobacco, severe, in sustained remission
  CC **F17.223** Nicotine dependence, chewing tobacco, with withdrawal
  F17.228 Nicotine dependence, chewing tobacco, with other nicotine-induced disorders
  F17.229 Nicotine dependence, chewing tobacco, with unspecified nicotine-induced disorders

+ **F17.29** Nicotine dependence, other tobacco product
  F17.290 Nicotine dependence, other tobacco product, uncomplicated
  AHA CC: 2Q, 2017, 28-29
  F17.291 Nicotine dependence, other tobacco product, in remission
  Tobacco use disorder, other tobacco product, mild, in early remission
  Tobacco use disorder, other tobacco product, mild, in sustained remission
  Tobacco use disorder, other tobacco product, moderate, in early remission
  Tobacco use disorder, other tobacco product, moderate, in sustained remission
  Tobacco use disorder, other tobacco product, severe, in early remission
  Tobacco use disorder, other tobacco product, severe, in sustained remission
  CC **F17.293** Nicotine dependence, other tobacco product, with withdrawal
  F17.298 Nicotine dependence, other tobacco product, with other nicotine-induced disorders
  F17.299 Nicotine dependence, other tobacco product, with unspecified nicotine-induced disorders

F18 Inhalant related disorders
  Includes: volatile solvents

+ **F18.1** Inhalant abuse
  Excludes1: *inhalant dependence (F18.2-)*
  inhalant use, unspecified (F18.9-)
  F18.10 Inhalant abuse, uncomplicated
  Inhalant use disorder, mild
  F18.11 Inhalant abuse, in remission
  Inhalant use disorder, mild, in early remission
  Inhalant use disorder, mild, in sustained remission
+ **F18.12** Inhalant abuse with intoxication
  F18.120 Inhalant abuse with intoxication, uncomplicated
  CC **F18.121** Inhalant abuse with intoxication delirium
  F18.129 Inhalant abuse with intoxication, unspecified
  F18.14 Inhalant abuse with inhalant-induced mood disorder
  Inhalant use disorder, mild, with inhalant-induced depressive disorder
+ **F18.15** Inhalant abuse with inhalant-induced psychotic disorder
  CC **F18.150** Inhalant abuse with inhalant-induced psychotic disorder with delusions
  CC **F18.151** Inhalant abuse with inhalant-induced psychotic disorder with hallucinations
  F18.159 Inhalant abuse with inhalant-induced psychotic disorder, unspecified
  CC **F18.17** Inhalant abuse with inhalant-induced dementia
  Inhalant use disorder, mild, with inhalant-induced major neurocognitive disorder
+ **F18.18** Inhalant abuse with other inhalant-induced disorders
  F18.180 Inhalant abuse with inhalant-induced anxiety disorder
  F18.188 Inhalant abuse with other inhalant-induced disorder
  Inhalant use disorder, mild, with inhalant-induced mild neurocognitive disorder
  F18.19 Inhalant abuse with unspecified inhalant-induced disorder

+ **F18.2** Inhalant dependence
  Excludes1: *inhalant abuse (F18.1-)*
  inhalant use, unspecified (F18.9-)
  CC **F18.20** Inhalant dependence, uncomplicated
  Inhalant use disorder, moderate
  Inhalant use disorder, severe
  F18.21 Inhalant dependence, in remission
  Inhalant use disorder, moderate, in early remission
  Inhalant use disorder, moderate, in sustained remission
  Inhalant use disorder, severe, in early remission
  Inhalant use disorder, severe, in sustained remission
+ **F18.22** Inhalant dependence with intoxication
  F18.220 Inhalant dependence with intoxication, uncomplicated
  CC **F18.221** Inhalant dependence with intoxication delirium
  F18.229 Inhalant dependence with intoxication, unspecified
  F18.24 Inhalant dependence with inhalant-induced mood disorder
  Inhalant use disorder, moderate, with inhalant-induced depressive disorder
  Inhalant use disorder, severe, with inhalant-induced depressive disorder
+ **F18.25** Inhalant dependence with inhalant-induced psychotic disorder
  CC **F18.250** Inhalant dependence with inhalant-induced psychotic disorder with delusions
  CC **F18.251** Inhalant dependence with inhalant-induced psychotic disorder with hallucinations
  CC **F18.259** Inhalant dependence with inhalant-induced psychotic disorder, unspecified
  CC **F18.27** Inhalant dependence with inhalant-induced dementia
  Inhalant use disorder, moderate, with inhalant-induced major neurocognitive disorder
  Inhalant use disorder, severe, with inhalant-induced major neurocognitive disorder

- **+ F18.28 Inhalant dependence with other inhalant-induced disorders**
  - CC **F18.280** Inhalant dependence with inhalant-induced anxiety disorder
  - CC **F18.288** Inhalant dependence with other inhalant-induced disorder
    - Inhalant use disorder, moderate, with inhalant-induced mild neurocognitive disorder
    - Inhalant use disorder, severe, with inhalant-induced mild neurocognitive disorder
- **F18.29** Inhalant dependence with unspecified inhalant-induced disorder
- **+ F18.9 Inhalant use, unspecified**
  - *Excludes1:* inhalant abuse (F18.1-)
    inhalant dependence (F18.2-)
  - Review coding guideline C.5.b.3
  - **F18.90** Inhalant use, unspecified, uncomplicated
  - **F18.91** Inhalant use, unspecified, in remission
  - **+ F18.92** Inhalant use, unspecified with intoxication
    - **F18.920** Inhalant use, unspecified with intoxication, uncomplicated
    - CC **F18.921** Inhalant use, unspecified with intoxication with delirium
    - **F18.929** Inhalant use, unspecified with intoxication, unspecified
  - **F18.94** Inhalant use, unspecified with inhalant-induced mood disorder
    - Inhalant-induced depressive disorder
  - **+ F18.95** Inhalant use, unspecified with inhalant-induced psychotic disorder
    - CC **F18.950** Inhalant use, unspecified with inhalant-induced psychotic disorder with delusions
    - CC **F18.951** Inhalant use, unspecified with inhalant-induced psychoticdisorder with hallucinations
    - **F18.959** Inhalant use, unspecified with inhalant-induced psychotic disorder, unspecified
  - CC **F18.97** Inhalant use, unspecified with inhalant-induced persisting dementia
    - Inhalant-induced major neurocognitive disorder
  - **+ F18.98** Inhalant use, unspecified with other inhalant-induced disorders
    - **F18.980** Inhalant use, unspecified with inhalant-induced anxiety disorder
    - **F18.988** Inhalant use, unspecified with other inhalant-induced disorder
      - Inhalant-induced mild neurocognitive disorder
  - **F18.99** Inhalant use, unspecified with unspecified inhalant-induced disorder

F19 Other psychoactive substance related disorders
Includes: polysubstance drug use (indiscriminate drug use)

- **+ F19.1 Other psychoactive substance abuse**
  - *Excludes1:* other psychoactive substance dependence (F19.2-)
    other psychoactive substance use, unspecified (F19.9-)
  - **F19.10** Other psychoactive substance abuse, uncomplicated
    - Other (or unknown) substance use disorder, mild
  - **F19.11** Other psychoactive substance abuse, in remission
    - Other (or unknown) substance use disorder, mild, in early remission
    - Other (or unknown) substance use disorder, mild, in sustained remission
  - **+ F19.12** Other psychoactive substance abuse with intoxication
    - **F19.120** Other psychoactive substance abuse with intoxication, uncomplicated
    - CC **F19.121** Other psychoactive substance abuse with intoxication delirium
    - **F19.122** Other psychoactive substance abuse with intoxication with perceptual disturbances
    - **F19.129** Other psychoactive substance abuse with intoxication, unspecified
  - **+ F19.13** Other psychoactive substance abuse with withdrawal
    - *AHA CC: 4Q, 2020, 16-17*
    - CC **F19.130** Other psychoactive substance abuse with withdrawal, uncomplicated
    - CC **F19.131** Other psychoactive substance abuse with withdrawal delirium
    - CC **F19.132** Other psychoactive substance abuse with withdrawal with perceptual disturbance
    - CC **F19.139** Other psychoactive substance abuse with withdrawal, unspecified
  - **F19.14** Other psychoactive substance abuse with psychoactive substance-induced mood disorder
    - Other (or unknown) substance use disorder, mild, with other (or known) substance-induced bipolar or related disorder
    - Other (or unknown) substance use disorder, mild, with other (or known) substance-induced depressive disorder
  - **+ F19.15** Other psychoactive substance abuse with psychoactive substance-induced psychotic disorder
    - CC **F19.150** Other psychoactive substance abuse with psychoactive substance-induced psychotic disorder with delusions
    - CC **F19.151** Other psychoactive substance abuse with psychoactive substance-induced psychotic disorder with hallucinations
    - **F19.159** Other psychoactive substance abuse with psychoactive substance-induced psychotic disorder, unspecified
  - **F19.16** Other psychoactive substance abuse with psychoactive substance-induced persisting amnestic disorder
  - CC **F19.17** Other psychoactive substance abuse with psychoactive substance-induced persisting dementia
    - Other (or unknown) substance use disorder, mild, with other (or known) substance-induced major neurocognitive disorder
  - **+ F19.18** Other psychoactive substance abuse with other psychoactive substance-induced disorders
    - **F19.180** Other psychoactive substance abuse with psychoactive substance-induced anxiety disorder
    - **F19.181** Other psychoactive substance abuse with psychoactive substance-induced sexual dysfunction
    - **F19.182** Other psychoactive substance abuse with psychoactive substance-induced sleep disorder
    - **F19.188** Other psychoactive substance abuse with other psychoactive substance-induced disorder
      - Other (or unknown) substance use disorder, mild, with other (or known) substance-induced mild neurocognitive disorder
      - Other (or unknown) substance use disorder, mild, with other (or known) substance-induced obsessive-compulsive disorder
  - **F19.19** Other psychoactive substance abuse with unspecified psychoactive substance-induced disorder
- **+ F19.2 Other psychoactive substance dependence**
  - *Excludes1:* other psychoactive substance abuse (F19.1-)
    other psychoactive substance use, unspecified (F19.9-)
  - CC **F19.20** Other psychoactive substance dependence, uncomplicated
    - Other (or unknown) substance use disorder, moderate
    - Other (or unknown) substance use disorder, severe

- **F19.21** Other psychoactive substance dependence, in remission
  - Other (or unknown) substance use disorder, moderate, in early remission
  - Other (or unknown) substance use disorder, moderate, in sustained remission
  - Other (or unknown) substance use disorder, severe, in early remission
  - Other (or unknown) substance use disorder, severe, in sustained remission
- **+ F19.22** Other psychoactive substance dependence with intoxication
  - *Excludes1:* other psychoactive substance dependence with withdrawal (F19.23-)
  - **F19.220** Other psychoactive substance dependence with intoxication, uncomplicated
  - CC **F19.221** Other psychoactive substance dependence with intoxication delirium
  - CC **F19.222** Other psychoactive substance dependence with intoxication with perceptual disturbance
  - **F19.229** Other psychoactive substance dependence with intoxication, unspecified
- **+ F19.23** Other psychoactive substance dependence with withdrawal
  - *Excludes1:* other psychoactive substance dependence with intoxication (F19.22-)
  - CC **F19.230** Other psychoactive substance dependence with withdrawal, uncomplicated
  - CC **F19.231** Other psychoactive substance dependence with withdrawal delirium
  - CC **F19.232** Other psychoactive substance dependence with withdrawal with perceptual disturbance
  - CC **F19.239** Other psychoactive substance dependence with withdrawal, unspecified
- **F19.24** Other psychoactive substance dependence with psychoactive substance-induced mood disorder
  - Other (or known) substance use disorder, moderate, with other (or unknown) substance-induced bipolar or related disorder
  - Other (or unknown) substance use disorder, moderate, with other (or unknown) substance-induced depressive disorder
  - Other (or unknown) substance use disorder, severe, with other (or unknown) substance-induced bipolar or related disorder
  - Other (or unknown) substance use disorder, severe, with other (or unknown) substance-induced depressive disorder
- **+ F19.25** Other psychoactive substance dependence with psychoactive substance-induced psychotic disorder
  - CC **F19.250** Other psychoactive substance dependence with psychoactive substance-induced psychotic disorder with delusions
  - CC **F19.251** Other psychoactive substance dependence with psychoactive substance-induced psychotic disorder with hallucinations
  - CC **F19.259** Other psychoactive substance dependence with psychoactive substance-induced psychotic disorder, unspecified
- CC **F19.26** Other psychoactive substance dependence with psychoactive substance-induced persisting amnestic disorder
- CC **F19.27** Other psychoactive substance dependence with psychoactive substance-induced persisting dementia
  - Other (or unknown) substance use disorder, moderate, with other (or known) substance-induced major neurocognitive disorder
  - Other (or unknown) substance use disorder, severe, with other (or known) substance-induced major neurocognitive disorder
- **+ F19.28** Other psychoactive substance dependence with other psychoactive substance-induced disorders
  - CC **F19.280** Other psychoactive substance dependence with psychoactive substance-induced anxiety disorder
  - CC **F19.281** Other psychoactive substance dependence with psychoactive substance-induced sexual dysfunction
  - CC **F19.282** Other psychoactive substance dependence with psychoactive substance-induced sleep disorder
  - CC **F19.288** Other psychoactive substance dependence with other psychoactive substance-induced disorder
    - Other (or unknown) substance use disorder, moderate, with other (or known) substance-induced mild neurocognitive disorder
    - Other (or unknown) substance use disorder, moderate, with other (or known) substance-induced obsessive-compulsive disorder
    - Other (or unknown) substance use disorder, severe, with other (or known) substance-induced mild neurocognitive disorder
    - Other (or unknown) substance use disorder, severe, with other (or known) substance-induced obsessive-compulsive disorder
- **F19.29** Other psychoactive substance dependence with unspecified psychoactive substance-induced disorder
- **+ F19.9** Other psychoactive substance use, unspecified
  - *Excludes1:* other psychoactive substance abuse (F19.1-)
    other psychoactive substance dependence (F19.2-)
  - Review coding guideline C.5.b.3
  - **F19.90** Other psychoactive substance use, unspecified, uncomplicated
  - **F19.91** Other psychoactive substance use, unspecified, in remission
- **+ F19.92** Other psychoactive substance use, unspecified with intoxication
  - *Excludes1:* other psychoactive substance use, unspecified with withdrawal (F19.93)
  - **F19.920** Other psychoactive substance use, unspecified with intoxication, uncomplicated
  - CC **F19.921** Other psychoactive substance use, unspecified with intoxication with delirium
    - Other (or unknown) substance-induced delirium
  - **F19.922** Other psychoactive substance use, unspecified with intoxication with perceptual disturbance
  - **F19.929** Other psychoactive substance use, unspecified with intoxication, unspecified
- **+ F19.93** Other psychoactive substance use, unspecified with withdrawal
  - *Excludes1:* other psychoactive substance use, unspecified with intoxication (F19.92-)
  - CC **F19.930** Other psychoactive substance use, unspecified with withdrawal, uncomplicated
  - CC **F19.931** Other psychoactive substance use, unspecified with withdrawal delirium
  - CC **F19.932** Other psychoactive substance use, unspecified with withdrawal with perceptual disturbance

- **CC F19.939** Other psychoactive substance use, unspecified with withdrawal, unspecified
- **F19.94** Other psychoactive substance use, unspecified with psychoactive substance-induced mood disorder
  - Other (or unknown) substance-induced bipolar or related disorder, without use disorder
  - Other (or unknown) substance-induced depressive disorder, without use disorder
- **+ F19.95** Other psychoactive substance use, unspecified with psychoactive substance-induced psychotic disorder
  - **CC F19.950** Other psychoactive substance use, unspecified with psychoactive substance-induced psychotic disorder with delusions
  - **CC F19.951** Other psychoactive substance use, unspecified with psychoactive substance-induced psychotic disorder with hallucinations
  - **F19.959** Other psychoactive substance use, unspecified with psychoactive substance-induced psychotic disorder, unspecified
    - Other (or unknown) substance-induced psychotic disorder, without use disorder
- **F19.96** Other psychoactive substance use, unspecified with psychoactive substance-induced persisting amnestic disorder
- **CC F19.97** Other psychoactive substance use, unspecified with psychoactive substance-induced persisting dementia
  - Other (or unknown) substance-induced major neurocognitive disorder, without use disorder
- **+ F19.98** Other psychoactive substance use, unspecified with other psychoactive substance-induced disorders
  - **F19.980** Other psychoactive substance use, unspecified with psychoactive substance-induced anxiety disorder
    - Other (or unknown) substance-induced anxiety disorder, without use disorder
  - **F19.981** Other psychoactive substance use, unspecified with psychoactive substance-induced sexual dysfunction
    - Other (or unknown) substance-induced sexual dysfunction, without use disorder
  - **F19.982** Other psychoactive substance use, unspecified with psychoactive substance-induced sleep disorder
    - Other (or unknown) substance-induced sleep disorder, without use disorder
  - **F19.988** Other psychoactive substance use, unspecified with other psychoactive substance-induced disorder
    - Other (or unknown) substance-induced mild neurocognitive disorder, without use disorder
    - Other (or unknown) substance-induced obsessive-compulsive or related disorder, without use disorder
- **F19.99** Other psychoactive substance use, unspecified with unspecified psychoactive substance-induced disorder

Schizophrenia, schizotypal, delusional, and other non-mood psychotic disorders (F20-F29)

F20 Schizophrenia
Excludes1: brief psychotic disorder (F23)
cyclic schizophrenia (F25.0)
mood [affective] disorders with psychotic symptoms (F30.2, F31.2, F31.5, F31.64, F32.3, F33.3)
schizoaffective disorder (F25.-)
schizophrenic reaction NOS (F23)
Excludes2: schizophrenic reaction in:
alcoholism (F10.15-, F10.25-, F10.95-)
brain disease (F06.2)
epilepsy (F06.2)
psychoactive drug use (F11-F19 with .15, .25, .95)
schizotypal disorder (F21)

- **CC F20.0** Paranoid schizophrenia
  - Paraphrenic schizophrenia
  - **Excludes1:** involutional paranoid state (F22)
    paranoia (F22)
- **CC F20.1** Disorganized schizophrenia
  - Hebephrenic schizophrenia
  - Hebephrenia
- **CC F20.2** Catatonic schizophrenia
  - Schizophrenic catalepsy
  - Schizophrenic catatonia
  - Schizophrenic flexibilitas cerea
  - **Excludes1:** catatonic stupor (R40.1)
- **F20.3** Undifferentiated schizophrenia
  - Atypical schizophrenia
  - **Excludes1:** acute schizophrenia-like psychotic disorder (F23)
  - **Excludes2:** post-schizophrenic depression (F32.89)
- **CC F20.5** Residual schizophrenia
  - Restzustand (schizophrenic)
  - Schizophrenic residual state
- **+ F20.8** Other schizophrenia
  - **CC F20.81** Schizophreniform disorder
    - Schizophreniform psychosis NOS
  - **CC F20.89** Other schizophrenia
    - Cenesthopathic schizophrenia
    - Simple schizophrenia
- **F20.9** Schizophrenia, unspecified
  - AHA CC: 2Q, 2019, 32

F21 Schizotypal disorder
Borderline schizophrenia
Latent schizophrenia
Latent schizophrenic reaction
Prepsychotic schizophrenia
Prodromal schizophrenia
Pseudoneurotic schizophrenia
Pseudopsychopathic schizophrenia
Schizotypal personality disorder
Excludes2: Asperger's syndrome (F84.5)
schizoid personality disorder (F60.1)
Valid 3-character code, no further characters required

F22 Delusional disorders
Delusional dysmorphophobia
Involutional paranoid state
Paranoia
Paranoia querulans
Paranoid psychosis
Paranoid state
Paraphrenia (late)
Sensitiver Beziehungswahn
Excludes1: mood [affective] disorders with psychotic symptoms (F30.2, F31.2, F31.5, F31.64, F32.3, F33.3)
paranoid schizophrenia (F20.0)
Excludes2: paranoid personality disorder (F60.0)
paranoid psychosis, psychogenic (F23)
paranoid reaction (F23)
Valid 3-character code, no further characters required

CC F23 Brief psychotic disorder
Paranoid reaction
Psychogenic paranoid psychosis
Excludes2: mood [affective] disorders with psychotic symptoms (F30.2, F31.2, F31.5, F31.64, F32.3, F33.3)
Valid 3-character code, no further characters required

F24 Shared psychotic disorder
Folie à deux
Induced paranoid disorder
Induced psychotic disorder
Valid 3-character code, no further characters required

F25 Schizoaffective disorders
Excludes1: mood [affective] disorders with psychotic symptoms (F30.2, F31.2, F31.5, F31.64, F32.3, F33.3)
schizophrenia (F20.-)
- **F25.0** Schizoaffective disorder, bipolar type
  - Cyclic schizophrenia
  - Schizoaffective disorder, manic type
  - Schizoaffective disorder, mixed type
  - Schizoaffective psychosis, bipolar type
- **F25.1** Schizoaffective disorder, depressive type
  - Schizoaffective psychosis, depressive type

F25.8 Other schizoaffective disorders
F25.9 Schizoaffective disorder, unspecified
Schizoaffective psychosis NOS

F28 Other psychotic disorder not due to a substance or known physiological condition
Chronic hallucinatory psychosis
Other specified schizophrenia spectrum and other psychotic disorder
Valid 3-character code, no further characters required

F29 Unspecified psychosis not due to a substance or known physiological condition
Psychosis NOS
Unspecified schizophrenia spectrum and other psychotic disorder
Excludes1: mental disorder NOS (F99)
unspecified mental disorder due to known physiological condition (F09)
Valid 3-character code, no further characters required

Mood [affective] disorders (F30-F39)

F30 Manic episode
Includes: bipolar disorder, single manic episode
mixed affective episode
Excludes1: bipolar disorder (F31.-)
major depressive disorder, single episode (F32.-)
major depressive disorder, recurrent (F33.-)

+ F30.1 Manic episode without psychotic symptoms
  CC F30.10 Manic episode without psychotic symptoms, unspecified
  CC F30.11 Manic episode without psychotic symptoms, mild
  CC F30.12 Manic episode without psychotic symptoms, moderate
  CC F30.13 Manic episode, severe, without psychotic symptoms
CC F30.2 Manic episode, severe with psychotic symptoms
  Manic stupor
  Mania with mood-congruent psychotic symptoms
  Mania with mood-incongruent psychotic symptoms
F30.3 Manic episode in partial remission
F30.4 Manic episode in full remission
F30.8 Other manic episodes
  Hypomania
CC F30.9 Manic episode, unspecified
  Mania NOS

F31 Bipolar disorder
Includes: bipolar I disorder
bipolar type I disorder
manic-depressive illness
manic-depressive psychosis
manic-depressive reaction
seasonal bipolar disorder
Excludes1: bipolar disorder, single manic episode (F30.-)
major depressive disorder, single episode (F32.-)
major depressive disorder, recurrent (F33.-)
Excludes2: cyclothymia (F34.0)

CC F31.0 Bipolar disorder, current episode hypomanic
+ F31.1 Bipolar disorder, current episode manic without psychotic features
  CC F31.10 Bipolar disorder, current episode manic without psychotic features, unspecified
  CC F31.11 Bipolar disorder, current episode manic without psychotic features, mild
  CC F31.12 Bipolar disorder, current episode manic without psychotic features, moderate
  CC F31.13 Bipolar disorder, current episode manic without psychotic features, severe
CC F31.2 Bipolar disorder, current episode manic severe with psychotic features
  Bipolar disorder, current episode manic with mood-congruent psychotic symptoms
  Bipolar disorder, current episode manic with mood-incongruent psychotic symptoms
  Bipolar I disorder, current or most recent episode manic, with psychotic features
+ F31.3 Bipolar disorder, current episode depressed, mild or moderate severity
  CC F31.30 Bipolar disorder, current episode depressed, mild or moderate severity, unspecified
  CC F31.31 Bipolar disorder, current episode depressed, mild
  CC F31.32 Bipolar disorder, current episode depressed, moderate
CC F31.4 Bipolar disorder, current episode depressed, severe, without psychotic features
CC F31.5 Bipolar disorder, current episode depressed, severe, with psychotic features
  Bipolar disorder, current episode depressed with mood-incongruent psychotic symptoms
  Bipolar disorder, current episode depressed with mood-congruent psychotic symptoms
  Bipolar I disorder, current or most recent episode depressed, with psychotic features
+ F31.6 Bipolar disorder, current episode mixed
  CC F31.60 Bipolar disorder, current episode mixed, unspecified
  CC F31.61 Bipolar disorder, current episode mixed, mild
  CC F31.62 Bipolar disorder, current episode mixed, moderate
  CC F31.63 Bipolar disorder, current episode mixed, severe, without psychotic features
  CC F31.64 Bipolar disorder, current episode mixed, severe, with psychotic features
    Bipolar disorder, current episode mixed with mood-congruent psychotic symptoms
    Bipolar disorder, current episode mixed with mood-incongruent psychotic symptoms
+ F31.7 Bipolar disorder, currently in remission
  F31.70 Bipolar disorder, currently in remission, most recent episode unspecified
  F31.71 Bipolar disorder, in partial remission, most recent episode hypomanic
  F31.72 Bipolar disorder, in full remission, most recent episode hypomanic
  F31.73 Bipolar disorder, in partial remission, most recent episode manic
  F31.74 Bipolar disorder, in full remission, most recent episode manic
  F31.75 Bipolar disorder, in partial remission, most recent episode depressed
  F31.76 Bipolar disorder, in full remission, most recent episode depressed
  F31.77 Bipolar disorder, in partial remission, most recent episode mixed
  F31.78 Bipolar disorder, in full remission, most recent episode mixed
+ F31.8 Other bipolar disorders
  CC F31.81 Bipolar II disorder
    Bipolar disorder, type 2
  CC F31.89 Other bipolar disorder
    Recurrent manic episodes NOS
F31.9 Bipolar disorder, unspecified
  Manic depression
  AHA CC: 1Q, 2020, 23

F32 Depressive episode
Includes: single episode of agitated depression
single episode of depressive reaction
single episode of major depression
single episode of psychogenic depression
single episode of reactive depression
single episode of vital depression
Excludes1: bipolar disorder (F31.-)
manic episode (F30.-)
recurrent depressive disorder (F33.-)
Excludes2: adjustment disorder (F43.2)

CC F32.0 Major depressive disorder, single episode, mild
CC F32.1 Major depressive disorder, single episode, moderate
CC F32.2 Major depressive disorder, single episode, severe without psychotic features
CC F32.3 Major depressive disorder, single episode, severe with psychotic features
  Single episode of major depression with mood-congruent psychotic symptoms
  Single episode of major depression with mood-incongruent psychotic symptoms
  Single episode of major depression with psychotic symptoms
  Single episode of psychogenic depressive psychosis
  Single episode of psychotic depression
  Single episode of reactive depressive psychosis
F32.4 Major depressive disorder, single episode, in partial remission
F32.5 Major depressive disorder, single episode, in full remission

+ F32.8 **Other depressive episodes**
AHA CC: 4Q, 2016, 14
♀ F32.81 **Premenstrual dysphoric disorder**
Excludes1: *premenstrual tension syndrome (N94.3)*
F32.89 **Other specified depressive episodes**
Atypical depression
Post-schizophrenic depression
Single episode of 'masked' depression NOS
F32.9 **Major depressive disorder, single episode, unspecified**
Major depression NOS
AHA CC: 4Q, 2013, 107-108; 1Q, 2021, 10-11
F32.A **Depression, unspecified**
Depression NOS
Depressive disorder NOS
AHA CC: 4Q, 2021, 9-10

F33 **Major depressive disorder, recurrent**
Includes: recurrent episodes of depressive reaction
recurrent episodes of endogenous depression
recurrent episodes of major depression
recurrent episodes of psychogenic depression
recurrent episodes of reactive depression
recurrent episodes of seasonal affective disorder
recurrent episodes of seasonal depressive disorder
recurrent episodes of vital depression
Excludes1: *bipolar disorder (F31.-)*
manic episode (F30.-)
CC F33.0 **Major depressive disorder, recurrent, mild**
CC F33.1 **Major depressive disorder, recurrent, moderate**
CC F33.2 **Major depressive disorder, recurrent severe without psychotic features**
CC F33.3 **Major depressive disorder, recurrent, severe with psychotic symptoms**
Endogenous depression with psychotic symptoms
Major depressive disorder, recurrent, with psychotic features
Recurrent severe episodes of major depression with mood-congruent psychotic symptoms
Recurrent severe episodes of major depression with mood-incongruent psychotic symptoms
Recurrent severe episodes of major depression with psychotic symptoms
Recurrent severe episodes of psychogenic depressive psychosis
Recurrent severe episodes of psychotic depression
Recurrent severe episodes of reactive depressive psychosis
+ F33.4 **Major depressive disorder, recurrent, in remission**
CC F33.40 **Major depressive disorder, recurrent, in remission, unspecified**
F33.41 **Major depressive disorder, recurrent, in partial remission**
F33.42 **Major depressive disorder, recurrent, in full remission**
CC F33.8 **Other recurrent depressive disorders**
Recurrent brief depressive episodes
CC F33.9 **Major depressive disorder, recurrent, unspecified**
Monopolar depression NOS

F34 **Persistent mood [affective] disorders**
F34.0 **Cyclothymic disorder**
Affective personality disorder
Cycloid personality
Cyclothymia
Cyclothymic personality
F34.1 **Dysthymic disorder**
Depressive neurosis
Depressive personality disorder
Dysthymia
Neurotic depression
Persistent depressive disorder
Persistent anxiety depression
Excludes2: *anxiety depression (mild or not persistent) (F41.8)*
+ F34.8 **Other persistent mood [affective] disorders**
AHA CC: 4Q, 2016, 14
CC F34.81 **Disruptive mood dysregulation disorder**
CC F34.89 **Other specified persistent mood disorders**
CC F34.9 **Persistent mood [affective] disorder, unspecified**

F39 **Unspecified mood [affective] disorder**
Affective psychosis NOS
Valid 3-character code, no further characters required

Anxiety, dissociative, stress-related, somatoform and other nonpsychotic mental disorders (F40-F48)

F40 **Phobic anxiety disorders**
+ F40.0 **Agoraphobia**
F40.00 **Agoraphobia, unspecified**
F40.01 **Agoraphobia with panic disorder**
Panic disorder with agoraphobia
Excludes1: *panic disorder without agoraphobia (F41.0)*
F40.02 **Agoraphobia without panic disorder**
+ F40.1 **Social phobias**
Anthropophobia
Social anxiety disorder
Social anxiety disorder of childhood
Social neurosis
F40.10 **Social phobia, unspecified**
F40.11 **Social phobia, generalized**
+ F40.2 **Specific (isolated) phobias**
Excludes2: *dysmorphophobia (nondelusional) (F45.22)*
nosophobia (F45.22)
+ F40.21 **Animal type phobia**
F40.210 **Arachnophobia**
Fear of spiders
F40.218 **Other animal type phobia**
+ F40.22 **Natural environment type phobia**
F40.220 **Fear of thunderstorms**
F40.228 **Other natural environment type phobia**
+ F40.23 **Blood, injection, injury type phobia**
F40.230 **Fear of blood**
F40.231 **Fear of injections and transfusions**
F40.232 **Fear of other medical care**
F40.233 **Fear of injury**
+ F40.24 **Situational type phobia**
F40.240 **Claustrophobia**
F40.241 **Acrophobia**
F40.242 **Fear of bridges**
F40.243 **Fear of flying**
F40.248 **Other situational type phobia**
+ F40.29 **Other specified phobia**
F40.290 **Androphobia**
Fear of men
F40.291 **Gynephobia**
Fear of women
F40.298 **Other specified phobia**
F40.8 **Other phobic anxiety disorders**
Phobic anxiety disorder of childhood
F40.9 **Phobic anxiety disorder, unspecified**
Phobia NOS
Phobic state NOS

F41 **Other anxiety disorders**
Excludes2: *anxiety in:*
acute stress reaction (F43.0)
transient adjustment reaction (F43.2)
neurasthenia (F48.8)
psychophysiologic disorders (F45.-)
separation anxiety (F93.0)
F41.0 **Panic disorder [episodic paroxysmal anxiety]**
Panic attack
Panic state
Excludes1: *panic disorder with agoraphobia (F40.01)*
F41.1 **Generalized anxiety disorder**
Anxiety neurosis
Anxiety reaction
Anxiety state
Overanxious disorder
Excludes2: *neurasthenia (F48.8)*
F41.3 **Other mixed anxiety disorders**
F41.8 **Other specified anxiety disorders**
Anxiety depression (mild or not persistent)
Anxiety hysteria
Mixed anxiety and depressive disorder
F41.9 **Anxiety disorder, unspecified**
Anxiety NOS
AHA CC: 1Q, 2021, 10-11

F42 Obsessive-compulsive disorder
Excludes2: obsessive-compulsive personality (disorder) (F60.5)
obsessive-compulsive symptoms occurring in depression (F32-F33)
obsessive-compulsive symptoms occurring in schizophrenia (F20.-)
AHA CC: 4Q, 2016, 14-15
- **F42.2** Mixed obsessional thoughts and acts
- **F42.3** Hoarding disorder
- **F42.4** Excoriation (skin-picking) disorder
  Excludes1: factitial dermatitis (L98.1)
  other specified behavioral and emotional disorders with onset usually occurring in early childhood and adolescence (F98.8)
- **F42.8** Other obsessive compulsive disorder
  Anancastic neurosis
  Obsessive-compulsive neurosis
- **F42.9** Obsessive-compulsive disorder, unspecified

F43 Reaction to severe stress, and adjustment disorders
- **F43.0** Acute stress reaction
  Acute crisis reaction
  Acute reaction to stress
  Combat and operational stress reaction
  Combat fatigue
  Crisis state
  Psychic shock
- **+ F43.1** Post-traumatic stress disorder (PTSD)
  Traumatic neurosis
  - **F43.10** Post-traumatic stress disorder, unspecified
  - **F43.11** Post-traumatic stress disorder, acute
  - **F43.12** Post-traumatic stress disorder, chronic
- **+ F43.2** Adjustment disorders
  Culture shock
  Grief reaction
  Hospitalism in children
  Excludes2: separation anxiety disorder of childhood (F93.0)
  - **F43.20** Adjustment disorder, unspecified
  - **F43.21** Adjustment disorder with depressed mood
    AHA CC: 1Q, 2014, 25
  - **F43.22** Adjustment disorder with anxiety
  - **F43.23** Adjustment disorder with mixed anxiety and depressed mood
  - **F43.24** Adjustment disorder with disturbance of conduct
  - **F43.25** Adjustment disorder with mixed disturbance of emotions and conduct
  - **F43.29** Adjustment disorder with other symptoms
- **+ F43.8** Other reactions to severe stress
  Other specified trauma and stressor-related disorder
  AHA CC: 4Q, 2022, 17
  - **F43.81** Prolonged grief disorder
    Complicated grief
    Complicated grief disorder
    Persistent complex bereavement disorder
  - **F43.89** Other reactions to severe stress
- **F43.9** Reaction to severe stress, unspecified
  Trauma and stressor-related disorder, NOS
  Unspecified trauma and stressor-related disorder

F44 Dissociative and conversion disorders
Includes: conversion hysteria
conversion reaction
hysteria
hysterical psychosis
Excludes2: malingering [conscious simulation] (Z76.5)
- **F44.0** Dissociative amnesia
  Excludes1: amnesia NOS (R41.3)
  anterograde amnesia (R41.1)
  dissociative amnesia with dissociative fugue (F44.1)
  retrograde amnesia (R41.2)
  Excludes2: alcohol-or other psychoactive substance-induced amnestic disorder (F10, F13, F19 with .26, .96)
  amnestic disorder due to known physiological condition (F04)
  postictal amnesia in epilepsy (G40.-)
- **F44.1** Dissociative fugue
  Dissociative amnesia with dissociative fugue
  Excludes2: postictal fugue in epilepsy (G40.-)
- **F44.2** Dissociative stupor
  Excludes1: catatonic stupor (R40.1)
  stupor NOS (R40.1)
  Excludes2: catatonic disorder due to known physiological condition (F06.1)
  depressive stupor (F32, F33)
  manic stupor (F30, F31)
- **F44.4** Conversion disorder with motor symptom or deficit
  Conversion disorder with abnormal movement
  Conversion disorder with speech symptoms
  Conversion disorder with swallowing symptoms
  Conversion disorder with weakness/paralysis
  Dissociative motor disorders
  Psychogenic aphonia
  Psychogenic dysphonia
- **F44.5** Conversion disorder with seizures or convulsions
  Conversion disorder with attacks or seizures
  Dissociative convulsions
  AHA CC: 1Q, 2019, 19
- **F44.6** Conversion disorder with sensory symptom or deficit
  Conversion disorder with anesthesia or sensory loss
  Conversion disorder with special sensory symptoms
  Dissociative anesthesia and sensory loss
  Psychogenic deafness
- **F44.7** Conversion disorder with mixed symptom presentation
- **+ F44.8** Other dissociative and conversion disorders
  - **F44.81** Dissociative identity disorder
    Multiple personality disorder
  - **F44.89** Other dissociative and conversion disorders
    Ganser's syndrome
    Psychogenic confusion
    Psychogenic twilight state
    Trance and possession disorders
- **F44.9** Dissociative and conversion disorder, unspecified
  Dissociative disorder NOS

F45 Somatoform disorders
Excludes2: dissociative and conversion disorders (F44.-)
factitious disorders (F68.1-, F68.A)
hair-plucking (F63.3)
lalling (F80.0)
lisping (F80.0)
malingering [conscious simulation] (Z76.5)
nail-biting (F98.8)
psychological or behavioral factors associated with disorders or diseases classified elsewhere (F54)
sexual dysfunction, not due to a substance or known physiological condition (F52.-)
thumb-sucking (F98.8)
tic disorders (in childhood and adolescence) (F95.-)
Tourette's syndrome (F95.2)
trichotillomania (F63.3)
- **F45.0** Somatization disorder
  Briquet's disorder
  Multiple psychosomatic disorder
- **F45.1** Undifferentiated somatoform disorder
  Somatic symptom disorder
  Undifferentiated psychosomatic disorder
- **+ F45.2** Hypochondriacal disorders
  Excludes2: delusional dysmorphophobia (F22)
  fixed delusions about bodily functions or shape (F22)
  - **F45.20** Hypochondriacal disorder, unspecified
  - **F45.21** Hypochondriasis
    Hypochondriacal neurosis
    Illness anxiety disorder
  - **F45.22** Body dysmorphic disorder
    Dysmorphophobia (nondelusional)
    Nosophobia
  - **F45.29** Other hypochondriacal disorders
- **+ F45.4** Pain disorders related to psychological factors
  Excludes1: pain NOS (R52)
  - **F45.41** Pain disorder exclusively related to psychological factors
    Somatoform pain disorder (persistent)
    Review coding guideline C.5.a
  - **F45.42** Pain disorder with related psychological factors
    Code also associated acute or chronic pain (G89.-)
    Review coding guideline C.5.a

F45.8 Other somatoform disorders
Psychogenic dysmenorrhea
Psychogenic dysphagia, including 'globus hystericus'
Psychogenic pruritus
Psychogenic torticollis
Somatoform autonomic dysfunction
Teeth grinding
Excludes1: sleep related teeth grinding (G47.63)
F45.9 Somatoform disorder, unspecified
Psychosomatic disorder NOS

F48 Other nonpsychotic mental disorders
F48.1 Depersonalization-derealization syndrome
F48.2 Pseudobulbar affect
Involuntary emotional expression disorder
Code first underlying cause, if known, such as:
amyotrophic lateral sclerosis (G12.21)
multiple sclerosis (G35)
sequelae of cerebrovascular disease (I69.-)
sequelae of traumatic intracranial injury (S06.-)
F48.8 Other specified nonpsychotic mental disorders
Dhat syndrome
Neurasthenia
Occupational neurosis, including writer's cramp
Psychasthenia
Psychasthenic neurosis
Psychogenic syncope
F48.9 Nonpsychotic mental disorder, unspecified
Neurosis NOS

Behavioral syndromes associated with physiological disturbances and physical factors (F50-F59)

F50 Eating disorders
Excludes1: anorexia NOS (R63.0)
feeding problems of newborn (P92.-)
polyphagia (R63.2)
Excludes2: feeding difficulties (R63.3-)
feeding disorder in infancy or childhood (F98.2-)
+ F50.0 Anorexia nervosa
Excludes1: loss of appetite (R63.0)
psychogenic loss of appetite (F50.89)
CC F50.00 Anorexia nervosa, unspecified
CC F50.01 Anorexia nervosa, restricting type
CC F50.02 Anorexia nervosa, binge eating/purging type
Excludes1: bulimia nervosa (F50.2)
AHA CC: 1Q, 2022, 13-14
CC F50.2 Bulimia nervosa
Bulimia NOS
Hyperorexia nervosa
Excludes1: anorexia nervosa, binge eating/purging type (F50.02)
+ F50.8 Other eating disorders
Excludes2: pica of infancy and childhood (F98.3)
AHA CC: 4Q, 2016, 15-16
F50.81 Binge eating disorder
F50.82 Avoidant/restrictive food intake disorder
AHA CC: 4Q, 2017, 9
F50.89 Other specified eating disorder
Pica in adults
Psychogenic loss of appetite
F50.9 Eating disorder, unspecified
Atypical anorexia nervosa
Atypical bulimia nervosa
Feeding or eating disorder, unspecified
Other specified feeding disorder

F51 Sleep disorders not due to a substance or known physiological condition
Excludes2: organic sleep disorders (G47.-)
+ F51.0 Insomnia not due to a substance or known physiological condition
Excludes2: alcohol related insomnia (F10.182, F10.282, F10.982)
drug-related insomnia (F11.182, F11.282, F11.982, F13.182, F13.282, F13.982, F14.182, F14.282, F14.982, F15.182, F15.282, F15.982, F19.182, F19.282, F19.982)
insomnia NOS (G47.0-)
insomnia due to known physiological condition (G47.0-)
organic insomnia (G47.0-)
sleep deprivation (Z72.820)
F51.01 Primary insomnia
Idiopathic insomnia
F51.02 Adjustment insomnia
F51.03 Paradoxical insomnia
F51.04 Psychophysiologic insomnia
F51.05 Insomnia due to other mental disorder
Code also associated mental disorder
F51.09 Other insomnia not due to a substance or known physiological condition
+ F51.1 Hypersomnia not due to a substance or known physiological condition
Excludes2: alcohol related hypersomnia (F10.182, F10.282, F10.982)
drug-related hypersomnia (F11.182, F11.282, F11.982, F13.182, F13.282, F13.982, F14.182, F14.282, F14.982, F15.182, F15.282, F15.982, F19.182, F19.282, F19.982)
hypersomnia NOS (G47.10)
hypersomnia due to known physiological condition (G47.10)
idiopathic hypersomnia (G47.11, G47.12)
narcolepsy (G47.4-)
F51.11 Primary hypersomnia
F51.12 Insufficient sleep syndrome
Excludes1: sleep deprivation (Z72.820)
F51.13 Hypersomnia due to other mental disorder
Code also associated mental disorder
F51.19 Other hypersomnia not due to a substance or known physiological condition
F51.3 Sleepwalking [somnambulism]
Non-rapid eye movement sleep arousal disorders, sleepwalking type
F51.4 Sleep terrors [night terrors]
Non-rapid eye movement sleep arousal disorders, sleep terror type
F51.5 Nightmare disorder
Dream anxiety disorder
F51.8 Other sleep disorders not due to a substance or known physiological condition
F51.9 Sleep disorder not due to a substance or known physiological condition, unspecified
Emotional sleep disorder NOS

F52 Sexual dysfunction not due to a substance or known physiological condition
Excludes2: Dhat syndrome (F48.8)
F52.0 Hypoactive sexual desire disorder
Lack or loss of sexual desire
Male hypoactive sexual desire disorder
Sexual anhedonia
Excludes1: decreased libido (R68.82)
F52.1 Sexual aversion disorder
Sexual aversion and lack of sexual enjoyment
+ F52.2 Sexual arousal disorders
Failure of genital response
♂ F52.21 Male erectile disorder
Erectile disorder
Psychogenic impotence
Excludes1: impotence of organic origin (N52.-)
impotence NOS (N52.-)
♀ F52.22 Female sexual arousal disorder
Female sexual interest/arousal disorder
+ F52.3 Orgasmic disorder
Inhibited orgasm
Psychogenic anorgasmy
♀ F52.31 Female orgasmic disorder
♂ F52.32 Male orgasmic disorder
Delayed ejaculation
♂ F52.4 Premature ejaculation
♀ F52.5 Vaginismus not due to a substance or known physiological condition
Psychogenic vaginismus
Excludes2: vaginismus (due to a known physiological condition) (N94.2)
F52.6 Dyspareunia not due to a substance or known physiological condition
Genito-pelvic pain penetration disorder
Psychogenic dyspareunia
Excludes2: dyspareunia (due to a known physiological condition) (N94.1-)

- **F52.8** Other sexual dysfunction not due to a substance or known physiological condition
  - Excessive sexual drive
  - Nymphomania
  - Satyriasis
- **F52.9** Unspecified sexual dysfunction not due to a substance or known physiological condition
  - Sexual dysfunction NOS

F53 Mental and behavioral disorders associated with the puerperium, not elsewhere classified
Excludes1: mood disorders with psychotic features (F30.2, F31.2, F31.5, F31.64, F32.3, F33.3)
postpartum dysphoria (O90.6)
psychosis in schizophrenia, schizotypal, delusional, and other psychotic disorders (F20-F29)

AHA CC: 4Q, 2018, 8-9

- **F53.0** Postpartum depression
  - Postnatal depression, NOS
  - Postpartum depression, NOS
- **F53.1** Puerperal psychosis
  - Postpartum psychosis
  - Puerperal psychosis, NOS

F54 Psychological and behavioral factors associated with disorders or diseases classified elsewhere
Psychological factors affecting physical conditions
Code first the associated physical disorder, such as:
  - asthma (J45.-)
  - dermatitis (L23-L25)
  - gastric ulcer (K25.-)
  - mucous colitis (K58.-)
  - ulcerative colitis (K51.-)
  - urticaria (L50.-)

Excludes2: tension-type headache (G44.2)
Valid 3-character code, no further characters required

F55 Abuse of non-psychoactive substances
Excludes2: abuse of psychoactive substances (F10-F19)
- **F55.0** Abuse of antacids
- **F55.1** Abuse of herbal or folk remedies
- **F55.2** Abuse of laxatives
- **F55.3** Abuse of steroids or hormones
- **F55.4** Abuse of vitamins
- **F55.8** Abuse of other non-psychoactive substances

F59 Unspecified behavioral syndromes associated with physiological disturbances and physical factors
Psychogenic physiological dysfunction NOS
Valid 3-character code, no further characters required

Disorders of adult personality and behavior (F60-F69)

F60 Specific personality disorders

- **F60.0** Paranoid personality disorder
  - Expansive paranoid personality (disorder)
  - Fanatic personality (disorder)
  - Querulant personality (disorder)
  - Paranoid personality (disorder)
  - Sensitive paranoid personality (disorder)

  Excludes2: paranoia (F22)
  paranoia querulans (F22)
  paranoid psychosis (F22)
  paranoid schizophrenia (F20.0)
  paranoid state (F22)

- **F60.1** Schizoid personality disorder

  Excludes2: Asperger's syndrome (F84.5)
  delusional disorder (F22)
  schizoid disorder of childhood (F84.5)
  schizophrenia (F20.-)
  schizotypal disorder (F21)

- **F60.2** Antisocial personality disorder
  - Amoral personality (disorder)
  - Asocial personality (disorder)
  - Dissocial personality disorder
  - Psychopathic personality (disorder)
  - Sociopathic personality (disorder)

  Excludes1: conduct disorders (F91.-)
  Excludes2: borderline personality disorder (F60.3)

- **F60.3** Borderline personality disorder
  - Aggressive personality (disorder)
  - Emotionally unstable personality disorder
  - Explosive personality (disorder)

  Excludes2: antisocial personality disorder (F60.2)

- **F60.4** Histrionic personality disorder
  - Hysterical personality (disorder)
  - Psychoinfantile personality (disorder)
- **F60.5** Obsessive-compulsive personality disorder
  - Anankastic personality (disorder)
  - Compulsive personality (disorder)
  - Obsessional personality (disorder)

  Excludes2: obsessive-compulsive disorder (F42.-)

- **F60.6** Avoidant personality disorder
  - Anxious personality disorder
- **F60.7** Dependent personality disorder
  - Asthenic personality (disorder)
  - Inadequate personality (disorder)
  - Passive personality (disorder)
- **+ F60.8** Other specific personality disorders
  - **F60.81** Narcissistic personality disorder
  - **F60.89** Other specific personality disorders
    - Eccentric personality disorder
    - 'Haltlose' type personality disorder
    - Immature personality disorder
    - Passive-aggressive personality disorder
    - Psychoneurotic personality disorder
    - Self-defeating personality disorder
- **F60.9** Personality disorder, unspecified
  - Character disorder NOS
  - Character neurosis NOS
  - Pathological personality NOS

F63 Impulse disorders
Excludes2: habitual excessive use of alcohol or psychoactive substances (F10-F19)
impulse disorders involving sexual behavior (F65.-)

- **F63.0** Pathological gambling
  - Compulsive gambling
  - Gambling disorder

  Excludes1: gambling and betting NOS (Z72.6)
  Excludes2: excessive gambling by manic patients (F30, F31)
  gambling in antisocial personality disorder (F60.2)

- **F63.1** Pyromania
  - Pathological fire-setting

  Excludes2: fire-setting (by) (in):
  adult with antisocial personality disorder (F60.2)
  alcohol or psychoactive substance intoxication (F10-F19)
  conduct disorders (F91.-)
  mental disorders due to known physiological condition (F01-F09)
  schizophrenia (F20.-)

- **F63.2** Kleptomania
  - Pathological stealing

  Excludes1: shoplifting as the reason for observation for suspected mental disorder (Z03.8)
  Excludes2: depressive disorder with stealing (F31-F33)
  stealing due to underlying mental condition-code to mental condition
  stealing in mental disorders due to known physiological condition (F01-F09)

- **F63.3** Trichotillomania
  - Hair plucking

  Excludes2: other stereotyped movement disorder (F98.4)

- **+ F63.8** Other impulse disorders
  - **F63.81** Intermittent explosive disorder
  - **F63.89** Other impulse disorders
- **F63.9** Impulse disorder, unspecified
  - Impulse control disorder NOS

F64 Gender identity disorders
AHA CC: 4Q, 2016, 16

- **F64.0** Transsexualism
  - Gender identify disorder in adolescence and adulthood
  - Gender dysphoria in adolescents and adults
  - Gender incongruence in adolescents and adults
  - Transgender

  Excludes1: gender identity disorder of childhood (F64.2)

- **F64.1** Dual role transvestism
  Use additional code to identify sex reassignment status (Z87.890)

  Excludes1: gender identity disorder in childhood (F64.2)
  Excludes2: fetishistic transvestism (F65.1)

- **F64.2 Gender identity disorder of childhood**
    Gender incongruence of childhood
    Gender dysphoria in children
    Excludes1: gender identity disorder in adolescence and
              adulthood (F64.0)
    Excludes2: sexual maturation disorder (F66)
- **F64.8 Other gender identity disorders**
    Other specified gender dysphoria
- **F64.9 Gender identity disorder, unspecified**
    Gender dysphoria, unspecified
    Gender incongruence, unspecified
    Gender-role disorder NOS

F65 Paraphilias
- **F65.0 Fetishism**
    Fetishistic disorder
- **F65.1 Transvestic fetishism**
    Fetishistic transvestism
    Transvestic disorder
- **F65.2 Exhibitionism**
    Exhibitionistic disorder
- **F65.3 Voyeurism**
    Voyeuristic disorder
- **F65.4 Pedophilia**
    Pedophilic disorder
- **+ F65.5 Sadomasochism**
    - **F65.50 Sadomasochism, unspecified**
    - **F65.51 Sexual masochism**
        Sexual masochism disorder
    - **F65.52 Sexual sadism**
        Sexual sadism disorder
- **+ F65.8 Other paraphilias**
    - **F65.81 Frotteurism**
        Frotteuristic disorder
    - **F65.89 Other paraphilias**
        Necrophilia
        Other specified paraphilic disorder
- **F65.9 Paraphilia, unspecified**
    Paraphillic disorder, unspecified
    Sexual deviation NOS

F66 Other sexual disorders
Sexual maturation disorder
Sexual relationship disorder
Valid 3-character code, no further characters required

F68 Other disorders of adult personality and behavior
- **+ F68.1 Factitious disorder imposed on self**
    Compensation neurosis
    Elaboration of physical symptoms for psychological reasons
    Hospital hopper syndrome
    Münchausen's syndrome
    Peregrinating patient
    Excludes2: factitial dermatitis (L98.1)
               person feigning illness (with obvious
                   motivation) (Z76.5)
    AHA CC: 4Q, 2018, 9
    Review coding guideline C.5.c
    - CC **F68.10 Factitious disorder imposed on self, unspecified**
    - **F68.11 Factitious disorder imposed on self with
              predominantly psychological signs and symptoms**
    - CC **F68.12 Factitious disorder imposed on self with
              predominantly physical signs and symptoms**
    - **F68.13 Factitious disorder imposed on self with combined
              psychological and physical signs and symptoms**
- CC **F68.A Factitious disorder imposed on another**
    Factitious disorder by proxy
    Münchaüsen's by proxy
    AHA CC: 4Q, 2018, 9
    Review coding guideline C.5.c
- **F68.8 Other specified disorders of adult personality and behavior**
- **F69 Unspecified disorder of adult personality and behavior**
    Valid 3-character code, no further characters required

Intellectual Disabilities (F70-F79)
Code first any associated physical or developmental disorders
Excludes1: borderline intellectual functioning, IQ above 70 to 84 (R41.83)

F70 Mild intellectual disabilities
IQ level 50-55 to approximately 70
Mild mental subnormality
Valid 3-character code, no further characters required

F71 Moderate intellectual disabilities
IQ level 35-40 to 50-55
Moderate mental subnormality
Valid 3-character code, no further characters required

CC F72 Severe intellectual disabilities
IQ 20-25 to 35-40
Severe mental subnormality
Valid 3-character code, no further characters required

CC F73 Profound intellectual disabilities
IQ level below 20-25
Profound mental subnormality
Valid 3-character code, no further characters required

F78 Other intellectual disabilities
- **+ F78.A Other genetic related intellectual disability**
    AHA CC: 4Q, 2021, 10-11
    - **F78.A1 SYNGAP1-related intellectual disability**
        Code also, if applicable, any associated:
          autism spectrum disorder (F84.0)
          autistic disorder (F84.0)
          encephalopathy (G93.4-)
          epilepsy and recurrent seizures (G40.-)
          other pervasive developmental disorders (F84.8)
          pervasive developmental disorder, NOS (F84.9)
    - **F78.A9 Other genetic related intellectual disability**
        Code also, if applicable, any associated disorders

F79 Unspecified intellectual disabilities
Mental deficiency NOS
Mental subnormality NOS
Valid 3-character code, no further characters required

Pervasive and specific developmental disorders (F80-F89)

F80 Specific developmental disorders of speech and language
- **F80.0 Phonological disorder**
    Dyslalia
    Functional speech articulation disorder
    Lalling
    Lisping
    Phonological developmental disorder
    Speech articulation developmental disorder
    Speech-sound disorder
    Excludes1: speech articulation impairment due to aphasia
                NOS (R47.01)
               speech articulation impairment due to apraxia
                (R48.2)
    Excludes2: speech articulation impairment due to hearing
                loss (F80.4)
               speech articulation impairment due
                to intellectual disabilities (F70-F79)
               speech articulation impairment with expressive
                language developmental disorder (F80.1)
               speech articulation impairment with mixed
                receptive expressive language developmental
                disorder (F80.2)
- **F80.1 Expressive language disorder**
    Developmental dysphasia or aphasia, expressive type
    Excludes1: mixed receptive-expressive language disorder
                (F80.2)
               dysphasia and aphasia NOS (R47.-)
    Excludes2: acquired aphasia with epilepsy [Landau-
                Kleffner] (G40.80-)
               selective mutism (F94.0)
               intellectual disabilities (F70-F79)
               pervasive developmental disorders (F84.-)
- **F80.2 Mixed receptive-expressive language disorder**
    Developmental dysphasia or aphasia, receptive type
    Developmental Wernicke's aphasia
    Excludes1: central auditory processing disorder (H93.25)
               dysphasia or aphasia NOS (R47.-)
               expressive language disorder (F80.1)
               expressive type dysphasia or aphasia (F80.1)
               word deafness (H93.25)
    Excludes2: acquired aphasia with epilepsy [Landau-
                Kleffner] (G40.80-)
               pervasive developmental disorders (F84.-)
               selective mutism (F94.0)
               intellectual disabilities (F70-F79)

F80.4 Speech and language development delay due to hearing loss
Code also type of hearing loss (H90.-, H91.-)

+ **F80.8** Other developmental disorders of speech and language
- **F80.81** Childhood onset fluency disorder
  - Cluttering NOS
  - Stuttering NOS
  - *Excludes1:* adult onset fluency disorder (F98.5)
    - fluency disorder in conditions classified elsewhere (R47.82)
    - fluency disorder (stuttering) following cerebrovascular disease (I69. with final characters -23)
- **F80.82** Social pragmatic communication disorder
  - *Excludes1:* Asperger's syndrome (F84.5)
    - autistic disorder (F84.0)
  - AHA CC: 4Q, 2016, 16
- **F80.89** Other developmental disorders of speech and language
  - AHA CC: 1Q, 2017, 27-28
- **F80.9** Developmental disorder of speech and language, unspecified
  - Communication disorder NOS
  - Language disorder NOS

F81 Specific developmental disorders of scholastic skills
- **F81.0** Specific reading disorder
  - 'Backward reading'
  - Developmental dyslexia
  - Specific learning disorder, with impairment in reading
  - Specific reading retardation
  - *Excludes1:* alexia NOS (R48.0)
    - dyslexia NOS (R48.0)
- **F81.2** Mathematics disorder
  - Developmental acalculia
  - Developmental arithmetical disorder
  - Developmental Gerstmann's syndrome
  - Specific learning disorder, with impairment in mathematics
  - *Excludes1:* acalculia NOS (R48.8)
  - *Excludes2:* arithmetical difficulties associated with a reading disorder (F81.0)
    - arithmetical difficulties associated with a spelling disorder (F81.81)
    - arithmetical difficulties due to inadequate teaching (Z55.8)
+ **F81.8** Other developmental disorders of scholastic skills
  - **F81.81** Disorder of written expression
    - Specific learning disorder, with impairment in written expression
    - Specific spelling disorder
  - **F81.89** Other developmental disorders of scholastic skills
- **F81.9** Developmental disorder of scholastic skills, unspecified
  - Knowledge acquisition disability NOS
  - Learning disability NOS
  - Learning disorder NOS
  - AHA CC: 4Q, 2022, 41

F82 Specific developmental disorder of motor function
- Clumsy child syndrome
- Developmental coordination disorder
- Developmental dyspraxia
- *Excludes1:* abnormalities of gait and mobility (R26.-)
  - lack of coordination (R27.-)
- *Excludes2:* lack of coordination secondary to intellectual disabilities (F70-F79)
- Valid 3-character code, no further characters required

F84 Pervasive developmental disorders
Code also any associated medical condition and intellectual disabilities.
- CC **F84.0** Autistic disorder
  - Autism spectrum disorder
  - Infantile autism
  - Infantile psychosis
  - Kanner's syndrome
  - *Excludes1:* Asperger's syndrome (F84.5)
  - AHA CC: 1Q, 2017, 27-28; 4Q, 2022, 41
- CC **F84.2** Rett's syndrome
  - *Excludes1:* Asperger's syndrome (F84.5)
    - Autistic disorder (F84.0)
    - Other childhood disintegrative disorder (F84.3)

- CC **F84.3** Other childhood disintegrative disorder
  - Dementia infantilis
  - Disintegrative psychosis
  - Heller's syndrome
  - Symbiotic psychosis
  - Use additional code to identify any associated neurological condition.
  - *Excludes1:* Asperger's syndrome (F84.5)
    - Autistic disorder (F84.0)
    - Rett's syndrome (F84.2)
- CC **F84.5** Asperger's syndrome
  - Asperger's disorder
  - Autistic psychopathy
  - Schizoid disorder of childhood
- CC **F84.8** Other pervasive developmental disorders
  - Overactive disorder associated with intellectual disabilities and stereotyped movements
- CC **F84.9** Pervasive developmental disorder, unspecified
  - Atypical autism

F88 Other disorders of psychological development
- Developmental agnosia
- Global developmental delay
- Other specified neurodevelopmental disorder
- Valid 3-character code, no further characters required

F89 Unspecified disorder of psychological development
- Developmental disorder NOS
- Neurodevelopmental disorder NOS
- Valid 3-character code, no further characters required

Behavioral and emotional disorders with onset usually occurring in childhood and adolescence (F90-F98)

NOTE Codes within categories F90-F98 may be used regardless of the age of a patient. These disorders generally have onset within the childhood or adolescent years, but may continue throughout life or not be diagnosed until adulthood

F90 Attention-deficit hyperactivity disorders
- *Includes:* attention deficit disorder with hyperactivity
  - attention deficit syndrome with hyperactivity
- *Excludes2:* anxiety disorders (F40.-, F41.-)
  - mood [affective] disorders (F30-F39)
  - pervasive developmental disorders (F84.-)
  - schizophrenia (F20.-)
- **F90.0** Attention-deficit hyperactivity disorder, predominantly inattentive type
  - Attention-deficit/hyperactivity disorder, predominantly inattentive presentation
- **F90.1** Attention-deficit hyperactivity disorder, predominantly hyperactive type
  - Attention-deficit/hyperactivity disorder, predominantly hyperactive impulsive presentation
- **F90.2** Attention-deficit hyperactivity disorder, combined type
  - Attention-deficit/hyperactivity disorder, combined presentation
- **F90.8** Attention-deficit hyperactivity disorder, other type
- **F90.9** Attention-deficit hyperactivity disorder, unspecified type
  - Attention-deficit hyperactivity disorder of childhood or adolescence NOS
  - Attention-deficit hyperactivity disorder NOS

F91 Conduct disorders
- *Excludes1:* antisocial behavior (Z72.81-)
  - antisocial personality disorder (F60.2)
- *Excludes2:* conduct problems associated with attention-deficit hyperactivity disorder (F90.-)
  - mood [affective] disorders (F30-F39)
  - pervasive developmental disorders (F84.-)
  - schizophrenia (F20.-)
- **F91.0** Conduct disorder confined to family context
- **F91.1** Conduct disorder, childhood-onset type
  - Unsocialized conduct disorder
  - Conduct disorder, solitary aggressive type
  - Unsocialized aggressive disorder
- **F91.2** Conduct disorder, adolescent-onset type
  - Socialized conduct disorder
  - Conduct disorder, group type
- **F91.3** Oppositional defiant disorder

F91.8 Other conduct disorders
- Other specified conduct disorder
- Other specified disruptive disorder

F91.9 Conduct disorder, unspecified
- Behavioral disorder NOS
- Conduct disorder NOS
- Disruptive behavior disorder NOS
- Disruptive disorder NOS

F93 Emotional disorders with onset specific to childhood

F93.0 Separation anxiety disorder of childhood
- *Excludes2:* mood [affective] disorders (F30-F39)
  - nonpsychotic mental disorders (F40-F48)
  - phobic anxiety disorder of childhood (F40.8)
  - social phobia (F40.1)

F93.8 Other childhood emotional disorders
- Identity disorder
- *Excludes2:* gender identity disorder of childhood (F64.2)

F93.9 Childhood emotional disorder, unspecified

F94 Disorders of social functioning with onset specific to childhood and adolescence

F94.0 Selective mutism
- Elective mutism
- *Excludes2:* pervasive developmental disorders (F84.-)
  - schizophrenia (F20.-)
  - specific developmental disorders of speech and language (F80.-)
  - transient mutism as part of separation anxiety in young children (F93.0)

F94.1 Reactive attachment disorder of childhood
- Use additional code to identify any associated failure to thrive or growth retardation
- *Excludes1:* disinhibited attachment disorder of childhood (F94.2)
  - normal variation in pattern of selective attachment
- *Excludes2:* Asperger's syndrome (F84.5)
  - maltreatment syndromes (T74.-)
  - sexual or physical abuse in childhood, resulting in psychosocial problems (Z62.81-)

F94.2 Disinhibited attachment disorder of childhood
- Affectionless psychopathy
- Institutional syndrome
- *Excludes1:* reactive attachment disorder of childhood (F94.1)
- *Excludes2:* Asperger's syndrome (F84.5)
  - attention-deficit hyperactivity disorders (F90.-)
  - hospitalism in children (F43.2-)

F94.8 Other childhood disorders of social functioning

F94.9 Childhood disorder of social functioning, unspecified

F95 Tic disorder

F95.0 Transient tic disorder
- Provisional tic disorder

F95.1 Chronic motor or vocal tic disorder

F95.2 Tourette's disorder
- Combined vocal and multiple motor tic disorder [de la Tourette]
- Tourette's syndrome

F95.8 Other tic disorders

F95.9 Tic disorder, unspecified
- Tic NOS

F98 Other behavioral and emotional disorders with onset usually occurring in childhood and adolescence

Excludes2: breath-holding spells (R06.89)
- gender identity disorder of childhood (F64.2)
- Kleine-Levin syndrome (G47.13)
- obsessive-compulsive disorder (F42.-)
- sleep disorders not due to a substance or known physiological condition (F51.-)

F98.0 Enuresis not due to a substance or known physiological condition
- Enuresis (primary) (secondary) of nonorganic origin
- Functional enuresis
- Psychogenic enuresis
- Urinary incontinence of nonorganic origin
- *Excludes1:* enuresis NOS (R32)

F98.1 Encopresis not due to a substance or known physiological condition
- Functional encopresis
- Incontinence of feces of nonorganic origin
- Psychogenic encopresis
- Use additional code to identify the cause of any coexisting constipation.
- *Excludes1:* encopresis NOS (R15.-)

+ **F98.2** Other feeding disorders of infancy and childhood
- *Excludes2:* anorexia nervosa and other eating disorders (F50.-)
  - feeding difficulties (R63.3-)
  - feeding problems of newborn (P92.-)
  - pica of infancy or childhood (F98.3)

   F98.21 Rumination disorder of infancy

   F98.29 Other feeding disorders of infancy and early childhood

F98.3 Pica of infancy and childhood

F98.4 Stereotyped movement disorders
- Stereotype/habit disorder
- *Excludes1:* abnormal involuntary movements (R25.-)
- *Excludes2:* compulsions in obsessive-compulsive disorder (F42.-)
  - hair plucking (F63.3)
  - movement disorders of organic origin (G20-G25)
  - nail-biting (F98.8)
  - nose-picking (F98.8)
  - stereotypies that are part of a broader psychiatric condition (F01-F95)
  - thumb-sucking (F98.8)
  - tic disorders (F95.-)
  - trichotillomania (F63.3)

F98.5 Adult onset fluency disorder
- *Excludes1:* childhood onset fluency disorder (F80.81)
  - dysphasia (R47.02)
  - fluency disorder in conditions classified elsewhere (R47.82)
  - fluency disorder (stuttering) following cerebrovascular disease (I69. with final characters -23)
  - tic disorders (F95.-)

F98.8 Other specified behavioral and emotional disorders with onset usually occurring in childhood and adolescence
- Excessive masturbation
- Nail-biting
- Nose-picking
- Thumb-sucking

F98.9 Unspecified behavioral and emotional disorders with onset usually occurring in childhood and adolescence

Unspecified mental disorder (F99)

F99 Mental disorder, not otherwise specified
- Mental illness NOS
- *Excludes1:* unspecified mental disorder due to known physiological condition (F09)
- Valid 3-character code, no further characters required

Chapter 6: Diseases of the Nervous System (G00-G99)

Excludes2: *certain conditions originating in the perinatal period (P04-P96)*
certain infectious and parasitic diseases (A00-B99)
complications of pregnancy, childbirth and the puerperium (O00-O9A)
congenital malformations, deformations, and chromosomal abnormalities (Q00-Q99)
endocrine, nutritional and metabolic diseases (E00-E88)
injury, poisoning and certain other consequences of external causes (S00-T88)
neoplasms (C00-D49)
symptoms, signs and abnormal clinical and laboratory findings, not elsewhere classified (R00-R94)

This chapter contains the following category blocks:
- G00-G09 Inflammatory diseases of the central nervous system
- G10-G14 Systemic atrophies primarily affecting the central nervous system
- G20-G26 Extrapyramidal and movement disorders
- G30-G32 Other degenerative diseases of the nervous system
- G35-G37 Demyelinating diseases of the central nervous system
- G40-G47 Episodic and paroxysmal disorders
- G50-G59 Nerve, nerve root and plexus disorders
- G60-G65 Polyneuropathies and other disorders of the peripheral nervous system
- G70-G73 Diseases of myoneural junction and muscle
- G80-G83 Cerebral palsy and other paralytic syndromes
- G89-G99 Other disorders of the nervous system

C. Chapter-Specific Coding Guidelines

In addition to general coding guidelines, there are guidelines for specific diagnoses and/or conditions in the classification. Unless otherwise indicated, these guidelines apply to all health care settings. Please refer to Section II for guidelines on the selection of principal diagnosis.

6. Chapter 6: Diseases of the Nervous System (G00-G99)

a. Dominant/nondominant side

Codes from category G81, Hemiplegia and hemiparesis, and subcategories, G83.1, Monoplegia of lower limb, G83.2, Monoplegia of upper limb, and G83.3, Monoplegia, unspecified, identify whether the dominant or nondominant side is affected. Should the affected side be documented, but not specified as dominant or nondominant, and the classification system does not indicate a default, code selection is as follows:

- For ambidextrous patients, the default should be dominant.
- If the left side is affected, the default is non-dominant.
- If the right side is affected, the default is dominant.

b. Pain-Category G89

1) General coding information

Codes in category G89, Pain, not elsewhere classified, may be used in conjunction with codes from other categories and chapters to provide more detail about acute or chronic pain and neoplasm-related pain, unless otherwise indicated below.

If the pain is not specified as acute or chronic, post-thoracotomy, post procedural, or neoplasm-related, do not assign codes from category G89.

A code from category G89 should not be assigned if the underlying (definitive) diagnosis is known, unless the reason for the encounter is pain control/management and not management of the underlying condition.

When an admission or encounter is for a procedure aimed at treating the underlying condition (e.g., spinal fusion, kyphoplasty), a code for the underlying condition (e.g., vertebral fracture, spinal stenosis) should be assigned as the principal diagnosis. No code from category G89 should be assigned.

(a) Category G89 Codes as Principal or First-Listed Diagnosis

Category G89 codes are acceptable as principal diagnosis or the first-listed code:

- When pain control or pain management is the reason for the admission/encounter (e.g., a patient with displaced intervertebral disc, nerve impingement and severe back pain presents for injection of steroid into the spinal canal). The underlying cause of the pain should be reported as an additional diagnosis, if known.
- When a patient is admitted for the insertion of a neurostimulator for pain control, assign the appropriate pain code as the principal or first-listed diagnosis. When an admission or encounter is for a procedure aimed at treating the underlying condition and a neurostimulator is inserted for pain control during the same admission/encounter, a code for the underlying condition should be assigned as the principal diagnosis and the appropriate pain code should be assigned as a secondary diagnosis.

(b) Use of Category G89 Codes in Conjunction with Site Specific Pain Codes

####### (i) Assigning Category G89 and Site-Specific Pain Codes

Codes from category G89 may be used in conjunction with codes that identify the site of pain (including codes from chapter 18) if the category G89 code provides additional information. For example, if the code describes the site of the pain, but does not fully describe whether the pain is acute or chronic, then both codes should be assigned.

####### (ii) Sequencing of Category G89 Codes with Site-Specific Pain Codes

The sequencing of category G89 codes with site-specific pain codes (including chapter 18 codes), is dependent on the circumstances of the encounter/admission as follows:

- If the encounter is for pain control or pain management, assign the code from category G89 followed by the code identifying the specific site of pain (e.g., encounter for pain management for acute neck pain from trauma is assigned code G89.11, Acute pain due to trauma, followed by code M54.2, Cervicalgia, to identify the site of pain).
- If the encounter is for any other reason except pain control or pain management, and a related definitive diagnosis has not been established (confirmed) by the provider, assign the code for the specific site of pain first, followed by the appropriate code from category G89.

2) Pain due to devices, implants and grafts

See Section I.C.19. Pain due to medical devices

3) Postoperative Pain

The provider's documentation should be used to guide the coding of postoperative pain, as well as *Section III. Reporting Additional Diagnoses and Section IV. Diagnostic Coding* and *Reporting in the Outpatient Setting.*

The default for post-thoracotomy and other postoperative pain not specified as acute or chronic is the code for the acute form.

Routine or expected postoperative pain immediately after surgery should not be coded.

(a) Postoperative pain not associated with specific postoperative complication

Postoperative pain not associated with a specific postoperative complication is assigned to the appropriate postoperative pain code in category G89.

(b) Postoperative pain associated with specific postoperative complication

Postoperative pain associated with a specific postoperative complication (such as painful wire sutures) is assigned to the appropriate code(s) found in Chapter 19, Injury, poisoning, and certain other consequences of external causes. If appropriate, use additional code(s) from category G89 to identify acute or chronic pain (G89.18 or G89.28).

4) Chronic pain

Chronic pain is classified to subcategory G89.2. There is no time frame defining when pain becomes chronic pain. The provider's documentation should be used to guide use of these codes.

5) Neoplasm Related Pain

Code G89.3 is assigned to pain documented as being related, associated or due to cancer, primary or secondary malignancy, or tumor. This code is assigned regardless of whether the pain is acute or chronic.

This code may be assigned as the principal or first-listed code when the stated reason for the admission/encounter is documented as pain control/pain management. The underlying neoplasm should be reported as an additional diagnosis.

When the reason for the admission/encounter is management of the neoplasm and the pain associated with the neoplasm is also documented, code G89.3 may be assigned as an additional diagnosis. It is not necessary to assign an additional code for the site of the pain.

See Section I.C.2 for instructions on the sequencing of neoplasms for all other stated reasons for the admission/encounter (except for pain control/pain management).

6) Chronic pain syndrome

Central pain syndrome (G89.0) and chronic pain syndrome (G89.4) are different than the term "chronic pain," and therefore codes should only be used when the provider has specifically documented this condition.

See Section I.C.5. Pain disorders related to psychological factors

Inflammatory diseases of the central nervous system (G00-G09)

G00 Bacterial meningitis, not elsewhere classified
Includes: bacterial arachnoiditis
bacterial leptomeningitis
bacterial meningitis
bacterial pachymeningitis
Excludes1: bacterial meningoencephalitis (G04.2)
bacterial meningomyelitis (G04.2)

MCC G00.0 Hemophilus meningitis
Meningitis due to Hemophilus influenzae

MCC G00.1 Pneumococcal meningitis
Mengtitis due to Streptococcal pneumoniae

MCC G00.2 Streptococcal meningitis
Use additional code to further identify organism (B95.0-B95.5)

MCC G00.3 Staphylococcal meningitis
Use additional code to further identify organism (B95.61-B95.8)

MCC G00.8 Other bacterial meningitis
Meningitis due to Escherichia coli
Meningitis due to Friedländer's bacillus
Meningitis due to Klebsiella
Use additional code to further identify organism (B96.-)

MCC G00.9 Bacterial meningitis, unspecified
Meningitis due to gram-negative bacteria, unspecified
Purulent meningitis NOS
Pyogenic meningitis NOS
Suppurative meningitis NOS

MCC G01 Meningitis in bacterial diseases classified elsewhere
Code first underlying disease
Excludes1: meningitis (in):
gonococcal (A54.81)
leptospirosis (A27.81)
listeriosis (A32.11)
Lyme disease (A69.21)
meningococcal (A39.0)
neurosyphilis (A52.13)
tuberculosis (A17.0)
meningoencephalitis and meningomyelitis in bacterial diseases classified elsewhere (G05)
Valid 3-character code, no further characters required

MCC G02 Meningitis in other infectious and parasitic diseases classified elsewhere
Code first underlying disease, such as:
African trypanosomiasis (B56.-)
poliovirus infection (A80.-)
Excludes1: candidal meningitis (B37.5)
coccidioidomycosis meningitis (B38.4)
cryptococcal meningitis (B45.1)
herpesviral [herpes simplex] meningitis (B00.3)
infectious mononucleosis complicated by meningitis (B27.- with fifth character 2)
measles complicated by meningitis (B05.1)
meningoencephalitis and meningomyelitis in other infectious and parasitic diseases classified elsewhere (G05)
mumps meningitis (B26.1)
rubella meningitis (B06.02)
varicella [chickenpox] meningitis (B01.0)
zoster meningitis (B02.1)
Valid 3-character code, no further characters required

G03 Meningitis due to other and unspecified causes
Includes: arachnoiditis NOS
leptomeningitis NOS
meningitis NOS
pachymeningitis NOS
Excludes1: meningoencephalitis (G04.-)
meningomyelitis (G04.-)

MCC G03.0 Nonpyogenic meningitis
Aseptic meningitis
Nonbacterial meningitis

CC G03.1 Chronic meningitis

CC G03.2 Benign recurrent meningitis [Mollaret]

MCC G03.8 Meningitis due to other specified causes

MCC G03.9 Meningitis, unspecified
Arachnoiditis (spinal) NOS

G04 Encephalitis, myelitis and encephalomyelitis
Includes: acute ascending myelitis
meningoencephalitis
meningomyelitis
Excludes1: encephalopathy NOS (G93.40)
Excludes2: acute transverse myelitis (G37.3)
alcoholic encephalopathy (G31.2)
multiple sclerosis (G35)
myalgic encephalomyelitis (G93.32)
subacute necrotizing myelitis (G37.4)
toxic encephalitis (G92.8)
toxic encephalopathy (G92.8)

+ G04.0 Acute disseminated encephalitis and encephalomyelitis (ADEM)
Excludes1: acute necrotizing hemorrhagic encephalopathy (G04.3-)
other noninfectious acute disseminated encephalomyelitis (noninfectious ADEM) (G04.81)

MCC G04.00 Acute disseminated encephalitis and encephalomyelitis, unspecified

MCC G04.01 Postinfectious acute disseminated encephalitis and encephalomyelitis (postinfectious ADEM)
Excludes1: post chickenpox encephalitis (B01.1)
post measles encephalitis (B05.0)
post measles myelitis (B05.1)

MCC G04.02 Postimmunization acute disseminated encephalitis, myelitis and encephalomyelitis
Encephalitis, post immunization
Encephalomyelitis, post immunization
Use additional code to identify the vaccine (T50.A-, T50.B-, T50.Z-)

CC G04.1 Tropical spastic paraplegia

MCC G04.2 Bacterial meningoencephalitis and meningomyelitis, not elsewhere classified

+ G04.3 Acute necrotizing hemorrhagic encephalopathy
Excludes1: acute disseminated encephalitis and encephalomyelitis (G04.0-)

MCC G04.30 Acute necrotizing hemorrhagic encephalopathy, unspecified

MCC G04.31 Postinfectious acute necrotizing hemorrhagic encephalopathy

MCC G04.32 Postimmunization acute necrotizing hemorrhagic encephalopathy
Use additional code to identify the vaccine (T50.A-, T50.B-, T50.Z-)

MCC G04.39 Other acute necrotizing hemorrhagic encephalopathy
Code also underlying etiology, if applicable

+ G04.8 Other encephalitis, myelitis and encephalomyelitis
Code also any associated seizure (G40.-, R56.9)

MCC G04.81 Other encephalitis and encephalomyelitis
Noninfectious acute disseminated encephalomyelitis (noninfectious ADEM)

MCC G04.82 Acute flaccid myelitis
Excludes1: transverse myelitis (G37.3)
AHA CC: 4Q, 2021, 11

MCC G04.89 Other myelitis
AHA CC: 1Q, 2020, 14

+ G04.9 Encephalitis, myelitis and encephalomyelitis, unspecified

MCC G04.90 Encephalitis and encephalomyelitis, unspecified
Ventriculitis (cerebral) NOS

MCC G04.91 Myelitis, unspecified

G05 Encephalitis, myelitis and encephalomyelitis in diseases classified elsewhere

Code first underlying disease, such as:
congenital toxoplasmosis encephalitis, myelitis and encephalomyelitis (P37.1)
cytomegaloviral encephalitis, myelitis and encephalomyelitis (B25.8)
encephalitis, myelitis and encephalomyelitis (in) systemic lupus erythematosus (M32.19)
eosinophilic meningoencephalitis (B83.2)
human immunodeficiency virus [HIV] disease (B20)
poliovirus (A80.-)
suppurative otitis media (H66.01-H66.4)
systemic lupus erythematosus (M32.19)
trichinellosis (B75)

Excludes1: adenoviral encephalitis, myelitis and encephalomyelitis (A85.1)
encephalitis, myelitis and encephalomyelitis (in) measles (B05.0)
enteroviral encephalitis, myelitis and encephalomyelitis (A85.0)
herpesviral [herpes simplex] encephalitis, myelitis and encephalomyelitis (B00.4)
listerial encephalitis, myelitis and encephalomyelitis (A32.12)
meningococcal encephalitis, myelitis and encephalomyelitis (A39.81)
mumps encephalitis, myelitis and encephalomyelitis (B26.2)
postchickenpox encephalitis, myelitis and encephalomyelitis (B01.1-)
rubella encephalitis, myelitis and encephalomyelitis (B06.01)
toxoplasmosis encephalitis, myelitis and encephalomyelitis (B58.2)
zoster encephalitis, myelitis and encephalomyelitis (B02.0)

MCC G05.3 Encephalitis and encephalomyelitis in diseases classified elsewhere
Meningoencephalitis in diseases classified elsewhere
Code first underlying disease

MCC G05.4 Myelitis in diseases classified elsewhere
Meningomyelitis in diseases classified elsewhere

G06 Intracranial and intraspinal abscess and granuloma

Use additional code (B95-B97) to identify infectious agent.

MCC G06.0 Intracranial abscess and granuloma
Brain [any part] abscess (embolic)
Cerebellar abscess (embolic)
Cerebral abscess (embolic)
Intracranial epidural abscess or granuloma
Intracranial extradural abscess or granuloma
Intracranial subdural abscess or granuloma
Otogenic abscess (embolic)
Excludes1: tuberculous intracranial abscess and granuloma (A17.81)

MCC G06.1 Intraspinal abscess and granuloma
Abscess (embolic) of spinal cord [any part]
Intraspinal epidural abscess or granuloma
Intraspinal extradural abscess or granuloma
Intraspinal subdural abscess or granuloma
Excludes1: tuberculous intraspinal abscess and granuloma (A17.81)

MCC G06.2 Extradural and subdural abscess, unspecified

G07 Intracranial and intraspinal abscess and granuloma in diseases classified elsewhere
MCC

Code first underlying disease such as:
schistosomiasis granuloma of brain (B65.-)
Excludes1: abscess of brain:
amebic (A06.6)
chromomycotic (B43.1)
gonococcal (A54.82)
tuberculous (A17.81)
tuberculoma of meninges (A17.1)

Valid 3-character code, no further characters required

MCC G08 Intracranial and intraspinal phlebitis and thrombophlebitis

Septic embolism of intracranial or intraspinal venous sinuses and veins
Septic endophlebitis of intracranial or intraspinal venous sinuses and veins
Septic phlebitis of intracranial or intraspinal venous sinuses and veins
Septic thrombophlebitis of intracranial or intraspinal venous sinuses and veins
Septic thrombosis of intracranial or intraspinal venous sinuses and veins

Excludes1: intracranial phlebitis and thrombophlebitis complicating:
abortion, ectopic or molar pregnancy (O00-O07, O08.7)
pregnancy, childbirth and the puerperium (O22.5, O87.3)
nonpyogenic intracranial phlebitis and thrombophlebitis (I67.6)

Excludes2: intracranial phlebitis and thrombophlebitis complicating nonpyogenic intraspinal phlebitis and thrombophlebitis (G95.1)

Valid 3-character code, no further characters required

G09 Sequelae of inflammatory diseases of central nervous system

NOTE Category G09 is to be used to indicate conditions whose primary classification is to G00-G08 as the cause of sequelae, themselves classifiable elsewhere. The 'sequelae' include conditions specified as residuals.

Code first condition resulting from (sequela) of inflammatory diseases of central nervous system

Valid 3-character code, no further characters required

Systemic atrophies primarily affecting the central nervous system (G10-G14)

CC G10 Huntington's disease

Huntington's chorea
Huntington's dementia

Use additional code, if applicable, to identify:
dementia with anxiety (F02.84, F02.A4, F02.B4, F02.C4)
dementia with behavioral disturbance (F02.81-, F02.A1-, F02.B1-, F02.C1-)
dementia with mood disturbance (F02.83, F02.A3, F02.B3, F02.C3)
dementia with psychotic disturbance (F02.82, F02.A2, F02.B2, F02.C2)
dementia without behavioral disturbance (F02.80, F02.A0, F02.B0, F02.C0)
mild neurocognitive disorder due to known physiological condition (F06.7-)

Valid 3-character code, no further characters required

G11 Hereditary ataxia

Excludes2: cerebral palsy (G80.-)
hereditary and idiopathic neuropathy (G60.-)
metabolic disorders (E70-E88)

CC G11.0 Congenital nonprogressive ataxia

+ G11.1 Early-onset cerebellar ataxia
AHA CC: 4Q, 2020, 17-18

CC G11.10 Early-onset cerebellar ataxia, unspecified

CC G11.11 Friedreich ataxia
Autosomal recessive Friedreich ataxia
Friedreich ataxia with retained reflexes

CC G11.19 Other early-onset cerebellar ataxia
Early-onset cerebellar ataxia with essential tremor
Early-onset cerebellar ataxia with myoclonus [Hunt's ataxia]
Early-onset cerebellar ataxia with retained tendon reflexes
X-linked recessive spinocerebellar ataxia

• CC G11.2 Late-onset cerebellar ataxia

CC G11.3 Cerebellar ataxia with defective DNA repair
Ataxia telangiectasia [Louis-Bar]
Excludes2: Cockayne's syndrome (Q87.19)
other disorders of purine and pyrimidine metabolism (E79.-)
xeroderma pigmentosum (Q82.19)

CC G11.4 Hereditary spastic paraplegia

CC G11.5 Hypomyelination - hypogonadotropic hypogonadism - hypodontia
4H syndrome
Pol III-related leukodystrophy

CC G11.6 Leukodystrophy with vanishing white matter disease

CC G11.8 Other hereditary ataxias

CC G11.9 Hereditary ataxia, unspecified
Hereditary cerebellar ataxia NOS
Hereditary cerebellar degeneration
Hereditary cerebellar disease
Hereditary cerebellar syndrome

G12 Spinal muscular atrophy and related syndromes

CC G12.0 Infantile spinal muscular atrophy, type I [Werdnig-Hoffman]

CC G12.1 Other inherited spinal muscular atrophy
 Adult form spinal muscular atrophy
 Childhood form, type II spinal muscular atrophy
 Distal spinal muscular atrophy
 Juvenile form, type III spinal muscular atrophy [Kugelberg-Welander]
 Progressive bulbar palsy of childhood [Fazio-Londe]
 Scapuloperoneal form spinal muscular atrophy

+ G12.2 Motor neuron disease
 CC G12.20 Motor neuron disease, unspecified
 • CC G12.21 Amyotrophic lateral sclerosis
 CC G12.22 Progressive bulbar palsy
 CC G12.23 Primary lateral sclerosis
  AHA CC: 4Q, 2017, 9-10
 CC G12.24 Familial motor neuron disease
  AHA CC: 4Q, 2017, 9-10
 CC G12.25 Progressive spinal muscle atrophy
  AHA CC: 4Q, 2017, 9-10
 CC G12.29 Other motor neuron disease

CC G12.8 Other spinal muscular atrophies and related syndromes
CC G12.9 Spinal muscular atrophy, unspecified

G13 Systemic atrophies primarily affecting central nervous system in diseases classified elsewhere

G13.0 Paraneoplastic neuromyopathy and neuropathy
 Carcinomatous neuromyopathy
 Sensorial paraneoplastic neuropathy [Denny Brown]
 Code first underlying neoplasm (C00-D49)

G13.1 Other systemic atrophy primarily affecting central nervous system in neoplastic disease
 Paraneoplastic limbic encephalopathy
 Code first underlying neoplasm (C00-D49)

G13.2 Systemic atrophy primarily affecting the central nervous system in myxedema
 Code first underlying disease, such as:
  hypothyroidism (E03.-)
  myxedematous congenital iodine deficiency (E00.1)

G13.8 Systemic atrophy primarily affecting central nervous system in other diseases classified elsewhere
 Code first underlying disease

G14 Postpolio syndrome
 Includes: postpolio myelitic syndrome
 Excludes1: *sequelae of poliomyelitis (B91)*
 Valid 3-character code, no further characters required

Extrapyramidal and movement disorders (G20-G26)

+ G20 Parkinson's disease
 Hemiparkinsonism
 Idiopathic Parkinsonism or Parkinson's disease
 Paralysis agitans
 Primary Parkinsonism or Parkinson's disease
 Use additional code, if applicable, to identify:
  dementia with anxiety (F02.84, F02.A4, F02.B4, F02.C4)
  dementia with behavioral disturbance (F02.81-, F02.A1-, F02.B1-, F02.C1-)
  dementia with mood disturbance (F02.83, F02.A3, F02.B3, F02.C3)
  dementia with psychotic disturbance (F02.82, F02.A2, F02.B2, F02.C2)
  dementia without behavioral disturbance (F02.80, F02.A0, F02.B0, F02.C0)
  mild neurocognitive disorder due to known physiological condition (F06.7-)
 AHA CC: 2Q, 2016, 6-7; 2Q, 2017, 7-8

+ G20.A Parkinson's disease without dyskinesia
 G20.A1 Parkinson's disease without dyskinesia, without mention of fluctuations
  Parkinson's disease NOS
  Parkinson's disease without dyskinesia, without mention of OFF episodes
 G20.A2 Parkinson's disease without dyskinesia, with fluctuations
  Parkinson's disease without dyskinesia, with OFF episodes

+ G20.B Parkinson's disease with dyskinesia
 Excludes1: *drug induced dystonia (G24.0-)*

 G20.B1 Parkinson's disease with dyskinesia, without mention of fluctuations
  Parkinson's disease with dyskinesia, without mention of OFF episodes
 G20.B2 Parkinson's disease with dyskinesia, with fluctuations
  Parkinson's disease with dyskinesia, with OFF episodes

G20.C Parkinsonism, unspecified
 Parkinsonism, NOS
 Excludes1: *Parkinson's disease NOS (G20.A1)*
  Parkinson's disease with dyskinesia (G20.B-)
  Parkinson's disease without dyskinesia (G20.A-)
  secondary parkinsonism (G21-)

G21 Secondary parkinsonism

 Excludes1: *dementia with Parkinsonism (G31.83)*
  Huntington's disease (G10)
  Shy-Drager syndrome (G90.3)
  syphilitic Parkinsonism (A52.19)

MCC G21.0 Malignant neuroleptic syndrome
 Use additional code for adverse effect, if applicable, to identify drug (T43.3X5, T43.4X5, T43.505, T43.595)
 Excludes1: *neuroleptic induced parkinsonism (G21.11)*

+ G21.1 Other drug-induced secondary parkinsonism
 CC G21.11 Neuroleptic induced parkinsonism
  Use additional code for adverse effect, if applicable, to identify drug (T43.3X5, T43.4X5, T43.505, T43.595)
  Excludes1: *malignant neuroleptic syndrome (G21.0)*
 CC G21.19 Other drug induced secondary parkinsonism
  Other medication-induced parkinsonism
  Use additional code for adverse effect, if applicable, to identify drug (T36-T50 with fifth or sixth character 5)

CC G21.2 Secondary parkinsonism due to other external agents
 Code first (T51-T65) to identify external agent

CC G21.3 Postencephalitic parkinsonism
CC G21.4 Vascular parkinsonism
CC G21.8 Other secondary parkinsonism
CC G21.9 Secondary parkinsonism, unspecified

G23 Other degenerative diseases of basal ganglia

 Excludes2: *multi-system degeneration of the autonomic nervous system (G90.3)*

CC G23.0 Hallervorden-Spatz disease
 Pigmentary pallidal degeneration
CC G23.1 Progressive supranuclear ophthalmoplegia [Steele-Richardson-Olszewski]
 Progressive supranuclear palsy
CC G23.2 Striatonigral degeneration
 G23.3 Hypomyelination with atrophy of the basal ganglia and cerebellum
  H-ABC
CC G23.8 Other specified degenerative diseases of basal ganglia
 Calcification of basal ganglia
CC G23.9 Degenerative disease of basal ganglia, unspecified

G24 Dystonia
 Includes: dyskinesia
 Excludes2: *athetoid cerebral palsy (G80.3)*

+ G24.0 Drug induced dystonia
 Use additional code for adverse effect, if applicable, to identify drug (T36-T50 with fifth or sixth character 5)
 G24.01 Drug induced subacute dyskinesia
  Drug induced blepharospasm
  Drug induced orofacial dyskinesia
  Neuroleptic induced tardive dyskinesia
  Tardive dyskinesia
 CC G24.02 Drug induced acute dystonia
  Acute dystonic reaction to drugs
  Neuroleptic induced acute dystonia
 CC G24.09 Other drug induced dystonia

G24.1 Genetic torsion dystonia
 Dystonia deformans progressiva
 Dystonia musculorum deformans
 Familial torsion dystonia
 Idiopathic familial dystonia
 Idiopathic (torsion) dystonia NOS
 (Schwalbe-) Ziehen-Oppenheim disease

CC G24.2 Idiopathic nonfamilial dystonia

G24.3 Spasmodic torticollis
  Excludes1: congenital torticollis (Q68.0)
    hysterical torticollis (F44.4)
    ocular torticollis (R29.891)
    psychogenic torticollis (F45.8)
    torticollis NOS (M43.6)
    traumatic recurrent torticollis (S13.4)
G24.4 Idiopathic orofacial dystonia
  Orofacial dyskinesia
  Excludes1: drug induced orofacial dyskinesia (G24.01)
G24.5 Blepharospasm
  Excludes1: drug induced blepharospasm (G24.01)
CC **G24.8 Other dystonia**
  Acquired torsion dystonia NOS
G24.9 Dystonia, unspecified
  Dyskinesia NOS

G25 Other extrapyramidal and movement disorders
  Excludes2: sleep related movement disorders (G47.6-)
  G25.0 Essential tremor
    Familial tremor
    Excludes1: tremor NOS (R25.1)
  G25.1 Drug-induced tremor
    Use additional code for adverse effect, if applicable, to identify drug (T36-T50 with fifth or sixth character 5)
  G25.2 Other specified forms of tremor
    Intention tremor
  G25.3 Myoclonus
    Drug-induced myoclonus
    Palatal myoclonus
    Use additional code for adverse effect, if applicable, to identify drug (T36-T50 with fifth or sixth character 5)
    Excludes1: facial myokymia (G51.4)
      myoclonic epilepsy (G40.-)
  G25.4 Drug-induced chorea
    Use additional code for adverse effect, if applicable, to identify drug (T36-T50 with fifth or sixth character 5)
  G25.5 Other chorea
    Chorea NOS
    Excludes1: chorea NOS with heart involvement (I02.0)
      Huntington's chorea (G10)
      rheumatic chorea (I02.-)
      Sydenham's chorea (I02.-)
  + **G25.6 Drug induced tics and other tics of organic origin**
    G25.61 Drug induced tics
      Use additional code for adverse effect, if applicable, to identify drug (T36-T50 with fifth or sixth character 5)
    G25.69 Other tics of organic origin
      Excludes1: habit spasm (F95.9)
        tic NOS (F95.9)
        Tourette's syndrome (F95.2)
  + **G25.7 Other and unspecified drug induced movement disorders**
    Use additional code for adverse effect, if applicable, to identify drug (T36-T50 with fifth or sixth character 5)
    G25.70 Drug induced movement disorder, unspecified
    G25.71 Drug induced akathisia
      Drug induced acathisia
      Neuroleptic induced acute akathisia
      Tardive akathisia
    G25.79 Other drug induced movement disorders
  + **G25.8 Other specified extrapyramidal and movement disorders**
    G25.81 Restless legs syndrome
  CC **G25.82 Stiff-man syndrome**
    G25.83 Benign shuddering attacks
    G25.89 Other specified extrapyramidal and movement disorders
  CC **G25.9 Extrapyramidal and movement disorder, unspecified**

G26 Extrapyramidal and movement disorders in diseases classified elsewhere
  Code first underlying disease
  Valid 3-character code, no further characters required

Other degenerative diseases of the nervous system (G30-G32)

G30 Alzheimer's disease
  Includes: Alzheimer's dementia senile and presenile forms
  Use additional code, if applicable, to identify:
    delirium, if applicable (F05)
    dementia with anxiety (F02.84, F02.A4, F02.B4, F02.C4)
    dementia with behavioral disturbance (F02.81-, F02.A1-, F02.B1-, F02.C1-)
    dementia with mood disturbance (F02.83, F02.A3, F02.B3, F02.C3)
    dementia with psychotic disturbance (F02.82, F02.A2, F02.B2, F02.C2)
    dementia without behavioral disturbance (F02.80, F02.A0, F02.B0, F02.C0)
    mild neurocognitive disorder due to known physiological condition (F06.7-)
  Excludes1: senile degeneration of brain NEC (G31.1)
    senile dementia NOS (F03)
    senility NOS (R41.81)
  G30.0 Alzheimer's disease with early onset
  • **G30.1 Alzheimer's disease with late onset**
    AHA CC: 4Q, 2022, 15
  G30.8 Other Alzheimer's disease
  G30.9 Alzheimer's disease, unspecified
    AHA CC: 4Q, 2012, 95-96; 2Q, 2016, 6; 1Q, 2017, 43-44

G31 Other degenerative diseases of nervous system, not elsewhere classified
  Use additional code, if applicable, for codes G31.0-G31.83, G31.85-G31.9, to identify:
    dementia with behavioral disturbance (F02.81-, F02.A1-, F02.B1-, F02.C1-)
    dementia with mood disturbance (F02.83, F02.A3, F02.B3, F02.C3)
    dementia with psychotic disturbance (F02.82, F02.A2, F02.B2, F02.C2)
    dementia without behavioral disturbance (F02.80, F02.A0, F02.B0, F02.C0)
    mild neurocognitive disorder due to known physiological condition (F06.7-)
  Excludes2: Reye's syndrome (G93.7)
  + **G31.0 Frontotemporal dementia**
    G31.01 Pick's disease
      Primary progressive aphasia
      Progressive isolated aphasia
    G31.09 Other frontotemporal neurocognitive disorder
      Frontal dementia
      Use additional code, if applicable, to identify mild neurocognitive disorders due to known physiological condition (F06.7-)
  G31.1 Senile degeneration of brain, not elsewhere classified
    Excludes1: Alzheimer's disease (G30.-)
      senility NOS (R41.81)
  G31.2 Degeneration of nervous system due to alcohol
    Alcoholic cerebellar ataxia
    Alcoholic cerebellar degeneration
    Alcoholic cerebral degeneration
    Alcoholic encephalopathy
    Dysfunction of the autonomic nervous system due to alcohol
    Code also associated alcoholism (F10.-)
  + **G31.8 Other specified degenerative diseases of nervous system**
    G31.80 Leukodystrophy, unspecified
    CC **G31.81 Alpers disease**
      Grey-matter degeneration
    CC **G31.82 Leigh's disease**
      Subacute necrotizing encephalopathy
    G31.83 Neurocognitive disorder with Lewy bodies
      Lewy body dementia
      Lewy body disease
      Use additional code, if applicable, to identify mild neurocognitive disorders due to known physiological condition (F06.7-)
      AHA CC: 4Q, 2016, 141
    G31.84 Mild cognitive impairment of uncertain or unknown etiology
      Mild cognitive disorder NOS
      Mild neurocognitive disorder of uncertain or unknown etiology
      Use additional code to identify presence of:
        alcohol abuse and dependence (F10.-)
        exposure to environmental tobacco smoke (Z77.22)
        history of tobacco dependence (Z87.891)
        hypertension (I10-I1A)
        occupational exposure to environmental tobacco smoke (Z57.31)
        tobacco dependence (F17.-)
        tobacco use (Z72.0)
      Excludes1: age related cognitive decline (R41.81)
        altered mental status (R41.82)

G31.85–G40.009

Chapter 6: Diseases of the Nervous System

        cerebral degeneration (G31.9)
        cerebrovascular diseases (I60-I69)
        change in mental status (R41.82)
        cognitive deficits following (sequelae of) cerebral hemorrhage or infarction (I69.01-, I69.11-, I69.21-, I69.31-, I69.81-, I69.91-)
        cognitive impairment due to intracranial or head injury (S06.-)
        dementia (F01.-, F02.-, F03)
        mild neurocognitive disorder due to a known physiological condition (F06.7-)
        neurologic neglect syndrome (R41.4)
        personality change, nonpsychotic (F68.8)
        AHA CC: 3Q, 2021, 3

  G31.85 Corticobasal degeneration
  G31.86 Alexander disease
  G31.89 Other specified degenerative diseases of nervous system
  G31.9 Degenerative disease of nervous system, unspecified
    AHA CC: 3Q, 2021, 3

G32 Other degenerative disorders of nervous system in diseases classified elsewhere

  CC G32.0 Subacute combined degeneration of spinal cord in diseases classified elsewhere
    Dana-Putnam syndrome
    Sclerosis of spinal cord (combined) (dorsolateral) (posterolateral)
    Code first underlying disease, such as:
      other dietary vitamin B12 Deficiency anemia (D51.3)
      vitamin B12 deficiency anemia due to intrinsic factor deficiency (D51.0)
      vitamin B12 deficiency anemia, unspecified (D51.8)
      vitamin B12 deficiency (E53.8)
    Excludes1: syphilitic combined degeneration of spinal cord (A52.11)

  + G32.8 Other specified degenerative disorders of nervous system in diseases classified elsewhere
    Code first underlying disease, such as:
      amyloidosis cerebral degeneration (E85.-)
      cerebral degeneration (due to) hypothyroidism (E00.0-E03.9)
      cerebral degeneration (due to) neoplasm (C00-D49)
      cerebral degeneration (due to) vitamin B deficiency, except thiamine (E52-E53.-)
      non-celiac gluten ataxia (M35.9)
    Excludes1: superior hemorrhagic polioencephalitis [Wernicke's encephalopathy] (E51.2)

  CC G32.81 Cerebellar ataxia in diseases classified elsewhere
    Code first underlying disease, such as:
      celiac disease (with gluten ataxia) (K90.0)
      cerebellar ataxia (in) neoplastic disease (paraneoplastic cerebellar degeneration) (C00-D49)
      non-celiac gluten ataxia (M35.9)
    Excludes1: systemic atrophy primarily affecting the central nervous system in alcoholic cerebellar ataxia (G31.2)
      systemic atrophy primarily affecting the central nervous system in myxedema (G13.2)

  G32.89 Other specified degenerative disorders of nervous system in diseases classified elsewhere
    Degenerative encephalopathy in diseases classified elsewhere

Demyelinating diseases of the central nervous system (G35-G37)

G35 Multiple sclerosis
  Disseminated multiple sclerosis
  Generalized multiple sclerosis
  Multiple sclerosis NOS
  Multiple sclerosis of brain stem
  Multiple sclerosis of cord
  AHA CC: 1Q, 2021, 7
  Valid 3-character code, no further characters required

G36 Other acute disseminated demyelination
  Excludes1: povstinfectious encephalitis and encephalomyelitis NOS (G04.01)
  CC G36.0 Neuromyelitis optica [Devic]
    Demyelination in optic neuritis
    Excludes1: optic neuritis NOS (H46)
  CC G36.1 Acute and subacute hemorrhagic leukoencephalitis [Hurst]
  CC G36.8 Other specified acute disseminated demyelination
  CC G36.9 Acute disseminated demyelination, unspecified

G37 Other demyelinating diseases of central nervous system
  CC G37.0 Diffuse sclerosis of central nervous system
    Periaxial encephalitis
    Schilder's disease
    Excludes1: X linked adrenoleukodystrophy (E71.52-)
  CC G37.1 Central demyelination of corpus callosum
  CC G37.2 Central pontine myelinolysis
    AHA CC: 2Q, 2022, 10-11
  CC G37.3 Acute transverse myelitis in demyelinating disease of central nervous system
    Acute transverse myelitis NOS
    Acute transverse myelopathy
    Excludes1: acute flaccid myelitis (G04.82)
      multiple sclerosis (G35)
      neuromyelitis optica [Devic] (G36.0)
  MCC G37.4 Subacute necrotizing myelitis of central nervous system
  CC G37.5 Concentric sclerosis [Balo] of central nervous system
  + G37.8 Other specified demyelinating diseases of central nervous system
    CC G37.81 Myelin oligodendrocyte glycoprotein antibody disease
      MOG antibody disease
      Code also associated manifestations, if known, such as:
        noninfectious acute disseminated encephalomyelitis (G04.81)
        neuromyelitis optica (G36.0)
    CC G37.89 Other specified demyelinating diseases of central nervous system
  CC G37.9 Demyelinating disease of central nervous system, unspecified

Episodic and paroxysmal disorders (G40-G47)

G40 Epilepsy and recurrent seizures
  NOTE the following terms are to be considered equivalent to intractable: pharmacoresistant (pharmacologically resistant), treatment resistant, refractory (medically) and poorly controlled
  Excludes1: conversion disorder with seizures (F44.5)
    convulsions NOS (R56.9)
    post traumatic seizures (R56.1)
    seizure (convulsive) NOS (R56.9)
    seizure of newborn (P90)
  Excludes2: hippocampal sclerosis (G93.81)
    mesial temporal sclerosis (G93.81)
    temporal sclerosis (G93.81)
    Todd's paralysis (G83.84)

  + G40.0 Localization-related (focal) (partial) idiopathic epilepsy and epileptic syndromes with seizures of localized onset
    Benign childhood epilepsy with centrotemporal EEG spikes
    Childhood epilepsy with occipital EEG paroxysms
    Excludes1: adult onset localization-related epilepsy (G40.1-, G40.2-)
    + G40.00 Localization-related (focal) (partial) idiopathic epilepsy and epileptic syndromes with seizures of localized onset, not intractable
      Localization-related (focal) (partial) idiopathic epilepsy and epileptic syndromes with seizures of localized onset without intractability
      CC G40.001 Localization-related (focal) (partial) idiopathic epilepsy and epileptic syndromes with seizures of localized onset, not intractable, with status epilepticus
      CC G40.009 Localization-related (focal) (partial) idiopathic epilepsy and epileptic syndromes with seizures of localized onset, not intractable, without status epilepticus
        Localization-related (focal) (partial) idiopathic epilepsy and epileptic syndromes with seizures of localized onset NOS

- **G40.01** Localization-related (focal) (partial) idiopathic epilepsy and epileptic syndromes with seizures of localized onset, intractable
  - CC **G40.011** Localization-related (focal) (partial) idiopathic epilepsy and epileptic syndromes with seizures of localized onset, intractable, with status epilepticus
  - CC **G40.019** Localization-related (focal) (partial) idiopathic epilepsy and epileptic syndromes with seizures of localized onset, intractable, without status epilepticus
- **G40.1** Localization-related (focal) (partial) symptomatic epilepsy and epileptic syndromes with simple partial seizures
  - Attacks without alteration of consciousness
  - Epilepsia partialis continua [Kozhevnikof]
  - Simple partial seizures developing into secondarily generalized seizures
  - **G40.10** Localization-related (focal) (partial) symptomatic epilepsy and epileptic syndromes with simple partial seizures, not intractable
    - Localization-related (focal) (partial) symptomatic epilepsy and epileptic syndromes with simple partial seizures without intractability
    - CC **G40.101** Localization-related (focal) (partial) symptomatic epilepsy and epileptic syndromes with simple partial seizures, not intractable, with status epilepticus
    - CC **G40.109** Localization-related (focal) (partial) symptomatic epilepsy and epileptic syndromes with simple partial seizures, not intractable, without status epilepticus
      - Localization-related (focal) (partial) symptomatic epilepsy and epileptic syndromes with simple partial seizures NOS
  - **G40.11** Localization-related (focal) (partial) symptomatic epilepsy and epileptic syndromes with simple partial seizures, intractable
    - CC **G40.111** Localization-related (focal) (partial) symptomatic epilepsy and epileptic syndromes with simple partial seizures, intractable, with status epilepticus
    - CC **G40.119** Localization-related (focal) (partial) symptomatic epilepsy and epileptic syndromes with simple partial seizures, intractable, without status epilepticus
- **G40.2** Localization-related (focal) (partial) symptomatic epilepsy and epileptic syndromes with complex partial seizures
  - Attacks with alteration of consciousness, often with automatisms
  - Complex partial seizures developing into secondarily generalized seizures
  - **G40.20** Localization-related (focal) (partial) symptomatic epilepsy and epileptic syndromes with complex partial seizures, not intractable
    - Localization-related (focal) (partial) symptomatic epilepsy and epileptic syndromes with complex partial seizures without intractability
    - CC **G40.201** Localization-related (focal) (partial) symptomatic epilepsy and epileptic syndromes with complex partial seizures, not intractable, with status epilepticus
    - CC **G40.209** Localization-related (focal) (partial) symptomatic epilepsy and epileptic syndromes with complex partial seizures, not intractable, without status epilepticus
      - Localization-related (focal) (partial) symptomatic epilepsy and epileptic syndromes with complex partial seizures NOS
  - **G40.21** Localization-related (focal) (partial) symptomatic epilepsy and epileptic syndromes with complex partial seizures, intractable
    - CC **G40.211** Localization-related (focal) (partial) symptomatic epilepsy and epileptic syndromes with complex partial seizures, intractable, with status epilepticus
    - CC **G40.219** Localization-related (focal) (partial) symptomatic epilepsy and epileptic syndromes with complex partial seizures, intractable, without status epilepticus
- **G40.3** Generalized idiopathic epilepsy and epileptic syndromes
  - Code also MERRF syndrome, if applicable (E88.42)
  - **G40.30** Generalized idiopathic epilepsy and epileptic syndromes, not intractable
    - Generalized idiopathic epilepsy and epileptic syndromes without intractability
    - MCC **G40.301** Generalized idiopathic epilepsy and epileptic syndromes, not intractable, with status epilepticus
    - **G40.309** Generalized idiopathic epilepsy and epileptic syndromes, not intractable, without status epilepticus
      - Generalized idiopathic epilepsy and epileptic syndromes NOS
  - **G40.31** Generalized idiopathic epilepsy and epileptic syndromes, intractable
    - MCC **G40.311** Generalized idiopathic epilepsy and epileptic syndromes, intractable, with status epilepticus
    - MCC **G40.319** Generalized idiopathic epilepsy and epileptic syndromes, intractable, without status epilepticus
- **G40.A** Absence epileptic syndrome
  - Childhood absence epilepsy [pyknolepsy]
  - Juvenile absence epilepsy
  - Absence epileptic syndrome, NOS
  - **G40.A0** Absence epileptic syndrome, not intractable
    - **G40.A01** Absence epileptic syndrome, not intractable, with status epilepticus
    - **G40.A09** Absence epileptic syndrome, not intractable, without status epilepticus
  - **G40.A1** Absence epileptic syndrome, intractable
    - CC **G40.A11** Absence epileptic syndrome, intractable, with status epilepticus
    - CC **G40.A19** Absence epileptic syndrome, intractable, without status epilepticus
- **G40.B** Juvenile myoclonic epilepsy [impulsive petit mal]
  - **G40.B0** Juvenile myoclonic epilepsy, not intractable
    - CC **G40.B01** Juvenile myoclonic epilepsy, not intractable, with status epilepticus
    - CC **G40.B09** Juvenile myoclonic epilepsy, not intractable, without status epilepticus
  - **G40.B1** Juvenile myoclonic epilepsy, intractable
    - CC **G40.B11** Juvenile myoclonic epilepsy, intractable, with status epilepticus
    - CC **G40.B19** Juvenile myoclonic epilepsy, intractable, without status epilepticus
- **G40.C** Lafora progressive myoclonus epilepsy
  - Lafora body disease
  - Code also, if applicable, associated conditions such as dementia (F02.8-)
  - **G40.C0** Lafora progressive myoclonus epilepsy, not intractable
    - CC **G40.C01** Lafora progressive myoclonus epilepsy, not intractable, with status epilepticus
    - CC **G40.C09** Lafora progressive myoclonus epilepsy, not intractable, without status epilepticus
      - Lafora progressive myoclonus epilepsy NOS
  - **G40.C1** Lafora progressive myoclonus epilepsy, intractable
    - CC **G40.C11** Lafora progressive myoclonus epilepsy, intractable, with status epilepticus
    - CC **G40.C19** Lafora progressive myoclonus epilepsy, intractable, without status epilepticus
- **G40.4** Other generalized epilepsy and epileptic syndromes
  - Epilepsy with grand mal seizures on awakening
  - Epilepsy with myoclonic absences
  - Epilepsy with myoclonic-astatic seizures
  - Grand mal seizure NOS
  - Nonspecific atonic epileptic seizures
  - Nonspecific clonic epileptic seizures
  - Nonspecific myoclonic epileptic seizures
  - Nonspecific tonic epileptic seizures
  - Nonspecific tonic-clonic epileptic seizures
  - Symptomatic early myoclonic encephalopathy

- **G40.40** Other generalized epilepsy and epileptic syndromes, not intractable
  - Other generalized epilepsy and epileptic syndromes without intractability
  - Other generalized epilepsy and epileptic syndromes NOS
  - **G40.401** Other generalized epilepsy and epileptic syndromes, not intractable, with status epilepticus
  - **G40.409** Other generalized epilepsy and epileptic syndromes, not intractable, without status epilepticus
- **G40.41** Other generalized epilepsy and epileptic syndromes, intractable
  - CC **G40.411** Other generalized epilepsy and epileptic syndromes, intractable, with status epilepticus
  - CC **G40.419** Other generalized epilepsy and epileptic syndromes, intractable, without status epilepticus
- **G40.42** Cyclin-Dependent Kinase-Like 5 Deficiency Disorder
  - CDKL5
  - Use additional code, if known, to identify associated manifestations, such as:
    - cortical blindness (H47.61-)
    - global developmental delay (F88)
  - *AHA CC: 4Q, 2020, 18-19*
- **G40.5** Epileptic seizures related to external causes
  - Epileptic seizures related to alcohol
  - Epileptic seizures related to drugs
  - Epileptic seizures related to hormonal changes
  - Epileptic seizures related to sleep deprivation
  - Epileptic seizures related to stress
  - Use additional code for adverse effect, if applicable, to identify drug (T36-T50 with fifth or sixth character 5)
  - Code also if applicable, associated epilepsy and recurrent seizures (G40.-)
  - **G40.50** Epileptic seizures related to external causes, not intractable
    - CC **G40.501** Epileptic seizures related to external causes, not intractable, with status epilepticus
    - CC **G40.509** Epileptic seizures related to external causes, not intractable, without status epilepticus
      - Epileptic seizures related to external causes, NOS
- **G40.8** Other epilepsy and recurrent seizures
  - Epilepsies and epileptic syndromes undetermined as to whether they are focal or generalized
  - Landau-Kleffner syndrome
  - **G40.80** Other epilepsy
    - CC **G40.801** Other epilepsy, not intractable, with status epilepticus
      - Other epilepsy without intractability with status epilepticus
    - CC **G40.802** Other epilepsy, not intractable, without status epilepticus
      - Other epilepsy NOS
      - Other epilepsy without intractability without status epilepticus
    - CC **G40.803** Other epilepsy, intractable, with status epilepticus
    - CC **G40.804** Other epilepsy, intractable, without status epilepticus
  - **G40.81** Lennox-Gastaut syndrome
    - CC **G40.811** Lennox-Gastaut syndrome, not intractable, with status epilepticus
    - CC **G40.812** Lennox-Gastaut syndrome, not intractable, without status epilepticus
    - CC **G40.813** Lennox-Gastaut syndrome, intractable, with status epilepticus
    - CC **G40.814** Lennox-Gastaut syndrome, intractable, without status epilepticus
  - **G40.82** Epileptic spasms
    - Infantile spasms
    - Salaam attacks
    - West's syndrome
    - CC **G40.821** Epileptic spasms, not intractable, with status epilepticus
    - CC **G40.822** Epileptic spasms, not intractable, without status epilepticus
    - CC **G40.823** Epileptic spasms, intractable, with status epilepticus
    - CC **G40.824** Epileptic spasms, intractable, without status epilepticus
  - **G40.83** Dravet syndrome
    - Polymorphic epilepsy in infancy (PMEI)
    - Severe myoclonic epilepsy in infancy (SMEI)
    - *AHA CC: 4Q, 2020, 19*
    - CC **G40.833** Dravet syndrome, intractable, with status epilepticus
    - CC **G40.834** Dravet syndrome, intractable, without status epilepticus
      - Dravet syndrome NOS
  - CC **G40.89** Other seizures
    - *Excludes1:* post traumatic seizures (R56.1)
      - recurrent seizures NOS (G40.909)
      - seizure NOS (R56.9)
- **G40.9** Epilepsy, unspecified
  - **G40.90** Epilepsy, unspecified, not intractable
    - Epilepsy, unspecified, without intractability
    - **G40.901** Epilepsy, unspecified, not intractable, with status epilepticus
    - **G40.909** Epilepsy, unspecified, not intractable, without status epilepticus
      - Epilepsy NOS
      - Epileptic convulsions NOS
      - Epileptic fits NOS
      - Epileptic seizures NOS
      - Recurrent seizures NOS
      - Seizure disorder NOS
      - *AHA CC: 2Q, 2021, 3-4*
  - **G40.91** Epilepsy, unspecified, intractable
    - Intractable seizure disorder NOS
    - CC **G40.911** Epilepsy, unspecified, intractable, with status epilepticus
    - CC **G40.919** Epilepsy, unspecified, intractable, without status epilepticus

G43 Migraine

NOTE The following terms are to be considered equivalent to intractable: pharmacoresistant (pharmacologically resistant), treatment resistant, refractory (medically) and poorly controlled

Use additional code for adverse effect, if applicable, to identify drug (T36-T50 with fifth or sixth character 5)

Excludes1: headache NOS (R51.9)
  lower half migraine (G44.00)
Excludes2: headache syndromes (G44.-)

- **G43.0** Migraine without aura
  - Common migraine
  - *Excludes1:* chronic migraine without aura (G43.7-)
  - **G43.00** Migraine without aura, not intractable
    - Migraine without aura without mention of refractory migraine
    - **G43.001** Migraine without aura, not intractable, with status migrainosus
    - **G43.009** Migraine without aura, not intractable, without status migrainosus
      - Migraine without aura NOS
  - **G43.01** Migraine without aura, intractable
    - Migraine without aura with refractory migraine
    - **G43.011** Migraine without aura, intractable, with status migrainosus
    - **G43.019** Migraine without aura, intractable, without status migrainosus
- **G43.1** Migraine with aura
  - Basilar migraine
  - Classical migraine
  - Migraine equivalents
  - Migraine preceded or accompanied by transient focal neurological phenomena
  - Migraine triggered seizures
  - Migraine with acute-onset aura
  - Migraine with aura without headache (migraine equivalents)
  - Migraine with prolonged aura
  - Migraine with typical aura
  - Retinal migraine

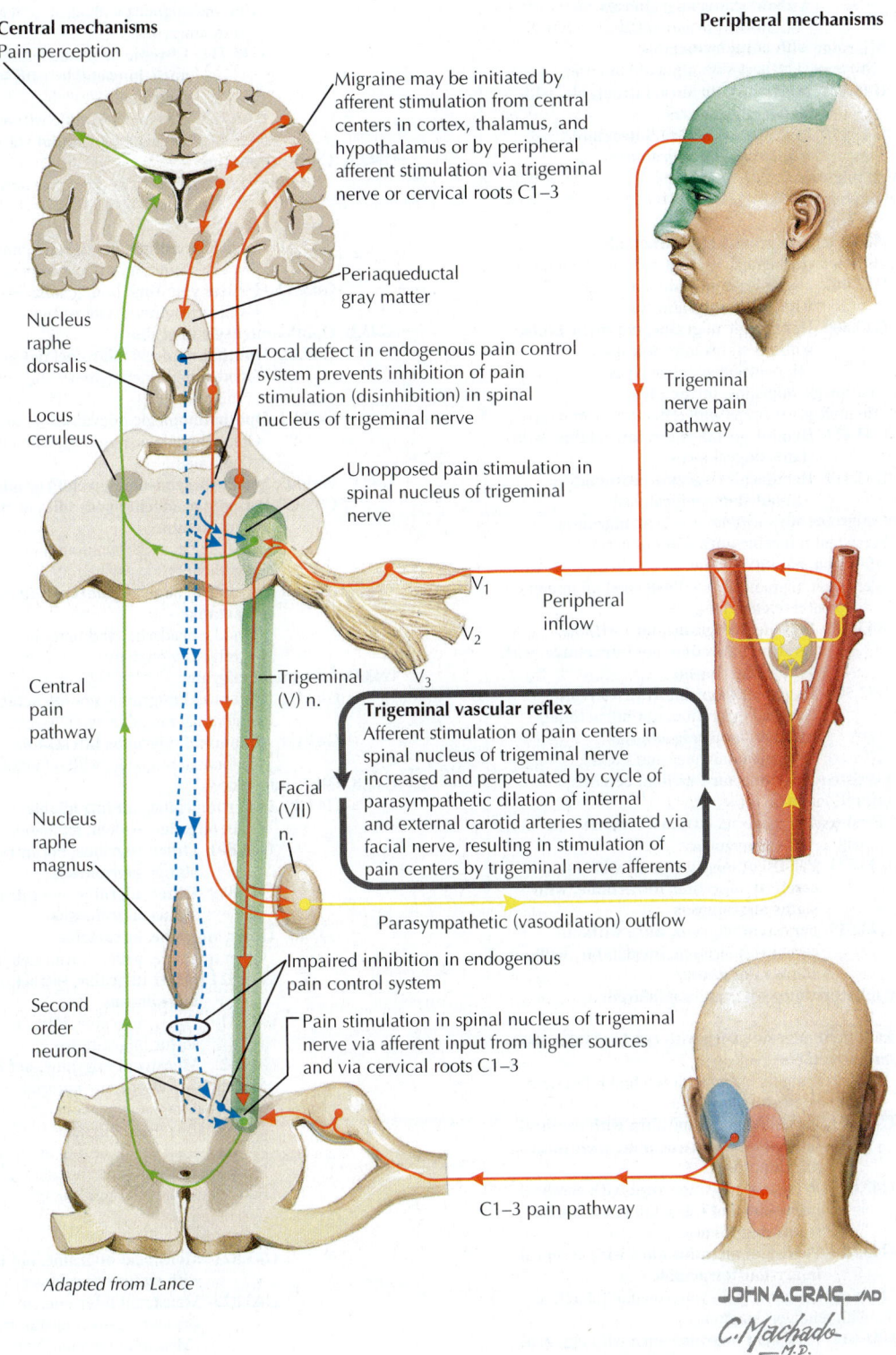

Code also any associated seizure (G40.-, R56.9)

Excludes1: chronic migraine with aura (G43.E-)
persistent migraine aura (G43.5-, G43.6-)

- G43.10 **Migraine with aura, not intractable**
  Migraine with aura without mention of refractory migraine
  - G43.101 Migraine with aura, not intractable, with status migrainosus
  - G43.109 Migraine with aura, not intractable, without status migrainosus
    Migraine with aura NOS
- G43.11 **Migraine with aura, intractable**
  Migraine with aura with refractory migraine
  - G43.111 Migraine with aura, intractable, with status migrainosus
  - G43.119 Migraine with aura, intractable, without status migrainosus

- G43.4 **Hemiplegic migraine**
  Familial migraine
  Sporadic migraine
  - G43.40 **Hemiplegic migraine, not intractable**
    Hemiplegic migraine without refractory migraine
    - G43.401 Hemiplegic migraine, not intractable, with status migrainosus
    - G43.409 Hemiplegic migraine, not intractable, without status migrainosus
      Hemiplegic migraine NOS
  - G43.41 **Hemiplegic migraine, intractable**
    Hemiplegic migraine with refractory migraine
    - G43.411 Hemiplegic migraine, intractable, with status migrainosus
    - G43.419 Hemiplegic migraine, intractable, without status migrainosus

- G43.5 **Persistent migraine aura without cerebral infarction**
  - G43.50 **Persistent migraine aura without cerebral infarction, not intractable**
    Persistent migraine aura without cerebral infarction, without refractory migraine
    - G43.501 Persistent migraine aura without cerebral infarction, not intractable, with status migrainosus
    - G43.509 Persistent migraine aura without cerebral infarction, not intractable, without status migrainosus
      Persistent migraine aura NOS
  - G43.51 **Persistent migraine aura without cerebral infarction, intractable**
    Persistent migraine aura without cerebral infarction, with refractory migraine
    - G43.511 Persistent migraine aura without cerebral infarction, intractable, with status migrainosus
    - G43.519 Persistent migraine aura without cerebral infarction, intractable, without status migrainosus

- G43.6 **Persistent migraine aura with cerebral infarction**
  Code also the type of cerebral infarction (I63.-)
  - G43.60 **Persistent migraine aura with cerebral infarction, not intractable**
    Persistent migraine aura with cerebral infarction, without refractory migraine
    - CC G43.601 Persistent migraine aura with cerebral infarction, not intractable, with status migrainosus
    - CC G43.609 Persistent migraine aura with cerebral infarction, not intractable, without status migrainosus
  - G43.61 **Persistent migraine aura with cerebral infarction, intractable**
    Persistent migraine aura with cerebral infarction, with refractory migraine
    - CC G43.611 Persistent migraine aura with cerebral infarction, intractable, with status migrainosus
    - CC G43.619 Persistent migraine aura with cerebral infarction, intractable, without status migrainosus

- G43.7 **Chronic migraine without aura**
  Transformed migraine
  Excludes1: migraine without aura (G43.0-)
  - G43.70 **Chronic migraine without aura, not intractable**
    Chronic migraine without aura, without refractory migraine
    - G43.701 Chronic migraine without aura, not intractable, with status migrainosus
    - G43.709 Chronic migraine without aura, not intractable, without status migrainosus
      Chronic migraine without aura NOS
  - G43.71 **Chronic migraine without aura, intractable**
    Chronic migraine without aura, with refractory migraine
    - G43.711 Chronic migraine without aura, intractable, with status migrainosus
    - G43.719 Chronic migraine without aura, intractable, without status migrainosus

- G43.A **Cyclical vomiting**
  Excludes1: cyclical vomiting syndrome unrelated to migraine (R11.15)
  AHA CC: 4Q, 2019, 15
  - G43.A0 Cyclical vomiting, in migraine, not intractable
    Cyclical vomiting, without refractory migraine
  - G43.A1 Cyclical vomiting, in migraine, intractable
    Cyclical vomiting, with refractory migraine

- G43.B **Ophthalmoplegic migraine**
  - G43.B0 Ophthalmoplegic migraine, not intractable
    Ophthalmoplegic migraine, without refractory migraine
  - G43.B1 Ophthalmoplegic migraine, intractable
    Ophthalmoplegic migraine, with refractory migraine

- G43.C **Periodic headache syndromes in child or adult**
  - G43.C0 Periodic headache syndromes in child or adult, not intractable
    Periodic headache syndromes in child or adult, without refractory migraine
  - G43.C1 Periodic headache syndromes in child or adult, intractable
    Periodic headache syndromes in child or adult, with refractory migraine

- G43.D **Abdominal migraine**
  - G43.D0 Abdominal migraine, not intractable
    Abdominal migraine, without refractory migraine
  - G43.D1 Abdominal migraine, intractable
    Abdominal migraine, with refractory migraine

- G43.8 **Other migraine**
  - G43.80 **Other migraine, not intractable**
    Other migraine, without refractory migraine
    - G43.801 Other migraine, not intractable, with status migrainosus
    - G43.809 Other migraine, not intractable, without status migrainosus
  - G43.81 **Other migraine, intractable**
    Other migraine, with refractory migraine
    - G43.811 Other migraine, intractable, with status migrainosus
    - G43.819 Other migraine, intractable, without status migrainosus
  - G43.82 **Menstrual migraine, not intractable**
    Menstrual headache, not intractable
    Menstrual migraine, without refractory migraine
    Menstrually related migraine, not intractable
    Pre-menstrual headache, not intractable
    Pre-menstrual migraine, not intractable
    Pure menstrual migraine, not intractable
    Code also associated premenstrual tension syndrome (N94.3)
    - ♀ G43.821 Menstrual migraine, not intractable, with status migrainosus
    - ♀ G43.829 Menstrual migraine, not intractable, without status migrainosus
      Menstrual migraine NOS
  - G43.83 **Menstrual migraine, intractable**
    Menstrual headache, intractable
    Menstrual migraine, with refractory migraine
    Menstrually related migraine, intractable
    Pre-menstrual headache, intractable
    Pre-menstrual migraine, intractable
    Pure menstrual migraine, intractable
    Code also associated premenstrual tension syndrome (N94.3)

♀ G43.831 Menstrual migraine, intractable, with status migrainosus
♀ G43.839 Menstrual migraine, intractable, without status migrainosus

+ G43.9 **Migraine, unspecified**
  + G43.90 Migraine, unspecified, not intractable
    Migraine, unspecified, without refractory migraine
    G43.901 Migraine, unspecified, not intractable, with status migrainosus
      Status migrainosus NOS
    G43.909 Migraine, unspecified, not intractable, without status migrainosus
      Migraine NOS
  + G43.91 Migraine, unspecified, intractable
    Migraine, unspecified, with refractory migraine
    G43.911 Migraine, unspecified, intractable, with status migrainosus
    G43.919 Migraine, unspecified, intractable, without status migrainosus

+ G43.E **Chronic migraine with aura**
  Excludes1: migraine with aura (G43.1-)
  + G43.E0 Chronic migraine with aura, not intractable
    Chronic migraine with aura, without refractory migraine
    G43.E01 Chronic migraine with aura, not intractable, with status migrainosus
    G43.E09 Chronic migraine with aura, not intractable, without status migrainosus
      Chronic migraine with aura NOS
  + G43.E1 Chronic migraine with aura, intractable
    Chronic migraine with aura, with refractory migraine
    G43.E11 Chronic migraine with aura, intractable, with status migrainosus
    G43.E19 Chronic migraine with aura, intractable, without status migrainosus

G44 **Other headache syndromes**
  Excludes1: headache NOS (R51.9)
  Excludes2: atypical facial pain (G50.1)
    headache due to lumbar puncture (G97.1)
    migraines (G43.-)
    trigeminal neuralgia (G50.0)
  + G44.0 **Cluster headaches and other trigeminal autonomic cephalgias (TAC)**
    + G44.00 Cluster headache syndrome, unspecified
      Ciliary neuralgia
      Cluster headache NOS
      Histamine cephalgia
      Lower half migraine
      Migrainous neuralgia
      G44.001 Cluster headache syndrome, unspecified, intractable
      G44.009 Cluster headache syndrome, unspecified, not intractable
        Cluster headache syndrome NOS
    + G44.01 Episodic cluster headache
      G44.011 Episodic cluster headache, intractable
      G44.019 Episodic cluster headache, not intractable
        Episodic cluster headache NOS
    + G44.02 Chronic cluster headache
      G44.021 Chronic cluster headache, intractable
      G44.029 Chronic cluster headache, not intractable
        Chronic cluster headache NOS
    + G44.03 Episodic paroxysmal hemicrania
      Paroxysmal hemicrania NOS
      G44.031 Episodic paroxysmal hemicrania, intractable
      G44.039 Episodic paroxysmal hemicrania, not intractable
        Episodic paroxysmal hemicrania NOS
    + G44.04 Chronic paroxysmal hemicrania
      G44.041 Chronic paroxysmal hemicrania, intractable
      G44.049 Chronic paroxysmal hemicrania, not intractable
        Chronic paroxysmal hemicrania NOS
    + G44.05 Short lasting unilateral neuralgiform headache with conjunctival injection and tearing (SUNCT)
      G44.051 Short lasting unilateral neuralgiform headache with conjunctival injection and tearing (SUNCT), intractable
      G44.059 Short lasting unilateral neuralgiform headache with conjunctival injection and tearing (SUNCT), not intractable
        Short lasting unilateral neuralgiform headache with conjunctival injection and tearing (SUNCT) NOS
    + G44.09 Other trigeminal autonomic cephalgias (TAC)
      G44.091 Other trigeminal autonomic cephalgias (TAC), intractable
      G44.099 Other trigeminal autonomic cephalgias (TAC), not intractable
  G44.1 **Vascular headache, not elsewhere classified**
    Excludes2: cluster headache (G44.0)
      complicated headache syndromes (G44.5-)
      drug-induced headache (G44.4-)
      migraine (G43.-)
      other specified headache syndromes (G44.8-)
      post-traumatic headache (G44.3-)
      tension-type headache (G44.2-)
  + G44.2 **Tension-type headache**
    + G44.20 Tension-type headache, unspecified
      G44.201 Tension-type headache, unspecified, intractable
      G44.209 Tension-type headache, unspecified, not intractable
        Tension headache NOS
    + G44.21 Episodic tension-type headache
      G44.211 Episodic tension-type headache, intractable
      G44.219 Episodic tension-type headache, not intractable
        Episodic tension-type headache NOS
    + G44.22 Chronic tension-type headache
      G44.221 Chronic tension-type headache, intractable
      G44.229 Chronic tension-type headache, not intractable
        Chronic tension-type headache NOS
  + G44.3 **Post-traumatic headache**
    + G44.30 Post-traumatic headache, unspecified
      G44.301 Post-traumatic headache, unspecified, intractable
      G44.309 Post-traumatic headache, unspecified, not intractable
        Post-traumatic headache NOS
    + G44.31 Acute post-traumatic headache
      G44.311 Acute post-traumatic headache, intractable
      G44.319 Acute post-traumatic headache, not intractable
        Acute post-traumatic headache NOS
    + G44.32 Chronic post-traumatic headache
      G44.321 Chronic post-traumatic headache, intractable
      G44.329 Chronic post-traumatic headache, not intractable
        Chronic post-traumatic headache NOS
  + G44.4 **Drug-induced headache, not elsewhere classified**
    Medication overuse headache
    Use additional code for adverse effect, if applicable, to identify drug (T36-T50 with fifth or sixth character 5)
    G44.40 Drug-induced headache, not elsewhere classified, not intractable
    G44.41 Drug-induced headache, not elsewhere classified, intractable
  + G44.5 **Complicated headache syndromes**
    G44.51 Hemicrania continua
    G44.52 New daily persistent headache (NDPH)
    G44.53 Primary thunderclap headache
    G44.59 Other complicated headache syndrome
  + G44.8 **Other specified headache syndromes**
    Excludes2: headache with orthostatic or positional component, not elsewhere classified (R51.0)
    G44.81 Hypnic headache
    G44.82 Headache associated with sexual activity
      Orgasmic headache
      Preorgasmic headache
    G44.83 Primary cough headache

Medial Views of Cerebrum

Sagittal section of brain in situ

Labels: Cingulate gyrus, Cingulate sulcus, Paracentral sulcus, Central sulcus (of Rolando), Paracentral lobule, Marginal sulcus, Corpus callosum, Precuneus, Superior sagittal sinus, Choroid plexus of 3rd ventricle, Stria medullaris of thalamus, Parietooccipital sulcus, Cuneus, Habenular commissure, Pineal body, Posterior commissure, Calcarine sulcus, Straight sinus in tentorium cerebelli, Great cerebral vein (of Galen), Superior colliculus, Inferior colliculus, Tectal (quadrigeminal) plate, Cerebellum, Superior medullary velum, 4th ventricle and choroid plexus, Inferior medullary velum, Medulla oblongata, Pons, Cerebral aqueduct (of Sylvius), Cerebral peduncle, Mammillary body, Hypophysis (pituitary gland), Tuber cinereum, Optic chiasm, Supraoptic recess, Lamina terminalis, Hypothalamic sulcus, Subcallosal gyrus, Anterior commissure, Subcallosal (parolfactory) area, Thalamus and 3rd ventricle, Interthalamic adhesion, Interventricular foramen (of Monro), Septum pellucidum, Fornix, Sulcus of corpus callosum, Medial frontal gyrus

Medial surface of cerebral hemisphere: brainstem excised

Labels: Cingulate gyrus, Mammillothalamic fasciculus, Mammillary body, Uncus, Optic nerve (II), Olfactory tract, Collateral sulcus, Rhinal sulcus, Medial occipitotemporal gyrus, Occipitotemporal sulcus, Lateral occipitotemporal gyrus, Parahippocampal gyrus, Dentate gyrus, Fimbria of hippocampus, Crus/Body/Column of fornix, Lingual gyrus, Calcarine sulcus, Cuneus, Parietooccipital sulcus, Isthmus of cingulate gyrus, Genu/Rostrum/Trunk/Splenium of corpus callosum

Chapter 6: Diseases of the Nervous System

© 2010 Elsevier Inc. All rights reserved. www.netterimages.com

622

Cranial Nerves: Schema

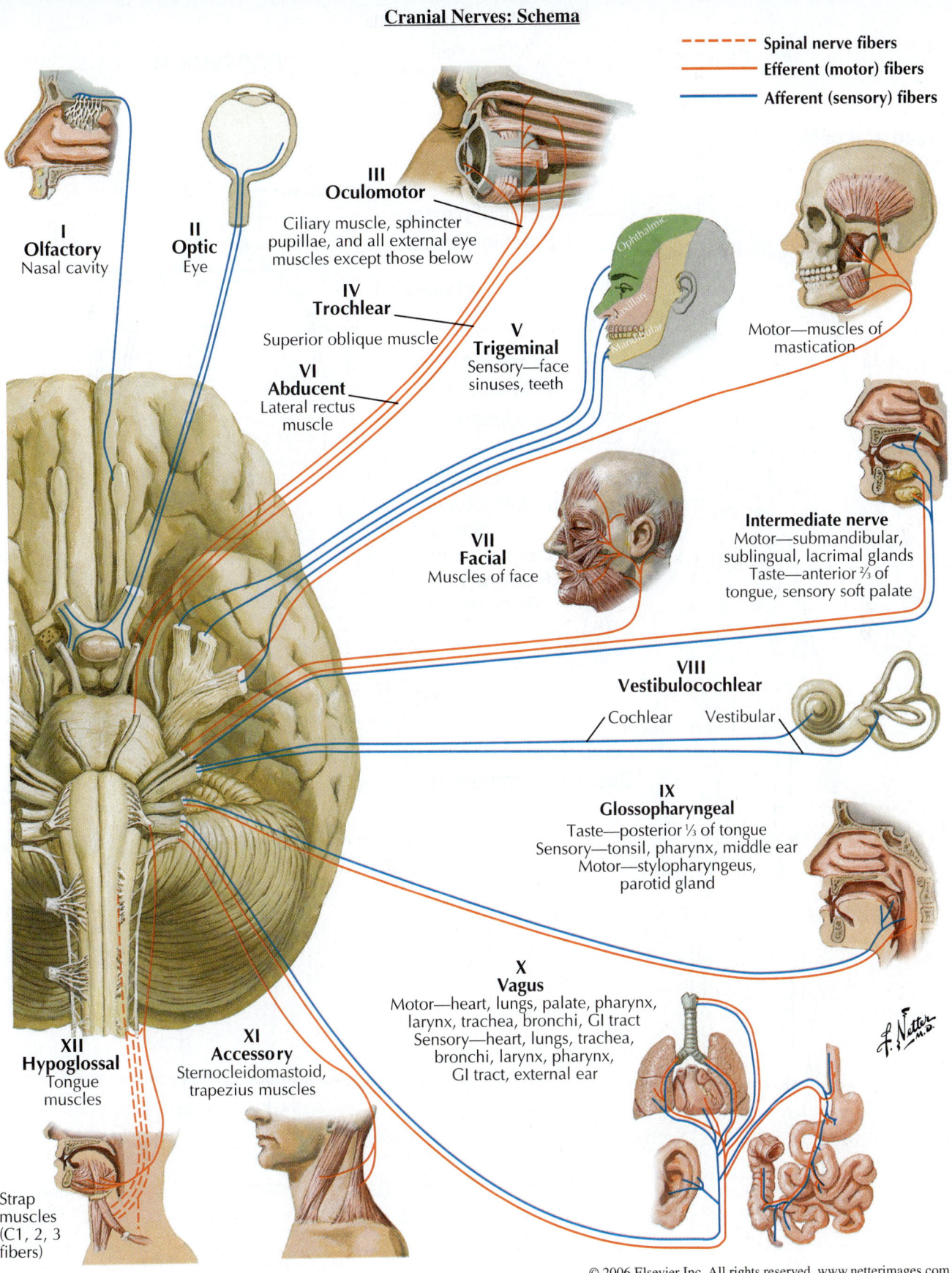

Peripheral Nervous System

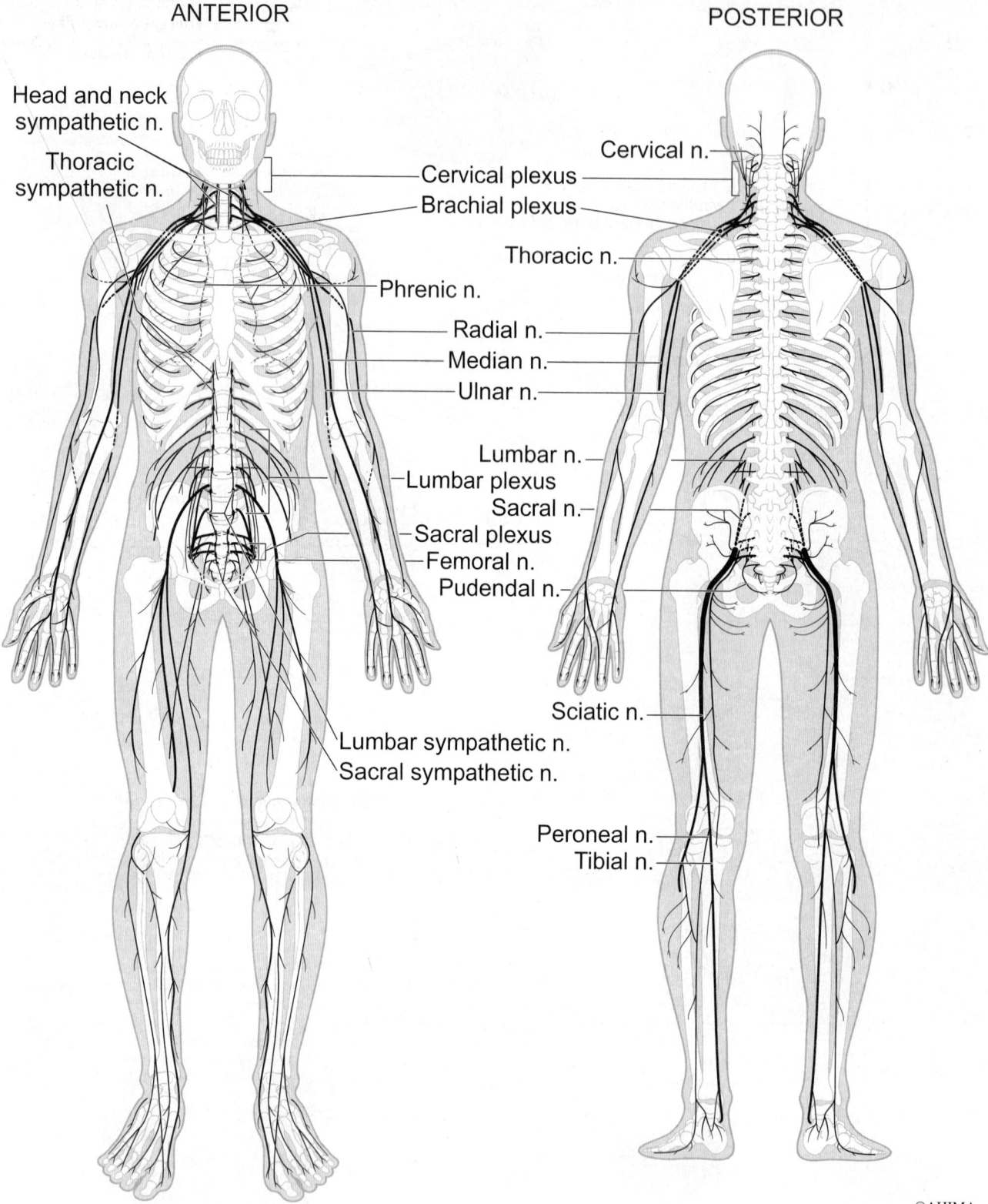

G44.84 Primary exertional headache
G44.85 Primary stabbing headache
G44.86 Cervicogenic headache
  Code also associated cervical spinal condition, if known
  AHA CC: 4Q, 2021, 11-12
G44.89 Other headache syndrome

G45 Transient cerebral ischemic attacks and related syndromes
Excludes1: neonatal cerebral ischemia (P91.0)
  transient retinal artery occlusion (H34.0-)
  AHA CC: 1Q, 2023, 37-38

CC G45.0 Vertebro-basilar artery syndrome
CC G45.1 Carotid artery syndrome (hemispheric)
CC G45.2 Multiple and bilateral precerebral artery syndromes
CC G45.3 Amaurosis fugax
G45.4 Transient global amnesia
  Excludes1: amnesia NOS (R41.3)
CC G45.8 Other transient cerebral ischemic attacks and related syndromes
CC G45.9 Transient cerebral ischemic attack, unspecified
  Spasm of cerebral artery
  TIA
  Transient cerebral ischemia NOS

G46 Vascular syndromes of brain in cerebrovascular diseases
Code first underlying cerebrovascular disease (I60-I69)

CC G46.0 Middle cerebral artery syndrome
CC G46.1 Anterior cerebral artery syndrome
CC G46.2 Posterior cerebral artery syndrome
G46.3 Brain stem stroke syndrome
  Benedikt syndrome
  Claude syndrome
  Foville syndrome
  Millard-Gubler syndrome
  Wallenberg syndrome
  Weber syndrome
G46.4 Cerebellar stroke syndrome
G46.5 Pure motor lacunar syndrome
G46.6 Pure sensory lacunar syndrome
G46.7 Other lacunar syndromes
G46.8 Other vascular syndromes of brain in cerebrovascular diseases

G47 Sleep disorders
Excludes2: nightmares (F51.5)
  nonorganic sleep disorders (F51.-)
  sleep terrors (F51.4)
  sleepwalking (F51.3)

+ G47.0 Insomnia
  Excludes2: alcohol related insomnia (F10.182, F10.282, F10.982)
    drug-related insomnia (F11.182, F11.282, F11.982, F13.182, F13.282, F13.982, F14.182, F14.282, F14.982, F15.182, F15.282, F15.982, F19.182, F19.282, F19.982)
    idiopathic insomnia (F51.01)
    insomnia due to a mental disorder (F51.05)
    insomnia not due to a substance or known physiological condition (F51.0-)
    nonorganic insomnia (F51.0-)
    primary insomnia (F51.01)
    sleep apnea (G47.3-)
  G47.00 Insomnia, unspecified
    Insomnia NOS
  G47.01 Insomnia due to medical condition
    Code also associated medical condition
  G47.09 Other insomnia

+ G47.1 Hypersomnia
  Excludes2: alcohol-related hypersomnia (F10.182, F10.282, F10.982)
    drug-related hypersomnia (F11.182, F11.282, F11.982, F13.182, F13.282, F13.982, F14.182, F14.282, F14.982, F15.182, F15.282, F15.982, F19.182, F19.282, F19.982)
    hypersomnia due to a mental disorder (F51.13)
    hypersomnia not due to a substance or known physiological condition (F51.1-)
    primary hypersomnia (F51.11)
    sleep apnea (G47.3-)
  G47.10 Hypersomnia, unspecified
    Hypersomnia NOS
  G47.11 Idiopathic hypersomnia with long sleep time
    Idiopathic hypersomnia NOS
  G47.12 Idiopathic hypersomnia without long sleep time
  G47.13 Recurrent hypersomnia
    Kleine-Levin syndrome
    Menstrual related hypersomnia
  G47.14 Hypersomnia due to medical condition
    Code also associated medical condition
  G47.19 Other hypersomnia

+ G47.2 Circadian rhythm sleep disorders
  Disorders of the sleep wake schedule
  Inversion of nyctohemeral rhythm
  Inversion of sleep rhythm
  G47.20 Circadian rhythm sleep disorder, unspecified type
    Sleep wake schedule disorder NOS
  G47.21 Circadian rhythm sleep disorder, delayed sleep phase type
    Delayed sleep phase syndrome
  G47.22 Circadian rhythm sleep disorder, advanced sleep phase type
  G47.23 Circadian rhythm sleep disorder, irregular sleep wake type
    Irregular sleep-wake pattern
  G47.24 Circadian rhythm sleep disorder, free running type
    Circadian rhythm sleep disorder, non-24-hour sleep-wake type
  G47.25 Circadian rhythm sleep disorder, jet lag type
  G47.26 Circadian rhythm sleep disorder, shift work type
  G47.27 Circadian rhythm sleep disorder in conditions classified elsewhere
    Code first underlying condition
  G47.29 Other circadian rhythm sleep disorder

+ G47.3 Sleep apnea
  Code also any associated underlying condition
  Excludes1: apnea NOS (R06.81)
    Cheyne-Stokes breathing (R06.3)
    pickwickian syndrome (E66.2)
    sleep apnea of newborn (P28.3-)
  G47.30 Sleep apnea, unspecified
    Sleep apnea NOS
  G47.31 Primary central sleep apnea
    Idiopathic central sleep apnea
  G47.32 High altitude periodic breathing
  G47.33 Obstructive sleep apnea (adult) (pediatric)
    Obstructive sleep apnea hypopnea
    Excludes1: obstructive sleep apnea of newborn (P28.3-)
  G47.34 Idiopathic sleep related nonobstructive alveolar hypoventilation
    Sleep related hypoxia
  G47.35 Congenital central alveolar hypoventilation syndrome
  G47.36 Sleep related hypoventilation in conditions classified elsewhere
    Sleep related hypoxemia in conditions classified elsewhere
    Code first underlying condition
  G47.37 Central sleep apnea in conditions classified elsewhere
    Code first underlying condition
  G47.39 Other sleep apnea

+ G47.4 Narcolepsy and cataplexy
  + G47.41 Narcolepsy
    G47.411 Narcolepsy with cataplexy
    G47.419 Narcolepsy without cataplexy
      Narcolepsy NOS
  + G47.42 Narcolepsy in conditions classified elsewhere
    Code first underlying condition
    G47.421 Narcolepsy in conditions classified elsewhere with cataplexy
    G47.429 Narcolepsy in conditions classified elsewhere without cataplexy

+ G47.5 Parasomnia
  Excludes1: alcohol induced parasomnia (F10.182, F10.282, F10.982)

drug induced parasomnia (F11.182, F11.282, F11.982, F13.182, F13.282, F13.982, F14.182, F14.282, F14.982, F15.182, F15.282, F15.982, F19.182, F19.282, F19.982)
parasomnia not due to a substance or known physiological condition (F51.8)

- G47.50 **Parasomnia, unspecified**
  - Parasomnia NOS
- G47.51 **Confusional arousals**
- G47.52 **REM sleep behavior disorder**
- G47.53 **Recurrent isolated sleep paralysis**
- G47.54 **Parasomnia in conditions classified elsewhere**
  - Code first underlying condition
- G47.59 **Other parasomnia**

+ G47.6 **Sleep related movement disorders**
  - **Excludes2:** restless legs syndrome (G25.81)
  - G47.61 **Periodic limb movement disorder**
  - G47.62 **Sleep related leg cramps**
  - G47.63 **Sleep related bruxism**
    - **Excludes1:** psychogenic bruxism (F45.8)
  - G47.69 **Other sleep related movement disorders**
- G47.8 **Other sleep disorders**
  - Other specified sleep-wake disorder
- G47.9 **Sleep disorder, unspecified**
  - Sleep disorder NOS
  - Unspecified sleep-wake disorder

Nerve, nerve root and plexus disorders (G50-G59)

Excludes1: current traumatic nerve, nerve root and plexus disorders - see Injury, nerve by body region
neuralgia NOS (M79.2)
neuritis NOS (M79.2)
peripheral neuritis in pregnancy (O26.82-)
radiculitis NOS (M54.1-)

G50 Disorders of trigeminal nerve
Includes: disorders of 5th cranial nerve
- G50.0 **Trigeminal neuralgia**
  - Syndrome of paroxysmal facial pain
  - Tic douloureux
- G50.1 **Atypical facial pain**
- G50.8 **Other disorders of trigeminal nerve**
- G50.9 **Disorder of trigeminal nerve, unspecified**

G51 Facial nerve disorders
Includes: disorders of 7th cranial nerve
- G51.0 **Bell's palsy**
  - Facial palsy
- G51.1 **Geniculate ganglionitis**
  - **Excludes1:** postherpetic geniculate ganglionitis (B02.21)
- G51.2 **Melkersson's syndrome**
  - Melkersson-Rosenthal syndrome
+ G51.3 **Clonic hemifacial spasm**
  - *AHA CC: 4Q, 2018, 10*
  - G51.31 **Clonic hemifacial spasm, right**
  - G51.32 **Clonic hemifacial spasm, left**
    - *AHA CC: 4Q, 2018, 10*
  - G51.33 **Clonic hemifacial spasm, bilateral**
  - G51.39 **Clonic hemifacial spasm, unspecified**
- G51.4 **Facial myokymia**
- G51.8 **Other disorders of facial nerve**
- G51.9 **Disorder of facial nerve, unspecified**

G52 Disorders of other cranial nerves
Excludes2: disorders of acoustic [8th] nerve (H93.3)
disorders of optic [2nd] nerve (H46, H47.0)
paralytic strabismus due to nerve palsy (H49.0-H49.2)
- G52.0 **Disorders of olfactory nerve**
  - Disorders of 1st cranial nerve
- G52.1 **Disorders of glossopharyngeal nerve**
  - Disorder of 9th cranial nerve
  - Glossopharyngeal neuralgia
- G52.2 **Disorders of vagus nerve**
  - Disorders of pneumogastric [10th] nerve
- G52.3 **Disorders of hypoglossal nerve**
  - Disorders of 12th cranial nerve
- G52.7 **Disorders of multiple cranial nerves**
  - Polyneuritis cranialis
- G52.8 **Disorders of other specified cranial nerves**
- G52.9 **Cranial nerve disorder, unspecified**

G53 Cranial nerve disorders in diseases classified elsewhere
Code first underlying disease, such as:
neoplasm (C00-D49)
Excludes1: multiple cranial nerve palsy in sarcoidosis (D86.82)
multiple cranial nerve palsy in syphilis (A52.15)
postherpetic geniculate ganglionitis (B02.21)
postherpetic trigeminal neuralgia (B02.22)
Valid 3-character code, no further characters required

G54 Nerve root and plexus disorders
Excludes1: current traumatic nerve root and plexus disorders - see nerve injury by body region
intervertebral disc disorders (M50-M51)
neuralgia or neuritis NOS (M79.2)
neuritis or radiculitis brachial NOS (M54.13)
neuritis or radiculitis lumbar NOS (M54.16)
neuritis or radiculitis lumbosacral NOS (M54.17)
neuritis or radiculitis thoracic NOS (M54.14)
radiculitis NOS (M54.10)
radiculopathy NOS (M54.10)
spondylosis (M47.-)
- G54.0 **Brachial plexus disorders**
  - Thoracic outlet syndrome
  - *AHA CC: 2Q, 2023, 8*
- G54.1 **Lumbosacral plexus disorders**
- G54.2 **Cervical root disorders, not elsewhere classified**
- G54.3 **Thoracic root disorders, not elsewhere classified**
- G54.4 **Lumbosacral root disorders, not elsewhere classified**
- G54.5 **Neuralgic amyotrophy**
  - Parsonage-Aldren-Turner syndrome
  - Shoulder-girdle neuritis
  - **Excludes1:** neuralgic amyotrophy in diabetes mellitus (E08-E13 with .44)
- G54.6 **Phantom limb syndrome with pain**
- G54.7 **Phantom limb syndrome without pain**
  - Phantom limb syndrome NOS
- G54.8 **Other nerve root and plexus disorders**
- G54.9 **Nerve root and plexus disorder, unspecified**

G55 Nerve root and plexus compressions in diseases classified elsewhere
Code first underlying disease, such as:
neoplasm (C00-D49)
Excludes1: nerve root compression (due to) (in) ankylosing spondylitis (M45.-)
nerve root compression (due to) (in) dorsopathies (M53.-, M54.-)
nerve root compression (due to) (in) intervertebral disc disorders (M50.1.-, M51.1.-)
nerve root compression (due to) (in) spondylopathies (M46.-, M48.-)
nerve root compression (due to) (in) spondylosis (M47.0-, M47.2-)
Valid 3-character code, no further characters required

G56 Mononeuropathies of upper limb
Excludes1: current traumatic nerve disorder - see nerve injury by body region
AHA CC: 4Q, 2016, 17-18
+ G56.0 **Carpal tunnel syndrome**
  - G56.00 **Carpal tunnel syndrome, unspecified upper limb**
  - G56.01 **Carpal tunnel syndrome, right upper limb**
  - G56.02 **Carpal tunnel syndrome, left upper limb**
  - G56.03 **Carpal tunnel syndrome, bilateral upper limbs**
+ G56.1 **Other lesions of median nerve**
  - G56.10 **Other lesions of median nerve, unspecified upper limb**
  - G56.11 **Other lesions of median nerve, right upper limb**
  - G56.12 **Other lesions of median nerve, left upper limb**
  - G56.13 **Other lesions of median nerve, bilateral upper limbs**
+ G56.2 **Lesion of ulnar nerve**
  - Tardy ulnar nerve palsy
  - G56.20 **Lesion of ulnar nerve, unspecified upper limb**
  - G56.21 **Lesion of ulnar nerve, right upper limb**
  - G56.22 **Lesion of ulnar nerve, left upper limb**
  - G56.23 **Lesion of ulnar nerve, bilateral upper limbs**
+ G56.3 **Lesion of radial nerve**
  - G56.30 **Lesion of radial nerve, unspecified upper limb**
  - G56.31 **Lesion of radial nerve, right upper limb**

G56.32 Lesion of radial nerve, left upper limb
G56.33 Lesion of radial nerve, bilateral upper limbs
+ **G56.4 Causalgia of upper limb**
Complex regional pain syndrome II of upper limb
Excludes1: *complex regional pain syndrome I of lower limb (G90.52-)*
complex regional pain syndrome I of upper limb (G90.51-)
complex regional pain syndrome II of lower limb (G57.7-)
reflex sympathetic dystrophy of lower limb (G90.52-)
reflex sympathetic dystrophy of upper limb (G90.51-)
G56.40 Causalgia of unspecified upper limb
G56.41 Causalgia of right upper limb
G56.42 Causalgia of left upper limb
G56.43 Causalgia of bilateral upper limbs
+ **G56.8 Other specified mononeuropathies of upper limb**
Interdigital neuroma of upper limb
G56.80 Other specified mononeuropathies of unspecified upper limb
G56.81 Other specified mononeuropathies of right upper limb
G56.82 Other specified mononeuropathies of left upper limb
G56.83 Other specified mononeuropathies of bilateral upper limbs
+ **G56.9 Unspecified mononeuropathy of upper limb**
G56.90 Unspecified mononeuropathy of unspecified upper limb
G56.91 Unspecified mononeuropathy of right upper limb
G56.92 Unspecified mononeuropathy of left upper limb
G56.93 Unspecified mononeuropathy of bilateral upper limbs

G57 Mononeuropathies of lower limb
Excludes1: *current traumatic nerve disorder - see nerve injury by body region*
AHA CC: 4Q, 2016, 17-18
+ **G57.0 Lesion of sciatic nerve**
Excludes1: *sciatica NOS (M54.3-)*
Excludes2: *sciatica attributed to intervertebral disc disorder (M51.1.-)*
G57.00 Lesion of sciatic nerve, unspecified lower limb
G57.01 Lesion of sciatic nerve, right lower limb
G57.02 Lesion of sciatic nerve, left lower limb
G57.03 Lesion of sciatic nerve, bilateral lower limbs
+ **G57.1 Meralgia paresthetica**
Lateral cutaneous nerve of thigh syndrome
G57.10 Meralgia paresthetica, unspecified lower limb
G57.11 Meralgia paresthetica, right lower limb
G57.12 Meralgia paresthetica, left lower limb
G57.13 Meralgia paresthetica, bilateral lower limbs
+ **G57.2 Lesion of femoral nerve**
G57.20 Lesion of femoral nerve, unspecified lower limb
G57.21 Lesion of femoral nerve, right lower limb
G57.22 Lesion of femoral nerve, left lower limb
G57.23 Lesion of femoral nerve, bilateral lower limbs
+ **G57.3 Lesion of lateral popliteal nerve**
Peroneal nerve palsy
G57.30 Lesion of lateral popliteal nerve, unspecified lower limb
G57.31 Lesion of lateral popliteal nerve, right lower limb
AHA CC: 3Q, 2020, 12
G57.32 Lesion of lateral popliteal nerve, left lower limb
G57.33 Lesion of lateral popliteal nerve, bilateral lower limbs
+ **G57.4 Lesion of medial popliteal nerve**
G57.40 Lesion of medial popliteal nerve, unspecified lower limb
G57.41 Lesion of medial popliteal nerve, right lower limb
G57.42 Lesion of medial popliteal nerve, left lower limb
G57.43 Lesion of medial popliteal nerve, bilateral lower limbs
+ **G57.5 Tarsal tunnel syndrome**
G57.50 Tarsal tunnel syndrome, unspecified lower limb
G57.51 Tarsal tunnel syndrome, right lower limb
G57.52 Tarsal tunnel syndrome, left lower limb
G57.53 Tarsal tunnel syndrome, bilateral lower limbs
+ **G57.6 Lesion of plantar nerve**
Morton's metatarsalgia
G57.60 Lesion of plantar nerve, unspecified lower limb
G57.61 Lesion of plantar nerve, right lower limb
G57.62 Lesion of plantar nerve, left lower limb
G57.63 Lesion of plantar nerve, bilateral lower limbs
+ **G57.7 Causalgia of lower limb**
Complex regional pain syndrome II of lower limb
Excludes1: *complex regional pain syndrome I of lower limb (G90.52-)*
complex regional pain syndrome I of upper limb (G90.51-)
complex regional pain syndrome II of upper limb (G56.4-)
reflex sympathetic dystrophy of lower limb (G90.52-)
reflex sympathetic dystrophy of upper limb (G90.51-)
G57.70 Causalgia of unspecified lower limb
G57.71 Causalgia of right lower limb
G57.72 Causalgia of left lower limb
G57.73 Causalgia of bilateral lower limbs
+ **G57.8 Other specified mononeuropathies of lower limb**
Interdigital neuroma of lower limb
G57.80 Other specified mononeuropathies of unspecified lower limb
G57.81 Other specified mononeuropathies of right lower limb
G57.82 Other specified mononeuropathies of left lower limb
G57.83 Other specified mononeuropathies of bilateral lower limbs
+ **G57.9 Unspecified mononeuropathy of lower limb**
G57.90 Unspecified mononeuropathy of unspecified limb
G57.91 Unspecified mononeuropathy of right lower limb
G57.92 Unspecified mononeuropathy of left lower limb
G57.93 Unspecified mononeuropathy of bilateral lower limbs

G58 Other mononeuropathies
G58.0 Intercostal neuropathy
G58.7 Mononeuritis multiplex
G58.8 Other specified mononeuropathies
G58.9 Mononeuropathy, unspecified

G59 Mononeuropathy in diseases classified elsewhere
Code first underlying disease
Excludes1: *diabetic mononeuropathy (E08-E13 with .41)*
syphilitic nerve paralysis (A52.19)
syphilitic neuritis (A52.15)
tuberculous mononeuropathy (A17.83)
Valid 3-character code, no further characters required

Polyneuropathies and other disorders of the peripheral nervous system (G60-G65)

Excludes1: *neuralgia NOS (M79.2)*
neuritis NOS (M79.2)
peripheral neuritis in pregnancy (O26.82-)
radiculitis NOS (M54.10)

G60 Hereditary and idiopathic neuropathy
G60.0 Hereditary motor and sensory neuropathy
Charcot-Marie-Tooth disease
Déjérine-Sottas disease
Hereditary motor and sensory neuropathy, types I-IV
Hypertrophic neuropathy of infancy
Peroneal muscular atrophy (axonal type) (hypertrophic type)
Roussy-Levy syndrome
CC G60.1 Refsum's disease
Infantile Refsum disease
G60.2 Neuropathy in association with hereditary ataxia
G60.3 Idiopathic progressive neuropathy
G60.8 Other hereditary and idiopathic neuropathies
Dominantly inherited sensory neuropathy
Morvan's disease
Nelaton's syndrome
Recessively inherited sensory neuropathy
G60.9 Hereditary and idiopathic neuropathy, unspecified

G61 Inflammatory polyneuropathy
CC **G61.0 Guillain-Barre syndrome**
Acute (post-)infective polyneuritis
Miller Fisher Syndrome
AHA CC: 2Q, 2014, 4; 3Q, 2020, 12

G61.1 Serum neuropathy
  Use additional code for adverse effect, if applicable, to identify serum (T50.-)
G61.8 Other inflammatory polyneuropathies
  CC **G61.81** Chronic inflammatory demyelinating polyneuritis
  G61.82 Multifocal motor neuropathy
    MMN
    AHA CC: 4Q, 2016, 18
  G61.89 Other inflammatory polyneuropathies
G61.9 Inflammatory polyneuropathy, unspecified

G62 Other and unspecified polyneuropathies

G62.0 Drug-induced polyneuropathy
  Use additional code for adverse effect, if applicable, to identify drug (T36-T50 with fifth or sixth character 5)
G62.1 Alcoholic polyneuropathy
  AHA CC: 3Q, 2019, 8
G62.2 Polyneuropathy due to other toxic agents
  Code first (T51-T65) to identify toxic agent
+ **G62.8** Other specified polyneuropathies
  CC **G62.81** Critical illness polyneuropathy
    Acute motor neuropathy
  G62.82 Radiation-induced polyneuropathy
    Use additional external cause code (W88-W90, X39.0-) to identify cause
  G62.89 Other specified polyneuropathies
    AHA CC: 2Q, 2016, 11
G62.9 Polyneuropathy, unspecified
  Neuropathy NOS

G63 Polyneuropathy in diseases classified elsewhere

Code first underlying disease, such as:
  amyloidosis (E85.-)
  endocrine disease, except diabetes (E00-E07, E15-E16, E20-E34)
  metabolic diseases (E70-E88)
  neoplasm (C00-D49)
  nutritional deficiency (E40-E64)
Excludes1: polyneuropathy (in):
  diabetes mellitus (E08-E13 with .42)
  diphtheria (A36.83)
  infectious mononucleosis complicated by polyneuropathy (B27.0-B27.9 with fifth character 1)
  Lyme disease (A69.22)
  mumps (B26.84)
  postherpetic (B02.23)
  rheumatoid arthritis (M05.5-)
  scleroderma (M34.83)
  systemic lupus erythematosus (M32.19)
AHA CC: 4Q, 2012, 99-101; 1Q, 2021, 7
Valid 3-character code, no further characters required

G64 Other disorders of peripheral nervous system

Disorder of peripheral nervous system NOS
Valid 3-character code, no further characters required

G65 Sequelae of inflammatory and toxic polyneuropathies

Code first condition resulting from (sequela) of inflammatory and toxic polyneuropathies
G65.0 Sequelae of Guillain-Barré syndrome
G65.1 Sequelae of other inflammatory polyneuropathy
G65.2 Sequelae of toxic polyneuropathy

Diseases of myoneural junction and muscle (G70-G73)

G70 Myasthenia gravis and other myoneural disorders

Excludes1: botulism (A05.1, A48.51-A48.52)
  transient neonatal myasthenia gravis (P94.0)
+ **G70.0** Myasthenia gravis
  G70.00 Myasthenia gravis without (acute) exacerbation
    Myasthenia gravis NOS
    AHA CC: 3Q, 2022, 15-16
  MCC **G70.01** Myasthenia gravis with (acute) exacerbation
    Myasthenia gravis in crisis
G70.1 Toxic myoneural disorders
  Code first (T51-T65) to identify toxic agent
G70.2 Congenital and developmental myasthenia
+ **G70.8** Other specified myoneural disorders
  CC **G70.80** Lambert-Eaton syndrome, unspecified
    Lambert-Eaton syndrome NOS
  CC **G70.81** Lambert-Eaton syndrome in disease classified elsewhere
    Code first underlying disease
    Excludes1: Lambert-Eaton syndrome in neoplastic disease (G73.1)
  G70.89 Other specified myoneural disorders
G70.9 Myoneural disorder, unspecified

G71 Primary disorders of muscles

Excludes2: arthrogryposis multiplex congenita (Q74.3)
  metabolic disorders (E70-E88)
  myositis (M60.-)
+ **G71.0** Muscular dystrophy
  AHA CC: 4Q, 2018, 11; 4Q, 2022, 17-18
  G71.00 Muscular dystrophy, unspecified
  G71.01 Duchenne or Becker muscular dystrophy
    Autosomal recessive, childhood type, muscular dystrophy resembling Duchenne or Becker muscular dystrophy
    Benign [Becker] muscular dystrophy
    Severe [Duchenne] muscular dystrophy
  G71.02 Facioscapulohumeral muscular dystrophy
    Scapulohumeral muscular dystrophy
    AHA CC: 4Q, 2018, 12-13
+ **G71.03** Limb girdle muscular dystrophies
  G71.031 Autosomal dominant limb girdle muscular dystrophy
    LGMD D4 calpain-3-related
    LGMD D5 collagen 6-related
    Limb girdle muscular dystrophy type 1
  G71.032 Autosomal recessive limb girdle muscular dystrophy due to calpain-3 dysfunction
    Limb girdle muscular dystrophy type 2A
    LGMD R1 calpain-3-related
    Primary calpainopathy
  G71.033 Limb girdle muscular dystrophy due to dysferlin dysfunction
    Dysferlinopathy
    LGMD R2 dysferlin-related
    Limb girdle muscular dystrophy type 2B
    Miyoshi Myopathy type 1
+ **G71.034** Limb girdle muscular dystrophy due to sarcoglycan dysfunction
    G71.0340 Limb girdle muscular dystrophy due to sarcoglycan dysfunction, unspecified
      Sarcoglycanopathy, NOS
    G71.0341 Limb girdle muscular dystrophy due to alpha sarcoglycan dysfunction
      Alpha sarcoglycanopathy
      Limb-girdle muscular dystrophy due to alpha-sarcoglycan deficiency
      Limb girdle muscular dystrophy type 2D
    G71.0342 Limb girdle muscular dystrophy due to beta sarcoglycan dysfunction
      Beta sarcoglycanopathy
      Limb girdle muscular dystrophy due to beta-sarcoglycan deficiency
      Limb girdle muscular dystrophy type 2E
    G71.0349 Limb girdle muscular dystrophy due to other sarcoglycan dysfunction
      Delta sarcoglycanopathy
      Delta-sarcoglycan-related LGMD R6
      Gamma sarcoglycanopathy
      Gamma-sarcoglycan-related LGMD R5
      Limb girdle muscular dystrophy type 2C
      Limb girdle muscular dystrophy type 2F
  G71.035 Limb girdle muscular dystrophy due to anoctamin-5 dysfunction
    Anoctamin-5-related LGMD R12
    Anoctaminopathy

Autosomal recessive limb girdle
muscular dystrophy type 2L
Miyoshi myopathy type 3
- **G71.038 Other limb girdle muscular dystrophy**
LGMD R9 FKRP-related
LGMD R22 collagen 6-related
Limb girdle muscular dystrophy due to fukutin related protein dysfunction
Limb girdle muscular dystrophy type 2I
Other autosomal recessive limb girdle muscular dystrophy
- **G71.039 Limb girdle muscular dystrophy, unspecified**
- **G71.09 Other specified muscular dystrophies**
Benign scapuloperoneal muscular dystrophy with early contractures [Emery-Dreifuss]
Congenital muscular dystrophy NOS
Congenital muscular dystrophy with specific morphological abnormalities of the muscle fiber
Distal muscular dystrophy
Ocular muscular dystrophy
Oculopharyngeal muscular dystrophy
Scapuloperoneal muscular dystrophy

+ **G71.1 Myotonic disorders**
- **G71.11 Myotonic muscular dystrophy**
Dystrophia myotonica [Steinert]
Myotonia atrophica
Myotonic dystrophy
Proximal myotonic myopathy (PROMM)
Steinert disease
- **G71.12 Myotonia congenita**
Acetazolamide responsive myotonia congenita
Dominant myotonia congenita [Thomsen disease]
Myotonia levior
Recessive myotonia congenita [Becker disease]
- **G71.13 Myotonic chondrodystrophy**
Chondrodystrophic myotonia
Congenital myotonic chondrodystrophy
Schwartz-Jampel disease
- **G71.14 Drug induced myotonia**
Use additional code for adverse effect, if applicable, to identify drug (T36-T50 with fifth or sixth character 5)
- **G71.19 Other specified myotonic disorders**
Myotonia fluctuans
Myotonia permanens
Neuromyotonia [Isaacs]
Paramyotonia congenita (of von Eulenburg)
Pseudomyotonia
Symptomatic myotonia

+ **G71.2 Congenital myopathies**
Excludes2: arthrogryposis multiplex congenita (Q74.3)
AHA CC: 4Q, 2020, 19-21
- CC **G71.20 Congenital myopathy, unspecified**
- CC **G71.21 Nemaline myopathy**
- + **G71.22 Centronuclear myopathy**
  - CC **G71.220 X-linked myotubular myopathy**
Myotubular (centronuclear) myopathy
  - CC **G71.228 Other centronuclear myopathy**
Autosomal centronuclear myopathy
Autosomal dominant centronuclear myopathy
Autosomal recessive centronuclear myopathy
Centronuclear myopathy, NOS
- CC **G71.29 Other congenital myopathy**
Central core disease
Minicore disease
Multicore disease
Multiminicore disease

- **G71.3 Mitochondrial myopathy, not elsewhere classified**
Excludes1: Kearns-Sayre syndrome (H49.81)
Leber's disease (H47.21)
Leigh's encephalopathy (G31.82)
mitochondrial metabolism disorders (E88.4.-)
Reye's syndrome (G93.7)
- **G71.8 Other primary disorders of muscles**
- **G71.9 Primary disorder of muscle, unspecified**
Hereditary myopathy NOS

G72 Other and unspecified myopathies
Excludes1: arthrogryposis multiplex congenita (Q74.3)
dermatopolymyositis (M33.-)
ischemic infarction of muscle (M62.2-)
myositis (M60.-)
polymyositis (M33.2.-)
- CC **G72.0 Drug-induced myopathy**
Use additional code for adverse effect, if applicable, to identify drug (T36-T50 with fifth or sixth character 5)
- CC **G72.1 Alcoholic myopathy**
Use additional code to identify alcoholism (F10.-)
- CC **G72.2 Myopathy due to other toxic agents**
Code first (T51-T65) to identify toxic agent
- **G72.3 Periodic paralysis**
Familial periodic paralysis
Hyperkalemic periodic paralysis (familial)
Hypokalemic periodic paralysis (familial)
Myotonic periodic paralysis (familial)
Normokalemic paralysis (familial)
Potassium sensitive periodic paralysis
Excludes1: paramyotonia congenita (of von Eulenburg) (G71.19)
- + **G72.4 Inflammatory and immune myopathies, not elsewhere classified**
  - **G72.41 Inclusion body myositis [IBM]**
  - **G72.49 Other inflammatory and immune myopathies, not elsewhere classified**
Inflammatory myopathy NOS
- + **G72.8 Other specified myopathies**
  - CC **G72.81 Critical illness myopathy**
Acute necrotizing myopathy
Acute quadriplegic myopathy
Intensive care (ICU) myopathy
Myopathy of critical illness
AHA CC: 3Q, 2020, 12
  - **G72.89 Other specified myopathies**
- **G72.9 Myopathy, unspecified**

G73 Disorders of myoneural junction and muscle in diseases classified elsewhere
- CC **G73.1 Lambert-Eaton syndrome in neoplastic disease**
Code first underlying neoplasm (C00-D49)
Excludes1: Lambert-Eaton syndrome not associated with neoplasm (G70.80-G70.81)
- CC **G73.3 Myasthenic syndromes in other diseases classified elsewhere**
Code first underlying disease, such as:
neoplasm (C00-D49)
thyrotoxicosis (E05.-)
- **G73.7 Myopathy in diseases classified elsewhere**
Code first underlying disease, such as:
hyperparathyroidism (E21.0, E21.3)
hypoparathyroidism (E20.-)
glycogen storage disease (E74.0-)
lipid storage disorders (E75.-)
Excludes1: myopathy in:
rheumatoid arthritis (M05.32)
sarcoidosis (D86.87)
scleroderma (M34.82)
Sjögren syndrome (M35.03)
systemic lupus erythematosus (M32.19)
Cerebral palsy and other paralytic syndromes (G80-G83)

G80 Cerebral palsy
Excludes1: hereditary spastic paraplegia (G11.4)
- MCC **G80.0 Spastic quadriplegic cerebral palsy**
Congenital spastic paralysis (cerebral)
- CC **G80.1 Spastic diplegic cerebral palsy**
Spastic cerebral palsy NOS
- CC **G80.2 Spastic hemiplegic cerebral palsy**
- CC **G80.3 Athetoid cerebral palsy**
Double athetosis (syndrome)
Dyskinetic cerebral palsy
Dystonic cerebral palsy
Vogt disease
- **G80.4 Ataxic cerebral palsy**
- **G80.8 Other cerebral palsy**
Mixed cerebral palsy syndromes
- **G80.9 Cerebral palsy, unspecified**
Cerebral palsy NOS

G81 Hemiplegia and hemiparesis

NOTE This category is to be used only when hemiplegia (complete) (incomplete) is reported without further specification, or is stated to be old or longstanding but of unspecified cause. The category is also for use in multiple coding to identify these types of hemiplegia resulting from any cause.

Excludes1: congenital cerebral palsy (G80.-)
hemiplegia and hemiparesis due to sequela of cerebrovascular disease (I69.05-, I69.15-, I69.25-, I69.35-, I69.85-, I69.95-)

Review coding guideline C.6.a

+ **G81.0 Flaccid hemiplegia**
  - CC G81.00 Flaccid hemiplegia affecting unspecified side
  - CC G81.01 Flaccid hemiplegia affecting right dominant side
  - CC G81.02 Flaccid hemiplegia affecting left dominant side
  - CC G81.03 Flaccid hemiplegia affecting right nondominant side
  - CC G81.04 Flaccid hemiplegia affecting left nondominant side

+ **G81.1 Spastic hemiplegia**
  - CC G81.10 Spastic hemiplegia affecting unspecified side
  - CC G81.11 Spastic hemiplegia affecting right dominant side
  - CC G81.12 Spastic hemiplegia affecting left dominant side
  - CC G81.13 Spastic hemiplegia affecting right nondominant side
  - CC G81.14 Spastic hemiplegia affecting left nondominant side

+ **G81.9 Hemiplegia, unspecified**
  - CC G81.90 Hemiplegia, unspecified affecting unspecified side
  - CC G81.91 Hemiplegia, unspecified affecting right dominant side
  - CC G81.92 Hemiplegia, unspecified affecting left dominant side
  - CC G81.93 Hemiplegia, unspecified affecting right nondominant side
  - CC G81.94 Hemiplegia, unspecified affecting left nondominant side

    AHA CC: 1Q, 2015, 26

G82 Paraplegia (paraparesis) and quadriplegia (quadriparesis)

NOTE This category is to be used only when the listed conditions are reported without further specification, or are stated to be old or longstanding but of unspecified cause. The category is also for use in multiple coding to identify these conditions resulting from any cause

Excludes1: congenital cerebral palsy (G80.-)
functional quadriplegia (R53.2)
hysterical paralysis (F44.4)

+ **G82.2 Paraplegia**
  Paralysis of both lower limbs NOS
  Paraparesis (lower) NOS
  Paraplegia (lower) NOS
  - CC G82.20 Paraplegia, unspecified

    AHA CC: 3Q, 2017, 3
  - CC G82.21 Paraplegia, complete
  - CC G82.22 Paraplegia, incomplete

+ **G82.5 Quadriplegia**
  - MCC G82.50 Quadriplegia, unspecified
  - MCC G82.51 Quadriplegia, C1-C4 complete
  - MCC G82.52 Quadriplegia, C1-C4 incomplete
  - MCC G82.53 Quadriplegia, C5-C7 complete
  - MCC G82.54 Quadriplegia, C5-C7 incomplete

G83 Other paralytic syndromes

NOTE This category is to be used only when the listed conditions are reported without further specification, or are stated to be old or longstanding but of unspecified cause. The category is also for use in multiple coding to identify these conditions resulting from any cause.

Includes: paralysis (complete) (incomplete), except as in G80-G82

- CC **G83.0 Diplegia of upper limbs**
  Diplegia (upper)
  Paralysis of both upper limbs

+ **G83.1 Monoplegia of lower limb**
  Paralysis of lower limb

  Excludes1: monoplegia of lower limbs due to sequela of cerebrovascular disease (I69.04-, I69.14-, I69.24-, I69.34-, I69.84-, I69.94-)

  Review coding guideline C.6.a
  - G83.10 Monoplegia of lower limb affecting unspecified side
  - G83.11 Monoplegia of lower limb affecting right dominant side
  - G83.12 Monoplegia of lower limb affecting left dominant side
  - G83.13 Monoplegia of lower limb affecting right nondominant side
  - G83.14 Monoplegia of lower limb affecting left nondominant side

+ **G83.2 Monoplegia of upper limb**
  Paralysis of upper limb

  Excludes1: monoplegia of upper limbs due to sequela of cerebrovascular disease (I69.03-, I69.13-, I69.23-, I69.33-, I69.83-, I69.93-)

  Review coding guideline C.6.a
  - G83.20 Monoplegia of upper limb affecting unspecified side
  - G83.21 Monoplegia of upper limb affecting right dominant side
  - G83.22 Monoplegia of upper limb affecting left dominant side
  - G83.23 Monoplegia of upper limb affecting right nondominant side
  - G83.24 Monoplegia of upper limb affecting left nondominant side

+ **G83.3 Monoplegia, unspecified**
  Review coding guideline C.6.a
  - G83.30 Monoplegia, unspecified affecting unspecified side
  - G83.31 Monoplegia, unspecified affecting right dominant side
  - G83.32 Monoplegia, unspecified affecting left dominant side
  - G83.33 Monoplegia, unspecified affecting right nondominant side
  - G83.34 Monoplegia, unspecified affecting left nondominant side

- CC **G83.4 Cauda equina syndrome**
  Neurogenic bladder due to cauda equina syndrome

  Excludes1: cord bladder NOS (G95.89)
  neurogenic bladder NOS (N31.9)

  AHA CC: 3Q, 2020, 24

- MCC **G83.5 Locked-in state**

+ **G83.8 Other specified paralytic syndromes**

  Excludes1: paralytic syndromes due to current spinal cord injury-code to spinal cord injury (S14, S24, S34)
  - G83.81 Brown-Séquard syndrome
  - G83.82 Anterior cord syndrome
  - G83.83 Posterior cord syndrome
  - G83.84 Todd's paralysis (postepileptic)
  - G83.89 Other specified paralytic syndromes

- **G83.9 Paralytic syndrome, unspecified**

Other disorders of the nervous system (G89-G99)

G89 Pain, not elsewhere classified

Code also related psychological factors associated with pain (F45.42)

Excludes1: generalized pain NOS (R52)
pain disorders exclusively related to psychological factors (F45.41)
pain NOS (R52)

Excludes2: atypical face pain (G50.1)
headache syndromes (G44.-)
localized pain, unspecified type - code to pain by site, such as:
abdomen pain (R10.-)
back pain (M54.9)
breast pain (N64.4)
chest pain (R07.1-R07.9)
ear pain (H92.0-)
eye pain (H57.1)
headache (R51.9)
joint pain (M25.5-)
limb pain (M79.6-)
lumbar region pain (M54.5-)
painful urination (R30.9)
pelvic and perineal pain (R10.2)
shoulder pain (M25.51-)
spine pain (M54.-)

throat pain (R07.0)
tongue pain (K14.6)
tooth pain (K08.8)
renal colic (N23)
migraines (G43.-)
myalgia (M79.1-)
pain from prosthetic devices, implants, and grafts (T82.84, T83.84, T84.84, T85.84-)
phantom limb syndrome with pain (G54.6)
vulvar vestibulitis (N94.810)
vulvodynia (N94.81-)

Review coding guideline C.5.a
Review coding guidelines C.6.b.1 and C.6.b.3
Review coding guideline C.19.g.2

G89.0 Central pain syndrome
Déjérine-Roussy syndrome
Myelopathic pain syndrome
Thalamic pain syndrome (hyperesthetic)
Review coding guideline C.6.b.6

+ **G89.1 Acute pain, not elsewhere classified**
    G89.11 Acute pain due to trauma
    G89.12 Acute post-thoracotomy pain
        Post-thoracotomy pain NOS
    G89.18 Other acute postprocedural pain
        Postoperative pain NOS
        Postprocedural pain NOS

+ **G89.2 Chronic pain, not elsewhere classified**
    Excludes1: *causalgia, lower limb (G57.7-)*
        causalgia, upper limb (G56.4-)
        central pain syndrome (G89.0)
        chronic pain syndrome (G89.4)
        complex regional pain syndrome II, lower limb (G57.7-)
        complex regional pain syndrome II, upper limb (G56.4-)
        neoplasm related chronic pain (G89.3)
        reflex sympathetic dystrophy (G90.5-)
    Review coding guideline C.6.b.4
    G89.21 Chronic pain due to trauma
    G89.22 Chronic post-thoracotomy pain
    G89.28 Other chronic postprocedural pain
        Other chronic postoperative pain
    G89.29 Other chronic pain

G89.3 Neoplasm related pain (acute) (chronic)
    Cancer associated pain
    Pain due to malignancy (primary) (secondary)
    Tumor associated pain
    Review coding guideline C.6.b.5

G89.4 Chronic pain syndrome
    Chronic pain associated with significant psychosocial dysfunction
    Review coding guideline C.6.b.6

G90 Disorders of autonomic nervous system
    Excludes1: *dysfunction of the autonomic nervous system due to alcohol (G31.2)*

+ **G90.0 Idiopathic peripheral autonomic neuropathy**
    G90.01 Carotid sinus syncope
        Carotid sinus syndrome
    G90.09 Other idiopathic peripheral autonomic neuropathy
        Idiopathic peripheral autonomic neuropathy NOS

G90.1 Familial dysautonomia [Riley-Day]
G90.2 Horner's syndrome
    Bernard(-Horner) syndrome
    Cervical sympathetic dystrophy or paralysis

CC **G90.3 Multi-system degeneration of the autonomic nervous system**
    Neurogenic orthostatic hypotension [Shy-Drager]
    Excludes1: *orthostatic hypotension NOS (I95.1)*

G90.4 Autonomic dysreflexia
    Use additional code to identify the cause, such as:
        fecal impaction (K56.41)
        pressure ulcer (pressure area) (L89.-)
        urinary tract infection (N39.0)

+ **G90.5 Complex regional pain syndrome I (CRPS I)**
    Reflex sympathetic dystrophy
    Excludes1: *causalgia of lower limb (G57.7-)*
        causalgia of upper limb (G56.4-)
        complex regional pain syndrome II of lower limb (G57.7-)
        complex regional pain syndrome II of upper limb (G56.4-)

    CC **G90.50 Complex regional pain syndrome I, unspecified**
+   **G90.51 Complex regional pain syndrome I of upper limb**
        CC **G90.511 Complex regional pain syndrome I of right upper limb**
        CC **G90.512 Complex regional pain syndrome I of left upper limb**
        CC **G90.513 Complex regional pain syndrome I of upper limb, bilateral**
        CC **G90.519 Complex regional pain syndrome I of unspecified upper limb**
+   **G90.52 Complex regional pain syndrome I of lower limb**
        CC **G90.521 Complex regional pain syndrome I of right lower limb**
        CC **G90.522 Complex regional pain syndrome I of left lower limb**
        CC **G90.523 Complex regional pain syndrome I of lower limb, bilateral**
        CC **G90.529 Complex regional pain syndrome I of unspecified lower limb**
    CC **G90.59 Complex regional pain syndrome I of other specified site**

G90.8 Other disorders of autonomic nervous system
    AHA CC: 2Q, 2023, 8-9

G90.9 Disorder of the autonomic nervous system, unspecified

G90.A Postural orthostatic tachycardia syndrome [POTS]
    Chronic orthostatic intolerance
    Postural tachycardia syndrome
    AHA CC: 4Q, 2022, 19-20

G90.B LMNB1-related autosomal dominant leukodystrophy

G91 Hydrocephalus
    Includes: acquired hydrocephalus
    Excludes1: *Arnold-Chiari syndrome with hydrocephalus (Q07.-)*
        congenital hydrocephalus (Q03.-)
        spina bifida with hydrocephalus (Q05.-)

CC **G91.0 Communicating hydrocephalus**
    Secondary normal pressure hydrocephalus

CC **G91.1 Obstructive hydrocephalus**

CC **G91.2 (Idiopathic) normal pressure hydrocephalus**
    Normal pressure hydrocephalus NOS

CC **G91.3 Post-traumatic hydrocephalus, unspecified**

G91.4 Hydrocephalus in diseases classified elsewhere
    Code first underlying condition, such as:
        congenital syphilis (A50.4-)
        neoplasm (C00-D49)
        plasminogen deficiency (E88.02)
    Excludes1: *hydrocephalus due to congenital toxoplasmosis (P37.1)*
    AHA CC: 3Q, 2014, 3-4

CC **G91.8 Other hydrocephalus**
CC **G91.9 Hydrocephalus, unspecified**

G92 Toxic encephalopathy
    AHA CC: 1Q, 2017, 39-40; 4Q, 2020, 14; 1Q, 2021, 13

+ **G92.0 Immune effector cell-associated neurotoxicity syndrome**
    Code first underlying cause such as:
        complications of immune effector cellular therapy (T80.82)
    Code also, if applicable, associated signs and symptoms, such as:
        cerebral edema (G93.6)
        unspecified convulsions (R56.9)
    AHA CC: 4Q, 2021, 12-14

    G92.00 Immune effector cell-associated neurotoxicity syndrome, grade unspecified
        ICANS, grade unspecified
    G92.01 Immune effector cell-associated neurotoxicity syndrome, grade 1
        ICANS, grade 1
    G92.02 Immune effector cell-associated neurotoxicity syndrome, grade 2
        ICANS, grade 2
    CC **G92.03 Immune effector cell-associated neurotoxicity syndrome, grade 3**
        ICANS, grade 3
    CC **G92.04 Immune effector cell-associated neurotoxicity syndrome, grade 4**
        ICANS, grade 4
    CC **G92.05 Immune effector cell-associated neurotoxicity syndrome, grade 5**
        ICANS, grade 5

MCC G92.8 Other toxic encephalopathy
  Toxic encephalitis
  Toxic metabolic encephalopathy
  Code first poisoning due to drug or toxin, if applicable, (T36-T65 with fifth or sixth character 1-4)
  Use additional code for adverse effect, if applicable, to identify drug (T36-T50 with fifth or sixth character 5)
  AHA CC: 4Q, 2021, 12-14; 2Q, 2022, 52-53

MCC G92.9 Unspecified toxic encephalopathy
  Code first poisoning due to drug or toxin, if applicable, (T36-T65 with fifth or sixth character 1-4)
  Use additional code for adverse effect, if applicable, to identify drug (T36-T50 with fifth or sixth character 5)
  AHA CC: 4Q, 2021, 12-14

G93 Other disorders of brain

G93.0 Cerebral cysts
  Arachnoid cyst
  Porencephalic cyst, acquired
  Excludes1: acquired periventricular cysts of newborn (P91.1)
    congenital cerebral cysts (Q04.6)

CC G93.1 Anoxic brain damage, not elsewhere classified
  Excludes1: cerebral anoxia due to anesthesia during labor and delivery (O74.3)
    cerebral anoxia due to anesthesia during the puerperium (O89.2)
    neonatal anoxia (P84)

G93.2 Benign intracranial hypertension
  Pseudotumor
  Excludes1: hypertensive encephalopathy (I67.4)
    obstructive hydrocephalus (G91.1)

+ G93.3 Postviral and related fatigue syndromes
  Use additional code, if applicable, for post COVID-19 condition, unspecified (U09.9)
  Excludes1: chronic fatigue NOS (R53.82)
    neurasthenia (F48.8)
  AHA CC: 4Q, 2022, 20

  G93.31 Postviral fatigue syndrome
  G93.32 Myalgic encephalomyelitis/chronic fatigue syndrome
    Chronic fatigue syndrome
    ME/CFS
    Myalgic encephalomyelitis
  G93.39 Other post infection and related fatigue syndromes

+ G93.4 Other and unspecified encephalopathy
  Excludes2: alcoholic encephalopathy (G31.2)
    encephalopathy in diseases classified elsewhere (G94)
    hypertensive encephalopathy (I67.4)
    toxic (metabolic) encephalopathy (G92.8)
  AHA CC: 2Q, 2017, 8-9

  CC G93.40 Encephalopathy, unspecified
  MCC G93.41 Metabolic encephalopathy
    Septic encephalopathy
    AHA CC: 3Q, 2015, 21; 3Q, 2016, 42
  CC G93.42 Megaloencephalic leukoencephalopathy with subcortical cysts
  CC G93.43 Leukoencephalopathy with calcifications and cysts
  • **CC G93.44 Adult-onset leukodystrophy with axonal spheroids**
    Adult-onset leukoencephalopathy with axonal spheroids and pigmented glia
  CC G93.49 Other encephalopathy
    Encephalopathy NEC
    AHA CC: 2Q, 2017, 9; 2Q, 2018, 22, 25; 4Q, 2018, 16; 2Q, 2021, 3-4

MCC G93.5 Compression of brain
  Arnold-Chiari type 1 compression of brain
  Compression of brain (stem)
  Herniation of brain (stem)
  Excludes1: traumatic compression of brain (S06.A-)
  AHA CC: 2Q, 2020, 31

MCC G93.6 Cerebral edema
  Excludes1: cerebral edema due to birth injury (P11.0)
    traumatic cerebral edema (S06.1-)
  AHA CC: 3Q, 2022, 9, 11

• **MCC G93.7 Reye's syndrome**
  Code first poisoning due to salicylates, if applicable (T39.0-, with sixth character 1-4)
  Use additional code for adverse effect due to salicylates, if applicable (T39.0-, with sixth character 5)

+ G93.8 Other specified disorders of brain
  G93.81 Temporal sclerosis
    Hippocampal sclerosis
    Mesial temporal sclerosis
  MCC G93.82 Brain death
  G93.89 Other specified disorders of brain
    Postradiation encephalopathy
    AHA CC: 4Q, 2016, 4-7; 3Q, 2019, 8-9; 2Q, 2020, 24

G93.9 Disorder of brain, unspecified

G94 Other disorders of brain in diseases classified elsewhere
  Code first underlying disease
  Excludes1: encephalopathy in congenital syphilis (A50.49)
    encephalopathy in influenza (J09.X9, J10.81, J11.81)
    encephalopathy in syphilis (A52.19)
    hydrocephalus in diseases classified elsewhere (G91.4)
  AHA CC: 2Q, 2017, 8-9
  Valid 3-character code, no further characters required

G95 Other and unspecified diseases of spinal cord
  Excludes2: myelitis (G04.-)

  CC G95.0 Syringomyelia and syringobulbia
  + G95.1 Vascular myelopathies
    Excludes2: intraspinal phlebitis and thrombophlebitis, except non-pyogenic (G08)

  MCC G95.11 Acute infarction of spinal cord (embolic) (nonembolic)
    Anoxia of spinal cord
    Arterial thrombosis of spinal cord
  MCC G95.19 Other vascular myelopathies
    Edema of spinal cord
    Hematomyelia
    Nonpyogenic intraspinal phlebitis and thrombophlebitis
    Subacute necrotic myelopathy

  + G95.2 Other and unspecified cord compression
    CC G95.20 Unspecified cord compression
    CC G95.29 Other cord compression

  + G95.8 Other specified diseases of spinal cord
    Excludes1: neurogenic bladder NOS (N31.9)
      neurogenic bladder due to cauda equina syndrome (G83.4)
      neuromuscular dysfunction of bladder without spinal cord lesion (N31.-)
    CC G95.81 Conus medullaris syndrome
    CC G95.89 Other specified diseases of spinal cord
      Cord bladder NOS
      Drug-induced myelopathy
      Radiation-induced myelopathy
      Excludes1: myelopathy NOS (G95.9)

  CC G95.9 Disease of spinal cord, unspecified
    Myelopathy NOS

G96 Other disorders of central nervous system

+ G96.0 Cerebrospinal fluid leak
  Excludes1: cerebrospinal fluid leak from spinal puncture (G97.0)
  Code also if applicable:
    intracranial hypotension (G96.81-)
  AHA CC: 2Q, 2018, 13; 4Q, 2020, 21-22

  CC G96.00 Cerebrospinal fluid leak, unspecified
    Code also if applicable:
      head injury (S00-S09)
  CC G96.01 Cranial cerebrospinal fluid leak, spontaneous
    Otorrhea due to spontaneous cerebrospinal fluid CSF leak
    Rhinorrhea due to spontaneous cerebrospinal fluid CSF leak
    Spontaneous cerebrospinal fluid leak from skull base
  CC G96.02 Spinal cerebrospinal fluid leak, spontaneous
    Spontaneous cerebrospinal fluid leak from spine
  CC G96.08 Other cranial cerebrospinal fluid leak
    Postoperative cranial cerebrospinal fluid leak
    Traumatic cranial cerebrospinal fluid leak
    Code also if applicable:
      head injury (S00 - S09)
  CC G96.09 Other spinal cerebrospinal fluid leak
    Other spinal CSF leak
    Postoperative spinal cerebrospinal fluid leak

Traumatic spinal cerebrospinal fluid leak
Code also if applicable:
head injury (S00 - S09)
AHA CC: 3Q, 2022, 24

+ **G96.1** Disorders of meninges, not elsewhere classified
  - CC **G96.11** Dural tear
    - **Excludes1:** *accidental puncture or laceration of dura during a procedure (G97.41)*
    - Code also intracranial hypotension, if applicable (G96.81-)
    - *AHA CC: 4Q, 2014, 24*
  - **G96.12** Meningeal adhesions (cerebral) (spinal)
  - + **G96.19** Other disorders of meninges, not elsewhere classified
    - *AHA CC: 4Q, 2020, 22*
    - **G96.191** Perineural cyst
      - Cervical nerve root cyst
      - Lumbar nerve root cyst
      - Sacral nerve root cyst
      - Tarlov cyst
      - Thoracic nerve root cyst
    - **G96.198** Other disorders of meninges, not elsewhere classified
+ **G96.8** Other specified disorders of central nervous system
  + **G96.81** Intracranial hypotension
    - Code also any associated diagnoses, such as:
      - Brachial amyotrophy (G54.5)
      - Cerebrospinal fluid leak from spine (G96.02)
      - Cranial nerve disorders in diseases classified elsewhere (G53)
      - Nerve root and compressions in diseases classified elsewhere (G55)
      - Nonpyogenic thrombosis of intracranial venous system (I67.6)
      - Nontraumatic intracerebral hemorrhage (I61.-)
      - Nontraumatic subdural hemorrhage (I62.0-)
      - Other and unspecified cord compression (G95.2-)
      - Other secondary parkinsonism (G21.8)
      - Reversible cerebrovascular vasoconstriction syndrome (I67.841)
      - Spinal cord herniation (G95.89)
      - Stroke (I63.-)
      - Syringomyelia (G95.0)
    - *AHA CC: 4Q, 2020, 23*
    - **G96.810** Intracranial hypotension, unspecified
    - **G96.811** Intracranial hypotension, spontaneous
      - *AHA CC: 4Q, 2020, 24*
    - **G96.819** Other intracranial hypotension
  - **G96.89** Other specified disorders of central nervous system
- **G96.9** Disorder of central nervous system, unspecified

G97 Intraoperative and postprocedural complications and disorders of nervous system, not elsewhere classified
- **Excludes2:** *intraoperative and postprocedural cerebrovascular infarction (I97.81-, I97.82-)*
- *AHA CC: 4Q, 2016, 9-10*
- CC **G97.0** Cerebrospinal fluid leak from spinal puncture
  - Code also any associated diagnoses or complications, such as:
    - intracranial hypotension following a procedure (G97.83-G97.84)
- **G97.1** Other reaction to spinal and lumbar puncture
  - Headache due to lumbar puncture
  - Other reaction to spinal dural puncture
  - Code also, if applicable, any associated headache with orthostatic component (R51.0)
- CC **G97.2** Intracranial hypotension following ventricular shunting
  - Code also any associated diagnoses or complications
+ **G97.3** Intraoperative hemorrhage and hematoma of a nervous system organ or structure complicating a procedure
  - **Excludes1:** *intraoperative hemorrhage and hematoma of a nervous system organ or structure due to accidental puncture and laceration during a procedure (G97.4-)*
  - CC **G97.31** Intraoperative hemorrhage and hematoma of a nervous system organ or structure complicating a nervous system procedure
  - CC **G97.32** Intraoperative hemorrhage and hematoma of a nervous system organ or structure complicating other procedure
+ **G97.4** Accidental puncture and laceration of a nervous system organ or structure during a procedure
  - CC **G97.41** Accidental puncture or laceration of dura during a procedure
    - Incidental (inadvertent) durotomy
    - Code also any associated diagnoses or complications
  - CC **G97.48** Accidental puncture and laceration of other nervous system organ or structure during a nervous system procedure
  - CC **G97.49** Accidental puncture and laceration of other nervous system organ or structure during other procedure
+ **G97.5** Postprocedural hemorrhage of a nervous system organ or structure following a procedure
  - CC **G97.51** Postprocedural hemorrhage of a nervous system organ or structure following a nervous system procedure
  - CC **G97.52** Postprocedural hemorrhage of a nervous system organ or structure following other procedure
+ **G97.6** Postprocedural hematoma and seroma of a nervous system organ or structure following a procedure
  - CC **G97.61** Postprocedural hematoma of a nervous system organ or structure following a nervous system procedure
    - *AHA CC: 3Q, 2020, 24*
  - CC **G97.62** Postprocedural hematoma of a nervous system organ or structure following other procedure
  - CC **G97.63** Postprocedural seroma of a nervous system organ or structure following a nervous system procedure
  - CC **G97.64** Postprocedural seroma of a nervous system organ or structure following other procedure
+ **G97.8** Other intraoperative and postprocedural complications and disorders of nervous system
  - Use additional code to further specify disorder
  - *AHA CC: 4Q, 2020, 23-24*
  - CC **G97.81** Other intraoperative complications of nervous system
  - CC **G97.82** Other postprocedural complications and disorders of nervous system
    - *AHA CC: 1Q, 2022, 34-35*
  - CC **G97.83** Intracranial hypotension following lumbar cerebrospinal fluid shunting
    - Code also any associated diagnoses or complications
  - CC **G97.84** Intracranial hypotension following other procedure
    - Code also, if applicable:
      - accidental puncture or laceration of dura during a procedure (G97.41)
      - cerebrospinal fluid leak from spinal puncture (G97.0)

G98 Other disorders of nervous system not elsewhere classified
- **Includes:** nervous system disorder NOS
- **G98.0** Neurogenic arthritis, not elsewhere classified
  - Nonsyphilitic neurogenic arthropathy NEC
  - Nonsyphilitic neurogenic spondylopathy NEC
  - **Excludes1:** *spondylopathy (in):*
    - *syringomyelia and syringobulbia (G95.0)*
    - *tabes dorsalis (A52.11)*
- **G98.8** Other disorders of nervous system
  - Nervous system disorder NOS

G99 Other disorders of nervous system in diseases classified elsewhere

CC G99.0 Autonomic neuropathy in diseases classified elsewhere
Code first underlying disease, such as:
   amyloidosis (E85.-)
   gout (M1A.-, M10.-)
   hyperthyroidism (E05.-)
Excludes1: diabetic autonomic neuropathy (E08-E13 with .43)

CC G99.2 Myelopathy in diseases classified elsewhere
Code first underlying disease, such as:
   neoplasm (C00-D49)
Excludes1: myelopathy in:
   intervertebral disease (M50.0-, M51.0-)
   spondylosis (M47.0-, M47.1-)
AHA CC: 3Q, 2018, 18-19

G99.8 Other specified disorders of nervous system in diseases classified elsewhere
Code first underlying disorder, such as:
   amyloidosis (E85.-)
   avitaminosis (E56.-)
Excludes1: nervous system involvement in:
   cysticercosis (B69.0)
   rubella (B06.0-)
   syphilis (A52.1-)

Chapter 7: Diseases of the Eye and Adnexa (H00-H59)

NOTE Use an external cause code following the code for the eye condition, if applicable, to identify the cause of the eye condition

Excludes2: *certain conditions originating in the perinatal period (P04-P96)*
certain infectious and parasitic diseases (A00-B99)
complications of pregnancy, childbirth and the puerperium (O00-O9A)
congenital malformations, deformations, and chromosomal abnormalities (Q00-Q99)
diabetes mellitus related eye conditions (E09.3-, E10.3-, E11.3-, E13.3-)
endocrine, nutritional and metabolic diseases (E00-E88)
injury (trauma) of eye and orbit (S05.-)
injury, poisoning and certain other consequences of external causes (S00-T88)
neoplasms (C00-D49)
symptoms, signs and abnormal clinical and laboratory findings, not elsewhere classified (R00-R94)
syphilis related eye disorders (A50.01, A50.3-, A51.43, A52.71)

This chapter contains the following category blocks:
- H00-H05 Disorders of eyelid, lacrimal system and orbit
- H10-H11 Disorders of conjunctiva
- H15-H22 Disorders of sclera, cornea, iris and ciliary body
- H25-H28 Disorders of lens
- H30-H36 Disorders of choroid and retina
- H40-H42 Glaucoma
- H43-H44 Disorders of vitreous body and globe
- H46-H47 Disorders of optic nerve and visual pathways
- H49-H52 Disorders of ocular muscles, binocular movement, accommodation and refraction
- H53-H54 Visual disturbances and blindness
- H55-H57 Other disorders of eye and adnexa
- H59 Intraoperative and postprocedural complications and disorders of eye and adnexa, not elsewhere classified

C. Chapter-Specific Coding Guidelines

In addition to general coding guidelines, there are guidelines for specific diagnoses and/or conditions in the classification. Unless otherwise indicated, these guidelines apply to all health care settings. Please refer to Section II for guidelines on the selection of principal diagnosis.

7. Chapter 7: Diseases of the Eye and Adnexa (H00-H59)

a. Glaucoma

1) Assigning Glaucoma Codes

Assign as many codes from category H40, Glaucoma, as needed to identify the type of glaucoma, the affected eye, and the glaucoma stage.

2) Bilateral glaucoma with same type and stage

When a patient has bilateral glaucoma and both eyes are documented as being the same type and stage, and there is a code for bilateral glaucoma, report only the code for the type of glaucoma, bilateral, with the seventh character for the stage.

When a patient has bilateral glaucoma and both eyes are documented as being the same type and stage, and the classification does not provide a code for bilateral glaucoma (i.e. subcategories H40.10, H40.11 and H40.20) report only one code for the type of glaucoma with the appropriate seventh character for the stage.

3) Bilateral glaucoma stage with different types or stages

When a patient has bilateral glaucoma and each eye is documented as having a different type or stage, and the classification distinguishes laterality, assign the appropriate code for each eye rather than the code for bilateral glaucoma.

When a patient has bilateral glaucoma and each eye is documented as having a different type, and the classification does not distinguish laterality (i.e. subcategories H40.10, H40.11 and H40.20), assign one code for each type of glaucoma with the appropriate seventh character for the stage.

When a patient has bilateral glaucoma and each eye is documented as having the same type, but different stage, and the classification does not distinguish laterality (i.e. subcategories H40.10, H40.11 and H40.20), assign a code for the type of glaucoma for each eye with the seventh character for the specific glaucoma stage documented for each eye.

4) Patient admitted with glaucoma and stage evolves during the admission

If a patient is admitted with glaucoma and the stage progresses during the admission, assign the code for highest stage documented.

5) Indeterminate stage glaucoma

Assignment of the seventh character "4" for "indeterminate stage" should be based on the clinical documentation. The seventh character "4" is used for glaucomas whose stage cannot be clinically determined. This seventh character should not be confused with the seventh character "0", unspecified, which should be assigned when there is no documentation regarding the stage of the glaucoma.

b. Blindness

If "blindness" or "low vision" of both eyes is documented but the visual impairment category is not documented, assign code H54.3, Unqualified visual loss, both eyes. If "blindness" or "low vision" in one eye is documented but the visual impairment category is not documented, assign a code from H54.6-, Unqualified visual loss, one eye. If "blindness" or "visual loss" is documented without any information about whether one or both eyes are affected, assign code H54.7, Unspecified visual loss.

Disorders of eyelid, lacrimal system and orbit (H00-H05)

Excludes2: *open wound of eyelid (S01.1-)*
superficial injury of eyelid (S00.1-, S00.2-)

H00 Hordeolum and chalazion

+ **H00.0 Hordeolum (externum) (internum) of eyelid**
  + **H00.01 Hordeolum externum**
    Hordeolum NOS
    Stye
    - H00.011 Hordeolum externum right upper eyelid
    - H00.012 Hordeolum externum right lower eyelid
    - H00.013 Hordeolum externum right eye, unspecified eyelid
    - H00.014 Hordeolum externum left upper eyelid
    - H00.015 Hordeolum externum left lower eyelid
    - H00.016 Hordeolum externum left eye, unspecified eyelid
    - H00.019 Hordeolum externum unspecified eye, unspecified eyelid
  + **H00.02 Hordeolum internum**
    Infection of meibomian gland
    - H00.021 Hordeolum internum right upper eyelid
    - H00.022 Hordeolum internum right lower eyelid
    - H00.023 Hordeolum internum right eye, unspecified eyelid
    - H00.024 Hordeolum internum left upper eyelid
    - H00.025 Hordeolum internum left lower eyelid
    - H00.026 Hordeolum internum left eye, unspecified eyelid
    - H00.029 Hordeolum internum unspecified eye, unspecified eyelid
  + **H00.03 Abscess of eyelid**
    Furuncle of eyelid
    - H00.031 Abscess of right upper eyelid
    - H00.032 Abscess of right lower eyelid
    - H00.033 Abscess of eyelid right eye, unspecified eyelid
    - H00.034 Abscess of left upper eyelid
    - H00.035 Abscess of left lower eyelid
    - H00.036 Abscess of eyelid left eye, unspecified eyelid
    - H00.039 Abscess of eyelid unspecified eye, unspecified eyelid
+ **H00.1 Chalazion**
  Meibomian (gland) cyst
  Excludes2: *infected meibomian gland (H00.02-)*
  - H00.11 Chalazion right upper eyelid
  - H00.12 Chalazion right lower eyelid
  - H00.13 Chalazion right eye, unspecified eyelid
  - H00.14 Chalazion left upper eyelid
  - H00.15 Chalazion left lower eyelid
  - H00.16 Chalazion left eye, unspecified eyelid
  - H00.19 Chalazion unspecified eye, unspecified eyelid

H01 Other inflammation of eyelid

+ **H01.0 Blepharitis**
  Excludes1: *blepharoconjunctivitis (H10.5-)*
  AHA CC: 4Q, 2018, 13
  + **H01.00 Unspecified blepharitis**
    - H01.001 Unspecified blepharitis right upper eyelid
    - H01.002 Unspecified blepharitis right lower eyelid
    - H01.003 Unspecified blepharitis right eye, unspecified eyelid
    - H01.004 Unspecified blepharitis left upper eyelid
    - H01.005 Unspecified blepharitis left lower eyelid

Chapter 7: Diseases of the Eye and Adnexa

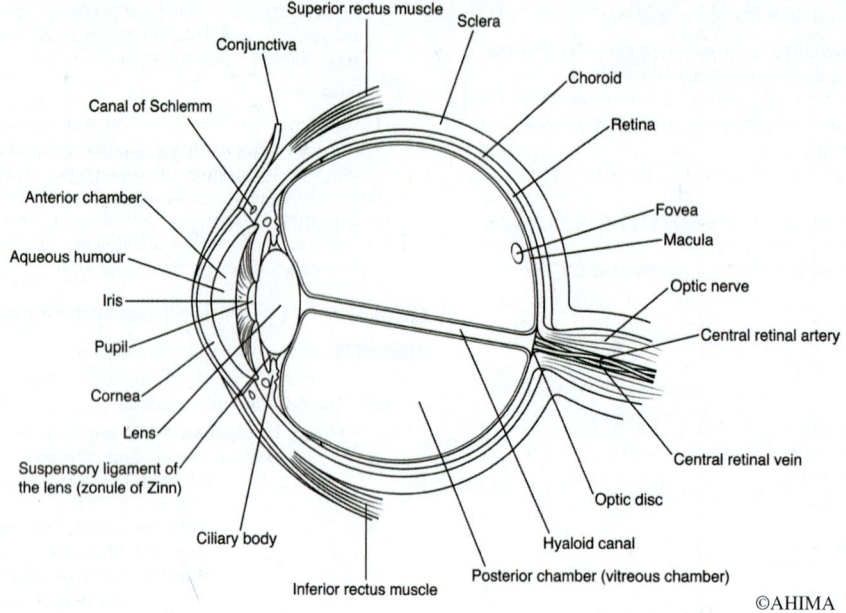

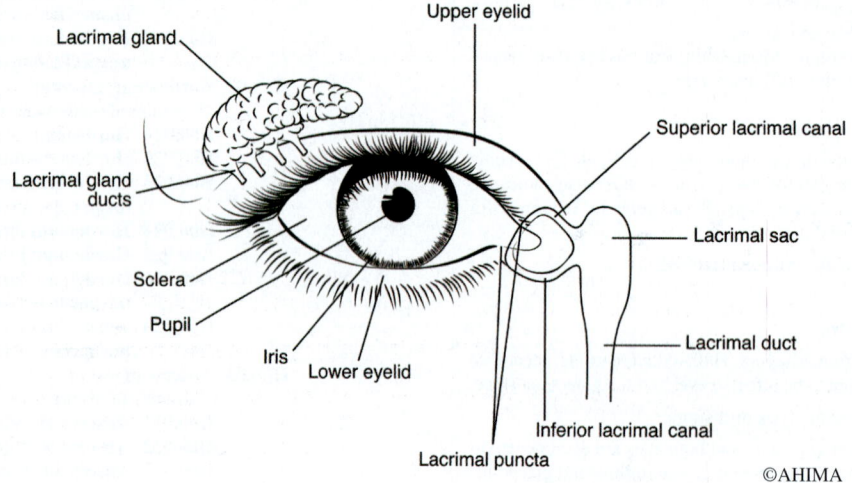

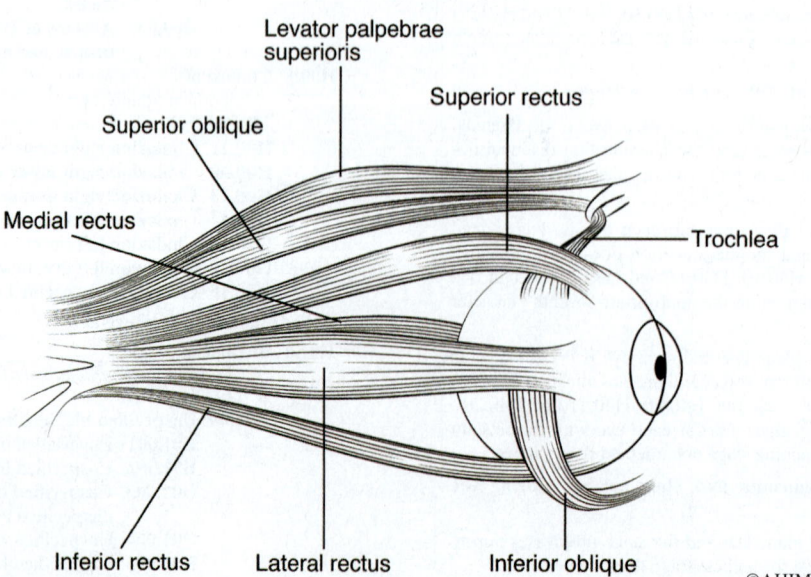

- **+ H01.006** Unspecified blepharitis left eye, unspecified eyelid
- **H01.009** Unspecified blepharitis unspecified eye, unspecified eyelid
- **H01.00A** Unspecified blepharitis right eye, upper and lower eyelids
- **H01.00B** Unspecified blepharitis left eye, upper and lower eyelids
- **+ H01.01** Ulcerative blepharitis
  - **H01.011** Ulcerative blepharitis right upper eyelid
  - **H01.012** Ulcerative blepharitis right lower eyelid
  - **H01.013** Ulcerative blepharitis right eye, unspecified eyelid
  - **H01.014** Ulcerative blepharitis left upper eyelid
  - **H01.015** Ulcerative blepharitis left lower eyelid
  - **H01.016** Ulcerative blepharitis left eye, unspecified eyelid
  - **H01.019** Ulcerative blepharitis unspecified eye, unspecified eyelid
  - **H01.01A** Ulcerative blepharitis right eye, upper and lower eyelids
  - **H01.01B** Ulcerative blepharitis left eye, upper and lower eyelids
- **+ H01.02** Squamous blepharitis
  - **H01.021** Squamous blepharitis right upper eyelid
  - **H01.022** Squamous blepharitis right lower eyelid
  - **H01.023** Squamous blepharitis right eye, unspecified eyelid
  - **H01.024** Squamous blepharitis left upper eyelid
  - **H01.025** Squamous blepharitis left lower eyelid
  - **H01.026** Squamous blepharitis left eye, unspecified eyelid
  - **H01.029** Squamous blepharitis unspecified eye, unspecified eyelid
  - **H01.02A** Squamous blepharitis right eye, upper and lower eyelids
  - **H01.02B** Squamous blepharitis left eye, upper and lower eyelids
- **+ H01.1** Noninfectious dermatoses of eyelid
  - **+ H01.11** Allergic dermatitis of eyelid
    Contact dermatitis of eyelid
    - **H01.111** Allergic dermatitis of right upper eyelid
    - **H01.112** Allergic dermatitis of right lower eyelid
    - **H01.113** Allergic dermatitis of right eye, unspecified eyelid
    - **H01.114** Allergic dermatitis of left upper eyelid
    - **H01.115** Allergic dermatitis of left lower eyelid
    - **H01.116** Allergic dermatitis of left eye, unspecified eyelid
    - **H01.119** Allergic dermatitis of unspecified eye, unspecified eyelid
  - **+ H01.12** Discoid lupus erythematosus of eyelid
    - **H01.121** Discoid lupus erythematosus of right upper eyelid
    - **H01.122** Discoid lupus erythematosus of right lower eyelid
    - **H01.123** Discoid lupus erythematosus of right eye, unspecified eyelid
    - **H01.124** Discoid lupus erythematosus of left upper eyelid
    - **H01.125** Discoid lupus erythematosus of left lower eyelid
    - **H01.126** Discoid lupus erythematosus of left eye, unspecified eyelid
    - **H01.129** Discoid lupus erythematosus of unspecified eye, unspecified eyelid
  - **+ H01.13** Eczematous dermatitis of eyelid
    - **H01.131** Eczematous dermatitis of right upper eyelid
    - **H01.132** Eczematous dermatitis of right lower eyelid
    - **H01.133** Eczematous dermatitis of right eye, unspecified eyelid
    - **H01.134** Eczematous dermatitis of left upper eyelid
    - **H01.135** Eczematous dermatitis of left lower eyelid
    - **H01.136** Eczematous dermatitis of left eye, unspecified eyelid
    - **H01.139** Eczematous dermatitis of unspecified eye, unspecified eyelid
  - **+ H01.14** Xeroderma of eyelid
    - **H01.141** Xeroderma of right upper eyelid
    - **H01.142** Xeroderma of right lower eyelid
    - **H01.143** Xeroderma of right eye, unspecified eyelid
    - **H01.144** Xeroderma of left upper eyelid
    - **H01.145** Xeroderma of left lower eyelid
    - **H01.146** Xeroderma of left eye, unspecified eyelid
    - **H01.149** Xeroderma of unspecified eye, unspecified eyelid
- **H01.8** Other specified inflammations of eyelid
- **H01.9** Unspecified inflammation of eyelid
  Inflammation of eyelid NOS
- **H02** Other disorders of eyelid

  Excludes1: *congenital malformations of eyelid (Q10.0-Q10.3)*

  - **+ H02.0** Entropion and trichiasis of eyelid
    - **+ H02.00** Unspecified entropion of eyelid
      - **H02.001** Unspecified entropion of right upper eyelid
      - **H02.002** Unspecified entropion of right lower eyelid
      - **H02.003** Unspecified entropion of right eye, unspecified eyelid
      - **H02.004** Unspecified entropion of left upper eyelid
      - **H02.005** Unspecified entropion of left lower eyelid
      - **H02.006** Unspecified entropion of left eye, unspecified eyelid
      - **H02.009** Unspecified entropion of unspecified eye, unspecified eyelid
    - **+ H02.01** Cicatricial entropion of eyelid
      - **H02.011** Cicatricial entropion of right upper eyelid
      - **H02.012** Cicatricial entropion of right lower eyelid
      - **H02.013** Cicatricial entropion of right eye, unspecified eyelid
      - **H02.014** Cicatricial entropion of left upper eyelid
      - **H02.015** Cicatricial entropion of left lower eyelid
      - **H02.016** Cicatricial entropion of left eye, unspecified eyelid
      - **H02.019** Cicatricial entropion of unspecified eye, unspecified eyelid
    - **+ H02.02** Mechanical entropion of eyelid
      - **H02.021** Mechanical entropion of right upper eyelid
      - **H02.022** Mechanical entropion of right lower eyelid
      - **H02.023** Mechanical entropion of right eye, unspecified eyelid
      - **H02.024** Mechanical entropion of left upper eyelid
      - **H02.025** Mechanical entropion of left lower eyelid
      - **H02.026** Mechanical entropion of left eye, unspecified eyelid
      - **H02.029** Mechanical entropion of unspecified eye, unspecified eyelid
    - **+ H02.03** Senile entropion of eyelid
      - **H02.031** Senile entropion of right upper eyelid
      - **H02.032** Senile entropion of right lower eyelid
      - **H02.033** Senile entropion of right eye, unspecified eyelid
      - **H02.034** Senile entropion of left upper eyelid
      - **H02.035** Senile entropion of left lower eyelid
      - **H02.036** Senile entropion of left eye, unspecified eyelid
      - **H02.039** Senile entropion of unspecified eye, unspecified eyelid
    - **+ H02.04** Spastic entropion of eyelid
      - **H02.041** Spastic entropion of right upper eyelid
      - **H02.042** Spastic entropion of right lower eyelid
      - **H02.043** Spastic entropion of right eye, unspecified eyelid
      - **H02.044** Spastic entropion of left upper eyelid
      - **H02.045** Spastic entropion of left lower eyelid
      - **H02.046** Spastic entropion of left eye, unspecified eyelid
      - **H02.049** Spastic entropion of unspecified eye, unspecified eyelid

- **H02.05 Trichiasis without entropion**
  - H02.051 Trichiasis without entropion right upper eyelid
  - H02.052 Trichiasis without entropion right lower eyelid
  - H02.053 Trichiasis without entropion right eye, unspecified eyelid
  - H02.054 Trichiasis without entropion left upper eyelid
  - H02.055 Trichiasis without entropion left lower eyelid
  - H02.056 Trichiasis without entropion left eye, unspecified eyelid
  - H02.059 Trichiasis without entropion unspecified eye, unspecified eyelid
- **H02.1 Ectropion of eyelid**
  - **H02.10 Unspecified ectropion of eyelid**
    - H02.101 Unspecified ectropion of right upper eyelid
    - H02.102 Unspecified ectropion of right lower eyelid
    - H02.103 Unspecified ectropion of right eye, unspecified eyelid
    - H02.104 Unspecified ectropion of left upper eyelid
    - H02.105 Unspecified ectropion of left lower eyelid
    - H02.106 Unspecified ectropion of left eye, unspecified eyelid
    - H02.109 Unspecified ectropion of unspecified eye, unspecified eyelid
  - **H02.11 Cicatricial ectropion of eyelid**
    - H02.111 Cicatricial ectropion of right upper eyelid
    - H02.112 Cicatricial ectropion of right lower eyelid
    - H02.113 Cicatricial ectropion of right eye, unspecified eyelid
    - H02.114 Cicatricial ectropion of left upper eyelid
    - H02.115 Cicatricial ectropion of left lower eyelid
    - H02.116 Cicatricial ectropion of left eye, unspecified eyelid
    - H02.119 Cicatricial ectropion of unspecified eye, unspecified eyelid
  - **H02.12 Mechanical ectropion of eyelid**
    - H02.121 Mechanical ectropion of right upper eyelid
    - H02.122 Mechanical ectropion of right lower eyelid
    - H02.123 Mechanical ectropion of right eye, unspecified eyelid
    - H02.124 Mechanical ectropion of left upper eyelid
    - H02.125 Mechanical ectropion of left lower eyelid
    - H02.126 Mechanical ectropion of left eye, unspecified eyelid
    - H02.129 Mechanical ectropion of unspecified eye, unspecified eyelid
  - **H02.13 Senile ectropion of eyelid**
    - H02.131 Senile ectropion of right upper eyelid
    - H02.132 Senile ectropion of right lower eyelid
    - H02.133 Senile ectropion of right eye, unspecified eyelid
    - H02.134 Senile ectropion of left upper eyelid
    - H02.135 Senile ectropion of left lower eyelid
    - H02.136 Senile ectropion of left eye, unspecified eyelid
    - H02.139 Senile ectropion of unspecified eye, unspecified eyelid
  - **H02.14 Spastic ectropion of eyelid**
    - H02.141 Spastic ectropion of right upper eyelid
    - H02.142 Spastic ectropion of right lower eyelid
    - H02.143 Spastic ectropion of right eye, unspecified eyelid
    - H02.144 Spastic ectropion of left upper eyelid
    - H02.145 Spastic ectropion of left lower eyelid
    - H02.146 Spastic ectropion of left eye, unspecified eyelid
    - H02.149 Spastic ectropion of unspecified eye, unspecified eyelid
- **H02.15 Paralytic ectropion of eyelid**
  AHA CC: 4Q, 2018, 13
  - H02.151 Paralytic ectropion of right upper eyelid
  - H02.152 Paralytic ectropion of right lower eyelid
  - H02.153 Paralytic ectropion of right eye, unspecified eyelid
  - H02.154 Paralytic ectropion of left upper eyelid
  - H02.155 Paralytic ectropion of left lower eyelid
  - H02.156 Paralytic ectropion of left eye, unspecified eyelid
  - H02.159 Paralytic ectropion of unspecified eye, unspecified eyelid
- **H02.2 Lagophthalmos**
  AHA CC: 4Q, 2018, 14
  - **H02.20 Unspecified lagophthalmos**
    - H02.201 Unspecified lagophthalmos right upper eyelid
    - H02.202 Unspecified lagophthalmos right lower eyelid
    - H02.203 Unspecified lagophthalmos right eye, unspecified eyelid
    - H02.204 Unspecified lagophthalmos left upper eyelid
    - H02.205 Unspecified lagophthalmos left lower eyelid
    - H02.206 Unspecified lagophthalmos left eye, unspecified eyelid
    - H02.209 Unspecified lagophthalmos unspecified eye, unspecified eyelid
    - H02.20A Unspecified lagophthalmos right eye, upper and lower eyelids
    - H02.20B Unspecified lagophthalmos left eye, upper and lower eyelids
    - H02.20C Unspecified lagophthalmos, bilateral, upper and lower eyelids
  - **H02.21 Cicatricial lagophthalmos**
    - H02.211 Cicatricial lagophthalmos right upper eyelid
    - H02.212 Cicatricial lagophthalmos right lower eyelid
    - H02.213 Cicatricial lagophthalmos right eye, unspecified eyelid
    - H02.214 Cicatricial lagophthalmos left upper eyelid
    - H02.215 Cicatricial lagophthalmos left lower eyelid
    - H02.216 Cicatricial lagophthalmos left eye, unspecified eyelid
    - H02.219 Cicatricial lagophthalmos unspecified eye, unspecified eyelid
    - H02.21A Cicatricial lagophthalmos right eye, upper and lower eyelids
    - H02.21B Cicatricial lagophthalmos left eye, upper and lower eyelids
    - H02.21C Cicatricial lagophthalmos, bilateral, upper and lower eyelids
  - **H02.22 Mechanical lagophthalmos**
    - H02.221 Mechanical lagophthalmos right upper eyelid
    - H02.222 Mechanical lagophthalmos right lower eyelid
    - H02.223 Mechanical lagophthalmos right eye, unspecified eyelid
    - H02.224 Mechanical lagophthalmos left upper eyelid
    - H02.225 Mechanical lagophthalmos left lower eyelid
    - H02.226 Mechanical lagophthalmos left eye, unspecified eyelid
    - H02.229 Mechanical lagophthalmos unspecified eye, unspecified eyelid
    - H02.22A Mechanical lagophthalmos right eye, upper and lower eyelids
    - H02.22B Mechanical lagophthalmos left eye, upper and lower eyelids
    - H02.22C Mechanical lagophthalmos, bilateral, upper and lower eyelids

- **+ H02.23 Paralytic lagophthalmos**
  - H02.231 Paralytic lagophthalmos right upper eyelid
  - H02.232 Paralytic lagophthalmos right lower eyelid
  - H02.233 Paralytic lagophthalmos right eye, unspecified eyelid
  - H02.234 Paralytic lagophthalmos left upper eyelid
  - H02.235 Paralytic lagophthalmos left lower eyelid
  - H02.236 Paralytic lagophthalmos left eye, unspecified eyelid
  - H02.239 Paralytic lagophthalmos unspecified eye, unspecified eyelid
  - H02.23A Paralytic lagophthalmos right eye, upper and lower eyelids
  - H02.23B Paralytic lagophthalmos left eye, upper and lower eyelids
  - H02.23C Paralytic lagophthalmos, bilateral, upper and lower eyelids
- **+ H02.3 Blepharochalasis**
  Pseudoptosis
  - H02.30 Blepharochalasis unspecified eye, unspecified eyelid
  - H02.31 Blepharochalasis right upper eyelid
  - H02.32 Blepharochalasis right lower eyelid
  - H02.33 Blepharochalasis right eye, unspecified eyelid
  - H02.34 Blepharochalasis left upper eyelid
  - H02.35 Blepharochalasis left lower eyelid
  - H02.36 Blepharochalasis left eye, unspecified eyelid
- **+ H02.4 Ptosis of eyelid**
  - **+ H02.40 Unspecified ptosis of eyelid**
    - H02.401 Unspecified ptosis of right eyelid
    - H02.402 Unspecified ptosis of left eyelid
    - H02.403 Unspecified ptosis of bilateral eyelids
    - H02.409 Unspecified ptosis of unspecified eyelid
  - **+ H02.41 Mechanical ptosis of eyelid**
    - H02.411 Mechanical ptosis of right eyelid
    - H02.412 Mechanical ptosis of left eyelid
    - H02.413 Mechanical ptosis of bilateral eyelids
    - H02.419 Mechanical ptosis of unspecified eyelid
  - **+ H02.42 Myogenic ptosis of eyelid**
    - H02.421 Myogenic ptosis of right eyelid
    - H02.422 Myogenic ptosis of left eyelid
    - H02.423 Myogenic ptosis of bilateral eyelids
    - H02.429 Myogenic ptosis of unspecified eyelid
  - **+ H02.43 Paralytic ptosis of eyelid**
    Neurogenic ptosis of eyelid
    - H02.431 Paralytic ptosis of right eyelid
    - H02.432 Paralytic ptosis of left eyelid
    - H02.433 Paralytic ptosis of bilateral eyelids
    - H02.439 Paralytic ptosis unspecified eyelid
- **+ H02.5 Other disorders affecting eyelid function**
  Excludes2: *blepharospasm (G24.5)*
  organic tic (G25.69)
  psychogenic tic (F95.-)
  - **+ H02.51 Abnormal innervation syndrome**
    - H02.511 Abnormal innervation syndrome right upper eyelid
    - H02.512 Abnormal innervation syndrome right lower eyelid
    - H02.513 Abnormal innervation syndrome right eye, unspecified eyelid
    - H02.514 Abnormal innervation syndrome left upper eyelid
    - H02.515 Abnormal innervation syndrome left lower eyelid
    - H02.516 Abnormal innervation syndrome left eye, unspecified eyelid
    - H02.519 Abnormal innervation syndrome unspecified eye, unspecified eyelid
  - **+ H02.52 Blepharophimosis**
    Ankyloblepharon
    - H02.521 Blepharophimosis right upper eyelid
    - H02.522 Blepharophimosis right lower eyelid
    - H02.523 Blepharophimosis right eye, unspecified eyelid
    - H02.524 Blepharophimosis left upper eyelid
    - H02.525 Blepharophimosis left lower eyelid
    - H02.526 Blepharophimosis left eye, unspecified eyelid
    - H02.529 Blepharophimosis unspecified eye, unspecified lid
  - **+ H02.53 Eyelid retraction**
    Eyelid lag
    - H02.531 Eyelid retraction right upper eyelid
    - H02.532 Eyelid retraction right lower eyelid
    - H02.533 Eyelid retraction right eye, unspecified eyelid
    - H02.534 Eyelid retraction left upper eyelid
    - H02.535 Eyelid retraction left lower eyelid
    - H02.536 Eyelid retraction left eye, unspecified eyelid
    - H02.539 Eyelid retraction unspecified eye, unspecified lid
  - H02.59 Other disorders affecting eyelid function
    Deficient blink reflex
    Sensory disorders
- **+ H02.6 Xanthelasma of eyelid**
  - H02.60 Xanthelasma of unspecified eye, unspecified eyelid
  - H02.61 Xanthelasma of right upper eyelid
  - H02.62 Xanthelasma of right lower eyelid
  - H02.63 Xanthelasma of right eye, unspecified eyelid
  - H02.64 Xanthelasma of left upper eyelid
  - H02.65 Xanthelasma of left lower eyelid
  - H02.66 Xanthelasma of left eye, unspecified eyelid
- **+ H02.7 Other and unspecified degenerative disorders of eyelid and periocular area**
  - H02.70 Unspecified degenerative disorders of eyelid and periocular area
  - **+ H02.71 Chloasma of eyelid and periocular area**
    Dyspigmentation of eyelid
    Hyperpigmentation of eyelid
    - H02.711 Chloasma of right upper eyelid and periocular area
    - H02.712 Chloasma of right lower eyelid and periocular area
    - H02.713 Chloasma of right eye, unspecified eyelid and periocular area
    - H02.714 Chloasma of left upper eyelid and periocular area
    - H02.715 Chloasma of left lower eyelid and periocular area
    - H02.716 Chloasma of left eye, unspecified eyelid and periocular area
    - H02.719 Chloasma of unspecified eye, unspecified eyelid and periocular area
  - **+ H02.72 Madarosis of eyelid and periocular area**
    Hypotrichosis of eyelid
    - H02.721 Madarosis of right upper eyelid and periocular area
    - H02.722 Madarosis of right lower eyelid and periocular area
    - H02.723 Madarosis of right eye, unspecified eyelid and periocular area
    - H02.724 Madarosis of left upper eyelid and periocular area
    - H02.725 Madarosis of left lower eyelid and periocular area
    - H02.726 Madarosis of left eye, unspecified eyelid and periocular area
    - H02.729 Madarosis of unspecified eye, unspecified eyelid and periocular area
  - **+ H02.73 Vitiligo of eyelid and periocular area**
    Hypopigmentation of eyelid
    - H02.731 Vitiligo of right upper eyelid and periocular area
    - H02.732 Vitiligo of right lower eyelid and periocular area
    - H02.733 Vitiligo of right eye, unspecified eyelid and periocular area
    - H02.734 Vitiligo of left upper eyelid and periocular area
    - H02.735 Vitiligo of left lower eyelid and periocular area
    - H02.736 Vitiligo of left eye, unspecified eyelid and periocular area
    - H02.739 Vitiligo of unspecified eye, unspecified eyelid and periocular area
  - H02.79 Other degenerative disorders of eyelid and periocular area

- **H02.8 Other specified disorders of eyelid**
  - **H02.81 Retained foreign body in eyelid**
    Use additional code to identify the type of retained foreign body (Z18.-)
    Excludes1: laceration of eyelid with foreign body (S01.12-)
    retained intraocular foreign body (H44.6-, H44.7-)
    superficial foreign body of eyelid and periocular area (S00.25-)
    - H02.811 Retained foreign body in right upper eyelid
    - H02.812 Retained foreign body in right lower eyelid
    - H02.813 Retained foreign body in right eye, unspecified eyelid
    - H02.814 Retained foreign body in left upper eyelid
    - H02.815 Retained foreign body in left lower eyelid
    - H02.816 Retained foreign body in left eye, unspecified eyelid
    - H02.819 Retained foreign body in unspecified eye, unspecified eyelid
  - **H02.82 Cysts of eyelid**
    Sebaceous cyst of eyelid
    - H02.821 Cysts of right upper eyelid
    - H02.822 Cysts of right lower eyelid
    - H02.823 Cysts of right eye, unspecified eyelid
    - H02.824 Cysts of left upper eyelid
    - H02.825 Cysts of left lower eyelid
    - H02.826 Cysts of left eye, unspecified eyelid
    - H02.829 Cysts of unspecified eye, unspecified eyelid
  - **H02.83 Dermatochalasis of eyelid**
    - H02.831 Dermatochalasis of right upper eyelid
    - H02.832 Dermatochalasis of right lower eyelid
    - H02.833 Dermatochalasis of right eye, unspecified eyelid
    - H02.834 Dermatochalasis of left upper eyelid
    - H02.835 Dermatochalasis of left lower eyelid
    - H02.836 Dermatochalasis of left eye, unspecified eyelid
    - H02.839 Dermatochalasis of unspecified eye, unspecified eyelid
  - **H02.84 Edema of eyelid**
    Hyperemia of eyelid
    - H02.841 Edema of right upper eyelid
    - H02.842 Edema of right lower eyelid
    - H02.843 Edema of right eye, unspecified eyelid
    - H02.844 Edema of left upper eyelid
    - H02.845 Edema of left lower eyelid
    - H02.846 Edema of left eye, unspecified eyelid
    - H02.849 Edema of unspecified eye, unspecified eyelid
  - **H02.85 Elephantiasis of eyelid**
    - H02.851 Elephantiasis of right upper eyelid
    - H02.852 Elephantiasis of right lower eyelid
    - H02.853 Elephantiasis of right eye, unspecified eyelid
    - H02.854 Elephantiasis of left upper eyelid
    - H02.855 Elephantiasis of left lower eyelid
    - H02.856 Elephantiasis of left eye, unspecified eyelid
    - H02.859 Elephantiasis of unspecified eye, unspecified eyelid
  - **H02.86 Hypertrichosis of eyelid**
    - H02.861 Hypertrichosis of right upper eyelid
    - H02.862 Hypertrichosis of right lower eyelid
    - H02.863 Hypertrichosis of right eye, unspecified eyelid
    - H02.864 Hypertrichosis of left upper eyelid
    - H02.865 Hypertrichosis of left lower eyelid
    - H02.866 Hypertrichosis of left eye, unspecified eyelid
    - H02.869 Hypertrichosis of unspecified eye, unspecified eyelid
- **H02.87 Vascular anomalies of eyelid**
  - H02.871 Vascular anomalies of right upper eyelid
  - H02.872 Vascular anomalies of right lower eyelid
  - H02.873 Vascular anomalies of right eye, unspecified eyelid
  - H02.874 Vascular anomalies of left upper eyelid
  - H02.875 Vascular anomalies of left lower eyelid
  - H02.876 Vascular anomalies of left eye, unspecified eyelid
  - H02.879 Vascular anomalies of unspecified eye, unspecified eyelid
- **H02.88 Meibomian gland dysfunction of eyelid**
  AHA CC: 4Q, 2018, 14-15
  - H02.881 Meibomian gland dysfunction right upper eyelid
  - H02.882 Meibomian gland dysfunction right lower eyelid
  - H02.883 Meibomian gland dysfunction of right eye, unspecified eyelid
  - H02.884 Meibomian gland dysfunction left upper eyelid
  - H02.885 Meibomian gland dysfunction left lower eyelid
  - H02.886 Meibomian gland dysfunction of left eye, unspecified eyelid
  - H02.889 Meibomian gland dysfunction of unspecified eye, unspecified eyelid
  - H02.88A Meibomian gland dysfunction right eye, upper and lower eyelids
  - H02.88B Meibomian gland dysfunction left eye, upper and lower eyelids
- H02.89 Other specified disorders of eyelid
  Hemorrhage of eyelid
- H02.9 **Unspecified disorder of eyelid**
  Disorder of eyelid NOS

H04 Disorders of lacrimal system
Excludes1: congenital malformations of lacrimal system (Q10.4-Q10.6)
- **H04.0 Dacryoadenitis**
  - **H04.00 Unspecified dacryoadenitis**
    - H04.001 Unspecified dacryoadenitis, right lacrimal gland
    - H04.002 Unspecified dacryoadenitis, left lacrimal gland
    - H04.003 Unspecified dacryoadenitis, bilateral lacrimal glands
    - H04.009 Unspecified dacryoadenitis, unspecified lacrimal gland
  - **H04.01 Acute dacryoadenitis**
    - H04.011 Acute dacryoadenitis, right lacrimal gland
    - H04.012 Acute dacryoadenitis, left lacrimal gland
    - H04.013 Acute dacryoadenitis, bilateral lacrimal glands
    - H04.019 Acute dacryoadenitis, unspecified lacrimal gland
  - **H04.02 Chronic dacryoadenitis**
    - H04.021 Chronic dacryoadenitis, right lacrimal gland
    - H04.022 Chronic dacryoadenitis, left lacrimal gland
    - H04.023 Chronic dacryoadenitis, bilateral lacrimal gland
    - H04.029 Chronic dacryoadenitis, unspecified lacrimal gland
  - **H04.03 Chronic enlargement of lacrimal gland**
    - H04.031 Chronic enlargement of right lacrimal gland
    - H04.032 Chronic enlargement of left lacrimal gland
    - H04.033 Chronic enlargement of bilateral lacrimal glands
    - H04.039 Chronic enlargement of unspecified lacrimal gland
- **H04.1 Other disorders of lacrimal gland**
  - **H04.11 Dacryops**
    - H04.111 Dacryops of right lacrimal gland
    - H04.112 Dacryops of left lacrimal gland
    - H04.113 Dacryops of bilateral lacrimal glands
    - H04.119 Dacryops of unspecified lacrimal gland

+ **H04.12 Dry eye syndrome**
  Tear film insufficiency, NOS
  H04.121 Dry eye syndrome of right lacrimal gland
  H04.122 Dry eye syndrome of left lacrimal gland
  H04.123 Dry eye syndrome of bilateral lacrimal glands
  H04.129 Dry eye syndrome of unspecified lacrimal gland

+ **H04.13 Lacrimal cyst**
  Lacrimal cystic degeneration
  H04.131 Lacrimal cyst, right lacrimal gland
  H04.132 Lacrimal cyst, left lacrimal gland
  H04.133 Lacrimal cyst, bilateral lacrimal glands
  H04.139 Lacrimal cyst, unspecified lacrimal gland

+ **H04.14 Primary lacrimal gland atrophy**
  H04.141 Primary lacrimal gland atrophy, right lacrimal gland
  H04.142 Primary lacrimal gland atrophy, left lacrimal gland
  H04.143 Primary lacrimal gland atrophy, bilateral lacrimal glands
  H04.149 Primary lacrimal gland atrophy, unspecified lacrimal gland

+ **H04.15 Secondary lacrimal gland atrophy**
  H04.151 Secondary lacrimal gland atrophy, right lacrimal gland
  H04.152 Secondary lacrimal gland atrophy, left lacrimal gland
  H04.153 Secondary lacrimal gland atrophy, bilateral lacrimal glands
  H04.159 Secondary lacrimal gland atrophy, unspecified lacrimal gland

+ **H04.16 Lacrimal gland dislocation**
  H04.161 Lacrimal gland dislocation, right lacrimal gland
  H04.162 Lacrimal gland dislocation, left lacrimal gland
  H04.163 Lacrimal gland dislocation, bilateral lacrimal glands
  H04.169 Lacrimal gland dislocation, unspecified lacrimal gland

H04.19 Other specified disorders of lacrimal gland

+ **H04.2 Epiphora**
  + **H04.20 Unspecified epiphora**
    H04.201 Unspecified epiphora, right side
    H04.202 Unspecified epiphora, left side
    H04.203 Unspecified epiphora, bilateral
    H04.209 Unspecified epiphora, unspecified side
  + **H04.21 Epiphora due to excess lacrimation**
    H04.211 Epiphora due to excess lacrimation, right lacrimal gland
    H04.212 Epiphora due to excess lacrimation, left lacrimal gland
    H04.213 Epiphora due to excess lacrimation, bilateral lacrimal glands
    H04.219 Epiphora due to excess lacrimation, unspecified lacrimal gland
  + **H04.22 Epiphora due to insufficient drainage**
    H04.221 Epiphora due to insufficient drainage, right side
    H04.222 Epiphora due to insufficient drainage, left side
    H04.223 Epiphora due to insufficient drainage, bilateral
    H04.229 Epiphora due to insufficient drainage, unspecified side

+ **H04.3 Acute and unspecified inflammation of lacrimal passages**
  Excludes1: neonatal dacryocystitis (P39.1)
  + **H04.30 Unspecified dacryocystitis**
    H04.301 Unspecified dacryocystitis of right lacrimal passage
    H04.302 Unspecified dacryocystitis of left lacrimal passage
    H04.303 Unspecified dacryocystitis of bilateral lacrimal passages
    H04.309 Unspecified dacryocystitis of unspecified lacrimal passage

+ **H04.31 Phlegmonous dacryocystitis**
  H04.311 Phlegmonous dacryocystitis of right lacrimal passage
  H04.312 Phlegmonous dacryocystitis of left lacrimal passage
  H04.313 Phlegmonous dacryocystitis of bilateral lacrimal passages
  H04.319 Phlegmonous dacryocystitis of unspecified lacrimal passage

+ **H04.32 Acute dacryocystitis**
  Acute dacryopericystitis
  H04.321 Acute dacryocystitis of right lacrimal passage
  H04.322 Acute dacryocystitis of left lacrimal passage
  H04.323 Acute dacryocystitis of bilateral lacrimal passages
  H04.329 Acute dacryocystitis of unspecified lacrimal passage

+ **H04.33 Acute lacrimal canaliculitis**
  H04.331 Acute lacrimal canaliculitis of right lacrimal passage
  H04.332 Acute lacrimal canaliculitis of left lacrimal passage
  H04.333 Acute lacrimal canaliculitis of bilateral lacrimal passages
  H04.339 Acute lacrimal canaliculitis of unspecified lacrimal passage

+ **H04.4 Chronic inflammation of lacrimal passages**
  + **H04.41 Chronic dacryocystitis**
    H04.411 Chronic dacryocystitis of right lacrimal passage
    H04.412 Chronic dacryocystitis of left lacrimal passage
    H04.413 Chronic dacryocystitis of bilateral lacrimal passages
    H04.419 Chronic dacryocystitis of unspecified lacrimal passage
  + **H04.42 Chronic lacrimal canaliculitis**
    H04.421 Chronic lacrimal canaliculitis of right lacrimal passage
    H04.422 Chronic lacrimal canaliculitis of left lacrimal passage
    H04.423 Chronic lacrimal canaliculitis of bilateral lacrimal passages
    H04.429 Chronic lacrimal canaliculitis of unspecified lacrimal passage
  + **H04.43 Chronic lacrimal mucocele**
    H04.431 Chronic lacrimal mucocele of right lacrimal passage
    H04.432 Chronic lacrimal mucocele of left lacrimal passage
    H04.433 Chronic lacrimal mucocele of bilateral lacrimal passages
    H04.439 Chronic lacrimal mucocele of unspecified lacrimal passage

+ **H04.5 Stenosis and insufficiency of lacrimal passages**
  + **H04.51 Dacryolith**
    H04.511 Dacryolith of right lacrimal passage
    H04.512 Dacryolith of left lacrimal passage
    H04.513 Dacryolith of bilateral lacrimal passages
    H04.519 Dacryolith of unspecified lacrimal passage
  + **H04.52 Eversion of lacrimal punctum**
    H04.521 Eversion of right lacrimal punctum
    H04.522 Eversion of left lacrimal punctum
    H04.523 Eversion of bilateral lacrimal punctum
    H04.529 Eversion of unspecified lacrimal punctum
  + **H04.53 Neonatal obstruction of nasolacrimal duct**
    Excludes1: congenital stenosis and stricture of lacrimal duct (Q10.5)
    • H04.531 Neonatal obstruction of right nasolacrimal duct
    • H04.532 Neonatal obstruction of left nasolacrimal duct
    • H04.533 Neonatal obstruction of bilateral nasolacrimal duct
    • H04.539 Neonatal obstruction of unspecified nasolacrimal duct

- **H04.54** Stenosis of lacrimal canaliculi
  - H04.541 Stenosis of right lacrimal canaliculi
  - H04.542 Stenosis of left lacrimal canaliculi
  - H04.543 Stenosis of bilateral lacrimal canaliculi
  - H04.549 Stenosis of unspecified lacrimal canaliculi
- **H04.55** Acquired stenosis of nasolacrimal duct
  - H04.551 Acquired stenosis of right nasolacrimal duct
  - H04.552 Acquired stenosis of left nasolacrimal duct
  - H04.553 Acquired stenosis of bilateral nasolacrimal duct
  - H04.559 Acquired stenosis of unspecified nasolacrimal duct
- **H04.56** Stenosis of lacrimal punctum
  - H04.561 Stenosis of right lacrimal punctum
  - H04.562 Stenosis of left lacrimal punctum
  - H04.563 Stenosis of bilateral lacrimal punctum
  - H04.569 Stenosis of unspecified lacrimal punctum
- **H04.57** Stenosis of lacrimal sac
  - H04.571 Stenosis of right lacrimal sac
  - H04.572 Stenosis of left lacrimal sac
  - H04.573 Stenosis of bilateral lacrimal sac
  - H04.579 Stenosis of unspecified lacrimal sac
- **H04.6** Other changes of lacrimal passages
  - **H04.61** Lacrimal fistula
    - H04.611 Lacrimal fistula right lacrimal passage
    - H04.612 Lacrimal fistula left lacrimal passage
    - H04.613 Lacrimal fistula bilateral lacrimal passages
    - H04.619 Lacrimal fistula unspecified lacrimal passage
  - H04.69 Other changes of lacrimal passages
- **H04.8** Other disorders of lacrimal system
  - **H04.81** Granuloma of lacrimal passages
    - H04.811 Granuloma of right lacrimal passage
    - H04.812 Granuloma of left lacrimal passage
    - H04.813 Granuloma of bilateral lacrimal passages
    - H04.819 Granuloma of unspecified lacrimal passage
  - H04.89 Other disorders of lacrimal system
- H04.9 Disorder of lacrimal system, unspecified

H05 Disorders of orbit

Excludes1: *congenital malformation of orbit (Q10.7)*

- **H05.0** Acute inflammation of orbit
  - H05.00 Unspecified acute inflammation of orbit
  - **H05.01** Cellulitis of orbit
    Abscess of orbit
    - CC H05.011 Cellulitis of right orbit
    - CC H05.012 Cellulitis of left orbit
    - CC H05.013 Cellulitis of bilateral orbits
    - CC H05.019 Cellulitis of unspecified orbit
  - **H05.02** Osteomyelitis of orbit
    - CC H05.021 Osteomyelitis of right orbit
    - CC H05.022 Osteomyelitis of left orbit
    - CC H05.023 Osteomyelitis of bilateral orbits
    - CC H05.029 Osteomyelitis of unspecified orbit
  - **H05.03** Periostitis of orbit
    - CC H05.031 Periostitis of right orbit
    - CC H05.032 Periostitis of left orbit
    - CC H05.033 Periostitis of bilateral orbits
    - CC H05.039 Periostitis of unspecified orbit
  - **H05.04** Tenonitis of orbit
    - H05.041 Tenonitis of right orbit
    - H05.042 Tenonitis of left orbit
    - H05.043 Tenonitis of bilateral orbits
    - H05.049 Tenonitis of unspecified orbit
- **H05.1** Chronic inflammatory disorders of orbit
  - H05.10 Unspecified chronic inflammatory disorders of orbit
  - **H05.11** Granuloma of orbit
    Pseudotumor (inflammatory) of orbit
    - H05.111 Granuloma of right orbit
    - H05.112 Granuloma of left orbit
    - H05.113 Granuloma of bilateral orbits
    - H05.119 Granuloma of unspecified orbit
  - **H05.12** Orbital myositis
    - H05.121 Orbital myositis, right orbit
    - H05.122 Orbital myositis, left orbit
    - H05.123 Orbital myositis, bilateral
    - H05.129 Orbital myositis, unspecified orbit
- **H05.2** Exophthalmic conditions
  - H05.20 Unspecified exophthalmos
  - **H05.21** Displacement (lateral) of globe
    - H05.211 Displacement (lateral) of globe, right eye
    - H05.212 Displacement (lateral) of globe, left eye
    - H05.213 Displacement (lateral) of globe, bilateral
    - H05.219 Displacement (lateral) of globe, unspecified eye
  - **H05.22** Edema of orbit
    Orbital congestion
    - H05.221 Edema of right orbit
    - H05.222 Edema of left orbit
    - H05.223 Edema of bilateral orbit
    - H05.229 Edema of unspecified orbit
  - **H05.23** Hemorrhage of orbit
    - H05.231 Hemorrhage of right orbit
    - H05.232 Hemorrhage of left orbit
    - H05.233 Hemorrhage of bilateral orbit
    - H05.239 Hemorrhage of unspecified orbit
  - **H05.24** Constant exophthalmos
    - H05.241 Constant exophthalmos, right eye
    - H05.242 Constant exophthalmos, left eye
    - H05.243 Constant exophthalmos, bilateral
    - H05.249 Constant exophthalmos, unspecified eye
  - **H05.25** Intermittent exophthalmos
    - H05.251 Intermittent exophthalmos, right eye
    - H05.252 Intermittent exophthalmos, left eye
    - H05.253 Intermittent exophthalmos, bilateral
    - H05.259 Intermittent exophthalmos, unspecified eye
  - **H05.26** Pulsating exophthalmos
    - H05.261 Pulsating exophthalmos, right eye
    - H05.262 Pulsating exophthalmos, left eye
    - H05.263 Pulsating exophthalmos, bilateral
    - H05.269 Pulsating exophthalmos, unspecified eye
- **H05.3** Deformity of orbit
  Excludes1: *congenital deformity of orbit (Q10.7)*
  hypertelorism (Q75.2)
  - H05.30 Unspecified deformity of orbit
  - **H05.31** Atrophy of orbit
    - H05.311 Atrophy of right orbit
    - H05.312 Atrophy of left orbit
    - H05.313 Atrophy of bilateral orbit
    - H05.319 Atrophy of unspecified orbit
  - **H05.32** Deformity of orbit due to bone disease
    Code also associated bone disease
    - H05.321 Deformity of right orbit due to bone disease
    - H05.322 Deformity of left orbit due to bone disease
    - H05.323 Deformity of bilateral orbits due to bone disease
    - H05.329 Deformity of unspecified orbit due to bone disease
  - **H05.33** Deformity of orbit due to trauma or surgery
    - H05.331 Deformity of right orbit due to trauma or surgery
    - H05.332 Deformity of left orbit due to trauma or surgery
    - H05.333 Deformity of bilateral orbits due to trauma or surgery
    - H05.339 Deformity of unspecified orbit due to trauma or surgery
  - **H05.34** Enlargement of orbit
    - H05.341 Enlargement of right orbit
    - H05.342 Enlargement of left orbit
    - H05.343 Enlargement of bilateral orbits
    - H05.349 Enlargement of unspecified orbit
  - **H05.35** Exostosis of orbit
    - H05.351 Exostosis of right orbit
    - H05.352 Exostosis of left orbit
    - H05.353 Exostosis of bilateral orbits
    - H05.359 Exostosis of unspecified orbit

- **H05.4** Enophthalmos
  - **H05.40** Unspecified enophthalmos
    - H05.401 Unspecified enophthalmos, right eye
    - H05.402 Unspecified enophthalmos, left eye
    - H05.403 Unspecified enophthalmos, bilateral
    - H05.409 Unspecified enophthalmos, unspecified eye
  - **H05.41** Enophthalmos due to atrophy of orbital tissue
    - H05.411 Enophthalmos due to atrophy of orbital tissue, right eye
    - H05.412 Enophthalmos due to atrophy of orbital tissue, left eye
    - H05.413 Enophthalmos due to atrophy of orbital tissue, bilateral
    - H05.419 Enophthalmos due to atrophy of orbital tissue, unspecified eye
  - **H05.42** Enophthalmos due to trauma or surgery
    - H05.421 Enophthalmos due to trauma or surgery, right eye
    - H05.422 Enophthalmos due to trauma or surgery, left eye
    - H05.423 Enophthalmos due to trauma or surgery, bilateral
    - H05.429 Enophthalmos due to trauma or surgery, unspecified eye
- **H05.5** Retained (old) foreign body following penetrating wound of orbit
  - Retrobulbar foreign body
  - *Use additional code to identify the type of retained foreign body (Z18.-)*
  - **Excludes1:** *current penetrating wound of orbit (S05.4-)*
  - **Excludes2:** *retained foreign body of eyelid (H02.81-)*
    retained intraocular foreign body (H44.6-, H44.7-)
  - H05.50 Retained (old) foreign body following penetrating wound of unspecified orbit
  - H05.51 Retained (old) foreign body following penetrating wound of right orbit
  - H05.52 Retained (old) foreign body following penetrating wound of left orbit
  - H05.53 Retained (old) foreign body following penetrating wound of bilateral orbits
- **H05.8** Other disorders of orbit
  - **H05.81** Cyst of orbit
    - Encephalocele of orbit
    - H05.811 Cyst of right orbit
    - H05.812 Cyst of left orbit
    - H05.813 Cyst of bilateral orbits
    - H05.819 Cyst of unspecified orbit
  - **H05.82** Myopathy of extraocular muscles
    - H05.821 Myopathy of extraocular muscles, right orbit
    - H05.822 Myopathy of extraocular muscles, left orbit
    - H05.823 Myopathy of extraocular muscles, bilateral
    - H05.829 Myopathy of extraocular muscles, unspecified orbit
  - H05.89 Other disorders of orbit
- H05.9 Unspecified disorder of orbit

Disorders of conjunctiva (H10-H11)

H10 Conjunctivitis
Excludes1: *keratoconjunctivitis (H16.2-)*
- **H10.0** Mucopurulent conjunctivitis
  - **H10.01** Acute follicular conjunctivitis
    - H10.011 Acute follicular conjunctivitis, right eye
    - H10.012 Acute follicular conjunctivitis, left eye
    - H10.013 Acute follicular conjunctivitis, bilateral
    - H10.019 Acute follicular conjunctivitis, unspecified eye
  - **H10.02** Other mucopurulent conjunctivitis
    - H10.021 Other mucopurulent conjunctivitis, right eye
    - H10.022 Other mucopurulent conjunctivitis, left eye
    - H10.023 Other mucopurulent conjunctivitis, bilateral
    - H10.029 Other mucopurulent conjunctivitis, unspecified eye
- **H10.1** Acute atopic conjunctivitis
  - Acute papillary conjunctivitis
  - H10.10 Acute atopic conjunctivitis, unspecified eye
  - H10.11 Acute atopic conjunctivitis, right eye
  - H10.12 Acute atopic conjunctivitis, left eye
  - H10.13 Acute atopic conjunctivitis, bilateral
- **H10.2** Other acute conjunctivitis
  - **H10.21** Acute toxic conjunctivitis
    - Acute chemical conjunctivitis
    - **Code first (T51-T65) to identify chemical and intent**
    - **Excludes1:** *burn and corrosion of eye and adnexa (T26.-)*
    - H10.211 Acute toxic conjunctivitis, right eye
    - H10.212 Acute toxic conjunctivitis, left eye
    - H10.213 Acute toxic conjunctivitis, bilateral
    - H10.219 Acute toxic conjunctivitis, unspecified eye
  - **H10.22** Pseudomembranous conjunctivitis
    - H10.221 Pseudomembranous conjunctivitis, right eye
    - H10.222 Pseudomembranous conjunctivitis, left eye
    - H10.223 Pseudomembranous conjunctivitis, bilateral
    - H10.229 Pseudomembranous conjunctivitis, unspecified eye
  - **H10.23** Serous conjunctivitis, except viral
    - **Excludes1:** *viral conjunctivitis (B30.-)*
    - H10.231 Serous conjunctivitis, except viral, right eye
    - H10.232 Serous conjunctivitis, except viral, left eye
    - H10.233 Serous conjunctivitis, except viral, bilateral
    - H10.239 Serous conjunctivitis, except viral, unspecified eye
- **H10.3** Unspecified acute conjunctivitis
  - **Excludes1:** *ophthalmia neonatorum NOS (P39.1)*
  - H10.30 Unspecified acute conjunctivitis, unspecified eye
  - H10.31 Unspecified acute conjunctivitis, right eye
  - H10.32 Unspecified acute conjunctivitis, left eye
  - H10.33 Unspecified acute conjunctivitis, bilateral
- **H10.4** Chronic conjunctivitis
  - **H10.40** Unspecified chronic conjunctivitis
    - H10.401 Unspecified chronic conjunctivitis, right eye
    - H10.402 Unspecified chronic conjunctivitis, left eye
    - H10.403 Unspecified chronic conjunctivitis, bilateral
    - H10.409 Unspecified chronic conjunctivitis, unspecified eye
  - **H10.41** Chronic giant papillary conjunctivitis
    - H10.411 Chronic giant papillary conjunctivitis, right eye
    - H10.412 Chronic giant papillary conjunctivitis, left eye
    - H10.413 Chronic giant papillary conjunctivitis, bilateral
    - H10.419 Chronic giant papillary conjunctivitis, unspecified eye
  - **H10.42** Simple chronic conjunctivitis
    - H10.421 Simple chronic conjunctivitis, right eye
    - H10.422 Simple chronic conjunctivitis, left eye
    - H10.423 Simple chronic conjunctivitis, bilateral
    - H10.429 Simple chronic conjunctivitis, unspecified eye
  - **H10.43** Chronic follicular conjunctivitis
    - H10.431 Chronic follicular conjunctivitis, right eye
    - H10.432 Chronic follicular conjunctivitis, left eye
    - H10.433 Chronic follicular conjunctivitis, bilateral
    - H10.439 Chronic follicular conjunctivitis, unspecified eye
  - H10.44 Vernal conjunctivitis
    - **Excludes1:** *vernal keratoconjunctivitis with limbar and corneal involvement (H16.26-)*
  - H10.45 Other chronic allergic conjunctivitis

- H10.5 Blepharoconjunctivitis
  - H10.50 Unspecified blepharoconjunctivitis
    - H10.501 Unspecified blepharoconjunctivitis, right eye
    - H10.502 Unspecified blepharoconjunctivitis, left eye
    - H10.503 Unspecified blepharoconjunctivitis, bilateral
    - H10.509 Unspecified blepharoconjunctivitis, unspecified eye
  - H10.51 Ligneous conjunctivitis
    Code also underlying condition if known, such as: plasminogen deficiency (E88.02)
    - H10.511 Ligneous conjunctivitis, right eye
    - H10.512 Ligneous conjunctivitis, left eye
    - H10.513 Ligneous conjunctivitis, bilateral
    - H10.519 Ligneous conjunctivitis, unspecified eye
  - H10.52 Angular blepharoconjunctivitis
    - H10.521 Angular blepharoconjunctivitis, right eye
    - H10.522 Angular blepharoconjunctivitis, left eye
    - H10.523 Angular blepharoconjunctivitis, bilateral
    - H10.529 Angular blepharoconjunctivitis, unspecified eye
  - H10.53 Contact blepharoconjunctivitis
    - H10.531 Contact blepharoconjunctivitis, right eye
    - H10.532 Contact blepharoconjunctivitis, left eye
    - H10.533 Contact blepharoconjunctivitis, bilateral
    - H10.539 Contact blepharoconjunctivitis, unspecified eye
- H10.8 Other conjunctivitis
  AHA CC: 4Q, 2018, 15
  - H10.81 Pingueculitis
    Excludes1: pinguecula (H11.15-)
    - H10.811 Pingueculitis, right eye
    - H10.812 Pingueculitis, left eye
    - H10.813 Pingueculitis, bilateral
    - H10.819 Pingueculitis, unspecified eye
  - H10.82 Rosacea conjunctivitis
    Code first underlying rosacea dermatitis (L71.-)
    - H10.821 Rosacea conjunctivitis, right eye
    - H10.822 Rosacea conjunctivitis, left eye
    - H10.823 Rosacea conjunctivitis, bilateral
      AHA CC: 4Q, 2018, 15
    - H10.829 Rosacea conjunctivitis, unspecified eye
  - H10.89 Other conjunctivitis
- H10.9 Unspecified conjunctivitis

H11 Other disorders of conjunctiva

Excludes1: keratoconjunctivitis (H16.2-)

- H11.0 Pterygium of eye
  Excludes1: pseudopterygium (H11.81-)
  - H11.00 Unspecified pterygium of eye
    - H11.001 Unspecified pterygium of right eye
    - H11.002 Unspecified pterygium of left eye
    - H11.003 Unspecified pterygium of eye, bilateral
    - H11.009 Unspecified pterygium of unspecified eye
  - H11.01 Amyloid pterygium
    - H11.011 Amyloid pterygium of right eye
    - H11.012 Amyloid pterygium of left eye
    - H11.013 Amyloid pterygium of eye, bilateral
    - H11.019 Amyloid pterygium of unspecified eye
  - H11.02 Central pterygium of eye
    - H11.021 Central pterygium of right eye
    - H11.022 Central pterygium of left eye
    - H11.023 Central pterygium of eye, bilateral
    - H11.029 Central pterygium of unspecified eye
  - H11.03 Double pterygium of eye
    - H11.031 Double pterygium of right eye
    - H11.032 Double pterygium of left eye
    - H11.033 Double pterygium of eye, bilateral
    - H11.039 Double pterygium of unspecified eye
  - H11.04 Peripheral pterygium of eye, stationary
    - H11.041 Peripheral pterygium, stationary, right eye
    - H11.042 Peripheral pterygium, stationary, left eye
    - H11.043 Peripheral pterygium, stationary, bilateral
    - H11.049 Peripheral pterygium, stationary, unspecified eye
  - H11.05 Peripheral pterygium of eye, progressive
    - H11.051 Peripheral pterygium, progressive, right eye
    - H11.052 Peripheral pterygium, progressive, left eye
    - H11.053 Peripheral pterygium, progressive, bilateral
    - H11.059 Peripheral pterygium, progressive, unspecified eye
  - H11.06 Recurrent pterygium of eye
    - H11.061 Recurrent pterygium of right eye
    - H11.062 Recurrent pterygium of left eye
    - H11.063 Recurrent pterygium of eye, bilateral
    - H11.069 Recurrent pterygium of unspecified eye
- H11.1 Conjunctival degenerations and deposits
  Excludes2: pseudopterygium (H11.81)
  - H11.10 Unspecified conjunctival degenerations
  - H11.11 Conjunctival deposits
    - H11.111 Conjunctival deposits, right eye
    - H11.112 Conjunctival deposits, left eye
    - H11.113 Conjunctival deposits, bilateral
    - H11.119 Conjunctival deposits, unspecified eye
  - H11.12 Conjunctival concretions
    - H11.121 Conjunctival concretions, right eye
    - H11.122 Conjunctival concretions, left eye
    - H11.123 Conjunctival concretions, bilateral
    - H11.129 Conjunctival concretions, unspecified eye
  - H11.13 Conjunctival pigmentations
    Conjunctival argyrosis [argyria]
    - H11.131 Conjunctival pigmentations, right eye
    - H11.132 Conjunctival pigmentations, left eye
    - H11.133 Conjunctival pigmentations, bilateral
    - H11.139 Conjunctival pigmentations, unspecified eye
  - H11.14 Conjunctival xerosis, unspecified
    Excludes1: xerosis of conjunctiva due to vitamin A deficiency (E50.0, E50.1)
    - H11.141 Conjunctival xerosis, unspecified, right eye
    - H11.142 Conjunctival xerosis, unspecified, left eye
    - H11.143 Conjunctival xerosis, unspecified, bilateral
    - H11.149 Conjunctival xerosis, unspecified, unspecified eye
  - H11.15 Pinguecula
    Excludes1: pingueculitis (H10.81-)
    - H11.151 Pinguecula, right eye
    - H11.152 Pinguecula, left eye
    - H11.153 Pinguecula, bilateral
    - H11.159 Pinguecula, unspecified eye
- H11.2 Conjunctival scars
  - H11.21 Conjunctival adhesions and strands (localized)
    - H11.211 Conjunctival adhesions and strands (localized), right eye
    - H11.212 Conjunctival adhesions and strands (localized), left eye
    - H11.213 Conjunctival adhesions and strands (localized), bilateral
    - H11.219 Conjunctival adhesions and strands (localized), unspecified eye
  - H11.22 Conjunctival granuloma
    - H11.221 Conjunctival granuloma, right eye
    - H11.222 Conjunctival granuloma, left eye
    - H11.223 Conjunctival granuloma, bilateral
    - H11.229 Conjunctival granuloma, unspecified
  - H11.23 Symblepharon
    - H11.231 Symblepharon, right eye
    - H11.232 Symblepharon, left eye
    - H11.233 Symblepharon, bilateral
    - H11.239 Symblepharon, unspecified eye
  - H11.24 Scarring of conjunctiva
    - H11.241 Scarring of conjunctiva, right eye
    - H11.242 Scarring of conjunctiva, left eye
    - H11.243 Scarring of conjunctiva, bilateral
    - H11.249 Scarring of conjunctiva, unspecified eye
- H11.3 Conjunctival hemorrhage
  Subconjunctival hemorrhage
  - H11.30 Conjunctival hemorrhage, unspecified eye
  - H11.31 Conjunctival hemorrhage, right eye
  - H11.32 Conjunctival hemorrhage, left eye
  - H11.33 Conjunctival hemorrhage, bilateral

- **H11.4** Other conjunctival vascular disorders and cysts
  - **H11.41** Vascular abnormalities of conjunctiva
    Conjunctival aneurysm
    - H11.411 Vascular abnormalities of conjunctiva, right eye
    - H11.412 Vascular abnormalities of conjunctiva, left eye
    - H11.413 Vascular abnormalities of conjunctiva, bilateral
    - H11.419 Vascular abnormalities of conjunctiva, unspecified eye
  - **H11.42** Conjunctival edema
    - H11.421 Conjunctival edema, right eye
    - H11.422 Conjunctival edema, left eye
    - H11.423 Conjunctival edema, bilateral
    - H11.429 Conjunctival edema, unspecified eye
  - **H11.43** Conjunctival hyperemia
    - H11.431 Conjunctival hyperemia, right eye
    - H11.432 Conjunctival hyperemia, left eye
    - H11.433 Conjunctival hyperemia, bilateral
    - H11.439 Conjunctival hyperemia, unspecified eye
  - **H11.44** Conjunctival cysts
    - H11.441 Conjunctival cysts, right eye
    - H11.442 Conjunctival cysts, left eye
    - H11.443 Conjunctival cysts, bilateral
    - H11.449 Conjunctival cysts, unspecified eye
- **H11.8** Other specified disorders of conjunctiva
  - **H11.81** Pseudopterygium of conjunctiva
    - H11.811 Pseudopterygium of conjunctiva, right eye
    - H11.812 Pseudopterygium of conjunctiva, left eye
    - H11.813 Pseudopterygium of conjunctiva, bilateral
    - H11.819 Pseudopterygium of conjunctiva, unspecified eye
  - **H11.82** Conjunctivochalasis
    - H11.821 Conjunctivochalasis, right eye
    - H11.822 Conjunctivochalasis, left eye
    - H11.823 Conjunctivochalasis, bilateral
    - H11.829 Conjunctivochalasis, unspecified eye
  - H11.89 Other specified disorders of conjunctiva
- H11.9 Unspecified disorder of conjunctiva

Disorders of sclera, cornea, iris and ciliary body (H15-H22)

- **H15** Disorders of sclera
  - **H15.0** Scleritis
    - **H15.00** Unspecified scleritis
      - H15.001 Unspecified scleritis, right eye
      - H15.002 Unspecified scleritis, left eye
      - H15.003 Unspecified scleritis, bilateral
      - H15.009 Unspecified scleritis, unspecified eye
    - **H15.01** Anterior scleritis
      - H15.011 Anterior scleritis, right eye
      - H15.012 Anterior scleritis, left eye
      - H15.013 Anterior scleritis, bilateral
      - H15.019 Anterior scleritis, unspecified eye
    - **H15.02** Brawny scleritis
      - H15.021 Brawny scleritis, right eye
      - H15.022 Brawny scleritis, left eye
      - H15.023 Brawny scleritis, bilateral
      - H15.029 Brawny scleritis, unspecified eye
    - **H15.03** Posterior scleritis
      Sclerotenonitis
      - H15.031 Posterior scleritis, right eye
      - H15.032 Posterior scleritis, left eye
      - H15.033 Posterior scleritis, bilateral
      - H15.039 Posterior scleritis, unspecified eye
    - **H15.04** Scleritis with corneal involvement
      - H15.041 Scleritis with corneal involvement, right eye
      - H15.042 Scleritis with corneal involvement, left eye
      - H15.043 Scleritis with corneal involvement, bilateral
      - H15.049 Scleritis with corneal involvement, unspecified eye
    - **H15.05** Scleromalacia perforans
      - H15.051 Scleromalacia perforans, right eye
      - H15.052 Scleromalacia perforans, left eye
      - H15.053 Scleromalacia perforans, bilateral
      - H15.059 Scleromalacia perforans, unspecified eye
    - **H15.09** Other scleritis
      Scleral abscess
      - H15.091 Other scleritis, right eye
      - H15.092 Other scleritis, left eye
      - H15.093 Other scleritis, bilateral
      - H15.099 Other scleritis, unspecified eye
  - **H15.1** Episcleritis
    - **H15.10** Unspecified episcleritis
      - H15.101 Unspecified episcleritis, right eye
      - H15.102 Unspecified episcleritis, left eye
      - H15.103 Unspecified episcleritis, bilateral
      - H15.109 Unspecified episcleritis, unspecified eye
    - **H15.11** Episcleritis periodica fugax
      - H15.111 Episcleritis periodica fugax, right eye
      - H15.112 Episcleritis periodica fugax, left eye
      - H15.113 Episcleritis periodica fugax, bilateral
      - H15.119 Episcleritis periodica fugax, unspecified eye
    - **H15.12** Nodular episcleritis
      - H15.121 Nodular episcleritis, right eye
      - H15.122 Nodular episcleritis, left eye
      - H15.123 Nodular episcleritis, bilateral
      - H15.129 Nodular episcleritis, unspecified eye
  - **H15.8** Other disorders of sclera
    Excludes2: *blue sclera (Q13.5)*
    degenerative myopia (H44.2-)
    - **H15.81** Equatorial staphyloma
      - H15.811 Equatorial staphyloma, right eye
      - H15.812 Equatorial staphyloma, left eye
      - H15.813 Equatorial staphyloma, bilateral
      - H15.819 Equatorial staphyloma, unspecified eye
    - **H15.82** Localized anterior staphyloma
      - H15.821 Localized anterior staphyloma, right eye
      - H15.822 Localized anterior staphyloma, left eye
      - H15.823 Localized anterior staphyloma, bilateral
      - H15.829 Localized anterior staphyloma, unspecified eye
    - **H15.83** Staphyloma posticum
      - H15.831 Staphyloma posticum, right eye
      - H15.832 Staphyloma posticum, left eye
      - H15.833 Staphyloma posticum, bilateral
      - H15.839 Staphyloma posticum, unspecified eye
    - **H15.84** Scleral ectasia
      - H15.841 Scleral ectasia, right eye
      - H15.842 Scleral ectasia, left eye
      - H15.843 Scleral ectasia, bilateral
      - H15.849 Scleral ectasia, unspecified eye
    - **H15.85** Ring staphyloma
      - H15.851 Ring staphyloma, right eye
      - H15.852 Ring staphyloma, left eye
      - H15.853 Ring staphyloma, bilateral
      - H15.859 Ring staphyloma, unspecified eye
    - H15.89 Other disorders of sclera
  - H15.9 Unspecified disorder of sclera
- **H16** Keratitis
  - **H16.0** Corneal ulcer
    - **H16.00** Unspecified corneal ulcer
      - H16.001 Unspecified corneal ulcer, right eye
      - H16.002 Unspecified corneal ulcer, left eye
      - H16.003 Unspecified corneal ulcer, bilateral
      - H16.009 Unspecified corneal ulcer, unspecified eye
    - **H16.01** Central corneal ulcer
      - H16.011 Central corneal ulcer, right eye
      - H16.012 Central corneal ulcer, left eye
      - H16.013 Central corneal ulcer, bilateral
      - H16.019 Central corneal ulcer, unspecified eye
    - **H16.02** Ring corneal ulcer
      - H16.021 Ring corneal ulcer, right eye
      - H16.022 Ring corneal ulcer, left eye
      - H16.023 Ring corneal ulcer, bilateral
      - H16.029 Ring corneal ulcer, unspecified eye

- **+ H16.03 Corneal ulcer with hypopyon**
  - H16.031 Corneal ulcer with hypopyon, right eye
  - H16.032 Corneal ulcer with hypopyon, left eye
  - H16.033 Corneal ulcer with hypopyon, bilateral
  - H16.039 Corneal ulcer with hypopyon, unspecified eye
- **+ H16.04 Marginal corneal ulcer**
  - H16.041 Marginal corneal ulcer, right eye
  - H16.042 Marginal corneal ulcer, left eye
  - H16.043 Marginal corneal ulcer, bilateral
  - H16.049 Marginal corneal ulcer, unspecified eye
- **+ H16.05 Mooren's corneal ulcer**
  - H16.051 Mooren's corneal ulcer, right eye
  - H16.052 Mooren's corneal ulcer, left eye
  - H16.053 Mooren's corneal ulcer, bilateral
  - H16.059 Mooren's corneal ulcer, unspecified eye
- **+ H16.06 Mycotic corneal ulcer**
  - H16.061 Mycotic corneal ulcer, right eye
  - H16.062 Mycotic corneal ulcer, left eye
  - H16.063 Mycotic corneal ulcer, bilateral
  - H16.069 Mycotic corneal ulcer, unspecified eye
- **+ H16.07 Perforated corneal ulcer**
  - H16.071 Perforated corneal ulcer, right eye
  - H16.072 Perforated corneal ulcer, left eye
  - H16.073 Perforated corneal ulcer, bilateral
  - H16.079 Perforated corneal ulcer, unspecified eye
- **+ H16.1 Other and unspecified superficial keratitis without conjunctivitis**
  - **+ H16.10 Unspecified superficial keratitis**
    - H16.101 Unspecified superficial keratitis, right eye
    - H16.102 Unspecified superficial keratitis, left eye
    - H16.103 Unspecified superficial keratitis, bilateral
    - H16.109 Unspecified superficial keratitis, unspecified eye
  - **+ H16.11 Macular keratitis**
    - Areolar keratitis
    - Nummular keratitis
    - Stellate keratitis
    - Striate keratitis
    - H16.111 Macular keratitis, right eye
    - H16.112 Macular keratitis, left eye
    - H16.113 Macular keratitis, bilateral
    - H16.119 Macular keratitis, unspecified eye
  - **+ H16.12 Filamentary keratitis**
    - H16.121 Filamentary keratitis, right eye
    - H16.122 Filamentary keratitis, left eye
    - H16.123 Filamentary keratitis, bilateral
    - H16.129 Filamentary keratitis, unspecified eye
  - **+ H16.13 Photokeratitis**
    - Snow blindness
    - Welders keratitis
    - H16.131 Photokeratitis, right eye
    - H16.132 Photokeratitis, left eye
    - H16.133 Photokeratitis, bilateral
    - H16.139 Photokeratitis, unspecified eye
  - **+ H16.14 Punctate keratitis**
    - H16.141 Punctate keratitis, right eye
    - H16.142 Punctate keratitis, left eye
    - H16.143 Punctate keratitis, bilateral
    - H16.149 Punctate keratitis, unspecified eye
- **+ H16.2 Keratoconjunctivitis**
  - **+ H16.20 Unspecified keratoconjunctivitis**
    - Superficial keratitis with conjunctivitis NOS
    - H16.201 Unspecified keratoconjunctivitis, right eye
    - H16.202 Unspecified keratoconjunctivitis, left eye
    - H16.203 Unspecified keratoconjunctivitis, bilateral
    - H16.209 Unspecified keratoconjunctivitis, unspecified eye
  - **+ H16.21 Exposure keratoconjunctivitis**
    - H16.211 Exposure keratoconjunctivitis, right eye
    - H16.212 Exposure keratoconjunctivitis, left eye
    - H16.213 Exposure keratoconjunctivitis, bilateral
    - H16.219 Exposure keratoconjunctivitis, unspecified eye
  - **+ H16.22 Keratoconjunctivitis sicca, not specified as Sjögren's**
    - *Excludes1: Sjögren's syndrome (M35.01)*
    - H16.221 Keratoconjunctivitis sicca, not specified as Sjögren's, right eye
    - H16.222 Keratoconjunctivitis sicca, not specified as Sjögren's, left eye
    - H16.223 Keratoconjunctivitis sicca, not specified as Sjögren's, bilateral
    - H16.229 Keratoconjunctivitis sicca, not specified as Sjögren's, unspecified eye
  - **+ H16.23 Neurotrophic keratoconjunctivitis**
    - H16.231 Neurotrophic keratoconjunctivitis, right eye
    - H16.232 Neurotrophic keratoconjunctivitis, left eye
    - H16.233 Neurotrophic keratoconjunctivitis, bilateral
    - H16.239 Neurotrophic keratoconjunctivitis, unspecified eye
  - **+ H16.24 Ophthalmia nodosa**
    - H16.241 Ophthalmia nodosa, right eye
    - H16.242 Ophthalmia nodosa, left eye
    - H16.243 Ophthalmia nodosa, bilateral
    - H16.249 Ophthalmia nodosa, unspecified eye
  - **+ H16.25 Phlyctenular keratoconjunctivitis**
    - H16.251 Phlyctenular keratoconjunctivitis, right eye
    - H16.252 Phlyctenular keratoconjunctivitis, left eye
    - H16.253 Phlyctenular keratoconjunctivitis, bilateral
    - H16.259 Phlyctenular keratoconjunctivitis, unspecified eye
  - **+ H16.26 Vernal keratoconjunctivitis, with limbar and corneal involvement**
    - *Excludes1: vernal conjunctivitis without limbar and corneal involvement (H10.44)*
    - H16.261 Vernal keratoconjunctivitis, with limbar and corneal involvement, right eye
    - H16.262 Vernal keratoconjunctivitis, with limbar and corneal involvement, left eye
    - H16.263 Vernal keratoconjunctivitis, with limbar and corneal involvement, bilateral
    - H16.269 Vernal keratoconjunctivitis, with limbar and corneal involvement, unspecified eye
  - **+ H16.29 Other keratoconjunctivitis**
    - H16.291 Other keratoconjunctivitis, right eye
    - H16.292 Other keratoconjunctivitis, left eye
    - H16.293 Other keratoconjunctivitis, bilateral
    - H16.299 Other keratoconjunctivitis, unspecified eye
- **+ H16.3 Interstitial and deep keratitis**
  - **+ H16.30 Unspecified interstitial keratitis**
    - H16.301 Unspecified interstitial keratitis, right eye
    - H16.302 Unspecified interstitial keratitis, left eye
    - H16.303 Unspecified interstitial keratitis, bilateral
    - H16.309 Unspecified interstitial keratitis, unspecified eye
  - **+ H16.31 Corneal abscess**
    - H16.311 Corneal abscess, right eye
    - H16.312 Corneal abscess, left eye
    - H16.313 Corneal abscess, bilateral
    - H16.319 Corneal abscess, unspecified eye
  - **+ H16.32 Diffuse interstitial keratitis**
    - Cogan's syndrome
    - H16.321 Diffuse interstitial keratitis, right eye
    - H16.322 Diffuse interstitial keratitis, left eye
    - H16.323 Diffuse interstitial keratitis, bilateral
    - H16.329 Diffuse interstitial keratitis, unspecified eye
  - **+ H16.33 Sclerosing keratitis**
    - H16.331 Sclerosing keratitis, right eye
    - H16.332 Sclerosing keratitis, left eye
    - H16.333 Sclerosing keratitis, bilateral
    - H16.339 Sclerosing keratitis, unspecified eye

+ H16.39 Other interstitial and deep keratitis
- H16.391 Other interstitial and deep keratitis, right eye
- H16.392 Other interstitial and deep keratitis, left eye
- H16.393 Other interstitial and deep keratitis, bilateral
- H16.399 Other interstitial and deep keratitis, unspecified eye

+ H16.4 Corneal neovascularization
+ H16.40 Unspecified corneal neovascularization
- H16.401 Unspecified corneal neovascularization, right eye
- H16.402 Unspecified corneal neovascularization, left eye
- H16.403 Unspecified corneal neovascularization, bilateral
- H16.409 Unspecified corneal neovascularization, unspecified eye

+ H16.41 Ghost vessels (corneal)
- H16.411 Ghost vessels (corneal), right eye
- H16.412 Ghost vessels (corneal), left eye
- H16.413 Ghost vessels (corneal), bilateral
- H16.419 Ghost vessels (corneal), unspecified eye

+ H16.42 Pannus (corneal)
- H16.421 Pannus (corneal), right eye
- H16.422 Pannus (corneal), left eye
- H16.423 Pannus (corneal), bilateral
- H16.429 Pannus (corneal), unspecified eye

+ H16.43 Localized vascularization of cornea
- H16.431 Localized vascularization of cornea, right eye
- H16.432 Localized vascularization of cornea, left eye
- H16.433 Localized vascularization of cornea, bilateral
- H16.439 Localized vascularization of cornea, unspecified eye

+ H16.44 Deep vascularization of cornea
- H16.441 Deep vascularization of cornea, right eye
- H16.442 Deep vascularization of cornea, left eye
- H16.443 Deep vascularization of cornea, bilateral
- H16.449 Deep vascularization of cornea, unspecified eye

H16.8 Other keratitis
H16.9 Unspecified keratitis

H17 Corneal scars and opacities

+ H17.0 Adherent leukoma
- H17.00 Adherent leukoma, unspecified eye
- H17.01 Adherent leukoma, right eye
- H17.02 Adherent leukoma, left eye
- H17.03 Adherent leukoma, bilateral

+ H17.1 Central corneal opacity
- H17.10 Central corneal opacity, unspecified eye
- H17.11 Central corneal opacity, right eye
- H17.12 Central corneal opacity, left eye
- H17.13 Central corneal opacity, bilateral

+ H17.8 Other corneal scars and opacities
+ H17.81 Minor opacity of cornea
  Corneal nebula
- H17.811 Minor opacity of cornea, right eye
- H17.812 Minor opacity of cornea, left eye
- H17.813 Minor opacity of cornea, bilateral
- H17.819 Minor opacity of cornea, unspecified eye

+ H17.82 Peripheral opacity of cornea
- H17.821 Peripheral opacity of cornea, right eye
- H17.822 Peripheral opacity of cornea, left eye
- H17.823 Peripheral opacity of cornea, bilateral
- H17.829 Peripheral opacity of cornea, unspecified eye

H17.89 Other corneal scars and opacities
H17.9 Unspecified corneal scar and opacity

H18 Other disorders of cornea

+ H18.0 Corneal pigmentations and deposits
+ H18.00 Unspecified corneal deposit
- H18.001 Unspecified corneal deposit, right eye
- H18.002 Unspecified corneal deposit, left eye
- H18.003 Unspecified corneal deposit, bilateral
- H18.009 Unspecified corneal deposit, unspecified eye

+ H18.01 Anterior corneal pigmentations
  Staehli's line
- H18.011 Anterior corneal pigmentations, right eye
- H18.012 Anterior corneal pigmentations, left eye
- H18.013 Anterior corneal pigmentations, bilateral
- H18.019 Anterior corneal pigmentations, unspecified eye

+ H18.02 Argentous corneal deposits
- H18.021 Argentous corneal deposits, right eye
- H18.022 Argentous corneal deposits, left eye
- H18.023 Argentous corneal deposits, bilateral
- H18.029 Argentous corneal deposits, unspecified eye

+ H18.03 Corneal deposits in metabolic disorders
  Code also associated metabolic disorder
- H18.031 Corneal deposits in metabolic disorders, right eye
- H18.032 Corneal deposits in metabolic disorders, left eye
- H18.033 Corneal deposits in metabolic disorders, bilateral
- H18.039 Corneal deposits in metabolic disorders, unspecified eye

+ H18.04 Kayser-Fleischer ring
  Code also associated Wilson's disease (E83.01)
- H18.041 Kayser-Fleischer ring, right eye
- H18.042 Kayser-Fleischer ring, left eye
- H18.043 Kayser-Fleischer ring, bilateral
- H18.049 Kayser-Fleischer ring, unspecified eye

+ H18.05 Posterior corneal pigmentations
  Krukenberg's spindle
- H18.051 Posterior corneal pigmentations, right eye
- H18.052 Posterior corneal pigmentations, left eye
- H18.053 Posterior corneal pigmentations, bilateral
- H18.059 Posterior corneal pigmentations, unspecified eye

+ H18.06 Stromal corneal pigmentations
  Hematocornea
- H18.061 Stromal corneal pigmentations, right eye
- H18.062 Stromal corneal pigmentations, left eye
- H18.063 Stromal corneal pigmentations, bilateral
- H18.069 Stromal corneal pigmentations, unspecified eye

+ H18.1 Bullous keratopathy
- H18.10 Bullous keratopathy, unspecified eye
- H18.11 Bullous keratopathy, right eye
- H18.12 Bullous keratopathy, left eye
- H18.13 Bullous keratopathy, bilateral

+ H18.2 Other and unspecified corneal edema
- H18.20 Unspecified corneal edema
+ H18.21 Corneal edema secondary to contact lens
  Excludes2: *other corneal disorders due to contact lens (H18.82-)*
- H18.211 Corneal edema secondary to contact lens, right eye
- H18.212 Corneal edema secondary to contact lens, left eye
- H18.213 Corneal edema secondary to contact lens, bilateral
- H18.219 Corneal edema secondary to contact lens, unspecified eye

- **+ H18.22 Idiopathic corneal edema**
  - H18.221 Idiopathic corneal edema, right eye
  - H18.222 Idiopathic corneal edema, left eye
  - H18.223 Idiopathic corneal edema, bilateral
  - H18.229 Idiopathic corneal edema, unspecified eye
- **+ H18.23 Secondary corneal edema**
  - H18.231 Secondary corneal edema, right eye
  - H18.232 Secondary corneal edema, left eye
  - H18.233 Secondary corneal edema, bilateral
  - H18.239 Secondary corneal edema, unspecified eye
- **+ H18.3 Changes of corneal membranes**
  - H18.30 Unspecified corneal membrane change
  - **+ H18.31 Folds and rupture in Bowman's membrane**
    - H18.311 Folds and rupture in Bowman's membrane, right eye
    - H18.312 Folds and rupture in Bowman's membrane, left eye
    - H18.313 Folds and rupture in Bowman's membrane, bilateral
    - H18.319 Folds and rupture in Bowman's membrane, unspecified eye
  - **+ H18.32 Folds in Descemet's membrane**
    - H18.321 Folds in Descemet's membrane, right eye
    - H18.322 Folds in Descemet's membrane, left eye
    - H18.323 Folds in Descemet's membrane, bilateral
    - H18.329 Folds in Descemet's membrane, unspecified eye
  - **+ H18.33 Rupture in Descemet's membrane**
    - H18.331 Rupture in Descemet's membrane, right eye
    - H18.332 Rupture in Descemet's membrane, left eye
    - H18.333 Rupture in Descemet's membrane, bilateral
    - H18.339 Rupture in Descemet's membrane, unspecified eye
- **+ H18.4 Corneal degeneration**
  - *Excludes1:* Mooren's ulcer (H16.0-)
    - recurrent erosion of cornea (H18.83-)
  - H18.40 Unspecified corneal degeneration
  - **+ H18.41 Arcus senilis**
    - Senile corneal changes
    - H18.411 Arcus senilis, right eye
    - H18.412 Arcus senilis, left eye
    - H18.413 Arcus senilis, bilateral
    - H18.419 Arcus senilis, unspecified eye
  - **+ H18.42 Band keratopathy**
    - H18.421 Band keratopathy, right eye
    - H18.422 Band keratopathy, left eye
    - H18.423 Band keratopathy, bilateral
    - H18.429 Band keratopathy, unspecified eye
  - H18.43 Other calcerous corneal degeneration
  - **+ H18.44 Keratomalacia**
    - *Excludes1:* keratomalacia due to vitamin A deficiency (E50.4)
    - H18.441 Keratomalacia, right eye
    - H18.442 Keratomalacia, left eye
    - H18.443 Keratomalacia, bilateral
    - H18.449 Keratomalacia, unspecified eye
  - **+ H18.45 Nodular corneal degeneration**
    - H18.451 Nodular corneal degeneration, right eye
    - H18.452 Nodular corneal degeneration, left eye
    - H18.453 Nodular corneal degeneration, bilateral
    - H18.459 Nodular corneal degeneration, unspecified eye
  - **+ H18.46 Peripheral corneal degeneration**
    - H18.461 Peripheral corneal degeneration, right eye
    - H18.462 Peripheral corneal degeneration, left eye
    - H18.463 Peripheral corneal degeneration, bilateral
    - H18.469 Peripheral corneal degeneration, unspecified eye
  - H18.49 Other corneal degeneration
- **+ H18.5 Hereditary corneal dystrophies**
  - AHA CC: 4Q, 2020, 24
  - **+ H18.50 Unspecified hereditary corneal dystrophies**
    - H18.501 Unspecified hereditary corneal dystrophies, right eye
    - H18.502 Unspecified hereditary corneal dystrophies, left eye
    - H18.503 Unspecified hereditary corneal dystrophies, bilateral
    - H18.509 Unspecified hereditary corneal dystrophies, unspecified eye
  - **+ H18.51 Endothelial corneal dystrophy**
    - Fuchs' dystrophy
    - H18.511 Endothelial corneal dystrophy, right eye
    - H18.512 Endothelial corneal dystrophy, left eye
    - H18.513 Endothelial corneal dystrophy, bilateral
    - H18.519 Endothelial corneal dystrophy, unspecified eye
  - **+ H18.52 Epithelial (juvenile) corneal dystrophy**
    - H18.521 Epithelial (juvenile) corneal dystrophy, right eye
    - H18.522 Epithelial (juvenile) corneal dystrophy, left eye
    - H18.523 Epithelial (juvenile) corneal dystrophy, bilateral
    - H18.529 Epithelial (juvenile) corneal dystrophy, unspecified eye
  - **+ H18.53 Granular corneal dystrophy**
    - H18.531 Granular corneal dystrophy, right eye
    - H18.532 Granular corneal dystrophy, left eye
    - H18.533 Granular corneal dystrophy, bilateral
    - H18.539 Granular corneal dystrophy, unspecified eye
  - **+ H18.54 Lattice corneal dystrophy**
    - H18.541 Lattice corneal dystrophy, right eye
    - H18.542 Lattice corneal dystrophy, left eye
    - H18.543 Lattice corneal dystrophy, bilateral
    - H18.549 Lattice corneal dystrophy, unspecified eye
  - **+ H18.55 Macular corneal dystrophy**
    - H18.551 Macular corneal dystrophy, right eye
    - H18.552 Macular corneal dystrophy, left eye
    - H18.553 Macular corneal dystrophy, bilateral
    - H18.559 Macular corneal dystrophy, unspecified eye
  - **+ H18.59 Other hereditary corneal dystrophies**
    - H18.591 Other hereditary corneal dystrophies, right eye
    - H18.592 Other hereditary corneal dystrophies, left eye
    - H18.593 Other hereditary corneal dystrophies, bilateral
    - H18.599 Other hereditary corneal dystrophies, unspecified eye
- **+ H18.6 Keratoconus**
  - **+ H18.60 Keratoconus, unspecified**
    - H18.601 Keratoconus, unspecified, right eye
    - H18.602 Keratoconus, unspecified, left eye
    - H18.603 Keratoconus, unspecified, bilateral
    - H18.609 Keratoconus, unspecified, unspecified eye
  - **+ H18.61 Keratoconus, stable**
    - H18.611 Keratoconus, stable, right eye
    - H18.612 Keratoconus, stable, left eye
    - H18.613 Keratoconus, stable, bilateral
    - H18.619 Keratoconus, stable, unspecified eye
  - **+ H18.62 Keratoconus, unstable**
    - Acute hydrops
    - H18.621 Keratoconus, unstable, right eye
    - H18.622 Keratoconus, unstable, left eye
    - H18.623 Keratoconus, unstable, bilateral
    - H18.629 Keratoconus, unstable, unspecified eye
- **+ H18.7 Other and unspecified corneal deformities**
  - *Excludes1:* congenital malformations of cornea (Q13.3-Q13.4)
  - H18.70 Unspecified corneal deformity
  - **+ H18.71 Corneal ectasia**
    - H18.711 Corneal ectasia, right eye
    - H18.712 Corneal ectasia, left eye
    - H18.713 Corneal ectasia, bilateral
    - H18.719 Corneal ectasia, unspecified eye
  - **+ H18.72 Corneal staphyloma**
    - H18.721 Corneal staphyloma, right eye
    - H18.722 Corneal staphyloma, left eye

H18.723 Corneal staphyloma, bilateral
H18.729 Corneal staphyloma, unspecified eye
+ H18.73 Descemetocele
H18.731 Descemetocele, right eye
H18.732 Descemetocele, left eye
H18.733 Descemetocele, bilateral
H18.739 Descemetocele, unspecified eye
+ H18.79 Other corneal deformities
H18.791 Other corneal deformities, right eye
H18.792 Other corneal deformities, left eye
H18.793 Other corneal deformities, bilateral
H18.799 Other corneal deformities, unspecified eye
+ H18.8 Other specified disorders of cornea
+ H18.81 Anesthesia and hypoesthesia of cornea
H18.811 Anesthesia and hypoesthesia of cornea, right eye
H18.812 Anesthesia and hypoesthesia of cornea, left eye
H18.813 Anesthesia and hypoesthesia of cornea, bilateral
H18.819 Anesthesia and hypoesthesia of cornea, unspecified eye
+ H18.82 Corneal disorder due to contact lens
Excludes2: *corneal edema due to contact lens (H18.21-)*
H18.821 Corneal disorder due to contact lens, right eye
H18.822 Corneal disorder due to contact lens, left eye
H18.823 Corneal disorder due to contact lens, bilateral
H18.829 Corneal disorder due to contact lens, unspecified eye
+ H18.83 Recurrent erosion of cornea
H18.831 Recurrent erosion of cornea, right eye
H18.832 Recurrent erosion of cornea, left eye
H18.833 Recurrent erosion of cornea, bilateral
H18.839 Recurrent erosion of cornea, unspecified eye
+ H18.89 Other specified disorders of cornea
H18.891 Other specified disorders of cornea, right eye
H18.892 Other specified disorders of cornea, left eye
H18.893 Other specified disorders of cornea, bilateral
H18.899 Other specified disorders of cornea, unspecified eye
H18.9 Unspecified disorder of cornea

H20 Iridocyclitis

+ H20.0 Acute and subacute iridocyclitis
Acute anterior uveitis
Acute cyclitis
Acute iritis
Subacute anterior uveitis
Subacute cyclitis
Subacute iritis
Excludes1: *iridocyclitis, iritis, uveitis (due to) (in) diabetes mellitus (E08-E13 with .39)*
iridocyclitis, iritis, uveitis (due to) (in) diphtheria (A36.89)
iridocyclitis, iritis, uveitis (due to) (in) gonococcal (A54.32)
iridocyclitis, iritis, uveitis (due to) (in) herpes (simplex) (B00.51)
iridocyclitis, iritis, uveitis (due to) (in) herpes zoster (B02.32)
iridocyclitis, iritis, uveitis (due to) (in) late congenital syphilis (A50.39)
iridocyclitis, iritis, uveitis (due to) (in) late syphilis (A52.71)
iridocyclitis, iritis, uveitis (due to) (in) sarcoidosis (D86.83)
iridocyclitis, iritis, uveitis (due to) (in) syphilis (A51.43)
iridocyclitis, iritis, uveitis (due to) (in) toxoplasmosis (B58.09)
iridocyclitis, iritis, uveitis (due to) (in) tuberculosis (A18.54)

CC H20.00 Unspecified acute and subacute iridocyclitis
+ H20.01 Primary iridocyclitis
CC H20.011 Primary iridocyclitis, right eye
CC H20.012 Primary iridocyclitis, left eye
CC H20.013 Primary iridocyclitis, bilateral
CC H20.019 Primary iridocyclitis, unspecified eye
+ H20.02 Recurrent acute iridocyclitis
CC H20.021 Recurrent acute iridocyclitis, right eye
CC H20.022 Recurrent acute iridocyclitis, left eye
CC H20.023 Recurrent acute iridocyclitis, bilateral
CC H20.029 Recurrent acute iridocyclitis, unspecified eye
+ H20.03 Secondary infectious iridocyclitis
CC H20.031 Secondary infectious iridocyclitis, right eye
CC H20.032 Secondary infectious iridocyclitis, left eye
CC H20.033 Secondary infectious iridocyclitis, bilateral
CC H20.039 Secondary infectious iridocyclitis, unspecified eye
+ H20.04 Secondary noninfectious iridocyclitis
H20.041 Secondary noninfectious iridocyclitis, right eye
H20.042 Secondary noninfectious iridocyclitis, left eye
H20.043 Secondary noninfectious iridocyclitis, bilateral
H20.049 Secondary noninfectious iridocyclitis, unspecified eye
+ H20.05 Hypopyon
H20.051 Hypopyon, right eye
H20.052 Hypopyon, left eye
H20.053 Hypopyon, bilateral
H20.059 Hypopyon, unspecified eye
+ H20.1 Chronic iridocyclitis
Use additional code for any associated cataract (H26.21-)
Excludes2: *posterior cyclitis (H30.2-)*
H20.10 Chronic iridocyclitis, unspecified eye
H20.11 Chronic iridocyclitis, right eye
H20.12 Chronic iridocyclitis, left eye
H20.13 Chronic iridocyclitis, bilateral
+ H20.2 Lens-induced iridocyclitis
H20.20 Lens-induced iridocyclitis, unspecified eye
H20.21 Lens-induced iridocyclitis, right eye
H20.22 Lens-induced iridocyclitis, left eye
H20.23 Lens-induced iridocyclitis, bilateral
+ H20.8 Other iridocyclitis
Excludes2: *glaucomatocyclitis crises (H40.4-)*
posterior cyclitis (H30.2-)
sympathetic uveitis (H44.13-)
+ H20.81 Fuchs' heterochromic cyclitis
H20.811 Fuchs' heterochromic cyclitis, right eye
H20.812 Fuchs' heterochromic cyclitis, left eye
H20.813 Fuchs' heterochromic cyclitis, bilateral
H20.819 Fuchs' heterochromic cyclitis, unspecified eye
+ H20.82 Vogt-Koyanagi syndrome
H20.821 Vogt-Koyanagi syndrome, right eye
H20.822 Vogt-Koyanagi syndrome, left eye
H20.823 Vogt-Koyanagi syndrome, bilateral
H20.829 Vogt-Koyanagi syndrome, unspecified eye
CC H20.9 Unspecified iridocyclitis
Uveitis NOS

H21 Other disorders of iris and ciliary body

Excludes2: *sympathetic uveitis (H44.1-)*
+ H21.0 Hyphema
Excludes1: *traumatic hyphema (S05.1-)*
H21.00 Hyphema, unspecified eye
H21.01 Hyphema, right eye
H21.02 Hyphema, left eye
H21.03 Hyphema, bilateral

- **H21.1 Other vascular disorders of iris and ciliary body**
  Neovascularization of iris or ciliary body
  Rubeosis iridis
  Rubeosis of iris
  - **H21.1X Other vascular disorders of iris and ciliary body**
    - H21.1X1 Other vascular disorders of iris and ciliary body, right eye
    - H21.1X2 Other vascular disorders of iris and ciliary body, left eye
    - H21.1X3 Other vascular disorders of iris and ciliary body, bilateral
    - H21.1X9 Other vascular disorders of iris and ciliary body, unspecified eye
- **H21.2 Degeneration of iris and ciliary body**
  - **H21.21 Degeneration of chamber angle**
    - H21.211 Degeneration of chamber angle, right eye
    - H21.212 Degeneration of chamber angle, left eye
    - H21.213 Degeneration of chamber angle, bilateral
    - H21.219 Degeneration of chamber angle, unspecified eye
  - **H21.22 Degeneration of ciliary body**
    - H21.221 Degeneration of ciliary body, right eye
    - H21.222 Degeneration of ciliary body, left eye
    - H21.223 Degeneration of ciliary body, bilateral
    - H21.229 Degeneration of ciliary body, unspecified eye
  - **H21.23 Degeneration of iris (pigmentary)**
    Translucency of iris
    - H21.231 Degeneration of iris (pigmentary), right eye
    - H21.232 Degeneration of iris (pigmentary), left eye
    - H21.233 Degeneration of iris (pigmentary), bilateral
    - H21.239 Degeneration of iris (pigmentary), unspecified eye
  - **H21.24 Degeneration of pupillary margin**
    - H21.241 Degeneration of pupillary margin, right eye
    - H21.242 Degeneration of pupillary margin, left eye
    - H21.243 Degeneration of pupillary margin, bilateral
    - H21.249 Degeneration of pupillary margin, unspecified eye
  - **H21.25 Iridoschisis**
    - H21.251 Iridoschisis, right eye
    - H21.252 Iridoschisis, left eye
    - H21.253 Iridoschisis, bilateral
    - H21.259 Iridoschisis, unspecified eye
  - **H21.26 Iris atrophy (essential) (progressive)**
    - H21.261 Iris atrophy (essential) (progressive), right eye
    - H21.262 Iris atrophy (essential) (progressive), left eye
    - H21.263 Iris atrophy (essential) (progressive), bilateral
    - H21.269 Iris atrophy (essential) (progressive), unspecified eye
  - **H21.27 Miotic pupillary cyst**
    - H21.271 Miotic pupillary cyst, right eye
    - H21.272 Miotic pupillary cyst, left eye
    - H21.273 Miotic pupillary cyst, bilateral
    - H21.279 Miotic pupillary cyst, unspecified eye
  - H21.29 Other iris atrophy
- **H21.3 Cyst of iris, ciliary body and anterior chamber**
  Excludes2: miotic pupillary cyst (H21.27-)
  - **H21.30 Idiopathic cysts of iris, ciliary body or anterior chamber**
    Cyst of iris, ciliary body or anterior chamber NOS
    - H21.301 Idiopathic cysts of iris, ciliary body or anterior chamber, right eye
    - H21.302 Idiopathic cysts of iris, ciliary body or anterior chamber, left eye
    - H21.303 Idiopathic cysts of iris, ciliary body or anterior chamber, bilateral
    - H21.309 Idiopathic cysts of iris, ciliary body or anterior chamber, unspecified eye
  - **H21.31 Exudative cysts of iris or anterior chamber**
    - H21.311 Exudative cysts of iris or anterior chamber, right eye
    - H21.312 Exudative cysts of iris or anterior chamber, left eye
    - H21.313 Exudative cysts of iris or anterior chamber, bilateral
    - H21.319 Exudative cysts of iris or anterior chamber, unspecified eye
  - **H21.32 Implantation cysts of iris, ciliary body or anterior chamber**
    - H21.321 Implantation cysts of iris, ciliary body or anterior chamber, right eye
    - H21.322 Implantation cysts of iris, ciliary body or anterior chamber, left eye
    - H21.323 Implantation cysts of iris, ciliary body or anterior chamber, bilateral
    - H21.329 Implantation cysts of iris, ciliary body or anterior chamber, unspecified eye
  - **H21.33 Parasitic cyst of iris, ciliary body or anterior chamber**
    - CC H21.331 Parasitic cyst of iris, ciliary body or anterior chamber, right eye
    - CC H21.332 Parasitic cyst of iris, ciliary body or anterior chamber, left eye
    - CC H21.333 Parasitic cyst of iris, ciliary body or anterior chamber, bilateral
    - CC H21.339 Parasitic cyst of iris, ciliary body or anterior chamber, unspecified eye
  - **H21.34 Primary cyst of pars plana**
    - H21.341 Primary cyst of pars plana, right eye
    - H21.342 Primary cyst of pars plana, left eye
    - H21.343 Primary cyst of pars plana, bilateral
    - H21.349 Primary cyst of pars plana, unspecified eye
  - **H21.35 Exudative cyst of pars plana**
    - H21.351 Exudative cyst of pars plana, right eye
    - H21.352 Exudative cyst of pars plana, left eye
    - H21.353 Exudative cyst of pars plana, bilateral
    - H21.359 Exudative cyst of pars plana, unspecified eye
- **H21.4 Pupillary membranes**
  Iris bombé
  Pupillary occlusion
  Pupillary seclusion
  Excludes1: congenital pupillary membranes (Q13.8)
  - H21.40 Pupillary membranes, unspecified eye
  - H21.41 Pupillary membranes, right eye
  - H21.42 Pupillary membranes, left eye
  - H21.43 Pupillary membranes, bilateral
- **H21.5 Other and unspecified adhesions and disruptions of iris and ciliary body**
  Excludes1: corectopia (Q13.2)
  - **H21.50 Unspecified adhesions of iris**
    Synechia (iris) NOS
    - H21.501 Unspecified adhesions of iris, right eye
    - H21.502 Unspecified adhesions of iris, left eye
    - H21.503 Unspecified adhesions of iris, bilateral
    - H21.509 Unspecified adhesions of iris and ciliary body, unspecified eye
  - **H21.51 Anterior synechiae (iris)**
    - H21.511 Anterior synechiae (iris), right eye
    - H21.512 Anterior synechiae (iris), left eye
    - H21.513 Anterior synechiae (iris), bilateral
    - H21.519 Anterior synechiae (iris), unspecified eye
  - **H21.52 Goniosynechiae**
    - H21.521 Goniosynechiae, right eye
    - H21.522 Goniosynechiae, left eye
    - H21.523 Goniosynechiae, bilateral
    - H21.529 Goniosynechiae, unspecified eye

- **+ H21.53 Iridodialysis**
  - H21.531 Iridodialysis, right eye
  - H21.532 Iridodialysis, left eye
  - H21.533 Iridodialysis, bilateral
  - H21.539 Iridodialysis, unspecified eye
- **+ H21.54 Posterior synechiae (iris)**
  - H21.541 Posterior synechiae (iris), right eye
  - H21.542 Posterior synechiae (iris), left eye
  - H21.543 Posterior synechiae (iris), bilateral
  - H21.549 Posterior synechiae (iris), unspecified eye
- **+ H21.55 Recession of chamber angle**
  - H21.551 Recession of chamber angle, right eye
  - H21.552 Recession of chamber angle, left eye
  - H21.553 Recession of chamber angle, bilateral
  - H21.559 Recession of chamber angle, unspecified eye
- **+ H21.56 Pupillary abnormalities**
  - Deformed pupil
  - Ectopic pupil
  - Rupture of sphincter, pupil
  - *Excludes1:* *congenital deformity of pupil (Q13.2-)*
  - H21.561 Pupillary abnormality, right eye
  - H21.562 Pupillary abnormality, left eye
  - H21.563 Pupillary abnormality, bilateral
  - H21.569 Pupillary abnormality, unspecified eye
- **+ H21.8 Other specified disorders of iris and ciliary body**
  - H21.81 Floppy iris syndrome
    - Intraoperative floppy iris syndrome (IFIS)
    - Use additional code for adverse effect, if applicable, to identify drug (T36-T50 with fifth or sixth character 5)
  - H21.82 Plateau iris syndrome (post-iridectomy) (postprocedural)
  - H21.89 Other specified disorders of iris and ciliary body
- **H21.9 Unspecified disorder of iris and ciliary body**
- **H22 Disorders of iris and ciliary body in diseases classified elsewhere**
  - Code first underlying disease, such as:
    - gout (M1A.-, M10.-)
    - leprosy (A30.-)
    - parasitic disease (B89)
  - *Valid 3-character code, no further characters required*

Disorders of lens (H25-H28)

- **H25 Age-related cataract**
  - Senile cataract
  - *Excludes2:* *capsular glaucoma with pseudoexfoliation of lens (H40.1-)*
  - **+ H25.0 Age-related incipient cataract**
    - **+ H25.01 Cortical age-related cataract**
      - H25.011 Cortical age-related cataract, right eye
      - H25.012 Cortical age-related cataract, left eye
      - H25.013 Cortical age-related cataract, bilateral
      - H25.019 Cortical age-related cataract, unspecified eye
    - **+ H25.03 Anterior subcapsular polar age-related cataract**
      - H25.031 Anterior subcapsular polar age-related cataract, right eye
      - H25.032 Anterior subcapsular polar age-related cataract, left eye
      - H25.033 Anterior subcapsular polar age-related cataract, bilateral
      - H25.039 Anterior subcapsular polar age-related cataract, unspecified eye
    - **+ H25.04 Posterior subcapsular polar age-related cataract**
      - H25.041 Posterior subcapsular polar age-related cataract, right eye
      - H25.042 Posterior subcapsular polar age-related cataract, left eye
      - H25.043 Posterior subcapsular polar age-related cataract, bilateral
      - H25.049 Posterior subcapsular polar age-related cataract, unspecified eye
  - **+ H25.09 Other age-related incipient cataract**
    - Coronary age-related cataract
    - Punctate age-related cataract
    - Water clefts
    - H25.091 Other age-related incipient cataract, right eye
    - H25.092 Other age-related incipient cataract, left eye
    - H25.093 Other age-related incipient cataract, bilateral
    - H25.099 Other age-related incipient cataract, unspecified eye
  - **+ H25.1 Age-related nuclear cataract**
    - Cataracta brunescens
    - Nuclear sclerosis cataract
    - H25.10 Age-related nuclear cataract, unspecified eye
    - H25.11 Age-related nuclear cataract, right eye
      - *AHA CC: 2Q, 2019, 31*
    - H25.12 Age-related nuclear cataract, left eye
      - *AHA CC: 1Q, 2016, 32-33*
    - H25.13 Age-related nuclear cataract, bilateral
      - *AHA CC: 1Q, 2016, 32-33*
  - **+ H25.2 Age-related cataract, morgagnian type**
    - Age-related hypermature cataract
    - H25.20 Age-related cataract, morgagnian type, unspecified eye
    - H25.21 Age-related cataract, morgagnian type, right eye
    - H25.22 Age-related cataract, morgagnian type, left eye
    - H25.23 Age-related cataract, morgagnian type, bilateral
  - **+ H25.8 Other age-related cataract**
    - **+ H25.81 Combined forms of age-related cataract**
      - H25.811 Combined forms of age-related cataract, right eye
      - H25.812 Combined forms of age-related cataract, left eye
      - H25.813 Combined forms of age-related cataract, bilateral
        - *AHA CC: 2Q, 2019, 30*
      - H25.819 Combined forms of age-related cataract, unspecified eye
    - H25.89 Other age-related cataract
  - **H25.9 Unspecified age-related cataract**
- **H26 Other cataract**
  - *Excludes1:* *congenital cataract (Q12.0)*
  - **+ H26.0 Infantile and juvenile cataract**
    - **+ H26.00 Unspecified infantile and juvenile cataract**
      - H26.001 Unspecified infantile and juvenile cataract, right eye
      - H26.002 Unspecified infantile and juvenile cataract, left eye
      - H26.003 Unspecified infantile and juvenile cataract, bilateral
      - H26.009 Unspecified infantile and juvenile cataract, unspecified eye
    - **+ H26.01 Infantile and juvenile cortical, lamellar, or zonular cataract**
      - H26.011 Infantile and juvenile cortical, lamellar, or zonular cataract, right eye
      - H26.012 Infantile and juvenile cortical, lamellar, or zonular cataract, left eye
      - H26.013 Infantile and juvenile cortical, lamellar, or zonular cataract, bilateral
      - H26.019 Infantile and juvenile cortical, lamellar, or zonular cataract, unspecified eye
    - **+ H26.03 Infantile and juvenile nuclear cataract**
      - H26.031 Infantile and juvenile nuclear cataract, right eye
      - H26.032 Infantile and juvenile nuclear cataract, left eye
      - H26.033 Infantile and juvenile nuclear cataract, bilateral
      - H26.039 Infantile and juvenile nuclear cataract, unspecified eye

- **H26.04** Anterior subcapsular polar infantile and juvenile cataract
  - H26.041 Anterior subcapsular polar infantile and juvenile cataract, right eye
  - H26.042 Anterior subcapsular polar infantile and juvenile cataract, left eye
  - H26.043 Anterior subcapsular polar infantile and juvenile cataract, bilateral
  - H26.049 Anterior subcapsular polar infantile and juvenile cataract, unspecified eye
- **H26.05** Posterior subcapsular polar infantile and juvenile cataract
  - H26.051 Posterior subcapsular polar infantile and juvenile cataract, right eye
  - H26.052 Posterior subcapsular polar infantile and juvenile cataract, left eye
  - H26.053 Posterior subcapsular polar infantile and juvenile cataract, bilateral
  - H26.059 Posterior subcapsular polar infantile and juvenile cataract, unspecified eye
- **H26.06** Combined forms of infantile and juvenile cataract
  - H26.061 Combined forms of infantile and juvenile cataract, right eye
  - H26.062 Combined forms of infantile and juvenile cataract, left eye
  - H26.063 Combined forms of infantile and juvenile cataract, bilateral
  - H26.069 Combined forms of infantile and juvenile cataract, unspecified eye
- H26.09 Other infantile and juvenile cataract
- **H26.1** Traumatic cataract

  Use additional code (Chapter 20) to identify external cause
  - **H26.10** Unspecified traumatic cataract
    - H26.101 Unspecified traumatic cataract, right eye
    - H26.102 Unspecified traumatic cataract, left eye
    - H26.103 Unspecified traumatic cataract, bilateral
    - H26.109 Unspecified traumatic cataract, unspecified eye
  - **H26.11** Localized traumatic opacities
    - H26.111 Localized traumatic opacities, right eye
    - H26.112 Localized traumatic opacities, left eye
    - H26.113 Localized traumatic opacities, bilateral
    - H26.119 Localized traumatic opacities, unspecified eye
  - **H26.12** Partially resolved traumatic cataract
    - H26.121 Partially resolved traumatic cataract, right eye
    - H26.122 Partially resolved traumatic cataract, left eye
    - H26.123 Partially resolved traumatic cataract, bilateral
    - H26.129 Partially resolved traumatic cataract, unspecified eye
  - **H26.13** Total traumatic cataract
    - H26.131 Total traumatic cataract, right eye
    - H26.132 Total traumatic cataract, left eye
    - H26.133 Total traumatic cataract, bilateral
    - H26.139 Total traumatic cataract, unspecified eye
- **H26.2** Complicated cataract
  - H26.20 Unspecified complicated cataract

    Cataracta complicata NOS
  - **H26.21** Cataract with neovascularization

    Code also, if applicable, associated condition, such as: chronic iridocyclitis (H20.1-)
    - H26.211 Cataract with neovascularization, right eye
    - H26.212 Cataract with neovascularization, left eye
    - H26.213 Cataract with neovascularization, bilateral
    - H26.219 Cataract with neovascularization, unspecified eye
  - **H26.22** Cataract secondary to ocular disorders (degenerative) (inflammatory)

    Code also associated ocular disorder
    - H26.221 Cataract secondary to ocular disorders (degenerative) (inflammatory), right eye
    - H26.222 Cataract secondary to ocular disorders (degenerative) (inflammatory), left eye
    - H26.223 Cataract secondary to ocular disorders (degenerative) (inflammatory), bilateral
    - H26.229 Cataract secondary to ocular disorders (degenerative) (inflammatory), unspecified eye
- **H26.23** Glaucomatous flecks (subcapsular)

  Code first underlying glaucoma (H40-H42)
  - H26.231 Glaucomatous flecks (subcapsular), right eye
  - H26.232 Glaucomatous flecks (subcapsular), left eye
  - H26.233 Glaucomatous flecks (subcapsular), bilateral
  - H26.239 Glaucomatous flecks (subcapsular), unspecified eye
- **H26.3** Drug-induced cataract

  Toxic cataract

  Use additional code for adverse effect, if applicable, to identify drug (T36-T50 with fifth or sixth character 5)
  - H26.30 Drug-induced cataract, unspecified eye
  - H26.31 Drug-induced cataract, right eye
  - H26.32 Drug-induced cataract, left eye
  - H26.33 Drug-induced cataract, bilateral
- **H26.4** Secondary cataract
  - H26.40 Unspecified secondary cataract
  - **H26.41** Soemmering's ring
    - H26.411 Soemmering's ring, right eye
    - H26.412 Soemmering's ring, left eye
    - H26.413 Soemmering's ring, bilateral
    - H26.419 Soemmering's ring, unspecified eye
  - **H26.49** Other secondary cataract
    - H26.491 Other secondary cataract, right eye
    - H26.492 Other secondary cataract, left eye

      AHA CC: 2Q, 2018, 14
    - H26.493 Other secondary cataract, bilateral
    - H26.499 Other secondary cataract, unspecified eye
- H26.8 Other specified cataract
- H26.9 Unspecified cataract

H27 Other disorders of lens

Excludes1: congenital lens malformations (Q12.-)
mechanical complications of intraocular lens implant (T85.2)
pseudophakia (Z96.1)

- **H27.0** Aphakia

  Acquired absence of lens
  Acquired aphakia
  Aphakia due to trauma

  Excludes1: cataract extraction status (Z98.4-)
  congenital absence of lens (Q12.3)
  congenital aphakia (Q12.3)
  - H27.00 Aphakia, unspecified eye
  - H27.01 Aphakia, right eye
  - H27.02 Aphakia, left eye
  - H27.03 Aphakia, bilateral
- **H27.1** Dislocation of lens
  - H27.10 Unspecified dislocation of lens
  - **H27.11** Subluxation of lens
    - H27.111 Subluxation of lens, right eye
    - H27.112 Subluxation of lens, left eye
    - H27.113 Subluxation of lens, bilateral
    - H27.119 Subluxation of lens, unspecified eye
  - **H27.12** Anterior dislocation of lens
    - H27.121 Anterior dislocation of lens, right eye
    - H27.122 Anterior dislocation of lens, left eye
    - H27.123 Anterior dislocation of lens, bilateral
    - H27.129 Anterior dislocation of lens, unspecified eye
  - **H27.13** Posterior dislocation of lens
    - H27.131 Posterior dislocation of lens, right eye
    - H27.132 Posterior dislocation of lens, left eye
    - H27.133 Posterior dislocation of lens, bilateral
    - H27.139 Posterior dislocation of lens, unspecified eye
- H27.8 Other specified disorders of lens
- H27.9 Unspecified disorder of lens

H28 Cataract in diseases classified elsewhere

Code first underlying disease, such as:
hypoparathyroidism (E20.-)
myotonia (G71.1-)
myxedema (E03.-)
protein-calorie malnutrition (E40-E46)

Excludes1: cataract in diabetes mellitus (E08.36, E09.36, E10.36, E11.36, E13.36)

Valid 3-character code, no further characters required

Disorders of choroid and retina (H30-H36)

H30 Chorioretinal inflammation

- **H30.0** Focal chorioretinal inflammation
  - Focal chorioretinitis
  - Focal choroiditis
  - Focal retinitis
  - Focal retinochoroiditis
  - **H30.00** Unspecified focal chorioretinal inflammation
    - Focal chorioretinitis NOS
    - Focal choroiditis NOS
    - Focal retinitis NOS
    - Focal retinochoroiditis NOS
    - **H30.001** Unspecified focal chorioretinal inflammation, right eye
    - **H30.002** Unspecified focal chorioretinal inflammation, left eye
    - **H30.003** Unspecified focal chorioretinal inflammation, bilateral
    - **H30.009** Unspecified focal chorioretinal inflammation, unspecified eye
  - **H30.01** Focal chorioretinal inflammation, juxtapapillary
    - **H30.011** Focal chorioretinal inflammation, juxtapapillary, right eye
    - **H30.012** Focal chorioretinal inflammation, juxtapapillary, left eye
    - **H30.013** Focal chorioretinal inflammation, juxtapapillary, bilateral
    - **H30.019** Focal chorioretinal inflammation, juxtapapillary, unspecified eye
  - **H30.02** Focal chorioretinal inflammation of posterior pole
    - **H30.021** Focal chorioretinal inflammation of posterior pole, right eye
    - **H30.022** Focal chorioretinal inflammation of posterior pole, left eye
    - **H30.023** Focal chorioretinal inflammation of posterior pole, bilateral
    - **H30.029** Focal chorioretinal inflammation of posterior pole, unspecified eye
  - **H30.03** Focal chorioretinal inflammation, peripheral
    - **H30.031** Focal chorioretinal inflammation, peripheral, right eye
    - **H30.032** Focal chorioretinal inflammation, peripheral, left eye
    - **H30.033** Focal chorioretinal inflammation, peripheral, bilateral
    - **H30.039** Focal chorioretinal inflammation, peripheral, unspecified eye
  - **H30.04** Focal chorioretinal inflammation, macular or paramacular
    - **H30.041** Focal chorioretinal inflammation, macular or paramacular, right eye
    - **H30.042** Focal chorioretinal inflammation, macular or paramacular, left eye
    - **H30.043** Focal chorioretinal inflammation, macular or paramacular, bilateral
    - **H30.049** Focal chorioretinal inflammation, macular or paramacular, unspecified eye
- **H30.1** Disseminated chorioretinal inflammation
  - Disseminated chorioretinitis
  - Disseminated choroiditis
  - Disseminated retinitis
  - Disseminated retinochoroiditis
  - **Excludes2:** exudative retinopathy (H35.02-)
  - **H30.10** Unspecified disseminated chorioretinal inflammation
    - Disseminated chorioretinitis NOS
    - Disseminated choroiditis NOS
    - Disseminated retinitis NOS
    - Disseminated retinochoroiditis NOS
    - CC **H30.101** Unspecified disseminated chorioretinal inflammation, right eye
    - CC **H30.102** Unspecified disseminated chorioretinal inflammation, left eye
    - CC **H30.103** Unspecified disseminated chorioretinal inflammation, bilateral
    - CC **H30.109** Unspecified disseminated chorioretinal inflammation, unspecified eye
  - **H30.11** Disseminated chorioretinal inflammation of posterior pole
    - CC **H30.111** Disseminated chorioretinal inflammation of posterior pole, right eye
    - CC **H30.112** Disseminated chorioretinal inflammation of posterior pole, left eye
    - CC **H30.113** Disseminated chorioretinal inflammation of posterior pole, bilateral
    - CC **H30.119** Disseminated chorioretinal inflammation of posterior pole, unspecified eye
  - **H30.12** Disseminated chorioretinal inflammation, peripheral
    - CC **H30.121** Disseminated chorioretinal inflammation, peripheral right eye
    - CC **H30.122** Disseminated chorioretinal inflammation, peripheral, left eye
    - CC **H30.123** Disseminated chorioretinal inflammation, peripheral, bilateral
    - CC **H30.129** Disseminated chorioretinal inflammation, peripheral, unspecified eye
  - **H30.13** Disseminated chorioretinal inflammation, generalized
    - CC **H30.131** Disseminated chorioretinal inflammation, generalized, right eye
    - CC **H30.132** Disseminated chorioretinal inflammation, generalized, left eye
    - CC **H30.133** Disseminated chorioretinal inflammation, generalized, bilateral
    - CC **H30.139** Disseminated chorioretinal inflammation, generalized, unspecified eye
  - **H30.14** Acute posterior multifocal placoid pigment epitheliopathy
    - CC **H30.141** Acute posterior multifocal placoid pigment epitheliopathy, right eye
    - CC **H30.142** Acute posterior multifocal placoid pigment epitheliopathy, left eye
    - CC **H30.143** Acute posterior multifocal placoid pigment epitheliopathy, bilateral
    - CC **H30.149** Acute posterior multifocal placoid pigment epitheliopathy, unspecified eye
- **H30.2** Posterior cyclitis
  - Pars planitis
  - **H30.20** Posterior cyclitis, unspecified eye
  - **H30.21** Posterior cyclitis, right eye
  - **H30.22** Posterior cyclitis, left eye
  - **H30.23** Posterior cyclitis, bilateral
- **H30.8** Other chorioretinal inflammations
  - **H30.81** Harada's disease
    - **H30.811** Harada's disease, right eye
    - **H30.812** Harada's disease, left eye
    - **H30.813** Harada's disease, bilateral
    - **H30.819** Harada's disease, unspecified eye
  - **H30.89** Other chorioretinal inflammations
    - CC **H30.891** Other chorioretinal inflammations, right eye
    - CC **H30.892** Other chorioretinal inflammations, left eye
    - CC **H30.893** Other chorioretinal inflammations, bilateral
    - CC **H30.899** Other chorioretinal inflammations, unspecified eye
- **H30.9** Unspecified chorioretinal inflammation
  - Chorioretinitis NOS
  - Choroiditis NOS
  - Neuroretinitis NOS
  - Retinitis NOS
  - Retinochoroiditis NOS
  - CC **H30.90** Unspecified chorioretinal inflammation, unspecified eye
  - CC **H30.91** Unspecified chorioretinal inflammation, right eye
  - CC **H30.92** Unspecified chorioretinal inflammation, left eye
  - CC **H30.93** Unspecified chorioretinal inflammation, bilateral

H31 Other disorders of choroid

- **+ H31.0 Chorioretinal scars**
  - *Excludes2:* postsurgical chorioretinal scars (H59.81-)
  - **+ H31.00 Unspecified chorioretinal scars**
    - H31.001 Unspecified chorioretinal scars, right eye
    - H31.002 Unspecified chorioretinal scars, left eye
    - H31.003 Unspecified chorioretinal scars, bilateral
    - H31.009 Unspecified chorioretinal scars, unspecified eye
  - **+ H31.01 Macula scars of posterior pole (postinflammatory) (post-traumatic)**
    - *Excludes1:* postprocedural chorioretinal scar (H59.81-)
    - H31.011 Macula scars of posterior pole (postinflammatory) (post-traumatic), right eye
    - H31.012 Macula scars of posterior pole (postinflammatory) (post-traumatic), left eye
    - H31.013 Macula scars of posterior pole (postinflammatory) (post-traumatic), bilateral
    - H31.019 Macula scars of posterior pole (postinflammatory) (post-traumatic), unspecified eye
  - **+ H31.02 Solar retinopathy**
    - H31.021 Solar retinopathy, right eye
    - H31.022 Solar retinopathy, left eye
    - H31.023 Solar retinopathy, bilateral
    - H31.029 Solar retinopathy, unspecified eye
  - **+ H31.09 Other chorioretinal scars**
    - H31.091 Other chorioretinal scars, right eye
    - H31.092 Other chorioretinal scars, left eye
    - H31.093 Other chorioretinal scars, bilateral
    - H31.099 Other chorioretinal scars, unspecified eye
- **+ H31.1 Choroidal degeneration**
  - *Excludes2:* angioid streaks of macula (H35.33)
  - **+ H31.10 Unspecified choroidal degeneration**
    - Choroidal sclerosis NOS
    - H31.101 Choroidal degeneration, unspecified, right eye
    - H31.102 Choroidal degeneration, unspecified, left eye
    - H31.103 Choroidal degeneration, unspecified, bilateral
    - H31.109 Choroidal degeneration, unspecified, unspecified eye
  - **+ H31.11 Age-related choroidal atrophy**
    - • H31.111 Age-related choroidal atrophy, right eye
    - • H31.112 Age-related choroidal atrophy, left eye
    - • H31.113 Age-related choroidal atrophy, bilateral
    - • H31.119 Age-related choroidal atrophy, unspecified eye
  - **+ H31.12 Diffuse secondary atrophy of choroid**
    - H31.121 Diffuse secondary atrophy of choroid, right eye
    - H31.122 Diffuse secondary atrophy of choroid, left eye
    - H31.123 Diffuse secondary atrophy of choroid, bilateral
    - H31.129 Diffuse secondary atrophy of choroid, unspecified eye
- **+ H31.2 Hereditary choroidal dystrophy**
  - *Excludes2:* hyperornithinemia (E72.4)
    - ornithinemia (E72.4)
  - H31.20 Hereditary choroidal dystrophy, unspecified
  - H31.21 Choroideremia
  - H31.22 Choroidal dystrophy (central areolar) (generalized) (peripapillary)
  - H31.23 Gyrate atrophy, choroid
  - H31.29 Other hereditary choroidal dystrophy
- **+ H31.3 Choroidal hemorrhage and rupture**
  - **+ H31.30 Unspecified choroidal hemorrhage**
    - H31.301 Unspecified choroidal hemorrhage, right eye
    - H31.302 Unspecified choroidal hemorrhage, left eye
    - H31.303 Unspecified choroidal hemorrhage, bilateral
    - H31.309 Unspecified choroidal hemorrhage, unspecified eye
  - **+ H31.31 Expulsive choroidal hemorrhage**
    - H31.311 Expulsive choroidal hemorrhage, right eye
    - H31.312 Expulsive choroidal hemorrhage, left eye
    - H31.313 Expulsive choroidal hemorrhage, bilateral
    - H31.319 Expulsive choroidal hemorrhage, unspecified eye
  - **+ H31.32 Choroidal rupture**
    - CC H31.321 Choroidal rupture, right eye
    - CC H31.322 Choroidal rupture, left eye
    - CC H31.323 Choroidal rupture, bilateral
    - CC H31.329 Choroidal rupture, unspecified eye
- **+ H31.4 Choroidal detachment**
  - **+ H31.40 Unspecified choroidal detachment**
    - CC H31.401 Unspecified choroidal detachment, right eye
    - CC H31.402 Unspecified choroidal detachment, left eye
    - CC H31.403 Unspecified choroidal detachment, bilateral
    - CC H31.409 Unspecified choroidal detachment, unspecified eye
  - **+ H31.41 Hemorrhagic choroidal detachment**
    - CC H31.411 Hemorrhagic choroidal detachment, right eye
    - CC H31.412 Hemorrhagic choroidal detachment, left eye
    - CC H31.413 Hemorrhagic choroidal detachment, bilateral
    - CC H31.419 Hemorrhagic choroidal detachment, unspecified eye
  - **+ H31.42 Serous choroidal detachment**
    - CC H31.421 Serous choroidal detachment, right eye
    - CC H31.422 Serous choroidal detachment, left eye
    - CC H31.423 Serous choroidal detachment, bilateral
    - CC H31.429 Serous choroidal detachment, unspecified eye
- H31.8 Other specified disorders of choroid
- H31.9 Unspecified disorder of choroid

H32 Chorioretinal disorders in diseases classified elsewhere

Code first underlying disease, such as:
  congenital toxoplasmosis (P37.1)
  histoplasmosis (B39.-)
  leprosy (A30.-)
Excludes1: chorioretinitis (in):
  toxoplasmosis (acquired) (B58.01)
  tuberculosis (A18.53)

Valid 3-character code, no further characters required

H33 Retinal detachments and breaks

Excludes1: detachment of retinal pigment epithelium (H35.72-, H35.73-)

- **H33.0** Retinal detachment with retinal break
  Rhegmatogenous retinal detachment
  Excludes1: serous retinal detachment (without retinal break) (H33.2-)
  - **H33.00** Unspecified retinal detachment with retinal break
    - H33.001 Unspecified retinal detachment with retinal break, right eye
    - H33.002 Unspecified retinal detachment with retinal break, left eye
    - H33.003 Unspecified retinal detachment with retinal break, bilateral
    - H33.009 Unspecified retinal detachment with retinal break, unspecified eye
  - **H33.01** Retinal detachment with single break
    - H33.011 Retinal detachment with single break, right eye
    - H33.012 Retinal detachment with single break, left eye
    - H33.013 Retinal detachment with single break, bilateral
    - H33.019 Retinal detachment with single break, unspecified eye
  - **H33.02** Retinal detachment with multiple breaks
    - H33.021 Retinal detachment with multiple breaks, right eye
    - H33.022 Retinal detachment with multiple breaks, left eye
    - H33.023 Retinal detachment with multiple breaks, bilateral
    - H33.029 Retinal detachment with multiple breaks, unspecified eye
  - **H33.03** Retinal detachment with giant retinal tear
    - H33.031 Retinal detachment with giant retinal tear, right eye
    - H33.032 Retinal detachment with giant retinal tear, left eye
    - H33.033 Retinal detachment with giant retinal tear, bilateral
    - H33.039 Retinal detachment with giant retinal tear, unspecified eye
  - **H33.04** Retinal detachment with retinal dialysis
    - H33.041 Retinal detachment with retinal dialysis, right eye
    - H33.042 Retinal detachment with retinal dialysis, left eye
    - H33.043 Retinal detachment with retinal dialysis, bilateral
    - H33.049 Retinal detachment with retinal dialysis, unspecified eye
  - **H33.05** Total retinal detachment
    - H33.051 Total retinal detachment, right eye
    - H33.052 Total retinal detachment, left eye
    - H33.053 Total retinal detachment, bilateral
    - H33.059 Total retinal detachment, unspecified eye
- **H33.1** Retinoschisis and retinal cysts
  Excludes1: congenital retinoschisis (Q14.1)
  microcystoid degeneration of retina (H35.42-)
  - **H33.10** Unspecified retinoschisis
    - H33.101 Unspecified retinoschisis, right eye
    - H33.102 Unspecified retinoschisis, left eye
    - H33.103 Unspecified retinoschisis, bilateral
    - H33.109 Unspecified retinoschisis, unspecified eye
  - **H33.11** Cyst of ora serrata
    - H33.111 Cyst of ora serrata, right eye
    - H33.112 Cyst of ora serrata, left eye
    - H33.113 Cyst of ora serrata, bilateral
    - H33.119 Cyst of ora serrata, unspecified eye
  - **H33.12** Parasitic cyst of retina
    - CC H33.121 Parasitic cyst of retina, right eye
    - CC H33.122 Parasitic cyst of retina, left eye
    - CC H33.123 Parasitic cyst of retina, bilateral
    - CC H33.129 Parasitic cyst of retina, unspecified eye
  - **H33.19** Other retinoschisis and retinal cysts
    Pseudocyst of retina
    - H33.191 Other retinoschisis and retinal cysts, right eye
    - H33.192 Other retinoschisis and retinal cysts, left eye
    - H33.193 Other retinoschisis and retinal cysts, bilateral
    - H33.199 Other retinoschisis and retinal cysts, unspecified eye
- **H33.2** Serous retinal detachment
  Retinal detachment NOS
  Retinal detachment without retinal break
  Excludes1: central serous chorioretinopathy (H35.71-)
  - CC H33.20 Serous retinal detachment, unspecified eye
  - CC H33.21 Serous retinal detachment, right eye
  - CC H33.22 Serous retinal detachment, left eye
  - CC H33.23 Serous retinal detachment, bilateral
- **H33.3** Retinal breaks without detachment
  Excludes1: chorioretinal scars after surgery for detachment (H59.81-)
  peripheral retinal degeneration without break (H35.4-)
  - **H33.30** Unspecified retinal break
    - H33.301 Unspecified retinal break, right eye
    - H33.302 Unspecified retinal break, left eye
    - H33.303 Unspecified retinal break, bilateral
    - H33.309 Unspecified retinal break, unspecified eye
  - **H33.31** Horseshoe tear of retina without detachment
    Operculum of retina without detachment
    - H33.311 Horseshoe tear of retina without detachment, right eye
    - H33.312 Horseshoe tear of retina without detachment, left eye
    - H33.313 Horseshoe tear of retina without detachment, bilateral
    - H33.319 Horseshoe tear of retina without detachment, unspecified eye
  - **H33.32** Round hole of retina without detachment
    - H33.321 Round hole, right eye
    - H33.322 Round hole, left eye
    - H33.323 Round hole, bilateral
    - H33.329 Round hole, unspecified eye
  - **H33.33** Multiple defects of retina without detachment
    - H33.331 Multiple defects of retina without detachment, right eye
    - H33.332 Multiple defects of retina without detachment, left eye
    - H33.333 Multiple defects of retina without detachment, bilateral
    - H33.339 Multiple defects of retina without detachment, unspecified eye
- **H33.4** Traction detachment of retina
  Proliferative vitreo-retinopathy with retinal detachment
  - CC H33.40 Traction detachment of retina, unspecified eye
  - CC H33.41 Traction detachment of retina, right eye
  - CC H33.42 Traction detachment of retina, left eye
  - CC H33.43 Traction detachment of retina, bilateral
- CC **H33.8** Other retinal detachments

H34 Retinal vascular occlusions

Excludes1: *amaurosis fugax (G45.3)*

- **H34.0 Transient retinal artery occlusion**
  - CC **H34.00** Transient retinal artery occlusion, unspecified eye
  - CC **H34.01** Transient retinal artery occlusion, right eye
  - CC **H34.02** Transient retinal artery occlusion, left eye
  - CC **H34.03** Transient retinal artery occlusion, bilateral
- **H34.1 Central retinal artery occlusion**
  - CC **H34.10** Central retinal artery occlusion, unspecified eye
  - CC **H34.11** Central retinal artery occlusion, right eye
  - CC **H34.12** Central retinal artery occlusion, left eye
  - CC **H34.13** Central retinal artery occlusion, bilateral
- **H34.2 Other retinal artery occlusions**
  - **H34.21 Partial retinal artery occlusion**
    - Hollenhorst's plaque
    - Retinal microembolism
    - CC **H34.211** Partial retinal artery occlusion, right eye
    - CC **H34.212** Partial retinal artery occlusion, left eye
    - CC **H34.213** Partial retinal artery occlusion, bilateral
    - CC **H34.219** Partial retinal artery occlusion, unspecified eye
  - **H34.23 Retinal artery branch occlusion**
    - CC **H34.231** Retinal artery branch occlusion, right eye
    - CC **H34.232** Retinal artery branch occlusion, left eye
    - CC **H34.233** Retinal artery branch occlusion, bilateral
    - CC **H34.239** Retinal artery branch occlusion, unspecified eye
- **H34.8 Other retinal vascular occlusions**
  - *AHA CC: 4Q, 2016, 19*
  - **H34.81 Central retinal vein occlusion**

    > One of the following 7th characters is to be assigned to codes in subcategory **H34.81** to designate the severity of the occlusion:
    > 0   with macular edema
    > 1   with retinal neovascularization
    > 2   stable
    >   Old central retinal vein occlusion

    - +7th CC **H34.811** Central retinal vein occlusion, right eye
    - +7th CC **H34.812** Central retinal vein occlusion, left eye
    - +7th CC **H34.813** Central retinal vein occlusion, bilateral
    - +7th CC **H34.819** Central retinal vein occlusion, unspecified eye
  - **H34.82 Venous engorgement**
    - Incipient retinal vein occlusion
    - Partial retinal vein occlusion
    - **H34.821** Venous engorgement, right eye
    - **H34.822** Venous engorgement, left eye
    - **H34.823** Venous engorgement, bilateral
    - **H34.829** Venous engorgement, unspecified eye
  - **H34.83 Tributary (branch) retinal vein occlusion**

    > One of the following 7th characters is to be assigned to codes in subcategory **H34.83** to designate the severity of the occlusion:
    > 0   with macular edema
    > 1   with retinal neovascularization
    > 2   stable
    >   Old central retinal vein occlusion

    - +7th **H34.831** Tributary (branch) retinal vein occlusion, right eye
    - +7th **H34.832** Tributary (branch) retinal vein occlusion, left eye
    - +7th **H34.833** Tributary (branch) retinal vein occlusion, bilateral
    - +7th **H34.839** Tributary (branch) retinal vein occlusion, unspecified eye
- CC **H34.9** Unspecified retinal vascular occlusion

H35 Other retinal disorders

Excludes2: *diabetic retinal disorders (E08.311-E08.359, E09.311-E09.359, E10.311-E10.359, E11.311-E11.359, E13.311-E13.359)*

- **H35.0 Background retinopathy and retinal vascular changes**
  - *Review coding guideline C.9.a.5*
  - Code also any associated hypertension (I10)
  - **H35.00** Unspecified background retinopathy
  - **H35.01 Changes in retinal vascular appearance**
    - Retinal vascular sheathing
    - **H35.011** Changes in retinal vascular appearance, right eye
    - **H35.012** Changes in retinal vascular appearance, left eye
    - **H35.013** Changes in retinal vascular appearance, bilateral
    - **H35.019** Changes in retinal vascular appearance, unspecified eye
  - **H35.02 Exudative retinopathy**
    - Coats retinopathy
    - **H35.021** Exudative retinopathy, right eye
    - **H35.022** Exudative retinopathy, left eye
    - **H35.023** Exudative retinopathy, bilateral
    - **H35.029** Exudative retinopathy, unspecified eye
  - **H35.03 Hypertensive retinopathy**
    - **H35.031** Hypertensive retinopathy, right eye
    - **H35.032** Hypertensive retinopathy, left eye
    - **H35.033** Hypertensive retinopathy, bilateral
    - **H35.039** Hypertensive retinopathy, unspecified eye
  - **H35.04 Retinal micro-aneurysms, unspecified**
    - **H35.041** Retinal micro-aneurysms, unspecified, right eye
    - **H35.042** Retinal micro-aneurysms, unspecified, left eye
    - **H35.043** Retinal micro-aneurysms, unspecified, bilateral
    - **H35.049** Retinal micro-aneurysms, unspecified, unspecified eye
  - **H35.05 Retinal neovascularization, unspecified**
    - **H35.051** Retinal neovascularization, unspecified, right eye
    - **H35.052** Retinal neovascularization, unspecified, left eye
    - **H35.053** Retinal neovascularization, unspecified, bilateral
    - **H35.059** Retinal neovascularization, unspecified, unspecified eye
  - **H35.06 Retinal vasculitis**
    - Eales disease
    - Retinal perivasculitis
    - **H35.061** Retinal vasculitis, right eye
    - **H35.062** Retinal vasculitis, left eye
    - **H35.063** Retinal vasculitis, bilateral
    - **H35.069** Retinal vasculitis, unspecified eye
  - **H35.07 Retinal telangiectasis**
    - **H35.071** Retinal telangiectasis, right eye
    - **H35.072** Retinal telangiectasis, left eye
    - **H35.073** Retinal telangiectasis, bilateral
    - **H35.079** Retinal telangiectasis, unspecified eye
  - **H35.09** Other intraretinal microvascular abnormalities
    - Retinal varices
- **H35.1 Retinopathy of prematurity**
  - **H35.10 Retinopathy of prematurity, unspecified**
    - Retinopathy of prematurity NOS

H35.101 Retinopathy of prematurity, unspecified, right eye
H35.102 Retinopathy of prematurity, unspecified, left eye
H35.103 Retinopathy of prematurity, unspecified, bilateral
H35.109 Retinopathy of prematurity, unspecified, unspecified eye
+ H35.11 **Retinopathy of prematurity, stage 0**
H35.111 Retinopathy of prematurity, stage 0, right eye
H35.112 Retinopathy of prematurity, stage 0, left eye
H35.113 Retinopathy of prematurity, stage 0, bilateral
H35.119 Retinopathy of prematurity, stage 0, unspecified eye
+ H35.12 **Retinopathy of prematurity, stage 1**
H35.121 Retinopathy of prematurity, stage 1, right eye
H35.122 Retinopathy of prematurity, stage 1, left eye
H35.123 Retinopathy of prematurity, stage 1, bilateral
H35.129 Retinopathy of prematurity, stage 1, unspecified eye
+ H35.13 **Retinopathy of prematurity, stage 2**
H35.131 Retinopathy of prematurity, stage 2, right eye
H35.132 Retinopathy of prematurity, stage 2, left eye
H35.133 Retinopathy of prematurity, stage 2, bilateral
H35.139 Retinopathy of prematurity, stage 2, unspecified eye
+ H35.14 **Retinopathy of prematurity, stage 3**
H35.141 Retinopathy of prematurity, stage 3, right eye
H35.142 Retinopathy of prematurity, stage 3, left eye
H35.143 Retinopathy of prematurity, stage 3, bilateral
H35.149 Retinopathy of prematurity, stage 3, unspecified eye
+ H35.15 **Retinopathy of prematurity, stage 4**
H35.151 Retinopathy of prematurity, stage 4, right eye
H35.152 Retinopathy of prematurity, stage 4, left eye
H35.153 Retinopathy of prematurity, stage 4, bilateral
H35.159 Retinopathy of prematurity, stage 4, unspecified eye
+ H35.16 **Retinopathy of prematurity, stage 5**
H35.161 Retinopathy of prematurity, stage 5, right eye
H35.162 Retinopathy of prematurity, stage 5, left eye
H35.163 Retinopathy of prematurity, stage 5, bilateral
H35.169 Retinopathy of prematurity, stage 5, unspecified eye
+ H35.17 **Retrolental fibroplasia**
H35.171 Retrolental fibroplasia, right eye
H35.172 Retrolental fibroplasia, left eye
H35.173 Retrolental fibroplasia, bilateral
H35.179 Retrolental fibroplasia, unspecified eye
+ H35.2 **Other non-diabetic proliferative retinopathy**
Proliferative vitreo-retinopathy
Thalassemia proliferative retinopathy
Excludes1: proliferative vitreo-retinopathy with retinal detachment (H33.4-)
Excludes2: proliferative sickle-cell retinopathy (H36.82-)

H35.20 Other non-diabetic proliferative retinopathy, unspecified eye
H35.21 Other non-diabetic proliferative retinopathy, right eye
H35.22 Other non-diabetic proliferative retinopathy, left eye
H35.23 Other non-diabetic proliferative retinopathy, bilateral
+ H35.3 **Degeneration of macula and posterior pole**
AHA CC: 4Q, 2016, 20-21
• H35.30 **Unspecified macular degeneration**
Age-related macular degeneration
+ H35.31 **Nonexudative age-related macular degeneration**
Atrophic age-related macular degeneration
Dry age-related macular degeneration

> One of the following 7th characters is to be assigned to codes in subcategory **H35.31** to designate the stage of the disease:
> 0 stage unspecified
> 1 early dry stage
> 2 intermediate dry stage
> 3 advanced atrophic without subfoveal involvement advanced dry stage
> 4 advanced atrophic with sobfoveal involvement

• +7th H35.311 Nonexudative age-related macular degeneration, right eye
AHA CC: 4Q, 2016, 21
• +7th H35.312 Nonexudative age-related macular degeneration, left eye
AHA CC: 4Q, 2016, 21
• +7th H35.313 Nonexudative age-related macular degeneration, bilateral
• +7th H35.319 Nonexudative age-related macular degeneration, unspecified eye
+ H35.32 **Exudative age-related macular degeneration**
Wet age-related macular degeneration

> One of the following 7th characters is to be assigned to codes in subcategory **H35.32** to designate the stage of the disease:
> 0 stage unspecified
> 1 with active choroidal neovascularization
> 2 with inactive choroidal neovascularization with involuted or regressed neovascularization
> 3 with inactive scar

• +7th H35.321 Exudative age-related macular degeneration, right eye
• +7th H35.322 Exudative age-related macular degeneration, left eye
• +7th H35.323 Exudative age-related macular degeneration, bilateral
• +7th H35.329 Exudative age-related macular degeneration, unspecified eye
H35.33 Angioid streaks of macula
+ H35.34 **Macular cyst, hole, or pseudohole**
H35.341 Macular cyst, hole, or pseudohole, right eye
H35.342 Macular cyst, hole, or pseudohole, left eye
H35.343 Macular cyst, hole, or pseudohole, bilateral
H35.349 Macular cyst, hole, or pseudohole, unspecified eye
+ H35.35 **Cystoid macular degeneration**
Excludes1: *cystoid macular edema following cataract surgery (H59.03-)*
H35.351 Cystoid macular degeneration, right eye
H35.352 Cystoid macular degeneration, left eye
H35.353 Cystoid macular degeneration, bilateral
H35.359 Cystoid macular degeneration, unspecified eye

- **+ H35.36 Drusen (degenerative) of macula**
  - H35.361 Drusen (degenerative) of macula, right eye
  - H35.362 Drusen (degenerative) of macula, left eye
    - *AHA CC: 4Q, 2016, 21*
  - H35.363 Drusen (degenerative) of macula, bilateral
    - *AHA CC: 4Q, 2016, 21; 1Q, 2017, 51*
  - H35.369 Drusen (degenerative) of macula, unspecified eye
- **+ H35.37 Puckering of macula**
  - H35.371 Puckering of macula, right eye
  - H35.372 Puckering of macula, left eye
  - H35.373 Puckering of macula, bilateral
  - H35.379 Puckering of macula, unspecified eye
- **+ H35.38 Toxic maculopathy**
  - Code first poisoning due to drug or toxin, if applicable (T36-T65 with fifth or sixth character 1-4)
  - Use additional code for adverse effect, if applicable, to identify drug (T36-T50 with fifth or sixth character 5)
  - H35.381 Toxic maculopathy, right eye
  - H35.382 Toxic maculopathy, left eye
  - H35.383 Toxic maculopathy, bilateral
  - H35.389 Toxic maculopathy, unspecified eye
- **+ H35.4 Peripheral retinal degeneration**
  - **Excludes1:** hereditary retinal degeneration (dystrophy) (H35.5-)
    - peripheral retinal degeneration with retinal break (H33.3-)
  - H35.40 Unspecified peripheral retinal degeneration
  - **+ H35.41 Lattice degeneration of retina**
    - Palisade degeneration of retina
    - H35.411 Lattice degeneration of retina, right eye
    - H35.412 Lattice degeneration of retina, left eye
    - H35.413 Lattice degeneration of retina, bilateral
    - H35.419 Lattice degeneration of retina, unspecified eye
  - **+ H35.42 Microcystoid degeneration of retina**
    - H35.421 Microcystoid degeneration of retina, right eye
    - H35.422 Microcystoid degeneration of retina, left eye
    - H35.423 Microcystoid degeneration of retina, bilateral
    - H35.429 Microcystoid degeneration of retina, unspecified eye
  - **+ H35.43 Paving stone degeneration of retina**
    - H35.431 Paving stone degeneration of retina, right eye
    - H35.432 Paving stone degeneration of retina, left eye
    - H35.433 Paving stone degeneration of retina, bilateral
    - H35.439 Paving stone degeneration of retina, unspecified eye
  - **+ H35.44 Age-related reticular degeneration of retina**
    - • H35.441 Age-related reticular degeneration of retina, right eye
    - • H35.442 Age-related reticular degeneration of retina, left eye
    - • H35.443 Age-related reticular degeneration of retina, bilateral
    - • H35.449 Age-related reticular degeneration of retina, unspecified eye
  - **+ H35.45 Secondary pigmentary degeneration**
    - H35.451 Secondary pigmentary degeneration, right eye
    - H35.452 Secondary pigmentary degeneration, left eye
    - H35.453 Secondary pigmentary degeneration, bilateral
    - H35.459 Secondary pigmentary degeneration, unspecified eye
- **+ H35.46 Secondary vitreoretinal degeneration**
  - H35.461 Secondary vitreoretinal degeneration, right eye
  - H35.462 Secondary vitreoretinal degeneration, left eye
  - H35.463 Secondary vitreoretinal degeneration, bilateral
  - H35.469 Secondary vitreoretinal degeneration, unspecified eye
- **+ H35.5 Hereditary retinal dystrophy**
  - **Excludes1:** dystrophies primarily involving Bruch's membrane (H31.1-)
  - H35.50 Unspecified hereditary retinal dystrophy
  - H35.51 Vitreoretinal dystrophy
  - H35.52 Pigmentary retinal dystrophy
    - Albipunctate retinal dystrophy
    - Retinitis pigmentosa
    - Tapetoretinal dystrophy
  - H35.53 Other dystrophies primarily involving the sensory retina
    - Stargardt's disease
  - H35.54 Dystrophies primarily involving the retinal pigment epithelium
    - Vitelliform retinal dystrophy
- **+ H35.6 Retinal hemorrhage**
  - H35.60 Retinal hemorrhage, unspecified eye
  - H35.61 Retinal hemorrhage, right eye
  - H35.62 Retinal hemorrhage, left eye
  - H35.63 Retinal hemorrhage, bilateral
- **+ H35.7 Separation of retinal layers**
  - **Excludes1:** retinal detachment (serous) (H33.2-)
    - rhegmatogenous retinal detachment (H33.0-)
  - CC H35.70 Unspecified separation of retinal layers
  - **+ H35.71 Central serous chorioretinopathy**
    - H35.711 Central serous chorioretinopathy, right eye
    - H35.712 Central serous chorioretinopathy, left eye
    - H35.713 Central serous chorioretinopathy, bilateral
    - H35.719 Central serous chorioretinopathy, unspecified eye
  - **+ H35.72 Serous detachment of retinal pigment epithelium**
    - CC H35.721 Serous detachment of retinal pigment epithelium, right eye
    - CC H35.722 Serous detachment of retinal pigment epithelium, left eye
    - CC H35.723 Serous detachment of retinal pigment epithelium, bilateral
    - CC H35.729 Serous detachment of retinal pigment epithelium, unspecified eye
  - **+ H35.73 Hemorrhagic detachment of retinal pigment epithelium**
    - CC H35.731 Hemorrhagic detachment of retinal pigment epithelium, right eye
    - CC H35.732 Hemorrhagic detachment of retinal pigment epithelium, left eye
    - CC H35.733 Hemorrhagic detachment of retinal pigment epithelium, bilateral
    - CC H35.739 Hemorrhagic detachment of retinal pigment epithelium, unspecified eye
- **+ H35.8 Other specified retinal disorders**
  - **Excludes2:** retinal hemorrhage (H35.6-)
  - H35.81 Retinal edema
    - Retinal cotton wool spots
  - CC H35.82 Retinal ischemia
  - H35.89 Other specified retinal disorders
- H35.9 Unspecified retinal disorder

H36 Retinal disorders in diseases classified elsewhere

Code first underlying disease, such as:
- lipid storage disorders (E75.-)
- sickle-cell disorders (D57.-)

Excludes1: arteriosclerotic retinopathy (H35.0-)
- diabetic retinopathy (E08.3-, E09.3-, E10.3-, E11.3-, E13.3-)

- **H36.8** Other retinal disorders in diseases classified elsewhere
  - **H36.81** Nonproliferative sickle-cell retinopathy
    - **H36.811** Nonproliferative sickle-cell retinopathy, right eye
    - **H36.812** Nonproliferative sickle-cell retinopathy, left eye
    - **H36.813** Nonproliferative sickle-cell retinopathy, bilateral
    - **H36.819** Nonproliferative sickle-cell retinopathy, unspecified eye
  - **H36.82** Proliferative sickle-cell retinopathy
    - **H36.821** Proliferative sickle-cell retinopathy, right eye
    - **H36.822** Proliferative sickle-cell retinopathy, left eye
    - **H36.823** Proliferative sickle-cell retinopathy, bilateral
    - **H36.829** Proliferative sickle-cell retinopathy, unspecified eye
  - **H36.89** Other retinal disorders in diseases classified elsewhere
    - Retinal dystrophy in lipid storage disorders

Glaucoma (H40-H42)

H40 Glaucoma

Excludes1: absolute glaucoma (H44.51-)
congenital glaucoma (Q15.0)
traumatic glaucoma due to birth injury (P15.3)

Review coding guideline C.7.a

- **H40.0** Glaucoma suspect
  - **H40.00** Preglaucoma, unspecified
    - **H40.001** Preglaucoma, unspecified, right eye
    - **H40.002** Preglaucoma, unspecified, left eye
    - **H40.003** Preglaucoma, unspecified, bilateral
    - **H40.009** Preglaucoma, unspecified, unspecified eye
  - **H40.01** Open angle with borderline findings, low risk
    - Open angle, low risk
    - **H40.011** Open angle with borderline findings, low risk, right eye
    - **H40.012** Open angle with borderline findings, low risk, left eye
    - **H40.013** Open angle with borderline findings, low risk, bilateral
    - **H40.019** Open angle with borderline findings, low risk, unspecified eye
  - **H40.02** Open angle with borderline findings, high risk
    - Open angle, high risk
    - **H40.021** Open angle with borderline findings, high risk, right eye
    - **H40.022** Open angle with borderline findings, high risk, left eye
    - **H40.023** Open angle with borderline findings, high risk, bilateral
    - **H40.029** Open angle with borderline findings, high risk, unspecified eye
  - **H40.03** Anatomical narrow angle
    - Primary angle closure suspect
    - **H40.031** Anatomical narrow angle, right eye
    - **H40.032** Anatomical narrow angle, left eye
    - **H40.033** Anatomical narrow angle, bilateral
    - **H40.039** Anatomical narrow angle, unspecified eye
  - **H40.04** Steroid responder
    - **H40.041** Steroid responder, right eye
    - **H40.042** Steroid responder, left eye
    - **H40.043** Steroid responder, bilateral
    - **H40.049** Steroid responder, unspecified eye
  - **H40.05** Ocular hypertension
    - **H40.051** Ocular hypertension, right eye
    - **H40.052** Ocular hypertension, left eye
    - **H40.053** Ocular hypertension, bilateral
    - **H40.059** Ocular hypertension, unspecified eye
  - **H40.06** Primary angle closure without glaucoma damage
    - **H40.061** Primary angle closure without glaucoma damage, right eye
    - **H40.062** Primary angle closure without glaucoma damage, left eye
    - **H40.063** Primary angle closure without glaucoma damage, bilateral
    - **H40.069** Primary angle closure without glaucoma damage, unspecified eye
- **H40.1** Open-angle glaucoma
  - AHA CC: 4Q, 2016, 22
  - **H40.10** Unspecified open-angle glaucoma
    - One of the following 7th characters is to be assigned to code **H40.10** to designate the stage of glaucoma
      - 0 stage unspecified
      - 1 mild stage
      - 2 moderate stage
      - 3 severe stage
      - 4 indeterminate stage
  - **H40.11** Primary open-angle glaucoma
    - Chronic simple glaucoma
    - One of the following 7th characters is to be assigned to each code in subcategory **H40.11** to designate the stage of glaucoma
      - 0 stage unspecified
      - 1 mild stage
      - 2 moderate stage
      - 3 severe stage
      - 4 indeterminate stage
    - **H40.111** Primary open-angle glaucoma, right eye
      - AHA CC: 2Q, 2019, 31
    - **H40.112** Primary open-angle glaucoma, left eye
    - **H40.113** Primary open-angle glaucoma, bilateral
    - **H40.119** Primary open-angle glaucoma, unspecified eye
  - **H40.12** Low-tension glaucoma
    - One of the following 7th characters is to be assigned to each code in subcategory **H40.12** to designate the stage of glaucoma
      - 0 stage unspecified
      - 1 mild stage
      - 2 moderate stage
      - 3 severe stage
      - 4 indeterminate stage
    - **H40.121** Low-tension glaucoma, right eye
    - **H40.122** Low-tension glaucoma, left eye
    - **H40.123** Low-tension glaucoma, bilateral
    - **H40.129** Low-tension glaucoma, unspecified eye
  - **H40.13** Pigmentary glaucoma
    - One of the following 7th characters is to be assigned to each code in subcategory **H40.13** to designate the stage of glaucoma
      - 0 stage unspecified
      - 1 mild stage
      - 2 moderate stage
      - 3 severe stage
      - 4 indeterminate stage
    - **H40.131** Pigmentary glaucoma, right eye
    - **H40.132** Pigmentary glaucoma, left eye
    - **H40.133** Pigmentary glaucoma, bilateral
    - **H40.139** Pigmentary glaucoma, unspecified eye
  - **H40.14** Capsular glaucoma with pseudoexfoliation of lens
    - One of the following 7th characters is to be assigned to each code in subcategory **H40.14** to designate the stage of glaucoma
      - 0 stage unspecified
      - 1 mild stage
      - 2 moderate stage
      - 3 severe stage
      - 4 indeterminate stage
    - **H40.141** Capsular glaucoma with pseudoexfoliation of lens, right eye
    - **H40.142** Capsular glaucoma with pseudoexfoliation of lens, left eye
    - **H40.143** Capsular glaucoma with pseudoexfoliation of lens, bilateral
    - **H40.149** Capsular glaucoma with pseudoexfoliation of lens, unspecified eye

- **H40.15** Residual stage of open-angle glaucoma
  - **H40.151** Residual stage of open-angle glaucoma, right eye
  - **H40.152** Residual stage of open-angle glaucoma, left eye
  - **H40.153** Residual stage of open-angle glaucoma, bilateral
  - **H40.159** Residual stage of open-angle glaucoma, unspecified eye
- **H40.2** Primary angle-closure glaucoma
  - *Excludes1:* aqueous misdirection (H40.83-)
  - malignant glaucoma (H40.83-)
  - **H40.20** Unspecified primary angle-closure glaucoma [X+7th]

    One of the following 7th characters is to be assigned to code **H40.20** to designate the stage of glaucoma
    - 0 stage unspecified
    - 1 mild stage
    - 2 moderate stage
    - 3 severe stage
    - 4 indeterminate stage

  - **H40.21** Acute angle-closure glaucoma
    - Acute angle-closure glaucoma attack
    - Acute angle-closure glaucoma crisis
    - **H40.211** Acute angle-closure glaucoma, right eye [CC]
    - **H40.212** Acute angle-closure glaucoma, left eye [CC]
    - **H40.213** Acute angle-closure glaucoma, bilateral [CC]
    - **H40.219** Acute angle-closure glaucoma, unspecified eye [CC]
  - **H40.22** Chronic angle-closure glaucoma
    - Chronic primary angle closure glaucoma

    One of the following 7th characters is to be assigned to each code in subcategory **H40.22** to designate the stage of glaucoma
    - 0 stage unspecified
    - 1 mild stage
    - 2 moderate stage
    - 3 severe stage
    - 4 indeterminate stage

    - **H40.221** Chronic angle-closure glaucoma, right eye [+7th]
    - **H40.222** Chronic angle-closure glaucoma, left eye [+7th]
    - **H40.223** Chronic angle-closure glaucoma, bilateral [+7th]
    - **H40.229** Chronic angle-closure glaucoma, unspecified eye [+7th]
  - **H40.23** Intermittent angle-closure glaucoma
    - **H40.231** Intermittent angle-closure glaucoma, right eye
    - **H40.232** Intermittent angle-closure glaucoma, left eye
    - **H40.233** Intermittent angle-closure glaucoma, bilateral
    - **H40.239** Intermittent angle-closure glaucoma, unspecified eye
  - **H40.24** Residual stage of angle-closure glaucoma
    - **H40.241** Residual stage of angle-closure glaucoma, right eye
    - **H40.242** Residual stage of angle-closure glaucoma, left eye
    - **H40.243** Residual stage of angle-closure glaucoma, bilateral
    - **H40.249** Residual stage of angle-closure glaucoma, unspecified eye
- **H40.3** Glaucoma secondary to eye trauma
  - Code also underlying condition

  One of the following 7th characters is to be assigned to each code in subcategory **H40.3** to designate the stage of glaucoma
  - 0 stage unspecified
  - 1 mild stage
  - 2 moderate stage
  - 3 severe stage
  - 4 indeterminate stage

  - **H40.30** Glaucoma secondary to eye trauma, unspecified eye [X+7th]
  - **H40.31** Glaucoma secondary to eye trauma, right eye [X+7th]
  - **H40.32** Glaucoma secondary to eye trauma, left eye [X+7th]
  - **H40.33** Glaucoma secondary to eye trauma, bilateral [X+7th]
- **H40.4** Glaucoma secondary to eye inflammation
  - Code also underlying condition

  One of the following 7th characters is to be assigned to each code in subcategory **H40.4** to designate the stage of glaucoma
  - 0 stage unspecified
  - 1 mild stage
  - 2 moderate stage
  - 3 severe stage
  - 4 indeterminate stage

  - **H40.40** Glaucoma secondary to eye inflammation, unspecified eye [X+7th]
  - **H40.41** Glaucoma secondary to eye inflammation, right eye [X+7th]
  - **H40.42** Glaucoma secondary to eye inflammation, left eye [X+7th]
  - **H40.43** Glaucoma secondary to eye inflammation, bilateral [X+7th]
- **H40.5** Glaucoma secondary to other eye disorders
  - Code also underlying eye disorder

  One of the following 7th characters is to be assigned to each code in subcategory **H40.5** to designate the stage of glaucoma
  - 0 stage unspecified
  - 1 mild stage
  - 2 moderate stage
  - 3 severe stage
  - 4 indeterminate stage

  - **H40.50** Glaucoma secondary to other eye disorders, unspecified eye [X+7th]
  - **H40.51** Glaucoma secondary to other eye disorders, right eye [X+7th]
  - **H40.52** Glaucoma secondary to other eye disorders, left eye [X+7th]
  - **H40.53** Glaucoma secondary to other eye disorders, bilateral [X+7th]
- **H40.6** Glaucoma secondary to drugs
  - Use additional code for adverse effect, if applicable, to identify drug (T36-T50 with fifth or sixth character 5)

  One of the following 7th characters is to be assigned to each code in subcategory **H40.6** to designate the stage of glaucoma
  - 0 stage unspecified
  - 1 mild stage
  - 2 moderate stage
  - 3 severe stage
  - 4 indeterminate stage

  - **H40.60** Glaucoma secondary to drugs, unspecified eye [X+7th]
  - **H40.61** Glaucoma secondary to drugs, right eye [X+7th]
  - **H40.62** Glaucoma secondary to drugs, left eye [X+7th]
  - **H40.63** Glaucoma secondary to drugs, bilateral [X+7th]
- **H40.8** Other glaucoma
  - **H40.81** Glaucoma with increased episcleral venous pressure
    - **H40.811** Glaucoma with increased episcleral venous pressure, right eye
    - **H40.812** Glaucoma with increased episcleral venous pressure, left eye
    - **H40.813** Glaucoma with increased episcleral venous pressure, bilateral
    - **H40.819** Glaucoma with increased episcleral venous pressure, unspecified eye
  - **H40.82** Hypersecretion glaucoma
    - **H40.821** Hypersecretion glaucoma, right eye
    - **H40.822** Hypersecretion glaucoma, left eye
    - **H40.823** Hypersecretion glaucoma, bilateral
    - **H40.829** Hypersecretion glaucoma, unspecified eye
  - **H40.83** Aqueous misdirection
    - Malignant glaucoma
    - **H40.831** Aqueous misdirection, right eye
    - **H40.832** Aqueous misdirection, left eye
    - **H40.833** Aqueous misdirection, bilateral
    - **H40.839** Aqueous misdirection, unspecified eye
  - **H40.89** Other specified glaucoma
- **H40.9** Unspecified glaucoma

H42 Glaucoma in diseases classified elsewhere

Code first underlying condition, such as:
- amyloidosis (E85.-)
- aniridia (Q13.1)
- glaucoma (in) diabetes mellitus (E08.39, E09.39, E10.39, E11.39, E13.39)
- Lowe's syndrome (E72.03)
- Reiger's anomaly (Q13.81)
- specified metabolic disorder (E70-E88)

Excludes1: *glaucoma (in) onchocerciasis (B73.02)*
glaucoma (in) syphilis (A52.71)
glaucoma (in) tuberculous (A18.59)
Valid 3-character code, no further characters required

Disorders of vitreous body and globe (H43-H44)

H43 Disorders of vitreous body
- **H43.0** Vitreous prolapse
  - **Excludes1:** *vitreous syndrome following cataract surgery (H59.0-)*
  - *traumatic vitreous prolapse (S05.2-)*
  - H43.00 Vitreous prolapse, unspecified eye
  - H43.01 Vitreous prolapse, right eye
  - H43.02 Vitreous prolapse, left eye
  - H43.03 Vitreous prolapse, bilateral
- **H43.1** Vitreous hemorrhage
  - H43.10 Vitreous hemorrhage, unspecified eye
  - H43.11 Vitreous hemorrhage, right eye
  - H43.12 Vitreous hemorrhage, left eye
  - H43.13 Vitreous hemorrhage, bilateral
- **H43.2** Crystalline deposits in vitreous body
  - H43.20 Crystalline deposits in vitreous body, unspecified eye
  - H43.21 Crystalline deposits in vitreous body, right eye
  - H43.22 Crystalline deposits in vitreous body, left eye
  - H43.23 Crystalline deposits in vitreous body, bilateral
- **H43.3** Other vitreous opacities
  - **H43.31** Vitreous membranes and strands
    - H43.311 Vitreous membranes and strands, right eye
    - H43.312 Vitreous membranes and strands, left eye
    - H43.313 Vitreous membranes and strands, bilateral
    - H43.319 Vitreous membranes and strands, unspecified eye
  - **H43.39** Other vitreous opacities
    - Vitreous floaters
    - H43.391 Other vitreous opacities, right eye
    - H43.392 Other vitreous opacities, left eye
    - H43.393 Other vitreous opacities, bilateral
    - H43.399 Other vitreous opacities, unspecified eye
- **H43.8** Other disorders of vitreous body
  - **Excludes1:** *proliferative vitreo-retinopathy with retinal detachment (H33.4-)*
  - **Excludes2:** *vitreous abscess (H44.02-)*
  - **H43.81** Vitreous degeneration
    - Vitreous detachment
    - H43.811 Vitreous degeneration, right eye
    - H43.812 Vitreous degeneration, left eye
    - H43.813 Vitreous degeneration, bilateral
    - H43.819 Vitreous degeneration, unspecified eye
  - **H43.82** Vitreomacular adhesion
    - Vitreomacular traction
    - H43.821 Vitreomacular adhesion, right eye
    - H43.822 Vitreomacular adhesion, left eye
    - H43.823 Vitreomacular adhesion, bilateral
    - H43.829 Vitreomacular adhesion, unspecified eye
  - H43.89 Other disorders of vitreous body
- **H43.9** Unspecified disorder of vitreous body

H44 Disorders of globe
Includes: disorders affecting multiple structures of eye
- **H44.0** Purulent endophthalmitis
  - Use additional code to identify organism
  - **Excludes1:** *bleb associated endophthalmitis (H59.4-)*
  - **H44.00** Unspecified purulent endophthalmitis
    - CC H44.001 Unspecified purulent endophthalmitis, right eye
    - CC H44.002 Unspecified purulent endophthalmitis, left eye
    - CC H44.003 Unspecified purulent endophthalmitis, bilateral
    - CC H44.009 Unspecified purulent endophthalmitis, unspecified eye
  - **H44.01** Panophthalmitis (acute)
    - CC H44.011 Panophthalmitis (acute), right eye
    - CC H44.012 Panophthalmitis (acute), left eye
    - CC H44.013 Panophthalmitis (acute), bilateral
    - CC H44.019 Panophthalmitis (acute), unspecified eye
  - **H44.02** Vitreous abscess (chronic)
    - CC H44.021 Vitreous abscess (chronic), right eye
    - CC H44.022 Vitreous abscess (chronic), left eye
    - CC H44.023 Vitreous abscess (chronic), bilateral
    - CC H44.029 Vitreous abscess (chronic), unspecified eye
- **H44.1** Other endophthalmitis
  - **Excludes1:** *bleb associated endophthalmitis (H59.4-)*
  - **Excludes2:** *ophthalmia nodosa (H16.2-)*
  - **H44.11** Panuveitis
    - CC H44.111 Panuveitis, right eye
    - CC H44.112 Panuveitis, left eye
    - CC H44.113 Panuveitis, bilateral
    - CC H44.119 Panuveitis, unspecified eye
  - **H44.12** Parasitic endophthalmitis, unspecified
    - CC H44.121 Parasitic endophthalmitis, unspecified, right eye
    - CC H44.122 Parasitic endophthalmitis, unspecified, left eye
    - CC H44.123 Parasitic endophthalmitis, unspecified, bilateral
    - CC H44.129 Parasitic endophthalmitis, unspecified, unspecified eye
  - **H44.13** Sympathetic uveitis
    - CC H44.131 Sympathetic uveitis, right eye
    - CC H44.132 Sympathetic uveitis, left eye
    - CC H44.133 Sympathetic uveitis, bilateral
    - CC H44.139 Sympathetic uveitis, unspecified eye
  - CC H44.19 Other endophthalmitis
- **H44.2** Degenerative myopia
  - Malignant myopia
  - *AHA CC: 4Q, 2017, 10-11*
  - H44.20 Degenerative myopia, unspecified eye
  - H44.21 Degenerative myopia, right eye
  - H44.22 Degenerative myopia, left eye
  - H44.23 Degenerative myopia, bilateral
  - **H44.2A** Degenerative myopia with choroidal neovascularization
    - Use additional code for any associated choroid disorders (H31.-)
    - H44.2A1 Degenerative myopia with choroidal neovascularization, right eye
    - H44.2A2 Degenerative myopia with choroidal neovascularization, left eye
    - H44.2A3 Degenerative myopia with choroidal neovascularization, bilateral eye
    - H44.2A9 Degenerative myopia with choroidal neovascularization, unspecified eye
  - **H44.2B** Degenerative myopia with macular hole
    - H44.2B1 Degenerative myopia with macular hole, right eye
    - H44.2B2 Degenerative myopia with macular hole, left eye
    - H44.2B3 Degenerative myopia with macular hole, bilateral eye
    - H44.2B9 Degenerative myopia with macular hole, unspecified eye
  - **H44.2C** Degenerative myopia with retinal detachment
    - Use additional code to identify the retinal detachment (H33.-)
    - H44.2C1 Degenerative myopia with retinal detachment, right eye
    - H44.2C2 Degenerative myopia with retinal detachment, left eye
    - H44.2C3 Degenerative myopia with retinal detachment, bilateral eye
    - H44.2C9 Degenerative myopia with retinal detachment, unspecified eye

- **+ H44.2D Degenerative myopia with foveoschisis**
  - H44.2D1 Degenerative myopia with foveoschisis, right eye
  - H44.2D2 Degenerative myopia with foveoschisis, left eye
  - H44.2D3 Degenerative myopia with foveoschisis, bilateral eye
  - H44.2D9 Degenerative myopia with foveoschisis, unspecified eye
- **+ H44.2E Degenerative myopia with other maculopathy**
  - H44.2E1 Degenerative myopia with other maculopathy, right eye
  - H44.2E2 Degenerative myopia with other maculopathy, left eye
  - H44.2E3 Degenerative myopia with other maculopathy, bilateral eye
  - H44.2E9 Degenerative myopia with other maculopathy, unspecified eye
- **+ H44.3 Other and unspecified degenerative disorders of globe**
  - H44.30 Unspecified degenerative disorder of globe
  - **+ H44.31 Chalcosis**
    - H44.311 Chalcosis, right eye
    - H44.312 Chalcosis, left eye
    - H44.313 Chalcosis, bilateral
    - H44.319 Chalcosis, unspecified eye
  - **+ H44.32 Siderosis of eye**
    - H44.321 Siderosis of eye, right eye
    - H44.322 Siderosis of eye, left eye
    - H44.323 Siderosis of eye, bilateral
    - H44.329 Siderosis of eye, unspecified eye
  - **+ H44.39 Other degenerative disorders of globe**
    - H44.391 Other degenerative disorders of globe, right eye
    - H44.392 Other degenerative disorders of globe, left eye
    - H44.393 Other degenerative disorders of globe, bilateral
    - H44.399 Other degenerative disorders of globe, unspecified eye
- **+ H44.4 Hypotony of eye**
  - H44.40 Unspecified hypotony of eye
  - **+ H44.41 Flat anterior chamber hypotony of eye**
    - H44.411 Flat anterior chamber hypotony of right eye
    - H44.412 Flat anterior chamber hypotony of left eye
    - H44.413 Flat anterior chamber hypotony of eye, bilateral
    - H44.419 Flat anterior chamber hypotony of unspecified eye
  - **+ H44.42 Hypotony of eye due to ocular fistula**
    - H44.421 Hypotony of right eye due to ocular fistula
    - H44.422 Hypotony of left eye due to ocular fistula
    - H44.423 Hypotony of eye due to ocular fistula, bilateral
    - H44.429 Hypotony of unspecified eye due to ocular fistula
  - **+ H44.43 Hypotony of eye due to other ocular disorders**
    - H44.431 Hypotony of eye due to other ocular disorders, right eye
    - H44.432 Hypotony of eye due to other ocular disorders, left eye
    - H44.433 Hypotony of eye due to other ocular disorders, bilateral
    - H44.439 Hypotony of eye due to other ocular disorders, unspecified eye
  - **+ H44.44 Primary hypotony of eye**
    - H44.441 Primary hypotony of right eye
    - H44.442 Primary hypotony of left eye
    - H44.443 Primary hypotony of eye, bilateral
    - H44.449 Primary hypotony of unspecified eye
- **+ H44.5 Degenerated conditions of globe**
  - H44.50 Unspecified degenerated conditions of globe
  - **+ H44.51 Absolute glaucoma**
    - H44.511 Absolute glaucoma, right eye
    - H44.512 Absolute glaucoma, left eye
    - H44.513 Absolute glaucoma, bilateral
    - H44.519 Absolute glaucoma, unspecified eye
  - **+ H44.52 Atrophy of globe**
    - Phthisis bulbi
    - H44.521 Atrophy of globe, right eye
    - H44.522 Atrophy of globe, left eye
    - H44.523 Atrophy of globe, bilateral
    - H44.529 Atrophy of globe, unspecified eye
  - **+ H44.53 Leucocoria**
    - H44.531 Leucocoria, right eye
    - H44.532 Leucocoria, left eye
    - H44.533 Leucocoria, bilateral
    - H44.539 Leucocoria, unspecified eye
- **+ H44.6 Retained (old) intraocular foreign body, magnetic**

  Use additional code to identify magnetic foreign body (Z18.11)

  Excludes1: current intraocular foreign body (S05.-)

  Excludes2: retained foreign body in eyelid (H02.81-)
  retained (old) foreign body following penetrating wound of orbit (H05.5-)
  retained (old) intraocular foreign body, nonmagnetic (H44.7-)
  - **+ H44.60 Unspecified retained (old) intraocular foreign body, magnetic**
    - H44.601 Unspecified retained (old) intraocular foreign body, magnetic, right eye
    - H44.602 Unspecified retained (old) intraocular foreign body, magnetic, left eye
    - H44.603 Unspecified retained (old) intraocular foreign body, magnetic, bilateral
    - H44.609 Unspecified retained (old) intraocular foreign body, magnetic, unspecified eye
  - **+ H44.61 Retained (old) magnetic foreign body in anterior chamber**
    - H44.611 Retained (old) magnetic foreign body in anterior chamber, right eye
    - H44.612 Retained (old) magnetic foreign body in anterior chamber, left eye
    - H44.613 Retained (old) magnetic foreign body in anterior chamber, bilateral
    - H44.619 Retained (old) magnetic foreign body in anterior chamber, unspecified eye
  - **+ H44.62 Retained (old) magnetic foreign body in iris or ciliary body**
    - H44.621 Retained (old) magnetic foreign body in iris or ciliary body, right eye
    - H44.622 Retained (old) magnetic foreign body in iris or ciliary body, left eye
    - H44.623 Retained (old) magnetic foreign body in iris or ciliary body, bilateral
    - H44.629 Retained (old) magnetic foreign body in iris or ciliary body, unspecified eye
  - **+ H44.63 Retained (old) magnetic foreign body in lens**
    - H44.631 Retained (old) magnetic foreign body in lens, right eye
    - H44.632 Retained (old) magnetic foreign body in lens, left eye
    - H44.633 Retained (old) magnetic foreign body in lens, bilateral
    - H44.639 Retained (old) magnetic foreign body in lens, unspecified eye
  - **+ H44.64 Retained (old) magnetic foreign body in posterior wall of globe**
    - H44.641 Retained (old) magnetic foreign body in posterior wall of globe, right eye
    - H44.642 Retained (old) magnetic foreign body in posterior wall of globe, left eye
    - H44.643 Retained (old) magnetic foreign body in posterior wall of globe, bilateral
    - H44.649 Retained (old) magnetic foreign body in posterior wall of globe, unspecified eye
  - **+ H44.65 Retained (old) magnetic foreign body in vitreous body**
    - H44.651 Retained (old) magnetic foreign body in vitreous body, right eye
    - H44.652 Retained (old) magnetic foreign body in vitreous body, left eye

H44.653 Retained (old) magnetic foreign body in vitreous body, bilateral
H44.659 Retained (old) magnetic foreign body in vitreous body, unspecified eye
+ H44.69 Retained (old) intraocular foreign body, magnetic, in other or multiple sites
H44.691 Retained (old) intraocular foreign body, magnetic, in other or multiple sites, right eye
H44.692 Retained (old) intraocular foreign body, magnetic, in other or multiple sites, left eye
H44.693 Retained (old) intraocular foreign body, magnetic, in other or multiple sites, bilateral
H44.699 Retained (old) intraocular foreign body, magnetic, in other or multiple sites, unspecified eye
+ H44.7 Retained (old) intraocular foreign body, nonmagnetic
Use additional code to identify nonmagnetic foreign body (Z18.01-Z18.10, Z18.12, Z18.2-Z18.9)
Excludes1: current intraocular foreign body (S05.-)
Excludes2: retained foreign body in eyelid (H02.81-)
retained (old) foreign body following penetrating wound of orbit (H05.5-)
retained (old) intraocular foreign body, magnetic (H44.6-)
+ H44.70 Unspecified retained (old) intraocular foreign body, nonmagnetic
H44.701 Unspecified retained (old) intraocular foreign body, nonmagnetic, right eye
H44.702 Unspecified retained (old) intraocular foreign body, nonmagnetic, left eye
H44.703 Unspecified retained (old) intraocular foreign body, nonmagnetic, bilateral
H44.709 Unspecified retained (old) intraocular foreign body, nonmagnetic, unspecified eye
Retained (old) intraocular foreign body NOS
+ H44.71 Retained (nonmagnetic) (old) foreign body in anterior chamber
H44.711 Retained (nonmagnetic) (old) foreign body in anterior chamber, right eye
H44.712 Retained (nonmagnetic) (old) foreign body in anterior chamber, left eye
H44.713 Retained (nonmagnetic) (old) foreign body in anterior chamber, bilateral
H44.719 Retained (nonmagnetic) (old) foreign body in anterior chamber, unspecified eye
+ H44.72 Retained (nonmagnetic) (old) foreign body in iris or ciliary body
H44.721 Retained (nonmagnetic) (old) foreign body in iris or ciliary body, right eye
H44.722 Retained (nonmagnetic) (old) foreign body in iris or ciliary body, left eye
H44.723 Retained (nonmagnetic) (old) foreign body in iris or ciliary body, bilateral
H44.729 Retained (nonmagnetic) (old) foreign body in iris or ciliary body, unspecified eye
+ H44.73 Retained (nonmagnetic) (old) foreign body in lens
H44.731 Retained (nonmagnetic) (old) foreign body in lens, right eye
H44.732 Retained (nonmagnetic) (old) foreign body in lens, left eye
H44.733 Retained (nonmagnetic) (old) foreign body in lens, bilateral
H44.739 Retained (nonmagnetic) (old) foreign body in lens, unspecified eye
+ H44.74 Retained (nonmagnetic) (old) foreign body in posterior wall of globe
H44.741 Retained (nonmagnetic) (old) foreign body in posterior wall of globe, right eye
H44.742 Retained (nonmagnetic) (old) foreign body in posterior wall of globe, left eye
H44.743 Retained (nonmagnetic) (old) foreign body in posterior wall of globe, bilateral
H44.749 Retained (nonmagnetic) (old) foreign body in posterior wall of globe, unspecified eye

+ H44.75 Retained (nonmagnetic) (old) foreign body in vitreous body
H44.751 Retained (nonmagnetic) (old) foreign body in vitreous body, right eye
H44.752 Retained (nonmagnetic) (old) foreign body in vitreous body, left eye
H44.753 Retained (nonmagnetic) (old) foreign body in vitreous body, bilateral
H44.759 Retained (nonmagnetic) (old) foreign body in vitreous body, unspecified eye
+ H44.79 Retained (old) intraocular foreign body, nonmagnetic, in other or multiple sites
H44.791 Retained (old) intraocular foreign body, nonmagnetic, in other or multiple sites, right eye
H44.792 Retained (old) intraocular foreign body, nonmagnetic, in other or multiple sites, left eye
H44.793 Retained (old) intraocular foreign body, nonmagnetic, in other or multiple sites, bilateral
H44.799 Retained (old) intraocular foreign body, nonmagnetic, in other or multiple sites, unspecified eye
+ H44.8 Other disorders of globe
+ H44.81 Hemophthalmos
H44.811 Hemophthalmos, right eye
H44.812 Hemophthalmos, left eye
H44.813 Hemophthalmos, bilateral
H44.819 Hemophthalmos, unspecified eye
+ H44.82 Luxation of globe
H44.821 Luxation of globe, right eye
H44.822 Luxation of globe, left eye
H44.823 Luxation of globe, bilateral
H44.829 Luxation of globe, unspecified eye
H44.89 Other disorders of globe
AHA CC: 1Q, 2022, 33
H44.9 Unspecified disorder of globe

Disorders of optic nerve and visual pathways (H46-H47)

H46 Optic neuritis
Excludes2: ischemic optic neuropathy (H47.01-)
neuromyelitis optica [Devic] (G36.0)
+ H46.0 Optic papillitis
CC H46.00 Optic papillitis, unspecified eye
CC H46.01 Optic papillitis, right eye
CC H46.02 Optic papillitis, left eye
CC H46.03 Optic papillitis, bilateral
+ H46.1 Retrobulbar neuritis
Retrobulbar neuritis NOS
Excludes1: syphilitic retrobulbar neuritis (A52.15)
CC H46.10 Retrobulbar neuritis, unspecified eye
CC H46.11 Retrobulbar neuritis, right eye
CC H46.12 Retrobulbar neuritis, left eye
CC H46.13 Retrobulbar neuritis, bilateral
H46.2 Nutritional optic neuropathy
H46.3 Toxic optic neuropathy
Code first (T51-T65) to identify cause
CC H46.8 Other optic neuritis
CC H46.9 Unspecified optic neuritis
H47 Other disorders of optic [2nd] nerve and visual pathways
+ H47.0 Disorders of optic nerve, not elsewhere classified
+ H47.01 Ischemic optic neuropathy
H47.011 Ischemic optic neuropathy, right eye
H47.012 Ischemic optic neuropathy, left eye
H47.013 Ischemic optic neuropathy, bilateral
H47.019 Ischemic optic neuropathy, unspecified eye
+ H47.02 Hemorrhage in optic nerve sheath
H47.021 Hemorrhage in optic nerve sheath, right eye
H47.022 Hemorrhage in optic nerve sheath, left eye
H47.023 Hemorrhage in optic nerve sheath, bilateral
H47.029 Hemorrhage in optic nerve sheath, unspecified eye

- **+ H47.03 Optic nerve hypoplasia**
  - H47.031 Optic nerve hypoplasia, right eye
  - H47.032 Optic nerve hypoplasia, left eye
  - H47.033 Optic nerve hypoplasia, bilateral
  - H47.039 Optic nerve hypoplasia, unspecified eye
- **+ H47.09 Other disorders of optic nerve, not elsewhere classified**
  - Compression of optic nerve
  - H47.091 Other disorders of optic nerve, not elsewhere classified, right eye
  - H47.092 Other disorders of optic nerve, not elsewhere classified, left eye
  - H47.093 Other disorders of optic nerve, not elsewhere classified, bilateral
  - H47.099 Other disorders of optic nerve, not elsewhere classified, unspecified eye
- **+ H47.1 Papilledema**
  - CC H47.10 Unspecified papilledema
  - CC H47.11 Papilledema associated with increased intracranial pressure
  - H47.12 Papilledema associated with decreased ocular pressure
  - H47.13 Papilledema associated with retinal disorder
  - **+ H47.14 Foster-Kennedy syndrome**
    - H47.141 Foster-Kennedy syndrome, right eye
    - H47.142 Foster-Kennedy syndrome, left eye
    - H47.143 Foster-Kennedy syndrome, bilateral
    - H47.149 Foster-Kennedy syndrome, unspecified eye
- **+ H47.2 Optic atrophy**
  - H47.20 Unspecified optic atrophy
  - **+ H47.21 Primary optic atrophy**
    - H47.211 Primary optic atrophy, right eye
    - H47.212 Primary optic atrophy, left eye
    - H47.213 Primary optic atrophy, bilateral
    - H47.219 Primary optic atrophy, unspecified eye
  - H47.22 Hereditary optic atrophy
    - Leber's optic atrophy
  - **+ H47.23 Glaucomatous optic atrophy**
    - H47.231 Glaucomatous optic atrophy, right eye
    - H47.232 Glaucomatous optic atrophy, left eye
    - H47.233 Glaucomatous optic atrophy, bilateral
    - H47.239 Glaucomatous optic atrophy, unspecified eye
  - **+ H47.29 Other optic atrophy**
    - Temporal pallor of optic disc
    - H47.291 Other optic atrophy, right eye
    - H47.292 Other optic atrophy, left eye
    - H47.293 Other optic atrophy, bilateral
    - H47.299 Other optic atrophy, unspecified eye
- **+ H47.3 Other disorders of optic disc**
  - **+ H47.31 Coloboma of optic disc**
    - H47.311 Coloboma of optic disc, right eye
    - H47.312 Coloboma of optic disc, left eye
    - H47.313 Coloboma of optic disc, bilateral
    - H47.319 Coloboma of optic disc, unspecified eye
  - **+ H47.32 Drusen of optic disc**
    - H47.321 Drusen of optic disc, right eye
    - H47.322 Drusen of optic disc, left eye
    - H47.323 Drusen of optic disc, bilateral
    - H47.329 Drusen of optic disc, unspecified eye
  - **+ H47.33 Pseudopapilledema of optic disc**
    - H47.331 Pseudopapilledema of optic disc, right eye
    - H47.332 Pseudopapilledema of optic disc, left eye
    - H47.333 Pseudopapilledema of optic disc, bilateral
    - H47.339 Pseudopapilledema of optic disc, unspecified eye
  - **+ H47.39 Other disorders of optic disc**
    - H47.391 Other disorders of optic disc, right eye
    - H47.392 Other disorders of optic disc, left eye
    - H47.393 Other disorders of optic disc, bilateral
    - H47.399 Other disorders of optic disc, unspecified eye
- **+ H47.4 Disorders of optic chiasm**
  - *Code also underlying condition*
  - CC H47.41 Disorders of optic chiasm in (due to) inflammatory disorders
  - CC H47.42 Disorders of optic chiasm in (due to) neoplasm
  - CC H47.43 Disorders of optic chiasm in (due to) vascular disorders
  - CC H47.49 Disorders of optic chiasm in (due to) other disorders
- **+ H47.5 Disorders of other visual pathways**
  - Disorders of optic tracts, geniculate nuclei and optic radiations
  - *Code also underlying condition*
  - **+ H47.51 Disorders of visual pathways in (due to) inflammatory disorders**
    - CC H47.511 Disorders of visual pathways in (due to) inflammatory disorders, right side
    - CC H47.512 Disorders of visual pathways in (due to) inflammatory disorders, left side
    - CC H47.519 Disorders of visual pathways in (due to) inflammatory disorders, unspecified side
  - **+ H47.52 Disorders of visual pathways in (due to) neoplasm**
    - CC H47.521 Disorders of visual pathways in (due to) neoplasm, right side
    - CC H47.522 Disorders of visual pathways in (due to) neoplasm, left side
    - CC H47.529 Disorders of visual pathways in (due to) neoplasm, unspecified side
  - **+ H47.53 Disorders of visual pathways in (due to) vascular disorders**
    - CC H47.531 Disorders of visual pathways in (due to) vascular disorders, right side
    - CC H47.532 Disorders of visual pathways in (due to) vascular disorders, left side
    - CC H47.539 Disorders of visual pathways in (due to) vascular disorders, unspecified side
- **+ H47.6 Disorders of visual cortex**
  - *Code also underlying condition*
  - **Excludes1:** *injury to visual cortex S04.04-*
  - **+ H47.61 Cortical blindness**
    - H47.611 Cortical blindness, right side of brain
    - H47.612 Cortical blindness, left side of brain
    - H47.619 Cortical blindness, unspecified side of brain
  - **+ H47.62 Disorders of visual cortex in (due to) inflammatory disorders**
    - CC H47.621 Disorders of visual cortex in (due to) inflammatory disorders, right side of brain
    - CC H47.622 Disorders of visual cortex in (due to) inflammatory disorders, left side of brain
    - CC H47.629 Disorders of visual cortex in (due to) inflammatory disorders, unspecified side of brain
  - **+ H47.63 Disorders of visual cortex in (due to) neoplasm**
    - CC H47.631 Disorders of visual cortex in (due to) neoplasm, right side of brain
    - CC H47.632 Disorders of visual cortex in (due to) neoplasm, left side of brain
    - CC H47.639 Disorders of visual cortex in (due to) neoplasm, unspecified side of brain
  - **+ H47.64 Disorders of visual cortex in (due to) vascular disorders**
    - CC H47.641 Disorders of visual cortex in (due to) vascular disorders, right side of brain
    - CC H47.642 Disorders of visual cortex in (due to) vascular disorders, left side of brain
    - CC H47.649 Disorders of visual cortex in (due to) vascular disorders, unspecified side of brain
- H47.9 Unspecified disorder of visual pathways

Disorders of ocular muscles, binocular movement, accommodation and refraction (H49-H52)

Excludes2: *nystagmus and other irregular eye movements (H55)*

H49 Paralytic strabismus

Excludes2: *internal ophthalmoplegia (H52.51-)*
internuclear ophthalmoplegia (H51.2-)
progressive supranuclear ophthalmoplegia (G23.1)

- **H49.0** Third [oculomotor] nerve palsy
  - H49.00 Third [oculomotor] nerve palsy, unspecified eye
  - H49.01 Third [oculomotor] nerve palsy, right eye
  - H49.02 Third [oculomotor] nerve palsy, left eye
  - H49.03 Third [oculomotor] nerve palsy, bilateral
- **H49.1** Fourth [trochlear] nerve palsy
  - H49.10 Fourth [trochlear] nerve palsy, unspecified eye
  - H49.11 Fourth [trochlear] nerve palsy, right eye
  - H49.12 Fourth [trochlear] nerve palsy, left eye
  - H49.13 Fourth [trochlear] nerve palsy, bilateral
- **H49.2** Sixth [abducent] nerve palsy
  - H49.20 Sixth [abducent] nerve palsy, unspecified eye
  - H49.21 Sixth [abducent] nerve palsy, right eye
  - H49.22 Sixth [abducent] nerve palsy, left eye
  - H49.23 Sixth [abducent] nerve palsy, bilateral
- **H49.3** Total (external) ophthalmoplegia
  - H49.30 Total (external) ophthalmoplegia, unspecified eye
  - H49.31 Total (external) ophthalmoplegia, right eye
  - H49.32 Total (external) ophthalmoplegia, left eye
  - H49.33 Total (external) ophthalmoplegia, bilateral
- **H49.4** Progressive external ophthalmoplegia
  - **Excludes1:** *Kearns-Sayre syndrome (H49.81-)*
  - H49.40 Progressive external ophthalmoplegia, unspecified eye
  - H49.41 Progressive external ophthalmoplegia, right eye
  - H49.42 Progressive external ophthalmoplegia, left eye
  - H49.43 Progressive external ophthalmoplegia, bilateral
- **H49.8** Other paralytic strabismus
  - **H49.81** Kearns-Sayre syndrome
    - Progressive external ophthalmoplegia with pigmentary retinopathy
    - Code also, if applicable, other manifestation, such as: heart block (I45.9)
    - CC H49.811 Kearns-Sayre syndrome, right eye
    - CC H49.812 Kearns-Sayre syndrome, left eye
    - CC H49.813 Kearns-Sayre syndrome, bilateral
    - CC H49.819 Kearns-Sayre syndrome, unspecified eye
  - **H49.88** Other paralytic strabismus
    - External ophthalmoplegia NOS
    - H49.881 Other paralytic strabismus, right eye
    - H49.882 Other paralytic strabismus, left eye
    - H49.883 Other paralytic strabismus, bilateral
    - H49.889 Other paralytic strabismus, unspecified eye
  - H49.9 Unspecified paralytic strabismus
- **H50 Other strabismus**
  - **H50.0** Esotropia
    - Convergent concomitant strabismus
    - **Excludes1:** *intermittent esotropia (H50.31-, H50.32)*
    - H50.00 Unspecified esotropia
    - **H50.01** Monocular esotropia
      - H50.011 Monocular esotropia, right eye
      - H50.012 Monocular esotropia, left eye
    - **H50.02** Monocular esotropia with A pattern
      - H50.021 Monocular esotropia with A pattern, right eye
      - H50.022 Monocular esotropia with A pattern, left eye
    - **H50.03** Monocular esotropia with V pattern
      - H50.031 Monocular esotropia with V pattern, right eye
      - H50.032 Monocular esotropia with V pattern, left eye
    - **H50.04** Monocular esotropia with other noncomitancies
      - H50.041 Monocular esotropia with other noncomitancies, right eye
      - H50.042 Monocular esotropia with other noncomitancies, left eye
    - H50.05 Alternating esotropia
    - H50.06 Alternating esotropia with A pattern
    - H50.07 Alternating esotropia with V pattern
    - H50.08 Alternating esotropia with other noncomitancies
  - **H50.1** Exotropia
    - Divergent concomitant strabismus
    - **Excludes1:** *intermittent exotropia (H50.33-, H50.34)*
    - H50.10 Unspecified exotropia
    - **H50.11** Monocular exotropia
      - H50.111 Monocular exotropia, right eye
      - H50.112 Monocular exotropia, left eye
    - **H50.12** Monocular exotropia with A pattern
      - H50.121 Monocular exotropia with A pattern, right eye
      - H50.122 Monocular exotropia with A pattern, left eye
    - **H50.13** Monocular exotropia with V pattern
      - H50.131 Monocular exotropia with V pattern, right eye
      - H50.132 Monocular exotropia with V pattern, left eye
    - **H50.14** Monocular exotropia with other noncomitancies
      - H50.141 Monocular exotropia with other noncomitancies, right eye
      - H50.142 Monocular exotropia with other noncomitancies, left eye
    - H50.15 Alternating exotropia
    - H50.16 Alternating exotropia with A pattern
    - H50.17 Alternating exotropia with V pattern
    - H50.18 Alternating exotropia with other noncomitancies
  - **H50.2** Vertical strabismus
    - Hypertropia
    - H50.21 Vertical strabismus, right eye
    - H50.22 Vertical strabismus, left eye
  - **H50.3** Intermittent heterotropia
    - H50.30 Unspecified intermittent heterotropia
    - **H50.31** Intermittent monocular esotropia
      - H50.311 Intermittent monocular esotropia, right eye
      - H50.312 Intermittent monocular esotropia, left eye
    - H50.32 Intermittent alternating esotropia
    - **H50.33** Intermittent monocular exotropia
      - H50.331 Intermittent monocular exotropia, right eye
      - H50.332 Intermittent monocular exotropia, left eye
    - H50.34 Intermittent alternating exotropia
  - **H50.4** Other and unspecified heterotropia
    - H50.40 Unspecified heterotropia
    - **H50.41** Cyclotropia
      - H50.411 Cyclotropia, right eye
      - H50.412 Cyclotropia, left eye
    - H50.42 Monofixation syndrome
    - H50.43 Accommodative component in esotropia
  - **H50.5** Heterophoria
    - H50.50 Unspecified heterophoria
    - H50.51 Esophoria
    - H50.52 Exophoria
    - H50.53 Vertical heterophoria
    - H50.54 Cyclophoria
    - H50.55 Alternating heterophoria
  - **H50.6** Mechanical strabismus
    - H50.60 Mechanical strabismus, unspecified
    - **H50.61** Brown's sheath syndrome
      - H50.611 Brown's sheath syndrome, right eye
      - H50.612 Brown's sheath syndrome, left eye
    - **H50.62** Inferior oblique muscle entrapment
      - H50.621 Inferior oblique muscle entrapment, right eye
      - H50.622 Inferior oblique muscle entrapment, left eye
      - H50.629 Inferior oblique muscle entrapment, unspecified eye
    - **H50.63** Inferior rectus muscle entrapment
      - H50.631 Inferior rectus muscle entrapment, right eye
      - H50.632 Inferior rectus muscle entrapment, left eye
      - H50.639 Inferior rectus muscle entrapment, unspecified eye
    - **H50.64** Lateral rectus muscle entrapment
      - H50.641 Lateral rectus muscle entrapment, right eye
      - H50.642 Lateral rectus muscle entrapment, left eye
      - H50.649 Lateral rectus muscle entrapment, unspecified eye

- **H50.65 Medial rectus muscle entrapment**
  - H50.651 Medial rectus muscle entrapment, right eye
  - H50.652 Medial rectus muscle entrapment, left eye
  - H50.659 Medial rectus muscle entrapment, unspecified eye
- **H50.66 Superior oblique muscle entrapment**
  - H50.661 Superior oblique muscle entrapment, right eye
  - H50.662 Superior oblique muscle entrapment, left eye
  - H50.669 Superior oblique muscle entrapment, unspecified eye
- **H50.67 Superior rectus muscle entrapment**
  - H50.671 Superior rectus muscle entrapment, right eye
  - H50.672 Superior rectus muscle entrapment, left eye
  - H50.679 Superior rectus muscle entrapment, unspecified eye
- **H50.68 Extraocular muscle entrapment, unspecified**
  - H50.681 Extraocular muscle entrapment, unspecified, right eye
  - H50.682 Extraocular muscle entrapment, unspecified, left eye
  - H50.689 Extraocular muscle entrapment, unspecified, unspecified eye
  - H50.69 Other mechanical strabismus
    - Strabismus due to adhesions
    - Traumatic limitation of duction of eye muscle
- **H50.8 Other specified strabismus**
  - **H50.81 Duane's syndrome**
    - H50.811 Duane's syndrome, right eye
    - H50.812 Duane's syndrome, left eye
  - H50.89 Other specified strabismus
  - H50.9 Unspecified strabismus

H51 Other disorders of binocular movement
- H51.0 Palsy (spasm) of conjugate gaze
- **H51.1 Convergence insufficiency and excess**
  - H51.11 Convergence insufficiency
  - H51.12 Convergence excess
- **H51.2 Internuclear ophthalmoplegia**
  - H51.20 Internuclear ophthalmoplegia, unspecified eye
  - H51.21 Internuclear ophthalmoplegia, right eye
  - H51.22 Internuclear ophthalmoplegia, left eye
  - H51.23 Internuclear ophthalmoplegia, bilateral
- H51.8 Other specified disorders of binocular movement
- H51.9 Unspecified disorder of binocular movement

H52 Disorders of refraction and accommodation
- **H52.0 Hypermetropia**
  - H52.00 Hypermetropia, unspecified eye
  - H52.01 Hypermetropia, right eye
  - H52.02 Hypermetropia, left eye
  - H52.03 Hypermetropia, bilateral
- **H52.1 Myopia**
  - **Excludes1:** degenerative myopia (H44.2-)
  - H52.10 Myopia, unspecified eye
  - H52.11 Myopia, right eye
  - H52.12 Myopia, left eye
  - H52.13 Myopia, bilateral
- **H52.2 Astigmatism**
  - **H52.20 Unspecified astigmatism**
    - H52.201 Unspecified astigmatism, right eye
    - H52.202 Unspecified astigmatism, left eye
    - H52.203 Unspecified astigmatism, bilateral
    - H52.209 Unspecified astigmatism, unspecified eye
  - **H52.21 Irregular astigmatism**
    - H52.211 Irregular astigmatism, right eye
    - H52.212 Irregular astigmatism, left eye
    - H52.213 Irregular astigmatism, bilateral
    - H52.219 Irregular astigmatism, unspecified eye
  - **H52.22 Regular astigmatism**
    - H52.221 Regular astigmatism, right eye
    - H52.222 Regular astigmatism, left eye
    - H52.223 Regular astigmatism, bilateral
    - H52.229 Regular astigmatism, unspecified eye
- **H52.3 Anisometropia and aniseikonia**
  - H52.31 Anisometropia
  - H52.32 Aniseikonia
- H52.4 Presbyopia
- **H52.5 Disorders of accommodation**
  - **H52.51 Internal ophthalmoplegia (complete) (total)**
    - H52.511 Internal ophthalmoplegia (complete) (total), right eye
    - H52.512 Internal ophthalmoplegia (complete) (total), left eye
    - H52.513 Internal ophthalmoplegia (complete) (total), bilateral
    - H52.519 Internal ophthalmoplegia (complete) (total), unspecified eye
  - **H52.52 Paresis of accommodation**
    - H52.521 Paresis of accommodation, right eye
    - H52.522 Paresis of accommodation, left eye
    - H52.523 Paresis of accommodation, bilateral
    - H52.529 Paresis of accommodation, unspecified eye
  - **H52.53 Spasm of accommodation**
    - H52.531 Spasm of accommodation, right eye
    - H52.532 Spasm of accommodation, left eye
    - H52.533 Spasm of accommodation, bilateral
    - H52.539 Spasm of accommodation, unspecified eye
- H52.6 Other disorders of refraction
- H52.7 Unspecified disorder of refraction

Visual disturbances and blindness (H53-H54)

H53 Visual disturbances
- **H53.0 Amblyopia ex anopsia**
  - **Excludes1:** amblyopia due to vitamin A deficiency (E50.5)
  - **H53.00 Unspecified amblyopia**
    - H53.001 Unspecified amblyopia, right eye
    - H53.002 Unspecified amblyopia, left eye
    - H53.003 Unspecified amblyopia, bilateral
    - H53.009 Unspecified amblyopia, unspecified eye
  - **H53.01 Deprivation amblyopia**
    - H53.011 Deprivation amblyopia, right eye
    - H53.012 Deprivation amblyopia, left eye
    - H53.013 Deprivation amblyopia, bilateral
    - H53.019 Deprivation amblyopia, unspecified eye
  - **H53.02 Refractive amblyopia**
    - H53.021 Refractive amblyopia, right eye
    - H53.022 Refractive amblyopia, left eye
    - H53.023 Refractive amblyopia, bilateral
    - H53.029 Refractive amblyopia, unspecified eye
  - **H53.03 Strabismic amblyopia**
    - **Excludes1:** strabismus (H50.-)
    - H53.031 Strabismic amblyopia, right eye
    - H53.032 Strabismic amblyopia, left eye
    - H53.033 Strabismic amblyopia, bilateral
    - H53.039 Strabismic amblyopia, unspecified eye
  - **H53.04 Amblyopia suspect**
    - *AHA CC: 4Q, 2016, 22-23*
    - H53.041 Amblyopia suspect, right eye
    - H53.042 Amblyopia suspect, left eye
    - H53.043 Amblyopia suspect, bilateral
    - H53.049 Amblyopia suspect, unspecified eye
- **H53.1 Subjective visual disturbances**
  - **Excludes1:** subjective visual disturbances due to vitamin A deficiency (E50.5)
    - visual hallucinations (R44.1)
  - H53.10 Unspecified subjective visual disturbances
  - H53.11 Day blindness
    - Hemeralopia
  - **H53.12 Transient visual loss**
    - Scintillating scotoma
    - **Excludes1:** amaurosis fugax (G45.3-)
      - transient retinal artery occlusion (H34.0-)
    - *AHA CC: 1Q, 2022, 30*
    - CC H53.121 Transient visual loss, right eye
    - CC H53.122 Transient visual loss, left eye
    - CC H53.123 Transient visual loss, bilateral
    - CC H53.129 Transient visual loss, unspecified eye
  - **H53.13 Sudden visual loss**
    - CC H53.131 Sudden visual loss, right eye
    - CC H53.132 Sudden visual loss, left eye

       CC H53.133 Sudden visual loss, bilateral
       CC H53.139 Sudden visual loss, unspecified eye
+ **H53.14 Visual discomfort**
    Asthenopia
    Photophobia
    H53.141 Visual discomfort, right eye
    H53.142 Visual discomfort, left eye
    H53.143 Visual discomfort, bilateral
    H53.149 Visual discomfort, unspecified
H53.15 Visual distortions of shape and size
    Metamorphopsia
H53.16 Psychophysical visual disturbances
H53.19 Other subjective visual disturbances
    Visual halos
H53.2 Diplopia
  Double vision
  AHA CC: 3Q, 2022, 10
+ **H53.3 Other and unspecified disorders of binocular vision**
  H53.30 Unspecified disorder of binocular vision
  H53.31 Abnormal retinal correspondence
  H53.32 Fusion with defective stereopsis
  H53.33 Simultaneous visual perception without fusion
  H53.34 Suppression of binocular vision
+ **H53.4 Visual field defects**
  H53.40 Unspecified visual field defects
+ **H53.41** Scotoma involving central area
    Central scotoma
    H53.411 Scotoma involving central area, right eye
    H53.412 Scotoma involving central area, left eye
    H53.413 Scotoma involving central area, bilateral
    H53.419 Scotoma involving central area, unspecified eye
+ **H53.42** Scotoma of blind spot area
    Enlarged blind spot
    H53.421 Scotoma of blind spot area, right eye
    H53.422 Scotoma of blind spot area, left eye
    H53.423 Scotoma of blind spot area, bilateral
    H53.429 Scotoma of blind spot area, unspecified eye
+ **H53.43** Sector or arcuate defects
    Arcuate scotoma
    Bjerrum scotoma
    H53.431 Sector or arcuate defects, right eye
    H53.432 Sector or arcuate defects, left eye
    H53.433 Sector or arcuate defects, bilateral
    H53.439 Sector or arcuate defects, unspecified eye
+ **H53.45** Other localized visual field defect
    Peripheral visual field defect
    Ring scotoma NOS
    Scotoma NOS
    H53.451 Other localized visual field defect, right eye
    H53.452 Other localized visual field defect, left eye
    H53.453 Other localized visual field defect, bilateral
    H53.459 Other localized visual field defect, unspecified eye
+ **H53.46** Homonymous bilateral field defects
    Homonymous hemianopsia
    Quadrant anopia
    Quadrant anopsia
    H53.461 Homonymous bilateral field defects, right side
    H53.462 Homonymous bilateral field defects, left side
    H53.469 Homonymous bilateral field defects, unspecified side
        Homonymous bilateral field defects NOS
  H53.47 Heteronymous bilateral field defects
    Heteronymous hemianop(s)ia
+ **H53.48** Generalized contraction of visual field
    H53.481 Generalized contraction of visual field, right eye
    H53.482 Generalized contraction of visual field, left eye
    H53.483 Generalized contraction of visual field, bilateral
    H53.489 Generalized contraction of visual field, unspecified eye
+ **H53.5 Color vision deficiencies**
  Color blindness
  Excludes2: *day blindness (H53.11)*
  H53.50 Unspecified color vision deficiencies
    Color blindness NOS
  H53.51 Achromatopsia
  H53.52 Acquired color vision deficiency
  H53.53 Deuteranomaly
    Deuteranopia
  H53.54 Protanomaly
    Protanopia
  H53.55 Tritanomaly
    Tritanopia
  H53.59 Other color vision deficiencies
+ **H53.6 Night blindness**
  Excludes1: *night blindness due to vitamin A deficiency (E50.5)*
  H53.60 Unspecified night blindness
  H53.61 Abnormal dark adaptation curve
  H53.62 Acquired night blindness
  H53.63 Congenital night blindness
  H53.69 Other night blindness
+ **H53.7 Vision sensitivity deficiencies**
  H53.71 Glare sensitivity
  H53.72 Impaired contrast sensitivity
H53.8 Other visual disturbances
H53.9 Unspecified visual disturbance

H54 Blindness and low vision

  NOTE For definition of visual impairment categories see table below
  Code first any associated underlying cause of the blindness
  Excludes1: *amaurosis fugax (G45.3)*
  AHA CC: 4Q, 2017, 11-12

+ **H54.0 Blindness, both eyes**
  Visual impairment categories 3, 4, 5 in both eyes.
  H54.0X Blindness, both eyes, different category levels
+   **H54.0X3** Blindness right eye, category 3
      H54.0X33 Blindness right eye category 3, blindness left eye category 3
      H54.0X34 Blindness right eye category 3, blindness left eye category 4
      H54.0X35 Blindness right eye category 3, blindness left eye category 5
+   **H54.0X4** Blindness right eye, category 4
      H54.0X43 Blindness right eye category 4, blindness left eye category 3
      H54.0X44 Blindness right eye category 4, blindness left eye category 4
      H54.0X45 Blindness right eye category 4, blindness left eye category 5
+   **H54.0X5** Blindness right eye, category 5
      H54.0X53 Blindness right eye category 5, blindness left eye category 3
      H54.0X54 Blindness right eye category 5, blindness left eye category 4
      H54.0X55 Blindness right eye category 5, blindness left eye category 5
+ **H54.1 Blindness, one eye, low vision other eye**
  Visual impairment categories 3, 4, 5 in one eye, with categories 1 or 2 in the other eye.
  H54.10 Blindness, one eye, low vision other eye, unspecified eyes
+ **H54.11** Blindness, right eye, low vision left eye
+   **H54.113** Blindness right eye category 3, low vision left eye
      H54.1131 Blindness right eye category 3, low vision left eye category 1
      H54.1132 Blindness right eye category 3, low vision left eye category 2
+   **H54.114** Blindness right eye category 4, low vision left eye
      H54.1141 Blindness right eye category 4, low vision left eye category 1
      H54.1142 Blindness right eye category 4, low vision left eye category 2

- H54.115 **Blindness right eye category 5, low vision left eye**
  - H54.1151 Blindness right eye category 5, low vision left eye category 1
  - H54.1152 Blindness right eye category 5, low vision left eye category 2
- + H54.12 **Blindness, left eye, low vision right eye**
  - + H54.121 **Low vision right eye category 1, blindness left eye**
    - H54.1213 Low vision right eye category 1, blindness left eye category 3
    - H54.1214 Low vision right eye category 1, blindness left eye category 4
    - H54.1215 Low vision right eye category 1, blindness left eye category 5
  - + H54.122 **Low vision right eye category 2, blindness left eye**
    - H54.1223 Low vision right eye category 2, blindness left eye category 3
    - H54.1224 Low vision right eye category 2, blindness left eye category 4
    - H54.1225 Low vision right eye category 2, blindness left eye category 5
- + H54.2 **Low vision, both eyes**
  Visual impairment categories 1 or 2 in both eyes.
  - + H54.2X **Low vision, both eyes, different category levels**
    - + H54.2X1 **Low vision, right eye, category 1**
      - H54.2X11 Low vision, right eye, category 1, low vision left eye category 1
      - H54.2X12 Low vision, right eye, category 1, low vision left eye category 2
    - + H54.2X2 **Low vision, right eye, category 2**
      - H54.2X21 Low vision, right eye, category 2, low vision left eye category 1
      - H54.2X22 Low vision, right eye, category 2, low vision left eye category 2
- H54.3 **Unqualified visual loss, both eyes**
  Visual impairment category 9 in both eyes.
  Review coding guideline C.7.b
- + H54.4 **Blindness, one eye**
  Visual impairment categories 3, 4, 5 in one eye [normal vision in other eye]
  - H54.40 Blindness, one eye, unspecified eye
  - + H54.41 **Blindness, right eye, normal vision left eye**
    - + H54.413 **Blindness, right eye, category 3**
      - H54.413A Blindness right eye category 3, normal vision left eye
    - + H54.414 **Blindness, right eye, category 4**
      - H54.414A Blindness right eye category 4, normal vision left eye
    - + H54.415 **Blindness, right eye, category 5**
      - H54.415A Blindness right eye category 5, normal vision left eye
  - + H54.42 **Blindness, left eye, normal vision right eye**
    - + H54.42A **Blindness, left eye, category 3-5**
      - H54.42A3 Blindness left eye category 3, normal vision right eye
      - H54.42A4 Blindness left eye category 4, normal vision right eye
      - H54.42A5 Blindness left eye category 5, normal vision right eye
- + H54.5 **Low vision, one eye**
  Visual impairment categories 1 or 2 in one eye [normal vision in other eye].
  - H54.50 Low vision, one eye, unspecified eye
  - + H54.51 **Low vision, right eye, normal vision left eye**
    - + H54.511 **Low vision, right eye, category 1**
      - H54.511A Low vision right eye category 1, normal vision left eye
    - + H54.512 **Low vision, right eye, category 2**
      - H54.512A Low vision right eye category 2, normal vision left eye
  - + H54.52 **Low vision, left eye, normal vision right eye**
    - + H54.52A **Low vision, left eye, category 1-2**
      - H54.52A1 Low vision left eye category 1, normal vision right eye
      - H54.52A2 Low vision left eye category 2, normal vision right eye
- + H54.6 **Unqualified visual loss, one eye**
  Visual impairment category 9 in one eye [normal vision in other eye].
  Review coding guideline C.7.b
  - H54.60 Unqualified visual loss, one eye, unspecified
  - H54.61 Unqualified visual loss, right eye, normal vision left eye
  - H54.62 Unqualified visual loss, left eye, normal vision right eye
- H54.7 **Unspecified visual loss**
  Visual impairment category 9 NOS
  Review coding guideline C.7.b
- H54.8 **Legal blindness, as defined in USA**
  Blindness NOS according to USA definition
  Excludes1: *legal blindness with specification of impairment level (H54.0-H54.7)*

  NOTE The table below gives a classification of severity of visual impairment recommended by a WHO Study Group on the Prevention of Blindness, Geneva, 6-10 November 1972.
  The term 'low vision' in category H54 comprises categories 1 and 2 of the table, the term 'blindness' categories 3, 4 and 5, and the term 'unqualified visual loss' category 9.
  If the extent of the visual field is taken into account, patients with a field no greater than 10 but greater than 5 around central fixation should be placed in category 3 and patients with a field no greater than 5 around central fixation should be placed in category 4, even if the central acuity is not impaired.

Category of visual impairment	Visual acuity with best possible correction	
	Maximum less than:	Minimum equal to or better than:
	6/18	6/60
3/10(0.3)	1/10(0.1)	
20/70	20/200	
	6/60	3/60
1/10(0.1)	1/20(0.05)	
20/200	20/400	
	3/60	1/60(finger counting at one meter)
1/20(0.05)	1/50(0.02)	
20/400	5/300(20/1200)	
	1/60(finger counting at one meter)	Light perception
1/50(0.02)		
5/300		
	No light perception	
	Undetermined or unspecified	

Note: Document 508 compliance requires all cells in the above table to be filled.

Other disorders of eye and adnexa (H55-H57)

H55 Nystagmus and other irregular eye movements
- **+ H55.0 Nystagmus**
  - H55.00 Unspecified nystagmus
  - H55.01 Congenital nystagmus
  - H55.02 Latent nystagmus
  - H55.03 Visual deprivation nystagmus
  - H55.04 Dissociated nystagmus
  - H55.09 Other forms of nystagmus
- **+ H55.8 Other irregular eye movements**
  - *AHA CC: 4Q, 2020, 25*
  - H55.81 Deficient saccadic eye movements
  - H55.82 Deficient smooth pursuit eye movements
  - H55.89 Other irregular eye movements

H57 Other disorders of eye and adnexa
- **+ H57.0 Anomalies of pupillary function**
  - H57.00 Unspecified anomaly of pupillary function
  - H57.01 Argyll Robertson pupil, atypical
    - **Excludes1:** syphilitic Argyll Robertson pupil (A52.19)
  - H57.02 Anisocoria
  - H57.03 Miosis
  - H57.04 Mydriasis
  - **+ H57.05 Tonic pupil**
    - H57.051 Tonic pupil, right eye
    - H57.052 Tonic pupil, left eye
    - H57.053 Tonic pupil, bilateral
    - H57.059 Tonic pupil, unspecified eye
  - H57.09 Other anomalies of pupillary function
- **+ H57.1 Ocular pain**
  - H57.10 Ocular pain, unspecified eye
  - H57.11 Ocular pain, right eyew
  - H57.12 Ocular pain, left eye
  - H57.13 Ocular pain, bilateral
- **+ H57.8 Other specified disorders of eye and adnexa**
  - *AHA CC: 4Q, 2018, 15-16*
  - **+ H57.81 Brow ptosis**
    - H57.811 Brow ptosis, right
    - H57.812 Brow ptosis, left
    - H57.813 Brow ptosis, bilateral
    - H57.819 Brow ptosis, unspecified
  - H57.89 Other specified disorders of eye and adnexa
  - **+ H57.8A Foreign body sensation eye (ocular)**
    - H57.8A1 Foreign body sensation, right eye
    - H57.8A2 Foreign body sensation, left eye
    - H57.8A3 Foreign body sensation, bilateral eyes
    - H57.8A9 Foreign body sensation, unspecified eye
- H57.9 Unspecified disorder of eye and adnexa

Intraoperative and postprocedural complications and disorders of eye and adnexa, not elsewhere classified (H59)

H59 Intraoperative and postprocedural complications and disorders of eye and adnexa, not elsewhere classified
- **Excludes1:** mechanical complication of intraocular lens (T85.2)
  mechanical complication of other ocular prosthetic devices, implants and grafts (T85.3)
  pseudophakia (Z96.1)
  secondary cataracts (H26.4-)
- **+ H59.0 Disorders of the eye following cataract surgery**
  - **+ H59.01 Keratopathy (bullous aphakic) following cataract surgery**
    - Vitreal corneal syndrome
    - Vitreous (touch) syndrome
    - CC H59.011 Keratopathy (bullous aphakic) following cataract surgery, right eye
    - CC H59.012 Keratopathy (bullous aphakic) following cataract surgery, left eye
    - CC H59.013 Keratopathy (bullous aphakic) following cataract surgery, bilateral
    - CC H59.019 Keratopathy (bullous aphakic) following cataract surgery, unspecified eye
  - **+ H59.02 Cataract (lens) fragments in eye following cataract surgery**
    - H59.021 Cataract (lens) fragments in eye following cataract surgery, right eye
    - H59.022 Cataract (lens) fragments in eye following cataract surgery, left eye
    - H59.023 Cataract (lens) fragments in eye following cataract surgery, bilateral
    - H59.029 Cataract (lens) fragments in eye following cataract surgery, unspecified eye
  - **+ H59.03 Cystoid macular edema following cataract surgery**
    - CC H59.031 Cystoid macular edema following cataract surgery, right eye
    - CC H59.032 Cystoid macular edema following cataract surgery, left eye
    - CC H59.033 Cystoid macular edema following cataract surgery, bilateral
    - CC H59.039 Cystoid macular edema following cataract surgery, unspecified eye
  - **+ H59.09 Other disorders of the eye following cataract surgery**
    - CC H59.091 Other disorders of the right eye following cataract surgery
    - CC H59.092 Other disorders of the left eye following cataract surgery
    - CC H59.093 Other disorders of the eye following cataract surgery, bilateral
    - CC H59.099 Other disorders of unspecified eye following cataract surgery
- **+ H59.1 Intraoperative hemorrhage and hematoma of eye and adnexa complicating a procedure**
  - **Excludes1:** intraoperative hemorrhage and hematoma of eye and adnexa due to accidental puncture or laceration during a procedure (H59.2-)
  - **+ H59.11 Intraoperative hemorrhage and hematoma of eye and adnexa complicating an ophthalmic procedure**
    - CC H59.111 Intraoperative hemorrhage and hematoma of right eye and adnexa complicating an ophthalmic procedure
    - CC H59.112 Intraoperative hemorrhage and hematoma of left eye and adnexa complicating an ophthalmic procedure
    - CC H59.113 Intraoperative hemorrhage and hematoma of eye and adnexa complicating an ophthalmic procedure, bilateral
    - CC H59.119 Intraoperative hemorrhage and hematoma of unspecified eye and adnexa complicating an ophthalmic procedure
  - **+ H59.12 Intraoperative hemorrhage and hematoma of eye and adnexa complicating other procedure**
    - CC H59.121 Intraoperative hemorrhage and hematoma of right eye and adnexa complicating other procedure
    - CC H59.122 Intraoperative hemorrhage and hematoma of left eye and adnexa complicating other procedure
    - CC H59.123 Intraoperative hemorrhage and hematoma of eye and adnexa complicating other procedure, bilateral
    - CC H59.129 Intraoperative hemorrhage and hematoma of unspecified eye and adnexa complicating other procedure
- **+ H59.2 Accidental puncture and laceration of eye and adnexa during a procedure**
  - **+ H59.21 Accidental puncture and laceration of eye and adnexa during an ophthalmic procedure**
    - CC H59.211 Accidental puncture and laceration of right eye and adnexa during an ophthalmic procedure
    - CC H59.212 Accidental puncture and laceration of left eye and adnexa during an ophthalmic procedure

- CC H59.213 Accidental puncture and laceration of eye and adnexa during an ophthalmic procedure, bilateral
- CC H59.219 Accidental puncture and laceration of unspecified eye and adnexa during an ophthalmic procedure
- + H59.22 Accidental puncture and laceration of eye and adnexa during other procedure
  - CC H59.221 Accidental puncture and laceration of right eye and adnexa during other procedure
  - CC H59.222 Accidental puncture and laceration of left eye and adnexa during other procedure
  - CC H59.223 Accidental puncture and laceration of eye and adnexa during other procedure, bilateral
  - CC H59.229 Accidental puncture and laceration of unspecified eye and adnexa during other procedure
- + H59.3 Postprocedural hemorrhage, hematoma and seroma of eye and adnexa following a procedure
  - AHA CC: 4Q, 2016, 9-10
  - + H59.31 Postprocedural hemorrhage of eye and adnexa following an ophthalmic procedure
    - CC H59.311 Postprocedural hemorrhage of right eye and adnexa following an ophthalmic procedure
    - CC H59.312 Postprocedural hemorrhage of left eye and adnexa following an ophthalmic procedure
    - CC H59.313 Postprocedural hemorrhage of eye and adnexa following an ophthalmic procedure, bilateral
    - CC H59.319 Postprocedural hemorrhage of unspecified eye and adnexa following an ophthalmic procedure
  - + H59.32 Postprocedural hemorrhage of eye and adnexa following other procedure
    - CC H59.321 Postprocedural hemorrhage of right eye and adnexa following other procedure
    - CC H59.322 Postprocedural hemorrhage of left eye and adnexa following other procedure
    - CC H59.323 Postprocedural hemorrhage of eye and adnexa following other procedure, bilateral
    - CC H59.329 Postprocedural hemorrhage of unspecified eye and adnexa following other procedure
  - + H59.33 Postprocedural hematoma of eye and adnexa following an ophthalmic procedure
    - CC H59.331 Postprocedural hematoma of right eye and adnexa following an ophthalmic procedure
    - CC H59.332 Postprocedural hematoma of left eye and adnexa following an ophthalmic procedure
    - CC H59.333 Postprocedural hematoma of eye and adnexa following an ophthalmic procedure, bilateral
    - CC H59.339 Postprocedural hematoma of unspecified eye and adnexa following an ophthalmic procedure
  - + H59.34 Postprocedural hematoma of eye and adnexa following other procedure
    - CC H59.341 Postprocedural hematoma of right eye and adnexa following other procedure
    - CC H59.342 Postprocedural hematoma of left eye and adnexa following other procedure
    - CC H59.343 Postprocedural hematoma of eye and adnexa following other procedure, bilateral
    - CC H59.349 Postprocedural hematoma of unspecified eye and adnexa following other procedure
  - + H59.35 Postprocedural seroma of eye and adnexa following an ophthalmic procedure
    - CC H59.351 Postprocedural seroma of right eye and adnexa following an ophthalmic procedure
    - CC H59.352 Postprocedural seroma of left eye and adnexa following an ophthalmic procedure
    - CC H59.353 Postprocedural seroma of eye and adnexa following an ophthalmic procedure, bilateral
    - CC H59.359 Postprocedural seroma of unspecified eye and adnexa following an ophthalmic procedure
  - + H59.36 Postprocedural seroma of eye and adnexa following other procedure
    - CC H59.361 Postprocedural seroma of right eye and adnexa following other procedure
    - CC H59.362 Postprocedural seroma of left eye and adnexa following other procedure
    - CC H59.363 Postprocedural seroma of eye and adnexa following other procedure, bilateral
    - CC H59.369 Postprocedural seroma of unspecified eye and adnexa following other procedure
- + H59.4 Inflammation (infection) of postprocedural bleb
  - Postprocedural blebitis
  - **Excludes1:** filtering (vitreous) bleb after glaucoma surgery status (Z98.83)
  - H59.40 Inflammation (infection) of postprocedural bleb, unspecified
  - H59.41 Inflammation (infection) of postprocedural bleb, stage 1
  - H59.42 Inflammation (infection) of postprocedural bleb, stage 2
  - H59.43 Inflammation (infection) of postprocedural bleb, stage 3
    - Bleb endophthalmitis
- + H59.8 Other intraoperative and postprocedural complications and disorders of eye and adnexa, not elsewhere classified
  - + H59.81 Chorioretinal scars after surgery for detachment
    - CC H59.811 Chorioretinal scars after surgery for detachment, right eye
    - CC H59.812 Chorioretinal scars after surgery for detachment, left eye
    - CC H59.813 Chorioretinal scars after surgery for detachment, bilateral
    - CC H59.819 Chorioretinal scars after surgery for detachment, unspecified eye
  - CC H59.88 Other intraoperative complications of eye and adnexa, not elsewhere classified
  - CC H59.89 Other postprocedural complications and disorders of eye and adnexa, not elsewhere classified
    - AHA CC: 3Q, 2020, 29

Chapter 8: Diseases of the Ear and Mastoid Process (H60-H95)

NOTE Use an external cause code following the code for the ear condition, if applicable, to identify the cause of the ear condition

Excludes2: *certain conditions originating in the perinatal period (P04-P96)*
certain infectious and parasitic diseases (A00-B99)
complications of pregnancy, childbirth and the puerperium (O00-O9A)
congenital malformations, deformations and chromosomal abnormalities (Q00-Q99)
endocrine, nutritional and metabolic diseases (E00-E88)
injury, poisoning and certain other consequences of external causes (S00-T88)
neoplasms (C00-D49)
symptoms, signs and abnormal clinical and laboratory findings, not elsewhere classified (R00-R94)

This chapter contains the following category blocks:
- H60-H62 Diseases of external ear
- H65-H75 Diseases of middle ear and mastoid
- H80-H83 Diseases of inner ear
- H90-H94 Other disorders of ear
- H95 Intraoperative and postprocedural complications and disorders of ear and mastoid process, not elsewhere classified

C. Chapter-Specific Coding Guidelines

In addition to general coding guidelines, there are guidelines for specific diagnoses and/or conditions in the classification. Unless otherwise indicated, these guidelines apply to all health care settings. Please refer to Section II for guidelines on the selection of principal diagnosis.

8. Chapter 8: Diseases of the Ear and Mastoid Process (H60-H95)

Reserved for future guideline expansion

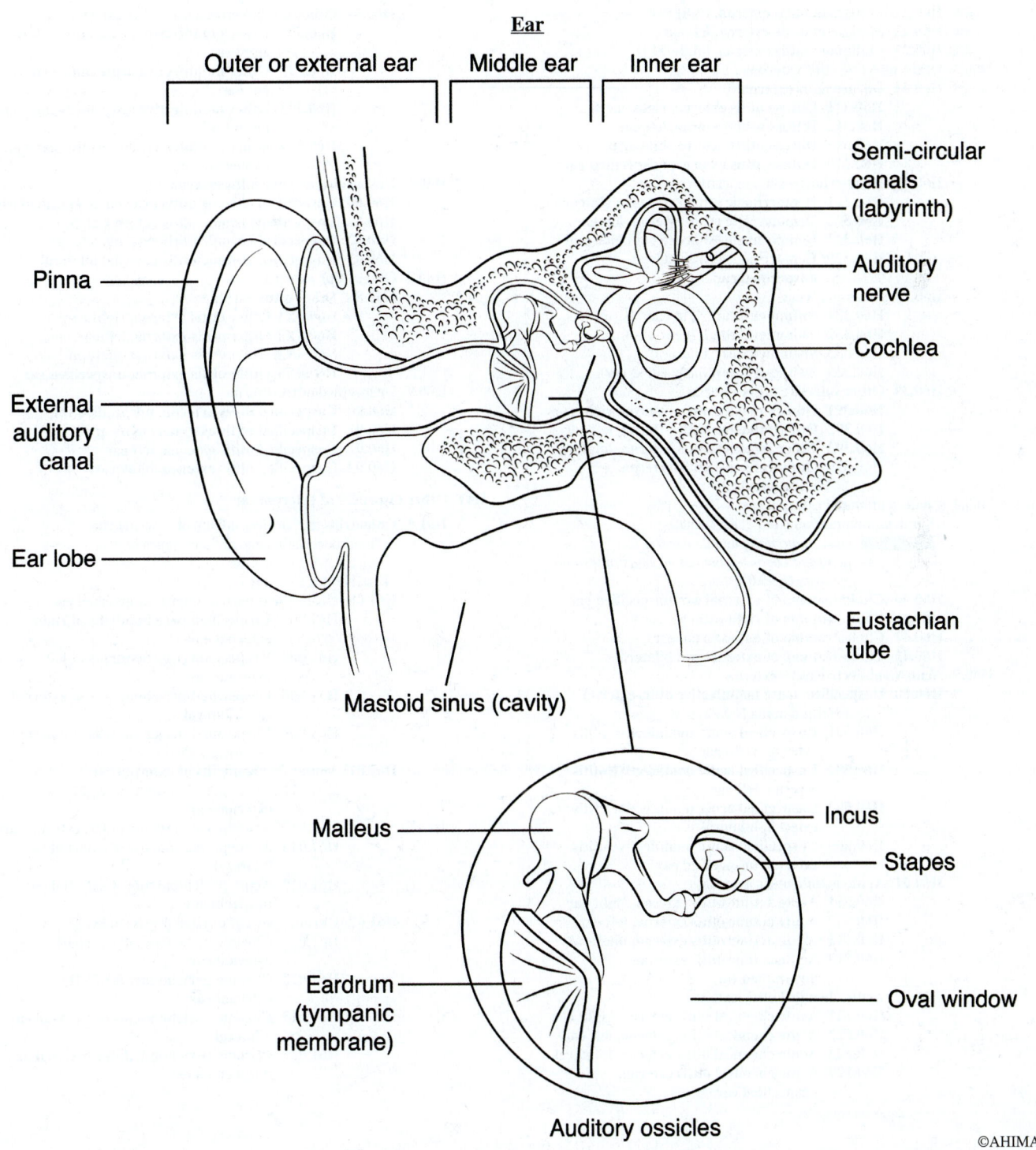

Diseases of external ear (H60-H62)

H60 Otitis externa

- **+ H60.0 Abscess of external ear**
  - Boil of external ear
  - Carbuncle of auricle or external auditory canal
  - Furuncle of external ear
  - H60.00 Abscess of external ear, unspecified ear
  - H60.01 Abscess of right external ear
  - H60.02 Abscess of left external ear
  - H60.03 Abscess of external ear, bilateral
- **+ H60.1 Cellulitis of external ear**
  - Cellulitis of auricle
  - Cellulitis of external auditory canal
  - H60.10 Cellulitis of external ear, unspecified ear
  - H60.11 Cellulitis of right external ear
  - H60.12 Cellulitis of left external ear
  - H60.13 Cellulitis of external ear, bilateral
- **+ H60.2 Malignant otitis externa**
  - CC H60.20 Malignant otitis externa, unspecified ear
  - CC H60.21 Malignant otitis externa, right ear
  - CC H60.22 Malignant otitis externa, left ear
  - CC H60.23 Malignant otitis externa, bilateral
- **+ H60.3 Other infective otitis externa**
  - **+ H60.31 Diffuse otitis externa**
    - H60.311 Diffuse otitis externa, right ear
    - H60.312 Diffuse otitis externa, left ear
    - H60.313 Diffuse otitis externa, bilateral
    - H60.319 Diffuse otitis externa, unspecified ear
  - **+ H60.32 Hemorrhagic otitis externa**
    - H60.321 Hemorrhagic otitis externa, right ear
    - H60.322 Hemorrhagic otitis externa, left ear
    - H60.323 Hemorrhagic otitis externa, bilateral
    - H60.329 Hemorrhagic otitis externa, unspecified ear
  - **+ H60.33 Swimmer's ear**
    - H60.331 Swimmer's ear, right ear
    - H60.332 Swimmer's ear, left ear
    - H60.333 Swimmer's ear, bilateral
    - H60.339 Swimmer's ear, unspecified ear
  - **+ H60.39 Other infective otitis externa**
    - H60.391 Other infective otitis externa, right ear
    - H60.392 Other infective otitis externa, left ear
    - H60.393 Other infective otitis externa, bilateral
    - H60.399 Other infective otitis externa, unspecified ear
- **+ H60.4 Cholesteatoma of external ear**
  - Keratosis obturans of external ear (canal)
  - **Excludes2:** cholesteatoma of middle ear (H71.-)
    recurrent cholesteatoma of postmastoidectomy cavity (H95.0-)
  - H60.40 Cholesteatoma of external ear, unspecified ear
  - H60.41 Cholesteatoma of right external ear
  - H60.42 Cholesteatoma of left external ear
  - H60.43 Cholesteatoma of external ear, bilateral
- **+ H60.5 Acute noninfective otitis externa**
  - **+ H60.50 Unspecified acute noninfective otitis externa**
    - Acute otitis externa NOS
    - H60.501 Unspecified acute noninfective otitis externa, right ear
    - H60.502 Unspecified acute noninfective otitis externa, left ear
    - H60.503 Unspecified acute noninfective otitis externa, bilateral
    - H60.509 Unspecified acute noninfective otitis externa, unspecified ear
  - **+ H60.51 Acute actinic otitis externa**
    - H60.511 Acute actinic otitis externa, right ear
    - H60.512 Acute actinic otitis externa, left ear
    - H60.513 Acute actinic otitis externa, bilateral
    - H60.519 Acute actinic otitis externa, unspecified ear
  - **+ H60.52 Acute chemical otitis externa**
    - H60.521 Acute chemical otitis externa, right ear
    - H60.522 Acute chemical otitis externa, left ear
    - H60.523 Acute chemical otitis externa, bilateral
    - H60.529 Acute chemical otitis externa, unspecified ear
  - **+ H60.53 Acute contact otitis externa**
    - H60.531 Acute contact otitis externa, right ear
    - H60.532 Acute contact otitis externa, left ear
    - H60.533 Acute contact otitis externa, bilateral
    - H60.539 Acute contact otitis externa, unspecified ear
  - **+ H60.54 Acute eczematoid otitis externa**
    - H60.541 Acute eczematoid otitis externa, right ear
    - H60.542 Acute eczematoid otitis externa, left ear
    - H60.543 Acute eczematoid otitis externa, bilateral
    - H60.549 Acute eczematoid otitis externa, unspecified ear
  - **+ H60.55 Acute reactive otitis externa**
    - H60.551 Acute reactive otitis externa, right ear
    - H60.552 Acute reactive otitis externa, left ear
    - H60.553 Acute reactive otitis externa, bilateral
    - H60.559 Acute reactive otitis externa, unspecified ear
  - **+ H60.59 Other noninfective acute otitis externa**
    - H60.591 Other noninfective acute otitis externa, right ear
    - H60.592 Other noninfective acute otitis externa, left ear
    - H60.593 Other noninfective acute otitis externa, bilateral
    - H60.599 Other noninfective acute otitis externa, unspecified ear
- **+ H60.6 Unspecified chronic otitis externa**
  - H60.60 Unspecified chronic otitis externa, unspecified ear
  - H60.61 Unspecified chronic otitis externa, right ear
  - H60.62 Unspecified chronic otitis externa, left ear
  - H60.63 Unspecified chronic otitis externa, bilateral
- **+ H60.8 Other otitis externa**
  - **+ H60.8X Other otitis externa**
    - H60.8X1 Other otitis externa, right ear
    - H60.8X2 Other otitis externa, left ear
    - H60.8X3 Other otitis externa, bilateral
    - H60.8X9 Other otitis externa, unspecified ear
- **+ H60.9 Unspecified otitis externa**
  - H60.90 Unspecified otitis externa, unspecified ear
  - H60.91 Unspecified otitis externa, right ear
  - H60.92 Unspecified otitis externa, left ear
  - H60.93 Unspecified otitis externa, bilateral

H61 Other disorders of external ear

- **+ H61.0 Chondritis and perichondritis of external ear**
  - Chondrodermatitis nodularis chronica helicis
  - Perichondritis of auricle
  - Perichondritis of pinna
  - **+ H61.00 Unspecified perichondritis of external ear**
    - H61.001 Unspecified perichondritis of right external ear
    - H61.002 Unspecified perichondritis of left external ear
    - H61.003 Unspecified perichondritis of external ear, bilateral
    - H61.009 Unspecified perichondritis of external ear, unspecified ear
  - **+ H61.01 Acute perichondritis of external ear**
    - H61.011 Acute perichondritis of right external ear
    - H61.012 Acute perichondritis of left external ear
    - H61.013 Acute perichondritis of external ear, bilateral
    - H61.019 Acute perichondritis of external ear, unspecified ear
  - **+ H61.02 Chronic perichondritis of external ear**
    - H61.021 Chronic perichondritis of right external ear
    - H61.022 Chronic perichondritis of left external ear
    - H61.023 Chronic perichondritis of external ear, bilateral
    - H61.029 Chronic perichondritis of external ear, unspecified ear

- **+ H61.03 Chondritis of external ear**
  Chondritis of auricle
  Chondritis of pinna
  - H61.031 Chondritis of right external ear
  - H61.032 Chondritis of left external ear
    AHA CC: 1Q, 2015, 18-19
  - H61.033 Chondritis of external ear, bilateral
  - H61.039 Chondritis of external ear, unspecified ear
- **+ H61.1 Noninfective disorders of pinna**
  Excludes2: *cauliflower ear (M95.1-)*
  gouty tophi of ear (M1A.-)
  - **+ H61.10 Unspecified noninfective disorders of pinna**
    Disorder of pinna NOS
    - H61.101 Unspecified noninfective disorders of pinna, right ear
    - H61.102 Unspecified noninfective disorders of pinna, left ear
    - H61.103 Unspecified noninfective disorders of pinna, bilateral
    - H61.109 Unspecified noninfective disorders of pinna, unspecified ear
  - **+ H61.11 Acquired deformity of pinna**
    Acquired deformity of auricle
    Excludes2: *cauliflower ear (M95.1-)*
    - H61.111 Acquired deformity of pinna, right ear
    - H61.112 Acquired deformity of pinna, left ear
    - H61.113 Acquired deformity of pinna, bilateral
    - H61.119 Acquired deformity of pinna, unspecified ear
  - **+ H61.12 Hematoma of pinna**
    Hematoma of auricle
    - H61.121 Hematoma of pinna, right ear
    - H61.122 Hematoma of pinna, left ear
    - H61.123 Hematoma of pinna, bilateral
    - H61.129 Hematoma of pinna, unspecified ear
  - **+ H61.19 Other noninfective disorders of pinna**
    - H61.191 Noninfective disorders of pinna, right ear
    - H61.192 Noninfective disorders of pinna, left ear
    - H61.193 Noninfective disorders of pinna, bilateral
    - H61.199 Noninfective disorders of pinna, unspecified ear
- **+ H61.2 Impacted cerumen**
  Wax in ear
  - H61.20 Impacted cerumen, unspecified ear
  - H61.21 Impacted cerumen, right ear
  - H61.22 Impacted cerumen, left ear
  - H61.23 Impacted cerumen, bilateral
- **+ H61.3 Acquired stenosis of external ear canal**
  Collapse of external ear canal
  Excludes1: *postprocedural stenosis of external ear canal (H95.81-)*
  - **+ H61.30 Acquired stenosis of external ear canal, unspecified**
    - H61.301 Acquired stenosis of right external ear canal, unspecified
    - H61.302 Acquired stenosis of left external ear canal, unspecified
    - H61.303 Acquired stenosis of external ear canal, unspecified, bilateral
    - H61.309 Acquired stenosis of external ear canal, unspecified, unspecified ear
  - **+ H61.31 Acquired stenosis of external ear canal secondary to trauma**
    - H61.311 Acquired stenosis of right external ear canal secondary to trauma
    - H61.312 Acquired stenosis of left external ear canal secondary to trauma
    - H61.313 Acquired stenosis of external ear canal secondary to trauma, bilateral
    - H61.319 Acquired stenosis of external ear canal secondary to trauma, unspecified ear
  - **+ H61.32 Acquired stenosis of external ear canal secondary to inflammation and infection**
    - H61.321 Acquired stenosis of right external ear canal secondary to inflammation and infection
    - H61.322 Acquired stenosis of left external ear canal secondary to inflammation and infection
    - H61.323 Acquired stenosis of external ear canal secondary to inflammation and infection, bilateral
    - H61.329 Acquired stenosis of external ear canal secondary to inflammation and infection, unspecified ear
  - **+ H61.39 Other acquired stenosis of external ear canal**
    - H61.391 Other acquired stenosis of right external ear canal
    - H61.392 Other acquired stenosis of left external ear canal
    - H61.393 Other acquired stenosis of external ear canal, bilateral
    - H61.399 Other acquired stenosis of external ear canal, unspecified ear
- **+ H61.8 Other specified disorders of external ear**
  - **+ H61.81 Exostosis of external canal**
    - H61.811 Exostosis of right external canal
    - H61.812 Exostosis of left external canal
    - H61.813 Exostosis of external canal, bilateral
    - H61.819 Exostosis of external canal, unspecified
  - **+ H61.89 Other specified disorders of external ear**
    - H61.891 Other specified disorders of right external ear
    - H61.892 Other specified disorders of left external ear
    - H61.893 Other specified disorders of external ear, bilateral
    - H61.899 Other specified disorders of external ear, unspecified ear
- **+ H61.9 Disorder of external ear, unspecified**
  - H61.90 Disorder of external ear, unspecified, unspecified ear
  - H61.91 Disorder of right external ear, unspecified
  - H61.92 Disorder of left external ear, unspecified
  - H61.93 Disorder of external ear, unspecified, bilateral

H62 Disorders of external ear in diseases classified elsewhere

- **+ H62.4 Otitis externa in other diseases classified elsewhere**
  Code first underlying disease, such as:
  erysipelas (A46)
  impetigo (L01.0-)
  Excludes1: *otitis externa (in):*
  candidiasis (B37.84)
  herpes viral [herpes simplex] (B00.1)
  herpes zoster (B02.8)
  - H62.40 Otitis externa in other diseases classified elsewhere, unspecified ear
  - H62.41 Otitis externa in other diseases classified elsewhere, right ear
  - H62.42 Otitis externa in other diseases classified elsewhere, left ear
  - H62.43 Otitis externa in other diseases classified elsewhere, bilateral
- **+ H62.8 Other disorders of external ear in diseases classified elsewhere**
  Code first underlying disease, such as:
  gout (M1A.-, M10.-)
  - **+ H62.8X Other disorders of external ear in diseases classified elsewhere**
    - H62.8X1 Other disorders of right external ear in diseases classified elsewhere
    - H62.8X2 Other disorders of left external ear in diseases classified elsewhere
    - H62.8X3 Other disorders of external ear in diseases classified elsewhere, bilateral
    - H62.8X9 Other disorders of external ear in diseases classified elsewhere, unspecified ear

Diseases of middle ear and mastoid (H65-H75)

H65 Nonsuppurative otitis media

Includes: nonsuppurative otitis media with myringitis

Use additional code for any associated perforated tympanic membrane (H72.-)

Use additional code, if applicable, to identify:
- exposure to environmental tobacco smoke (Z77.22)
- exposure to tobacco smoke in the perinatal period (P96.81)
- history of tobacco dependence (Z87.891)
- infectious agent (B95-B97)
- occupational exposure to environmental tobacco smoke (Z57.31)
- tobacco dependence (F17.-)
- tobacco use (Z72.0)

- **+ H65.0 Acute serous otitis media**
  Acute and subacute secretory otitis
  - H65.00 Acute serous otitis media, unspecified ear
  - H65.01 Acute serous otitis media, right ear
  - H65.02 Acute serous otitis media, left ear
  - H65.03 Acute serous otitis media, bilateral
  - H65.04 Acute serous otitis media, recurrent, right ear
  - H65.05 Acute serous otitis media, recurrent, left ear
  - H65.06 Acute serous otitis media, recurrent, bilateral
  - H65.07 Acute serous otitis media, recurrent, unspecified ear

- **+ H65.1 Other acute nonsuppurative otitis media**
  Excludes1: otitic barotrauma (T70.0)
  otitis media (acute) NOS (H66.9)

  - **+ H65.11 Acute and subacute allergic otitis media (mucoid) (sanguinous) (serous)**
    - H65.111 Acute and subacute allergic otitis media (mucoid) (sanguinous) (serous), right ear
    - H65.112 Acute and subacute allergic otitis media (mucoid) (sanguinous) (serous), left ear
    - H65.113 Acute and subacute allergic otitis media (mucoid) (sanguinous) (serous), bilateral
    - H65.114 Acute and subacute allergic otitis media (mucoid) (sanguinous) (serous), recurrent, right ear
    - H65.115 Acute and subacute allergic otitis media (mucoid) (sanguinous) (serous), recurrent, left ear
    - H65.116 Acute and subacute allergic otitis media (mucoid) (sanguinous) (serous), recurrent, bilateral
    - H65.117 Acute and subacute allergic otitis media (mucoid) (sanguinous) (serous), recurrent, unspecified ear
    - H65.119 Acute and subacute allergic otitis media (mucoid) (sanguinous) (serous), unspecified ear

  - **+ H65.19 Other acute nonsuppurative otitis media**
    Acute and subacute mucoid otitis media
    Acute and subacute nonsuppurative otitis media NOS
    Acute and subacute sanguinous otitis media
    Acute and subacute seromucinous otitis media
    - H65.191 Other acute nonsuppurative otitis media, right ear
    - H65.192 Other acute nonsuppurative otitis media, left ear
    - H65.193 Other acute nonsuppurative otitis media, bilateral
    - H65.194 Other acute nonsuppurative otitis media, recurrent, right ear
    - H65.195 Other acute nonsuppurative otitis media, recurrent, left ear
    - H65.196 Other acute nonsuppurative otitis media, recurrent, bilateral
    - H65.197 Other acute nonsuppurative otitis media recurrent, unspecified ear
    - H65.199 Other acute nonsuppurative otitis media, unspecified ear

- **+ H65.2 Chronic serous otitis media**
  Chronic tubotympanal catarrh
  - H65.20 Chronic serous otitis media, unspecified ear
  - H65.21 Chronic serous otitis media, right ear
  - H65.22 Chronic serous otitis media, left ear
  - H65.23 Chronic serous otitis media, bilateral

- **+ H65.3 Chronic mucoid otitis media**
  Chronic mucinous otitis media
  Chronic secretory otitis media
  Chronic transudative otitis media
  Glue ear
  Excludes1: adhesive middle ear disease (H74.1)
  - H65.30 Chronic mucoid otitis media, unspecified ear
  - H65.31 Chronic mucoid otitis media, right ear
  - H65.32 Chronic mucoid otitis media, left ear
  - H65.33 Chronic mucoid otitis media, bilateral

- **+ H65.4 Other chronic nonsuppurative otitis media**
  - **+ H65.41 Chronic allergic otitis media**
    - H65.411 Chronic allergic otitis media, right ear
    - H65.412 Chronic allergic otitis media, left ear
    - H65.413 Chronic allergic otitis media, bilateral
    - H65.419 Chronic allergic otitis media, unspecified ear

  - **+ H65.49 Other chronic nonsuppurative otitis media**
    Chronic exudative otitis media
    Chronic nonsuppurative otitis media NOS
    Chronic otitis media with effusion (nonpurulent)
    Chronic seromucinous otitis media
    - H65.491 Other chronic nonsuppurative otitis media, right ear
    - H65.492 Other chronic nonsuppurative otitis media, left ear
    - H65.493 Other chronic nonsuppurative otitis media, bilateral
    - H65.499 Other chronic nonsuppurative otitis media, unspecified ear

- **+ H65.9 Unspecified nonsuppurative otitis media**
  Allergic otitis media NOS
  Catarrhal otitis media NOS
  Exudative otitis media NOS
  Mucoid otitis media NOS
  Otitis media with effusion (nonpurulent) NOS
  Secretory otitis media NOS
  Seromucinous otitis media NOS
  Serous otitis media NOS
  Transudative otitis media NOS
  - H65.90 Unspecified nonsuppurative otitis media, unspecified ear
  - H65.91 Unspecified nonsuppurative otitis media, right ear
  - H65.92 Unspecified nonsuppurative otitis media, left ear
  - H65.93 Unspecified nonsuppurative otitis media, bilateral

H66 Suppurative and unspecified otitis media

Includes: suppurative and unspecified otitis media with myringitis

Use additional code to identify:
- exposure to environmental tobacco smoke (Z77.22)
- exposure to tobacco smoke in the perinatal period (P96.81)
- history of tobacco dependence (Z87.891)
- occupational exposure to environmental tobacco smoke (Z57.31)
- tobacco dependence (F17.-)
- tobacco use (Z72.0)

- **+ H66.0 Acute suppurative otitis media**
  - **+ H66.00 Acute suppurative otitis media without spontaneous rupture of ear drum**
    - H66.001 Acute suppurative otitis media without spontaneous rupture of ear drum, right ear
    - H66.002 Acute suppurative otitis media without spontaneous rupture of ear drum, left ear
    - H66.003 Acute suppurative otitis media without spontaneous rupture of ear drum, bilateral
    - H66.004 Acute suppurative otitis media without spontaneous rupture of ear drum, recurrent, right ear
    - H66.005 Acute suppurative otitis media without spontaneous rupture of ear drum, recurrent, left ear
    - H66.006 Acute suppurative otitis media without spontaneous rupture of ear drum, recurrent, bilateral
    - H66.007 Acute suppurative otitis media without spontaneous rupture of ear drum, recurrent, unspecified ear
    - H66.009 Acute suppurative otitis media without spontaneous rupture of ear drum, unspecified ear

- **+ H66.01 Acute suppurative otitis media with spontaneous rupture of ear drum**
  - H66.011 Acute suppurative otitis media with spontaneous rupture of ear drum, right ear
  - H66.012 Acute suppurative otitis media with spontaneous rupture of ear drum, left ear
  - H66.013 Acute suppurative otitis media with spontaneous rupture of ear drum, bilateral
  - H66.014 Acute suppurative otitis media with spontaneous rupture of ear drum, recurrent, right ear
  - H66.015 Acute suppurative otitis media with spontaneous rupture of ear drum, recurrent, left ear
  - H66.016 Acute suppurative otitis media with spontaneous rupture of ear drum, recurrent, bilateral
  - H66.017 Acute suppurative otitis media with spontaneous rupture of ear drum, recurrent, unspecified ear
  - H66.019 Acute suppurative otitis media with spontaneous rupture of ear drum, unspecified ear
- **+ H66.1 Chronic tubotympanic suppurative otitis media**
  - Benign chronic suppurative otitis media
  - Chronic tubotympanic disease
  - Use additional code for any associated perforated tympanic membrane (H72.-)
  - H66.10 Chronic tubotympanic suppurative otitis media, unspecified
  - H66.11 Chronic tubotympanic suppurative otitis media, right ear
  - H66.12 Chronic tubotympanic suppurative otitis media, left ear
  - H66.13 Chronic tubotympanic suppurative otitis media, bilateral
- **+ H66.2 Chronic atticoantral suppurative otitis media**
  - Chronic atticoantral disease
  - Use additional code for any associated perforated tympanic membrane (H72.-)
  - H66.20 Chronic atticoantral suppurative otitis media, unspecified
  - H66.21 Chronic atticoantral suppurative otitis media, right ear
  - H66.22 Chronic atticoantral suppurative otitis media, left ear
  - H66.23 Chronic atticoantral suppurative otitis media, bilateral
- **+ H66.3 Other chronic suppurative otitis media**
  - Chronic suppurative otitis media NOS
  - Use additional code for any associated perforated tympanic membrane (H72.-)
  - **Excludes1:** tuberculous otitis media (A18.6)
  - **+ H66.3X Other chronic suppurative otitis media**
    - H66.3X1 Other chronic suppurative otitis media, right ear
    - H66.3X2 Other chronic suppurative otitis media, left ear
    - H66.3X3 Other chronic suppurative otitis media, bilateral
    - H66.3X9 Other chronic suppurative otitis media, unspecified ear
- **+ H66.4 Suppurative otitis media, unspecified**
  - Purulent otitis media NOS
  - Use additional code for any associated perforated tympanic membrane (H72.-)
  - H66.40 Suppurative otitis media, unspecified, unspecified ear
  - H66.41 Suppurative otitis media, unspecified, right ear
  - H66.42 Suppurative otitis media, unspecified, left ear
  - H66.43 Suppurative otitis media, unspecified, bilateral
- **+ H66.9 Otitis media, unspecified**
  - Otitis media NOS
  - Acute otitis media NOS
  - Chronic otitis media NOS
  - Use additional code for any associated perforated tympanic membrane (H72.-)
  - H66.90 Otitis media, unspecified, unspecified ear
  - H66.91 Otitis media, unspecified, right ear
  - H66.92 Otitis media, unspecified, left ear
    - *AHA CC: 4Q, 2020, 11-12*
  - H66.93 Otitis media, unspecified, bilateral

H67 Otitis media in diseases classified elsewhere
Code first underlying disease, such as:
  plasminogen deficiency (E88.02)
  viral disease NEC (B00-B34)

Use additional code for any associated perforated tympanic membrane (H72.-)

Excludes1: otitis media in:
  influenza (J09.X9, J10.83, J11.83)
  measles (B05.3)
  scarlet fever (A38.0)
  tuberculosis (A18.6)

- **H67.1** Otitis media in diseases classified elsewhere, right ear
- **H67.2** Otitis media in diseases classified elsewhere, left ear
- **H67.3** Otitis media in diseases classified elsewhere, bilateral
- **H67.9** Otitis media in diseases classified elsewhere, unspecified ear

H68 Eustachian salpingitis and obstruction
- **+ H68.0 Eustachian salpingitis**
  - **+ H68.00 Unspecified Eustachian salpingitis**
    - H68.001 Unspecified Eustachian salpingitis, right ear
    - H68.002 Unspecified Eustachian salpingitis, left ear
    - H68.003 Unspecified Eustachian salpingitis, bilateral
    - H68.009 Unspecified Eustachian salpingitis, unspecified ear
  - **+ H68.01 Acute Eustachian salpingitis**
    - H68.011 Acute Eustachian salpingitis, right ear
    - H68.012 Acute Eustachian salpingitis, left ear
    - H68.013 Acute Eustachian salpingitis, bilateral
    - H68.019 Acute Eustachian salpingitis, unspecified ear
  - **+ H68.02 Chronic Eustachian salpingitis**
    - H68.021 Chronic Eustachian salpingitis, right ear
    - H68.022 Chronic Eustachian salpingitis, left ear
    - H68.023 Chronic Eustachian salpingitis, bilateral
    - H68.029 Chronic Eustachian salpingitis, unspecified ear
- **+ H68.1 Obstruction of Eustachian tube**
  - Stenosis of Eustachian tube
  - Stricture of Eustachian tube
  - **+ H68.10 Unspecified obstruction of Eustachian tube**
    - H68.101 Unspecified obstruction of Eustachian tube, right ear
    - H68.102 Unspecified obstruction of Eustachian tube, left ear
    - H68.103 Unspecified obstruction of Eustachian tube, bilateral
    - H68.109 Unspecified obstruction of Eustachian tube, unspecified ear
  - **+ H68.11 Osseous obstruction of Eustachian tube**
    - H68.111 Osseous obstruction of Eustachian tube, right ear
    - H68.112 Osseous obstruction of Eustachian tube, left ear
    - H68.113 Osseous obstruction of Eustachian tube, bilateral
    - H68.119 Osseous obstruction of Eustachian tube, unspecified ear
  - **+ H68.12 Intrinsic cartilagenous obstruction of Eustachian tube**
    - H68.121 Intrinsic cartilagenous obstruction of Eustachian tube, right ear
    - H68.122 Intrinsic cartilagenous obstruction of Eustachian tube, left ear
    - H68.123 Intrinsic cartilagenous obstruction of Eustachian tube, bilateral
    - H68.129 Intrinsic cartilagenous obstruction of Eustachian tube, unspecified ear

- **H68.13 Extrinsic cartilagenous obstruction of Eustachian tube**
  Compression of Eustachian tube
  - H68.131 Extrinsic cartilagenous obstruction of Eustachian tube, right ear
  - H68.132 Extrinsic cartilagenous obstruction of Eustachian tube, left ear
  - H68.133 Extrinsic cartilagenous obstruction of Eustachian tube, bilateral
  - H68.139 Extrinsic cartilagenous obstruction of Eustachian tube, unspecified ear

H69 Other and unspecified disorders of Eustachian tube
- **H69.0 Patulous Eustachian tube**
  - H69.00 Patulous Eustachian tube, unspecified ear
  - H69.01 Patulous Eustachian tube, right ear
  - H69.02 Patulous Eustachian tube, left ear
  - H69.03 Patulous Eustachian tube, bilateral
- **H69.8 Other specified disorders of Eustachian tube**
  - H69.80 Other specified disorders of Eustachian tube, unspecified ear
  - H69.81 Other specified disorders of Eustachian tube, right ear
  - H69.82 Other specified disorders of Eustachian tube, left ear
  - H69.83 Other specified disorders of Eustachian tube, bilateral
- **H69.9 Unspecified Eustachian tube disorder**
  - H69.90 Unspecified Eustachian tube disorder, unspecified ear
  - H69.91 Unspecified Eustachian tube disorder, right ear
  - H69.92 Unspecified Eustachian tube disorder, left ear
  - H69.93 Unspecified Eustachian tube disorder, bilateral

H70 Mastoiditis and related conditions
- **H70.0 Acute mastoiditis**
  Abscess of mastoid
  Empyema of mastoid
  - **H70.00 Acute mastoiditis without complications**
    - CC H70.001 Acute mastoiditis without complications, right ear
    - CC H70.002 Acute mastoiditis without complications, left ear
    - CC H70.003 Acute mastoiditis without complications, bilateral
    - CC H70.009 Acute mastoiditis without complications, unspecified ear
  - **H70.01 Subperiosteal abscess of mastoid**
    - CC H70.011 Subperiosteal abscess of mastoid, right ear
    - CC H70.012 Subperiosteal abscess of mastoid, left ear
    - CC H70.013 Subperiosteal abscess of mastoid, bilateral
    - CC H70.019 Subperiosteal abscess of mastoid, unspecified ear
  - **H70.09 Acute mastoiditis with other complications**
    - CC H70.091 Acute mastoiditis with other complications, right ear
    - CC H70.092 Acute mastoiditis with other complications, left ear
    - CC H70.093 Acute mastoiditis with other complications, bilateral
    - CC H70.099 Acute mastoiditis with other complications, unspecified ear
- **H70.1 Chronic mastoiditis**
  Caries of mastoid
  Fistula of mastoid
  Excludes1: *tuberculous mastoiditis (A18.03)*
  - H70.10 Chronic mastoiditis, unspecified ear
  - H70.11 Chronic mastoiditis, right ear
  - H70.12 Chronic mastoiditis, left ear
  - H70.13 Chronic mastoiditis, bilateral
- **H70.2 Petrositis**
  Inflammation of petrous bone
  - **H70.20 Unspecified petrositis**
    - H70.201 Unspecified petrositis, right ear
    - H70.202 Unspecified petrositis, left ear
    - H70.203 Unspecified petrositis, bilateral
    - H70.209 Unspecified petrositis, unspecified ear
  - **H70.21 Acute petrositis**
    - H70.211 Acute petrositis, right ear
    - H70.212 Acute petrositis, left ear
    - H70.213 Acute petrositis, bilateral
    - H70.219 Acute petrositis, unspecified ear
  - **H70.22 Chronic petrositis**
    - H70.221 Chronic petrositis, right ear
    - H70.222 Chronic petrositis, left ear
    - H70.223 Chronic petrositis, bilateral
    - H70.229 Chronic petrositis, unspecified ear
- **H70.8 Other mastoiditis and related conditions**
  Excludes1: *preauricular sinus and cyst (Q18.1)*
  sinus, fistula, and cyst of branchial cleft (Q18.0)
  - **H70.81 Postauricular fistula**
    - H70.811 Postauricular fistula, right ear
    - H70.812 Postauricular fistula, left ear
    - H70.813 Postauricular fistula, bilateral
    - H70.819 Postauricular fistula, unspecified ear
  - **H70.89 Other mastoiditis and related conditions**
    - H70.891 Other mastoiditis and related conditions, right ear
    - H70.892 Other mastoiditis and related conditions, left ear
    - H70.893 Other mastoiditis and related conditions, bilateral
    - H70.899 Other mastoiditis and related conditions, unspecified ear
- **H70.9 Unspecified mastoiditis**
  - H70.90 Unspecified mastoiditis, unspecified ear
  - H70.91 Unspecified mastoiditis, right ear
  - H70.92 Unspecified mastoiditis, left ear
  - H70.93 Unspecified mastoiditis, bilateral

H71 Cholesteatoma of middle ear
Excludes2: *cholesteatoma of external ear (H60.4-)*
recurrent cholesteatoma of postmastoidectomy cavity (H95.0-)
- **H71.0 Cholesteatoma of attic**
  - H71.00 Cholesteatoma of attic, unspecified ear
  - H71.01 Cholesteatoma of attic, right ear
  - H71.02 Cholesteatoma of attic, left ear
    AHA CC: 3Q, 2021, 8-9
  - H71.03 Cholesteatoma of attic, bilateral
- **H71.1 Cholesteatoma of tympanum**
  - H71.10 Cholesteatoma of tympanum, unspecified ear
  - H71.11 Cholesteatoma of tympanum, right ear
  - H71.12 Cholesteatoma of tympanum, left ear
  - H71.13 Cholesteatoma of tympanum, bilateral
- **H71.2 Cholesteatoma of mastoid**
  - H71.20 Cholesteatoma of mastoid, unspecified ear
  - H71.21 Cholesteatoma of mastoid, right ear
  - H71.22 Cholesteatoma of mastoid, left ear
    AHA CC: 3Q, 2021, 8-9
  - H71.23 Cholesteatoma of mastoid, bilateral
- **H71.3 Diffuse cholesteatosis**
  AHA CC: 3Q, 2021, 8-9
  - H71.30 Diffuse cholesteatosis, unspecified ear
  - H71.31 Diffuse cholesteatosis, right ear
  - H71.32 Diffuse cholesteatosis, left ear
  - H71.33 Diffuse cholesteatosis, bilateral
- **H71.9 Unspecified cholesteatoma**
  - H71.90 Unspecified cholesteatoma, unspecified ear
  - H71.91 Unspecified cholesteatoma, right ear
  - H71.92 Unspecified cholesteatoma, left ear
  - H71.93 Unspecified cholesteatoma, bilateral

H72 Perforation of tympanic membrane
Includes: persistent post-traumatic perforation of ear drum
postinflammatory perforation of ear drum
Code first any associated otitis media (H65.-, H66.1-, H66.2-, H66.3-, H66.4-, H66.9-, H67.-)
Excludes1: *acute suppurative otitis media with rupture of the tympanic membrane (H66.01-)*
traumatic rupture of ear drum (S09.2-)
- **H72.0 Central perforation of tympanic membrane**
  - H72.00 Central perforation of tympanic membrane, unspecified ear
  - H72.01 Central perforation of tympanic membrane, right ear

- H72.02 Central perforation of tympanic membrane, left ear
- H72.03 Central perforation of tympanic membrane, bilateral
- **+ H72.1 Attic perforation of tympanic membrane**
  Perforation of pars flaccida
  - H72.10 Attic perforation of tympanic membrane, unspecified ear
  - H72.11 Attic perforation of tympanic membrane, right ear
  - H72.12 Attic perforation of tympanic membrane, left ear
  - H72.13 Attic perforation of tympanic membrane, bilateral
- **+ H72.2 Other marginal perforations of tympanic membrane**
  - **+ H72.2X Other marginal perforations of tympanic membrane**
    - H72.2X1 Other marginal perforations of tympanic membrane, right ear
    - H72.2X2 Other marginal perforations of tympanic membrane, left ear
    - H72.2X3 Other marginal perforations of tympanic membrane, bilateral
    - H72.2X9 Other marginal perforations of tympanic membrane, unspecified ear
- **+ H72.8 Other perforations of tympanic membrane**
  - **+ H72.81 Multiple perforations of tympanic membrane**
    - H72.811 Multiple perforations of tympanic membrane, right ear
    - H72.812 Multiple perforations of tympanic membrane, left ear
    - H72.813 Multiple perforations of tympanic membrane, bilateral
    - H72.819 Multiple perforations of tympanic membrane, unspecified ear
  - **+ H72.82 Total perforations of tympanic membrane**
    - H72.821 Total perforations of tympanic membrane, right ear
    - H72.822 Total perforations of tympanic membrane, left ear
    - H72.823 Total perforations of tympanic membrane, bilateral
    - H72.829 Total perforations of tympanic membrane, unspecified ear
- **+ H72.9 Unspecified perforation of tympanic membrane**
  - H72.90 Unspecified perforation of tympanic membrane, unspecified ear
  - H72.91 Unspecified perforation of tympanic membrane, right ear
  - H72.92 Unspecified perforation of tympanic membrane, left ear
  - H72.93 Unspecified perforation of tympanic membrane, bilateral

H73 Other disorders of tympanic membrane

- **+ H73.0 Acute myringitis**
  Excludes1: acute myringitis with otitis media (H65, H66)
  - **+ H73.00 Unspecified acute myringitis**
    Acute tympanitis NOS
    - H73.001 Acute myringitis, right ear
    - H73.002 Acute myringitis, left ear
    - H73.003 Acute myringitis, bilateral
    - H73.009 Acute myringitis, unspecified ear
  - **+ H73.01 Bullous myringitis**
    - H73.011 Bullous myringitis, right ear
    - H73.012 Bullous myringitis, left ear
    - H73.013 Bullous myringitis, bilateral
    - H73.019 Bullous myringitis, unspecified ear
  - **+ H73.09 Other acute myringitis**
    - H73.091 Other acute myringitis, right ear
    - H73.092 Other acute myringitis, left ear
    - H73.093 Other acute myringitis, bilateral
    - H73.099 Other acute myringitis, unspecified ear
- **+ H73.1 Chronic myringitis**
  Chronic tympanitis
  Excludes1: chronic myringitis with otitis media (H65, H66)
  - H73.10 Chronic myringitis, unspecified ear
  - H73.11 Chronic myringitis, right ear
  - H73.12 Chronic myringitis, left ear
  - H73.13 Chronic myringitis, bilateral
- **+ H73.2 Unspecified myringitis**
  - H73.20 Unspecified myringitis, unspecified ear
  - H73.21 Unspecified myringitis, right ear
  - H73.22 Unspecified myringitis, left ear
  - H73.23 Unspecified myringitis, bilateral
- **+ H73.8 Other specified disorders of tympanic membrane**
  - **+ H73.81 Atrophic flaccid tympanic membrane**
    - H73.811 Atrophic flaccid tympanic membrane, right ear
    - H73.812 Atrophic flaccid tympanic membrane, left ear
    - H73.813 Atrophic flaccid tympanic membrane, bilateral
    - H73.819 Atrophic flaccid tympanic membrane, unspecified ear
  - **+ H73.82 Atrophic nonflaccid tympanic membrane**
    - H73.821 Atrophic nonflaccid tympanic membrane, right ear
    - H73.822 Atrophic nonflaccid tympanic membrane, left ear
    - H73.823 Atrophic nonflaccid tympanic membrane, bilateral
    - H73.829 Atrophic nonflaccid tympanic membrane, unspecified ear
  - **+ H73.89 Other specified disorders of tympanic membrane**
    - H73.891 Other specified disorders of tympanic membrane, right ear
    - H73.892 Other specified disorders of tympanic membrane, left ear
    - H73.893 Other specified disorders of tympanic membrane, bilateral
    - H73.899 Other specified disorders of tympanic membrane, unspecified ear
- **+ H73.9 Unspecified disorder of tympanic membrane**
  - H73.90 Unspecified disorder of tympanic membrane, unspecified ear
  - H73.91 Unspecified disorder of tympanic membrane, right ear
  - H73.92 Unspecified disorder of tympanic membrane, left ear
  - H73.93 Unspecified disorder of tympanic membrane, bilateral

H74 Other disorders of middle ear mastoid

Excludes2: mastoiditis (H70.-)

- **+ H74.0 Tympanosclerosis**
  - H74.01 Tympanosclerosis, right ear
  - H74.02 Tympanosclerosis, left ear
  - H74.03 Tympanosclerosis, bilateral
  - H74.09 Tympanosclerosis, unspecified ear
- **+ H74.1 Adhesive middle ear disease**
  Adhesive otitis
  Excludes1: glue ear (H65.3-)
  - H74.11 Adhesive right middle ear disease
  - H74.12 Adhesive left middle ear disease
  - H74.13 Adhesive middle ear disease, bilateral
  - H74.19 Adhesive middle ear disease, unspecified ear
- **+ H74.2 Discontinuity and dislocation of ear ossicles**
  - H74.20 Discontinuity and dislocation of ear ossicles, unspecified ear
  - H74.21 Discontinuity and dislocation of right ear ossicles
  - H74.22 Discontinuity and dislocation of left ear ossicles
  - H74.23 Discontinuity and dislocation of ear ossicles, bilateral
- **+ H74.3 Other acquired abnormalities of ear ossicles**
  - **+ H74.31 Ankylosis of ear ossicles**
    - H74.311 Ankylosis of ear ossicles, right ear
    - H74.312 Ankylosis of ear ossicles, left ear
    - H74.313 Ankylosis of ear ossicles, bilateral
    - H74.319 Ankylosis of ear ossicles, unspecified ear
  - **+ H74.32 Partial loss of ear ossicles**
    - H74.321 Partial loss of ear ossicles, right ear
    - H74.322 Partial loss of ear ossicles, left ear
    - H74.323 Partial loss of ear ossicles, bilateral
    - H74.329 Partial loss of ear ossicles, unspecified ear
  - **+ H74.39 Other acquired abnormalities of ear ossicles**
    - H74.391 Other acquired abnormalities of right ear ossicles

H74.392 Other acquired abnormalities of left ear ossicles
H74.393 Other acquired abnormalities of ear ossicles, bilateral
H74.399 Other acquired abnormalities of ear ossicles, unspecified ear

+ **H74.4 Polyp of middle ear**
H74.40 Polyp of middle ear, unspecified ear
H74.41 Polyp of right middle ear
H74.42 Polyp of left middle ear
H74.43 Polyp of middle ear, bilateral

+ **H74.8 Other specified disorders of middle ear and mastoid**
  + **H74.8X Other specified disorders of middle ear and mastoid**
    H74.8X1 Other specified disorders of right middle ear and mastoid
    H74.8X2 Other specified disorders of left middle ear and mastoid
    H74.8X3 Other specified disorders of middle ear and mastoid, bilateral
    H74.8X9 Other specified disorders of middle ear and mastoid, unspecified ear

+ **H74.9 Unspecified disorder of middle ear and mastoid**
  H74.90 Unspecified disorder of middle ear and mastoid, unspecified ear
  H74.91 Unspecified disorder of right middle ear and mastoid
  H74.92 Unspecified disorder of left middle ear and mastoid
  H74.93 Unspecified disorder of middle ear and mastoid, bilateral

H75 Other disorders of middle ear and mastoid in diseases classified elsewhere

Code first underlying disease

+ **H75.0 Mastoiditis in infectious and parasitic diseases classified elsewhere**

  Excludes1: mastoiditis (in):
  syphilis (A52.77)
  tuberculosis (A18.03)

  H75.00 Mastoiditis in infectious and parasitic diseases classified elsewhere, unspecified ear
  H75.01 Mastoiditis in infectious and parasitic diseases classified elsewhere, right ear
  H75.02 Mastoiditis in infectious and parasitic diseases classified elsewhere, left ear
  H75.03 Mastoiditis in infectious and parasitic diseases classified elsewhere, bilateral

+ **H75.8 Other specified disorders of middle ear and mastoid in diseases classified elsewhere**
  H75.80 Other specified disorders of middle ear and mastoid in diseases classified elsewhere, unspecified ear
  H75.81 Other specified disorders of right middle ear and mastoid in diseases classified elsewhere
  H75.82 Other specified disorders of left middle ear and mastoid in diseases classified elsewhere
  H75.83 Other specified disorders of middle ear and mastoid in diseases classified elsewhere, bilateral

Diseases of inner ear (H80-H83)

H80 Otosclerosis

Includes: Otospongiosis

+ **H80.0 Otosclerosis involving oval window, nonobliterative**
  H80.00 Otosclerosis involving oval window, nonobliterative, unspecified ear
  H80.01 Otosclerosis involving oval window, nonobliterative, right ear
  H80.02 Otosclerosis involving oval window, nonobliterative, left ear
  H80.03 Otosclerosis involving oval window, nonobliterative, bilateral

+ **H80.1 Otosclerosis involving oval window, obliterative**
  H80.10 Otosclerosis involving oval window, obliterative, unspecified ear
  H80.11 Otosclerosis involving oval window, obliterative, right ear
  H80.12 Otosclerosis involving oval window, obliterative, left ear
  H80.13 Otosclerosis involving oval window, obliterative, bilateral

+ **H80.2 Cochlear otosclerosis**
  Otosclerosis involving otic capsule
  Otosclerosis involving round window
  H80.20 Cochlear otosclerosis, unspecified ear
  H80.21 Cochlear otosclerosis, right ear
  H80.22 Cochlear otosclerosis, left ear
  H80.23 Cochlear otosclerosis, bilateral

+ **H80.8 Other otosclerosis**
  H80.80 Other otosclerosis, unspecified ear
  H80.81 Other otosclerosis, right ear
  H80.82 Other otosclerosis, left ear
  H80.83 Other otosclerosis, bilateral

+ **H80.9 Unspecified otosclerosis**
  H80.90 Unspecified otosclerosis, unspecified ear
  H80.91 Unspecified otosclerosis, right ear
  H80.92 Unspecified otosclerosis, left ear
  H80.93 Unspecified otosclerosis, bilateral

H81 Disorders of vestibular function

Excludes1: epidemic vertigo (A88.1)
vertigo NOS (R42)

+ **H81.0 Ménière's disease**
  Labyrinthine hydrops
  Ménière's syndrome or vertigo
  H81.01 Ménière's disease, right ear
  H81.02 Ménière's disease, left ear
  H81.03 Ménière's disease, bilateral
  H81.09 Ménière's disease, unspecified ear

+ **H81.1 Benign paroxysmal vertigo**
  H81.10 Benign paroxysmal vertigo, unspecified ear
  H81.11 Benign paroxysmal vertigo, right ear
  H81.12 Benign paroxysmal vertigo, left ear
  H81.13 Benign paroxysmal vertigo, bilateral

+ **H81.2 Vestibular neuronitis**
  H81.20 Vestibular neuronitis, unspecified ear
  H81.21 Vestibular neuronitis, right ear
  H81.22 Vestibular neuronitis, left ear
  H81.23 Vestibular neuronitis, bilateral

+ **H81.3 Other peripheral vertigo**
  + **H81.31 Aural vertigo**
    H81.311 Aural vertigo, right ear
    H81.312 Aural vertigo, left ear
    H81.313 Aural vertigo, bilateral
    H81.319 Aural vertigo, unspecified ear
  + **H81.39 Other peripheral vertigo**
    Lermoyez' syndrome
    Otogenic vertigo
    Peripheral vertigo NOS
    H81.391 Other peripheral vertigo, right ear
    H81.392 Other peripheral vertigo, left ear
    H81.393 Other peripheral vertigo, bilateral
    H81.399 Other peripheral vertigo, unspecified ear

H81.4 Vertigo of central origin
Central positional nystagmus
AHA CC: 4Q, 2019, 4

+ **H81.8 Other disorders of vestibular function**
  + **H81.8X Other disorders of vestibular function**
    H81.8X1 Other disorders of vestibular function, right ear
    H81.8X2 Other disorders of vestibular function, left ear
    H81.8X3 Other disorders of vestibular function, bilateral
    H81.8X9 Other disorders of vestibular function, unspecified ear
    AHA CC: 2Q, 2022, 12-13

+ **H81.9 Unspecified disorder of vestibular function**
  Vertiginous syndrome NOS
  H81.90 Unspecified disorder of vestibular function, unspecified ear
  H81.91 Unspecified disorder of vestibular function, right ear
  H81.92 Unspecified disorder of vestibular function, left ear
  H81.93 Unspecified disorder of vestibular function, bilateral

H82 Vertiginous syndromes in diseases classified elsewhere
   Code first underlying disease
   Excludes1: *epidemic vertigo (A88.1)*
   H82.1 Vertiginous syndromes in diseases classified elsewhere, right ear
   H82.2 Vertiginous syndromes in diseases classified elsewhere, left ear
   H82.3 Vertiginous syndromes in diseases classified elsewhere, bilateral
   H82.9 Vertiginous syndromes in diseases classified elsewhere, unspecified ear

H83 Other diseases of inner ear
   + **H83.0** Labyrinthitis
      H83.01 Labyrinthitis, right ear
      H83.02 Labyrinthitis, left ear
      H83.03 Labyrinthitis, bilateral
      H83.09 Labyrinthitis, unspecified ear
   + **H83.1** Labyrinthine fistula
      H83.11 Labyrinthine fistula, right ear
      H83.12 Labyrinthine fistula, left ear
      H83.13 Labyrinthine fistula, bilateral
      H83.19 Labyrinthine fistula, unspecified ear
   + **H83.2** Labyrinthine dysfunction
      Labyrinthine hypersensitivity
      Labyrinthine hypofunction
      Labyrinthine loss of function
      + **H83.2X** Labyrinthine dysfunction
         H83.2X1 Labyrinthine dysfunction, right ear
         H83.2X2 Labyrinthine dysfunction, left ear
         H83.2X3 Labyrinthine dysfunction, bilateral
         H83.2X9 Labyrinthine dysfunction, unspecified ear
   + **H83.3** Noise effects on inner ear
      Acoustic trauma of inner ear
      Noise-induced hearing loss of inner ear
      + **H83.3X** Noise effects on inner ear
         H83.3X1 Noise effects on right inner ear
         H83.3X2 Noise effects on left inner ear
         H83.3X3 Noise effects on inner ear, bilateral
         H83.3X9 Noise effects on inner ear, unspecified ear
   + **H83.8** Other specified diseases of inner ear
      + **H83.8X** Other specified diseases of inner ear
         H83.8X1 Other specified diseases of right inner ear
         H83.8X2 Other specified diseases of left inner ear
         H83.8X3 Other specified diseases of inner ear, bilateral
         H83.8X9 Other specified diseases of inner ear, unspecified ear
   + **H83.9** Unspecified disease of inner ear
      H83.90 Unspecified disease of inner ear, unspecified ear
      H83.91 Unspecified disease of right inner ear
      H83.92 Unspecified disease of left inner ear
      H83.93 Unspecified disease of inner ear, bilateral

Other disorders of ear (H90-H94)

H90 Conductive and sensorineural hearing loss
   Excludes1: *deaf nonspeaking NEC (H91.3)*
      deafness NOS (H91.9-)
      hearing loss NOS (H91.9-)
      noise-induced hearing loss (H83.3-)
      ototoxic hearing loss (H91.0-)
      sudden (idiopathic) hearing loss (H91.2-)
   H90.0 Conductive hearing loss, bilateral
   + **H90.1** Conductive hearing loss, unilateral with unrestricted hearing on the contralateral side
      H90.11 Conductive hearing loss, unilateral, right ear, with unrestricted hearing on the contralateral side
      H90.12 Conductive hearing loss, unilateral, left ear, with unrestricted hearing on the contralateral side
   H90.2 Conductive hearing loss, unspecified
      Conductive deafness NOS
   H90.3 Sensorineural hearing loss, bilateral
   + **H90.4** Sensorineural hearing loss, unilateral with unrestricted hearing on the contralateral side
      H90.41 Sensorineural hearing loss, unilateral, right ear, with unrestricted hearing on the contralateral side
      H90.42 Sensorineural hearing loss, unilateral, left ear, with unrestricted hearing on the contralateral side
   H90.5 Unspecified sensorineural hearing loss
      Central hearing loss NOS
      Congenital deafness NOS
      Neural hearing loss NOS
      Perceptive hearing loss NOS
      Sensorineural deafness NOS
      Sensory hearing loss NOS
      Excludes1: *abnormal auditory perception (H93.2-)*
         psychogenic deafness (F44.6)
   H90.6 Mixed conductive and sensorineural hearing loss, bilateral
      AHA CC: 2Q, 2015, 7
   + **H90.7** Mixed conductive and sensorineural hearing loss, unilateral with unrestricted hearing on the contralateral side
      H90.71 Mixed conductive and sensorineural hearing loss, unilateral, right ear, with unrestricted hearing on the contralateral side
      H90.72 Mixed conductive and sensorineural hearing loss, unilateral, left ear, with unrestricted hearing on the contralateral side
   H90.8 Mixed conductive and sensorineural hearing loss, unspecified
   + **H90.A** Conductive and sensorineural hearing loss with restricted hearing on the contralateral side
      AHA CC: 4Q, 2016, 23-24
      + **H90.A1** Conductive hearing loss, unilateral, with restricted hearing on the contralateral side
         H90.A11 Conductive hearing loss, unilateral, right ear with restricted hearing on the contralateral side
         H90.A12 Conductive hearing loss, unilateral, left ear with restricted hearing on the contralateral side
         AHA CC: 4Q, 2016, 24-25
      + **H90.A2** Sensorineural hearing loss, unilateral, with restricted hearing on the contralateral side
         H90.A21 Sensorineural hearing loss, unilateral, right ear, with restricted hearing on the contralateral side
         AHA CC: 4Q, 2016, 24-25
         H90.A22 Sensorineural hearing loss, unilateral, left ear, with restricted hearing on the contralateral side
      + **H90.A3** Mixed conductive and sensorineural hearing loss, unilateral with restricted hearing on the contralateral side
         H90.A31 Mixed conductive and sensorineural hearing loss, unilateral, right ear with restricted hearing on the contralateral side
         H90.A32 Mixed conductive and sensorineural hearing, unilateral, left ear with restricted hearing on the contralateral side

H91 Other and unspecified hearing loss
   Excludes1: *abnormal auditory perception (H93.2-)*
      hearing loss as classified in H90.-
      impacted cerumen (H61.2-)
      noise-induced hearing loss (H83.3-)
      psychogenic deafness (F44.6)
      transient ischemic deafness (H93.01-)

- **H91.0 Ototoxic hearing loss**
  Code first poisoning due to drug or toxin, if applicable (T36-T65 with fifth or sixth character 1-4)
  Use additional code for adverse effect, if applicable, to identify drug (T36-T50 with fifth or sixth character 5)
  - H91.01 Ototoxic hearing loss, right ear
  - H91.02 Ototoxic hearing loss, left ear
  - H91.03 Ototoxic hearing loss, bilateral
  - H91.09 Ototoxic hearing loss, unspecified ear
- **H91.1 Presbycusis**
  Presbyacusia
  - H91.10 Presbycusis, unspecified ear
  - H91.11 Presbycusis, right ear
  - H91.12 Presbycusis, left ear
  - H91.13 Presbycusis, bilateral
- **H91.2 Sudden idiopathic hearing loss**
  Sudden hearing loss NOS
  - H91.20 Sudden idiopathic hearing loss, unspecified ear
  - H91.21 Sudden idiopathic hearing loss, right ear
  - H91.22 Sudden idiopathic hearing loss, left ear
  - H91.23 Sudden idiopathic hearing loss, bilateral
- H91.3 Deaf nonspeaking, not elsewhere classified
- **H91.8 Other specified hearing loss**
  - **H91.8X Other specified hearing loss**
    - H91.8X1 Other specified hearing loss, right ear
    - H91.8X2 Other specified hearing loss, left ear
    - H91.8X3 Other specified hearing loss, bilateral
    - H91.8X9 Other specified hearing loss, unspecified ear
- **H91.9 Unspecified hearing loss**
  Deafness NOS
  High frequency deafness
  Low frequency deafness
  - H91.90 Unspecified hearing loss, unspecified ear
  - H91.91 Unspecified hearing loss, right ear
  - H91.92 Unspecified hearing loss, left ear
  - H91.93 Unspecified hearing loss, bilateral

H92 Otalgia and effusion of ear

- **H92.0 Otalgia**
  - H92.01 Otalgia, right ear
  - H92.02 Otalgia, left ear
  - H92.03 Otalgia, bilateral
  - H92.09 Otalgia, unspecified ear
- **H92.1 Otorrhea**
  Excludes1: leakage of cerebrospinal fluid through ear (G96.0)
  - H92.10 Otorrhea, unspecified ear
  - H92.11 Otorrhea, right ear
  - H92.12 Otorrhea, left ear
  - H92.13 Otorrhea, bilateral
- **H92.2 Otorrhagia**
  Excludes1: traumatic otorrhagia - code to injury
  - H92.20 Otorrhagia, unspecified ear
  - H92.21 Otorrhagia, right ear
  - H92.22 Otorrhagia, left ear
  - H92.23 Otorrhagia, bilateral

H93 Other disorders of ear, not elsewhere classified

- **H93.0 Degenerative and vascular disorders of ear**
  Excludes1: presbycusis (H91.1)
  - **H93.01 Transient ischemic deafness**
    - H93.011 Transient ischemic deafness, right ear
    - H93.012 Transient ischemic deafness, left ear
    - H93.013 Transient ischemic deafness, bilateral
    - H93.019 Transient ischemic deafness, unspecified ear
  - **H93.09 Unspecified degenerative and vascular disorders of ear**
    - H93.091 Unspecified degenerative and vascular disorders of right ear
    - H93.092 Unspecified degenerative and vascular disorders of left ear
    - H93.093 Unspecified degenerative and vascular disorders of ear, bilateral
    - H93.099 Unspecified degenerative and vascular disorders of unspecified ear
- **H93.1 Tinnitus**
  - H93.11 Tinnitus, right ear
  - H93.12 Tinnitus, left ear
  - H93.13 Tinnitus, bilateral
  - H93.19 Tinnitus, unspecified ear
- **H93.A Pulsatile tinnitus**
  AHA CC: 4Q, 2016, 25-26
  - H93.A1 Pulsatile tinnitus, right ear
    AHA CC: 4Q, 2016, 26; 2Q, 2023, 18-19
  - H93.A2 Pulsatile tinnitus, left ear
  - H93.A3 Pulsatile tinnitus, bilateral
  - H93.A9 Pulsatile tinnitus, unspecified ear
- **H93.2 Other abnormal auditory perceptions**
  Excludes2: auditory hallucinations (R44.0)
  - **H93.21 Auditory recruitment**
    - H93.211 Auditory recruitment, right ear
    - H93.212 Auditory recruitment, left ear
    - H93.213 Auditory recruitment, bilateral
    - H93.219 Auditory recruitment, unspecified ear
  - **H93.22 Diplacusis**
    - H93.221 Diplacusis, right ear
    - H93.222 Diplacusis, left ear
    - H93.223 Diplacusis, bilateral
    - H93.229 Diplacusis, unspecified ear
  - **H93.23 Hyperacusis**
    - H93.231 Hyperacusis, right ear
    - H93.232 Hyperacusis, left ear
    - H93.233 Hyperacusis, bilateral
    - H93.239 Hyperacusis, unspecified ear
  - **H93.24 Temporary auditory threshold shift**
    - H93.241 Temporary auditory threshold shift, right ear
    - H93.242 Temporary auditory threshold shift, left ear
    - H93.243 Temporary auditory threshold shift, bilateral
    - H93.249 Temporary auditory threshold shift, unspecified ear
  - H93.25 Central auditory processing disorder
    Congenital auditory imperception
    Word deafness
    Excludes1: mixed receptive-expressive language disorder (F80.2)
  - **H93.29 Other abnormal auditory perceptions**
    - H93.291 Other abnormal auditory perceptions, right ear
    - H93.292 Other abnormal auditory perceptions, left ear
    - H93.293 Other abnormal auditory perceptions, bilateral
    - H93.299 Other abnormal auditory perceptions, unspecified ear
- **H93.3 Disorders of acoustic nerve**
  Disorder of 8th cranial nerve
  Excludes1: acoustic neuroma (D33.3)
  syphilitic acoustic neuritis (A52.15)
  - **H93.3X Disorders of acoustic nerve**
    - H93.3X1 Disorders of right acoustic nerve
    - H93.3X2 Disorders of left acoustic nerve
    - H93.3X3 Disorders of bilateral acoustic nerves
    - H93.3X9 Disorders of unspecified acoustic nerve
- **H93.8 Other specified disorders of ear**
  - **H93.8X Other specified disorders of ear**
    - H93.8X1 Other specified disorders of right ear
    - H93.8X2 Other specified disorders of left ear
    - H93.8X3 Other specified disorders of ear, bilateral
    - H93.8X9 Other specified disorders of ear, unspecified ear
- **H93.9 Unspecified disorder of ear**
  - H93.90 Unspecified disorder of ear, unspecified ear
  - H93.91 Unspecified disorder of right ear
  - H93.92 Unspecified disorder of left ear
  - H93.93 Unspecified disorder of ear, bilateral

H94 Other disorders of ear in diseases classified elsewhere

+ **H94.0** Acoustic neuritis in infectious and parasitic diseases classified elsewhere

  Code first underlying disease, such as:
  parasitic disease (B65-B89)

  Excludes1: acoustic neuritis (in):
  herpes zoster (B02.29)
  syphilis (A52.15)

  H94.00 Acoustic neuritis in infectious and parasitic diseases classified elsewhere, unspecified ear
  H94.01 Acoustic neuritis in infectious and parasitic diseases classified elsewhere, right ear
  H94.02 Acoustic neuritis in infectious and parasitic diseases classified elsewhere, left ear
  H94.03 Acoustic neuritis in infectious and parasitic diseases classified elsewhere, bilateral

+ **H94.8** Other specified disorders of ear in diseases classified elsewhere

  Code first underlying disease, such as:
  congenital syphilis (A50.0)

  Excludes1: aural myiasis (B87.4)
  syphilitic labyrinthitis (A52.79)

  H94.80 Other specified disorders of ear in diseases classified elsewhere, unspecified ear
  H94.81 Other specified disorders of right ear in diseases classified elsewhere
  H94.82 Other specified disorders of left ear in diseases classified elsewhere
  H94.83 Other specified disorders of ear in diseases classified elsewhere, bilateral

Intraoperative and postprocedural complications and disorders of ear and mastoid process, not elsewhere classified (H95)

H95 Intraoperative and postprocedural complications and disorders of ear and mastoid process, not elsewhere classified

AHA CC: 4Q, 2016, 9-10

+ **H95.0** Recurrent cholesteatoma of postmastoidectomy cavity
  H95.00 Recurrent cholesteatoma of postmastoidectomy cavity, unspecified ear
  H95.01 Recurrent cholesteatoma of postmastoidectomy cavity, right ear
  H95.02 Recurrent cholesteatoma of postmastoidectomy cavity, left ear
  H95.03 Recurrent cholesteatoma of postmastoidectomy cavity, bilateral ears

+ **H95.1** Other disorders of ear and mastoid process following mastoidectomy
  + **H95.11** Chronic inflammation of postmastoidectomy cavity
    H95.111 Chronic inflammation of postmastoidectomy cavity, right ear
    H95.112 Chronic inflammation of postmastoidectomy cavity, left ear
    H95.113 Chronic inflammation of postmastoidectomy cavity, bilateral ears
    H95.119 Chronic inflammation of postmastoidectomy cavity, unspecified ear
  + **H95.12** Granulation of postmastoidectomy cavity
    H95.121 Granulation of postmastoidectomy cavity, right ear
    H95.122 Granulation of postmastoidectomy cavity, left ear
    H95.123 Granulation of postmastoidectomy cavity, bilateral ears
    H95.129 Granulation of postmastoidectomy cavity, unspecified ear
  + **H95.13** Mucosal cyst of postmastoidectomy cavity
    H95.131 Mucosal cyst of postmastoidectomy cavity, right ear
    H95.132 Mucosal cyst of postmastoidectomy cavity, left ear
    H95.133 Mucosal cyst of postmastoidectomy cavity, bilateral ears
    H95.139 Mucosal cyst of postmastoidectomy cavity, unspecified ear
  + **H95.19** Other disorders following mastoidectomy
    H95.191 Other disorders following mastoidectomy, right ear
    H95.192 Other disorders following mastoidectomy, left ear
    H95.193 Other disorders following mastoidectomy, bilateral ears
    H95.199 Other disorders following mastoidectomy, unspecified ear

+ **H95.2** Intraoperative hemorrhage and hematoma of ear and mastoid process complicating a procedure

  Excludes1: intraoperative hemorrhage and hematoma of ear and mastoid process due to accidental puncture or laceration during a procedure (H95.3-)

  CC **H95.21** Intraoperative hemorrhage and hematoma of ear and mastoid process complicating a procedure on the ear and mastoid process
  CC **H95.22** Intraoperative hemorrhage and hematoma of ear and mastoid process complicating other procedure

+ **H95.3** Accidental puncture and laceration of ear and mastoid process during a procedure
  CC **H95.31** Accidental puncture and laceration of the ear and mastoid process during a procedure on the ear and mastoid process
  CC **H95.32** Accidental puncture and laceration of the ear and mastoid process during other procedure

+ **H95.4** Postprocedural hemorrhage of ear and mastoid process following a procedure
  CC **H95.41** Postprocedural hemorrhage of ear and mastoid process following a procedure on the ear and mastoid process
  CC **H95.42** Postprocedural hemorrhage of ear and mastoid process following other procedure

+ **H95.5** Postprocedural hematoma and seroma of ear and mastoid process following a procedure
  CC **H95.51** Postprocedural hematoma of ear and mastoid process following a procedure on the ear and mastoid process
  CC **H95.52** Postprocedural hematoma of ear and mastoid process following other procedure
  CC **H95.53** Postprocedureal seroma of ear and mastoid process following a procedure on the ear and mastoid process
  CC **H95.54** Postprocedureal seroma of ear and mastoid process following other procedure

+ **H95.8** Other intraoperative and postprocedural complications and disorders of the ear and mastoid process, not elsewhere classified

  Excludes2: postprocedural complications and disorders following mastoidectomy (H95.0-, H95.1-)

  + **H95.81** Postprocedural stenosis of external ear canal
    CC **H95.811** Postprocedural stenosis of right external ear canal
    CC **H95.812** Postprocedural stenosis of left external ear canal
    CC **H95.813** Postprocedural stenosis of external ear canal, bilateral
    CC **H95.819** Postprocedural stenosis of unspecified external ear canal
  CC **H95.88** Other intraoperative complications and disorders of the ear and mastoid process, not elsewhere classified

  Use additional code, if applicable, to further specify disorder

  CC **H95.89** Other postprocedural complications and disorders of the ear and mastoid process, not elsewhere classified

  Use additional code, if applicable, to further specify disorder

Chapter 9: Diseases of the Circulatory System (I00-I99)

Excludes2: certain conditions originating in the perinatal period (P04-P96)
certain infectious and parasitic diseases (A00-B99)
complications of pregnancy, childbirth and the puerperium (O00-O9A)
congenital malformations, deformations, and chromosomal abnormalities (Q00-Q99)
endocrine, nutritional and metabolic diseases (E00-E88)
injury, poisoning and certain other consequences of external causes (S00-T88)
neoplasms (C00-D49)
symptoms, signs and abnormal clinical and laboratory findings, not elsewhere classified (R00-R94)
systemic connective tissue disorders (M30-M36)
transient cerebral ischemic attacks and related syndromes (G45.-)

This chapter contains the following category blocks:
- I00-I02 Acute rheumatic fever
- I05-I09 Chronic rheumatic heart diseases
- I10-I1A Hypertensive diseases
- I20-I25 Ischemic heart diseases
- I26-I28 Pulmonary heart disease and diseases of pulmonary circulation
- I30-I5A Other forms of heart disease
- I60-I69 Cerebrovascular diseases
- I70-I79 Diseases of arteries, arterioles and capillaries
- I80-I89 Diseases of veins, lymphatic vessels and lymph nodes, not elsewhere classified
- I95-I99 Other and unspecified disorders of the circulatory system

C. Chapter-Specific Coding Guidelines

In addition to general coding guidelines, there are guidelines for specific diagnoses and/or conditions in the classification. Unless otherwise indicated, these guidelines apply to all health care settings. Please refer to Section II for guidelines on the selection of principal diagnosis.

9. Chapter 9: Diseases of the Circulatory System (I00-I99)

a. Hypertension

The classification presumes a causal relationship between hypertension and heart involvement and between hypertension and kidney involvement, as the two conditions are linked by the term "with" in the Alphabetic Index. These conditions should be coded as related even in the absence of provider documentation explicitly linking them, unless the documentation clearly states the conditions are unrelated.

For hypertension and conditions not specifically linked by relational terms such as "with," "associated with" or "due to" in the classification, provider documentation must link the conditions in order to code them as related.

1) Hypertension with Heart Disease

Hypertension with heart conditions classified to I50.- or I51.4-I51.7, I51.89, I51.9, are assigned to, a code from category I11, Hypertensive heart disease. Use an additional code(s) from category I50, Heart failure, to identify the type(s) of heart failure in those patients with heart failure.

The same heart conditions (I50.-, I51.4-I51.7, I51.89, I51.9) with hypertension are coded separately if the provider has documented they are unrelated to the hypertension. Sequence according to the circumstances of the admission/encounter.

2) Hypertensive Chronic Kidney Disease

Assign codes from category I12, Hypertensive chronic kidney disease, when both hypertension and a condition classifiable to category N18, Chronic kidney disease (CKD), are present. CKD should not be coded as hypertensive if the provider indicates the CKD is not related to the hypertension.

The appropriate code from category N18 should be used as a secondary code with a code from category I12 to identify the stage of chronic kidney disease.

See Section I.C.14. Chronic kidney disease.

If a patient has hypertensive chronic kidney disease and acute renal failure, the acute renal failure should also be coded. Sequence according to the circumstances of the admission/encounter.

3) Hypertensive Heart and Chronic Kidney Disease

Assign codes from combination category I13, Hypertensive heart and chronic kidney disease, when there is hypertension with both heart and kidney involvement. If heart failure is present, assign an additional code from category I50 to identify the type of heart failure.

The appropriate code from category N18, Chronic kidney disease, should be used as a secondary code with a code from category I13 to identify the stage of chronic kidney disease.

See Section I.C.14. Chronic kidney disease.

The codes in category I13, Hypertensive heart and chronic kidney disease, are combination codes that include hypertension, heart disease and chronic kidney disease. The Includes note at I13 specifies that the conditions included at I11 and I12 are included together in I13. If a patient has hypertension, heart disease and chronic kidney disease then a code from I13 should be used, not individual codes for hypertension, heart disease and chronic kidney disease, or codes from I11 or I12.

For patients with both acute renal failure and chronic kidney disease the acute renal failure should also be coded. Sequence according to the circumstances of the admission/encounter.

4) Hypertensive Cerebrovascular Disease

For hypertensive cerebrovascular disease, first assign the appropriate code from categories I60-I69, followed by the appropriate hypertension code.

5) Hypertensive Retinopathy

Subcategory H35.0, Background retinopathy and retinal vascular changes, should be used with a code from category I10 – I15, Hypertensive disease to include the systemic hypertension. The sequencing is based on the reason for the encounter.

6) Hypertension, Secondary

Secondary hypertension is due to an underlying condition. Two codes are required: one to identify the underlying etiology and one from category I15 to identify the hypertension. Sequencing of codes is determined by the reason for admission/encounter.

7) Hypertension, Transient

Assign code R03.0, Elevated blood pressure reading without diagnosis of hypertension, unless patient has an established diagnosis of hypertension. Assign code O13.-, Gestational [pregnancy-induced] hypertension without significant proteinuria, or O14.-, Pre-eclampsia, for transient hypertension of pregnancy.

8) Hypertension, Controlled

This diagnostic statement usually refers to an existing state of hypertension under control by therapy. Assign the appropriate code from categories I10-I15, Hypertensive diseases.

9) Hypertension, Uncontrolled

Uncontrolled hypertension may refer to untreated hypertension or hypertension not responding to current therapeutic regimen. In either case, assign the appropriate code from categories I10-I15, Hypertensive diseases.

10) Hypertensive Crisis

Assign a code from category I16, Hypertensive crisis, for documented hypertensive urgency, hypertensive emergency or unspecified hypertensive crisis. Code also any identified hypertensive disease (I10-I15). The sequencing is based on the reason for the encounter.

11) Pulmonary Hypertension

Pulmonary hypertension is classified to category I27, Other pulmonary heart diseases. For secondary pulmonary hypertension (I27.1, I27.2-), code also any associated conditions or adverse effects of drugs or toxins. The sequencing is based on the reason for the encounter, except for adverse effects of drugs (See Section I.C.19.e).

12) Hypertension, Resistant

Resistant hypertension refers to blood pressure of a patient with hypertension that remains above goal in spite of the use of antihypertensive medications. Assign ode I1A.0 Resistant hypertension, as an additional code when apparent treatment resistant hypertension, treatment resistant hypertension, or true resistant hypertension is documented by the provider. A code for the specific type of existing hypertension is sequenced first, if known.

b. Atherosclerotic Coronary Artery Disease and Angina

ICD-10-CM has combination codes for atherosclerotic heart disease with angina pectoris. The subcategories for these codes are I25.11, Atherosclerotic heart disease of native coronary artery with angina pectoris and I25.7, Atherosclerosis of coronary artery bypass graft(s) and coronary artery of transplanted heart with angina pectoris.

When using one of these combination codes it is not necessary to use an additional code for angina pectoris. A causal relationship can be assumed in a patient with both atherosclerosis and angina pectoris, unless the documentation indicates the angina is due to something other than the atherosclerosis.

If a patient with coronary artery disease is admitted due to an acute myocardial infarction (AMI), the AMI should be sequenced before the coronary artery disease.

See Section I.C.9. Acute myocardial infarction (AMI)

c. **Intraoperative and Postprocedural Cerebrovascular Accident**

Medical record documentation should clearly specify the cause- and-effect relationship between the medical intervention and the cerebrovascular accident in order to assign a code for intraoperative or postprocedural cerebrovascular accident.

Proper code assignment depends on whether it was an infarction or hemorrhage and whether it occurred intraoperatively or postoperatively. If it was a cerebral hemorrhage, code assignment depends on the type of procedure performed.

d. **Sequelae of Cerebrovascular Disease**

1) **Category I69, Sequelae of Cerebrovascular disease**

   Category I69 is used to indicate conditions classifiable to categories I60-I67 as the causes of sequela (neurologic deficits), themselves classified elsewhere. These "late effects" include neurologic deficits that persist after initial onset of conditions classifiable to categories I60-I67. The neurologic deficits caused by cerebrovascular disease may be present from the onset or may arise at any time after the onset of the condition classifiable to categories I60-I67.

   Codes from category I69, Sequelae of cerebrovascular disease, that specify hemiplegia, hemiparesis and monoplegia identify whether the dominant or nondominant side is affected. Should the affected side be documented, but not specified as dominant or nondominant, and the classification system does not indicate a default, code selection is as follows:

   - For ambidextrous patients, the default should be dominant.
   - If the left side is affected, the default is non-dominant.
   - If the right side is affected, the default is dominant.

2) **Codes from category I69 with codes from I60-I67**

   Codes from category I69 may be assigned on a health care record with codes from I60-I67, if the patient has a current cerebrovascular disease and deficits from an old cerebrovascular disease.

3) **Codes from category I69 and Personal history of transient ischemic attack (TIA) and cerebral infarction (Z86.73)**

   Codes from category I69 should not be assigned if the patient does not have neurologic deficits.

   See Section I.C.21. 4. History (of) for use of personal history codes

e. **Acute myocardial infarction (AMI)**

1) **ST elevation myocardial infarction (STEMI) and non ST elevation myocardial infarction (NSTEMI)**

   The ICD-10-CM codes for type 1 acute myocardial infarction (AMI) identify the site, such as anterolateral wall or true posterior wall. Subcategories I21.0-I21.2 and code I21.3 are used for type 1 ST elevation myocardial infarction (STEMI). Code I21.4, Non-ST elevation (NSTEMI) myocardial infarction, is used for type 1 non ST elevation myocardial infarction (NSTEMI) and nontransmural MIs.

   If a type 1 NSTEMI evolves to STEMI, assign the STEMI code. If a type 1 STEMI converts to NSTEMI due to thrombolytic therapy, it is still coded as STEMI.

   For encounters occurring while the myocardial infarction is equal to, or less than, four weeks old, including transfers to another acute setting or a postacute setting, and the myocardial infarction meets the definition for "other diagnoses" (see Section III, Reporting Additional Diagnoses), codes from category I21 may continue to be reported. For encounters after the 4 week time frame and the patient is still receiving care related to the myocardial infarction, the appropriate aftercare code should be assigned, rather than a code from category I21. For old or healed myocardial infarctions not requiring further care, code I25.2, Old myocardial infarction, may be assigned.

2) **Acute myocardial infarction, unspecified**

   Code I21.9, Acute myocardial infarction, unspecified, is the default for unspecified acute myocardial infarction or unspecified type. If only type 1 STEMI or transmural MI without the site is documented, assign code I21.3, ST elevation (STEMI) myocardial infarction of unspecified site.

3) **AMI documented as nontransmural or subendocardial but site provided**

   If an AMI is documented as nontransmural or subendocardial, but the site is provided, it is still coded as a subendocardial AMI.

   See Section I.C.21.3 for information on coding status post administration of tPA in a different facility within the last 24 hours.

4) **Subsequent acute myocardial infarction**

   A code from category I22, Subsequent ST elevation (STEMI) and non-ST elevation (NSTEMI) myocardial infarction, is to be used when a patient who has suffered a type 1 or unspecified AMI has a new AMI within the 4 week time frame of the initial AMI. A code from category I22 must be used in conjunction with a code from category I21. The sequencing of the I22 and I21 codes depends on the circumstances of the encounter.

   Do not assign code I22 for subsequent myocardial infarctions other than type 1 or unspecified. For subsequent type 2 AMI assign only code I21.A1. For subsequent type 4 or type 5 AMI, assign only code I21.A9.

   If a subsequent myocardial infarction of one type occurs within 4 weeks of a myocardial infarction of a different type, assign the appropriate codes from category I21 to identify each type. Do not assign a code from I22. Codes from category I22 should only be assigned if both the initial and subsequent myocardial infarctions are type 1 or unspecified.

5) **Other Types of Myocardial Infarction**

   The ICD-10-CM provides codes for different types of myocardial infarction. Type 1 myocardial infarctions are assigned to codes I21.0-I21.4.

   Type 2 myocardial infarction (myocardial infarction due to demand ischemia or secondary to ischemic imbalance) is assigned to code I21.A1, Myocardial infarction type 2 with the underlying cause coded first. Do not assign code I24.8, Other forms of acute ischemic heart disease, for the demand ischemia. If a type 2 AMI is described as NSTEMI or STEMI, only assign code I21.A1. Codes I21.0-I21.4 should only be assigned for type 1 AMIs.

   Acute myocardial infarctions type 3, 4a, 4b, 4c and 5 are assigned to code I21.A9, Other myocardial infarction type.

   The "Code also" and "Code first" notes should be followed related to complications, and for coding of postprocedural myocardial infarctions during or following cardiac surgery.

   Add a new guideline here.

6) **Myocardial Infarction with Coronary Microvascular Dysfunction**

   Coronary microvascular dysfunction (CMD) is a condition that impacts the microvasculature by restricting microvascular flow and increasing microvascular resistance. Code I21.B, Myocardial infarction with coronary microvascular dysfunction, is assigned for myocardial infarction with coronary microvascular disease, myocardial infarction with coronary microvascular dysfunction, and myocardial infarction with non-obstructive coronary arteries (MINOCA) with microvascular disease.

Acute rheumatic fever (I00-I02)

I00 Rheumatic fever without heart involvement

   Includes: arthritis, rheumatic, acute or subacute
   Excludes1: *rheumatic fever with heart involvement (I01.0-I01.9)*
   Valid 3-character code, no further characters required

I01 Rheumatic fever with heart involvement

   Excludes1: *chronic diseases of rheumatic origin (I05-I09) unless rheumatic fever is also present or there is evidence of reactivation or activity of the rheumatic process.*

   CC **I01.0 Acute rheumatic pericarditis**
   Any condition in I00 with pericarditis
   Rheumatic pericarditis (acute)
   Excludes1: *acute pericarditis not specified as rheumatic (I30.-)*

   CC **I01.1 Acute rheumatic endocarditis**
   Any condition in I00 with endocarditis or valvulitis
   Acute rheumatic valvulitis

   CC **I01.2 Acute rheumatic myocarditis**
   Any condition in I00 with myocarditis

   CC **I01.8 Other acute rheumatic heart disease**
   Any condition in I00 with other or multiple types of heart involvement
   Acute rheumatic pancarditis

   CC **I01.9 Acute rheumatic heart disease, unspecified**
   Any condition in I00 with unspecified type of heart involvement
   Rheumatic carditis, acute
   Rheumatic heart disease, active or acute

I02 Rheumatic chorea

   Includes: Sydenham's chorea
   Excludes1: *chorea NOS (G25.5)*
   Huntington's chorea (G10)

   CC **I02.0 Rheumatic chorea with heart involvement**
   Chorea NOS with heart involvement
   Rheumatic chorea with heart involvement of any type classifiable under I01.-

   CC **I02.9 Rheumatic chorea without heart involvement**
   Rheumatic chorea NOS

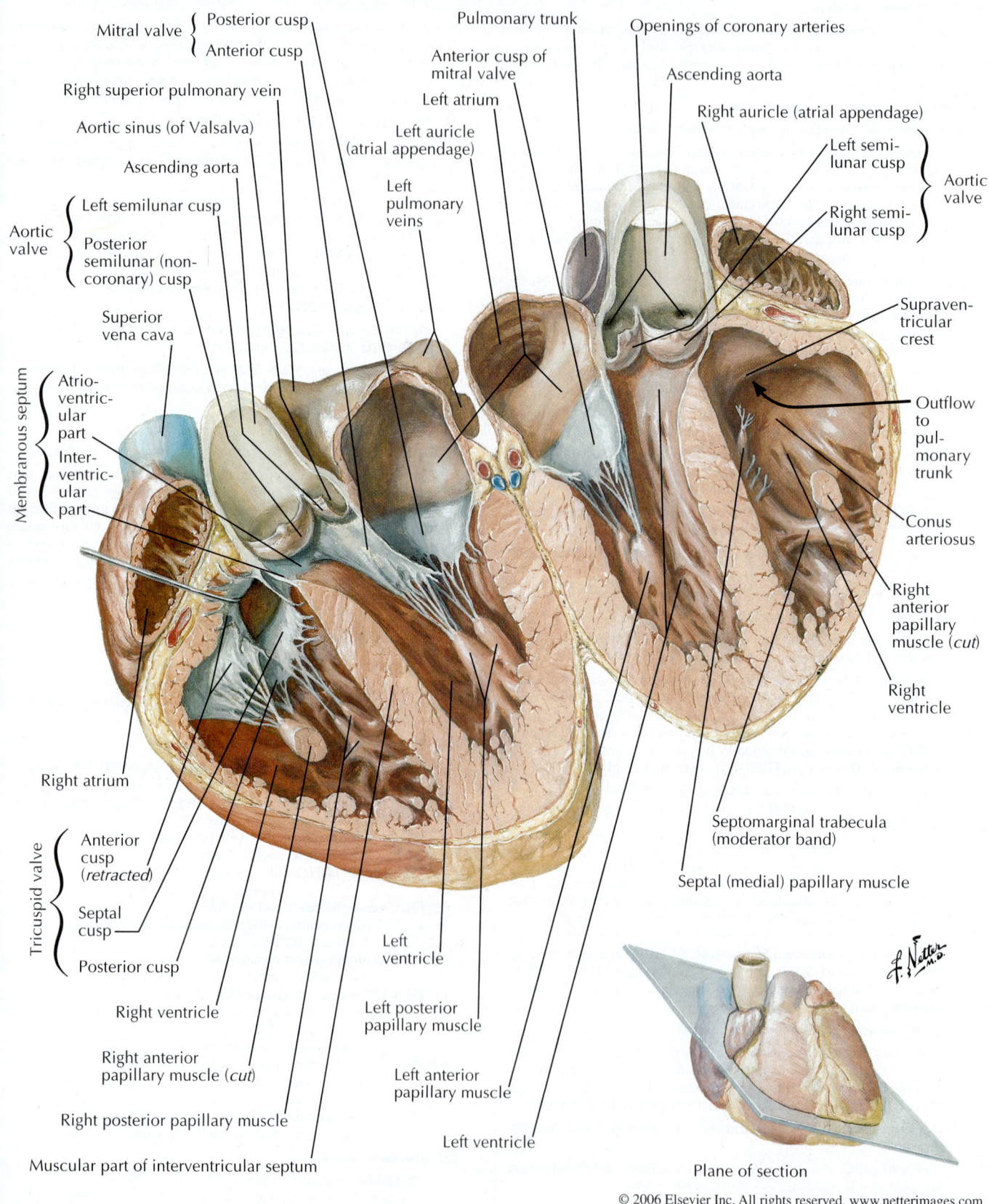

Veins

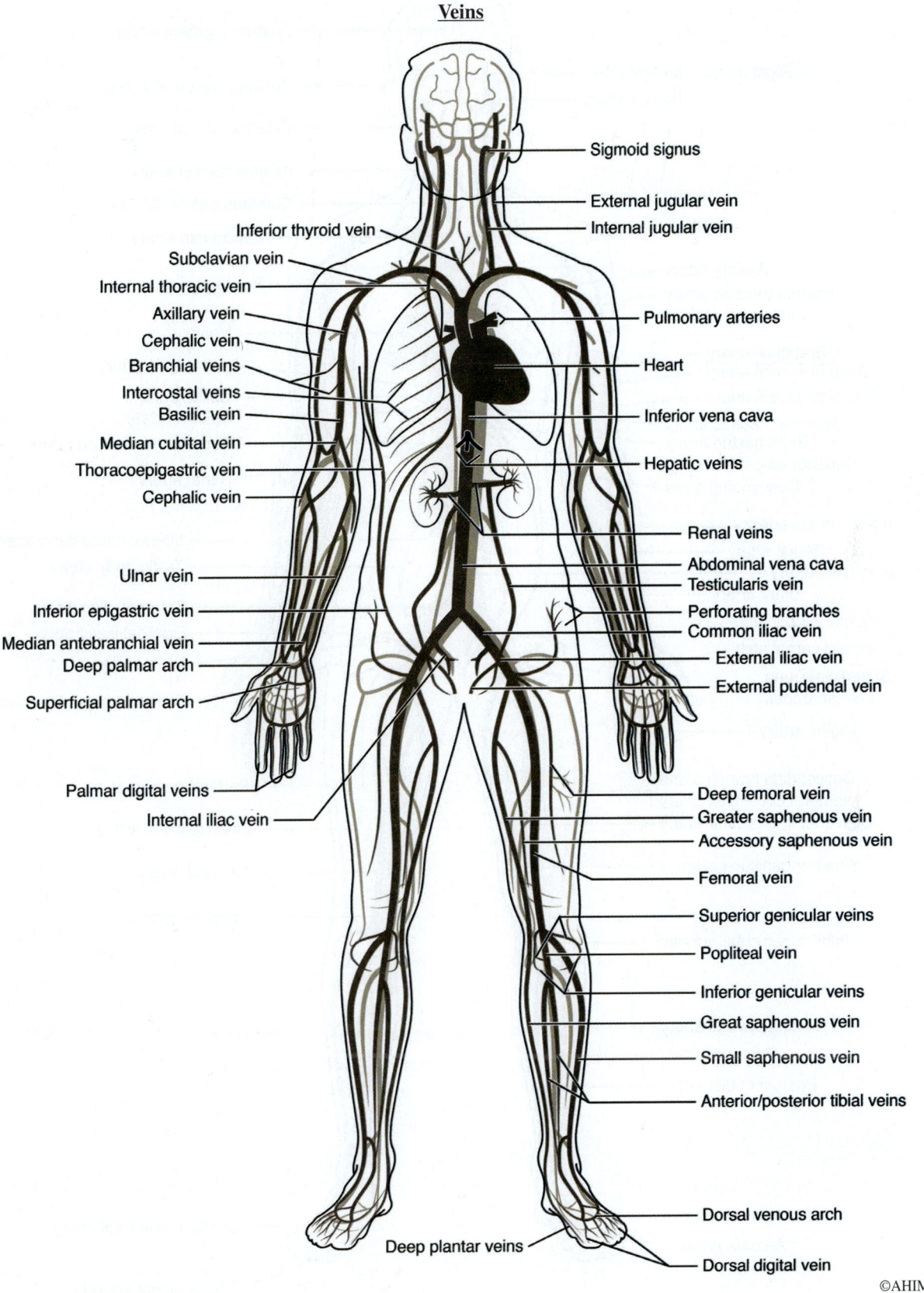

685

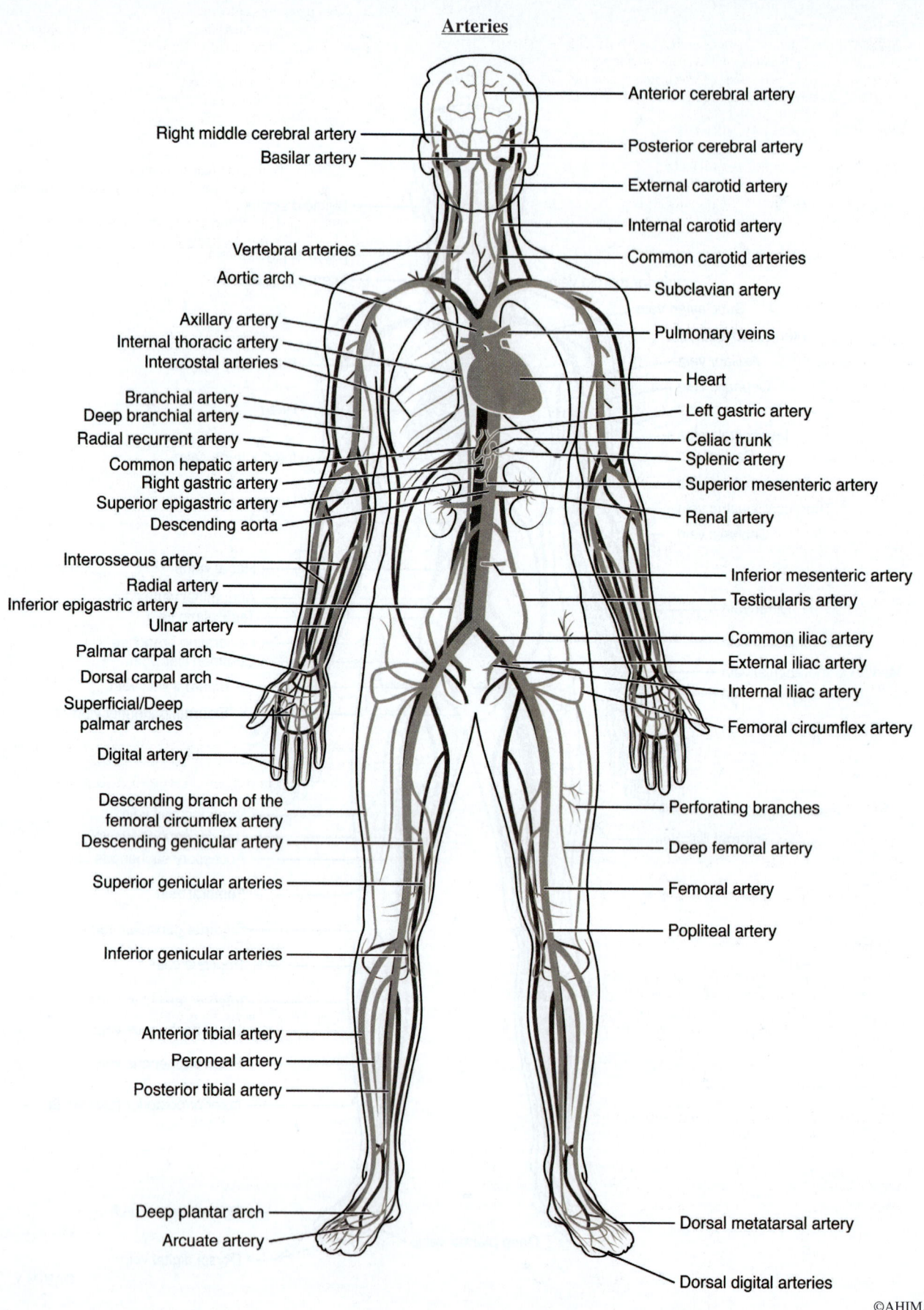

Chronic rheumatic heart diseases (I05-I09)

I05 Rheumatic mitral valve diseases
Includes: conditions classifiable to both I05.0 and I05.2-I05.9, whether specified as rheumatic or not
Excludes1: mitral valve disease specified as nonrheumatic (I34.-)
mitral valve disease with aortic and/or tricuspid valve involvement (I08.-)

- **I05.0 Rheumatic mitral stenosis**
  Mitral (valve) obstruction (rheumatic)
- **I05.1 Rheumatic mitral insufficiency**
  Rheumatic mitral incompetence
  Rheumatic mitral regurgitation
  Excludes1: mitral insufficiency not specified as rheumatic (I34.0)
- **I05.2 Rheumatic mitral stenosis with insufficiency**
  Rheumatic mitral stenosis with incompetence or regurgitation
- **I05.8 Other rheumatic mitral valve diseases**
  Rheumatic mitral (valve) failure
- **I05.9 Rheumatic mitral valve disease, unspecified**
  Rheumatic mitral (valve) disorder (chronic) NOS

I06 Rheumatic aortic valve diseases
Excludes1: aortic valve disease not specified as rheumatic (I35.-)
aortic valve disease with mitral and/or tricuspid valve involvement (I08.-)

- **I06.0 Rheumatic aortic stenosis**
  Rheumatic aortic (valve) obstruction
- **I06.1 Rheumatic aortic insufficiency**
  Rheumatic aortic incompetence
  Rheumatic aortic regurgitation
- **I06.2 Rheumatic aortic stenosis with insufficiency**
  Rheumatic aortic stenosis with incompetence or regurgitation
- **I06.8 Other rheumatic aortic valve diseases**
- **I06.9 Rheumatic aortic valve disease, unspecified**
  Rheumatic aortic (valve) disease NOS

I07 Rheumatic tricuspid valve diseases
Includes: rheumatic tricuspid valve diseases specified as rheumatic or unspecified
Excludes1: tricuspid valve disease specified as nonrheumatic (I36.-)
tricuspid valve disease with aortic and/or mitral valve involvement (I08.-)

- **I07.0 Rheumatic tricuspid stenosis**
  Tricuspid (valve) stenosis (rheumatic)
- **I07.1 Rheumatic tricuspid insufficiency**
  Tricuspid (valve) insufficiency (rheumatic)
- **I07.2 Rheumatic tricuspid stenosis and insufficiency**
- **I07.8 Other rheumatic tricuspid valve diseases**
- **I07.9 Rheumatic tricuspid valve disease, unspecified**
  Rheumatic tricuspid valve disorder NOS

I08 Multiple valve diseases
Includes: multiple valve diseases specified as rheumatic or unspecified
Excludes1: endocarditis, valve unspecified (I38)
multiple valve disease specified a nonrheumatic (I34.-, I35.-, I36.-, I37.-, I38., Q22.-, Q23.-, Q24.8-)
rheumatic heart disease NOS (I09.1)

- **I08.0 Rheumatic disorders of both mitral and aortic valves**
  Involvement of both mitral and aortic valves specified as rheumatic or unspecified
  AHA CC: 2Q, 2019, 5
- **I08.1 Rheumatic disorders of both mitral and tricuspid valves**
- **I08.2 Rheumatic disorders of both aortic and tricuspid valves**
- **I08.3 Combined rheumatic disorders of mitral, aortic and tricuspid valves**
- **I08.8 Other rheumatic multiple valve diseases**
- **I08.9 Rheumatic multiple valve disease, unspecified**

I09 Other rheumatic heart diseases
- CC **I09.0 Rheumatic myocarditis**
  Excludes1: myocarditis not specified as rheumatic (I51.4)
- **I09.1 Rheumatic diseases of endocardium, valve unspecified**
  Rheumatic endocarditis (chronic)
  Rheumatic valvulitis (chronic)
  Excludes1: endocarditis, valve unspecified (I38)
- CC **I09.2 Chronic rheumatic pericarditis**
  Adherent pericardium, rheumatic
  Chronic rheumatic mediastinopericarditis
  Chronic rheumatic myopericarditis
  Excludes1: chronic pericarditis not specified as rheumatic (I31.-)
- + **I09.8 Other specified rheumatic heart diseases**
  - CC **I09.81 Rheumatic heart failure**
    Use additional code to identify type of heart failure (I50.-)
  - **I09.89 Other specified rheumatic heart diseases**
    Rheumatic disease of pulmonary valve
- **I09.9 Rheumatic heart disease, unspecified**
  Rheumatic carditis
  Excludes1: rheumatoid carditis (M05.31)

Hypertensive diseases (I10-I1A)
Use additional code to identify:
exposure to environmental tobacco smoke (Z77.22)
history of tobacco dependence (Z87.891)
occupational exposure to environmental tobacco smoke (Z57.31)
tobacco dependence (F17.-)
tobacco use (Z72.0)

Excludes1: neonatal hypertension (P29.2)
primary pulmonary hypertension (I27.0)
Excludes2: hypertensive disease complicating pregnancy, childbirth and the puerperium (O10-O11, O13-O16)
Review coding guidelines C.9, C.9.a.5, C.9.a.8 and C.9.a.9

I10 Essential (primary) hypertension
Includes: high blood pressure
hypertension (arterial) (benign) (essential) (malignant) (primary) (systemic)
Excludes1: hypertensive disease complicating pregnancy, childbirth and the puerperium (O10-O11, O13-O16)
Excludes2: essential (primary) hypertension involving vessels of brain (I60-I69)
essential (primary) hypertension involving vessels of eye (H35.0-)
AHA CC: 4Q, 2013, 128; 4Q, 2016, 27-28; 2Q, 2018, 9-10
Valid 3-character code, no further characters required

I11 Hypertensive heart disease
Includes: any condition in I50.-or I51.4-I51.7, I51.89, I51.9 due to hypertension
Review coding guidelines C.9.a.1 and C.9.a.3
- **I11.0 Hypertensive heart disease with heart failure**
  Hypertensive heart failure
  Use additional code to identify type of heart failure (I50.-)
  AHA CC: 1Q, 2017, 47
- **I11.9 Hypertensive heart disease without heart failure**
  Hypertensive heart disease NOS

I12 Hypertensive chronic kidney disease
Includes: any condition in N18 and N26 - due to hypertension
arteriosclerosis of kidney
arteriosclerotic nephritis (chronic) (interstitial)
hypertensive nephropathy
nephrosclerosis
Excludes1: hypertension due to kidney disease (I15.0, I15.1)
renovascular hypertension (I15.0)
secondary hypertension (I15.-)
Excludes2: acute kidney failure (N17.-)
Review coding guidelines C.9.a.2 and C.9.a.3
- CC **I12.0 Hypertensive chronic kidney disease with stage 5 chronic kidney disease or end stage renal disease**
  Use additional code to identify the stage of chronic kidney disease (N18.5, N18.6)

Hypertension and CHF

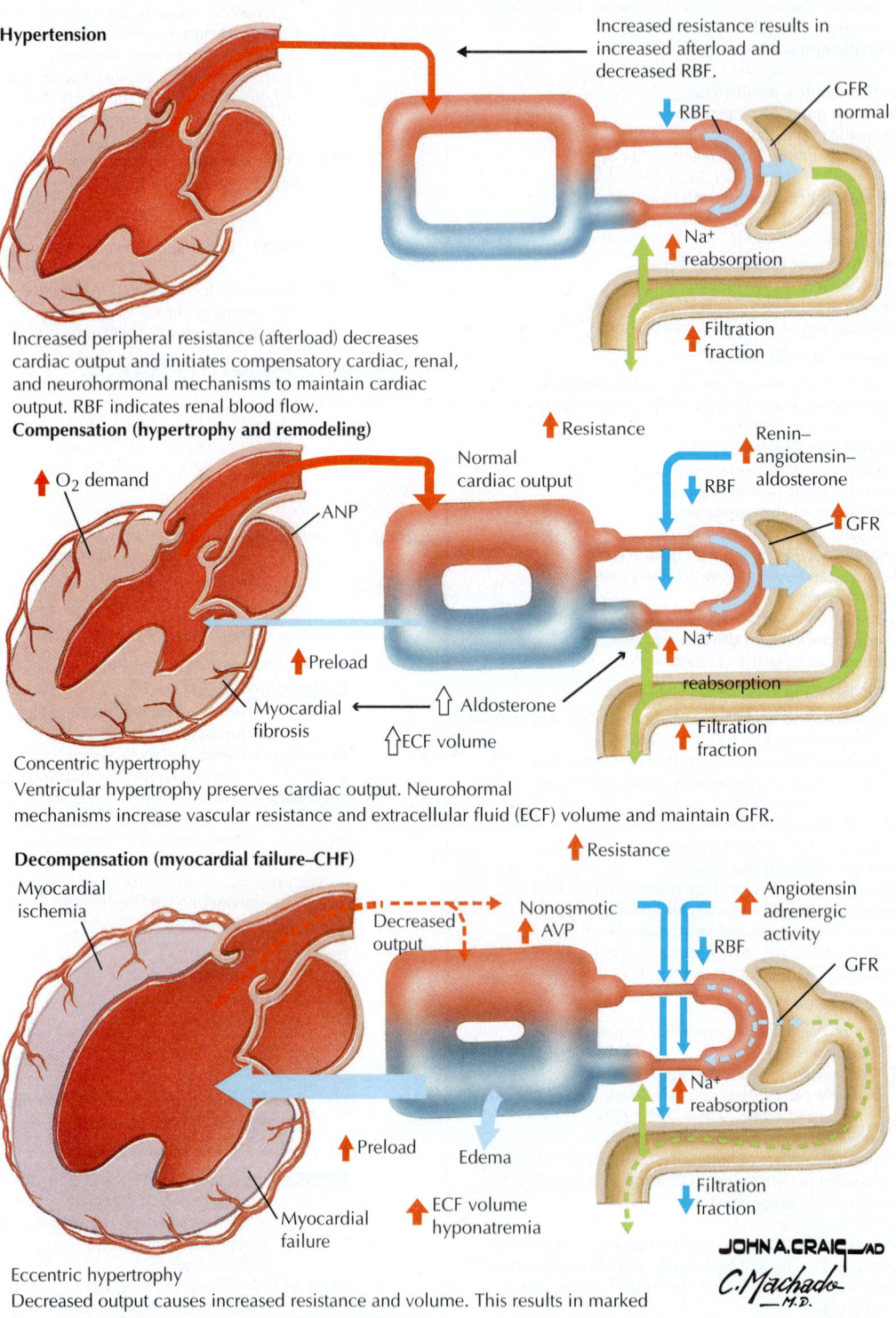

Hypertension

Increased resistance results in increased afterload and decreased RBF.

Increased peripheral resistance (afterload) decreases cardiac output and initiates compensatory cardiac, renal, and neurohormonal mechanisms to maintain cardiac output. RBF indicates renal blood flow.

Compensation (hypertrophy and remodeling)

Concentric hypertrophy
Ventricular hypertrophy preserves cardiac output. Neurohormal mechanisms increase vascular resistance and extracellular fluid (ECF) volume and maintain GFR.

Decompensation (myocardial failure–CHF)

Eccentric hypertrophy
Decreased output causes increased resistance and volume. This results in marked decrease in cardiac output, renal perfusion, and GFR.

© 2004 Elsevier Inc. All rights reserved. www.netterimages.com

The Kidneys in Congestive Heart Failure (CHF)

Effects of Left Heart Failure on Renal Blood Flow and Tubular Function

Distribution of renal blood flow in CHF

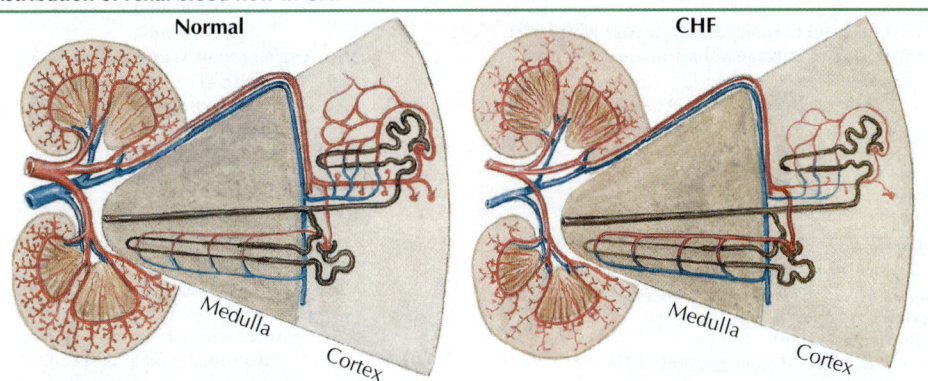

20% to 25% of cardiac output flows through kidneys: blood flows largely through cortical glomeruli, partially through juxtamedullary glomeruli

<10% of cardiac output flows through kidneys: redistribution of blood flow from cortical to juxtamedullary glomeruli

Tubular function in CHF

Low perfusion pressure activates tubuloglomerular feedback and renin release, causing afferent arteriole dilation and efferent arteriole constriction in order to maintain GFR. If hypoperfusion is severe, GFR may decline.

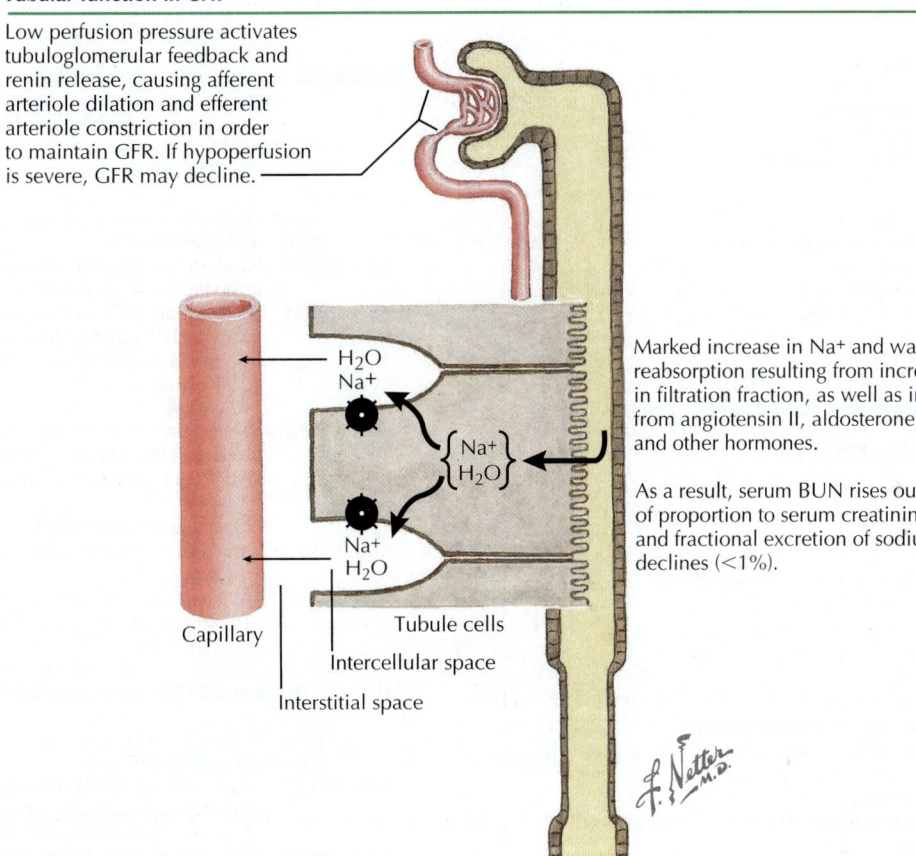

Marked increase in Na+ and water reabsorption resulting from increase in filtration fraction, as well as input from angiotensin II, aldosterone, and other hormones.

As a result, serum BUN rises out of proportion to serum creatinine, and fractional excretion of sodium declines (<1%).

I12.9 Hypertensive chronic kidney disease with stage 1 through stage 4 chronic kidney disease, or unspecified chronic kidney disease
  Hypertensive chronic kidney disease NOS
  Hypertensive renal disease NOS
  Use additional code to identify the stage of chronic kidney disease (N18.1-N18.4, N18.9)
  AHA CC: 4Q, 2018, 88-89; 4Q, 2022, 5-6

I13 Hypertensive heart and chronic kidney disease
  Includes: any condition in I11.- with any condition in I12.-
    cardiorenal disease
    cardiovascular renal disease
  Review coding guideline C.9.a.3

CC **I13.0** Hypertensive heart and chronic kidney disease with heart failure and stage 1 through stage 4 chronic kidney disease, or unspecified chronic kidney disease
  Use additional code to identify type of heart failure (I50.-)
  Use additional code to identify stage of chronic kidney disease (N18.1-N18.4, N18.9)

+ **I13.1** Hypertensive heart and chronic kidney disease without heart failure
  I13.10 Hypertensive heart and chronic kidney disease without heart failure, with stage 1 through stage 4 chronic kidney disease, or unspecified chronic kidney disease
    Hypertensive heart disease and hypertensive chronic kidney disease NOS
    Use additional code to identify the stage of chronic kidney disease (N18.1-N18.4, N18.9)

CC I13.11 Hypertensive heart and chronic kidney disease without heart failure, with stage 5 chronic kidney disease, or end stage renal disease
Use additional code to identify the stage of chronic kidney disease (N18.5, N18.6)

CC I13.2 Hypertensive heart and chronic kidney disease with heart failure and with stage 5 chronic kidney disease, or end stage renal disease
Use additional code to identify type of heart failure (I50.-)
Use additional code to identify the stage of chronic kidney disease (N18.5, N18.6)

I15 Secondary hypertension
Code also underlying condition
Excludes1: postprocedural hypertension (I97.3)
Excludes2: secondary hypertension involving vessels of brain (I60-I69)
secondary hypertension involving vessels of eye (H35.0-)
Review coding guideline C.9.a.6

- **I15.0** Renovascular hypertension
- **I15.1** Hypertension secondary to other renal disorders
  AHA CC: 3Q, 2016, 22-23
- **I15.2** Hypertension secondary to endocrine disorders
- **I15.8** Other secondary hypertension
- **I15.9** Secondary hypertension, unspecified

I16 Hypertensive crisis
Code also any identified hypertensive disease (I10-I15, I1A)
Review coding guideline C.9.a.10
AHA CC: 4Q, 2016, 26-28

- **I16.0** Hypertensive urgency
  AHA CC: 4Q, 2016, 27-28
- **CC I16.1** Hypertensive emergency
  AHA CC: 4Q, 2016, 27-28
- **CC I16.9** Hypertensive crisis, unspecified

I1A Other hypertension

- **I1A.0** Resistant hypertension
  Apparent treatment resistant hypertension
  Treatment resistant hypertension
  True resistant hypertension
  Code first specific type of existing hypertension, if known, such as:
  essential hypertension (I10)
  secondary hypertension (I15.-)
  Review coding guideline C.9.a.12

Ischemic heart diseases (I20-I25)
Code also the presence of hypertension (I10-I1A)

I20 Angina pectoris
Use additional code to identify:
exposure to environmental tobacco smoke (Z77.22)
history of tobacco dependence (Z87.891)
occupational exposure to environmental tobacco smoke (Z57.31)
tobacco dependence (F17.-)
tobacco use (Z72.0)
Excludes1: angina pectoris with atherosclerotic heart disease of native coronary arteries (I25.1-)
atherosclerosis of coronary artery bypass graft(s) and coronary artery of transplanted heart with angina pectoris (I25.7-)
postinfarction angina (I23.7)

- **CC I20.0** Unstable angina
  Accelerated angina
  Crescendo angina
  De novo effort angina
  Intermediate coronary syndrome
  Preinfarction syndrome
  Worsening effort angina
- **CC I20.1** Angina pectoris with documented spasm
  Angiospastic angina
  Prinzmetal angina
  Spasm-induced angina
  Variant angina
- **CC I20.2** Refractory angina pectoris
  AHA CC: 4Q, 2022, 20-22
- **+ I20.8** Other forms of angina pectoris
  Use additional code(s) for symptoms associated with angina equivalent
  - **I20.81** Angina pectoris with coronary microvascular dysfunction
    Angina pectoris with coronary microvascular disease

- **I20.89** Other forms of angina pectoris
  Angina equivalent
  Angina of effort
  Coronary slow flow syndrome
  Stable angina
  Stenocardia
- **I20.9** Angina pectoris, unspecified
  Angina NOS
  Anginal syndrome
  Cardiac angina
  Ischemic chest pain

I21 Acute myocardial infarction
Includes: cardiac infarction
coronary (artery) embolism
coronary (artery) occlusion
coronary (artery) rupture
coronary (artery) thrombosis
infarction of heart, myocardium, or ventricle
myocardial infarction specified as acute or with a stated duration of 4 weeks (28 days) or less from onset
Use additional code, if applicable, to identify:
exposure to environmental tobacco smoke (Z77.22)
history of tobacco dependence (Z87.891)
occupational exposure to environmental tobacco smoke (Z57.31)
status post administration of tPA (rtPA) in a different facility within the last 24 hours prior to admission to current facility (Z92.82)
tobacco dependence (F17.-)
tobacco use (Z72.0)
Excludes2: old myocardial infarction (I25.2)
postmyocardial infarction syndrome (I24.1)
subsequent type 1 myocardial infarction (I22.-)
AHA CC: 1Q, 2013, 25; 4Q, 2016, 140

- **+ I21.0** ST elevation (STEMI) myocardial infarction of anterior wall
  Type 1 ST elevation myocardial infarction of anterior wall
  Review coding guideline C.9.e.1
  - **MCC I21.01** ST elevation (STEMI) myocardial infarction involving left main coronary artery
  - **MCC I21.02** ST elevation (STEMI) myocardial infarction involving left anterior descending coronary artery
    ST elevation (STEMI) myocardial infarction involving diagonal coronary artery
    AHA CC: 1Q, 2013, 25-26
  - **MCC I21.09** ST elevation (STEMI) myocardial infarction involving other coronary artery of anterior wall
    Acute transmural myocardial infarction of anterior wall
    Anteroapical transmural (Q wave) infarction (acute)
    Anterolateral transmural (Q wave) infarction (acute)
    Anteroseptal transmural (Q wave) infarction (acute)
    Transmural (Q wave) infarction (acute) (of) anterior (wall) NOS
    AHA CC: 4Q, 2012, 102-104

- **+ I21.1** ST elevation (STEMI) myocardial infarction of inferior wall
  Type 1 ST elevation myocardial infarction of inferior wall
  Review coding guideline C.9.e.1
  - **MCC I21.11** ST elevation (STEMI) myocardial infarction involving right coronary artery
    Inferoposterior transmural (Q wave) infarction (acute)
  - **MCC I21.19** ST elevation (STEMI) myocardial infarction involving other coronary artery of inferior wall
    Acute transmural myocardial infarction of inferior wall
    Inferolateral transmural (Q wave) infarction (acute)
    Transmural (Q wave) infarction (acute) (of) diaphragmatic wall
    Transmural (Q wave) infarction (acute) (of) inferior (wall) NOS
    Excludes2: ST elevation (STEMI) myocardial infarction involving left circumflex coronary artery (I21.21)
    AHA CC: 4Q, 2012, 97

- **+ I21.2** ST elevation (STEMI) myocardial infarction of other sites
  Type 1 ST elevation myocardial infarction of other sites
  Review coding guideline C.9.e.1
  - **MCC I21.21** ST elevation (STEMI) myocardial infarction involving left circumflex coronary artery
    ST elevation (STEMI) myocardial infarction involving oblique marginal coronary artery

Localization of Anterior and Posterior Infarcts

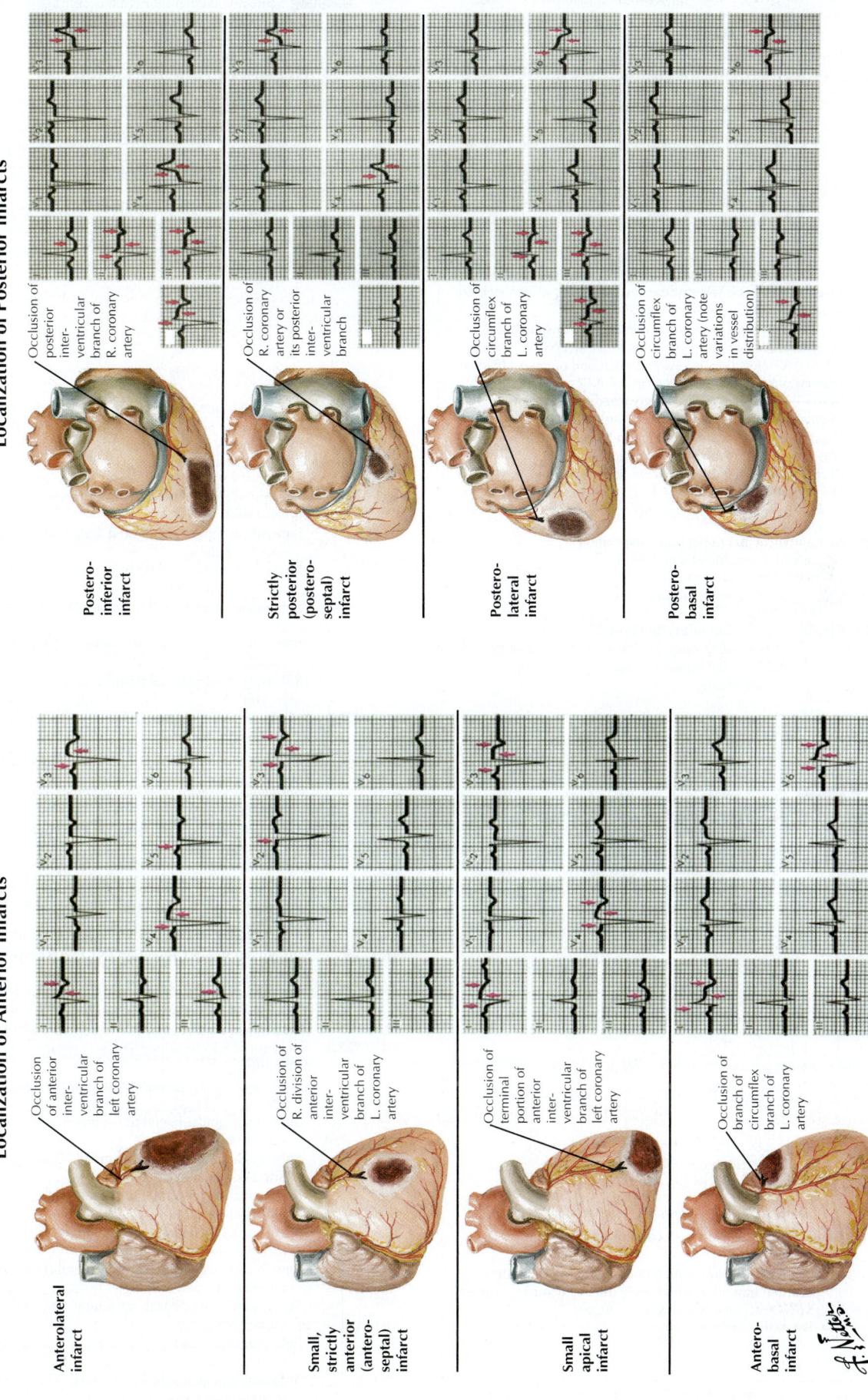

Localization of Posterior Infarcts

- Posteroinferior infarct — Occlusion of posterior interventricular branch of R. coronary artery
- Strictly posterior (posteroseptal) infarct — Occlusion of R. coronary artery or its posterior interventricular branch
- Posterolateral infarct — Occlusion of circumflex branch of L. coronary artery
- Posterobasal infarct — Occlusion of circumflex branch of L. coronary artery (note variations in vessel distribution)

Localization of Anterior Infarcts

- Anterolateral infarct — Occlusion of anterior interventricular branch of left coronary artery
- Small, strictly anterior (anteroseptal) infarct — Occlusion of R. division of anterior interventricular branch of L. coronary artery
- Small apical infarct — Occlusion of terminal portion of anterior interventricular branch of left coronary artery
- Anterobasal infarct — Occlusion of branch of circumflex branch of L. coronary artery

MCC I21.29 ST elevation (STEMI) myocardial infarction involving other sites
    Acute transmural myocardial infarction of other sites
    Apical-lateral transmural (Q wave) infarction (acute)
    Basal-lateral transmural (Q wave) infarction (acute)
    High lateral transmural (Q wave) infarction (acute)
    Lateral (wall) NOS transmural (Q wave) infarction (acute)
    Posterior (true) transmural (Q wave) infarction (acute)
    Posterobasal transmural (Q wave) infarction (acute)
    Posterolateral transmural (Q wave) infarction (acute)
    Posteroseptal transmural (Q wave) infarction (acute)
    Septal transmural (Q wave) infarction (acute) NOS

MCC I21.3 ST elevation (STEMI) myocardial infarction of unspecified site
    Acute transmural myocardial infarction of unspecified site
    Transmural (Q wave) myocardial infarction NOS
    Type 1 ST elevation myocardial infarction of unspecified site
    Review coding guidelines C.9.e.1 and C.9.e.2

MCC I21.4 Non-ST elevation (NSTEMI) myocardial infarction
    Acute subendocardial myocardial infarction
    Non-Q wave myocardial infarction NOS
    Nontransmural myocardial infarction NOS
    Type 1 non-ST elevation myocardial infarction
    Review coding guideline C.9.e.1
    AHA CC: 2Q, 2015, 16-17; 1Q, 2017, 44-45; 3Q, 2021, 6-7; 2Q, 2023, 29

MCC I21.9 Acute myocardial infarction, unspecified
    Myocardial infarction (acute) NOS
    Review coding guideline C.9.e.5

+ I21.A Other type of myocardial infarction
    AHA CC: 4Q, 2017, 12-14

MCC I21.A1 Myocardial infarction type 2
    Myocardial infarction due to demand ischemia
    Myocardial infarction secondary to ischemic imbalance
    Code first the underlying cause, such as:
      anemia (D50.0-D64.9)
      chronic obstructive pulmonary disease (J44.-)
      paroxysmal tachycardia (I47.0-I47.9)
      shock (R57.0-R57.9)

MCC I21.A9 Other myocardial infarction type
    Myocardial infarction associated with revascularization procedure
    Myocardial infarction type 3
    Myocardial infarction type 4a
    Myocardial infarction type 4b
    Myocardial infarction type 4c
    Myocardial infarction type 5
    Code first, if applicable, postprocedural myocardial infarction following cardiac surgery (I97.190), or postprocedural myocardial infarction during cardiac surgery (I97.790)
    Code also complication, if known and applicable, such as:
      (acute) stent occlusion (T82.897-)
      (acute) stent stenosis (T82.855-)
      (acute) stent thrombosis (T82.867-)
      cardiac arrest due to underlying cardiac condition (I46.2)
      complication of percutaneous coronary intervention (PCI) (I97.89)
      occlusion of coronary artery bypass graft (T82.218-)
    AHA CC: 2Q, 2019, 32-33; 3Q, 2021, 6-7

MCC I21.B Myocardial infarction with coronary microvascular dysfunction
    Myocardial infarction with coronary microvascular disease
    Myocardial infarction with nonobstructive coronary arteries [MINOCA] with microvascular disease
    Review coding guideline C.9.e.6

I22 Subsequent ST elevation (STEMI) and non-ST elevation (NSTEMI) myocardial infarction
    Includes: acute myocardial infarction occurring within four weeks (28 days) of a previous acute myocardial infarction, regardless of site
      cardiac infarction
      coronary (artery) embolism
      coronary (artery) occlusion
      coronary (artery) rupture
      coronary (artery) thrombosis
      infarction of heart, myocardium, or ventricle
      recurrent myocardial infarction
      reinfarction of myocardium
      rupture of heart, myocardium, or ventricle
      subsequent type 1 myocardial infarction
    Use additional code, if applicable, to identify:
      exposure to environmental tobacco smoke (Z77.22)
      history of tobacco dependence (Z87.891)
      occupational exposure to environmental tobacco smoke (Z57.31)
      status post administration of tPA (rtPA) in a different facility within the last 24 hours prior to admission to current facility (Z92.82)
      tobacco dependence (F17.-)
      tobacco use (Z72.0)
    Excludes1: subsequent myocardial infarction, type 2 (I21.A1)
      subsequent myocardial infarction of other type (type 3) (type 4) (type 5) (I21.A9)
    Review coding guideline C.9.e.4
    AHA CC: 1Q, 2013, 25

MCC I22.0 Subsequent ST elevation (STEMI) myocardial infarction of anterior wall
    Subsequent acute transmural myocardial infarction of anterior wall
    Subsequent transmural (Q wave) infarction (acute)(of) anterior (wall) NOS
    Subsequent anteroapical transmural (Q wave) infarction (acute)
    Subsequent anterolateral transmural (Q wave) infarction (acute)
    Subsequent anteroseptal transmural (Q wave) infarction (acute)

MCC I22.1 Subsequent ST elevation (STEMI) myocardial infarction of inferior wall
    Subsequent acute transmural myocardial infarction of inferior wall
    Subsequent transmural (Q wave) infarction (acute)(of) diaphragmatic wall
    Subsequent transmural (Q wave) infarction (acute)(of) inferior (wall) NOS
    Subsequent inferolateral transmural (Q wave) infarction (acute)
    Subsequent inferoposterior transmural (Q wave) infarction (acute)
    AHA CC: 4Q, 2012, 102-104

MCC I22.2 Subsequent non-ST elevation (NSTEMI) myocardial infarction
    Subsequent acute subendocardial myocardial infarction
    Subsequent non-Q wave myocardial infarction NOS
    Subsequent nontransmural myocardial infarction NOS

MCC I22.8 Subsequent ST elevation (STEMI) myocardial infarction of other sites
    Subsequent acute transmural myocardial infarction of other sites
    Subsequent apical-lateral transmural (Q wave) myocardial infarction (acute)
    Subsequent basal-lateral transmural (Q wave) myocardial infarction (acute)
    Subsequent high lateral transmural (Q wave) myocardial infarction (acute)
    Subsequent transmural (Q wave) myocardial infarction (acute)(of) lateral (wall) NOS
    Subsequent posterior (true) transmural (Q wave) myocardial infarction (acute)
    Subsequent posterobasal transmural (Q wave) myocardial infarction (acute)
    Subsequent posterolateral transmural (Q wave) myocardial infarction (acute)
    Subsequent posteroseptal transmural (Q wave) myocardial infarction (acute)
    Subsequent septal NOS transmural (Q wave) myocardial infarction (acute)

MCC **I22.9** **Subsequent ST elevation (STEMI) myocardial infarction of unspecified site**
Subsequent acute myocardial infarction of unspecified site
Subsequent myocardial infarction (acute) NOS

I23 **Certain current complications following ST elevation (STEMI) and non-ST elevation (NSTEMI) myocardial infarction (within the 28 day period)**

- CC **I23.0** **Hemopericardium as current complication following acute myocardial infarction**
Excludes1: hemopericardium not specified as current complication following acute myocardial infarction (I31.2)

- CC **I23.1** **Atrial septal defect as current complication following acute myocardial infarction**
Excludes1: acquired atrial septal defect not specified as current complication following acute myocardial infarction (I51.0)

- CC **I23.2** **Ventricular septal defect as current complication following acute myocardial infarction**
Excludes1: acquired ventricular septal defect not specified as current complication following acute myocardial infarction (I51.0)

- CC **I23.3** **Rupture of cardiac wall without hemopericardium as current complication following acute myocardial infarction**
AHA CC: 2Q, 2017, 11-12

MCC **I23.4** **Rupture of chordae tendineae as current complication following acute myocardial infarction**
Excludes1: rupture of chordae tendineae not specified as current complication following acute myocardial infarction (I51.1)

MCC **I23.5** **Rupture of papillary muscle as current complication following acute myocardial infarction**
Excludes1: rupture of papillary muscle not specified as current complication following acute myocardial infarction (I51.2)

- CC **I23.6** **Thrombosis of atrium, auricular appendage, and ventricle as current complications following acute myocardial infarction**
Excludes1: thrombosis of atrium, auricular appendage, and ventricle not specified as current complication following acute myocardial infarction (I51.3)

- CC **I23.7** **Postinfarction angina**
AHA CC: 2Q, 2015, 16-17

- CC **I23.8** **Other current complications following acute myocardial infarction**

I24 **Other acute ischemic heart diseases**
Excludes1: angina pectoris (I20.-)
transient myocardial ischemia in newborn (P29.4)
Excludes2: non-ischemic myocardial injury (I5A)

CC **I24.0** **Acute coronary thrombosis not resulting in myocardial infarction**
Acute coronary (artery) (vein) embolism not resulting in myocardial infarction
Acute coronary (artery) (vein) occlusion not resulting in myocardial infarction
Acute coronary (artery) (vein) thromboembolism not resulting in myocardial infarction
Excludes1: atherosclerotic heart disease (I25.1-)

CC **I24.1** **Dressler's syndrome**
Postmyocardial infarction syndrome
Excludes1: postinfarction angina (I23.7)

+ **I24.8** **Other forms of acute ischemic heart disease**
Excludes1: myocardial infarction due to demand ischemia (I21.A1)

CC **I24.81** **Acute coronary microvascular dysfunction**
Acute (presentation of) coronary microvascular disease

CC **I24.89** **Other forms of acute ischemic heart disease**

CC **I24.9** **Acute ischemic heart disease, unspecified**
Excludes1: ischemic heart disease (chronic) NOS (I25.9)

I25 **Chronic ischemic heart disease**
Use additional code to identify:
chronic total occlusion of coronary artery (I25.82)
exposure to environmental tobacco smoke (Z77.22)
history of tobacco dependence (Z87.891)
occupational exposure to environmental tobacco smoke (Z57.31)
tobacco dependence (F17.-)
tobacco use (Z72.0)
Excludes2: non-ischemic myocardial injury (I5A)

+ **I25.1** **Atherosclerotic heart disease of native coronary artery**
Atherosclerotic cardiovascular disease
Coronary (artery) atheroma
Coronary (artery) atherosclerosis
Coronary (artery) disease
Coronary (artery) sclerosis
Use additional code, if applicable, to identify:
coronary atherosclerosis due to calcified coronary lesion (I25.84)
coronary atherosclerosis due to lipid rich plaque (I25.83)
Excludes2: atheroembolism (I75.-)
atherosclerosis of coronary artery bypass graft(s) and transplanted heart (I25.7-)

- **I25.10** **Atherosclerotic heart disease of native coronary artery without angina pectoris**
Atherosclerotic heart disease NOS
AHA CC: 4Q, 2012, 92-92; 4Q, 2013, 128;3Q, 2021, 6-8

Great Vessels of the Heart

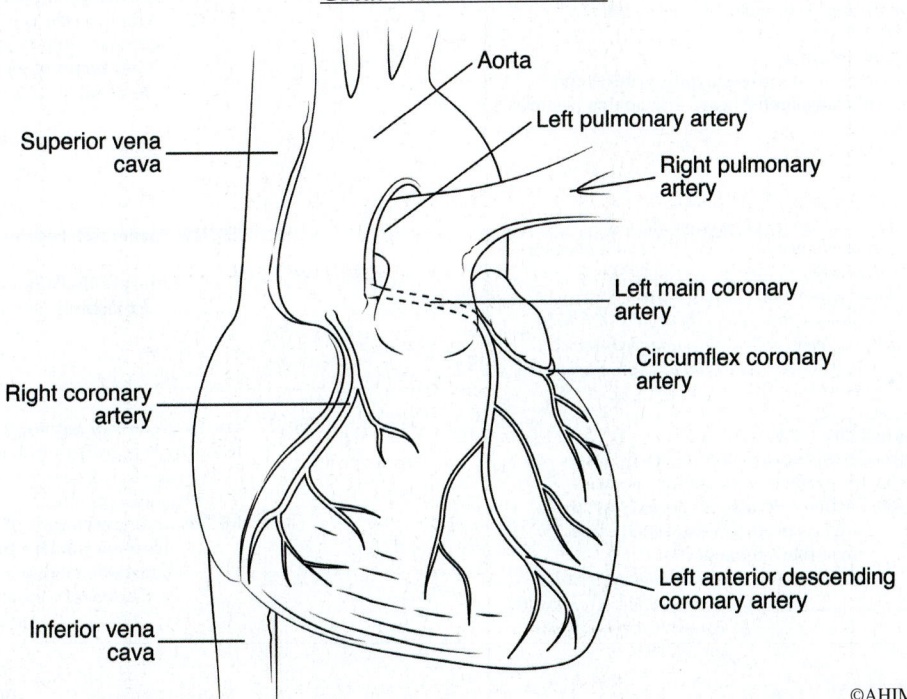

©AHIMA

I25.11–I25.720 — Chapter 9: Diseases of the Circulatory System

- **+ I25.11** Atherosclerotic heart disease of native coronary artery with angina pectoris
  Review coding guideline C.9.b
  - **CC I25.110** Atherosclerotic heart disease of native coronary artery with unstable angina pectoris
    Excludes1: unstable angina without atherosclerotic heart disease (I20.0)
  - **I25.111** Atherosclerotic heart disease of native coronary artery with angina pectoris with documented spasm
    Excludes1: angina pectoris with documented spasm without atherosclerotic heart disease (I20.1)
  - **CC I25.112** Atherosclerotic heart disease of native coronary artery with refractory angina pectoris
    AHA CC: 4Q, 2022, 20-22
  - **I25.118** Atherosclerotic heart disease of native coronary artery with other forms of angina pectoris
    Excludes1: other forms of angina pectoris without atherosclerotic heart disease (I20.8-)
    AHA CC: 2Q, 2015, 16-17
  - **I25.119** Atherosclerotic heart disease of native coronary artery with unspecified angina pectoris
    Atherosclerotic heart disease with angina NOS
    Atherosclerotic heart disease with ischemic chest pain
    Excludes1: unspecified angina pectoris without atherosclerotic heart disease (I20.9)

- **I25.2** Old myocardial infarction
  Healed myocardial infarction
  Past myocardial infarction diagnosed by ECG or other investigation, but currently presenting no symptoms
- **CC I25.3** Aneurysm of heart
  Mural aneurysm
  Ventricular aneurysm
- **+ I25.4** Coronary artery aneurysm and dissection
  - **I25.41** Coronary artery aneurysm
    Coronary arteriovenous fistula, acquired
    Excludes1: congenital coronary (artery) aneurysm (Q24.5)
  - **MCC I25.42** Coronary artery dissection
- **I25.5** Ischemic cardiomyopathy
  Excludes2: coronary atherosclerosis (I25.1-, I25.7-)
  AHA CC: 3Q, 2022, 17-18
- **I25.6** Silent myocardial ischemia
- **+ I25.7** Atherosclerosis of coronary artery bypass graft(s) and coronary artery of transplanted heart with angina pectoris
  Use additional code, if applicable, to identify:
    coronary atherosclerosis due to calcified coronary lesion (I25.84)
    coronary atherosclerosis due to lipid rich plaque (I25.83)
  Excludes1: atherosclerosis of bypass graft(s) of transplanted heart without angina pectoris (I25.812)
    atherosclerosis of coronary artery bypass graft(s) without angina pectoris (I25.810)
    atherosclerosis of native coronary artery of transplanted heart without angina pectoris (I25.811)
  AHA CC: 4Q, 2022, 20-22
  Review coding guideline C.9.b
  - **+ I25.70** Atherosclerosis of coronary artery bypass graft(s), unspecified, with angina pectoris
    - **CC I25.700** Atherosclerosis of coronary artery bypass graft(s), unspecified, with unstable angina pectoris
      Excludes1: unstable angina pectoris without atherosclerosis of coronary artery bypass graft (I20.0)
    - **I25.701** Atherosclerosis of coronary artery bypass graft(s), unspecified, with angina pectoris with documented spasm
      Excludes1: angina pectoris with documented spasm without atherosclerosis of coronary artery bypass graft (I20.1)
    - **CC I25.702** Atherosclerosis of coronary artery bypass graft(s), unspecified, with refractory angina pectoris
      AHA CC: 4Q, 2022, 21-22
    - **I25.708** Atherosclerosis of coronary artery bypass graft(s), unspecified, with other forms of angina pectoris
      Excludes1: other forms of angina pectoris without atherosclerosis of coronary artery bypass graft (I20.8-)
    - **I25.709** Atherosclerosis of coronary artery bypass graft(s), unspecified, with unspecified angina pectoris
      Excludes1: unspecified angina pectoris without atherosclerosis of coronary artery bypass graft (I20.9)
  - **+ I25.71** Atherosclerosis of autologous vein coronary artery bypass graft(s) with angina pectoris
    - **CC I25.710** Atherosclerosis of autologous vein coronary artery bypass graft(s) with unstable angina pectoris
      Excludes1: unstable angina without atherosclerosis of autologous vein coronary artery bypass graft(s) (I20.0)
      Excludes2: embolism or thrombus of coronary artery bypass graft(s) (T82.8-)
    - **CC I25.711** Atherosclerosis of autologous vein coronary artery bypass graft(s) with angina pectoris with documented spasm
      Excludes1: angina pectoris with documented spasm without atherosclerosis of autologous vein coronary artery bypass graft(s) (I20.1)
    - **CC I25.712** Atherosclerosis of autologous vein coronary artery bypass graft(s) with refractory angina pectoris
    - **CC I25.718** Atherosclerosis of autologous vein coronary artery bypass graft(s) with other forms of angina pectoris
      Excludes1: other forms of angina pectoris without atherosclerosis of autologous vein coronary artery bypass graft(s) (I20.8-)
    - **CC I25.719** Atherosclerosis of autologous vein coronary artery bypass graft(s) with unspecified angina pectoris
      Excludes1: unspecified angina pectoris without atherosclerosis of autologous vein coronary artery bypass graft(s) (I20.9)
  - **+ I25.72** Atherosclerosis of autologous artery coronary artery bypass graft(s) with angina pectoris
    Atherosclerosis of internal mammary artery graft with angina pectoris
    - **CC I25.720** Atherosclerosis of autologous artery coronary artery bypass graft(s) with unstable angina pectoris
      Excludes1: unstable angina without atherosclerosis of autologous artery coronary artery bypass graft(s) (I20.0)

Pathologic Changes in CAD; Types and Degrees of Coronary Atherosclerotic Narrowing or Occlusion

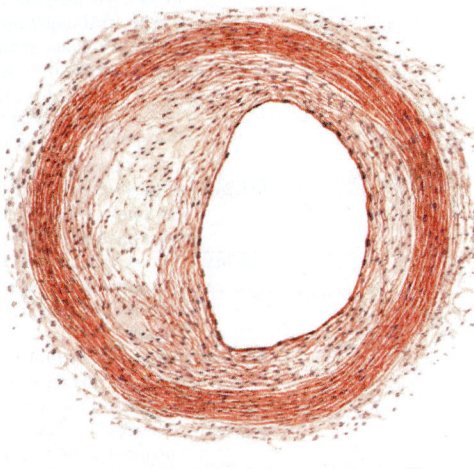

Moderate atherosclerotic narrowing of lumen

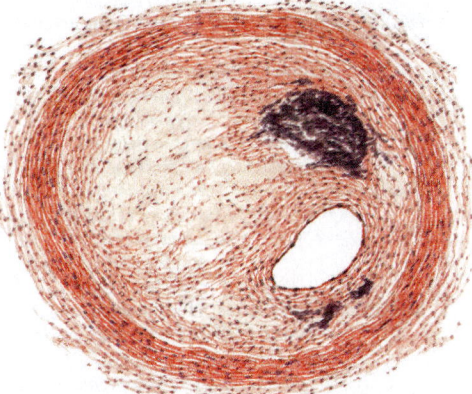

Almost complete occlusion by intimal atherosclerosis with calcium deposition

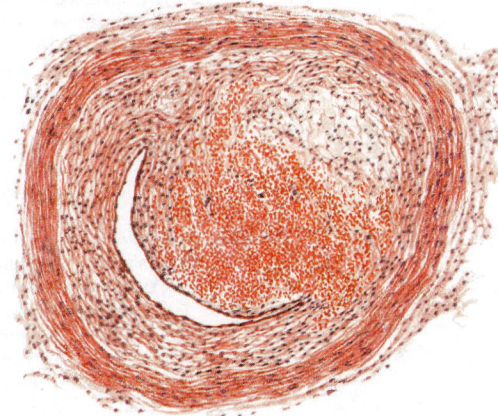

Hemorrhage into atheroma, leaving only a slit-like lumen

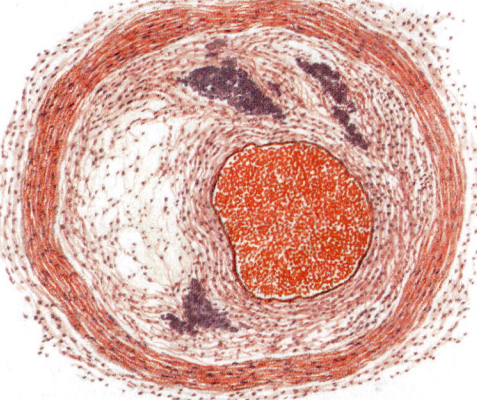

Complete occlusion by thrombus in lumen greatly narrowed by atheroma

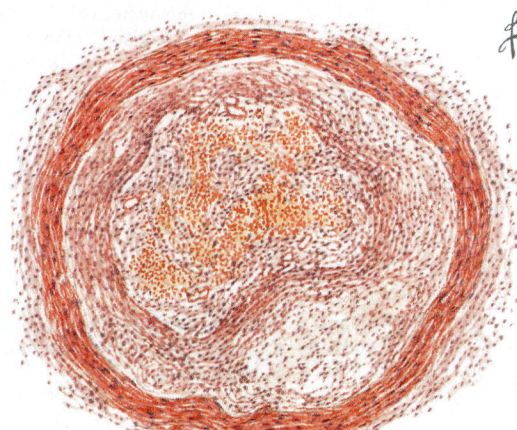

Organization of thrombus

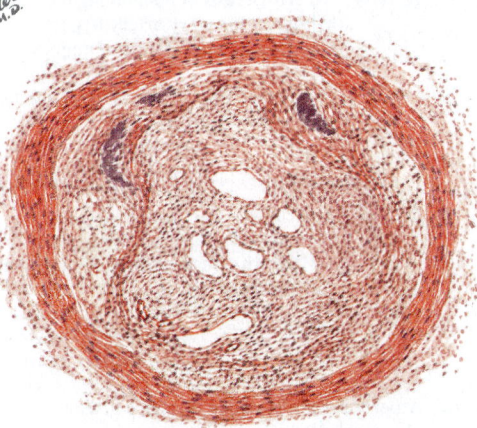

Organization with recanalization may occur

I25.721–I25.810 Chapter 9: Diseases of the Circulatory System

- **CC I25.721** Atherosclerosis of autologous artery coronary artery bypass graft(s) with angina pectoris with documented spasm
  Excludes1: angina pectoris with documented spasm without atherosclerosis of autologous artery coronary artery bypass graft(s) (I20.1)
- **CC I25.722** Atherosclerosis of autologous artery coronary artery bypass graft(s) with refractory angina pectoris
- **CC I25.728** Atherosclerosis of autologous artery coronary artery bypass graft(s) with other forms of angina pectoris
  Excludes1: other forms of angina pectoris without atherosclerosis of autologous artery coronary artery bypass graft(s) (I20.8-)
- **CC I25.729** Atherosclerosis of autologous artery coronary artery bypass graft(s) with unspecified angina pectoris
  Excludes1: unspecified angina pectoris without atherosclerosis of autologous artery coronary artery bypass graft(s) (I20.9)

+ **I25.73** Atherosclerosis of nonautologous biological coronary artery bypass graft(s) with angina pectoris
  - **CC I25.730** Atherosclerosis of nonautologous biological coronary artery bypass graft(s) with unstable angina pectoris
    Excludes1: unstable angina without atherosclerosis of nonautologous biological coronary artery bypass graft(s) (I20.0)
  - **CC I25.731** Atherosclerosis of nonautologous biological coronary artery bypass graft(s) with angina pectoris with documented spasm
    Excludes1: angina pectoris with documented spasm without atherosclerosis of nonautologous biological coronary artery bypass graft(s) (I20.1)
  - **CC I25.732** Atherosclerosis of nonautologous biological coronary artery bypass graft(s) with refractory angina pectoris
  - **CC I25.738** Atherosclerosis of nonautologous biological coronary artery bypass graft(s) with other forms of angina pectoris
    Excludes1: other forms of angina pectoris without atherosclerosis of nonautologous biological coronary artery bypass graft(s) (I20.8-)
  - **CC I25.739** Atherosclerosis of nonautologous biological coronary artery bypass graft(s) with unspecified angina pectoris
    Excludes1: unspecified angina pectoris without atherosclerosis of nonautologous biological coronary artery bypass graft(s) (I20.9)

+ **I25.75** Atherosclerosis of native coronary artery of transplanted heart with angina pectoris
  Excludes1: atherosclerosis of native coronary artery of transplanted heart without angina pectoris (I25.811)
  - **CC I25.750** Atherosclerosis of native coronary artery of transplanted heart with unstable angina
  - **CC I25.751** Atherosclerosis of native coronary artery of transplanted heart with angina pectoris with documented spasm
  - **CC I25.752** Atherosclerosis of native coronary artery of transplanted heart with refractory angina pectoris
  - **CC I25.758** Atherosclerosis of native coronary artery of transplanted heart with other forms of angina pectoris
  - **CC I25.759** Atherosclerosis of native coronary artery of transplanted heart with unspecified angina pectoris

+ **I25.76** Atherosclerosis of bypass graft of coronary artery of transplanted heart with angina pectoris
  Excludes1: atherosclerosis of bypass graft of coronary artery of transplanted heart without angina pectoris (I25.812)
  - **CC I25.760** Atherosclerosis of bypass graft of coronary artery of transplanted heart with unstable angina
  - **CC I25.761** Atherosclerosis of bypass graft of coronary artery of transplanted heart with angina pectoris with documented spasm
  - **CC I25.762** Atherosclerosis of bypass graft of coronary artery of transplanted heart with refractory angina pectoris
  - **CC I25.768** Atherosclerosis of bypass graft of coronary artery of transplanted heart with other forms of angina pectoris
  - **CC I25.769** Atherosclerosis of bypass graft of coronary artery of transplanted heart with unspecified angina pectoris

+ **I25.79** Atherosclerosis of other coronary artery bypass graft(s) with angina pectoris
  - **CC I25.790** Atherosclerosis of other coronary artery bypass graft(s) with unstable angina pectoris
    Excludes1: unstable angina without atherosclerosis of other coronary artery bypass graft(s) (I20.0)
  - **CC I25.791** Atherosclerosis of other coronary artery bypass graft(s) with angina pectoris with documented spasm
    Excludes1: angina pectoris with documented spasm without atherosclerosis of other coronary artery bypass graft(s) (I20.1)
  - **CC I25.792** Atherosclerosis of other coronary artery bypass graft(s) with refractory angina pectoris
  - **CC I25.798** Atherosclerosis of other coronary artery bypass graft(s) with other forms of angina pectoris
    Excludes1: other forms of angina pectoris without atherosclerosis of other coronary artery bypass graft(s) (I20.8-)
  - **CC I25.799** Atherosclerosis of other coronary artery bypass graft(s) with unspecified angina pectoris
    Excludes1: unspecified angina pectoris without atherosclerosis of other coronary artery bypass graft(s) (I20.9)

+ **I25.8** Other forms of chronic ischemic heart disease
  + **I25.81** Atherosclerosis of other coronary vessels without angina pectoris
    Use additional code, if applicable, to identify:
    coronary atherosclerosis due to calcified coronary lesion (I25.84)
    coronary atherosclerosis due to lipid rich plaque (I25.83)
    Excludes2: atherosclerotic heart disease of native coronary artery without angina pectoris (I25.10)
    - **CC I25.810** Atherosclerosis of coronary artery bypass graft(s) without angina pectoris
      Atherosclerosis of coronary artery bypass graft NOS

Excludes1: atherosclerosis of coronary bypass graft(s) with angina pectoris (I25.70-I25.73-, I25.79-)

- **CC I25.811 Atherosclerosis of native coronary artery of transplanted heart without angina pectoris**
  Atherosclerosis of native coronary artery of transplanted heart NOS
  Excludes1: atherosclerosis of native coronary artery of transplanted heart with angina pectoris (I25.75-)
- **CC I25.812 Atherosclerosis of bypass graft of coronary artery of transplanted heart without angina pectoris**
  Atherosclerosis of bypass graft of transplanted heart NOS
  Excludes1: atherosclerosis of bypass graft of transplanted heart with angina pectoris (I25.76)

I25.82 Chronic total occlusion of coronary artery
  Complete occlusion of coronary artery
  Total occlusion of coronary artery
  Code first coronary atherosclerosis (I25.1-, I25.7-, I25.81-)
  Excludes1: acute coronary occlusion with myocardial infarction (I21.0-I21.B, I22.-)
  acute coronary occlusion without myocardial infarction (I24.0)
  AHA CC: 3Q, 2018, 5-6

- **I25.83 Coronary atherosclerosis due to lipid rich plaque**
  Code first coronary atherosclerosis (I25.1-, I25.7-, I25.81-)

I25.84 Coronary atherosclerosis due to calcified coronary lesion
  Coronary atherosclerosis due to severely calcified coronary lesion
  Code first coronary atherosclerosis (I25.1-, I25.7-, I25.81-)

I25.85 Chronic coronary microvascular dysfunction
  Chronic (presentation of) coronary microvascular disease
  Coronary microvascular dysfunction NOS

I25.89 Other forms of chronic ischemic heart disease

I25.9 Chronic ischemic heart disease, unspecified
  Ischemic heart disease (chronic) NOS

Pulmonary heart disease and diseases of pulmonary circulation (I26-I28)

I26 Pulmonary embolism
Includes: pulmonary (acute) (artery)(vein) infarction
pulmonary (acute) (artery)(vein) thromboembolism
pulmonary (acute) (artery)(vein) thrombosis
Excludes1: cor pulmonale without embolism (I27.81)
Excludes2: chronic pulmonary embolism (I27.82)
personal history of pulmonary embolism (Z86.711)
pulmonary embolism due to trauma (T79.0, T79.1)
pulmonary embolism due to complications of surgical and medical care (T80.0, T81.7-, T82.8-)
pulmonary embolism complicating abortion, ectopic or molar pregnancy (O00-O07, O08.2)
pulmonary embolism complicating pregnancy, childbirth and the puerperium (O88.-)
septic (non-pulmonary) arterial embolism (I76)

+ **I26.0 Pulmonary embolism with acute cor pulmonale**
  MCC I26.01 Septic pulmonary embolism with acute cor pulmonale
    Code first underlying infection
  MCC I26.02 Saddle embolus of pulmonary artery with acute cor pulmonale
    HAC see Appendix B for HAC conditional logic
  MCC I26.09 Other pulmonary embolism with acute cor pulmonale
    HAC see Appendix B for HAC conditional logic

+ **I26.9 Pulmonary embolism without acute cor pulmonale**
  MCC I26.90 Septic pulmonary embolism without acute cor pulmonale
    Code first underlying infection

MCC I26.92 Saddle embolus of pulmonary artery without acute cor pulmonale
  HAC see Appendix B for HAC conditional logic

MCC I26.93 Single subsegmental pulmonary embolism without acute cor pulmonale
  Subsegmental pulmonary embolism NOS
  AHA CC: 4Q, 2019, 6-7
  HAC see Appendix B for HAC conditional logic

MCC I26.94 Multiple subsegmental pulmonary emboli without acute cor pulmonale
  AHA CC: 4Q, 2019, 6-7; 2Q, 2021, 9-10; 2Q, 2022, 13
  HAC see Appendix B for HAC conditional logic

MCC I26.99 Other pulmonary embolism without acute cor pulmonale
  Acute pulmonary embolism NOS
  Pulmonary embolism NOS
  AHA CC: 2Q, 2019, 22-23; 3Q, 2020, 10-11; 2Q, 2022, 13
  HAC see Appendix B for HAC conditional logic

I27 Other pulmonary heart diseases
Review coding guideline C.9.a.11

CC I27.0 Primary pulmonary hypertension
  Heritable pulmonary arterial hypertension
  Idiopathic pulmonary arterial hypertension
  Primary group 1 pulmonary hypertension
  Primary pulmonary arterial hypertension
  Excludes1: persistent pulmonary hypertension of newborn (P29.30)
  pulmonary hypertension NOS (I27.20)
  secondary pulmonary arterial hypertension (I27.21)
  secondary pulmonary hypertension (I27.29)
  AHA CC: 4Q, 2017, 14-15

CC I27.1 Kyphoscoliotic heart disease

+ **I27.2 Other secondary pulmonary hypertension**
  Code also associated underlying condition
  Excludes1: Eisenmenger's syndrome (I27.83)
  AHA CC: 4Q, 2014, 21-22; 2Q, 2016, 8; 4Q, 2017, 14-15

  I27.20 Pulmonary hypertension, unspecified
    Pulmonary hypertension NOS

  I27.21 Secondary pulmonary arterial hypertension
    (Associated) (drug-induced) (toxin-induced) pulmonary arterial hypertension NOS
    (Associated) (drug-induced) (toxin-induced) (secondary) group 1 pulmonary hypertension
    Code also associated conditions if applicable, or adverse effects of drugs or toxins, such as:
    adverse effect of appetite depressants (T50.5X5)
    congenital heart disease (Q20-Q28)
    human immunodeficiency virus [HIV] disease (B20)
    polymyositis (M33.2-)
    portal hypertension (K76.6)
    rheumatoid arthritis (M05.-)
    schistosomiasis (B65.-)
    Sjögren syndrome (M35.0-)
    systemic sclerosis (M34.-)

  I27.22 Pulmonary hypertension due to left heart disease
    Group 2 pulmonary hypertension
    Code also associated left heart disease, if known, such as:
    multiple valve disease (I08.-)
    rheumatic mitral valve diseases (I05.-)
    rheumatic aortic valve diseases (I06.-)

  I27.23 Pulmonary hypertension due to lung diseases and hypoxia
    Group 3 pulmonary hypertension
    Code also associated lung disease, if known, such as:
    bronchiectasis (J47.-)
    cystic fibrosis with pulmonary manifestations (E84.0)
    interstitial lung disease (J84.-)
    pleural effusion (J90)
    sleep apnea (G47.3-)

  I27.24 Chronic thromboembolic pulmonary hypertension
    Group 4 pulmonary hypertension
    Code also associated pulmonary embolism, if applicable (I26.-, I27.82)

  I27.29 Other secondary pulmonary hypertension
    Group 5 pulmonary hypertension

Pulmonary hypertension with unclear multifactorial mechanisms
Pulmonary hypertension due to hematologic disorders
Pulmonary hypertension due to metabolic disorders
Pulmonary hypertension due to other systemic disorders
Code also other associated disorders, if known, such as:
chronic myeloid leukemia (C92.10-C92.22)
essential thrombocythemia (D47.3)
Gaucher disease (E75.22)
hypertensive chronic kidney disease with end stage renal disease (I12.0, I13.11, I13.2)
hyperthyroidism (E05.-)
hypothyroidism (E00-E03)
polycythemia vera (D45)
sarcoidosis (D86.-)

+ **I27.8 Other specified pulmonary heart diseases**
  I27.81 Cor pulmonale (chronic)
  Cor pulmonale NOS
  Code also, if applicable, right heart failure (I50.81-)
  Excludes1: acute cor pulmonale (I26.0-)
  AHA CC: 4Q, 2014, 21-22
  CC **I27.82 Chronic pulmonary embolism**
  Use additional code, if applicable, for associated long-term (current) use of anticoagulants (Z79.01)
  Excludes1: personal history of pulmonary embolism (Z86.711)
  AHA CC: 2Q, 2021, 9-10
  I27.83 Eisenmenger's syndrome
  Eisenmenger's complex
  (Irreversible) Eisenmenger's disease
  Pulmonary hypertension with right to left shunt related to congenital heart disease
  Code also underlying heart defect, if known, such as:
  atrial septal defect (Q21.1-)
  Eisenmenger's defect (Q21.8)
  patent ductus arteriosus (Q25.0)
  ventricular septal defect (Q21.0)
  I27.89 Other specified pulmonary heart diseases

I27.9 Pulmonary heart disease, unspecified
Chronic cardiopulmonary disease

I28 Other diseases of pulmonary vessels
CC **I28.0 Arteriovenous fistula of pulmonary vessels**
Excludes1: congenital arteriovenous fistula (Q25.72)
CC **I28.1 Aneurysm of pulmonary artery**
Excludes1: congenital aneurysm (Q25.79)
congenital arteriovenous aneurysm (Q25.72)
I28.8 Other diseases of pulmonary vessels
Pulmonary arteritis
Pulmonary endarteritis
Rupture of pulmonary vessels
Stenosis of pulmonary vessels
Stricture of pulmonary vessels
I28.9 Disease of pulmonary vessels, unspecified

Other forms of heart disease (I30-I5A)

I30 Acute pericarditis
Includes: acute mediastinopericarditis
acute myopericarditis
acute pericardial effusion
acute pleuropericarditis
acute pneumopericarditis
Excludes1: Dressler's syndrome (I24.1)
rheumatic pericarditis (acute) (I01.0)
viral pericarditis due to Coxsackie virus (B33.23)
CC **I30.0 Acute nonspecific idiopathic pericarditis**
CC **I30.1 Infective pericarditis**
Pneumococcal pericarditis
Pneumopyopericardium
Purulent pericarditis
Pyopericarditis
Pyopericardium
Pyopneumopericardium
Staphylococcal pericarditis
Streptococcal pericarditis
Suppurative pericarditis
Viral pericarditis
Use additional code (B95-B97) to identify infectious agent
CC **I30.8 Other forms of acute pericarditis**
CC **I30.9 Acute pericarditis, unspecified**

I31 Other diseases of pericardium
Excludes1: diseases of pericardium specified as rheumatic (I09.2)
postcardiotomy syndrome (I97.0)
traumatic injury to pericardium (S26.-)
CC **I31.0 Chronic adhesive pericarditis**
Accretio cordis
Adherent pericardium
Adhesive mediastinopericarditis
CC **I31.1 Chronic constrictive pericarditis**
Concretio cordis
Pericardial calcification
CC **I31.2 Hemopericardium, not elsewhere classified**
Excludes1: hemopericardium as current complication following acute myocardial infarction (I23.0)
malignant pericardial effusion (I31.31)
+ **I31.3 Pericardial effusion (noninflammatory)**
Excludes1: acute pericardial effusion (I30.9)
AHA CC: 1Q, 2019, 16; 4Q, 2022, 22-23
CC **I31.31 Malignant pericardial effusion in diseases classified elsewhere**
Code first underlying neoplasm (C00-D49)
AHA CC: 4Q, 2022, 22-23
CC **I31.39 Other pericardial effusion (noninflammatory)**
Chylopericardium
CC **I31.4 Cardiac tamponade**
Code first underlying cause
CC **I31.8 Other specified diseases of pericardium**
Epicardial plaques
Focal pericardial adhesions
CC **I31.9 Disease of pericardium, unspecified**
Pericarditis (chronic) NOS

CC **I32 Pericarditis in diseases classified elsewhere**
Code first underlying disease
Excludes1: pericarditis (in):
coxsackie (virus) (B33.23)
gonococcal (A54.83)
meningococcal (A39.53)
rheumatoid (arthritis) (M05.31)
syphilitic (A52.06)
systemic lupus erythematosus (M32.12)
tuberculosis (A18.84)
Valid 3-character code, no further characters required

I33 Acute and subacute endocarditis
Excludes1: acute rheumatic endocarditis (I01.1)
endocarditis NOS (I38)
MCC **I33.0 Acute and subacute infective endocarditis**
Bacterial endocarditis (acute) (subacute)
Infective endocarditis (acute) (subacute) NOS
Endocarditis lenta (acute) (subacute)
Malignant endocarditis (acute) (subacute)
Purulent endocarditis (acute) (subacute)
Septic endocarditis (acute) (subacute)
Ulcerative endocarditis (acute) (subacute)
Vegetative endocarditis (acute) (subacute)
Use additional code (B95-B97) to identify infectious agent
MCC **I33.9 Acute and subacute endocarditis, unspecified**
Acute endocarditis NOS
Acute myoendocarditis NOS
Acute periendocarditis NOS
Subacute endocarditis NOS
Subacute myoendocarditis NOS
Subacute periendocarditis NOS

I34 Nonrheumatic mitral valve disorders
Excludes1: mitral valve disease (I05.9)
mitral valve failure (I05.8)
mitral valve stenosis (I05.0)
mitral valve disorder of unspecified cause with diseases of aortic and/or tricuspid valve(s) (I08.-)
mitral valve disorder of unspecified cause with mitral stenosis or obstruction (I05.0)
mitral valve disorder specified as congenital (Q23.2, Q23.9)
mitral valve disorder specified as rheumatic (I05.-)
I34.0 Nonrheumatic mitral (valve) insufficiency
Nonrheumatic mitral (valve) incompetence NOS
Nonrheumatic mitral (valve) regurgitation NOS
Code also, if applicable:
nonrheumatic mitral (valve) annulus calcification (I34.81)

I34.1 Nonrheumatic mitral (valve) prolapse
　　Floppy nonrheumatic mitral valve syndrome
　　Excludes1: *Marfan's syndrome (Q87.4-)*
I34.2 Nonrheumatic mitral (valve) stenosis
　　Code also, if applicable:
　　　nonrheumatic mitral (valve) annulus calcification (I34.81)
+ I34.8 Other nonrheumatic mitral valve disorders
　　AHA CC: 4Q, 2022, 23
　　I34.81 Nonrheumatic mitral (valve) annulus calcification
　　　　Nonrheumatic mitral (valve) annular calcification
　　　　Mitral (valve) annulus calcification NOS
　　　　Code also, if applicable:
　　　　　nonrheumatic mitral (valve) insufficiency (I34.0)
　　　　　nonrheumatic mitral (valve) stenosis (I34.2)
　　I34.89 Other nonrheumatic mitral valve disorders
I34.9 Nonrheumatic mitral valve disorder, unspecified

I35 **Nonrheumatic aortic valve disorders**
　　Excludes1: *aortic valve disorder of unspecified cause but with diseases of mitral and/or tricuspid valve(s) (I08.-)*
　　　　aortic valve disorder specified as congenital (Q23.0, Q23.1)
　　　　aortic valve disorder specified as rheumatic (I06.-)
　　　　hypertrophic subaortic stenosis (I42.1)
I35.0 Nonrheumatic aortic (valve) stenosis
I35.1 Nonrheumatic aortic (valve) insufficiency
　　Nonrheumatic aortic (valve) incompetence NOS
　　Nonrheumatic aortic (valve) regurgitation NOS
I35.2 Nonrheumatic aortic (valve) stenosis with insufficiency
I35.8 Other nonrheumatic aortic valve disorders
I35.9 Nonrheumatic aortic valve disorder, unspecified

I36 **Nonrheumatic tricuspid valve disorders**
　　Excludes1: *tricuspid valve disorders of unspecified cause (I07.-)*
　　　　tricuspid valve disorders specified as congenital (Q22.4, Q22.8, Q22.9)
　　　　tricuspid valve disorders specified as rheumatic (I07.-)
　　　　tricuspid valve disorders with aortic and/or mitral valve involvement (I08.-)
I36.0 Nonrheumatic tricuspid (valve) stenosis
I36.1 Nonrheumatic tricuspid (valve) insufficiency
　　Nonrheumatic tricuspid (valve) incompetence
　　Nonrheumatic tricuspid (valve) regurgitation
I36.2 Nonrheumatic tricuspid (valve) stenosis with insufficiency
I36.8 Other nonrheumatic tricuspid valve disorders
I36.9 Nonrheumatic tricuspid valve disorder, unspecified

I37 **Nonrheumatic pulmonary valve disorders**
　　Excludes1: *pulmonary valve disorder specified as congenital (Q22.1, Q22.2, Q22.3)*
　　　　pulmonary valve disorder specified as rheumatic (I09.89)
I37.0 Nonrheumatic pulmonary valve stenosis
I37.1 Nonrheumatic pulmonary valve insufficiency
　　Nonrheumatic pulmonary valve incompetence
　　Nonrheumatic pulmonary valve regurgitation
I37.2 Nonrheumatic pulmonary valve stenosis with insufficiency
I37.8 Other nonrheumatic pulmonary valve disorders
I37.9 Nonrheumatic pulmonary valve disorder, unspecified

CC I38 **Endocarditis, valve unspecified**
　　Includes: endocarditis (chronic) NOS
　　　　valvular incompetence NOS
　　　　valvular insufficiency NOS
　　　　valvular regurgitation NOS
　　　　valvular stenosis NOS
　　　　valvulitis (chronic) NOS
　　Excludes1: *congenital insufficiency of cardiac valve NOS (Q24.8)*
　　　　congenital stenosis of cardiac valve NOS (Q24.8)
　　　　endocardial fibroelastosis (I42.4)
　　　　endocarditis specified as rheumatic (I09.1)
　　Valid 3-character code, no further characters required

CC I39 **Endocarditis and heart valve disorders in diseases classified elsewhere**
　　Code first underlying disease, such as:
　　　Q fever (A78)
　　Excludes1: *endocardial involvement in:*
　　　　candidiasis (B37.6)
　　　　gonococcal infection (A54.83)
　　　　Libman-Sacks disease (M32.11)
　　　　listerosis (A32.82)
　　　　meningococcal infection (A39.51)
　　　　rheumatoid arthritis (M05.31)
　　　　syphilis (A52.03)
　　　　tuberculosis (A18.84)
　　　　typhoid fever (A01.02)
　　Valid 3-character code, no further characters required

I40 **Acute myocarditis**
　　Includes: subacute myocarditis
　　Excludes1: *acute rheumatic myocarditis (I01.2)*
MCC I40.0 Infective myocarditis
　　Septic myocarditis
　　Use additional code (B95-B97) to identify infectious agent
MCC I40.1 Isolated myocarditis
　　Fiedler's myocarditis
　　Giant cell myocarditis
　　Idiopathic myocarditis
MCC I40.8 Other acute myocarditis
MCC I40.9 Acute myocarditis, unspecified

MCC I41 **Myocarditis in diseases classified elsewhere**
　　Code first underlying disease, such as:
　　　typhus (A75.0-A75.9)
　　Excludes1: *myocarditis (in):*
　　　　Chagas' disease (chronic) (B57.2)
　　　　acute (B57.0)
　　　　coxsackie (virus) infection (B33.22)
　　　　diphtheritic (A36.81)
　　　　gonococcal (A54.83)
　　　　influenzal (J09.X9, J10.82, J11.82)
　　　　meningococcal (A39.52)
　　　　mumps (B26.82)
　　　　rheumatoid arthritis (M05.31)
　　　　sarcoid (D86.85)
　　　　syphilis (A52.06)
　　　　toxoplasmosis (B58.81)
　　　　tuberculous (A18.84)
　　Valid 3-character code, no further characters required

I42 **Cardiomyopathy**
　　Includes: myocardiopathy
　　Code first pre-existing cardiomyopathy complicating pregnancy and puerperium (O99.4)
　　Excludes2: *ischemic cardiomyopathy (I25.5)*
　　　　peripartum cardiomyopathy (O90.3)
　　　　ventricular hypertrophy (I51.7)
CC I42.0 Dilated cardiomyopathy
　　Congestive cardiomyopathy
CC I42.1 Obstructive hypertrophic cardiomyopathy
　　Hypertrophic subaortic stenosis (idiopathic)
CC I42.2 Other hypertrophic cardiomyopathy
　　Nonobstructive hypertrophic cardiomyopathy
CC I42.3 Endomyocardial (eosinophilic) disease
　　Endomyocardial (tropical) fibrosis
　　Löffler's endocarditis
CC I42.4 Endocardial fibroelastosis
　　Congenital cardiomyopathy
　　Elastomyofibrosis
CC I42.5 Other restrictive cardiomyopathy
　　Constrictive cardiomyopathy NOS
CC I42.6 Alcoholic cardiomyopathy
　　Code also presence of alcoholism (F10.-)
CC I42.7 Cardiomyopathy due to drug and external agent
　　Code first poisoning due to drug or toxin, if applicable (T36-T65 with fifth or sixth character 1-4)
　　Use additional code for adverse effect, if applicable, to identify drug (T36-T50 with fifth or sixth character 5)
　　AHA CC: 3Q, 2021, 8
CC I42.8 Other cardiomyopathies
CC I42.9 Cardiomyopathy, unspecified
　　Cardiomyopathy (primary) (secondary) NOS

CC I43 **Cardiomyopathy in diseases classified elsewhere**
　　Code first underlying disease, such as:
　　　amyloidosis (E85.-)
　　　glycogen storage disease (E74.0-)
　　　gout (M10.0-)
　　　thyrotoxicosis (E05.0-E05.9-)
　　Excludes1: *cardiomyopathy (in):*
　　　　coxsackie (virus) (B33.24)
　　　　diphtheria (A36.81)
　　　　sarcoidosis (D86.85)
　　　　tuberculosis (A18.84)
　　Valid 3-character code, no further characters required

Chapter 9: Diseases of the Circulatory System

I44 Atrioventricular and left bundle-branch block
- **I44.0** Atrioventricular block, first degree
- **I44.1** Atrioventricular block, second degree
  - Atrioventricular block, type I and II
  - Möbitz block, type I and II
  - Second degree block, type I and II
  - Wenckebach's block
- CC **I44.2** Atrioventricular block, complete
  - Complete heart block NOS
  - Third degree block
  - *AHA CC: 2Q, 2019, 4*
- + **I44.3** Other and unspecified atrioventricular block
  - Atrioventricular block NOS
  - **I44.30** Unspecified atrioventricular block
  - **I44.39** Other atrioventricular block
- **I44.4** Left anterior fascicular block
- **I44.5** Left posterior fascicular block
- + **I44.6** Other and unspecified fascicular block
  - **I44.60** Unspecified fascicular block
    - Left bundle-branch hemiblock NOS
  - **I44.69** Other fascicular block
- **I44.7** Left bundle-branch block, unspecified

I45 Other conduction disorders
- **I45.0** Right fascicular block
- + **I45.1** Other and unspecified right bundle-branch block
  - **I45.10** Unspecified right bundle-branch block
    - Right bundle-branch block NOS
  - **I45.19** Other right bundle-branch block
- CC **I45.2** Bifascicular block
- CC **I45.3** Trifascicular block
- **I45.4** Nonspecific intraventricular block
  - Bundle-branch block NOS
- **I45.5** Other specified heart block
  - Sinoatrial block
  - Sinoauricular block
  - **Excludes1:** heart block NOS (I45.9)
- **I45.6** Pre-excitation syndrome
  - Accelerated atrioventricular conduction
  - Accessory atrioventricular conduction
  - Anomalous atrioventricular excitation
  - Lown-Ganong-Levine syndrome
  - Pre-excitation atrioventricular conduction
  - Wolff-Parkinson-White syndrome
- + **I45.8** Other specified conduction disorders
  - **I45.81** Long QT syndrome
  - CC **I45.89** Other specified conduction disorders
    - Atrioventricular [AV] dissociation
    - Interference dissociation
    - Isorhythmic dissociation
    - Nonparoxysmal AV nodal tachycardia
    - *AHA CC: 2Q, 2013, 31-32*
- **I45.9** Conduction disorder, unspecified
  - Heart block NOS
  - Stokes-Adams syndrome

I46 Cardiac arrest
- **Excludes2:** cardiogenic shock (R57.0)
- MCC **I46.2** Cardiac arrest due to underlying cardiac condition
  - Code first underlying cardiac condition
- MCC **I46.8** Cardiac arrest due to other underlying condition
  - Code first underlying condition
- MCC **I46.9** Cardiac arrest, cause unspecified
  - *AHA CC: 3Q, 2020, 26*

I47 Paroxysmal tachycardia
Code first tachycardia complicating:
- abortion or ectopic or molar pregnancy (O00-O07, O08.8)
- obstetric surgery and procedures (O75.4)

Excludes1: tachycardia NOS (R00.0)
- sinoauricular tachycardia NOS (R00.0)
- sinus [sinusal] tachycardia NOS (R00.0)

- CC **I47.0** Re-entry ventricular arrhythmia
- + **I47.1** Supraventricular tachycardia
  - CC **I47.10** Supraventricular tachycardia, unspecified
  - CC **I47.11** Inappropriate sinus tachycardia, so stated
    - IST
  - CC **I47.19** Other supraventricular tachycardia
    - Atrial (paroxysmal) tachycardia
    - Atrioventricular [AV] (paroxysmal) tachycardia
    - Atrioventricular re-entrant (nodal) tachycardia [AVNRT] [AVRT]
    - Junctional (paroxysmal) tachycardia
    - Nodal (paroxysmal) tachycardia
- + **I47.2** Ventricular tachycardia
  - *AHA CC: 3Q, 2013, 23-24; 3Q, 2021, 11-12; 4Q, 2022, 23-24*
  - CC **I47.20** Ventricular tachycardia, unspecified
  - CC **I47.21** Torsades de pointes
    - Code also, if applicable, long QT syndrome (I45.81)
    - Use additional code for adverse effect, if applicable, to identify drug (T36-T50 with fifth or sixth character 5)
    - *AHA CC: 4Q, 2022, 24*
  - CC **I47.29** Other ventricular tachycardia
- **I47.9** Paroxysmal tachycardia, unspecified
  - Bouveret (-Hoffman) syndrome

I48 Atrial fibrillation and flutter
AHA CC: 4Q, 2019, 7
- **I48.0** Paroxysmal atrial fibrillation
- + **I48.1** Persistent atrial fibrillation
  - **Excludes1:** Permanent atrial fibrillation (I48.21)
  - *AHA CC: 2Q, 2019, 3-4*
  - CC **I48.11** Longstanding persistent atrial fibrillation
  - CC **I48.19** Other persistent atrial fibrillation
    - Chronic persistent atrial fibrillation
    - Persistent atrial fibrillation, NOS
- + **I48.2** Chronic atrial fibrillation
  - *AHA CC: 4Q, 2013, 128; 3Q, 2018, 6*
  - CC **I48.20** Chronic atrial fibrillation, unspecified
    - **Excludes1:** Chronic persistent atrial fibrillation (I48.19)
  - CC **I48.21** Permanent atrial fibrillation
- **I48.3** Typical atrial flutter
  - Type I atrial flutter
- CC **I48.4** Atypical atrial flutter
  - Type II atrial flutter
- + **I48.9** Unspecified atrial fibrillation and atrial flutter
  - **I48.91** Unspecified atrial fibrillation
  - CC **I48.92** Unspecified atrial flutter

I49 Other cardiac arrhythmias
Code first cardiac arrhythmia complicating:
- abortion or ectopic or molar pregnancy (O00-O07, O08.8)
- obstetric surgery and procedures (O75.4)

Excludes1: neonatal dysrhythmia (P29.1-)
- sinoatrial bradycardia (R00.1)
- sinus bradycardia (R00.1)
- vagal bradycardia (R00.1)

Excludes2: bradycardia NOS (R00.1)

- + **I49.0** Ventricular fibrillation and flutter
  - MCC **I49.01** Ventricular fibrillation
  - MCC **I49.02** Ventricular flutter
- **I49.1** Atrial premature depolarization
  - Atrial premature beats
- CC **I49.2** Junctional premature depolarization
- **I49.3** Ventricular premature depolarization
  - *AHA CC: 2Q, 2020, 23-24*
- + **I49.4** Other and unspecified premature depolarization
  - **I49.40** Unspecified premature depolarization
    - Premature beats NOS
  - **I49.49** Other premature depolarization
    - Ectopic beats
    - Extrasystoles
    - Extrasystolic arrhythmias
    - Premature contractions
- **I49.5** Sick sinus syndrome
  - Tachycardia-bradycardia syndrome
  - *AHA CC: 1Q, 2019, 33-34*
- **I49.8** Other specified cardiac arrhythmias
  - Brugada syndrome
  - Coronary sinus rhythm disorder
  - Ectopic rhythm disorder
  - Nodal rhythm disorder
- **I49.9** Cardiac arrhythmia, unspecified
  - Arrhythmia (cardiac) NOS

I50 Heart failure

Code first:
- heart failure complicating abortion or ectopic or molar pregnancy O00-O07, O08.8
- heart failure due to hypertension (I11.0)
- heart failure due to hypertension with chronic kidney disease (I13.-)
- heart failure following surgery (I97.13-)
- obstetrics surgery and procedures (O75.4)
- rheumatic heart failure (I09.81)

Excludes2: cardiac arrest (I46.-)
neonatal cardiac failure (P29.0)

Review coding guidelines C.9.a.1 and C.9.a.3
AHA CC: 1Q, 2017, 47

CC I50.1 Left ventricular failure, unspecified
- Cardiac asthma
- Edema of lung with heart disease NOS
- Edema of lung with heart failure
- Left heart failure
- Pulmonary edema with heart disease NOS
- Pulmonary edema with heart failure

Excludes1: edema of lung without heart disease or heart failure (J81.-)
pulmonary edema without heart disease or failure (J81.-)

+ I50.2 Systolic (congestive) heart failure
- Heart failure with reduced ejection fraction [HFrEF]
- Systolic left ventricular heart failure

Code also end stage heart failure, if applicable (I50.84)

Excludes1: combined systolic (congestive) and diastolic (congestive) heart failure (I50.4-)

- **CC I50.20** Unspecified systolic (congestive) heart failure
- **MCC I50.21** Acute systolic (congestive) heart failure
- **CC I50.22** Chronic systolic (congestive) heart failure
- **MCC I50.23** Acute on chronic systolic (congestive) heart failure
  AHA CC: 2Q, 2013, 33

+ I50.3 Diastolic (congestive) heart failure
- Diastolic left ventricular heart failure
- Heart failure with normal ejection fraction
- Heart failure with preserved ejection fraction [HFpEF]

Code also end stage heart failure, if applicable (I50.84)

Excludes1: combined systolic (congestive) and diastolic (congestive) heart failure (I50.4-)

- **CC I50.30** Unspecified diastolic (congestive) heart failure
- **MCC I50.31** Acute diastolic (congestive) heart failure
  AHA CC: 1Q, 2017, 46
- **CC I50.32** Chronic diastolic (congestive) heart failure
  AHA CC: 3Q, 2020, 32
- **MCC I50.33** Acute on chronic diastolic (congestive) heart failure

+ I50.4 Combined systolic (congestive) and diastolic (congestive) heart failure
- Combined systolic and diastolic left ventricular heart failure
- Heart failure with reduced ejection fraction and diastolic dysfunction

Code also end stage heart failure, if applicable (I50.84)

- **CC I50.40** Unspecified combined systolic (congestive) and diastolic (congestive) heart failure
- **MCC I50.41** Acute combined systolic (congestive) and diastolic (congestive) heart failure
- **CC I50.42** Chronic combined systolic (congestive) and diastolic (congestive) heart failure
- **MCC I50.43** Acute on chronic combined systolic (congestive) and diastolic (congestive) heart failure

+ I50.8 Other heart failure
AHA CC: 4Q, 2017, 15-16

+ I50.81 Right heart failure
Right ventricular failure

- **I50.810** Right heart failure, unspecified
  - Right heart failure without mention of left heart failure
  - Right ventricular failure NOS
- **I50.811** Acute right heart failure
  - Acute isolated right heart failure
  - Acute (isolated) right ventricular failure
- **I50.812** Chronic right heart failure
  - Chronic isolated right heart failure
  - Chronic (isolated) right ventricular failure
- **I50.813** Acute on chronic right heart failure
  - Acute on chronic isolated right heart failure
  - Acute on chronic (isolated) right ventricular failure
  - Acute decompensation of chronic (isolated) right ventricular failure
  - Acute exacerbation of chronic (isolated) right ventricular failure
- **I50.814** Right heart failure, unspecified
  - Right ventricular failure secondary to left ventricular failure

Code also the type of left ventricular failure, if known (I50.2-I50.43)

Excludes1: right heart failure with but not due to left heart failure (I50.82)

I50.82 Biventricular heart failure
Code also the type of left ventricular failure as systolic, diastolic, or combined, if known (I50.2-I50.43)

I50.83 High output heart failure

I50.84 End stage heart failure
Stage D heart failure

Code also the type of heart failure as systolic, diastolic, or combined, if known (I50.2-I50.43)
AHA CC: 3Q, 2022, 16-17

I50.89 Heart failure, unspecified

I50.9 Heart failure, unspecified
- Cardiac, heart or myocardial failure NOS
- Congestive heart disease
- Congestive heart failure NOS

Excludes2: fluid overload unrelated to congestive heart failure (E87.70)

AHA CC: 4Q, 2012, 92-93; 4Q, 2014, 21-22; 1Q, 2017, 46

I51 Complications and ill-defined descriptions of heart disease

Excludes1: any condition in I51.4-I51.9 due to hypertension (I11.-)
any condition in I51.4-I51.9 due to hypertension and chronic kidney disease (I13.-)
heart disease specified as rheumatic (I00-I09)

• CC I51.0 Cardiac septal defect, acquired
- Acquired septal atrial defect (old)
- Acquired septal auricular defect (old)
- Acquired septal ventricular defect (old)

Excludes1: cardiac septal defect as current complication following acute myocardial infarction (I23.1, I23.2)

MCC I51.1 Rupture of chordae tendineae, not elsewhere classified
Excludes1: rupture of chordae tendineae as current complication following acute myocardial infarction (I23.4)

MCC I51.2 Rupture of papillary muscle, not elsewhere classified
Excludes1: rupture of papillary muscle as current complication following acute myocardial infarction (I23.5)

I51.3 Intracardiac thrombosis, not elsewhere classified
- Apical thrombosis (old)
- Atrial thrombosis (old)
- Auricular thrombosis (old)
- Mural thrombosis (old)
- Ventricular thrombosis (old)

Excludes1: intracardiac thrombosis as current complication following acute myocardial infarction (I23.6)

AHA CC: 1Q, 2013, 24

I51.4 Myocarditis, unspecified
- Chronic (interstitial) myocarditis
- Myocardial fibrosis
- Myocarditis NOS

Excludes1: acute or subacute myocarditis (I40.-)
Review coding guideline C.9.a.1

I51.5 Myocardial degeneration
- Fatty degeneration of heart or myocardium
- Myocardial disease
- Senile degeneration of heart or myocardium

Review coding guideline C.9.a.1

I51.7 Cardiomegaly
- Cardiac dilatation
- Cardiac hypertrophy
- Ventricular dilatation

Review coding guideline C.9.a.1

I51.8–I62.9

+ **I51.8** **Other ill-defined heart diseases**
  Review coding guideline C.9.a.1
  CC **I51.81** **Takotsubo syndrome**
  Reversible left ventricular dysfunction following sudden emotional stress
  Stress induced cardiomyopathy
  Takotsubo cardiomyopathy
  Transient left ventricular apical ballooning syndrome
  AHA CC: 2Q, 2018, 9-10
  I51.89 **Other ill-defined heart diseases**
  Carditis (acute)(chronic)
  Pancarditis (acute)(chronic)
  AHA CC: 2Q, 2019, 5-6
  I51.9 **Heart disease, unspecified**
  Review coding guideline C.9.a.1

I52 **Other heart disorders in diseases classified elsewhere**
  Code first underlying disease, such as:
    congenital syphilis (A50.5)
    mucopolysaccharidosis (E76.3)
    schistosomiasis (B65.0-B65.9)
  Excludes1: *heart disease (in):*
    gonococcal infection (A54.83)
    meningococcal infection (A39.50)
    rheumatoid arthritis (M05.31)
    syphilis (A52.06)
  Valid 3-character code, no further characters required

CC **I5A** **Non-ischemic myocardial injury (non-traumatic)**
  Acute (non-ischemic) myocardial injury
  Chronic (non-ischemic) myocardial injury
  Unspecified (non-ischemic) myocardial injury
  Code first the underlying cause, if known and applicable, such as:
    acute kidney failure (N17.-)
    acute myocarditis (I40.-)
    cardiomyopathy (I42.-)
    chronic kidney disease (CKD) (N18.-)
    heart failure (I50.-)
    hypertensive urgency (I16.0)
    nonrheumatic aortic valve disorders (I35.-)
    paroxysmal tachycardia (I47.-)
    pulmonary embolism (I26.-)
    pulmonary hypertension (I27.0, I27.2-)
    sepsis (A41.-)
    takotsubo syndrome (I51.81)
  Excludes1: *acute myocardial infarction (I21.-)*
    injury of heart (S26.-)
  Excludes2: *other acute ischemic heart diseases (I24.-)*
    AHA CC: 4Q, 2021, 14-15
  Valid 3-character code, no further characters required

Cerebrovascular diseases (I60-I69)

Use additional code to identify presence of:
  alcohol abuse and dependence (F10.-)
  exposure to environmental tobacco smoke (Z77.22)
  history of tobacco dependence (Z87.891)
  hypertension (I10-I1A)
  occupational exposure to environmental tobacco smoke (Z57.31)
  tobacco dependence (F17.-)
  tobacco use (Z72.0)
Excludes1: *traumatic intracranial hemorrhage (S06.-)*
Review coding guidelines C.9.a.4 and C.9.d

I60 **Nontraumatic subarachnoid hemorrhage**
  Use Additional code, if known, to indicate National Institutes of Health Stroke Scale (NIHSS) score (R29.7-)
  Excludes1: *syphilitic ruptured cerebral aneurysm (A52.05)*
  Excludes2: *sequelae of subarachnoid hemorrhage (I69.0-)*
  + **I60.0** **Nontraumatic subarachnoid hemorrhage from carotid siphon and bifurcation**
    MCC **I60.00** Nontraumatic subarachnoid hemorrhage from unspecified carotid siphon and bifurcation
    MCC **I60.01** Nontraumatic subarachnoid hemorrhage from right carotid siphon and bifurcation
    MCC **I60.02** Nontraumatic subarachnoid hemorrhage from left carotid siphon and bifurcation
  + **I60.1** **Nontraumatic subarachnoid hemorrhage from middle cerebral artery**
    MCC **I60.10** Nontraumatic subarachnoid hemorrhage from unspecified middle cerebral artery
    MCC **I60.11** Nontraumatic subarachnoid hemorrhage from right middle cerebral artery
    MCC **I60.12** Nontraumatic subarachnoid hemorrhage from left middle cerebral artery
  MCC **I60.2** Nontraumatic subarachnoid hemorrhage from anterior communicating artery
  + **I60.3** **Nontraumatic subarachnoid hemorrhage from posterior communicating artery**
    MCC **I60.30** Nontraumatic subarachnoid hemorrhage from unspecified posterior communicating artery
    MCC **I60.31** Nontraumatic subarachnoid hemorrhage from right posterior communicating artery
    MCC **I60.32** Nontraumatic subarachnoid hemorrhage from left posterior communicating artery
  MCC **I60.4** Nontraumatic subarachnoid hemorrhage from basilar artery
  + **I60.5** **Nontraumatic subarachnoid hemorrhage from vertebral artery**
    MCC **I60.50** Nontraumatic subarachnoid hemorrhage from unspecified vertebral artery
    MCC **I60.51** Nontraumatic subarachnoid hemorrhage from right vertebral artery
    MCC **I60.52** Nontraumatic subarachnoid hemorrhage from left vertebral artery
  MCC **I60.6** Nontraumatic subarachnoid hemorrhage from other intracranial arteries
  MCC **I60.7** Nontraumatic subarachnoid hemorrhage from unspecified intracranial artery
    Ruptured (congenital) berry aneurysm
    Ruptured (congenital) cerebral aneurysm
    Subarachnoid hemorrhage (nontraumatic) from cerebral artery NOS
    Subarachnoid hemorrhage (nontraumatic) from communicating artery NOS
    Excludes1: *berry aneurysm, nonruptured (I67.1)*
  MCC **I60.8** Other nontraumatic subarachnoid hemorrhage
    Meningeal hemorrhage
    Rupture of cerebral arteriovenous malformation
  MCC **I60.9** Nontraumatic subarachnoid hemorrhage, unspecified

I61 **Nontraumatic intracerebral hemorrhage**
  Use Additional code, if known, to indicate National Institutes of Health Stroke Scale (NIHSS) score (R29.7-)
  Excludes2: *sequelae of intracerebral hemorrhage (I69.1-)*
  AHA CC: 2Q, 2017, 10
  MCC **I61.0** Nontraumatic intracerebral hemorrhage in hemisphere, subcortical
    Deep intracerebral hemorrhage (nontraumatic)
  MCC **I61.1** Nontraumatic intracerebral hemorrhage in hemisphere, cortical
    Cerebral lobe hemorrhage (nontraumatic)
    Superficial intracerebral hemorrhage (nontraumatic)
  MCC **I61.2** Nontraumatic intracerebral hemorrhage in hemisphere, unspecified
  MCC **I61.3** Nontraumatic intracerebral hemorrhage in brain stem
  MCC **I61.4** Nontraumatic intracerebral hemorrhage in cerebellum
  MCC **I61.5** Nontraumatic intracerebral hemorrhage, intraventricular
  MCC **I61.6** Nontraumatic intracerebral hemorrhage, multiple localized
  MCC **I61.8** Other nontraumatic intracerebral hemorrhage
  MCC **I61.9** Nontraumatic intracerebral hemorrhage, unspecified
    AHA CC: 3Q, 2022, 9-10

I62 **Other and unspecified nontraumatic intracranial hemorrhage**
  Use Additional code, if known, to indicate National Institutes of Health Stroke Scale (NIHSS) score (R29.7-)
  Excludes2: *sequelae of intracranial hemorrhage (I69.2)*
  + **I62.0** **Nontraumatic subdural hemorrhage**
    MCC **I62.00** Nontraumatic subdural hemorrhage, unspecified
    MCC **I62.01** Nontraumatic acute subdural hemorrhage
    MCC **I62.02** Nontraumatic subacute subdural hemorrhage
    MCC **I62.03** Nontraumatic chronic subdural hemorrhage
  MCC **I62.1** Nontraumatic extradural hemorrhage
    Nontraumatic epidural hemorrhage
  CC **I62.9** Nontraumatic intracranial hemorrhage, unspecified

I63 Cerebral infarction

Includes: occlusion and stenosis of cerebral and precerebral arteries, resulting in cerebral infarction

Use additional code, if applicable, to identify status post administration of tPA (rtPA) in a different facility within the last 24 hours prior to admission to current facility (Z92.82)

Use additional code, if known, to indicate National Institutes of Health Stroke Scale (NIHSS) score (R29.7-)

Excludes1: neonatal cerebral infarction (P91.82-)
Excludes2: chronic, without residual deficits (sequelae) (Z86.73)
sequelae of cerebral infarction (I69.3-)

AHA CC: 4Q, 2016, 28

- **+ I63.0 Cerebral infarction due to thrombosis of precerebral arteries**
  - MCC **I63.00** Cerebral infarction due to thrombosis of unspecified precerebral artery
  - **+ I63.01 Cerebral infarction due to thrombosis of vertebral artery**
    - MCC **I63.011** Cerebral infarction due to thrombosis of right vertebral artery
    - MCC **I63.012** Cerebral infarction due to thrombosis of left vertebral artery
    - MCC **I63.013** Cerebral infarction due to thrombosis of bilateral vertebral arteries
    - MCC **I63.019** Cerebral infarction due to thrombosis of unspecified vertebral artery
  - MCC **I63.02** Cerebral infarction due to thrombosis of basilar artery
  - **+ I63.03 Cerebral infarction due to thrombosis of carotid artery**
    - MCC **I63.031** Cerebral infarction due to thrombosis of right carotid artery
    - MCC **I63.032** Cerebral infarction due to thrombosis of left carotid artery
    - MCC **I63.033** Cerebral infarction due to thrombosis of bilateral carotid arteries
    - MCC **I63.039** Cerebral infarction due to thrombosis of unspecified carotid artery
  - MCC **I63.09** Cerebral infarction due to thrombosis of other precerebral artery
- **+ I63.1 Cerebral infarction due to embolism of precerebral arteries**
  - MCC **I63.10** Cerebral infarction due to embolism of unspecified precerebral artery
  - **+ I63.11 Cerebral infarction due to embolism of vertebral artery**
    - MCC **I63.111** Cerebral infarction due to embolism of right vertebral artery
    - MCC **I63.112** Cerebral infarction due to embolism of left vertebral artery
    - MCC **I63.113** Cerebral infarction due to embolism of bilateral vertebral arteries
    - MCC **I63.119** Cerebral infarction due to embolism of unspecified vertebral artery
  - MCC **I63.12** Cerebral infarction due to embolism of basilar artery
  - **+ I63.13 Cerebral infarction due to embolism of carotid artery**
    - MCC **I63.131** Cerebral infarction due to embolism of right carotid artery
    - MCC **I63.132** Cerebral infarction due to embolism of left carotid artery
    - MCC **I63.133** Cerebral infarction due to embolism of bilateral carotid arteries
    - MCC **I63.139** Cerebral infarction due to embolism of unspecified carotid artery
  - MCC **I63.19** Cerebral infarction due to embolism of other precerebral artery
- **+ I63.2 Cerebral infarction due to unspecified occlusion or stenosis of precerebral arteries**
  - MCC **I63.20** Cerebral infarction due to unspecified occlusion or stenosis of unspecified precerebral arteries
  - **+ I63.21 Cerebral infarction due to unspecified occlusion or stenosis of vertebral arteries**
    - MCC **I63.211** Cerebral infarction due to unspecified occlusion or stenosis of right vertebral artery
    - MCC **I63.212** Cerebral infarction due to unspecified occlusion or stenosis of left vertebral artery
    - MCC **I63.213** Cerebral infarction due to unspecified occlusion or stenosis of bilateral vertebral arteries
    - MCC **I63.219** Cerebral infarction due to unspecified occlusion or stenosis of unspecified vertebral artery
  - MCC **I63.22** Cerebral infarction due to unspecified occlusion or stenosis of basilar artery
  - **+ I63.23 Cerebral infarction due to unspecified occlusion or stenosis of carotid arteries**
    - MCC **I63.231** Cerebral infarction due to unspecified occlusion or stenosis of right carotid arteries
      AHA CC: 3Q, 2020, 28-29
    - MCC **I63.232** Cerebral infarction due to unspecified occlusion or stenosis of left carotid arteries
    - MCC **I63.233** Cerebral infarction due to unspecified occlusion or stenosis of bilateral carotid arteries
    - MCC **I63.239** Cerebral infarction due to unspecified occlusion or stenosis of unspecified carotid artery
  - MCC **I63.29** Cerebral infarction due to unspecified occlusion or stenosis of other precerebral arteries
- **+ I63.3 Cerebral infarction due to thrombosis of cerebral arteries**
  - MCC **I63.30** Cerebral infarction due to thrombosis of unspecified cerebral artery
  - **+ I63.31 Cerebral infarction due to thrombosis of middle cerebral artery**
    - MCC **I63.311** Cerebral infarction due to thrombosis of right middle cerebral artery
    - MCC **I63.312** Cerebral infarction due to thrombosis of left middle cerebral artery
    - MCC **I63.313** Cerebral infarction due to thrombosis of bilateral middle cerebral arteries
    - MCC **I63.319** Cerebral infarction due to thrombosis of unspecified middle cerebral artery
  - **+ I63.32 Cerebral infarction due to thrombosis of anterior cerebral artery**
    - MCC **I63.321** Cerebral infarction due to thrombosis of right anterior cerebral artery
    - MCC **I63.322** Cerebral infarction due to thrombosis of left anterior cerebral artery
    - MCC **I63.323** Cerebral infarction due to thrombosis of bilateral anterior cerebral arteries
    - MCC **I63.329** Cerebral infarction due to thrombosis of unspecified anterior cerebral artery
  - **+ I63.33 Cerebral infarction due to thrombosis of posterior cerebral artery**
    - MCC **I63.331** Cerebral infarction due to thrombosis of right posterior cerebral artery
    - MCC **I63.332** Cerebral infarction due to thrombosis of left posterior cerebral artery
    - MCC **I63.333** Cerebral infarction due to thrombosis of bilateral posterior cerebral arteries
    - MCC **I63.339** Cerebral infarction due to thrombosis of unspecified posterior cerebral artery
  - **+ I63.34 Cerebral infarction due to thrombosis of cerebellar artery**
    - MCC **I63.341** Cerebral infarction due to thrombosis of right cerebellar artery
    - MCC **I63.342** Cerebral infarction due to thrombosis of left cerebellar artery
    - MCC **I63.343** Cerebral infarction due to thrombosis of bilateral cerebellar arteries
    - MCC **I63.349** Cerebral infarction due to thrombosis of unspecified cerebellar artery
  - MCC **I63.39** Cerebral infarction due to thrombosis of other cerebral artery

- **I63.4 Cerebral infarction due to embolism of cerebral arteries**
  - MCC **I63.40** Cerebral infarction due to embolism of unspecified cerebral artery
  - **I63.41** Cerebral infarction due to embolism of middle cerebral artery
    - MCC **I63.411** Cerebral infarction due to embolism of right middle cerebral artery
    - MCC **I63.412** Cerebral infarction due to embolism of left middle cerebral artery
    - MCC **I63.413** Cerebral infarction due to embolism of bilateral middle cerebral arteries
    - MCC **I63.419** Cerebral infarction due to embolism of unspecified middle cerebral artery
  - **I63.42** Cerebral infarction due to embolism of anterior cerebral artery
    - MCC **I63.421** Cerebral infarction due to embolism of right anterior cerebral artery
    - MCC **I63.422** Cerebral infarction due to embolism of left anterior cerebral artery
    - MCC **I63.423** Cerebral infarction due to embolism of bilateral anterior cerebral arteries
    - MCC **I63.429** Cerebral infarction due to embolism of unspecified anterior cerebral artery
  - **I63.43** Cerebral infarction due to embolism of posterior cerebral artery
    - MCC **I63.431** Cerebral infarction due to embolism of right posterior cerebral artery
    - MCC **I63.432** Cerebral infarction due to embolism of left posterior cerebral artery
    - MCC **I63.433** Cerebral infarction due to embolism of bilateral posterior cerebral arteries
    - MCC **I63.439** Cerebral infarction due to embolism of unspecified posterior cerebral artery
  - **I63.44** Cerebral infarction due to embolism of cerebellar artery
    - MCC **I63.441** Cerebral infarction due to embolism of right cerebellar artery
    - MCC **I63.442** Cerebral infarction due to embolism of left cerebellar artery
    - MCC **I64.443** Cerebral infarction due to embolism of bilateral cerebellar arteries
    - MCC **I63.449** Cerebral infarction due to embolism of unspecified cerebellar artery
  - MCC **I63.49** Cerebral infarction due to embolism of other cerebral artery
- **I63.5 Cerebral infarction due to unspecified occlusion or stenosis of cerebral arteries**
  - MCC **I63.50** Cerebral infarction due to unspecified occlusion or stenosis of unspecified cerebral artery
  - **I63.51** Cerebral infarction due to unspecified occlusion or stenosis of middle cerebral artery
    - MCC **I63.511** Cerebral infarction due to unspecified occlusion or stenosis of right middle cerebral artery
    - MCC **I63.512** Cerebral infarction due to unspecified occlusion or stenosis of left middle cerebral artery
    - MCC **I63.513** Cerebral infarction due to unspecified occlusion or stenosis of bilateral middle cerebral arteries
    - MCC **I63.519** Cerebral infarction due to unspecified occlusion or stenosis of unspecified middle cerebral artery
  - **I63.52** Cerebral infarction due to unspecified occlusion or stenosis of anterior cerebral artery
    - MCC **I63.521** Cerebral infarction due to unspecified occlusion or stenosis of right anterior cerebral artery
    - MCC **I63.522** Cerebral infarction due to unspecified occlusion or stenosis of left anterior cerebral artery
    - MCC **I63.523** Cerebral infarction due to unspecified occlusion or stenosis of bilateral anterior cerebral arteries
    - MCC **I63.529** Cerebral infarction due to unspecified occlusion or stenosis of unspecified anterior cerebral artery
  - **I63.53** Cerebral infarction due to unspecified occlusion or stenosis of posterior cerebral artery
    - MCC **I63.531** Cerebral infarction due to unspecified occlusion or stenosis of right posterior cerebral artery
    - MCC **I63.532** Cerebral infarction due to unspecified occlusion or stenosis of left posterior cerebral artery
      - *AHA CC: 2Q, 2017, 10*
    - MCC **I63.533** Cerebral infarction due to unspecified occlusion or stenosis of bilateral posterior cerebral arteries
    - MCC **I63.539** Cerebral infarction due to unspecified occlusion or stenosis of unspecified posterior cerebral artery
  - **I63.54** Cerebral infarction due to unspecified occlusion or stenosis of cerebellar artery
    - MCC **I63.541** Cerebral infarction due to unspecified occlusion or stenosis of right cerebellar artery
    - MCC **I63.542** Cerebral infarction due to unspecified occlusion or stenosis of left cerebellar artery
    - MCC **I63.543** Cerebral infarction due to unspecified occlusion or stenosis of bilateral cerebellar arteries
    - MCC **I63.549** Cerebral infarction due to unspecified occlusion or stenosis of unspecified cerebellar artery
  - MCC **I63.59** Cerebral infarction due to unspecified occlusion or stenosis of other cerebral artery
- MCC **I63.6** Cerebral infarction due to cerebral venous thrombosis, nonpyogenic
- **I63.8 Other cerebral infarction**
  - *AHA CC: 2Q, 2017, 9-10; 4Q, 2018, 16*
  - MCC **I63.81** Other cerebral infarction due to occlusion or stenosis of small artery
    - Lacunar infarction
    - *AHA CC: 4Q, 2018, 16; 3Q, 2020, 27-28*
  - MCC **I63.89** Other cerebral infarction
    - *AHA CC: 1Q, 2022, 25*
- MCC **I63.9** Cerebral infarction, unspecified
  - Stroke NOS
  - **Excludes2:** transient cerebral ischemic attacks and related syndromes (G45.-)
  - *AHA CC: 1Q, 2015, 26; 4Q, 2016, 61-62*

I65 Occlusion and stenosis of precerebral arteries, not resulting in cerebral infarction

Includes: embolism of precerebral artery
narrowing of precerebral artery
obstruction (complete) (partial) of precerebral artery
thrombosis of precerebral artery

Excludes1: insufficiency, NOS, of precerebral artery (G45.-)
insufficiency of precerebral arteries causing cerebral infarction (I63.0-I63.2)

- **I65.0 Occlusion and stenosis of vertebral artery**
  - **I65.01** Occlusion and stenosis of right vertebral artery
  - **I65.02** Occlusion and stenosis of left vertebral artery
  - **I65.03** Occlusion and stenosis of bilateral vertebral arteries
  - **I65.09** Occlusion and stenosis of unspecified vertebral artery
- **I65.1** Occlusion and stenosis of basilar artery
- **I65.2 Occlusion and stenosis of carotid artery**
  - **I65.21** Occlusion and stenosis of right carotid artery
  - **I65.22** Occlusion and stenosis of left carotid artery
    - *AHA CC: 3Q, 2020, 28-29*
  - **I65.23** Occlusion and stenosis of bilateral carotid arteries
    - *AHA CC: 2Q, 2018, 9; 1Q, 2021, 4*
  - **I65.29** Occlusion and stenosis of unspecified carotid artery
- **I65.8** Occlusion and stenosis of other precerebral arteries
- **I65.9** Occlusion and stenosis of unspecified precerebral artery
  - Occlusion and stenosis of precerebral artery NOS

I66 **Occlusion and stenosis of cerebral arteries, not resulting in cerebral infarction**

> **Includes:** embolism of cerebral artery
> narrowing of cerebral artery
> obstruction (complete) (partial) of cerebral artery
> thrombosis of cerebral artery
>
> **Excludes1:** Occlusion and stenosis of cerebral artery causing cerebral infarction (I63.3-I63.5)

- **I66.0** Occlusion and stenosis of middle cerebral artery
  - **I66.01** Occlusion and stenosis of right middle cerebral artery
  - **I66.02** Occlusion and stenosis of left middle cerebral artery
  - **I66.03** Occlusion and stenosis of bilateral middle cerebral arteries
  - **I66.09** Occlusion and stenosis of unspecified middle cerebral artery
- **I66.1** Occlusion and stenosis of anterior cerebral artery
  - **I66.11** Occlusion and stenosis of right anterior cerebral artery
  - **I66.12** Occlusion and stenosis of left anterior cerebral artery
  - **I66.13** Occlusion and stenosis of bilateral anterior cerebral arteries
  - **I66.19** Occlusion and stenosis of unspecified anterior cerebral artery
- **I66.2** Occlusion and stenosis of posterior cerebral artery
  - **I66.21** Occlusion and stenosis of right posterior cerebral artery
  - **I66.22** Occlusion and stenosis of left posterior cerebral artery
  - **I66.23** Occlusion and stenosis of bilateral posterior cerebral arteries
  - **I66.29** Occlusion and stenosis of unspecified posterior cerebral artery
- **I66.3** Occlusion and stenosis of cerebellar arteries
- **I66.8** Occlusion and stenosis of other cerebral arteries
  Occlusion and stenosis of perforating arteries
- **I66.9** Occlusion and stenosis of unspecified cerebral artery

I67 **Other cerebrovascular diseases**

> **Excludes1:** Occlusion and stenosis of cerebral artery causing cerebral infarction (I63.3-I63.5-)
> Occlusion and stenosis of precerebral artery causing cerebral infarction (I63.2-)
>
> **Excludes2:** sequelae of the listed conditions (I69.8)

- **MCC I67.0** Dissection of cerebral arteries, nonruptured
  Excludes1: ruptured cerebral arteries (I60.7)
  AHA CC: 3Q, 2021, 5
- **I67.1** Cerebral aneurysm, nonruptured
  Cerebral aneurysm NOS
  Cerebral arteriovenous fistula, acquired
  Internal carotid artery aneurysm, intracranial portion
  Internal carotid artery aneurysm, NOS
  Excludes1: congenital cerebral aneurysm, nonruptured (Q28.-)
  ruptured cerebral aneurysm (I60.7)
- **I67.2** Cerebral atherosclerosis
  Atheroma of cerebral and precerebral arteries
- **CC I67.3** Progressive vascular leukoencephalopathy
  Binswanger's disease
- **CC I67.4** Hypertensive encephalopathy
  Code also, if applicable, associated hypertensive conditions such as:
  essential (primary) hypertension (I10)
  hypertensive chronic kidney disease (I12.-)
  hypertensive heart and chronic kidney disease (I13.-)
  hypertensive heart disease (I11.-)
  Excludes2: insufficiency, NOS, of precerebral arteries (G45.2)
- **CC I67.5** Moyamoya disease
- **CC I67.6** Nonpyogenic thrombosis of intracranial venous system
  Nonpyogenic thrombosis of cerebral vein
  Nonpyogenic thrombosis of intracranial venous sinus
  Excludes1: nonpyogenic thrombosis of intracranial venous system causing infarction (I63.6)
- **CC I67.7** Cerebral arteritis, not elsewhere classified
  Granulomatous angiitis of the nervous system
  Excludes1: allergic granulomatous angiitis (M30.1)
- **I67.8** Other specified cerebrovascular diseases
  AHA CC: 4Q, 2018, 17
  - **CC I67.81** Acute cerebrovascular insufficiency
    Acute cerebrovascular insufficiency unspecified as to location or reversibility
  - **CC I67.82** Cerebral ischemia
    Chronic cerebral ischemia
  - **MCC I67.83** Posterior reversible encephalopathy syndrome
    PRES
  - **I67.84** Cerebral vasospasm and vasoconstriction
    - **CC I67.841** Reversible cerebrovascular vasoconstriction syndrome
      Call-Fleming syndrome
      Code first underlying condition, if applicable, such as eclampsia (O15.00-O15.9)
    - **CC I67.848** Other cerebrovascular vasospasm and vasoconstriction
  - **I67.85** Hereditary cerebrovascular diseases
    - **CC I67.850** Cerebral autosomal dominant arteriopathy with subcortical infarcts and leukoencephalopathy
      CADASIL
      Code also any associated diagnoses, such as:
      epilepsy (G40.-)
      stroke (I63.-)
      vascular dementia (F01.-)
    - **CC I67.858** Other hereditary cerebrovascular disease
  - **CC I67.89** Other cerebrovascular disease
    AHA CC: 2Q, 2023, 18-19
- **I67.9** Cerebrovascular disease, unspecified

I68 **Cerebrovascular disorders in diseases classified elsewhere**

- **I68.0** Cerebral amyloid angiopathy
  Code first underlying amyloidosis (E85.-)
- **CC I68.2** Cerebral arteritis in other diseases classified elsewhere
  Code first underlying disease
  Excludes1: cerebral arteritis (in):
  listerosis (A32.89)
  systemic lupus erythematosus (M32.19)
  syphilis (A52.04)
  tuberculosis (A18.89)
- **I68.8** Other cerebrovascular disorders in diseases classified elsewhere
  Code first underlying disease
  Excludes1: syphilitic cerebral aneurysm (A52.05)

I69 **Sequelae of cerebrovascular disease**

> **NOTE** Category I69 is to be used to indicate conditions in I60-I67 as the cause of sequelae. The 'sequelae' include conditions specified as such or as residuals which may occur at any time after the onset of the causal condition
>
> **Excludes1:** personal history of cerebral infarction without residual deficit (Z86.73)
> personal history of prolonged reversible ischemic neurologic deficit (PRIND) (Z86.73)
> personal history of reversible ischemic neurologcial deficit (RIND) (Z86.73)
> sequelae of traumatic intracranial injury (S06.-)
>
> *Review coding guideline C.9.d*
> *AHA CC: 4Q, 2016, 28*

- **I69.0** Sequelae of nontraumatic subarachnoid hemorrhage
  - **I69.00** Unspecified sequelae of nontraumatic subarachnoid hemorrhage
  - **I69.01** Cognitive deficits following nontraumatic subarachnoid hemorrhage
    - **I69.010** Attention and concentration deficit following nontraumatic subarachnoid hemorrhage
    - **I69.011** Memory deficit following nontraumatic subarachnoid hemorrhage
    - **I69.012** Visuospatial deficit and spatial neglect following nontraumatic subarachnoid hemorrhage
    - **I69.013** Psychomotor deficit following nontraumatic subarachnoid hemorrhage
    - **I69.014** Frontal lobe and executive function deficit following nontraumatic subarachnoid hemorrhage
    - **I69.015** Cognitive social or emotional deficit following nontraumatic subarachnoid hemorrhage

- **I69.018** Other symptoms and signs involving cognitive functions following nontraumatic subarachnoid hemorrhage
- **I69.019** Unspecified symptoms and signs involving cognitive functions following nontraumatic subarachnoid hemorrhage

+ I69.02 Speech and language deficits following nontraumatic subarachnoid hemorrhage
- **I69.020** Aphasia following nontraumatic subarachnoid hemorrhage
- **I69.021** Dysphasia following nontraumatic subarachnoid hemorrhage
- **I69.022** Dysarthria following nontraumatic subarachnoid hemorrhage
- **I69.023** Fluency disorder following nontraumatic subarachnoid hemorrhage
   - Stuttering following nontraumatic subarachnoid hemorrhage
- **I69.028** Other speech and language deficits following nontraumatic subarachnoid hemorrhage

+ I69.03 Monoplegia of upper limb following nontraumatic subarachnoid hemorrhage
- **I69.031** Monoplegia of upper limb following nontraumatic subarachnoid hemorrhage affecting right dominant side
- **I69.032** Monoplegia of upper limb following nontraumatic subarachnoid hemorrhage affecting left dominant side
- **I69.033** Monoplegia of upper limb following nontraumatic subarachnoid hemorrhage affecting right non-dominant side
- **I69.034** Monoplegia of upper limb following nontraumatic subarachnoid hemorrhage affecting left non-dominant side
- **I69.039** Monoplegia of upper limb following nontraumatic subarachnoid hemorrhage affecting unspecified side

+ I69.04 Monoplegia of lower limb following nontraumatic subarachnoid hemorrhage
- **I69.041** Monoplegia of lower limb following nontraumatic subarachnoid hemorrhage affecting right dominant side
- **I69.042** Monoplegia of lower limb following nontraumatic subarachnoid hemorrhage affecting left dominant side
- **I69.043** Monoplegia of lower limb following nontraumatic subarachnoid hemorrhage affecting right non-dominant side
- **I69.044** Monoplegia of lower limb following nontraumatic subarachnoid hemorrhage affecting left non-dominant side
- **I69.049** Monoplegia of lower limb following nontraumatic subarachnoid hemorrhage affecting unspecified side

+ I69.05 Hemiplegia and hemiparesis following nontraumatic subarachnoid hemorrhage
- CC **I69.051** Hemiplegia and hemiparesis following nontraumatic subarachnoid hemorrhage affecting right dominant side
- CC **I69.052** Hemiplegia and hemiparesis following nontraumatic subarachnoid hemorrhage affecting left dominant side
- CC **I69.053** Hemiplegia and hemiparesis following nontraumatic subarachnoid hemorrhage affecting right non-dominant side
- CC **I69.054** Hemiplegia and hemiparesis following nontraumatic subarachnoid hemorrhage affecting left non-dominant side
- CC **I69.059** Hemiplegia and hemiparesis following nontraumatic subarachnoid hemorrhage affecting unspecified side

+ I69.06 Other paralytic syndrome following nontraumatic subarachnoid hemorrhage
   Use additional code to identify type of paralytic syndrome, such as:
   locked-in state (G83.5)
   quadriplegia (G82.5-)
   Excludes1: hemiplegia/hemiparesis following nontraumatic subarachnoid hemorrhage (I69.05-)
   monoplegia of lower limb following nontraumatic subarachnoid hemorrhage (I69.04-)
   monoplegia of upper limb following nontraumatic subarachnoid hemorrhage (I69.03-)
- **I69.061** Other paralytic syndrome following nontraumatic subarachnoid hemorrhage affecting right dominant side
- **I69.062** Other paralytic syndrome following nontraumatic subarachnoid hemorrhage affecting left dominant side
- **I69.063** Other paralytic syndrome following nontraumatic subarachnoid hemorrhage affecting right non-dominant side
- **I69.064** Other paralytic syndrome following nontraumatic subarachnoid hemorrhage affecting left non-dominant side
- **I69.065** Other paralytic syndrome following nontraumatic subarachnoid hemorrhage, bilateral
- **I69.069** Other paralytic syndrome following nontraumatic subarachnoid hemorrhage affecting unspecified side

+ I69.09 Other sequelae of nontraumatic subarachnoid hemorrhage
- **I69.090** Apraxia following nontraumatic subarachnoid hemorrhage
- **I69.091** Dysphagia following nontraumatic subarachnoid hemorrhage
   Use additional code to identify the type of dysphagia, if known (R13.11-R13.19)
- **I69.092** Facial weakness following nontraumatic subarachnoid hemorrhage
   Facial droop following nontraumatic subarachnoid hemorrhage
- **I69.093** Ataxia following nontraumatic subarachnoid hemorrhage
- **I69.098** Other sequelae following nontraumatic subarachnoid hemorrhage
   Alterations of sensation following nontraumatic subarachnoid hemorrhage
   Disturbance of vision following nontraumatic subarachnoid hemorrhage
   Use additional code to identify the sequelae

+ I69.1 Sequelae of nontraumatic intracerebral hemorrhage
- **I69.10** Unspecified sequelae of nontraumatic intracerebral hemorrhage

+ I69.11 Cognitive deficits following nontraumatic intracerebral hemorrhage
- **I69.110** Attention and concentration deficit following nontraumatic intracerebral hemorrhage
- **I69.111** Memory deficit following nontraumatic intracerebral hemorrhage
- **I69.112** Visuospatial deficit and spatial neglect following nontraumatic intracerebral hemorrhage
- **I69.113** Psychomotor deficit following nontraumatic intracerebral hemorrhage
- **I69.114** Frontal lobe and executive function deficit following nontraumatic intracerebral hemorrhage

- **I69.115** Cognitive social or emotional deficit following nontraumatic intracerebral hemorrhage
- **I69.118** Other symptoms and signs involving cognitive functions following nontraumatic intracerebral hemorrhage
- **I69.119** Unspecified symptoms and signs involving cognitive functions following nontraumatic intracerebral hemorrhage

+ **I69.12** Speech and language deficits following nontraumatic intracerebral hemorrhage
- **I69.120** Aphasia following nontraumatic intracerebral hemorrhage
- **I69.121** Dysphasia following nontraumatic intracerebral hemorrhage
- **I69.122** Dysarthria following nontraumatic intracerebral hemorrhage
- **I69.123** Fluency disorder following nontraumatic intracerebral hemorrhage
  - Stuttering following nontraumatic intracerebral hemorrhage
- **I69.128** Other speech and language deficits following nontraumatic intracerebral hemorrhage

+ **I69.13** Monoplegia of upper limb following nontraumatic intracerebral hemorrhage
- **I69.131** Monoplegia of upper limb following nontraumatic intracerebral hemorrhage affecting right dominant side
- **I69.132** Monoplegia of upper limb following nontraumatic intracerebral hemorrhage affecting left dominant side
- **I69.133** Monoplegia of upper limb following nontraumatic intracerebral hemorrhage affecting right non-dominant side
- **I69.134** Monoplegia of upper limb following nontraumatic intracerebral hemorrhage affecting left non-dominant side
- **I69.139** Monoplegia of upper limb following nontraumatic intracerebral hemorrhage affecting unspecified side

+ **I69.14** Monoplegia of lower limb following nontraumatic intracerebral hemorrhage
- **I69.141** Monoplegia of lower limb following nontraumatic intracerebral hemorrhage affecting right dominant side
- **I69.142** Monoplegia of lower limb following nontraumatic intracerebral hemorrhage affecting left dominant side
- **I69.143** Monoplegia of lower limb following nontraumatic intracerebral hemorrhage affecting right non-dominant side
- **I69.144** Monoplegia of lower limb following nontraumatic intracerebral hemorrhage affecting left non-dominant side
- **I69.149** Monoplegia of lower limb following nontraumatic intracerebral hemorrhage affecting unspecified side

+ **I69.15** Hemiplegia and hemiparesis following nontraumatic intracerebral hemorrhage
- CC **I69.151** Hemiplegia and hemiparesis following nontraumatic intracerebral hemorrhage affecting right dominant side
- CC **I69.152** Hemiplegia and hemiparesis following nontraumatic intracerebral hemorrhage affecting left dominant side
- CC **I69.153** Hemiplegia and hemiparesis following nontraumatic intracerebral hemorrhage affecting right non-dominant side
- CC **I69.154** Hemiplegia and hemiparesis following nontraumatic intracerebral hemorrhage affecting left non-dominant side
- CC **I69.159** Hemiplegia and hemiparesis following nontraumatic intracerebral hemorrhage affecting unspecified side

+ **I69.16** Other paralytic syndrome following nontraumatic intracerebral hemorrhage
  Use additional code to identify type of paralytic syndrome, such as:
   locked-in state (G83.5)
   quadriplegia (G82.5-)
  Excludes1: hemiplegia/hemiparesis following nontraumatic intracerebral hemorrhage (I69.15-)
   monoplegia of lower limb following nontraumatic intracerebral hemorrhage (I69.14-)
   monoplegia of upper limb following nontraumatic intracerebral hemorrhage (I69.13-)
- **I69.161** Other paralytic syndrome following nontraumatic intracerebral hemorrhage affecting right dominant side
- **I69.162** Other paralytic syndrome following nontraumatic intracerebral hemorrhage affecting left dominant side
- **I69.163** Other paralytic syndrome following nontraumatic intracerebral hemorrhage affecting right non-dominant side
- **I69.164** Other paralytic syndrome following nontraumatic intracerebral hemorrhage affecting left non-dominant side
- **I69.165** Other paralytic syndrome following nontraumatic intracerebral hemorrhage, bilateral
- **I69.169** Other paralytic syndrome following nontraumatic intracerebral hemorrhage affecting unspecified side

+ **I69.19** Other sequelae of nontraumatic intracerebral hemorrhage
- **I69.190** Apraxia following nontraumatic intracerebral hemorrhage
- **I69.191** Dysphagia following nontraumatic intracerebral hemorrhage
  Use additional code to identify the type of dysphagia, if known (R13.11-R13.19)
- **I69.192** Facial weakness following nontraumatic intracerebral hemorrhage
  Facial droop following nontraumatic intracerebral hemorrhage
- **I69.193** Ataxia following nontraumatic intracerebral hemorrhage
- **I69.198** Other sequelae of nontraumatic intracerebral hemorrhage
  Alteration of sensations following nontraumatic intracerebral hemorrhage
  Disturbance of vision following nontraumatic intracerebral hemorrhage
  Use additional code to identify the sequelae

+ **I69.2** Sequelae of other nontraumatic intracranial hemorrhage
- **I69.20** Unspecified sequelae of other nontraumatic intracranial hemorrhage

+ **I69.21** Cognitive deficits following other nontraumatic intracranial hemorrhage
- **I69.210** Attention and concentration deficit following other nontraumatic intracranial hemorrhage
- **I69.211** Memory deficit following other nontraumatic intracranial hemorrhage
- **I69.212** Visuospatial deficit and spatial neglect following other nontraumatic intracranial hemorrhage
- **I69.213** Psychomotor deficit following other nontraumatic intracranial hemorrhage
- **I69.214** Frontal lobe and executive function deficit following other nontraumatic intracranial hemorrhage
- **I69.215** Cognitive social or emotional deficit following other nontraumatic intracranial hemorrhage

- **I69.218** Other symptoms and signs involving cognitive functions following other nontraumatic intracranial hemorrhage
- **I69.219** Unspecified symptoms and signs involving cognitive functions following other nontraumatic intracranial hemorrhage

+ **I69.22** Speech and language deficits following other nontraumatic intracranial hemorrhage
  - **I69.220** Aphasia following other nontraumatic intracranial hemorrhage
  - **I69.221** Dysphasia following other nontraumatic intracranial hemorrhage
  - **I69.222** Dysarthria following other nontraumatic intracranial hemorrhage
  - **I69.223** Fluency disorder following other nontraumatic intracranial hemorrhage
    Stuttering following other nontraumatic intracranial hemorrhage
  - **I69.228** Other speech and language deficits following other nontraumatic intracranial hemorrhage

+ **I69.23** Monoplegia of upper limb following other nontraumatic intracranial hemorrhage
  - **I69.231** Monoplegia of upper limb following other nontraumatic intracranial hemorrhage affecting right dominant side
  - **I69.232** Monoplegia of upper limb following other nontraumatic intracranial hemorrhage affecting left dominant side
  - **I69.233** Monoplegia of upper limb following other nontraumatic intracranial hemorrhage affecting right non-dominant side
  - **I69.234** Monoplegia of upper limb following other nontraumatic intracranial hemorrhage affecting left non-dominant side
  - **I69.239** Monoplegia of upper limb following other nontraumatic intracranial hemorrhage affecting unspecified side

+ **I69.24** Monoplegia of lower limb following other nontraumatic intracranial hemorrhage
  - **I69.241** Monoplegia of lower limb following other nontraumatic intracranial hemorrhage affecting right dominant side
  - **I69.242** Monoplegia of lower limb following other nontraumatic intracranial hemorrhage affecting left dominant side
  - **I69.243** Monoplegia of lower limb following other nontraumatic intracranial hemorrhage affecting right non-dominant side
  - **I69.244** Monoplegia of lower limb following other nontraumatic intracranial hemorrhage affecting left non-dominant side
  - **I69.249** Monoplegia of lower limb following other nontraumatic intracranial hemorrhage affecting unspecified side

+ **I69.25** Hemiplegia and hemiparesis following other nontraumatic intracranial hemorrhage
  - CC **I69.251** Hemiplegia and hemiparesis following other nontraumatic intracranial hemorrhage affecting right dominant side
  - CC **I69.252** Hemiplegia and hemiparesis following other nontraumatic intracranial hemorrhage affecting left dominant side
  - CC **I69.253** Hemiplegia and hemiparesis following other nontraumatic intracranial hemorrhage affecting right non-dominant side
  - CC **I69.254** Hemiplegia and hemiparesis following other nontraumatic intracranial hemorrhage affecting left non-dominant side
  - CC **I69.259** Hemiplegia and hemiparesis following other nontraumatic intracranial hemorrhage affecting unspecified side

+ **I69.26** Other paralytic syndrome following other nontraumatic intracranial hemorrhage
  Use additional code to identify type of paralytic syndrome, such as:
    locked-in state (G83.5)
    quadriplegia (G82.5-)
  Excludes1: hemiplegia/hemiparesis following other nontraumatic intracranial hemorrhage (I69.25-)
    monoplegia of lower limb following other nontraumatic intracranial hemorrhage (I69.24-)
    monoplegia of upper limb following other nontraumatic intracranial hemorrhage (I69.23-)
  - **I69.261** Other paralytic syndrome following other nontraumatic intracranial hemorrhage affecting right dominant side
  - **I69.262** Other paralytic syndrome following other nontraumatic intracranial hemorrhage affecting left dominant side
  - **I69.263** Other paralytic syndrome following other nontraumatic intracranial hemorrhage affecting right non-dominant side
  - **I69.264** Other paralytic syndrome following other nontraumatic intracranial hemorrhage affecting left non-dominant side
  - **I69.265** Other paralytic syndrome following other nontraumatic intracranial hemorrhage, bilateral
  - **I69.269** Other paralytic syndrome following other nontraumatic intracranial hemorrhage affecting unspecified side

+ **I69.29** Other sequelae of other nontraumatic intracranial hemorrhage
  - **I69.290** Apraxia following other nontraumatic intracranial hemorrhage
  - **I69.291** Dysphagia following other nontraumatic intracranial hemorrhage
    Use additional code to identify the type of dysphagia, if known (R13.11-R13.19)
  - **I69.292** Facial weakness following other nontraumatic intracranial hemorrhage
    Facial droop following other nontraumatic intracranial hemorrhage
  - **I69.293** Ataxia following other nontraumatic intracranial hemorrhage
  - **I69.298** Other sequelae of other nontraumatic intracranial hemorrhage
    Alteration of sensation following other nontraumatic intracranial hemorrhage
    Disturbance of vision following other nontraumatic intracranial hemorrhage
    Use additional code to identify the sequelae

+ **I69.3** Sequelae of cerebral infarction
  Sequelae of stroke NOS
  AHA CC: 4Q, 2012, 95; 4Q, 2013, 127-128
  - **I69.30** Unspecified sequelae of cerebral infarction
  + **I69.31** Cognitive deficits following cerebral infarction
    - **I69.310** Attention and concentration deficit following cerebral infarction
    - **I69.311** Memory deficit following cerebral infarction
    - **I69.312** Visuospatial deficit and spatial neglect following cerebral infarction
    - **I69.313** Psychomotor deficit following cerebral infarction

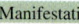

I69.314 Frontal lobe and executive function deficit following cerebral infarction
I69.315 Cognitive social or emotional deficit following cerebral infarction
I69.318 Other symptoms and signs involving cognitive functions following cerebral infarction
I69.319 Unspecified symptoms and signs involving cognitive functions following cerebral infarction

+ I69.32 Speech and language deficits following cerebral infarction
I69.320 Aphasia following cerebral infarction
AHA CC: 4Q, 2013, 128
I69.321 Dysphasia following cerebral infarction
AHA CC: 4Q, 2012, 91
I69.322 Dysarthria following cerebral infarction
Excludes2: *transient ischemic attach (TIA) (G45.9)*
I69.323 Fluency disorder following cerebral infarction
Stuttering following cerebral hemorrhage
I69.328 Other speech and language deficits following cerebral infarction

+ I69.33 Monoplegia of upper limb following cerebral infarction
AHA CC: 1Q, 2017, 47-48
I69.331 Monoplegia of upper limb following cerebral infarction affecting right dominant side
I69.332 Monoplegia of upper limb following cerebral infarction affecting left dominant side
I69.333 Monoplegia of upper limb following cerebral infarction affecting right non-dominant side
I69.334 Monoplegia of upper limb following cerebral infarction affecting left non-dominant side
I69.339 Monoplegia of upper limb following cerebral infarction affecting unspecified side

+ I69.34 Monoplegia of lower limb following cerebral infarction
AHA CC: 1Q, 2017, 47-48
I69.341 Monoplegia of lower limb following cerebral infarction affecting right dominant side
I69.342 Monoplegia of lower limb following cerebral infarction affecting left dominant side
I69.343 Monoplegia of lower limb following cerebral infarction affecting right non-dominant side
I69.344 Monoplegia of lower limb following cerebral infarction affecting left non-dominant side
I69.349 Monoplegia of lower limb following cerebral infarction affecting unspecified side

+ I69.35 Hemiplegia and hemiparesis following cerebral infarction
CC I69.351 Hemiplegia and hemiparesis following cerebral infarction affecting right dominant side
Excludes2: *transient ischemic attach (TIA) (G45.9)*
AHA CC: 4Q, 2013, 128; 1Q, 2015, 25
CC I69.352 Hemiplegia and hemiparesis following cerebral infarction affecting left dominant side
CC I69.353 Hemiplegia and hemiparesis following cerebral infarction affecting right non-dominant side
CC I69.354 Hemiplegia and hemiparesis following cerebral infarction affecting left non-dominant side
AHA CC: 4Q, 2012, 91
CC I69.359 Hemiplegia and hemiparesis following cerebral infarction affecting unspecified side

+ I69.36 Other paralytic syndrome following cerebral infarction
Use additional code to identify type of paralytic syndrome, such as:
locked-in state (G83.5)
quadriplegia (G82.5-)
Excludes1: *hemiplegia/hemiparesis following cerebral infarction (I69.35-)
monoplegia of lower limb following cerebral infarction (I69.34-)
monoplegia of upper limb following cerebral infarction (I69.33-)*
I69.361 Other paralytic syndrome following cerebral infarction affecting right dominant side
I69.362 Other paralytic syndrome following cerebral infarction affecting left dominant side
I69.363 Other paralytic syndrome following cerebral infarction affecting right non-dominant side
I69.364 Other paralytic syndrome following cerebral infarction affecting left non-dominant side
I69.365 Other paralytic syndrome following cerebral infarction, bilateral
I69.369 Other paralytic syndrome following cerebral infarction affecting unspecified side

+ I69.39 Other sequelae of cerebral infarction
I69.390 Apraxia following cerebral infarction
I69.391 Dysphagia following cerebral infarction
Use additional code to identify the type of dysphagia, if known (R13.11-R13.19)
I69.392 Facial weakness following cerebral infarction
Facial droop following cerebral infarction
I69.393 Ataxia following cerebral infarction
I69.398 Other sequelae of cerebral infarction
Alteration of sensation following cerebral infarction
Disturbance of vision following cerebral infarction
Use additional code to identify the sequelae
AHA CC: 2Q, 2020, 29

+ I69.8 Sequelae of other cerebrovascular diseases
Excludes1: *sequelae of traumatic intracranial injury (S06.-)*
I69.80 Unspecified sequelae of other cerebrovascular disease
+ I69.81 Cognitive deficits following other cerebrovascular disease
I69.810 Attention and concentration deficit following other cerebrovascular disease
I69.811 Memory deficit following other cerebrovascular disease
I69.812 Visuospatial deficit and spatial neglect following other cerebrovascular disease
I69.813 Psychomotor deficit following other cerebrovascular disease
I69.814 Frontal lobe and executive function deficit following other cerebrovascular disease
I69.815 Cognitive social or emotional deficit following other cerebrovascular disease
I69.818 Other symptoms and signs involving cognitive functions following other cerebrovascular disease
I69.819 Unspecified symptoms and signs involving cognitive functions following other cerebrovascular disease

+ I69.82 Speech and language deficits following other cerebrovascular disease
I69.820 Aphasia following other cerebrovascular disease
I69.821 Dysphasia following other cerebrovascular disease
I69.822 Dysarthria following other cerebrovascular disease

I69.823 **Fluency disorder following other cerebrovascular disease**
Stuttering following other cerebrovascular disease hemorrhage

I69.828 **Other speech and language deficits following other cerebrovascular disease**
AHA CC: 3Q, 2019, 8-9

+ I69.83 **Monoplegia of upper limb following other cerebrovascular disease**

I69.831 **Monoplegia of upper limb following other cerebrovascular disease affecting right dominant side**

I69.832 **Monoplegia of upper limb following other cerebrovascular disease affecting left dominant side**

I69.833 **Monoplegia of upper limb following other cerebrovascular disease affecting right non-dominant side**

I69.834 **Monoplegia of upper limb following other cerebrovascular disease affecting left non-dominant side**

I69.839 **Monoplegia of upper limb following other cerebrovascular disease affecting unspecified side**

+ I69.84 **Monoplegia of lower limb following other cerebrovascular disease**

I69.841 **Monoplegia of lower limb following other cerebrovascular disease affecting right dominant side**

I69.842 **Monoplegia of lower limb following other cerebrovascular disease affecting left dominant side**

I69.843 **Monoplegia of lower limb following other cerebrovascular disease affecting right non-dominant side**

I69.844 **Monoplegia of lower limb following other cerebrovascular disease affecting left non-dominant side**

I69.849 **Monoplegia of lower limb following other cerebrovascular disease affecting unspecified side**

+ I69.85 **Hemiplegia and hemiparesis following other cerebrovascular disease**

CC I69.851 **Hemiplegia and hemiparesis following other cerebrovascular disease affecting right dominant side**

CC I69.852 **Hemiplegia and hemiparesis following other cerebrovascular disease affecting left dominant side**

CC I69.853 **Hemiplegia and hemiparesis following other cerebrovascular disease affecting right non-dominant side**

CC I69.854 **Hemiplegia and hemiparesis following other cerebrovascular disease affecting left non-dominant side**

CC I69.859 **Hemiplegia and hemiparesis following other cerebrovascular disease affecting unspecified side**

+ I69.86 **Other paralytic syndrome following other cerebrovascular disease**
Use additional code to identify type of paralytic syndrome, such as:
locked-in state (G83.5)
quadriplegia (G82.5-)
Excludes1: hemiplegia/hemiparesis following other cerebrovascular disease (I69.85-)
monoplegia of lower limb following other cerebrovascular disease (I69.84-)
monoplegia of upper limb following other cerebrovascular disease (I69.83-)

I69.861 **Other paralytic syndrome following other cerebrovascular disease affecting right dominant side**

I69.862 **Other paralytic syndrome following other cerebrovascular disease affecting left dominant side**

I69.863 **Other paralytic syndrome following other cerebrovascular disease affecting right non-dominant side**

I69.864 **Other paralytic syndrome following other cerebrovascular disease affecting left non-dominant side**

I69.865 **Other paralytic syndrome following other cerebrovascular disease, bilateral**

I69.869 **Other paralytic syndrome following other cerebrovascular disease affecting unspecified side**

+ I69.89 **Other sequelae of other cerebrovascular disease**

I69.890 **Apraxia following other cerebrovascular disease**

I69.891 **Dysphagia following other cerebrovascular disease**
Use additional code to identify the type of dysphagia, if known (R13.11-R13.19)

I69.892 **Facial weakness following other cerebrovascular disease**
Facial droop following other cerebrovascular disease

I69.893 **Ataxia following other cerebrovascular disease**

I69.898 **Other sequelae of other cerebrovascular disease**
Alteration of sensation following other cerebrovascular disease
Disturbance of vision following other cerebrovascular disease
Use additional code to identify the sequelae

+ I69.9 **Sequelae of unspecified cerebrovascular diseases**
Excludes1: sequelae of stroke (I69.3)
sequelae of traumatic intracranial injury (S06.-)

I69.90 **Unspecified sequelae of unspecified cerebrovascular disease**

+ I69.91 **Cognitive deficits following unspecified cerebrovascular disease**

I69.910 **Attention and concentration deficit following unspecified cerebrovascular disease**

I69.911 **Memory deficit following unspecified cerebrovascular disease**

I69.912 **Visuospatial deficit and spatial neglect following unspecified cerebrovascular disease**

I69.913 **Psychomotor deficit following unspecified cerebrovascular disease**

I69.914 **Frontal lobe and executive function deficit following unspecified cerebrovascular disease**

I69.915 **Cognitive social or emotional deficit following unspecified cerebrovascular disease**

I69.918 **Other symptoms and signs involving cognitive functions following unspecified cerebrovascular disease**

I69.919 **Unspecified symptoms and signs involving cognitive functions following unspecified cerebrovascular disease**

+ I69.92 **Speech and language deficits following unspecified cerebrovascular disease**

I69.920 **Aphasia following unspecified cerebrovascular disease**

I69.921 **Dysphasia following unspecified cerebrovascular disease**

I69.922 **Dysarthria following unspecified cerebrovascular disease**

I69.923 **Fluency disorder following unspecified cerebrovascular disease**
Stuttering following unspecified cerebrovascular disease

I69.928 **Other speech and language deficits following unspecified cerebrovascular disease**

+ **I69.93** Monoplegia of upper limb following unspecified cerebrovascular disease
  - **I69.931** Monoplegia of upper limb following unspecified cerebrovascular disease affecting right dominant side
  - **I69.932** Monoplegia of upper limb following unspecified cerebrovascular disease affecting left dominant side
  - **I69.933** Monoplegia of upper limb following unspecified cerebrovascular disease affecting right non-dominant side
  - **I69.934** Monoplegia of upper limb following unspecified cerebrovascular disease affecting left non-dominant side
  - **I69.939** Monoplegia of upper limb following unspecified cerebrovascular disease affecting unspecified side

+ **I69.94** Monoplegia of lower limb following unspecified cerebrovascular disease
  - **I69.941** Monoplegia of lower limb following unspecified cerebrovascular disease affecting right dominant side
  - **I69.942** Monoplegia of lower limb following unspecified cerebrovascular disease affecting left dominant side
  - **I69.943** Monoplegia of lower limb following unspecified cerebrovascular disease affecting right non-dominant side
  - **I69.944** Monoplegia of lower limb following unspecified cerebrovascular disease affecting left non-dominant side
  - **I69.949** Monoplegia of lower limb following unspecified cerebrovascular disease affecting unspecified side

+ **I69.95** Hemiplegia and hemiparesis following unspecified cerebrovascular disease
  - CC **I69.951** Hemiplegia and hemiparesis following unspecified cerebrovascular disease affecting right dominant side
  - CC **I69.952** Hemiplegia and hemiparesis following unspecified cerebrovascular disease affecting left dominant side
  - CC **I69.953** Hemiplegia and hemiparesis following unspecified cerebrovascular disease affecting right non-dominant side
  - CC **I69.954** Hemiplegia and hemiparesis following unspecified cerebrovascular disease affecting left non-dominant side
  - CC **I69.959** Hemiplegia and hemiparesis following unspecified cerebrovascular disease affecting unspecified side

+ **I69.96** Other paralytic syndrome following unspecified cerebrovascular disease
  Use additional code to identify type of paralytic syndrome, such as:
    locked-in state (G83.5)
    quadriplegia (G82.5-)
  Excludes1: hemiplegia/hemiparesis following unspecified cerebrovascular disease (I69.95-)
    monoplegia of lower limb following unspecified cerebrovascular disease (I69.94-)
    monoplegia of upper limb following unspecified cerebrovascular disease (I69.93-)
  - **I69.961** Other paralytic syndrome following unspecified cerebrovascular disease affecting right dominant side
  - **I69.962** Other paralytic syndrome following unspecified cerebrovascular disease affecting left dominant side
  - **I69.963** Other paralytic syndrome following unspecified cerebrovascular disease affecting right non-dominant side
  - **I69.964** Other paralytic syndrome following unspecified cerebrovascular disease affecting left non-dominant side
  - **I69.965** Other paralytic syndrome following unspecified cerebrovascular disease, bilateral
  - **I69.969** Other paralytic syndrome following unspecified cerebrovascular disease affecting unspecified side

+ **I69.99** Other sequelae of unspecified cerebrovascular disease
  - **I69.990** Apraxia following unspecified cerebrovascular disease
  - **I69.991** Dysphagia following unspecified cerebrovascular disease
    Use additional code to identify the type of dysphagia, if known (R13.11-R13.19)
  - **I69.992** Facial weakness following unspecified cerebrovascular disease
    Facial droop following unspecified cerebrovascular disease
  - **I69.993** Ataxia following unspecified cerebrovascular disease
  - **I69.998** Other sequelae following unspecified cerebrovascular disease
    Alteration in sensation following unspecified cerebrovascular disease
    Disturbance of vision following unspecified cerebrovascular disease
    Use additional code to identify the sequelae

Diseases of arteries, arterioles and capillaries (I70-I79)

I70 **Atherosclerosis**
  Includes: arteriolosclerosis
    arterial degeneration
    arteriosclerosis
    arteriosclerotic vascular disease
    arteriovascular degeneration
    atheroma
    endarteritis deformans or obliterans
    senile arteritis
    senile endarteritis
    vascular degeneration
  Use additional code to identify:
    exposure to environmental tobacco smoke (Z77.22)
    history of tobacco dependence (Z87.891)
    occupational exposure to environmental tobacco smoke (Z57.31)
    tobacco dependence (F17.-)
    tobacco use (Z72.0)
  Excludes2: arteriosclerotic cardiovascular disease (I25.1-)
    arteriosclerotic heart disease (I25.1-)
    atheroembolism (I75.-)
    cerebral atherosclerosis (I67.2)
    coronary atherosclerosis (I25.1-)
    mesenteric atherosclerosis (K55.1)
    precerebral atherosclerosis (I67.2)
    primary pulmonary atherosclerosis (I27.0)
  AHA CC: 4Q, 2020, 98-99

- **I70.0** Atherosclerosis of aorta
- **I70.1** Atherosclerosis of renal artery
    Goldblatt's kidney
    Excludes2: atherosclerosis of renal arterioles (I12.-)
+ **I70.2** Atherosclerosis of native arteries of the extremities
    Mönckeberg's (medial) sclerosis
    Use additional code, if applicable, to identify chronic total occlusion of artery of extremity (I70.92)
    Excludes2: atherosclerosis of bypass graft of extremities (I70.30-I70.79)
    AHA CC: 3Q, 2018, 4
  + **I70.20** Unspecified atherosclerosis of native arteries of extremities
    - **I70.201** Unspecified atherosclerosis of native arteries of extremities, right leg
    - **I70.202** Unspecified atherosclerosis of native arteries of extremities, left leg
    - **I70.203** Unspecified atherosclerosis of native arteries of extremities, bilateral legs
    - **I70.208** Unspecified atherosclerosis of native arteries of extremities, other extremity
    - **I70.209** Unspecified atherosclerosis of native arteries of extremities, unspecified extremity

I70.21–I70.299 — Chapter 9: Diseases of the Circulatory System

- **+ I70.21 Atherosclerosis of native arteries of extremities with intermittent claudication**
  - I70.211 Atherosclerosis of native arteries of extremities with intermittent claudication, right leg
  - I70.212 Atherosclerosis of native arteries of extremities with intermittent claudication, left leg
  - I70.213 Atherosclerosis of native arteries of extremities with intermittent claudication, bilateral legs
  - I70.218 Atherosclerosis of native arteries of extremities with intermittent claudication, other extremity
  - I70.219 Atherosclerosis of native arteries of extremities with intermittent claudication, unspecified extremity

- **+ I70.22 Atherosclerosis of native arteries of extremities with rest pain**
  - **Includes:** any condition classifiable to I70.21-
    chronic limb-threatening ischemia NOS of native arteries of the extremities
    chronic limb-threatening ischemia of native arteries of the extremities with rest pain
    critical limb ischemia NOS of native arteries of the extremities
    critical limb ischemia of native arteries of the extremities with rest pain
  - I70.221 Atherosclerosis of native arteries of extremities with rest pain, right leg
  - I70.222 Atherosclerosis of native arteries of extremities with rest pain, left leg
  - I70.223 Atherosclerosis of native arteries of extremities with rest pain, bilateral legs
  - I70.228 Atherosclerosis of native arteries of extremities with rest pain, other extremity
  - I70.229 Atherosclerosis of native arteries of extremities with rest pain, unspecified extremity

- **+ I70.23 Atherosclerosis of native arteries of right leg with ulceration**
  - **Includes:** any condition classifiable to I70.211 and I70.221
    chronic limb-threatening ischemia of native arteries of right leg with ulceration
    critical limb ischemia of native arteries of right leg with ulceration
  - *Use additional code to identify severity of ulcer (L97.-)*
  - I70.231 Atherosclerosis of native arteries of right leg with ulceration of thigh
  - I70.232 Atherosclerosis of native arteries of right leg with ulceration of calf
  - I70.233 Atherosclerosis of native arteries of right leg with ulceration of ankle
  - I70.234 Atherosclerosis of native arteries of right leg with ulceration of heel and midfoot
    Atherosclerosis of native arteries of right leg with ulceration of plantar surface of midfoot
  - I70.235 Atherosclerosis of native arteries of right leg with ulceration of other part of foot
    Atherosclerosis of native arteries of right leg extremities with ulceration of toe
  - I70.238 Atherosclerosis of native arteries of right leg with ulceration of other part of lower leg
  - I70.239 Atherosclerosis of native arteries of right leg with ulceration of unspecified site

- **+ I70.24 Atherosclerosis of native arteries of left leg with ulceration**
  - **Includes:** any condition classifiable to I70.212 and I70.222
    chronic limb-threatening ischemia of native arteries of left leg with ulceration
    critical limb ischemia of native arteries of left leg with ulceration
  - *Use additional code to identify severity of ulcer (L97.-)*
  - I70.241 Atherosclerosis of native arteries of left leg with ulceration of thigh
  - I70.242 Atherosclerosis of native arteries of left leg with ulceration of calf
  - I70.243 Atherosclerosis of native arteries of left leg with ulceration of ankle
  - I70.244 Atherosclerosis of native arteries of left leg with ulceration of heel and midfoot
    Atherosclerosis of native arteries of left leg with ulceration of plantar surface of midfoot
  - I70.245 Atherosclerosis of native arteries of left leg with ulceration of other part of foot
    Atherosclerosis of native arteries of left leg extremities with ulceration of toe
  - I70.248 Atherosclerosis of native arteries of left leg with ulceration of other part of lower leg
  - I70.249 Atherosclerosis of native arteries of left leg with ulceration of unspecified site

- **I70.25 Atherosclerosis of native arteries of other extremities with ulceration**
  - **Includes:** any condition classifiable to I70.218 and I70.228
  - *Use additional code to identify the severity of the ulcer (L98.49-)*

- **+ I70.26 Atherosclerosis of native arteries of extremities with gangrene**
  - **Includes:** any condition classifiable to I70.21-, I70.22-, I70.23-, I70.24-, and I70.25-
    chronic limb-threatening ischemia of native arteries of extremities with gangrene
    critical limb ischemia of native arteries of extremities with gangrene
  - *Use additional code to identify the severity of any ulcer (L97.-, L98.49-), if applicable*
  - CC I70.261 Atherosclerosis of native arteries of extremities with gangrene, right leg
  - CC I70.262 Atherosclerosis of native arteries of extremities with gangrene, left leg
  - CC I70.263 Atherosclerosis of native arteries of extremities with gangrene, bilateral legs
  - CC I70.268 Atherosclerosis of native arteries of extremities with gangrene, other extremity
  - CC I70.269 Atherosclerosis of native arteries of extremities with gangrene, unspecified extremity

- **+ I70.29 Other atherosclerosis of native arteries of extremities**
  - I70.291 Other atherosclerosis of native arteries of extremities, right leg
  - I70.292 Other atherosclerosis of native arteries of extremities, left leg
  - I70.293 Other atherosclerosis of native arteries of extremities, bilateral legs
  - I70.298 Other atherosclerosis of native arteries of extremities, other extremity
  - I70.299 Other atherosclerosis of native arteries of extremities, unspecified extremity

+ **I70.3** Atherosclerosis of unspecified type of bypass graft(s) of the extremities
  Use additional code, if applicable, to identify chronic total occlusion of artery of extremity (I70.92)
  Excludes1: embolism or thrombus of bypass graft(s) of extremities (T82.8-)

+ **I70.30** Unspecified atherosclerosis of unspecified type of bypass graft(s) of the extremities
  - **I70.301** Unspecified atherosclerosis of unspecified type of bypass graft(s) of the extremities, right leg
  - **I70.302** Unspecified atherosclerosis of unspecified type of bypass graft(s) of the extremities, left leg
  - **I70.303** Unspecified atherosclerosis of unspecified type of bypass graft(s) of the extremities, bilateral legs
  - **I70.308** Unspecified atherosclerosis of unspecified type of bypass graft(s) of the extremities, other extremity
  - **I70.309** Unspecified atherosclerosis of unspecified type of bypass graft(s) of the extremities, unspecified extremity

+ **I70.31** Atherosclerosis of unspecified type of bypass graft(s) of the extremities with intermittent claudication
  - **I70.311** Atherosclerosis of unspecified type of bypass graft(s) of the extremities with intermittent claudication, right leg
  - **I70.312** Atherosclerosis of unspecified type of bypass graft(s) of the extremities with intermittent claudication, left leg
  - **I70.313** Atherosclerosis of unspecified type of bypass graft(s) of the extremities with intermittent claudication, bilateral legs
  - **I70.318** Atherosclerosis of unspecified type of bypass graft(s) of the extremities with intermittent claudication, other extremity
  - **I70.319** Atherosclerosis of unspecified type of bypass graft(s) of the extremities with intermittent claudication, unspecified extremity

+ **I70.32** Atherosclerosis of unspecified type of bypass graft(s) of the extremities with rest pain
  Includes: any condition classifiable to I70.31-
  chronic limb-threatening ischemia NOS of unspecified type of bypass graft(s) of the extremities
  chronic limb-threatening ischemia of unspecified type of bypass graft(s) of the extremities with rest pain
  critical limb ischemia NOS of unspecified type of bypass graft(s) of the extremities
  critical limb ischemia of unspecified type of bypass graft(s) of the extremities with rest pain
  - **I70.321** Atherosclerosis of unspecified type of bypass graft(s) of the extremities with rest pain, right leg
  - **I70.322** Atherosclerosis of unspecified type of bypass graft(s) of the extremities with rest pain, left leg
  - **I70.323** Atherosclerosis of unspecified type of bypass graft(s) of the extremities with rest pain, bilateral legs
  - **I70.328** Atherosclerosis of unspecified type of bypass graft(s) of the extremities with rest pain, other extremity
  - **I70.329** Atherosclerosis of unspecified type of bypass graft(s) of the extremities with rest pain, unspecified extremity

+ **I70.33** Atherosclerosis of unspecified type of bypass graft(s) of the right leg with ulceration
  Includes: any condition classifiable to I70.311 and I70.321
  chronic limb-threatening ischemia of unspecified type of bypass graft(s) of right leg with ulceration
  critical limb ischemia of unspecified type of bypass graft(s) of right leg with ulceration
  Use additional code to identify severity of ulcer (L97.-)
  - CC **I70.331** Atherosclerosis of unspecified type of bypass graft(s) of the right leg with ulceration of thigh
  - CC **I70.332** Atherosclerosis of unspecified type of bypass graft(s) of the right leg with ulceration of calf
  - CC **I70.333** Atherosclerosis of unspecified type of bypass graft(s) of the right leg with ulceration of ankle
  - CC **I70.334** Atherosclerosis of unspecified type of bypass graft(s) of the right leg with ulceration of heel and midfoot
    Atherosclerosis of unspecified type of bypass graft(s) of right leg with ulceration of plantar surface of midfoot
  - **I70.335** Atherosclerosis of unspecified type of bypass graft(s) of the right leg with ulceration of other part of foot
    Atherosclerosis of unspecified type of bypass graft(s) of the right leg with ulceration of toe
  - CC **I70.338** Atherosclerosis of unspecified type of bypass graft(s) of the right leg with ulceration of other part of lower leg
  - CC **I70.339** Atherosclerosis of unspecified type of bypass graft(s) of the right leg with ulceration of unspecified site

+ **I70.34** Atherosclerosis of unspecified type of bypass graft(s) of the left leg with ulceration
  Includes: any condition classifiable to I70.312 and I70.322
  chronic limb-threatening ischemia of unspecified type of bypass graft(s) of left leg with ulceration
  critical limb ischemia of unspecified type of bypass graft(s) of left leg with ulceration
  Use additional code to identify severity of ulcer (L97.-)
  - CC **I70.341** Atherosclerosis of unspecified type of bypass graft(s) of the left leg with ulceration of thigh
  - CC **I70.342** Atherosclerosis of unspecified type of bypass graft(s) of the left leg with ulceration of calf
  - CC **I70.343** Atherosclerosis of unspecified type of bypass graft(s) of the left leg with ulceration of ankle
  - CC **I70.344** Atherosclerosis of unspecified type of bypass graft(s) of the left leg with ulceration of heel and midfoot
    Atherosclerosis of unspecified type of bypass graft(s) of left leg with ulceration of plantar surface of midfoot
  - **I70.345** Atherosclerosis of unspecified type of bypass graft(s) of the left leg with ulceration of other part of foot
    Atherosclerosis of unspecified type of bypass graft(s) of the left leg with ulceration of toe
  - CC **I70.348** Atherosclerosis of unspecified type of bypass graft(s) of the left leg with ulceration of other part of lower leg
  - CC **I70.349** Atherosclerosis of unspecified type of bypass graft(s) of the left leg with ulceration of unspecified site

- **I70.35** Atherosclerosis of unspecified type of bypass graft(s) of other extremity with ulceration
  Includes: any condition classifiable to I70.318 and I70.328
  Use additional code to identify severity of ulcer (L98.49-)
- +**I70.36** Atherosclerosis of unspecified type of bypass graft(s) of the extremities with gangrene
  Includes: any condition classifiable to I70.31-, I70.32-, I70.33-, I70.34-, I70.35
  chronic limb-threatening ischemia of unspecified type of bypass graft(s) of the extremities with gangrene
  critical limb ischemia of unspecified type of bypass graft(s) of the extremities with gangrene
  Use additional code to identify the severity of any ulcer (L97.-, L98.49-), if applicable
  - CC **I70.361** Atherosclerosis of unspecified type of bypass graft(s) of the extremities with gangrene, right leg
  - CC **I70.362** Atherosclerosis of unspecified type of bypass graft(s) of the extremities with gangrene, left leg
  - CC **I70.363** Atherosclerosis of unspecified type of bypass graft(s) of the extremities with gangrene, bilateral legs
  - CC **I70.368** Atherosclerosis of unspecified type of bypass graft(s) of the extremities with gangrene, other extremity
  - CC **I70.369** Atherosclerosis of unspecified type of bypass graft(s) of the extremities with gangrene, unspecified extremity
- +**I70.39** Other atherosclerosis of unspecified type of bypass graft(s) of the extremities
  - **I70.391** Other atherosclerosis of unspecified type of bypass graft(s) of the extremities, right leg
  - **I70.392** Other atherosclerosis of unspecified type of bypass graft(s) of the extremities, left leg
  - **I70.393** Other atherosclerosis of unspecified type of bypass graft(s) of the extremities, bilateral legs
  - **I70.398** Other atherosclerosis of unspecified type of bypass graft(s) of the extremities, other extremity
  - **I70.399** Other atherosclerosis of unspecified type of bypass graft(s) of the extremities, unspecified extremity
- +**I70.4** Atherosclerosis of autologous vein bypass graft(s) of the extremities
  Use additional code, if applicable, to identify chronic total occlusion of artery of extremity (I70.92)
  - +**I70.40** Unspecified atherosclerosis of autologous vein bypass graft(s) of the extremities
    - **I70.401** Unspecified atherosclerosis of autologous vein bypass graft(s) of the extremities, right leg
    - **I70.402** Unspecified atherosclerosis of autologous vein bypass graft(s) of the extremities, left leg
    - **I70.403** Unspecified atherosclerosis of autologous vein bypass graft(s) of the extremities, bilateral legs
    - **I70.408** Unspecified atherosclerosis of autologous vein bypass graft(s) of the extremities, other extremity
    - **I70.409** Unspecified atherosclerosis of autologous vein bypass graft(s) of the extremities, unspecified extremity
  - +**I70.41** Atherosclerosis of autologous vein bypass graft(s) of the extremities with intermittent claudication
    - **I70.411** Atherosclerosis of autologous vein bypass graft(s) of the extremities with intermittent claudication, right leg
    - **I70.412** Atherosclerosis of autologous vein bypass graft(s) of the extremities with intermittent claudication, left leg
    - **I70.413** Atherosclerosis of autologous vein bypass graft(s) of the extremities with intermittent claudication, bilateral legs
    - **I70.418** Atherosclerosis of autologous vein bypass graft(s) of the extremities with intermittent claudication, other extremity
    - **I70.419** Atherosclerosis of autologous vein bypass graft(s) of the extremities with intermittent claudication, unspecified extremity
  - +**I70.42** Atherosclerosis of autologous vein bypass graft(s) of the extremities with rest pain
    Includes: any condition classifiable to I70.41-
    chronic limb-threatening ischemia NOS of autologous vein bypass graft(s) of the extremities
    chronic limb-threatening ischemia of autologous vein bypass graft(s) of the extremities with rest pain
    critical limb ischemia NOS of autologous vein bypass graft(s) of the extremities
    critical limb ischemia of autologous vein bypass graft(s) of the extremities with rest pain
    - **I70.421** Atherosclerosis of autologous vein bypass graft(s) of the extremities with rest pain, right leg
    - **I70.422** Atherosclerosis of autologous vein bypass graft(s) of the extremities with rest pain, left leg
    - **I70.423** Atherosclerosis of autologous vein bypass graft(s) of the extremities with rest pain, bilateral legs
    - **I70.428** Atherosclerosis of autologous vein bypass graft(s) of the extremities with rest pain, other extremity
    - **I70.429** Atherosclerosis of autologous vein bypass graft(s) of the extremities with rest pain, unspecified extremity
  - +**I70.43** Atherosclerosis of autologous vein bypass graft(s) of the right leg with ulceration
    Includes: any condition classifiable to I70.411 and I70.421
    chronic limb-threatening ischemia of autologous vein bypass graft(s) of right leg with ulceration
    critical limb ischemia of autologous vein bypass graft(s) of right leg with ulceration
    Use additional code to identify severity of ulcer (L97.-)
    - CC **I70.431** Atherosclerosis of autologous vein bypass graft(s) of the right leg with ulceration of thigh
    - CC **I70.432** Atherosclerosis of autologous vein bypass graft(s) of the right leg with ulceration of calf
    - CC **I70.433** Atherosclerosis of autologous vein bypass graft(s) of the right leg with ulceration of ankle
    - CC **I70.434** Atherosclerosis of autologous vein bypass graft(s) of the right leg with ulceration of heel and midfoot
      Atherosclerosis of autologous vein bypass graft(s) of right leg with ulceration of plantar surface of midfoot
    - **I70.435** Atherosclerosis of autologous vein bypass graft(s) of the right leg with ulceration of other part of foot
      Atherosclerosis of autologous vein bypass graft(s) of right leg with ulceration of toe
    - CC **I70.438** Atherosclerosis of autologous vein bypass graft(s) of the right leg with ulceration of other part of lower leg
    - CC **I70.439** Atherosclerosis of autologous vein bypass graft(s) of the right leg with ulceration of unspecified site

- **+ I70.44** **Atherosclerosis of autologous vein bypass graft(s) of the left leg with ulceration**
  - **Includes:** any condition classifiable to I70.412 and I70.422
    - chronic limb-threatening ischemia of autologous vein bypass graft(s) of left leg with ulceration
    - critical limb ischemia of autologous vein bypass graft(s) of left leg with ulceration
  - **Use additional code to identify severity of ulcer (L97.-)**
  - • CC **I70.441** Atherosclerosis of autologous vein bypass graft(s) of the left leg with ulceration of thigh
  - • CC **I70.442** Atherosclerosis of autologous vein bypass graft(s) of the left leg with ulceration of calf
  - • CC **I70.443** Atherosclerosis of autologous vein bypass graft(s) of the left leg with ulceration of ankle
  - • CC **I70.444** Atherosclerosis of autologous vein bypass graft(s) of the left leg with ulceration of heel and midfoot
    - Atherosclerosis of autologous vein bypass graft(s) of left leg with ulceration of plantar surface of midfoot
  - • **I70.445** Atherosclerosis of autologous vein bypass graft(s) of the left leg with ulceration of other part of foot
    - Atherosclerosis of autologous vein bypass graft(s) of left leg with ulceration of toe
  - • CC **I70.448** Atherosclerosis of autologous vein bypass graft(s) of the left leg with ulceration of other part of lower leg
  - • CC **I70.449** Atherosclerosis of autologous vein bypass graft(s) of the left leg with ulceration of unspecified site
- • **I70.45** **Atherosclerosis of autologous vein bypass graft(s) of other extremity with ulceration**
  - **Includes:** any condition classifiable to I70.418, I70.428, and I70.438
  - **Use additional code to identify severity of ulcer (L98.49)**
- **+ I70.46** **Atherosclerosis of autologous vein bypass graft(s) of the extremities with gangrene**
  - **Includes:** any condition classifiable to I70.41-, I70.42-, and I70.43-, I70.44-, I70.45
    - chronic limb-threatening ischemia of autologous vein bypass graft(s) of the extremities with gangrene
    - critical limb ischemia of autologous vein bypass graft(s) of the extremities with gangrene
  - **Use additional code to identify the severity of any ulcer (L97.-, L98.49-), if applicable**
  - • CC **I70.461** Atherosclerosis of autologous vein bypass graft(s) of the extremities with gangrene, right leg
  - • CC **I70.462** Atherosclerosis of autologous vein bypass graft(s) of the extremities with gangrene, left leg
  - • CC **I70.463** Atherosclerosis of autologous vein bypass graft(s) of the extremities with gangrene, bilateral legs
  - • CC **I70.468** Atherosclerosis of autologous vein bypass graft(s) of the extremities with gangrene, other extremity
  - • CC **I70.469** Atherosclerosis of autologous vein bypass graft(s) of the extremities with gangrene, unspecified extremity
- **+ I70.49** **Other atherosclerosis of autologous vein bypass graft(s) of the extremities**
  - • **I70.491** Other atherosclerosis of autologous vein bypass graft(s) of the extremities, right leg
  - • **I70.492** Other atherosclerosis of autologous vein bypass graft(s) of the extremities, left leg
  - • **I70.493** Other atherosclerosis of autologous vein bypass graft(s) of the extremities, bilateral legs
  - • **I70.498** Other atherosclerosis of autologous vein bypass graft(s) of the extremities, other extremity
  - • **I70.499** Other atherosclerosis of autologous vein bypass graft(s) of the extremities, unspecified extremity
- **+ I70.5** **Atherosclerosis of nonautologous biological bypass graft(s) of the extremities**
  - **Use additional code, if applicable, to identify chronic total occlusion of artery of extremity (I70.92)**
  - **+ I70.50** **Unspecified atherosclerosis of nonautologous biological bypass graft(s) of the extremities**
    - • **I70.501** Unspecified atherosclerosis of nonautologous biological bypass graft(s) of the extremities, right leg
    - • **I70.502** Unspecified atherosclerosis of nonautologous biological bypass graft(s) of the extremities, left leg
    - • **I70.503** Unspecified atherosclerosis of nonautologous biological bypass graft(s) of the extremities, bilateral legs
    - • **I70.508** Unspecified atherosclerosis of nonautologous biological bypass graft(s) of the extremities, other extremity
    - • **I70.509** Unspecified atherosclerosis of nonautologous biological bypass graft(s) of the extremities, unspecified extremity
  - **+ I70.51** **Atherosclerosis of nonautologous biological bypass graft(s) of the extremities intermittent claudication**
    - • **I70.511** Atherosclerosis of nonautologous biological bypass graft(s) of the extremities with intermittent claudication, right leg
    - • **I70.512** Atherosclerosis of nonautologous biological bypass graft(s) of the extremities with intermittent claudication, left leg
    - • **I70.513** Atherosclerosis of nonautologous biological bypass graft(s) of the extremities with intermittent claudication, bilateral legs
    - • **I70.518** Atherosclerosis of nonautologous biological bypass graft(s) of the extremities with intermittent claudication, other extremity
    - • **I70.519** Atherosclerosis of nonautologous biological bypass graft(s) of the extremities with intermittent claudication, unspecified extremity
  - **+ I70.52** **Atherosclerosis of nonautologous biological bypass graft(s) of the extremities with rest pain**
    - **Includes:** any condition classifiable to I70.51-
      - chronic limb-threatening ischemia NOS of nonautologous vein bypass graft(s) of the extremities
      - chronic limb-threatening ischemia of nonautologous vein bypass graft(s) of the extremities with rest pain
      - critical limb ischemia NOS of nonautologous vein bypass graft(s) of the extremities
      - critical limb ischemia of nonautologous vein bypass graft(s) of the extremities with rest pain
    - • **I70.521** Atherosclerosis of nonautologous biological bypass graft(s) of the extremities with rest pain, right leg
    - • **I70.522** Atherosclerosis of nonautologous biological bypass graft(s) of the extremities with rest pain, left leg
    - • **I70.523** Atherosclerosis of nonautologous biological bypass graft(s) of the extremities with rest pain, bilateral legs

- **I70.528** Atherosclerosis of nonautologous biological bypass graft(s) of the extremities with rest pain, other extremity
- **I70.529** Atherosclerosis of nonautologous biological bypass graft(s) of the extremities with rest pain, unspecified extremity

+ **I70.53** Atherosclerosis of nonautologous biological bypass graft(s) of the right leg with ulceration
  - **Includes:** any condition classifiable to I70.511 and I70.521
    chronic limb-threatening ischemia of nonautologous vein bypass graft(s) of right leg with ulceration
    critical limb ischemia of nonautologous vein bypass graft(s) of right leg with ulceration
  - Use additional code to identify severity of ulcer (L97.-)
  - CC **I70.531** Atherosclerosis of nonautologous biological bypass graft(s) of the right leg with ulceration of thigh
  - CC **I70.532** Atherosclerosis of nonautologous biological bypass graft(s) of the right leg with ulceration of calf
  - CC **I70.533** Atherosclerosis of nonautologous biological bypass graft(s) of the right leg with ulceration of ankle
  - CC **I70.534** Atherosclerosis of nonautologous biological bypass graft(s) of the right leg with ulceration of heel and midfoot
    Atherosclerosis of nonautologous biological bypass graft(s) of right leg with ulceration of plantar surface of midfoot
  - **I70.535** Atherosclerosis of nonautologous biological bypass graft(s) of the right leg with ulceration of other part of foot
    Atherosclerosis of nonautologous biological bypass graft(s) of the right leg with ulceration of toe
  - CC **I70.538** Atherosclerosis of nonautologous biological bypass graft(s) of the right leg with ulceration of other part of lower leg
  - CC **I70.539** Atherosclerosis of nonautologous biological bypass graft(s) of the right leg with ulceration of unspecified site

+ **I70.54** Atherosclerosis of nonautologous biological bypass graft(s) of the left leg with ulceration
  - **Includes:** any condition classifiable to I70.512 and I70.522
    chronic limb-threatening ischemia of nonautologous vein bypass graft(s) of left leg with ulceration
    critical limb ischemia of nonautologous vein bypass graft(s) of left leg with ulceration
  - Use additional code to identify severity of ulcer (L97.-)
  - CC **I70.541** Atherosclerosis of nonautologous biological bypass graft(s) of the left leg with ulceration of thigh
  - CC **I70.542** Atherosclerosis of nonautologous biological bypass graft(s) of the left leg with ulceration of calf
  - CC **I70.543** Atherosclerosis of nonautologous biological bypass graft(s) of the left leg with ulceration of ankle
  - CC **I70.544** Atherosclerosis of nonautologous biological bypass graft(s) of the left leg with ulceration of heel and midfoot
    Atherosclerosis of nonautologous biological bypass graft(s) of left leg with ulceration of plantar surface of midfoot
  - **I70.545** Atherosclerosis of nonautologous biological bypass graft(s) of the left leg with ulceration of other part of foot
    Atherosclerosis of nonautologous biological bypass graft(s) of the left leg with ulceration of toe
  - CC **I70.548** Atherosclerosis of nonautologous biological bypass graft(s) of the left leg with ulceration of other part of lower leg
  - CC **I70.549** Atherosclerosis of nonautologous biological bypass graft(s) of the left leg with ulceration of unspecified site

- **I70.55** Atherosclerosis of nonautologous biological bypass graft(s) of other extremity with ulceration
  - **Includes:** any condition classifiable to I70.518, I70.528, and I70.538
  - Use additional code to identify severity of ulcer (L98.49)

+ **I70.56** Atherosclerosis of nonautologous biological bypass graft(s) of the extremities with gangrene
  - **Includes:** any condition classifiable to I70.51-, I70.52-, and I70.53-, I70.54-, I70.55
    chronic limb-threatening ischemia of nonautologous vein bypass graft(s) of the extremities with gangrene
    critical limb ischemia of nonautologous vein bypass graft(s) of the extremities with gangrene
  - Use additional code to identify the severity of any ulcer (L97.-, L98.49-), if applicable
  - CC **I70.561** Atherosclerosis of nonautologous biological bypass graft(s) of the extremities with gangrene, right leg
  - CC **I70.562** Atherosclerosis of nonautologous biological bypass graft(s) of the extremities with gangrene, left leg
  - CC **I70.563** Atherosclerosis of nonautologous biological bypass graft(s) of the extremities with gangrene, bilateral legs
  - CC **I70.568** Atherosclerosis of nonautologous biological bypass graft(s) of the extremities with gangrene, other extremity
  - CC **I70.569** Atherosclerosis of nonautologous biological bypass graft(s) of the extremities with gangrene, unspecified extremity

+ **I70.59** Other atherosclerosis of nonautologous biological bypass graft(s) of the extremities
  - **I70.591** Other atherosclerosis of nonautologous biological bypass graft(s) of the extremities, right leg
  - **I70.592** Other atherosclerosis of nonautologous biological bypass graft(s) of the extremities, left leg
  - **I70.593** Other atherosclerosis of nonautologous biological bypass graft(s) of the extremities, bilateral legs
  - **I70.598** Other atherosclerosis of nonautologous biological bypass graft(s) of the extremities, other extremity
  - **I70.599** Other atherosclerosis of nonautologous biological bypass graft(s) of the extremities, unspecified extremity

+ **I70.6** Atherosclerosis of nonbiological bypass graft(s) of the extremities
  - Use additional code, if applicable, to identify chronic total occlusion of artery of extremity (I70.92)

+ **I70.60** Unspecified atherosclerosis of nonbiological bypass graft(s) of the extremities
  - **I70.601** Unspecified atherosclerosis of nonbiological bypass graft(s) of the extremities, right leg
  - **I70.602** Unspecified atherosclerosis of nonbiological bypass graft(s) of the extremities, left leg
  - **I70.603** Unspecified atherosclerosis of nonbiological bypass graft(s) of the extremities, bilateral legs

- **I70.608** Unspecified atherosclerosis of nonbiological bypass graft(s) of the extremities, other extremity
- **I70.609** Unspecified atherosclerosis of nonbiological bypass graft(s) of the extremities, unspecified extremity

+ **I70.61** Atherosclerosis of nonbiological bypass graft(s) of the extremities with intermittent claudication
  - **I70.611** Atherosclerosis of nonbiological bypass graft(s) of the extremities with intermittent claudication, right leg
  - **I70.612** Atherosclerosis of nonbiological bypass graft(s) of the extremities with intermittent claudication, left leg
  - **I70.613** Atherosclerosis of nonbiological bypass graft(s) of the extremities with intermittent claudication, bilateral legs
  - **I70.618** Atherosclerosis of nonbiological bypass graft(s) of the extremities with intermittent claudication, other extremity
  - **I70.619** Atherosclerosis of nonbiological bypass graft(s) of the extremities with intermittent claudication, unspecified extremity

+ **I70.62** Atherosclerosis of nonbiological bypass graft(s) of the extremities with rest pain
    Includes: any condition classifiable to I70.61-
    chronic limb-threatening ischemia NOS of nonbiological bypass graft(s) of the extremities
    chronic limb-threatening ischemia of nonbiological bypass graft(s) of the extremities with rest pain
    critical limb ischemia NOS of nonbiological bypass graft(s) of the extremities
    critical limb ischemia of nonbiological bypass graft(s) of the extremities with rest pain
  - **I70.621** Atherosclerosis of nonbiological bypass graft(s) of the extremities with rest pain, right leg
  - **I70.622** Atherosclerosis of nonbiological bypass graft(s) of the extremities with rest pain, left leg
  - **I70.623** Atherosclerosis of nonbiological bypass graft(s) of the extremities with rest pain, bilateral legs
  - **I70.628** Atherosclerosis of nonbiological bypass graft(s) of the extremities with rest pain, other extremity
  - **I70.629** Atherosclerosis of nonbiological bypass graft(s) of the extremities with rest pain, unspecified extremity

+ **I70.63** Atherosclerosis of nonbiological bypass graft(s) of the right leg with ulceration
    Includes: any condition classifiable to I70.611 and I70.621
    chronic limb-threatening ischemia of nonbiological bypass graft(s) of the right leg with ulceration
    critical limb ischemia of nonbiological bypass graft(s) of the right leg with ulceration
    Use additional code to identify severity of ulcer (L97.-)
  - CC **I70.631** Atherosclerosis of nonbiological bypass graft(s) of the right leg with ulceration of thigh
  - CC **I70.632** Atherosclerosis of nonbiological bypass graft(s) of the right leg with ulceration of calf
  - CC **I70.633** Atherosclerosis of nonbiological bypass graft(s) of the right leg with ulceration of ankle
  - CC **I70.634** Atherosclerosis of nonbiological bypass graft(s) of the right leg with ulceration of heel and midfoot
    Atherosclerosis of nonbiological bypass graft(s) of right leg with ulceration of plantar surface of midfoot
  - **I70.635** Atherosclerosis of nonbiological bypass graft(s) of the right leg with ulceration of other part of foot
    Atherosclerosis of nonbiological bypass graft(s) of the right leg with ulceration of toe
  - CC **I70.638** Atherosclerosis of nonbiological bypass graft(s) of the right leg with ulceration of other part of lower leg
  - CC **I70.639** Atherosclerosis of nonbiological bypass graft(s) of the right leg with ulceration of unspecified site

+ **I70.64** Atherosclerosis of nonbiological bypass graft(s) of the left leg with ulceration
    Includes: any condition classifiable to I70.612 and I70.622
    chronic limb-threatening ischemia of nonbiological bypass graft(s) of the left leg with ulceration
    critical limb ischemia of nonbiological bypass graft(s) of the left leg with ulceration
    Use additional code to identify severity of ulcer (L97.-)
  - CC **I70.641** Atherosclerosis of nonbiological bypass graft(s) of the left leg with ulceration of thigh
  - CC **I70.642** Atherosclerosis of nonbiological bypass graft(s) of the left leg with ulceration of calf
  - CC **I70.643** Atherosclerosis of nonbiological bypass graft(s) of the left leg with ulceration of ankle
  - CC **I70.644** Atherosclerosis of nonbiological bypass graft(s) of the left leg with ulceration of heel and midfoot
    Atherosclerosis of nonbiological bypass graft(s) of left leg with ulceration of plantar surface of midfoot
  - **I70.645** Atherosclerosis of nonbiological bypass graft(s) of the left leg with ulceration of other part of foot
    Atherosclerosis of nonbiological bypass graft(s) of the left leg with ulceration of toe
  - CC **I70.648** Atherosclerosis of nonbiological bypass graft(s) of the left leg with ulceration of other part of lower leg
  - CC **I70.649** Atherosclerosis of nonbiological bypass graft(s) of the left leg with ulceration of unspecified site

- **I70.65** Atherosclerosis of nonbiological bypass graft(s) of other extremity with ulceration
    Includes: any condition classifiable to I70.618 and I70.628
    Use additional code to identify severity of ulcer (L98.49)

+ **I70.66** Atherosclerosis of nonbiological bypass graft(s) of the extremities with gangrene
    Includes: any condition classifiable to I70.61-, I70.62-, I70.63-, I70.64-, I70.65
    chronic limb-threatening ischemia of nonbiological bypass graft(s) of the extremities with gangrene
    critical limb ischemia of nonbiological bypass graft(s) of the extremities with gangrene
    Use additional code to identify the severity of any ulcer (L97.-, L98.49-), if applicable
  - CC **I70.661** Atherosclerosis of nonbiological bypass graft(s) of the extremities with gangrene, right leg
  - CC **I70.662** Atherosclerosis of nonbiological bypass graft(s) of the extremities with gangrene, left leg
  - CC **I70.663** Atherosclerosis of nonbiological bypass graft(s) of the extremities with gangrene, bilateral legs

- CC **I70.668** Atherosclerosis of nonbiological bypass graft(s) of the extremities with gangrene, other extremity
- CC **I70.669** Atherosclerosis of nonbiological bypass graft(s) of the extremities with gangrene, unspecified extremity

+ **I70.69** Other atherosclerosis of nonbiological bypass graft(s) of the extremities
  - **I70.691** Other atherosclerosis of nonbiological bypass graft(s) of the extremities, right leg
  - **I70.692** Other atherosclerosis of nonbiological bypass graft(s) of the extremities, left leg
  - **I70.693** Other atherosclerosis of nonbiological bypass graft(s) of the extremities, bilateral legs
  - **I70.698** Other atherosclerosis of nonbiological bypass graft(s) of the extremities, other extremity
  - **I70.699** Other atherosclerosis of nonbiological bypass graft(s) of the extremities, unspecified extremity

+ **I70.7** Atherosclerosis of other type of bypass graft(s) of the extremities
  Use additional code, if applicable, to identify chronic total occlusion of artery of extremity (I70.92)

  + **I70.70** Unspecified atherosclerosis of other type of bypass graft(s) of the extremities
    - **I70.701** Unspecified atherosclerosis of other type of bypass graft(s) of the extremities, right leg
    - **I70.702** Unspecified atherosclerosis of other type of bypass graft(s) of the extremities, left leg
    - **I70.703** Unspecified atherosclerosis of other type of bypass graft(s) of the extremities, bilateral legs
    - **I70.708** Unspecified atherosclerosis of other type of bypass graft(s) of the extremities, other extremity
    - **I70.709** Unspecified atherosclerosis of other type of bypass graft(s) of the extremities, unspecified extremity

  + **I70.71** Atherosclerosis of other type of bypass graft(s) of the extremities with intermittent claudication
    - **I70.711** Atherosclerosis of other type of bypass graft(s) of the extremities with intermittent claudication, right leg
    - **I70.712** Atherosclerosis of other type of bypass graft(s) of the extremities with intermittent claudication, left leg
    - **I70.713** Atherosclerosis of other type of bypass graft(s) of the extremities with intermittent claudication, bilateral legs
    - **I70.718** Atherosclerosis of other type of bypass graft(s) of the extremities with intermittent claudication, other extremity
    - **I70.719** Atherosclerosis of other type of bypass graft(s) of the extremities with intermittent claudication, unspecified extremity

  + **I70.72** Atherosclerosis of other type of bypass graft(s) of the extremities with rest pain
    Includes: any condition classifiable to I70.71-
    chronic limb-threatening ischemia NOS of other type of bypass graft(s) of the extremities
    chronic limb-threatening ischemia of other type of bypass graft(s) of the extremities with rest pain
    critical limb ischemia NOS of other type of bypass graft(s) of the extremities
    critical limb ischemia of other type of bypass graft(s) of the extremities with rest pain
    - **I70.721** Atherosclerosis of other type of bypass graft(s) of the extremities with rest pain, right leg
    - **I70.722** Atherosclerosis of other type of bypass graft(s) of the extremities with rest pain, left leg
    - **I70.723** Atherosclerosis of other type of bypass graft(s) of the extremities with rest pain, bilateral legs
    - **I70.728** Atherosclerosis of other type of bypass graft(s) of the extremities with rest pain, other extremity
    - **I70.729** Atherosclerosis of other type of bypass graft(s) of the extremities with rest pain, unspecified extremity

  + **I70.73** Atherosclerosis of other type of bypass graft(s) of the right leg with ulceration
    Includes: any condition classifiable to I70.711 and I70.721
    chronic limb-threatening ischemia of other type of bypass graft(s) of the right leg with ulceration
    critical limb ischemia of other type of bypass graft(s) of the right leg with ulceration
    Use additional code to identify severity of ulcer (L97.-)
    - CC **I70.731** Atherosclerosis of other type of bypass graft(s) of the right leg with ulceration of thigh
    - CC **I70.732** Atherosclerosis of other type of bypass graft(s) of the right leg with ulceration of calf
    - CC **I70.733** Atherosclerosis of other type of bypass graft(s) of the right leg with ulceration of ankle
    - CC **I70.734** Atherosclerosis of other type of bypass graft(s) of the right leg with ulceration of heel and midfoot
      Atherosclerosis of other type of bypass graft(s) of right leg with ulceration of plantar surface of midfoot
    - **I70.735** Atherosclerosis of other type of bypass graft(s) of the right leg with ulceration of other part of foot
      Atherosclerosis of other type of bypass graft(s) of right leg with ulceration of toe
    - CC **I70.738** Atherosclerosis of other type of bypass graft(s) of the right leg with ulceration of other part of lower leg
    - CC **I70.739** Atherosclerosis of other type of bypass graft(s) of the right leg with ulceration of unspecified site

  + **I70.74** Atherosclerosis of other type of bypass graft(s) of the left leg with ulceration
    Includes: any condition classifiable to I70.712 and I70.722
    chronic limb-threatening ischemia of other type of bypass graft(s) of the left leg with ulceration
    critical limb ischemia of other type of bypass graft(s) of the left leg with ulceration
    Use additional code to identify severity of ulcer (L97.-)
    - CC **I70.741** Atherosclerosis of other type of bypass graft(s) of the left leg with ulceration of thigh
    - CC **I70.742** Atherosclerosis of other type of bypass graft(s) of the left leg with ulceration of calf
    - CC **I70.743** Atherosclerosis of other type of bypass graft(s) of the left leg with ulceration of ankle
    - CC **I70.744** Atherosclerosis of other type of bypass graft(s) of the left leg with ulceration of heel and midfoot
      Atherosclerosis of other type of bypass graft(s) of left leg with ulceration of plantar surface of midfoot
    - **I70.745** Atherosclerosis of other type of bypass graft(s) of the left leg with ulceration of other part of foot
      Atherosclerosis of other type of bypass graft(s) of left leg with ulceration of toe

- CC **I70.748** Atherosclerosis of other type of bypass graft(s) of the left leg with ulceration of other part of lower leg
- CC **I70.749** Atherosclerosis of other type of bypass graft(s) of the left leg with ulceration of unspecified site
- **I70.75** Atherosclerosis of other type of bypass graft(s) of other extremity with ulceration
  - **Includes:** any condition classifiable to I70.718 and I70.728
  - Use additional code to identify severity of ulcer (L98.49)
+ **I70.76** Atherosclerosis of other type of bypass graft(s) of the extremities with gangrene
  - **Includes:** any condition classifiable to I70.71-, I70.72-, I70.73-, I70.74-, I70.75
    chronic limb-threatening ischemia of other type of bypass graft(s) of the extremities with gangrene
    critical limb ischemia of other type of bypass graft(s) of the extremities with gangrene
  - Use additional code to identify the severity of any ulcer (L97.-, L98.49-), if applicable
  - CC **I70.761** Atherosclerosis of other type of bypass graft(s) of the extremities with gangrene, right leg
  - CC **I70.762** Atherosclerosis of other type of bypass graft(s) of the extremities with gangrene, left leg
  - CC **I70.763** Atherosclerosis of other type of bypass graft(s) of the extremities with gangrene, bilateral legs
  - CC **I70.768** Atherosclerosis of other type of bypass graft(s) of the extremities with gangrene, other extremity
  - CC **I70.769** Atherosclerosis of other type of bypass graft(s) of the extremities with gangrene, unspecified extremity
+ **I70.79** Other atherosclerosis of other type of bypass graft(s) of the extremities
  - **I70.791** Other atherosclerosis of other type of bypass graft(s) of the extremities, right leg
  - **I70.792** Other atherosclerosis of other type of bypass graft(s) of the extremities, left leg
  - **I70.793** Other atherosclerosis of other type of bypass graft(s) of the extremities, bilateral legs
  - **I70.798** Other atherosclerosis of other type of bypass graft(s) of the extremities, other extremity
  - **I70.799** Other atherosclerosis of other type of bypass graft(s) of the extremities, unspecified extremity
- **I70.8** Atherosclerosis of other arteries
+ **I70.9** Other and unspecified atherosclerosis
  - **I70.90** Unspecified atherosclerosis
  - **I70.91** Generalized atherosclerosis
  - CC **I70.92** Chronic total occlusion of artery of the extremities
    Complete occlusion of artery of the extremities
    Total occlusion of artery of the extremities
    Code first atherosclerosis of arteries of the extremities (I70.2-, I70.3-, I70.4-, I70.5-, I70.6-, I70.7-)

I71 Aortic aneurysm and dissection

Code first, if applicable:
syphilitic aortic aneurysm (A52.01)
traumatic aortic aneurysm (S25.09, S35.09)
AHA CC: 4Q, 2022, 24-26

+ **I71.0** Dissection of aorta
  - MCC **I71.00** Dissection of unspecified site of aorta
  + **I71.01** Dissection of thoracic aorta
    - MCC **I71.010** Dissection of ascending aorta
    - MCC **I71.011** Dissection of aortic arch
    - MCC **I71.012** Dissection of descending thoracic aorta
    - MCC **I71.019** Dissection of thoracic aorta, unspecified
  - MCC **I71.02** Dissection of abdominal aorta
  - MCC **I71.03** Dissection of thoracoabdominal aorta
+ **I71.1** Thoracic aortic aneurysm, ruptured
  - MCC **I71.10** Thoracic aortic aneurysm, ruptured, unspecified
  - MCC **I71.11** Aneurysm of the ascending aorta, ruptured
  - MCC **I71.12** Aneurysm of the aortic arch, ruptured
  - MCC **I71.13** Aneurysm of the descending thoracic aorta, ruptured
+ **I71.2** Thoracic aortic aneurysm, without rupture
  - **I71.20** Thoracic aortic aneurysm, without rupture, unspecified
  - **I71.21** Aneurysm of the ascending aorta, without rupture
  - **I71.22** Aneurysm of the aortic arch, without rupture
  - **I71.23** Aneurysm of the descending thoracic aorta, without rupture
+ **I71.3** Abdominal aortic aneurysm, ruptured
  - MCC **I71.30** Abdominal aortic aneurysm, ruptured, unspecified
  - MCC **I71.31** Pararenal abdominal aortic aneurysm, ruptured
  - MCC **I71.32** Juxtarenal abdominal aortic aneurysm, ruptured
  - MCC **I71.33** Infrarenal abdominal aortic aneurysm, ruptured
+ **I71.4** Abdominal aortic aneurysm, without rupture
  - **I71.40** Abdominal aortic aneurysm, without rupture, unspecified
  - **I71.41** Pararenal abdominal aortic aneurysm, without rupture
  - **I71.42** Juxtarenal abdominal aortic aneurysm, without rupture
  - **I71.43** Infrarenal abdominal aortic aneurysm, without rupture
+ **I71.5** Thoracoabdominal aortic aneurysm, ruptured
  - MCC **I71.50** Thoracoabdominal aortic aneurysm, ruptured, unspecified
  - MCC **I71.51** Supraceliac aneurysm of the thoracoabdominal aorta, ruptured
  - MCC **I71.52** Paravisceral aneurysm of the thoracoabdominal aorta, ruptured
+ **I71.6** Thoracoabdominal aortic aneurysm, without rupture
  - **I71.60** Thoracoabdominal aortic aneurysm, without rupture, unspecified
  - **I71.61** Supraceliac aneurysm of the thoracoabdominal aorta, without rupture
  - **I71.62** Paravisceral aneurysm of the thoracoabdominal aorta, without rupture
- **I71.8** Aortic aneurysm of unspecified site, ruptured
  Rupture of aorta NOS
- **I71.9** Aortic aneurysm of unspecified site, without rupture
  Aneurysm of aorta
  Dilatation of aorta
  Hyaline necrosis of aorta

I72 Other aneurysm

Includes: aneurysm (cirsoid) (false) (ruptured)
Excludes2: acquired aneurysm (I77.0)
aneurysm (of) aorta (I71.-)
aneurysm (of) arteriovenous NOS (Q27.3-)
carotid artery dissection (I77.71)
cerebral (nonruptured) aneurysm (I67.1)
coronary aneurysm (I25.4)
coronary artery dissection (I25.42)
dissection of artery NEC (I77.79)
dissection of precerebral artery, congenital (nonruptured) (Q28.1)
heart aneurysm (I25.3)
iliac artery dissection (I77.72)
precerebral artery, congenital (nonruptured) (Q28.1)
pulmonary artery aneurysm (I28.1)
renal artery dissection (I77.73)
retinal aneurysm (H35.0)
ruptured cerebral aneurysm (I60.7)
varicose aneurysm (I77.0)
vertebral artery dissection (I77.74)

- **I72.0** Aneurysm of carotid artery
  Aneurysm of common carotid artery
  Aneurysm of external carotid artery
  Aneurysm of internal carotid artery, extracranial portion
  Excludes1: aneurysm of internal carotid artery, intracranial portion (I67.1)
  aneurysm of internal carotid artery NOS (I67.1)
- **I72.1** Aneurysm of artery of upper extremity
- **I72.2** Aneurysm of renal artery

Chapter 9: Diseases of the Circulatory System

I72.3 Aneurysm of iliac artery
I72.4 Aneurysm of artery of lower extremity
  AHA CC: 2Q, 2019, 21-22
I72.5 Aneurysm of other precerebral arteries
  Aneurysm of basilar artery (trunk)
  Excludes2: aneurysm of carotid artery (I72.0)
    aneurysm of vertebral artery (I72.6)
    dissection of carotid artery (I77.71)
    dissection of other precerebral arteries (I77.75)
    dissection of vertebral artery (I77.74)
  AHA CC: 4Q, 2016, 28-29
I72.6 Aneurysm of vertebral artery
  Excludes2: dissection of vertebral artery (I77.74)
  AHA CC: 4Q, 2016, 28-29
I72.8 Aneurysm of other specified arteries
I72.9 Aneurysm of unspecified site

I73 Other peripheral vascular diseases
  Excludes2: chilblains (T69.1)
    frostbite (T33-T34)
    immersion hand or foot (T69.0-)
    spasm of cerebral artery (G45.9)
  + **I73.0** Raynaud's syndrome
    Raynaud's disease
    Raynaud's phenomenon (secondary)
    I73.00 Raynaud's syndrome without gangrene
    CC **I73.01** Raynaud's syndrome with gangrene
  I73.1 Thromboangiitis obliterans [Buerger's disease]
  + **I73.8** Other specified peripheral vascular diseases
    Excludes1: diabetic (peripheral) angiopathy (E08-E13 with .51-.52)
    I73.81 Erythromelalgia
    I73.89 Other specified peripheral vascular diseases
      Acrocyanosis
      Erythrocyanosis
      Simple acroparesthesia [Schultze's type]
      Vasomotor acroparesthesia [Nothnagel's type]
  I73.9 Peripheral vascular disease, unspecified
    Intermittent claudication
    Peripheral angiopathy NOS
    Spasm of artery
    Excludes1: atherosclerosis of the extremities (I70.2--I70.7-)

I74 Arterial embolism and thrombosis
  Includes: embolic infarction
    embolic occlusion
    thrombotic infarction
    thrombotic occlusion
  Code first embolism and thrombosis complicating abortion or ectopic or molar pregnancy (O00-O07, O08.2)
    embolism and thrombosis complicating pregnancy, childbirth and the puerperium (O88.-)
  Excludes2: atheroembolism (I75.-)
    basilar embolism and thrombosis (I63.0-I63.2, I65.1)
    carotid embolism and thrombosis (I63.0-I63.2, I65.2)
    cerebral embolism and thrombosis (I63.3-I63.5, I66.-)
    coronary embolism and thrombosis (I21-I25)
    mesenteric embolism and thrombosis (K55.0-)
    ophthalmic embolism and thrombosis (H34.-)
    precerebral embolism and thrombosis NOS (I63.0-I63.2, I65.9)
    pulmonary embolism and thrombosis (I26.-)
    renal embolism and thrombosis (N28.0)
    retinal embolism and thrombosis (H34.-)
    septic embolism and thrombosis (I76)
    vertebral embolism and thrombosis (I63.0-I63.2, I65.0)
  + **I74.0** Embolism and thrombosis of abdominal aorta
    MCC **I74.01** Saddle embolus of abdominal aorta
    CC **I74.09** Other arterial embolism and thrombosis of abdominal aorta
      Aortic bifurcation syndrome
      Aortoiliac obstruction
      Leriche's syndrome
  + **I74.1** Embolism and thrombosis of other and unspecified parts of aorta
    CC **I74.10** Embolism and thrombosis of unspecified parts of aorta
    CC **I74.11** Embolism and thrombosis of thoracic aorta
    CC **I74.19** Embolism and thrombosis of other parts of aorta
  CC **I74.2** Embolism and thrombosis of arteries of the upper extremities

CC **I74.3** Embolism and thrombosis of arteries of the lower extremities
CC **I74.4** Embolism and thrombosis of arteries of extremities, unspecified
  Peripheral arterial embolism NOS
CC **I74.5** Embolism and thrombosis of iliac artery
  AHA CC: 2Q, 2023, 7
CC **I74.8** Embolism and thrombosis of other arteries
CC **I74.9** Embolism and thrombosis of unspecified artery

I75 Atheroembolism
  Includes: atherothrombotic microembolism
    cholesterol embolism
  + **I75.0** Atheroembolism of extremities
    + **I75.01** Atheroembolism of upper extremity
      CC **I75.011** Atheroembolism of right upper extremity
      CC **I75.012** Atheroembolism of left upper extremity
      CC **I75.013** Atheroembolism of bilateral upper extremities
      CC **I75.019** Atheroembolism of unspecified upper extremity
    + **I75.02** Atheroembolism of lower extremity
      CC **I75.021** Atheroembolism of right lower extremity
      CC **I75.022** Atheroembolism of left lower extremity
      CC **I75.023** Atheroembolism of bilateral lower extremities
      CC **I75.029** Atheroembolism of unspecified lower extremity
  + **I75.8** Atheroembolism of other sites
    CC **I75.81** Atheroembolism of kidney
      Use additional code for any associated acute kidney failure and chronic kidney disease (N17.-, N18.-)
    CC **I75.89** Atheroembolism of other site

CC I76 Septic arterial embolism
  Code first underlying infection, such as:
    infective endocarditis (I33.0)
    lung abscess (J85.-)
  Use additional code to identify the site of the embolism (I74.-)
  Excludes2: septic pulmonary embolism (I26.01, I26.90)
  Valid 3-character code, no further characters required

I77 Other disorders of arteries and arterioles
  Excludes2: collagen (vascular) diseases (M30-M36)
    hypersensitivity angiitis (M31.0)
    pulmonary artery (I28.-)
  I77.0 Arteriovenous fistula, acquired
    Aneurysmal varix
    Arteriovenous aneurysm, acquired
    Excludes1: arteriovenous aneurysm NOS (Q27.3-)
      presence of arteriovenous shunt (fistula) for dialysis (Z99.2)
      traumatic - see injury of blood vessel by body region
    Excludes2: cerebral (I67.1)
      coronary (I25.4)
  I77.1 Stricture of artery
    Narrowing of artery
    AHA CC: 3Q, 2021, 12-13
  CC **I77.2** Rupture of artery
    Erosion of artery
    Fistula of artery
    Ulcer of artery
    Excludes1: traumatic rupture of artery - see injury of blood vessel by body region
  I77.3 Arterial fibromuscular dysplasia
    Fibromuscular hyperplasia (of) carotid artery
    Fibromuscular hyperplasia (of) renal artery
  CC **I77.4** Celiac artery compression syndrome
    AHA CC: 3Q, 2021, 12-13
  CC **I77.5** Necrosis of artery
  I77.6 Arteritis, unspecified
    Aortitis NOS
    Endarteritis NOS
    Excludes1: arteritis or endarteritis:
      aortic arch (M31.4)
      cerebral NEC (I67.7)
      coronary (I25.89)
      deformans (I70.-)
      giant cell (M31.5, M31.6)

720

obliterans (I70.-)
senile (I70.-)
+ **I77.7** **Other arterial dissection**
  Excludes2: dissection of aorta (I71.0-)
  dissection of coronary artery (I25.42)
  MCC **I77.70** Dissection of unspecified artery
  AHA CC: 4Q, 2016, 28-29
  MCC **I77.71** Dissection of carotid artery
  MCC **I77.72** Dissection of iliac artery
  MCC **I77.73** Dissection of renal artery
  MCC **I77.74** Dissection of vertebral artery
  Excludes2: aneurysm of vertebral artery (I72.6)
  MCC **I77.75** Dissection of other precerebral arteries
  Dissection of basilar artery (trunk)
  Excludes2: aneurysm of carotid artery (I72.0)
  aneurysm of other precerebral arteries (I72.5)
  aneurysm of vertebral artery (I72.6)
  dissection of carotid artery (I77.71)
  dissection of vertebral artery (I77.74)
  AHA CC: 4Q, 2016, 28-29
  MCC **I77.76** Dissection of artery of upper extremity
  AHA CC: 4Q, 2016, 28-29
  MCC **I77.77** Dissection of artery of lower extremity
  AHA CC: 4Q, 2016, 28-29
  MCC **I77.79** Dissection of other specified artery
+ **I77.8** **Other specified disorders of arteries and arterioles**
  + **I77.81** Aortic ectasia
    Ectasis aorta
    Excludes1: aortic aneurysm and dissection (I71.-)
    I77.810 Thoracic aortic ectasia
    I77.811 Abdominal aortic ectasia
    I77.812 Thoracoabdominal aortic ectasia
    I77.819 Aortic ectasia, unspecified site
  I77.82 Antineutrophilic cytoplasmic antibody [ANCA] vasculitis
    ANCA associated vasculitis
    ANCA positive vasculitis
    Excludes2: eosinophilic granulomatosis with polyangiitis (M30.1)
    granulomatosis with polyangiitis (M31.3-)
    microscopic polyangiitis (M31.7)
    AHA CC: 4Q, 2022, 26-27
  I77.89 Other specified disorders of arteries and arterioles
    AHA CC: 1Q, 2021, 23
I77.9 **Disorder of arteries and arterioles, unspecified**
  AHA CC: 1Q, 2021, 4

I78 **Diseases of capillaries**
  I78.0 Hereditary hemorrhagic telangiectasia
    Rendu-Osler-Weber disease
  I78.1 Nevus, non-neoplastic
    Araneus nevus
    Senile nevus
    Spider nevus
    Stellar nevus
    Excludes1: nevus NOS (D22.-)
    vascular NOS (Q82.5)
    Excludes2: blue nevus (D22.-)
    flammeus nevus (Q82.5)
    hairy nevus (D22.-)
    melanocytic nevus (D22.-)
    pigmented nevus (D22.-)
    portwine nevus (Q82.5)
    sanguineous nevus (Q82.5)
    strawberry nevus (Q82.5)
    verrucous nevus (Q82.5)
  I78.8 Other diseases of capillaries
  I78.9 Disease of capillaries, unspecified

I79 **Disorders of arteries, arterioles and capillaries in diseases classified elsewhere**
  I79.0 Aneurysm of aorta in diseases classified elsewhere
    Code first underlying disease
    Excludes1: syphilitic aneurysm (A52.01)
  I79.1 Aortitis in diseases classified elsewhere
    Code first underlying disease
    Excludes1: syphilitic aortitis (A52.02)
  I79.8 Other disorders of arteries, arterioles and capillaries in diseases classified elsewhere
    Code first underlying disease, such as:
    amyloidosis (E85.-)

Excludes1: diabetic (peripheral) angiopathy (E08-E13 with .51-.52)
syphilitic endarteritis (A52.09)
tuberculous endarteritis (A18.89)

Diseases of veins, lymphatic vessels and lymph nodes, not elsewhere classified (I80-I89)

I80 **Phlebitis and thrombophlebitis**
  Includes: endophlebitis
  inflammation, vein
  periphlebitis
  suppurative phlebitis
  Code first phlebitis and thrombophlebitis complicating abortion, ectopic or molar pregnancy (O00-O07, O08.7)
  phlebitis and thrombophlebitis complicating pregnancy, childbirth and the puerperium (O22.-, O87.-)
  Excludes1: venous embolism and thrombosis of lower extremities (I82.4-, I82.5-, I82.81-)
+ **I80.0** Phlebitis and thrombophlebitis of superficial vessels of lower extremities
    Phlebitis and thrombophlebitis of femoropopliteal vein
    I80.00 Phlebitis and thrombophlebitis of superficial vessels of unspecified lower extremity
    I80.01 Phlebitis and thrombophlebitis of superficial vessels of right lower extremity
    I80.02 Phlebitis and thrombophlebitis of superficial vessels of left lower extremity
    I80.03 Phlebitis and thrombophlebitis of superficial vessels of lower extremities, bilateral
+ **I80.1** Phlebitis and thrombophlebitis of femoral vein
    Phlebitis and thrombophlebitis of common femoral vein
    Phlebitis and thrombophlebitis of deep femoral vein
    CC **I80.10** Phlebitis and thrombophlebitis of unspecified femoral vein
    CC **I80.11** Phlebitis and thrombophlebitis of right femoral vein
    CC **I80.12** Phlebitis and thrombophlebitis of left femoral vein
    CC **I80.13** Phlebitis and thrombophlebitis of femoral vein, bilateral
+ **I80.2** Phlebitis and thrombophlebitis of other and unspecified deep vessels of lower extremities
    + **I80.20** Phlebitis and thrombophlebitis of unspecified deep vessels of lower extremities
      CC **I80.201** Phlebitis and thrombophlebitis of unspecified deep vessels of right lower extremity
      CC **I80.202** Phlebitis and thrombophlebitis of unspecified deep vessels of left lower extremity
      CC **I80.203** Phlebitis and thrombophlebitis of unspecified deep vessels of lower extremities, bilateral
      CC **I80.209** Phlebitis and thrombophlebitis of unspecified deep vessels of unspecified lower extremity
    + **I80.21** Phlebitis and thrombophlebitis of iliac vein
      Phlebitis and thrombophlebitis of common iliac vein
      Phlebitis and thrombophlebitis of external iliac vein
      Phlebitis and thrombophlebitis of internal iliac vein
      CC **I80.211** Phlebitis and thrombophlebitis of right iliac vein
      CC **I80.212** Phlebitis and thrombophlebitis of left iliac vein
      CC **I80.213** Phlebitis and thrombophlebitis of iliac vein, bilateral
      CC **I80.219** Phlebitis and thrombophlebitis of unspecified iliac vein
    + **I80.22** Phlebitis and thrombophlebitis of popliteal vein
      CC **I80.221** Phlebitis and thrombophlebitis of right popliteal vein
      CC **I80.222** Phlebitis and thrombophlebitis of left popliteal vein
      CC **I80.223** Phlebitis and thrombophlebitis of popliteal vein, bilateral
      CC **I80.229** Phlebitis and thrombophlebitis of unspecified popliteal vein

- **+ I80.23** Phlebitis and thrombophlebitis of tibial vein
  - Phlebitis and thrombophlebitis of anterior tibial vein
  - Phlebitis and thrombophlebitis of posterior tibial vein
  - **CC I80.231** Phlebitis and thrombophlebitis of right tibial vein
  - **CC I80.232** Phlebitis and thrombophlebitis of left tibial vein
  - **CC I80.233** Phlebitis and thrombophlebitis of tibial vein, bilateral
  - **CC I80.239** Phlebitis and thrombophlebitis of unspecified tibial vein
- **+ I80.24** Phlebitis and thrombophlebitis of peroneal vein
  - *AHA CC: 4Q, 2019, 8*
  - **CC I80.241** Phlebitis and thrombophlebitis of right peroneal vein
  - **CC I80.242** Phlebitis and thrombophlebitis of left peroneal vein
  - **CC I80.243** Phlebitis and thrombophlebitis of peroneal vein, bilateral
  - **CC I80.249** Phlebitis and thrombophlebitis of unspecified peroneal vein
- **+ I80.25** Phlebitis and thrombophlebitis of calf muscular vein
  - Phlebitis and thrombophlebitis of calf muscular vein, NOS
  - Phlebitis and thrombophlebitis of gastocnemial vein
  - Phlebitis and thrombophlebitis of soleal vein
  - *AHA CC: 4Q, 2019, 8*
  - **I80.251** Phlebitis and thrombophlebitis of right calf muscular vein
  - **I80.252** Phlebitis and thrombophlebitis of left calf muscular vein
  - **I80.253** Phlebitis and thrombophlebitis of calf muscular vein, bilateral
  - **I80.259** Phlebitis and thrombophlebitis of unspecified calf muscular vein
- **+ I80.29** Phlebitis and thrombophlebitis of other deep vessels of lower extremities
  - **CC I80.291** Phlebitis and thrombophlebitis of other deep vessels of right lower extremity
  - **CC I80.292** Phlebitis and thrombophlebitis of other deep vessels of left lower extremity
  - **CC I80.293** Phlebitis and thrombophlebitis of other deep vessels of lower extremity, bilateral
  - **CC I80.299** Phlebitis and thrombophlebitis of other deep vessels of unspecified lower extremity
- **I80.3** Phlebitis and thrombophlebitis of lower extremities, unspecified
- **I80.8** Phlebitis and thrombophlebitis of other sites
- **I80.9** Phlebitis and thrombophlebitis of unspecified site

MCC I81 Portal vein thrombosis
Portal (vein) obstruction
Excludes2: hepatic vein thrombosis (I82.0)
phlebitis of portal vein (K75.1)
Valid 3-character code, no further characters required

I82 Other venous embolism and thrombosis
Code first venous embolism and thrombosis complicating:
abortion, ectopic or molar pregnancy (O00-O07, O08.7)
pregnancy, childbirth and the puerperium (O22.-, O87.-)
Excludes2: venous embolism and thrombosis (of):
cerebral (I63.6, I67.6)
coronary (I21-I25)
intracranial and intraspinal, septic or NOS (G08)
intracranial, nonpyogenic (I67.6)
intraspinal, nonpyogenic (G95.1)
mesenteric (K55.0-)
portal (I81)
pulmonary (I26.-)

- **MCC I82.0** Budd-Chiari syndrome
  - Hepatic vein thrombosis
- **CC I82.1** Thrombophlebitis migrans
- **+ I82.2** Embolism and thrombosis of vena cava and other thoracic veins
  - **+ I82.21** Embolism and thrombosis of superior vena cava
    - **CC I82.210** Acute embolism and thrombosis of superior vena cava
      - Embolism and thrombosis of superior vena cava NOS
    - **CC I82.211** Chronic embolism and thrombosis of superior vena cava
  - **+ I82.22** Embolism and thrombosis of inferior vena cava
    - **MCC I82.220** Acute embolism and thrombosis of inferior vena cava
      - Embolism and thrombosis of inferior vena cava NOS
    - **MCC I82.221** Chronic embolism and thrombosis of inferior vena cava
  - **+ I82.29** Embolism and thrombosis of other thoracic veins
    - Embolism and thrombosis of brachiocephalic (innominate) vein
    - **CC I82.290** Acute embolism and thrombosis of other thoracic veins
    - **CC I82.291** Chronic embolism and thrombosis of other thoracic veins
- **CC I82.3** Embolism and thrombosis of renal vein
- **+ I82.4** Acute embolism and thrombosis of deep veins of lower extremity
  - *AHA CC: 4Q, 2019, 8-10*
  - **+ I82.40** Acute embolism and thrombosis of unspecified deep veins of lower extremity
    - Deep vein thrombosis NOS
    - DVT NOS
    - **Excludes1:** acute embolism and thrombosis of unspecified deep veins of distal lower extremity (I82.4Z-)
      acute embolism and thrombosis of unspecified deep veins of proximal lower extremity (I82.4Y-)
    - **CC I82.401** Acute embolism and thrombosis of unspecified deep veins of right lower extremity
      - **HAC** see Appendix B for HAC conditional logic
    - **CC I82.402** Acute embolism and thrombosis of unspecified deep veins of left lower extremity
      - **HAC** see Appendix B for HAC conditional logic
    - **CC I82.403** Acute embolism and thrombosis of unspecified deep veins of lower extremity, bilateral
      - **HAC** see Appendix B for HAC conditional logic
    - **CC I82.409** Acute embolism and thrombosis of unspecified deep veins of unspecified lower extremity
      - **HAC** see Appendix B for HAC conditional logic
  - **+ I82.41** Acute embolism and thrombosis of femoral vein
    - Acute embolism and thrombosis of common femoral vein
    - Acute embolism and thrombosis of deep femoral vein
    - **CC I82.411** Acute embolism and thrombosis of right femoral vein
      - **HAC** see Appendix B for HAC conditional logic
    - **CC I82.412** Acute embolism and thrombosis of left femoral vein
      - **HAC** see Appendix B for HAC conditional logic
    - **CC I82.413** Acute embolism and thrombosis of femoral vein, bilateral
      - **HAC** see Appendix B for HAC conditional logic
    - **CC I82.419** Acute embolism and thrombosis of unspecified femoral vein
      - **HAC** see Appendix B for HAC conditional logic
  - **+ I82.42** Acute embolism and thrombosis of iliac vein
    - Acute embolism and thrombosis of common iliac vein
    - Acute embolism and thrombosis of external iliac vein
    - Acute embolism and thrombosis of internal iliac vein
    - **CC I82.421** Acute embolism and thrombosis of right iliac vein
      - **HAC** see Appendix B for HAC conditional logic

- CC **I82.422** Acute embolism and thrombosis of left iliac vein
  - HAC see Appendix B for HAC conditional logic
- CC **I82.423** Acute embolism and thrombosis of iliac vein, bilateral
  - HAC see Appendix B for HAC conditional logic
- CC **I82.429** Acute embolism and thrombosis of unspecified iliac vein
  - HAC see Appendix B for HAC conditional logic
- \+ **I82.43** Acute embolism and thrombosis of popliteal vein
  - CC **I82.431** Acute embolism and thrombosis of right popliteal vein
    - HAC see Appendix B for HAC conditional logic
  - CC **I82.432** Acute embolism and thrombosis of left popliteal vein
    - HAC see Appendix B for HAC conditional logic
  - CC **I82.433** Acute embolism and thrombosis of popliteal vein, bilateral
    - HAC see Appendix B for HAC conditional logic
  - CC **I82.439** Acute embolism and thrombosis of unspecified popliteal vein
    - HAC see Appendix B for HAC conditional logic
- \+ **I82.44** Acute embolism and thrombosis of tibial vein
  - Acute embolism and thrombosis of anterior tibial vein
  - Acute embolism and thrombosis of posterior tibial vein
  - CC **I82.441** Acute embolism and thrombosis of right tibial vein
    - HAC see Appendix B for HAC conditional logic
  - CC **I82.442** Acute embolism and thrombosis of left tibial vein
    - HAC see Appendix B for HAC conditional logic
  - CC **I82.443** Acute embolism and thrombosis of tibial vein, bilateral
    - HAC see Appendix B for HAC conditional logic
  - CC **I82.449** Acute embolism and thrombosis of unspecified tibial vein
    - HAC see Appendix B for HAC conditional logic
- \+ **I82.45** Acute embolism and thrombosis of peroneal vein
  - CC **I82.451** Acute embolism and thrombosis of right peroneal vein
    - HAC see Appendix B for HAC conditional logic
  - CC **I82.452** Acute embolism and thrombosis of left peroneal vein
    - HAC see Appendix B for HAC conditional logic
  - CC **I82.453** Acute embolism and thrombosis of peroneal vein, bilateral
    - HAC see Appendix B for HAC conditional logic
  - CC **I82.459** Acute embolism and thrombosis of unspecified peroneal vein
    - HAC see Appendix B for HAC conditional logic
- \+ **I82.46** Acute embolism and thrombosis of calf muscular vein
  - Acute embolism and thrombosis of calf muscular vein, NOS
  - Acute embolism and thrombosis of gastocnemial vein
  - Acute embolism and thrombosis of soleal vein
  - **I82.461** Acute embolism and thrombosis of right calf muscular vein
  - **I82.462** Acute embolism and thrombosis of left calf muscular vein
  - **I82.463** Acute embolism and thrombosis of calf muscular vein, bilateral
  - **I82.469** Acute embolism and thrombosis of unspecified calf muscular vein

- \+ **I82.49** Acute embolism and thrombosis of other specified deep vein of lower extremity
  - CC **I82.491** Acute embolism and thrombosis of other specified deep vein of right lower extremity
    - HAC see Appendix B for HAC conditional logic
  - CC **I82.492** Acute embolism and thrombosis of other specified deep vein of left lower extremity
    - HAC see Appendix B for HAC conditional logic
  - CC **I82.493** Acute embolism and thrombosis of other specified deep vein of lower extremity, bilateral
    - HAC see Appendix B for HAC conditional logic
  - CC **I82.499** Acute embolism and thrombosis of other specified deep vein of unspecified lower extremity
    - HAC see Appendix B for HAC conditional logic
- \+ **I82.4Y** Acute embolism and thrombosis of unspecified deep veins of proximal lower extremity
  - Acute embolism and thrombosis of deep vein of thigh NOS
  - Acute embolism and thrombosis of deep vein of upper leg NOS
  - CC **I82.4Y1** Acute embolism and thrombosis of unspecified deep veins of right proximal lower extremity
    - HAC see Appendix B for HAC conditional logic
  - CC **I82.4Y2** Acute embolism and thrombosis of unspecified deep veins of left proximal lower extremity
    - HAC see Appendix B for HAC conditional logic
  - CC **I82.4Y3** Acute embolism and thrombosis of unspecified deep veins of proximal lower extremity, bilateral
    - HAC see Appendix B for HAC conditional logic
  - CC **I82.4Y9** Acute embolism and thrombosis of unspecified deep veins of unspecified proximal lower extremity
    - HAC see Appendix B for HAC conditional logic
- \+ **I82.4Z** Acute embolism and thrombosis of unspecified deep veins of distal lower extremity
  - Acute embolism and thrombosis of deep vein of calf NOS
  - Acute embolism and thrombosis of deep vein of lower leg NOS
  - CC **I82.4Z1** Acute embolism and thrombosis of unspecified deep veins of right distal lower extremity
    - HAC see Appendix B for HAC conditional logic
  - CC **I82.4Z2** Acute embolism and thrombosis of unspecified deep veins of left distal lower extremity
    - HAC see Appendix B for HAC conditional logic
  - CC **I82.4Z3** Acute embolism and thrombosis of unspecified deep veins of distal lower extremity, bilateral
    - HAC see Appendix B for HAC conditional logic
  - CC **I82.4Z9** Acute embolism and thrombosis of unspecified deep veins of unspecified distal lower extremity
    - HAC see Appendix B for HAC conditional logic
- \+ **I82.5** Chronic embolism and thrombosis of deep veins of lower extremity
  - Use additional code, if applicable, for associated long-term (current) use of anticoagulants (Z79.01)
  - **Excludes1:** personal history of venous embolism and thrombosis (Z86.718)
  - AHA CC: 4Q, 2019, 8-10

- **I82.50** Chronic embolism and thrombosis of unspecified deep veins of lower extremity
  Excludes1: *chronic embolism and thrombosis of unspecified deep veins of distal lower extremity (I82.5Z-)*
  chronic embolism and thrombosis of unspecified deep veins of proximal lower extremity (I82.5Y-)
  - CC **I82.501** Chronic embolism and thrombosis of unspecified deep veins of right lower extremity
  - CC **I82.502** Chronic embolism and thrombosis of unspecified deep veins of left lower extremity
  - CC **I82.503** Chronic embolism and thrombosis of unspecified deep veins of lower extremity, bilateral
  - CC **I82.509** Chronic embolism and thrombosis of unspecified deep veins of unspecified lower extremity
- **I82.51** Chronic embolism and thrombosis of femoral vein
  Chronic embolism and thrombosis of common femoral vein
  Chronic embolism and thrombosis of deep femoral vein
  - CC **I82.511** Chronic embolism and thrombosis of right femoral vein
  - CC **I82.512** Chronic embolism and thrombosis of left femoral vein
  - CC **I82.513** Chronic embolism and thrombosis of femoral vein, bilateral
  - CC **I82.519** Chronic embolism and thrombosis of unspecified femoral vein
- **I82.52** Chronic embolism and thrombosis of iliac vein
  Chronic embolism and thrombosis of common iliac vein
  Chronic embolism and thrombosis of external iliac vein
  Chronic embolism and thrombosis of internal iliac vein
  - CC **I82.521** Chronic embolism and thrombosis of right iliac vein
  - CC **I82.522** Chronic embolism and thrombosis of left iliac vein
  - CC **I82.523** Chronic embolism and thrombosis of iliac vein, bilateral
  - CC **I82.529** Chronic embolism and thrombosis of unspecified iliac vein
- **I82.53** Chronic embolism and thrombosis of popliteal vein
  - CC **I82.531** Chronic embolism and thrombosis of right popliteal vein
  - CC **I82.532** Chronic embolism and thrombosis of left popliteal vein
  - CC **I82.533** Chronic embolism and thrombosis of popliteal vein, bilateral
  - CC **I82.539** Chronic embolism and thrombosis of unspecified popliteal vein
- **I82.54** Chronic embolism and thrombosis of tibial vein
  Chronic embolism and thrombosis of anterior tibial vein
  Chronic embolism and thrombosis of posterior tibial vein
  - CC **I82.541** Chronic embolism and thrombosis of right tibial vein
  - CC **I82.542** Chronic embolism and thrombosis of left tibial vein
  - CC **I82.543** Chronic embolism and thrombosis of tibial vein, bilateral
  - CC **I82.549** Chronic embolism and thrombosis of unspecified tibial vein
- **I82.55** Acute embolism and thrombosis of peroneal vein
  - CC **I82.551** Chronic embolism and thrombosis of right peroneal vein
  - CC **I82.552** Chronic embolism and thrombosis of left peroneal vein
  - CC **I82.553** Chronic embolism and thrombosis of peroneal vein, bilateral
  - CC **I82.559** Chronic embolism and thrombosis of unspecified peroneal vein
- **I82.56** Acute embolism and thrombosis of calf muscular vein
  Acute embolism and thrombosis of calf muscular vein, NOS
  Acute embolism and thrombosis of gastocnemial vein
  Acute embolism and thrombosis of soleal vein
  - **I82.561** Chronic embolism and thrombosis of right calf muscular vein
  - **I82.562** Chronic embolism and thrombosis of left calf muscular vein
  - **I82.563** Chronic embolism and thrombosis of calf muscular vein, bilateral
  - **I82.569** Chronic embolism and thrombosis of unspecified calf muscular vein
- **I82.59** Chronic embolism and thrombosis of other specified deep vein of lower extremity
  - CC **I82.591** Chronic embolism and thrombosis of other specified deep vein of right lower extremity
  - CC **I82.592** Chronic embolism and thrombosis of other specified deep vein of left lower extremity
  - CC **I82.593** Chronic embolism and thrombosis of other specified deep vein of lower extremity, bilateral
  - CC **I82.599** Chronic embolism and thrombosis of other specified deep vein of unspecified lower extremity
- **I82.5Y** Chronic embolism and thrombosis of unspecified deep veins of proximal lower extremity
  Chronic embolism and thrombosis of deep veins of thigh NOS
  Chronic embolism and thrombosis of deep veins of upper leg NOS
  - CC **I82.5Y1** Chronic embolism and thrombosis of unspecified deep veins of right proximal lower extremity
  - CC **I82.5Y2** Chronic embolism and thrombosis of unspecified deep veins of left proximal lower extremity
  - CC **I82.5Y3** Chronic embolism and thrombosis of unspecified deep veins of proximal lower extremity, bilateral
  - CC **I82.5Y9** Chronic embolism and thrombosis of unspecified deep veins of unspecified proximal lower extremity
- **I82.5Z** Chronic embolism and thrombosis of unspecified deep veins of distal lower extremity
  Chronic embolism and thrombosis of deep veins of calf NOS
  Chronic embolism and thrombosis of deep veins of lower leg NOS
  - CC **I82.5Z1** Chronic embolism and thrombosis of unspecified deep veins of right distal lower extremity
  - CC **I82.5Z2** Chronic embolism and thrombosis of unspecified deep veins of left distal lower extremity
  - CC **I82.5Z3** Chronic embolism and thrombosis of unspecified deep veins of distal lower extremity, bilateral
  - CC **I82.5Z9** Chronic embolism and thrombosis of unspecified deep veins of unspecified distal lower extremity
- **I82.6** Acute embolism and thrombosis of veins of upper extremity
  - **I82.60** Acute embolism and thrombosis of unspecified veins of upper extremity
    - CC **I82.601** Acute embolism and thrombosis of unspecified veins of right upper extremity
    - CC **I82.602** Acute embolism and thrombosis of unspecified veins of left upper extremity
    - CC **I82.603** Acute embolism and thrombosis of unspecified veins of upper extremity, bilateral
    - CC **I82.609** Acute embolism and thrombosis of unspecified veins of unspecified upper extremity

- **+ I82.61** Acute embolism and thrombosis of superficial veins of upper extremity
  - Acute embolism and thrombosis of antecubital vein
  - Acute embolism and thrombosis of basilic vein
  - Acute embolism and thrombosis of cephalic vein
  - **CC I82.611** Acute embolism and thrombosis of superficial veins of right upper extremity
  - **CC I82.612** Acute embolism and thrombosis of superficial veins of left upper extremity
  - **CC I82.613** Acute embolism and thrombosis of superficial veins of upper extremity, bilateral
  - **CC I82.619** Acute embolism and thrombosis of superficial veins of unspecified upper extremity
- **+ I82.62** Acute embolism and thrombosis of deep veins of upper extremity
  - Acute embolism and thrombosis of brachial vein
  - Acute embolism and thrombosis of radial vein
  - Acute embolism and thrombosis of ulnar vein
  - **CC I82.621** Acute embolism and thrombosis of deep veins of right upper extremity
  - **CC I82.622** Acute embolism and thrombosis of deep veins of left upper extremity
  - **CC I82.623** Acute embolism and thrombosis of deep veins of upper extremity, bilateral
  - **CC I82.629** Acute embolism and thrombosis of deep veins of unspecified upper extremity
- **+ I82.7** Chronic embolism and thrombosis of veins of upper extremity
  - Use additional code, if applicable, for associated long-term (current) use of anticoagulants (Z79.01)
  - **Excludes1:** personal history of venous embolism and thrombosis (Z86.718)
  - **+ I82.70** Chronic embolism and thrombosis of unspecified veins of upper extremity
    - **CC I82.701** Chronic embolism and thrombosis of unspecified veins of right upper extremity
    - **CC I82.702** Chronic embolism and thrombosis of unspecified veins of left upper extremity
    - **CC I82.703** Chronic embolism and thrombosis of unspecified veins of upper extremity, bilateral
    - **CC I82.709** Chronic embolism and thrombosis of unspecified veins of unspecified upper extremity
  - **+ I82.71** Chronic embolism and thrombosis of superficial veins of upper extremity
    - Chronic embolism and thrombosis of antecubital vein
    - Chronic embolism and thrombosis of basilic vein
    - Chronic embolism and thrombosis of cephalic vein
    - **CC I82.711** Chronic embolism and thrombosis of superficial veins of right upper extremity
    - **CC I82.712** Chronic embolism and thrombosis of superficial veins of left upper extremity
    - **CC I82.713** Chronic embolism and thrombosis of superficial veins of upper extremity, bilateral
    - **CC I82.719** Chronic embolism and thrombosis of superficial veins of unspecified upper extremity
  - **+ I82.72** Chronic embolism and thrombosis of deep veins of upper extremity
    - Chronic embolism and thrombosis of brachial vein
    - Chronic embolism and thrombosis of radial vein
    - Chronic embolism and thrombosis of ulnar vein
    - **CC I82.721** Chronic embolism and thrombosis of deep veins of right upper extremity
    - **CC I82.722** Chronic embolism and thrombosis of deep veins of left upper extremity
    - **CC I82.723** Chronic embolism and thrombosis of deep veins of upper extremity, bilateral
    - **CC I82.729** Chronic embolism and thrombosis of deep veins of unspecified upper extremity
- **+ I82.A** Embolism and thrombosis of axillary vein
  - **+ I82.A1** Acute embolism and thrombosis of axillary vein
    - **CC I82.A11** Acute embolism and thrombosis of right axillary vein
    - **CC I82.A12** Acute embolism and thrombosis of left axillary vein
    - **CC I82.A13** Acute embolism and thrombosis of axillary vein, bilateral
    - **CC I82.A19** Acute embolism and thrombosis of unspecified axillary vein
  - **+ I82.A2** Chronic embolism and thrombosis of axillary vein
    - **CC I82.A21** Chronic embolism and thrombosis of right axillary vein
    - **CC I82.A22** Chronic embolism and thrombosis of left axillary vein
    - **CC I82.A23** Chronic embolism and thrombosis of axillary vein, bilateral
    - **CC I82.A29** Chronic embolism and thrombosis of unspecified axillary vein
- **+ I82.B** Embolism and thrombosis of subclavian vein
  - **+ I82.B1** Acute embolism and thrombosis of subclavian≈vein
    - **CC I82.B11** Acute embolism and thrombosis of right subclavian vein
    - **CC I82.B12** Acute embolism and thrombosis of left subclavian vein
    - **CC I82.B13** Acute embolism and thrombosis of subclavian vein, bilateral
    - **CC I82.B19** Acute embolism and thrombosis of unspecified subclavian vein
  - **+ I82.B2** Chronic embolism and thrombosis of subclavian vein
    - **CC I82.B21** Chronic embolism and thrombosis of right subclavian vein
    - **CC I82.B22** Chronic embolism and thrombosis of left subclavian vein
    - **CC I82.B23** Chronic embolism and thrombosis of subclavian vein, bilateral
    - **CC I82.B29** Chronic embolism and thrombosis of unspecified subclavian vein
- **+ I82.C** Embolism and thrombosis of internal jugular vein
  - **+ I82.C1** Acute embolism and thrombosis of internal jugular vein
    - **CC I82.C11** Acute embolism and thrombosis of right internal jugular vein
    - **CC I82.C12** Acute embolism and thrombosis of left internal jugular vein
    - **CC I82.C13** Acute embolism and thrombosis of internal jugular vein, bilateral
    - **CC I82.C19** Acute embolism and thrombosis of unspecified internal jugular vein
  - **+ I82.C2** Chronic embolism and thrombosis of internal jugular vein
    - **CC I82.C21** Chronic embolism and thrombosis of right internal jugular vein
    - **CC I82.C22** Chronic embolism and thrombosis of left internal jugular vein
    - **CC I82.C23** Chronic embolism and thrombosis of internal jugular vein, bilateral
    - **CC I82.C29** Chronic embolism and thrombosis of unspecified internal jugular vein
- **+ I82.8** Embolism and thrombosis of other specified veins
  - Use additional code, if applicable, for associated long-term (current) use of anticoagulants (Z79.01)
  - **+ I82.81** Embolism and thrombosis of superficial veins of lower extremities
    - Embolism and thrombosis of saphenous vein (greater) (lesser)
    - **CC I82.811** Embolism and thrombosis of superficial veins of right lower extremity
    - **CC I82.812** Embolism and thrombosis of superficial veins of left lower extremity
    - **CC I82.813** Embolism and thrombosis of superficial veins of lower extremities, bilateral
    - **CC I82.819** Embolism and thrombosis of superficial veins of unspecified lower extremity
  - **+ I82.89** Embolism and thrombosis of other specified veins
    - **CC I82.890** Acute embolism and thrombosis of other specified veins
    - **CC I82.891** Chronic embolism and thrombosis of other specified veins
- **+ I82.9** Embolism and thrombosis of unspecified vein
  - **CC I82.90** Acute embolism and thrombosis of unspecified vein
    - Embolism of vein NOS
    - Thrombosis (vein) NOS

CC	**I82.91**	Chronic embolism and thrombosis of unspecified vein
I83		**Varicose veins of lower extremities**

> **Excludes2:** varicose veins complicating pregnancy (O22.0-)
> varicose veins complicating the puerperium (O87.4)

- **+ I83.0 Varicose veins of lower extremities with ulcer**
  Use additional code to identify severity of ulcer (L97.-)
  - **+ I83.00 Varicose veins of unspecified lower extremity with ulcer**
    - **I83.001** Varicose veins of unspecified lower extremity with ulcer of thigh
    - **I83.002** Varicose veins of unspecified lower extremity with ulcer of calf
    - **I83.003** Varicose veins of unspecified lower extremity with ulcer of ankle
    - **I83.004** Varicose veins of unspecified lower extremity with ulcer of heel and midfoot
      Varicose veins of unspecified lower extremity with ulcer of plantar surface of midfoot
    - **I83.005** Varicose veins of unspecified lower extremity with ulcer other part of foot
      Varicose veins of unspecified lower extremity with ulcer of toe
    - **I83.008** Varicose veins of unspecified lower extremity with ulcer other part of lower leg
    - **I83.009** Varicose veins of unspecified lower extremity with ulcer of unspecified site
  - **+ I83.01 Varicose veins of right lower extremity with ulcer**
    - **I83.011** Varicose veins of right lower extremity with ulcer of thigh
    - **I83.012** Varicose veins of right lower extremity with ulcer of calf
    - **I83.013** Varicose veins of right lower extremity with ulcer of ankle
    - **I83.014** Varicose veins of right lower extremity with ulcer of heel and midfoot
      Varicose veins of right lower extremity with ulcer of plantar surface of midfoot
    - **I83.015** Varicose veins of right lower extremity with ulcer other part of foot
      Varicose veins of right lower extremity with ulcer of toe
    - **I83.018** Varicose veins of right lower extremity with ulcer other part of lower leg
    - **I83.019** Varicose veins of right lower extremity with ulcer of unspecified site
  - **+ I83.02 Varicose veins of left lower extremity with ulcer**
    - **I83.021** Varicose veins of left lower extremity with ulcer of thigh
    - **I83.022** Varicose veins of left lower extremity with ulcer of calf
    - **I83.023** Varicose veins of left lower extremity with ulcer of ankle
    - **I83.024** Varicose veins of left lower extremity with ulcer of heel and midfoot
      Varicose veins of left lower extremity with ulcer of plantar surface of midfoot
    - **I83.025** Varicose veins of left lower extremity with ulcer other part of foot
      Varicose veins of left lower extremity with ulcer of toe
    - **I83.028** Varicose veins of left lower extremity with ulcer other part of lower leg
    - **I83.029** Varicose veins of left lower extremity with ulcer of unspecified site
- **+ I83.1 Varicose veins of lower extremities with inflammation**
  - **I83.10** Varicose veins of unspecified lower extremity with inflammation
  - **I83.11** Varicose veins of right lower extremity with inflammation
  - **I83.12** Varicose veins of left lower extremity with inflammation
- **+ I83.2 Varicose veins of lower extremities with both ulcer and inflammation**
  Use additional code to identify severity of ulcer (L97.-)
  - **+ I83.20 Varicose veins of unspecified lower extremity with both ulcer and inflammation**
    - CC **I83.201** Varicose veins of unspecified lower extremity with both ulcer of thigh and inflammation
    - CC **I83.202** Varicose veins of unspecified lower extremity with both ulcer of calf and inflammation
    - CC **I83.203** Varicose veins of unspecified lower extremity with both ulcer of ankle and inflammation
    - CC **I83.204** Varicose veins of unspecified lower extremity with both ulcer of heel and midfoot and inflammation
      Varicose veins of unspecified lower extremity with both ulcer of plantar surface of midfoot and inflammation
    - CC **I83.205** Varicose veins of unspecified lower extremity with both ulcer other part of foot and inflammation
      Varicose veins of unspecified lower extremity with both ulcer of toe and inflammation
    - CC **I83.208** Varicose veins of unspecified lower extremity with both ulcer of other part of lower extremity and inflammation
    - CC **I83.209** Varicose veins of unspecified lower extremity with both ulcer of unspecified site and inflammation
  - **+ I83.21 Varicose veins of right lower extremity with both ulcer and inflammation**
    - CC **I83.211** Varicose veins of right lower extremity with both ulcer of thigh and inflammation
    - CC **I83.212** Varicose veins of right lower extremity with both ulcer of calf and inflammation
    - CC **I83.213** Varicose veins of right lower extremity with both ulcer of ankle and inflammation
    - CC **I83.214** Varicose veins of right lower extremity with both ulcer of heel and midfoot and inflammation
      Varicose veins of right lower extremity with both ulcer of plantar surface of midfoot and inflammation
    - CC **I83.215** Varicose veins of right lower extremity with both ulcer other part of foot and inflammation
      Varicose veins of right lower extremity with both ulcer of toe and inflammation
    - CC **I83.218** Varicose veins of right lower extremity with both ulcer of other part of lower extremity and inflammation
    - CC **I83.219** Varicose veins of right lower extremity with both ulcer of unspecified site and inflammation
  - **+ I83.22 Varicose veins of left lower extremity with both ulcer and inflammation**
    - CC **I83.221** Varicose veins of left lower extremity with both ulcer of thigh and inflammation
    - CC **I83.222** Varicose veins of left lower extremity with both ulcer of calf and inflammation
    - CC **I83.223** Varicose veins of left lower extremity with both ulcer of ankle and inflammation
    - CC **I83.224** Varicose veins of left lower extremity with both ulcer of heel and midfoot and inflammation
      Varicose veins of left lower extremity with both ulcer of plantar surface of midfoot and inflammation
    - CC **I83.225** Varicose veins of left lower extremity with both ulcer other part of foot and inflammation
      Varicose veins of left lower extremity with both ulcer of toe and inflammation

- **CC** **I83.228** Varicose veins of left lower extremity with both ulcer of other part of lower extremity and inflammation
- **CC** **I83.229** Varicose veins of left lower extremity with both ulcer of unspecified site and inflammation

+ **I83.8** Varicose veins of lower extremities with other complications
  + **I83.81** Varicose veins of lower extremities with pain
    - **I83.811** Varicose veins of right lower extremity with pain
    - **I83.812** Varicose veins of left lower extremity with pain
    - **I83.813** Varicose veins of bilateral lower extremities with pain
    - **I83.819** Varicose veins of unspecified lower extremity with pain
  + **I83.89** Varicose veins of lower extremities with other complications
    Varicose veins of lower extremities with edema
    Varicose veins of lower extremities with swelling
    - **I83.891** Varicose veins of right lower extremity with other complications
    - **I83.892** Varicose veins of left lower extremity with other complications
    - **I83.893** Varicose veins of bilateral lower extremities with other complications
    - **I83.899** Varicose veins of unspecified lower extremity with other complications

+ **I83.9** Asymptomatic varicose veins of lower extremities
  Phlebectasia of lower extremities
  Varicose veins of lower extremities
  Varix of lower extremities
  - **I83.90** Asymptomatic varicose veins of unspecified lower extremity
    Varicose veins NOS
  - **I83.91** Asymptomatic varicose veins of right lower extremity
  - **I83.92** Asymptomatic varicose veins of left lower extremity
  - **I83.93** Asymptomatic varicose veins of bilateral lower extremities

I85 Esophageal varices
Use additional code to identify:
alcohol abuse and dependence (F10.-)

+ **I85.0** Esophageal varices
  Idiopathic esophageal varices
  Primary esophageal varices
  - **CC** **I85.00** Esophageal varices without bleeding
    Esophageal varices NOS
  - **MCC** **I85.01** Esophageal varices with bleeding

+ **I85.1** Secondary esophageal varices
  Esophageal varices secondary to alcoholic liver disease
  Esophageal varices secondary to cirrhosis of liver
  Esophageal varices secondary to schistosomiasis
  Esophageal varices secondary to toxic liver disease
  Code first underlying disease
  - **CC** **I85.10** Secondary esophageal varices without bleeding
  - **MCC** **I85.11** Secondary esophageal varices with bleeding

I86 Varicose veins of other sites
Excludes1: varicose veins of unspecified site (I83.9-)
Excludes2: retinal varices (H35.0-)
- **I86.0** Sublingual varices
- ♂ **I86.1** Scrotal varices
  Varicocele
- **I86.2** Pelvic varices
- ♀ **I86.3** Vulval varices
  Excludes1: vulval varices complicating childbirth and the puerperium (O87.8)
  vulval varices complicating pregnancy (O22.1-)
- **I86.4** Gastric varices
- **I86.8** Varicose veins of other specified sites
  Varicose ulcer of nasal septum

I87 Other disorders of veins
+ **I87.0** Postthrombotic syndrome
  Chronic venous hypertension due to deep vein thrombosis
  Postphlebitic syndrome
  Excludes1: chronic venous hypertension without deep vein thrombosis (I87.3-)

+ **I87.00** Postthrombotic syndrome without complications
  Asymptomatic Postthrombotic syndrome
  - **I87.001** Postthrombotic syndrome without complications of right lower extremity
  - **I87.002** Postthrombotic syndrome without complications of left lower extremity
  - **I87.003** Postthrombotic syndrome without complications of bilateral lower extremity
  - **I87.009** Postthrombotic syndrome without complications of unspecified extremity
    Postthrombotic syndrome NOS

+ **I87.01** Postthrombotic syndrome with ulcer
  Use additional code to specify site and severity of ulcer (L97.-)
  - **CC** **I87.011** Postthrombotic syndrome with ulcer of right lower extremity
  - **CC** **I87.012** Postthrombotic syndrome with ulcer of left lower extremity
  - **CC** **I87.013** Postthrombotic syndrome with ulcer of bilateral lower extremity
  - **CC** **I87.019** Postthrombotic syndrome with ulcer of unspecified lower extremity

+ **I87.02** Postthrombotic syndrome with inflammation
  - **I87.021** Postthrombotic syndrome with inflammation of right lower extremity
  - **I87.022** Postthrombotic syndrome with inflammation of left lower extremity
  - **I87.023** Postthrombotic syndrome with inflammation of bilateral lower extremity
  - **I87.029** Postthrombotic syndrome with inflammation of unspecified lower extremity

+ **I87.03** Postthrombotic syndrome with ulcer and inflammation
  Use additional code to specify site and severity of ulcer (L97.-)
  - **CC** **I87.031** Postthrombotic syndrome with ulcer and inflammation of right lower extremity
  - **CC** **I87.032** Postthrombotic syndrome with ulcer and inflammation of left lower extremity
  - **CC** **I87.033** Postthrombotic syndrome with ulcer and inflammation of bilateral lower extremity
  - **CC** **I87.039** Postthrombotic syndrome with ulcer and inflammation of unspecified lower extremity

+ **I87.09** Postthrombotic syndrome with other complications
  - **I87.091** Postthrombotic syndrome with other complications of right lower extremity
  - **I87.092** Postthrombotic syndrome with other complications of left lower extremity
  - **I87.093** Postthrombotic syndrome with other complications of bilateral lower extremity
  - **I87.099** Postthrombotic syndrome with other complications of unspecified lower extremity

CC **I87.1** Compression of vein
  Stricture of vein
  Vena cava syndrome (inferior) (superior)
  Excludes2: compression of pulmonary vein (I28.8)
  AHA CC: 2Q, 2023, 8

I87.2 Venous insufficiency (chronic) (peripheral)
  Stasis dermatitis
  Use Additional code, if applicable, to specify site and severity of ulcer (L97.-)
  Code also, if applicable, associated hypertensive conditions such as:
  essential (primary) hypertension (I10)
  hypertensive chronic kidney disease (I12.-)
  hypertensive heart and chronic kidney disease (I13.-)
  hypertensive heart disease (I11.-)
  Excludes1: stasis dermatitis with varicose veins of lower extremities (I83.1-, I83.2-)

+ **I87.3** Chronic venous hypertension (idiopathic)
  Stasis edema

Excludes1: chronic venous hypertension due to deep vein thrombosis (I87.0-)
varicose veins of lower extremities (I83.-)

+ **I87.30 Chronic venous hypertension (idiopathic) without complications**
Asymptomatic chronic venous hypertension (idiopathic)
- I87.301 Chronic venous hypertension (idiopathic) without complications of right lower extremity
- I87.302 Chronic venous hypertension (idiopathic) without complications of left lower extremity
- I87.303 Chronic venous hypertension (idiopathic) without complications of bilateral lower extremity
- I87.309 Chronic venous hypertension (idiopathic) without complications of unspecified lower extremity
  Chronic venous hypertension NOS

+ **I87.31 Chronic venous hypertension (idiopathic) with ulcer**
Use additional code to specify site and severity of ulcer (L97.-)
- CC I87.311 Chronic venous hypertension (idiopathic) with ulcer of right lower extremity
- CC I87.312 Chronic venous hypertension (idiopathic) with ulcer of left lower extremity
- CC I87.313 Chronic venous hypertension (idiopathic) with ulcer of bilateral lower extremity
- CC I87.319 Chronic venous hypertension (idiopathic) with ulcer of unspecified lower extremity

+ **I87.32 Chronic venous hypertension (idiopathic) with inflammation**
- I87.321 Chronic venous hypertension (idiopathic) with inflammation of right lower extremity
- I87.322 Chronic venous hypertension (idiopathic) with inflammation of left lower extremity
- I87.323 Chronic venous hypertension (idiopathic) with inflammation of bilateral lower extremity
- I87.329 Chronic venous hypertension (idiopathic) with inflammation of unspecified lower extremity

+ **I87.33 Chronic venous hypertension (idiopathic) with ulcer and inflammation**
Use additional code to specify site and severity of ulcer (L97.-)
- CC I87.331 Chronic venous hypertension (idiopathic) with ulcer and inflammation of right lower extremity
- CC I87.332 Chronic venous hypertension (idiopathic) with ulcer and inflammation of left lower extremity
- CC I87.333 Chronic venous hypertension (idiopathic) with ulcer and inflammation of bilateral lower extremity
- CC I87.339 Chronic venous hypertension (idiopathic) with ulcer and inflammation of unspecified lower extremity

+ **I87.39 Chronic venous hypertension (idiopathic) with other complications**
- I87.391 Chronic venous hypertension (idiopathic) with other complications of right lower extremity
- I87.392 Chronic venous hypertension (idiopathic) with other complications of left lower extremity
- I87.393 Chronic venous hypertension (idiopathic) with other complications of bilateral lower extremity
- I87.399 Chronic venous hypertension (idiopathic) with other complications of unspecified lower extremity

I87.8 Other specified disorders of veins
Phlebosclerosis
Venofibrosis

I87.9 Disorder of vein, unspecified

I88 Nonspecific lymphadenitis

Excludes1: acute lymphadenitis, except mesenteric (L04.-)
enlarged lymph nodes NOS (R59.-)
human immunodeficiency virus [HIV] disease resulting in generalized lymphadenopathy (B20)

I88.0 Nonspecific mesenteric lymphadenitis
Mesenteric lymphadenitis (acute)(chronic)

I88.1 Chronic lymphadenitis, except mesenteric
Adenitis
Lymphadenitis

I88.8 Other nonspecific lymphadenitis

I88.9 Nonspecific lymphadenitis, unspecified
Lymphadenitis NOS

I89 Other noninfective disorders of lymphatic vessels and lymph nodes

Excludes1: chylocele, tunica vaginalis (nonfilarial) NOS (N50.89)
enlarged lymph nodes NOS (R59.-)
filarial chylocele (B74.-)
hereditary lymphedema (Q82.0)

I89.0 Lymphedema, not elsewhere classified
Elephantiasis (nonfilarial) NOS
Lymphangiectasis
Obliteration, lymphatic vessel
Praecox lymphedema
Secondary lymphedema
Excludes1: postmastectomy lymphedema (I97.2)

I89.1 Lymphangitis
Chronic lymphangitis
Lymphangitis NOS
Subacute lymphangitis
Excludes1: acute lymphangitis (L03.-)

I89.8 Other specified noninfective disorders of lymphatic vessels and lymph nodes
Chylocele (nonfilarial)
Chylous ascites
Chylous cyst
Lipomelanotic reticulosis
Lymph node or vessel fistula
Lymph node or vessel infarction
Lymph node or vessel rupture

I89.9 Noninfective disorder of lymphatic vessels and lymph nodes, unspecified
Disease of lymphatic vessels NOS

Other and unspecified disorders of the circulatory system (I95-I99)

I95 Hypotension

Excludes1: cardiovascular collapse (R57.9)
maternal hypotension syndrome (O26.5-)
nonspecific low blood pressure reading NOS (R03.1)

I95.0 Idiopathic hypotension

I95.1 Orthostatic hypotension
Hypotension, postural
Excludes1: neurogenic orthostatic hypotension [Shy-Drager] (G90.3)
orthostatic hypotension due to drugs (I95.2)
AHA CC: 2Q, 2023, 8-9

I95.2 Hypotension due to drugs
Orthostatic hypotension due to drugs
Use additional code for adverse effect, if applicable, to identify drug (T36-T50 with fifth or sixth character 5)

I95.3 Hypotension of hemodialysis
Intra-dialytic hypotension

I95.8 Other hypotension
- I95.81 Postprocedural hypotension
- I95.89 Other hypotension
  Chronic hypotension

I95.9 Hypotension, unspecified

CC I96 Gangrene, not elsewhere classified

Gangrenous cellulitis
Excludes1: gangrene in atherosclerosis of native arteries of the extremities (I70.26)

gangrene in hernia (K40.1, K40.4, K41.1, K41.4, K42.1, K43.1-, K44.1, K45.1, K46.1)
gangrene in other peripheral vascular diseases (I73.-)
gangrene of certain specified sites - see Alphabetical Index
gas gangrene (A48.0)
pyoderma gangrenosum (L88)

Excludes2: *gangrene in diabetes mellitus (E08-E13 with .52)*
AHA CC: Q2, 2013, 34-35; 3Q, 2017, 6; 3Q, 2018, 3-4
Valid 3-character code, no further characters required

I97 Intraoperative and postprocedural complications and disorders of circulatory system, not elsewhere classified

Excludes2: *postprocedural shock (T81.1-)*
AHA CC: 1Q, 2021, 13-14

- **I97.0 Postcardiotomy syndrome**
- **+ I97.1 Other postprocedural cardiac functional disturbances**
    Excludes2: *acute pulmonary insufficiency following thoracic surgery (J95.1)*
    intraoperative cardiac functional disturbances (I97.7-)
    - **+ I97.11 Postprocedural cardiac insufficiency**
        - CC **I97.110** Postprocedural cardiac insufficiency following cardiac surgery
        - CC **I97.111** Postprocedural cardiac insufficiency following other surgery
    - **+ I97.12 Postprocedural cardiac arrest**
        - CC **I97.120** Postprocedural cardiac arrest following cardiac surgery
        - CC **I97.121** Postprocedural cardiac arrest following other surgery
    - **+ I97.13 Postprocedural heart failure**
        Use additional code to identify the heart failure (I50.-)
        - CC **I97.130** Postprocedural heart failure following cardiac surgery
        - CC **I97.131** Postprocedural heart failure following other surgery
    - **+ I97.19 Other postprocedural cardiac functional disturbances**
        Use additional code, if applicable, to further specify disorder
        - CC **I97.190** Other postprocedural cardiac functional disturbances following cardiac surgery
            Use additional code, if applicable, for type 4 or type 5 myocardial infarction, to further specify disorder
            AHA CC: 2Q, 2019, 32-33
        - CC **I97.191** Other postprocedural cardiac functional disturbances following other surgery
- • **I97.2 Postmastectomy lymphedema syndrome**
    Elephantiasis due to mastectomy
    Obliteration of lymphatic vessels
- **I97.3 Postprocedural hypertension**
- **+ I97.4 Intraoperative hemorrhage and hematoma of a circulatory system organ or structure complicating a procedure**
    Excludes1: *intraoperative hemorrhage and hematoma of a circulatory system organ or structure due to accidental puncture and laceration during a procedure (I97.5-)*
    Excludes2: *intraoperative cerebrovascular hemorrhage complicating a procedure (G97.3-)*
    - **+ I97.41 Intraoperative hemorrhage and hematoma of a circulatory system organ or structure complicating a circulatory system procedure**
        - CC **I97.410** Intraoperative hemorrhage and hematoma of a circulatory system organ or structure complicating a cardiac catheterization
        - CC **I97.411** Intraoperative hemorrhage and hematoma of a circulatory system organ or structure complicating a cardiac bypass
        - CC **I97.418** Intraoperative hemorrhage and hematoma of a circulatory system organ or structure complicating other circulatory system procedure
    - CC **I97.42** Intraoperative hemorrhage and hematoma of a circulatory system organ or structure complicating other procedure
        AHA CC: 4Q, 2016, 100-101
- **+ I97.5 Accidental puncture and laceration of a circulatory system organ or structure during a procedure**
    Excludes2: *accidental puncture and laceration of brain during a procedure (G97.4-)*
    - CC **I97.51** Accidental puncture and laceration of a circulatory system organ or structure during a circulatory system procedure
        AHA CC: 2Q, 2019, 24
    - CC **I97.52** Accidental puncture and laceration of a circulatory system organ or structure during other procedure
- **+ I97.6 Postprocedural hemorrhage, hematoma and seroma of a circulatory system organ or structure following a procedure**
    Excludes2: *postprocedural cerebrovascular hemorrhage complicating a procedure (G97.5-)*
    AHA CC: 4Q, 2016, 9-10
    - **+ I97.61 Postprocedural hemorrhage of a circulatory system organ or structure following a circulatory system procedure**
        - CC **I97.610** Postprocedural hemorrhage of a circulatory system organ or structure following a cardiac catheterization
        - CC **I97.611** Postprocedural hemorrhage of a circulatory system organ or structure following cardiac bypass
        - CC **I97.618** Postprocedural hemorrhage of a circulatory system organ or structure following other circulatory system procedure
    - **+ I97.62 Postprocedural hemorrhage, hematoma and seroma of a circulatory system organ or structure following other procedure**
        - CC **I97.620** Postprocedural hemorrhage of a circulatory system organ or structure following other procedure
        - CC **I97.621** Postprocedural hematoma of a circulatory system organ or structure following other procedure
        - CC **I97.622** Postprocedural seroma of a circulatory system organ or structure following other procedure
    - **+ I97.63 Postprocedural hematoma of a circulatory system organ or structure following a circulatory system procedure**
        - CC **I97.630** Postprocedural hematoma of a circulatory system organ or structure following a cardiac catheterization
        - CC **I97.631** Postprocedural hematoma of a circulatory system organ or structure following cardiac bypass
        - CC **I97.638** Postprocedural hematoma of a circulatory system organ or structure following other circulatory system procedure
    - **I97.64 Postprocedural seroma of a circulatory system organ or structure following a circulatory system procedure**
        - CC **I97.640** Postprocedural seroma of a circulatory system organ or structure following a cardiac catheterization
        - CC **I97.641** Postprocedural seroma of a circulatory system organ or structure following cardiac bypass
        - CC **I97.648** Postprocedural seroma of a circulatory system organ or structure following other circulatory system procedure
- **+ I97.7 Intraoperative cardiac functional disturbances**
    Excludes2: *acute pulmonary insufficiency following thoracic surgery (J95.1)*
    postprocedural cardiac functional disturbances (I97.1-)
    - **+ I97.71 Intraoperative cardiac arrest**
        - CC **I97.710** Intraoperative cardiac arrest during cardiac surgery
        - CC **I97.711** Intraoperative cardiac arrest during other surgery

- **+ I97.79** Other intraoperative cardiac functional disturbances
  Use additional code, if applicable, to further specify disorder
  - CC **I97.790** Other intraoperative cardiac functional disturbances during cardiac surgery
  - CC **I97.791** Other intraoperative cardiac functional disturbances during other surgery
- **+ I97.8** Other intraoperative and postprocedural complications and disorders of the circulatory system, not elsewhere classified
  Use additional code, if applicable, to further specify disorder
  - **+ I97.81** Intraoperative cerebrovascular infarction
    - CC **I97.810** Intraoperative cerebrovascular infarction cardiac surgery
    - CC **I97.811** Intraoperative cerebrovascular infarction during other surgery
  - **+ I97.82** Postprocedural cerebrovascular infarction
    - CC **I97.820** Postprocedural cerebrovascular infarction following cardiac surgery
    - CC **I97.821** Postprocedural cerebrovascular infarction following other surgery
  - CC **I97.88** Other intraoperative complications of the circulatory system, not elsewhere classified
  - CC **I97.89** Other postprocedural complications and disorders of the circulatory system, not elsewhere classified
    AHA CC: 3Q, 2020, 4, 7-8; 3Q, 2021, 33

I99 Other and unspecified disorders of circulatory system
- **I99.8** Other disorder of circulatory system
- **I99.9** Unspecified disorder of circulatory system

Chapter 10: Diseases of the Respiratory System (J00-J99)

NOTE When a respiratory condition is described as occurring in more than one site and is not specifically indexed, it should be classified to the lower anatomic site (e.g. tracheobronchitis to bronchitis in J40).

Use additional code, where applicable, to identify:
 exposure to environmental tobacco smoke (Z77.22)
 exposure to tobacco smoke in the perinatal period (P96.81)
 history of tobacco dependence (Z87.891)
 occupational exposure to environmental tobacco smoke (Z57.31)
 tobacco dependence (F17.-)
 tobacco use (Z72.0)

Excludes2: certain conditions originating in the perinatal period (P04-P96)
 certain infectious and parasitic diseases (A00-B99)
 complications of pregnancy, childbirth and the puerperium (O00-O9A)
 congenital malformations, deformations and chromosomal abnormalities (Q00-Q99)
 endocrine, nutritional and metabolic diseases (E00-E88)
 injury, poisoning and certain other consequences of external causes (S00-T88)
 neoplasms (C00-D49)
 smoke inhalation (T59.81-)
 symptoms, signs and abnormal clinical and laboratory findings, not elsewhere classified (R00-R94)

This chapter contains the following category blocks:
 J00-J06 Acute upper respiratory infections
 J09-J18 Influenza and pneumonia
 J20-J22 Other acute lower respiratory infections
 J30-J39 Other diseases of upper respiratory tract
 J40-J4A Chronic lower respiratory diseases
 J60-J70 Lung diseases due to external agents
 J80-J84 Other respiratory diseases principally affecting the interstitium
 J85-J86 Suppurative and necrotic conditions of the lower respiratory tract
 J90-J94 Other diseases of the pleura
 J95   Intraoperative and postprocedural complications and disorders of respiratory system, not elsewhere classified
 J96-J99 Other diseases of the respiratory system

C. Chapter-Specific Coding Guidelines

In addition to general coding guidelines, there are guidelines for specific diagnoses and/or conditions in the classification. Unless otherwise indicated, these guidelines apply to all health care settings. Please refer to Section II for guidelines on the selection of principal diagnosis.

10. Chapter 10: Diseases of the Respiratory System (J00-J99), U07.0

a. Chronic Obstructive Pulmonary Disease [COPD] and Asthma

1) Acute exacerbation of chronic obstructive bronchitis and asthma

The codes in categories J44 and J45 distinguish between uncomplicated cases and those in acute exacerbation. An acute exacerbation is a worsening or a decompensation of a chronic condition. An acute exacerbation is not equivalent to an infection superimposed on a chronic condition, though an exacerbation may be triggered by an infection.

b. Acute Respiratory Failure

1) Acute respiratory failure as principal diagnosis

A code from subcategory J96.0, Acute respiratory failure, or subcategory J96.2, Acute and chronic respiratory failure, may be assigned as a principal diagnosis when it is the condition established after study to be chiefly responsible for occasioning the admission to the hospital, and the selection is supported by the Alphabetic Index and Tabular List. However, chapter-specific coding guidelines (such as obstetrics, poisoning, HIV, newborn) that provide sequencing direction take precedence.

2) Acute respiratory failure as secondary diagnosis

Respiratory failure may be listed as a secondary diagnosis if it occurs after admission, or if it is present on admission, but does not meet the definition of principal diagnosis.

3) Sequencing of acute respiratory failure and another acute condition

When a patient is admitted with respiratory failure and another acute condition, (e.g., myocardial infarction, cerebrovascular accident, aspiration pneumonia), the principal diagnosis will not be the same in every situation. This applies whether the other acute condition is a respiratory or nonrespiratory condition. Selection of the principal diagnosis will be dependent on the circumstances of admission. If both the respiratory failure and the other acute condition are equally responsible for occasioning the admission to the hospital, and there are no chapter-specific sequencing rules, the guideline regarding two or more diagnoses that equally meet the definition for principal diagnosis *(Section II, C.)* may be applied in these situations.

If the documentation is not clear as to whether acute respiratory failure and another condition are equally responsible for occasioning the admission, query the provider for clarification.

c. Influenza due to certain identified influenza viruses

Code only confirmed cases of influenza due to certain identified influenza viruses (category J09), and due to other identified influenza virus (category J10). This is an exception to the hospital inpatient guideline Section II, H. (Uncertain Diagnosis).

In this context, "confirmation" does not require documentation of positive laboratory testing specific for avian or other novel influenza A or other identified influenza virus. However, coding should be based on the provider's diagnostic statement that the patient has avian influenza, or other novel influenza A, for category J09, or has another particular identified strain of influenza, such as H1N1 or H3N2, but not identified as novel or variant, for category J10.

If the provider records "suspected" or "possible" or "probable" avian influenza, or novel influenza, or other identified influenza, then the appropriate influenza code from category J11, Influenza due to unidentified influenza virus, should be assigned. A code from category J09, Influenza due to certain identified influenza viruses, should not be assigned nor should a code from category J10, Influenza due to other identified influenza virus.

d. Ventilator associated Pneumonia

1) Documentation of Ventilator associated Pneumonia

As with all procedural or postprocedural complications, code assignment is based on the provider's documentation of the relationship between the condition and the procedure.

Code J95.851, Ventilator associated pneumonia, should be assigned only when the provider has documented ventilator associated pneumonia (VAP). An additional code to identify the organism (e.g., Pseudomonas aeruginosa, code B96.5) should also be assigned. Do not assign an additional code from categories J12-J18 to identify the type of pneumonia.

Code J95.851 should not be assigned for cases where the patient has pneumonia and is on a mechanical ventilator and the provider has not specifically stated that the pneumonia is ventilator-associated pneumonia. If the documentation is unclear as to whether the patient has a pneumonia that is a complication attributable to the mechanical ventilator, query the provider.

2) Ventilator associated Pneumonia Develops after Admission

A patient may be admitted with one type of pneumonia (e.g., code J13, Pneumonia due to Streptococcus pneumonia) and subsequently develop VAP. In this instance, the principal diagnosis would be the appropriate code from categories J12-J18 for the pneumonia diagnosed at the time of admission. Code J95.851, Ventilator associated pneumonia, would be assigned as an additional diagnosis when the provider has also documented the presence of ventilator associated pneumonia.

e. Vaping-related disorders

For patients presenting with condition(s) related to vaping, assign code U07.0, Vaping-related disorder, as the principal diagnosis. For lung injury due to vaping, assign only code U07.0. Assign additional codes for other manifestations, such as acute respiratory failure (subcategory J96.0-) or pneumonitis (code J68.0)

Associated respiratory signs and symptoms due to vaping, such as cough, shortness of breath, etc., are not coded separately, when a definitive diagnosis has been established. However, it would be appropriate to code separately any gastrointestinal symptoms, such as diarrhea and abdominal pain.

See Section I.C.1.g.1.c.i. for Pneumonia confirmed as due to COVID-19

Acute upper respiratory infections (J00-J06)

Excludes1: chronic obstructive pulmonary disease with acute lower respiratory infection (J44.0)

J00 Acute nasopharyngitis [common cold]

Acute rhinitis
Coryza (acute)
Infective nasopharyngitis NOS
Infective rhinitis
Nasal catarrh, acute
Nasopharyngitis NOS
Excludes1: acute pharyngitis (J02.-)
 acute sore throat NOS (J02.9)
 influenza virus with other respiratory manifestations (J09.X2, J10.1, J11.1)
 pharyngitis NOS (J02.9)
 rhinitis NOS (J31.0)
 sore throat NOS (J02.9)

Nose and Sinuses

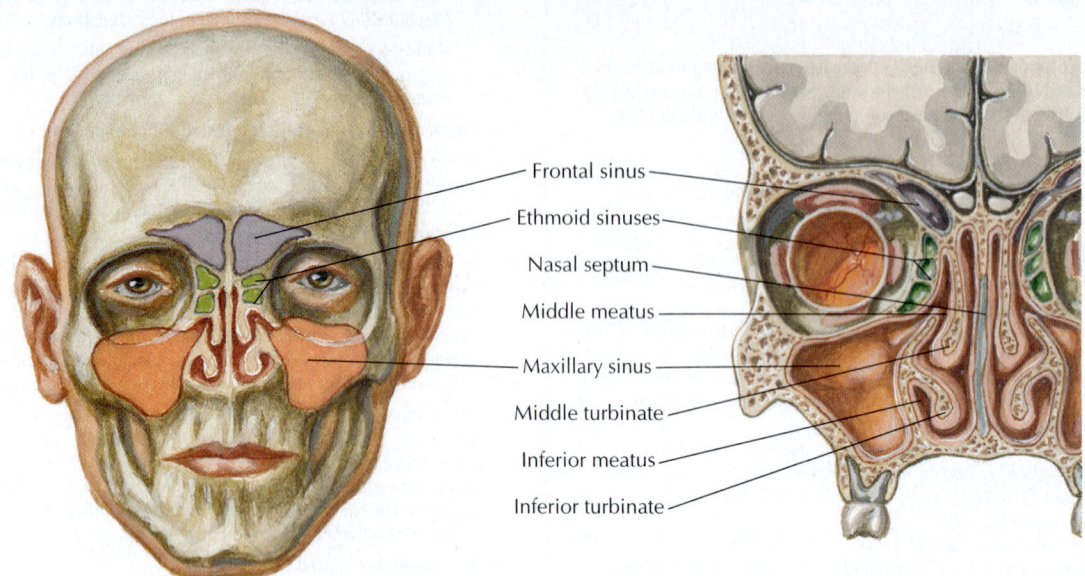

Anatomy of nasal cavity and sinuses

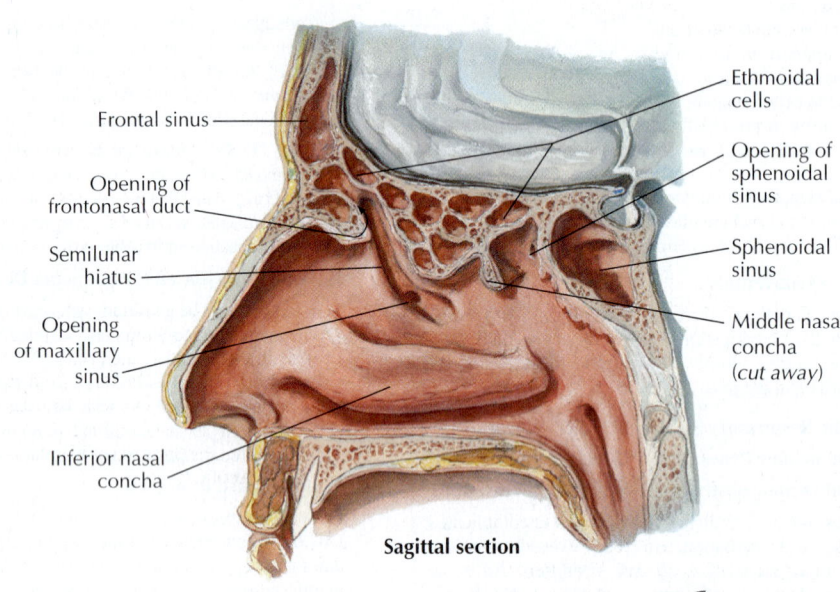

Paranasal sinuses

© Elsevier Inc. All rights reserved. www.netterimages.com

Excludes2: allergic rhinitis (J30.1-J30.9)
chronic pharyngitis (J31.2)
chronic rhinitis (J31.0)
chronic sore throat (J31.2)
nasopharyngitis, chronic (J31.1)
vasomotor rhinitis (J30.0)

Valid 3-character code, no further characters required

J01 Acute sinusitis

  Includes: acute abscess of sinus
  acute empyema of sinus
  acute infection of sinus
  acute inflammation of sinus
  acute suppuration of sinus

  Use additional code (B95-B97) to identify infectious agent
  Excludes1: sinusitis NOS (J32.9)
  Excludes2: chronic sinusitis (J32.0-J32.8)

+ J01.0 Acute maxillary sinusitis
    Acute antritis
    J01.00 Acute maxillary sinusitis, unspecified
    J01.01 Acute recurrent maxillary sinusitis
+ J01.1 Acute frontal sinusitis
    J01.10 Acute frontal sinusitis, unspecified
    J01.11 Acute recurrent frontal sinusitis
+ J01.2 Acute ethmoidal sinusitis
    J01.20 Acute ethmoidal sinusitis, unspecified
    J01.21 Acute recurrent ethmoidal sinusitis
+ J01.3 Acute sphenoidal sinusitis
    J01.30 Acute sphenoidal sinusitis, unspecified
    J01.31 Acute recurrent sphenoidal sinusitis
+ J01.4 Acute pansinusitis
    J01.40 Acute pansinusitis, unspecified
    J01.41 Acute recurrent pansinusitis

+ **J01.8** Other acute sinusitis
    J01.80 Other acute sinusitis
        Acute sinusitis involving more than one sinus but not pansinusitis
    J01.81 Other acute recurrent sinusitis
        Acute recurrent sinusitis involving more than one sinus but not pansinusitis
+ **J01.9** Acute sinusitis, unspecified
    J01.90 Acute sinusitis, unspecified
    J01.91 Acute recurrent sinusitis, unspecified

J02 Acute pharyngitis

Includes: acute sore throat
Excludes1: acute laryngopharyngitis (J06.0)
    peritonsillar abscess (J36)
    pharyngeal abscess (J39.1)
    retropharyngeal abscess (J39.0)
Excludes2: chronic pharyngitis (J31.2)

J02.0 Streptococcal pharyngitis
    Septic pharyngitis
    Streptococcal sore throat
    Excludes2: scarlet fever (A38.-)
J02.8 Acute pharyngitis due to other specified organisms
    Use additional code (B95-B97) to identify infectious agent
    Excludes1: acute pharyngitis due to coxsackie virus (B08.5)
        acute pharyngitis due to gonococcus (A54.5)
        acute pharyngitis due to herpes [simplex] virus (B00.2)
        acute pharyngitis due to infectious mononucleosis (B27.-)
        enteroviral vesicular pharyngitis (B08.5)
J02.9 Acute pharyngitis, unspecified
    Gangrenous pharyngitis (acute)
    Infective pharyngitis (acute) NOS
    Pharyngitis (acute) NOS
    Sore throat (acute) NOS
    Suppurative pharyngitis (acute)
    Ulcerative pharyngitis (acute)
    Excludes1: influenza virus with other respiratory manifestations (J09.X2, J10.1, J11.1)

J03 Acute tonsillitis

Excludes1: acute sore throat (J02.-)
    hypertrophy of tonsils (J35.1)
    peritonsillar abscess (J36)
    sore throat NOS (J02.9)
    streptococcal sore throat (J02.0)
Excludes2: chronic tonsillitis (J35.0)

+ **J03.0** Streptococcal tonsillitis
    J03.00 Acute streptococcal tonsillitis, unspecified
    J03.01 Acute recurrent streptococcal tonsillitis
+ **J03.8** Acute tonsillitis due to other specified organisms
    Use additional code (B95-B97) to identify infectious agent
    Excludes1: diphtheritic tonsillitis (A36.0)
        herpesviral pharyngotonsillitis (B00.2)
        streptococcal tonsillitis (J03.0)
        tuberculous tonsillitis (A15.8)
        Vincent's tonsillitis (A69.1)
    J03.80 Acute tonsillitis due to other specified organisms
    J03.81 Acute recurrent tonsillitis due to other specified organisms
+ **J03.9** Acute tonsillitis, unspecified
    Follicular tonsillitis (acute)
    Gangrenous tonsillitis (acute)
    Infective tonsillitis (acute)
    Tonsillitis (acute) NOS
    Ulcerative tonsillitis (acute)
    Excludes1: influenza virus with other respiratory manifestations (J09.X2, J10.1, J11.1)
    J03.90 Acute tonsillitis, unspecified
    J03.91 Acute recurrent tonsillitis, unspecified

J04 Acute laryngitis and tracheitis

Code also influenza, if present, such as:
    influenza due to identified novel influenza A virus with other respiratory manifestations (J09.X2)
    influenza due to other identified influenza virus with other respiratory manifestations (J10.1)
    influenza due to unidentified influenza virus with other respiratory manifestations (J11.1)
Use additional code (B95-B97) to identify infectious agent

Excludes1: acute obstructive laryngitis [croup] and epiglottitis (J05.-)
Excludes2: laryngismus (stridulus) (J38.5)

J04.0 Acute laryngitis
    Edematous laryngitis (acute)
    Laryngitis (acute) NOS
    Subglottic laryngitis (acute)
    Suppurative laryngitis (acute)
    Ulcerative laryngitis (acute)
    Excludes1: acute obstructive laryngitis (J05.0)
    Excludes2: chronic laryngitis (J37.0)
+ **J04.1** Acute tracheitis
    Acute viral tracheitis
    Catarrhal tracheitis (acute)
    Tracheitis (acute) NOS
    Excludes2: chronic tracheitis (J42)
    J04.10 Acute tracheitis without obstruction
    MCC J04.11 Acute tracheitis with obstruction
J04.2 Acute laryngotracheitis
    Laryngotracheitis NOS
    Tracheitis (acute) with laryngitis (acute)
    Excludes1: acute obstructive laryngotracheitis (J05.0)
    Excludes2: chronic laryngotracheitis (J37.1)
+ **J04.3** Supraglottitis, unspecified
    J04.30 Supraglottitis, unspecified, without obstruction
    MCC J04.31 Supraglottitis, unspecified, with obstruction

J05 Acute obstructive laryngitis [croup] and epiglottitis

Code also, influenza, if present, such as:
    influenza due to identified novel influenza A virus with other respiratory manifestations (J09.X2)
    influenza due to other identified influenza virus with other respiratory manifestations (J10.1)
    influenza due to unidentified influenza virus with other respiratory manifestations (J11.1)
Use additional code (B95-B97) to identify infectious agent

J05.0 Acute obstructive laryngitis [croup]
    Obstructive laryngitis (acute) NOS
    Obstructive laryngotracheitis NOS
+ **J05.1** Acute epiglottitis
    Excludes2: epiglottitis, chronic (J37.0)
    CC J05.10 Acute epiglottitis without obstruction
        Epiglottitis NOS
    MCC J05.11 Acute epiglottitis with obstruction

J06 Acute upper respiratory infections of multiple and unspecified sites

Excludes1: acute respiratory infection NOS (J22)
    influenza virus with other respiratory manifestations (J09.X2, J10.1, J11.1)
    streptococcal pharyngitis (J02.0)

J06.0 Acute laryngopharyngitis
J06.9 Acute upper respiratory infection, unspecified
    Upper respiratory disease, acute
    Upper respiratory infection NOS
    Use additional code (B95-B97) to identify infectious agent, if known, such as:
        respiratory syncytial virus (RSV) (B97.4)

Influenza and pneumonia (J09-J18)

Use Additional code, if applicable, to identify resistance to antimicrobial drugs (Z16.-)

Excludes2: allergic or eosinophilic pneumonia (J82)
    aspiration pneumonia NOS (J69.0)
    meconium pneumonia (P24.01)
    neonatal aspiration pneumonia (P24.-)
    pneumonia due to solids and liquids (J69-)
    congenital pneumonia (P23.9)
    lipid pneumonia (J69.1)
    rheumatic pneumonia (I00)
    ventilator associated pneumonia (J95.851)

J09 Influenza due to certain identified influenza viruses

Excludes1: influenza A/H1N1 (J10.-)
    influenza due to other identified influenza virus (J10.-)
    influenza due to unidentified influenza virus (J11.-)
    seasonal influenza due to other identified influenza virus (J10.-)
    seasonal influenza due to unidentified influenza virus (J11.-)
Review coding guideline C.10.c

+ **J09.X** Influenza due to identified novel influenza A virus
    Avian influenza
    Bird influenza

+, +7th, X + 7th   ● Newborn   ● Pediatric   ● Maternity   ● Adult   ♀ Female   ♂ Male   Manifestation   Unacceptable PDX   HCC   CC   MCC   HAC

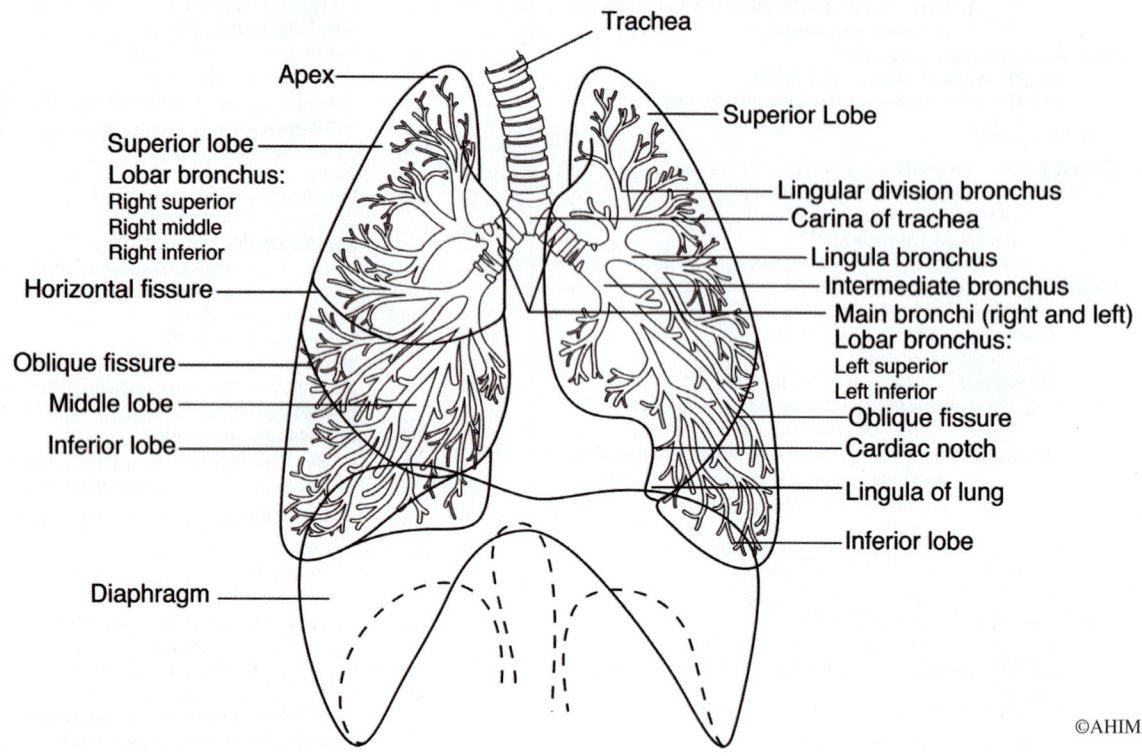

Influenza A/H5N1
Influenza of other animal origin, not bird or swine
Swine influenza virus (viruses that normally cause infections in pigs)

MCC J09.X1 Influenza due to identified novel influenza A virus with pneumonia
Code also if applicable, associated:
lung abscess (J85.1)
other specified type of pneumonia

J09.X2 Influenza due to identified novel influenza A virus with other respiratory manifestations
Influenza due to identified novel influenza A virus NOS
Influenza due to identified novel influenza A virus with laryngitis
Influenza due to identified novel influenza A virus with pharyngitis
Influenza due to identified novel influenza A virus with upper respiratory symptoms
Use additional code, if applicable, for associated:
pleural effusion (J91.8)
sinusitis (J01.-)

J09.X3 Influenza due to identified novel influenza A virus with gastrointestinal manifestations
Influenza due to identified novel influenza A virus gastroenteritis
Excludes1: 'intestinal flu' [viral gastroenteritis] (A08.-)

J09.X9 Influenza due to identified novel influenza A virus with other manifestations
Influenza due to identified novel influenza A virus with encephalopathy
Influenza due to identified novel influenza A virus with myocarditis
Influenza due to identified novel influenza A virus with otitis media
Use additional code to identify manifestation

J10 Influenza due to other identified influenza virus
Includes: influenza A (non-novel)
influenza B
influenza C

Excludes1: influenza due to avian influenza virus (J09.X-)
influenza due to swine flu (J09.X-)
influenza due to unidentifed influenza virus (J11.-)
Review coding guideline C.10.c

+ J10.0 Influenza due to other identified influenza virus with pneumonia
Code also associated lung abscess, if applicable (J85.1)

MCC J10.00 Influenza due to other identified influenza virus with unspecified type of pneumonia

MCC J10.01 Influenza due to other identified influenza virus with the same other identified influenza virus pneumonia

MCC J10.08 Influenza due to other identified influenza virus with other specified pneumonia
Code also other specified type of pneumonia
AHA CC: 4Q, 2017, 96

J10.1 Influenza due to other identified influenza virus with other respiratory manifestations
Influenza due to other identified influenza virus NOS
Influenza due to other identified influenza virus with laryngitis
Influenza due to other identified influenza virus with pharyngitis
Influenza due to other identified influenza virus with upper respiratory symptoms
Use additional code for associated pleural effusion, if applicable (J91.8)
Use additional code for associated sinusitis, if applicable (J01.-)
AHA CC: 3Q, 2016, 10-11

J10.2 Influenza due to other identified influenza virus with gastrointestinal manifestations
Influenza due to other identified influenza virus gastroenteritis
Excludes1: 'intestinal flu' [viral gastroenteritis] (A08.-)

+ J10.8 Influenza due to other identified influenza virus with other manifestations

J10.81 Influenza due to other identified influenza virus with encephalopathy

J10.82 Influenza due to other identified influenza virus with myocarditis

- **J10.83** Influenza due to other identified influenza virus with otitis media
  - *Use additional code for any associated perforated tympanic membrane (H72.-)*
- **J10.89** Influenza due to other identified influenza virus with other manifestations
  - *Use additional codes to identify the manifestations*

J11 Influenza due to unidentified influenza virus

- **+ J11.0** Influenza due to unidentified influenza virus with pneumonia
  - *Code also associated lung abscess, if applicable (J85.1)*
  - **MCC J11.00** Influenza due to unidentified influenza virus with unspecified type of pneumonia
    - Influenza with pneumonia NOS
    - *AHA CC: 3Q, 2016, 11-12*
  - **MCC J11.08** Influenza due to unidentified influenza virus with specified pneumonia
    - *Code also other specified type of pneumonia*
- **J11.1** Influenza due to unidentified influenza virus with other respiratory manifestations
  - Influenza NOS
  - Influenzal laryngitis NOS
  - Influenzal pharyngitis NOS
  - Influenza with upper respiratory symptoms NOS
  - *Use additional code for associated pleural effusion, if applicable (J91.8)*
  - *Use additional code for associated sinusitis, if applicable (J01.-)*
- **J11.2** Influenza due to unidentified influenza virus with gastrointestinal manifestations
  - Influenza gastroenteritis NOS
  - **Excludes1:** *'intestinal flu' [viral gastroenteritis] (A08.-)*
- **+ J11.8** Influenza due to unidentified influenza virus with other manifestations
  - **J11.81** Influenza due to unidentified influenza virus with encephalopathy
    - Influenzal encephalopathy NOS
  - **J11.82** Influenza due to unidentified influenza virus with myocarditis
    - Influenzal myocarditis NOS
  - **J11.83** Influenza due to unidentified influenza virus with otitis media
    - Influenzal otitis media NOS
    - *Use additional code for any associated perforated tympanic membrane (H72.-)*
  - **J11.89** Influenza due to unidentified influenza virus with other manifestations
    - *Use additional codes to identify the manifestations*

J12 Viral pneumonia, not elsewhere classified

Includes: bronchopneumonia due to viruses other than influenza viruses

Code first associated influenza, if applicable (J09.X1, J10.0-, J11.0-)

Code also associated abscess, if applicable (J85.1)

Excludes1: aspiration pneumonia due to anesthesia during labor and delivery (O74.0)
aspiration pneumonia due to anesthesia during pregnancy (O29)
aspiration pneumonia due to anesthesia during puerperium (O89.0)
aspiration pneumonia due to solids and liquids (J69.-)
aspiration pneumonia NOS (J69.0)
congenital pneumonia (P23.0)
congenital rubella pneumonitis (P35.0)
interstitial pneumonia NOS (J84.9)
lipid pneumonia (J69.1)
neonatal aspiration pneumonia (P24.-)

- **MCC J12.0** Adenoviral pneumonia
- **MCC J12.1** Respiratory syncytial virus pneumonia
  - RSV pneumonia
- **MCC J12.2** Parainfluenza virus pneumonia
- **MCC J12.3** Human metapneumovirus pneumonia
- **+ J12.8** Other viral pneumonia
  - **MCC J12.81** Pneumonia due to SARS-associated coronavirus
    - Severe acute respiratory syndrome NOS
  - **MCC J12.82** Pneumonia due to coronavirus disease 2019
    - Pneumonia due to 2019 novel coronavirus (SARS-CoV-2)
    - Pneumonia due to COVID-19
    - *Code first COVID-19 (U07.1)*
    - *AHA CC: 1Q, 2021, 33-34, 41-42, 46-49*
  - **MCC J12.89** Other viral pneumonia
    - *AHA CC: 1Q, 2020, 34-36; 2Q, 2020, 8,11; 1Q, 2021, 33-34*
    - *Review coding guideline C.1.g.1.c.i*
- **MCC J12.9** Viral pneumonia, unspecified

MCC J13 Pneumonia due to Streptococcus pneumoniae

Bronchopneumonia due to S. pneumoniae
Code first associated influenza, if applicable (J09.X1, J10.0-, J11.0-)

Code also associated abscess, if applicable (J85.1)
Excludes1: congenital pneumonia due to S. pneumoniae (P23.6)
lobar pneumonia, unspecified organism (J18.1)
pneumonia due to other streptococci (J15.3-J15.4)
Valid 3-character code, no further characters required

MCC J14 Pneumonia due to Hemophilus influenzae

Bronchopneumonia due to H. influenzae
Code first associated influenza, if applicable (J09.X1, J10.0-, J11.0-)

Code also associated abscess, if applicable (J85.1)
Excludes1: congenital pneumonia due to H. influenzae (P23.6)
Valid 3-character code, no further characters required

J15 Bacterial pneumonia, not elsewhere classified

Includes: bronchopneumonia due to bacteria other than S. pneumoniae and H. influenzae
Code first associated influenza, if applicable (J09.X1, J10.0-, J11.0-)

Code also associated abscess, if applicable (J85.1)
Excludes1: chlamydial pneumonia (J16.0)
congenital pneumonia (P23.-)
Legionnaires' disease (A48.1)
spirochetal pneumonia (A69.8)

- **MCC J15.0** Pneumonia due to Klebsiella pneumoniae
- **MCC J15.1** Pneumonia due to Pseudomonas
- **+ J15.2** Pneumonia due to staphylococcus
  - **MCC J15.20** Pneumonia due to staphylococcus, unspecified
  - **+ J15.21** Pneumonia due to staphylococcus aureus
    - **MCC J15.211** Pneumonia due to Methicillin susceptible Staphylococcus aureus
      - MSSA pneumonia
      - Pneumonia due to Staphylococcus aureus NOS
    - **MCC J15.212** Pneumonia due to Methicillin resistant Staphylococcus aureus
      - *Review coding guideline C.1.e.1.a*
  - **MCC J15.29** Pneumonia due to other staphylococcus
- **MCC J15.3** Pneumonia due to streptococcus, group B
- **MCC J15.4** Pneumonia due to other streptococci
  - **Excludes1:** pneumonia due to streptococcus, group B (J15.3)
    pneumonia due to Streptococcus pneumoniae (J13)
- **MCC J15.5** Pneumonia due to Escherichia coli
- **+ J15.6** Pneumonia due to other Gram-negative bacteria
  - *AHA CC: 2Q, 2020, 29*
  - **MCC J15.61** Pneumonia due to Acinetobacter baumannii
  - **MCC J15.69** Pneumonia due to other Gram-negative bacteria
    - Pneumonia due to other aerobic Gram-negative bacteria
    - Pneumonia due to Serratia marcescens
- **MCC J15.7** Pneumonia due to Mycoplasma pneumoniae
- **MCC J15.8** Pneumonia due to other specified bacteria
- **MCC J15.9** Unspecified bacterial pneumonia
  - Pneumonia due to gram-positive bacteria
  - *AHA CC: 4Q, 2017, 96*

J16 Pneumonia due to other infectious organisms, not elsewhere classified

Code first associated influenza, if applicable (J09.X1, J10.0-, J11.0-)

Code also associated abscess, if applicable (J85.1)
Excludes1: congenital pneumonia (P23.-)
ornithosis (A70)
pneumocystosis (B59)
pneumonia NOS (J18.9)

- **MCC J16.0** Chlamydial pneumonia
- **MCC J16.8** Pneumonia due to other specified infectious organisms

MCC J17 **Pneumonia in diseases classified elsewhere**
Code first underlying disease, such as:
Q fever (A78)
rheumatic fever (I00)
schistosomiasis (B65.0-B65.9)
Excludes1: candidial pneumonia (B37.1)
chlamydial pneumonia (J16.0)
gonorrheal pneumonia (A54.84)
histoplasmosis pneumonia (B39.0-B39.2)
measles pneumonia (B05.2)
nocardiosis pneumonia (A43.0)
pneumocystosis (B59)
pneumonia due to Pneumocystis carinii (B59)
pneumonia due to Pneumocystis jiroveci (B59)
pneumonia in actinomycosis (A42.0)
pneumonia in anthrax (A22.1)
pneumonia in ascariasis (B77.81)
pneumonia in aspergillosis (B44.0-B44.1)
pneumonia in coccidioidomycosis (B38.0-B38.2)
pneumonia in cytomegalovirus disease(B25.0)
pneumonia in toxoplasmosis (B58.3)
rubella pneumonia (B06.81)
salmonella pneumonia (A02.22)
spirochetal infection NEC with pneumonia (A69.8)
tularemia pneumonia (A21.2)
typhoid fever with pneumonia (A01.03)
varicella pneumonia (B01.2)
whooping cough with pneumonia (A37 with fifth-character 1)
Valid 3-character code, no further characters required

J18 **Pneumonia, unspecified organism**
Code first associated influenza, if applicable (J09.X1, J10.0-, J11.0-)
Excludes1: abscess of lung with pneumonia (J85.1)
aspiration pneumonia due to anesthesia during labor and delivery (O74.0)
aspiration pneumonia due to anesthesia during pregnancy (O29)
aspiration pneumonia due to anesthesia during puerperium (O89.0)
aspiration pneumonia due to solids and liquids (J69.-)
aspiration pneumonia NOS (J69.0)
congenital pneumonia (P23.0)
drug-induced interstitial lung disorder (J70.2-J70.4)
interstitial pneumonia NOS (J84.9)
lipid pneumonia (J69.1)
neonatal aspiration pneumonia (P24.-)
pneumonitis due to external agents (J67-J70)
pneumonitis due to fumes and vapors (J68.0)
usual interstitial pneumonia (J84.178)

MCC J18.0 **Bronchopneumonia, unspecified organism**
Excludes1: hypostatic bronchopneumonia (J18.2)
lipid pneumonia (J69.1)
Excludes2: acute bronchiolitis (J21.-)
chronic bronchiolitis (J44.9)
MCC J18.1 **Lobar pneumonia, unspecified organism**
AHA CC: 3Q, 2016, 15
CC J18.2 **Hypostatic pneumonia, unspecified organism**
Hypostatic bronchopneumonia
Passive pneumonia
MCC J18.8 **Other pneumonia, unspecified organism**
MCC J18.9 **Pneumonia, unspecified organism**
AHA CC: 4Q, 2012, 94; 3Q, 2014, 4; 3Q, 2016, 15-16; 1Q, 2019, 35-36; 3Q, 2019, 15; 2Q, 2020, 28

Other acute lower respiratory infections (J20-J22)

Excludes2: chronic obstructive pulmonary disease with acute lower respiratory infection (J44.0)

J20 **Acute bronchitis**
Includes: acute and subacute bronchitis (with) bronchospasm
acute and subacute bronchitis (with) tracheitis
acute and subacute bronchitis (with) tracheobronchitis, acute
acute and subacute fibrinous bronchitis
acute and subacute membranous bronchitis
acute and subacute purulent bronchitis
acute and subacute septic bronchitis
Excludes1: bronchitis NOS (J40)
tracheobronchitis NOS (J40)
Excludes2: acute bronchitis with bronchiectasis (J47.0)
acute bronchitis with chronic obstructive asthma (J44.0)
acute bronchitis with chronic obstructive pulmonary disease (J44.0)
allergic bronchitis NOS (J45.909-)
bronchitis due to chemicals, fumes and vapors (J68.0)
chronic bronchitis NOS (J42)
chronic mucopurulent bronchitis (J41.1)
chronic obstructive bronchitis (J44.-)
chronic obstructive tracheobronchitis (J44.-)
chronic simple bronchitis (J41.0)
chronic tracheobronchitis (J42)
J20.0 **Acute bronchitis due to Mycoplasma pneumoniae**
J20.1 **Acute bronchitis due to Hemophilus influenzae**
J20.2 **Acute bronchitis due to streptococcus**
J20.3 **Acute bronchitis due to coxsackievirus**
J20.4 **Acute bronchitis due to parainfluenza virus**
J20.5 **Acute bronchitis due to respiratory syncytial virus**
Acute bronchitis due to RSV
J20.6 **Acute bronchitis due to rhinovirus**
AHA CC: 3Q, 2016, 10
J20.7 **Acute bronchitis due to echovirus**
J20.8 **Acute bronchitis due to other specified organisms**
AHA CC: 3Q, 2016, 10-11; 1Q, 2020, 34-36; 4Q, 2020, 11-12
Review coding guideline C.1.g.1.c.ii
J20.9 **Acute bronchitis, unspecified**
AHA CC: 3Q, 2016, 16; 1Q, 2019, 35

J21 **Acute bronchiolitis**
Includes: acute bronchiolitis with bronchospasm
Excludes2: respiratory bronchiolitis interstitial lung disease (J84.115)
CC J21.0 **Acute bronchiolitis due to respiratory syncytial virus**
Acute bronchiolitis due to RSV
CC J21.1 **Acute bronchiolitis due to human metapneumovirus**
CC J21.8 **Acute bronchiolitis due to other specified organisms**
CC J21.9 **Acute bronchiolitis, unspecified**
Bronchiolitis (acute)
Excludes1: chronic bronchiolitis (J44.-)

J22 **Unspecified acute lower respiratory infection**
Acute (lower) respiratory (tract) infection NOS
Excludes1: upper respiratory infection (acute) (J06.9)
AHA CC: 1Q, 2020, 22-23, 34-36
Review coding guideline C.1.g.1.c.iii
Valid 3-character code, no further characters required

Other diseases of upper respiratory tract (J30-J39)

J30 **Vasomotor and allergic rhinitis**
Includes: spasmodic rhinorrhea
Excludes1: allergic rhinitis with asthma (bronchial) (J45.909)
rhinitis NOS (J31.0)
J30.0 **Vasomotor rhinitis**
J30.1 **Allergic rhinitis due to pollen**
Allergy NOS due to pollen
Hay fever
Pollinosis
J30.2 **Other seasonal allergic rhinitis**
J30.5 **Allergic rhinitis due to food**
+ **J30.8** **Other allergic rhinitis**
J30.81 **Allergic rhinitis due to animal (cat) (dog) hair and dander**
J30.89 **Other allergic rhinitis**
Perennial allergic rhinitis
J30.9 **Allergic rhinitis, unspecified**

J31 **Chronic rhinitis, nasopharyngitis and pharyngitis**

J31.0 Chronic rhinitis
- Atrophic rhinitis (chronic)
- Granulomatous rhinitis (chronic)
- Hypertrophic rhinitis (chronic)
- Obstructive rhinitis (chronic)
- Ozena
- Purulent rhinitis (chronic)
- Rhinitis (chronic) NOS
- Ulcerative rhinitis (chronic)

Excludes1: allergic rhinitis (J30.1-J30.9)
vasomotor rhinitis (J30.0)

J31.1 Chronic nasopharyngitis
Excludes2: acute nasopharyngitis (J00)

J31.2 Chronic pharyngitis
- Chronic sore throat
- Atrophic pharyngitis (chronic)
- Granular pharyngitis (chronic)
- Hypertrophic pharyngitis (chronic)

Excludes2: acute pharyngitis (J02.9)

J32 Chronic sinusitis

Includes:
- sinus abscess
- sinus empyema
- sinus infection
- sinus suppuration

Use additional code to identify:
infectious agent (B95-B97)

Excludes2: acute sinusitis (J01.-)

J32.0 Chronic maxillary sinusitis
- Antritis (chronic)
- Maxillary sinusitis NOS

J32.1 Chronic frontal sinusitis
- Frontal sinusitis NOS

J32.2 Chronic ethmoidal sinusitis
- Ethmoidal sinusitis NOS

Excludes1: Woakes' ethmoiditis (J33.1)

J32.3 Chronic sphenoidal sinusitis
- Sphenoidal sinusitis NOS

J32.4 Chronic pansinusitis
- Pansinusitis NOS

J32.8 Other chronic sinusitis
- Sinusitis (chronic) involving more than one sinus but not pansinusitis

J32.9 Chronic sinusitis, unspecified
- Sinusitis (chronic) NOS

J33 Nasal polyp

Excludes1: adenomatous polyps (D14.0)

J33.0 Polyp of nasal cavity
- Choanal polyp
- Nasopharyngeal polyp

J33.1 Polypoid sinus degeneration
- Woakes' syndrome or ethmoiditis

J33.8 Other polyp of sinus
- Accessory polyp of sinus
- Ethmoidal polyp of sinus
- Maxillary polyp of sinus
- Sphenoidal polyp of sinus

J33.9 Nasal polyp, unspecified

J34 Other and unspecified disorders of nose and nasal sinuses

Excludes2: varicose ulcer of nasal septum (I86.8)

J34.0 Abscess, furuncle and carbuncle of nose
- Cellulitis of nose
- Necrosis of nose
- Ulceration of nose

J34.1 Cyst and mucocele of nose and nasal sinus

J34.2 Deviated nasal septum
- Deflection or deviation of septum (nasal) (acquired)

Excludes1: congenital deviated nasal septum (Q67.4)

J34.3 Hypertrophy of nasal turbinates

+ **J34.8 Other specified disorders of nose and nasal sinuses**

J34.81 Nasal mucositis (ulcerative)
Code also type of associated therapy, such as:
antineoplastic and immunosuppressive drugs (T45.1X-)
radiological procedure and radiotherapy (Y84.2)

Excludes2: gastrointestinal mucositis (ulcerative) (K92.81)
mucositis (ulcerative) of vagina and vulva (N76.81)
oral mucositis (ulcerative) (K12.3-)

J34.89 Other specified disorders of nose and nasal sinuses
- Perforation of nasal septum NOS
- Rhinolith

J34.9 Unspecified disorder of nose and nasal sinuses

J35 Chronic diseases of tonsils and adenoids

+ **J35.0 Chronic tonsillitis and adenoiditis**

Excludes2: acute tonsillitis (J03.-)

J35.01 Chronic tonsillitis
J35.02 Chronic adenoiditis
J35.03 Chronic tonsillitis and adenoiditis

J35.1 Hypertrophy of tonsils
- Enlargement of tonsils

Excludes1: hypertrophy of tonsils with tonsillitis (J35.0-)

J35.2 Hypertrophy of adenoids
- Enlargement of adenoids

Excludes1: hypertrophy of adenoids with adenoiditis (J35.0-)

J35.3 Hypertrophy of tonsils with hypertrophy of adenoids

Excludes1: hypertrophy of tonsils and adenoids with tonsillitis and adenoiditis (J35.03)

J35.8 Other chronic diseases of tonsils and adenoids
- Adenoid vegetations
- Amygdalolith
- Calculus, tonsil
- Cicatrix of tonsil (and adenoid)
- Tonsillar tag
- Ulcer of tonsil

J35.9 Chronic disease of tonsils and adenoids, unspecified
- Disease (chronic) of tonsils and adenoids NOS

CC J36 Peritonsillar abscess

Includes:
- abscess of tonsil
- peritonsillar cellulitis
- quinsy

Use additional code (B95-B97) to identify infectious agent

Excludes1: acute tonsillitis (J03.-)
chronic tonsillitis (J35.0)
retropharyngeal abscess (J39.0)
tonsillitis NOS (J03.9-)

Valid 3-character code, no further characters required

J37 Chronic laryngitis and laryngotracheitis

Use additional code to identify:
exposure to environmental tobacco smoke (Z77.22)
exposure to tobacco smoke in the perinatal period (P96.81)
history of tobacco dependence (Z87.891)
infectious agent (B95-B97)
occupational exposure to environmental tobacco smoke (Z57.31)
tobacco dependence (F17.-)
tobacco use (Z72.0)

J37.0 Chronic laryngitis
- Catarrhal laryngitis
- Hypertrophic laryngitis
- Sicca laryngitis

Excludes2: acute laryngitis (J04.0)
obstructive (acute) laryngitis (J05.0)

J37.1 Chronic laryngotracheitis
- Laryngitis, chronic, with tracheitis (chronic)
- Tracheitis, chronic, with laryngitis

Excludes1: chronic tracheitis (J42)
Excludes2: acute laryngotracheitis (J04.2)
acute tracheitis (J04.1)

J38 Diseases of vocal cords and larynx, not elsewhere classified

Excludes1: congenital laryngeal stridor (P28.89)
obstructive laryngitis (acute) (J05.0)
postprocedural subglottic stenosis (J95.5)
stridor (R06.1)
ulcerative laryngitis (J04.0)

- **+ J38.0 Paralysis of vocal cords and larynx**
  Laryngoplegia
  Paralysis of glottis
  - **J38.00** Paralysis of vocal cords and larynx, unspecified
  - **J38.01** Paralysis of vocal cords and larynx, unilateral
  - **J38.02** Paralysis of vocal cords and larynx, bilateral
- **J38.1 Polyp of vocal cord and larynx**
  Excludes1: adenomatous polyps (D14.1)
- **J38.2 Nodules of vocal cords**
  Chorditis (fibrinous)(nodosa)(tuberosa)
  Singer's nodes
  Teacher's nodes
- **J38.3 Other diseases of vocal cords**
  Abscess of vocal cords
  Cellulitis of vocal cords
  Granuloma of vocal cords
  Leukokeratosis of vocal cords
  Leukoplakia of vocal cords
- **J38.4 Edema of larynx**
  Edema (of) glottis
  Subglottic edema
  Supraglottic edema
  Excludes1: acute obstructive laryngitis [croup] (J05.0)
  edematous laryngitis (J04.0)
- **J38.5 Laryngeal spasm**
  Laryngismus (stridulus)
- **J38.6 Stenosis of larynx**
- **J38.7 Other diseases of larynx**
  Abscess of larynx
  Cellulitis of larynx
  Disease of larynx NOS
  Necrosis of larynx
  Pachyderma of larynx
  Perichondritis of larynx
  Ulcer of larynx

J39 Other diseases of upper respiratory tract

Excludes1: acute respiratory infection NOS (J22)
acute upper respiratory infection (J06.9)
upper respiratory inflammation due to chemicals, gases, fumes or vapors (J68.2)

- **CC J39.0 Retropharyngeal and parapharyngeal abscess**
  Peripharyngeal abscess
  Excludes1: peritonsillar abscess (J36)
- **CC J39.1 Other abscess of pharynx**
  Cellulitis of pharynx
  Nasopharyngeal abscess
- **J39.2 Other diseases of pharynx**
  Cyst of pharynx
  Edema of pharynx
  Excludes2: chronic pharyngitis (J31.2)
  ulcerative pharyngitis (J02.9)
- **J39.3 Upper respiratory tract hypersensitivity reaction, site unspecified**
  Excludes1: hypersensitivity reaction of upper respiratory tract, such as:
  extrinsic allergic alveolitis (J67.9)
  pneumoconiosis (J60-J67.9)
- **J39.8 Other specified diseases of upper respiratory tract**
  AHA CC: 1Q, 2023, 30
- **J39.9 Disease of upper respiratory tract, unspecified**

Chronic lower respiratory diseases (J40-J4A)

Excludes1: bronchitis due to chemicals, gases, fumes and vapors (J68.0)
Excludes2: cystic fibrosis (E84.-)

J40 Bronchitis, not specified as acute or chronic
Bronchitis NOS
Bronchitis with tracheitis NOS
Catarrhal bronchitis
Tracheobronchitis NOS

Use additional code to identify:
exposure to environmental tobacco smoke (Z77.22)
exposure to tobacco smoke in the perinatal period (P96.81)
history of tobacco dependence (Z87.891)
occupational exposure to environmental tobacco smoke (Z57.31)
tobacco dependence (F17.-)
tobacco use (Z72.0)

Excludes1: allergic bronchitis NOS (J45.909-)
asthmatic bronchitis NOS (J45.9-)
acute bronchitis (J20.-)
bronchitis due to chemicals, gases, fumes and vapors (J68.0)

AHA CC: 1Q, 2020 34-36
Review coding guideline C.1.g.1.c.ii
Valid 3-character code, no further characters required

J41 Simple and mucopurulent chronic bronchitis

Use additional code to identify:
exposure to environmental tobacco smoke (Z77.22)
exposure to tobacco smoke in the perinatal period (P96.81)
history of tobacco dependence (Z87.891)
occupational exposure to environmental tobacco smoke (Z57.31)
tobacco dependence (F17.-)
tobacco use (Z72.0)

Excludes2: chronic bronchitis NOS (J42)
chronic obstructive bronchitis (J44.-)

- **J41.0 Simple chronic bronchitis**
- **J41.1 Mucopurulent chronic bronchitis**
- **J41.8 Mixed simple and mucopurulent chronic bronchitis**

J42 Unspecified chronic bronchitis
Chronic bronchitis NOS
Chronic tracheitis
Chronic tracheobronchitis

Use additional code to identify:
exposure to environmental tobacco smoke (Z77.22)
exposure to tobacco smoke in the perinatal period (P96.81)
history of tobacco dependence (Z87.891)
occupational exposure to environmental tobacco smoke (Z57.31)
tobacco dependence (F17.-)
tobacco use (Z72.0)

Excludes1: bronchiolitis obliterans and bronchiolitis obliterans syndrome (J44.81)
chronic asthmatic bronchitis (J44.-)
chronic bronchitis with airways obstruction (J44.-)
chronic emphysematous bronchitis (J44.-)
chronic obstructive pulmonary disease NOS (J44.9)
simple and mucopurulent chronic bronchitis (J41.-)

Valid 3-character code, no further characters required

J43 Emphysema

Excludes1: compensatory emphysema (J98.3)
emphysema due to inhalation of chemicals, gases, fumes or vapors (J68.4)
interstitial emphysema (J98.2)
mediastinal emphysema (J98.2)
neonatal interstitial emphysema (P25.0)
surgical (subcutaneous) emphysema (T81.82)

Excludes2: emphysema with chronic (obstructive) bronchitis (J44.-)
emphysematous (obstructive) bronchitis (J44.-)
traumatic subcutaneous emphysema (T79.7)

- **J43.0 Unilateral pulmonary emphysema [MacLeod's syndrome]**
  Swyer-James syndrome
  Unilateral emphysema
  Unilateral hyperlucent lung
  Unilateral pulmonary artery functional hypoplasia
  Unilateral transparency of lung
- **J43.1 Panlobular emphysema**
  Panacinar emphysema
- **J43.2 Centrilobular emphysema**
- **J43.8 Other emphysema**
- **J43.9 Emphysema, unspecified**
  Bullous emphysema (lung)(pulmonary)
  Emphysema (lung)(pulmonary) NOS
  Emphysematous bleb
  Vesicular emphysema (lung)(pulmonary)

  AHA CC: 4Q, 2017, 97-98; 1Q, 2019, 34-37

Chronic Obstructive Pulmonary Disease

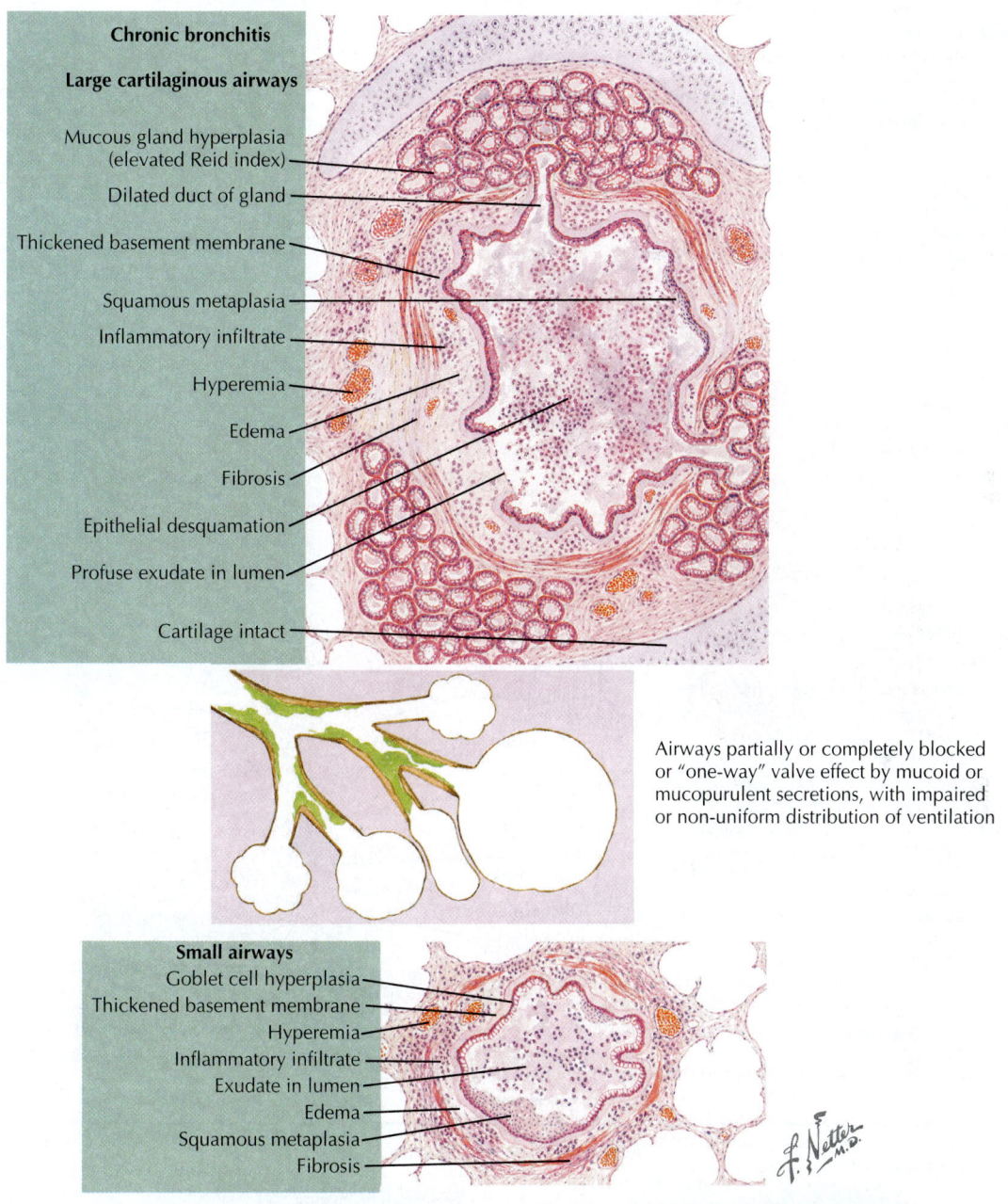

J44 Other chronic obstructive pulmonary disease

Includes: asthma with chronic obstructive pulmonary disease
chronic asthmatic (obstructive) bronchitis
chronic bronchitis with airway obstruction
chronic bronchitis with emphysema
chronic emphysematous bronchitis
chronic obstructive asthma
chronic obstructive bronchitis
chronic obstructive tracheobronchitis

Code also type of asthma, if applicable (J45.-)

Excludes1: chronic bronchitis NOS (J42)
chronic simple and mucopurulent bronchitis (J41.-)
chronic tracheitis (J42)
chronic tracheobronchitis (J42)

Excludes2: bronchiectasis (J47.-)
emphysema without chronic bronchitis (J43.-)

Review coding guideline C.10.a.1

CC J44.0 Chronic obstructive pulmonary disease with (acute) lower respiratory infection
Code also to identify the infection
AHA CC: 3Q, 2016, 15-16; 4Q, 2017, 96

CC J44.1 Chronic obstructive pulmonary disease with (acute) exacerbation
Decompensated COPD
Decompensated COPD with (acute) exacerbation

Excludes2: chronic obstructive pulmonary disease [COPD] with acute bronchitis (J44.0)
lung diseases due to external agents (J60-J70)
AHA CC: 1Q, 2016, 36; 3Q, 2016, 15-16; 1Q, 2017, 26; 4Q, 2017, 96
Code also to identify the infection

+ J44.8 Other specified chronic obstructive pulmonary disease

J44.81 Bronchiolitis obliterans and bronchiolitis obliterans syndrome
Obliterative bronchiolitis
Code first, if applicable:
complication of bone marrow transplant (T86.09)
complication of stem cell transplant (T86.5)
heart-lung transplant rejection (T86.31)
lung transplant rejection (T86.810)
other complications of heart-lung transplant (T86.39)
other complications of lung transplant (T86.818)
Code also, if applicable, associated conditions, such as:
chronic graft-versus-host disease (D89.811)
chronic lung allograft dysfunction (J4A.-)
chronic respiratory conditions due to chemicals, gases, fumes and vapors (J68.4)

J44.89 Other specified chronic obstructive pulmonary disease
Chronic asthmatic (obstructive) bronchitis
Chronic emphysematous bronchitis

Pathology of Asthma

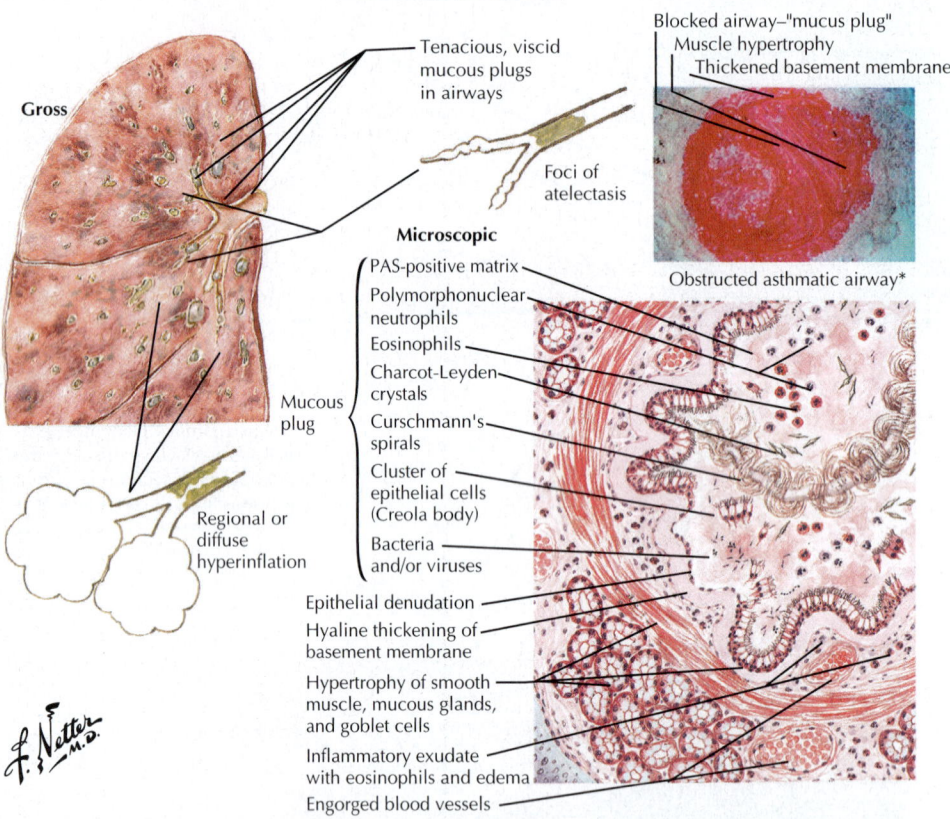

Microscopy of Airway

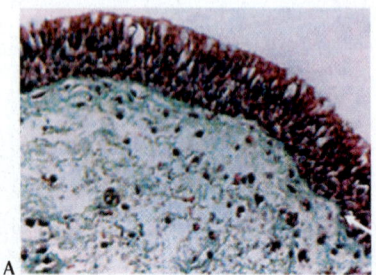
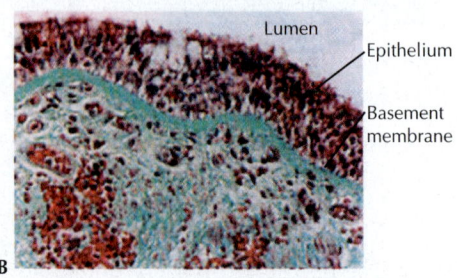

(**A**) Normal airway. (**B**) Asthmatic airway before therapy with high-dose inhaled steroids demonstrating remodeling.

© 2008 Elsevier Inc. All rights reserved. www.netterimages.com

J44.9 Chronic obstructive pulmonary disease, unspecified
Chronic obstructive airway disease NOS
Chronic obstructive lung disease NOS
Excludes2: *lung diseases due to external agents (J60-J70)*
AHA CC: 4Q, 2013, 109, 129; 4Q, 2014, 21-22; 1Q, 2016, 36-37; 1Q, 2017, 24-25; 4Q, 2017, 96-97

J45 Asthma
Includes: allergic (predominantly) asthma
allergic bronchitis NOS
allergic rhinitis with asthma
atopic asthma
extrinsic allergic asthma
hay fever with asthma
idiosyncratic asthma
intrinsic nonallergic asthma
nonallergic asthma
Use additional code to identify:
eosinophilic asthma (J82.83)
exposure to environmental tobacco smoke (Z77.22)
exposure to tobacco smoke in the perinatal period (P96.81)
history of tobacco dependence (Z87.891)
occupational exposure to environmental tobacco smoke (Z57.31)
tobacco dependence (F17.-)
tobacco use (Z72.0)
Excludes1: *detergent asthma (J69.8)*
eosinophilic asthma (J82)
miner's asthma (J60)
wheezing NOS (R06.2)
wood asthma (J67.8)
Excludes2: *asthma with chronic obstructive pulmonary disease (J44.9)*
chronic asthmatic (obstructive) bronchitis (J44.9)
chronic obstructive asthma (J44.9)
AHA CC: 1Q, 2019, 36-37
Review coding guideline C.10.a.1

+ **J45.2 Mild intermittent asthma**
  J45.20 Mild intermittent asthma, uncomplicated
  Mild intermittent asthma NOS
  CC **J45.21** Mild intermittent asthma with (acute) exacerbation
  CC **J45.22** Mild intermittent asthma with status asthmaticus
+ **J45.3 Mild persistent asthma**
  J45.30 Mild persistent asthma, uncomplicated
  Mild persistent asthma NOS
  CC **J45.31** Mild persistent asthma with (acute) exacerbation
  AHA CC: 1Q, 2016, 35
  CC **J45.32** Mild persistent asthma with status asthmaticus
+ **J45.4 Moderate persistent asthma**
  J45.40 Moderate persistent asthma, uncomplicated
  Moderate persistent asthma NOS
  CC **J45.41** Moderate persistent asthma with (acute) exacerbation
  AHA CC: 1Q, 2017, 26
  CC **J45.42** Moderate persistent asthma with status asthmaticus
+ **J45.5 Severe persistent asthma**
  J45.50 Severe persistent asthma, uncomplicated
  Severe persistent asthma NOS
  CC **J45.51** Severe persistent asthma with (acute) exacerbation
  AHA CC: 4Q, 2020, 27
  CC **J45.52** Severe persistent asthma with status asthmaticus
+ **J45.9 Other and unspecified asthma**
  + **J45.90 Unspecified asthma**
    Asthmatic bronchitis NOS
    Childhood asthma NOS
    Late onset asthma
    CC **J45.901** Unspecified asthma with (acute) exacerbation
    AHA CC: 4Q, 2017, 96-97
    CC **J45.902** Unspecified asthma with status asthmaticus
    J45.909 Unspecified asthma, uncomplicated
    Asthma NOS
    Excludes2: *lung diseases due to external agents (J60-J70)*
    AHA CC: 1Q, 2023, 17
  + **J45.99 Other asthma**
    J45.990 Exercise induced bronchospasm
    J45.991 Cough variant asthma
    J45.998 Other asthma

J47 Bronchiectasis
Includes: bronchiolectasis
Use additional code to identify:
exposure to environmental tobacco smoke (Z77.22)
exposure to tobacco smoke in the perinatal period (P96.81)
history of tobacco dependence (Z87.891)
occupational exposure to environmental tobacco smoke (Z57.31)
tobacco dependence (F17.-)
tobacco use (Z72.0)
Excludes1: *congenital bronchiectasis (Q33.4)*
tuberculous bronchiectasis (current disease) (A15.0)
CC **J47.0 Bronchiectasis with acute lower respiratory infection**
Bronchiectasis with acute bronchitis
Code also to identify infection, if applicable
CC **J47.1 Bronchiectasis with (acute) exacerbation**
AHA CC: 1Q, 2021, 23-24
J47.9 Bronchiectasis, uncomplicated
Bronchiectasis NOS

+ **J4A Chronic lung allograft dysfunction**
Code first, if applicable:
heart-lung transplant rejection (T86.31)
lung transplant rejection (T86.810)
other complications of heart-lung transplant (T86.39)
other complications of lung transplant (T86.818)
Code also, if applicable, bronchiolitis obliterans syndrome (J44.81)
J4A.0 Restrictive allograft syndrome
Code also, if applicable, for mixed chronic lung allograft dysfunction, bronchiolitis obliterans syndrome (J44.81)
J4A.8 Other chronic lung allograft dysfunction
J4A.9 Chronic lung allograft dysfunction, unspecified

Lung diseases due to external agents (J60-J70)

Excludes2: *asthma (J45.-)*
malignant neoplasm of bronchus and lung (C34.-)

• **J60 Coalworker's pneumoconiosis**
Anthracosilicosis
Anthracosis
Black lung disease
Coalworker's lung
Excludes1: *coalworker pneumoconiosis with tuberculosis, any type in A15 (J65)*
Valid 3-character code, no further characters required

• **J61 Pneumoconiosis due to asbestos and other mineral fibers**
Asbestosis
Excludes1: *pleural plaque with asbestosis (J92.0)*
pneumoconiosis with tuberculosis, any type in A15 (J65)
Valid 3-character code, no further characters required

J62 Pneumoconiosis due to dust containing silica
Includes: silicotic fibrosis (massive) of lung
Excludes1: *pneumoconiosis with tuberculosis, any type in A15 (J65)*
J62.0 Pneumoconiosis due to talc dust
J62.8 Pneumoconiosis due to other dust containing silica
Silicosis NOS

J63 Pneumoconiosis due to other inorganic dusts
Excludes1: *pneumoconiosis with tuberculosis, any type in A15 (J65)*
J63.0 Aluminosis (of lung)
J63.1 Bauxite fibrosis (of lung)
J63.2 Berylliosis
J63.3 Graphite fibrosis (of lung)
J63.4 Siderosis
J63.5 Stannosis
J63.6 Pneumoconiosis due to other specified inorganic dusts

J64 Unspecified pneumoconiosis
Excludes1: *pneumonoconiosis with tuberculosis, any type in A15 (J65)*
Valid 3-character code, no further characters required

J65 Pneumoconiosis associated with tuberculosis
Any condition in J60-J64 with tuberculosis, any type in A15
Silicotuberculosis
Valid 3-character code, no further characters required

J66 Airway disease due to specific organic dust
Excludes2: *allergic alveolitis (J67.-)*
asbestosis (J61)
bagassosis (J67.1)
farmer's lung (J67.0)
hypersensitivity pneumonitis due to organic dust (J67.-)
reactive airways dysfunction syndrome (J68.3)

J66.0	**Byssinosis**
	Airway disease due to cotton dust
J66.1	**Flax-dressers' disease**
J66.2	**Cannabinosis**
J66.8	**Airway disease due to other specific organic dusts**

J67 Hypersensitivity pneumonitis due to organic dust

    Includes: allergic alveolitis and pneumonitis due to inhaled organic dust and particles of fungal, actinomycetic or other origin

    Excludes1: pneumonitis due to inhalation of chemicals, gases, fumes or vapors (J68.0)

J67.0	**Farmer's lung**
	Harvester's lung
	Haymaker's lung
	Moldy hay disease
J67.1	**Bagassosis**
	Bagasse disease
	Bagasse pneumonitis
J67.2	**Bird fancier's lung**
	Budgerigar fancier's disease or lung
	Pigeon fancier's disease or lung
J67.3	**Suberosis**
	Corkhandler's disease or lung
	Corkworker's disease or lung
J67.4	**Maltworker's lung**
	Alveolitis due to Aspergillus clavatus
J67.5	**Mushroom-worker's lung**
J67.6	**Maple-bark-stripper's lung**
	Alveolitis due to Cryptostroma corticale
	Cryptostromosis
CC **J67.7**	**Air conditioner and humidifier lung**
	Allergic alveolitis due to fungal, thermophilic actinomycetes and other organisms growing in ventilation [air conditioning] systems
CC **J67.8**	**Hypersensitivity pneumonitis due to other organic dusts**
	Cheese-washer's lung
	Coffee-worker's lung
	Fish-meal worker's lung
	Furrier's lung
	Sequoiosis
CC **J67.9**	**Hypersensitivity pneumonitis due to unspecified organic dust**
	Allergic alveolitis (extrinsic) NOS
	Hypersensitivity pneumonitis NOS

J68 Respiratory conditions due to inhalation of chemicals, gases, fumes and vapors

    Code first (T51-T65) to identify cause

    Use additional code to identify associated respiratory conditions, such as: acute respiratory failure (J96.0-)

CC **J68.0**	**Bronchitis and pneumonitis due to chemicals, gases, fumes and vapors**
	Chemical bronchitis (acute)
	AHA CC: 2Q, 2019, 31-32
	Review coding guideline C.11.e
MCC **J68.1**	**Pulmonary edema due to chemicals, gases, fumes and vapors**
	Chemical pulmonary edema (acute) (chronic)
	Excludes1: pulmonary edema (acute) (chronic) NOS (J81.-)
J68.2	**Upper respiratory inflammation due to chemicals, fumes and vapors, not elsewhere classified**
J68.3	**Other acute and subacute respiratory conditions due to chemicals, gases, fumes and vapors**
	Reactive airways dysfunction syndrome
J68.4	**Chronic respiratory conditions due to chemicals, gases, fumes and vapors**
	Code also, if applicable, chronic conditions, such as:
	emphysema (J43.-)
	obliterative bronchiolitis (J44.81)
	pulmonary fibrosis (J84.10)
	Excludes1: chronic pulmonary edema due to chemicals, gases, fumes and vapors (J68.1)
J68.8	**Other respiratory conditions due to chemicals, gases, fumes and vapors**
J68.9	**Unspecified respiratory condition due to chemicals, gases, fumes and vapors**

J69 Pneumonitis due to solids and liquids

    Excludes1: neonatal aspiration syndromes (P24.-)
             postprocedural pneumonitis (J95.4)

    AHA CC: 2Q, 2020, 11, 28-29

MCC **J69.0**	**Pneumonitis due to inhalation of food and vomit**
	Aspiration pneumonia NOS
	Aspiration pneumonia (due to) food (regurgitated)
	Aspiration pneumonia (due to) gastric secretions
	Aspiration pneumonia (due to) milk
	Aspiration pneumonia (due to) vomit
	Code also any associated foreign body in respiratory tract (T17.-)
	Excludes1: chemical pneumonitis due to anesthesia (J95.4)
	obstetric aspiration pneumonitis (O74.0)
	AHA CC: 1Q, 2017, 24; 2Q, 2019, 6-7, 31-32
MCC **J69.1**	**Pneumonitis due to inhalation of oils and essences**
	Exogenous lipoid pneumonia
	Lipid pneumonia NOS
	Code first (T51-T65) to identify substance
	Excludes1: endogenous lipoid pneumonia (J84.89)
MCC **J69.8**	**Pneumonitis due to inhalation of other solids and liquids**
	Pneumonitis due to aspiration of blood
	Pneumonitis due to aspiration of detergent
	Code first (T51-T65) to identify substance

J70 Respiratory conditions due to other external agents

CC **J70.0**	**Acute pulmonary manifestations due to radiation**
	Radiation pneumonitis
	Use additional code (W88-W90, X39.0-) to identify the external cause
CC **J70.1**	**Chronic and other pulmonary manifestations due to radiation**
	Fibrosis of lung following radiation
	Use additional code (W88-W90, X39.0-) to identify the external cause
J70.2	**Acute drug-induced interstitial lung disorders**
	Use additional code for adverse effect, if applicable, to identify drug (T36-T50 with fifth or sixth character 5)
	AHA CC: 2Q, 2019, 28
	Excludes1: interstitial pneumonia NOS (J84.9)
	lymphoid interstitial pneumonia (J84.2)
J70.3	**Chronic drug-induced interstitial lung disorders**
	Use additional code for adverse effect, if applicable, to identify drug (T36-T50 with fifth or sixth character 5)
	Excludes1: interstitial pneumonia NOS (J84.9)
	lymphoid interstitial pneumonia (J84.2)
J70.4	**Drug-induced interstitial lung disorders, unspecified**
	Use additional code for adverse effect, if applicable, to identify drug (T36-T50 with fifth or sixth character 5)
	AHA CC: 2Q, 2019, 28
	Excludes1: interstitial pneumonia NOS (J84.9)
	lymphoid interstitial pneumonia (J84.2)
J70.5	**Respiratory conditions due to smoke inhalation**
	Code first smoke inhalation (T59.81-)
	Excludes2: smoke inhalation due to chemicals, gases, fumes and vapors (J68.9)
J70.8	**Respiratory conditions due to other specified external agents**
	Code first (T51-T65) to identify the external agent
J70.9	**Respiratory conditions due to unspecified external agent**
	Code first (T51-T65) to identify the external agent

Other respiratory diseases principally affecting the interstitium (J80-J84)

MCC J80 Acute respiratory distress syndrome

    Acute respiratory distress syndrome in adult or child
    Adult hyaline membrane disease
    Excludes1: respiratory distress syndrome in newborn (perinatal) (P22.0)
    AHA CC: 1Q, 2017, 26-27; 1Q, 2020, 34-36; 4Q, 2020, 96-97; 2Q, 2021, 23
    Review coding guideline C.1.g.1.c.iv
    Valid 3-character code, no further characters required

J81 Pulmonary edema

    Use additional code to identify:
        exposure to environmental tobacco smoke (Z77.22)
        history of tobacco dependence (Z87.891)
        occupational exposure to environmental tobacco smoke (Z57.31)
        tobacco dependence (F17.-)
        tobacco use (Z72.0)
    Excludes1: chemical (acute) pulmonary edema (J68.1)
              hypostatic pneumonia (J18.2)
              passive pneumonia (J18.2)
              pulmonary edema due to external agents (J60-J70)
              pulmonary edema with heart disease NOS (I50.1)
              pulmonary edema with heart failure (I50.1)

MCC **J81.0** Acute pulmonary edema
　　Acute edema of lung
　　AHA CC: 3Q, 2020, 27; 1Q, 2023, 25-26
CC **J81.1** Chronic pulmonary edema
　　Pulmonary congestion (chronic) (passive)
　　Pulmonary edema NOS

J82 Pulmonary eosinophilia, not elsewhere classified
　　Excludes2: *pulmonary eosinophilia due to aspergillosis (B44.-)*
　　　　pulmonary eosinophilia due to drugs (J70.2-J70.4)
　　　　pulmonary eosinophilia due to specified parasitic infection (B50-B83)
　　　　pulmonary eosinophilia due to systemic connective tissue disorders (M30-M36)
　　　　pulmonary infiltrate NOS (R91.8)
+ J82.8 Pulmonary eosinophilia, not elsewhere classified
　　AHA CC: 4Q, 2020, 25-27
　　CC **J82.81** Chronic eosinophilic pneumonia
　　　　Eosinophilic pneumonia, NOS
　　CC **J82.82** Acute eosinophilic pneumonia
　　CC **J82.83** Eosinophilic asthma
　　　　Code first asthma, by type, such as:
　　　　　mild intermittent asthma (J45.2-)
　　　　　mild persistent asthma (J45.3-)
　　　　　moderate persistent asthma (J45.4-)
　　　　　severe persistent asthma (J45.5-)
　　　　AHA CC: 4Q, 2020, 27
　　CC **J82.89** Other pulmonary eosinophilia, not elsewhere classified
　　　　Allergic pneumonia
　　　　Löffler's pneumonia
　　　　Tropical (pulmonary) eosinophilia NOS

J84 Other interstitial pulmonary diseases
　　Excludes1: *drug-induced interstitial lung disorders (J70.2-J70.4)*
　　　　interstitial emphysema (J98.2)
　　Excludes2: *lung diseases due to external agents (J60-J70)*
+ J84.0 Alveolar and parieto-alveolar conditions
　　CC **J84.01** Alveolar proteinosis
　　CC **J84.02** Pulmonary alveolar microlithiasis
　　CC **J84.03** Idiopathic pulmonary hemosiderosis
　　　　Essential brown induration of lung
　　　　Code first underlying disease, such as:
　　　　　disorders of iron metabolism (E83.1-)
　　　　Excludes1: *acute idiopathic pulmonary hemorrhage in infants [AIPHI] (R04.81)*
　　CC **J84.09** Other alveolar and parieto-alveolar conditions
+ J84.1 Other interstitial pulmonary diseases with fibrosis
　　Excludes1: *pulmonary fibrosis (chronic) due to inhalation of chemicals, gases, fumes or vapors (J68.4)*
　　　　pulmonary fibrosis (chronic) following radiation (J70.1)
　　J84.10 Pulmonary fibrosis, unspecified
　　　　Capillary fibrosis of lung
　　　　Cirrhosis of lung (chronic) NOS
　　　　Fibrosis of lung (atrophic) (chronic) (confluent) (massive) (perialveolar) (peribronchial) NOS
　　　　Induration of lung (chronic) NOS
　　　　Postinflammatory pulmonary fibrosis
　　+ J84.11 Idiopathic interstitial pneumonia
　　　　Excludes1: *lymphoid interstitial pneumonia (J84.2)*
　　　　　pneumocystis pneumonia (B59)
　　　　J84.111 Idiopathic interstitial pneumonia, not otherwise specified
　　　　J84.112 Idiopathic pulmonary fibrosis
　　　　　　Cryptogenic fibrosing alveolitis
　　　　　　Idiopathic fibrosing alveolitis
　　　　J84.113 Idiopathic non-specific interstitial pneumonitis
　　　　　　Excludes1: *non-specific interstitial pneumonia NOS, or due to known underlying cause (J84.89)*
　　　　CC **J84.114** Acute interstitial pneumonitis
　　　　　　Hamman-Rich syndrome
　　　　　　Excludes1: *pneumocystis pneumonia (B59)*
　　　　J84.115 Respiratory bronchiolitis interstitial lung disease
　　　　CC **J84.116** Cryptogenic organizing pneumonia
　　　　　　Excludes1: *organizing pneumonia NOS, or due to known underlying cause (J84.89)*
　　　　CC **J84.117** Desquamative interstitial pneumonia
　　J84.17 Other interstitial pulmonary diseases with fibrosis in diseases classified elsewhere
　　　　AHA CC: 4Q, 2020, 27-28
　　　　J84.170 Interstitial lung disease with progressive fibrotic phenotype in diseases classified elsewhere
　　　　　　Progressive fibrotic interstitial lung disease
　　　　　　Code first underlying disease, such as:
　　　　　　　lung diseases due to external agents (J60-J70)
　　　　　　　rheumatoid arthritis (M05.00-M06.9)
　　　　　　　sarcoidosis (D86.-)
　　　　　　　systemic connective tissue disorders (M30-M36)
　　　　J84.178 Other interstitial pulmonary diseases with fibrosis in diseases classified elsewhere
　　　　　　Interstitial pneumonia (nonspecific) (usual) due to collagen vascular disease
　　　　　　Interstitial pneumonia (nonspecific) (usual) in diseases classified elsewhere
　　　　　　Organizing pneumonia due to collagen vascular disease
　　　　　　Organizing pneumonia in diseases classified elsewhere
　　　　　　Code first underlying diseases, such as:
　　　　　　　progressive systemic sclerosis (M34.0)
　　　　　　　rheumatoid arthritis (M05.00-M06.9)
　　　　　　　systemic lupus erythematosus (M32.0-M32.9)
　　CC **J84.2** Lymphoid interstitial pneumonia
　　　　Lymphoid interstitial pneumonitis
+ J84.8 Other specified interstitial pulmonary diseases
　　Excludes1: *exogenous lipoid pneumonia (J69.1)*
　　　　unspecified lipoid pneumonia (J69.1)
　　MCC **J84.81** Lymphangioleiomyomatosis
　　　　Lymphangiomyomatosis
　　● **CC** **J84.82** Adult pulmonary Langerhans cell histiocytosis
　　　　Adult PLCH
　　MCC **J84.83** Surfactant mutations of the lung
　　+ J84.84 Other interstitial lung diseases of childhood
　　　　MCC **J84.841** Neuroendocrine cell hyperplasia of infancy
　　　　MCC **J84.842** Pulmonary interstitial glycogenosis
　　　　MCC **J84.843** Alveolar capillary dysplasia with vein misalignment
　　　　MCC **J84.848** Other interstitial lung diseases of childhood
　　J84.89 Other specified interstitial pulmonary diseases
　　　　Endogenous lipoid pneumonia
　　　　Interstitial pneumonitis
　　　　Non-specific interstitial pneumonitis NOS
　　　　Organizing pneumonia NOS
　　　　Code first if applicable:
　　　　　poisoning due to drug or toxin (T51-T65 with fifth or sixth character to indicate intent), for toxic pneumonopathy
　　　　　underlying cause of pneumonopathy, if known
　　　　Use additional code, for adverse effect, to identify drug (T36-T50 with fifth or sixth character 5), if drug-induced
　　　　Excludes1: *cryptogenic organizing pneumonia (J84.116)*
　　　　　idiopathic non-specific interstitial pneumonitis (J84.113)
　　　　　lipoid pneumonia, exogenous or unspecified (J69.1)
　　　　　lymphoid interstitial pneumonia (J84.2)
　　　　AHA CC: 2Q, 2019, 28; 1Q, 2021, 48; 4Q, 2021, 106-107
CC **J84.9** Interstitial pulmonary disease, unspecified
　　Interstitial pneumonia NOS

Suppurative and necrotic conditions of the lower respiratory tract (J85-J86)

J85 Abscess of lung and mediastinum
Use additional code (B95-B97) to identify infectious agent
- MCC **J85.0** Gangrene and necrosis of lung
- MCC **J85.1** Abscess of lung with pneumonia
  Code also the type of pneumonia
- MCC **J85.2** Abscess of lung without pneumonia
  Abscess of lung NOS
- MCC **J85.3** Abscess of mediastinum

J86 Pyothorax
Use additional code (B95-B97) to identify infectious agent
Excludes1: abscess of lung (J85.-)
pyothorax due to tuberculosis (A15.6)
- MCC **J86.0** Pyothorax with fistula
  Bronchocutaneous fistula
  Bronchopleural fistula
  Hepatopleural fistula
  Mediastinal fistula
  Pleural fistula
  Thoracic fistula
  Any condition classifiable to J86.9 with fistula
- MCC **J86.9** Pyothorax without fistula
  Abscess of pleura
  Abscess of thorax
  Empyema (chest) (lung) (pleura)
  Fibrinopurulent pleurisy
  Purulent pleurisy
  Pyopneumothorax
  Septic pleurisy
  Seropurulent pleurisy
  Suppurative pleurisy

Other diseases of the pleura (J90-J94)

CC J90 Pleural effusion, not elsewhere classified
Encysted pleurisy
Pleural effusion NOS
Pleurisy with effusion (exudative) (serous)
Excludes1: chylous (pleural) effusion (J94.0)
malignant pleural effusion (J91.0)
pleurisy NOS (R09.1)
tuberculous pleural effusion (A15.6)
Valid 3-character code, no further characters required

J91 Pleural effusion in conditions classified elsewhere
Excludes2: pleural effusion in heart failure (I50.-)
pleural effusion in systemic lupus erythematosus (M32.13)
- CC **J91.0** Malignant pleural effusion
  Code first underlying neoplasm (C00-D49)
  AHA CC: 3Q, 2022, 14-15
- CC **J91.8** Pleural effusion in other conditions classified elsewhere
  Code first underlying disease, such as:
  filariasis (B74.0-B74.9)
  influenza (J09.X2, J10.1, J11.1)
  AHA CC: 2Q, 2015, 15-16

J92 Pleural plaque
Includes: pleural thickening
- **J92.0** Pleural plaque with presence of asbestos
- **J92.9** Pleural plaque without asbestos
  Pleural plaque NOS

J93 Pneumothorax and air leak
Excludes1: congenital or perinatal pneumothorax (P25.1)
postprocedural air leak (J95.812)
postprocedural pneumothorax (J95.811)
traumatic pneumothorax (S27.0)
tuberculous (current disease) pneumothorax (A15.-)
pyopneumothorax (J86.-)
- MCC **J93.0** Spontaneous tension pneumothorax
- + **J93.1** Other spontaneous pneumothorax
  - CC **J93.11** Primary spontaneous pneumothorax
  - CC **J93.12** Secondary spontaneous pneumothorax
    Code first underlying condition, such as:
    catamenial pneumothorax due to endometriosis (N80.B-)
    cystic fibrosis (E84.-)
    eosinophilic pneumonia (J82.81-J82.82)
    lymphangioleiomyomatosis (J84.81)
    malignant neoplasm of bronchus and lung (C34.-)
    Marfan syndrome (Q87.4-)
    pneumonia due to Pneumocystis carinii (B59)
    secondary malignant neoplasm of lung (C78.0-)
    spontaneous rupture of the esophagus (K22.3)
- + **J93.8** Other pneumothorax and air leak
  - CC **J93.81** Chronic pneumothorax
  - CC **J93.82** Other air leak
    Persistent air leak
  - CC **J93.83** Other pneumothorax
    Acute pneumothorax
    Spontaneous pneumothorax NOS
    AHA CC: 3Q, 2020, 9-10
- CC **J93.9** Pneumothorax, unspecified
  Pneumothorax NOS

J94 Other pleural conditions
Excludes1: pleurisy NOS (R09.1)
traumatic hemopneumothorax (S27.2)
traumatic hemothorax (S27.1)
tuberculous pleural conditions (current disease) (A15.-)
- CC **J94.0** Chylous effusion
  Chyliform effusion
- **J94.1** Fibrothorax
- CC **J94.2** Hemothorax
  Hemopneumothorax
- CC **J94.8** Other specified pleural conditions
  Hydropneumothorax
  Hydrothorax
  AHA CC: 1Q, 2021, 48-49
- **J94.9** Pleural condition, unspecified

Intraoperative and postprocedural complications and disorders of respiratory system, not elsewhere classified (J95)

J95 Intraoperative and postprocedural complications and disorders of respiratory system, not elsewhere classified
Excludes2: aspiration pneumonia (J69.-)
emphysema (subcutaneous) resulting from a procedure (T81.82)
hypostatic pneumonia (J18.2)
pulmonary manifestations due to radiation (J70.0-J70.1)
- + **J95.0** Tracheostomy complications
  - CC **J95.00** Unspecified tracheostomy complication
  - CC **J95.01** Hemorrhage from tracheostomy stoma
  - CC **J95.02** Infection of tracheostomy stoma
    Use additional code to identify type of infection, such as:
    cellulitis of neck (L03.221)
    sepsis (A40, A41.-)
  - CC **J95.03** Malfunction of tracheostomy stoma
    Mechanical complication of tracheostomy stoma
    Obstruction of tracheostomy airway
    Tracheal stenosis due to tracheostomy
  - CC **J95.04** Tracheo-esophageal fistula following tracheostomy
  - CC **J95.09** Other tracheostomy complication
- MCC **J95.1** Acute pulmonary insufficiency following thoracic surgery
  Excludes2: Functional disturbances following cardiac surgery (I97.0, I97.1-)

MCC **J95.2** Acute pulmonary insufficiency following nonthoracic surgery
- *Excludes2:* Functional disturbances following cardiac surgery (I97.0, I97.1-)

MCC **J95.3** Chronic pulmonary insufficiency following surgery
- *Excludes2:* Functional disturbances following cardiac surgery (I97.0, I97.1-)

CC **J95.4** Chemical pneumonitis due to anesthesia
- Mendelson's syndrome
- Postprocedural aspiration pneumonia
- Use additional code for adverse effect, if applicable, to identify drug (T41.- with fifth or sixth character 5)
- *Excludes1:* aspiration pneumonitis due to anesthesia complicating labor and delivery (O74.0)
  - aspiration pneumonitis due to anesthesia complicating pregnancy (O29)
  - aspiration pneumonitis due to anesthesia complicating the puerperium (O89.01)

CC **J95.5** Postprocedural subglottic stenosis

+ **J95.6** Intraoperative hemorrhage and hematoma of a respiratory system organ or structure complicating a procedure
- *Excludes1:* intraoperative hemorrhage and hematoma of a respiratory system organ or structure due to accidental puncture and laceration during procedure (J95.7-)

CC **J95.61** Intraoperative hemorrhage and hematoma of a respiratory system organ or structure complicating a respiratory system procedure

CC **J95.62** Intraoperative hemorrhage and hematoma of a respiratory system organ or structure complicating other procedure

+ **J95.7** Accidental puncture and laceration of a respiratory system organ or structure during a procedure
- *Excludes2:* postprocedural pneumothorax (J95.811)

CC **J95.71** Accidental puncture and laceration of a respiratory system organ or structure during a respiratory system procedure

CC **J95.72** Accidental puncture and laceration of a respiratory system organ or structure during other procedure

+ **J95.8** Other intraoperative and postprocedural complications and disorders of respiratory system, not elsewhere classified
- *AHA CC: 4Q, 2016, 9-10*

+ **J95.81** Postprocedural pneumothorax and air leak

CC **J95.811** Postprocedural pneumothorax
- *AHA CC: 1Q, 2021, 48-49*
- **HAC** see Appendix B for HAC conditional logic

CC **J95.812** Postprocedural air leak

+ **J95.82** Postprocedural respiratory failure
- *Excludes1:* Respiratory failure in other conditions (J96.-)

MCC **J95.821** Acute postprocedural respiratory failure
- Postprocedural respiratory failure NOS

MCC **J95.822** Acute and chronic postprocedural respiratory failure

+ **J95.83** Postprocedural hemorrhage of a respiratory system organ or structure following a procedure

CC **J95.830** Postprocedural hemorrhage of a respiratory system organ or structure following a respiratory system procedure

CC **J95.831** Postprocedural hemorrhage of a respiratory system organ or structure following other procedure
- *AHA CC: 2Q, 2023, 28*

CC **J95.84** Transfusion-related acute lung injury (TRALI)

+ **J95.85** Complication of respirator [ventilator]

CC **J95.850** Mechanical complication of respirator
- *Excludes1:* encounter for respirator [ventilator] dependence during power failure (Z99.12)

CC **J95.851** Ventilator associated pneumonia
- Ventilator associated pneumonitis
- Use additional code to identify the organism, if known (B95.-, B96.-, B97.-)
- *Excludes1:* ventilator lung in newborn (P27.8)
- Review coding guideline C.10.d.1
- *AHA CC: 1Q, 2017, 25; 2Q, 2020, 17-18*

CC **J95.859** Other complication of respirator [ventilator]
- *AHA CC: 1Q, 2021, 48-49*

+ **J95.86** Postprocedural hematoma and seroma of a respiratory system organ or structure following a procedure

CC **J95.860** Postprocedural hematoma of a respiratory system organ or structure following a respiratory system procedure

CC **J95.861** Postprocedural hematoma of a respiratory system organ or structure following other procedure

CC **J95.862** Postprocedural seroma of a respiratory system organ or structure following a respiratory system procedure

CC **J95.863** Postprocedural seroma of a respiratory system organ or structure following other procedure

CC **J95.87** Transfusion-associated dyspnea (TAD)
- *Excludes1:* transfusion associated circulatory overload (TACO) (E87.71)
  - transfusion-related acute lung injury (TRALI) (J95.84)
- *AHA CC: 4Q, 2022, 27*

CC **J95.88** Other intraoperative complications of respiratory system, not elsewhere classified

CC **J95.89** Other postprocedural complications and disorders of respiratory system, not elsewhere classified
- Use additional code to identify disorder, such as:
  - aspiration pneumonia (J69.-)
  - bacterial or viral pneumonia (J12-J18)
- *Excludes2:* acute pulmonary insufficiency following thoracic surgery (J95.1)
  - postprocedural subglottic stenosis (J95.5)

Other diseases of the respiratory system (J96-J99)

J96 Respiratory failure, not elsewhere classified
- *Excludes1:* acute respiratory distress syndrome (J80)
  - cardiorespiratory failure (R09.2)
  - newborn respiratory distress syndrome (P22.0)
  - postprocedural respiratory failure (J95.82-)
  - respiratory arrest (R09.2)
  - respiratory arrest of newborn (P28.81)
  - respiratory failure of newborn (P28.5)

+ **J96.0** Acute respiratory failure
- *AHA CC: 1Q, 2021, 34*
- Review coding guideline C.10.b and C.11.e

MCC **J96.00** Acute respiratory failure, unspecified whether with hypoxia or hypercapnia
- *AHA CC: 4Q, 2013, 121; 3Q, 2016, 14*

MCC **J96.01** Acute respiratory failure with hypoxia
- *AHA CC: 3Q, 2020, 12*

MCC **J96.02** Acute respiratory failure with hypercapnia
- Acute respiratory acidosis

+ **J96.1** Chronic respiratory failure

CC **J96.10** Chronic respiratory failure, unspecified whether with hypoxia or hypercapnia
- *AHA CC: 1Q, 2015, 21; 1Q, 2021, 45-46; 4Q, 2021, 105-106*

CC **J96.11** Chronic respiratory failure with hypoxia
- *AHA CC: 4Q, 2013, 129*

CC **J96.12** Chronic respiratory failure with hypercapnia
- Chronic respiratory acidosis

+ **J96.2** Acute and chronic respiratory failure
- Acute on chronic respiratory failure
- Review coding guideline C.10.b

MCC **J96.20** Acute and chronic respiratory failure, unspecified whether with hypoxia or hypercapnia

MCC **J96.21** Acute and chronic respiratory failure with hypoxia

MCC **J96.22** Acute and chronic respiratory failure with hypercapnia

+ **J96.9** Respiratory failure, unspecified

MCC **J96.90** Respiratory failure, unspecified, unspecified whether with hypoxia or hypercapnia

MCC **J96.91** Respiratory failure, unspecified with hypoxia

MCC **J96.92** Respiratory failure, unspecified with hypercapnia

J98 Other respiratory disorders
Use additional code to identify:
exposure to environmental tobacco smoke (Z77.22)
exposure to tobacco smoke in the perinatal period (P96.81)
history of tobacco dependence (Z87.891)
occupational exposure to environmental tobacco smoke (Z57.31)
tobacco dependence (F17.-)
tobacco use (Z72.0)
Excludes1: newborn apnea (P28.4-)
newborn sleep apnea (P28.3-)
Excludes2: apnea NOS (R06.81)
sleep apnea (G47.3-)

+ **J98.0 Diseases of bronchus, not elsewhere classified**
    J98.01 Acute bronchospasm
        Excludes1: acute bronchiolitis with bronchospasm (J21.-)
            acute bronchitis with bronchospasm (J20.-)
            asthma (J45.-)
            exercise induced bronchospasm (J45.990)
    J98.09 Other diseases of bronchus, not elsewhere classified
        Broncholithiasis
        Calcification of bronchus
        Stenosis of bronchus
        Tracheobronchial collapse
        Tracheobronchial dyskinesia
        Ulcer of bronchus
        AHA CC: 3Q, 2022, 8-9

+ **J98.1 Pulmonary collapse**
    Excludes1: therapeutic collapse of lung status (Z98.3)
  CC **J98.11 Atelectasis**
        Excludes1: newborn atelectasis tuberculous atelectasis (current disease) (A15)
  CC **J98.19 Other pulmonary collapse**

J98.2 Interstitial emphysema
    Mediastinal emphysema
    Excludes1: emphysema NOS (J43.9)
        emphysema in newborn (P25.0)
        surgical emphysema (subcutaneous) (T81.82)
        traumatic subcutaneous emphysema (T79.7)

J98.3 Compensatory emphysema

J98.4 Other disorders of lung
    Calcification of lung
    Cystic lung disease (acquired)
    Lung disease NOS
    Pulmolithiasis
    Excludes1: acute interstitial pneumonitis (J84.114)
        pulmonary insufficiency following surgery (J95.1-J95.2)

+ **J98.5 Diseases of mediastinum, not elsewhere classified**
    Excludes2: abscess of mediastinum (J85.3)
    AHA CC: 4Q, 2016, 29
  MCC **J98.51 Mediastinitis**
        Code first underlying condition, if applicable, such as postoperative mediastinitis (T81.-)
  MCC **J98.59 Other diseases of mediastinum, not elsewhere classified**
        Fibrosis of mediastinum
        Hernia of mediastinum
        Retraction of mediastinum

J98.6 Disorders of diaphragm
    Diaphragmatitis
    Paralysis of diaphragm
    Relaxation of diaphragm
    Excludes1: congenital malformation of diaphragm NEC (Q79.1)
        congenital diaphragmatic hernia (Q79.0)
    Excludes2: diaphragmatic hernia (K44.-)

J98.8 Other specified respiratory disorders
    AHA CC: 1Q, 2020, 34-36
    Review coding guideline C.1.g.1.c.iii

J98.9 Respiratory disorder, unspecified
    Respiratory disease (chronic) NOS

J99 Respiratory disorders in diseases classified elsewhere
Code first underlying disease, such as:
    amyloidosis (E85.-)
    ankylosing spondylitis (M45.-)
    congenital syphilis (A50-)
    cryoglobulinemia (D89.1)
    early congenital syphilis (A50.0-)
    plasminogen deficiency (E88.02)
    schistosomiasis (B65.0-B65.9)
Excludes1: respiratory disorders in:
    amebiasis (A06.5)
    blastomycosis (B40.0-B40.2)
    candidiasis (B37.1)
    coccidioidomycosis (B38.0-B38.2)
    cystic fibrosis with pulmonary manifestations (E84.0)
    dermatomyositis (M33.01, M33.11)
    histoplasmosis (B39.0-B39.2)
    late syphilis (A52.72, A52.73)
    polymyositis (M33.21)
    Sjögren syndrome (M35.02)
    systemic lupus erythematosus (M32.13)
    systemic sclerosis (M34.81)
    Wegener's granulomatosis (M31.30-M31.31)
Valid 3-character code, no further characters required

Chapter 11: Diseases of the Digestive System (K00-K95)

Excludes2: certain conditions originating in the perinatal period (P04-P96)
certain infectious and parasitic diseases (A00-B99)
complications of pregnancy, childbirth and the puerperium (O00-O9A)
congenital malformations, deformations and chromosomal abnormalities (Q00-Q99)
endocrine, nutritional and metabolic diseases (E00-E88)
injury, poisoning and certain other consequences of external causes (S00-T88)
neoplasms (C00-D49)
symptoms, signs and abnormal clinical and laboratory findings, not elsewhere classified (R00-R94)

This chapter contains the following category blocks:
- K00-K14 Diseases of oral cavity and salivary glands
- K20-K31 Diseases of esophagus, stomach and duodenum
- K35-K38 Diseases of appendix
- K40-K46 Hernia
- K50-K52 Noninfective enteritis and colitis
- K55-K64 Other diseases of intestines
- K65-K68 Diseases of peritoneum and retroperitoneum
- K70-K77 Diseases of liver
- K80-K87 Disorders of gallbladder, biliary tract and pancreas
- K90-K95 Other diseases of the digestive system

C. Chapter-Specific Coding Guidelines

In addition to general coding guidelines, there are guidelines for specific diagnoses and/or conditions in the classification. Unless otherwise indicated, these guidelines apply to all health care settings. Please refer to Section II for guidelines on the selection of principal diagnosis.

11. Chapter 11: Diseases of the Digestive System (K00-K95)

Reserved for future guideline expansion

Diseases of oral cavity and salivary glands (K00-K14)

K00 Disorders of tooth development and eruption

Excludes2: embedded and impacted teeth (K01.-)

K00.0 Anodontia
Hypodontia
Oligodontia
Excludes1: acquired absence of teeth (K08.1-)

K00.1 Supernumerary teeth
Distomolar
Fourth molar
Mesiodens
Paramolar
Supplementary teeth
Excludes2: supernumerary roots (K00.2)

K00.2 Abnormalities of size and form of teeth
Concrescence of teeth
Fusion of teeth
Gemination of teeth
Dens evaginatus
Dens in dente
Dens invaginatus
Enamel pearls
Macrodontia
Microdontia
Peg-shaped [conical] teeth
Supernumerary roots
Taurodontism
Tuberculum paramolare
Excludes1: abnormalities of teeth due to congenital syphilis (A50.5)
tuberculum Carabelli, which is regarded as a normal variation and should not be coded

K00.3 Mottled teeth
Dental fluorosis
Mottling of enamel
Nonfluoride enamel opacities
Excludes2: deposits [accretions] on teeth (K03.6)

K00.4 Disturbances in tooth formation
Aplasia and hypoplasia of cementum
Dilaceration of tooth
Enamel hypoplasia (neonatal) (postnatal) (prenatal)
Regional odontodysplasia
Turner's tooth
Excludes1: Hutchinson's teeth and mulberry molars in congenital syphilis (A50.5)
Excludes2: mottled teeth (K00.3)

K00.5 Hereditary disturbances in tooth structure, not elsewhere classified
Amelogenesis imperfecta
Dentinogenesis imperfecta
Odontogenesis imperfecta
Dentinal dysplasia
Shell teeth

Oral Cavity

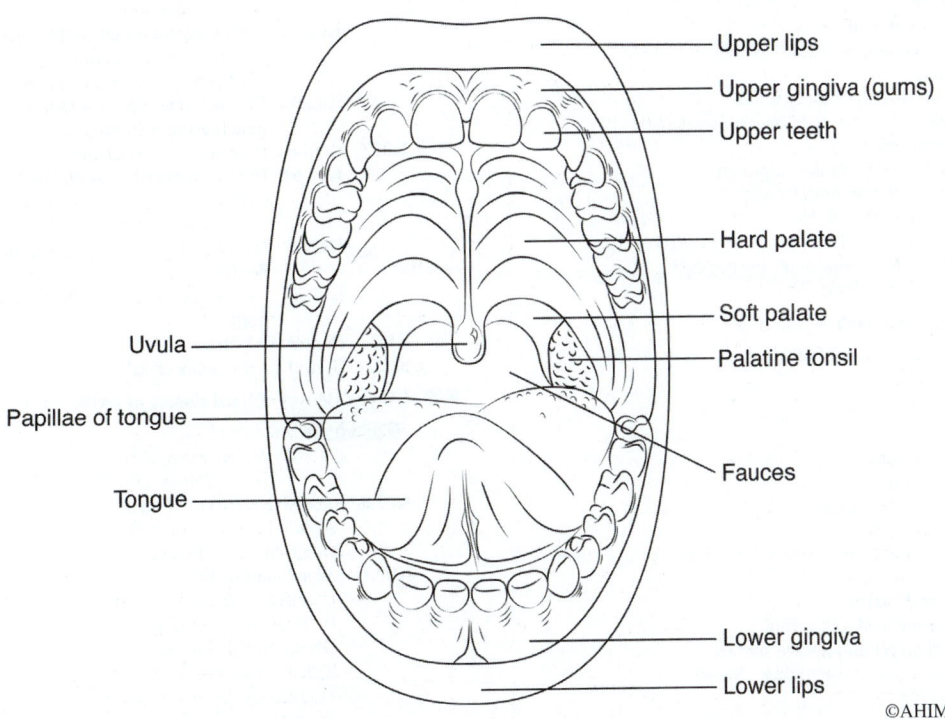

©AHIMA

Glands of the Oral Cavity

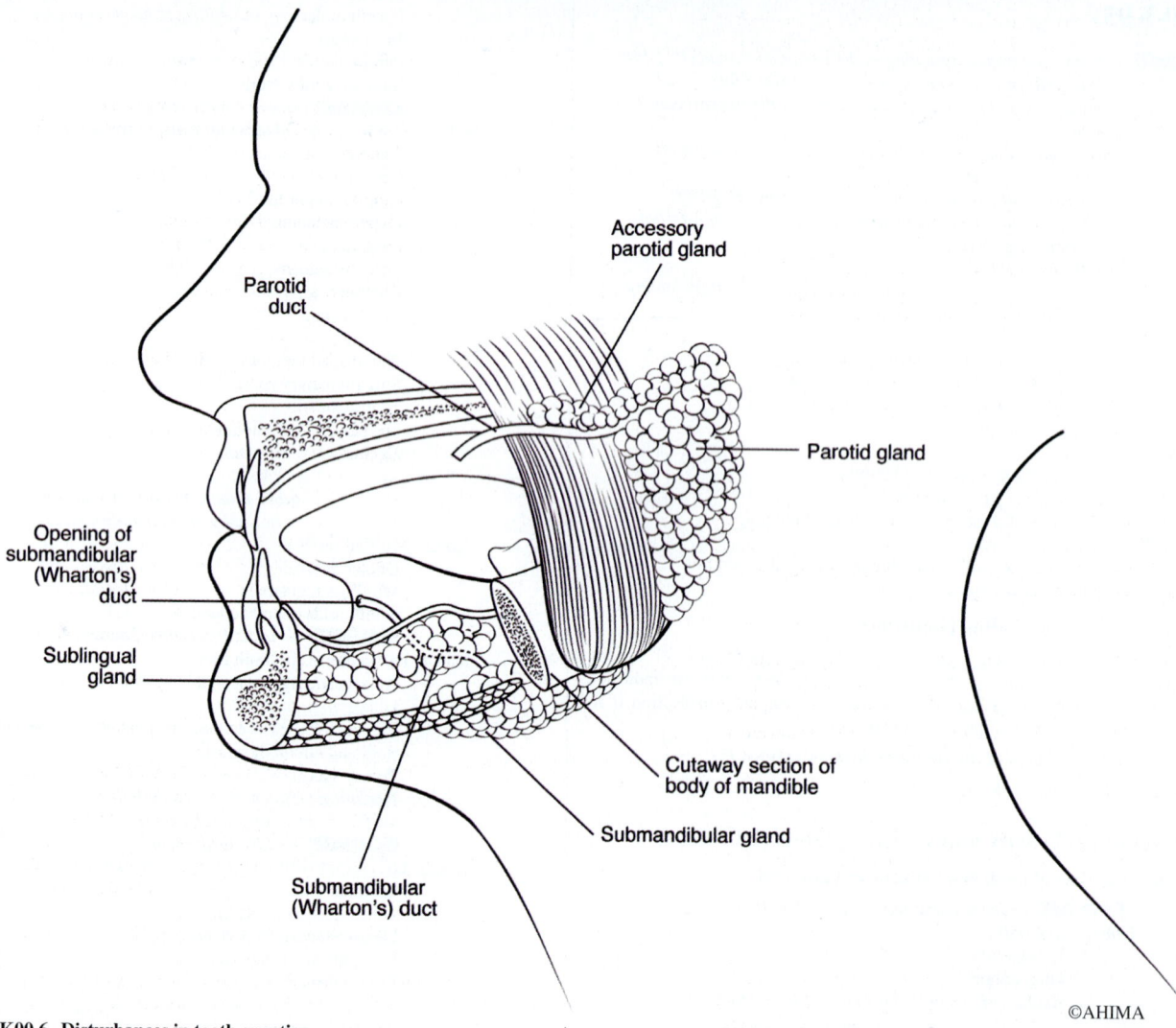

©AHIMA

K00.6 Disturbances in tooth eruption
Dentia praecox
Natal tooth
Neonatal tooth
Premature eruption of tooth
Premature shedding of primary [deciduous] tooth
Prenatal teeth
Retained [persistent] primary tooth
Excludes2: embedded and impacted teeth (K01.-)
K00.7 Teething syndrome
K00.8 Other disorders of tooth development
Color changes during tooth formation
Intrinsic staining of teeth NOS
Excludes2: posteruptive color changes (K03.7)
K00.9 Disorder of tooth development, unspecified
Disorder of odontogenesis NOS

K01 Embedded and impacted teeth
Excludes1: abnormal position of fully erupted teeth (M26.3-)
K01.0 Embedded teeth
K01.1 Impacted teeth

K02 Dental caries
Includes: caries of dentine
dental cavities
early childhood caries
pre-eruptive caries
recurrent caries (dentino enamel junction) (enamel) (to the pulp) tooth decay
K02.3 Arrested dental caries
Arrested coronal and root caries
+ **K02.5** Dental caries on pit and fissure surface
Dental caries on chewing surface of tooth

K02.51 Dental caries on pit and fissure surface limited to enamel
White spot lesions [initial caries] on pit and fissure surface of tooth
K02.52 Dental caries on pit and fissure surface penetrating into dentin
Primary dental caries, cervical origin
K02.53 Dental caries on pit and fissure surface penetrating into pulp
+ **K02.6** Dental caries on smooth surface
K02.61 Dental caries on smooth surface limited to enamel
White spot lesions [initial caries] on smooth surface of tooth
K02.62 Dental caries on smooth surface penetrating into dentin
K02.63 Dental caries on smooth surface penetrating into pulp
K02.7 Dental root caries
K02.9 Dental caries, unspecified

K03 Other diseases of hard tissues of teeth
Excludes2: bruxism (F45.8)
dental caries (K02.-)
teeth-grinding NOS (F45.8)
K03.0 Excessive attrition of teeth
Approximal wear of teeth
Occlusal wear of teeth
K03.1 Abrasion of teeth
Dentifrice abrasion of teeth
Habitual abrasion of teeth
Occupational abrasion of teeth
Ritual abrasion of teeth
Traditional abrasion of teeth
Wedge defect NOS

K03.2 Erosion of teeth
 Erosion of teeth due to diet
 Erosion of teeth due to drugs and medicaments
 Erosion of teeth due to persistent vomiting
 Erosion of teeth NOS
 Idiopathic erosion of teeth
 Occupational erosion of teeth

K03.3 Pathological resorption of teeth
 Internal granuloma of pulp
 Resorption of teeth (external)

K03.4 Hypercementosis
 Cementation hyperplasia

K03.5 Ankylosis of teeth

K03.6 Deposits [accretions] on teeth
 Betel deposits [accretions] on teeth
 Black deposits [accretions] on teeth
 Extrinsic staining of teeth NOS
 Green deposits [accretions] on teeth
 Materia alba deposits [accretions] on teeth
 Orange deposits [accretions] on teeth
 Staining of teeth NOS
 Subgingival dental calculus
 Supragingival dental calculus
 Tobacco deposits [accretions] on teeth

K03.7 Posteruptive color changes of dental hard tissues
 Excludes2: deposits [accretions] on teeth (K03.6)

+ **K03.8** Other specified diseases of hard tissues of teeth
  K03.81 Cracked tooth
   Excludes1: asymptomatic craze lines in enamel - omit code
    broken or fractured tooth due to trauma (S02.5)
  K03.89 Other specified diseases of hard tissues of teeth

K03.9 Disease of hard tissues of teeth, unspecified

K04 Diseases of pulp and periapical tissues
 AHA CC: 4Q, 2016, 29-30

+ **K04.0** Pulpitis
  Acute pulpitis
  Chronic (hyperplastic) (ulcerative) pulpitis
  CC **K04.01** Reversible pulpitis
  CC **K04.02** Irreversible pulpitis

K04.1 Necrosis of pulp
 Pulpal gangrene

K04.2 Pulp degeneration
 Denticles
 Pulpal calcifications
 Pulpal stones

K04.3 Abnormal hard tissue formation in pulp
 Secondary or irregular dentine

CC **K04.4** Acute apical periodontitis of pulpal origin
 Acute apical periodontitis NOS
 Excludes1: acute periodontitis (K05.2-)

K04.5 Chronic apical periodontitis
 Apical or periapical granuloma
 Apical periodontitis NOS
 Excludes1: chronic periodontitis (K05.3-)

K04.6 Periapical abscess with sinus
 Dental abscess with sinus
 Dentoalveolar abscess with sinus

K04.7 Periapical abscess without sinus
 Dental abscess without sinus
 Dentoalveolar abscess without sinus

K04.8 Radicular cyst
 Apical (periodontal) cyst
 Periapical cyst
 Residual radicular cyst
 Excludes2: lateral periodontal cyst (K09.0)

+ **K04.9** Other and unspecified diseases of pulp and periapical tissues
  K04.90 Unspecified diseases of pulp and periapical tissues
  K04.99 Other diseases of pulp and periapical tissues

K05 Gingivitis and periodontal diseases
 Use additional code to identify:
  alcohol abuse and dependence (F10.-)
  exposure to environmental tobacco smoke (Z77.22)
  exposure to tobacco smoke in the perinatal period (P96.81)
  history of tobacco dependence (Z87.891)
  occupational exposure to environmental tobacco smoke (Z57.31)
  tobacco dependence (F17.-)
  tobacco use (Z72.0)
 AHA CC: 4Q, 2016, 29-30

+ **K05.0** Acute gingivitis
  Excludes1: acute necrotizing ulcerative gingivitis (A69.1)
   herpesviral [herpes simplex] gingivostomatitis (B00.2)
  K05.00 Acute gingivitis, plaque induced
   Acute gingivitis NOS
   Plaque induced gingival disease
  K05.01 Acute gingivitis, non-plaque induced

+ **K05.1** Chronic gingivitis
  Desquamative gingivitis (chronic)
  Gingivitis (chronic) NOS
  Hyperplastic gingivitis (chronic)
  Pregnancy associated gingivitis
  Simple marginal gingivitis (chronic)
  Ulcerative gingivitis (chronic)
  Code first, if applicable, diseases of the digestive system complicating pregnancy (O99.61-)
  K05.10 Chronic gingivitis, plaque induced
   Chronic gingivitis NOS
   Gingivitis NOS
  K05.11 Chronic gingivitis, non-plaque induced

+ **K05.2** Aggressive periodontitis
  Acute pericoronitis
  Excludes1: acute apical periodontitis (K04.4)
   periapical abscess (K04.7)
   periapical abscess with sinus (K04.6)
  K05.20 Aggressive periodontitis, unspecified
  + **K05.21** Aggressive periodontitis, localized
   Periodontal abscess
    K05.211 Aggressive periodontitis, localized, slight
    K05.212 Aggressive periodontitis, localized, moderate
    K05.213 Aggressive periodontitis, localized, severe
    K05.219 Aggressive periodontitis, localized, unspecified severity
  + **K05.22** Aggressive periodontitis, generalized
    K05.221 Aggressive periodontitis, generalized, slight
    K05.222 Aggressive periodontitis, generalized, moderate
    K05.223 Aggressive periodontitis, generalized, severe
    K05.229 Aggressive periodontitis, generalized, unspecified severity

+ **K05.3** Chronic periodontitis
  Chronic pericoronitis
  Complex periodontitis
  Periodontitis NOS
  Simplex periodontitis
  Excludes1: chronic apical periodontitis (K04.5)
  K05.30 Chronic periodontitis, unspecified
  + **K05.31** Chronic periodontitis, localized
    K05.311 Chronic periodontitis, localized, slight
    K05.312 Chronic periodontitis, localized, moderate
    K05.313 Chronic periodontitis, localized, severe
    K05.319 Chronic periodontitis, localized, unspecified severity
  + **K05.32** Chronic periodontitis, generalized
    K05.321 Chronic periodontitis, generalized, slight
    K05.322 Chronic periodontitis, generalized, moderate
    K05.323 Chronic periodontitis, generalized, severe
    K05.329 Chronic periodontitis, generalized, unspecified severity

K05.4 Periodontosis
 Juvenile periodontosis

K05.5 Other periodontal diseases
 Combined periodontic-endodontic lesion
 Narrow gingival width (of periodontal soft tissue)
 Excludes2: leukoplakia of gingiva (K13.21)

K05.6 Periodontal disease, unspecified

K06 Other disorders of gingiva and edentulous alveolar ridge

Excludes2: acute gingivitis (K05.0)
atrophy of edentulous alveolar ridge (K08.2)
chronic gingivitis (K05.1)
gingivitis NOS (K05.1)

AHA CC: 4Q, 2016, 29-30

K06.0 Gingival recession
Gingival recession (postinfective) (postprocedural)
AHA CC: 4Q, 2017, 16

- **+ K06.01 Gingival recession, localized**
  - K06.010 Localized gingival recession, unspecified
    - Localized gingival recession, NOS
  - K06.011 Localized gingival recession, minimal
  - K06.012 Localized gingival recession, moderate
  - K06.013 Localized gingival recession, severe
- **+ K06.02 Gingival recession, generalized**
  - K06.020 Generalized gingival recession, unspecified
    - Generalized gingival recession, NOS
  - K06.021 Generalized gingival recession, minimal
  - K06.022 Generalized gingival recession, moderate
  - K06.023 Generalized gingival recession, severe

K06.1 Gingival enlargement
Gingival fibromatosis

K06.2 Gingival and edentulous alveolar ridge lesions associated with trauma
Irritative hyperplasia of edentulous ridge [denture hyperplasia]
Use additional code (Chapter 20) to identify external cause or denture status (Z97.2)

K06.3 Horizontal alveolar bone loss

K06.8 Other specified disorders of gingiva and edentulous alveolar ridge
Fibrous epulis
Flabby alveolar ridge
Giant cell epulis
Peripheral giant cell granuloma of gingiva
Pyogenic granuloma of gingiva
Vertical ridge deficiency
Excludes2: gingival cyst (K09.0)

K06.9 Disorder of gingiva and edentulous alveolar ridge, unspecified

K08 Other disorders of teeth and supporting structures

Excludes2: dentofacial anomalies [including malocclusion] (M26.-)
disorders of jaw (M27.-)

AHA CC: 4Q, 2016, 29-30

K08.0 Exfoliation of teeth due to systemic causes
Code also underlying systemic condition

+ K08.1 Complete loss of teeth
Acquired loss of teeth, complete
Excludes1: congenital absence of teeth (K00.0)
exfoliation of teeth due to systemic causes (K08.0)
partial loss of teeth (K08.4-)

- **+ K08.10 Complete loss of teeth, unspecified cause**
  - K08.101 Complete loss of teeth, unspecified cause, class I
  - K08.102 Complete loss of teeth, unspecified cause, class II
  - K08.103 Complete loss of teeth, unspecified cause, class III
  - K08.104 Complete loss of teeth, unspecified cause, class IV
  - K08.109 Complete loss of teeth, unspecified cause, unspecified class
    - Edentulism NOS
- **+ K08.11 Complete loss of teeth due to trauma**
  - K08.111 Complete loss of teeth due to trauma, class I
  - K08.112 Complete loss of teeth due to trauma, class II
  - K08.113 Complete loss of teeth due to trauma, class III
  - K08.114 Complete loss of teeth due to trauma, class IV
  - K08.119 Complete loss of teeth due to trauma, unspecified class
- **+ K08.12 Complete loss of teeth due to periodontal diseases**
  - K08.121 Complete loss of teeth due to periodontal diseases, class I
  - K08.122 Complete loss of teeth due to periodontal diseases, class II
  - K08.123 Complete loss of teeth due to periodontal diseases, class III
  - K08.124 Complete loss of teeth due to periodontal diseases, class IV
  - K08.129 Complete loss of teeth due to periodontal diseases, unspecified class
- **+ K08.13 Complete loss of teeth due to caries**
  - K08.131 Complete loss of teeth due to caries, class I
  - K08.132 Complete loss of teeth due to caries, class II
  - K08.133 Complete loss of teeth due to caries, class III
  - K08.134 Complete loss of teeth due to caries, class IV
  - K08.139 Complete loss of teeth due to caries, unspecified class
- **+ K08.19 Complete loss of teeth due to other specified cause**
  - K08.191 Complete loss of teeth due to other specified cause, class I
  - K08.192 Complete loss of teeth due to other specified cause, class II
  - K08.193 Complete loss of teeth due to other specified cause, class III
  - K08.194 Complete loss of teeth due to other specified cause, class IV
  - K08.199 Complete loss of teeth due to other specified cause, unspecified class

+ K08.2 Atrophy of edentulous alveolar ridge
- **K08.20 Unspecified atrophy of edentulous alveolar ridge**
  - Atrophy of the mandible NOS
  - Atrophy of the maxilla NOS
- **K08.21 Minimal atrophy of the mandible**
  - Minimal atrophy of the edentulous mandible
- **K08.22 Moderate atrophy of the mandible**
  - Moderate atrophy of the edentulous mandible
- **K08.23 Severe atrophy of the mandible**
  - Severe atrophy of the edentulous mandible
- **K08.24 Minimal atrophy of maxilla**
  - Minimal atrophy of the edentulous maxilla
- **K08.25 Moderate atrophy of the maxilla**
  - Moderate atrophy of the edentulous maxilla
- **K08.26 Severe atrophy of the maxilla**
  - Severe atrophy of the edentulous maxilla

K08.3 Retained dental root

+ K08.4 Partial loss of teeth
Acquired loss of teeth, partial
Excludes1: complete loss of teeth (K08.1-)
congenital absence of teeth (K00.0)
Excludes2: exfoliation of teeth due to systemic causes (K08.0)

- **+ K08.40 Partial loss of teeth, unspecified cause**
  - K08.401 Partial loss of teeth, unspecified cause, class I
  - K08.402 Partial loss of teeth, unspecified cause, class II
  - K08.403 Partial loss of teeth, unspecified cause, class III
  - K08.404 Partial loss of teeth, unspecified cause, class IV
  - K08.409 Partial loss of teeth, unspecified cause, unspecified class
    - Tooth extraction status NOS
- **+ K08.41 Partial loss of teeth due to trauma**
  - K08.411 Partial loss of teeth due to trauma, class I
  - K08.412 Partial loss of teeth due to trauma, class II
  - K08.413 Partial loss of teeth due to trauma, class III
  - K08.414 Partial loss of teeth due to trauma, class IV
  - K08.419 Partial loss of teeth due to trauma, unspecified class

- **+ K08.42** Partial loss of teeth due to periodontal diseases
  - K08.421 Partial loss of teeth due to periodontal diseases, class I
  - K08.422 Partial loss of teeth due to periodontal diseases, class II
  - K08.423 Partial loss of teeth due to periodontal diseases, class III
  - K08.424 Partial loss of teeth due to periodontal diseases, class IV
  - K08.429 Partial loss of teeth due to periodontal diseases, unspecified class
- **+ K08.43** Partial loss of teeth due to caries
  - K08.431 Partial loss of teeth due to caries, class I
  - K08.432 Partial loss of teeth due to caries, class II
  - K08.433 Partial loss of teeth due to caries, class III
  - K08.434 Partial loss of teeth due to caries, class IV
  - K08.439 Partial loss of teeth due to caries, unspecified class
- **+ K08.49** Partial loss of teeth due to other specified cause
  - K08.491 Partial loss of teeth due to other specified cause, class I
  - K08.492 Partial loss of teeth due to other specified cause, class II
  - K08.493 Partial loss of teeth due to other specified cause, class III
  - K08.494 Partial loss of teeth due to other specified cause, class IV
  - K08.499 Partial loss of teeth due to other specified cause, unspecified class
- **+ K08.5** Unsatisfactory restoration of tooth
  - Defective bridge, crown, filling
  - Defective dental restoration
  - **Excludes1:** dental restoration status (Z98.811)
  - **Excludes2:** endosseous dental implant failure (M27.6-)
    unsatisfactory endodontic treatment (M27.5-)
  - K08.50 Unsatisfactory restoration of tooth, unspecified
    - Defective dental restoration NOS
  - K08.51 Open restoration margins of tooth
    - Dental restoration failure of marginal integrity
    - Open margin on tooth restoration
    - Poor gingival margin to tooth restoration
  - K08.52 Unrepairable overhanging of dental restorative materials
    - Overhanging of tooth restoration
  - **+ K08.53** Fractured dental restorative material
    - **Excludes1:** cracked tooth (K03.81)
      traumatic fracture of tooth (S02.5)
    - K08.530 Fractured dental restorative material without loss of material
    - K08.531 Fractured dental restorative material with loss of material
    - K08.539 Fractured dental restorative material, unspecified
  - K08.54 Contour of existing restoration of tooth biologically incompatible with oral health
    - Dental restoration failure of periodontal anatomical integrity
    - Unacceptable contours of existing restoration of tooth
    - Unacceptable morphology of existing restoration of tooth
  - K08.55 Allergy to existing dental restorative material
    - Use additional code to identify the specific type of allergy
  - K08.56 Poor aesthetic of existing restoration of tooth
    - Dental restoration aesthetically inadequate or displeasing
  - K08.59 Other unsatisfactory restoration of tooth
    - Other defective dental restoration
- **+ K08.8** Other specified disorders of teeth and supporting structures
  - K08.81 Primary occlusal trauma
  - K08.82 Secondary occlusal trauma
  - K08.89 Other specified disorders of teeth and supporting structures
    - Enlargement of alveolar ridge NOS
    - Insufficient anatomic crown height
    - Insufficient clinical crown length
    - Irregular alveolar process
    - Toothache NOS
- **K08.9** Disorder of teeth and supporting structures, unspecified

K09 Cysts of oral region, not elsewhere classified
  Includes: lesions showing histological features both of aneurysmal cyst and of another fibro-osseous lesion
  Excludes2: cysts of jaw (M27.0-, M27.4-)
    radicular cyst (K04.8)
- **K09.0** Developmental odontogenic cysts
  - Dentigerous cyst
  - Eruption cyst
  - Follicular cyst
  - Gingival cyst
  - Lateral periodontal cyst
  - Primordial cyst
  - **Excludes2:** keratocysts (D16.4, D16.5)
    odontogenic keratocystic tumors (D16.4, D16.5)
- **K09.1** Developmental (nonodontogenic) cysts of oral region
  - Cyst (of) incisive canal
  - Cyst (of) palatine of papilla
  - Globulomaxillary cyst
  - Median palatal cyst
  - Nasoalveolar cyst
  - Nasolabial cyst
  - Nasopalatine duct cyst
- **K09.8** Other cysts of oral region, not elsewhere classified
  - Dermoid cyst
  - Epidermoid cyst
  - Lymphoepithelial cyst
  - Epstein's pearl
- **K09.9** Cyst of oral region, unspecified

K11 Diseases of salivary glands
  Use additional code to identify:
    alcohol abuse and dependence (F10.-)
    exposure to environmental tobacco smoke (Z77.22)
    exposure to tobacco smoke in the perinatal period (P96.81)
    history of tobacco dependence (Z87.891)
    occupational exposure to environmental tobacco smoke (Z57.31)
    tobacco dependence (F17.-)
    tobacco use (Z72.0)
- **K11.0** Atrophy of salivary gland
- **K11.1** Hypertrophy of salivary gland
- **+ K11.2** Sialoadenitis
  - Parotitis
  - **Excludes1:** epidemic parotitis (B26.-)
    mumps (B26.-)
    uveoparotid fever [Heerfordt] (D86.89)
  - K11.20 Sialoadenitis, unspecified
  - K11.21 Acute sialoadenitis
    - **Excludes1:** acute recurrent sialoadenitis (K11.22)
  - K11.22 Acute recurrent sialoadenitis
  - K11.23 Chronic sialoadenitis
- CC **K11.3** Abscess of salivary gland
- CC **K11.4** Fistula of salivary gland
  - **Excludes1:** congenital fistula of salivary gland (Q38.4)
- **K11.5** Sialolithiasis
  - Calculus of salivary gland or duct
  - Stone of salivary gland or duct
- **K11.6** Mucocele of salivary gland
  - Mucous extravasation cyst of salivary gland
  - Mucous retention cyst of salivary gland
  - Ranula
- **K11.7** Disturbances of salivary secretion
  - Hypoptyalism
  - Ptyalism
  - Xerostomia
  - **Excludes2:** dry mouth NOS (R68.2)
- **K11.8** Other diseases of salivary glands
  - Benign lymphoepithelial lesion of salivary gland
  - Mikulicz' disease
  - Necrotizing sialometaplasia
  - Sialectasia
  - Stenosis of salivary duct
  - Stricture of salivary duct
  - **Excludes1:** Sjögren syndrome (M35.0-)
- **K11.9** Disease of salivary gland, unspecified
  - Sialoadenopathy NOS

K12 Stomatitis and related lesions
Use additional code to identify:
alcohol abuse and dependence (F10.-)
exposure to environmental tobacco smoke (Z77.22)
exposure to tobacco smoke in the perinatal period (P96.81)
history of tobacco dependence (Z87.891)
occupational exposure to environmental tobacco smoke (Z57.31)
tobacco dependence (F17.-)
tobacco use (Z72.0)

Excludes1: cancrum oris (A69.0)
cheilitis (K13.0)
gangrenous stomatitis (A69.0)
herpesviral [herpes simplex] gingivostomatitis (B00.2)
noma (A69.0)

K12.0 Recurrent oral aphthae
Aphthous stomatitis (major) (minor)
Bednar's aphthae
Periadenitis mucosa necrotica recurrens
Recurrent aphthous ulcer
Stomatitis herpetiformis

K12.1 Other forms of stomatitis
Stomatitis NOS
Denture stomatitis
Ulcerative stomatitis
Vesicular stomatitis

Excludes1: acute necrotizing ulcerative stomatitis (A69.1)
Vincent's stomatitis (A69.1)

CC K12.2 Cellulitis and abscess of mouth
Cellulitis of mouth (floor)
Submandibular abscess

Excludes2: abscess of salivary gland (K11.3)
abscess of tongue (K14.0)
periapical abscess (K04.6-K04.7)
periodontal abscess (K05.21)
peritonsillar abscess (J36)

+ K12.3 Oral mucositis (ulcerative)
Mucositis (oral) (oropharyneal)

Excludes2: gastrointestinal mucositis (ulcerative) (K92.81)
mucositis (ulcerative) of vagina and vulva (N76.81)
nasal mucositis (ulcerative) (J34.81)

K12.30 Oral mucositis (ulcerative), unspecified
K12.31 Oral mucositis (ulcerative) due to antineoplastic therapy
Use additional code for adverse effect, if applicable, to identify antineoplastic and immunosuppressive drugs (T45.1X5)

Use additional code for other antineoplastic therapy, such as: radiological procedure and radiotherapy (Y84.2)

K12.32 Oral mucositis (ulcerative) due to other drugs
Use additional code for adverse effect, if applicable, to identify drug (T36-T50 with fifth or sixth character 5)

K12.33 Oral mucositis (ulcerative) due to radiation
Use additional external cause code (W88-W90, X39.0-) to identify cause

K12.39 Other oral mucositis (ulcerative)
Viral oral mucositis (ulcerative)

K13 Other diseases of lip and oral mucosa
Includes: epithelial disturbances of tongue
Use additional code to identify:
alcohol abuse and dependence (F10.-)
exposure to environmental tobacco smoke (Z77.22)
exposure to tobacco smoke in the perinatal period (P96.81)
history of tobacco dependence (Z87.891)
occupational exposure to environmental tobacco smoke (Z57.31)
tobacco dependence (F17.-)
tobacco use (Z72.0)

Excludes2: certain disorders of gingiva and edentulous alveolar ridge (K05-K06)
cysts of oral region (K09.-)
diseases of tongue (K14.-)
stomatitis and related lesions (K12.-)

K13.0 Diseases of lips
Abscess of lips
Angular cheilitis
Cellulitis of lips
Cheilitis NOS
Cheilodynia
Cheilosis
Exfoliative cheilitis
Fistula of lips
Glandular cheilitis
Hypertrophy of lips
Perlèche NEC

Excludes1: ariboflavinosis (E53.0)
cheilitis due to radiation-related disorders (L55-L59)
congenital fistula of lips (Q38.0)
congenital hypertrophy of lips (Q18.6)
Perlèche due to candidiasis (B37.83)
Perlèche due to riboflavin deficiency (E53.0)

K13.1 Cheek and lip biting
+ K13.2 Leukoplakia and other disturbances of oral epithelium, including tongue

Excludes1: carcinoma in situ of oral epithelium (D00.0-)
hairy leukoplakia (K13.3)

K13.21 Leukoplakia of oral mucosa, including tongue
Leukokeratosis of oral mucosa
Leukoplakia of gingiva, lips, tongue

Excludes1: hairy leukoplakia (K13.3)
leukokeratosis nicotina palati (K13.24)

K13.22 Minimal keratinized residual ridge mucosa
Minimal keratinization of alveolar ridge mucosa
K13.23 Excessive keratinized residual ridge mucosa
Excessive keratinization of alveolar ridge mucosa
K13.24 Leukokeratosis nicotina palati
Smoker's palate
K13.29 Other disturbances of oral epithelium, including tongue
Erythroplakia of mouth or tongue
Focal epithelial hyperplasia of mouth or tongue
Leukoedema of mouth or tongue
Other oral epithelium disturbances

K13.3 Hairy leukoplakia
K13.4 Granuloma and granuloma-like lesions of oral mucosa
Eosinophilic granuloma
Granuloma pyogenicum
Verrucous xanthoma
K13.5 Oral submucous fibrosis
Submucous fibrosis of tongue
K13.6 Irritative hyperplasia of oral mucosa
Excludes2: irritative hyperplasia of edentulous ridge [denture hyperplasia] (K06.2)

+ K13.7 Other and unspecified lesions of oral mucosa
K13.70 Unspecified lesions of oral mucosa
K13.79 Other lesions of oral mucosa
Focal oral mucinosis
AHA CC: 2Q, 2022, 7-8

K14 Diseases of tongue
Use additional code to identify:
alcohol abuse and dependence (F10.-)
exposure to environmental tobacco smoke (Z77.22)
history of tobacco dependence (Z87.891)
occupational exposure to environmental tobacco smoke (Z57.31)
tobacco dependence (F17.-)
tobacco use (Z72.0)

Excludes2: erythroplakia (K13.29)
focal epithelial hyperplasia (K13.29)
leukedema of tongue (K13.29)
leukoplakia of tongue (K13.21)
hairy leukoplakia (K13.3)
macroglossia (congenital) (Q38.2)
submucous fibrosis of tongue (K13.5)

K14.0 Glossitis
Abscess of tongue
Ulceration (traumatic) of tongue

Excludes1: atrophic glossitis (K14.4)

K14.1 **Geographic tongue**
Benign migratory glossitis
Glossitis areata exfoliativa
K14.2 **Median rhomboid glossitis**
K14.3 **Hypertrophy of tongue papillae**
Black hairy tongue
Coated tongue
Hypertrophy of foliate papillae
Lingua villosa nigra
K14.4 **Atrophy of tongue papillae**
Atrophic glossitis
K14.5 **Plicated tongue**
Fissured tongue
Furrowed tongue
Scrotal tongue
Excludes1: fissured tongue, congenital (Q38.3)
K14.6 **Glossodynia**
Glossopyrosis
Painful tongue
K14.8 **Other diseases of tongue**
Atrophy of tongue
Crenated tongue
Enlargement of tongue
Glossocele
Glossoptosis
Hypertrophy of tongue
K14.9 **Disease of tongue, unspecified**
Glossopathy NOS

Diseases of esophagus, stomach and duodenum (K20-K31)

Excludes2: hiatus hernia (K44.-)

K20 Esophagitis

Use additional code to identify:
alcohol abuse and dependence (F10.-)
Excludes1: erosion of esophagus (K22.1-)
esophagitis with gastro-esophageal reflux disease (K21.0-)
reflux esophagitis (K21.0-)
ulcerative esophagitis (K22.1-)
Excludes2: eosinophilic gastritis or gastroenteritis (K52.81)

K20.0 **Eosinophilic esophagitis**
AHA CC: 4Q, 2020, 9-10
+ K20.8 **Other esophagitis**
AHA CC: 4Q, 2020, 28-29
K20.80 Other esophagitis without bleeding
Abscess of esophagus
Other esophagitis NOS
MCC K20.81 Other esophagitis with bleeding
+ K20.9 **Esophagitis, unspecified**
AHA CC: 4Q, 2020, 28-29
K20.90 Esophagitis, unspecified without bleeding
Esophagitis NOS
MCC K20.91 Esophagitis, unspecified with bleeding

K21 Gastro-esophageal reflux disease

Excludes1: newborn esophageal reflux (P78.83)
+ K21.0 **Gastro-esophageal reflux disease with esophagitis**
AHA CC: 4Q, 2020, 28-29
K21.00 Gastro-esophageal reflux disease with esophagitis, without bleeding
Reflux esophagitis
MCC K21.01 Gastro-esophageal reflux disease with esophagitis, with bleeding
K21.9 **Gastro-esophageal reflux disease without esophagitis**
Esophageal reflux NOS
CC AHA: 1Q, 2016, 18

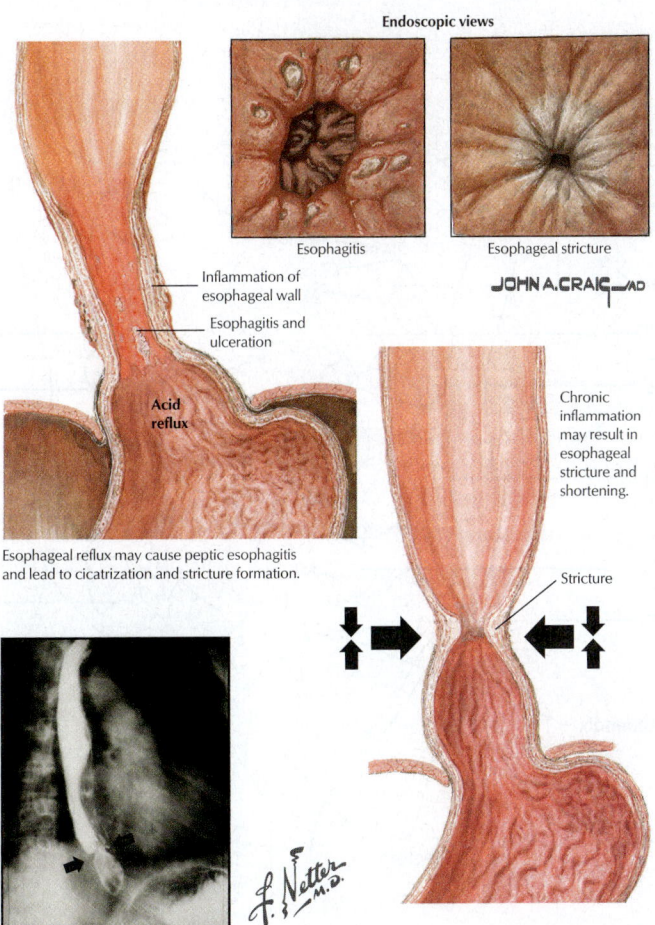

Gastroesophageal Reflux Disease

Endoscopic views

Esophagitis

Esophageal stricture

Inflammation of esophageal wall
Esophagitis and ulceration
Acid reflux

Esophageal reflux may cause peptic esophagitis and lead to cicatrization and stricture formation.

Chronic inflammation may result in esophageal stricture and shortening.

Stricture

Barium study shows esophageal stricture.

© 2005 Elsevier Inc. All rights reserved. www.netterimages.com

Gastrointestinal System Side View

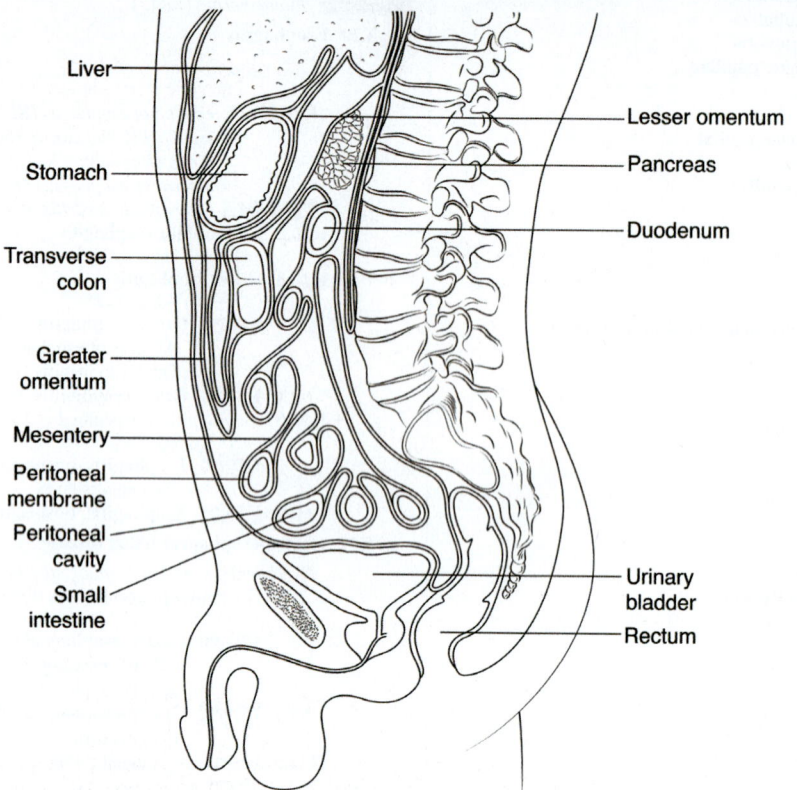

©AHIMA

Gastrointestinal System Front View

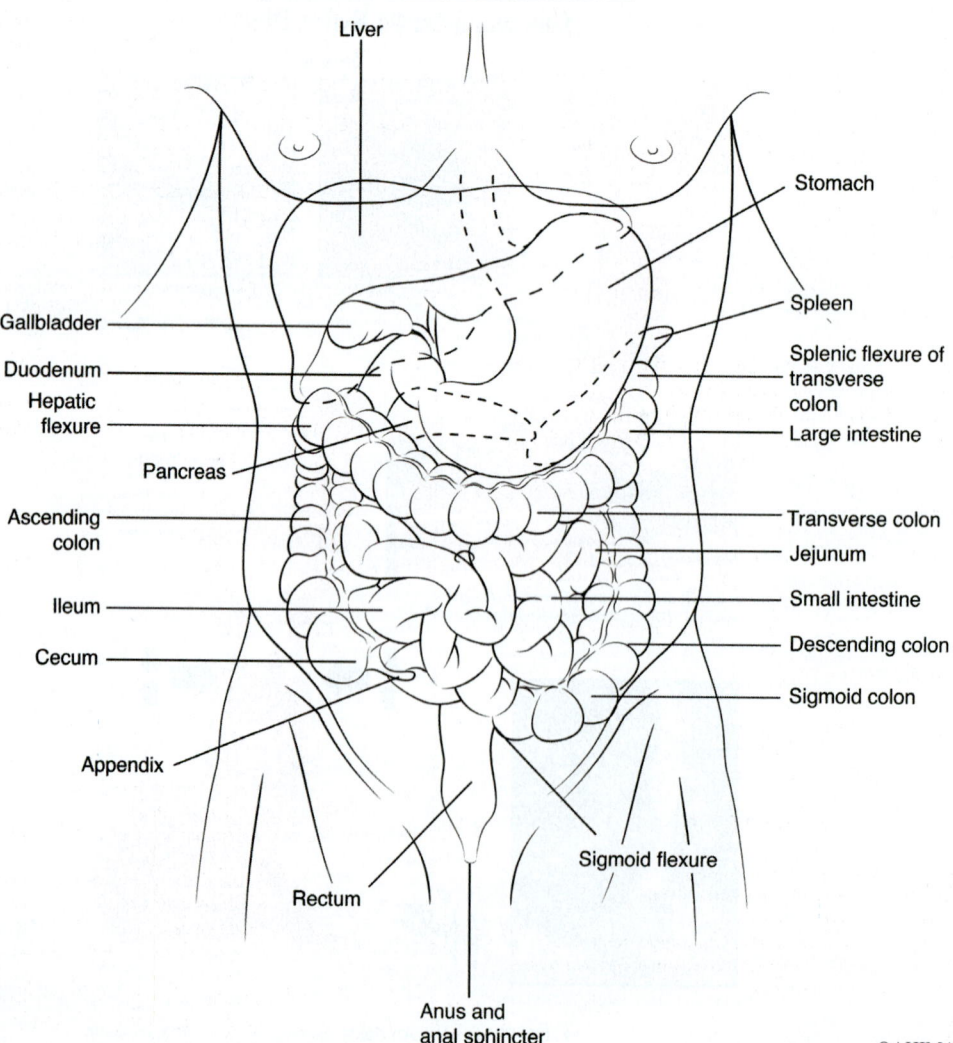

©AHIMA

Upper Gastrointestinal System

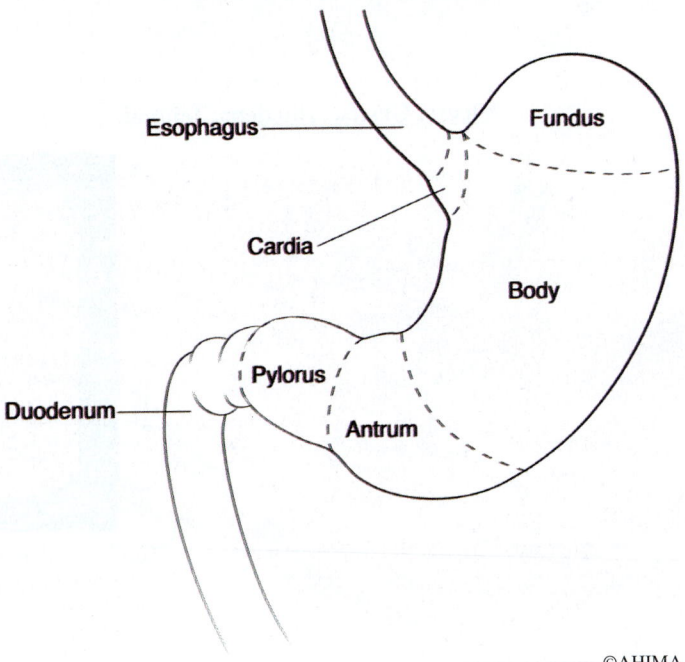

©AHIMA

K22 Other diseases of esophagus
  Excludes2: esophageal varices (I85.-)
  K22.0 Achalasia of cardia
    Achalasia NOS
    Cardiospasm
    Excludes1: congenital cardiospasm (Q39.5)
+ **K22.1 Ulcer of esophagus**
    Barrett's ulcer
    Erosion of esophagus
    Fungal ulcer of esophagus
    Peptic ulcer of esophagus
    Ulcer of esophagus due to ingestion of chemicals
    Ulcer of esophagus due to ingestion of drugs and medicaments
    Ulcerative esophagitis
    Code first poisoning due to drug or toxin, if applicable (T36-T65 with fifth or sixth character 1-4)
    Use additional code for adverse effect, if applicable, to identify drug (T36-T50 with fifth or sixth character 5)
    Excludes1: Barrett's esophagus (K22.7-)
  CC **K22.10 Ulcer of esophagus without bleeding**
    Ulcer of esophagus NOS
  MCC **K22.11 Ulcer of esophagus with bleeding**
    Excludes2: bleeding esophageal varices (I85.01, I85.11)
    AHA CC: 3Q, 2018, 22-23; 1Q, 2023, 20
  K22.2 Esophageal obstruction
    Compression of esophagus
    Constriction of esophagus
    Stenosis of esophagus
    Stricture of esophagus
    Excludes1: congenital stenosis or stricture of esophagus (Q39.3)
  MCC **K22.3 Perforation of esophagus**
    Rupture of esophagus
    Excludes1: traumatic perforation of (thoracic) esophagus (S27.8-)
  K22.4 Dyskinesia of esophagus
    Corkscrew esophagus
    Diffuse esophageal spasm
    Spasm of esophagus
    Excludes1: cardiospasm (K22.0)
  K22.5 Diverticulum of esophagus, acquired
    Esophageal pouch, acquired
    Excludes1: diverticulum of esophagus (congenital) (Q39.6)
  MCC **K22.6 Gastro-esophageal laceration-hemorrhage syndrome**
    Mallory-Weiss syndrome

+ **K22.7 Barrett's esophagus**
    Barrett's disease
    Barrett's syndrome
    Excludes1: Barrett's ulcer (K22.1)
      malignant neoplasm of esophagus (C15.-)
    K22.70 Barrett's esophagus without dysplasia
      Barrett's esophagus NOS
  + **K22.71 Barrett's esophagus with dysplasia**
      K22.710 Barrett's esophagus with low grade dysplasia
      K22.711 Barrett's esophagus with high grade dysplasia
      K22.719 Barrett's esophagus with dysplasia, unspecified
+ **K22.8 Other specified diseases of esophagus**
    Excludes2: esophageal varices (I85.-)
      Paterson-Kelly syndrome (D50.1)
    AHA CC: 1Q, 2020, 16; 4Q, 2021, 15
    K22.81 Esophageal polyp
      Excludes1: benign neoplasm of esophagus (D13.0)
    K22.82 Esophagogastric junction polyp
      Excludes1: benign neoplasm of stomach (D13.1)
    K22.89 Other specified disease of esophagus
      Hemorrhage of esophagus NOS
  K22.9 Disease of esophagus, unspecified
K23 Disorders of esophagus in diseases classified elsewhere
    Code first underlying disease, such as:
      congenital syphilis (A50.5)
    Excludes1: late syphilis (A52.79)
      megaesophagus due to Chagas' disease (B57.31)
      tuberculosis (A18.83)
    Valid 3-character code, no further characters required
K25 Gastric ulcer
    Includes: erosion (acute) of stomach
      pylorus ulcer (peptic)
      stomach ulcer (peptic)
    Use additional code to identify:
      alcohol abuse and dependence (F10.-)
    Excludes1: acute gastritis (K29.0-)
      peptic ulcer NOS (K27.-)
  MCC **K25.0 Acute gastric ulcer with hemorrhage**
    AHA CC: 1Q, 2023, 16
  MCC **K25.1 Acute gastric ulcer with perforation**
  MCC **K25.2 Acute gastric ulcer with both hemorrhage and perforation**
  CC **K25.3 Acute gastric ulcer without hemorrhage or perforation**
  MCC **K25.4 Chronic or unspecified gastric ulcer with hemorrhage**
    AHA CC: 3Q, 2017, 27
  MCC **K25.5 Chronic or unspecified gastric ulcer with perforation**
  MCC **K25.6 Chronic or unspecified gastric ulcer with both hemorrhage and perforation**

Ulcers: Gastric, Duodena, Jejunal

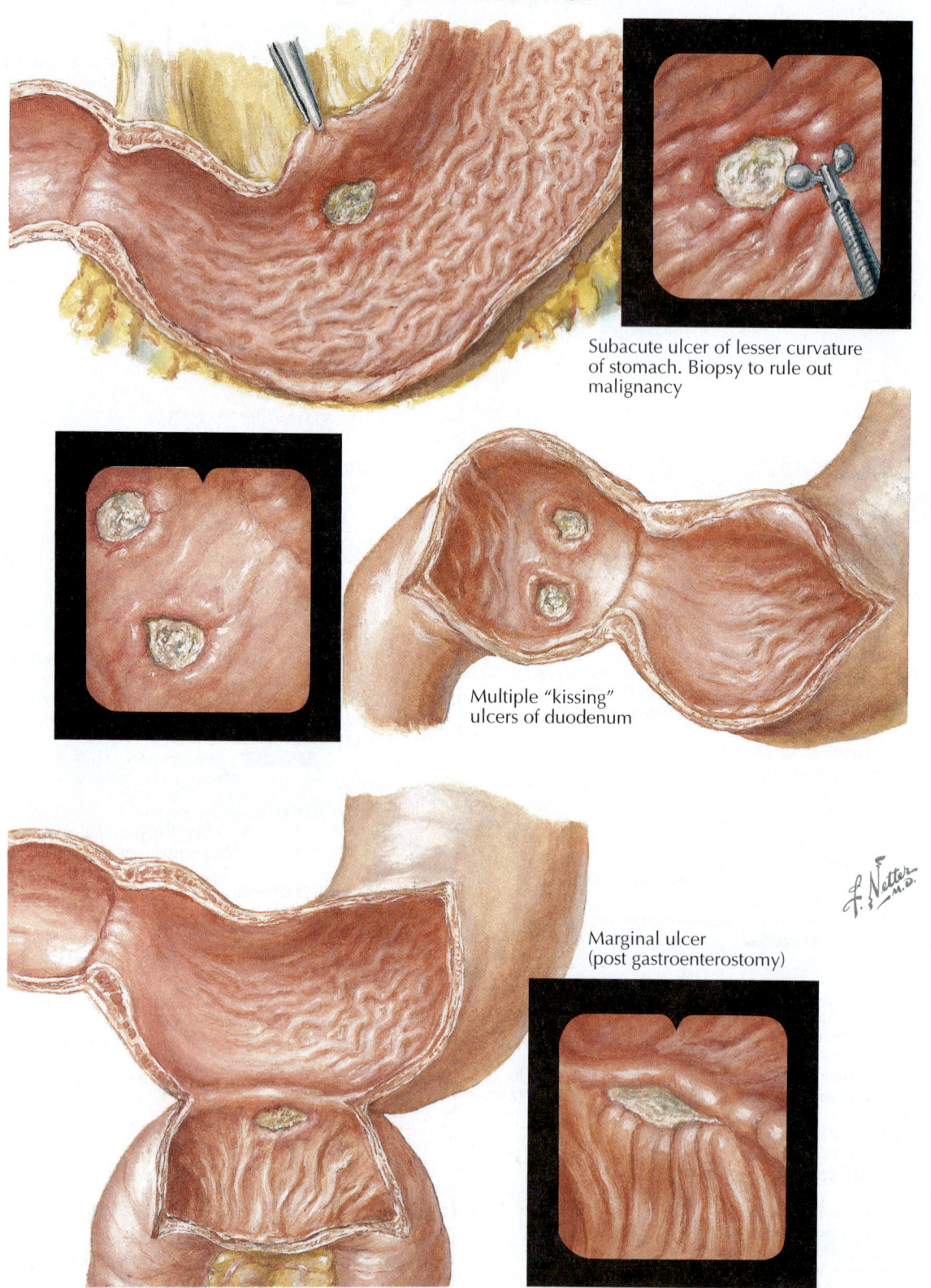

Subacute ulcer of lesser curvature of stomach. Biopsy to rule out malignancy

Multiple "kissing" ulcers of duodenum

Marginal ulcer (post gastroenterostomy)

- K25.7 Chronic gastric ulcer without hemorrhage or perforation
- K25.9 Gastric ulcer, unspecified as acute or chronic, without hemorrhage or perforation
  AHA CC: 1Q, 2021, 11-12

K26 Duodenal ulcer
Includes: erosion (acute) of duodenum
duodenum ulcer (peptic)
postpyloric ulcer (peptic)
Use additional code to identify:
alcohol abuse and dependence (F10.-)
Excludes1: peptic ulcer NOS (K27.-)
- MCC K26.0 Acute duodenal ulcer with hemorrhage
- K26.1 Acute duodenal ulcer with perforation
- K26.2 Acute duodenal ulcer with both hemorrhage and perforation
- CC K26.3 Acute duodenal ulcer without hemorrhage or perforation
- MCC K26.4 Chronic or unspecified duodenal ulcer with hemorrhage
  CC AHA: 1Q, 2016, 14
- MCC K26.5 Chronic or unspecified duodenal ulcer with perforation
- MCC K26.6 Chronic or unspecified duodenal ulcer with both hemorrhage and perforation
- K26.7 Chronic duodenal ulcer without hemorrhage or perforation
  AHA CC: 2Q, 2023, 11
- K26.9 Duodenal ulcer, unspecified as acute or chronic, without hemorrhage or perforation

K27 Peptic ulcer, site unspecified
Includes: gastroduodenal ulcer NOS
peptic ulcer NOS
Use additional code to identify:
alcohol abuse and dependence (F10.-)
Excludes1: peptic ulcer of newborn (P78.82)
- MCC K27.0 Acute peptic ulcer, site unspecified, with hemorrhage
- MCC K27.1 Acute peptic ulcer, site unspecified, with perforation
- K27.2 Acute peptic ulcer, site unspecified, with both hemorrhage and perforation
- CC K27.3 Acute peptic ulcer, site unspecified, without hemorrhage or perforation
- MCC K27.4 Chronic or unspecified peptic ulcer, site unspecified, with hemorrhage
- MCC K27.5 Chronic or unspecified peptic ulcer, site unspecified, with perforation
- MCC K27.6 Chronic or unspecified peptic ulcer, site unspecified, with both hemorrhage and perforation
- K27.7 Chronic peptic ulcer, site unspecified, without hemorrhage or perforation
- K27.9 Peptic ulcer, site unspecified, unspecified as acute or chronic, without hemorrhage or perforation

K28 Gastrojejunal ulcer
Includes: anastomotic ulcer (peptic) or erosion
gastrocolic ulcer (peptic) or erosion
gastrointestinal ulcer (peptic) or erosion
gastrojejunal ulcer (peptic) or erosion
jejunal ulcer (peptic) or erosion
marginal ulcer (peptic) or erosion
stomal ulcer (peptic) or erosion
Use additional code to identify:
alcohol abuse and dependence (F10.-)
Excludes1: primary ulcer of small intestine (K63.3)
- MCC K28.0 Acute gastrojejunal ulcer with hemorrhage
- MCC K28.1 Acute gastrojejunal ulcer with perforation
- MCC K28.2 Acute gastrojejunal ulcer with both hemorrhage and perforation
- CC K28.3 Acute gastrojejunal ulcer without hemorrhage or perforation
- MCC K28.4 Chronic or unspecified gastrojejunal ulcer with hemorrhage
- MCC K28.5 Chronic or unspecified gastrojejunal ulcer with perforation
- MCC K28.6 Chronic or unspecified gastrojejunal ulcer with both hemorrhage and perforation
- K28.7 Chronic gastrojejunal ulcer without hemorrhage or perforation
- K28.9 Gastrojejunal ulcer, unspecified as acute or chronic, without hemorrhage or perforation

K29 Gastritis and duodenitis
Excludes1: eosinophilic gastritis or gastroenteritis (K52.81)
Zollinger-Ellison syndrome (E16.4)
- + K29.0 Acute gastritis
  Use additional code to identify:
  alcohol abuse and dependence (F10.-)
  Excludes1: erosion (acute) of stomach (K25.-)
  - K29.00 Acute gastritis without bleeding
  - MCC K29.01 Acute gastritis with bleeding
- + K29.2 Alcoholic gastritis
  Use additional code to identify:
  alcohol abuse and dependence (F10.-)
  - K29.20 Alcoholic gastritis without bleeding
  - MCC K29.21 Alcoholic gastritis with bleeding
- + K29.3 Chronic superficial gastritis
  - K29.30 Chronic superficial gastritis without bleeding
  - MCC K29.31 Chronic superficial gastritis with bleeding
- + K29.4 Chronic atrophic gastritis
  Gastric atrophy
  - K29.40 Chronic atrophic gastritis without bleeding
  - MCC K29.41 Chronic atrophic gastritis with bleeding
- + K29.5 Unspecified chronic gastritis
  Chronic antral gastritis
  Chronic fundal gastritis
  - K29.50 Unspecified chronic gastritis without bleeding
  - MCC K29.51 Unspecified chronic gastritis with bleeding
- + K29.6 Other gastritis
  Giant hypertrophic gastritis
  Granulomatous gastritis
  Ménétrier's disease
  - K29.60 Other gastritis without bleeding
  - MCC K29.61 Other gastritis with bleeding
- + K29.7 Gastritis, unspecified
  - K29.70 Gastritis, unspecified, without bleeding
  - MCC K29.71 Gastritis, unspecified, with bleeding
- + K29.8 Duodenitis
  - K29.80 Duodenitis without bleeding
  - MCC K29.81 Duodenitis with bleeding
    AHA CC: 3Q, 2018, 22-23
- + K29.9 Gastroduodenitis, unspecified
  - K29.90 Gastroduodenitis, unspecified, without bleeding
  - MCC K29.91 Gastroduodenitis, unspecified, with bleeding

K30 Functional dyspepsia
Indigestion
Excludes1: dyspepsia NOS (R10.13)
heartburn (R12)
nervous dyspepsia (F45.8)
neurotic dyspepsia (F45.8)
psychogenic dyspepsia (F45.8)
Valid 3-character code, no further characters required

K31 Other diseases of stomach and duodenum
Includes: functional disorders of stomach
Excludes2: diabetic gastroparesis (E08.43, E09.43, E10.43, E11.43, E13.43)
diverticulum of duodenum (K57.00-K57.13)
- K31.0 Acute dilatation of stomach
  Acute distention of stomach
- ● K31.1 Adult hypertrophic pyloric stenosis
  Pyloric stenosis NOS
  Excludes1: congenital or infantile pyloric stenosis (Q40.0)
- K31.2 Hourglass stricture and stenosis of stomach
  Excludes1: congenital hourglass stomach (Q40.2)
  hourglass contraction of stomach (K31.89)
- K31.3 Pylorospasm, not elsewhere classified
  Excludes1: congenital or infantile pylorospasm (Q40.0)
  neurotic pylorospasm (F45.8)
  psychogenic pylorospasm (F45.8)v
- K31.4 Gastric diverticulum
  Excludes1: congenital diverticulum of stomach (Q40.2)
- CC K31.5 Obstruction of duodenum
  Constriction of duodenum
  Duodenal ileus (chronic)
  Stenosis of duodenum
  Stricture of duodenum
  Volvulus of duodenum
  Excludes1: congenital stenosis of duodenum (Q41.0)
- CC K31.6 Fistula of stomach and duodenum
  Gastrocolic fistula
  Gastrojejunocolic fistula
- K31.7 Polyp of stomach and duodenum
  Excludes1: adenomatous polyp of stomach (D13.1)
  AHA CC: 1Q, 2020, 16
- + K31.8 Other specified diseases of stomach and duodenum
  - + K31.81 Angiodysplasia of stomach and duodenum
    - MCC K31.811 Angiodysplasia of stomach and duodenum with bleeding
      AHA CC: 1Q, 2023, 16

K31.819 Angiodysplasia of stomach and duodenum without bleeding
　　Angiodysplasia of stomach and duodenum NOS
MCC K31.82 Dieulafoy lesion (hemorrhagic) of stomach and duodenum
　　Excludes2: *Dieulafoy lesion of intestine (K63.81)*
K31.83 Achlorhydria
K31.84 Gastroparesis
　　Gastroparalysis
　　Code first underlying disease, if known, such as:
　　　anorexia nervosa (F50.0-)
　　　diabetes mellitus (E08.43, E09.43, E10.43, E11.43, E13.43)
　　　scleroderma (M34.-)
　　AHA CC: 4Q, 2013, 114-115
K31.89 Other diseases of stomach and duodenum
　　AHA CC: 1Q, 2017, 28; 1Q, 2020, 15
K31.9 Disease of stomach and duodenum, unspecified
+ K31.A Gastric intestinal metaplasia
　　AHA CC: 4Q, 2021, 15-16
　K31.A0 Gastric intestinal metaplasia, unspecified
　　　Gastric intestinal metaplasia definite for dysplasia
　　　Gastric intestinal metaplasia NOS
+ K31.A1 Gastric intestinal metaplasia without dysplasia
　　K31.A11 Gastric intestinal metaplasia without dysplasia, involving the antrum
　　K31.A12 Gastric intestinal metaplasia without dysplasia, involving the body (corpus)
　　K31.A13 Gastric intestinal metaplasia without dysplasia, involving the fundus
　　K31.A14 Gastric intestinal metaplasia without dysplasia, involving the cardia
　　K31.A15 Gastric intestinal metaplasia without dysplasia, involving the multiple sites
　　K31.A19 Gastric intestinal metaplasia without dysplasia, unspecified site
+ K31.A2 Gastric intestinal metaplasia with dysplasia
　　K31.A21 Gastric intestinal metaplasia with low grade dysplasia
　　K31.A22 Gastric intestinal metaplasia with high grade dysplasia
　　K31.A29 Gastric intestinal metaplasia with dysplasia, unspecified

Diseases of appendix (K35-K38)

K35 Acute appendicitis
+ K35.2 Acute appendicitis with generalized peritonitis
　　AHA CC: 4Q, 2018, 17-18
　+ K35.20 Acute appendicitis with generalized peritonitis, without abscess
　　　AHA CC: 4Q, 2018, 18
　　CC K35.200 Acute appendicitis with generalized peritonitis, without perforation or abscess
　　　(Acute) appendicitis with generalized peritonitis without rupture or perforation of appendix NOS
　　CC K35.201 Acute appendicitis with generalized peritonitis, with perforation, without abscess
　　　Appendicitis (acute) with generalized (diffuse) peritonitis following rupture or perforation of appendix NOS
　　CC K35.209 Acute appendicitis with generalized peritonitis, without abscess, unspecified as to perforation
　　　(Acute) appendicitis with generalized peritonitis NOS
　+ K35.21 Acute appendicitis with generalized peritonitis, with abscess
　　MCC K35.210 Acute appendicitis with generalized peritonitis, without perforation, with abscess
　　　(Acute) appendicitis with generalized peritonitis without rupture or perforation of appendix, with abscess
　　MCC K35.211 Acute appendicitis with generalized peritonitis, with perforation and abscess
　　　Appendicitis (acute) with generalized (diffuse) peritonitis following rupture or perforation of appendix, with abscess
　　MCC K35.219 Acute appendicitis with generalized peritonitis, with abscess, unspecified as to perforation
　　　(Acute) appendicitis with generalized peritonitis and abscess NOS
+ K35.3 Acute appendicitis with localized peritonitis
　　AHA CC: 4Q, 2018, 17-18
　CC K35.30 Acute appendicitis with localized peritonitis, without perforation or gangrene
　　　Acute appendicitis with localized peritonitis NOS
　CC K35.31 Acute appendicitis with localized peritonitis and gangrene, without perforation
　MCC K35.32 Acute appendicitis with perforation, localized peritonitis, and gangrene, without abscess
　　　(Acute) appendicitis with perforation NOS
　　　Perforated appendix NOS
　　　Ruptured appendix (with localized peritonitis) NOS
　　　AHA CC: 4Q, 2018, 18; 1Q, 2020, 16
　MCC K35.33 Acute appendicitis with perforation, localized peritonitis, and gangrene, with abscess
　　　(Acute) appendicitis with (peritoneal) abscess NOS
　　　Ruptured appendix with localized peritonitis and abscess
+ K35.8 Other and unspecified acute appendicitis
　CC K35.80 Unspecified acute appendicitis
　　　Acute appendicitis NOS
　　　Acute appendicitis without (localized) (generalized) peritonitis
　+ K35.89 Other acute appendicitis
　　　AHA CC: 4Q, 2018, 17-18
　　CC K35.890 Other acute appendicitis without perforation or gangrene
　　CC K35.891 Other acute appendicitis without perforation, with gangrene
　　　(Acute) appendicitis with gangrene NOS

Abdominal Wall: Inguinal Hernia

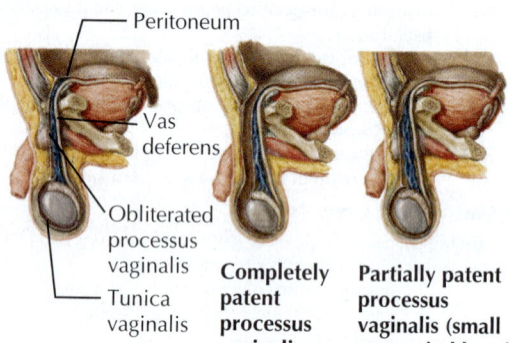

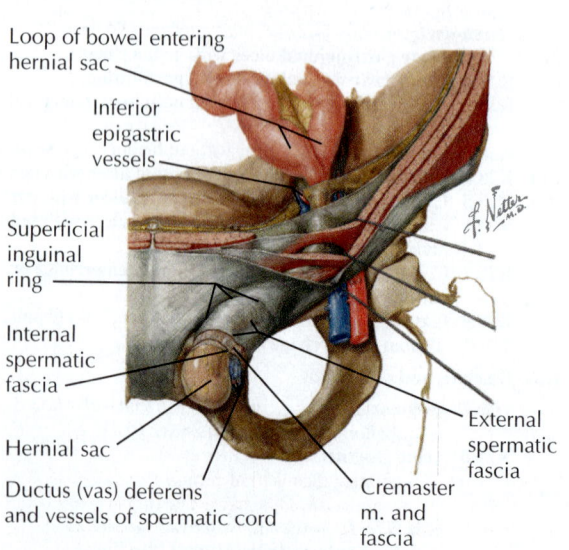

© 2017 Elsevier Inc. All rights reserved. www.netterimages.com

K36 Other appendicitis
  Chronic appendicitis
  Recurrent appendicitis
  Valid 3-character code, no further characters required

K37 Unspecified appendicitis
  Excludes1: unspecified appendicitis with peritonitis (K35.2-, K35.3-)
  Valid 3-character code, no further characters required

K38 Other diseases of appendix
  K38.0 Hyperplasia of appendix
  K38.1 Appendicular concretions
    Fecalith of appendix
    Stercolith of appendix
  K38.2 Diverticulum of appendix
  K38.3 Fistula of appendix
  K38.8 Other specified diseases of appendix
    Intussusception of appendix
  K38.9 Disease of appendix, unspecified

Hernia (K40-K46)

NOTE Hernia with both gangrene and obstruction is classified to hernia with gangrene.

Includes: acquired hernia
  congenital [except diaphragmatic or hiatus] hernia
  recurrent hernia

K40 Inguinal hernia
  Includes: bubonocele
    direct inguinal hernia
    double inguinal hernia
    indirect inguinal hernia
    inguinal hernia NOS
    oblique inguinal hernia
    scrotal hernia

  + **K40.0** Bilateral inguinal hernia, with obstruction, without gangrene
      Inguinal hernia (bilateral) causing obstruction without gangrene
      Incarcerated inguinal hernia (bilateral) without gangrene
      Irreducible inguinal hernia (bilateral) without gangrene
      Strangulated inguinal hernia (bilateral) without gangrene
    CC **K40.00** Bilateral inguinal hernia, with obstruction, without gangrene, not specified as recurrent
        Bilateral inguinal hernia, with obstruction, without gangrene NOS
    CC **K40.01** Bilateral inguinal hernia, with obstruction, without gangrene, recurrent
  + **K40.1** Bilateral inguinal hernia, with gangrene
    MCC **K40.10** Bilateral inguinal hernia, with gangrene, not specified as recurrent
        Bilateral inguinal hernia, with gangrene NOS
    MCC **K40.11** Bilateral inguinal hernia, with gangrene, recurrent
  + **K40.2** Bilateral inguinal hernia, without obstruction or gangrene
    K40.20 Bilateral inguinal hernia, without obstruction or gangrene, not specified as recurrent
        Bilateral inguinal hernia NOS
    K40.21 Bilateral inguinal hernia, without obstruction or gangrene, recurrent
  + **K40.3** Unilateral inguinal hernia, with obstruction, without gangrene
      Inguinal hernia (unilateral) causing obstruction without gangrene
      Incarcerated inguinal hernia (unilateral) without gangrene
      Irreducible inguinal hernia (unilateral) without gangrene
      Strangulated inguinal hernia (unilateral) without gangrene
    CC **K40.30** Unilateral inguinal hernia, with obstruction, without gangrene, not specified as recurrent
        Inguinal hernia, with obstruction NOS
        Unilateral inguinal hernia, with obstruction, without gangrene NOS
    CC **K40.31** Unilateral inguinal hernia, with obstruction, without gangrene, recurrent
  + **K40.4** Unilateral inguinal hernia, with gangrene
    MCC **K40.40** Unilateral inguinal hernia, with gangrene, not specified as recurrent
        Inguinal hernia with gangrene NOS
        Unilateral inguinal hernia with gangrene NOS
    MCC **K40.41** Unilateral inguinal hernia, with gangrene, recurrent
  + **K40.9** Unilateral inguinal hernia, without obstruction or gangrene
    K40.90 Unilateral inguinal hernia, without obstruction or gangrene, not specified as recurrent
        Inguinal hernia NOS
        Unilateral inguinal hernia NOS
        AHA CC: 3Q, 2021, 31
    K40.91 Unilateral inguinal hernia, without obstruction or gangrene, recurrent
        AHA CC: 3Q, 2021, 31

K41 Femoral hernia
  + **K41.0** Bilateral femoral hernia, with obstruction, without gangrene
      Femoral hernia (bilateral) causing obstruction, without gangrene
      Incarcerated femoral hernia (bilateral), without gangrene
      Irreducible femoral hernia (bilateral), without gangrene
      Strangulated femoral hernia (bilateral), without gangrene
    CC **K41.00** Bilateral femoral hernia, with obstruction, without gangrene, not specified as recurrent
        Bilateral femoral hernia, with obstruction, without gangrene NOS
    CC **K41.01** Bilateral femoral hernia, with obstruction, without gangrene, recurrent
  + **K41.1** Bilateral femoral hernia, with gangrene
    MCC **K41.10** Bilateral femoral hernia, with gangrene, not specified as recurrent
        Bilateral femoral hernia, with gangrene NOS
    MCC **K41.11** Bilateral femoral hernia, with gangrene, recurrent
  + **K41.2** Bilateral femoral hernia, without obstruction or gangrene
    K41.20 Bilateral femoral hernia, without obstruction or gangrene, not specified as recurrent
        Bilateral femoral hernia NOS
    K41.21 Bilateral femoral hernia, without obstruction or gangrene, recurrent
  + **K41.3** Unilateral femoral hernia, with obstruction, without gangrene
      Femoral hernia (unilateral) causing obstruction, without gangrene
      Incarcerated femoral hernia (unilateral), without gangrene
      Irreducible femoral hernia (unilateral), without gangrene
      Strangulated femoral hernia (unilateral), without gangrene
    CC **K41.30** Unilateral femoral hernia, with obstruction, without gangrene, not specified as recurrent
        Femoral hernia, with obstruction NOS
        Unilateral femoral hernia, with obstruction NOS
    CC **K41.31** Unilateral femoral hernia, with obstruction, without gangrene, recurrent
        AHA CC: 3Q, 2021, 30
  + **K41.4** Unilateral femoral hernia, with gangrene
    CC **K41.40** Unilateral femoral hernia, with gangrene, not specified as recurrent
        Femoral hernia, with gangrene NOS
        Unilateral femoral hernia, with gangrene NOS
    CC **K41.41** Unilateral femoral hernia, with gangrene, recurrent
  + **K41.9** Unilateral femoral hernia, without obstruction or gangrene
    K41.90 Unilateral femoral hernia, without obstruction or gangrene, not specified as recurrent
        Femoral hernia NOS
        Unilateral femoral hernia NOS
        AHA CC: 3Q, 2021, 30
    K41.91 Unilateral femoral hernia, without obstruction or gangrene, recurrent

K42 Umbilical hernia
  Includes: paraumbilical hernia
  Excludes1: omphalocele (Q79.2)
  K42.0 Umbilical hernia with obstruction, without gangrene
      Umbilical hernia causing obstruction, without gangrene
      Incarcerated umbilical hernia, without gangrene
      Irreducible umbilical hernia, without gangrene
      Strangulated umbilical hernia, without gangrene
  K42.1 Umbilical hernia with gangrene
      Gangrenous umbilical hernia
  K42.9 Umbilical hernia without obstruction or gangrene
      Umbilical hernia NOS

K43 Ventral hernia
  K43.0 Incisional hernia with obstruction, without gangrene
      Incisional hernia causing obstruction, without gangrene
      Incarcerated incisional hernia, without gangrene

Irreducible incisional hernia, without gangrene
Strangulated incisional hernia, without gangrene

K43.1 Incisional hernia with gangrene
Gangrenous incisional hernia
AHA CC: 2Q, 2020, 22

K43.2 Incisional hernia without obstruction or gangrene
Incisional hernia NOS

K43.3 Parastomal hernia with obstruction, without gangrene
Incarcerated parastomal hernia, without gangrene
Irreducible parastomal hernia, without gangrene
Parastomal hernia causing obstruction, without gangrene
Strangulated parastomal hernia, without gangrene

K43.4 Parastomal hernia with gangrene
Gangrenous parastomal hernia

K43.5 Parastomal hernia without obstruction or gangrene
Parastomal hernia NOS

K43.6 Other and unspecified ventral hernia with obstruction, without gangrene
Epigastric hernia causing obstruction, without gangrene
Hypogastric hernia causing obstruction, without gangrene
Incarcerated epigastric hernia without gangrene
Incarcerated hypogastric hernia without gangrene
Incarcerated midline hernia without gangrene
Incarcerated spigelian hernia without gangrene
Incarcerated subxiphoid hernia without gangrene
Irreducible epigastric hernia without gangrene
Irreducible hypogastric hernia without gangrene
Irreducible midline hernia without gangrene
Irreducible spigelian hernia without gangrene
Irreducible subxiphoid hernia without gangrene
Midline hernia causing obstruction, without gangrene
Spigelian hernia causing obstruction, without gangrene
Strangulated epigastric hernia without gangrene
Strangulated hypogastric hernia without gangrene
Strangulated midline hernia without gangrene
Strangulated spigelian hernia without gangrene
Strangulated subxiphoid hernia without gangrene
Subxiphoid hernia causing obstruction, without gangrene

K43.7 Other and unspecified ventral hernia with gangrene
Any condition listed under K43.6 specified as gangrenous

K43.9 Ventral hernia without obstruction or gangrene
Epigastric hernia
Ventral hernia NOS

K44 Diaphragmatic hernia
Includes: hiatus hernia (esophageal) (sliding)
paraesophageal hernia
Excludes1: *congenital diaphragmatic hernia (Q79.0)*
congenital hiatus hernia (Q40.1)

K44.0 Diaphragmatic hernia with obstruction, without gangrene
Diaphragmatic hernia causing obstruction
Incarcerated diaphragmatic hernia
Irreducible diaphragmatic hernia
Strangulated diaphragmatic hernia
AHA CC: 2Q, 2022, 13-14

K44.1 Diaphragmatic hernia with gangrene
Gangrenous diaphragmatic hernia

K44.9 Diaphragmatic hernia without obstruction or gangrene
Diaphragmatic hernia NOS

K45 Other abdominal hernia
Includes: abdominal hernia, specified site NEC
lumbar hernia
obturator hernia
pudendal hernia
retroperitoneal hernia
sciatic hernia

K45.0 Other specified abdominal hernia with obstruction, without gangrene
Other specified abdominal hernia causing obstruction
Other specified incarcerated abdominal hernia
Other specified irreducible abdominal hernia
Other specified strangulated abdominal hernia

K45.1 Other specified abdominal hernia with gangrene
Any condition listed under K45 specified as gangrenous

K45.8 Other specified abdominal hernia without obstruction or gangrene

K46 Unspecified abdominal hernia
Includes: enterocele
epiplocele
hernia NOS
interstitial hernia
intestinal hernia
intra-abdominal hernia
Excludes1: *vaginal enterocele (N81.5)*

K46.0 Unspecified abdominal hernia with obstruction, without gangrene
Unspecified abdominal hernia causing obstruction
Unspecified incarcerated abdominal hernia
Unspecified irreducible abdominal hernia
Unspecified strangulated abdominal hernia

K46.1 Unspecified abdominal hernia with gangrene
Any condition listed under K46 specified as gangrenous

K46.9 Unspecified abdominal hernia without obstruction or gangrene
Abdominal hernia NOS

Noninfective enteritis and colitis (K50-K52)

Includes: noninfective inflammatory bowel disease
Excludes1: *irritable bowel syndrome (K58.-)*
megacolon (K59.3-)

K50 Crohn's disease [regional enteritis]
Includes: granulomatous enteritis
Use additional code to identify manifestations, such as:
pyoderma gangrenosum (L88)
Excludes1: *ulcerative colitis (K51.-)*

K50.0 Crohn's disease of small intestine
Crohn's disease [regional enteritis] of duodenum
Crohn's disease [regional enteritis] of ileum
Crohn's disease [regional enteritis] of jejunum
Regional ileitis
Terminal ileitis
Excludes1: *Crohn's disease of both small and large intestine (K50.8-)*

CC K50.00 Crohn's disease of small intestine without complications

K50.01 Crohn's disease of small intestine with complications

CC K50.011 Crohn's disease of small intestine with rectal bleeding

CC K50.012 Crohn's disease of small intestine with intestinal obstruction

CC K50.013 Crohn's disease of small intestine with fistula

CC K50.014 Crohn's disease of small intestine with abscess
AHA CC: 4Q, 2012, 104

CC K50.018 Crohn's disease of small intestine with other complication

CC K50.019 Crohn's disease of small intestine with unspecified complications

K50.1 Crohn's disease of large intestine
Crohn's disease [regional enteritis] of colon
Crohn's disease [regional enteritis] of large bowel
Crohn's disease [regional enteritis] of rectum
Granulomatous colitis
Regional colitis
Excludes1: *Crohn's disease of both small and large intestine (K50.8)*

CC K50.10 Crohn's disease of large intestine without complications

K50.11 Crohn's disease of large intestine with complications

CC K50.111 Crohn's disease of large intestine with rectal bleeding

CC K50.112 Crohn's disease of large intestine with intestinal obstruction

CC K50.113 Crohn's disease of large intestine with fistula

CC K50.114 Crohn's disease of large intestine with abscess
AHA CC: 4Q, 2012, 104

CC K50.118 Crohn's disease of large intestine with other complication

CC K50.119 Crohn's disease of large intestine with unspecified complications

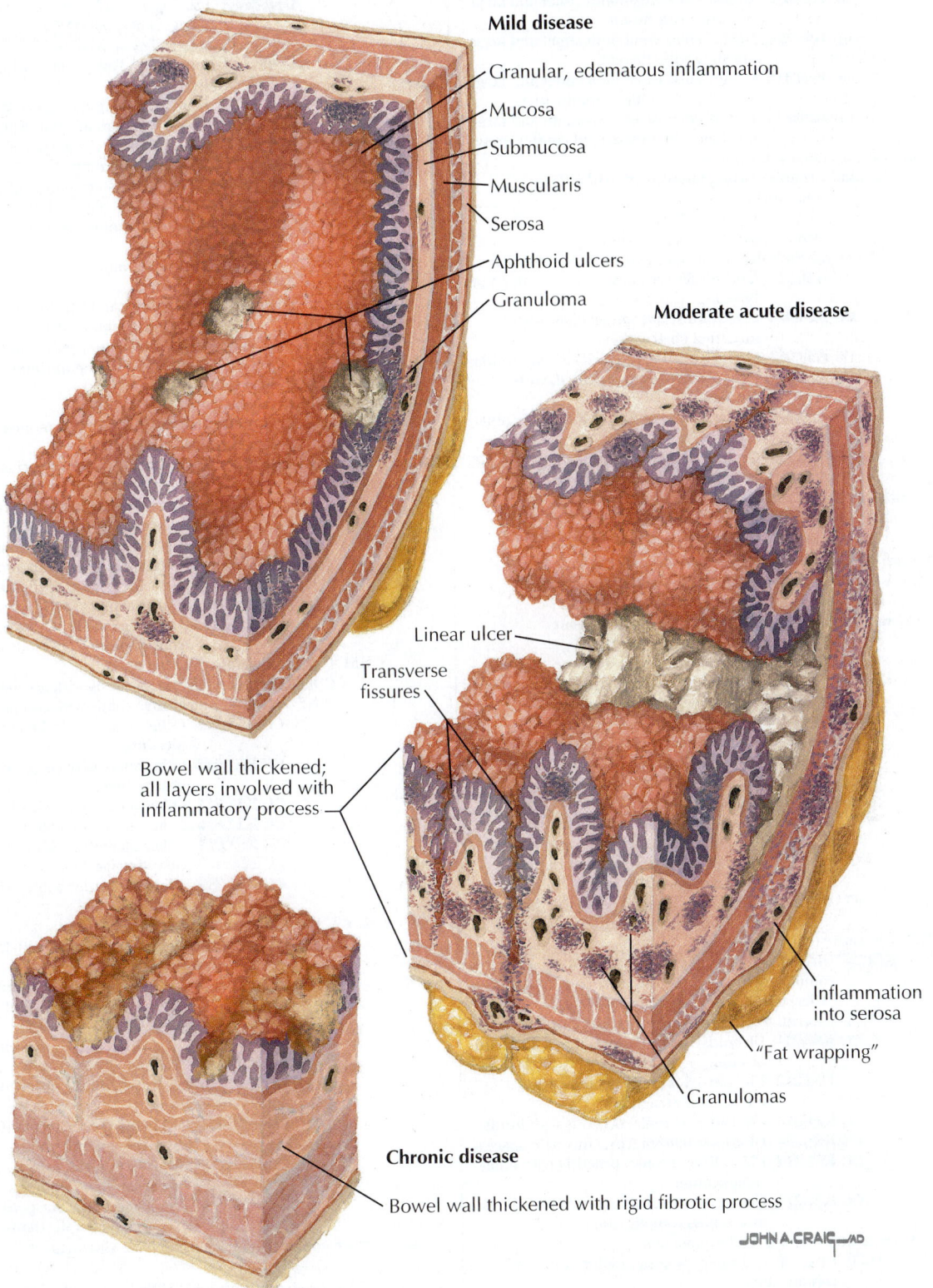

Inflammatory Bowel Disease: Progression of Inflammatory Process in Chron's Disease

- **K50.8** Crohn's disease of both small and large intestine
  - CC **K50.80** Crohn's disease of both small and large intestine without complications
  - **K50.81** Crohn's disease of both small and large intestine with complications
    - CC **K50.811** Crohn's disease of both small and large intestine with rectal bleeding
    - CC **K50.812** Crohn's disease of both small and large intestine with intestinal obstruction
    - CC **K50.813** Crohn's disease of both small and large intestine with fistula
    - CC **K50.814** Crohn's disease of both small and large intestine with abscess
    - CC **K50.818** Crohn's disease of both small and large intestine with other complication
    - CC **K50.819** Crohn's disease of both small and large intestine with unspecified complications
- **K50.9** Crohn's disease, unspecified
  - CC **K50.90** Crohn's disease, unspecified, without complications
    - Crohn's disease NOS
    - Regional enteritis NOS
  - **K50.91** Crohn's disease, unspecified, with complications
    - CC **K50.911** Crohn's disease, unspecified, with rectal bleeding
    - CC **K50.912** Crohn's disease, unspecified, with intestinal obstruction
    - CC **K50.913** Crohn's disease, unspecified, with fistula
    - CC **K50.914** Crohn's disease, unspecified, with abscess
    - CC **K50.918** Crohn's disease, unspecified, with other complication
    - CC **K50.919** Crohn's disease, unspecified, with unspecified complications

K51 Ulcerative colitis

Use additional code to identify manifestations, such as: pyoderma gangrenosum (L88)

Excludes1: Crohn's disease [regional enteritis] (K50.-)

- **K51.0** Ulcerative (chronic) pancolitis
  - Backwash ileitis
  - CC **K51.00** Ulcerative (chronic) pancolitis without complications
    - Ulcerative (chronic) pancolitis NOS
  - **K51.01** Ulcerative (chronic) pancolitis with complications
    - CC **K51.011** Ulcerative (chronic) pancolitis with rectal bleeding
    - CC **K51.012** Ulcerative (chronic) pancolitis with intestinal obstruction
    - CC **K51.013** Ulcerative (chronic) pancolitis with fistula
    - CC **K51.014** Ulcerative (chronic) pancolitis with abscess
    - CC **K51.018** Ulcerative (chronic) pancolitis with other complication
    - CC **K51.019** Ulcerative (chronic) pancolitis with unspecified complications
- **K51.2** Ulcerative (chronic) proctitis
  - CC **K51.20** Ulcerative (chronic) proctitis without complications
    - Ulcerative (chronic) proctitis NOS
  - **K51.21** Ulcerative (chronic) proctitis with complications
    - CC **K51.211** Ulcerative (chronic) proctitis with rectal bleeding
    - **K51.212** Ulcerative (chronic) proctitis with intestinal obstruction
    - CC **K51.213** Ulcerative (chronic) proctitis with fistula
    - CC **K51.214** Ulcerative (chronic) proctitis with abscess
    - CC **K51.218** Ulcerative (chronic) proctitis with other complication
    - CC **K51.219** Ulcerative (chronic) proctitis with unspecified complications
- **K51.3** Ulcerative (chronic) rectosigmoiditis
  - CC **K51.30** Ulcerative (chronic) rectosigmoiditis without complications
    - Ulcerative (chronic) rectosigmoiditis NOS
  - **K51.31** Ulcerative (chronic) rectosigmoiditis with complications
    - CC **K51.311** Ulcerative (chronic) rectosigmoiditis with rectal bleeding
    - CC **K51.312** Ulcerative (chronic) rectosigmoiditis with intestinal obstruction
    - CC **K51.313** Ulcerative (chronic) rectosigmoiditis with fistula
    - CC **K51.314** Ulcerative (chronic) rectosigmoiditis with abscess
    - CC **K51.318** Ulcerative (chronic) rectosigmoiditis with other complication
    - CC **K51.319** Ulcerative (chronic) rectosigmoiditis with unspecified complications
- **K51.4** Inflammatory polyps of colon
  - **Excludes2:** adenomatous polyp of colon (D12.6)
    polyposis of colon (D12.6)
    polyps of colon NOS (K63.5)
  - CC **K51.40** Inflammatory polyps of colon without complications
    - Inflammatory polyps of colon NOS
  - **K51.41** Inflammatory polyps of colon with complications
    - CC **K51.411** Inflammatory polyps of colon with rectal bleeding
    - CC **K51.412** Inflammatory polyps of colon with intestinal obstruction
    - CC **K51.413** Inflammatory polyps of colon with fistula
    - CC **K51.414** Inflammatory polyps of colon with abscess
    - CC **K51.418** Inflammatory polyps of colon with other complication
    - CC **K51.419** Inflammatory polyps of colon with unspecified complications
- **K51.5** Left sided colitis
  - Left hemicolitis
  - CC **K51.50** Left sided colitis without complications
    - Left sided colitis NOS
  - **K51.51** Left sided colitis with complications
    - CC **K51.511** Left sided colitis with rectal bleeding
    - CC **K51.512** Left sided colitis with intestinal obstruction
    - CC **K51.513** Left sided colitis with fistula
    - CC **K51.514** Left sided colitis with abscess
    - CC **K51.518** Left sided colitis with other complication
    - CC **K51.519** Left sided colitis with unspecified complications
- **K51.8** Other ulcerative colitis
  - CC **K51.80** Other ulcerative colitis without complications
  - **K51.81** Other ulcerative colitis with complications
    - CC **K51.811** Other ulcerative colitis with rectal bleeding
    - CC **K51.812** Other ulcerative colitis with intestinal obstruction
    - CC **K51.813** Other ulcerative colitis with fistula
    - CC **K51.814** Other ulcerative colitis with abscess
    - CC **K51.818** Other ulcerative colitis with other complication
    - CC **K51.819** Other ulcerative colitis with unspecified complications
- **K51.9** Ulcerative colitis, unspecified
  - CC **K51.90** Ulcerative colitis, unspecified, without complications
  - **K51.91** Ulcerative colitis, unspecified, with complications
    - CC **K51.911** Ulcerative colitis, unspecified with rectal bleeding
    - CC **K51.912** Ulcerative colitis, unspecified with intestinal obstruction
    - CC **K51.913** Ulcerative colitis, unspecified with fistula
    - CC **K51.914** Ulcerative colitis, unspecified with abscess
    - CC **K51.918** Ulcerative colitis, unspecified with other complication
    - CC **K51.919** Ulcerative colitis, unspecified with unspecified complications

K52 Other and unspecified noninfective gastroenteritis and colitis

AHA CC: 4Q, 2016, 30-31

- CC **K52.0** Gastroenteritis and colitis due to radiation
- CC **K52.1** Toxic gastroenteritis and colitis
  - Drug-induced gastroenteritis and colitis
  - Code first (T51-T65) to identify toxic agent
  - Use additional code for adverse effect, if applicable, to identify drug (T36-T50 with fifth or sixth character 5)
  - AHA CC: 1Q, 2019, 17

+ **K52.2 Allergic and dietetic gastroenteritis and colitis**
　　Food hypersensitivity gastroenteritis or colitis
　　Use additional code to identify type of food allergy (Z91.01-, Z91.02-)
　　Excludes2: *allergic eosinophilic colitis (K52.82)*
　　　　　　　allergic eosinophilic esophagitis (K20.0)
　　　　　　　allergic eosinophilic gastritis (K52.81)
　　　　　　　allergic eosinophilic gastroenteritis (K52.81)
　　K52.21 Food protein-induced enterocolitis syndrome
　　　　FPIES
　　　　Use additional code for hypovolemic shock, if present (R57.1)
　　K52.22 Food protein-induced enteropathy
　　K52.29 Other allergic and dietetic gastroenteritis and colitis
　　　　Allergic proctocolitis
　　　　Food hypersensitivity gastroenteritis or colitis
　　　　Food-induced eosinophilic proctocolitis
　　　　Food protein-induced proctocolitis
　　　　Immediate gastrointestinal hypersensitivity
　　　　Milk protein-induced proctocolitis
K52.3 Indeterminate colitis
　　Colonic inflammatory bowel disease unclassified (IBDU)
　　Excludes1: *unspecified colitis (K52.9)*
+ **K52.8 Other specified noninfective gastroenteritis and colitis**
　　K52.81 Eosinophilic gastritis or gastroenteritis
　　　　Eosinophilic enteritis
　　　　Excludes2: *eosinophilic esophagitis (K20.0)*
　　K52.82 Eosinophilic colitis
　　　　Excludes2: *allergic protocolitis (K52.29)*
　　　　　　　　food-induced eosinophilic proctocolitis (K52.29)
　　　　　　　　food protein-induced enterocolitis syndrome (FPIES) (K52.21)
　　　　　　　　food protein-induced proctocolitis (K52.29)
　　　　　　　　milk protein induced proctocolitis (K52.29)
+ **K52.83 Microscopic colitis**
　　K52.831 Collagenous colitis
　　K52.832 Lymphocytic colitis
　　K52.838 Other microscopic colitis
　　K52.839 Microscopic colitis, unspecified
　　K52.89 Other specified noninfective gastroenteritis and colitis
　　　　AHA CC: 1Q, 2019, 20-21
K52.9 Noninfective gastroenteritis and colitis, unspecified
　　Colitis NOS
　　Enteritis NOS
　　Gastroenteritis NOS
　　Ileitis NOS
　　Jejunitis NOS
　　Sigmoiditis NOS
　　Excludes1: *diarrhea NOS (R19.7)*
　　　　　　　functional diarrhea (K59.1)
　　　　　　　infectious gastroenteritis and colitis NOS (A09)
　　　　　　　neonatal diarrhea (noninfective) (P78.3)
　　　　　　　psychogenic diarrhea (F45.8)
　　AHA CC: 3Q, 2021, 3-4

Other diseases of intestines (K55-K64)

K55 Vascular disorders of intestine
Excludes1: *necrotizing enterocolitis of newborn (P77.-)*
Excludes2: *angioectasia (angiodysplasia) duodenum (K31.81-)*
AHA CC: 4Q, 2016, 32-33

+ **K55.0 Acute vascular disorders of intestine**
　　Infarction of appendices epiploicae
　　Mesenteric (artery) (vein) embolism
　　Mesenteric (artery) (vein) infarction
　　Mesenteric (artery) (vein) thrombosis
+ **K55.01 Acute (reversible) ischemia of small intestine**
　　MCC **K55.011** Focal (segmental) acute (reversible) ischemia of small intestine
　　MCC **K55.012** Diffuse acute (reversible) ischemia of small intestine
　　MCC **K55.019** Acute (reversible) ischemia of small intestine, extent unspecified

+ **K55.02 Acute infarction of small intestine**
　　Gangrene of small intestine
　　Necrosis of small intestine
　　MCC **K55.021** Focal (segmental) acute infarction of small intestine
　　MCC **K55.022** Diffuse acute infarction of small intestine
　　MCC **K55.029** Acute infarction of small intestine, extent unspecified
+ **K55.03 Acute (reversible) ischemia of large intestine**
　　Acute fulminant ischemic colitis
　　Subacute ischemic colitis
　　MCC **K55.031** Focal (segmental) acute (reversible) ischemia of large intestine
　　MCC **K55.032** Diffuse acute (reversible) ischemia of large intestine
　　MCC **K55.039** Acute (reversible) ischemia of large intestine, extent unspecified
　　AHA CC: 4Q, 2019, 68
+ **K55.04 Acute infarction of large intestine**
　　Gangrene of large intestine
　　Necrosis of large intestine
　　MCC **K55.041** Focal (segmental) acute infarction of large intestine
　　MCC **K55.042** Diffuse acute infarction of large intestine
　　MCC **K55.049** Acute infarction of large intestine, extent unspecified
+ **K55.05 Acute (reversible) ischemia of intestine, part unspecified**
　　MCC **K55.051** Focal (segmental) acute (reversible) ischemia of intestine, part unspecified
　　MCC **K55.052** Diffuse acute (reversible) ischemia of intestine, part unspecified
　　MCC **K55.059** Acute (reversible) ischemia of intestine, part and extent unspecified
+ **K55.06 Acute infarction of intestine, part unspecified**
　　Acute intestinal infarction
　　Gangrene of intestine
　　Necrosis of intestine
　　MCC **K55.061** Focal (segmental) acute infarction of intestine, part unspecified
　　MCC **K55.062** Diffuse acute infarction of intestine, part unspecified
　　MCC **K55.069** Acute infarction of intestine, part and extent unspecified
CC **K55.1 Chronic vascular disorders of intestine**
　　Chronic ischemic colitis
　　Chronic ischemic enteritis
　　Chronic ischemic enterocolitis
　　Ischemic stricture of intestine
　　Mesenteric atherosclerosis
　　Mesenteric vascular insufficiency
+ **K55.2 Angiodysplasia of colon**
　　K55.20 Angiodysplasia of colon without hemorrhage
　　MCC **K55.21 Angiodysplasia of colon with hemorrhage**
　　　　AHA CC: 3Q, 2018, 21
+ **K55.3 Necrotizing enterocolitis**
　　Excludes1: *necrotizing enterocolitis of newborn (P77.-)*
　　Excludes2: *necrotizing enterocolitis due to Clostridium difficile (A04.7-)*
　　MCC **K55.30 Necrotizing enterocolitis, unspecified**
　　　　Necrotizing enterocolitis, NOS
　　MCC **K55.31 Stage 1 necrotizing enterocolitis**
　　　　Necrotizing enterocolitis without pneumatosis, without perforation
　　MCC **K55.32 Stage 2 necrotizing enterocolitis**
　　　　Necrotizing enterocolitis with pneumatosis, without perforation
　　MCC **K55.33 Stage 3 necrotizing enterocolitis**
　　　　Necrotizing enterocolitis with perforation
　　　　Necrotizing enterocolitis with pneumatosis and perforation
CC **K55.8 Other vascular disorders of intestine**
CC **K55.9 Vascular disorder of intestine, unspecified**
　　Ischemic colitis
　　Ischemic enteritis
　　Ischemic enterocolitis

K56 Paralytic ileus and intestinal obstruction without hernia

Excludes1: congenital stricture or stenosis of intestine (Q41-Q42)
cystic fibrosis with meconium ileus (E84.11)
ischemic stricture of intestine (K55.1)
meconium ileus NOS (P76.0)
neonatal intestinal obstructions classifiable to P76.-
obstruction of duodenum (K31.5)
postprocedural intestinal obstruction (K91.3-)

Excludes2: stenosis of anus or rectum (K62.4)

- CC **K56.0 Paralytic ileus**
  Paralysis of bowel
  Paralysis of colon
  Paralysis of intestine
  Excludes1: gallstone ileus (K56.3)
  ileus NOS (K56.7)
  obstructive ileus NOS (K56.69-)

- CC **K56.1 Intussusception**
  Intussusception or invagination of bowel
  Intussusception or invagination of colon
  Intussusception or invagination of intestine
  Intussusception or invagination of rectum
  Excludes2: intussusception of appendix (K38.8)

- MCC **K56.2 Volvulus**
  Strangulation of colon or intestine
  Torsion of colon or intestine
  Twist of colon or intestine
  Excludes2: volvulus of duodenum (K31.5)

- **K56.3 Gallstone ileus**
  Obstruction of intestine by gallstone

- + **K56.4 Other impaction of intestine**
  K56.41 Fecal impaction
  Excludes2: constipation (K59.0-)
  incomplete defecation (R15.0)
  - CC **K56.49 Other impaction of intestine**

- + **K56.5 Intestinal adhesions [bands] with obstruction (postinfection)**
  Abdominal hernia due to adhesions with obstruction
  Peritoneal adhesions [bands] with intestinal obstruction (postinfection)
  AHA CC: 4Q, 2017, 16-17
  - CC **K56.50 Intestinal adhesions [bands], unspecified as to partial versus complete obstruction**
    Intestinal adhesions with obstruction NOS
  - CC **K56.51 Intestinal adhesions [bands], with partial obstruction**
    Intestinal adhesions with incomplete obstruction
  - CC **K56.52 Intestinal adhesions [bands] with complete obstruction**

- + **K56.6 Other and unspecified intestinal obstruction**
  AHA CC: 4Q, 2017, 16-17
  - + **K56.60 Unspecified intestinal obstruction**
    - CC **K56.600 Partial intestinal obstruction, unspecified as to cause**
      Incomplete intestinal obstruction, NOS
    - CC **K56.601 Complete intestinal obstruction, unspecified as to cause**
    - CC **K56.609 Unspecified intestinal obstruction, unspecified as to partial versus complete obstruction**
      Intestinal obstruction NOS
  - + **K56.69 Other intestinal obstruction**
    Enterostenosis NOS
    Obstructive ileus NOS
    Occlusion of colon or intestine NOS
    Stenosis of colon or intestine NOS
    Stricture of colon or intestine NOS
    - CC **K56.690 Other partial intestinal obstruction**
      Other incomplete intestinal obstruction
    - CC **K56.691 Other complete intestinal obstruction**
    - CC **K56.699 Other intestinal obstruction unspecified as to partial versus complete obstruction**
      Other intestinal obstruction, NEC

- CC **K56.7 Ileus, unspecified**
  Excludes1: obstructive ileus (K56.69-)
  Excludes2: intestinal obstruction with hernia (K40-K46)
  AHA CC: 1Q, 2017, 40-41

K57 Diverticular disease of intestine

Excludes1: congenital diverticulum of intestine (Q43.8)
Meckel's diverticulum (Q43.0)
Excludes2: diverticulum of appendix (K38.2)
Code also if applicable peritonitis K65.-

- + **K57.0 Diverticulitis of small intestine with perforation and abscess**
  Excludes1: diverticulitis of both small and large intestine with perforation and abscess (K57.4-)
  - CC **K57.00 Diverticulitis of small intestine with perforation and abscess without bleeding**
  - MCC **K57.01 Diverticulitis of small intestine with perforation and abscess with bleeding**

- + **K57.1 Diverticular disease of small intestine without perforation or abscess**
  Excludes1: diverticular disease of both small and large intestine without perforation or abscess (K57.5-)
  - **K57.10 Diverticulosis of small intestine without perforation or abscess without bleeding**
    Diverticular disease of small intestine NOS
  - MCC **K57.11 Diverticulosis of small intestine without perforation or abscess with bleeding**
  - CC **K57.12 Diverticulitis of small intestine without perforation or abscess without bleeding**
  - MCC **K57.13 Diverticulitis of small intestine without perforation or abscess with bleeding**

- + **K57.2 Diverticulitis of large intestine with perforation and abscess**
  Excludes1: diverticulitis of both small and large intestine with perforation and abscess (K57.4-)
  - CC **K57.20 Diverticulitis of large intestine with perforation and abscess without bleeding**
    AHA CC: 1Q, 2022, 26-27
  - MCC **K57.21 Diverticulitis of large intestine with perforation and abscess with bleeding**

- + **K57.3 Diverticular disease of large intestine without perforation or abscess**
  Excludes1: diverticular disease of both small and large intestine without perforation or abscess (K57.5-)
  - **K57.30 Diverticulosis of large intestine without perforation or abscess without bleeding**
    Diverticular disease of colon NOS
  - MCC **K57.31 Diverticulosis of large intestine without perforation or abscess with bleeding**
    AHA CC: 3Q, 2018, 21-22
  - CC **K57.32 Diverticulitis of large intestine without perforation or abscess without bleeding**
  - MCC **K57.33 Diverticulitis of large intestine without perforation or abscess with bleeding**

- + **K57.4 Diverticulitis of both small and large intestine with perforation and abscess**
  - CC **K57.40 Diverticulitis of both small and large intestine with perforation and abscess without bleeding**
  - MCC **K57.41 Diverticulitis of both small and large intestine with perforation and abscess with bleeding**

- + **K57.5 Diverticular disease of both small and large intestine without perforation or abscess**
  - **K57.50 Diverticulosis of both small and large intestine without perforation or abscess without bleeding**
    Diverticular disease of both small and large intestine NOS
  - MCC **K57.51 Diverticulosis of both small and large intestine without perforation or abscess with bleeding**
  - CC **K57.52 Diverticulitis of both small and large intestine without perforation or abscess without bleeding**
  - MCC **K57.53 Diverticulitis of both small and large intestine without perforation or abscess with bleeding**

- + **K57.8 Diverticulitis of intestine, part unspecified, with perforation and abscess**
  - CC **K57.80 Diverticulitis of intestine, part unspecified, with perforation and abscess without bleeding**
  - MCC **K57.81 Diverticulitis of intestine, part unspecified, with perforation and abscess with bleeding**

- + **K57.9 Diverticular disease of intestine, part unspecified, without perforation or abscess**
  - **K57.90 Diverticulosis of intestine, part unspecified, without perforation or abscess without bleeding**
    Diverticular disease of intestine NOS
    AHA CC: 1Q, 2021, 11-12

MCC K57.91 Diverticulosis of intestine, part unspecified, without perforation or abscess with bleeding
CC K57.92 Diverticulitis of intestine, part unspecified, without perforation or abscess without bleeding
MCC K57.93 Diverticulitis of intestine, part unspecified, without perforation or abscess with bleeding

K58 Irritable bowel syndrome
Includes: irritable colon
spastic colon

K58.0 Irritable bowel syndrome with diarrhea
K58.1 Irritable bowel syndrome with constipation
AHA CC: 4Q, 2016, 32-33
K58.2 Mixed irritable bowel syndrome
AHA CC: 4Q, 2016, 32-33
K58.8 Other irritable bowel syndrome
AHA CC: 4Q, 2016, 32-33
K58.9 Irritable bowel syndrome without diarrhea
Irritable bowel syndrome NOS

K59 Other functional intestinal disorders
Excludes1: *change in bowel habit NOS (R19.4)*
intestinal malabsorption (K90.-)
psychogenic intestinal disorders (F45.8)
Excludes2: *functional disorders of stomach (K31.-)*

+ K59.0 Constipation
Excludes1: *fecal impaction (K56.41)*
Excludes2: *incomplete defecation (R15.0)*
K59.00 Constipation, unspecified
K59.01 Slow transit constipation
K59.02 Outlet dysfunction constipation
AHA CC: 1Q, 2023, 24
K59.03 Drug induced constipation
Use additional code for adverse effect, if applicable, to identify drug (T36-T50 with fifth or sixth character 5)
AHA CC: 4Q, 2016, 33
K59.04 Chronic idiopathic constipation
Functional constipation
AHA CC: 4Q, 2016, 33
K59.09 Other constipation
Chronic constipation
K59.1 Functional diarrhea
Excludes1: *diarrhea NOS (R19.7)*
irritable bowel syndrome with diarrhea (K58.0)
CC K59.2 Neurogenic bowel, not elsewhere classified
+ K59.3 Megacolon, not elsewhere classified
Dilatation of colon
Code first, if applicable (T51-T65) to identify toxic agent
Excludes1: *congenital megacolon (aganglionic) (Q43.1)*
megacolon (due to) (in) Chagas' disease (B57.32)
megacolon (due to) (in) Clostridium difficile (A04.7-)
megacolon (due to) (in) Hirschsprung's disease (Q43.1)
AHA CC: 4Q, 2016, 33-34
CC K59.31 Toxic megacolon
CC K59.39 Other megacolon
Megacolon NOS
K59.4 Anal spasm
Proctalgia fugax
+ K59.8 Other specified functional intestinal disorders
AHA CC: 4Q, 2020, 29-30
K59.81 Ogilvie syndrome
Acute colonic pseudo-obstruction (ACPO)
K59.89 Other specified functional intestinal disorders
Atony of colon
Pseudo-obstruction (acute) (chronic) of intestine
K59.9 Functional intestinal disorder, unspecified

K60 Fissure and fistula of anal and rectal regions
Excludes1: *fissure and fistula of anal and rectal regions with abscess or cellulitis (K61.-)*
Excludes2: *anal sphincter tear (healed) (nontraumatic) (old) (K62.81)*
K60.0 Acute anal fissure
K60.1 Chronic anal fissure
K60.2 Anal fissure, unspecified
K60.3 Anal fistula
K60.4 Rectal fistula
Fistula of rectum to skin
Excludes1: *rectovaginal fistula (N82.3)*
vesicorectal fistual (N32.1)
K60.5 Anorectal fistula

K61 Abscess of anal and rectal regions
Includes: abscess of anal and rectal regions
cellulitis of anal and rectal regions
CC K61.0 Anal abscess
Perianal abscess
Excludes2: *intrasphincteric abscess (K61.4)*
CC K61.1 Rectal abscess
Perirectal abscess
Excludes1: *ischiorectal abscess (K61.39)*
CC K61.2 Anorectal abscess
+ K61.3 Ischiorectal abscess
AHA CC: 4Q, 2018, 19
CC K61.31 Horseshoe abscess
CC K61.32 Ischiorectal abscess, NOS
K61.39 Other ischiorectal abscess
Abscess of ischiorectal fossa
Ischiorectal abscess, NOS
CC K61.4 Intrasphincteric abscess
Intersphincteric abscess
AHA CC: 4Q, 2018, 19
CC K61.5 Supralevator abscess
AHA CC: 4Q, 2018, 19

K62 Other diseases of anus and rectum
Includes: anal canal
Excludes2: *colostomy and enterostomy malfunction (K94.0-, K94.1-)*
fecal incontinence (R15.-)
hemorrhoids (K64.-)
K62.0 Anal polyp
K62.1 Rectal polyp
Excludes1: *adenomatous polyp (D12.8)*
K62.2 Anal prolapse
Prolapse of anal canal
K62.3 Rectal prolapse
Prolapse of rectal mucosa
K62.4 Stenosis of anus and rectum
Stricture of anus (sphincter)
AHA CC: 2Q, 2019, 13
CC K62.5 Hemorrhage of anus and rectum
Excludes1: *gastrointestinal bleeding NOS (K92.2)*
melena (K92.1)
neonatal rectal hemorrhage (P54.2)
AHA CC: 1Q, 2019, 21
CC K62.6 Ulcer of anus and rectum
Solitary ulcer of anus and rectum
Stercoral ulcer of anus and rectum
Excludes1: *fissure and fistula of anus and rectum (K60.-)*
ulcerative colitis (K51.-)
K62.7 Radiation proctitis
Use additional code to identify the type of radiation (W88.-) or radiation therapy (Y84.2)
AHA CC: 1Q, 2019, 21
+ K62.8 Other specified diseases of anus and rectum
Excludes2: *ulcerative proctitis (K51.2)*
K62.81 Anal sphincter tear (healed) (nontraumatic) (old)
Tear of anus, nontraumatic
Use additional code for any associated fecal incontinence (R15.-)
Excludes2: *anal fissure (K60.-)*
anal sphincter tear (healed) (old) complicating delivery (O34.7-)
traumatic tear of anal sphincter (S31.831)
K62.82 Dysplasia of anus
Anal intraepithelial neoplasia I and II (AIN I and II) (histologically confirmed)
Dysplasia of anus NOS
Mild and moderate dysplasia of anus (histologically confirmed)
Excludes1: *abnormal results from anal cytologic examination without histologic confirmation (R85.61-)*
anal intraepithelial neoplasia III (D01.3)
carcinoma in situ of anus (D01.3)
HGSIL of anus (R85.613)
severe dysplasia of anus (D01.3)

K62.89 Other specified diseases of anus and rectum
  Proctitis NOS
  Use additional code for any associated fecal incontinence (R15.-)
K62.9 Disease of anus and rectum, unspecified

K63 Other diseases of intestine

CC **K63.0** Abscess of intestine
  Excludes1: *abscess of intestine with Crohn's disease (K50.014, K50.114, K50.814, K50.914,)*
    abscess of intestine with diverticular disease (K57.0, K57.2, K57.4, K57.8)
    abscess of intestine with ulcerative colitis (K51.014, K51.214, K51.314, K51.414, K51.514, K51.814, K51.914)
  Excludes2: *abscess of anal and rectal regions (K61.-)*
    abscess of appendix (K35.3-)

MCC **K63.1** Perforation of intestine (nontraumatic)
  Perforation (nontraumatic) of rectum
  Excludes1: *perforation (nontraumatic) of duodenum (K26.-)*
    perforation (nontraumatic) of intestine with diverticular disease (K57.0, K57.2, K57.4, K57.8)
  Excludes2: *perforation (nontraumatic) of appendix (K35.2-, K35.3-)*
  AHA CC: 2Q, 2020, 22

CC **K63.2** Fistula of intestine
  Excludes1: *fistula of duodenum (K31.6)*
    fistula of intestine with Crohn's disease (K50.013, K50.113, K50.813, K50.913,)
    fistula of intestine with ulcerative colitis (K51.013, K51.213, K51.313, K51.413, K51.513, K51.813, K51.913)
  Excludes2: *fistula of anal and rectal regions (K60.-)*
    fistula of appendix (K38.3)
    intestinal-genital fistula, female (N82.2-N82.4)
    vesicointestinal fistula (N32.1)
  AHA CC: 3Q, 2017, 4-5

CC **K63.3** Ulcer of intestine
  Primary ulcer of small intestine
  Excludes1: *duodenal ulcer (K26.-)*
    gastrointestinal ulcer (K28.-)
    gastrojejunal ulcer (K28.-)
    jejunal ulcer (K28.-)
    peptic ulcer, site unspecified (K27.-)
    ulcer of intestine with perforation (K63.1)
    ulcer of anus or rectum (K62.6)
    ulcerative colitis (K51.-)

CC **K63.4** Enteroptosis
K63.5 Polyp of colon
  Excludes2: *adenomatous polyp of colon (D12.-)*
    inflammatory polyp of colon (K51.4-)
    polyposis of colon (D12.6)
  AHA CC: 2Q, 2015, 14; 1Q, 2017, 15-16; 1Q, 2019, 33

+ **K63.8** Other specified diseases of intestine
  MCC **K63.81** Dieulafoy lesion of intestine
    Excludes2: *Dieulafoy lesion of stomach and duodenum (K31.82)*
  + **K63.82** Intestinal microbial overgrowth
    + **K63.821** Small intestinal bacterial overgrowth
      K63.8211 Small intestinal bacterial overgrowth, hydrogen-subtype
      K63.8212 Small intestinal bacterial overgrowth, hydrogen sulfide-subtype
      K63.8219 Small intestinal bacterial overgrowth, unspecified
    K63.822 Small intestinal fungal overgrowth
    K63.829 Intestinal methanogen overgrowth, unspecified
  K63.89 Other specified diseases of intestine
K63.9 Disease of intestine, unspecified

K64 Hemorrhoids and perianal venous thrombosis

  Includes: piles
  Excludes1: *hemorrhoids complicating childbirth and the puerperium (O87.2)*
    hemorrhoids complicating pregnancy (O22.4)

K64.0 First degree hemorrhoids
  Grade/stage I hemorrhoids
  Hemorrhoids (bleeding) without prolapse outside of anal canal
K64.1 Second degree hemorrhoids
  Grade/stage II hemorrhoids
  Hemorrhoids (bleeding) that prolapse with straining, but retract spontaneously
K64.2 Third degree hemorrhoids
  Grade/stage III hemorrhoids
  Hemorrhoids (bleeding) that prolapse with straining and require manual replacement back inside anal canal
K64.3 Fourth degree hemorrhoids
  Grade/stage IV hemorrhoids
  Hemorrhoids (bleeding) with prolapsed tissue that cannot be manually replaced
K64.4 Residual hemorrhoidal skin tags
  External hemorrhoids, NOS
  Skin tags of anus
K64.5 Perianal venous thrombosis
  External hemorrhoids with thrombosis
  Perianal hematoma
  Thrombosed hemorrhoids NOS
K64.8 Other hemorrhoids
  Internal hemorrhoids, without mention of degree
  Prolapsed hemorrhoids, degree not specified
  AHA CC: 3Q, 2018, 22
K64.9 Unspecified hemorrhoids
  Hemorrhoids (bleeding) NOS
  Hemorrhoids (bleeding) without mention of degree

Diseases of peritoneum and retroperitoneum (K65-K68)

K65 Peritonitis

  Use additional code (B95-B97), to identify infectious agent, if known

  Code also if applicable diverticular disease of intestine (K57.-)
  Excludes1: *acute appendicitis with generalized peritonitis (K35.2-)*
    aseptic peritonitis (T81.6)
    benign paroxysmal peritonitis (E85.0)
    chemical peritonitis (T81.6)
    gonococcal peritonitis (A54.85)
    neonatal peritonitis (P78.0-P78.1)
    pelvic peritonitis, female (N73.3-N73.5)
    periodic familial peritonitis (E85.0)
    peritonitis due to talc or other foreign substance (T81.6)
    peritonitis in chlamydia (A74.81)
    peritonitis in diphtheria (A36.89)
    peritonitis in syphilis (late) (A52.74)
    peritonitis in tuberculosis (A18.31)
    peritonitis with or following abortion or ectopic or molar pregnancy (O00-O07, O08.0)
    peritonitis with or following appendicitis (K35.-)
    puerperal peritonitis (O85)
    retroperitoneal infections (K68.-)

MCC **K65.0** Generalized (acute) peritonitis
  Pelvic peritonitis (acute), male
  Subphrenic peritonitis (acute)
  Suppurative peritonitis (acute)
MCC **K65.1** Peritoneal abscess
  Abdominopelvic abscess
  Abscess (of) omentum
  Abscess (of) peritoneum
  Mesenteric abscess
  Retrocecal abscess
  Subdiaphragmatic abscess
  Subhepatic abscess
  Subphrenic abscess
  AHA CC: 1Q, 2019, 15-16; 1Q, 2022, 26
MCC **K65.2** Spontaneous bacterial peritonitis
  Excludes1: *bacterial peritonitis NOS (K65.9)*
MCC **K65.3** Choleperitonitis
  Peritonitis due to bile

CC **K65.4** **Sclerosing mesenteritis**
　　　　Fat necrosis of peritoneum
　　　　(Idiopathic) sclerosing mesenteric fibrosis
　　　　Mesenteric lipodystrophy
　　　　Mesenteric panniculitis
　　　　Retractile mesenteritis
MCC **K65.8** **Other peritonitis**
　　　　Chronic proliferative peritonitis
　　　　Peritonitis due to urine
MCC **K65.9** **Peritonitis, unspecified**
　　　　Bacterial peritonitis NOS
　　　　AHA CC: 2Q, 2013, 31; 1Q, 2022, 27

K66 **Other disorders of peritoneum**
　　Excludes2: ascites (R18.-)
　　　　　　　peritoneal effusion (chronic) (R18.8)
　　K66.0 **Peritoneal adhesions (postprocedural) (postinfection)**
　　　　Adhesions (of) abdominal (wall)
　　　　Adhesions (of) diaphragm
　　　　Adhesions (of) intestine
　　　　Adhesions (of) male pelvis
　　　　Adhesions (of) omentum
　　　　Adhesions (of) stomach
　　　　Adhesive bands
　　　　Mesenteric adhesions
　　　　Excludes1: female pelvic adhesions [bands] (N73.6)
　　　　　　　　peritoneal adhesions with intestinal obstruction (K56.5-)
MCC **K66.1** **Hemoperitoneum**
　　　　Peritoneal hematoma
　　　　Peritoneal hemorrhage
　　　　Excludes1: traumatic hemoperitoneum (S36.8-)
　　　　Excludes2: retroperitoneal hematoma (K68.3)
　　　　　　　　retroperitoneal hemorrhage (K68.3)
　　　　AHA CC: 1Q, 2022, 22-23
　　K66.8 **Other specified disorders of peritoneum**
　　K66.9 **Disorder of peritoneum, unspecified**

MCC **K67** **Disorders of peritoneum in infectious diseases classified elsewhere**
　　Code first underlying disease, such as:
　　　　congenital syphilis (A50.0)
　　　　helminthiasis (B65.0-B83.9)
　　Excludes1: peritonitis in chlamydia (A74.81)
　　　　　　　peritonitis in diphtheria (A36.89)
　　　　　　　peritonitis in gonococcal (A54.85)
　　　　　　　peritonitis in syphilis (late) (A52.74)
　　　　　　　peritonitis in tuberculosis (A18.31)
　　Valid 3-character code, no further characters required

K68 **Disorders of retroperitoneum**
　+ **K68.1** **Retroperitoneal abscess**
　　CC **K68.11** **Postprocedural retroperitoneal abscess**
　　　　Excludes2: infection following procedure (T81.4-)
　　　　HAC see Appendix B for HAC conditional logic
　　MCC **K68.12** **Psoas muscle abscess**
　　MCC **K68.19** **Other retroperitoneal abscess**
　　　　AHA CC: 1Q, 2019, 15-16; 2Q, 2023, 27-28
　MCC **K68.2** **Retroperitoneal fibrosis**
　　　　Code also, if applicable, associated obstruction of ureter (N13.5)
　MCC **K68.3** **Retroperitoneal hematoma**
　　　　Retroperitoneal hemorrhage
　MCC **K68.9** **Other disorders of retroperitoneum**

Diseases of liver (K70-K77)

Excludes1: jaundice NOS (R17)
Excludes2: hemochromatosis (E83.11-)
　　　　　　Reye's syndrome (G93.7)
　　　　　　viral hepatitis (B15-B19)
　　　　　　Wilson's disease (E83.01)

K70 **Alcoholic liver disease**
　　Use additional code to identify:
　　　　alcohol abuse and dependence (F10.-)
　• **K70.0** **Alcoholic fatty liver**
　+ **K70.1** **Alcoholic hepatitis**
　　• **K70.10** **Alcoholic hepatitis without ascites**
　　　K70.11 **Alcoholic hepatitis with ascites**
　• **K70.2** **Alcoholic fibrosis and sclerosis of liver**
　+ **K70.3** **Alcoholic cirrhosis of liver**
　　　　Alcoholic cirrhosis NOS
　　• **K70.30** **Alcoholic cirrhosis of liver without ascites**
　　• **K70.31** **Alcoholic cirrhosis of liver with ascites**
　+ **K70.4** **Alcoholic hepatic failure**
　　　　Acute alcoholic hepatic failure
　　　　Alcoholic hepatic failure NOS
　　　　Chronic alcoholic hepatic failure
　　　　Subacute alcoholic hepatic failure
　　• **K70.40** **Alcoholic hepatic failure without coma**
　　• **MCC** **K70.41** **Alcoholic hepatic failure with coma**
　• **K70.9** **Alcoholic liver disease, unspecified**

K71 **Toxic liver disease**
　　Includes: drug-induced idiosyncratic (unpredictable) liver disease
　　　　　　drug-induced toxic (predictable) liver disease
　　Code first poisoning due to drug or toxin, if applicable (T36-T65 with fifth or sixth character 1-4)
　　Use additional code for adverse effect, if applicable, to identify drug (T36-T50 with fifth or sixth character 5)
　　Excludes2: alcoholic liver disease (K70.-)
　　　　　　　Budd-Chiari syndrome (I82.0)
　K71.0 **Toxic liver disease with cholestasis**
　　　　Cholestasis with hepatocyte injury
　　　　'Pure' cholestasis
　+ **K71.1** **Toxic liver disease with hepatic necrosis**
　　　　Hepatic failure (acute) (chronic) due to drugs
　　　K71.10 **Toxic liver disease with hepatic necrosis, without coma**
　　MCC **K71.11** **Toxic liver disease with hepatic necrosis, with coma**
　　K71.2 **Toxic liver disease with acute hepatitis**
　　K71.3 **Toxic liver disease with chronic persistent hepatitis**
　　K71.4 **Toxic liver disease with chronic lobular hepatitis**
　+ **K71.5** **Toxic liver disease with chronic active hepatitis**
　　　　Toxic liver disease with lupoid hepatitis
　　　K71.50 **Toxic liver disease with chronic active hepatitis without ascites**
　　　K71.51 **Toxic liver disease with chronic active hepatitis with ascites**
　　K71.6 **Toxic liver disease with hepatitis, not elsewhere classified**
　　K71.7 **Toxic liver disease with fibrosis and cirrhosis of liver**
　　K71.8 **Toxic liver disease with other disorders of liver**
　　　　Toxic liver disease with focal nodular hyperplasia
　　　　Toxic liver disease with hepatic granulomas
　　　　Toxic liver disease with peliosis hepatis
　　　　Toxic liver disease with veno-occlusive disease of liver
　　K71.9 **Toxic liver disease, unspecified**

K72 **Hepatic failure, not elsewhere classified**
　　Includes: fulminant hepatitis NEC, with hepatic failure
　　　　　　liver (cell) necrosis with hepatic failure
　　　　　　malignant hepatitis NEC, with hepatic failure
　　　　　　yellow liver atrophy or dystrophy
　　Excludes1: alcoholic hepatic failure (K70.4)
　　　　　　　hepatic failure with toxic liver disease (K71.1-)
　　　　　　　icterus of newborn (P55-P59)
　　　　　　　postprocedural hepatic failure (K91.82)
　　Excludes2: hepatic failure complicating abortion or ectopic or molar pregnancy (O00-O07, O08.8)
　　　　　　　hepatic failure complicating pregnancy, childbirth and the puerperium (O26.6-)
　　　　　　　viral hepatitis with hepatic coma (B15-B19)
　+ **K72.0** **Acute and subacute hepatic failure**
　　　　Acute non-viral hepatitis NOS
　　　AHA CC: 2Q, 2014, 13
　　MCC **K72.00** **Acute and subacute hepatic failure without coma**
　　　AHA CC: 1Q, 2021, 13
　　MCC **K72.01** **Acute and subacute hepatic failure with coma**
　+ **K72.1** **Chronic hepatic failure**
　　　　End stage liver disease
　　　K72.10 **Chronic hepatic failure without coma**
　　　　AHA CC: 1Q, 2017, 41; 1Q, 2021, 13
　　MCC **K72.11** **Chronic hepatic failure with coma**
　+ **K72.9** **Hepatic failure, unspecified**
　　　K72.90 **Hepatic failure, unspecified without coma**
　　　　AHA CC: 2Q, 2016, 35; 4Q, 2018, 21; 1Q, 2022, 52-53
　　MCC **K72.91** **Hepatic failure, unspecified with coma**
　　　　Hepatic coma NOS

K73 **Chronic hepatitis, not elsewhere classified**
　　Excludes1: alcoholic hepatitis (chronic) (K70.1-)
　　　　　　　drug-induced hepatitis (chronic) (K71.-)
　　　　　　　granulomatous hepatitis (chronic) NEC (K75.3)
　　　　　　　reactive, nonspecific hepatitis (chronic) (K75.2)
　　　　　　　viral hepatitis (chronic) (B15-B19)

767

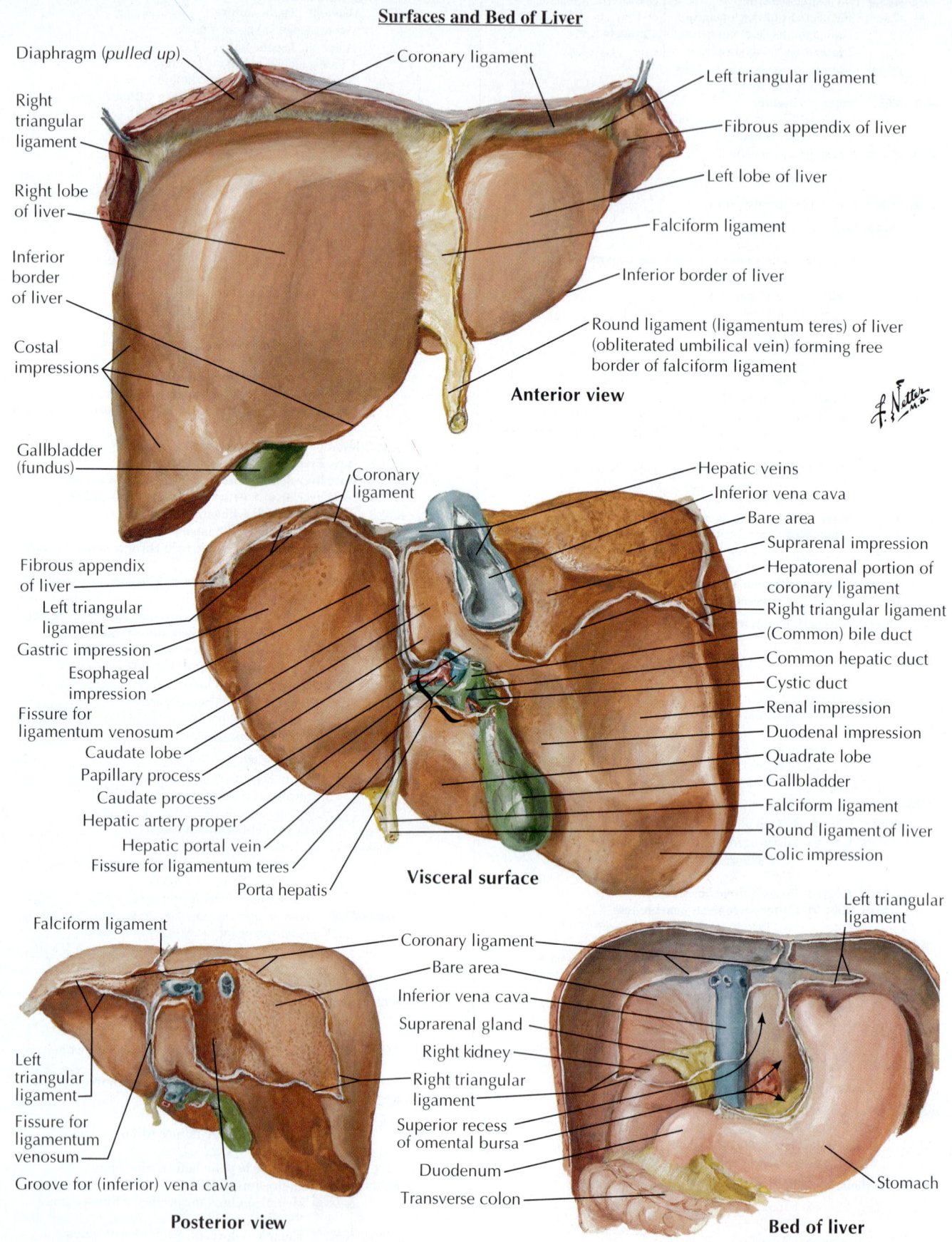

K73.0 Chronic persistent hepatitis, not elsewhere classified
K73.1 Chronic lobular hepatitis, not elsewhere classified
K73.2 Chronic active hepatitis, not elsewhere classified
K73.8 Other chronic hepatitis, not elsewhere classified
K73.9 Chronic hepatitis, unspecified

K74 Fibrosis and cirrhosis of liver
Code also, if applicable, viral hepatitis (acute) (chronic) (B15-B19)
Excludes1: alcoholic cirrhosis (of liver) (K70.3)
alcoholic fibrosis of liver (K70.2)
cardiac sclerosis of liver (K76.1)
cirrhosis (of liver) with toxic liver disease (K71.7)
congenital cirrhosis (of liver) (P78.81)
pigmentary cirrhosis (of liver) (E83.110)

+ **K74.0** Hepatic fibrosis
Code first underlying liver disease such as:
nonalcoholic steatohepatitis (NASH) (K57.81)
AHA CC: 4Q, 2020, 30-31
K74.00 Hepatic fibrosis, unspecified
K74.01 Hepatic fibrosis, early fibrosis
Hepatic fibrosis, stage F1 or stage F2
K74.02 Hepatic fibrosis, advanced fibrosis
Hepatic fibrosis, stage 3
Excludes1: cirrhosis of liver (K74.6-)
hepatic fibrosis, stage F4 (K74.6-)
K74.1 Hepatic sclerosis
K74.2 Hepatic fibrosis with hepatic sclerosis
K74.3 Primary biliary cirrhosis
Chronic nonsuppurative destructive cholangitis
Primary biliary cholangitis
Excludes2: primary sclerosing cholangitis (K83.01)
K74.4 Secondary biliary cirrhosis
K74.5 Biliary cirrhosis, unspecified
+ **K74.6** Other and unspecified cirrhosis of liver
K74.60 Unspecified cirrhosis of liver
Cirrhosis (of liver) NOS
AHA CC: 1Q, 2018, 4-5
K74.69 Other cirrhosis of liver
Cryptogenic cirrhosis (of liver)
Macronodular cirrhosis (of liver)
Micronodular cirrhosis (of liver)
Mixed type cirrhosis (of liver)
Portal cirrhosis (of liver)
Postnecrotic cirrhosis (of liver)

K75 Other inflammatory liver diseases
Excludes2: toxic liver disease (K71.-)
MCC **K75.0** Abscess of liver
Cholangitic hepatic abscess
Hematogenic hepatic abscess
Hepatic abscess NOS
Lymphogenic hepatic abscess
Pylephlebitic hepatic abscess
Excludes1: amebic liver abscess (A06.4)
cholangitis without liver abscess (K83.09)
pylephlebitis without liver abscess (K75.1)
Excludes2: acute or subacute hepatitis NOS (B17.9)
acute or subacute non-viral hepatitis (K72.0)
chronic hepatitis NEC (K73.8)
MCC **K75.1** Phlebitis of portal vein
Pylephlebitis
Excludes1: pylephlebitic liver abscess (K75.0)
K75.2 Nonspecific reactive hepatitis
Excludes1: acute or subacute hepatitis (K72.0-)
chronic hepatitis NEC (K73.-)
viral hepatitis (B15-B19)
K75.3 Granulomatous hepatitis, not elsewhere classified
Excludes1: acute or subacute hepatitis (K72.0-)
chronic hepatitis NEC (K73.-)
viral hepatitis (B15-B19)
K75.4 Autoimmune hepatitis
Lupoid hepatitis NEC
+ **K75.8** Other specified inflammatory liver diseases
K75.81 Nonalcoholic steatohepatitis (NASH)
Use additional code, if applicable, hepatic fibrosis (K74.0)
K75.89 Other specified inflammatory liver diseases
K75.9 Inflammatory liver disease, unspecified
Hepatitis NOS
Excludes1: acute or subacute hepatitis (K72.0-)
chronic hepatitis NEC (K73.-)
viral hepatitis (B15-B19)

K76 Other diseases of liver
Excludes2: alcoholic liver disease (K70.-)
amyloid degeneration of liver (E85.-)
cystic disease of liver (congenital) (Q44.6)
hepatic vein thrombosis (I82.0)
hepatomegaly NOS (R16.0)
pigmentary cirrhosis (of liver) (E83.110)
portal vein thrombosis (I81)
toxic liver disease (K71.-)
K76.0 Fatty (change of) liver, not elsewhere classified
Nonalcoholic fatty liver disease (NAFLD)
Excludes1: nonalcoholic steatohepatitis (NASH) (K75.81)
K76.1 Chronic passive congestion of liver
Cardiac cirrhosis
Cardiac sclerosis
MCC **K76.2** Central hemorrhagic necrosis of liver
Excludes1: liver necrosis with hepatic failure (K72.-)
MCC **K76.3** Infarction of liver
K76.4 Peliosis hepatis
Hepatic angiomatosis
K76.5 Hepatic veno-occlusive disease
Excludes1: Budd-Chiari syndrome (I82.0)
CC **K76.6** Portal hypertension
Use additional code for any associated complications, such as:
portal hypertensive gastropathy (K31.89)
AHA CC: 1Q, 2020, 15
MCC **K76.7** Hepatorenal syndrome
Excludes1: hepatorenal syndrome following labor and delivery (O90.41)
postprocedural hepatorenal syndrome (K91.83)
+ **K76.8** Other specified diseases of liver
AHA CC: 4Q, 2022, 27-28
K76.81 Hepatopulmonary syndrome
Code first underlying liver disease, such as:
alcoholic cirrhosis of liver (K70.3-)
cirrhosis of liver without mention of alcohol (K74.6-)
K76.82 Hepatic encephalopathy
Hepatic encephalopathy, NOS
Hepatic encephalopathy without coma
Hepatocerebral intoxication
Portal-systemic encephalopathy
Code also underlying liver disease, such as:
acute and subacute hepatic failure without coma (K72.00)
alcoholic hepatic failure without coma (K70.40)
chronic hepatic failure without coma (K72.10)
hepatic failure with toxic liver disease without coma (K71.10)
hepatic failure without coma (K72.90)
icterus of newborn (P55-P59)
postprocedural hepatic failure (K91.82)
viral hepatitis without hepatic coma (B15.9, B16.1, B16.9, B17.10, B19.10, B19.20, B19.9)
Excludes1: acute and subacute hepatic failure with coma (K72.01)
alcoholic hepatic failure with coma (K70.41)
chronic hepatic failure with coma (K72.11)
hepatic failure with coma (K72.91)
K76.89 Other specified diseases of liver
Cyst (simple) of liver
Focal nodular hyperplasia of liver
Hepatoptosis
AHA CC: 3Q, 2022, 7; 1Q, 2023, 27
K76.9 Liver disease, unspecified

CC K77 Liver disorders in diseases classified elsewhere
Code first underlying disease, such as:
amyloidosis (E85.-)
congenital syphilis (A50.0, A50.5)
congenital toxoplasmosis (P37.1)
infectious mononucleosis with liver disease (B27.0-B27.9 with fifth character 9)
schistosomiasis (B65.0-B65.9)
Excludes1: alcoholic hepatitis (K70.1-)
alcoholic liver disease (K70.-)
cytomegaloviral hepatitis (B25.1)
herpesviral [herpes simplex] hepatitis (B00.81)
mumps hepatitis (B26.81)
sarcoidosis with liver disease (D86.89)

Cholelithiasis (Gallstones)

Sudden obstruction (biliary colic)

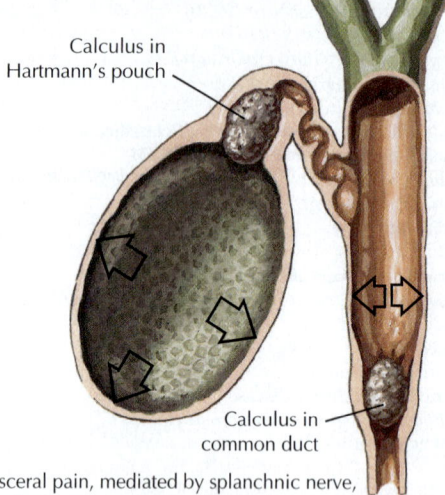

Calculus in Hartmann's pouch
Calculus in common duct

Visceral pain, mediated by splanchnic nerve, results from increased intraluminal pressure and distention caused by sudden calculous obstruction of cystic or common duct.

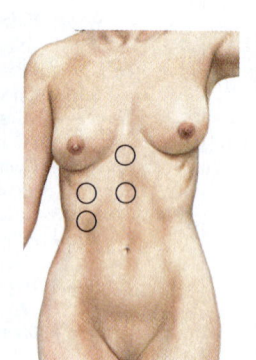

Sites of pain in biliary colic

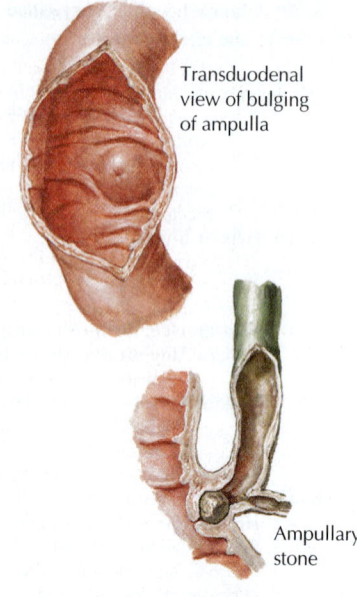

Transduodenal view of bulging of ampulla

Ampullary stone

Persistent obstruction (acute cholecystitis)

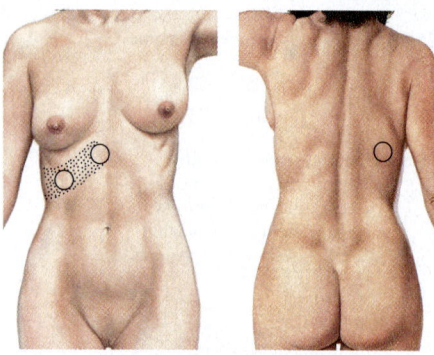

Sites of pain and hyperesthesia in acute cholecystitis

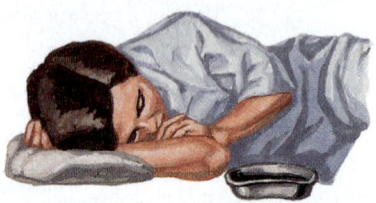

Patient lies motionless because jarring or respiration increases pain. Nausea is common.

Edema, ischemia, and transmural inflammation

Parietal epigastric or right upper quadrant pain results from ischemia and inflammation of gallbladder wall caused by persistent calculous obstruction of cystic duct. Prostaglandins are released.

© Elsevier Inc. All rights reserved. www.netterimages.com

secondary syphilis with liver disease (A51.45)
syphilis (late) with liver disease (A52.74)
toxoplasmosis (acquired) hepatitis (B58.1)
tuberculosis with liver disease (A18.83)
Valid 3-character code, no further characters required

Disorders of gallbladder, biliary tract and pancreas (K80-K87)

K80 Cholelithiasis

Excludes1: *retained cholelithiasis following cholecystectomy (K91.86)*

+ **K80.0** Calculus of gallbladder with acute cholecystitis
Any condition listed in K80.2 with acute cholecystitis
Use additional code if applicable for associated gangrene of gallbladder (K82.A1), or perforation of gallbladder (K82.A2)

CC **K80.00** Calculus of gallbladder with acute cholecystitis without obstruction
AHA CC: 4Q, 2018, 20; 2Q, 2023, 11-12

CC **K80.01** Calculus of gallbladder with acute cholecystitis with obstruction

+ **K80.1** Calculus of gallbladder with other cholecystitis
Use additional code if applicable for associated gangrene of gallbladder (K82.A1), or perforation of gallbladder (K82.A2)

CC **K80.10** Calculus of gallbladder with chronic cholecystitis without obstruction
Cholelithiasis with cholecystitis NOS

CC **K80.11** Calculus of gallbladder with chronic cholecystitis with obstruction

CC **K80.12** Calculus of gallbladder with acute and chronic cholecystitis without obstruction

CC **K80.13** Calculus of gallbladder with acute and chronic cholecystitis with obstruction

CC **K80.18** Calculus of gallbladder with other cholecystitis without obstruction

- **CC K80.19 Calculus of gallbladder with other cholecystitis with obstruction**
- **+ K80.2 Calculus of gallbladder without cholecystitis**
  - Cholecystolithiasis without cholecystitis
  - Cholelithiasis (without cholecystitis)
  - Colic (recurrent) of gallbladder (without cholecystitis)
  - Gallstone (impacted) of cystic duct (without cholecystitis)
  - Gallstone (impacted) of gallbladder (without cholecystitis)
  - **K80.20 Calculus of gallbladder without cholecystitis without obstruction**
  - **CC K80.21 Calculus of gallbladder without cholecystitis with obstruction**
- **+ K80.3 Calculus of bile duct with cholangitis**
  - Any condition listed in K80.5 with cholangitis
  - **CC K80.30 Calculus of bile duct with cholangitis, unspecified, without obstruction**
  - **CC K80.31 Calculus of bile duct with cholangitis, unspecified, with obstruction**
  - **CC K80.32 Calculus of bile duct with acute cholangitis without obstruction**
  - **CC K80.33 Calculus of bile duct with acute cholangitis with obstruction**
  - **CC K80.34 Calculus of bile duct with chronic cholangitis without obstruction**
  - **CC K80.35 Calculus of bile duct with chronic cholangitis with obstruction**
  - **CC K80.36 Calculus of bile duct with acute and chronic cholangitis without obstruction**
  - **CC K80.37 Calculus of bile duct with acute and chronic cholangitis with obstruction**
- **+ K80.4 Calculus of bile duct with cholecystitis**
  - Any condition listed in K80.5 with cholecystitis (with cholangitis)
  - Code also, if applicable, fistula of bile duct (K83.3)
  - Use additional code if applicable for associated gangrene of gallbladder (K82.A1), or perforation of gallbladder (K82.A2)
  - **CC K80.40 Calculus of bile duct with cholecystitis, unspecified, without obstruction**
  - **CC K80.41 Calculus of bile duct with cholecystitis, unspecified, with obstruction**
    - *AHA CC: 1Q, 2019, 17-18*
  - **CC K80.42 Calculus of bile duct with acute cholecystitis without obstruction**
  - **CC K80.43 Calculus of bile duct with acute cholecystitis with obstruction**
  - **CC K80.44 Calculus of bile duct with chronic cholecystitis without obstruction**
  - **CC K80.45 Calculus of bile duct with chronic cholecystitis with obstruction**
  - **CC K80.46 Calculus of bile duct with acute and chronic cholecystitis without obstruction**
  - **CC K80.47 Calculus of bile duct with acute and chronic cholecystitis with obstruction**
- **+ K80.5 Calculus of bile duct without cholangitis or cholecystitis**
  - Choledocholithiasis (without cholangitis or cholecystitis)
  - Gallstone (impacted) of bile duct NOS (without cholangitis or cholecystitis)
  - Gallstone (impacted) of common duct (without cholangitis or cholecystitis)
  - Gallstone (impacted) of hepatic duct (without cholangitis or cholecystitis)
  - Hepatic cholelithiasis (without cholangitis or cholecystitis)
  - Hepatic colic (recurrent) (without cholangitis or cholecystitis)
  - **K80.50 Calculus of bile duct without cholangitis or cholecystitis without obstruction**
  - **CC K80.51 Calculus of bile duct without cholangitis or cholecystitis with obstruction**
- **+ K80.6 Calculus of gallbladder and bile duct with cholecystitis**
  - Use additional code if applicable for associated gangrene of gallbladder (K82.A1), or perforation of gallbladder (K82.A2)
  - **CC K80.60 Calculus of gallbladder and bile duct with cholecystitis, unspecified, without obstruction**
  - **CC K80.61 Calculus of gallbladder and bile duct with cholecystitis, unspecified, with obstruction**
  - **CC K80.62 Calculus of gallbladder and bile duct with acute cholecystitis without obstruction**
  - **CC K80.63 Calculus of gallbladder and bile duct with acute cholecystitis with obstruction**
- **CC K80.64 Calculus of gallbladder and bile duct with chronic cholecystitis without obstruction**
- **CC K80.65 Calculus of gallbladder and bile duct with chronic cholecystitis with obstruction**
- **CC K80.66 Calculus of gallbladder and bile duct with acute and chronic cholecystitis without obstruction**
- **MCC K80.67 Calculus of gallbladder and bile duct with acute and chronic cholecystitis with obstruction**
- **+ K80.7 Calculus of gallbladder and bile duct without cholecystitis**
  - **K80.70 Calculus of gallbladder and bile duct without cholecystitis without obstruction**
  - **CC K80.71 Calculus of gallbladder and bile duct without cholecystitis with obstruction**
- **+ K80.8 Other cholelithiasis**
  - **K80.80 Other cholelithiasis without obstruction**
  - **CC K80.81 Other cholelithiasis with obstruction**

K81 Cholecystitis

Excludes1: cholecystitis with cholelithiasis (K80.-)
Use additional code if applicable for associated gangrene of gallbladder (K82.A1), or perforation of gallbladder (K82.A2)

- **K81.0 Acute cholecystitis**
  - Abscess of gallbladder
  - Angiocholecystitis
  - Emphysematous (acute) cholecystitis
  - Empyema of gallbladder
  - Gangrene of gallbladder
  - Gangrenous cholecystitis
  - Suppurative cholecystitis
- **K81.1 Chronic cholecystitis**
- **CC K81.2 Acute cholecystitis with chronic cholecystitis**
- **K81.9 Cholecystitis, unspecified**

K82 Other diseases of gallbladder

Excludes1: nonvisualization of gallbladder (R93.2)
postcholecystectomy syndrome (K91.5)

- **CC K82.0 Obstruction of gallbladder**
  - Occlusion of cystic duct or gallbladder without cholelithiasis
  - Stenosis of cystic duct or gallbladder without cholelithiasis
  - Stricture of cystic duct or gallbladder without cholelithiasis
  - *Excludes1:* obstruction of gallbladder with cholelithiasis (K80.-)
- **CC K82.1 Hydrops of gallbladder**
  - Mucocele of gallbladder
- **MCC K82.2 Perforation of gallbladder**
  - Rupture of cystic duct or gallbladder
  - *Exlcudes1:* Perforation of gallbladder in cholecystitis (K82.A2)
- **CC K82.3 Fistula of gallbladder**
  - Cholecystocolic fistula
  - Cholecystoduodenal fistula
- **K82.4 Cholesterolosis of gallbladder**
  - Strawberry gallbladder
  - *Excludes1:* cholesterolosis of gallbladder with cholecystitis (K81.-)
  - cholesterolosis of gallbladder with cholelithiasis (K80.-)
- **K82.8 Other specified diseases of gallbladder**
  - Adhesions of cystic duct or gallbladder
  - Atrophy of cystic duct or gallbladder
  - Cyst of cystic duct or gallbladder
  - Dyskinesia of cystic duct or gallbladder
  - Hypertrophy of cystic duct or gallbladder
  - Nonfunctioning of cystic duct or gallbladder
  - Ulcer of cystic duct or gallbladder
- **K82.9 Disease of gallbladder, unspecified**
- **+ K82.A Disorders of gallbladder in diseases classified elsewhere**
  - Code first the type of cholecystitis (K81.-), or cholelithiasis with cholecystitis (K80.00-K80.19, K80.40-K80.47, K80.60-K80.67)
  - **K82.A1 Gangrene of gallbladder in cholecystitis**
    - *AHA CC: 4Q, 2018, 19-20*
  - **CC K82.A2 Perforation of gallbladder in cholecystitis**
    - *AHA CC: 4Q, 2018, 19-20*

K83 Other diseases of biliary tract

Excludes1: postcholecystectomy syndrome (K91.5)
Excludes2: conditions involving the gallbladder (K81-K82)
conditions involving the cystic duct (K81-K82)

- **+ K83.0 Cholangitis**
  - *Excludes1:* cholangitic liver abscess (K75.0)

Acute Pancreatitis

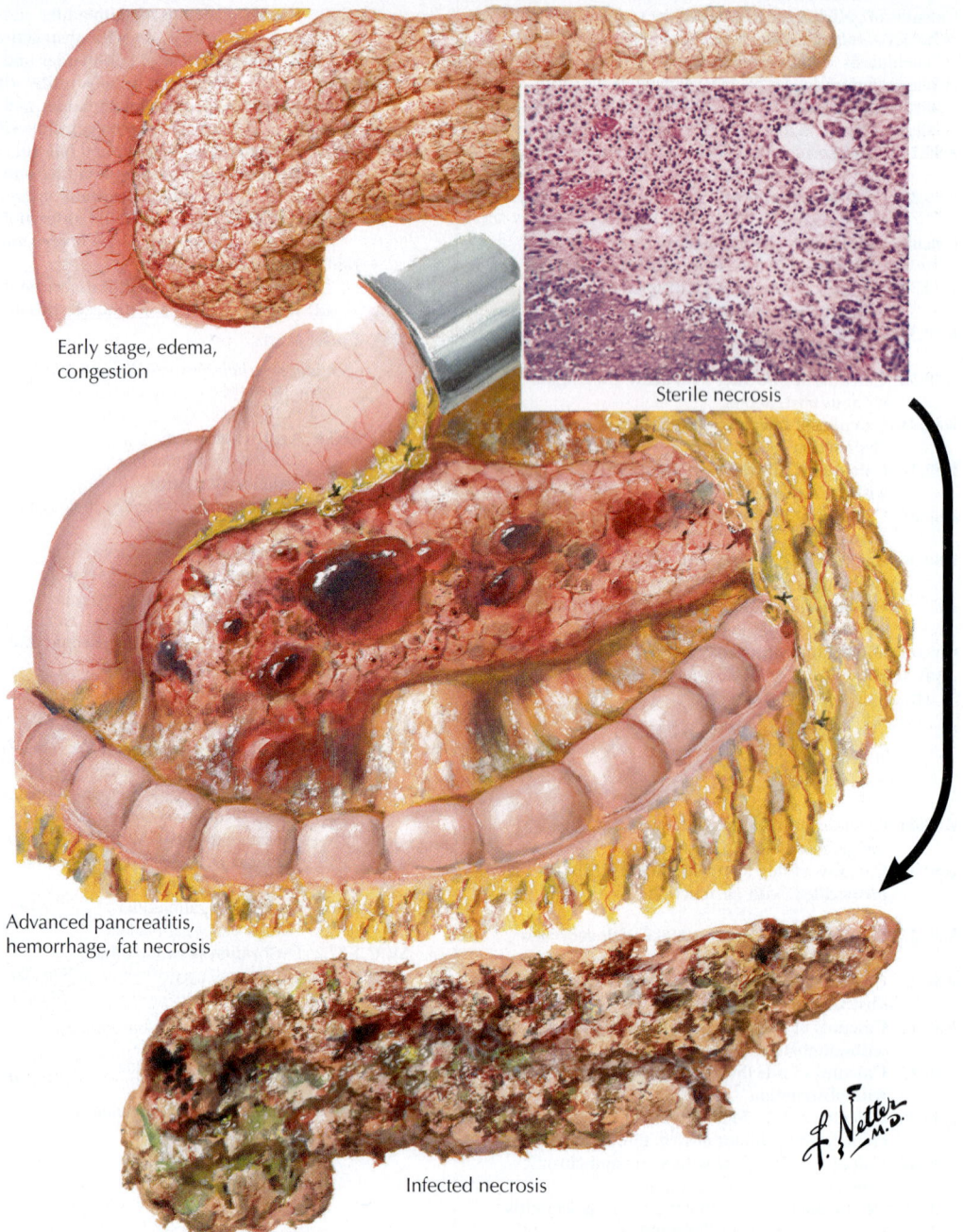

Early stage, edema, congestion

Sterile necrosis

Advanced pancreatitis, hemorrhage, fat necrosis

Infected necrosis

© 2020 Elsevier Inc. All rights reserved. www.netterimages.com

        cholangitis with choledocholithiasis (K80.3-, K80.4-)
Excludes2: *chronic nonsuppurative destructive cholangitis (K74.3)*
        primary biliary cholangitis (K74.3)
        primary biliary cirrhosis (K74.3)
        AHA CC: 4Q, 2018, 20
CC K83.01 Primary sclerosing cholangitis
        AHA CC: 4Q, 2018, 21
CC K83.09 Other cholangitis
        Ascending cholangitis
        Cholangitis NOS
        Primary cholangitis
        Recurrent cholangitis
        Sclerosing cholangitis
        Secondary cholangitis
        Stenosing cholangitis
        Suppurative cholangitis
MCC K83.1 Obstruction of bile duct
        Occlusion of bile duct without cholelithiasis
        Stenosis of bile duct without cholelithiasis
        Stricture of bile duct without cholelithiasis
Excludes1: *congenital obstruction of bile duct (Q44.3)*
        obstruction of bile duct with cholelithiasis (K80.-)
        CC AHA: 1Q, 2016, 18-19
MCC K83.2 Perforation of bile duct
        Rupture of bile duct
CC K83.3 Fistula of bile duct
        Choledochoduodenal fistula
        AHA CC: 1Q, 2019, 17-18
K83.4 Spasm of sphincter of Oddi
K83.5 Biliary cyst
K83.8 Other specified diseases of biliary tract
        Adhesions of biliary tract
        Atrophy of biliary tract
        Hypertrophy of biliary tract
        Ulcer of biliary tract
K83.9 Disease of biliary tract, unspecified

K85 Acute pancreatitis
        Includes: acute (recurrent) pancreatitis
                  subacute pancreatitis
        AHA CC: 4Q, 2016, 34

- **+ K85.0** Idiopathic acute pancreatitis
  - **MCC K85.00** Idiopathic acute pancreatitis without necrosis or infection
  - **MCC K85.01** Idiopathic acute pancreatitis with uninfected necrosis
  - **MCC K85.02** Idiopathic acute pancreatitis with infected necrosis
- **+ K85.1** Biliary acute pancreatitis
  - Gallstone pancreatitis
  - **MCC K85.10** Biliary acute pancreatitis without necrosis or infection
    - *AHA CC: 2Q, 2023, 11-12*
  - **MCC K85.11** Biliary acute pancreatitis with uninfected necrosis
  - **MCC K85.12** Biliary acute pancreatitis with infected necrosis
- **+ K85.2** Alcohol induced acute pancreatitis
  - **Excludes2:** *alcohol induced chronic pancreatitis (K86.0)*
  - **MCC K85.20** Alcohol induced acute pancreatitis without necrosis or infection
    - *AHA CC: 1Q, 2020, 9*
  - **MCC K85.21** Alcohol induced acute pancreatitis with uninfected necrosis
  - **MCC K85.22** Alcohol induced acute pancreatitis with infected necrosis
- **+ K85.3** Drug induced acute pancreatitis
  - Use additional code for adverse effect, if applicable, to identify drug (T36-T50 with fifth or sixth character 5)
  - Use additional code to identify drug abuse and dependence (F11.-F17.-)
  - **MCC K85.30** Drug induced acute pancreatitis without necrosis or infection
  - **MCC K85.31** Drug induced acute pancreatitis with uninfected necrosis
  - **MCC K85.32** Drug induced acute pancreatitis with infected necrosis
- **+ K85.8** Other acute pancreatitis
  - **MCC K85.80** Other acute pancreatitis without necrosis or infection
  - **MCC K85.81** Other acute pancreatitis with uninfected necrosis
  - **MCC K85.82** Other acute pancreatitis with infected necrosis
- **+ K85.9** Acute pancreatitis, unspecified
  - Pancreatitis NOS
  - **MCC K85.90** Acute pancreatitis without necrosis or infection, unspecified
  - **MCC K85.91** Acute pancreatitis with uninfected necrosis, unspecified
  - **MCC K85.92** Acute pancreatitis with infected necrosis, unspecified

K86 Other diseases of pancreas
- **Excludes2:** *fibrocystic disease of pancreas (E84.-)*
  islet cell tumor (of pancreas) (D13.7)
  pancreatic steatorrhea (K90.3)
- **CC K86.0** Alcohol-induced chronic pancreatitis
  - Use additional code to identify:
    alcohol abuse and dependence (F10.-)
  - Code also exocrine pancreatic insufficiency (K86.81)
  - **Excludes2:** *alcohol induced acute pancreatitis (K85.2-)*
- **CC K86.1** Other chronic pancreatitis
  - Chronic pancreatitis NOS
  - Infectious chronic pancreatitis
  - Recurrent chronic pancreatitis
  - Relapsing chronic pancreatitis
  - Code also exocrine pancreatic insufficiency (K86.81)
- **CC K86.2** Cyst of pancreas
- **CC K86.3** Pseudocyst of pancreas
- **+ K86.8** Other specified diseases of pancreas
  - *AHA CC: 4Q, 2016, 33*
  - **K86.81** Exocrine pancreatic insufficiency
  - **K86.89** Other specified diseases of pancreas
    - Aseptic pancreatic necrosis, unrelated to acute pancreatitis
    - Atrophy of pancreas
    - Calculus of pancreas
    - Cirrhosis of pancreas
    - Fibrosis of pancreas
    - Pancreatic fat necrosis, unrelated to acute pancreatitis
    - Pancreatic infantilism
    - Pancreatic necrosis NOS, unrelated to acute pancreatitis
- **K86.9** Disease of pancreas, unspecified

K87 Disorders of gallbladder, biliary tract and pancreas in diseases classified elsewhere
- Code first underlying disease
- **Excludes1:** *cytomegaloviral pancreatitis (B25.2)*
  mumps pancreatitis (B26.3)
  syphilitic gallbladder (A52.74)
  syphilitic pancreas (A52.74)
  tuberculosis of gallbladder (A18.83)
  tuberculosis of pancreas (A18.83)
- Valid 3-character code, no further characters required

Other diseases of the digestive system (K90-K95)

K90 Intestinal malabsorption
- **Excludes1:** *intestinal malabsorption following gastrointestinal surgery (K91.2)*
- **K90.0** Celiac disease
  - Celiac disease with steatorrhea
  - Celiac gluten-sensitive enteropathy
  - Nontropical sprue
  - Code also exocrine pancreatic insufficiency (K86.81)
  - Use additional code for associated disorders including:
    dermatitis herpetiformis (L13.0)
    gluten ataxia (G32.81)
- **CC K90.1** Tropical sprue
  - Sprue NOS
  - Tropical steatorrhea
- **CC K90.2** Blind loop syndrome, not elsewhere classified
  - Blind loop syndrome NOS
  - **Excludes1:** *congenital blind loop syndrome (Q43.8)*
    postsurgical blind loop syndrome (K91.2)
- **CC K90.3** Pancreatic steatorrhea
- **+ K90.4** Other malabsorption due to intolerance
  - **Excludes2:** *celiac gluten-sensitive enteropathy (K90.0)*
    lactose intolerance (E73.-)
  - **CC K90.41** Non-celiac gluten sensitivity
    - Gluten sensitivity NOS
    - Non-celiac gluten sensitive enteropathy
    - *AHA CC: 4Q, 2016, 35-36*
  - **CC K90.49** Malabsorption due to intolerance, not elsewhere classified
    - Malabsorption due to intolerance to carbohydrate
    - Malabsorption due to intolerance to fat
    - Malabsorption due to intolerance to protein
    - Malabsorption due to intolerance to starch
- **+ K90.8** Other intestinal malabsorption
  - **CC K90.81** Whipple's disease
  - **+ K90.82** Short bowel syndrome
    - Short gut syndrome
    - **CC K90.821** Short bowel syndrome with colon in continuity
      - Short bowel syndrome with colonic continuity
    - **CC K90.822** Short bowel syndrome without colon in continuity
      - Short bowel syndrome without colonic continuity
    - **CC K90.829** Short bowel syndrome, unspecified
  - **CC K90.83** Intestinal failure
  - **CC K90.89** Other intestinal malabsorption
- **CC K90.9** Intestinal malabsorption, unspecified
  - *AHA CC: 4Q, 2017, 108-109*

K91 Intraoperative and postprocedural complications and disorders of digestive system, not elsewhere classified
- **Excludes2:** *complications of artificial opening of digestive system (K94.-)*
  complications of bariatric procedures (K95.-)
  gastrojejunal ulcer (K28.-)
  postprocedural (radiation) retroperitoneal abscess (K68.11)
  radiation colitis (K52.0)
  radiation gastroenteritis (K52.0)
  radiation proctitis (K62.7)
- *AHA CC: 4Q, 2016, 9-10*
- **K91.0** Vomiting following gastrointestinal surgery
- **K91.1** Postgastric surgery syndromes
  - Dumping syndrome
  - Postgastrectomy syndrome
  - Postvagotomy syndrome

- **CC K91.2 Postsurgical malabsorption, not elsewhere classified**
  Postsurgical blind loop syndrome
  Excludes1: malabsorption osteomalacia in adults (M83.2)
  malabsorption osteoporosis, postsurgical (M80.8-, M81.8)
- **+ K91.3 Postprocedural intestinal obstruction**
  AHA CC: 4Q, 2017, 16-17
  - **CC K91.30 Postprocedural intestinal obstruction, unspecified as to partial versus complete**
    Postprocedural intestinal obstruction NOS
  - **CC K91.31 Postprocedural partial intestinal obstruction**
    Postprocedural incomplete intestinal obstruction
  - **CC K91.32 Postprocedural complete intestinal obstruction**
- **K91.5 Postcholecystectomy syndrome**
- **+ K91.6 Intraoperative hemorrhage and hematoma of a digestive system organ or structure complicating a procedure**
  Excludes1: intraoperative hemorrhage and hematoma of a digestive system organ or structure due to accidental puncture and laceration during a procedure (K91.7-)
  - **CC K91.61 Intraoperative hemorrhage and hematoma of a digestive system organ or structure complicating a digestive system procedure**
    AHA CC: 1Q, 2020, 19-20
  - **CC K91.62 Intraoperative hemorrhage and hematoma of a digestive system organ or structure complicating other procedure**
- **+ K91.7 Accidental puncture and laceration of a digestive system organ or structure during a procedure**
  - **CC K91.71 Accidental puncture and laceration of a digestive system organ or structure during a digestive system procedure**
    AHA CC: 2Q, 2021, 11-12
  - **CC K91.72 Accidental puncture and laceration of a digestive system organ or structure during other procedure**
    AHA CC: 2Q, 2019, 23-24
- **+ K91.8 Other intraoperative and postprocedural complications and disorders of digestive system**
  - **CC K91.81 Other intraoperative complications of digestive system**
  - **CC K91.82 Postprocedural hepatic failure**
  - **CC K91.83 Postprocedural hepatorenal syndrome**
  - **+ K91.84 Postprocedural hemorrhage of a digestive system organ or structure following a procedure**
    - **CC K91.840 Postprocedural hemorrhage of a digestive system organ or structure following a digestive system procedure**
      AHA CC: 1Q, 2016, 15
    - **CC K91.841 Postprocedural hemorrhage of a digestive system organ or structure following other procedure**
  - **+ K91.85 Complications of intestinal pouch**
    - **CC K91.850 Pouchitis**
      Inflammation of internal ileoanal pouch
    - **CC K91.858 Other complications of intestinal pouch**
      AHA CC: 2Q, 2019, 13
  - **CC K91.86 Retained cholelithiasis following cholecystectomy**
  - **+ K91.87 Postprocedural hematoma and seroma of a digestive system organ or structure following a procedure**
    - **CC K91.870 Postprocedural hematoma of a digestive system organ or structure following a digestive system procedure**
      AHA CC: 1Q, 2022, 24
    - **CC K91.871 Postprocedural hematoma of a digestive system organ or structure following other procedure**
    - **CC K91.872 Postprocedural seroma of a digestive system organ or structure following a digestive system procedure**
    - **CC K91.873 Postprocedural seroma of a digestive system organ or structure following other procedure**
  - **CC K91.89 Other postprocedural complications and disorders of digestive system**
    Use additional code, if applicable, to further specify disorder
    Excludes2: postprocedural retroperitoneal abscess (K68.11)
    AHA CC: 1Q, 2017, 40-41; 2Q, 2020, 22-23

K92 Other diseases of digestive system
Excludes1: neonatal gastrointestinal hemorrhage (P54.0-P54.3)
- **CC K92.0 Hematemesis**
- **CC K92.1 Melena**
  Excludes1: occult blood in feces (R19.5)
- **CC K92.2 Gastrointestinal hemorrhage, unspecified**
  Gastric hemorrhage NOS
  Intestinal hemorrhage NOS
  Excludes1: acute hemorrhagic gastritis (K29.01)
  hemorrhage of anus and rectum (K62.5)
  angiodysplasia of stomach with hemorrhage (K31.811)
  diverticular disease with hemorrhage (K57.-)
  gastritis and duodenitis with hemorrhage (K29.-)
  peptic ulcer with hemorrhage (K25-K28)
  AHA CC: 1Q, 2021, 11-12
- **+ K92.8 Other specified diseases of the digestive system**
  - **CC K92.81 Gastrointestinal mucositis (ulcerative)**
    Code also type of associated therapy, such as:
    antineoplastic and immunosuppressive drugs (T45.1X-)
    radiological procedure and radiotherapy (Y84.2)
    Excludes2: mucositis (ulcerative) of vagina and vulva (N76.81)
    nasal mucositis (ulcerative) (J34.81)
    oral mucositis (ulcerative) (K12.3-)
  - **K92.89 Other specified diseases of the digestive system**
- **K92.9 Disease of digestive system, unspecified**

K94 Complications of artificial openings of the digestive system
- **+ K94.0 Colostomy complications**
  - **K94.00 Colostomy complication, unspecified**
  - **CC K94.01 Colostomy hemorrhage**
  - **CC K94.02 Colostomy infection**
    Use additional code to specify type of infection, such as:
    cellulitis of abdominal wall (L03.311)
    sepsis (A40.-, A41.-)
  - **CC K94.03 Colostomy malfunction**
    Mechanical complication of colostomy
  - **K94.09 Other complications of colostomy**
- **+ K94.1 Enterostomy complications**
  - **K94.10 Enterostomy complication, unspecified**
  - **CC K94.11 Enterostomy hemorrhage**
  - **CC K94.12 Enterostomy infection**
    Use additional code to specify type of infection, such as:
    cellulitis of abdominal wall (L03.311)
    sepsis (A40.-, A41.-)
  - **CC K94.13 Enterostomy malfunction**
    Mechanical complication of enterostomy
    AHA CC: 4Q, 2021, 17-18
  - **CC K94.19 Other complications of enterostomy**
- **+ K94.2 Gastrostomy complications**
  - **K94.20 Gastrostomy complication, unspecified**
  - **K94.21 Gastrostomy hemorrhage**
  - **CC K94.22 Gastrostomy infection**
    Use additional code to specify type of infection, such as:
    cellulitis of abdominal wall (L03.311)
    sepsis (A40.-, A41.-)
  - **CC K94.23 Gastrostomy malfunction**
    Mechanical complication of gastrostomy
    AHA CC: 1Q, 2019, 26
  - **K94.29 Other complications of gastrostomy**
- **+ K94.3 Esophagostomy complications**
  - **CC K94.30 Esophagostomy complications, unspecified**
  - **CC K94.31 Esophagostomy hemorrhage**
  - **CC K94.32 Esophagostomy infection**
    Use additional code to identify the infection
  - **CC K94.33 Esophagostomy malfunction**
    Mechanical complication of esophagostomy
  - **CC K94.39 Other complications of esophagostomy**

+ **K95** **Complications of bariatric procedures**
  + **K95.0** **Complications of gastric band procedure**
    - CC **K95.01** **Infection due to gastric band procedure**
      Use additional code to specify type of infection or organism, such as:
      bacterial and viral infectious agents (B95.-, B96.-)
      cellulitis of abdominal wall (L03.311)
      sepsis (A40.-, A41.-)
      HAC see Appendix B for HAC conditional logic
    - CC **K95.09** **Other complications of gastric band procedure**
      Use additional code, if applicable, to further specify complication

+ **K95.8** **Complications of other bariatric procedure**
  Excludes1: *complications of gastric band surgery (K95.0-)*
  - CC **K95.81** **Infection due to other bariatric procedure**
    Use additional code to specify type of infection or organism, such as:
    bacterial and viral infectious agents (B95.-, B96.-)
    cellulitis of abdominal wall (L03.311)
    sepsis (A40.-, A41.-)
    HAC see Appendix B for HAC conditional logic
  - CC **K95.89** **Other complications of other bariatric procedure**
    Use additional code, if applicable, to further specify complication

Chapter 12: Diseases of the Skin and Subcutaneous Tissue (L00-L99)

Excludes2: certain conditions originating in the perinatal period (P04-P96)
certain infectious and parasitic diseases (A00-B99)
complications of pregnancy, childbirth and the puerperium (O00-O9A)
congenital malformations, deformations, and chromosomal abnormalities (Q00-Q99)
endocrine, nutritional and metabolic diseases (E00-E88)
lipomelanotic reticulosis (I89.8)
neoplasms (C00-D49)
symptoms, signs and abnormal clinical and laboratory findings, not elsewhere classified (R00-R94)
systemic connective tissue disorders (M30-M36)
viral warts (B07.-)

This chapter contains the following category blocks:
L00-L08 Infections of the skin and subcutaneous tissue
L10-L14 Bullous disorders
L20-L30 Dermatitis and eczema
L40-L45 Papulosquamous disorders
L49-L54 Urticaria and erythema
L55-L59 Radiation-related disorders of the skin and subcutaneous tissue
L60-L75 Disorders of skin appendages
L76   Intraoperative and postprocedural complications of skin and subcutaneous tissue
L80-L99 Other disorders of the skin and subcutaneous tissue

C. Chapter-Specific Coding Guidelines

In addition to general coding guidelines, there are guidelines for specific diagnoses and/or conditions in the classification. Unless otherwise indicated, these guidelines apply to all health care settings. Please refer to Section II for guidelines on the selection of principal diagnosis.

12. Chapter 12: Diseases of the Skin and Subcutaneous Tissue (L00-L99)

   a. Pressure ulcer stage codes

   1) **Pressure ulcer stages**

   Codes in category L89, Pressure ulcer, identify the site and stage of the pressure ulcer.

   The ICD-10-CM classifies pressure ulcer stages based on severity, which is designated by stages 1-4 deep tissue pressure injury, unspecified stage and unstageable.

   Assign as many codes from category L89 as needed to identify all the pressure ulcers the patient has, if applicable.

   See Section I.B.14 for pressure ulcer stage documentation by clinicians other than patient's provider.

   2) **Unstageable pressure ulcers**

   Assignment of the code for unstageable pressure ulcer (L89.--0) should be based on the clinical documentation. These codes are used for pressure ulcers whose stage cannot be clinically determined (e.g., the ulcer is covered by eschar or has been treated with a skin or muscle graft) and pressure ulcers that are documented as deep tissue injury but not documented as due to trauma. This code should not be confused with the codes for unspecified stage (L89.--9). When there is no documentation regarding the stage of the pressure ulcer, assign the appropriate code for unspecified stage (L89.--9).

   If during an encounter, the stage of an unstageable pressure ulcer is revealed after debridement, assign only the code for the stage revealed following debridement.

   3) **Documented pressure ulcer stage**

   Assignment of the pressure ulcer stage code should be guided by clinical documentation of the stage or documentation of the terms found in the Alphabetic Index. For clinical terms describing the stage that are not found in the Alphabetic Index, and there is no documentation of the stage, the provider should be queried.

   4) **Patients admitted with pressure ulcers documented as healed**

   No code is assigned if the documentation states that the pressure ulcer is completely healed at the time of admission.

   5) **Patients admitted with pressure ulcers documented as healing**

   Pressure ulcers described as healing should be assigned the appropriate pressure ulcer stage code based on the documentation in the medical record. If the documentation does not provide information about the stage of the healing pressure ulcer, assign the appropriate code for unspecified stage.

   If the documentation is unclear as to whether the patient has a current (new) pressure ulcer or if the patient is being treated for a healing pressure ulcer, query the provider.

   For ulcers that were present on admission but healed at the time of discharge, assign the code for the site and stage of the pressure ulcer at the time of admission.

   6) **Patient admitted with pressure ulcer evolving into another stage during the admission**

   If a patient is admitted to an inpatient hospital with a pressure ulcer at one stage and it progresses to a higher stage, two separate codes should be assigned: one code for the site and stage of the ulcer on admission and a second code for the same ulcer site and the highest stage reported during the stay.

   7) **Pressure-induced deep tissue damage**

   For pressure-induced deep tissue damage or deep tissue pressure injury, assign only the appropriate code for pressure-induced deep tissue damage (L89.--6).

   b. Non-Pressure Chronic Ulcers

   1) **Patients admitted with non-pressure ulcers documented as healed**

   No code is assigned if the documentation states that the non-pressure ulcer is completely healed at the time of admission.

   2) **Patients admitted with non-pressure ulcers documented as healing**

   Non-pressure ulcers described as healing should be assigned the appropriate non-pressure ulcer code based on the documentation in the medical record. If the documentation does not provide information about the severity of the healing non-pressure ulcer, assign the appropriate code unspecified severity.

   If the documentation is unclear as to whether the patient has a current (new) non-pressure ulcer or if the patient is being treated for a healing non-pressure ulcer, query the provider.

   For ulcers that were present on admission but healed at the time of discharge, assign the code for the site and severity of the non-pressure ulcer at the time of admission.

   3) **Patient admitted with non-pressure ulcer that progresses to another severity level during the admission**

   If a patient is admitted to an inpatient hospital with a non-pressure ulcer at one severity level and it progresses to a higher severity level, two separate codes should be assigned; one code for the site and severity level of the ulcer on admission and a second code for the same ulcer site and the highest severity level reported during the stay.

   See Section I.B.14 for pressure ulcer stage documentation by clinicians other than patient's provider.

Infections of the skin and subcutaneous tissue (L00-L08)

Use additional code (B95-B97) to identify infectious agent

Excludes2: hordeolum (H00.0)
infective dermatitis (L30.3)
local infections of skin classified in Chapter 1
lupus panniculitis (L93.2)
panniculitis NOS (M79.3)
panniculitis of neck and back (M54.0-)
Perlèche NOS (K13.0)
Perlèche due to candidiasis (B37.0)
Perlèche due to riboflavin deficiency (E53.0)
pyogenic granuloma (L98.0)
relapsing panniculitis [Weber-Christian] (M35.6)
viral warts (B07.-)
zoster (B02.-)

L00 Staphylococcal scalded skin syndrome
Ritter's disease
Use additional code to identify percentage of skin exfoliation (L49.-)
Excludes1: bullous impetigo (L01.03)
pemphigus neonatorum (L01.03)
toxic epidermal necrolysis [Lyell] (L51.2)
Valid 3-character code, no further characters required

L01 Impetigo
Excludes1: impetigo herpetiformis (L40.1)

+ **L01.0 Impetigo**
Impetigo contagiosa
Impetigo vulgaris
  L01.00 Impetigo, unspecified
  Impetigo NOS
  L01.01 Non-bullous impetigo
  L01.02 Bockhart's impetigo
  Impetigo follicularis
  Perifolliculitis NOS
  Superficial pustular perifolliculitis

Cross-Section of the Skin Showing Layers and Types of Infection

Skin compartments: Epidermis, Dermis, Subcutaneous tissue, Deep fascia, Muscle, Bone

Labels: Vesicle, Crust, Hair follicle, Bullae, Sebaceous gland, Lymphatic vessel, Artery, Vein, Sweat gland

Infection site — Etiologic organisms

- (Epidermis): *Staphylococcus aureus*
- Group A β-hemolytic Streptococcus (common)
  Group C and G Streptococcus (uncommon)
  Staphylococcus aureus, Streptococcus pneumoniae,
  Enterococci or aerobic Gram-negative bacilli (rare)
- Folliculitis / furuncles: *Staphylococcus aureus*
- Group A B-hemolytic Streptococcus (most common)
  Group B, C and G Streptococcus (common)
  Staphylococcus aureus (uncommon)
  H. Influenzae (rare)
  Other (rare)
- Necrotizing fasciitis: Streptococcus pyogenes; Enterococci Gram-negative bacilli
- Myositis

J. Chovan

© 2008 Elsevier Inc. All rights reserved. www.netterimages.com

---

L01.03 Bullous impetigo
   Impetigo neonatorum
   Pemphigus neonatorum
L01.09 Other impetigo
   Ulcerative impetigo
L01.1 Impetiginization of other dermatoses
L02 Cutaneous abscess, furuncle and carbuncle
   Use additional code to identify organism (B95-B96)
   Excludes2: abscess of anus and rectal regions (K61.-)
      abscess of female genital organs (external) (N76.4)
      abscess of male genital organs (external) (N48.2, N49.-)
+ **L02.0 Cutaneous abscess, furuncle and carbuncle of face**
   Excludes2: abscess of ear, external (H60.0)
      abscess of eyelid (H00.0)
      abscess of head [any part, except face] (L02.8)
      abscess of lacrimal gland (H04.0)
      abscess of lacrimal passages (H04.3)
      abscess of mouth (K12.2)
      abscess of nose (J34.0)
      abscess of orbit (H05.0)
      submandibular abscess (K12.2)
   CC **L02.01 Cutaneous abscess of face**
   L02.02 Furuncle of face
      Boil of face
      Folliculitis of face
   L02.03 Carbuncle of face

+ **L02.1 Cutaneous abscess, furuncle and carbuncle of neck**
   CC **L02.11 Cutaneous abscess of neck**
   L02.12 Furuncle of neck
      Boil of neck
      Folliculitis of neck
   L02.13 Carbuncle of neck
+ **L02.2 Cutaneous abscess, furuncle and carbuncle of trunk**
   Excludes1: non-newborn omphalitis (L08.82)
      omphalitis of newborn (P38.-)
   Excludes2: abscess of breast (N61.1)
      abscess of buttocks (L02.3)
      abscess of female external genital organs
         (N76.4)
      abscess of male external genital organs
         (N48.2, N49.-)
      abscess of hip (L02.4)
   CC **L02.21 Cutaneous abscess of trunk**
      CC **L02.211 Cutaneous abscess of abdominal wall**
      CC **L02.212 Cutaneous abscess of back [any part, except buttock]**
      CC **L02.213 Cutaneous abscess of chest wall**
      CC **L02.214 Cutaneous abscess of groin**
      CC **L02.215 Cutaneous abscess of perineum**
      CC **L02.216 Cutaneous abscess of umbilicus**
      CC **L02.219 Cutaneous abscess of trunk, unspecified**

+, +7th, X + 7th   • Newborn   • Pediatric   • Maternity   • Adult   ♀ Female   ♂ Male   Manifestation   Unacceptable PDX   HCC   CC   MCC   HAC

- **+ L02.22 Furuncle of trunk**
  - Boil of trunk
  - Folliculitis of trunk
  - L02.221 Furuncle of abdominal wall
  - L02.222 Furuncle of back [any part, except buttock]
  - L02.223 Furuncle of chest wall
  - L02.224 Furuncle of groin
  - L02.225 Furuncle of perineum
  - L02.226 Furuncle of umbilicus
  - L02.229 Furuncle of trunk, unspecified
- **+ L02.23 Carbuncle of trunk**
  - L02.231 Carbuncle of abdominal wall
  - L02.232 Carbuncle of back [any part, except buttock]
  - L02.233 Carbuncle of chest wall
  - L02.234 Carbuncle of groin
  - L02.235 Carbuncle of perineum
  - L02.236 Carbuncle of umbilicus
  - L02.239 Carbuncle of trunk, unspecified
- **+ L02.3 Cutaneous abscess, furuncle and carbuncle of buttock**
  - **Excludes1:** pilonidal cyst with abscess (L05.01)
  - CC L02.31 Cutaneous abscess of buttock
    - Cutaneous abscess of gluteal region
  - L02.32 Furuncle of buttock
    - Boil of buttock
    - Folliculitis of buttock
    - Furuncle of gluteal region
  - L02.33 Carbuncle of buttock
    - Carbuncle of gluteal region
- **+ L02.4 Cutaneous abscess, furuncle and carbuncle of limb**
  - **Excludes2:** Cutaneous abscess, furuncle and carbuncle of groin (L02.214, L02.224, L02.234)
    Cutaneous abscess, furuncle and carbuncle of hand (L02.5-)
    Cutaneous abscess, furuncle and carbuncle of foot (L02.6-)
  - **+ L02.41 Cutaneous abscess of limb**
    - CC L02.411 Cutaneous abscess of right axilla
    - CC L02.412 Cutaneous abscess of left axilla
    - CC L02.413 Cutaneous abscess of right upper limb
    - CC L02.414 Cutaneous abscess of left upper limb
    - CC L02.415 Cutaneous abscess of right lower limb
    - CC L02.416 Cutaneous abscess of left lower limb
    - CC L02.419 Cutaneous abscess of limb, unspecified
  - **+ L02.42 Furuncle of limb**
    - Boil of limb
    - Folliculitis of limb
    - L02.421 Furuncle of right axilla
    - L02.422 Furuncle of left axilla
    - L02.423 Furuncle of right upper limb
    - L02.424 Furuncle of left upper limb
    - L02.425 Furuncle of right lower limb
    - L02.426 Furuncle of left lower limb
    - L02.429 Furuncle of limb, unspecified
  - **+ L02.43 Carbuncle of limb**
    - L02.431 Carbuncle of right axilla
    - L02.432 Carbuncle of left axilla
    - L02.433 Carbuncle of right upper limb
    - L02.434 Carbuncle of left upper limb
    - L02.435 Carbuncle of right lower limb
    - L02.436 Carbuncle of left lower limb
    - L02.439 Carbuncle of limb, unspecified
- **+ L02.5 Cutaneous abscess, furuncle and carbuncle of hand**
  - **+ L02.51 Cutaneous abscess of hand**
    - CC L02.511 Cutaneous abscess of right hand
    - CC L02.512 Cutaneous abscess of left hand
    - CC L02.519 Cutaneous abscess of unspecified hand
  - **+ L02.52 Furuncle hand**
    - Boil of hand
    - Folliculitis of hand
    - L02.521 Furuncle right hand
    - L02.522 Furuncle left hand
    - L02.529 Furuncle unspecified hand
  - **+ L02.53 Carbuncle of hand**
    - L02.531 Carbuncle of right hand
    - L02.532 Carbuncle of left hand
    - L02.539 Carbuncle of unspecified hand
- **+ L02.6 Cutaneous abscess, furuncle and carbuncle of foot**
  - **+ L02.61 Cutaneous abscess of foot**
    - CC L02.611 Cutaneous abscess of right foot
    - CC L02.612 Cutaneous abscess of left foot
    - CC L02.619 Cutaneous abscess of unspecified foot
  - **+ L02.62 Furuncle of foot**
    - Boil of foot
    - Folliculitis of foot
    - L02.621 Furuncle of right foot
    - L02.622 Furuncle of left foot
    - L02.629 Furuncle of unspecified foot
  - **+ L02.63 Carbuncle of foot**
    - L02.631 Carbuncle of right foot
    - L02.632 Carbuncle of left foot
    - L02.639 Carbuncle of unspecified foot
- **+ L02.8 Cutaneous abscess, furuncle and carbuncle of other sites**
  - **+ L02.81 Cutaneous abscess of other sites**
    - CC L02.811 Cutaneous abscess of head [any part, except face]
    - CC L02.818 Cutaneous abscess of other sites
  - **+ L02.82 Furuncle of other sites**
    - Boil of other sites
    - Folliculitis of other sites
    - L02.821 Furuncle of head [any part, except face]
    - L02.828 Furuncle of other sites
  - **+ L02.83 Carbuncle of other sites**
    - L02.831 Carbuncle of head [any part, except face]
    - L02.838 Carbuncle of other sites
- **+ L02.9 Cutaneous abscess, furuncle and carbuncle, unspecified**
  - CC L02.91 Cutaneous abscess, unspecified
  - L02.92 Furuncle, unspecified
    - Boil NOS
    - Furunculosis NOS
  - L02.93 Carbuncle, unspecified

L03 Cellulitis and acute lymphangitis

Excludes2: cellulitis of anal and rectal region (K61.-)
cellulitis of external auditory canal (H60.1)
cellulitis of eyelid (H00.0)
cellulitis of female external genital organs (N76.4)
cellulitis of lacrimal apparatus (H04.3)
cellulitis of male external genital organs (N48.2, N49.-)
cellulitis of mouth (K12.2)
cellulitis of nose (J34.0)
eosinophilic cellulitis [Wells] (L98.3)
febrile neutrophilic dermatosis [Sweet] (L98.2)
lymphangitis (chronic) (subacute) (I89.1)

- **+ L03.0 Cellulitis and acute lymphangitis of finger and toe**
  - Infection of nail
  - Onychia
  - Paronychia
  - Perionychia
  - **+ L03.01 Cellulitis of finger**
    - Felon
    - Whitlow
    - **Excludes1:** herpetic whitlow (B00.89)
    - L03.011 Cellulitis of right finger
      - *AHA CC: 4Q, 2020, 11*
    - L03.012 Cellulitis of left finger
    - L03.019 Cellulitis of unspecified finger
  - **+ L03.02 Acute lymphangitis of finger**
    - Hangnail with lymphangitis of finger
    - L03.021 Acute lymphangitis of right finger
    - L03.022 Acute lymphangitis of left finger
    - L03.029 Acute lymphangitis of unspecified finger
  - **+ L03.03 Cellulitis of toe**
    - L03.031 Cellulitis of right toe
    - L03.032 Cellulitis of left toe
    - L03.039 Cellulitis of unspecified toe
  - **+ L03.04 Acute lymphangitis of toe**
    - Hangnail with lymphangitis of toe
    - L03.041 Acute lymphangitis of right toe
    - L03.042 Acute lymphangitis of left toe
    - L03.049 Acute lymphangitis of unspecified toe

- **L03.1 Cellulitis and acute lymphangitis of other parts of limb**
  - **L03.11 Cellulitis of other parts of limb**
    - *Excludes2:* cellulitis of fingers (L03.01-)
      cellulitis of toes (L03.03-)
      groin (L03.314)
    - CC L03.111 Cellulitis of right axilla
    - CC L03.112 Cellulitis of left axilla
    - CC L03.113 Cellulitis of right upper limb
    - CC L03.114 Cellulitis of left upper limb
      AHA CC: 1Q, 2019, 13
    - CC L03.115 Cellulitis of right lower limb
    - CC L03.116 Cellulitis of left lower limb
    - CC L03.119 Cellulitis of unspecified part of limb
  - **L03.12 Acute lymphangitis of other parts of limb**
    - *Excludes2:* acute lymphangitis of fingers (L03.2-)
      acute lymphangitis of toes (L03.04-)
      acute lymphangitis of groin (L03.324)
    - CC L03.121 Acute lymphangitis of right axilla
    - CC L03.122 Acute lymphangitis of left axilla
    - CC L03.123 Acute lymphangitis of right upper limb
    - CC L03.124 Acute lymphangitis of left upper limb
    - CC L03.125 Acute lymphangitis of right lower limb
    - CC L03.126 Acute lymphangitis of left lower limb
    - CC L03.129 Acute lymphangitis of unspecified part of limb
- **L03.2 Cellulitis and acute lymphangitis of face and neck**
  - **L03.21 Cellulitis and acute lymphangitis of face**
    - CC L03.211 Cellulitis of face
      - *Excludes2:* abscess of orbit (H05.01-)
        cellulitis of ear (H60.1-)
        cellulitis of eyelid (H00.0-)
        cellulitis of head (L03.81)
        cellulitis of lacrimal apparatus (H04.3)
        cellulitis of lip (K13.0)
        cellulitis of mouth (K12.2)
        cellulitis of nose (internal) (J34.0)
        cellulitis of orbit (H05.01-)
        cellulitis of scalp (L03.81)
      - *AHA CC: 4Q, 2013, 123*
    - CC L03.212 Acute lymphangitis of face
    - CC L03.213 Periorbital cellulitis
      Preseptal cellulitis
      AHA CC: 4Q, 2016, 36
  - **L03.22 Cellulitis and acute lymphangitis of neck**
    - CC L03.221 Cellulitis of neck
    - CC L03.222 Acute lymphangitis of neck
- **L03.3 Cellulitis and acute lymphangitis of trunk**
  - **L03.31 Cellulitis of trunk**
    - *Excludes2:* cellulitis of anal and rectal regions (K61.-)
      cellulitis of breast NOS (N61.0)
      cellulitis of female external genital organs (N76.4)
      cellulitis of male external genital organs (N48.2, N49.-)
      omphalitis of newborn (P38.-)
      puerperal cellulitis of breast (O91.2)
    - CC L03.311 Cellulitis of abdominal wall
      - *Excludes2:* cellulitis of umbilicus (L03.316)
        cellulitis of groin (L03.314)
    - CC L03.312 Cellulitis of back [any part except buttock]
    - CC L03.313 Cellulitis of chest wall
    - CC L03.314 Cellulitis of groin
    - CC L03.315 Cellulitis of perineum
    - CC L03.316 Cellulitis of umbilicus
    - CC L03.317 Cellulitis of buttock
    - CC L03.319 Cellulitis of trunk, unspecified
  - **L03.32 Acute lymphangitis of trunk**
    - CC L03.321 Acute lymphangitis of abdominal wall
    - CC L03.322 Acute lymphangitis of back [any part except buttock]
    - CC L03.323 Acute lymphangitis of chest wall
    - CC L03.324 Acute lymphangitis of groin
    - CC L03.325 Acute lymphangitis of perineum
    - CC L03.326 Acute lymphangitis of umbilicus
    - CC L03.327 Acute lymphangitis of buttock
    - CC L03.329 Acute lymphangitis of trunk, unspecified

- **L03.8 Cellulitis and acute lymphangitis of other sites**
  - **L03.81 Cellulitis of other sites**
    - CC L03.811 Cellulitis of head [any part, except face]
      Cellulitis of scalp
      - *Excludes2:* cellulitis of face (L03.211)
    - CC L03.818 Cellulitis of other sites
  - **L03.89 Acute lymphangitis of other sites**
    - CC L03.891 Acute lymphangitis of head [any part, except face]
    - CC L03.898 Acute lymphangitis of other sites
- **L03.9 Cellulitis and acute lymphangitis, unspecified**
  - CC L03.90 Cellulitis, unspecified
  - CC L03.91 Acute lymphangitis, unspecified
    - *Excludes1:* lymphangitis NOS (I89.1)

L04 Acute lymphadenitis
  Includes: abscess (acute) of lymph nodes, except mesenteric
  acute lymphadenitis, except mesenteric
  Excludes1: chronic or subacute lymphadenitis, except mesenteric (I88.1)
  enlarged lymph nodes (R59.-)
  human immunodeficiency virus [HIV] disease resulting in generalized lymphadenopathy (B20)
  lymphadenitis NOS (I88.9)
  nonspecific mesenteric lymphadenitis (I88.0)
  - L04.0 Acute lymphadenitis of face, head and neck
  - L04.1 Acute lymphadenitis of trunk
  - L04.2 Acute lymphadenitis of upper limb
    Acute lymphadenitis of axilla
    Acute lymphadenitis of shoulder
  - L04.3 Acute lymphadenitis of lower limb
    Acute lymphadenitis of hip
    - *Excludes2:* acute lymphadenitis of groin (L04.1)
  - L04.8 Acute lymphadenitis of other sites
  - L04.9 Acute lymphadenitis, unspecified

L05 Pilonidal cyst and sinus
  - **L05.0 Pilonidal cyst and sinus with abscess**
    - CC L05.01 Pilonidal cyst with abscess
      Pilonidal abscess
      Pilonidal dimple with abscess
      Postanal dimple with abscess
      - *Excludes2:* congenital sacral dimple (Q82.6)
        parasacral dimple (Q82.6)
    - CC L05.02 Pilonidal sinus with abscess
      Coccygeal fistula with abscess
      Coccygeal sinus with abscess
      Pilonidal fistula with abscess
  - **L05.9 Pilonidal cyst and sinus without abscess**
    - L05.91 Pilonidal cyst without abscess
      Pilonidal dimple
      Postanal dimple
      Pilonidal cyst NOS
      - *Excludes2:* congenital sacral dimple (Q82.6)
        parasacral dimple (Q82.6)
    - L05.92 Pilonidal sinus without abscess
      Coccygeal fistula
      Coccygeal sinus without abscess
      Pilonidal fistula

L08 Other local infections of skin and subcutaneous tissue
  - L08.0 Pyoderma
    Dermatitis gangrenosa
    Purulent dermatitis
    Septic dermatitis
    Suppurative dermatitis
    - *Excludes1:* pyoderma gangrenosum (L88)
      pyoderma vegetans (L08.81)
  - CC L08.1 Erythrasma
  - **L08.8 Other specified local infections of the skin and subcutaneous tissue**
    - L08.81 Pyoderma vegetans
      - *Excludes1:* pyoderma gangrenosum (L88)
        pyoderma NOS (L08.0)
    - L08.82 Omphalitis not of newborn
      - *Excludes1:* omphalitis of newborn (P38.-)
    - L08.89 Other specified local infections of the skin and subcutaneous tissue
  - L08.9 Local infection of the skin and subcutaneous tissue, unspecified

Bullous disorders (L10-L14)

Excludes1: benign familial pemphigus [Hailey-Hailey] (Q82.8)
staphylococcal scalded skin syndrome (L00)
toxic epidermal necrolysis [Lyell] (L51.2)

L10 Pemphigus

Excludes1: pemphigus neonatorum (L01.03)

- CC **L10.0** Pemphigus vulgaris
- CC **L10.1** Pemphigus vegetans
- CC **L10.2** Pemphigus foliaceous
- CC **L10.3** Brazilian pemphigus [fogo selvagem]
- CC **L10.4** Pemphigus erythematosus
  Senear-Usher syndrome
- CC **L10.5** Drug-induced pemphigus
  Use additional code for adverse effect, if applicable, to identify drug (T36-T50 with fifth or sixth character 5)
- + **L10.8** Other pemphigus
  - CC **L10.81** Paraneoplastic pemphigus
  - CC **L10.89** Other pemphigus
- CC **L10.9** Pemphigus, unspecified

L11 Other acantholytic disorders

- **L11.0** Acquired keratosis follicularis
  Excludes1: keratosis follicularis (congenital) [Darier-White] (Q82.8)
- **L11.1** Transient acantholytic dermatosis [Grover]
- **L11.8** Other specified acantholytic disorders
- **L11.9** Acantholytic disorder, unspecified

L12 Pemphigoid

Excludes1: herpes gestationis (O26.4-)
impetigo herpetiformis (L40.1)

- CC **L12.0** Bullous pemphigoid
- **L12.1** Cicatricial pemphigoid
  Benign mucous membrane pemphigoid
- • **L12.2** Chronic bullous disease of childhood
  Juvenile dermatitis herpetiformis
- + **L12.3** Acquired epidermolysis bullosa
  Excludes1: epidermolysis bullosa (congenital) (Q81.-)
  - CC **L12.30** Acquired epidermolysis bullosa, unspecified
  - CC **L12.31** Epidermolysis bullosa due to drug
    Use additional code for adverse effect, if applicable, to identify drug (T36-T50 with fifth or sixth character 5)
  - CC **L12.35** Other acquired epidermolysis bullosa
- CC **L12.8** Other pemphigoid
- CC **L12.9** Pemphigoid, unspecified

L13 Other bullous disorders

- **L13.0** Dermatitis herpetiformis
  Duhring's disease
  Hydroa herpetiformis
  Excludes1: juvenile dermatitis herpetiformis (L12.2)
  senile dermatitis herpetiformis (L12.0)
- **L13.1** Subcorneal pustular dermatitis
  Sneddon-Wilkinson disease
- **L13.8** Other specified bullous disorders
- **L13.9** Bullous disorder, unspecified

L14 Bullous disorders in diseases classified elsewhere

Code first underlying disease
Valid 3-character code, no further characters required

Dermatitis and eczema (L20-L30)

NOTE In this block the terms dermatitis and eczema are used synonymously and interchangeably.

Excludes2: chronic (childhood) granulomatous disease (D71)
dermatitis gangrenosa (L08.0)
dermatitis herpetiformis (L13.0)
dry skin dermatitis (L85.3)
factitial dermatitis (L98.1)
perioral dermatitis (L71.0)
radiation-related disorders of the skin and subcutaneous tissue (L55-L59)
stasis dermatitis (I87.2)

L20 Atopic dermatitis

- **L20.0** Besnier's prurigo
- + **L20.8** Other atopic dermatitis
  Excludes2: circumscribed neurodermatitis (L28.0)
  - **L20.81** Atopic neurodermatitis
    Diffuse neurodermatitis
  - **L20.82** Flexural eczema
  - • **L20.83** Infantile (acute) (chronic) eczema
  - **L20.84** Intrinsic (allergic) eczema
  - **L20.89** Other atopic dermatitis
- **L20.9** Atopic dermatitis, unspecified

L21 Seborrheic dermatitis

Excludes2: infective dermatitis (L30.3)
seborrheic keratosis (L82.-)

- **L21.0** Seborrhea capitis
  Cradle cap
  AHA CC: 1Q, 2018, 6
- • **L21.1** Seborrheic infantile dermatitis
- **L21.8** Other seborrheic dermatitis
- **L21.9** Seborrheic dermatitis, unspecified
  Seborrhea NOS

L22 Diaper dermatitis

Diaper erythema
Diaper rash
Psoriasiform diaper rash
AHA CC: 4Q, 2021, 18
Valid 3-character code, no further characters required

L23 Allergic contact dermatitis

Excludes1: allergy NOS (T78.40)
contact dermatitis NOS (L25.9)
dermatitis NOS (L30.9)
Excludes2: dermatitis due to substances taken internally (L27.-)
dermatitis of eyelid (H01.1-)
diaper dermatitis (L22)
eczema of external ear (H60.5-)
irritant contact dermatitis (L24.-)
perioral dermatitis (L71.0)
radiation-related disorders of the skin and subcutaneous tissue (L55-L59)

- **L23.0** Allergic contact dermatitis due to metals
  Allergic contact dermatitis due to chromium
  Allergic contact dermatitis due to nickel
- **L23.1** Allergic contact dermatitis due to adhesives
- **L23.2** Allergic contact dermatitis due to cosmetics
- **L23.3** Allergic contact dermatitis due to drugs in contact with skin
  Use additional code for adverse effect, if applicable, to identify drug (T36-T50 with fifth or sixth character 5)
  Excludes2: dermatitis due to ingested drugs and medicaments (L27.0-L27.1)
- **L23.4** Allergic contact dermatitis due to dyes
- **L23.5** Allergic contact dermatitis due to other chemical products
  Allergic contact dermatitis due to cement
  Allergic contact dermatitis due to insecticide
  Allergic contact dermatitis due to plastic
  Allergic contact dermatitis due to rubber
- **L23.6** Allergic contact dermatitis due to food in contact with the skin
  Excludes2: dermatitis due to ingested food (L27.2)
- **L23.7** Allergic contact dermatitis due to plants, except food
  Excludes2: allergy NOS due to pollen (J30.1)
- + **L23.8** Allergic contact dermatitis due to other agents
  - **L23.81** Allergic contact dermatitis due to animal (cat) (dog) dander
    Allergic contact dermatitis due to animal (cat) (dog) hair
  - **L23.89** Allergic contact dermatitis due to other agents
- **L23.9** Allergic contact dermatitis, unspecified cause
  Allergic contact eczema NOS

L24 Irritant contact dermatitis
> *Excludes1:* allergy NOS (T78.40)
> contact dermatitis NOS (L25.9)
> dermatitis NOS (L30.9)
> *Excludes2:* allergic contact dermatitis (L23.-)
> dermatitis due to substances taken internally (L27.-)
> dermatitis of eyelid (H01.1-)
> diaper dermatitis (L22)
> eczema of external ear (H60.5-)
> perioral dermatitis (L71.0)
> radiation-related disorders of the skin and subcutaneous tissue (L55-L59)

- **L24.0** Irritant contact dermatitis due to detergents
- **L24.1** Irritant contact dermatitis due to oils and greases
- **L24.2** Irritant contact dermatitis due to solvents
  - Irritant contact dermatitis due to chlorocompound
  - Irritant contact dermatitis due to cyclohexane
  - Irritant contact dermatitis due to ester
  - Irritant contact dermatitis due to glycol
  - Irritant contact dermatitis due to hydrocarbon
  - Irritant contact dermatitis due to ketone
- **L24.3** Irritant contact dermatitis due to cosmetics
- **L24.4** Irritant contact dermatitis due to drugs in contact with skin
  > Use additional code for adverse effect, if applicable, to identify drug (T36-T50 with fifth or sixth character 5)
- **L24.5** Irritant contact dermatitis due to other chemical products
  - Irritant contact dermatitis due to cement
  - Irritant contact dermatitis due to insecticide
  - Irritant contact dermatitis due to plastic
  - Irritant contact dermatitis due to rubber
- **L24.6** Irritant contact dermatitis due to food in contact with skin
  > *Excludes2:* dermatitis due to ingested food (L27.2)
- **L24.7** Irritant contact dermatitis due to plants, except food
  > *Excludes2:* allergy NOS to pollen (J30.1)
- + **L24.8** Irritant contact dermatitis due to other agents
  - **L24.81** Irritant contact dermatitis due to metals
    - Irritant contact dermatitis due to chromium
    - Irritant contact dermatitis due to nickel
  - **L24.89** Irritant contact dermatitis due to other agents
    - Irritant contact dermatitis due to dyes
- **L24.9** Irritant contact dermatitis, unspecified cause
  - Irritant contact eczema NOS
- + **L24.A** Irritant contact dermatitis due to friction or contact with body fluids
  > *Excludes1:* irritant contact dermatitis related to stoma or fistula (L24.B-)
  > *Excludes2:* erythema intertrigo (L30.4)
  > *AHA CC: 4Q, 2021, 16-18*
  - **L24.A0** Irritant contact dermatitis due to friction or contact with body fluids, unspecified
  - **L24.A1** Irritant contact dermatitis due to saliva
  - **L24.A2** Irritant contact dermatitis due to fecal, urinary or dual incontinence
    > *Excludes1:* diaper dermatitis (L22)
    > *AHA CC: 4Q, 2021, 18*
  - **L24.A9** Irritant contact dermatitis due to friction or contact with other specified body fluids
    - Irritant contact dermatitis related to endotracheal tube
    - Wound fluids, exudate
- + **L24.B** Irritant contact dermatitis related to stoma or fistula
  > Use additional code to identify any artificial opening status (Z93.-), if applicable, for contact dermatitis related to stoma secretions
  > *AHA CC: 4Q, 2021, 16-18*
  - **L24.B0** Irritant contact dermatitis related to unspecified stoma or fistula
    - Irritant contact dermatitis related to fistula NOS
    - Irritant contact dermatitis related to stoma NOS
  - **L24.B1** Irritant contact dermatitis related to digestive stoma or fistula
    - Irritant contact dermatitis related to gastrostomy
    - Irritant contact dermatitis related to jejunostomy
    - Irritant contact dermatitis related to saliva or spit fistula
  - **L24.B2** Irritant contact dermatitis related to respiratory stoma or fistula
    - Irritant contact dermatitis related tracheostomy
  - **L24.B3** Irritant contact dermatitis related to fecal or urinary stoma or fistula
    - Irritant contact dermatitis related to colostomy
    - Irritant contact dermatitis related to enterocutaneous fistua
    - Irritant contact dermatitis related to ileostomy
  > *AHA CC: 4Q, 2021, 17-19*

L25 Unspecified contact dermatitis
> *Excludes1:* allergic contact dermatitis (L23.-)
> allergy NOS (T78.40)
> dermatitis NOS (L30.9)
> irritant contact dermatitis (L24.-)
> *Excludes2:* dermatitis due to ingested substances (L27.-)
> dermatitis of eyelid (H01.1-)
> eczema of external ear (H60.5-)
> perioral dermatitis (L71.0)
> radiation-related disorders of the skin and subcutaneous tissue (L55-L59)

- **L25.0** Unspecified contact dermatitis due to cosmetics
- **L25.1** Unspecified contact dermatitis due to drugs in contact with skin
  > Use additional code for adverse effect, if applicable, to identify drug (T36-T50 with fifth or sixth character 5)
  > *Excludes2:* dermatitis due to ingested drugs and medicaments (L27.0-L27.1)
- **L25.2** Unspecified contact dermatitis due to dyes
- **L25.3** Unspecified contact dermatitis due to other chemical products
  - Unspecified contact dermatitis due to cement
  - Unspecified contact dermatitis due to insecticide
- **L25.4** Unspecified contact dermatitis due to food in contact with skin
  > *Excludes2:* dermatitis due to ingested food (L27.2)
- **L25.5** Unspecified contact dermatitis due to plants, except food
  > *Excludes1:* nettle rash (L50.9)
  > *Excludes2:* allergy NOS due to pollen (J30.1)
- **L25.8** Unspecified contact dermatitis due to other agents
- **L25.9** Unspecified contact dermatitis, unspecified cause
  - Contact dermatitis (occupational) NOS
  - Contact eczema (occupational) NOS

L26 Exfoliative dermatitis
- Hebra's pityriasis
> *Excludes1:* Ritter's disease (L00)
> **Valid 3-character code, no further characters required**

L27 Dermatitis due to substances taken internally
> *Excludes1:* allergy NOS (T78.40)
> *Excludes2:* adverse food reaction, except dermatitis (T78.0-T78.1)
> contact dermatitis (L23-L25)
> drug photoallergic response (L56.1)
> drug phototoxic response (L56.0)
> urticaria (L50.-)

- **L27.0** Generalized skin eruption due to drugs and medicaments taken internally
  > Use additional code for adverse effect, if applicable, to identify drug (T36-T50 with fifth or sixth character 5)
- **L27.1** Localized skin eruption due to drugs and medicaments taken internally
  > Use additional code for adverse effect, if applicable, to identify drug (T36-T50 with fifth or sixth character 5)
- **L27.2** Dermatitis due to ingested food
  > *Excludes2:* dermatitis due to food in contact with skin (L23.6, L24.6, L25.4)
- **L27.8** Dermatitis due to other substances taken internally
- **L27.9** Dermatitis due to unspecified substance taken internally

L28 Lichen simplex chronicus and prurigo
- **L28.0** Lichen simplex chronicus
  - Circumscribed neurodermatitis
  - Lichen NOS
- **L28.1** Prurigo nodularis
- **L28.2** Other prurigo
  - Prurigo NOS
  - Prurigo Hebra
  - Prurigo mitis
  - Urticaria papulosa

L29 Pruritus
Excludes1: neurotic excoriation (L98.1)
psychogenic pruritus (F45.8)
- L29.0 Pruritus ani
- ♂ L29.1 Pruritus scroti
- ♀ L29.2 Pruritus vulvae
- L29.3 Anogenital pruritus, unspecified
- L29.8 Other pruritus
- L29.9 Pruritus, unspecified
  Itch NOS

L30 Other and unspecified dermatitis
Excludes2: contact dermatitis (L23-L25)
dry skin dermatitis (L85.3)
small plaque parapsoriasis (L41.3)
stasis dermatitis (I87.2)
- L30.0 Nummular dermatitis
- L30.1 Dyshidrosis [pompholyx]
- L30.2 Cutaneous autosensitization
  Candidid [levurid]
  Dermatophytid
  Eczematid
- L30.3 Infective dermatitis
  Infectious eczematoid dermatitis
- L30.4 Erythema intertrigo
- L30.5 Pityriasis alba
- L30.8 Other specified dermatitis
- L30.9 Dermatitis, unspecified
  Eczema NOS

Papulosquamous disorders (L40-L45)

L40 Psoriasis
- L40.0 Psoriasis vulgaris
  Nummular psoriasis
  Plaque psoriasis
- L40.1 Generalized pustular psoriasis
  Impetigo herpetiformis
  Von Zumbusch's disease
- L40.2 Acrodermatitis continua
- L40.3 Pustulosis palmaris et plantaris
- L40.4 Guttate psoriasis
- + L40.5 Arthropathic psoriasis
  - L40.50 Arthropathic psoriasis, unspecified
  - L40.51 Distal interphalangeal psoriatic arthropathy
  - L40.52 Psoriatic arthritis mutilans
  - L40.53 Psoriatic spondylitis
  - L40.54 Psoriatic juvenile arthropathy
  - L40.59 Other psoriatic arthropathy
- L40.8 Other psoriasis
  Flexural psoriasis
- L40.9 Psoriasis, unspecified

L41 Parapsoriasis
Excludes1: poikiloderma vasculare atrophicans (L94.5)
- L41.0 Pityriasis lichenoides et varioliformis acuta
  Mucha-Habermann disease
- L41.1 Pityriasis lichenoides chronica
- L41.3 Small plaque parapsoriasis
- L41.4 Large plaque parapsoriasis
- L41.5 Retiform parapsoriasis
- L41.8 Other parapsoriasis
- L41.9 Parapsoriasis, unspecified

L42 Pityriasis rosea
Valid 3-character code, no further characters required

L43 Lichen planus
Excludes1: lichen planopilaris (L66.1)
- L43.0 Hypertrophic lichen planus
- L43.1 Bullous lichen planus
- L43.2 Lichenoid drug reaction
  Use additional code for adverse effect, if applicable, to identify drug (T36-T50 with fifth or sixth character 5)
- L43.3 Subacute (active) lichen planus
  Lichen planus tropicus
- L43.8 Other lichen planus
- L43.9 Lichen planus, unspecified

L44 Other papulosquamous disorders
- L44.0 Pityriasis rubra pilaris
- L44.1 Lichen nitidus
- L44.2 Lichen striatus
- L44.3 Lichen ruber moniliformis
- L44.4 Infantile papular acrodermatitis [Gianotti-Crosti]
- L44.8 Other specified papulosquamous disorders
- L44.9 Papulosquamous disorder, unspecified

L45 Papulosquamous disorders in diseases classified elsewhere
Code first underlying disease.
Valid 3-character code, no further characters required

Urticaria and erythema (L49-L54)
Excludes1: Lyme disease (A69.2-)
rosacea (L71.-)

L49 Exfoliation due to erythematous conditions according to extent of body surface involved
Code first erythematous condition causing exfoliation, such as:
Ritter's disease (L00)
(Staphylococcal) scalded skin syndrome (L00)
Stevens-Johnson syndrome (L51.1)
Stevens-Johnson syndrome-toxic epidermal necrolysis overlap syndrome (L51.3)
Toxic epidermal necrolysis (L51.2)
- L49.0 Exfoliation due to erythematous condition involving less than 10 percent of body surface
  Exfoliation due to erythematous condition NOS
- L49.1 Exfoliation due to erythematous condition involving 10-19 percent of body surface
- L49.2 Exfoliation due to erythematous condition involving 20-29 percent of body surface
- CC L49.3 Exfoliation due to erythematous condition involving 30-39 percent of body surface
- CC L49.4 Exfoliation due to erythematous condition involving 40-49 percent of body surface
- CC L49.5 Exfoliation due to erythematous condition involving 50-59 percent of body surface
- CC L49.6 Exfoliation due to erythematous condition involving 60-69 percent of body surface
- CC L49.7 Exfoliation due to erythematous condition involving 70-79 percent of body surface
- CC L49.8 Exfoliation due to erythematous condition involving 80-89 percent of body surface
- CC L49.9 Exfoliation due to erythematous condition involving 90 or more percent of body surface

L50 Urticaria
Excludes1: allergic contact dermatitis (L23.-)
angioneurotic edema (T78.3)
giant urticaria (T78.3)
hereditary angio-edema (D84.1)
Quincke's edema (T78.3)
serum urticaria (T80.6-)
solar urticaria (L56.3)
urticaria neonatorum (P83.8)
urticaria papulosa (L28.2)
urticaria pigmentosa (D47.01)
- L50.0 Allergic urticaria
- L50.1 Idiopathic urticaria
- L50.2 Urticaria due to cold and heat
  Excludes2: familial cold urticaria (M04.2)
- L50.3 Dermatographic urticaria
- L50.4 Vibratory urticaria
- L50.5 Cholinergic urticaria
- L50.6 Contact urticaria
- L50.8 Other urticaria
  Chronic urticaria
  Recurrent periodic urticaria
- L50.9 Urticaria, unspecified

L51 Erythema multiforme

Use additional code for adverse effect, if applicable, to identify drug (T36-T50 with fifth or sixth character 5)

Use additional code to identify associated manifestations, such as:
arthropathy associated with dermatological disorders (M14.8-)
conjunctival edema (H11.42)
conjunctivitis (H10.22-)
corneal scars and opacities (H17.-)
corneal ulcer (H16.0-)
edema of eyelid (H02.84-)
inflammation of eyelid (H01.8)
keratoconjunctivitis sicca (H16.22-)
mechanical lagophthalmos (H02.22-)
stomatitis (K12.-)
symblepharon (H11.23-)

Use additional code to identify percentage of skin exfoliation (L49.-)

Excludes1: staphylococcal scalded skin syndrome (L00)
Ritter's disease (L00)

- L51.0 Nonbullous erythema multiforme
- CC L51.1 Stevens-Johnson syndrome
- CC L51.2 Toxic epidermal necrolysis [Lyell]
- CC L51.3 Stevens-Johnson syndrome-toxic epidermal necrolysis overlap syndrome
  SJS-TEN overlap syndrome
- L51.8 Other erythema multiforme
- L51.9 Erythema multiforme, unspecified
  Erythema iris
  Erythema multiforme major NOS
  Erythema multiforme minor NOS
  Herpes iris

L52 Erythema nodosum

Excludes1: tuberculous erythema nodosum (A18.4)
Valid 3-character code, no further characters required

L53 Other erythematous conditions

Excludes1: erythema ab igne (L59.0)
erythema due to external agents in contact with skin (L23-L25)
erythema intertrigo (L30.4)

- CC L53.0 Toxic erythema
  Code first poisoning due to drug or toxin, if applicable (T36-T65 with fifth or sixth character 1-4)
  Use additional code for adverse effect, if applicable, to identify drug (T36-T50 with fifth or sixth character 5)
  Excludes1: neonatal erythema toxicum (P83.1)
- CC L53.1 Erythema annulare centrifugum
- CC L53.2 Erythema marginatum
- CC L53.3 Other chronic figurate erythema
- L53.8 Other specified erythematous conditions
- L53.9 Erythematous condition, unspecified
  Erythema NOS
  Erythroderma NOS

L54 Erythema in diseases classified elsewhere

Code first underlying disease
Valid 3-character code, no further characters required

Radiation-related disorders of the skin and subcutaneous tissue (L55-L59)

L55 Sunburn

- L55.0 Sunburn of first degree
- L55.1 Sunburn of second degree
- L55.2 Sunburn of third degree
- L55.9 Sunburn, unspecified

L56 Other acute skin changes due to ultraviolet radiation

Use additional code to identify the source of the ultraviolet radiation (W89, X32)

- L56.0 Drug phototoxic response
  Use additional code for adverse effect, if applicable, to identify drug (T36-T50 with fifth or sixth character 5)
- L56.1 Drug photoallergic response
  Use additional code for adverse effect, if applicable, to identify drug (T36-T50 with fifth or sixth character 5)
- L56.2 Photocontact dermatitis [berloque dermatitis]
- L56.3 Solar urticaria
- L56.4 Polymorphous light eruption
- L56.5 Disseminated superficial actinic porokeratosis (DSAP)
- L56.8 Other specified acute skin changes due to ultraviolet radiation
- L56.9 Acute skin change due to ultraviolet radiation, unspecified

L57 Skin changes due to chronic exposure to nonionizing radiation

Use additional code to identify the source of the ultraviolet radiation (W89), or other nonionizing radiation (W90)

- L57.0 Actinic keratosis
  Keratosis NOS
  Senile keratosis
  Solar keratosis
- L57.1 Actinic reticuloid
- L57.2 Cutis rhomboidalis nuchae
- L57.3 Poikiloderma of Civatte
- L57.4 Cutis laxa senilis
  Elastosis senilis
- L57.5 Actinic granuloma
- L57.8 Other skin changes due to chronic exposure to nonionizing radiation
  Farmer's skin
  Sailor's skin
  Solar dermatitis
- L57.9 Skin changes due to chronic exposure to nonionizing radiation, unspecified

L58 Radiodermatitis

Use additional code to identify the source of the radiation (W88, W90)

- L58.0 Acute radiodermatitis
- L58.1 Chronic radiodermatitis
- L58.9 Radiodermatitis, unspecified

L59 Other disorders of skin and subcutaneous tissue related to radiation

- L59.0 Erythema ab igne [dermatitis ab igne]
- L59.8 Other specified disorders of the skin and subcutaneous tissue related to radiation
  AHA CC: 1Q, 2017, 33-34
- L59.9 Disorder of the skin and subcutaneous tissue related to radiation, unspecified

Disorders of skin appendages (L60-L75)

Excludes1: congenital malformations of integument (Q84.-)

L60 Nail disorders

Excludes2: clubbing of nails (R68.3)
onychia and paronychia (L03.0-)

- L60.0 Ingrowing nail
- L60.1 Onycholysis
- L60.2 Onychogryphosis
- L60.3 Nail dystrophy
- L60.4 Beau's lines
- L60.5 Yellow nail syndrome
- L60.8 Other nail disorders
- L60.9 Nail disorder, unspecified

L62 Nail disorders in diseases classified elsewhere

Code first underlying disease, such as:
pachydermoperiostosis (M89.4-)
Valid 3-character code, no further characters required

L63 Alopecia areata

- L63.0 Alopecia (capitis) totalis
- L63.1 Alopecia universalis
- L63.2 Ophiasis
- L63.8 Other alopecia areata
- L63.9 Alopecia areata, unspecified

L64 Androgenic alopecia

Includes: male-pattern baldness

- L64.0 Drug-induced androgenic alopecia
  Use additional code for adverse effect, if applicable, to identify drug (T36-T50 with fifth or sixth character 5)
- L64.8 Other androgenic alopecia
- L64.9 Androgenic alopecia, unspecified

L65 Other nonscarring hair loss
Use additional code for adverse effect, if applicable, to identify drug (T36-T50 with fifth or sixth character 5)
Excludes1: *trichotillomania (F63.3)*
- L65.0 Telogen effluvium
- L65.1 Anagen effluvium
- L65.2 Alopecia mucinosa
- L65.8 Other specified nonscarring hair loss
- L65.9 Nonscarring hair loss, unspecified
  Alopecia NOS

L66 Cicatricial alopecia [scarring hair loss]
- L66.0 Pseudopelade
- L66.1 Lichen planopilaris
  Follicular lichen planus
- L66.2 Folliculitis decalvans
- L66.3 Perifolliculitis capitis abscedens
- L66.4 Folliculitis ulerythematosa reticulata
- L66.8 Other cicatricial alopecia
  AHA CC: 1Q, 2015, 19
- L66.9 Cicatricial alopecia, unspecified

L67 Hair color and hair shaft abnormalities
Excludes1: *monilethrix (Q84.1)*
pili annulati (Q84.1)
telogen effluvium (L65.0)
- L67.0 Trichorrhexis nodosa
- L67.1 Variations in hair color
  Canities
  Greyness, hair (premature)
  Heterochromia of hair
  Poliosis circumscripta, acquired
  Poliosis NOS
- L67.8 Other hair color and hair shaft abnormalities
  Fragilitas crinium
- L67.9 Hair color and hair shaft abnormality, unspecified

L68 Hypertrichosis
Includes: excess hair
Excludes1: *congenital hypertrichosis (Q84.2)*
persistent lanugo (Q84.2)
- L68.0 Hirsutism
- L68.1 Acquired hypertrichosis lanuginosa
- L68.2 Localized hypertrichosis
- L68.3 Polytrichia
- L68.8 Other hypertrichosis
- L68.9 Hypertrichosis, unspecified

L70 Acne
Excludes2: *acne keloid (L73.0)*
- L70.0 Acne vulgaris
- L70.1 Acne conglobata
- L70.2 Acne varioliformis
  Acne necrotica miliaris
- L70.3 Acne tropica
- L70.4 Infantile acne
- L70.5 Acné excoriée
  Acné exocoriée des jeunes filles
  Picker's acne
- L70.8 Other acne
- L70.9 Acne, unspecified

L71 Rosacea
Use additional code for adverse effect, if applicable, to identify drug (T36-T50 with fifth or sixth character 5)
- L71.0 Perioral dermatitis
- L71.1 Rhinophyma
- L71.8 Other rosacea
  AHA CC: 4Q, 2018, 15
- L71.9 Rosacea, unspecified

L72 Follicular cysts of skin and subcutaneous tissue
- L72.0 Epidermal cyst
- + L72.1 Pilar and trichodermal cyst
  - L72.11 Pilar cyst
  - L72.12 Trichodermal cyst
    Trichilemmal (proliferating) cyst
- L72.2 Steatocystoma multiplex
- L72.3 Sebaceous cyst
  Excludes2: *pilar cyst (L72.11)*
  trichilemmal (proliferating) cyst (L72.12)
- L72.8 Other follicular cysts of the skin and subcutaneous tissue
- L72.9 Follicular cyst of the skin and subcutaneous tissue, unspecified

L73 Other follicular disorders
- L73.0 Acne keloid
- L73.1 Pseudofolliculitis barbae
- L73.2 Hidradenitis suppurativa
- L73.8 Other specified follicular disorders
  Sycosis barbae
- L73.9 Follicular disorder, unspecified

L74 Eccrine sweat disorders
Excludes2: *generalized hyperhidrosis (R61)*
- L74.0 Miliaria rubra
- L74.1 Miliaria crystallina
- L74.2 Miliaria profunda
  Miliaria tropicalis
- L74.3 Miliaria, unspecified
- L74.4 Anhidrosis
  Hypohidrosis
- + L74.5 Focal hyperhidrosis
  - + L74.51 Primary focal hyperhidrosis
    - L74.510 Primary focal hyperhidrosis, axilla
    - L74.511 Primary focal hyperhidrosis, face
    - L74.512 Primary focal hyperhidrosis, palms
    - L74.513 Primary focal hyperhidrosis, soles
    - L74.519 Primary focal hyperhidrosis, unspecified
  - L74.52 Secondary focal hyperhidrosis
    Frey's syndrome
- L74.8 Other eccrine sweat disorders
- L74.9 Eccrine sweat disorder, unspecified
  Sweat gland disorder NOS

L75 Apocrine sweat disorders
Excludes1: *dyshidrosis (L30.1)*
hidradenitis suppurativa (L73.2)
- L75.0 Bromhidrosis
- L75.1 Chromhidrosis
- L75.2 Apocrine miliaria
  Fox-Fordyce disease
- L75.8 Other apocrine sweat disorders
- L75.9 Apocrine sweat disorder, unspecified

Intraoperative and postprocedural complications of skin and subcutaneous tissue (L76)

L76 Intraoperative and postprocedural complications of skin and subcutaneous tissue
AHA CC: 4Q, 2016, 9-10
- + L76.0 Intraoperative hemorrhage and hematoma of skin and subcutaneous tissue complicating a procedure
  Excludes1: *intraoperative hemorrhage and hematoma of skin and subcutaneous tissue due to accidental puncture and laceration during a procedure (L76.1-)*
  - CC L76.01 Intraoperative hemorrhage and hematoma of skin and subcutaneous tissue complicating a dermatologic procedure
  - CC L76.02 Intraoperative hemorrhage and hematoma of skin and subcutaneous tissue complicating other procedure
- + L76.1 Accidental puncture and laceration of skin and subcutaneous tissue during a procedure
  - CC L76.11 Accidental puncture and laceration of skin and subcutaneous tissue during a dermatologic procedure
  - CC L76.12 Accidental puncture and laceration of skin and subcutaneous tissue during other procedure
- + L76.2 Postprocedural hemorrhage of skin and subcutaneous tissue following a procedure
  - CC L76.21 Postprocedural hemorrhage of skin and subcutaneous tissue following a dermatologic procedure
  - CC L76.22 Postprocedural hemorrhage of skin and subcutaneous tissue following other procedure

+ **L76.3** Postprocedural hematoma and seroma of skin and subcutaneous tissue following a procedure
- CC **L76.31** Postprocedural hematoma of skin and subcutaneous tissue following a dermatologic procedure
- CC **L76.32** Postprocedural hematoma of skin and subcutaneous tissue following other procedure
- CC **L76.33** Postprocedural seroma of skin and subcutaneous tissue following a dermatologic procedure
- CC **L76.34** Postprocedural seroma of skin and subcutaneous tissue following other procedure

+ **L76.8** Other intraoperative and postprocedural complications of skin and subcutaneous tissue
Use additional code, if applicable, to further specify disorder
- **L76.81** Other intraoperative complications of skin and subcutaneous tissue
- **L76.82** Other postprocedural complications of skin and subcutaneous tissue
  AHA CC: 3Q, 2017, 6

Other disorders of the skin and subcutaneous tissue (L80-L99)

L80 Vitiligo
Excludes2: vitiligo of eyelids (H02.73-)
vitiligo of vulva (N90.89)
Valid 3-character code, no further characters required

L81 Other disorders of pigmentation
Excludes1: birthmark NOS (Q82.5)
Peutz-Jeghers syndrome (Q85.89)
Excludes2: nevus - see Alphabetical Index
- **L81.0** Postinflammatory hyperpigmentation
- **L81.1** Chloasma
- **L81.2** Freckles
- **L81.3** Café au lait spots
- **L81.4** Other melanin hyperpigmentation
  Lentigo
- **L81.5** Leukoderma, not elsewhere classified
- **L81.6** Other disorders of diminished melanin formation
- **L81.7** Pigmented purpuric dermatosis
  Angioma serpiginosum
- **L81.8** Other specified disorders of pigmentation
  Iron pigmentation
  Tattoo pigmentation
- **L81.9** Disorder of pigmentation, unspecified

L82 Seborrheic keratosis
Includes: basal cell papilloma
dermatosis papulosa nigra
Leser-Trélat disease
Excludes2: seborrheic dermatitis (L21.-)
- **L82.0** Inflamed seborrheic keratosis
  AHA CC: 3Q, 2021, 10-11; 2Q, 2023, 12
- **L82.1** Other seborrheic keratosis
  Seborrheic keratosis NOS

L83 Acanthosis nigricans
Confluent and reticulated papillomatosis
Valid 3-character code, no further characters required

L84 Corns and callosities
Callus
Clavus
Valid 3-character code, no further characters required

L85 Other epidermal thickening
Excludes2: hypertrophic disorders of the skin (L91.-)
- **L85.0** Acquired ichthyosis
  Excludes1: congenital ichthyosis (Q80.-)
- **L85.1** Acquired keratosis [keratoderma] palmaris et plantaris
  Excludes1: inherited keratosis palmaris et plantaris (Q82.8)
- **L85.2** Keratosis punctata (palmaris et plantaris)
- **L85.3** Xerosis cutis
  Dry skin dermatitis
- **L85.8** Other specified epidermal thickening
  Cutaneous horn
- **L85.9** Epidermal thickening, unspecified

L86 Keratoderma in diseases classified elsewhere
Code first underlying disease, such as:
Reiter's disease (M02.3-)
Excludes1: gonococcal keratoderma (A54.89)
gonococcal keratosis (A54.89)
keratoderma due to vitamin A deficiency (E50.8)
keratosis due to vitamin A deficiency (E50.8)
xeroderma due to vitamin A deficiency (E50.8)
Valid 3-character code, no further characters required

L87 Transepidermal elimination disorders
Excludes1: granuloma annulare (perforating) (L92.0)
- **L87.0** Keratosis follicularis et parafollicularis in cutem penetrans
  Kyrle disease
  Hyperkeratosis follicularis penetrans
- **L87.1** Reactive perforating collagenosis
- **L87.2** Elastosis perforans serpiginosa
- **L87.8** Other transepidermal elimination disorders
- **L87.9** Transepidermal elimination disorder, unspecified

CC **L88** Pyoderma gangrenosum
Phagedenic pyoderma
Excludes1: dermatitis gangrenosa (L08.0)
Valid 3-character code, no further characters required

L89 Pressure ulcer
Includes: bed sore
decubitus ulcer
plaster ulcer
pressure area
pressure sore
Code first any associated gangrene (I96)
Excludes2: decubitus (trophic) ulcer of cervix (uteri) (N86)
diabetic ulcers (E08.621, E08.622, E09.621, E09.622, E10.621, E10.622, E11.621, E11.622, E13.621, E13.622)
non-pressure chronic ulcer of skin (L97.-)
skin infections (L00-L08)
varicose ulcer (I83.0, I83.2)
AHA CC: 2Q, 2018, 21-22; 4Q, 2019, 10-11
Review coding guidelines B.14 and C.12.a

+ **L89.0** Pressure ulcer of elbow
  + **L89.00** Pressure ulcer of unspecified elbow
    - **L89.000** Pressure ulcer of unspecified elbow, unstageable
    - **L89.001** Pressure ulcer of unspecified elbow, stage 1
      Healing pressure ulcer of unspecified elbow, stage 1
      Pressure pre-ulcer skin changes limited to persistent focal edema, unspecified elbow
    - **L89.002** Pressure ulcer of unspecified elbow, stage 2
      Healing pressure ulcer of unspecified elbow, stage 2
      Pressure ulcer with abrasion, blister, partial thickness skin loss involving epidermis and/or dermis, unspecified elbow
    - MCC **L89.003** Pressure ulcer of unspecified elbow, stage 3
      Healing pressure ulcer of unspecified elbow, stage 3
      Pressure ulcer with full thickness skin loss involving damage or necrosis of subcutaneous tissue, unspecified elbow
      HAC see Appendix B for HAC conditional logic
    - MCC **L89.004** Pressure ulcer of unspecified elbow, stage 4
      Healing pressure ulcer of unspecified elbow, stage 4
      Pressure ulcer with necrosis of soft tissues through to underlying muscle, tendon, or bone, unspecified elbow
      HAC see Appendix B for HAC conditional logic

Pressure Ulcer

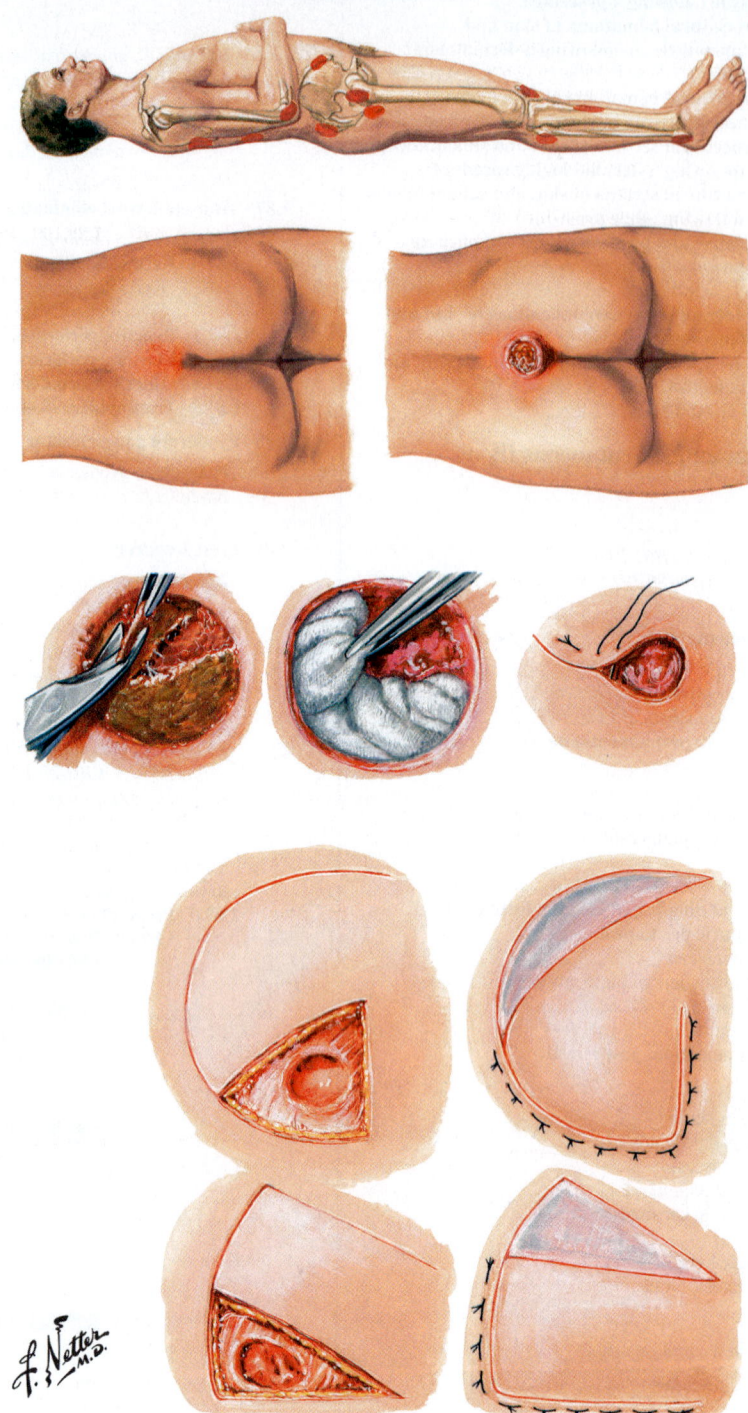

L89.006 Pressure-induced deep tissue damage of unspecified elbow	**L89.012** Pressure ulcer of right elbow, stage 2
L89.009 Pressure ulcer of unspecified elbow, unspecified stage	Healing pressure ulcer of right elbow, stage 2
Healing pressure ulcer of elbow NOS	Pressure ulcer with abrasion, blister, partial thickness skin loss involving epidermis and/or dermis, right elbow
Healing pressure ulcer of unspecified elbow, unspecified stage	MCC **L89.013** Pressure ulcer of right elbow, stage 3
+ **L89.01** Pressure ulcer of right elbow	Healing pressure ulcer of right elbow, stage 3
L89.010 Pressure ulcer of right elbow, unstageable	Pressure ulcer with full thickness skin loss involving damage or necrosis of subcutaneous tissue, right elbow
L89.011 Pressure ulcer of right elbow, stage 1	HAC see Appendix B for HAC conditional logic
Healing pressure ulcer of right elbow, stage 1	
Pressure pre-ulcer skin changes limited to persistent focal edema, right elbow	

MCC L89.014 **Pressure ulcer of right elbow, stage 4**
  Healing pressure ulcer of right elbow, stage 4
  Pressure ulcer with necrosis of soft tissues through to underlying muscle, tendon, or bone, right elbow
  HAC see Appendix B for HAC conditional logic

L89.016 Pressure-induced deep tissue damage of right elbow

L89.019 Pressure ulcer of right elbow, unspecified stage
  Healing pressure ulcer of right elbow NOS

+ **L89.02 Pressure ulcer of left elbow**
  L89.020 Pressure ulcer of left elbow, unstageable
  L89.021 Pressure ulcer of left elbow, stage 1
    Healing pressure ulcer of left elbow, stage 1
    Pressure pre-ulcer skin changes limited to persistent focal edema, left elbow
  L89.022 Pressure ulcer of left elbow, stage 2
    Healing pressure ulcer of left elbow, stage 2
    Pressure ulcer with abrasion, blister, partial thickness skin loss involving epidermis and/or dermis, left elbow
  MCC L89.023 **Pressure ulcer of left elbow, stage 3**
    Healing pressure ulcer of left elbow, stage 3
    Pressure ulcer with full thickness skin loss involving damage or necrosis of subcutaneous tissue, left elbow
    HAC see Appendix B for HAC conditional logic
  MCC L89.024 **Pressure ulcer of left elbow, stage 4**
    Healing pressure ulcer of left elbow, stage 4
    Pressure ulcer with necrosis of soft tissues through to underlying muscle, tendon, or bone, left elbow
    HAC see Appendix B for HAC conditional logic
  L89.026 Pressure-induced deep tissue damage of left elbow
  L89.029 Pressure ulcer of left elbow, unspecified stage
    Healing pressure ulcer of left elbow NOS

+ **L89.1 Pressure ulcer of back**
  + **L89.10 Pressure ulcer of unspecified part of back**
    L89.100 Pressure ulcer of unspecified part of back, unstageable
    L89.101 Pressure ulcer of unspecified part of back, stage 1
      Healing pressure ulcer of unspecified part of back, stage 1
      Pressure pre-ulcer skin changes limited to persistent focal edema, unspecified part of back
    L89.102 Pressure ulcer of unspecified part of back, stage 2
      Healing pressure ulcer of unspecified part of back, stage 2
      Pressure ulcer with abrasion, blister, partial thickness skin loss involving epidermis and/or dermis, unspecified part of back
    MCC L89.103 **Pressure ulcer of unspecified part of back, stage 3**
      Healing pressure ulcer of unspecified part of back, stage 3
      Pressure ulcer with full thickness skin loss involving damage or necrosis of subcutaneous tissue, unspecified part of back
      HAC see Appendix B for HAC conditional logic

MCC L89.104 **Pressure ulcer of unspecified part of back, stage 4**
  Healing pressure ulcer of unspecified part of back, stage 4
  Pressure ulcer with necrosis of soft tissues through to underlying muscle, tendon, or bone, unspecified part of back
  HAC see Appendix B for HAC conditional logic

L89.106 Pressure-induced deep tissue damage of unspecified part of back

L89.109 Pressure ulcer of unspecified part of back, unspecified stage
  Healing pressure ulcer of unspecified part of back NOS
  Healing pressure ulcer of unspecified part of back, unspecified stage

+ **L89.11 Pressure ulcer of right upper back**
  Pressure ulcer of right shoulder blade
  L89.110 Pressure ulcer of right upper back, unstageable
  L89.111 Pressure ulcer of right upper back, stage 1
    Healing pressure ulcer of right upper back, stage 1
    Pressure pre-ulcer skin changes limited to persistent focal edema, right upper back
  L89.112 Pressure ulcer of right upper back, stage 2
    Healing pressure ulcer of right upper back, stage 2
    Pressure ulcer with abrasion, blister, partial thickness skin loss involving epidermis and/or dermis, right upper back
  MCC L89.113 **Pressure ulcer of right upper back, stage 3**
    Healing pressure ulcer of right upper back, stage 3
    Pressure ulcer with full thickness skin loss involving damage or necrosis of subcutaneous tissue, right upper back
    HAC see Appendix B for HAC conditional logic
  MCC L89.114 **Pressure ulcer of right upper back, stage 4**
    Healing pressure ulcer of right upper back, stage 4
    Pressure ulcer with necrosis of soft tissues through to underlying muscle, tendon, or bone, right upper back
    HAC see Appendix B for HAC conditional logic
  L89.116 Pressure-induced deep tissue damage of right upper back
  L89.119 Pressure ulcer of right upper back, unspecified stage
    Healing pressure ulcer of right upper back NOS
    Healing pressure ulcer of right upper back, unspecified stage

+ **L89.12 Pressure ulcer of left upper back**
  Pressure ulcer of left shoulder blade
  L89.120 Pressure ulcer of left upper back, unstageable
  L89.121 Pressure ulcer of left upper back, stage 1
    Healing pressure ulcer of left upper back, stage 1
    Pressure pre-ulcer skin changes limited to persistent focal edema, left upper back
  L89.122 Pressure ulcer of left upper back, stage 2
    Healing pressure ulcer of left upper back, stage 2
    Pressure ulcer with abrasion, blister, partial thickness skin loss involving epidermis and/or dermis, left upper back

L89.123–L89.159

Chapter 12: Diseases of the Skin and Subcutaneous Tissue

- **MCC L89.123** Pressure ulcer of left upper back, stage 3
  - Healing pressure ulcer of left upper back, stage 3
  - Pressure ulcer with full thickness skin loss involving damage or necrosis of subcutaneous tissue, left upper back
  - **HAC** see Appendix B for HAC conditional logic
- **MCC L89.124** Pressure ulcer of left upper back, stage 4
  - Healing pressure ulcer of left upper back, stage 4
  - Pressure ulcer with necrosis of soft tissues through to underlying muscle, tendon, or bone, left upper back
  - **HAC** see Appendix B for HAC conditional logic
- **L89.126** Pressure-induced deep tissue damage of left upper back
- **L89.129** Pressure ulcer of left upper back, unspecified stage
  - Healing pressure ulcer of left upper back NOS
  - Healing pressure ulcer of left upper back, unspecified stage

+ L89.13 Pressure ulcer of right lower back
- **L89.130** Pressure ulcer of right lower back, unstageable
- **L89.131** Pressure ulcer of right lower back, stage 1
  - Healing pressure ulcer of right lower back, stage 1
  - Pressure pre-ulcer skin changes limited to persistent focal edema, right lower back
- **L89.132** Pressure ulcer of right lower back, stage 2
  - Healing pressure ulcer of right lower back, stage 2
  - Pressure ulcer with abrasion, blister, partial thickness skin loss involving epidermis and/or dermis, right lower back
- **MCC L89.133** Pressure ulcer of right lower back, stage 3
  - Healing pressure ulcer of right lower back, stage 3
  - Pressure ulcer with full thickness skin loss involving damage or necrosis of subcutaneous tissue, right lower back
  - **HAC** see Appendix B for HAC conditional logic
- **MCC L89.134** Pressure ulcer of right lower back, stage 4
  - Healing pressure ulcer of right lower back, stage 4
  - Pressure ulcer with necrosis of soft tissues through to underlying muscle, tendon, or bone, right lower back
  - **HAC** see Appendix B for HAC conditional logic
- **L89.136** Pressure-induced deep tissue damage of right lower back
- **L89.139** Pressure ulcer of right lower back, unspecified stage
  - Healing pressure ulcer of right lower back NOS
  - Healing pressure ulcer of right lower back, unspecified stage

+ L89.14 Pressure ulcer of left lower back
- **L89.140** Pressure ulcer of left lower back, unstageable
- **L89.141** Pressure ulcer of left lower back, stage 1
  - Healing pressure ulcer of left lower back, stage 1
  - Pressure pre-ulcer skin changes limited to persistent focal edema, left lower back
- **L89.142** Pressure ulcer of left lower back, stage 2
  - Healing pressure ulcer of left lower back, stage 2
  - Pressure ulcer with abrasion, blister, partial thickness skin loss involving epidermis and/or dermis, left lower back
- **MCC L89.143** Pressure ulcer of left lower back, stage 3
  - Healing pressure ulcer of left lower back, stage 3
  - Pressure ulcer with full thickness skin loss involving damage or necrosis of subcutaneous tissue, left lower back
  - **HAC** see Appendix B for HAC conditional logic
- **MCC L89.144** Pressure ulcer of left lower back, stage 4
  - Healing pressure ulcer of left lower back, stage 4
  - Pressure ulcer with necrosis of soft tissues through to underlying muscle, tendon, or bone, left lower back
  - **HAC** see Appendix B for HAC conditional logic
- **L89.146** Pressure-induced deep tissue damage of left lower back
- **L89.149** Pressure ulcer of left lower back, unspecified stage
  - Healing pressure ulcer of left lower back NOS
  - Healing pressure ulcer of left lower back, unspecified stage

+ L89.15 Pressure ulcer of sacral region
  - Pressure ulcer of coccyx
  - Pressure ulcer of tailbone
- **L89.150** Pressure ulcer of sacral region, unstageable
- **L89.151** Pressure ulcer of sacral region, stage 1
  - Healing pressure ulcer of sacral region, stage 1
  - Pressure pre-ulcer skin changes limited to persistent focal edema, sacral region
- **L89.152** Pressure ulcer of sacral region, stage 2
  - Healing pressure ulcer of sacral region, stage 2
  - Pressure ulcer with abrasion, blister, partial thickness skin loss involving epidermis and/or dermis, sacral region
- **MCC L89.153** Pressure ulcer of sacral region, stage 3
  - Healing pressure ulcer of sacral region, stage 3
  - Pressure ulcer with full thickness skin loss involving damage or necrosis of subcutaneous tissue, sacral region
  - *AHA CC: 3Q, 2021, 10*
  - **HAC** see Appendix B for HAC conditional logic
- **MCC L89.154** Pressure ulcer of sacral region, stage 4
  - Healing pressure ulcer of sacral region, stage 4
  - Pressure ulcer with necrosis of soft tissues through to underlying muscle, tendon, or bone, sacral region
  - *AHA CC: 1Q, 2021, 24; 2Q, 2022, 8-9*
  - **HAC** see Appendix B for HAC conditional logic
- **L89.156** Pressure-induced deep tissue damage of sacral region
- **L89.159** Pressure ulcer of sacral region, unspecified stage
  - Healing pressure ulcer of sacral region NOS
  - Healing pressure ulcer of sacral region, unspecified stage

- **L89.2 Pressure ulcer of hip**
  - **L89.20 Pressure ulcer of unspecified hip**
    - **L89.200** Pressure ulcer of unspecified hip, unstageable
    - **L89.201** Pressure ulcer of unspecified hip, stage 1
      - Healing pressure ulcer of unspecified hip back, stage 1
      - Pressure pre-ulcer skin changes limited to persistent focal edema, unspecified hip
    - **L89.202** Pressure ulcer of unspecified hip, stage 2
      - Healing pressure ulcer of unspecified hip, stage 2
      - Pressure ulcer with abrasion, blister, partial thickness skin loss involving epidermis and/or dermis, unspecified hip
    - MCC **L89.203** Pressure ulcer of unspecified hip, stage 3
      - Healing pressure ulcer of unspecified hip, stage 3
      - Pressure ulcer with full thickness skin loss involving damage or necrosis of subcutaneous tissue, unspecified hip
      - HAC see Appendix B for HAC conditional logic
    - MCC **L89.204** Pressure ulcer of unspecified hip, stage 4
      - Healing pressure ulcer of unspecified hip, stage 4
      - Pressure ulcer with necrosis of soft tissues through to underlying muscle, tendon, or bone, unspecified hip
      - HAC see Appendix B for HAC conditional logic
    - **L89.206** Pressure-induced deep tissue damage of unspecified hip
    - **L89.209** Pressure ulcer of unspecified hip, unspecified stage
      - Healing pressure ulcer of unspecified hip NOS
      - Healing pressure ulcer of unspecified hip, unspecified stage
  - **L89.21 Pressure ulcer of right hip**
    - **L89.210** Pressure ulcer of right hip, unstageable
    - **L89.211** Pressure ulcer of right hip, stage 1
      - Healing pressure ulcer of right hip back, stage 1
      - Pressure pre-ulcer skin changes limited to persistent focal edema, right hip
    - **L89.212** Pressure ulcer of right hip, stage 2
      - Healing pressure ulcer of right hip, stage 2
      - Pressure ulcer with abrasion, blister, partial thickness skin loss involving epidermis and/or dermis, right hip
    - MCC **L89.213** Pressure ulcer of right hip, stage 3
      - Healing pressure ulcer of right hip, stage 3
      - Pressure ulcer with full thickness skin loss involving damage or necrosis of subcutaneous tissue, right hip
      - HAC see Appendix B for HAC conditional logic
    - MCC **L89.214** Pressure ulcer of right hip, stage 4
      - Healing pressure ulcer of right hip, stage 4
      - Pressure ulcer with necrosis of soft tissues through to underlying muscle, tendon, or bone, right hip
      - HAC see Appendix B for HAC conditional logic
    - **L89.216** Pressure-induced deep tissue damage of right hip
    - **L89.219** Pressure ulcer of right hip, unspecified stage
      - Healing pressure ulcer of right hip NOS
      - Healing pressure ulcer of right hip, unspecified stage
  - **L89.22 Pressure ulcer of left hip**
    - **L89.220** Pressure ulcer of left hip, unstageable
    - **L89.221** Pressure ulcer of left hip, stage 1
      - Healing pressure ulcer of left hip back, stage 1
      - Pressure pre-ulcer skin changes limited to persistent focal edema, left hip
    - **L89.222** Pressure ulcer of left hip, stage 2
      - Healing pressure ulcer of left hip, stage 2
      - Pressure ulcer with abrasion, blister, partial thickness skin loss involving epidermis and/or dermis, left hip
    - MCC **L89.223** Pressure ulcer of left hip, stage 3
      - Healing pressure ulcer of left hip, stage 3
      - Pressure ulcer with full thickness skin loss involving damage or necrosis of subcutaneous tissue, left hip
      - HAC see Appendix B for HAC conditional logic
    - MCC **L89.224** Pressure ulcer of left hip, stage 4
      - Healing pressure ulcer of left hip, stage 4
      - Pressure ulcer with necrosis of soft tissues through to underlying muscle, tendon, or bone, left hip
      - HAC see Appendix B for HAC conditional logic
    - **L89.226** Pressure-induced deep tissue damage of left hip
    - **L89.229** Pressure ulcer of left hip, unspecified stage
      - Healing pressure ulcer of left hip NOS
      - Healing pressure ulcer of left hip, unspecified stage
- **L89.3 Pressure ulcer of buttock**
  - **L89.30 Pressure ulcer of unspecified buttock**
    - **L89.300** Pressure ulcer of unspecified buttock, unstageable
    - **L89.301** Pressure ulcer of unspecified buttock, stage 1
      - Healing pressure ulcer of unspecified buttock, stage 1
      - Pressure pre-ulcer skin changes limited to persistent focal edema, unspecified buttock
    - **L89.302** Pressure ulcer of unspecified buttock, stage 2
      - Healing pressure ulcer of unspecified buttock, stage 2
      - Pressure ulcer with abrasion, blister, partial thickness skin loss involving epidermis and/or dermis, unspecified buttock
    - MCC **L89.303** Pressure ulcer of unspecified buttock, stage 3
      - Healing pressure ulcer of unspecified buttock, stage 3
      - Pressure ulcer with full thickness skin loss involving damage or necrosis of subcutaneous tissue, unspecified buttock
      - HAC see Appendix B for HAC conditional logic
    - MCC **L89.304** Pressure ulcer of unspecified buttock, stage 4
      - Healing pressure ulcer of unspecified buttock, stage 4
      - Pressure ulcer with necrosis of soft tissues through to underlying muscle, tendon, or bone, unspecified buttock
      - HAC see Appendix B for HAC conditional logic
    - **L89.306** Pressure-induced deep tissue damage of unspecified buttock
    - **L89.309** Pressure ulcer of unspecified buttock, unspecified stage
      - Healing pressure ulcer of unspecified buttock NOS
      - Healing pressure ulcer of unspecified buttock, unspecified stage

+ L89.31 Pressure ulcer of right buttock
 L89.310 Pressure ulcer of right buttock, unstageable
 L89.311 Pressure ulcer of right buttock, stage 1
  Healing pressure ulcer of right buttock, stage 1
  Pressure pre-ulcer skin changes limited to persistent focal edema, right buttock
 L89.312 Pressure ulcer of right buttock, stage 2
  Healing pressure ulcer of right buttock, stage 2
  Pressure ulcer with abrasion, blister, partial thickness skin loss involving epidermis and/or dermis, right buttock
 MCC **L89.313 Pressure ulcer of right buttock, stage 3**
  Healing pressure ulcer of right buttock, stage 3
  Pressure ulcer with full thickness skin loss involving damage or necrosis of subcutaneous tissue, right buttock
  HAC see Appendix B for HAC conditional logic
 MCC **L89.314 Pressure ulcer of right buttock, stage 4**
  Healing pressure ulcer of right buttock, stage 4
  Pressure ulcer with necrosis of soft tissues through to underlying muscle, tendon, or bone, right buttock
  HAC see Appendix B for HAC conditional logic
 L89.316 Pressure-induced deep tissue damage of right buttock
 L89.319 Pressure ulcer of right buttock, unspecified stage
  Healing pressure ulcer of right buttock NOS
  Healing pressure ulcer of right buttock, unspecified stage

+ L89.32 Pressure ulcer of left buttock
 L89.320 Pressure ulcer of left buttock, unstageable
 L89.321 Pressure ulcer of left buttock, stage 1
  Healing pressure ulcer of left buttock, stage 1
  Pressure pre-ulcer skin changes limited to persistent focal edema, left buttock
 L89.322 Pressure ulcer of left buttock, stage 2
  Healing pressure ulcer of left buttock, stage 2
  Pressure ulcer with abrasion, blister, partial thickness skin loss involving epidermis and/or dermis, left buttock
 MCC **L89.323 Pressure ulcer of left buttock, stage 3**
  Healing pressure ulcer of left buttock, stage 3
  Pressure ulcer with full thickness skin loss involving damage or necrosis of subcutaneous tissue, left buttock
  HAC see Appendix B for HAC conditional logic
 MCC **L89.324 Pressure ulcer of left buttock, stage 4**
  Healing pressure ulcer of left buttock, stage 4
  Pressure ulcer with necrosis of soft tissues through to underlying muscle, tendon, or bone, left buttock
  HAC see Appendix B for HAC conditional logic
 L89.326 Pressure-induced deep tissue damage of left buttock
 L89.329 Pressure ulcer of left buttock, unspecified stage
  Healing pressure ulcer of left buttock NOS
  Healing pressure ulcer of left buttock, unspecified stage

+ L89.4 Pressure ulcer of contiguous site of back, buttock and hip
 L89.40 Pressure ulcer of contiguous site of back, buttock and hip, unspecified stage
  Healing pressure ulcer of contiguous site of back, buttock and hip NOS
  Healing pressure ulcer of contiguous site of back, buttock and hip, unspecified stage
 L89.41 **Pressure ulcer of contiguous site of back, buttock and hip, stage 1**
  Healing pressure ulcer of contiguous site of back, buttock and hip, stage 1
  Pressure pre-ulcer skin changes limited to persistent focal edema, contiguous site of back, buttock and hip
 L89.42 **Pressure ulcer of contiguous site of back, buttock and hip, stage 2**
  Healing pressure ulcer of contiguous site of back, buttock and hip, stage 2
  Pressure ulcer with abrasion, blister, partial thickness skin loss involving epidermis and/or dermis, contiguous site of back, buttock and hip
 MCC L89.43 **Pressure ulcer of contiguous site of back, buttock and hip, stage 3**
  Healing pressure ulcer of contiguous site of back, buttock and hip, stage 3
  Pressure ulcer with full thickness skin loss involving damage or necrosis of subcutaneous tissue, contiguous site of back, buttock and hip
  HAC see Appendix B for HAC conditional logic
 MCC L89.44 **Pressure ulcer of contiguous site of back, buttock and hip, stage 4**
  Healing pressure ulcer of contiguous site of back, buttock and hip, stage 4
  Pressure ulcer with necrosis of soft tissues through to underlying muscle, tendon, or bone, contiguous site of back, buttock and hip
  HAC see Appendix B for HAC conditional logic
 L89.45 **Pressure ulcer of contiguous site of back, buttock and hip, unstageable**
 L89.46 Pressure-induced deep tissue damage of contiguous site of back, buttock and hip

+ L89.5 Pressure ulcer of ankle
 + L89.50 Pressure ulcer of unspecified ankle
  L89.500 Pressure ulcer of unspecified ankle, unstageable
  L89.501 Pressure ulcer of unspecified ankle, stage 1
   Healing pressure ulcer of unspecified ankle, stage 1
   Pressure pre-ulcer skin changes limited to persistent focal edema, unspecified ankle
  L89.502 **Pressure ulcer of unspecified ankle, stage 2**
   Healing pressure ulcer of unspecified ankle, stage 2
   Pressure ulcer with abrasion, blister, partial thickness skin loss involving epidermis and/or dermis, unspecified ankle
  MCC L89.503 **Pressure ulcer of unspecified ankle, stage 3**
   Healing pressure ulcer of unspecified ankle, stage 3
   Pressure ulcer with full thickness skin loss involving damage or necrosis of subcutaneous tissue, unspecified ankle
   HAC see Appendix B for HAC conditional logic
  MCC L89.504 **Pressure ulcer of unspecified ankle, stage 4**
   Healing pressure ulcer of unspecified ankle, stage 4
   Pressure ulcer with necrosis of soft tissues through to underlying muscle, tendon, or bone, unspecified ankle
   HAC see Appendix B for HAC conditional logic

L89.506 **Pressure-induced deep tissue damage of unspecified ankle**
L89.509 **Pressure ulcer of unspecified ankle, unspecified stage**
  Healing pressure ulcer of unspecified ankle NOS
  Healing pressure ulcer of unspecified ankle, unspecified stage

+ L89.51 **Pressure ulcer of right ankle**
  L89.510 **Pressure ulcer of right ankle, unstageable**
  L89.511 **Pressure ulcer of right ankle, stage 1**
    Healing pressure ulcer of right ankle, stage 1
    Pressure pre-ulcer skin changes limited to persistent focal edema, right ankle
  L89.512 **Pressure ulcer of right ankle, stage 2**
    Healing pressure ulcer of right ankle, stage 2
    Pressure ulcer with abrasion, blister, partial thickness skin loss involving epidermis and/or dermis, right ankle
  MCC L89.513 **Pressure ulcer of right ankle, stage 3**
    Healing pressure ulcer of right ankle, stage 3
    Pressure ulcer with full thickness skin loss involving damage or necrosis of subcutaneous tissue, right ankle
    HAC see Appendix B for HAC conditional logic
  MCC L89.514 **Pressure ulcer of right ankle, stage 4**
    Healing pressure ulcer of right ankle, stage 4
    Pressure ulcer with necrosis of soft tissues through to underlying muscle, tendon, or bone, right ankle
    HAC see Appendix B for HAC conditional logic
  L89.516 **Pressure-induced deep tissue damage of right ankle**
  L89.519 **Pressure ulcer of right ankle, unspecified stage**
    Healing pressure ulcer of right ankle NOS
    Healing pressure ulcer of right ankle, unspecified stage

+ L89.52 **Pressure ulcer of left ankle**
  L89.520 **Pressure ulcer of left ankle, unstageable**
  L89.521 **Pressure ulcer of left ankle, stage 1**
    Healing pressure ulcer of left ankle, stage 1
    Pressure pre-ulcer skin changes limited to persistent focal edema, left ankle
  L89.522 **Pressure ulcer of left ankle, stage 2**
    Healing pressure ulcer of left ankle, stage 2
    Pressure ulcer with abrasion, blister, partial thickness skin loss involving epidermis and/or dermis, left ankle
  MCC L89.523 **Pressure ulcer of left ankle, stage 3**
    Healing pressure ulcer of left ankle, stage 3
    Pressure ulcer with full thickness skin loss involving damage or necrosis of subcutaneous tissue, left ankle
    HAC see Appendix B for HAC conditional logic
  MCC L89.524 **Pressure ulcer of left ankle, stage 4**
    Healing pressure ulcer of left ankle, stage 4
    Pressure ulcer with necrosis of soft tissues through to underlying muscle, tendon, or bone, left ankle
    HAC see Appendix B for HAC conditional logic

L89.526 **Pressure-induced deep tissue damage of left ankle**
L89.529 **Pressure ulcer of left ankle, unspecified stage**
  Healing pressure ulcer of left ankle NOS
  Healing pressure ulcer of left ankle, unspecified stage

+ L89.6 **Pressure ulcer of heel**
+ L89.60 **Pressure ulcer of unspecified heel**
  L89.600 **Pressure ulcer of unspecified heel, unstageable**
  L89.601 **Pressure ulcer of unspecified heel, stage 1**
    Healing pressure ulcer of unspecified heel, stage 1
    Pressure pre-ulcer skin changes limited to persistent focal edema, unspecified heel
  L89.602 **Pressure ulcer of unspecified heel, stage 2**
    Healing pressure ulcer of unspecified heel, stage 2
    Pressure ulcer with abrasion, blister, partial thickness skin loss involving epidermis and/or dermis, unspecified heel
  MCC L89.603 **Pressure ulcer of unspecified heel, stage 3**
    Healing pressure ulcer of unspecified heel, stage 3
    Pressure ulcer with full thickness skin loss involving damage or necrosis of subcutaneous tissue, unspecified heel
    HAC see Appendix B for HAC conditional logic
  MCC L89.604 **Pressure ulcer of unspecified heel, stage 4**
    Healing pressure ulcer of unspecified heel, stage 4
    Pressure ulcer with necrosis of soft tissues through to underlying muscle, tendon, or bone, unspecified heel
    HAC see Appendix B for HAC conditional logic
  L89.606 **Pressure-induced deep tissue damage of unspecified heel**
  L89.609 **Pressure ulcer of unspecified heel, unspecified stage**
    Healing pressure ulcer of unspecified heel NOS
    Healing pressure ulcer of unspecified heel, unspecified stage

+ L89.61 **Pressure ulcer of right heel**
  L89.610 **Pressure ulcer of right heel, unstageable**
  L89.611 **Pressure ulcer of right heel, stage 1**
    Healing pressure ulcer of right heel, stage 1
    Pressure pre-ulcer skin changes limited to persistent focal edema, right heel
  L89.612 **Pressure ulcer of right heel, stage 2**
    Healing pressure ulcer of right heel, stage 2
    Pressure ulcer with abrasion, blister, partial thickness skin loss involving epidermis and/or dermis, right heel
  MCC L89.613 **Pressure ulcer of right heel, stage 3**
    Healing pressure ulcer of right heel, stage 3
    Pressure ulcer with full thickness skin loss involving damage or necrosis of subcutaneous tissue, right heel
    HAC see Appendix B for HAC conditional logic
  MCC L89.614 **Pressure ulcer of right heel, stage 4**
    Healing pressure ulcer of right heel, stage 4
    Pressure ulcer with necrosis of soft tissues through to underlying muscle, tendon, or bone, right heel
    HAC see Appendix B for HAC conditional logic

L89.616 Pressure-induced deep tissue damage of right heel
L89.619 Pressure ulcer of right heel, unspecified stage
    Healing pressure ulcer of right heel NOS
    Healing pressure ulcer of right heel, unspecified stage

+ **L89.62 Pressure ulcer of left heel**
  L89.620 Pressure ulcer of left heel, unstageable
  L89.621 Pressure ulcer of left heel, stage 1
    Healing pressure ulcer of left heel, stage 1
    Pressure pre-ulcer skin changes limited to persistent focal edema, left heel
  L89.622 Pressure ulcer of left heel, stage 2
    Healing pressure ulcer of left heel, stage 2
    Pressure ulcer with abrasion, blister, partial thickness skin loss involving epidermis and/or dermis, left heel
    AHA CC: 4Q, 2016, 144
  MCC L89.623 Pressure ulcer of left heel, stage 3
    Healing pressure ulcer of left heel, stage 3
    Pressure ulcer with full thickness skin loss involving damage or necrosis of subcutaneous tissue, left heel
    AHA CC: 4Q, 2016, 144; 3Q, 2018, 3-4
    HAC see Appendix B for HAC conditional logic
  MCC L89.624 Pressure ulcer of left heel, stage 4
    Healing pressure ulcer of left heel, stage 4
    Pressure ulcer with necrosis of soft tissues through to underlying muscle, tendon, or bone, left heel
    HAC see Appendix B for HAC conditional logic
  L89.626 Pressure-induced deep tissue damage of left heel
  L89.629 Pressure ulcer of left heel, unspecified stage
    Healing pressure ulcer of left heel NOS
    Healing pressure ulcer of left heel, unspecified stage

+ **L89.8 Pressure ulcer of other site**
  + **L89.81 Pressure ulcer of head**
    Pressure ulcer of face
    L89.810 Pressure ulcer of head, unstageable
    L89.811 Pressure ulcer of head, stage 1
      Healing pressure ulcer of head, stage 1
      Pressure pre-ulcer skin changes limited to persistent focal edema, head
    L89.812 Pressure ulcer of head, stage 2
      Healing pressure ulcer of head, stage 2
      Pressure ulcer with abrasion, blister, partial thickness skin loss involving epidermis and/or dermis, head
    MCC L89.813 Pressure ulcer of head, stage 3
      Healing pressure ulcer of head, stage 3
      Pressure ulcer with full thickness skin loss involving damage or necrosis of subcutaneous tissue, head
      HAC see Appendix B for HAC conditional logic
    MCC L89.814 Pressure ulcer of head, stage 4
      Healing pressure ulcer of head, stage 4
      Pressure ulcer with necrosis of soft tissues through to underlying muscle, tendon, or bone, head
      HAC see Appendix B for HAC conditional logic
    L89.816 Pressure-induced deep tissue damage of head
    L89.819 Pressure ulcer of head, unspecified stage
      Healing pressure ulcer of head NOS
      Healing pressure ulcer of head, unspecified stage

+ **L89.89 Pressure ulcer of other site**
  L89.890 Pressure ulcer of other site, unstageable
  L89.891 Pressure ulcer of other site, stage 1
    Healing pressure ulcer of other site, stage 1
    Pressure pre-ulcer skin changes limited to persistent focal edema, other site
  L89.892 Pressure ulcer of other site, stage 2
    Healing pressure ulcer of other site, stage 2
    Pressure ulcer with abrasion, blister, partial thickness skin loss involving epidermis and/or dermis, other site
  MCC L89.893 Pressure ulcer of other site, stage 3
    Healing pressure ulcer of other site, stage 3
    Pressure ulcer with full thickness skin loss involving damage or necrosis of subcutaneous tissue, other site
    HAC see Appendix B for HAC conditional logic
  MCC L89.894 Pressure ulcer of other site, stage 4
    Healing pressure ulcer of other site, stage 4
    Pressure ulcer with necrosis of soft tissues through to underlying muscle, tendon, or bone, other site
    HAC see Appendix B for HAC conditional logic
  L89.896 Pressure-induced deep tissue damage of other site
  L89.899 Pressure ulcer of other site, unspecified stage
    Healing pressure ulcer of other site NOS
    Healing pressure ulcer of other site, unspecified stage

+ **L89.9 Pressure ulcer of unspecified site**
  L89.90 Pressure ulcer of unspecified site, unspecified stage
    Healing pressure ulcer of unspecified site NOS
    Healing pressure ulcer of unspecified site, unspecified stage
  L89.91 Pressure ulcer of unspecified site, stage 1
    Healing pressure ulcer of unspecified site, stage 1
    Pressure pre-ulcer skin changes limited to persistent focal edema, unspecified site
  L89.92 Pressure ulcer of unspecified site, stage 2
    Healing pressure ulcer of unspecified site, stage 2
    Pressure ulcer with abrasion, blister, partial thickness skin loss involving epidermis and/or dermis, unspecified site
  MCC L89.93 Pressure ulcer of unspecified site, stage 3
    Healing pressure ulcer of unspecified site, stage 3
    Pressure ulcer with full thickness skin loss involving damage or necrosis of subcutaneous tissue, unspecified site
    HAC see Appendix B for HAC conditional logic
  MCC L89.94 Pressure ulcer of unspecified site, stage 4
    Healing pressure ulcer of unspecified site, stage 4
    Pressure ulcer with necrosis of soft tissues through to underlying muscle, tendon, or bone, unspecified site
    HAC see Appendix B for HAC conditional logic
  L89.95 Pressure ulcer of unspecified site, unstageable
  L89.96 Pressure-induced deep tissue damage of unspecified site

L90 Atrophic disorders of skin
  L90.0 Lichen sclerosus et atrophicus
    Excludes2: lichen sclerosus of external female genital organs (N90.4)
    lichen sclerosus of external male genital organs (N48.0)
  L90.1 Anetoderma of Schweninger-Buzzi
  L90.2 Anetoderma of Jadassohn-Pellizzari
  L90.3 Atrophoderma of Pasini and Pierini
  L90.4 Acrodermatitis chronica atrophicans

L90.5 Scar conditions and fibrosis of skin
  Adherent scar (skin)
  Cicatrix
  Disfigurement of skin due to scar
  Fibrosis of skin NOS
  Scar NOS
  Excludes2: *hypertrophic scar (L91.0)*
  keloid scar (L91.0)
  AHA CC: 1Q, 2015, 19; 2Q, 2016, 5
L90.6 Striae atrophicae
L90.8 Other atrophic disorders of skin
L90.9 Atrophic disorder of skin, unspecified

L91 Hypertrophic disorders of skin

L91.0 Hypertrophic scar
  Keloid
  Keloid scar
  Excludes2: *acne keloid (L73.0)*
  scar NOS (L90.5)
L91.8 Other hypertrophic disorders of the skin
L91.9 Hypertrophic disorder of the skin, unspecified

L92 Granulomatous disorders of skin and subcutaneous tissue

  Excludes2: *actinic granuloma (L57.5)*
L92.0 Granuloma annulare
  Perforating granuloma annulare
L92.1 Necrobiosis lipoidica, not elsewhere classified
  Excludes1: *necrobiosis lipoidica associated with diabetes mellitus (E08-E13 with .620)*
L92.2 Granuloma faciale [eosinophilic granuloma of skin]
L92.3 Foreign body granuloma of the skin and subcutaneous tissue
  Use additional code to identify the type of retained foreign body (Z18.-)
L92.8 Other granulomatous disorders of the skin and subcutaneous tissue
L92.9 Granulomatous disorder of the skin and subcutaneous tissue, unspecified
  Excludes2: *umbilical granuloma (P83.81)*

L93 Lupus erythematosus

Use additional code for adverse effect, if applicable, to identify drug (T36-T50 with fifth or sixth character 5)
  Excludes1: *lupus exedens (A18.4)*
  lupus vulgaris (A18.4)
  scleroderma (M34.-)
  systemic lupus erythematosus (M32.-)
L93.0 Discoid lupus erythematosus
  Lupus erythematosus NOS
L93.1 Subacute cutaneous lupus erythematosus
L93.2 Other local lupus erythematosus
  Lupus erythematosus profundus
  Lupus panniculitis

L94 Other localized connective tissue disorders

  Excludes1: *systemic connective tissue disorders (M30-M36)*
L94.0 Localized scleroderma [morphea]
  Circumscribed scleroderma
L94.1 Linear scleroderma
  En coup de sabre lesion
L94.2 Calcinosis cutis
L94.3 Sclerodactyly
L94.4 Gottron's papules
L94.5 Poikiloderma vasculare atrophicans
L94.6 Ainhum
L94.8 Other specified localized connective tissue disorders
L94.9 Localized connective tissue disorder, unspecified

L95 Vasculitis limited to skin, not elsewhere classified

  Excludes1: *angioma serpiginosum (L81.7)*
  Henoch(-Schönlein) purpura (D69.0)
  hypersensitivity angiitis (M31.0)
  lupus panniculitis (L93.2)
  panniculitis NOS (M79.3)
  panniculitis of neck and back (M54.0-)
  polyarteritis nodosa (M30.0)
  relapsing panniculitis (M35.6)
  rheumatoid vasculitis (M05.2)
  serum sickness (T80.6-)
  urticaria (L50.-)
  Wegener's granulomatosis (M31.3-)
L95.0 Livedoid vasculitis
  Atrophie blanche (en plaque)
L95.1 Erythema elevatum diutinum
L95.8 Other vasculitis limited to the skin
L95.9 Vasculitis limited to the skin, unspecified

L97 Non-pressure chronic ulcer of lower limb, not elsewhere classified

  Includes: chronic ulcer of skin of lower limb NOS
  non-healing ulcer of skin
  non-infected sinus of skin
  trophic ulcer NOS
  tropical ulcer NOS
  ulcer of skin of lower limb NOS
Code first any associated underlying condition, such as:
  any associated gangrene (I96)
  atherosclerosis of the lower extremities (I70.23-, I70.24-, I70.33-, I70.34-, I70.43-, I70.44-, I70.53-, I70.54-, I70.63-, I70.64-, I70.73-, I70.74-)
  chronic venous hypertension (I87.31-, I87.33-)
  diabetic ulcers (E08.621, E08.622, E09.621, E09.622, E10.621, E10.622, E11.621, E11.622, E13.621, E13.622)
  postphlebitic syndrome (I87.01-, I87.03-)
  postthrombotic syndrome (I87.01-, I87.03-)
  varicose ulcer (I83.0-, I83.2-)
  Excludes2: *pressure ulcer (pressure area) (L89.-)*
  skin infections (L00-L08)
  specific infections classified to A00-B99
  AHA CC: 4Q, 2017, 17
  Review coding guidelines B.14 and C.12.b
+ **L97.1 Non-pressure chronic ulcer of thigh**
  + **L97.10 Non-pressure chronic ulcer of unspecified thigh**
    CC **L97.101** Non-pressure chronic ulcer of unspecified thigh limited to breakdown of skin
    CC **L97.102** Non-pressure chronic ulcer of unspecified thigh with fat layer exposed
    CC **L97.103** Non-pressure chronic ulcer of unspecified thigh with necrosis of muscle
    CC **L97.104** Non-pressure chronic ulcer of unspecified thigh with necrosis of bone
    CC **L97.105** Non-pressure chronic ulcer of unspecified thigh with muscle involvement without evidence of necrosis
    CC **L97.106** Non-pressure chronic ulcer of unspecified thigh with bone involvement without evidence of necrosis
    CC **L97.108** Non-pressure chronic ulcer of unspecified thigh with other specified severity
    CC **L97.109** Non-pressure chronic ulcer of unspecified thigh with unspecified severity

- **L97.11** Non-pressure chronic ulcer of right thigh
  - CC **L97.111** Non-pressure chronic ulcer of right thigh limited to breakdown of skin
  - CC **L97.112** Non-pressure chronic ulcer of right thigh with fat layer exposed
  - CC **L97.113** Non-pressure chronic ulcer of right thigh with necrosis of muscle
  - CC **L97.114** Non-pressure chronic ulcer of right thigh with necrosis of bone
  - CC **L97.115** Non-pressure chronic ulcer of right thigh with muscle involvement without evidence of necrosis
  - CC **L97.116** Non-pressure chronic ulcer of right thigh with bone involvement without evidence of necrosis
  - CC **L97.118** Non-pressure chronic ulcer of right thigh with other specified severity
  - CC **L97.119** Non-pressure chronic ulcer of right thigh with unspecified severity
- **L97.12** Non-pressure chronic ulcer of left thigh
  - CC **L97.121** Non-pressure chronic ulcer of left thigh limited to breakdown of skin
  - CC **L97.122** Non-pressure chronic ulcer of left thigh with fat layer exposed
  - CC **L97.123** Non-pressure chronic ulcer of left thigh with necrosis of muscle
  - CC **L97.124** Non-pressure chronic ulcer of left thigh with necrosis of bone
  - CC **L97.125** Non-pressure chronic ulcer of left thigh with muscle involvement without evidence of necrosis
  - CC **L97.126** Non-pressure chronic ulcer of left thigh with bone involvement without evidence of necrosis
  - CC **L97.128** Non-pressure chronic ulcer of left thigh with other specified severity
  - CC **L97.129** Non-pressure chronic ulcer of left thigh with unspecified severity
- **L97.2** Non-pressure chronic ulcer of calf
  - **L97.20** Non-pressure chronic ulcer of unspecified calf
    - CC **L97.201** Non-pressure chronic ulcer of unspecified calf limited to breakdown of skin
    - CC **L97.202** Non-pressure chronic ulcer of unspecified calf with fat layer exposed
    - CC **L97.203** Non-pressure chronic ulcer of unspecified calf with necrosis of muscle
    - CC **L97.204** Non-pressure chronic ulcer of unspecified calf with necrosis of bone
    - CC **L97.205** Non-pressure chronic ulcer of unspecified calf with muscle involvement without evidence of necrosis
    - CC **L97.206** Non-pressure chronic ulcer of unspecified calf with bone involvement without evidence of necrosis
    - CC **L97.208** Non-pressure chronic ulcer of unspecified calf with other specified severity
    - CC **L97.209** Non-pressure chronic ulcer of unspecified calf with unspecified severity
  - **L97.21** Non-pressure chronic ulcer of right calf
    - CC **L97.211** Non-pressure chronic ulcer of right calf limited to breakdown of skin
    - CC **L97.212** Non-pressure chronic ulcer of right calf with fat layer exposed
    - CC **L97.213** Non-pressure chronic ulcer of right calf with necrosis of muscle
    - CC **L97.214** Non-pressure chronic ulcer of right calf with necrosis of bone
    - CC **L97.215** Non-pressure chronic ulcer of right calf with muscle involvement without evidence of necrosis
    - CC **L97.216** Non-pressure chronic ulcer of right calf with bone involvement without evidence of necrosis
    - CC **L97.218** Non-pressure chronic ulcer of right calf with other specified severity
    - CC **L97.219** Non-pressure chronic ulcer of right calf with unspecified severity
  - **L97.22** Non-pressure chronic ulcer of left calf
    - CC **L97.221** Non-pressure chronic ulcer of left calf limited to breakdown of skin
    - CC **L97.222** Non-pressure chronic ulcer of left calf with fat layer exposed
      - *AHA CC: 1Q, 2016, 12-13*
    - CC **L97.223** Non-pressure chronic ulcer of left calf with necrosis of muscle
    - CC **L97.224** Non-pressure chronic ulcer of left calf with necrosis of bone
    - CC **L97.225** Non-pressure chronic ulcer of left calf with muscle involvement without evidence of necrosis
    - CC **L97.226** Non-pressure chronic ulcer of left calf with bone involvement without evidence of necrosis
    - CC **L97.228** Non-pressure chronic ulcer of left calf with other specified severity
    - CC **L97.229** Non-pressure chronic ulcer of left calf with unspecified severity
- **L97.3** Non-pressure chronic ulcer of ankle
  - **L97.30** Non-pressure chronic ulcer of unspecified ankle
    - CC **L97.301** Non-pressure chronic ulcer of unspecified ankle limited to breakdown of skin
    - CC **L97.302** Non-pressure chronic ulcer of unspecified ankle with fat layer exposed
    - CC **L97.303** Non-pressure chronic ulcer of unspecified ankle with necrosis of muscle
    - CC **L97.304** Non-pressure chronic ulcer of unspecified ankle with necrosis of bone
    - CC **L97.305** Non-pressure chronic ulcer of unspecified ankle with muscle involvement without evidence of necrosis
    - CC **L97.306** Non-pressure chronic ulcer of unspecified ankle with bone involvement without evidence of necrosis
    - CC **L97.308** Non-pressure chronic ulcer of unspecified ankle with other specified severity
    - CC **L97.309** Non-pressure chronic ulcer of unspecified ankle with unspecified severity
  - **L97.31** Non-pressure chronic ulcer of right ankle
    - CC **L97.311** Non-pressure chronic ulcer of right ankle limited to breakdown of skin
    - CC **L97.312** Non-pressure chronic ulcer of right ankle with fat layer exposed
    - CC **L97.313** Non-pressure chronic ulcer of right ankle with necrosis of muscle
    - CC **L97.314** Non-pressure chronic ulcer of right ankle with necrosis of bone
    - CC **L97.315** Non-pressure chronic ulcer of right ankle with muscle involvement without evidence of necrosis
      - *AHA CC: 4Q, 2017, 17*
    - CC **L97.316** Non-pressure chronic ulcer of right ankle with bone involvement without evidence of necrosis
    - CC **L97.318** Non-pressure chronic ulcer of right ankle with other specified severity
    - CC **L97.319** Non-pressure chronic ulcer of right ankle with unspecified severity

- **L97.32** Non-pressure chronic ulcer of left ankle
  - CC **L97.321** Non-pressure chronic ulcer of left ankle limited to breakdown of skin
  - CC **L97.322** Non-pressure chronic ulcer of left ankle with fat layer exposed
    - *AHA CC: 1Q, 2021, 7-8*
  - CC **L97.323** Non-pressure chronic ulcer of left ankle with necrosis of muscle
  - CC **L97.324** Non-pressure chronic ulcer of left ankle with necrosis of bone
  - CC **L97.325** Non-pressure chronic ulcer of left ankle with muscle involvement without evidence of necrosis
  - CC **L97.326** Non-pressure chronic ulcer of left ankle with bone involvement without evidence of necrosis
  - CC **L97.328** Non-pressure chronic ulcer of left ankle with other specified severity
  - CC **L97.329** Non-pressure chronic ulcer of left ankle with unspecified severity
- **L97.4** Non-pressure chronic ulcer of heel and midfoot
  Non-pressure chronic ulcer of plantar surface of midfoot
  - **L97.40** Non-pressure chronic ulcer of unspecified heel and midfoot
    - CC **L97.401** Non-pressure chronic ulcer of unspecified heel and midfoot limited to breakdown of skin
    - CC **L97.402** Non-pressure chronic ulcer of unspecified heel and midfoot with fat layer exposed
    - CC **L97.403** Non-pressure chronic ulcer of unspecified heel and midfoot with necrosis of muscle
    - CC **L97.404** Non-pressure chronic ulcer of unspecified heel and midfoot with necrosis of bone
    - CC **L97.405** Non-pressure chronic ulcer of unspecified heel and midfoot with muscle involvement without evidence of necrosis
    - CC **L97.406** Non-pressure chronic ulcer of unspecified heel and midfoot with bone involvement without evidence of necrosis
    - CC **L97.408** Non-pressure chronic ulcer of unspecified heel and midfoot with other specified severity
    - CC **L97.409** Non-pressure chronic ulcer of unspecified heel and midfoot with unspecified severity
  - **L97.41** Non-pressure chronic ulcer of right heel and midfoot
    - CC **L97.411** Non-pressure chronic ulcer of right heel and midfoot limited to breakdown of skin
    - CC **L97.412** Non-pressure chronic ulcer of right heel and midfoot with fat layer exposed
      - *AHA CC: 2Q, 2020, 19*
    - CC **L97.413** Non-pressure chronic ulcer of right heel and midfoot with necrosis of muscle
    - CC **L97.414** Non-pressure chronic ulcer of right heel and midfoot with necrosis of bone
    - CC **L97.415** Non-pressure chronic ulcer of right heel and midfoot with muscle involvement without evidence of necrosis
    - CC **L97.416** Non-pressure chronic ulcer of right heel and midfoot with bone involvement without evidence of necrosis
    - CC **L97.418** Non-pressure chronic ulcer of right heel and midfoot with other specified severity
    - CC **L97.419** Non-pressure chronic ulcer of right heel and midfoot with unspecified severity
- **L97.42** Non-pressure chronic ulcer of left heel and midfoot
  - CC **L97.421** Non-pressure chronic ulcer of left heel and midfoot limited to breakdown of skin
  - CC **L97.422** Non-pressure chronic ulcer of left heel and midfoot with fat layer exposed
  - CC **L97.423** Non-pressure chronic ulcer of left heel and midfoot with necrosis of muscle
  - CC **L97.424** Non-pressure chronic ulcer of left heel and midfoot with necrosis of bone
  - CC **L97.425** Non-pressure chronic ulcer of left heel and midfoot with muscle involvement without evidence of necrosis
  - CC **L97.426** Non-pressure chronic ulcer of left heel and midfoot with bone involvement without evidence of necrosis
  - CC **L97.428** Non-pressure chronic ulcer of left heel and midfoot with other specified severity
  - CC **L97.429** Non-pressure chronic ulcer of left heel and midfoot with unspecified severity
- **L97.5** Non-pressure chronic ulcer of other part of foot
  Non-pressure chronic ulcer of toe
  - **L97.50** Non-pressure chronic ulcer of other part of unspecified foot
    - **L97.501** Non-pressure chronic ulcer of other part of unspecified foot limited to breakdown of skin
    - **L97.502** Non-pressure chronic ulcer of other part of unspecified foot with fat layer exposed
    - **L97.503** Non-pressure chronic ulcer of other part of unspecified foot with necrosis of muscle
    - **L97.504** Non-pressure chronic ulcer of other part of unspecified foot with necrosis of bone
    - CC **L97.505** Non-pressure chronic ulcer of other part of unspecified foot with muscle involvement without evidence of necrosis
    - CC **L97.506** Non-pressure chronic ulcer of other part of unspecified foot with bone involvement without evidence of necrosis
    - CC **L97.508** Non-pressure chronic ulcer of other part of unspecified foot with other specified severity
    - **L97.509** Non-pressure chronic ulcer of other part of unspecified foot with unspecified severity
  - **L97.51** Non-pressure chronic ulcer of other part of right foot
    - **L97.511** Non-pressure chronic ulcer of other part of right foot limited to breakdown of skin
      - *AHA CC: 1Q, 2020, 12*
    - **L97.512** Non-pressure chronic ulcer of other part of right foot with fat layer exposed
      - *AHA CC: 2Q, 2020, 19-20*
    - **L97.513** Non-pressure chronic ulcer of other part of right foot with necrosis of muscle
    - **L97.514** Non-pressure chronic ulcer of other part of right foot with necrosis of bone
    - CC **L97.515** Non-pressure chronic ulcer of other part of right foot with muscle involvement without evidence of necrosis
    - CC **L97.516** Non-pressure chronic ulcer of other part of right foot with bone involvement without evidence of necrosis
    - CC **L97.518** Non-pressure chronic ulcer of other part of right foot with other specified severity
    - **L97.519** Non-pressure chronic ulcer of other part of right foot with unspecified severity

+ **L97.52** Non-pressure chronic ulcer of other part of left foot
- **L97.521** Non-pressure chronic ulcer of other part of left foot limited to breakdown of skin
- **L97.522** Non-pressure chronic ulcer of other part of left foot with fat layer exposed
- **L97.523** Non-pressure chronic ulcer of other part of left foot with necrosis of muscle
- **L97.524** Non-pressure chronic ulcer of other part of left foot with necrosis of bone
- CC **L97.525** Non-pressure chronic ulcer of other part of left foot with muscle involvement without evidence of necrosis
- CC **L97.526** Non-pressure chronic ulcer of other part of left foot with bone involvement without evidence of necrosis
- CC **L97.528** Non-pressure chronic ulcer of other part of left foot with other specified severity
- **L97.529** Non-pressure chronic ulcer of other part of left foot with unspecified severity

+ **L97.8** Non-pressure chronic ulcer of other part of lower leg
  + **L97.80** Non-pressure chronic ulcer of other part of unspecified lower leg
    - CC **L97.801** Non-pressure chronic ulcer of other part of unspecified lower leg limited to breakdown of skin
    - CC **L97.802** Non-pressure chronic ulcer of other part of unspecified lower leg with fat layer exposed
    - CC **L97.803** Non-pressure chronic ulcer of other part of unspecified lower leg with necrosis of muscle
    - CC **L97.804** Non-pressure chronic ulcer of other part of unspecified lower leg with necrosis of bone
    - CC **L97.805** Non-pressure chronic ulcer of other part of unspecified lower leg with muscle involvement without evidence of necrosis
    - CC **L97.806** Non-pressure chronic ulcer of other part of unspecified lower leg with bone involvement without evidence of necrosis
    - CC **L97.808** Non-pressure chronic ulcer of other part of unspecified lower leg with other specified severity
    - CC **L97.809** Non-pressure chronic ulcer of other part of unspecified lower leg with unspecified severity
  + **L97.81** Non-pressure chronic ulcer of other part of right lower leg
    - CC **L97.811** Non-pressure chronic ulcer of other part of right lower leg limited to breakdown of skin
    - CC **L97.812** Non-pressure chronic ulcer of other part of right lower leg with fat layer exposed
    - CC **L97.813** Non-pressure chronic ulcer of other part of right lower leg with necrosis of muscle
    - CC **L97.814** Non-pressure chronic ulcer of other part of right lower leg with necrosis of bone
    - CC **L97.815** Non-pressure chronic ulcer of other part of right lower leg with muscle involvement without evidence of necrosis
    - CC **L97.816** Non-pressure chronic ulcer of other part of right lower leg with bone involvement without evidence of necrosis
    - CC **L97.818** Non-pressure chronic ulcer of other part of right lower leg with other specified severity
    - CC **L97.819** Non-pressure chronic ulcer of other part of right lower leg with unspecified severity

+ **L97.82** Non-pressure chronic ulcer of other part of left lower leg
  - CC **L97.821** Non-pressure chronic ulcer of other part of left lower leg limited to breakdown of skin
  - CC **L97.822** Non-pressure chronic ulcer of other part of left lower leg with fat layer exposed
  - CC **L97.823** Non-pressure chronic ulcer of other part of left lower leg with necrosis of muscle
  - CC **L97.824** Non-pressure chronic ulcer of other part of left lower leg with necrosis of bone
  - CC **L97.825** Non-pressure chronic ulcer of other part of left lower leg with muscle involvement without evidence of necrosis
  - CC **L97.826** Non-pressure chronic ulcer of other part of left lower leg with bone involvement without evidence of necrosis
  - CC **L97.828** Non-pressure chronic ulcer of other part of left lower leg with other specified severity
  - CC **L97.829** Non-pressure chronic ulcer of other part of left lower leg with unspecified severity

+ **L97.9** Non-pressure chronic ulcer of unspecified part of lower leg
  + **L97.90** Non-pressure chronic ulcer of unspecified part of unspecified lower leg
    - CC **L97.901** Non-pressure chronic ulcer of unspecified part of unspecified lower leg limited to breakdown of skin
    - CC **L97.902** Non-pressure chronic ulcer of unspecified part of unspecified lower leg with fat layer exposed
    - CC **L97.903** Non-pressure chronic ulcer of unspecified part of unspecified lower leg with necrosis of muscle
    - CC **L97.904** Non-pressure chronic ulcer of unspecified part of unspecified lower leg with necrosis of bone
    - CC **L97.905** Non-pressure chronic ulcer of unspecified part of unspecified lower leg with muscle involvement without evidence of necrosis
    - CC **L97.906** Non-pressure chronic ulcer of unspecified part of unspecified lower leg with bone involvement without evidence of necrosis
    - CC **L97.908** Non-pressure chronic ulcer of unspecified part of unspecified lower leg with other specified severity
    - CC **L97.909** Non-pressure chronic ulcer of unspecified part of unspecified lower leg with unspecified severity
  + **L97.91** Non-pressure chronic ulcer of unspecified part of right lower leg
    - CC **L97.911** Non-pressure chronic ulcer of unspecified part of right lower leg limited to breakdown of skin
    - CC **L97.912** Non-pressure chronic ulcer of unspecified part of right lower leg with fat layer exposed
    - CC **L97.913** Non-pressure chronic ulcer of unspecified part of right lower leg with necrosis of muscle
    - CC **L97.914** Non-pressure chronic ulcer of unspecified part of right lower leg with necrosis of bone
    - CC **L97.915** Non-pressure chronic ulcer of unspecified part of right lower leg with muscle involvement without evidence of necrosis
    - CC **L97.916** Non-pressure chronic ulcer of unspecified part of right lower leg with bone involvement without evidence of necrosis

- **CC L97.918** Non-pressure chronic ulcer of unspecified part of right lower leg with other specified severity
- **CC L97.919** Non-pressure chronic ulcer of unspecified part of right lower leg with unspecified severity
- **+ L97.92** Non-pressure chronic ulcer of unspecified part of left lower leg
  - **CC L97.921** Non-pressure chronic ulcer of unspecified part of left lower leg limited to breakdown of skin
  - **CC L97.922** Non-pressure chronic ulcer of unspecified part of left lower leg with fat layer exposed
  - **CC L97.923** Non-pressure chronic ulcer of unspecified part of left lower leg with necrosis of muscle
  - **CC L97.924** Non-pressure chronic ulcer of unspecified part of left lower leg with necrosis of bone
  - **CC L97.925** Non-pressure chronic ulcer of unspecified part of left lower leg with muscle involvement without evidence of necrosis
  - **CC L97.926** Non-pressure chronic ulcer of unspecified part of left lower leg with bone involvement without evidence of necrosis
  - **CC L97.928** Non-pressure chronic ulcer of unspecified part of left lower leg with other specified severity
  - **CC L97.929** Non-pressure chronic ulcer of unspecified part of left lower leg with unspecified severity

L98 Other disorders of skin and subcutaneous tissue, not elsewhere classified

- **L98.0 Pyogenic granuloma**
  - *Excludes2:* pyogenic granuloma of gingiva (K06.8)
    pyogenic granuloma of maxillary alveolar ridge (K04.5)
    pyogenic granuloma of oral mucosa (K13.4)
- **L98.1 Factitial dermatitis**
  Neurotic excoriation
  Excludes1: Excoriation (skin-picking) disorder (F42.4)
- **L98.2 Febrile neutrophilic dermatosis [Sweet]**
- **CC L98.3 Eosinophilic cellulitis [Wells]**
- **+ L98.4 Non-pressure chronic ulcer of skin, not elsewhere classified**
  Chronic ulcer of skin NOS
  Tropical ulcer NOS
  Ulcer of skin NOS
  Excludes2: pressure ulcer (pressure area) (L89.-)
    gangrene (I96)
    skin infections (L00-L08)
    specific infections classified to A00-B99
    ulcer of lower limb NEC (L97.-)
    varicose ulcer (I83.0-I83.93)
  AHA CC: 4Q, 2017, 17
  - **+ L98.41 Non-pressure chronic ulcer of buttock**
    - **L98.411** Non-pressure chronic ulcer of buttock limited to breakdown of skin
    - **L98.412** Non-pressure chronic ulcer of buttock with fat layer exposed
    - **L98.413** Non-pressure chronic ulcer of buttock with necrosis of muscle
    - **L98.414** Non-pressure chronic ulcer of buttock with necrosis of bone
    - **CC L98.415** Non-pressure chronic ulcer of buttock with muscle involvement without evidence of necrosis
    - **CC L98.416** Non-pressure chronic ulcer of buttock with bone involvement without evidence of necrosis
    - **CC L98.418** Non-pressure chronic ulcer of buttock with other specified severity
    - **L98.419** Non-pressure chronic ulcer of buttock with unspecified severity
  - **+ L98.42 Non-pressure chronic ulcer of back**
    - **L98.421** Non-pressure chronic ulcer of back limited to breakdown of skin
    - **L98.422** Non-pressure chronic ulcer of back with fat layer exposed
    - **L98.423** Non-pressure chronic ulcer of back with necrosis of muscle
    - **L98.424** Non-pressure chronic ulcer of back with necrosis of bone
    - **CC L98.425** Non-pressure chronic ulcer of back with muscle involvement without evidence of necrosis
    - **CC L98.426** Non-pressure chronic ulcer of back with bone involvement without evidence of necrosis
    - **CC L98.428** Non-pressure chronic ulcer of back with other specified severity
    - **L98.429** Non-pressure chronic ulcer of back with unspecified severity
  - **+ L98.49 Non-pressure chronic ulcer of skin of other sites**
    Non-pressure chronic ulcer of skin NOS
    - **L98.491** Non-pressure chronic ulcer of skin of other sites limited to breakdown of skin
    - **L98.492** Non-pressure chronic ulcer of skin of other sites with fat layer exposed
    - **L98.493** Non-pressure chronic ulcer of skin of other sites with necrosis of muscle
    - **L98.494** Non-pressure chronic ulcer of skin of other sites with necrosis of bone
    - **CC L98.495** Non-pressure chronic ulcer of skin of other sites with muscle involvement without evidence of necrosis
    - **CC L98.496** Non-pressure chronic ulcer of skin of other sites with bone involvement without evidence of necrosis
    - **CC L98.498** Non-pressure chronic ulcer of skin of other sites with other specified severity
    - **L98.499** Non-pressure chronic ulcer of skin of other sites with unspecified severity
- **L98.5 Mucinosis of the skin**
  Focal mucinosis
  Lichen myxedematosus
  Reticular erythematous mucinosis
  Excludes1: focal oral mucinosis (K13.79)
    myxedema (E03.9)
- **L98.6 Other infiltrative disorders of the skin and subcutaneous tissue**
  Excludes1: hyalinosis cutis et mucosae (E78.89)
- **L98.7 Excessive and redundant skin and subcutaneous tissue**
  Loose or sagging skin following bariatric surgery weight loss
  Loose or sagging skin following dietary weight loss
  Loose or sagging skin, NOS
  Excludes2: acquired excess or redundant skin of eyelid (H02.3-)
    congenital excess or redundant skin or eyelid (Q10.3)
    skin changes due to chronic exposure to nonionizing radiation (L57.-)
  AHA CC: 4Q, 2016, 36; 3Q, 2022, 11
- **L98.8 Other specified disorders of the skin and subcutaneous tissue**
  AHA CC: 2Q, 2013, 32-33
- **L98.9 Disorder of the skin and subcutaneous tissue, unspecified**

L99 Other disorders of skin and subcutaneous tissue in diseases classified elsewhere

Code first underlying disease, such as:
  amyloidosis (E85.-)
Excludes1: skin disorders in diabetes (E08-E13 with .62-)
  skin disorders in gonorrhea (A54.89)
  skin disorders in syphilis (A51.31, A52.79)
AHA CC: 1Q, 2021, 39-40
Valid 3-character code, no further characters required

Chapter 13: Diseases of the Musculoskeletal System and Connective Tissue (M00-M99)

Intervertebral Joint

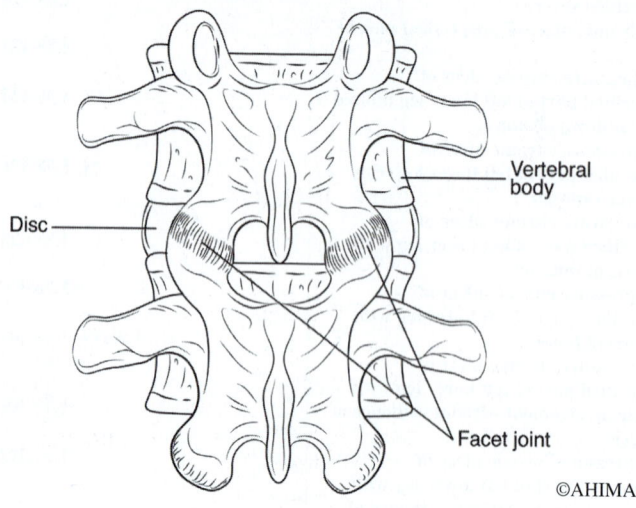

Shoulder Joint

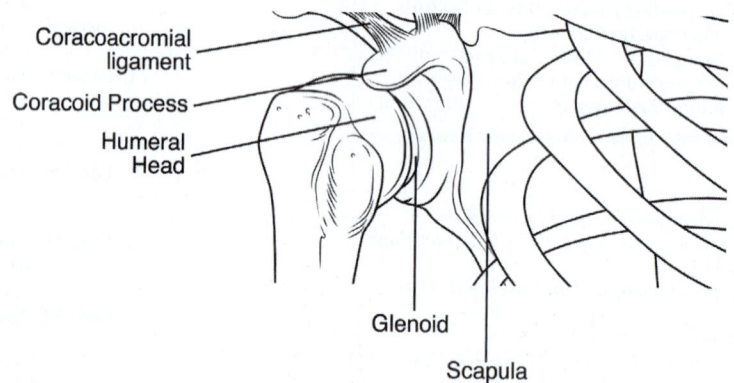

Elbow

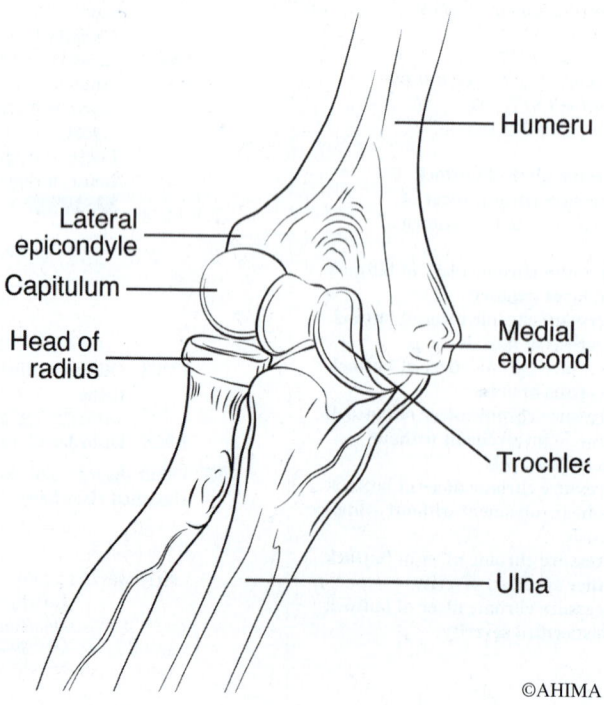

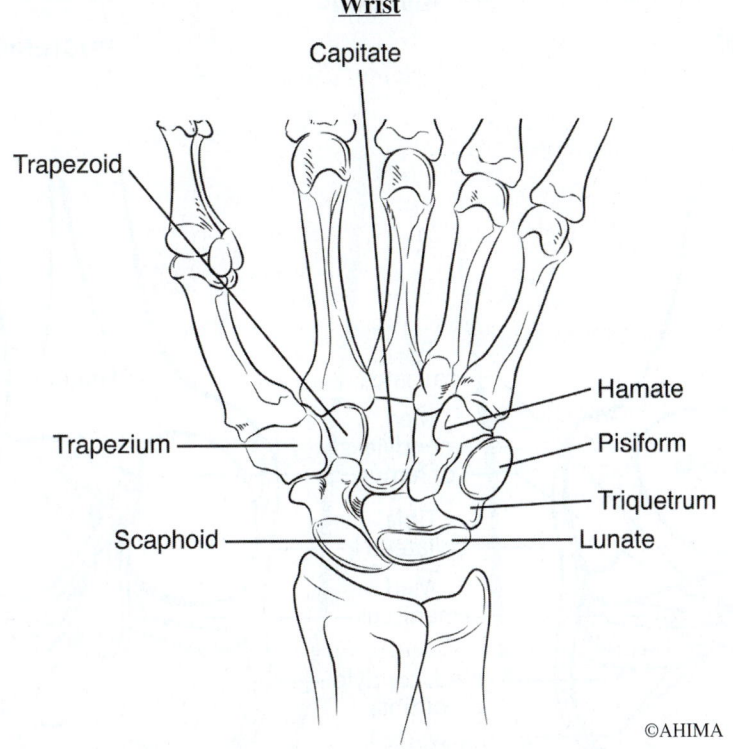

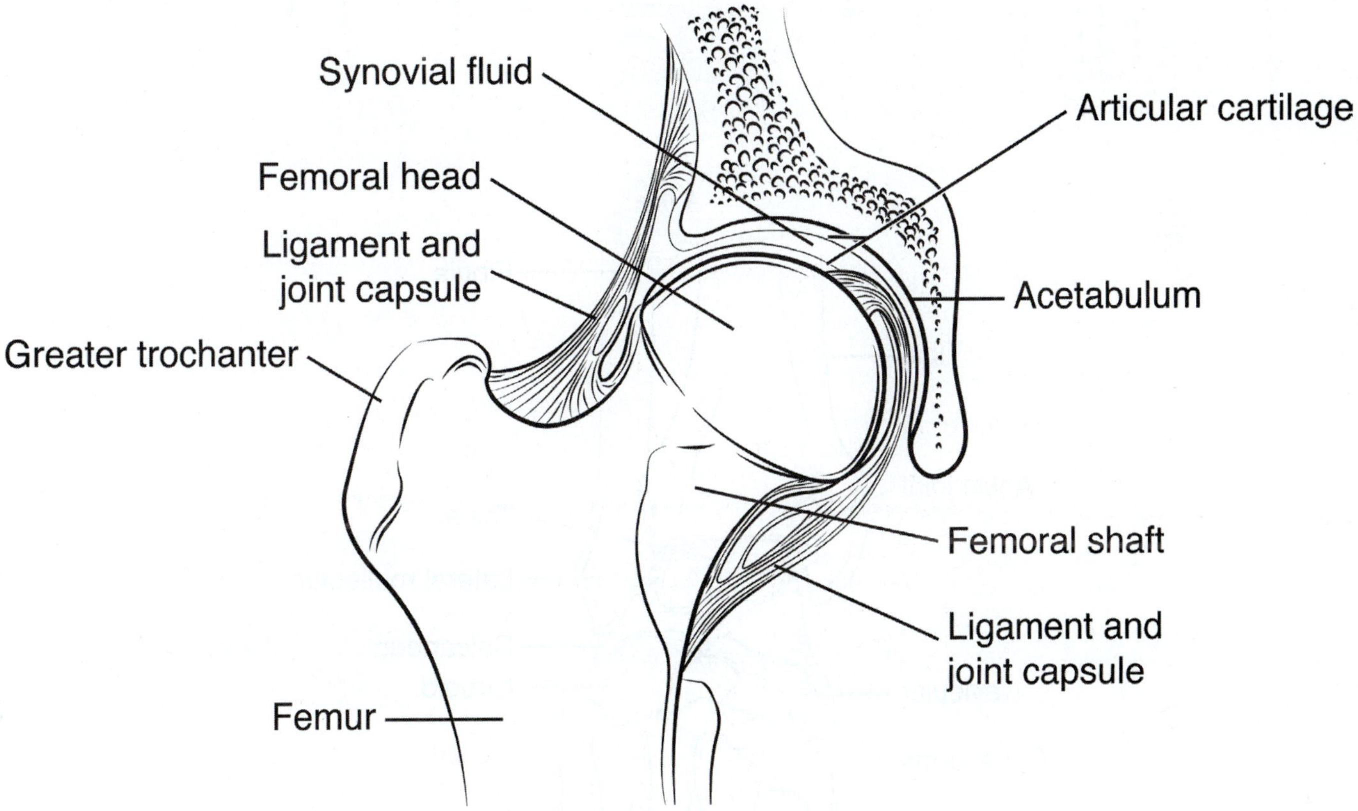

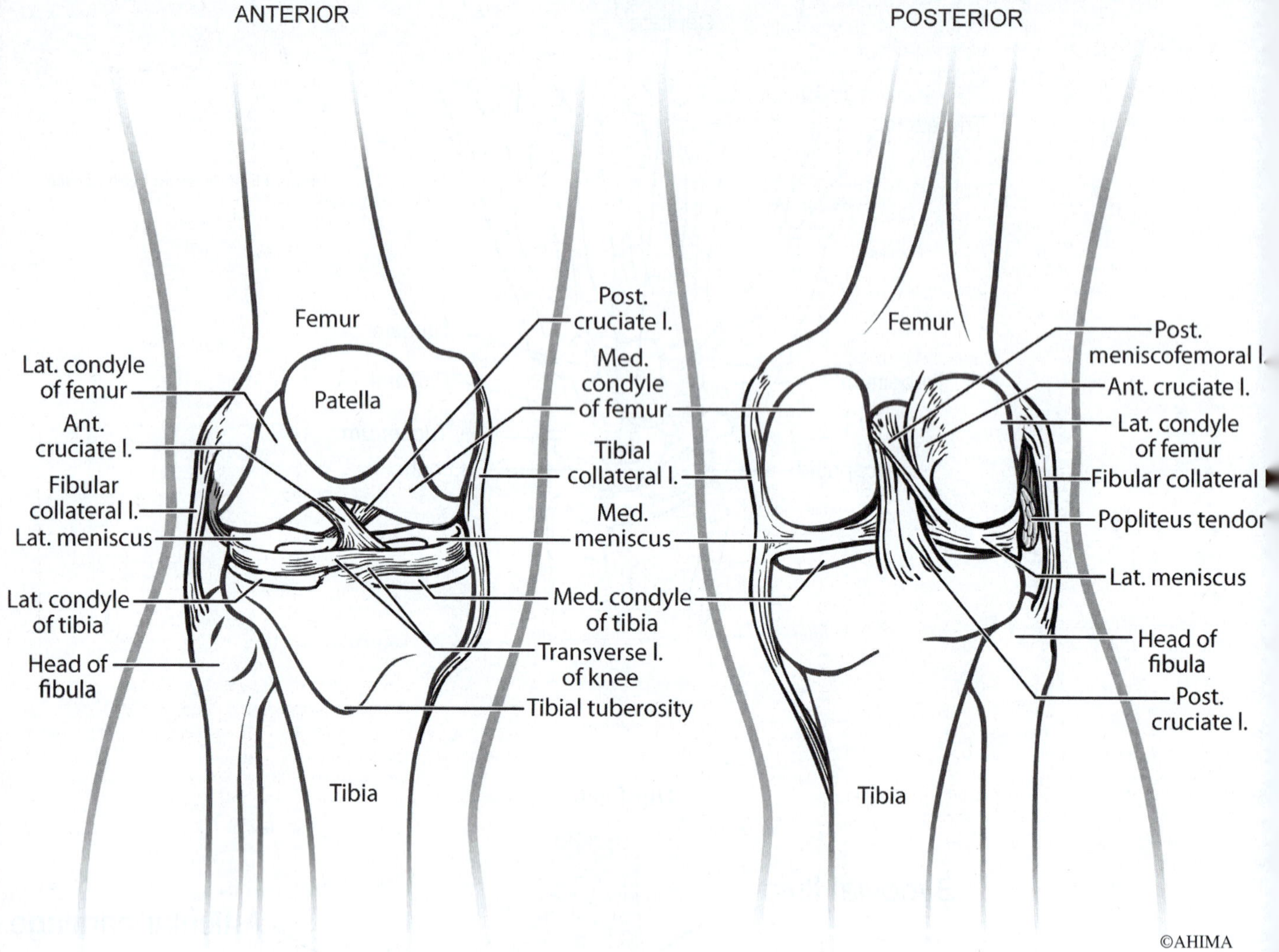

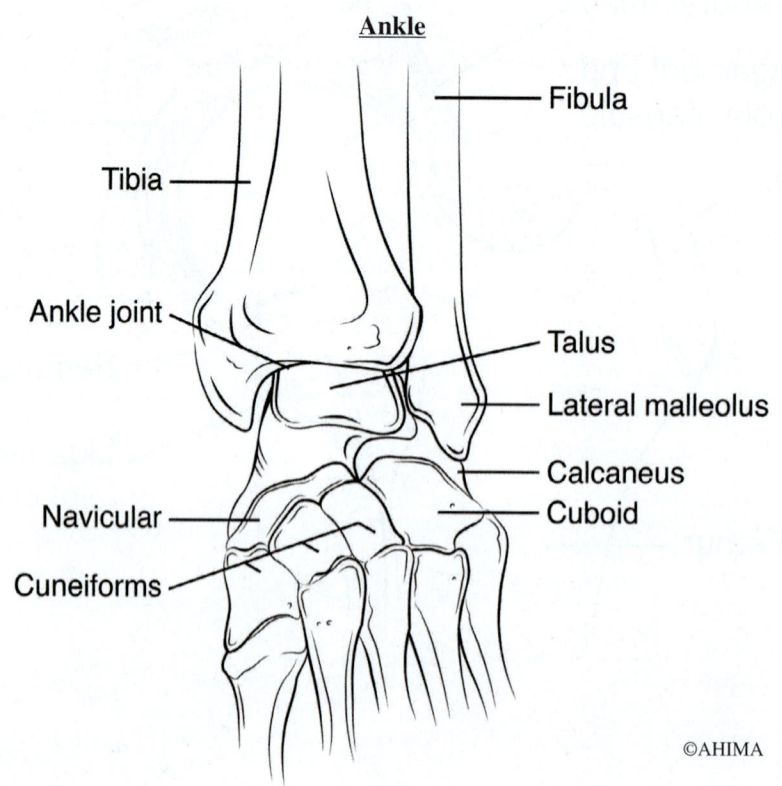

Chapter 13: Diseases of the Musculoskeletal System and Connective Tissue (M00-M99)

NOTE Use an external cause code following the code for the musculoskeletal condition, if applicable, to identify the cause of the musculoskeletal condition

Excludes2: arthropathic psoriasis (L40.5-)
certain conditions originating in the perinatal period (P04-P96)
certain infectious and parasitic diseases (A00-B99)
compartment syndrome (traumatic) (T79.A-)
complications of pregnancy, childbirth and the puerperium (O00-O9A)
congenital malformations, deformations, and chromosomal abnormalities (Q00-Q99)
endocrine, nutritional and metabolic diseases (E00-E88)
injury, poisoning and certain other consequences of external causes (S00-T88)
neoplasms (C00-D49)
symptoms, signs and abnormal clinical and laboratory findings, not elsewhere classified (R00-R94)

This chapter contains the following category blocks:
- M00-M02 Infectious arthropathies
- M04 Autoinflammatory syndromes
- M05-M14 Inflammatory polyarthropathies
- M15-M19 Osteoarthritis
- M20-M25 Other joint disorders
- M26-M27 Dentofacial anomalies [including malocclusion] and other disorders of jaw
- M30-M36 Systemic connective tissue disorders
- M40-M43 Deforming dorsopathies
- M45-M49 Spondylopathies
- M50-M54 Other dorsopathies
- M60-M63 Disorders of muscles
- M65-M67 Disorders of synovium and tendon
- M70-M79 Other soft tissue disorders
- M80-M85 Disorders of bone density and structure
- M86-M90 Other osteopathies
- M91-M94 Chondropathies
- M95 Other disorders of the musculoskeletal system and connective tissue
- M96 Intraoperative and postprocedural complications and disorders of musculoskeletal system, not elsewhere classified
- M97 Periprosthetic fracture around internal prosthetic joint
- M99 Biomechanical lesions, not elsewhere classified

C. Chapter-Specific Coding Guidelines

In addition to general coding guidelines, there are guidelines for specific diagnoses and/or conditions in the classification. Unless otherwise indicated, these guidelines apply to all health care settings. Please refer to Section II for guidelines on the selection of principal diagnosis.

13. Chapter 13: Diseases of the Musculoskeletal System and Connective Tissue (M00-M99)

a. Site and laterality

Most of the codes within Chapter 13 have site and laterality designations. The site represents the bone, joint or the muscle involved. For some conditions where more than one bone, joint or muscle is usually involved, such as osteoarthritis, there is a "multiple sites" code available. For categories where no multiple site code is provided and more than one bone, joint or muscle is involved, multiple codes should be used to indicate the different sites involved.

1) Bone versus joint

For certain conditions, the bone may be affected at the upper or lower end, (e.g., avascular necrosis of bone, M87, Osteoporosis, M80, M81). Though the portion of the bone affected may be at the joint, the site designation will be the bone, not the joint.

b. Acute traumatic versus chronic or recurrent musculoskeletal conditions

Many musculoskeletal conditions are a result of previous injury or trauma to a site, or are recurrent conditions. Bone, joint or muscle conditions that are the result of a healed injury are usually found in chapter 13. Recurrent bone, joint or muscle conditions are also usually found in chapter 13. Any current, acute injury should be coded to the appropriate injury code from chapter 19. Chronic or recurrent conditions should generally be coded with a code from chapter 13. If it is difficult to determine from the documentation in the record which code is best to describe a condition, query the provider.

c. Coding of Pathologic Fractures

7th character A is for use as long as the patient is receiving active treatment for the fracture. While the patient may be seen by a new or different provider over the course of treatment for a pathological fracture, assignment of the 7th character is based on whether the patient is undergoing active treatment and not whether the provider is seeing the patient for the first time.

7th character, D is to be used for encounters after the patient has completed active treatment for the fracture and is receiving routine care for the fracture during the healing or recovery phase. The other 7th characters, listed under each subcategory in the Tabular List, are to be used for subsequent encounters for routine care of fractures during the healing and recovery phase as well as treatment of problems associated with the healing, such as malunions, nonunions, and sequelae.

Care for complications of surgical treatment for fracture repairs during the healing or recovery phase should be coded with the appropriate complication codes.

See Section I.C.19. Coding of traumatic fractures.

d. Osteoporosis

Osteoporosis is a systemic condition, meaning that all bones of the musculoskeletal system are affected. Therefore, site is not a component of the codes under category M81, Osteoporosis without current pathological fracture. The site codes under category M80, Osteoporosis with current pathological fracture, identify the site of the fracture, not the osteoporosis.

1) Osteoporosis without pathological fracture

Category M81, Osteoporosis without current pathological fracture, is for use for patients with osteoporosis who do not currently have a pathologic fracture due to the osteoporosis, even if they have had a fracture in the past. For patients with a history of osteoporosis fractures, status code Z87.310, Personal history of (healed) osteoporosis fracture, should follow the code from M81.

2) Osteoporosis with current pathological fracture

Category M80, Osteoporosis with current pathological fracture, is for patients who have a current pathologic fracture at the time of an encounter. The codes under M80 identify the site of the fracture. A code from category M80, not a traumatic fracture code, should be used for any patient with known osteoporosis who suffers a fracture, even if the patient had a minor fall or trauma, if that fall or trauma would not usually break a normal, healthy bone.

e. Multisystem Inflammatory Syndrome

See Section I.C.1.g.1.l for Multisystem Inflammatory Syndrome

ARTHROPATHIES (M00-M25)

Includes: Disorders affecting predominantly peripheral (limb) joints

Infectious arthropathies (M00-M02)

NOTE This block comprises arthropathies due to microbiological agents. Distinction is made between the following types of etiological relationship:
a) direct infection of joint, where organisms invade synovial tissue and microbial antigen is present in the joint;
b) indirect infection, which may be of two types: a reactive arthropathy, where microbial infection of the body is established but neither organisms nor antigens can be identified in the joint, and a postinfective arthropathy, where microbial antigen is present but recovery of an organism is inconstant and evidence of local multiplication is lacking.

M00 Pyogenic arthritis

Excludes2: infection and inflammatory reaction due to internal joint prosthesis (T84.5-)

+ **M00.0 Staphylococcal arthritis and polyarthritis**
  Use additional code (B95.61-B95.8) to identify bacterial agent
  - CC **M00.00** Staphylococcal arthritis, unspecified joint
  + **M00.01** Staphylococcal arthritis, shoulder
    - **M00.011** Staphylococcal arthritis, right shoulder
    - **M00.012** Staphylococcal arthritis, left shoulder
    - CC **M00.019** Staphylococcal arthritis, unspecified shoulder
  + **M00.02** Staphylococcal arthritis, elbow
    - **M00.021** Staphylococcal arthritis, right elbow
    - **M00.022** Staphylococcal arthritis, left elbow
    - CC **M00.029** Staphylococcal arthritis, unspecified elbow

801

+ **M00.03 Staphylococcal arthritis, wrist**
  Staphylococcal arthritis of carpal bones
  - **M00.031** Staphylococcal arthritis, right wrist
  - **M00.032** Staphylococcal arthritis, left wrist
  - CC **M00.039** Staphylococcal arthritis, unspecified wrist
+ **M00.04 Staphylococcal arthritis, hand**
  Staphylococcal arthritis of metacarpus and phalanges
  - **M00.041** Staphylococcal arthritis, right hand
  - **M00.042** Staphylococcal arthritis, left hand
  - CC **M00.049** Staphylococcal arthritis, unspecified hand
+ **M00.05 Staphylococcal arthritis, hip**
  - **M00.051** Staphylococcal arthritis, right hip
  - **M00.052** Staphylococcal arthritis, left hip
  - CC **M00.059** Staphylococcal arthritis, unspecified hip
+ **M00.06 Staphylococcal arthritis, knee**
  - **M00.061** Staphylococcal arthritis, right knee
  - **M00.062** Staphylococcal arthritis, left knee
  - CC **M00.069** Staphylococcal arthritis, unspecified knee
+ **M00.07 Staphylococcal arthritis, ankle and foot**
  Staphylococcal arthritis, tarsus, metatarsus and phalanges
  - **M00.071** Staphylococcal arthritis, right ankle and foot
  - **M00.072** Staphylococcal arthritis, left ankle and foot
  - CC **M00.079** Staphylococcal arthritis, unspecified ankle and foot
- CC **M00.08** Staphylococcal arthritis, vertebrae
- CC **M00.09** Staphylococcal polyarthritis
+ **M00.1 Pneumococcal arthritis and polyarthritis**
  - CC **M00.10** Pneumococcal arthritis, unspecified joint
  + **M00.11 Pneumococcal arthritis, shoulder**
    - CC **M00.111** Pneumococcal arthritis, right shoulder
    - CC **M00.112** Pneumococcal arthritis, left shoulder
    - CC **M00.119** Pneumococcal arthritis, unspecified shoulder
  + **M00.12 Pneumococcal arthritis, elbow**
    - CC **M00.121** Pneumococcal arthritis, right elbow
    - CC **M00.122** Pneumococcal arthritis, left elbow
    - CC **M00.129** Pneumococcal arthritis, unspecified elbow
  + **M00.13 Pneumococcal arthritis, wrist**
    Pneumococcal arthritis of carpal bones
    - CC **M00.131** Pneumococcal arthritis, right wrist
    - CC **M00.132** Pneumococcal arthritis, left wrist
    - CC **M00.139** Pneumococcal arthritis, unspecified wrist
  + **M00.14 Pneumococcal arthritis, hand**
    Pneumococcal arthritis of metacarpus and phalanges
    - CC **M00.141** Pneumococcal arthritis, right hand
    - CC **M00.142** Pneumococcal arthritis, left hand
    - CC **M00.149** Pneumococcal arthritis, unspecified hand
  + **M00.15 Pneumococcal arthritis, hip**
    - CC **M00.151** Pneumococcal arthritis, right hip
    - CC **M00.152** Pneumococcal arthritis, left hip
    - CC **M00.159** Pneumococcal arthritis, unspecified hip
  + **M00.16 Pneumococcal arthritis, knee**
    - CC **M00.161** Pneumococcal arthritis, right knee
    - CC **M00.162** Pneumococcal arthritis, left knee
    - CC **M00.169** Pneumococcal arthritis, unspecified knee
  + **M00.17 Pneumococcal arthritis, ankle and foot**
    Pneumococcal arthritis, tarsus, metatarsus and phalanges
    - CC **M00.171** Pneumococcal arthritis, right ankle and foot
    - CC **M00.172** Pneumococcal arthritis, left ankle and foot
    - CC **M00.179** Pneumococcal arthritis, unspecified ankle and foot
  - CC **M00.18** Pneumococcal arthritis, vertebrae
  - CC **M00.19** Pneumococcal polyarthritis

+ **M00.2 Other streptococcal arthritis and polyarthritis**
  Use additional code (B95.0-B95.2, B95.4-B95.5) to identify bacterial agent
  - CC **M00.20** Other streptococcal arthritis, unspecified joint
  + **M00.21 Other streptococcal arthritis, shoulder**
    - CC **M00.211** Other streptococcal arthritis, right shoulder
    - CC **M00.212** Other streptococcal arthritis, left shoulder
    - CC **M00.219** Other streptococcal arthritis, unspecified shoulder
  + **M00.22 Other streptococcal arthritis, elbow**
    - CC **M00.221** Other streptococcal arthritis, right elbow
    - CC **M00.222** Other streptococcal arthritis, left elbow
    - CC **M00.229** Other streptococcal arthritis, unspecified elbow
  + **M00.23 Other streptococcal arthritis, wrist**
    Other streptococcal arthritis of carpal bones
    - CC **M00.231** Other streptococcal arthritis, right wrist
    - CC **M00.232** Other streptococcal arthritis, left wrist
    - CC **M00.239** Other streptococcal arthritis, unspecified wrist
  + **M00.24 Other streptococcal arthritis, hand**
    Other streptococcal arthritis metacarpus and phalanges
    - CC **M00.241** Other streptococcal arthritis, right hand
    - CC **M00.242** Other streptococcal arthritis, left hand
    - CC **M00.249** Other streptococcal arthritis, unspecified hand
  + **M00.25 Other streptococcal arthritis, hip**
    - CC **M00.251** Other streptococcal arthritis, right hip
    - CC **M00.252** Other streptococcal arthritis, left hip
    - CC **M00.259** Other streptococcal arthritis, unspecified hip
  + **M00.26 Other streptococcal arthritis, knee**
    - CC **M00.261** Other streptococcal arthritis, right knee
    - CC **M00.262** Other streptococcal arthritis, left knee
    - CC **M00.269** Other streptococcal arthritis, unspecified knee
  + **M00.27 Other streptococcal arthritis, ankle and foot**
    Other streptococcal arthritis, tarsus, metatarsus and phalanges
    - CC **M00.271** Other streptococcal arthritis, right ankle and foot
    - CC **M00.272** Other streptococcal arthritis, left ankle and foot
    - CC **M00.279** Other streptococcal arthritis, unspecified ankle and foot
  - CC **M00.28** Other streptococcal arthritis, vertebrae
  - CC **M00.29** Other streptococcal polyarthritis
+ **M00.8 Arthritis and polyarthritis due to other bacteria**
  Use additional code (B96) to identify bacteria
  - CC **M00.80** Arthritis due to other bacteria, unspecified joint
  + **M00.81 Arthritis due to other bacteria, shoulder**
    - CC **M00.811** Arthritis due to other bacteria, right shoulder
    - CC **M00.812** Arthritis due to other bacteria, left shoulder
    - CC **M00.819** Arthritis due to other bacteria, unspecified shoulder
  + **M00.82 Arthritis due to other bacteria, elbow**
    - CC **M00.821** Arthritis due to other bacteria, right elbow
    - CC **M00.822** Arthritis due to other bacteria, left elbow
    - CC **M00.829** Arthritis due to other bacteria, unspecified elbow
  + **M00.83 Arthritis due to other bacteria, wrist**
    Arthritis due to other bacteria, carpal bones
    - CC **M00.831** Arthritis due to other bacteria, right wrist
    - CC **M00.832** Arthritis due to other bacteria, left wrist
    - CC **M00.839** Arthritis due to other bacteria, unspecified wrist

- **+ M00.84** Arthritis due to other bacteria, hand
  Arthritis due to other bacteria, metacarpus and phalanges
  - **CC M00.841** Arthritis due to other bacteria, right hand
  - **CC M00.842** Arthritis due to other bacteria, left hand
  - **CC M00.849** Arthritis due to other bacteria, unspecified hand
- **+ M00.85** Arthritis due to other bacteria, hip
  - **CC M00.851** Arthritis due to other bacteria, right hip
  - **CC M00.852** Arthritis due to other bacteria, left hip
  - **CC M00.859** Arthritis due to other bacteria, unspecified hip
- **+ M00.86** Arthritis due to other bacteria, knee
  - **CC M00.861** Arthritis due to other bacteria, right knee
  - **CC M00.862** Arthritis due to other bacteria, left knee
    AHA CC: 3Q, 2019, 16-17
  - **CC M00.869** Arthritis due to other bacteria, unspecified knee
- **+ M00.87** Arthritis due to other bacteria, ankle and foot
  Arthritis due to other bacteria, tarsus, metatarsus, and phalanges
  - **CC M00.871** Arthritis due to other bacteria, right ankle and foot
  - **CC M00.872** Arthritis due to other bacteria, left ankle and foot
  - **CC M00.879** Arthritis due to other bacteria, unspecified ankle and foot
- **CC M00.88** Arthritis due to other bacteria, vertebrae
- **CC M00.89** Polyarthritis due to other bacteria
- **CC M00.9** Pyogenic arthritis, unspecified
  Infective arthritis NOS

M01 Direct infections of joint in infectious and parasitic diseases classified elsewhere

Code first underlying disease, such as:
 leprosy [Hansen's disease] (A30.-)
 mycoses (B35-B49)
 O'nyong-nyong fever (A92.1)
 paratyphoid fever (A01.1-A01.4)

Excludes1: arthropathy in Lyme disease (A69.23)
 gonococcal arthritis (A54.42)
 meningococcal arthritis (A39.83)
 mumps arthritis (B26.85)
 postinfective arthropathy (M02.-)
 postmeningococcal arthritis (39.84)
 reactive arthritis (M02.3)
 rubella arthritis (B06.82)
 sarcoidosis arthritis (D86.86)
 tuberculosis arthritis (A18.01-A18.02)
 typhoid fever arthritis (A01.04)

- **+ M01.X** Direct infection of joint in infectious and parasitic diseases classified elsewhere
  - **CC M01.X0** Direct infection of unspecified joint in infectious and parasitic diseases classified elsewhere
  - **+ M01.X1** Direct infection of shoulder joint in infectious and parasitic diseases classified elsewhere
    - **CC M01.X11** Direct infection of right shoulder in infectious and parasitic diseases classified elsewhere
    - **CC M01.X12** Direct infection of left shoulder in infectious and parasitic diseases classified elsewhere
    - **CC M01.X19** Direct infection of unspecified shoulder in infectious and parasitic diseases classified elsewhere
  - **+ M01.X2** Direct infection of elbow in infectious and parasitic diseases classified elsewhere
    - **CC M01.X21** Direct infection of right elbow in infectious and parasitic diseases classified elsewhere
    - **CC M01.X22** Direct infection of left elbow in infectious and parasitic diseases classified elsewhere
    - **CC M01.X29** Direct infection of unspecified elbow in infectious and parasitic diseases classified elsewhere
  - **+ M01.X3** Direct infection of wrist in infectious and parasitic diseases classified elsewhere
    Direct infection of carpal bones in infectious and parasitic diseases classified elsewhere
    - **CC M01.X31** Direct infection of right wrist in infectious and parasitic diseases classified elsewhere
    - **CC M01.X32** Direct infection of left wrist in infectious and parasitic diseases classified elsewhere
    - **CC M01.X39** Direct infection of unspecified wrist in infectious and parasitic diseases classified elsewhere
  - **+ M01.X4** Direct infection of hand in infectious and parasitic diseases classified elsewhere
    Direct infection of metacarpus and phalanges in infectious and parasitic diseases classified elsewhere
    - **CC M01.X41** Direct infection of right hand in infectious and parasitic diseases classified elsewhere
    - **CC M01.X42** Direct infection of left hand in infectious and parasitic diseases classified elsewhere
    - **CC M01.X49** Direct infection of unspecified hand in infectious and parasitic diseases classified elsewhere
  - **+ M01.X5** Direct infection of hip in infectious and parasitic diseases classified elsewhere
    - **CC M01.X51** Direct infection of right hip in infectious and parasitic diseases classified elsewhere
    - **CC M01.X52** Direct infection of left hip in infectious and parasitic diseases classified elsewhere
    - **CC M01.X59** Direct infection of unspecified hip in infectious and parasitic diseases classified elsewhere
  - **+ M01.X6** Direct infection of knee in infectious and parasitic diseases classified elsewhere
    - **CC M01.X61** Direct infection of right knee in infectious and parasitic diseases classified elsewhere
    - **CC M01.X62** Direct infection of left knee in infectious and parasitic diseases classified elsewhere
    - **CC M01.X69** Direct infection of unspecified knee in infectious and parasitic diseases classified elsewhere
  - **+ M01.X7** Direct infection of ankle and foot in infectious and parasitic diseases classified elsewhere
    Direct infection of tarsus, metatarsus and phalanges in infectious and parasitic diseases classified elsewhere
    - **CC M01.X71** Direct infection of right ankle and foot in infectious and parasitic diseases classified elsewhere
    - **CC M01.X72** Direct infection of left ankle and foot in infectious and parasitic diseases classified elsewhere
    - **CC M01.X79** Direct infection of unspecified ankle and foot in infectious and parasitic diseases classified elsewhere
  - **CC M01.X8** Direct infection of vertebrae in infectious and parasitic diseases classified elsewhere
  - **CC M01.X9** Direct infection of multiple joints in infectious and parasitic diseases classified elsewhere

M02 Postinfective and reactive arthropathies

Code first underlying disease, such as:
congenital syphilis [Clutton's joints] (A50.5)
enteritis due to Yersinia enterocolitica (A04.6)
infective endocarditis (I33.0)
viral hepatitis (B15-B19)

Excludes1: Behçet's disease (M35.2)
direct infections of joint in infectious and parasitic diseases classified elsewhere (M01.-)
postmeningcoccal arthritis (A39.84)
mumps arthritis (B26.85)
rubella arthritis (B06.82)
syphilis arthritis (late) (A52.77)
rheumatic fever (I00)
tabetic arthropathy [Charcôt's] (A52.16)

- **M02.0 Arthropathy following intestinal bypass**
  - M02.00 Arthropathy following intestinal bypass, unspecified site
  - **M02.01 Arthropathy following intestinal bypass, shoulder**
    - M02.011 Arthropathy following intestinal bypass, right shoulder
    - M02.012 Arthropathy following intestinal bypass, left shoulder
    - M02.019 Arthropathy following intestinal bypass, unspecified shoulder
  - **M02.02 Arthropathy following intestinal bypass, elbow**
    - M02.021 Arthropathy following intestinal bypass, right elbow
    - M02.022 Arthropathy following intestinal bypass, left elbow
    - M02.029 Arthropathy following intestinal bypass, unspecified elbow
  - **M02.03 Arthropathy following intestinal bypass, wrist**
    Arthropathy following intestinal bypass, carpal bones
    - M02.031 Arthropathy following intestinal bypass, right wrist
    - M02.032 Arthropathy following intestinal bypass, left wrist
    - M02.039 Arthropathy following intestinal bypass, unspecified wrist
  - **M02.04 Arthropathy following intestinal bypass, hand**
    Arthropathy following intestinal bypass, metacarpals and phalanges
    - M02.041 Arthropathy following intestinal bypass, right hand
    - M02.042 Arthropathy following intestinal bypass, left hand
    - M02.049 Arthropathy following intestinal bypass, unspecified hand
  - **M02.05 Arthropathy following intestinal bypass, hip**
    - M02.051 Arthropathy following intestinal bypass, right hip
    - M02.052 Arthropathy following intestinal bypass, left hip
    - M02.059 Arthropathy following intestinal bypass, unspecified hip
  - **M02.06 Arthropathy following intestinal bypass, knee**
    - M02.061 Arthropathy following intestinal bypass, right knee
    - M02.062 Arthropathy following intestinal bypass, left knee
    - M02.069 Arthropathy following intestinal bypass, unspecified knee
  - **M02.07 Arthropathy following intestinal bypass, ankle and foot**
    Arthropathy following intestinal bypass, tarsus, metatarsus and phalanges
    - M02.071 Arthropathy following intestinal bypass, right ankle and foot
    - M02.072 Arthropathy following intestinal bypass, left ankle and foot
    - M02.079 Arthropathy following intestinal bypass, unspecified ankle and foot
  - M02.08 Arthropathy following intestinal bypass, vertebrae
  - M02.09 Arthropathy following intestinal bypass, multiple sites

- **M02.1 Postdysenteric arthropathy**
  - CC M02.10 Postdysenteric arthropathy, unspecified site
  - **M02.11 Postdysenteric arthropathy, shoulder**
    - CC M02.111 Postdysenteric arthropathy, right shoulder
    - CC M02.112 Postdysenteric arthropathy, left shoulder
    - CC M02.119 Postdysenteric arthropathy, unspecified shoulder
  - **M02.12 Postdysenteric arthropathy, elbow**
    - CC M02.121 Postdysenteric arthropathy, right elbow
    - CC M02.122 Postdysenteric arthropathy, left elbow
    - CC M02.129 Postdysenteric arthropathy, unspecified elbow
  - **M02.13 Postdysenteric arthropathy, wrist**
    Postdysenteric arthropathy, carpal bones
    - CC M02.131 Postdysenteric arthropathy, right wrist
    - CC M02.132 Postdysenteric arthropathy, left wrist
    - CC M02.139 Postdysenteric arthropathy, unspecified wrist
  - **M02.14 Postdysenteric arthropathy, hand**
    Postdysenteric arthropathy, metacarpus and phalanges
    - CC M02.141 Postdysenteric arthropathy, right hand
    - CC M02.142 Postdysenteric arthropathy, left hand
    - CC M02.149 Postdysenteric arthropathy, unspecified hand
  - **M02.15 Postdysenteric arthropathy, hip**
    - CC M02.151 Postdysenteric arthropathy, right hip
    - CC M02.152 Postdysenteric arthropathy, left hip
    - CC M02.159 Postdysenteric arthropathy, unspecified hip
  - **M02.16 Postdysenteric arthropathy, knee**
    - CC M02.161 Postdysenteric arthropathy, right knee
    - CC M02.162 Postdysenteric arthropathy, left knee
    - CC M02.169 Postdysenteric arthropathy, unspecified knee
  - **M02.17 Postdysenteric arthropathy, ankle and foot**
    Postdysenteric arthropathy, tarsus, metatarsus and phalanges
    - CC M02.171 Postdysenteric arthropathy, right ankle and foot
    - CC M02.172 Postdysenteric arthropathy, left ankle and foot
    - CC M02.179 Postdysenteric arthropathy, unspecified ankle and foot
  - CC M02.18 Postdysenteric arthropathy, vertebrae
  - CC M02.19 Postdysenteric arthropathy, multiple sites

- **M02.2 Postimmunization arthropathy**
  - M02.20 Postimmunization arthropathy, unspecified site
  - **M02.21 Postimmunization arthropathy, shoulder**
    - M02.211 Postimmunization arthropathy, right shoulder
    - M02.212 Postimmunization arthropathy, left shoulder
    - M02.219 Postimmunization arthropathy, unspecified shoulder
  - **M02.22 Postimmunization arthropathy, elbow**
    - M02.221 Postimmunization arthropathy, right elbow
    - M02.222 Postimmunization arthropathy, left elbow
    - M02.229 Postimmunization arthropathy, unspecified elbow
  - **M02.23 Postimmunization arthropathy, wrist**
    Postimmunization arthropathy, carpal bones
    - M02.231 Postimmunization arthropathy, right wrist
    - M02.232 Postimmunization arthropathy, left wrist
    - M02.239 Postimmunization arthropathy, unspecified wrist
  - **M02.24 Postimmunization arthropathy, hand**
    Postimmunization arthropathy, metacarpus and phalanges
    - M02.241 Postimmunization arthropathy, right hand

M02.242 Postimmunization arthropathy, left hand
M02.249 Postimmunization arthropathy, unspecified hand
+ M02.25 Postimmunization arthropathy, hip
M02.251 Postimmunization arthropathy, right hip
M02.252 Postimmunization arthropathy, left hip
M02.259 Postimmunization arthropathy, unspecified hip
+ M02.26 Postimmunization arthropathy, knee
M02.261 Postimmunization arthropathy, right knee
M02.262 Postimmunization arthropathy, left knee
M02.269 Postimmunization arthropathy, unspecified knee
+ M02.27 Postimmunization arthropathy, ankle and foot
Postimmunization arthropathy, tarsus, metatarsus and phalanges
M02.271 Postimmunization arthropathy, right ankle and foot
M02.272 Postimmunization arthropathy, left ankle and foot
M02.279 Postimmunization arthropathy, unspecified ankle and foot
M02.28 Postimmunization arthropathy, vertebrae
M02.29 Postimmunization arthropathy, multiple sites
+ M02.3 Reiter's disease
Reactive arthritis
CC M02.30 Reiter's disease, unspecified site
+ M02.31 Reiter's disease, shoulder
CC M02.311 Reiter's disease, right shoulder
CC M02.312 Reiter's disease, left shoulder
CC M02.319 Reiter's disease, unspecified shoulder
+ M02.32 Reiter's disease, elbow
CC M02.321 Reiter's disease, right elbow
CC M02.322 Reiter's disease, left elbow
CC M02.329 Reiter's disease, unspecified elbow
+ M02.33 Reiter's disease, wrist
Reiter's disease, carpal bones
CC M02.331 Reiter's disease, right wrist
CC M02.332 Reiter's disease, left wrist
CC M02.339 Reiter's disease, unspecified wrist
+ M02.34 Reiter's disease, hand
Reiter's disease, metacarpus and phalanges
CC M02.341 Reiter's disease, right hand
CC M02.342 Reiter's disease, left hand
CC M02.349 Reiter's disease, unspecified hand
+ M02.35 Reiter's disease, hip
CC M02.351 Reiter's disease, right hip
CC M02.352 Reiter's disease, left hip
CC M02.359 Reiter's disease, unspecified hip
+ M02.36 Reiter's disease, knee
CC M02.361 Reiter's disease, right knee
CC M02.362 Reiter's disease, left knee
CC M02.369 Reiter's disease, unspecified knee
+ M02.37 Reiter's disease, ankle and foot
Reiter's disease, tarsus, metatarsus and phalanges
CC M02.371 Reiter's disease, right ankle and foot
CC M02.372 Reiter's disease, left ankle and foot
CC M02.379 Reiter's disease, unspecified ankle and foot
CC M02.38 Reiter's disease, vertebrae
CC M02.39 Reiter's disease, multiple sites
+ M02.8 Other reactive arthropathies
CC M02.80 Other reactive arthropathies, unspecified site
+ M02.81 Other reactive arthropathies, shoulder
CC M02.811 Other reactive arthropathies, right shoulder
CC M02.812 Other reactive arthropathies, left shoulder
CC M02.819 Other reactive arthropathies, unspecified shoulder
+ M02.82 Other reactive arthropathies, elbow
CC M02.821 Other reactive arthropathies, right elbow
CC M02.822 Other reactive arthropathies, left elbow
CC M02.829 Other reactive arthropathies, unspecified elbow

+ M02.83 Other reactive arthropathies, wrist
Other reactive arthropathies, carpal bones
CC M02.831 Other reactive arthropathies, right wrist
CC M02.832 Other reactive arthropathies, left wrist
CC M02.839 Other reactive arthropathies, unspecified wrist
+ M02.84 Other reactive arthropathies, hand
Other reactive arthropathies, metacarpus and phalanges
CC M02.841 Other reactive arthropathies, right hand
CC M02.842 Other reactive arthropathies, left hand
CC M02.849 Other reactive arthropathies, unspecified hand
+ M02.85 Other reactive arthropathies, hip
CC M02.851 Other reactive arthropathies, right hip
CC M02.852 Other reactive arthropathies, left hip
CC M02.859 Other reactive arthropathies, unspecified hip
+ M02.86 Other reactive arthropathies, knee
CC M02.861 Other reactive arthropathies, right knee
CC M02.862 Other reactive arthropathies, left knee
CC M02.869 Other reactive arthropathies, unspecified knee
+ M02.87 Other reactive arthropathies, ankle and foot
Other reactive arthropathies, tarsus, metatarsus and phalanges
CC M02.871 Other reactive arthropathies, right ankle and foot
CC M02.872 Other reactive arthropathies, left ankle and foot
CC M02.879 Other reactive arthropathies, unspecified ankle and foot
CC M02.88 Other reactive arthropathies, vertebrae
CC M02.89 Other reactive arthropathies, multiple sites
M02.9 Reactive arthropathy, unspecified

Autoinflammatory syndromes (M04)

M04 Autoinflammatory syndromes
Excludes2: Crohn's disease (K50.-)
AHA CC: 4Q, 2016, 37
M04.1 Periodic fever syndromes
Familial Mediterranean fever
Hyperimmunoglobin D syndrome
Mevalonate kinase deficiency
Tumor necrosis factor receptor associated periodic syndrome [TRAPS]
M04.2 Cryopyrin-associated periodic syndromes
Chronic infantile neurological, cutaneous and articular syndrome [CINCA]
Familial cold autoinflammatory syndrome
Familial cold urticaria
Muckle-Wells syndrome
Neonatal onset multisystemic inflammatory disorder [NOMID]
M04.8 Other autoinflammatory syndromes
Blau syndrome
Deficiency of interleukin 1 receptor antagonist [DIRA]
Majeed syndrome
Periodic fever, aphthous stomatitis, pharyngitis, and adenopathy syndrome [PFAPA]
Pyogenic arthritis, pyoderma gangrenosum, and acne syndrome [PAPA]
M04.9 Autoinflammatory syndrome, unspecified

Inflammatory polyarthropathies (M05-M14)

M05 Rheumatoid arthritis with rheumatoid factor
Excludes1: rheumatic fever (I00)
juvenile rheumatoid arthritis (M08.-)
rheumatoid arthritis of spine (M45.-)
AHA CC: 4Q, 2020, 31-32
+ M05.0 Felty's syndrome
Rheumatoid arthritis with splenoadenomegaly and leukopenia
M05.00 Felty's syndrome, unspecified site

- **M05.01 Felty's syndrome, shoulder**
  - M05.011 Felty's syndrome, right shoulder
  - M05.012 Felty's syndrome, left shoulder
  - M05.019 Felty's syndrome, unspecified shoulder
- **M05.02 Felty's syndrome, elbow**
  - M05.021 Felty's syndrome, right elbow
  - M05.022 Felty's syndrome, left elbow
  - M05.029 Felty's syndrome, unspecified elbow
- **M05.03 Felty's syndrome, wrist**
  - Felty's syndrome, carpal bones
  - M05.031 Felty's syndrome, right wrist
  - M05.032 Felty's syndrome, left wrist
  - M05.039 Felty's syndrome, unspecified wrist
- **M05.04 Felty's syndrome, hand**
  - Felty's syndrome, metacarpus and phalanges
  - M05.041 Felty's syndrome, right hand
  - M05.042 Felty's syndrome, left hand
  - M05.049 Felty's syndrome, unspecified hand
- **M05.05 Felty's syndrome, hip**
  - M05.051 Felty's syndrome, right hip
  - M05.052 Felty's syndrome, left hip
  - M05.059 Felty's syndrome, unspecified hip
- **M05.06 Felty's syndrome, knee**
  - M05.061 Felty's syndrome, right knee
  - M05.062 Felty's syndrome, left knee
  - M05.069 Felty's syndrome, unspecified knee
- **M05.07 Felty's syndrome, ankle and foot**
  - Felty's syndrome, tarsus, metatarsus and phalanges
  - M05.071 Felty's syndrome, right ankle and foot
  - M05.072 Felty's syndrome, left ankle and foot
  - M05.079 Felty's syndrome, unspecified ankle and foot
- M05.09 Felty's syndrome, multiple sites
- **M05.1 Rheumatoid lung disease with rheumatoid arthritis**
  - M05.10 Rheumatoid lung disease with rheumatoid arthritis of unspecified site
  - **M05.11 Rheumatoid lung disease with rheumatoid arthritis of shoulder**
    - M05.111 Rheumatoid lung disease with rheumatoid arthritis of right shoulder
    - M05.112 Rheumatoid lung disease with rheumatoid arthritis of left shoulder
    - M05.119 Rheumatoid lung disease with rheumatoid arthritis of unspecified shoulder
  - **M05.12 Rheumatoid lung disease with rheumatoid arthritis of elbow**
    - M05.121 Rheumatoid lung disease with rheumatoid arthritis of right elbow
    - M05.122 Rheumatoid lung disease with rheumatoid arthritis of left elbow
    - M05.129 Rheumatoid lung disease with rheumatoid arthritis of unspecified elbow
  - **M05.13 Rheumatoid lung disease with rheumatoid arthritis of wrist**
    - Rheumatoid lung disease with rheumatoid arthritis, carpal bones
    - M05.131 Rheumatoid lung disease with rheumatoid arthritis of right wrist
    - M05.132 Rheumatoid lung disease with rheumatoid arthritis of left wrist
    - M05.139 Rheumatoid lung disease with rheumatoid arthritis of unspecified wrist
  - **M05.14 Rheumatoid lung disease with rheumatoid arthritis of hand**
    - Rheumatoid lung disease with rheumatoid arthritis, metacarpus and phalanges
    - M05.141 Rheumatoid lung disease with rheumatoid arthritis of right hand
    - M05.142 Rheumatoid lung disease with rheumatoid arthritis of left hand
    - M05.149 Rheumatoid lung disease with rheumatoid arthritis of unspecified hand
  - **M05.15 Rheumatoid lung disease with rheumatoid arthritis of hip**
    - M05.151 Rheumatoid lung disease with rheumatoid arthritis of right hip
    - M05.152 Rheumatoid lung disease with rheumatoid arthritis of left hip
    - M05.159 Rheumatoid lung disease with rheumatoid arthritis of unspecified hip
  - **M05.16 Rheumatoid lung disease with rheumatoid arthritis of knee**
    - M05.161 Rheumatoid lung disease with rheumatoid arthritis of right knee
    - M05.162 Rheumatoid lung disease with rheumatoid arthritis of left knee
    - M05.169 Rheumatoid lung disease with rheumatoid arthritis of unspecified knee
  - **M05.17 Rheumatoid lung disease with rheumatoid arthritis of ankle and foot**
    - Rheumatoid lung disease with rheumatoid arthritis, tarsus, metatarsus and phalanges
    - M05.171 Rheumatoid lung disease with rheumatoid arthritis of right ankle and foot
    - M05.172 Rheumatoid lung disease with rheumatoid arthritis of left ankle and foot
    - M05.179 Rheumatoid lung disease with rheumatoid arthritis of unspecified ankle and foot
  - M05.19 Rheumatoid lung disease with rheumatoid arthritis of multiple sites
- **M05.2 Rheumatoid vasculitis with rheumatoid arthritis**
  - M05.20 Rheumatoid vasculitis with rheumatoid arthritis of unspecified site
  - **M05.21 Rheumatoid vasculitis with rheumatoid arthritis of shoulder**
    - M05.211 Rheumatoid vasculitis with rheumatoid arthritis of right shoulder
    - M05.212 Rheumatoid vasculitis with rheumatoid arthritis of left shoulder
    - M05.219 Rheumatoid vasculitis with rheumatoid arthritis of unspecified shoulder
  - **M05.22 Rheumatoid vasculitis with rheumatoid arthritis of elbow**
    - M05.221 Rheumatoid vasculitis with rheumatoid arthritis of right elbow
    - M05.222 Rheumatoid vasculitis with rheumatoid arthritis of left elbow
    - M05.229 Rheumatoid vasculitis with rheumatoid arthritis of unspecified elbow
  - **M05.23 Rheumatoid vasculitis with rheumatoid arthritis of wrist**
    - Rheumatoid vasculitis with rheumatoid arthritis, carpal bones
    - M05.231 Rheumatoid vasculitis with rheumatoid arthritis of right wrist
    - M05.232 Rheumatoid vasculitis with rheumatoid arthritis of left wrist
    - M05.239 Rheumatoid vasculitis with rheumatoid arthritis of unspecified wrist
  - **M05.24 Rheumatoid vasculitis with rheumatoid arthritis of hand**
    - Rheumatoid vasculitis with rheumatoid arthritis, metacarpus and phalanges
    - M05.241 Rheumatoid vasculitis with rheumatoid arthritis of right hand
    - M05.242 Rheumatoid vasculitis with rheumatoid arthritis of left hand
    - M05.249 Rheumatoid vasculitis with rheumatoid arthritis of unspecified hand
  - **M05.25 Rheumatoid vasculitis with rheumatoid arthritis of hip**
    - M05.251 Rheumatoid vasculitis with rheumatoid arthritis of right hip
    - M05.252 Rheumatoid vasculitis with rheumatoid arthritis of left hip
    - M05.259 Rheumatoid vasculitis with rheumatoid arthritis of unspecified hip

- **+ M05.26 Rheumatoid vasculitis with rheumatoid arthritis of knee**
  - M05.261 Rheumatoid vasculitis with rheumatoid arthritis of right knee
  - M05.262 Rheumatoid vasculitis with rheumatoid arthritis of left knee
  - M05.269 Rheumatoid vasculitis with rheumatoid arthritis of unspecified knee
- **+ M05.27 Rheumatoid vasculitis with rheumatoid arthritis of ankle and foot**
  - Rheumatoid vasculitis with rheumatoid arthritis, tarsus, metatarsus and phalanges
  - M05.271 Rheumatoid vasculitis with rheumatoid arthritis of right ankle and foot
  - M05.272 Rheumatoid vasculitis with rheumatoid arthritis of left ankle and foot
  - M05.279 Rheumatoid vasculitis with rheumatoid arthritis of unspecified ankle and foot
- **M05.29 Rheumatoid vasculitis with rheumatoid arthritis of multiple sites**
- **+ M05.3 Rheumatoid heart disease with rheumatoid arthritis**
  - Rheumatoid carditis
  - Rheumatoid endocarditis
  - Rheumatoid myocarditis
  - Rheumatoid pericarditis
  - M05.30 Rheumatoid heart disease with rheumatoid arthritis of unspecified site
- **+ M05.31 Rheumatoid heart disease with rheumatoid arthritis of shoulder**
  - M05.311 Rheumatoid heart disease with rheumatoid arthritis of right shoulder
  - M05.312 Rheumatoid heart disease with rheumatoid arthritis of left shoulder
  - M05.319 Rheumatoid heart disease with rheumatoid arthritis of unspecified shoulder
- **+ M05.32 Rheumatoid heart disease with rheumatoid arthritis of elbow**
  - M05.321 Rheumatoid heart disease with rheumatoid arthritis of right elbow
  - M05.322 Rheumatoid heart disease with rheumatoid arthritis of left elbow
  - M05.329 Rheumatoid heart disease with rheumatoid arthritis of unspecified elbow
- **+ M05.33 Rheumatoid heart disease with rheumatoid arthritis of wrist**
  - Rheumatoid heart disease with rheumatoid arthritis, carpal bones
  - M05.331 Rheumatoid heart disease with rheumatoid arthritis of right wrist
  - M05.332 Rheumatoid heart disease with rheumatoid arthritis of left wrist
  - M05.339 Rheumatoid heart disease with rheumatoid arthritis of unspecified wrist
- **+ M05.34 Rheumatoid heart disease with rheumatoid arthritis of hand**
  - Rheumatoid heart disease with rheumatoid arthritis, metacarpus and phalanges
  - M05.341 Rheumatoid heart disease with rheumatoid arthritis of right hand
  - M05.342 Rheumatoid heart disease with rheumatoid arthritis of left hand
  - M05.349 Rheumatoid heart disease with rheumatoid arthritis of unspecified hand
- **+ M05.35 Rheumatoid heart disease with rheumatoid arthritis of hip**
  - M05.351 Rheumatoid heart disease with rheumatoid arthritis of right hip
  - M05.352 Rheumatoid heart disease with rheumatoid arthritis of left hip
  - M05.359 Rheumatoid heart disease with rheumatoid arthritis of unspecified hip
- **+ M05.36 Rheumatoid heart disease with rheumatoid arthritis of knee**
  - M05.361 Rheumatoid heart disease with rheumatoid arthritis of right knee
  - M05.362 Rheumatoid heart disease with rheumatoid arthritis of left knee
  - M05.369 Rheumatoid heart disease with rheumatoid arthritis of unspecified knee
- **+ M05.37 Rheumatoid heart disease with rheumatoid arthritis of ankle and foot**
  - Rheumatoid heart disease with rheumatoid arthritis, tarsus, metatarsus and phalanges
  - M05.371 Rheumatoid heart disease with rheumatoid arthritis of right ankle and foot
  - M05.372 Rheumatoid heart disease with rheumatoid arthritis of left ankle and foot
  - M05.379 Rheumatoid heart disease with rheumatoid arthritis of unspecified ankle and foot
- **M05.39 Rheumatoid heart disease with rheumatoid arthritis of multiple sites**
- **+ M05.4 Rheumatoid myopathy with rheumatoid arthritis**
  - CC M05.40 Rheumatoid myopathy with rheumatoid arthritis of unspecified site
- **+ M05.41 Rheumatoid myopathy with rheumatoid arthritis of shoulder**
  - CC M05.411 Rheumatoid myopathy with rheumatoid arthritis of right shoulder
  - CC M05.412 Rheumatoid myopathy with rheumatoid arthritis of left shoulder
  - CC M05.419 Rheumatoid myopathy with rheumatoid arthritis of unspecified shoulder
- **+ M05.42 Rheumatoid myopathy with rheumatoid arthritis of elbow**
  - CC M05.421 Rheumatoid myopathy with rheumatoid arthritis of right elbow
  - CC M05.422 Rheumatoid myopathy with rheumatoid arthritis of left elbow
  - CC M05.429 Rheumatoid myopathy with rheumatoid arthritis of unspecified elbow
- **+ M05.43 Rheumatoid myopathy with rheumatoid arthritis of wrist**
  - Rheumatoid myopathy with rheumatoid arthritis, carpal bones
  - CC M05.431 Rheumatoid myopathy with rheumatoid arthritis of right wrist
  - CC M05.432 Rheumatoid myopathy with rheumatoid arthritis of left wrist
  - CC M05.439 Rheumatoid myopathy with rheumatoid arthritis of unspecified wrist
- **+ M05.44 Rheumatoid myopathy with rheumatoid arthritis of hand**
  - Rheumatoid myopathy with rheumatoid arthritis, metacarpus and phalanges
  - CC M05.441 Rheumatoid myopathy with rheumatoid arthritis of right hand
  - CC M05.442 Rheumatoid myopathy with rheumatoid arthritis of left hand
  - CC M05.449 Rheumatoid myopathy with rheumatoid arthritis of unspecified hand
- **+ M05.45 Rheumatoid myopathy with rheumatoid arthritis of hip**
  - CC M05.451 Rheumatoid myopathy with rheumatoid arthritis of right hip
  - CC M05.452 Rheumatoid myopathy with rheumatoid arthritis of left hip
  - CC M05.459 Rheumatoid myopathy with rheumatoid arthritis of unspecified hip
- **+ M05.46 Rheumatoid myopathy with rheumatoid arthritis of knee**
  - CC M05.461 Rheumatoid myopathy with rheumatoid arthritis of right knee
  - CC M05.462 Rheumatoid myopathy with rheumatoid arthritis of left knee
  - CC M05.469 Rheumatoid myopathy with rheumatoid arthritis of unspecified knee
- **+ M05.47 Rheumatoid myopathy with rheumatoid arthritis of ankle and foot**
  - Rheumatoid myopathy with rheumatoid arthritis, tarsus, metatarsus and phalanges
  - CC M05.471 Rheumatoid myopathy with rheumatoid arthritis of right ankle and foot

CC **M05.472** Rheumatoid myopathy with rheumatoid arthritis of left ankle and foot
CC **M05.479** Rheumatoid myopathy with rheumatoid arthritis of unspecified ankle and foot
CC **M05.49** Rheumatoid myopathy with rheumatoid arthritis of multiple sites

+ **M05.5** Rheumatoid polyneuropathy with rheumatoid arthritis
  - **M05.50** Rheumatoid polyneuropathy with rheumatoid arthritis of unspecified site
  + **M05.51** Rheumatoid polyneuropathy with rheumatoid arthritis of shoulder
    - **M05.511** Rheumatoid polyneuropathy with rheumatoid arthritis of right shoulder
    - **M05.512** Rheumatoid polyneuropathy with rheumatoid arthritis of left shoulder
    - **M05.519** Rheumatoid polyneuropathy with rheumatoid arthritis of unspecified shoulder
  + **M05.52** Rheumatoid polyneuropathy with rheumatoid arthritis of elbow
    - **M05.521** Rheumatoid polyneuropathy with rheumatoid arthritis of right elbow
    - **M05.522** Rheumatoid polyneuropathy with rheumatoid arthritis of left elbow
    - **M05.529** Rheumatoid polyneuropathy with rheumatoid arthritis of unspecified elbow
  + **M05.53** Rheumatoid polyneuropathy with rheumatoid arthritis of wrist
    Rheumatoid polyneuropathy with rheumatoid arthritis, carpal bones
    - **M05.531** Rheumatoid polyneuropathy with rheumatoid arthritis of right wrist
    - **M05.532** Rheumatoid polyneuropathy with rheumatoid arthritis of left wrist
    - **M05.539** Rheumatoid polyneuropathy with rheumatoid arthritis of unspecified wrist
  + **M05.54** Rheumatoid polyneuropathy with rheumatoid arthritis of hand
    Rheumatoid polyneuropathy with rheumatoid arthritis, metacarpus and phalanges
    - **M05.541** Rheumatoid polyneuropathy with rheumatoid arthritis of right hand
    - **M05.542** Rheumatoid polyneuropathy with rheumatoid arthritis of left hand
    - **M05.549** Rheumatoid polyneuropathy with rheumatoid arthritis of unspecified hand
  + **M05.55** Rheumatoid polyneuropathy with rheumatoid arthritis of hip
    - **M05.551** Rheumatoid polyneuropathy with rheumatoid arthritis of right hip
    - **M05.552** Rheumatoid polyneuropathy with rheumatoid arthritis of left hip
    - **M05.559** Rheumatoid polyneuropathy with rheumatoid arthritis of unspecified hip
  + **M05.56** Rheumatoid polyneuropathy with rheumatoid arthritis of knee
    - **M05.561** Rheumatoid polyneuropathy with rheumatoid arthritis of right knee
    - **M05.562** Rheumatoid polyneuropathy with rheumatoid arthritis of left knee
    - **M05.569** Rheumatoid polyneuropathy with rheumatoid arthritis of unspecified knee
  + **M05.57** Rheumatoid polyneuropathy with rheumatoid arthritis of ankle and foot
    Rheumatoid polyneuropathy with rheumatoid arthritis, tarsus, metatarsus and phalanges
    - **M05.571** Rheumatoid polyneuropathy with rheumatoid arthritis of right ankle and foot
    - **M05.572** Rheumatoid polyneuropathy with rheumatoid arthritis of left ankle and foot
    - **M05.579** Rheumatoid polyneuropathy with rheumatoid arthritis of unspecified ankle and foot
  - **M05.59** Rheumatoid polyneuropathy with rheumatoid arthritis of multiple sites

+ **M05.6** Rheumatoid arthritis with involvement of other organs and systems
  - **M05.60** Rheumatoid arthritis of unspecified site with involvement of other organs and systems
  + **M05.61** Rheumatoid arthritis of shoulder with involvement of other organs and systems
    - **M05.611** Rheumatoid arthritis of right shoulder with involvement of other organs and systems
    - **M05.612** Rheumatoid arthritis of left shoulder with involvement of other organs and systems
    - **M05.619** Rheumatoid arthritis of unspecified shoulder with involvement of other organs and systems
  + **M05.62** Rheumatoid arthritis of elbow with involvement of other organs and systems
    - **M05.621** Rheumatoid arthritis of right elbow with involvement of other organs and systems
    - **M05.622** Rheumatoid arthritis of left elbow with involvement of other organs and systems
    - **M05.629** Rheumatoid arthritis of unspecified elbow with involvement of other organs and systems
  + **M05.63** Rheumatoid arthritis of wrist with involvement of other organs and systems
    Rheumatoid arthritis of carpal bones with involvement of other organs and systems
    - **M05.631** Rheumatoid arthritis of right wrist with involvement of other organs and systems
    - **M05.632** Rheumatoid arthritis of left wrist with involvement of other organs and systems
    - **M05.639** Rheumatoid arthritis of unspecified wrist with involvement of other organs and systems
  + **M05.64** Rheumatoid arthritis of hand with involvement of other organs and systems
    Rheumatoid arthritis of metacarpus and phalanges with involvement of other organs and systems
    - **M05.641** Rheumatoid arthritis of right hand with involvement of other organs and systems
    - **M05.642** Rheumatoid arthritis of left hand with involvement of other organs and systems
    - **M05.649** Rheumatoid arthritis of unspecified hand with involvement of other organs and systems
  + **M05.65** Rheumatoid arthritis of hip with involvement of other organs and systems
    - **M05.651** Rheumatoid arthritis of right hip with involvement of other organs and systems
    - **M05.652** Rheumatoid arthritis of left hip with involvement of other organs and systems
    - **M05.659** Rheumatoid arthritis of unspecified hip with involvement of other organs and systems
  + **M05.66** Rheumatoid arthritis of knee with involvement of other organs and systems
    - **M05.661** Rheumatoid arthritis of right knee with involvement of other organs and systems
    - **M05.662** Rheumatoid arthritis of left knee with involvement of other organs and systems
    - **M05.669** Rheumatoid arthritis of unspecified knee with involvement of other organs and systems

- **M05.67** Rheumatoid arthritis of ankle and foot with involvement of other organs and systems
  Rheumatoid arthritis of tarsus, metatarsus and phalanges with involvement of other organs and systems
  - **M05.671** Rheumatoid arthritis of right ankle and foot with involvement of other organs and systems
  - **M05.672** Rheumatoid arthritis of left ankle and foot with involvement of other organs and systems
  - **M05.679** Rheumatoid arthritis of unspecified ankle and foot with involvement of other organs and systems
  - **M05.69** Rheumatoid arthritis of multiple sites with involvement of other organs and systems
- **M05.7** Rheumatoid arthritis with rheumatoid factor without organ or systems involvement
  - **M05.70** Rheumatoid arthritis with rheumatoid factor of unspecified site without organ or systems involvement
  - **M05.71** Rheumatoid arthritis with rheumatoid factor of shoulder without organ or systems involvement
    - **M05.711** Rheumatoid arthritis with rheumatoid factor of right shoulder without organ or systems involvement
    - **M05.712** Rheumatoid arthritis with rheumatoid factor of left shoulder without organ or systems involvement
    - **M05.719** Rheumatoid arthritis with rheumatoid factor of unspecified shoulder without organ or systems involvement
  - **M05.72** Rheumatoid arthritis with rheumatoid factor of elbow without organ or systems involvement
    - **M05.721** Rheumatoid arthritis with rheumatoid factor of right elbow without organ or systems involvement
    - **M05.722** Rheumatoid arthritis with rheumatoid factor of left elbow without organ or systems involvement
    - **M05.729** Rheumatoid arthritis with rheumatoid factor of unspecified elbow without organ or systems involvement
  - **M05.73** Rheumatoid arthritis with rheumatoid factor of wrist without organ or systems involvement
    - **M05.731** Rheumatoid arthritis with rheumatoid factor of right wrist without organ or systems involvement
    - **M05.732** Rheumatoid arthritis with rheumatoid factor of left wrist without organ or systems involvement
    - **M05.739** Rheumatoid arthritis with rheumatoid factor of unspecified wrist without organ or systems involvement
  - **M05.74** Rheumatoid arthritis with rheumatoid factor of hand without organ or systems involvement
    - **M05.741** Rheumatoid arthritis with rheumatoid factor of right hand without organ or systems involvement
    - **M05.742** Rheumatoid arthritis with rheumatoid factor of left hand without organ or systems involvement
    - **M05.749** Rheumatoid arthritis with rheumatoid factor of unspecified hand without organ or systems involvement
  - **M05.75** Rheumatoid arthritis with rheumatoid factor of hip without organ or systems involvement
    - **M05.751** Rheumatoid arthritis with rheumatoid factor of right hip without organ or systems involvement
    - **M05.752** Rheumatoid arthritis with rheumatoid factor of left hip without organ or systems involvement
    - **M05.759** Rheumatoid arthritis with rheumatoid factor of unspecified hip without organ or systems involvement
  - **M05.76** Rheumatoid arthritis with rheumatoid factor of knee without organ or systems involvement
    - **M05.761** Rheumatoid arthritis with rheumatoid factor of right knee without organ or systems involvement
    - **M05.762** Rheumatoid arthritis with rheumatoid factor of left knee without organ or systems involvement
    - **M05.769** Rheumatoid arthritis with rheumatoid factor of unspecified knee without organ or systems involvement
  - **M05.77** Rheumatoid arthritis with rheumatoid factor of ankle and foot without organ or systems involvement
    - **M05.771** Rheumatoid arthritis with rheumatoid factor of right ankle and foot without organ or systems involvement
    - **M05.772** Rheumatoid arthritis with rheumatoid factor of left ankle and foot without organ or systems involvement
    - **M05.779** Rheumatoid arthritis with rheumatoid factor of unspecified ankle and foot without organ or systems involvement
  - **M05.79** Rheumatoid arthritis with rheumatoid factor of multiple sites without organ or systems involvement
  - **M05.7A** Rheumatoid arthritis with rheumatoid factor of other specified site without organ or systems involvement
- **M05.8** Other rheumatoid arthritis with rheumatoid factor
  - **M05.80** Other rheumatoid arthritis with rheumatoid factor of unspecified site
  - **M05.81** Other rheumatoid arthritis with rheumatoid factor of shoulder
    - **M05.811** Other rheumatoid arthritis with rheumatoid factor of right shoulder
    - **M05.812** Other rheumatoid arthritis with rheumatoid factor of left shoulder
    - **M05.819** Other rheumatoid arthritis with rheumatoid factor of unspecified shoulder
  - **M05.82** Other rheumatoid arthritis with rheumatoid factor of elbow
    - **M05.821** Other rheumatoid arthritis with rheumatoid factor of right elbow
    - **M05.822** Other rheumatoid arthritis with rheumatoid factor of left elbow
    - **M05.829** Other rheumatoid arthritis with rheumatoid factor of unspecified elbow
  - **M05.83** Other rheumatoid arthritis with rheumatoid factor of wrist
    - **M05.831** Other rheumatoid arthritis with rheumatoid factor of right wrist
    - **M05.832** Other rheumatoid arthritis with rheumatoid factor of left wrist
    - **M05.839** Other rheumatoid arthritis with rheumatoid factor of unspecified wrist
  - **M05.84** Other rheumatoid arthritis with rheumatoid factor of hand
    - **M05.841** Other rheumatoid arthritis with rheumatoid factor of right hand
    - **M05.842** Other rheumatoid arthritis with rheumatoid factor of left hand
    - **M05.849** Other rheumatoid arthritis with rheumatoid factor of unspecified hand
  - **M05.85** Other rheumatoid arthritis with rheumatoid factor of hip
    - **M05.851** Other rheumatoid arthritis with rheumatoid factor of right hip
    - **M05.852** Other rheumatoid arthritis with rheumatoid factor of left hip
    - **M05.859** Other rheumatoid arthritis with rheumatoid factor of unspecified hip

- M05.86 Other rheumatoid arthritis with rheumatoid factor of knee
  - M05.861 Other rheumatoid arthritis with rheumatoid factor of right knee
  - M05.862 Other rheumatoid arthritis with rheumatoid factor of left knee
  - M05.869 Other rheumatoid arthritis with rheumatoid factor of unspecified knee
- M05.87 Other rheumatoid arthritis with rheumatoid factor of ankle and foot
  - M05.871 Other rheumatoid arthritis with rheumatoid factor of right ankle and foot
  - M05.872 Other rheumatoid arthritis with rheumatoid factor of left ankle and foot
  - M05.879 Other rheumatoid arthritis with rheumatoid factor of unspecified ankle and foot
- M05.89 Other rheumatoid arthritis with rheumatoid factor of multiple sites
- M05.8A Other rheumatoid arthritis with rheumatoid factor of other specified site
- M05.9 Rheumatoid arthritis with rheumatoid factor, unspecified

M06 Other rheumatoid arthritis
AHA CC: 4Q, 2020, 31-32

- M06.0 Rheumatoid arthritis without rheumatoid factor
  - M06.00 Rheumatoid arthritis without rheumatoid factor, unspecified site
  - M06.01 Rheumatoid arthritis without rheumatoid factor, shoulder
    - M06.011 Rheumatoid arthritis without rheumatoid factor, right shoulder
    - M06.012 Rheumatoid arthritis without rheumatoid factor, left shoulder
    - M06.019 Rheumatoid arthritis without rheumatoid factor, unspecified shoulder
  - M06.02 Rheumatoid arthritis without rheumatoid factor, elbow
    - M06.021 Rheumatoid arthritis without rheumatoid factor, right elbow
    - M06.022 Rheumatoid arthritis without rheumatoid factor, left elbow
    - M06.029 Rheumatoid arthritis without rheumatoid factor, unspecified elbow
  - M06.03 Rheumatoid arthritis without rheumatoid factor, wrist
    - M06.031 Rheumatoid arthritis without rheumatoid factor, right wrist
    - M06.032 Rheumatoid arthritis without rheumatoid factor, left wrist
    - M06.039 Rheumatoid arthritis without rheumatoid factor, unspecified wrist
  - M06.04 Rheumatoid arthritis without rheumatoid factor, hand
    - M06.041 Rheumatoid arthritis without rheumatoid factor, right hand
    - M06.042 Rheumatoid arthritis without rheumatoid factor, left hand
    - M06.049 Rheumatoid arthritis without rheumatoid factor, unspecified hand
  - M06.05 Rheumatoid arthritis without rheumatoid factor, hip
    - M06.051 Rheumatoid arthritis without rheumatoid factor, right hip
    - M06.052 Rheumatoid arthritis without rheumatoid factor, left hip
    - M06.059 Rheumatoid arthritis without rheumatoid factor, unspecified hip
  - M06.06 Rheumatoid arthritis without rheumatoid factor, knee
    - M06.061 Rheumatoid arthritis without rheumatoid factor, right knee
    - M06.062 Rheumatoid arthritis without rheumatoid factor, left knee
    - M06.069 Rheumatoid arthritis without rheumatoid factor, unspecified knee
  - M06.07 Rheumatoid arthritis without rheumatoid factor, ankle and foot
    - M06.071 Rheumatoid arthritis without rheumatoid factor, right ankle and foot
    - M06.072 Rheumatoid arthritis without rheumatoid factor, left ankle and foot
    - M06.079 Rheumatoid arthritis without rheumatoid factor, unspecified ankle and foot
  - M06.08 Rheumatoid arthritis without rheumatoid factor, vertebrae
  - M06.09 Rheumatoid arthritis without rheumatoid factor, multiple sites
  - M06.0A Rheumatoid arthritis without rheumatoid factor, other specified site
- M06.1 Adult-onset Still's disease
  - **Excludes1:** Still's disease NOS (M08.2-)
- M06.2 Rheumatoid bursitis
  - M06.20 Rheumatoid bursitis, unspecified site
  - M06.21 Rheumatoid bursitis, shoulder
    - M06.211 Rheumatoid bursitis, right shoulder
    - M06.212 Rheumatoid bursitis, left shoulder
    - M06.219 Rheumatoid bursitis, unspecified shoulder
  - M06.22 Rheumatoid bursitis, elbow
    - M06.221 Rheumatoid bursitis, right elbow
    - M06.222 Rheumatoid bursitis, left elbow
    - M06.229 Rheumatoid bursitis, unspecified elbow
  - M06.23 Rheumatoid bursitis, wrist
    - M06.231 Rheumatoid bursitis, right wrist
    - M06.232 Rheumatoid bursitis, left wrist
    - M06.239 Rheumatoid bursitis, unspecified wrist
  - M06.24 Rheumatoid bursitis, hand
    - M06.241 Rheumatoid bursitis, right hand
    - M06.242 Rheumatoid bursitis, left hand
    - M06.249 Rheumatoid bursitis, unspecified hand
  - M06.25 Rheumatoid bursitis, hip
    - M06.251 Rheumatoid bursitis, right hip
    - M06.252 Rheumatoid bursitis, left hip
    - M06.259 Rheumatoid bursitis, unspecified hip
  - M06.26 Rheumatoid bursitis, knee
    - M06.261 Rheumatoid bursitis, right knee
    - M06.262 Rheumatoid bursitis, left knee
    - M06.269 Rheumatoid bursitis, unspecified knee
  - M06.27 Rheumatoid bursitis, ankle and foot
    - M06.271 Rheumatoid bursitis, right ankle and foot
    - M06.272 Rheumatoid bursitis, left ankle and foot
    - M06.279 Rheumatoid bursitis, unspecified ankle and foot
  - M06.28 Rheumatoid bursitis, vertebrae
  - M06.29 Rheumatoid bursitis, multiple sites
- M06.3 Rheumatoid nodule
  - M06.30 Rheumatoid nodule, unspecified site
  - M06.31 Rheumatoid nodule, shoulder
    - M06.311 Rheumatoid nodule, right shoulder
    - M06.312 Rheumatoid nodule, left shoulder
    - M06.319 Rheumatoid nodule, unspecified shoulder
  - M06.32 Rheumatoid nodule, elbow
    - M06.321 Rheumatoid nodule, right elbow
    - M06.322 Rheumatoid nodule, left elbow
    - M06.329 Rheumatoid nodule, unspecified elbow
  - M06.33 Rheumatoid nodule, wrist
    - M06.331 Rheumatoid nodule, right wrist
    - M06.332 Rheumatoid nodule, left wrist
    - M06.339 Rheumatoid nodule, unspecified wrist
  - M06.34 Rheumatoid nodule, hand
    - M06.341 Rheumatoid nodule, right hand
    - M06.342 Rheumatoid nodule, left hand
    - M06.349 Rheumatoid nodule, unspecified hand
  - M06.35 Rheumatoid nodule, hip
    - M06.351 Rheumatoid nodule, right hip
    - M06.352 Rheumatoid nodule, left hip
    - M06.359 Rheumatoid nodule, unspecified hip
  - M06.36 Rheumatoid nodule, knee
    - M06.361 Rheumatoid nodule, right knee
    - M06.362 Rheumatoid nodule, left knee
    - M06.369 Rheumatoid nodule, unspecified knee
  - M06.37 Rheumatoid nodule, ankle and foot
    - M06.371 Rheumatoid nodule, right ankle and foot
    - M06.372 Rheumatoid nodule, left ankle and foot
    - M06.379 Rheumatoid nodule, unspecified ankle and foot

M06.38 Rheumatoid nodule, vertebrae
M06.39 Rheumatoid nodule, multiple sites
M06.4 Inflammatory polyarthropathy
   Excludes1: polyarthritis NOS (M13.0)
+ **M06.8** Other specified rheumatoid arthritis
   M06.80 Other specified rheumatoid arthritis, unspecified site
   + **M06.81** Other specified rheumatoid arthritis, shoulder
      M06.811 Other specified rheumatoid arthritis, right shoulder
      M06.812 Other specified rheumatoid arthritis, left shoulder
      M06.819 Other specified rheumatoid arthritis, unspecified shoulder
   + **M06.82** Other specified rheumatoid arthritis, elbow
      M06.821 Other specified rheumatoid arthritis, right elbow
      M06.822 Other specified rheumatoid arthritis, left elbow
      M06.829 Other specified rheumatoid arthritis, unspecified elbow
   + **M06.83** Other specified rheumatoid arthritis, wrist
      M06.831 Other specified rheumatoid arthritis, right wrist
      M06.832 Other specified rheumatoid arthritis, left wrist
      M06.839 Other specified rheumatoid arthritis, unspecified wrist
   + **M06.84** Other specified rheumatoid arthritis, hand
      M06.841 Other specified rheumatoid arthritis, right hand
      M06.842 Other specified rheumatoid arthritis, left hand
      M06.849 Other specified rheumatoid arthritis, unspecified hand
   + **M06.85** Other specified rheumatoid arthritis, hip
      M06.851 Other specified rheumatoid arthritis, right hip
      M06.852 Other specified rheumatoid arthritis, left hip
      M06.859 Other specified rheumatoid arthritis, unspecified hip
   + **M06.86** Other specified rheumatoid arthritis, knee
      M06.861 Other specified rheumatoid arthritis, right knee
      M06.862 Other specified rheumatoid arthritis, left knee
      M06.869 Other specified rheumatoid arthritis, unspecified knee
   + **M06.87** Other specified rheumatoid arthritis, ankle and foot
      M06.871 Other specified rheumatoid arthritis, right ankle and foot
      M06.872 Other specified rheumatoid arthritis, left ankle and foot
      M06.879 Other specified rheumatoid arthritis, unspecified ankle and foot
   M06.88 Other specified rheumatoid arthritis, vertebrae
   M06.89 Other specified rheumatoid arthritis, multiple sites
   M06.8A Other specified rheumatoid arthritis, other specified site
M06.9 Rheumatoid arthritis, unspecified

M07 Enteropathic arthropathies
   Code also associated enteropathy, such as:
      regional enteritis [Crohn's disease] (K50.-)
      ulcerative colitis (K51.-)
   Excludes1: psoriatic arthropathies (L40.5-)
+ **M07.6** Enteropathic arthropathies
   M07.60 Enteropathic arthropathies, unspecified site
   + **M07.61** Enteropathic arthropathies, shoulder
      M07.611 Enteropathic arthropathies, right shoulder
      M07.612 Enteropathic arthropathies, left shoulder
      M07.619 Enteropathic arthropathies, unspecified shoulder
   + **M07.62** Enteropathic arthropathies, elbow
      M07.621 Enteropathic arthropathies, right elbow
      M07.622 Enteropathic arthropathies, left elbow
      M07.629 Enteropathic arthropathies, unspecified elbow
   + **M07.63** Enteropathic arthropathies, wrist
      M07.631 Enteropathic arthropathies, right wrist
      M07.632 Enteropathic arthropathies, left wrist
      M07.639 Enteropathic arthropathies, unspecified wrist
   + **M07.64** Enteropathic arthropathies, hand
      M07.641 Enteropathic arthropathies, right hand
      M07.642 Enteropathic arthropathies, left hand
      M07.649 Enteropathic arthropathies, unspecified hand
   + **M07.65** Enteropathic arthropathies, hip
      M07.651 Enteropathic arthropathies, right hip
      M07.652 Enteropathic arthropathies, left hip
      M07.659 Enteropathic arthropathies, unspecified hip
   + **M07.66** Enteropathic arthropathies, knee
      M07.661 Enteropathic arthropathies, right knee
      M07.662 Enteropathic arthropathies, left knee
      M07.669 Enteropathic arthropathies, unspecified knee
   + **M07.67** Enteropathic arthropathies, ankle and foot
      M07.671 Enteropathic arthropathies, right ankle and foot
      M07.672 Enteropathic arthropathies, left ankle and foot
      M07.679 Enteropathic arthropathies, unspecified ankle and foot
   M07.68 Enteropathic arthropathies, vertebrae
   M07.69 Enteropathic arthropathies, multiple sites

M08 Juvenile arthritis
   Code also any associated underlying condition, such as:
      regional enteritis [Crohn's disease] (K50.-)
      ulcerative colitis (K51.-)
   Excludes1: arthropathy in Whipple's disease (M14.8)
      Felty's syndrome (M05.0)
      juvenile dermatomyositis (M33.0-)
      psoriatic juvenile arthropathy (L40.54)
   AHA CC: 4Q, 2020, 31-32
+ **M08.0** Unspecified juvenile rheumatoid arthritis
   Juvenile rheumatoid arthritis with or without rheumatoid factor
   M08.00 Unspecified juvenile rheumatoid arthritis of unspecified site
   + **M08.01** Unspecified juvenile rheumatoid arthritis, shoulder
      M08.011 Unspecified juvenile rheumatoid arthritis, right shoulder
      M08.012 Unspecified juvenile rheumatoid arthritis, left shoulder
      M08.019 Unspecified juvenile rheumatoid arthritis, unspecified shoulder
   + **M08.02** Unspecified juvenile rheumatoid arthritis of elbow
      M08.021 Unspecified juvenile rheumatoid arthritis, right elbow
      M08.022 Unspecified juvenile rheumatoid arthritis, left elbow
      M08.029 Unspecified juvenile rheumatoid arthritis, unspecified elbow
   + **M08.03** Unspecified juvenile rheumatoid arthritis, wrist
      M08.031 Unspecified juvenile rheumatoid arthritis, right wrist
      M08.032 Unspecified juvenile rheumatoid arthritis, left wrist
      M08.039 Unspecified juvenile rheumatoid arthritis, unspecified wrist
   + **M08.04** Unspecified juvenile rheumatoid arthritis, hand
      M08.041 Unspecified juvenile rheumatoid arthritis, right hand
      M08.042 Unspecified juvenile rheumatoid arthritis, left hand
      M08.049 Unspecified juvenile rheumatoid arthritis, unspecified hand
   + **M08.05** Unspecified juvenile rheumatoid arthritis, hip
      M08.051 Unspecified juvenile rheumatoid arthritis, right hip

- **M08.052** Unspecified juvenile rheumatoid arthritis, left hip
- **M08.059** Unspecified juvenile rheumatoid arthritis, unspecified hip
- \+ **M08.06** Unspecified juvenile rheumatoid arthritis, knee
  - **M08.061** Unspecified juvenile rheumatoid arthritis, right knee
  - **M08.062** Unspecified juvenile rheumatoid arthritis, left knee
  - **M08.069** Unspecified juvenile rheumatoid arthritis, unspecified knee
- \+ **M08.07** Unspecified juvenile rheumatoid arthritis, ankle and foot
  - **M08.071** Unspecified juvenile rheumatoid arthritis, right ankle and foot
  - **M08.072** Unspecified juvenile rheumatoid arthritis, left ankle and foot
  - **M08.079** Unspecified juvenile rheumatoid arthritis, unspecified ankle and foot
- **M08.08** Unspecified juvenile rheumatoid arthritis, vertebrae
- **M08.09** Unspecified juvenile rheumatoid arthritis, multiple sites
- **M08.0A** Unspecified juvenile rheumatoid arthritis, other specified site
- **M08.1** Juvenile ankylosing spondylitis
  - *Excludes1:* ankylosing spondylitis in adults (M45.0-)
- \+ **M08.2** Juvenile rheumatoid arthritis with systemic onset
  - Still's disease NOS
  - *Excludes1:* adult-onset Still's disease (M06.1-)
  - **M08.20** Juvenile rheumatoid arthritis with systemic onset, unspecified site
  - \+ **M08.21** Juvenile rheumatoid arthritis with systemic onset, shoulder
    - **M08.211** Juvenile rheumatoid arthritis with systemic onset, right shoulder
    - **M08.212** Juvenile rheumatoid arthritis with systemic onset, left shoulder
    - **M08.219** Juvenile rheumatoid arthritis with systemic onset, unspecified shoulder
  - \+ **M08.22** Juvenile rheumatoid arthritis with systemic onset, elbow
    - **M08.221** Juvenile rheumatoid arthritis with systemic onset, right elbow
    - **M08.222** Juvenile rheumatoid arthritis with systemic onset, left elbow
    - **M08.229** Juvenile rheumatoid arthritis with systemic onset, unspecified elbow
  - \+ **M08.23** Juvenile rheumatoid arthritis with systemic onset, wrist
    - **M08.231** Juvenile rheumatoid arthritis with systemic onset, right wrist
    - **M08.232** Juvenile rheumatoid arthritis with systemic onset, left wrist
    - **M08.239** Juvenile rheumatoid arthritis with systemic onset, unspecified wrist
  - \+ **M08.24** Juvenile rheumatoid arthritis with systemic onset, hand
    - **M08.241** Juvenile rheumatoid arthritis with systemic onset, right hand
    - **M08.242** Juvenile rheumatoid arthritis with systemic onset, left hand
    - **M08.249** Juvenile rheumatoid arthritis with systemic onset, unspecified hand
  - \+ **M08.25** Juvenile rheumatoid arthritis with systemic onset, hip
    - **M08.251** Juvenile rheumatoid arthritis with systemic onset, right hip
    - **M08.252** Juvenile rheumatoid arthritis with systemic onset, left hip
    - **M08.259** Juvenile rheumatoid arthritis with systemic onset, unspecified hip
  - \+ **M08.26** Juvenile rheumatoid arthritis with systemic onset, knee
    - **M08.261** Juvenile rheumatoid arthritis with systemic onset, right knee
    - **M08.262** Juvenile rheumatoid arthritis with systemic onset, left knee
    - **M08.269** Juvenile rheumatoid arthritis with systemic onset, unspecified knee
  - \+ **M08.27** Juvenile rheumatoid arthritis with systemic onset, ankle and foot
    - **M08.271** Juvenile rheumatoid arthritis with systemic onset, right ankle and foot
    - **M08.272** Juvenile rheumatoid arthritis with systemic onset, left ankle and foot
    - **M08.279** Juvenile rheumatoid arthritis with systemic onset, unspecified ankle and foot
  - **M08.28** Juvenile rheumatoid arthritis with systemic onset, vertebrae
  - **M08.29** Juvenile rheumatoid arthritis with systemic onset, multiple sites
  - **M08.2A** Juvenile rheumatoid arthritis with systemic onset, other specified site
- **M08.3** Juvenile rheumatoid polyarthritis (seronegative)
- \+ **M08.4** Pauciarticular juvenile rheumatoid arthritis
  - **M08.40** Pauciarticular juvenile rheumatoid arthritis, unspecified site
  - \+ **M08.41** Pauciarticular juvenile rheumatoid arthritis, shoulder
    - **M08.411** Pauciarticular juvenile rheumatoid arthritis, right shoulder
    - **M08.412** Pauciarticular juvenile rheumatoid arthritis, left shoulder
    - **M08.419** Pauciarticular juvenile rheumatoid arthritis, unspecified shoulder
  - \+ **M08.42** Pauciarticular juvenile rheumatoid arthritis, elbow
    - **M08.421** Pauciarticular juvenile rheumatoid arthritis, right elbow
    - **M08.422** Pauciarticular juvenile rheumatoid arthritis, left elbow
    - **M08.429** Pauciarticular juvenile rheumatoid arthritis, unspecified elbow
  - \+ **M08.43** Pauciarticular juvenile rheumatoid arthritis, wrist
    - **M08.431** Pauciarticular juvenile rheumatoid arthritis, right wrist
    - **M08.432** Pauciarticular juvenile rheumatoid arthritis, left wrist
    - **M08.439** Pauciarticular juvenile rheumatoid arthritis, unspecified wrist
  - \+ **M08.44** Pauciarticular juvenile rheumatoid arthritis, hand
    - **M08.441** Pauciarticular juvenile rheumatoid arthritis, right hand
    - **M08.442** Pauciarticular juvenile rheumatoid arthritis, left hand
    - **M08.449** Pauciarticular juvenile rheumatoid arthritis, unspecified hand
  - \+ **M08.45** Pauciarticular juvenile rheumatoid arthritis, hip
    - **M08.451** Pauciarticular juvenile rheumatoid arthritis, right hip
    - **M08.452** Pauciarticular juvenile rheumatoid arthritis, left hip
    - **M08.459** Pauciarticular juvenile rheumatoid arthritis, unspecified hip
  - \+ **M08.46** Pauciarticular juvenile rheumatoid arthritis, knee
    - **M08.461** Pauciarticular juvenile rheumatoid arthritis, right knee
    - **M08.462** Pauciarticular juvenile rheumatoid arthritis, left knee
    - **M08.469** Pauciarticular juvenile rheumatoid arthritis, unspecified knee
  - \+ **M08.47** Pauciarticular juvenile rheumatoid arthritis, ankle and foot
    - **M08.471** Pauciarticular juvenile rheumatoid arthritis, right ankle and foot
    - **M08.472** Pauciarticular juvenile rheumatoid arthritis, left ankle and foot
    - **M08.479** Pauciarticular juvenile rheumatoid arthritis, unspecified ankle and foot
  - **M08.48** Pauciarticular juvenile rheumatoid arthritis, vertebrae
  - **M08.4A** Pauciarticular juvenile rheumatoid arthritis, other specified site

- **M08.8 Other juvenile arthritis**
  - M08.80 Other juvenile arthritis, unspecified site
  - **M08.81 Other juvenile arthritis, shoulder**
    - M08.811 Other juvenile arthritis, right shoulder
    - M08.812 Other juvenile arthritis, left shoulder
    - M08.819 Other juvenile arthritis, unspecified shoulder
  - **M08.82 Other juvenile arthritis, elbow**
    - M08.821 Other juvenile arthritis, right elbow
    - M08.822 Other juvenile arthritis, left elbow
    - M08.829 Other juvenile arthritis, unspecified elbow
  - **M08.83 Other juvenile arthritis, wrist**
    - M08.831 Other juvenile arthritis, right wrist
    - M08.832 Other juvenile arthritis, left wrist
    - M08.839 Other juvenile arthritis, unspecified wrist
  - **M08.84 Other juvenile arthritis, hand**
    - M08.841 Other juvenile arthritis, right hand
    - M08.842 Other juvenile arthritis, left hand
    - M08.849 Other juvenile arthritis, unspecified hand
  - **M08.85 Other juvenile arthritis, hip**
    - M08.851 Other juvenile arthritis, right hip
    - M08.852 Other juvenile arthritis, left hip
    - M08.859 Other juvenile arthritis, unspecified hip
  - **M08.86 Other juvenile arthritis, knee**
    - M08.861 Other juvenile arthritis, right knee
    - M08.862 Other juvenile arthritis, left knee
    - M08.869 Other juvenile arthritis, unspecified knee
  - **M08.87 Other juvenile arthritis, ankle and foot**
    - M08.871 Other juvenile arthritis, right ankle and foot
    - M08.872 Other juvenile arthritis, left ankle and foot
    - M08.879 Other juvenile arthritis, unspecified ankle and foot
  - M08.88 Other juvenile arthritis, other specified site
    Other juvenile arthritis, vertebrae
  - M08.89 Other juvenile arthritis, multiple sites
- **M08.9 Juvenile arthritis, unspecified**
  - *Excludes1:* juvenile rheumatoid arthritis, unspecified (M08.0-)
  - M08.90 Juvenile arthritis, unspecified, unspecified site
  - **M08.91 Juvenile arthritis, unspecified, shoulder**
    - M08.911 Juvenile arthritis, unspecified, right shoulder
    - M08.912 Juvenile arthritis, unspecified, left shoulder
    - M08.919 Juvenile arthritis, unspecified, unspecified shoulder
  - **M08.92 Juvenile arthritis, unspecified, elbow**
    - M08.921 Juvenile arthritis, unspecified, right elbow
    - M08.922 Juvenile arthritis, unspecified, left elbow
    - M08.929 Juvenile arthritis, unspecified, unspecified elbow
  - **M08.93 Juvenile arthritis, unspecified, wrist**
    - M08.931 Juvenile arthritis, unspecified, right wrist
    - M08.932 Juvenile arthritis, unspecified, left wrist
    - M08.939 Juvenile arthritis, unspecified, unspecified wrist
  - **M08.94 Juvenile arthritis, unspecified, hand**
    - M08.941 Juvenile arthritis, unspecified, right hand
    - M08.942 Juvenile arthritis, unspecified, left hand
    - M08.949 Juvenile arthritis, unspecified, unspecified hand
  - **M08.95 Juvenile arthritis, unspecified, hip**
    - M08.951 Juvenile arthritis, unspecified, right hip
    - M08.952 Juvenile arthritis, unspecified, left hip
    - M08.959 Juvenile arthritis, unspecified, unspecified hip
  - **M08.96 Juvenile arthritis, unspecified, knee**
    - M08.961 Juvenile arthritis, unspecified, right knee
    - M08.962 Juvenile arthritis, unspecified, left knee
    - M08.969 Juvenile arthritis, unspecified, unspecified knee
  - **M08.97 Juvenile arthritis, unspecified, ankle and foot**
    - M08.971 Juvenile arthritis, unspecified, right ankle and foot
    - M08.972 Juvenile arthritis, unspecified, left ankle and foot
    - M08.979 Juvenile arthritis, unspecified, unspecified ankle and foot
  - M08.98 Juvenile arthritis, unspecified, vertebrae
  - M08.99 Juvenile arthritis, unspecified, multiple sites
  - M08.9A Juvenile arthritis, unspecified, other specified site

M1A Chronic gout

Use additional code to identify:
Autonomic neuropathy in diseases classified elsewhere (G99.0)
Calculus of urinary tract in diseases classified elsewhere (N22)
Cardiomyopathy in diseases classified elsewhere (I43)
Disorders of external ear in diseases classified elsewhere (H61.1-, H62.8-)
Disorders of iris and ciliary body in diseases classified elsewhere (H22)
Glomerular disorders in diseases classified elsewhere (N08)

Excludes1: gout NOS (M10.-)
Excludes2: acute gout (M10.-)

The appropriate 7th character is to be added to each code from category M1A
0   without tophus (tophi)
1   with tophus (tophi)

- **M1A.0 Idiopathic chronic gout**
  Chronic gouty bursitis
  Primary chronic gout
  - X+7th M1A.00 Idiopathic chronic gout, unspecified site
  - **M1A.01 Idiopathic chronic gout, shoulder**
    - +7th M1A.011 Idiopathic chronic gout, right shoulder
    - +7th M1A.012 Idiopathic chronic gout, left shoulder
    - +7th M1A.019 Idiopathic chronic gout, unspecified shoulder
  - **M1A.02 Idiopathic chronic gout, elbow**
    - +7th M1A.021 Idiopathic chronic gout, right elbow
    - +7th M1A.022 Idiopathic chronic gout, left elbow
    - +7th M1A.029 Idiopathic chronic gout, unspecified elbow
  - **M1A.03 Idiopathic chronic gout, wrist**
    - +7th M1A.031 Idiopathic chronic gout, right wrist
    - +7th M1A.032 Idiopathic chronic gout, left wrist
    - +7th M1A.039 Idiopathic chronic gout, unspecified wrist
  - **M1A.04 Idiopathic chronic gout, hand**
    - +7th M1A.041 Idiopathic chronic gout, right hand
    - +7th M1A.042 Idiopathic chronic gout, left hand
    - +7th M1A.049 Idiopathic chronic gout, unspecified hand
  - **M1A.05 Idiopathic chronic gout, hip**
    - +7th M1A.051 Idiopathic chronic gout, right hip
    - +7th M1A.052 Idiopathic chronic gout, left hip
    - +7th M1A.059 Idiopathic chronic gout, unspecified hip
  - **M1A.06 Idiopathic chronic gout, knee**
    - +7th M1A.061 Idiopathic chronic gout, right knee
    - +7th M1A.062 Idiopathic chronic gout, left knee
    - +7th M1A.069 Idiopathic chronic gout, unspecified knee
  - **M1A.07 Idiopathic chronic gout, ankle and foot**
    - +7th M1A.071 Idiopathic chronic gout, right ankle and foot
    - +7th M1A.072 Idiopathic chronic gout, left ankle and foot
    - +7th M1A.079 Idiopathic chronic gout, unspecified ankle and foot
  - X+7th M1A.08 Idiopathic chronic gout, vertebrae
  - M1A.09 Idiopathic chronic gout, multiple sites
- **M1A.1 Lead-induced chronic gout**
  Code first toxic effects of lead and its compounds (T56.0-)
  - X+7th M1A.10 Lead-induced chronic gout, unspecified site
  - **M1A.11 Lead-induced chronic gout, shoulder**
    - +7th M1A.111 Lead-induced chronic gout, right shoulder
    - +7th M1A.112 Lead-induced chronic gout, left shoulder
    - +7th M1A.119 Lead-induced chronic gout, unspecified shoulder

- **+ M1A.12 Lead-induced chronic gout, elbow**
  - +7th M1A.121 Lead-induced chronic gout, right elbow
  - +7th M1A.122 Lead-induced chronic gout, left elbow
  - +7th M1A.129 Lead-induced chronic gout, unspecified elbow
- **+ M1A.13 Lead-induced chronic gout, wrist**
  - +7th M1A.131 Lead-induced chronic gout, right wrist
  - +7th M1A.132 Lead-induced chronic gout, left wrist
  - +7th M1A.139 Lead-induced chronic gout, unspecified wrist
- **+ M1A.14 Lead-induced chronic gout, hand**
  - +7th M1A.141 Lead-induced chronic gout, right hand
  - +7th M1A.142 Lead-induced chronic gout, left hand
  - +7th M1A.149 Lead-induced chronic gout, unspecified hand
- **+ M1A.15 Lead-induced chronic gout, hip**
  - +7th M1A.151 Lead-induced chronic gout, right hip
  - +7th M1A.152 Lead-induced chronic gout, left hip
  - +7th M1A.159 Lead-induced chronic gout, unspecified hip
- **+ M1A.16 Lead-induced chronic gout, knee**
  - +7th M1A.161 Lead-induced chronic gout, right knee
  - +7th M1A.162 Lead-induced chronic gout, left knee
  - +7th M1A.169 Lead-induced chronic gout, unspecified knee
- **+ M1A.17 Lead-induced chronic gout, ankle and foot**
  - +7th M1A.171 Lead-induced chronic gout, right ankle and foot
  - +7th M1A.172 Lead-induced chronic gout, left ankle and foot
  - +7th M1A.179 Lead-induced chronic gout, unspecified ankle and foot
- X+7th **M1A.18 Lead-induced chronic gout, vertebrae**
- X+7th **M1A.19 Lead-induced chronic gout, multiple sites**
- **+ M1A.2 Drug-induced chronic gout**
  - Use additional code for adverse effect, if applicable, to identify drug (T36-T50 with fifth or sixth character 5)
- X+7th **M1A.20 Drug-induced chronic gout, unspecified site**
- **+ M1A.21 Drug-induced chronic gout, shoulder**
  - +7th M1A.211 Drug-induced chronic gout, right shoulder
  - +7th M1A.212 Drug-induced chronic gout, left shoulder
  - +7th M1A.219 Drug-induced chronic gout, unspecified shoulder
- **+ M1A.22 Drug-induced chronic gout, elbow**
  - +7th M1A.221 Drug-induced chronic gout, right elbow
  - +7th M1A.222 Drug-induced chronic gout, left elbow
  - +7th M1A.229 Drug-induced chronic gout, unspecified elbow
- **+ M1A.23 Drug-induced chronic gout, wrist**
  - +7th M1A.231 Drug-induced chronic gout, right wrist
  - +7th M1A.232 Drug-induced chronic gout, left wrist
  - +7th M1A.239 Drug-induced chronic gout, unspecified wrist
- **+ M1A.24 Drug-induced chronic gout, hand**
  - +7th M1A.241 Drug-induced chronic gout, right hand
  - +7th M1A.242 Drug-induced chronic gout, left hand
  - +7th M1A.249 Drug-induced chronic gout, unspecified hand
- **+ M1A.25 Drug-induced chronic gout, hip**
  - +7th M1A.251 Drug-induced chronic gout, right hip
  - +7th M1A.252 Drug-induced chronic gout, left hip
  - +7th M1A.259 Drug-induced chronic gout, unspecified hip
- **+ M1A.26 Drug-induced chronic gout, knee**
  - +7th M1A.261 Drug-induced chronic gout, right knee
  - +7th M1A.262 Drug-induced chronic gout, left knee
  - +7th M1A.269 Drug-induced chronic gout, unspecified knee
- **+ M1A.27 Drug-induced chronic gout, ankle and foot**
  - +7th M1A.271 Drug-induced chronic gout, right ankle and foot
  - +7th M1A.272 Drug-induced chronic gout, left ankle and foot
  - +7th M1A.279 Drug-induced chronic gout, unspecified ankle and foot
- X+7th **M1A.28 Drug-induced chronic gout, vertebrae**
- X+7th **M1A.29 Drug-induced chronic gout, multiple sites**

- **+ M1A.3 Chronic gout due to renal impairment**
  - Code first associated renal disease
- X+7th **M1A.30 Chronic gout due to renal impairment, unspecified site**
- **+ M1A.31 Chronic gout due to renal impairment, shoulder**
  - +7th M1A.311 Chronic gout due to renal impairment, right shoulder
  - +7th M1A.312 Chronic gout due to renal impairment, left shoulder
  - +7th M1A.319 Chronic gout due to renal impairment, unspecified shoulder
- **+ M1A.32 Chronic gout due to renal impairment, elbow**
  - +7th M1A.321 Chronic gout due to renal impairment, right elbow
  - +7th M1A.322 Chronic gout due to renal impairment, left elbow
  - +7th M1A.329 Chronic gout due to renal impairment, unspecified elbow
- **+ M1A.33 Chronic gout due to renal impairment, wrist**
  - +7th M1A.331 Chronic gout due to renal impairment, right wrist
  - +7th M1A.332 Chronic gout due to renal impairment, left wrist
  - +7th M1A.339 Chronic gout due to renal impairment, unspecified wrist
- **+ M1A.34 Chronic gout due to renal impairment, hand**
  - +7th M1A.341 Chronic gout due to renal impairment, right hand
  - +7th M1A.342 Chronic gout due to renal impairment, left hand
  - +7th M1A.349 Chronic gout due to renal impairment, unspecified hand
- **+ M1A.35 Chronic gout due to renal impairment, hip**
  - +7th M1A.351 Chronic gout due to renal impairment, right hip
  - +7th M1A.352 Chronic gout due to renal impairment, left hip
  - +7th M1A.359 Chronic gout due to renal impairment, unspecified hip
- **+ M1A.36 Chronic gout due to renal impairment, knee**
  - +7th M1A.361 Chronic gout due to renal impairment, right knee
  - +7th M1A.362 Chronic gout due to renal impairment, left knee
  - +7th M1A.369 Chronic gout due to renal impairment, unspecified knee
- **+ M1A.37 Chronic gout due to renal impairment, ankle and foot**
  - +7th M1A.371 Chronic gout due to renal impairment, right ankle and foot
  - +7th M1A.372 Chronic gout due to renal impairment, left ankle and foot
  - +7th M1A.379 Chronic gout due to renal impairment, unspecified ankle and foot
- X+7th **M1A.38 Chronic gout due to renal impairment, vertebrae**
- X+7th **M1A.39 Chronic gout due to renal impairment, multiple sites**
- **+ M1A.4 Other secondary chronic gout**
  - Code first associated condition
- X+7th **M1A.40 Other secondary chronic gout, unspecified site**
- **+ M1A.41 Other secondary chronic gout, shoulder**
  - +7th M1A.411 Other secondary chronic gout, right shoulder
  - +7th M1A.412 Other secondary chronic gout, left shoulder
  - +7th M1A.419 Other secondary chronic gout, unspecified shoulder
- **+ M1A.42 Other secondary chronic gout, elbow**
  - +7th M1A.421 Other secondary chronic gout, right elbow
  - +7th M1A.422 Other secondary chronic gout, left elbow
  - +7th M1A.429 Other secondary chronic gout, unspecified elbow

- **+ M1A.43 Other secondary chronic gout, wrist**
  - +7th M1A.431 Other secondary chronic gout, right wrist
  - +7th M1A.432 Other secondary chronic gout, left wrist
  - +7th M1A.439 Other secondary chronic gout, unspecified wrist
- **+ M1A.44 Other secondary chronic gout, hand**
  - +7th M1A.441 Other secondary chronic gout, right hand
  - +7th M1A.442 Other secondary chronic gout, left hand
  - +7th M1A.449 Other secondary chronic gout, unspecified hand
- **+ M1A.45 Other secondary chronic gout, hip**
  - +7th M1A.451 Other secondary chronic gout, right hip
  - +7th M1A.452 Other secondary chronic gout, left hip
  - +7th M1A.459 Other secondary chronic gout, unspecified hip
- **+ M1A.46 Other secondary chronic gout, knee**
  - +7th M1A.461 Other secondary chronic gout, right knee
  - +7th M1A.462 Other secondary chronic gout, left knee
  - +7th M1A.469 Other secondary chronic gout, unspecified knee
- **+ M1A.47 Other secondary chronic gout, ankle and foot**
  - +7th M1A.471 Other secondary chronic gout, right ankle and foot
  - +7th M1A.472 Other secondary chronic gout, left ankle and foot
  - +7th M1A.479 Other secondary chronic gout, unspecified ankle and foot
- X+7th M1A.48 Other secondary chronic gout, vertebrae
- X+7th M1A.49 Other secondary chronic gout, multiple sites
- X+7th **M1A.9 Chronic gout, unspecified**

M10 Gout

Acute gout
Gout attack
Gout flare
Podagra

Use additional code to identify:
  Autonomic neuropathy in diseases classified elsewhere (G99.0)
  Calculus of urinary tract in diseases classified elsewhere (N22)
  Cardiomyopathy in diseases classified elsewhere (I43)
  Disorders of external ear in diseases classified elsewhere (H61.1-, H62.8-)
  Disorders of iris and ciliary body in diseases classified elsewhere (H22)
  Glomerular disorders in diseases classified elsewhere (N08)

Excludes2: chronic gout (M1A.-)

- **+ M10.0 Idiopathic gout**
  Gouty bursitis
  Primary gout
  - M10.00 Idiopathic gout, unspecified site
  - + M10.01 Idiopathic gout, shoulder
    - M10.011 Idiopathic gout, right shoulder
    - M10.012 Idiopathic gout, left shoulder
    - M10.019 Idiopathic gout, unspecified shoulder
  - + M10.02 Idiopathic gout, elbow
    - M10.021 Idiopathic gout, right elbow
    - M10.022 Idiopathic gout, left elbow
    - M10.029 Idiopathic gout, unspecified elbow
  - + M10.03 Idiopathic gout, wrist
    - M10.031 Idiopathic gout, right wrist
    - M10.032 Idiopathic gout, left wrist
    - M10.039 Idiopathic gout, unspecified wrist
  - + M10.04 Idiopathic gout, hand
    - M10.041 Idiopathic gout, right hand
    - M10.042 Idiopathic gout, left hand
    - M10.049 Idiopathic gout, unspecified hand
  - + M10.05 Idiopathic gout, hip
    - M10.051 Idiopathic gout, right hip
    - M10.052 Idiopathic gout, left hip
    - M10.059 Idiopathic gout, unspecified hip
  - + M10.06 Idiopathic gout, knee
    - M10.061 Idiopathic gout, right knee
    - M10.062 Idiopathic gout, left knee
    - M10.069 Idiopathic gout, unspecified knee
  - + M10.07 Idiopathic gout, ankle and foot
    - M10.071 Idiopathic gout, right ankle and foot
    - M10.072 Idiopathic gout, left ankle and foot
    - M10.079 Idiopathic gout, unspecified ankle and foot
  - M10.08 Idiopathic gout, vertebrae
  - M10.09 Idiopathic gout, multiple sites
- **+ M10.1 Lead-induced gout**
  Code first toxic effects of lead and its compounds (T56.0-)
  - M10.10 Lead-induced gout, unspecified site
  - + M10.11 Lead-induced gout, shoulder
    - M10.111 Lead-induced gout, right shoulder
    - M10.112 Lead-induced gout, left shoulder
    - M10.119 Lead-induced gout, unspecified shoulder
  - + M10.12 Lead-induced gout, elbow
    - M10.121 Lead-induced gout, right elbow
    - M10.122 Lead-induced gout, left elbow
    - M10.129 Lead-induced gout, unspecified elbow
  - + M10.13 Lead-induced gout, wrist
    - M10.131 Lead-induced gout, right wrist
    - M10.132 Lead-induced gout, left wrist
    - M10.139 Lead-induced gout, unspecified wrist
  - + M10.14 Lead-induced gout, hand
    - M10.141 Lead-induced gout, right hand
    - M10.142 Lead-induced gout, left hand
    - M10.149 Lead-induced gout, unspecified hand
  - + M10.15 Lead-induced gout, hip
    - M10.151 Lead-induced gout, right hip
    - M10.152 Lead-induced gout, left hip
    - M10.159 Lead-induced gout, unspecified hip
  - + M10.16 Lead-induced gout, knee
    - M10.161 Lead-induced gout, right knee
    - M10.162 Lead-induced gout, left knee
    - M10.169 Lead-induced gout, unspecified knee
  - + M10.17 Lead-induced gout, ankle and foot
    - M10.171 Lead-induced gout, right ankle and foot
    - M10.172 Lead-induced gout, left ankle and foot
    - M10.179 Lead-induced gout, unspecified ankle and foot
  - M10.18 Lead-induced gout, vertebrae
  - M10.19 Lead-induced gout, multiple sites
- **+ M10.2 Drug-induced gout**
  Use additional code for adverse effect, if applicable, to identify drug (T36-T50 with fifth or sixth character 5)
  - M10.20 Drug-induced gout, unspecified site
  - + M10.21 Drug-induced gout, shoulder
    - M10.211 Drug-induced gout, right shoulder
    - M10.212 Drug-induced gout, left shoulder
    - M10.219 Drug-induced gout, unspecified shoulder
  - + M10.22 Drug-induced gout, elbow
    - M10.221 Drug-induced gout, right elbow
    - M10.222 Drug-induced gout, left elbow
    - M10.229 Drug-induced gout, unspecified elbow
  - + M10.23 Drug-induced gout, wrist
    - M10.231 Drug-induced gout, right wrist
    - M10.232 Drug-induced gout, left wrist
    - M10.239 Drug-induced gout, unspecified wrist
  - + M10.24 Drug-induced gout, hand
    - M10.241 Drug-induced gout, right hand
    - M10.242 Drug-induced gout, left hand
    - M10.249 Drug-induced gout, unspecified hand
  - + M10.25 Drug-induced gout, hip
    - M10.251 Drug-induced gout, right hip
    - M10.252 Drug-induced gout, left hip
    - M10.259 Drug-induced gout, unspecified hip
  - + M10.26 Drug-induced gout, knee
    - M10.261 Drug-induced gout, right knee
    - M10.262 Drug-induced gout, left knee
    - M10.269 Drug-induced gout, unspecified knee
  - + M10.27 Drug-induced gout, ankle and foot
    - M10.271 Drug-induced gout, right ankle and foot
    - M10.272 Drug-induced gout, left ankle and foot
    - M10.279 Drug-induced gout, unspecified ankle and foot
  - M10.28 Drug-induced gout, vertebrae
  - M10.29 Drug-induced gout, multiple sites

+ **M10.3 Gout due to renal impairment**
Code first associated renal disease
M10.30 Gout due to renal impairment, unspecified site
+ M10.31 Gout due to renal impairment, shoulder
M10.311 Gout due to renal impairment, right shoulder
M10.312 Gout due to renal impairment, left shoulder
M10.319 Gout due to renal impairment, unspecified shoulder
+ M10.32 Gout due to renal impairment, elbow
M10.321 Gout due to renal impairment, right elbow
M10.322 Gout due to renal impairment, left elbow
M10.329 Gout due to renal impairment, unspecified elbow
+ M10.33 Gout due to renal impairment, wrist
M10.331 Gout due to renal impairment, right wrist
M10.332 Gout due to renal impairment, left wrist
M10.339 Gout due to renal impairment, unspecified wrist
+ M10.34 Gout due to renal impairment, hand
M10.341 Gout due to renal impairment, right hand
M10.342 Gout due to renal impairment, left hand
M10.349 Gout due to renal impairment, unspecified hand
+ M10.35 Gout due to renal impairment, hip
M10.351 Gout due to renal impairment, right hip
M10.352 Gout due to renal impairment, left hip
M10.359 Gout due to renal impairment, unspecified hip
+ M10.36 Gout due to renal impairment, knee
M10.361 Gout due to renal impairment, right knee
M10.362 Gout due to renal impairment, left knee
M10.369 Gout due to renal impairment, unspecified knee
+ M10.37 Gout due to renal impairment, ankle and foot
M10.371 Gout due to renal impairment, right ankle and foot
M10.372 Gout due to renal impairment, left ankle and foot
M10.379 Gout due to renal impairment, unspecified ankle and foot
M10.38 Gout due to renal impairment, vertebrae
M10.39 Gout due to renal impairment, multiple sites
+ **M10.4 Other secondary gout**
Code first associated condition
M10.40 Other secondary gout, unspecified site
+ M10.41 Other secondary gout, shoulder
M10.411 Other secondary gout, right shoulder
M10.412 Other secondary gout, left shoulder
M10.419 Other secondary gout, unspecified shoulder
+ M10.42 Other secondary gout, elbow
M10.421 Other secondary gout, right elbow
M10.422 Other secondary gout, left elbow
M10.429 Other secondary gout, unspecified elbow
+ M10.43 Other secondary gout, wrist
M10.431 Other secondary gout, right wrist
M10.432 Other secondary gout, left wrist
M10.439 Other secondary gout, unspecified wrist
+ M10.44 Other secondary gout, hand
M10.441 Other secondary gout, right hand
M10.442 Other secondary gout, left hand
M10.449 Other secondary gout, unspecified hand
+ M10.45 Other secondary gout, hip
M10.451 Other secondary gout, right hip
M10.452 Other secondary gout, left hip
M10.459 Other secondary gout, unspecified hip
+ M10.46 Other secondary gout, knee
M10.461 Other secondary gout, right knee
M10.462 Other secondary gout, left knee
M10.469 Other secondary gout, unspecified knee

+ M10.47 Other secondary gout, ankle and foot
M10.471 Other secondary gout, right ankle and foot
M10.472 Other secondary gout, left ankle and foot
M10.479 Other secondary gout, unspecified ankle and foot
M10.48 Other secondary gout, vertebrae
M10.49 Other secondary gout, multiple sites
M10.9 Gout, unspecified
Gout NOS

M11 Other crystal arthropathies

+ **M11.0 Hydroxyapatite deposition disease**
M11.00 Hydroxyapatite deposition disease, unspecified site
+ M11.01 Hydroxyapatite deposition disease, shoulder
M11.011 Hydroxyapatite deposition disease, right shoulder
M11.012 Hydroxyapatite deposition disease, left shoulder
M11.019 Hydroxyapatite deposition disease, unspecified shoulder
+ M11.02 Hydroxyapatite deposition disease, elbow
M11.021 Hydroxyapatite deposition disease, right elbow
M11.022 Hydroxyapatite deposition disease, left elbow
M11.029 Hydroxyapatite deposition disease, unspecified elbow
+ M11.03 Hydroxyapatite deposition disease, wrist
M11.031 Hydroxyapatite deposition disease, right wrist
M11.032 Hydroxyapatite deposition disease, left wrist
M11.039 Hydroxyapatite deposition disease, unspecified wrist
+ M11.04 Hydroxyapatite deposition disease, hand
M11.041 Hydroxyapatite deposition disease, right hand
M11.042 Hydroxyapatite deposition disease, left hand
M11.049 Hydroxyapatite deposition disease, unspecified hand
+ M11.05 Hydroxyapatite deposition disease, hip
M11.051 Hydroxyapatite deposition disease, right hip
M11.052 Hydroxyapatite deposition disease, left hip
M11.059 Hydroxyapatite deposition disease, unspecified hip
+ M11.06 Hydroxyapatite deposition disease, knee
M11.061 Hydroxyapatite deposition disease, right knee
M11.062 Hydroxyapatite deposition disease, left knee
M11.069 Hydroxyapatite deposition disease, unspecified knee
+ M11.07 Hydroxyapatite deposition disease, ankle and foot
M11.071 Hydroxyapatite deposition disease, right ankle and foot
M11.072 Hydroxyapatite deposition disease, left ankle and foot
M11.079 Hydroxyapatite deposition disease, unspecified ankle and foot
M11.08 Hydroxyapatite deposition disease, vertebrae
M11.09 Hydroxyapatite deposition disease, multiple sites
+ **M11.1 Familial chondrocalcinosis**
M11.10 Familial chondrocalcinosis, unspecified site
+ M11.11 Familial chondrocalcinosis, shoulder
M11.111 Familial chondrocalcinosis, right shoulder
M11.112 Familial chondrocalcinosis, left shoulder
M11.119 Familial chondrocalcinosis, unspecified shoulder
+ M11.12 Familial chondrocalcinosis, elbow
M11.121 Familial chondrocalcinosis, right elbow
M11.122 Familial chondrocalcinosis, left elbow
M11.129 Familial chondrocalcinosis, unspecified elbow

- **+ M11.13 Familial chondrocalcinosis, wrist**
  - M11.131 Familial chondrocalcinosis, right wrist
  - M11.132 Familial chondrocalcinosis, left wrist
  - M11.139 Familial chondrocalcinosis, unspecified wrist
- **+ M11.14 Familial chondrocalcinosis, hand**
  - M11.141 Familial chondrocalcinosis, right hand
  - M11.142 Familial chondrocalcinosis, left hand
  - M11.149 Familial chondrocalcinosis, unspecified hand
- **+ M11.15 Familial chondrocalcinosis, hip**
  - M11.151 Familial chondrocalcinosis, right hip
  - M11.152 Familial chondrocalcinosis, left hip
  - M11.159 Familial chondrocalcinosis, unspecified hip
- **+ M11.16 Familial chondrocalcinosis, knee**
  - M11.161 Familial chondrocalcinosis, right knee
  - M11.162 Familial chondrocalcinosis, left knee
  - M11.169 Familial chondrocalcinosis, unspecified knee
- **+ M11.17 Familial chondrocalcinosis, ankle and foot**
  - M11.171 Familial chondrocalcinosis, right ankle and foot
  - M11.172 Familial chondrocalcinosis, left ankle and foot
  - M11.179 Familial chondrocalcinosis, unspecified ankle and foot
- M11.18 Familial chondrocalcinosis, vertebrae
- M11.19 Familial chondrocalcinosis, multiple sites
- **+ M11.2 Other chondrocalcinosis**
  - Chondrocalcinosis NOS
  - M11.20 Other chondrocalcinosis, unspecified site
  - **+ M11.21 Other chondrocalcinosis, shoulder**
    - M11.211 Other chondrocalcinosis, right shoulder
    - M11.212 Other chondrocalcinosis, left shoulder
    - M11.219 Other chondrocalcinosis, unspecified shoulder
  - **+ M11.22 Other chondrocalcinosis, elbow**
    - M11.221 Other chondrocalcinosis, right elbow
    - M11.222 Other chondrocalcinosis, left elbow
    - M11.229 Other chondrocalcinosis, unspecified elbow
  - **+ M11.23 Other chondrocalcinosis, wrist**
    - M11.231 Other chondrocalcinosis, right wrist
    - M11.232 Other chondrocalcinosis, left wrist
    - M11.239 Other chondrocalcinosis, unspecified wrist
  - **+ M11.24 Other chondrocalcinosis, hand**
    - M11.241 Other chondrocalcinosis, right hand
    - M11.242 Other chondrocalcinosis, left hand
    - M11.249 Other chondrocalcinosis, unspecified hand
  - **+ M11.25 Other chondrocalcinosis, hip**
    - M11.251 Other chondrocalcinosis, right hip
    - M11.252 Other chondrocalcinosis, left hip
    - M11.259 Other chondrocalcinosis, unspecified hip
  - **+ M11.26 Other chondrocalcinosis, knee**
    - M11.261 Other chondrocalcinosis, right knee
    - M11.262 Other chondrocalcinosis, left knee
      - *AHA CC: 3Q, 2018, 20*
    - M11.269 Other chondrocalcinosis, unspecified knee
  - **+ M11.27 Other chondrocalcinosis, ankle and foot**
    - M11.271 Other chondrocalcinosis, right ankle and foot
    - M11.272 Other chondrocalcinosis, left ankle and foot
    - M11.279 Other chondrocalcinosis, unspecified ankle and foot
  - M11.28 Other chondrocalcinosis, vertebrae
  - M11.29 Other chondrocalcinosis, multiple sites
- **+ M11.8 Other specified crystal arthropathies**
  - M11.80 Other specified crystal arthropathies, unspecified site
  - **+ M11.81 Other specified crystal arthropathies, shoulder**
    - M11.811 Other specified crystal arthropathies, right shoulder
    - M11.812 Other specified crystal arthropathies, left shoulder
    - M11.819 Other specified crystal arthropathies, unspecified shoulder
  - **+ M11.82 Other specified crystal arthropathies, elbow**
    - M11.821 Other specified crystal arthropathies, right elbow
    - M11.822 Other specified crystal arthropathies, left elbow
    - M11.829 Other specified crystal arthropathies, unspecified elbow
  - **+ M11.83 Other specified crystal arthropathies, wrist**
    - M11.831 Other specified crystal arthropathies, right wrist
    - M11.832 Other specified crystal arthropathies, left wrist
    - M11.839 Other specified crystal arthropathies, unspecified wrist
  - **+ M11.84 Other specified crystal arthropathies, hand**
    - M11.841 Other specified crystal arthropathies, right hand
    - M11.842 Other specified crystal arthropathies, left hand
    - M11.849 Other specified crystal arthropathies, unspecified hand
  - **+ M11.85 Other specified crystal arthropathies, hip**
    - M11.851 Other specified crystal arthropathies, right hip
    - M11.852 Other specified crystal arthropathies, left hip
    - M11.859 Other specified crystal arthropathies, unspecified hip
  - **+ M11.86 Other specified crystal arthropathies, knee**
    - M11.861 Other specified crystal arthropathies, right knee
    - M11.862 Other specified crystal arthropathies, left knee
    - M11.869 Other specified crystal arthropathies, unspecified knee
  - **+ M11.87 Other specified crystal arthropathies, ankle and foot**
    - M11.871 Other specified crystal arthropathies, right ankle and foot
    - M11.872 Other specified crystal arthropathies, left ankle and foot
    - M11.879 Other specified crystal arthropathies, unspecified ankle and foot
  - M11.88 Other specified crystal arthropathies, vertebrae
  - M11.89 Other specified crystal arthropathies, multiple sites
- M11.9 Crystal arthropathy, unspecified

M12 Other and unspecified arthropathy

Excludes1: arthrosis (M15-M19)
cricoarytenoid arthropathy (J38.7)

- **+ M12.0 Chronic postrheumatic arthropathy [Jaccoud]**
  - M12.00 Chronic postrheumatic arthropathy [Jaccoud], unspecified site
  - **+ M12.01 Chronic postrheumatic arthropathy [Jaccoud], shoulder**
    - M12.011 Chronic postrheumatic arthropathy [Jaccoud], right shoulder
    - M12.012 Chronic postrheumatic arthropathy [Jaccoud], left shoulder
    - M12.019 Chronic postrheumatic arthropathy [Jaccoud], unspecified shoulder
  - **+ M12.02 Chronic postrheumatic arthropathy [Jaccoud], elbow**
    - M12.021 Chronic postrheumatic arthropathy [Jaccoud], right elbow
    - M12.022 Chronic postrheumatic arthropathy [Jaccoud], left elbow
    - M12.029 Chronic postrheumatic arthropathy [Jaccoud], unspecified elbow
  - **+ M12.03 Chronic postrheumatic arthropathy [Jaccoud], wrist**
    - M12.031 Chronic postrheumatic arthropathy [Jaccoud], right wrist
    - M12.032 Chronic postrheumatic arthropathy [Jaccoud], left wrist
    - M12.039 Chronic postrheumatic arthropathy [Jaccoud], unspecified wrist

- **+ M12.04 Chronic postrheumatic arthropathy [Jaccoud], hand**
  - **M12.041** Chronic postrheumatic arthropathy [Jaccoud], right hand
  - **M12.042** Chronic postrheumatic arthropathy [Jaccoud], left hand
  - **M12.049** Chronic postrheumatic arthropathy [Jaccoud], unspecified hand
- **+ M12.05 Chronic postrheumatic arthropathy [Jaccoud], hip**
  - **M12.051** Chronic postrheumatic arthropathy [Jaccoud], right hip
  - **M12.052** Chronic postrheumatic arthropathy [Jaccoud], left hip
  - **M12.059** Chronic postrheumatic arthropathy [Jaccoud], unspecified hip
- **+ M12.06 Chronic postrheumatic arthropathy [Jaccoud], knee**
  - **M12.061** Chronic postrheumatic arthropathy [Jaccoud], right knee
  - **M12.062** Chronic postrheumatic arthropathy [Jaccoud], left knee
  - **M12.069** Chronic postrheumatic arthropathy [Jaccoud], unspecified knee
- **+ M12.07 Chronic postrheumatic arthropathy [Jaccoud], ankle and foot**
  - **M12.071** Chronic postrheumatic arthropathy [Jaccoud], right ankle and foot
  - **M12.072** Chronic postrheumatic arthropathy [Jaccoud], left ankle and foot
  - **M12.079** Chronic postrheumatic arthropathy [Jaccoud], unspecified ankle and foot
- **M12.08** Chronic postrheumatic arthropathy [Jaccoud], other specified site
  - Chronic postrheumatic arthropathy [Jaccoud], vertebrae
- **M12.09** Chronic postrheumatic arthropathy [Jaccoud], multiple sites
- **+ M12.1 Kaschin-Beck disease**
  - Osteochondroarthrosis deformans endemica
  - **M12.10** Kaschin-Beck disease, unspecified site
- **+ M12.11 Kaschin-Beck disease, shoulder**
  - M12.111 Kaschin-Beck disease, right shoulder
  - M12.112 Kaschin-Beck disease, left shoulder
  - M12.119 Kaschin-Beck disease, unspecified shoulder
- **+ M12.12 Kaschin-Beck disease, elbow**
  - M12.121 Kaschin-Beck disease, right elbow
  - M12.122 Kaschin-Beck disease, left elbow
  - M12.129 Kaschin-Beck disease, unspecified elbow
- **+ M12.13 Kaschin-Beck disease, wrist**
  - M12.131 Kaschin-Beck disease, right wrist
  - M12.132 Kaschin-Beck disease, left wrist
  - M12.139 Kaschin-Beck disease, unspecified wrist
- **+ M12.14 Kaschin-Beck disease, hand**
  - M12.141 Kaschin-Beck disease, right hand
  - M12.142 Kaschin-Beck disease, left hand
  - M12.149 Kaschin-Beck disease, unspecified hand
- **+ M12.15 Kaschin-Beck disease, hip**
  - M12.151 Kaschin-Beck disease, right hip
  - M12.152 Kaschin-Beck disease, left hip
  - M12.159 Kaschin-Beck disease, unspecified hip
- **+ M12.16 Kaschin-Beck disease, knee**
  - M12.161 Kaschin-Beck disease, right knee
  - M12.162 Kaschin-Beck disease, left knee
  - M12.169 Kaschin-Beck disease, unspecified knee
- **+ M12.17 Kaschin-Beck disease, ankle and foot**
  - M12.171 Kaschin-Beck disease, right ankle and foot
  - M12.172 Kaschin-Beck disease, left ankle and foot
  - M12.179 Kaschin-Beck disease, unspecified ankle and foot
- **M12.18** Kaschin-Beck disease, vertebrae
- **M12.19** Kaschin-Beck disease, multiple sites

- **+ M12.2 Villonodular synovitis (pigmented)**
  - **M12.20** Villonodular synovitis (pigmented), unspecified site
- **+ M12.21 Villonodular synovitis (pigmented), shoulder**
  - M12.211 Villonodular synovitis (pigmented), right shoulder
  - M12.212 Villonodular synovitis (pigmented), left shoulder
  - M12.219 Villonodular synovitis (pigmented), unspecified shoulder
- **+ M12.22 Villonodular synovitis (pigmented), elbow**
  - M12.221 Villonodular synovitis (pigmented), right elbow
  - M12.222 Villonodular synovitis (pigmented), left elbow
  - M12.229 Villonodular synovitis (pigmented), unspecified elbow
- **+ M12.23 Villonodular synovitis (pigmented), wrist**
  - M12.231 Villonodular synovitis (pigmented), right wrist
  - M12.232 Villonodular synovitis (pigmented), left wrist
  - M12.239 Villonodular synovitis (pigmented), unspecified wrist
- **+ M12.24 Villonodular synovitis (pigmented), hand**
  - M12.241 Villonodular synovitis (pigmented), right hand
  - M12.242 Villonodular synovitis (pigmented), left hand
  - M12.249 Villonodular synovitis (pigmented), unspecified hand
- **+ M12.25 Villonodular synovitis (pigmented), hip**
  - M12.251 Villonodular synovitis (pigmented), right hip
  - M12.252 Villonodular synovitis (pigmented), left hip
  - M12.259 Villonodular synovitis (pigmented), unspecified hip
- **+ M12.26 Villonodular synovitis (pigmented), knee**
  - M12.261 Villonodular synovitis (pigmented), right knee
  - M12.262 Villonodular synovitis (pigmented), left knee
  - M12.269 Villonodular synovitis (pigmented), unspecified knee
- **+ M12.27 Villonodular synovitis (pigmented), ankle and foot**
  - M12.271 Villonodular synovitis (pigmented), right ankle and foot
  - M12.272 Villonodular synovitis (pigmented), left ankle and foot
  - M12.279 Villonodular synovitis (pigmented), unspecified ankle and foot
- **M12.28** Villonodular synovitis (pigmented), other specified site
  - Villonodular synovitis (pigmented), vertebrae
- **M12.29** Villonodular synovitis (pigmented), multiple sites
- **+ M12.3 Palindromic rheumatism**
  - **M12.30** Palindromic rheumatism, unspecified site
- **+ M12.31 Palindromic rheumatism, shoulder**
  - M12.311 Palindromic rheumatism, right shoulder
  - M12.312 Palindromic rheumatism, left shoulder
  - M12.319 Palindromic rheumatism, unspecified shoulder
- **+ M12.32 Palindromic rheumatism, elbow**
  - M12.321 Palindromic rheumatism, right elbow
  - M12.322 Palindromic rheumatism, left elbow
  - M12.329 Palindromic rheumatism, unspecified elbow
- **+ M12.33 Palindromic rheumatism, wrist**
  - M12.331 Palindromic rheumatism, right wrist
  - M12.332 Palindromic rheumatism, left wrist
  - M12.339 Palindromic rheumatism, unspecified wrist
- **+ M12.34 Palindromic rheumatism, hand**
  - M12.341 Palindromic rheumatism, right hand
  - M12.342 Palindromic rheumatism, left hand
  - M12.349 Palindromic rheumatism, unspecified hand

+ M12.35 Palindromic rheumatism, hip
   M12.351 Palindromic rheumatism, right hip
   M12.352 Palindromic rheumatism, left hip
   M12.359 Palindromic rheumatism, unspecified hip
+ M12.36 Palindromic rheumatism, knee
   M12.361 Palindromic rheumatism, right knee
   M12.362 Palindromic rheumatism, left knee
   M12.369 Palindromic rheumatism, unspecified knee
+ M12.37 Palindromic rheumatism, ankle and foot
   M12.371 Palindromic rheumatism, right ankle and foot
   M12.372 Palindromic rheumatism, left ankle and foot
   M12.379 Palindromic rheumatism, unspecified ankle and foot
  M12.38 Palindromic rheumatism, other specified site
       Palindromic rheumatism, vertebrae
  M12.39 Palindromic rheumatism, multiple sites
+ M12.4 Intermittent hydrarthrosis
  M12.40 Intermittent hydrarthrosis, unspecified site
+ M12.41 Intermittent hydrarthrosis, shoulder
   M12.411 Intermittent hydrarthrosis, right shoulder
   M12.412 Intermittent hydrarthrosis, left shoulder
   M12.419 Intermittent hydrarthrosis, unspecified shoulder
+ M12.42 Intermittent hydrarthrosis, elbow
   M12.421 Intermittent hydrarthrosis, right elbow
   M12.422 Intermittent hydrarthrosis, left elbow
   M12.429 Intermittent hydrarthrosis, unspecified elbow
+ M12.43 Intermittent hydrarthrosis, wrist
   M12.431 Intermittent hydrarthrosis, right wrist
   M12.432 Intermittent hydrarthrosis, left wrist
   M12.439 Intermittent hydrarthrosis, unspecified wrist
+ M12.44 Intermittent hydrarthrosis, hand
   M12.441 Intermittent hydrarthrosis, right hand
   M12.442 Intermittent hydrarthrosis, left hand
   M12.449 Intermittent hydrarthrosis, unspecified hand
+ M12.45 Intermittent hydrarthrosis, hip
   M12.451 Intermittent hydrarthrosis, right hip
   M12.452 Intermittent hydrarthrosis, left hip
   M12.459 Intermittent hydrarthrosis, unspecified hip
+ M12.46 Intermittent hydrarthrosis, knee
   M12.461 Intermittent hydrarthrosis, right knee
   M12.462 Intermittent hydrarthrosis, left knee
   M12.469 Intermittent hydrarthrosis, unspecified knee
+ M12.47 Intermittent hydrarthrosis, ankle and foot
   M12.471 Intermittent hydrarthrosis, right ankle and foot
   M12.472 Intermittent hydrarthrosis, left ankle and foot
   M12.479 Intermittent hydrarthrosis, unspecified ankle and foot
  M12.48 Intermittent hydrarthrosis, other site
  M12.49 Intermittent hydrarthrosis, multiple sites
+ M12.5 Traumatic arthropathy
   Excludes1: current injury-see Alphabetic Index
          post-traumatic osteoarthritis of first carpometacarpal joint (M18.2-M18.3)
          post-traumatic osteoarthritis of hip (M16.4-M16.5)
          post-traumatic osteoarthritis of knee (M17.2-M17.3)
          post-traumatic osteoarthritis NOS (M19.1-)
          post-traumatic osteoarthritis of other single joints (M19.1-)
  M12.50 Traumatic arthropathy, unspecified site
+ M12.51 Traumatic arthropathy, shoulder
   M12.511 Traumatic arthropathy, right shoulder
   M12.512 Traumatic arthropathy, left shoulder
   M12.519 Traumatic arthropathy, unspecified shoulder
+ M12.52 Traumatic arthropathy, elbow
   M12.521 Traumatic arthropathy, right elbow
   M12.522 Traumatic arthropathy, left elbow
   M12.529 Traumatic arthropathy, unspecified elbow
+ M12.53 Traumatic arthropathy, wrist
   M12.531 Traumatic arthropathy, right wrist
   M12.532 Traumatic arthropathy, left wrist
   M12.539 Traumatic arthropathy, unspecified wrist
+ M12.54 Traumatic arthropathy, hand
   M12.541 Traumatic arthropathy, right hand
   M12.542 Traumatic arthropathy, left hand
   M12.549 Traumatic arthropathy, unspecified hand
+ M12.55 Traumatic arthropathy, hip
   M12.551 Traumatic arthropathy, right hip
   M12.552 Traumatic arthropathy, left hip
         AHA CC: 1Q, 2015, 17-18
   M12.559 Traumatic arthropathy, unspecified hip
+ M12.56 Traumatic arthropathy, knee
   M12.561 Traumatic arthropathy, right knee
   M12.562 Traumatic arthropathy, left knee
   M12.569 Traumatic arthropathy, unspecified knee
+ M12.57 Traumatic arthropathy, ankle and foot
   M12.571 Traumatic arthropathy, right ankle and foot
   M12.572 Traumatic arthropathy, left ankle and foot
   M12.579 Traumatic arthropathy, unspecified ankle and foot
  M12.58 Traumatic arthropathy, other specified site
       Traumatic arthropathy, vertebrae
  M12.59 Traumatic arthropathy, multiple sites
+ M12.8 Other specific arthropathies, not elsewhere classified
       Transient arthropathy
  M12.80 Other specific arthropathies, not elsewhere classified, unspecified site
+ M12.81 Other specific arthropathies, not elsewhere classified, shoulder
   M12.811 Other specific arthropathies, not elsewhere classified, right shoulder
   M12.812 Other specific arthropathies, not elsewhere classified, left shoulder
   M12.819 Other specific arthropathies, not elsewhere classified, unspecified shoulder
+ M12.82 Other specific arthropathies, not elsewhere classified, elbow
   M12.821 Other specific arthropathies, not elsewhere classified, right elbow
   M12.822 Other specific arthropathies, not elsewhere classified, left elbow
   M12.829 Other specific arthropathies, not elsewhere classified, unspecified elbow
+ M12.83 Other specific arthropathies, not elsewhere classified, wrist
   M12.831 Other specific arthropathies, not elsewhere classified, right wrist
   M12.832 Other specific arthropathies, not elsewhere classified, left wrist
   M12.839 Other specific arthropathies, not elsewhere classified, unspecified wrist
+ M12.84 Other specific arthropathies, not elsewhere classified, hand
   M12.841 Other specific arthropathies, not elsewhere classified, right hand
   M12.842 Other specific arthropathies, not elsewhere classified, left hand
   M12.849 Other specific arthropathies, not elsewhere classified, unspecified hand
+ M12.85 Other specific arthropathies, not elsewhere classified, hip
   M12.851 Other specific arthropathies, not elsewhere classified, right hip
   M12.852 Other specific arthropathies, not elsewhere classified, left hip
   M12.859 Other specific arthropathies, not elsewhere classified, unspecified hip

- **M12.86** Other specific arthropathies, not elsewhere classified, knee
  - M12.861 Other specific arthropathies, not elsewhere classified, right knee
  - M12.862 Other specific arthropathies, not elsewhere classified, left knee
  - M12.869 Other specific arthropathies, not elsewhere classified, unspecified knee
- **M12.87** Other specific arthropathies, not elsewhere classified, ankle and foot
  - M12.871 Other specific arthropathies, not elsewhere classified, right ankle and foot
  - M12.872 Other specific arthropathies, not elsewhere classified, left ankle and foot
  - M12.879 Other specific arthropathies, not elsewhere classified, unspecified ankle and foot
- **M12.88** Other specific arthropathies, not elsewhere classified, other specified site
  - Other specific arthropathies, not elsewhere classified, vertebrae
- **M12.89** Other specific arthropathies, not elsewhere classified, multiple sites
- **M12.9** Arthropathy, unspecified

M13 Other arthritis

Excludes1: arthrosis (M15-M19)
osteoarthritis (M15-M19)

- **M13.0** Polyarthritis, unspecified
- **M13.1** Monoarthritis, not elsewhere classified
  - M13.10 Monoarthritis, not elsewhere classified, unspecified site
  - **M13.11** Monoarthritis, not elsewhere classified, shoulder
    - M13.111 Monoarthritis, not elsewhere classified, right shoulder
    - M13.112 Monoarthritis, not elsewhere classified, left shoulder
    - M13.119 Monoarthritis, not elsewhere classified, unspecified shoulder
  - **M13.12** Monoarthritis, not elsewhere classified, elbow
    - M13.121 Monoarthritis, not elsewhere classified, right elbow
    - M13.122 Monoarthritis, not elsewhere classified, left elbow
    - M13.129 Monoarthritis, not elsewhere classified, unspecified elbow
  - **M13.13** Monoarthritis, not elsewhere classified, wrist
    - M13.131 Monoarthritis, not elsewhere classified, right wrist
    - M13.132 Monoarthritis, not elsewhere classified, left wrist
    - M13.139 Monoarthritis, not elsewhere classified, unspecified wrist
  - **M13.14** Monoarthritis, not elsewhere classified, hand
    - M13.141 Monoarthritis, not elsewhere classified, right hand
    - M13.142 Monoarthritis, not elsewhere classified, left hand
    - M13.149 Monoarthritis, not elsewhere classified, unspecified hand
  - **M13.15** Monoarthritis, not elsewhere classified, hip
    - M13.151 Monoarthritis, not elsewhere classified, right hip
    - M13.152 Monoarthritis, not elsewhere classified, left hip
    - M13.159 Monoarthritis, not elsewhere classified, unspecified hip
  - **M13.16** Monoarthritis, not elsewhere classified, knee
    - M13.161 Monoarthritis, not elsewhere classified, right knee
    - M13.162 Monoarthritis, not elsewhere classified, left knee
    - M13.169 Monoarthritis, not elsewhere classified, unspecified knee
  - **M13.17** Monoarthritis, not elsewhere classified, ankle and foot
    - M13.171 Monoarthritis, not elsewhere classified, right ankle and foot
    - M13.172 Monoarthritis, not elsewhere classified, left ankle and foot
    - M13.179 Monoarthritis, not elsewhere classified, unspecified ankle and foot

- **M13.8** Other specified arthritis
  - Allergic arthritis
  - *Excludes1:* osteoarthritis (M15-M19)
  - M13.80 Other specified arthritis, unspecified site
  - **M13.81** Other specified arthritis, shoulder
    - M13.811 Other specified arthritis, right shoulder
    - M13.812 Other specified arthritis, left shoulder
    - M13.819 Other specified arthritis, unspecified shoulder
  - **M13.82** Other specified arthritis, elbow
    - M13.821 Other specified arthritis, right elbow
    - M13.822 Other specified arthritis, left elbow
    - M13.829 Other specified arthritis, unspecified elbow
  - **M13.83** Other specified arthritis, wrist
    - M13.831 Other specified arthritis, right wrist
    - M13.832 Other specified arthritis, left wrist
    - M13.839 Other specified arthritis, unspecified wrist
  - **M13.84** Other specified arthritis, hand
    - M13.841 Other specified arthritis, right hand
    - M13.842 Other specified arthritis, left hand
    - M13.849 Other specified arthritis, unspecified hand
  - **M13.85** Other specified arthritis, hip
    - M13.851 Other specified arthritis, right hip
    - M13.852 Other specified arthritis, left hip
    - M13.859 Other specified arthritis, unspecified hip
  - **M13.86** Other specified arthritis, knee
    - M13.861 Other specified arthritis, right knee
    - M13.862 Other specified arthritis, left knee
    - M13.869 Other specified arthritis, unspecified knee
  - **M13.87** Other specified arthritis, ankle and foot
    - M13.871 Other specified arthritis, right ankle and foot
    - M13.872 Other specified arthritis, left ankle and foot
    - M13.879 Other specified arthritis, unspecified ankle and foot
  - M13.88 Other specified arthritis, other site
  - M13.89 Other specified arthritis, multiple sites

M14 Arthropathies in other diseases classified elsewhere

Excludes1: arthropathy in:
diabetes mellitus (E08-E13 with .61-)
hematological disorders (M36.2-M36.3)
hypersensitivity reactions (M36.4)
neoplastic disease (M36.1)
neurosyphillis (A52.16)
sarcoidosis (D86.86)
enteropathic arthropathies (M07.-)
juvenile psoriatic arthropathy (L40.54)
lipoid dermatoarthritis (E78.81)

- **M14.6** Charcôt's joint
  - Neuropathic arthropathy
  - *Excludes1:* Charcôt's joint in diabetes mellitus (E08-E13 with .610)
    Charcôt's joint in tabes dorsalis (A52.16)
  - M14.60 Charcôt's joint, unspecified site
  - **M14.61** Charcôt's joint, shoulder
    - M14.611 Charcôt's joint, right shoulder
    - M14.612 Charcôt's joint, left shoulder
    - M14.619 Charcôt's joint, unspecified shoulder
  - **M14.62** Charcôt's joint, elbow
    - M14.621 Charcôt's joint, right elbow
    - M14.622 Charcôt's joint, left elbow
    - M14.629 Charcôt's joint, unspecified elbow
  - **M14.63** Charcôt's joint, wrist
    - M14.631 Charcôt's joint, right wrist
    - M14.632 Charcôt's joint, left wrist
    - M14.639 Charcôt's joint, unspecified wrist
  - **M14.64** Charcôt's joint, hand
    - M14.641 Charcôt's joint, right hand
    - M14.642 Charcôt's joint, left hand
    - M14.649 Charcôt's joint, unspecified hand
  - **M14.65** Charcôt's joint, hip
    - M14.651 Charcôt's joint, right hip
    - M14.652 Charcôt's joint, left hip
    - M14.659 Charcôt's joint, unspecified hip

- + M14.66 Charcôt's joint, knee
    - M14.661 Charcôt's joint, right knee
    - M14.662 Charcôt's joint, left knee
    - M14.669 Charcôt's joint, unspecified knee
- + M14.67 Charcôt's joint, ankle and foot
    - M14.671 Charcôt's joint, right ankle and foot
    - M14.672 Charcôt's joint, left ankle and foot
    - M14.679 Charcôt's joint, unspecified ankle and foot
- M14.68 Charcôt's joint, vertebrae
- M14.69 Charcôt's joint, multiple sites
- + M14.8 Arthropathies in other specified diseases classified elsewhere

    Code first underlying disease, such as:
    amyloidosis (E85.-)
    erythema multiforme (L51.-)
    erythema nodosum (L52)
    hemochromatosis (E83.11-)
    hyperparathyroidism (E21.-)
    hypothyroidism (E00-E03)
    sickle-cell disorders (D57.-)
    thyrotoxicosis [hyperthyroidism] (E05.-)
    Whipple's disease (K90.81)

    - M14.80 Arthropathies in other specified diseases classified elsewhere, unspecified site
    - + M14.81 Arthropathies in other specified diseases classified elsewhere, shoulder
        - M14.811 Arthropathies in other specified diseases classified elsewhere, right shoulder
        - M14.812 Arthropathies in other specified diseases classified elsewhere, left shoulder
        - M14.819 Arthropathies in other specified diseases classified elsewhere, unspecified shoulder
    - + M14.82 Arthropathies in other specified diseases classified elsewhere, elbow
        - M14.821 Arthropathies in other specified diseases classified elsewhere, right elbow
        - M14.822 Arthropathies in other specified diseases classified elsewhere, left elbow
        - M14.829 Arthropathies in other specified diseases classified elsewhere, unspecified elbow
    - + M14.83 Arthropathies in other specified diseases classified elsewhere, wrist
        - M14.831 Arthropathies in other specified diseases classified elsewhere, right wrist
        - M14.832 Arthropathies in other specified diseases classified elsewhere, left wrist
        - M14.839 Arthropathies in other specified diseases classified elsewhere, unspecified wrist
    - + M14.84 Arthropathies in other specified diseases classified elsewhere, hand
        - M14.841 Arthropathies in other specified diseases classified elsewhere, right hand
        - M14.842 Arthropathies in other specified diseases classified elsewhere, left hand
        - M14.849 Arthropathies in other specified diseases classified elsewhere, unspecified hand
    - + M14.85 Arthropathies in other specified diseases classified elsewhere, hip
        - M14.851 Arthropathies in other specified diseases classified elsewhere, right hip
        - M14.852 Arthropathies in other specified diseases classified elsewhere, left hip
        - M14.859 Arthropathies in other specified diseases classified elsewhere, unspecified hip
    - + M14.86 Arthropathies in other specified diseases classified elsewhere, knee
        - M14.861 Arthropathies in other specified diseases classified elsewhere, right knee
        - M14.862 Arthropathies in other specified diseases classified elsewhere, left knee
        - M14.869 Arthropathies in other specified diseases classified elsewhere, unspecified knee
    - + M14.87 Arthropathies in other specified diseases classified elsewhere, ankle and foot
        - M14.871 Arthropathies in other specified diseases classified elsewhere, right ankle and foot
        - M14.872 Arthropathies in other specified diseases classified elsewhere, left ankle and foot
        - M14.879 Arthropathies in other specified diseases classified elsewhere, unspecified ankle and foot
    - M14.88 Arthropathies in other specified diseases classified elsewhere, vertebrae
    - M14.89 Arthropathies in other specified diseases classified elsewhere, multiple sites

Osteoarthritis (M15-M19)

Excludes2: osteoarthritis of spine (M47.-)

M15 Polyosteoarthritis

Includes: arthritis of multiple sites
Excludes1: bilateral involvement of single joint (M16-M19)

- M15.0 Primary generalized (osteo)arthritis
- M15.1 Heberden's nodes (with arthropathy)
    Interphalangeal distal osteoarthritis
- M15.2 Bouchard's nodes (with arthropathy)
    Juxtaphalangeal distal osteoarthritis
- M15.3 Secondary multiple arthritis
    Post-traumatic polyosteoarthritis
- M15.4 Erosive (osteo)arthritis
- M15.8 Other polyosteoarthritis
- M15.9 Polyosteoarthritis, unspecified
    Generalized osteoarthritis NOS

M16 Osteoarthritis of hip

- M16.0 Bilateral primary osteoarthritis of hip
    AHA CC: 4Q, 2016, 146; 2Q, 2018, 15
- + M16.1 Unilateral primary osteoarthritis of hip
    Primary osteoarthritis of hip NOS
    - M16.10 Unilateral primary osteoarthritis, unspecified hip
    - M16.11 Unilateral primary osteoarthritis, right hip
    - M16.12 Unilateral primary osteoarthritis, left hip
- M16.2 Bilateral osteoarthritis resulting from hip dysplasia
- + M16.3 Unilateral osteoarthritis resulting from hip dysplasia
    Dysplastic osteoarthritis of hip NOS
    - M16.30 Unilateral osteoarthritis resulting from hip dysplasia, unspecified hip
    - M16.31 Unilateral osteoarthritis resulting from hip dysplasia, right hip
    - M16.32 Unilateral osteoarthritis resulting from hip dysplasia, left hip
- M16.4 Bilateral post-traumatic osteoarthritis of hip
- + M16.5 Unilateral post-traumatic osteoarthritis of hip
    Post-traumatic osteoarthritis of hip NOS
    - M16.50 Unilateral post-traumatic osteoarthritis, unspecified hip
    - M16.51 Unilateral post-traumatic osteoarthritis, right hip
    - M16.52 Unilateral post-traumatic osteoarthritis, left hip
- M16.6 Other bilateral secondary osteoarthritis of hip
- M16.7 Other unilateral secondary osteoarthritis of hip
    Secondary osteoarthritis of hip NOS
- M16.9 Osteoarthritis of hip, unspecified

M17 Osteoarthritis of knee

- M17.0 Bilateral primary osteoarthritis of knee
- + M17.1 Unilateral primary osteoarthritis of knee
    Primary osteoarthritis of knee NOS
    - M17.10 Unilateral primary osteoarthritis, unspecified knee
        AHA CC: 4Q, 2016, 147
    - M17.11 Unilateral primary osteoarthritis, right knee
    - M17.12 Unilateral primary osteoarthritis, left knee
        AHA CC: 4Q, 2016, 146
- M17.2 Bilateral post-traumatic osteoarthritis of knee
- + M17.3 Unilateral post-traumatic osteoarthritis of knee
    Post-traumatic osteoarthritis of knee NOS
    - M17.30 Unilateral post-traumatic osteoarthritis, unspecified knee
    - M17.31 Unilateral post-traumatic osteoarthritis, right knee
    - M17.32 Unilateral post-traumatic osteoarthritis, left knee
- M17.4 Other bilateral secondary osteoarthritis of knee
- M17.5 Other unilateral secondary osteoarthritis of knee
    Secondary osteoarthritis of knee NOS
- M17.9 Osteoarthritis of knee, unspecified

Pathology in Osteoarthritis

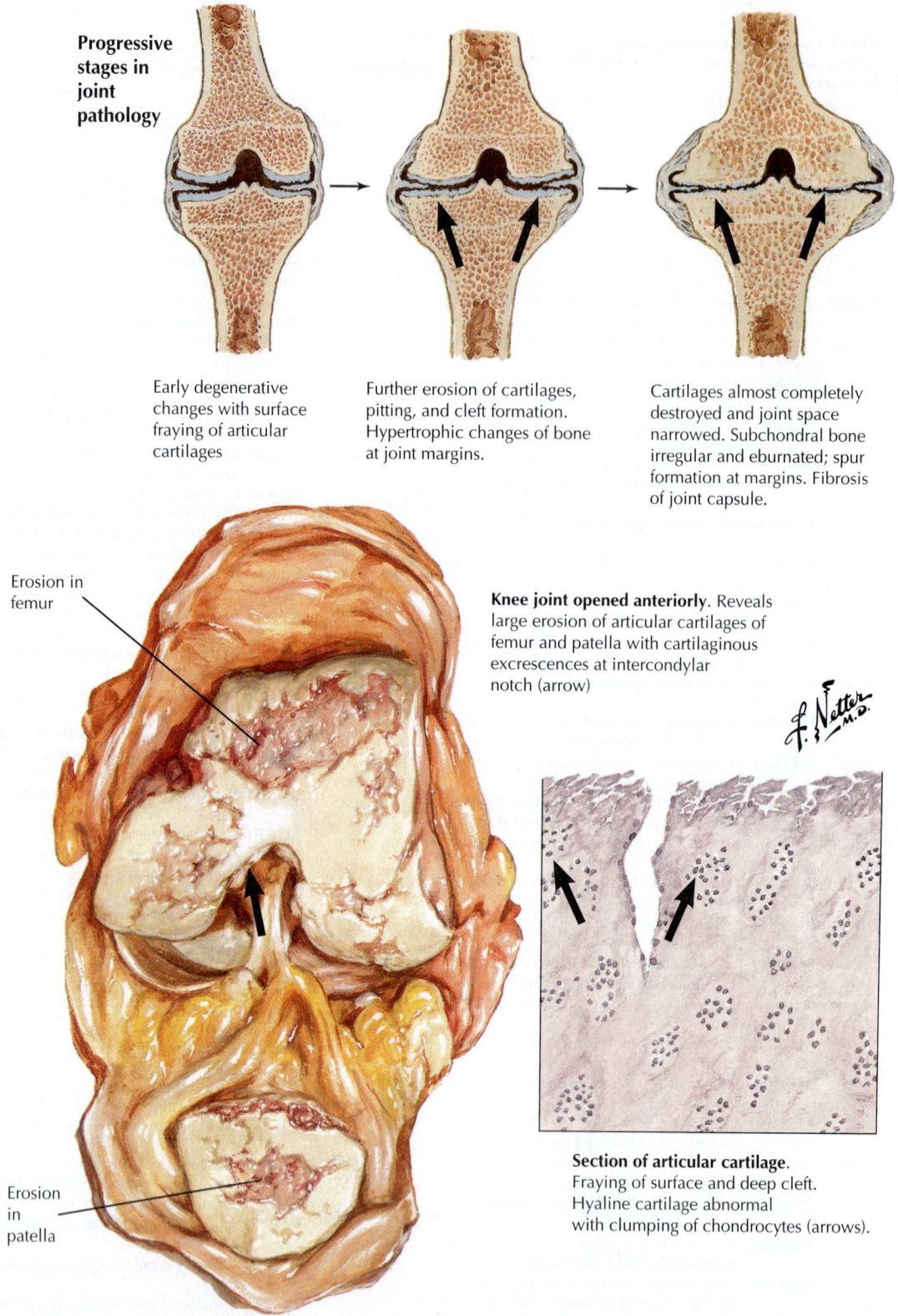

Progressive stages in joint pathology

Early degenerative changes with surface fraying of articular cartilages

Further erosion of cartilages, pitting, and cleft formation. Hypertrophic changes of bone at joint margins.

Cartilages almost completely destroyed and joint space narrowed. Subchondral bone irregular and eburnated; spur formation at margins. Fibrosis of joint capsule.

Erosion in femur

Erosion in patella

Knee joint opened anteriorly. Reveals large erosion of articular cartilages of femur and patella with cartilaginous excrescences at intercondylar notch (arrow)

Section of articular cartilage. Fraying of surface and deep cleft. Hyaline cartilage abnormal with clumping of chondrocytes (arrows).

M18 Osteoarthritis of first carpometacarpal joint
- M18.0 Bilateral primary osteoarthritis of first carpometacarpal joints
- + M18.1 Unilateravl primary osteoarthritis of first carpometacarpal joint
  - Primary osteoarthritis of first carpometacarpal joint NOS
  - M18.10 Unilateral primary osteoarthritis of first carpometacarpal joint, unspecified hand
  - M18.11 Unilateral primary osteoarthritis of first carpometacarpal joint, right hand
  - M18.12 Unilateral primary osteoarthritis of first carpometacarpal joint, left hand
- M18.2 Bilateral post-traumatic osteoarthritis of first carpometacarpal joints
- + M18.3 Unilateral post-traumatic osteoarthritis of first carpometacarpal joint
  - Post-traumatic osteoarthritis of first carpometacarpal joint NOS
  - M18.30 Unilateral post-traumatic osteoarthritis of first carpometacarpal joint, unspecified hand
  - M18.31 Unilateral post-traumatic osteoarthritis of first carpometacarpal joint, right hand
  - M18.32 Unilateral post-traumatic osteoarthritis of first carpometacarpal joint, left hand
- M18.4 Other bilateral secondary osteoarthritis of first carpometacarpal joints
- + M18.5 Other unilateral secondary osteoarthritis of first carpometacarpal joint
  - Secondary osteoarthritis of first carpometacarpal joint NOS
  - M18.50 Other unilateral secondary osteoarthritis of first carpometacarpal joint, unspecified hand
  - M18.51 Other unilateral secondary osteoarthritis of first carpometacarpal joint, right hand
  - M18.52 Other unilateral secondary osteoarthritis of first carpometacarpal joint, left hand
- M18.9 Osteoarthritis of first carpometacarpal joint, unspecified

M19 Other and unspecified osteoarthritis

Excludes1: polyarthritis (M15.-)
Excludes2: arthrosis of spine (M47.-)
hallux rigidus (M20.2)
osteoarthritis of spine (M47.-)
AHA CC: 4Q, 2020, 31-32

- + M19.0 Primary osteoarthritis of other joints
  - + M19.01 Primary osteoarthritis, shoulder
    - M19.011 Primary osteoarthritis, right shoulder
      AHA CC: 4Q, 2016, 145
    - M19.012 Primary osteoarthritis, left shoulder
    - M19.019 Primary osteoarthritis, unspecified shoulder
  - + M19.02 Primary osteoarthritis, elbow
    - M19.021 Primary osteoarthritis, right elbow
    - M19.022 Primary osteoarthritis, left elbow
    - M19.029 Primary osteoarthritis, unspecified elbow
  - + M19.03 Primary osteoarthritis, wrist
    - M19.031 Primary osteoarthritis, right wrist
    - M19.032 Primary osteoarthritis, left wrist
    - M19.039 Primary osteoarthritis, unspecified wrist
  - + M19.04 Primary osteoarthritis, hand
    - **Excludes2:** primary osteoarthritis of first carpometacarpal joint (M18.0-, M18.1-)
    - M19.041 Primary osteoarthritis, right hand
    - M19.042 Primary osteoarthritis, left hand
    - M19.049 Primary osteoarthritis, unspecified hand
  - + M19.07 Primary osteoarthritis ankle and foot
    - M19.071 Primary osteoarthritis, right ankle and foot
    - M19.072 Primary osteoarthritis, left ankle and foot
    - M19.079 Primary osteoarthritis, unspecified ankle and foot
  - M19.09 Primary osteoarthritis, other specified site
- + M19.1 Post-traumatic osteoarthritis of other joints
  - + M19.11 Post-traumatic osteoarthritis, shoulder
    - M19.111 Post-traumatic osteoarthritis, right shoulder
    - M19.112 Post-traumatic osteoarthritis, left shoulder
    - M19.119 Post-traumatic osteoarthritis, unspecified shoulder
  - + M19.12 Post-traumatic osteoarthritis, elbow
    - M19.121 Post-traumatic osteoarthritis, right elbow
    - M19.122 Post-traumatic osteoarthritis, left elbow
    - M19.129 Post-traumatic osteoarthritis, unspecified elbow
  - + M19.13 Post-traumatic osteoarthritis, wrist
    - M19.131 Post-traumatic osteoarthritis, right wrist
    - M19.132 Post-traumatic osteoarthritis, left wrist
    - M19.139 Post-traumatic osteoarthritis, unspecified wrist
  - + M19.14 Post-traumatic osteoarthritis, hand
    - **Excludes2:** post-traumatic osteoarthritis of first carpometacarpal joint (M18.2-, M18.3-)
    - M19.141 Post-traumatic osteoarthritis, right hand
    - M19.142 Post-traumatic osteoarthritis, left hand
    - M19.149 Post-traumatic osteoarthritis, unspecified hand
  - + M19.17 Post-traumatic osteoarthritis, ankle and foot
    - M19.171 Post-traumatic osteoarthritis, right ankle and foot
    - M19.172 Post-traumatic osteoarthritis, left ankle and foot
    - M19.179 Post-traumatic osteoarthritis, unspecified ankle and foot
  - M19.19 Post-traumatic osteoarthritis, other specified site
- + M19.2 Secondary osteoarthritis of other joints
  - + M19.21 Secondary osteoarthritis, shoulder
    - M19.211 Secondary osteoarthritis, right shoulder
    - M19.212 Secondary osteoarthritis, left shoulder
    - M19.219 Secondary osteoarthritis, unspecified shoulder
  - + M19.22 Secondary osteoarthritis, elbow
    - M19.221 Secondary osteoarthritis, right elbow
    - M19.222 Secondary osteoarthritis, left elbow
    - M19.229 Secondary osteoarthritis, unspecified elbow
  - + M19.23 Secondary osteoarthritis, wrist
    - M19.231 Secondary osteoarthritis, right wrist
    - M19.232 Secondary osteoarthritis, left wrist
    - M19.239 Secondary osteoarthritis, unspecified wrist
  - + M19.24 Secondary osteoarthritis, hand
    - M19.241 Secondary osteoarthritis, right hand
    - M19.242 Secondary osteoarthritis, left hand
    - M19.249 Secondary osteoarthritis, unspecified hand
  - + M19.27 Secondary osteoarthritis, ankle and foot
    - M19.271 Secondary osteoarthritis, right ankle and foot
    - M19.272 Secondary osteoarthritis, left ankle and foot
    - M19.279 Secondary osteoarthritis, unspecified ankle and foot
  - M19.29 Secondary osteoarthritis, other specified site
- + M19.9 Osteoarthritis, unspecified site
  - M19.90 Unspecified osteoarthritis, unspecified site
    - Arthrosis NOS
    - Arthritis NOS
    - Osteoarthritis NOS
    AHA CC: 4Q, 2016, 147
  - M19.91 Primary osteoarthritis, unspecified site
    - Primary osteoarthritis NOS
  - M19.92 Post-traumatic osteoarthritis, unspecified site
    - Post-traumatic osteoarthritis NOS
  - M19.93 Secondary osteoarthritis, unspecified site
    - Secondary osteoarthritis NOS

Other joint disorders (M20-M25)

Excludes2: *joints of the spine (M40-M54)*

M20 Acquired deformities of fingers and toes

Excludes1: *acquired absence of fingers and toes (Z89.-)*
congenital absence of fingers and toes (Q71.3-, Q72.3-)
congenital deformities and malformations of fingers and toes (Q66.-, Q68-Q70, Q74.-)

- M20.0 Deformity of finger(s)
  Excludes1: *clubbing of fingers (R68.3)*
  palmar fascial fibromatosis [Dupuytren] (M72.0)
  trigger finger (M65.3)
  - M20.00 Unspecified deformity of finger(s)
    - M20.001 Unspecified deformity of right finger(s)
    - M20.002 Unspecified deformity of left finger(s)
    - M20.009 Unspecified deformity of unspecified finger(s)
  - M20.01 Mallet finger
    - M20.011 Mallet finger of right finger(s)
    - M20.012 Mallet finger of left finger(s)
    - M20.019 Mallet finger of unspecified finger(s)
  - M20.02 Boutonnière deformity
    - M20.021 Boutonnière deformity of right finger(s)
    - M20.022 Boutonnière deformity of left finger(s)
    - M20.029 Boutonnière deformity of unspecified finger(s)
  - M20.03 Swan-neck deformity
    - M20.031 Swan-neck deformity of right finger(s)
    - M20.032 Swan-neck deformity of left finger(s)
    - M20.039 Swan-neck deformity of unspecified finger(s)
  - M20.09 Other deformity of finger(s)
    - M20.091 Other deformity of right finger(s)
    - M20.092 Other deformity of left finger(s)
    - M20.099 Other deformity of finger(s), unspecified finger(s)
- M20.1 Hallux valgus (acquired)
  Excludes2: *bunion (M21.6-)*
  - M20.10 Hallux valgus (acquired), unspecified foot
  - M20.11 Hallux valgus (acquired), right foot
  - M20.12 Hallux valgus (acquired), left foot
- M20.2 Hallux rigidus
  - M20.20 Hallux rigidus, unspecified foot
  - M20.21 Hallux rigidus, right foot
  - M20.22 Hallux rigidus, left foot
- M20.3 Hallux varus (acquired)
  - M20.30 Hallux varus (acquired), unspecified foot
  - M20.31 Hallux varus (acquired), right foot
  - M20.32 Hallux varus (acquired), left foot
- M20.4 Other hammer toe(s) (acquired)
  - M20.40 Other hammer toe(s) (acquired), unspecified foot
  - M20.41 Other hammer toe(s) (acquired), right foot
  - M20.42 Other hammer toe(s) (acquired), left foot
- M20.5 Other deformities of toe(s) (acquired)
  - M20.5X Other deformities of toe(s) (acquired)
    - M20.5X1 Other deformities of toe(s) (acquired), right foot
    - M20.5X2 Other deformities of toe(s) (acquired), left foot
    - M20.5X9 Other deformities of toe(s) (acquired), unspecified foot
- M20.6 Acquired deformities of toe(s), unspecified
  - M20.60 Acquired deformities of toe(s), unspecified, unspecified foot
  - M20.61 Acquired deformities of toe(s), unspecified, right foot
  - M20.62 Acquired deformities of toe(s), unspecified, left foot

M21 Other acquired deformities of limbs

Excludes1: *acquired absence of limb (Z89.-)*
congenital absence of limbs (Q71-Q73)
congenital deformities and malformations of limbs (Q65-Q66, Q68-Q74)

Excludes2: *acquired deformities of fingers or toes (M20.-)*
coxa plana (M91.2)

- M21.0 Valgus deformity, not elsewhere classified
  Excludes1: *metatarsus valgus (Q66.6)*
  talipes calcaneovalgus (Q66.4-)
  - M21.00 Valgus deformity, not elsewhere classified, unspecified site
  - M21.02 Valgus deformity, not elsewhere classified, elbow
    Cubitus valgus
    - M21.021 Valgus deformity, not elsewhere classified, right elbow
    - M21.022 Valgus deformity, not elsewhere classified, left elbow
    - M21.029 Valgus deformity, not elsewhere classified, unspecified elbow
  - M21.05 Valgus deformity, not elsewhere classified, hip
    - M21.051 Valgus deformity, not elsewhere classified, right hip
    - M21.052 Valgus deformity, not elsewhere classified, left hip
    - M21.059 Valgus deformity, not elsewhere classified, unspecified hip
  - M21.06 Valgus deformity, not elsewhere classified, knee
    Genu valgum
    Knock knee
    - M21.061 Valgus deformity, not elsewhere classified, right knee
    - M21.062 Valgus deformity, not elsewhere classified, left knee
    - M21.069 Valgus deformity, not elsewhere classified, unspecified knee
  - M21.07 Valgus deformity, not elsewhere classified, ankle
    - M21.071 Valgus deformity, not elsewhere classified, right ankle
    - M21.072 Valgus deformity, not elsewhere classified, left ankle
    - M21.079 Valgus deformity, not elsewhere classified, unspecified ankle
- M21.1 Varus deformity, not elsewhere classified
  Excludes1: *metatarsus varus (Q66.22-)*
  tibia vara (M92.51-)
  - M21.10 Varus deformity, not elsewhere classified, unspecified site
  - M21.12 Varus deformity, not elsewhere classified, elbow
    Cubitus varus, elbow
    - M21.121 Varus deformity, not elsewhere classified, right elbow
    - M21.122 Varus deformity, not elsewhere classified, left elbow
    - M21.129 Varus deformity, not elsewhere classified, unspecified elbow
  - M21.15 Varus deformity, not elsewhere classified, hip
    - M21.151 Varus deformity, not elsewhere classified, right hip
    - M21.152 Varus deformity, not elsewhere classified, left hip
    - M21.159 Varus deformity, not elsewhere classified, unspecified
  - M21.16 Varus deformity, not elsewhere classified, knee
    Bow leg
    Genu varum
    - M21.161 Varus deformity, not elsewhere classified, right knee
    - M21.162 Varus deformity, not elsewhere classified, left knee
    - M21.169 Varus deformity, not elsewhere classified, unspecified knee
  - M21.17 Varus deformity, not elsewhere classified, ankle
    - M21.171 Varus deformity, not elsewhere classified, right ankle
    - M21.172 Varus deformity, not elsewhere classified, left ankle
    - M21.179 Varus deformity, not elsewhere classified, unspecified ankle
- M21.2 Flexion deformity
  - M21.20 Flexion deformity, unspecified site
  - M21.21 Flexion deformity, shoulder
    - M21.211 Flexion deformity, right shoulder
    - M21.212 Flexion deformity, left shoulder
    - M21.219 Flexion deformity, unspecified shoulder

- **+ M21.22 Flexion deformity, elbow**
  - M21.221 Flexion deformity, right elbow
  - M21.222 Flexion deformity, left elbow
  - M21.229 Flexion deformity, unspecified elbow
- **+ M21.23 Flexion deformity, wrist**
  - M21.231 Flexion deformity, right wrist
  - M21.232 Flexion deformity, left wrist
  - M21.239 Flexion deformity, unspecified wrist
- **+ M21.24 Flexion deformity, finger joints**
  - M21.241 Flexion deformity, right finger joints
  - M21.242 Flexion deformity, left finger joints
  - M21.249 Flexion deformity, unspecified finger joints
- **+ M21.25 Flexion deformity, hip**
  - M21.251 Flexion deformity, right hip
  - M21.252 Flexion deformity, left hip
  - M21.259 Flexion deformity, unspecified hip
- **+ M21.26 Flexion deformity, knee**
  - M21.261 Flexion deformity, right knee
  - M21.262 Flexion deformity, left knee
  - M21.269 Flexion deformity, unspecified knee
- **+ M21.27 Flexion deformity, ankle and toes**
  - M21.271 Flexion deformity, right ankle and toes
  - M21.272 Flexion deformity, left ankle and toes
  - M21.279 Flexion deformity, unspecified ankle and toes
- **+ M21.3 Wrist or foot drop (acquired)**
  - **+ M21.33 Wrist drop (acquired)**
    - M21.331 Wrist drop, right wrist
    - M21.332 Wrist drop, left wrist
    - M21.339 Wrist drop, unspecified wrist
  - **+ M21.37 Foot drop (acquired)**
    - M21.371 Foot drop, right foot
    - M21.372 Foot drop, left foot
    - M21.379 Foot drop, unspecified foot
- **+ M21.4 Flat foot [pes planus] (acquired)**
  - *Excludes1:* congenital pes planus (Q66.5-)
  - M21.40 Flat foot [pes planus] (acquired), unspecified foot
  - M21.41 Flat foot [pes planus] (acquired), right foot
  - M21.42 Flat foot [pes planus] (acquired), left foot
- **+ M21.5 Acquired clawhand, clubhand, clawfoot and clubfoot**
  - *Excludes1:* clubfoot, not specified as acquired (Q66.89)
  - **+ M21.51 Acquired clawhand**
    - M21.511 Acquired clawhand, right hand
    - M21.512 Acquired clawhand, left hand
    - M21.519 Acquired clawhand, unspecified hand
  - **+ M21.52 Acquired clubhand**
    - M21.521 Acquired clubhand, right hand
    - M21.522 Acquired clubhand, left hand
    - M21.529 Acquired clubhand, unspecified hand
  - **+ M21.53 Acquired clawfoot**
    - M21.531 Acquired clawfoot, right foot
    - M21.532 Acquired clawfoot, left foot
    - M21.539 Acquired clawfoot, unspecified foot
  - **+ M21.54 Acquired clubfoot**
    - M21.541 Acquired clubfoot, right foot
    - M21.542 Acquired clubfoot, left foot
    - M21.549 Acquired clubfoot, unspecified foot
- **+ M21.6 Other acquired deformities of foot**
  - *Excludes2:* deformities of toe (acquired) (M20.1-M20.6-)
  - AHA CC: 4Q, 2016, 38
  - **+ M21.61 Bunion**
    - M21.611 Bunion of right foot
    - M21.612 Bunion of left foot
    - M21.619 Bunion of unspecified foot
  - **+ M21.62 Bunionette**
    - M21.621 Bunionette of right foot
    - M21.622 Bunionette of left foot
    - M21.629 Bunionette of unspecified foot
  - **+ M21.6X Other acquired deformities of foot**
    - M21.6X1 Other acquired deformities of right foot
    - M21.6X2 Other acquired deformities of left foot
    - M21.6X9 Other acquired deformities of unspecified foot
- **+ M21.7 Unequal limb length (acquired)**
  - **NOTE** The site used should correspond to the shorter limb
  - M21.70 Unequal limb length (acquired), unspecified site
  - **+ M21.72 Unequal limb length (acquired), humerus**
    - M21.721 Unequal limb length (acquired), right humerus
    - M21.722 Unequal limb length (acquired), left humerus
    - M21.729 Unequal limb length (acquired), unspecified humerus
  - **+ M21.73 Unequal limb length (acquired), ulna and radius**
    - M21.731 Unequal limb length (acquired), right ulna
    - M21.732 Unequal limb length (acquired), left ulna
    - M21.733 Unequal limb length (acquired), right radius
    - M21.734 Unequal limb length (acquired), left radius
    - M21.739 Unequal limb length (acquired), unspecified ulna and radius
  - **+ M21.75 Unequal limb length (acquired), femur**
    - M21.751 Unequal limb length (acquired), right femur
    - M21.752 Unequal limb length (acquired), left femur
    - M21.759 Unequal limb length (acquired), unspecified femur
  - **+ M21.76 Unequal limb length (acquired), tibia and fibula**
    - M21.761 Unequal limb length (acquired), right tibia
    - M21.762 Unequal limb length (acquired), left tibia
    - M21.763 Unequal limb length (acquired), right fibula
    - M21.764 Unequal limb length (acquired), left fibula
    - M21.769 Unequal limb length (acquired), unspecified tibia and fibula
- **+ M21.8 Other specified acquired deformities of limbs**
  - *Excludes2:* coxa plana (M91.2)
  - M21.80 Other specified acquired deformities of unspecified limb
  - **+ M21.82 Other specified acquired deformities of upper arm**
    - M21.821 Other specified acquired deformities of right upper arm
    - M21.822 Other specified acquired deformities of left upper arm
    - M21.829 Other specified acquired deformities of unspecified upper arm
  - **+ M21.83 Other specified acquired deformities of forearm**
    - M21.831 Other specified acquired deformities of right forearm
    - M21.832 Other specified acquired deformities of left forearm
    - M21.839 Other specified acquired deformities of unspecified forearm
  - **+ M21.85 Other specified acquired deformities of thigh**
    - M21.851 Other specified acquired deformities of right thigh
    - M21.852 Other specified acquired deformities of left thigh
    - M21.859 Other specified acquired deformities of unspecified thigh
  - **+ M21.86 Other specified acquired deformities of lower leg**
    - M21.861 Other specified acquired deformities of right lower leg
    - M21.862 Other specified acquired deformities of left lower leg
    - M21.869 Other specified acquired deformities of unspecified lower leg
- **+ M21.9 Unspecified acquired deformity of limb and hand**
  - M21.90 Unspecified acquired deformity of unspecified limb
  - **+ M21.92 Unspecified acquired deformity of upper arm**
    - M21.921 Unspecified acquired deformity of right upper arm
    - M21.922 Unspecified acquired deformity of left upper arm
    - M21.929 Unspecified acquired deformity of unspecified upper arm
  - **+ M21.93 Unspecified acquired deformity of forearm**
    - M21.931 Unspecified acquired deformity of right forearm
    - M21.932 Unspecified acquired deformity of left forearm
    - M21.939 Unspecified acquired deformity of unspecified forearm

- **+ M21.94 Unspecified acquired deformity of hand**
  - M21.941 Unspecified acquired deformity of hand, right hand
  - M21.942 Unspecified acquired deformity of hand, left hand
  - M21.949 Unspecified acquired deformity of hand, unspecified hand
- **+ M21.95 Unspecified acquired deformity of thigh**
  - M21.951 Unspecified acquired deformity of right thigh
  - M21.952 Unspecified acquired deformity of left thigh
  - M21.959 Unspecified acquired deformity of unspecified thigh
- **+ M21.96 Unspecified acquired deformity of lower leg**
  - M21.961 Unspecified acquired deformity of right lower leg
  - M21.962 Unspecified acquired deformity of left lower leg
  - M21.969 Unspecified acquired deformity of unspecified lower leg

M22 Disorder of patella

Excludes2: *traumatic dislocation of patella (S83.0-)*

- **+ M22.0 Recurrent dislocation of patella**
  - M22.00 Recurrent dislocation of patella, unspecified knee
  - M22.01 Recurrent dislocation of patella, right knee
  - M22.02 Recurrent dislocation of patella, left knee
- **+ M22.1 Recurrent subluxation of patella**
  - Incomplete dislocation of patella
  - M22.10 Recurrent subluxation of patella, unspecified knee
  - M22.11 Recurrent subluxation of patella, right knee
  - M22.12 Recurrent subluxation of patella, left knee
- **+ M22.2 Patellofemoral disorders**
  - **+ M22.2X Patellofemoral disorders**
    - M22.2X1 Patellofemoral disorders, right knee
    - M22.2X2 Patellofemoral disorders, left knee
    - M22.2X9 Patellofemoral disorders, unspecified knee
- **+ M22.3 Other derangements of patella**
  - **+ M22.3X Other derangements of patella**
    - M22.3X1 Other derangements of patella, right knee
    - M22.3X2 Other derangements of patella, left knee
    - M22.3X9 Other derangements of patella, unspecified knee
- **+ M22.4 Chondromalacia patellae**
  - M22.40 Chondromalacia patellae, unspecified knee
  - M22.41 Chondromalacia patellae, right knee
  - M22.42 Chondromalacia patellae, left knee
- **+ M22.8 Other disorders of patella**
  - **+ M22.8X Other disorders of patella**
    - M22.8X1 Other disorders of patella, right knee
    - M22.8X2 Other disorders of patella, left knee
    - M22.8X9 Other disorders of patella, unspecified knee
- **+ M22.9 Unspecified disorder of patella**
  - M22.90 Unspecified disorder of patella, unspecified knee
  - M22.91 Unspecified disorder of patella, right knee
  - M22.92 Unspecified disorder of patella, left knee

M23 Internal derangement of knee

Excludes1: *ankylosis (M24.66)*
deformity of knee (M21.-)
osteochondritis dissecans (M93.2)

Excludes2: *current injury - see injury of knee and lower leg (S80-S89)*
recurrent dislocation or subluxation of joints (M24.4)
recurrent dislocation or subluxation of patella (M22.0-M22.1)

- **+ M23.0 Cystic meniscus**
  - **+ M23.00 Cystic meniscus, unspecified meniscus**
    - Cystic meniscus, unspecified lateral meniscus
    - Cystic meniscus, unspecified medial meniscus
    - M23.000 Cystic meniscus, unspecified lateral meniscus, right knee
    - M23.001 Cystic meniscus, unspecified lateral meniscus, left knee
    - M23.002 Cystic meniscus, unspecified lateral meniscus, unspecified knee
    - M23.003 Cystic meniscus, unspecified medial meniscus, right knee
    - M23.004 Cystic meniscus, unspecified medial meniscus, left knee
    - M23.005 Cystic meniscus, unspecified medial meniscus, unspecified knee
    - M23.006 Cystic meniscus, unspecified meniscus, right knee
    - M23.007 Cystic meniscus, unspecified meniscus, left knee
    - M23.009 Cystic meniscus, unspecified meniscus, unspecified knee
  - **+ M23.01 Cystic meniscus, anterior horn of medial meniscus**
    - M23.011 Cystic meniscus, anterior horn of medial meniscus, right knee
    - M23.012 Cystic meniscus, anterior horn of medial meniscus, left knee
    - M23.019 Cystic meniscus, anterior horn of medial meniscus, unspecified knee
  - **+ M23.02 Cystic meniscus, posterior horn of medial meniscus**
    - M23.021 Cystic meniscus, posterior horn of medial meniscus, right knee
    - M23.022 Cystic meniscus, posterior horn of medial meniscus, left knee
    - M23.029 Cystic meniscus, posterior horn of medial meniscus, unspecified knee
  - **+ M23.03 Cystic meniscus, other medial meniscus**
    - M23.031 Cystic meniscus, other medial meniscus, right knee
    - M23.032 Cystic meniscus, other medial meniscus, left knee
    - M23.039 Cystic meniscus, other medial meniscus, unspecified knee
  - **+ M23.04 Cystic meniscus, anterior horn of lateral meniscus**
    - M23.041 Cystic meniscus, anterior horn of lateral meniscus, right knee
    - M23.042 Cystic meniscus, anterior horn of lateral meniscus, left knee
    - M23.049 Cystic meniscus, anterior horn of lateral meniscus, unspecified knee
  - **+ M23.05 Cystic meniscus, posterior horn of lateral meniscus**
    - M23.051 Cystic meniscus, posterior horn of lateral meniscus, right knee
    - M23.052 Cystic meniscus, posterior horn of lateral meniscus, left knee
    - M23.059 Cystic meniscus, posterior horn of lateral meniscus, unspecified knee
  - **+ M23.06 Cystic meniscus, other lateral meniscus**
    - M23.061 Cystic meniscus, other lateral meniscus, right knee
    - M23.062 Cystic meniscus, other lateral meniscus, left knee
    - M23.069 Cystic meniscus, other lateral meniscus, unspecified knee
- **+ M23.2 Derangement of meniscus due to old tear or injury**
  - Old bucket-handle tear
  - **+ M23.20 Derangement of unspecified meniscus due to old tear or injury**
    - Derangement of unspecified lateral meniscus due to old tear or injury
    - Derangement of unspecified medial meniscus due to old tear or injury
    - M23.200 Derangement of unspecified lateral meniscus due to old tear or injury, right knee
    - M23.201 Derangement of unspecified lateral meniscus due to old tear or injury, left knee
    - M23.202 Derangement of unspecified lateral meniscus due to old tear or injury, unspecified knee
    - M23.203 Derangement of unspecified medial meniscus due to old tear or injury, right knee
    - M23.204 Derangement of unspecified medial meniscus due to old tear or injury, left knee

M23.205 Derangement of unspecified medial meniscus due to old tear or injury, unspecified knee
M23.206 Derangement of unspecified meniscus due to old tear or injury, right knee
M23.207 Derangement of unspecified meniscus due to old tear or injury, left knee
M23.209 Derangement of unspecified meniscus due to old tear or injury, unspecified knee
+ M23.21 Derangement of anterior horn of medial meniscus due to old tear or injury
    M23.211 Derangement of anterior horn of medial meniscus due to old tear or injury, right knee
    M23.212 Derangement of anterior horn of medial meniscus due to old tear or injury, left knee
    M23.219 Derangement of anterior horn of medial meniscus due to old tear or injury, unspecified knee
+ M23.22 Derangement of posterior horn of medial meniscus due to old tear or injury
    M23.221 Derangement of posterior horn of medial meniscus due to old tear or injury, right knee
    M23.222 Derangement of posterior horn of medial meniscus due to old tear or injury, left knee
    M23.229 Derangement of posterior horn of medial meniscus due to old tear or injury, unspecified knee
+ M23.23 Derangement of other medial meniscus due to old tear or injury
    M23.231 Derangement of other medial meniscus due to old tear or injury, right knee
    M23.232 Derangement of other medial meniscus due to old tear or injury, left knee
    M23.239 Derangement of other medial meniscus due to old tear or injury, unspecified knee
+ M23.24 Derangement of anterior horn of lateral meniscus due to old tear or injury
    M23.241 Derangement of anterior horn of lateral meniscus due to old tear or injury, right knee
    M23.242 Derangement of anterior horn of lateral meniscus due to old tear or injury, left knee
    M23.249 Derangement of anterior horn of lateral meniscus due to old tear or injury, unspecified knee
+ M23.25 Derangement of posterior horn of lateral meniscus due to old tear or injury
    M23.251 Derangement of posterior horn of lateral meniscus due to old tear or injury, right knee
    M23.252 Derangement of posterior horn of lateral meniscus due to old tear or injury, left knee
    M23.259 Derangement of posterior horn of lateral meniscus due to old tear or injury, unspecified knee
+ M23.26 Derangement of other lateral meniscus due to old tear or injury
    M23.261 Derangement of other lateral meniscus due to old tear or injury, right knee
    M23.262 Derangement of other lateral meniscus due to old tear or injury, left knee
    M23.269 Derangement of other lateral meniscus due to old tear or injury, unspecified knee
+ M23.3 Other meniscus derangements
    Degenerate meniscus
    Detached meniscus
    Retained meniscus
+ M23.30 Other meniscus derangements, unspecified meniscus
    Other meniscus derangements, unspecified lateral meniscus
    Other meniscus derangements, unspecified medial meniscus
    M23.300 Other meniscus derangements, unspecified lateral meniscus, right knee
    M23.301 Other meniscus derangements, unspecified lateral meniscus, left knee
    M23.302 Other meniscus derangements, unspecified lateral meniscus, unspecified knee
    M23.303 Other meniscus derangements, unspecified medial meniscus, right knee
    M23.304 Other meniscus derangements, unspecified medial meniscus, left knee
    M23.305 Other meniscus derangements, unspecified medial meniscus, unspecified knee
    M23.306 Other meniscus derangements, unspecified meniscus, right knee
    M23.307 Other meniscus derangements, unspecified meniscus, left knee
    M23.309 Other meniscus derangements, unspecified meniscus, unspecified knee
+ M23.31 Other meniscus derangements, anterior horn of medial meniscus
    M23.311 Other meniscus derangements, anterior horn of medial meniscus, right knee
    M23.312 Other meniscus derangements, anterior horn of medial meniscus, left knee
    M23.319 Other meniscus derangements, anterior horn of medial meniscus, unspecified knee
+ M23.32 Other meniscus derangements, posterior horn of medial meniscus
    M23.321 Other meniscus derangements, posterior horn of medial meniscus, right knee
    M23.322 Other meniscus derangements, posterior horn of medial meniscus, left knee
    M23.329 Other meniscus derangements, posterior horn of medial meniscus, unspecified knee
+ M23.33 Other meniscus derangements, other medial meniscus
    M23.331 Other meniscus derangements, other medial meniscus, right knee
    M23.332 Other meniscus derangements, other medial meniscus, left knee
    M23.339 Other meniscus derangements, other medial meniscus, unspecified knee
+ M23.34 Other meniscus derangements, anterior horn of lateral meniscus
    M23.341 Other meniscus derangements, anterior horn of lateral meniscus, right knee
    M23.342 Other meniscus derangements, anterior horn of lateral meniscus, left knee
    M23.349 Other meniscus derangements, anterior horn of lateral meniscus, unspecified knee
+ M23.35 Other meniscus derangements, posterior horn of lateral meniscus
    M23.351 Other meniscus derangements, posterior horn of lateral meniscus, right knee
    M23.352 Other meniscus derangements, posterior horn of lateral meniscus, left knee
    M23.359 Other meniscus derangements, posterior horn of lateral meniscus, unspecified knee
+ M23.36 Other meniscus derangements, other lateral meniscus
    M23.361 Other meniscus derangements, other lateral meniscus, right knee
    M23.362 Other meniscus derangements, other lateral meniscus, left knee
    M23.369 Other meniscus derangements, other lateral meniscus, unspecified knee
+ M23.4 Loose body in knee
    M23.40 Loose body in knee, unspecified knee
    M23.41 Loose body in knee, right knee
    M23.42 Loose body in knee, left knee
+ M23.5 Chronic instability of knee
    M23.50 Chronic instability of knee, unspecified knee
    M23.51 Chronic instability of knee, right knee
    M23.52 Chronic instability of knee, left knee

- **+ M23.6 Other spontaneous disruption of ligament(s) of knee**
    - **+ M23.60 Other spontaneous disruption of unspecified ligament of knee**
        - M23.601 Other spontaneous disruption of unspecified ligament of right knee
        - M23.602 Other spontaneous disruption of unspecified ligament of left knee
        - M23.609 Other spontaneous disruption of unspecified ligament of unspecified knee
    - **+ M23.61 Other spontaneous disruption of anterior cruciate ligament of knee**
        - M23.611 Other spontaneous disruption of anterior cruciate ligament of right knee
        - M23.612 Other spontaneous disruption of anterior cruciate ligament of left knee
        - M23.619 Other spontaneous disruption of anterior cruciate ligament of unspecified knee
    - **+ M23.62 Other spontaneous disruption of posterior cruciate ligament of knee**
        - M23.621 Other spontaneous disruption of posterior cruciate ligament of right knee
        - M23.622 Other spontaneous disruption of posterior cruciate ligament of left knee
        - M23.629 Other spontaneous disruption of posterior cruciate ligament of unspecified knee
    - **+ M23.63 Other spontaneous disruption of medial collateral ligament of knee**
        - M23.631 Other spontaneous disruption of medial collateral ligament of right knee
        - M23.632 Other spontaneous disruption of medial collateral ligament of left knee
        - M23.639 Other spontaneous disruption of medial collateral ligament of unspecified knee
    - **+ M23.64 Other spontaneous disruption of lateral collateral ligament of knee**
        - M23.641 Other spontaneous disruption of lateral collateral ligament of right knee
        - M23.642 Other spontaneous disruption of lateral collateral ligament of left knee
        - M23.649 Other spontaneous disruption of lateral collateral ligament of unspecified knee
    - **+ M23.67 Other spontaneous disruption of capsular ligament of knee**
        - M23.671 Other spontaneous disruption of capsular ligament of right knee
        - M23.672 Other spontaneous disruption of capsular ligament of left knee
        - M23.679 Other spontaneous disruption of capsular ligament of unspecified knee
- **+ M23.8 Other internal derangements of knee**
    - Laxity of ligament of knee
    - Snapping knee
    - **+ M23.8X Other internal derangements of knee**
        - M23.8X1 Other internal derangements of right knee
        - M23.8X2 Other internal derangements of left knee
        - M23.8X9 Other internal derangements of unspecified knee
- **+ M23.9 Unspecified internal derangement of knee**
    - M23.90 Unspecified internal derangement of unspecified knee
    - M23.91 Unspecified internal derangement of right knee
    - M23.92 Unspecified internal derangement of left knee

M24 Other specific joint derangements

Excludes1: current injury - see injury of joint by body region
Excludes2: ganglion (M67.4)
  snapping knee (M23.8-)
  temporomandibular joint disorders (M26.6-)

AHA CC: 4Q, 2020, 31-32

- **+ M24.0 Loose body in joint**
    - **Excludes2:** loose body in knee (M23.4)
    - M24.00 Loose body in unspecified joint
    - **+ M24.01 Loose body in shoulder**
        - M24.011 Loose body in right shoulder
        - M24.012 Loose body in left shoulder
        - M24.019 Loose body in unspecified shoulder
    - **+ M24.02 Loose body in elbow**
        - M24.021 Loose body in right elbow
        - M24.022 Loose body in left elbow
        - M24.029 Loose body in unspecified elbow
    - **+ M24.03 Loose body in wrist**
        - M24.031 Loose body in right wrist
        - M24.032 Loose body in left wrist
        - M24.039 Loose body in unspecified wrist
    - **+ M24.04 Loose body in finger joints**
        - M24.041 Loose body in right finger joint(s)
        - M24.042 Loose body in left finger joint(s)
        - M24.049 Loose body in unspecified finger joint(s)
    - **+ M24.05 Loose body in hip**
        - M24.051 Loose body in right hip
        - M24.052 Loose body in left hip
        - M24.059 Loose body in unspecified hip
    - **+ M24.07 Loose body in ankle and toe joints**
        - M24.071 Loose body in right ankle
        - M24.072 Loose body in left ankle
        - M24.073 Loose body in unspecified ankle
        - M24.074 Loose body in right toe joint(s)
        - M24.075 Loose body in left toe joint(s)
        - M24.076 Loose body in unspecified toe joints
    - M24.08 Loose body, other site
- **+ M24.1 Other articular cartilage disorders**
    - **Excludes2:** chondrocalcinosis (M11.1-, M11.2-)
      internal derangement of knee (M23.-)
      metastatic calcification (E83.59)
      ochronosis (E70.29)
    - M24.10 Other articular cartilage disorders, unspecified site
    - **+ M24.11 Other articular cartilage disorders, shoulder**
        - M24.111 Other articular cartilage disorders, right shoulder
        - M24.112 Other articular cartilage disorders, left shoulder
        - M24.119 Other articular cartilage disorders, unspecified shoulder
    - **+ M24.12 Other articular cartilage disorders, elbow**
        - M24.121 Other articular cartilage disorders, right elbow
        - M24.122 Other articular cartilage disorders, left elbow
        - M24.129 Other articular cartilage disorders, unspecified elbow
    - **+ M24.13 Other articular cartilage disorders, wrist**
        - M24.131 Other articular cartilage disorders, right wrist
        - M24.132 Other articular cartilage disorders, left wrist
        - M24.139 Other articular cartilage disorders, unspecified wrist
    - **+ M24.14 Other articular cartilage disorders, hand**
        - M24.141 Other articular cartilage disorders, right hand
        - M24.142 Other articular cartilage disorders, left hand
        - M24.149 Other articular cartilage disorders, unspecified hand
    - **+ M24.15 Other articular cartilage disorders, hip**
        - M24.151 Other articular cartilage disorders, right hip
        - M24.152 Other articular cartilage disorders, left hip
        - M24.159 Other articular cartilage disorders, unspecified hip
    - **+ M24.17 Other articular cartilage disorders, ankle and foot**
        - M24.171 Other articular cartilage disorders, right ankle
        - M24.172 Other articular cartilage disorders, left ankle
        - M24.173 Other articular cartilage disorders, unspecified ankle
        - M24.174 Other articular cartilage disorders, right foot
        - M24.175 Other articular cartilage disorders, left foot
        - M24.176 Other articular cartilage disorders, unspecified foot
    - M24.19 Other articular cartilage disorders, other specified site

- **M24.2** **Disorder of ligament**
  Instability secondary to old ligament injury
  Ligamentous laxity NOS
  Excludes1: *familial ligamentous laxity (M35.7)*
  Excludes2: *internal derangement of knee (M23.5-M23.8X9)*
  - M24.20 Disorder of ligament, unspecified site
  - + M24.21 Disorder of ligament, shoulder
    - M24.211 Disorder of ligament, right shoulder
    - M24.212 Disorder of ligament, left shoulder
    - M24.219 Disorder of ligament, unspecified shoulder
  - + M24.22 Disorder of ligament, elbow
    - M24.221 Disorder of ligament, right elbow
    - M24.222 Disorder of ligament, left elbow
    - M24.229 Disorder of ligament, unspecified elbow
  - + M24.23 Disorder of ligament, wrist
    - M24.231 Disorder of ligament, right wrist
    - M24.232 Disorder of ligament, left wrist
    - M24.239 Disorder of ligament, unspecified wrist
  - + M24.24 Disorder of ligament, hand
    - M24.241 Disorder of ligament, right hand
    - M24.242 Disorder of ligament, left hand
    - M24.249 Disorder of ligament, unspecified hand
  - + M24.25 Disorder of ligament, hip
    - M24.251 Disorder of ligament, right hip
    - M24.252 Disorder of ligament, left hip
    - M24.259 Disorder of ligament, unspecified hip
  - + M24.27 Disorder of ligament, ankle and foot
    - M24.271 Disorder of ligament, right ankle
    - M24.272 Disorder of ligament, left ankle
    - M24.273 Disorder of ligament, unspecified ankle
    - M24.274 Disorder of ligament, right foot
    - M24.275 Disorder of ligament, left foot
    - M24.276 Disorder of ligament, unspecifiedfoot
  - M24.28 Disorder of ligament, vertebrae
    AHA CC: 2Q, 2023, 13-14
  - M24.29 Disorder of ligament, other specified site
- + **M24.3** **Pathological dislocation of joint, not elsewhere classified**
  Excludes1: *congenital dislocation or displacement of joint- see congenital malformations and deformations of the musculoskeletal system (Q65-Q79)*
  current injury - see injury of joints and ligaments by body region
  recurrent dislocation of joint (M24.4-)
  - M24.30 Pathological dislocation of unspecified joint, not elsewhere classified
  - + M24.31 Pathological dislocation of shoulder, not elsewhere classified
    - M24.311 Pathological dislocation of right shoulder, not elsewhere classified
    - M24.312 Pathological dislocation of left shoulder, not elsewhere classified
    - M24.319 Pathological dislocation of unspecified shoulder, not elsewhere classified
  - + M24.32 Pathological dislocation of elbow, not elsewhere classified
    - M24.321 Pathological dislocation of right elbow, not elsewhere classified
    - M24.322 Pathological dislocation of left elbow, not elsewhere classified
    - M24.329 Pathological dislocation of unspecified elbow, not elsewhere classified
  - + M24.33 Pathological dislocation of wrist, not elsewhere classified
    - M24.331 Pathological dislocation of right wrist, not elsewhere classified
    - M24.332 Pathological dislocation of left wrist, not elsewhere classified
    - M24.339 Pathological dislocation of unspecified wrist, not elsewhere classified
  - + M24.34 Pathological dislocation of hand, not elsewhere classified
    - M24.341 Pathological dislocation of right hand, not elsewhere classified
    - M24.342 Pathological dislocation of left hand, not elsewhere classified
    - M24.349 Pathological dislocation of unspecified hand, not elsewhere classified
  - + M24.35 Pathological dislocation of hip, not elsewhere classified
    - M24.351 Pathological dislocation of right hip, not elsewhere classified
      AHA CC: 1Q, 2022, 32
    - M24.352 Pathological dislocation of left hip, not elsewhere classified
      AHA CC: 1Q, 2022, 32
    - M24.359 Pathological dislocation of unspecified hip, not elsewhere classified
  - + M24.36 Pathological dislocation of knee, not elsewhere classified
    - M24.361 Pathological dislocation of right knee, not elsewhere classified
    - M24.362 Pathological dislocation of left knee, not elsewhere classified
    - M24.369 Pathological dislocation of unspecified knee, not elsewhere classified
  - + M24.37 Pathological dislocation of ankle and foot, not elsewhere classified
    - M24.371 Pathological dislocation of right ankle, not elsewhere classified
    - M24.372 Pathological dislocation of left ankle, not elsewhere classified
    - M24.373 Pathological dislocation of unspecified ankle, not elsewhere classified
    - M24.374 Pathological dislocation of right foot, not elsewhere classified
    - M24.375 Pathological dislocation of left foot, not elsewhere classified
    - M24.376 Pathological dislocation of unspecified foot, not elsewhere classified
  - M24.39 Pathological dislocation of other specified joint, not elsewhere classified
- + **M24.4** **Recurrent dislocation of joint**
  Recurrent subluxation of joint
  Excludes2: *recurrent dislocation of patella (M22.0-M22.1)*
  recurrent vertebral dislocation (M43.3-, M43.4, M43.5-)
  - M24.40 Recurrent dislocation, unspecified joint
  - + M24.41 Recurrent dislocation, shoulder
    - M24.411 Recurrent dislocation, right shoulder
    - M24.412 Recurrent dislocation, left shoulder
    - M24.419 Recurrent dislocation, unspecified shoulder
  - + M24.42 Recurrent dislocation, elbow
    - M24.421 Recurrent dislocation, right elbow
    - M24.422 Recurrent dislocation, left elbow
    - M24.429 Recurrent dislocation, unspecified elbow
  - + M24.43 Recurrent dislocation, wrist
    - M24.431 Recurrent dislocation, right wrist
    - M24.432 Recurrent dislocation, left wrist
    - M24.439 Recurrent dislocation, unspecified wrist
  - + M24.44 Recurrent dislocation, hand and finger(s)
    - M24.441 Recurrent dislocation, right hand
    - M24.442 Recurrent dislocation, left hand
    - M24.443 Recurrent dislocation, unspecified hand
    - M24.444 Recurrent dislocation, right finger
    - M24.445 Recurrent dislocation, left finger
    - M24.446 Recurrent dislocation, unspecified finger
  - + M24.45 Recurrent dislocation, hip
    - M24.451 Recurrent dislocation, right hip
    - M24.452 Recurrent dislocation, left hip
    - M24.459 Recurrent dislocation, unspecified hip
  - + M24.46 Recurrent dislocation, knee
    - M24.461 Recurrent dislocation, right knee
    - M24.462 Recurrent dislocation, left knee
    - M24.469 Recurrent dislocation, unspecified knee
  - + M24.47 Recurrent dislocation, ankle, foot and toes
    - M24.471 Recurrent dislocation, right ankle
    - M24.472 Recurrent dislocation, left ankle
    - M24.473 Recurrent dislocation, unspecified ankle
    - M24.474 Recurrent dislocation, right foot
    - M24.475 Recurrent dislocation, left foot
    - M24.476 Recurrent dislocation, unspecified foot
    - M24.477 Recurrent dislocation, right toe(s)
    - M24.478 Recurrent dislocation, left toe(s)
    - M24.479 Recurrent dislocation, unspecified toe(s)
  - M24.49 Recurrent dislocation, other specified joint

- **M24.5 Contracture of joint**
  - *Excludes1:* contracture of muscle without contracture of joint (M62.4-)
    contracture of tendon (sheath) without contracture of joint (M62.4-)
    Dupuytren's contracture (M72.0)
  - *Excludes2:* acquired deformities of limbs (M20-M21)
  - AHA CC: 2Q, 2016, 6
  - M24.50 Contracture, unspecified joint
  - M24.51 Contracture, shoulder
    - M24.511 Contracture, right shoulder
    - M24.512 Contracture, left shoulder
    - M24.519 Contracture, unspecified shoulder
  - M24.52 Contracture, elbow
    - M24.521 Contracture, right elbow
    - M24.522 Contracture, left elbow
    - M24.529 Contracture, unspecified elbow
  - M24.53 Contracture, wrist
    - M24.531 Contracture, right wrist
    - M24.532 Contracture, left wrist
    - M24.539 Contracture, unspecified wrist
  - M24.54 Contracture, hand
    - M24.541 Contracture, right hand
    - M24.542 Contracture, left hand
    - M24.549 Contracture, unspecified hand
  - M24.55 Contracture, hip
    - M24.551 Contracture, right hip
    - M24.552 Contracture, left hip
    - M24.559 Contracture, unspecified hip
  - M24.56 Contracture, knee
    - M24.561 Contracture, right knee
    - M24.562 Contracture, left knee
    - M24.569 Contracture, unspecified knee
  - M24.57 Contracture, ankle and foot
    - M24.571 Contracture, right ankle
    - M24.572 Contracture, left ankle
    - M24.573 Contracture, unspecified ankle
    - M24.574 Contracture, right foot
    - M24.575 Contracture, left foot
    - M24.576 Contracture, unspecified foot
  - M24.59 Contracture, other specified joint
- **M24.6 Ankylosis of joint**
  - *Excludes1:* stiffness of joint without ankylosis (M25.6-)
  - *Excludes2:* spine (M43.2-)
  - M24.60 Ankylosis, unspecified joint
  - M24.61 Ankylosis, shoulder
    - M24.611 Ankylosis, right shoulder
    - M24.612 Ankylosis, left shoulder
    - M24.619 Ankylosis, unspecified shoulder
  - M24.62 Ankylosis, elbow
    - M24.621 Ankylosis, right elbow
    - M24.622 Ankylosis, left elbow
    - M24.629 Ankylosis, unspecified elbow
  - M24.63 Ankylosis, wrist
    - M24.631 Ankylosis, right wrist
    - M24.632 Ankylosis, left wrist
    - M24.639 Ankylosis, unspecified wrist
  - M24.64 Ankylosis, hand
    - M24.641 Ankylosis, right hand
    - M24.642 Ankylosis, left hand
    - M24.649 Ankylosis, unspecified hand
  - M24.65 Ankylosis, hip
    - M24.651 Ankylosis, right hip
    - M24.652 Ankylosis, left hip
    - M24.659 Ankylosis, unspecified hip
  - M24.66 Ankylosis, knee
    - M24.661 Ankylosis, right knee
    - M24.662 Ankylosis, left knee
    - M24.669 Ankylosis, unspecified knee
  - M24.67 Ankylosis, ankle and foot
    - M24.671 Ankylosis, right ankle
    - M24.672 Ankylosis, left ankle
    - M24.673 Ankylosis, unspecified ankle
    - M24.674 Ankylosis, right foot
    - M24.675 Ankylosis, left foot
    - M24.676 Ankylosis, unspecified foot
  - M24.69 Ankylosis, other specified joint
- M24.7 Protrusio acetabuli

- **M24.8 Other specific joint derangements, not elsewhere classified**
  - *Excludes2:* iliotibial band syndrome (M76.3)
  - M24.80 Other specific joint derangements of unspecified joint, not elsewhere classified
  - M24.81 Other specific joint derangements of shoulder, not elsewhere classified
    - M24.811 Other specific joint derangements of right shoulder, not elsewhere classified
    - M24.812 Other specific joint derangements of left shoulder, not elsewhere classified
    - M24.819 Other specific joint derangements of unspecified shoulder, not elsewhere classified
  - M24.82 Other specific joint derangements of elbow, not elsewhere classified
    - M24.821 Other specific joint derangements of right elbow, not elsewhere classified
    - M24.822 Other specific joint derangements of left elbow, not elsewhere classified
    - M24.829 Other specific joint derangements of unspecified elbow, not elsewhere classified
  - M24.83 Other specific joint derangements of wrist, not elsewhere classified
    - M24.831 Other specific joint derangements of right wrist, not elsewhere classified
    - M24.832 Other specific joint derangements of left wrist, not elsewhere classified
    - M24.839 Other specific joint derangements of unspecified wrist, not elsewhere classified
  - M24.84 Other specific joint derangements of hand, not elsewhere classified
    - M24.841 Other specific joint derangements of right hand, not elsewhere classified
    - M24.842 Other specific joint derangements of left hand, not elsewhere classified
    - M24.849 Other specific joint derangements of unspecified hand, not elsewhere classified
  - M24.85 Other specific joint derangements of hip, not elsewhere classified
    - Irritable hip
    - M24.851 Other specific joint derangements of right hip, not elsewhere classified
    - M24.852 Other specific joint derangements of left hip, not elsewhere classified
    - M24.859 Other specific joint derangements of unspecified hip, not elsewhere classified
  - M24.87 Other specific joint derangements of ankle and foot, not elsewhere classified
    - M24.871 Other specific joint derangements of right ankle, not elsewhere classified
    - M24.872 Other specific joint derangements of left ankle, not elsewhere classified
    - M24.873 Other specific joint derangements of unspecified ankle, not elsewhere classified
    - M24.874 Other specific joint derangements of right foot, not elsewhere classified
    - M24.875 Other specific joint derangements left foot, not elsewhere classified
    - M24.876 Other specific joint derangements of unspecified foot, not elsewhere classified
  - M24.89 Other specific joint derangement of other specified joint, not elsewhere classified
- M24.9 Joint derangement, unspecified

M25 Other joint disorder, not elsewhere classified

Excludes2: abnormality of gait and mobility (R26.-)
acquired deformities of limb (M20-M21)
calcification of bursa (M71.4-)
calcification of shoulder (joint) (M75.3)
calcification of tendon (M65.2-)
difficulty in walking (R26.2)
temporomandibular joint disorder (M26.6-)

AHA CC: 4Q, 2020, 31-32

- **M25.0 Hemarthrosis**
  - *Excludes1:* current injury - see injury of joint by body region
    hemophilic arthropathy (M36.2)
  - CC M25.00 Hemarthrosis, unspecified joint

+ **M25.01** Hemarthrosis, shoulder
    CC **M25.011** Hemarthrosis, right shoulder
    CC **M25.012** Hemarthrosis, left shoulder
    CC **M25.019** Hemarthrosis, unspecified shoulder
+ **M25.02** Hemarthrosis, elbow
    CC **M25.021** Hemarthrosis, right elbow
    CC **M25.022** Hemarthrosis, left elbow
    CC **M25.029** Hemarthrosis, unspecified elbow
+ **M25.03** Hemarthrosis, wrist
    CC **M25.031** Hemarthrosis, right wrist
    CC **M25.032** Hemarthrosis, left wrist
    CC **M25.039** Hemarthrosis, unspecified wrist
+ **M25.04** Hemarthrosis, hand
    CC **M25.041** Hemarthrosis, right hand
    CC **M25.042** Hemarthrosis, left hand
    CC **M25.049** Hemarthrosis, unspecified hand
+ **M25.05** Hemarthrosis, hip
    CC **M25.051** Hemarthrosis, right hip
    CC **M25.052** Hemarthrosis, left hip
    CC **M25.059** Hemarthrosis, unspecified hip
+ **M25.06** Hemarthrosis, knee
    CC **M25.061** Hemarthrosis, right knee
    CC **M25.062** Hemarthrosis, left knee
    CC **M25.069** Hemarthrosis, unspecified knee
+ **M25.07** Hemarthrosis, ankle and foot
    CC **M25.071** Hemarthrosis, right ankle
    CC **M25.072** Hemarthrosis, left ankle
    CC **M25.073** Hemarthrosis, unspecified ankle
    CC **M25.074** Hemarthrosis, right foot
    CC **M25.075** Hemarthrosis, left foot
    CC **M25.076** Hemarthrosis, unspecified foot
CC **M25.08** Hemarthrosis, other specified site
    Hemarthrosis, vertebrae
+ **M25.1** Fistula of joint
    M25.10 Fistula, unspecified joint
+ **M25.11** Fistula, shoulder
    M25.111 Fistula, right shoulder
    M25.112 Fistula, left shoulder
    M25.119 Fistula, unspecified shoulder
+ **M25.12** Fistula, elbow
    M25.121 Fistula, right elbow
    M25.122 Fistula, left elbow
    M25.129 Fistula, unspecified elbow
+ **M25.13** Fistula, wrist
    M25.131 Fistula, right wrist
    M25.132 Fistula, left wrist
    M25.139 Fistula, unspecified wrist
+ **M25.14** Fistula, hand
    M25.141 Fistula, right hand
    M25.142 Fistula, left hand
    M25.149 Fistula, unspecified hand
+ **M25.15** Fistula, hip
    M25.151 Fistula, right hip
    M25.152 Fistula, left hip
    M25.159 Fistula, unspecified hip
+ **M25.16** Fistula, knee
    M25.161 Fistula, right knee
    M25.162 Fistula, left knee
    M25.169 Fistula, unspecified knee
+ **M25.17** Fistula, ankle and foot
    M25.171 Fistula, right ankle
    M25.172 Fistula, left ankle
    M25.173 Fistula, unspecified ankle
    M25.174 Fistula, right foot
    M25.175 Fistula, left foot
    M25.176 Fistula, unspecified foot
M25.18 Fistula, other specified site
    Fistula, vertebrae
+ **M25.2** Flail joint
    M25.20 Flail joint, unspecified joint
+ **M25.21** Flail joint, shoulder
    M25.211 Flail joint, right shoulder
    M25.212 Flail joint, left shoulder
    M25.219 Flail joint, unspecified shoulder
+ **M25.22** Flail joint, elbow
    M25.221 Flail joint, right elbow
    M25.222 Flail joint, left elbow
    M25.229 Flail joint, unspecified elbow
+ **M25.23** Flail joint, wrist
    M25.231 Flail joint, right wrist
    M25.232 Flail joint, left wrist
    M25.239 Flail joint, unspecified wrist
+ **M25.24** Flail joint, hand
    M25.241 Flail joint, right hand
    M25.242 Flail joint, left hand
    M25.249 Flail joint, unspecified hand
+ **M25.25** Flail joint, hip
    M25.251 Flail joint, right hip
    M25.252 Flail joint, left hip
    M25.259 Flail joint, unspecified hip
+ **M25.26** Flail joint, knee
    M25.261 Flail joint, right knee
    M25.262 Flail joint, left knee
    M25.269 Flail joint, unspecified knee
+ **M25.27** Flail joint, ankle and foot
    M25.271 Flail joint, right ankle and foot
    M25.272 Flail joint, left ankle and foot
    M25.279 Flail joint, unspecified ankle and foot
M25.28 Flail joint, other site
+ **M25.3** Other instability of joint
    Excludes1: *instability of joint secondary to old ligament injury (M24.2-)*
    instability of joint secondary to removal of joint prosthesis (M96.8-)
    Excludes2: *spinal instabilities (M53.2-)*
    M25.30 Other instability, unspecified joint
+ **M25.31** Other instability, shoulder
    M25.311 Other instability, right shoulder
    M25.312 Other instability, left shoulder
    M25.319 Other instability, unspecified shoulder
+ **M25.32** Other instability, elbow
    M25.321 Other instability, right elbow
    M25.322 Other instability, left elbow
    M25.329 Other instability, unspecified elbow
+ **M25.33** Other instability, wrist
    M25.331 Other instability, right wrist
    M25.332 Other instability, left wrist
    M25.339 Other instability, unspecified wrist
+ **M25.34** Other instability, hand
    M25.341 Other instability, right hand
    M25.342 Other instability, left hand
    M25.349 Other instability, unspecified hand
+ **M25.35** Other instability, hip
    M25.351 Other instability, right hip
    M25.352 Other instability, left hip
    M25.359 Other instability, unspecified hip
+ **M25.36** Other instability, knee
    M25.361 Other instability, right knee
    M25.362 Other instability, left knee
    M25.369 Other instability, unspecified knee
+ **M25.37** Other instability, ankle and foot
    M25.371 Other instability, right ankle
    M25.372 Other instability, left ankle
    M25.373 Other instability, unspecified ankle
    M25.374 Other instability, right foot
    M25.375 Other instability, left foot
    M25.376 Other instability, unspecified foot
M25.39 Other instability, other specified joint
+ **M25.4** Effusion of joint
    Excludes1: *hydrarthrosis in yaws (A66.6)*
    intermittent hydrarthrosis (M12.4-)
    other infective (teno)synovitis (M65.1-)
    M25.40 Effusion, unspecified joint
+ **M25.41** Effusion, shoulder
    M25.411 Effusion, right shoulder
    M25.412 Effusion, left shoulder
    M25.419 Effusion, unspecified shoulder
+ **M25.42** Effusion, elbow
    M25.421 Effusion, right elbow
    M25.422 Effusion, left elbow
    M25.429 Effusion, unspecified elbow
+ **M25.43** Effusion, wrist
    M25.431 Effusion, right wrist
    M25.432 Effusion, left wrist
    M25.439 Effusion, unspecified wrist

+ M25.44 Effusion, hand
    M25.441 Effusion, right hand
    M25.442 Effusion, left hand
    M25.449 Effusion, unspecified hand
+ M25.45 Effusion, hip
    M25.451 Effusion, right hip
    M25.452 Effusion, left hip
    M25.459 Effusion, unspecified hip
+ M25.46 Effusion, knee
    M25.461 Effusion, right knee
    M25.462 Effusion, left knee
    M25.469 Effusion, unspecified knee
+ M25.47 Effusion, ankle and foot
    M25.471 Effusion, right ankle
    M25.472 Effusion, left ankle
    M25.473 Effusion, unspecified ankle
    M25.474 Effusion, right foot
    M25.475 Effusion, left foot
    M25.476 Effusion, unspecified foot
  M25.48 Effusion, other site
+ M25.5 Pain in joint
    Excludes2: pain in hand (M79.64-)
                  pain in fingers (M79.64-)
                    pain in foot (M79.67-)
                    pain in limb (M79.6-)
                    pain in toes (M79.67-)
    AHA CC: 4Q, 2016, 38
  M25.50 Pain in unspecified joint
+ M25.51 Pain in shoulder
    M25.511 Pain in right shoulder
    M25.512 Pain in left shoulder
    M25.519 Pain in unspecified shoulder
+ M25.52 Pain in elbow
    M25.521 Pain in right elbow
    M25.522 Pain in left elbow
    M25.529 Pain in unspecified elbow
+ M25.53 Pain in wrist
    M25.531 Pain in right wrist
    M25.532 Pain in left wrist
    M25.539 Pain in unspecified wrist
+ M25.54 Pain in joints of hand
    M25.541 Pain in joints of right hand
    M25.542 Pain in joints of left hand
    M25.549 Pain in joints of unspecified hand
            Pain in joints of hand NOS
+ M25.55 Pain in hip
    M25.551 Pain in right hip
    M25.552 Pain in left hip
    M25.559 Pain in unspecified hip
+ M25.56 Pain in knee
    M25.561 Pain in right knee
    M25.562 Pain in left knee
    M25.569 Pain in unspecified knee
+ M25.57 Pain in ankle and joints of foot
    M25.571 Pain in right ankle and joints of right foot
    M25.572 Pain in left ankle and joints of left foot
    M25.579 Pain in unspecified ankle and joints of unspecified foot
  M25.59 Pain in other specified joint
+ M25.6 Stiffness of joint, not elsewhere classified
    Excludes1: ankylosis of joint (M24.6-)
                    contracture of joint (M24.5-)
  M25.60 Stiffness of unspecified joint, not elsewhere classified
+ M25.61 Stiffness of shoulder, not elsewhere classified
    M25.611 Stiffness of right shoulder, not elsewhere classified
    M25.612 Stiffness of left shoulder, not elsewhere classified
    M25.619 Stiffness of unspecified shoulder, not elsewhere classified
+ M25.62 Stiffness of elbow, not elsewhere classified
    M25.621 Stiffness of right elbow, not elsewhere classified
    M25.622 Stiffness of left elbow, not elsewhere classified
    M25.629 Stiffness of unspecified elbow, not elsewhere classified
+ M25.63 Stiffness of wrist, not elsewhere classified
    M25.631 Stiffness of right wrist, not elsewhere classified
    M25.632 Stiffness of left wrist, not elsewhere classified
    M25.639 Stiffness of unspecified wrist, not elsewhere classified
+ M25.64 Stiffness of hand, not elsewhere classified
    M25.641 Stiffness of right hand, not elsewhere classified
    M25.642 Stiffness of left hand, not elsewhere classified
    M25.649 Stiffness of unspecified hand, not elsewhere classified
+ M25.65 Stiffness of hip, not elsewhere classified
    M25.651 Stiffness of right hip, not elsewhere classified
    M25.652 Stiffness of left hip, not elsewhere classified
    M25.659 Stiffness of unspecified hip, not elsewhere classified
+ M25.66 Stiffness of knee, not elsewhere classified
    M25.661 Stiffness of right knee, not elsewhere classified
    M25.662 Stiffness of left knee, not elsewhere classified
    M25.669 Stiffness of unspecified knee, not elsewhere classified
+ M25.67 Stiffness of ankle and foot, not elsewhere classified
    M25.671 Stiffness of right ankle, not elsewhere classified
    M25.672 Stiffness of left ankle, not elsewhere classified
    M25.673 Stiffness of unspecified ankle, not elsewhere classified
    M25.674 Stiffness of right foot, not elsewhere classified
    M25.675 Stiffness of left foot, not elsewhere classified
    M25.676 Stiffness of unspecified foot, not elsewhere classified
  M25.69 Stiffness of other specified joint, not elsewhere classified
+ M25.7 Osteophyte
  M25.70 Osteophyte, unspecified joint
+ M25.71 Osteophyte, shoulder
    M25.711 Osteophyte, right shoulder
    M25.712 Osteophyte, left shoulder
    M25.719 Osteophyte, unspecified shoulder
+ M25.72 Osteophyte, elbow
    M25.721 Osteophyte, right elbow
    M25.722 Osteophyte, left elbow
    M25.729 Osteophyte, unspecified elbow
+ M25.73 Osteophyte, wrist
    M25.731 Osteophyte, right wrist
    M25.732 Osteophyte, left wrist
    M25.739 Osteophyte, unspecified wrist
+ M25.74 Osteophyte, hand
    M25.741 Osteophyte, right hand
    M25.742 Osteophyte, left hand
    M25.749 Osteophyte, unspecified hand
+ M25.75 Osteophyte, hip
    M25.751 Osteophyte, right hip
    M25.752 Osteophyte, left hip
    M25.759 Osteophyte, unspecified hip
+ M25.76 Osteophyte, knee
    M25.761 Osteophyte, right knee
    M25.762 Osteophyte, left knee
    M25.769 Osteophyte, unspecified knee
+ M25.77 Osteophyte, ankle and foot
    M25.771 Osteophyte, right ankle
    M25.772 Osteophyte, left ankle
    M25.773 Osteophyte, unspecified ankle
    M25.774 Osteophyte, right foot
    M25.775 Osteophyte, left foot
    M25.776 Osteophyte, unspecified foot
  M25.78 Osteophyte, vertebrae

- **M25.8 Other specified joint disorders**
  - M25.80 Other specified joint disorders, unspecified joint
  - **M25.81 Other specified joint disorders, shoulder**
    - M25.811 Other specified joint disorders, right shoulder
    - M25.812 Other specified joint disorders, left shoulder
      AHA CC: 3Q, 2022, 18-19
    - M25.819 Other specified joint disorders, unspecified shoulder
  - **M25.82 Other specified joint disorders, elbow**
    - M25.821 Other specified joint disorders, right elbow
    - M25.822 Other specified joint disorders, left elbow
    - M25.829 Other specified joint disorders, unspecified elbow
  - **M25.83 Other specified joint disorders, wrist**
    - M25.831 Other specified joint disorders, right wrist
    - M25.832 Other specified joint disorders, left wrist
    - M25.839 Other specified joint disorders, unspecified wrist
  - **M25.84 Other specified joint disorders, hand**
    - M25.841 Other specified joint disorders, right hand
    - M25.842 Other specified joint disorders, left hand
    - M25.849 Other specified joint disorders, unspecified hand
  - **M25.85 Other specified joint disorders, hip**
    - M25.851 Other specified joint disorders, right hip
    - M25.852 Other specified joint disorders, left hip
      AHA CC: 4Q, 2014, 25
    - M25.859 Other specified joint disorders, unspecified hip
  - **M25.86 Other specified joint disorders, knee**
    - M25.861 Other specified joint disorders, right knee
    - M25.862 Other specified joint disorders, left knee
    - M25.869 Other specified joint disorders, unspecified knee
  - **M25.87 Other specified joint disorders, ankle and foot**
    - M25.871 Other specified joint disorders, right ankle and foot
    - M25.872 Other specified joint disorders, left ankle and foot
    - M25.879 Other specified joint disorders, unspecified ankle and foot
- M25.9 Joint disorder, unspecified

Dentofacial anomalies [including malocclusion] and other disorders of jaw (M26-M27)

Excludes1: hemifacial atrophy or hypertrophy (Q67.4)
unilateral condylar hyperplasia or hypoplasia (M27.8)

M26 Dentofacial anomalies [including malocclusion]

- **M26.0 Major anomalies of jaw size**
  - **Excludes1:** acromegaly (E22.0)
    Robin's syndrome (Q87.0)
  - M26.00 Unspecified anomaly of jaw size
  - M26.01 Maxillary hyperplasia
  - M26.02 Maxillary hypoplasia
    AHA CC: 3Q, 2014, 23-24
  - M26.03 Mandibular hyperplasia
  - M26.04 Mandibular hypoplasia
  - M26.05 Macrogenia
  - M26.06 Microgenia
  - M26.07 Excessive tuberosity of jaw
    Entire maxillary tuberosity
  - M26.09 Other specified anomalies of jaw size
- **M26.1 Anomalies of jaw-cranial base relationship**
  - M26.10 Unspecified anomaly of jaw-cranial base relationship
  - M26.11 Maxillary asymmetry
  - M26.12 Other jaw asymmetry
  - M26.19 Other specified anomalies of jaw-cranial base relationship
    AHA CC: 1Q, 2020, 21
- **M26.2 Anomalies of dental arch relationship**
  - M26.20 Unspecified anomaly of dental arch relationship
  - **M26.21 Malocclusion, Angle's class**
    - M26.211 Malocclusion, Angle's class I
      Neutro-occlusion
    - M26.212 Malocclusion, Angle's class II
      Disto-occlusion Division I
      Disto-occlusion Division II
    - M26.213 Malocclusion, Angle's class III
      Mesio-occlusion
    - M26.219 Malocclusion, Angle's class, unspecified
  - **M26.22 Open occlusal relationship**
    - M26.220 Open anterior occlusal relationship
      Anterior open bite
    - M26.221 Open posterior occlusal relationship
      Posterior open bite
  - M26.23 Excessive horizontal overlap
    Excessive horizontal overjet
  - M26.24 Reverse articulation
    Crossbite (anterior) (posterior)
  - M26.25 Anomalies of interarch distance
  - M26.29 Other anomalies of dental arch relationship
    Midline deviation of dental arch
    Overbite (excessive) deep
    Overbite (excessive) horizontal
    Overbite (excessive) vertical
    Posterior lingual occlusion of mandibular teeth
- **M26.3 Anomalies of tooth position of fully erupted tooth or teeth**
  - **Excludes2:** embedded and impacted teeth (K01.-)
  - M26.30 Unspecified anomaly of tooth position of fully erupted tooth or teeth
    Abnormal spacing of fully erupted tooth or teeth NOS
    Displacement of fully erupted tooth or teeth NOS
    Transposition of fully erupted tooth or teeth NOS
  - M26.31 Crowding of fully erupted teeth
  - M26.32 Excessive spacing of fully erupted teeth
    Diastema of fully erupted tooth or teeth NOS
  - M26.33 Horizontal displacement of fully erupted tooth or teeth
    Tipped tooth or teeth
    Tipping of fully erupted tooth
  - M26.34 Vertical displacement of fully erupted tooth or teeth
    Extruded tooth
    Infraeruption of tooth or teeth
    Supraeruption of tooth or teeth
  - M26.35 Rotation of fully erupted tooth or teeth
  - M26.36 Insufficient interocclusal distance of fully erupted teeth (ridge)
    Lack of adequate intermaxillary vertical dimension of fully erupted teeth
  - M26.37 Excessive interocclusal distance of fully erupted teeth
    Excessive intermaxillary vertical dimension of fully erupted teeth
    Loss of occlusal vertical dimension of fully erupted teeth
  - M26.39 Other anomalies of tooth position of fully erupted tooth or teeth
- M26.4 Malocclusion, unspecified
- **M26.5 Dentofacial functional abnormalities**
  - **Excludes1:** bruxism (F45.8)
    teeth-grinding NOS (F45.8)
  - M26.50 Dentofacial functional abnormalities, unspecified
  - M26.51 Abnormal jaw closure
  - M26.52 Limited mandibular range of motion
  - M26.53 Deviation in opening and closing of the mandible
  - M26.54 Insufficient anterior guidance
    Insufficient anterior occlusal guidance
  - M26.55 Centric occlusion maximum intercuspation discrepancy
    Excludes1: centric occlusion NOS (M26.59)
  - M26.56 Non-working side interference
    Balancing side interference
  - M26.57 Lack of posterior occlusal support
  - M26.59 Other dentofacial functional abnormalities
    Centric occlusion (of teeth) NOS
    Malocclusion due to abnormal swallowing
    Malocclusion due to mouth breathing
    Malocclusion due to tongue, lip or finger habits

- **M26.6 Temporomandibular joint disorders**
    Excludes2: current temporomandibular joint dislocation (S03.0)
    current temporomandibular joint sprain (S03.4)
    AHA CC: 4Q, 2016, 38-39
    - **M26.60 Temporomandibular joint disorder, unspecified**
        - M26.601 Right temporomandibular joint disorder, unspecified
        - M26.602 Left temporomandibular joint disorder, unspecified
        - M26.603 Bilateral temporomandibular joint disorder, unspecified
        - M26.609 Unspecified temporomandibular joint disorder, unspecified side
            Temporomandibular joint disorder NOS
    - **M26.61 Adhesions and ankylosis of temporomandibular joint**
        - M26.611 Adhesions and ankylosis of right temporomandibular joint
        - M26.612 Adhesions and ankylosis of left temporomandibular joint
        - M26.613 Adhesions and ankylosis of bilateral temporomandibular joint
        - M26.619 Adhesions and ankylosis of temporomandibular joint, unspecified side
    - **M26.62 Arthralgia of temporomandibular joint**
        - M26.621 Arthralgia of right temporomandibular joint
        - M26.622 Arthralgia of left temporomandibular joint
        - M26.623 Arthralgia of bilateral temporomandibular joint
        - M26.629 Arthralgia of temporomandibular joint, unspecified side
    - **M26.63 Articular disc disorder of temporomandibular joint**
        - M26.631 Articular disc disorder of right temporomandibular joint
        - M26.632 Articular disc disorder of left temporomandibular joint
        - M26.633 Articular disc disorder of bilateral temporomandibular joint
        - M26.639 Articular disc disorder of temporomandibular joint, unspecified side
    - **M26.64 Arthritis of temporomandibular joint**
        AHA CC: 4Q, 2020, 32
        - M26.641 Arthritis of right temporomandibular joint
        - M26.642 Arthritis of left temporomandibular joint
        - M26.643 Arthritis of bilateral temporomandibular joint
        - M26.649 Arthritis of unspecified temporomandibular joint
    - **M26.65 Arthropathy of temporomandibular joing**
        AHA CC: 4Q, 2020, 32
        - M26.651 Arthropathy of right temporomandibular joint
        - M26.652 Arthropathy of left temporomandibular joint
        - M26.653 Arthropathy of bilateral temporomandibular joint
        - M26.659 Arthropathy of unspecified temporomandibular joint
    - M26.69 Other specified disorders of temporomandibular joint
- **M26.7 Dental alveolar anomalies**
    - M26.70 Unspecified alveolar anomaly
    - M26.71 Alveolar maxillary hyperplasia
    - M26.72 Alveolar mandibular hyperplasia
    - M26.73 Alveolar maxillary hypoplasia
    - M26.74 Alveolar mandibular hypoplasia
    - M26.79 Other specified alveolar anomalies
- **M26.8 Other dentofacial anomalies**
    - M26.81 Anterior soft tissue impingement
        Anterior soft tissue impingement on teeth
    - M26.82 Posterior soft tissue impingement
        Posterior soft tissue impingement on teeth
    - M26.89 Other dentofacial anomalies
- **M26.9 Dentofacial anomaly, unspecified**

M27 Other diseases of jaws
- **M27.0 Developmental disorders of jaws**
    Latent bone cyst of jaw
    Stafne's cyst
    Torus mandibularis
    Torus palatinus
- **M27.1 Giant cell granuloma, central**
    Giant cell granuloma NOS
    Excludes1: peripheral giant cell granuloma (K06.8)
- **M27.2 Inflammatory conditions of jaws**
    Osteitis of jaw(s)
    Osteomyelitis (neonatal) jaw(s)
    Osteoradionecrosis jaw(s)
    Periostitis jaw(s)
    Sequestrum of jaw bone
    Use additional code (W88-W90, X39.0) to identify radiation, if radiation-induced
    Excludes2: osteonecrosis of jaw due to drug (M87.180)
- **M27.3 Alveolitis of jaws**
    Alveolar osteitis
    Dry socket
- **M27.4 Other and unspecified cysts of jaw**
    Excludes1: cysts of oral region (K09.-)
    latent bone cyst of jaw (M27.0)
    Stafne's cyst (M27.0)
    - **M27.40 Unspecified cyst of jaw**
        Cyst of jaw NOS
    - **M27.49 Other cysts of jaw**
        Aneurysmal cyst of jaw
        Hemorrhagic cyst of jaw
        Traumatic cyst of jaw
- **M27.5 Periradicular pathology associated with previous endodontic treatment**
    - M27.51 Perforation of root canal space due to endodontic treatment
    - M27.52 Endodontic overfill
    - M27.53 Endodontic underfill
    - M27.59 Other periradicular pathology associated with previous endodontic treatment
- **M27.6 Endosseous dental implant failure**
    - **M27.61 Osseointegration failure of dental implant**
        Hemorrhagic complications of dental implant placement
        Iatrogenic osseointegration failure of dental implant
        Osseointegration failure of dental implant due to complications of systemic disease
        Osseointegration failure of dental implant due to poor bone quality
        Pre-integration failure of dental implant NOS
        Pre-osseointegration failure of dental implant
    - **M27.62 Post-osseointegration biological failure of dental implant**
        Failure of dental implant due to lack of attached gingiva
        Failure of dental implant due to occlusal trauma (caused by poor prosthetic design)
        Failure of dental implant due to parafunctional habits
        Failure of dental implant due to periodontal infection (peri-implantitis)
        Failure of dental implant due to poor oral hygiene
        Iatrogenic post-osseointegration failure of dental implant
        Post-osseointegration failure of dental implant due to complications of systemic disease
    - **M27.63 Post-osseointegration mechanical failure of dental implant**
        Failure of dental prosthesis causing loss of dental implant
        Fracture of dental implant
        Excludes2: cracked tooth (K03.81)
        fractured dental restorative material with loss of material (K08.531)
        fractured dental restorative material without loss of material (K08.530)
        fractured tooth (S02.5)
    - **M27.69 Other endosseous dental implant failure**
        Dental implant failure NOS

M27.8 Other specified diseases of jaws
- Cherubism
- Exostosis
- Fibrous dysplasia
- Unilateral condylar hyperplasia
- Unilateral condylar hypoplasia
- **Excludes1:** jaw pain (R68.84)

M27.9 Disease of jaws, unspecified

Systemic connective tissue disorders (M30-M36)

Includes: autoimmune disease NOS
collagen (vascular) disease NOS
systemic autoimmune disease
systemic collagen (vascular) disease

Excludes1: autoimmune disease, single organ or single cell-type -code to relevant condition category

M30 Polyarteritis nodosa and related conditions
Excludes1: microscopic polyarteritis (M31.7)
- CC **M30.0** Polyarteritis nodosa
- CC **M30.1** Polyarteritis with lung involvement [Churg-Strauss]
  - Allergic granulomatous angiitis
  - Eosinophilic granulomatosis with polyangiitis [EGPA]
  - *AHA CC: 1Q, 2021, 23*
- CC **M30.2** Juvenile polyarteritis
- CC **M30.3** Mucocutaneous lymph node syndrome [Kawasaki]
- CC **M30.8** Other conditions related to polyarteritis nodosa
  - Polyangiitis overlap syndrome

M31 Other necrotizing vasculopathies
- CC **M31.0** Hypersensitivity angiitis
  - Goodpasture's syndrome
- + **M31.1** Thrombotic microangiopathy
  - *AHA CC: 4Q, 2021, 19*
  - MCC **M31.10** Thrombotic microangiopathy, unspecified
  - MCC **M31.11** Hematopoietic stem cell transplantation-associated thrombotic microangiopathy [HSCT-TMA]
    - Transplant-associated thrombotic microangiopathy [TA-TMA]
    - Code first if applicable:
      - complications of bone marrow transplant (T86.0-)
      - complications of stem cell transplant (T86.5)
    - Use additional code to identify specific organ dysfunction, such as:
      - acute kidney failure (N17.-)
      - acute respiratory distress syndrome (J80)
      - capillary leak syndrome (I78.8)
      - diffuse alveolar hemorrhage (R04.89)
      - encephalopathy (metabolic) (septic) G93.41
      - fluid overload, unspecified (E87.70)
      - graft versus host disease (D89.81-)
      - hemolytic uremic syndrome (D59.3-)
      - hepatic failure (K72.-)
      - hepatic veno-occlusive disease (K76.5)
      - idiopathic interstitial pneumonia (J84.11-)
      - sinusoidal obstruction syndrome (K76.5)
  - MCC **M31.19** Other thrombotic microangiopathy
    - Thrombotic thrombocytopenic purpura
- CC **M31.2** Lethal midline granuloma
- + **M31.3** Wegener's granulomatosis
  - Granulomatosis with polyangiitis
  - Necrotizing respiratory granulomatosis
  - *AHA CC: 1Q, 2021, 23*
  - CC **M31.30** Wegener's granulomatosis without renal involvement
    - Wegener's granulomatosis NOS
    - *AHA CC: 2Q, 2021, 10*
  - CC **M31.31** Wegener's granulomatosis with renal involvement
- CC **M31.4** Aortic arch syndrome [Takayasu]
- **M31.5** Giant cell arteritis with polymyalgia rheumatica
- **M31.6** Other giant cell arteritis
- CC **M31.7** Microscopic polyangiitis
  - Microscopic polyarteritis
  - **Excludes1:** polyarteritis nodosa (M30.0)
  - *AHA CC: 1Q, 2021, 23*
- CC **M31.8** Other specified necrotizing vasculopathies
  - Hypocomplementemic vasculitis
  - Septic vasculitis
- CC **M31.9** Necrotizing vasculopathy, unspecified

M32 Systemic lupus erythematosus (SLE)
Excludes1: lupus erythematosus (discoid) (NOS) (L93.0)
AHA CC: 3Q, 2018, 14-15
- **M32.0** Drug-induced systemic lupus erythematosus
  - Use additional code for adverse effect, if applicable, to identify drug (T36-T50 with fifth or sixth character 5)
- + **M32.1** Systemic lupus erythematosus with organ or system involvement
  - **M32.10** Systemic lupus erythematosus, organ or system involvement unspecified
  - CC **M32.11** Endocarditis in systemic lupus erythematosus
    - Libman-Sacks disease
  - CC **M32.12** Pericarditis in systemic lupus erythematosus
    - Lupus pericarditis
  - **M32.13** Lung involvement in systemic lupus erythematosus
    - Pleural effusion due to systemic lupus erythematosus
  - **M32.14** Glomerular disease in systemic lupus erythematosus
    - Lupus renal disease NOS
    - *AHA CC: 4Q, 2013, 125*
  - **M32.15** Tubulo-interstitial nephropathy in systemic lupus erythematosus
  - **M32.19** Other organ or system involvement in systemic lupus erythematosus
    - Use Additional code(s) to identify organ or system involvement, such as encephalitis (G05.3)
- **M32.8** Other forms of systemic lupus erythematosus
- **M32.9** Systemic lupus erythematosus, unspecified
  - SLE NOS
  - Systemic lupus erythematosus NOS
  - Systemic lupus erythematosus without organ involvement
  - *AHA CC: 3Q, 2018, 14-15; 4Q, 2020, 11*

M33 Dermatopolymyositis
- + **M33.0** Juvenile dermatomyositis
  - CC **M33.00** Juvenile dermatomyositis, organ involvement unspecified
  - CC **M33.01** Juvenile dermatomyositis with respiratory involvement
  - CC **M33.02** Juvenile dermatomyositis with myopathy
  - CC **M33.03** Juvenile dermatomyositis without myopathy
    - *AHA CC: 4Q, 2017, 18*
  - CC **M33.09** Juvenile dermatomyositis with other organ involvement
- + **M33.1** Other dermatomyositis
  - Adult dematomyositis
  - CC **M33.10** Other dermatomyositis, organ involvement unspecified
  - CC **M33.11** Other dermatomyositis with respiratory involvement
  - CC **M33.12** Other dermatomyositis with myopathy
  - CC **M33.13** Other dermatomyositis without myopathy
    - Dermatomyositis NOS
    - *AHA CC: 4Q, 2017, 18*
  - CC **M33.19** Other dermatomyositis with other organ involvement
- + **M33.2** Polymyositis
  - CC **M33.20** Polymyositis, organ involvement unspecified
  - CC **M33.21** Polymyositis with respiratory involvement
  - CC **M33.22** Polymyositis with myopathy
  - CC **M33.29** Polymyositis with other organ involvement
- + **M33.9** Dermatopolymyositis, unspecified
  - CC **M33.90** Dermatopolymyositis, unspecified, organ involvement unspecified
  - CC **M33.91** Dermatopolymyositis, unspecified with respiratory involvement
  - CC **M33.92** Dermatopolymyositis, unspecified with myopathy
  - CC **M33.93** Dermatopolymyositis, unspecified without myopathy
    - *AHA CC: 4Q, 2017, 18*
  - CC **M33.99** Dermatopolymyositis, unspecified with other organ involvement

M34 Systemic sclerosis [scleroderma]
Excludes1: circumscribed scleroderma (L94.0)
neonatal scleroderma (P83.88)
- **M34.0** Progressive systemic sclerosis
- **M34.1** CR(E)ST syndrome
  - Combination of calcinosis, Raynaud's phenomenon, esophageal dysfunction, sclerodactyly, telangiectasia

M34.2 Systemic sclerosis induced by drug and chemical
   Code first poisoning due to drug or toxin, if applicable (T36-T65 with fifth or sixth character 1-4)
   Use additional code for adverse effect, if applicable, to identify drug (T36-T50 with fifth or sixth character 5)

+ **M34.8** Other forms of systemic sclerosis
   CC **M34.81** Systemic sclerosis with lung involvement
      Code also if applicable:
         other interstitial pulmonary diseases (J84.89)
         secondary pulmonary arterial hypertension (I27.21)
   CC **M34.82** Systemic sclerosis with myopathy
   M34.83 Systemic sclerosis with polyneuropathy
   M34.89 Other systemic sclerosis
M34.9 Systemic sclerosis, unspecified

M35 Other systemic involvement of connective tissue
   Excludes1: reactive perforating collagenosis (L87.1)
+ **M35.0** Sjögren syndrome
      Sicca syndrome
      Use additional code to identify associated manifestations
      Excludes1: dry mouth, unspecified (R68.2)
      AHA CC: 4Q, 2021, 20
   M35.00 Sjögren syndrome, unspecified
   M35.01 Sjögren syndrome with keratoconjunctivitis
   M35.02 Sjögren syndrome with lung involvement
   CC **M35.03** Sjögren syndrome with myopathy
   M35.04 Sjögren syndrome with tubulo-interstitial nephropathy
      Renal tubular acidosis in sicca syndrome
   M35.05 Sjögren syndrome with inflammatory arthritis
   M35.06 Sjögren syndrome with peripheral nervous system involvement
   CC **M35.07** Sjögren syndrome with central nervous system involvement
   M35.08 Sjögren syndrome with gastrointestinal involvement
   M35.0A Sjögren syndrome with glomerular disease
   M35.0B Sjögren syndrome with vasculitis
   M35.0C Sjögren syndrome with dental involvement
   M35.09 Sjögren syndrome with other organ involvement
CC **M35.1** Other overlap syndromes
      Mixed connective tissue disease
      Excludes1: polyangiitis overlap syndrome (M30.8)
CC **M35.2** Behçet's disease
M35.3 Polymyalgia rheumatica
      Excludes1: polymyalgia rheumatica with giant cell arteritis (M31.5)
M35.4 Diffuse (eosinophilic) fasciitis
CC **M35.5** Multifocal fibrosclerosis
M35.6 Relapsing panniculitis [Weber-Christian]
      Excludes1: lupus panniculitis (L93.2)
         panniculitis NOS (M79.3-)
M35.7 Hypermobility syndrome
      Familial ligamentous laxity
      Excludes1: ligamentous laxity, NOS (M24.2-)
      Excludes2: Ehlers-Danlos syndromes (Q79.6-)
M35.8 Other specified systemic involvement of connective tissue
      AHA CC: 3Q, 2020, 13-14; 1Q, 2021, 36-37
   CC **M35.81** Multisystem inflammatory syndrome
      MIS-A
      MIS-C
      Multisystem inflammatory syndrome in adults
      Multisystem inflammatory syndrome in children
      Pediatric inflammatory multisystem syndrome
      PIMS
      Code first, if applicable, COVID-19 (U07.1)

      Code also any associated complications such as:
         acute hepatic failure (K72.0-)
         acute kidney failure (N17.-)
         acute myocarditis (I40.-)
         acute respiratory distress syndrome (J80)
         cardiac arrhythmia (I47-I49.-)
         pneumonia due to COVID-19 (J12.82)
         severe sepsis (R65.2-)
         viral cardiomyopathy (B33.24)
         viral pericarditis (B33.23)

      Use additional code, if applicable, for:
         exposure to COVID-19 or SARS-CoV-2 infection (Z20.822)
         personal history of COVID-19 (Z86.16)
         post COVID-19 condition (U09.9)
      AHA CC: 1Q, 2021, 36-37, 41-42; 4Q, 2021, 102
   CC **M35.89** Other specified systemic involvement of connective tissue
   M35.9 Systemic involvement of connective tissue, unspecified
      Autoimmune disease (systemic) NOS
      Collagen (vascular) disease NOS

M36 Systemic disorders of connective tissue in diseases classified elsewhere
   Excludes2: arthropathies in diseases classified elsewhere (M14.-)
CC **M36.0** Dermato(poly)myositis in neoplastic disease
      Code first underlying neoplasm (C00-D49)
M36.1 Arthropathy in neoplastic disease
      Code first underlying neoplasm, such as:
         leukemia (C91-C95)
         malignant histiocytosis (C96.A)
         multiple myeloma (C90.0)
M36.2 Hemophilic arthropathy
      Hemarthrosis in hemophilic arthropathy
      Code first underlying disease, such as:
         factor VIII deficiency (D66)
            with vascular defect (D68.0-)
         factor IX deficiency (D67)
         hemophilia (classical) (D66)
         hemophilia B (D67)
         hemophilia C (D68.1)
M36.3 Arthropathy in other blood disorders
M36.4 Arthropathy in hypersensitivity reactions classified elsewhere
      Code first underlying disease, such as:
         Henoch (-Schönlein) purpura (D69.0)
         serum sickness (T80.6-)
M36.8 Systemic disorders of connective tissue in other diseases classified elsewhere
      Code first underlying disease, such as:
         alkaptonuria (E70.29)
         hypogammaglobulinemia (D80.-)
         ochronosis (E70.29)

DORSOPATHIES (M40-M54)

Deforming dorsopathies (M40-M43)

M40 Kyphosis and lordosis
   Code first underlying disease
   Excludes1: congenital kyphosis and lordosis (Q76.4)
      kyphoscoliosis (M41.-)
      postprocedural kyphosis and lordosis (M96.-)
+ **M40.0** Postural kyphosis
   Excludes1: osteochondrosis of spine (M42.-)
   M40.00 Postural kyphosis, site unspecified
   M40.03 Postural kyphosis, cervicothoracic region
   M40.04 Postural kyphosis, thoracic region
   M40.05 Postural kyphosis, thoracolumbar region
+ **M40.1** Other secondary kyphosis
   M40.10 Other secondary kyphosis, site unspecified
   M40.12 Other secondary kyphosis, cervical region
   M40.13 Other secondary kyphosis, cervicothoracic region
   M40.14 Other secondary kyphosis, thoracic region
   M40.15 Other secondary kyphosis, thoracolumbar region
+ **M40.2** Other and unspecified kyphosis
   + **M40.20** Unspecified kyphosis
      M40.202 Unspecified kyphosis, cervical region
      M40.203 Unspecified kyphosis, cervicothoracic region
      M40.204 Unspecified kyphosis, thoracic region
      M40.205 Unspecified kyphosis, thoracolumbar region
      M40.209 Unspecified kyphosis, site unspecified
   + **M40.29** Other kyphosis
      M40.292 Other kyphosis, cervical region
      M40.293 Other kyphosis, cervicothoracic region
      M40.294 Other kyphosis, thoracic region
      M40.295 Other kyphosis, thoracolumbar region
      M40.299 Other kyphosis, site unspecified

+ **M40.3 Flatback syndrome**
    M40.30 Flatback syndrome, site unspecified
    M40.35 Flatback syndrome, thoracolumbar region
    M40.36 Flatback syndrome, lumbar region
    M40.37 Flatback syndrome, lumbosacral region

+ **M40.4 Postural lordosis**
    Acquired lordosis
    M40.40 Postural lordosis, site unspecified
    M40.45 Postural lordosis, thoracolumbar region
    M40.46 Postural lordosis, lumbar region
    M40.47 Postural lordosis, lumbosacral region

+ **M40.5 Lordosis, unspecified**
    M40.50 Lordosis, unspecified, site unspecified
    M40.55 Lordosis, unspecified, thoracolumbar region
    M40.56 Lordosis, unspecified, lumbar region
    M40.57 Lordosis, unspecified, lumbosacral region

M41 Scoliosis
Includes: kyphoscoliosis
Excludes1: congenital scoliosis NOS (Q67.5)
    congenital scoliosis due to bony malformation (Q76.3)
    postural congenital scoliosis (Q67.5)
    kyphoscoliotic heart disease (I27.1)
Excludes2: postprocedural scoliosis (M96.89)
    postradiation scoliosis (M96.5)

+ **M41.0 Infantile idiopathic scoliosis**
    M41.00 Infantile idiopathic scoliosis, site unspecified
    M41.02 Infantile idiopathic scoliosis, cervical region
    M41.03 Infantile idiopathic scoliosis, cervicothoracic region
    M41.04 Infantile idiopathic scoliosis, thoracic region
        AHA CC: 4Q, 2014, 26-27
    M41.05 Infantile idiopathic scoliosis, thoracolumbar region
    M41.06 Infantile idiopathic scoliosis, lumbar region
    M41.07 Infantile idiopathic scoliosis, lumbosacral region
    M41.08 Infantile idiopathic scoliosis, sacral and sacrococcygeal region

+ **M41.1 Juvenile and adolescent idiopathic scoliosis**
  + **M41.11 Juvenile idiopathic scoliosis**
        M41.112 Juvenile idiopathic scoliosis, cervical region
        M41.113 Juvenile idiopathic scoliosis, cervicothoracic region
        M41.114 Juvenile idiopathic scoliosis, thoracic region
        M41.115 Juvenile idiopathic scoliosis, thoracolumbar region
        M41.116 Juvenile idiopathic scoliosis, lumbar region
        M41.117 Juvenile idiopathic scoliosis, lumbosacral region
        M41.119 Juvenile idiopathic scoliosis, site unspecified
          AHA CC: 4Q, 2014, 28-29
  + **M41.12 Adolescent idiopathic scoliosis**
        M41.122 Adolescent idiopathic scoliosis, cervical region
        M41.123 Adolescent idiopathic scoliosis, cervicothoracic region
        M41.124 Adolescent idiopathic scoliosis, thoracic region
        M41.125 Adolescent idiopathic scoliosis, thoracolumbar region
        M41.126 Adolescent idiopathic scoliosis, lumbar region
        M41.127 Adolescent idiopathic scoliosis, lumbosacral region
        M41.129 Adolescent idiopathic scoliosis, site unspecified

+ **M41.2 Other idiopathic scoliosis**
    M41.20 Other idiopathic scoliosis, site unspecified
    M41.22 Other idiopathic scoliosis, cervical region
    M41.23 Other idiopathic scoliosis, cervicothoracic region
    M41.24 Other idiopathic scoliosis, thoracic region
    M41.25 Other idiopathic scoliosis, thoracolumbar region
    M41.26 Other idiopathic scoliosis, lumbar region
    M41.27 Other idiopathic scoliosis, lumbosacral region

+ **M41.3 Thoracogenic scoliosis**
    M41.30 Thoracogenic scoliosis, site unspecified
    M41.34 Thoracogenic scoliosis, thoracic region
    M41.35 Thoracogenic scoliosis, thoracolumbar region

+ **M41.4 Neuromuscular scoliosis**
    Scoliosis secondary to cerebral palsy, Friedreich's ataxia, poliomyelitis and other neuromuscular disorders
    Code also underlying condition
    M41.40 Neuromuscular scoliosis, site unspecified
    M41.41 Neuromuscular scoliosis, occipito-atlanto-axial region
    M41.42 Neuromuscular scoliosis, cervical region
    M41.43 Neuromuscular scoliosis, cervicothoracic region
    M41.44 Neuromuscular scoliosis, thoracic region
    M41.45 Neuromuscular scoliosis, thoracolumbar region
        AHA CC: 4Q, 2014, 27-28
    M41.46 Neuromuscular scoliosis, lumbar region
    M41.47 Neuromuscular scoliosis, lumbosacral region

+ **M41.5 Other secondary scoliosis**
    Code first underlying disease
        AHA CC: 1Q, 2019, 19
    M41.50 Other secondary scoliosis, site unspecified
    M41.52 Other secondary scoliosis, cervical region
    M41.53 Other secondary scoliosis, cervicothoracic region
    M41.54 Other secondary scoliosis, thoracic region
    M41.55 Other secondary scoliosis, thoracolumbar region
    M41.56 Other secondary scoliosis, lumbar region
    M41.57 Other secondary scoliosis, lumbosacral region

+ **M41.8 Other forms of scoliosis**
    M41.80 Other forms of scoliosis, site unspecified
    M41.82 Other forms of scoliosis, cervical region
    M41.83 Other forms of scoliosis, cervicothoracic region
    M41.84 Other forms of scoliosis, thoracic region
    M41.85 Other forms of scoliosis, thoracolumbar region
    M41.86 Other forms of scoliosis, lumbar region
    M41.87 Other forms of scoliosis, lumbosacral region

M41.9 Scoliosis, unspecified
    AHA CC: 1Q, 2022, 30

M42 Spinal osteochondrosis
+ **M42.0 Juvenile osteochondrosis of spine**
    Calvé's disease
    Scheuermann's disease
    Excludes1: postural kyphosis (M40.0)
    M42.00 Juvenile osteochondrosis of spine, site unspecified
    M42.01 Juvenile osteochondrosis of spine, occipito-atlanto-axial region
    M42.02 Juvenile osteochondrosis of spine, cervical region
    M42.03 Juvenile osteochondrosis of spine, cervicothoracic region
    M42.04 Juvenile osteochondrosis of spine, thoracic region
    M42.05 Juvenile osteochondrosis of spine, thoracolumbar region
    M42.06 Juvenile osteochondrosis of spine, lumbar region
    M42.07 Juvenile osteochondrosis of spine, lumbosacral region
    M42.08 Juvenile osteochondrosis of spine, sacral and sacrococcygeal region
    M42.09 Juvenile osteochondrosis of spine, multiple sites in spine

+ **M42.1 Adult osteochondrosis of spine**
    • M42.10 Adult osteochondrosis of spine, site unspecified
    • M42.11 Adult osteochondrosis of spine, occipito-atlanto-axial region
    • M42.12 Adult osteochondrosis of spine, cervical region
    • M42.13 Adult osteochondrosis of spine, cervicothoracic region
    • M42.14 Adult osteochondrosis of spine, thoracic region
    • M42.15 Adult osteochondrosis of spine, thoracolumbar region
    • M42.16 Adult osteochondrosis of spine, lumbar region
    • M42.17 Adult osteochondrosis of spine, lumbosacral region
    • M42.18 Adult osteochondrosis of spine, sacral and sacrococcygeal region
    • M42.19 Adult osteochondrosis of spine, multiple sites in spine

M42.9 Spinal osteochondrosis, unspecified

M43 Other deforming dorsopathies

Excludes1: congenital spondylolysis and spondylolisthesis (Q76.2)
hemivertebra (Q76.3-Q76.4)
Klippel-Feil syndrome (Q76.1)
lumbarization and sacralization (Q76.4)
platyspondylisis (Q76.4)
spina bifida occulta (Q76.0)
spinal curvature in osteoporosis (M80.-)
spinal curvature in Paget's disease of bone [osteitis deformans] (M88.-)

+ **M43.0 Spondylolysis**
Excludes1: congenital spondylolysis (Q76.2)
spondylolisthesis (M43.1)
- M43.00 Spondylolysis, site unspecified
- M43.01 Spondylolysis, occipito-atlanto-axial region
- M43.02 Spondylolysis, cervical region
- M43.03 Spondylolysis, cervicothoracic region
- M43.04 Spondylolysis, thoracic region
- M43.05 Spondylolysis, thoracolumbar region
- M43.06 Spondylolysis, lumbar region
- M43.07 Spondylolysis, lumbosacral region
- M43.08 Spondylolysis, sacral and sacrococcygeal region
- M43.09 Spondylolysis, multiple sites in spine

+ **M43.1 Spondylolisthesis**
Excludes1: acute traumatic of lumbosacral region (S33.1)
acute traumatic of sites other than lumbosacral- code to Fracture, vertebra, by region
congenital spondylolisthesis (Q76.2)
AHA CC: 2Q, 2020, 21
- M43.10 Spondylolisthesis, site unspecified
- M43.11 Spondylolisthesis, occipito-atlanto-axial region
- M43.12 Spondylolisthesis, cervical region
- M43.13 Spondylolisthesis, cervicothoracic region
- M43.14 Spondylolisthesis, thoracic region
- M43.15 Spondylolisthesis, thoracolumbar region
- M43.16 Spondylolisthesis, lumbar region
AHA CC: 3Q, 2018, 18
- M43.17 Spondylolisthesis, lumbosacral region
- M43.18 Spondylolisthesis, sacral and sacrococcygeal region
- M43.19 Spondylolisthesis, multiple sites in spine

+ **M43.2 Fusion of spine**
Ankylosis of spinal joint
Excludes1: ankylosing spondylitis (M45.0-)
congenital fusion of spine (Q76.4)
Excludes2: arthrodesis status (Z98.1)
pseudoarthrosis after fusion or arthrodesis (M96.0)
- M43.20 Fusion of spine, site unspecified
- M43.21 Fusion of spine, occipito-atlanto-axial region
- M43.22 Fusion of spine, cervical region
- M43.23 Fusion of spine, cervicothoracic region
- M43.24 Fusion of spine, thoracic region
- M43.25 Fusion of spine, thoracolumbar region
- M43.26 Fusion of spine, lumbar region
- M43.27 Fusion of spine, lumbosacral region
- M43.28 Fusion of spine, sacral and sacrococcygeal region

M43.3 Recurrent atlantoaxial dislocation with myelopathy
M43.4 Other recurrent atlantoaxial dislocation

+ **M43.5 Other recurrent vertebral dislocation**
Excludes1: biomechanical lesions NEC (M99.-)
+ M43.5X Other recurrent vertebral dislocation
- M43.5X2 Other recurrent vertebral dislocation, cervical region
- M43.5X3 Other recurrent vertebral dislocation, cervicothoracic region
- M43.5X4 Other recurrent vertebral dislocation, thoracic region
- M43.5X5 Other recurrent vertebral dislocation, thoracolumbar region
- M43.5X6 Other recurrent vertebral dislocation, lumbar region
- M43.5X7 Other recurrent vertebral dislocation, lumbosacral region
- M43.5X8 Other recurrent vertebral dislocation, sacral and sacrococcygeal region
- M43.5X9 Other recurrent vertebral dislocation, site unspecified

M43.6 Torticollis
Excludes1: congenital (sternomastoid) torticollis (Q68.0)
current injury - see Injury, of spine, by body region
ocular torticollis (R29.891)
psychogenic torticollis (F45.8)
spasmodic torticollis (G24.3)
torticollis due to birth injury (P15.2)

+ **M43.8 Other specified deforming dorsopathies**
Excludes2: kyphosis and lordosis (M40.-)
scoliosis (M41.-)
+ M43.8X Other specified deforming dorsopathies
- M43.8X1 Other specified deforming dorsopathies, occipito-atlanto-axial region
- M43.8X2 Other specified deforming dorsopathies, cervical region
- M43.8X3 Other specified deforming dorsopathies, cervicothoracic region
- M43.8X4 Other specified deforming dorsopathies, thoracic region
- M43.8X5 Other specified deforming dorsopathies, thoracolumbar region
- M43.8X6 Other specified deforming dorsopathies, lumbar region
- M43.8X7 Other specified deforming dorsopathies, lumbosacral region
- M43.8X8 Other specified deforming dorsopathies, sacral and sacrococcygeal region
- M43.8X9 Other specified deforming dorsopathies, site unspecified

M43.9 Deforming dorsopathy, unspecified
Curvature of spine NOS

Spondylopathies (M45-M49)

M45 Ankylosing spondylitis
Rheumatoid arthritis of spine
Excludes1: arthropathy in Reiter's disease (M02.3-)
juvenile (ankylosing) spondylitis (M08.1)
Excludes2: Behçet's disease (M35.2)
AHA CC: 4Q, 2021, 21-22
- **M45.0** Ankylosing spondylitis of multiple sites in spine
- **M45.1** Ankylosing spondylitis of occipito-atlanto-axial region
- **M45.2** Ankylosing spondylitis of cervical region
- **M45.3** Ankylosing spondylitis of cervicothoracic region
- **M45.4** Ankylosing spondylitis of thoracic region
- **M45.5** Ankylosing spondylitis of thoracolumbar region
- **M45.6** Ankylosing spondylitis lumbar region
- **M45.7** Ankylosing spondylitis of lumbosacral region
- **M45.8** Ankylosing spondylitis sacral and sacrococcygeal region
- **M45.9** Ankylosing spondylitis of unspecified sites in spine

+ **M45.A Non-radiographic axial spondyloarthritis**
- M45.A0 Non-radiographic axial spondyloarthritis of unspecified sites in spine
- M45.A1 Non-radiographic axial spondyloarthritis of occipito-atlanto-axial region
- M45.A2 Non-radiographic axial spondyloarthritis of cervical region
- M45.A3 Non-radiographic axial spondyloarthritis of cerviothoracic region
- M45.A4 Non-radiographic axial spondyloarthritis of throacic region
- M45.A5 Non-radiographic axial spondyloarthritis of thoracolumbar region
- M45.A6 Non-radiographic axial spondyloarthritis of lumbar region
- M45.A7 Non-radiographic axial spondyloarthritis of lumbosacral region
- M45.A8 Non-radiographic axial spondyloarthritis of sacral and sacrococcygeal region
- M45.AB Non-radiographic axial spondyloarthritis of multiple sites in spine

M46 Other inflammatory spondylopathies

+ **M46.0 Spinal enthesopathy**
Disorder of ligamentous or muscular attachments of spine
- **M46.00** Spinal enthesopathy, site unspecified
- **M46.01** Spinal enthesopathy, occipito-atlanto-axial region
- **M46.02** Spinal enthesopathy, cervical region
- **M46.03** Spinal enthesopathy, cervicothoracic region
- **M46.04** Spinal enthesopathy, thoracic region

- **M46.05** Spinal enthesopathy, thoracolumbar region
- **M46.06** Spinal enthesopathy, lumbar region
- **M46.07** Spinal enthesopathy, lumbosacral region
- **M46.08** Spinal enthesopathy, sacral and sacrococcygeal region
- **M46.09** Spinal enthesopathy, multiple sites in spine
- **M46.1** Sacroiliitis, not elsewhere classified
  AHA CC: 2Q, 2020, 14
- **+ M46.2** Osteomyelitis of vertebra
  - CC **M46.20** Osteomyelitis of vertebra, site unspecified
  - CC **M46.21** Osteomyelitis of vertebra, occipito-atlanto-axial region
  - CC **M46.22** Osteomyelitis of vertebra, cervical region
  - CC **M46.23** Osteomyelitis of vertebra, cervicothoracic region
  - CC **M46.24** Osteomyelitis of vertebra, thoracic region
  - CC **M46.25** Osteomyelitis of vertebra, thoracolumbar region
  - CC **M46.26** Osteomyelitis of vertebra, lumbar region
  - CC **M46.27** Osteomyelitis of vertebra, lumbosacral region
  - CC **M46.28** Osteomyelitis of vertebra, sacral and sacrococcygeal region
- **+ M46.3** Infection of intervertebral disc (pyogenic)
  Use additional code (B95-B97) to identify infectious agent
  - CC **M46.30** Infection of intervertebral disc (pyogenic), site unspecified
  - CC **M46.31** Infection of intervertebral disc (pyogenic), occipito-atlanto-axial region
  - CC **M46.32** Infection of intervertebral disc (pyogenic), cervical region
  - CC **M46.33** Infection of intervertebral disc (pyogenic), cervicothoracic region
  - CC **M46.34** Infection of intervertebral disc (pyogenic), thoracic region
  - CC **M46.35** Infection of intervertebral disc (pyogenic), thoracolumbar region
  - CC **M46.36** Infection of intervertebral disc (pyogenic), lumbar region
  - CC **M46.37** Infection of intervertebral disc (pyogenic), lumbosacral region
  - CC **M46.38** Infection of intervertebral disc (pyogenic), sacral and sacrococcygeal region
  - CC **M46.39** Infection of intervertebral disc (pyogenic), multiple sites in spine
- **+ M46.4** Discitis, unspecified
  - **M46.40** Discitis, unspecified, site unspecified
  - **M46.41** Discitis, unspecified, occipito-atlanto-axial region
  - **M46.42** Discitis, unspecified, cervical region
  - **M46.43** Discitis, unspecified, cervicothoracic region
  - **M46.44** Discitis, unspecified, thoracic region
  - **M46.45** Discitis, unspecified, thoracolumbar region
  - **M46.46** Discitis, unspecified, lumbar region
  - **M46.47** Discitis, unspecified, lumbosacral region
  - **M46.48** Discitis, unspecified, sacral and sacrococcygeal region
  - **M46.49** Discitis, unspecified, multiple sites in spine
- **+ M46.5** Other infective spondylopathies
  - **M46.50** Other infective spondylopathies, site unspecified
  - **M46.51** Other infective spondylopathies, occipito-atlanto-axial region
  - **M46.52** Other infective spondylopathies, cervical region
  - **M46.53** Other infective spondylopathies, cervicothoracic region
  - **M46.54** Other infective spondylopathies, thoracic region
  - **M46.55** Other infective spondylopathies, thoracolumbar region
  - **M46.56** Other infective spondylopathies, lumbar region
  - **M46.57** Other infective spondylopathies, lumbosacral region
  - **M46.58** Other infective spondylopathies, sacral and sacrococcygeal region
  - **M46.59** Other infective spondylopathies, multiple sites in spine
- **+ M46.8** Other specified inflammatory spondylopathies
  - **M46.80** Other specified inflammatory spondylopathies, site unspecified
  - **M46.81** Other specified inflammatory spondylopathies, occipito-atlanto-axial region
  - **M46.82** Other specified inflammatory spondylopathies, cervical region
  - **M46.83** Other specified inflammatory spondylopathies, cervicothoracic region
  - **M46.84** Other specified inflammatory spondylopathies, thoracic region
  - **M46.85** Other specified inflammatory spondylopathies, thoracolumbar region
  - **M46.86** Other specified inflammatory spondylopathies, lumbar region
  - **M46.87** Other specified inflammatory spondylopathies, lumbosacral region
  - **M46.88** Other specified inflammatory spondylopathies, sacral and sacrococcygeal region
  - **M46.89** Other specified inflammatory spondylopathies, multiple sites in spine
- **+ M46.9** Unspecified inflammatory spondylopathy
  - **M46.90** Unspecified inflammatory spondylopathy, site unspecified
  - **M46.91** Unspecified inflammatory spondylopathy, occipito-atlanto-axial region
  - **M46.92** Unspecified inflammatory spondylopathy, cervical region
  - **M46.93** Unspecified inflammatory spondylopathy, cervicothoracic region
  - **M46.94** Unspecified inflammatory spondylopathy, thoracic region
  - **M46.95** Unspecified inflammatory spondylopathy, thoracolumbar region
  - **M46.96** Unspecified inflammatory spondylopathy, lumbar region
  - **M46.97** Unspecified inflammatory spondylopathy, lumbosacral region
  - **M46.98** Unspecified inflammatory spondylopathy, sacral and sacrococcygeal region
  - **M46.99** Unspecified inflammatory spondylopathy, multiple sites in spine

M47 Spondylosis

Includes: arthrosis or osteoarthritis of spine
degeneration of facet joints

- **+ M47.0** Anterior spinal and vertebral artery compression syndromes
  - **+ M47.01** Anterior spinal artery compression syndromes
    - CC **M47.011** Anterior spinal artery compression syndromes, occipito-atlanto-axial region
    - CC **M47.012** Anterior spinal artery compression syndromes, cervical region
    - CC **M47.013** Anterior spinal artery compression syndromes, cervicothoracic region
    - CC **M47.014** Anterior spinal artery compression syndromes, thoracic region
    - CC **M47.015** Anterior spinal artery compression syndromes, thoracolumbar region
    - CC **M47.016** Anterior spinal artery compression syndromes, lumbar region
    - CC **M47.019** Anterior spinal artery compression syndromes, site unspecified
  - **+ M47.02** Vertebral artery compression syndromes
    - CC **M47.021** Vertebral artery compression syndromes, occipito-atlanto-axial region
    - CC **M47.022** Vertebral artery compression syndromes, cervical region
      AHA CC: 1Q, 2023, 37-38
    - CC **M47.029** Vertebral artery compression syndromes, site unspecified
- **+ M47.1** Other spondylosis with myelopathy
  Spondylogenic compression of spinal cord
  Excludes1: vertebral subluxation (M43.3-M43.5X9)
  - CC **M47.10** Other spondylosis with myelopathy, site unspecified
  - CC **M47.11** Other spondylosis with myelopathy, occipito-atlanto-axial region
  - CC **M47.12** Other spondylosis with myelopathy, cervical region
    AHA CC: 1Q, 2020, 17
  - CC **M47.13** Other spondylosis with myelopathy, cervicothoracic region
  - CC **M47.14** Other spondylosis with myelopathy, thoracic region
  - CC **M47.15** Other spondylosis with myelopathy, thoracolumbar region
  - CC **M47.16** Other spondylosis with myelopathy, lumbar region
- **+ M47.2** Other spondylosis with radiculopathy

M47.20 Other spondylosis with radiculopathy, site unspecified
M47.21 Other spondylosis with radiculopathy, occipito-atlanto-axial region
M47.22 Other spondylosis with radiculopathy, cervical region
  AHA CC: 1Q, 2020, 17
M47.23 Other spondylosis with radiculopathy, cervicothoracic region
M47.24 Other spondylosis with radiculopathy, thoracic region
M47.25 Other spondylosis with radiculopathy, thoracolumbar region
M47.26 Other spondylosis with radiculopathy, lumbar region
M47.27 Other spondylosis with radiculopathy, lumbosacral region
M47.28 Other spondylosis with radiculopathy, sacral and sacrococcygeal region

+ M47.8 Other spondylosis
  + M47.81 Spondylosis without myelopathy or radiculopathy
    M47.811 Spondylosis without myelopathy or radiculopathy, occipito-atlanto-axial region
    M47.812 Spondylosis without myelopathy or radiculopathy, cervical region
      AHA CC: 2Q, 2018, 14-15; 3Q, 2019, 10-11
    M47.813 Spondylosis without myelopathy or radiculopathy, cervicothoracic region
    M47.814 Spondylosis without myelopathy or radiculopathy, thoracic region
    M47.815 Spondylosis without myelopathy or radiculopathy, thoracolumbar region
    M47.816 Spondylosis without myelopathy or radiculopathy, lumbar region
    M47.817 Spondylosis without myelopathy or radiculopathy, lumbosacral region
    M47.818 Spondylosis without myelopathy or radiculopathy, sacral and sacrococcygeal region
    M47.819 Spondylosis without myelopathy or radiculopathy, site unspecified
  + M47.89 Other spondylosis
    M47.891 Other spondylosis, occipito-atlanto-axial region
    M47.892 Other spondylosis, cervical region
    M47.893 Other spondylosis, cervicothoracic region
    M47.894 Other spondylosis, thoracic region
    M47.895 Other spondylosis, thoracolumbar region
    M47.896 Other spondylosis, lumbar region
    M47.897 Other spondylosis, lumbosacral region
    M47.898 Other spondylosis, sacral and sacrococcygeal region
    M47.899 Other spondylosis, site unspecified
M47.9 Spondylosis, unspecified

M48 Other spondylopathies

+ M48.0 Spinal stenosis
  Caudal stenosis
  M48.00 Spinal stenosis, site unspecified
  M48.01 Spinal stenosis, occipito-atlanto-axial region
  M48.02 Spinal stenosis, cervical region
    AHA CC: 3Q, 2018, 18-19; 1Q, 2020, 17
  M48.03 Spinal stenosis, cervicothoracic region
  M48.04 Spinal stenosis, thoracic region
  M48.05 Spinal stenosis, thoracolumbar region
  + M48.06 Spinal stenosis, lumbar region
    AHA CC: 3Q, 2017, 24
    M48.061 Spinal stenosis, lumbar region without neurogenic claudication
      Spinal stenosis, lumbar region NOS
      AHA CC: 4Q, 2017, 18-19; 3Q, 2018, 19-20
    M48.062 Spinal stenosis, lumbar region with neurogenic claudication
      AHA CC: 4Q, 2017, 18-19
  M48.07 Spinal stenosis, lumbosacral region
    AHA CC: 3Q, 2018, 19-20
  M48.08 Spinal stenosis, sacral and sacrococcygeal region
+ M48.1 Ankylosing hyperostosis [Forestier]
  Diffuse idiopathic skeletal hyperostosis [DISH]
  M48.10 Ankylosing hyperostosis [Forestier], site unspecified
  M48.11 Ankylosing hyperostosis [Forestier], occipito-atlanto-axial region
  M48.12 Ankylosing hyperostosis [Forestier], cervical region
  M48.13 Ankylosing hyperostosis [Forestier], cervicothoracic region
  M48.14 Ankylosing hyperostosis [Forestier], thoracic region
  M48.15 Ankylosing hyperostosis [Forestier], thoracolumbar region
  M48.16 Ankylosing hyperostosis [Forestier], lumbar region
  M48.17 Ankylosing hyperostosis [Forestier], lumbosacral region
  M48.18 Ankylosing hyperostosis [Forestier], sacral and sacrococcygeal region
  M48.19 Ankylosing hyperostosis [Forestier], multiple sites in spine
+ M48.2 Kissing spine
  M48.20 Kissing spine, site unspecified
  M48.21 Kissing spine, occipito-atlanto-axial region
  M48.22 Kissing spine, cervical region
  M48.23 Kissing spine, cervicothoracic region
  M48.24 Kissing spine, thoracic region
  M48.25 Kissing spine, thoracolumbar region
  M48.26 Kissing spine, lumbar region
  M48.27 Kissing spine, lumbosacral region
+ M48.3 Traumatic spondylopathy
  CC M48.30 Traumatic spondylopathy, site unspecified
  CC M48.31 Traumatic spondylopathy, occipito-atlanto-axial region
  CC M48.32 Traumatic spondylopathy, cervical region
  CC M48.33 Traumatic spondylopathy, cervicothoracic region
  CC M48.34 Traumatic spondylopathy, thoracic region
  CC M48.35 Traumatic spondylopathy, thoracolumbar region
  CC M48.36 Traumatic spondylopathy, lumbar region
  CC M48.37 Traumatic spondylopathy, lumbosacral region
  CC M48.38 Traumatic spondylopathy, sacral and sacrococcygeal region
+ M48.4 Fatigue fracture of vertebra
  Stress fracture of vertebra
  Excludes1: pathological fracture NOS (M84.4-)
    pathological fracture of vertebra due to neoplasm (M84.58)
    pathological fracture of vertebra due to other diagnosis (M84.68)
    pathological fracture of vertebra due to osteoporosis (M80.-)
    traumatic fracture of vertebrae (S12.0-S12.3-, S22.0-, S32.0-)

The appropriate 7th character is to be added to each code from subcategory **M48.4**:
A initial encounter for fracture
D subsequent encounter for fracture with routine healing
G subsequent encounter for fracture with delayed healing
S sequela of fracture

X+7th M48.40 Fatigue fracture of vertebra, site unspecified
X+7th M48.41 Fatigue fracture of vertebra, occipito-atlanto-axial region
X+7th M48.42 Fatigue fracture of vertebra, cervical region
X+7th M48.43 Fatigue fracture of vertebra, cervicothoracic region
X+7th M48.44 Fatigue fracture of vertebra, thoracic region
X+7th M48.45 Fatigue fracture of vertebra, thoracolumbar region
X+7th M48.46 Fatigue fracture of vertebra, lumbar region
X+7th M48.47 Fatigue fracture of vertebra, lumbosacral region
X+7th M48.48 Fatigue fracture of vertebra, sacral and sacrococcygeal region

Lumbar Spinal Stenosis

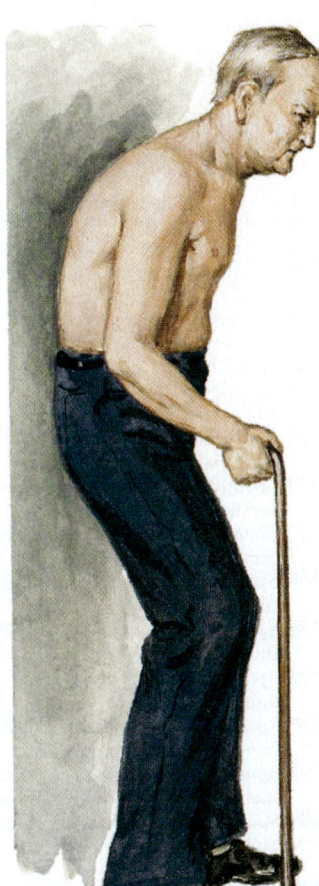

Patient assumes characteristic bent-over posture, with neck, spine, hips, and knees flexed; back is flat or convex, with absence of normal lordotic curvature. Pressure on cauda equina and resultant pain thus relieved.

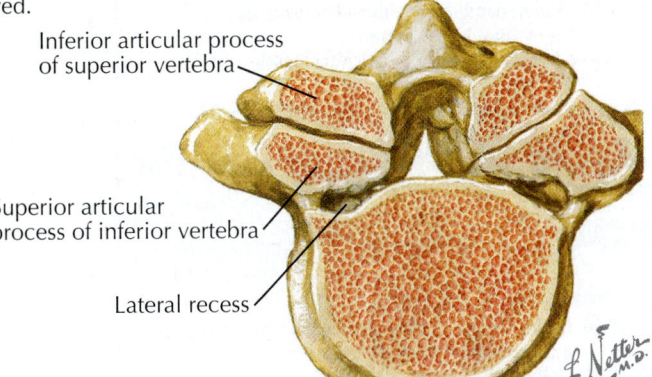

Inferior articular process of superior vertebra

Superior articular process of inferior vertebra

Lateral recess

Central spinal canal narrowed by enlargement of inferior articular process of superior vertebra. Lateral recesses narrowed by subluxation and osteophytic enlargement of superior articular processes of inferior vertebra.

Vertebrae approximated due to loss of disc height. Subluxated superior articular process of inferior vertebra has encroached on foramen. Internal disruption of disc shown in cut section.

Vascular vs. Neurogenic Claudication		
Evaluation	Vascular	Neurogenic
Walking distance	Fixed	Variable
Palliative factors	Standing	Sitting/Bending
Provocative factors	Walking	Walking/Standing
Walking uphill	Painful	Painless
Bicycle test	Positive (painful)	Negative (painless)
Pulses	Absent	Present
Skin	Loss of hair/shiny	Normal
Weakness	Rarely	Occasionally
Back pain	Occasionally	Commonly
Back motion	Normal	Limited
Pain character	Cramping/distal-to-proximal	Numbness/aching/proximal-to-distal
Atrophy	Uncommon	Occasionally

© 2023. Netter illustration used with permission of Elsevier Inc. All rights reserved. www.netterimages.com

+ M48.5 Collapsed vertebra, not elsewhere classified
Collapsed vertebra NOS
Compression fracture of vertebra NOS
Wedging of vertebra NOS
Excludes1: current injury - see Injury of spine, by body region
fatigue fracture of vertebra (M48.4)
pathological fracture of vertebra due to neoplasm (M84.58)
pathological fracture of vertebra due to other diagnosis (M84.68)
pathological fracture of vertebra due to osteoporosis (M80.-)
pathological fracture NOS (M84.4-)
stress fracture of vertebra (M48.4-)
traumatic fracture of vertebra (S12.-, S22.-, S32.-)

> The appropriate 7th character is to be added to each code from subcategory **M48.5**:
> A initial encounter for fracture
> D subsequent encounter for fracture with routine healing
> G subsequent encounter for fracture with delayed healing
> S sequela of fracture

CC X+7th **M48.50** Collapsed vertebra, not elsewhere classified, site unspecified
CC X+7th **M48.51** Collapsed vertebra, not elsewhere classified, occipito-atlanto-axial region
CC X+7th **M48.52** Collapsed vertebra, not elsewhere classified, cervical region
CC X+7th **M48.53** Collapsed vertebra, not elsewhere classified, cervicothoracic region
CC X+7th **M48.54** Collapsed vertebra, not elsewhere classified, thoracic region
CC X+7th **M48.55** Collapsed vertebra, not elsewhere classified, thoracolumbar region
CC X+7th **M48.56** Collapsed vertebra, not elsewhere classified, lumbar region
CC X+7th **M48.57** Collapsed vertebra, not elsewhere classified, lumbosacral region
CC X+7th **M48.58** Collapsed vertebra, not elsewhere classified, sacral and sacrococcygeal region

+ M48.8 Other specified spondylopathies
Ossification of posterior longitudinal ligament
+ M48.8X Other specified spondylopathies
M48.8X1 Other specified spondylopathies, occipito-atlanto-axial region
M48.8X2 Other specified spondylopathies, cervical region
M48.8X3 Other specified spondylopathies, cervicothoracic region
M48.8X4 Other specified spondylopathies, thoracic region
M48.8X5 Other specified spondylopathies, thoracolumbar region
M48.8X6 Other specified spondylopathies, lumbar region
M48.8X7 Other specified spondylopathies, lumbosacral region
M48.8X8 Other specified spondylopathies, sacral and sacrococcygeal region
M48.8X9 Other specified spondylopathies, site unspecified

M48.9 Spondylopathy, unspecified

M49 Spondylopathies in diseases classified elsewhere
Includes: curvature of spine in diseases classified elsewhere
deformity of spine in diseases classified elsewhere
kyphosis in diseases classified elsewhere
scoliosis in diseases classified elsewhere
spondylopathy in diseases classified elsewhere
Code first *underlying disease, such as:*
brucellosis (A23.-)
Charcot-Marie-Tooth disease (G60.0)
enterobacterial infections (A01-A04)
osteitis fibrosa cystica (E21.0)
Excludes1: curvature of spine in tuberculosis [Pott's] (A18.01)
enteropathic arthropathies (M07.-)
gonococcal spondylitis (A54.41)
neuropathic [tabes dorsalis] spondylitis (A52.11)
neuropathic spondylopathy in syringomyelia (G95.0)
neuropathic spondylopathy in tabes dorsalis (A52.11)
nonsyphilitic neuropathic spondylopathy NEC (G98.0)
spondylitis in syphilis (acquired) (A52.77)
tuberculous spondylitis (A18.01)
typhoid fever spondylitis (A01.05)

+ M49.8 Spondylopathy in diseases classified elsewhere
M49.80 Spondylopathy in diseases classified elsewhere, site unspecified
M49.81 Spondylopathy in diseases classified elsewhere, occipito-atlanto-axial region
M49.82 Spondylopathy in diseases classified elsewhere, cervical region
M49.83 Spondylopathy in diseases classified elsewhere, cervicothoracic region
M49.84 Spondylopathy in diseases classified elsewhere, thoracic region
M49.85 Spondylopathy in diseases classified elsewhere, thoracolumbar region
M49.86 Spondylopathy in diseases classified elsewhere, lumbar region
M49.87 Spondylopathy in diseases classified elsewhere, lumbosacral region
M49.88 Spondylopathy in diseases classified elsewhere, sacral and sacrococcygeal region
M49.89 Spondylopathy in diseases classified elsewhere, multiple sites in spine

Other dorsopathies (M50-M54)

Excludes1: current injury - see injury of spine by body region
discitis NOS (M46.4-)

M50 Cervical disc disorders
Includes: cervicothoracic disc disorders with cervicalgia
cervicothoracic disc disorders

+ M50.0 Cervical disc disorder with myelopathy
CC **M50.00** Cervical disc disorder with myelopathy, unspecified cervical region
CC **M50.01** Cervical disc disorder with myelopathy, high cervical region
C2-C3 disc disorder with myelopathy
C3-C4 disc disorder with myelopathy
AHA CC: 1Q, 2016, 17

+ M50.02 Cervical disc disorder with myelopathy, mid-cervical region
AHA CC: 4Q, 2016, 39-40
CC **M50.020** Cervical disc disorder with myelopathy, mid-cervical region, unspecified level
CC **M50.021** Cervical disc disorder at C4-C5 level with myelopathy
C4-C5 disc disorder with myelopathy
CC **M50.022** Cervical disc disorder at C5-C6 level with myelopathy
C5-C6 disc disorder with myelopathy
AHA CC: 3Q, 2018, 19
CC **M50.023** Cervical disc disorder at C6-C7 level with myelopathy
C6-C7 disc disorder with myelopathy
CC **M50.03** Cervical disc disorder with myelopathy, cervicothoracic region
C7-T1 disc disorder with myelopathy

Lumbar Disk Herniation: Clinical Manifestation

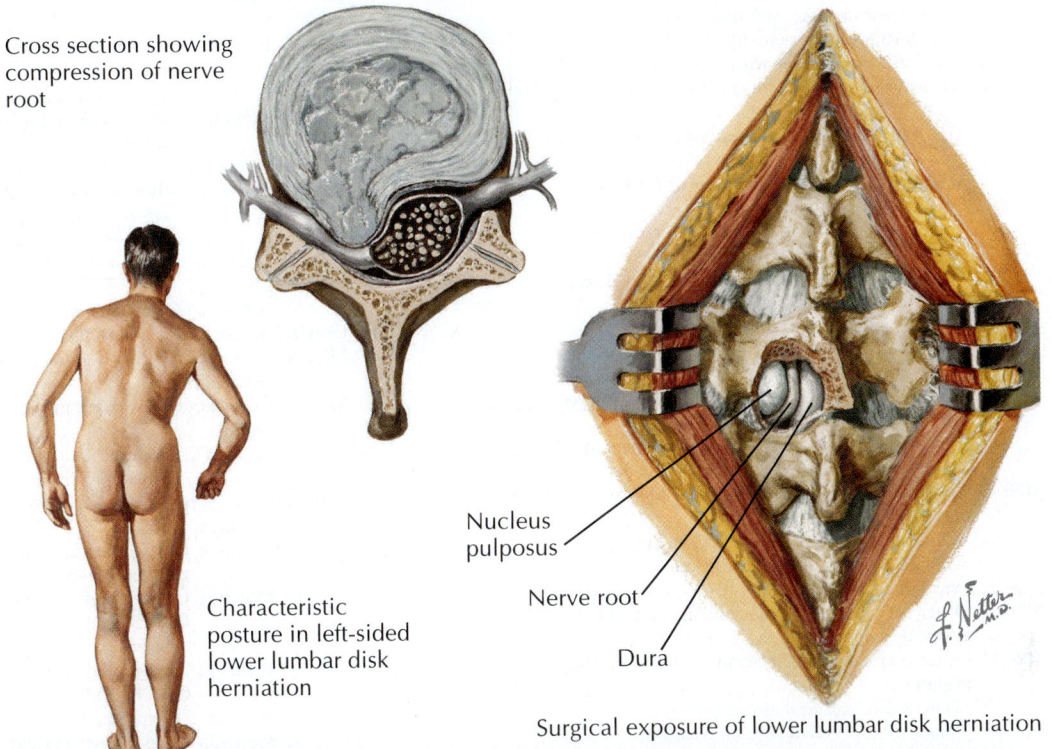

Level of herniation	Pain	Numbness	Weakness	Atrophy	Reflexes
L4-5 disk; 5th lumbar nerve root	Over sacroiliac joint, hip, lateral thigh and leg	Lateral leg, first 3 toes	Dorsiflexion of great toe and foot; difficulty walking on heels; foot drop may occur	Minor	Changes uncommon in knee and ankle jerks, but internal hamstring reflex diminished or absent
L5-S1 disk; 1st sacral nerve root	Over sacroiliac joint, hip, posterolateral thigh and leg to heel	Back of calf, lateral heel, foot to toe	Plantar flexion of foot and great toe may be affected; difficulty walking on toes	Gastrocnemius and soleus	Ankle jerk diminished or absent

Clinical features of herniated lumbar nucleus pulposus

- **M50.1 Cervical disc disorder with radiculopathy**
  Excludes2: brachial radiculitis NOS (M54.13)
  - M50.10 Cervical disc disorder with radiculopathy, unspecified cervical region
  - M50.11 Cervical disc disorder with radiculopathy, high cervical region
    - C2-C3 disc disorder with radiculopathy
    - C3 radiculopathy due to disc disorder
    - C3-C4 disc disorder with radiculopathy
    - C4 radiculopathy due to disc disorder
  - **M50.12 Cervical disc disorder with radiculopathy, mid-cervical region**
    AHA CC: 4Q, 2016, 39-40
    - M50.120 Mid-cervical disc disorder, unspecified level
    - M50.121 Cervical disc disorder at C4-C5 level with radiculopathy
      - C4-C5 disc disorder with radiculopathy
      - C5 radiculopathy due to disc disorder
    - M50.122 Cervical disc disorder at C5-C6 level with radiculopathy
      - C5-C6 disc disorder with radiculopathy
      - C6 radiculopathy due to disc disorder
      AHA CC: 3Q, 2018, 19
    - M50.123 Cervical disc disorder at C6-C7 level with radiculopathy
      - C6-C7 disc disorder with radiculopathy
      - C7 radiculopathy due to disc disorder
  - M50.13 Cervical disc disorder with radiculopathy, cervicothoracic region
    - C7-T1 disc disorder with radiculopathy
    - C8 radiculopathy due to disc disorder
- **M50.2 Other cervical disc displacement**
  - M50.20 Other cervical disc displacement, unspecified cervical region
  - M50.21 Other cervical disc displacement, high cervical region
    - Other C2-C3 cervical disc displacement
    - Other C3-C4 cervical disc displacement
    AHA CC: 4Q, 2021, 11-12
  - **M50.22 Other cervical disc displacement, mid-cervical region**
    - M50.220 Other cervical disc displacement, mid-cervical region, unspecified level
    - M50.221 Other cervical disc displacement at C4-C5 level
      - Other C4-C5 cervical disc displacement
    - M50.222 Other cervical disc displacement at C5-C6 level
      - Other C5-C6 cervical disc displacement
    - M50.223 Other cervical disc displacement at C6-C7 level
      - Other C6-C7 cervical disc displacement
  - M50.23 Other cervical disc displacement, cervicothoracic region
    - Other C7-T1 cervical disc displacement
- **M50.3 Other cervical disc degeneration**
  - M50.30 Other cervical disc degeneration, unspecified cervical region
  - M50.31 Other cervical disc degeneration, high cervical region
    - Other C2-C3 cervical disc degeneration
    - Other C3-C4 cervical disc degeneration
  - **M50.32 Other cervical disc degeneration, mid-cervical region**
    - M50.320 Other cervical disc degeneration, mid-cervical region, unspecified level
    - M50.321 Other cervical disc degeneration at C4-C5 level
      - Other C4-C5 cervical disc degeneration
    - M50.322 Other cervical disc degeneration at C5-C6 level
      - Other C5-C6 cervical disc degeneration
    - M50.323 Other cervical disc degeneration at C6-C7 level
      - Other C6-C7 cervical disc degeneration
  - M50.33 Other cervical disc degeneration, cervicothoracic region
    - Other C7-T1 cervical disc degeneration

- **M50.8 Other cervical disc disorders**
  - M50.80 Other cervical disc disorders, unspecified cervical region
  - M50.81 Other cervical disc disorders, high cervical region
    - Other C2-C3 cervical disc disorders
    - Other C3-C4 cervical disc disorders
  - **M50.82 Other cervical disc disorders, mid-cervical region**
    - M50.820 Other cervical disc disorders, mid-cervical region, unspecified level
    - M50.821 Other cervical disc disorders at C4-C5 level
      - Other C4-C5 cervical disc disorders
    - M50.822 Other cervical disc disorders at C5-C6 level
      - Other C5-C6 cervical disc disorders
    - M50.823 Other cervical disc disorders at C6-C7 level
      - Other C6-C7 cervical disc disorders
  - M50.83 Other cervical disc disorders, cervicothoracic region
    - Other C7-T1 cervical disc disorders
- **M50.9 Cervical disc disorder, unspecified**
  - M50.90 Cervical disc disorder, unspecified, unspecified cervical region
  - M50.91 Cervical disc disorder, unspecified, high cervical region
    - Other C2-C3 cervical disc disorder, unspecified
    - Other C3-C4 cervical disc disorder, unspecified
  - **M50.92 Cervical disc disorder, unspecified, mid-cervical region**
    - M50.920 Unspecified cervical disc disorder, mid-cervical region, unspecified level
    - M50.921 Unspecified cervical disc disorder at C4-C5 level
      - Unspecified C4-C5 cervical disc disorder
    - M50.922 Unspecified cervical disc disorder at C5-C6 level
      - Unspecified C5-C6 cervical disc disorder
    - M50.923 Unspecified cervical disc disorder at C6-C7 level
      - Unspecified C6-C7 cervical disc disorder
  - M50.93 Cervical disc disorder, unspecified, cervicothoracic region
    - Other C7-T1 cervical disc disorder, unspecified

M51 Thoracic, thoracolumbar, and lumbosacral intervertebral disc disorders

Excludes2: cervical and cervicothoracic disc disorders (M50.-)
sacral and sacrococcygeal disorders (M53.3)

- **M51.0 Thoracic, thoracolumbar and lumbosacral intervertebral disc disorders with myelopathy**
  - CC M51.04 Intervertebral disc disorders with myelopathy, thoracic region
  - CC M51.05 Intervertebral disc disorders with myelopathy, thoracolumbar region
  - CC M51.06 Intervertebral disc disorders with myelopathy, lumbar region
- **M51.1 Thoracic, thoracolumbar and lumbosacral intervertebral disc disorders with radiculopathy**
  Sciatica due to intervertebral disc disorder
  Excludes1: lumbar radiculitis NOS (M54.16)
  sciatica NOS (M54.3)
  - M51.14 Intervertebral disc disorders with radiculopathy, thoracic region
  - M51.15 Intervertebral disc disorders with radiculopathy, thoracolumbar region
  - M51.16 Intervertebral disc disorders with radiculopathy, lumbar region
  - M51.17 Intervertebral disc disorders with radiculopathy, lumbosacral region
- **M51.2 Other thoracic, thoracolumbar and lumbosacral intervertebral disc displacement**
  Lumbago due to displacement of intervertebral disc
  - M51.24 Other intervertebral disc displacement, thoracic region
  - M51.25 Other intervertebral disc displacement, thoracolumbar region

M51.26 Other intervertebral disc displacement, lumbar region
M51.27 Other intervertebral disc displacement, lumbosacral region
+ **M51.3 Other thoracic, thoracolumbar and lumbosacral intervertebral disc degeneration**
M51.34 Other intervertebral disc degeneration, thoracic region
M51.35 Other intervertebral disc degeneration, thoracolumbar region
M51.36 Other intervertebral disc degeneration, lumbar region
AHA CC: 2Q, 2018, 15
M51.37 Other intervertebral disc degeneration, lumbosacral region
AHA CC: 1Q, 2022, 26
+ **M51.4 Schmorl's nodes**
M51.44 Schmorl's nodes, thoracic region
M51.45 Schmorl's nodes, thoracolumbar region
M51.46 Schmorl's nodes, lumbar region
M51.47 Schmorl's nodes, lumbosacral region
+ **M51.8 Other thoracic, thoracolumbar and lumbosacral intervertebral disc disorders**
M51.84 Other intervertebral disc disorders, thoracic region
M51.85 Other intervertebral disc disorders, thoracolumbar region
M51.86 Other intervertebral disc disorders, lumbar region
M51.87 Other intervertebral disc disorders, lumbosacral region
M51.9 Unspecified thoracic, thoracolumbar and lumbosacral intervertebral disc disorder
+ **M51.A Other lumbar and lumbosacral annulus fibrosus disc defects**
AHA CC: 4Q, 2022, 28-29
M51.A0 Intervertebral annulus fibrosus defect, lumbar region, unspecified size
Code first, if applicable, lumbar disc herniation (M51.06, M51.16, M51.26)
M51.A1 Intervertebral annulus fibrosus defect, small, lumbar region
Code first, if applicable, lumbar disc herniation (M51.06, M51.16, M51.26)
M51.A2 Intervertebral annulus fibrosus defect, large, lumbar region
Code first, if applicable, lumbar disc herniation (M51.06, M51.16, M51.26)
M51.A3 Intervertebral annulus fibrosus defect, lumbosacral region, unspecified size
Code first, if applicable, lumbosacral disc herniation (M51.17, M51.27)
M51.A4 Intervertebral annulus fibrosus defect, small, lumbosacral region
Code first, if applicable, lumbosacral disc herniation (M51.17, M51.27)
M51.A5 Intervertebral annulus fibrosus defect, large, lumbosacral region
Code first, if applicable, lumbosacral disc herniation (M51.17, M51.27)

M53 Other and unspecified dorsopathies, not elsewhere classified
M53.0 Cervicocranial syndrome
Posterior cervical sympathetic syndrome
M53.1 Cervicobrachial syndrome
Excludes2: cervical disc disorder (M50.-)
thoracic outlet syndrome (G54.0)
+ **M53.2 Spinal instabilities**
+ **M53.2X Spinal instabilities**
M53.2X1 Spinal instabilities, occipito-atlanto-axial region
M53.2X2 Spinal instabilities, cervical region
M53.2X3 Spinal instabilities, cervicothoracic region
M53.2X4 Spinal instabilities, thoracic region
M53.2X5 Spinal instabilities, thoracolumbar region
M53.2X6 Spinal instabilities, lumbar region
M53.2X7 Spinal instabilities, lumbosacral region
M53.2X8 Spinal instabilities, sacral and sacrococcygeal region
M53.2X9 Spinal instabilities, site unspecified
M53.3 Sacrococcygeal disorders, not elsewhere classified
Coccygodynia
+ **M53.8 Other specified dorsopathies**
M53.80 Other specified dorsopathies, site unspecified
M53.81 Other specified dorsopathies, occipito-atlanto-axial region
M53.82 Other specified dorsopathies, cervical region
M53.83 Other specified dorsopathies, cervicothoracic region
M53.84 Other specified dorsopathies, thoracic region
M53.85 Other specified dorsopathies, thoracolumbar region
M53.86 Other specified dorsopathies, lumbar region
M53.87 Other specified dorsopathies, lumbosacral region
M53.88 Other specified dorsopathies, sacral and sacrococcygeal region
M53.9 Dorsopathy, unspecified

M54 Dorsalgia
Excludes1: psychogenic dorsalgia (F45.41)
+ **M54.0 Panniculitis affecting regions of neck and back**
Excludes1: lupus panniculitis (L93.2)
panniculitis NOS (M79.3)
relapsing [Weber-Christian] panniculitis (M35.6)
M54.00 Panniculitis affecting regions of neck and back, site unspecified
M54.01 Panniculitis affecting regions of neck and back, occipito-atlanto-axial region
M54.02 Panniculitis affecting regions of neck and back, cervical region
M54.03 Panniculitis affecting regions of neck and back, cervicothoracic region
M54.04 Panniculitis affecting regions of neck and back, thoracic region
M54.05 Panniculitis affecting regions of neck and back, thoracolumbar region
M54.06 Panniculitis affecting regions of neck and back, lumbar region
M54.07 Panniculitis affecting regions of neck and back, lumbosacral region
M54.08 Panniculitis affecting regions of neck and back, sacral and sacrococcygeal region
M54.09 Panniculitis affecting regions, neck and back, multiple sites in spine
+ **M54.1 Radiculopathy**
Brachial neuritis or radiculitis NOS
Lumbar neuritis or radiculitis NOS
Lumbosacral neuritis or radiculitis NOS
Thoracic neuritis or radiculitis NOS
Radiculitis NOS
Excludes1: neuralgia and neuritis NOS (M79.2)
radiculopathy with cervical disc disorder (M50.1)
radiculopathy with lumbar and other intervertebral disc disorder (M51.1-)
radiculopathy with spondylosis (M47.2-)
M54.10 Radiculopathy, site unspecified
M54.11 Radiculopathy, occipito-atlanto-axial region
M54.12 Radiculopathy, cervical region
AHA CC: 3Q, 2018, 18-19
M54.13 Radiculopathy, cervicothoracic region
M54.14 Radiculopathy, thoracic region
M54.15 Radiculopathy, thoracolumbar region
M54.16 Radiculopathy, lumbar region
AHA CC: 3Q, 2018, 18
M54.17 Radiculopathy, lumbosacral region
M54.18 Radiculopathy, sacral and sacrococcygeal region
M54.2 Cervicalgia
Excludes1: cervicalgia due to intervertebral cervical disc disorder (M50.-)
+ **M54.3 Sciatica**
Excludes1: lesion of sciatic nerve (G57.0)
sciatica due to intervertebral disc disorder (M51.1-)
sciatica with lumbago (M54.4-)
M54.30 Sciatica, unspecified side
M54.31 Sciatica, right side
M54.32 Sciatica, left side
+ **M54.4 Lumbago with sciatica**
Excludes1: lumbago with sciatica due to intervertebral disc disorder (M51.1-)
M54.40 Lumbago with sciatica, unspecified side
M54.41 Lumbago with sciatica, right side
M54.42 Lumbago with sciatica, left side
AHA CC: 2Q, 2016, 7

+ **M54.5 Low back pain**
  Excludes1: low back strain (S39.012)
      lumbago due to intervertebral disc displacement
       (M51.2-)
      lumbago with sciatica (M54.4-)
  AHA CC: 4Q, 2021, 22
  M54.50 Low pack pain, unspecified
    Loin pain
    Lumbago NOS
  M54.51 Vertebrogenic low back pain
    Low back vertebral endplate pain
  AHA CC: 4Q, 2021, 22
  M54.59 Other low back pain
M54.6 Pain in thoracic spine
  Excludes1: pain in thoracic spine due to intervertebral disc
      disorder (M51.-)
+ **M54.8 Other dorsalgia**
  Excludes1: dorsalgia in thoracic region (M54.6)
      low back pain (M54.5-)
  M54.81 Occipital neuralgia
  M54.89 Other dorsalgia
M54.9 Dorsalgia, unspecified
  Backache NOS
  Back pain NOS

SOFT TISSUE DISORDERS (M60-M79)

Disorders of muscles (M60-M63)

Excludes1: dermatopolymyositis (M33.-)
    muscular dystrophies and myopathies (G71-G72)
    myopathy in amyloidosis (E85.-)
    myopathy in polyarteritis nodosa (M30.0)
    myopathy in rheumatoid arthritis (M05.32)
    myopathy in scleroderma (M34.-)
    myopathy in Sjögren's syndrome (M35.03)
    myopathy in systemic lupus erythematosus (M32.-)

M60 Myositis
  Excludes2: inclusion body myositis [IBM] (G72.41)
+ **M60.0 Infective myositis**
  Tropical pyomyositis
  Use additional code (B95-B97) to identify infectious agent
+ **M60.00 Infective myositis, unspecified site**
  CC **M60.000 Infective myositis, unspecified right arm**
    Infective myositis, right upper limb NOS
  CC **M60.001 Infective myositis, unspecified left arm**
    Infective myositis, left upper limb NOS
  CC **M60.002 Infective myositis, unspecified arm**
    Infective myositis, upper limb NOS
  CC **M60.003 Infective myositis, unspecified right leg**
    Infective myositis, right lower limb NOS
  CC **M60.004 Infective myositis, unspecified left leg**
    Infective myositis, left lower limb NOS
  CC **M60.005 Infective myositis, unspecified leg**
    Infective myositis, lower limb NOS
  CC **M60.009 Infective myositis, unspecified site**
+ **M60.01 Infective myositis, shoulder**
  CC **M60.011 Infective myositis, right shoulder**
  CC **M60.012 Infective myositis, left shoulder**
  CC **M60.019 Infective myositis, unspecified shoulder**
+ **M60.02 Infective myositis, upper arm**
  CC **M60.021 Infective myositis, right upper arm**
  CC **M60.022 Infective myositis, left upper arm**
  CC **M60.029 Infective myositis, unspecified upper arm**
+ **M60.03 Infective myositis, forearm**
  CC **M60.031 Infective myositis, right forearm**
  CC **M60.032 Infective myositis, left forearm**
  CC **M60.039 Infective myositis, unspecified forearm**
+ **M60.04 Infective myositis, hand and fingers**
  CC **M60.041 Infective myositis, right hand**
  CC **M60.042 Infective myositis, left hand**
  CC **M60.043 Infective myositis, unspecified hand**
  CC **M60.044 Infective myositis, right finger(s)**
  CC **M60.045 Infective myositis, left finger(s)**
  CC **M60.046 Infective myositis, unspecified finger(s)**
+ **M60.05 Infective myositis, thigh**
  CC **M60.051 Infective myositis, right thigh**
  CC **M60.052 Infective myositis, left thigh**
  CC **M60.059 Infective myositis, unspecified thigh**

+ **M60.06 Infective myositis, lower leg**
  CC **M60.061 Infective myositis, right lower leg**
  CC **M60.062 Infective myositis, left lower leg**
  CC **M60.069 Infective myositis, unspecified lower leg**
+ **M60.07 Infective myositis, ankle, foot and toes**
  CC **M60.070 Infective myositis, right ankle**
  CC **M60.071 Infective myositis, left ankle**
  CC **M60.072 Infective myositis, unspecified ankle**
  CC **M60.073 Infective myositis, right foot**
  CC **M60.074 Infective myositis, left foot**
  CC **M60.075 Infective myositis, unspecified foot**
  CC **M60.076 Infective myositis, right toe(s)**
  CC **M60.077 Infective myositis, left toe(s)**
  CC **M60.078 Infective myositis, unspecified toe(s)**
 CC **M60.08 Infective myositis, other site**
 CC **M60.09 Infective myositis, multiple sites**
+ **M60.1 Interstitial myositis**
  M60.10 Interstitial myositis of unspecified site
+ **M60.11 Interstitial myositis, shoulder**
  M60.111 Interstitial myositis, right shoulder
  M60.112 Interstitial myositis, left shoulder
  M60.119 Interstitial myositis, unspecified shoulder
+ **M60.12 Interstitial myositis, upper arm**
  M60.121 Interstitial myositis, right upper arm
  M60.122 Interstitial myositis, left upper arm
  M60.129 Interstitial myositis, unspecified upper arm
+ **M60.13 Interstitial myositis, forearm**
  M60.131 Interstitial myositis, right forearm
  M60.132 Interstitial myositis, left forearm
  M60.139 Interstitial myositis, unspecified forearm
+ **M60.14 Interstitial myositis, hand**
  M60.141 Interstitial myositis, right hand
  M60.142 Interstitial myositis, left hand
  M60.149 Interstitial myositis, unspecified hand
+ **M60.15 Interstitial myositis, thigh**
  M60.151 Interstitial myositis, right thigh
  M60.152 Interstitial myositis, left thigh
  M60.159 Interstitial myositis, unspecified thigh
+ **M60.16 Interstitial myositis, lower leg**
  M60.161 Interstitial myositis, right lower leg
  M60.162 Interstitial myositis, left lower leg
  M60.169 Interstitial myositis, unspecified lower leg
+ **M60.17 Interstitial myositis, ankle and foot**
  M60.171 Interstitial myositis, right ankle and foot
  M60.172 Interstitial myositis, left ankle and foot
  M60.179 Interstitial myositis, unspecified ankle and foot
 M60.18 Interstitial myositis, other site
 M60.19 Interstitial myositis, multiple sites
+ **M60.2 Foreign body granuloma of soft tissue, not elsewhere classified**
  Use additional code to identify the type of retained foreign body (Z18.-)
  Excludes1: foreign body granuloma of skin and
      subcutaneous tissue (L92.3)
  M60.20 Foreign body granuloma of soft tissue, not elsewhere classified, unspecified site
+ **M60.21 Foreign body granuloma of soft tissue, not elsewhere classified, shoulder**
  M60.211 Foreign body granuloma of soft tissue, not elsewhere classified, right shoulder
  M60.212 Foreign body granuloma of soft tissue, not elsewhere classified, left shoulder
  M60.219 Foreign body granuloma of soft tissue, not elsewhere classified, unspecified shoulder
+ **M60.22 Foreign body granuloma of soft tissue, not elsewhere classified, upper arm**
  M60.221 Foreign body granuloma of soft tissue, not elsewhere classified, right upper arm
  M60.222 Foreign body granuloma of soft tissue, not elsewhere classified, left upper arm
  M60.229 Foreign body granuloma of soft tissue, not elsewhere classified, unspecified upper arm

- **+ M60.23** Foreign body granuloma of soft tissue, not elsewhere classified, forearm
  - M60.231 Foreign body granuloma of soft tissue, not elsewhere classified, right forearm
  - M60.232 Foreign body granuloma of soft tissue, not elsewhere classified, left forearm
  - M60.239 Foreign body granuloma of soft tissue, not elsewhere classified, unspecified forearm
- **+ M60.24** Foreign body granuloma of soft tissue, not elsewhere classified, hand
  - M60.241 Foreign body granuloma of soft tissue, not elsewhere classified, right hand
  - M60.242 Foreign body granuloma of soft tissue, not elsewhere classified, left hand
  - M60.249 Foreign body granuloma of soft tissue, not elsewhere classified, unspecified hand
- **+ M60.25** Foreign body granuloma of soft tissue, not elsewhere classified, thigh
  - M60.251 Foreign body granuloma of soft tissue, not elsewhere classified, right thigh
  - M60.252 Foreign body granuloma of soft tissue, not elsewhere classified, left thigh
  - M60.259 Foreign body granuloma of soft tissue, not elsewhere classified, unspecified thigh
- **+ M60.26** Foreign body granuloma of soft tissue, not elsewhere classified, lower leg
  - M60.261 Foreign body granuloma of soft tissue, not elsewhere classified, right lower leg
  - M60.262 Foreign body granuloma of soft tissue, not elsewhere classified, left lower leg
  - M60.269 Foreign body granuloma of soft tissue, not elsewhere classified, unspecified lower leg
- **+ M60.27** Foreign body granuloma of soft tissue, not elsewhere classified, ankle and foot
  - M60.271 Foreign body granuloma of soft tissue, not elsewhere classified, right ankle and foot
  - M60.272 Foreign body granuloma of soft tissue, not elsewhere classified, left ankle and foot
  - M60.279 Foreign body granuloma of soft tissue, not elsewhere classified, unspecified ankle and foot
- M60.28 Foreign body granuloma of soft tissue, not elsewhere classified, other site
- **+ M60.8** Other myositis
  - M60.80 Other myositis, unspecified site
  - **+ M60.81** Other myositis shoulder
    - M60.811 Other myositis, right shoulder
    - M60.812 Other myositis, left shoulder
    - M60.819 Other myositis, unspecified shoulder
  - **+ M60.82** Other myositis, upper arm
    - M60.821 Other myositis, right upper arm
    - M60.822 Other myositis, left upper arm
    - M60.829 Other myositis, unspecified upper arm
  - **+ M60.83** Other myositis, forearm
    - M60.831 Other myositis, right forearm
    - M60.832 Other myositis, left forearm
    - M60.839 Other myositis, unspecified forearm
  - **+ M60.84** Other myositis, hand
    - M60.841 Other myositis, right hand
    - M60.842 Other myositis, left hand
    - M60.849 Other myositis, unspecified hand
  - **+ M60.85** Other myositis, thigh
    - M60.851 Other myositis, right thigh
    - M60.852 Other myositis, left thigh
    - M60.859 Other myositis, unspecified thigh
  - **+ M60.86** Other myositis, lower leg
    - M60.861 Other myositis, right lower leg
    - M60.862 Other myositis, left lower leg
    - M60.869 Other myositis, unspecified lower leg
  - **+ M60.87** Other myositis, ankle and foot
    - M60.871 Other myositis, right ankle and foot
    - M60.872 Other myositis, left ankle and foot
    - M60.879 Other myositis, unspecified ankle and foot
  - M60.88 Other myositis, other site
  - M60.89 Other myositis, multiple sites
- M60.9 Myositis, unspecified

M61 Calcification and ossification of muscle
- **+ M61.0** Myositis ossificans traumatica
  - M61.00 Myositis ossificans traumatica, unspecified site
  - **+ M61.01** Myositis ossificans traumatica, shoulder
    - M61.011 Myositis ossificans traumatica, right shoulder
    - M61.012 Myositis ossificans traumatica, left shoulder
    - M61.019 Myositis ossificans traumatica, unspecified shoulder
  - **+ M61.02** Myositis ossificans traumatica, upper arm
    - M61.021 Myositis ossificans traumatica, right upper arm
    - M61.022 Myositis ossificans traumatica, left upper arm
    - M61.029 Myositis ossificans traumatica, unspecified upper arm
  - **+ M61.03** Myositis ossificans traumatica, forearm
    - M61.031 Myositis ossificans traumatica, right forearm
    - M61.032 Myositis ossificans traumatica, left forearm
    - M61.039 Myositis ossificans traumatica, unspecified forearm
  - **+ M61.04** Myositis ossificans traumatica, hand
    - M61.041 Myositis ossificans traumatica, right hand
    - M61.042 Myositis ossificans traumatica, left hand
    - M61.049 Myositis ossificans traumatica, unspecified hand
  - **+ M61.05** Myositis ossificans traumatica, thigh
    - M61.051 Myositis ossificans traumatica, right thigh
    - M61.052 Myositis ossificans traumatica, left thigh
    - M61.059 Myositis ossificans traumatica, unspecified thigh
  - **+ M61.06** Myositis ossificans traumatica, lower leg
    - M61.061 Myositis ossificans traumatica, right lower leg
    - M61.062 Myositis ossificans traumatica, left lower leg
    - M61.069 Myositis ossificans traumatica, unspecified lower leg
  - **+ M61.07** Myositis ossificans traumatica, ankle and foot
    - M61.071 Myositis ossificans traumatica, right ankle and foot
    - M61.072 Myositis ossificans traumatica, left ankle and foot
    - M61.079 Myositis ossificans traumatica, unspecified ankle and foot
  - M61.08 Myositis ossificans traumatica, other site
  - M61.09 Myositis ossificans traumatica, multiple sites
- **+ M61.1** Myositis ossificans progressiva
  Fibrodysplasia ossificans progressiva
  - M61.10 Myositis ossificans progressiva, unspecified site
  - **+ M61.11** Myositis ossificans progressiva, shoulder
    - M61.111 Myositis ossificans progressiva, right shoulder
    - M61.112 Myositis ossificans progressiva, left shoulder
    - M61.119 Myositis ossificans progressiva, unspecified shoulder
  - **+ M61.12** Myositis ossificans progressiva, upper arm
    - M61.121 Myositis ossificans progressiva, right upper arm
    - M61.122 Myositis ossificans progressiva, left upper arm
    - M61.129 Myositis ossificans progressiva, unspecified arm
  - **+ M61.13** Myositis ossificans progressiva, forearm
    - M61.131 Myositis ossificans progressiva, right forearm
    - M61.132 Myositis ossificans progressiva, left forearm
    - M61.139 Myositis ossificans progressiva, unspecified forearm
  - **+ M61.14** Myositis ossificans progressiva, hand and finger(s)
    - M61.141 Myositis ossificans progressiva, right hand
    - M61.142 Myositis ossificans progressiva, left hand

M61.143 Myositis ossificans progressiva, unspecified hand
M61.144 Myositis ossificans progressiva, right finger(s)
M61.145 Myositis ossificans progressiva, left finger(s)
M61.146 Myositis ossificans progressiva, unspecified finger(s)
+ M61.15 Myositis ossificans progressiva, thigh
M61.151 Myositis ossificans progressiva, right thigh
M61.152 Myositis ossificans progressiva, left thigh
M61.159 Myositis ossificans progressiva, unspecified thigh
+ M61.16 Myositis ossificans progressiva, lower leg
M61.161 Myositis ossificans progressiva, right lower leg
M61.162 Myositis ossificans progressiva, left lower leg
M61.169 Myositis ossificans progressiva, unspecified lower leg
+ M61.17 Myositis ossificans progressiva, ankle, foot and toe(s)
M61.171 Myositis ossificans progressiva, right ankle
M61.172 Myositis ossificans progressiva, left ankle
M61.173 Myositis ossificans progressiva, unspecified ankle
M61.174 Myositis ossificans progressiva, right foot
M61.175 Myositis ossificans progressiva, left foot
M61.176 Myositis ossificans progressiva, unspecified foot
M61.177 Myositis ossificans progressiva, right toe(s)
M61.178 Myositis ossificans progressiva, left toe(s)
M61.179 Myositis ossificans progressiva, unspecified toe(s)
M61.18 Myositis ossificans progressiva, other site
M61.19 Myositis ossificans progressiva, multiple sites
+ M61.2 Paralytic calcification and ossification of muscle
  Myositis ossificans associated with quadriplegia or paraplegia
M61.20 Paralytic calcification and ossification of muscle, unspecified site
+ M61.21 Paralytic calcification and ossification of muscle, shoulder
M61.211 Paralytic calcification and ossification of muscle, right shoulder
M61.212 Paralytic calcification and ossification of muscle, left shoulder
M61.219 Paralytic calcification and ossification of muscle, unspecified shoulder
+ M61.22 Paralytic calcification and ossification of muscle, upper arm
M61.221 Paralytic calcification and ossification of muscle, right upper arm
M61.222 Paralytic calcification and ossification of muscle, left upper arm
M61.229 Paralytic calcification and ossification of muscle, unspecified upper arm
+ M61.23 Paralytic calcification and ossification of muscle, forearm
M61.231 Paralytic calcification and ossification of muscle, right forearm
M61.232 Paralytic calcification and ossification of muscle, left forearm
M61.239 Paralytic calcification and ossification of muscle, unspecified forearm
+ M61.24 Paralytic calcification and ossification of muscle, hand
M61.241 Paralytic calcification and ossification of muscle, right hand
M61.242 Paralytic calcification and ossification of muscle, left hand
M61.249 Paralytic calcification and ossification of muscle, unspecified hand
+ M61.25 Paralytic calcification and ossification of muscle, thigh
M61.251 Paralytic calcification and ossification of muscle, right thigh
M61.252 Paralytic calcification and ossification of muscle, left thigh
M61.259 Paralytic calcification and ossification of muscle, unspecified thigh
+ M61.26 Paralytic calcification and ossification of muscle, lower leg
M61.261 Paralytic calcification and ossification of muscle, right lower leg
M61.262 Paralytic calcification and ossification of muscle, left lower leg
M61.269 Paralytic calcification and ossification of muscle, unspecified lower leg
+ M61.27 Paralytic calcification and ossification of muscle, ankle and foot
M61.271 Paralytic calcification and ossification of muscle, right ankle and foot
M61.272 Paralytic calcification and ossification of muscle, left ankle and foot
M61.279 Paralytic calcification and ossification of muscle, unspecified ankle and foot
M61.28 Paralytic calcification and ossification of muscle, other site
M61.29 Paralytic calcification and ossification of muscle, multiple sites
+ M61.3 Calcification and ossification of muscles associated with burns
  Myositis ossificans associated with burns
M61.30 Calcification and ossification of muscles associated with burns, unspecified site
+ M61.31 Calcification and ossification of muscles associated with burns, shoulder
M61.311 Calcification and ossification of muscles associated with burns, right shoulder
M61.312 Calcification and ossification of muscles associated with burns, left shoulder
M61.319 Calcification and ossification of muscles associated with burns, unspecified shoulder
+ M61.32 Calcification and ossification of muscles associated with burns, upper arm
M61.321 Calcification and ossification of muscles associated with burns, right upper arm
M61.322 Calcification and ossification of muscles associated with burns, left upper arm
M61.329 Calcification and ossification of muscles associated with burns, unspecified upper arm
+ M61.33 Calcification and ossification of muscles associated with burns, forearm
M61.331 Calcification and ossification of muscles associated with burns, right forearm
M61.332 Calcification and ossification of muscles associated with burns, left forearm
M61.339 Calcification and ossification of muscles associated with burns, unspecified forearm
+ M61.34 Calcification and ossification of muscles associated with burns, hand
M61.341 Calcification and ossification of muscles associated with burns, right hand
M61.342 Calcification and ossification of muscles associated with burns, left hand
M61.349 Calcification and ossification of muscles associated with burns, unspecified hand
+ M61.35 Calcification and ossification of muscles associated with burns, thigh
M61.351 Calcification and ossification of muscles associated with burns, right thigh
M61.352 Calcification and ossification of muscles associated with burns, left thigh
M61.359 Calcification and ossification of muscles associated with burns, unspecified thigh
+ M61.36 Calcification and ossification of muscles associated with burns, lower leg
M61.361 Calcification and ossification of muscles associated with burns, right lower leg
M61.362 Calcification and ossification of muscles associated with burns, left lower leg
M61.369 Calcification and ossification of muscles associated with burns, unspecified lower leg

- **M61.37** Calcification and ossification of muscles associated with burns, ankle and foot
  - M61.371 Calcification and ossification of muscles associated with burns, right ankle and foot
  - M61.372 Calcification and ossification of muscles associated with burns, left ankle and foot
  - M61.379 Calcification and ossification of muscles associated with burns, unspecified ankle and foot
- M61.38 Calcification and ossification of muscles associated with burns, other site
- M61.39 Calcification and ossification of muscles associated with burns, multiple sites
- **M61.4** Other calcification of muscle
  - **Excludes1:** *calcific tendinitis NOS (M65.2-)*
    calcific tendinitis of shoulder (M75.3)
  - M61.40 Other calcification of muscle, unspecified site
  - **M61.41** Other calcification of muscle, shoulder
    - M61.411 Other calcification of muscle, right shoulder
    - M61.412 Other calcification of muscle, left shoulder
    - M61.419 Other calcification of muscle, unspecified shoulder
  - **M61.42** Other calcification of muscle, upper arm
    - M61.421 Other calcification of muscle, right upper arm
    - M61.422 Other calcification of muscle, left upper arm
    - M61.429 Other calcification of muscle, unspecified upper arm
  - **M61.43** Other calcification of muscle, forearm
    - M61.431 Other calcification of muscle, right forearm
    - M61.432 Other calcification of muscle, left forearm
    - M61.439 Other calcification of muscle, unspecified forearm
  - **M61.44** Other calcification of muscle, hand
    - M61.441 Other calcification of muscle, right hand
    - M61.442 Other calcification of muscle, left hand
    - M61.449 Other calcification of muscle, unspecified hand
  - **M61.45** Other calcification of muscle, thigh
    - M61.451 Other calcification of muscle, right thigh
    - M61.452 Other calcification of muscle, left thigh
    - M61.459 Other calcification of muscle, unspecified thigh
  - **M61.46** Other calcification of muscle, lower leg
    - M61.461 Other calcification of muscle, right lower leg
    - M61.462 Other calcification of muscle, left lower leg
    - M61.469 Other calcification of muscle, unspecified lower leg
  - **M61.47** Other calcification of muscle, ankle and foot
    - M61.471 Other calcification of muscle, right ankle and foot
    - M61.472 Other calcification of muscle, left ankle and foot
    - M61.479 Other calcification of muscle, unspecified ankle and foot
  - M61.48 Other calcification of muscle, other site
  - M61.49 Other calcification of muscle, multiple sites
- **M61.5** Other ossification of muscle
  - M61.50 Other ossification of muscle, unspecified site
  - **M61.51** Other ossification of muscle, shoulder
    - M61.511 Other ossification of muscle, right shoulder
    - M61.512 Other ossification of muscle, left shoulder
    - M61.519 Other ossification of muscle, unspecified shoulder
  - **M61.52** Other ossification of muscle, upper arm
    - M61.521 Other ossification of muscle, right upper arm
    - M61.522 Other ossification of muscle, left upper arm
    - M61.529 Other ossification of muscle, unspecified upper arm
  - **M61.53** Other ossification of muscle, forearm
    - M61.531 Other ossification of muscle, right forearm
    - M61.532 Other ossification of muscle, left forearm
    - M61.539 Other ossification of muscle, unspecified forearm
  - **M61.54** Other ossification of muscle, hand
    - M61.541 Other ossification of muscle, right hand
    - M61.542 Other ossification of muscle, left hand
    - M61.549 Other ossification of muscle, unspecified hand
  - **M61.55** Other ossification of muscle, thigh
    - M61.551 Other ossification of muscle, right thigh
    - M61.552 Other ossification of muscle, left thigh
    - M61.559 Other ossification of muscle, unspecified thigh
  - **M61.56** Other ossification of muscle, lower leg
    - M61.561 Other ossification of muscle, right lower leg
    - M61.562 Other ossification of muscle, left lower leg
    - M61.569 Other ossification of muscle, unspecified lower leg
  - **M61.57** Other ossification of muscle, ankle and foot
    - M61.571 Other ossification of muscle, right ankle and foot
    - M61.572 Other ossification of muscle, left ankle and foot
    - M61.579 Other ossification of muscle, unspecified ankle and foot
  - M61.58 Other ossification of muscle, other site
  - M61.59 Other ossification of muscle, multiple sites
- M61.9 Calcification and ossification of muscle, unspecified

M62 Other disorders of muscle
- **Excludes1:** *alcoholic myopathy (G72.1)*
  cramp and spasm (R25.2)
  drug-induced myopathy (G72.0)
  myalgia (M79.1-)
  stiff-man syndrome (G25.82)
- **Excludes2:** *nontraumatic hematoma of muscle (M79.81)*
- **M62.0** Separation of muscle (nontraumatic)
  Diastasis of muscle
  - **Excludes1:** *diastasis recti complicating pregnancy, labor and delivery (O71.8)*
    traumatic separation of muscle- see strain of muscle by body region
  - M62.00 Separation of muscle (nontraumatic), unspecified site
  - **M62.01** Separation of muscle (nontraumatic), shoulder
    - M62.011 Separation of muscle (nontraumatic), right shoulder
    - M62.012 Separation of muscle (nontraumatic), left shoulder
    - M62.019 Separation of muscle (nontraumatic), unspecified shoulder
  - **M62.02** Separation of muscle (nontraumatic), upper arm
    - M62.021 Separation of muscle (nontraumatic), right upper arm
    - M62.022 Separation of muscle (nontraumatic), left upper arm
    - M62.029 Separation of muscle (nontraumatic), unspecified upper arm
  - **M62.03** Separation of muscle (nontraumatic), forearm
    - M62.031 Separation of muscle (nontraumatic), right forearm
    - M62.032 Separation of muscle (nontraumatic), left forearm
    - M62.039 Separation of muscle (nontraumatic), unspecified forearm

- **+ M62.04 Separation of muscle (nontraumatic), hand**
  - M62.041 Separation of muscle (nontraumatic), right hand
  - M62.042 Separation of muscle (nontraumatic), left hand
  - M62.049 Separation of muscle (nontraumatic), unspecified hand
- **+ M62.05 Separation of muscle (nontraumatic), thigh**
  - M62.051 Separation of muscle (nontraumatic), right thigh
  - M62.052 Separation of muscle (nontraumatic), left thigh
  - M62.059 Separation of muscle (nontraumatic), unspecified thigh
- **+ M62.06 Separation of muscle (nontraumatic), lower leg**
  - M62.061 Separation of muscle (nontraumatic), right lower leg
  - M62.062 Separation of muscle (nontraumatic), left lower leg
  - M62.069 Separation of muscle (nontraumatic), unspecified lower leg
- **+ M62.07 Separation of muscle (nontraumatic), ankle and foot**
  - M62.071 Separation of muscle (nontraumatic), right ankle and foot
  - M62.072 Separation of muscle (nontraumatic), left ankle and foot
  - M62.079 Separation of muscle (nontraumatic), unspecified ankle and foot
- M62.08 Separation of muscle (nontraumatic), other site
- **+ M62.1 Other rupture of muscle (nontraumatic)**
  - *Excludes1:* traumatic rupture of muscle - see strain of muscle by body region
  - *Excludes2:* rupture of tendon (M66.-)
  - M62.10 Other rupture of muscle (nontraumatic), unspecified site
- **+ M62.11 Other rupture of muscle (nontraumatic), shoulder**
  - M62.111 Other rupture of muscle (nontraumatic), right shoulder
  - M62.112 Other rupture of muscle (nontraumatic), left shoulder
  - M62.119 Other rupture of muscle (nontraumatic), unspecified shoulder
- **+ M62.12 Other rupture of muscle (nontraumatic), upper arm**
  - M62.121 Other rupture of muscle (nontraumatic), right upper arm
  - M62.122 Other rupture of muscle (nontraumatic), left upper arm
  - M62.129 Other rupture of muscle (nontraumatic), unspecified upper arm
- **+ M62.13 Other rupture of muscle (nontraumatic), forearm**
  - M62.131 Other rupture of muscle (nontraumatic), right forearm
  - M62.132 Other rupture of muscle (nontraumatic), left forearm
  - M62.139 Other rupture of muscle (nontraumatic), unspecified forearm
- **+ M62.14 Other rupture of muscle (nontraumatic), hand**
  - M62.141 Other rupture of muscle (nontraumatic), right hand
  - M62.142 Other rupture of muscle (nontraumatic), left hand
  - M62.149 Other rupture of muscle (nontraumatic), unspecified hand
- **+ M62.15 Other rupture of muscle (nontraumatic), thigh**
  - M62.151 Other rupture of muscle (nontraumatic), right thigh
  - M62.152 Other rupture of muscle (nontraumatic), left thigh
  - M62.159 Other rupture of muscle (nontraumatic), unspecified thigh
- **+ M62.16 Other rupture of muscle (nontraumatic), lower leg**
  - M62.161 Other rupture of muscle (nontraumatic), right lower leg
  - M62.162 Other rupture of muscle (nontraumatic), left lower leg
  - M62.169 Other rupture of muscle (nontraumatic), unspecified lower leg
- **+ M62.17 Other rupture of muscle (nontraumatic), ankle and foot**
  - M62.171 Other rupture of muscle (nontraumatic), right ankle and foot
  - M62.172 Other rupture of muscle (nontraumatic), left ankle and foot
  - M62.179 Other rupture of muscle (nontraumatic), unspecified ankle and foot
- M62.18 Other rupture of muscle (nontraumatic), other site
- **+ M62.2 Nontraumatic ischemic infarction of muscle**
  - *Excludes1:* compartment syndrome (traumatic) (T79.A-)
    nontraumatic compartment syndrome (M79.A-)
    traumatic ischemia of muscle (T79.6)
    rhabdomyolysis (M62.82)
    Volkmann's ischemic contracture (T79.6)
  - M62.20 Nontraumatic ischemic infarction of muscle, unspecified site
- **+ M62.21 Nontraumatic ischemic infarction of muscle, shoulder**
  - M62.211 Nontraumatic ischemic infarction of muscle, right shoulder
  - M62.212 Nontraumatic ischemic infarction of muscle, left shoulder
  - M62.219 Nontraumatic ischemic infarction of muscle, unspecified shoulder
- **+ M62.22 Nontraumatic ischemic infarction of muscle, upper arm**
  - M62.221 Nontraumatic ischemic infarction of muscle, right upper arm
  - M62.222 Nontraumatic ischemic infarction of muscle, left upper arm
  - M62.229 Nontraumatic ischemic infarction of muscle, unspecified upper arm
- **+ M62.23 Nontraumatic ischemic infarction of muscle, forearm**
  - M62.231 Nontraumatic ischemic infarction of muscle, right forearm
  - M62.232 Nontraumatic ischemic infarction of muscle, left forearm
  - M62.239 Nontraumatic ischemic infarction of muscle, unspecified forearm
- **+ M62.24 Nontraumatic ischemic infarction of muscle, hand**
  - M62.241 Nontraumatic ischemic infarction of muscle, right hand
  - M62.242 Nontraumatic ischemic infarction of muscle, left hand
  - M62.249 Nontraumatic ischemic infarction of muscle, unspecified hand
- **+ M62.25 Nontraumatic ischemic infarction of muscle, thigh**
  - M62.251 Nontraumatic ischemic infarction of muscle, right thigh
  - M62.252 Nontraumatic ischemic infarction of muscle, left thigh
  - M62.259 Nontraumatic ischemic infarction of muscle, unspecified thigh
- **+ M62.26 Nontraumatic ischemic infarction of muscle, lower leg**
  - M62.261 Nontraumatic ischemic infarction of muscle, right lower leg
  - M62.262 Nontraumatic ischemic infarction of muscle, left lower leg
  - M62.269 Nontraumatic ischemic infarction of muscle, unspecified lower leg
- **+ M62.27 Nontraumatic ischemic infarction of muscle, ankle and foot**
  - M62.271 Nontraumatic ischemic infarction of muscle, right ankle and foot
  - M62.272 Nontraumatic ischemic infarction of muscle, left ankle and foot
  - M62.279 Nontraumatic ischemic infarction of muscle, unspecified ankle and foot
- M62.28 Nontraumatic ischemic infarction of muscle, other site
- **M62.3 Immobility syndrome (paraplegic)**

- **M62.4 Contracture of muscle**
  Contracture of tendon (sheath)
  Excludes1: *contracture of joint (M24.5-)*
  M62.40 Contracture of muscle, unspecified site
  - M62.41 Contracture of muscle, shoulder
    M62.411 Contracture of muscle, right shoulder
    M62.412 Contracture of muscle, left shoulder
    M62.419 Contracture of muscle, unspecified shoulder
  - M62.42 Contracture of muscle, upper arm
    M62.421 Contracture of muscle, right upper arm
    M62.422 Contracture of muscle, left upper arm
    M62.429 Contracture of muscle, unspecified upper arm
  - M62.43 Contracture of muscle, forearm
    M62.431 Contracture of muscle, right forearm
    M62.432 Contracture of muscle, left forearm
    M62.439 Contracture of muscle, unspecified forearm
  - M62.44 Contracture of muscle, hand
    M62.441 Contracture of muscle, right hand
    M62.442 Contracture of muscle, left hand
    M62.449 Contracture of muscle, unspecified hand
  - M62.45 Contracture of muscle, thigh
    M62.451 Contracture of muscle, right thigh
    M62.452 Contracture of muscle, left thigh
    M62.459 Contracture of muscle, unspecified thigh
  - M62.46 Contracture of muscle, lower leg
    M62.461 Contracture of muscle, right lower leg
    M62.462 Contracture of muscle, left lower leg
      AHA CC: 2Q, 2023, 14
    M62.469 Contracture of muscle, unspecified lower leg
  - M62.47 Contracture of muscle, ankle and foot
    M62.471 Contracture of muscle, right ankle and foot
    M62.472 Contracture of muscle, left ankle and foot
    M62.479 Contracture of muscle, unspecified ankle and foot
  M62.48 Contracture of muscle, other site
  M62.49 Contracture of muscle, multiple sites
- **M62.5 Muscle wasting and atrophy, not elsewhere classified**
  Disuse atrophy NEC
  Excludes1: *neuralgic amyotrophy (G54.5)*
  progressive muscular atrophy (G12.21)
  sarcopenia (M62.84)
  Excludes2: *pelvic muscle wasting (N81.84)*
  M62.50 Muscle wasting and atrophy, not elsewhere classified, unspecified site
  - M62.51 Muscle wasting and atrophy, not elsewhere classified, shoulder
    M62.511 Muscle wasting and atrophy, not elsewhere classified, right shoulder
    M62.512 Muscle wasting and atrophy, not elsewhere classified, left shoulder
    M62.519 Muscle wasting and atrophy, not elsewhere classified, unspecified shoulder
  - M62.52 Muscle wasting and atrophy, not elsewhere classified, upper arm
    M62.521 Muscle wasting and atrophy, not elsewhere classified, right upper arm
    M62.522 Muscle wasting and atrophy, not elsewhere classified, left upper arm
    M62.529 Muscle wasting and atrophy, not elsewhere classified, unspecified upper arm
  - M62.53 Muscle wasting and atrophy, not elsewhere classified, forearm
    M62.531 Muscle wasting and atrophy, not elsewhere classified, right forearm
    M62.532 Muscle wasting and atrophy, not elsewhere classified, left forearm
    M62.539 Muscle wasting and atrophy, not elsewhere classified, unspecified forearm
  - M62.54 Muscle wasting and atrophy, not elsewhere classified, hand
    M62.541 Muscle wasting and atrophy, not elsewhere classified, right hand
    M62.542 Muscle wasting and atrophy, not elsewhere classified, left hand
    M62.549 Muscle wasting and atrophy, not elsewhere classified, unspecified hand
  - M62.55 Muscle wasting and atrophy, not elsewhere classified, thigh
    M62.551 Muscle wasting and atrophy, not elsewhere classified, right thigh
    M62.552 Muscle wasting and atrophy, not elsewhere classified, left thigh
    M62.559 Muscle wasting and atrophy, not elsewhere classified, unspecified thigh
  - M62.56 Muscle wasting and atrophy, not elsewhere classified, lower leg
    M62.561 Muscle wasting and atrophy, not elsewhere classified, right lower leg
    M62.562 Muscle wasting and atrophy, not elsewhere classified, left lower leg
    M62.569 Muscle wasting and atrophy, not elsewhere classified, unspecified lower leg
  - M62.57 Muscle wasting and atrophy, not elsewhere classified, ankle and foot
    M62.571 Muscle wasting and atrophy, not elsewhere classified, right ankle and foot
    M62.572 Muscle wasting and atrophy, not elsewhere classified, left ankle and foot
    M62.579 Muscle wasting and atrophy, not elsewhere classified, unspecified ankle and foot
  M62.58 Muscle wasting and atrophy, not elsewhere classified, other site
  M62.59 Muscle wasting and atrophy, not elsewhere classified, multiple sites
  - M62.5A Muscle wasting and atrophy, not elsewhere classified, back
    AHA CC: 4Q, 2022, 29
    M62.5A0 Muscle wasting and atrophy, not elsewhere classified, back, cervical
    M62.5A1 Muscle wasting and atrophy, not elsewhere classified, back, thoracic
    M62.5A2 Muscle wasting and atrophy, not elsewhere classified, back, lumbosacral
    M62.5A9 Muscle wasting and atrophy, not elsewhere classified, back, unspecified level
- **M62.8 Other specified disorders of muscle**
  Excludes2: *nontraumatic hematoma of muscle (M79.81)*
  M62.81 Muscle weakness (generalized)
    Excludes1: *muscle weakness in sarcopenia (M62.84)*
  CC M62.82 Rhabdomyolysis
    Excludes1: *traumatic rhabdomyolysis (T79.6)*
    AHA CC: 2Q, 2019, 12-13
  - M62.83 Muscle spasm
    M62.830 Muscle spasm of back
    M62.831 Muscle spasm of calf
      Charley-horse
    M62.838 Other muscle spasm
  M62.84 Sarcopenia
    Age-related sarcopenia
    Code first underlying disease, if applicable, such as: disorders of myoneural junction and muscle disease
      in diseases classified elsewhere (G73.-)
      other and unspecified myopathies (G72.-)
      primary disorders of muscles (G71.-)
    AHA CC: 4Q, 2016, 41
  M62.89 Other specified disorders of muscle
    Muscle (sheath) hernia
  M62.9 Disorder of muscle, unspecified

M63 Disorders of muscle in diseases classified elsewhere

Code first underlying disease, such as:
  leprosy (A30.-)
  neoplasm (C49.-, C79.89, D21.-, D48.1-)
  schistosomiasis (B65.-)
  trichinellosis (B75)
Excludes1: *myopathy in cysticercosis (B69.81)*
  myopathy in endocrine diseases (G73.7)
  myopathy in metabolic diseases (G73.7)
  myopathy in sarcoidosis (D86.87)
  myopathy in secondary syphilis (A51.49)
  myopathy in syphilis (late) (A52.78)
  myopathy in toxoplasmosis (B58.82)
  myopathy in tuberculosis (A18.09)

- **M63.8 Disorders of muscle in diseases classified elsewhere**
  - **M63.80** Disorders of muscle in diseases classified elsewhere, unspecified site
  - **M63.81** Disorders of muscle in diseases classified elsewhere, shoulder
    - **M63.811** Disorders of muscle in diseases classified elsewhere, right shoulder
    - **M63.812** Disorders of muscle in diseases classified elsewhere, left shoulder
    - **M63.819** Disorders of muscle in diseases classified elsewhere, unspecified shoulder
  - **M63.82** Disorders of muscle in diseases classified elsewhere, upper arm
    - **M63.821** Disorders of muscle in diseases classified elsewhere, right upper arm
    - **M63.822** Disorders of muscle in diseases classified elsewhere, left upper arm
    - **M63.829** Disorders of muscle in diseases classified elsewhere, unspecified upper arm
  - **M63.83** Disorders of muscle in diseases classified elsewhere, forearm
    - **M63.831** Disorders of muscle in diseases classified elsewhere, right forearm
    - **M63.832** Disorders of muscle in diseases classified elsewhere, left forearm
    - **M63.839** Disorders of muscle in diseases classified elsewhere, unspecified forearm
  - **M63.84** Disorders of muscle in diseases classified elsewhere, hand
    - **M63.841** Disorders of muscle in diseases classified elsewhere, right hand
    - **M63.842** Disorders of muscle in diseases classified elsewhere, left hand
    - **M63.849** Disorders of muscle in diseases classified elsewhere, unspecified hand
  - **M63.85** Disorders of muscle in diseases classified elsewhere, thigh
    - **M63.851** Disorders of muscle in diseases classified elsewhere, right thigh
    - **M63.852** Disorders of muscle in diseases classified elsewhere, left thigh
    - **M63.859** Disorders of muscle in diseases classified elsewhere, unspecified thigh
  - **M63.86** Disorders of muscle in diseases classified elsewhere, lower leg
    - **M63.861** Disorders of muscle in diseases classified elsewhere, right lower leg
    - **M63.862** Disorders of muscle in diseases classified elsewhere, left lower leg
    - **M63.869** Disorders of muscle in diseases classified elsewhere, unspecified lower leg
  - **M63.87** Disorders of muscle in diseases classified elsewhere, ankle and foot
    - **M63.871** Disorders of muscle in diseases classified elsewhere, right ankle and foot
    - **M63.872** Disorders of muscle in diseases classified elsewhere, left ankle and foot
    - **M63.879** Disorders of muscle in diseases classified elsewhere, unspecified ankle and foot
  - **M63.88** Disorders of muscle in diseases classified elsewhere, other site
  - **M63.89** Disorders of muscle in diseases classified elsewhere, multiple sites

Disorders of synovium and tendon (M65-M67)

M65 Synovitis and tenosynovitis

Excludes1: chronic crepitant synovitis of hand and wrist (M70.0-)
current injury - see injury of ligament or tendon by body region
soft tissue disorders related to use, overuse and pressure (M70.-)

- **M65.0 Abscess of tendon sheath**
  Use additional code (B95-B96) to identify bacterial agent
  - **M65.00** Abscess of tendon sheath, unspecified site
  - **M65.01** Abscess of tendon sheath, shoulder
    - **M65.011** Abscess of tendon sheath, right shoulder
    - **M65.012** Abscess of tendon sheath, left shoulder
    - **M65.019** Abscess of tendon sheath, unspecified shoulder
  - **M65.02** Abscess of tendon sheath, upper arm
    - **M65.021** Abscess of tendon sheath, right upper arm
    - **M65.022** Abscess of tendon sheath, left upper arm
    - **M65.029** Abscess of tendon sheath, unspecified upper arm
  - **M65.03** Abscess of tendon sheath, forearm
    - **M65.031** Abscess of tendon sheath, right forearm
    - **M65.032** Abscess of tendon sheath, left forearm
    - **M65.039** Abscess of tendon sheath, unspecified forearm
  - **M65.04** Abscess of tendon sheath, hand
    - **M65.041** Abscess of tendon sheath, right hand
    - **M65.042** Abscess of tendon sheath, left hand
    - **M65.049** Abscess of tendon sheath, unspecified hand
  - **M65.05** Abscess of tendon sheath, thigh
    - **M65.051** Abscess of tendon sheath, right thigh
    - **M65.052** Abscess of tendon sheath, left thigh
    - **M65.059** Abscess of tendon sheath, unspecified thigh
  - **M65.06** Abscess of tendon sheath, lower leg
    - **M65.061** Abscess of tendon sheath, right lower leg
    - **M65.062** Abscess of tendon sheath, left lower leg
    - **M65.069** Abscess of tendon sheath, unspecified lower leg
  - **M65.07** Abscess of tendon sheath, ankle and foot
    - **M65.071** Abscess of tendon sheath, right ankle and foot
    - **M65.072** Abscess of tendon sheath, left ankle and foot
    - **M65.079** Abscess of tendon sheath, unspecified ankle and foot
  - **M65.08** Abscess of tendon sheath, other site
- **M65.1 Other infective (teno)synovitis**
  - **M65.10** Other infective (teno)synovitis, unspecified site
  - **M65.11** Other infective (teno)synovitis, shoulder
    - **M65.111** Other infective (teno)synovitis, right shoulder
    - **M65.112** Other infective (teno)synovitis, left shoulder
    - **M65.119** Other infective (teno)synovitis, unspecified shoulder
  - **M65.12** Other infective (teno)synovitis, elbow
    - **M65.121** Other infective (teno)synovitis, right elbow
    - **M65.122** Other infective (teno)synovitis, left elbow
    - **M65.129** Other infective (teno)synovitis, unspecified elbow
  - **M65.13** Other infective (teno)synovitis, wrist
    - **M65.131** Other infective (teno)synovitis, right wrist
    - **M65.132** Other infective (teno)synovitis, left wrist
    - **M65.139** Other infective (teno)synovitis, unspecified wrist
  - **M65.14** Other infective (teno)synovitis, hand
    - **M65.141** Other infective (teno)synovitis, right hand
    - **M65.142** Other infective (teno)synovitis, left hand
    - **M65.149** Other infective (teno)synovitis, unspecified hand
  - **M65.15** Other infective (teno)synovitis, hip
    - **M65.151** Other infective (teno)synovitis, right hip
    - **M65.152** Other infective (teno)synovitis, left hip
    - **M65.159** Other infective (teno)synovitis, unspecified hip
  - **M65.16** Other infective (teno)synovitis, knee
    - **M65.161** Other infective (teno)synovitis, right knee
    - **M65.162** Other infective (teno)synovitis, left knee
    - **M65.169** Other infective (teno)synovitis, unspecified knee

- **+ M65.17 Other infective (teno)synovitis, ankle and foot**
  - M65.171 Other infective (teno)synovitis, right ankle and foot
  - M65.172 Other infective (teno)synovitis, left ankle and foot
  - M65.179 Other infective (teno)synovitis, unspecified ankle and foot
- M65.18 Other infective (teno)synovitis, other site
- M65.19 Other infective (teno)synovitis, multiple sites
- **+ M65.2 Calcific tendinitis**
  - *Excludes1:* tendinitis as classified in M75-M77
    calcified tendinitis of shoulder (M75.3)
  - M65.20 Calcific tendinitis, unspecified site
  - **+ M65.22 Calcific tendinitis, upper arm**
    - M65.221 Calcific tendinitis, right upper arm
    - M65.222 Calcific tendinitis, left upper arm
    - M65.229 Calcific tendinitis, unspecified upper arm
  - **+ M65.23 Calcific tendinitis, forearm**
    - M65.231 Calcific tendinitis, right forearm
    - M65.232 Calcific tendinitis, left forearm
    - M65.239 Calcific tendinitis, unspecified forearm
  - **+ M65.24 Calcific tendinitis, hand**
    - M65.241 Calcific tendinitis, right hand
    - M65.242 Calcific tendinitis, left hand
    - M65.249 Calcific tendinitis, unspecified hand
  - **+ M65.25 Calcific tendinitis, thigh**
    - M65.251 Calcific tendinitis, right thigh
    - M65.252 Calcific tendinitis, left thigh
    - M65.259 Calcific tendinitis, unspecified thigh
  - **+ M65.26 Calcific tendinitis, lower leg**
    - M65.261 Calcific tendinitis, right lower leg
    - M65.262 Calcific tendinitis, left lower leg
    - M65.269 Calcific tendinitis, unspecified lower leg
  - **+ M65.27 Calcific tendinitis, ankle and foot**
    - M65.271 Calcific tendinitis, right ankle and foot
    - M65.272 Calcific tendinitis, left ankle and foot
    - M65.279 Calcific tendinitis, unspecified ankle and foot
  - M65.28 Calcific tendinitis, other site
  - M65.29 Calcific tendinitis, multiple sites
- **+ M65.3 Trigger finger**
  - Nodular tendinous disease
  - M65.30 Trigger finger, unspecified finger
  - **+ M65.31 Trigger thumb**
    - M65.311 Trigger thumb, right thumb
    - M65.312 Trigger thumb, left thumb
    - M65.319 Trigger thumb, unspecified thumb
  - **+ M65.32 Trigger finger, index finger**
    - M65.321 Trigger finger, right index finger
    - M65.322 Trigger finger, left index finger
    - M65.329 Trigger finger, unspecified index finger
  - **+ M65.33 Trigger finger, middle finger**
    - M65.331 Trigger finger, right middle finger
    - M65.332 Trigger finger, left middle finger
    - M65.339 Trigger finger, unspecified middle finger
  - **+ M65.34 Trigger finger, ring finger**
    - M65.341 Trigger finger, right ring finger
    - M65.342 Trigger finger, left ring finger
    - M65.349 Trigger finger, unspecified ring finger
  - **+ M65.35 Trigger finger, little finger**
    - M65.351 Trigger finger, right little finger
    - M65.352 Trigger finger, left little finger
    - M65.359 Trigger finger, unspecified little finger
- M65.4 Radial styloid tenosynovitis [de Quervain]
- **+ M65.8 Other synovitis and tenosynovitis**
  - M65.80 Other synovitis and tenosynovitis, unspecified site
  - **+ M65.81 Other synovitis and tenosynovitis, shoulder**
    - M65.811 Other synovitis and tenosynovitis, right shoulder
    - M65.812 Other synovitis and tenosynovitis, left shoulder
    - M65.819 Other synovitis and tenosynovitis, unspecified shoulder
  - **+ M65.82 Other synovitis and tenosynovitis, upper arm**
    - M65.821 Other synovitis and tenosynovitis, right upper arm
    - M65.822 Other synovitis and tenosynovitis, left upper arm
    - M65.829 Other synovitis and tenosynovitis, unspecified upper arm
  - **+ M65.83 Other synovitis and tenosynovitis, forearm**
    - M65.831 Other synovitis and tenosynovitis, right forearm
    - M65.832 Other synovitis and tenosynovitis, left forearm
    - M65.839 Other synovitis and tenosynovitis, unspecified forearm
  - **+ M65.84 Other synovitis and tenosynovitis, hand**
    - M65.841 Other synovitis and tenosynovitis, right hand
    - M65.842 Other synovitis and tenosynovitis, left hand
    - M65.849 Other synovitis and tenosynovitis, unspecified hand
  - **+ M65.85 Other synovitis and tenosynovitis, thigh**
    - M65.851 Other synovitis and tenosynovitis, right thigh
    - M65.852 Other synovitis and tenosynovitis, left thigh
    - M65.859 Other synovitis and tenosynovitis, unspecified thigh
  - **+ M65.86 Other synovitis and tenosynovitis, lower leg**
    - M65.861 Other synovitis and tenosynovitis, right lower leg
    - M65.862 Other synovitis and tenosynovitis, left lower leg
    - M65.869 Other synovitis and tenosynovitis, unspecified lower leg
  - **+ M65.87 Other synovitis and tenosynovitis, ankle and foot**
    - M65.871 Other synovitis and tenosynovitis, right ankle and foot
    - M65.872 Other synovitis and tenosynovitis, left ankle and foot
    - M65.879 Other synovitis and tenosynovitis, unspecified ankle and foot
  - M65.88 Other synovitis and tenosynovitis, other site
  - M65.89 Other synovitis and tenosynovitis, multiple sites
- M65.9 Synovitis and tenosynovitis, unspecified

M66 Spontaneous rupture of synovium and tendon

Includes: rupture that occurs when a normal force is applied to tissues that are inferred to have less than normal strength

Excludes2: rotator cuff syndrome (M75.1-)
rupture where an abnormal force is applied to normal tissue - see injury of tendon by body region

- M66.0 Rupture of popliteal cyst
- **+ M66.1 Rupture of synovium**
  - Rupture of synovial cyst
  - *Excludes2:* rupture of popliteal cyst (M66.0)
  - M66.10 Rupture of synovium, unspecified joint
  - **+ M66.11 Rupture of synovium, shoulder**
    - M66.111 Rupture of synovium, right shoulder
    - M66.112 Rupture of synovium, left shoulder
    - M66.119 Rupture of synovium, unspecified shoulder
  - **+ M66.12 Rupture of synovium, elbow**
    - M66.121 Rupture of synovium, right elbow
    - M66.122 Rupture of synovium, left elbow
    - M66.129 Rupture of synovium, unspecified elbow
  - **+ M66.13 Rupture of synovium, wrist**
    - M66.131 Rupture of synovium, right wrist
    - M66.132 Rupture of synovium, left wrist
    - M66.139 Rupture of synovium, unspecified wrist
  - **+ M66.14 Rupture of synovium, hand and fingers**
    - M66.141 Rupture of synovium, right hand
    - M66.142 Rupture of synovium, left hand
    - M66.143 Rupture of synovium, unspecified hand
    - M66.144 Rupture of synovium, right finger(s)
    - M66.145 Rupture of synovium, left finger(s)
    - M66.146 Rupture of synovium, unspecified finger(s)
  - **+ M66.15 Rupture of synovium, hip**
    - M66.151 Rupture of synovium, right hip
    - M66.152 Rupture of synovium, left hip
    - M66.159 Rupture of synovium, unspecified hip
  - **+ M66.17 Rupture of synovium, ankle, foot and toes**
    - M66.171 Rupture of synovium, right ankle
    - M66.172 Rupture of synovium, left ankle
    - M66.173 Rupture of synovium, unspecified ankle
    - M66.174 Rupture of synovium, right foot

M66.175 Rupture of synovium, left foot
M66.176 Rupture of synovium, unspecified foot
M66.177 Rupture of synovium, right toe(s)
M66.178 Rupture of synovium, left toe(s)
M66.179 Rupture of synovium, unspecified toe(s)
M66.18 Rupture of synovium, other site
+ M66.2 Spontaneous rupture of extensor tendons
  M66.20 Spontaneous rupture of extensor tendons, unspecified site
  + M66.21 Spontaneous rupture of extensor tendons, shoulder
    M66.211 Spontaneous rupture of extensor tendons, right shoulder
    M66.212 Spontaneous rupture of extensor tendons, left shoulder
    M66.219 Spontaneous rupture of extensor tendons, unspecified shoulder
  + M66.22 Spontaneous rupture of extensor tendons, upper arm
    M66.221 Spontaneous rupture of extensor tendons, right upper arm
    M66.222 Spontaneous rupture of extensor tendons, left upper arm
    M66.229 Spontaneous rupture of extensor tendons, unspecified upper arm
  + M66.23 Spontaneous rupture of extensor tendons, forearm
    M66.231 Spontaneous rupture of extensor tendons, right forearm
    M66.232 Spontaneous rupture of extensor tendons, left forearm
    M66.239 Spontaneous rupture of extensor tendons, unspecified forearm
  + M66.24 Spontaneous rupture of extensor tendons, hand
    M66.241 Spontaneous rupture of extensor tendons, right hand
    M66.242 Spontaneous rupture of extensor tendons, left hand
    M66.249 Spontaneous rupture of extensor tendons, unspecified hand
  + M66.25 Spontaneous rupture of extensor tendons, thigh
    M66.251 Spontaneous rupture of extensor tendons, right thigh
    M66.252 Spontaneous rupture of extensor tendons, left thigh
    M66.259 Spontaneous rupture of extensor tendons, unspecified thigh
  + M66.26 Spontaneous rupture of extensor tendons, lower leg
    M66.261 Spontaneous rupture of extensor tendons, right lower leg
    M66.262 Spontaneous rupture of extensor tendons, left lower leg
    M66.269 Spontaneous rupture of extensor tendons, unspecified lower leg
  + M66.27 Spontaneous rupture of extensor tendons, ankle and foot
    M66.271 Spontaneous rupture of extensor tendons, right ankle and foot
    M66.272 Spontaneous rupture of extensor tendons, left ankle and foot
    M66.279 Spontaneous rupture of extensor tendons, unspecified ankle and foot
  M66.28 Spontaneous rupture of extensor tendons, other site
  M66.29 Spontaneous rupture of extensor tendons, multiple sites
+ M66.3 Spontaneous rupture of flexor tendons
  M66.30 Spontaneous rupture of flexor tendons, unspecified site
  + M66.31 Spontaneous rupture of flexor tendons, shoulder
    M66.311 Spontaneous rupture of flexor tendons, right shoulder
    M66.312 Spontaneous rupture of flexor tendons, left shoulder
    M66.319 Spontaneous rupture of flexor tendons, unspecified shoulder
  + M66.32 Spontaneous rupture of flexor tendons, upper arm
    M66.321 Spontaneous rupture of flexor tendons, right upper arm
    M66.322 Spontaneous rupture of flexor tendons, left upper arm
    M66.329 Spontaneous rupture of flexor tendons, unspecified upper arm
  + M66.33 Spontaneous rupture of flexor tendons, forearm
    M66.331 Spontaneous rupture of flexor tendons, right forearm
    M66.332 Spontaneous rupture of flexor tendons, left forearm
    M66.339 Spontaneous rupture of flexor tendons, unspecified forearm
  + M66.34 Spontaneous rupture of flexor tendons, hand
    M66.341 Spontaneous rupture of flexor tendons, right hand
    M66.342 Spontaneous rupture of flexor tendons, left hand
    M66.349 Spontaneous rupture of flexor tendons, unspecified hand
  + M66.35 Spontaneous rupture of flexor tendons, thigh
    M66.351 Spontaneous rupture of flexor tendons, right thigh
    M66.352 Spontaneous rupture of flexor tendons, left thigh
    M66.359 Spontaneous rupture of flexor tendons, unspecified thigh
  + M66.36 Spontaneous rupture of flexor tendons, lower leg
    M66.361 Spontaneous rupture of flexor tendons, right lower leg
    M66.362 Spontaneous rupture of flexor tendons, left lower leg
    M66.369 Spontaneous rupture of flexor tendons, unspecified lower leg
  + M66.37 Spontaneous rupture of flexor tendons, ankle and foot
    M66.371 Spontaneous rupture of flexor tendons, right ankle and foot
    M66.372 Spontaneous rupture of flexor tendons, left ankle and foot
    M66.379 Spontaneous rupture of flexor tendons, unspecified ankle and foot
  M66.38 Spontaneous rupture of flexor tendons, other site
  M66.39 Spontaneous rupture of flexor tendons, multiple sites
+ M66.8 Spontaneous rupture of other tendons
  M66.80 Spontaneous rupture of other tendons, unspecified site
  + M66.81 Spontaneous rupture of other tendons, shoulder
    M66.811 Spontaneous rupture of other tendons, right shoulder
    M66.812 Spontaneous rupture of other tendons, left shoulder
    M66.819 Spontaneous rupture of other tendons, unspecified shoulder
  + M66.82 Spontaneous rupture of other tendons, upper arm
    M66.821 Spontaneous rupture of other tendons, right upper arm
    M66.822 Spontaneous rupture of other tendons, left upper arm
    M66.829 Spontaneous rupture of other tendons, unspecified upper arm
  + M66.83 Spontaneous rupture of other tendons, forearm
    M66.831 Spontaneous rupture of other tendons, right forearm
    M66.832 Spontaneous rupture of other tendons, left forearm
    M66.839 Spontaneous rupture of other tendons, unspecified forearm
  + M66.84 Spontaneous rupture of other tendons, hand
    M66.841 Spontaneous rupture of other tendons, right hand
    M66.842 Spontaneous rupture of other tendons, left hand
    M66.849 Spontaneous rupture of other tendons, unspecified hand

+ M66.85 Spontaneous rupture of other tendons, thigh
　　　　M66.851 Spontaneous rupture of other tendons, right thigh
　　　　M66.852 Spontaneous rupture of other tendons, left thigh
　　　　M66.859 Spontaneous rupture of other tendons, unspecified thigh
+ M66.86 Spontaneous rupture of other tendons, lower leg
　　　　M66.861 Spontaneous rupture of other tendons, right lower leg
　　　　M66.862 Spontaneous rupture of other tendons, left lower leg
　　　　M66.869 Spontaneous rupture of other tendons, unspecified lower leg
+ M66.87 Spontaneous rupture of other tendons, ankle and foot
　　　　M66.871 Spontaneous rupture of other tendons, right ankle and foot
　　　　M66.872 Spontaneous rupture of other tendons, left ankle and foot
　　　　M66.879 Spontaneous rupture of other tendons, unspecified ankle and foot
　　M66.88 Spontaneous rupture of other tendons, other sites
　　M66.89 Spontaneous rupture of other tendons, multiple sites
　M66.9 Spontaneous rupture of unspecified tendon
　　　Rupture at musculotendinous junction, nontraumatic

M67 Other disorders of synovium and tendon

Excludes1: *palmar fascial fibromatosis [Dupuytren] (M72.0)*
　　　　　tendinitis NOS (M77.9-)
　　　　　xanthomatosis localized to tendons (E78.2)

+ M67.0 Short Achilles tendon (acquired)
　　M67.00 Short Achilles tendon (acquired), unspecified ankle
　　M67.01 Short Achilles tendon (acquired), right ankle
　　M67.02 Short Achilles tendon (acquired), left ankle
+ M67.2 Synovial hypertrophy, not elsewhere classified
　　Excludes1: *villonodular synovitis (pigmented) (M12.2-)*
　　M67.20 Synovial hypertrophy, not elsewhere classified, unspecified site
+ 　M67.21 Synovial hypertrophy, not elsewhere classified, shoulder
　　　　M67.211 Synovial hypertrophy, not elsewhere classified, right shoulder
　　　　M67.212 Synovial hypertrophy, not elsewhere classified, left shoulder
　　　　M67.219 Synovial hypertrophy, not elsewhere classified, unspecified shoulder
+ 　M67.22 Synovial hypertrophy, not elsewhere classified, upper arm
　　　　M67.221 Synovial hypertrophy, not elsewhere classified, right upper arm
　　　　M67.222 Synovial hypertrophy, not elsewhere classified, left upper arm
　　　　M67.229 Synovial hypertrophy, not elsewhere classified, unspecified upper arm
+ 　M67.23 Synovial hypertrophy, not elsewhere classified, forearm
　　　　M67.231 Synovial hypertrophy, not elsewhere classified, right forearm
　　　　M67.232 Synovial hypertrophy, not elsewhere classified, left forearm
　　　　M67.239 Synovial hypertrophy, not elsewhere classified, unspecified forearm
+ 　M67.24 Synovial hypertrophy, not elsewhere classified, hand
　　　　M67.241 Synovial hypertrophy, not elsewhere classified, right hand
　　　　M67.242 Synovial hypertrophy, not elsewhere classified, left hand
　　　　M67.249 Synovial hypertrophy, not elsewhere classified, unspecified hand
+ 　M67.25 Synovial hypertrophy, not elsewhere classified, thigh
　　　　M67.251 Synovial hypertrophy, not elsewhere classified, right thigh
　　　　M67.252 Synovial hypertrophy, not elsewhere classified, left thigh
　　　　M67.259 Synovial hypertrophy, not elsewhere classified, unspecified thigh

+ 　M67.26 Synovial hypertrophy, not elsewhere classified, lower leg
　　　　M67.261 Synovial hypertrophy, not elsewhere classified, right lower leg
　　　　M67.262 Synovial hypertrophy, not elsewhere classified, left lower leg
　　　　M67.269 Synovial hypertrophy, not elsewhere classified, unspecified lower leg
+ 　M67.27 Synovial hypertrophy, not elsewhere classified, ankle and foot
　　　　M67.271 Synovial hypertrophy, not elsewhere classified, right ankle and foot
　　　　M67.272 Synovial hypertrophy, not elsewhere classified, left ankle and foot
　　　　M67.279 Synovial hypertrophy, not elsewhere classified, unspecified ankle and foot
　　M67.28 Synovial hypertrophy, not elsewhere classified, other site
　　M67.29 Synovial hypertrophy, not elsewhere classified, multiple sites
+ M67.3 Transient synovitis
　　Toxic synovitis
　　Excludes1: *palindromic rheumatism (M12.3-)*
　　M67.30 Transient synovitis, unspecified site
+ 　M67.31 Transient synovitis, shoulder
　　　　M67.311 Transient synovitis, right shoulder
　　　　M67.312 Transient synovitis, left shoulder
　　　　M67.319 Transient synovitis, unspecified shoulder
+ 　M67.32 Transient synovitis, elbow
　　　　M67.321 Transient synovitis, right elbow
　　　　M67.322 Transient synovitis, left elbow
　　　　M67.329 Transient synovitis, unspecified elbow
+ 　M67.33 Transient synovitis, wrist
　　　　M67.331 Transient synovitis, right wrist
　　　　M67.332 Transient synovitis, left wrist
　　　　M67.339 Transient synovitis, unspecified wrist
+ 　M67.34 Transient synovitis, hand
　　　　M67.341 Transient synovitis, right hand
　　　　M67.342 Transient synovitis, left hand
　　　　M67.349 Transient synovitis, unspecified hand
+ 　M67.35 Transient synovitis, hip
　　　　M67.351 Transient synovitis, right hip
　　　　M67.352 Transient synovitis, left hip
　　　　M67.359 Transient synovitis, unspecified hip
+ 　M67.36 Transient synovitis, knee
　　　　M67.361 Transient synovitis, right knee
　　　　M67.362 Transient synovitis, left knee
　　　　M67.369 Transient synovitis, unspecified knee
+ 　M67.37 Transient synovitis, ankle and foot
　　　　M67.371 Transient synovitis, right ankle and foot
　　　　M67.372 Transient synovitis, left ankle and foot
　　　　M67.379 Transient synovitis, unspecified ankle and foot
　　M67.38 Transient synovitis, other site
　　M67.39 Transient synovitis, multiple sites
+ M67.4 Ganglion
　　Ganglion of joint or tendon (sheath)
　　Excludes1: *ganglion in yaws (A66.6)*
　　Excludes2: *cyst of bursa (M71.2-M71.3)*
　　　　　cyst of synovium (M71.2-M71.3)
　　M67.40 Ganglion, unspecified site
+ 　M67.41 Ganglion, shoulder
　　　　M67.411 Ganglion, right shoulder
　　　　M67.412 Ganglion, left shoulder
　　　　M67.419 Ganglion, unspecified shoulder
+ 　M67.42 Ganglion, elbow
　　　　M67.421 Ganglion, right elbow
　　　　M67.422 Ganglion, left elbow
　　　　M67.429 Ganglion, unspecified elbow
+ 　M67.43 Ganglion, wrist
　　　　M67.431 Ganglion, right wrist
　　　　M67.432 Ganglion, left wrist
　　　　M67.439 Ganglion, unspecified wrist
+ 　M67.44 Ganglion, hand
　　　　M67.441 Ganglion, right hand
　　　　M67.442 Ganglion, left hand
　　　　M67.449 Ganglion, unspecified hand

- **M67.45** Ganglion, hip
  - M67.451 Ganglion, right hip
  - M67.452 Ganglion, left hip
  - M67.459 Ganglion, unspecified hip
- **M67.46** Ganglion, knee
  - M67.461 Ganglion, right knee
  - M67.462 Ganglion, left knee
  - M67.469 Ganglion, unspecified knee
- **M67.47** Ganglion, ankle and foot
  - M67.471 Ganglion, right ankle and foot
  - M67.472 Ganglion, left ankle and foot
  - M67.479 Ganglion, unspecified ankle and foot
- M67.48 Ganglion, other site
- M67.49 Ganglion, multiple sites

- **M67.5** Plica syndrome
  - Plica knee
  - M67.50 Plica syndrome, unspecified knee
  - M67.51 Plica syndrome, right knee
  - M67.52 Plica syndrome, left knee

- **M67.8** Other specified disorders of synovium and tendon
  - M67.80 Other specified disorders of synovium and tendon, unspecified site
  - **M67.81** Other specified disorders of synovium and tendon, shoulder
    - M67.811 Other specified disorders of synovium, right shoulder
    - M67.812 Other specified disorders of synovium, left shoulder
    - M67.813 Other specified disorders of tendon, right shoulder
    - M67.814 Other specified disorders of tendon, left shoulder
    - M67.819 Other specified disorders of synovium and tendon, unspecified shoulder
  - **M67.82** Other specified disorders of synovium and tendon, elbow
    - M67.821 Other specified disorders of synovium, right elbow
    - M67.822 Other specified disorders of synovium, left elbow
    - M67.823 Other specified disorders of tendon, right elbow
    - M67.824 Other specified disorders of tendon, left elbow
    - M67.829 Other specified disorders of synovium and tendon, unspecified elbow
  - **M67.83** Other specified disorders of synovium and tendon, wrist
    - M67.831 Other specified disorders of synovium, right wrist
    - M67.832 Other specified disorders of synovium, left wrist
    - M67.833 Other specified disorders of tendon, right wrist
    - M67.834 Other specified disorders of tendon, left wrist
    - M67.839 Other specified disorders of synovium and tendon, unspecified wrist
  - **M67.84** Other specified disorders of synovium and tendon, hand
    - M67.841 Other specified disorders of synovium, right hand
    - M67.842 Other specified disorders of synovium, left hand
    - M67.843 Other specified disorders of tendon, right hand
    - M67.844 Other specified disorders of tendon, left hand
    - M67.849 Other specified disorders of synovium and tendon, unspecified hand
  - **M67.85** Other specified disorders of synovium and tendon, hip
    - M67.851 Other specified disorders of synovium, right hip
    - M67.852 Other specified disorders of synovium, left hip
    - M67.853 Other specified disorders of tendon, right hip
    - M67.854 Other specified disorders of tendon, left hip
    - M67.859 Other specified disorders of synovium and tendon, unspecified hip
  - **M67.86** Other specified disorders of synovium and tendon, knee
    - M67.861 Other specified disorders of synovium, right knee
    - M67.862 Other specified disorders of synovium, left knee
    - M67.863 Other specified disorders of tendon, right knee
    - M67.864 Other specified disorders of tendon, left knee
    - M67.869 Other specified disorders of synovium and tendon, unspecified knee
  - **M67.87** Other specified disorders of synovium and tendon, ankle and foot
    - M67.871 Other specified disorders of synovium, right ankle and foot
    - M67.872 Other specified disorders of synovium, left ankle and foot
    - M67.873 Other specified disorders of tendon, right ankle and foot
    - M67.874 Other specified disorders of tendon, left ankle and foot
    - M67.879 Other specified disorders of synovium and tendon, unspecified ankle and foot
  - M67.88 Other specified disorders of synovium and tendon, other site
  - M67.89 Other specified disorders of synovium and tendon, multiple sites

- **M67.9** Unspecified disorder of synovium and tendon
  - M67.90 Unspecified disorder of synovium and tendon, unspecified site
  - **M67.91** Unspecified disorder of synovium and tendon, shoulder
    - M67.911 Unspecified disorder of synovium and tendon, right shoulder
    - M67.912 Unspecified disorder of synovium and tendon, left shoulder
    - M67.919 Unspecified disorder of synovium and tendon, unspecified shoulder
  - **M67.92** Unspecified disorder of synovium and tendon, upper arm
    - M67.921 Unspecified disorder of synovium and tendon, right upper arm
    - M67.922 Unspecified disorder of synovium and tendon, left upper arm
    - M67.929 Unspecified disorder of synovium and tendon, unspecified upper arm
  - **M67.93** Unspecified disorder of synovium and tendon, forearm
    - M67.931 Unspecified disorder of synovium and tendon, right forearm
    - M67.932 Unspecified disorder of synovium and tendon, left forearm
    - M67.939 Unspecified disorder of synovium and tendon, unspecified forearm
  - **M67.94** Unspecified disorder of synovium and tendon, hand
    - M67.941 Unspecified disorder of synovium and tendon, right hand
    - M67.942 Unspecified disorder of synovium and tendon, left hand
    - M67.949 Unspecified disorder of synovium and tendon, unspecified hand
  - **M67.95** Unspecified disorder of synovium and tendon, thigh
    - M67.951 Unspecified disorder of synovium and tendon, right thigh
    - M67.952 Unspecified disorder of synovium and tendon, left thigh
    - M67.959 Unspecified disorder of synovium and tendon, unspecified thigh

- **+ M67.96** Unspecified disorder of synovium and tendon, lower leg
  - M67.961 Unspecified disorder of synovium and tendon, right lower leg
  - M67.962 Unspecified disorder of synovium and tendon, left lower leg
  - M67.969 Unspecified disorder of synovium and tendon, unspecified lower leg
- **+ M67.97** Unspecified disorder of synovium and tendon, ankle and foot
  - M67.971 Unspecified disorder of synovium and tendon, right ankle and foot
  - M67.972 Unspecified disorder of synovium and tendon, left ankle and foot
  - M67.979 Unspecified disorder of synovium and tendon, unspecified ankle and foot
- M67.98 Unspecified disorder of synovium and tendon, other site
- M67.99 Unspecified disorder of synovium and tendon, multiple sites

Other soft tissue disorders (M70-M79)

M70 Soft tissue disorders related to use, overuse and pressure

Includes: soft tissue disorders of occupational origin
Use additional external cause code to identify activity causing disorder (Y93.-)
- **Excludes1:** bursitis NOS (M71.9-)
- **Excludes2:** bursitis of shoulder (M75.5)
  - enthesopathies (M76-M77)
  - pressure ulcer (pressure area) (L89.-)

- **+ M70.0** Crepitant synovitis (acute) (chronic) of hand and wrist
  - **+ M70.03** Crepitant synovitis (acute) (chronic), wrist
    - M70.031 Crepitant synovitis (acute) (chronic), right wrist
    - M70.032 Crepitant synovitis (acute) (chronic), left wrist
    - M70.039 Crepitant synovitis (acute) (chronic), unspecified wrist
  - **+ M70.04** Crepitant synovitis (acute) (chronic), hand
    - M70.041 Crepitant synovitis (acute) (chronic), right hand
    - M70.042 Crepitant synovitis (acute) (chronic), left hand
    - M70.049 Crepitant synovitis (acute) (chronic), unspecified hand
- **+ M70.1** Bursitis of hand
  - M70.10 Bursitis, unspecified hand
  - M70.11 Bursitis, right hand
  - M70.12 Bursitis, left hand
- **+ M70.2** Olecranon bursitis
  - M70.20 Olecranon bursitis, unspecified elbow
  - M70.21 Olecranon bursitis, right elbow
  - M70.22 Olecranon bursitis, left elbow
- **+ M70.3** Other bursitis of elbow
  - M70.30 Other bursitis of elbow, unspecified elbow
  - M70.31 Other bursitis of elbow, right elbow
  - M70.32 Other bursitis of elbow, left elbow
- **+ M70.4** Prepatellar bursitis
  - M70.40 Prepatellar bursitis, unspecified knee
  - M70.41 Prepatellar bursitis, right knee
  - M70.42 Prepatellar bursitis, left knee
- **+ M70.5** Other bursitis of knee
  - M70.50 Other bursitis of knee, unspecified knee
  - M70.51 Other bursitis of knee, right knee
  - M70.52 Other bursitis of knee, left knee
- **+ M70.6** Trochanteric bursitis
  - Trochanteric tendinitis
  - M70.60 Trochanteric bursitis, unspecified hip
  - M70.61 Trochanteric bursitis, right hip
  - M70.62 Trochanteric bursitis, left hip
- **+ M70.7** Other bursitis of hip
  - Ischial bursitis
  - M70.70 Other bursitis of hip, unspecified hip
  - M70.71 Other bursitis of hip, right hip
  - M70.72 Other bursitis of hip, left hip

- **+ M70.8** Other soft tissue disorders related to use, overuse and pressure
  - M70.80 Other soft tissue disorders related to use, overuse and pressure of unspecified site
  - **+ M70.81** Other soft tissue disorders related to use, overuse and pressure of shoulder
    - M70.811 Other soft tissue disorders related to use, overuse and pressure, right shoulder
    - M70.812 Other soft tissue disorders related to use, overuse and pressure, left shoulder
    - M70.819 Other soft tissue disorders related to use, overuse and pressure, unspecified shoulder
  - **+ M70.82** Other soft tissue disorders related to use, overuse and pressure of upper arm
    - M70.821 Other soft tissue disorders related to use, overuse and pressure, right upper arm
    - M70.822 Other soft tissue disorders related to use, overuse and pressure, left upper arm
    - M70.829 Other soft tissue disorders related to use, overuse and pressure, unspecified upper arms
  - **+ M70.83** Other soft tissue disorders related to use, overuse and pressure of forearm
    - M70.831 Other soft tissue disorders related to use, overuse and pressure, right forearm
    - M70.832 Other soft tissue disorders related to use, overuse and pressure, left forearm
    - M70.839 Other soft tissue disorders related to use, overuse and pressure, unspecified forearm
  - **+ M70.84** Other soft tissue disorders related to use, overuse and pressure of hand
    - M70.841 Other soft tissue disorders related to use, overuse and pressure, right hand
    - M70.842 Other soft tissue disorders related to use, overuse and pressure, left hand
    - M70.849 Other soft tissue disorders related to use, overuse and pressure, unspecified hand
  - **+ M70.85** Other soft tissue disorders related to use, overuse and pressure of thigh
    - M70.851 Other soft tissue disorders related to use, overuse and pressure, right thigh
    - M70.852 Other soft tissue disorders related to use, overuse and pressure, left thigh
    - M70.859 Other soft tissue disorders related to use, overuse and pressure, unspecified thigh
  - **+ M70.86** Other soft tissue disorders related to use, overuse and pressure lower leg
    - M70.861 Other soft tissue disorders related to use, overuse and pressure, right lower leg
    - M70.862 Other soft tissue disorders related to use, overuse and pressure, left lower leg
    - M70.869 Other soft tissue disorders related to use, overuse and pressure, unspecified leg
  - **+ M70.87** Other soft tissue disorders related to use, overuse and pressure of ankle and foot
    - M70.871 Other soft tissue disorders related to use, overuse and pressure, right ankle and foot
    - M70.872 Other soft tissue disorders related to use, overuse and pressure, left ankle and foot
    - M70.879 Other soft tissue disorders related to use, overuse and pressure, unspecified ankle and foot
  - M70.88 Other soft tissue disorders related to use, overuse and pressure other site
  - M70.89 Other soft tissue disorders related to use, overuse and pressure multiple sites

- **M70.9** Unspecified soft tissue disorder related to use, overuse and pressure
  - M70.90 Unspecified soft tissue disorder related to use, overuse and pressure of unspecified site
  - **+ M70.91** Unspecified soft tissue disorder related to use, overuse and pressure of shoulder
    - M70.911 Unspecified soft tissue disorder related to use, overuse and pressure, right shoulder
    - M70.912 Unspecified soft tissue disorder related to use, overuse and pressure, left shoulder
    - M70.919 Unspecified soft tissue disorder related to use, overuse and pressure, unspecified shoulder
  - **+ M70.92** Unspecified soft tissue disorder related to use, overuse and pressure of upper arm
    - M70.921 Unspecified soft tissue disorder related to use, overuse and pressure, right upper arm
    - M70.922 Unspecified soft tissue disorder related to use, overuse and pressure, left upper arm
    - M70.929 Unspecified soft tissue disorder related to use, overuse and pressure, unspecified upper arm
  - **+ M70.93** Unspecified soft tissue disorder related to use, overuse and pressure of forearm
    - M70.931 Unspecified soft tissue disorder related to use, overuse and pressure, right forearm
    - M70.932 Unspecified soft tissue disorder related to use, overuse and pressure, left forearm
    - M70.939 Unspecified soft tissue disorder related to use, overuse and pressure, unspecified forearm
  - **+ M70.94** Unspecified soft tissue disorder related to use, overuse and pressure of hand
    - M70.941 Unspecified soft tissue disorder related to use, overuse and pressure, right hand
    - M70.942 Unspecified soft tissue disorder related to use, overuse and pressure, left hand
    - M70.949 Unspecified soft tissue disorder related to use, overuse and pressure, unspecified hand
  - **+ M70.95** Unspecified soft tissue disorder related to use, overuse and pressure of thigh
    - M70.951 Unspecified soft tissue disorder related to use, overuse and pressure, right thigh
    - M70.952 Unspecified soft tissue disorder related to use, overuse and pressure, left thigh
    - M70.959 Unspecified soft tissue disorder related to use, overuse and pressure, unspecified thigh
  - **+ M70.96** Unspecified soft tissue disorder related to use, overuse and pressure lower leg
    - M70.961 Unspecified soft tissue disorder related to use, overuse and pressure, right lower leg
    - M70.962 Unspecified soft tissue disorder related to use, overuse and pressure, left lower leg
    - M70.969 Unspecified soft tissue disorder related to use, overuse and pressure, unspecified lower leg
  - **+ M70.97** Unspecified soft tissue disorder related to use, overuse and pressure of ankle and foot
    - M70.971 Unspecified soft tissue disorder related to use, overuse and pressure, right ankle and foot
    - M70.972 Unspecified soft tissue disorder related to use, overuse and pressure, left ankle and foot
    - M70.979 Unspecified soft tissue disorder related to use, overuse and pressure, unspecified ankle and foot
  - M70.98 Unspecified soft tissue disorder related to use, overuse and pressure other
  - M70.99 Unspecified soft tissue disorder related to use, overuse and pressure multiple sites

M71 Other bursopathies

Excludes1: bunion (M20.1)
bursitis related to use, overuse or pressure (M70.-)
enthesopathies (M76-M77)

- **+ M71.0** Abscess of bursa
  Use additional code (B95.-, B96.-) to identify causative organism
  - M71.00 Abscess of bursa, unspecified site
  - **+ M71.01** Abscess of bursa, shoulder
    - M71.011 Abscess of bursa, right shoulder
    - M71.012 Abscess of bursa, left shoulder
    - M71.019 Abscess of bursa, unspecified shoulder
  - **+ M71.02** Abscess of bursa, elbow
    - M71.021 Abscess of bursa, right elbow
    - M71.022 Abscess of bursa, left elbow
    - M71.029 Abscess of bursa, unspecified elbow
  - **+ M71.03** Abscess of bursa, wrist
    - M71.031 Abscess of bursa, right wrist
    - M71.032 Abscess of bursa, left wrist
    - M71.039 Abscess of bursa, unspecified wrist
  - **+ M71.04** Abscess of bursa, hand
    - M71.041 Abscess of bursa, right hand
    - M71.042 Abscess of bursa, left hand
    - M71.049 Abscess of bursa, unspecified hand
  - **+ M71.05** Abscess of bursa, hip
    - M71.051 Abscess of bursa, right hip
    - M71.052 Abscess of bursa, left hip
    - M71.059 Abscess of bursa, unspecified hip
  - **+ M71.06** Abscess of bursa, knee
    - M71.061 Abscess of bursa, right knee
    - M71.062 Abscess of bursa, left knee
    - M71.069 Abscess of bursa, unspecified knee
  - **+ M71.07** Abscess of bursa, ankle and foot
    - M71.071 Abscess of bursa, right ankle and foot
    - M71.072 Abscess of bursa, left ankle and foot
    - M71.079 Abscess of bursa, unspecified ankle and foot
  - M71.08 Abscess of bursa, other site
  - M71.09 Abscess of bursa, multiple sites
- **+ M71.1** Other infective bursitis
  Use additional code (B95.-, B96.-) to identify causative organism
  - M71.10 Other infective bursitis, unspecified site
  - **+ M71.11** Other infective bursitis, shoulder
    - M71.111 Other infective bursitis, right shoulder
    - M71.112 Other infective bursitis, left shoulder
    - M71.119 Other infective bursitis, unspecified shoulder
  - **+ M71.12** Other infective bursitis, elbow
    - M71.121 Other infective bursitis, right elbow
    - M71.122 Other infective bursitis, left elbow
    - M71.129 Other infective bursitis, unspecified elbow
  - **+ M71.13** Other infective bursitis, wrist
    - M71.131 Other infective bursitis, right wrist
    - M71.132 Other infective bursitis, left wrist
    - M71.139 Other infective bursitis, unspecified wrist
  - **+ M71.14** Other infective bursitis, hand
    - M71.141 Other infective bursitis, right hand
    - M71.142 Other infective bursitis, left hand
    - M71.149 Other infective bursitis, unspecified hand
  - **+ M71.15** Other infective bursitis, hip
    - M71.151 Other infective bursitis, right hip
    - M71.152 Other infective bursitis, left hip
    - M71.159 Other infective bursitis, unspecified hip
  - **+ M71.16** Other infective bursitis, knee
    - M71.161 Other infective bursitis, right knee
    - M71.162 Other infective bursitis, left knee
    - M71.169 Other infective bursitis, unspecified knee
  - **+ M71.17** Other infective bursitis, ankle and foot
    - M71.171 Other infective bursitis, right ankle and foot
    - M71.172 Other infective bursitis, left ankle and foot
    - M71.179 Other infective bursitis, unspecified ankle and foot
  - M71.18 Other infective bursitis, other site
  - M71.19 Other infective bursitis, multiple sites

+ **M71.2 Synovial cyst of popliteal space [Baker]**
  Excludes1: *synovial cyst of popliteal space with rupture (M66.0)*
  M71.20 Synovial cyst of popliteal space [Baker], unspecified knee
  M71.21 Synovial cyst of popliteal space [Baker], right knee
  M71.22 Synovial cyst of popliteal space [Baker], left knee
+ **M71.3 Other bursal cyst**
  Synovial cyst NOS
  Excludes1: *synovial cyst with rupture (M66.1-)*
  M71.30 Other bursal cyst, unspecified site
  + M71.31 Other bursal cyst, shoulder
    M71.311 Other bursal cyst, right shoulder
    M71.312 Other bursal cyst, left shoulder
    M71.319 Other bursal cyst, unspecified shoulder
  + M71.32 Other bursal cyst, elbow
    M71.321 Other bursal cyst, right elbow
    M71.322 Other bursal cyst, left elbow
    M71.329 Other bursal cyst, unspecified elbow
  + M71.33 Other bursal cyst, wrist
    M71.331 Other bursal cyst, right wrist
    M71.332 Other bursal cyst, left wrist
    M71.339 Other bursal cyst, unspecified wrist
  + M71.34 Other bursal cyst, hand
    M71.341 Other bursal cyst, right hand
    M71.342 Other bursal cyst, left hand
    M71.349 Other bursal cyst, unspecified hand
  + M71.35 Other bursal cyst, hip
    M71.351 Other bursal cyst, right hip
    M71.352 Other bursal cyst, left hip
    M71.359 Other bursal cyst, unspecified hip
  + M71.37 Other bursal cyst, ankle and foot
    M71.371 Other bursal cyst, right ankle and foot
    M71.372 Other bursal cyst, left ankle and foot
    M71.379 Other bursal cyst, unspecified ankle and foot
  M71.38 Other bursal cyst, other site
  M71.39 Other bursal cyst, multiple sites
+ **M71.4 Calcium deposit in bursa**
  Excludes2: *calcium deposit in bursa of shoulder (M75.3)*
  M71.40 Calcium deposit in bursa, unspecified site
  + M71.42 Calcium deposit in bursa, elbow
    M71.421 Calcium deposit in bursa, right elbow
    M71.422 Calcium deposit in bursa, left elbow
    M71.429 Calcium deposit in bursa, unspecified elbow
  + M71.43 Calcium deposit in bursa, wrist
    M71.431 Calcium deposit in bursa, right wrist
    M71.432 Calcium deposit in bursa, left wrist
    M71.439 Calcium deposit in bursa, unspecified wrist
  + M71.44 Calcium deposit in bursa, hand
    M71.441 Calcium deposit in bursa, right hand
    M71.442 Calcium deposit in bursa, left hand
    M71.449 Calcium deposit in bursa, unspecified hand
  + M71.45 Calcium deposit in bursa, hip
    M71.451 Calcium deposit in bursa, right hip
    M71.452 Calcium deposit in bursa, left hip
    M71.459 Calcium deposit in bursa, unspecified hip
  + M71.46 Calcium deposit in bursa, knee
    M71.461 Calcium deposit in bursa, right knee
    M71.462 Calcium deposit in bursa, left knee
    M71.469 Calcium deposit in bursa, unspecified knee
  + M71.47 Calcium deposit in bursa, ankle and foot
    M71.471 Calcium deposit in bursa, right ankle and foot
    M71.472 Calcium deposit in bursa, left ankle and foot
    M71.479 Calcium deposit in bursa, unspecified ankle and foot
  M71.48 Calcium deposit in bursa, other site
  M71.49 Calcium deposit in bursa, multiple sites

+ **M71.5 Other bursitis, not elsewhere classified**
  Excludes1: *bursitis NOS (M71.9-)*
  Excludes2: *bursitis of shoulder (M75.5)*
  bursitis of tibial collateral [Pellegrini-Stieda] (M76.4-)
  M71.50 Other bursitis, not elsewhere classified, unspecified site
  + M71.52 Other bursitis, not elsewhere classified, elbow
    M71.521 Other bursitis, not elsewhere classified, right elbow
    M71.522 Other bursitis, not elsewhere classified, left elbow
    M71.529 Other bursitis, not elsewhere classified, unspecified elbow
  + M71.53 Other bursitis, not elsewhere classified, wrist
    M71.531 Other bursitis, not elsewhere classified, right wrist
    M71.532 Other bursitis, not elsewhere classified, left wrist
    M71.539 Other bursitis, not elsewhere classified, unspecified wrist
  + M71.54 Other bursitis, not elsewhere classified, hand
    M71.541 Other bursitis, not elsewhere classified, right hand
    M71.542 Other bursitis, not elsewhere classified, left hand
    M71.549 Other bursitis, not elsewhere classified, unspecified hand
  + M71.55 Other bursitis, not elsewhere classified, hip
    M71.551 Other bursitis, not elsewhere classified, right hip
    M71.552 Other bursitis, not elsewhere classified, left hip
    M71.559 Other bursitis, not elsewhere classified, unspecified hip
  + M71.56 Other bursitis, not elsewhere classified, knee
    M71.561 Other bursitis, not elsewhere classified, right knee
    M71.562 Other bursitis, not elsewhere classified, left knee
    M71.569 Other bursitis, not elsewhere classified, unspecified knee
  + M71.57 Other bursitis, not elsewhere classified, ankle and foot
    M71.571 Other bursitis, not elsewhere classified, right ankle and foot
    M71.572 Other bursitis, not elsewhere classified, left ankle and foot
    M71.579 Other bursitis, not elsewhere classified, unspecified ankle and foot
  M71.58 Other bursitis, not elsewhere classified, other site
+ **M71.8 Other specified bursopathies**
  M71.80 Other specified bursopathies, unspecified site
  + M71.81 Other specified bursopathies, shoulder
    M71.811 Other specified bursopathies, right shoulder
    M71.812 Other specified bursopathies, left shoulder
    M71.819 Other specified bursopathies, unspecified shoulder
  + M71.82 Other specified bursopathies, elbow
    M71.821 Other specified bursopathies, right elbow
    M71.822 Other specified bursopathies, left elbow
    M71.829 Other specified bursopathies, unspecified elbow
  + M71.83 Other specified bursopathies, wrist
    M71.831 Other specified bursopathies, right wrist
    M71.832 Other specified bursopathies, left wrist
    M71.839 Other specified bursopathies, unspecified wrist
  + M71.84 Other specified bursopathies, hand
    M71.841 Other specified bursopathies, right hand
    M71.842 Other specified bursopathies, left hand
    M71.849 Other specified bursopathies, unspecified hand

+ **M71.85 Other specified bursopathies, hip**
　　M71.851 Other specified bursopathies, right hip
　　M71.852 Other specified bursopathies, left hip
　　M71.859 Other specified bursopathies, unspecified hip
+ **M71.86 Other specified bursopathies, knee**
　　M71.861 Other specified bursopathies, right knee
　　M71.862 Other specified bursopathies, left knee
　　M71.869 Other specified bursopathies, unspecified knee
+ **M71.87 Other specified bursopathies, ankle and foot**
　　M71.871 Other specified bursopathies, right ankle and foot
　　M71.872 Other specified bursopathies, left ankle and foot
　　M71.879 Other specified bursopathies, unspecified ankle and foot
　M71.88 Other specified bursopathies, other site
　M71.89 Other specified bursopathies, multiple sites
M71.9 Bursopathy, unspecified
　Bursitis NOS

M72 Fibroblastic disorders

　Excludes2: *retroperitoneal fibromatosis (D48.3)*
- **M72.0** Palmar fascial fibromatosis [Dupuytren]
M72.1 Knuckle pads
M72.2 Plantar fascial fibromatosis
　Plantar fasciitis
M72.4 Pseudosarcomatous fibromatosis
　Nodular fasciitis
MCC **M72.6** Necrotizing fasciitis
　Use additional code (B95.-, B96.-) to identify causative organism
M72.8 Other fibroblastic disorders
　Abscess of fascia
　Fasciitis NEC
　Other infective fasciitis
　Use additional code to (B95.-, B96.-) identify causative organism
　　Excludes1: *diffuse (eosinophilic) fasciitis (M35.4)*
　　　　necrotizing fasciitis (M72.6)
　　　　nodular fasciitis (M72.4)
　　　　perirenal fasciitis NOS (N13.5)
　　　　perirenal fasciitis with infection (N13.6)
　　　　plantar fasciitis (M72.2)
M72.9 Fibroblastic disorder, unspecified
　Fasciitis NOS
　Fibromatosis NOS

M75 Shoulder lesions

　Excludes2: *shoulder-hand syndrome (M89.0-)*
+ **M75.0 Adhesive capsulitis of shoulder**
　Frozen shoulder
　Periarthritis of shoulder
　M75.00 Adhesive capsulitis of unspecified shoulder
　M75.01 Adhesive capsulitis of right shoulder
　M75.02 Adhesive capsulitis of left shoulder
+ **M75.1 Rotator cuff tear or rupture, not specified as traumatic**
　Rotator cuff syndrome
　Supraspinatus tear or rupture, not specified as traumatic
　Supraspinatus syndrome
　　Excludes1: *tear of rotator cuff, traumatic (S46.01-)*
+ **M75.10 Unspecified rotator cuff tear or rupture, not specified as traumatic**
　　M75.100 Unspecified rotator cuff tear or rupture of unspecified shoulder, not specified as traumatic
　　M75.101 Unspecified rotator cuff tear or rupture of right shoulder, not specified as traumatic
　　M75.102 Unspecified rotator cuff tear or rupture of left shoulder, not specified as traumatic
+ **M75.11 Incomplete rotator cuff tear or rupture not specified as traumatic**
　　M75.110 Incomplete rotator cuff tear or rupture of unspecified shoulder, not specified as traumatic
　　M75.111 Incomplete rotator cuff tear or rupture of right shoulder, not specified as traumatic
　　M75.112 Incomplete rotator cuff tear or rupture of left shoulder, not specified as traumatic
+ **M75.12 Complete rotator cuff tear or rupture not specified as traumatic**
　　M75.120 Complete rotator cuff tear or rupture of unspecified shoulder, not specified as traumatic
　　M75.121 Complete rotator cuff tear or rupture of right shoulder, not specified as traumatic
　　M75.122 Complete rotator cuff tear or rupture of left shoulder, not specified as traumatic
+ **M75.2 Bicipital tendinitis**
　M75.20 Bicipital tendinitis, unspecified shoulder
　M75.21 Bicipital tendinitis, right shoulder
　M75.22 Bicipital tendinitis, left shoulder
+ **M75.3 Calcific tendinitis of shoulder**
　Calcified bursa of shoulder
　M75.30 Calcific tendinitis of unspecified shoulder
　M75.31 Calcific tendinitis of right shoulder
　M75.32 Calcific tendinitis of left shoulder
+ **M75.4 Impingement syndrome of shoulder**
　AHA CC: 3Q, 2022, 18-19
　M75.40 Impingement syndrome of unspecified shoulder
　M75.41 Impingement syndrome of right shoulder
　M75.42 Impingement syndrome of left shoulder
+ **M75.5 Bursitis of shoulder**
　M75.50 Bursitis of unspecified shoulder
　M75.51 Bursitis of right shoulder
　M75.52 Bursitis of left shoulder
+ **M75.8 Other shoulder lesions**
　M75.80 Other shoulder lesions, unspecified shoulder
　M75.81 Other shoulder lesions, right shoulder
　M75.82 Other shoulder lesions, left shoulder
+ **M75.9 Shoulder lesion, unspecified**
　M75.90 Shoulder lesion, unspecified, unspecified shoulder
　M75.91 Shoulder lesion, unspecified, right shoulder
　M75.92 Shoulder lesion, unspecified, left shoulder

M76 Enthesopathies, lower limb, excluding foot

　Excludes2: *bursitis due to use, overuse and pressure (M70.-)*
　　　enthesopathies of ankle and foot (M77.5-)
+ **M76.0 Gluteal tendinitis**
　M76.00 Gluteal tendinitis, unspecified hip
　M76.01 Gluteal tendinitis, right hip
　M76.02 Gluteal tendinitis, left hip
+ **M76.1 Psoas tendinitis**
　M76.10 Psoas tendinitis, unspecified hip
　M76.11 Psoas tendinitis, right hip
　M76.12 Psoas tendinitis, left hip
+ **M76.2 Iliac crest spur**
　M76.20 Iliac crest spur, unspecified hip
　M76.21 Iliac crest spur, right hip
　M76.22 Iliac crest spur, left hip
+ **M76.3 Iliotibial band syndrome**
　M76.30 Iliotibial band syndrome, unspecified leg
　M76.31 Iliotibial band syndrome, right leg
　M76.32 Iliotibial band syndrome, left leg
+ **M76.4 Tibial collateral bursitis [Pellegrini-Stieda]**
　M76.40 Tibial collateral bursitis [Pellegrini-Stieda], unspecified leg
　M76.41 Tibial collateral bursitis [Pellegrini-Stieda], right leg
　M76.42 Tibial collateral bursitis [Pellegrini-Stieda], left leg
+ **M76.5 Patellar tendinitis**
　M76.50 Patellar tendinitis, unspecified knee
　M76.51 Patellar tendinitis, right knee
　M76.52 Patellar tendinitis, left knee

+ **M76.6 Achilles tendinitis**
Achilles bursitis
M76.60 Achilles tendinitis, unspecified leg
M76.61 Achilles tendinitis, right leg
M76.62 Achilles tendinitis, left leg
+ **M76.7 Peroneal tendinitis**
M76.70 Peroneal tendinitis, unspecified leg
M76.71 Peroneal tendinitis, right leg
M76.72 Peroneal tendinitis, left leg
+ **M76.8 Other specified enthesopathies of lower limb, excluding foot**
+ M76.81 Anterior tibial syndrome
M76.811 Anterior tibial syndrome, right leg
M76.812 Anterior tibial syndrome, left leg
M76.819 Anterior tibial syndrome, unspecified leg
+ M76.82 Posterior tibial tendinitis
M76.821 Posterior tibial tendinitis, right leg
M76.822 Posterior tibial tendinitis, left leg
M76.829 Posterior tibial tendinitis, unspecified leg
+ M76.89 Other specified enthesopathies of lower limb, excluding foot
M76.891 Other specified enthesopathies of right lower limb, excluding foot
M76.892 Other specified enthesopathies of left lower limb, excluding foot
M76.899 Other specified enthesopathies of unspecified lower limb, excluding foot
M76.9 Unspecified enthesopathy, lower limb, excluding foot

M77 Other enthesopathies

Excludes1: bursitis NOS (M71.9-)
Excludes2: bursitis due to use, overuse and pressure (M70.-)
osteophyte (M25.7)
spinal enthesopathy (M46.0-)
+ **M77.0 Medial epicondylitis**
M77.00 Medial epicondylitis, unspecified elbow
M77.01 Medial epicondylitis, right elbow
M77.02 Medial epicondylitis, left elbow
+ **M77.1 Lateral epicondylitis**
Tennis elbow
M77.10 Lateral epicondylitis, unspecified elbow
M77.11 Lateral epicondylitis, right elbow
M77.12 Lateral epicondylitis, left elbow
+ **M77.2 Periarthritis of wrist**
M77.20 Periarthritis, unspecified wrist
M77.21 Periarthritis, right wrist
M77.22 Periarthritis, left wrist
+ **M77.3 Calcaneal spur**
M77.30 Calcaneal spur, unspecified foot
M77.31 Calcaneal spur, right foot
M77.32 Calcaneal spur, left foot
+ **M77.4 Metatarsalgia**
Excludes1: Morton's metatarsalgia (G57.6)
M77.40 Metatarsalgia, unspecified foot
M77.41 Metatarsalgia, right foot
M77.42 Metatarsalgia, left foot
+ **M77.5 Other enthesopathy of foot and ankle**
M77.50 Other enthesopathy of unspecified foot and ankle
M77.51 Other enthesopathy of right foot and ankle
M77.52 Other enthesopathy of left foot and ankle
M77.8 Other enthesopathies, not elsewhere classified
M77.9 Enthesopathy, unspecified
Bone spur NOS
Capsulitis NOS
Periarthritis NOS
Tendinitis NOS

M79 Other and unspecified soft tissue disorders, not elsewhere classified

Excludes1: psychogenic rheumatism (F45.8)
soft tissue pain, psychogenic (F45.41)
M79.0 Rheumatism, unspecified
Excludes1: fibromyalgia (M79.7)
palindromic rheumatism (M12.3-)

+ **M79.1 Myalgia**
Myofascial pain syndrome
Excludes1: fibromyalgia (M79.7)
myositis (M60.-)
AHA CC: 4Q, 2018, 21
M79.10 Myalgia, unspecified site
M79.11 Myalgia of mastication muscle
M79.12 Myalgia of auxiliary muscles, head and neck
M79.18 Myalgia, other site
M79.2 Neuralgia and neuritis, unspecified
Excludes1: brachial radiculitis NOS (M54.1)
lumbosacral radiculitis NOS (M54.1)
mononeuropathies (G56-G58)
radiculitis NOS (M54.1)
sciatica (M54.3-M54.4)
M79.3 Panniculitis, unspecified
Excludes1: lupus panniculitis (L93.2)
neck and back panniculitis (M54.0-)
relapsing [Weber-Christian] panniculitis (M35.6)
M79.4 Hypertrophy of (infrapatellar) fat pad
M79.5 Residual foreign body in soft tissue
Excludes1: foreign body granuloma of skin and subcutaneous tissue (L92.3)
foreign body granuloma of soft tissue (M60.2-)
AHA CC: 2Q, 2023, 27-28
+ **M79.6 Pain in limb, hand, foot, fingers and toes**
Excludes2: pain in joint (M25.5-)
+ M79.60 Pain in limb, unspecified
M79.601 Pain in right arm
Pain in right upper limb NOS
M79.602 Pain in left arm
Pain in left upper limb NOS
M79.603 Pain in arm, unspecified
Pain in upper limb NOS
M79.604 Pain in right leg
Pain in right lower limb NOS
M79.605 Pain in left leg
Pain in left lower limb NOS
M79.606 Pain in leg, unspecified
Pain in lower limb NOS
M79.609 Pain in unspecified limb
Pain in limb NOS
+ M79.62 Pain in upper arm
Pain in axillary region
M79.621 Pain in right upper arm
M79.622 Pain in left upper arm
M79.629 Pain in unspecified upper arm
+ M79.63 Pain in forearm
M79.631 Pain in right forearm
M79.632 Pain in left forearm
M79.639 Pain in unspecified forearm
+ M79.64 Pain in hand and fingers
M79.641 Pain in right hand
M79.642 Pain in left hand
M79.643 Pain in unspecified hand
M79.644 Pain in right finger(s)
M79.645 Pain in left finger(s)
M79.646 Pain in unspecified finger(s)
+ M79.65 Pain in thigh
M79.651 Pain in right thigh
M79.652 Pain in left thigh
M79.659 Pain in unspecified thigh
+ M79.66 Pain in lower leg
M79.661 Pain in right lower leg
M79.662 Pain in left lower leg
M79.669 Pain in unspecified lower leg
+ M79.67 Pain in foot and toes
M79.671 Pain in right foot
M79.672 Pain in left foot
M79.673 Pain in unspecified foot
M79.674 Pain in right toe(s)
M79.675 Pain in left toe(s)
M79.676 Pain in unspecified toe(s)
M79.7 Fibromyalgia
Fibromyositis
Fibrositis
Myofibrositis

Osteoporosis

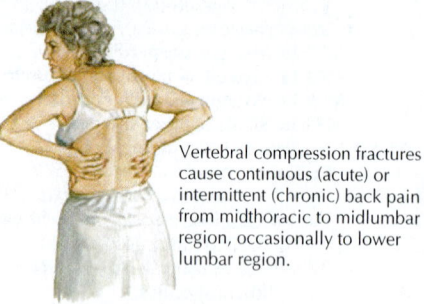

Axial

Vertebral compression fractures cause continuous (acute) or intermittent (chronic) back pain from midthoracic to midlumbar region, occasionally to lower lumbar region.

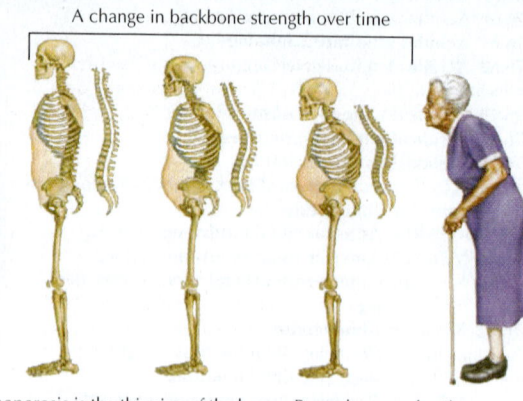

A change in backbone strength over time

Osteoporosis is the thinning of the bones. Bones become fragile and loss of height is common as the back bones begin to collapse.

Characteristics of Osteoporosis	
Characteristic	Description
Etiology	Postmenopausal women, genetics, vitamin D synthesis deficiency, idiopathic
Prevalence	Approximately 10 million Americans (8 million of them women), white
Risk factors	Family history, white female, increasing age, estrogen deficiency, vitamin D deficiency, low calcium intake, smoking, excessive alcohol use, inactive lifestyle
Complications	Vertebral compression fractures, fracture of proximal femur or humerus, ribs, and distal radius (Colles' fracture)

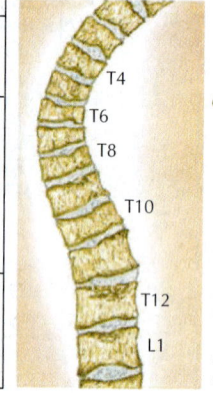

Multiple compression fractures of lower thoracic and upper lumbar vertebrae in patient with severe osteoporosis

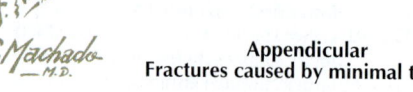

Appendicular
Fractures caused by minimal trauma

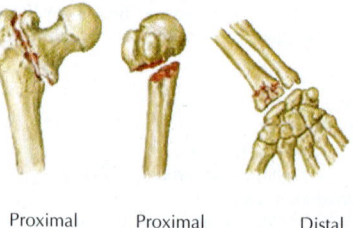

Proximal femur   Proximal humerus   Distal radius

Most common types

© Elsevier Inc. All rights reserved. www.netterimages.com

+ **M79.A Nontraumatic compartment syndrome**
   Code first if applicable, associated postprocedural complication
   Excludes1: compartment syndrome NOS (T79.A-)
                fibromyalgia (M79.7)
                nontraumatic ischemic infarction of muscle (M62.2-)
                traumatic compartment syndrome (T79.A-)
+ **M79.A1 Nontraumatic compartment syndrome of upper extremity**
   Nontraumatic compartment syndrome of shoulder, arm, forearm, wrist, hand, and fingers
   CC **M79.A11** Nontraumatic compartment syndrome of right upper extremity
   CC **M79.A12** Nontraumatic compartment syndrome of left upper extremity
   CC **M79.A19** Nontraumatic compartment syndrome of unspecified upper extremity
+ **M79.A2 Nontraumatic compartment syndrome of lower extremity**
   Nontraumatic compartment syndrome of hip, buttock, thigh, leg, foot, and toes
   CC **M79.A21** Nontraumatic compartment syndrome of right lower extremity
   CC **M79.A22** Nontraumatic compartment syndrome of left lower extremity
   CC **M79.A29** Nontraumatic compartment syndrome of unspecified lower extremity
CC **M79.A3 Nontraumatic compartment syndrome of abdomen**
CC **M79.A9 Nontraumatic compartment syndrome of other sites**
+ **M79.8 Other specified soft tissue disorders**
   M79.81 Nontraumatic hematoma of soft tissue
      Nontraumatic hematoma of muscle
      Nontraumatic seroma of muscle and soft tissue
   M79.89 Other specified soft tissue disorders
      Polyalgia
M79.9 Soft tissue disorder, unspecified

OSTEOPATHIES AND CHONDROPATHIES (M80-M94)
Disorders of bone density and structure (M80-M85)

M80 Osteoporosis with current pathological fracture
   Includes: osteoporosis with current fragility fracture
   Use additional code to identify major osseous defect, if applicable (M89.7-)
   Excludes1: collapsed vertebra NOS (M48.5)
                pathological fracture NOS (M84.4)
                wedging of vertebra NOS (M48.5)
   Excludes2: personal history of (healed) osteoporosis fracture (Z87.310)

The appropriate 7th character is to be added to each code from category M80:
A   initial encounter for fracture
D   subsequent encounter for fracture with routine healing
G   subsequent encounter for fracture with delayed healing
K   subsequent encounter for fracture with nonunion
P   subsequent encounter for fracture with malunion
S   sequela

Review coding guideline C.13.c
Review coding guideline C.19.c.1

+ **M80.0 Age-related osteoporosis with current pathological fracture**
   Involutional osteoporosis with current pathological fracture
   Osteoporosis NOS with current pathological fracture
   Postmenopausal osteoporosis with current pathological fracture
   Senile osteoporosis with current pathological fracture

- CC X+7th **M80.00** Age-related osteoporosis with current pathological fracture, unspecified site
  + **M80.01** Age-related osteoporosis with current pathological fracture, shoulder
    - CC +7th **M80.011** Age-related osteoporosis with current pathological fracture, right shoulder
    - CC +7th **M80.012** Age-related osteoporosis with current pathological fracture, left shoulder
    - CC +7th **M80.019** Age-related osteoporosis with current pathological fracture, unspecified shoulder
  + **M80.02** Age-related osteoporosis with current pathological fracture, humerus
    - CC +7th **M80.021** Age-related osteoporosis with current pathological fracture, right humerus
    - CC +7th **M80.022** Age-related osteoporosis with current pathological fracture, left humerus
    - CC +7th **M80.029** Age-related osteoporosis with current pathological fracture, unspecified humerus
  + **M80.03** Age-related osteoporosis with current pathological fracture, forearm
    Age-related osteoporosis with current pathological fracture of wrist
    - CC +7th **M80.031** Age-related osteoporosis with current pathological fracture, right forearm
    - CC +7th **M80.032** Age-related osteoporosis with current pathological fracture, left forearm
    - CC +7th **M80.039** Age-related osteoporosis with current pathological fracture, unspecified forearm
  + **M80.04** Age-related osteoporosis with current pathological fracture, hand
    - CC +7th **M80.041** Age-related osteoporosis with current pathological fracture, right hand
    - CC +7th **M80.042** Age-related osteoporosis with current pathological fracture, left hand
    - CC +7th **M80.049** Age-related osteoporosis with current pathological fracture, unspecified hand
  + **M80.05** Age-related osteoporosis with current pathological fracture, femur
    Age-related osteoporosis with current pathological fracture of hip
    - CC +7th **M80.051** Age-related osteoporosis with current pathological fracture, right femur
      AHA CC: 2Q, 2018, 12
    - CC +7th **M80.052** Age-related osteoporosis with current pathological fracture, left femur
    - CC +7th **M80.059** Age-related osteoporosis with current pathological fracture, unspecified femur
  + **M80.06** Age-related osteoporosis with current pathological fracture, lower leg
    - CC +7th **M80.061** Age-related osteoporosis with current pathological fracture, right lower leg
    - CC +7th **M80.062** Age-related osteoporosis with current pathological fracture, left lower leg
    - CC +7th **M80.069** Age-related osteoporosis with current pathological fracture, unspecified lower leg
  + **M80.07** Age-related osteoporosis with current pathological fracture, ankle and foot
    - CC +7th **M80.071** Age-related osteoporosis with current pathological fracture, right ankle and foot
    - CC +7th **M80.072** Age-related osteoporosis with current pathological fracture, left ankle and foot
    - CC +7th **M80.079** Age-related osteoporosis with current pathological fracture, unspecified ankle and foot
- CC X+7th **M80.08** Age-related osteoporosis with current pathological fracture, vertebra(e)
- CC X+7th **M80.0A** Age-related osteoporosis with current pathological fracture, other site
  AHA CC: 4Q, 2020, 32-33
  + **M80.0B** Age-related osteoporosis with current pathological fracture, pelvis
    - CC X+7th **M80.0B1** Age-related osteoporosis with current pathological fracture, right pelvis
    - CC X+7th **M80.0B2** Age-related osteoporosis with current pathological fracture, left pelvis
    - CC X+7th **M80.0B9** Age-related osteoporosis with current pathological fracture, unspecified pelvis

+ **M80.8** Other osteoporosis with current pathological fracture
  Drug-induced osteoporosis with current pathological fracture
  Idiopathic osteoporosis with current pathological fracture
  Osteoporosis of disuse with current pathological fracture
  Postoophorectomy osteoporosis with current pathological fracture
  Postsurgical malabsorption osteoporosis with current pathological fracture
  Post-traumatic osteoporosis with current pathological fracture
  Use additional code for adverse effect, if applicable, to identify drug (T36-T50 with fifth or sixth character 5)
  - CC X+7th **M80.80** Other osteoporosis with current pathological fracture, unspecified site
  + **M80.81** Other osteoporosis with pathological fracture, shoulder
    - CC +7th **M80.811** Other osteoporosis with current pathological fracture, right shoulder
    - CC +7th **M80.812** Other osteoporosis with current pathological fracture, left shoulder
    - CC +7th **M80.819** Other osteoporosis with current pathological fracture, unspecified shoulder
  + **M80.82** Other osteoporosis with current pathological fracture, humerus
    - CC +7th **M80.821** Other osteoporosis with current pathological fracture, right humerus
    - CC +7th **M80.822** Other osteoporosis with current pathological fracture, left humerus
    - CC +7th **M80.829** Other osteoporosis with current pathological fracture, unspecified humerus
  + **M80.83** Other osteoporosis with current pathological fracture, forearm
    Other osteoporosis with current pathological fracture of wrist
    - CC +7th **M80.831** Other osteoporosis with current pathological fracture, right forearm
    - CC +7th **M80.832** Other osteoporosis with current pathological fracture, left forearm
    - CC +7th **M80.839** Other osteoporosis with current pathological fracture, unspecified forearm
  + **M80.84** Other osteoporosis with current pathological fracture, hand
    - CC +7th **M80.841** Other osteoporosis with current pathological fracture, right hand
    - CC +7th **M80.842** Other osteoporosis with current pathological fracture, left hand
    - CC +7th **M80.849** Other osteoporosis with current pathological fracture, unspecified hand
  + **M80.85** Other osteoporosis with current pathological fracture, femur
    Other osteoporosis with current pathological fracture of hip
    - CC +7th **M80.851** Other osteoporosis with current pathological fracture, right femur
    - CC +7th **M80.852** Other osteoporosis with current pathological fracture, left femur
    - CC +7th **M80.859** Other osteoporosis with current pathological fracture, unspecified femur
  + **M80.86** Other osteoporosis with current pathological fracture, lower leg
    - CC +7th **M80.861** Other osteoporosis with current pathological fracture, right lower leg
    - CC +7th **M80.862** Other osteoporosis with current pathological fracture, left lower leg
    - CC +7th **M80.869** Other osteoporosis with current pathological fracture, unspecified lower leg
  + **M80.87** Other osteoporosis with current pathological fracture, ankle and foot
    - CC +7th **M80.871** Other osteoporosis with current pathological fracture, right ankle and foot
    - CC +7th **M80.872** Other osteoporosis with current pathological fracture, left ankle and foot
    - CC +7th **M80.879** Other osteoporosis with current pathological fracture, unspecified ankle and foot

CC X+7th **M80.88** Other osteoporosis with current pathological fracture, vertebra(e)
CC X+7th **M80.8A** Other osteoporosis with current pathological fracture, other site
AHA CC: 4Q, 2020, 32
+ **M80.8B** Other osteoporosis with current pathological fracture, pelvis
CC X+7th **M80.8B1** Other osteoporosis with current pathological fracture, right pelvis
CC X+7th **M80.8B2** Other osteoporosis with current pathological fracture, left pelvis
CC X+7th **M80.8B9** Other osteoporosis with current pathological fracture, unspecified pelvis

M81 Osteoporosis without current pathological fracture

Use additional code to identify:
major osseous defect, if applicable (M89.7-)
personal history of (healed) osteoporosis fracture, if applicable (Z87.310)
Excludes1: osteoporosis with current pathological fracture (M80.-)
Sudeck's atrophy (M89.0)
Review coding guideline C.13.d

- **M81.0 Age-related osteoporosis without current pathological fracture**
  Involutional osteoporosis without current pathological fracture
  Osteoporosis NOS
  Postmenopausal osteoporosis without current pathological fracture
  Senile osteoporosis without current pathological fracture
- **M81.6 Localized osteoporosis [Lequesne]**
  Excludes1: Sudeck's atrophy (M89.0)
- **M81.8 Other osteoporosis without current pathological fracture**
  Drug-induced osteoporosis without current pathological fracture
  Idiopathic osteoporosis without current pathological fracture
  Osteoporosis of disuse without current pathological fracture
  Postoophorectomy osteoporosis without current pathological fracture
  Postsurgical malabsorption osteoporosis without current pathological fracture
  Post-traumatic osteoporosis without current pathological fracture
  Use additional code for adverse effect, if applicable, to identify drug (T36-T50 with fifth or sixth character 5)

M83 Adult osteomalacia

Excludes1: infantile and juvenile osteomalacia (E55.0)
renal osteodystrophy (N25.0)
rickets (active) (E55.0)
rickets (active) sequelae (E64.3)
vitamin D-resistant osteomalacia (E83.31)
vitamin D-resistant rickets (active) (E83.31)

- ♀ **M83.0 Puerperal osteomalacia**
- **M83.1 Senile osteomalacia**
- **M83.2 Adult osteomalacia due to malabsorption**
  Postsurgical malabsorption osteomalacia in adults
- **M83.3 Adult osteomalacia due to malnutrition**
  M83.4 Aluminum bone disease
- **M83.5 Other drug-induced osteomalacia in adults**
  Use additional code for adverse effect, if applicable, to identify drug (T36-T50 with fifth or sixth character 5)
- **M83.8 Other adult osteomalacia**
- **M83.9 Adult osteomalacia, unspecified**

M84 Disorder of continuity of bone

Excludes2: traumatic fracture of bone-see fracture, by site

+ **M84.3 Stress fracture**
  Fatigue fracture
  March fracture
  Stress fracture NOS
  Stress reaction
  external cause code(s) to identify the cause of the stress fracture
  Excludes1: pathological fracture NOS (M84.4.-)
  pathological fracture due to osteoporosis (M80.-)
  traumatic fracture (S12.-, S22.-, S32.-, S42.-, S52.-, S62.-, S72.-, S82.-, S92.-)
  Excludes2: personal history of (healed) stress (fatigue) fracture (Z87.312)
  stress fracture of vertebra (M48.4-)

The appropriate 7th character is to be added to each code from subcategory M84.3:
A initial encounter for fracture
D subsequent encounter for fracture with routine healing
G subsequent encounter for fracture with delayed healing
K subsequent encounter for fracture with nonunion
P subsequent encounter for fracture with malunion
S sequela

CC X+7th **M84.30** Stress fracture, unspecified site
+ **M84.31** Stress fracture, shoulder
CC +7th **M84.311** Stress fracture, right shoulder
CC +7th **M84.312** Stress fracture, left shoulder
CC +7th **M84.319** Stress fracture, unspecified shoulder
+ **M84.32** Stress fracture, humerus
CC +7th **M84.321** Stress fracture, right humerus
CC +7th **M84.322** Stress fracture, left humerus
CC +7th **M84.329** Stress fracture, unspecified humerus
+ **M84.33** Stress fracture, ulna and radius
CC +7th **M84.331** Stress fracture, right ulna
CC +7th **M84.332** Stress fracture, left ulna
CC +7th **M84.333** Stress fracture, right radius
CC +7th **M84.334** Stress fracture, left radius
CC +7th **M84.339** Stress fracture, unspecified ulna and radius
+ **M84.34** Stress fracture, hand and fingers
CC +7th **M84.341** Stress fracture, right hand
CC +7th **M84.342** Stress fracture, left hand
CC +7th **M84.343** Stress fracture, unspecified hand
CC +7th **M84.344** Stress fracture, right finger(s)
CC +7th **M84.345** Stress fracture, left finger(s)
CC +7th **M84.346** Stress fracture, unspecified finger(s)
+ **M84.35** Stress fracture, pelvis and femur
Stress fracture, hip
CC +7th **M84.350** Stress fracture, pelvis
CC +7th **M84.351** Stress fracture, right femur
CC +7th **M84.352** Stress fracture, left femur
CC +7th **M84.353** Stress fracture, unspecified femur
CC +7th **M84.359** Stress fracture, hip, unspecified
+ **M84.36** Stress fracture, tibia and fibula
CC +7th **M84.361** Stress fracture, right tibia
CC +7th **M84.362** Stress fracture, left tibia
CC +7th **M84.363** Stress fracture, right fibula
CC +7th **M84.364** Stress fracture, left fibula
CC +7th **M84.369** Stress fracture, unspecified tibia and fibula
+ **M84.37** Stress fracture, ankle, foot and toes
CC +7th **M84.371** Stress fracture, right ankle
CC +7th **M84.372** Stress fracture, left ankle
CC +7th **M84.373** Stress fracture, unspecified ankle
CC +7th **M84.374** Stress fracture, right foot
CC +7th **M84.375** Stress fracture, left foot
CC +7th **M84.376** Stress fracture, unspecified foot
CC +7th **M84.377** Stress fracture, right toe(s)
CC +7th **M84.378** Stress fracture, left toe(s)
CC +7th **M84.379** Stress fracture, unspecified toe(s)
CC X+7th **M84.38** Stress fracture, other site
Excludes2: stress fracture of vertebra (M48.4-)

+ M84.4 Pathological fracture, not elsewhere classified
Chronic fracture
Pathological fracture NOS
Excludes1: collapsed vertebra NEC (M48.5)
pathological fracture in neoplastic disease (M84.5-)
pathological fracture in osteoporosis (M80.-)
pathological fracture in other disease (M84.6-)
stress fracture (M84.3-)
traumatic fracture (S12.-, S22.-, S32.-, S42.-, S52.-, S62.-, S72.-, S82.-, S92.-)
Excludes2: personal history of (healed) pathological fracture (Z87.311)

The appropriate 7th character is to be added to each code from subcategory **M84.4**:
A   initial encounter for fracture
D   subsequent encounter for fracture with routine healing
G   subsequent encounter for fracture with delayed healing
K   subsequent encounter for fracture with nonunion
P   subsequent encounter for fracture with malunion
S   sequela

CC X+7th   M84.40 Pathological fracture, unspecified site
+ M84.41 Pathological fracture, shoulder
  CC +7th M84.411 Pathological fracture, right shoulder
  CC +7th M84.412 Pathological fracture, left shoulder
  CC +7th M84.419 Pathological fracture, unspecified shoulder
+ M84.42 Pathological fracture, humerus
  CC +7th M84.421 Pathological fracture, right humerus
  CC +7th M84.422 Pathological fracture, left humerus
  CC +7th M84.429 Pathological fracture, unspecified humerus
+ M84.43 Pathological fracture, ulna and radius
  CC +7th M84.431 Pathological fracture, right ulna
  CC +7th M84.432 Pathological fracture, left ulna
  CC +7th M84.433 Pathological fracture, right radius
  CC +7th M84.434 Pathological fracture, left radius
  CC +7th M84.439 Pathological fracture, unspecified ulna and radius
+ M84.44 Pathological fracture, hand and fingers
  CC +7th M84.441 Pathological fracture, right hand
  CC +7th M84.442 Pathological fracture, left hand
  CC +7th M84.443 Pathological fracture, unspecified hand
  CC +7th M84.444 Pathological fracture, right finger(s)
  CC +7th M84.445 Pathological fracture, left finger(s)
  CC +7th M84.446 Pathological fracture, unspecified finger(s)
+ M84.45 Pathological fracture, femur and pelvis
  CC +7th M84.451 Pathological fracture, right femur
  CC +7th M84.452 Pathological fracture, left femur
  CC +7th M84.453 Pathological fracture, unspecified femur
  CC +7th M84.454 Pathological fracture, pelvis
         AHA CC: 4Q, 2016, 42-43
  CC +7th M84.459 Pathological fracture, hip, unspecified
+ M84.46 Pathological fracture, tibia and fibula
  CC +7th M84.461 Pathological fracture, right tibia
  CC +7th M84.462 Pathological fracture, left tibia
  CC +7th M84.463 Pathological fracture, right fibula
  CC +7th M84.464 Pathological fracture, left fibula
  CC +7th M84.469 Pathological fracture, unspecified tibia and fibula
+ M84.47 Pathological fracture, ankle, foot and toes
  CC +7th M84.471 Pathological fracture, right ankle
  CC +7th M84.472 Pathological fracture, left ankle
  CC +7th M84.473 Pathological fracture, unspecified ankle
  CC +7th M84.474 Pathological fracture, right foot
  CC +7th M84.475 Pathological fracture, left foot
  CC +7th M84.476 Pathological fracture, unspecified foot
  CC +7th M84.477 Pathological fracture, right toe(s)
  CC +7th M84.478 Pathological fracture, left toe(s)
  CC +7th M84.479 Pathological fracture, unspecified toe(s)
CC X+7th   M84.48 Pathological fracture, other site

+ M84.5 Pathological fracture in neoplastic disease
Code also underlying neoplasm

The appropriate 7th character is to be added to each code from subcategory **M84.5**:
A   initial encounter for fracture
D   subsequent encounter for fracture with routine healing
G   subsequent encounter for fracture with delayed healing
K   subsequent encounter for fracture with nonunion
P   subsequent encounter for fracture with malunion
S   sequela

Review coding guideline C.2.l.6

CC X+7th   M84.50 Pathological fracture in neoplastic disease, unspecified site
+ M84.51 Pathological fracture in neoplastic disease, shoulder
  CC +7th M84.511 Pathological fracture in neoplastic disease, right shoulder
  CC +7th M84.512 Pathological fracture in neoplastic disease, left shoulder
  CC +7th M84.519 Pathological fracture in neoplastic disease, unspecified shoulder
+ M84.52 Pathological fracture in neoplastic disease, humerus
  CC +7th M84.521 Pathological fracture in neoplastic disease, right humerus
  CC +7th M84.522 Pathological fracture in neoplastic disease, left humerus
  CC +7th M84.529 Pathological fracture in neoplastic disease, unspecified humerus
+ M84.53 Pathological fracture in neoplastic disease, ulna and radius
  CC +7th M84.531 Pathological fracture in neoplastic disease, right ulna
  CC +7th M84.532 Pathological fracture in neoplastic disease, left ulna
  CC +7th M84.533 Pathological fracture in neoplastic disease, right radius
  CC +7th M84.534 Pathological fracture in neoplastic disease, left radius
  CC +7th M84.539 Pathological fracture in neoplastic disease, unspecified ulna and radius
+ M84.54 Pathological fracture in neoplastic disease, hand
  CC +7th M84.541 Pathological fracture in neoplastic disease, right hand
  CC +7th M84.542 Pathological fracture in neoplastic disease, left hand
  CC +7th M84.549 Pathological fracture in neoplastic disease, unspecified hand
+ M84.55 Pathological fracture in neoplastic disease, pelvis and femur
  CC +7th M84.550 Pathological fracture in neoplastic disease, pelvis
  CC +7th M84.551 Pathological fracture in neoplastic disease, right femur
  CC +7th M84.552 Pathological fracture in neoplastic disease, left femur
  CC +7th M84.553 Pathological fracture in neoplastic disease, unspecified femur
  CC +7th M84.559 Pathological fracture in neoplastic disease, hip, unspecified
+ M84.56 Pathological fracture in neoplastic disease, tibia and fibula
  CC +7th M84.561 Pathological fracture in neoplastic disease, right tibia
  CC +7th M84.562 Pathological fracture in neoplastic disease, left tibia
  CC +7th M84.563 Pathological fracture in neoplastic disease, right fibula
  CC +7th M84.564 Pathological fracture in neoplastic disease, left fibula
  CC +7th M84.569 Pathological fracture in neoplastic disease, unspecified tibia and fibula
+ M84.57 Pathological fracture in neoplastic disease, ankle and foot
  CC +7th M84.571 Pathological fracture in neoplastic disease, right ankle
  CC +7th M84.572 Pathological fracture in neoplastic disease, left ankle

CC +7th	M84.573	Pathological fracture in neoplastic disease, unspecified ankle
CC +7th	M84.574	Pathological fracture in neoplastic disease, right foot
CC +7th	M84.575	Pathological fracture in neoplastic disease, left foot
CC +7th	M84.576	Pathological fracture in neoplastic disease, unspecified foot
CC X+7th	M84.58	Pathological fracture in neoplastic disease, other specified site
		Pathological fracture in neoplastic disease, vertebrae

+ **M84.6 Pathological fracture in other disease**
  Code also underlying condition
  Excludes1: *pathological fracture in osteoporosis (M80.-)*

> The appropriate 7th character is to be added to each code from subcategory **M84.6**:
> A initial encounter for fracture
> D subsequent encounter for fracture with routine healing
> G subsequent encounter for fracture with delayed healing
> K subsequent encounter for fracture with nonunion
> P subsequent encounter for fracture with malunion
> S sequela

CC X+7th	M84.60	Pathological fracture in other disease, unspecified site
+	M84.61	Pathological fracture in other disease, shoulder
CC +7th	M84.611	Pathological fracture in other disease, right shoulder
CC +7th	M84.612	Pathological fracture in other disease, left shoulder
CC +7th	M84.619	Pathological fracture in other disease, unspecified shoulder
+	M84.62	Pathological fracture in other disease, humerus
CC +7th	M84.621	Pathological fracture in other disease, right humerus
CC +7th	M84.622	Pathological fracture in other disease, left humerus
CC +7th	M84.629	Pathological fracture in other disease, unspecified humerus
+	M84.63	Pathological fracture in other disease, ulna and radius
CC +7th	M84.631	Pathological fracture in other disease, right ulna
CC +7th	M84.632	Pathological fracture in other disease, left ulna
CC +7th	M84.633	Pathological fracture in other disease, right radius
CC +7th	M84.634	Pathological fracture in other disease, left radius
CC +7th	M84.639	Pathological fracture in other disease, unspecified ulna and radius
+	M84.64	Pathological fracture in other disease, hand
CC +7th	M84.641	Pathological fracture in other disease, right hand
CC +7th	M84.642	Pathological fracture in other disease, left hand
CC +7th	M84.649	Pathological fracture in other disease, unspecified hand
+	M84.65	Pathological fracture in other disease, pelvis and femur
	M84.650	Pathological fracture in other disease, pelvis
CC +7th	**M84.651**	Pathological fracture in other disease, right femur
CC +7th	**M84.652**	Pathological fracture in other disease, left femur
CC +7th	**M84.653**	Pathological fracture in other disease, unspecified femur
CC +7th	**M84.659**	Pathological fracture in other disease, hip, unspecified
+	M84.66	Pathological fracture in other disease, tibia and fibula
CC +7th	M84.661	Pathological fracture in other disease, right tibia
CC +7th	M84.662	Pathological fracture in other disease, left tibia
CC +7th	M84.663	Pathological fracture in other disease, right fibula
CC +7th	M84.664	Pathological fracture in other disease, left fibula
CC +7th	M84.669	Pathological fracture in other disease, unspecified tibia and fibula
+	M84.67	Pathological fracture in other disease, ankle and foot
CC +7th	M84.671	Pathological fracture in other disease, right ankle
CC +7th	M84.672	Pathological fracture in other disease, left ankle
CC +7th	M84.673	Pathological fracture in other disease, unspecified ankle
CC +7th	M84.674	Pathological fracture in other disease, right foot
CC +7th	M84.675	Pathological fracture in other disease, left foot
CC +7th	M84.676	Pathological fracture in other disease, unspecified foot
CC X+7th	M84.68	Pathological fracture in other disease, other site

+ **M84.7 Nontraumatic fracture, not elsewhere classified**
  + **M84.75 Atypical femoral fracture**
    AHA CC: 4Q, 2016, 41-42

> The appropriate 7th character is to be added to each code from subcategory **M84.75**:
> A initial encounter for fracture
> D subsequent encounter for fracture with routine healing
> G subsequent encounter for fracture with delayed healing
> K subsequent encounter for fracture with nonunion
> P subsequent encounter for fracture with malunion
> S sequela

CC +7th	**M84.750**	Atypical femoral fracture, unspecified
CC +7th	**M84.751**	Incomplete atypical femoral fracture, right leg
CC +7th	**M84.752**	Incomplete atypical femoral fracture, left leg
CC +7th	**M84.753**	Incomplete atypical femoral fracture, unspecified leg
CC +7th	**M84.754**	Complete transverse atypical femoral fracture, right leg
CC +7th	**M84.755**	Complete transverse atypical femoral fracture, left leg
CC +7th	**M84.756**	Complete transverse atypical femoral fracture, unspecified leg
CC +7th	**M84.757**	Complete oblique atypical femoral fracture, right leg
CC +7th	**M84.758**	Complete oblique atypical femoral fracture, left leg
CC +7th	**M84.759**	Complete oblique atypical femoral fracture, unspecified leg

+ **M84.8 Other disorders of continuity of bone**
  M84.80 Other disorders of continuity of bone, unspecified site
  + M84.81 Other disorders of continuity of bone, shoulder
    M84.811 Other disorders of continuity of bone, right shoulder
    M84.812 Other disorders of continuity of bone, left shoulder
    M84.819 Other disorders of continuity of bone, unspecified shoulder
  + M84.82 Other disorders of continuity of bone, humerus
    M84.821 Other disorders of continuity of bone, right humerus
    M84.822 Other disorders of continuity of bone, left humerus
    M84.829 Other disorders of continuity of bone, unspecified humerus
  + M84.83 Other disorders of continuity of bone, ulna and radius
    M84.831 Other disorders of continuity of bone, right ulna
    M84.832 Other disorders of continuity of bone, left ulna
    M84.833 Other disorders of continuity of bone, right radius
    M84.834 Other disorders of continuity of bone, left radius
    M84.839 Other disorders of continuity of bone, unspecified ulna and radius

+ M84.84 Other disorders of continuity of bone, hand
 M84.841 Other disorders of continuity of bone, right hand
 M84.842 Other disorders of continuity of bone, left hand
 M84.849 Other disorders of continuity of bone, unspecified hand
+ M84.85 Other disorders of continuity of bone, pelvic region and thigh
 M84.851 Other disorders of continuity of bone, right pelvic region and thigh
 M84.852 Other disorders of continuity of bone, left pelvic region and thigh
 M84.859 Other disorders of continuity of bone, unspecified pelvic region and thigh
+ M84.86 Other disorders of continuity of bone, tibia and fibula
 M84.861 Other disorders of continuity of bone, right tibia
 M84.862 Other disorders of continuity of bone, left tibia
 M84.863 Other disorders of continuity of bone, right fibula
 M84.864 Other disorders of continuity of bone, left fibula
 M84.869 Other disorders of continuity of bone, unspecified tibia and fibula
+ M84.87 Other disorders of continuity of bone, ankle and foot
 M84.871 Other disorders of continuity of bone, right ankle and foot
 M84.872 Other disorders of continuity of bone, left ankle and foot
 M84.879 Other disorders of continuity of bone, unspecified ankle and foot
 M84.88 Other disorders of continuity of bone, other site
 M84.9 Disorder of continuity of bone, unspecified

M85 Other disorders of bone density and structure

Excludes1: *osteogenesis imperfecta (Q78.0)*
osteopetrosis (Q78.2)
osteopoikilosis (Q78.8)
polyostotic fibrous dysplasia (Q78.1)

+ M85.0 Fibrous dysplasia (monostotic)
 Excludes2: *fibrous dysplasia of jaw (M27.8)*
 M85.00 Fibrous dysplasia (monostotic), unspecified site
+ M85.01 Fibrous dysplasia (monostotic), shoulder
 M85.011 Fibrous dysplasia (monostotic), right shoulder
 M85.012 Fibrous dysplasia (monostotic), left shoulder
 M85.019 Fibrous dysplasia (monostotic), unspecified shoulder
+ M85.02 Fibrous dysplasia (monostotic), upper arm
 M85.021 Fibrous dysplasia (monostotic), right upper arm
 M85.022 Fibrous dysplasia (monostotic), left upper arm
 M85.029 Fibrous dysplasia (monostotic), unspecified upper arm
+ M85.03 Fibrous dysplasia (monostotic), forearm
 M85.031 Fibrous dysplasia (monostotic), right forearm
 M85.032 Fibrous dysplasia (monostotic), left forearm
 M85.039 Fibrous dysplasia (monostotic), unspecified forearm
+ M85.04 Fibrous dysplasia (monostotic), hand
 M85.041 Fibrous dysplasia (monostotic), right hand
 M85.042 Fibrous dysplasia (monostotic), left hand
 M85.049 Fibrous dysplasia (monostotic), unspecified hand
+ M85.05 Fibrous dysplasia (monostotic), thigh
 M85.051 Fibrous dysplasia (monostotic), right thigh
 M85.052 Fibrous dysplasia (monostotic), left thigh
 M85.059 Fibrous dysplasia (monostotic), unspecified thigh
+ M85.06 Fibrous dysplasia (monostotic), lower leg
 M85.061 Fibrous dysplasia (monostotic), right lower leg
 M85.062 Fibrous dysplasia (monostotic), left lower leg
 M85.069 Fibrous dysplasia (monostotic), unspecified lower leg
+ M85.07 Fibrous dysplasia (monostotic), ankle and foot
 M85.071 Fibrous dysplasia (monostotic), right ankle and foot
 M85.072 Fibrous dysplasia (monostotic), left ankle and foot
 M85.079 Fibrous dysplasia (monostotic), unspecified ankle and foot
 M85.08 Fibrous dysplasia (monostotic), other site
 M85.09 Fibrous dysplasia (monostotic), multiple sites
+ M85.1 Skeletal fluorosis
 M85.10 Skeletal fluorosis, unspecified site
+ M85.11 Skeletal fluorosis, shoulder
 M85.111 Skeletal fluorosis, right shoulder
 M85.112 Skeletal fluorosis, left shoulder
 M85.119 Skeletal fluorosis, unspecified shoulder
+ M85.12 Skeletal fluorosis, upper arm
 M85.121 Skeletal fluorosis, right upper arm
 M85.122 Skeletal fluorosis, left upper arm
 M85.129 Skeletal fluorosis, unspecified upper arm
+ M85.13 Skeletal fluorosis, forearm
 M85.131 Skeletal fluorosis, right forearm
 M85.132 Skeletal fluorosis, left forearm
 M85.139 Skeletal fluorosis, unspecified forearm
+ M85.14 Skeletal fluorosis, hand
 M85.141 Skeletal fluorosis, right hand
 M85.142 Skeletal fluorosis, left hand
 M85.149 Skeletal fluorosis, unspecified hand
+ M85.15 Skeletal fluorosis, thigh
 M85.151 Skeletal fluorosis, right thigh
 M85.152 Skeletal fluorosis, left thigh
 M85.159 Skeletal fluorosis, unspecified thigh
+ M85.16 Skeletal fluorosis, lower leg
 M85.161 Skeletal fluorosis, right lower leg
 M85.162 Skeletal fluorosis, left lower leg
 M85.169 Skeletal fluorosis, unspecified lower leg
+ M85.17 Skeletal fluorosis, ankle and foot
 M85.171 Skeletal fluorosis, right ankle and foot
 M85.172 Skeletal fluorosis, left ankle and foot
 M85.179 Skeletal fluorosis, unspecified ankle and foot
 M85.18 Skeletal fluorosis, other site
 M85.19 Skeletal fluorosis, multiple sites
 M85.2 Hyperostosis of skull
+ M85.3 Osteitis condensans
 M85.30 Osteitis condensans, unspecified site
+ M85.31 Osteitis condensans, shoulder
 M85.311 Osteitis condensans, right shoulder
 M85.312 Osteitis condensans, left shoulder
 M85.319 Osteitis condensans, unspecified shoulder
+ M85.32 Osteitis condensans, upper arm
 M85.321 Osteitis condensans, right upper arm
 M85.322 Osteitis condensans, left upper arm
 M85.329 Osteitis condensans, unspecified upper arm
+ M85.33 Osteitis condensans, forearm
 M85.331 Osteitis condensans, right forearm
 M85.332 Osteitis condensans, left forearm
 M85.339 Osteitis condensans, unspecified forearm
+ M85.34 Osteitis condensans, hand
 M85.341 Osteitis condensans, right hand
 M85.342 Osteitis condensans, left hand
 M85.349 Osteitis condensans, unspecified hand
+ M85.35 Osteitis condensans, thigh
 M85.351 Osteitis condensans, right thigh
 M85.352 Osteitis condensans, left thigh
 M85.359 Osteitis condensans, unspecified thigh
+ M85.36 Osteitis condensans, lower leg
 M85.361 Osteitis condensans, right lower leg
 M85.362 Osteitis condensans, left lower leg
 M85.369 Osteitis condensans, unspecified lower leg

+ M85.37 Osteitis condensans, ankle and foot
    M85.371 Osteitis condensans, right ankle and foot
    M85.372 Osteitis condensans, left ankle and foot
    M85.379 Osteitis condensans, unspecified ankle and foot
M85.38 Osteitis condensans, other site
M85.39 Osteitis condensans, multiple sites

+ **M85.4 Solitary bone cyst**
    Excludes2: *solitary cyst of jaw (M27.4)*
M85.40 Solitary bone cyst, unspecified site
+ M85.41 Solitary bone cyst, shoulder
    M85.411 Solitary bone cyst, right shoulder
    M85.412 Solitary bone cyst, left shoulder
    M85.419 Solitary bone cyst, unspecified shoulder
+ M85.42 Solitary bone cyst, humerus
    M85.421 Solitary bone cyst, right humerus
    M85.422 Solitary bone cyst, left humerus
    M85.429 Solitary bone cyst, unspecified humerus
+ M85.43 Solitary bone cyst, ulna and radius
    M85.431 Solitary bone cyst, right ulna and radius
    M85.432 Solitary bone cyst, left ulna and radius
    M85.439 Solitary bone cyst, unspecified ulna and radius
+ M85.44 Solitary bone cyst, hand
    M85.441 Solitary bone cyst, right hand
    M85.442 Solitary bone cyst, left hand
    M85.449 Solitary bone cyst, unspecified hand
+ M85.45 Solitary bone cyst, pelvis
    M85.451 Solitary bone cyst, right pelvis
    M85.452 Solitary bone cyst, left pelvis
    M85.459 Solitary bone cyst, unspecified pelvis
+ M85.46 Solitary bone cyst, tibia and fibula
    M85.461 Solitary bone cyst, right tibia and fibula
    M85.462 Solitary bone cyst, left tibia and fibula
    M85.469 Solitary bone cyst, unspecified tibia and fibula
+ M85.47 Solitary bone cyst, ankle and foot
    M85.471 Solitary bone cyst, right ankle and foot
    M85.472 Solitary bone cyst, left ankle and foot
    M85.479 Solitary bone cyst, unspecified ankle and foot
M85.48 Solitary bone cyst, other site

+ **M85.5 Aneurysmal bone cyst**
    Excludes2: *aneurysmal cyst of jaw (M27.4)*
M85.50 Aneurysmal bone cyst, unspecified site
+ M85.51 Aneurysmal bone cyst, shoulder
    M85.511 Aneurysmal bone cyst, right shoulder
    M85.512 Aneurysmal bone cyst, left shoulder
    M85.519 Aneurysmal bone cyst, unspecified shoulder
+ M85.52 Aneurysmal bone cyst, upper arm
    M85.521 Aneurysmal bone cyst, right upper arm
    M85.522 Aneurysmal bone cyst, left upper arm
    M85.529 Aneurysmal bone cyst, unspecified upper arm
+ M85.53 Aneurysmal bone cyst, forearm
    M85.531 Aneurysmal bone cyst, right forearm
    M85.532 Aneurysmal bone cyst, left forearm
    M85.539 Aneurysmal bone cyst, unspecified forearm
+ M85.54 Aneurysmal bone cyst, hand
    M85.541 Aneurysmal bone cyst, right hand
    M85.542 Aneurysmal bone cyst, left hand
    M85.549 Aneurysmal bone cyst, unspecified hand
+ M85.55 Aneurysmal bone cyst, thigh
    M85.551 Aneurysmal bone cyst, right thigh
    M85.552 Aneurysmal bone cyst, left thigh
    M85.559 Aneurysmal bone cyst, unspecified thigh
+ M85.56 Aneurysmal bone cyst, lower leg
    M85.561 Aneurysmal bone cyst, right lower leg
    M85.562 Aneurysmal bone cyst, left lower leg
    M85.569 Aneurysmal bone cyst, unspecified lower leg
+ M85.57 Aneurysmal bone cyst, ankle and foot
    M85.571 Aneurysmal bone cyst, right ankle and foot
    M85.572 Aneurysmal bone cyst, left ankle and foot
    M85.579 Aneurysmal bone cyst, unspecified ankle and foot
M85.58 Aneurysmal bone cyst, other site
M85.59 Aneurysmal bone cyst, multiple sites

+ **M85.6 Other cyst of bone**
    Excludes1: *cyst of jaw NEC (M27.4)*
        osteitis fibrosa cystica generalisata [von Recklinghausen's disease of bone] (E21.0)
M85.60 Other cyst of bone, unspecified site
+ M85.61 Other cyst of bone, shoulder
    M85.611 Other cyst of bone, right shoulder
    M85.612 Other cyst of bone, left shoulder
    M85.619 Other cyst of bone, unspecified shoulder
+ M85.62 Other cyst of bone, upper arm
    M85.621 Other cyst of bone, right upper arm
    M85.622 Other cyst of bone, left upper arm
    M85.629 Other cyst of bone, unspecified upper arm
+ M85.63 Other cyst of bone, forearm
    M85.631 Other cyst of bone, right forearm
    M85.632 Other cyst of bone, left forearm
    M85.639 Other cyst of bone, unspecified forearm
+ M85.64 Other cyst of bone, hand
    M85.641 Other cyst of bone, right hand
    M85.642 Other cyst of bone, left hand
    M85.649 Other cyst of bone, unspecified hand
+ M85.65 Other cyst of bone, thigh
    M85.651 Other cyst of bone, right thigh
    M85.652 Other cyst of bone, left thigh
    M85.659 Other cyst of bone, unspecified thigh
+ M85.66 Other cyst of bone, lower leg
    M85.661 Other cyst of bone, right lower leg
    M85.662 Other cyst of bone, left lower leg
    M85.669 Other cyst of bone, unspecified lower leg
+ M85.67 Other cyst of bone, ankle and foot
    M85.671 Other cyst of bone, right ankle and foot
    M85.672 Other cyst of bone, left ankle and foot
    M85.679 Other cyst of bone, unspecified ankle and foot
M85.68 Other cyst of bone, other site
M85.69 Other cyst of bone, multiple sites

+ **M85.8 Other specified disorders of bone density and structure**
    Hyperostosis of bones, except skull
    Osteosclerosis, acquired
    Excludes1: *diffuse idiopathic skeletal hyperostosis [DISH] (M48.1)*
        osteosclerosis congenita (Q77.4)
        osteosclerosis fragilitas (generalista) (Q78.2)
        osteosclerosis myelofibrosis (D75.81)
M85.80 Other specified disorders of bone density and structure, unspecified site
+ M85.81 Other specified disorders of bone density and structure, shoulder
    M85.811 Other specified disorders of bone density and structure, right shoulder
    M85.812 Other specified disorders of bone density and structure, left shoulder
    M85.819 Other specified disorders of bone density and structure, unspecified shoulder
+ M85.82 Other specified disorders of bone density and structure, upper arm
    M85.821 Other specified disorders of bone density and structure, right upper arm
    M85.822 Other specified disorders of bone density and structure, left upper arm
    M85.829 Other specified disorders of bone density and structure, unspecified upper arm

+ **M85.83** Other specified disorders of bone density and structure, forearm
- **M85.831** Other specified disorders of bone density and structure, right forearm
- **M85.832** Other specified disorders of bone density and structure, left forearm
- **M85.839** Other specified disorders of bone density and structure, unspecified forearm

+ **M85.84** Other specified disorders of bone density and structure, hand
- **M85.841** Other specified disorders of bone density and structure, right hand
- **M85.842** Other specified disorders of bone density and structure, left hand
- **M85.849** Other specified disorders of bone density and structure, unspecified hand

+ **M85.85** Other specified disorders of bone density and structure, thigh
- **M85.851** Other specified disorders of bone density and structure, right thigh
- **M85.852** Other specified disorders of bone density and structure, left thigh
- **M85.859** Other specified disorders of bone density and structure, unspecified thigh

+ **M85.86** Other specified disorders of bone density and structure, lower leg
- **M85.861** Other specified disorders of bone density and structure, right lower leg
- **M85.862** Other specified disorders of bone density and structure, left lower leg
- **M85.869** Other specified disorders of bone density and structure, unspecified lower leg

+ **M85.87** Other specified disorders of bone density and structure, ankle and foot
- **M85.871** Other specified disorders of bone density and structure, right ankle and foot
- **M85.872** Other specified disorders of bone density and structure, left ankle and foot
- **M85.879** Other specified disorders of bone density and structure, unspecified ankle and foot

M85.88 Other specified disorders of bone density and structure, other site
M85.89 Other specified disorders of bone density and structure, multiple sites
M85.9 Disorder of bone density and structure, unspecified
AHA CC: 3Q, 2021, 11

Other osteopathies (M86-M90)

Excludes1: *postprocedural osteopathies (M96.-)*

M86 Osteomyelitis

Use additional code (B95-B97) to identify infectious agent

Use additional code to identify major osseous defect, if applicable (M89.7-)

Excludes1: *osteomyelitis due to:*
echinococcus (B67.2)
gonococcus (A54.43)
salmonella (A02.24)

Excludes2: *ostemyelitis of:*
orbit (H05.0-)
petrous bone (H70.2-)
vertebra (M46.2-)

+ **M86.0** Acute hematogenous osteomyelitis
- CC **M86.00** Acute hematogenous osteomyelitis, unspecified site
+ **M86.01** Acute hematogenous osteomyelitis, shoulder
  - CC **M86.011** Acute hematogenous osteomyelitis, right shoulder
  - CC **M86.012** Acute hematogenous osteomyelitis, left shoulder
  - CC **M86.019** Acute hematogenous osteomyelitis, unspecified shoulder

+ **M86.02** Acute hematogenous osteomyelitis, humerus
  - CC **M86.021** Acute hematogenous osteomyelitis, right humerus
  - CC **M86.022** Acute hematogenous osteomyelitis, left humerus
  - CC **M86.029** Acute hematogenous osteomyelitis, unspecified humerus

+ **M86.03** Acute hematogenous osteomyelitis, radius and ulna
  - CC **M86.031** Acute hematogenous osteomyelitis, right radius and ulna
  - CC **M86.032** Acute hematogenous osteomyelitis, left radius and ulna
  - CC **M86.039** Acute hematogenous osteomyelitis, unspecified radius and ulna

+ **M86.04** Acute hematogenous osteomyelitis, hand
  - CC **M86.041** Acute hematogenous osteomyelitis, right hand
  - CC **M86.042** Acute hematogenous osteomyelitis, left hand
  - CC **M86.049** Acute hematogenous osteomyelitis, unspecified hand

+ **M86.05** Acute hematogenous osteomyelitis, femur
  - CC **M86.051** Acute hematogenous osteomyelitis, right femur
  - CC **M86.052** Acute hematogenous osteomyelitis, left femur
  - CC **M86.059** Acute hematogenous osteomyelitis, unspecified femur

+ **M86.06** Acute hematogenous osteomyelitis, tibia and fibula
  - CC **M86.061** Acute hematogenous osteomyelitis, right tibia and fibula
  - CC **M86.062** Acute hematogenous osteomyelitis, left tibia and fibula
  - CC **M86.069** Acute hematogenous osteomyelitis, unspecified tibia and fibula

+ **M86.07** Acute hematogenous osteomyelitis, ankle and foot
  - CC **M86.071** Acute hematogenous osteomyelitis, right ankle and foot
  - CC **M86.072** Acute hematogenous osteomyelitis, left ankle and foot
  - CC **M86.079** Acute hematogenous osteomyelitis, unspecified ankle and foot

CC **M86.08** Acute hematogenous osteomyelitis, other sites
CC **M86.09** Acute hematogenous osteomyelitis, multiple sites

+ **M86.1** Other acute osteomyelitis
- CC **M86.10** Other acute osteomyelitis, unspecified site
+ **M86.11** Other acute osteomyelitis, shoulder
  - CC **M86.111** Other acute osteomyelitis, right shoulder
  - CC **M86.112** Other acute osteomyelitis, left shoulder
  - CC **M86.119** Other acute osteomyelitis, unspecified shoulder

+ **M86.12** Other acute osteomyelitis, humerus
  - CC **M86.121** Other acute osteomyelitis, right humerus
  - CC **M86.122** Other acute osteomyelitis, left humerus
  - CC **M86.129** Other acute osteomyelitis, unspecified humerus

+ **M86.13** Other acute osteomyelitis, radius and ulna
  - CC **M86.131** Other acute osteomyelitis, right radius and ulna
  - CC **M86.132** Other acute osteomyelitis, left radius and ulna
  - CC **M86.139** Other acute osteomyelitis, unspecified radius and ulna

+ **M86.14** Other acute osteomyelitis, hand
  - CC **M86.141** Other acute osteomyelitis, right hand
  - CC **M86.142** Other acute osteomyelitis, left hand
  - CC **M86.149** Other acute osteomyelitis, unspecified hand

+ **M86.15** Other acute osteomyelitis, femur
  - CC **M86.151** Other acute osteomyelitis, right femur
  - CC **M86.152** Other acute osteomyelitis, left femur
  - CC **M86.159** Other acute osteomyelitis, unspecified femur

- **+ M86.16** Other acute osteomyelitis, tibia and fibula
  - CC **M86.161** Other acute osteomyelitis, right tibia and fibula
  - CC **M86.162** Other acute osteomyelitis, left tibia and fibula
  - CC **M86.169** Other acute osteomyelitis, unspecified tibia and fibula
- **+ M86.17** Other acute osteomyelitis, ankle and foot
  - CC **M86.171** Other acute osteomyelitis, right ankle and foot
    - *AHA CC: 1Q, 2020, 12*
  - CC **M86.172** Other acute osteomyelitis, left ankle and foot
  - CC **M86.179** Other acute osteomyelitis, unspecified ankle and foot
- CC **M86.18** Other acute osteomyelitis, other site
- CC **M86.19** Other acute osteomyelitis, multiple sites
- **+ M86.2** Subacute osteomyelitis
  - CC **M86.20** Subacute osteomyelitis, unspecified site
  - **+ M86.21** Subacute osteomyelitis, shoulder
    - CC **M86.211** Subacute osteomyelitis, right shoulder
    - CC **M86.212** Subacute osteomyelitis, left shoulder
    - CC **M86.219** Subacute osteomyelitis, unspecified shoulder
  - **+ M86.22** Subacute osteomyelitis, humerus
    - CC **M86.221** Subacute osteomyelitis, right humerus
    - CC **M86.222** Subacute osteomyelitis, left humerus
    - CC **M86.229** Subacute osteomyelitis, unspecified humerus
  - **+ M86.23** Subacute osteomyelitis, radius and ulna
    - CC **M86.231** Subacute osteomyelitis, right radius and ulna
    - CC **M86.232** Subacute osteomyelitis, left radius and ulna
    - CC **M86.239** Subacute osteomyelitis, unspecified radius and ulna
  - **+ M86.24** Subacute osteomyelitis, hand
    - CC **M86.241** Subacute osteomyelitis, right hand
    - CC **M86.242** Subacute osteomyelitis, left hand
    - CC **M86.249** Subacute osteomyelitis, unspecified hand
  - **+ M86.25** Subacute osteomyelitis, femur
    - CC **M86.251** Subacute osteomyelitis, right femur
    - CC **M86.252** Subacute osteomyelitis, left femur
    - CC **M86.259** Subacute osteomyelitis, unspecified femur
  - **+ M86.26** Subacute osteomyelitis, tibia and fibula
    - CC **M86.261** Subacute osteomyelitis, right tibia and fibula
    - CC **M86.262** Subacute osteomyelitis, left tibia and fibula
    - CC **M86.269** Subacute osteomyelitis, unspecified tibia and fibula
  - **+ M86.27** Subacute osteomyelitis, ankle and foot
    - CC **M86.271** Subacute osteomyelitis, right ankle and foot
    - CC **M86.272** Subacute osteomyelitis, left ankle and foot
    - CC **M86.279** Subacute osteomyelitis, unspecified ankle and foot
  - CC **M86.28** Subacute osteomyelitis, other site
  - CC **M86.29** Subacute osteomyelitis, multiple sites
- **+ M86.3** Chronic multifocal osteomyelitis
  - CC **M86.30** Chronic multifocal osteomyelitis, unspecified site
  - **+ M86.31** Chronic multifocal osteomyelitis, shoulder
    - CC **M86.311** Chronic multifocal osteomyelitis, right shoulder
    - CC **M86.312** Chronic multifocal osteomyelitis, left shoulder
    - CC **M86.319** Chronic multifocal osteomyelitis, unspecified shoulder
  - **+ M86.32** Chronic multifocal osteomyelitis, humerus
    - CC **M86.321** Chronic multifocal osteomyelitis, right humerus
    - CC **M86.322** Chronic multifocal osteomyelitis, left humerus
    - CC **M86.329** Chronic multifocal osteomyelitis, unspecified humerus
- **+ M86.33** Chronic multifocal osteomyelitis, radius and ulna
  - CC **M86.331** Chronic multifocal osteomyelitis, right radius and ulna
  - CC **M86.332** Chronic multifocal osteomyelitis, left radius and ulna
  - CC **M86.339** Chronic multifocal osteomyelitis, unspecified radius and ulna
- **+ M86.34** Chronic multifocal osteomyelitis, hand
  - CC **M86.341** Chronic multifocal osteomyelitis, right hand
  - CC **M86.342** Chronic multifocal osteomyelitis, left hand
  - CC **M86.349** Chronic multifocal osteomyelitis, unspecified hand
- **+ M86.35** Chronic multifocal osteomyelitis, femur
  - CC **M86.351** Chronic multifocal osteomyelitis, right femur
  - CC **M86.352** Chronic multifocal osteomyelitis, left femur
  - CC **M86.359** Chronic multifocal osteomyelitis, unspecified femur
- **+ M86.36** Chronic multifocal osteomyelitis, tibia and fibula
  - CC **M86.361** Chronic multifocal osteomyelitis, right tibia and fibula
  - CC **M86.362** Chronic multifocal osteomyelitis, left tibia and fibula
  - CC **M86.369** Chronic multifocal osteomyelitis, unspecified tibia and fibula
- **+ M86.37** Chronic multifocal osteomyelitis, ankle and foot
  - CC **M86.371** Chronic multifocal osteomyelitis, right ankle and foot
  - CC **M86.372** Chronic multifocal osteomyelitis, left ankle and foot
  - CC **M86.379** Chronic multifocal osteomyelitis, unspecified ankle and foot
- CC **M86.38** Chronic multifocal osteomyelitis, other site
- CC **M86.39** Chronic multifocal osteomyelitis, multiple sites
- **+ M86.4** Chronic osteomyelitis with draining sinus
  - CC **M86.40** Chronic osteomyelitis with draining sinus, unspecified site
  - **+ M86.41** Chronic osteomyelitis with draining sinus, shoulder
    - CC **M86.411** Chronic osteomyelitis with draining sinus, right shoulder
    - CC **M86.412** Chronic osteomyelitis with draining sinus, left shoulder
    - CC **M86.419** Chronic osteomyelitis with draining sinus, unspecified shoulder
  - **+ M86.42** Chronic osteomyelitis with draining sinus, humerus
    - CC **M86.421** Chronic osteomyelitis with draining sinus, right humerus
    - CC **M86.422** Chronic osteomyelitis with draining sinus, left humerus
    - CC **M86.429** Chronic osteomyelitis with draining sinus, unspecified humerus
  - **+ M86.43** Chronic osteomyelitis with draining sinus, radius and ulna
    - CC **M86.431** Chronic osteomyelitis with draining sinus, right radius and ulna
    - CC **M86.432** Chronic osteomyelitis with draining sinus, left radius and ulna
    - CC **M86.439** Chronic osteomyelitis with draining sinus, unspecified radius and ulna
  - **+ M86.44** Chronic osteomyelitis with draining sinus, hand
    - CC **M86.441** Chronic osteomyelitis with draining sinus, right hand
    - CC **M86.442** Chronic osteomyelitis with draining sinus, left hand
    - CC **M86.449** Chronic osteomyelitis with draining sinus, unspecified hand
  - **+ M86.45** Chronic osteomyelitis with draining sinus, femur
    - CC **M86.451** Chronic osteomyelitis with draining sinus, right femur
    - CC **M86.452** Chronic osteomyelitis with draining sinus, left femur
    - CC **M86.459** Chronic osteomyelitis with draining sinus, unspecified femur

- **+ M86.46** Chronic osteomyelitis with draining sinus, tibia and fibula
  - CC **M86.461** Chronic osteomyelitis with draining sinus, right tibia and fibula
  - CC **M86.462** Chronic osteomyelitis with draining sinus, left tibia and fibula
  - CC **M86.469** Chronic osteomyelitis with draining sinus, unspecified tibia and fibula
- **+ M86.47** Chronic osteomyelitis with draining sinus, ankle and foot
  - CC **M86.471** Chronic osteomyelitis with draining sinus, right ankle and foot
  - CC **M86.472** Chronic osteomyelitis with draining sinus, left ankle and foot
  - CC **M86.479** Chronic osteomyelitis with draining sinus, unspecified ankle and foot
- CC **M86.48** Chronic osteomyelitis with draining sinus, other site
- CC **M86.49** Chronic osteomyelitis with draining sinus, multiple sites
- **+ M86.5** Other chronic hematogenous osteomyelitis
  - CC **M86.50** Other chronic hematogenous osteomyelitis, unspecified site
  - **+ M86.51** Other chronic hematogenous osteomyelitis, shoulder
    - CC **M86.511** Other chronic hematogenous osteomyelitis, right shoulder
    - CC **M86.512** Other chronic hematogenous osteomyelitis, left shoulder
    - CC **M86.519** Other chronic hematogenous osteomyelitis, unspecified shoulder
  - **+ M86.52** Other chronic hematogenous osteomyelitis, humerus
    - CC **M86.521** Other chronic hematogenous osteomyelitis, right humerus
    - CC **M86.522** Other chronic hematogenous osteomyelitis, left humerus
    - CC **M86.529** Other chronic hematogenous osteomyelitis, unspecified humerus
  - **+ M86.53** Other chronic hematogenous osteomyelitis, radius and ulna
    - CC **M86.531** Other chronic hematogenous osteomyelitis, right radius and ulna
    - CC **M86.532** Other chronic hematogenous osteomyelitis, left radius and ulna
    - CC **M86.539** Other chronic hematogenous osteomyelitis, unspecified radius and ulna
  - **+ M86.54** Other chronic hematogenous osteomyelitis, hand
    - CC **M86.541** Other chronic hematogenous osteomyelitis, right hand
    - CC **M86.542** Other chronic hematogenous osteomyelitis, left hand
    - CC **M86.549** Other chronic hematogenous osteomyelitis, unspecified hand
  - **+ M86.55** Other chronic hematogenous osteomyelitis, femur
    - CC **M86.551** Other chronic hematogenous osteomyelitis, right femur
    - CC **M86.552** Other chronic hematogenous osteomyelitis, left femur
    - CC **M86.559** Other chronic hematogenous osteomyelitis, unspecified femur
  - **+ M86.56** Other chronic hematogenous osteomyelitis, tibia and fibula
    - CC **M86.561** Other chronic hematogenous osteomyelitis, right tibia and fibula
    - CC **M86.562** Other chronic hematogenous osteomyelitis, left tibia and fibula
    - CC **M86.569** Other chronic hematogenous osteomyelitis, unspecified tibia and fibula
  - **+ M86.57** Other chronic hematogenous osteomyelitis, ankle and foot
    - CC **M86.571** Other chronic hematogenous osteomyelitis, right ankle and foot
    - CC **M86.572** Other chronic hematogenous osteomyelitis, left ankle and foot
    - CC **M86.579** Other chronic hematogenous osteomyelitis, unspecified ankle and foot
  - CC **M86.58** Other chronic hematogenous osteomyelitis, other site
  - CC **M86.59** Other chronic hematogenous osteomyelitis, multiple sites
- **+ M86.6** Other chronic osteomyelitis
  - CC **M86.60** Other chronic osteomyelitis, unspecified site
  - **+ M86.61** Other chronic osteomyelitis, shoulder
    - CC **M86.611** Other chronic osteomyelitis, right shoulder
    - CC **M86.612** Other chronic osteomyelitis, left shoulder
    - CC **M86.619** Other chronic osteomyelitis, unspecified shoulder
  - **+ M86.62** Other chronic osteomyelitis, humerus
    - CC **M86.621** Other chronic osteomyelitis, right humerus
    - CC **M86.622** Other chronic osteomyelitis, left humerus
    - CC **M86.629** Other chronic osteomyelitis, unspecified humerus
  - **+ M86.63** Other chronic osteomyelitis, radius and ulna
    - CC **M86.631** Other chronic osteomyelitis, right radius and ulna
    - CC **M86.632** Other chronic osteomyelitis, left radius and ulna
    - CC **M86.639** Other chronic osteomyelitis, unspecified radius and ulna
  - **+ M86.64** Other chronic osteomyelitis, hand
    - CC **M86.641** Other chronic osteomyelitis, right hand
    - CC **M86.642** Other chronic osteomyelitis, left hand
    - CC **M86.649** Other chronic osteomyelitis, unspecified hand
  - **+ M86.65** Other chronic osteomyelitis, thigh
    - CC **M86.651** Other chronic osteomyelitis, right thigh
    - CC **M86.652** Other chronic osteomyelitis, left thigh
    - CC **M86.659** Other chronic osteomyelitis, unspecified thigh
  - **+ M86.66** Other chronic osteomyelitis, tibia and fibula
    - CC **M86.661** Other chronic osteomyelitis, right tibia and fibula
    - CC **M86.662** Other chronic osteomyelitis, left tibia and fibula
    - CC **M86.669** Other chronic osteomyelitis, unspecified tibia and fibula
  - **+ M86.67** Other chronic osteomyelitis, ankle and foot
    - CC **M86.671** Other chronic osteomyelitis, right ankle and foot
      - *AHA CC: 1Q, 2016, 13*
    - CC **M86.672** Other chronic osteomyelitis, left ankle and foot
    - CC **M86.679** Other chronic osteomyelitis, unspecified ankle and foot
  - CC **M86.68** Other chronic osteomyelitis, other site
  - CC **M86.69** Other chronic osteomyelitis, multiple sites
- **+ M86.8** Other osteomyelitis
  - Brodie's abscess
  - **+ M86.8X** Other osteomyelitis
    - CC **M86.8X0** Other osteomyelitis, multiple sites
    - CC **M86.8X1** Other osteomyelitis, shoulder
    - CC **M86.8X2** Other osteomyelitis, upper arm
    - CC **M86.8X3** Other osteomyelitis, forearm
    - CC **M86.8X4** Other osteomyelitis, hand
    - CC **M86.8X5** Other osteomyelitis, thigh
    - CC **M86.8X6** Other osteomyelitis, lower leg
    - CC **M86.8X7** Other osteomyelitis, ankle and foot
    - CC **M86.8X8** Other osteomyelitis, other site
      - *AHA CC: 1Q, 2022, 31*
    - CC **M86.8X9** Other osteomyelitis, unspecified sites
- CC **M86.9** Osteomyelitis, unspecified
  - Infection of bone NOS
  - Periostitis without osteomyelitis

M87 Osteonecrosis

Includes: avascular necrosis of bone

Use additional code to identify major osseous defect, if applicable (M89.7-)

Excludes1: juvenile osteonecrosis (M91-M92)
osteochondropathies (M90-M93)

- **M87.0 Idiopathic aseptic necrosis of bone**
  - CC **M87.00** Idiopathic aseptic necrosis of unspecified bone
  - **M87.01 Idiopathic aseptic necrosis of shoulder**
    Idiopathic aseptic necrosis of clavicle and scapula
    - CC **M87.011** Idiopathic aseptic necrosis of right shoulder
    - CC **M87.012** Idiopathic aseptic necrosis of left shoulder
    - CC **M87.019** Idiopathic aseptic necrosis of unspecified shoulder
  - **M87.02 Idiopathic aseptic necrosis of humerus**
    - CC **M87.021** Idiopathic aseptic necrosis of right humerus
    - CC **M87.022** Idiopathic aseptic necrosis of left humerus
    - CC **M87.029** Idiopathic aseptic necrosis of unspecified humerus
  - **M87.03 Idiopathic aseptic necrosis of radius, ulna and carpus**
    - CC **M87.031** Idiopathic aseptic necrosis of right radius
    - CC **M87.032** Idiopathic aseptic necrosis of left radius
    - CC **M87.033** Idiopathic aseptic necrosis of unspecified radius
    - CC **M87.034** Idiopathic aseptic necrosis of right ulna
    - CC **M87.035** Idiopathic aseptic necrosis of left ulna
    - CC **M87.036** Idiopathic aseptic necrosis of unspecified ulna
    - CC **M87.037** Idiopathic aseptic necrosis of right carpus
    - CC **M87.038** Idiopathic aseptic necrosis of left carpus
    - CC **M87.039** Idiopathic aseptic necrosis of unspecified carpus
  - **M87.04 Idiopathic aseptic necrosis of hand and fingers**
    Idiopathic aseptic necrosis of metacarpals and phalanges of hands
    - CC **M87.041** Idiopathic aseptic necrosis of right hand
    - CC **M87.042** Idiopathic aseptic necrosis of left hand
    - CC **M87.043** Idiopathic aseptic necrosis of unspecified hand
    - CC **M87.044** Idiopathic aseptic necrosis of right finger(s)
    - CC **M87.045** Idiopathic aseptic necrosis of left finger(s)
    - CC **M87.046** Idiopathic aseptic necrosis of unspecified finger(s)
  - **M87.05 Idiopathic aseptic necrosis of pelvis and femur**
    - CC **M87.050** Idiopathic aseptic necrosis of pelvis
    - CC **M87.051** Idiopathic aseptic necrosis of right femur
    - CC **M87.052** Idiopathic aseptic necrosis of left femur
    - CC **M87.059** Idiopathic aseptic necrosis of unspecified femur
      Idiopathic aseptic necrosis of hip NOS
  - **M87.06 Idiopathic aseptic necrosis of tibia and fibula**
    - CC **M87.061** Idiopathic aseptic necrosis of right tibia
    - CC **M87.062** Idiopathic aseptic necrosis of left tibia
    - CC **M87.063** Idiopathic aseptic necrosis of unspecified tibia
    - CC **M87.064** Idiopathic aseptic necrosis of right fibula
    - CC **M87.065** Idiopathic aseptic necrosis of left fibula
    - CC **M87.066** Idiopathic aseptic necrosis of unspecified fibula
  - **M87.07 Idiopathic aseptic necrosis of ankle, foot and toes**
    Idiopathic aseptic necrosis of metatarsus, tarsus, and phalanges of toes
    - CC **M87.071** Idiopathic aseptic necrosis of right ankle
    - CC **M87.072** Idiopathic aseptic necrosis of left ankle
    - CC **M87.073** Idiopathic aseptic necrosis of unspecified ankle
    - CC **M87.074** Idiopathic aseptic necrosis of right foot
    - CC **M87.075** Idiopathic aseptic necrosis of left foot
    - CC **M87.076** Idiopathic aseptic necrosis of unspecified foot
    - CC **M87.077** Idiopathic aseptic necrosis of right toe(s)
    - CC **M87.078** Idiopathic aseptic necrosis of left toe(s)
    - CC **M87.079** Idiopathic aseptic necrosis of unspecified toe(s)
  - CC **M87.08** Idiopathic aseptic necrosis of bone, other site
  - CC **M87.09** Idiopathic aseptic necrosis of bone, multiple sites
- **M87.1 Osteonecrosis due to drugs**
  Use additional code for adverse effect, if applicable, to identify drug (T36-T50 with fifth or sixth character 5)
  - CC **M87.10** Osteonecrosis due to drugs, unspecified bone
  - **M87.11 Osteonecrosis due to drugs, shoulder**
    - CC **M87.111** Osteonecrosis due to drugs, right shoulder
    - CC **M87.112** Osteonecrosis due to drugs, left shoulder
    - CC **M87.119** Osteonecrosis due to drugs, unspecified shoulder
  - **M87.12 Osteonecrosis due to drugs, humerus**
    - CC **M87.121** Osteonecrosis due to drugs, right humerus
    - CC **M87.122** Osteonecrosis due to drugs, left humerus
    - CC **M87.129** Osteonecrosis due to drugs, unspecified humerus
  - **M87.13 Osteonecrosis due to drugs of radius, ulna and carpus**
    - CC **M87.131** Osteonecrosis due to drugs of right radius
    - CC **M87.132** Osteonecrosis due to drugs of left radius
    - CC **M87.133** Osteonecrosis due to drugs of unspecified radius
    - CC **M87.134** Osteonecrosis due to drugs of right ulna
    - CC **M87.135** Osteonecrosis due to drugs of left ulna
    - CC **M87.136** Osteonecrosis due to drugs of unspecified ulna
    - CC **M87.137** Osteonecrosis due to drugs of right carpus
    - CC **M87.138** Osteonecrosis due to drugs of left carpus
    - CC **M87.139** Osteonecrosis due to drugs of unspecified carpus
  - **M87.14 Osteonecrosis due to drugs, hand and fingers**
    - CC **M87.141** Osteonecrosis due to drugs, right hand
    - CC **M87.142** Osteonecrosis due to drugs, left hand
    - CC **M87.143** Osteonecrosis due to drugs, unspecified hand
    - CC **M87.144** Osteonecrosis due to drugs, right finger(s)
    - CC **M87.145** Osteonecrosis due to drugs, left finger(s)
    - CC **M87.146** Osteonecrosis due to drugs, unspecified finger(s)
  - **M87.15 Osteonecrosis due to drugs, pelvis and femur**
    - CC **M87.150** Osteonecrosis due to drugs, pelvis
    - CC **M87.151** Osteonecrosis due to drugs, right femur
    - CC **M87.152** Osteonecrosis due to drugs, left femur
    - CC **M87.159** Osteonecrosis due to drugs, unspecified femur
  - **M87.16 Osteonecrosis due to drugs, tibia and fibula**
    - CC **M87.161** Osteonecrosis due to drugs, right tibia
    - CC **M87.162** Osteonecrosis due to drugs, left tibia
    - CC **M87.163** Osteonecrosis due to drugs, unspecified tibia
    - CC **M87.164** Osteonecrosis due to drugs, right fibula
    - CC **M87.165** Osteonecrosis due to drugs, left fibula
    - CC **M87.166** Osteonecrosis due to drugs, unspecified fibula
  - **M87.17 Osteonecrosis due to drugs, ankle, foot and toes**
    - CC **M87.171** Osteonecrosis due to drugs, right ankle
    - CC **M87.172** Osteonecrosis due to drugs, left ankle
    - CC **M87.173** Osteonecrosis due to drugs, unspecified ankle
    - CC **M87.174** Osteonecrosis due to drugs, right foot
    - CC **M87.175** Osteonecrosis due to drugs, left foot
    - CC **M87.176** Osteonecrosis due to drugs, unspecified foot

- CC M87.177 Osteonecrosis due to drugs, right toe(s)
- CC M87.178 Osteonecrosis due to drugs, left toe(s)
- CC M87.179 Osteonecrosis due to drugs, unspecified toe(s)
- \+ M87.18 Osteonecrosis due to drugs, other site
  - CC M87.180 Osteonecrosis due to drugs, jaw
  - CC M87.188 Osteonecrosis due to drugs, other site
- CC M87.19 Osteonecrosis due to drugs, multiple sites
- \+ M87.2 Osteonecrosis due to previous trauma
  - CC M87.20 Osteonecrosis due to previous trauma, unspecified bone
  - \+ M87.21 Osteonecrosis due to previous trauma, shoulder
    - CC M87.211 Osteonecrosis due to previous trauma, right shoulder
    - CC M87.212 Osteonecrosis due to previous trauma, left shoulder
    - CC M87.219 Osteonecrosis due to previous trauma, unspecified shoulder
  - \+ M87.22 Osteonecrosis due to previous trauma, humerus
    - CC M87.221 Osteonecrosis due to previous trauma, right humerus
    - CC M87.222 Osteonecrosis due to previous trauma, left humerus
    - CC M87.229 Osteonecrosis due to previous trauma, unspecified humerus
  - \+ M87.23 Osteonecrosis due to previous trauma of radius, ulna and carpus
    - CC M87.231 Osteonecrosis due to previous trauma of right radius
    - CC M87.232 Osteonecrosis due to previous trauma of left radius
    - CC M87.233 Osteonecrosis due to previous trauma of unspecified radius
    - CC M87.234 Osteonecrosis due to previous trauma of right ulna
    - CC M87.235 Osteonecrosis due to previous trauma of left ulna
    - CC M87.236 Osteonecrosis due to previous trauma of unspecified ulna
    - CC M87.237 Osteonecrosis due to previous trauma of right carpus
    - CC M87.238 Osteonecrosis due to previous trauma of left carpus
    - CC M87.239 Osteonecrosis due to previous trauma of unspecified carpus
  - \+ M87.24 Osteonecrosis due to previous trauma, hand and fingers
    - CC M87.241 Osteonecrosis due to previous trauma, right hand
    - CC M87.242 Osteonecrosis due to previous trauma, left hand
    - CC M87.243 Osteonecrosis due to previous trauma, unspecified hand
    - CC M87.244 Osteonecrosis due to previous trauma, right finger(s)
    - CC M87.245 Osteonecrosis due to previous trauma, left finger(s)
    - CC M87.246 Osteonecrosis due to previous trauma, unspecified finger(s)
  - \+ M87.25 Osteonecrosis due to previous trauma, pelvis and femur
    - CC M87.250 Osteonecrosis due to previous trauma, pelvis
    - CC M87.251 Osteonecrosis due to previous trauma, right femur
    - CC M87.252 Osteonecrosis due to previous trauma, left femur
    - CC M87.256 Osteonecrosis due to previous trauma, unspecified femur
  - \+ M87.26 Osteonecrosis due to previous trauma, tibia and fibula
    - CC M87.261 Osteonecrosis due to previous trauma, right tibia
    - CC M87.262 Osteonecrosis due to previous trauma, left tibia
    - CC M87.263 Osteonecrosis due to previous trauma, unspecified tibia
    - CC M87.264 Osteonecrosis due to previous trauma, right fibula
    - CC M87.265 Osteonecrosis due to previous trauma, left fibula
    - CC M87.266 Osteonecrosis due to previous trauma, unspecified fibula
  - \+ M87.27 Osteonecrosis due to previous trauma, ankle, foot and toes
    - CC M87.271 Osteonecrosis due to previous trauma, right ankle
    - CC M87.272 Osteonecrosis due to previous trauma, left ankle
    - CC M87.273 Osteonecrosis due to previous trauma, unspecified ankle
    - CC M87.274 Osteonecrosis due to previous trauma, right foot
    - CC M87.275 Osteonecrosis due to previous trauma, left foot
    - CC M87.276 Osteonecrosis due to previous trauma, unspecified foot
    - CC M87.277 Osteonecrosis due to previous trauma, right toe(s)
    - CC M87.278 Osteonecrosis due to previous trauma, left toe(s)
    - CC M87.279 Osteonecrosis due to previous trauma, unspecified toe(s)
  - CC M87.28 Osteonecrosis due to previous trauma, other site
  - CC M87.29 Osteonecrosis due to previous trauma, multiple sites
- \+ M87.3 Other secondary osteonecrosis
  - CC M87.30 Other secondary osteonecrosis, unspecified bone
  - \+ M87.31 Other secondary osteonecrosis, shoulder
    - CC M87.311 Other secondary osteonecrosis, right shoulder
    - CC M87.312 Other secondary osteonecrosis, left shoulder
    - CC M87.319 Other secondary osteonecrosis, unspecified shoulder
  - \+ M87.32 Other secondary osteonecrosis, humerus
    - CC M87.321 Other secondary osteonecrosis, right humerus
    - CC M87.322 Other secondary osteonecrosis, left humerus
    - CC M87.329 Other secondary osteonecrosis, unspecified humerus
  - \+ M87.33 Other secondary osteonecrosis of radius, ulna and carpus
    - CC M87.331 Other secondary osteonecrosis of right radius
    - CC M87.332 Other secondary osteonecrosis of left radius
    - CC M87.333 Other secondary osteonecrosis of unspecified radius
    - CC M87.334 Other secondary osteonecrosis of right ulna
    - CC M87.335 Other secondary osteonecrosis of left ulna
    - CC M87.336 Other secondary osteonecrosis of unspecified ulna
    - CC M87.337 Other secondary osteonecrosis of right carpus
    - CC M87.338 Other secondary osteonecrosis of left carpus
    - CC M87.339 Other secondary osteonecrosis of unspecified carpus
  - \+ M87.34 Other secondary osteonecrosis, hand and fingers
    - CC M87.341 Other secondary osteonecrosis, right hand
    - CC M87.342 Other secondary osteonecrosis, left hand
    - CC M87.343 Other secondary osteonecrosis, unspecified hand
    - CC M87.344 Other secondary osteonecrosis, right finger(s)
    - CC M87.345 Other secondary osteonecrosis, left finger(s)
    - CC M87.346 Other secondary osteonecrosis, unspecified finger(s)

- **+ M87.35 Other secondary osteonecrosis, pelvis and femur**
  - CC M87.350 Other secondary osteonecrosis, pelvis
  - CC M87.351 Other secondary osteonecrosis, right femur
  - CC M87.352 Other secondary osteonecrosis, left femur
  - CC M87.353 Other secondary osteonecrosis, unspecified femur
- **+ M87.36 Other secondary osteonecrosis, tibia and fibula**
  - CC M87.361 Other secondary osteonecrosis, right tibia
  - CC M87.362 Other secondary osteonecrosis, left tibia
  - CC M87.363 Other secondary osteonecrosis, unspecified tibia
  - CC M87.364 Other secondary osteonecrosis, right fibula
  - CC M87.365 Other secondary osteonecrosis, left fibula
  - CC M87.366 Other secondary osteonecrosis, unspecified fibula
- **+ M87.37 Other secondary osteonecrosis, ankle and foot**
  - CC M87.371 Other secondary osteonecrosis, right ankle
  - CC M87.372 Other secondary osteonecrosis, left ankle
  - CC M87.373 Other secondary osteonecrosis, unspecified ankle
  - CC M87.374 Other secondary osteonecrosis, right foot
  - CC M87.375 Other secondary osteonecrosis, left foot
  - CC M87.376 Other secondary osteonecrosis, unspecified foot
  - CC M87.377 Other secondary osteonecrosis, right toe(s)
  - CC M87.378 Other secondary osteonecrosis, left toe(s)
  - CC M87.379 Other secondary osteonecrosis, unspecified toe(s)
- CC M87.38 Other secondary osteonecrosis, other site
- CC M87.39 Other secondary osteonecrosis, multiple sites
- **+ M87.8 Other osteonecrosis**
  - CC M87.80 Other osteonecrosis, unspecified bone
  - **+ M87.81 Other osteonecrosis, shoulder**
    - CC M87.811 Other osteonecrosis, right shoulder
    - CC M87.812 Other osteonecrosis, left shoulder
    - CC M87.819 Other osteonecrosis, unspecified shoulder
  - **+ M87.82 Other osteonecrosis, humerus**
    - CC M87.821 Other osteonecrosis, right humerus
    - CC M87.822 Other osteonecrosis, left humerus
    - CC M87.829 Other osteonecrosis, unspecified humerus
  - **+ M87.83 Other osteonecrosis of radius, ulna and carpus**
    - CC M87.831 Other osteonecrosis of right radius
    - CC M87.832 Other osteonecrosis of left radius
    - CC M87.833 Other osteonecrosis of unspecified radius
    - CC M87.834 Other osteonecrosis of right ulna
    - CC M87.835 Other osteonecrosis of left ulna
    - CC M87.836 Other osteonecrosis of unspecified ulna
    - CC M87.837 Other osteonecrosis of right carpus
    - CC M87.838 Other osteonecrosis of left carpus
    - CC M87.839 Other osteonecrosis of unspecified carpus
  - **+ M87.84 Other osteonecrosis, hand and fingers**
    - CC M87.841 Other osteonecrosis, right hand
    - CC M87.842 Other osteonecrosis, left hand
    - CC M87.843 Other osteonecrosis, unspecified hand
    - CC M87.844 Other osteonecrosis, right finger(s)
    - CC M87.845 Other osteonecrosis, left finger(s)
    - CC M87.849 Other osteonecrosis, unspecified finger(s)
  - **+ M87.85 Other osteonecrosis, pelvis and femur**
    - CC M87.850 Other osteonecrosis, pelvis
    - CC M87.851 Other osteonecrosis, right femur
    - CC M87.852 Other osteonecrosis, left femur
    - CC M87.859 Other osteonecrosis, unspecified femur
  - **+ M87.86 Other osteonecrosis, tibia and fibula**
    - CC M87.861 Other osteonecrosis, right tibia
    - CC M87.862 Other osteonecrosis, left tibia
    - CC M87.863 Other osteonecrosis, unspecified tibia
    - CC M87.864 Other osteonecrosis, right fibula
    - CC M87.865 Other osteonecrosis, left fibula
    - CC M87.869 Other osteonecrosis, unspecified fibula
  - **+ M87.87 Other osteonecrosis, ankle, foot and toes**
    - CC M87.871 Other osteonecrosis, right ankle
    - CC M87.872 Other osteonecrosis, left ankle
    - CC M87.873 Other osteonecrosis, unspecified ankle
    - CC M87.874 Other osteonecrosis, right foot
    - CC M87.875 Other osteonecrosis, left foot
    - CC M87.876 Other osteonecrosis, unspecified foot
    - CC M87.877 Other osteonecrosis, right toe(s)
    - CC M87.878 Other osteonecrosis, left toe(s)
    - CC M87.879 Other osteonecrosis, unspecified toe(s)
  - CC M87.88 Other osteonecrosis, other site
  - CC M87.89 Other osteonecrosis, multiple sites
- CC **M87.9 Osteonecrosis, unspecified**
  - Necrosis of bone NOS

M88 Osteitis deformans [Paget's disease of bone]

Excludes1: *osteitis deformans in neoplastic disease (M90.6)*

- **M88.0 Osteitis deformans of skull**
- **M88.1 Osteitis deformans of vertebrae**
- **+ M88.8 Osteitis deformans of other bones**
  - **+ M88.81 Osteitis deformans of shoulder**
    - M88.811 Osteitis deformans of right shoulder
    - M88.812 Osteitis deformans of left shoulder
    - M88.819 Osteitis deformans of unspecified shoulder
  - **+ M88.82 Osteitis deformans of upper arm**
    - M88.821 Osteitis deformans of right upper arm
    - M88.822 Osteitis deformans of left upper arm
    - M88.829 Osteitis deformans of unspecified upper arm
  - **+ M88.83 Osteitis deformans of forearm**
    - M88.831 Osteitis deformans of right forearm
    - M88.832 Osteitis deformans of left forearm
    - M88.839 Osteitis deformans of unspecified forearm
  - **+ M88.84 Osteitis deformans of hand**
    - M88.841 Osteitis deformans of right hand
    - M88.842 Osteitis deformans of left hand
    - M88.849 Osteitis deformans of unspecified hand
  - **+ M88.85 Osteitis deformans of thigh**
    - M88.851 Osteitis deformans of right thigh
    - M88.852 Osteitis deformans of left thigh
    - M88.859 Osteitis deformans of unspecified thigh
  - **+ M88.86 Osteitis deformans of lower leg**
    - M88.861 Osteitis deformans of right lower leg
    - M88.862 Osteitis deformans of left lower leg
    - M88.869 Osteitis deformans of unspecified lower leg
  - **+ M88.87 Osteitis deformans of ankle and foot**
    - M88.871 Osteitis deformans of right ankle and foot
    - M88.872 Osteitis deformans of left ankle and foot
    - M88.879 Osteitis deformans of unspecified ankle and foot
  - **M88.88 Osteitis deformans of other bones**
    - **Excludes2:** *osteitis deformans of skull (M88.0)*
      osteitis deformans of vertebrae (M88.1)
  - **M88.89 Osteitis deformans of multiple sites**
- **M88.9 Osteitis deformans of unspecified bone**

M89 Other disorders of bone

- **+ M89.0 Algoneurodystrophy**
  - Shoulder-hand syndrome
  - Sudeck's atrophy
  - **Excludes1:** *causalgia, lower limb (G57.7-)*
    causalgia, upper limb (G56.4-)
    complex regional pain syndrome II, lower limb (G57.7-)
    complex regional pain syndrome II, upper limb (G56.4-)
    reflex sympathetic dystrophy (G90.5-)
  - M89.00 Algoneurodystrophy, unspecified site
  - **+ M89.01 Algoneurodystrophy, shoulder**
    - M89.011 Algoneurodystrophy, right shoulder
    - M89.012 Algoneurodystrophy, left shoulder
    - M89.019 Algoneurodystrophy, unspecified shoulder

- **M89.02 Algoneurodystrophy, upper arm**
  - M89.021 Algoneurodystrophy, right upper arm
  - M89.022 Algoneurodystrophy, left upper arm
  - M89.029 Algoneurodystrophy, unspecified upper arm
- **M89.03 Algoneurodystrophy, forearm**
  - M89.031 Algoneurodystrophy, right forearm
  - M89.032 Algoneurodystrophy, left forearm
  - M89.039 Algoneurodystrophy, unspecified forearm
- **M89.04 Algoneurodystrophy, hand**
  - M89.041 Algoneurodystrophy, right hand
  - M89.042 Algoneurodystrophy, left hand
  - M89.049 Algoneurodystrophy, unspecified hand
- **M89.05 Algoneurodystrophy, thigh**
  - M89.051 Algoneurodystrophy, right thigh
  - M89.052 Algoneurodystrophy, left thigh
  - M89.059 Algoneurodystrophy, unspecified thigh
- **M89.06 Algoneurodystrophy, lower leg**
  - M89.061 Algoneurodystrophy, right lower leg
  - M89.062 Algoneurodystrophy, left lower leg
  - M89.069 Algoneurodystrophy, unspecified lower leg
- **M89.07 Algoneurodystrophy, ankle and foot**
  - M89.071 Algoneurodystrophy, right ankle and foot
  - M89.072 Algoneurodystrophy, left ankle and foot
  - M89.079 Algoneurodystrophy, unspecified ankle and foot
- M89.08 Algoneurodystrophy, other site
- M89.09 Algoneurodystrophy, multiple sites
- **M89.1 Physeal arrest**
  Arrest of growth plate
  Epiphyseal arrest
  Growth plate arrest
  - **M89.12 Physeal arrest, humerus**
    - M89.121 Complete physeal arrest, right proximal humerus
    - M89.122 Complete physeal arrest, left proximal humerus
    - M89.123 Partial physeal arrest, right proximal humerus
    - M89.124 Partial physeal arrest, left proximal humerus
    - M89.125 Complete physeal arrest, right distal humerus
    - M89.126 Complete physeal arrest, left distal humerus
    - M89.127 Partial physeal arrest, right distal humerus
    - M89.128 Partial physeal arrest, left distal humerus
    - M89.129 Physeal arrest, humerus, unspecified
  - **M89.13 Physeal arrest, forearm**
    - M89.131 Complete physeal arrest, right distal radius
    - M89.132 Complete physeal arrest, left distal radius
    - M89.133 Partial physeal arrest, right distal radius
    - M89.134 Partial physeal arrest, left distal radius
    - M89.138 Other physeal arrest of forearm
    - M89.139 Physeal arrest, forearm, unspecified
  - **M89.15 Physeal arrest, femur**
    - M89.151 Complete physeal arrest, right proximal femur
    - M89.152 Complete physeal arrest, left proximal femur
    - M89.153 Partial physeal arrest, right proximal femur
    - M89.154 Partial physeal arrest, left proximal femur
    - M89.155 Complete physeal arrest, right distal femur
    - M89.156 Complete physeal arrest, left distal femur
    - M89.157 Partial physeal arrest, right distal femur
    - M89.158 Partial physeal arrest, left distal femur
    - M89.159 Physeal arrest, femur, unspecified
  - **M89.16 Physeal arrest, lower leg**
    - M89.160 Complete physeal arrest, right proximal tibia
    - M89.161 Complete physeal arrest, left proximal tibia
    - M89.162 Partial physeal arrest, right proximal tibia
    - M89.163 Partial physeal arrest, left proximal tibia
    - M89.164 Complete physeal arrest, right distal tibia
    - M89.165 Complete physeal arrest, left distal tibia
    - M89.166 Partial physeal arrest, right distal tibia
    - M89.167 Partial physeal arrest, left distal tibia
    - M89.168 Other physeal arrest of lower leg
    - M89.169 Physeal arrest, lower leg, unspecified
  - M89.18 Physeal arrest, other site
- **M89.2 Other disorders of bone development and growth**
  - M89.20 Other disorders of bone development and growth, unspecified site
  - **M89.21 Other disorders of bone development and growth, shoulder**
    - M89.211 Other disorders of bone development and growth, right shoulder
    - M89.212 Other disorders of bone development and growth, left shoulder
    - M89.219 Other disorders of bone development and growth, unspecified shoulder
  - **M89.22 Other disorders of bone development and growth, humerus**
    - M89.221 Other disorders of bone development and growth, right humerus
    - M89.222 Other disorders of bone development and growth, left humerus
    - M89.229 Other disorders of bone development and growth, unspecified humerus
  - **M89.23 Other disorders of bone development and growth, ulna and radius**
    - M89.231 Other disorders of bone development and growth, right ulna
    - M89.232 Other disorders of bone development and growth, left ulna
    - M89.233 Other disorders of bone development and growth, right radius
    - M89.234 Other disorders of bone development and growth, left radius
    - M89.239 Other disorders of bone development and growth, unspecified ulna and radius
  - **M89.24 Other disorders of bone development and growth, hand**
    - M89.241 Other disorders of bone development and growth, right hand
    - M89.242 Other disorders of bone development and growth, left hand
    - M89.249 Other disorders of bone development and growth, unspecified hand
  - **M89.25 Other disorders of bone development and growth, femur**
    - M89.251 Other disorders of bone development and growth, right femur
    - M89.252 Other disorders of bone development and growth, left femur
    - M89.259 Other disorders of bone development and growth, unspecified femur
  - **M89.26 Other disorders of bone development and growth, tibia and fibula**
    - M89.261 Other disorders of bone development and growth, right tibia
    - M89.262 Other disorders of bone development and growth, left tibia
    - M89.263 Other disorders of bone development and growth, right fibula
    - M89.264 Other disorders of bone development and growth, left fibula
    - M89.269 Other disorders of bone development and growth, unspecified lower leg

- **+ M89.27 Other disorders of bone development and growth, ankle and foot**
  - M89.271 Other disorders of bone development and growth, right ankle and foot
  - M89.272 Other disorders of bone development and growth, left ankle and foot
  - M89.279 Other disorders of bone development and growth, unspecified ankle and foot
- M89.28 Other disorders of bone development and growth, other site
- M89.29 Other disorders of bone development and growth, multiple sites
- **+ M89.3 Hypertrophy of bone**
  - M89.30 Hypertrophy of bone, unspecified site
  - **+ M89.31 Hypertrophy of bone, shoulder**
    - M89.311 Hypertrophy of bone, right shoulder
    - M89.312 Hypertrophy of bone, left shoulder
    - M89.319 Hypertrophy of bone, unspecified shoulder
  - **+ M89.32 Hypertrophy of bone, humerus**
    - M89.321 Hypertrophy of bone, right humerus
    - M89.322 Hypertrophy of bone, left humerus
    - M89.329 Hypertrophy of bone, unspecified humerus
  - **+ M89.33 Hypertrophy of bone, ulna and radius**
    - M89.331 Hypertrophy of bone, right ulna
    - M89.332 Hypertrophy of bone, left ulna
    - M89.333 Hypertrophy of bone, right radius
    - M89.334 Hypertrophy of bone, left radius
    - M89.339 Hypertrophy of bone, unspecified ulna and radius
  - **+ M89.34 Hypertrophy of bone, hand**
    - M89.341 Hypertrophy of bone, right hand
    - M89.342 Hypertrophy of bone, left hand
    - M89.349 Hypertrophy of bone, unspecified hand
  - **+ M89.35 Hypertrophy of bone, femur**
    - M89.351 Hypertrophy of bone, right femur
    - M89.352 Hypertrophy of bone, left femur
    - M89.359 Hypertrophy of bone, unspecified femur
  - **+ M89.36 Hypertrophy of bone, tibia and fibula**
    - M89.361 Hypertrophy of bone, right tibia
    - M89.362 Hypertrophy of bone, left tibia
    - M89.363 Hypertrophy of bone, right fibula
    - M89.364 Hypertrophy of bone, left fibula
    - M89.369 Hypertrophy of bone, unspecified tibia and fibula
  - **+ M89.37 Hypertrophy of bone, ankle and foot**
    - M89.371 Hypertrophy of bone, right ankle and foot
    - M89.372 Hypertrophy of bone, left ankle and foot
    - M89.379 Hypertrophy of bone, unspecified ankle and foot
  - M89.38 Hypertrophy of bone, other site
  - M89.39 Hypertrophy of bone, multiple sites
- **+ M89.4 Other hypertrophic osteoarthropathy**
  Marie-Bamberger disease
  Pachydermoperiostosis
  - M89.40 Other hypertrophic osteoarthropathy, unspecified site
  - **+ M89.41 Other hypertrophic osteoarthropathy, shoulder**
    - M89.411 Other hypertrophic osteoarthropathy, right shoulder
    - M89.412 Other hypertrophic osteoarthropathy, left shoulder
    - M89.419 Other hypertrophic osteoarthropathy, unspecified shoulder
  - **+ M89.42 Other hypertrophic osteoarthropathy, upper arm**
    - M89.421 Other hypertrophic osteoarthropathy, right upper arm
    - M89.422 Other hypertrophic osteoarthropathy, left upper arm
    - M89.429 Other hypertrophic osteoarthropathy, unspecified upper arm
  - **+ M89.43 Other hypertrophic osteoarthropathy, forearm**
    - M89.431 Other hypertrophic osteoarthropathy, right forearm
    - M89.432 Other hypertrophic osteoarthropathy, left forearm
    - M89.439 Other hypertrophic osteoarthropathy, unspecified forearm
  - **+ M89.44 Other hypertrophic osteoarthropathy, hand**
    - M89.441 Other hypertrophic osteoarthropathy, right hand
    - M89.442 Other hypertrophic osteoarthropathy, left hand
    - M89.449 Other hypertrophic osteoarthropathy, unspecified hand
  - **+ M89.45 Other hypertrophic osteoarthropathy, thigh**
    - M89.451 Other hypertrophic osteoarthropathy, right thigh
    - M89.452 Other hypertrophic osteoarthropathy, left thigh
    - M89.459 Other hypertrophic osteoarthropathy, unspecified thigh
  - **+ M89.46 Other hypertrophic osteoarthropathy, lower leg**
    - M89.461 Other hypertrophic osteoarthropathy, right lower leg
    - M89.462 Other hypertrophic osteoarthropathy, left lower leg
    - M89.469 Other hypertrophic osteoarthropathy, unspecified lower leg
  - **+ M89.47 Other hypertrophic osteoarthropathy, ankle and foot**
    - M89.471 Other hypertrophic osteoarthropathy, right ankle and foot
    - M89.472 Other hypertrophic osteoarthropathy, left ankle and foot
    - M89.479 Other hypertrophic osteoarthropathy, unspecified ankle and foot
  - M89.48 Other hypertrophic osteoarthropathy, other site
  - M89.49 Other hypertrophic osteoarthropathy, multiple sites
- **+ M89.5 Osteolysis**
  Use additional code to identify major osseous defect, if applicable (M89.7-)
  Excludes2: periprosthetic osteolysis of internal prosthetic joint (T84.05-)
  - M89.50 Osteolysis, unspecified site
  - **+ M89.51 Osteolysis, shoulder**
    - M89.511 Osteolysis, right shoulder
    - M89.512 Osteolysis, left shoulder
    - M89.519 Osteolysis, unspecified shoulder
  - **+ M89.52 Osteolysis, upper arm**
    - M89.521 Osteolysis, right upper arm
    - M89.522 Osteolysis, left upper arm
    - M89.529 Osteolysis, unspecified upper arm
  - **+ M89.53 Osteolysis, forearm**
    - M89.531 Osteolysis, right forearm
    - M89.532 Osteolysis, left forearm
    - M89.539 Osteolysis, unspecified forearm
  - **+ M89.54 Osteolysis, hand**
    - M89.541 Osteolysis, right hand
    - M89.542 Osteolysis, left hand
    - M89.549 Osteolysis, unspecified hand
  - **+ M89.55 Osteolysis, thigh**
    - M89.551 Osteolysis, right thigh
    - M89.552 Osteolysis, left thigh
    - M89.559 Osteolysis, unspecified thigh
  - **+ M89.56 Osteolysis, lower leg**
    - M89.561 Osteolysis, right lower leg
    - M89.562 Osteolysis, left lower leg
    - M89.569 Osteolysis, unspecified lower leg
  - **+ M89.57 Osteolysis, ankle and foot**
    - M89.571 Osteolysis, right ankle and foot
    - M89.572 Osteolysis, left ankle and foot
    - M89.579 Osteolysis, unspecified ankle and foot
  - M89.58 Osteolysis, other site
  - M89.59 Osteolysis, multiple sites
- **+ M89.6 Osteopathy after poliomyelitis**
  Use additional code (B91) to identify previous poliomyelitis
  Excludes1: postpolio syndrome (G14)
  - M89.60 Osteopathy after poliomyelitis, unspecified site
  - **+ M89.61 Osteopathy after poliomyelitis, shoulder**
    - M89.611 Osteopathy after poliomyelitis, right shoulder
    - M89.612 Osteopathy after poliomyelitis, left shoulder
    - M89.619 Osteopathy after poliomyelitis, unspecified shoulder

- **+ M89.62 Osteopathy after poliomyelitis, upper arm**
  - M89.621 Osteopathy after poliomyelitis, right upper arm
  - M89.622 Osteopathy after poliomyelitis, left upper arm
  - M89.629 Osteopathy after poliomyelitis, unspecified upper arm
- **+ M89.63 Osteopathy after poliomyelitis, forearm**
  - M89.631 Osteopathy after poliomyelitis, right forearm
  - M89.632 Osteopathy after poliomyelitis, left forearm
  - M89.639 Osteopathy after poliomyelitis, unspecified forearm
- **+ M89.64 Osteopathy after poliomyelitis, hand**
  - M89.641 Osteopathy after poliomyelitis, right hand
  - M89.642 Osteopathy after poliomyelitis, left hand
  - M89.649 Osteopathy after poliomyelitis, unspecified hand
- **+ M89.65 Osteopathy after poliomyelitis, thigh**
  - M89.651 Osteopathy after poliomyelitis, right thigh
  - M89.652 Osteopathy after poliomyelitis, left thigh
  - M89.659 Osteopathy after poliomyelitis, unspecified thigh
- **+ M89.66 Osteopathy after poliomyelitis, lower leg**
  - M89.661 Osteopathy after poliomyelitis, right lower leg
  - M89.662 Osteopathy after poliomyelitis, left lower leg
  - M89.669 Osteopathy after poliomyelitis, unspecified lower leg
- **+ M89.67 Osteopathy after poliomyelitis, ankle and foot**
  - M89.671 Osteopathy after poliomyelitis, right ankle and foot
  - M89.672 Osteopathy after poliomyelitis, left ankle and foot
  - M89.679 Osteopathy after poliomyelitis, unspecified ankle and foot
- **M89.68 Osteopathy after poliomyelitis, other site**
- **M89.69 Osteopathy after poliomyelitis, multiple sites**
- **+ M89.7 Major osseous defect**
  - Code first underlying disease, if known, such as:
    - aseptic necrosis of bone (M87.-)
    - malignant neoplasm of bone (C40.-)
    - osteolysis (M89.5-)
    - osteomyelitis (M86.-)
    - osteonecrosis (M87.-)
    - osteoporosis (M80.-, M81.-)
    - periprosthetic osteolysis (T84.05-)
  - M89.70 Major osseous defect, unspecified site
- **+ M89.71 Major osseous defect, shoulder region**
  - Major osseous defect clavicle or scapula
  - M89.711 Major osseous defect, right shoulder region
  - M89.712 Major osseous defect, left shoulder region
  - M89.719 Major osseous defect, unspecified shoulder region
- **+ M89.72 Major osseous defect, humerus**
  - M89.721 Major osseous defect, right humerus
  - M89.722 Major osseous defect, left humerus
  - M89.729 Major osseous defect, unspecified humerus
- **+ M89.73 Major osseous defect, forearm**
  - Major osseous defect of radius and ulna
  - M89.731 Major osseous defect, right forearm
  - M89.732 Major osseous defect, left forearm
  - M89.739 Major osseous defect, unspecified forearm
- **+ M89.74 Major osseous defect, hand**
  - Major osseous defect of carpus, fingers, metacarpus
  - M89.741 Major osseous defect, right hand
  - M89.742 Major osseous defect, left hand
  - M89.749 Major osseous defect, unspecified hand
- **+ M89.75 Major osseous defect, pelvic region and thigh**
  - Major osseous defect of femur and pelvis
  - M89.751 Major osseous defect, right pelvic region and thigh
  - M89.752 Major osseous defect, left pelvic region and thigh
  - M89.759 Major osseous defect, unspecified pelvic region and thigh
- **+ M89.76 Major osseous defect, lower leg**
  - Major osseous defect of fibula and tibia
  - M89.761 Major osseous defect, right lower leg
  - M89.762 Major osseous defect, left lower leg
  - M89.769 Major osseous defect, unspecified lower leg
- **+ M89.77 Major osseous defect, ankle and foot**
  - Major osseous defect of metatarsus, tarsus, toes
  - M89.771 Major osseous defect, right ankle and foot
  - M89.772 Major osseous defect, left ankle and foot
  - M89.779 Major osseous defect, unspecified ankle and foot
- **M89.78 Major osseous defect, other site**
- **M89.79 Major osseous defect, multiple sites**
- **+ M89.8 Other specified disorders of bone**
  - Infantile cortical hyperostoses
  - Post-traumatic subperiosteal ossification
  - *AHA CC: 2Q, 2022, 10*
  - **+ M89.8X Other specified disorders of bone**
    - M89.8X0 Other specified disorders of bone, multiple sites
    - M89.8X1 Other specified disorders of bone, shoulder
    - M89.8X2 Other specified disorders of bone, upper arm
    - M89.8X3 Other specified disorders of bone, forearm
      - *AHA CC: 3Q, 2019, 9-10*
    - M89.8X4 Other specified disorders of bone, hand
    - M89.8X5 Other specified disorders of bone, thigh
    - M89.8X6 Other specified disorders of bone, lower leg
    - M89.8X7 Other specified disorders of bone, ankle and foot
    - M89.8X8 Other specified disorders of bone, other site
      - *AHA CC: 2Q, 2023, 18-19*
    - M89.8X9 Other specified disorders of bone, unspecified site
- **M89.9 Disorder of bone, unspecified**

M90 Osteopathies in diseases classified elsewhere

Excludes1: osteochondritis, osteomyelitis, and osteopathy (in):
- cryptococcosis (B45.3)
- diabetes mellitus (E08-E13 with .69-)
- gonococcal (A54.43)
- neurogenic syphilis (A52.11)
- renal osteodystrophy (N25.0)
- salmonellosis (A02.24)
- secondary syphilis (A51.46)
- syphilis (late) (A52.77)

- **+ M90.5 Osteonecrosis in diseases classified elsewhere**
  - Code first underlying disease, such as:
    - caisson disease (T70.3)
    - hemoglobinopathy (D50-D64)
  - **CC M90.50** Osteonecrosis in diseases classified elsewhere, unspecified site
  - **+ M90.51** Osteonecrosis in diseases classified elsewhere, shoulder
    - **CC M90.511** Osteonecrosis in diseases classified elsewhere, right shoulder
    - **CC M90.512** Osteonecrosis in diseases classified elsewhere, left shoulder
    - **CC M90.519** Osteonecrosis in diseases classified elsewhere, unspecified shoulder
  - **+ M90.52** Osteonecrosis in diseases classified elsewhere, upper arm
    - **CC M90.521** Osteonecrosis in diseases classified elsewhere, right upper arm
    - **CC M90.522** Osteonecrosis in diseases classified elsewhere, left upper arm
    - **CC M90.529** Osteonecrosis in diseases classified elsewhere, unspecified upper arm

Knee Injuries and Problems

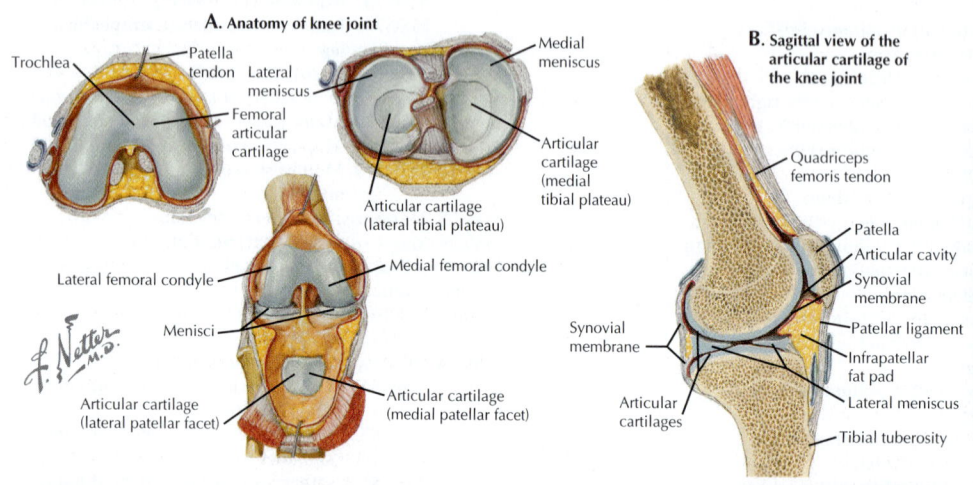

A. Anatomy of knee joint

B. Sagittal view of the articular cartilage of the knee joint

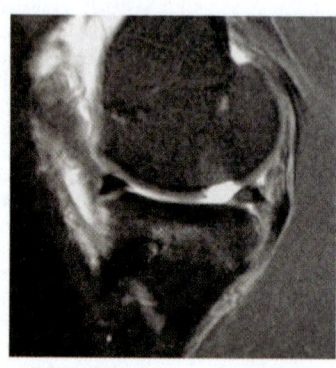

D. Chondromalacia

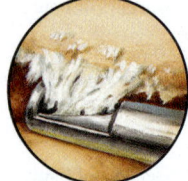
Shaving chondroplasty

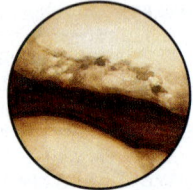
Appearance immediately after shaving chondroplasty

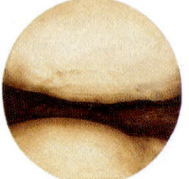
Appearance after several months

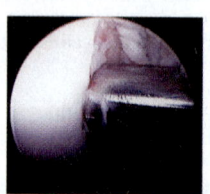

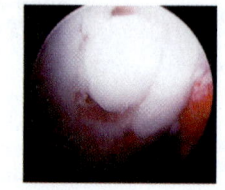

F. Osteochondritis dissecans

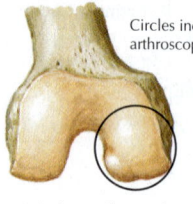
1. Articular cartilage surface irregular but intact over defect in the subchondral bone.

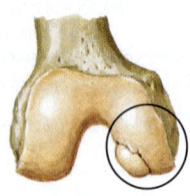
2. Early separation of osteochondral defect.

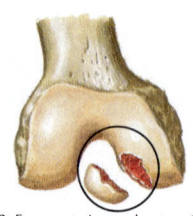
3. Fragmentation and separation of osteochondral defect.

Circles indicate arthroscopic view

G. Radiologic appearance of OCD lesion in skeletally immature patient

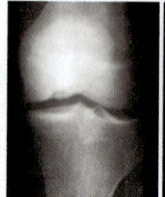
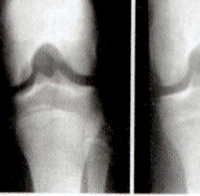

Initial lesion   Healing lesion   Healed lesion

H. Treatment of OCD

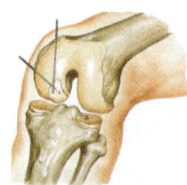
1. Retrograde drilling of OCD lesion

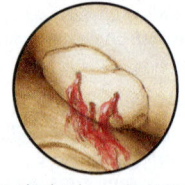
2. Bleeding bone after drilling

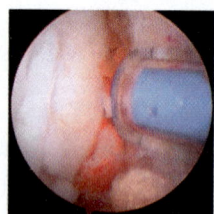
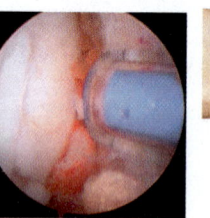
3. Arthroscopic image of OCD fragment fixed in place with osteochondral plug.

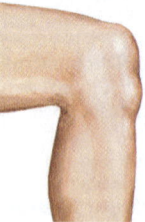
Classic appearance of tibial tuberosity.

I. Osgood-Schlatter disease

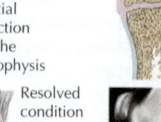
Initial traction at the apophysis

Resolved condition with classic enlargement of tibial tuberosity.

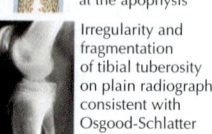
Fragmentation at the apophysis

Irregularity and fragmentation of tibial tuberosity on plain radiographs consistent with Osgood-Schlatter disease.

© 2009 Elsevier Inc. All rights reserved. www.netterimages.com

- **+ M90.53** Osteonecrosis in diseases classified elsewhere, forearm
  - CC **M90.531** Osteonecrosis in diseases classified elsewhere, right forearm
  - CC **M90.532** Osteonecrosis in diseases classified elsewhere, left forearm
  - CC **M90.539** Osteonecrosis in diseases classified elsewhere, unspecified forearm
- **+ M90.54** Osteonecrosis in diseases classified elsewhere, hand
  - CC **M90.541** Osteonecrosis in diseases classified elsewhere, right hand
  - CC **M90.542** Osteonecrosis in diseases classified elsewhere, left hand
  - CC **M90.549** Osteonecrosis in diseases classified elsewhere, unspecified hand
- **+ M90.55** Osteonecrosis in diseases classified elsewhere, thigh
  - CC **M90.551** Osteonecrosis in diseases classified elsewhere, right thigh
  - CC **M90.552** Osteonecrosis in diseases classified elsewhere, left thigh
  - CC **M90.559** Osteonecrosis in diseases classified elsewhere, unspecified thigh
- **+ M90.56** Osteonecrosis in diseases classified elsewhere, lower leg
  - CC **M90.561** Osteonecrosis in diseases classified elsewhere, right lower leg
  - CC **M90.562** Osteonecrosis in diseases classified elsewhere, left lower leg
  - CC **M90.569** Osteonecrosis in diseases classified elsewhere, unspecified lower leg
- **+ M90.57** Osteonecrosis in diseases classified elsewhere, ankle and foot
  - CC **M90.571** Osteonecrosis in diseases classified elsewhere, right ankle and foot
  - CC **M90.572** Osteonecrosis in diseases classified elsewhere, left ankle and foot
  - CC **M90.579** Osteonecrosis in diseases classified elsewhere, unspecified ankle and foot
- CC **M90.58** Osteonecrosis in diseases classified elsewhere, other site
- CC **M90.59** Osteonecrosis in diseases classified elsewhere, multiple sites
- **+ M90.6** Osteitis deformans in neoplastic diseases
  Osteitis deformans in malignant neoplasm of bone
  Code first the neoplasm (C40.-, C41.-)
  Excludes1: osteitis deformans [Paget's disease of bone] (M88.-)
  - **M90.60** Osteitis deformans in neoplastic diseases, unspecified site
  - **+ M90.61** Osteitis deformans in neoplastic diseases, shoulder
    - **M90.611** Osteitis deformans in neoplastic diseases, right shoulder
    - **M90.612** Osteitis deformans in neoplastic diseases, left shoulder
    - **M90.619** Osteitis deformans in neoplastic diseases, unspecified shoulder
  - **+ M90.62** Osteitis deformans in neoplastic diseases, upper arm
    - **M90.621** Osteitis deformans in neoplastic diseases, right upper arm
    - **M90.622** Osteitis deformans in neoplastic diseases, left upper arm
    - **M90.629** Osteitis deformans in neoplastic diseases, unspecified upper arm
  - **+ M90.63** Osteitis deformans in neoplastic diseases, forearm
    - **M90.631** Osteitis deformans in neoplastic diseases, right forearm
    - **M90.632** Osteitis deformans in neoplastic diseases, left forearm
    - **M90.639** Osteitis deformans in neoplastic diseases, unspecified forearm
  - **+ M90.64** Osteitis deformans in neoplastic diseases, hand
    - **M90.641** Osteitis deformans in neoplastic diseases, right hand
    - **M90.642** Osteitis deformans in neoplastic diseases, left hand
    - **M90.649** Osteitis deformans in neoplastic diseases, unspecified hand
  - **+ M90.65** Osteitis deformans in neoplastic diseases, thigh
    - **M90.651** Osteitis deformans in neoplastic diseases, right thigh
    - **M90.652** Osteitis deformans in neoplastic diseases, left thigh
    - **M90.659** Osteitis deformans in neoplastic diseases, unspecified thigh
  - **+ M90.66** Osteitis deformans in neoplastic diseases, lower leg
    - **M90.661** Osteitis deformans in neoplastic diseases, right lower leg
    - **M90.662** Osteitis deformans in neoplastic diseases, left lower leg
    - **M90.669** Osteitis deformans in neoplastic diseases, unspecified lower leg
  - **+ M90.67** Osteitis deformans in neoplastic diseases, ankle and foot
    - **M90.671** Osteitis deformans in neoplastic diseases, right ankle and foot
    - **M90.672** Osteitis deformans in neoplastic diseases, left ankle and foot
    - **M90.679** Osteitis deformans in neoplastic diseases, unspecified ankle and foot
  - **M90.68** Osteitis deformans in neoplastic diseases, other site
  - **M90.69** Osteitis deformans in neoplastic diseases, multiple sites
- **+ M90.8** Osteopathy in diseases classified elsewhere
  Code first underlying disease, such as:
  rickets (E55.0)
  vitamin-D-resistant rickets (E83.31)
  - **M90.80** Osteopathy in diseases classified elsewhere, unspecified site
  - **+ M90.81** Osteopathy in diseases classified elsewhere, shoulder
    - **M90.811** Osteopathy in diseases classified elsewhere, right shoulder
    - **M90.812** Osteopathy in diseases classified elsewhere, left shoulder
    - **M90.819** Osteopathy in diseases classified elsewhere, unspecified shoulder
  - **+ M90.82** Osteopathy in diseases classified elsewhere, upper arm
    - **M90.821** Osteopathy in diseases classified elsewhere, right upper arm
    - **M90.822** Osteopathy in diseases classified elsewhere, left upper arm
    - **M90.829** Osteopathy in diseases classified elsewhere, unspecified upper arm
  - **+ M90.83** Osteopathy in diseases classified elsewhere, forearm
    - **M90.831** Osteopathy in diseases classified elsewhere, right forearm
    - **M90.832** Osteopathy in diseases classified elsewhere, left forearm
    - **M90.839** Osteopathy in diseases classified elsewhere, unspecified forearm
  - **+ M90.84** Osteopathy in diseases classified elsewhere, hand
    - **M90.841** Osteopathy in diseases classified elsewhere, right hand
    - **M90.842** Osteopathy in diseases classified elsewhere, left hand
    - **M90.849** Osteopathy in diseases classified elsewhere, unspecified hand
  - **+ M90.85** Osteopathy in diseases classified elsewhere, thigh
    - **M90.851** Osteopathy in diseases classified elsewhere, right thigh
    - **M90.852** Osteopathy in diseases classified elsewhere, left thigh
    - **M90.859** Osteopathy in diseases classified elsewhere, unspecified thigh
  - **+ M90.86** Osteopathy in diseases classified elsewhere, lower leg
    - **M90.861** Osteopathy in diseases classified elsewhere, right lower leg
    - **M90.862** Osteopathy in diseases classified elsewhere, left lower leg
    - **M90.869** Osteopathy in diseases classified elsewhere, unspecified lower leg

- **M90.87** Osteopathy in diseases classified elsewhere, ankle and foot
  - **M90.871** Osteopathy in diseases classified elsewhere, right ankle and foot
  - **M90.872** Osteopathy in diseases classified elsewhere, left ankle and foot
  - **M90.879** Osteopathy in diseases classified elsewhere, unspecified ankle and foot
- **M90.88** Osteopathy in diseases classified elsewhere, other site
- **M90.89** Osteopathy in diseases classified elsewhere, multiple sites

Chondropathies (M91-M94)

Excludes1: postprocedural chondropathies (M96.-)

M91 Juvenile osteochondrosis of hip and pelvis

Excludes1: slipped upper femoral epiphysis (nontraumatic) (M93.0-)

- **M91.0** Juvenile osteochondrosis of pelvis
  - Osteochondrosis (juvenile) of acetabulum
  - Osteochondrosis (juvenile) of iliac crest [Buchanan]
  - Osteochondrosis (juvenile) of ischiopubic synchondrosis [van Neck]
  - Osteochondrosis (juvenile) of symphysis pubis [Pierson]
- + **M91.1** Juvenile osteochondrosis of head of femur [Legg-Calvé-Perthes]
  - **M91.10** Juvenile osteochondrosis of head of femur [Legg-Calvé-Perthes], unspecified leg
  - **M91.11** Juvenile osteochondrosis of head of femur [Legg-Calvé-Perthes], right leg
  - **M91.12** Juvenile osteochondrosis of head of femur [Legg-Calvé-Perthes], left leg
- + **M91.2** Coxa plana
  - Hip deformity due to previous juvenile osteochondrosis
  - **M91.20** Coxa plana, unspecified hip
  - **M91.21** Coxa plana, right hip
  - **M91.22** Coxa plana, left hip
- + **M91.3** Pseudocoxalgia
  - **M91.30** Pseudocoxalgia, unspecified hip
  - **M91.31** Pseudocoxalgia, right hip
  - **M91.32** Pseudocoxalgia, left hip
- + **M91.4** Coxa magna
  - **M91.40** Coxa magna, unspecified hip
  - **M91.41** Coxa magna, right hip
  - **M91.42** Coxa magna, left hip
- + **M91.8** Other juvenile osteochondrosis of hip and pelvis
  - Juvenile osteochondrosis after reduction of congenital dislocation of hip
  - **M91.80** Other juvenile osteochondrosis of hip and pelvis, unspecified leg
  - **M91.81** Other juvenile osteochondrosis of hip and pelvis, right leg
  - **M91.82** Other juvenile osteochondrosis of hip and pelvis, left leg
- + **M91.9** Juvenile osteochondrosis of hip and pelvis, unspecified
  - **M91.90** Juvenile osteochondrosis of hip and pelvis, unspecified, unspecified leg
  - **M91.91** Juvenile osteochondrosis of hip and pelvis, unspecified, right leg
  - **M91.92** Juvenile osteochondrosis of hip and pelvis, unspecified, left leg

M92 Other juvenile osteochondrosis

- + **M92.0** Juvenile osteochondrosis of humerus
  - Osteochondrosis (juvenile) of capitulum of humerus [Panner]
  - Osteochondrosis (juvenile) of head of humerus [Haas]
  - **M92.00** Juvenile osteochondrosis of humerus, unspecified arm
  - **M92.01** Juvenile osteochondrosis of humerus, right arm
  - **M92.02** Juvenile osteochondrosis of humerus, left arm
- + **M92.1** Juvenile osteochondrosis of radius and ulna
  - Osteochondrosis (juvenile) of lower ulna [Burns]
  - Osteochondrosis (juvenile) of radial head [Brailsford]
  - **M92.10** Juvenile osteochondrosis of radius and ulna, unspecified arm
  - **M92.11** Juvenile osteochondrosis of radius and ulna, right arm
  - **M92.12** Juvenile osteochondrosis of radius and ulna, left arm
- + **M92.2** Juvenile osteochondrosis, hand
  - + **M92.20** Unspecified juvenile osteochondrosis, hand
    - **M92.201** Unspecified juvenile osteochondrosis, right hand
    - **M92.202** Unspecified juvenile osteochondrosis, left hand
    - **M92.209** Unspecified juvenile osteochondrosis, unspecified hand
  - + **M92.21** Osteochondrosis (juvenile) of carpal lunate [Kienböck]
    - **M92.211** Osteochondrosis (juvenile) of carpal lunate [Kienböck], right hand
    - **M92.212** Osteochondrosis (juvenile) of carpal lunate [Kienböck], left hand
    - **M92.219** Osteochondrosis (juvenile) of carpal lunate [Kienböck], unspecified hand
  - + **M92.22** Osteochondrosis (juvenile) of metacarpal heads [Mauclaire]
    - **M92.221** Osteochondrosis (juvenile) of metacarpal heads [Mauclaire], right hand
    - **M92.222** Osteochondrosis (juvenile) of metacarpal heads [Mauclaire], left hand
    - **M92.229** Osteochondrosis (juvenile) of metacarpal heads [Mauclaire], unspecified hand
  - + **M92.29** Other juvenile osteochondrosis, hand
    - **M92.291** Other juvenile osteochondrosis, right hand
    - **M92.292** Other juvenile osteochondrosis, left hand
    - **M92.299** Other juvenile osteochondrosis, unspecified hand
- + **M92.3** Other juvenile osteochondrosis, upper limb
  - **M92.30** Other juvenile osteochondrosis, unspecified upper limb
  - **M92.31** Other juvenile osteochondrosis, right upper limb
  - **M92.32** Other juvenile osteochondrosis, left upper limb
- + **M92.4** Juvenile osteochondrosis of patella
  - Osteochondrosis (juvenile) of primary patellar center [Köhler]
  - Osteochondrosis (juvenile) of secondary patellar centre [Sinding Larsen]
  - **M92.40** Juvenile osteochondrosis of patella, unspecified knee
  - **M92.41** Juvenile osteochondrosis of patella, right knee
  - **M92.42** Juvenile osteochondrosis of patella, left knee
- + **M92.5** Juvenile osteochondrosis of tibia and fibula tubercle
  - *AHA CC: 4Q, 2020, 33-34*
  - + **M92.50** Unspecified juvenile osteochondrosis of tibia and fibula
    - **M92.501** Unspecified juvenile osteochondrosis, right leg
    - **M92.502** Unspecified juvenile osteochondrosis, left leg
    - **M92.503** Unspecified juvenile osteochondrosis, bilateral leg
    - **M92.509** Unspecified juvenile osteochondrosis, unspecified leg
  - + **M92.51** Juvenile osteochondrosis of proximal tibia
    - Blount disease
    - Tibia vara
    - **M92.511** Juvenile osteochondrosis of proximal tibia, right leg
    - **M92.512** Juvenile osteochondrosis of proximal tibia, left leg
    - **M92.513** Juvenile osteochondrosis of proximal tibia, bilateral
    - **M92.519** Juvenile osteochondrosis of proximal tibia, unspecified leg
  - + **M92.52** Juvenile osteochondrosis of tibia tubercle
    - Osgood-Schlatter disease
    - **M92.521** Juvenile osteochondrosis of tibia tubercle, right leg
    - **M92.522** Juvenile osteochondrosis of tibia tubercle, left leg
    - **M92.523** Juvenile osteochondrosis of tibia tubercle, bilateral
    - **M92.529** Juvenile osteochondrosis of tibia tubercle, unspecified leg

- **+ M92.59 Other juvenile osteochondrosis of tibia and fibula**
  - M92.591 Other juvenile osteochondrosis of tibia and fibula, right leg
  - M92.592 Other juvenile osteochondrosis of tibia and fibula, left leg
  - M92.593 Other juvenile osteochondrosis of tibia and fibula, bilateral
  - M92.599 Other juvenile osteochondrosis of tibia and fibula, unspecified leg
- **+ M92.6 Juvenile osteochondrosis of tarsus**
  - Osteochondrosis (juvenile) of calcaneum [Sever]
  - Osteochondrosis (juvenile) of os tibiale externum [Haglund]
  - Osteochondrosis (juvenile) of talus [Diaz]
  - Osteochondrosis (juvenile) of tarsal navicular [Köhler]
  - M92.60 Juvenile osteochondrosis of tarsus, unspecified ankle
  - M92.61 Juvenile osteochondrosis of tarsus, right ankle
  - M92.62 Juvenile osteochondrosis of tarsus, left ankle
- **+ M92.7 Juvenile osteochondrosis of metatarsus**
  - Osteochondrosis (juvenile) of fifth metatarsus [Iselin]
  - Osteochondrosis (juvenile) of second metatarsus [Freiberg]
  - M92.70 Juvenile osteochondrosis of metatarsus, unspecified foot
  - M92.71 Juvenile osteochondrosis of metatarsus, right foot
  - M92.72 Juvenile osteochondrosis of metatarsus, left foot
- **M92.8 Other specified juvenile osteochondrosis**
  - Calcaneal apophysitis
- **M92.9 Juvenile osteochondrosis, unspecified**
  - Juvenile apophysitis NOS
  - Juvenile epiphysitis NOS
  - Juvenile osteochondritis NOS
  - Juvenile osteochondrosis NOS

M93 Other osteochondropathies

Excludes2: *osteochondrosis of spine (M42.-)*

- **+ M93.0 Slipped upper femoral epiphysis (nontraumatic)**
  - Slipped capital femoral epiphysis (SCFE)
  - Slipped upper femoral epiphysis (SUFE)
  - Use additional code for associated chondrolysis (M94.3)
  - *AHA CC: 4Q, 2022, 30-31*
  - **+ M93.00 Unspecified slipped upper femoral epiphysis (nontraumatic)**
    - M93.001 Unspecified slipped upper femoral epiphysis (nontraumatic), right hip
    - M93.002 Unspecified slipped upper femoral epiphysis (nontraumatic), left hip
    - M93.003 Unspecified slipped upper femoral epiphysis (nontraumatic), unspecified hip
    - M93.004 Unspecified slipped upper femoral epiphysis (nontraumatic), bilateral hips
  - **+ M93.01 Acute slipped upper femoral epiphysis, stable (nontraumatic)**
    - M93.011 Acute slipped upper femoral epiphysis, stable (nontraumatic), right hip
    - M93.012 Acute slipped upper femoral epiphysis, stable (nontraumatic), left hip
    - M93.013 Acute slipped upper femoral epiphysis, stable (nontraumatic), unspecified hip
    - M93.014 Acute slipped upper femoral epiphysis, stable (nontraumatic), bilateral hips
  - **+ M93.02 Chronic slipped upper femoral epiphysis, stable (nontraumatic)**
    - M93.021 Chronic slipped upper femoral epiphysis, stable (nontraumatic), right hip
    - M93.022 Chronic slipped upper femoral epiphysis, stable (nontraumatic), left hip
    - M93.023 Chronic slipped upper femoral epiphysis, stable (nontraumatic), unspecified hip
    - M93.024 Chronic slipped upper femoral epiphysis, stable (nontraumatic), bilateral hips
  - **+ M93.03 Acute on chronic slipped upper femoral epiphysis, stable (nontraumatic)**
    - M93.031 Acute on chronic slipped upper femoral epiphysis, stable (nontraumatic), right hip
    - M93.032 Acute on chronic slipped upper femoral epiphysis, stable (nontraumatic), left hip
    - M93.033 Acute on chronic slipped upper femoral epiphysis, stable (nontraumatic), unspecified hip
    - M93.034 Acute on chronic slipped upper femoral epiphysis, stable (nontraumatic), bilateral hips
  - **+ M93.04 Acute slipped upper femoral epiphysis, unstable (nontraumatic)**
    - M93.041 Acute slipped upper femoral epiphysis, unstable (nontraumatic), right hip
    - M93.042 Acute slipped upper femoral epiphysis, unstable (nontraumatic), left hip
    - M93.043 Acute slipped upper femoral epiphysis, unstable (nontraumatic), unspecified hip
    - M93.044 Acute slipped upper femoral epiphysis, unstable (nontraumatic), bilateral hips
  - **+ M93.05 Acute on chronic slipped upper femoral epiphysis, unstable (nontraumatic)**
    - M93.051 Acute on chronic slipped upper femoral epiphysis, unstable (nontraumatic), right hip
    - M93.052 Acute on chronic slipped upper femoral epiphysis, unstable (nontraumatic), left hip
    - M93.053 Acute on chronic slipped upper femoral epiphysis, unstable (nontraumatic), unspecified hip
    - M93.054 Acute on chronic slipped upper femoral epiphysis, unstable (nontraumatic), bilateral hips
  - **+ M93.06 Acute slipped upper femoral epiphysis, unspecified stability (nontraumatic)**
    - M93.061 Acute slipped upper femoral epiphysis, unspecified stability (nontraumatic), right hip
    - M93.062 Acute slipped upper femoral epiphysis, unspecified stability (nontraumatic), left hip
    - M93.063 Acute slipped upper femoral epiphysis, unspecified stability (nontraumatic), unspecified hip
    - M93.064 Acute slipped upper femoral epiphysis, unspecified stability (nontraumatic), bilateral hips
  - **+ M93.07 Acute on chronic slipped upper femoral epiphysis, unspecified stability (nontraumatic)**
    - M93.071 Acute on chronic slipped upper femoral epiphysis, unspecified stability (nontraumatic), right hip
    - M93.072 Acute on chronic slipped upper femoral epiphysis, unspecified stability (nontraumatic), left hip
    - M93.073 Acute on chronic slipped upper femoral epiphysis, unspecified stability (nontraumatic), unspecified hip
    - M93.074 Acute on chronic slipped upper femoral epiphysis, unspecified stability (nontraumatic), bilateral hips
- **• M93.1 Kienböck's disease of adults**
  - Adult osteochondrosis of carpal lunates
- **+ M93.2 Osteochondritis dissecans**
  - M93.20 Osteochondritis dissecans of unspecified site
  - **+ M93.21 Osteochondritis dissecans of shoulder**
    - M93.211 Osteochondritis dissecans, right shoulder
    - M93.212 Osteochondritis dissecans, left shoulder
    - M93.219 Osteochondritis dissecans, unspecified shoulder
  - **+ M93.22 Osteochondritis dissecans of elbow**
    - M93.221 Osteochondritis dissecans, right elbow
    - M93.222 Osteochondritis dissecans, left elbow
    - M93.229 Osteochondritis dissecans, unspecified elbow
  - **+ M93.23 Osteochondritis dissecans of wrist**
    - M93.231 Osteochondritis dissecans, right wrist
    - M93.232 Osteochondritis dissecans, left wrist
    - M93.239 Osteochondritis dissecans, unspecified wrist
  - **+ M93.24 Osteochondritis dissecans of joints of hand**
    - M93.241 Osteochondritis dissecans, joints of right hand
    - M93.242 Osteochondritis dissecans, joints of left hand
    - M93.249 Osteochondritis dissecans, joints of unspecified hand

- **+ M93.25 Osteochondritis dissecans of hip**
  - M93.251 Osteochondritis dissecans, right hip
  - M93.252 Osteochondritis dissecans, left hip
  - M93.259 Osteochondritis dissecans, unspecified hip
- **+ M93.26 Osteochondritis dissecans knee**
  - M93.261 Osteochondritis dissecans, right knee
  - M93.262 Osteochondritis dissecans, left knee
  - M93.269 Osteochondritis dissecans, unspecified knee
- **+ M93.27 Osteochondritis dissecans of ankle and joints of foot**
  - M93.271 Osteochondritis dissecans, right ankle and joints of right foot
  - M93.272 Osteochondritis dissecans, left ankle and joints of left foot
  - M93.279 Osteochondritis dissecans, unspecified ankle and joints of foot
- M93.28 Osteochondritis dissecans other site
- M93.29 Osteochondritis dissecans multiple sites
- **+ M93.8 Other specified osteochondropathies**
  - M93.80 Other specified osteochondropathies of unspecified site
  - **+ M93.81 Other specified osteochondropathies of shoulder**
    - M93.811 Other specified osteochondropathies, right shoulder
    - M93.812 Other specified osteochondropathies, left shoulder
    - M93.819 Other specified osteochondropathies, unspecified shoulder
  - **+ M93.82 Other specified osteochondropathies of upper arm**
    - M93.821 Other specified osteochondropathies, right upper arm
    - M93.822 Other specified osteochondropathies, left upper arm
    - M93.829 Other specified osteochondropathies, unspecified upper arm
  - **+ M93.83 Other specified osteochondropathies of forearm**
    - M93.831 Other specified osteochondropathies, right forearm
    - M93.832 Other specified osteochondropathies, left forearm
    - M93.839 Other specified osteochondropathies, unspecified forearm
  - **+ M93.84 Other specified osteochondropathies of hand**
    - M93.841 Other specified osteochondropathies, right hand
    - M93.842 Other specified osteochondropathies, left hand
    - M93.849 Other specified osteochondropathies, unspecified hand
  - **+ M93.85 Other specified osteochondropathies of thigh**
    - M93.851 Other specified osteochondropathies, right thigh
    - M93.852 Other specified osteochondropathies, left thigh
    - M93.859 Other specified osteochondropathies, unspecified thigh
  - **+ M93.86 Other specified osteochondropathies lower leg**
    - M93.861 Other specified osteochondropathies, right lower leg
    - M93.862 Other specified osteochondropathies, left lower leg
    - M93.869 Other specified osteochondropathies, unspecified lower leg
  - **+ M93.87 Other specified osteochondropathies of ankle and foot**
    - M93.871 Other specified osteochondropathies, right ankle and foot
    - M93.872 Other specified osteochondropathies, left ankle and foot
    - M93.879 Other specified osteochondropathies, unspecified ankle and foot
  - M93.88 Other specified osteochondropathies other
  - M93.89 Other specified osteochondropathies multiple sites
- **+ M93.9 Osteochondropathy, unspecified**
  - Apophysitis NOS
  - Epiphysitis NOS
  - Osteochondritis NOS
  - Osteochondrosis NOS
  - M93.90 Osteochondropathy, unspecified of unspecified site
  - **+ M93.91 Osteochondropathy, unspecified of shoulder**
    - M93.911 Osteochondropathy, unspecified, right shoulder
    - M93.912 Osteochondropathy, unspecified, left shoulder
    - M93.919 Osteochondropathy, unspecified, unspecified shoulder
  - **+ M93.92 Osteochondropathy, unspecified of upper arm**
    - M93.921 Osteochondropathy, unspecified, right upper arm
    - M93.922 Osteochondropathy, unspecified, left upper arm
    - M93.929 Osteochondropathy, unspecified, unspecified upper arm
  - **+ M93.93 Osteochondropathy, unspecified of forearm**
    - M93.931 Osteochondropathy, unspecified, right forearm
    - M93.932 Osteochondropathy, unspecified, left forearm
    - M93.939 Osteochondropathy, unspecified, unspecified forearm
  - **+ M93.94 Osteochondropathy, unspecified of hand**
    - M93.941 Osteochondropathy, unspecified, right hand
    - M93.942 Osteochondropathy, unspecified, left hand
    - M93.949 Osteochondropathy, unspecified, unspecified hand
  - **+ M93.95 Osteochondropathy, unspecified of thigh**
    - M93.951 Osteochondropathy, unspecified, right thigh
    - M93.952 Osteochondropathy, unspecified, left thigh
    - M93.959 Osteochondropathy, unspecified, unspecified thigh
  - **+ M93.96 Osteochondropathy, unspecified lower leg**
    - M93.961 Osteochondropathy, unspecified, right lower leg
    - M93.962 Osteochondropathy, unspecified, left lower leg
    - M93.969 Osteochondropathy, unspecified, unspecified lower leg
  - **+ M93.97 Osteochondropathy, unspecified of ankle and foot**
    - M93.971 Osteochondropathy, unspecified, right ankle and foot
    - M93.972 Osteochondropathy, unspecified, left ankle and foot
    - M93.979 Osteochondropathy, unspecified, unspecified ankle and foot
  - M93.98 Osteochondropathy, unspecified other
  - M93.99 Osteochondropathy, unspecified multiple sites

M94 Other disorders of cartilage
- M94.0 Chondrocostal junction syndrome [Tietze]
  - Costochondritis
- M94.1 Relapsing polychondritis
- **+ M94.2 Chondromalacia**
  - **Excludes1:** *chondromalacia patellae (M22.4)*
  - M94.20 Chondromalacia, unspecified site
  - **+ M94.21 Chondromalacia, shoulder**
    - M94.211 Chondromalacia, right shoulder
    - M94.212 Chondromalacia, left shoulder
    - M94.219 Chondromalacia, unspecified shoulder
  - **+ M94.22 Chondromalacia, elbow**
    - M94.221 Chondromalacia, right elbow
    - M94.222 Chondromalacia, left elbow
    - M94.229 Chondromalacia, unspecified elbow
  - **+ M94.23 Chondromalacia, wrist**
    - M94.231 Chondromalacia, right wrist
    - M94.232 Chondromalacia, left wrist
    - M94.239 Chondromalacia, unspecified wrist
  - **+ M94.24 Chondromalacia, joints of hand**
    - M94.241 Chondromalacia, joints of right hand
    - M94.242 Chondromalacia, joints of left hand
    - M94.249 Chondromalacia, joints of unspecified hand
  - **+ M94.25 Chondromalacia, hip**
    - M94.251 Chondromalacia, right hip
    - M94.252 Chondromalacia, left hip
    - M94.259 Chondromalacia, unspecified hip

- **M94.26 Chondromalacia, knee**
  - M94.261 Chondromalacia, right knee
  - M94.262 Chondromalacia, left knee
  - M94.269 Chondromalacia, unspecified knee
- **M94.27 Chondromalacia, ankle and joints of foot**
  - M94.271 Chondromalacia, right ankle and joints of right foot
  - M94.272 Chondromalacia, left ankle and joints of left foot
  - M94.279 Chondromalacia, unspecified ankle and joints of foot
- M94.28 Chondromalacia, other site
- M94.29 Chondromalacia, multiple sites

M94.3 Chondrolysis
  Code first any associated slipped upper femoral epiphysis (nontraumatic) (M93.0-)
- **M94.35 Chondrolysis, hip**
  - M94.351 Chondrolysis, right hip
  - M94.352 Chondrolysis, left hip
  - M94.359 Chondrolysis, unspecified hip

M94.8 Other specified disorders of cartilage
- **M94.8X Other specified disorders of cartilage**
  - M94.8X0 Other specified disorders of cartilage, multiple sites
  - M94.8X1 Other specified disorders of cartilage, shoulder
  - M94.8X2 Other specified disorders of cartilage, upper arm
  - M94.8X3 Other specified disorders of cartilage, forearm
  - M94.8X4 Other specified disorders of cartilage, hand
  - M94.8X5 Other specified disorders of cartilage, thigh
  - M94.8X6 Other specified disorders of cartilage, lower leg
  - M94.8X7 Other specified disorders of cartilage, ankle and foot
  - M94.8X8 Other specified disorders of cartilage, other site
  - M94.8X9 Other specified disorders of cartilage, unspecified sites

M94.9 Disorder of cartilage, unspecified

Other disorders of the musculoskeletal system and connective tissue (M95)

M95 Other acquired deformities of musculoskeletal system and connective tissue
  Excludes2: acquired absence of limbs and organs (Z89-Z90)
  acquired deformities of limbs (M20-M21)
  congenital malformations and deformations of the musculoskeletal system (Q65-Q79)
  deforming dorsopathies (M40-M43)
  dentofacial anomalies [including malocclusion] (M26.-)
  postprocedural musculoskeletal disorders (M96.-)

- **M95.0 Acquired deformity of nose**
  Excludes2: deviated nasal septum (J34.2)
- **M95.1 Cauliflower ear**
  Excludes2: other acquired deformities of ear (H61.1)
  - M95.10 Cauliflower ear, unspecified ear
  - M95.11 Cauliflower ear, right ear
  - M95.12 Cauliflower ear, left ear
- **M95.2 Other acquired deformity of head**
  AHA CC: 1Q, 2022, 34-35; 1Q, 2023, 30-31
- **M95.3 Acquired deformity of neck**
- **M95.4 Acquired deformity of chest and rib**
  AHA CC: 4Q, 2014, 26-27
- **M95.5 Acquired deformity of pelvis**
  Excludes1: maternal care for known or suspected disproportion (O33.-)
- **M95.8 Other specified acquired deformities of musculoskeletal system**
- **M95.9 Acquired deformity of musculoskeletal system, unspecified**

Intraoperative and postprocedural complications and disorders of musculoskeletal system, not elsewhere classified (M96)

M96 Intraoperative and postprocedural complications and disorders of musculoskeletal system, not elsewhere classified
  Excludes2: arthropathy following intestinal bypass (M02.0-)
  complications of internal orthopedic prosthetic devices, implants and grafts (T84.-)
  disorders associated with osteoporosis (M80)
  periprosthetic fracture around internal prosthetic joint (M97.-)
  presence of functional implants and other devices (Z96-Z97)

- CC **M96.0 Pseudarthrosis after fusion or arthrodesis**
- **M96.1 Postlaminectomy syndrome, not elsewhere classified**
- **M96.2 Postradiation kyphosis**
- **M96.3 Postlaminectomy kyphosis**
- **M96.4 Postsurgical lordosis**
- **M96.5 Postradiation scoliosis**
- **M96.6 Fracture of bone following insertion of orthopedic implant, joint prosthesis, or bone plate**
  Intraoperative fracture of bone during insertion of orthopedic implant, joint prosthesis, or bone plate
  Excludes2: complication of internal orthopedic devices, implants or grafts (T84.-)
  - **M96.62 Fracture of humerus following insertion of orthopedic implant, joint prosthesis, or bone plate**
    - CC M96.621 Fracture of humerus following insertion of orthopedic implant, joint prosthesis, or bone plate, right arm
    - CC M96.622 Fracture of humerus following insertion of orthopedic implant, joint prosthesis, or bone plate, left arm
    - CC M96.629 Fracture of humerus following insertion of orthopedic implant, joint prosthesis, or bone plate, unspecified arm
  - **M96.63 Fracture of radius or ulna following insertion of orthopedic implant, joint prosthesis, or bone plate**
    - CC M96.631 Fracture of radius or ulna following insertion of orthopedic implant, joint prosthesis, or bone plate, right arm
    - CC M96.632 Fracture of radius or ulna following insertion of orthopedic implant, joint prosthesis, or bone plate, left arm
    - CC M96.639 Fracture of radius or ulna following insertion of orthopedic implant, joint prosthesis, or bone plate, unspecified arm
  - CC **M96.65 Fracture of pelvis following insertion of orthopedic implant, joint prosthesis, or bone plate**
  - **M96.66 Fracture of femur following insertion of orthopedic implant, joint prosthesis, or bone plate**
    - CC M96.661 Fracture of femur following insertion of orthopedic implant, joint prosthesis, or bone plate, right leg
    - CC M96.662 Fracture of femur following insertion of orthopedic implant, joint prosthesis, or bone plate, left leg
    - CC M96.669 Fracture of femur following insertion of orthopedic implant, joint prosthesis, or bone plate, unspecified leg
  - **M96.67 Fracture of tibia or fibula following insertion of orthopedic implant, joint prosthesis, or bone plate**
    - CC M96.671 Fracture of tibia or fibula following insertion of orthopedic implant, joint prosthesis, or bone plate, right leg
    - CC M96.672 Fracture of tibia or fibula following insertion of orthopedic implant, joint prosthesis, or bone plate, left leg
    - CC M96.679 Fracture of tibia or fibula following insertion of orthopedic implant, joint prosthesis, or bone plate, unspecified leg
  - CC **M96.69 Fracture of other bone following insertion of orthopedic implant, joint prosthesis, or bone plate**
- **M96.8 Other intraoperative and postprocedural complications and disorders of musculoskeletal system, not elsewhere classified**
  AHA CC: 4Q, 2016, 9-10

- **M96.81** Intraoperative hemorrhage and hematoma of a musculoskeletal structure complicating a procedure
  Excludes1: intraoperative hemorrhage and hematoma of a musculoskeletal structure due to accidental puncture and laceration during a procedure (M96.82)
  - CC **M96.810** Intraoperative hemorrhage and hematoma of a musculoskeletal structure complicating a musculoskeletal system procedure
  - CC **M96.811** Intraoperative hemorrhage and hematoma of a musculoskeletal structure complicating other procedure
- **M96.82** Accidental puncture and laceration of a musculoskeletal structure during a procedure
  - CC **M96.820** Accidental puncture and laceration of a musculoskeletal structure during a musculoskeletal system procedure
  - CC **M96.821** Accidental puncture and laceration of a musculoskeletal structure during other procedure
- **M96.83** Postprocedural hemorrhage of a musculoskeletal structure following a procedure
  - CC **M96.830** Postprocedural hemorrhage of a musculoskeletal structure following a musculoskeletal system procedure
  - CC **M96.831** Postprocedural hemorrhage of a musculoskeletal structure following other procedure
- **M96.84** Postprocedural hematoma and seroma of a musculoskeletal structure following a procedure
  - CC **M96.840** Postprocedural hematoma of a musculoskeletal structure following a musculoskeletal system procedure
  - CC **M96.841** Postprocedural hematoma of a musculoskeletal structure following other procedure
    AHA CC: 4Q, 2016, 9-10
  - CC **M96.842** Postprocedural seroma of a musculoskeletal structure following a musculoskeletal system procedure
  - CC **M96.843** Postprocedural seroma of a musculoskeletal structure following other procedure
    AHA CC: 3Q, 2018, 6; 2Q, 2023, 13
- CC **M96.89** Other intraoperative and postprocedural complications and disorders of the musculoskeletal system
  Instability of joint secondary to removal of joint prosthesis
  Use additional code, if applicable, to further specify disorder
  AHA CC: 1Q, 2021, 5-6; 2Q, 2022, 14; 2Q, 2023, 14
- **M96.A** Fracture of ribs, sternum and thorax associated with compression of the chest and cardiopulmonary resuscitation
  AHA CC: 4Q, 2022, 31-33
  - CC **M96.A1** Fracture of sternum associated with chest compression and cardiopulmonary resuscitation
    Fracture of xiphoid process associated with chest compression and cardiopulmonary resuscitation
  - CC **M96.A2** Fracture of one rib associated with chest compression and cardiopulmonary resuscitation
  - CC **M96.A3** Multiple fractures of ribs associated with chest compression and cardiopulmonary resuscitation
    AHA CC: 4Q, 2022, 32-33
  - MCC **M96.A4** Flail chest associated with chest compression and cardiopulmonary resuscitation
  - CC **M96.A9** Other fracture associated with chest compression and cardiopulmonary resuscitation

Periprosthetic fracture around internal prosthetic joint (M97)

M97 Periprosthetic fracture around internal prosthetic joint

Code first, if known, the specific type and cause of fracture, such as traumatic or pathological

Excludes2: fracture of bone following insertion of orthopedic implant, joint prosthesis or bone plate (M96.6-)
breakage (fracture) of prosthetic joint (T84.01-)

AHA CC: 4Q, 2016, 42-43

The appropriate 7th character is to be added to each code from category M97:
A initial encounter
D subsequent encounter
S sequela

- **M97.0** Periprosthetic fracture around internal prosthetic hip joint
  - CC X+7th **M97.01** Periprosthetic fracture around internal prosthetic right hip joint
    AHA CC: 4Q, 2016, 42-43
  - CC X+7th **M97.02** Periprosthetic fracture around internal prosthetic left hip joint
- **M97.1** Periprosthetic fracture around internal prosthetic knee joint
  - CC X+7th **M97.11** Periprosthetic fracture around internal prosthetic right knee joint
  - CC X+7th **M97.12** Periprosthetic fracture around internal prosthetic left knee joint
- **M97.2** Periprosthetic fracture around internal prosthetic ankle joint
  - CC X+7th **M97.21** Periprosthetic fracture around internal prosthetic right ankle joint
  - CC X+7th **M97.22** Periprosthetic fracture around internal prosthetic left ankle joint
- **M97.3** Periprosthetic fracture around internal prosthetic shoulder joint
  - CC X+7th **M97.31** Periprosthetic fracture around internal prosthetic right shoulder joint
  - CC X+7th **M97.32** Periprosthetic fracture around internal prosthetic left shoulder joint
- **M97.4** Periprosthetic fracture around internal prosthetic elbow joint
  - CC X+7th **M97.41** Periprosthetic fracture around internal prosthetic right elbow joint
  - CC X+7th **M97.42** Periprosthetic fracture around internal prosthetic left elbow joint
- CC X+7th **M97.8** Periprosthetic fracture around other internal prosthetic joint
  Periprosthetic fracture around internal prosthetic finger joint
  Periprosthetic fracture around internal prosthetic spinal joint
  Periprosthetic fracture around internal prosthetic toe joint
  Periprosthetic fracture around internal prosthetic wrist joint
  Use additional code to identify the joint (Z96.6-)
- CC X+7th **M97.9** Periprosthetic fracture around unspecified internal prosthetic joint

Biomechanical lesions, not elsewhere classified (M99)

M99 Biomechanical lesions, not elsewhere classified

NOTE This category should not be used if the condition can be classified elsewhere.

- **M99.0** Segmental and somatic dysfunction
  - **M99.00** Segmental and somatic dysfunction of head region
  - **M99.01** Segmental and somatic dysfunction of cervical region
  - **M99.02** Segmental and somatic dysfunction of thoracic region
  - **M99.03** Segmental and somatic dysfunction of lumbar region
  - **M99.04** Segmental and somatic dysfunction of sacral region
  - **M99.05** Segmental and somatic dysfunction of pelvic region
  - **M99.06** Segmental and somatic dysfunction of lower extremity
  - **M99.07** Segmental and somatic dysfunction of upper extremity
  - **M99.08** Segmental and somatic dysfunction of rib cage
  - **M99.09** Segmental and somatic dysfunction of abdomen and other regions

+ **M99.1 Subluxation complex (vertebral)**
    CC **M99.10** Subluxation complex (vertebral) of head region
        HAC see Appendix B for HAC conditional logic
    CC **M99.11** Subluxation complex (vertebral) of cervical region
        HAC see Appendix B for HAC conditional logic
    M99.12 Subluxation complex (vertebral) of thoracic region
    M99.13 Subluxation complex (vertebral) of lumbar region
    M99.14 Subluxation complex (vertebral) of sacral region
    M99.15 Subluxation complex (vertebral) of pelvic region
    M99.16 Subluxation complex (vertebral) of lower extremity
    M99.17 Subluxation complex (vertebral) of upper extremity
    CC **M99.18** Subluxation complex (vertebral) of rib cage
        HAC see Appendix B for HAC conditional logic
    M99.19 Subluxation complex (vertebral) of abdomen and other regions
+ **M99.2 Subluxation stenosis of neural canal**
    M99.20 Subluxation stenosis of neural canal of head region
    M99.21 Subluxation stenosis of neural canal of cervical region
    M99.22 Subluxation stenosis of neural canal of thoracic region
    M99.23 Subluxation stenosis of neural canal of lumbar region
    M99.24 Subluxation stenosis of neural canal of sacral region
    M99.25 Subluxation stenosis of neural canal of pelvic region
    M99.26 Subluxation stenosis of neural canal of lower extremity
    M99.27 Subluxation stenosis of neural canal of upper extremity
    M99.28 Subluxation stenosis of neural canal of rib cage
    M99.29 Subluxation stenosis of neural canal of abdomen and other regions
+ **M99.3 Osseous stenosis of neural canal**
    M99.30 Osseous stenosis of neural canal of head region
    M99.31 Osseous stenosis of neural canal of cervical region
    M99.32 Osseous stenosis of neural canal of thoracic region
    M99.33 Osseous stenosis of neural canal of lumbar region
    M99.34 Osseous stenosis of neural canal of sacral region
    M99.35 Osseous stenosis of neural canal of pelvic region
    M99.36 Osseous stenosis of neural canal of lower extremity
    M99.37 Osseous stenosis of neural canal of upper extremity
    M99.38 Osseous stenosis of neural canal of rib cage
    M99.39 Osseous stenosis of neural canal of abdomen and other regions
+ **M99.4 Connective tissue stenosis of neural canal**
    M99.40 Connective tissue stenosis of neural canal of head region
    M99.41 Connective tissue stenosis of neural canal of cervical region
    M99.42 Connective tissue stenosis of neural canal of thoracic region
    M99.43 Connective tissue stenosis of neural canal of lumbar region
    M99.44 Connective tissue stenosis of neural canal of sacral region
    M99.45 Connective tissue stenosis of neural canal of pelvic region
    M99.46 Connective tissue stenosis of neural canal of lower extremity
    M99.47 Connective tissue stenosis of neural canal of upper extremity
    M99.48 Connective tissue stenosis of neural canal of rib cage
    M99.49 Connective tissue stenosis of neural canal of abdomen and other regions
+ **M99.5 Intervertebral disc stenosis of neural canal**
    M99.50 Intervertebral disc stenosis of neural canal of head region
    M99.51 Intervertebral disc stenosis of neural canal of cervical region
    M99.52 Intervertebral disc stenosis of neural canal of thoracic region
    M99.53 Intervertebral disc stenosis of neural canal of lumbar region
    M99.54 Intervertebral disc stenosis of neural canal of sacral region
    M99.55 Intervertebral disc stenosis of neural canal of pelvic region
    M99.56 Intervertebral disc stenosis of neural canal of lower extremity
    M99.57 Intervertebral disc stenosis of neural canal of upper extremity
    M99.58 Intervertebral disc stenosis of neural canal of rib cage
    M99.59 Intervertebral disc stenosis of neural canal of abdomen and other regions
+ **M99.6 Osseous and subluxation stenosis of intervertebral foramina**
    M99.60 Osseous and subluxation stenosis of intervertebral foramina of head region
    M99.61 Osseous and subluxation stenosis of intervertebral foramina of cervical region
    M99.62 Osseous and subluxation stenosis of intervertebral foramina of thoracic region
    M99.63 Osseous and subluxation stenosis of intervertebral foramina of lumbar region
    M99.64 Osseous and subluxation stenosis of intervertebral foramina of sacral region
    M99.65 Osseous and subluxation stenosis of intervertebral foramina of pelvic region
    M99.66 Osseous and subluxation stenosis of intervertebral foramina of lower extremity
    M99.67 Osseous and subluxation stenosis of intervertebral foramina of upper extremity
    M99.68 Osseous and subluxation stenosis of intervertebral foramina of rib cage
    M99.69 Osseous and subluxation stenosis of intervertebral foramina of abdomen and other regions
+ **M99.7 Connective tissue and disc stenosis of intervertebral foramina**
    M99.70 Connective tissue and disc stenosis of intervertebral foramina of head region
    M99.71 Connective tissue and disc stenosis of intervertebral foramina of cervical region
    M99.72 Connective tissue and disc stenosis of intervertebral foramina of thoracic region
    M99.73 Connective tissue and disc stenosis of intervertebral foramina of lumbar region
    M99.74 Connective tissue and disc stenosis of intervertebral foramina of sacral region
    M99.75 Connective tissue and disc stenosis of intervertebral foramina of pelvic region
    M99.76 Connective tissue and disc stenosis of intervertebral foramina of lower extremity
    M99.77 Connective tissue and disc stenosis of intervertebral foramina of upper extremity
    M99.78 Connective tissue and disc stenosis of intervertebral foramina of rib cage
    M99.79 Connective tissue and disc stenosis of intervertebral foramina of abdomen and other regions
+ **M99.8 Other biomechanical lesions**
    M99.80 Other biomechanical lesions of head region
    M99.81 Other biomechanical lesions of cervical region
    M99.82 Other biomechanical lesions of thoracic region
    M99.83 Other biomechanical lesions of lumbar region
    M99.84 Other biomechanical lesions of sacral region
    M99.85 Other biomechanical lesions of pelvic region
    M99.86 Other biomechanical lesions of lower extremity
    M99.87 Other biomechanical lesions of upper extremity
    M99.88 Other biomechanical lesions of rib cage
    M99.89 Other biomechanical lesions of abdomen and other regions
M99.9 Biomechanical lesion, unspecified

Chapter 14: Diseases of the Genitourinary System (N00-N99)

Excludes2: *certain conditions originating in the perinatal period (P04-P96)*
certain infectious and parasitic diseases (A00-B99)
complications of pregnancy, childbirth and the puerperium (O00-O9A)
congenital malformations, deformations and chromosomal abnormalities (Q00-Q99)
endocrine, nutritional and metabolic diseases (E00-E88)
injury, poisoning and certain other consequences of external causes (S00-T88)
neoplasms (C00-D49)
symptoms, signs and abnormal clinical and laboratory findings, not elsewhere classified (R00-R94)

This chapter contains the following category blocks:
N00-N08 Glomerular diseases
N10-N16 Renal tubulo-interstitial diseases
N17-N19 Acute kidney failure and chronic kidney disease
N20-N23 Urolithiasis
N25-N29 Other disorders of kidney and ureter
N30-N39 Other diseases of the urinary system
N40-N53 Diseases of male genital organs
N60-N65 Disorders of breast
N70-N77 Inflammatory diseases of female pelvic organs
N80-N98 Noninflammatory disorders of female genital tract
N99   Intraoperative and postprocedural complications and disorders of genitourinary system, not elsewhere classified

C. Chapter-Specific Coding Guidelines

In addition to general coding guidelines, there are guidelines for specific diagnoses and/or conditions in the classification. Unless otherwise indicated, these guidelines apply to all health care settings. Please refer to Section II for guidelines on the selection of principal diagnosis.

14. Chapter 14: Diseases of the Genitourinary System (N00-N99)
   a. Chronic kidney disease
      1) Stages of chronic kidney disease (CKD)

The ICD-10-CM classifies CKD based on severity. The severity of CKD is designated by stages 1-5. Stage 2, code N18.2, equates to mild CKD; stage 3, code N18.3, equates to moderate CKD; and stage 4, code N18.4, equates to severe CKD. Code N18.6, End stage renal disease (ESRD), is assigned when the provider has documented end-stage-renal disease (ESRD).

If both a stage of CKD and ESRD are documented, assign code N18.6 only.

      2) Chronic kidney disease and kidney transplant status

Patients who have undergone kidney transplant may still have some form of chronic kidney disease (CKD) because the kidney transplant may not fully restore kidney function. Therefore, the presence of CKD alone does not constitute a transplant complication. Assign the appropriate N18 code for the patient's stage of CKD and code Z94.0, Kidney transplant status. If a transplant complication such as failure or rejection or other transplant complication is documented, see section I.C.19.g for information on coding complications of a kidney transplant. If the documentation is unclear as to whether the patient has a complication of the transplant, query the provider.

      3) Chronic kidney disease with other conditions

Patients with CKD may also suffer from other serious conditions, most commonly diabetes mellitus and hypertension. The sequencing of the CKD code in relationship to codes for other contributing conditions is based on the conventions in the Tabular List.

See I.C.9. Hypertensive chronic kidney disease.

See I.C.19. Chronic kidney disease and kidney transplant complications.

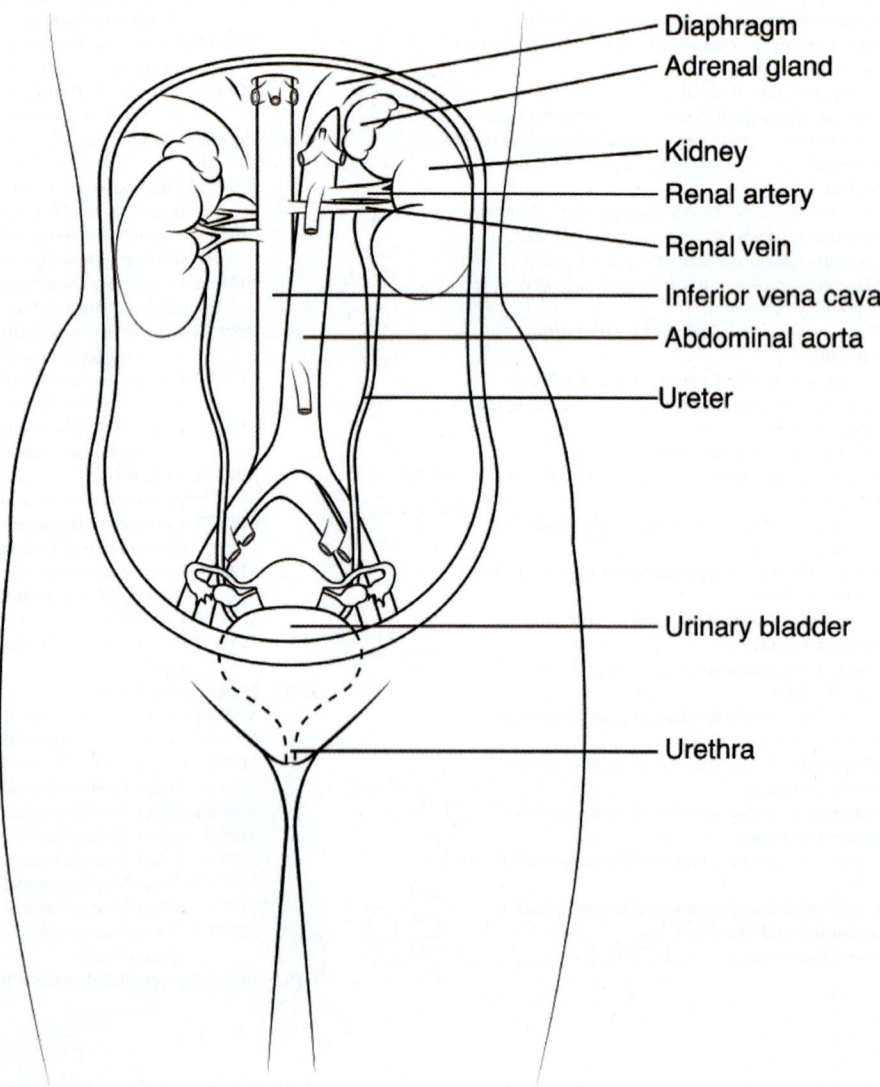

Urinary System

©AHIMA

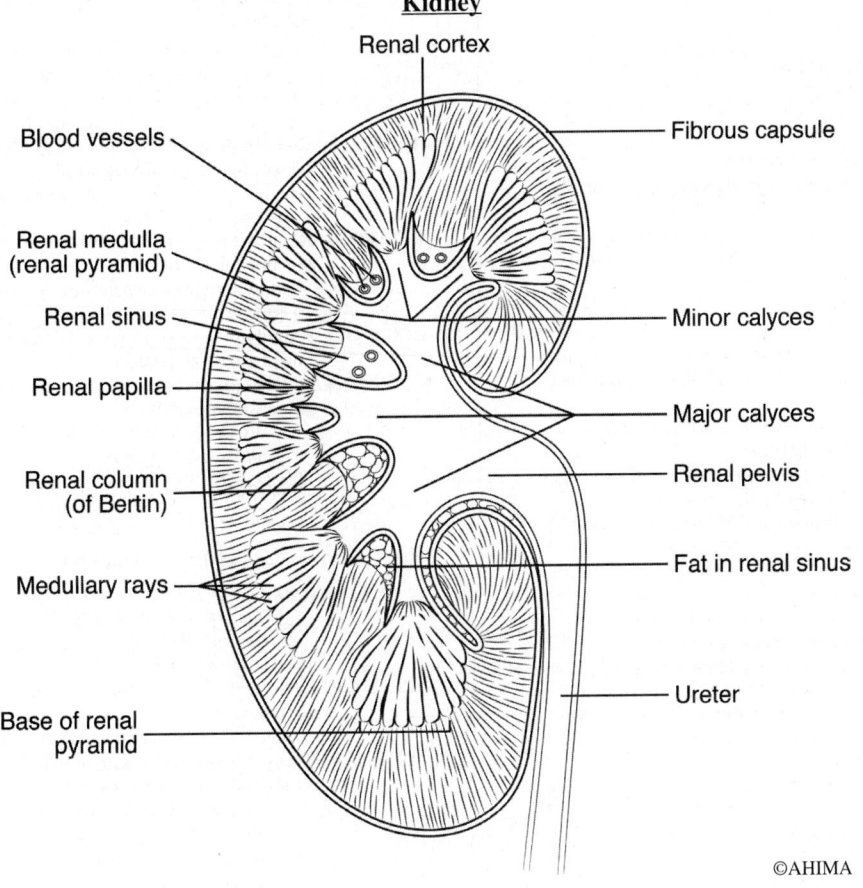

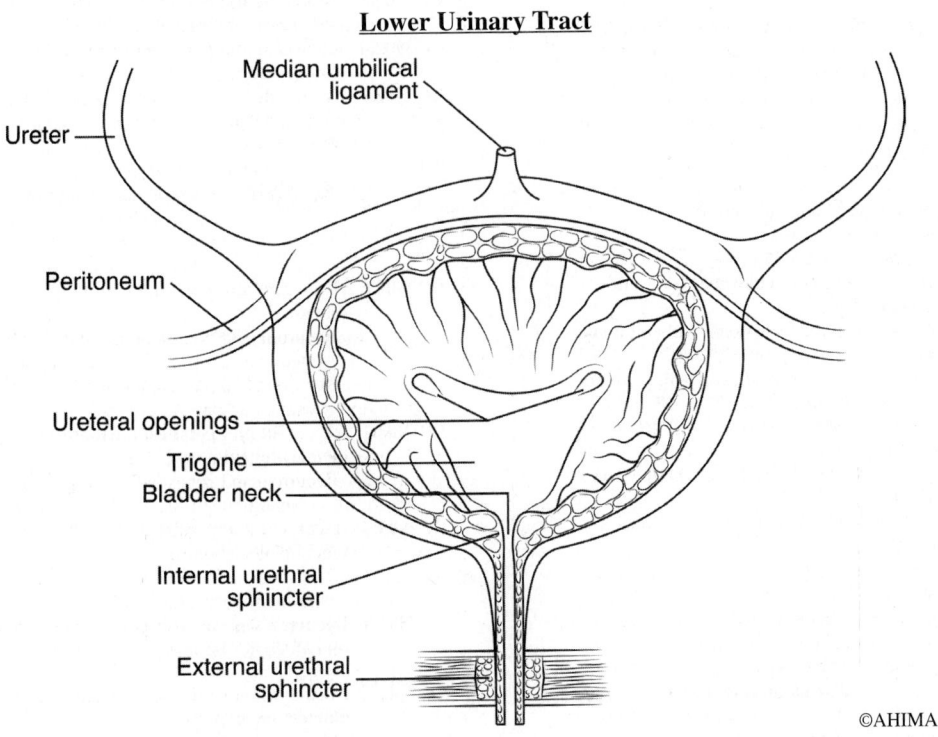

Glomerular diseases (N00-N08)

Code also any associated kidney failure (N17-N19)

Excludes1: hypertensive chronic kidney disease (I12.-)

AHA CC: 4Q, 2020, 34-35

N00 Acute nephritic syndrome
  Includes: acute glomerular disease
  acute glomerulonephritis
  acute nephritis
  Excludes1: acute tubulo-interstitial nephritis (N10)
  nephritic syndrome NOS (N05.-)

MCC **N00.0 Acute nephritic syndrome with minor glomerular abnormality**
  Acute nephritic syndrome with minimal change lesion

MCC **N00.1 Acute nephritic syndrome with focal and segmental glomerular lesions**
  Acute nephritic syndrome with focal and segmental hyalinosis
  Acute nephritic syndrome with focal and segmental sclerosis
  Acute nephritic syndrome with focal glomerulonephritis

MCC **N00.2 Acute nephritic syndrome with diffuse membranous glomerulonephritis**

MCC **N00.3 Acute nephritic syndrome with diffuse mesangial proliferative glomerulonephritis**

MCC **N00.4 Acute nephritic syndrome with diffuse endocapillary proliferative glomerulonephritis**

MCC **N00.5 Acute nephritic syndrome with diffuse mesangiocapillary glomerulonephritis**
  Acute nephritic syndrome with membranoproliferative glomerulonephritis, types 1 and 3, or NOS
  Excludes1: Acute nephritic syndrome with C3 glomerulonephritis (N00.A)
  Acute nephritic syndrome with C3 glomerulopathy (N00.A)

MCC **N00.6 Acute nephritic syndrome with dense deposit disease**
  Acute nephritic syndrome with membranoproliferative glomerulonephritis, type 2
  Acute nephritic syndrome with C3 glomerulopathy with dense deposit disease

MCC **N00.7 Acute nephritic syndrome with diffuse crescentic glomerulonephritis**
  Acute nephritic syndrome with extracapillary glomerulonephritis

MCC **N00.8 Acute nephritic syndrome with other morphologic changes**
  Acute nephritic syndrome with proliferative glomerulonephritis NOS

MCC **N00.9 Acute nephritic syndrome with unspecified morphologic changes**

MCC **N00.A Acute nephritic syndrome with C3 glomerulonephritis**
  Acute nephritic syndrome with C3 glomerulopathy, NOS
  Excludes1: Acute nephritic syndrome (with C3 glomerulopathy) with dense deposit disease (N00.6)

N01 Rapidly progressive nephritic syndrome
  Includes: rapidly progressive glomerular disease
  rapidly progressive glomerulonephritis
  rapidly progressive nephritis
  Excludes1: nephritic syndrome NOS (N05.-)

MCC **N01.0 Rapidly progressive nephritic syndrome with minor glomerular abnormality**
  Rapidly progressive nephritic syndrome with minimal change lesion

MCC **N01.1 Rapidly progressive nephritic syndrome with focal and segmental glomerular lesions**
  Rapidly progressive nephritic syndrome with focal and segmental hyalinosis
  Rapidly progressive nephritic syndrome with focal and segmental sclerosis
  Rapidly progressive nephritic syndrome with focal glomerulonephritis

MCC **N01.2 Rapidly progressive nephritic syndrome with diffuse membranous glomerulonephritis**

MCC **N01.3 Rapidly progressive nephritic syndrome with diffuse mesangial proliferative glomerulonephritis**

MCC **N01.4 Rapidly progressive nephritic syndrome with diffuse endocapillary proliferative glomerulonephritis**

MCC **N01.5 Rapidly progressive nephritic syndrome with diffuse mesangiocapillary glomerulonephritis**
  Rapidly progressive nephritic syndrome with membranoproliferative glomerulonephritis, types 1 and 3, or NOS
  Excludes1: Rapidly progressive nephritic syndrome with C3 glomerulonephritis (N01.A)
  Rapidly progressive nephritic syndrome with C3 glomerulopathy (N01.A)

MCC **N01.6 Rapidly progressive nephritic syndrome with dense deposit disease**
  Rapidly progressive nephritic syndrome with membranoproliferative glomerulonephritis, type 2
  Rapidly progressive nephritic syndrome with C3 glomerulopathy with dense deposit disease

MCC **N01.7 Rapidly progressive nephritic syndrome with diffuse crescentic glomerulonephritis**
  Rapidly progressive nephritic syndrome with extracapillary glomerulonephritis

MCC **N01.8 Rapidly progressive nephritic syndrome with other morphologic changes**
  Rapidly progressive nephritic syndrome with proliferative glomerulonephritis NOS

MCC **N01.9 Rapidly progressive nephritic syndrome with unspecified morphologic changes**

MCC **N01.A Rapidly progressive nephritic syndrome with C3 glomerulonephritis**
  Rapidly progressive nephritic syndrome with C3 glomerulopathy, NOS
  Excludes1: Rapidly progressive nephritic syndrome (with C3 glomerulopathy) with dense deposit disease (N01.6)

N02 Recurrent and persistent hematuria
  Excludes1: acute cystitis with hematuria (N30.01)
  hematuria NOS (R31.9)
  hematuria not associated with specified morphologic lesions (R31.-)

CC **N02.0 Recurrent and persistent hematuria with minor glomerular abnormality**
  Recurrent and persistent hematuria with minimal change lesion

CC **N02.1 Recurrent and persistent hematuria with focal and segmental glomerular lesions**
  Recurrent and persistent hematuria with focal and segmental hyalinosis
  Recurrent and persistent hematuria with focal and segmental sclerosis
  Recurrent and persistent hematuria with focal glomerulonephritis

CC **N02.2 Recurrent and persistent hematuria with diffuse membranous glomerulonephritis**

CC **N02.3 Recurrent and persistent hematuria with diffuse mesangial proliferative glomerulonephritis**

CC **N02.4 Recurrent and persistent hematuria with diffuse endocapillary proliferative glomerulonephritis**

CC **N02.5 Recurrent and persistent hematuria with diffuse mesangiocapillary glomerulonephritis**
  Recurrent and persistent hematuria with membranoproliferative glomerulonephritis, types 1 and 3, or NOS
  Excludes1: Recurrent and persistent hematuria with C3 glomerulonephritis (N02.A)
  Recurrent and persistent hematuria with C3 glomerulopathy (N02.A)

CC **N02.6 Recurrent and persistent hematuria with dense deposit disease**
  Recurrent and persistent hematuria with membranoproliferative glomerulonephritis, type 2
  Recurrent and persistent hematuria with C3 glomerulopathy with dense deposit disease

CC **N02.7 Recurrent and persistent hematuria with diffuse crescentic glomerulonephritis**
  Recurrent and persistent hematuria with extracapillary glomerulonephritis

CC **N02.8 Recurrent and persistent hematuria with other morphologic changes**
  Recurrent and persistent hematuria with proliferative glomerulonephritis NOS

CC **N02.9 Recurrent and persistent hematuria with unspecified morphologic changes**
  AHA CC: 2Q, 2017, 5

CC **N02.A Recurrent and persistent hematuria with C3 glomerulonephritis**
  Recurrent and persistent hematuria with C3 glomerulopathy
  Excludes1: Recurrent and persistent hematuria (with C3 glomerulopathy) with dense deposit disease (N02.6)

- **+ N02.B Recurrent and persistent immunoglobulin A nephropathy**
  - CC **N02.B1** Recurrent and persistent immunoglobulin A nephropathy with glomerular lesion
  - CC **N02.B2** Recurrent and persistent immunoglobulin A nephropathy with focal and segmental glomerular lesion
    Recurrent and persistent immunoglobulin A nephropathy with focal and segmental hyalinosis or sclerosis
  - CC **N02.B3** Recurrent and persistent immunoglobulin A nephropathy with diffuse membranoproliferative glomerulonephritis
  - CC **N02.B4** Recurrent and persistent immunoglobulin A nephropathy with diffuse membranous glomerulonephritis
  - CC **N02.B5** Recurrent and persistent immunoglobulin A nephropathy with diffuse mesangial proliferative glomerulonephritis
  - CC **N02.B6** Recurrent and persistent immunoglobulin A nephropathy with diffuse mesangiocapillary glomerulonephritis
  - CC **N02.B9** Other recurrent and persistent immunoglobulin A nephropathy

N03 Chronic nephritic syndrome

Includes: chronic glomerular disease
chronic glomerulonephritis
chronic nephritis

Excludes1: chronic tubulo-interstitial nephritis (N11.-)
diffuse sclerosing glomerulonephritis (N05.8-)
nephritic syndrome NOS (N05.-)

- CC **N03.0** Chronic nephritic syndrome with minor glomerular abnormality
  Chronic nephritic syndrome with minimal change lesion
- CC **N03.1** Chronic nephritic syndrome with focal and segmental glomerular lesions
  Chronic nephritic syndrome with focal and segmental hyalinosis
  Chronic nephritic syndrome with focal and segmental sclerosis
  Chronic nephritic syndrome with focal glomerulonephritis
- CC **N03.2** Chronic nephritic syndrome with diffuse membranous glomerulonephritis
- CC **N03.3** Chronic nephritic syndrome with diffuse mesangial proliferative glomerulonephritis
- CC **N03.4** Chronic nephritic syndrome with diffuse endocapillary proliferative glomerulonephritis
- CC **N03.5** Chronic nephritic syndrome with diffuse mesangiocapillary glomerulonephritis
  Chronic nephritic syndrome with membranoproliferative glomerulonephritis, types 1 and 3, or NOS
  Excludes1: Chronic nephritic syndrome with C3 glomerulonephritis (N03.A)
  Chronic nephritic syndrome with C3 glomerulopathy (N03.A)
- CC **N03.6** Chronic nephritic syndrome with dense deposit disease
  Chronic nephritic syndrome with membranoproliferative glomerulonephritis, type 2
  Chronic nephritic syndrome with C3 glomerulopathy with dense deposit disease
- CC **N03.7** Chronic nephritic syndrome with diffuse crescentic glomerulonephritis
  Chronic nephritic syndrome with extracapillary glomerulonephritis
- CC **N03.8** Chronic nephritic syndrome with other morphologic changes
  Chronic nephritic syndrome with proliferative glomerulonephritis NOS
- CC **N03.9** Chronic nephritic syndrome with unspecified morphologic changes
- CC **N03.A** Chronic nephritic syndrome with C3 glomerulonephritis
  Chronic nephritic syndrome with C3 glomerulopathy
  Excludes1: Chronic nephritic syndrome (with C3 glomerulopathy) with dense deposit disease (N03.6)

N04 Nephrotic syndrome

Includes: congenital nephrotic syndrome
lipoid nephrosis

- CC **N04.0** Nephrotic syndrome with minor glomerular abnormality
  Nephrotic syndrome with minimal change lesion
- CC **N04.1** Nephrotic syndrome with focal and segmental glomerular lesions
  Nephrotic syndrome with focal and segmental hyalinosis
  Nephrotic syndrome with focal and segmental sclerosis
  Nephrotic syndrome with focal glomerulonephritis
- + **N04.2** Nephrotic syndrome with diffuse membranous glomerulonephritis
  - CC **N04.20** Nephrotic syndrome with diffuse membranous glomerulonephritis, unspecified
    Membranous nephropathy NOS with nephrotic syndrome
  - CC **N04.21** Primary membranous nephropathy with nephrotic syndrome
    Idiopathic membranous nephropathy with nephrotic syndrome
  - CC **N04.22** Secondary membranous nephropathy with nephrotic syndrome
    Code first, if applicable, other disease or disorder or poisoning causing membranous nephropathy
    Use Additional code, if applicable, for adverse effect of drug causing membranous nephropathy
  - CC **N04.29** Other nephrotic syndrome with diffuse membranous glomerulonephritis
- CC **N04.3** Nephrotic syndrome with diffuse mesangial proliferative glomerulonephritis
- CC **N04.4** Nephrotic syndrome with diffuse endocapillary proliferative glomerulonephritis
- CC **N04.5** Nephrotic syndrome with diffuse mesangiocapillary glomerulonephritis
  Nephrotic syndrome with membranoproliferative glomerulonephritis, types 1 and 3, or NOS
  Excludes1: Nephrotic syndrome with C3 glomerulonephritis (N04.A)
  Nephrotic syndrome with C3 glomerulopathy (N04.A)
- CC **N04.6** Nephrotic syndrome with dense deposit disease
  Nephrotic syndrome with membranoproliferative glomerulonephritis, type 2
  Nephrotic syndrome with C3 glomerulopathy with dense deposit disease
- CC **N04.7** Nephrotic syndrome with diffuse crescentic glomerulonephritis
  Nephrotic syndrome with extracapillary glomerulonephritis
- CC **N04.8** Nephrotic syndrome with other morphologic changes
  Nephrotic syndrome with proliferative glomerulonephritis NOS
- CC **N04.9** Nephrotic syndrome with unspecified morphologic changes
- CC **N04.A** Nephrotic syndrome with C3 glomerulonephritis
  Nephrotic syndrome with C3 glomerulopathy
  Excludes1: Nephrotic syndrome (with C3 glomerulopathy) with dense deposit disease (N04.6)

N05 Unspecified nephritic syndrome

Includes: glomerular disease NOS
glomerulonephritis NOS
nephritis NOS
nephropathy NOS and renal disease NOS with morphological lesion specified in .0-.8

Excludes1: nephropathy NOS with no stated morphological lesion (N28.9)
renal disease NOS with no stated morphological lesion (N28.9)
tubulo-interstitial nephritis NOS (N12)

- **N05.0** Unspecified nephritic syndrome with minor glomerular abnormality
  Unspecified nephritic syndrome with minimal change lesion
- **N05.1** Unspecified nephritic syndrome with focal and segmental glomerular lesions
  Unspecified nephritic syndrome with focal and segmental hyalinosis
  Unspecified nephritic syndrome with focal and segmental sclerosis
  Unspecified nephritic syndrome with focal glomerulonephritis
- CC **N05.2** Unspecified nephritic syndrome with diffuse membranous glomerulonephritis
- CC **N05.3** Unspecified nephritic syndrome with diffuse mesangial proliferative glomerulonephritis

CC N05.4 Unspecified nephritic syndrome with diffuse endocapillary proliferative glomerulonephritis

CC N05.5 Unspecified nephritic syndrome with diffuse mesangiocapillary glomerulonephritis
Unspecified nephritic syndrome with membranoproliferative glomerulonephritis, types 1 and 3, or NOS
Excludes1: Unspecified nephritic syndrome with C3 glomerulonephritis (N05.A)
Unspecified nephritic syndrome with C3 glomerulopathy (N05.A)

N05.6 Unspecified nephritic syndrome with dense deposit disease
Unspecified nephritic syndrome with membranoproliferative glomerulonephritis, type 2
Unspecified nephritic syndrome with C3 glomerulopathy with dense deposit disease

N05.7 Unspecified nephritic syndrome with diffuse crescentic glomerulonephritis
Unspecified nephritic syndrome with extracapillary glomerulonephritis

N05.8 Unspecified nephritic syndrome with other morphologic changes
Unspecified nephritic syndrome with proliferative glomerulonephritis NOS

N05.9 Unspecified nephritic syndrome with unspecified morphologic changes

CC N05.A Unspecified nephritic syndrome with C3 glomerulonephritis
Unspecified nephritic syndrome with C3 glomerulopathy
Excludes1: Unspecified nephritic syndrome (with C3 glomerulopathy) with dense deposit disease (N05.6)

N06 Isolated proteinuria with specified morphological lesion
Excludes1: Proteinuria not associated with specific morphologic lesions (R80.0)

N06.0 Isolated proteinuria with minor glomerular abnormality
Isolated proteinuria with minimal change lesion

N06.1 Isolated proteinuria with focal and segmental glomerular lesions
Isolated proteinuria with focal and segmental hyalinosis
Isolated proteinuria with focal and segmental sclerosis
Isolated proteinuria with focal glomerulonephritis

+ N06.2 Isolated proteinuria with diffuse membranous glomerulonephritis

CC N06.20 Isolated proteinuria with diffuse membranous glomerulonephritis, unspecified
Membranous nephropathy, NOS
Excludes1: membranous nephropathy NOS with nephrotic syndrome (N04.20)

CC N06.21 Primary membranous nephropathy with isolated proteinuria
Idiopathic membranous nephropathy (with isolated proteinuria)
Primary membranous nephropathy, NOS
Excludes1: primary membranous nephropathy with nephrotic syndrome (N04.21)

CC N06.22 Secondary membranous nephropathy with isolated proteinuria
Secondary membranous nephropathy, NOS
Code first, if applicable, other disease or disorder or poisoning causing membranous nephropathy

Use Additional code, if applicable, for adverse effect of drug causing membranous nephropathy
Excludes1: secondary membranous nephropathy with nephrotic syndrome (N04.22)

CC N06.29 Other isolated proteinuria with diffuse membranous glomerulonephritis

CC N06.3 Isolated proteinuria with diffuse mesangial proliferative glomerulonephritis

CC N06.4 Isolated proteinuria with diffuse endocapillary proliferative glomerulonephritis

CC N06.5 Isolated proteinuria with diffuse mesangiocapillary glomerulonephritis
Isolated proteinuria with membranoproliferative glomerulonephritis, types 1 and 3, or NOS
Excludes1: Isolated proteinuria with C3 glomerulonephritis (N06.A)
Isolated proteinuria with C3 glomerulopathy (N06.A)

N06.6 Isolated proteinuria with dense deposit disease
Isolated proteinuria with membranoproliferative glomerulonephritis, type 2
Isolated proteinuria with C3 glomerulopathy with dense deposit disease

N06.7 Isolated proteinuria with diffuse crescentic glomerulonephritis
Isolated proteinuria with extracapillary glomerulonephritis

N06.8 Isolated proteinuria with other morphologic lesion
Isolated proteinuria with proliferative glomerulonephritis NOS

N06.9 Isolated proteinuria with unspecified morphologic lesion

CC N06.A Isolated proteinuria with C3 glomerulonephritis
Isolated proteinuria with C3 glomerulopathy
Excludes1: Isolated proteinuria (with C3 glomerulopathy) with dense deposit disease (N06.6)

N07 Hereditary nephropathy, not elsewhere classified
Excludes2: Alport's syndrome (Q87.81-)
hereditary amyloid nephropathy (E85.-)
nail patella syndrome (Q87.2)
non-neuropathic heredofamilial amyloidosis (E85.-)

N07.0 Hereditary nephropathy, not elsewhere classified with minor glomerular abnormality
Hereditary nephropathy, not elsewhere classified with minimal change lesion

N07.1 Hereditary nephropathy, not elsewhere classified with focal and segmental glomerular lesions
Hereditary nephropathy, not elsewhere classified with focal and segmental hyalinosis
Hereditary nephropathy, not elsewhere classified with focal and segmental sclerosis
Hereditary nephropathy, not elsewhere classified with focal glomerulonephritis

CC N07.2 Hereditary nephropathy, not elsewhere classified with diffuse membranous glomerulonephritis

CC N07.3 Hereditary nephropathy, not elsewhere classified with diffuse mesangial proliferative glomerulonephritis

CC N07.4 Hereditary nephropathy, not elsewhere classified with diffuse endocapillary proliferative glomerulonephritis

CC N07.5 Hereditary nephropathy, not elsewhere classified with diffuse mesangiocapillary glomerulonephritis
Hereditary nephropathy, not elsewhere classified with membranoproliferative glomerulonephritis, types 1 and 3, or NOS
Excludes1: Hereditary nephropathy, not elsewhere classified with C3 glomerulonephritis (N07.A)
Hereditary nephropathy, not elsewhere classified with C3 glomerulopathy (N07.A)

N07.6 Hereditary nephropathy, not elsewhere classified with dense deposit disease
Hereditary nephropathy, not elsewhere classified with membranoproliferative glomerulonephritis, type 2
Hereditary nephropathy, not elsewhere classified with C3 glomerulopathy with dense deposit disease

N07.7 Hereditary nephropathy, not elsewhere classified with diffuse crescentic glomerulonephritis
Hereditary nephropathy, not elsewhere classified with extracapillary glomerulonephritis

N07.8 Hereditary nephropathy, not elsewhere classified with other morphologic lesions
Hereditary nephropathy, not elsewhere classified with proliferative glomerulonephritis NOS

N07.9 Hereditary nephropathy, not elsewhere classified with unspecified morphologic lesions

CC N07.A Hereditary nephropathy, not elsewhere classified with C3 glomerulonephritis
Hereditary nephropathy, not elsewhere classified with C3 glomerulopathy
Excludes1: Hereditary nephropathy, not elsewhere classified (with C3 glomerulopathy) with dense deposit disease (N07.6)

N08 Glomerular disorders in diseases classified elsewhere
Glomerulonephritis
Nephritis
Nephropathy
Code first underlying disease, such as:
amyloidosis (E85.-)
congenital syphilis (A50.5)
cryoglobulinemia (D89.1)

disseminated intravascular coagulation (D65)
gout (M1A.-, M10.-)
microscopic polyangiitis (M31.7)
multiple myeloma (C90.0-)
sepsis (A40.0-A41.9)
sickle-cell disease (D57.0-D57.8)

Excludes1: glomerulonephritis, nephritis and nephropathy (in):
antiglomerular basement membrane disease (M31.0)
diabetes (E08-E13 with .21)
gonococcal (A54.21)
Goodpasture's syndrome (M31.0)
hemolytic-uremic syndrome (D59.3-)
lupus (M32.14)
mumps (B26.83)
syphilis (A52.75)
systemic lupus erythematosus (M32.14)
Wegener's granulomatosis (M31.31)
pyelonephritis in diseases classified elsewhere (N16)
renal tubulo-interstitial disorders classified elsewhere (N16)

Valid 3-character code, no further characters required

Renal tubulo-interstitial diseases (N10-N16)

Includes: pyelonephritis

Excludes1: pyeloureteritis cystica (N28.85)

CC N10 Acute pyelonephritis
Acute infectious interstitial nephritis
Acute pyelitis
Acute tubulo-interstitial nephritis
Hemoglobin nephrosis
Myoglobin nephrosis
Use additional code (B95-B97), to identify infectious agent
AHA CC: 3Q, 2019, 13-14; 3Q, 2020, 25-26
HAC see Appendix B for HAC conditional logic
Valid 3-character code, no further characters required

N11 Chronic tubulo-interstitial nephritis
Includes: chronic infectious interstitial nephritis
chronic pyelitis
chronic pyelonephritis
Use additional code (B95-B97), to identify infectious agent

- **N11.0 Nonobstructive reflux-associated chronic pyelonephritis**
  Pyelonephritis (chronic) associated with (vesicoureteral) reflux
  Excludes1: vesicoureteral reflux NOS (N13.70)

- **CC N11.1 Chronic obstructive pyelonephritis**
  Pyelonephritis (chronic) associated with anomaly of pelviureteric junction
  Pyelonephritis (chronic) associated with anomaly of pyeloureteric junction
  Pyelonephritis (chronic) associated with crossing of vessel
  Pyelonephritis (chronic) associated with kinking of ureter
  Pyelonephritis (chronic) associated with obstruction of ureter
  Pyelonephritis (chronic) associated with stricture of pelviureteric junction
  Pyelonephritis (chronic) associated with stricture of ureter
  Excludes1: calculous pyelonephritis (N20.9)
  obstructive uropathy (N13.-)

- **CC N11.8 Other chronic tubulo-interstitial nephritis**
  Nonobstructive chronic pyelonephritis NOS

- **CC N11.9 Chronic tubulo-interstitial nephritis, unspecified**
  Chronic interstitial nephritis NOS
  Chronic pyelitis NOS
  Chronic pyelonephritis NOS
  HAC see Appendix B for HAC conditional logic

CC N12 Tubulo-interstitial nephritis, not specified as acute or chronic
Interstitial nephritis NOS
Pyelitis NOS
Pyelonephritis NOS
Excludes1: calculous pyelonephritis (N20.9)
HAC see Appendix B for HAC conditional logic
Valid 3-character code, no further characters required

N13 Obstructive and reflux uropathy
Excludes2: calculus of kidney and ureter without hydronephrosis (N20.-)
congenital obstructive defects of renal pelvis and ureter (Q62.0-Q62.3)
hydronephrosis with ureteropelvic junction obstruction (Q62.11)
obstructive pyelonephritis (N11.1)

- **CC N13.0 Hydronephrosis with ureteropelvic junction obstruction**
  Hydronephrosis due to acquired occlusion of ureteropelvic junction
  Excludes2: Hydronephrosis with ureteropelvic junction obstruction due to calculus (N13.2)
  AHA CC: 4Q, 2016, 43

- **CC N13.1 Hydronephrosis with ureteral stricture, not elsewhere classified**
  Excludes1: hydronephrosis with ureteral stricture with infection (N13.6)

- **N13.2 Hydronephrosis with renal and ureteral calculous obstruction**
  Excludes1: hydronephrosis with renal and ureteral calculous obstruction with infection (N13.6)

- **+ N13.3 Other and unspecified hydronephrosis**
  Excludes1: hydronephrosis with infection (N13.6)
  - **CC N13.30 Unspecified hydronephrosis**
  - **CC N13.39 Other hydronephrosis**

- **CC N13.4 Hydroureter**
  Excludes1: congenital hydroureter (Q62.3-)
  hydroureter with infection (N13.6)
  vesicoureteral-reflux with hydroureter (N13.73-)

- **N13.5 Crossing vessel and stricture of ureter without hydronephrosis**
  Kinking and stricture of ureter without hydronephrosis
  Excludes1: Crossing vessel and stricture of ureter without hydronephrosis with infection (N13.6)

- **CC N13.6 Pyonephrosis**
  Conditions in N13.0-N13.5 with infection
  Obstructive uropathy with infection
  Use additional code (B95-B97), to identify infectious agent
  AHA CC: 2Q, 2018, 21
  HAC see Appendix B for HAC conditional logic

- **+ N13.7 Vesicoureteral-reflux**
  Excludes1: reflux-associated pyelonephritis (N11.0)
  - **N13.70 Vesicoureteral-reflux, unspecified**
    Vesicoureteral-reflux NOS
  - **N13.71 Vesicoureteral-reflux without reflux nephropathy**
  - **+ N13.72 Vesicoureteral-reflux with reflux nephropathy without hydroureter**
    - **N13.721 Vesicoureteral-reflux with reflux nephropathy without hydroureter, unilateral**
    - **N13.722 Vesicoureteral-reflux with reflux nephropathy without hydroureter, bilateral**
    - **N13.729 Vesicoureteral-reflux with reflux nephropathy without hydroureter, unspecified**
  - **+ N13.73 Vesicoureteral-reflux with reflux nephropathy with hydroureter**
    - **N13.731 Vesicoureteral-reflux with reflux nephropathy with hydroureter, unilateral**
    - **N13.732 Vesicoureteral-reflux with reflux nephropathy with hydroureter, bilateral**
    - **N13.739 Vesicoureteral-reflux with reflux nephropathy with hydroureter, unspecified**

- **CC N13.8 Other obstructive and reflux uropathy**
  Urinary tract obstruction due to specified cause
  Code first, if applicable, any causal condition, such as:
  enlarged prostate (N40.1)

- **N13.9 Obstructive and reflux uropathy, unspecified**
  Urinary tract obstruction NOS

N14 Drug- and heavy-metal-induced tubulo-interstitial and tubular conditions
Code first poisoning due to drug or toxin, if applicable (T36-T65 with fifth or sixth character 1-4)
Use additional code for adverse effect, if applicable, to identify drug (T36-T50 with fifth or sixth character 5)

- **N14.0 Analgesic nephropathy**
- **+ N14.1 Nephropathy induced by other drugs, medicaments and biological substances**
  AHA CC: 3Q, 2021, 9-10; 4Q, 2022, 33
  - **N14.11 Contrast-induced nephropathy**
    Contrast medium, radiography nephropathy
    Excludes2: acute kidney failure (N17.-)
    AHA CC: 4Q, 2022, 33
  - **N14.19 Nephropathy induced by other drugs, medicaments and biological substances**

N14.2 Nephropathy induced by unspecified drug, medicament or biological substance
N14.3 Nephropathy induced by heavy metals
N14.4 Toxic nephropathy, not elsewhere classified

N15 Other renal tubulo-interstitial diseases

N15.0 Balkan nephropathy
Balkan endemic nephropathy

MCC N15.1 Renal and perinephric abscess
HAC see Appendix B for HAC conditional logic

N15.8 Other specified renal tubulo-interstitial diseases

N15.9 Renal tubulo-interstitial disease, unspecified
Infection of kidney NOS
Excludes1: urinary tract infection NOS (N39.0)

N16 Renal tubulo-interstitial disorders in diseases classified elsewhere

Pyelonephritis
Tubulo-interstitial nephritis
Code first underlying disease, such as:
 brucellosis (A23.0-A23.9)
 cryoglobulinemia (D89.1)
 glycogen storage disease (E74.0-)
 leukemia (C91-C95)
 lymphoma (C81.0-C85.9, C96.0-C96.9)
 multiple myeloma (C90.0-)
 sepsis (A40.0-A41.9)
 Wilson's disease (E83.01)
Excludes1: diphtheritic pyelonephritis and tubulo-interstitial nephritis (A36.84)
 pyelonephritis and tubulo-interstitial nephritis in candidiasis (B37.49)
 pyelonephritis and tubulo-interstitial nephritis in cystinosis (E72.04)
 pyelonephritis and tubulo-interstitial nephritis in salmonella infection (A02.25)
 pyelonephritis and tubulo-interstitial nephritis in sarcoidosis (D86.84)
 pyelonephritis and tubulo-interstitial nephritis in Sjögren's syndrome (M35.04)
 pyelonephritis and tubulo-interstitial nephritis in systemic lupus erythematosus (M32.15)
 pyelonephritis and tubulo-interstitial nephritis in toxoplasmosis (B58.83)
 renal tubular degeneration in diabetes (E08-E13 with .29)
 syphilitic pyelonephritis and tubulo-interstitial nephritis (A52.75)

Valid 3-character code, no further characters required

Acute kidney failure and chronic kidney disease (N17-N19)

Excludes2: congenital renal failure (P96.0)
 drug- and heavy-metal-induced tubulo-interstitial and tubular conditions (N14.-)
 extrarenal uremia (R39.2)
 hemolytic-uremic syndrome (D59.3-)
 hepatorenal syndrome (K76.7)
 postpartum hepatorenal syndrome (O90.41)
 posttraumatic renal failure (T79.5)
 prerenal uremia (R39.2)
 renal failure complicating abortion or ectopic or molar pregnancy (O00-O07, O08.4)
 renal failure following labor and delivery (O90.41)
 renal failure postprocedural (N99.0)

N17 Acute kidney failure
Code also associated underlying condition
Excludes1: posttraumatic renal failure (T79.5)

MCC N17.0 Acute kidney failure with tubular necrosis
Acute tubular necrosis
Renal tubular necrosis
Tubular necrosis NOS
AHA CC: 3Q, 2020, 22; 3Q, 2021, 10; 4Q, 2022, 33

MCC N17.1 Acute kidney failure with acute cortical necrosis
Acute cortical necrosis
Cortical necrosis NOS
Renal cortical necrosis

N17.2 Acute kidney failure with medullary necrosis
Medullary [papillary] necrosis NOS
Acute medullary [papillary] necrosis
Renal medullary [papillary] necrosis

CC N17.8 Other acute kidney failure

CC N17.9 Acute kidney failure, unspecified
Acute kidney injury (nontraumatic)
Excludes2: traumatic kidney injury (S37.0-)
AHA CC: 2Q, 2019, 7, 24-26

N18 Chronic kidney disease (CKD)
Code first any associated:
 diabetic chronic kidney disease (E08.22, E09.22, E10.22, E11.22, E13.22)
 hypertensive chronic kidney disease (I12.-, I13.-)
Use additional code to identify kidney transplant status, if applicable, (Z94.0)
Review coding guidelines C.9.a.2 and C.9.a.3
Review coding guidelines C.14.a.1 and C.14.a.2

N18.1 Chronic kidney disease, stage 1
N18.2 Chronic kidney disease, stage 2 (mild)
+ N18.3 Chronic kidney disease, stage 3 (moderate)
AHA CC: 4Q, 2020, 35
 N18.30 Chronic kidney disease, stage 3 unspecified
 AHA CC: 4Q, 2022, 5-6
 N18.31 Chronic kidney disease, stage 3a
 N18.32 Chronic kidney disease, stage 3b
CC N18.4 Chronic kidney disease, stage 4 (severe)
AHA CC: 4Q, 2022, 14; 1Q, 2023, 17-18
CC N18.5 Chronic kidney disease, stage 5
Excludes1: chronic kidney disease, stage 5 requiring chronic dialysis (N18.6)
MCC N18.6 End stage renal disease
Chronic kidney disease requiring chronic dialysis
Use additional code to identify dialysis status (Z99.2)
AHA CC: 4Q, 2013, 125; 3Q, 2016, 22-23; 3Q, 2022, 15-16
N18.9 Chronic kidney disease, unspecified
Chronic renal disease
Chronic renal failure NOS
Chronic renal insufficiency
Chronic uremia NOS
Diffuse sclerosing glomerulonephritis NOS
AHA CC: 4Q, 2018, 88-89

N19 Unspecified kidney failure
Uremia NOS
Excludes1: acute kidney failure (N17.-)
 chronic kidney disease (N18.-)
 chronic uremia (N18.9)
 extrarenal uremia (R39.2)
 prerenal uremia (R39.2)
 renal insufficiency (acute) (N28.9)
 uremia of newborn (P96.0)

Valid 3-character code, no further characters required

Urolithiasis (N20-N23)

N20 Calculus of kidney and ureter
Calculous pyelonephritis
Excludes1: nephrocalcinosis (E83.59)
 that with hydronephrosis (N13.2)

N20.0 Calculus of kidney
Nephrolithiasis NOS
Renal calculus
Renal stone
Staghorn calculus
Stone in kidney
AHA CC: 1Q, 2017, 5; 3Q, 2019, 13-14

CC N20.1 Calculus of ureter
Calculus of the ureteropelvic junction
Ureteric stone
AHA CC: 3Q, 2016, 23-24

CC N20.2 Calculus of kidney with calculus of ureter
AHA CC: 2Q, 2015, 8-9

N20.9 Urinary calculus, unspecified

N21 Calculus of lower urinary tract
Includes: calculus of lower urinary tract with cystitis and urethritis

N21.0 Calculus in bladder
Calculus in diverticulum of bladder
Urinary bladder stone
Excludes2: staghorn calculus (N20.0)

N21.1 Calculus in urethra
Excludes2: calculus of prostate (N42.0)

N21.8 Other lower urinary tract calculus

N21.9 Calculus of lower urinary tract, unspecified
Excludes1: calculus of urinary tract NOS (N20.9)

N22 Calculus of urinary tract in diseases classified elsewhere
   Code first underlying disease, such as:
      gout (M1A.-, M10.-)
      schistosomiasis (B65.0-B65.9)
   Valid 3-character code, no further characters required

N23 Unspecified renal colic
   Valid 3-character code, no further characters required

Other disorders of kidney and ureter (N25-N29)

Excludes2: disorders of kidney and ureter with urolithiasis (N20-N23)

N25 Disorders resulting from impaired renal tubular function
   N25.0 Renal osteodystrophy
      Azotemic osteodystrophy
      Phosphate-losing tubular disorders
      Renal rickets
      Renal short stature
      Excludes2: metabolic disorders classifiable to E70-E88
   CC **N25.1 Nephrogenic diabetes insipidus**
      Excludes1: diabetes insipidus NOS (E23.2)
   + **N25.8 Other disorders resulting from impaired renal tubular function**
      CC **N25.81 Secondary hyperparathyroidism of renal origin**
         Excludes1: secondary hyperparathyroidism, non-renal (E21.1)
         Excludes2: metabolic disorders classifiable to E70-E88
      N25.89 Other disorders resulting from impaired renal tubular function
         Hypokalemic nephropathy
         Lightwood-Albright syndrome
         Renal tubular acidosis NOS
   N25.9 Disorder resulting from impaired renal tubular function, unspecified

N26 Unspecified contracted kidney
   Excludes1: contracted kidney due to hypertension (I12.-)
      diffuse sclerosing glomerulonephritis (N05.8.-)
      hypertensive nephrosclerosis (arteriolar) (arteriosclerotic) (I12.-)
      small kidney of unknown cause (N27.-)
   N26.1 Atrophy of kidney (terminal)
   N26.2 Page kidney
   N26.9 Renal sclerosis, unspecified

N27 Small kidney of unknown cause
   Includes: oligonephronia
   N27.0 Small kidney, unilateral
   N27.1 Small kidney, bilateral
   N27.9 Small kidney, unspecified

N28 Other disorders of kidney and ureter, not elsewhere classified
   CC **N28.0 Ischemia and infarction of kidney**
      Renal artery embolism
      Renal artery obstruction
      Renal artery occlusion
      Renal artery thrombosis
      Renal infarct
      Excludes1: atherosclerosis of renal artery (extrarenal part) (I70.1)
         congenital stenosis of renal artery (Q27.1)
         Goldblatt's kidney (I70.1)
   N28.1 Cyst of kidney, acquired
      Cyst (multiple) (solitary) of kidney (acquired)
      Excludes1: cystic kidney disease (congenital) (Q61.-)
   + **N28.8 Other specified disorders of kidney and ureter**
      Excludes1: hydroureter (N13.4)
         ureteric stricture with hydronephrosis (N13.1)
         ureteric stricture without hydronephrosis (N13.5)

      N28.81 Hypertrophy of kidney
      N28.82 Megaloureter
      N28.83 Nephroptosis
   CC **N28.84 Pyelitis cystica**
      HAC see Appendix B for HAC conditional logic
   CC **N28.85 Pyeloureteritis cystica**
      HAC see Appendix B for HAC conditional logic
   CC **N28.86 Ureteritis cystica**
      HAC see Appendix B for HAC conditional logic
      N28.89 Other specified disorders of kidney and ureter
   N28.9 Disorder of kidney and ureter, unspecified
      Nephropathy NOS
      Renal disease (acute) NOS
      Renal insufficiency (acute)
      Excludes1: chronic renal insufficiency (N18.9)
         unspecified nephritic syndrome (N05.-)
      AHA CC: 1Q, 2016, 13

N29 Other disorders of kidney and ureter in diseases classified elsewhere
   Code first underlying disease, such as:
      amyloidosis (E85.-)
      nephrocalcinosis (E83.59)
      schistosomiasis (B65.0-B65.9)
   Excludes1: disorders of kidney and ureter in:
      cystinosis (E72.0)
      gonorrhea (A54.21)
      syphilis (A52.75)
      tuberculosis (A18.11)
   Valid 3-character code, no further characters required

Other diseases of the urinary system (N30-N39)

Excludes2: urinary infection (complicating):
   abortion or ectopic or molar pregnancy (O00-O07, O08.8)
   pregnancy, childbirth and the puerperium (O23.-, O75.3, O86.2-)

N30 Cystitis
   Use additional code to identify infectious agent (B95-B97)
   Excludes1: prostatocystitis (N41.3)
   + **N30.0 Acute cystitis**
      Excludes1: irradiation cystitis (N30.4-)
         trigonitis (N30.3-)
      CC **N30.00 Acute cystitis without hematuria**
         HAC see Appendix B for HAC conditional logic
      CC **N30.01 Acute cystitis with hematuria**
         HAC see Appendix B for HAC conditional logic
   + **N30.1 Interstitial cystitis (chronic)**
      N30.10 Interstitial cystitis (chronic) without hematuria
      N30.11 Interstitial cystitis (chronic) with hematuria
   + **N30.2 Other chronic cystitis**
      N30.20 Other chronic cystitis without hematuria
      N30.21 Other chronic cystitis with hematuria
   + **N30.3 Trigonitis**
      Urethrotrigonitis
      N30.30 Trigonitis without hematuria
      N30.31 Trigonitis with hematuria
   + **N30.4 Irradiation cystitis**
      CC **N30.40 Irradiation cystitis without hematuria**
      CC **N30.41 Irradiation cystitis with hematuria**
   + **N30.8 Other cystitis**
      Abscess of bladder
      N30.80 Other cystitis without hematuria
      N30.81 Other cystitis with hematuria
   + **N30.9 Cystitis, unspecified**
      N30.90 Cystitis, unspecified without hematuria
      N30.91 Cystitis, unspecified with hematuria

N31 Neuromuscular dysfunction of bladder, not elsewhere classified
   Use additional code to identify any associated urinary incontinence (N39.3-N39.4-)
   Excludes1: cord bladder NOS (G95.89)
      neurogenic bladder due to cauda equina syndrome (G83.4)
      neuromuscular dysfunction due to spinal cord lesion (G95.89)

893

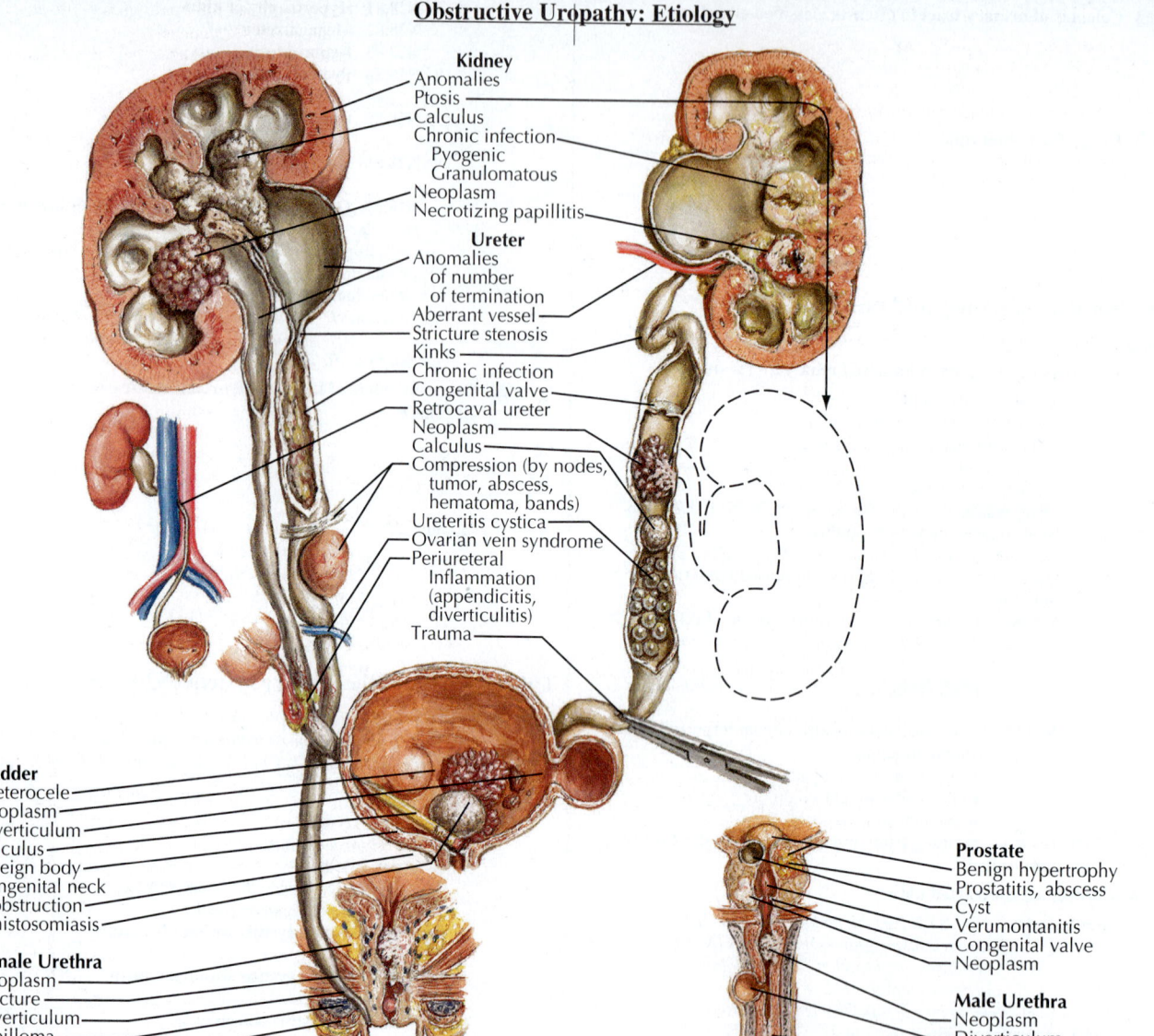

Obstructive Uropathy: Etiology

© 2008 Elsevier Inc. All rights reserved. www.netterimages.com

- N31.0 Uninhibited neuropathic bladder, not elsewhere classified
- N31.1 Reflex neuropathic bladder, not elsewhere classified
- N31.2 Flaccid neuropathic bladder, not elsewhere classified
  - Atonic (motor) (sensory) neuropathic bladder
  - Autonomous neuropathic bladder
  - Nonreflex neuropathic bladder
- N31.8 Other neuromuscular dysfunction of bladder
- N31.9 Neuromuscular dysfunction of bladder, unspecified
  - Neurogenic bladder dysfunction NOS

N32 Other disorders of bladder

Excludes2: *calculus of bladder (N21.0)*
cystocele (N81.1-)
hernia or prolapse of bladder, female (N81.1-)

- N32.0 Bladder-neck obstruction
  - Bladder-neck stenosis (acquired)
  - **Excludes1:** *congenital bladder-neck obstruction (Q64.3-)*
- CC N32.1 Vesicointestinal fistula
  - Vesicorectal fistula
- CC N32.2 Vesical fistula, not elsewhere classified
  - **Excludes1:** *fistula between bladder and female genital tract (N82.0-N82.1)*
- N32.3 Diverticulum of bladder
  - **Excludes1:** *congenital diverticulum of bladder (Q64.6)*
  - *diverticulitis of bladder (N30.8-)*

+ N32.8 Other specified disorders of bladder
- N32.81 Overactive bladder
  - Detrusor muscle hyperactivity
  - **Excludes1:** *frequent urination due to specified bladder condition-code to condition*
- N32.89 Other specified disorders of bladder
  - Bladder hemorrhage
  - Bladder hypertrophy
  - Calcified bladder
  - Contracted bladder
- N32.9 Bladder disorder, unspecified

N33 Bladder disorders in diseases classified elsewhere

Code first underlying disease, such as:
schistosomiasis (B65.0-B65.9)

Excludes1: *bladder disorder in syphilis (A52.76)*
bladder disorder in tuberculosis (A18.12)
candidal cystitis (B37.41)
chlamydial cystitis (A56.01)
cystitis in gonorrhea (A54.01)
cystitis in neurogenic bladder (N31.-)
diphtheritic cystitis (A36.85)
syphilitic cystitis (A52.76)
trichomonal cystitis (A59.03)

Valid 3-character code, no further characters required

N34 Urethritis and urethral syndrome
Use additional code (B95-B97), to identify infectious agent.
Excludes2: Reiter's disease (M02.3-)
urethritis in diseases with a predominantly sexual mode of transmission (A50-A64)
urethrotrigonitis (N30.3-)

CC N34.0 Urethral abscess
Abscess (of) Cowper's gland
Abscess (of) Littré's gland
Abscess (of) urethral (gland)
Periurethral abscess
Excludes1: urethral caruncle (N36.2)
HAC see Appendix B for HAC conditional logic

N34.1 Nonspecific urethritis
Nongonococcal urethritis
Nonvenereal urethritis

N34.2 Other urethritis
Meatitis, urethral
Postmenopausal urethritis
Ulcer of urethra (meatus)
Urethritis NOS

N34.3 Urethral syndrome, unspecified

N35 Urethral stricture
Excludes1: congenital urethral stricture (Q64.3-)
postprocedural urethral stricture (N99.1-)

+ **N35.0 Post-traumatic urethral stricture**
Urethral stricture due to injury
Excludes1: postprocedural urethral stricture (N99.1-)

+ **N35.01 Post-traumatic urethral stricture, male**
- ♂ N35.010 Post-traumatic urethral stricture, male, meatal
- ♂ N35.011 Post-traumatic bulbous urethral stricture
- ♂ N35.012 Post-traumatic membranous urethral stricture
- ♂ N35.013 Post-traumatic anterior urethral stricture
- ♂ N35.014 Post-traumatic urethral stricture, male, unspecified
- ♂ N35.016 Post-traumatic urethral stricture, male, overlapping sites
  AHA CC: 4Q, 2018, 21-22

+ **N35.02 Post-traumatic urethral stricture, female**
- ♀ N35.021 Urethral stricture due to childbirth
- ♀ N35.028 Other post-traumatic urethral stricture, female

+ **N35.1 Postinfective urethral stricture, not elsewhere classified**
Excludes1: urethral stricture associated with schistosomiasis (B65.-, N29)
gonococcal urethral stricture (A54.01)
syphilitic urethral stricture (A52.76)

+ **N35.11 Postinfective urethral stricture, not elsewhere classified, male**
- ♂ N35.111 Postinfective urethral stricture, not elsewhere classified, male, meatal
- ♂ N35.112 Postinfective bulbous urethral stricture, not elsewhere classified, male
- ♂ N35.113 Postinfective membranous urethral stricture, not elsewhere classified, male
- ♂ N35.114 Postinfective anterior urethral stricture, not elsewhere classified, male
- ♂ N35.116 Postinfective urethral stricture, not elsewhere classified, male, overlapping sites
  AHA CC: 4Q, 2018, 21-22
- ♂ N35.119 Postinfective urethral stricture, not elsewhere classified, male, unspecified
- ♀ N35.12 Postinfective urethral stricture, not elsewhere classified, female

+ **N35.8 Other urethral stricture**
Excludes1: postprocedural urethral stricture (N99.1-)

+ **N35.81 Other urethral stricture, male**
AHA CC: 4Q, 2018, 21-22
- ♂ N35.811 Other urethral stricture, male, meatal
- ♂ N35.812 Other bulbous urethral stricture, male
- ♂ N35.813 Other membranous urethral stricture, male
- ♂ N35.814 Other anterior urethral stricture, male
- ♂ N35.816 Other urethral stricture, male, overlapping sites
- ♂ N35.819 Other urethral stricture, male, unspecified site
- ♀ N35.82 Other urethral stricture, female
  AHA CC: 4Q, 2018, 21-22

+ **N35.9 Urethral stricture, unspecified**
+ **N35.91 Urethral stricture, unspecified, male**
AHA CC: 4Q, 2018, 21-22
- ♂ N35.911 Unspecified urethral stricture, male, meatal
- ♂ N35.912 Unspecified bulbous urethral stricture, male
- ♂ N35.913 Unspecified membranous urethral stricture, male
- ♂ N35.914 Unspecified anterior urethral stricture, male
- ♂ N35.916 Unspecified urethral stricture, male, overlapping sites
- ♂ N35.919 Unspecified urethral stricture, male, unspecified site
  Pinhole meatus NOS
  Urethral stricture NOS
- ♀ N35.92 Unspecified urethral stricture, female
  AHA CC: 4Q, 2018, 21-22

N36 Other disorders of urethra

CC N36.0 Urethral fistula
Urethroperineal fistula
Urethrorectal fistula
Urinary fistula NOS
Excludes1: urethroscrotal fistula (N50.89)
urethrovaginal fistula (N82.1)
urethrovesicovaginal fistula (N82.1)

N36.1 Urethral diverticulum

N36.2 Urethral caruncle

+ **N36.4 Urethral functional and muscular disorders**
Use additional code to identify associated urinary stress incontinence (N39.3)
- **N36.41 Hypermobility of urethra**
- **N36.42 Intrinsic sphincter deficiency (ISD)**
- **N36.43 Combined hypermobility of urethra and intrinsic sphincter deficiency**
- **N36.44 Muscular disorders of urethra**
  Bladder sphincter dyssynergy

N36.5 Urethral false passage

N36.8 Other specified disorders of urethra
Excludes1: congenital urethrocele (Q64.7)
female urethrocele (N81.0)

N36.9 Urethral disorder, unspecified

N37 Urethral disorders in diseases classified elsewhere
Code first underlying disease
Excludes1: urethritis (in):
candidal infection (B37.41)
chlamydial (A56.01)
gonorrhea (A54.01)
syphilis (A52.76)
trichomonal infection (A59.03)
tuberculosis (A18.13)
Valid 3-character code, no further characters required

N39 Other disorders of urinary system
Excludes2: hematuria NOS (R31.-)
recurrent or persistent hematuria (N02.-)
recurrent or persistent hematuria with specified morphological lesion (N02.-)
proteinuria NOS (R80.-)

CC N39.0 Urinary tract infection, site not specified
Use additional code (B95-B97), to identify infectious agent
Excludes1: candidiasis of urinary tract (B37.4-)
neonatal urinary tract infection (P39.3)
pyuria (R82.81)
urinary tract infection of specified site, such as:
cystitis (N30.-)
urethritis (N34.-)
HAC see Appendix B for HAC conditional logic
AHA CC: 4Q, 2012, 94; 1Q, 2018, 16; 2Q, 2018, 22

Ureteral Strictures

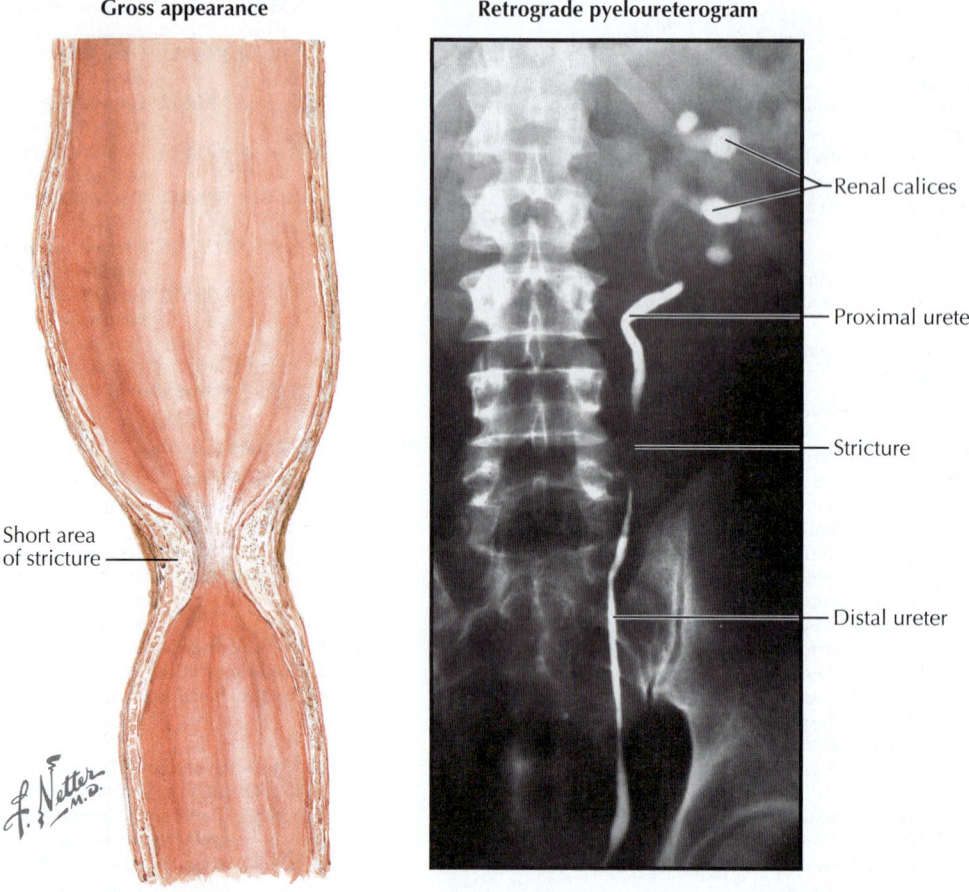

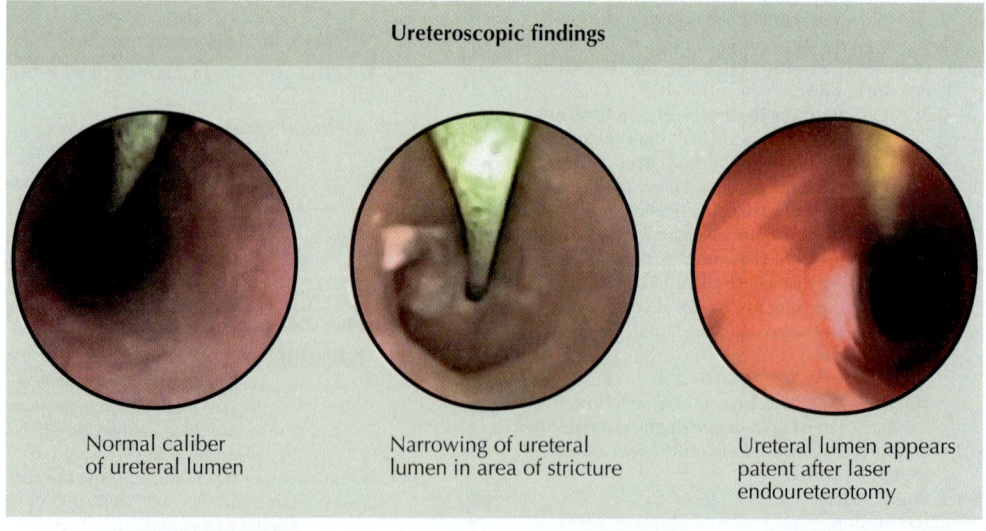

N39.3 Stress incontinence (female) (male)
  Code also any associated overactive bladder (N32.81)
  Excludes1: mixed incontinence (N39.46)
  AHA CC: 4Q, 2021, 18
+ **N39.4** Other specified urinary incontinence
  Code also any associated overactive bladder (N32.81)
  Excludes1: enuresis NOS (R32)
    functional urinary incontinence (R39.81)
    urinary incontinence associated with cognitive impairment (R39.81)
    urinary incontinence NOS (R32)
    urinary incontinence of nonorganic origin (F98.0)
  N39.41 Urge incontinence
    Excludes1: mixed incontinence (N39.46)
  N39.42 Incontinence without sensory awareness
    Insensible (urinary) incontinence
  N39.43 Post-void dribbling
  N39.44 Nocturnal enuresis
    Excludes2: nocturnal polyuria (R35.81)
  N39.45 Continuous leakage
  N39.46 Mixed incontinence
    Urge and stress incontinence
+ **N39.49** Other specified urinary incontinence
    AHA CC: 4Q, 2016, 44
    N39.490 Overflow incontinence
    N39.491 Coital incontinence
    N39.492 Postural (urinary) incontinence
    N39.498 Other specified urinary incontinence
      Reflex incontinence
      Total incontinence
N39.8 Other specified disorders of urinary system
N39.9 Disorder of urinary system, unspecified

Diseases of male genital organs (N40-N53)

N40 Benign prostatic hyperplasia
  Includes: adenofibromatous hypertrophy of prostate
    benign hypertrophy of the prostate
    benign prostatic hypertrophy
    BPH
    enlarged prostate
    nodular prostate
    polyp of prostate
  Excludes1: benign neoplasms of prostate (adenoma, benign) (fibroadenoma) (fibroma) (myoma) (D29.1)
  Excludes2: malignant neoplasm of prostate (C61)
● ♂ **N40.0** Benign prostatic hyperplasia without lower urinary tract symptoms
    Enlarged prostate without LUTS
    Enlarged prostate NOS
● ♂ **N40.1** Benign prostatic hyperplasia with lower urinary tract symptoms
    Enlarged prostate with LUTS
    Use additional code for associated symptoms, when specified:
      incomplete bladder emptying (R39.14)
      nocturia (R35.1)
      straining on urination (R39.16)
      urinary frequency (R35.0)
      urinary hesitancy (R39.11)
      urinary incontinence (N39.4-)
      urinary obstruction (N13.8)
      urinary retention (R33.8)
      urinary urgency (R39.15)
      weak urinary stream (R39.12)
● ♂ **N40.2** Nodular prostate without lower urinary tract symptoms
    Nodular prostate without LUTS
● ♂ **N40.3** Nodular prostate with lower urinary tract symptoms
    Use additional code for associated symptoms, when specified:
      incomplete bladder emptying (R39.14)
      nocturia (R35.1)
      straining on urination (R39.16)
      urinary frequency (R35.0)
      urinary hesitancy (R39.11)
      urinary incontinence (N39.4-)
      urinary obstruction (N13.8)
      urinary retention (R33.8)
      urinary urgency (R39.15)
      weak urinary stream (R39.12)

N41 Inflammatory diseases of prostate
  Use additional code (B95-B97), to identify infectious agent
● CC ♂ **N41.0** Acute prostatitis
● ♂ **N41.1** Chronic prostatitis
● CC ♂ **N41.2** Abscess of prostate
● ♂ **N41.3** Prostatocystitis
● ♂ **N41.4** Granulomatous prostatitis
● ♂ **N41.8** Other inflammatory diseases of prostate
● ♂ **N41.9** Inflammatory disease of prostate, unspecified
    Prostatitis NOS

N42 Other and unspecified disorders of prostate
● ♂ **N42.0** Calculus of prostate
    Prostatic stone
● ♂ **N42.1** Congestion and hemorrhage of prostate
    Excludes1: enlarged prostate (N40.-)
      hematuria (R31.-)
      hyperplasia of prostate (N40.-)
      inflammatory diseases of prostate (N41.-)
+ **N42.3** Dysplasia of prostate
    AHA CC: 4Q, 2016, 44
    ♂ **N42.30** Unspecified dysplasia of prostate
    ♂ **N42.31** Prostatic intraepithelial neoplasia
      PIN
      Prostatic intraepithelial neoplasia I (PIN I)
      Prostatic intraepithelial neoplasia II (PIN II)
      Excludes1: prostatic intraepithelial neoplasia III (PIN III) (D07.5)
    ♂ **N42.32** Atypical small acinar proliferation of prostate
    ♂ **N42.39** Other dysplasia of prostate
+ **N42.8** Other specified disorders of prostate
  ● ♂ **N42.81** Prostatodynia syndrome
      Painful prostate syndrome
  ● ♂ **N42.82** Prostatosis syndrome
  ● ♂ **N42.83** Cyst of prostate
  ● ♂ **N42.89** Other specified disorders of prostate
● ♂ **N42.9** Disorder of prostate, unspecified

N43 Hydrocele and spermatocele
  Includes: hydrocele of spermatic cord, testis or tunica vaginalis
  Excludes1: congenital hydrocele (P83.5)
  ♂ **N43.0** Encysted hydrocele
  CC ♂ **N43.1** Infected hydrocele
    Use additional code (B95-B97), to identify infectious agent
  ♂ **N43.2** Other hydrocele
  ♂ **N43.3** Hydrocele, unspecified
+ **N43.4** Spermatocele of epididymis
    Spermatic cyst
    ♂ **N43.40** Spermatocele of epididymis, unspecified
    ♂ **N43.41** Spermatocele of epididymis, single
    ♂ **N43.42** Spermatocele of epididymis, multiple

N44 Noninflammatory disorders of testis
+ **N44.0** Torsion of testis
    CC ♂ **N44.00** Torsion of testis, unspecified
    CC ♂ **N44.01** Extravaginal torsion of spermatic cord
    CC ♂ **N44.02** Intravaginal torsion of spermatic cord
      Torsion of spermatic cord NOS
    CC ♂ **N44.03** Torsion of appendix testis
    CC ♂ **N44.04** Torsion of appendix epididymis
  ♂ **N44.1** Cyst of tunica albuginea testis
  ♂ **N44.2** Benign cyst of testis
  ♂ **N44.8** Other noninflammatory disorders of the testis

N45 Orchitis and epididymitis
  Use additional code (B95-B97), to identify infectious agent
  ♂ **N45.1** Epididymitis
  ♂ **N45.2** Orchitis
  ♂ **N45.3** Epididymo-orchitis
  CC ♂ **N45.4** Abscess of epididymis or testis

N46 Male infertility
  Excludes1: vasectomy status (Z98.52)
+ **N46.0** Azoospermia
    Absolute male infertility
    Male infertility due to germinal (cell) aplasia
    Male infertility due to spermatogenic arrest (complete)
  ● ♂ **N46.01** Organic azoospermia
      Azoospermia NOS

Male Reproductive System

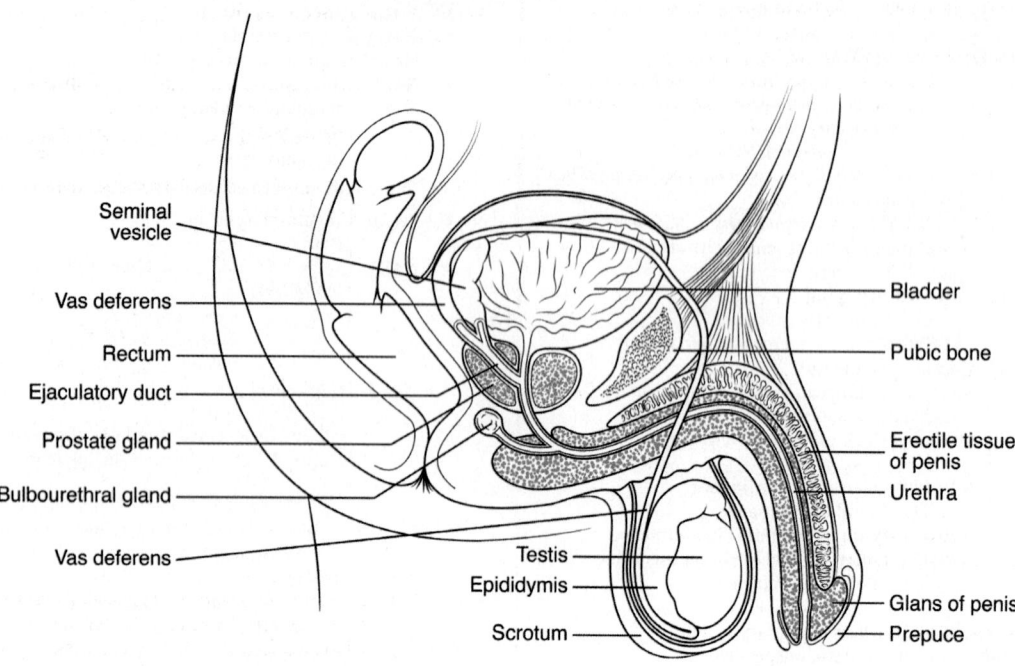

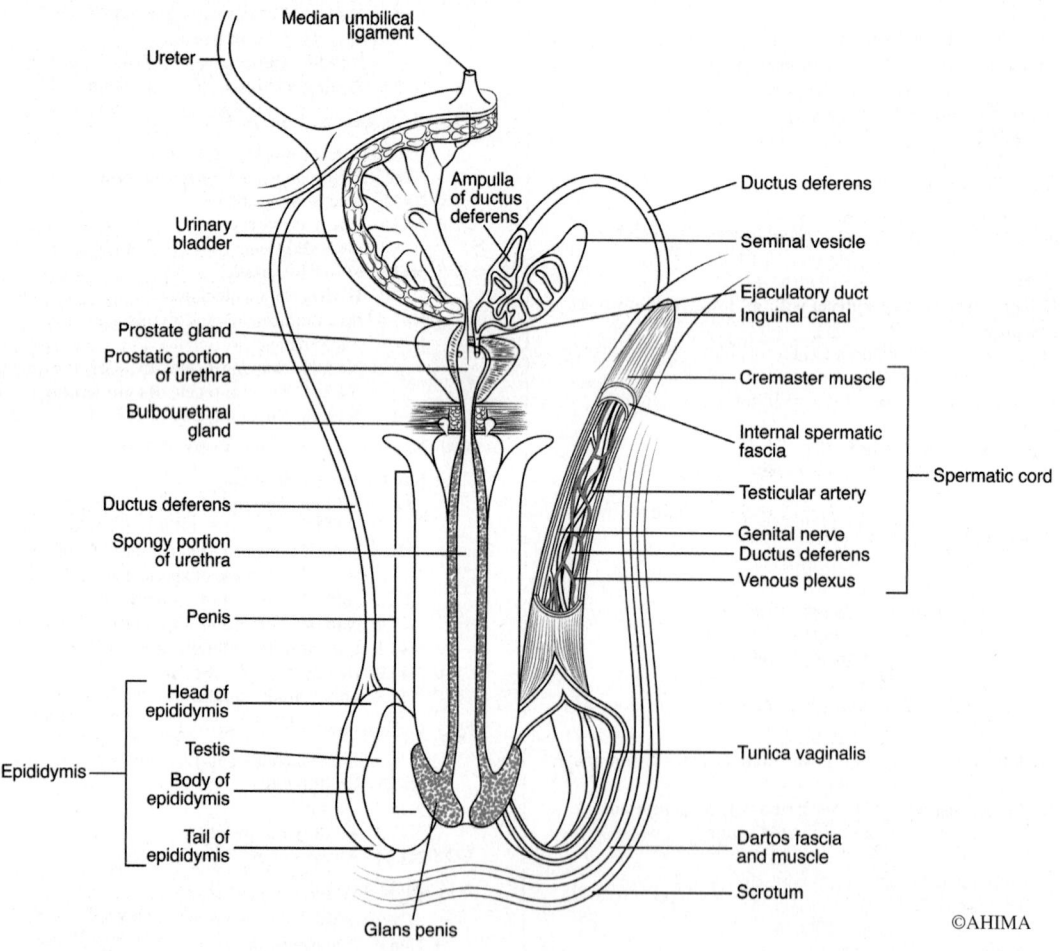

©AHIMA

- **+ N46.02 Azoospermia due to extratesticular causes**
  Code also associated cause
  - ♂ **N46.021** Azoospermia due to drug therapy
  - ♂ **N46.022** Azoospermia due to infection
  - ♂ **N46.023** Azoospermia due to obstruction of efferent ducts
  - ♂ **N46.024** Azoospermia due to radiation
  - ♂ **N46.025** Azoospermia due to systemic disease
  - ♂ **N46.029** Azoospermia due to other extratesticular causes
- **+ N46.1 Oligospermia**
  Male infertility due to germinal cell desquamation
  Male infertility due to hypospermatogenesis
  Male infertility due to incomplete spermatogenic arrest
  - ♂ **N46.11** Organic oligospermia
    Oligospermia NOS
  - **+ N46.12** Oligospermia due to extratesticular causes
    Code also associated cause
    - ♂ **N46.121** Oligospermia due to drug therapy
    - ♂ **N46.122** Oligospermia due to infection
    - ♂ **N46.123** Oligospermia due to obstruction of efferent ducts
    - ♂ **N46.124** Oligospermia due to radiation
    - ♂ **N46.125** Oligospermia due to systemic disease
    - ♂ **N46.129** Oligospermia due to other extratesticular causes
- ♂ **N46.8** Other male infertility
- ♂ **N46.9** Male infertility, unspecified

N47 Disorders of prepuce
- ♂ **N47.0** Adherent prepuce, newborn
- ♂ **N47.1** Phimosis
- ♂ **N47.2** Paraphimosis
- ♂ **N47.3** Deficient foreskin
- ♂ **N47.4** Benign cyst of prepuce
- ♂ **N47.5** Adhesions of prepuce and glans penis
- ♂ **N47.6** Balanoposthitis
  Use additional code (B95-B97), to identify infectious agent
  Excludes1: *balanitis (N48.1)*
- ♂ **N47.7** Other inflammatory diseases of prepuce
  Use additional code (B95-B97), to identify infectious agent
- ♂ **N47.8** Other disorders of prepuce

N48 Other disorders of penis
- ♂ **N48.0** Leukoplakia of penis
  Balanitis xerotica obliterans
  Kraurosis of penis
  Lichen sclerosus of external male genital organs
  Excludes1: *carcinoma in situ of penis (D07.4)*
- ♂ **N48.1** Balanitis
  Use additional code (B95-B97), to identify infectious agent
  Excludes1: *amebic balanitis (A06.8)*
  balanitis xerotica obliterans (N48.0)
  candidal balanitis (B37.42)
  gonococcal balanitis (A54.23)
  herpesviral [herpes simplex] balanitis (A60.01)
- **+ N48.2** Other inflammatory disorders of penis
  Use additional code (B95-B97), to identify infectious agent
  Excludes1: *balanitis (N48.1)*
  balanitis xerotica obliterans (N48.0)
  balanoposthitis (N47.6)
  - ♂ **N48.21** Abscess of corpus cavernosum and penis
  - ♂ **N48.22** Cellulitis of corpus cavernosum and penis
  - ♂ **N48.29** Other inflammatory disorders of penis
- **+ N48.3** Priapism
  Painful erection
  Code first underlying cause
  - CC ♂ **N48.30** Priapism, unspecified
  - CC ♂ **N48.31** Priapism due to trauma
  - CC ♂ **N48.32** Priapism due to disease classified elsewhere
  - CC ♂ **N48.33** Priapism, drug-induced
  - CC ♂ **N48.39** Other priapism
- ♂ **N48.5** Ulcer of penis
- ♂ **N48.6** Induration penis plastica
  Peyronie's disease
  Plastic induration of penis
- **+ N48.8** Other specified disorders of penis
  - ♂ **N48.81** Thrombosis of superficial vein of penis
  - ♂ **N48.82** Acquired torsion of penis
    Acquired torsion of penis NOS
    Excludes1: *congenital torsion of penis (Q55.63)*
  - ♂ **N48.83** Acquired buried penis
    Excludes1: *congenital hidden penis (Q55.64)*
  - ♂ **N48.89** Other specified disorders of penis
- ♂ **N48.9** Disorder of penis, unspecified

N49 Inflammatory disorders of male genital organs, not elsewhere classified
Use additional code (B95-B97), to identify infectious agent
Excludes1: *inflammation of penis (N48.1, N48.2-)*
orchitis and epididymitis (N45.-)
- ♂ **N49.0** Inflammatory disorders of seminal vesicle
  Vesiculitis NOS
- ♂ **N49.1** Inflammatory disorders of spermatic cord, tunica vaginalis and vas deferens
  Vasitis
- ♂ **N49.2** Inflammatory disorders of scrotum
- ♂ **N49.3** Fournier gangrene
  AHA CC: 2Q, 2020, 18
- ♂ **N49.8** Inflammatory disorders of other specified male genital organs
  Inflammation of multiple sites in male genital organs
- ♂ **N49.9** Inflammatory disorder of unspecified male genital organ
  Abscess of unspecified male genital organ
  Boil of unspecified male genital organ
  Carbuncle of unspecified male genital organ
  Cellulitis of unspecified male genital organ

N50 Other and unspecified disorders of male genital organs
Excludes2: *torsion of testis (N44.0-)*
- ♂ **N50.0** Atrophy of testis
- ♂ **N50.1** Vascular disorders of male genital organs
  Hematocele, NOS, of male genital organs
  Hemorrhage of male genital organs
  Thrombosis of male genital organs
- ♂ **N50.3** Cyst of epididymis
- **+ N50.8** Other specified disorders of male genital organs
  AHA CC: 4Q, 2016, 45
  - **+ N50.81** Testicular pain
    - ♂ **N50.811** Right testicular pain
    - ♂ **N50.812** Left testicular pain
    - ♂ **N50.819** Testicular pain, unspecified
  - ♂ **N50.82** Scrotal pain
  - ♂ **N50.89** Other specified disorders of the male genital organs
    Atrophy of scrotum, seminal vesicle, spermatic cord, tunica vaginalis and vas deferens
    Chylocele, tunica vaginalis (nonfilarial) NOS
    Edema of scrotum, seminal vesicle, spermatic cord, tunica vaginalis and vas deferens
    Hypertrophy of scrotum, seminal vesicle, spermatic cord, tunica vaginalis and vas deferens
    Stricture of spermatic cord, tunical vaginalis, and vas deferens
    Ulcer of scrotum, seminal vesicle, spermatic cord, testis, tunica vaginalis and vas deferens
    Urethroscrotal fistula
- ♂ **N50.9** Disorder of male genital organs, unspecified

♂ N51 Disorders of male genital organs in diseases classified elsewhere
Code first underlying disease, such as:
filariasis (B74.0-B74.9)
Excludes1: *amebic balanitis (A06.8)*
candidal balanitis (B37.42)
gonococcal balanitis (A54.23)
gonococcal prostatitis (A54.22)
herpesviral [herpes simplex] balanitis (A60.01)
trichomonal prostatitis (A59.02)
tuberculous prostatitis (A18.14)
Valid 3-character code, no further characters required

N52 Male erectile dysfunction
Excludes1: *psychogenic impotence (F52.21)*
- **+ N52.0** Vasculogenic erectile dysfunction
  - ♂ **N52.01** Erectile dysfunction due to arterial insufficiency
  - ♂ **N52.02** Corporo-venous occlusive erectile dysfunction
  - ♂ **N52.03** Combined arterial insufficiency and corporo-venous occlusive erectile dysfunction
- ♂ CC **N52.1** Erectile dysfunction due to diseases classified elsewhere
  Code first underlying disease
- ♂ CC **N52.2** Drug-induced erectile dysfunction

- ♂ **N52.3 Postprocedural erectile dysfunction**
  AHA CC: 4Q, 2016, 45
  - ♂ N52.31 Erectile dysfunction following radical prostatectomy
  - ♂ N52.32 Erectile dysfunction following radical cystectomy
  - ♂ N52.33 Erectile dysfunction following urethral surgery
  - ♂ N52.34 Erectile dysfunction following simple prostatectomy
  - ♂ N52.35 Erectile dysfunction following radiation therapy
  - ♂ N52.36 Erectile dysfunction following interstitial seed therapy
  - ♂ N52.37 Erectile dysfunction following prostate ablative therapy
    Erectile dysfunction following cryotherapy
    Erectile dysfunction following other prostate ablative therapies
    Erectile dysfunction following ultrasound ablative therapies
  - ♂ N52.39 Other and unspecified postprocedural erectile dysfunction
- ♂ N52.8 Other male erectile dysfunction
- ♂ N52.9 Male erectile dysfunction, unspecified
  Impotence NOS

N53 Other male sexual dysfunction
Excludes1: *psychogenic sexual dysfunction (F52.-)*
- **N53.1 Ejaculatory dysfunction**
  Excludes1: *premature ejaculation (F52.4)*
  - ♂ N53.11 Retarded ejaculation
  - ♂ N53.12 Painful ejaculation
  - ♂ N53.13 Anejaculatory orgasm
  - ♂ N53.14 Retrograde ejaculation
  - ♂ N53.19 Other ejaculatory dysfunction
    Ejaculatory dysfunction NOS
- ♂ N53.8 Other male sexual dysfunction
- ♂ N53.9 Unspecified male sexual dysfunction

Disorders of breast (N60-N65)
Excludes1: *disorders of breast associated with childbirth (O91-O92)*

N60 Benign mammary dysplasia
Includes: fibrocystic mastopathy
- **N60.0 Solitary cyst of breast**
  Cyst of breast
  - N60.01 Solitary cyst of right breast
  - N60.02 Solitary cyst of left breast
  - N60.09 Solitary cyst of unspecified breast
- **N60.1 Diffuse cystic mastopathy**
  Cystic breast
  Fibrocystic disease of breast
  Excludes1: *diffuse cystic mastopathy with epithelial proliferation (N60.3-)*
  - N60.11 Diffuse cystic mastopathy of right breast
  - N60.12 Diffuse cystic mastopathy of left breast
  - N60.19 Diffuse cystic mastopathy of unspecified breast
- **N60.2 Fibroadenosis of breast**
  Adenofibrosis of breast
  Excludes2: *fibroadenoma of breast (D24.-)*
  - N60.21 Fibroadenosis of right breast
  - N60.22 Fibroadenosis of left breast
  - N60.29 Fibroadenosis of unspecified breast
- **N60.3 Fibrosclerosis of breast**
  Cystic mastopathy with epithelial proliferation
  - N60.31 Fibrosclerosis of right breast
  - N60.32 Fibrosclerosis of left breast
  - N60.39 Fibrosclerosis of unspecified breast
- **N60.4 Mammary duct ectasia**
  - N60.41 Mammary duct ectasia of right breast
  - N60.42 Mammary duct ectasia of left breast
  - N60.49 Mammary duct ectasia of unspecified breast
- **N60.8 Other benign mammary dysplasias**
  - N60.81 Other benign mammary dysplasias of right breast
  - N60.82 Other benign mammary dysplasias of left breast
  - N60.89 Other benign mammary dysplasias of unspecified breast
- **N60.9 Unspecified benign mammary dysplasia**
  - N60.91 Unspecified benign mammary dysplasia of right breast
  - N60.92 Unspecified benign mammary dysplasia of left breast
  - N60.99 Unspecified benign mammary dysplasia of unspecified breast

N61 Inflammatory disorders of breast
Excludes1: *inflammatory carcinoma of breast (C50.9)*
inflammatory disorder of breast associated with childbirth (O91.-)
neonatal infective mastitis (P39.0)
thrombophlebitis of breast [Mondor's disease] (I80.8)
- **N61.0 Mastitis without abscess**
  Infective mastitis (acute) (nonpuerperal) (subacute)
  Mastitis (acute) (nonpuerperal) (subacute) NOS
  Cellulitis (acute) (nonpuerperal) (subacute) of breast NOS
  Cellulitis (acute) (nonpuerperal) (subacute) of nipple NOS
- **N61.1 Abscess of the breast and nipple**
  Abscess (acute) (chronic) (nonpuerperal) of areola
  Abscess (acute) (chronic) (nonpuerperal) of breast
  Carbuncle of breast
  Mastitis with abscess
- **N61.2 Granulomatous mastitis**
  AHA CC: 4Q, 2020, 35
  - N61.20 Granulomatous mastitis, unspecified breast
  - N61.21 Granulomatous mastitis, right breast
  - N61.22 Granulomatous mastitis, left breast
  - N61.23 Granulomatous mastitis, bilateral breast

N62 Hypertrophy of breast
Gynecomastia
Hypertrophy of breast NOS
Massive pubertal hypertrophy of breast
Excludes1: *breast engorgement of newborn (P83.4)*
disproportion of reconstructed breast (N65.1)
Valid 3-character code, no further characters required

N63 Unspecified lump in breast
Nodule(s) NOS in breast
AHA CC: 4Q, 2017, 19
- N63.0 Unspecified lump in unspecified breast
- **N63.1 Unspecified lump in the right breast**
  - N63.10 Unspecified lump in the right breast, unspecified quadrant
    AHA CC: 3Q, 2022, 8
  - N63.11 Unspecified lump in the right breast, upper outer quadrant
  - N63.12 Unspecified lump in the right breast, upper inner quadrant
  - N63.13 Unspecified lump in the right breast, lower outer quadrant
  - N63.14 Unspecified lump in the right breast, lower inner quadrant
  - N63.15 Unspecified lump in the right breast, overlapping quadrants
    AHA CC: 4Q, 2019, 12
- **N63.2 Unspecified lump in the left breast**
  - N63.20 Unspecified lump in the left breast, unspecified quadrant
  - N63.21 Unspecified lump in the left breast, upper outer quadrant
  - N63.22 Unspecified lump in the left breast, upper inner quadrant
  - N63.23 Unspecified lump in the left breast, lower outer quadrant
  - N63.24 Unspecified lump in the left breast, lower inner quadrant
  - N63.25 Unspecified lump in the left breast, overlapping quadrants
    AHA CC: 4Q, 2019, 12
- **N63.3 Unspecified lump in axillary tail**
  - N63.31 Unspecified lump in axillary tail of the right breast
  - N63.32 Unspecified lump in axillary tail of the left breast
- **N63.4 Unspecified lump in breast, subareolar**
  - N63.41 Unspecified lump in right breast, subareolar
  - N63.42 Unspecified lump in left breast, subareolar

N64 Other disorders of breast
Excludes2: *mechanical complication of breast prosthesis and implant (T85.4-)*
- N64.0 Fissure and fistula of nipple
- **N64.1 Fat necrosis of breast**
  Fat necrosis (segmental) of breast
  Code first breast necrosis due to breast graft (T85.898)

Breast

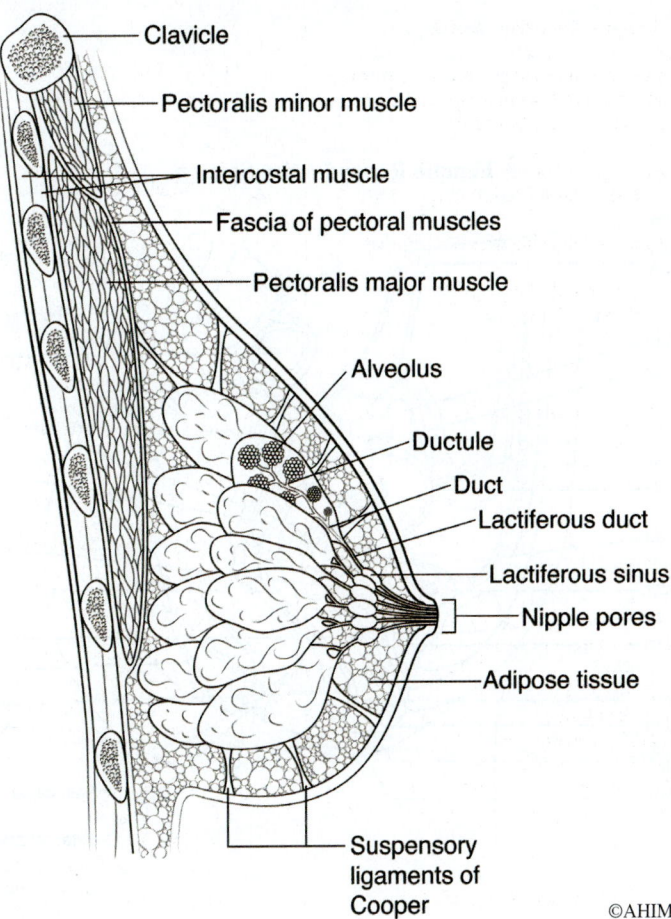

N64.2 Atrophy of breast
N64.3 Galactorrhea not associated with childbirth
N64.4 Mastodynia
+ N64.5 Other signs and symptoms in breast
  Excludes2: *abnormal findings on diagnostic imaging of breast (R92.-)*
  N64.51 Induration of breast
  N64.52 Nipple discharge
  Excludes1: *abnormal findings in nipple discharge (R89.-)*
  N64.53 Retraction of nipple
  N64.59 Other signs and symptoms in breast
+ N64.8 Other specified disorders of breast
  • N64.81 Ptosis of breast
    Excludes1: *ptosis of native breast in relation to reconstructed breast (N65.1)*
  • N64.82 Hypoplasia of breast
    Micromastia
    Excludes1: *congenital absence of breast (Q83.0)*
    hypoplasia of native breast in relation to reconstructed breast (N65.1)
  N64.89 Other specified disorders of breast
    Galactocele
    Subinvolution of breast (postlactational)
    AHA CC: 1Q, 2018, 3-4; 1Q, 2019, 32
  N64.9 Disorder of breast, unspecified
N65 **Deformity and disproportion of reconstructed breast**
  • N65.0 Deformity of reconstructed breast
    Contour irregularity in reconstructed breast
    Excess tissue in reconstructed breast
    Misshapen reconstructed breast
  • N65.1 Disproportion of reconstructed breast
    Breast asymmetry between native breast and reconstructed breast
    Disproportion between native breast and reconstructed breast

Inflammatory diseases of female pelvic organs (N70-N77)

Excludes1: *inflammatory diseases of female pelvic organs complicating: abortion or ectopic or molar pregnancy (O00-O07, O08.0) pregnancy, childbirth and the puerperium (O23.-, O75.3, O85, O86.-)*

N70 **Salpingitis and oophoritis**
  Includes: abscess (of) fallopian tube
    abscess (of) ovary
    pyosalpinx
    salpingo-oophoritis
    tubo-ovarian abscess
    tubo-ovarian inflammatory disease
  Use additional code (B95-B97), to identify infectious agent
  Excludes1: *gonococcal infection (A54.24)*
    tuberculous infection (A18.17)
+ N70.0 Acute salpingitis and oophoritis
  ♀ CC N70.01 Acute salpingitis
  ♀ CC N70.02 Acute oophoritis
  ♀ CC N70.03 Acute salpingitis and oophoritis
+ N70.1 Chronic salpingitis and oophoritis
    Hydrosalpinx
  ♀ N70.11 Chronic salpingitis
  ♀ N70.12 Chronic oophoritis
  ♀ N70.13 Chronic salpingitis and oophoritis
+ N70.9 Salpingitis and oophoritis, unspecified
  ♀ N70.91 Salpingitis, unspecified
  ♀ N70.92 Oophoritis, unspecified
  ♀ N70.93 Salpingitis and oophoritis, unspecified

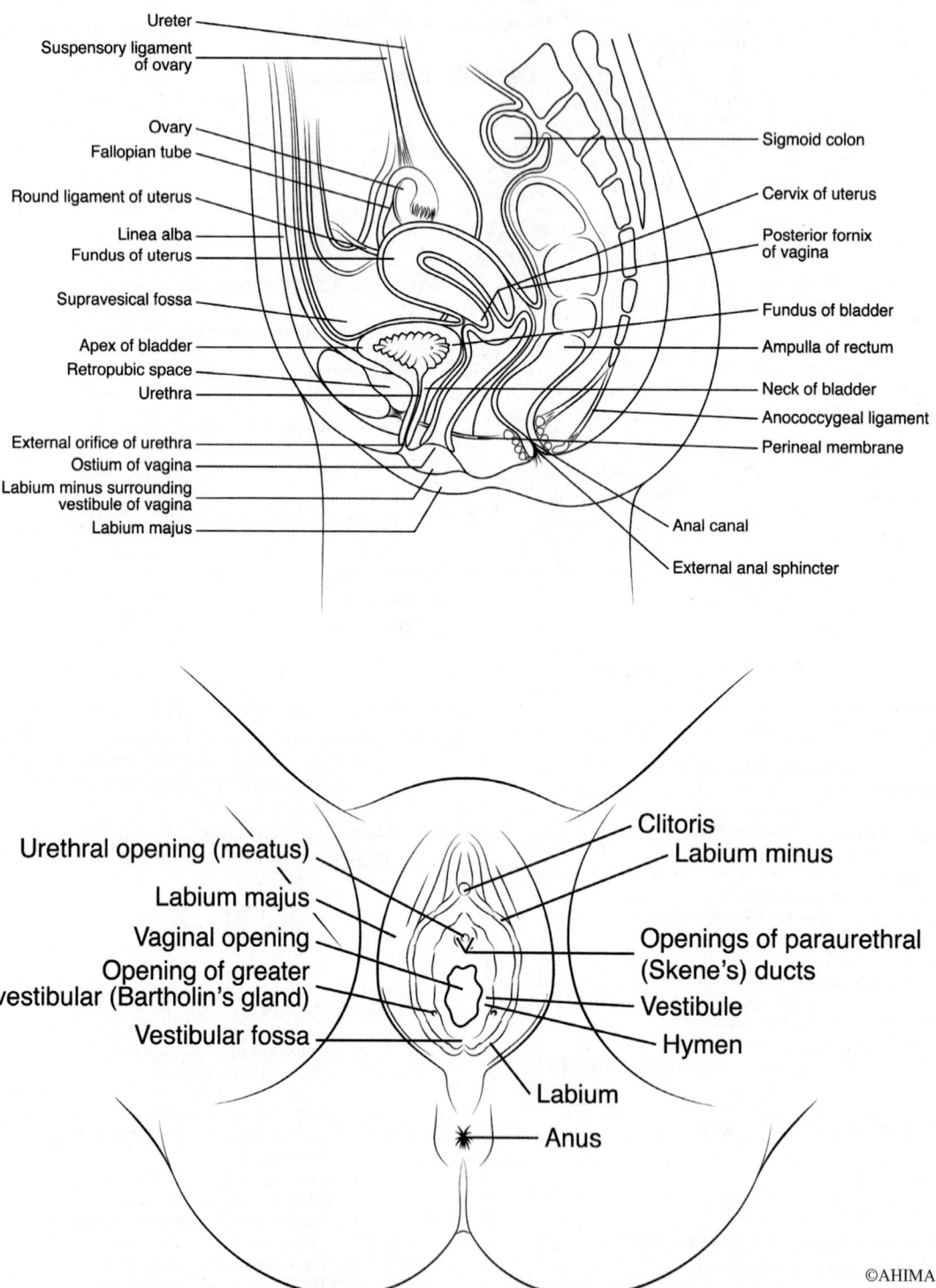

N71 **Inflammatory disease of uterus, except cervix**
    Includes: endo (myo) metritis
                   metritis
                     myometritis
                     pyometra
                     uterine abscess
    Use additional code (B95-B97), to identify infectious agent
    Excludes1: hyperplastic endometritis (N85.0-)
                   infection of uterus following delivery (O85, O86.-)
    ♀ CC **N71.0** Acute inflammatory disease of uterus
      ♀ **N71.1** Chronic inflammatory disease of uterus
      ♀ **N71.9** Inflammatory disease of uterus, unspecified
♀ **N72** **Inflammatory disease of cervix uteri**
    Includes: cervicitis (with or without erosion or ectropion)
                     endocervicitis (with or without erosion or ectropion)
                     exocervicitis (with or without erosion or ectropion)
    Use additional code (B95-B97), to identify infectious agent
    Excludes1: erosion and ectropion of cervix without cervicitis (N86)
    Valid 3-character code, no further characters required
N73 **Other female pelvic inflammatory diseases**
    Use additional code (B95-B97), to identify infectious agent
  ♀ CC **N73.0** Acute parametritis and pelvic cellulitis
           Abscess of broad ligament
           Abscess of parametrium
           Pelvic cellulitis, female
    ♀ **N73.1** Chronic parametritis and pelvic cellulitis
           Any condition in N73.0 specified as chronic
           Excludes1: tuberculous parametritis and pelvic cellultis (A18.17)
    ♀ **N73.2** Unspecified parametritis and pelvic cellulitis
           Any condition in N73.0 unspecified whether acute or chronic
  ♀ MCC **N73.3** Female acute pelvic peritonitis
  ♀ CC **N73.4** Female chronic pelvic peritonitis
           Excludes1: tuberculous pelvic (female) peritonitis (A18.17)
    ♀ **N73.5** Female pelvic peritonitis, unspecified
    ♀ **N73.6** Female pelvic peritoneal adhesions (postinfective)
           Excludes2: postprocedural pelvic peritoneal adhesions
                           (N99.4)
           AHA CC: 1Q, 2014, 6
    ♀ **N73.8** Other specified female pelvic inflammatory diseases
    ♀ **N73.9** Female pelvic inflammatory disease, unspecified
           Female pelvic infection or inflammation NOS
♀ **N74** **Female pelvic inflammatory disorders in diseases classified elsewhere**
    Code first underlying disease
    Excludes1: chlamydial cervicitis (A56.02)
                   chlamydial pelvic inflammatory disease (A56.11)
                   gonococcal cervicitis (A54.03)
                   gonococcal pelvic inflammatory disease (A54.24)
                   herpesviral [herpes simplex] cervicitis (A60.03)
                   herpesviral [herpes simplex] pelvic inflammatory
                      disease (A60.09)
                   syphilitic cervicitis (A52.76)
                   syphilitic pelvic inflammatory disease (A52.76)
                   trichomonal cervicitis (A59.09)
                   tuberculous cervicitis (A18.16)
                   tuberculous pelvic inflammatory disease (A18.17)
    Valid 3-character code, no further characters required
N75 **Diseases of Bartholin's gland**
    ♀ **N75.0** Cyst of Bartholin's gland
  ♀ CC **N75.1** Abscess of Bartholin's gland
    ♀ **N75.8** Other diseases of Bartholin's gland
           Bartholinitis
    ♀ **N75.9** Disease of Bartholin's gland, unspecified
N76 **Other inflammation of vagina and vulva**
    Use additional code (B95-B97), to identify infectious agent
    Excludes2: senile (atrophic) vaginitis (N95.2)
                   vulvar vestibulitis (N94.810)
    ♀ **N76.0** Acute vaginitis
           Acute vulvovaginitis
           Vaginitis NOS
           Vulvovaginitis NOS
    ♀ **N76.1** Subacute and chronic vaginitis
           Chronic vulvovaginitis
           Subacute vulvovaginitis
    ♀ **N76.2** Acute vulvitis
           Vulvitis NOS
    ♀ **N76.3** Subacute and chronic vulvitis
  ♀ CC **N76.4** Abscess of vulva
           Furuncle of vulva
    ♀ **N76.5** Ulceration of vagina
    ♀ **N76.6** Ulceration of vulva
  + ♀ **N76.8** Other specified inflammation of vagina and vulva
  ♀ CC **N76.81** Mucositis (ulcerative) of vagina and vulva
           Code also type of associated therapy, such as:
           antineoplastic and immunosuppressive
           drugs (T45.1X-)
           radiological procedure and radiotherapy (Y84.2)
           Excludes2: gastrointestinal mucositis (ulcerative)
                        (K92.81)
                     nasal mucositis (ulcerative) (J34.81)
                     oral mucositis (ulcerative) (K12.3-)
    ♀ **N76.82** Fournier disease of vagina and vulva
           Fournier gangrene of vagina and vulva
           Code also, if applicable, diabetes mellitus (E08-E13
           with .9)
           Excludes1: gangrene in diabetes mellitus
                        (E08-E13 with .52)
           AHA CC: 4Q, 2022, 34
    ♀ **N76.89** Other specified inflammation of vagina and vulva
N77 **Vulvovaginal ulceration and inflammation in diseases classified elsewhere**
    ♀ **N77.0** Ulceration of vulva in diseases classified elsewhere
           Code first underlying disease, such as:
           Behçet's disease (M35.2)
           Excludes1: ulceration of vulva in gonococcal infection
                        (A54.02)
                     ulceration of vulva in herpesviral [herpes
                        simplex] infection (A60.04)
                     ulceration of vulva in syphilis (A51.0)
                     ulceration of vulva in tuberculosis (A18.18)
    ♀ **N77.1** Vaginitis, vulvitis and vulvovaginitis in diseases classified elsewhere
           Code first underlying disease, such as:
           pinworm (B80)
           Excludes1: candidal vulvovaginitis (B37.3-)
                     chlamydial vulvovaginitis (A56.02)
                     gonococcal vulvovaginitis (A54.02)
                     herpesviral [herpes simplex] vulvovaginitis
                        (A60.04)
                     trichomonal vulvovaginitis (A59.01)
                     tuberculous vulvovaginitis (A18.18)
                     vulvovaginitis in early syphilis (A51.0)
                     vulvovaginitis in late syphilis (A52.76)

Noninflammatory disorders of female genital tract (N80-N98)

N80 **Endometriosis**
    AHA CC: 4Q, 2022, 34-36
  + **N80.0** Endometriosis of uterus
           Endometriosis of the cervix
           Excludes1: stromal endometriosis (D39.0)
    ♀ **N80.00** Endometriosis of the uterus, unspecified
    ♀ **N80.01** Superficial endometriosis of the uterus
    ♀ **N80.02** Deep endometriosis of the uterus
           Deep retrocervical endometriosis
    ♀ **N80.03** Adenomyosis of the uterus
           Adenomyosis NOS
  + **N80.1** Endometriosis of ovary
    + **N80.10** Endometriosis of ovary, unspecified depth
      ♀ **N80.101** Endometriosis of right ovary,
                unspecified depth
      ♀ **N80.102** Endometriosis of left ovary, unspecified
                depth
      ♀ **N80.103** Endometriosis of bilateral ovaries,
                unspecified depth
      ♀ **N80.109** Endometriosis of ovary, unspecified
                side, unspecified depth
                Endometriosis of ovary NOS
    + **N80.11** Superficial endometriosis of the ovary
      ♀ **N80.111** Superficial endometriosis of right ovary
                AHA CC: 4Q, 2022, 35-36
      ♀ **N80.112** Superficial endometriosis of left ovary
      ♀ **N80.113** Superficial endometriosis of bilateral
                ovaries
      ♀ **N80.119** Superficial endometriosis of ovary,
                unspecified ovary

Vaginal Prolapse

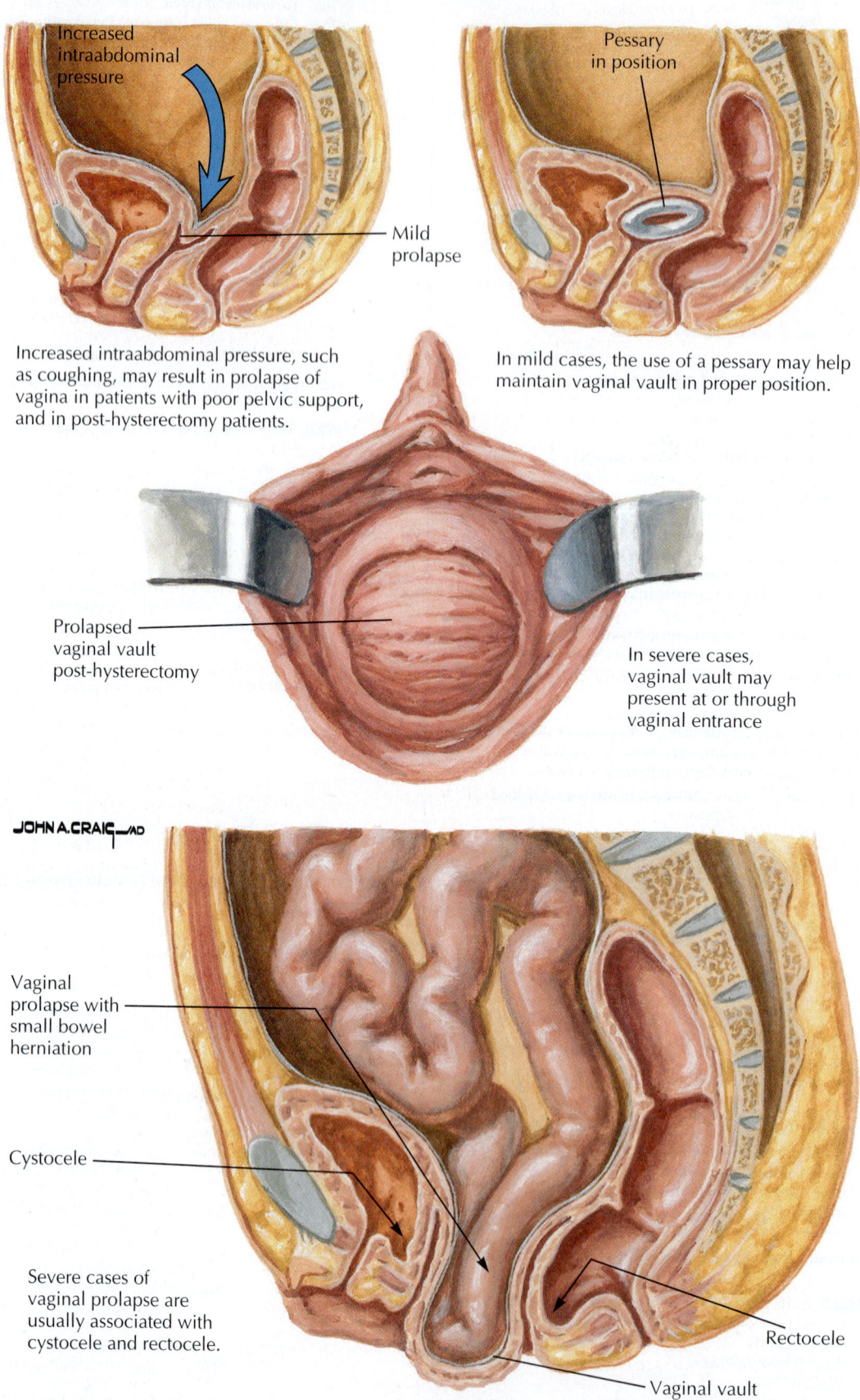

Increased intraabdominal pressure, such as coughing, may result in prolapse of vagina in patients with poor pelvic support, and in post-hysterectomy patients.

In mild cases, the use of a pessary may help maintain vaginal vault in proper position.

In severe cases, vaginal vault may present at or through vaginal entrance

Severe cases of vaginal prolapse are usually associated with cystocele and rectocele.

- **N80.12 Deep endometriosis of ovary**
  - Deep ovarian endometriosis
  - Endometrioma
  - ♀ N80.121 Deep endometriosis of right ovary
  - ♀ N80.122 Deep endometriosis of left ovary
  - ♀ N80.123 Deep endometriosis of bilateral ovaries
  - ♀ N80.129 Deep endometriosis of ovary, unspecified ovary
- **N80.2 Endometriosis of fallopian tube**
  - **N80.20 Endometriosis of fallopian tube, unspecified depth**
    - ♀ N80.201 Endometriosis of right fallopian tube, unspecified depth
    - ♀ N80.202 Endometriosis of left fallopian tube, unspecified depth
    - ♀ N80.203 Endometriosis of bilateral fallopian tubes, unspecified depth
    - ♀ N80.209 Endometriosis of unspecified fallopian tube, unspecified depth
      - Endometriosis fallopian tube NOS
  - **N80.21 Superficial endometriosis of fallopian tube**
    - ♀ N80.211 Superficial endometriosis of right fallopian tube
    - ♀ N80.212 Superficial endometriosis of left fallopian tube
    - ♀ N80.213 Superficial endometriosis of bilateral fallopian tubes
    - ♀ N80.219 Superficial endometriosis of unspecified fallopian tube
  - **N80.22 Deep endometriosis of the fallopian tube**
    - Deep endometriosis involving muscular wall of fallopian tube
    - ♀ N80.221 Deep endometriosis of right fallopian tube
    - ♀ N80.222 Deep endometriosis of left fallopian tube
    - ♀ N80.223 Deep endometriosis of bilateral fallopian tubes
    - ♀ N80.229 Deep endometriosis of unspecified fallopian tube
- **N80.3 Endometriosis of pelvic peritoneum**
  - **N80.30 Endometriosis of pelvic peritoneum, unspecified**
    - Endometriosis of the retroperitoneum NOS
  - **N80.31 Endometriosis of the anterior cul-de-sac**
    - ♀ N80.311 Superficial endometriosis of the anterior cul-de-sac
    - ♀ N80.312 Deep endometriosis of the anterior cul-de-sac
    - ♀ N80.319 Endometriosis of the anterior cul-de-sac, unspecified depth
      - Endometriosis of the anterior cul-de-sac NOS
  - **N80.32 Endometriosis of the posterior cul-de-sac**
    - ♀ N80.321 Superficial endometriosis of the posterior cul-de-sac
    - ♀ N80.322 Deep endometriosis of the posterior cul-de-sac
    - ♀ N80.329 Endometriosis of the posterior cul-de-sac, unspecified depth
      - Endometriosis of the posterior cul-de-sac NOS
  - **N80.33 Superficial endometriosis of the pelvic sidewall**
    - ♀ N80.331 Superficial endometriosis of the right pelvic sidewall
    - ♀ N80.332 Superficial endometriosis of the left pelvic sidewall
    - ♀ N80.333 Superficial endometriosis of bilateral pelvic sidewall
    - ♀ N80.339 Superficial endometriosis of pelvic sidewall, unspecified side
  - **N80.34 Deep endometriosis of the pelvic sidewall**
    - ♀ N80.341 Deep endometriosis of the right pelvic sidewall
    - ♀ N80.342 Deep endometriosis of the left pelvic sidewall
    - ♀ N80.343 Deep endometriosis of the bilateral pelvic sidewall
    - ♀ N80.349 Deep endometriosis of the pelvic sidewall, unspecified side
      - AHA CC: 4Q, 2022, 36
  - **N80.35 Endometriosis of the pelvic sidewall, unspecified depth**
    - ♀ N80.351 Endometriosis of the right pelvic sidewall, unspecified depth
    - ♀ N80.352 Endometriosis of the left pelvic sidewall, unspecified depth
    - ♀ N80.353 Endometriosis of bilateral pelvic sidewall, unspecified depth
    - ♀ N80.359 Endometriosis of pelvic sidewall, unspecified side, unspecified depth
      - Endometriosis of the pelvic sidewall NOS
  - **N80.36 Superficial endometriosis of the pelvic brim**
    - ♀ N80.361 Superficial endometriosis of the right pelvic brim
    - ♀ N80.362 Superficial endometriosis of the left pelvic brim
    - ♀ N80.363 Superficial endometriosis of bilateral pelvic brim
    - ♀ N80.369 Superficial endometriosis of the pelvic brim, unspecified side
  - **N80.37 Deep endometriosis of the pelvic brim**
    - ♀ N80.371 Deep endometriosis of the right pelvic brim
    - ♀ N80.372 Deep endometriosis of the left pelvic brim
    - ♀ N80.373 Deep endometriosis of bilateral pelvic brim
    - ♀ N80.379 Deep endometriosis of the pelvic brim, unspecified side
  - **N80.38 Endometriosis of the pelvic brim, unspecified depth**
    - ♀ N80.381 Endometriosis of the right pelvic brim, unspecified depth
    - ♀ N80.382 Endometriosis of the left pelvic brim, unspecified depth
    - ♀ N80.383 Endometriosis of bilateral pelvic brim, unspecified depth
    - ♀ N80.389 Endometriosis of the pelvic brim, unspecified side, unspecified depth
      - Endometriosis of the pelvic brim NOS
  - **N80.3A Superficial endometriosis of the uterosacral ligament(s)**
    - ♀ N80.3A1 Superficial endometriosis of the right uterosacral ligament
    - ♀ N80.3A2 Superficial endometriosis of the left uterosacral ligament
    - ♀ N80.3A3 Superficial endometriosis of the bilateral uterosacral ligament(s)
    - ♀ N80.3A9 Superficial endometriosis of the uterosacral ligament(s), unspecified side
  - **N80.3B Deep endometriosis of the uterosacral ligament(s)**
    - ♀ N80.3B1 Deep endometriosis of the right uterosacral ligament
    - ♀ N80.3B2 Deep endometriosis of the left uterosacral ligament
    - ♀ N80.3B3 Deep endometriosis of bilateral uterosacral ligament(s)
    - ♀ N80.3B9 Deep endometriosis of the uterosacral ligament(s), unspecified side
  - **N80.3C Endometriosis of the uterosacral ligament(s), unspecified depth**
    - ♀ N80.3C1 Endometriosis of the right uterosacral ligament, unspecified depth
    - ♀ N80.3C2 Endometriosis of the left uterosacral ligament, unspecified depth
    - ♀ N80.3C3 Endometriosis of bilateral uterosacral ligament(s), unspecified depth
    - ♀ N80.3C9 Endometriosis of the uterosacral ligament(s), unspecified side, unspecified depth
      - Endometriosis of the uterosacral ligament(s) NOS
  - **N80.39 Endometriosis of other pelvic peritoneum**
    - ♀ N80.391 Superficial endometriosis of the pelvic peritoneum, other specified sites
    - ♀ N80.392 Deep endometriosis of the pelvic peritoneum, other specified sites
    - ♀ N80.399 Endometriosis of the pelvic peritoneum, other specified sites, unspecified depth

- **N80.4 Endometriosis of rectovaginal septum and vagina**
  - ♀ **N80.40** Endometriosis of rectovaginal septum, unspecified involvement of vagina
    - Endometriosis of the rectovaginal septum, NOS
  - ♀ **N80.41** Endometriosis of rectovaginal septum without involvement of vagina
  - ♀ **N80.42** Endometriosis of rectovaginal septum with involvement of vagina
- **N80.5 Endometriosis of intestine**
  - ♀ **N80.50** Endometriosis of intestine, unspecified
  - **N80.51** Endometriosis of the rectum
    - ♀ **N80.511** Superficial endometriosis of the rectum
    - ♀ **N80.512** Deep endometriosis of the rectum
      - Deep endometriosis of the rectum, multifocal
    - ♀ **N80.519** Endometriosis of the rectum, unspecified depth
      - Endometriosis of the rectum NOS
  - **N80.52** Endometriosis of the sigmoid colon
    - ♀ **N80.521** Superficial endometriosis of the sigmoid colon
    - ♀ **N80.522** Deep endometriosis of the sigmoid colon
    - ♀ **N80.529** Endometriosis of the sigmoid colon, unspecified depth
      - Endometriosis of the sigmoid colon NOS
  - **N80.53** Endometriosis of the cecum
    - ♀ **N80.531** Superficial endometriosis of the cecum
    - ♀ **N80.532** Deep endometriosis of the cecum
    - ♀ **N80.539** Endometriosis of the cecum, unspecified depth
      - Endometriosis of the cecum NOS
  - **N80.54** Endometriosis of the appendix
    - ♀ **N80.541** Superficial endometriosis of the appendix
    - ♀ **N80.542** Deep endometriosis of the appendix
    - ♀ **N80.549** Endometriosis of the appendix, unspecified depth
      - Endometriosis of the appendix NOS
  - **N80.55** Endometriosis of other parts of the colon
    - Endometriosis of descending colon
    - Endometriosis of transverse colon
    - ♀ **N80.551** Superficial endometriosis of other parts of the colon
    - ♀ **N80.552** Deep endometriosis of other parts of the colon
    - ♀ **N80.559** Endometriosis of other parts of the colon, unspecified depth
      - Endometriosis of colon NOS
  - **N80.56** Endometriosis of the small intestine
    - ♀ **N80.561** Superficial endometriosis of the small intestine
    - ♀ **N80.562** Deep endometriosis of the small intestine
      - Deep endometriosis of the small intestine, multifocal
    - ♀ **N80.569** Endometriosis of the small intestine, unspecified depth
      - Endometriosis of the small intestine NOS
- **N80.A Endometriosis of bladder and ureters**
  - ♀ **N80.A0** Endometriosis of bladder, unspecified depth
    - Endometriosis of bladder NOS
  - ♀ **N80.A1** Superficial endometriosis of bladder
  - ♀ **N80.A2** Deep endometriosis of bladder
  - **N80.A4** Superficial endometriosis of ureter
    - Extrinsic endometriosis of ureter
    - Code also, if applicable, obstructive and reflux uropathy (N13.-)
    - ♀ **N80.A41** Superficial endometriosis of right ureter
    - ♀ **N80.A42** Superficial endometriosis of left ureter
    - ♀ **N80.A43** Superficial endometriosis of bilateral ureters
    - ♀ **N80.A49** Superficial endometriosis of unspecified ureter
  - **N80.A5** Deep endometriosis of ureter
    - Intrinsic endometriosis of ureter
    - Code also, if applicable, obstructive and reflux uropathy (N13.-)
    - ♀ **N80.A51** Deep endometriosis of right ureter
    - ♀ **N80.A52** Deep endometriosis of left ureter
    - ♀ **N80.A53** Deep endometriosis of bilateral ureters
    - ♀ **N80.A59** Deep endometriosis of unspecified ureter
  - **N80.A6** Endometriosis of ureter, unspecified depth
    - Code also, if applicable, obstructive and reflux uropathy (N13.-)
    - ♀ **N80.A61** Endometriosis of right ureter, unspecified depth
    - ♀ **N80.A62** Endometriosis of left ureter, unspecified depth
    - ♀ **N80.A63** Endometriosis of bilateral ureters, unspecified depth
    - ♀ **N80.A69** Endometriosis of unspecified ureter, unspecified depth
- **N80.B Endometriosis of cardiothoracic space**
  - Endometriosis of thorax
  - Code also, if applicable:
    - catamenial hemothorax (J94.2)
    - catamenial pneumothorax (J93.12)
  - ♀ **N80.B1** Endometriosis of pleura
  - ♀ **N80.B2** Endometriosis of lung
  - **N80.B3** Endometriosis of diaphragm
    - ♀ **N80.B31** Superficial endometriosis of diaphragm
    - ♀ **N80.B32** Deep endometriosis of diaphragm
    - ♀ **N80.B39** Endometriosis of diaphragm, unspecified depth
      - Endometriosis of the diaphragm NOS
  - ♀ **N80.B4** Endometriosis of the pericardial space
  - ♀ **N80.B5** Endometriosis of the mediastinal space
  - ♀ **N80.B6** Endometriosis of cardiothoracic space
- **N80.C Endometriosis of the abdomen**
  - ♀ **N80.C0** Endometriosis of the abdomen, unspecified
    - Endometriosis of the abdomen NOS
  - **N80.C1** Endometriosis of the anterior abdominal wall
    - ♀ **N80.C10** Endometriosis of the anterior abdominal wall, subcutaneous tissue
    - ♀ **N80.C11** Endometriosis of the anterior abdominal wall, fascia and muscular layers
    - ♀ **N80.C19** Endometriosis of the anterior abdominal wall, unspecified depth
      - Endometriosis of the anterior abdominal wall NOS
  - ♀ **N80.C2** Endometriosis of the umbilicus
  - ♀ **N80.C3** Endometriosis of the inguinal canal
  - ♀ **N80.C4** Endometriosis of extra-pelvic abdominal peritoneum
  - ♀ **N80.C9** Endometriosis of other site of abdomen
- **N80.D Endometriosis of the pelvic nerves**
  - Endometriosis of the nerves of the retroperitoneum
  - ♀ **N80.D0** Endometriosis of the pelvic nerves, unspecified
    - Endometriosis of nerve of the retroperitoneum, NOS
  - ♀ **N80.D1** Endometriosis of the sacral splanchnic nerves
    - Endometriosis of the pelvic splanchnic nerves
  - ♀ **N80.D2** Endometriosis of the sacral nerve roots
  - ♀ **N80.D3** Endometriosis of the obturator nerve
  - ♀ **N80.D4** Endometriosis of the sciatic nerve
  - ♀ **N80.D5** Endometriosis of the pudendal nerve
  - ♀ **N80.D6** Endometriosis of the femoral nerve
  - ♀ **N80.D9** Endometriosis of other pelvic nerve
    - Endometriosis of the other nerves of the retroperitoneum
- ♀ **N80.6** Endometriosis in cutaneous scar
- ♀ **N80.8** Other endometriosis
  - Endometriosis of other site
- ♀ **N80.9** Endometriosis, unspecified

N81 Female genital prolapse
See page 896 for Vaginal Prolapse illustration.

Excludes1: genital prolapse complicating pregnancy, labor or delivery (O34.5-)
prolapse and hernia of ovary and fallopian tube (N83.4-)
prolapse of vaginal vault after hysterectomy (N99.3)

- ♀ **N81.0** Urethrocele
  - **Excludes1:** urethrocele with cystocele (N81.1-)
    urethrocele with prolapse of uterus (N81.2-N81.4)

- **N81.1 Cystocele**
  - Cystocele with urethrocele
  - Cystourethrocele
  - *Excludes1:* cystocele with prolapse of uterus (N81.2-N81.4)
  - ♀ **N81.10 Cystocele, unspecified**
    - Prolapse of (anterior) vaginal wall NOS
  - ♀ **N81.11 Cystocele, midline**
  - ♀ **N81.12 Cystocele, lateral**
    - Paravaginal cystocele
- ♀ **N81.2 Incomplete uterovaginal prolapse**
  - First degree uterine prolapse
  - Prolapse of cervix NOS
  - Second degree uterine prolapse
  - *Excludes1:* cervical stump prolapse (N81.85)
- ♀ **N81.3 Complete uterovaginal prolapse**
  - Procidentia (uteri) NOS
  - Third degree uterine prolapse
- ♀ **N81.4 Uterovaginal prolapse, unspecified**
  - Prolapse of uterus NOS
- ♀ **N81.5 Vaginal enterocele**
  - *Excludes1:* enterocele with prolapse of uterus (N81.2-N81.4)
- ♀ **N81.6 Rectocele**
  - Prolapse of posterior vaginal wall
  - Use additional code for any associated fecal incontinence, if applicable (R15.-)
  - *Excludes1:* rectocele with prolapse of uterus (N81.2-N81.4)
  - *Excludes2:* perineocele (N81.81)
    - rectal prolapse (K62.3)
- **N81.8 Other female genital prolapse**
  - ♀ **N81.81 Perineocele**
  - ♀ **N81.82 Incompetence or weakening of pubocervical tissue**
  - ♀ **N81.83 Incompetence or weakening of rectovaginal tissue**
  - ♀ **N81.84 Pelvic muscle wasting**
    - Disuse atrophy of pelvic muscles and anal sphincter
  - ♀ **N81.85 Cervical stump prolapse**
  - ♀ **N81.89 Other female genital prolapse**
    - Deficient perineum
    - Old laceration of muscles of pelvic floor
- ♀ **N81.9 Female genital prolapse, unspecified**

N82 Fistulae involving female genital tract
Excludes1: vesicointestinal fistulae (N32.1)
- ♀ CC **N82.0 Vesicovaginal fistula**
- ♀ CC **N82.1 Other female urinary-genital tract fistulae**
  - Cervicovesical fistula
  - Ureterovaginal fistula
  - Urethrovaginal fistula
  - Uteroureteric fistula
  - Uterovesical fistula
  - AHA CC: 3Q, 2017, 3-4
- ♀ CC **N82.2 Fistula of vagina to small intestine**
- ♀ CC **N82.3 Fistula of vagina to large intestine**
  - Rectovaginal fistula
- ♀ CC **N82.4 Other female intestinal-genital tract fistulae**
  - Intestinouterine fistula
- ♀ CC **N82.5 Female genital tract-skin fistulae**
  - Uterus to abdominal wall fistula
  - Vaginoperineal fistula
- ♀ CC **N82.8 Other female genital tract fistulae**
- ♀ CC **N82.9 Female genital tract fistula, unspecified**

N83 Noninflammatory disorders of ovary, fallopian tube and broad ligament
Excludes2: hydrosalpinx (N70.1-)
AHA CC: 4Q, 2016, 46
- **N83.0 Follicular cyst of ovary**
  - Cyst of graafian follicle
  - Hemorrhagic follicular cyst (of ovary)
  - ♀ **N83.00 Follicular cyst of ovary, unspecified side**
  - ♀ **N83.01 Follicular cyst of right ovary**
  - ♀ **N83.02 Follicular cyst of left ovary**
- **N83.1 Corpus luteum cyst**
  - Hemorrhagic corpus luteum cyst
  - ♀ **N83.10 Corpus luteum cyst of ovary, unspecified side**
  - ♀ **N83.11 Corpus luteum cyst of right ovary**
  - ♀ **N83.12 Corpus luteum cyst of left ovary**
    - AHA CC: 1Q, 2022, 23
- **N83.2 Other and unspecified ovarian cysts**
  - *Excludes1:* developmental ovarian cyst (Q50.1)
    - neoplastic ovarian cyst (D27.-)
    - polycystic ovarian syndrome (E28.2)
    - Stein-Leventhal syndrome (E28.2)
  - **N83.20 Unspecified ovarian cysts**
    - ♀ **N83.201 Unspecified ovarian cyst, right side**
    - ♀ **N83.202 Unspecified ovarian cyst, left side**
      - AHA CC: 1Q, 2022, 23
    - ♀ **N83.209 Unspecified ovarian cyst, unspecified side**
      - Ovarian cyst, NOS
  - **N83.29 Other ovarian cysts**
    - Retention cyst of ovary
    - Simple cyst of ovary
    - ♀ **N83.291 Other ovarian cyst, right side**
    - ♀ **N83.292 Other ovarian cyst, left side**
    - ♀ **N83.299 Other ovarian cyst, unspecified side**
- **N83.3 Acquired atrophy of ovary and fallopian tube**
  - **N83.31 Acquired atrophy of ovary**
    - ♀ **N83.311 Acquired atrophy of right ovary**
    - ♀ **N83.312 Acquired atrophy of left ovary**
    - ♀ **N83.319 Acquired atrophy of ovary, unspecified side**
      - Acquired atrophy of ovary, NOS
  - **N83.32 Acquired atrophy of fallopian tube**
    - ♀ **N83.321 Acquired atrophy of right fallopian tube**
    - ♀ **N83.322 Acquired atrophy of left fallopian tube**
    - ♀ **N83.329 Acquired atrophy of fallopian tube, unspecified side**
      - Acquired atrophy of fallopian tube, NOS
  - **N83.33 Acquired atrophy of ovary and fallopian tube**
    - ♀ **N83.331 Acquired atrophy of right ovary and fallopian tube**
    - ♀ **N83.332 Acquired atrophy of left ovary and fallopian tube**
    - ♀ **N83.339 Acquired atrophy of ovary and fallopian tube, unspecified side**
      - Acquired atrophy of ovary and fallopian tube, NOS
- **N83.4 Prolapse and hernia of ovary and fallopian tube**
  - ♀ **N83.40 Prolapse and hernia of ovary and fallopian tube, unspecified side**
    - Prolapse and hernia of ovary and fallopian tube, NOS
  - ♀ **N83.41 Prolapse and hernia of right ovary and fallopian tube**
  - ♀ **N83.42 Prolapse and hernia of left ovary and fallopian tube**
- **N83.5 Torsion of ovary, ovarian pedicle and fallopian tube**
  - Torsion of accessory tube
  - **N83.51 Torsion of ovary and ovarian pedicle**
    - ♀ CC **N83.511 Torsion of right ovary and ovarian pedicle**
    - ♀ CC **N83.512 Torsion of left ovary and ovarian pedicle**
    - ♀ CC **N83.519 Torsion of ovary and ovarian pedicle, unspecified side**
      - Torsion of ovary and ovarian pedicle, NOS
  - **N83.52 Torsion of fallopian tube**
    - Torsion of hydatid of Morgagni
    - ♀ CC **N83.521 Torsion of right fallopian tube**
    - ♀ CC **N83.522 Torsion of left fallopian tube**
    - ♀ CC **N83.529 Torsion of fallopian tube, unspecified side**
      - Torsion of fallopian tube, NOS
  - ♀ CC **N83.53 Torsion of ovary, ovarian pedicle and fallopian tube**
- ♀ **N83.6 Hematosalpinx**
  - *Excludes1:* hematosalpinx (with) (in):
    - hematocolpos (N89.7)
    - hematometra (N85.7)
    - tubal pregnancy (O00.1-)
- ♀ **N83.7 Hematoma of broad ligament**
- ♀ **N83.8 Other noninflammatory disorders of ovary, fallopian tube and broad ligament**
  - Broad ligament laceration syndrome [Allen-Masters]
- ♀ **N83.9 Noninflammatory disorder of ovary, fallopian tube and broad ligament, unspecified**

N84 Polyp of female genital tract
Excludes1: adenomatous polyp (D28.-)
placental polyp (O90.89)

- ♀ **N84.0 Polyp of corpus uteri**
  Polyp of endometrium
  Polyp of uterus NOS
  Excludes1: polypoid endometrial hyperplasia (N85.0-)
- ♀ **N84.1 Polyp of cervix uteri**
  Mucous polyp of cervix
- ♀ **N84.2 Polyp of vagina**
- ♀ **N84.3 Polyp of vulva**
  Polyp of labia
- ♀ **N84.8 Polyp of other parts of female genital tract**
- ♀ **N84.9 Polyp of female genital tract, unspecified**

N85 Other noninflammatory disorders of uterus, except cervix
Excludes1: endometriosis (N80.-)
inflammatory diseases of uterus (N71.-)
noninflammatory disorders of cervix, except malposition (N86-N88)
polyp of corpus uteri (N84.0)
uterine prolapse (N81.-)

- + **N85.0 Endometrial hyperplasia**
  - ♀ **N85.00 Endometrial hyperplasia, unspecified**
    Hyperplasia (adenomatous) (cystic) (glandular) of endometrium
    Hyperplastic endometritis
  - ♀ **N85.01 Benign endometrial hyperplasia**
    Endometrial hyperplasia (complex) (simple) without atypia
  - ♀ **N85.02 Endometrial intraepithelial neoplasia [EIN]**
    Endometrial hyperplasia with atypia
    Excludes1: malignant neoplasm of endometrium (with endometrial intraepithelial neoplasia [EIN]) (C54.1)
- ♀ **N85.2 Hypertrophy of uterus**
  Bulky or enlarged uterus
  Excludes1: puerperal hypertrophy of uterus (O90.89)
- ♀ **N85.3 Subinvolution of uterus**
  Excludes1: puerperal subinvolution of uterus (O90.89)
- ♀ **N85.4 Malposition of uterus**
  Anteversion of uterus
  Retroflexion of uterus
  Retroversion of uterus
  Excludes1: malposition of uterus complicating pregnancy, labor or delivery (O34.5-, O65.5)
- ♀ **N85.5 Inversion of uterus**
  Excludes1: current obstetric trauma (O71.2)
  postpartum inversion of uterus (O71.2)
- ♀ **N85.6 Intrauterine synechiae**
- ♀ **N85.7 Hematometra**
  Hematosalpinx with hematometra
  Excludes1: hematometra with hematocolpos (N89.7)
- ♀ **N85.8 Other specified noninflammatory disorders of uterus**
  Atrophy of uterus, acquired
  Fibrosis of uterus NOS
- ♀ **N85.9 Noninflammatory disorder of uterus, unspecified**
  Disorder of uterus NOS
- **N85.A Isthmocele**
  Isthmocele (non-pregnant state)
  Code also any associated conditions such as:
  abnormal uterine and vaginal bleeding, unspecified (N93.9)
  female infertility of uterine origin (N97.2)
  pelvic and perineal pain (R10.2)
  Excludes1: maternal care for cesarean scar defect (isthmocele) (O34.22)
  AHA CC: 4Q, 2022, 36-37

♀ N86 Erosion and ectropion of cervix uteri
Decubitus (trophic) ulcer of cervix
Eversion of cervix
Excludes1: erosion and ectropion of cervix with cervicitis (N72)
Valid 3-character code, no further characters required

N87 Dysplasia of cervix uteri
Excludes1: abnormal results from cervical cytologic examination without histologic confirmation (R87.61-)
carcinoma in situ of cervix uteri (D06.-)
cervical intraepithelial neoplasia III [CIN III] (D06.-)
HGSIL of cervix (R87.613)
severe dysplasia of cervix uteri (D06.-)

- ♀ **N87.0 Mild cervical dysplasia**
  Cervical intraepithelial neoplasia I [CIN I]
- ♀ **N87.1 Moderate cervical dysplasia**
  Cervical intraepithelial neoplasia II [CIN II]
- ♀ **N87.9 Dysplasia of cervix uteri, unspecified**
  Anaplasia of cervix
  Cervical atypism
  Cervical dysplasia NOS

N88 Other noninflammatory disorders of cervix uteri
Excludes2: inflammatory disease of cervix (N72)
polyp of cervix (N84.1)

- ♀ **N88.0 Leukoplakia of cervix uteri**
- ♀ **N88.1 Old laceration of cervix uteri**
  Adhesions of cervix
  Excludes1: current obstetric trauma (O71.3)
- ♀ **N88.2 Stricture and stenosis of cervix uteri**
  Excludes1: stricture and stenosis of cervix uteri complicating labor (O65.5)
- ♀ **N88.3 Incompetence of cervix uteri**
  Investigation and management of (suspected) cervical incompetence in a nonpregnant woman
  Excludes1: cervical incompetence complicating pregnancy (O34.3-)
- ♀ **N88.4 Hypertrophic elongation of cervix uteri**
- ♀ **N88.8 Other specified noninflammatory disorders of cervix uteri**
  Excludes1: current obstetric trauma (O71.3)
- ♀ **N88.9 Noninflammatory disorder of cervix uteri, unspecified**

N89 Other noninflammatory disorders of vagina
Excludes1: abnormal results from vaginal cytologic examination without histologic confirmation (R87.62-)
carcinoma in situ of vagina (D07.2)
HGSIL of vagina (R87.623)
inflammation of vagina (N76.-)
senile (atrophic) vaginitis (N95.2)
severe dysplasia of vagina (D07.2)
trichomonal leukorrhea (A59.00)
vaginal intraepithelial neoplasia [VAIN], grade III (D07.2)

- ♀ **N89.0 Mild vaginal dysplasia**
  Vaginal intraepithelial neoplasia [VAIN], grade I
- ♀ **N89.1 Moderate vaginal dysplasia**
  Vaginal intraepithelial neoplasia [VAIN], grade II
- ♀ **N89.3 Dysplasia of vagina, unspecified**
- ♀ **N89.4 Leukoplakia of vagina**
- ♀ **N89.5 Stricture and atresia of vagina**
  Vaginal adhesions
  Vaginal stenosis
  Excludes1: congenital atresia or stricture (Q52.4)
  postprocedural adhesions of vagina (N99.2)
- ♀ **N89.6 Tight hymenal ring**
  Rigid hymen
  Tight introitus
  Excludes1: imperforate hymen (Q52.3)
- ♀ **N89.7 Hematocolpos**
  Hematocolpos with hematometra or hematosalpinx
  AHA CC: 4Q, 2016, 58-59
- ♀ **N89.8 Other specified noninflammatory disorders of vagina**
  Leukorrhea NOS
  Old vaginal laceration
  Pessary ulcer of vagina
  Excludes1: current obstetric trauma (O70.-, O71.4, O71.7-O71.8)
  old laceration involving muscles of pelvic floor (N81.8)
- ♀ **N89.9 Noninflammatory disorder of vagina, unspecified**

N90 Other noninflammatory disorders of vulva and perineum
Excludes1: anogenital (venereal) warts (A63.0)
carcinoma in situ of vulva (D07.1)
condyloma acuminatum (A63.0)
current obstetric trauma (O70.-, O71.7-O71.8)
inflammation of vulva (N76.-)
severe dysplasia of vulva (D07.1)
vulvar intraepithelial neoplasm III [VIN III] (D07.1)

- ♀ **N90.0 Mild vulvar dysplasia**
  Vulvar intraepithelial neoplasia [VIN], grade I
- ♀ **N90.1 Moderate vulvar dysplasia**
  Vulvar intraepithelial neoplasia [VIN], grade II
- ♀ **N90.3 Dysplasia of vulva, unspecified**

- **N90.4 Leukoplakia of vulva**
  - Dystrophy of vulva
  - Kraurosis of vulva
  - Lichen sclerosus of external female genital organs
- **N90.5 Atrophy of vulva**
  - Stenosis of vulva
- **N90.6 Hypertrophy of vulva**
  - *AHA CC: 4Q, 2016, 46*
  - **N90.60 Unspecified hypertrophy of vulva**
    - Unspecified hypertrophy of labia
  - **N90.61 Childhood asymmetric labium majus enlargement**
    - CALME
  - **N90.69 Other specified hypertrophy of vulva**
    - Other specified hypertrophy of labia
- **N90.7 Vulvar cyst**
- **N90.8 Other specified noninflammatory disorders of vulva and perineum**
  - **N90.81 Female genital mutilation status**
    - Female genital cutting status
    - **N90.810 Female genital mutilation status, unspecified**
      - Female genital cutting status, unspecified
      - Female genital mutilation status NOS
    - **N90.811 Female genital mutilation Type I status**
      - Clitorectomy status
      - Female genital cutting Type I status
    - **N90.812 Female genital mutilation Type II status**
      - Clitorectomy with excision of labia minora status
      - Female genital cutting Type II status
    - **N90.813 Female genital mutilation Type III status**
      - Female genital cutting Type III status
      - Infibulation status
    - **N90.818 Other female genital mutilation status**
      - Female genital cutting Type IV status
      - Female genital mutilation Type IV status
      - Other female genital cutting status
  - **N90.89 Other specified noninflammatory disorders of vulva and perineum**
    - Adhesions of vulva
    - Hypertrophy of clitoris
- **N90.9 Noninflammatory disorder of vulva and perineum, unspecified**

N91 Absent, scanty and rare menstruation
Excludes1: *ovarian dysfunction (E28.-)*
- **N91.0 Primary amenorrhea**
- **N91.1 Secondary amenorrhea**
- **N91.2 Amenorrhea, unspecified**
- **N91.3 Primary oligomenorrhea**
- **N91.4 Secondary oligomenorrhea**
- **N91.5 Oligomenorrhea, unspecified**
  - Hypomenorrhea NOS

N92 Excessive, frequent and irregular menstruation
Excludes1: *postmenopausal bleeding (N95.0)*
precocious puberty (menstruation) (E30.1)
- **N92.0 Excessive and frequent menstruation with regular cycle**
  - Heavy periods NOS
  - Menorrhagia NOS
  - Polymenorrhea
- **N92.1 Excessive and frequent menstruation with irregular cycle**
  - Irregular intermenstrual bleeding
  - Irregular, shortened intervals between menstrual bleeding
  - Menometrorrhagia
  - Metrorrhagia
- **N92.2 Excessive menstruation at puberty**
  - Excessive bleeding associated with onset of menstrual periods
  - Pubertal menorrhagia
  - Puberty bleeding
- **N92.3 Ovulation bleeding**
  - Regular intermenstrual bleeding
- **N92.4 Excessive bleeding in the premenopausal period**
  - Climacteric menorrhagia or metrorrhagia
  - Menopausal menorrhagia or metrorrhagia
  - Perimenopausal bleeding
  - Perimenopausal menorrhagia or metrorrhagia
  - Preclimacteric menorrhagia or metrorrhagia
  - Premenopausal menorrhagia or metrorrhagia
- **N92.5 Other specified irregular menstruation**
- **N92.6 Irregular menstruation, unspecified**
  - Irregular bleeding NOS
  - Irregular periods NOS
  - **Excludes1:** *irregular menstruation with:*
    lengthened intervals or scanty bleeding (N91.3-N91.5)
    shortened intervals or excessive bleeding (N92.1)

N93 Other abnormal uterine and vaginal bleeding
Excludes1: *neonatal vaginal hemorrhage (P54.6)*
precocious puberty (menstruation) (E30.1)
pseudomenses (P54.6)
- **N93.0 Postcoital and contact bleeding**
- **N93.1 Pre-pubertal vaginal bleeding**
  - *AHA CC: 4Q, 2016, 47*
- **N93.8 Other specified abnormal uterine and vaginal bleeding**
  - Dysfunctional or functional uterine or vaginal bleeding NOS
- **N93.9 Abnormal uterine and vaginal bleeding, unspecified**

N94 Pain and other conditions associated with female genital organs and menstrual cycle
- **N94.0 Mittelschmerz**
- **N94.1 Dyspareunia**
  - **Excludes1:** *psychogenic dyspareunia (F52.6)*
  - *AHA CC: 4Q, 2016, 47*
  - **N94.10 Unspecified dyspareunia**
  - **N94.11 Superficial (introital) dyspareunia**
  - **N94.12 Deep dyspareunia**
  - **N94.19 Other specified dyspareunia**
- **N94.2 Vaginismus**
  - **Excludes1:** *psychogenic vaginismus (F52.5)*
- **N94.3 Premenstrual tension syndrome**
  - Code also associated menstrual migraine (G43.82-, G43.83-)
  - **Excludes1:** *Premenstrual dysphoric disorder (F32.81)*
- **N94.4 Primary dysmenorrhea**
- **N94.5 Secondary dysmenorrhea**
- **N94.6 Dysmenorrhea, unspecified**
  - **Excludes1:** *psychogenic dysmenorrhea (F45.8)*
- **N94.8 Other specified conditions associated with female genital organs and menstrual cycle**
  - **N94.81 Vulvodynia**
    - **N94.810 Vulvar vestibulitis**
    - **N94.818 Other vulvodynia**
    - **N94.819 Vulvodynia, unspecified**
      - Vulvodynia NOS
  - **N94.89 Other specified conditions associated with female genital organs and menstrual cycle**
- **N94.9 Unspecified condition associated with female genital organs and menstrual cycle**

N95 Menopausal and other perimenopausal disorders
Menopausal and other perimenopausal disorders due to naturally occurring (age-related) menopause and perimenopause
Excludes1: *excessive bleeding in the premenopausal period (N92.4)*
menopausal and perimenopausal disorders due to artificial or premature menopause (E89.4-, E28.31-)
premature menopause (E28.31-)
Excludes2: *postmenopausal osteoporosis (M81.0-)*
postmenopausal osteoporosis with current pathological fracture (M80.0-)
postmenopausal urethritis (N34.2)
- **N95.0 Postmenopausal bleeding**
- **N95.1 Menopausal and female climacteric states**
  - Symptoms such as flushing, sleeplessness, headache, lack of concentration, associated with natural (age-related) menopause
  - Use additional code for associated symptoms
  - **Excludes1:** *asymptomatic menopausal state (Z78.0)*
  symptoms associated with artificial menopause (E89.41)
  symptoms associated with premature menopause (E28.310)
- **N95.2 Postmenopausal atrophic vaginitis**
  - Senile (atrophic) vaginitis
- **N95.8 Other specified menopausal and perimenopausal disorders**
- **N95.9 Unspecified menopausal and perimenopausal disorder**

N96 Recurrent pregnancy loss
Investigation or care in a nonpregnant woman with history of recurrent pregnancy loss
Excludes1: recurrent pregancy loss with current pregnancy (O26.2-)
Valid 3-character code, no further characters required

N97 Female infertility
Includes: inability to achieve a pregnancy
sterility, female NOS
Excludes2: female infertility associated with:
hypopituitarism (E23.0)
incompetence of cervix uteri (N88.3)
Stein-Leventhal syndrome (E28.2)

- **N97.0** Female infertility associated with anovulation
  AHA CC: 2Q, 2022, 16
- **N97.1** Female infertility of tubal origin
  Female infertility associated with congenital anomaly of tube
  Female infertility due to tubal block
  Female infertility due to tubal occlusion
  Female infertility due to tubal stenosis
- **N97.2** Female infertility of uterine origin
  Female infertility associated with congenital anomaly of uterus
  Female infertility due to nonimplantation of ovum
- **N97.8** Female infertility of other origin
  AHA CC: 2Q, 2022, 15-16
- **N97.9** Female infertility, unspecified

N98 Complications associated with artificial fertilization
- CC **N98.0** Infection associated with artificial insemination
- CC **N98.1** Hyperstimulation of ovaries
  Hyperstimulation of ovaries NOS
  Hyperstimulation of ovaries associated with induced ovulation
- CC **N98.2** Complications of attempted introduction of fertilized ovum following in vitro fertilization
- CC **N98.3** Complications of attempted introduction of embryo in embryo transfer
- CC **N98.8** Other complications associated with artificial fertilization
- **N98.9** Complication associated with artificial fertilization, unspecified

Intraoperative and postprocedural complications and disorders of genitourinary system, not elsewhere classified (N99)

N99 Intraoperative and postprocedural complications and disorders of genitourinary system, not elsewhere classified
Excludes2: irradiation cystitis (N30.4-)
postoophorectomy osteoporosis with current pathological fracture (M80.8-)
postoophorectomy osteoporosis without current pathological fracture (M81.8)

- **N99.0** Postprocedural (acute) (chronic) kidney failure
  Use additional code to type of kidney disease
- **+ N99.1** Postprocedural urethral stricture
  Postcatheterization urethral stricture
  - **+ N99.11** Postprocedural urethral stricture, male
    - ♂ **N99.110** Postprocedural urethral stricture, male, meatal
    - ♂ **N99.111** Postprocedural bulbous urethral stricture, male
    - ♂ **N99.112** Postprocedural membranous urethral stricture, male
    - ♂ **N99.113** Postprocedural anterior bulbous urethral stricture, male
      AHA CC: 4Q, 2016, 47-48
    - ♂ **N99.114** Postprocedural urethral stricture, male, unspecified
    - ♂ **N99.115** Postprocedural fossa navicularis urethral stricture
      AHA CC: 4Q, 2016, 47-48
    - ♂ **N99.116** Postprocedural urethral stricture, male, overlapping sites
      AHA CC: 4Q, 2018, 21-22
  - ♀ **N99.12** Postprocedural urethral stricture, female
- ♀ **N99.2** Postprocedural adhesions of vagina
- ♀ **N99.3** Prolapse of vaginal vault after hysterectomy
- **N99.4** Postprocedural pelvic peritoneal adhesions
  Excludes2: pelvic peritoneal adhesions NOS (N73.6)
  postinfective pelvic peritoneal adhesions (N73.6)

- **+ N99.5** Complications of stoma of urinary tract
  Excludes2: mechanical complication of urinary catheter (T83.0-)
  AHA CC: 4Q, 2016, 48
  - **+ N99.51** Complication of cystostomy
    - CC **N99.510** Cystostomy hemorrhage
    - CC **N99.511** Cystostomy infection
    - CC **N99.512** Cystostomy malfunction
    - CC **N99.518** Other cystostomy complication
  - **+ N99.52** Complication of incontinent external stoma of urinary tract
    - **N99.520** Hemorrhage of incontinent external stoma of urinary tract
    - **N99.521** Infection of incontinent external stoma of urinary tract
      AHA CC: 4Q, 2016, 48
    - **N99.522** Malfunction of incontinent external stoma of urinary tract
    - **N99.523** Herniation of incontinent stoma of urinary tract
    - **N99.524** Stenosis of incontinent stoma of urinary tract
    - **N99.528** Other complication of incontinent external stoma of urinary tract
  - **+ N99.53** Complication of continent stoma of urinary tract
    - **N99.530** Hemorrhage of continent stoma of urinary tract
    - **N99.531** Infection of continent stoma of urinary tract
    - **N99.532** Malfunction of continent stoma of urinary tract
    - **N99.533** Herniation of continent stoma of urinary tract
    - **N99.534** Stenosis of continent stoma of urinary tract
    - **N99.538** Other complication of continent stoma of urinary tract
- **+ N99.6** Intraoperative hemorrhage and hematoma of a genitourinary system organ or structure complicating a procedure
  Excludes1: intraoperative hemorrhage and hematoma of a genitourinary system organ or structure due to accidental puncture or laceration during a procedure (N99.7-)
  - **N99.61** Intraoperative hemorrhage and hematoma of a genitourinary system organ or structure complicating a genitourinary system procedure
  - CC **N99.62** Intraoperative hemorrhage and hematoma of a genitourinary system organ or structure complicating other procedure
- **+ N99.7** Accidental puncture and laceration of a genitourinary system organ or structure during a procedure
  - CC **N99.71** Accidental puncture and laceration of a genitourinary system organ or structure during a genitourinary system procedure
  - CC **N99.72** Accidental puncture and laceration of a genitourinary system organ or structure during other procedure
- **+ N99.8** Other intraoperative and postprocedural complications and disorders of genitourinary system
  AHA CC: 4Q, 2016, 9-10
  - **N99.81** Other intraoperative complications of genitourinary system
  - **+ N99.82** Postprocedural hemorrhage of a genitourinary system organ or structure following a procedure
    - CC **N99.820** Postprocedural hemorrhage of a genitourinary system organ or structure following a genitourinary system procedure
    - CC **N99.821** Postprocedural hemorrhage of a genitourinary system organ or structure following other procedure
  - ♀ **N99.83** Residual ovary syndrome
  - **+ N99.84** Postprocedural hematoma and seroma of a genitourinary system organ or structure following a procedure
    - CC **N99.840** Postprocedural hematoma of a genitourinary system organ or structure following a genitourinary system procedure

CC **N99.841** Postprocedural hematoma of a genitourinary system organ or structure following other procedure

CC **N99.842** Postprocedural seroma of a genitourinary system organ or structure following a genitourinary system procedure

CC **N99.843** Postprocedural seroma of a genitourinary system organ or structure following other procedure

♀ **N99.85** Post endometrial ablation syndrome
AHA CC: 4Q, 2019, 12

N99.89 Other postprocedural complications and disorders of genitourinary system

Chapter 15: Pregnancy, Childbirth and the Puerperium (O00-O9A)

NOTE Codes from this chapter are for use only on maternal records, never on newborn records
Codes from this chapter are for use for conditions related to or aggravated by the pregnancy, childbirth, or by the puerperium (maternal causes or obstetric causes)

NOTE Trimesters are counted from the first day of the last menstrual period. They are defined as follows:
1st trimester- less than 14 weeks 0 days
2nd trimester- 14 weeks 0 days to less than 28 weeks 0 days
3rd trimester- 28 weeks 0 days until delivery

Use additional code, if applicable, from category Z3A, Weeks of gestation, to identify the specific week of the pregnancy, if known

Excludes1: supervision of normal pregnancy (Z34.-)

Excludes2: mental and behavioral disorders associated with the puerperium (F53.-)
obstetrical tetanus (A34)
postpartum necrosis of pituitary gland (E23.0)
puerperal osteomalacia (M83.0)

This chapter contains the following category blocks:
O00-O08	Pregnancy with abortive outcome
O09	Supervision of high risk pregnancy
O10-O16	Edema, proteinuria and hypertensive disorders in pregnancy, childbirth and the puerperium
O20-O29	Other maternal disorders predominantly related to pregnancy
O30-O48	Maternal care related to the fetus and amniotic cavity and possible delivery problems
O60-O77	Complications of labor and delivery
O80-O82	Encounter for delivery
O85-O92	Complications predominantly related to the puerperium
O94-O9A	Other obstetric conditions, not elsewhere classified

C. Chapter-Specific Coding Guidelines

In addition to general coding guidelines, there are guidelines for specific diagnoses and/or conditions in the classification. Unless otherwise indicated, these guidelines apply to all health care settings. Please refer to Section II for guidelines on the selection of principal diagnosis.

15. Chapter 15: Pregnancy, Childbirth and the Puerperium (O00-O9A)

a. General Rules for Obstetric Cases

1) Codes from chapter 15 and sequencing priority

Obstetric cases require codes from chapter 15, codes in the range O00-O9A, Pregnancy, Childbirth, and the Puerperium. Chapter 15 codes have sequencing priority over codes from other chapters. Additional codes from other chapters may be used in conjunction with chapter 15 codes to further specify conditions. Should the provider document that the pregnancy is incidental to the encounter, then code Z33.1, Pregnant state, incidental, should be used in place of any chapter 15 codes. It is the provider's responsibility to state that the condition being treated is not affecting the pregnancy.

2) Chapter 15 codes used only on the maternal record

Chapter 15 codes are to be used only on the maternal record, never on the record of the newborn.

3) Final character for trimester

The majority of codes in Chapter 15 have a final character indicating the trimester of pregnancy. The timeframes for the trimesters are indicated at the beginning of the chapter. If trimester is not a component of a code it is because the condition always occurs in a specific trimester, or the concept of trimester of pregnancy is not applicable. Certain codes have characters for only certain trimesters because the condition does not occur in all trimesters, but it may occur in more than just one.

Assignment of the final character for trimester should be based on the provider's documentation of the trimester (or number of weeks) for the current admission/encounter. This applies to the assignment of trimester for pre-existing conditions as well as those that develop during or are due to the pregnancy. The provider's documentation of the number of weeks may be used to assign the appropriate code identifying the trimester.

Whenever delivery occurs during the current admission, and there is an "in childbirth" option for the obstetric complication being coded, the "in childbirth" code should be assigned. When the classification does not provide an obstetric code with an "in childbirth" option, it is appropriate to assign a code describing the current trimester.

4) Selection of trimester for inpatient admissions that encompass more than one trimester

In instances when a patient is admitted to a hospital for complications of pregnancy during one trimester and remains in the hospital into a subsequent trimester, the trimester character for the antepartum complication code should be assigned on the basis of the trimester when the complication developed, not the trimester of the discharge. If the condition developed prior to the current admission/encounter or represents a pre-existing condition, the trimester character for the trimester at the time of the admission/encounter should be assigned.

5) Unspecified trimester

Each category that includes codes for trimester has a code for "unspecified trimester." The "unspecified trimester" code should rarely be used, such as when the documentation in the record is insufficient to determine the trimester and it is not possible to obtain clarification.

6) 7th character for Fetus Identification

Where applicable, a 7th character is to be assigned for certain categories (O31, O32, O33.3 - O33.6, O35, O36, O40, O41, O60.1, O60.2, O64, and O69) to identify the fetus for which the complication code applies.

Assign 7th character "0":
- For single gestations
- When the documentation in the record is insufficient to determine the fetus affected and it is not possible to obtain clarification.
- When it is not possible to clinically determine which fetus is affected.

7) Completed weeks of gestation

In ICD-10-CM, "completed" weeks of gestation refers to full weeks. For example, if the provider documents gestation at 39 weeks and 6 days, the code for 39 weeks of gestation should be assigned, as the patient has not yet reached 40 completed weeks.

b. Selection of OB Principal or First-listed Diagnosis

1) Routine outpatient prenatal visits

For routine outpatient prenatal visits when no complications are present, a code from category Z34, Encounter for supervision of normal pregnancy, should be used as the first-listed diagnosis. These codes should not be used in conjunction with chapter 15 codes.

2) Supervision of High-Risk Pregnancy

Codes from category O09, Supervision of high-risk pregnancy, are intended for use only during the prenatal period. For complications during the labor or delivery episode as a result of a high-risk pregnancy, assign the applicable complication codes from Chapter 15. If there are no complications during the labor or delivery episode, assign code O80, Encounter for full-term uncomplicated delivery.

For routine prenatal outpatient visits for patients with high-risk pregnancies, a code from category O09, Supervision of high-risk pregnancy, should be used as the first-listed diagnosis. Secondary chapter 15 codes may be used in conjunction with these codes if appropriate.

3) Episodes when no delivery occurs

In episodes when no delivery occurs, the principal diagnosis should correspond to the principal complication of the pregnancy which necessitated the encounter. Should more than one complication exist, all of which are treated or monitored, any of the complications codes may be sequenced first.

4) When a delivery occurs

When an obstetric patient is admitted and delivers during that admission, the condition that prompted the admission should be sequenced as the principal diagnosis. If multiple conditions prompted the admission, sequence the one most related to the delivery as the principal diagnosis. A code for any complication of the delivery should be assigned as an additional diagnosis. In cases of cesarean delivery, if the patient was admitted with a condition that resulted in the performance of a cesarean procedure, that condition should be selected as the principal diagnosis. If the reason for the admission was unrelated to the condition resulting in the cesarean delivery, the condition related to the reason for the admission should be selected as the principal diagnosis.

5) Outcome of delivery

A code from category Z37, Outcome of delivery, should be included on every maternal record when a delivery has occurred. These codes are not to be used on subsequent records or on the newborn record.

c. Pre-existing conditions versus conditions due to the pregnancy

Certain categories in Chapter 15 distinguish between conditions of the mother that existed prior to pregnancy (pre-existing) and those that are a direct result of pregnancy. When assigning codes from Chapter 15, it is important to assess if a condition was pre-existing prior to pregnancy or developed during or due to the pregnancy in order to assign the correct code.

Categories that do not distinguish between pre-existing and pregnancy-related conditions may be used for either. It is acceptable to use codes specifically for the puerperium with codes complicating pregnancy and childbirth if a condition arises postpartum during the delivery encounter.

d. Pre-existing hypertension in pregnancy

Category O10, Pre-existing hypertension complicating pregnancy, childbirth and the puerperium, includes codes for hypertensive heart and hypertensive chronic kidney disease. When assigning one of the O10 codes that includes hypertensive heart disease or hypertensive chronic kidney disease, it is necessary to add a secondary code from the appropriate hypertension category to specify the type of heart failure or chronic kidney disease.

See Section I.C.9. Hypertension.

e. Fetal Conditions Affecting the Management of the Mother

1) Codes from categories O35 and O36

Codes from categories O35, Maternal care for known or suspected fetal abnormality and damage, and O36, Maternal care for other fetal problems, are assigned only when the fetal condition is actually responsible for modifying the management of the mother, i.e., by requiring diagnostic studies, additional observation, special care, or termination of pregnancy. The fact that the fetal condition exists does not justify assigning a code from this series to the mother's record.

2) In utero surgery

In cases when surgery is performed on the fetus, a diagnosis code from category O35, Maternal care for known or suspected fetal abnormality and damage, should be assigned identifying the fetal condition. Assign the appropriate procedure code for the procedure performed.

No code from Chapter 16, the perinatal codes, should be used on the mother's record to identify fetal conditions. Surgery performed in utero on a fetus is still to be coded as an obstetric encounter.

f. HIV Infection in Pregnancy, Childbirth and the Puerperium

During pregnancy, childbirth or the puerperium, a patient admitted because of an HIV-related illness should receive a principal diagnosis from subcategory O98.7-, Human immunodeficiency [HIV] disease complicating pregnancy, childbirth and the puerperium, followed by the code(s) for the HIV-related illness(es).

Patients with asymptomatic HIV infection status admitted during pregnancy, childbirth, or the puerperium should receive codes of O98.7- and Z21, Asymptomatic human immunodeficiency virus [HIV] infection status.

g. Diabetes mellitus in pregnancy

Diabetes mellitus is a significant complicating factor in pregnancy. Pregnant women who are diabetic should be assigned a code from category O24, Diabetes mellitus in pregnancy, childbirth, and the puerperium, first, followed by the appropriate diabetes code(s) (E08-E13) from Chapter 4.

h. Long term use of insulin and oral hypoglycemics

See section I.C.4.a.3 for information on the long term use of insulin and oral hypoglycemic.

i. Gestational (pregnancy induced) diabetes

Gestational (pregnancy induced) diabetes can occur during the second and third trimester of pregnancy in patients who were not diabetic prior to pregnancy. Gestational diabetes can cause complications in the pregnancy similar to those of pre-existing diabetes mellitus. It also puts the patient at greater risk of developing diabetes after the pregnancy. Codes for gestational diabetes are in subcategory O24.4, Gestational diabetes mellitus. No other code from category O24, Diabetes mellitus in pregnancy, childbirth, and the puerperium, should be used with a code from O24.4

The codes under subcategory O24.4 include diet controlled, insulin controlled, and controlled by oral hypoglycemic drugs. If a patient with gestational diabetes is treated with both diet and insulin, only the code for insulin-controlled is required. If a patient with gestational diabetes is treated with both diet and oral hypoglycemic medications, only the code for "controlled by oral hypoglycemic drugs" is required. Code Z79.4, Long-term (current) use of insulin, Z79.84, Long-term (current) use of oral hypoglycemic drugs, and Z79.85, Long-term (current) use of injectable non-insulin antidiabetic drugs, should not be assigned with codes from subcategory O24.4.

An abnormal glucose tolerance in pregnancy is assigned a code from subcategory O99.81, Abnormal glucose complicating pregnancy, childbirth, and the puerperium.

j. Sepsis and septic shock complicating abortion, pregnancy, childbirth and the puerperium

When assigning a chapter 15 code for sepsis complicating abortion, pregnancy, childbirth, and the puerperium, a code for the specific type of infection should be assigned as an additional diagnosis. If severe sepsis is present, a code from subcategory R65.2, Severe sepsis, and code(s) for associated organ dysfunction(s) should also be assigned as additional diagnoses.

k. Puerperal sepsis

Code O85, Puerperal sepsis, should be assigned with a secondary code to identify the causal organism (e.g., for a bacterial infection, assign a code from category B95-B96, Bacterial infections in conditions classified elsewhere). A code from category A40, Streptococcal sepsis, or A41, Other sepsis, should not be used for puerperal sepsis. If applicable, use additional codes to identify severe sepsis (R65.2-) and any associated acute organ dysfunction.

Code O85 should not be assigned for sepsis following an obstetrical procedure (*See Section I.C.1.d.5b., Sepsis due to a postprocedural infection*).

l. Alcohol, tobacco and drug use during pregnancy, childbirth and the puerperium

1) Alcohol use during pregnancy, childbirth and the puerperium

Codes under subcategory O99.31, Alcohol use complicating pregnancy, childbirth, and the puerperium, should be assigned for any pregnancy case when a patient uses alcohol during the pregnancy or postpartum. A secondary code from category F10, Alcohol related disorders, should also be assigned to identify manifestations of the alcohol use.

2) Tobacco use during pregnancy, childbirth and the puerperium

Codes under subcategory O99.33, Smoking (tobacco) complicating pregnancy, childbirth, and the puerperium, should be assigned for any pregnancy case when a mother uses any type of tobacco product during the pregnancy or postpartum. A secondary code from category F17, Nicotine dependence, should also be assigned to identify the type of nicotine dependence.

3) Drug use during pregnancy, childbirth and the puerperium

Codes under subcategory O99.32, Drug use complicating pregnancy, childbirth, and the puerperium, should be assigned for any pregnancy case when a patient uses drugs during the pregnancy or postpartum. This can involve illegal drugs, or inappropriate use or abuse of prescription drugs. Secondary code(s) from categories F11-F16 and F18-F19 should also be assigned to identify manifestations of the drug use.

m. Poisoning, toxic effects, adverse effects and underdosing in a pregnant patient

A code from subcategory O9A.2, Injury, poisoning and certain other consequences of external causes complicating pregnancy, childbirth, and the puerperium, should be sequenced first, followed by the appropriate injury, poisoning, toxic effect, adverse effect or underdosing code, and then the additional code(s) that specifies the condition caused by the poisoning, toxic effect, adverse effect or underdosing.

See Section I.C.19. Adverse effects, poisoning, underdosing and toxic effects.

n. Normal Delivery, Code O80

1) Encounter for full term uncomplicated delivery

Code O80 should be assigned when a patient is admitted for a full-term normal delivery and delivers a single, healthy infant without any complications antepartum, during the delivery, or postpartum during the delivery episode. Code O80 is always a principal diagnosis. It is not to be used if any other code from chapter 15 is needed to describe a current complication of the antenatal, delivery, or postnatal period. Additional codes from other chapters may be used with code O80 if they are not related to or are in any way complicating the pregnancy.

2) Uncomplicated delivery with resolved antepartum complication

Code O80 may be used if the patient had a complication at some point during the pregnancy., but the complication is not present at the time of the admission for delivery.

3) Outcome of delivery for O80

Z37.0, Single live birth, is the only outcome of delivery code appropriate for use with O80.

o. The Peripartum and Postpartum Periods

1) Peripartum and Postpartum periods

The postpartum period begins immediately after delivery and continues for six weeks following delivery. The peripartum period is defined as the last month of pregnancy to five months postpartum.

2) Peripartum and postpartum complication

A postpartum complication is any complication occurring within the six-week period.

3) Pregnancy-related complications after 6 week period

Chapter 15 codes may also be used to describe pregnancy-related complications after the peripartum or postpartum period if the provider documents that a condition is pregnancy related.

4) Admission for routine postpartum care following delivery outside hospital

When the mother delivers outside the hospital prior to admission and is admitted for routine postpartum care and no complications are noted, code Z39.0, Encounter for care and examination of mother immediately after delivery, should be assigned as the principal diagnosis.

5) Pregnancy associated cardiomyopathy

Pregnancy associated cardiomyopathy, code O90.3, is unique in that it may be diagnosed in the third trimester of pregnancy but may continue to progress months after delivery. For this reason, it is referred to as peripartum cardiomyopathy. Code O90.3 is only for use when the cardiomyopathy develops as a result of pregnancy in a woman who did not have pre-existing heart disease.

p. Code O94, Sequelae of complication of pregnancy, childbirth, and the puerperium

1) Code O94

Code O94, Sequelae of complication of pregnancy, childbirth, and the puerperium, is for use in those cases when an initial complication of a pregnancy develops a sequelae requiring care or treatment at a future date.

2) After the initial postpartum period

This code may be used at any time after the initial postpartum period.

3) Sequencing of Code O94

This code, like all sequela codes, is to be sequenced following the code describing the sequelae of the complication.

q. Termination of Pregnancy and Spontaneous abortions

1) Abortion with Liveborn Fetus

When an attempted termination of pregnancy results in a liveborn fetus, assign code Z33.2, Encounter for elective termination of pregnancy and a code from category Z37, Outcome of Delivery.

2) Retained Products of Conception following an abortion

Subsequent encounters for retained products of conception following a spontaneous abortion or elective termination of pregnancy, without complications are assigned O03.4, Incomplete spontaneous, abortion without complication, or codes O07.4, Failed attempted termination of pregnancy without complication. This advice is appropriate even when the patient was discharged previously with a discharge diagnosis of complete abortion. If the patient has a specific complication associated with the spontaneous abortion or elective termination of pregnancy in addition to retained products of conception, assign the appropriate complication code (e.g., O03.-, O04.-, O07.-) instead of code O03.4 or O07.4.

3) Complications leading to abortion

Codes from Chapter 15 may be used as additional codes to identify any documented complications of the pregnancy in conjunction with codes in categories in O04, O07 and O08.

4) Hemorrhage following elective abortion

For hemorrhage post elective abortion, assign code O04.6, Delayed or excessive hemorrhage following (induced) termination of pregnancy. Do not assign code O72.1, Other immediate postpartum hemorrhage, as this code should not be assigned for post abortion conditions.

r. Abuse in a pregnant patient

For suspected or confirmed cases of abuse of a pregnant patient, a code(s) from subcategories O9A.3, Physical abuse complicating pregnancy, childbirth, and the puerperium, O9A.4, Sexual abuse complicating pregnancy, childbirth, and the puerperium, and O9A.5, Psychological abuse complicating pregnancy, childbirth, and the puerperium, should be sequenced first, followed by the appropriate codes (if applicable) to identify any associated current injury due to physical abuse, sexual abuse, and the perpetrator of abuse.

See Section I.C.19. Adult and child abuse, neglect and other maltreatment.

s. COVID-19 infection in pregnancy, childbirth, and the puerperium

During pregnancy, childbirth or the puerperium, when COVID-19 is the reason for admission/encounter, code O98.5-, Other viral diseases complicating pregnancy, childbirth and the puerperium, should be sequenced as the principal/first-listed diagnosis, and code U07.1, COVID-19, and the appropriate codes for associated manifestation(s) should be assigned as additional diagnoses. Codes from Chapter 15 always take sequencing priority.

If the reason for admission/encounter is unrelated to COVID-19 but the patient tests positive for COVID-19 during the admission/encounter, the appropriate code for the reason for admission/encounter should be sequenced as the principal/first-listed diagnosis, and code O98.5- and U07.1, as well as the appropriate codes for associated COVID-19 manifestations, should be assigned as additional diagnoses.

Pregnancy with abortive outcome (O00-O08)

Excludes1: continuing pregnancy in multiple gestation after abortion of one fetus or more (O31.1-, O31.3-)

O00 Ectopic pregnancy

Includes: ruptured ectopic pregnancy

Use additional code from category O08 to identify any associated complication

AHA CC: 4Q, 2016, 48-50

+ **O00.0 Abdominal pregnancy**

Excludes1: maternal care for viable fetus in abdominal pregnancy (O36.7-)

• ♀ CC **O00.00** Abdominal pregnancy without intrauterine pregnancy
Abdominal pregnancy NOS

• ♀ CC **O00.01** Abdominal pregnancy with intrauterine pregnancy

+ **O00.1 Tubal pregnancy**
Fallopian pregnancy
Rupture of (fallopian) tube due to pregnancy
Tubal abortion
AHA CC: 4Q, 2017, 20

+ **O00.10** Tubal pregnancy without intrauterine pregnancy
Tubal pregnancy NOS

• ♀ CC **O00.101** Right tubal pregnancy without intrauterine pregnancy

• ♀ CC **O00.102** Left tubal pregnancy without intrauterine pregnancy

• ♀ CC **O00.109** Unspecified tubal pregnancy without intrauterine pregnancy

+ **O00.11** Tubal pregnancy with intrauterine pregnancy

• ♀ CC **O00.111** Right tubal pregnancy with intrauterine pregnancy

• ♀ CC **O00.112** Left tubal pregnancy with intrauterine pregnancy

• ♀ CC **O00.119** Unspecified tubal pregnancy with intrauterine pregnancy

+ **O00.2 Ovarian pregnancy**
AHA CC: 4Q, 2017, 20

+ **O00.20** Ovarian pregnancy without intrauterine pregnancy
Ovarian pregnancy NOS

• ♀ CC **O00.201** Right ovarian pregnancy without intrauterine pregnancy

• ♀ CC **O00.202** Left ovarian pregnancy without intrauterine pregnancy

• ♀ CC **O00.209** Unspecified ovarian pregnancy without intrauterine pregnancy

+ **O00.21** Ovarian pregnancy with intrauterine pregnancy

• ♀ CC **O00.211** Right ovarian pregnancy with intrauterine pregnancy

• ♀ CC **O00.212** Left ovarian pregnancy with intrauterine pregnancy

• ♀ CC **O00.219** Unspecified ovarian pregnancy with intrauterine pregnancy

+ **O00.8 Other ectopic pregnancy**
Cervical pregnancy
Cornual pregnancy
Intraligamentous pregnancy
Mural pregnancy

• ♀ CC **O00.80** Other ectopic pregnancy without intrauterine pregnancy
Other ectopic pregnancy NOS

• ♀ CC **O00.81** Other ectopic pregnancy with intrauterine pregnancy

+ **O00.9 Ectopic pregnancy, unspecified**

• ♀ CC **O00.90** Unspecified ectopic pregnancy without intrauterine pregnancy
Ectopic pregnancy NOS

• ♀ CC **O00.91** Unspecified ectopic pregnancy with intrauterine pregnancy

O01 Hydatidiform mole

Use additional code from category O08 to identify any associated complication

Excludes1: chorioadenoma (destruens) (D39.2)
malignant hydatidiform mole (D39.2)

• ♀ **O01.0** Classical hydatidiform mole
Complete hydatidiform mole

• ♀ **O01.1** Incomplete and partial hydatidiform mole

• ♀ **O01.9** Hydatidiform mole, unspecified
Trophoblastic disease NOS
Vesicular mole NOS

Ectopic Pregnancy I - Tubal Pregnancy

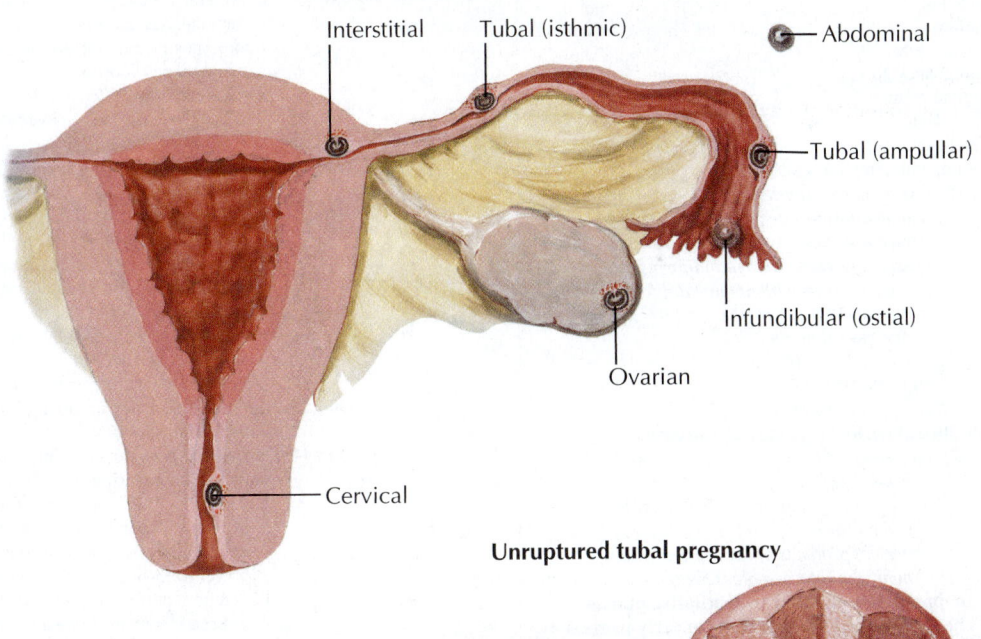

Unruptured tubal pregnancy

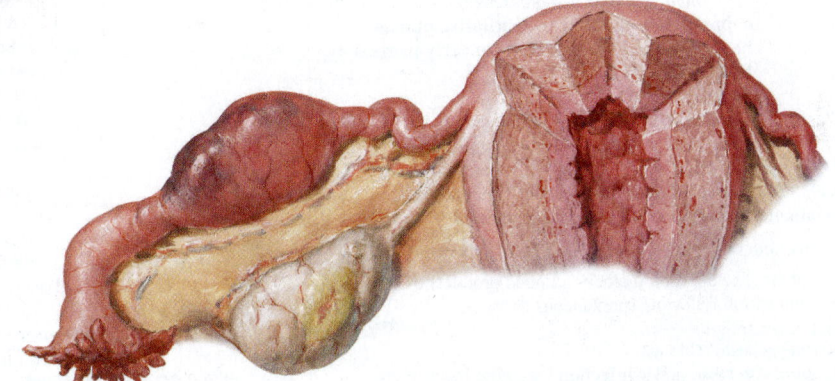

Section through tubal pregnancy

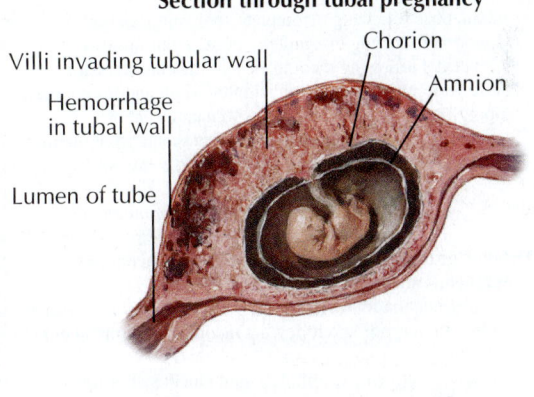

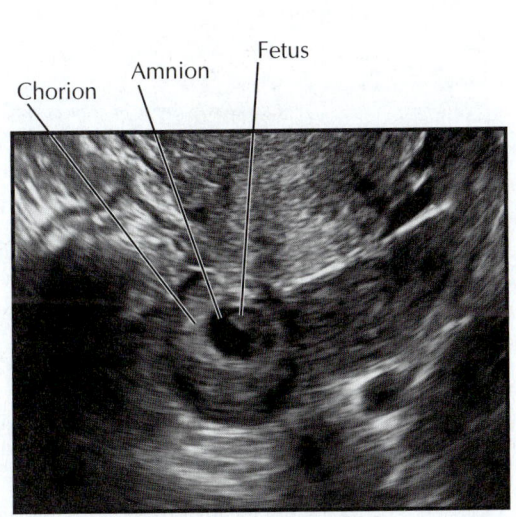

Ultrasonographic view of adnexa

O02 Other abnormal products of conception
Use additional code from category O08 to identify any associated complication
Excludes1: papyraceous fetus (O31.0-)

- ♀ **O02.0 Blighted ovum and nonhydatidiform mole**
  Carneous mole
  Fleshy mole
  Intrauterine mole NOS
  Molar pregnancy NEC
  Pathological ovum
- ♀ **O02.1 Missed abortion**
  Early fetal death, before completion of 20 weeks of gestation, with retention of dead fetus
  Excludes1: failed induced abortion (O07.-)
  fetal death (intrauterine) (late) (O36.4)
  missed abortion with blighted ovum (O02.0)
  missed abortion with hydatidiform mole (O01.-)
  missed abortion with nonhydatidiform (O02.0)
  missed abortion with other abnormal products of conception (O02.8-)
  missed delivery (O36.4)
  stillbirth (P95)
  AHA CC: 3Q, 2019, 11-12; 2Q, 2022, 3-4
+ **O02.8 Other specified abnormal products of conception**
  Excludes1: abnormal products of conception with blighted ovum (O02.0)
  abnormal products of conception with hydatidiform mole (O01.-)
  abnormal products of conception with nonhydatidiform mole (O02.0)
  - ♀ **O02.81 Inappropriate change in quantitative human chorionic gonadotropin (hCG) in early pregnancy**
    Biochemical pregnancy
    Chemical pregnancy
    Inappropriate level of quantitative human chorionic gonadotropin (hCG) for gestational age in early pregnancy
  - ♀ **O02.89 Other abnormal products of conception**
- ♀ **O02.9 Abnormal product of conception, unspecified**

O03 Spontaneous abortion
NOTE Incomplete abortion includes retained products of conception following spontaneous abortion
Includes: miscarriage
Review coding guideline C.15.q.2

- ♀ CC **O03.0 Genital tract and pelvic infection following incomplete spontaneous abortion**
  Endometritis following incomplete spontaneous abortion
  Oophoritis following incomplete spontaneous abortion
  Parametritis following incomplete spontaneous abortion
  Pelvic peritonitis following incomplete spontaneous abortion
  Salpingitis following incomplete spontaneous abortion
  Salpingo-oophoritis following incomplete spontaneous abortion
  Excludes1: sepsis following incomplete spontaneous abortion (O03.37)
  urinary tract infection following incomplete spontaneous abortion (O03.38)
- ♀ **O03.1 Delayed or excessive hemorrhage following incomplete spontaneous abortion**
  Afibrinogenemia following incomplete spontaneous abortion
  Defibrination syndrome following incomplete spontaneous abortion
  Hemolysis following incomplete spontaneous abortion
  Intravascular coagulation following incomplete spontaneous abortion
  AHA CC: 1Q, 2022, 19
- ♀ MCC **O03.2 Embolism following incomplete spontaneous abortion**
  Air embolism following incomplete spontaneous abortion
  Amniotic fluid embolism following incomplete spontaneous abortion
  Blood-clot embolism following incomplete spontaneous abortion
  Embolism NOS following incomplete spontaneous abortion
  Fat embolism following incomplete spontaneous abortion
  Pulmonary embolism following incomplete spontaneous abortion
  Pyemic embolism following incomplete spontaneous abortion
  Septic or septicopyemic embolism following incomplete spontaneous abortion
  Soap embolism following incomplete spontaneous abortion
  Review coding guideline C.15.j

+ **O03.3 Other and unspecified complications following incomplete spontaneous abortion**
  - ♀ CC **O03.30 Unspecified complication following incomplete spontaneous abortion**
  - ♀ MCC **O03.31 Shock following incomplete spontaneous abortion**
    Circulatory collapse following incomplete spontaneous abortion
    Shock (postprocedural) following incomplete spontaneous abortion
    Excludes1: shock due to infection following incomplete spontaneous abortion (O03.37)
  - ♀ MCC **O03.32 Renal failure following incomplete spontaneous abortion**
    Kidney failure (acute) following incomplete spontaneous abortion
    Oliguria following incomplete spontaneous abortion
    Renal shutdown following incomplete spontaneous abortion
    Renal tubular necrosis following incomplete spontaneous abortion
    Uremia following incomplete spontaneous abortion
  - ♀ CC **O03.33 Metabolic disorder following incomplete spontaneous abortion**
  - ♀ CC **O03.34 Damage to pelvic organs following incomplete spontaneous abortion**
    Laceration, perforation, tear or chemical damage of bladder following incomplete spontaneous abortion
    Laceration, perforation, tear or chemical damage of bowel following incomplete spontaneous abortion
    Laceration, perforation, tear or chemical damage of broad ligament following incomplete spontaneous abortion
    Laceration, perforation, tear or chemical damage of cervix following incomplete spontaneous abortion
    Laceration, perforation, tear or chemical damage of periurethral tissue following incomplete spontaneous abortion
    Laceration, perforation, tear or chemical damage of uterus following incomplete spontaneous abortion
    Laceration, perforation, tear or chemical damage of vagina following incomplete spontaneous abortion
  - ♀ CC **O03.35 Other venous complications following incomplete spontaneous abortion**
  - ♀ CC **O03.36 Cardiac arrest following incomplete spontaneous abortion**
  - ♀ CC **O03.37 Sepsis following incomplete spontaneous abortion**
    Use additional code to identify infectious agent (B95-B97)
    Use additional code to identify severe sepsis, if applicable (R65.2-)
    Excludes1: septic or septicopyemic embolism following incomplete spontaneous abortion (O03.2)
    Review coding guideline C.15.j
  - ♀ CC **O03.38 Urinary tract infection following incomplete spontaneous abortion**
    Cystitis following incomplete spontaneous abortion
  - ♀ CC **O03.39 Incomplete spontaneous abortion with other complications**
- ♀ **O03.4 Incomplete spontaneous abortion without complication**
  AHA CC: 1Q, 2023, 17
- ♀ CC **O03.5 Genital tract and pelvic infection following complete or unspecified spontaneous abortion**
  Endometritis following complete or unspecified spontaneous abortion
  Oophoritis following complete or unspecified spontaneous abortion
  Parametritis following complete or unspecified spontaneous abortion
  Pelvic peritonitis following complete or unspecified spontaneous abortion
  Salpingitis following complete or unspecified spontaneous abortion
  Salpingo-oophoritis following complete or unspecified spontaneous abortion
  Excludes1: sepsis following complete or unspecified spontaneous abortion (O03.87)
  urinary tract infection following complete or unspecified spontaneous abortion (O03.88)

- ♀ **O03.6** **Delayed or excessive hemorrhage following complete or unspecified spontaneous abortion**
  - Afibrinogenemia following complete or unspecified spontaneous abortion
  - Defibrination syndrome following complete or unspecified spontaneous abortion
  - Hemolysis following complete or unspecified spontaneous abortion
  - Intravascular coagulation following complete or unspecified spontaneous abortion
  - *AHA CC: 1Q, 2022, 19*
- ♀ CC **O03.7** **Embolism following complete or unspecified spontaneous abortion**
  - Air embolism following complete or unspecified spontaneous abortion
  - Amniotic fluid embolism following complete or unspecified spontaneous abortion
  - Blood-clot embolism following complete or unspecified spontaneous abortion
  - Embolism NOS following complete or unspecified spontaneous abortion
  - Fat embolism following complete or unspecified spontaneous abortion
  - Pulmonary embolism following complete or unspecified spontaneous abortion
  - Pyemic embolism following complete or unspecified spontaneous abortion
  - Septic or septicopyemic embolism following complete or unspecified spontaneous abortion
  - Soap embolism following complete or unspecified spontaneous abortion
- + **O03.8** **Other and unspecified complications following complete or unspecified spontaneous abortion**
  - ♀ CC **O03.80** **Unspecified complication following complete or unspecified spontaneous abortion**
  - ♀ MCC **O03.81** **Shock following complete or unspecified spontaneous abortion**
    - Circulatory collapse following complete or unspecified spontaneous abortion
    - Shock (postprocedural) following complete or unspecified spontaneous abortion
    - **Excludes1:** shock due to infection following complete or unspecified spontaneous abortion (O03.87)
  - ♀ MCC **O03.82** **Renal failure following complete or unspecified spontaneous abortion**
    - Kidney failure (acute) following complete or unspecified spontaneous abortion
    - Oliguria following complete or unspecified spontaneous abortion
    - Renal shutdown following complete or unspecified spontaneous abortion
    - Renal tubular necrosis following complete or unspecified spontaneous abortion
    - Uremia following complete or unspecified spontaneous abortion
  - ♀ CC **O03.83** **Metabolic disorder following complete or unspecified spontaneous abortion**
  - ♀ CC **O03.84** **Damage to pelvic organs following complete or unspecified spontaneous abortion**
    - Laceration, perforation, tear or chemical damage of bladder following complete or unspecified spontaneous abortion
    - Laceration, perforation, tear or chemical damage of bowel following complete or unspecified spontaneous abortion
    - Laceration, perforation, tear or chemical damage of broad ligament following complete or unspecified spontaneous abortion
    - Laceration, perforation, tear or chemical damage of cervix following complete or unspecified spontaneous abortion
    - Laceration, perforation, tear or chemical damage of periurethral tissue following complete or unspecified spontaneous abortion
    - Laceration, perforation, tear or chemical damage of uterus following complete or unspecified spontaneous abortion
    - Laceration, perforation, tear or chemical damage of vagina following complete or unspecified spontaneous abortion
  - ♀ CC **O03.85** **Other venous complications following complete or unspecified spontaneous abortion**
  - ♀ CC **O03.86** **Cardiac arrest following complete or unspecified spontaneous abortion**
  - ♀ CC **O03.87** **Sepsis following complete or unspecified spontaneous abortion**
    - Use additional code to identify infectious agent (B95-B97)
    - Use additional code to identify severe sepsis, if applicable (R65.2-)
    - **Excludes1:** septic or septicopyemic embolism following complete or unspecified spontaneous abortion (O03.7)
    - *Review coding guideline C.15.j*
  - ♀ CC **O03.88** **Urinary tract infection following complete or unspecified spontaneous abortion**
    - Cystitis following complete or unspecified spontaneous abortion
  - ♀ CC **O03.89** **Complete or unspecified spontaneous abortion with other complications**
- ♀ **O03.9** **Complete or unspecified spontaneous abortion without complication**
  - Miscarriage NOS
  - Spontaneous abortion NOS

O04 **Complications following (induced) termination of pregnancy**
  - **Includes:** complications following (induced) termination of pregnancy
  - **Excludes2:** encounter for elective termination of pregnancy, uncomplicated (Z33.2)
    - failed attempted termination of pregnancy (O07.-)
- ♀ CC **O04.5** **Genital tract and pelvic infection following (induced) termination of pregnancy**
  - Endometritis following (induced) termination of pregnancy
  - Oophoritis following (induced) termination of pregnancy
  - Parametritis following (induced) termination of pregnancy
  - Pelvic peritonitis following (induced) termination of pregnancy
  - Salpingitis following (induced) termination of pregnancy
  - Salpingo-oophoritis following (induced) termination of pregnancy
  - **Excludes1:** sepsis following (induced) termination of pregnancy (O04.87)
    - urinary tract infection following (induced) termination of pregnancy (O04.88)
- ♀ **O04.6** **Delayed or excessive hemorrhage following (induced) termination of pregnancy**
  - Afibrinogenemia following (induced) termination of pregnancy
  - Defibrination syndrome following (induced) termination of pregnancy
  - Hemolysis following (induced) termination of pregnancy
  - Intravascular coagulation following (induced) termination of pregnancy
  - *AHA CC: 3Q, 2019, 11-12; 2Q, 2023, 15-16*
- ♀ MCC **O04.7** **Embolism following (induced) termination of pregnancy**
  - Air embolism following (induced) termination of pregnancy
  - Amniotic fluid embolism following (induced) termination of pregnancy
  - Blood-clot embolism following (induced) termination of pregnancy
  - Embolism NOS following (induced) termination of pregnancy
  - Fat embolism following (induced) termination of pregnancy
  - Pulmonary embolism following (induced) termination of pregnancy
  - Pyemic embolism following (induced) termination of pregnancy
  - Septic or septicopyemic embolism following (induced) termination of pregnancy
  - Soap embolism following (induced) termination of pregnancy
- + **O04.8** **(Induced) termination of pregnancy with other and unspecified complications**
  - ♀ CC **O04.80** **(Induced) termination of pregnancy with unspecified complications**
  - ♀ MCC **O04.81** **Shock following (induced) termination of pregnancy**
    - Circulatory collapse following (induced) termination of pregnancy
    - Shock (postprocedural) following (induced) termination of pregnancy
    - **Excludes1:** shock due to infection following (induced) termination of pregnancy (O04.87)

- ♀ MCC **O04.82** Renal failure following (induced) termination of pregnancy
  - Kidney failure (acute) following (induced) termination of pregnancy
  - Oliguria following (induced) termination of pregnancy
  - Renal shutdown following (induced) termination of pregnancy
  - Renal tubular necrosis following (induced) termination of pregnancy
  - Uremia following (induced) termination of pregnancy
- ♀ CC **O04.83** Metabolic disorder following (induced) termination of pregnancy
- ♀ CC **O04.84** Damage to pelvic organs following (induced) termination of pregnancy
  - Laceration, perforation, tear or chemical damage of bladder following (induced) termination of pregnancy
  - Laceration, perforation, tear or chemical damage of bowel following (induced) termination of pregnancy
  - Laceration, perforation, tear or chemical damage of broad ligament following (induced) termination of pregnancy
  - Laceration, perforation, tear or chemical damage of cervix following (induced) termination of pregnancy
  - Laceration, perforation, tear or chemical damage of periurethral tissue following (induced) termination of pregnancy
  - Laceration, perforation, tear or chemical damage of uterus following (induced) termination of pregnancy
  - Laceration, perforation, tear or chemical damage of vagina following (induced) termination of pregnancy
- ♀ CC **O04.85** Other venous complications following (induced) termination of pregnancy
- ♀ CC **O04.86** Cardiac arrest following (induced) termination of pregnancy
- ♀ CC **O04.87** Sepsis following (induced) termination of pregnancy
  - Use additional code to identify infectious agent (B95-B97)
  - Use additional code to identify severe sepsis, if applicable (R65.2-)
  - **Excludes1:** septic or septicopyemic embolism following (induced) termination of pregnancy (O04.7)
  - Review coding guideline C.15.j
- ♀ CC **O04.88** Urinary tract infection following (induced) termination of pregnancy
  - Cystitis following (induced) termination of pregnancy
- ♀ CC **O04.89** (Induced) termination of pregnancy with other complications

O07 Failed attempted termination of pregnancy
Includes: failure of attempted induction of termination of pregnancy
incomplete elective abortion
Excludes1: incomplete spontaneous abortion (O03.0-)

- ♀ CC **O07.0** Genital tract and pelvic infection following failed attempted termination of pregnancy
  - Endometritis following failed attempted termination of pregnancy
  - Oophoritis following failed attempted termination of pregnancy
  - Parametritis following failed attempted termination of pregnancy
  - Pelvic peritonitis following failed attempted termination of pregnancy
  - Salpingitis following failed attempted termination of pregnancy
  - Salpingo-oophoritis following failed attempted termination of pregnancy
  - **Excludes1:** sepsis following failed attempted termination of pregnancy (O07.37)
    urinary tract infection following failed attempted termination of pregnancy (O07.38)
- ♀ CC **O07.1** Delayed or excessive hemorrhage following failed attempted termination of pregnancy
  - Afibrinogenemia following failed attempted termination of pregnancy
  - Defibrination syndrome following failed attempted termination of pregnancy
  - Hemolysis following failed attempted termination of pregnancy
  - Intravascular coagulation following failed attempted termination of pregnancy
- ♀ MCC **O07.2** Embolism following failed attempted termination of pregnancy
  - Air embolism following failed attempted termination of pregnancy
  - Amniotic fluid embolism following failed attempted termination of pregnancy
  - Blood-clot embolism following failed attempted termination of pregnancy
  - Embolism NOS following failed attempted termination of pregnancy
  - Fat embolism following failed attempted termination of pregnancy
  - Pulmonary embolism following failed attempted termination of pregnancy
  - Pyemic embolism following failed attempted termination of pregnancy
  - Septic or septicopyemic embolism following failed attempted termination of pregnancy
  - Soap embolism following failed attempted termination of pregnancy
- + **O07.3** Failed attempted termination of pregnancy with other and unspecified complications
  - ♀ CC **O07.30** Failed attempted termination of pregnancy with unspecified complications
  - ♀ MCC **O07.31** Shock following failed attempted termination of pregnancy
    - Circulatory collapse following failed attempted termination of pregnancy
    - Shock (postprocedural) following failed attempted termination of pregnancy
    - **Excludes1:** shock due to infection following failed attempted termination of pregnancy (O07.37)
  - ♀ MCC **O07.32** Renal failure following failed attempted termination of pregnancy
    - Kidney failure (acute) following failed attempted termination of pregnancy
    - Oliguria following failed attempted termination of pregnancy
    - Renal shutdown following failed attempted termination of pregnancy
    - Renal tubular necrosis following failed attempted termination of pregnancy
    - Uremia following failed attempted termination of pregnancy
  - ♀ CC **O07.33** Metabolic disorder following failed attempted termination of pregnancy
  - ♀ CC **O07.34** Damage to pelvic organs following failed attempted termination of pregnancy
    - Laceration, perforation, tear or chemical damage of bladder following failed attempted termination of pregnancy
    - Laceration, perforation, tear or chemical damage of bowel following failed attempted termination of pregnancy
    - Laceration, perforation, tear or chemical damage of broad ligament following failed attempted termination of pregnancy
    - Laceration, perforation, tear or chemical damage of cervix following failed attempted termination of pregnancy
    - Laceration, perforation, tear or chemical damage of periurethral tissue following failed attempted termination of pregnancy
    - Laceration, perforation, tear or chemical damage of uterus following failed attempted termination of pregnancy
    - Laceration, perforation, tear or chemical damage of vagina following failed attempted termination of pregnancy

- ♀ CC **O07.35** Other venous complications following failed attempted termination of pregnancy
- ♀ CC **O07.36** Cardiac arrest following failed attempted termination of pregnancy
- ♀ CC **O07.37** Sepsis following failed attempted termination of pregnancy

  Use additional code (B95-B97), to identify infectious agent

  Use additional code (R65.2-) to identify severe sepsis, if applicable

  Excludes1: septic or septicopyemic embolism following failed attempted termination of pregnancy (O07.2)

  Review coding guideline C.15.j

- ♀ CC **O07.38** Urinary tract infection following failed attempted termination of pregnancy

  Cystitis following failed attempted termination of pregnancy

- ♀ CC **O07.39** Failed attempted termination of pregnancy with other complications
- ♀ CC **O07.4** Failed attempted termination of pregnancy without complication

  Review coding guideline C.15.q.2

O08 Complications following ectopic and molar pregnancy

This category is for use with categories O00-O02 to identify any associated complications

- ♀ CC **O08.0** Genital tract and pelvic infection following ectopic and molar pregnancy

  Endometritis following ectopic and molar pregnancy
  Oophoritis following ectopic and molar pregnancy
  Parametritis following ectopic and molar pregnancy
  Pelvic peritonitis following ectopic and molar pregnancy
  Salpingitis following ectopic and molar pregnancy
  Salpingo-oophoritis following ectopic and molar pregnancy

  Excludes1: sepsis following ectopic and molar pregnancy (O08.82)
  urinary tract infection (O08.83)

- ♀ CC **O08.1** Delayed or excessive hemorrhage following ectopic and molar pregnancy

  Afibrinogenemia following ectopic and molar pregnancy
  Defibrination syndrome following ectopic and molar pregnancy
  Hemolysis following ectopic and molar pregnancy
  Intravascular coagulation following ectopic and molar pregnancy

  Excludes1: delayed or excessive hemorrhage due to incomplete abortion (O03.1)

- ♀ MCC **O08.2** Embolism following ectopic and molar pregnancy

  Air embolism following ectopic and molar pregnancy
  Amniotic fluid embolism following ectopic and molar pregnancy
  Blood-clot embolism following ectopic and molar pregnancy
  Embolism NOS following ectopic and molar pregnancy
  Fat embolism following ectopic and molar pregnancy
  Pulmonary embolism following ectopic and molar pregnancy
  Pyemic embolism following ectopic and molar pregnancy
  Septic or septicopyemic embolism following ectopic and molar pregnancy
  Soap embolism following ectopic and molar pregnancy

- ♀ MCC **O08.3** Shock following ectopic and molar pregnancy

  Circulatory collapse following ectopic and molar pregnancy
  Shock (postprocedural) following ectopic and molar pregnancy

  Excludes1: shock due to infection following ectopic and molar pregnancy (O08.82)

- ♀ MCC **O08.4** Renal failure following ectopic and molar pregnancy

  Kidney failure (acute) following ectopic and molar pregnancy
  Oliguria following ectopic and molar pregnancy
  Renal shutdown following ectopic and molar pregnancy
  Renal tubular necrosis following ectopic and molar pregnancy
  Uremia following ectopic and molar pregnancy

- ♀ CC **O08.5** Metabolic disorders following an ectopic and molar pregnancy
- ♀ CC **O08.6** Damage to pelvic organs and tissues following an ectopic and molar pregnancy

  Laceration, perforation, tear or chemical damage of bladder following an ectopic and molar pregnancy
  Laceration, perforation, tear or chemical damage of bowel following an ectopic and molar pregnancy
  Laceration, perforation, tear or chemical damage of broad ligament following an ectopic and molar pregnancy
  Laceration, perforation, tear or chemical damage of cervix following an ectopic and molar pregnancy
  Laceration, perforation, tear or chemical damage of periurethral tissue following an ectopic and molar pregnancy
  Laceration, perforation, tear or chemical damage of uterus following an ectopic and molar pregnancy
  Laceration, perforation, tear or chemical damage of vagina following an ectopic and molar pregnancy

- ♀ CC **O08.7** Other venous complications following an ectopic and molar pregnancy
- + **O08.8** Other complications following an ectopic and molar pregnancy
  - ♀ CC **O08.81** Cardiac arrest following an ectopic and molar pregnancy
  - ♀ CC **O08.82** Sepsis following ectopic and molar pregnancy

    Use additional code (B95-B97), to identify infectious agent

    Use additional code (R65.2-) to identify severe sepsis, if applicable

    Excludes1: septic or septicopyemic embolism following ectopic and molar pregnancy (O08.2)

    Review coding guideline C.15.j

  - ♀ CC **O08.83** Urinary tract infection following an ectopic and molar pregnancy

    Cystitis following an ectopic and molar pregnancy

  - ♀ CC **O08.89** Other complications following an ectopic and molar pregnancy

- ♀ CC **O08.9** Unspecified complication following an ectopic and molar pregnancy

Supervision of high risk pregnancy (O09)

O09 Supervision of high risk pregnancy

  Review coding guideline C.15.b.2
  AHA CC: 4Q, 2016, 48-50

- + **O09.0** Supervision of pregnancy with history of infertility
  - ♀ **O09.00** Supervision of pregnancy with history of infertility, unspecified trimester
  - ♀ **O09.01** Supervision of pregnancy with history of infertility, first trimester
  - ♀ **O09.02** Supervision of pregnancy with history of infertility, second trimester
  - ♀ **O09.03** Supervision of pregnancy with history of infertility, third trimester
- + **O09.1** Supervision of pregnancy with history of ectopic pregnancy
  - ♀ **O09.10** Supervision of pregnancy with history of ectopic pregnancy, unspecified trimester
  - ♀ **O09.11** Supervision of pregnancy with history of ectopic pregnancy, first trimester
  - ♀ **O09.12** Supervision of pregnancy with history of ectopic pregnancy, second trimester
  - ♀ **O09.13** Supervision of pregnancy with history of ectopic pregnancy, third trimester
- + **O09.A** Supervision of pregnancy with history of molar pregnancy
  - ♀ **O09.A0** Supervision of pregnancy with history of molar pregnancy, unspecified trimester
  - ♀ **O09.A1** Supervision of pregnancy with history of molar pregnancy, first trimester
  - ♀ **O09.A2** Supervision of pregnancy with history of molar pregnancy, second trimester
  - ♀ **O09.A3** Supervision of pregnancy with history of molar pregnancy, third trimester

- **O09.2 Supervision of pregnancy with other poor reproductive or obstetric history**

  Excludes2: pregnancy care for patient with history of recurrent pregnancy loss (O26.2-)

  - **O09.21 Supervision of pregnancy with history of pre-term labor**
    - ♀ **O09.211** Supervision of pregnancy with history of pre-term labor, first trimester
    - ♀ **O09.212** Supervision of pregnancy with history of pre-term labor, second trimester
    - ♀ **O09.213** Supervision of pregnancy with history of pre-term labor, third trimester
    - ♀ **O09.219** Supervision of pregnancy with history of pre-term labor, unspecified trimester
  - **O09.29 Supervision of pregnancy with other poor reproductive or obstetric history**

    Supervision of pregnancy with history of neonatal death

    Supervision of pregnancy with history of stillbirth

    - ♀ **O09.291** Supervision of pregnancy with other poor reproductive or obstetric history, first trimester
    - ♀ **O09.292** Supervision of pregnancy with other poor reproductive or obstetric history, second trimester
    - ♀ **O09.293** Supervision of pregnancy with other poor reproductive or obstetric history, third trimester
    - ♀ **O09.299** Supervision of pregnancy with other poor reproductive or obstetric history, unspecified trimester

- **O09.3 Supervision of pregnancy with insufficient antenatal care**

  Supervision of concealed pregnancy

  Supervision of hidden pregnancy

  - ♀ **O09.30** Supervision of pregnancy with insufficient antenatal care, unspecified trimester
  - ♀ **O09.31** Supervision of pregnancy with insufficient antenatal care, first trimester
  - ♀ **O09.32** Supervision of pregnancy with insufficient antenatal care, second trimester
  - ♀ **O09.33** Supervision of pregnancy with insufficient antenatal care, third trimester

- **O09.4 Supervision of pregnancy with grand multiparity**
  - ♀ **O09.40** Supervision of pregnancy with grand multiparity, unspecified trimester
  - ♀ **O09.41** Supervision of pregnancy with grand multiparity, first trimester
  - ♀ **O09.42** Supervision of pregnancy with grand multiparity, second trimester
  - ♀ **O09.43** Supervision of pregnancy with grand multiparity, third trimester

- **O09.5 Supervision of elderly primigravida and multigravida**

  Pregnancy for a female 35 years and older at expected date of delivery

  - **O09.51 Supervision of elderly primigravida**
    - ♀ **O09.511** Supervision of elderly primigravida, first trimester
    - ♀ **O09.512** Supervision of elderly primigravida, second trimester
    - ♀ **O09.513** Supervision of elderly primigravida, third trimester
    - ♀ **O09.519** Supervision of elderly primigravida, unspecified trimester
  - **O09.52 Supervision of elderly multigravida**
    - ♀ **O09.521** Supervision of elderly multigravida, first trimester
    - ♀ **O09.522** Supervision of elderly multigravida, second trimester
    - ♀ **O09.523** Supervision of elderly multigravida, third trimester
    - ♀ **O09.529** Supervision of elderly multigravida, unspecified trimester

- **O09.6 Supervision of young primigravida and multigravida**

  Supervision of pregnancy for a female less than 16 years old at expected date of delivery

  - **O09.61 Supervision of young primigravida**
    - ♀ **O09.611** Supervision of young primigravida, first trimester
    - ♀ **O09.612** Supervision of young primigravida, second trimester
    - ♀ **O09.613** Supervision of young primigravida, third trimester
    - ♀ **O09.619** Supervision of young primigravida, unspecified trimester
  - **O09.62 Supervision of young multigravida**
    - ♀ **O09.621** Supervision of young multigravida, first trimester
    - ♀ **O09.622** Supervision of young multigravida, second trimester
    - ♀ **O09.623** Supervision of young multigravida, third trimester
    - ♀ **O09.629** Supervision of young multigravida, unspecified trimester

- **O09.7 Supervision of high risk pregnancy due to social problems**
  - ♀ **O09.70** Supervision of high risk pregnancy due to social problems, unspecified trimester
  - ♀ **O09.71** Supervision of high risk pregnancy due to social problems, first trimester
  - ♀ **O09.72** Supervision of high risk pregnancy due to social problems, second trimester
  - ♀ **O09.73** Supervision of high risk pregnancy due to social problems, third trimester

- **O09.8 Supervision of other high risk pregnancies**
  - **O09.81 Supervision of pregnancy resulting from assisted reproductive technology**

    Supervision of pregnancy resulting from in-vitro fertilization

    Excludes2: gestational carrier status (Z33.3)

    - ♀ **O09.811** Supervision of pregnancy resulting from assisted reproductive technology, first trimester
    - ♀ **O09.812** Supervision of pregnancy resulting from assisted reproductive technology, second trimester
    - ♀ **O09.813** Supervision of pregnancy resulting from assisted reproductive technology, third trimester
    - ♀ **O09.819** Supervision of pregnancy resulting from assisted reproductive technology, unspecified trimester
  - **O09.82 Supervision of pregnancy with history of in utero procedure during previous pregnancy**
    - ♀ **O09.821** Supervision of pregnancy with history of in utero procedure during previous pregnancy, first trimester
    - ♀ **O09.822** Supervision of pregnancy with history of in utero procedure during previous pregnancy, second trimester
    - ♀ **O09.823** Supervision of pregnancy with history of in utero procedure during previous pregnancy, third trimester
    - ♀ **O09.829** Supervision of pregnancy with history of in utero procedure during previous pregnancy, unspecified trimester

      Excludes1: supervision of pregnancy affected by in utero procedure during current pregnancy (O35.7)
  - **O09.89 Supervision of other high risk pregnancies**
    - ♀ **O09.891** Supervision of other high risk pregnancies, first trimester
    - ♀ **O09.892** Supervision of other high risk pregnancies, second trimester
    - ♀ **O09.893** Supervision of other high risk pregnancies, third trimester
    - ♀ **O09.899** Supervision of other high risk pregnancies, unspecified trimester

- **O09.9 Supervision of high risk pregnancy, unspecified**
  - ♀ **O09.90** Supervision of high risk pregnancy, unspecified, unspecified trimester
  - ♀ **O09.91** Supervision of high risk pregnancy, unspecified, first trimester
  - ♀ **O09.92** Supervision of high risk pregnancy, unspecified, second trimester
  - ♀ **O09.93** Supervision of high risk pregnancy, unspecified, third trimester

Edema, proteinuria and hypertensive disorders in pregnancy, childbirth and the puerperium (O10-O16)

O10 Pre-existing hypertension complicating pregnancy, childbirth and the puerperium

Includes: pre-existing hypertension with pre-existing proteinuria complicating pregnancy, childbirth and the puerperium

Excludes2: pre-existing hypertension with superimposed pre-eclampsia complicating pregnancy, childbirth and the puerperium (O11.-)

Review coding guideline C.15.d

- **O10.0** Pre-existing essential hypertension complicating pregnancy, childbirth and the puerperium
  Any condition in I10 specified as a reason for obstetric care during pregnancy, childbirth or the puerperium
  - **O10.01** Pre-existing essential hypertension complicating pregnancy,
    - CC **O10.011** Pre-existing essential hypertension complicating pregnancy, first trimester
    - CC **O10.012** Pre-existing essential hypertension complicating pregnancy, second trimester
    - CC **O10.013** Pre-existing essential hypertension complicating pregnancy, third trimester
    - **O10.019** Pre-existing essential hypertension complicating pregnancy, unspecified trimester
  - CC **O10.02** Pre-existing essential hypertension complicating childbirth
  - **O10.03** Pre-existing essential hypertension complicating the puerperium
- **O10.1** Pre-existing hypertensive heart disease complicating pregnancy, childbirth and the puerperium
  Any condition in I11 specified as a reason for obstetric care during pregnancy, childbirth or the puerperium
  Use additional code from I11 to identify the type of hypertensive heart disease
  - **O10.11** Pre-existing hypertensive heart disease complicating pregnancy
    - **O10.111** Pre-existing hypertensive heart disease complicating pregnancy, first trimester
    - **O10.112** Pre-existing hypertensive heart disease complicating pregnancy, second trimester
    - **O10.113** Pre-existing hypertensive heart disease complicating pregnancy, third trimester
    - **O10.119** Pre-existing hypertensive heart disease complicating pregnancy, unspecified trimester
  - **O10.12** Pre-existing hypertensive heart disease complicating childbirth
  - **O10.13** Pre-existing hypertensive heart disease complicating the puerperium
- **O10.2** Pre-existing hypertensive chronic kidney disease complicating pregnancy, childbirth and the puerperium
  Any condition in I12 specified as a reason for obstetric care during pregnancy, childbirth or the puerperium
  Use additional code from I12 to identify the type of hypertensive chronic kidney disease
  - **O10.21** Pre-existing hypertensive chronic kidney disease complicating pregnancy
    - **O10.211** Pre-existing hypertensive chronic kidney disease complicating pregnancy, first trimester
    - **O10.212** Pre-existing hypertensive chronic kidney disease complicating pregnancy, second trimester
    - **O10.213** Pre-existing hypertensive chronic kidney disease complicating pregnancy, third trimester
    - **O10.219** Pre-existing hypertensive chronic kidney disease complicating pregnancy, unspecified trimester
  - **O10.22** Pre-existing hypertensive chronic kidney disease complicating childbirth
  - **O10.23** Pre-existing hypertensive chronic kidney disease complicating the puerperium
- **O10.3** Pre-existing hypertensive heart and chronic kidney disease complicating pregnancy, childbirth and the puerperium
  Any condition in I13 specified as a reason for obstetric care during pregnancy, childbirth or the puerperium
  Use additional code from I13 to identify the type of hypertensive heart and chronic kidney disease
  - **O10.31** Pre-existing hypertensive heart and chronic kidney disease complicating pregnancy
    - **O10.311** Pre-existing hypertensive heart and chronic kidney disease complicating pregnancy, first trimester
    - **O10.312** Pre-existing hypertensive heart and chronic kidney disease complicating pregnancy, second trimester
    - **O10.313** Pre-existing hypertensive heart and chronic kidney disease complicating pregnancy, third trimester
    - **O10.319** Pre-existing hypertensive heart and chronic kidney disease complicating pregnancy, unspecified trimester
  - **O10.32** Pre-existing hypertensive heart and chronic kidney disease complicating childbirth
  - **O10.33** Pre-existing hypertensive heart and chronic kidney disease complicating the puerperium
- **O10.4** Pre-existing secondary hypertension complicating pregnancy, childbirth and the puerperium
  Any condition in I15 specified as a reason for obstetric care during pregnancy, childbirth or the puerperium
  Use additional code from I15 to identify the type of secondary hypertension
  - **O10.41** Pre-existing secondary hypertension complicating pregnancy
    - CC **O10.411** Pre-existing secondary hypertension complicating pregnancy, first trimester
    - CC **O10.412** Pre-existing secondary hypertension complicating pregnancy, second trimester
    - CC **O10.413** Pre-existing secondary hypertension complicating pregnancy, third trimester
    - **O10.419** Pre-existing secondary hypertension complicating pregnancy, unspecified trimester
  - MCC **O10.42** Pre-existing secondary hypertension complicating childbirth
  - CC **O10.43** Pre-existing secondary hypertension complicating the puerperium
- **O10.9** Unspecified pre-existing hypertension complicating pregnancy, childbirth and the puerperium
  - **O10.91** Unspecified pre-existing hypertension complicating pregnancy
    - CC **O10.911** Unspecified pre-existing hypertension complicating pregnancy, first trimester
    - CC **O10.912** Unspecified pre-existing hypertension complicating pregnancy, second trimester
    - CC **O10.913** Unspecified pre-existing hypertension complicating pregnancy, third trimester
    - **O10.919** Unspecified pre-existing hypertension complicating pregnancy, unspecified trimester
  - CC **O10.92** Unspecified pre-existing hypertension complicating childbirth
  - **O10.93** Unspecified pre-existing hypertension complicating the puerperium

O11 Pre-existing hypertension with pre-eclampsia

Includes: conditions in O10 complicated by pre-eclampsia
pre-eclampsia superimposed pre-existing hypertension

Use additional code from O10 to identify the type of hypertension
AHA CC: 4Q, 2016, 50

- MCC **O11.1** Pre-existing hypertension with pre-eclampsia, first trimester
- MCC **O11.2** Pre-existing hypertension with pre-eclampsia, second trimester
- MCC **O11.3** Pre-existing hypertension with pre-eclampsia, third trimester

- ♀ **O11.4** Pre-existing hypertension with pre-eclampsia, complicating childbirth
- ♀ **O11.5** Pre-existing hypertension with pre-eclampsia, complicating the puerperium
- ♀ **O11.9** Pre-existing hypertension with pre-eclampsia, unspecified trimester

O12 Gestational [pregnancy-induced] edema and proteinuria without hypertension

AHA CC: 4Q, 2016, 50

+ **O12.0** Gestational edema
    - ♀ **O12.00** Gestational edema, unspecified trimester
    - ♀ **O12.01** Gestational edema, first trimester
    - ♀ **O12.02** Gestational edema, second trimester
    - ♀ **O12.03** Gestational edema, third trimester
    - ♀ **O12.04** Gestational edema, complicating childbirth
    - ♀ **O12.05** Gestational edema, complicating the puerperium
+ **O12.1** Gestational proteinuria
    - ♀ **O12.10** Gestational proteinuria, unspecified trimester
    - ♀ CC **O12.11** Gestational proteinuria, first trimester
    - ♀ CC **O12.12** Gestational proteinuria, second trimester
    - ♀ CC **O12.13** Gestational proteinuria, third trimester
    - ♀ **O12.14** Gestational proteinuria, complicating childbirth
    - ♀ **O12.15** Gestational proteinuria, complicating the puerperium
+ **O12.2** Gestational edema with proteinuria
    - ♀ **O12.20** Gestational edema with proteinuria, unspecified trimester
    - ♀ CC **O12.21** Gestational edema with proteinuria, first trimester
    - ♀ CC **O12.22** Gestational edema with proteinuria, second trimester
    - ♀ CC **O12.23** Gestational edema with proteinuria, third trimester
    - ♀ **O12.24** Gestational edema with proteinuria, complicating childbirth
    - ♀ **O12.25** Gestational edema with proteinuria, complicating the puerperium

O13 Gestational [pregnancy-induced] hypertension without significant proteinuria

Includes: gestational hypertension NOS
transient hypertension of pregnancy
Review coding guideline C.9.a.7
AHA CC: 4Q, 2016, 50

- ♀ **O13.1** Gestational [pregnancy-induced] hypertension without significant proteinuria, first trimester
- ♀ **O13.2** Gestational [pregnancy-induced] hypertension without significant proteinuria, second trimester
- ♀ **O13.3** Gestational [pregnancy-induced] hypertension without significant proteinuria, third trimester
- ♀ **O13.4** Gestational [pregnancy-induced] hypertension without significant proteinuria, complicating childbirth
- ♀ **O13.5** Gestational [pregnancy-induced] hypertension without significant proteinuria, complicating the puerperium
- ♀ **O13.9** Gestational [pregnancy-induced] hypertension without significant proteinuria, unspecified trimester

O14 Pre-eclampsia

Excludes1: *pre-existing hypertension with pre-eclampsia (O11)*
Review coding guideline C.9.a.7
AHA CC: 4Q, 2016, 50

+ **O14.0** Mild to moderate pre-eclampsia
    - ♀ **O14.00** Mild to moderate pre-eclampsia, unspecified trimester
    - ♀ CC **O14.02** Mild to moderate pre-eclampsia, second trimester
    - ♀ CC **O14.03** Mild to moderate pre-eclampsia, third trimester
    - ♀ **O14.04** Mild to moderate pre-eclampsia, complicating childbirth
        AHA CC: 2Q, 2019, 8
    - ♀ **O14.05** Mild to moderate pre-eclampsia, complicating the puerperium
    + **O14.1** Severe pre-eclampsia
        Excludes1: *HELLP syndrome (O14.2-)*
        AHA CC: 3Q, 2019, 12
        - ♀ **O14.10** Severe pre-eclampsia, unspecified trimester
        - ♀ MCC **O14.12** Severe pre-eclampsia, second trimester
        - ♀ MCC **O14.13** Severe pre-eclampsia, third trimester
        - ♀ **O14.14** Severe pre-eclampsia complicating childbirth
        - ♀ **O14.15** Severe pre-eclampsia, complicating the puerperium

+ **O14.2** HELLP syndrome
    Severe pre-eclampsia with hemolysis, elevated liver enzymes and low platelet count (HELLP)
    - ♀ **O14.20** HELLP syndrome (HELLP), unspecified trimester
    - ♀ MCC **O14.22** HELLP syndrome (HELLP), second trimester
    - ♀ MCC **O14.23** HELLP syndrome (HELLP), third trimester
    - ♀ **O14.24** HELLP syndrome, complicating childbirth
    - ♀ **O14.25** HELLP syndrome, complicating the puerperium
+ **O14.9** Unspecified pre-eclampsia
    - ♀ **O14.90** Unspecified pre-eclampsia, unspecified trimester
    - ♀ CC **O14.92** Unspecified pre-eclampsia, second trimester
    - ♀ CC **O14.93** Unspecified pre-eclampsia, third trimester
    - ♀ **O14.94** Unspecified pre-eclampsia, complicating childbirth
    - ♀ **O14.95** Unspecified pre-eclampsia, complicating the puerperium

O15 Eclampsia

Includes: convulsions following conditions in O10-O14 and O16

+ **O15.0** Eclampsia complicating pregnancy
    AHA CC: 4Q, 2016, 50
    - ♀ **O15.00** Eclampsia complicating pregnancy, unspecified trimester
    - ♀ MCC **O15.02** Eclampsia complicating pregnancy, second trimester
    - ♀ MCC **O15.03** Eclampsia complicating pregnancy, third trimester
- ♀ MCC **O15.1** Eclampsia complicating labor
- ♀ MCC **O15.2** Eclampsia complicating the puerperium
- ♀ **O15.9** Eclampsia, unspecified as to time period
    Eclampsia NOS

O16 Unspecified maternal hypertension

AHA CC: 4Q, 2016, 50

- ♀ CC **O16.1** Unspecified maternal hypertension, first trimester
- ♀ CC **O16.2** Unspecified maternal hypertension, second trimester
- ♀ CC **O16.3** Unspecified maternal hypertension, third trimester
- ♀ **O16.4** Unspecified maternal hypertension, complicating childbirth
- ♀ **O16.5** Unspecified maternal hypertension, complicating the puerperium
- ♀ **O16.9** Unspecified maternal hypertension, unspecified trimester

Other maternal disorders predominantly related to pregnancy (O20-O29)

Excludes2: *maternal care related to the fetus and amniotic cavity and possible delivery problems (O30-O48)*
maternal diseases classifiable elsewhere but complicating pregnancy, labor and delivery, and the puerperium (O98-O99)

O20 Hemorrhage in early pregnancy

Includes: hemorrhage before completion of 20 weeks gestation
Excludes1: *pregnancy with abortive outcome (O00-O08)*

- ♀ CC **O20.0** Threatened abortion
    Hemorrhage specified as due to threatened abortion
- ♀ **O20.8** Other hemorrhage in early pregnancy
- ♀ CC **O20.9** Hemorrhage in early pregnancy, unspecified

O21 Excessive vomiting in pregnancy

- ♀ **O21.0** Mild hyperemesis gravidarum
    Hyperemesis gravidarum, mild or unspecified, starting before the end of the 20th week of gestation
- ♀ **O21.1** Hyperemesis gravidarum with metabolic disturbance
    Hyperemesis gravidarum, starting before the end of the 20th week of gestation, with metabolic disturbance such as carbohydrate depletion
    Hyperemesis gravidarum, starting before the end of the 20th week of gestation, with metabolic disturbance such as dehydration
    Hyperemesis gravidarum, starting before the end of the 20th week of gestation, with metabolic disturbance such as electrolyte imbalance
- ♀ **O21.2** Late vomiting of pregnancy
    Excessive vomiting starting after 20 completed weeks of gestation
- ♀ **O21.8** Other vomiting complicating pregnancy
    Vomiting due to diseases classified elsewhere, complicating pregnancy
    Use additional code, to identify cause.
- ♀ **O21.9** Vomiting of pregnancy, unspecified

Preeclampsia/Eclampsia

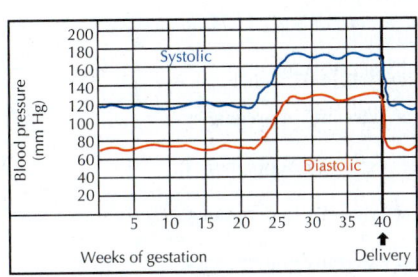

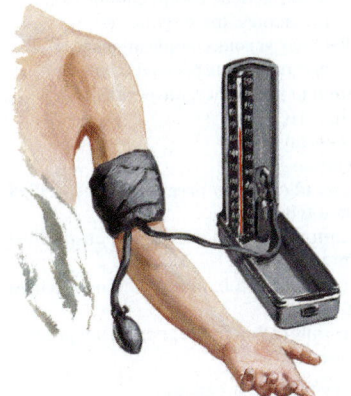

Elevated blood pressure

Preeclampsia-eclampsia is characterized by increase in blood pressure above 160 mm Hg systolic and/or 110 mm Hg diastolic after 20th week of gestation, accompanied by proteinuria, elevation of serum transaminases, and additional clinical findings, which usually resolve within 24–48 hours postpartum.

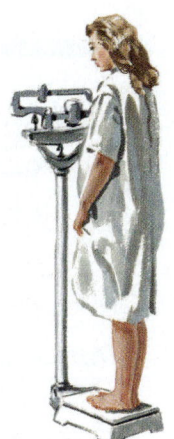

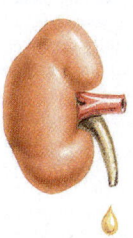 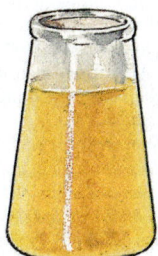
Proteinuria seen in preeclampsia and eclampsia

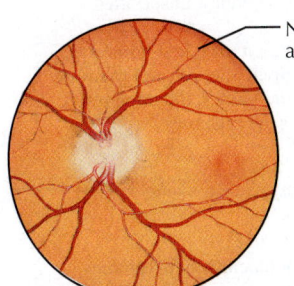
Narrowed retinal arterioles

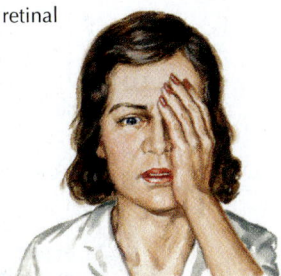
Visual changes and persistent headaches are common complaints.

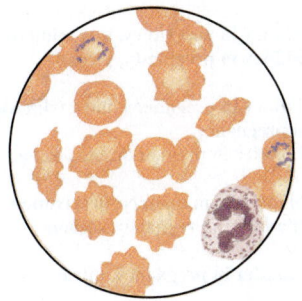
Microangiopathic hemolytic anemia and thrombocytopenia often noted

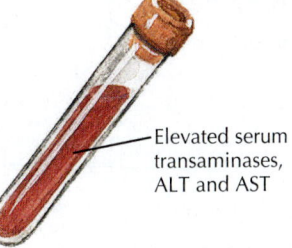
Elevated serum transaminases, ALT and AST

Elevated serum transaminases common in preeclampsia-eclampsia

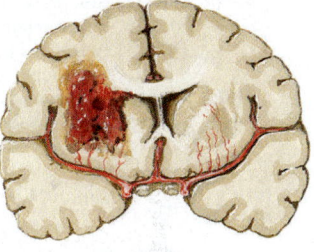
Cerebral infarction or hemorrhage most common cause of death

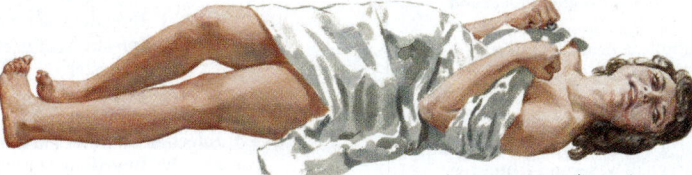
Convulsion in true eclampsia

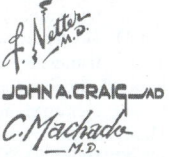

© 2023. Netter illustration used with permission of Elsevier Inc. All rights reserved. www.netterimages.com

Chapter 15: Pregnancy, Childbirth and the Puerperium

O22 Venous complications and hemorrhoids in pregnancy

Excludes1: venous complications of:
- abortion NOS (O03.9)
- ectopic or molar pregnancy (O08.7)
- failed attempted abortion (O07.35)
- induced abortion (O04.85)
- spontaneous abortion (O03.89)

Excludes2: obstetric pulmonary embolism (O88.-)
venous complications and hemorrhoids of childbirth and the puerperium (O87.-)

- **+ O22.0 Varicose veins of lower extremity in pregnancy**
  Varicose veins NOS in pregnancy
  - ♀ O22.00 Varicose veins of lower extremity in pregnancy, unspecified trimester
  - ♀ O22.01 Varicose veins of lower extremity in pregnancy, first trimester
  - ♀ O22.02 Varicose veins of lower extremity in pregnancy, second trimester
  - ♀ O22.03 Varicose veins of lower extremity in pregnancy, third trimester
- **+ O22.1 Genital varices in pregnancy**
  Perineal varices in pregnancy
  Vaginal varices in pregnancy
  Vulval varices in pregnancy
  - ♀ O22.10 Genital varices in pregnancy, unspecified trimester
  - ♀ O22.11 Genital varices in pregnancy, first trimester
  - ♀ O22.12 Genital varices in pregnancy, second trimester
  - ♀ O22.13 Genital varices in pregnancy, third trimester
- **+ O22.2 Superficial thrombophlebitis in pregnancy**
  Phlebitis in pregnancy NOS
  Thrombophlebitis of legs in pregnancy
  Thrombosis in pregnancy NOS
  Use additional code to identify the superficial thrombophlebitis (I80.0-)
  - ♀ CC O22.20 Superficial thrombophlebitis in pregnancy, unspecified trimester
  - ♀ CC O22.21 Superficial thrombophlebitis in pregnancy, first trimester
  - ♀ CC O22.22 Superficial thrombophlebitis in pregnancy, second trimester
  - ♀ CC O22.23 Superficial thrombophlebitis in pregnancy, third trimester
- **+ O22.3 Deep phlebothrombosis in pregnancy**
  Deep vein thrombosis, antepartum
  Use additional code to identify the deep vein thrombosis (I82.4-, I82.5-, I82.62-, I82.72-)
  Use additional code, if applicable, for associated long-term (current) use of anticoagulants (Z79.01)
  - ♀ CC O22.30 Deep phlebothrombosis in pregnancy, unspecified trimester
  - ♀ MCC O22.31 Deep phlebothrombosis in pregnancy, first trimester
  - ♀ MCC O22.32 Deep phlebothrombosis in pregnancy, second trimester
  - ♀ MCC O22.33 Deep phlebothrombosis in pregnancy, third trimester
- **+ O22.4 Hemorrhoids in pregnancy**
  - ♀ CC O22.40 Hemorrhoids in pregnancy, unspecified trimester
  - ♀ CC O22.41 Hemorrhoids in pregnancy, first trimester
  - ♀ CC O22.42 Hemorrhoids in pregnancy, second trimester
  - ♀ CC O22.43 Hemorrhoids in pregnancy, third trimester
- **+ O22.5 Cerebral venous thrombosis in pregnancy**
  Cerebrovenous sinus thrombosis in pregnancy
  - ♀ CC O22.50 Cerebral venous thrombosis in pregnancy, unspecified trimester
  - ♀ CC O22.51 Cerebral venous thrombosis in pregnancy, first trimester
  - ♀ CC O22.52 Cerebral venous thrombosis in pregnancy, second trimester
  - ♀ CC O22.53 Cerebral venous thrombosis in pregnancy, third trimester
- **+ O22.8 Other venous complications in pregnancy**
  - **+ O22.8X Other venous complications in pregnancy**
    - ♀ CC O22.8X1 Other venous complications in pregnancy, first trimester
    - ♀ CC O22.8X2 Other venous complications in pregnancy, second trimester
    - ♀ CC O22.8X3 Other venous complications in pregnancy, third trimester
    - ♀ CC O22.8X9 Other venous complications in pregnancy, unspecified trimester
- **+ O22.9 Venous complication in pregnancy, unspecified**
  Gestational phlebitis NOS
  Gestational phlebopathy NOS
  Gestational thrombosis NOS
  - ♀ CC O22.90 Venous complication in pregnancy, unspecified, unspecified trimester
  - ♀ O22.91 Venous complication in pregnancy, unspecified, first trimester
  - ♀ O22.92 Venous complication in pregnancy, unspecified, second trimester
  - ♀ O22.93 Venous complication in pregnancy, unspecified, third trimester

O23 Infections of genitourinary tract in pregnancy

Use additional code to identify organism (B95.-, B96.-)

Excludes2: gonococcal infections complicating pregnancy, childbirth and the puerperium (O98.2)
infections with a predominantly sexual mode of transmission NOS complicating pregnancy, childbirth and the puerperium (O98.3)
syphilis complicating pregnancy, childbirth and the puerperium (O98.1)
tuberculosis of genitourinary system complicating pregnancy, childbirth and the puerperium (O98.0)
venereal disease NOS complicating pregnancy, childbirth and the puerperium (O98.3)

- **+ O23.0 Infections of kidney in pregnancy**
  Pyelonephritis in pregnancy
  - ♀ O23.00 Infections of kidney in pregnancy, unspecified trimester
  - ♀ CC O23.01 Infections of kidney in pregnancy, first trimester
  - ♀ CC O23.02 Infections of kidney in pregnancy, second trimester
  - ♀ CC O23.03 Infections of kidney in pregnancy, third trimester
- **+ O23.1 Infections of bladder in pregnancy**
  - ♀ O23.10 Infections of bladder in pregnancy, unspecified trimester
  - ♀ CC O23.11 Infections of bladder in pregnancy, first trimester
  - ♀ CC O23.12 Infections of bladder in pregnancy, second trimester
  - ♀ CC O23.13 Infections of bladder in pregnancy, third trimester
- **+ O23.2 Infections of urethra in pregnancy**
  - ♀ O23.20 Infections of urethra in pregnancy, unspecified trimester
  - ♀ CC O23.21 Infections of urethra in pregnancy, first trimester
  - ♀ CC O23.22 Infections of urethra in pregnancy, second trimester
  - ♀ CC O23.23 Infections of urethra in pregnancy, third trimester
- **+ O23.3 Infections of other parts of urinary tract in pregnancy**
  - ♀ O23.30 Infections of other parts of urinary tract in pregnancy, unspecified trimester
  - ♀ CC O23.31 Infections of other parts of urinary tract in pregnancy, first trimester
  - ♀ CC O23.32 Infections of other parts of urinary tract in pregnancy, second trimester
  - ♀ CC O23.33 Infections of other parts of urinary tract in pregnancy, third trimester
- **+ O23.4 Unspecified infection of urinary tract in pregnancy**
  - ♀ O23.40 Unspecified infection of urinary tract in pregnancy, unspecified trimester
  - ♀ CC O23.41 Unspecified infection of urinary tract in pregnancy, first trimester
  - ♀ CC O23.42 Unspecified infection of urinary tract in pregnancy, second trimester
  - ♀ CC O23.43 Unspecified infection of urinary tract in pregnancy, third trimester
    AHA CC: 2Q, 2018, 20

- **+ O23.5 Infections of the genital tract in pregnancy**
  - **+ O23.51 Infection of cervix in pregnancy**
    - ● ♀ CC **O23.511** Infections of cervix in pregnancy, first trimester
    - ● ♀ CC **O23.512** Infections of cervix in pregnancy, second trimester
    - ● ♀ CC **O23.513** Infections of cervix in pregnancy, third trimester
    - ● ♀ **O23.519** Infections of cervix in pregnancy, unspecified trimester
  - **+ O23.52 Salpingo-oophoritis in pregnancy**
    Oophoritis in pregnancy
    Salpingitis in pregnancy
    - ● ♀ CC **O23.521** Salpingo-oophoritis in pregnancy, first trimester
    - ● ♀ CC **O23.522** Salpingo-oophoritis in pregnancy, second trimester
    - ● ♀ CC **O23.523** Salpingo-oophoritis in pregnancy, third trimester
    - ● ♀ **O23.529** Salpingo-oophoritis in pregnancy, unspecified trimester
  - **+ O23.59 Infection of other part of genital tract in pregnancy**
    - ● ♀ CC **O23.591** Infection of other part of genital tract in pregnancy, first trimester
    - ● ♀ CC **O23.592** Infection of other part of genital tract in pregnancy, second trimester
    - ● ♀ CC **O23.593** Infection of other part of genital tract in pregnancy, third trimester
      AHA CC: 1Q, 2022, 20
    - ● ♀ **O23.599** Infection of other part of genital tract in pregnancy, unspecified trimester
- **+ O23.9 Unspecified genitourinary tract infection in pregnancy**
  Genitourinary tract infection in pregnancy NOS
  - ● ♀ **O23.90** Unspecified genitourinary tract infection in pregnancy, unspecified trimester
  - ● ♀ CC **O23.91** Unspecified genitourinary tract infection in pregnancy, first trimester
  - ● ♀ CC **O23.92** Unspecified genitourinary tract infection in pregnancy, second trimester
  - ● ♀ CC **O23.93** Unspecified genitourinary tract infection in pregnancy, third trimester

O24 Diabetes mellitus in pregnancy, childbirth, and the puerperium
Review coding guideline C.15.g

- **+ O24.0 Pre-existing type 1 diabetes mellitus, in pregnancy, childbirth and the puerperium**
  Juvenile onset diabetes mellitus, in pregnancy, childbirth and the puerperium
  Ketosis-prone diabetes mellitus in pregnancy, childbirth and the puerperium
  Use additional code from category E10 to further identify any manifestations
  - **+ O24.01 Pre-existing type 1 diabetes mellitus, in pregnancy**
    - ● ♀ CC **O24.011** Pre-existing type 1 diabetes mellitus, in pregnancy, first trimester
    - ● ♀ CC **O24.012** Pre-existing type 1 diabetes mellitus, in pregnancy, second trimester
    - ● ♀ CC **O24.013** Pre-existing type 1 diabetes mellitus, in pregnancy, third trimester
    - ● ♀ CC **O24.019** Pre-existing type 1 diabetes mellitus, in pregnancy, unspecified trimester
  - ● ♀ MCC **O24.02** Pre-existing type 1 diabetes mellitus, in childbirth
  - ● ♀ CC **O24.03** Pre-existing type 1 diabetes mellitus, in the puerperium
- **+ O24.1 Pre-existing type 2 diabetes mellitus, in pregnancy, childbirth and the puerperium**
  Insulin-resistant diabetes mellitus in pregnancy, childbirth and the puerperium
  Use additional code (for):
  from category E11 to further identify any manifestations
  long-term (current) use of insulin (Z79.4)
  - **+ O24.11 Pre-existing type 2 diabetes mellitus, in pregnancy**
    - ● ♀ CC **O24.111** Pre-existing type 2 diabetes mellitus, in pregnancy, first trimester
    - ● ♀ CC **O24.112** Pre-existing type 2 diabetes mellitus, in pregnancy, second trimester
    - ● ♀ CC **O24.113** Pre-existing type 2 diabetes mellitus, in pregnancy, third trimester
    - ● ♀ CC **O24.119** Pre-existing type 2 diabetes mellitus, in pregnancy, unspecified trimester
  - ● ♀ MCC **O24.12** Pre-existing type 2 diabetes mellitus, in childbirth
  - ● ♀ CC **O24.13** Pre-existing type 2 diabetes mellitus, in the puerperium
- **+ O24.3 Unspecified pre-existing diabetes mellitus in pregnancy, childbirth and the puerperium**
  Use additional code (for):
  from category E11 to further identify any manifestation
  long-term (current) use of insulin (Z79.4)
  - **+ O24.31 Unspecified pre-existing diabetes mellitus in pregnancy**
    - ● ♀ CC **O24.311** Unspecified pre-existing diabetes mellitus in pregnancy, first trimester
    - ● ♀ CC **O24.312** Unspecified pre-existing diabetes mellitus in pregnancy, second trimester
    - ● ♀ CC **O24.313** Unspecified pre-existing diabetes mellitus in pregnancy, third trimester
    - ● ♀ CC **O24.319** Unspecified pre-existing diabetes mellitus in pregnancy, unspecified trimester
  - ● ♀ MCC **O24.32** Unspecified pre-existing diabetes mellitus in childbirth
  - ● ♀ CC **O24.33** Unspecified pre-existing diabetes mellitus in the puerperium
- **+ O24.4 Gestational diabetes mellitus**
  Diabetes mellitus arising in pregnancy
  Gestational diabetes mellitus NOS
  Review coding guideline C.15.i
  AHA CC: 4Q, 2016, 50
  - **+ O24.41 Gestational diabetes mellitus in pregnancy**
    - ● ♀ **O24.410** Gestational diabetes mellitus in pregnancy, diet controlled
    - ● ♀ **O24.414** Gestational diabetes mellitus in pregnancy, insulin controlled
    - ● ♀ **O24.415** Gestational diabetes mellitus in pregnancy, controlled by oral hypoglycemic drugs
      Gestational diabetes mellitus in pregnancy, controlled by oral antidiabetic drugs
    - ● ♀ **O24.419** Gestational diabetes mellitus in pregnancy, unspecified control
      AHA CC: 4Q, 2015, 34; 3Q, 2020, 30-31
  - **+ O24.42 Gestational diabetes mellitus in childbirth**
    - ● ♀ **O24.420** Gestational diabetes mellitus in childbirth, diet controlled
    - ● ♀ **O24.424** Gestational diabetes mellitus in childbirth, insulin controlled
    - ● ♀ **O24.425** Gestational diabetes mellitus in childbirth, controlled by oral hypoglycemic drugs
      Gestational diabetes mellitus in childbirth, controlled by oral antidiabetic drugs
    - ● ♀ **O24.429** Gestational diabetes mellitus in childbirth, unspecified control
  - **+ O24.43 Gestational diabetes mellitus in the puerperium**
    - ● ♀ **O24.430** Gestational diabetes mellitus in the puerperium, diet controlled
    - ● ♀ **O24.434** Gestational diabetes mellitus in the puerperium, insulin controlled
    - ● ♀ **O24.435** Gestational diabetes mellitus in puerperium, controlled by oral hypoglycemic drugs
      Gestational diabetes mellitus in puerperium, controlled by oral antidiabetic drugs
    - ● ♀ **O24.439** Gestational diabetes mellitus in the puerperium, unspecified control
- **+ O24.8 Other pre-existing diabetes mellitus in pregnancy, childbirth, and the puerperium**
  Use additional code (for):
  from categories E08, E09 and E13 to further identify any manifestation
  long-term (current) use of insulin (Z79.4)
  - **+ O24.81 Other pre-existing diabetes mellitus in pregnancy**
    - ● ♀ CC **O24.811** Other pre-existing diabetes mellitus in pregnancy, first trimester
    - ● ♀ CC **O24.812** Other pre-existing diabetes mellitus in pregnancy, second trimester
    - ● ♀ CC **O24.813** Other pre-existing diabetes mellitus in pregnancy, third trimester
    - ● ♀ CC **O24.819** Other pre-existing diabetes mellitus in pregnancy, unspecified trimester
  - ● ♀ MCC **O24.82** Other pre-existing diabetes mellitus in childbirth

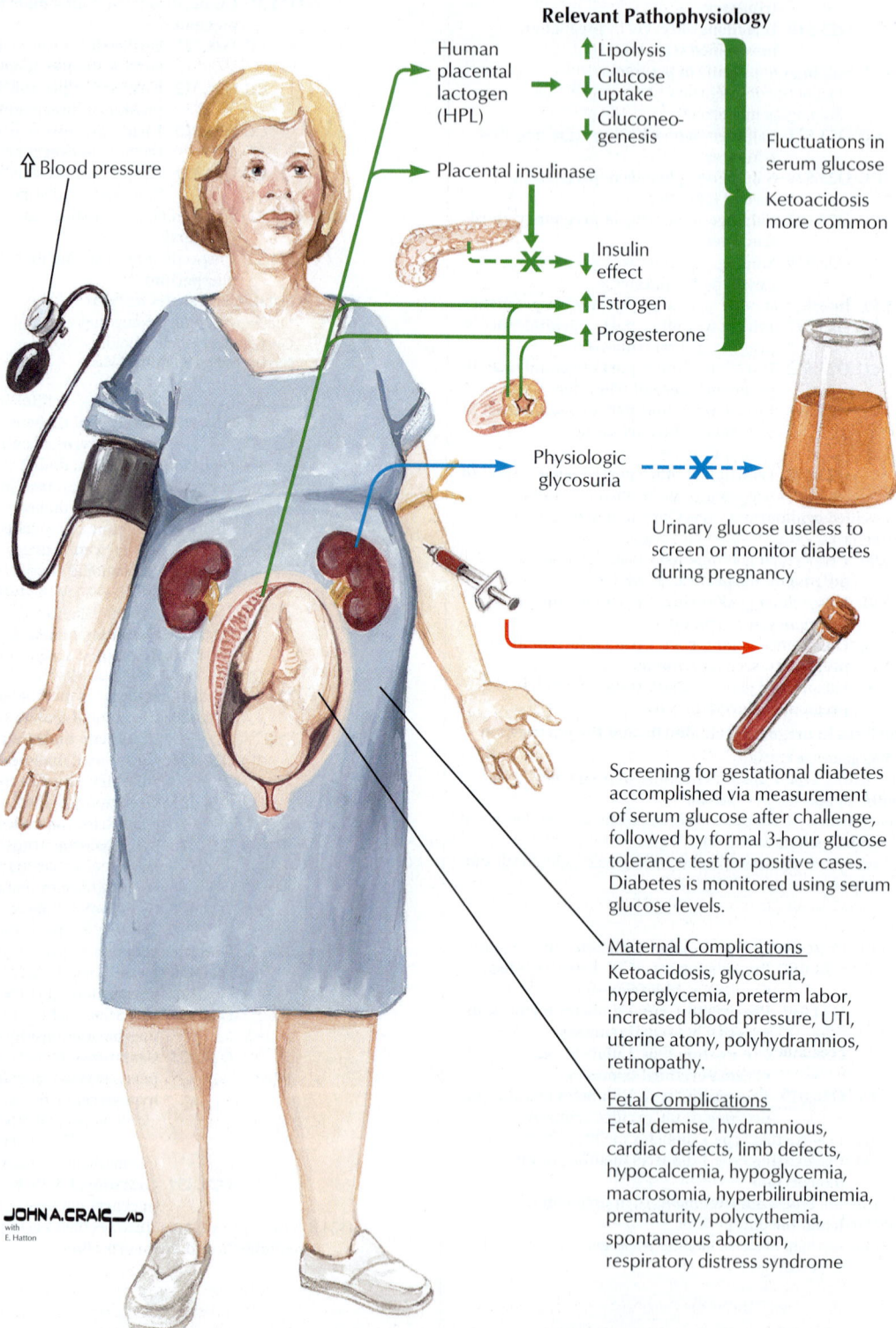

- ♀ CC **O24.83** Other pre-existing diabetes mellitus in the puerperium
+ **O24.9** Unspecified diabetes mellitus in pregnancy, childbirth and the puerperium
  Use additional code for long-term (current) use of insulin (Z79.4)
  + **O24.91** Unspecified diabetes mellitus in pregnancy
    - ♀ CC **O24.911** Unspecified diabetes mellitus in pregnancy, first trimester
    - ♀ CC **O24.912** Unspecified diabetes mellitus in pregnancy, second trimester
    - ♀ CC **O24.913** Unspecified diabetes mellitus in pregnancy, third trimester
    - ♀ CC **O24.919** Unspecified diabetes mellitus in pregnancy, unspecified trimester
  - ♀ **O24.92** Unspecified diabetes mellitus in childbirth
  - ♀ CC **O24.93** Unspecified diabetes mellitus in the puerperium

O25 Malnutrition in pregnancy, childbirth and the puerperium
+ **O25.1** Malnutrition in pregnancy
  - ♀ **O25.10** Malnutrition in pregnancy, unspecified trimester
  - ♀ **O25.11** Malnutrition in pregnancy, first trimester
  - ♀ **O25.12** Malnutrition in pregnancy, second trimester
  - ♀ **O25.13** Malnutrition in pregnancy, third trimester
- ♀ **O25.2** Malnutrition in childbirth
- ♀ **O25.3** Malnutrition in the puerperium

O26 Maternal care for other conditions predominantly related to pregnancy
+ **O26.0** Excessive weight gain in pregnancy
  Excludes2: gestational edema (O12.0, O12.2)
  - ♀ **O26.00** Excessive weight gain in pregnancy, unspecified trimester
  - ♀ **O26.01** Excessive weight gain in pregnancy, first trimester
  - ♀ **O26.02** Excessive weight gain in pregnancy, second trimester
  - ♀ **O26.03** Excessive weight gain in pregnancy, third trimester
+ **O26.1** Low weight gain in pregnancy
  - ♀ **O26.10** Low weight gain in pregnancy, unspecified trimester
  - ♀ **O26.11** Low weight gain in pregnancy, first trimester
  - ♀ **O26.12** Low weight gain in pregnancy, second trimester
  - ♀ **O26.13** Low weight gain in pregnancy, third trimester
+ **O26.2** Pregnancy care for patient with recurrent pregnancy loss
  - ♀ **O26.20** Pregnancy care for patient with recurrent pregnancy loss, unspecified trimester
  - ♀ **O26.21** Pregnancy care for patient with recurrent pregnancy loss, first trimester
  - ♀ **O26.22** Pregnancy care for patient with recurrent pregnancy loss, second trimester
  - ♀ **O26.23** Pregnancy care for patient with recurrent pregnancy loss, third trimester
+ **O26.3** Retained intrauterine contraceptive device in pregnancy
  - ♀ **O26.30** Retained intrauterine contraceptive device in pregnancy, unspecified trimester
  - ♀ **O26.31** Retained intrauterine contraceptive device in pregnancy, first trimester
  - ♀ **O26.32** Retained intrauterine contraceptive device in pregnancy, second trimester
  - ♀ **O26.33** Retained intrauterine contraceptive device in pregnancy, third trimester
+ **O26.4** Herpes gestationis
  - ♀ **O26.40** Herpes gestationis, unspecified trimester
  - ♀ **O26.41** Herpes gestationis, first trimester
  - ♀ **O26.42** Herpes gestationis, second trimester
  - ♀ **O26.43** Herpes gestationis, third trimester
+ **O26.5** Maternal hypotension syndrome
  Supine hypotensive syndrome
  - ♀ **O26.50** Maternal hypotension syndrome, unspecified trimester
  - ♀ **O26.51** Maternal hypotension syndrome, first trimester
  - ♀ **O26.52** Maternal hypotension syndrome, second trimester
  - ♀ **O26.53** Maternal hypotension syndrome, third trimester
+ **O26.6** Liver and biliary tract disorders in pregnancy, childbirth and the puerperium
  Use additional code to identify the specific disorder
  Excludes2: hepatorenal syndrome following labor and delivery (O90.41)
  + **O26.61** Liver and biliary tract disorders in pregnancy
    - ♀ CC **O26.611** Liver and biliary tract disorders in pregnancy, first trimester
    - ♀ CC **O26.612** Liver and biliary tract disorders in pregnancy, second trimester
    - ♀ CC **O26.613** Liver and biliary tract disorders in pregnancy, third trimester
    - ♀ **O26.619** Liver and biliary tract disorders in pregnancy, unspecified trimester
  - ♀ CC **O26.62** Liver and biliary tract disorders in childbirth
    AHA CC: 1Q, 2023, 27
  - ♀ **O26.63** Liver and biliary tract disorders in the puerperium
  + **O26.64** Intrahepatic cholestasis of pregnancy
    - ♀ CC **O26.641** Intrahepatic cholestasis of pregnancy, first trimester
    - ♀ CC **O26.642** Intrahepatic cholestasis of pregnancy, second trimester
    - ♀ CC **O26.643** Intrahepatic cholestasis of pregnancy, third trimester
    - ♀ **O26.649** Intrahepatic cholestasis of pregnancy, unspecified trimester
+ **O26.7** Subluxation of symphysis (pubis) in pregnancy, childbirth and the puerperium
  Excludes1: traumatic separation of symphysis (pubis) during childbirth (O71.6)
  + **O26.71** Subluxation of symphysis (pubis) in pregnancy
    - ♀ **O26.711** Subluxation of symphysis (pubis) in pregnancy, first trimester
    - ♀ **O26.712** Subluxation of symphysis (pubis) in pregnancy, second trimester
    - ♀ **O26.713** Subluxation of symphysis (pubis) in pregnancy, third trimester
    - ♀ **O26.719** Subluxation of symphysis (pubis) in pregnancy, unspecified trimester
  - ♀ **O26.72** Subluxation of symphysis (pubis) in childbirth
  - ♀ **O26.73** Subluxation of symphysis (pubis) in the puerperium
+ **O26.8** Other specified pregnancy related conditions
  + **O26.81** Pregnancy related exhaustion and fatigue
    - ♀ **O26.811** Pregnancy related exhaustion and fatigue, first trimester
    - ♀ **O26.812** Pregnancy related exhaustion and fatigue, second trimester
    - ♀ **O26.813** Pregnancy related exhaustion and fatigue, third trimester
    - ♀ **O26.819** Pregnancy related exhaustion and fatigue, unspecified trimester
  + **O26.82** Pregnancy related peripheral neuritis
    - ♀ **O26.821** Pregnancy related peripheral neuritis, first trimester
    - ♀ **O26.822** Pregnancy related peripheral neuritis, second trimester
    - ♀ **O26.823** Pregnancy related peripheral neuritis, third trimester
    - ♀ **O26.829** Pregnancy related peripheral neuritis, unspecified trimester
  + **O26.83** Pregnancy related renal disease
    Use additional code to identify the specific disorder
    - ♀ CC **O26.831** Pregnancy related renal disease, first trimester
    - ♀ CC **O26.832** Pregnancy related renal disease, second trimester
    - ♀ CC **O26.833** Pregnancy related renal disease, third trimester
    - ♀ **O26.839** Pregnancy related renal disease, unspecified trimester
  + **O26.84** Uterine size-date discrepancy complicating pregnancy
    Excludes1: encounter for suspected problem with fetal growth ruled out (Z03.74)
    - ♀ **O26.841** Uterine size-date discrepancy, first trimester
    - ♀ **O26.842** Uterine size-date discrepancy, second trimester
    - ♀ **O26.843** Uterine size-date discrepancy, third trimester
    - ♀ **O26.849** Uterine size-date discrepancy, unspecified trimester

- **+ O26.85 Spotting complicating pregnancy**
  - ♀ O26.851 Spotting complicating pregnancy, first trimester
  - ♀ O26.852 Spotting complicating pregnancy, second trimester
  - ♀ O26.853 Spotting complicating pregnancy, third trimester
  - ♀ O26.859 Spotting complicating pregnancy, unspecified trimester
- ♀ O26.86 Pruritic urticarial papules and plaques of pregnancy (PUPPP)
  Polymorphic eruption of pregnancy
- **+ O26.87 Cervical shortening**
  Excludes1: encounter for suspected cervical shortening ruled out (Z03.75)
  - ♀ CC O26.872 Cervical shortening, second trimester
  - ♀ CC O26.873 Cervical shortening, third trimester
  - ♀ CC O26.879 Cervical shortening, unspecified trimester
- **+ O26.89 Other specified pregnancy related conditions**
  Use Additional code, if applicable, to identify specific condition such as insulin resistance (E88.81-)
  - ♀ O26.891 Other specified pregnancy related conditions, first trimester
  - ♀ O26.892 Other specified pregnancy related conditions, second trimester
  - ♀ O26.893 Other specified pregnancy related conditions, third trimester
    AHA CC: 3Q, 2015, 40
  - ♀ O26.899 Other specified pregnancy related conditions, unspecified trimester
- **+ O26.9 Pregnancy related conditions, unspecified**
  - ♀ O26.90 Pregnancy related conditions, unspecified, unspecified trimester
  - ♀ O26.91 Pregnancy related conditions, unspecified, first trimester
  - ♀ O26.92 Pregnancy related conditions, unspecified, second trimester
  - ♀ O26.93 Pregnancy related conditions, unspecified, third trimester

O28 Abnormal findings on antenatal screening of mother
Excludes1: diagnostic findings classified elsewhere - see Alphabetical Index
- ♀ O28.0 Abnormal hematological finding on antenatal screening of mother
- ♀ O28.1 Abnormal biochemical finding on antenatal screening of mother
- ♀ O28.2 Abnormal cytological finding on antenatal screening of mother
- ♀ O28.3 Abnormal ultrasonic finding on antenatal screening of mother
  AHA CC: 4Q, 2016, 4-7
- ♀ O28.4 Abnormal radiological finding on antenatal screening of mother
- ♀ O28.5 Abnormal chromosomal and genetic finding on antenatal screening of mother
- ♀ O28.8 Other abnormal findings on antenatal screening of mother
- ♀ O28.9 Unspecified abnormal findings on antenatal screening of mother

O29 Complications of anesthesia during pregnancy
Includes: maternal complications arising from the administration of a general, regional or local anesthetic, analgesic or other sedation during pregnancy
Use additional code, if necessary, to identify the complication
Excludes2: complications of anesthesia during labor and delivery (O74.-)
complications of anesthesia during the puerperium (O89.-)
- **+ O29.0 Pulmonary complications of anesthesia during pregnancy**
  - **+ O29.01 Aspiration pneumonitis due to anesthesia during pregnancy**
    Inhalation of stomach contents or secretions NOS due to anesthesia during pregnancy
    Mendelson's syndrome due to anesthesia during pregnancy
    - ♀ O29.011 Aspiration pneumonitis due to anesthesia during pregnancy, first trimester
    - ♀ O29.012 Aspiration pneumonitis due to anesthesia during pregnancy, second trimester
    - ♀ O29.013 Aspiration pneumonitis due to anesthesia during pregnancy, third trimester
    - ♀ O29.019 Aspiration pneumonitis due to anesthesia during pregnancy, unspecified trimester
  - **+ O29.02 Pressure collapse of lung due to anesthesia during pregnancy**
    - ♀ O29.021 Pressure collapse of lung due to anesthesia during pregnancy, first trimester
    - ♀ O29.022 Pressure collapse of lung due to anesthesia during pregnancy, second trimester
    - ♀ O29.023 Pressure collapse of lung due to anesthesia during pregnancy, third trimester
    - ♀ O29.029 Pressure collapse of lung due to anesthesia during pregnancy, unspecified trimester
  - **+ O29.09 Other pulmonary complications of anesthesia during pregnancy**
    - ♀ O29.091 Other pulmonary complications of anesthesia during pregnancy, first trimester
    - ♀ O29.092 Other pulmonary complications of anesthesia during pregnancy, second trimester
    - ♀ O29.093 Other pulmonary complications of anesthesia during pregnancy, third trimester
    - ♀ O29.099 Other pulmonary complications of anesthesia during pregnancy, unspecified trimester
- **+ O29.1 Cardiac complications of anesthesia during pregnancy**
  - **+ O29.11 Cardiac arrest due to anesthesia during pregnancy**
    - ♀ O29.111 Cardiac arrest due to anesthesia during pregnancy, first trimester
    - ♀ O29.112 Cardiac arrest due to anesthesia during pregnancy, second trimester
    - ♀ O29.113 Cardiac arrest due to anesthesia during pregnancy, third trimester
    - ♀ O29.119 Cardiac arrest due to anesthesia during pregnancy, unspecified trimester
  - **+ O29.12 Cardiac failure due to anesthesia during pregnancy**
    - ♀ O29.121 Cardiac failure due to anesthesia during pregnancy, first trimester
    - ♀ O29.122 Cardiac failure due to anesthesia during pregnancy, second trimester
    - ♀ O29.123 Cardiac failure due to anesthesia during pregnancy, third trimester
    - ♀ O29.129 Cardiac failure due to anesthesia during pregnancy, unspecified trimester
  - **+ O29.19 Other cardiac complications of anesthesia during pregnancy**
    - ♀ O29.191 Other cardiac complications of anesthesia during pregnancy, first trimester
    - ♀ O29.192 Other cardiac complications of anesthesia during pregnancy, second trimester
    - ♀ O29.193 Other cardiac complications of anesthesia during pregnancy, third trimester
    - ♀ O29.199 Other cardiac complications of anesthesia during pregnancy, unspecified trimester
- **+ O29.2 Central nervous system complications of anesthesia during pregnancy**
  - **+ O29.21 Cerebral anoxia due to anesthesia during pregnancy**
    - ♀ O29.211 Cerebral anoxia due to anesthesia during pregnancy, first trimester
    - ♀ O29.212 Cerebral anoxia due to anesthesia during pregnancy, second trimester
    - ♀ O29.213 Cerebral anoxia due to anesthesia during pregnancy, third trimester
    - ♀ O29.219 Cerebral anoxia due to anesthesia during pregnancy, unspecified trimester

- **+ O29.29** Other central nervous system complications of anesthesia during pregnancy
  - ♀ **O29.291** Other central nervous system complications of anesthesia during pregnancy, first trimester
  - ♀ **O29.292** Other central nervous system complications of anesthesia during pregnancy, second trimester
  - ♀ **O29.293** Other central nervous system complications of anesthesia during pregnancy, third trimester
  - ♀ **O29.299** Other central nervous system complications of anesthesia during pregnancy, unspecified trimester
- **+ O29.3** Toxic reaction to local anesthesia during pregnancy
  - **+ O29.3X** Toxic reaction to local anesthesia during pregnancy
    - ♀ **O29.3X1** Toxic reaction to local anesthesia during pregnancy, first trimester
    - ♀ **O29.3X2** Toxic reaction to local anesthesia during pregnancy, second trimester
    - ♀ **O29.3X3** Toxic reaction to local anesthesia during pregnancy, third trimester
    - ♀ **O29.3X9** Toxic reaction to local anesthesia during pregnancy, unspecified trimester
- **+ O29.4** Spinal and epidural anesthesia induced headache during pregnancy
  - ♀ **O29.40** Spinal and epidural anesthesia induced headache during pregnancy, unspecified trimester
  - ♀ **O29.41** Spinal and epidural anesthesia induced headache during pregnancy, first trimester
  - ♀ **O29.42** Spinal and epidural anesthesia induced headache during pregnancy, second trimester
  - ♀ **O29.43** Spinal and epidural anesthesia induced headache during pregnancy, third trimester
- **+ O29.5** Other complications of spinal and epidural anesthesia during pregnancy
  - **+ O29.5X** Other complications of spinal and epidural anesthesia during pregnancy
    - ♀ **O29.5X1** Other complications of spinal and epidural anesthesia during pregnancy, first trimester
    - ♀ **O29.5X2** Other complications of spinal and epidural anesthesia during pregnancy, second trimester
    - ♀ **O29.5X3** Other complications of spinal and epidural anesthesia during pregnancy, third trimester
    - ♀ **O29.5X9** Other complications of spinal and epidural anesthesia during pregnancy, unspecified trimester
- **+ O29.6** Failed or difficult intubation for anesthesia during pregnancy
  - ♀ **O29.60** Failed or difficult intubation for anesthesia during pregnancy, unspecified trimester
  - ♀ **O29.61** Failed or difficult intubation for anesthesia during pregnancy, first trimester
  - ♀ **O29.62** Failed or difficult intubation for anesthesia during pregnancy, second trimester
  - ♀ **O29.63** Failed or difficult intubation for anesthesia during pregnancy, third trimester
- **+ O29.8** Other complications of anesthesia during pregnancy
  - **+ O29.8X** Other complications of anesthesia during pregnancy
    - ♀ **O29.8X1** Other complications of anesthesia during pregnancy, first trimester
    - ♀ **O29.8X2** Other complications of anesthesia during pregnancy, second trimester
    - ♀ **O29.8X3** Other complications of anesthesia during pregnancy, third trimester
    - ♀ **O29.8X9** Other complications of anesthesia during pregnancy, unspecified trimester
- **+ O29.9** Unspecified complication of anesthesia during pregnancy
  - ♀ **O29.90** Unspecified complication of anesthesia during pregnancy, unspecified trimester
  - ♀ **O29.91** Unspecified complication of anesthesia during pregnancy, first trimester
  - ♀ **O29.92** Unspecified complication of anesthesia during pregnancy, second trimester
  - ♀ **O29.93** Unspecified complication of anesthesia during pregnancy, third trimester

Maternal care related to the fetus and amniotic cavity and possible delivery problems (O30-O48)

O30 Multiple gestation

Code also any complications specific to multiple gestation

- **+ O30.0** Twin pregnancy
  - **+ O30.00** Twin pregnancy, unspecified number of placenta and unspecified number of amniotic sacs
    - ♀ **O30.001** Twin pregnancy, unspecified number of placenta and unspecified number of amniotic sacs, first trimester
    - ♀ **O30.002** Twin pregnancy, unspecified number of placenta and unspecified number of amniotic sacs, second trimester
    - ♀ **O30.003** Twin pregnancy, unspecified number of placenta and unspecified number of amniotic sacs, third trimester
    - ♀ **O30.009** Twin pregnancy, unspecified number of placenta and unspecified number of amniotic sacs, unspecified trimester
  - **+ O30.01** Twin pregnancy, monochorionic/monoamniotic
    Twin pregnancy, one placenta, one amniotic sac
    Excludes1: *conjoined twins (O30.02-)*
    - ♀ **O30.011** Twin pregnancy, monochorionic/monoamniotic, first trimester
    - ♀ **O30.012** Twin pregnancy, monochorionic/monoamniotic, second trimester
    - ♀ **O30.013** Twin pregnancy, monochorionic/monoamniotic, third trimester
    - ♀ **O30.019** Twin pregnancy, monochorionic/monoamniotic, unspecified trimester
  - **+ O30.02** Conjoined twin pregnancy
    - ♀ **O30.021** Conjoined twin pregnancy, first trimester
    - ♀ **O30.022** Conjoined twin pregnancy, second trimester
    - ♀ **O30.023** Conjoined twin pregnancy, third trimester
    - ♀ **O30.029** Conjoined twin pregnancy, unspecified trimester
  - **+ O30.03** Twin pregnancy, monochorionic/diamniotic
    Twin pregnancy, one placenta, two amniotic sacs
    - ♀ **O30.031** Twin pregnancy, monochorionic/diamniotic, first trimester
    - ♀ **O30.032** Twin pregnancy, monochorionic/diamniotic, second trimester
    - ♀ **O30.033** Twin pregnancy, monochorionic/diamniotic, third trimester
    - ♀ **O30.039** Twin pregnancy, monochorionic/diamniotic, unspecified trimester
  - **+ O30.04** Twin pregnancy, dichorionic/diamniotic
    Twin pregnancy, two placentae, two amniotic sacs
    - ♀ **O30.041** Twin pregnancy, dichorionic/diamniotic, first trimester
    - ♀ **O30.042** Twin pregnancy, dichorionic/diamniotic, second trimester
    - ♀ **O30.043** Twin pregnancy, dichorionic/diamniotic, third trimester
    - ♀ **O30.049** Twin pregnancy, dichorionic/diamniotic, unspecified trimester
  - **+ O30.09** Twin pregnancy, unable to determine number of placenta and number of amniotic sacs
    - ♀ **O30.091** Twin pregnancy, unable to determine number of placenta and number of amniotic sacs, first trimester
    - ♀ **O30.092** Twin pregnancy, unable to determine number of placenta and number of amniotic sacs, second trimester
    - ♀ **O30.093** Twin pregnancy, unable to determine number of placenta and number of amniotic sacs, third trimester
    - ♀ **O30.099** Twin pregnancy, unable to determine number of placenta and number of amniotic sacs, unspecified trimester

+ **O30.1 Triplet pregnancy**
  + **O30.10** Triplet pregnancy, unspecified number of placenta and unspecified number of amniotic sacs
    - ♀ CC **O30.101** Triplet pregnancy, unspecified number of placenta and unspecified number of amniotic sacs, first trimester
    - ♀ CC **O30.102** Triplet pregnancy, unspecified number of placenta and unspecified number of amniotic sacs, second trimester
    - ♀ CC **O30.103** Triplet pregnancy, unspecified number of placenta and unspecified number of amniotic sacs, third trimester
      AHA CC: 2Q, 2016, 8
    - ♀ **O30.109** Triplet pregnancy, unspecified number of placenta and unspecified number of amniotic sacs, unspecified trimester
  + **O30.11** Triplet pregnancy with two or more monochorionic fetuses
    - ♀ CC **O30.111** Triplet pregnancy with two or more monochorionic fetuses, first trimester
    - ♀ CC **O30.112** Triplet pregnancy with two or more monochorionic fetuses, second trimester
    - ♀ CC **O30.113** Triplet pregnancy with two or more monochorionic fetuses, third trimester
    - ♀ **O30.119** Triplet pregnancy with two or more monochorionic fetuses, unspecified trimester
  + **O30.12** Triplet pregnancy with two or more monoamniotic fetuses
    - ♀ CC **O30.121** Triplet pregnancy with two or more monoamniotic fetuses, first trimester
    - ♀ CC **O30.122** Triplet pregnancy with two or more monoamniotic fetuses, second trimester
    - ♀ CC **O30.123** Triplet pregnancy with two or more monoamniotic fetuses, third trimester
    - ♀ **O30.129** Triplet pregnancy with two or more monoamniotic fetuses, unspecified trimester
  + **O30.13** Triplet pregnancy, trichorionic/trimniotic
    AHA CC: 4Q, 2018, 22
    - ♀ CC **O30.131** Triplet pregnancy, trichorionic/triamniotic, first trimester
    - ♀ CC **O30.132** Triplet pregnancy, trichorionic/triamniotic, second trimester
    - ♀ CC **O30.133** Triplet pregnancy, trichorionic/triamniotic, third trimester
    - ♀ **O30.139** Triplet pregnancy, trichorionic/triamniotic, unspecified trimester
  + **O30.19** Triplet pregnancy, unable to determine number of placenta and number of amniotic sacs
    - ♀ CC **O30.191** Triplet pregnancy, unable to determine number of placenta and number of amniotic sacs, first trimester
    - ♀ CC **O30.192** Triplet pregnancy, unable to determine number of placenta and number of amniotic sacs, second trimester
    - ♀ CC **O30.193** Triplet pregnancy, unable to determine number of placenta and number of amniotic sacs, third trimester
    - ♀ **O30.199** Triplet pregnancy, unable to determine number of placenta and number of amniotic sacs, unspecified trimester
+ **O30.2 Quadruplet pregnancy**
  + **O30.20** Quadruplet pregnancy, unspecified number of placenta and unspecified number of amniotic sacs
    - ♀ CC **O30.201** Quadruplet pregnancy, unspecified number of placenta and unspecified number of amniotic sacs, first trimester
    - ♀ CC **O30.202** Quadruplet pregnancy, unspecified number of placenta and unspecified number of amniotic sacs, second trimester
    - ♀ CC **O30.203** Quadruplet pregnancy, unspecified number of placenta and unspecified number of amniotic sacs, third trimester
    - ♀ **O30.209** Quadruplet pregnancy, unspecified number of placenta and unspecified number of amniotic sacs, unspecified trimester
  + **O30.21** Quadruplet pregnancy with two or more monochorionic fetuses
    - ♀ CC **O30.211** Quadruplet pregnancy with two or more monochorionic fetuses, first trimester
    - ♀ CC **O30.212** Quadruplet pregnancy with two or more monochorionic fetuses, second trimester
    - ♀ CC **O30.213** Quadruplet pregnancy with two or more monochorionic fetuses, third trimester
    - ♀ **O30.219** Quadruplet pregnancy with two or more monochorionic fetuses, unspecified trimester
  + **O30.22** Quadruplet pregnancy with two or more monoamniotic fetuses
    - ♀ CC **O30.221** Quadruplet pregnancy with two or more monoamniotic fetuses, first trimester
    - ♀ CC **O30.222** Quadruplet pregnancy with two or more monoamniotic fetuses, second trimester
    - ♀ CC **O30.223** Quadruplet pregnancy with two or more monoamniotic fetuses, third trimester
    - ♀ **O30.229** Quadruplet pregnancy with two or more monoamniotic fetuses, unspecified trimester
  + **O30.23** Quadruplet pregnancy, quadrachorionic/quadra-amniotic
    AHA CC: 4Q, 2018, 22
    - ♀ CC **O30.231** Quadruplet pregnancy, quadrachorionic/quadra-amniotic, first trimester
    - ♀ CC **O30.232** Quadruplet pregnancy, quadrachorionic/quadra-amniotic, second trimester
    - ♀ CC **O30.233** Quadruplet pregnancy, quadrachorionic/quadra-amniotic, third trimester
    - ♀ **O30.239** Quadruplet pregnancy, quadrachorionic/quadra-amniotic, unspecified trimester
  + **O30.29** Quadruplet pregnancy, unable to determine number of placenta and number of amniotic sacs
    - ♀ CC **O30.291** Quadruplet pregnancy, unable to determine number of placenta and number of amniotic sacs, first trimester
    - ♀ CC **O30.292** Quadruplet pregnancy, unable to determine number of placenta and number of amniotic sacs, second trimester
    - ♀ CC **O30.293** Quadruplet pregnancy, unable to determine number of placenta and number of amniotic sacs, third trimester
    - ♀ **O30.299** Quadruplet pregnancy, unable to determine number of placenta and number of amniotic sacs, unspecified trimester
+ **O30.8 Other specified multiple gestation**
  Multiple gestation pregnancy greater then quadruplets
  + **O30.80** Other specified multiple gestation, unspecified number of placenta and unspecified number of amniotic sacs
    - ♀ CC **O30.801** Other specified multiple gestation, unspecified number of placenta and unspecified number of amniotic sacs, first trimester
    - ♀ CC **O30.802** Other specified multiple gestation, unspecified number of placenta and unspecified number of amniotic sacs, second trimester
    - ♀ CC **O30.803** Other specified multiple gestation, unspecified number of placenta and unspecified number of amniotic sacs, third trimester
    - ♀ **O30.809** Other specified multiple gestation, unspecified number of placenta and unspecified number of amniotic sacs, unspecified trimester

- **+ O30.81** Other specified multiple gestation with two or more monochorionic fetuses
  - ● ♀ CC **O30.811** Other specified multiple gestation with two or more monochorionic fetuses, first trimester
  - ● ♀ CC **O30.812** Other specified multiple gestation with two or more monochorionic fetuses, second trimester
  - ● ♀ CC **O30.813** Other specified multiple gestation with two or more monochorionic fetuses, third trimester
  - ● ♀ **O30.819** Other specified multiple gestation with two or more monochorionic fetuses, unspecified trimester
- **+ O30.82** Other specified multiple gestation with two or more monoamniotic fetuses
  - ● ♀ CC **O30.821** Other specified multiple gestation with two or more monoamniotic fetuses, first trimester
  - ● ♀ CC **O30.822** Other specified multiple gestation with two or more monoamniotic fetuses, second trimester
  - ● ♀ CC **O30.823** Other specified multiple gestation with two or more monoamniotic fetuses, third trimester
  - ● ♀ **O30.829** Other specified multiple gestation with two or more monoamniotic fetuses, unspecified trimester
- **+ O30.83** Other specified multiple gestation, number of chorions and amnions are both equal to the number of fetuses
  Pentachorionic, penta-amniotic pregnancy (quintuplets)
  Hexachorionic, hexa-amniotic pregnancy (sextuplets)
  Heptachorionic, hepta-amniotic pregnancy (septuplets)
  AHA CC: 4Q, 2018, 22
  - ● ♀ CC **O30.831** Other specified multiple gestation, number of chorions and amnions are both equal to the number of fetuses, first trimester
  - ● ♀ CC **O30.832** Other specified multiple gestation, number of chorions and amnions are both equal to the number of fetuses, second trimester
  - ● ♀ CC **O30.833** Other specified multiple gestation, number of chorions and amnions are both equal to the number of fetuses, third trimester
  - ● ♀ **O30.839** Other specified multiple gestation, number of chorions and amnions are both equal to the number of fetuses, unspecified trimester
- **+ O30.89** Other specified multiple gestation, unable to determine number of placenta and number of amniotic sacs
  - ● ♀ CC **O30.891** Other specified multiple gestation, unable to determine number of placenta and number of amniotic sacs, first trimester
  - ● ♀ CC **O30.892** Other specified multiple gestation, unable to determine number of placenta and number of amniotic sacs, second trimester
  - ● ♀ CC **O30.893** Other specified multiple gestation, unable to determine number of placenta and number of amniotic sacs, third trimester
  - ● ♀ **O30.899** Other specified multiple gestation, unable to determine number of placenta and number of amniotic sacs, unspecified trimester
- **+ O30.9** Multiple gestation, unspecified
  Multiple pregnancy NOS
  - ● ♀ **O30.90** Multiple gestation, unspecified, unspecified trimester
  - ● ♀ **O30.91** Multiple gestation, unspecified, first trimester
  - ● ♀ **O30.92** Multiple gestation, unspecified, second trimester
  - ● ♀ **O30.93** Multiple gestation, unspecified, third trimester

O31 Complications specific to multiple gestation

Excludes2: delayed delivery of second twin, triplet, etc. (O63.2)
malpresentation of one fetus or more (O32.9)
placental transfusion syndromes (O43.0-)

One of the following 7th characters is to be assigned to each code under category O31. 7th character 0 is for single gestations and multiple gestations where the fetus is unspecified. 7th characters 1 through 9 are for cases of multiple gestations to identify the fetus for which the code applies. The appropriate code from category O30, Multiple gestation, must also be assigned when assigning a code from category O31 that has a 7th character of 1 through 9.

0 - not applicable or unspecified
1 - fetus 1
2 - fetus 2
3 - fetus 3
4 - fetus 4
5 - fetus 5
9 - other fetus

- **+ O31.0** Papyraceous fetus
  Fetus compressus
  - ● ♀ X+7th **O31.00** Papyraceous fetus, unspecified trimester
  - ● ♀ X+7th **O31.01** Papyraceous fetus, first trimester
  - ● ♀ X+7th **O31.02** Papyraceous fetus, second trimester
  - ● ♀ X+7th **O31.03** Papyraceous fetus, third trimester
- **+ O31.1** Continuing pregnancy after spontaneous abortion of one fetus or more
  - ● ♀ X+7th **O31.10** Continuing pregnancy after spontaneous abortion of one fetus or more, unspecified trimester
  - ● ♀ X+7th **O31.11** Continuing pregnancy after spontaneous abortion of one fetus or more, first trimester
  - ● ♀ X+7th **O31.12** Continuing pregnancy after spontaneous abortion of one fetus or more, second trimester
  - ● ♀ X+7th **O31.13** Continuing pregnancy after spontaneous abortion of one fetus or more, third trimester
- **+ O31.2** Continuing pregnancy after intrauterine death of one fetus or more
  - ● ♀ X+7th **O31.20** Continuing pregnancy after intrauterine death of one fetus or more, unspecified trimester
  - ● ♀ X+7th **O31.21** Continuing pregnancy after intrauterine death of one fetus or more, first trimester
  - ● ♀ X+7th **O31.22** Continuing pregnancy after intrauterine death of one fetus or more, second trimester
  - ● ♀ X+7th **O31.23** Continuing pregnancy after intrauterine death of one fetus or more, third trimester
- **+ O31.3** Continuing pregnancy after elective fetal reduction of one fetus or more
  Continuing pregnancy after selective termination of one fetus or more
  - ● ♀ X+7th **O31.30** Continuing pregnancy after elective fetal reduction of one fetus or more, unspecified trimester
  - ● ♀ X+7th **O31.31** Continuing pregnancy after elective fetal reduction of one fetus or more, first trimester
  - ● ♀ X+7th **O31.32** Continuing pregnancy after elective fetal reduction of one fetus or more, second trimester
  - ● ♀ X+7th **O31.33** Continuing pregnancy after elective fetal reduction of one fetus or more, third trimester
- **+ O31.8** Other complications specific to multiple gestation
  - **+ O31.8X** Other complications specific to multiple gestation
    - ● ♀ CC +7th **O31.8X1** Other complications specific to multiple gestation, first trimester
    - ● ♀ +7th **O31.8X2** Other complications specific to multiple gestation, second trimester
    - ● ♀ +7th **O31.8X3** Other complications specific to multiple gestation, third trimester
    - ● ♀ +7th **O31.8X9** Other complications specific to multiple gestation, unspecified trimester

O32 Maternal care for malpresentation of fetus

Includes: the listed conditions as a reason for observation, hospitalization or other obstetric care of the mother, or for cesarean delivery before onset of labor

Excludes1: malpresentation of fetus with obstructed labor (O64.-)

One of the following 7th characters is to be assigned to each code under category O32. 7th character 0 is for single gestations and multiple gestations where the fetus is unspecified. 7th characters 1 through 9 are for cases of multiple gestations to identify the fetus for which the code applies. The appropriate code from category O30, Multiple gestation, must also be assigned when assigning a code from category O32 that has a 7th character of 1 through 9.
- 0 - not applicable or unspecified
- 1 - fetus 1
- 2 - fetus 2
- 3 - fetus 3
- 4 - fetus 4
- 5 - fetus 5
- 9 - other fetus

- ♀ X+7th **O32.0** Maternal care for unstable lie
- ♀ X+7th **O32.1** Maternal care for breech presentation
  - Maternal care for buttocks presentation
  - Maternal care for complete breech
  - Maternal care for frank breech
  - **Excludes1:** footling presentation (O32.8)
  - incomplete breech (O32.8)
- ♀ X+7th **O32.2** Maternal care for transverse and oblique lie
  - Maternal care for oblique presentation
  - Maternal care for transverse presentation
- ♀ X+7th **O32.3** Maternal care for face, brow and chin presentation
- ♀ X+7th **O32.4** Maternal care for high head at term
  - Maternal care for failure of head to enter pelvic brim
- ♀ X+7th **O32.6** Maternal care for compound presentation
- ♀ X+7th **O32.8** Maternal care for other malpresentation of fetus
  - Maternal care for footling presentation
  - Maternal care for incomplete breech
- ♀ X+7th **O32.9** Maternal care for malpresentation of fetus, unspecified

O33 Maternal care for disproportion

Includes: the listed conditions as a reason for observation, hospitalization or other obstetric care of the mother, or for cesarean delivery before onset of labor

Excludes1: disproportion with obstructed labor (O65-O66)

- ♀ CC **O33.0** Maternal care for disproportion due to deformity of maternal pelvic bones
  - Maternal care for disproportion due to pelvic deformity causing disproportion NOS
- ♀ **O33.1** Maternal care for disproportion due to generally contracted pelvis
  - Maternal care for disproportion due to contracted pelvis NOS causing disproportion
- ♀ **O33.2** Maternal care for disproportion due to inlet contraction of pelvis
  - Maternal care for disproportion due to inlet contraction (pelvis) causing disproportion
- ♀ +7th **O33.3** Maternal care for disproportion due to outlet contraction of pelvis
  - Maternal care for disproportion due to mid-cavity contraction (pelvis)
  - Maternal care for disproportion due to outlet contraction (pelvis)

One of the following 7th characters is to be assigned to code O33.3. 7th character 0 is for single gestations and multiple gestations where the fetus is unspecified. 7th characters 1 through 9 are for cases of multiple gestations to identify the fetus for which the code applies. The appropriate code from category O30, Multiple gestation, must also be assigned when assigning code O33.3 with a 7th character of 1 through 9.
- 0 - not applicable or unspecified
- 1 - fetus 1
- 2 - fetus 2
- 3 - fetus 3
- 4 - fetus 4
- 5 - fetus 5
- 9 - other fetus

- ♀ X+7th **O33.4** Maternal care for disproportion of mixed maternal and fetal origin

One of the following 7th characters is to be assigned to code O33.4. 7th character 0 is for single gestations and multiple gestations where the fetus is unspecified. 7th characters 1 through 9 are for cases of multiple gestations to identify the fetus for which the code applies. The appropriate code from category O30, Multiple gestation, must also be assigned when assigning code O33.4 with a 7th character of 1 through 9.
- 0 - not applicable or unspecified
- 1 - fetus 1
- 2 - fetus 2
- 3 - fetus 3
- 4 - fetus 4
- 5 - fetus 5
- 9 - other fetus

- ♀ X+7th **O33.5** Maternal care for disproportion due to unusually large fetus
  - Maternal care for disproportion due to disproportion of fetal origin with normally formed fetus
  - Maternal care for disproportion due to fetal disproportion NOS

One of the following 7th characters is to be assigned to code O33.5. 7th character 0 is for single gestations and multiple gestations where the fetus is unspecified. 7th characters 1 through 9 are for cases of multiple gestations to identify the fetus for which the code applies. The appropriate code from category O30, Multiple gestation, must also be assigned when assigning code O33.5 with a 7th character of 1 through 9.
- 0 - not applicable or unspecified
- 1 - fetus 1
- 2 - fetus 2
- 3 - fetus 3
- 4 - fetus 4
- 5 - fetus 5
- 9 - other fetus

- ♀ X+7th **O33.6** Maternal care for disproportion due to hydrocephalic fetus

One of the following 7th characters is to be assigned to code O33.6. 7th character 0 is for single gestations and multiple gestations where the fetus is unspecified. 7th characters 1 through 9 are for cases of multiple gestations to identify the fetus for which the code applies. The appropriate code from category O30, Multiple gestation, must also be assigned when assigning code O33.6 with a 7th character of 1 through 9.
- 0 - not applicable or unspecified
- 1 - fetus 1
- 2 - fetus 2
- 3 - fetus 3
- 4 - fetus 4
- 5 - fetus 5
- 9 - other fetus

- ♀ X+7th **O33.7** Maternal care for disproportion due to other fetal deformities
  - Maternal care for disproportion due to fetal ascites
  - Maternal care for disproportion due to fetal hydrops
  - Maternal care for disproportion due to fetal meningomyelocele
  - Maternal care for disproportion due to fetal sacral teratoma
  - Maternal care for disproportion due to fetal tumor
  - **Excludes1:** obstructed labor due to other fetal deformities (O66.3)
  - *AHA CC: 4Q, 2016, 51*

One of the following 7th characters is to be assigned to code O33.7. 7th character 0 is for single gestations and multiple gestations where the fetus is unspecified. 7th characters 1 through 9 are for cases of multiple gestations to identify the fetus for which the code applies. The appropriate code from category O30, Multiple gestation, must also be assigned when assigning code O33.7 with a 7th character of 1 through 9.
- 0 - not applicable or unspecified
- 1 - fetus 1
- 2 - fetus 2
- 3 - fetus 3
- 4 - fetus 4
- 5 - fetus 5
- 9 - other fetus

- ♀ **O33.8** Maternal care for disproportion of other origin
- ♀ **O33.9** Maternal care for disproportion, unspecified
  - Maternal care for disproportion due to cephalopelvic disproportion NOS
  - Maternal care for disproportion due to fetopelvic disproportion NOS

O34 Maternal care for abnormality of pelvic organs
  Includes: the listed conditions as a reason for hospitalization or other obstetric care of the mother, or for cesarean delivery before onset of labor
  Code first any associated obstructed labor (O65.5)
  Use additional code for specific condition

+ **O34.0 Maternal care for congenital malformation of uterus**
    Maternal care for double uterus
    Maternal care for uterus bicornis
  • ♀ **O34.00** Maternal care for unspecified congenital malformation of uterus, unspecified trimester
  • ♀ **O34.01** Maternal care for unspecified congenital malformation of uterus, first trimester
  • ♀ **O34.02** Maternal care for unspecified congenital malformation of uterus, second trimester
  • ♀ **O34.03** Maternal care for unspecified congenital malformation of uterus, third trimester

+ **O34.1 Maternal care for benign tumor of corpus uteri**
    Excludes2: maternal care for benign tumor of cervix (O34.4-)
              maternal care for malignant neoplasm of uterus (O9A.1-)
  • ♀ **O34.10** Maternal care for benign tumor of corpus uteri, unspecified trimester
  • ♀ **O34.11** Maternal care for benign tumor of corpus uteri, first trimester
  • ♀ **O34.12** Maternal care for benign tumor of corpus uteri, second trimester
  • ♀ **O34.13** Maternal care for benign tumor of corpus uteri, third trimester

+ **O34.2 Maternal care due to uterine scar from previous surgery**
  + **O34.21 Maternal care for scar from previous cesarean delivery**
      AHA CC: 4Q, 2016, 51-52
    • ♀ **O34.211** Maternal care for low transverse scar from previous cesarean delivery
        AHA CC: 3Q, 2018, 23-24
    • ♀ **O34.212** Maternal care for vertical scar from previous cesarean delivery
        Maternal care for classical scar from previous cesarean delivery
    • ♀ **O34.218** Maternal care for other type scar from previous cesarean delivery
        Mid-transverse T incision
        AHA CC: 4Q, 2020, 36
    • ♀ **O34.219** Maternal care for unspecified type scar from previous cesarean delivery
        AHA CC: 3Q, 2018, 23
  • ♀ **O34.22** Maternal care for cesarean scar defect (isthmocele)
      AHA CC: 4Q, 2020, 36
  • ♀ **O34.29** Maternal care due to uterine scar from other previous surgery
      Maternal care due to uterine scar from other transmural uterine

+ **O34.3 Maternal care for cervical incompetence**
    Maternal care for cerclage with or without cervical incompetence
    Maternal care for Shirodkar suture with or without cervical incompetence
  • ♀ **O34.30** Maternal care for cervical incompetence, unspecified trimester
  • ♀ MCC **O34.31** Maternal care for cervical incompetence, first trimester
  • ♀ MCC **O34.32** Maternal care for cervical incompetence, second trimester
  • ♀ MCC **O34.33** Maternal care for cervical incompetence, third trimester

+ **O34.4 Maternal care for other abnormalities of cervix**
  • ♀ **O34.40** Maternal care for other abnormalities of cervix, unspecified trimester
  • ♀ **O34.41** Maternal care for other abnormalities of cervix, first trimester
  • ♀ **O34.42** Maternal care for other abnormalities of cervix, second trimester
  • ♀ **O34.43** Maternal care for other abnormalities of cervix, third trimester

+ **O34.5 Maternal care for other abnormalities of gravid uterus**
  + **O34.51 Maternal care for incarceration of gravid uterus**
    • ♀ **O34.511** Maternal care for incarceration of gravid uterus, first trimester
    • ♀ **O34.512** Maternal care for incarceration of gravid uterus, second trimester
    • ♀ **O34.513** Maternal care for incarceration of gravid uterus, third trimester
    • ♀ **O34.519** Maternal care for incarceration of gravid uterus, unspecified trimester
  + **O34.52 Maternal care for prolapse of gravid uterus**
    • ♀ **O34.521** Maternal care for prolapse of gravid uterus, first trimester
    • ♀ **O34.522** Maternal care for prolapse of gravid uterus, second trimester
    • ♀ **O34.523** Maternal care for prolapse of gravid uterus, third trimester
    • ♀ **O34.529** Maternal care for prolapse of gravid uterus, unspecified trimester
  + **O34.53 Maternal care for retroversion of gravid uterus**
    • ♀ **O34.531** Maternal care for retroversion of gravid uterus, first trimester
    • ♀ **O34.532** Maternal care for retroversion of gravid uterus, second trimester
    • ♀ **O34.533** Maternal care for retroversion of gravid uterus, third trimester
    • ♀ **O34.539** Maternal care for retroversion of gravid uterus, unspecified trimester
  + **O34.59 Maternal care for other abnormalities of gravid uterus**
    • ♀ **O34.591** Maternal care for other abnormalities of gravid uterus, first trimester
    • ♀ **O34.592** Maternal care for other abnormalities of gravid uterus, second trimester
    • ♀ **O34.593** Maternal care for other abnormalities of gravid uterus, third trimester
    • ♀ **O34.599** Maternal care for other abnormalities of gravid uterus, unspecified trimester

O34.6 Maternal care for abnormality of vagina
    Excludes2: maternal care for vaginal varices in pregnancy (O22.1-)
  • ♀ **O34.60** Maternal care for abnormality of vagina, unspecified trimester
  • ♀ **O34.61** Maternal care for abnormality of vagina, first trimester
  • ♀ **O34.62** Maternal care for abnormality of vagina, second trimester
  • ♀ **O34.63** Maternal care for abnormality of vagina, third trimester

+ **O34.7 Maternal care for abnormality of vulva and perineum**
    Excludes2: maternal care for perineal and vulval varices in pregnancy (O22.1-)
  • ♀ **O34.70** Maternal care for abnormality of vulva and perineum, unspecified trimester
  • ♀ **O34.71** Maternal care for abnormality of vulva and perineum, first trimester
  • ♀ **O34.72** Maternal care for abnormality of vulva and perineum, second trimester
  • ♀ **O34.73** Maternal care for abnormality of vulva and perineum, third trimester

+ **O34.8 Maternal care for other abnormalities of pelvic organs**
  • ♀ **O34.80** Maternal care for other abnormalities of pelvic organs, unspecified trimester
  • ♀ **O34.81** Maternal care for other abnormalities of pelvic organs, first trimester
  • ♀ **O34.82** Maternal care for other abnormalities of pelvic organs, second trimester
  • ♀ **O34.83** Maternal care for other abnormalities of pelvic organs, third trimester

+ **O34.9 Maternal care for abnormality of pelvic organ, unspecified**
  • ♀ **O34.90** Maternal care for abnormality of pelvic organ, unspecified, unspecified trimester
  • ♀ **O34.91** Maternal care for abnormality of pelvic organ, unspecified, first trimester
  • ♀ **O34.92** Maternal care for abnormality of pelvic organ, unspecified, second trimester
  • ♀ **O34.93** Maternal care for abnormality of pelvic organ, unspecified, third trimester

O35 Maternal care for known or suspected fetal abnormality and damage

Includes: the listed conditions in the fetus as a reason for hospitalization or other obstetric care to the mother, or for termination of pregnancy

Code also any associated maternal condition

Excludes1: encounter for suspected maternal and fetal conditions ruled out (Z03.7-)

One of the following 7th characters is to be assigned to each code under category O35. 7th character 0 is for single gestations and multiple gestations where the fetus is unspecified. 7th characters 1 through 9 are for cases of multiple gestations to identify the fetus for which the code applies. The appropriate code from category O30, Multiple gestation, must also be assigned when assigning a code from category O35 that has a 7th character of 1 through 9.
- 0 - not applicable or unspecified
- 1 - fetus 1
- 2 - fetus 2
- 3 - fetus 3
- 4 - fetus 4
- 5 - fetus 5
- 9 - other fetus

Review coding guideline C.15.e

AHA CC: 4Q, 2022, 37

- ♀+ **O35.0** Maternal care for (suspected) central nervous system malformation in fetus
  Excludes2: chromosomal abnormality in fetus (O35.1-)
  - ♀ X+7th **O35.00** Maternal care for (suspected) central nervous system malformation or damage in fetus, unspecified
  - ♀ X+7th **O35.01** Maternal care for (suspected) central nervous system malformation or damage in fetus, agenesis of the corpus callosum
  - ♀ X+7th **O35.02** Maternal care for (suspected) central nervous system malformation or damage in fetus, anencephaly
  - ♀ X+7th **O35.03** Maternal care for (suspected) central nervous system malformation or damage in fetus, choroid plexus cysts
  - ♀ X+7th **O35.04** Maternal care for (suspected) central nervous system malformation or damage in fetus, encephalocele
  - ♀ X+7th **O35.05** Maternal care for (suspected) central nervous system malformation or damage in fetus, holoprosencephaly
  - ♀ X+7th **O35.06** Maternal care for (suspected) central nervous system malformation or damage in fetus, hydrocephaly
    Maternal care for fetal hydrocephalus
  - ♀ X+7th **O35.07** Maternal care for (suspected) central nervous system malformation or damage in fetus, microcephaly
  - ♀ X+7th **O35.08** Maternal care for (suspected) central nervous system malformation or damage in fetus, spina bifida
  - ♀ X+7th **O35.09** Maternal care for (suspected) other central nervous system malformation or damage in fetus
- ♀+ **O35.1** Maternal care for (suspected) chromosomal abnormality in fetus
  - ♀ X+7th **O35.10** Maternal care for (suspected) chromosomal abnormality in fetus, unspecified
    AHA CC: 2Q, 2023, 15-16
  - ♀ X+7th **O35.11** Maternal care for (suspected) chromosomal abnormality in fetus, Trisomy 13
  - ♀ X+7th **O35.12** Maternal care for (suspected) chromosomal abnormality in fetus, Trisomy 18
  - ♀ X+7th **O35.13** Maternal care for (suspected) chromosomal abnormality in fetus, Trisomy 21
  - ♀ X+7th **O35.14** Maternal care for (suspected) chromosomal abnormality in fetus, Turner Syndrome
  - ♀ X+7th **O35.15** Maternal care for (suspected) chromosomal abnormality in fetus, sex chromosome abnormality
  - ♀ X+7th **O35.19** Maternal care for (suspected) chromosomal abnormality in fetus, other chromosomal abnormality
- ♀ X+7th **O35.A** Maternal care for other (suspected) fetal abnormality and damage, fetal facial anomalies
- ♀ X+7th **O35.B** Maternal care for other (suspected) fetal abnormality and damage, fetal cardiac anomalies
- ♀ X+7th **O35.C** Maternal care for other (suspected) fetal abnormality and damage, fetal pulmonary anomalies
- ♀ X+7th **O35.D** Maternal care for other (suspected) fetal abnormality and damage, fetal gastrointestinal anomalies
- ♀ X+7th **O35.E** Maternal care for other (suspected) fetal abnormality and damage, fetal genitourinary anomalies
- ♀ X+7th **O35.F** Maternal care for other (suspected) fetal abnormality and damage, fetal musculoskeletal anomalies of trunk
  Excludes2: maternal care for other (suspected) fetal abnormality and damage, fetal lower extremities anomalies (O35.H)
  maternal care for other (suspected) fetal abnormality and damage, fetal upper extremities anomalies (O35.G)
- ♀ X+7th **O35.G** Maternal care for other (suspected) fetal abnormality and damage, fetal upper extremities anomalies
- ♀ X+7th **O35.H** Maternal care for other (suspected) fetal abnormality and damage, fetal lower extremities anomalies
- ♀ X+7th **O35.2** Maternal care for (suspected) hereditary disease in fetus
  Excludes2: chromosomal abnormality in fetus (O35.1-)
- ♀ X+7th **O35.3** Maternal care for (suspected) damage to fetus from viral disease in mother
  Maternal care for damage to fetus from maternal cytomegalovirus infection
  Maternal care for damage to fetus from maternal rubella
  AHA CC: 4Q, 2016, 4-7
- ♀ X+7th **O35.4** Maternal care for (suspected) damage to fetus from alcohol
- ♀ X+7th **O35.5** Maternal care for (suspected) damage to fetus by drugs
  Maternal care for damage to fetus from drug addiction
- ♀ X+7th **O35.6** Maternal care for (suspected) damage to fetus by radiation
- ♀ X+7th **O35.7** Maternal care for (suspected) damage to fetus by other medical procedures
  Maternal care for damage to fetus by amniocentesis
  Maternal care for damage to fetus by biopsy procedures
  Maternal care for damage to fetus by hematological investigation
  Maternal care for damage to fetus by intrauterine contraceptive device
  Maternal care for damage to fetus by intrauterine surgery
- ♀ X+7th **O35.8** Maternal care for other (suspected) fetal abnormality and damage
  Maternal care for damage to fetus from maternal listeriosis
  Maternal care for damage to fetus from maternal toxoplasmosis
- ♀ X+7th **O35.9** Maternal care for (suspected) fetal abnormality and damage, unspecified

O36 Maternal care for other fetal problems

Includes: the listed conditions in the fetus as a reason for hospitalization or other obstetric care of the mother, or for termination of pregnancy

Excludes1: encounter for suspected maternal and fetal conditions ruled out (Z03.7-)
placental transfusion syndromes (O43.0-)

Excludes2: labor and delivery complicated by fetal stress (O77.-)

One of the following 7th characters is to be assigned to each code under category O36. 7th character 0 is for single gestations and multiple gestations where the fetus is unspecified. 7th characters 1 through 9 are for cases of multiple gestations to identify the fetus for which the code applies. The appropriate code from category O30, Multiple gestation, must also be assigned when assigning a code from category O36 that has a 7th character of 1 through 9.
- 0 - not applicable or unspecified
- 1 - fetus 1
- 2 - fetus 2
- 3 - fetus 3
- 4 - fetus 4
- 5 - fetus 5
- 9 - other fetus

Review coding guideline C.15.e

- **O36.0 Maternal care for rhesus isoimmunization**
  Maternal care for Rh incompatibility (with hydrops fetalis)
  - **O36.01 Maternal care for anti-D [Rh] antibodies**
    - ♀ CC +7th O36.011 Maternal care for anti-D [Rh] antibodies, first trimester
    - ♀ CC +7th O36.012 Maternal care for anti-D [Rh] antibodies, second trimester
    - ♀ CC +7th O36.013 Maternal care for anti-D [Rh] antibodies, third trimester
      AHA CC: 4Q, 2014, 17-18
    - ♀ +7th O36.019 Maternal care for anti-D [Rh] antibodies, unspecified trimester
  - **O36.09 Maternal care for other rhesus isoimmunization**
    - ♀ CC +7th O36.091 Maternal care for other rhesus isoimmunization, first trimester
    - ♀ CC +7th O36.092 Maternal care for other rhesus isoimmunization, second trimester
    - ♀ CC +7th O36.093 Maternal care for other rhesus isoimmunization, third trimester
    - ♀ +7th O36.099 Maternal care for other rhesus isoimmunization, unspecified trimester
- **O36.1 Maternal care for other isoimmunization**
  Maternal care for ABO isoimmunization
  - **O36.11 Maternal care for Anti-A sensitization**
    Maternal care for isoimmunization NOS (with hydrops fetalis)
    - ♀ +7th O36.111 Maternal care for Anti-A sensitization, first trimester
    - ♀ +7th O36.112 Maternal care for Anti-A sensitization, second trimester
    - ♀ +7th O36.113 Maternal care for Anti-A sensitization, third trimester
    - ♀ +7th O36.119 Maternal care for Anti-A sensitization, unspecified trimester
  - **O36.19 Maternal care for other isoimmunization**
    Maternal care for Anti-B sensitization
    - ♀ +7th O36.191 Maternal care for other isoimmunization, first trimester
    - ♀ +7th O36.192 Maternal care for other isoimmunization, second trimester
    - ♀ +7th O36.193 Maternal care for other isoimmunization, third trimester
    - ♀ +7th O36.199 Maternal care for other isoimmunization, unspecified trimester
- **O36.2 Maternal care for hydrops fetalis**
  Maternal care for hydrops fetalis NOS
  Maternal care for hydrops fetalis not associated with isoimmunization
  Excludes1: hydrops fetalis associated with ABO isoimmunization (O36.1-)
  hydrops fetalis associated with rhesus isoimmunization (O36.0-)
  - ♀ X+7th O36.20 Maternal care for hydrops fetalis, unspecified trimester
  - ♀ X+7th O36.21 Maternal care for hydrops fetalis, first trimester
  - ♀ X+7th O36.22 Maternal care for hydrops fetalis, second trimester
  - ♀ X+7th O36.23 Maternal care for hydrops fetalis, third trimester
- ♀ CC **O36.4 Maternal care for intrauterine death**
  X+7th
  Maternal care for intrauterine fetal death NOS
  Maternal care for intrauterine fetal death after completion of 20 weeks of gestation
  Maternal care for late fetal death
  Maternal care for missed delivery
  Excludes1: missed abortion (O02.1) stillbirth (P95)
  AHA CC: 2Q, 2022, 3-4
- **O36.5 Maternal care for known or suspected poor fetal growth**
  - **O36.51 Maternal care for known or suspected placental insufficiency**
    - ♀ +7th O36.511 Maternal care for known or suspected placental insufficiency, first trimester
    - ♀ +7th O36.512 Maternal care for known or suspected placental insufficiency, second trimester
    - ♀ +7th O36.513 Maternal care for known or suspected placental insufficiency, third trimester
    - ♀ +7th O36.519 Maternal care for known or suspected placental insufficiency, unspecified trimester
  - **O36.59 Maternal care for other known or suspected poor fetal growth**
    Maternal care for known or suspected light-for-dates NOS
    Maternal care for known or suspected small-for-dates NOS
    - ♀ +7th O36.591 Maternal care for other known or suspected poor fetal growth, first trimester
    - ♀ +7th O36.592 Maternal care for other known or suspected poor fetal growth, second trimester
    - ♀ +7th O36.593 Maternal care for other known or suspected poor fetal growth, third trimester
    - ♀ +7th O36.599 Maternal care for other known or suspected poor fetal growth, unspecified trimester
- **O36.6 Maternal care for excessive fetal growth**
  Maternal care for known or suspected large-for-dates
  - ♀ X+7th O36.60 Maternal care for excessive fetal growth, unspecified trimester
  - ♀ X+7th O36.61 Maternal care for excessive fetal growth, first trimester
  - ♀ X+7th O36.62 Maternal care for excessive fetal growth, second trimester
  - ♀ X+7th O36.63 Maternal care for excessive fetal growth, third trimester
- **O36.7 Maternal care for viable fetus in abdominal pregnancy**
  - ♀ X+7th O36.70 Maternal care for viable fetus in abdominal pregnancy, unspecified trimester
  - ♀ X+7th O36.71 Maternal care for viable fetus in abdominal pregnancy, first trimester
  - ♀ X+7th O36.72 Maternal care for viable fetus in abdominal pregnancy, second trimester
  - ♀ X+7th O36.73 Maternal care for viable fetus in abdominal pregnancy, third trimester
- **O36.8 Maternal care for other specified fetal problems**
  - ♀ X+7th O36.80 Pregnancy with inconclusive fetal viability
    Encounter to determine fetal viability of pregnancy
    AHA CC: 2Q, 2019, 29
  - **O36.81 Decreased fetal movements**
    - ♀ +7th O36.812 Decreased fetal movements, second trimester
    - ♀ +7th O36.813 Decreased fetal movements, third trimester
    - ♀ +7th O36.819 Decreased fetal movements, unspecified trimester
  - **O36.82 Fetal anemia and thrombocytopenia**
    - ♀ +7th O36.821 Fetal anemia and thrombocytopenia, first trimester
    - ♀ +7th O36.822 Fetal anemia and thrombocytopenia, second trimester
    - ♀ +7th O36.823 Fetal anemia and thrombocytopenia, third trimester
    - ♀ +7th O36.829 Fetal anemia and thrombocytopenia, unspecified trimester
  - **O36.83 Maternal care for abnormalities of the fetal heart rate or rhythm**
    Maternal care for depressed fetal heart rate tones
    Maternal care for fetal bradycardia
    Maternal care for fetal heart rate abnormal variability
    Maternal care for fetal heart rate decelerations
    Maternal care for fetal heart rate irregularity
    Maternal care for fetal tachycardia
    Maternal care for non-reassuring fetal heart rate or rhythm
    AHA CC: 4Q, 2017, 20
    - ♀ +7th O36.831 Maternal care for abnormalities of the fetal heart rate or rhythm, first trimester
    - ♀ +7th O36.832 Maternal care for abnormalities of the fetal heart rate or rhythm, second trimester
    - ♀ +7th O36.833 Maternal care for abnormalities of the fetal heart rate or rhythm, third trimester
    - ♀ +7th O36.839 Maternal care for abnormalities of the fetal heart rate or rhythm, unspecified trimester

- **+ O36.89 Maternal care for other specified fetal problems**
  - ● ♀ +7th **O36.891** Maternal care for other specified fetal problems, first trimester
  - ● ♀ +7th **O36.892** Maternal care for other specified fetal problems, second trimester
  - ● ♀ +7th **O36.893** Maternal care for other specified fetal problems, third trimester
  - ● ♀ +7th **O36.899** Maternal care for other specified fetal problems, unspecified trimester
- **+ O36.9 Maternal care for fetal problem, unspecified**
  - ● ♀ X+7th **O36.90** Maternal care for fetal problem, unspecified, unspecified trimester
  - ● ♀ X+7th **O36.91** Maternal care for fetal problem, unspecified, first trimester
  - ● ♀ X+7th **O36.92** Maternal care for fetal problem, unspecified, second trimester
  - ● ♀ X+7th **O36.93** Maternal care for fetal problem, unspecified, third trimester

O40 Polyhydramnios

Includes: hydramnios
Excludes1: encounter for suspected maternal and fetal conditions ruled out (Z03.7-)

> One of the following 7th characters is to be assigned to each code under category O40. 7th character 0 is for single gestations and multiple gestations where the fetus is unspecified. 7th characters 1 through 9 are for cases of multiple gestations to identify the fetus for which the code applies. The appropriate code from category O30, Multiple gestation, must also be assigned when assigning a code from category O40 that has a 7th character of 1 through 9.
> 0 - not applicable or unspecified
> 1 - fetus 1
> 2 - fetus 2
> 3 - fetus 3
> 4 - fetus 4
> 5 - fetus 5
> 9 - other fetus

- ● ♀ X+7th **O40.1** Polyhydramnios, first trimester
- ● ♀ X+7th **O40.2** Polyhydramnios, second trimester
- ● ♀ X+7th **O40.3** Polyhydramnios, third trimester
- ● ♀ X+7th **O40.9** Polyhydramnios, unspecified trimester

O41 Other disorders of amniotic fluid and membranes

Excludes1: encounter for suspected maternal and fetal conditions ruled out (Z03.7-)

> One of the following 7th characters is to be assigned to each code under category O41. 7th character 0 is for single gestations and multiple gestations where the fetus is unspecified. 7th characters 1 through 9 are for cases of multiple gestations to identify the fetus for which the code applies. The appropriate code from category O30, Multiple gestation, must also be assigned when assigning a code from category O41 that has a 7th character of 1 through 9.
> 0 - not applicable or unspecified
> 1 - fetus 1
> 2 - fetus 2
> 3 - fetus 3
> 4 - fetus 4
> 5 - fetus 5
> 9 - other fetus

- **+ O41.0 Oligohydramnios**
  Oligohydramnios without rupture of membranes
  - ● ♀ X+7th **O41.00** Oligohydramnios, unspecified trimester
  - ● ♀ CC X+7th **O41.01** Oligohydramnios, first trimester
  - ● ♀ CC X+7th **O41.02** Oligohydramnios, second trimester
  - ● ♀ CC X+7th **O41.03** Oligohydramnios, third trimester
- **+ O41.1 Infection of amniotic sac and membranes**
  - **+ O41.10** Infection of amniotic sac and membranes, unspecified
    - ● ♀ MCC +7th **O41.101** Infection of amniotic sac and membranes, unspecified, first trimester
    - ● ♀ MCC +7th **O41.102** Infection of amniotic sac and membranes, unspecified, second trimester
    - ● ♀ MCC +7th **O41.103** Infection of amniotic sac and membranes, unspecified, third trimester
    - ● ♀ +7th **O41.109** Infection of amniotic sac and membranes, unspecified, unspecified trimester
  - **+ O41.12 Chorioamnionitis**
    AHA CC: 2Q, 2019, 34-35
    - ● ♀ MCC +7th **O41.121** Chorioamnionitis, first trimester
    - ● ♀ MCC +7th **O41.122** Chorioamnionitis, second trimester
    - ● ♀ MCC +7th **O41.123** Chorioamnionitis, third trimester
    - ● ♀ +7th **O41.129** Chorioamnionitis, unspecified trimester
  - **+ O41.14 Placentitis**
    - ● ♀ MCC +7th **O41.141** Placentitis, first trimester
    - ● ♀ MCC +7th **O41.142** Placentitis, second trimester
    - ● ♀ MCC +7th **O41.143** Placentitis, third trimester
    - ● ♀ +7th **O41.149** Placentitis, unspecified trimester
- **+ O41.8 Other specified disorders of amniotic fluid and membranes**
  - **+ O41.8X** Other specified disorders of amniotic fluid and membranes
    - ● ♀ +7th **O41.8X1** Other specified disorders of amniotic fluid and membranes, first trimester
    - ● ♀ +7th **O41.8X2** Other specified disorders of amniotic fluid and membranes, second trimester
    - ● ♀ +7th **O41.8X3** Other specified disorders of amniotic fluid and membranes, third trimester
    - ● ♀ +7th **O41.8X9** Other specified disorders of amniotic fluid and membranes, unspecified trimester
- **+ O41.9 Disorder of amniotic fluid and membranes, unspecified**
  - ● ♀ X+7th **O41.90** Disorder of amniotic fluid and membranes, unspecified, unspecified trimester
  - ● ♀ X+7th **O41.91** Disorder of amniotic fluid and membranes, unspecified, first trimester
  - ● ♀ X+7th **O41.92** Disorder of amniotic fluid and membranes, unspecified, second trimester
  - ● ♀ X+7th **O41.93** Disorder of amniotic fluid and membranes, unspecified, third trimester

O42 Premature rupture of membranes

- **+ O42.0 Premature rupture of membranes, onset of labor within 24 hours of rupture**
  - ● ♀ **O42.00** Premature rupture of membranes, onset of labor within 24 hours of rupture, unspecified weeks of gestation
  - **+ O42.01** Preterm premature rupture of membranes, onset of labor within 24 hours of rupture
    Premature rupture of membranes before 37 completed weeks of gestation, onset of labor within 24 hours of rupture
    - ● ♀ **O42.011** Preterm premature rupture of membranes, onset of labor within 24 hours of rupture, first trimester
    - ● ♀ **O42.012** Preterm premature rupture of membranes, onset of labor within 24 hours of rupture, second trimester
    - ● ♀ **O42.013** Preterm premature rupture of membranes, onset of labor within 24 hours of rupture, third trimester
    - ● ♀ **O42.019** Preterm premature rupture of membranes, onset of labor within 24 hours of rupture, unspecified trimester
  - ● ♀ **O42.02** Full-term premature rupture of membranes, onset of labor within 24 hours of rupture
    Premature rupture of membranes at or after 37 completed weeks of gestation, onset of labor within 24 hours of rupture
- **+ O42.1 Premature rupture of membranes, onset of labor more than 24 hours following rupture**
  - ● ♀ **O42.10** Premature rupture of membranes, onset of labor more than 24 hours following rupture, unspecified weeks of gestation
  - **+ O42.11** Preterm premature rupture of membranes, onset of labor more than 24 hours following rupture
    Premature rupture of membranes before 37 completed weeks of gestation
    - ● ♀ **O42.111** Preterm premature rupture of membranes, onset of labor more than 24 hours following rupture, first trimester
    - ● ♀ **O42.112** Preterm premature rupture of membranes, onset of labor more than 24 hours following rupture, second trimester
    - ● ♀ **O42.113** Preterm premature rupture of membranes, onset of labor more than 24 hours following rupture, third trimester
    - ● ♀ **O42.119** Preterm premature rupture of membranes, onset of labor more than 24 hours following rupture, unspecified trimester

- ♀ **O42.12** Full-term premature rupture of membranes, onset of labor more than 24 hours following rupture
  Premature rupture of membranes at or after 37 completed weeks of gestation, onset of labor more than 24 hours following rupture
+ **O42.9** Premature rupture of membranes, unspecified as to length of time between rupture and onset of labor
  - ♀ **O42.90** Premature rupture of membranes, unspecified as to length of time between rupture and onset of labor, unspecified weeks of gestation
  + **O42.91** Preterm premature rupture of membranes, unspecified as to length of time between rupture and onset of labor
    Premature rupture of membranes before 37 completed weeks of gestation
    - ♀ **O42.911** Preterm premature rupture of membranes, unspecified as to length of time between rupture and onset of labor, first trimester
    - ♀ **O42.912** Preterm premature rupture of membranes, unspecified as to length of time between rupture and onset of labor, second trimester
    - **MCC** ♀ **O42.913** Preterm premature rupture of membranes, unspecified as to length of time between rupture and onset of labor, third trimester
    - ♀ **O42.919** Preterm premature rupture of membranes, unspecified as to length of time between rupture and onset of labor, unspecified trimester
  - ♀ **O42.92** Full-term premature rupture of membranes, unspecified as to length of time between rupture and onset of labor
    Premature rupture of membranes at or after 37 completed weeks of gestation, unspecified as to length of time between rupture and onset of labor

O43 Placental disorders
Excludes2: maternal care for poor fetal growth due to placental insufficiency (O36.5-)
  placenta previa (O44.-)
  placental polyp (O90.89)
  placentitis (O41.14-)
  premature separation of placenta [abruptio placentae] (O45.-)

+ **O43.0** Placental transfusion syndromes
  + **O43.01** Fetomaternal placental transfusion syndrome
    Maternofetal placental transfusion syndrome
    - ♀ **O43.011** Fetomaternal placental transfusion syndrome, first trimester
    - ♀ **O43.012** Fetomaternal placental transfusion syndrome, second trimester
    - ♀ **O43.013** Fetomaternal placental transfusion syndrome, third trimester
    - ♀ **O43.019** Fetomaternal placental transfusion syndrome, unspecified trimester
  + **O43.02** Fetus-to-fetus placental transfusion syndrome
    - ♀ **O43.021** Fetus-to-fetus placental transfusion syndrome, first trimester
    - ♀ **O43.022** Fetus-to-fetus placental transfusion syndrome, second trimester
    - ♀ **O43.023** Fetus-to-fetus placental transfusion syndrome, third trimester
    - ♀ **O43.029** Fetus-to-fetus placental transfusion syndrome, unspecified trimester
+ **O43.1** Malformation of placenta
  + **O43.10** Malformation of placenta, unspecified
    Abnormal placenta NOS
    - ♀ **O43.101** Malformation of placenta, unspecified, first trimester
    - ♀ **O43.102** Malformation of placenta, unspecified, second trimester
    - ♀ **O43.103** Malformation of placenta, unspecified, third trimester
    - ♀ **O43.109** Malformation of placenta, unspecified, unspecified trimester
  + **O43.11** Circumvallate placenta
    - ♀ **O43.111** Circumvallate placenta, first trimester
    - ♀ **O43.112** Circumvallate placenta, second trimester
    - ♀ **O43.113** Circumvallate placenta, third trimester
    - ♀ **O43.119** Circumvallate placenta, unspecified trimester
  + **O43.12** Velamentous insertion of umbilical cord
    - ♀ **O43.121** Velamentous insertion of umbilical cord, first trimester
    - ♀ **O43.122** Velamentous insertion of umbilical cord, second trimester
    - ♀ **O43.123** Velamentous insertion of umbilical cord, third trimester
    - ♀ **O43.129** Velamentous insertion of umbilical cord, unspecified trimester
  + **O43.19** Other malformation of placenta
    - ♀ **O43.191** Other malformation of placenta, first trimester
    - ♀ **O43.192** Other malformation of placenta, second trimester
    - ♀ **O43.193** Other malformation of placenta, third trimester
    - ♀ **O43.199** Other malformation of placenta, unspecified trimester
+ **O43.2** Morbidly adherent placenta
  Code also associated third stage postpartum hemorrhage, if applicable (O72.0)
  Excludes1: retained placenta (O73.-)
  + **O43.21** Placenta accreta
    - ♀ **O43.211** Placenta accreta, first trimester
    - **MCC** ♀ **O43.212** Placenta accreta, second trimester
    - ♀ **O43.213** Placenta accreta, third trimester
    - ♀ **O43.219** accreta, unspecified trimester
  + **O43.22** Placenta increta
    - ♀ **O43.221** Placenta increta, first trimester
    - ♀ **O43.222** Placenta increta, second trimester
      AHA CC: 1Q, 2022, 20-21
    - ♀ **O43.223** Placenta increta, third trimester
    - ♀ **O43.229** Placenta increta, unspecified trimester
  + **O43.23** Placenta percreta
    - ♀ **O43.231** Placenta percreta, first trimester
    - ♀ **O43.232** Placenta percreta, second trimester
    - ♀ **O43.233** Placenta percreta, third trimester
    - ♀ **O43.239** Placenta percreta, unspecified trimester
+ **O43.8** Other placental disorders
  + **O43.81** Placental infarction
    - ♀ **O43.811** Placental infarction, first trimester
    - ♀ **O43.812** Placental infarction, second trimester
    - ♀ **O43.813** Placental infarction, third trimester
    - ♀ **O43.819** Placental infarction, unspecified trimester
  + **O43.89** Other placental disorders
    Placental dysfunction
    - ♀ **O43.891** Other placental disorders, first trimester
    - ♀ **O43.892** Other placental disorders, second trimester
    - ♀ **O43.893** Other placental disorders, third trimester
    - ♀ **O43.899** Other placental disorders, unspecified trimester
+ **O43.9** Unspecified placental disorder
  - ♀ **O43.90** Unspecified placental disorder, unspecified trimester
  - ♀ **O43.91** Unspecified placental disorder, first trimester
  - ♀ **O43.92** Unspecified placental disorder, second trimester
  - ♀ **O43.93** Unspecified placental disorder, third trimester

O44 Placenta previa
AHA CC: 4Q, 2016, 52-53
+ **O44.0** Complete placenta previa NOS or without hemorrhage
  Placenta previa NOS
  - ♀ **O44.00** Complete placenta previa NOS or without hemorrhage, unspecified trimester
  - ♀ CC **O44.01** Complete placenta previa NOS or without hemorrhage, first trimester
  - ♀ CC **O44.02** Complete placenta previa NOS or without hemorrhage, second trimester
  - ♀ CC **O44.03** Complete placenta previa NOS or without hemorrhage, third trimester
+ **O44.1** Complete placenta previa with hemorrhage
  Excludes1: labor and delivery complicated by hemorrhage from vasa previa (O69.4)
  - ♀ **O44.10** Complete placenta previa with hemorrhage, unspecified trimester

- • ♀ MCC **O44.11** Complete placenta previa with hemorrhage, first trimester
- • ♀ MCC **O44.12** Complete placenta previa with hemorrhage, second trimester
- • ♀ MCC **O44.13** Complete placenta previa with hemorrhage, third trimester
- + **O44.2** Partial placenta previa without hemorrhage
  Marginal placenta previa, NOS or without hemorrhage
  - • ♀ **O44.20** Partial placenta previa NOS or without hemorrhage, unspecified trimester
  - • ♀ CC **O44.21** Partial placenta previa NOS or without hemorrhage, first trimester
  - • ♀ CC **O44.22** Partial placenta previa NOS or without hemorrhage, second trimester
  - • ♀ CC **O44.23** Partial placenta previa NOS or without hemorrhage, third trimester
- + **O44.3** Partial placenta previa with hemorrhage
  Marginal placenta previa with hemorrhage
  - • ♀ **O44.30** Partial placenta previa with hemorrhage, unspecified trimester
  - • ♀ MCC **O44.31** Partial placenta previa with hemorrhage, first trimester
  - • ♀ MCC **O44.32** Partial placenta previa with hemorrhage, second trimester
  - • ♀ MCC **O44.33** Partial placenta previa with hemorrhage, third trimester
- + **O44.4** Low lying placenta NOS or without hemorrhage
  Low implantation of placenta NOS or without hemorrhage
  - • ♀ **O44.40** Low lying placenta NOS or without hemorrhage, unspecified trimester
  - • ♀ CC **O44.41** Low lying placenta NOS or without hemorrhage, first trimester
  - • ♀ CC **O44.42** Low lying placenta NOS or without hemorrhage, second trimester
  - • ♀ CC **O44.43** Low lying placenta NOS or without hemorrhage, third trimester
- + **O44.5** Low lying placenta with hemorrhage
  Low implantation of placenta with hemorrhage
  - • ♀ **O44.50** Low lying placenta with hemorrhage, unspecified trimester
  - • ♀ MCC **O44.51** Low lying placenta with hemorrhage, first trimester
  - • ♀ MCC **O44.52** Low lying placenta with hemorrhage, second trimester
  - • ♀ MCC **O44.53** Low lying placenta with hemorrhage, third trimester

O45 Premature separation of placenta [abruptio placentae]
- + **O45.0** Premature separation of placenta with coagulation defect
  - + **O45.00** Premature separation of placenta with coagulation defect, unspecified
    - • ♀ MCC **O45.001** Premature separation of placenta with coagulation defect, unspecified, first trimester
    - • ♀ MCC **O45.002** Premature separation of placenta with coagulation defect, unspecified, second trimester
    - • ♀ MCC **O45.003** Premature separation of placenta with coagulation defect, unspecified, third trimester
    - • ♀ **O45.009** Premature separation of placenta with coagulation defect, unspecified, unspecified trimester
  - + **O45.01** Premature separation of placenta with afibrinogenemia
    Premature separation of placenta with hypofibrinogenemia
    - • ♀ MCC **O45.011** Premature separation of placenta with afibrinogenemia, first trimester
    - • ♀ MCC **O45.012** Premature separation of placenta with afibrinogenemia, second trimester
    - • ♀ MCC **O45.013** Premature separation of placenta with afibrinogenemia, third trimester
    - • ♀ **O45.019** Premature separation of placenta with afibrinogenemia, unspecified trimester
  - + **O45.02** Premature separation of placenta with disseminated intravascular coagulation
    - • ♀ MCC **O45.021** Premature separation of placenta with disseminated intravascular coagulation, first trimester
    - • ♀ MCC **O45.022** Premature separation of placenta with disseminated intravascular coagulation, second trimester
    - • ♀ MCC **O45.023** Premature separation of placenta with disseminated intravascular coagulation, third trimester
    - • ♀ **O45.029** Premature separation of placenta with disseminated intravascular coagulation, unspecified trimester
  - **O45.09** Premature separation of placenta with other coagulation defect
    - • ♀ MCC **O45.091** Premature separation of placenta with other coagulation defect, first trimester
    - • ♀ MCC **O45.092** Premature separation of placenta with other coagulation defect, second trimester
    - • ♀ MCC **O45.093** Premature separation of placenta with other coagulation defect, third trimester
    - • ♀ **O45.099** Premature separation of placenta with other coagulation defect, unspecified trimester
- + **O45.8** Other premature separation of placenta
  - + **O45.8X** Other premature separation of placenta
    - • ♀ MCC **O45.8X1** Other premature separation of placenta, first trimester
    - • ♀ MCC **O45.8X2** Other premature separation of placenta, second trimester
    - • ♀ MCC **O45.8X3** Other premature separation of placenta, third trimester
    - • ♀ **O45.8X9** Other premature separation of placenta, unspecified trimester
- + **O45.9** Premature separation of placenta, unspecified
  Abruptio placentae NOS
  - • ♀ **O45.90** Premature separation of placenta, unspecified, unspecified trimester
  - • ♀ MCC **O45.91** Premature separation of placenta, unspecified, first trimester
  - • ♀ MCC **O45.92** Premature separation of placenta, unspecified, second trimester
  - • ♀ MCC **O45.93** Premature separation of placenta, unspecified, third trimester

O46 Antepartum hemorrhage, not elsewhere classified
Excludes1: hemorrhage in early pregnancy (O20.-)
intrapartum hemorrhage NEC (O67.-)
placenta previa (O44.-)
premature separation of placenta [abruptio placentae] (O45.-)
- + **O46.0** Antepartum hemorrhage with coagulation defect
  - + **O46.00** Antepartum hemorrhage with coagulation defect, unspecified
    - • ♀ MCC **O46.001** Antepartum hemorrhage with coagulation defect, unspecified, first trimester
    - • ♀ MCC **O46.002** Antepartum hemorrhage with coagulation defect, unspecified, second trimester
    - • ♀ MCC **O46.003** Antepartum hemorrhage with coagulation defect, unspecified, third trimester
    - • ♀ **O46.009** Antepartum hemorrhage with coagulation defect, unspecified, unspecified trimester
  - + **O46.01** Antepartum hemorrhage with afibrinogenemia
    Antepartum hemorrhage with hypofibrinogenemia
    - • ♀ MCC **O46.011** Antepartum hemorrhage with afibrinogenemia, first trimester
    - • ♀ MCC **O46.012** Antepartum hemorrhage with afibrinogenemia, second trimester
    - • ♀ MCC **O46.013** Antepartum hemorrhage with afibrinogenemia, third trimester
    - • ♀ **O46.019** Antepartum hemorrhage with afibrinogenemia, unspecified trimester
  - + **O46.02** Antepartum hemorrhage with disseminated intravascular coagulation
    - • ♀ MCC **O46.021** Antepartum hemorrhage with disseminated intravascular coagulation, first trimester
    - • ♀ MCC **O46.022** Antepartum hemorrhage with disseminated intravascular coagulation, second trimester

- ♀ MCC **O46.023** Antepartum hemorrhage with disseminated intravascular coagulation, third trimester
  - ♀ **O46.029** Antepartum hemorrhage with disseminated intravascular coagulation, unspecified trimester
- + **O46.09** Antepartum hemorrhage with other coagulation defect
  - ♀ MCC **O46.091** Antepartum hemorrhage with other coagulation defect, first trimester
  - ♀ MCC **O46.092** Antepartum hemorrhage with other coagulation defect, second trimester
  - ♀ MCC **O46.093** Antepartum hemorrhage with other coagulation defect, third trimester
  - ♀ **O46.099** Antepartum hemorrhage with other coagulation defect, unspecified trimester
- + **O46.8** Other antepartum hemorrhage
  - + **O46.8X** Other antepartum hemorrhage
    - ♀ **O46.8X1** Other antepartum hemorrhage, first trimester
    - ♀ **O46.8X2** Other antepartum hemorrhage, second trimester
    - ♀ **O46.8X3** Other antepartum hemorrhage, third trimester
    - ♀ **O46.8X9** Other antepartum hemorrhage, unspecified trimester
- + **O46.9** Antepartum hemorrhage, unspecified
  - ♀ **O46.90** Antepartum hemorrhage, unspecified, unspecified trimester
  - ♀ **O46.91** Antepartum hemorrhage, unspecified, first trimester
  - ♀ **O46.92** Antepartum hemorrhage, unspecified, second trimester
  - ♀ **O46.93** Antepartum hemorrhage, unspecified, third trimester

O47 False labor
Includes: Braxton Hicks contractions
threatened labor
Excludes1: preterm labor (O60.-)

- + **O47.0** False labor before 37 completed weeks of gestation
  - ♀ **O47.00** False labor before 37 completed weeks of gestation, unspecified trimester
  - ♀ CC **O47.02** False labor before 37 completed weeks of gestation, second trimester
  - ♀ CC **O47.03** False labor before 37 completed weeks of gestation, third trimester
- ♀ CC **O47.1** False labor at or after 37 completed weeks of gestation
  AHA CC: 1Q, 2021, 10
- ♀ **O47.9** False labor, unspecified

O48 Late pregnancy

- ♀ **O48.0** Post-term pregnancy
  Pregnancy over 40 completed weeks to 42 completed weeks gestation
  AHA CC: 2Q, 2022, 3-4
- ♀ **O48.1** Prolonged pregnancy
  Pregnancy which has advanced beyond 42 completed weeks gestation
  AHA CC: 2Q, 2022, 3-4

Complications of labor and delivery (O60-O77)

O60 Preterm labor
Includes: onset (spontaneous) of labor before 37 completed weeks of gestation
Excludes1: false labor (O47.0-)
threatened labor NOS (O47.0-)

- + **O60.0** Preterm labor without delivery
  - ♀ **O60.00** Preterm labor without delivery, unspecified trimester
  - ♀ MCC **O60.02** Preterm labor without delivery, second trimester
  - ♀ MCC **O60.03** Preterm labor without delivery, third trimester
- + **O60.1** Preterm labor with preterm delivery

One of the following 7th characters is to be assigned to each code under subcategory **O60.1**. 7th character 0 is for single gestations and multiple gestations where the fetus is unspecified. 7th characters 1 through 9 are for cases of multiple gestations to identify the fetus for which the code applies. The appropriate code from category O30, Multiple gestation, must also be assigned when assigning a code from subcategory O60.1 that has a 7th character of 1 through 9.
0 - not applicable or unspecified
1 - fetus 1
2 - fetus 2
3 - fetus 3
4 - fetus 4
5 - fetus 5
9 - other fetus

- ♀ CC X+7th **O60.10** Preterm labor with preterm delivery, unspecified trimester
  Preterm labor with delivery NOS
- ♀ MCC X+7th **O60.12** Preterm labor second trimester with preterm delivery second trimester
- ♀ MCC X+7th **O60.13** Preterm labor second trimester with preterm delivery third trimester
- ♀ MCC X+7th **O60.14** Preterm labor third trimester with preterm delivery third trimester
  AHA CC: 2Q, 2016, 10-11
- + **O60.2** Term delivery with preterm labor

One of the following 7th characters is to be assigned to each code under subcategory **O60.2**. 7th character 0 is for single gestations and multiple gestations where the fetus is unspecified. 7th characters 1 through 9 are for cases of multiple gestations to identify the fetus for which the code applies. The appropriate code from category O30, Multiple gestation, must also be assigned when assigning a code from subcategory O60.2 that has a 7th character of 1 through 9.
0 - not applicable or unspecified
1 - fetus 1
2 - fetus 2
3 - fetus 3
4 - fetus 4
5 - fetus 5
9 - other fetus

- ♀ CC X+7th **O60.20** Term delivery with preterm labor, unspecified trimester
- ♀ MCC X+7th **O60.22** Term delivery with preterm labor, second trimester
- ♀ MCC X+7th **O60.23** Term delivery with preterm labor, third trimester

O61 Failed induction of labor
- ♀ **O61.0** Failed medical induction of labor
  Failed induction (of labor) by oxytocin
  Failed induction (of labor) by prostaglandins
- ♀ **O61.1** Failed instrumental induction of labor
  Failed mechanical induction (of labor)
  Failed surgical induction (of labor)
- ♀ **O61.8** Other failed induction of labor
- ♀ **O61.9** Failed induction of labor, unspecified

O62 Abnormalities of forces of labor
- ♀ **O62.0** Primary inadequate contractions
  Failure of cervical dilatation
  Primary hypotonic uterine dysfunction
  Uterine inertia during latent phase of labor
- ♀ **O62.1** Secondary uterine inertia
  Arrested active phase of labor
  Secondary hypotonic uterine dysfunction
- ♀ **O62.2** Other uterine inertia
  Atony of uterus without hemorrhage
  Atony of uterus NOS
  Desultory labor
  Hypotonic uterine dysfunction NOS
  Irregular labor
  Poor contractions
  Slow slope active phase of labor
  Uterine inertia NOS
  Excludes1: atony of uterus with hemorrhage (postpartum) (O72.1)
  postpartum atony of uterus without hemorrhage (O75.89)

- ● ♀ **O62.3** Precipitate labor
- ● ♀ **O62.4** Hypertonic, incoordinate, and prolonged uterine contractions
  - Cervical spasm
  - Contraction ring dystocia
  - Dyscoordinate labor
  - Hour-glass contraction of uterus
  - Hypertonic uterine dysfunction
  - Incoordinate uterine action
  - Tetanic contractions
  - Uterine dystocia NOS
  - Uterine spasm
  - **Excludes1:** *dystocia (fetal) (maternal) NOS (O66.9)*
- ● ♀ **O62.8** Other abnormalities of forces of labor
- ● ♀ **O62.9** Abnormality of forces of labor, unspecified

O63 Long labor
- ● ♀ **O63.0** Prolonged first stage (of labor)
- ● ♀ **O63.1** Prolonged second stage (of labor)
- ● ♀ **O63.2** Delayed delivery of second twin, triplet, etc.
- ● CC **O63.9** Long labor, unspecified
  - Prolonged labor NOS

O64 Obstructed labor due to malposition and malpresentation of fetus

> One of the following 7th characters is to be assigned to each code under category O64. 7th character 0 is for single gestations and multiple gestations where the fetus is unspecified. 7th characters 1 through 9 are for cases of multiple gestations to identify the fetus for which the code applies. The appropriate code from category O30, Multiple gestation, must also be assigned when assigning a code from category O64 that has a 7th character of 1 through 9.
>
> 0 - not applicable or unspecified
> 1 - fetus 1
> 2 - fetus 2
> 3 - fetus 3
> 4 - fetus 4
> 5 - fetus 5
> 9 - other fetus

- ● ♀ X+7th **O64.0** Obstructed labor due to incomplete rotation of fetal head
  - Deep transverse arrest
  - Obstructed labor due to persistent occipitoiliac (position)
  - Obstructed labor due to persistent occipitoposterior (position)
  - Obstructed labor due to persistent occipitosacral (position)
  - Obstructed labor due to persistent occipitotransverse (position)
- ● ♀ X+7th **O64.1** Obstructed labor due to breech presentation
  - Obstructed labor due to buttocks presentation
  - Obstructed labor due to complete breech presentation
  - Obstructed labor due to frank breech presentation
- ● ♀ X+7th **O64.2** Obstructed labor due to face presentation
  - Obstructed labor due to chin presentation
- ● ♀ X+7th **O64.3** Obstructed labor due to brow presentation
- ● ♀ X+7th **O64.4** Obstructed labor due to shoulder presentation
  - Prolapsed arm
  - **Excludes1:** *impacted shoulders (O66.0)*
    shoulder dystocia (O66.0)
- ● ♀ X+7th **O64.5** Obstructed labor due to compound presentation
- ● ♀ X+7th **O64.8** Obstructed labor due to other malposition and malpresentation
  - Obstructed labor due to footling presentation
  - Obstructed labor due to incomplete breech presentation
- ● ♀ X+7th **O64.9** Obstructed labor due to malposition and malpresentation, unspecified

O65 Obstructed labor due to maternal pelvic abnormality
- ● ♀ **O65.0** Obstructed labor due to deformed pelvis
- ● ♀ **O65.1** Obstructed labor due to generally contracted pelvis
- ● ♀ **O65.2** Obstructed labor due to pelvic inlet contraction
- ● ♀ **O65.3** Obstructed labor due to pelvic outlet and mid-cavity contraction
- ● ♀ **O65.4** Obstructed labor due to fetopelvic disproportion, unspecified
  - **Excludes1:** *dystocia due to abnormality of fetus (O66.2-O66.3)*
- ● ♀ **O65.5** Obstructed labor due to abnormality of maternal pelvic organs
  - Obstructed labor due to conditions listed in O34.-
  - Use additional code to identify abnormality of pelvic organs O34.-
- ● ♀ **O65.8** Obstructed labor due to other maternal pelvic abnormalities
- ● ♀ **O65.9** Obstructed labor due to maternal pelvic abnormality, unspecified

O66 Other obstructed labor
- ● ♀ **O66.0** Obstructed labor due to shoulder dystocia
  - Impacted shoulders
- ● ♀ **O66.1** Obstructed labor due to locked twins
- ● ♀ **O66.2** Obstructed labor due to unusually large fetus
- ● ♀ **O66.3** Obstructed labor due to other abnormalities of fetus
  - Dystocia due to fetal ascites
  - Dystocia due to fetal hydrops
  - Dystocia due to fetal meningomyelocele
  - Dystocia due to fetal sacral teratoma
  - Dystocia due to fetal tumor
  - Dystocia due to hydrocephalic fetus
  - Use additional code to identify cause of obstruction
- + **O66.4** Failed trial of labor
  - ● ♀ **O66.40** Failed trial of labor, unspecified
  - ● ♀ **O66.41** Failed attempted vaginal birth after previous cesarean delivery
    - Code first rupture of uterus, if applicable (O71.0-, O71.1)
- ● ♀ **O66.5** Attempted application of vacuum extractor and forceps
  - Attempted application of vacuum or forceps, with subsequent delivery by forceps or cesarean delivery
- ● ♀ **O66.6** Obstructed labor due to other multiple fetuses
- ● ♀ **O66.8** Other specified obstructed labor
  - Use additional code to identify cause of obstruction
- ● ♀ **O66.9** Obstructed labor, unspecified
  - Dystocia NOS
  - Fetal dystocia NOS
  - Maternal dystocia NOS

O67 Labor and delivery complicated by intrapartum hemorrhage, not elsewhere classified
Excludes1: *antepartum hemorrhage NEC (O46.-)*
placenta previa (O44.-)
premature separation of placenta [abruptio placentae] (O45.-)
Excludes2: *postpartum hemorrhage (O72.-)*
- ● ♀ MCC **O67.0** Intrapartum hemorrhage with coagulation defect
  - Intrapartum hemorrhage (excessive) associated with afibrinogenemia
  - Intrapartum hemorrhage (excessive) associated with disseminated intravascular coagulation
  - Intrapartum hemorrhage (excessive) associated with hyperfibrinolysis
  - Intrapartum hemorrhage (excessive) associated with hypofibrinogenemia
- ● ♀ **O67.8** Other intrapartum hemorrhage
  - Excessive intrapartum hemorrhage
- ● ♀ **O67.9** Intrapartum hemorrhage, unspecified

● ♀ CC O68 Labor and delivery complicated by abnormality of fetal acid-base balance
- Fetal acidemia complicating labor and delivery
- Fetal acidosis complicating labor and delivery
- Fetal alkalosis complicating labor and delivery
- Fetal metabolic acidemia complicating labor and delivery
- **Excludes1:** *fetal stress NOS (O77.9)*
  labor and delivery complicated by electrocardiographic evidence of fetal stress (O77.8)
  labor and delivery complicated by ultrasonic evidence of fetal stress (O77.8)
- **Excludes2:** *abnormality in fetal heart rate or rhythm (O76)*
  labor and delivery complicated by meconium in amniotic fluid (O77.0)

Valid 3-character code, no further characters required

O69 Labor and delivery complicated by umbilical cord complications

One of the following 7th characters is to be assigned to each code under category O69. 7th character 0 is for single gestations and multiple gestations where the fetus is unspecified. 7th characters 1 through 9 are for cases of multiple gestations to identify the fetus for which the code applies. The appropriate code from category O30, Multiple gestation, must also be assigned when assigning a code from category O69 that has a 7th character of 1 through 9.
0 - not applicable or unspecified
1 - fetus 1
2 - fetus 2
3 - fetus 3
4 - fetus 4
5 - fetus 5
9 - other fetus

- X+7th **O69.0** Labor and delivery complicated by prolapse of cord
- X+7th **O69.1** Labor and delivery complicated by cord around neck, with compression
  - *Excludes1:* labor and delivery complicated by cord around neck, without compression (O69.81)
- X+7th **O69.2** Labor and delivery complicated by other cord entanglement, with compression
  - Labor and delivery complicated by compression of cord NOS
  - Labor and delivery complicated by entanglement of cords of twins in monoamniotic sac
  - Labor and delivery complicated by knot in cord
  - *Excludes1:* labor and delivery complicated by other cord entanglement, without compression (O69.82)
- X+7th **O69.3** Labor and delivery complicated by short cord
- X+7th **O69.4** Labor and delivery complicated by vasa previa
  - Labor and delivery complicated by hemorrhage from vasa previa
- X+7th **O69.5** Labor and delivery complicated by vascular lesion of cord
  - Labor and delivery complicated by cord bruising
  - Labor and delivery complicated by cord hematoma
  - Labor and delivery complicated by thrombosis of umbilical vessels
- X+7th **O69.8** Labor and delivery complicated by other cord complications
  - X+7th **O69.81** Labor and delivery complicated by cord around neck, without compression
  - X+7th **O69.82** Labor and delivery complicated by other cord entanglement, without compression
  - X+7th **O69.89** Labor and delivery complicated by other cord complications
    - *AHA CC: 2Q, 2023, 29*
- X+7th **O69.9** Labor and delivery complicated by cord complication, unspecified

O70 Perineal laceration during delivery

Includes: episiotomy extended by laceration
Excludes1: obstetric high vaginal laceration alone (O71.4)

- **O70.0** First degree perineal laceration during delivery
  - Perineal laceration, rupture or tear involving fourchette during delivery
  - Perineal laceration, rupture or tear involving labia during delivery
  - Perineal laceration, rupture or tear involving skin during delivery
  - Perineal laceration, rupture or tear involving vagina during delivery
  - Perineal laceration, rupture or tear involving vulva during delivery
  - Slight perineal laceration, rupture or tear during delivery
- **O70.1** Second degree perineal laceration during delivery
  - Perineal laceration, rupture or tear during delivery as in O70.0, also involving pelvic floor
  - Perineal laceration, rupture or tear during delivery as in O70.0, also involving perineal muscles
  - Perineal laceration, rupture or tear during delivery as in O70.0, also involving vaginal muscles
  - *Excludes1:* perineal laceration involving anal sphincter (O70.2)
  - *AHA CC: 2Q, 2016, 34*
- + **O70.2** Third degree perineal laceration during delivery
  - Perineal laceration, rupture or tear during delivery as in O70.1, also involving anal sphincter
  - Perineal laceration, rupture or tear during delivery as in O70.1, also involving rectovaginal septum
  - Perineal laceration, rupture or tear during delivery as in O70.1, also involving sphincter NOS
  - *Excludes1:* anal sphincter tear during delivery without third degree perineal laceration (O70.4)
    - perineal laceration involving anal or rectal mucosa (O70.3)
  - *AHA CC: 4Q, 2016, 53-54*
  - CC **O70.20** Third degree perineal laceration during delivery, unspecified
  - CC **O70.21** Third degree perineal laceration during delivery, IIIa
    - Third degree perineal laceration during delivery with less than 50% of external anal sphincter (EAS) thickness torn
  - CC **O70.22** Third degree perineal laceration during delivery, IIIb
    - Third degree perineal laceration during delivery with more than 50% of external anal sphincter (EAS) thickness torn
  - CC **O70.23** Third degree perineal laceration during delivery, IIIc
    - Third degree perineal laceration during delivery with both external anal sphincter (EAS) and internal anal sphincter (IAS) torn
- CC **O70.3** Fourth degree perineal laceration during delivery
  - Perineal laceration, rupture or tear during delivery as in O70.2, also involving anal mucosa
  - Perineal laceration, rupture or tear during delivery as in O70.2, also involving rectal mucosa
- CC **O70.4** Anal sphincter tear complicating delivery, not associated with third degree perineal laceration
  - *Excludes1:* anal sphincter tear with third degree perineal laceration (O70.2)
- **O70.9** Perineal laceration during delivery, unspecified

O71 Other obstetric trauma

Includes: obstetric damage from instruments

- + **O71.0** Rupture of uterus (spontaneous) before onset of labor
  - *Excludes1:* disruption of (current) cesarean delivery wound (O90.0)
    - laceration of uterus, NEC (O71.81)
  - **O71.00** Rupture of uterus before onset of labor, unspecified trimester
  - MCC **O71.02** Rupture of uterus before onset of labor, second trimester
  - MCC **O71.03** Rupture of uterus before onset of labor, third trimester
- MCC **O71.1** Rupture of uterus during labor
  - Rupture of uterus not stated as occurring before onset of labor
  - *Excludes1:* disruption of cesarean delivery wound (O90.0)
    - laceration of uterus, NEC (O71.81)
- CC **O71.2** Postpartum inversion of uterus
- CC **O71.3** Obstetric laceration of cervix
  - Annular detachment of cervix
- CC **O71.4** Obstetric high vaginal laceration alone
  - Laceration of vaginal wall without perineal laceration
  - *Excludes1:* obstetric high vaginal laceration with perineal laceration (O70.-)
- CC **O71.5** Other obstetric injury to pelvic organs
  - Obstetric injury to bladder
  - Obstetric injury to urethra
  - *Excludes2:* obstetric periurethral trauma (O71.82)
- CC **O71.6** Obstetric damage to pelvic joints and ligaments
  - Obstetric avulsion of inner symphyseal cartilage
  - Obstetric damage to coccyx
  - Obstetric traumatic separation of symphysis (pubis)
- CC **O71.7** Obstetric hematoma of pelvis
  - Obstetric hematoma of perineum
  - Obstetric hematoma of vagina
  - Obstetric hematoma of vulva
- + **O71.8** Other specified obstetric trauma
  - **O71.81** Laceration of uterus, not elsewhere classified

- ♀ **O71.82** Other specified trauma to perineum and vulva
  Obstetric periurethral trauma
  AHA CC: 4Q, 2014, 18-19
- ♀ **O71.89** Other specified obstetric trauma
- ♀ **O71.9** Obstetric trauma, unspecified

O72 Postpartum hemorrhage

Includes: hemorrhage after delivery of fetus or infant

- ♀ CC **O72.0** Third-stage hemorrhage
  Hemorrhage associated with retained, trapped or adherent placenta
  Retained placenta NOS
  Code also type of adherent placenta (O43.2-)
- ♀ CC **O72.1** Other immediate postpartum hemorrhage
  Hemorrhage following delivery of placenta
  Postpartum hemorrhage (atonic) NOS
  Uterine atony with hemorrhage
  Excludes1: *uterine atony NOS (O62.2)*
  uterine atony without hemorrhage (O62.2)
  postpartum atony of uterus without hemorrhage (O75.89)
  AHA CC: 2Q, 2023, 15-16
- ♀ CC **O72.2** Delayed and secondary postpartum hemorrhage
  Hemorrhage associated with retained portions of placenta or membranes after the first 24 hours following delivery of placenta
  Retained products of conception NOS, following delivery
- ♀ **O72.3** Postpartum coagulation defects
  Postpartum afibrinogenemia
  Postpartum fibrinolysis

O73 Retained placenta and membranes, without hemorrhage

Excludes1: *placenta accreta (O43.21-)*
placenta increta (O43.22-)
placenta percreta (O43.23-)

- ♀ **O73.0** Retained placenta without hemorrhage
  Adherent placenta, without hemorrhage
  Trapped placenta without hemorrhage
- ♀ **O73.1** Retained portions of placenta and membranes, without hemorrhage
  Retained products of conception following delivery, without hemorrhage

O74 Complications of anesthesia during labor and delivery

Includes: maternal complications arising from the administration of a general, regional or local anesthetic, analgesic or other sedation during labor and delivery

Use additional code, if applicable, to identify specific complication

- ♀ **O74.0** Aspiration pneumonitis due to anesthesia during labor and delivery
  Inhalation of stomach contents or secretions NOS due to anesthesia during labor and delivery
  Mendelson's syndrome due to anesthesia during labor and delivery
- ♀ **O74.1** Other pulmonary complications of anesthesia during labor and delivery
- ♀ **O74.2** Cardiac complications of anesthesia during labor and delivery
- ♀ **O74.3** Central nervous system complications of anesthesia during labor and delivery
- ♀ **O74.4** Toxic reaction to local anesthesia during labor and delivery
- ♀ **O74.5** Spinal and epidural anesthesia-induced headache during labor and delivery
- ♀ **O74.6** Other complications of spinal and epidural anesthesia during labor and delivery
- ♀ **O74.7** Failed or difficult intubation for anesthesia during labor and delivery
- ♀ **O74.8** Other complications of anesthesia during labor and delivery
- ♀ **O74.9** Complication of anesthesia during labor and delivery, unspecified

O75 Other complications of labor and delivery, not elsewhere classified

Excludes2: *puerperal (postpartum) infection (O86.-)*
puerperal (postpartum) sepsis (O85)

- ♀ **O75.0** Maternal distress during labor and delivery
- ♀ MCC **O75.1** Shock during or following labor and delivery
  Obstetric shock following labor and delivery
- ♀ CC **O75.2** Pyrexia during labor, not elsewhere classified
- ♀ MCC **O75.3** Other infection during labor
  Sepsis during labor
  Use additional code (B95-B97), to identify infectious agent
  Review coding guideline C.15.j
- ♀ **O75.4** Other complications of obstetric surgery and procedures
  Cardiac arrest following obstetric surgery or procedures
  Cardiac failure following obstetric surgery or procedures
  Cerebral anoxia following obstetric surgery or procedures
  Pulmonary edema following obstetric surgery or procedures
  Use additional code to identify specific complication
  Excludes2: *complications of anesthesia during labor and delivery (O74.-)*
  disruption of obstetrical (surgical) wound (O90.0-O90.1)
  hematoma of obstetrical (surgical) wound (O90.2)
  infection of obstetrical (surgical) wound (O86.0-)
- ♀ **O75.5** Delayed delivery after artificial rupture of membranes
- + **O75.8** Other specified complications of labor and delivery
  - ♀ **O75.81** Maternal exhaustion complicating labor and delivery
  - ♀ **O75.82** Onset (spontaneous) of labor after 37 completed weeks of gestation but before 39 completed weeks gestation, with delivery by (planned) cesarean section
    Delivery by (planned) cesarean section occurring after 37 completed weeks of gestation but before 39 completed weeks gestation due to (spontaneous) onset of labor
    Code first to specify reason for planned cesarean section such as:
    cephalopelvic disproportion (normally formed fetus) (O33.9)
    previous cesarean delivery (O34.21-)
    AHA CC: 2Q, 2022, 3-4
  - ♀ **O75.89** Other specified complications of labor and delivery
- ♀ **O75.9** Complication of labor and delivery, unspecified

O76 Abnormality in fetal heart rate and rhythm complicating labor and delivery

Depressed fetal heart rate tones complicating labor and delivery
Fetal bradycardia complicating labor and delivery
Fetal heart rate decelerations complicating labor and delivery
Fetal heart rate irregularity complicating labor and delivery
Fetal heart rate abnormal variability complicating labor and delivery
Fetal tachycardia complicating labor and delivery
Non-reassuring fetal heart rate or rhythm complicating labor and delivery

Excludes1: *fetal stress NOS (O77.9)*
labor and delivery complicated by electrocardiographic evidence of fetal stress (O77.8)
labor and delivery complicated by ultrasonic evidence of fetal stress (O77.8)

Excludes2: *fetal metabolic acidemia (O68)*
other fetal stress (O77.0-O77.1)
AHA CC: 4Q, 2013, 118
Valid 3-character code, no further characters required

O77 Other fetal stress complicating labor and delivery

- ♀ **O77.0** Labor and delivery complicated by meconium in amniotic fluid
  AHA CC: 4Q, 2013, 118; 2Q, 2022, 16-17
- ♀ **O77.1** Fetal stress in labor or delivery due to drug administration
- ♀ **O77.8** Labor and delivery complicated by other evidence of fetal stress
  Labor and delivery complicated by electrocardiographic evidence of fetal stress
  Labor and delivery complicated by ultrasonic evidence of fetal stress
  Excludes1: *abnormality of fetal acid-base balance (O68)*
  abnormality in fetal heart rate or rhythm (O76)
  fetal metabolic acidemia (O68)
- ♀ **O77.9** Labor and delivery complicated by fetal stress, unspecified
  Excludes1: *abnormality of fetal acid-base balance (O68)*
  abnormality in fetal heart rate or rhythm (O76)
  fetal metabolic acidemia (O68)

Encounter for delivery (O80-O82)

- ♀ **O80** **Encounter for full-term uncomplicated delivery**

    Delivery requiring minimal or no assistance, with or without episiotomy, without fetal manipulation [e.g., rotation version] or instrumentation [forceps] of a spontaneous, cephalic, vaginal, full-term, single, live-born infant. This code is for use as a single diagnosis code and is not to be used with any other code from chapter 15.
    Use additional code to indicate outcome of delivery (Z37.0)
    AHA CC: 2Q, 2014, 9; 4Q, 2016, 150
    Review coding guideline C.15.n
    Valid 3-character code, no further characters required

- ♀ **O82** **Encounter for cesarean delivery without indication**

    Use additional code to indicate outcome of delivery (Z37.0)
    Valid 3-character code, no further characters required

Complications predominantly related to the puerperium (O85-O92)

Excludes2: mental and behavioral disorders associated with the puerperium (F53.-)
obstetrical tetanus (A34)
puerperal osteomalacia (M83.0)

O85 **Puerperal sepsis**
MCC
- ♀ Postpartum sepsis
    Puerperal peritonitis
    Puerperal pyemia
    Use additional code (B95-B97), to identify infectious agent
    Use additional code (R65.2-) to identify severe sepsis, if applicable
    Excludes1: fever of unknown origin following delivery (O86.4)
    genital tract infection following delivery (O86.1-)
    obstetric pyemic and septic embolism (O88.3-)
    puerperal septic thrombophlebitis (O86.81)
    urinary tract infection following delivery (O86.2-)
    Excludes2: sepsis during labor (O75.3)
    Review coding guideline C.15.k
    Valid 3-character code, no further characters required

O86 **Other puerperal infections**
    Use additional code (B95-B97), to identify infectious agent
    Excludes2: infection during labor (O75.3)
    obstetrical tetanus (A34)
+ **O86.0** **Infection of obstetric surgical wound**
    Infected cesarean delivery wound following delivery
    Infected perineal repair following delivery
    Excludes1: complications of procedures, not elsewhere classified (T81.4-)
    postprocedural fever NOS (R50.82)
    postprocedural retroperitoneal abscess (K68.11)
    AHA CC: 4Q, 2018, 22-23
    Review coding guideline C.1.d.5
  - ♀ **O86.00** Infection of obstetric surgical wound, unspecified
  - ♀ **O86.01** Infection of obstetric surgical wound, superficial incisional site
    Subcutaneous abscess following an obstetrical procedure
    Stitch abscess following an obstetrical procedure
  - ♀ **O86.02** Infection of obstetric surgical wound, deep incisional site
    Intramuscular abscess following an obstetrical procedure
    Sub-fascial abscess following an obstetrical procedure
    AHA CC: 4Q, 2018, 23; 2Q, 2020, 32-33
  - ♀ **O86.03** Infection of obstetric surgical wound, organ and space site
    Intraabdominal abscess following an obstetrical procedure
    Subphrenic abscess following an obstetrical procedure
  - ♀ MCC **O86.04** Sepsis following an obstetrical procedure
    Use additional code to identify the sepsis
    AHA CC: 4Q, 2018, 23; 2Q, 2019, 39; 2Q, 2020, 32-33
  - ♀ **O86.09** Infection of obstetric surgical wound, other surgical site

+ **O86.1** **Other infection of genital tract following delivery**
  - ♀ CC **O86.11** Cervicitis following delivery
  - ♀ CC **O86.12** Endometritis following delivery
  - ♀ CC **O86.13** Vaginitis following delivery
  - ♀ CC **O86.19** Other infection of genital tract following delivery
+ **O86.2** **Urinary tract infection following delivery**
  - ♀ CC **O86.20** Urinary tract infection following delivery, unspecified
    Puerperal urinary tract infection NOS
    AHA CC: 2Q, 2022, 5
  - ♀ CC **O86.21** Infection of kidney following delivery
  - ♀ CC **O86.22** Infection of bladder following delivery
    Infection of urethra following delivery
  - ♀ CC **O86.29** Other urinary tract infection following delivery
- ♀ CC **O86.4** **Pyrexia of unknown origin following delivery**
    Puerperal infection NOS following delivery
    Puerperal pyrexia NOS following delivery
    Excludes2: pyrexia during labor (O75.2)
+ **O86.8** **Other specified puerperal infections**
  - ♀ MCC **O86.81** Puerperal septic thrombophlebitis
  - ♀ MCC **O86.89** Other specified puerperal infections

O87 **Venous complications and hemorrhoids in the puerperium**
    Includes: venous complications in labor, delivery and the puerperium
    Excludes2: obstetric embolism (O88.-)
    puerperal septic thrombophlebitis (O86.81)
    venous complications in pregnancy (O22.-)
- ♀ CC **O87.0** Superficial thrombophlebitis in the puerperium
    Puerperal phlebitis NOS
    Puerperal thrombosis NOS
    Use Additional code, if applicable, to identify the superficial vein thrombosis, such as thrombosis of superficial vessels of lower extremities (I80.0-)
- ♀ MCC **O87.1** Deep phlebothrombosis in the puerperium
    Deep vein thrombosis, postpartum
    Pelvic thrombophlebitis, postpartum
    Use additional code to identify the deep vein thrombosis (I82.4-, I82.5-, I82.62-, I82.72-)
    Use additional code, if applicable, for associated long-term (current) use of anticoagulants (Z79.01)
- ♀ CC **O87.2** Hemorrhoids in the puerperium
- ♀ CC **O87.3** Cerebral venous thrombosis in the puerperium
    Cerebrovenous sinus thrombosis in the puerperium
- ♀ **O87.4** Varicose veins of lower extremity in the puerperium
- ♀ CC **O87.8** Other venous complications in the puerperium
    Genital varices in the puerperium
- ♀ **O87.9** Venous complication in the puerperium, unspecified
    Puerperal phlebopathy NOS

O88 **Obstetric embolism**
    Excludes1: embolism complicating abortion NOS (O03.2)
    embolism complicating ectopic or molar pregnancy (O08.2)
    embolism complicating failed attempted abortion (O07.2)
    embolism complicating induced abortion (O04.7)
    embolism complicating spontaneous abortion (O03.2, O03.7)
+ **O88.0** **Obstetric air embolism**
    + **O88.01** Obstetric air embolism in pregnancy
      - ♀ MCC **O88.011** Air embolism in pregnancy, first trimester
      - ♀ MCC **O88.012** Air embolism in pregnancy, second trimester
      - ♀ MCC **O88.013** Air embolism in pregnancy, third trimester
      - ♀ **O88.019** Air embolism in pregnancy, unspecified trimester
    - ♀ MCC **O88.02** Air embolism in childbirth
    - ♀ MCC **O88.03** Air embolism in the puerperium
+ **O88.1** **Amniotic fluid embolism**
    Anaphylactoid syndrome in pregnancy
    + **O88.11** Amniotic fluid embolism in pregnancy
      - ♀ MCC **O88.111** Amniotic fluid embolism in pregnancy, first trimester
      - ♀ MCC **O88.112** Amniotic fluid embolism in pregnancy, second trimester
      - ♀ MCC **O88.113** Amniotic fluid embolism in pregnancy, third trimester
      - ♀ **O88.119** Amniotic fluid embolism in pregnancy, unspecified trimester

- ♀ MCC **O88.12** Amniotic fluid embolism in childbirth
- ♀ MCC **O88.13** Amniotic fluid embolism in the puerperium
- **+ O88.2** Obstetric thromboembolism
  - **+ O88.21** Thromboembolism in pregnancy
    - Obstetric (pulmonary) embolism NOS
    - ♀ MCC **O88.211** Thromboembolism in pregnancy, first trimester
    - ♀ MCC **O88.212** Thromboembolism in pregnancy, second trimester
    - ♀ MCC **O88.213** Thromboembolism in pregnancy, third trimester
    - ♀ **O88.219** Thromboembolism in pregnancy, unspecified trimester
  - ♀ MCC **O88.22** Thromboembolism in childbirth
  - ♀ MCC **O88.23** Thromboembolism in the puerperium
    - Puerperal (pulmonary) embolism NOS
- **+ O88.3** Obstetric pyemic and septic embolism
  - **+ O88.31** Pyemic and septic embolism in pregnancy
    - ♀ MCC **O88.311** Pyemic and septic embolism in pregnancy, first trimester
    - ♀ MCC **O88.312** Pyemic and septic embolism in pregnancy, second trimester
    - ♀ MCC **O88.313** Pyemic and septic embolism in pregnancy, third trimester
    - ♀ **O88.319** Pyemic and septic embolism in pregnancy, unspecified trimester
  - ♀ MCC **O88.32** Pyemic and septic embolism in childbirth
  - ♀ MCC **O88.33** Pyemic and septic embolism in the puerperium
- **+ O88.8** Other obstetric embolism
  - Obstetric fat embolism
  - **+ O88.81** Other embolism in pregnancy
    - ♀ MCC **O88.811** Other embolism in pregnancy, first trimester
    - ♀ MCC **O88.812** Other embolism in pregnancy, second trimester
    - ♀ MCC **O88.813** Other embolism in pregnancy, third trimester
    - ♀ CC **O88.819** Other embolism in pregnancy, unspecified trimester
  - ♀ MCC **O88.82** Other embolism in childbirth
  - ♀ MCC **O88.83** Other embolism in the puerperium

O89 Complications of anesthesia during the puerperium

Includes: maternal complications arising from the administration of a general, regional or local anesthetic, analgesic or other sedation during the puerperium

Use additional code, if applicable, to identify specific complication

- **+ O89.0** Pulmonary complications of anesthesia during the puerperium
  - ♀ **O89.01** Aspiration pneumonitis due to anesthesia during the puerperium
    - Inhalation of stomach contents or secretions NOS due to anesthesia during the puerperium
    - Mendelson's syndrome due to anesthesia during the puerperium
  - ♀ **O89.09** Other pulmonary complications of anesthesia during the puerperium
- ♀ **O89.1** Cardiac complications of anesthesia during the puerperium
- ♀ **O89.2** Central nervous system complications of anesthesia during the puerperium
- ♀ **O89.3** Toxic reaction to local anesthesia during the puerperium
- ♀ **O89.4** Spinal and epidural anesthesia-induced headache during the puerperium
- ♀ **O89.5** Other complications of spinal and epidural anesthesia during the puerperium
- ♀ **O89.6** Failed or difficult intubation for anesthesia during the puerperium
- ♀ **O89.8** Other complications of anesthesia during the puerperium
- ♀ **O89.9** Complication of anesthesia during the puerperium, unspecified

O90 Complications of the puerperium, not elsewhere classified

- ♀ **O90.0** Disruption of cesarean delivery wound
  - Dehiscence of cesarean delivery wound
  - **Excludes1:** rupture of uterus (spontaneous) before onset of labor (O71.0-)
    - rupture of uterus during labor (O71.1)
- ♀ **O90.1** Disruption of perineal obstetric wound
  - Disruption of wound of episiotomy
  - Disruption of wound of perineal laceration
  - Secondary perineal tear
- ♀ **O90.2** Hematoma of obstetric wound
- ♀ MCC **O90.3** Peripartum cardiomyopathy
  - Conditions in I42.- arising during pregnancy and the puerperium
  - **Excludes1:** pre-existing heart disease complicating pregnancy and the puerperium (O99.4-)
  - AHA CC: 3Q, 2022, 16-17
  - Review coding guideline C.15.o.5
- **+ O90.4** Postpartum acute kidney failure
  - **Excludes1:** non-anuria and oliguria (R34)
  - ♀ MCC **O90.41** Hepatorenal syndrome following labor and delivery
  - ♀ MCC **O90.49** Other postpartum acute kidney failure
    - Postpartum acute kidney failure
    - Puerperal anuria
    - Puerperal oliguria
- ♀ **O90.5** Postpartum thyroiditis
- ♀ **O90.6** Postpartum mood disturbance
  - Postpartum blues
  - Postpartum dysphoria
  - Postpartum sadness
  - **Excludes1:** postpartum depression (F53.0)
    - puerperal psychosis (F53.1)
- **+ O90.8** Other complications of the puerperium, not elsewhere classified
  - ♀ **O90.81** Anemia of the puerperium
    - Postpartum anemia NOS
    - **Excludes1:** pre-existing anemia complicating the puerperium (O99.03)
  - ♀ **O90.89** Other complications of the puerperium, not elsewhere classified
    - Placental polyp
- ♀ **O90.9** Complication of the puerperium, unspecified

O91 Infections of breast associated with pregnancy, the puerperium and lactation

Use additional code to identify infection

- **+ O91.0** Infection of nipple associated with pregnancy, the puerperium and lactation
  - **+ O91.01** Infection of nipple associated with pregnancy
    - Gestational abscess of nipple
    - ♀ **O91.011** Infection of nipple associated with pregnancy, first trimester
    - ♀ **O91.012** Infection of nipple associated with pregnancy, second trimester
    - ♀ **O91.013** Infection of nipple associated with pregnancy, third trimester
    - ♀ **O91.019** Infection of nipple associated with pregnancy, unspecified trimester
  - ♀ **O91.02** Infection of nipple associated with the puerperium
    - Puerperal abscess of nipple
  - ♀ **O91.03** Infection of nipple associated with lactation
    - Abscess of nipple associated with lactation
- **+ O91.1** Abscess of breast associated with pregnancy, the puerperium and lactation
  - **+ O91.11** Abscess of breast associated with pregnancy
    - Gestational mammary abscess
    - Gestational purulent mastitis
    - Gestational subareolar abscess
    - ♀ **O91.111** Abscess of breast associated with pregnancy, first trimester
    - ♀ **O91.112** Abscess of breast associated with pregnancy, second trimester
    - ♀ **O91.113** Abscess of breast associated with pregnancy, third trimester
    - ♀ **O91.119** Abscess of breast associated with pregnancy, unspecified trimester
  - ♀ **O91.12** Abscess of breast associated with the puerperium
    - Puerperal mammary abscess
    - Puerperal purulent mastitis
    - Puerperal subareolar abscess
  - ♀ **O91.13** Abscess of breast associated with lactation
    - Mammary abscess associated with lactation
    - Purulent mastitis associated with lactation
    - Subareolar abscess associated with lactation
- **+ O91.2** Nonpurulent mastitis associated with pregnancy, the puerperium and lactation
  - **+ O91.21** Nonpurulent mastitis associated with pregnancy
    - Gestational interstitial mastitis
    - Gestational lymphangitis of breast
    - Gestational mastitis NOS
    - Gestational parenchymatous mastitis

- ♀ **O91.211** Nonpurulent mastitis associated with pregnancy, first trimester
- ♀ **O91.212** Nonpurulent mastitis associated with pregnancy, second trimester
- ♀ **O91.213** Nonpurulent mastitis associated with pregnancy, third trimester
- ♀ **O91.219** Nonpurulent mastitis associated with pregnancy, unspecified trimester
- ♀ **O91.22** Nonpurulent mastitis associated with the puerperium
   - Puerperal interstitial mastitis
   - Puerperal lymphangitis of breast
   - Puerperal mastitis NOS
   - Puerperal parenchymatous mastitis
- ♀ **O91.23** Nonpurulent mastitis associated with lactation
   - Interstitial mastitis associated with lactation
   - Lymphangitis of breast associated with lactation
   - Mastitis NOS associated with lactation
   - Parenchymatous mastitis associated with lactation

O92 Other disorders of breast and disorders of lactation associated with pregnancy and the puerperium

- **O92.0** Retracted nipple associated with pregnancy, the puerperium, and lactation
   - **O92.01** Retracted nipple associated with pregnancy
     - ♀ **O92.011** Retracted nipple associated with pregnancy, first trimester
     - ♀ **O92.012** Retracted nipple associated with pregnancy, second trimester
     - ♀ **O92.013** Retracted nipple associated with pregnancy, third trimester
     - ♀ **O92.019** Retracted nipple associated with pregnancy, unspecified trimester
   - ♀ **O92.02** Retracted nipple associated with the puerperium
   - ♀ **O92.03** Retracted nipple associated with lactation
- **O92.1** Cracked nipple associated with pregnancy, the puerperium, and lactation
   - Fissure of nipple, gestational or puerperal
   - **O92.11** Cracked nipple associated with pregnancy
     - ♀ **O92.111** Cracked nipple associated with pregnancy, first trimester
     - ♀ **O92.112** Cracked nipple associated with pregnancy, second trimester
     - ♀ **O92.113** Cracked nipple associated with pregnancy, third trimester
     - ♀ **O92.119** Cracked nipple associated with pregnancy, unspecified trimester
   - ♀ **O92.12** Cracked nipple associated with the puerperium
   - ♀ **O92.13** Cracked nipple associated with lactation
- **O92.2** Other and unspecified disorders of breast associated with pregnancy and the puerperium
   - ♀ **O92.20** Unspecified disorder of breast associated with pregnancy and the puerperium
   - ♀ **O92.29** Other disorders of breast associated with pregnancy and the puerperium
- ♀ **O92.3** Agalactia
   - Primary agalactia
   - **Excludes1:** *Elective agalactia (O92.5)*
     Secondary agalactia (O92.5)
     Therapeutic agalactia (O92.5)
- ♀ **O92.4** Hypogalactia
- ♀ **O92.5** Suppressed lactation
   - Elective agalactia
   - Secondary agalactia
   - Therapeutic agalactia
   - **Excludes1:** *primary agalactia (O92.3)*
- ♀ **O92.6** Galactorrhea
- **O92.7** Other and unspecified disorders of lactation
   - ♀ **O92.70** Unspecified disorders of lactation
   - ♀ **O92.79** Other disorders of lactation
     - Puerperal galactocele

Other obstetric conditions, not elsewhere classified (O94-O9A)

- ♀ **O94** Sequelae of complication of pregnancy, childbirth, and the puerperium
   - **NOTE** This category is to be used to indicate conditions in O00-O77.-, O85-O94 and O98-O9A.- as the cause of late effects. The sequelae include conditions specified as such, or as late effects, which may occur at any time after the puerperium
   - Code first condition resulting from (sequela) of complication of pregnancy, childbirth, and the puerperium
   - AHA CC: 3Q, 2022, 17-18
   - Review coding guideline C.15.p
   - *Valid 3-character code, no further characters required*

O98 Maternal infectious and parasitic diseases classifiable elsewhere but complicating pregnancy, childbirth and the puerperium
   - **Includes:** the listed conditions when complicating the pregnant state, when aggravated by the pregnancy, or as a reason for obstetric care
   - Use additional code (Chapter 1), to identify specific infectious or parasitic disease
   - **Excludes2:** *herpes gestationis (O26.4-)*
     infectious carrier state (O99.82-, O99.83-)
     obstetrical tetanus (A34)
     puerperal infection (O86.-)
     puerperal sepsis (O85)
     when the reason for maternal care is that the disease is known or suspected to have affected the fetus (O35-O36)
- **O98.0** Tuberculosis complicating pregnancy, childbirth and the puerperium
   - Conditions in A15-A19
   - **O98.01** Tuberculosis complicating pregnancy
     - ♀ CC **O98.011** Tuberculosis complicating pregnancy, first trimester
     - ♀ CC **O98.012** Tuberculosis complicating pregnancy, second trimester
     - ♀ CC **O98.013** Tuberculosis complicating pregnancy, third trimester
     - ♀ **O98.019** Tuberculosis complicating pregnancy, unspecified trimester
   - ♀ CC **O98.02** Tuberculosis complicating childbirth
   - ♀ CC **O98.03** Tuberculosis complicating the puerperium
- **O98.1** Syphilis complicating pregnancy, childbirth and the puerperium
   - Conditions in A50-A53
   - **O98.11** Syphilis complicating pregnancy
     - ♀ CC **O98.111** Syphilis complicating pregnancy, first trimester
     - ♀ CC **O98.112** Syphilis complicating pregnancy, second trimester
     - ♀ CC **O98.113** Syphilis complicating pregnancy, third trimester
     - ♀ **O98.119** Syphilis complicating pregnancy, unspecified trimester
   - ♀ CC **O98.12** Syphilis complicating childbirth
   - ♀ CC **O98.13** Syphilis complicating the puerperium
- **O98.2** Gonorrhea complicating pregnancy, childbirth and the puerperium
   - Conditions in A54.-
   - **O98.21** Gonorrhea complicating pregnancy
     - ♀ CC **O98.211** Gonorrhea complicating pregnancy, first trimester
     - ♀ CC **O98.212** Gonorrhea complicating pregnancy, second trimester
     - ♀ CC **O98.213** Gonorrhea complicating pregnancy, third trimester
     - ♀ **O98.219** Gonorrhea complicating pregnancy, unspecified trimester
   - ♀ CC **O98.22** Gonorrhea complicating childbirth
   - ♀ CC **O98.23** Gonorrhea complicating the puerperium
- **O98.3** Other infections with a predominantly sexual mode of transmission complicating pregnancy, childbirth and the puerperium
   - Conditions in A55-A64
   - **O98.31** Other infections with a predominantly sexual mode of transmission complicating pregnancy
     - ♀ CC **O98.311** Other infections with a predominantly sexual mode of transmission complicating pregnancy, first trimester
     - ♀ CC **O98.312** Other infections with a predominantly sexual mode of transmission complicating pregnancy, second trimester
     - ♀ CC **O98.313** Other infections with a predominantly sexual mode of transmission complicating pregnancy, third trimester
     - ♀ **O98.319** Other infections with a predominantly sexual mode of transmission complicating pregnancy, unspecified trimester

- ♀ CC **O98.32** Other infections with a predominantly sexual mode of transmission complicating childbirth
  AHA CC: 1Q, 2020, 20
- ♀ CC **O98.33** Other infections with a predominantly sexual mode of transmission complicating the puerperium
+ **O98.4** Viral hepatitis complicating pregnancy, childbirth and the puerperium
  Conditions in B15-B19
  + **O98.41** Viral hepatitis complicating pregnancy
    - ♀ CC **O98.411** Viral hepatitis complicating pregnancy, first trimester
    - ♀ CC **O98.412** Viral hepatitis complicating pregnancy, second trimester
    - ♀ CC **O98.413** Viral hepatitis complicating pregnancy, third trimester
    - ♀ **O98.419** Viral hepatitis complicating pregnancy, unspecified trimester
  - ♀ CC **O98.42** Viral hepatitis complicating childbirth
  - ♀ CC **O98.43** Viral hepatitis complicating the puerperium
+ **O98.5** Other viral diseases complicating pregnancy, childbirth and the puerperium
  Conditions in A80-B09, B25-B34, R87.81-, R87.82-
  Excludes1: *human immunodeficiency virus [HIV] disease complicating pregnancy, childbirth and the puerperium (O98.7-)*
  Review coding guideline C.15.s
  + **O98.51** Other viral diseases complicating pregnancy
    - ♀ CC **O98.511** Other viral diseases complicating pregnancy, first trimester
    - ♀ CC **O98.512** Other viral diseases complicating pregnancy, second trimester
      AHA CC: 4Q, 2016, 4-7
    - ♀ CC **O98.513** Other viral diseases complicating pregnancy, third trimester
      AHA CC: 4Q, 2016, 4-7
    - ♀ **O98.519** Other viral diseases complicating pregnancy, unspecified trimester
  - ♀ CC **O98.52** Other viral diseases complicating childbirth
  - ♀ CC **O98.53** Other viral diseases complicating the puerperium
+ **O98.6** Protozoal diseases complicating pregnancy, childbirth and the puerperium
  Conditions in B50-B64
  + **O98.61** Protozoal diseases complicating pregnancy
    - ♀ CC **O98.611** Protozoal diseases complicating pregnancy, first trimester
    - ♀ CC **O98.612** Protozoal diseases complicating pregnancy, second trimester
    - ♀ CC **O98.613** Protozoal diseases complicating pregnancy, third trimester
    - ♀ **O98.619** Protozoal diseases complicating pregnancy, unspecified trimester
  - ♀ CC **O98.62** Protozoal diseases complicating childbirth
  - ♀ CC **O98.63** Protozoal diseases complicating the puerperium
+ **O98.7** Human immunodeficiency virus [HIV] disease complicating pregnancy, childbirth and the puerperium
  Use additional code to identify the type of HIV disease:
    Acquired immune deficiency syndrome (AIDS) (B20)
    Asymptomatic HIV status (Z21)
    HIV positive NOS (Z21)
    Symptomatic HIV disease (B20)
  Review coding guideline C.1.a.2.g
  Review coding guideline C.15.f
  + **O98.71** Human immunodeficiency virus [HIV] disease complicating pregnancy
    - ♀ CC **O98.711** Human immunodeficiency virus [HIV] disease complicating pregnancy, first trimester
    - ♀ CC **O98.712** Human immunodeficiency virus [HIV] disease complicating pregnancy, second trimester
    - ♀ CC **O98.713** Human immunodeficiency virus [HIV] disease complicating pregnancy, third trimester
    - ♀ **O98.719** Human immunodeficiency virus [HIV] disease complicating pregnancy, unspecified trimester
  - ♀ CC **O98.72** Human immunodeficiency virus [HIV] disease complicating childbirth
  - ♀ CC **O98.73** Human immunodeficiency virus [HIV] disease complicating the puerperium

+ **O98.8** Other maternal infectious and parasitic diseases complicating pregnancy, childbirth and the puerperium
  + **O98.81** Other maternal infectious and parasitic diseases complicating pregnancy
    - ♀ CC **O98.811** Other maternal infectious and parasitic diseases complicating pregnancy, first trimester
    - ♀ CC **O98.812** Other maternal infectious and parasitic diseases complicating pregnancy, second trimester
    - ♀ CC **O98.813** Other maternal infectious and parasitic diseases complicating pregnancy, third trimester
    - ♀ **O98.819** Other maternal infectious and parasitic diseases complicating pregnancy, unspecified trimester
  - ♀ CC **O98.82** Other maternal infectious and parasitic diseases complicating childbirth
    AHA CC: 1Q, 2020, 10
  - ♀ CC **O98.83** Other maternal infectious and parasitic diseases complicating the puerperium
    AHA CC: 2Q, 2022, 5
+ **O98.9** Unspecified maternal infectious and parasitic disease complicating pregnancy, childbirth and the puerperium
  + **O98.91** Unspecified maternal infectious and parasitic disease complicating pregnancy
    - ♀ CC **O98.911** Unspecified maternal infectious and parasitic disease complicating pregnancy, first trimester
    - ♀ CC **O98.912** Unspecified maternal infectious and parasitic disease complicating pregnancy, second trimester
    - ♀ CC **O98.913** Unspecified maternal infectious and parasitic disease complicating pregnancy, third trimester
    - ♀ **O98.919** Unspecified maternal infectious and parasitic disease complicating pregnancy, unspecified trimester
  - ♀ CC **O98.92** Unspecified maternal infectious and parasitic disease complicating childbirth
  - ♀ CC **O98.93** Unspecified maternal infectious and parasitic disease complicating the puerperium

O99 Other maternal diseases classifiable elsewhere but complicating pregnancy, childbirth and the puerperium
  Includes: conditions which complicate the pregnant state, are aggravated by the pregnancy or are a main reason for obstetric care
  Use additional code to identify specific condition
  Excludes2: *when the reason for maternal care is that the condition is known or suspected to have affected the fetus (O35-O36)*
+ **O99.0** Anemia complicating pregnancy, childbirth and the puerperium
  Conditions in D50-D64
  Excludes1: *anemia arising in the puerperium (O90.81)*
  postpartum anemia NOS (O90.81)
  + **O99.01** Anemia complicating pregnancy
    - ♀ **O99.011** Anemia complicating pregnancy, first trimester
    - ♀ **O99.012** Anemia complicating pregnancy, second trimester
    - ♀ **O99.013** Anemia complicating pregnancy, third trimester
    - ♀ **O99.019** Anemia complicating pregnancy, unspecified trimester
  - ♀ **O99.02** Anemia complicating childbirth
  - ♀ **O99.03** Anemia complicating the puerperium
    Excludes1: *postpartum anemia not pre-existing prior to delivery (O90.81)*
+ **O99.1** Other diseases of the blood and blood-forming organs and certain disorders involving the immune mechanism complicating pregnancy, childbirth and the puerperium
  Conditions in D65-D89
  Excludes1: *hemorrhage with coagulation defects (O45.-, O46.0-, O67.0, O72.3)*
  + **O99.11** Other diseases of the blood and blood-forming organs and certain disorders involving the immune mechanism complicating pregnancy

- ♀ CC **O99.111** Other diseases of the blood and blood-forming organs and certain disorders involving the immune mechanism complicating pregnancy, first trimester
- ♀ CC **O99.112** Other diseases of the blood and blood-forming organs and certain disorders involving the immune mechanism complicating pregnancy, second trimester
- ♀ CC **O99.113** Other diseases of the blood and blood-forming organs and certain disorders involving the immune mechanism complicating pregnancy, third trimester
- ♀ CC **O99.119** Other diseases of the blood and blood-forming organs and certain disorders involving the immune mechanism complicating pregnancy, unspecified trimester
- ♀ CC **O99.12** Other diseases of the blood and blood-forming organs and certain disorders involving the immune mechanism complicating childbirth
- ♀ CC **O99.13** Other diseases of the blood and blood-forming organs and certain disorders involving the immune mechanism complicating the puerperium

+ **O99.2** Endocrine, nutritional and metabolic diseases complicating pregnancy, childbirth and the puerperium
Conditions in E00-E89
Excludes2: *diabetes mellitus (O24.-)*
malnutrition (O25.-)
postpartum thyroiditis (O90.5)

+ **O99.21** Obesity complicating pregnancy, childbirth, and the puerperium
Use additional code to identify the type of obesity (E66.-)
- ♀ **O99.210** Obesity complicating pregnancy, unspecified trimester
- ♀ **O99.211** Obesity complicating pregnancy, first trimester
- ♀ **O99.212** Obesity complicating pregnancy, second trimester
- ♀ **O99.213** Obesity complicating pregnancy, third trimester
- ♀ **O99.214** Obesity complicating childbirth
AHA CC: 4Q, 2018, 80; 2Q, 2021, 10-11
- ♀ **O99.215** Obesity complicating the puerperium

+ **O99.28** Other endocrine, nutritional and metabolic diseases complicating pregnancy, childbirth and the puerperium
- ♀ **O99.280** Endocrine, nutritional and metabolic diseases complicating pregnancy, unspecified trimester
- ♀ **O99.281** Endocrine, nutritional and metabolic diseases complicating pregnancy, first trimester
- ♀ **O99.282** Endocrine, nutritional and metabolic diseases complicating pregnancy, second trimester
- ♀ **O99.283** Endocrine, nutritional and metabolic diseases complicating pregnancy, third trimester
- ♀ **O99.284** Endocrine, nutritional and metabolic diseases complicating childbirth
AHA CC: 1Q, 2021, 8-9
- ♀ **O99.285** Endocrine, nutritional and metabolic diseases complicating the puerperium

+ **O99.3** Mental disorders and diseases of the nervous system complicating pregnancy, childbirth and the puerperium

+ **O99.31** Alcohol use complicating pregnancy, childbirth, and the puerperium
Use additional code(s) from F10 to identify manifestations of the alcohol use
Review coding guideline C.15.I.1
- ♀ **O99.310** Alcohol use complicating pregnancy, unspecified trimester
- ♀ **O99.311** Alcohol use complicating pregnancy, first trimester
- ♀ **O99.312** Alcohol use complicating pregnancy, second trimester
- ♀ **O99.313** Alcohol use complicating pregnancy, third trimester
- ♀ **O99.314** Alcohol use complicating childbirth
- ♀ **O99.315** Alcohol use complicating the puerperium

+ **O99.32** Drug use complicating pregnancy, childbirth, and the puerperium
Use additional code(s) from F11-F16 and F18-F19 to identify manifestations of the drug use
AHA CC: 2Q, 2018, 10-11
Review coding guideline C.15.I.3
- ♀ **O99.320** Drug use complicating pregnancy, unspecified trimester
- ♀ CC **O99.321** Drug use complicating pregnancy, first trimester
- ♀ CC **O99.322** Drug use complicating pregnancy, second trimester
- ♀ CC **O99.323** Drug use complicating pregnancy, third trimester
- ♀ CC **O99.324** Drug use complicating childbirth
- ♀ CC **O99.325** Drug use complicating the puerperium

+ **O99.33** Tobacco use disorder complicating pregnancy, childbirth, and the puerperium
Smoking complicating pregnancy, childbirth, and the puerperium
Use additional code from category F17 to identify type of tobacco nicotine dependence
Review coding guideline C.15.I.2
- ♀ **O99.330** Smoking (tobacco) complicating pregnancy, unspecified trimester
- ♀ **O99.331** Smoking (tobacco) complicating pregnancy, first trimester
- ♀ **O99.332** Smoking (tobacco) complicating pregnancy, second trimester
- ♀ **O99.333** Smoking (tobacco) complicating pregnancy, third trimester
- ♀ **O99.334** Smoking (tobacco) complicating childbirth
- ♀ **O99.335** Smoking (tobacco) complicating the puerperium

+ **O99.34** Other mental disorders complicating pregnancy, childbirth, and the puerperium
Conditions in F01-F09, F20-F52 and F54-F99
Excludes2: *postpartum mood disturbance (O90.6)*
postnatal psychosis (F53.1)
puerperal psychosis (F53.1)
- ♀ **O99.340** Other mental disorders complicating pregnancy, unspecified trimester
- ♀ **O99.341** Other mental disorders complicating pregnancy, first trimester
- ♀ **O99.342** Other mental disorders complicating pregnancy, second trimester
- ♀ **O99.343** Other mental disorders complicating pregnancy, third trimester
- ♀ **O99.344** Other mental disorders complicating childbirth
- ♀ **O99.345** Other mental disorders complicating the puerperium
AHA CC: 4Q, 2018, 8-9

+ **O99.35** Diseases of the nervous system complicating pregnancy, childbirth, and the puerperium
Conditions in G00-G99
Excludes2: *pregnancy related peripheral neuritis (O26.8-)*
- ♀ **O99.350** Diseases of the nervous system complicating pregnancy, unspecified trimester
- ♀ **O99.351** Diseases of the nervous system complicating pregnancy, first trimester
- ♀ **O99.352** Diseases of the nervous system complicating pregnancy, second trimester
- ♀ **O99.353** Diseases of the nervous system complicating pregnancy, third trimester
- ♀ CC **O99.354** Diseases of the nervous system complicating childbirth
- ♀ CC **O99.355** Diseases of the nervous system complicating the puerperium

- **O99.4 Diseases of the circulatory system complicating pregnancy, childbirth and the puerperium**
  Conditions in I00-I99
  Excludes1: peripartum cardiomyopathy (O90.3)
  Excludes2: hypertensive disorders (O10-O16)
  obstetric embolism (O88.-)
  venous complications and cerebrovenous sinus thrombosis in labor, childbirth and the puerperium (O87.-)
  venous complications and cerebrovenous sinus thrombosis in pregnancy (O22.-)
  - **O99.41 Diseases of the circulatory system complicating pregnancy**
    AHA CC: 2Q, 2016, 8
    - ♀ CC **O99.411** Diseases of the circulatory system complicating pregnancy, first trimester
    - ♀ CC **O99.412** Diseases of the circulatory system complicating pregnancy, second trimester
    - ♀ CC **O99.413** Diseases of the circulatory system complicating pregnancy, third trimester
    - ♀ **O99.419** Diseases of the circulatory system complicating pregnancy, unspecified trimester
  - ♀ MCC **O99.42** Diseases of the circulatory system complicating childbirth
  - ♀ CC **O99.43** Diseases of the circulatory system complicating the puerperium
- **O99.5 Diseases of the respiratory system complicating pregnancy, childbirth and the puerperium**
  Conditions in J00-J99
  - **O99.51 Diseases of the respiratory system complicating pregnancy**
    - ♀ **O99.511** Diseases of the respiratory system complicating pregnancy, first trimester
    - ♀ **O99.512** Diseases of the respiratory system complicating pregnancy, second trimester
    - ♀ **O99.513** Diseases of the respiratory system complicating pregnancy, third trimester
    - ♀ **O99.519** Diseases of the respiratory system complicating pregnancy, unspecified trimester
  - ♀ **O99.52** Diseases of the respiratory system complicating childbirth
  - ♀ **O99.53** Diseases of the respiratory system complicating the puerperium
- **O99.6 Diseases of the digestive system complicating pregnancy, childbirth and the puerperium**
  Conditions in K00-K93
  Excludes2: liver and biliary tract disorders in pregnancy, childbirth and the puerperium (O26.6-)
  hemorrhoids in pregnancy (O22.4-)
  - **O99.61 Diseases of the digestive system complicating pregnancy**
    - ♀ **O99.611** Diseases of the digestive system complicating pregnancy, first trimester
    - ♀ **O99.612** Diseases of the digestive system complicating pregnancy, second trimester
    - ♀ **O99.613** Diseases of the digestive system complicating pregnancy, third trimester
    - ♀ **O99.619** Diseases of the digestive system complicating pregnancy, unspecified trimester
  - ♀ **O99.62** Diseases of the digestive system complicating childbirth
  - ♀ **O99.63** Diseases of the digestive system complicating the puerperium
- **O99.7 Diseases of the skin and subcutaneous tissue complicating pregnancy, childbirth and the puerperium**
  Conditions in L00-L99
  Excludes2: herpes gestationis (O26.4)
  pruritic urticarial papules and plaques of pregnancy (PUPPP) (O26.86)
  - **O99.71 Diseases of the skin and subcutaneous tissue complicating pregnancy**
    - ♀ **O99.711** Diseases of the skin and subcutaneous tissue complicating pregnancy, first trimester
    - ♀ **O99.712** Diseases of the skin and subcutaneous tissue complicating pregnancy, second trimester
    - ♀ **O99.713** Diseases of the skin and subcutaneous tissue complicating pregnancy, third trimester
    - ♀ **O99.719** Diseases of the skin and subcutaneous tissue complicating pregnancy, unspecified trimester
  - ♀ **O99.72** Diseases of the skin and subcutaneous tissue complicating childbirth
  - ♀ **O99.73** Diseases of the skin and subcutaneous tissue complicating the puerperium
- **O99.8 Other specified diseases and conditions complicating pregnancy, childbirth and the puerperium**
  Conditions in D00-D48, H00-H95, M00-N99, and Q00-Q99
  Use additional code to identify condition
  Excludes2: genitourinary infections in pregnancy (O23.-)
  infection of genitourinary tract following delivery (O86.1-O86.4)
  malignant neoplasm complicating pregnancy, childbirth and the puerperium (O9A.1-)
  maternal care for known or suspected abnormality of maternal pelvic organs (O34.-)
  postpartum acute kidney failure (O90.49)
  traumatic injuries in pregnancy (O9A.2-)
  - **O99.81 Abnormal glucose complicating pregnancy, childbirth and the puerperium**
    Excludes1: gestational diabetes (O24.4-)
    Review coding guideline C.15.i
    - ♀ **O99.810** Abnormal glucose complicating pregnancy
    - ♀ **O99.814** Abnormal glucose complicating childbirth
    - ♀ **O99.815** Abnormal glucose complicating the puerperium
  - **O99.82 Streptococcus B carrier state complicating pregnancy, childbirth and the puerperium**
    Excludes1: Carrier of streptococcus group B (GBS) in a nonpregnant woman (Z22.330)
    - ♀ **O99.820** Streptococcus B carrier state complicating pregnancy
    - ♀ **O99.824** Streptococcus B carrier state complicating childbirth
      AHA CC: 2Q, 2019, 9
    - ♀ **O99.825** Streptococcus B carrier state complicating the puerperium
  - **O99.83 Other infection carrier state complicating pregnancy, childbirth and the puerperium**
    Use additional code to identify the carrier state (Z22.-)
    - ♀ CC **O99.830** Other infection carrier state complicating pregnancy
    - ♀ CC **O99.834** Other infection carrier state complicating childbirth
    - ♀ CC **O99.835** Other infection carrier state complicating the puerperium
  - **O99.84 Bariatric surgery status complicating pregnancy, childbirth and the puerperium**
    Gastric banding status complicating pregnancy, childbirth and the puerperium
    Gastric bypass status for obesity complicating pregnancy, childbirth and the puerperium
    Obesity surgery status complicating pregnancy, childbirth and the puerperium
    - ♀ **O99.840** Bariatric surgery status complicating pregnancy, unspecified trimester
    - ♀ **O99.841** Bariatric surgery status complicating pregnancy, first trimester
    - ♀ **O99.842** Bariatric surgery status complicating pregnancy, second trimester
    - ♀ **O99.843** Bariatric surgery status complicating pregnancy, third trimester
    - ♀ **O99.844** Bariatric surgery status complicating childbirth
    - ♀ **O99.845** Bariatric surgery status complicating the puerperium

- **+ O99.89 Other specified diseases and conditions complicating pregnancy, childbirth and the puerperium**
  AHA CC: 4Q, 2020, 36-37
  - ● ♀ O99.891 Other specified diseases and conditions complicating pregnancy
  - ● ♀ O99.892 Other specified diseases and conditions complicating childbirth
  - ● ♀ O99.893 Other specified diseases and conditions complicating puerperium

O9A Maternal malignant neoplasms, traumatic injuries and abuse classifiable elsewhere but complicating pregnancy, childbirth and the puerperium

- **+ O9A.1 Malignant neoplasm complicating pregnancy, childbirth and the puerperium**
  Conditions in C00-C96
  Use additional code to identify neoplasm
  Excludes2: maternal care for benign tumor of corpus uteri (O34.1-)
  maternal care for benign tumor of cervix (O34.4-)
  Review coding guideline C.2.l.3
  - **+ O9A.11 Malignant neoplasm complicating pregnancy**
    - ● ♀ O9A.111 Malignant neoplasm complicating pregnancy, first trimester
    - ● ♀ O9A.112 Malignant neoplasm complicating pregnancy, second trimester
    - ● ♀ O9A.113 Malignant neoplasm complicating pregnancy, third trimester
    - ● ♀ O9A.119 Malignant neoplasm complicating pregnancy, unspecified trimester
  - ● ♀ O9A.12 Malignant neoplasm complicating childbirth
  - ● ♀ O9A.13 Malignant neoplasm complicating the puerperium
    AHA CC: 3Q, 2015, 19-20
- **+ O9A.2 Injury, poisoning and certain other consequences of external causes complicating pregnancy, childbirth and the puerperium**
  Conditions in S00-T88, except T74 and T76
  Use additional code(s) to identify the injury or poisoning
  Excludes2: physical, sexual and psychological abuse complicating pregnancy, childbirth and the puerperium (O9A.3-, O9A.4-, O9A.5-)
  Review coding guideline C.15.m
  - **+ O9A.21 Injury, poisoning and certain other consequences of external causes complicating pregnancy**
    - ● ♀ O9A.211 Injury, poisoning and certain other consequences of external causes complicating pregnancy, first trimester
    - ● ♀ O9A.212 Injury, poisoning and certain other consequences of external causes complicating pregnancy, second trimester
    - ● ♀ O9A.213 Injury, poisoning and certain other consequences of external causes complicating pregnancy, third trimester
    - ● ♀ O9A.219 Injury, poisoning and certain other consequences of external causes complicating pregnancy, unspecified trimester
  - ● ♀ O9A.22 Injury, poisoning and certain other consequences of external causes complicating childbirth
  - ● ♀ O9A.23 Injury, poisoning and certain other consequences of external causes complicating the puerperium
- **+ O9A.3 Physical abuse complicating pregnancy, childbirth and the puerperium**
  Conditions in T74.11 or T76.11
  Use additional code (if applicable):
  to identify any associated current injury due to physical abuse
  to identify the perpetrator of abuse (Y07.-)
  Excludes2: sexual abuse complicating pregnancy, childbirth and the puerperium (O9A.4)
  Review coding guideline C.15.r
  - **+ O9A.31 Physical abuse complicating pregnancy**
    - ● ♀ O9A.311 Physical abuse complicating pregnancy, first trimester
    - ● ♀ O9A.312 Physical abuse complicating pregnancy, second trimester
    - ● ♀ O9A.313 Physical abuse complicating pregnancy, third trimester
    - ● ♀ O9A.319 Physical abuse complicating pregnancy, unspecified trimester
  - ● ♀ O9A.32 Physical abuse complicating childbirth
  - ● ♀ O9A.33 Physical abuse complicating the puerperium
- **+ O9A.4 Sexual abuse complicating pregnancy, childbirth and the puerperium**
  Conditions in T74.21 or T76.21
  Use additional code (if applicable):
  to identify any associated current injury due to sexual abuse
  to identify the perpetrator of abuse (Y07.-)
  Review coding guideline C.15.r
  - **+ O9A.41 Sexual abuse complicating pregnancy**
    - ● ♀ O9A.411 Sexual abuse complicating pregnancy, first trimester
    - ● ♀ O9A.412 Sexual abuse complicating pregnancy, second trimester
    - ● ♀ O9A.413 Sexual abuse complicating pregnancy, third trimester
    - ● ♀ O9A.419 Sexual abuse complicating pregnancy, unspecified trimester
  - ● ♀ O9A.42 Sexual abuse complicating childbirth
  - ● ♀ O9A.43 Sexual abuse complicating the puerperium
- **+ O9A.5 Psychological abuse complicating pregnancy, childbirth and the puerperium**
  Conditions in T74.31 or T76.31
  Use additional code to identify the perpetrator of abuse (Y07.-)
  Review coding guideline C.15.r
  - **+ O9A.51 Psychological abuse complicating pregnancy**
    - ● ♀ O9A.511 Psychological abuse complicating pregnancy, first trimester
    - ● ♀ O9A.512 Psychological abuse complicating pregnancy, second trimester
    - ● ♀ O9A.513 Psychological abuse complicating pregnancy, third trimester
    - ● ♀ O9A.519 Psychological abuse complicating pregnancy, unspecified trimester
  - ● ♀ O9A.52 Psychological abuse complicating childbirth
  - ● ♀ O9A.53 Psychological abuse complicating the puerperium

Chapter 16: Certain Conditions Originating in the Perinatal Period (P00-P96)

NOTE Codes from this chapter are for use on newborn records only, never on maternal records

Includes: conditions that have their origin in the fetal or perinatal period (before birth through the first 28 days after birth) even if morbidity occurs later

Excludes2: congenital malformations, deformations and chromosomal abnormalities (Q00-Q99)
endocrine, nutritional and metabolic diseases (E00-E88)
injury, poisoning and certain other consequences of external causes (S00-T88)
neoplasms (C00-D49)
tetanus neonatorum (A33)

This chapter contains the following category blocks:
- P00-P04 Newborn affected by maternal factors and by complications of pregnancy, labor, and delivery
- P05-P08 Disorders of newborn related to length of gestation and fetal growth
- P09 Abnormal findings on neonatal screening
- P10-P15 Birth trauma
- P19-P29 Respiratory and cardiovascular disorders specific to the perinatal period
- P35-P39 Infections specific to the perinatal period
- P50-P61 Hemorrhagic and hematological disorders of newborn
- P70-P74 Transitory endocrine and metabolic disorders specific to newborn
- P76-P78 Digestive system disorders of newborn
- P80-P83 Conditions involving the integument and temperature regulation of newborn
- P84 Other problems with newborn
- P90-P96 Other disorders originating in the perinatal period

C. Chapter-Specific Coding Guidelines

In addition to general coding guidelines, there are guidelines for specific diagnoses and/or conditions in the classification. Unless otherwise indicated, these guidelines apply to all health care settings. Please refer to Section II for guidelines on the selection of principal diagnosis.

16. Chapter 16: Certain Conditions Originating in the Perinatal Period (P00-P96)

For coding and reporting purposes the perinatal period is defined as before birth through the 28th day following birth. The following guidelines are provided for reporting purposes

a. General Perinatal Rules

1) Use of Chapter 16 Codes

Codes in this chapter are <u>never</u> for use on the maternal record. Codes from Chapter 15, the obstetric chapter, are never permitted on the newborn record. Chapter 16 codes may be used throughout the life of the patient if the condition is still present.

2) Principal Diagnosis for Birth Record

When coding the birth episode in a newborn record, assign a code from category Z38, Liveborn infants according to place of birth and type of delivery, as the principal diagnosis. A code from category Z38 is assigned only once, to a newborn at the time of birth. If a newborn is transferred to another institution, a code from category Z38 should not be used at the receiving hospital.

A code from category Z38 is used only on the newborn record, not on the mother's record.

3) Use of Codes from other Chapters with Codes from Chapter 16

Codes from other chapters may be used with codes from chapter 16 if the codes from the other chapters provide more specific detail. Codes for signs and symptoms may be assigned when a definitive diagnosis has not been established. If the reason for the encounter is a perinatal condition, the code from chapter 16 should be sequenced first.

4) Use of Chapter 16 Codes after the Perinatal Period

Should a condition originate in the perinatal period, and continue throughout the life of the patient, the perinatal code should continue to be used regardless of the patient's age.

5) Birth process or community acquired conditions

If a newborn has a condition that may be either due to the birth process or community acquired and the documentation does not indicate which it is, the default is due to the birth process and the code from Chapter 16 should be used. If the condition is community-acquired, a code from Chapter 16 should not be assigned.

For COVID-19 infection in a newborn, see guideline I.C.16.h

6) Code all clinically significant conditions

All clinically significant conditions noted on routine newborn examination should be coded. A condition is clinically significant if it requires:
- clinical evaluation; or
- therapeutic treatment; or
- diagnostic procedures; or
- extended length of hospital stay; or
- increased nursing care and/or monitoring; or
- has implications for future health care needs

Note: The perinatal guidelines listed above are the same as the general coding guidelines for "additional diagnoses", except for the final point regarding implications for future health care needs. Codes should be assigned for conditions that have been specified by the provider as having implications for future health care needs.

b. Observation and Evaluation of Newborns for Suspected Conditions not Found

1) Use of Z05 codes

Assign a code from category Z05, Observation and evaluation of newborns and infants for suspected diseases and conditions ruled out, to identify those instances when a healthy newborn is evaluated for a suspected condition/disease that is determined after study not to be present. Do not use a code from category Z05 when the patient is documented to have signs or symptoms of a suspected problem; in such cases code the sign or symptom.

2) Z05 on Other than the Birth Record

A code from category Z05 may also be assigned as a principal or first-listed code for readmissions or encounters when the code from category Z38 code no longer applies. Codes from category Z05 are fur use only for healthy newborns and infants for which no condition after study is found to be present.

3) Z05 on a birth record

A code from category Z05 is to be used as a secondary code after the code from category Z38, Liveborn infants according to place of birth and type of delivery.

c. Coding Additional Perinatal Diagnoses

1) Assigning codes for conditions that require treatment

Assign codes for conditions that require treatment or further investigation, prolong the length of stay, or require resource utilization.

2) Codes for conditions specified as having implications for future health care needs

Assign codes for conditions that have been specified by the provider as having implications for future health care needs.

Note: This guideline should not be used for adult patients.

d. Prematurity and Fetal Growth Retardation

Providers utilize different criteria in determining prematurity. A code for prematurity should not be assigned unless it is documented. Assignment of codes in categories P05, Disorders of newborn related to slow fetal growth and fetal malnutrition, and P07, Disorders of newborn related to short gestation and low birth weight, not elsewhere classified, should be based on the recorded birth weight and estimated gestational age.

When both birth weight and gestational age are available, two codes from category P07 should be assigned, with the code for birth weight sequenced before the code for gestational age.

e. Low birth weight and immaturity status

Codes from category P07, Disorders of newborn related to short gestation and low birth weight, not elsewhere classified, are for use for a child or adult who was premature or had a low birth weight as a newborn and this is affecting the patient's current health status.

See Section I.C.21. Factors influencing health status and contact with health services, Status.

f. Bacterial Sepsis of Newborn

Category P36, Bacterial sepsis of newborn, includes congenital sepsis. If a perinate is documented as having sepsis without documentation of congenital or community acquired, the default is congenital and a code from category P36 should be assigned. If the P36 code includes the causal organism, an additional code from category B95, Streptococcus, Staphylococcus, and Enterococcus as the cause of diseases classified elsewhere, or B96, Other bacterial agents as the cause of diseases classified elsewhere, should not be assigned. If the P36 code does not include the causal organism, assign an additional code from category B96. If applicable, use additional codes to identify severe sepsis (R65.2-) and any associated acute organ dysfunction.

g. Stillbirth

Code P95, Stillbirth, is only for use in institutions that maintain separate records for stillbirths. No other code should be used with P95. Code P95 should not be used on the mother's record.

h. COVID-19 Infection in Newborn

For a newborn that tests positive for COVID-19, assign code U07.1, COVID-19, and the appropriate codes for associated manifestation(s) in neonates/newborns in the absence of documentation indicating a specific type of transmission. For a newborn that tests positive for COVID-19 and the provider documents the condition was contracted in utero or during the birth process, assign codes P35.8, Other congenital viral diseases, and U07.1, COVID-19. When coding the birth episode in a newborn record, the appropriate code from category Z38, Liveborn infants according to place of birth and type of delivery, should be assigned as the principal diagnosis.

Newborn affected by maternal factors and by complications of pregnancy, labor, and delivery (P00-P04)

NOTE These codes are for use when the listed maternal conditions are specified as the cause of confirmed morbidity or potential morbidity which have their origin in the perinatal period (before birth through the first 28 days after birth).

AHA CC: 4Q, 2016, 54-55

P00 Newborn affected by maternal conditions that may be unrelated to present pregnancy

Code first any current condition in newborn

Excludes2: encounter for observation for newborn for suspected diseases and conditions ruled out (Z05.-)
newborn affected by maternal complications of pregnancy (P01.-)
newborn affected by maternal endocrine and metabolic disorders (P70-P74)
newborn affected by noxious substances transmitted via placenta or breast milk (P04.-)

P00.0 Newborn affected by maternal hypertensive disorders
Newborn affected by maternal conditions classifiable to O10-O11, O13-O16

P00.1 Newborn affected by maternal renal and urinary tract diseases
Newborn affected by maternal conditions classifiable to N00-N39

P00.2 Newborn affected by maternal infectious and parasitic diseases
Newborn affected by maternal infectious disease classifiable to A00-B99, J09 and J10

Excludes1: maternal genital tract or other localized infections (P00.8)
Excludes2: infections specific to the perinatal period (P35-P39)
newborn affected by (positive) maternal group B streptococcus (GBS) colonization (P00.82)

AHA CC: 3Q, 2015, 20; 2Q, 2019, 10

P00.3 Newborn affected by other maternal circulatory and respiratory diseases
Newborn affected by maternal conditions classifiable to I00-I99, J00-J99, Q20-Q34 and not included in P00.0, P00.2

P00.4 Newborn affected by maternal nutritional disorders
Newborn affected by maternal disorders classifiable to E40-E64
Maternal malnutrition NOS

P00.5 Newborn affected by maternal injury
Newborn affected by maternal conditions classifiable to O9A.2-

P00.6 Newborn affected by surgical procedure on mother
Newborn affected by amniocentesis

Excludes1: Cesarean delivery for present delivery (P03.4)
damage to placenta from amniocentesis, Cesarean delivery or surgical induction (P02.1)
previous surgery to uterus or pelvic organs (P03.89)
Excludes2: newborn affected by complication of (fetal) intrauterine procedure (P96.5)

P00.7 Newborn affected by other medical procedures on mother, not elsewhere classified
Newborn affected by radiation to mother

Excludes1: damage to placenta from amniocentesis, cesarean delivery or surgical induction (P02.1)
newborn affected by other complications of labor and delivery (P03.-)

+ **P00.8 Newborn affected by other maternal conditions**
  P00.81 Newborn affected by periodontal disease in mother
  P00.82 Newborn affected by (positive) maternal group B streptococcus (GBS) colonization
  Contact with positive maternal group B streptococcus
  AHA CC: 4Q, 2021, 23

P00.89 Newborn affected by other maternal conditions
Newborn affected by conditions classifiable to T80-T88
Newborn affected by maternal genital tract or other localized infections
Newborn affected by maternal systemic lupus erythematosus

Use additional code to identify infectious agent, if known

Excludes2: newborn affected by positive maternal group B streptococcus (GBS) colonization (P00.82)

AHA CC: 2Q, 2019, 9

P00.9 Newborn affected by unspecified maternal condition

P01 Newborn affected by maternal complications of pregnancy

Code first any current condition in newborn

Excludes2: encounter for observation of newborn for suspected diseases and conditions ruled out (Z05.-)

P01.0 Newborn affected by incompetent cervix
P01.1 Newborn affected by premature rupture of membranes
P01.2 Newborn affected by oligohydramnios
Excludes1: oligohydramnios due to premature rupture of membranes (P01.1)

P01.3 Newborn affected by polyhydramnios
Newborn affected by hydramnios

P01.4 Newborn affected by ectopic pregnancy
Newborn affected by abdominal pregnancy

P01.5 Newborn affected by multiple pregnancy
Newborn affected by triplet (pregnancy)
Newborn affected by twin (pregnancy)

P01.6 Newborn affected by maternal death

P01.7 Newborn affected by malpresentation before labor
Newborn affected by breech presentation before labor
Newborn affected by external version before labor
Newborn affected by face presentation before labor
Newborn affected by transverse lie before labor
Newborn affected by unstable lie before labor

P01.8 Newborn affected by other maternal complications of pregnancy

P01.9 Newborn affected by maternal complication of pregnancy, unspecified

P02 Newborn affected by complications of placenta, cord and membranes

Code first any current condition in newborn

Excludes2: encounter for observation of newborn for suspected diseases and conditions ruled out (Z05.-)

P02.0 Newborn affected by placenta previa
P02.1 Newborn affected by other forms of placental separation and hemorrhage
Newborn affected by abruptio placenta
Newborn affected by accidental hemorrhage
Newborn affected by antepartum hemorrhage
Newborn affected by damage to placenta from amniocentesis, cesarean delivery or surgical induction
Newborn affected by maternal blood loss
Newborn affected by premature separation of placenta

+ **P02.2 Newborn affected by other and unspecified morphological and functional abnormalities of placenta**
  P02.20 Newborn affected by unspecified morphological and functional abnormalities of placenta
  P02.29 Newborn affected by other morphological and functional abnormalities of placenta
  Newborn affected by placental dysfunction
  Newborn affected by placental infarction
  Newborn affected by placental insufficiency

P02.3 Newborn affected by placental transfusion syndromes
Newborn affected by placental and cord abnormalities resulting in twin-to-twin or other transplacental transfusion

P02.4 Newborn affected by prolapsed cord
P02.5 Newborn affected by other compression of umbilical cord
Newborn affected by umbilical cord (tightly) around neck
Newborn affected by entanglement of umbilical cord
Newborn affected by knot in umbilical cord

+ **P02.6 Newborn affected by other and unspecified conditions of umbilical cord**
  P02.60 Newborn affected by unspecified conditions of umbilical cord

P02.69	**Newborn affected by other conditions of umbilical cord**	

Newborn affected by short umbilical cord
Newborn affected by vasa previa
Excludes1: newborn affected by single umbilical artery (Q27.0)

+ **P02.7 Newborn affected by chorioamnionitis**
AHA CC: 4Q, 2018, 23-24

- **P02.70 Newborn affected by fetal inflammatory response syndrome**
  Newborn affected by FIRS
- **P02.78 Newborn affected by other conditions from chorioamnionitis**
  Newborn affected by amnionitis
  Newborn affected by membranitis
  Newborn affected by placentitis

P02.8 Newborn affected by other abnormalities of membranes

P02.9 Newborn affected by abnormality of membranes, unspecified

P03 Newborn affected by other complications of labor and delivery

Code first any current condition in newborn
Excludes2: encounter for observation of newborn for suspected diseases and conditions ruled out (Z05.-)

P03.0 Newborn affected by breech delivery and extraction

P03.1 Newborn affected by other malpresentation, malposition and disproportion during labor and delivery
Newborn affected by contracted pelvis
Newborn affected by conditions classifiable to O64-O66
Newborn affected by persistent occipitoposterior
Newborn affected by transverse lie

P03.2 Newborn affected by forceps delivery

P03.3 Newborn affected by delivery by vacuum extractor [ventouse]

P03.4 Newborn affected by Cesarean delivery

P03.5 Newborn affected by precipitate delivery
Newborn affected by rapid second stage

P03.6 Newborn affected by abnormal uterine contractions
Newborn affected by conditions classifiable to O62.-, except O62.3
Newborn affected by hypertonic labor
Newborn affected by uterine inertia

+ **P03.8 Newborn affected by other specified complications of labor and delivery**

  + **P03.81 Newborn affected by abnormality in fetal (intrauterine) heart rate or rhythm**
    Excludes1: neonatal cardiac dysrhythmia (P29.1-)
    - **P03.810 Newborn affected by abnormality in fetal (intrauterine) heart rate or rhythm before the onset of labor**
    - **P03.811 Newborn affected by abnormality in fetal (intrauterine) heart rate or rhythm during labor**
    - **P03.819 Newborn affected by abnormality in fetal (intrauterine) heart rate or rhythm, unspecified as to time of onset**
  - **P03.82 Meconium passage during delivery**
    Excludes1: meconium aspiration (P24.00, P24.01)
    meconium staining (P96.83)
  - **P03.89 Newborn affected by other specified complications of labor and delivery**
    Newborn affected by abnormality of maternal soft tissues
    Newborn affected by conditions classifiable to O60-O75 and by procedures used in labor and delivery not included in P02.- and P03.0-P03.6
    Newborn affected by induction of labor

P03.9 Newborn affected by complication of labor and delivery, unspecified

P04 Newborn affected by noxious substances transmitted via placenta or breast milk

Includes: nonteratogenic effects of substances transmitted via placenta
Code first any current condition in newborn, if applicable
Excludes2: congenital malformations (Q00-Q99)
encounter for observation of newborn for suspected diseases and conditions ruled out (Z05.-)
neonatal jaundice from excessive hemolysis due to drugs or toxins transmitted from mother (P58.4)
newborn in contact with and (suspected) exposures hazardous to health not transmitted via placenta or breast milk (Z77.-)
AHA CC: 4Q, 2018, 24-25

P04.0 Newborn affected by maternal anesthesia and analgesia in pregnancy, labor and delivery
Newborn affected by reactions and intoxications from maternal opiates and tranquilizers administered for procedures during pregnancy or labor and delivery
Excludes2: newborn affected by other maternal medication (P04.1-)

+ **P04.1 Newborn affected by other maternal medication**
Code first, if applicable, withdrawal symptoms from maternal use of drugs of addiction (P96.1)
withdrawal symptoms from therapeutic use of drugs in newborn (P96.2)
Excludes1: dysmorphism due to warfarin (Q86.2)
fetal hydantoin syndrome (Q86.1)
Excludes2: maternal anesthesia and analgesia in pregnancy, labor and delivery (P04.0)
maternal use of drugs of addition (P04.4-)
AHA CC: 4Q, 2016, 54-55; 4Q, 2018, 24-25

- **P04.11 Newborn affected by maternal antineoplastic chemotherapy**
- **P04.12 Newborn affected by maternal cytotoxic drugs**
- **P04.13 Newborn affected by maternal use of anticonvulsants**
- **P04.14 Newborn affected by maternal use of opiates**
- **P04.15 Newborn affected by maternal use of antidepressants**
- **P04.16 Newborn affected by maternal use of amphetamines**
- **P04.17 Newborn affected by maternal use of sedative-hypnotics**
- **P04.1A Newborn affected by maternal use of anxiolytics**
- **P04.18 Newborn affected by other maternal medication**
- **P04.19 Newborn affected by maternal use of unspecified medication**

P04.2 Newborn affected by maternal use of tobacco
Newborn affected by exposure in utero to tobacco smoke
Excludes2: newborn exposure to environmental tobacco smoke (P96.81)

P04.3 Newborn affected by maternal use of alcohol
Excludes1: fetal alcohol syndrome (Q86.0)

+ **P04.4 Newborn affected by maternal use of drugs of addiction**
AHA CC: 4Q, 2018, 25

- **P04.40 Newborn affected by maternal use of unspecified drugs of addiction**
- **P04.41 Newborn affected by maternal use of cocaine**
- **P04.42 Newborn affected by maternal use of hallucinogens**
  Excludes2: newborn affected by other maternal medication (P04.1-)
- **P04.49 Newborn affected by maternal use of other drugs of addiction**
  Excludes2: newborn affected by maternal anesthesia and analgesia (P04.0)
  withdrawal symptoms from maternal use
  of drugs of addiction (P96.1)

P04.5 Newborn affected by maternal use of nutritional chemical substances

P04.6 Newborn affected by maternal exposure to environmental chemical substances

+ **P04.8 Newborn affected by other maternal noxious substances**
AHA CC: 4Q, 2018, 25

- **P04.81 Newborn affected by maternal use of cannabis**
- **P04.89 Newborn affected by other maternal noxious substances**

P04.9 Newborn affected by maternal noxious substance, unspecified

Disorders of newborn related to length of gestation and fetal growth (P05-P08)

P05 Disorders of newborn related to slow fetal growth and fetal malnutrition

Review coding guideline C.16.d

+ **P05.0 Newborn light for gestational age**
Newborn light-for-dates
Weight below but length above 10th percentile for gestational age
- P05.00 Newborn light for gestational age, unspecified weight
- P05.01 Newborn light for gestational age, less than 500 grams
- P05.02 Newborn light for gestational age, 500-749 grams
- P05.03 Newborn light for gestational age, 750-999 grams
- P05.04 Newborn light for gestational age, 1000-1249 grams
- P05.05 Newborn light for gestational age, 1250-1499 grams
- P05.06 Newborn light for gestational age, 1500-1749 grams
- P05.07 Newborn light for gestational age, 1750-1999 grams
- P05.08 Newborn light for gestational age, 2000-2499 grams
- P05.09 Newborn light for gestational age, 2500 grams and over
    Newborn light for gestational age, other
    AHA CC: 4Q, 2016, 55-56

+ **P05.1 Newborn small for gestational age**
Newborn small-and-light-for-dates
Newborn small-for-dates
Weight and length below 10th percentile for gestational age
- P05.10 Newborn small for gestational age, unspecified weight
- P05.11 Newborn small for gestational age, less than 500 grams
- P05.12 Newborn small for gestational age, 500-749 grams
- P05.13 Newborn small for gestational age, 750-999 grams
- P05.14 Newborn small for gestational age, 1000-1249 grams
- P05.15 Newborn small for gestational age, 1250-1499 grams
- P05.16 Newborn small for gestational age, 1500-1749 grams
- P05.17 Newborn small for gestational age, 1750-1999 grams
- P05.18 Newborn small for gestational age, 2000-2499 grams
- P05.19 Newborn small for gestational age, other
    Newborn small for gestational age, 2500 grams and over
    AHA CC: 4Q, 2016, 55-56

P05.2 Newborn affected by fetal (intrauterine) malnutrition not light or small for gestational age
Infant, not light or small for gestational age, showing signs of fetal malnutrition, such as dry, peeling skin and loss of subcutaneous tissue
Excludes1: newborn affected by fetal malnutrition with light for gestational age (P05.0-)
newborn affected by fetal malnutrition with small for gestational age (P05.1-)

P05.9 Newborn affected by slow intrauterine growth, unspecified
Newborn affected by fetal growth retardation NOS

P07 Disorders of newborn related to short gestation and low birth weight, not elsewhere classified

NOTE When both birth weight and gestational age of the newborn are available, both should be coded with birth weight sequenced before gestational age

Includes: the listed conditions, without further specification, as the cause of morbidity or additional care, in newborn

Review coding guidelines C.16.d and C.16.e

+ **P07.0 Extremely low birth weight newborn**
Newborn birth weight 999 g. or less
Excludes1: low birth weight due to slow fetal growth and fetal malnutrition (P05.-)
- P07.00 Extremely low birth weight newborn, unspecified weight
- P07.01 Extremely low birth weight newborn, less than 500 grams
- P07.02 Extremely low birth weight newborn, 500-749 grams
- P07.03 Extremely low birth weight newborn, 750-999 grams

+ **P07.1 Other low birth weight newborn**
Newborn birth weight 1000-2499 g.
Excludes1: low birth weight due to slow fetal growth and fetal malnutrition (P05.-)
- P07.10 Other low birth weight newborn, unspecified weight
- P07.14 Other low birth weight newborn, 1000-1249 grams
- P07.15 Other low birth weight newborn, 1250-1499 grams
- P07.16 Other low birth weight newborn, 1500-1749 grams
- P07.17 Other low birth weight newborn, 1750-1999 grams
- P07.18 Other low birth weight newborn, 2000-2499 grams

+ **P07.2 Extreme immaturity of newborn**
Less than 28 completed weeks (less than 196 completed days) of gestation.
- P07.20 Extreme immaturity of newborn, unspecified weeks of gestation
    Gestational age less than 28 completed weeks NOS
- P07.21 Extreme immaturity of newborn, gestational age less than 23 completed weeks
    Extreme immaturity of newborn, gestational age less than 23 weeks, 0 days
- P07.22 Extreme immaturity of newborn, gestational age 23 completed weeks
    Extreme immaturity of newborn, gestational age 23 weeks, 0 days through 23 weeks, 6 days
- P07.23 Extreme immaturity of newborn, gestational age 24 completed weeks
    Extreme immaturity of newborn, gestational age 24 weeks, 0 days through 24 weeks, 6 days
- P07.24 Extreme immaturity of newborn, gestational age 25 completed weeks
    Extreme immaturity of newborn, gestational age 25 weeks, 0 days through 25 weeks, 6 days
- P07.25 Extreme immaturity of newborn, gestational age 26 completed weeks
    Extreme immaturity of newborn, gestational age 26 weeks, 0 days through 26 weeks, 6 days
- P07.26 Extreme immaturity of newborn, gestational age 27 completed weeks
    Extreme immaturity of newborn, gestational age 27 weeks, 0 days through 27 weeks, 6 days

+ **P07.3 Preterm [premature] newborn [other]**
28 completed weeks or more but less than 37 completed weeks (196 completed days but less than 259 completed days) of gestation.
Prematurity NOS
- P07.30 Preterm newborn, unspecified weeks of gestation
- P07.31 Preterm newborn, gestational age 28 completed weeks
    Preterm newborn, gestational age 28 weeks, 0 days through 28 weeks, 6 days
- P07.32 Preterm newborn, gestational age 29 completed weeks
    Preterm newborn, gestational age 29 weeks, 0 days through 29 weeks, 6 days
- P07.33 Preterm newborn, gestational age 30 completed weeks
    Preterm newborn, gestational age 30 weeks, 0 days through 30 weeks, 6 days
- P07.34 Preterm newborn, gestational age 31 completed weeks
    Preterm newborn, gestational age 31 weeks, 0 days through 31 weeks, 6 days
- P07.35 Preterm newborn, gestational age 32 completed weeks
    Preterm newborn, gestational age 32 weeks, 0 days through 32 weeks, 6 days
- P07.36 Preterm newborn, gestational age 33 completed weeks
    Preterm newborn, gestational age 33 weeks, 0 days through 33 weeks, 6 days
- P07.37 Preterm newborn, gestational age 34 completed weeks
    Preterm newborn, gestational age 34 weeks, 0 days through 34 weeks, 6 days
    AHA CC: 2Q, 2017, 7

P07.38 Preterm newborn, gestational age 35 completed weeks
Preterm newborn, gestational age 35 weeks, 0 days through 35 weeks, 6 days
P07.39 Preterm newborn, gestational age 36 completed weeks
Preterm newborn, gestational age 36 weeks, 0 days through 36 weeks, 6 days
AHA CC: 3Q, 2017, 26

P08 Disorders of newborn related to long gestation and high birth weight

NOTE When both birth weight and gestational age of the newborn are available, priority of assignment should be given to birth weight

Includes: the listed conditions, without further specification, as causes of morbidity or additional care, in newborn

P08.0 Exceptionally large newborn baby
Usually implies a birth weight of 4500 g. or more
Excludes1: syndrome of infant of diabetic mother (P70.1)
syndrome of infant of mother with gestational diabetes (P70.0)

P08.1 Other heavy for gestational age newborn
Other newborn heavy- or large-for-dates regardless of period of gestation
Usually implies a birth weight of 4000 g. to 4499 g.
Excludes1: newborn with a birth weight of 4500 or more (P08.0)
syndrome of infant of diabetic mother (P70.1)
syndrome of infant of mother with gestational diabetes (P70.0)

+ P08.2 Late newborn, not heavy for gestational age
P08.21 Post-term newborn
Newborn with gestation period over 40 completed weeks to 42 completed weeks
AHA CC: 1Q, 2014, 14
P08.22 Prolonged gestation of newborn
Newborn with gestation period over 42 completed weeks (294 days or more), not heavy- or large-for-dates.
Postmaturity NOS
AHA CC: 1Q, 2014, 14

Abnormal findings on neonatal screening (P09)

P09 Abnormal findings on neonatal screening

Includes: Abnormal findings on state mandated newborn screens
Failed newborn screening
Excludes2: nonspecific serologic evidence of human immunodeficiency virus [HIV] (R75)
AHA CC: 4Q, 2021, 24

P09.1 Abnormal findings on neonatal screening for inborn errors of metabolism
P09.2 Abnormal findings on neonatal screening for congenital endocrine disease
Abnormal findings on neonatal screening for congenital adrenal hyperplasia
Abnormal findings on neonatal screening for hypothyroidism screen
P09.3 Abnormal findings on neonatal screening for congenital hematologic disorders
Abnormal findings for hemoglobinopathy screening
Abnormal findings on red cell membrane defects screen
Abnormal findings on sickle cell screen
P09.4 Abnormal findings on neonatal screening for cystic fibrosis
P09.5 Abnormal findings on neonatal screening for critical congenital heart disease
Neonatal congenital heart disease screening failure
P09.6 Abnormal findings on neonatal screening for neonatal hearing loss
Excludes2: encounter for hearing examination following failed hearing screening (Z01.110)
P09.8 Other abnormal findings on neonatal screening
P09.9 Abnormal findings on neonatal screening, unspecified

Birth trauma (P10-P15)

P10 Intracranial laceration and hemorrhage due to birth injury

Excludes1: intracranial hemorrhage of newborn NOS (P52.9)
intracranial hemorrhage of newborn due to anoxia or hypoxia (P52.-)
nontraumatic intracranial hemorrhage of newborn (P52.-)

MCC P10.0 Subdural hemorrhage due to birth injury
Subdural hematoma (localized) due to birth injury
Excludes1: subdural hemorrhage accompanying tentorial tear (P10.4)
MCC P10.1 Cerebral hemorrhage due to birth injury
CC P10.2 Intraventricular hemorrhage due to birth injury
MCC P10.3 Subarachnoid hemorrhage due to birth injury
MCC P10.4 Tentorial tear due to birth injury
MCC P10.8 Other intracranial lacerations and hemorrhages due to birth injury
MCC P10.9 Unspecified intracranial laceration and hemorrhage due to birth injury

P11 Other birth injuries to central nervous system

MCC P11.0 Cerebral edema due to birth injury
P11.1 Other specified brain damage due to birth injury
MCC P11.2 Unspecified brain damage due to birth injury
P11.3 Birth injury to facial nerve
Facial palsy due to birth injury
P11.4 Birth injury to other cranial nerves
P11.5 Birth injury to spine and spinal cord
Fracture of spine due to birth injury
MCC P11.9 Birth injury to central nervous system, unspecified

P12 Birth injury to scalp

P12.0 Cephalhematoma due to birth injury
P12.1 Chignon (from vacuum extraction) due to birth injury
CC P12.2 Epicranial subaponeurotic hemorrhage due to birth injury
Subgaleal hemorrhage
P12.3 Bruising of scalp due to birth injury
P12.4 Injury of scalp of newborn due to monitoring equipment
Sampling incision of scalp of newborn
Scalp clip (electrode) injury of newborn
+ P12.8 Other birth injuries to scalp
P12.81 Caput succedaneum
P12.89 Other birth injuries to scalp
P12.9 Birth injury to scalp, unspecified

P13 Birth injury to skeleton

Excludes2: birth injury to spine (P11.5)
P13.0 Fracture of skull due to birth injury
P13.1 Other birth injuries to skull
Excludes1: cephalhematoma (P12.0)
P13.2 Birth injury to femur
P13.3 Birth injury to other long bones
P13.4 Fracture of clavicle due to birth injury
P13.8 Birth injuries to other parts of skeleton
P13.9 Birth injury to skeleton, unspecified

P14 Birth injury to peripheral nervous system

P14.0 Erb's paralysis due to birth injury
P14.1 Klumpke's paralysis due to birth injury
P14.2 Phrenic nerve paralysis due to birth injury
P14.3 Other brachial plexus birth injuries
P14.8 Birth injuries to other parts of peripheral nervous system
P14.9 Birth injury to peripheral nervous system, unspecified

P15 Other birth injuries

P15.0 Birth injury to liver
Rupture of liver due to birth injury
P15.1 Birth injury to spleen
Rupture of spleen due to birth injury
P15.2 Sternomastoid injury due to birth injury
P15.3 Birth injury to eye
Subconjunctival hemorrhage due to birth injury
Traumatic glaucoma due to birth injury
P15.4 Birth injury to face
Facial congestion due to birth injury
P15.5 Birth injury to external genitalia
P15.6 Subcutaneous fat necrosis due to birth injury
P15.8 Other specified birth injuries
P15.9 Birth injury, unspecified

Respiratory and cardiovascular disorders specific to the perinatal period (P19-P29)

P19 Metabolic acidemia in newborn
  Includes: metabolic acidemia in newborn
  P19.0 Metabolic acidemia in newborn first noted before onset of labor
  P19.1 Metabolic acidemia in newborn first noted during labor
  P19.2 Metabolic acidemia noted at birth
  P19.9 Metabolic acidemia in newborn, unspecified

P22 Respiratory distress of newborn
  MCC P22.0 Respiratory distress syndrome of newborn
      Cardiorespiratory distress syndrome of newborn
      Hyaline membrane disease
      Idiopathic respiratory distress syndrome [IRDS or RDS] of newborn
      Pulmonary hypoperfusion syndrome
      Respiratory distress syndrome, type I
      Excludes2: respiratory arrest of newborn (P28.81)
          respiratory failure of newborn NOS (P28.5)
      AHA CC: 2Q, 2019, 29
  P22.1 Transient tachypnea of newborn
      Idiopathic tachypnea of newborn
      Respiratory distress syndrome, type II
      Wet lung syndrome
  P22.8 Other respiratory distress of newborn
      Excludes1: respiratory arrest of newborn (P28.81)
          respiratory failure of newborn NOS (P28.5)
  P22.9 Respiratory distress of newborn, unspecified
      Excludes1: respiratory arrest of newborn (P28.81)
          respiratory failure of newborn NOS (P28.5)

P23 Congenital pneumonia
  Includes: infective pneumonia acquired in utero or during birth
  Excludes1: neonatal pneumonia resulting from aspiration (P24.-)
  MCC P23.0 Congenital pneumonia due to viral agent
      Use additional code (B97) to identify organism
      Excludes1: congenital rubella pneumonitis (P35.0)
  MCC P23.1 Congenital pneumonia due to Chlamydia
  MCC P23.2 Congenital pneumonia due to staphylococcus
  MCC P23.3 Congenital pneumonia due to streptococcus, group B
  MCC P23.4 Congenital pneumonia due to Escherichia coli
  P23.5 Congenital pneumonia due to Pseudomonas
  MCC P23.6 Congenital pneumonia due to other bacterial agents
      Congenital pneumonia due to Hemophilus influenzae
      Congenital pneumonia due to Klebsiella pneumoniae
      Congenital pneumonia due to Mycoplasma
      Congenital pneumonia due to Streptococcus, except group B
      Use additional code (B95-B96) to identify organism
  MCC P23.8 Congenital pneumonia due to other organisms
  MCC P23.9 Congenital pneumonia, unspecified

P24 Neonatal aspiration
  Includes: aspiration in utero and during delivery
  + P24.0 Meconium aspiration
      Excludes1: meconium passage (without aspiration) during delivery (P03.82)
          meconium staining (P96.83)
      P24.00 Meconium aspiration without respiratory symptoms
          Meconium aspiration NOS
      MCC P24.01 Meconium aspiration with respiratory symptoms
          Meconium aspiration pneumonia
          Meconium aspiration pneumonitis
          Meconium aspiration syndrome NOS
          Use additional code to identify any secondary pulmonary hypertension, if applicable (I27.2-)
  + P24.1 Neonatal aspiration of (clear) amniotic fluid and mucus
      Neonatal aspiration of liquor (amnii)
      P24.10 Neonatal aspiration of (clear) amniotic fluid and mucus without respiratory symptoms
          Neonatal aspiration of amniotic fluid and mucus NOS
      MCC P24.11 Neonatal aspiration of (clear) amniotic fluid and mucus with respiratory symptoms
          Neonatal aspiration of amniotic fluid and mucus with pneumonia
          Neonatal aspiration of amniotic fluid and mucus with pneumonitis
          Use additional code to identify any secondary pulmonary hypertension, if applicable (I27.2-)
  + P24.2 Neonatal aspiration of blood
      P24.20 Neonatal aspiration of blood without respiratory symptoms
          Neonatal aspiration of blood NOS
      MCC P24.21 Neonatal aspiration of blood with respiratory symptoms
          Neonatal aspiration of blood with pneumonia
          Neonatal aspiration of blood with pneumonitis
          Use additional code to identify any secondary pulmonary hypertension, if applicable (I27.2-)
  + P24.3 Neonatal aspiration of milk and regurgitated food
      Neonatal aspiration of stomach contents
      P24.30 Neonatal aspiration of milk and regurgitated food without respiratory symptoms
          Neonatal aspiration of milk and regurgitated food NOS
      MCC P24.31 Neonatal aspiration of milk and regurgitated food with respiratory symptoms
          Neonatal aspiration of milk and regurgitated food with pneumonia
          Neonatal aspiration of milk and regurgitated food with pneumonitis
          Use additional code to identify any secondary pulmonary hypertension, if applicable (I27.2-)
  + P24.8 Other neonatal aspiration
      P24.80 Other neonatal aspiration without respiratory symptoms
          Neonatal aspiration NEC
      MCC P24.81 Other neonatal aspiration with respiratory symptoms
          Neonatal aspiration pneumonia NEC
          Neonatal aspiration with pneumonitis NEC
          Neonatal aspiration with pneumonia NOS
          Neonatal aspiration with pneumonitis NOS
          Use additional code to identify any secondary pulmonary hypertension, if applicable (I27.2-)
  P24.9 Neonatal aspiration, unspecified

P25 Interstitial emphysema and related conditions originating in the perinatal period
  MCC P25.0 Interstitial emphysema originating in the perinatal period
  MCC P25.1 Pneumothorax originating in the perinatal period
  MCC P25.2 Pneumomediastinum originating in the perinatal period
  MCC P25.3 Pneumopericardium originating in the perinatal period
  MCC P25.8 Other conditions related to interstitial emphysema originating in the perinatal period

P26 Pulmonary hemorrhage originating in the perinatal period
  Excludes1: acute idiopathic hemorrhage in infants over 28 days old (R04.81)
  MCC P26.0 Tracheobronchial hemorrhage originating in the perinatal period
  MCC P26.1 Massive pulmonary hemorrhage originating in the perinatal period
  MCC P26.8 Other pulmonary hemorrhages originating in the perinatal period
  MCC P26.9 Unspecified pulmonary hemorrhage originating in the perinatal period

P27 Chronic respiratory disease originating in the perinatal period
  Excludes2: respiratory distress of newborn (P22.0-P22.9)
  MCC P27.0 Wilson-Mikity syndrome
      Pulmonary dysmaturity
  MCC P27.1 Bronchopulmonary dysplasia originating in the perinatal period
  MCC P27.8 Other chronic respiratory diseases originating in the perinatal period
      Congenital pulmonary fibrosis
      Ventilator lung in newborn
  MCC P27.9 Unspecified chronic respiratory disease originating in the perinatal period

P28 Other respiratory conditions originating in the perinatal period
  Code also, if applicable, congenital malformations of the respiratory system (Q30-Q34)
  CC P28.0 Primary atelectasis of newborn
      Primary failure to expand terminal respiratory units
      Pulmonary hypoplasia associated with short gestation
      Pulmonary immaturity NOS
  + P28.1 Other and unspecified atelectasis of newborn
      CC P28.10 Unspecified atelectasis of newborn
          Atelectasis of newborn NOS

CC **P28.11** Resorption atelectasis without respiratory distress syndrome
  Excludes1: resorption atelectasis with respiratory distress syndrome (P22.0)
CC **P28.19** Other atelectasis of newborn
  Partial atelectasis of newborn
  Secondary atelectasis of newborn
CC **P28.2** Cyanotic attacks of newborn
  Excludes1: apnea of newborn (P28.3- -P28.4-)
+ **P28.3** Primary sleep apnea of newborn
  Sleep apnea of newborn NOS
  Excludes2: other apnea of newborn (P28.4-)
  AHA CC: 4Q, 2022, 38-39
CC **P28.30** Primary sleep apnea of newborn, unspecified
  Transient oxygen desaturation spells of newborn during sleep
CC **P28.31** Primary central sleep apnea of newborn
CC **P28.32** Primary obstructive sleep apnea of newborn
CC **P28.33** Primary mixed sleep apnea of newborn
CC **P28.39** Other primary sleep apnea of newborn
+ **P28.4** Other apnea of newborn
  Excludes2: primary sleep apnea of newborn (P28.3-)
CC **P28.40** Unspecified apnea of newborn
  Apnea of newborn, NOS
  Transient oxygen desaturation spells of newborn
CC **P28.41** Central neonatal apnea of newborn
CC **P28.42** Obstructive apnea of newborn
CC **P28.43** Mixed neonatal apnea of newborn
CC **P28.49** Other apnea of newborn
  Apnea of prematurity
MCC **P28.5** Respiratory failure of newborn
  Excludes2: respiratory arrest of newborn (P28.81)
    respiratory distress of newborn (P22.0-)
  AHA CC: 2Q, 2019, 29
+ **P28.8** Other specified respiratory conditions of newborn
  MCC **P28.81** Respiratory arrest of newborn
    AHA CC: 2Q, 2017, 6-7
  P28.89 Other specified respiratory conditions of newborn
    Congenital laryngeal stridor
    Sniffles in newborn
    Snuffles in newborn
    Excludes1: early congenital syphilitic rhinitis (A50.05)
P28.9 Respiratory condition of newborn, unspecified
  Respiratory depression in newborn

P29 Cardiovascular disorders originating in the perinatal period
  Excludes2: congenital malformations of the circulatory system (Q20-Q28)
P29.0 Neonatal cardiac failure
  Code also associated underlying condition
+ **P29.1** Neonatal cardiac dysrhythmia
  P29.11 Neonatal tachycardia
  P29.12 Neonatal bradycardia
P29.2 Neonatal hypertension
+ **P29.3** Persistent fetal circulation
  AHA CC: 4Q, 2017, 20-21
  MCC **P29.30** Pulmonary hypertension of newborn
    Persistent pulmonary hypertension of newborn
  MCC **P29.38** Other persistent fetal circulation
    Delayed closure of ductus arteriosus
P29.4 Transient myocardial ischemia in newborn
+ **P29.8** Other cardiovascular disorders originating in the perinatal period
  MCC **P29.81** Cardiac arrest of newborn
  P29.89 Other cardiovascular disorders originating in the perinatal period
    AHA CC: 4Q, 2014, 23
P29.9 Cardiovascular disorder originating in the perinatal period, unspecified

Infections specific to the perinatal period (P35-P39)

Infections acquired in utero, during birth via the umbilicus, or during the first 28 days after birth

Excludes2: asymptomatic human immunodeficiency virus [HIV] infection status (Z21)
  congenital gonococcal infection (A54.-)
  congenital pneumonia (P23.-)
  congenital syphilis (A50.-)
  human immunodeficiency virus [HIV] disease (B20)
  infant botulism (A48.51)
  infectious diseases not specific to the perinatal period (A00-B99, J09, J10.-)
  intestinal infectious disease (A00-A09)
  laboratory evidence of human immunodeficiency virus [HIV] (R75)
  tetanus neonatorum (A33)

P35 Congenital viral diseases
  Includes: infections acquired in utero or during birth
  CC **P35.0** Congenital rubella syndrome
    Congenital rubella pneumonitis
  MCC **P35.1** Congenital cytomegalovirus infection
  MCC **P35.2** Congenital herpesviral [herpes simplex] infection
  MCC **P35.3** Congenital viral hepatitis
  MCC **P35.4** Congenital Zika virus disease
    Use additional code to identify manifestations of congenital Zika virus disease
    AHA CC: 4Q, 2018, 25-26
  MCC **P35.8** Other congenital viral diseases
    Congenital varicella [chickenpox]
    AHA CC: 4Q, 2016, 4-7; 2Q, 2020, 13
    Review coding guideline C.16.h
  MCC **P35.9** Congenital viral disease, unspecified

P36 Bacterial sepsis of newborn
  Includes: congenital sepsis
  Use additional code(s), if applicable, to identify severe sepsis (R65.2-) and associated acute organ dysfunction(s)
  Review coding guideline C.1.d and C.16.f
  MCC **P36.0** Sepsis of newborn due to streptococcus, group B
  + **P36.1** Sepsis of newborn due to other and unspecified streptococci
    MCC **P36.10** Sepsis of newborn due to unspecified streptococci
    MCC **P36.19** Sepsis of newborn due to other streptococci
  MCC **P36.2** Sepsis of newborn due to Staphylococcus aureus
  + **P36.3** Sepsis of newborn due to other and unspecified staphylococci
    MCC **P36.30** Sepsis of newborn due to unspecified staphylococci
    MCC **P36.39** Sepsis of newborn due to other staphylococci
  MCC **P36.4** Sepsis of newborn due to Escherichia coli
  MCC **P36.5** Sepsis of newborn due to anaerobes
  MCC **P36.8** Other bacterial sepsis of newborn
    Use additional code from category B96 to identify organism
  MCC **P36.9** Bacterial sepsis of newborn, unspecified

P37 Other congenital infectious and parasitic diseases
  Excludes2: congenital syphilis (A50.-)
    infectious neonatal diarrhea (A00-A09)
    necrotizing enterocolitis in newborn (P77.-)
    noninfectious neonatal diarrhea (P78.3)
    ophthalmia neonatorum due to gonococcus (A54.31)
    tetanus neonatorum (A33)
  MCC **P37.0** Congenital tuberculosis
  MCC **P37.1** Congenital toxoplasmosis
    Hydrocephalus due to congenital toxoplasmosis
  MCC **P37.2** Neonatal (disseminated) listeriosis
  MCC **P37.3** Congenital falciparum malaria
  MCC **P37.4** Other congenital malaria
  P37.5 Neonatal candidiasis
  MCC **P37.8** Other specified congenital infectious and parasitic diseases
  MCC **P37.9** Congenital infectious or parasitic disease, unspecified

P38 Omphalitis of newborn

> **Excludes1:** omphalitis not of newborn (L08.82)
> tetanus omphalitis (A33)
> umbilical hemorrhage of newborn (P51.-)

CC **P38.1** Omphalitis with mild hemorrhage
CC **P38.9** Omphalitis without hemorrhage
  Omphalitis of newborn NOS

P39 Other infections specific to the perinatal period

> Use additional code to identify organism or specific infection

CC **P39.0** Neonatal infective mastitis
> **Excludes1:** breast engorgement of newborn (P83.4)
> noninfective mastitis of newborn (P83.4)

P39.1 Neonatal conjunctivitis and dacryocystitis
  Neonatal chlamydial conjunctivitis
  Ophthalmia neonatorum NOS
> **Excludes1:** gonococcal conjunctivitis (A54.31)

CC **P39.2** Intra-amniotic infection affecting newborn, not elsewhere classified
CC **P39.3** Neonatal urinary tract infection
CC **P39.4** Neonatal skin infection
  Neonatal pyoderma
> **Excludes1:** pemphigus neonatorum (L00)
> staphylococcal scalded skin syndrome (L00)

CC **P39.8** Other specified infections specific to the perinatal period
CC **P39.9** Infection specific to the perinatal period, unspecified

Hemorrhagic and hematological disorders of newborn (P50-P61)

> **Excludes1:** congenital stenosis and stricture of bile ducts (Q44.3)
> Crigler-Najjar syndrome (E80.5)
> Dubin-Johnson syndrome (E80.6)
> Gilbert syndrome (E80.4)
> hereditary hemolytic anemias (D55-D58)

P50 Newborn affected by intrauterine (fetal) blood loss

> **Excludes1:** congenital anemia from intrauterine (fetal) blood loss (P61.3)

P50.0 Newborn affected by intrauterine (fetal) blood loss from vasa previa
P50.1 Newborn affected by intrauterine (fetal) blood loss from ruptured cord
P50.2 Newborn affected by intrauterine (fetal) blood loss from placenta
P50.3 Newborn affected by hemorrhage into co-twin
P50.4 Newborn affected by hemorrhage into maternal circulation
P50.5 Newborn affected by intrauterine (fetal) blood loss from cut end of co-twin's cord
P50.8 Newborn affected by other intrauterine (fetal) blood loss
P50.9 Newborn affected by intrauterine (fetal) blood loss, unspecified
  Newborn affected by fetal hemorrhage NOS

P51 Umbilical hemorrhage of newborn

> **Excludes1:** omphalitis with mild hemorrhage (P38.1)
> umbilical hemorrhage from cut end of co-twins cord (P50.5)

P51.0 Massive umbilical hemorrhage of newborn
P51.8 Other umbilical hemorrhages of newborn
  Slipped umbilical ligature NOS
P51.9 Umbilical hemorrhage of newborn, unspecified

P52 Intracranial nontraumatic hemorrhage of newborn

> **Includes:** intracranial hemorrhage due to anoxia or hypoxia
> **Excludes1:** intracranial hemorrhage due to birth injury (P10.-)
> intracranial hemorrhage due to other injury (S06.-)

CC **P52.0** Intraventricular (nontraumatic) hemorrhage, grade 1, of newborn
  Subependymal hemorrhage (without intraventricular extension)
  Bleeding into germinal matrix
CC **P52.1** Intraventricular (nontraumatic) hemorrhage, grade 2, of newborn
  Subependymal hemorrhage with intraventricular extension
  Bleeding into ventricle
+ **P52.2** Intraventricular (nontraumatic) hemorrhage, grade 3 and grade 4, of newborn
  MCC **P52.21** Intraventricular (nontraumatic) hemorrhage, grade 3, of newborn
    Subependymal hemorrhage with intraventricular extension with enlargement of ventricle
  MCC **P52.22** Intraventricular (nontraumatic) hemorrhage, grade 4, of newborn
    Bleeding into cerebral cortex
    Subependymal hemorrhage with intracerebral extension
CC **P52.3** Unspecified intraventricular (nontraumatic) hemorrhage of newborn
MCC **P52.4** Intracerebral (nontraumatic) hemorrhage of newborn
MCC **P52.5** Subarachnoid (nontraumatic) hemorrhage of newborn
MCC **P52.6** Cerebellar (nontraumatic) and posterior fossa hemorrhage of newborn
MCC **P52.8** Other intracranial (nontraumatic) hemorrhages of newborn
MCC **P52.9** Intracranial (nontraumatic) hemorrhage of newborn, unspecified

CC **P53 Hemorrhagic disease of newborn**
  Vitamin K deficiency of newborn
  Valid 3-character code, no further characters required

P54 Other neonatal hemorrhages

> **Excludes1:** newborn affected by (intrauterine) blood loss (P50.-)
> pulmonary hemorrhage originating in the perinatal period (P26.-)

P54.0 Neonatal hematemesis
> **Excludes1:** neonatal hematemesis due to swallowed maternal blood (P78.2)

MCC **P54.1** Neonatal melena
> **Excludes1:** neonatal melena due to swallowed maternal blood (P78.2)

MCC **P54.2** Neonatal rectal hemorrhage
MCC **P54.3** Other neonatal gastrointestinal hemorrhage
CC **P54.4** Neonatal adrenal hemorrhage
P54.5 Neonatal cutaneous hemorrhage
  Neonatal bruising
  Neonatal ecchymoses
  Neonatal petechiae
  Neonatal superficial hematomata
> **Excludes2:** bruising of scalp due to birth injury (P12.3)
> cephalhematoma due to birth injury (P12.0)

♀ **P54.6** Neonatal vaginal hemorrhage
  Neonatal pseudomenses
P54.8 Other specified neonatal hemorrhages
P54.9 Neonatal hemorrhage, unspecified

P55 Hemolytic disease of newborn

P55.0 Rh isoimmunization of newborn
P55.1 ABO isoimmunization of newborn
  AHA CC: 3Q, 2015, 20
P55.8 Other hemolytic diseases of newborn
  AHA CC: 3Q, 2018, 24
P55.9 Hemolytic disease of newborn, unspecified

P56 Hydrops fetalis due to hemolytic disease

> **Excludes1:** hydrops fetalis NOS (P83.2)

MCC **P56.0** Hydrops fetalis due to isoimmunization
+ **P56.9** Hydrops fetalis due to other and unspecified hemolytic disease
  MCC **P56.90** Hydrops fetalis due to unspecified hemolytic disease
  MCC **P56.99** Hydrops fetalis due to other hemolytic disease

P57 Kernicterus

MCC **P57.0** Kernicterus due to isoimmunization
MCC **P57.8** Other specified kernicterus
> **Excludes1:** Crigler-Najjar syndrome (E80.5)

MCC **P57.9** Kernicterus, unspecified

P58 Neonatal jaundice due to other excessive hemolysis

> **Excludes1:** jaundice due to isoimmunization (P55-P57)

P58.0 Neonatal jaundice due to bruising
P58.1 Neonatal jaundice due to bleeding
P58.2 Neonatal jaundice due to infection
P58.3 Neonatal jaundice due to polycythemia
+ **P58.4** Neonatal jaundice due to drugs or toxins transmitted from mother or given to newborn
  Code first poisoning due to drug or toxin, if applicable (T36-T65 with fifth or sixth character 1-4)

  Use additional code for adverse effect, if applicable, to identify drug (T36-T50 with fifth or sixth character 5)

P58.41 Neonatal jaundice due to drugs or toxins transmitted from mother
P58.42 Neonatal jaundice due to drugs or toxins given to newborn
P58.5 Neonatal jaundice due to swallowed maternal blood
P58.8 Neonatal jaundice due to other specified excessive hemolysis
P58.9 Neonatal jaundice due to excessive hemolysis, unspecified

P59 Neonatal jaundice from other and unspecified causes
  Excludes1: jaundice due to inborn errors of metabolism (E70-E88)
  kernicterus (P57.-)
  P59.0 Neonatal jaundice associated with preterm delivery
    Hyperbilirubinemia of prematurity
    Jaundice due to delayed conjugation associated with preterm delivery
  MCC P59.1 Inspissated bile syndrome
  + P59.2 Neonatal jaundice from other and unspecified hepatocellular damage
    Excludes1: congenital viral hepatitis (P35.3)
    MCC P59.20 Neonatal jaundice from unspecified hepatocellular damage
    MCC P59.29 Neonatal jaundice from other hepatocellular damage
      Neonatal giant cell hepatitis
      Neonatal (idiopathic) hepatitis
  P59.3 Neonatal jaundice from breast milk inhibitor
  P59.8 Neonatal jaundice from other specified causes
  P59.9 Neonatal jaundice, unspecified
    Neonatal physiological jaundice (intense)(prolonged) NOS
    AHA CC: 3Q, 2015, 20

P60 Disseminated intravascular coagulation of newborn
MCC
  Defibrination syndrome of newborn
  Valid 3-character code, no further characters required

P61 Other perinatal hematological disorders
  Excludes1: transient hypogammaglobulinemia of infancy (D80.7)
  MCC P61.0 Transient neonatal thrombocytopenia
    Neonatal thrombocytopenia due to exchange transfusion
    Neonatal thrombocytopenia due to idiopathic maternal thrombocytopenia
    Neonatal thrombocytopenia due to isoimmunization
  P61.1 Polycythemia neonatorum
  CC P61.2 Anemia of prematurity
  CC P61.3 Congenital anemia from fetal blood loss
  CC P61.4 Other congenital anemias, not elsewhere classified
    Congenital anemia NOS
  MCC P61.5 Transient neonatal neutropenia
    Excludes1: congenital neutropenia (nontransient) (D70.0)
  CC P61.6 Other transient neonatal disorders of coagulation
  P61.8 Other specified perinatal hematological disorders
  P61.9 Perinatal hematological disorder, unspecified

Transitory endocrine and metabolic disorders specific to newborn (P70-P74)
Includes: transitory endocrine and metabolic disturbances caused by the infant's response to maternal endocrine and metabolic factors, or its adjustment to extrauterine environment

P70 Transitory disorders of carbohydrate metabolism specific to newborn
  P70.0 Syndrome of infant of mother with gestational diabetes
    Newborn (with hypoglycemia) affected by maternal gestational diabetes
    Excludes1: newborn (with hypoglycemia) affected by maternal (pre-existing) diabetes mellitus (P70.1)
    syndrome of infant of a diabetic mother (P70.1)
  P70.1 Syndrome of infant of a diabetic mother
    Newborn (with hypoglycemia) affected by maternal (pre-existing) diabetes mellitus
    Excludes1: newborn (with hypoglycemia) affected by maternal gestational diabetes (P70.0)
    syndrome of infant of mother with gestational diabetes (P70.0)
  CC P70.2 Neonatal diabetes mellitus
  P70.3 Iatrogenic neonatal hypoglycemia
  P70.4 Other neonatal hypoglycemia
    Transitory neonatal hypoglycemia

  CC P70.8 Other transitory disorders of carbohydrate metabolism of newborn
  P70.9 Transitory disorder of carbohydrate metabolism of newborn, unspecified

P71 Transitory neonatal disorders of calcium and magnesium metabolism
  CC P71.0 Cow's milk hypocalcemia in newborn
  CC P71.1 Other neonatal hypocalcemia
    Excludes1: neonatal hypoparathyroidism (P71.4)
  CC P71.2 Neonatal hypomagnesemia
  CC P71.3 Neonatal tetany without calcium or magnesium deficiency
    Neonatal tetany NOS
  CC P71.4 Transitory neonatal hypoparathyroidism
  CC P71.8 Other transitory neonatal disorders of calcium and magnesium metabolism
    AHA CC: 4Q, 2016, 54-55
  CC P71.9 Transitory neonatal disorder of calcium and magnesium metabolism, unspecified

P72 Other transitory neonatal endocrine disorders
  Excludes1: congenital hypothyroidism with or without goiter (E03.0-E03.1)
    dyshormogenetic goiter (E07.1)
    Pendred's syndrome (E07.1)
  CC P72.0 Neonatal goiter, not elsewhere classified
    Transitory congenital goiter with normal functioning
  CC P72.1 Transitory neonatal hyperthyroidism
    Neonatal thyrotoxicosis
  CC P72.2 Other transitory neonatal disorders of thyroid function, not elsewhere classified
    Transitory neonatal hypothyroidism
  CC P72.8 Other specified transitory neonatal endocrine disorders
  P72.9 Transitory neonatal endocrine disorder, unspecified

P74 Other transitory neonatal electrolyte and metabolic disturbances
  MCC P74.0 Late metabolic acidosis of newborn
    Excludes1: (fetal) metabolic acidosis of newborn (P19)
  P74.1 Dehydration of newborn
  + P74.2 Disturbances of sodium balance of newborn
    AHA CC: 2Q, 2018, 6; 4Q, 2018, 27
    P74.21 Hypernatremia of newborn
    P74.22 Hyponatremia of newborn
  + P74.3 Disturbances of potassium balance of newborn
    AHA CC: 4Q, 2018, 27
    P74.31 Hyperkalemia of newborn
    P74.32 Hypokalemia of newborn
  + P74.4 Other transitory electrolyte disturbances of newborn
    AHA CC: 4Q, 2018, 27
    CC P74.41 Alkalosis of newborn
      Hyperbicarbonatemia
    + P74.42 Disturbances of chlorine balance of newborn
      P74.421 Hyperchloremia of newborn
        Hyperchloremic metabolic acidosis
        Excludes2: late metabolic acidosis of the newborn (P74.0)
      P74.422 Hypochloremia of newborn
    P74.49 Other transitory electrolyte disturbance of newborn
  CC P74.5 Transitory tyrosinemia of newborn
  CC P74.6 Transitory hyperammonemia of newborn
  CC P74.8 Other transitory metabolic disturbances of newborn
    Amino-acid metabolic disorders described as transitory
  P74.9 Transitory metabolic disturbance of newborn, unspecified

Digestive system disorders of newborn (P76-P78)

P76 Other intestinal obstruction of newborn
  P76.0 Meconium plug syndrome
    Meconium ileus NOS
    Excludes1: meconium ileus in cystic fibrosis (E84.11)
  CC P76.1 Transitory ileus of newborn
    Excludes1: Hirschsprung's disease (Q43.1)
  P76.2 Intestinal obstruction due to inspissated milk
  P76.8 Other specified intestinal obstruction of newborn
    Excludes1: intestinal obstruction classifiable to K56.-
  P76.9 Intestinal obstruction of newborn, unspecified

P77 Necrotizing enterocolitis of newborn
  MCC P77.1 Stage 1 necrotizing enterocolitis in newborn
    Necrotizing enterocolitis without pneumatosis, without perforation

MCC **P77.2** **Stage 2 necrotizing enterocolitis in newborn**
  Necrotizing enterocolitis with pneumatosis, without perforation
MCC **P77.3** **Stage 3 necrotizing enterocolitis in newborn**
  Necrotizing enterocolitis with perforation
  Necrotizing enterocolitis with pneumatosis and perforation
MCC **P77.9** **Necrotizing enterocolitis in newborn, unspecified**
  Necrotizing enterocolitis in newborn, NOS

P78 **Other perinatal digestive system disorders**
  Excludes1: cystic fibrosis (E84.0-E84.9)
    neonatal gastrointestinal hemorrhages (P54.0-P54.3)
  MCC **P78.0** **Perinatal intestinal perforation**
    Meconium peritonitis
  P78.1 **Other neonatal peritonitis**
    Neonatal peritonitis NOS
  P78.2 **Neonatal hematemesis and melena due to swallowed maternal blood**
  P78.3 **Noninfective neonatal diarrhea**
    Neonatal diarrhea NOS
  + **P78.8** **Other specified perinatal digestive system disorders**
    P78.81 **Congenital cirrhosis (of liver)**
    P78.82 **Peptic ulcer of newborn**
    P78.83 **Newborn esophageal reflux**
      Neonatal esophageal reflux
    P78.84 **Gestational alloimmune liver disease**
      GALD
      Neonatal hemochromatosis
      Excludes1: hemochromatosis (E83.11-)
      AHA CC: 4Q, 2017, 21
    P78.89 **Other specified perinatal digestive system disorders**
  P78.9 **Perinatal digestive system disorder, unspecified**

Conditions involving the integument and temperature regulation of newborn (P80-P83)

P80 **Hypothermia of newborn**
  P80.0 **Cold injury syndrome**
    Severe and usually chronic hypothermia associated with a pink flushed appearance, edema and neurological and biochemical abnormalities.
    Excludes1: mild hypothermia of newborn (P80.8)
  P80.8 **Other hypothermia of newborn**
    Mild hypothermia of newborn
  P80.9 **Hypothermia of newborn, unspecified**

P81 **Other disturbances of temperature regulation of newborn**
  P81.0 **Environmental hyperthermia of newborn**
  P81.8 **Other specified disturbances of temperature regulation of newborn**
  P81.9 **Disturbance of temperature regulation of newborn, unspecified**
    Fever of newborn NOS

P83 **Other conditions of integument specific to newborn**
  Excludes1: congenital malformations of skin and integument (Q80-Q84)
    hydrops fetalis due to hemolytic disease (P56.-)
    neonatal skin infection (P39.4)
    staphylococcal scalded skin syndrome (L00)
  Excludes2: cradle cap (L21.0)
    diaper [napkin] dermatitis (L22)
  CC **P83.0** **Sclerema neonatorum**
  P83.1 **Neonatal erythema toxicum**
  MCC **P83.2** **Hydrops fetalis not due to hemolytic disease**
    Hydrops fetalis NOS
  + **P83.3** **Other and unspecified edema specific to newborn**
    CC **P83.30** **Unspecified edema specific to newborn**
    CC **P83.39** **Other edema specific to newborn**
  P83.4 **Breast engorgement of newborn**
    Noninfective mastitis of newborn
  ♂ **P83.5** **Congenital hydrocele**
  P83.6 **Umbilical polyp of newborn**
  + **P83.8** **Other specified conditions of integument specific to newborn**
    AHA CC: 4Q, 2017, 21-22
    P83.81 **Umbilical granuloma**
      Excludes2: granulomatous disorder of the skin and subcutaneous tissue, unspecified (L92.9)
    P83.88 **Other specified conditions of integument specific to newborn**
      Bronze baby syndrome
      Neonatal scleroderma
      Urticaria neonatorum
  P83.9 **Condition of the integument specific to newborn, unspecified**

Other problems with newborn (P84)

P84 **Other problems with newborn**
  Acidemia of newborn
  Acidosis of newborn
  Anoxia of newborn NOS
  Asphyxia of newborn NOS
  Hypercapnia of newborn
  Hypoxemia of newborn
  Hypoxia of newborn NOS
  Mixed metabolic and respiratory acidosis of newborn
  Excludes1: intracranial hemorrhage due to anoxia or hypoxia (P52.-)
    hypoxic ischemic encephalopathy [HIE] (P91.6-)
    late metabolic acidosis of newborn (P74.0)
  Valid 3-character code, no further characters required

Other disorders originating in the perinatal period (P90-P96)

MCC **P90** **Convulsions of newborn**
  Excludes1: benign myoclonic epilepsy in infancy (G40.3-)
    benign neonatal convulsions (familial) (G40.3-)
  Valid 3-character code, no further characters required

P91 **Other disturbances of cerebral status of newborn**
  MCC **P91.0** **Neonatal cerebral ischemia**
    Excludes1: Neonatal cerebral infarction (P91.82-)
  MCC **P91.1** **Acquired periventricular cysts of newborn**
  MCC **P91.2** **Neonatal cerebral leukomalacia**
    Periventricular leukomalacia
  MCC **P91.3** **Neonatal cerebral irritability**
  MCC **P91.4** **Neonatal cerebral depression**
  MCC **P91.5** **Neonatal coma**
  + **P91.6** **Hypoxic ischemic encephalopathy [HIE]**
    Excludes1: neonatal cerebral depression (P91.4)
      neonatal cerebral irritability (P91.3)
      neonatal coma (P91.5)
    AHA CC: 4Q, 2017, 22
    CC **P91.60** **Hypoxic ischemic encephalopathy [HIE], unspecified**
    CC **P91.61** **Mild hypoxic ischemic encephalopathy [HIE]**
    CC **P91.62** **Moderate hypoxic ischemic encephalopathy [HIE]**
    MCC **P91.63** **Severe hypoxic ischemic encephalopathy [HIE]**
  + **P91.8** **Other specified disturbances of cerebral status of newborn**
    + **P91.81** **Neonatal encephalopathy**
      AHA CC: 4Q, 2017, 22
      P91.811 **Neonatal encephalopathy in diseases classified elsewhere**
        Code first underlying condition, if known, such as:
        congenital cirrhosis (of liver) (P78.81)
        intracranial nontraumatic hemorrhage of newborn (P52.-)
        kernicterus (P57.-)
      P91.819 **Neonatal encephalopathy, unspecified**
    + **P91.82** **Neonatal cerebral infarction**
      Neonatal stroke
      Perinatal arterial ischemic stroke
      Perinatal cerebral infarction
      Excludes1: cerebral infarction (I63.-)
      Excludes2: intracranial hemorrhage of newborn (P52.-)
      AHA CC: 4Q, 2020, 37-38
      MCC **P91.821** **Neonatal cerebral infarction, right side of brain**
      MCC **P91.822** **Neonatal cerebral infarction, left side of brain**
        AHA CC: 4Q, 2020, 38
      MCC **P91.823** **Neonatal cerebral infarction, bilateral**
      MCC **P91.829** **Neonatal cerebral infarction, unspecified side**
    P91.88 **Other specified disturbances of cerebral status of newborn**
  P91.9 **Disturbance of cerebral status of newborn, unspecified**

P92 Feeding problems of newborn
Excludes1: eating disorders (F50.-)
Excludes2: feeding problems in child over 28 days old (R63.3-)

+ **P92.0 Vomiting of newborn**
  Excludes1: vomiting of child over 28 days old (R11.-)
  MCC **P92.01 Bilious vomiting of newborn**
  Excludes1: bilious vomiting in child over 28 days old (R11.14)
  P92.09 Other vomiting of newborn
  Excludes1: regurgitation of food in newborn (P92.1)

P92.1 Regurgitation and rumination of newborn
P92.2 Slow feeding of newborn
P92.3 Underfeeding of newborn
P92.4 Overfeeding of newborn
P92.5 Neonatal difficulty in feeding at breast
   AHA CC: 3Q, 2016, 19; 1Q, 2017, 28-29
P92.6 Failure to thrive in newborn
   Excludes1: failure to thrive in child over 28 days old (R62.51)
P92.8 Other feeding problems of newborn
P92.9 Feeding problem of newborn, unspecified

P93 Reactions and intoxications due to drugs administered to newborn
Includes: reactions and intoxications due to drugs administered to fetus affecting newborn
Excludes1: jaundice due to drugs or toxins transmitted from mother or given to newborn (P58.4-)
reactions and intoxications from maternal opiates, tranquilizers and other medication (P04.0-P04.1, P04.4-)
withdrawal symptoms from maternal use of drugs of addiction (P96.1)
withdrawal symptoms from therapeutic use of drugs in newborn (P96.2)

CC **P93.0 Grey baby syndrome**
   Grey syndrome from chloramphenicol administration in newborn
CC **P93.8 Other reactions and intoxications due to drugs administered to newborn**
   Use additional code for adverse effect, if applicable, to identify drug (T36-T50 with fifth or sixth character 5)

P94 Disorders of muscle tone of newborn
CC **P94.0 Transient neonatal myasthenia gravis**
   Excludes1: myasthenia gravis (G70.0)
P94.1 Congenital hypertonia
P94.2 Congenital hypotonia
   Floppy baby syndrome, unspecified
P94.8 Other disorders of muscle tone of newborn
P94.9 Disorder of muscle tone of newborn, unspecified

P95 Stillbirth
Deadborn fetus NOS
Fetal death of unspecified cause
Stillbirth NOS
Excludes1: maternal care for intrauterine death (O36.4)
missed abortion (O02.1)
outcome of delivery, stillbirth (Z37.1, Z37.3, Z37.4, Z37.7)
Review coding guideline C.16.g
Valid 3-character code, no further characters required

P96 Other conditions originating in the perinatal period
P96.0 Congenital renal failure
   Uremia of newborn
CC **P96.1 Neonatal withdrawal symptoms from maternal use of drugs of addiction**
   Drug withdrawal syndrome in infant of dependent mother
   Neonatal abstinence syndrome
   Excludes1: reactions and intoxications from maternal opiates and tranquilizers administered during labor and delivery (P04.0)
   AHA CC: 4Q, 2018, 24-25
CC **P96.2 Withdrawal symptoms from therapeutic use of drugs in newborn**
P96.3 Wide cranial sutures of newborn
   Neonatal craniotabes
P96.5 Complication to newborn due to (fetal) intrauterine procedure
   Excludes2: newborn affected by amniocentesis (P00.6)
+ **P96.8 Other specified conditions originating in the perinatal period**
   P96.81 Exposure to (parental) (environmental) tobacco smoke in the perinatal period
      Excludes2: newborn affected by in utero exposure to tobacco (P04.2)
         exposure to environmental tobacco smoke after the perinatal period (Z77.22)
   P96.82 Delayed separation of umbilical cord
   P96.83 Meconium staining
      Excludes1: meconium aspiration (P24.00, P24.01)
         meconium passage during delivery (P03.82)
   P96.89 Other specified conditions originating in the perinatal period
      Use additional code to specify condition
P96.9 Condition originating in the perinatal period, unspecified
   Congenital debility NOS

Chapter 17: Congenital Malformations, Deformations and Chromosomal Abnormalities (Q00-Q99)

NOTE Codes from this chapter are not for use on maternal records
Excludes2: *inborn errors of metabolism (E70-E88)*

This chapter contains the following category blocks:
- Q00-Q07 Congenital malformations of the nervous system
- Q10-Q18 Congenital malformations of eye, ear, face and neck
- Q20-Q28 Congenital malformations of the circulatory system
- Q30-Q34 Congenital malformations of the respiratory system
- Q35-Q37 Cleft lip and cleft palate
- Q38-Q45 Other congenital malformations of the digestive system
- Q50-Q56 Congenital malformations of genital organs
- Q60-Q64 Congenital malformations of the urinary system
- Q65-Q79 Congenital malformations and deformations of the musculoskeletal system
- Q80-Q89 Other congenital malformations
- Q90-Q99 Chromosomal abnormalities, not elsewhere classified

C. Chapter-Specific Coding Guidelines

In addition to general coding guidelines, there are guidelines for specific diagnoses and/or conditions in the classification. Unless otherwise indicated, these guidelines apply to all health care settings. Please refer to Section II for guidelines on the selection of principal diagnosis.

17. **Chapter 17: Congenital Malformations, Deformations and Chromosomal Abnormalities (Q00-Q99)**

Assign an appropriate code(s) from categories Q00-Q99, Congenital malformations, deformations, and chromosomal abnormalities when a malformation/deformation or chromosomal abnormality is documented. A malformation/deformation or chromosomal abnormality may be the principal/first-listed diagnosis on a record or a secondary diagnosis.

When a malformation/deformation or chromosomal abnormality does not have a unique code assignment, assign additional code(s) for any manifestations that may be present.

When the code assignment specifically identifies the malformation/deformation/or chromosomal abnormality, manifestations that are an inherent component of the anomaly should not be coded separately. Additional codes should be assigned for manifestations that are not an inherent component.

Codes from Chapter 17 may be used throughout the life of the patient. If a congenital malformation or deformity has been corrected, a personal history code should be used to identify the history of the malformation or deformity. Although present at birth, a malformation/deformation or chromosomal abnormality may not be identified until later in life. Whenever the condition is diagnosed by the provider, it is appropriate to assign a code from codes Q00-Q99. For the birth admission, the appropriate code from category Z38, Liveborn infants, according to place of birth and type of delivery, should be sequenced as the principal diagnosis, followed by any congenital anomaly codes, Q00-Q99.

Congenital malformations of the nervous system (Q00-Q07)

Q00 Anencephaly and similar malformations
   MCC **Q00.0** Anencephaly
        Acephaly
        Acrania
        Amyelencephaly
        Hemianencephaly
        Hemicephaly
   MCC **Q00.1** Craniorachischisis
   MCC **Q00.2** Iniencephaly

Q01 Encephalocele
   Includes: Arnold-Chiari syndrome, type III
         encephalocystocele
         encephalomyelocele
         hydroencephalocele
         hydromeningocele, cranial
         meningocele, cerebral
         meningoencephalocele
   Excludes1: *Meckel-Gruber syndrome (Q61.9)*
   CC **Q01.0** Frontal encephalocele
   CC **Q01.1** Nasofrontal encephalocele
   CC **Q01.2** Occipital encephalocele
   CC **Q01.8** Encephalocele of other sites
   CC **Q01.9** Encephalocele, unspecified

Q02 Microcephaly
   Includes: hydromicrocephaly
         micrencephalon
   Excludes1: *Meckel-Gruber syndrome (Q61.9)*
   Code first, if applicable, congenital Zika virus disease
   AHA CC: 4Q, 2016, 4-7; 4Q, 2018, 26
   Valid 3-character code, no further characters required

Q03 Congenital hydrocephalus
   Includes: hydrocephalus in newborn
   Excludes1: *Arnold-Chiari syndrome, type II (Q07.0-)*
        acquired hydrocephalus (G91.-)
        hydrocephalus due to congenital toxoplasmosis (P37.1)
        hydrocephalus with spina bifida (Q05.0-Q05.4)
   Q03.0 Malformations of aqueduct of Sylvius
        Anomaly of aqueduct of Sylvius
        Obstruction of aqueduct of Sylvius, congenital
        Stenosis of aqueduct of Sylvius
   Q03.1 Atresia of foramina of Magendie and Luschka
        Dandy-Walker syndrome
   Q03.8 Other congenital hydrocephalus
   Q03.9 Congenital hydrocephalus, unspecified

Q04 Other congenital malformations of brain
   Excludes1: *cyclopia (Q87.0)*
        macrocephaly (Q75.3)
   MCC **Q04.0** Congenital malformations of corpus callosum
        Agenesis of corpus callosum
   MCC **Q04.1** Arhinencephaly
   MCC **Q04.2** Holoprosencephaly
   MCC **Q04.3** Other reduction deformities of brain
        Absence of part of brain
        Agenesis of part of brain
        Agyria
        Aplasia of part of brain
        Hydranencephaly
        Hypoplasia of part of brain
        Lissencephaly
        Microgyria
        Pachygyria
   Excludes1: *congenital malformations of corpus callosum (Q04.0)*
   CC **Q04.4** Septo-optic dysplasia of brain
   CC **Q04.5** Megalencephaly
   CC **Q04.6** Congenital cerebral cysts
        Porencephaly
        Schizencephaly
   Excludes1: *acquired porencephalic cyst (G93.0)*
   CC **Q04.8** Other specified congenital malformations of brain
        Arnold-Chiari syndrome, type IV
        Macrogyria
   Q04.9 Congenital malformation of brain, unspecified
        Congenital anomaly NOS of brain
        Congenital deformity NOS of brain
        Congenital disease or lesion NOS of brain
        Multiple anomalies NOS of brain, congenital

Q05 Spina bifida
   Includes: hydromeningocele (spinal)
         meningocele (spinal)
         meningomyelocele
         myelocele
         myelomeningocele
         rachischisis
         spina bifida (aperta)(cystica)
         syringomyelocele
   Use additional code for any associated paraplegia (paraparesis) (G82.2-)
   Excludes1: *Arnold-Chiari syndrome, type II (Q07.0-)*
        spina bifida occulta (Q76.0)
   CC **Q05.0** Cervical spina bifida with hydrocephalus
   CC **Q05.1** Thoracic spina bifida with hydrocephalus
        Dorsal spina bifida with hydrocephalus
        Thoracolumbar spina bifida with hydrocephalus
   CC **Q05.2** Lumbar spina bifida with hydrocephalus
        Lumbosacral spina bifida with hydrocephalus
   CC **Q05.3** Sacral spina bifida with hydrocephalus
   CC **Q05.4** Unspecified spina bifida with hydrocephalus
   Q05.5 Cervical spina bifida without hydrocephalus

Chapter 17: Congenital Malformations, Deformations and Chromosomal Abnormalities

- **Q05.6** **Thoracic spina bifida without hydrocephalus**
  - Dorsal spina bifida NOS
  - Thoracolumbar spina bifida NOS
- **Q05.7** **Lumbar spina bifida without hydrocephalus**
  - Lumbosacral spina bifida NOS
- **Q05.8** **Sacral spina bifida without hydrocephalus**
- **Q05.9** **Spina bifida, unspecified**

Q06 Other congenital malformations of spinal cord
- **Q06.0** **Amyelia**
- **Q06.1** **Hypoplasia and dysplasia of spinal cord**
  - Atelomyelia
  - Myelatelia
  - Myelodysplasia of spinal cord
- **Q06.2** **Diastematomyelia**
- **Q06.3** **Other congenital cauda equina malformations**
- **Q06.4** **Hydromyelia**
  - Hydrorachis
- **Q06.8** **Other specified congenital malformations of spinal cord**
- **Q06.9** **Congenital malformation of spinal cord, unspecified**
  - Congenital anomaly NOS of spinal cord
  - Congenital deformity NOS of spinal cord
  - Congenital disease or lesion NOS of spinal cord

Q07 Other congenital malformations of nervous system

Excludes2: congenital central alveolar hypoventilation syndrome (G47.35)
  familial dysautonomia [Riley-Day] (G90.1)
  neurofibromatosis (nonmalignant) (Q85.0-)

- **+ Q07.0** **Arnold-Chiari syndrome**
  - Arnold-Chiari syndrome, type II
  - **Excludes1:** Arnold-Chiari syndrome, type III (Q01.-)
    Arnold-Chiari syndrome, type IV (Q04.8)
  - **Q07.00** **Arnold-Chiari syndrome without spina bifida or hydrocephalus**
  - **Q07.01** **Arnold-Chiari syndrome with spina bifida**
  - CC **Q07.02** **Arnold-Chiari syndrome with hydrocephalus**
  - CC **Q07.03** **Arnold-Chiari syndrome with spina bifida and hydrocephalus**
- **Q07.8** **Other specified congenital malformations of nervous system**
  - Agenesis of nerve
  - Displacement of brachial plexus
  - Jaw-winking syndrome
  - Marcus Gunn's syndrome
- **Q07.9** **Congenital malformation of nervous system, unspecified**
  - Congenital anomaly NOS of nervous system
  - Congenital deformity NOS of nervous system
  - Congenital disease or lesion NOS of nervous system

Congenital malformations of eye, ear, face and neck (Q10-Q18)

Excludes2: cleft lip and cleft palate (Q35-Q37)
  congenital malformation of cervical spine (Q05.0, Q05.5, Q67.5, Q76.0-Q76.4)
  congenital malformation of larynx (Q31.-)
  congenital malformation of lip NEC (Q38.0)
  congenital malformation of nose (Q30.-)
  congenital malformation of parathyroid gland (Q89.2)
  congenital malformation of thyroid gland (Q89.2)

Q10 Congenital malformations of eyelid, lacrimal apparatus and orbit

Excludes1: cryptophthalmos NOS (Q11.2)
  cryptophthalmos syndrome (Q87.0)

- **Q10.0** **Congenital ptosis**
- **Q10.1** **Congenital ectropion**
- **Q10.2** **Congenital entropion**
- **Q10.3** **Other congenital malformations of eyelid**
  - Ablepharon
  - Blepharophimosis, congenital
  - Coloboma of eyelid
  - Congenital absence or agenesis of cilia
  - Congenital absence or agenesis of eyelid
  - Congenital accessory eyelid
  - Congenital accessory eye muscle
  - Congenital malformation of eyelid NOS
- **Q10.4** **Absence and agenesis of lacrimal apparatus**
  - Congenital absence of punctum lacrimale
- **Q10.5** **Congenital stenosis and stricture of lacrimal duct**
- **Q10.6** **Other congenital malformations of lacrimal apparatus**
  - Congenital malformation of lacrimal apparatus NOS
- **Q10.7** **Congenital malformation of orbit**

Q11 Anophthalmos, microphthalmos and macrophthalmos
- **Q11.0** **Cystic eyeball**
- **Q11.1** **Other anophthalmos**
  - Anophthalmos NOS
  - Agenesis of eye
  - Aplasia of eye
- **Q11.2** **Microphthalmos**
  - Cryptophthalmos NOS
  - Dysplasia of eye
  - Hypoplasia of eye
  - Rudimentary eye
  - **Excludes1:** cryptophthalmos syndrome (Q87.0)
- **Q11.3** **Macrophthalmos**
  - **Excludes1:** macrophthalmos in congenital glaucoma (Q15.0)

Q12 Congenital lens malformations
- CC **Q12.0** **Congenital cataract**
- CC **Q12.1** **Congenital displaced lens**
- CC **Q12.2** **Coloboma of lens**
- **Q12.3** **Congenital aphakia**
- **Q12.4** **Spherophakia**
- **Q12.8** **Other congenital lens malformations**
  - Microphakia
- **Q12.9** **Congenital lens malformation, unspecified**

Q13 Congenital malformations of anterior segment of eye
- **Q13.0** **Coloboma of iris**
  - Coloboma NOS
- **Q13.1** **Absence of iris**
  - Aniridia
  - Use additional code for associated glaucoma (H42)
- **Q13.2** **Other congenital malformations of iris**
  - Anisocoria, congenital
  - Atresia of pupil
  - Congenital malformation of iris NOS
  - Corectopia
- **Q13.3** **Congenital corneal opacity**
- **Q13.4** **Other congenital corneal malformations**
  - Congenital malformation of cornea NOS
  - Microcornea
  - Peter's anomaly
- **Q13.5** **Blue sclera**
- **Q13.8** **Other congenital malformations of anterior segment of eye**
  - **Q13.81** **Rieger's anomaly**
    - Use additional code for associated glaucoma (H42)
  - **Q13.89** **Other congenital malformations of anterior segment of eye**
- **Q13.9** **Congenital malformation of anterior segment of eye, unspecified**

Q14 Congenital malformations of posterior segment of eye

Excludes2: optic nerve hypoplasia (H47.03-)

- **Q14.0** **Congenital malformation of vitreous humor**
  - Congenital vitreous opacity
- **Q14.1** **Congenital malformation of retina**
  - Congenital retinal aneurysm
- **Q14.2** **Congenital malformation of optic disc**
  - Coloboma of optic disc
- **Q14.3** **Congenital malformation of choroid**
- **Q14.8** **Other congenital malformations of posterior segment of eye**
  - Coloboma of the fundus
- **Q14.9** **Congenital malformation of posterior segment of eye, unspecified**

Q15 Other congenital malformations of eye

Excludes1: congenital nystagmus (H55.01)
  ocular albinism (E70.31-)
  optic nerve hypoplasia (H47.03-)
  retinitis pigmentosa (H35.52)

- **Q15.0** **Congenital glaucoma**
  - Axenfeld's anomaly
  - Buphthalmos
  - Glaucoma of childhood
  - Glaucoma of newborn
  - Hydrophthalmos
  - Keratoglobus, congenital, with glaucoma
  - Macrocornea with glaucoma
  - Macrophthalmos in congenital glaucoma
  - Megalocornea with glaucoma

Q15.8 Other specified congenital malformations of eye
Q15.9 Congenital malformation of eye, unspecified
    Congenital anomaly of eye
    Congenital deformity of eye

Q16 Congenital malformations of ear causing impairment of hearing

Excludes1: *congenital deafness (H90.-)*

Q16.0 Congenital absence of (ear) auricle
Q16.1 Congenital absence, atresia and stricture of auditory canal (external)
    Congenital atresia or stricture of osseous meatus
Q16.2 Absence of eustachian tube
Q16.3 Congenital malformation of ear ossicles
    Congenital fusion of ear ossicles
Q16.4 Other congenital malformations of middle ear
    Congenital malformation of middle ear NOS
Q16.5 Congenital malformation of inner ear
    Congenital anomaly of membranous labyrinth
    Congenital anomaly of organ of Corti
Q16.9 Congenital malformation of ear causing impairment of hearing, unspecified
    Congenital absence of ear NOS

Q17 Other congenital malformations of ear

Excludes1: *congenital malformations of ear with impairment of hearing (Q16.0-Q16.9)*
preauricular sinus (Q18.1)

Q17.0 Accessory auricle
    Accessory tragus
    Polyotia
    Preauricular appendage or tag
    Supernumerary ear
    Supernumerary lobule
Q17.1 Macrotia
Q17.2 Microtia
Q17.3 Other misshapen ear
    Pointed ear
Q17.4 Misplaced ear
    Low-set ears
    Excludes1: *cervical auricle (Q18.2)*
Q17.5 Prominent ear
    Bat ear
Q17.8 Other specified congenital malformations of ear
    Congenital absence of lobe of ear
Q17.9 Congenital malformation of ear, unspecified
    Congenital anomaly of ear NOS

Q18 Other congenital malformations of face and neck

Excludes1: *cleft lip and cleft palate (Q35-Q37)*
conditions classified to (Q67.0-Q67.4)
congenital malformations of skull and face bones (Q75.-)
cyclopia (Q87.0)
dentofacial anomalies [including malocclusion] (M26.-)
malformation syndromes affecting facial appearance (Q87.0)
persistent thyroglossal duct (Q89.2)

Q18.0 Sinus, fistula and cyst of branchial cleft
    Branchial vestige
Q18.1 Preauricular sinus and cyst
    Fistula of auricle, congenital
    Cervicoaural fistula
Q18.2 Other branchial cleft malformations
    Branchial cleft malformation NOS
    Cervical auricle
    Otocephaly
Q18.3 Webbing of neck
    Pterygium colli
Q18.4 Macrostomia
Q18.5 Microstomia
Q18.6 Macrocheilia
    Hypertrophy of lip, congenital
Q18.7 Microcheilia
Q18.8 Other specified congenital malformations of face and neck
    Medial cyst of face and neck
    Medial fistula of face and neck
    Medial sinus of face and neck
Q18.9 Congenital malformation of face and neck, unspecified
    Congenital anomaly NOS of face and neck

Congenital malformations of the circulatory system (Q20-Q28)

Q20 Congenital malformations of cardiac chambers and connections

Excludes1: *dextrocardia with situs inversus (Q89.3)*
mirror-image atrial arrangement with situs inversus (Q89.3)

MCC Q20.0 Common arterial trunk
    Persistent truncus arteriosus
    Excludes1: *aortic septal defect (Q21.4)*
MCC Q20.1 Double outlet right ventricle
    Taussig-Bing syndrome
MCC Q20.2 Double outlet left ventricle
MCC Q20.3 Discordant ventriculoarterial connection
    Dextrotransposition of aorta
    Transposition of great vessels (complete)
MCC Q20.4 Double inlet ventricle
    Common ventricle
    Cor triloculare biatriatum
    Single ventricle
CC Q20.5 Discordant atrioventricular connection
    Corrected transposition
    Levotransposition
    Ventricular inversion
Q20.6 Isomerism of atrial appendages
    Isomerism of atrial appendages with asplenia or polysplenia
Q20.8 Other congenital malformations of cardiac chambers and connections
    Cor binoculare
Q20.9 Congenital malformation of cardiac chambers and connections, unspecified

Q21 Congenital malformations of cardiac septa

Excludes1: *acquired cardiac septal defect (I51.0)*
AHA CC: 4Q, 2022, 39-40

CC Q21.0 Ventricular septal defect
    Roger's disease
+ Q21.1 Atrial septal defect
    Excludes2: *ostium primum atrial septal defect (type I) (Q21.20)*
    CC Q21.10 Atrial septal defect, unspecified
    CC Q21.11 Secundum atrial septal defect
        Fenestrated atrial septum
        Patent or persistent ostium secundum defect (type II)
    CC Q21.12 Patent foramen ovale
        Persistent foramen ovale
    CC Q21.13 Coronary sinus atrial septal defect
        Coronary sinus defect
        Unroofed coronary sinus
    CC Q21.14 Superior sinus venosus atrial septal defect
        Superior vena cava type atrial septal defect
    CC Q21.15 Inferior sinus venosus atrial septal defect
        Inferior vena cava type atrial septal defect
    CC Q21.16 Sinus venosus atrial septal defect, unspecified
        Sinus venosus defect, NOS
    CC Q21.19 Other specified atrial septal defect
        Common atrium
        Other specified atrial septal abnormality
+ Q21.2 Atrioventricular septal defect
    Atrioventricular canal defect
    Endocardial cushion defect
    Ostium primum atrial septal defect (type I)
    CC Q21.20 Atrioventricular septal defect, unspecified as to partial or complete
        Atrioventricular canal, NOS
        Endocardial cushion defect NOS
        Ostium primum atrial septal defect (type I) NOS
    CC Q21.21 Partial atrioventricular septal defect
        Incomplete atrioventricular canal
        Incomplete atrioventricular septal defect
        Incomplete endocardial cushion defect
        Ostium primum atrial septal defect (type I) with separate atrioventricular valves
        Partial atrioventricular canal
        Partial endocardial cushion defect

CC Q21.22 Transitional atrioventricular septal defect
Intermediate atrioventricular canal
Intermediate atrioventricular septal defect
Intermediate endocardial cushion defect
Ostium primum atrial septal defect (type I) with separate atrioventricular valves and a small or restrictive inlet VSD
Transitional atrioventricular canal
Transitional endocardial cushion defect

CC Q21.23 Complete atrioventricular septal defect
Common atrioventricular canal
Common atrioventricular septal defect
Common endocardial cushion defect
Ostium primum atrial septal defect (type I) with common atrioventricular valve and a moderate or larger inlet VSD

MCC Q21.3 Tetralogy of Fallot
Ventricular septal defect with pulmonary stenosis or atresia, dextroposition of aorta and hypertrophy of right ventricle.
AHA CC: 3Q, 2014, 16-17

Q21.4 Aortopulmonary septal defect
Aortic septal defect
Aortopulmonary window

Q21.8 Other congenital malformations of cardiac septa
Eisenmenger's defect
Pentalogy of Fallot
Code also, if applicable:
Eisenmenger's complex (I27.83)
Eisenmenger's syndrome (I27.83)

Q21.9 Congenital malformation of cardiac septum, unspecified
Septal (heart) defect NOS

Q22 Congenital malformations of pulmonary and tricuspid valves

MCC Q22.0 Pulmonary valve atresia
CC Q22.1 Congenital pulmonary valve stenosis
CC Q22.2 Congenital pulmonary valve insufficiency
Congenital pulmonary valve regurgitation
CC Q22.3 Other congenital malformations of pulmonary valve
Congenital malformation of pulmonary valve NOS
Supernumerary cusps of pulmonary valve
MCC Q22.4 Congenital tricuspid stenosis
Congenital tricuspid atresia
MCC Q22.5 Ebstein's anomaly
MCC Q22.6 Hypoplastic right heart syndrome
MCC Q22.8 Other congenital malformations of tricuspid valve
MCC Q22.9 Congenital malformation of tricuspid valve, unspecified

Q23 Congenital malformations of aortic and mitral valves

Q23.0 Congenital stenosis of aortic valve
Congenital aortic atresia
Congenital aortic stenosis NOS
Excludes1: congenital stenosis of aortic valve in hypoplastic left heart syndrome (Q23.4)
congenital subaortic stenosis (Q24.4)
supravalvular aortic stenosis (congenital) (Q25.3)

Q23.1 Congenital insufficiency of aortic valve
Bicuspid aortic valve
Congenital aortic insufficiency
Q23.2 Congenital mitral stenosis
Congenital mitral atresia
CC Q23.3 Congenital mitral insufficiency
MCC Q23.4 Hypoplastic left heart syndrome
CC Q23.8 Other congenital malformations of aortic and mitral valves
CC Q23.9 Congenital malformation of aortic and mitral valves, unspecified

Q24 Other congenital malformations of heart

Excludes1: endocardial fibroelastosis (I42.4)
CC Q24.0 Dextrocardia
Excludes1: dextrocardia with situs inversus (Q89.3)
isomerism of atrial appendages (with asplenia or polysplenia) (Q20.6)
mirror-image atrial arrangement with situs inversus (Q89.3)

CC Q24.1 Levocardia
MCC Q24.2 Cor triatriatum
CC Q24.3 Pulmonary infundibular stenosis
Subvalvular pulmonic stenosis

MCC Q24.4 Congenital subaortic stenosis
CC Q24.5 Malformation of coronary vessels
Congenital coronary (artery) aneurysm
MCC Q24.6 Congenital heart block
Q24.8 Other specified congenital malformations of heart
Congenital diverticulum of left ventricle
Congenital malformation of myocardium
Congenital malformation of pericardium
Malposition of heart
Uhl's disease
Q24.9 Congenital malformation of heart, unspecified
Congenital anomaly of heart
Congenital disease of heart

Q25 Congenital malformations of great arteries

CC Q25.0 Patent ductus arteriosus
Patent ductus Botallo
Persistent ductus arteriosus
CC Q25.1 Coarctation of aorta
Coarctation of aorta (preductal) (postductal)
Stenosis of aorta
AHA CC: 4Q, 2016, 56-57
+ Q25.2 Atresia of aorta
AHA CC: 4Q, 2016, 56-57
CC Q25.21 Interruption of aortic arch
Atresia of aortic arch
CC Q25.29 Other atresia of aorta
Atresia of aorta
CC Q25.3 Supravalvular aortic stenosis
Excludes1: congenital aortic stenosis NOS (Q23.0)
congenital stenosis of aortic valve (Q23.0)
+ Q25.4 Other congenital malformations of aorta
Excludes1: hypoplasia of aorta in hypoplastic left heart syndrome (Q23.4)
AHA CC: 4Q, 2016, 57
CC Q25.40 Congenital malformation of aorta unspecified
CC Q25.41 Absence and aplasia of aorta
CC Q25.42 Hypoplasia of aorta
CC Q25.43 Congenital aneurysm of aorta
Congenital aneurysm of aortic root
Congenital aneurysm of aortic sinus
CC Q25.44 Congenital dilation of aorta
CC Q25.45 Double aortic arch
Vascular ring of aorta
CC Q25.46 Tortuous aortic arch
Persistent convolutions of aortic arch
CC Q25.47 Right aortic arch
Persistent right aortic arch
CC Q25.48 Anomalous origin of subclavian artery
CC Q25.49 Other congenital malformations of aorta
Aortic arch
Bovine arch
MCC Q25.5 Atresia of pulmonary artery
MCC Q25.6 Stenosis of pulmonary artery
Supravalvular pulmonary stenosis
+ Q25.7 Other congenital malformations of pulmonary artery
MCC Q25.71 Coarctation of pulmonary artery
MCC Q25.72 Congenital pulmonary arteriovenous malformation
Congenital pulmonary arteriovenous aneurysm
MCC Q25.79 Other congenital malformations of pulmonary artery
Aberrant pulmonary artery
Agenesis of pulmonary artery
Congenital aneurysm of pulmonary artery
Congenital anomaly of pulmonary artery
Hypoplasia of pulmonary artery
Q25.8 Other congenital malformations of other great arteries
CC Q25.9 Congenital malformation of great arteries, unspecified

Q26 Congenital malformations of great veins

CC Q26.0 Congenital stenosis of vena cava
Congenital stenosis of vena cava (inferior)(superior)
CC Q26.1 Persistent left superior vena cava
CC Q26.2 Total anomalous pulmonary venous connection
Total anomalous pulmonary venous return [TAPVR], subdiaphragmatic
Total anomalous pulmonary venous return [TAPVR], supradiaphragmatic

CC	Q26.3	Partial anomalous pulmonary venous connection
		Partial anomalous pulmonary venous return
CC	Q26.4	Anomalous pulmonary venous connection, unspecified
	Q26.5	Anomalous portal venous connection
	Q26.6	Portal vein-hepatic artery fistula
CC	Q26.8	Other congenital malformations of great veins
		Absence of vena cava (inferior) (superior)
		Azygos continuation of inferior vena cava
		Persistent left posterior cardinal vein
		Scimitar syndrome
CC	Q26.9	Congenital malformation of great vein, unspecified
		Congenital anomaly of vena cava (inferior) (superior) NOS

Q27 Other congenital malformations of peripheral vascular system

Excludes2: anomalies of cerebral and precerebral vessels (Q28.0-Q28.3)
anomalies of coronary vessels (Q24.5)
anomalies of pulmonary artery (Q25.5-Q25.7)
congenital retinal aneurysm (Q14.1)
hemangioma and lymphangioma (D18.-)

	Q27.0	Congenital absence and hypoplasia of umbilical artery
		Single umbilical artery
	Q27.1	Congenital renal artery stenosis
	Q27.2	Other congenital malformations of renal artery
		Congenital malformation of renal artery NOS
		Multiple renal arteries
+	Q27.3	Arteriovenous malformation (peripheral)
		Arteriovenous aneurysm

Excludes1: acquired arteriovenous aneurysm (I77.0)
Excludes2: arteriovenous malformation of cerebral vessels (Q28.2)
arteriovenous malformation of precerebral vessels (Q28.0)

CC	Q27.30	Arteriovenous malformation, site unspecified
	Q27.31	Arteriovenous malformation of vessel of upper limb
	Q27.32	Arteriovenous malformation of vessel of lower limb
	Q27.33	Arteriovenous malformation of digestive system vessel
	Q27.34	Arteriovenous malformation of renal vessel
	Q27.39	Arteriovenous malformation, other site
CC	Q27.4	Congenital phlebectasia
	Q27.8	Other specified congenital malformations of peripheral vascular system
		Absence of peripheral vascular system
		Atresia of peripheral vascular system
		Congenital aneurysm (peripheral)
		Congenital stricture, artery
		Congenital varix

Excludes1: arteriovenous malformation (Q27.3-)

	Q27.9	Congenital malformation of peripheral vascular system, unspecified
		Anomaly of artery or vein NOS

Q28 Other congenital malformations of circulatory system

Excludes1: congenital aneurysm NOS (Q27.8)
congenital coronary aneurysm (Q24.5)
ruptured cerebral arteriovenous malformation (I60.8)
ruptured malformation of precerebral vessels (I72.0)
Excludes2: congenital peripheral aneurysm (Q27.8)
congenital pulmonary aneurysm (Q25.79)
congenital retinal aneurysm (Q14.1)

CC	Q28.0	Arteriovenous malformation of precerebral vessels
		Congenital arteriovenous precerebral aneurysm (nonruptured)
CC	Q28.1	Other malformations of precerebral vessels
		Congenital malformation of precerebral vessels NOS
		Congenital precerebral aneurysm (nonruptured)
MCC	Q28.2	Arteriovenous malformation of cerebral vessels
		Arteriovenous malformation of brain NOS
		Congenital arteriovenous cerebral aneurysm (nonruptured)
MCC	Q28.3	Other malformations of cerebral vessels
		Congenital cerebral aneurysm (nonruptured)
		Congenital malformation of cerebral vessels NOS
		Developmental venous anomaly
CC	Q28.8	Other specified congenital malformations of circulatory system
		Congenital aneurysm, specified site NEC
		Spinal vessel anomaly
CC	Q28.9	Congenital malformation of circulatory system, unspecified

Congenital malformations of the respiratory system (Q30-Q34)

Q30 Congenital malformations of nose

Excludes1: congenital deviation of nasal septum (Q67.4)

	Q30.0	Choanal atresia
		Atresia of nares (anterior) (posterior)
		Congenital stenosis of nares (anterior) (posterior)
	Q30.1	Agenesis and underdevelopment of nose
		Congenital absent of nose
	Q30.2	Fissured, notched and cleft nose
	Q30.3	Congenital perforated nasal septum
	Q30.8	Other congenital malformations of nose
		Accessory nose
		Congenital anomaly of nasal sinus wall
		AHA CC: 2Q, 2022, 17
	Q30.9	Congenital malformation of nose, unspecified

Q31 Congenital malformations of larynx

Excludes1: congenital laryngeal stridor NOS (P28.89)

	Q31.0	Web of larynx
		Glottic web of larynx
		Subglottic web of larynx
		Web of larynx NOS
CC	Q31.1	Congenital subglottic stenosis
CC	Q31.2	Laryngeal hypoplasia
CC	Q31.3	Laryngocele
CC	Q31.5	Congenital laryngomalacia
CC	Q31.8	Other congenital malformations of larynx
		Absence of larynx
		Agenesis of larynx
		Atresia of larynx
		Congenital cleft thyroid cartilage
		Congenital fissure of epiglottis
		Congenital stenosis of larynx NEC
		Posterior cleft of cricoid cartilage
CC	Q31.9	Congenital malformation of larynx, unspecified

Q32 Congenital malformations of trachea and bronchus

Excludes1: congenital bronchiectasis (Q33.4)

CC	Q32.0	Congenital tracheomalacia
CC	Q32.1	Other congenital malformations of trachea
		Atresia of trachea
		Congenital anomaly of tracheal cartilage
		Congenital dilatation of trachea
		Congenital malformation of trachea
		Congenital stenosis of trachea
		Congenital tracheocele
CC	Q32.2	Congenital bronchomalacia
CC	Q32.3	Congenital stenosis of bronchus
CC	Q32.4	Other congenital malformations of bronchus
		Absence of bronchus
		Agenesis of bronchus
		Atresia of bronchus
		Congenital diverticulum of bronchus
		Congenital malformation of bronchus NOS

Q33 Congenital malformations of lung

CC	Q33.0	Congenital cystic lung
		Congenital cystic lung disease
		Congenital honeycomb lung
		Congenital polycystic lung disease

Excludes1: cystic fibrosis (E84.0)
cystic lung disease, acquired or unspecified (J98.4)

	Q33.1	Accessory lobe of lung
		Azygos lobe (fissured), lung
MCC	Q33.2	Sequestration of lung
MCC	Q33.3	Agenesis of lung
		Congenital absence of lung (lobe)
CC	Q33.4	Congenital bronchiectasis
	Q33.5	Ectopic tissue in lung
MCC	Q33.6	Congenital hypoplasia and dysplasia of lung

Excludes1: pulmonary hypoplasia associated with short gestation (P28.0)

	Q33.8	Other congenital malformations of lung
	Q33.9	Congenital malformation of lung, unspecified

Q34 Other congenital malformations of respiratory system
  Excludes2: congenital central alveolar hypoventilation syndrome (G47.35)
  Q34.0 Anomaly of pleura
  Q34.1 Congenital cyst of mediastinum
  Q34.8 Other specified congenital malformations of respiratory system
    Atresia of nasopharynx
  Q34.9 Congenital malformation of respiratory system, unspecified
    Congenital absence of respiratory system
    Congenital anomaly of respiratory system NOS

Cleft lip and cleft palate (Q35-Q37)

Use additional code to identify associated malformation of the nose (Q30.2)
Excludes2: Robin's syndrome (Q87.0)

Q35 Cleft palate
  Includes: fissure of palate
    palatoschisis
  Excludes1: cleft palate with cleft lip (Q37.-)
  Q35.1 Cleft hard palate
  Q35.3 Cleft soft palate
  Q35.5 Cleft hard palate with cleft soft palate
  Q35.7 Cleft uvula
  Q35.9 Cleft palate, unspecified
    Cleft palate NOS

Q36 Cleft lip
  Includes: cheiloschisis
    congenital fissure of lip
    harelip
    labium leporinum
  Excludes1: cleft lip with cleft palate (Q37.-)
  Q36.0 Cleft lip, bilateral
  Q36.1 Cleft lip, median
  Q36.9 Cleft lip, unilateral
    Cleft lip NOS

Q37 Cleft palate with cleft lip
  Includes: cheilopalatoschisis
  Q37.0 Cleft hard palate with bilateral cleft lip
  Q37.1 Cleft hard palate with unilateral cleft lip
    Cleft hard palate with cleft lip NOS
  Q37.2 Cleft soft palate with bilateral cleft lip
  Q37.3 Cleft soft palate with unilateral cleft lip
    Cleft soft palate with cleft lip NOS
  Q37.4 Cleft hard and soft palate with bilateral cleft lip
  Q37.5 Cleft hard and soft palate with unilateral cleft lip
    Cleft hard and soft palate with cleft lip NOS
  Q37.8 Unspecified cleft palate with bilateral cleft lip
  Q37.9 Unspecified cleft palate with unilateral cleft lip
    Cleft palate with cleft lip NOS

Other congenital malformations of the digestive system (Q38-Q45)

Q38 Other congenital malformations of tongue, mouth and pharynx
  Excludes1: dentofacial anomalies (M26.-)
    macrostomia (Q18.4)
    microstomia (Q18.5)
  Q38.0 Congenital malformations of lips, not elsewhere classified
    Congenital fistula of lip
    Congenital malformation of lip NOS
    Van der Woude's syndrome
    Excludes1: cleft lip (Q36.-)
      cleft lip with cleft palate (Q37.-)
      macrocheilia (Q18.6)
      microcheilia (Q18.7)
  Q38.1 Ankyloglossia
    Tongue tie
  Q38.2 Macroglossia
    Congenital hypertrophy of tongue

Q38.3 Other congenital malformations of tongue
    Aglossia
    Bifid tongue
    Congenital adhesion of tongue
    Congenital fissure of tongue
    Congenital malformation of tongue NOS
    Double tongue
    Hypoglossia
    Hypoplasia of tongue
    Microglossia
  Q38.4 Congenital malformations of salivary glands and ducts
    Atresia of salivary glands and ducts
    Congenital absence of salivary glands and ducts
    Congenital accessory salivary glands and ducts
    Congenital fistula of salivary gland
  Q38.5 Congenital malformations of palate, not elsewhere classified
    Congenital absence of uvula
    Congenital malformation of palate NOS
    Congenital high arched palate
    Excludes1: cleft palate (Q35.-)
      cleft palate with cleft lip (Q37.-)
  Q38.6 Other congenital malformations of mouth
    Congenital malformation of mouth NOS
  Q38.7 Congenital pharyngeal pouch
    Congenital diverticulum of pharynx
    Excludes1: pharyngeal pouch syndrome (D82.1)
  Q38.8 Other congenital malformations of pharynx
    Congenital malformation of pharynx NOS
    Imperforate pharynx

Q39 Congenital malformations of esophagus
  MCC **Q39.0** Atresia of esophagus without fistula
    Atresia of esophagus NOS
  MCC **Q39.1** Atresia of esophagus with tracheo-esophageal fistula
    Atresia of esophagus with broncho-esophageal fistula
  MCC **Q39.2** Congenital tracheo-esophageal fistula without atresia
    Congenital tracheo-esophageal fistula NOS
  MCC **Q39.3** Congenital stenosis and stricture of esophagus
  MCC **Q39.4** Esophageal web
  CC **Q39.5** Congenital dilatation of esophagus
    Congenital cardiospasm
  CC **Q39.6** Congenital diverticulum of esophagus
    Congenital esophageal pouch
  CC **Q39.8** Other congenital malformations of esophagus
    Congenital absence of esophagus
    Congenital displacement of esophagus
    Congenital duplication of esophagus
  CC **Q39.9** Congenital malformation of esophagus, unspecified

Q40 Other congenital malformations of upper alimentary tract
  Q40.0 Congenital hypertrophic pyloric stenosis
    Congenital or infantile constriction
    Congenital or infantile hypertrophy
    Congenital or infantile spasm
    Congenital or infantile stenosis
    Congenital or infantile stricture
  Q40.1 Congenital hiatus hernia
    Congenital displacement of cardia through esophageal hiatus
    Excludes1: congenital diaphragmatic hernia (Q79.0)
  Q40.2 Other specified congenital malformations of stomach
    Congenital displacement of stomach
    Congenital diverticulum of stomach
    Congenital hourglass stomach
    Congenital duplication of stomach
    Megalogastria
    Microgastria
  Q40.3 Congenital malformation of stomach, unspecified
  Q40.8 Other specified congenital malformations of upper alimentary tract
  Q40.9 Congenital malformation of upper alimentary tract, unspecified
    Congenital anomaly of upper alimentary tract
    Congenital deformity of upper alimentary tract

Q41 Congenital absence, atresia and stenosis of small intestine
    Includes: congenital obstruction, occlusion or stricture of small intestine or intestine NOS
    Excludes1: cystic fibrosis with intestinal manifestation (E84.11)
          meconium ileus NOS (without cystic fibrosis) (P76.0)
- CC **Q41.0** Congenital absence, atresia and stenosis of duodenum
- CC **Q41.1** Congenital absence, atresia and stenosis of jejunum
  - Apple peel syndrome
  - Imperforate jejunum
- CC **Q41.2** Congenital absence, atresia and stenosis of ileum
- CC **Q41.8** Congenital absence, atresia and stenosis of other specified parts of small intestine
- CC **Q41.9** Congenital absence, atresia and stenosis of small intestine, part unspecified
  - Congenital absence, atresia and stenosis of intestine NOS

Q42 Congenital absence, atresia and stenosis of large intestine
    Includes: congenital obstruction, occlusion and stricture of large intestine
- CC **Q42.0** Congenital absence, atresia and stenosis of rectum with fistula
- CC **Q42.1** Congenital absence, atresia and stenosis of rectum without fistula
  - Imperforate rectum
- CC **Q42.2** Congenital absence, atresia and stenosis of anus with fistula
- CC **Q42.3** Congenital absence, atresia and stenosis of anus without fistula
  - Imperforate anus
- CC **Q42.8** Congenital absence, atresia and stenosis of other parts of large intestine
- CC **Q42.9** Congenital absence, atresia and stenosis of large intestine, part unspecified

Q43 Other congenital malformations of intestine
- **Q43.0** Meckel's diverticulum (displaced) (hypertrophic)
  - Persistent omphalomesenteric duct
  - Persistent vitelline duct
- CC **Q43.1** Hirschsprung's disease
  - Aganglionosis
  - Congenital (aganglionic) megacolon
- CC **Q43.2** Other congenital functional disorders of colon
  - Congenital dilatation of colon
- CC **Q43.3** Congenital malformations of intestinal fixation
  - Congenital omental, anomalous adhesions [bands]
  - Congenital peritoneal adhesions [bands]
  - Incomplete rotation of cecum and colon
  - Insufficient rotation of cecum and colon
  - Jackson's membrane
  - Malrotation of colon
  - Rotation failure of cecum and colon
  - Universal mesentery
- CC **Q43.4** Duplication of intestine
- CC **Q43.5** Ectopic anus
- CC **Q43.6** Congenital fistula of rectum and anus
  - **Excludes1:** congenital fistula of anus with absence, atresia and stenosis (Q42.2)
  -     congenital fistula of rectum with absence, atresia and stenosis (Q42.0)
  -     congenital rectovaginal fistula (Q52.2)
  -     congenital urethrorectal fistula (Q64.73)
  -     pilonidal fistula or sinus (L05.-)
- CC **Q43.7** Persistent cloaca
  - Cloaca NOS
- CC **Q43.8** Other specified congenital malformations of intestine
  - Congenital blind loop syndrome
  - Congenital diverticulitis, colon
  - Congenital diverticulum, intestine
  - Dolichocolon
  - Megaloappendix
  - Megaloduodenum
  - Microcolon
  - Transposition of appendix
  - Transposition of colon
  - Transposition of intestine
  - *AHA CC: 2Q, 2013, 31*
- CC **Q43.9** Congenital malformation of intestine, unspecified

Q44 Congenital malformations of gallbladder, bile ducts and liver
- CC **Q44.0** Agenesis, aplasia and hypoplasia of gallbladder
  - Congenital absence of gallbladder
- CC **Q44.1** Other congenital malformations of gallbladder
  - Congenital malformation of gallbladder NOS
  - Intrahepatic gallbladder
- MCC **Q44.2** Atresia of bile ducts
- MCC **Q44.3** Congenital stenosis and stricture of bile ducts
- CC **Q44.4** Choledochal cyst
- CC **Q44.5** Other congenital malformations of bile ducts
  - Accessory hepatic duct
  - Biliary duct duplication
  - Congenital malformation of bile duct NOS
  - Cystic duct duplication
- CC **Q44.6** Cystic disease of liver
  - Fibrocystic disease of liver
- + **Q44.7** Other congenital malformations of liver
  - Code also, if applicable, associated malformations affecting other systems
  - CC **Q44.70** Other congenital malformation of liver, unspecified
    - Congenital malformation of liver, NOS
  - CC **Q44.71** Alagille syndrome
    - Alagille-Watson syndrome
  - CC **Q44.79** Other congenital malformations of liver
    - Accessory liver
    - Congenital absence of liver
    - Congenital hepatomegaly

Q45 Other congenital malformations of digestive system
    Excludes2: congenital diaphragmatic hernia (Q79.0)
          congenital hiatus hernia (Q40.1)
- CC **Q45.0** Agenesis, aplasia and hypoplasia of pancreas
  - Congenital absence of pancreas
- CC **Q45.1** Annular pancreas
- CC **Q45.2** Congenital pancreatic cyst
- **Q45.3** Other congenital malformations of pancreas and pancreatic duct
  - Accessory pancreas
  - Congenital malformation of pancreas or pancreatic duct NOS
  - **Excludes1:** congenital diabetes mellitus (E10.-)
  -     cystic fibrosis (E84.0-E84.9)
  -     fibrocystic disease of pancreas (E84.-)
  -     neonatal diabetes mellitus (P70.2)
- **Q45.8** Other specified congenital malformations of digestive system
  - Absence (complete) (partial) of alimentary tract NOS
  - Duplication of digestive system
  - Malposition, congenital of digestive system
- **Q45.9** Congenital malformation of digestive system, unspecified
  - Congenital anomaly of digestive system
  - Congenital deformity of digestive system

Congenital malformations of genital organs (Q50-Q56)

Excludes1: androgen insensitivity syndrome (E34.5-)
    syndromes associated with anomalies in the number and form of chromosomes (Q90-Q99)

Q50 Congenital malformations of ovaries, fallopian tubes and broad ligaments
- + **Q50.0** Congenital absence of ovary
  - **Excludes1:** Turner's syndrome (Q96.-)
  - ♀ **Q50.01** Congenital absence of ovary, unilateral
  - ♀ **Q50.02** Congenital absence of ovary, bilateral
- ♀ **Q50.1** Developmental ovarian cyst
- ♀ **Q50.2** Congenital torsion of ovary
- + **Q50.3** Other congenital malformations of ovary
  - ♀ **Q50.31** Accessory ovary
  - ♀ **Q50.32** Ovarian streak
    - 46, XX with streak gonads
  - ♀ **Q50.39** Other congenital malformation of ovary
    - Congenital malformation of ovary NOS
- ♀ **Q50.4** Embryonic cyst of fallopian tube
  - Fimbrial cyst
- ♀ **Q50.5** Embryonic cyst of broad ligament
  - Epoophoron cyst
  - Parovarian cyst

Q50.6 Other congenital malformations of fallopian tube and broad ligament
  Absence of fallopian tube and broad ligament
  Accessory fallopian tube and broad ligament
  Atresia of fallopian tube and broad ligament
  Congenital malformation of fallopian tube or broad ligament NOS

Q51 Congenital malformations of uterus and cervix

Q51.0 Agenesis and aplasia of uterus
  Congenital absence of uterus
+ **Q51.1** Doubling of uterus with doubling of cervix and vagina
  Q51.10 Doubling of uterus with doubling of cervix and vagina without obstruction
    Doubling of uterus with doubling of cervix and vagina NOS
  Q51.11 Doubling of uterus with doubling of cervix and vagina with obstruction
+ **Q51.2** Other doubling of uterus
  Doubling of uterus NOS
  Septate uterus
  AHA CC: 4Q, 2018, 27
  Q51.21 Complete doubling of uterus
    Complete septate uterus
  Q51.22 Partial doubling of uterus
    Partial septate uterus
  Q51.28 Other and unspecified doubling of uterus
    Septate uterus NOS
Q51.3 Bicornate uterus
  Bicornate uterus, complete or partial
Q51.4 Unicornate uterus
  Unicornate uterus with or without a separate uterine horn
  Uterus with only one functioning horn
Q51.5 Agenesis and aplasia of cervix
  Congenital absence of cervix
Q51.6 Embryonic cyst of cervix
Q51.7 Congenital fistulae between uterus and digestive and urinary tracts
+ **Q51.8** Other congenital malformations of uterus and cervix
  + **Q51.81** Other congenital malformations of uterus
    Q51.810 Arcuate uterus
      Arcuatus uterus
    Q51.811 Hypoplasia of uterus
    Q51.818 Other congenital malformations of uterus
      Müllerian anomaly of uterus NEC
  + **Q51.82** Other congenital malformations of cervix
    Q51.820 Cervical duplication
    Q51.821 Hypoplasia of cervix
    Q51.828 Other congenital malformations of cervix
Q51.9 Congenital malformation of uterus and cervix, unspecified

Q52 Other congenital malformations of female genitalia

Q52.0 Congenital absence of vagina
  Vaginal agenesis, total or partial
+ **Q52.1** Doubling of vagina
  Excludes1: *doubling of vagina with doubling of uterus and cervix (Q51.1-)*
  Q52.10 Doubling of vagina, unspecified
    Septate vagina NOS
  Q52.11 Transverse vaginal septum
  + **Q52.12** Longitudinal vaginal septum
    AHA CC: 4Q, 2016, 58-59
    Q52.120 Longitudinal vaginal septum, nonobstructing
    Q52.121 Longitudinal vaginal septum, obstructing, right side
    Q52.122 Longitudinal vaginal septum, obstructing, left side
    Q52.123 Longitudinal vaginal septum, microperforate, right side
    Q52.124 Longitudinal vaginal septum, microperforate, left side
    AHA CC: 4Q, 2016, 58-59
    Q52.129 Other and unspecified longitudinal vaginal septum
Q52.2 Congenital rectovaginal fistula
  Excludes1: *cloaca (Q43.7)*
Q52.3 Imperforate hymen

Q52.4 Other congenital malformations of vagina
  Canal of Nuck cyst, congenital
  Congenital malformation of vagina NOS
  Embryonic vaginal cyst
  Gartner's duct cyst
Q52.5 Fusion of labia
Q52.6 Congenital malformation of clitoris
+ **Q52.7** Other and unspecified congenital malformations of vulva
  Q52.70 Unspecified congenital malformations of vulva
    Congenital malformation of vulva NOS
  Q52.71 Congenital absence of vulva
  Q52.79 Other congenital malformations of vulva
    Congenital cyst of vulva
Q52.8 Other specified congenital malformations of female genitalia
Q52.9 Congenital malformation of female genitalia, unspecified

Q53 Undescended and ectopic testicle
AHA CC: 4Q, 2017, 22-23
+ **Q53.0** Ectopic testis
  Q53.00 Ectopic testis, unspecified
  Q53.01 Ectopic testis, unilateral
  Q53.02 Ectopic testes, bilateral
+ **Q53.1** Undescended testicle, unilateral
  Q53.10 Unspecified undescended testicle, unilateral
  + **Q53.11** Abdominal testis, unilateral
    Q53.111 Unilateral intraabdominal testis
    Q53.112 Unilateral inguinal testis
  Q53.12 Ectopic perineal testis, unilateral
  Q53.13 Unilateral high scrotal testis
+ **Q53.2** Undescended testicle, bilateral
  Q53.20 Undescended testicle, unspecified, bilateral
  + **Q53.21** Abdominal testis, bilateral
    Q53.211 Bilateral intraabdominal testes
    Q53.212 Bilateral inguinal testes
  Q53.22 Ectopic perineal testis, bilateral
  Q53.23 Bilateral high scrotal testes
Q53.9 Undescended testicle, unspecified
  Cryptorchism NOS

Q54 Hypospadias
Excludes1: *epispadias (Q64.0)*
Q54.0 Hypospadias, balanic
  Hypospadias, coronal
  Hypospadias, glandular
Q54.1 Hypospadias, penile
Q54.2 Hypospadias, penoscrotal
Q54.3 Hypospadias, perineal
Q54.4 Congenital chordee
  Chordee without hypospadias
Q54.8 Other hypospadias
  Hypospadias with intersex state
Q54.9 Hypospadias, unspecified

Q55 Other congenital malformations of male genital organs
Excludes1: *congenital hydrocele (P83.5)*
  hypospadias (Q54.-)
Q55.0 Absence and aplasia of testis
  Monorchism
Q55.1 Hypoplasia of testis and scrotum
  Fusion of testes
+ **Q55.2** Other and unspecified congenital malformations of testis and scrotum
  Q55.20 Unspecified congenital malformations of testis and scrotum
    Congenital malformation of testis or scrotum NOS
  Q55.21 Polyorchism
  Q55.22 Retractile testis
  Q55.23 Scrotal transposition
  Q55.29 Other congenital malformations of testis and scrotum
Q55.3 Atresia of vas deferens
  Code first any associated cystic fibrosis (E84.-)
Q55.4 Other congenital malformations of vas deferens, epididymis, seminal vesicles and prostate
  Absence or aplasia of prostate
  Absence or aplasia of spermatic cord
  Congenital malformation of vas deferens, epididymis, seminal vesicles or prostate NOS
Q55.5 Congenital absence and aplasia of penis

- **+ Q55.6 Other congenital malformations of penis**
  - ♂ Q55.61 Curvature of penis (lateral)
  - ♂ Q55.62 Hypoplasia of penis
    - Micropenis
  - ♂ Q55.63 Congenital torsion of penis
    - **Excludes1:** acquired torsion of penis (N48.82)
  - ♂ Q55.64 Hidden penis
    - Buried penis
    - Concealed penis
    - **Excludes1:** acquired buried penis (N48.83)
  - ♂ Q55.69 Other congenital malformation of penis
    - Congenital malformation of penis NOS
- ♂ **Q55.7 Congenital vasocutaneous fistula**
- ♂ **Q55.8 Other specified congenital malformations of male genital organs**
- ♂ **Q55.9 Congenital malformation of male genital organ, unspecified**
  - Congenital anomaly of male genital organ
  - Congenital deformity of male genital organ

Q56 Indeterminate sex and pseudohermaphroditism

Excludes1: 46,XX true hermaphrodite (Q99.1)
androgen insensitivity syndrome (E34.5-)
chimera 46,XX/46,XY true hermaphrodite (Q99.0)
female pseudohermaphroditism with adrenocortical disorder (E25.-)
pseudohermaphroditism with specified chromosomal anomaly (Q96-Q99)
pure gonadal dysgenesis (Q99.1)

- **Q56.0 Hermaphroditism, not elsewhere classified**
  - Ovotestis
- ♂ **Q56.1 Male pseudohermaphroditism, not elsewhere classified**
  - 46, XY with streak gonads
  - Male pseudohermaphroditism NOS
- ♀ **Q56.2 Female pseudohermaphroditism, not elsewhere classified**
  - Female pseudohermaphroditism NOS
- **Q56.3 Pseudohermaphroditism, unspecified**
- **Q56.4 Indeterminate sex, unspecified**
  - Ambiguous genitalia

Congenital malformations of the urinary system (Q60-Q64)

Q60 Renal agenesis and other reduction defects of kidney

Includes: congenital absence of kidney
congenital atrophy of kidney
infantile atrophy of kidney

- CC **Q60.0 Renal agenesis, unilateral**
- CC **Q60.1 Renal agenesis, bilateral**
- CC **Q60.2 Renal agenesis, unspecified**
- CC **Q60.3 Renal hypoplasia, unilateral**
- CC **Q60.4 Renal hypoplasia, bilateral**
- CC **Q60.5 Renal hypoplasia, unspecified**
- CC **Q60.6 Potter's syndrome**

Q61 Cystic kidney disease

Excludes1: acquired cyst of kidney (N28.1)
Potter's syndrome (Q60.6)

- + **Q61.0 Congenital renal cyst**
  - CC **Q61.00 Congenital renal cyst, unspecified**
    - Cyst of kidney NOS (congenital)
  - CC **Q61.01 Congenital single renal cyst**
  - CC **Q61.02 Congenital multiple renal cysts**
- + **Q61.1 Polycystic kidney, infantile type**
  - Polycystic kidney, autosomal recessive
  - CC **Q61.11 Cystic dilatation of collecting ducts**
  - CC **Q61.19 Other polycystic kidney, infantile type**
- CC **Q61.2 Polycystic kidney, adult type**
  - Polycystic kidney, autosomal dominant
- CC **Q61.3 Polycystic kidney, unspecified**
  - *AHA CC: 3Q, 2016, 22-23*
- CC **Q61.4 Renal dysplasia**
  - Multicystic dysplastic kidney
  - Multicystic kidney (development)
  - Multicystic kidney disease
  - Multicystic renal dysplasia
  - **Excludes1:** polycystic kidney disease (Q61.11-Q61.3)
- CC **Q61.5 Medullary cystic kidney**
  - Nephronophthisis
  - Sponge kidney NOS
- CC **Q61.8 Other cystic kidney diseases**
  - Fibrocystic kidney
  - Fibrocystic renal degeneration or disease
- CC **Q61.9 Cystic kidney disease, unspecified**
  - Meckel-Gruber syndrome

Q62 Congenital obstructive defects of renal pelvis and congenital malformations of ureter

- CC **Q62.0 Congenital hydronephrosis**
- + **Q62.1 Congenital occlusion of ureter**
  - Atresia and stenosis of ureter
  - CC **Q62.10 Congenital occlusion of ureter, unspecified**
  - CC **Q62.11 Congenital occlusion of ureteropelvic junction**
  - CC **Q62.12 Congenital occlusion of ureterovesical orifice**
- **Q62.2 Congenital megaureter**
  - Congenital dilatation of ureter
- + **Q62.3 Other obstructive defects of renal pelvis and ureter**
  - CC **Q62.31 Congenital ureterocele, orthotopic**
  - CC **Q62.32 Cecoureterocele**
    - Ectopic ureterocele
  - CC **Q62.39 Other obstructive defects of renal pelvis and ureter**
    - Ureteropelvic junction obstruction NOS
- **Q62.4 Agenesis of ureter**
  - Congenital absence ureter
- **Q62.5 Duplication of ureter**
  - Accessory ureter
  - Double ureter
- + **Q62.6 Malposition of ureter**
  - **Q62.60 Malposition of ureter, unspecified**
  - **Q62.61 Deviation of ureter**
  - **Q62.62 Displacement of ureter**
  - **Q62.63 Anomalous implantation of ureter**
    - Ectopia of ureter
    - Ectopic ureter
  - **Q62.69 Other malposition of ureter**
- **Q62.7 Congenital vesico-uretero-renal reflux**
- **Q62.8 Other congenital malformations of ureter**
  - Anomaly of ureter NOS

Q63 Other congenital malformations of kidney

Excludes1: congenital nephrotic syndrome (N04.-)

- **Q63.0 Accessory kidney**
- **Q63.1 Lobulated, fused and horseshoe kidney**
- **Q63.2 Ectopic kidney**
  - Congenital displaced kidney
  - Malrotation of kidney
- **Q63.3 Hyperplastic and giant kidney**
  - Compensatory hypertrophy of kidney
- **Q63.8 Other specified congenital malformations of kidney**
  - Congenital renal calculi
- **Q63.9 Congenital malformation of kidney, unspecified**

Q64 Other congenital malformations of urinary system

- **Q64.0 Epispadias**
  - **Excludes1:** hypospadias (Q54.-)
- + **Q64.1 Exstrophy of urinary bladder**
  - CC **Q64.10 Exstrophy of urinary bladder, unspecified**
    - Ectopia vesicae
  - CC **Q64.11 Supravesical fissure of urinary bladder**
  - CC **Q64.12 Cloacal exstrophy of urinary bladder**
  - CC **Q64.19 Other exstrophy of urinary bladder**
    - Extroversion of bladder
- CC **Q64.2 Congenital posterior urethral valves**
- + **Q64.3 Other atresia and stenosis of urethra and bladder neck**
  - CC **Q64.31 Congenital bladder neck obstruction**
    - Congenital obstruction of vesicourethral orifice
  - CC **Q64.32 Congenital stricture of urethra**
  - CC **Q64.33 Congenital stricture of urinary meatus**
  - CC **Q64.39 Other atresia and stenosis of urethra and bladder neck**
    - Atresia and stenosis of urethra and bladder neck NOS
- **Q64.4 Malformation of urachus**
  - Cyst of urachus
  - Patent urachus
  - Prolapse of urachus
- **Q64.5 Congenital absence of bladder and urethra**
- **Q64.6 Congenital diverticulum of bladder**
- + **Q64.7 Other and unspecified congenital malformations of bladder and urethra**
  - **Excludes1:** congenital prolapse of bladder (mucosa) (Q79.4)

Q64.70 Unspecified congenital malformation of bladder and urethra
Malformation of bladder or urethra NOS
Q64.71 Congenital prolapse of urethra
Q64.72 Congenital prolapse of urinary meatus
Q64.73 Congenital urethrorectal fistula
Q64.74 Double urethra
Q64.75 Double urinary meatus
Q64.79 Other congenital malformations of bladder and urethra
Q64.8 Other specified congenital malformations of urinary system
Q64.9 Congenital malformation of urinary system, unspecified
Congenital anomaly NOS of urinary system
Congenital deformity NOS of urinary system

Congenital malformations and deformations of the musculoskeletal system (Q65-Q79)

Q65 Congenital deformities of hip
Excludes1: clicking hip (R29.4)
+ Q65.0 Congenital dislocation of hip, unilateral
Q65.00 Congenital dislocation of unspecified hip, unilateral
Q65.01 Congenital dislocation of right hip, unilateral
Q65.02 Congenital dislocation of left hip, unilateral
Q65.1 Congenital dislocation of hip, bilateral
Q65.2 Congenital dislocation of hip, unspecified
+ Q65.3 Congenital partial dislocation of hip, unilateral
Q65.30 Congenital partial dislocation of unspecified hip, unilateral
Q65.31 Congenital partial dislocation of right hip, unilateral
Q65.32 Congenital partial dislocation of left hip, unilateral
Q65.4 Congenital partial dislocation of hip, bilateral
Q65.5 Congenital partial dislocation of hip, unspecified
Q65.6 Congenital unstable hip
Congenital dislocatable hip
+ Q65.8 Other congenital deformities of hip
Q65.81 Congenital coxa valga
Q65.82 Congenital coxa vara
Q65.89 Other specified congenital deformities of hip
Anteversion of femoral neck
Congenital acetabular dysplasia
Q65.9 Congenital deformity of hip, unspecified

Q66 Congenital deformities of feet
Excludes1: reduction defects of feet (Q72.-)
valgus deformities (acquired) (M21.0-)
varus deformities (acquired) (M21.1-)
AHA CC: 4Q, 2019, 13
+ Q66.0 Congenital talipes equinovarus
Q66.00 Congenital talipes equinovarus, unspecified foot
Q66.01 Congenital talipes equinovarus, right foot
Q66.02 Congenital talipes equinovarus, left foot
+ Q66.1 Congenital talipes calcaneovarus
Q66.10 Congenital talipes calcaneovarus, unspecified foot
Q66.11 Congenital talipes calcaneovarus, right foot
Q66.12 Congenital talipes calcaneovarus, left foot
+ Q66.2 Congenital metatarsus (primus) varus
AHA CC: 4Q, 2016, 59
+ Q66.21 Congenital metatarsus primus varus
Q66.211 Congenital metatarsus primus varus, right foot
Q66.212 Congenital metatarsus primus varus, left foot
Q66.219 Congenital metatarsus primus varus, unspecified foot
+ Q66.22 Congenital metatarsus adductus
Congenital metatarsus varus
Q66.221 Congenital metatarsus adductus, right foot
Q66.222 Congenital metatarsus adductus, left foot
Q66.229 Congenital metatarsus adductus, unspecified foot
+ Q66.3 Other congenital varus deformities of feet
Hallux varus, congenital
Q66.30 Other congenital varus deformities of feet, unspecified foot
Q66.31 Other congenital varus deformities of feet, right foot
Q66.32 Other congenital varus deformities of feet, left foot
+ Q66.4 Congenital talipes calcaneovalgus
Q66.40 Congenital talipes calcaneovalgus, unspecified foot
Q66.41 Congenital talipes calcaneovalgus, right foot
Q66.42 Congenital talipes calcaneovalgus, left foot
+ Q66.5 Congenital pes planus
Congenital flat foot
Congenital rigid flat foot
Congenital spastic (everted) flat foot
Excludes1: pes planus, acquired (M21.4)
Q66.50 Congenital pes planus, unspecified foot
Q66.51 Congenital pes planus, right foot
Q66.52 Congenital pes planus, left foot
Q66.6 Other congenital valgus deformities of feet
Congenital metatarsus valgus
+ Q66.7 Congenital pes cavus
Q66.70 Congenital pes cavus, unspecified foot
Q66.71 Congenital pes cavus, right foot
Q66.72 Congenital pes cavus, left foot
+ Q66.8 Other congenital deformities of feet
Q66.80 Congenital vertical talus deformity, unspecified foot
Q66.81 Congenital vertical talus deformity, right foot
Q66.82 Congenital vertical talus deformity, left foot
Q66.89 Other specified congenital deformities of feet
Congenital asymmetric talipes
Congenital clubfoot NOS
Congenital talipes NOS
Congenital tarsal coalition
Hammer toe, congenital
+ Q66.9 Congenital deformity of feet, unspecified
Q66.90 Congenital deformity of feet, unspecified, unspecified foot
Q66.91 Congenital deformity of feet, unspecified, right foot
Q66.92 Congenital deformity of feet, unspecified, left foot

Q67 Congenital musculoskeletal deformities of head, face, spine and chest
Excludes1: congenital malformation syndromes classified to Q87.-
Potter's syndrome (Q60.6)
Q67.0 Congenital facial asymmetry
Q67.1 Congenital compression facies
Q67.2 Dolichocephaly
Excludes1: sagittal craniosynostosis (Q75.01)
Q67.3 Plagiocephaly
Excludes1: coronal craniosynostosis (Q75.02-)
lambdoid craniosynostosis (Q75.04-)
Q67.4 Other congenital deformities of skull, face and jaw
Congenital depressions in skull
Congenital hemifacial atrophy or hypertrophy
Deviation of nasal septum, congenital
Squashed or bent nose, congenital
Excludes1: dentofacial anomalies [including malocclusion] (M26.-)
syphilitic saddle nose (A50.5)
CC Q67.5 Congenital deformity of spine
Congenital postural scoliosis
Congenital scoliosis NOS
Excludes1: infantile idiopathic scoliosis (M41.0)
scoliosis due to congenital bony malformation (Q76.3)
AHA CC: 4Q, 2014, 26
Q67.6 Pectus excavatum
Congenital funnel chest
Q67.7 Pectus carinatum
Congenital pigeon chest
CC Q67.8 Other congenital deformities of chest
Congenital deformity of chest wall NOS

Q68 Other congenital musculoskeletal deformities
Excludes1: reduction defects of limb(s) (Q71-Q73)
Excludes2: congenital myotonic chondrodystrophy (G71.13)
Q68.0 Congenital deformity of sternocleidomastoid muscle
Congenital contracture of sternocleidomastoid (muscle)
Congenital (sternomastoid) torticollis
Sternomastoid tumor (congenital)
CC Q68.1 Congenital deformity of finger(s) and hand
Congenital clubfinger
Spade-like hand (congenital)
Q68.2 Congenital deformity of knee
Congenital dislocation of knee
Congenital genu recurvatum

- **Q68.3** Congenital bowing of femur
  - *Excludes1:* anteversion of femur (neck) (Q65.89)
- **Q68.4** Congenital bowing of tibia and fibula
- **Q68.5** Congenital bowing of long bones of leg, unspecified
- **Q68.6** Discoid meniscus
- **Q68.8** Other specified congenital musculoskeletal deformities
  - Congenital deformity of clavicle
  - Congenital deformity of elbow
  - Congenital deformity of forearm
  - Congenital deformity of scapula
  - Congenital deformity of wrist
  - Congenital dislocation of elbow
  - Congenital dislocation of shoulder
  - Congenital dislocation of wrist

Q69 Polydactyly
- **Q69.0** Accessory finger(s)
- **Q69.1** Accessory thumb(s)
- **Q69.2** Accessory toe(s)
  - Accessory hallux
- **Q69.9** Polydactyly, unspecified
  - Supernumerary digit(s) NOS

Q70 Syndactyly
- **+ Q70.0** Fused fingers
  - Complex syndactyly of fingers with synostosis
  - **Q70.00** Fused fingers, unspecified hand
  - **Q70.01** Fused fingers, right hand
  - **Q70.02** Fused fingers, left hand
  - **Q70.03** Fused fingers, bilateral
- **+ Q70.1** Webbed fingers
  - Simple syndactyly of fingers without synostosis
  - **Q70.10** Webbed fingers, unspecified hand
  - **Q70.11** Webbed fingers, right hand
  - **Q70.12** Webbed fingers, left hand
  - **Q70.13** Webbed fingers, bilateral
- **+ Q70.2** Fused toes
  - Complex syndactyly of toes with synostosis
  - **Q70.20** Fused toes, unspecified foot
  - **Q70.21** Fused toes, right foot
  - **Q70.22** Fused toes, left foot
  - **Q70.23** Fused toes, bilateral
- **+ Q70.3** Webbed toes
  - Simple syndactyly of toes without synostosis
  - **Q70.30** Webbed toes, unspecified foot
  - **Q70.31** Webbed toes, right foot
  - **Q70.32** Webbed toes, left foot
  - **Q70.33** Webbed toes, bilateral
- **Q70.4** Polysyndactyly, unspecified
  - *Excludes1:* specified syndactyly of hand and feet - code to specified conditions (Q70.0-Q70.3-)
- **Q70.9** Syndactyly, unspecified
  - Symphalangy NOS

Q71 Reduction defects of upper limb
- **+ Q71.0** Congenital complete absence of upper limb
  - **Q71.00** Congenital complete absence of unspecified upper limb
  - **Q71.01** Congenital complete absence of right upper limb
  - **Q71.02** Congenital complete absence of left upper limb
  - **Q71.03** Congenital complete absence of upper limb, bilateral
- **+ Q71.1** Congenital absence of upper arm and forearm with hand present
  - **Q71.10** Congenital absence of unspecified upper arm and forearm with hand present
  - **Q71.11** Congenital absence of right upper arm and forearm with hand present
  - **Q71.12** Congenital absence of left upper arm and forearm with hand present
  - **Q71.13** Congenital absence of upper arm and forearm with hand present, bilateral
- **+ Q71.2** Congenital absence of both forearm and hand
  - **Q71.20** Congenital absence of both forearm and hand, unspecified upper limb
  - **Q71.21** Congenital absence of both forearm and hand, right upper limb
  - **Q71.22** Congenital absence of both forearm and hand, left upper limb
  - **Q71.23** Congenital absence of both forearm and hand, bilateral
- **+ Q71.3** Congenital absence of hand and finger
  - **Q71.30** Congenital absence of unspecified hand and finger
  - **Q71.31** Congenital absence of right hand and finger
  - **Q71.32** Congenital absence of left hand and finger
  - **Q71.33** Congenital absence of hand and finger, bilateral
- **+ Q71.4** Longitudinal reduction defect of radius
  - Clubhand (congenital)
  - Radial clubhand
  - **Q71.40** Longitudinal reduction defect of unspecified radius
  - **Q71.41** Longitudinal reduction defect of right radius
  - **Q71.42** Longitudinal reduction defect of left radius
  - **Q71.43** Longitudinal reduction defect of radius, bilateral
- **+ Q71.5** Longitudinal reduction defect of ulna
  - **Q71.50** Longitudinal reduction defect of unspecified ulna
  - **Q71.51** Longitudinal reduction defect of right ulna
  - **Q71.52** Longitudinal reduction defect of left ulna
  - **Q71.53** Longitudinal reduction defect of ulna, bilateral
- **+ Q71.6** Lobster-claw hand
  - **Q71.60** Lobster-claw hand, unspecified hand
  - **Q71.61** Lobster-claw right hand
  - **Q71.62** Lobster-claw left hand
  - **Q71.63** Lobster-claw hand, bilateral
- **+ Q71.8** Other reduction defects of upper limb
  - **+ Q71.81** Congenital shortening of upper limb
    - **Q71.811** Congenital shortening of right upper limb
    - **Q71.812** Congenital shortening of left upper limb
    - **Q71.813** Congenital shortening of upper limb, bilateral
    - **Q71.819** Congenital shortening of unspecified upper limb
  - **+ Q71.89** Other reduction defects of upper limb
    - **Q71.891** Other reduction defects of right upper limb
    - **Q71.892** Other reduction defects of left upper limb
    - **Q71.893** Other reduction defects of upper limb, bilateral
    - **Q71.899** Other reduction defects of unspecified upper limb
- **+ Q71.9** Unspecified reduction defect of upper limb
  - **Q71.90** Unspecified reduction defect of unspecified upper limb
  - **Q71.91** Unspecified reduction defect of right upper limb
  - **Q71.92** Unspecified reduction defect of left upper limb
  - **Q71.93** Unspecified reduction defect of upper limb, bilateral

Q72 Reduction defects of lower limb
- **+ Q72.0** Congenital complete absence of lower limb
  - **Q72.00** Congenital complete absence of unspecified lower limb
  - **Q72.01** Congenital complete absence of right lower limb
  - **Q72.02** Congenital complete absence of left lower limb
  - **Q72.03** Congenital complete absence of lower limb, bilateral
- **+ Q72.1** Congenital absence of thigh and lower leg with foot present
  - **Q72.10** Congenital absence of unspecified thigh and lower leg with foot present
  - **Q72.11** Congenital absence of right thigh and lower leg with foot present
  - **Q72.12** Congenital absence of left thigh and lower leg with foot present
  - **Q72.13** Congenital absence of thigh and lower leg with foot present, bilateral
- **+ Q72.2** Congenital absence of both lower leg and foot
  - **Q72.20** Congenital absence of both lower leg and foot, unspecified lower limb
  - **Q72.21** Congenital absence of both lower leg and foot, right lower limb
  - **Q72.22** Congenital absence of both lower leg and foot, left lower limb
  - **Q72.23** Congenital absence of both lower leg and foot, bilateral
- **+ Q72.3** Congenital absence of foot and toe(s)
  - **Q72.30** Congenital absence of unspecified foot and toe(s)
  - **Q72.31** Congenital absence of right foot and toe(s)
  - **Q72.32** Congenital absence of left foot and toe(s)
  - **Q72.33** Congenital absence of foot and toe(s), bilateral

- **Q72.4 Longitudinal reduction defect of femur**
  Proximal femoral focal deficiency
  - Q72.40 Longitudinal reduction defect of unspecified femur
  - Q72.41 Longitudinal reduction defect of right femur
  - Q72.42 Longitudinal reduction defect of left femur
  - Q72.43 Longitudinal reduction defect of femur, bilateral
- **Q72.5 Longitudinal reduction defect of tibia**
  - Q72.50 Longitudinal reduction defect of unspecified tibia
  - Q72.51 Longitudinal reduction defect of right tibia
  - Q72.52 Longitudinal reduction defect of left tibia
  - Q72.53 Longitudinal reduction defect of tibia, bilateral
- **Q72.6 Longitudinal reduction defect of fibula**
  - Q72.60 Longitudinal reduction defect of unspecified fibula
  - Q72.61 Longitudinal reduction defect of right fibula
  - Q72.62 Longitudinal reduction defect of left fibula
  - Q72.63 Longitudinal reduction defect of fibula, bilateral
- **Q72.7 Split foot**
  - Q72.70 Split foot, unspecified lower limb
  - Q72.71 Split foot, right lower limb
  - Q72.72 Split foot, left lower limb
  - Q72.73 Split foot, bilateral
- **Q72.8 Other reduction defects of lower limb**
  - **Q72.81 Congenital shortening of lower limb**
    - Q72.811 Congenital shortening of right lower limb
    - Q72.812 Congenital shortening of left lower limb
    - Q72.813 Congenital shortening of lower limb, bilateral
    - Q72.819 Congenital shortening of unspecified lower limb
  - **Q72.89 Other reduction defects of lower limb**
    - Q72.891 Other reduction defects of right lower limb
    - Q72.892 Other reduction defects of left lower limb
    - Q72.893 Other reduction defects of lower limb, bilateral
    - Q72.899 Other reduction defects of unspecified lower limb
- **Q72.9 Unspecified reduction defect of lower limb**
  - Q72.90 Unspecified reduction defect of unspecified lower limb
  - Q72.91 Unspecified reduction defect of right lower limb
  - Q72.92 Unspecified reduction defect of left lower limb
  - Q72.93 Unspecified reduction defect of lower limb, bilateral

Q73 Reduction defects of unspecified limb
- **Q73.0 Congenital absence of unspecified limb(s)**
  Amelia NOS
- **Q73.1 Phocomelia, unspecified limb(s)**
  Phocomelia NOS
- **Q73.8 Other reduction defects of unspecified limb(s)**
  Longitudinal reduction deformity of unspecified limb(s)
  Ectromelia of limb NOS
  Hemimelia of limb NOS
  Reduction defect of limb NOS

Q74 Other congenital malformations of limb(s)
Excludes1: polydactyly (Q69.-)
reduction defect of limb (Q71-Q73)
syndactyly (Q70.-)
- **Q74.0 Other congenital malformations of upper limb(s), including shoulder girdle**
  Accessory carpal bones
  Cleidocranial dysostosis
  Congenital pseudarthrosis of clavicle
  Macrodactylia (fingers)
  Madelung's deformity
  Radioulnar synostosis
  Sprengel's deformity
  Triphalangeal thumb
- **Q74.1 Congenital malformation of knee**
  Congenital absence of patella
  Congenital dislocation of patella
  Congenital genu valgum
  Congenital genu varum
  Rudimentary patella
  Excludes1: congenital dislocation of knee (Q68.2)
  congenital genu recurvatum (Q68.2)
  nail patella syndrome (Q87.2)
- **Q74.2 Other congenital malformations of lower limb(s), including pelvic girdle**
  Congenital fusion of sacroiliac joint
  Congenital malformation of ankle joint
  Congenital malformation of sacroiliac joint
  Excludes1: anteversion of femur (neck) (Q65.89)
- CC **Q74.3 Arthrogryposis multiplex congenita**
- **Q74.8 Other specified congenital malformations of limb(s)**
- **Q74.9 Unspecified congenital malformation of limb(s)**
  Congenital anomaly of limb(s) NOS

Q75 Other congenital malformations of skull and face bones
Excludes1: congenital malformation of face NOS (Q18.-)
congenital malformation syndromes classified to (Q87.-)
dentofacial anomalies [including malocclusion] (M26.-)
musculoskeletal deformities of head and face (Q67.0-Q67.4)
skull defects associated with congenital anomalies of brain such as:
anencephaly (Q00.0)
encephalocele (Q01.-)
hydrocephalus (Q03.-)
microcephaly (Q02)
- **Q75.0 Craniosynostosis**
  - **Q75.00 Craniosynostosis unspecified**
    Craniosynostosis NOS
    - Q75.001 Craniosynostosis unspecified, unilateral
    - Q75.002 Craniosynostosis unspecified, bilateral
    - Q75.009 Craniosynostosis unspecified
      Imperfect fusion of skull
  - **Q75.01 Sagittal craniosynostosis**
    Non-deformational dolichocephaly
    Non-deformational scaphocephaly
    Excludes1: plagiocephaly (Q67.3)
  - **Q75.02 Coronal craniosynostosis**
    Non-deformational anterior plagiocephaly
    Excludes1: dolichocephaly (Q67.2)
    - Q75.021 Coronal craniosynostosis unilateral
      Non-deformational anterior plagiocephaly
    - Q75.022 Coronal craniosynostosis bilateral
      Non-deformational brachycephaly
    - Q75.029 Coronal craniosynostosis unspecified
  - **Q75.03 Metopic craniosynostosis**
    Trigonocephaly
  - **Q75.04 Lambdoid craniosynostosis**
    Non-deformational posterior plagiocephaly
    Excludes1: dolichocephaly (Q67.2)
    - Q75.041 Lambdoid craniosynostosis, unilateral
    - Q75.042 Lambdoid craniosynostosis, bilateral
    - Q75.049 Lambdoid craniosynostosis, unspecified
  - **Q75.05 Multi-suture craniosynostosis**
    - Q75.051 Cloverleaf skull
      Kleeblattschaedel skull
    - Q75.052 Pansynostosis
    - Q75.058 Other multi-suture craniosynostosis
      Excludes1: coronal craniosynostosis, bilateral (Q75.022)
      lambdoid craniosynostosis, bilateral (Q75.042)
  - Q75.08 Other single-suture craniosynostosis
- **Q75.1 Craniofacial dysostosis**
  Crouzon's disease
- **Q75.2 Hypertelorism**
- **Q75.3 Macrocephaly**
  AHA CC: 4Q, 2022, 41
- **Q75.4 Mandibulofacial dysostosis**
  Franceschetti syndrome
  Treacher Collins syndrome
- **Q75.5 Oculomandibular dysostosis**
- **Q75.8 Other specified congenital malformations of skull and face bones**
  Absence of skull bone, congenital
  Congenital deformity of forehead
  Platybasia
- **Q75.9 Congenital malformation of skull and face bones, unspecified**
  Congenital anomaly of face bones NOS
  Congenital anomaly of skull NOS

Q76 Congenital malformations of spine and bony thorax

Excludes1: *congenital musculoskeletal deformities of spine and chest (Q67.5-Q67.8)*

- **Q76.0 Spina bifida occulta**
  Excludes1: *meningocele (spinal) (Q05.-)*
  spina bifida (aperta) (cystica) (Q05.-)
- **Q76.1 Klippel-Feil syndrome**
  Cervical fusion syndrome
- **Q76.2 Congenital spondylolisthesis**
  Congenital spondylolysis
  Excludes1: *spondylolisthesis (acquired) (M43.1-)*
  spondylolysis (acquired) (M43.0-)
- CC **Q76.3 Congenital scoliosis due to congenital bony malformation**
  Hemivertebra fusion or failure of segmentation with scoliosis
- + **Q76.4 Other congenital malformations of spine, not associated with scoliosis**
  - + **Q76.41 Congenital kyphosis**
    - Q76.411 Congenital kyphosis, occipito-atlanto-axial region
    - Q76.412 Congenital kyphosis, cervical region
    - Q76.413 Congenital kyphosis, cervicothoracic region
    - Q76.414 Congenital kyphosis, thoracic region
    - Q76.415 Congenital kyphosis, thoracolumbar region
    - Q76.419 Congenital kyphosis, unspecified region
  - + **Q76.42 Congenital lordosis**
    - CC Q76.425 Congenital lordosis, thoracolumbar region
    - CC Q76.426 Congenital lordosis, lumbar region
    - CC Q76.427 Congenital lordosis, lumbosacral region
    - CC Q76.428 Congenital lordosis, sacral and sacrococcygeal region
    - CC Q76.429 Congenital lordosis, unspecified region
  - **Q76.49 Other congenital malformations of spine, not associated with scoliosis**
    Congenital absence of vertebra NOS
    Congenital fusion of spine NOS
    Congenital malformation of lumbosacral (joint) (region) NOS
    Congenital malformation of spine NOS
    Hemivertebra NOS
    Malformation of spine NOS
    Platyspondylisis NOS
    Supernumerary vertebra NOS
- **Q76.5 Cervical rib**
  Supernumerary rib in cervical region
- CC **Q76.6 Other congenital malformations of ribs**
  Accessory rib
  Congenital absence of rib
  Congenital fusion of ribs
  Congenital malformation of ribs NOS
  Excludes1: *short rib syndrome (Q77.2)*
- CC **Q76.7 Congenital malformation of sternum**
  Congenital absence of sternum
  Sternum bifidum
- CC **Q76.8 Other congenital malformations of bony thorax**
- CC **Q76.9 Congenital malformation of bony thorax, unspecified**

Q77 Osteochondrodysplasia with defects of growth of tubular bones and spine

Excludes1: *mucopolysaccharidosis (E76.0-E76.3)*
Excludes2: *congenital myotonic chondrodystrophy (G71.13)*

- **Q77.0 Achondrogenesis**
  Hypochondrogenesis
- **Q77.1 Thanatophoric short stature**
- CC **Q77.2 Short rib syndrome**
  Asphyxiating thoracic dysplasia [Jeune]
- **Q77.3 Chondrodysplasia punctata**
  Excludes1: *Rhizomelic chondrodysplasia punctata (E71.43)*
- **Q77.4 Achondroplasia**
  Hypochondroplasia
  Osteosclerosis congenita
- **Q77.5 Diastrophic dysplasia**
- **Q77.6 Chondroectodermal dysplasia**
  Ellis-van Creveld syndrome
- **Q77.7 Spondyloepiphyseal dysplasia**
- **Q77.8 Other osteochondrodysplasia with defects of growth of tubular bones and spine**
- **Q77.9 Osteochondrodysplasia with defects of growth of tubular bones and spine, unspecified**

Q78 Other osteochondrodysplasias

Excludes2: *congenital myotonic chondrodystrophy (G71.13)*

- CC **Q78.0 Osteogenesis imperfecta**
  Fragilitas ossium
  Osteopsathyrosis
- **Q78.1 Polyostotic fibrous dysplasia**
  Albright(-McCune)(-Sternberg) syndrome
- CC **Q78.2 Osteopetrosis**
  Albers-Schönberg syndrome
  Osteosclerosis NOS
- **Q78.3 Progressive diaphyseal dysplasia**
  Camurati-Engelmann syndrome
- **Q78.4 Enchondromatosis**
  Maffucci's syndrome
  Ollier's disease
- **Q78.5 Metaphyseal dysplasia**
  Pyle's syndrome
- **Q78.6 Multiple congenital exostoses**
  Diaphyseal aclasis
- **Q78.8 Other specified osteochondrodysplasias**
  Osteopoikilosis
- **Q78.9 Osteochondrodysplasia, unspecified**
  Chondrodystrophy NOS
  Osteodystrophy NOS

Q79 Congenital malformations of musculoskeletal system, not elsewhere classified

Excludes2: *congenital (sternomastoid) torticollis (Q68.0)*

- MCC **Q79.0 Congenital diaphragmatic hernia**
  Excludes1: *congenital hiatus hernia (Q40.1)*
- MCC **Q79.1 Other congenital malformations of diaphragm**
  Absence of diaphragm
  Congenital malformation of diaphragm NOS
  Eventration of diaphragm
- MCC **Q79.2 Exomphalos**
  Omphalocele
  Excludes1: *umbilical hernia (K42.-)*
- MCC **Q79.3 Gastroschisis**
- MCC **Q79.4 Prune belly syndrome**
  Congenital prolapse of bladder mucosa
  Eagle-Barrett syndrome
- + **Q79.5 Other congenital malformations of abdominal wall**
  Excludes1: *umbilical hernia (K42.-)*
  - MCC **Q79.51 Congenital hernia of bladder**
  - MCC **Q79.59 Other congenital malformations of abdominal wall**
- + **Q79.6 Ehlers-Danlos syndromes**
  AHA CC: 4Q, 2019, 13-14
  - CC **Q79.60 Ehlers-Danlos Syndrome, unspecified**
  - CC **Q79.61 Classical Ehlers-Danlos syndrome**
    Classical EDS (cEDS)
  - CC **Q79.62 Hypermobile Ehlers-Danlos syndrome**
    Hypermobile EDS (hEDS)
  - CC **Q79.63 Vascular Ehlers-Danlas syndrome**
    Vascular EDS (vEDS)
  - CC **Q79.69 Other Ehlers-Danlos syndromes**
- **Q79.8 Other congenital malformations of musculoskeletal system**
  Absence of muscle
  Absence of tendon
  Accessory muscle
  Amyotrophia congenita
  Congenital constricting bands
  Congenital shortening of tendon
  Poland syndrome
- **Q79.9 Congenital malformation of musculoskeletal system, unspecified**
  Congenital anomaly of musculoskeletal system NOS
  Congenital deformity of musculoskeletal system NOS

Other congenital malformations (Q80-Q89)

Q80 Congenital ichthyosis

Excludes1: *Refsum's disease (G60.1)*

- **Q80.0 Ichthyosis vulgaris**
- **Q80.1 X-linked ichthyosis**

Q80.2 Lamellar ichthyosis
  Collodion baby
Q80.3 Congenital bullous ichthyosiform erythroderma
Q80.4 Harlequin fetus
Q80.8 Other congenital ichthyosis
Q80.9 Congenital ichthyosis, unspecified

Q81 Epidermolysis bullosa

Q81.0 Epidermolysis bullosa simplex
  Excludes1: Cockayne's syndrome (Q87.19)
Q81.1 Epidermolysis bullosa letalis
  Herlitz' syndrome
Q81.2 Epidermolysis bullosa dystrophica
Q81.8 Other epidermolysis bullosa
Q81.9 Epidermolysis bullosa, unspecified

Q82 Other congenital malformations of skin

Excludes1: acrodermatitis enteropathica (E83.2)
  congenital erythropoietic porphyria (E80.0)
  pilonidal cyst or sinus (L05.-)
  Sturge-Weber (-Dimitri) syndrome (Q85.89)

Q82.0 Hereditary lymphedema
Q82.1 Xeroderma pigmentosum
Q82.2 Congenital cutaneous mastocytosis
  Congenital diffuse cutaneous mastocytosis
  Congenital maculopapular cutaneous mastocytosis
  Congenital urticaria pigmentosa
  Excludes1: cutaneous mastocytosis NOS (D47.01)
    diffuse cutaneous mastocytosis (with onset after newborn period) (D47.01)
    malignant mastocytosis (C96.2-)
    systemic mastocytosis (D47.02)
    urticaria pigmentosa (non-congenital) (with onset after newborn period) (D47.01)
  AHA CC: 4Q, 2017, 5
Q82.3 Incontinentia pigmenti
Q82.4 Ectodermal dysplasia (anhidrotic)
  Excludes1: Ellis-van Creveld syndrome (Q77.6)
Q82.5 Congenital non-neoplastic nevus
  Birthmark NOS
  Flammeus Nevus
  Portwine Nevus
  Sanguineous Nevus
  Strawberry Nevus
  Vascular Nevus NOS
  Verrucous Nevus
  Excludes2: Café au lait spots (L81.3)
    lentigo (L81.4)
    nevus NOS (D22.-)
    araneus nevus (I78.1)
    melanocytic nevus (D22.-)
    pigmented nevus (D22.-)
    spider nevus (I78.1)
    stellar nevus (I78.1)
Q82.6 Congenital sacral dimple
  Parasacral dimple
  Excludes2: pilonidal cyst with abscess (L05.01)
    pilonidal cyst without abscess (L05.91)
  AHA CC: 4Q, 2016, 60
Q82.8 Other specified congenital malformations of skin
  Abnormal palmar creases
  Accessory skin tags
  Benign familial pemphigus [Hailey-Hailey]
  Congenital poikiloderma
  Cutis laxa (hyperelastica)
  Dermatoglyphic anomalies
  Inherited keratosis palmaris et plantaris
  Keratosis follicularis [Darier-White]
  Excludes1: Ehlers-Danlos syndromes (Q79.6-)
  AHA CC: 1Q, 2016, 17
Q82.9 Congenital malformation of skin, unspecified

Q83 Congenital malformations of breast

Excludes2: absence of pectoral muscle (Q79.8)
  hypoplasia of breast (N64.82)
  micromastia (N64.82)

Q83.0 Congenital absence of breast with absent nipple
Q83.1 Accessory breast
  Supernumerary breast
Q83.2 Absent nipple

Q83.3 Accessory nipple
  Supernumerary nipple
Q83.8 Other congenital malformations of breast
Q83.9 Congenital malformation of breast, unspecified

Q84 Other congenital malformations of integument

Q84.0 Congenital alopecia
  Congenital atrichosis
Q84.1 Congenital morphological disturbances of hair, not elsewhere classified
  Beaded hair
  Monilethrix
  Pili annulati
  Excludes1: Menkes' kinky hair syndrome (E83.09)
Q84.2 Other congenital malformations of hair
  Congenital hypertrichosis
  Congenital malformation of hair NOS
  Persistent lanugo
Q84.3 Anonychia
  Excludes1: nail patella syndrome (Q87.2)
Q84.4 Congenital leukonychia
Q84.5 Enlarged and hypertrophic nails
  Congenital onychauxis
  Pachyonychia
Q84.6 Other congenital malformations of nails
  Congenital clubnail
  Congenital koilonychia
  Congenital malformation of nail NOS
Q84.8 Other specified congenital malformations of integument
  Aplasia cutis congenita
Q84.9 Congenital malformation of integument, unspecified
  Congenital anomaly of integument NOS
  Congenital deformity of integument NOS

Q85 Phakomatoses, not elsewhere classified

Excludes1: ataxia telangiectasia [Louis-Bar] (G11.3)
  familial dysautonomia [Riley-Day] (G90.1)

+ **Q85.0** Neurofibromatosis (nonmalignant)
  Q85.00 Neurofibromatosis, unspecified
  Q85.01 Neurofibromatosis, type 1
    Von Recklinghausen disease
  Q85.02 Neurofibromatosis, type 2
    Acoustic neurofibromatosis
  Q85.03 Schwannomatosis
  Q85.09 Other neurofibromatosis
CC **Q85.1** Tuberous sclerosis
  Bourneville's disease
  Epiloia
+ **Q85.8** Other phakomatoses, not elsewhere classified
  Excludes1: Meckel-Gruber syndrome (Q61.9)
  AHA CC: 3Q, 2021, 12; 4Q, 2022, 40-41
  CC **Q85.81** PTEN hamartoma tumor syndrome
    PHTS
    PTEN related Cowden syndrome
    Code also, if applicable, genetic susceptibility to malignant neoplasm (Z15.0-)
    AHA CC: 4Q, 2022, 41
  CC **Q85.82** Other Cowden syndrome
  CC **Q85.83** Von Hippel-Lindau syndrome
    Code also manifestations
    AHA CC: 2Q, 2023, 16
  CC **Q85.89** Other phakomatoses, not elsewhere classified
    Peutz-Jeghers syndrome
    Sturge-Weber(-Dimitri) syndrome
CC **Q85.9** Phakomatosis, unspecified
  Hamartosis NOS

Q86 Congenital malformation syndromes due to known exogenous causes, not elsewhere classified

Excludes2: iodine-deficiency-related hypothyroidism (E00-E02)
  nonteratogenic effects of substances transmitted via placenta or breast milk (P04.-)

Q86.0 Fetal alcohol syndrome (dysmorphic)
Q86.1 Fetal hydantoin syndrome
  Meadow's syndrome
Q86.2 Dysmorphism due to warfarin
Q86.8 Other congenital malformation syndromes due to known exogenous causes

Q87 Other specified congenital malformation syndromes affecting multiple systems

Use additional code(s) to identify all associated manifestations

- **Q87.0 Congenital malformation syndromes predominantly affecting facial appearance**
  - Acrocephalopolysyndactyly
  - Acrocephalosyndactyly [Apert]
  - Cryptophthalmos syndrome
  - Cyclopia
  - Goldenhar syndrome
  - Moebius syndrome
  - Oro-facial-digital syndrome
  - Robin syndrome
  - Whistling face

+ **Q87.1 Congenital malformation syndromes predominantly associated with short stature**
  - *Excludes1:* Ellis-van Creveld syndrome (Q77.6)
    Smith-Lemli-Opitz syndrome (E78.72)
  - AHA CC: 4Q, 2019, 14-15
  - CC **Q87.11 Prader-Willi syndrome**
  - CC **Q87.19 Other congenital malformation syndromes predominantly associated with short stature**
    - Aarskog syndrome
    - Cockayne syndrome
    - De Lange syndrome
    - Dubowitz syndrome
    - Noonan syndrome
    - Robinow-Silverman-Smith syndrome
    - Russell-Silver syndrome
    - Seckel syndrome

- CC **Q87.2 Congenital malformation syndromes predominantly involving limbs**
  - Holt-Oram syndrome
  - Klippel-Trenaunay-Weber syndrome
  - Nail patella syndrome
  - Rubinstein-Taybi syndrome
  - Sirenomelia syndrome
  - Thrombocytopenia with absent radius [TAR] syndrome
  - VATER syndrome

- CC **Q87.3 Congenital malformation syndromes involving early overgrowth**
  - Beckwith-Wiedemann syndrome
  - Sotos syndrome
  - Weaver syndrome

+ **Q87.4 Marfan syndrome**
  - CC **Q87.40 Marfan syndrome, unspecified**
  - + **Q87.41 Marfan syndrome with cardiovascular manifestations**
    - CC **Q87.410 Marfan syndrome with aortic dilation**
    - CC **Q87.418 Marfan syndrome with other cardiovascular manifestations**
  - CC **Q87.42 Marfan syndrome with ocular manifestations**
  - CC **Q87.43 Marfan syndrome with skeletal manifestation**

- CC **Q87.5 Other congenital malformation syndromes with other skeletal changes**

+ **Q87.8 Other specified congenital malformation syndromes, not elsewhere classified**
  - *Excludes1:* Zellweger syndrome (E71.510)
  - CC **Q87.81 Alport syndrome**
    - Use additional code to identify stage of chronic kidney disease (N18.1-N18.6)
  - CC **Q87.82 Arterial tortuosity syndrome**
    - AHA CC: 4Q, 2016, 60-61
  - CC **Q87.83 Bardet-Biedl syndrome**
  - CC **Q87.84 Laurence-Moon syndrome**
  - CC **Q87.85 MED13L syndrome**
    - Asadollahi-Rauch syndrome
    - Mediator complex subunit 13L syndrome
    - Code also, if applicable, any associated manifestations such as:
      - autism spectrum disorder (F84.0-)
      - congenital malformations of cardiac septa (Q21.-)
      - epilepsy and recurrent seizures (G40.-)
      - intellectual disability (F70-F79)
  - CC **Q87.89 Other specified congenital malformation syndromes, not elsewhere classified**

Q89 Other congenital malformations, not elsewhere classified

+ **Q89.0 Congenital absence and malformations of spleen**
  - *Excludes1:* isomerism of atrial appendages (with asplenia or polysplenia) (Q20.6)
  - CC **Q89.01 Asplenia (congenital)**
  - CC **Q89.09 Congenital malformations of spleen**
    - Congenital splenomegaly

- **Q89.1 Congenital malformations of adrenal gland**
  - *Excludes1:* adrenogenital disorders (E25.-)
    congenital adrenal hyperplasia (E25.0)

- **Q89.2 Congenital malformations of other endocrine glands**
  - Congenital malformation of parathyroid or thyroid gland
  - Persistent thyroglossal duct
  - Thyroglossal cyst
  - *Excludes1:* congenital goiter (E03.0)
    congenital hypothyroidism (E03.1)

- CC **Q89.3 Situs inversus**
  - Dextrocardia with situs inversus
  - Mirror-image atrial arrangement with situs inversus
  - Situs inversus or transversus abdominalis
  - Situs inversus or transversus thoracis
  - Transposition of abdominal viscera
  - Transposition of thoracic viscera
  - *Excludes1:* dextrocardia NOS (Q24.0)

- MCC **Q89.4 Conjoined twins**
  - Craniopagus
  - Dicephaly
  - Pygopagus
  - Thoracopagus

- CC **Q89.7 Multiple congenital malformations, not elsewhere classified**
  - Multiple congenital anomalies NOS
  - Multiple congenital deformities NOS
  - *Excludes1:* congenital malformation syndromes affecting multiple systems (Q87.-)

- CC **Q89.8 Other specified congenital malformations**
  - Use additional code(s) to identify all associated manifestations
  - AHA CC: 3Q, 2021, 12

- **Q89.9 Congenital malformation, unspecified**
  - Congenital anomaly NOS
  - Congenital deformity NOS

Chromosomal abnormalities, not elsewhere classified (Q90-Q99)

Excludes2: mitochondrial metabolic disorders (E88.4-)

Q90 Down syndrome

Code also associated physical condition(s), such as atrioventricular septal defect (Q21.2-)

Use additional code(s) to identify any associated degree of intellectual disabilities (F70-F79)

- **Q90.0 Trisomy 21, nonmosaicism (meiotic nondisjunction)**
- **Q90.1 Trisomy 21, mosaicism (mitotic nondisjunction)**
- **Q90.2 Trisomy 21, translocation**
- **Q90.9 Down syndrome, unspecified**
  - Trisomy 21 NOS

Q91 Trisomy 18 and Trisomy 13

- CC **Q91.0 Trisomy 18, nonmosaicism (meiotic nondisjunction)**
- CC **Q91.1 Trisomy 18, mosaicism (mitotic nondisjunction)**
- CC **Q91.2 Trisomy 18, translocation**
- CC **Q91.3 Trisomy 18, unspecified**
- CC **Q91.4 Trisomy 13, nonmosaicism (meiotic nondisjunction)**
- CC **Q91.5 Trisomy 13, mosaicism (mitotic nondisjunction)**
- CC **Q91.6 Trisomy 13, translocation**
- CC **Q91.7 Trisomy 13, unspecified**

Q92 Other trisomies and partial trisomies of the autosomes, not elsewhere classified

Includes: unbalanced translocations and insertions
Excludes1: trisomies of chromosomes 13, 18, 21 (Q90-Q91)

- **Q92.0 Whole chromosome trisomy, nonmosaicism (meiotic nondisjunction)**
- **Q92.1 Whole chromosome trisomy, mosaicism (mitotic nondisjunction)**
- **Q92.2 Partial trisomy**
  - Less than whole arm duplicated
  - Whole arm or more duplicated
  - *Excludes1:* partial trisomy due to unbalanced translocation (Q92.5)
- **Q92.5 Duplications with other complex rearrangements**
  - Partial trisomy due to unbalanced translocations
  - Code also any associated deletions due to unbalanced translocations, inversions and insertions (Q93.7)

+ Q92.6 Marker chromosomes
- Trisomies due to dicentrics
- Trisomies due to extra rings
- Trisomies due to isochromosomes
- Individual with marker heterochromatin
  - **Q92.61** Marker chromosomes in normal individual
  - **Q92.62** Marker chromosomes in abnormal individual

Q92.7 Triploidy and polyploidy

Q92.8 Other specified trisomies and partial trisomies of autosomes
- Duplications identified by fluorescence in situ hybridization (FISH)
- Duplications identified by in situ hybridization (ISH)
- Duplications seen only at prometaphase

Q92.9 Trisomy and partial trisomy of autosomes, unspecified

Q93 Monosomies and deletions from the autosomes, not elsewhere classified

- **Q93.0** Whole chromosome monosomy, nonmosaicism (meiotic nondisjunction)
- **Q93.1** Whole chromosome monosomy, mosaicism (mitotic nondisjunction)
- **Q93.2** Chromosome replaced with ring, dicentric or isochromosome
- CC **Q93.3** Deletion of short arm of chromosome 4
  - Wolff-Hirschorn syndrome
- CC **Q93.4** Deletion of short arm of chromosome 5
  - Cri-du-chat syndrome
- + **Q93.5** Other deletions of part of a chromosome
  - *AHA CC: 4Q, 2018, 28*
  - CC **Q93.51** Angelman syndrome
  - CC **Q93.52** Phelan-McDermid syndrome
    - 22q13.3 deletion syndrome
    - Use Additional code(s) to identify any associated conditions, such as:
      - autism spectrum disorder (F84.0)
      - degree of intellectual disabilities (F70-F79)
      - epilepsy and recurrent seizures (G40.-)
      - lymphedema (I89.0)
  - CC **Q93.59** Other deletions of part of a chromosome
- CC **Q93.7** Deletions with other complex rearrangements
  - Deletions due to unbalanced translocations, inversions and insertions
  - Code also any associated duplications due to unbalanced translocations, inversions and insertions (Q92.5)
- + **Q93.8** Other deletions from the autosomes
  - MCC **Q93.81** Velo-cardio-facial syndrome
    - Deletion 22q11.2
    - *AHA CC: 3Q, 2019, 14-15*
  - CC **Q93.82** Williams syndrome
    - *AHA CC: 4Q, 2018, 28-29*
  - CC **Q93.88** Other microdeletions
    - Miller-Dieker syndrome
    - Smith-Magenis syndrome
  - CC **Q93.89** Other deletions from the autosomes
    - Deletions identified by fluorescence in situ hybridization (FISH)
    - Deletions identified by in situ hybridization (ISH)
    - Deletions seen only at prometaphase
- CC **Q93.9** Deletion from autosomes, unspecified

Q95 Balanced rearrangements and structural markers, not elsewhere classified

Includes: Robertsonian and balanced reciprocal translocations and insertions

- **Q95.0** Balanced translocation and insertion in normal individual
- **Q95.1** Chromosome inversion in normal individual
- **Q95.2** Balanced autosomal rearrangement in abnormal individual
- **Q95.3** Balanced sex/autosomal rearrangement in abnormal individual
- **Q95.5** Individual with autosomal fragile site
- **Q95.8** Other balanced rearrangements and structural markers
- **Q95.9** Balanced rearrangement and structural marker, unspecified

Q96 Turner's syndrome

Excludes1: Noonan syndrome (Q87.19)

- ♀ **Q96.0** Karyotype 45, X
- ♀ **Q96.1** Karyotype 46, X iso (Xq)
  - Karyotype 46, isochromosome Xq
- ♀ **Q96.2** Karyotype 46, X with abnormal sex chromosome, except iso (Xq)
  - Karyotype 46, X with abnormal sex chromosome, except isochromosome Xq
- ♀ **Q96.3** Mosaicism, 45, X/46, XX or XY
- ♀ **Q96.4** Mosaicism, 45, X/other cell line(s) with abnormal sex chromosome
- ♀ **Q96.8** Other variants of Turner's syndrome
- ♀ **Q96.9** Turner's syndrome, unspecified

Q97 Other sex chromosome abnormalities, female phenotype, not elsewhere classified

Excludes1: Turner's syndrome (Q96.-)

- ♀ **Q97.0** Karyotype 47, XXX
- ♀ **Q97.1** Female with more than three X chromosomes
- ♀ **Q97.2** Mosaicism, lines with various numbers of X chromosomes
- ♀ **Q97.3** Female with 46, XY karyotype
- ♀ **Q97.8** Other specified sex chromosome abnormalities, female phenotype
- ♀ **Q97.9** Sex chromosome abnormality, female phenotype, unspecified

Q98 Other sex chromosome abnormalities, male phenotype, not elsewhere classified

- ♂ **Q98.0** Klinefelter syndrome karyotype 47, XXY
- ♂ **Q98.1** Klinefelter syndrome, male with more than two X chromosomes
- ♂ **Q98.3** Other male with 46, XX karyotype
- ♂ **Q98.4** Klinefelter syndrome, unspecified
- ♂ **Q98.5** Karyotype 47, XYY
- ♂ **Q98.6** Male with structurally abnormal sex chromosome
- ♂ **Q98.7** Male with sex chromosome mosaicism
- ♂ **Q98.8** Other specified sex chromosome abnormalities, male phenotype
- ♂ **Q98.9** Sex chromosome abnormality, male phenotype, unspecified

Q99 Other chromosome abnormalities, not elsewhere classified

- **Q99.0** Chimera 46, XX/46, XY
  - Chimera 46, XX/46, XY true hermaphrodite
- **Q99.1** 46, XX true hermaphrodite
  - 46, XX with streak gonads
  - 46, XY with streak gonads
  - Pure gonadal dysgenesis
- **Q99.2** Fragile X chromosome
  - Fragile X syndrome
- **Q99.8** Other specified chromosome abnormalities
- **Q99.9** Chromosomal abnormality, unspecified

Chapter 18: Symptoms, Signs and Abnormal Clinical and Laboratory Findings, Not Elsewhere Classified (R00-R99)

NOTE This chapter includes symptoms, signs, abnormal results of clinical or other investigative procedures, and ill-defined conditions regarding which no diagnosis classifiable elsewhere is recorded.

Signs and symptoms that point rather definitely to a given diagnosis have been assigned to a category in other chapters of the classification. In general, categories in this chapter include the less well-defined conditions and symptoms that, without the necessary study of the case to establish a final diagnosis, point perhaps equally to two or more diseases or to two or more systems of the body. Practically all categories in the chapter could be designated 'not otherwise specified', 'unknown etiology' or 'transient'. The Alphabetical Index should be consulted to determine which symptoms and signs are to be allocated here and which to other chapters. The residual subcategories, numbered .8, are generally provided for other relevant symptoms that cannot be allocated elsewhere in the classification.

The conditions and signs or symptoms included in categories R00-R94 consist of:
(a) cases for which no more specific diagnosis can be made even after all the facts bearing on the case have been investigated;
(b) signs or symptoms existing at the time of initial encounter that proved to be transient and whose causes could not be determined;
(c) provisional diagnosis in a patient who failed to return for further investigation or care;
(d) cases referred elsewhere for investigation or treatment before the diagnosis was made;
(e) cases in which a more precise diagnosis was not available for any other reason;
(f) certain symptoms, for which supplementary information is provided, that represent important problems in medical care in their own right.

Excludes2: *abnormal findings on antenatal screening of mother (O28.-)*
certain conditions originating in the perinatal period (P04-P96)
signs and symptoms classified in the body system chapters
signs and symptoms of breast (N63, N64.5)

This chapter contains the following category blocks:
- R00-R09 Symptoms and signs involving the circulatory and respiratory systems
- R10-R19 Symptoms and signs involving the digestive system and abdomen
- R20-R23 Symptoms and signs involving the skin and subcutaneous tissue
- R25-R29 Symptoms and signs involving the nervous and musculoskeletal systems
- R30-R39 Symptoms and signs involving the genitourinary system
- R40-R46 Symptoms and signs involving cognition, perception, emotional state and behavior
- R47-R49 Symptoms and signs involving speech and voice
- R50-R69 General symptoms and signs
- R70-R79 Abnormal findings on examination of blood, without diagnosis
- R80-R82 Abnormal findings on examination of urine, without diagnosis
- R83-R89 Abnormal findings on examination of other body fluids, substances and tissues, without diagnosis
- R90-R94 Abnormal findings on diagnostic imaging and in function studies, without diagnosis
- R97 Abnormal tumor markers
- R99 Ill-defined and unknown cause of mortality

C. Chapter-Specific Coding Guidelines

In addition to general coding guidelines, there are guidelines for specific diagnoses and/or conditions in the classification. Unless otherwise indicated, these guidelines apply to all health care settings. Please refer to Section II for guidelines on the selection of principal diagnosis.

18. Chapter 18: Symptoms, Signs, and Abnormal Clinical and Laboratory Findings, Not Elsewhere Classified (R00-R99)

Chapter 18 includes symptoms, signs, abnormal results of clinical or other investigative procedures, and ill-defined conditions regarding which no diagnosis classifiable elsewhere is recorded. Signs and symptoms that point to a specific diagnosis have been assigned to a category in other chapters of the classification.

a. Use of symptom codes

Codes that describe symptoms and signs are acceptable for reporting purposes when a related definitive diagnosis has not been established (confirmed) by the provider.

b. Use of a symptom code with a definitive diagnosis code

Codes for signs and symptoms may be reported in addition to a related definitive diagnosis when the sign or symptom is not routinely associated with that diagnosis, such as the various signs and symptoms associated with complex syndromes. The definitive diagnosis code should be sequenced before the symptom code.

Signs or symptoms that are associated routinely with a disease process should not be assigned as additional codes, unless otherwise instructed by the classification.

c. Combination codes that include symptoms

ICD-10-CM contains a number of combination codes that identify both the definitive diagnosis and common symptoms of that diagnosis. When using one of these combination codes, an additional code should not be assigned for the symptom.

d. Repeated falls

Code R29.6, Repeated falls, is for use for encounters when a patient has recently fallen and the reason for the fall is being investigated.

Code Z91.81, History of falling, is for use when a patient has fallen in the past and is at risk for future falls. When appropriate, both codes R29.6 and Z91.81 may be assigned together.

e. Coma

Code R40.20, Unspecified coma, **should** be assigned **when the underlying cause of the coma is not known, or the cause is a traumatic brain injury and the coma scale is not documented in the medical record.**

Do not report codes for unspecified coma, individual or total Glasgow coma scale scores for a patient with a medically induced coma or a sedated patient.

1) **Coma Scale**

The coma scale codes (R40.21-to R40.24-) can be used in conjunction with traumatic brain injury codes. These codes **cannot be used with code R40.2A, Nontraumatic coma due to underlying condition. They** are primarily for use by trauma registries, but they may be used in any setting where this information is collected. The coma scale codes should be sequenced after the diagnosis code(s).

These codes, one from each subcategory, are needed to complete the scale. The 7th character indicates when the scale was recorded. The 7th character should match for all three codes.

At a minimum, report the initial score documented on presentation at your facility. This may be a score from the emergency medicine technician (EMT) or in the emergency department. If desired, a facility may choose to capture multiple coma scale scores.

Assign code R40.24, Glasgow coma scale, total score, when only the total score is documented in the medical record and not the individual score(s).

If multiple coma scores are captured within the first 24 hours after hospital admission, assign only the code for the score at the time of admission. ICD-10-CM does not classify coma scores that are reported after admission but less than 24 hours later. *See Section I.B.14 for coma scale documentation by clinicians other than the patient's provider.*

f. Functional quadriplegia

GUIDELINE HAS BEEN DELETED EFFECTIVE OCTOBER 1, 2017

g. SIRS due to Non-Infectious Process

The systemic inflammatory response syndrome (SIRS) can develop as a result of certain non-infectious disease processes, such as trauma, malignant neoplasm, or pancreatitis. When SIRS is documented with a noninfectious condition, and no subsequent infection is documented, the code for the underlying condition, such as an injury, should be assigned, followed by code R65.10, Systemic inflammatory response syndrome (SIRS) of non-infectious origin without acute organ dysfunction, or code R65.11, Systemic inflammatory response syndrome (SIRS) of non-infectious origin with acute organ dysfunction. If an associated acute organ dysfunction is documented, the appropriate code(s) for the specific type of organ dysfunction(s) should be assigned in addition to code R65.11. If acute organ dysfunction is documented, but it cannot be determined if the acute organ dysfunction is associated with SIRS or due to another condition (e.g., directly due to the trauma), the provider should be queried.

h. Death NOS

Code R99, Ill-defined and unknown cause of mortality, is only for use in the very limited circumstance when a patient who has already died is brought into an emergency department or other healthcare facility and is pronounced dead upon arrival. It does not represent the discharge disposition of death.

i. NIHSS Stroke Scale

The NIH stroke scale (NIHSS) codes (R29.7--) can be used in conjunction with acute stroke codes (I60-I63) to identify the patient's neurological status and the severity of the stroke. The stroke scale codes should be sequenced after the acute stroke diagnosis code(s).

At a minimum, report the initial score documented. If desired, a facility may choose to capture multiple stroke scale scores.

See Section I.B.14 for NIHSS stroke scale documentation by clinicians other than patient's provider.

Symptoms and signs involving the circulatory and respiratory systems (R00-R09)

R00 Abnormalities of heart beat

    Excludes1: abnormalities originating in the perinatal period (P29.1-)
    Excludes2: specified arrhythmias (I47-I49)

  R00.0 **Tachycardia, unspecified**
    Rapid heart beat
    Sinoauricular tachycardia NOS
    Sinus [sinusal] tachycardia NOS
    Excludes1: inappropriate sinus tachycardia, so stated (I47.11)
        neonatal tachycardia (P29.11)
        paroxysmal tachycardia (I47.-)
    AHA CC: 4Q, 2022, 46-47

  R00.1 **Bradycardia, unspecified**
    Sinoatrial bradycardia
    Sinus bradycardia
    Slow heart beat
    Systolic murmur NOS
    Vagal bradycardia
    Use additional code for adverse effect, if applicable, to identify drug (T36-T50 with fifth or sixth character 5)
    Excludes1: neonatal bradycardia (P29.12)
    AHA CC: 2Q, 2020, 23-24

  R00.2 **Palpitations**
    Awareness of heart beat

  R00.8 **Other abnormalities of heart beat**
  R00.9 **Unspecified abnormalities of heart beat**

R01 Cardiac murmurs and other cardiac sounds

    Excludes1: cardiac murmurs and sounds originating in the perinatal period (P29.8)

  R01.0 **Benign and innocent cardiac murmurs**
    Functional cardiac murmur

  R01.1 **Cardiac murmur, unspecified**
    Cardiac bruit NOS
    Heart murmur NOS
    Systolic murmur NOS

  R01.2 **Other cardiac sounds**
    Cardiac dullness, increased or decreased
    Precordial friction

R03 Abnormal blood-pressure reading, without diagnosis

  R03.0 **Elevated blood-pressure reading, without diagnosis of hypertension**
    NOTE This category is to be used to record an episode of elevated blood pressure in a patient in whom no formal diagnosis of hypertension has been made, or as an isolated incidental finding.
    Review coding guideline C.9.a.7

  R03.1 **Nonspecific low blood-pressure reading**
    Excludes1: hypotension (I95.-)
        maternal hypotension syndrome (O26.5-)
        neurogenic orthostatic hypotension (G90.3)

R04 Hemorrhage from respiratory passages

  R04.0 **Epistaxis**
    Hemorrhage from nose
    Nosebleed
    AHA CC: 4Q, 2018, 38; 2Q, 2023, 28

  R04.1 **Hemorrhage from throat**
    Excludes2: hemoptysis (R04.2)

  CC R04.2 **Hemoptysis**
    Blood-stained sputum
    Cough with hemorrhage
    AHA CC: 4Q, 2013, 118

+ R04.8 **Hemorrhage from other sites in respiratory passages**
  CC R04.81 **Acute idiopathic pulmonary hemorrhage in infants**
    AIPHI
    Acute idiopathic hemorrhage in infants over 28 days old
    Excludes1: perinatal pulmonary hemorrhage (P26.-)
        von Willebrand disease (D68.0-)
  CC R04.89 **Hemorrhage from other sites in respiratory passages**
    Pulmonary hemorrhage NOS

CC R04.9 **Hemorrhage from respiratory passages, unspecified**

R05 Cough

    Excludes1: paroxysmal cough due to Bordetella pertussis (A37.0-)
        smoker's cough (J41.0)
    Excludes2: cough with hemorrhage (R04.2)
    AHA CC: 2Q, 2016, 34; 1Q, 2020, 34-36; 4Q, 2021, 24-25

  R05.1 **Acute cough**
  R05.2 **Subacute cough**
  R05.3 **Chronic cough**
    Persistent cough
    Refractory cough
    Unexplained cough
  R05.4 **Cough syncope**
    Code first syncope and collapse (R55)
  R05.8 **Other specified cough**
  R05.9 **Cough, unspecified**

R06 Abnormalities of breathing

    Excludes1: acute respiratory distress syndrome (J80)
        respiratory arrest (R09.2)
        respiratory arrest of newborn (P28.81)
        respiratory distress syndrome of newborn (P22.-)
        respiratory failure (J96.-)
        respiratory failure of newborn (P28.5)

+ R06.0 **Dyspnea**
    Excludes1: tachypnea NOS (R06.82)
        transient tachypnea of newborn (P22.1)
  R06.00 **Dyspnea, unspecified**
    AHA CC: 1Q, 2017, 26-27
  R06.01 **Orthopnea**
  R06.02 **Shortness of breath**
    AHA CC: 1Q, 2020, 34-36
  R06.03 **Acute respiratory distress**
    AHA CC: 4Q, 2017, 23
  R06.09 **Other forms of dyspnea**

  R06.1 **Stridor**
    Excludes1: congenital laryngeal stridor (P28.89)
        laryngismus (stridulus) (J38.5)

  R06.2 **Wheezing**
    Excludes1: Asthma (J45.-)
    AHA CC: 2Q, 2016, 34

CC R06.3 **Periodic breathing**
    Cheyne-Stokes breathing

  R06.4 **Hyperventilation**
    Excludes1: psychogenic hyperventilation (F45.8)

  R06.5 **Mouth breathing**
    Excludes2: dry mouth NOS (R68.2)

  R06.6 **Hiccough**
    Excludes1: psychogenic hiccough (F45.8)

  R06.7 **Sneezing**

+ R06.8 **Other abnormalities of breathing**
  R06.81 **Apnea, not elsewhere classified**
    Apnea NOS
    Excludes1: apnea (of) newborn (P28.4-)
        sleep apnea (G47.3-)
        sleep apnea of newborn (primary) (P28.3-)
  R06.82 **Tachypnea, not elsewhere classified**
    Tachypnea NOS
    Excludes1: transitory tachypnea of newborn (P22.1)
  R06.83 **Snoring**
  R06.89 **Other abnormalities of breathing**
    Breath-holding (spells)
    Sighing

  R06.9 **Unspecified abnormalities of breathing**

R07 Pain in throat and chest
> *Excludes1:* epidemic myalgia (B33.0)
> *Excludes2:* jaw pain (R68.84)
>   pain in breast (N64.4)

- **R07.0 Pain in throat**
  > *Excludes1:* chronic sore throat (J31.2)
  >   sore throat (acute) NOS (J02.9)
  > *Excludes2:* dysphagia (R13.1-)
  >   pain in neck (M54.2)
- **R07.1 Chest pain on breathing**
  Painful respiration
- **R07.2 Precordial pain**
- + **R07.8 Other chest pain**
  - **R07.81 Pleurodynia**
    Pleurodynia NOS
    > *Excludes1:* epidemic pleurodynia (B33.0)
  - **R07.82 Intercostal pain**
  - **R07.89 Other chest pain**
    Anterior chest-wall pain NOS
    AHA CC: 1Q, 2021, 42
- **R07.9 Chest pain, unspecified**

R09 Other symptoms and signs involving the circulatory and respiratory system
> *Excludes1:* acute respiratory distress syndrome (J80)
>   respiratory arrest of newborn (P28.81)
>   respiratory distress syndrome of newborn (P22.0)
>   respiratory failure (J96.-)
>   respiratory failure of newborn (P28.5)

- + **R09.0 Asphyxia and hypoxemia**
  > *Excludes1:* asphyxia due to carbon monoxide (T58.-)
  >   asphyxia due to foreign body in respiratory tract (T17.-)
  >   birth (intrauterine) asphyxia (P84)
  >   hyperventilation (R06.4)
  >   traumatic asphyxia (T71.-)
  > *Excludes2:* hypercapnia (R06.89)
  - **CC R09.01 Asphyxia**
  - **R09.02 Hypoxemia**
    AHA CC: 3Q, 2019, 15
- **R09.1 Pleurisy**
  > *Excludes1:* pleurisy with effusion (J90)
- **MCC R09.2 Respiratory arrest**
  Cardiorespiratory failure
  > *Excludes1:* cardiac arrest (I46.-)
  >   respiratory arrest of newborn (P28.81)
  >   respiratory distress of newborn (P22.0)
  >   respiratory failure (J96.-)
  >   respiratory failure of newborn (P28.5)
  >   respiratory insufficiency (R06.89)
  >   respiratory insufficiency of newborn (P28.5)
- **R09.3 Abnormal sputum**
  Abnormal amount of sputum
  Abnormal color of sputum
  Abnormal odor of sputum
  Excessive sputum
  > *Excludes1:* blood-stained sputum (R04.2)
- + **R09.8 Other specified symptoms and signs involving the circulatory and respiratory systems**
  - **R09.81 Nasal congestion**
  - **R09.82 Postnasal drip**
  - **R09.89 Other specified symptoms and signs involving the circulatory and respiratory systems**
    Bruit (arterial)
    Abnormal chest percussion
    Friction sounds in chest
    Chest tympany
    Choking sensation
    Rales
    Weak pulse
    > *Excludes2:* foreign body in throat (T17.2-)
    >   wheezing (R06.2)
    AHA CC: 1Q, 2021, 42
- + **R09.A Foreign body sensation of the circulatory and respiratory system**
  - **R09.A0 Foreign body sensation, unspecified**
  - **R09.A1 Foreign body sensation, nose**
  - **R09.A2 Foreign body sensation, throat**
    Foreign body sensation globus
  - **R09.A9 Foreign body sensation, other site**

Symptoms and signs involving the digestive system and abdomen (R10-R19)

> *Excludes2:* congenital or infantile pylorospasm (Q40.0)
>   gastrointestinal hemorrhage (K92.0-K92.2)
>   intestinal obstruction (K56.-)
>   newborn gastrointestinal hemorrhage (P54.0-P54.3)
>   newborn intestinal obstruction (P76.-)
>   pylorospasm (K31.3)
>   signs and symptoms involving the urinary system (R30-R39)
>   symptoms referable to female genital organs (N94.-)
>   symptoms referable to male genital organs male (N48-N50)

R10 Abdominal and pelvic pain
> *Excludes1:* renal colic (N23)
> *Excludes2:* dorsalgia (M54.-)
>   flatulence and related conditions (R14.-)

- **R10.0 Acute abdomen**
  Severe abdominal pain (generalized) (with abdominal rigidity)
  > *Excludes1:* abdominal rigidity NOS (R19.3)
  >   generalized abdominal pain NOS (R10.84)
  >   localized abdominal pain (R10.1-R10.3-)
- + **R10.1 Pain localized to upper abdomen**
  - **R10.10 Upper abdominal pain, unspecified**
  - **R10.11 Right upper quadrant pain**
  - **R10.12 Left upper quadrant pain**
  - **R10.13 Epigastric pain**
    Dyspepsia
    > *Excludes1:* functional dyspepsia (K30)
- **R10.2 Pelvic and perineal pain**
  > *Excludes1:* vulvodynia (N94.81)
- + **R10.3 Pain localized to other parts of lower abdomen**
  - **R10.30 Lower abdominal pain, unspecified**
  - **R10.31 Right lower quadrant pain**
  - **R10.32 Left lower quadrant pain**
  - **R10.33 Periumbilical pain**
- + **R10.8 Other abdominal pain**
  - + **R10.81 Abdominal tenderness**
    Abdominal tenderness NOS
    - **R10.811 Right upper quadrant abdominal tenderness**
    - **R10.812 Left upper quadrant abdominal tenderness**
    - **R10.813 Right lower quadrant abdominal tenderness**
    - **R10.814 Left lower quadrant abdominal tenderness**
    - **R10.815 Periumbilic abdominal tenderness**
    - **R10.816 Epigastric abdominal tenderness**
    - **R10.817 Generalized abdominal tenderness**
    - **R10.819 Abdominal tenderness, unspecified site**
  - + **R10.82 Rebound abdominal tenderness**
    - **R10.821 Right upper quadrant rebound abdominal tenderness**
    - **R10.822 Left upper quadrant rebound abdominal tenderness**
    - **R10.823 Right lower quadrant rebound abdominal tenderness**
    - **R10.824 Left lower quadrant rebound abdominal tenderness**
    - **R10.825 Periumbilic rebound abdominal tenderness**
    - **R10.826 Epigastric rebound abdominal tenderness**
    - **R10.827 Generalized rebound abdominal tenderness**
    - **R10.829 Rebound abdominal tenderness, unspecified site**
  - • **R10.83 Colic**
    Colic NOS
    Infantile colic
    > *Excludes1:* colic in adult and child over 12 months old (R10.84)
  - **R10.84 Generalized abdominal pain**
    > *Excludes1:* generalized abdominal pain associated with acute abdomen (R10.0)
- **R10.9 Unspecified abdominal pain**

R11 Nausea and vomiting
   Excludes1: cyclical vomiting associated with migraine (G43.A-)
            excessive vomiting in pregnancy (O21.-)
            hematemesis (K92.0)
            neonatal hematemesis (P54.0)
            newborn vomiting (P92.0-)
            psychogenic vomiting (F50.89)
            vomiting associated with bulimia nervosa (F50.2)
            vomiting following gastrointestinal surgery (K91.0)
   AHA CC: 1Q, 2017, 28
   R11.0 Nausea
         Nausea NOS
         Nausea without vomiting
   + **R11.1 Vomiting**
      R11.10 Vomiting, unspecified
            Vomiting NOS
      R11.11 Vomiting without nausea
      R11.12 Projectile vomiting
      R11.13 Vomiting of fecal matter
      R11.14 Bilious vomiting
            Bilious emesis
      R11.15 Cyclical vomiting syndrome unrelated to migraine
            Cyclic vomiting syndrome NOS
            Persistent vomiting
         Excludes1: cyclical vomiting in migraine (G43.A-)
         Excludes2: bulimia nervosa (F50.2)
                  diabetes mellitus due to underlying condition (E08.-)
         AHA CC: 4Q, 2019, 15
   R11.2 Nausea with vomiting, unspecified
         Persistent nausea with vomiting NOS
         AHA CC: 1Q, 2020, 8

R12 Heartburn
   Excludes1: dyspepsia NOS (R10.13)
            functional dyspepsia (K30)
   Valid 3-character code, no further characters required

R13 Aphagia and dysphagia
   R13.0 Aphagia
         Inability to swallow
         Excludes1: psychogenic aphagia (F50.9)
   + **R13.1 Dysphagia**
         Code first if applicable, dysphagia following cerebrovascular disease (I69. with final characters -91)
         Excludes1: psychogenic dysphagia (F45.8)
      R13.10 Dysphagia, unspecified
            Difficulty in swallowing NOS
      R13.11 Dysphagia, oral phase
      R13.12 Dysphagia, oropharyngeal phase
      R13.13 Dysphagia, pharyngeal phase
      R13.14 Dysphagia, pharyngoesophageal phase
      R13.19 Other dysphagia
            Cervical dysphagia
            Neurogenic dysphagia

R14 Flatulence and related conditions
   Excludes1: psychogenic aerophagy (F45.8)
   R14.0 Abdominal distension (gaseous)
         Bloating
         Tympanites (abdominal) (intestinal)
   R14.1 Gas pain
   R14.2 Eructation
   R14.3 Flatulence

R15 Fecal incontinence
   Includes: encopresis NOS
   Excludes1: fecal incontinence of nonorganic origin (F98.1)
   R15.0 Incomplete defecation
         Excludes1: constipation (K59.0-)
                  fecal impaction (K56.41)
   R15.1 Fecal smearing
         Fecal soiling
   R15.2 Fecal urgency
   R15.9 Full incontinence of feces
         Fecal incontinence NOS
         AHA CC: 4Q, 2021, 18

R16 Hepatomegaly and splenomegaly, not elsewhere classified
   R16.0 Hepatomegaly, not elsewhere classified
         Hepatomegaly NOS
   R16.1 Splenomegaly, not elsewhere classified
         Splenomegaly NOS
   R16.2 Hepatomegaly with splenomegaly, not elsewhere classified
         Hepatosplenomegaly NOS

R17 Unspecified jaundice
   Excludes1: neonatal jaundice (P55, P57-P59)
   Valid 3-character code, no further characters required

CC **R18 Ascites**
   Includes: fluid in peritoneal cavity
   Excludes1: ascites in alcoholic cirrhosis (K70.31)
            ascites in alcoholic hepatitis (K70.11)
            ascites in toxic liver disease with chronic active hepatitis (K71.51)
   CC **R18.0 Malignant ascites**
         Code first malignancy, such as:
            malignant neoplasm of ovary (C56.-)
            secondary malignant neoplasm of retroperitoneum and peritoneum (C78.6)
   CC **R18.8 Other ascites**
         Ascites NOS
         Peritoneal effusion (chronic)
         AHA CC: 1Q, 2018, 4-5

R19 Other symptoms and signs involving the digestive system and abdomen
   Excludes1: acute abdomen (R10.0)
   + **R19.0 Intra-abdominal and pelvic swelling, mass and lump**
         Excludes1: abdominal distension (gaseous) (R14.-)
                  ascites (R18.-)
      R19.00 Intra-abdominal and pelvic swelling, mass and lump, unspecified site
      R19.01 Right upper quadrant abdominal swelling, mass and lump
      R19.02 Left upper quadrant abdominal swelling, mass and lump
      R19.03 Right lower quadrant abdominal swelling, mass and lump
      R19.04 Left lower quadrant abdominal swelling, mass and lump
      R19.05 Periumbilic swelling, mass or lump
            Diffuse or generalized umbilical swelling or mass
      R19.06 Epigastric swelling, mass or lump
      R19.07 Generalized intra-abdominal and pelvic swelling, mass and lump
            Diffuse or generalized intra-abdominal swelling or mass NOS
            Diffuse or generalized pelvic swelling or mass NOS
      R19.09 Other intra-abdominal and pelvic swelling, mass and lump
   + **R19.1 Abnormal bowel sounds**
      R19.11 Absent bowel sounds
      R19.12 Hyperactive bowel sounds
      R19.15 Other abnormal bowel sounds
            Abnormal bowel sounds NOS
   R19.2 Visible peristalsis
         Hyperperistalsis
   + **R19.3 Abdominal rigidity**
         Excludes1: abdominal rigidity with severe abdominal pain (R10.0)
      R19.30 Abdominal rigidity, unspecified site
      R19.31 Right upper quadrant abdominal rigidity
      R19.32 Left upper quadrant abdominal rigidity
      R19.33 Right lower quadrant abdominal rigidity
      R19.34 Left lower quadrant abdominal rigidity
      R19.35 Periumbilic abdominal rigidity
      R19.36 Epigastric abdominal rigidity
      R19.37 Generalized abdominal rigidity
   R19.4 Change in bowel habit
         Excludes1: constipation (K59.0-)
                  functional diarrhea (K59.1)
   R19.5 Other fecal abnormalities
         Abnormal stool color
         Bulky stools
         Mucus in stools
         Occult blood in feces
         Occult blood in stools
         Excludes1: melena (K92.1)
                  neonatal melena (P54.1)
         AHA CC: 1Q, 2019, 32; 1Q, 2021, 9-10
   R19.6 Halitosis

R19.7 Diarrhea, unspecified
Diarrhea NOS
Excludes1: functional diarrhea (K59.1)
neonatal diarrhea (P78.3)
psychogenic diarrhea (F45.8)
AHA CC: 3Q, 2021, 3-4

R19.8 Other specified symptoms and signs involving the digestive system and abdomen

Symptoms and signs involving the skin and subcutaneous tissue (R20-R23)

Excludes2: symptoms relating to breast (N64.4-N64.5)

R20 Disturbances of skin sensation
Excludes1: dissociative anesthesia and sensory loss (F44.6)
psychogenic disturbances (F45.8)

R20.0 Anesthesia of skin
R20.1 Hypoesthesia of skin
R20.2 Paresthesia of skin
Formication
Pins and needles
Tingling skin
Excludes1: acroparesthesia (I73.8)
R20.3 Hyperesthesia
R20.8 Other disturbances of skin sensation
R20.9 Unspecified disturbances of skin sensation

R21 Rash and other nonspecific skin eruption
Includes: rash NOS
Excludes1: specified type of rash- code to condition vesicular eruption (R23.8)
Valid 3-character code, no further characters required

R22 Localized swelling, mass and lump of skin and subcutaneous tissue
Includes: subcutaneous nodules (localized)(superficial)
Excludes1: abnormal findings on diagnostic imaging (R90-R93)
edema (R60.-)
enlarged lymph nodes (R59.-)
localized adiposity (E65)
swelling of joint (M25.4-)
R22.0 Localized swelling, mass and lump, head
R22.1 Localized swelling, mass and lump, neck
R22.2 Localized swelling, mass and lump, trunk
Excludes1: intra-abdominal or pelvic mass and lump (R19.0-)
intra-abdominal or pelvic swelling (R19.0-)
Excludes2: breast mass and lump (N63)
AHA CC: 3Q, 2022, 8
+ **R22.3 Localized swelling, mass and lump, upper limb**
R22.30 Localized swelling, mass and lump, unspecified upper limb
R22.31 Localized swelling, mass and lump, right upper limb
R22.32 Localized swelling, mass and lump, left upper limb
R22.33 Localized swelling, mass and lump, upper limb, bilateral
+ **R22.4 Localized swelling, mass and lump, lower limb**
R22.40 Localized swelling, mass and lump, unspecified lower limb
R22.41 Localized swelling, mass and lump, right lower limb
R22.42 Localized swelling, mass and lump, left lower limb
R22.43 Localized swelling, mass and lump, lower limb, bilateral
R22.9 Localized swelling, mass and lump, unspecified

R23 Other skin changes
R23.0 Cyanosis
Excludes1: acrocyanosis (I73.8)
cyanotic attacks of newborn (P28.2)
R23.1 Pallor
Clammy skin
R23.2 Flushing
Excessive blushing
Code first, if applicable, menopausal and female climacteric states (N95.1)

R23.3 Spontaneous ecchymoses
Petechiae
Excludes1: ecchymoses of newborn (P54.5)
purpura (D69.-)
R23.4 Changes in skin texture
Desquamation of skin
Induration of skin
Scaling of skin
Excludes1: epidermal thickening NOS (L85.9)
R23.8 Other skin changes
R23.9 Unspecified skin changes

Symptoms and signs involving the nervous and musculoskeletal systems (R25-R29)

R25 Abnormal involuntary movements
Excludes1: specific movement disorders (G20-G26)
stereotyped movement disorders (F98.4)
tic disorders (F95.-)
R25.0 Abnormal head movements
R25.1 Tremor, unspecified
Excludes1: chorea NOS (G25.5)
essential tremor (G25.0)
hysterical tremor (F44.4)
intention tremor (G25.2)
R25.2 Cramp and spasm
Excludes2: carpopedal spasm (R29.0)
charley-horse (M62.831)
infantile spasms (G40.4-)
muscle spasm of back (M62.830)
muscle spasm of calf (M62.831)
R25.3 Fasciculation
Twitching NOS
R25.8 Other abnormal involuntary movements
R25.9 Unspecified abnormal involuntary movements

R26 Abnormalities of gait and mobility
Excludes1: ataxia NOS (R27.0)
hereditary ataxia (G11.-)
locomotor (syphilitic) ataxia (A52.11)
immobility syndrome (paraplegic) (M62.3)
R26.0 Ataxic gait
Staggering gait
AHA CC: 2Q, 2022, 12-13
R26.1 Paralytic gait
Spastic gait
R26.2 Difficulty in walking, not elsewhere classified
Excludes1: falling (R29.6)
unsteadiness on feet (R26.81)
AHA CC: 2Q, 2016, 7
R26.8 Other abnormalities of gait and mobility
R26.81 Unsteadiness on feet
R26.89 Other abnormalities of gait and mobility
AHA CC: 2Q, 2020, 29
R26.9 Unspecified abnormalities of gait and mobility

R27 Other lack of coordination
Excludes1: ataxic gait (R26.0)
hereditary ataxia (G11.-)
vertigo NOS (R42)
R27.0 Ataxia, unspecified
Excludes1: ataxia following cerebrovascular disease (I69. with final characters -93)
AHA CC: 3Q, 2022, 10
R27.8 Other lack of coordination
R27.9 Unspecified lack of coordination

R29 Other symptoms and signs involving the nervous and musculoskeletal systems
CC **R29.0 Tetany**
Carpopedal spasm
Excludes1: hysterical tetany (F44.5)
neonatal tetany (P71.3)
parathyroid tetany (E20.9)
post-thyroidectomy tetany (E89.2)
CC **R29.1 Meningismus**
R29.2 Abnormal reflex
Excludes2: abnormal pupillary reflex (H57.0)
hyperactive gag reflex (J39.2)
vasovagal reaction or syncope (R55)
R29.3 Abnormal posture

R29.4 Clicking hip
   Excludes1: congenital deformities of hip (Q65.-)
CC **R29.5** Transient paralysis
   Code first any associated spinal cord injury (S14.0, S14.1-, S24.0, S24.1-, S34.0-, S34.1-)
   Excludes1: transient ischemic attack (G45.9)
R29.6 Repeated falls
   Falling
   Tendency to fall
   Excludes2: at risk for falling (Z91.81)
      history of falling (Z91.81)
   Review coding guideline C.18.d
   AHA CC: 2Q, 2016, 6-7
+ **R29.7** National Institutes of Health Stroke Scale (NIHSS) score
   Code first the type of cerebral infarction (I63.-)
   Review coding guidelines B.14 and C.18.i
   AHA CC: 4Q, 2016, 61-62
   + **R29.70** NIHSS score 0-9
      R29.700 NIHSS score 0
      R29.701 NIHSS score 1
      R29.702 NIHSS score 2
      R29.703 NIHSS score 3
      R29.704 NIHSS score 4
      R29.705 NIHSS score 5
      R29.706 NIHSS score 6
      R29.707 NIHSS score 7
      R29.708 NIHSS score 8
      R29.709 NIHSS score 9
   + **R29.71** NIHSS score 10-19
      R29.710 NIHSS score 10
      R29.711 NIHSS score 11
      R29.712 NIHSS score 12
      R29.713 NIHSS score 13
      R29.714 NIHSS score 14
      R29.715 NIHSS score 15
      R29.716 NIHSS score 16
      R29.717 NIHSS score 17
      R29.718 NIHSS score 18
      R29.719 NIHSS score 19
   + **R29.72** NIHSS score 20-29
      R29.720 NIHSS score 20
      R29.721 NIHSS score 21
      R29.722 NIHSS score 22
      R29.723 NIHSS score 23
      R29.724 NIHSS score 24
      R29.725 NIHSS score 25
      R29.726 NIHSS score 26
      R29.727 NIHSS score 27
      R29.728 NIHSS score 28
      R29.729 NIHSS score 29
   + **R29.73** NIHSS score 30-39
      R29.730 NIHSS score 30
         AHA CC: 4Q, 2016, 61-62
      R29.731 NIHSS score 31
      R29.732 NIHSS score 32
      R29.733 NIHSS score 33
      R29.734 NIHSS score 34
      R29.735 NIHSS score 35
      R29.736 NIHSS score 36
      R29.737 NIHSS score 37
      R29.738 NIHSS score 38
      R29.739 NIHSS score 39
   + **R29.74** NIHSS score 40-42
      R29.740 NIHSS score 40
      R29.741 NIHSS score 41
      R29.742 NIHSS score 42
+ **R29.8** Other symptoms and signs involving the nervous and musculoskeletal systems
   + **R29.81** Other symptoms and signs involving the nervous system
      R29.810 Facial weakness
         Facial droop
         Excludes1: Bell's palsy (G51.0)
            facial weakness following cerebrovascular disease (I69. with final characters -92)
         AHA CC: 3Q, 2022, 9
      R29.818 Other symptoms and signs involving the nervous system
   + **R29.89** Other symptoms and signs involving the musculoskeletal system
      Excludes2: pain in limb (M79.6-)
      R29.890 Loss of height
         Excludes1: osteoporosis (M80-M81)
      R29.891 Ocular torticollis
         Excludes1: congenital (sternomastoid) torticollis (Q68.0)
            psychogenic torticollis (F45.8)
            spasmodic torticollis (G24.3)
            torticollis due to birth injury (P15.8)
            torticollis NOS (M43.6)
      R29.898 Other symptoms and signs involving the musculoskeletal system
+ **R29.9** Unspecified symptoms and signs involving the nervous and musculoskeletal systems
   R29.90 Unspecified symptoms and signs involving the nervous system
   R29.91 Unspecified symptoms and signs involving the musculoskeletal system

Symptoms and signs involving the genitourinary system (R30-R39)

R30 Pain associated with micturition
   Excludes1: psychogenic pain associated with micturition (F45.8)
   R30.0 Dysuria
      Strangury
   R30.1 Vesical tenesmus
   R30.9 Painful micturition, unspecified
      Painful urination NOS

R31 Hematuria
   Excludes1: hematuria included with underlying conditions, such as:
      acute cystitis with hematuria (N30.01)
      recurrent and persistent hematuria in glomerular diseases (N02.-)
   R31.0 Gross hematuria
      AHA CC: 1Q, 2017, 17-18
   R31.1 Benign essential microscopic hematuria
   + **R31.2** Other microscopic hematuria
      AHA CC: 4Q, 2016, 62
      R31.21 Asymptomatic microscopic hematuria
         AMH
         AHA CC: 4Q, 2016, 62
      R31.29 Other microscopic hematuria
   R31.9 Hematuria, unspecified
      AHA CC: 1Q, 2017, 6

R32 Unspecified urinary incontinence
   Enuresis NOS
   Excludes1: functional urinary incontinence (R39.81)
      nonorganic enuresis (F98.0)
      stress incontinence and other specified urinary incontinence (N39.3-N39.4-)
      urinary incontinence associated with cognitive impairment (R39.81)
   AHA CC: 4Q, 2021, 18
   Valid 3-character code, no further characters required

R33 Retention of urine
   Excludes1: psychogenic retention of urine (F45.8)
   R33.0 Drug induced retention of urine
      Use additional code for adverse effect, if applicable, to identify drug (T36-T50 with fifth or sixth character 5)
   R33.8 Other retention of urine
      Code first if applicable, any causal condition, such as: enlarged prostate (N40.1)
   R33.9 Retention of urine, unspecified

R34 Anuria and oliguria
   Excludes1: anuria and oliguria complicating abortion or ectopic or molar pregnancy (O00-O07, O08.4)
      anuria and oliguria complicating pregnancy (O26.83-)
      anuria and oliguria complicating the puerperium (O90.49)
   Valid 3-character code, no further characters required

R35 Polyuria
   Code first if applicable, any causal condition, such as:
     enlarged prostate (N40.1)
   Excludes1: psychogenic polyuria (F45.8)
   R35.0 Frequency of micturition
   R35.1 Nocturia
 + **R35.8 Other polyuria**
     AHA CC: 4Q, 2021, 26
     R35.81 Nocturnal polyuria
        Excludes2: nocturnal enuresis (N39.44)
     R35.89 Other polyuria
        Polyuria NOS

R36 Urethral discharge
   R36.0 Urethral discharge without blood
 ♂ **R36.1 Hematospermia**
   R36.9 Urethral discharge, unspecified
     Penile discharge NOS
     Urethrorrhea

R37 Sexual dysfunction, unspecified
   Valid 3-character code, no further characters required

R39 Other and unspecified symptoms and signs involving the genitourinary system
 CC **R39.0 Extravasation of urine**
 + **R39.1 Other difficulties with micturition**
     Code first if applicable, any causal condition, such as:
       enlarged prostate (N40.1)
     R39.11 Hesitancy of micturition
     R39.12 Poor urinary stream
        Weak urinary steam
     R39.13 Splitting of urinary stream
     R39.14 Feeling of incomplete bladder emptying
     R39.15 Urgency of urination
        Excludes1: urge incontinence (N39.41, N39.46)
     R39.16 Straining to void
   + **R39.19 Other difficulties with micturition**
        AHA CC: 4Q, 2016, 63
        R39.191 Need to immediately re-void
        R39.192 Position dependent micturition
        R39.198 Other difficulties with micturition
   R39.2 Extrarenal uremia
     Prerenal uremia
     Excludes1: uremia NOS (N19)
 + **R39.8 Other symptoms and signs involving the genitourinary system**
     AHA CC: 4Q, 2016, 64
     R39.81 Functional urinary incontinence
        Urinary incontinence due to cognitive impairment, or severe physical disability or immobility
        Excludes1: stress incontinence and other specified urinary incontinence (N39.3-N39.4-)
          urinary incontinence NOS (R32)
     R39.82 Chronic bladder pain
        AHA CC: 4Q, 2016, 64
     ♂ **R39.83 Unilateral non-palpable testicle**
        AHA CC: 4Q, 2017, 22-23
     ♂ **R39.84 Bilateral non-palpable testicles**
        AHA CC: 4Q, 2017, 22-23
     R39.89 Other symptoms and signs involving the genitourinary system
   R39.9 Unspecified symptoms and signs involving the genitourinary system

Symptoms and signs involving cognition, perception, emotional state and behavior (R40-R46)
Excludes2: symptoms and signs constituting part of a pattern of mental disorder (F01-F99)

R40 Somnolence, stupor and coma
   Excludes1: neonatal coma (P91.5)
     somnolence, stupor and coma in diabetes (E08-E13)
     somnolence, stupor and coma in hepatic failure (K72.-)
     somnolence, stupor and coma in hypoglycemia (nondiabetic) (E15)
   R40.0 Somnolence
     Drowsiness
     Excludes1: coma (R40.2-)
   R40.1 Stupor
     Catatonic stupor
     Semicoma
     Excludes1: catatonic schizophrenia (F20.2)
       coma (R40.2-)
       depressive stupor (F31-F33)
       dissociative stupor (F44.2)
       manic stupor (F30.2)
 + **R40.2 Coma**
     Code first any associated:
       fracture of skull (S02.-)
       intracranial injury (S06.-)
     NOTE One code from each subcategory, R40.21-R40.23, is required to complete the coma scale
     Review coding guidelines B.14 and C.18.e
     AHA CC: 1Q, 2014, 19-20; 2Q, 2015, 17-18
 MCC X+7th **R40.20 Unspecified coma**
     Coma NOS
     Unconsciousness NOS
     AHA CC: 2Q, 2021, 5; 4Q, 2021, 112-113
 + **R40.21 Coma scale, eyes open**
     AHA CC: 4Q, 2017, 25

The appropriate 7th character is to be added to each code from subcategory **R40.21-**:
0 unspecified time
1 in the field [EMT or ambulance]
2 at arrival to emergency department
3 at hospital admission
4 24 hours or more after hospital admission

 MCC +7th **R40.211 Coma scale, eyes open, never**
        Coma scale eye opening score of 1
 MCC +7th **R40.212 Coma scale, eyes open, to pain**
        Coma scale eye opening score of 2
 +7th **R40.213 Coma scale, eyes open, to sound**
        Coma scale eye opening score of 3
 +7th **R40.214 Coma scale, eyes open, spontaneous**
        Coma scale eye opening score of 4
 + **R40.22 Coma scale, best verbal response**
     AHA CC: 4Q, 2017, 23-25

The appropriate 7th character is to be added to each code from subcategory **R40.22-**:
0 unspecified time
1 in the field [EMT or ambulance]
2 at arrival to emergency department
3 at hospital admission
4 24 hours or more after hospital admission

 MCC +7th **R40.221 Coma scale, best verbal response, none**
        Coma scale verbal score of 1
 MCC +7th **R40.222 Coma scale, best verbal response, incomprehensible words**
        Coma scale verbal score of 2
        Incomprehensible sounds (2-5 years of age)
        Moans/grunts to pain (<2 years of age)
 +7th **R40.223 Coma scale, best verbal response, inappropriate words**
        Coma scale verbal score of 3
        Inappropriate crying or screaming (<2 years of age)
        Screaming (2-5 years of age)
 +7th **R40.224 Coma scale, best verbal response, confused conversation**
        Coma scale verbal score of 4
        Inappropriate words (2-5 years of age)
        Irritable cries (<2 years of age)
 +7th **R40.225 Coma scale, best verbal response, oriented**
        Coma scale verbal score of 5
        Cooing or babbling or crying appropriately (<2 years of age)
        Uses appropriate words (2-5 years of age)

+ R40.23   Coma scale, best motor response
AHA CC: 4Q, 2017, 23-25

The appropriate 7th character is to be added to each code from subcategory **R40.23-**:
- 0   unspecified time
- 1   in the field [EMT or ambulance]
- 2   at arrival to emergency department
- 3   at hospital admission
- 4   24 hours or more after hospital admission

MCC +7th **R40.231   Coma scale, best motor response, none**
  Coma scale motor score of 1

MCC +7th **R40.232   Coma scale, best motor response, extension**
  Abnormal extensor posturing to pain or noxious stimuli (<2 years of age)
  Coma scale motor score of 2
  Extensor posturing to pain or noxious stimuli (2-5 years of age)

+7th **R40.233   Coma scale, best motor response, abnormal flexion**
  Abnormal flexure posturing to pain or noxious stimuli (2-5 years of age)
  Coma scale motor score of 3
  Flexion/decorticate posturing (<2 years of age)

MCC +7th **R40.234   Coma scale, best motor response, flexion withdrawal**
  Coma scale motor score of 4
  Withdraws from pain or noxious stimuli (2-5 years of age)

+7th **R40.235   Coma scale, best motor response, localizes pain**
  Coma scale motor score of 5
  Localizes pain (2-5 years of age)
  Withdraws to touch (<2 years of age)

+7th **R40.236   Coma scale, best motor response, obeys commands**
  Coma scale motor score of 6
  Normal or spontaneous movement (<2 years of age)
  Obeys commands (2-5 years of age)

+ **R40.24   Glasgow coma scale, total score**
  NOTE   Assign a code from subcategory R40.24, when only the total coma score is documented.
  AHA CC: 4Q, 2016, 64-65

The appropriate 7th character is to be added to each code from subcategory **R40.24-**:
- 0   unspecified time
- 1   in the field [EMT or ambulance]
- 2   at arrival to emergency department
- 3   at hospital admission
- 4   24 hours or more after hospital admission

+7th **R40.241   Glasgow coma scale score 13-15**
+7th **R40.242   Glasgow coma scale score 9-12**
+7th **R40.243   Glasgow coma scale score 3-8**
+7th **R40.244   Other coma, without documented Glasgow coma scale score, or with partial score reported**
  AHA CC: 3Q, 2020, 46

MCC **R40.2A   Nontraumatic coma due to underlying condition**
  Secondary coma
  Code first underlying condition

CC **R40.3   Persistent vegetative state**

R40.4   Transient alteration of awareness
  AHA CC: 2Q, 2020, 24

R41   Other symptoms and signs involving cognitive functions and awareness
  Excludes1: dissociative [conversion] disorders (F44.-)
  mild cognitive impairment of uncertain or unknown etiology (G31.84)

R41.0   Disorientation, unspecified
  Confusion NOS
  Delirium NOS
  AHA CC: 4Q, 2016, 74-76; 2Q, 2019, 34; 2Q, 2022, 11-12

R41.1   Anterograde amnesia
R41.2   Retrograde amnesia
R41.3   Other amnesia
  Amnesia NOS
  Memory loss NOS
  Excludes1: amnestic disorder due to known physiologic condition (F04)
  amnestic syndrome due to psychoactive substance use (F10-F19 with 5th character .6)
  mild memory disturbance due to known physiological condition (F06.8)
  transient global amnesia (G45.4)

CC **R41.4   Neurologic neglect syndrome**
  Asomatognosia
  Hemi-akinesia
  Hemi-inattention
  Hemispatial neglect
  Left-sided neglect
  Sensory neglect
  Visuospatial neglect
  Excludes1: visuospatial deficit (R41.842)

+ **R41.8   Other symptoms and signs involving cognitive functions and awareness**

  • **R41.81   Age-related cognitive decline**
    Senility NOS

  R41.82   Altered mental status, unspecified
    Change in mental status NOS
    Excludes1: altered level of consciousness (R40.-)
    altered mental status due to known condition - code to condition
    delirium NOS (R41.0)
    AHA CC: 4Q, 2012, 98

  R41.83   Borderline intellectual functioning
    IQ level 71 to 84
    Excludes1: intellectual disabilities (F70-F79)

+ **R41.84   Other specified cognitive deficit**
    Excludes1: cognitive deficits as sequelae of cerebrovascular disease (I69.01-, I69.11-, I19.21-, I69.31-, I59.81-, I69.91-)

  R41.840   Attention and concentration deficit
    Excludes1: attention-deficit hyperactivity disorders (F90.-)

  R41.841   Cognitive communication deficit
  R41.842   Visuospatial deficit
  R41.843   Psychomotor deficit
  R41.844   Frontal lobe and executive function deficit

  R41.89   Other symptoms and signs involving cognitive functions and awareness
    Anosognosia

R41.9   Unspecified symptoms and signs involving cognitive functions and awareness
  Unspecified neurocognitive disorder

R42   Dizziness and giddiness
  Light-headedness
  Vertigo NOS
  Excludes1: vertiginous syndromes (H81.-)
  vertigo from infrasound (T75.23)
  Valid 3-character code, no further characters required

R43   Disturbances of smell and taste
  R43.0   Anosmia
  R43.1   Parosmia
  R43.2   Parageusia
  R43.8   Other disturbances of smell and taste
    Mixed disturbance of smell and taste
  R43.9   Unspecified disturbances of smell and taste

R44   Other symptoms and signs involving general sensations and perceptions
  Excludes1: alcoholic hallucinations (F10.151, F10.251, F10.951)
  hallucinations in drug psychosis (F11-F19 with fifth to sixth characters 51)
  hallucinations in mood disorders with psychotic symptoms (F30.2, F31.5, F32.3, F33.3)
  hallucinations in schizophrenia, schizotypal and delusional disorders (F20-F29)
  Excludes2: disturbances of skin sensation (R20.-)

- **CC R44.0** Auditory hallucinations
- **R44.1** Visual hallucinations
- **CC R44.2** Other hallucinations
- **CC R44.3** Hallucinations, unspecified
  - *AHA CC: 2Q, 2022, 11-12*
- **R44.8** Other symptoms and signs involving general sensations and perceptions
- **R44.9** Unspecified symptoms and signs involving general sensations and perceptions

R45 Symptoms and signs involving emotional state

- **R45.0** Nervousness
  - Nervous tension
- **R45.1** Restlessness and agitation
- **R45.2** Unhappiness
- **R45.3** Demoralization and apathy
  - *Excludes1:* anhedonia (R45.84)
- **R45.4** Irritability and anger
- **R45.5** Hostility
- **R45.6** Violent behavior
- **R45.7** State of emotional shock and stress, unspecified
- **+ R45.8** Other symptoms and signs involving emotional state
  - **R45.81** Low self-esteem
  - **R45.82** Worries
  - **R45.83** Excessive crying of child, adolescent or adult
    - *Excludes1:* excessive crying of infant (baby) (R68.11)
  - **R45.84** Anhedonia
  - **+ R45.85** Homicidal and suicidal ideations
    - *Excludes1:* suicide attempt (T14.91)
    - **R45.850** Homicidal ideations
    - **CC R45.851** Suicidal ideations
      - *AHA CC: 1Q, 2022, 29*
  - **R45.86** Emotional lability
  - **R45.87** Impulsiveness
  - **R45.88** Nonsuicidal self-harm
    - Nonsuicidal self-injury
    - Nonsuicidal self-mutilation
    - Self-inflicted injury without suicidal intent
    - Code also injury, if known
    - *AHA CC: 4Q, 2021, 26-27, 33*
  - **R45.89** Other symptoms and signs involving emotional state
    - Flat affect
    - Loneliness

R46 Symptoms and signs involving appearance and behavior

Excludes1: appearance and behavior in schizophrenia, schizotypal and delusional disorders (F20-F29)
mental and behavioral disorders (F01-F99)

- **R46.0** Very low level of personal hygiene
- **R46.1** Bizarre personal appearance
- **R46.2** Strange and inexplicable behavior
- **R46.3** Overactivity
- **R46.4** Slowness and poor responsiveness
  - *Excludes1:* stupor (R40.1)
- **R46.5** Suspiciousness and marked evasiveness
- **R46.6** Undue concern and preoccupation with stressful events
- **R46.7** Verbosity and circumstantial detail obscuring reason for contact
- **+ R46.8** Other symptoms and signs involving appearance and behavior
  - **R46.81** Obsessive-compulsive behavior
    - *Excludes1:* obsessive-compulsive disorder (F42.-)
  - **R46.89** Other symptoms and signs involving appearance and behavior

Symptoms and signs involving speech and voice (R47-R49)

R47 Speech disturbances, not elsewhere classified

Excludes1: autism (F84.0)
cluttering (F80.81)
specific developmental disorders of speech and language (F80.-)
stuttering (F80.81)

- **+ R47.0** Dysphasia and aphasia
  - **CC R47.01** Aphasia
    - *Excludes1:* aphasia following cerebrovascular disease (I69. with final characters -20)
      progressive isolated aphasia (G31.01)
    - *AHA CC: 3Q, 2022, 9*
  - **R47.02** Dysphasia
    - *Excludes1:* dysphasia following cerebrovascular disease (I69. with final characters -21)
- **R47.1** Dysarthria and anarthria
  - *Excludes1:* dysarthria following cerebrovascular disease (I69. with final characters -22)
  - *AHA CC: 3Q, 2022, 9*
- **+ R47.8** Other speech disturbances
  - *Excludes1:* dysarthria following cerebrovascular disease (I69. with final characters -28)
  - **R47.81** Slurred speech
  - **R47.82** Fluency disorder in conditions classified elsewhere
    - Stuttering in conditions classified elsewhere
    - Code first underlying disease or condition, such as: Parkinson's disease (G20.-)
    - *Excludes1:* adult onset fluency disorder (F98.5)
      childhood onset fluency disorder (F80.81)
      fluency disorder (stuttering) following cerebrovascular disease (I69. with final characters -23)
  - **R47.89** Other speech disturbances
- **R47.9** Unspecified speech disturbances

R48 Dyslexia and other symbolic dysfunctions, not elsewhere classified

Excludes1: specific developmental disorders of scholastic skills (F81.-)

- **R48.0** Dyslexia and alexia
- **R48.1** Agnosia
  - Astereognosia (astereognosis)
  - Autotopagnosia
  - *Excludes1:* visual object agnosia (R48.3)
- **R48.2** Apraxia
  - *Excludes1:* apraxia following cerebrovascular disease (I69. with final characters -90)
- **R48.3** Visual agnosia
  - Prosopagnosia
  - Simultanagnosia (asimultagnosia)
- **R48.8** Other symbolic dysfunctions
  - Acalculia
  - Agraphia
  - *AHA CC: 1Q, 2017, 27-28*
- **R48.9** Unspecified symbolic dysfunctions

R49 Voice and resonance disorders

Excludes1: psychogenic voice and resonance disorders (F44.4)

- **R49.0** Dysphonia
  - Hoarseness
- **R49.1** Aphonia
  - Loss of voice
- **+ R49.2** Hypernasality and hyponasality
  - **R49.21** Hypernasality
  - **R49.22** Hyponasality
- **R49.8** Other voice and resonance disorders
- **R49.9** Unspecified voice and resonance disorder
  - Change in voice NOS
  - Resonance disorder NOS

General symptoms and signs (R50-R69)

R50 Fever of other and unknown origin

Excludes1: chills without fever (R68.83)
febrile convulsions (R56.0-)
fever of unknown origin during labor (O75.2)
fever of unknown origin in newborn (P81.9)
hypothermia due to illness (R68.0)
malignant hyperthermia due to anesthesia (T88.3)
puerperal pyrexia NOS (O86.4)

- **R50.2** Drug induced fever
  - Use additional code for adverse effect, if applicable, to identify drug (T36-T50 with fifth or sixth character 5)
  - *Excludes1:* postvaccination (postimmunization) fever (R50.83)
- **+ R50.8** Other specified fever
  - **R50.81** Fever presenting with conditions classified elsewhere
    - Code first underlying condition when associated fever is present, such as with:
      leukemia (C91-C95)
      neutropenia (D70.-)
      sickle-cell disease (D57.-)
    - *AHA CC: 4Q, 2014, 22-23; 2Q, 2019, 24-25; 3Q, 2020, 22-23*

R50.82 **Postprocedural fever**
    Excludes1: postprocedural infection (T81.4-)
                 posttransfusion fever (R50.84)
                 postvaccination (postimmunization)
                   fever (R50.83)

R50.83 **Postvaccination fever**
    Postimmunization fever

R50.84 **Febrile nonhemolytic transfusion reaction**
    FNHTR
    Posttransfusion fever

R50.9 **Fever, unspecified**
    Fever NOS
    Fever of unknown origin [FUO]
    Fever with chills
    Fever with rigors
    Hyperpyrexia NOS
    Persistent fever
    Pyrexia NOS
    AHA CC: 1Q, 2020, 34-36

R51 Headache
    Excludes2: atypical face pain (G50.1)
                 migraine and other headache syndromes (G43-G44)
                 trigeminal neuralgia (G50.0)
    AHA CC: 4Q, 2020, 38-39

R51.0 **Headache with orthostatic component, not elsewhere classified**
    Headache with positional component, not elsewhere classified

R51.9 **Headache, unspecified**
    Facial pain NOS

R52 Pain, unspecified
    Acute pain NOS
    Generalized pain NOS
    Pain NOS
    Excludes1: acute and chronic pain, not elsewhere classified (G89.-)
                 localized pain, unspecified type - code to pain by site, such as:
                     abdomen pain (R10.-)
                     back pain (M54.9)
                     breast pain (N64.4)
                     chest pain (R07.1-R07.9)
                     ear pain (H92.0-)
                     eye pain (H57.1)
                     headache (R51.9)
                     joint pain (M25.5-)
                     limb pain (M79.6-)
                     lumbar region pain (M54.5-)
                     pelvic and perineal pain (R10.2)
                     shoulder pain (M25.51-)
                     spine pain (M54.-)
                     throat pain (R07.0)
                     tongue pain (K14.6)
                     tooth pain (K08.8)
                     renal colic (N23)
                 pain disorders exclusively related to psychological factors (F45.41)
    Valid 3-character code, no further characters required

R53 Malaise and fatigue

R53.0 **Neoplastic (malignant) related fatigue**
    Code first associated neoplasm

R53.1 **Weakness**
    Asthenia NOS
    Excludes1: age-related weakness (R54)
                 muscle weakness (generalized) (M62.81)
                 sarcopenia (M62.84)
                 senile asthenia (R54)
    AHA CC: 1Q, 2017, 7; 4Q, 2021, 102-103

MCC R53.2 **Functional quadriplegia**
    Complete immobility due to severe physical disability or frailty
    Excludes1: frailty NOS (R54)
                 hysterical paralysis (F44.4)
                 immobility syndrome (M62.3)
                 neurologic quadriplegia (G82.5-)
                 quadriplegia (G82.50)
    Review coding guideline C.18.f
    AHA CC: 2Q, 2016, 6; 4Q, 2022, 15

+ R53.8 **Other malaise and fatigue**
    Excludes1: combat exhaustion and fatigue (F43.0)
                 congenital debility (P96.9)
                 exhaustion and fatigue due to excessive exertion (T73.3)
                 exhaustion and fatigue due to exposure (T73.2)
                 exhaustion and fatigue due to heat (T67.-)
                 exhaustion and fatigue due to pregnancy (O26.8-)
                 exhaustion and fatigue due to recurrent depressive episode (F33)
                 exhaustion and fatigue due to senile debility (R54)

R53.81 **Other malaise**
    Chronic debility
    Debility NOS
    General physical deterioration
    Malaise NOS
    Nervous debility
    Excludes1: age-related physical debility (R54)
    AHA CC: 1Q, 2021, 43

R53.82 **Chronic fatigue, unspecified**
    Excludes1: chronic fatigue syndrome (G93.32)
                 myalgic encephalomyelitis (G93.32)
                 other post infection and related fatigue syndromes (G93.39)
                 postviral fatigue syndrome (G93.31)

R53.83 **Other fatigue**
    Fatigue NOS
    Lack of energy
    Lethargy
    Tiredness
    Excludes2: exhaustion and fatigue due to depressive episode (F32.-)
    AHA CC: 1Q, 2017, 7

• R54 Age-related physical debility
    Frailty
    Old age
    Senescence
    Senile asthenia
    Senile debility
    Excludes1: age-related cognitive decline (R41.81)
                 sarcopenia (M62.84)
                 senile psychosis (F03)
                 senility NOS (R41.81)
    Valid 3-character code, no further characters required

R55 Syncope and collapse
    Blackout
    Fainting
    Vasovagal attack
    Excludes1: cardiogenic shock (R57.0)
                 carotid sinus syncope (G90.01)
                 heat syncope (T67.1)
                 neurocirculatory asthenia (F45.8)
                 neurogenic orthostatic hypotension (G90.3)
                 orthostatic hypotension (I95.1)
                 postprocedural shock (T81.1-)
                 psychogenic syncope (F48.8)
                 shock NOS (R57.9)
                 shock complicating or following abortion or ectopic or molar pregnancy (O00-O07, O08.3)
                 shock complicating or following labor and delivery (O75.1)
                 Stokes-Adams attack (I45.9)
                 unconsciousness NOS (R40.2-)
    Valid 3-character code, no further characters required

R56 Convulsions, not elsewhere classified
    Excludes1: dissociative convulsions and seizures (F44.5)
                 epileptic convulsions and seizures (G40.-)
                 newborn convulsions and seizures (P90)

+ R56.0 **Febrile convulsions**

CC R56.00 **Simple febrile convulsions**
    Febrile convulsion NOS
    Febrile seizure NOS

CC R56.01 **Complex febrile convulsions**
    Atypical febrile seizure
    Complex febrile seizure
    Complicated febrile seizure
    Excludes1: status epilepticus (G40.901)

CC R56.1 **Post traumatic seizures**
    Excludes1: post traumatic epilepsy (G40.-)

R56.9 Unspecified convulsions
Convulsion disorder
Fit NOS
Recurrent convulsions
Seizure(s) (convulsive) NOS
AHA CC: 4Q, 2019, 17-18; 1Q, 2021, 3; 4Q, 2022, 46

R57 Shock, not elsewhere classified
Excludes1: anaphylactic shock NOS (T78.2)
anaphylactic reaction or shock due to adverse food reaction (T78.0-)
anaphylactic shock due to adverse effect of correct drug or medicament properly administered (T88.6)
anaphylactic shock due to serum (T80.5-)
electric shock (T75.4)
obstetric shock (O75.1)
postprocedural shock (T81.1-)
psychic shock (F43.0)
shock complicating or following ectopic or molar pregnancy (O00-O07, O08.3)
shock due to anesthesia (T88.2)
shock due to lightning (T75.01)
traumatic shock (T79.4)
toxic shock syndrome (A48.3)

MCC **R57.0** Cardiogenic shock
Excludes2: septic shock (R65.21)
AHA CC: 3Q, 2020, 26

MCC **R57.1** Hypovolemic shock
AHA CC: 2Q, 2019, 7-8

MCC **R57.8** Other shock
CC **R57.9** Shock, unspecified
Failure of peripheral circulation NOS

R58 Hemorrhage, not elsewhere classified
Hemorrhage NOS
Excludes1: hemorrhage included with underlying conditions, such as:
acute duodenal ulcer with hemorrhage (K26.0)
acute gastritis with bleeding (K29.01)
ulcerative enterocolitis with rectal bleeding (K51.01)
Valid 3-character code, no further characters required

R59 Enlarged lymph nodes
Includes: swollen glands
Excludes1: lymphadenitis NOS (I88.9)
acute lymphadenitis (L04.-)
chronic lymphadenitis (I88.1)
mesenteric (acute) (chronic) lymphadenitis (I88.0)
R59.0 Localized enlarged lymph nodes
R59.1 Generalized enlarged lymph nodes
Lymphadenopathy NOS
R59.9 Enlarged lymph nodes, unspecified

R60 Edema, not elsewhere classified
Excludes1: angioneurotic edema (T78.3)
ascites (R18.-)
cerebral edema (G93.6)
cerebral edema due to birth injury (P11.0)
edema of larynx (J38.4)
edema of nasopharynx (J39.2)
edema of pharynx (J39.2)
gestational edema (O12.0-)
hereditary edema (Q82.0)
hydrops fetalis NOS (P83.2)
hydrothorax (J94.8)
hydrops fetalis NOS (P83.2)
newborn edema (P83.3)
pulmonary edema (J81.-)
R60.0 Localized edema
R60.1 Generalized edema
Excludes2: nutritional edema (E40-E46)
R60.9 Edema, unspecified
Fluid retention NOS

R61 Generalized hyperhidrosis
Excessive sweating
Night sweats
Secondary hyperhidrosis
Code first if applicable, menopausal and female climacteric states (N95.1)
Excludes1: focal (primary) (secondary) hyperhidrosis (L74.5-)
Frey's syndrome (L74.52)
localized (primary) (secondary) hyperhidrosis (L74.5-)
Valid 3-character code, no further characters required

R62 Lack of expected normal physiological development in childhood and adults
Excludes1: delayed puberty (E30.0)
gonadal dysgenesis (Q99.1)
hypopituitarism (E23.0)
• **R62.0** Delayed milestone in childhood
Delayed attainment of expected physiological developmental stage
Late talker
Late walker
+ **R62.5** Other and unspecified lack of expected normal physiological development in childhood
Excludes1: HIV disease resulting in failure to thrive (B20)
physical retardation due to malnutrition (E45)
R62.50 Unspecified lack of expected normal physiological development in childhood
Infantilism NOS
• **R62.51** Failure to thrive (child)
Failure to gain weight
Excludes1: failure to thrive in child under 28 days old (P92.6)
AHA CC: 4Q, 2018, 82
R62.52 Short stature (child)
Lack of growth
Physical retardation
Short stature NOS
Excludes1: short stature due to endocrine disorder (E34.3-)
R62.59 Other lack of expected normal physiological development in childhood
• **R62.7** Adult failure to thrive

R63 Symptoms and signs concerning food and fluid intake
Excludes1: bulimia NOS (F50.2)
R63.0 Anorexia
Loss of appetite
Excludes1: anorexia nervosa (F50.0-)
loss of appetite of nonorganic origin (F50.89)
AHA CC: 4Q, 2021, 102-103
R63.1 Polydipsia
Excessive thirst
R63.2 Polyphagia
Excessive eating
Hyperalimentation NOS
+ **R63.3** Feeding difficulties
Excludes2: eating disorders (F50.-)
feeding problems of newborn (P92.-)
infant feeding disorder of nonorganic origin (F98.2-)
AHA CC: 4Q, 2021, 27-28
R63.30 Feeding difficulties, unspecified
AHA CC: 4Q, 2021, 102-103
• **R63.31** Pediatric feeding disorder, acute
Pediatric feeding dysfunction, acute
Code also, if applicable, associated conditions such as:
aspiration pneumonia (J69.0)
dysphagia (R13.1-)
gastro-esophageal reflux disease (K21.-)
malnutrition (E40-E46)
• **R63.32** Pediatric feeding disorder, chronic
Pediatric feeding dysfunction, chronic
Code also, if applicable, associated conditions such as:
aspiration pneumonia (J69.0)
dysphagia (R13.1-)
gastro-esophageal reflux disease (K21.-)
malnutrition (E40-E46)
R63.39 Other feeding difficulties
Feeding problem (elderly) (infant) NOS
Picky eater
R63.4 Abnormal weight loss
R63.5 Abnormal weight gain
Excludes1: excessive weight gain in pregnancy (O26.0-)
obesity (E66.-)

Sepsis

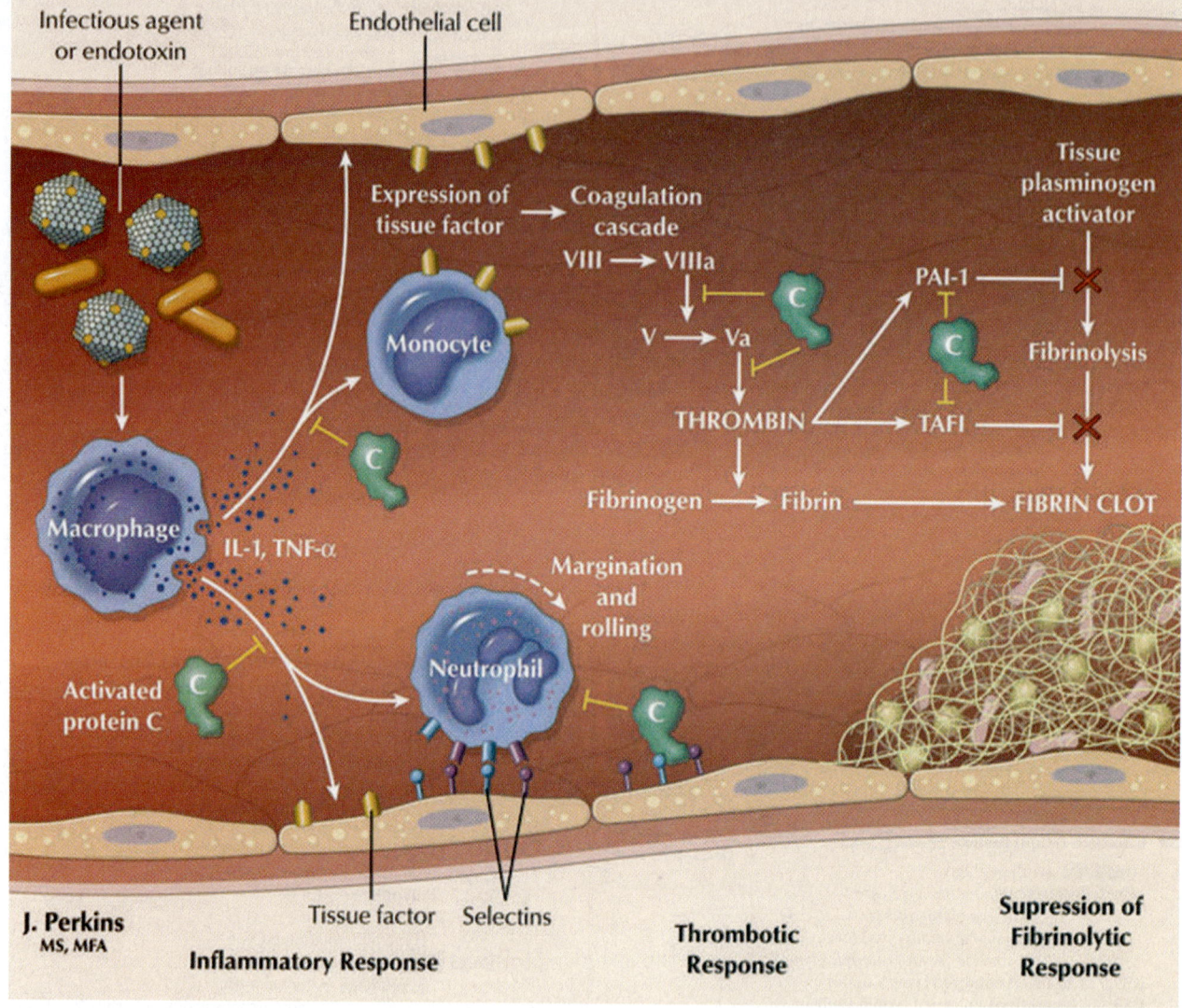

R63.6 Underweight
Use additional code to identify body mass index (BMI), if known (Z68.-)
Excludes1: *abnormal weight loss (R63.4)*
anorexia nervosa (F50.0-)
malnutrition (E40-E46)

R63.8 Other symptoms and signs concerning food and fluid intake

CC **R64** Cachexia
Wasting syndrome
Excludes1: *abnormal weight loss (R63.4)*
cachexia due to underlying condition (E88.A)
nutritional marasmus (E41)
AHA CC: 3Q, 2017, 24-25
Valid 3-character code, no further characters required

R65 Symptoms and signs specifically associated with systemic inflammation and infection
See page 966 for Sepsis illustration.

+ R65.1 Systemic inflammatory response syndrome (SIRS) of non-infectious origin
Code first underlying condition, such as:
heatstroke (T67.0-)
injury and trauma (S00-T88)
Excludes1: *sepsis- code to infection*
severe sepsis (R65.2)

CC **R65.10** Systemic inflammatory response syndrome (SIRS) of non-infectious origin without acute organ dysfunction
Systemic inflammatory response syndrome (SIRS) NOS
AHA CC: 2Q, 2019, 24-26, 38
Review coding guideline C.18.g

MCC **R65.11** Systemic inflammatory response syndrome (SIRS) of non-infectious origin with acute organ dysfunction
Use additional code to identify specific acute organ dysfunction, such as:
acute kidney failure (N17.-)
acute respiratory failure (J96.0-)
critical illness myopathy (G72.81)
critical illness polyneuropathy (G62.81)
disseminated intravascular coagulopathy [DIC] (D65)
encephalopathy (metabolic) (septic) (G93.41)
hepatic failure (K72.0-)
Review coding guideline C.18.g

+ **R65.2 Severe sepsis**
   Infection with associated acute organ dysfunction
   Sepsis with acute organ dysfunction
   Sepsis with multiple organ dysfunction
   Systemic inflammatory response syndrome due to infectious process with acute organ dysfunction
   Code first underlying infection, such as:
      infection following a procedure (T81.4-)
      infections following infusion, transfusion and therapeutic injection (T80.2-)
      puerperal sepsis (O85)
      sepsis following complete or unspecified spontaneous abortion (O03.87)
      sepsis following ectopic and molar pregnancy (O08.82)
      sepsis following incomplete spontaneous abortion (O03.37)
      sepsis following (induced) termination of pregnancy (O04.87)
      sepsis NOS (A41.9)

   Use additional code to identify specific acute organ dysfunction, such as:
      acute kidney failure (N17.-)
      acute respiratory failure (J96.0-)
      critical illness myopathy (G72.81)
      critical illness polyneuropathy (G62.81)
      disseminated intravascular coagulopathy [DIC] (D65)
      encephalopathy (metabolic) (septic) (G93.41)
      hepatic failure (K72.0-)
   AHA CC: 4Q, 2017, 98-99
   Review coding guideline C.1.d

   MCC **R65.20 Severe sepsis without septic shock**
      Severe sepsis NOS
      AHA CC: 3Q, 2016, 14; 2Q, 2020, 17-18
   MCC **R65.21 Severe sepsis with septic shock**
      Review coding guideline C.1.d.2 and C.1.d.5.c

R68 Other general symptoms and signs

   R68.0 Hypothermia, not associated with low environmental temperature
      Excludes1: hypothermia NOS (accidental) (T68)
                  hypothermia due to anesthesia (T88.51)
                  hypothermia due to low environmental temperature (T68)
                  newborn hypothermia (P80.-)

+ **R68.1 Nonspecific symptoms peculiar to infancy**
      Excludes1: colic, infantile (R10.83)
                  neonatal cerebral irritability (P91.3)
                  teething syndrome (K00.7)

   • **R68.11 Excessive crying of infant (baby)**
      Excludes1: excessive crying of child, adolescent, or adult (R45.83)

   • **R68.12 Fussy infant (baby)**
      Irritable infant

   • **R68.13 Apparent life threatening event in infant (ALTE)**
      Apparent life threatening event in newborn
      Brief resolved unexplained event (BRUE)
      Code first confirmed diagnosis, if known

      Use additional code(s) for associated signs and symptoms if no confirmed diagnosis established, or if signs and symptoms are not associated routinely with confirmed diagnosis, or provide additional information for cause of ALTE

   • **R68.19 Other nonspecific symptoms peculiar to infancy**

   R68.2 Dry mouth, unspecified
      Excludes1: dry mouth due to dehydration (E86.0)
                  dry mouth due to Sjögren syndrome (M35.0-)
                  salivary gland hyposecretion (K11.7)

   R68.3 Clubbing of fingers
      Clubbing of nails
      Excludes1: congenital clubfinger (Q68.1)

+ **R68.8 Other general symptoms and signs**
      R68.81 Early satiety
   • **R68.82 Decreased libido**
      Decreased sexual desire
      R68.83 Chills (without fever)
      Chills NOS
      Excludes1: chills with fever (R50.9)

   R68.84 Jaw pain
      Mandibular pain
      Maxilla pain
      Excludes1: temporomandibular joint arthralgia (M26.62-)

   R68.89 Other general symptoms and signs

R69 Illness, unspecified
   Unknown and unspecified cases of morbidity
   Valid 3-character code, no further characters required

Abnormal findings on examination of blood, without diagnosis (R70-R79)

Excludes2: abnormal findings on antenatal screening of mother (O28.-)
            abnormalities of lipids (E78.-)
            abnormalities of platelets and thrombocytes (D69.-)
            abnormalities of white blood cells classified elsewhere (D70-D72)
            coagulation hemorrhagic disorders (D65-D68)
            diagnostic abnormal findings classified elsewhere - see Alphabetic Index
            hemorrhagic and hematological disorders of newborn (P50-P61)

R70 Elevated erythrocyte sedimentation rate and abnormality of plasma viscosity
   R70.0 Elevated erythrocyte sedimentation rate
   R70.1 Abnormal plasma viscosity

R71 Abnormality of red blood cells
   Excludes1: anemias (D50-D64)
               anemia of premature infant (P61.2)
               benign (familial) polycythemia (D75.0)
               congenital anemias (P61.2-P61.4)
               newborn anemia due to isoimmunization (P55.-)
               polycythemia neonatorum (P61.1)
               polycythemia NOS (D75.1)
               polycythemia vera (D45)
               secondary polycythemia (D75.1)

   CC **R71.0 Precipitous drop in hematocrit**
      Drop (precipitous) in hemoglobin
      Drop in hematocrit
   R71.8 Other abnormality of red blood cells
      Abnormal red-cell morphology NOS
      Abnormal red-cell volume NOS
      Anisocytosis
      Poikilocytosis

R73 Elevated blood glucose level
   Excludes1: diabetes mellitus (E08-E13)
               diabetes mellitus in pregnancy, childbirth and the puerperium (O24.-)
               neonatal disorders (P70.0-P70.2)
               postsurgical hypoinsulinemia (E89.1)

+ **R73.0 Abnormal glucose**
   Excludes1: abnormal glucose in pregnancy (O99.81-)
               diabetes mellitus (E08-E13)
               dysmetabolic syndrome X (E88.81-)
               gestational diabetes (O24.4-)
               glycosuria (R81)
               hypoglycemia (E16.2)

   R73.01 Impaired fasting glucose
      Elevated fasting glucose
   R73.02 Impaired glucose tolerance (oral)
      Elevated glucose tolerance
   R73.03 Prediabetes
      Latent diabetes
      AHA CC: 4Q, 2016, 65
   R73.09 Other abnormal glucose
      Abnormal glucose NOS
      Abnormal non-fasting glucose tolerance
   R73.9 Hyperglycemia, unspecified

R74 Abnormal serum enzyme levels
+ **R74.0 Nonspecific elevation of levels of transaminase and lactic acid dehydrogenase [LDH]**
   AHA CC: 4Q, 2020, 39
   R74.01 Elevation of levels of liver transaminase levels
      Elevation of levels of alanine transaminase (ALT)
      Elevation of levels of aspartate transaminase (AST)
   R74.02 Elevation of levels of lactic acid dehydrogenase [LDH]

R74.8 Abnormal levels of other serum enzymes
    Abnormal level of acid phosphatase
    Abnormal level of alkaline phosphatase
    Abnormal level of amylase
    Abnormal level of lipase [triacylglycerol lipase]
    AHA CC: 2Q, 2019, 6
R74.9 Abnormal serum enzyme level, unspecified

R75 Inconclusive laboratory evidence of human immunodeficiency virus [HIV]
    Nonconclusive HIV-test finding in infants
    Excludes1: asymptomatic human immunodeficiency virus [HIV] infection status (Z21)
            human immunodeficiency virus [HIV] disease (B20)
    Review coding guidelines C.1.a.2.e and C.1.a.2.f
    Valid 3-character code, no further characters required

R76 Other abnormal immunological findings in serum
  R76.0 Raised antibody titer
    Excludes1: isoimmunization in pregnancy (O36.0-O36.1)
            isoimmunization affecting newborn (P55.-)
    AHA CC: 1Q, 2021, 6-7
  + **R76.1 Nonspecific reaction to test for tuberculosis**
    R76.11 Nonspecific reaction to tuberculin skin test without active tuberculosis
        Abnormal result of Mantoux test
        PPD positive
        Tuberculin (skin test) positive
        Tuberculin (skin test) reactor
        Excludes1: nonspecific reaction to cell mediated immunity measurement of gamma interferon antigen response without active tuberculosis (R76.12)
    R76.12 Nonspecific reaction to cell mediated immunity measurement of gamma interferon antigen response without active tuberculosis
        Nonspecific reaction to QuantiFERON-TB test (QFT) without active tuberculosis
        Excludes1: nonspecific reaction to tuberculin skin test without active tuberculosis (R76.11)
            positive tuberculin skin test (R76.11)
  R76.8 Other specified abnormal immunological findings in serum
    Raised level of immunoglobulins NOS
    AHA CC: 1Q, 2021, 6-7
  R76.9 Abnormal immunological finding in serum, unspecified

R77 Other abnormalities of plasma proteins
    Excludes1: disorders of plasma-protein metabolism (E88.0-)
  R77.0 Abnormality of albumin
  R77.1 Abnormality of globulin
    Hyperglobulinemia NOS
  R77.2 Abnormality of alphafetoprotein
  R77.8 Other specified abnormalities of plasma proteins
  R77.9 Abnormality of plasma protein, unspecified
    AHA CC: 2Q, 2019, 6

R78 Findings of drugs and other substances, not normally found in blood
    Use additional code to identify the any retained foreign body, if applicable (Z18.-)
    Excludes2: mental or behavioral disorders due to psychoactive substance use (F10-F19)
  R78.0 Finding of alcohol in blood
    external cause code (Y90.-), for detail regarding alcohol level.
  R78.1 Finding of opiate drug in blood
  R78.2 Finding of cocaine in blood
  R78.3 Finding of hallucinogen in blood
  R78.4 Finding of other drugs of addictive potential in blood
  R78.5 Finding of other psychotropic drug in blood
  R78.6 Finding of steroid agent in blood
  + **R78.7 Finding of abnormal level of heavy metals in blood**
    R78.71 Abnormal lead level in blood
        Excludes1: lead poisoning (T56.0-)
    R78.79 Finding of abnormal level of heavy metals in blood
  + **R78.8 Finding of other specified substances, not normally found in blood**
    CC **R78.81 Bacteremia**
        Excludes1: sepsis-code to specified infection

R78.89 Finding of other specified substances, not normally found in blood
    Finding of abnormal level of lithium in blood
R78.9 Finding of unspecified substance, not normally found in blood

R79 Other abnormal findings of blood chemistry
    Use additional code to identify any retained foreign body, if applicable (Z18.-)
    Excludes1: asymptomatic hyperuricemia (E79.0)
        hyperglycemia NOS (R73.9)
        hypoglycemia NOS (E16.2)
        neonatal hypoglycemia (P70.3-P70.4)
        specific findings indicating disorder of amino-acid metabolism (E70-E72)
        specific findings indicating disorder of carbohydrate metabolism (E73-E74)
        specific findings indicating disorder of lipid metabolism (E75.-)
  R79.0 Abnormal level of blood mineral
    Abnormal blood level of cobalt
    Abnormal blood level of copper
    Abnormal blood level of iron
    Abnormal blood level of magnesium
    Abnormal blood level of mineral NEC
    Abnormal blood level of zinc
    Excludes1: abnormal level of lithium (R78.89)
        disorders of mineral metabolism (E83.-)
        neonatal hypomagnesemia (P71.2)
        nutritional mineral deficiency (E58-E61)
  R79.1 Abnormal coagulation profile
    Abnormal or prolonged bleeding time
    Abnormal or prolonged coagulation time
    Abnormal or prolonged partial thromboplastin time [PTT]
    Abnormal or prolonged prothrombin time [PT]
    Low von Willebrand factor
    Excludes2: abnormality of fluid, electrolyte or acid-base balance (E86-E87)
        coagulation defects (D68.-)
  + **R79.8 Other specified abnormal findings of blood chemistry**
    R79.81 Abnormal blood-gas level
    R79.82 Elevated C-reactive protein (CRP)
    R79.83 Abnormal findings of blood amino-acid level
        Homocysteinemia
        Excludes1: disorders of amino-acid metabolism (E70-E72)
        AHA CC: 4Q, 2021, 28
    R79.89 Other specified abnormal findings of blood chemistry
        AHA CC: 2Q, 2019, 6
  R79.9 Abnormal finding of blood chemistry, unspecified

Abnormal findings on examination of urine, without diagnosis (R80-R82)

Excludes1: abnormal findings on antenatal screening of mother (O28.-)
    diagnostic abnormal findings classified elsewhere - see Alphabetical Index
    specific findings indicating disorder of amino-acid metabolism (E70-E72)
    specific findings indicating disorder of carbohydrate metabolism (E73-E74)

R80 Proteinuria
    Excludes1: gestational proteinuria (O12.1-)
  R80.0 Isolated proteinuria
    Idiopathic proteinuria
    Excludes1: isolated proteinuria with specific morphological lesion (N06.-)
  R80.1 Persistent proteinuria, unspecified
  R80.2 Orthostatic proteinuria, unspecified
    Postural proteinuria
  R80.3 Bence Jones proteinuria
  R80.8 Other proteinuria
  R80.9 Proteinuria, unspecified
    Albuminuria NOS

R81 Glycosuria
  Excludes1: renal glycosuria (E74.818)
  Valid 3-character code, no further characters required

R82 Other and unspecified abnormal findings in urine
  Includes: chromoabnormalities in urine
  Use additional code to identify any retained foreign body, if applicable (Z18.-)
  Excludes2: hematuria (R31.-)

CC **R82.0 Chyluria**
  Excludes1: filarial chyluria (B74.-)
CC **R82.1 Myoglobinuria**
  R82.2 Biliuria
  R82.3 Hemoglobinuria
  Excludes1: hemoglobinuria due to hemolysis from external causes NEC (D59.6)
  hemoglobinuria due to paroxysmal nocturnal [Marchiafava-Micheli] (D59.5)
  R82.4 Acetonuria
  Ketonuria
  R82.5 Elevated urine levels of drugs, medicaments and biological substances
  Elevated urine levels of catecholamines
  Elevated urine levels of indoleacetic acid
  Elevated urine levels of 17-ketosteroids
  Elevated urine levels of steroids
  R82.6 Abnormal urine levels of substances chiefly nonmedicinal as to source
  Abnormal urine level of heavy metals
+ **R82.7 Abnormal findings on microbiological examination of urine**
  Excludes1: colonization status (Z22.-)
  AHA CC: 4Q, 2016, 65
  R82.71 Bacteriuria
  R82.79 Other abnormal findings on microbiological examination of urine
  Positive culture findings of urine
+ **R82.8 Abnormal findings on cytological and histological examination of urine**
  AHA CC: 4Q, 2019, 16
  R82.81 Pyuria
  Sterile pyuria
  AHA CC: 4Q, 2019, 16
  R82.89 Other abnormal findings on cytological and histological examination of urine
+ **R82.9 Other and unspecified abnormal findings in urine**
  R82.90 Unspecified abnormal findings in urine
  R82.91 Other chromoabnormalities of urine
  Chromoconversion (dipstick)
  Idiopathic dipstick converts positive for blood with no cellular forms in sediment
  Excludes1: hemoglobinuria (R82.3)
  myoglobinuria (R82.1)
+ **R82.99 Other abnormal findings in urine**
  AHA CC: 4Q, 2018, 29-30
  R82.991 Hypocitraturia
  R82.992 Hyperoxaluria
  Excludes1: Primary hyperoxaluria (E72.53)
  R82.993 Hyperuricosuria
  R82.994 Hypercalciuria
  Idiopathic hypercalciuria
  R82.998 Other abnormal findings in urine
  Cells and casts in urine
  Crystalluria
  Melanuria

Abnormal findings on examination of other body fluids, substances and tissues, without diagnosis (R83-R89)

Excludes1: abnormal findings on antenatal screening of mother (O28.-)
diagnostic abnormal findings classified elsewhere - see Alphabetical Index
Excludes2: abnormal findings on examination of blood, without diagnosis (R70-R79)
abnormal findings on examination of urine, without diagnosis (R80-R82)
abnormal tumor markers (R97.-)

R83 Abnormal findings in cerebrospinal fluid
  R83.0 Abnormal level of enzymes in cerebrospinal fluid
  R83.1 Abnormal level of hormones in cerebrospinal fluid
  R83.2 Abnormal level of other drugs, medicaments and biological substances in cerebrospinal fluid
  R83.3 Abnormal level of substances chiefly nonmedicinal as to source in cerebrospinal fluid
  R83.4 Abnormal immunological findings in cerebrospinal fluid
  R83.5 Abnormal microbiological findings in cerebrospinal fluid
  Positive culture findings in cerebrospinal fluid
  Excludes1: colonization status (Z22.-)
  R83.6 Abnormal cytological findings in cerebrospinal fluid
  R83.8 Other abnormal findings in cerebrospinal fluid
  Abnormal chromosomal findings in cerebrospinal fluid
  R83.9 Unspecified abnormal finding in cerebrospinal fluid

R84 Abnormal findings in specimens from respiratory organs and thorax
  Includes: abnormal findings in bronchial washings
  abnormal findings in nasal secretions
  abnormal findings in pleural fluid
  abnormal findings in sputum
  abnormal findings in throat scrapings
  Excludes1: blood-stained sputum (R04.2)
  R84.0 Abnormal level of enzymes in specimens from respiratory organs and thorax
  R84.1 Abnormal level of hormones in specimens from respiratory organs and thorax
  R84.2 Abnormal level of other drugs, medicaments and biological substances in specimens from respiratory organs and thorax
  R84.3 Abnormal level of substances chiefly nonmedicinal as to source in specimens from respiratory organs and thorax
  R84.4 Abnormal immunological findings in specimens from respiratory organs and thorax
  R84.5 Abnormal microbiological findings in specimens from respiratory organs and thorax
  Positive culture findings in specimens from respiratory organs and thorax
  Excludes1: colonization status (Z22.-)
  R84.6 Abnormal cytological findings in specimens from respiratory organs and thorax
  R84.7 Abnormal histological findings in specimens from respiratory organs and thorax
  R84.8 Other abnormal findings in specimens from respiratory organs and thorax
  Abnormal chromosomal findings in specimens from respiratory organs and thorax
  R84.9 Unspecified abnormal finding in specimens from respiratory organs and thorax

R85 Abnormal findings in specimens from digestive organs and abdominal cavity
  Includes: abnormal findings in peritoneal fluid
  abnormal findings in saliva
  Excludes1: cloudy peritoneal dialysis effluent (R88.0)
  fecal abnormalities (R19.5)
  R85.0 Abnormal level of enzymes in specimens from digestive organs and abdominal cavity
  R85.1 Abnormal level of hormones in specimens from digestive organs and abdominal cavity
  R85.2 Abnormal level of other drugs, medicaments and biological substances in specimens from digestive organs and abdominal cavity
  R85.3 Abnormal level of substances chiefly nonmedicinal as to source in specimens from digestive organs and abdominal cavity
  R85.4 Abnormal immunological findings in specimens from digestive organs and abdominal cavity
  R85.5 Abnormal microbiological findings in specimens from digestive organs and abdominal cavity
  Positive culture findings in specimens from digestive organs and abdominal cavity
  Excludes1: colonization status (Z22.-)

+ **R85.6 Abnormal cytological findings in specimens from digestive organs and abdominal cavity**
  + **R85.61 Abnormal cytologic smear of anus**
    Excludes1: abnormal cytological findings in specimens from other digestive organs and abdominal cavity (R85.69)
    carcinoma in situ of anus (histologically confirmed) (D01.3)
    anal intraepithelial neoplasia I [AIN I] (K62.82)
    anal intraepithelial neoplasia II [AIN II] (K62.82)
    anal intraepithelial neoplasia III [AIN III] (D01.3)
    dysplasia (mild) (moderate) of anus (histologically confirmed) (K62.82)
    severe dysplasia of anus (histologically confirmed) (D01.3)
    Excludes2: anal high risk human papillomavirus (HPV) DNA test positive (R85.81)
    anal low risk human papillomavirus (HPV) DNA test positive (R85.82)
    - **R85.610** Atypical squamous cells of undetermined significance on cytologic smear of anus (ASC-US)
    - **R85.611** Atypical squamous cells cannot exclude high grade squamous intraepithelial lesion on cytologic smear of anus (ASC-H)
    - **R85.612** Low grade squamous intraepithelial lesion on cytologic smear of anus (LGSIL)
    - **R85.613** High grade squamous intraepithelial lesion on cytologic smear of anus (HGSIL)
    - **R85.614** Cytologic evidence of malignancy on smear of anus
    - **R85.615** Unsatisfactory cytologic smear of anus
      Inadequate sample of cytologic smear of anus
    - **R85.616** Satisfactory anal smear but lacking transformation zone
    - **R85.618** Other abnormal cytological findings on specimens from anus
    - **R85.619** Unspecified abnormal cytological findings in specimens from anus
      Abnormal anal cytology NOS
      Atypical glandular cells of anus NOS
  - **R85.69 Abnormal cytological findings in specimens from other digestive organs and abdominal cavity**
- **R85.7 Abnormal histological findings in specimens from digestive organs and abdominal cavity**
+ **R85.8 Other abnormal findings in specimens from digestive organs and abdominal cavity**
  - **R85.81 Anal high risk human papillomavirus (HPV) DNA test positive**
    Excludes1: anogenital warts due to human papillomavirus (HPV) (A63.0)
    condyloma acuminatum (A63.0)
  - **R85.82 Anal low risk human papillomavirus (HPV) DNA test positive**
    Use additional code for associated human papillomavirus (B97.7)
  - **R85.89 Other abnormal findings in specimens from digestive organs and abdominal cavity**
    Abnormal chromosomal findings in specimens from digestive organs and abdominal cavity
- **R85.9 Unspecified abnormal finding in specimens from digestive organs and abdominal cavity**

R86 Abnormal findings in specimens from male genital organs
  Includes: abnormal findings in prostatic secretions
  abnormal findings in semen, seminal fluid
  abnormal spermatozoa
  Excludes1: azoospermia (N46.0-)
  oligospermia (N46.1-)
  ♂ **R86.0 Abnormal level of enzymes in specimens from male genital organs**
  ♂ **R86.1 Abnormal level of hormones in specimens from male genital organs**
  ♂ **R86.2 Abnormal level of other drugs, medicaments and biological substances in specimens from male genital organs**
  ♂ **R86.3 Abnormal level of substances chiefly nonmedicinal as to source in specimens from male genital organs**
  ♂ **R86.4 Abnormal immunological findings in specimens from male genital organs**
  ♂ **R86.5 Abnormal microbiological findings in specimens from male genital organs**
    Positive culture findings in specimens from male genital organs
    Excludes1: colonization status (Z22.-)
  ♂ **R86.6 Abnormal cytological findings in specimens from male genital organs**
  ♂ **R86.7 Abnormal histological findings in specimens from male genital organs**
  ♂ **R86.8 Other abnormal findings in specimens from male genital organs**
    Abnormal chromosomal findings in specimens from male genital organs
  ♂ **R86.9 Unspecified abnormal finding in specimens from male genital organs**

R87 Abnormal findings in specimens from female genital organs
  Includes: abnormal findings in secretion and smears from cervix uteri
  abnormal findings in secretion and smears from vagina
  abnormal findings in secretion and smears from vulva
  ♀ **R87.0 Abnormal level of enzymes in specimens from female genital organs**
  ♀ **R87.1 Abnormal level of hormones in specimens from female genital organs**
  ♀ **R87.2 Abnormal level of other drugs, medicaments and biological substances in specimens from female genital organs**
  ♀ **R87.3 Abnormal level of substances chiefly nonmedicinal as to source in specimens from female genital organs**
  ♀ **R87.4 Abnormal immunological findings in specimens from female genital organs**
  ♀ **R87.5 Abnormal microbiological findings in specimens from female genital organs**
    Positive culture findings in specimens from female genital organs
    Excludes1: colonization status (Z22.-)
  + **R87.6 Abnormal cytological findings in specimens from female genital organs**
    + **R87.61 Abnormal cytological findings in specimens from cervix uteri**
      Excludes1: abnormal cytological findings in specimens from other female genital organs (R87.69)
      abnormal cytological findings in specimens from vagina (R87.62-)
      carcinoma in situ of cervix uteri (histologically confirmed) (D06.-)
      cervical intraepithelial neoplasia I [CIN I] (N87.0)
      cervical intraepithelial neoplasia II [CIN II] (N87.1)
      cervical intraepithelial neoplasia III [CIN III] (D06.-)
      dysplasia (mild) (moderate) of cervix uteri (histologically confirmed) (N87.-)
      severe dysplasia of cervix uteri (histologically confirmed) (D06.-)
      Excludes2: cervical high risk human papillomavirus (HPV) DNA test positive (R87.810)
      cervical low risk human papillomavirus (HPV) DNA test positive (R87.820)
      ♀ **R87.610** Atypical squamous cells of undetermined significance on cytologic smear of cervix (ASC-US)
      ♀ **R87.611** Atypical squamous cells cannot exclude high grade squamous intraepithelial lesion on cytologic smear of cervix (ASC-H)

- ♀ **R87.612** Low grade squamous intraepithelial lesion on cytologic smear of cervix (LGSIL)
- ♀ **R87.613** High grade squamous intraepithelial lesion on cytologic smear of cervix (HGSIL)
- ♀ **R87.614** Cytologic evidence of malignancy on smear of cervix
- ♀ **R87.615** Unsatisfactory cytologic smear of cervix
  - Inadequate sample of cytologic smear of cervix
- ♀ **R87.616** Satisfactory cervical smear but lacking transformation zone
- ♀ **R87.618** Other abnormal cytological findings on specimens from cervix uteri
- ♀ **R87.619** Unspecified abnormal cytological findings in specimens from cervix uteri
  - Abnormal cervical cytology NOS
  - Abnormal Papanicolaou smear of cervix NOS
  - Abnormal thin preparation smear of cervix NOS
  - Atypical endocervical cells of cervix NOS
  - Atypical endometrial cells of cervix NOS
  - Atypical glandular cells of cervix NOS
- + **R87.62** Abnormal cytological findings in specimens from vagina
  - *Use additional code to identify acquired absence of uterus and cervix, if applicable (Z90.71-)*
  - **Excludes1:** abnormal cytological findings in specimens from cervix uteri (R87.61-)
    - abnormal cytological findings in specimens from other female genital organs (R87.69)
    - carcinoma in situ of vagina (histologically confirmed) (D07.2)
    - vaginal intraepithelial neoplasia I [VAIN I] (N89.0)
    - vaginal intraepithelial neoplasia II [VAIN II] (N89.1)
    - vaginal intraepithelial neoplasia III [VAIN III] (D07.2)
    - dysplasia (mild) (moderate) of vagina (histologically confirmed) (N89.-)
    - severe dysplasia of vagina (histologically confirmed) (D07.2)
  - **Excludes2:** vaginal high risk human papillomavirus (HPV) DNA test positive (R87.811)
    - vaginal low risk human papillomavirus (HPV) DNA test positive (R87.821)
  - ♀ **R87.620** Atypical squamous cells of undetermined significance on cytologic smear of vagina (ASC-US)
  - ♀ **R87.621** Atypical squamous cells cannot exclude high grade squamous intraepithelial lesion on cytologic smear of vagina (ASC-H)
  - ♀ **R87.622** Low grade squamous intraepithelial lesion on cytologic smear of vagina (LGSIL)
  - ♀ **R87.623** High grade squamous intraepithelial lesion on cytologic smear of vagina (HGSIL)
  - ♀ **R87.624** Cytologic evidence of malignancy on smear of vagina
  - ♀ **R87.625** Unsatisfactory cytologic smear of vagina
    - Inadequate sample of cytologic smear of vagina
  - ♀ **R87.628** Other abnormal cytological findings on specimens from vagina
  - ♀ **R87.629** Unspecified abnormal cytological findings in specimens from vagina
    - Abnormal Papanicolaou smear of vagina NOS
    - Abnormal thin preparation smear of vagina NOS
    - Abnormal vaginal cytology NOS
    - Atypical endocervical cells of vagina NOS
    - Atypical endometrial cells of vagina NOS
    - Atypical glandular cells of vagina NOS
- ♀ **R87.69** Abnormal cytological findings in specimens from other female genital organs
  - Abnormal cytological findings in specimens from female genital organs NOS
  - **Excludes1:** dysplasia of vulva (histologically confirmed) (N90.0-N90.3)
- ♀ **R87.7** Abnormal histological findings in specimens from female genital organs
  - **Excludes1:** carcinoma in situ (histologically confirmed) of female genital organs (D06-D07.3)
    - cervical intraepithelial neoplasia I [CIN I] (N87.0)
    - cervical intraepithelial neoplasia II [CIN II] (N87.1)
    - cervical intraepithelial neoplasia III [CIN III] (D06.-)
    - dysplasia (mild) (moderate) of cervix uteri (histologically confirmed) (N87.-)
    - dysplasia (mild) (moderate) of vagina (histologically confirmed) (N89.-)
    - vaginal intraepithelial neoplasia I [VAIN I] (N89.0)
    - vaginal intraepithelial neoplasia II [VAIN II] (N89.1)
    - vaginal intraepithelial neoplasia III [VAIN III] (D07.2)
    - severe dysplasia of cervix uteri (histologically confirmed) (D06.-)
    - severe dysplasia of vagina (histologically confirmed) (D07.2)
- + **R87.8** Other abnormal findings in specimens from female genital organs
  - + **R87.81** High risk human papillomavirus (HPV) DNA test positive from female genital organs
    - **Excludes1:** anogenital warts due to human papillomavirus (HPV) (A63.0)
      - condyloma acuminatum (A63.0)
    - ♀ **R87.810** Cervical high risk human papillomavirus (HPV) DNA test positive
    - ♀ **R87.811** Vaginal high risk human papillomavirus (HPV) DNA test positive
  - + **R87.82** Low risk human papillomavirus (HPV) DNA test positive from female genital organs
    - *Use additional code for associated human papillomavirus (B97.7)*
    - ♀ **R87.820** Cervical low risk human papillomavirus (HPV) DNA test positive
    - ♀ **R87.821** Vaginal low risk human papillomavirus (HPV) DNA test positive
  - ♀ **R87.89** Other abnormal findings in specimens from female genital organs
    - Abnormal chromosomal findings in specimens from female genital organs
- ♀ **R87.9** Unspecified abnormal finding in specimens from female genital organs

R88 Abnormal findings in other body fluids and substances
- **R88.0** Cloudy (hemodialysis) (peritoneal) dialysis effluent
- **R88.8** Abnormal findings in other body fluids and substances

R89 Abnormal findings in specimens from other organs, systems and tissues
- **Includes:** abnormal findings in nipple discharge
  - abnormal findings in synovial fluid
  - abnormal findings in wound secretions
- **R89.0** Abnormal level of enzymes in specimens from other organs, systems and tissues
- **R89.1** Abnormal level of hormones in specimens from other organs, systems and tissues

R89.2 **Abnormal level of other drugs, medicants and biological substances in specimens from other organs, systems and tissues**

R89.3 **Abnormal level of substances chiefly nonmedicinal as to source in specimens from other organs, systems and tissues**

R89.4 **Abnormal immunological findings in specimens from other organs, systems and tissues**

R89.5 **Abnormal microbiological findings in specimens from other organs, systems and tissues**
Positive culture findings in specimens from other organs, systems and tissues
Excludes1: colonization status (Z22.-)

R89.6 **Abnormal cytological findings in specimens from other organs, systems and tissues**

R89.7 **Abnormal histological findings in specimens from other organs, systems and tissues**

R89.8 **Other abnormal findings in specimens from other organs, systems and tissues**
Abnormal chromosomal findings in specimens from other organs, systems and tissues

R89.9 **Unspecified abnormal finding in specimens from other organs, systems and tissues**

Abnormal findings on diagnostic imaging and in function studies, without diagnosis (R90-R94)

Includes: nonspecific abnormal findings on diagnostic imaging by computerized axial tomography [CAT scan]
nonspecific abnormal findings on diagnostic imaging by magnetic resonance imaging [MRI][NMR]
nonspecific abnormal findings on diagnostic imaging by positron emission tomography [PET scan]
nonspecific abnormal findings on diagnostic imaging by thermography
nonspecific abnormal findings on diagnostic imaging by ultrasound [echogram]
nonspecific abnormal findings on diagnostic imaging by X-ray examination

Excludes1: abnormal findings on antenatal screening of mother (O28.-)
diagnostic abnormal findings classified elsewhere - see Alphabetical Index

R90 Abnormal findings on diagnostic imaging of central nervous system

R90.0 **Intracranial space-occupying lesion found on diagnostic imaging of central nervous system**

+ R90.8 **Other abnormal findings on diagnostic imaging of central nervous system**
R90.81 Abnormal echoencephalogram
R90.82 White matter disease, unspecified
R90.89 Other abnormal findings on diagnostic imaging of central nervous system
Other cerebrovascular abnormality found on diagnostic imaging of central nervous system

R91 Abnormal findings on diagnostic imaging of lung

R91.1 **Solitary pulmonary nodule**
Coin lesion lung
Solitary pulmonary nodule, subsegmental branch of the bronchial tree

R91.8 **Other nonspecific abnormal finding of lung field**
Lung mass NOS found on diagnostic imaging of lung
Pulmonary infiltrate NOS
Shadow, lung

R92 Abnormal and inconclusive findings on diagnostic imaging of breast

R92.0 **Mammographic microcalcification found on diagnostic imaging of breast**
Excludes2: mammographic calcification (calculus) found on diagnostic imaging of breast (R92.1)

R92.1 **Mammographic calcification found on diagnostic imaging of breast**
Mammographic calculus found on diagnostic imaging of breast

R92.2 **Inconclusive mammogram**
Inconclusive mammogram NEC
Inconclusive mammography NEC
AHA CC: 1Q, 2015, 24

+ R92.3 **Mammographic density found on imaging of breast**
Code also, if applicable, inconclusive mammogram (R92.2)
R92.30 Dense breasts, unspecified
Dense breasts NOS
Low density

+ R92.31 **Mammographic fatty tissue density of breast**
Breast Imaging Reporting and Data System (BI-RADS): A
Breast Imaging Reporting and Data System (BI-RADS): 1
R92.311 Mammographic fatty tissue density, right breast
R92.312 Mammographic fatty tissue density, left breast
R92.313 Mammographic fatty tissue density, bilateral breasts

+ R92.32 **Mammographic fibroglandular density of breast**
Breast Imaging Reporting and Data System (BI-RADS): B
Breast Imaging Reporting and Data System (BI-RADS): 2
R92.321 Mammographic fibroglandular density, right breast
R92.322 Mammographic fibroglandular density, left breast
R92.323 Mammographic fibroglandular density, bilateral breasts

+ R92.33 **Mammographic heterogeneous density of breast**
Breast Imaging Reporting and Data System (BI-RADS): C
Breast Imaging Reporting and Data System (BI-RADS): 3
R92.331 Mammographic heterogeneous density, right breast
R92.332 Mammographic heterogeneous density, left breast
R92.333 Mammographic heterogeneous density, bilateral breasts

+ R92.34 **Mammographic extreme density of breast**
Breast Imaging Reporting and Data System (BI-RADS): D
Breast Imaging Reporting and Data System (BI-RADS): 4
R92.341 Mammographic extreme density, right breast
R92.342 Mammographic extreme density, left breast
R92.343 Mammographic extreme density, bilateral breasts

R92.8 **Other abnormal and inconclusive findings on diagnostic imaging of breast**

R93 Abnormal findings on diagnostic imaging of other body structures

R93.0 **Abnormal findings on diagnostic imaging of skull and head, not elsewhere classified**
Excludes1: intracranial space-occupying lesion found on diagnostic imaging (R90.0)

R93.1 **Abnormal findings on diagnostic imaging of heart and coronary circulation**
Abnormal echocardiogram NOS
Abnormal heart shadow

R93.2 **Abnormal findings on diagnostic imaging of liver and biliary tract**
Nonvisualization of gallbladder

R93.3 **Abnormal findings on diagnostic imaging of other parts of digestive tract**

+ R93.4 **Abnormal findings on diagnostic imaging of urinary organs**
Excludes2: hypertrophy of kidney (N28.81)
AHA CC: 4Q, 2016, 66
R93.41 **Abnormal radiologic findings on diagnostic imaging of of renal pelvis, ureter, or bladder**
Filling defect of bladder found on diagnostic imaging
Filling defect of renal pelvis found on diagnostic imaging
Filling defect of ureter found on diagnostic imaging

- **R93.42** Abnormal radiologic findings on diagnostic imaging of kidney
  - **R93.421** Abnormal radiologic findings on diagnostic imaging of right kidney
  - **R93.422** Abnormal radiologic findings on diagnostic imaging of left kidney
  - **R93.429** Abnormal radiologic findings on diagnostic imaging of unspecified kidney
- **R93.49** Abnormal radiologic findings on diagnostic imaging of other urinary organs
- **R93.5** Abnormal findings on diagnostic imaging of other abdominal regions, including retroperitoneum
- **R93.6** Abnormal findings on diagnostic imaging of limbs
  - *Excludes2:* abnormal finding in skin and subcutaneous tissue (R93.8-)
  - AHA CC: 1Q, 2020, 14-15
- **R93.7** Abnormal findings on diagnostic imaging of other parts of musculoskeletal system
  - *Excludes2:* abnormal findings on diagnostic imaging of skull (R93.0)
- + **R93.8** Abnormal findings on diagnostic imaging of other specified body structures
  - AHA CC: 4Q, 2018, 30
  - + **R93.81** Abnormal radiologic findings on diagnostic imaging of testis
    - ♂ **R93.811** Abnormal radiologic findings on diagnostic imaging of right testicle
    - ♂ **R93.812** Abnormal radiologic findings on diagnostic imaging of left testicle
    - ♂ **R93.813** Abnormal radiologic findings on diagnostic imaging of testicles, bilateral
    - ♂ **R93.819** Abnormal radiologic findings on diagnostic imaging of unspecified testicle
  - **R93.89** Abnormal findings on diagnostic imaging of other specified body structures
    - Abnormal findings by radioisotope localization of placenta
    - Abnormal radiological finding in skin and subcutaneous tissue
    - Mediastinal shift
- **R93.9** Diagnostic imaging inconclusive due to excess body fat of patient

R94 Abnormal results of function studies

Includes: abnormal results of radionuclide [radioisotope] uptake studies
abnormal results of scintigraphy

- + **R94.0** Abnormal results of function studies of central nervous system
  - **R94.01** Abnormal electroencephalogram [EEG]
  - **R94.02** Abnormal brain scan
  - **R94.09** Abnormal results of other function studies of central nervous system
- + **R94.1** Abnormal results of function studies of peripheral nervous system and special senses
  - + **R94.11** Abnormal results of function studies of eye
    - **R94.110** Abnormal electro-oculogram [EOG]
    - **R94.111** Abnormal electroretinogram [ERG]
      - Abnormal retinal function study
    - **R94.112** Abnormal visually evoked potential [VEP]
    - **R94.113** Abnormal oculomotor study
    - **R94.118** Abnormal results of other function studies of eye
  - + **R94.12** Abnormal results of function studies of ear and other special senses
    - **R94.120** Abnormal auditory function study
      - AHA CC: 3Q, 2016, 17
    - **R94.121** Abnormal vestibular function study
    - **R94.128** Abnormal results of other function studies of ear and other special senses
  - + **R94.13** Abnormal results of function studies of peripheral nervous system
    - **R94.130** Abnormal response to nerve stimulation, unspecified
    - **R94.131** Abnormal electromyogram [EMG]
      - *Excludes1:* electromyogram of eye (R94.113)
    - **R94.138** Abnormal results of other function studies of peripheral nervous system
- **R94.2** Abnormal results of pulmonary function studies
  - Reduced ventilatory capacity
  - Reduced vital capacity
- + **R94.3** Abnormal results of cardiovascular function studies
  - **R94.30** Abnormal result of cardiovascular function study, unspecified
  - **R94.31** Abnormal electrocardiogram [ECG] [EKG]
    - *Excludes1:* long QT syndrome (I45.81)
  - **R94.39** Abnormal result of other cardiovascular function study
    - Abnormal electrophysiological intracardiac studies
    - Abnormal phonocardiogram
    - Abnormal vectorcardiogram
    - AHA CC: 1Q, 2023, 25
- **R94.4** Abnormal results of kidney function studies
  - Abnormal renal function test
- **R94.5** Abnormal results of liver function studies
- **R94.6** Abnormal results of thyroid function studies
- **R94.7** Abnormal results of other endocrine function studies
  - *Excludes2:* abnormal glucose (R73.0-)
- **R94.8** Abnormal results of function studies of other organs and systems
  - Abnormal basal metabolic rate [BMR]
  - Abnormal bladder function test
  - Abnormal splenic function test

Abnormal tumor markers (R97)

R97 Abnormal tumor markers

Elevated tumor associated antigens [TAA]
Elevated tumor specific antigens [TSA]

- **R97.0** Elevated carcinoembryonic antigen [CEA]
- **R97.1** Elevated cancer antigen 125 [CA 125]
- + **R97.2** Elevated prostate specific antigen [PSA]
  - AHA CC: 4Q, 2016, 66
  - ♂ **R97.20** Elevated prostate specific antigen [PSA]
  - ♂ **R97.21** Rising PSA following treatment for malignant neoplasm of prostate
    - AHA CC: 2Q, 2023, 5-6
- **R97.8** Other abnormal tumor markers

Ill-defined and unknown cause of mortality (R99)

R99 Ill-defined and unknown cause of mortality

Death (unexplained) NOS
Unspecified cause of mortality
Review coding guideline C.18.h
Valid 3-character code, no further characters required

Chapter 19: Injury, Poisoning and Certain Other Consequences of External Causes (S00-T88)

Muscles

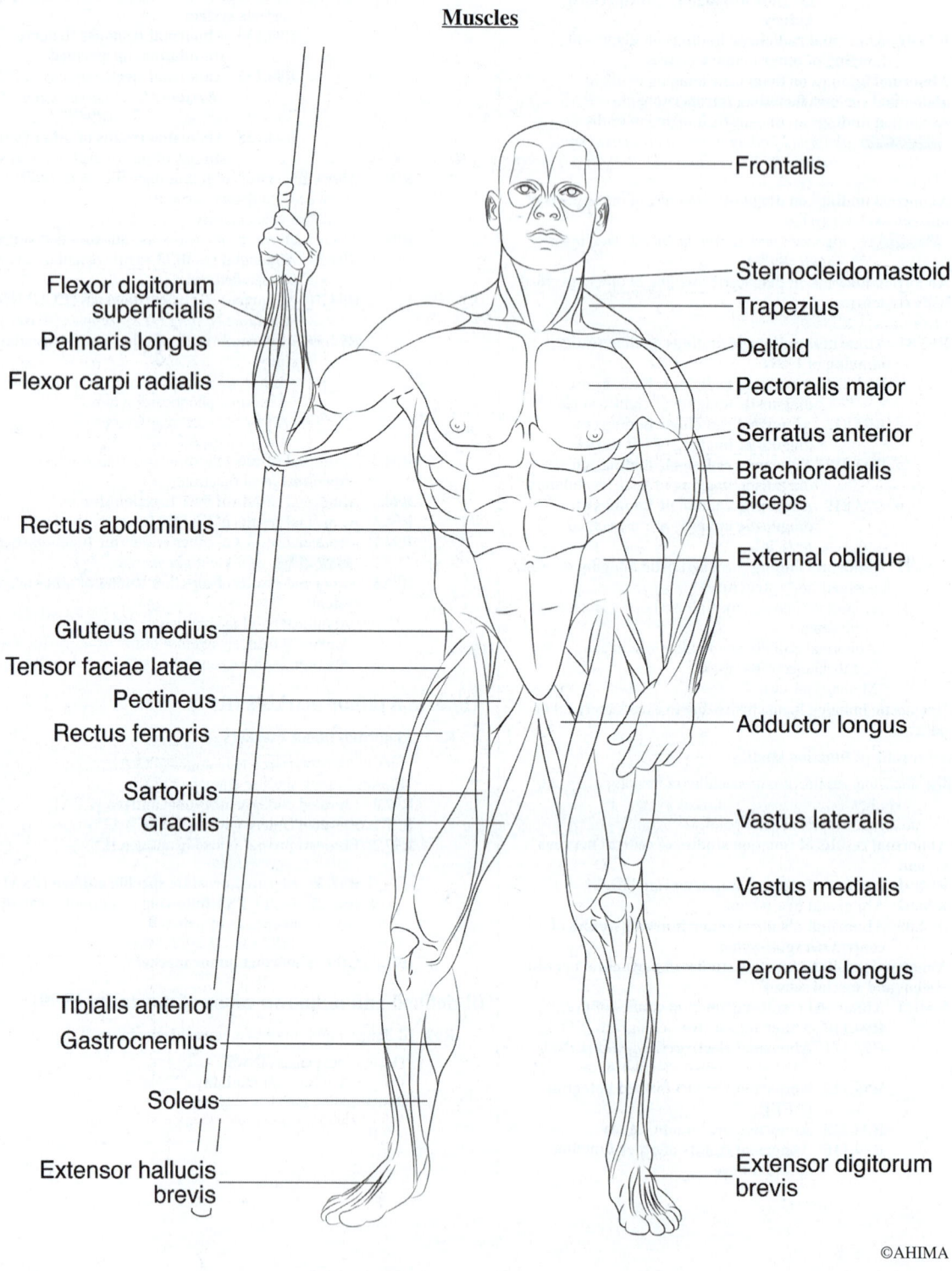

©AHIMA

Skeleton - Front and Side Views

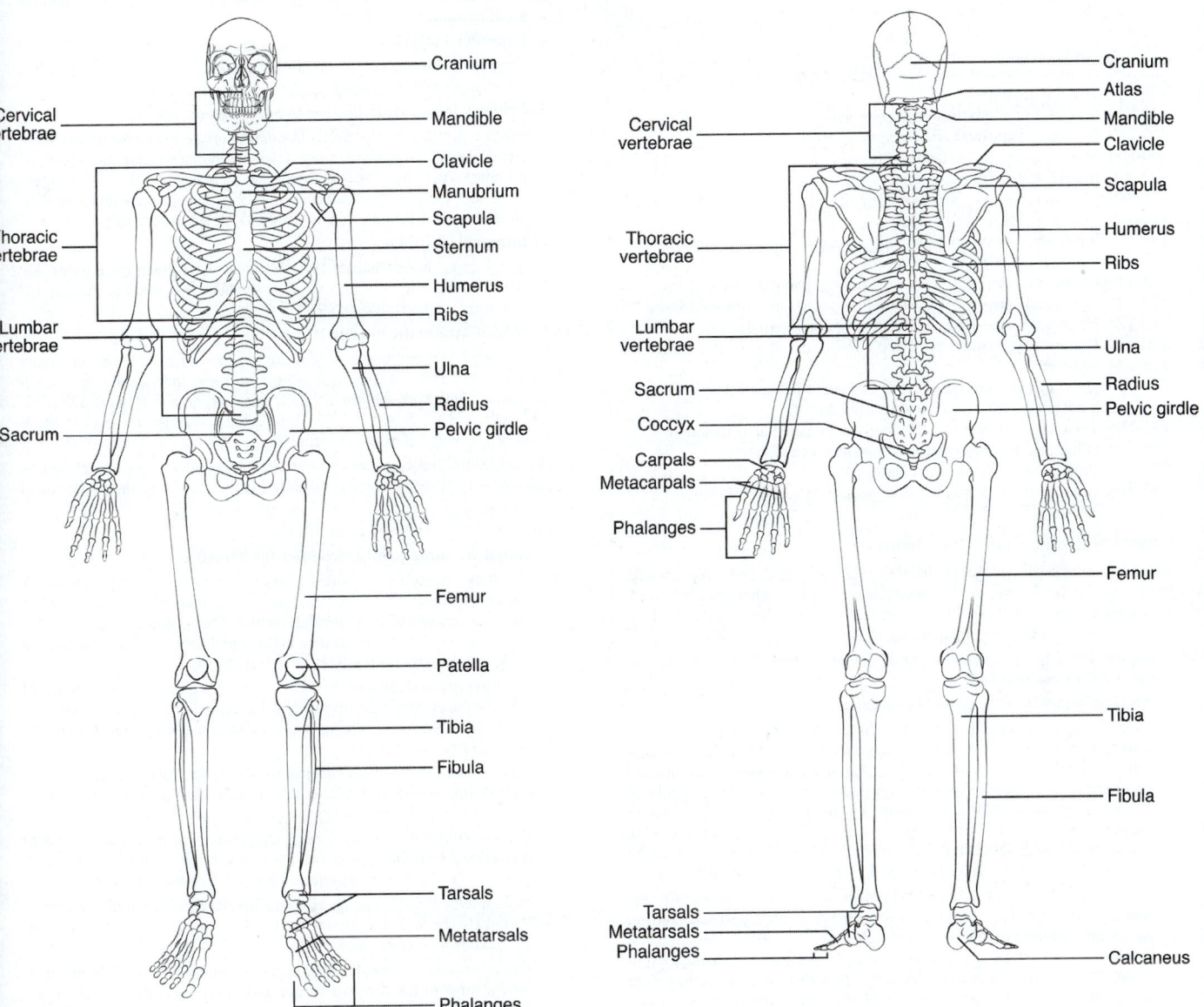

©AHIMA

Chapter 19: Injury, Poisoning and Certain Other Consequences of External Causes (S00-T88)

NOTE Use secondary code(s) from Chapter 20, External causes of morbidity, to indicate cause of injury. Codes within the T-section that include the external cause do not require an additional external cause code

Use additional code to identify any retained foreign body, if applicable (Z18.-)

Excludes1: birth trauma (P10-P15)
obstetric trauma (O70-O71)

NOTE The chapter uses the S-section for coding different types of injuries related to single body regions and the T-section to cover injuries to unspecified body regions as well as poisoning and certain other consequences of external causes.
AHA CC: 1Q, 2015, 3-21

This chapter contains the following category blocks:

S00-S09	Injuries to the head
S10-S19	Injuries to the neck
S20-S29	Injuries to the thorax
S30-S39	Injuries to the abdomen, lower back, lumbar spine, pelvis and external genitals
S40-S49	Injuries to the shoulder and upper arm
S50-S59	Injuries to the elbow and forearm
S60-S69	Injuries to the wrist, hand and fingers
S70-S79	Injuries to the hip and thigh
S80-S89	Injuries to the knee and lower leg
S90-S99	Injuries to the ankle and foot
T07	Injuries involving multiple body regions
T14	Injury of unspecified body region
T15-T19	Effects of foreign body entering through natural orifice
T20-T25	Burns and corrosions of external body surface, specified by site
T26-T28	Burns and corrosions confined to eye and internal organs
T30-T32	Burns and corrosions of multiple and unspecified body regions
T33-T34	Frostbite
T36-T50	Poisoning by, adverse effect of and underdosing of drugs, medicaments and biological substances
T51-T65	Toxic effects of substances chiefly nonmedicinal as to source
T66-T78	Other and unspecified effects of external causes
T79	Certain early complications of trauma
T80-T88	Complications of surgical and medical care, not elsewhere classified

C. Chapter-Specific Coding Guidelines

In addition to general coding guidelines, there are guidelines for specific diagnoses and/or conditions in the classification. Unless otherwise indicated, these guidelines apply to all health care settings. Please refer to Section II for guidelines on the selection of principal diagnosis.

19. Chapter 19: Injury, Poisoning and Certain Other Consequences of External Causes (S00-T88)

a. Application of 7th Characters in Chapter 19

Most categories in chapter 19 have a 7th character requirement for each applicable code. Most categories in this chapter have three 7th character values (with the exception of fractures): A, initial encounter, D, subsequent encounter and S, sequela. Categories for traumatic fractures have additional 7th character values. While the patient may be seen by a new or different provider over the course of treatment for an injury, assignment of the 7th character is based on whether the patient is undergoing active treatment and not whether the provider is seeing the patient for the first time.

For complication codes, active treatment refers to treatment for the condition described by the code, even though it may be related to an earlier precipitating problem. For example, code T84.50XA, Infection and inflammatory reaction due to unspecified internal joint prosthesis, initial encounter, is used when active treatment is provided for the infection, even though the condition relates to the prosthetic device, implant or graft that was placed at a previous encounter.

7th character "A", initial encounter is used for each encounter where the patient is receiving active treatment for the condition.

7th character "D" subsequent encounter is used for encounters after the patient has completed active treatment of the condition and is receiving routine care for the condition during the healing or recovery phase.

The aftercare Z codes should not be used for aftercare for conditions such as injuries or poisonings, where 7th characters are provided to identify subsequent care. For example, for aftercare of an injury, assign the acute injury code with the 7th character "D" (subsequent encounter).

7th character "S", sequela, is for use for complications or conditions that arise as a direct result of a condition, such as scar formation after a burn. The scars are sequelae of the burn. When using 7th character "S", it is necessary to use both the injury code that precipitated the sequela and the code for the sequela itself. The "S" is added only to the injury code, not the sequela code. The 7th character "S" identifies the injury responsible for the sequela. The specific type of sequela (e.g. scar) is sequenced first, followed by the injury code.

See Section I.B.10 Sequela (Late Effects)

b. Coding of Injuries

When coding injuries, assign separate codes for each injury unless a combination code is provided, in which case the combination code is assigned. Codes from category T07, Unspecified multiple injuries should not be assigned in the inpatient setting unless information for a more specific code is not available. Traumatic injury codes (S00-T14.9) are not to be used for normal, healing surgical wounds or to identify complications of surgical wounds.

The code for the most serious injury, as determined by the provider and the focus of treatment, is sequenced first.

1) Superficial injuries

Superficial injuries such as abrasions or contusions are not coded when associated with more severe injuries of the same site.

2) Primary injury with damage to nerves/blood vessels

When a primary injury results in minor damage to peripheral nerves or blood vessels, the primary injury is sequenced first with additional code(s) for injuries to nerves and spinal cord (such as category S04), and/or injury to blood vessels (such as category S15). When the primary injury is to the blood vessels or nerves, that injury should be sequenced first.

3) Iatrogenic injuries

Injury codes from Chapter 19 should not be assigned for injuries that occur during, or as a result of, a medical intervention. Assign the appropriate complication code(s).

c. Coding of Traumatic Fractures

The principles of multiple coding of injuries should be followed in coding fractures. Fractures of specified sites are coded individually by site in accordance with both the provisions within categories S02, S12, S22, S32, S42, S49, S52, S59, S62, S72, S79, S82, S89 and S92 and the level of detail furnished by medical record content.

A fracture not indicated as open or closed should be coded to closed. A fracture not indicated whether displaced or not displaced should be coded to displaced.

More specific guidelines are as follows:

1) Initial vs. Subsequent Encounter for Fractures

Traumatic fractures are coded using the appropriate 7th character for initial encounter (A, B, C) for each encounter where the patient is receiving active treatment for the fracture. The appropriate 7th character for initial encounter should also be assigned for a patient who delayed seeking treatment for the fracture or nonunion.

Fractures are coded using the appropriate 7th character for subsequent care for encounters after the patient has completed active treatment of the fracture and is receiving routine care for the fracture during the healing or recovery phase.

Care for complications of surgical treatment for fracture repairs during the healing or recovery phase should be coded with the appropriate complication codes.

Care of complications of fractures, such as malunion and nonunion, should be reported with the appropriate 7th character for subsequent care with nonunion (K, M, N,) or subsequent care with malunion (P, Q, R).

Malunion/nonunion: The appropriate 7th character for initial encounter should also be assigned for a patient who delayed seeking treatment for the fracture or nonunion.

The open fracture designations in the assignment of the 7th character for fractures of the forearm, femur and lower leg, including ankle are based on the Gustilo open fracture classification. When the Gustilo classification type is not specified for an open fracture, the 7th character for open fracture type I or II should be assigned (B, E, H, M, Q).

A code from category M80, not a traumatic fracture code, should be used for any patient with known osteoporosis who suffers a fracture, even if the patient had a minor fall or trauma, if that fall or trauma would not usually break a normal, healthy bone.

See Section I.C.13. Osteoporosis.

The aftercare Z codes should not be used for aftercare for traumatic fractures. For aftercare of a traumatic fracture, assign the acute fracture code with the appropriate 7th character.

2) Multiple fractures sequencing

Multiple fractures are sequenced in accordance with the severity of the fracture.

3) **Physeal fractures**

For physeal fractures, assign only the code identifying the type of physeal fracture. Do not assign a separate code to identify the specific bone that is fractured.

d. **Coding of Burns and Corrosions**

The ICD-10-CM makes a distinction between burns and corrosions. The burn codes are for thermal burns, except sunburns, that come from a heat source, such as a fire or hot appliance. The burn codes are also for burns resulting from electricity and radiation. Corrosions are burns due to chemicals. The guidelines are the same for burns and corrosions.

Current burns (T20-T25) are classified by depth, extent and by agent (X code). Burns are classified by depth as first degree (erythema), second degree (blistering), and third degree (full-thickness involvement). Burns of the eye and internal organs (T26-T28) are classified by site, but not by degree.

1) **Sequencing of burn and related condition codes**

Sequence first the code that reflects the highest degree of burn when more than one burn is present.

a. When the reason for the admission or encounter is for treatment of external multiple burns, sequence first the code that reflects the burn of the highest degree.

b. When a patient has both internal and external burns, the circumstances of admission govern the selection of the principal diagnosis or first-listed diagnosis.

c. When a patient is admitted for burn injuries and other related conditions such as smoke inhalation and/or respiratory failure, the circumstances of admission govern the selection of the principal or first-listed diagnosis.

2) **Burns of the same anatomical site**

Classify burns of the same anatomical site and on the same site but of different degrees to the subcategory identifying the highest degree recorded in the diagnosis (e.g., for second and third degree burns of right thigh, assign only code T24.311-).

3) **Non-healing burns**

Non-healing burns are coded as acute burns.

Necrosis of burned skin should be coded as a non-healed burn.

4) **Infected Burn**

For any documented infected burn site, use an additional code for the infection.

5) **Assign separate codes for each burn site**

When coding burns, assign separate codes for each burn site. Category T30, Burn and corrosion, body region unspecified is extremely vague and should rarely be used.

Codes for burns of "multiple sites" should only be assigned when the medical record documentation does not specify the individual sites.

6) **Burns and Corrosions Classified According to Extent of Body Surface Involved**

Assign codes from category T31, Burns classified according to extent of body surface involved, or T32, Corrosions classified according to extent of body surface involved, for acute burns or corrosions when the site of the burn or corrosion is not specified or when there is a need for additional data. It is advisable to use category T31 as additional coding when needed to provide data for evaluating burn mortality, such as that needed by burn units. It is also advisable to use category T31 as an additional code for reporting purposes when there is mention of a third-degree burn involving 20 percent or more of the body surface. Codes from categories T31 and T32 should not be used for sequelae of burns or corrosions.

Categories T31 and T32 are based on the classic "rule of nines" in estimating body surface involved: head and neck are assigned nine percent, each arm nine percent, each leg 18 percent, the anterior trunk 18 percent, posterior trunk 18 percent, and genitalia one percent. Providers may change these percentage assignments where necessary to accommodate infants and children who have proportionately larger heads than adults, and patients who have large buttocks, thighs, or abdomen that involve burns.

7) **Encounters for treatment of sequela of burns**

Encounters for the treatment of the late effects of burns or corrosions (i.e., scars or joint contractures) should be coded with a burn or corrosion code with the 7th character "S" for sequela.

8) **Sequelae with a late effect code and current burn**

When appropriate, both a code for a current burn or corrosion with 7th character "A" or "D" and a burn or corrosion code with 7th character "S" may be assigned on the same record (when both a current burn and sequelae of an old burn exist). Burns and corrosions do not heal at the same rate and a current healing wound may still exist with sequela of a healed burn or corrosion. *See Section I.B.10 Sequela (Late Effects)*

9) **Use of an external cause code with burns and corrosions**

An external cause code should be used with burns and corrosions to identify the source and intent of the burn, as well as the place where it occurred.

e. **Adverse Effects, Poisoning, Underdosing and Toxic Effects**

Codes in categories T36-T65 are combination codes that include the substance that was taken as well as the intent. No additional external cause code is required for poisonings, toxic effects, adverse effects and underdosing codes.

1) **Do not code directly from the Table of Drugs**

Do not code directly from the Table of Drugs and Chemicals. Always refer back to the Tabular List.

2) **Use as many codes as necessary to describe**

Use as many codes as necessary to describe completely all drugs, medicinal or biological substances.

3) **If the same code would describe the causative agent**

If the same code would describe the causative agent for more than one adverse reaction, poisoning, toxic effect or underdosing, assign the code only once.

4) **If two or more drugs, medicinal or biological substances**

If two or more drugs, medicinal or biological substances are taken, code each individually unless a combination code is listed in the Table of Drugs and Chemicals.

If multiple unspecified drugs, medicinal or biological substances were taken, assign the appropriate code from subcategory T50.91, Poisoning by, adverse effect of and underdosing of multiple unspecified drugs, medicaments and biological substances.

5) **The occurrence of drug toxicity is classified in ICD-10-CM as follows:**

(a) **Adverse Effect**

When coding an adverse effect of a drug that has been correctly prescribed and properly administered, assign the appropriate code for the nature of the adverse effect followed by the appropriate code for the adverse effect of the drug (T36-T50). The code for the drug should have a 5th or 6th character "5" (for example T36.0X5-) Examples of the nature of an adverse effect are tachycardia, delirium, gastrointestinal hemorrhaging, vomiting, hypokalemia, hepatitis, renal failure, or respiratory failure.

(b) **Poisoning**

When coding a poisoning or reaction to the improper use of a medication (e.g., overdose, wrong substance given or taken in error, wrong route of administration), first assign the appropriate code from categories T36-T50. The poisoning codes have an associated intent as their 5th or 6th character (accidental, intentional self-harm, assault and undetermined.) If the intent of the poisoning is unknown or unspecified, code the intent as accidental intent. The undetermined intent is only for use if the documentation in the record specifies that the intent cannot be determined. Use additional code(s) for all manifestations of poisonings.

If there is also a diagnosis of abuse or dependence of the substance, the abuse or dependence is assigned as an additional code.

Examples of poisoning include:

(i) Error was made in drug prescription

Errors made in drug prescription or in the administration of the drug by provider, nurse, patient, or other person.

(ii) Overdose of a drug intentionally taken

If an overdose of a drug was intentionally taken or administered and resulted in drug toxicity, it would be coded as a poisoning.

(iii) Nonprescribed drug taken with correctly prescribed and properly administered drug

If a nonprescribed drug or medicinal agent was taken in combination with a correctly prescribed and properly administered drug, any drug toxicity or other reaction resulting from the interaction of the two drugs would be classified as a poisoning.

(iv) Interaction of drug(s) and alcohol

When a reaction results from the interaction of a drug(s) and alcohol, this would be classified as poisoning.

See Section I.C.4. if poisoning is the result of insulin pump malfunctions.

(c) **Underdosing**

Underdosing refers to taking less of a medication than is prescribed by a provider or a manufacturer's instruction. Discontinuing the use of a prescribed medication on the patient's own initiative (not directed by the patient's provider) is also classified as an underdosing. For underdosing, assign the code from categories T36-T50 (fifth or sixth character "6").

Documentation of a change in the patient's condition is not required in order to assign an underdosing code. Documentation that the patient is taking less of a medication than is prescribed or discontinued the prescribed medication is sufficient for code assignment.

Codes for underdosing should never be assigned as principal or first-listed codes. If a patient has a relapse or exacerbation of the medical condition for which the drug is prescribed because of the reduction in dose, then the medical condition itself should be coded.

Noncompliance (Z91.12-, Z91.13-, Z91.14- **and Z91.A4-**) or complication of care (Y63.6-Y63.9) codes are to be used with an underdosing code to indicate intent, if known.

(d) Toxic Effects

When a harmful substance is ingested or comes in contact with a person, this is classified as a toxic effect. The toxic effect codes are in categories T51-T65.

Toxic effect codes have an associated intent: accidental, intentional self-harm, assault and undetermined.

For Sequela (Late Effects) see Section I.B.10. Sequela

f. Adult and child abuse, neglect and other maltreatment

Sequence first the appropriate code from categories T74.- (Adult and child abuse, neglect and other maltreatment, confirmed) or T76.- (Adult and child abuse, neglect and other maltreatment, suspected) for abuse, neglect and other maltreatment, followed by any accompanying mental health or injury code(s).

If the documentation in the medical record states abuse or neglect it is coded as confirmed (T74.-). It is coded as suspected if it is documented as suspected (T76.-).

For cases of confirmed abuse or neglect an external cause code from the assault section (X92-Y09) should be added to identify the cause of any physical injuries. A perpetrator code (Y07) should be added when the perpetrator of the abuse is known. For suspected cases of abuse or neglect, do not report external cause or perpetrator code.

If a suspected case of abuse, neglect or mistreatment is ruled out during an encounter code Z04.71, Encounter for examination and observation following alleged physical adult abuse, ruled out, or code Z04.72, Encounter for examination and observation following alleged child physical abuse, ruled out, should be used, not a code from T76.

If a suspected case of alleged rape or sexual abuse is ruled out during an encounter code Z04.41, Encounter for examination and observation following alleged adult rape or code Z04.42, Encounter for examination and observation following alleged child rape, should be used, not a code from T76.

If a suspected case of forced sexual exploitation or forced labor exploitation is ruled out during an encounter, code Z04.81, Encounter for examination and observation of victim following forced sexual exploitation, or code Z04.82, Encounter for examination and observation of victim following forced labor exploitation, should be used, not a code from T76.

See Section I.C.15. Abuse in a pregnant patient.

g. Complications of care

1) General guidelines for complications of care

(a) Documentation of complications of care

See Section I.B.16. for information on documentation of complications of care.

2) Pain due to medical devices

Pain associated with devices, implants or grafts left in a surgical site (for example painful hip prosthesis) is assigned to the appropriate code(s) found in Chapter 19, Injury, poisoning, and certain other consequences of external causes. Specific codes for pain due to medical devices are found in the T code section of the ICD-10-CM. Use additional code(s) from category G89 to identify acute or chronic pain due to presence of the device, implant or graft (G89.18 or G89.28).

3) Transplant complications

(a) Transplant complications other than kidney

Codes under category T86, Complications of transplanted organs and tissues, are for use for both complications and rejection of transplanted organs. A transplant complication code is only assigned if the complication affects the function of the transplanted organ. Two codes are required to fully describe a transplant complication: the appropriate code from category T86 and a secondary code that identifies the complication.

Pre-existing conditions or conditions that develop after the transplant are not coded as complications unless they affect the function of the transplanted organs.

See I.C.21. for transplant organ removal status.

See I.C.2. for malignant neoplasm associated with transplanted organ.

See I.C.1.d.4 for sequencing of sepsis due to infection in transplanted organ

(b) Kidney transplant complications

Patients who have undergone kidney transplant may still have some form of chronic kidney disease (CKD) because the kidney transplant may not fully restore kidney function. Code T86.1- should be assigned for documented complications of a kidney transplant, such as transplant failure or rejection or other transplant complication. Code T86.1- should not be assigned for post kidney transplant patients who have chronic kidney (CKD) unless a transplant complication such as transplant failure or rejection is documented. If the documentation is unclear as to whether the patient has a complication of the transplant, query the provider.

Conditions that affect the function of the transplanted kidney, other than CKD, should be assigned a code from subcategory T86.1, Complications of transplanted organ, Kidney, and a secondary code that identifies the complication.

For patients with CKD following a kidney transplant, but who do not have a complication such as failure or rejection, *see section I.C.14. Chronic kidney disease and kidney transplant status.*

See I.C.1.d.4 for sequencing of sepsis due to infection in transplanted organ

4) Complication codes that include the external cause

As with certain other T codes, some of the complications of care codes have the external cause included in the code. The code includes the nature of the complication as well as the type of procedure that caused the complication. No external cause code indicating the type of procedure is necessary for these codes.

5) Complications of care codes within the body system chapters

Intraoperative and postprocedural complication codes are found within the body system chapters with codes specific to the organs and structures of that body system. These codes should be sequenced first, followed by a code(s) for the specific complication, if applicable.

Complication codes from the body system chapters should be assigned for intraoperative and postprocedural complications (e.g., the appropriate complication code from chapter 9 would be assigned for a vascular intraoperative or postprocedural complication) unless the complication is specifically indexed to a T code in chapter 19.

Injuries to the head (S00-S09)

Includes: injuries of ear
injuries of eye
injuries of face [any part]
injuries of gum
injuries of jaw
injuries of oral cavity
injuries of palate
injuries of periocular area
injuries of scalp
injuries of temporomandibular joint area
injuries of tongue
injuries of tooth

Code also for any associated infection

Excludes2: burns and corrosions (T20-T32)
effects of foreign body in ear (T16)
effects of foreign body in larynx (T17.3)
effects of foreign body in mouth NOS (T18.0)
effects of foreign body in nose (T17.0-T17.1)
effects of foreign body in pharynx (T17.2)
effects of foreign body on external eye (T15.-)
frostbite (T33-T34)
insect bite or sting, venomous (T63.4)

S00 Superficial injury of head

Excludes1: diffuse cerebral contusion (S06.2-)
focal cerebral contusion (S06.3-)
injury of eye and orbit (S05.-)
open wound of head (S01.-)

The appropriate 7th character is to be added to each code from category S00
A   initial encounter
D   subsequent encounter
S   sequela

- **S00.0 Superficial injury of scalp**
  - X+7th S00.00 Unspecified superficial injury of scalp
  - X+7th S00.01 Abrasion of scalp
  - X+7th S00.02 Blister (nonthermal) of scalp
  - X+7th S00.03 Contusion of scalp
    Bruise of scalp
    Hematoma of scalp
  - X+7th S00.04 External constriction of part of scalp
  - X+7th S00.05 Superficial foreign body of scalp
    Splinter in the scalp
  - X+7th S00.06 Insect bite (nonvenomous) of scalp
  - X+7th S00.07 Other superficial bite of scalp
    Excludes1: *open bite of scalp (S01.05)*
- **S00.1 Contusion of eyelid and periocular area**
  Black eye
  Excludes2: *contusion of eyeball and orbital tissues (S05.1-)*
  - X+7th S00.10 Contusion of unspecified eyelid and periocular area
  - X+7th S00.11 Contusion of right eyelid and periocular area
  - X+7th S00.12 Contusion of left eyelid and periocular area
- **S00.2 Other and unspecified superficial injuries of eyelid and periocular area**
  Excludes2: *superficial injury of conjunctiva and cornea (S05.0-)*
  - S00.20 Unspecified superficial injury of eyelid and periocular area
    - +7th S00.201 Unspecified superficial injury of right eyelid and periocular area
    - +7th S00.202 Unspecified superficial injury of left eyelid and periocular area
    - +7th S00.209 Unspecified superficial injury of unspecified eyelid and periocular area
  - S00.21 Abrasion of eyelid and periocular area
    - +7th S00.211 Abrasion of right eyelid and periocular area
    - +7th S00.212 Abrasion of left eyelid and periocular area
    - +7th S00.219 Abrasion of unspecified eyelid and periocular area
  - S00.22 Blister (nonthermal) of eyelid and periocular area
    - +7th S00.221 Blister (nonthermal) of right eyelid and periocular area
    - +7th S00.222 Blister (nonthermal) of left eyelid and periocular area
    - +7th S00.229 Blister (nonthermal) of unspecified eyelid and periocular area
  - S00.24 External constriction of eyelid and periocular area
    - +7th S00.241 External constriction of right eyelid and periocular area
    - +7th S00.242 External constriction of left eyelid and periocular area
    - +7th S00.249 External constriction of unspecified eyelid and periocular area
  - S00.25 Superficial foreign body of eyelid and periocular area
    Splinter of eyelid and periocular area
    Excludes2: *retained foreign body in eyelid (H02.81-)*
    - +7th S00.251 Superficial foreign body of right eyelid and periocular area
    - +7th S00.252 Superficial foreign body of left eyelid and periocular area
    - +7th S00.259 Superficial foreign body of unspecified eyelid and periocular area
  - S00.26 Insect bite (nonvenomous) of eyelid and periocular area
    - +7th S00.261 Insect bite (nonvenomous) of right eyelid and periocular area
    - +7th S00.262 Insect bite (nonvenomous) of left eyelid and periocular area
    - +7th S00.269 Insect bite (nonvenomous) of unspecified eyelid and periocular area
  - S00.27 Other superficial bite of eyelid and periocular area
    Excludes1: *open bite of eyelid and periocular area (S01.15)*
    - +7th S00.271 Other superficial bite of right eyelid and periocular area
    - +7th S00.272 Other superficial bite of left eyelid and periocular area
    - +7th S00.279 Other superficial bite of unspecified eyelid and periocular area

- **S00.3 Superficial injury of nose**
  - X+7th S00.30 Unspecified superficial injury of nose
  - X+7th S00.31 Abrasion of nose
  - X+7th S00.32 Blister (nonthermal) of nose
  - X+7th S00.33 Contusion of nose
    Bruise of nose
    Hematoma of nose
  - X+7th S00.34 External constriction of nose
  - X+7th S00.35 Superficial foreign body of nose
    Splinter in the nose
  - X+7th S00.36 Insect bite (nonvenomous) of nose
  - X+7th S00.37 Other superficial bite of nose
    Excludes1: *open bite of nose (S01.25)*
- **S00.4 Superficial injury of ear**
  - S00.40 Unspecified superficial injury of ear
    - +7th S00.401 Unspecified superficial injury of right ear
    - +7th S00.402 Unspecified superficial injury of left ear
    - +7th S00.409 Unspecified superficial injury of unspecified ear
  - S00.41 Abrasion of ear
    - +7th S00.411 Abrasion of right ear
    - +7th S00.412 Abrasion of left ear
    - +7th S00.419 Abrasion of unspecified ear
  - S00.42 Blister (nonthermal) of ear
    - +7th S00.421 Blister (nonthermal) of right ear
    - +7th S00.422 Blister (nonthermal) of left ear
    - +7th S00.429 Blister (nonthermal) of unspecified ear
  - S00.43 Contusion of ear
    Bruise of ear
    Hematoma of ear
    - +7th S00.431 Contusion of right ear
    - +7th S00.432 Contusion of left ear
    - +7th S00.439 Contusion of unspecified ear
  - S00.44 External constriction of ear
    - +7th S00.441 External constriction of right ear
    - +7th S00.442 External constriction of left ear
    - +7th S00.449 External constriction of unspecified ear
  - S00.45 Superficial foreign body of ear
    Splinter in the ear
    - +7th S00.451 Superficial foreign body of right ear
    - +7th S00.452 Superficial foreign body of left ear
    - +7th S00.459 Superficial foreign body of unspecified ear
  - S00.46 Insect bite (nonvenomous) of ear
    - +7th S00.461 Insect bite (nonvenomous) of right ear
    - +7th S00.462 Insect bite (nonvenomous) of left ear
    - +7th S00.469 Insect bite (nonvenomous) of unspecified ear
  - S00.47 Other superficial bite of ear
    Excludes1: *open bite of ear (S01.35)*
    - +7th S00.471 Other superficial bite of right ear
    - +7th S00.472 Other superficial bite of left ear
    - +7th S00.479 Other superficial bite of unspecified ear
- **S00.5 Superficial injury of lip and oral cavity**
  - S00.50 Unspecified superficial injury of lip and oral cavity
    - +7th S00.501 Unspecified superficial injury of lip
    - +7th S00.502 Unspecified superficial injury of oral cavity
  - S00.51 Abrasion of lip and oral cavity
    - +7th S00.511 Abrasion of lip
    - +7th S00.512 Abrasion of oral cavity
  - S00.52 Blister (nonthermal) of lip and oral cavity
    - +7th S00.521 Blister (nonthermal) of lip
    - +7th S00.522 Blister (nonthermal) of oral cavity
  - S00.53 Contusion of lip and oral cavity
    - +7th S00.531 Contusion of lip
      Bruise of lip
      Hematoma of lip
    - +7th S00.532 Contusion of oral cavity
      Bruise of oral cavity
      Hematoma of oral cavity
  - S00.54 External constriction of lip and oral cavity
    - +7th S00.541 External constriction of lip
    - +7th S00.542 External constriction of oral cavity
  - S00.55 Superficial foreign body of lip and oral cavity
    - +7th S00.551 Superficial foreign body of lip
      Splinter of lip and oral cavity
    - +7th S00.552 Superficial foreign body of oral cavity
      Splinter of lip and oral cavity

- **+ S00.56** Insect bite (nonvenomous) of lip and oral cavity
  - **+7th S00.561** Insect bite (nonvenomous) of lip
  - **+7th S00.562** Insect bite (nonvenomous) of oral cavity
- **+ S00.57** Other superficial bite of lip and oral cavity
  - **+7th S00.571** Other superficial bite of lip
    - **Excludes1:** open bite of lip (S01.551)
  - **+7th S00.572** Other superficial bite of oral cavity
    - **Excludes1:** open bite of oral cavity (S01.552)
- **+ S00.8** Superficial injury of other parts of head
  - Superficial injuries of face [any part]
  - **X+7th S00.80** Unspecified superficial injury of other part of head
  - **X+7th S00.81** Abrasion of other part of head
  - **X+7th S00.82** Blister (nonthermal) of other part of head
  - **X+7th S00.83** Contusion of other part of head
    - Bruise of other part of head
    - Hematoma of other part of head
  - **X+7th S00.84** External constriction of other part of head
  - **X+7th S00.85** Superficial foreign body of other part of head
    - Splinter in other part of head
  - **X+7th S00.86** Insect bite (nonvenomous) of other part of head
  - **X+7th S00.87** Other superficial bite of other part of head
    - **Excludes1:** open bite of other part of head (S01.85)
- **+ S00.9** Superficial injury of unspecified part of head
  - **X+7th S00.90** Unspecified superficial injury of unspecified part of head
  - **X+7th S00.91** Abrasion of unspecified part of head
  - **X+7th S00.92** Blister (nonthermal) of unspecified part of head
  - **X+7th S00.93** Contusion of unspecified part of head
    - Bruise of head
    - Hematoma of head
  - **X+7th S00.94** External constriction of unspecified part of head
  - **X+7th S00.95** Superficial foreign body of unspecified part of head
    - Splinter of head
  - **X+7th S00.96** Insect bite (nonvenomous) of unspecified part of head
  - **X+7th S00.97** Other superficial bite of unspecified part of head
    - **Excludes1:** open bite of head (S01.95)

S01 Open wound of head

Code also any associated:
injury of cranial nerve (S04.-)
injury of muscle and tendon of head (S09.1-)
intracranial injury (S06.-)
wound infection
Excludes1: open skull fracture (S02.- with 7th character B)
Excludes2: injury of eye and orbit (S05.-)
traumatic amputation of part of head (S08.-)

> The appropriate 7th character is to be added to each code from category S01
> A   initial encounter
> D   subsequent encounter
> S   sequela

- **+ S01.0** Open wound of scalp
  - **Excludes1:** avulsion of scalp (S08.0-)
  - **X+7th S01.00** Unspecified open wound of scalp
  - **X+7th S01.01** Laceration without foreign body of scalp
  - **X+7th S01.02** Laceration with foreign body of scalp
    - AHA CC: 1Q, 2015, 3-21
  - **X+7th S01.03** Puncture wound without foreign body of scalp
  - **X+7th S01.04** Puncture wound with foreign body of scalp
  - **X+7th S01.05** Open bite of scalp
    - Bite of scalp NOS
    - **Excludes1:** superficial bite of scalp (S00.06, S00.07-)
- **+ S01.1** Open wound of eyelid and periocular area
  - Open wound of eyelid and periocular area with or without involvement of lacrimal passages
  - **+ S01.10** Unspecified open wound of eyelid and periocular area
    - **CC +7th S01.101** Unspecified open wound of right eyelid and periocular area
    - **CC +7th S01.102** Unspecified open wound of left eyelid and periocular area
    - **CC +7th S01.109** Unspecified open wound of unspecified eyelid and periocular area
  - **+ S01.11** Laceration without foreign body of eyelid and periocular area
    - **+7th S01.111** Laceration without foreign body of right eyelid and periocular area
    - **+7th S01.112** Laceration without foreign body of left eyelid and periocular area
    - **+7th S01.119** Laceration without foreign body of unspecified eyelid and periocular area
  - **+ S01.12** Laceration with foreign body of eyelid and periocular area
    - **+7th S01.121** Laceration with foreign body of right eyelid and periocular area
    - **+7th S01.122** Laceration with foreign body of left eyelid and periocular area
    - **+7th S01.129** Laceration with foreign body of unspecified eyelid and periocular area
  - **+ S01.13** Puncture wound without foreign body of eyelid and periocular area
    - **+7th S01.131** Puncture wound without foreign body of right eyelid and periocular area
    - **+7th S01.132** Puncture wound without foreign body of left eyelid and periocular area
    - **+7th S01.139** Puncture wound without foreign body of unspecified eyelid and periocular area
  - **+ S01.14** Puncture wound with foreign body of eyelid and periocular area
    - **+7th S01.141** Puncture wound with foreign body of right eyelid and periocular area
    - **+7th S01.142** Puncture wound with foreign body of left eyelid and periocular area
    - **+7th S01.149** Puncture wound with foreign body of unspecified eyelid and periocular area
  - **+ S01.15** Open bite of eyelid and periocular area
    - Bite of eyelid and periocular area NOS
    - **Excludes1:** superficial bite of eyelid and periocular area (S00.26, S00.27)
    - **+7th S01.151** Open bite of right eyelid and periocular area
    - **+7th S01.152** Open bite of left eyelid and periocular area
    - **+7th S01.159** Open bite of unspecified eyelid and periocular area
- **+ S01.2** Open wound of nose
  - **X+7th S01.20** Unspecified open wound of nose
  - **X+7th S01.21** Laceration without foreign body of nose
    - AHA CC: 1Q, 2015, 3-21
  - **X+7th S01.22** Laceration with foreign body of nose
  - **X+7th S01.23** Puncture wound without foreign body of nose
  - **X+7th S01.24** Puncture wound with foreign body of nose
  - **X+7th S01.25** Open bite of nose
    - Bite of nose NOS
    - **Excludes1:** superficial bite of nose (S00.36, S00.37)
- **+ S01.3** Open wound of ear
  - **+ S01.30** Unspecified open wound of ear
    - **+7th S01.301** Unspecified open wound of right ear
    - **+7th S01.302** Unspecified open wound of left ear
    - **+7th S01.309** Unspecified open wound of unspecified ear
  - **+ S01.31** Laceration without foreign body of ear
    - **+7th S01.311** Laceration without foreign body of right ear
    - **+7th S01.312** Laceration without foreign body of left ear
    - **+7th S01.319** Laceration without foreign body of unspecified ear
  - **+ S01.32** Laceration with foreign body of ear
    - **+7th S01.321** Laceration with foreign body of right ear
    - **+7th S01.322** Laceration with foreign body of left ear
    - **+7th S01.329** Laceration with foreign body of unspecified ear
  - **+ S01.33** Puncture wound without foreign body of ear
    - **+7th S01.331** Puncture wound without foreign body of right ear
    - **+7th S01.332** Puncture wound without foreign body of left ear
    - **+7th S01.339** Puncture wound without foreign body of unspecified ear

- **+ S01.34 Puncture wound with foreign body of ear**
  - +7th S01.341 Puncture wound with foreign body of right ear
  - +7th S01.342 Puncture wound with foreign body of left ear
  - +7th S01.349 Puncture wound with foreign body of unspecified ear
- **+ S01.35 Open bite of ear**
  - Bite of ear NOS
  - *Excludes1:* *superficial bite of ear (S00.46, S00.47)*
  - +7th S01.351 Open bite of right ear
  - +7th S01.352 Open bite of left ear
  - +7th S01.359 Open bite of unspecified ear
- **+ S01.4 Open wound of cheek and temporomandibular area**
  - **+ S01.40 Unspecified open wound of cheek and temporomandibular area**
    - +7th S01.401 Unspecified open wound of right cheek and temporomandibular area
    - +7th S01.402 Unspecified open wound of left cheek and temporomandibular area
    - +7th S01.409 Unspecified open wound of unspecified cheek and temporomandibular area
  - **+ S01.41 Laceration without foreign body of cheek and temporomandibular area**
    - +7th S01.411 Laceration without foreign body of right cheek and temporomandibular area
      - *AHA CC: 1Q, 2015, 3-21*
    - +7th S01.412 Laceration without foreign body of left cheek and temporomandibular area
    - +7th S01.419 Laceration without foreign body of unspecified cheek and temporomandibular area
  - **+ S01.42 Laceration with foreign body of cheek and temporomandibular area**
    - +7th S01.421 Laceration with foreign body of right cheek and temporomandibular area
    - +7th S01.422 Laceration with foreign body of left cheek and temporomandibular area
    - +7th S01.429 Laceration with foreign body of unspecified cheek and temporomandibular area
  - **+ S01.43 Puncture wound without foreign body of cheek and temporomandibular area**
    - +7th S01.431 Puncture wound without foreign body of right cheek and temporomandibular area
    - +7th S01.432 Puncture wound without foreign body of left cheek and temporomandibular area
    - +7th S01.439 Puncture wound without foreign body of unspecified cheek and temporomandibular area
  - **+ S01.44 Puncture wound with foreign body of cheek and temporomandibular area**
    - +7th S01.441 Puncture wound with foreign body of right cheek and temporomandibular area
    - +7th S01.442 Puncture wound with foreign body of left cheek and temporomandibular area
    - +7th S01.449 Puncture wound with foreign body of unspecified cheek and temporomandibular area
  - **+ S01.45 Open bite of cheek and temporomandibular area**
    - Bite of cheek and temporomandibular area NOS
    - *Excludes2:* *superficial bite of cheek and temporomandibular area (S00.86, S00.87)*
    - +7th S01.451 Open bite of right cheek and temporomandibular area
    - +7th S01.452 Open bite of left cheek and temporomandibular area
    - +7th S01.459 Open bite of unspecified cheek and temporomandibular area
- **+ S01.5 Open wound of lip and oral cavity**
  - *Excludes2:* *tooth dislocation (S03.2)*
  - *tooth fracture (S02.5)*
  - **+ S01.50 Unspecified open wound of lip and oral cavity**
    - +7th S01.501 Unspecified open wound of lip
    - +7th S01.502 Unspecified open wound of oral cavity
  - **+ S01.51 Laceration of lip and oral cavity without foreign body**
    - +7th S01.511 Laceration without foreign body of lip
    - +7th S01.512 Laceration without foreign body of oral cavity
  - **+ S01.52 Laceration of lip and oral cavity with foreign body**
    - +7th S01.521 Laceration with foreign body of lip
    - +7th S01.522 Laceration with foreign body of oral cavity
  - **+ S01.53 Puncture wound of lip and oral cavity without foreign body**
    - +7th S01.531 Puncture wound without foreign body of lip
    - +7th S01.532 Puncture wound without foreign body of oral cavity
  - **+ S01.54 Puncture wound of lip and oral cavity with foreign body**
    - +7th S01.541 Puncture wound with foreign body of lip
    - +7th S01.542 Puncture wound with foreign body of oral cavity
  - **+ S01.55 Open bite of lip and oral cavity**
    - +7th S01.551 Open bite of lip
      - Bite of lip NOS
      - *Excludes1:* *superficial bite of lip (S00.571)*
    - +7th S01.552 Open bite of oral cavity
      - Bite of oral cavity NOS
      - *Excludes1:* *superficial bite of oral cavity (S00.572)*
- **+ S01.8 Open wound of other parts of head**
  - X+7th S01.80 Unspecified open wound of other part of head
  - X+7th S01.81 Laceration without foreign body of other part of head
  - X+7th S01.82 Laceration with foreign body of other part of head
  - X+7th S01.83 Puncture wound without foreign body of other part of head
  - X+7th S01.84 Puncture wound with foreign body of other part of head
  - X+7th S01.85 Open bite of other part of head
    - Bite of other part of head NOS
    - *Excludes1:* *superficial bite of other part of head (S00.87)*
- **+ S01.9 Open wound of unspecified part of head**
  - X+7th S01.90 Unspecified open wound of unspecified part of head
  - X+7th S01.91 Laceration without foreign body of unspecified part of head
  - X+7th S01.92 Laceration with foreign body of unspecified part of head
  - X+7th S01.93 Puncture wound without foreign body of unspecified part of head
  - X+7th S01.94 Puncture wound with foreign body of unspecified part of head
  - X+7th S01.95 Open bite of unspecified part of head
    - Bite of head NOS
    - *Excludes1:* *superficial bite of head NOS (S00.97)*

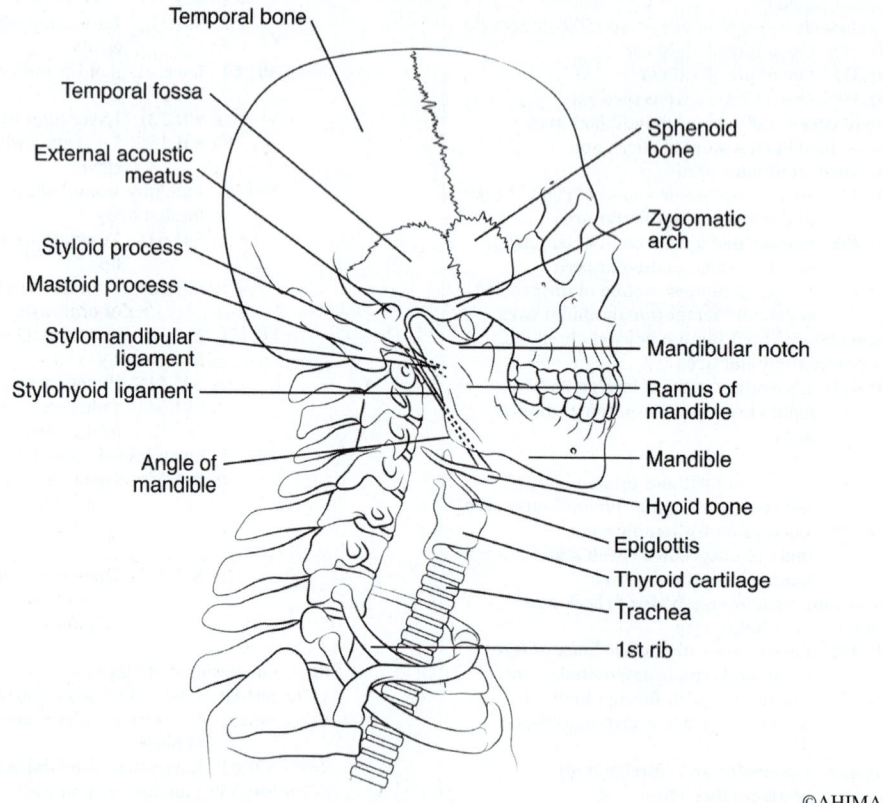

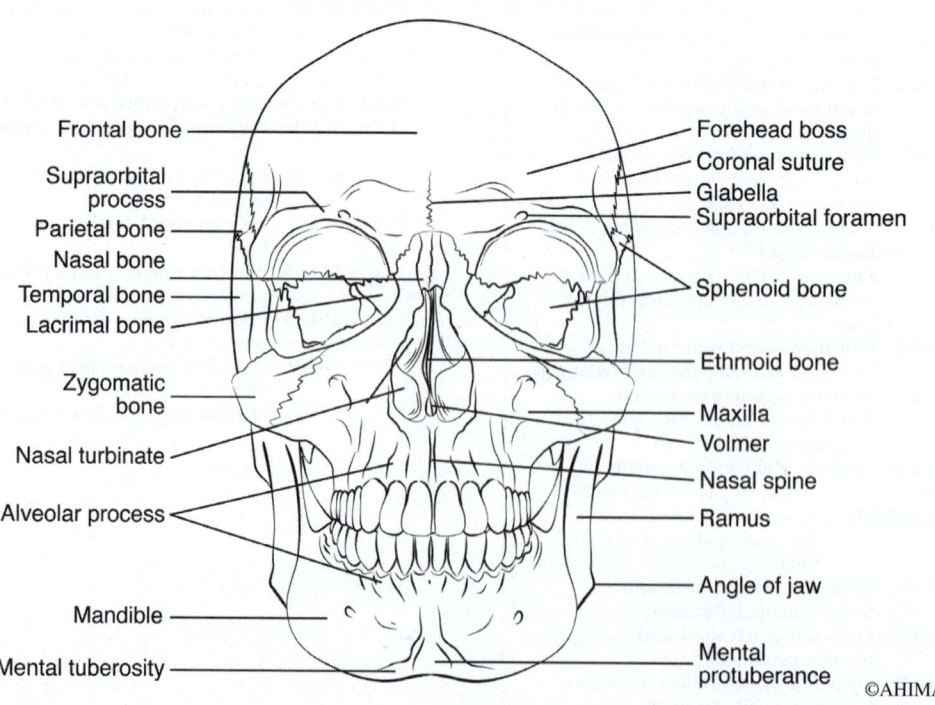

S02 **Fracture of skull and facial bones**

NOTE A fracture not indicated as open or closed should be coded to closed

Code also any associated intracranial injury (S06.-)

Review coding guideline C.19.c

AHA CC: 4Q, 2016, 66-67

The appropriate 7th character is to be added to each code from category S02
- A initial encounter for closed fracture
- B initial encounter for open fracture
- D subsequent encounter for fracture with routine healing
- G subsequent encounter for fracture with delayed healing
- K subsequent encounter for fracture with nonunion
- S sequela

X+7th **S02.0** **Fracture of vault of skull**
CC MCC
Fracture of frontal bone
Fracture of parietal bone
HAC 7th characters A & B see Appendix B for HAC conditional logic

+ **S02.1** **Fracture of base of skull**
Excludes2: lateral orbital wall (S02.84-)
medial orbital wall (S02.83-)
orbital floor (S02.3-)
AHA CC: 4Q, 2019, 16

+ **S02.10** **Unspecified fracture of base of skull**

CC MCC +7th **S02.101** **Fracture of base of skull, right side**
HAC 7th characters A & B see Appendix B for HAC conditional logic

CC MCC +7th **S02.102** **Fracture of base of skull, left side**
HAC 7th characters A & B see Appendix B for HAC conditional logic

CC MCC +7th **S02.109** **Fracture of base of skull, unspecified side**
HAC 7th characters A & B see Appendix B for HAC conditional logic

+ **S02.11** **Fracture of occiput**

CC MCC +7th **S02.110** **Type I occipital condyle fracture, unspecified side**
HAC 7th characters A & B see Appendix B for HAC conditional logic

CC MCC +7th **S02.111** **Type II occipital condyle fracture, unspecified side**
HAC 7th characters A & B see Appendix B for HAC conditional logic

CC MCC +7th **S02.112** **Type III occipital condyle fracture, unspecified side**
HAC 7th characters A & B see Appendix B for HAC conditional logic

CC MCC +7th **S02.113** **Unspecified occipital condyle fracture**
HAC 7th characters A & B see Appendix B for HAC conditional logic

CC MCC +7th **S02.118** **Other fracture of occiput, unspecified side**
HAC 7th characters A & B see Appendix B for HAC conditional logic

CC MCC +7th **S02.119** **Unspecified fracture of occiput**
HAC 7th characters A & B see Appendix B for HAC conditional logic

CC MCC +7th **S02.11A** **Type I occipital condyle fracture, right side**
HAC 7th characters A & B see Appendix B for HAC conditional logic

CC MCC +7th **S02.11B** **Type I occipital condyle fracture, left side**
HAC 7th characters A & B see Appendix B for HAC conditional logic

CC MCC +7th **S02.11C** **Type II occipital condyle fracture, right side**
HAC 7th characters A & B see Appendix B for HAC conditional logic

CC MCC +7th **S02.11D** **Type II occipital condyle fracture, left side**
HAC 7th characters A & B see Appendix B for HAC conditional logic

CC MCC +7th **S02.11E** **Type III occipital condyle fracture, right side**
HAC 7th characters A & B see Appendix B for HAC conditional logic

CC MCC +7th **S02.11F** **Type III occipital condyle fracture, left side**
HAC 7th characters A & B see Appendix B for HAC conditional logic

CC MCC +7th **S02.11G** **Other fracture or occiput, right side**
HAC 7th characters A & B see Appendix B for HAC conditional logic

CC MCC +7th **S02.11H** **Other fracture or occiput, left side**
HAC 7th characters A & B see Appendix B for HAC conditional logic

+ **S02.12** **Fracture of orbital roof**

CC MCC **S02.121** **Fracture of orbital roof, right side**
HAC 7th characters A & B see Appendix B for HAC conditional logic

CC MCC **S02.122** **Fracture of orbital roof, left side**
HAC 7th characters A & B see Appendix B for HAC conditional logic

CC MCC **S02.129** **Fracture of orbital roof, unspecified side**
HAC 7th characters A & B see Appendix B for HAC conditional logic

CC MCC X+7th **S02.19** **Other fracture of base of skull**
Fracture of anterior fossa of base of skull
Fracture of ethmoid sinus
Fracture of frontal sinus
Fracture of middle fossa of base of skull
Fracture of posterior fossa of base of skull
Fracture of sphenoid
Fracture of temporal bone
HAC 7th characters A & B see Appendix B for HAC conditional logic

CC X+7th **S02.2** **Fracture of nasal bones**
HAC 7th character B see Appendix B for HAC conditional logic

+ **S02.3** **Fracture of orbital floor**
Excludes1: orbit NOS (S02.85)
Excludes2: lateral orbital wall (S02.84-)
medial orbital wall (S02.83-)
orbital roof (S02.1-)

CC X+7th **S02.30** **Fracture of orbital floor, unspecified side**
HAC 7th characters A & B see Appendix B for HAC conditional logic

CC X+7th **S02.31** **Fracture of orbital floor, right side**
HAC 7th characters A & B see Appendix B for HAC conditional logic

CC X+7th **S02.32** **Fracture of orbital floor, left side**
HAC 7th characters A & B see Appendix B for HAC conditional logic

+ **S02.4** **Fracture of malar, maxillary and zygoma bones**
Fracture of superior maxilla
Fracture of upper jaw (bone)
Fracture of zygomatic process of temporal bone

+ **S02.40** **Fracture of malar, maxillary and zygoma bones, unspecified**

CC +7th **S02.400** **Malar fracture, unspecified side**
HAC 7th characters A & B see Appendix B for HAC conditional logic

CC +7th **S02.401** **Maxillary fracture, unspecified side**
HAC 7th characters A & B see Appendix B for HAC conditional logic

CC +7th **S02.402** **Zygomatic fracture, unspecified side**
HAC 7th characters A & B see Appendix B for HAC conditional logic

CC +7th **S02.40A** **Malar fracture, right side**
HAC 7th characters A & B see Appendix B for HAC conditional logic

CC +7th **S02.40B** **Malar fracture, left side**
HAC 7th characters A & B see Appendix B for HAC conditional logic

CC +7th **S02.40C** **Maxillary fracture, right side**
HAC 7th characters A & B see Appendix B for HAC conditional logic

CC +7th **S02.40D** **Maxillary fracture, left side**
HAC 7th characters A & B see Appendix B for HAC conditional logic

CC +7th **S02.40E** **Zygomatic fracture, right side**
HAC 7th characters A & B see Appendix B for HAC conditional logic

CC +7th **S02.40F** **Zygomatic fracture, left side**
HAC 7th characters A & B see Appendix B for HAC conditional logic

+ **S02.41** **LeFort fracture**

CC +7th **S02.411** **LeFort I fracture**
HAC 7th characters A & B see Appendix B for HAC conditional logic

CC +7th **S02.412** **LeFort II fracture**
HAC 7th characters A & B see Appendix B for HAC conditional logic

CC +7th **S02.413** **LeFort III fracture**
HAC 7th characters A & B see Appendix B for HAC conditional logic

CC X+7th **S02.42** **Fracture of alveolus of maxilla**
HAC 7th characters A & B see Appendix B for HAC conditional logic

CC X+7th **S02.5** **Fracture of tooth (traumatic)**
Broken tooth
Excludes1: cracked tooth (nontraumatic) (K03.81)

S02.6 Fracture of mandible
Fracture of lower jaw (bone)

S02.60 Fracture of mandible, unspecified
- **S02.600** Fracture of unspecified part of body of mandible, unspecified side
  HAC 7th characters A & B see Appendix B for HAC conditional logic
- **S02.601** Fracture of unspecified part of body of right mandible
  HAC 7th characters A & B see Appendix B for HAC conditional logic
- **S02.602** Fracture of unspecified part of body of left mandible
  HAC 7th characters A & B see Appendix B for HAC conditional logic
- **S02.609** Fracture of mandible, unspecified
  HAC 7th characters A & B see Appendix B for HAC conditional logic

S02.61 Fracture of condylar process of mandible
- **S02.610** Fracture of condylar process of mandible, unspecified side
  HAC 7th characters A & B see Appendix B for HAC conditional logic
- **S02.611** Fracture of condylar process of right mandible
  AHA CC: 1Q, 2021, 6
  HAC 7th characters A & B see Appendix B for HAC conditional logic
- **S02.612** Fracture of condylar process of left mandible
  HAC 7th characters A & B see Appendix B for HAC conditional logic

S02.62 Fracture of subcondylar process of mandible
- **S02.620** Fracture of subcondylar process of mandible, unspecified side
  HAC 7th characters A & B see Appendix B for HAC conditional logic
- **S02.621** Fracture of subcondylar process of right mandible
  HAC 7th characters A & B see Appendix B for HAC conditional logic
- **S02.622** Fracture of subcondylar process of left mandible
  HAC 7th characters A & B see Appendix B for HAC conditional logic

S02.63 Fracture of coronoid process of mandible
- **S02.630** Fracture of coronoid process of mandible, unspecified side
  HAC 7th characters A & B see Appendix B for HAC conditional logic
- **S02.631** Fracture of coronoid process of right mandible
  HAC 7th characters A & B see Appendix B for HAC conditional logic
- **S02.632** Fracture of coronoid process of left mandible
  HAC 7th characters A & B see Appendix B for HAC conditional logic

S02.64 Fracture of ramus of mandible
- **S02.640** Fracture of ramus of mandible, unspecified side
  HAC 7th characters A & B see Appendix B for HAC conditional logic
- **S02.641** Fracture of ramus of right mandible
  HAC 7th characters A & B see Appendix B for HAC conditional logic
- **S02.642** Fracture of ramus of left mandible
  HAC 7th characters A & B see Appendix B for HAC conditional logic

S02.65 Fracture of angle of mandible
- **S02.650** Fracture of angle of mandible, unspecified side
  HAC 7th characters A & B see Appendix B for HAC conditional logic
- **S02.651** Fracture of angle of right mandible
  HAC 7th characters A & B see Appendix B for HAC conditional logic
- **S02.652** Fracture of angle of left mandible
  HAC 7th characters A & B see Appendix B for HAC conditional logic

S02.66 Fracture of symphysis of mandible
AHA CC: 1Q, 2021, 6
HAC 7th characters A & B see Appendix B for HAC conditional logic

S02.67 Fracture of alveolus of mandible
- **S02.670** Fracture of alveolus of mandible, unspecified side
  HAC 7th characters A & B see Appendix B for HAC conditional logic
- **S02.671** Fracture of alveolus of right mandible
  HAC 7th characters A & B see Appendix B for HAC conditional logic
- **S02.672** Fracture of alveolus of left mandible
  HAC 7th characters A & B see Appendix B for HAC conditional logic

S02.69 Fracture of mandible of other specified site
HAC 7th characters A & B see Appendix B for HAC conditional logic

S02.8 Fractures of other specified skull and facial bones
Fracture of palate
Excludes2: *fracture of orbital floor (S02.3-)*
fracture of orbital roof (S02.12-)
AHA CC: 4Q, 2019, 16-17

- **S02.80** Fracture of other specified skull and facial bones, unspecified side
  HAC 7th characters A & B see Appendix B for HAC conditional logic
- **S02.81** Fracture of other specified skull and facial bones, right side
  HAC 7th characters A & B see Appendix B for HAC conditional logic
- **S02.82** Fracture of other specified skull and facial bones, left side
  HAC 7th characters A & B see Appendix B for HAC conditional logic

S02.83 Fracture of medial orbital wall
Excludes2: *orbital floor (S02.3-)*
orbital roof (S02.12-)
- **S02.831** Fracture of medial orbital wall, right side
  HAC 7th characters A & B see Appendix B for HAC conditional logic
- **S02.832** Fracture of medical orbital wall, left side
  HAC 7th characters A & B see Appendix B for HAC conditional logic
- **S03.839** Fracture of medical orbital wall, unspecified side
  HAC 7th characters A & B see Appendix B for HAC conditional logic

S02.84 Fracture of lateral orbital wall
Excludes2: *orbital floor (S02.3-)*
orbital roof (S02.12-)
- **S02.841** Fracture of lateral orbital wall, right side
  HAC 7th characters A & B see Appendix B for HAC conditional logic
- **S02.842** Fracture of lateral orbital wall, left side
  HAC 7th characters A & B see Appendix B for HAC conditional logic
- **S02.849** Fracture of lateral orbital wall, unspecified side
  HAC 7th characters A & B see Appendix B for HAC conditional logic

S02.85 Fracture of orbit, unspecified
Fracture of orbit NOS
Fracture of orbit wall NOS
Excludes1: *lateral orbital wall (S02.84-)*
medial orbital wall (S02.83-)
orbital floor (S02.3-)
orbital roof (S02.12-)
HAC 7th characters A & B see Appendix B for HAC conditional logic

S02.9 Fracture of unspecified skull and facial bones
- **S02.91** Unspecified fracture of skull
  AHA CC: 2Q, 2020, 24
  HAC 7th characters A & B see Appendix B for HAC conditional logic
- **S02.92** Unspecified fracture of facial bones
  HAC 7th characters A & B see Appendix B for HAC conditional logic

S03 Dislocation and sprain of joints and ligaments of head

Includes:
avulsion of joint (capsule) or ligament of head
laceration of cartilage, joint (capsule) or ligament of head
sprain of cartilage, joint (capsule) or ligament of head
traumatic hemarthrosis of joint or ligament of head
traumatic rupture of joint or ligament of head
traumatic subluxation of joint or ligament of head
traumatic tear of joint or ligament of head

Code also any associated open wound

Excludes2: Strain of muscle or tendon of head (S09.1)

The appropriate 7th character is to be added to each code from category S03
A initial encounter
D subsequent encounter
S sequela

+ **S03.0 Dislocation of jaw**
Dislocation of jaw (cartilage) (meniscus)
Dislocation of mandible
Dislocation of temporomandibular (joint)
AHA CC: 4Q, 2016, 67
- X+7th S03.00 Dislocation of jaw, unspecified side
- X+7th S03.01 Dislocation of jaw, right side
- X+7th S03.02 Dislocation of jaw, left side
- X+7th S03.03 Dislocation of jaw, bilateral

X+7th **S03.1 Dislocation of septal cartilage of nose**
X+7th **S03.2 Dislocation of tooth**

+ **S03.4 Sprain of jaw**
Sprain of temporomandibular (joint) (ligament)
AHA CC: 4Q, 2016, 67
- X+7th S03.40 Sprain of jaw, unspecified side
- X+7th S03.41 Sprain of jaw, right side
- X+7th S03.42 Sprain of jaw, left side
- X+7th S03.43 Sprain of jaw, bilateral

X+7th **S03.8 Sprain of joints and ligaments of other parts of head**
X+7th **S03.9 Sprain of joints and ligaments of unspecified parts of head**

S04 Injury of cranial nerve

The selection of side should be based on the side of the body being affected

Code first any associated intracranial injury (S06.-)

Code also any associated:
open wound of head (S01.-)
skull fracture (S02.-)

The appropriate 7th character is to be added to each code from category S04
A initial encounter
D subsequent encounter
S sequela

+ **S04.0 Injury of optic nerve and pathways**
Use additional code to identify any visual field defect or blindness (H53.4-, H54.-)

+ **S04.01 Injury of optic nerve**
Injury of 2nd cranial nerve
- CC +7th S04.011 Injury of optic nerve, right eye
- CC +7th S04.012 Injury of optic nerve, left eye
- CC +7th S04.019 Injury of optic nerve, unspecified eye
Injury of optic nerve NOS

CC X+7th **S04.02 Injury of optic chiasm**

+ **S04.03 Injury of optic tract and pathways**
Injury of optic radiation
- CC +7th S04.031 Injury of optic tract and pathways, right side
- CC +7th S04.032 Injury of optic tract and pathways, left side
- CC +7th S04.039 Injury of optic tract and pathways, unspecified side
Injury of optic tract and pathways NOS

+ **S04.04 Injury of visual cortex**
- CC +7th S04.041 Injury of visual cortex, right side
- CC +7th S04.042 Injury of visual cortex, left side
- CC +7th S04.049 Injury of visual cortex, unspecified side
Injury of visual cortex NOS

+ **S04.1 Injury of oculomotor nerve**
Injury of 3rd cranial nerve
- CC X+7th S04.10 Injury of oculomotor nerve, unspecified side
- CC X+7th S04.11 Injury of oculomotor nerve, right side
- CC X+7th S04.12 Injury of oculomotor nerve, left side

+ **S04.2 Injury of trochlear nerve**
Injury of 4th cranial nerve
- CC X+7th S04.20 Injury of trochlear nerve, unspecified side
- CC X+7th S04.21 Injury of trochlear nerve, right side
- CC X+7th S04.22 Injury of trochlear nerve, left side

+ **S04.3 Injury of trigeminal nerve**
Injury of 5th cranial nerve
- CC X+7th S04.30 Injury of trigeminal nerve, unspecified side
- CC X+7th S04.31 Injury of trigeminal nerve, right side
- CC X+7th S04.32 Injury of trigeminal nerve, left side

+ **S04.4 Injury of abducent nerve**
Injury of 6th cranial nerve
- CC X+7th S04.40 Injury of abducent nerve, unspecified side
- CC X+7th S04.41 Injury of abducent nerve, right side
- CC X+7th S04.42 Injury of abducent nerve, left side

+ **S04.5 Injury of facial nerve**
Injury of 7th cranial nerve
- CC X+7th S04.50 Injury of facial nerve, unspecified side
- CC X+7th S04.51 Injury of facial nerve, right side
- CC X+7th S04.52 Injury of facial nerve, left side

+ **S04.6 Injury of acoustic nerve**
Injury of auditory nerve
Injury of 8th cranial nerve
- CC X+7th S04.60 Injury of acoustic nerve, unspecified side
- CC X+7th S04.61 Injury of acoustic nerve, right side
- CC X+7th S04.62 Injury of acoustic nerve, left side

+ **S04.7 Injury of accessory nerve**
Injury of 11th cranial nerve
- CC X+7th S04.70 Injury of accessory nerve, unspecified side
- CC X+7th S04.71 Injury of accessory nerve, right side
- CC X+7th S04.72 Injury of accessory nerve, left side

+ **S04.8 Injury of other cranial nerves**
+ **S04.81 Injury of olfactory [1st] nerve**
- CC +7th S04.811 Injury of olfactory [1st] nerve, right side
- CC +7th S04.812 Injury of olfactory [1st] nerve, left side
- CC +7th S04.819 Injury of olfactory [1st] nerve, unspecified side

+ **S04.89 Injury of other cranial nerves**
Injury of vagus [10th] nerve
- CC +7th S04.891 Injury of other cranial nerves, right side
- CC +7th S04.892 Injury of other cranial nerves, left side
- CC +7th S04.899 Injury of other cranial nerves, unspecified side

CC X+7th **S04.9 Injury of unspecified cranial nerve**

S05 Injury of eye and orbit

Includes: open wound of eye and orbit

Excludes2: 2nd cranial [optic] nerve injury (S04.0-)
3rd cranial [oculomotor] nerve injury (S04.1-)
open wound of eyelid and periocular area (S01.1-)
orbital bone fracture (S02.1-, S02.3-, S02.8-)
superficial injury of eyelid (S00.1-S00.2)

The appropriate 7th character is to be added to each code from category S05
A initial encounter
D subsequent encounter
S sequela

+ **S05.0 Injury of conjunctiva and corneal abrasion without foreign body**

Excludes1: foreign body in conjunctival sac (T15.1)
foreign body in cornea (T15.0)

- X+7th S05.00 Injury of conjunctiva and corneal abrasion without foreign body, unspecified eye
- X+7th S05.01 Injury of conjunctiva and corneal abrasion without foreign body, right eye
- X+7th S05.02 Injury of conjunctiva and corneal abrasion without foreign body, left eye

+ **S05.1 Contusion of eyeball and orbital tissues**
Traumatic hyphema

Excludes2: black eye NOS (S00.1)
contusion of eyelid and periocular area (S00.1)

- X+7th S05.10 Contusion of eyeball and orbital tissues, unspecified eye
- X+7th S05.11 Contusion of eyeball and orbital tissues, right eye
- X+7th S05.12 Contusion of eyeball and orbital tissues, left eye

+ **S05.2 Ocular laceration and rupture with prolapse or loss of intraocular tissue**
- CC X+7th S05.20 Ocular laceration and rupture with prolapse or loss of intraocular tissue, unspecified eye

CC X+7th	S05.21	Ocular laceration and rupture with prolapse or loss of intraocular tissue, right eye	
CC X+7th	S05.22	Ocular laceration and rupture with prolapse or loss of intraocular tissue, left eye	
+	S05.3	Ocular laceration without prolapse or loss of intraocular tissue	
		Laceration of eye NOS	
CC X+7th	S05.30	Ocular laceration without prolapse or loss of intraocular tissue, unspecified eye	
CC X+7th	S05.31	Ocular laceration without prolapse or loss of intraocular tissue, right eye	
CC X+7th	S05.32	Ocular laceration without prolapse or loss of intraocular tissue, left eye	
+	S05.4	Penetrating wound of orbit with or without foreign body	

Excludes2: retained (old) foreign body following penetrating wound in orbit (H05.5-)

CC X+7th	S05.40	Penetrating wound of orbit with or without foreign body, unspecified eye
CC X+7th	S05.41	Penetrating wound of orbit with or without foreign body, right eye
CC X+7th	S05.42	Penetrating wound of orbit with or without foreign body, left eye
+ S05.5		Penetrating wound with foreign body of eyeball

Excludes2: retained (old) intraocular foreign body (H44.6-, H44.7)

CC X+7th	S05.50	Penetrating wound with foreign body of unspecified eyeball
CC X+7th	S05.51	Penetrating wound with foreign body of right eyeball
CC X+7th	S05.52	Penetrating wound with foreign body of left eyeball
+ S05.6		Penetrating wound without foreign body of eyeball
		Ocular penetration NOS
X+7th	S05.60	Penetrating wound without foreign body of unspecified eyeball
X+7th	S05.61	Penetrating wound without foreign body of right eyeball
X+7th	S05.62	Penetrating wound without foreign body of left eyeball
+ S05.7		Avulsion of eye
		Traumatic enucleation
CC X+7th	S05.70	Avulsion of unspecified eye
CC X+7th	S05.71	Avulsion of right eye
CC X+7th	S05.72	Avulsion of left eye
CC + S05.8		Other injuries of eye and orbit
		Lacrimal duct injury
+	S05.8X	Other injuries of eye and orbit
+7th	S05.8X1	Other injuries of right eye and orbit
+7th	S05.8X2	Other injuries of left eye and orbit
+7th	S05.8X9	Other injuries of unspecified eye and orbit
+ S05.9		Unspecified injury of eye and orbit
		Injury of eye NOS
X+7th	S05.90	Unspecified injury of unspecified eye and orbit
CC X+7th	S05.91	Unspecified injury of right eye and orbit
CC X+7th	S05.92	Unspecified injury of left eye and orbit

S06 Intracranial injury

Includes: traumatic brain injury

Code also any associated:
  open wound of head (S01.-)
  skull fracture (S02.-)
Use additional code, if applicable, to identify mild neurocognitive disorders due to known physiological condition (F06.7-)

Excludes1: head injury NOS (S09.90)

AHA CC: 4Q, 2017, 25; 4Q, 2022, 42-45

The appropriate 7th character is to be added to each code from category S06
  A initial encounter
  D subsequent encounter
  S sequela

NOTE 7th characters D and S do not apply to codes in category S06 with 6th character 7 - death due to brain injury prior to regaining consciousness, or 8 - death due to other cause prior to regaining consciousness.

+ S06.0		Concussion
		Commotio cerebri

Excludes1: concussion with other intracranial injuries classified in category S06.1- to S06.6-, and S06.81- to S06.89-, code to specified intracranial injury

AHA CC: 4Q, 2016, 67-68

+ S06.0X		Concussion
+7th S06.0X0		Concussion without loss of consciousness
		HAC 7th character A see Appendix B for HAC conditional logic
CC +7th S06.0X1		Concussion with loss of consciousness of 30 minutes or less
		Concussion with brief loss of consciousness
		HAC 7th character A see Appendix B for HAC conditional logic
CC +7th S06.0XA		Concussion with loss of consciousness status unknown
		Concussion NOS
		HAC 7th character A see Appendix B for HAC conditional logic
CC +7th S06.0X9		Concussion with loss of consciousness of unspecified duration
		HAC 7th character A see Appendix B for HAC conditional logic
+ S06.1		Traumatic cerebral edema
		Diffuse traumatic cerebral edema
		Focal traumatic cerebral edema
+ S06.1X		Traumatic cerebral edema
MCC +7th S06.1X0		Traumatic cerebral edema without loss of consciousness
		HAC 7th character A see Appendix B for HAC conditional logic
		AHA CC: 1Q, 2015, 3-21
MCC +7th S06.1X1		Traumatic cerebral edema with loss of consciousness of 30 minutes or less
		Traumatic cerebral edema with brief loss of consciousness
		HAC 7th character A see Appendix B for HAC conditional logic
MCC +7th S06.1X2		Traumatic cerebral edema with loss of consciousness of 31 minutes to 59 minutes
		HAC 7th character A see Appendix B for HAC conditional logic
MCC +7th S06.1X3		Traumatic cerebral edema with loss of consciousness of 1 hour to 5 hours 59 minutes
		HAC 7th character A see Appendix B for HAC conditional logic
MCC +7th S06.1X4		Traumatic cerebral edema with loss of consciousness of 6 hours to 24 hours
		HAC 7th character A see Appendix B for HAC conditional logic
MCC +7th S06.1X5		Traumatic cerebral edema with loss of consciousness greater than 24 hours with return to pre-existing conscious level
		HAC 7th character A see Appendix B for HAC conditional logic
MCC +7th S06.1X6		Traumatic cerebral edema with loss of consciousness greater than 24 hours without return to pre-existing conscious level with patient surviving
		HAC 7th character A see Appendix B for HAC conditional logic
MCC +7th S06.1X7		Traumatic cerebral edema with loss of consciousness of any duration with death due to brain injury prior to regaining consciousness
		HAC 7th character A see Appendix B for HAC conditional logic
MCC +7th S06.1X8		Traumatic cerebral edema with loss of consciousness of any duration with death due to other cause prior to regaining consciousness
		HAC 7th character A see Appendix B for HAC conditional logic
MCC +7th S06.1XA		Traumatic cerebral edema with loss of consciousness status unknown
		Traumatic cerebral edema NOS
		HAC 7th character A see Appendix B for HAC conditional logic
MCC +7th S06.1X9		Traumatic cerebral edema with loss of consciousness of unspecified duration
		HAC 7th character A see Appendix B for HAC conditional logic

CC + S06.2 Diffuse traumatic brain injury
Diffuse axonal brain injury
Use additional code, if applicable, for traumatic brain compression or herniation (S06.A-)
Excludes1: traumatic diffuse cerebral edema (S06.1X-)

+ S06.2X Diffuse traumatic brain injury

+7th S06.2X0 Diffuse traumatic brain injury without loss of consciousness
HAC 7th character A see Appendix B for HAC conditional logic

+7th S06.2X1 Diffuse traumatic brain injury with loss of consciousness of 30 minutes or less
Diffuse traumatic brain injury with brief loss of consciousness
HAC 7th character A see Appendix B for HAC conditional logic

+7th S06.2X2 Diffuse traumatic brain injury with loss of consciousness of 31 minutes to 59 minutes
HAC 7th character A see Appendix B for HAC conditional logic

+7th S06.2X3 Diffuse traumatic brain injury with loss of consciousness of 1 hour to 5 hours 59 minutes
HAC 7th character A see Appendix B for HAC conditional logic

+7th S06.2X4 Diffuse traumatic brain injury with loss of consciousness of 6 hours to 24 hours
HAC 7th character A see Appendix B for HAC conditional logic

+7th S06.2X5 Diffuse traumatic brain injury with loss of consciousness greater than 24 hours with return to pre-existing conscious levels
HAC 7th character A see Appendix B for HAC conditional logic

MCC +7th S06.2X6 Diffuse traumatic brain injury with loss of consciousness greater than 24 hours without return to pre-existing conscious level with patient surviving
HAC 7th character A see Appendix B for HAC conditional logic

MCC +7th S06.2X7 Diffuse traumatic brain injury with loss of consciousness of any duration with death due to brain injury prior to regaining consciousness
HAC 7th character A see Appendix B for HAC conditional logic

MCC +7th S06.2X8 Diffuse traumatic brain injury with loss of consciousness of any duration with death due to other cause prior to regaining consciousness
HAC 7th character A see Appendix B for HAC conditional logic

CC +7th S06.2XA Diffuse traumatic brain injury with loss of consciousness status unknown
Diffuse traumatic brain injury NOS
HAC 7th character A see Appendix B for HAC conditional logic

+7th S06.2X9 Diffuse traumatic brain injury with loss of consciousness of unspecified duration
HAC 7th character A see Appendix B for HAC conditional logic

+ S06.3 Focal traumatic brain injury
Use additional code, if applicable, for traumatic brain compression or herniation (S06.A-)
Excludes2: any condition classifiable to S06.4-S06.6 focal cerebral edema (S06.1)

+ S06.30 Unspecified focal traumatic brain injury

+7th S06.300 Unspecified focal traumatic brain injury without loss of consciousness

CC +7th S06.301 Unspecified focal traumatic brain injury with loss of consciousness of 30 minutes or less
Unspecified focal traumatic brain injury with brief loss of consciousness
HAC 7th character A see Appendix B for HAC conditional logic

CC +7th S06.302 Unspecified focal traumatic brain injury with loss of consciousness of 31 minutes to 59 minutes
HAC 7th character A see Appendix B for HAC conditional logic

CC +7th S06.303 Unspecified focal traumatic brain injury with loss of consciousness of 1 hour to 5 hours 59 minutes
HAC 7th character A see Appendix B for HAC conditional logic

CC +7th S06.304 Unspecified focal traumatic brain injury with loss of consciousness of 6 hours to 24 hours
HAC 7th character A see Appendix B for HAC conditional logic

CC +7th S06.305 Unspecified focal traumatic brain injury with loss of consciousness greater than 24 hours with return to pre-existing conscious level
HAC 7th character A see Appendix B for HAC conditional logic

MCC +7th S06.306 Unspecified focal traumatic brain injury with loss of consciousness greater than 24 hours without return to pre-existing conscious level with patient surviving
HAC 7th character A see Appendix B for HAC conditional logic

MCC +7th S06.307 Unspecified focal traumatic brain injury with loss of consciousness of any duration with death due to brain injury prior to regaining consciousness
HAC 7th character A see Appendix B for HAC conditional logic

MCC +7th S06.308 Unspecified focal traumatic brain injury with loss of consciousness of any duration with death due to other cause prior to regaining consciousness
HAC 7th character A see Appendix B for HAC conditional logic

CC +7th S06.30A Unspecified focal traumatic brain injury with loss of consciousness status unknown
Unspecified focal traumatic brain injury NOS
HAC 7th character A see Appendix B for HAC conditional logic

CC +7th S06.309 Unspecified focal traumatic brain injury with loss of consciousness of unspecified duration
HAC 7th character A see Appendix B for HAC conditional logic

+ S06.31 Contusion and laceration of right cerebrum

MCC +7th S06.310 Contusion and laceration of right cerebrum without loss of consciousness
HAC 7th character A see Appendix B for HAC conditional logic

MCC +7th S06.311 Contusion and laceration of right cerebrum with loss of consciousness of 30 minutes or less
Contusion and laceration of right cerebrum with brief loss of consciousness
HAC 7th character A see Appendix B for HAC conditional logic

MCC +7th S06.312 Contusion and laceration of right cerebrum with loss of consciousness of 31 minutes to 59 minutes
HAC 7th character A see Appendix B for HAC conditional logic

MCC +7th S06.313 Contusion and laceration of right cerebrum with loss of consciousness of 1 hour to 5 hours 59 minutes
HAC 7th character A see Appendix B for HAC conditional logic

MCC +7th S06.314 Contusion and laceration of right cerebrum with loss of consciousness of 6 hours to 24 hours
HAC 7th character A see Appendix B for HAC conditional logic

MCC +7th S06.315 Contusion and laceration of right cerebrum with loss of consciousness greater than 24 hours with return to pre-existing conscious level
HAC 7th character A see Appendix B for HAC conditional logic

MCC +7th S06.316 Contusion and laceration of right cerebrum with loss of consciousness greater than 24 hours without return to pre-existing conscious level with patient surviving
HAC 7th character A see Appendix B for HAC conditional logic

MCC +7th S06.317 Contusion and laceration of right cerebrum with loss of consciousness of any duration with death due to brain injury prior to regaining consciousness
HAC 7th character A see Appendix B for HAC conditional logic

MCC +7th S06.318 Contusion and laceration of right cerebrum with loss of consciousness of any duration with death due to other cause prior to regaining consciousness
> **HAC** 7th character A see Appendix B for HAC conditional logic

MCC +7th S06.31A Contusion and laceration of right cerebrum with loss of consciousness status unknown
> Contusion and laceration of right cerebrum NOS
> **HAC** 7th character A see Appendix B for HAC conditional logic

MCC +7th S06.319 Contusion and laceration of right cerebrum with loss of consciousness of unspecified duration
> **HAC** 7th character A see Appendix B for HAC conditional logic

+ S06.32 Contusion and laceration of left cerebrum

MCC +7th S06.320 Contusion and laceration of left cerebrum without loss of consciousness
> **HAC** 7th character A see Appendix B for HAC conditional logic

MCC +7th S06.321 Contusion and laceration of left cerebrum with loss of consciousness of 30 minutes or less
> Contusion and laceration of left cerebrum with brief loss of consciousness
> **HAC** 7th character A see Appendix B for HAC conditional logic

MCC +7th S06.322 Contusion and laceration of left cerebrum with loss of consciousness of 31 minutes to 59 minutes
> **HAC** 7th character A see Appendix B for HAC conditional logic

MCC +7th S06.323 Contusion and laceration of left cerebrum with loss of consciousness of 1 hour to 5 hours 59 minutes
> **HAC** 7th character A see Appendix B for HAC conditional logic

MCC +7th S06.324 Contusion and laceration of left cerebrum with loss of consciousness of 6 hours to 24 hours
> **HAC** 7th character A see Appendix B for HAC conditional logic

MCC +7th S06.325 Contusion and laceration of left cerebrum with loss of consciousness greater than 24 hours with return to pre-existing conscious level
> **HAC** 7th character A see Appendix B for HAC conditional logic

MCC +7th S06.326 Contusion and laceration of left cerebrum with loss of consciousness greater than 24 hours without return to pre-existing conscious level with patient surviving
> **HAC** 7th character A see Appendix B for HAC conditional logic

MCC +7th S06.327 Contusion and laceration of left cerebrum with loss of consciousness of any duration with death due to brain injury prior to regaining consciousness
> **HAC** 7th character A see Appendix B for HAC conditional logic

MCC +7th S06.328 Contusion and laceration of left cerebrum with loss of consciousness of any duration with death due to other cause prior to regaining consciousness
> **HAC** 7th character A see Appendix B for HAC conditional logic

MCC +7th S06.32A Contusion and laceration of left cerebrum with loss of consciousness status unknown
> Contusion and laceration of left cerebrum NOS
> **HAC** 7th character A see Appendix B for HAC conditional logic

MCC +7th S06.329 Contusion and laceration of left cerebrum with loss of consciousness of unspecified duration
> **HAC** 7th character A see Appendix B for HAC conditional logic

+ S06.33 Contusion and laceration of cerebrum, unspecified

MCC +7th S06.330 Contusion and laceration of cerebrum, unspecified, without loss of consciousness
> **HAC** 7th character A see Appendix B for HAC conditional logic

MCC +7th S06.331 Contusion and laceration of cerebrum, unspecified, with loss of consciousness of 30 minutes or less
> Contusion and laceration of cerebrum, unspecified, with brief loss of consciousness
> **HAC** 7th character A see Appendix B for HAC conditional logic

MCC +7th S06.332 Contusion and laceration of cerebrum, unspecified, with loss of consciousness of 31 minutes to 59 minutes
> **HAC** 7th character A see Appendix B for HAC conditional logic

MCC +7th S06.333 Contusion and laceration of cerebrum, unspecified, with loss of consciousness of 1 hour to 5 hours 59 minutes
> **HAC** 7th character A see Appendix B for HAC conditional logic

MCC +7th S06.334 Contusion and laceration of cerebrum, unspecified, with loss of consciousness of 6 hours to 24 hours
> **HAC** 7th character A see Appendix B for HAC conditional logic

MCC +7th S06.335 Contusion and laceration of cerebrum, unspecified, with loss of consciousness greater than 24 hours with return to pre-existing conscious level
> **HAC** 7th character A see Appendix B for HAC conditional logic

MCC +7th S06.336 Contusion and laceration of cerebrum, unspecified, with loss of consciousness greater than 24 hours without return to pre-existing conscious level with patient surviving
> **HAC** 7th character A see Appendix B for HAC conditional logic

MCC +7th S06.337 Contusion and laceration of cerebrum, unspecified, with loss of consciousness of any duration with death due to brain injury prior to regaining consciousness
> **HAC** 7th character A see Appendix B for HAC conditional logic

MCC +7th S06.338 Contusion and laceration of cerebrum, unspecified, with loss of consciousness of any duration with death due to other cause prior to regaining consciousness
> **HAC** 7th character A see Appendix B for HAC conditional logic

MCC +7th S06.33A Contusion and laceration of cerebrum, unspecified, with loss of consciousness status unknown
> Contusion and laceration of cerebrum NOS
> **HAC** 7th character A see Appendix B for HAC conditional logic

MCC +7th S06.339 Contusion and laceration of cerebrum, unspecified, with loss of consciousness of unspecified duration
> **HAC** 7th character A see Appendix B for HAC conditional logic

+ S06.34 Traumatic hemorrhage of right cerebrum
> Traumatic intracerebral hemorrhage and hematoma of right cerebrum

MCC +7th S06.340 Traumatic hemorrhage of right cerebrum without loss of consciousness
> **HAC** 7th character A see Appendix B for HAC conditional logic
> *AHA CC: 1Q, 2015, 3-21*

MCC +7th S06.341 Traumatic hemorrhage of right cerebrum with loss of consciousness of 30 minutes or less
> Traumatic hemorrhage of right cerebrum with loss of consciousness
> **HAC** 7th character A see Appendix B for HAC conditional logic

MCC +7th S06.342 Traumatic hemorrhage of right cerebrum with loss of consciousness of 31 minutes to 59 minutes
> **HAC** 7th character A see Appendix B for HAC conditional logic

MCC +7th S06.343 Traumatic hemorrhage of right cerebrum with loss of consciousness of 1 hours to 5 hours 59 minutes
   HAC 7th character A see Appendix B for HAC conditional logic

MCC +7th S06.344 Traumatic hemorrhage of right cerebrum with loss of consciousness of 6 hours to 24 hours
   HAC 7th character A see Appendix B for HAC conditional logic

MCC +7th S06.345 Traumatic hemorrhage of right cerebrum with loss of consciousness greater than 24 hours with return to pre-existing conscious level
   HAC 7th character A see Appendix B for HAC conditional logic

MCC +7th S06.346 Traumatic hemorrhage of right cerebrum with loss of consciousness greater than 24 hours without return to pre-existing conscious level with patient surviving
   HAC 7th character A see Appendix B for HAC conditional logic

MCC +7th S06.347 Traumatic hemorrhage of right cerebrum with loss of consciousness of any duration with death due to brain injury prior to regaining consciousness
   HAC 7th character A see Appendix B for HAC conditional logic

MCC +7th S06.348 Traumatic hemorrhage of right cerebrum with loss of consciousness of any duration with death due to other cause prior to regaining consciousness
   HAC 7th character A see Appendix B for HAC conditional logic

MCC +7th S06.34A Traumatic hemorrhage of right cerebrum with loss of consciousness status unknown
   Traumatic hemorrhage of right cerebrum NOS
   HAC 7th character A see Appendix B for HAC conditional logic

MCC +7th S06.349 Traumatic hemorrhage of right cerebrum with loss of consciousness of unspecified duration
   HAC 7th character A see Appendix B for HAC conditional logic

+ S06.35 Traumatic hemorrhage of left cerebrum
   Traumatic intracerebral hemorrhage and hematoma of left cerebrum

MCC +7th S06.350 Traumatic hemorrhage of left cerebrum without loss of consciousness
   HAC 7th character A see Appendix B for HAC conditional logic

MCC +7th S06.351 Traumatic hemorrhage of left cerebrum with loss of consciousness of 30 minutes or less
   Traumatic hemorrhage of left cerebrum with brief loss of consciousness
   HAC 7th character A see Appendix B for HAC conditional logic

MCC +7th S06.352 Traumatic hemorrhage of left cerebrum with loss of consciousness of 31 minutes to 59 minutes
   HAC 7th character A see Appendix B for HAC conditional logic

MCC +7th S06.353 Traumatic hemorrhage of left cerebrum with loss of consciousness of 1 hours to 5 hours 59 minutes
   HAC 7th character A see Appendix B for HAC conditional logic

MCC +7th S06.354 Traumatic hemorrhage of left cerebrum with loss of consciousness of 6 hours to 24 hours
   HAC 7th character A see Appendix B for HAC conditional logic

MCC +7th S06.355 Traumatic hemorrhage of left cerebrum with loss of consciousness greater than 24 hours with return to pre-existing conscious level
   HAC 7th character A see Appendix B for HAC conditional logic

MCC +7th S06.356 Traumatic hemorrhage of left cerebrum with loss of consciousness greater than 24 hours without return to pre-existing conscious level with patient surviving
   HAC 7th character A see Appendix B for HAC conditional logic

MCC +7th S06.357 Traumatic hemorrhage of left cerebrum with loss of consciousness of≈any duration with death due to brain injury prior to regaining consciousness
   HAC 7th character A see Appendix B for HAC conditional logic

MCC +7th S06.358 Traumatic hemorrhage of left cerebrum with loss of consciousness of any duration with death due to other cause prior to regaining consciousness
   HAC 7th character A see Appendix B for HAC conditional logic

MCC +7th S06.35A Traumatic hemorrhage of left cerebrum with loss of consciousness status unknown
   Traumatic hemorrhage of left cerebrum NOS
   HAC 7th character A see Appendix B for HAC conditional logic

MCC +7th S06.359 Traumatic hemorrhage of left cerebrum with loss of consciousness of unspecified duration
   HAC 7th character A see Appendix B for HAC conditional logic

+ S06.36 Traumatic hemorrhage of cerebrum, unspecified
   Traumatic intracerebral hemorrhage and hematoma, unspecified

MCC +7th S06.360 Traumatic hemorrhage of cerebrum, unspecified, without loss of consciousness
   HAC 7th character A see Appendix B for HAC conditional logic

MCC +7th S06.361 Traumatic hemorrhage of cerebrum, unspecified, with loss of consciousness of 30 minutes or less
   Traumatic hemorrhage of cerebrum, unspecified, with brief loss of consciousness
   HAC 7th character A see Appendix B for HAC conditional logic

MCC +7th S06.362 Traumatic hemorrhage of cerebrum, unspecified, with loss of consciousness of 31 minutes to 59 minutes
   HAC 7th character A see Appendix B for HAC conditional logic

MCC +7th S06.363 Traumatic hemorrhage of cerebrum, unspecified, with loss of consciousness of 1 hours to 5 hours 59 minutes
   HAC 7th character A see Appendix B for HAC conditional logic

MCC +7th S06.364 Traumatic hemorrhage of cerebrum, unspecified, with loss of consciousness of 6 hours to 24 hours
   HAC 7th character A see Appendix B for HAC conditional logic

MCC +7th S06.365 Traumatic hemorrhage of cerebrum, unspecified, with loss of consciousness greater than 24 hours with return to pre-existing conscious level
   HAC 7th character A see Appendix B for HAC conditional logic

MCC +7th S06.366 Traumatic hemorrhage of cerebrum, unspecified, with loss of consciousness greater than 24 hours without return to pre-existing conscious level with patient surviving
   HAC 7th character A see Appendix B for HAC conditional logic

MCC +7th S06.367 Traumatic hemorrhage of cerebrum, unspecified, with loss of consciousness of any duration with death due to brain injury prior to regaining consciousness
   HAC 7th character A see Appendix B for HAC conditional logic

MCC +7th S06.368 Traumatic hemorrhage of cerebrum, unspecified, with loss of consciousness of any duration with death due to other cause prior to regaining consciousness
   HAC 7th character A see Appendix B for HAC conditional logic

MCC +7th S06.36A Traumatic hemorrhage of cerebrum, unspecified, with loss of consciousness status unknown
  Traumatic hemorrhage of cerebrum NOS
  HAC 7th character A see Appendix B for HAC conditional logic

MCC +7th S06.369 Traumatic hemorrhage of cerebrum, unspecified, with loss of consciousness of unspecified duration
  HAC 7th character A see Appendix B for HAC conditional logic

+ S06.37 Contusion, laceration, and hemorrhage of cerebellum

MCC +7th S06.370 Contusion, laceration, and hemorrhage of cerebellum without loss of consciousness
  HAC 7th character A see Appendix B for HAC conditional logic

CC +7th S06.371 Contusion, laceration, and hemorrhage of cerebellum with loss of consciousness of 30 minutes or less
  Contusion, laceration, and hemorrhage of cerebellum with brief loss of consciousness
  HAC 7th character A see Appendix B for HAC conditional logic

CC +7th S06.372 Contusion, laceration, and hemorrhage of cerebellum with loss of consciousness of 31 minutes to 59 minutes
  HAC 7th character A see Appendix B for HAC conditional logic

CC +7th S06.373 Contusion, laceration, and hemorrhage of cerebellum with loss of consciousness of 1 hour to 5 hours 59 minutes
  HAC 7th character A see Appendix B for HAC conditional logic

CC +7th S06.374 Contusion, laceration, and hemorrhage of cerebellum with loss of consciousness of 6 hours to 24 hours
  HAC 7th character A see Appendix B for HAC conditional logic

CC +7th S06.375 Contusion, laceration, and hemorrhage of cerebellum with loss of consciousness greater than 24 hours with return to pre-existing conscious level
  HAC 7th character A see Appendix B for HAC conditional logic

MCC +7th S06.376 Contusion, laceration, and hemorrhage of cerebellum with loss of consciousness greater than 24 hours without return to pre-existing conscious level with patient surviving
  HAC 7th character A see Appendix B for HAC conditional logic

MCC +7th S06.377 Contusion, laceration, and hemorrhage of cerebellum with loss of consciousness of any duration with death due to brain injury prior to regaining consciousness
  HAC 7th character A see Appendix B for HAC conditional logic

MCC +7th S06.378 Contusion, laceration, and hemorrhage of cerebellum with loss of consciousness of any duration with death due to other cause prior to regaining consciousness
  HAC 7th character A see Appendix B for HAC conditional logic

MCC +7th S06.37A Contusion, laceration, and hemorrhage of cerebellum with loss of consciousness status unknown
  Contusion, laceration, and hemorrhage of cerebellum NOS
  HAC 7th character A see Appendix B for HAC conditional logic

CC +7th S06.379 Contusion, laceration, and hemorrhage of cerebellum with loss of consciousness of unspecified duration
  HAC 7th character A see Appendix B for HAC conditional logic

+ S06.38 Contusion, laceration, and hemorrhage of brainstem

MCC +7th S06.380 Contusion, laceration, and hemorrhage of brainstem without loss of consciousness
  HAC 7th character A see Appendix B for HAC conditional logic

CC +7th S06.381 Contusion, laceration, and hemorrhage of brainstem with loss of consciousness of 30 minutes or less
  Contusion, laceration, and hemorrhage of brainstem with brief loss of consciousness
  HAC 7th character A see Appendix B for HAC conditional logic

CC +7th S06.382 Contusion, laceration, and hemorrhage of brainstem with loss of consciousness of 31 minutes to 59 minutes
  HAC 7th character A see Appendix B for HAC conditional logic

CC +7th S06.383 Contusion, laceration, and hemorrhage of brainstem with loss of consciousness of 1 hour to 5 hours 59 minutes
  HAC 7th character A see Appendix B for HAC conditional logic

CC +7th S06.384 Contusion, laceration, and hemorrhage of brainstem with loss of consciousness of 6 hours to 24 hours
  HAC 7th character A see Appendix B for HAC conditional logic

CC +7th S06.385 Contusion, laceration, and hemorrhage of brainstem with loss of consciousness greater than 24 hours with return to pre-existing conscious level
  HAC 7th character A see Appendix B for HAC conditional logic

MCC +7th S06.386 Contusion, laceration, and hemorrhage of brainstem with loss of consciousness greater than 24 hours without return to pre-existing conscious level with patient surviving
  HAC 7th character A see Appendix B for HAC conditional logic

MCC +7th S06.387 Contusion, laceration, and hemorrhage of brainstem with loss of consciousness of any duration with death due to brain injury prior to regaining consciousness
  HAC 7th character A see Appendix B for HAC conditional logic

MCC +7th S06.388 Contusion, laceration, and hemorrhage of brainstem with loss of consciousness of any duration with death due to other cause prior to regaining consciousness
  HAC 7th character A see Appendix B for HAC conditional logic

MCC +7th S06.38A Contusion, laceration, and hemorrhage of brainstem with loss of consciousness status unknown
  Contusion, laceration, and hemorrhage of brainstem NOS
  HAC 7th character A see Appendix B for HAC conditional logic

CC +7th S06.389 Contusion, laceration, and hemorrhage of brainstem with loss of consciousness of unspecified duration
  HAC 7th character A see Appendix B for HAC conditional logic

+ S06.4 Epidural hemorrhage
  Extradural hemorrhage NOS
  Extradural hemorrhage (traumatic)

+ S06.4X Epidural hemorrhage

MCC +7th S06.4X0 Epidural hemorrhage without loss of consciousness
  HAC 7th character A see Appendix B for HAC conditional logic

MCC +7th S06.4X1 Epidural hemorrhage with loss of consciousness of 30 minutes or less
  Epidural hemorrhage with brief loss of consciousness
  HAC 7th character A see Appendix B for HAC conditional logic

MCC +7th S06.4X2 Epidural hemorrhage with loss of consciousness of 31 minutes to 59 minutes
  HAC 7th character A see Appendix B for HAC conditional logic

MCC +7th S06.4X3 Epidural hemorrhage with loss of consciousness of 1 hour to 5 hours 59 minutes
  HAC 7th character A see Appendix B for HAC conditional logic

MCC +7th S06.4X4 Epidural hemorrhage with loss of consciousness of 6 hours to 24 hours
  HAC 7th character A see Appendix B for HAC conditional logic

MCC +7th S06.4X5 Epidural hemorrhage with loss of consciousness greater than 24 hours with return to pre-existing conscious level
  HAC 7th character A see Appendix B for HAC conditional logic

MCC +7th S06.4X6 Epidural hemorrhage with loss of consciousness greater than 24 hours without return to pre-existing conscious level with patient surviving
  HAC 7th character A see Appendix B for HAC conditional logic

MCC +7th S06.4X7 Epidural hemorrhage with loss of consciousness of any duration with death due to brain injury prior to regaining consciousness
  HAC 7th character A see Appendix B for HAC conditional logic

MCC +7th S06.4X8 Epidural hemorrhage with loss of consciousness of any duration with death due to other causes prior to regaining consciousness
  HAC 7th character A see Appendix B for HAC conditional logic

MCC +7th S06.4XA Epidural hemorrhage with loss of consciousness status unknown
  Epidural hemorrhage NOS
  HAC 7th character A see Appendix B for HAC conditional logic

MCC +7th S06.4X9 Epidural hemorrhage with loss of consciousness of unspecified duration
  HAC 7th character A see Appendix B for HAC conditional logic

+ **S06.5** Traumatic subdural hemorrhage
  Use additional code, if applicable, for traumatic brain compression or herniation (S06.A-)
+ **S06.5X** Traumatic subdural hemorrhage

MCC +7th S06.5X0 Traumatic subdural hemorrhage without loss of consciousness
  HAC 7th character A see Appendix B for HAC conditional logic
  AHA CC: 3Q, 2015, 37; 2Q, 2018, 13; 1Q, 2021, 4-5

MCC +7th S06.5X1 Traumatic subdural hemorrhage with loss of consciousness of 30 minutes or less
  Traumatic subdural hemorrhage with brief loss of consciousness
  HAC 7th character A see Appendix B for HAC conditional logic

MCC +7th S06.5X2 Traumatic subdural hemorrhage with loss of consciousness of 31 minutes to 59 minutes
  HAC 7th character A see Appendix B for HAC conditional logic

MCC +7th S06.5X3 Traumatic subdural hemorrhage with loss of consciousness of 1 hour to 5 hours 59 minutes
  HAC 7th character A see Appendix B for HAC conditional logic

MCC +7th S06.5X4 Traumatic subdural hemorrhage with loss of consciousness of 6 hours to 24 hours
  HAC 7th character A see Appendix B for HAC conditional logic

MCC +7th S06.5X5 Traumatic subdural hemorrhage with loss of consciousness greater than 24 hours with return to pre-existing conscious level
  HAC 7th character A see Appendix B for HAC conditional logic

MCC +7th S06.5X6 Traumatic subdural hemorrhage with loss of consciousness greater than 24 hours without return to pre-existing conscious level with patient surviving
  AHA CC: 2Q, 2021, 5
  HAC 7th character A see Appendix B for HAC conditional logic

MCC +7th S06.5X7 Traumatic subdural hemorrhage with loss of consciousness of any duration with death due to brain injury before regaining consciousness
  HAC 7th character A see Appendix B for HAC conditional logic

MCC +7th S06.5X8 Traumatic subdural hemorrhage with loss of consciousness of any duration with death due to other cause before regaining consciousness
  HAC 7th character A see Appendix B for HAC conditional logic

MCC +7th S06.5XA Traumatic subdural hemorrhage with loss of consciousness status unknown
  Traumatic subdural hemorrhage NOS
  HAC 7th character A see Appendix B for HAC conditional logic
  AHA CC: 4Q, 2022, 44-45

MCC +7th S06.5X9 Traumatic subdural hemorrhage with loss of consciousness of unspecified duration
  HAC 7th character A see Appendix B for HAC conditional logic

+ **S06.6** Traumatic subarachnoid hemorrhage
  Use additional code, if applicable, for traumatic brain compression or herniation (S06.A-)
+ **S06.6X** Traumatic subarachnoid hemorrhage

MCC +7th S06.6X0 Traumatic subarachnoid hemorrhage without loss of consciousness
  HAC 7th character A see Appendix B for HAC conditional logic
  AHA CC: 3Q, 2015, 37

MCC +7th S06.6X1 Traumatic subarachnoid hemorrhage with loss of consciousness of 30 minutes or less
  Traumatic subarachnoid hemorrhage with brief loss of consciousness
  HAC 7th character A see Appendix B for HAC conditional logic

MCC +7th S06.6X2 Traumatic subarachnoid hemorrhage with loss of consciousness of 31 minutes to 59 minutes
  HAC 7th character A see Appendix B for HAC conditional logic

MCC +7th S06.6X3 Traumatic subarachnoid hemorrhage with loss of consciousness of 1 hour to 5 hours 59 minutes
  HAC 7th character A see Appendix B for HAC conditional logic

MCC +7th S06.6X4 Traumatic subarachnoid hemorrhage with loss of consciousness of 6 hours to 24 hours
  HAC 7th character A see Appendix B for HAC conditional logic

MCC +7th S06.6X5 Traumatic subarachnoid hemorrhage with loss of consciousness greater than 24 hours with return to pre-existing conscious level
  HAC 7th character A see Appendix B for HAC conditional logic

MCC +7th S06.6X6 Traumatic subarachnoid hemorrhage with loss of consciousness greater than 24 hours without return to pre-existing conscious level with patient surviving
  AHA CC: 2Q, 2021, 5
  HAC 7th character A see Appendix B for HAC conditional logic

MCC +7th S06.6X7 Traumatic subarachnoid hemorrhage with loss of consciousness of any duration with death due to brain injury prior to regaining consciousness
  HAC 7th character A see Appendix B for HAC conditional logic

MCC +7th S06.6X8 Traumatic subarachnoid hemorrhage with loss of consciousness of any duration with death due to other cause prior to regaining consciousness
  HAC 7th character A see Appendix B for HAC conditional logic

MCC +7th S06.6XA Traumatic subarachnoid hemorrhage with loss of consciousness status unknown
  Traumatic subarachnoid hemorrhage NOS
  HAC 7th character A see Appendix B for HAC conditional logic
  AHA CC: 4Q, 2022, 44-45

MCC +7th S06.6X9 Traumatic subarachnoid hemorrhage with loss of consciousness of unspecified duration
  HAC 7th character A see Appendix B for HAC conditional logic

- **+ S06.8 Other specified intracranial injuries**
  - **+ S06.81 Injury of right internal carotid artery, intracranial portion, not elsewhere classified**
    - **+7th S06.810** Injury of right internal carotid artery, intracranial portion, not elsewhere classified without loss of consciousness
    - **CC +7th S06.811** Injury of right internal carotid artery, intracranial portion, not elsewhere classified with loss of consciousness of 30 minutes or less
      - Injury of right internal carotid artery, intracranial portion, not elsewhere classified with brief loss of consciousness
      - **HAC** 7th character A see Appendix B for HAC conditional logic
    - **CC +7th S06.812** Injury of right internal carotid artery, intracranial portion, not elsewhere classified with loss of consciousness of 31 minutes to 59 minutes
      - **HAC** 7th character A see Appendix B for HAC conditional logic
    - **CC +7th S06.813** Injury of right internal carotid artery, intracranial portion, not elsewhere classified with loss of consciousness of 1 hour to 5 hours 59 minutes
      - **HAC** 7th character A see Appendix B for HAC conditional logic
    - **CC +7th S06.814** Injury of right internal carotid artery, intracranial portion, not elsewhere classified with loss of consciousness of 6 hours to 24 hours
      - **HAC** 7th character A see Appendix B for HAC conditional logic
    - **CC +7th S06.815** Injury of right internal carotid artery, intracranial portion, not elsewhere classified with loss of consciousness greater than 24 hours with return to pre-existing conscious level
      - **HAC** 7th character A see Appendix B for HAC conditional logic
    - **MCC +7th S06.816** Injury of right internal carotid artery, intracranial portion, not elsewhere classified with loss of consciousness greater than 24 hours without return to pre-existing conscious level with patient surviving
      - **HAC** 7th character A see Appendix B for HAC conditional logic
    - **MCC +7th S06.817** Injury of right internal carotid artery, intracranial portion, not elsewhere classified with loss of consciousness of any duration with death due to brain injury prior to regaining consciousness
      - **HAC** 7th character A see Appendix B for HAC conditional logic
    - **MCC +7th S06.818** Injury of right internal carotid artery, intracranial portion, not elsewhere classified with loss of consciousness of any duration with death due to other cause prior to regaining consciousness
      - **HAC** 7th character A see Appendix B for HAC conditional logic
    - **CC +7th S06.81A** Injury of right internal carotid artery, intracranial portion, not elsewhere classified with loss of consciousness status unknown
      - Injury of right internal carotid artery, intracranial portion, not elsewhere classified NOS
      - **HAC** 7th character A see Appendix B for HAC conditional logic
    - **CC +7th S06.819** Injury of right internal carotid artery, intracranial portion, not elsewhere classified with loss of consciousness of unspecified duration
      - **HAC** 7th character A see Appendix B for HAC conditional logic
  - **+ S06.82 Injury of left internal carotid artery, intracranial portion, not elsewhere classified**
    - **+7th S06.820** Injury of left internal carotid artery, intracranial portion, not elsewhere classified without loss of consciousness
    - **CC +7th S06.821** Injury of left internal carotid artery, intracranial portion, not elsewhere classified with loss of consciousness of 30 minutes or less
      - Injury of left internal carotid artery, intracranial portion, not elsewhere classified with brief loss of consciousness
      - **HAC** 7th character A see Appendix B for HAC conditional logic
    - **CC +7th S06.822** Injury of left internal carotid artery, intracranial portion, not elsewhere classified with loss of consciousness of 31 minutes to 59 minutes
      - **HAC** 7th character A see Appendix B for HAC conditional logic
    - **CC +7th S06.823** Injury of left internal carotid artery, intracranial portion, not elsewhere classified with loss of consciousness of 1 hour to 5 hours 59 minutes
      - **HAC** 7th character A see Appendix B for HAC conditional logic
    - **CC +7th S06.824** Injury of left internal carotid artery, intracranial portion, not elsewhere classified with loss of consciousness of 6 hours to 24 hours
      - **HAC** 7th character A see Appendix B for HAC conditional logic
    - **CC +7th S06.825** Injury of left internal carotid artery, intracranial portion, not elsewhere classified with loss of consciousness greater than 24 hours with return to pre-existing conscious level
      - **HAC** 7th character A see Appendix B for HAC conditional logic
    - **MCC +7th S06.826** Injury of left internal carotid artery, intracranial portion, not elsewhere classified with loss of consciousness greater than 24 hours without return to pre-existing conscious level with patient surviving
      - **HAC** 7th character A see Appendix B for HAC conditional logic
    - **MCC +7th S06.827** Injury of left internal carotid artery, intracranial portion, not elsewhere classified with loss of consciousness of any duration with death due to brain injury prior to regaining consciousness
      - **HAC** 7th character A see Appendix B for HAC conditional logic
    - **MCC +7th S06.828** Injury of left internal carotid artery, intracranial portion, not elsewhere classified with loss of consciousness of any duration with death due to other cause prior to regaining consciousness
      - **HAC** 7th character A see Appendix B for HAC conditional logic
    - **CC +7th S06.82A** Injury of left internal carotid artery, intracranial portion, not elsewhere classified with loss of consciousness status unknown
      - Injury of left internal carotid artery, intracranial portion, not elsewhere classified NOS
      - **HAC** 7th character A see Appendix B for HAC conditional logic
    - **CC +7th S06.829** Injury of left internal carotid artery, intracranial portion, not elsewhere classified with loss of consciousness of unspecified duration
      - **HAC** 7th character A see Appendix B for HAC conditional logic

+ S06.8A Primary blast injury of brain, not elsewhere classified
Code also, if applicable, focal traumatic brain injury (S03.3-)
Excludes2: traumatic cerebral edema (S06.1)

CC +7th S06.8A0 Primary blast injury of brain, not elsewhere classified without loss of consciousness
HAC 7th character A see Appendix B for HAC conditional logic

CC +7th S06.8A1 Primary blast injury of brain, not elsewhere classified with loss of consciousness of 30 minutes or less
Primary blast injury of brain, not elsewhere classified with brief loss of consciousness
HAC 7th character A see Appendix B for HAC conditional logic

CC +7th S06.8A2 Primary blast injury of brain, not elsewhere classified with loss of consciousness of 31 minutes to 59 minutes
HAC 7th character A see Appendix B for HAC conditional logic

CC +7th S06.8A3 Primary blast injury of brain, not elsewhere classified with loss of consciousness of 1 hour to 5 hours 59 minutes
HAC 7th character A see Appendix B for HAC conditional logic

CC +7th S06.8A4 Primary blast injury of brain, not elsewhere classified with loss of consciousness of 6 hours to 24 hours
HAC 7th character A see Appendix B for HAC conditional logic

CC +7th S06.8A5 Primary blast injury of brain, not elsewhere classified with loss of consciousness greater than 24 hours with return to pre-existing conscious level
HAC 7th character A see Appendix B for HAC conditional logic

MCC +7th S06.8A6 Primary blast injury of brain, not elsewhere classified with loss of consciousness greater than 24 hours without return to pre-existing conscious level with patient surviving
HAC 7th character A see Appendix B for HAC conditional logic

MCC +7th S06.8A7 Primary blast injury of brain, not elsewhere classified with loss of consciousness of any duration with death due to brain injury prior to regaining consciousness
HAC 7th character A see Appendix B for HAC conditional logic

MCC +7th S06.8A8 Primary blast injury of brain, not elsewhere classified with loss of consciousness of any duration with death due to other cause prior to regaining consciousness
HAC 7th character A see Appendix B for HAC conditional logic

CC +7th S06.8AA Primary blast injury of brain, not elsewhere classified with loss of consciousness status unknown
Primary blast injury of brain NOS
HAC 7th character A see Appendix B for HAC conditional logic

CC +7th S06.8A9 Primary blast injury of brain, not elsewhere classified with loss of consciousness of unspecified duration
HAC 7th character A see Appendix B for HAC conditional logic

+ S06.89 Other specified intracranial injury
Excludes1: concussion (S06.0X-)

+7th S06.890 Other specified intracranial injury without loss of consciousness

CC +7th S06.891 Other specified intracranial injury with loss of consciousness of 30 minutes or less
Other specified intracranial injury with brief loss of consciousness
HAC 7th character A see Appendix B for HAC conditional logic

CC +7th S06.892 Other specified intracranial injury with loss of consciousness of 31 minutes to 59 minutes
HAC 7th character A see Appendix B for HAC conditional logic

CC +7th S06.893 Other specified intracranial injury with loss of consciousness of 1 hour to 5 hours 59 minutes
HAC 7th character A see Appendix B for HAC conditional logic

CC +7th S06.894 Other specified intracranial injury with loss of consciousness of 6 hours to 24 hours
HAC 7th character A see Appendix B for HAC conditional logic

CC +7th S06.895 Other specified intracranial injury with loss of consciousness greater than 24 hours with return to pre-existing conscious level
HAC 7th character A see Appendix B for HAC conditional logic

MCC +7th S06.896 Other specified intracranial injury with loss of consciousness greater than 24 hours without return to pre-existing conscious level with patient surviving
HAC 7th character A see Appendix B for HAC conditional logic

MCC +7th S06.897 Other specified intracranial injury with loss of consciousness of any duration with death due to brain injury prior to regaining consciousness
HAC 7th character A see Appendix B for HAC conditional logic

MCC +7th S06.898 Other specified intracranial injury with loss of consciousness of any duration with death due to other cause prior to regaining consciousness
HAC 7th character A see Appendix B for HAC conditional logic

CC +7th S06.89A Other specified intracranial injury with loss of consciousness status unknown
HAC 7th character A see Appendix B for HAC conditional logic

CC +7th S06.899 Other specified intracranial injury with loss of consciousness of unspecified duration
HAC 7th character A see Appendix B for HAC conditional logic

CC + S06.9 Unspecified intracranial injury
Brain injury NOS
Head injury NOS with loss of consciousness
Traumatic brain injury NOS
Excludes1: conditions classifiable to S06.0- to S06.8- code to specified intracranial injury
head injury NOS (S09.90)

+ S06.9X Unspecified intracranial injury

+7th S06.9X0 Unspecified intracranial injury without loss of consciousness
AHA CC: 2Q, 2020, 31
HAC 7th character A see Appendix B for HAC conditional logic

+7th S06.9X1 Unspecified intracranial injury with loss of consciousness of 30 minutes or less
Unspecified intracranial injury with brief loss of consciousness
HAC 7th character A see Appendix B for HAC conditional logic

+7th S06.9X2 Unspecified intracranial injury with loss of consciousness of 31 minutes to 59 minutes
HAC 7th character A see Appendix B for HAC conditional logic

+7th S06.9X3 Unspecified intracranial injury with loss of consciousness of 1 hour to 5 hours 59 minutes
HAC 7th character A see Appendix B for HAC conditional logic

+7th S06.9X4 Unspecified intracranial injury with loss of consciousness of 6 hours to 24 hours
HAC 7th character A see Appendix B for HAC conditional logic

+7th S06.9X5 Unspecified intracranial injury with loss of consciousness greater than 24 hours with return to pre-existing conscious level
HAC 7th character A see Appendix B for HAC conditional logic

MCC +7th S06.9X6 Unspecified intracranial injury with loss of consciousness greater than 24 hours without return to pre-existing conscious level with patient surviving
  HAC 7th character A see Appendix B for HAC conditional logic

MCC +7th S06.9X7 Unspecified intracranial injury with loss of consciousness of any duration with death due to brain injury prior to regaining consciousness
  HAC 7th character A see Appendix B for HAC conditional logic

MCC +7th S06.9X8 Unspecified intracranial injury with loss of consciousness of any duration with death due to other cause prior to regaining consciousness
  HAC 7th character A see Appendix B for HAC conditional logic

CC +7th S06.9XA Unspecified intracranial injury with loss of consciousness status unknown
  HAC 7th character A see Appendix B for HAC conditional logic

+7th S06.9X9 Unspecified intracranial injury with loss of consciousness of unspecified duration
  HAC 7th character A see Appendix B for HAC conditional logic

+ **S06.A** Traumatic brain compression and herniation
  Traumatic cerebral compression
  Code first the underlying traumatic brain injury, such as:
    diffuse traumatic brain injury (S06.2-)
    focal traumatic brain injury (S06.3-)
    traumatic subdural hemorrhage (S06.5-)
    traumatic subarachnoid hemorrhage (S06.6-)
  AHA CC: 4Q, 2021, 29

  MCC S06.A0 Traumatic brain compression without herniation
    Traumatic brain compression NOS
    Traumatic cerebral compression NOS
    HAC 7th character A see Appendix B for HAC conditional logic

  MCC S06.A1 Traumatic brain compression with herniation
    Traumatic brain herniation
    Traumatic brainstem compression with herniation
    Traumatic cerebellar compression with herniation
    Traumatic cerebral compression with herniation
    HAC 7th character A see Appendix B for HAC conditional logic

S07 Crushing injury of head
  Use additional code for all associated injuries, such as:
    intracranial injuries (S06.-)
    skull fractures (S02.-)

  The appropriate 7th character is to be added to each code from category S07
    A initial encounter
    D subsequent encounter
    S sequela

CC X+7th S07.0 Crushing injury of face
  HAC 7th character A see Appendix B for HAC conditional logic
CC X+7th S07.1 Crushing injury of skull
  HAC 7th character A see Appendix B for HAC conditional logic
CC X+7th S07.8 Crushing injury of other parts of head
  HAC 7th character A see Appendix B for HAC conditional logic
CC X+7th S07.9 Crushing injury of head, part unspecified
  HAC 7th character A see Appendix B for HAC conditional logic

S08 Avulsion and traumatic amputation of part of head
  An amputation not identified as partial or complete should be coded to complete

  The appropriate 7th character is to be added to each code from category S08
    A initial encounter
    D subsequent encounter
    S sequela

X+7th S08.0 Avulsion of scalp
+ **S08.1** Traumatic amputation of ear
  + **S08.11** Complete traumatic amputation of ear
    +7th S08.111 Complete traumatic amputation of right ear
    +7th S08.112 Complete traumatic amputation of left ear
    +7th S08.119 Complete traumatic amputation of unspecified ear
  + **S08.12** Partial traumatic amputation of ear
    +7th S08.121 Partial traumatic amputation of right ear
    +7th S08.122 Partial traumatic amputation of left ear
    +7th S08.129 Partial traumatic amputation of unspecified ear
+ **S08.8** Traumatic amputation of other parts of head
  + **S08.81** Traumatic amputation of nose
    +7th S08.811 Complete traumatic amputation of nose
    +7th S08.812 Partial traumatic amputation of nose
  X+7th S08.89 Traumatic amputation of other parts of head

S09 Other and unspecified injuries of head

  The appropriate 7th character is to be added to each code from category S09
    A initial encounter
    D subsequent encounter
    S sequela

CC X+7th S09.0 Injury of blood vessels of head, not elsewhere classified
  Excludes1: *injury of cerebral blood vessels (S06.-)*
    injury of precerebral blood vessels (S15.-)

+ **S09.1** Injury of muscle and tendon of head
  Code also any associated open wound (S01.-)
  Excludes2: *sprain to joints and ligament of head (S03.9)*
  X+7th S09.10 Unspecified injury of muscle and tendon of head
    Injury of muscle and tendon of head NOS
  X+7th S09.11 Strain of muscle and tendon of head
  X+7th S09.12 Laceration of muscle and tendon of head
  X+7th S09.19 Other specified injury of muscle and tendon of head

+ **S09.2** Traumatic rupture of ear drum
  Excludes1: *traumatic rupture of ear drum due to blast injury (S09.31-)*
  CC X+7th S09.20 Traumatic rupture of unspecified ear drum
  CC X+7th S09.21 Traumatic rupture of right ear drum
  CC X+7th S09.22 Traumatic rupture of left ear drum

+ **S09.3** Other specified and unspecified injury of middle and inner ear
  Excludes1: *injury to ear NOS (S09.91-)*
  Excludes2: *injury to external ear (S00.4-, S01.3-, S08.1-)*
  + **S09.30** Unspecified injury of middle and inner ear
    CC +7th S09.301 Unspecified injury of right middle and inner ear
    CC +7th S09.302 Unspecified injury of left middle and inner ear
    CC +7th S09.309 Unspecified injury of unspecified middle and inner ear
  + **S09.31** Primary blast injury of ear
    Blast injury of ear NOS
    CC +7th S09.311 Primary blast injury of right ear
    CC +7th S09.312 Primary blast injury of left ear
    CC +7th S09.313 Primary blast injury of ear, bilateral
    CC +7th S09.319 Primary blast injury of unspecified ear
  + **S09.39** Other specified injury of middle and inner ear
    Secondary blast injury to ear
    CC +7th S09.391 Other specified injury of right middle and inner ear
    CC +7th S09.392 Other specified injury of left middle and inner ear
    CC +7th S09.399 Other specified injury of unspecified middle and inner ear

X+7th S09.8 Other specified injuries of head
+ **S09.9** Unspecified injury of face and head
  X+7th S09.90 Unspecified injury of head
    Head injury NOS
    Excludes1: *brain injury NOS (S06.9-)*
      head injury NOS with loss of consciousness (S06.9-)
      intracranial injury NOS (S06.9-)
  X+7th S09.91 Unspecified injury of ear
    Injury of ear NOS
  X+7th S09.92 Unspecified injury of nose
    Injury of nose NOS
  X+7th S09.93 Unspecified injury of face
    Injury of face NOS

Vertebrae

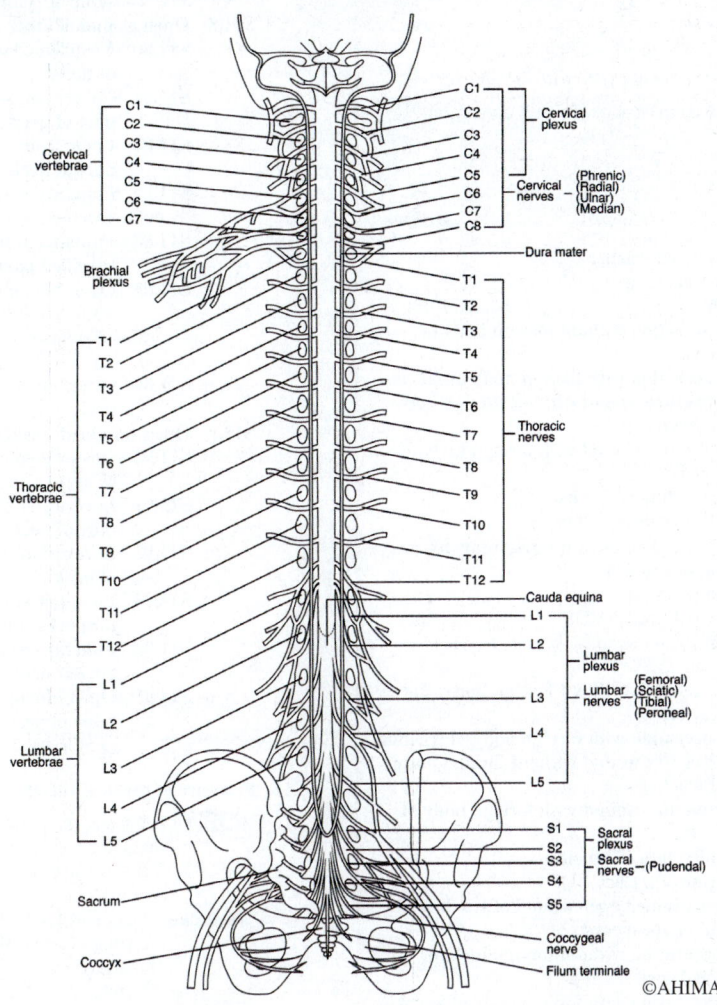

Injuries to the neck (S10-S19)

Includes: injuries of nape
injuries of supraclavicular region
injuries of throat

Excludes2: *burns and corrosions (T20-T32)*
effects of foreign body in esophagus (T18.1)
effects of foreign body in larynx (T17.3)
effects of foreign body in pharynx (T17.2)
effects of foreign body in trachea (T17.4)
frostbite (T33-T34)
insect bite or sting, venomous (T63.4)

S10 Superficial injury of neck

The appropriate 7th character is to be added to each code from category S10
A initial encounter
D subsequent encounter
S sequela

X+7th **S10.0 Contusion of throat**
Contusion of cervical esophagus
Contusion of larynx
Contusion of pharynx
Contusion of trachea

+ **S10.1 Other and unspecified superficial injuries of throat**
X+7th S10.10 Unspecified superficial injuries of throat
X+7th S10.11 Abrasion of throat
X+7th S10.12 Blister (nonthermal) of throat
X+7th S10.14 External constriction of part of throat
X+7th S10.15 Superficial foreign body of throat
Splinter in the throat
X+7th S10.16 Insect bite (nonvenomous) of throat
X+7th S10.17 Other superficial bite of throat
Excludes1: *open bite of throat (S11.85)*

+ **S10.8 Superficial injury of other specified parts of neck**
X+7th S10.80 Unspecified superficial injury of other specified part of neck
X+7th S10.81 Abrasion of other specified part of neck
X+7th S10.82 Blister (nonthermal) of other specified part of neck
X+7th S10.83 Contusion of other specified part of neck
X+7th S10.84 External constriction of other specified part of neck
X+7th S10.85 Superficial foreign body of other specified part of neck
Splinter in other specified part of neck
X+7th S10.86 Insect bite of other specified part of neck
X+7th S10.87 Other superficial bite of other specified part of neck
Excludes1: *open bite of other specified parts of neck (S11.85)*

+ **S10.9 Superficial injury of unspecified part of neck**
X+7th S10.90 Unspecified superficial injury of unspecified part of neck
X+7th S10.91 Abrasion of unspecified part of neck
X+7th S10.92 Blister (nonthermal) of unspecified part of neck
X+7th S10.93 Contusion of unspecified part of neck
X+7th S10.94 External constriction of unspecified part of neck
X+7th S10.95 Superficial foreign body of unspecified part of neck
X+7th S10.96 Insect bite of unspecified part of neck
X+7th S10.97 Other superficial bite of unspecified part of neck

S11 Open wound of neck

Code also any associated:
spinal cord injury (S14.0, S14.1-)
wound infection

Excludes2: open fracture of vertebra (S12.- with 7th character B)

The appropriate 7th character is to be added to each code from category S11
- A initial encounter
- D subsequent encounter
- S sequela

+ **S11.0 Open wound of larynx and trachea**
  + **S11.01 Open wound of larynx**
    Excludes2: open wound of vocal cord (S11.03)
    - MCC +7th S11.011 Laceration without foreign body of larynx
    - MCC +7th S11.012 Laceration with foreign body of larynx
    - MCC +7th S11.013 Puncture wound without foreign body of larynx
    - MCC +7th S11.014 Puncture wound with foreign body of larynx
    - MCC +7th S11.015 Open bite of larynx
      Bite of larynx NOS
    - MCC +7th S11.019 Unspecified open wound of larynx
  + **S11.02 Open wound of trachea**
    Open wound of cervical trachea
    Open wound of trachea NOS
    Excludes2: open wound of thoracic trachea (S27.5-)
    - MCC +7th S11.021 Laceration without foreign body of trachea
    - MCC +7th S11.022 Laceration with foreign body of trachea
    - MCC +7th S11.023 Puncture wound without foreign body of trachea
    - MCC +7th S11.024 Puncture wound with foreign body of trachea
    - MCC +7th S11.025 Open bite of trachea
      Bite of trachea NOS
    - MCC +7th S11.029 Unspecified open wound of trachea
  + **S11.03 Open wound of vocal cord**
    - MCC +7th S11.031 Laceration without foreign body of vocal cord
    - MCC +7th S11.032 Laceration with foreign body of vocal cord
    - MCC +7th S11.033 Puncture wound without foreign body of vocal cord
    - MCC +7th S11.034 Puncture wound with foreign body of vocal cord
    - MCC +7th S11.035 Open bite of vocal cord
      Bite of vocal cord NOS
    - MCC +7th S11.039 Unspecified open wound of vocal cord

+ **S11.1 Open wound of thyroid gland**
  - CC X+7th S11.10 Unspecified open wound of thyroid gland
  - CC X+7th S11.11 Laceration without foreign body of thyroid gland
  - CC X+7th S11.12 Laceration with foreign body of thyroid gland
  - CC X+7th S11.13 Puncture wound without foreign body of thyroid gland
  - CC X+7th S11.14 Puncture wound with foreign body of thyroid gland
  - CC X+7th S11.15 Open bite of thyroid gland
    Bite of thyroid gland NOS

+ **S11.2 Open wound of pharynx and cervical esophagus**
  Excludes1: open wound of esophagus NOS (S27.8-)
  - CC X+7th S11.20 Unspecified open wound of pharynx and cervical esophagus
  - CC X+7th S11.21 Laceration without foreign body of pharynx and cervical esophagus
  - CC X+7th S11.22 Laceration with foreign body of pharynx and cervical esophagus
  - CC X+7th S11.23 Puncture wound without foreign body of pharynx and cervical esophagus
  - CC X+7th S11.24 Puncture wound with foreign body of pharynx and cervical esophagus
  - CC X+7th S11.25 Open bite of pharynx and cervical esophagus
    Bite of pharynx and cervical esophagus NOS

+ **S11.8 Open wound of other specified parts of neck**
  - X+7th S11.80 Unspecified open wound of other specified part of neck
  - X+7th S11.81 Laceration without foreign body of other specified part of neck
  - X+7th S11.82 Laceration with foreign body of other specified part of neck
  - X+7th S11.83 Puncture wound without foreign body of other specified part of neck
  - X+7th S11.84 Puncture wound with foreign body of other specified part of neck
  - X+7th S11.85 Open bite of other specified part of neck
    Bite of other specified part of neck NOS
    Excludes1: superficial bite of other specified part of neck (S10.87)
  - X+7th S11.89 Other open wound of other specified part of neck

+ **S11.9 Open wound of unspecified part of neck**
  - X+7th S11.90 Unspecified open wound of unspecified part of neck
  - X+7th S11.91 Laceration without foreign body of unspecified part of neck
  - X+7th S11.92 Laceration with foreign body of unspecified part of neck
  - X+7th S11.93 Puncture wound without foreign body of unspecified part of neck
  - X+7th S11.94 Puncture wound with foreign body of unspecified part of neck
  - X+7th S11.95 Open bite of unspecified part of neck
    Bite of neck NOS
    Excludes1: superficial bite of neck (S10.97)

S12 Fracture of cervical vertebra and other parts of neck

NOTE A fracture not indicated as displaced or nondisplaced should be coded to displaced
A fracture not indicated as open or closed should be coded to closed

Includes: fracture of cervical neural arch
fracture of cervical spine
fracture of cervical spinous process
fracture of cervical transverse process
fracture of cervical vertebral arch
fracture of neck

Code first any associated cervical spinal cord injury (S14.0, S14.1-)

The appropriate 7th character is to be added to all codes from subcategories S12.0-S12.6
- A initial encounter for closed fracture
- B initial encounter for open fracture
- D subsequent encounter for fracture with routine healing
- G subsequent encounter for fracture with delayed healing
- K subsequent encounter for fracture with nonunion
- S sequela

Review coding guideline C.19.c

+ **S12.0 Fracture of first cervical vertebra**
  Atlas
  + **S12.00 Unspecified fracture of first cervical vertebra**
    - CC MCC +7th S12.000 Unspecified displaced fracture of first cervical vertebra
      HAC 7th characters A & B see Appendix B for HAC conditional logic
    - CC MCC +7th S12.001 Unspecified nondisplaced fracture of first cervical vertebra
      HAC 7th characters A & B see Appendix B for HAC conditional logic
  - CC MCC X+7th S12.01 Stable burst fracture of first cervical vertebra
    HAC 7th characters A & B see Appendix B for HAC conditional logic
  - CC MCC X+7th S12.02 Unstable burst fracture of first cervical vertebra
    HAC 7th characters A & B see Appendix B for HAC conditional logic

- **+ S12.03 Posterior arch fracture of first cervical vertebra**
  - CC MCC +7th **S12.030** Displaced posterior arch fracture of first cervical vertebra
    - HAC⁷ 7th characters A & B see Appendix B for HAC conditional logic
  - CC MCC +7th **S12.031** Nondisplaced posterior arch fracture of first cervical vertebra
    - HAC⁷ 7th characters A & B see Appendix B for HAC conditional logic
- **+ S12.04 Lateral mass fracture of first cervical vertebra**
  - CC MCC +7th **S12.040** Displaced lateral mass fracture of first cervical vertebra
    - HAC⁷ 7th characters A & B see Appendix B for HAC conditional logic
  - CC MCC +7th **S12.041** Nondisplaced lateral mass fracture of first cervical vertebra
    - HAC⁷ 7th characters A & B see Appendix B for HAC conditional logic
- **+ S12.09 Other fracture of first cervical vertebra**
  - CC MCC +7th **S12.090** Other displaced fracture of first cervical vertebra
    - HAC⁷ 7th characters A & B see Appendix B for HAC conditional logic
  - CC MCC +7th **S12.091** Other nondisplaced fracture of first cervical vertebra
    - HAC⁷ 7th characters A & B see Appendix B for HAC conditional logic
- **+ S12.1 Fracture of second cervical vertebra**
  - Axis
  - **+ S12.10 Unspecified fracture of second cervical vertebra**
    - CC MCC +7th **S12.100** Unspecified displaced fracture of second cervical vertebra
      - HAC⁷ 7th characters A & B see Appendix B for HAC conditional logic
    - CC MCC +7th **S12.101** Unspecified nondisplaced fracture of second cervical vertebra
      - HAC⁷ 7th characters A & B see Appendix B for HAC conditional logic
  - **+ S12.11 Type II dens fracture**
    - CC MCC +7th **S12.110** Anterior displaced Type II dens fracture
      - HAC⁷ 7th characters A & B see Appendix B for HAC conditional logic
    - CC MCC +7th **S12.111** Posterior displaced Type II dens fracture
      - HAC⁷ 7th characters A & B see Appendix B for HAC conditional logic
    - CC MCC +7th **S12.112** Nondisplaced Type II dens fracture
      - HAC⁷ 7th characters A & B see Appendix B for HAC conditional logic
  - **+ S12.12 Other dens fracture**
    - CC MCC +7th **S12.120** Other displaced dens fracture
      - HAC⁷ 7th characters A & B see Appendix B for HAC conditional logic
    - CC MCC +7th **S12.121** Other nondisplaced dens fracture
      - HAC⁷ 7th characters A & B see Appendix B for HAC conditional logic
  - **+ S12.13 Unspecified traumatic spondylolisthesis of second cervical vertebra**
    - CC MCC +7th **S12.130** Unspecified traumatic displaced spondylolisthesis of second cervical vertebra
      - HAC⁷ 7th characters A & B see Appendix B for HAC conditional logic
    - CC MCC +7th **S12.131** Unspecified traumatic nondisplaced spondylolisthesis of second cervical vertebra
      - HAC⁷ 7th characters A & B see Appendix B for HAC conditional logic
  - CC MCC X+7th **S12.14** Type III traumatic spondylolisthesis of second cervical vertebra
    - HAC⁷ 7th characters A & B see Appendix B for HAC conditional logic
  - **+ S12.15 Other traumatic spondylolisthesis of second cervical vertebra**
    - CC MCC +7th **S12.150** Other traumatic displaced spondylolisthesis of second cervical vertebra
      - HAC⁷ 7th characters A & B see Appendix B for HAC conditional logic
    - CC MCC +7th **S12.151** Other traumatic nondisplaced spondylolisthesis of second cervical vertebra
      - HAC⁷ 7th characters A & B see Appendix B for HAC conditional logic
- **+ S12.19 Other fracture of second cervical vertebra**
  - CC MCC +7th **S12.190** Other displaced fracture of second cervical vertebra
    - HAC⁷ 7th characters A & B see Appendix B for HAC conditional logic
  - CC MCC +7th **S12.191** Other nondisplaced fracture of second cervical vertebra
    - HAC⁷ 7th characters A & B see Appendix B for HAC conditional logic
- **+ S12.2 Fracture of third cervical vertebra**
  - **+ S12.20 Unspecified fracture of third cervical vertebra**
    - CC MCC +7th **S12.200** Unspecified displaced fracture of third cervical vertebra
      - HAC⁷ 7th characters A & B see Appendix B for HAC conditional logic
    - CC MCC +7th **S12.201** Unspecified nondisplaced fracture of third cervical vertebra
      - HAC⁷ 7th characters A & B see Appendix B for HAC conditional logic
  - **+ S12.23 Unspecified traumatic spondylolisthesis of third cervical vertebra**
    - CC MCC +7th **S12.230** Unspecified traumatic displaced spondylolisthesis of third cervical vertebra
      - HAC⁷ 7th characters A & B see Appendix B for HAC conditional logic
    - CC MCC +7th **S12.231** Unspecified traumatic nondisplaced spondylolisthesis of third cervical vertebra
      - HAC⁷ 7th characters A & B see Appendix B for HAC conditional logic
  - CC MCC X+7th **S12.24** Type III traumatic spondylolisthesis of third cervical vertebra
    - HAC⁷ 7th characters A & B see Appendix B for HAC conditional logic
  - **+ S12.25 Other traumatic spondylolisthesis of third cervical vertebra**
    - CC MCC +7th **S12.250** Other traumatic displaced spondylolisthesis of third cervical vertebra
      - HAC⁷ 7th characters A & B see Appendix B for HAC conditional logic
    - CC MCC +7th **S12.251** Other traumatic nondisplaced spondylolisthesis of third cervical vertebra
      - HAC⁷ 7th characters A & B see Appendix B for HAC conditional logic
  - **+ S12.29 Other fracture of third cervical vertebra**
    - CC MCC +7th **S12.290** Other displaced fracture of third cervical vertebra
      - HAC⁷ 7th characters A & B see Appendix B for HAC conditional logic
    - CC MCC +7th **S12.291** Other nondisplaced fracture of third cervical vertebra
      - HAC⁷ 7th characters A & B see Appendix B for HAC conditional logic
- **+ S12.3 Fracture of fourth cervical vertebra**
  - **+ S12.30 Unspecified fracture of fourth cervical vertebra**
    - CC MCC +7th **S12.300** Unspecified displaced fracture of fourth cervical vertebra
      - HAC⁷ 7th characters A & B see Appendix B for HAC conditional logic
    - CC MCC +7th **S12.301** Unspecified nondisplaced fracture of fourth cervical vertebra
      - HAC⁷ 7th characters A & B see Appendix B for HAC conditional logic
  - **+ S12.33 Unspecified traumatic spondylolisthesis of fourth cervical vertebra**
    - CC MCC +7th **S12.330** Unspecified traumatic displaced spondylolisthesis of fourth cervical vertebra
      - HAC⁷ 7th characters A & B see Appendix B for HAC conditional logic
    - CC MCC +7th **S12.331** Unspecified traumatic nondisplaced spondylolisthesis of fourth cervical vertebra
      - HAC⁷ 7th characters A & B see Appendix B for HAC conditional logic
  - CC MCC X+7th **S12.34** Type III traumatic spondylolisthesis of fourth cervical vertebra
    - HAC⁷ 7th characters A & B see Appendix B for HAC conditional logic

+, +7th, X + 7th • Newborn • Pediatric • Maternity • Adult ♀ Female ♂ Male Manifestation Unacceptable PDX HCC CC MCC HAC

S12.35–S12.691

- **+ S12.35** Other traumatic spondylolisthesis of fourth cervical vertebra
  - **CC MCC +7th S12.350** Other traumatic displaced spondylolisthesis of fourth cervical vertebra
    - *HAC* 7th characters A & B see Appendix B for HAC conditional logic
  - **CC MCC +7th S12.351** Other traumatic nondisplaced spondylolisthesis of fourth cervical vertebra
    - *HAC* 7th characters A & B see Appendix B for HAC conditional logic
- **+ S12.39** Other fracture of fourth cervical vertebra
  - **CC MCC +7th S12.390** Other displaced fracture of fourth cervical vertebra
    - *HAC* 7th characters A & B see Appendix B for HAC conditional logic
  - **CC MCC +7th S12.391** Other nondisplaced fracture of fourth cervical vertebra
    - *HAC* 7th characters A & B see Appendix B for HAC conditional logic

- **+ S12.4** Fracture of fifth cervical vertebra
  - **+ S12.40** Unspecified fracture of fifth cervical vertebra
    - **CC MCC +7th S12.400** Unspecified displaced fracture of fifth cervical vertebra
      - *HAC* 7th characters A & B see Appendix B for HAC conditional logic
    - **CC MCC +7th S12.401** Unspecified nondisplaced fracture of fifth cervical vertebra
      - *HAC* 7th characters A & B see Appendix B for HAC conditional logic
  - **+ S12.43** Unspecified traumatic spondylolisthesis of fifth cervical vertebra
    - **CC MCC +7th S12.430** Unspecified traumatic displaced spondylolisthesis of fifth cervical vertebra
      - *HAC* 7th characters A & B see Appendix B for HAC conditional logic
    - **CC MCC +7th S12.431** Unspecified traumatic nondisplaced spondylolisthesis of fifth cervical vertebra
      - *HAC* 7th characters A & B see Appendix B for HAC conditional logic
  - **CC MCC X+7th S12.44** Type III traumatic spondylolisthesis of fifth cervical vertebra
    - *HAC* 7th characters A & B see Appendix B for HAC conditional logic
  - **+ S12.45** Other traumatic spondylolisthesis of fifth cervical vertebra
    - **CC MCC +7th S12.450** Other traumatic displaced spondylolisthesis of fifth cervical vertebra
      - *HAC* 7th characters A & B see Appendix B for HAC conditional logic
    - **CC MCC +7th S12.451** Other traumatic nondisplaced spondylolisthesis of fifth cervical vertebra
      - *HAC* 7th characters A & B see Appendix B for HAC conditional logic
  - **+ S12.49** Other fracture of fifth cervical vertebra
    - **CC MCC +7th S12.490** Other displaced fracture of fifth cervical vertebra
      - *HAC* 7th characters A & B see Appendix B for HAC conditional logic
    - **CC MCC +7th S12.491** Other nondisplaced fracture of fifth cervical vertebra
      - *HAC* 7th characters A & B see Appendix B for HAC conditional logic

- **+ S12.5** Fracture of sixth cervical vertebra
  - **+ S12.50** Unspecified fracture of sixth cervical vertebra
    - **CC MCC +7th S12.500** Unspecified displaced fracture of sixth cervical vertebra
      - *HAC* 7th characters A & B see Appendix B for HAC conditional logic
    - **CC MCC +7th S12.501** Unspecified nondisplaced fracture of sixth cervical vertebra
      - *HAC* 7th characters A & B see Appendix B for HAC conditional logic
  - **+ S12.53** Unspecified traumatic spondylolisthesis of sixth cervical vertebra
    - **CC MCC +7th S12.530** Unspecified traumatic displaced spondylolisthesis of sixth cervical vertebra
      - *HAC* 7th characters A & B see Appendix B for HAC conditional logic
    - **CC MCC +7th S12.531** Unspecified traumatic nondisplaced spondylolisthesis of sixth cervical vertebra
      - *HAC* 7th characters A & B see Appendix B for HAC conditional logic
  - **CC MCC X+7th S12.54** Type III traumatic spondylolisthesis of sixth cervical vertebra
    - *HAC* 7th characters A & B see Appendix B for HAC conditional logic
  - **+ S12.55** Other traumatic spondylolisthesis of sixth cervical vertebra
    - **CC MCC +7th S12.550** Other traumatic displaced spondylolisthesis of sixth cervical vertebra
      - *HAC* 7th characters A & B see Appendix B for HAC conditional logic
    - **CC MCC +7th S12.551** Other traumatic nondisplaced spondylolisthesis of sixth cervical vertebra
      - *HAC* 7th characters A & B see Appendix B for HAC conditional logic
  - **+ S12.59** Other fracture of sixth cervical vertebra
    - **CC MCC +7th S12.590** Other displaced fracture of sixth cervical vertebra
      - *HAC* 7th characters A & B see Appendix B for HAC conditional logic
    - **CC MCC +7th S12.591** Other nondisplaced fracture of sixth cervical vertebra
      - *HAC* 7th characters A & B see Appendix B for HAC conditional logic

- **+ S12.6** Fracture of seventh cervical vertebra
  - **+ S12.60** Unspecified fracture of seventh cervical vertebra
    - **CC MCC +7th S12.600** Unspecified displaced fracture of seventh cervical vertebra
      - *HAC* 7th characters A & B see Appendix B for HAC conditional logic
    - **CC MCC +7th S12.601** Unspecified nondisplaced fracture of seventh cervical vertebra
      - *HAC* 7th characters A & B see Appendix B for HAC conditional logic
  - **+ S12.63** Unspecified traumatic spondylolisthesis of seventh cervical vertebra
    - **CC MCC +7th S12.630** Unspecified traumatic displaced spondylolisthesis of seventh cervical vertebra
      - *HAC* 7th characters A & B see Appendix B for HAC conditional logic
    - **CC MCC +7th S12.631** Unspecified traumatic nondisplaced spondylolisthesis of seventh cervical vertebra
      - *HAC* 7th characters A & B see Appendix B for HAC conditional logic
  - **CC MCC X+7th S12.64** Type III traumatic spondylolisthesis of seventh cervical vertebra
    - *HAC* 7th characters A & B see Appendix B for HAC conditional logic
  - **+ S12.65** Other traumatic spondylolisthesis of seventh cervical vertebra
    - **CC MCC +7th S12.650** Other traumatic displaced spondylolisthesis of seventh cervical vertebra
      - *HAC* 7th characters A & B see Appendix B for HAC conditional logic
    - **CC MCC +7th S12.651** Other traumatic nondisplaced spondylolisthesis of seventh cervical vertebra
      - *HAC* 7th characters A & B see Appendix B for HAC conditional logic
  - **+ S12.69** Other fracture of seventh cervical vertebra
    - **CC MCC +7th S12.690** Other displaced fracture of seventh cervical vertebra
      - *HAC* 7th characters A & B see Appendix B for HAC conditional logic
    - **CC MCC +7th S12.691** Other nondisplaced fracture of seventh cervical vertebra
      - *HAC* 7th characters A & B see Appendix B for HAC conditional logic

X+7th S12.8 Fracture of other parts of neck
MCC

> The appropriate 7th character is to be added to code **S12.8**
> A initial encounter
> D subsequent encounter
> S sequela

Hyoid bone
Larynx
Thyroid cartilage
Trachea
HAC 7th character A see Appendix B for HAC conditional logic

CC X+7th S12.9 Fracture of neck, unspecified

> The appropriate 7th character is to be added to code **S12.9**
> A initial encounter
> D subsequent encounter
> S sequela

Fracture of neck NOS
Fracture of cervical spine NOS
Fracture of cervical vertebra NOS
HAC 7th character A see Appendix B for HAC conditional logic

S13 Dislocation and sprain of joints and ligaments at neck level

Includes: avulsion of joint or ligament at neck level
laceration of cartilage, joint or ligament at neck level
sprain of cartilage, joint or ligament at neck level
traumatic hemarthrosis of joint or ligament at neck level
traumatic rupture of joint or ligament at neck level
traumatic subluxation of joint or ligament at neck level
traumatic tear of joint or ligament at neck level

Code also any associated open wound
Excludes2: strain of muscle or tendon at neck level (S16.1)

> The appropriate 7th character is to be added to each code from category S13
> A initial encounter
> D subsequent encounter
> S sequela

CC X+7th S13.0 Traumatic rupture of cervical intervertebral disc
Excludes1: rupture or displacement (nontraumatic) of cervical intervertebral disc NOS (M50.-)
HAC 7th character A see Appendix B for HAC conditional logic

+ S13.1 Subluxation and dislocation of cervical vertebrae
Code also any associated:
open wound of neck (S11.-)
spinal cord injury (S14.1-)
Excludes2: fracture of cervical vertebrae (S12.0-S12.3-)

  + S13.10 Subluxation and dislocation of unspecified cervical vertebrae

    CC +7th S13.100 Subluxation of unspecified cervical vertebrae
HAC 7th character A see Appendix B for HAC conditional logic

    CC +7th S13.101 Dislocation of unspecified cervical vertebrae
HAC 7th character A see Appendix B for HAC conditional logic

  + S13.11 Subluxation and dislocation of C0/C1 cervical vertebrae
Subluxation and dislocation of atlantooccipital joint
Subluxation and dislocation of atloidooccipital joint
Subluxation and dislocation of occipitoatloid joint

    CC +7th S13.110 Subluxation of C0/C1 cervical vertebrae
HAC 7th character A see Appendix B for HAC conditional logic

    CC +7th S13.111 Dislocation of C0/C1 cervical vertebrae
HAC 7th character A see Appendix B for HAC conditional logic

  + S13.12 Subluxation and dislocation of C1/C2 cervical vertebrae
Subluxation and dislocation of atlantoaxial joint

    CC +7th S13.120 Subluxation of C1/C2 cervical vertebrae
HAC 7th character A see Appendix B for HAC conditional logic

    CC +7th S13.121 Dislocation of C1/C2 cervical vertebrae
HAC 7th character A see Appendix B for HAC conditional logic

  + S13.13 Subluxation and dislocation of C2/C3 cervical vertebrae

    CC +7th S13.130 Subluxation of C2/C3 cervical vertebrae
HAC 7th character A see Appendix B for HAC conditional logic

    CC +7th S13.131 Dislocation of C2/C3 cervical vertebrae
HAC 7th character A see Appendix B for HAC conditional logic

  + S13.14 Subluxation and dislocation of C3/C4 cervical vertebrae

    CC +7th S13.140 Subluxation of C3/C4 cervical vertebrae
HAC 7th character A see Appendix B for HAC conditional logic

    CC +7th S13.141 Dislocation of C3/C4 cervical vertebrae
HAC 7th character A see Appendix B for HAC conditional logic

  + S13.15 Subluxation and dislocation of C4/C5 cervical vertebrae

    CC +7th S13.150 Subluxation of C4/C5 cervical vertebrae
HAC 7th character A see Appendix B for HAC conditional logic

    CC +7th S13.151 Dislocation of C4/C5 cervical vertebrae
HAC 7th character A see Appendix B for HAC conditional logic

  + S13.16 Subluxation and dislocation of C5/C6 cervical vertebrae

    CC +7th S13.160 Subluxation of C5/C6 cervical vertebrae
HAC 7th character A see Appendix B for HAC conditional logic

    CC +7th S13.161 Dislocation of C5/C6 cervical vertebrae
HAC 7th character A see Appendix B for HAC conditional logic

  + S13.17 Subluxation and dislocation of C6/C7 cervical vertebrae

    CC +7th S13.170 Subluxation of C6/C7 cervical vertebrae
HAC 7th character A see Appendix B for HAC conditional logic

    CC +7th S13.171 Dislocation of C6/C7 cervical vertebrae
HAC 7th character A see Appendix B for HAC conditional logic

  + S13.18 Subluxation and dislocation of C7/T1 cervical vertebrae

    CC +7th S13.180 Subluxation of C7/T1 cervical vertebrae
HAC 7th character A see Appendix B for HAC conditional logic

    CC +7th S13.181 Dislocation of C7/T1 cervical vertebrae
HAC 7th character A see Appendix B for HAC conditional logic

+ S13.2 Dislocation of other and unspecified parts of neck

  CC X+7th S13.20 Dislocation of unspecified parts of neck
HAC 7th character A see Appendix B for HAC conditional logic

  CC X+7th S13.29 Dislocation of other parts of neck
HAC 7th character A see Appendix B for HAC conditional logic

X+7th S13.4 Sprain of ligaments of cervical spine
Sprain of anterior longitudinal (ligament), cervical
Sprain of atlanto-axial (joints)
Sprain of atlanto-occipital (joints)
Whiplash injury of cervical spine

X+7th S13.5 Sprain of thyroid region
Sprain of cricoarytenoid (joint) (ligament)
Sprain of cricothyroid (joint) (ligament)
Sprain of thyroid cartilage

X+7th S13.8 Sprain of joints and ligaments of other parts of neck
X+7th S13.9 Sprain of joints and ligaments of unspecified parts of neck

S14 Injury of nerves and spinal cord at neck level

NOTE Code to highest level of cervical cord injury
Code also any associated:
fracture of cervical vertebra (S12.0--S12.6.-)
open wound of neck (S11.-)
transient paralysis (R29.5)

> The appropriate 7th character is to be added to each code from category S14
> A initial encounter
> D subsequent encounter
> S sequela

MCC X+7th S14.0 Concussion and edema of cervical spinal cord

+ S14.1 Other and unspecified injuries of cervical spinal cord

  + S14.10 Unspecified injury of cervical spinal cord

    MCC +7th S14.101 Unspecified injury at C1 level of cervical spinal cord
HAC 7th character A see Appendix B for HAC conditional logic

    MCC +7th S14.102 Unspecified injury at C2 level of cervical spinal cord
HAC 7th character A see Appendix B for HAC conditional logic

    MCC +7th S14.103 Unspecified injury at C3 level of cervical spinal cord
HAC 7th character A see Appendix B for HAC conditional logic

MCC +7th S14.104 Unspecified injury at C4 level of cervical spinal cord
  HAC 7th character A see Appendix B for HAC conditional logic

MCC +7th S14.105 Unspecified injury at C5 level of cervical spinal cord
  HAC 7th character A see Appendix B for HAC conditional logic

MCC +7th S14.106 Unspecified injury at C6 level of cervical spinal cord
  HAC 7th character A see Appendix B for HAC conditional logic

MCC +7th S14.107 Unspecified injury at C7 level of cervical spinal cord
  HAC 7th character A see Appendix B for HAC conditional logic

MCC +7th S14.108 Unspecified injury at C8 level of cervical spinal cord

+7th S14.109 Unspecified injury at unspecified level of cervical spinal cord
  Injury of cervical spinal cord NOS
  HAC 7th character A see Appendix B for HAC conditional logic

+ S14.11 Complete lesion of cervical spinal cord

MCC +7th S14.111 Complete lesion at C1 level of cervical spinal cord
  HAC 7th character A see Appendix B for HAC conditional logic

MCC +7th S14.112 Complete lesion at C2 level of cervical spinal cord
  HAC 7th character A see Appendix B for HAC conditional logic

MCC +7th S14.113 Complete lesion at C3 level of cervical spinal cord
  HAC 7th character A see Appendix B for HAC conditional logic

MCC +7th S14.114 Complete lesion at C4 level of cervical spinal cord
  HAC 7th character A see Appendix B for HAC conditional logic

MCC +7th S14.115 Complete lesion at C5 level of cervical spinal cord
  HAC 7th character A see Appendix B for HAC conditional logic

MCC +7th S14.116 Complete lesion at C6 level of cervical spinal cord
  HAC 7th character A see Appendix B for HAC conditional logic

MCC +7th S14.117 Complete lesion at C7 level of cervical spinal cord
  HAC 7th character A see Appendix B for HAC conditional logic

MCC +7th S14.118 Complete lesion at C8 level of cervical spinal cord

+7th S14.119 Complete lesion at unspecified level of cervical spinal cord

+ S14.12 Central cord syndrome of cervical spinal cord

MCC +7th S14.121 Central cord syndrome at C1 level of cervical spinal cord
  HAC 7th character A see Appendix B for HAC conditional logic

MCC +7th S14.122 Central cord syndrome at C2 level of cervical spinal cord
  HAC 7th character A see Appendix B for HAC conditional logic

MCC +7th S14.123 Central cord syndrome at C3 level of cervical spinal cord
  HAC 7th character A see Appendix B for HAC conditional logic

MCC +7th S14.124 Central cord syndrome at C4 level of cervical spinal cord
  HAC 7th character A see Appendix B for HAC conditional logic

MCC +7th S14.125 Central cord syndrome at C5 level of cervical spinal cord
  HAC 7th character A see Appendix B for HAC conditional logic

MCC +7th S14.126 Central cord syndrome at C6 level of cervical spinal cord
  HAC 7th character A see Appendix B for HAC conditional logic

MCC +7th S14.127 Central cord syndrome at C7 level of cervical spinal cord
  HAC 7th character A see Appendix B for HAC conditional logic

MCC +7th S14.128 Central cord syndrome at C8 level of cervical spinal cord

+7th S14.129 Central cord syndrome at unspecified level of cervical spinal cord

+ S14.13 Anterior cord syndrome of cervical spinal cord

MCC +7th S14.131 Anterior cord syndrome at C1 level of cervical spinal cord
  HAC 7th character A see Appendix B for HAC conditional logic

MCC +7th S14.132 Anterior cord syndrome at C2 level of cervical spinal cord
  HAC 7th character A see Appendix B for HAC conditional logic

MCC +7th S14.133 Anterior cord syndrome at C3 level of cervical spinal cord
  HAC 7th character A see Appendix B for HAC conditional logic

MCC +7th S14.134 Anterior cord syndrome at C4 level of cervical spinal cord
  HAC 7th character A see Appendix B for HAC conditional logic

MCC +7th S14.135 Anterior cord syndrome at C5 level of cervical spinal cord
  HAC 7th character A see Appendix B for HAC conditional logic

MCC +7th S14.136 Anterior cord syndrome at C6 level of cervical spinal cord
  HAC 7th character A see Appendix B for HAC conditional logic

MCC +7th S14.137 Anterior cord syndrome at C7 level of cervical spinal cord
  HAC 7th character A see Appendix B for HAC conditional logic

MCC +7th S14.138 Anterior cord syndrome at C8 level of cervical spinal cord

+7th S14.139 Anterior cord syndrome at unspecified level of cervical spinal cord

+ S14.14 Brown-Séquard syndrome of cervical spinal cord

MCC +7th S14.141 Brown-Séquard syndrome at C1 level of cervical spinal cord

MCC +7th S14.142 Brown-Séquard syndrome at C2 level of cervical spinal cord

MCC +7th S14.143 Brown-Séquard syndrome at C3 level of cervical spinal cord

MCC +7th S14.144 Brown-Séquard syndrome at C4 level of cervical spinal cord

MCC +7th S14.145 Brown-Séquard syndrome at C5 level of cervical spinal cord

MCC +7th S14.146 Brown-Séquard syndrome at C6 level of cervical spinal cord

MCC +7th S14.147 Brown-Séquard syndrome at C7 level of cervical spinal cord

MCC +7th S14.148 Brown-Séquard syndrome at C8 level of cervical spinal cord

+7th S14.149 Brown-Séquard syndrome at unspecified level of cervical spinal cord

+ S14.15 Other incomplete lesions of cervical spinal cord
  Incomplete lesion of cervical spinal cord NOS
  Posterior cord syndrome of cervical spinal cord

MCC +7th S14.151 Other incomplete lesion at C1 level of cervical spinal cord
  HAC 7th character A see Appendix B for HAC conditional logic

MCC +7th S14.152 Other incomplete lesion at C2 level of cervical spinal cord
  HAC 7th character A see Appendix B for HAC conditional logic

MCC +7th S14.153 Other incomplete lesion at C3 level of cervical spinal cord
  HAC 7th character A see Appendix B for HAC conditional logic

MCC +7th S14.154 Other incomplete lesion at C4 level of cervical spinal cord
  HAC 7th character A see Appendix B for HAC conditional logic

MCC +7th S14.155 Other incomplete lesion at C5 level of cervical spinal cord
  HAC 7th character A see Appendix B for HAC conditional logic

MCC +7th S14.156 Other incomplete lesion at C6 level of cervical spinal cord
 HAC 7th character A see Appendix B for HAC conditional logic
MCC +7th S14.157 Other incomplete lesion at C7 level of cervical spinal cord
 HAC 7th character A see Appendix B for HAC conditional logic
MCC +7th S14.158 Other incomplete lesion at C8 level of cervical spinal cord
+7th S14.159 Other incomplete lesion at unspecified level of cervical spinal cord
X+7th S14.2 Injury of nerve root of cervical spine
X+7th S14.3 Injury of brachial plexus
X+7th S14.4 Injury of peripheral nerves of neck
X+7th S14.5 Injury of cervical sympathetic nerves
X+7th S14.8 Injury of other specified nerves of neck
X+7th S14.9 Injury of unspecified nerves of neck

S15 Injury of blood vessels at neck level
Code also any associated open wound (S11.-)

> The appropriate 7th character is to be added to each code from category S15
> A initial encounter
> D subsequent encounter
> S sequela

+ S15.0 Injury of carotid artery of neck
 Injury of carotid artery (common) (external) (internal, extracranial portion)
 Injury of carotid artery NOS
 Excludes1: injury of internal carotid artery, intracranial portion (S06.8)
 + S15.00 Unspecified injury of carotid artery
  CC +7th S15.001 Unspecified injury of right carotid artery
  CC +7th S15.002 Unspecified injury of left carotid artery
  CC +7th S15.009 Unspecified injury of unspecified carotid artery
 + S15.01 Minor laceration of carotid artery
  Incomplete transection of carotid artery
  Laceration of carotid artery NOS
  Superficial laceration of carotid artery
  CC +7th S15.011 Minor laceration of right carotid artery
  CC +7th S15.012 Minor laceration of left carotid artery
  CC +7th S15.019 Minor laceration of unspecified carotid artery
 + S15.02 Major laceration of carotid artery
  Complete transection of carotid artery
  Traumatic rupture of carotid artery
  CC +7th S15.021 Major laceration of right carotid artery
  CC +7th S15.022 Major laceration of left carotid artery
  CC +7th S15.029 Major laceration of unspecified carotid artery
 + S15.09 Other specified injury of carotid artery
  CC +7th S15.091 Other specified injury of right carotid artery
  CC +7th S15.092 Other specified injury of left carotid artery
  CC +7th S15.099 Other specified injury of unspecified carotid artery
+ S15.1 Injury of vertebral artery
 + S15.10 Unspecified injury of vertebral artery
  CC +7th S15.101 Unspecified injury of right vertebral artery
  CC +7th S15.102 Unspecified injury of left vertebral artery
  CC +7th S15.109 Unspecified injury of unspecified vertebral artery
 + S15.11 Minor laceration of vertebral artery
  Incomplete transection of vertebral artery
  Laceration of vertebral artery NOS
  Superficial laceration of vertebral artery
  CC +7th S15.111 Minor laceration of right vertebral artery
  CC +7th S15.112 Minor laceration of left vertebral artery
  CC +7th S15.119 Minor laceration of unspecified vertebral artery
 + S15.12 Major laceration of vertebral artery
  Complete transection of vertebral artery
  Traumatic rupture of vertebral artery
  CC +7th S15.121 Major laceration of right vertebral artery
  CC +7th S15.122 Major laceration of left vertebral artery
  CC +7th S15.129 Major laceration of unspecified vertebral artery
 + S15.19 Other specified injury of vertebral artery
  CC +7th S15.191 Other specified injury of right vertebral artery
  CC +7th S15.192 Other specified injury of left vertebral artery
  CC +7th S15.199 Other specified injury of unspecified vertebral artery
+ S15.2 Injury of external jugular vein
 + S15.20 Unspecified injury of external jugular vein
  CC +7th S15.201 Unspecified injury of right external jugular vein
  CC +7th S15.202 Unspecified injury of left external jugular vein
  CC +7th S15.209 Unspecified injury of unspecified external jugular vein
 + S15.21 Minor laceration of external jugular vein
  Incomplete transection of external jugular vein
  Laceration of external jugular vein NOS
  Superficial laceration of external jugular vein
  CC +7th S15.211 Minor laceration of right external jugular vein
  CC +7th S15.212 Minor laceration of left external jugular vein
  CC +7th S15.219 Minor laceration of unspecified external jugular vein
 + S15.22 Major laceration of external jugular vein
  Complete transection of external jugular vein
  Traumatic rupture of external jugular vein
  CC +7th S15.221 Major laceration of right external jugular vein
  CC +7th S15.222 Major laceration of left external jugular vein
  CC +7th S15.229 Major laceration of unspecified external jugular vein
 + S15.29 Other specified injury of external jugular vein
  CC +7th S15.291 Other specified injury of right external jugular vein
  CC +7th S15.292 Other specified injury of left external jugular vein
  CC +7th S15.299 Other specified injury of unspecified external jugular vein
+ S15.3 Injury of internal jugular vein
 + S15.30 Unspecified injury of internal jugular vein
  CC +7th S15.301 Unspecified injury of right internal jugular vein
  CC +7th S15.302 Unspecified injury of left internal jugular vein
  CC +7th S15.309 Unspecified injury of unspecified internal jugular vein
 + S15.31 Minor laceration of internal jugular vein
  Incomplete transection of internal jugular vein
  Laceration of internal jugular vein NOS
  Superficial laceration of internal jugular vein
  CC +7th S15.311 Minor laceration of right internal jugular vein
  CC +7th S15.312 Minor laceration of left internal jugular vein
  CC +7th S15.319 Minor laceration of unspecified internal jugular vein
 + S15.32 Major laceration of internal jugular vein
  Complete transection of internal jugular vein
  Traumatic rupture of internal jugular vein
  CC +7th S15.321 Major laceration of right internal jugular vein
  CC +7th S15.322 Major laceration of left internal jugular vein
  CC +7th S15.329 Major laceration of unspecified internal jugular vein

- **+ S15.39** Other specified injury of internal jugular vein
  - **CC +7th S15.391** Other specified injury of right internal jugular vein
  - **CC +7th S15.392** Other specified injury of left internal jugular vein
  - **CC +7th S15.399** Other specified injury of unspecified internal jugular vein
- **CC S15.8** Injury of other specified blood vessels at neck level
- **CC S15.9** Injury of unspecified blood vessel at neck level

S16 Injury of muscle, fascia and tendon at neck level

Code also any associated open wound (S11.-)

Excludes2: *sprain of joint or ligament at neck level (S13.9)*

The appropriate 7th character is to be added to each code from category S16
- A initial encounter
- D subsequent encounter
- S sequela

- **X+7th S16.1** Strain of muscle, fascia and tendon at neck level
- **X+7th S16.2** Laceration of muscle, fascia and tendon at neck level
- **X+7th S16.8** Other specified injury of muscle, fascia and tendon at neck level
- **X+7th S16.9** Unspecified injury of muscle, fascia and tendon at neck level

S17 Crushing injury of neck

Use additional code for all associated injuries, such as:
- injury of blood vessels (S15.-)
- open wound of neck (S11.-)
- spinal cord injury (S14.0, S14.1-)
- vertebral fracture (S12.0--S12.3-)

The appropriate 7th character is to be added to each code from category S17
- A initial encounter
- D subsequent encounter
- S sequela

- **CC S17.0** Crushing injury of larynx and trachea
  - **X+7th HAC** 7th character A see Appendix B for HAC conditional logic
- **CC S17.8** Crushing injury of other specified parts of neck
  - **X+7th HAC** 7th character A see Appendix B for HAC conditional logic
- **CC S17.9** Crushing injury of neck, part unspecified
  - **X+7th HAC** 7th character A see Appendix B for HAC conditional logic

S19 Other specified and unspecified injuries of neck

The appropriate 7th character is to be added to each code from category S19
- A initial encounter
- D subsequent encounter
- S sequela

- **+ S19.8** Other specified injuries of neck
  - **X+7th S19.80** Other specified injuries of unspecified part of neck
  - **X+7th S19.81** Other specified injuries of larynx
  - **X+7th S19.82** Other specified injuries of cervical trachea
    - **Excludes2:** *other specified injury of thoracic trachea (S27.5-)*
  - **X+7th S19.83** Other specified injuries of vocal cord
  - **X+7th S19.84** Other specified injuries of thyroid gland
  - **X+7th S19.85** Other specified injuries of pharynx and cervical esophagus
    - *AHA CC: 1Q, 2022, 27-28*
  - **X+7th S19.89** Other specified injuries of other specified part of neck
- **X+7th S19.9** Unspecified injury of neck

Injuries to the thorax (S20-S29)

Includes: injuries of breast
injuries of chest (wall)
injuries of interscapular area

Excludes2: *burns and corrosions (T20-T32)*
effects of foreign body in bronchus (T17.5)
effects of foreign body in esophagus (T18.1)
effects of foreign body in lung (T17.8)
effects of foreign body in trachea (T17.4)
frostbite (T33-T34)
injuries of axilla
injuries of clavicle
injuries of scapular region
injuries of shoulder
insect bite or sting, venomous (T63.4)

S20 Superficial injury of thorax

The appropriate 7th character is to be added to each code from category S20
- A initial encounter
- D subsequent encounter
- S sequela

AHA CC: 4Q, 2020, 39

- **+ S20.0** Contusion of breast
  - **X+7th S20.00** Contusion of breast, unspecified breast
  - **X+7th S20.01** Contusion of right breast
  - **X+7th S20.02** Contusion of left breast
- **+ S20.1** Other and unspecified superficial injuries of breast
  - **+ S20.10** Unspecified superficial injuries of breast
    - **+7th S20.101** Unspecified superficial injuries of breast, right breast
    - **+7th S20.102** Unspecified superficial injuries of breast, left breast
    - **+7th S20.109** Unspecified superficial injuries of breast, unspecified breast
  - **+ S20.11** Abrasion of breast
    - **+7th S20.111** Abrasion of breast, right breast
    - **+7th S20.112** Abrasion of breast, left breast
    - **+7th S20.119** Abrasion of breast, unspecified breast
  - **+ S20.12** Blister (nonthermal) of breast
    - **+7th S20.121** Blister (nonthermal) of breast, right breast
    - **+7th S20.122** Blister (nonthermal) of breast, left breast
    - **+7th S20.129** Blister (nonthermal) of breast, unspecified breast
  - **+ S20.14** External constriction of part of breast
    - **+7th S20.141** External constriction of part of breast, right breast
    - **+7th S20.142** External constriction of part of breast, left breast
    - **+7th S20.149** External constriction of part of breast, unspecified breast
  - **+ S20.15** Superficial foreign body of breast
    Splinter in the breast
    - **+7th S20.151** Superficial foreign body of breast, right breast
    - **+7th S20.152** Superficial foreign body of breast, left breast
    - **+7th S20.159** Superficial foreign body of breast, unspecified breast
  - **+ S20.16** Insect bite (nonvenomous) of breast
    - **+7th S20.161** Insect bite (nonvenomous) of breast, right breast
    - **+7th S20.162** Insect bite (nonvenomous) of breast, left breast
    - **+7th S20.169** Insect bite (nonvenomous) of breast, unspecified breast
  - **+ S20.17** Other superficial bite of breast
    Excludes1: *open bite of breast (S21.05-)*
    - **+7th S20.171** Other superficial bite of breast, right breast
    - **+7th S20.172** Other superficial bite of breast, left breast
    - **+7th S20.179** Other superficial bite of breast, unspecified breast

- **S20.2 Contusion of thorax**
  - X+7th **S20.20** Contusion of thorax, unspecified
  - +**S20.21** Contusion of front wall of thorax
    - +7th S20.211 Contusion of right front wall of thorax
    - +7th S20.212 Contusion of left front wall of thorax
    - +7th S20.213 Contusion of bilateral front wall of thorax
    - +7th S20.214 Contusion of middle front wall of thorax
    - +7th S20.219 Contusion of unspecified front wall of thorax
  - +**S20.22** Contusion of back wall of thorax
    - +7th S20.221 Contusion of right back wall of thorax
    - +7th S20.222 Contusion of left back wall of thorax
    - +7th S20.223 Contusion of bilateral back wall of thorax
    - +7th S20.224 Contusion of middle back wall of thorax
    - +7th S20.229 Contusion of unspecified back wall of thorax
- **S20.3 Other and unspecified superficial injuries of front wall of thorax**
  - +**S20.30** Unspecified superficial injuries of front wall of thorax
    - +7th S20.301 Unspecified superficial injuries of right front wall of thorax
    - +7th S20.302 Unspecified superficial injuries of left front wall of thorax
    - +7th S20.303 Unspecified superficial injuries of bilateral front wall of thorax
    - +7th S20.304 Unspecified superficial injuries of middle front wall of thorax
    - +7th S20.309 Unspecified superficial injuries of unspecified front wall of thorax
  - +**S20.31** Abrasion of front wall of thorax
    - +7th S20.311 Abrasion of right front wall of thorax
    - +7th S20.312 Abrasion of left front wall of thorax
    - +7th S20.313 Abrasion of bilateral front wall of thorax
    - +7th S20.314 Abrasion of middle front wall of thorax
    - +7th S20.319 Abrasion of unspecified front wall of thorax
  - +**S20.32** Blister (nonthermal) of front wall of thorax
    - +7th S20.321 Blister (nonthermal) of right front wall of thorax
    - +7th S20.322 Blister (nonthermal) of left front wall of thorax
    - +7th S20.323 Blister (nonthermal) of bilateral front wall of thorax
    - +7th S20.324 Blister (nonthermal) of middle front wall of thorax
    - +7th S20.329 Blister (nonthermal) of unspecified front wall of thorax
  - +**S20.34** External constriction of front wall of thorax
    - +7th S20.341 External constriction of right front wall of thorax
    - +7th S20.342 External constriction of left front wall of thorax
    - +7th S20.343 External constriction of bilateral front wall of thorax
    - +7th S20.344 External constriction of middle front wall of thorax
    - +7th S20.349 External constriction of unspecified front wall of thorax
  - +**S20.35** Superficial foreign body of front wall of thorax
    Splinter in front wall of thorax
    - +7th S20.351 Superficial foreign body of right front wall of thorax
    - +7th S20.352 Superficial foreign body of left front wall of thorax
    - +7th S20.353 Superficial foreign body of bilateral front wall of thorax
    - +7th S20.354 Superficial foreign body of middle front wall of thorax
    - +7th S20.359 Superficial foreign body of unspecified front wall of thorax
  - +**S20.36** Insect bite (nonvenomous) of front wall of thorax
    - +7th S20.361 Insect bite (nonvenomous) of right front wall of thorax
    - +7th S20.362 Insect bite (nonvenomous) of left front wall of thorax
    - +7th S20.363 Insect bite (nonvenomous) of bilateral front wall of thorax
    - +7th S20.364 Insect bite (nonvenomous) of middle front wall of thorax
    - +7th S20.369 Insect bite (nonvenomous) of unspecified front wall of thorax
  - +**S20.37** Other superficial bite of front wall of thorax
    Excludes1: *open bite of front wall of thorax (S21.14)*
    - +7th S20.371 Other superficial bite of right front wall of thorax
    - +7th S20.372 Other superficial bite of left front wall of thorax
    - +7th S20.373 Other superficial bite of bilateral front wall of thorax
    - +7th S20.374 Other superficial bite of middle front wall of thorax
    - +7th S20.379 Other superficial bite of unspecified front wall of thorax
- **S20.4 Other and unspecified superficial injuries of back wall of thorax**
  - +**S20.40** Unspecified superficial injuries of back wall of thorax
    - +7th S20.401 Unspecified superficial injuries of right back wall of thorax
    - +7th S20.402 Unspecified superficial injuries of left back wall of thorax
    - +7th S20.409 Unspecified superficial injuries of unspecified back wall of thorax
  - +**S20.41** Abrasion of back wall of thorax
    - +7th S20.411 Abrasion of right back wall of thorax
    - +7th S20.412 Abrasion of left back wall of thorax
    - +7th S20.419 Abrasion of unspecified back wall of thorax
  - +**S20.42** Blister (nonthermal) of back wall of thorax
    - +7th S20.421 Blister (nonthermal) of right back wall of thorax
    - +7th S20.422 Blister (nonthermal) of left back wall of thorax
    - +7th S20.429 Blister (nonthermal) of unspecified back wall of thorax
  - +**S20.44** External constriction of back wall of thorax
    - +7th S20.441 External constriction of right back wall of thorax
    - +7th S20.442 External constriction of left back wall of thorax
    - +7th S20.449 External constriction of unspecified back wall of thorax
  - +**S20.45** Superficial foreign body of back wall of thorax
    Splinter of back wall of thorax
    - +7th S20.451 Superficial foreign body of right back wall of thorax
    - +7th S20.452 Superficial foreign body of left back wall of thorax
    - +7th S20.459 Superficial foreign body of unspecified back wall of thorax
  - +**S20.46** Insect bite (nonvenomous) of back wall of thorax
    - +7th S20.461 Insect bite (nonvenomous) of right back wall of thorax
    - +7th S20.462 Insect bite (nonvenomous) of left back wall of thorax
    - +7th S20.469 Insect bite (nonvenomous) of unspecified back wall of thorax
  - +**S20.47** Other superficial bite of back wall of thorax
    Excludes1: *open bite of back wall of thorax (S21.24)*
    - +7th S20.471 Other superficial bite of right back wall of thorax
    - +7th S20.472 Other superficial bite of left back wall of thorax
    - +7th S20.479 Other superficial bite of unspecified back wall of thorax
- **S20.9 Superficial injury of unspecified parts of thorax**
  Excludes1: *contusion of thorax NOS (S20.20)*
  - X+7th **S20.90** Unspecified superficial injury of unspecified parts of thorax
    Superficial injury of thoracic wall NOS
  - X+7th **S20.91** Abrasion of unspecified parts of thorax
  - X+7th **S20.92** Blister (nonthermal) of unspecified parts of thorax

X+7th S20.94 External constriction of unspecified parts of thorax
X+7th S20.95 Superficial foreign body of unspecified parts of thorax
Splinter in thorax NOS
X+7th S20.96 Insect bite (nonvenomous) of unspecified parts of thorax
X+7th S20.97 Other superficial bite of unspecified parts of thorax
Excludes1: open bite of thorax NOS (S21.95)

S21 Open wound of thorax

Code also any associated injury, such as:
 injury of heart (S26.-)
 injury of intrathoracic organs (S27.-)
 rib fracture (S22.3-, S22.4-)
 spinal cord injury (S24.0-, S24.1-)
 traumatic hemothorax (S27.1)
 traumatic hemopneumothorax (S27.3)
 traumatic pneumothorax (S27.0)
 wound infection
Excludes1: traumatic amputation (partial) of thorax (S28.1)

The appropriate 7th character is to be added to each code from category S21
 A initial encounter
 D subsequent encounter
 S sequela

+ **S21.0** Open wound of breast
  + **S21.00** Unspecified open wound of breast
    +7th **S21.001** Unspecified open wound of right breast
    +7th **S21.002** Unspecified open wound of left breast
    +7th **S21.009** Unspecified open wound of unspecified breast
  + **S21.01** Laceration without foreign body of breast
    +7th **S21.011** Laceration without foreign body of right breast
    +7th **S21.012** Laceration without foreign body of left breast
    +7th **S21.019** Laceration without foreign body of unspecified breast
  + **S21.02** Laceration with foreign body of breast
    +7th **S21.021** Laceration with foreign body of right breast
    +7th **S21.022** Laceration with foreign body of left breast
    +7th **S21.029** Laceration with foreign body of unspecified breast
  + **S21.03** Puncture wound without foreign body of breast
    +7th **S21.031** Puncture wound without foreign body of right breast
    +7th **S21.032** Puncture wound without foreign body of left breast
    +7th **S21.039** Puncture wound without foreign body of unspecified breast
  + **S21.04** Puncture wound with foreign body of breast
    +7th **S21.041** Puncture wound with foreign body of right breast
    +7th **S21.042** Puncture wound with foreign body of left breast
    +7th **S21.049** Puncture wound with foreign body of unspecified breast
  + **S21.05** Open bite of breast
    Bite of breast NOS
    Excludes1: superficial bite of breast (S20.17)
    S21.051 Open bite of right breast
    S21.052 Open bite of left breast
    S21.059 Open bite of unspecified breast
+ **S21.1** Open wound of front wall of thorax without penetration into thoracic cavity
  Open wound of chest without penetration into thoracic cavity
  + **S21.10** Unspecified open wound of front wall of thorax without penetration into thoracic cavity
    CC +7th **S21.101** Unspecified open wound of right front wall of thorax without penetration into thoracic cavity
    CC +7th **S21.102** Unspecified open wound of left front wall of thorax without penetration into thoracic cavity
    CC +7th **S21.109** Unspecified open wound of unspecified front wall of thorax without penetration into thoracic cavity
  + **S21.11** Laceration without foreign body of front wall of thorax without penetration into thoracic cavity
    CC +7th **S21.111** Laceration without foreign body of right front wall of thorax without penetration into thoracic cavity
    CC +7th **S21.112** Laceration without foreign body of left front wall of thorax without penetration into thoracic cavity
    CC +7th **S21.119** Laceration without foreign body of unspecified front wall of thorax without penetration into thoracic cavity
  + **S21.12** Laceration with foreign body of front wall of thorax without penetration into thoracic cavity
    CC +7th **S21.121** Laceration with foreign body of right front wall of thorax without penetration into thoracic cavity
    CC +7th **S21.122** Laceration with foreign body of left front wall of thorax without penetration into thoracic cavity
    CC +7th **S21.129** Laceration with foreign body of unspecified front wall of thorax without penetration into thoracic cavity
  + **S21.13** Puncture wound without foreign body of front wall of thorax without penetration into thoracic cavity
    CC +7th **S21.131** Puncture wound without foreign body of right front wall of thorax without penetration into thoracic cavity
    CC +7th **S21.132** Puncture wound without foreign body of left front wall of thorax without penetration into thoracic cavity
    CC +7th **S21.139** Puncture wound without foreign body of unspecified front wall of thorax without penetration into thoracic cavity
  + **S21.14** Puncture wound with foreign body of front wall of thorax without penetration into thoracic cavity
    CC +7th **S21.141** Puncture wound with foreign body of right front wall of thorax without penetration into thoracic cavity
    CC +7th **S21.142** Puncture wound with foreign body of left front wall of thorax without penetration into thoracic cavity
    CC +7th **S21.149** Puncture wound with foreign body of unspecified front wall of thorax without penetration into thoracic cavity
  + **S21.15** Open bite of front wall of thorax without penetration into thoracic cavity
    Bite of front wall of thorax NOS
    Excludes1: superficial bite of front wall of thorax (S20.37)
    CC +7th **S21.151** Open bite of right front wall of thorax without penetration into thoracic cavity
    CC +7th **S21.152** Open bite of left front wall of thorax without penetration into thoracic cavity
    CC +7th **S21.159** Open bite of unspecified front wall of thorax without penetration into thoracic cavity
+ **S21.2** Open wound of back wall of thorax without penetration into thoracic cavity
  + **S21.20** Unspecified open wound of back wall of thorax without penetration into thoracic cavity
    +7th **S21.201** Unspecified open wound of right back wall of thorax without penetration into thoracic cavity
    +7th **S21.202** Unspecified open wound of left back wall of thorax without penetration into thoracic cavity
    +7th **S21.209** Unspecified open wound of unspecified back wall of thorax without penetration into thoracic cavity
  + **S21.21** Laceration without foreign body of back wall of thorax without penetration into thoracic cavity
    +7th **S21.211** Laceration without foreign body of right back wall of thorax without penetration into thoracic cavity

- +7th **S21.212** Laceration without foreign body of left back wall of thorax without penetration into thoracic cavity
- +7th **S21.219** Laceration without foreign body of unspecified back wall of thorax without penetration into thoracic cavity
- + **S21.22** Laceration with foreign body of back wall of thorax without penetration into thoracic cavity
  - +7th **S21.221** Laceration with foreign body of right back wall of thorax without penetration into thoracic cavity
  - +7th **S21.222** Laceration with foreign body of left back wall of thorax without penetration into thoracic cavity
  - +7th **S21.229** Laceration with foreign body of unspecified back wall of thorax without penetration into thoracic cavity
- + **S21.23** Puncture wound without foreign body of back wall of thorax without penetration into thoracic cavity
  - +7th **S21.231** Puncture wound without foreign body of right back wall of thorax without penetration into thoracic cavity
  - +7th **S21.232** Puncture wound without foreign body of left back wall of thorax without penetration into thoracic cavity
  - +7th **S21.239** Puncture wound without foreign body of unspecified back wall of thorax without penetration into thoracic cavity
- + **S21.24** Puncture wound with foreign body of back wall of thorax without penetration into thoracic cavity
  - +7th **S21.241** Puncture wound with foreign body of right back wall of thorax without penetration into thoracic cavity
  - +7th **S21.242** Puncture wound with foreign body of left back wall of thorax without penetration into thoracic cavity
  - +7th **S21.249** Puncture wound with foreign body of unspecified back wall of thorax without penetration into thoracic cavity
- + **S21.25** Open bite of back wall of thorax without penetration into thoracic cavity
  Bite of back wall of thorax NOS
  Excludes1: *superficial bite of back wall of thorax (S20.47)*
  - +7th **S21.251** Open bite of right back wall of thorax without penetration into thoracic cavity
  - +7th **S21.252** Open bite of left back wall of thorax without penetration into thoracic cavity
  - +7th **S21.259** Open bite of unspecified back wall of thorax without penetration into thoracic cavity
- + **S21.3** Open wound of front wall of thorax with penetration into thoracic cavity
  Open wound of chest with penetration into thoracic cavity
  - + **S21.30** Unspecified open wound of front wall of thorax with penetration into thoracic cavity
    - MCC +7th **S21.301** Unspecified open wound of right front wall of thorax with penetration into thoracic cavity
    - MCC +7th **S21.302** Unspecified open wound of left front wall of thorax with penetration into thoracic cavity
    - MCC +7th **S21.309** Unspecified open wound of unspecified front wall of thorax with penetration into thoracic cavity
  - + **S21.31** Laceration without foreign body of front wall of thorax with penetration into thoracic cavity
    - MCC +7th **S21.311** Laceration without foreign body of right front wall of thorax with penetration into thoracic cavity
    - MCC +7th **S21.312** Laceration without foreign body of left front wall of thorax with penetration into thoracic cavity
    - MCC +7th **S21.319** Laceration without foreign body of unspecified front wall of thorax with penetration into thoracic cavity

- + **S21.32** Laceration with foreign body of front wall of thorax with penetration into thoracic cavity
  - MCC +7th **S21.321** Laceration with foreign body of right front wall of thorax with penetration into thoracic cavity
  - MCC +7th **S21.322** Laceration with foreign body of left front wall of thorax with penetration into thoracic cavity
  - MCC +7th **S21.329** Laceration with foreign body of unspecified front wall of thorax with penetration into thoracic cavity
- + **S21.33** Puncture wound without foreign body of front wall of thorax with penetration into thoracic cavity
  - MCC +7th **S21.331** Puncture wound without foreign body of right front wall of thorax with penetration into thoracic cavity
  - MCC +7th **S21.332** Puncture wound without foreign body of left front wall of thorax with penetration into thoracic cavity
  - MCC +7th **S21.339** Puncture wound without foreign body of unspecified front wall of thorax with penetration into thoracic cavity
- + **S21.34** Puncture wound with foreign body of front wall of thorax with penetration into thoracic cavity
  - MCC +7th **S21.341** Puncture wound with foreign body of right front wall of thorax with penetration into thoracic cavity
  - MCC +7th **S21.342** Puncture wound with foreign body of left front wall of thorax with penetration into thoracic cavity
  - MCC +7th **S21.349** Puncture wound with foreign body of unspecified front wall of thorax with penetration into thoracic cavity
- + **S21.35** Open bite of front wall of thorax with penetration into thoracic cavity
  Excludes1: *superficial bite of front wall of thorax (S20.37)*
  - MCC +7th **S21.351** Open bite of right front wall of thorax with penetration into thoracic cavity
  - MCC +7th **S21.352** Open bite of left front wall of thorax with penetration into thoracic cavity
  - MCC +7th **S21.359** Open bite of unspecified front wall of thorax with penetration into thoracic cavity
- + **S21.4** Open wound of back wall of thorax with penetration into thoracic cavity
  - + **S21.40** Unspecified open wound of back wall of thorax with penetration into thoracic cavity
    - MCC +7th **S21.401** Unspecified open wound of right back wall of thorax with penetration into thoracic cavity
    - MCC +7th **S21.402** Unspecified open wound of left back wall of thorax with penetration into thoracic cavity
    - MCC +7th **S21.409** Unspecified open wound of unspecified back wall of thorax with penetration into thoracic cavity
  - + **S21.41** Laceration without foreign body of back wall of thorax with penetration into thoracic cavity
    - MCC +7th **S21.411** Laceration without foreign body of right back wall of thorax with penetration into thoracic cavity
    - MCC +7th **S21.412** Laceration without foreign body of left back wall of thorax with penetration into thoracic cavity
    - MCC +7th **S21.419** Laceration without foreign body of unspecified back wall of thorax with penetration into thoracic cavity
  - + **S21.42** Laceration with foreign body of back wall of thorax with penetration into thoracic cavity
    - MCC +7th **S21.421** Laceration with foreign body of right back wall of thorax with penetration into thoracic cavity
    - MCC +7th **S21.422** Laceration with foreign body of left back wall of thorax with penetration into thoracic cavity

MCC +7th S21.429 Laceration with foreign body of unspecified back wall of thorax with penetration into thoracic cavity

+ S21.43 Puncture wound without foreign body of back wall of thorax with penetration into thoracic cavity

MCC +7th S21.431 Puncture wound without foreign body of right back wall of thorax with penetration into thoracic cavity

MCC +7th S21.432 Puncture wound without foreign body of left back wall of thorax with penetration into thoracic cavity

MCC +7th S21.439 Puncture wound without foreign body of unspecified back wall of thorax with penetration into thoracic cavity

+ S21.44 Puncture wound with foreign body of back wall of thorax with penetration into thoracic cavity

MCC +7th S21.441 Puncture wound with foreign body of right back wall of thorax with penetration into thoracic cavity

MCC +7th S21.442 Puncture wound with foreign body of left back wall of thorax with penetration into thoracic cavity

MCC +7th S21.449 Puncture wound with foreign body of unspecified back wall of thorax with penetration into thoracic cavity

+ S21.45 Open bite of back wall of thorax with penetration into thoracic cavity
　　Bite of back wall of thorax NOS
　　Excludes1: superficial bite of back wall of thorax (S20.47)

MCC +7th S21.451 Open bite of right back wall of thorax with penetration into thoracic cavity

MCC +7th S21.452 Open bite of left back wall of thorax with penetration into thoracic cavity

MCC +7th S21.459 Open bite of unspecified back wall of thorax with penetration into thoracic cavity

+ S21.9 Open wound of unspecified part of thorax
　　Open wound of thoracic wall NOS

CC X+7th S21.90 Unspecified open wound of unspecified part of thorax

CC X+7th S21.91 Laceration without foreign body of unspecified part of thorax

CC X+7th S21.92 Laceration with foreign body of unspecified part of thorax

CC X+7th S21.93 Puncture wound without foreign body of unspecified part of thorax

CC X+7th S21.94 Puncture wound with foreign body of unspecified part of thorax

CC X+7th S21.95 Open bite of unspecified part of thorax
　　Excludes1: superficial bite of thorax (S20.97)

See page 1007 for Vertebrae Illustration.

S22 Fracture of rib(s), sternum and thoracic spine

NOTE A fracture not indicated as displaced or nondisplaced should be coded to displaced
A fracture not indicated as open or closed should be coded to closed

Includes: fracture of thoracic neural arch
fracture of thoracic spinous process
fracture of thoracic transverse process
fracture of thoracic vertebra
fracture of thoracic vertebral arch

Code also, if applicable, any associated:
injury of intrathoracic organ (S27.-)
spinal cord injury (S24.0-, S24.1-)

Excludes1: transection of thorax (S28.1)
Excludes2: fracture of clavicle (S42.0-)
fracture of scapula (S42.1-)

The appropriate 7th character is to be added to each code from category S22
A   initial encounter for closed fracture
B   initial encounter for open fracture
D   subsequent encounter for fracture with routine healing
G   subsequent encounter for fracture with delayed healing
K   subsequent encounter for fracture with nonunion
S   sequela

Review coding guideline C.19.c

+ S22.0 Fracture of thoracic vertebra

+ S22.00 Fracture of unspecified thoracic vertebra

CC MCC +7th S22.000 Wedge compression fracture of unspecified thoracic vertebra
　　HAC 7th characters A & B see Appendix B for HAC conditional logic

CC MCC +7th S22.001 Stable burst fracture of unspecified thoracic vertebra
　　HAC 7th characters A & B see Appendix B for HAC conditional logic

CC MCC +7th S22.002 Unstable burst fracture of unspecified thoracic vertebra
　　HAC 7th characters A & B see Appendix B for HAC conditional logic

CC MCC +7th S22.008 Other fracture of unspecified thoracic vertebra
　　HAC 7th characters A & B see Appendix B for HAC conditional logic

CC MCC +7th S22.009 Unspecified fracture of unspecified thoracic vertebra
　　HAC 7th characters A & B see Appendix B for HAC conditional logic

+ S22.01 Fracture of first thoracic vertebra

CC MCC +7th S22.010 Wedge compression fracture of first thoracic vertebra
　　HAC 7th characters A & B see Appendix B for HAC conditional logic

CC MCC +7th S22.011 Stable burst fracture of first thoracic vertebra
　　HAC 7th characters A & B see Appendix B for HAC conditional logic

CC MCC +7th S22.012 Unstable burst fracture of first thoracic vertebra
　　HAC 7th characters A & B see Appendix B for HAC conditional logic

CC MCC +7th S22.018 Other fracture of first thoracic vertebra
　　HAC 7th characters A & B see Appendix B for HAC conditional logic

CC MCC +7th S22.019 Unspecified fracture of first thoracic vertebra
　　HAC 7th characters A & B see Appendix B for HAC conditional logic

+ S22.02 Fracture of second thoracic vertebra

CC MCC +7th S22.020 Wedge compression fracture of second thoracic vertebra
　　HAC 7th characters A & B see Appendix B for HAC conditional logic

CC MCC +7th S22.021 Stable burst fracture of second thoracic vertebra
　　HAC 7th characters A & B see Appendix B for HAC conditional logic

CC MCC +7th S22.022 Unstable burst fracture of second thoracic vertebra
　　HAC 7th characters A & B see Appendix B for HAC conditional logic

CC MCC +7th S22.028 Other fracture of second thoracic vertebra
　　HAC 7th characters A & B see Appendix B for HAC conditional logic

CC MCC +7th S22.029 Unspecified fracture of second thoracic vertebra
　　HAC 7th characters A & B see Appendix B for HAC conditional logic

+ S22.03 Fracture of third thoracic vertebra

CC MCC +7th S22.030 Wedge compression fracture of third thoracic vertebra
　　HAC 7th characters A & B see Appendix B for HAC conditional logic

CC MCC +7th S22.031 Stable burst fracture of third thoracic vertebra
　　HAC 7th characters A & B see Appendix B for HAC conditional logic

CC MCC +7th S22.032 Unstable burst fracture of third thoracic vertebra
　　HAC 7th characters A & B see Appendix B for HAC conditional logic

CC MCC +7th S22.038 Other fracture of third thoracic vertebra
　　HAC 7th characters A & B see Appendix B for HAC conditional logic

CC MCC +7th S22.039 Unspecified fracture of third thoracic vertebra
　　HAC 7th characters A & B see Appendix B for HAC conditional logic

+	S22.04	Fracture of fourth thoracic vertebra
CC MCC +7th	S22.040	Wedge compression fracture of fourth thoracic vertebra
		HAC 7th characters A & B see Appendix B for HAC conditional logic
CC MCC +7th	S22.041	Stable burst fracture of fourth thoracic vertebra
		HAC 7th characters A & B see Appendix B for HAC conditional logic
CC MCC +7th	S22.042	Unstable burst fracture of fourth thoracic vertebra
		HAC 7th characters A & B see Appendix B for HAC conditional logic
CC MCC +7th	S22.048	Other fracture of fourth thoracic vertebra
		HAC 7th characters A & B see Appendix B for HAC conditional logic
CC MCC +7th	S22.049	Unspecified fracture of fourth thoracic vertebra
		HAC 7th characters A & B see Appendix B for HAC conditional logic
+	S22.05	Fracture of T5-T6 vertebra
CC MCC +7th	S22.050	Wedge compression fracture of T5-T6 vertebra
		HAC 7th characters A & B see Appendix B for HAC conditional logic
CC MCC +7th	S22.051	Stable burst fracture of T5-T6 vertebra
		HAC 7th characters A & B see Appendix B for HAC conditional logic
CC MCC +7th	S22.052	Unstable burst fracture of T5-T6 vertebra
		HAC 7th characters A & B see Appendix B for HAC conditional logic
CC MCC +7th	S22.058	Other fracture of T5-T6 vertebra
		HAC 7th characters A & B see Appendix B for HAC conditional logic
CC MCC +7th	S22.059	Unspecified fracture of T5-T6 vertebra
		HAC 7th characters A & B see Appendix B for HAC conditional logic
+	S22.06	Fracture of T7-T8 vertebra
CC MCC +7th	S22.060	Wedge compression fracture of T7-T8 vertebra
		HAC 7th characters A & B see Appendix B for HAC conditional logic
CC MCC +7th	S22.061	Stable burst fracture of T7-T8 vertebra
		HAC 7th characters A & B see Appendix B for HAC conditional logic
CC MCC +7th	S22.062	Unstable burst fracture of T7-T8 vertebra
		HAC 7th characters A & B see Appendix B for HAC conditional logic
CC MCC +7th	S22.068	Other fracture of T7-T8 thoracic vertebra
		HAC 7th characters A & B see Appendix B for HAC conditional logic
CC MCC +7th	S22.069	Unspecified fracture of T7-T8 vertebra
		HAC 7th characters A & B see Appendix B for HAC conditional logic
+	S22.07	Fracture of T9-T10 vertebra
CC MCC +7th	S22.070	Wedge compression fracture of T9-T10 vertebra
		HAC 7th characters A & B see Appendix B for HAC conditional logic
CC MCC +7th	S22.071	Stable burst fracture of T9-T10 vertebra
		HAC 7th characters A & B see Appendix B for HAC conditional logic
CC MCC +7th	S22.072	Unstable burst fracture of T9-T10 vertebra
		HAC 7th characters A & B see Appendix B for HAC conditional logic
CC MCC +7th	S22.078	Other fracture of T9-T10 vertebra
		HAC 7th characters A & B see Appendix B for HAC conditional logic
CC MCC +7th	S22.079	Unspecified fracture of T9-T10 vertebra
		HAC 7th characters A & B see Appendix B for HAC conditional logic
+	S22.08	Fracture of T11-T12 vertebra
CC MCC +7th	S22.080	Wedge compression fracture of T11-T12 vertebra
		HAC 7th characters A & B see Appendix B for HAC conditional logic
CC MCC +7th	S22.081	Stable burst fracture of T11-T12 vertebra
		HAC 7th characters A & B see Appendix B for HAC conditional logic
CC MCC +7th	S22.082	Unstable burst fracture of T11-T12 vertebra
		HAC 7th characters A & B see Appendix B for HAC conditional logic
CC MCC +7th	S22.088	Other fracture of T11-T12 vertebra
		HAC 7th characters A & B see Appendix B for HAC conditional logic
CC MCC +7th	S22.089	Unspecified fracture of T11-T12 vertebra
		HAC 7th characters A & B see Appendix B for HAC conditional logic
+	S22.2	Fracture of sternum
MCC X+7th	S22.20	Unspecified fracture of sternum
		HAC 7th characters A & B see Appendix B for HAC conditional logic
CC MCC X+7th	S22.21	Fracture of manubrium
		HAC 7th characters A & B see Appendix B for HAC conditional logic
CC MCC X+7th	S22.22	Fracture of body of sternum
		HAC 7th characters A & B see Appendix B for HAC conditional logic
CC MCC X+7th	S22.23	Sternal manubrial dissociation
		HAC 7th characters A & B see Appendix B for HAC conditional logic
CC MCC X+7th	S22.24	Fracture of xiphoid process
		HAC 7th characters A & B see Appendix B for HAC conditional logic
+	S22.3	Fracture of one rib
CC MCC X+7th	S22.31	Fracture of one rib, right side
		HAC 7th characters A & B see Appendix B for HAC conditional logic
CC MCC X+7th	S22.32	Fracture of one rib, left side
		HAC 7th characters A & B see Appendix B for HAC conditional logic
CC MCC X+7th	S22.39	Fracture of one rib, unspecified side
		HAC 7th characters A & B see Appendix B for HAC conditional logic
+	S22.4	Multiple fractures of ribs
		Fractures of two or more ribs
		Excludes1: flail chest (S22.5-)
CC MCC X+7th	S22.41	Multiple fractures of ribs, right side
		HAC 7th characters A & B see Appendix B for HAC conditional logic
CC MCC X+7th	S22.42	Multiple fractures of ribs, left side
		HAC 7th characters A & B see Appendix B for HAC conditional logic
CC MCC X+7th	S22.43	Multiple fractures of ribs, bilateral
		HAC 7th characters A & B see Appendix B for HAC conditional logic
CC MCC X+7th	S22.49	Multiple fractures of ribs, unspecified side
		HAC 7th characters A & B see Appendix B for HAC conditional logic
X+7th	S22.5	Flail chest
		HAC 7th characters A & B see Appendix B for HAC conditional logic
X+7th	S22.9	Fracture of bony thorax, part unspecified
		HAC 7th characters A & B see Appendix B for HAC conditional logic

S23 Dislocation and sprain of joints and ligaments of thorax

Includes: avulsion of joint or ligament of thorax
laceration of cartilage, joint or ligament of thorax
sprain of cartilage, joint or ligament of thorax
traumatic hemarthrosis of joint or ligament of thorax
traumatic rupture of joint or ligament of thorax
traumatic subluxation of joint or ligament of thorax
traumatic tear of joint or ligament of thorax

Code also any associated open wound

Excludes2: dislocation, sprain of sternoclavicular joint (S43.2, S43.6)
strain of muscle or tendon of thorax (S29.01-)

The appropriate 7th character is to be added to each code from category S23
A initial encounter
D subsequent encounter
S sequela

X+7th	S23.0	Traumatic rupture of thoracic intervertebral disc
		Excludes1: rupture or displacement (nontraumatic) of thoracic intervertebral disc NOS (M51.- with fifth character 4)

- **S23.1 Subluxation and dislocation of thoracic vertebra**
  Code also any associated:
  open wound of thorax (S21.-)
  spinal cord injury (S24.0-, S24.1-)
  Excludes2: fracture of thoracic vertebrae (S22.0-)
  - **+ S23.10 Subluxation and dislocation of unspecified thoracic vertebra**
    - +7th S23.100 Subluxation of unspecified thoracic vertebra
    - +7th S23.101 Dislocation of unspecified thoracic vertebra
  - **+ S23.11 Subluxation and dislocation of T1/T2 thoracic vertebra**
    - +7th S23.110 Subluxation of T1/T2 thoracic vertebra
    - +7th S23.111 Dislocation of T1/T2 thoracic vertebra
  - **+ S23.12 Subluxation and dislocation of T2/T3-T3/T4 thoracic vertebra**
    - +7th S23.120 Subluxation of T2/T3 thoracic vertebra
    - +7th S23.121 Dislocation of T2/T3 thoracic vertebra
    - +7th S23.122 Subluxation of T3/T4 thoracic vertebra
    - +7th S23.123 Dislocation of T3/T4 thoracic vertebra
  - **+ S23.13 Subluxation and dislocation of T4/T5-T5/T6 thoracic vertebra**
    - +7th S23.130 Subluxation of T4/T5 thoracic vertebra
    - +7th S23.131 Dislocation of T4/T5 thoracic vertebra
    - +7th S23.132 Subluxation of T5/T6 thoracic vertebra
    - +7th S23.133 Dislocation of T5/T6 thoracic vertebra
  - **+ S23.14 Subluxation and dislocation of T6/T7-T7/T8 thoracic vertebra**
    - +7th S23.140 Subluxation of T6/T7 thoracic vertebra
    - +7th S23.141 Dislocation of T6/T7 thoracic vertebra
    - +7th S23.142 Subluxation of T7/T8 thoracic vertebra
    - +7th S23.143 Dislocation of T7/T8 thoracic vertebra
  - **+ S23.15 Subluxation and dislocation of T8/T9-T9/T10 thoracic vertebra**
    - +7th S23.150 Subluxation of T8/T9 thoracic vertebra
    - +7th S23.151 Dislocation of T8/T9 thoracic vertebra
    - +7th S23.152 Subluxation of T9/T10 thoracic vertebra
    - +7th S23.153 Dislocation of T9/T10 thoracic vertebra
  - **+ S23.16 Subluxation and dislocation of T10/T11-T11/T12 thoracic vertebra**
    - +7th S23.160 Subluxation of T10/T11 thoracic vertebra
    - +7th S23.161 Dislocation of T10/T11 thoracic vertebra
    - +7th S23.162 Subluxation of T11/T12 thoracic vertebra
    - +7th S23.163 Dislocation of T11/T12 thoracic vertebra
  - **+ S23.17 Subluxation and dislocation of T12/L1 thoracic vertebra**
    - +7th S23.170 Subluxation of T12/L1 thoracic vertebra
    - +7th S23.171 Dislocation of T12/L1 thoracic vertebra
- **+ S23.2 Dislocation of other and unspecified parts of thorax**
  - X+7th S23.20 Dislocation of unspecified part of thorax
  - X+7th S23.29 Dislocation of other parts of thorax
- X+7th **S23.3 Sprain of ligaments of thoracic spine**
- **+ S23.4 Sprain of ribs and sternum**
  - X+7th S23.41 Sprain of ribs
  - **+ S23.42 Sprain of sternum**
    - +7th S23.420 Sprain of sternoclavicular (joint) (ligament)
    - +7th S23.421 Sprain of chondrosternal joint
    - +7th S23.428 Other sprain of sternum
    - +7th S23.429 Unspecified sprain of sternum
- X+7th **S23.8 Sprain of other specified parts of thorax**
- X+7th **S23.9 Sprain of unspecified parts of thorax**

S24 Injury of nerves and spinal cord at thorax level

NOTE Code to highest level of thoracic spinal cord injury
Injuries to the spinal cord (S24.0 and S24.1) refer to the cord level and not bone level injury, and can affect nerve roots at and below the level given.

Code also any associated:
fracture of thoracic vertebra (S22.0-)
open wound of thorax (S21.-)
transient paralysis (R29.5)
Excludes2: injury of brachial plexus (S14.3)

The appropriate 7th character is to be added to each code from category S24
- A initial encounter
- D subsequent encounter
- S sequela

- MCC X+7th **S24.0 Concussion and edema of thoracic spinal cord**
- **+ S24.1 Other and unspecified injuries of thoracic spinal cord**
  - **+ S24.10 Unspecified injury of thoracic spinal cord**
    - MCC +7th S24.101 Unspecified injury at T1 level of thoracic spinal cord
      - HAC 7th character A see Appendix B for HAC conditional logic
    - MCC +7th S24.102 Unspecified injury at T2-T6 level of thoracic spinal cord
      - HAC 7th character A see Appendix B for HAC conditional logic
    - MCC +7th S24.103 Unspecified injury at T7-T10 level of thoracic spinal cord
      - HAC 7th character A see Appendix B for HAC conditional logic
    - MCC +7th S24.104 Unspecified injury at T11-T12 level of thoracic spinal cord
      - HAC 7th character A see Appendix B for HAC conditional logic
    - +7th S24.109 Unspecified injury at unspecified level of thoracic spinal cord
      Injury of thoracic spinal cord NOS
      - HAC 7th character A see Appendix B for HAC conditional logic
  - **+ S24.11 Complete lesion of thoracic spinal cord**
    - MCC +7th S24.111 Complete lesion at T1 level of thoracic spinal cord
      - HAC 7th character A see Appendix B for HAC conditional logic
    - MCC +7th S24.112 Complete lesion at T2-T6 level of thoracic spinal cord
      - HAC 7th character A see Appendix B for HAC conditional logic
    - MCC +7th S24.113 Complete lesion at T7-T10 level of thoracic spinal cord
      - HAC 7th character A see Appendix B for HAC conditional logic
    - MCC +7th S24.114 Complete lesion at T11-T12 level of thoracic spinal cord
      - HAC 7th character A see Appendix B for HAC conditional logic
    - +7th S24.119 Complete lesion at unspecified level of thoracic spinal cord
  - **+ S24.13 Anterior cord syndrome of thoracic spinal cord**
    - MCC +7th S24.131 Anterior cord syndrome at T1 level of thoracic spinal cord
      - HAC 7th character A see Appendix B for HAC conditional logic
    - MCC +7th S24.132 Anterior cord syndrome at T2-T6 level of thoracic spinal cord
      - HAC 7th character A see Appendix B for HAC conditional logic
    - MCC +7th S24.133 Anterior cord syndrome at T7-T10 level of thoracic spinal cord
      - HAC 7th character A see Appendix B for HAC conditional logic
    - MCC +7th S24.134 Anterior cord syndrome at T11-T12 level of thoracic spinal cord
      - HAC 7th character A see Appendix B for HAC conditional logic
    - +7th S24.139 Anterior cord syndrome at unspecified level of thoracic spinal cord

- **+ S24.14** Brown-Séquard syndrome of thoracic spinal cord
  - **MCC +7th S24.141** Brown-Séquard syndrome at T1 level of thoracic spinal cord
  - **MCC +7th S24.142** Brown-Séquard syndrome at T2-T6 level of thoracic spinal cord
  - **MCC +7th S24.143** Brown-Séquard syndrome at T7-T10 level of thoracic spinal cord
  - **MCC +7th S24.144** Brown-Séquard syndrome at T11-T12 level of thoracic spinal cord
  - **+7th S24.149** Brown-Séquard syndrome at unspecified level of thoracic spinal cord
- **+ S24.15** Other incomplete lesions of thoracic spinal cord
  - Incomplete lesion of thoracic spinal cord NOS
  - Posterior cord syndrome of thoracic spinal cord
  - **MCC +7th S24.151** Other incomplete lesion at T1 level of thoracic spinal cord
    - **HAC** 7th character A see Appendix B for HAC conditional logic
  - **MCC +7th S24.152** Other incomplete lesion at T2-T6 level of thoracic spinal cord
    - **HAC** 7th character A see Appendix B for HAC conditional logic
  - **MCC +7th S24.153** Other incomplete lesion at T7-T10 level of thoracic spinal cord
    - **HAC** 7th character A see Appendix B for HAC conditional logic
  - **MCC +7th S24.154** Other incomplete lesion at T11-T12 level of thoracic spinal cord
    - **HAC** 7th character A see Appendix B for HAC conditional logic
  - **+7th S24.159** Other incomplete lesion at unspecified level of thoracic spinal cord
- **X+7th S24.2** Injury of nerve root of thoracic spine
- **X+7th S24.3** Injury of peripheral nerves of thorax
- **X+7th S24.4** Injury of thoracic sympathetic nervous system
  - Injury of cardiac plexus
  - Injury of esophageal plexus
  - Injury of pulmonary plexus
  - Injury of stellate ganglion
  - Injury of thoracic sympathetic ganglion
- **X+7th S24.8** Injury of other specified nerves of thorax
- **X+7th S24.9** Injury of unspecified nerve of thorax

S25 Injury of blood vessels of thorax

Code also any associated open wound (S21.-)

> The appropriate 7th character is to be added to each code from category S25
> A initial encounter
> D subsequent encounter
> S sequela

- **+ S25.0** Injury of thoracic aorta
  - Injury of aorta NOS
  - **MCC X+7th S25.00** Unspecified injury of thoracic aorta
  - **MCC X+7th S25.01** Minor laceration of thoracic aorta
    - Incomplete transection of thoracic aorta
    - Laceration of thoracic aorta NOS
    - Superficial laceration of thoracic aorta
  - **MCC X+7th S25.02** Major laceration of thoracic aorta
    - Complete transection of thoracic aorta
    - Traumatic rupture of thoracic aorta
  - **MCC X+7th S25.09** Other specified injury of thoracic aorta
- **+ S25.1** Injury of innominate or subclavian artery
  - **+ S25.10** Unspecified injury of innominate or subclavian artery
    - **MCC +7th S25.101** Unspecified injury of right innominate or subclavian artery
    - **MCC +7th S25.102** Unspecified injury of left innominate or subclavian artery
    - **MCC +7th S25.109** Unspecified injury of unspecified innominate or subclavian artery
  - **+ S25.11** Minor laceration of innominate or subclavian artery
    - Incomplete transection of innominate or subclavian artery
    - Laceration of innominate or subclavian artery NOS
    - Superficial laceration of innominate or subclavian artery
    - **MCC +7th S25.111** Minor laceration of right innominate or subclavian artery
    - **MCC +7th S25.112** Minor laceration of left innominate or subclavian artery
    - **MCC +7th S25.119** Minor laceration of unspecified innominate or subclavian artery
  - **+ S25.12** Major laceration of innominate or subclavian artery
    - Complete transection of innominate or subclavian artery
    - Traumatic rupture of innominate or subclavian artery
    - **MCC +7th S25.121** Major laceration of right innominate or subclavian artery
    - **MCC +7th S25.122** Major laceration of left innominate or subclavian artery
    - **MCC +7th S25.129** Major laceration of unspecified innominate or subclavian artery
  - **+ S25.19** Other specified injury of innominate or subclavian artery
    - **MCC +7th S25.191** Other specified injury of right innominate or subclavian artery
    - **MCC +7th S25.192** Other specified injury of left innominate or subclavian artery
    - **MCC +7th S25.199** Other specified injury of unspecified innominate or subclavian artery
- **+ S25.2** Injury of superior vena cava
  - Injury of vena cava NOS
  - **MCC X+7th S25.20** Unspecified injury of superior vena cava
  - **MCC X+7th S25.21** Minor laceration of superior vena cava
    - Incomplete transection of superior vena cava
    - Laceration of superior vena cava NOS
    - Superficial laceration of superior vena cava
  - **MCC X+7th S25.22** Major laceration of superior vena cava
    - Complete transection of superior vena cava
    - Traumatic rupture of superior vena cava
  - **MCC X+7th S25.29** Other specified injury of superior vena cava
- **+ S25.3** Injury of innominate or subclavian vein
  - **+ S25.30** Unspecified injury of innominate or subclavian vein
    - **MCC +7th S25.301** Unspecified injury of right innominate or subclavian vein
    - **MCC +7th S25.302** Unspecified injury of left innominate or subclavian vein
    - **MCC +7th S25.309** Unspecified injury of unspecified innominate or subclavian vein
  - **+ S25.31** Minor laceration of innominate or subclavian vein
    - Incomplete transection of innominate or subclavian vein
    - Laceration of innominate or subclavian vein NOS
    - Superficial laceration of innominate or subclavian vein
    - **MCC +7th S25.311** Minor laceration of right innominate or subclavian vein
    - **MCC +7th S25.312** Minor laceration of left innominate or subclavian vein
    - **MCC +7th S25.319** Minor laceration of unspecified innominate or subclavian vein
  - **+ S25.32** Major laceration of innominate or subclavian vein
    - Complete transection of innominate or subclavian vein
    - Traumatic rupture of innominate or subclavian vein
    - **MCC +7th S25.321** Major laceration of right innominate or subclavian vein
    - **MCC +7th S25.322** Major laceration of left innominate or subclavian vein
    - **MCC +7th S25.329** Major laceration of unspecified innominate or subclavian vein
  - **+ S25.39** Other specified injury of innominate or subclavian vein
    - **MCC +7th S25.391** Other specified injury of right innominate or subclavian vein
    - **MCC +7th S25.392** Other specified injury of left innominate or subclavian vein
    - **MCC +7th S25.399** Other specified injury of unspecified innominate or subclavian vein

- **+ S25.4 Injury of pulmonary blood vessels**
  - **+ S25.40 Unspecified injury of pulmonary blood vessels**
    - MCC +7th S25.401 Unspecified injury of right pulmonary blood vessels
    - MCC +7th S25.402 Unspecified injury of left pulmonary blood vessels
    - MCC +7th S25.409 Unspecified injury of unspecified pulmonary blood vessels
  - **+ S25.41 Minor laceration of pulmonary blood vessels**
    - Incomplete transection of pulmonary blood vessels
    - Laceration of pulmonary blood vessels NOS
    - Superficial laceration of pulmonary blood vessels
    - MCC +7th S25.411 Minor laceration of right pulmonary blood vessels
    - MCC +7th S25.412 Minor laceration of left pulmonary blood vessels
    - MCC +7th S25.419 Minor laceration of unspecified pulmonary blood vessels
  - **+ S25.42 Major laceration of pulmonary blood vessels**
    - Complete transection of pulmonary blood vessels
    - Traumatic rupture of pulmonary blood vessels
    - MCC +7th S25.421 Major laceration of right pulmonary blood vessels
    - MCC +7th S25.422 Major laceration of left pulmonary blood vessels
    - MCC +7th S25.429 Major laceration of unspecified pulmonary blood vessels
  - **+ S25.49 Other specified injury of pulmonary blood vessels**
    - MCC +7th S25.491 Other specified injury of right pulmonary blood vessels
    - MCC +7th S25.492 Other specified injury of left pulmonary blood vessels
    - MCC +7th S25.499 Other specified injury of unspecified pulmonary blood vessels
- **+ S25.5 Injury of intercostal blood vessels**
  - **+ S25.50 Unspecified injury of intercostal blood vessels**
    - CC +7th S25.501 Unspecified injury of intercostal blood vessels, right side
    - CC +7th S25.502 Unspecified injury of intercostal blood vessels, left side
    - CC +7th S25.509 Unspecified injury of intercostal blood vessels, unspecified side
  - **+ S25.51 Laceration of intercostal blood vessels**
    - CC +7th S25.511 Laceration of intercostal blood vessels, right side
    - CC +7th S25.512 Laceration of intercostal blood vessels, left side
    - CC +7th S25.519 Laceration of intercostal blood vessels, unspecified side
  - **+ S25.59 Other specified injury of intercostal blood vessels**
    - CC +7th S25.591 Other specified injury of intercostal blood vessels, right side
    - CC +7th S25.592 Other specified injury of intercostal blood vessels, left side
    - CC +7th S25.599 Other specified injury of intercostal blood vessels, unspecified side
- **+ S25.8 Injury of other blood vessels of thorax**
  - Injury of azygos vein
  - Injury of mammary artery or vein
  - **+ S25.80 Unspecified injury of other blood vessels of thorax**
    - CC +7th S25.801 Unspecified injury of other blood vessels of thorax, right side
    - CC +7th S25.802 Unspecified injury of other blood vessels of thorax, left side
    - CC +7th S25.809 Unspecified injury of other blood vessels of thorax, unspecified side
  - **+ S25.81 Laceration of other blood vessels of thorax**
    - CC +7th S25.811 Laceration of other blood vessels of thorax, right side
    - CC +7th S25.812 Laceration of other blood vessels of thorax, left side
    - CC +7th S25.819 Laceration of other blood vessels of thorax, unspecified side
  - **+ S25.89 Other specified injury of other blood vessels of thorax**
    - CC +7th S25.891 Other specified injury of other blood vessels of thorax, right side
    - CC +7th S25.892 Other specified injury of other blood vessels of thorax, left side
    - CC +7th S25.899 Other specified injury of other blood vessels of thorax, unspecified side
- **+ S25.9 Injury of unspecified blood vessel of thorax**
  - CC X+7th S25.90 Unspecified injury of unspecified blood vessel of thorax
  - CC X+7th S25.91 Laceration of unspecified blood vessel of thorax
  - CC X+7th S25.99 Other specified injury of unspecified blood vessel of thorax

S26 Injury of heart

Code also any associated:
  open wound of thorax (S21.-)
  traumatic hemopneumothorax (S27.2)
  traumatic hemothorax (S27.1)
  traumatic pneumothorax (S27.0)

> The appropriate 7th character is to be added to each code from category S26
> A initial encounter
> D subsequent encounter
> S sequela

- **+ S26.0 Injury of heart with hemopericardium**
  - CC X+7th S26.00 Unspecified injury of heart with hemopericardium
  - CC X+7th S26.01 Contusion of heart with hemopericardium
  - **+ S26.02 Laceration of heart with hemopericardium**
    - MCC +7th S26.020 Mild laceration of heart with hemopericardium
      - Laceration of heart without penetration of heart chamber
    - MCC +7th S26.021 Moderate laceration of heart with hemopericardium
      - Laceration of heart with penetration of heart chamber
    - MCC +7th S26.022 Major laceration of heart with hemopericardium
      - Laceration of heart with penetration of multiple heart chambers
  - CC X+7th S26.09 Other injury of heart with hemopericardium
- **+ S26.1 Injury of heart without hemopericardium**
  - CC X+7th S26.10 Unspecified injury of heart without hemopericardium
  - CC X+7th S26.11 Contusion of heart without hemopericardium
  - MCC X+7th S26.12 Laceration of heart without hemopericardium
  - CC X+7th S26.19 Other injury of heart without hemopericardium
- **+ S26.9 Injury of heart, unspecified with or without hemopericardium**
  - CC X+7th S26.90 Unspecified injury of heart, unspecified with or without hemopericardium
  - CC X+7th S26.91 Contusion of heart, unspecified with or without hemopericardium
  - MCC X+7th S26.92 Laceration of heart, unspecified with or without hemopericardium
    - Laceration of heart NOS
  - CC X+7th S26.99 Other injury of heart, unspecified with or without hemopericardium

S27 Injury of other and unspecified intrathoracic organs

Code also associated open wound of thorax (S21.-)
Excludes2: injury of cervical esophagus (S10-S19)
  injury of trachea (cervical) (S10-S19)

> The appropriate 7th character is to be added to each code from category S27
> A initial encounter
> D subsequent encounter
> S sequela

- CC X+7th S27.0 Traumatic pneumothorax
  - **Excludes1:** spontaneous pneumothorax (J93.-)
- MCC S27.1 Traumatic hemothorax
- MCC S27.2 Traumatic hemopneumothorax

- **S27.3 Other and unspecified injuries of lung**
  - **+ S27.30 Unspecified injury of lung**
    - **CC +7th** S27.301 Unspecified injury of lung, unilateral
    - **CC +7th** S27.302 Unspecified injury of lung, bilateral
    - **CC +7th** S27.309 Unspecified injury of lung, unspecified
  - **+ S27.31 Primary blast injury of lung**
    Blast injury of lung NOS
    - **CC +7th** S27.311 Primary blast injury of lung, unilateral
    - **CC +7th** S27.312 Primary blast injury of lung, bilateral
    - **CC +7th** S27.319 Primary blast injury of lung, unspecified
  - **+ S27.32 Contusion of lung**
    - **CC +7th** S27.321 Contusion of lung, unilateral
    - **CC +7th** S27.322 Contusion of lung, bilateral
    - **CC +7th** S27.329 Contusion of lung, unspecified
  - **+ S27.33 Laceration of lung**
    - **MCC +7th** S27.331 Laceration of lung, unilateral
    - **MCC +7th** S27.332 Laceration of lung, bilateral
    - **MCC +7th** S27.339 Laceration of lung, unspecified
  - **+ S27.39 Other injuries of lung**
    Secondary blast injury of lung
    - **CC +7th** S27.391 Other injuries of lung, unilateral
    - **CC +7th** S27.392 Other injuries of lung, bilateral
    - **CC +7th** S27.399 Other injuries of lung, unspecified
- **S27.4 Injury of bronchus**
  - **+ S27.40 Unspecified injury of bronchus**
    - **MCC +7th** S27.401 Unspecified injury of bronchus, unilateral
    - **MCC +7th** S27.402 Unspecified injury of bronchus, bilateral
    - **MCC +7th** S27.409 Unspecified injury of bronchus, unspecified
  - **+ S27.41 Primary blast injury of bronchus**
    Blast injury of bronchus NOS
    - **MCC +7th** S27.411 Primary blast injury of bronchus, unilateral
    - **MCC +7th** S27.412 Primary blast injury of bronchus, bilateral
    - **MCC +7th** S27.419 Primary blast injury of bronchus, unspecified
  - **+ S27.42 Contusion of bronchus**
    - **MCC +7th** S27.421 Contusion of bronchus, unilateral
    - **MCC +7th** S27.422 Contusion of bronchus, bilateral
    - **MCC +7th** S27.429 Contusion of bronchus, unspecified
  - **+ S27.43 Laceration of bronchus**
    - **MCC +7th** S27.431 Laceration of bronchus, unilateral
    - **MCC +7th** S27.432 Laceration of bronchus, bilateral
    - **MCC +7th** S27.439 Laceration of bronchus, unspecified
  - **+ S27.49 Other injury of bronchus**
    Secondary blast injury of bronchus
    - **MCC +7th** S27.491 Other injury of bronchus, unilateral
    - **MCC +7th** S27.492 Other injury of bronchus, bilateral
    - **MCC +7th** S27.499 Other injury of bronchus, unspecified
- **S27.5 Injury of thoracic trachea**
  - **CC X+7th** S27.50 Unspecified injury of thoracic trachea
  - **CC X+7th** S27.51 Primary blast injury of thoracic trachea
    Blast injury of thoracic trachea NOS
  - **CC X+7th** S27.52 Contusion of thoracic trachea
  - **CC X+7th** S27.53 Laceration of thoracic trachea
  - **CC X+7th** S27.59 Other injury of thoracic trachea
    Secondary blast injury of thoracic trachea
- **S27.6 Injury of pleura**
  - **CC X+7th** S27.60 Unspecified injury of pleura
  - **CC X+7th** S27.63 Laceration of pleura
  - **CC X+7th** S27.69 Other injury of pleura
- **+ S27.8 Injury of other specified intrathoracic organs**
  - **+ S27.80 Injury of diaphragm**
    - **CC +7th** S27.802 Contusion of diaphragm
    - **CC +7th** S27.803 Laceration of diaphragm
    - **CC +7th** S27.808 Other injury of diaphragm
    - **CC +7th** S27.809 Unspecified injury of diaphragm
  - **+ S27.81 Injury of esophagus (thoracic part)**
    - **MCC +7th** S27.812 Contusion of esophagus (thoracic part)
    - **MCC +7th** S27.813 Laceration of esophagus (thoracic part)
    - **MCC +7th** S27.818 Other injury of esophagus (thoracic part)
    - **MCC +7th** S27.819 Unspecified injury of esophagus (thoracic part)
  - **+ S27.89 Injury of other specified intrathoracic organs**
    Injury of lymphatic thoracic duct
    Injury of thymus gland
    - **CC +7th** S27.892 Contusion of other specified intrathoracic organs
    - **CC +7th** S27.893 Laceration of other specified intrathoracic organs
    - **CC +7th** S27.898 Other injury of other specified intrathoracic organs
    - **CC +7th** S27.899 Unspecified injury of other specified intrathoracic organs
- **CC X+7th S27.9 Injury of unspecified intrathoracic organ**

- **S28 Crushing injury of thorax, and traumatic amputation of part of thorax**

  The appropriate 7th character is to be added to each code from category S28
  A initial encounter
  D subsequent encounter
  S sequela

  - **X+7th S28.0 Crushed chest**
    Use additional code for all associated injuries
    Excludes1: *flail chest (S22.5)*
  - **CC X+7th S28.1 Traumatic amputation (partial) of part of thorax, except breast**
  - **+ S28.2 Traumatic amputation of breast**
    - **+ S28.21 Complete traumatic amputation of breast**
      Traumatic amputation of breast NOS
      - **+7th** S28.211 Complete traumatic amputation of right breast
      - **+7th** S28.212 Complete traumatic amputation of left breast
      - **+7th** S28.219 Complete traumatic amputation of unspecified breast
    - **+ S28.22 Partial traumatic amputation of breast**
      - **+7th** S28.221 Partial traumatic amputation of right breast
      - **+7th** S28.222 Partial traumatic amputation of left breast
      - **+7th** S28.229 Partial traumatic amputation of unspecified breast

- **S29 Other and unspecified injuries of thorax**

  Code also any associated open wound (S21.-)

  The appropriate 7th character is to be added to each code from category S29
  A initial encounter
  D subsequent encounter
  S sequela

  - **+ S29.0 Injury of muscle and tendon at thorax level**
    - **+ S29.00 Unspecified injury of muscle and tendon of thorax**
      - **+7th** S29.001 Unspecified injury of muscle and tendon of front wall of thorax
      - **+7th** S29.002 Unspecified injury of muscle and tendon of back wall of thorax
      - **+7th** S29.009 Unspecified injury of muscle and tendon of unspecified wall of thorax
    - **+ S29.01 Strain of muscle and tendon of thorax**
      - **+7th** S29.011 Strain of muscle and tendon of front wall of thorax
      - **+7th** S29.012 Strain of muscle and tendon of back wall of thorax
      - **+7th** S29.019 Strain of muscle and tendon of unspecified wall of thorax
    - **+ S29.02 Laceration of muscle and tendon of thorax**
      - **CC +7th** S29.021 Laceration of muscle and tendon of front wall of thorax
      - **+7th** S29.022 Laceration of muscle and tendon of back wall of thorax
      - **CC +7th** S29.029 Laceration of muscle and tendon of unspecified wall of thorax
    - **+ S29.09 Other injury of muscle and tendon of thorax**
      - **+7th** S29.091 Other injury of muscle and tendon of front wall of thorax
      - **+7th** S29.092 Other injury of muscle and tendon of back wall of thorax
      - **+7th** S29.099 Other injury of muscle and tendon of unspecified wall of thorax
  - **X+7th S29.8 Other specified injuries of thorax**
  - **X+7th S29.9 Unspecified injury of thorax**

Injuries to the abdomen, lower back, lumbar spine, pelvis and external genitals (S30-S39)

Includes: injuries to the abdominal wall
injuries to the anus
injuries to the buttock
injuries to the external genitalia
injuries to the flank
injuries to the groin

Excludes2: burns and corrosions (T20-T32)
effects of foreign body in anus and rectum (T18.5)
effects of foreign body in genitourinary tract (T19.-)
effects of foreign body in stomach, small intestine and colon (T18.2-T18.4)
frostbite (T33-T34)
insect bite or sting, venomous (T63.4)

S30 Superficial injury of abdomen, lower back, pelvis and external genitals

Excludes2: superficial injury of hip (S70.-)

The appropriate 7th character is to be added to each code from category S30
A initial encounter
D subsequent encounter
S sequela

- X+7th **S30.0** Contusion of lower back and pelvis
  Contusion of buttock
- X+7th **S30.1** Contusion of abdominal wall
  Contusion of flank
  Contusion of groin
- + **S30.2** Contusion of external genital organs
  - + **S30.20** Contusion of unspecified external genital organ
    - ♂ +7th **S30.201** Contusion of unspecified external genital organ, male
    - ♀ +7th **S30.202** Contusion of unspecified external genital organ, female
  - ♂ X+7th **S30.21** Contusion of penis
  - ♂ X+7th **S30.22** Contusion of scrotum and testes
  - ♀ X+7th **S30.23** Contusion of vagina and vulva
- X+7th **S30.3** Contusion of anus
- + **S30.8** Other superficial injuries of abdomen, lower back, pelvis and external genitals
  - + **S30.81** Abrasion of abdomen, lower back, pelvis and external genitals
    - +7th **S30.810** Abrasion of lower back and pelvis
    - +7th **S30.811** Abrasion of abdominal wall
    - ♂ +7th **S30.812** Abrasion of penis
    - ♂ +7th **S30.813** Abrasion of scrotum and testes
    - ♀ +7th **S30.814** Abrasion of vagina and vulva
    - ♂ +7th **S30.815** Abrasion of unspecified external genital organs, male
    - ♀ +7th **S30.816** Abrasion of unspecified external genital organs, female
    - +7th **S30.817** Abrasion of anus
  - + **S30.82** Blister (nonthermal) of abdomen, lower back, pelvis and external genitals
    - +7th **S30.820** Blister (nonthermal) of lower back and pelvis
    - +7th **S30.821** Blister (nonthermal) of abdominal wall
    - ♂ +7th **S30.822** Blister (nonthermal) of penis
    - ♂ +7th **S30.823** Blister (nonthermal) of scrotum and testes
    - ♀ +7th **S30.824** Blister (nonthermal) of vagina and vulva
    - ♂ +7th **S30.825** Blister (nonthermal) of unspecified external genital organs, male
    - ♀ +7th **S30.826** Blister (nonthermal) of unspecified external genital organs, female
    - +7th **S30.827** Blister (nonthermal) of anus
  - + **S30.84** External constriction of abdomen, lower back, pelvis and external genitals
    - +7th **S30.840** External constriction of lower back and pelvis
    - +7th **S30.841** External constriction of abdominal wall
    - ♂ +7th **S30.842** External constriction of penis
      Hair tourniquet syndrome of penis
      Use additional cause code to identify the constricting item (W49.0-)
    - ♂ +7th **S30.843** External constriction of scrotum and testes
    - ♀ +7th **S30.844** External constriction of vagina and vulva
    - ♂ +7th **S30.845** External constriction of unspecified external genital organs, male
    - ♀ +7th **S30.846** External constriction of unspecified external genital organs, female
  - + **S30.85** Superficial foreign body of abdomen, lower back, pelvis and external genitals
    Splinter in the abdomen, lower back, pelvis and external genitals
    - +7th **S30.850** Superficial foreign body of lower back and pelvis
    - +7th **S30.851** Superficial foreign body of abdominal wall
    - ♂ +7th **S30.852** Superficial foreign body of penis
    - ♂ +7th **S30.853** Superficial foreign body of scrotum and testes
    - ♀ +7th **S30.854** Superficial foreign body of vagina and vulva
    - ♂ +7th **S30.855** Superficial foreign body of unspecified external genital organs, male
    - ♀ +7th **S30.856** Superficial foreign body of unspecified external genital organs, female
    - +7th **S30.857** Superficial foreign body of anus
  - + **S30.86** Insect bite (nonvenomous) of abdomen, lower back, pelvis and external genitals
    - +7th **S30.860** Insect bite (nonvenomous) of lower back and pelvis
    - +7th **S30.861** Insect bite (nonvenomous) of abdominal wall
    - ♂ +7th **S30.862** Insect bite (nonvenomous) of penis
    - ♂ +7th **S30.863** Insect bite (nonvenomous) of scrotum and testes
    - ♀ +7th **S30.864** Insect bite (nonvenomous) of vagina and vulva
    - ♂ +7th **S30.865** Insect bite (nonvenomous) of unspecified external genital organs, male
    - ♀ +7th **S30.866** Insect bite (nonvenomous) of unspecified external genital organs, female
    - +7th **S30.867** Insect bite (nonvenomous) of anus
  - + **S30.87** Other superficial bite of abdomen, lower back, pelvis and external genitals
    Excludes1: open bite of abdomen, lower back, pelvis and external genitals (S31.05, S31.15, S31.25, S31.35, S31.45, S31.55)
    - +7th **S30.870** Other superficial bite of lower back and pelvis
    - +7th **S30.871** Other superficial bite of abdominal wall
    - ♂ +7th **S30.872** Other superficial bite of penis
    - ♂ +7th **S30.873** Other superficial bite of scrotum and testes
    - ♀ +7th **S30.874** Other superficial bite of vagina and vulva
    - ♂ +7th **S30.875** Other superficial bite of unspecified external genital organs, male
    - ♀ +7th **S30.876** Other superficial bite of unspecified external genital organs, female
    - +7th **S30.877** Other superficial bite of anus
- + **S30.9** Unspecified superficial injury of abdomen, lower back, pelvis and external genitals
  - X+7th **S30.91** Unspecified superficial injury of lower back and pelvis
  - X+7th **S30.92** Unspecified superficial injury of abdominal wall
  - ♂ X+7th **S30.93** Unspecified superficial injury of penis
  - ♂ X+7th **S30.94** Unspecified superficial injury of scrotum and testes
  - ♀ X+7th **S30.95** Unspecified superficial injury of vagina and vulva
  - ♂ X+7th **S30.96** Unspecified superficial injury of unspecified external genital organs, male
  - ♀ X+7th **S30.97** Unspecified superficial injury of unspecified external genital organs, female
  - X+7th **S30.98** Unspecified superficial injury of anus

S31 Open wound of abdomen, lower back, pelvis and external genitals

Code also any associated:
spinal cord injury (S24.0, S24.1-, S34.0-, S34.1-)
wound infection

Excludes1: *traumatic amputation of part of abdomen, lower back and pelvis (S38.2-, S38.3)*

Excludes2: *open wound of hip (S71.00-S71.02)*
open fracture of pelvis (S32.1--S32.9 with 7th character B)

The appropriate 7th character is to be added to each code from category S31
- A initial encounter
- D subsequent encounter
- S sequela

+ **S31.0 Open wound of lower back and pelvis**
  + **S31.00 Unspecified open wound of lower back and pelvis**
    - +7th **S31.000** Unspecified open wound of lower back and pelvis without penetration into retroperitoneum
      Unspecified open wound of lower back and pelvis NOS
    - MCC +7th **S31.001** Unspecified open wound of lower back and pelvis with penetration into retroperitoneum
  + **S31.01 Laceration without foreign body of lower back and pelvis**
    - +7th **S31.010** Laceration without foreign body of lower back and pelvis without penetration into retroperitoneum
      Laceration without foreign body of lower back and pelvis NOS
    - MCC +7th **S31.011** Laceration without foreign body of lower back and pelvis with penetration into retroperitoneum
  + **S31.02 Laceration with foreign body of lower back and pelvis**
    - +7th **S31.020** Laceration with foreign body of lower back and pelvis without penetration into retroperitoneum
      Laceration with foreign body of lower back and pelvis NOS
    - MCC +7th **S31.021** Laceration with foreign body of lower back and pelvis with penetration into retroperitoneum
  + **S31.03 Puncture wound without foreign body of lower back and pelvis**
    - +7th **S31.030** Puncture wound without foreign body of lower back and pelvis without penetration into retroperitoneum
      Puncture wound without foreign body of lower back and pelvis NOS
    - MCC +7th **S31.031** Puncture wound without foreign body of lower back and pelvis with penetration into retroperitoneum
  + **S31.04 Puncture wound with foreign body of lower back and pelvis**
    - +7th **S31.040** Puncture wound with foreign body of lower back and pelvis without penetration into retroperitoneum
      Puncture wound with foreign body of lower back and pelvis NOS
    - MCC +7th **S31.041** Puncture wound with foreign body of lower back and pelvis with penetration into retroperitoneum
  + **S31.05 Open bite of lower back and pelvis**
    Bite of lower back and pelvis NOS
    Excludes1: *superficial bite of lower back and pelvis (S30.860, S30.870)*
    - +7th **S31.050** Open bite of lower back and pelvis without penetration into retroperitoneum
      Open bite of lower back and pelvis NOS
    - MCC +7th **S31.051** Open bite of lower back and pelvis with penetration into retroperitoneum

+ **S31.1 Open wound of abdominal wall without penetration into peritoneal cavity**
  Open wound of abdominal wall NOS
  Excludes2: *open wound of abdominal wall with penetration into peritoneal cavity (S31.6-)*
  + **S31.10 Unspecified open wound of abdominal wall without penetration into peritoneal cavity**
    - +7th **S31.100** Unspecified open wound of abdominal wall, right upper quadrant without penetration into peritoneal cavity
    - +7th **S31.101** Unspecified open wound of abdominal wall, left upper quadrant without penetration into peritoneal cavity
    - +7th **S31.102** Unspecified open wound of abdominal wall, epigastric region without penetration into peritoneal cavity
    - +7th **S31.103** Unspecified open wound of abdominal wall, right lower quadrant without penetration into peritoneal cavity
    - +7th **S31.104** Unspecified open wound of abdominal wall, left lower quadrant without penetration into peritoneal cavity
    - +7th **S31.105** Unspecified open wound of abdominal wall, periumbilic region without penetration into peritoneal cavity
    - +7th **S31.109** Unspecified open wound of abdominal wall, unspecified quadrant without penetration into peritoneal cavity
      Unspecified open wound of abdominal wall NOS
  + **S31.11 Laceration without foreign body of abdominal wall without penetration into peritoneal cavity**
    - +7th **S31.110** Laceration without foreign body of abdominal wall, right upper quadrant without penetration into peritoneal cavity
    - +7th **S31.111** Laceration without foreign body of abdominal wall, left upper quadrant without penetration into peritoneal cavity
    - +7th **S31.112** Laceration without foreign body of abdominal wall, epigastric region without penetration into peritoneal cavity
    - +7th **S31.113** Laceration without foreign body of abdominal wall, right lower quadrant without penetration into peritoneal cavity
    - +7th **S31.114** Laceration without foreign body of abdominal wall, left lower quadrant without penetration into peritoneal cavity
    - +7th **S31.115** Laceration without foreign body of abdominal wall, periumbilic region without penetration into peritoneal cavity
    - +7th **S31.119** Laceration without foreign body of abdominal wall, unspecified quadrant without penetration into peritoneal cavity
  + **S31.12 Laceration with foreign body of abdominal wall without penetration into peritoneal cavity**
    - +7th **S31.120** Laceration of abdominal wall with foreign body, right upper quadrant without penetration into peritoneal cavity
    - +7th **S31.121** Laceration of abdominal wall with foreign body, left upper quadrant without penetration into peritoneal cavity
    - +7th **S31.122** Laceration of abdominal wall with foreign body, epigastric region without penetration into peritoneal cavity
    - +7th **S31.123** Laceration of abdominal wall with foreign body, right lower quadrant without penetration into peritoneal cavity
    - +7th **S31.124** Laceration of abdominal wall with foreign body, left lower quadrant without penetration into peritoneal cavity

- +7th **S31.125** Laceration of abdominal wall with foreign body, periumbilic region without penetration into peritoneal cavity
- +7th **S31.129** Laceration of abdominal wall with foreign body, unspecified quadrant without penetration into peritoneal cavity
- **+ S31.13** Puncture wound of abdominal wall without foreign body without penetration into peritoneal cavity
  - +7th **S31.130** Puncture wound of abdominal wall without foreign body, right upper quadrant without penetration into peritoneal cavity
  - +7th **S31.131** Puncture wound of abdominal wall without foreign body, left upper quadrant without penetration into peritoneal cavity
  - +7th **S31.132** Puncture wound of abdominal wall without foreign body, epigastric region without penetration into peritoneal cavity
  - +7th **S31.133** Puncture wound of abdominal wall without foreign body, right lower quadrant without penetration into peritoneal cavity
  - +7th **S31.134** Puncture wound of abdominal wall without foreign body, left lower quadrant without penetration into peritoneal cavity
  - +7th **S31.135** Puncture wound of abdominal wall without foreign body, periumbilic region without penetration into peritoneal cavity
  - +7th **S31.139** Puncture wound of abdominal wall without foreign body, unspecified quadrant without penetration into peritoneal cavity
- **+ S31.14** Puncture wound of abdominal wall with foreign body without penetration into peritoneal cavity
  - +7th **S31.140** Puncture wound of abdominal wall with foreign body, right upper quadrant without penetration into peritoneal cavity
  - +7th **S31.141** Puncture wound of abdominal wall with foreign body, left upper quadrant without penetration into peritoneal cavity
  - +7th **S31.142** Puncture wound of abdominal wall with foreign body, epigastric region without penetration into peritoneal cavity
  - +7th **S31.143** Puncture wound of abdominal wall with foreign body, right lower quadrant without penetration into peritoneal cavity
  - +7th **S31.144** Puncture wound of abdominal wall with foreign body, left lower quadrant without penetration into peritoneal cavity
  - +7th **S31.145** Puncture wound of abdominal wall with foreign body, periumbilic region without penetration into peritoneal cavity
  - +7th **S31.149** Puncture wound of abdominal wall with foreign body, unspecified quadrant without penetration into peritoneal cavity
- **+ S31.15** Open bite of abdominal wall without penetration into peritoneal cavity
  Bite of abdominal wall NOS
  Excludes1: *superficial bite of abdominal wall (S30.871)*
  - +7th **S31.150** Open bite of abdominal wall, right upper quadrant without penetration into peritoneal cavity
  - +7th **S31.151** Open bite of abdominal wall, left upper quadrant without penetration into peritoneal cavity
  - +7th **S31.152** Open bite of abdominal wall, epigastric region without penetration into peritoneal cavity
  - +7th **S31.153** Open bite of abdominal wall, right lower quadrant without penetration into peritoneal cavity
  - +7th **S31.154** Open bite of abdominal wall, left lower quadrant without penetration into peritoneal cavity
  - +7th **S31.155** Open bite of abdominal wall, periumbilic region without penetration into peritoneal cavity
  - +7th **S31.159** Open bite of abdominal wall, unspecified quadrant without penetration into peritoneal cavity
- **+ S31.2** Open wound of penis
  - ♂ X+7th **S31.20** Unspecified open wound of penis
  - ♂ X+7th **S31.21** Laceration without foreign body of penis
  - ♂ X+7th **S31.22** Laceration with foreign body of penis
  - ♂ X+7th **S31.23** Puncture wound without foreign body of penis
  - ♂ X+7th **S31.24** Puncture wound with foreign body of penis
  - ♂ X+7th **S31.25** Open bite of penis
    Bite of penis NOS
    Excludes1: *superficial bite of penis (S30.862, S30.872)*
- **+ S31.3** Open wound of scrotum and testes
  - ♂ X+7th **S31.30** Unspecified open wound of scrotum and testes
  - ♂ X+7th **S31.31** Laceration without foreign body of scrotum and testes
  - ♂ X+7th **S31.32** Laceration with foreign body of scrotum and testes
  - ♂ X+7th **S31.33** Puncture wound without foreign body of scrotum and testes
  - ♂ X+7th **S31.34** Puncture wound with foreign body of scrotum and testes
  - ♂ X+7th **S31.35** Open bite of scrotum and testes
    Bite of scrotum and testes NOS
    Excludes1: *superficial bite of scrotum and testes (S30.863, S30.873)*
- **+ S31.4** Open wound of vagina and vulva
  Excludes1: *injury to vagina and vulva during delivery (O70.-, O71.4)*
  - ♀ X+7th **S31.40** Unspecified open wound of vagina and vulva
  - ♀ X+7th **S31.41** Laceration without foreign body of vagina and vulva
  - ♀ X+7th **S31.42** Laceration with foreign body of vagina and vulva
  - ♀ X+7th **S31.43** Puncture wound without foreign body of vagina and vulva
  - ♀ X+7th **S31.44** Puncture wound with foreign body of vagina and vulva
  - ♀ X+7th **S31.45** Open bite of vagina and vulva
    Bite of vagina and vulva NOS
    Excludes1: *superficial bite of vagina and vulva (S30.864, S30.874)*
- **+ S31.5** Open wound of unspecified external genital organs
  Excludes1: *traumatic amputation of external genital organs (S38.21, S38.22)*
  - **+ S31.50** Unspecified open wound of unspecified external genital organs
    - ♂ +7th **S31.501** Unspecified open wound of unspecified external genital organs, male
    - ♀ +7th **S31.502** Unspecified open wound of unspecified external genital organs, female
  - **+ S31.51** Laceration without foreign body of unspecified external genital organs
    - ♂ +7th **S31.511** Laceration without foreign body of unspecified external genital organs, male
    - ♀ +7th **S31.512** Laceration without foreign body of unspecified external genital organs, female
  - **+ S31.52** Laceration with foreign body of unspecified external genital organs
    - ♂ +7th **S31.521** Laceration with foreign body of unspecified external genital organs, male
    - ♀ +7th **S31.522** Laceration with foreign body of unspecified external genital organs, female

+ **S31.53** Puncture wound without foreign body of unspecified external genital organs
 ♂ +7th **S31.531** Puncture wound without foreign body of unspecified external genital organs, male
 ♀ +7th **S31.532** Puncture wound without foreign body of unspecified external genital organs, female
+ **S31.54** Puncture wound with foreign body of unspecified external genital organs
 ♂ +7th **S31.541** Puncture wound with foreign body of unspecified external genital organs, male
 ♀ +7th **S31.542** Puncture wound with foreign body of unspecified external genital organs, female
+ **S31.55** Open bite of unspecified external genital organs
 Bite of unspecified external genital organs NOS
 Excludes1: *superficial bite of unspecified external genital organs (S30.865, S30.866, S30.875, S30.876)*
 ♂ +7th **S31.551** Open bite of unspecified external genital organs, male
 ♀ +7th **S31.552** Open bite of unspecified external genital organs, female
+ **S31.6** Open wound of abdominal wall with penetration into peritoneal cavity
 + **S31.60** Unspecified open wound of abdominal wall with penetration into peritoneal cavity
  MCC +7th **S31.600** Unspecified open wound of abdominal wall, right upper quadrant with penetration into peritoneal cavity
  MCC +7th **S31.601** Unspecified open wound of abdominal wall, left upper quadrant with penetration into peritoneal cavity
  MCC +7th **S31.602** Unspecified open wound of abdominal wall, epigastric region with penetration into peritoneal cavity
  MCC +7th **S31.603** Unspecified open wound of abdominal wall, right lower quadrant with penetration into peritoneal cavity
  MCC +7th **S31.604** Unspecified open wound of abdominal wall, left lower quadrant with penetration into peritoneal cavity
  MCC +7th **S31.605** Unspecified open wound of abdominal wall, periumbilic region with penetration into peritoneal cavity
  MCC +7th **S31.609** Unspecified open wound of abdominal wall, unspecified quadrant with penetration into peritoneal cavity
 + **S31.61** Laceration without foreign body of abdominal wall with penetration into peritoneal cavity
  MCC +7th **S31.610** Laceration without foreign body of abdominal wall, right upper quadrant with penetration into peritoneal cavity
  MCC +7th **S31.611** Laceration without foreign body of abdominal wall, left upper quadrant with penetration into peritoneal cavity
  MCC +7th **S31.612** Laceration without foreign body of abdominal wall, epigastric region with penetration into peritoneal cavity
  MCC +7th **S31.613** Laceration without foreign body of abdominal wall, right lower quadrant with penetration into peritoneal cavity
   AHA CC: 4Q, 2015, 37-38
  MCC +7th **S31.614** Laceration without foreign body of abdominal wall, left lower quadrant with penetration into peritoneal cavity
  MCC +7th **S31.615** Laceration without foreign body of abdominal wall, periumbilic region with penetration into peritoneal cavity
  MCC +7th **S31.619** Laceration without foreign body of abdominal wall, unspecified quadrant with penetration into peritoneal cavity
 + **S31.62** Laceration with foreign body of abdominal wall with penetration into peritoneal cavity
  MCC +7th **S31.620** Laceration with foreign body of abdominal wall, right upper quadrant with penetration into peritoneal cavity
  MCC +7th **S31.621** Laceration with foreign body of abdominal wall, left upper quadrant with penetration into peritoneal cavity
  MCC +7th **S31.622** Laceration with foreign body of abdominal wall, epigastric region with penetration into peritoneal cavity
  MCC +7th **S31.623** Laceration with foreign body of abdominal wall, right lower quadrant with penetration into peritoneal cavity
  MCC +7th **S31.624** Laceration with foreign body of abdominal wall, left lower quadrant with penetration into peritoneal cavity
  MCC +7th **S31.625** Laceration with foreign body of abdominal wall, periumbilic region with penetration into peritoneal cavity
  MCC +7th **S31.629** Laceration with foreign body of abdominal wall, unspecified quadrant with penetration into peritoneal cavity
 + **S31.63** Puncture wound without foreign body of abdominal wall with penetration into peritoneal cavity
  MCC +7th **S31.630** Puncture wound without foreign body of abdominal wall, right upper quadrant with penetration into peritoneal cavity
  MCC +7th **S31.631** Puncture wound without foreign body of abdominal wall, left upper quadrant with penetration into peritoneal cavity
  MCC +7th **S31.632** Puncture wound without foreign body of abdominal wall, epigastric region with penetration into peritoneal cavity
  MCC +7th **S31.633** Puncture wound without foreign body of abdominal wall, right lower quadrant with penetration into peritoneal cavity
  MCC +7th **S31.634** Puncture wound without foreign body of abdominal wall, left lower quadrant with penetration into peritoneal cavity
  MCC +7th **S31.635** Puncture wound without foreign body of abdominal wall, periumbilic region with penetration into peritoneal cavity
  MCC +7th **S31.639** Puncture wound without foreign body of abdominal wall, unspecified quadrant with penetration into peritoneal cavity
 + **S31.64** Puncture wound with foreign body of abdominal wall with penetration into peritoneal cavity
  MCC +7th **S31.640** Puncture wound with foreign body of abdominal wall, right upper quadrant with penetration into peritoneal cavity
  MCC +7th **S31.641** Puncture wound with foreign body of abdominal wall, left upper quadrant with penetration into peritoneal cavity
  MCC +7th **S31.642** Puncture wound with foreign body of abdominal wall, epigastric region with penetration into peritoneal cavity
  MCC +7th **S31.643** Puncture wound with foreign body of abdominal wall, right lower quadrant with penetration into peritoneal cavity
  MCC +7th **S31.644** Puncture wound with foreign body of abdominal wall, left lower quadrant with penetration into peritoneal cavity
  MCC +7th **S31.645** Puncture wound with foreign body of abdominal wall, periumbilic region with penetration into peritoneal cavity

MCC +7th S31.649 Puncture wound with foreign body of abdominal wall, unspecified quadrant with penetration into peritoneal cavity
+ S31.65 Open bite of abdominal wall with penetration into peritoneal cavity
    Excludes1: *superficial bite of abdominal wall (S30.861, S30.871)*
MCC +7th S31.650 Open bite of abdominal wall, right upper quadrant with penetration into peritoneal cavity
MCC +7th S31.651 Open bite of abdominal wall, left upper quadrant with penetration into peritoneal cavity
MCC +7th S31.652 Open bite of abdominal wall, epigastric region with penetration into peritoneal cavity
MCC +7th S31.653 Open bite of abdominal wall, right lower quadrant with penetration into peritoneal cavity
MCC +7th S31.654 Open bite of abdominal wall, left lower quadrant with penetration into peritoneal cavity
MCC +7th S31.655 Open bite of abdominal wall, periumbilic region with penetration into peritoneal cavity
MCC +7th S31.659 Open bite of abdominal wall, unspecified quadrant with penetration into peritoneal cavity
+ S31.8 Open wound of other parts of abdomen, lower back and pelvis
  + S31.80 Open wound of unspecified buttock
    +7th S31.801 Laceration without foreign body of unspecified buttock
    +7th S31.802 Laceration with foreign body of unspecified buttock
    +7th S31.803 Puncture wound without foreign body of unspecified buttock
    +7th S31.804 Puncture wound with foreign body of unspecified buttock
    +7th S31.805 Open bite of unspecified buttock
        Bite of buttock NOS
        Excludes1: *superficial bite of buttock (S30.870)*
    +7th S31.809 Unspecified open wound of unspecified buttock
  + S31.81 Open wound of right buttock
    +7th S31.811 Laceration without foreign body of right buttock
    +7th S31.812 Laceration with foreign body of right buttock
    +7th S31.813 Puncture wound without foreign body of right buttock
    +7th S31.814 Puncture wound with foreign body of right buttock
    +7th S31.815 Open bite of right buttock
        Bite of right buttock NOS
        Excludes1: *superficial bite of buttock (S30.870)*
    +7th S31.819 Unspecified open wound of right buttock
  + S31.82 Open wound of left buttock
    +7th S31.821 Laceration without foreign body of left buttock
    +7th S31.822 Laceration with foreign body of left buttock
    +7th S31.823 Puncture wound without foreign body of left buttock
    +7th S31.824 Puncture wound with foreign body of left buttock
    +7th S31.825 Open bite of left buttock
        Bite of left buttock NOS
        Excludes1: *superficial bite of buttock (S30.870)*
    +7th S31.829 Unspecified open wound of left buttock
+ S31.83 Open wound of anus
  +7th S31.831 Laceration without foreign body of anus
  +7th S31.832 Laceration with foreign body of anus

+7th S31.833 Puncture wound without foreign body of anus
+7th S31.834 Puncture wound with foreign body of anus
+7th S31.835 Open bite of anus
    Bite of anus NOS
    Excludes1: *superficial bite of anus (S30.877)*
+7th S31.839 Unspecified open wound of anus

See page 1007 for Vertebrae Illustration.

S32 Fracture of lumbar spine and pelvis
NOTE A fracture not indicated as displaced or nondisplaced should be coded to displaced
A fracture not indicated as opened or closed should be coded to closed
Includes: fracture of lumbosacral neural arch
fracture of lumbosacral spinous process
fracture of lumbosacral transverse process
fracture of lumbosacral vertebra
fracture of lumbosacral vertebral arch
Code first any associated spinal cord and spinal nerve injury (S34.-)
Excludes1: *transection of abdomen (S38.3)*
Excludes2: *fracture of hip NOS (S72.0-)*

The appropriate 7th character is to be added to each code from category S32
A initial encounter for closed fracture
B initial encounter for open fracture
D subsequent encounter for fracture with routine healing
G subsequent encounter for fracture with delayed healing
K subsequent encounter for fracture with nonunion
S sequela

Review coding guideline C.19.c
+ S32.0 Fracture of lumbar vertebra
  Fracture of lumbar spine NOS
  + S32.00 Fracture of unspecified lumbar vertebra
    CC MCC +7th **S32.000** Wedge compression fracture of unspecified lumbar vertebra
        HAC 7th characters A & B see Appendix B for HAC conditional logic
    CC MCC +7th **S32.001** Stable burst fracture of unspecified lumbar vertebra
        HAC 7th characters A & B see Appendix B for HAC conditional logic
    CC MCC +7th **S32.002** Unstable burst fracture of unspecified lumbar vertebra
        HAC 7th characters A & B see Appendix B for HAC conditional logic
    CC MCC +7th **S32.008** Other fracture of unspecified lumbar vertebra
        HAC 7th characters A & B see Appendix B for HAC conditional logic
    CC MCC +7th **S32.009** Unspecified fracture of unspecified lumbar vertebra
        HAC 7th characters A & B see Appendix B for HAC conditional logic
  + S32.01 Fracture of first lumbar vertebra
    CC MCC +7th **S32.010** Wedge compression fracture of first lumbar vertebra
        HAC 7th characters A & B see Appendix B for HAC conditional logic
    CC MCC +7th **S32.011** Stable burst fracture of first lumbar vertebra
        HAC 7th characters A & B see Appendix B for HAC conditional logic
    CC MCC +7th **S32.012** Unstable burst fracture of first lumbar vertebra
        HAC 7th characters A & B see Appendix B for HAC conditional logic
    CC MCC +7th **S32.018** Other fracture of first lumbar vertebra
        HAC 7th characters A & B see Appendix B for HAC conditional logic
    CC MCC +7th **S32.019** Unspecified fracture of first lumbar vertebra
        HAC 7th characters A & B see Appendix B for HAC conditional logic
  + S32.02 Fracture of second lumbar vertebra
    CC MCC +7th **S32.020** Wedge compression fracture of second lumbar vertebra
        HAC 7th characters A & B see Appendix B for HAC conditional logic

CC MCC +7th	S32.021	Stable burst fracture of second lumbar vertebra	
		HAC 7th characters A & B see Appendix B for HAC conditional logic	
CC MCC +7th	S32.022	Unstable burst fracture of second lumbar vertebra	
		HAC 7th characters A & B see Appendix B for HAC conditional logic	
CC MCC +7th	S32.028	Other fracture of second lumbar vertebra	
		HAC 7th characters A & B see Appendix B for HAC conditional logic	
CC MCC +7th	S32.029	Unspecified fracture of second lumbar vertebra	
		HAC 7th characters A & B see Appendix B for HAC conditional logic	
+	S32.03	Fracture of third lumbar vertebra	
CC MCC +7th	S32.030	Wedge compression fracture of third lumbar vertebra	
		HAC 7th characters A & B see Appendix B for HAC conditional logic	
CC MCC +7th	S32.031	Stable burst fracture of third lumbar vertebra	
		HAC 7th characters A & B see Appendix B for HAC conditional logic	
CC MCC +7th	S32.032	Unstable burst fracture of third lumbar vertebra	
		HAC 7th characters A & B see Appendix B for HAC conditional logic	
CC MCC +7th	S32.038	Other fracture of third lumbar vertebra	
		HAC 7th characters A & B see Appendix B for HAC conditional logic	
CC MCC +7th	S32.039	Unspecified fracture of third lumbar vertebra	
		HAC 7th characters A & B see Appendix B for HAC conditional logic	
+	S32.04	Fracture of fourth lumbar vertebra	
CC MCC +7th	S32.040	Wedge compression fracture of fourth lumbar vertebra	
		HAC 7th characters A & B see Appendix B for HAC conditional logic	
CC MCC +7th	S32.041	Stable burst fracture of fourth lumbar vertebra	
		HAC 7th characters A & B see Appendix B for HAC conditional logic	
CC MCC +7th	S32.042	Unstable burst fracture of fourth lumbar vertebra	
		HAC 7th characters A & B see Appendix B for HAC conditional logic	
CC MCC +7th	S32.048	Other fracture of fourth lumbar vertebra	
		HAC 7th characters A & B see Appendix B for HAC conditional logic	
CC MCC +7th	S32.049	Unspecified fracture of fourth lumbar vertebra	
		HAC 7th characters A & B see Appendix B for HAC conditional logic	
+	S32.05	Fracture of fifth lumbar vertebra	
CC MCC +7th	S32.050	Wedge compression fracture of fifth lumbar vertebra	
		HAC 7th characters A & B see Appendix B for HAC conditional logic	
CC MCC +7th	S32.051	Stable burst fracture of fifth lumbar vertebra	
		HAC 7th characters A & B see Appendix B for HAC conditional logic	
CC MCC +7th	S32.052	Unstable burst fracture of fifth lumbar vertebra	
		HAC 7th characters A & B see Appendix B for HAC conditional logic	
CC MCC +7th	S32.058	Other fracture of fifth lumbar vertebra	
		HAC 7th characters A & B see Appendix B for HAC conditional logic	
CC MCC +7th	S32.059	Unspecified fracture of fifth lumbar vertebra	
		HAC 7th characters A & B see Appendix B for HAC conditional logic	

+	S32.1	Fracture of sacrum	
	NOTE	For vertical fractures, code to most medial fracture extension. Use two codes if both a vertical and transverse fracture are present	
		Code also any associated fracture of pelvic ring (S32.8-)	
CC MCC X+7th	S32.10	Unspecified fracture of sacrum	
		HAC 7th characters A & B see Appendix B for HAC conditional logic	
+	S32.11	Zone I fracture of sacrum	
		Vertical sacral ala fracture of sacrum	
CC MCC +7th	S32.110	Nondisplaced Zone I fracture of sacrum	
		HAC 7th characters A & B see Appendix B for HAC conditional logic	
CC MCC +7th	S32.111	Minimally displaced Zone I fracture of sacrum	
		HAC 7th characters A & B see Appendix B for HAC conditional logic	
CC MCC +7th	S32.112	Severely displaced Zone I fracture of sacrum	
		HAC 7th characters A & B see Appendix B for HAC conditional logic	
CC MCC +7th	S32.119	Unspecified Zone I fracture of sacrum	
		HAC 7th characters A & B see Appendix B for HAC conditional logic	
+	S32.12	Zone II fracture of sacrum	
		Vertical foraminal region fracture of sacrum	
CC MCC +7th	S32.120	Nondisplaced Zone II fracture of sacrum	
		HAC 7th characters A & B see Appendix B for HAC conditional logic	
CC MCC +7th	S32.121	Minimally displaced Zone II fracture of sacrum	
		HAC 7th characters A & B see Appendix B for HAC conditional logic	
CC MCC +7th	S32.122	Severely displaced Zone II fracture of sacrum	
		HAC 7th characters A & B see Appendix B for HAC conditional logic	
CC MCC +7th	S32.129	Unspecified Zone II fracture of sacrum	
		HAC 7th characters A & B see Appendix B for HAC conditional logic	
+	S32.13	Zone III fracture of sacrum	
		Vertical fracture into spinal canal region of sacrum	
CC MCC +7th	S32.130	Nondisplaced Zone III fracture of sacrum	
		HAC 7th characters A & B see Appendix B for HAC conditional logic	
CC MCC +7th	S32.131	Minimally displaced Zone III fracture of sacrum	
		HAC 7th characters A & B see Appendix B for HAC conditional logic	
CC MCC +7th	S32.132	Severely displaced Zone III fracture of sacrum	
		HAC 7th characters A & B see Appendix B for HAC conditional logic	
CC MCC +7th	S32.139	Unspecified Zone III fracture of sacrum	
		HAC 7th characters A & B see Appendix B for HAC conditional logic	
CC MCC X+7th	S32.14	Type 1 fracture of sacrum	
		Transverse flexion fracture of sacrum without displacement	
		HAC 7th characters A & B see Appendix B for HAC conditional logic	
CC MCC X+7th	S32.15	Type 2 fracture of sacrum	
		Transverse flexion fracture of sacrum with posterior displacement	
		HAC 7th characters A & B see Appendix B for HAC conditional logic	
CC MCC X+7th	S32.16	Type 3 fracture of sacrum	
		Transverse extension fracture of sacrum with anterior displacement	
		HAC 7th characters A & B see Appendix B for HAC conditional logic	
CC MCC X+7th	S32.17	Type 4 fracture of sacrum	
		Transverse segmental comminution of upper sacrum	
		HAC 7th characters A & B see Appendix B for HAC conditional logic	
CC MCC X+7th	S32.19	Other fracture of sacrum	
		HAC 7th characters A & B see Appendix B for HAC conditional logic	

X +7th **S32.2**	**Fracture of coccyx**	
	HAC 7th characters A & B see Appendix B for HAC conditional logic	
+ **S32.3**	**Fracture of ilium**	
	Excludes1: fracture of ilium with associated disruption of pelvic ring (S32.8-)	
+ **S32.30**	**Unspecified fracture of ilium**	
CC MCC +7th **S32.301**	Unspecified fracture of right ilium	
CC MCC +7th **S32.302**	Unspecified fracture of left ilium	
CC MCC +7th **S32.309**	Unspecified fracture of unspecified ilium	
+ **S32.31**	**Avulsion fracture of ilium**	
CC MCC +7th **S32.311**	Displaced avulsion fracture of right ilium	
CC MCC +7th **S32.312**	Displaced avulsion fracture of left ilium	
CC MCC +7th **S32.313**	Displaced avulsion fracture of unspecified ilium	
CC MCC +7th **S32.314**	Nondisplaced avulsion fracture of right ilium	
CC MCC +7th **S32.315**	Nondisplaced avulsion fracture of left ilium	
CC MCC +7th **S32.316**	Nondisplaced avulsion fracture of unspecified ilium	
+ **S32.39**	**Other fracture of ilium**	
CC MCC +7th **S32.391**	Other fracture of right ilium	
CC MCC +7th **S32.392**	Other fracture of left ilium	
CC MCC +7th **S32.399**	Other fracture of unspecified ilium	
+ **S32.4**	**Fracture of acetabulum**	
	Code also any associated fracture of pelvic ring (S32.8-)	
+ **S32.40**	**Unspecified fracture of acetabulum**	
CC +7th **S32.401**	Unspecified fracture of right acetabulum	
CC +7th **S32.402**	Unspecified fracture of left acetabulum	
CC +7th **S32.409**	Unspecified fracture of unspecified acetabulum	
S32.41	**Fracture of anterior wall of acetabulum**	
CC MCC +7th **S32.411**	Displaced fracture of anterior wall of right acetabulum	
CC MCC +7th **S32.412**	Displaced fracture of anterior wall of left acetabulum	
CC MCC +7th **S32.413**	Displaced fracture of anterior wall of unspecified acetabulum	
CC MCC +7th **S32.414**	Nondisplaced fracture of anterior wall of right acetabulum	
CC MCC +7th **S32.415**	Nondisplaced fracture of anterior wall of left acetabulum	
CC MCC +7th **S32.416**	Nondisplaced fracture of anterior wall of unspecified acetabulum	
+ **S32.42**	**Fracture of posterior wall of acetabulum**	
CC MCC +7th **S32.421**	Displaced fracture of posterior wall of right acetabulum	
CC MCC +7th **S32.422**	Displaced fracture of posterior wall of left acetabulum	
CC MCC +7th **S32.423**	Displaced fracture of posterior wall of unspecified acetabulum	
CC MCC +7th **S32.424**	Nondisplaced fracture of posterior wall of right acetabulum	
CC MCC +7th **S32.425**	Nondisplaced fracture of posterior wall of left acetabulum	
CC MCC +7th **S32.426**	Nondisplaced fracture of posterior wall of unspecified acetabulum	
+ **S32.43**	**Fracture of anterior column [iliopubic] of acetabulum**	
CC MCC +7th **S32.431**	Displaced fracture of anterior column [iliopubic] of right acetabulum	
CC MCC +7th **S32.432**	Displaced fracture of anterior column [iliopubic] of left acetabulum	
CC MCC +7th **S32.433**	Displaced fracture of anterior column [iliopubic] of unspecified acetabulum	
CC MCC +7th **S32.434**	Nondisplaced fracture of anterior column [iliopubic] of right acetabulum	
CC MCC +7th **S32.435**	Nondisplaced fracture of anterior column [iliopubic] of left acetabulum	
CC MCC +7th **S32.436**	Nondisplaced fracture of anterior column [iliopubic] of unspecified acetabulum	
+ **S32.44**	**Fracture of posterior column [ilioischial] of acetabulum**	
CC MCC +7th **S32.441**	Displaced fracture of posterior column [ilioischial] of right acetabulum	
CC MCC +7th **S32.442**	Displaced fracture of posterior column [ilioischial] of left acetabulum	
CC MCC +7th **S32.443**	Displaced fracture of posterior column [ilioischial] of unspecified acetabulum	
CC MCC +7th **S32.444**	Nondisplaced fracture of posterior column [ilioischial] of right acetabulum	
CC MCC +7th **S32.445**	Nondisplaced fracture of posterior column [ilioischial] of left acetabulum	
CC MCC +7th **S32.446**	Nondisplaced fracture of posterior column [ilioischial] of unspecified acetabulum	

(Each code above with +7th is annotated: HAC 7th characters A & B see Appendix B for HAC conditional logic)

- **+ S32.45 Transverse fracture of acetabulum**
  - CC MCC +7th **S32.451** Displaced transverse fracture of right acetabulum
    - HAC 7th characters A & B see Appendix B for HAC conditional logic
  - CC MCC +7th **S32.452** Displaced transverse fracture of left acetabulum
    - HAC 7th characters A & B see Appendix B for HAC conditional logic
  - CC MCC +7th **S32.453** Displaced transverse fracture of unspecified acetabulum
    - HAC 7th characters A & B see Appendix B for HAC conditional logic
  - CC MCC +7th **S32.454** Nondisplaced transverse fracture of right acetabulum
    - HAC 7th characters A & B see Appendix B for HAC conditional logic
  - CC MCC +7th **S32.455** Nondisplaced transverse fracture of left acetabulum
    - HAC 7th characters A & B see Appendix B for HAC conditional logic
  - CC MCC +7th **S32.456** Nondisplaced transverse fracture of unspecified acetabulum
    - HAC 7th characters A & B see Appendix B for HAC conditional logic

- **+ S32.46 Associated transverse-posterior fracture of acetabulum**
  - CC MCC +7th **S32.461** Displaced associated transverse-posterior fracture of right acetabulum
    - HAC 7th characters A & B see Appendix B for HAC conditional logic
  - CC MCC +7th **S32.462** Displaced associated transverse-posterior fracture of left acetabulum
    - HAC 7th characters A & B see Appendix B for HAC conditional logic
  - CC MCC +7th **S32.463** Displaced associated transverse-posterior fracture of unspecified acetabulum
    - HAC 7th characters A & B see Appendix B for HAC conditional logic
  - CC MCC +7th **S32.464** Nondisplaced associated transverse-posterior fracture of right acetabulum
    - HAC 7th characters A & B see Appendix B for HAC conditional logic
  - CC MCC +7th **S32.465** Nondisplaced associated transverse-posterior fracture of left acetabulum
    - HAC 7th characters A & B see Appendix B for HAC conditional logic
  - CC MCC +7th **S32.466** Nondisplaced associated transverse-posterior fracture of unspecified acetabulum
    - HAC 7th characters A & B see Appendix B for HAC conditional logic

- **+ S32.47 Fracture of medial wall of acetabulum**
  - CC MCC +7th **S32.471** Displaced fracture of medial wall of right acetabulum
    - HAC 7th characters A & B see Appendix B for HAC conditional logic
  - CC MCC +7th **S32.472** Displaced fracture of medial wall of left acetabulum
    - HAC 7th characters A & B see Appendix B for HAC conditional logic
  - CC MCC +7th **S32.473** Displaced fracture of medial wall of unspecified acetabulum
    - HAC 7th characters A & B see Appendix B for HAC conditional logic
  - CC MCC +7th **S32.474** Nondisplaced fracture of medial wall of right acetabulum
    - HAC 7th characters A & B see Appendix B for HAC conditional logic
  - CC MCC +7th **S32.475** Nondisplaced fracture of medial wall of left acetabulum
    - HAC 7th characters A & B see Appendix B for HAC conditional logic
  - CC MCC +7th **S32.476** Nondisplaced fracture of medial wall of unspecified acetabulum
    - HAC 7th characters A & B see Appendix B for HAC conditional logic

- **+ S32.48 Dome fracture of acetabulum**
  - CC MCC +7th **S32.481** Displaced dome fracture of right acetabulum
    - HAC 7th characters A & B see Appendix B for HAC conditional logic
  - CC MCC +7th **S32.482** Displaced dome fracture of left acetabulum
    - HAC 7th characters A & B see Appendix B for HAC conditional logic
  - CC MCC +7th **S32.483** Displaced dome fracture of unspecified acetabulum
    - HAC 7th characters A & B see Appendix B for HAC conditional logic
  - CC MCC +7th **S32.484** Nondisplaced dome fracture of right acetabulum
    - HAC 7th characters A & B see Appendix B for HAC conditional logic
  - CC MCC +7th **S32.485** Nondisplaced dome fracture of left acetabulum
    - HAC 7th characters A & B see Appendix B for HAC conditional logic
  - CC MCC +7th **S32.486** Nondisplaced dome fracture of unspecified acetabulum
    - HAC 7th characters A & B see Appendix B for HAC conditional logic

- **+ S32.49 Other specified fracture of acetabulum**
  - CC MCC +7th **S32.491** Other specified fracture of right acetabulum
    - HAC 7th characters A & B see Appendix B for HAC conditional logic
  - CC MCC +7th **S32.492** Other specified fracture of left acetabulum
    - HAC 7th characters A & B see Appendix B for HAC conditional logic
  - CC MCC +7th **S32.499** Other specified fracture of unspecified acetabulum
    - HAC 7th characters A & B see Appendix B for HAC conditional logic

- **+ S32.5 Fracture of pubis**
  - **Excludes1:** *fracture of pubis with associated disruption of pelvic ring (S32.8-)*
  - **+ S32.50 Unspecified fracture of pubis**
    - CC MCC +7th **S32.501** Unspecified fracture of right pubis
      - HAC 7th characters A & B see Appendix B for HAC conditional logic
    - CC MCC +7th **S32.502** Unspecified fracture of left pubis
      - HAC 7th characters A & B see Appendix B for HAC conditional logic
    - CC MCC +7th **S32.509** Unspecified fracture of unspecified pubis
      - HAC 7th characters A & B see Appendix B for HAC conditional logic
  - **+ S32.51 Fracture of superior rim of pubis**
    - CC MCC +7th **S32.511** Fracture of superior rim of right pubis
      - HAC 7th characters A & B see Appendix B for HAC conditional logic
    - CC MCC +7th **S32.512** Fracture of superior rim of left pubis
      - HAC 7th characters A & B see Appendix B for HAC conditional logic
    - CC MCC +7th **S32.519** Fracture of superior rim of unspecified pubis
      - HAC 7th characters A & B see Appendix B for HAC conditional logic
  - **+ S32.59 Other specified fracture of pubis**
    - CC MCC +7th **S32.591** Other specified fracture of right pubis
      - HAC 7th characters A & B see Appendix B for HAC conditional logic
    - CC MCC +7th **S32.592** Other specified fracture of left pubis
      - HAC 7th characters A & B see Appendix B for HAC conditional logic
    - CC MCC +7th **S32.599** Other specified fracture of unspecified pubis
      - HAC 7th characters A & B see Appendix B for HAC conditional logic

- **+ S32.6 Fracture of ischium**
  - **Excludes1:** *fracture of ischium with associated disruption of pelvic ring (S32.8-)*
  - **+ S32.60 Unspecified fracture of ischium**
    - CC MCC +7th **S32.601** Unspecified fracture of right ischium
      - HAC 7th characters A & B see Appendix B for HAC conditional logic
    - CC MCC +7th **S32.602** Unspecified fracture of left ischium
      - HAC 7th characters A & B see Appendix B for HAC conditional logic
    - CC MCC +7th **S32.609** Unspecified fracture of unspecified ischium
      - HAC 7th characters A & B see Appendix B for HAC conditional logic

+ **S32.61** Avulsion fracture of ischium

CC MCC +7th **S32.611** Displaced avulsion fracture of right ischium
- HAC 7th characters A & B see Appendix B for HAC conditional logic

CC MCC +7th **S32.612** Displaced avulsion fracture of left ischium
- HAC 7th characters A & B see Appendix B for HAC conditional logic

CC MCC +7th **S32.613** Displaced avulsion fracture of unspecified ischium
- HAC 7th characters A & B see Appendix B for HAC conditional logic

CC MCC +7th **S32.614** Nondisplaced avulsion fracture of right ischium
- HAC 7th characters A & B see Appendix B for HAC conditional logic

CC MCC +7th **S32.615** Nondisplaced avulsion fracture of left ischium
- HAC 7th characters A & B see Appendix B for HAC conditional logic

CC MCC +7th **S32.616** Nondisplaced avulsion fracture of unspecified ischium
- HAC 7th characters A & B see Appendix B for HAC conditional logic

+ **S32.69** Other specified fracture of ischium

CC MCC +7th **S32.691** Other specified fracture of right ischium
- HAC 7th characters A & B see Appendix B for HAC conditional logic

CC MCC +7th **S32.692** Other specified fracture of left ischium
- HAC 7th characters A & B see Appendix B for HAC conditional logic

+ **S32.8** Fracture of other parts of pelvis
  Code also any associated:
  fracture of acetabulum (S32.4-)
  sacral fracture (S32.1-)

+ **S32.81** Multiple fractures of pelvis with disruption of pelvic ring
  Multiple pelvic fractures with disruption of pelvic circle

CC MCC +7th **S32.810** Multiple fractures of pelvis with stable disruption of pelvic ring
- HAC 7th characters A & B see Appendix B for HAC conditional logic

CC MCC +7th **S32.811** Multiple fractures of pelvis with unstable disruption of pelvic ring
- HAC 7th characters A & B see Appendix B for HAC conditional logic

CC MCC X+7th **S32.82** Multiple fractures of pelvis without disruption of pelvic ring
  Multiple pelvic fractures without disruption of pelvic circle
- HAC 7th characters A & B see Appendix B for HAC conditional logic

CC MCC X+7th **S32.89** Fracture of other parts of pelvis
- HAC 7th characters A & B see Appendix B for HAC conditional logic

X+7th **S32.9** Fracture of unspecified parts of lumbosacral spine and pelvis
MCC
CC
  Fracture of lumbosacral spine NOS
  Fracture of pelvis NOS
- HAC 7th characters A & B see Appendix B for HAC conditional logic

S33 Dislocation and sprain of joints and ligaments of lumbar spine and pelvis

Includes: avulsion of joint or ligament of lumbar spine and pelvis
laceration of cartilage, joint or ligament of lumbar spine and pelvis
sprain of cartilage, joint or ligament of lumbar spine and pelvis
traumatic hemarthrosis of joint or ligament of lumbar spine and pelvis
traumatic rupture of joint or ligament of lumbar spine and pelvis
traumatic subluxation of joint or ligament of lumbar spine and pelvis
traumatic tear of joint or ligament of lumbar spine and pelvis

Code also any associated open wound

Excludes1: nontraumatic rupture or displacement of lumbar intervertebral disc NOS (M51.-)
obstetric damage to pelvic joints and ligaments (O71.6)
Excludes2: dislocation and sprain of joints and ligaments of hip (S73.-)
strain of muscle of lower back and pelvis (S39.01-)

The appropriate 7th character is to be added to each code from category S33
A initial encounter
D subsequent encounter
S sequela

X+7th **S33.0** Traumatic rupture of lumbar intervertebral disc
Excludes1: rupture or displacement (nontraumatic) of lumbar intervertebral disc NOS (M51.- with fifth character 6)

+ **S33.1** Subluxation and dislocation of lumbar vertebra
  Code also any associated:
  open wound of abdomen, lower back and pelvis (S31)
  spinal cord injury (S24.0, S24.1-, S34.0-, S34.1-)
  Excludes2: fracture of lumbar vertebrae (S32.0-)

+ **S33.10** Subluxation and dislocation of unspecified lumbar vertebra
  +7th **S33.100** Subluxation of unspecified lumbar vertebra
  +7th **S33.101** Dislocation of unspecified lumbar vertebra

+ **S33.11** Subluxation and dislocation of L1/L2 lumbar vertebra
  +7th **S33.110** Subluxation of L1/L2 lumbar vertebra
  +7th **S33.111** Dislocation of L1/L2 lumbar vertebra

+ **S33.12** Subluxation and dislocation of L2/L3 lumbar vertebra
  +7th **S33.120** Subluxation of L2/L3 lumbar vertebra
  +7th **S33.121** Dislocation of L2/L3 lumbar vertebra

+ **S33.13** Subluxation and dislocation of L3/L4 lumbar vertebra
  +7th **S33.130** Subluxation of L3/L4 lumbar vertebra
  +7th **S33.131** Dislocation of L3/L4 lumbar vertebra

+ **S33.14** Subluxation and dislocation of L4/L5 lumbar vertebra
  +7th **S33.140** Subluxation of L4/L5 lumbar vertebra
  +7th **S33.141** Dislocation of L4/L5 lumbar vertebra

X+7th **S33.2** Dislocation of sacroiliac and sacrococcygeal joint

+ **S33.3** Dislocation of other and unspecified parts of lumbar spine and pelvis
  X+7th **S33.30** Dislocation of unspecified parts of lumbar spine and pelvis
  X+7th **S33.39** Dislocation of other parts of lumbar spine and pelvis

X+7th **S33.4** Traumatic rupture of symphysis pubis
X+7th **S33.5** Sprain of ligaments of lumbar spine
X+7th **S33.6** Sprain of sacroiliac joint
X+7th **S33.8** Sprain of other parts of lumbar spine and pelvis
X+7th **S33.9** Sprain of unspecified parts of lumbar spine and pelvis

S34 Injury of lumbar and sacral spinal cord and nerves at abdomen, lower back and pelvis level

NOTE Code to highest level of lumbar cord injury
Injuries to the spinal cord (S34.0 and S34.1) refer to the cord level and not bone level injury, and can affect nerve roots at and below the level given.

Code also any associated:
fracture of vertebra (S22.0-, S32.0-)
open wound of abdomen, lower back and pelvis (S31.-)
transient paralysis (R29.5)

The appropriate 7th character is to be added to each code from category S34
A initial encounter
D subsequent encounter
S sequela

+ **S34.0** Concussion and edema of lumbar and sacral spinal cord
MCC X+7th **S34.01** Concussion and edema of lumbar spinal cord
MCC X+7th **S34.02** Concussion and edema of sacral spinal cord
  Concussion and edema of conus medullaris

- **S34.1** Other and unspecified injury of lumbar and sacral spinal cord
  - **S34.10** Unspecified injury to lumbar spinal cord
    - MCC +7th **S34.101** Unspecified injury to L1 level of lumbar spinal cord
      - Unspecified injury to lumbar spinal cord level 1
      - HAC 7th character A see Appendix B for HAC conditional logic
    - MCC +7th **S34.102** Unspecified injury to L2 level of lumbar spinal cord
      - Unspecified injury to lumbar spinal cord level 2
      - HAC 7th character A see Appendix B for HAC conditional logic
    - MCC +7th **S34.103** Unspecified injury to L3 level of lumbar spinal cord
      - Unspecified injury to lumbar spinal cord level 3
      - HAC 7th character A see Appendix B for HAC conditional logic
    - MCC +7th **S34.104** Unspecified injury to L4 level of lumbar spinal cord
      - Unspecified injury to lumbar spinal cord level 4
      - HAC 7th character A see Appendix B for HAC conditional logic
    - MCC +7th **S34.105** Unspecified injury to L5 level of lumbar spinal cord
      - Unspecified injury to lumbar spinal cord level 5
      - HAC 7th character A see Appendix B for HAC conditional logic
    - MCC +7th **S34.109** Unspecified injury to unspecified level of lumbar spinal cord
      - HAC 7th character A see Appendix B for HAC conditional logic
  - **S34.11** Complete lesion of lumbar spinal cord
    - MCC +7th **S34.111** Complete lesion of L1 level of lumbar spinal cord
      - Complete lesion of lumbar spinal cord level 1
      - HAC 7th character A see Appendix B for HAC conditional logic
    - MCC +7th **S34.112** Complete lesion of L2 level of lumbar spinal cord
      - Complete lesion of lumbar spinal cord level 2
      - HAC 7th character A see Appendix B for HAC conditional logic
    - MCC +7th **S34.113** Complete lesion of L3 level of lumbar spinal cord
      - Complete lesion of lumbar spinal cord level 3
      - HAC 7th character A see Appendix B for HAC conditional logic
    - MCC +7th **S34.114** Complete lesion of L4 level of lumbar spinal cord
      - Complete lesion of lumbar spinal cord level 4
      - HAC 7th character A see Appendix B for HAC conditional logic
    - MCC +7th **S34.115** Complete lesion of L5 level of lumbar spinal cord
      - Complete lesion of lumbar spinal cord level 5
      - HAC 7th character A see Appendix B for HAC conditional logic
    - MCC +7th **S34.119** Complete lesion of unspecified level of lumbar spinal cord
      - HAC 7th character A see Appendix B for HAC conditional logic
  - **S34.12** Incomplete lesion of lumbar spinal cord
    - MCC +7th **S34.121** Incomplete lesion of L1 level of lumbar spinal cord
      - Incomplete lesion of lumbar spinal cord level 1
      - HAC 7th character A see Appendix B for HAC conditional logic
    - MCC +7th **S34.122** Incomplete lesion of L2 level of lumbar spinal cord
      - Incomplete lesion of lumbar spinal cord level 2
      - HAC 7th character A see Appendix B for HAC conditional logic
    - MCC +7th **S34.123** Incomplete lesion of L3 level of lumbar spinal cord
      - Incomplete lesion of lumbar spinal cord level 3
      - HAC 7th character A see Appendix B for HAC conditional logic
    - MCC +7th **S34.124** Incomplete lesion of L4 level of lumbar spinal cord
      - Incomplete lesion of lumbar spinal cord level 4
      - HAC 7th character A see Appendix B for HAC conditional logic
    - MCC +7th **S34.125** Incomplete lesion of L5 level of lumbar spinal cord
      - Incomplete lesion of lumbar spinal cord level 5
      - HAC 7th character A see Appendix B for HAC conditional logic
    - MCC +7th **S34.129** Incomplete lesion of unspecified level of lumbar spinal cord
      - HAC 7th character A see Appendix B for HAC conditional logic
  - **S34.13** Other and unspecified injury of sacral spinal cord
    - Other injury to conus medullaris
    - MCC +7th **S34.131** Complete lesion of sacral spinal cord
      - Complete lesion of conus medullaris
      - HAC 7th character A see Appendix B for HAC conditional logic
    - MCC +7th **S34.132** Incomplete lesion of sacral spinal cord
      - Incomplete lesion of conus medullaris
      - HAC 7th character A see Appendix B for HAC conditional logic
    - MCC +7th **S34.139** Unspecified injury to sacral spinal cord
      - Unspecified injury of conus medullaris
      - HAC 7th character A see Appendix B for HAC conditional logic
- **S34.2** Injury of nerve root of lumbar and sacral spine
  - X+7th **S34.21** Injury of nerve root of lumbar spine
  - X+7th **S34.22** Injury of nerve root of sacral spine
- MCC X+7th **S34.3** Injury of cauda equina
  - HAC 7th character A see Appendix B for HAC conditional logic
- X+7th **S34.4** Injury of lumbosacral plexus
- X+7th **S34.5** Injury of lumbar, sacral and pelvic sympathetic nerves
  - Injury of celiac ganglion or plexus
  - Injury of hypogastric plexus
  - Injury of mesenteric plexus (inferior) (superior)
  - Injury of splanchnic nerve
- X+7th **S34.6** Injury of peripheral nerve(s) at abdomen, lower back and pelvis level
- X+7th **S34.8** Injury of other nerves at abdomen, lower back and pelvis level
- X+7th **S34.9** Injury of unspecified nerves at abdomen, lower back and pelvis level

S35 Injury of blood vessels at abdomen, lower back and pelvis level

Code also any associated open wound (S31.-)

The appropriate 7th character is to be added to each code from category S35
- A   initial encounter
- D   subsequent encounter
- S   sequela

- **S35.0** Injury of abdominal aorta
  - **Excludes1:** injury of aorta NOS (S25.0)
  - MCC X+7th **S35.00** Unspecified injury of abdominal aorta
  - MCC X+7th **S35.01** Minor laceration of abdominal aorta
    - Incomplete transection of abdominal aorta
    - Laceration of abdominal aorta NOS
    - Superficial laceration of abdominal aorta
  - MCC X+7th **S35.02** Major laceration of abdominal aorta
    - Complete transection of abdominal aorta
    - Traumatic rupture of abdominal aorta
  - MCC X+7th **S35.09** Other injury of abdominal aorta
- **S35.1** Injury of inferior vena cava
  - Injury of hepatic vein
  - **Excludes1:** injury of vena cava NOS (S25.2)
  - MCC X+7th **S35.10** Unspecified injury of inferior vena cava
  - MCC X+7th **S35.11** Minor laceration of inferior vena cava
    - Incomplete transection of inferior vena cava
    - Laceration of inferior vena cava NOS
    - Superficial laceration of inferior vena cava

1043

MCC X+7th	S35.12	Major laceration of inferior vena cava	
		Complete transection of inferior vena cava	
		Traumatic rupture of inferior vena cava	
MCC X+7th	S35.19	Other injury of inferior vena cava	
+	S35.2	Injury of celiac or mesenteric artery and branches	
+	S35.21	Injury of celiac artery	
MCC +7th	S35.211	Minor laceration of celiac artery	
		Incomplete transection of celiac artery	
		Laceration of celiac artery NOS	
		Superficial laceration of celiac artery	
MCC +7th	S35.212	Major laceration of celiac artery	
		Complete transection of celiac artery	
		Traumatic rupture of celiac artery	
MCC +7th	S35.218	Other injury of celiac artery	
MCC +7th	S35.219	Unspecified injury of celiac artery	
+	S35.22	Injury of superior mesenteric artery	
MCC +7th	S35.221	Minor laceration of superior mesenteric artery	
		Incomplete transection of superior mesenteric artery	
		Laceration of superior mesenteric artery NOS	
		Superficial laceration of superior mesenteric artery	
MCC +7th	S35.222	Major laceration of superior mesenteric artery	
		Complete transection of superior mesenteric artery	
		Traumatic rupture of superior mesenteric artery	
MCC +7th	S35.228	Other injury of superior mesenteric artery	
MCC +7th	S35.229	Unspecified injury of superior mesenteric artery	
+	S35.23	Injury of inferior mesenteric artery	
MCC +7th	S35.231	Minor laceration of inferior mesenteric artery	
		Incomplete transection of inferior mesenteric artery	
		Laceration of inferior mesenteric artery NOS	
		Superficial laceration of inferior mesenteric artery	
MCC +7th	S35.232	Major laceration of inferior mesenteric artery	
		Complete transection of inferior mesenteric artery	
		Traumatic rupture of inferior mesenteric artery	
MCC +7th	S35.238	Other injury of inferior mesenteric artery	
MCC +7th	S35.239	Unspecified injury of inferior mesenteric artery	
+	S35.29	Injury of branches of celiac and mesenteric artery	
		Injury of gastric artery	
		Injury of gastroduodenal artery	
		Injury of hepatic artery	
		Injury of splenic artery	
MCC +7th	S35.291	Minor laceration of branches of celiac and mesenteric artery	
		Incomplete transection of branches of celiac and mesenteric artery	
		Laceration of branches of celiac and mesenteric artery NOS	
		Superficial laceration of branches of celiac and mesenteric artery	
MCC +7th	S35.292	Major laceration of branches of celiac and mesenteric artery	
		Complete transection of branches of celiac and mesenteric artery	
		Traumatic rupture of branches of celiac and mesenteric artery	
MCC +7th	S35.298	Other injury of branches of celiac and mesenteric artery	
MCC +7th	S35.299	Unspecified injury of branches of celiac and mesenteric artery	
+	S35.3	Injury of portal or splenic vein and branches	
+	S35.31	Injury of portal vein	
MCC +7th	S35.311	Laceration of portal vein	
MCC +7th	S35.318	Other specified injury of portal vein	
MCC +7th	S35.319	Unspecified injury of portal vein	
+	S35.32	Injury of splenic vein	
MCC +7th	S35.321	Laceration of splenic vein	
MCC +7th	S35.328	Other specified injury of splenic vein	
MCC +7th	S35.329	Unspecified injury of splenic vein	
+	S35.33	Injury of superior mesenteric vein	
MCC +7th	S35.331	Laceration of superior mesenteric vein	
MCC +7th	S35.338	Other specified injury of superior mesenteric vein	
MCC +7th	S35.339	Unspecified injury of superior mesenteric vein	
+	S35.34	Injury of inferior mesenteric vein	
MCC +7th	S35.341	Laceration of inferior mesenteric vein	
MCC +7th	S35.348	Other specified injury of inferior mesenteric vein	
MCC +7th	S35.349	Unspecified injury of inferior mesenteric vein	
+	S35.4	Injury of renal blood vessels	
+	S35.40	Unspecified injury of renal blood vessel	
MCC +7th	S35.401	Unspecified injury of right renal artery	
MCC +7th	S35.402	Unspecified injury of left renal artery	
MCC +7th	S35.403	Unspecified injury of unspecified renal artery	
MCC +7th	S35.404	Unspecified injury of right renal vein	
MCC +7th	S35.405	Unspecified injury of left renal vein	
MCC +7th	S35.406	Unspecified injury of unspecified renal vein	
+	S35.41	Laceration of renal blood vessel	
MCC +7th	S35.411	Laceration of right renal artery	
MCC +7th	S35.412	Laceration of left renal artery	
MCC +7th	S35.413	Laceration of unspecified renal artery	
MCC +7th	S35.414	Laceration of right renal vein	
MCC +7th	S35.415	Laceration of left renal vein	
MCC +7th	S35.416	Laceration of unspecified renal vein	
+	S35.49	Other specified injury of renal blood vessel	
MCC +7th	S35.491	Other specified injury of right renal artery	
MCC +7th	S35.492	Other specified injury of left renal artery	
MCC +7th	S35.493	Other specified injury of unspecified renal artery	
MCC +7th	S35.494	Other specified injury of right renal vein	
MCC +7th	S35.495	Other specified injury of left renal vein	
MCC +7th	S35.496	Other specified injury of unspecified renal vein	
+	S35.5	Injury of iliac blood vessels	
MCC X+7th	S35.50	Injury of unspecified iliac blood vessel(s)	
+	S35.51	Injury of iliac artery or vein	
		Injury of hypogastric artery or vein	
MCC +7th	S35.511	Injury of right iliac artery	
MCC +7th	S35.512	Injury of left iliac artery	
MCC +7th	S35.513	Injury of unspecified iliac artery	
MCC +7th	S35.514	Injury of right iliac vein	
MCC +7th	S35.515	Injury of left iliac vein	
MCC +7th	S35.516	Injury of unspecified iliac vein	
+	S35.53	Injury of uterine artery or vein	
♀ CC +7th	S35.531	Injury of right uterine artery	
♀ CC +7th	S35.532	Injury of left uterine artery	
♀ CC +7th	S35.533	Injury of unspecified uterine artery	
♀ CC +7th	S35.534	Injury of right uterine vein	
♀ CC +7th	S35.535	Injury of left uterine vein	
♀ CC +7th	S35.536	Injury of unspecified uterine vein	
MCC X+7th	S35.59	Injury of other iliac blood vessels	
CC +	S35.8	Injury of other blood vessels at abdomen, lower back and pelvis level	
		Injury of ovarian artery or vein	
+	S35.8X	Injury of other blood vessels at abdomen, lower back and pelvis level	
+7th	S35.8X1	Laceration of other blood vessels at abdomen, lower back and pelvis level	
+7th	S35.8X8	Other specified injury of other blood vessels at abdomen, lower back and pelvis level	
+7th	S35.8X9	Unspecified injury of other blood vessels at abdomen, lower back and pelvis level	
+	S35.9	Injury of unspecified blood vessel at abdomen, lower back and pelvis level	
CC X+7th	S35.90	Unspecified injury of unspecified blood vessel at abdomen, lower back and pelvis level	

| CC X+7th | S35.91 | Laceration of unspecified blood vessel at abdomen, lower back and pelvis level |
| CC X+7th | S35.99 | Other specified injury of unspecified blood vessel at abdomen, lower back and pelvis level |

S36 Injury of intra-abdominal organs
Code also any associated open wound (S31.-)

> The appropriate 7th character is to be added to each code from category S36
> A initial encounter
> D subsequent encounter
> S sequela

- **+ S36.0 Injury of spleen**
  - CC X+7th S36.00 Unspecified injury of spleen
  - + S36.02 Contusion of spleen
    - CC +7th S36.020 Minor contusion of spleen
      Contusion of spleen less than 2 cm
    - CC +7th S36.021 Major contusion of spleen
      Contusion of spleen greater than 2 cm
    - CC +7th S36.029 Unspecified contusion of spleen
  - + S36.03 Laceration of spleen
    - CC +7th S36.030 Superficial (capsular) laceration of spleen
      Laceration of spleen less than 1 cm
      Minor laceration of spleen
      AHA CC: 1Q, 2015, 3-21
    - MCC +7th S36.031 Moderate laceration of spleen
      Laceration of spleen 1 to 3 cm
      AHA CC: 1Q, 2015, 3-21; 1Q, 2022, 22-23
    - MCC +7th S36.032 Major laceration of spleen
      Avulsion of spleen
      Laceration of spleen greater than 3 cm
      Massive laceration of spleen
      Multiple moderate lacerations of spleen
      Stellate laceration of spleen
    - CC +7th S36.039 Unspecified laceration of spleen
  - CC X+7th S36.09 Other injury of spleen
- **+ S36.1 Injury of liver and gallbladder and bile duct**
  - + S36.11 Injury of liver
    - CC +7th S36.112 Contusion of liver
    - CC +7th S36.113 Laceration of liver, unspecified degree
    - CC +7th S36.114 Minor laceration of liver
      Laceration involving capsule only, or, without significant involvement of hepatic parenchyma [i.e., less than 1 cm deep]
    - MCC +7th S36.115 Moderate laceration of liver
      Laceration involving parenchyma but without major disruption of parenchyma [i.e., less than 10 cm long and less than 3 cm deep]
    - MCC +7th S36.116 Major laceration of liver
      Laceration with significant disruption of hepatic parenchyma [i.e., greater than 10 cm long and 3 cm deep]
      Multiple moderate lacerations, with or without hematoma
      Stellate laceration of liver
    - CC +7th S36.118 Other injury of liver
    - CC +7th S36.119 Unspecified injury of liver
  - + S36.12 Injury of gallbladder
    - CC +7th S36.122 Contusion of gallbladder
    - CC +7th S36.123 Laceration of gallbladder
    - CC +7th S36.128 Other injury of gallbladder
    - CC +7th S36.129 Unspecified injury of gallbladder
  - CC X+7th S36.13 Injury of bile duct
- **+ S36.2 Injury of pancreas**
  - + S36.20 Unspecified injury of pancreas
    - CC +7th S36.200 Unspecified injury of head of pancreas
    - CC +7th S36.201 Unspecified injury of body of pancreas
    - CC +7th S36.202 Unspecified injury of tail of pancreas
    - CC +7th S36.209 Unspecified injury of unspecified part of pancreas
  - + S36.22 Contusion of pancreas
    - CC S36.220 Contusion of head of pancreas
    - CC S36.221 Contusion of body of pancreas
    - CC S36.222 Contusion of tail of pancreas
    - CC S36.229 Contusion of unspecified part of pancreas
  - + S36.23 Laceration of pancreas, unspecified degree
    - CC +7th S36.230 Laceration of head of pancreas, unspecified degree
    - CC +7th S36.231 Laceration of body of pancreas, unspecified degree
    - CC +7th S36.232 Laceration of tail of pancreas, unspecified degree
    - CC +7th S36.239 Laceration of unspecified part of pancreas, unspecified degree
  - + S36.24 Minor laceration of pancreas
    - CC +7th S36.240 Minor laceration of head of pancreas
    - CC +7th S36.241 Minor laceration of body of pancreas
    - CC +7th S36.242 Minor laceration of tail of pancreas
    - CC +7th S36.249 Minor laceration of unspecified part of pancreas
  - + S36.25 Moderate laceration of pancreas
    - CC +7th S36.250 Moderate laceration of head of pancreas
    - CC +7th S36.251 Moderate laceration of body of pancreas
    - CC +7th S36.252 Moderate laceration of tail of pancreas
    - CC +7th S36.259 Moderate laceration of unspecified part of pancreas
  - + S36.26 Major laceration of pancreas
    - CC +7th S36.260 Major laceration of head of pancreas
    - CC +7th S36.261 Major laceration of body of pancreas
    - CC +7th S36.262 Major laceration of tail of pancreas
    - CC +7th S36.269 Major laceration of unspecified part of pancreas
  - + S36.29 Other injury of pancreas
    - CC +7th S36.290 Other injury of head of pancreas
    - CC +7th S36.291 Other injury of body of pancreas
    - CC +7th S36.292 Other injury of tail of pancreas
    - CC +7th S36.299 Other injury of unspecified part of pancreas
- **+ S36.3 Injury of stomach**
  - CC X+7th S36.30 Unspecified injury of stomach
  - CC X+7th S36.32 Contusion of stomach
  - CC X+7th S36.33 Laceration of stomach
  - CC X+7th S36.39 Other injury of stomach
- **+ S36.4 Injury of small intestine**
  - + S36.40 Unspecified injury of small intestine
    - CC +7th S36.400 Unspecified injury of duodenum
    - CC +7th S36.408 Unspecified injury of other part of small intestine
    - CC +7th S36.409 Unspecified injury of unspecified part of small intestine
  - + S36.41 Primary blast injury of small intestine
    Blast injury of small intestine NOS
    - CC +7th S36.410 Primary blast injury of duodenum
    - CC +7th S36.418 Primary blast injury of other part of small intestine
    - CC +7th S36.419 Primary blast injury of unspecified part of small intestine
  - + S36.42 Contusion of small intestine
    - CC +7th S36.420 Contusion of duodenum
    - CC +7th S36.428 Contusion of other part of small intestine
    - CC +7th S36.429 Contusion of unspecified part of small intestine
  - + S36.43 Laceration of small intestine
    - CC +7th S36.430 Laceration of duodenum
    - CC +7th S36.438 Laceration of other part of small intestine
    - CC +7th S36.439 Laceration of unspecified part of small intestine
  - + S36.49 Other injury of small intestine
    - CC +7th S36.490 Other injury of duodenum
    - CC +7th S36.498 Other injury of other part of small intestine
    - CC +7th S36.499 Other injury of unspecified part of small intestine
- **S36.5 Injury of colon**
  Excludes2: *injury of rectum (S36.6-)*
  - + S36.50 Unspecified injury of colon
    - CC +7th S36.500 Unspecified injury of ascending [right] colon
    - CC +7th S36.501 Unspecified injury of transverse colon
    - CC +7th S36.502 Unspecified injury of descending [left] colon
    - CC +7th S36.503 Unspecified injury of sigmoid colon
    - CC +7th S36.508 Unspecified injury of other part of colon
    - CC +7th S36.509 Unspecified injury of unspecified part of colon

Shoulder

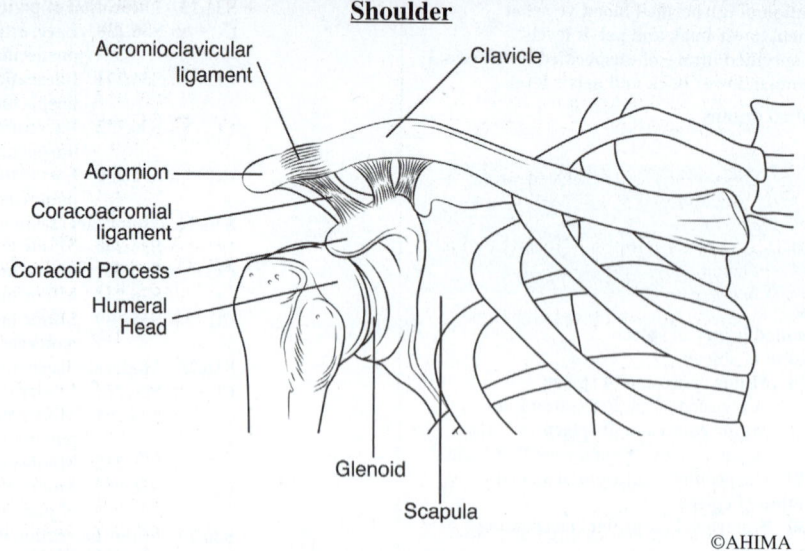

Shoulder Tendons

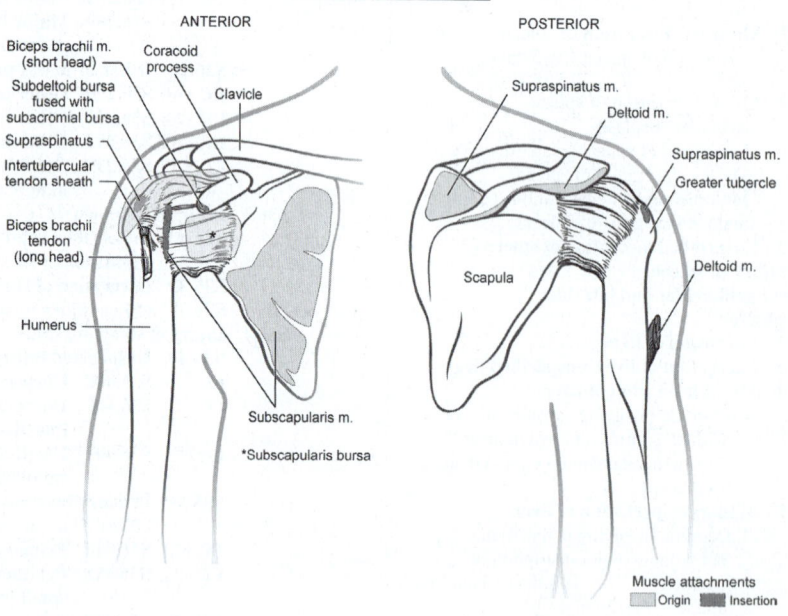

Shoulder Ligaments

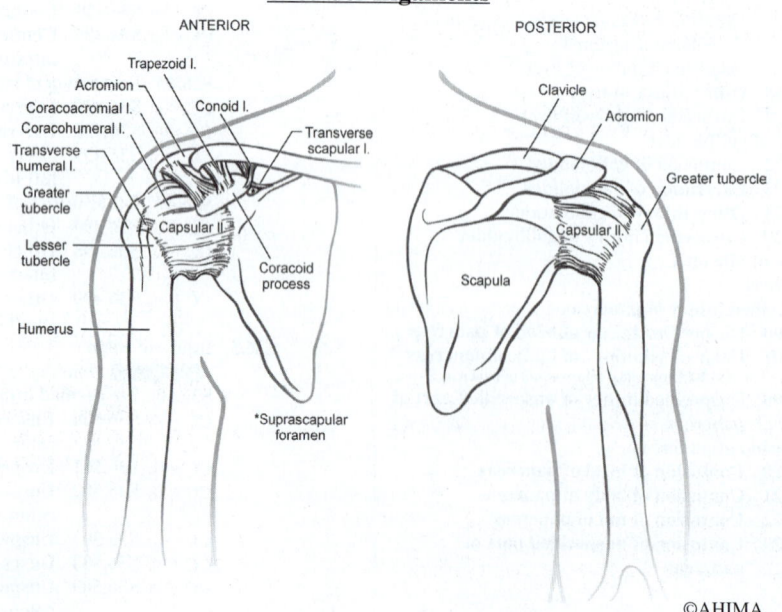

- **+ S36.51** Primary blast injury of colon
  Blast injury of colon NOS
  - CC +7th **S36.510** Primary blast injury of ascending [right] colon
  - CC +7th **S36.511** Primary blast injury of transverse colon
  - CC +7th **S36.512** Primary blast injury of descending [left] colon
  - CC +7th **S36.513** Primary blast injury of sigmoid colon
  - CC +7th **S36.518** Primary blast injury of other part of colon
  - CC +7th **S36.519** Primary blast injury of unspecified part of colon
- **+ S36.52** Contusion of colon
  - CC +7th **S36.520** Contusion of ascending [right] colon
  - CC +7th **S36.521** Contusion of transverse colon
  - CC +7th **S36.522** Contusion of descending [left] colon
  - CC +7th **S36.523** Contusion of sigmoid colon
  - CC +7th **S36.528** Contusion of other part of colon
  - CC +7th **S36.529** Contusion of unspecified part of colon
- **+ S36.53** Laceration of colon
  - CC +7th **S36.530** Laceration of ascending [right] colon
  - CC +7th **S36.531** Laceration of transverse colon
  - CC +7th **S36.532** Laceration of descending [left] colon
  - CC +7th **S36.533** Laceration of sigmoid colon
  - CC +7th **S36.538** Laceration of other part of colon
  - CC +7th **S36.539** Laceration of unspecified part of colon
- **+ S36.59** Other injury of colon
  Secondary blast injury of colon
  - CC +7th **S36.590** Other injury of ascending [right] colon
  - CC +7th **S36.591** Other injury of transverse colon
  - CC +7th **S36.592** Other injury of descending [left] colon
  - CC +7th **S36.593** Other injury of sigmoid colon
  - CC +7th **S36.598** Other injury of other part of colon
  - CC +7th **S36.599** Other injury of unspecified part of colon
- **+ S36.6** Injury of rectum
- CC X+7th **S36.60** Unspecified injury of rectum
- CC X+7th **S36.61** Primary blast injury of rectum
  Blast injury of rectum NOS
- CC X+7th **S36.62** Contusion of rectum
- CC X+7th **S36.63** Laceration of rectum
- CC X+7th **S36.69** Other injury of rectum
  Secondary blast injury of rectum
- **+ S36.8** Injury of other intra-abdominal organs
- CC X+7th **S36.81** Injury of peritoneum
  - **+ S36.89** Injury of other intra-abdominal organs
    Injury of retroperitoneum
    - CC +7th **S36.892** Contusion of other intra-abdominal organs
    - CC +7th **S36.893** Laceration of other intra-abdominal organs
    - CC +7th **S36.898** Other injury of other intra-abdominal organs
    - CC +7th **S36.899** Unspecified injury of other intra-abdominal organs
- **+ S36.9** Injury of unspecified intra-abdominal organ
- CC X+7th **S36.90** Unspecified injury of unspecified intra-abdominal organ
- CC X+7th **S36.92** Contusion of unspecified intra-abdominal organ
- CC X+7th **S36.93** Laceration of unspecified intra-abdominal organ
- CC X+7th **S36.99** Other injury of unspecified intra-abdominal organ

S37 Injury of urinary and pelvic organs
Code also any associated open wound (S31.-)
Excludes1: obstetric trauma to pelvic organs (O71.-)
Excludes2: injury of peritoneum (S36.81)
  injury of retroperitoneum (S36.89-)

The appropriate 7th character is to be added to each code from category S37
A initial encounter
D subsequent encounter
S sequela

- **+ S37.0** Injury of kidney
  Excludes2: acute kidney injury (nontraumatic) (N17.9)
  - **+ S37.00** Unspecified injury of kidney
    - CC +7th **S37.001** Unspecified injury of right kidney
    - CC +7th **S37.002** Unspecified injury of left kidney
    - CC +7th **S37.009** Unspecified injury of unspecified kidney
  - **+ S37.01** Minor contusion of kidney
    Contusion of kidney less than 2 cm
    Contusion of kidney NOS
    - CC +7th **S37.011** Minor contusion of right kidney
    - CC +7th **S37.012** Minor contusion of left kidney
    - CC +7th **S37.019** Minor contusion of unspecified kidney
  - **+ S37.02** Major contusion of kidney
    Contusion of kidney greater than 2 cm
    - CC +7th **S37.021** Major contusion of right kidney
    - CC +7th **S37.022** Major contusion of left kidney
    - CC +7th **S37.029** Major contusion of unspecified kidney
  - **+ S37.03** Laceration of kidney, unspecified degree
    - CC +7th **S37.031** Laceration of right kidney, unspecified degree
    - CC +7th **S37.032** Laceration of left kidney, unspecified degree
    - CC +7th **S37.039** Laceration of unspecified kidney, unspecified degree
  - **+ S37.04** Minor laceration of kidney
    Laceration of kidney less than 1 cm
    - CC +7th **S37.041** Minor laceration of right kidney
    - CC +7th **S37.042** Minor laceration of left kidney
    - CC +7th **S37.049** Minor laceration of unspecified kidney
  - **+ S37.05** Moderate laceration of kidney
    Laceration of kidney 1 to 3 cm
    - CC +7th **S37.051** Moderate laceration of right kidney
    - CC +7th **S37.052** Moderate laceration of left kidney
    - CC +7th **S37.059** Moderate laceration of unspecified kidney
  - **+ S37.06** Major laceration of kidney
    Avulsion of kidney
    Laceration of kidney greater than 3 cm
    Massive laceration of kidney
    Multiple moderate lacerations of kidney
    Stellate laceration of kidney
    - MCC +7th **S37.061** Major laceration of right kidney
    - MCC +7th **S37.062** Major laceration of left kidney
    - MCC +7th **S37.069** Major laceration of unspecified kidney
  - **+ S37.09** Other injury of kidney
    - MCC +7th **S37.091** Other injury of right kidney
    - MCC +7th **S37.092** Other injury of left kidney
    - MCC +7th **S37.099** Other injury of unspecified kidney
- **+ S37.1** Injury of ureter
- CC X+7th **S37.10** Unspecified injury of ureter
- CC X+7th **S37.12** Contusion of ureter
- CC X+7th **S37.13** Laceration of ureter
- CC X+7th **S37.19** Other injury of ureter
- **+ S37.2** Injury of bladder
- CC X+7th **S37.20** Unspecified injury of bladder
- CC X+7th **S37.22** Contusion of bladder
- CC X+7th **S37.23** Laceration of bladder
- CC X+7th **S37.29** Other injury of bladder
- **+ S37.3** Injury of urethra
- CC X+7th **S37.30** Unspecified injury of urethra
- CC X+7th **S37.32** Contusion of urethra
- CC X+7th **S37.33** Laceration of urethra
- CC X+7th **S37.39** Other injury of urethra
- **+ S37.4** Injury of ovary
  - **+ S37.40** Unspecified injury of ovary
    - ♀ +7th **S37.401** Unspecified injury of ovary, unilateral
    - ♀ +7th **S37.402** Unspecified injury of ovary, bilateral
    - ♀ +7th **S37.409** Unspecified injury of ovary, unspecified
  - **+ S37.42** Contusion of ovary
    - ♀ +7th **S37.421** Contusion of ovary, unilateral
    - ♀ +7th **S37.422** Contusion of ovary, bilateral
    - ♀ +7th **S37.429** Contusion of ovary, unspecified
  - **+ S37.43** Laceration of ovary
    - ♀ +7th **S37.431** Laceration of ovary, unilateral
    - ♀ +7th **S37.432** Laceration of ovary, bilateral
    - ♀ +7th **S37.439** Laceration of ovary, unspecified
  - **+ S37.49** Other injury of ovary
    - ♀ +7th **S37.491** Other injury of ovary, unilateral
    - ♀ +7th **S37.492** Other injury of ovary, bilateral
    - ♀ +7th **S37.499** Other injury of ovary, unspecified

- **+ S37.5 Injury of fallopian tube**
  - **+ S37.50 Unspecified injury of fallopian tube**
    - ♀ +7th S37.501 Unspecified injury of fallopian tube, unilateral
    - ♀ +7th S37.502 Unspecified injury of fallopian tube, bilateral
    - ♀ +7th S37.509 Unspecified injury of fallopian tube, unspecified
  - **+ S37.51 Primary blast injury of fallopian tube**
    Blast injury of fallopian tube NOS
    - ♀ +7th S37.511 Primary blast injury of fallopian tube, unilateral
    - ♀ +7th S37.512 Primary blast injury of fallopian tube, bilateral
    - ♀ +7th S37.519 Primary blast injury of fallopian tube, unspecified
  - **+ S37.52 Contusion of fallopian tube**
    - ♀ +7th S37.521 Contusion of fallopian tube, unilateral
    - ♀ +7th S37.522 Contusion of fallopian tube, bilateral
    - ♀ +7th S37.529 Contusion of fallopian tube, unspecified
  - **+ S37.53 Laceration of fallopian tube**
    - ♀ +7th S37.531 Laceration of fallopian tube, unilateral
    - ♀ +7th S37.532 Laceration of fallopian tube, bilateral
    - ♀ +7th S37.539 Laceration of fallopian tube, unspecified
  - **+ S37.59 Other injury of fallopian tube**
    Secondary blast injury of fallopian tube
    - ♀ +7th S37.591 Other injury of fallopian tube, unilateral
    - ♀ +7th S37.592 Other injury of fallopian tube, bilateral
    - ♀ +7th S37.599 Other injury of fallopian tube, unspecified
- **+ S37.6 Injury of uterus**
  - **Excludes1:** injury to gravid uterus (O9A.2-)
    injury to uterus during delivery (O71.-)
  - ♀ CC X+7th S37.60 Unspecified injury of uterus
  - ♀ CC X+7th S37.62 Contusion of uterus
  - ♀ CC X+7th S37.63 Laceration of uterus
  - ♀ CC X+7th S37.69 Other injury of uterus
- **+ S37.8 Injury of other urinary and pelvic organs**
  - **+ S37.81 Injury of adrenal gland**
    - CC +7th S37.812 Contusion of adrenal gland
    - CC +7th S37.813 Laceration of adrenal gland
    - CC +7th S37.818 Other injury of adrenal gland
    - CC +7th S37.819 Unspecified injury of adrenal gland
  - **+ S37.82 Injury of prostate**
    - ♂ +7th S37.822 Contusion of prostate
    - ♂ +7th S37.823 Laceration of prostate
    - ♂ +7th S37.828 Other injury of prostate
    - ♂ +7th S37.829 Unspecified injury of prostate
  - **+ S37.89 Injury of other urinary and pelvic organ**
    - CC +7th S37.892 Contusion of other urinary and pelvic organ
    - CC +7th S37.893 Laceration of other urinary and pelvic organ
    - CC +7th S37.898 Other injury of other urinary and pelvic organ
    - CC +7th S37.899 Unspecified injury of other urinary and pelvic organ
- **+ S37.9 Injury of unspecified urinary and pelvic organ**
  - CC X+7th S37.90 Unspecified injury of unspecified urinary and pelvic organ
  - CC X+7th S37.92 Contusion of unspecified urinary and pelvic organ
  - CC X+7th S37.93 Laceration of unspecified urinary and pelvic organ
  - CC X+7th S37.99 Other injury of unspecified urinary and pelvic organ

S38 Crushing injury and traumatic amputation of abdomen, lower back, pelvis and external genitals

An amputation not identified as partial or complete should be coded to complete

> The appropriate 7th character is to be added to each code from category S38
> A initial encounter
> D subsequent encounter
> S sequela

- **+ S38.0 Crushing injury of external genital organs**
  Use additional code for any associated injuries
  - **+ S38.00 Crushing injury of unspecified external genital organs**
    - ♂ +7th S38.001 Crushing injury of unspecified external genital organs, male
    - ♀ +7th S38.002 Crushing injury of unspecified external genital organs, female
  - ♂ X+7th S38.01 Crushing injury of penis
  - ♂ X+7th S38.02 Crushing injury of scrotum and testis
  - ♀ X+7th S38.03 Crushing injury of vulva
- X+7th **S38.1 Crushing injury of abdomen, lower back, and pelvis**
  Use additional code for all associated injuries, such as:
  fracture of thoracic or lumbar spine and pelvis (S22.0-, S32.-)
  injury to intra-abdominal organs (S36.-)
  injury to urinary and pelvic organs (S37.-)
  open wound of abdominal wall (S31.-)
  spinal cord injury (S34.0, S34.1-)
  Excludes2: crushing injury of external genital organs (S38.0-)
- **+ S38.2 Traumatic amputation of external genital organs**
  - **+ S38.21 Traumatic amputation of female external genital organs**
    Traumatic amputation of clitoris
    Traumatic amputation of labium (majus) (minus)
    Traumatic amputation of vulva
    - ♀ +7th S38.211 Complete traumatic amputation of female external genital organs
    - ♀ +7th S38.212 Partial traumatic amputation of female external genital organs
  - **+ S38.22 Traumatic amputation of penis**
    - ♂ +7th S38.221 Complete traumatic amputation of penis
    - ♂ +7th S38.222 Partial traumatic amputation of penis
  - **+ S38.23 Traumatic amputation of scrotum and testis**
    - ♂ +7th S38.231 Complete traumatic amputation of scrotum and testis
    - ♂ +7th S38.232 Partial traumatic amputation of scrotum and testis
- X+7th **S38.3 Transection (partial) of abdomen**

S39 Other and unspecified injuries of abdomen, lower back, pelvis and external genitals

Code also any associated open wound (S31.-)
Excludes2: sprain of joints and ligaments of lumbar spine and pelvis (S33.-)

> The appropriate 7th character is to be added to each code from category S39
> A initial encounter
> D subsequent encounter
> S sequela

- **+ S39.0 Injury of muscle, fascia and tendon of abdomen, lower back and pelvis**
  - **+ S39.00 Unspecified injury of muscle, fascia and tendon of abdomen, lower back and pelvis**
    - +7th S39.001 Unspecified injury of muscle, fascia and tendon of abdomen
    - +7th S39.002 Unspecified injury of muscle, fascia and tendon of lower back
    - +7th S39.003 Unspecified injury of muscle, fascia and tendon of pelvis

- **+ S39.01** Strain of muscle, fascia and tendon of abdomen, lower back and pelvis
  - **+7th S39.011** Strain of muscle, fascia and tendon of abdomen
  - **+7th S39.012** Strain of muscle, fascia and tendon of lower back
    AHA CC: 4Q, 2016, 73-74
  - **+7th S39.013** Strain of muscle, fascia and tendon of pelvis
- **+ S39.02** Laceration of muscle, fascia and tendon of abdomen, lower back and pelvis
  - **+7th S39.021** Laceration of muscle, fascia and tendon of abdomen
  - **+7th S39.022** Laceration of muscle, fascia and tendon of lower back
  - **+7th S39.023** Laceration of muscle, fascia and tendon of pelvis
- **+ S39.09** Other injury of muscle, fascia and tendon of abdomen, lower back and pelvis
  - **+7th S39.091** Other injury of muscle, fascia and tendon of abdomen
  - **+7th S39.092** Other injury of muscle, fascia and tendon of lower back
  - **+7th S39.093** Other injury of muscle, fascia and tendon of pelvis
- **+ S39.8** Other specified injuries of abdomen, lower back, pelvis and external genitals
  - **X+7th S39.81** Other specified injuries of abdomen
  - **X+7th S39.82** Other specified injuries of lower back
  - **X+7th S39.83** Other specified injuries of pelvis
  - **+ S39.84** Other specified injuries of external genitals
    - **♂ X+7th S39.840** Fracture of corpus cavernosum penis
    - **X+7th S39.848** Other specified injuries of external genitals
- **+ S39.9** Unspecified injury of abdomen, lower back, pelvis and external genitals
  - **X+7th S39.91** Unspecified injury of abdomen
  - **X+7th S39.92** Unspecified injury of lower back
  - **X+7th S39.93** Unspecified injury of pelvis
  - **X+7th S39.94** Unspecified injury of external genitals

Injuries to the shoulder and upper arm (S40-S49)

Includes: injuries of axilla
injuries of scapular region

Excludes2: and corrosions (T20-T32)
frostbite (T33-T34)
injuries of elbow (S50-S59)
insect bite or sting, venomous (T63.4)

S40 Superficial injury of shoulder and upper arm

The appropriate 7th character is to be added to each code from category S40
A initial encounter
D subsequent encounter
S sequela

- **+ S40.0** Contusion of shoulder and upper arm
  - **+ S40.01** Contusion of shoulder
    - **+7th S40.011** Contusion of right shoulder
    - **+7th S40.012** Contusion of left shoulder
    - **+7th S40.019** Contusion of unspecified shoulder
  - **+ S40.02** Contusion of upper arm
    - **+7th S40.021** Contusion of right upper arm
    - **+7th S40.022** Contusion of left upper arm
    - **+7th S40.029** Contusion of unspecified upper arm
- **+ S40.2** Other superficial injuries of shoulder
  - **+ S40.21** Abrasion of shoulder
    - **+7th S40.211** Abrasion of right shoulder
    - **+7th S40.212** Abrasion of left shoulder
    - **+7th S40.219** Abrasion of unspecified shoulder
  - **+ S40.22** Blister (nonthermal) of shoulder
    - **+7th S40.221** Blister (nonthermal) of right shoulder
    - **+7th S40.222** Blister (nonthermal) of left shoulder
    - **+7th S40.229** Blister (nonthermal) of unspecified shoulder
  - **+ S40.24** External constriction of shoulder
    - **+7th S40.241** External constriction of right shoulder
    - **+7th S40.242** External constriction of left shoulder
    - **+7th S40.249** External constriction of unspecified shoulder
  - **+ S40.25** Superficial foreign body of shoulder
    Splinter in the shoulder
    - **+7th S40.251** Superficial foreign body of right shoulder
    - **+7th S40.252** Superficial foreign body of left shoulder
    - **+7th S40.259** Superficial foreign body of unspecified shoulder
  - **+ S40.26** Insect bite (nonvenomous) of shoulder
    - **+7th S40.261** Insect bite (nonvenomous) of right shoulder
    - **+7th S40.262** Insect bite (nonvenomous) of left shoulder
    - **+7th S40.269** Insect bite (nonvenomous) of unspecified shoulder
  - **+ S40.27** Other superficial bite of shoulder
    Excludes1: open bite of shoulder (S41.05)
    - **+7th S40.271** Other superficial bite of right shoulder
    - **+7th S40.272** Other superficial bite of left shoulder
    - **+7th S40.279** Other superficial bite of unspecified shoulder
- **+ S40.8** Other superficial injuries of upper arm
  - **+ S40.81** Abrasion of upper arm
    - **+7th S40.811** Abrasion of right upper arm
    - **+7th S40.812** Abrasion of left upper arm
    - **+7th S40.819** Abrasion of unspecified upper arm
  - **+ S40.82** Blister (nonthermal) of upper arm
    - **+7th S40.821** Blister (nonthermal) of right upper arm
    - **+7th S40.822** Blister (nonthermal) of left upper arm
    - **+7th S40.829** Blister (nonthermal) of unspecified upper arm
  - **+ S40.84** External constriction of upper arm
    - **+7th S40.841** External constriction of right upper arm
    - **+7th S40.842** External constriction of left upper arm
    - **+7th S40.849** External constriction of unspecified upper arm
  - **+ S40.85** Superficial foreign body of upper arm
    Splinter in the upper arm
    - **+7th S40.851** Superficial foreign body of right upper arm
    - **+7th S40.852** Superficial foreign body of left upper arm
    - **+7th S40.859** Superficial foreign body of unspecified upper arm
  - **+ S40.86** Insect bite (nonvenomous) of upper arm
    - **+7th S40.861** Insect bite (nonvenomous) of right upper arm
    - **+7th S40.862** Insect bite (nonvenomous) of left upper arm
    - **+7th S40.869** Insect bite (nonvenomous) of unspecified upper arm
  - **+ S40.87** Other superficial bite of upper arm
    Excludes1: open bite of upper arm (S41.14)
    Excludes2: other superficial bite of shoulder (S40.27-)
    - **+7th S40.871** Other superficial bite of right upper arm
    - **+7th S40.872** Other superficial bite of left upper arm
    - **+7th S40.879** Other superficial bite of unspecified upper arm
- **+ S40.9** Unspecified superficial injury of shoulder and upper arm
  - **+ S40.91** Unspecified superficial injury of shoulder
    - **+7th S40.911** Unspecified superficial injury of right shoulder
    - **+7th S40.912** Unspecified superficial injury of left shoulder
    - **+7th S40.919** Unspecified superficial injury of unspecified shoulder
  - **+ S40.92** Unspecified superficial injury of upper arm
    - **+7th S40.921** Unspecified superficial injury of right upper arm
    - **+7th S40.922** Unspecified superficial injury of left upper arm
    - **+7th S40.929** Unspecified superficial injury of unspecified upper arm

S41 Open wound of shoulder and upper arm
 Code also any associated wound infection
 Excludes1: traumatic amputation of shoulder and upper arm (S48.-)
 Excludes2: open fracture of shoulder and upper arm (S42.- with 7th character B or C)

The appropriate 7th character is to be added to each code from category S41
 A initial encounter
 D subsequent encounter
 S sequela

+ **S41.0 Open wound of shoulder**
  + **S41.00 Unspecified open wound of shoulder**
    +7th S41.001 Unspecified open wound of right shoulder
    +7th S41.002 Unspecified open wound of left shoulder
    +7th S41.009 Unspecified open wound of unspecified shoulder
  + **S41.01 Laceration without foreign body of shoulder**
    +7th S41.011 Laceration without foreign body of right shoulder
    +7th S41.012 Laceration without foreign body of left shoulder
    +7th S41.019 Laceration without foreign body of unspecified shoulder
  + **S41.02 Laceration with foreign body of shoulder**
    +7th S41.021 Laceration with foreign body of right shoulder
    +7th S41.022 Laceration with foreign body of left shoulder
    +7th S41.029 Laceration with foreign body of unspecified shoulder
  + **S41.03 Puncture wound without foreign body of shoulder**
    +7th S41.031 Puncture wound without foreign body of right shoulder
    +7th S41.032 Puncture wound without foreign body of left shoulder
    +7th S41.039 Puncture wound without foreign body of unspecified shoulder
  + **S41.04 Puncture wound with foreign body of shoulder**
    +7th S41.041 Puncture wound with foreign body of right shoulder
    +7th S41.042 Puncture wound with foreign body of left shoulder
    +7th S41.049 Puncture wound with foreign body of unspecified shoulder
  + **S41.05 Open bite of shoulder**
    Bite of shoulder NOS
    Excludes1: superficial bite of shoulder (S40.27)
    +7th S41.051 Open bite of right shoulder
    +7th S41.052 Open bite of left shoulder
    +7th S41.059 Open bite of unspecified shoulder
+ **S41.1 Open wound of upper arm**
  + **S41.10 Unspecified open wound of upper arm**
    +7th S41.101 Unspecified open wound of right upper arm
    +7th S41.102 Unspecified open wound of left upper arm
    +7th S41.109 Unspecified open wound of unspecified upper arm
  + **S41.11 Laceration without foreign body of upper arm**
    S41.111 Laceration without foreign body of right upper arm
    S41.112 Laceration without foreign body of left upper arm
    S41.119 Laceration without foreign body of unspecified upper arm
  + **S41.12 Laceration with foreign body of upper arm**
    +7th S41.121 Laceration with foreign body of right upper arm
    +7th S41.122 Laceration with foreign body of left upper arm
    +7th S41.129 Laceration with foreign body of unspecified upper arm
  + **S41.13 Puncture wound without foreign body of upper arm**
    +7th S41.131 Puncture wound without foreign body of right upper arm
    +7th S41.132 Puncture wound without foreign body of left upper arm
    +7th S41.139 Puncture wound without foreign body of unspecified upper arm
  + **S41.14 Puncture wound with foreign body of upper arm**
    +7th S41.141 Puncture wound with foreign body of right upper arm
    +7th S41.142 Puncture wound with foreign body of left upper arm
    +7th S41.149 Puncture wound with foreign body of unspecified upper arm
  + **S41.15 Open bite of upper arm**
    Bite of upper arm NOS
    Excludes1: superficial bite of upper arm (S40.87)
    +7th S41.151 Open bite of right upper arm
    +7th S41.152 Open bite of left upper arm
    +7th S41.159 Open bite of unspecified upper arm

S42 Fracture of shoulder and upper arm
 NOTE A fracture not indicated as displaced or nondisplaced should be coded to displaced
  A fracture not indicated as open or closed should be coded to closed unless otherwise indicated.
 Excludes1: traumatic amputation of shoulder and upper arm (S48.-)
 Excludes2: periprosthetic fracture around internal prosthetic shoulder joint (M97.3)

The appropriate 7th character is to be added to all codes from category S42
 A initial encounter for closed fracture
 B initial encounter for open fracture
 D subsequent encounter for fracture with routine healing
 G subsequent encounter for fracture with delayed healing
 K subsequent encounter for fracture with nonunion
 P subsequent encounter for fracture with malunion
 S sequela

 Review coding guideline C.19.c
+ **S42.0 Fracture of clavicle**
  + **S42.00 Fracture of unspecified part of clavicle**
    CC +7th S42.001 Fracture of unspecified part of right clavicle
      HAC 7th character B see Appendix B for HAC conditional logic
    CC +7th S42.002 Fracture of unspecified part of left clavicle
      HAC 7th character B see Appendix B for HAC conditional logic
    CC +7th S42.009 Fracture of unspecified part of unspecified clavicle
      HAC 7th character B see Appendix B for HAC conditional logic
  + **S42.01 Fracture of sternal end of clavicle**
    CC +7th S42.011 Anterior displaced fracture of sternal end of right clavicle
      HAC 7th character B see Appendix B for HAC conditional logic
    CC +7th S42.012 Anterior displaced fracture of sternal end of left clavicle
      HAC 7th character B see Appendix B for HAC conditional logic
    CC +7th S42.013 Anterior displaced fracture of sternal end of unspecified clavicle
      Displaced fracture of sternal end of clavicle NOS
      HAC 7th character B see Appendix B for HAC conditional logic
    CC +7th S42.014 Posterior displaced fracture of sternal end of right clavicle
      HAC 7th character B see Appendix B for HAC conditional logic
    CC +7th S42.015 Posterior displaced fracture of sternal end of left clavicle
      HAC 7th character B see Appendix B for HAC conditional logic
    CC +7th S42.016 Posterior displaced fracture of sternal end of unspecified clavicle
      HAC 7th character B see Appendix B for HAC conditional logic

CC +7th	S42.017	Nondisplaced fracture of sternal end of right clavicle
		HAC 7th character B see Appendix B for HAC conditional logic
CC +7th	S42.018	Nondisplaced fracture of sternal end of left clavicle
		HAC 7th character B see Appendix B for HAC conditional logic
CC +7th	S42.019	Nondisplaced fracture of sternal end of unspecified clavicle
		HAC 7th character B see Appendix B for HAC conditional logic

+ **S42.02 Fracture of shaft of clavicle**

CC +7th	S42.021	Displaced fracture of shaft of right clavicle
		HAC 7th character B see Appendix B for HAC conditional logic
CC +7th	S42.022	Displaced fracture of shaft of left clavicle
		HAC 7th character B see Appendix B for HAC conditional logic
CC +7th	S42.023	Displaced fracture of shaft of unspecified clavicle
		HAC 7th character B see Appendix B for HAC conditional logic
CC +7th	S42.024	Nondisplaced fracture of shaft of right clavicle
		HAC 7th character B see Appendix B for HAC conditional logic
CC +7th	S42.025	Nondisplaced fracture of shaft of left clavicle
		HAC 7th character B see Appendix B for HAC conditional logic
CC +7th	S42.026	Nondisplaced fracture of shaft of unspecified clavicle
		HAC 7th character B see Appendix B for HAC conditional logic

+ **S42.03 Fracture of lateral end of clavicle**
Fracture of acromial end of clavicle

CC +7th	S42.031	Displaced fracture of lateral end of right clavicle
		HAC 7th character B see Appendix B for HAC conditional logic
CC +7th	S42.032	Displaced fracture of lateral end of left clavicle
		HAC 7th character B see Appendix B for HAC conditional logic
CC +7th	S42.033	Displaced fracture of lateral end of unspecified clavicle
		HAC 7th character B see Appendix B for HAC conditional logic
CC +7th	S42.034	Nondisplaced fracture of lateral end of right clavicle
		HAC 7th character B see Appendix B for HAC conditional logic
CC +7th	S42.035	Nondisplaced fracture of lateral end of left clavicle
		HAC 7th character B see Appendix B for HAC conditional logic
CC +7th	S42.036	Nondisplaced fracture of lateral end of unspecified clavicle
		HAC 7th character B see Appendix B for HAC conditional logic

+ **S42.1 Fracture of scapula**
+ **S42.10 Fracture of unspecified part of scapula**

CC +7th	S42.101	Fracture of unspecified part of scapula, right shoulder
		HAC 7th character B see Appendix B for HAC conditional logic
CC +7th	S42.102	Fracture of unspecified part of scapula, left shoulder
		HAC 7th character B see Appendix B for HAC conditional logic
CC +7th	S42.109	Fracture of unspecified part of scapula, unspecified shoulder
		HAC 7th character B see Appendix B for HAC conditional logic

+ **S42.11 Fracture of body of scapula**

CC +7th	S42.111	Displaced fracture of body of scapula, right shoulder
		HAC 7th character B see Appendix B for HAC conditional logic
CC +7th	S42.112	Displaced fracture of body of scapula, left shoulder
		HAC 7th character B see Appendix B for HAC conditional logic
CC +7th	S42.113	Displaced fracture of body of scapula, unspecified shoulder
		HAC 7th character B see Appendix B for HAC conditional logic
CC +7th	S42.114	Nondisplaced fracture of body of scapula, right shoulder
		HAC 7th character B see Appendix B for HAC conditional logic
CC +7th	S42.115	Nondisplaced fracture of body of scapula, left shoulder
		HAC 7th character B see Appendix B for HAC conditional logic
CC +7th	S42.116	Nondisplaced fracture of body of scapula, unspecified shoulder
		HAC 7th character B see Appendix B for HAC conditional logic

+ **S42.12 Fracture of acromial process**

CC +7th	S42.121	Displaced fracture of acromial process, right shoulder
		HAC 7th character B see Appendix B for HAC conditional logic
CC +7th	S42.122	Displaced fracture of acromial process, left shoulder
		HAC 7th character B see Appendix B for HAC conditional logic
CC +7th	S42.123	Displaced fracture of acromial process, unspecified shoulder
		HAC 7th character B see Appendix B for HAC conditional logic
CC +7th	S42.124	Nondisplaced fracture of acromial process, right shoulder
		HAC 7th character B see Appendix B for HAC conditional logic
CC +7th	S42.125	Nondisplaced fracture of acromial process, left shoulder
		HAC 7th character B see Appendix B for HAC conditional logic
CC +7th	S42.126	Nondisplaced fracture of acromial process, unspecified shoulder
		HAC 7th character B see Appendix B for HAC conditional logic

+ **S42.13 Fracture of coracoid process**

CC +7th	S42.131	Displaced fracture of coracoid process, right shoulder
		HAC 7th character B see Appendix B for HAC conditional logic
CC +7th	S42.132	Displaced fracture of coracoid process, left shoulder
		HAC 7th character B see Appendix B for HAC conditional logic
CC +7th	S42.133	Displaced fracture of coracoid process, unspecified shoulder
		HAC 7th character B see Appendix B for HAC conditional logic
CC +7th	S42.134	Nondisplaced fracture of coracoid process, right shoulder
		HAC 7th character B see Appendix B for HAC conditional logic
CC +7th	S42.135	Nondisplaced fracture of coracoid process, left shoulder
		HAC 7th character B see Appendix B for HAC conditional logic
CC +7th	S42.136	Nondisplaced fracture of coracoid process, unspecified shoulder
		HAC 7th character B see Appendix B for HAC conditional logic

+ **S42.14 Fracture of glenoid cavity of scapula**

CC +7th	S42.141	Displaced fracture of glenoid cavity of scapula, right shoulder
		HAC 7th character B see Appendix B for HAC conditional logic
CC +7th	S42.142	Displaced fracture of glenoid cavity of scapula, left shoulder
		HAC 7th character B see Appendix B for HAC conditional logic
CC +7th	S42.143	Displaced fracture of glenoid cavity of scapula, unspecified shoulder
		HAC 7th character B see Appendix B for HAC conditional logic
CC +7th	S42.144	Nondisplaced fracture of glenoid cavity of scapula, right shoulder
		HAC 7th character B see Appendix B for HAC conditional logic

- **CC +7th S42.145** Nondisplaced fracture of glenoid cavity of scapula, left shoulder
  - **HAC** 7th character B see Appendix B for HAC conditional logic
- **CC +7th S42.146** Nondisplaced fracture of glenoid cavity of scapula, unspecified shoulder
  - **HAC** 7th character B see Appendix B for HAC conditional logic
- **+ S42.15** Fracture of neck of scapula
  - **CC +7th S42.151** Displaced fracture of neck of scapula, right shoulder
    - **HAC** 7th character B see Appendix B for HAC conditional logic
  - **CC +7th S42.152** Displaced fracture of neck of scapula, left shoulder
    - **HAC** 7th character B see Appendix B for HAC conditional logic
  - **CC +7th S42.153** Displaced fracture of neck of scapula, unspecified shoulder
    - **HAC** 7th character B see Appendix B for HAC conditional logic
  - **CC +7th S42.154** Nondisplaced fracture of neck of scapula, right shoulder
    - **HAC** 7th character B see Appendix B for HAC conditional logic
  - **CC +7th S42.155** Nondisplaced fracture of neck of scapula, left shoulder
    - **HAC** 7th character B see Appendix B for HAC conditional logic
  - **CC +7th S42.156** Nondisplaced fracture of neck of scapula, unspecified shoulder
    - **HAC** 7th character B see Appendix B for HAC conditional logic
- **+ S42.19** Fracture of other part of scapula
  - **CC +7th S42.191** Fracture of other part of scapula, right shoulder
    - **HAC** 7th character B see Appendix B for HAC conditional logic
  - **CC +7th S42.192** Fracture of other part of scapula, left shoulder
    - **HAC** 7th character B see Appendix B for HAC conditional logic
  - **CC +7th S42.199** Fracture of other part of scapula, unspecified shoulder
    - **HAC** 7th character B see Appendix B for HAC conditional logic
- **+ S42.2** Fracture of upper end of humerus
  - Fracture of proximal end of humerus
  - *Excludes2:* fracture of shaft of humerus (S42.3-)
    physeal fracture of upper end of humerus (S49.0-)
  - **+ S42.20** Unspecified fracture of upper end of humerus
    - **CC MCC +7th S42.201** Unspecified fracture of upper end of right humerus
      - **HAC** 7th characters A & B see Appendix B for HAC conditional logic
    - **CC MCC +7th S42.202** Unspecified fracture of upper end of left humerus
      - **HAC** 7th characters A & B see Appendix B for HAC conditional logic
    - **CC MCC +7th S42.209** Unspecified fracture of upper end of unspecified humerus
      - **HAC** 7th characters A & B see Appendix B for HAC conditional logic
  - **+ S42.21** Unspecified fracture of surgical neck of humerus
    - Fracture of neck of humerus NOS
    - **CC MCC +7th S42.211** Unspecified displaced fracture of surgical neck of right humerus
      - **HAC** 7th characters A & B see Appendix B for HAC conditional logic
    - **CC MCC +7th S42.212** Unspecified displaced fracture of surgical neck of left humerus
    - **CC MCC +7th S42.213** Unspecified displaced fracture of surgical neck of unspecified humerus
      - **HAC** 7th characters A & B see Appendix B for HAC conditional logic
    - **CC MCC +7th S42.214** Unspecified nondisplaced fracture of surgical neck of right humerus
      - **HAC** 7th characters A & B see Appendix B for HAC conditional logic
    - **CC MCC +7th S42.215** Unspecified nondisplaced fracture of surgical neck of left humerus
      - **HAC** 7th characters A & B see Appendix B for HAC conditional logic
    - **CC MCC +7th S42.216** Unspecified nondisplaced fracture of surgical neck of unspecified humerus
      - **HAC** 7th characters A & B see Appendix B for HAC conditional logic
  - **+ S42.22** 2-part fracture of surgical neck of humerus
    - **CC MCC +7th S42.221** 2-part displaced fracture of surgical neck of right humerus
      - **HAC** 7th characters A & B see Appendix B for HAC conditional logic
    - **CC MCC +7th S42.222** 2-part displaced fracture of surgical neck of left humerus
      - **HAC** 7th characters A & B see Appendix B for HAC conditional logic
    - **CC MCC +7th S42.223** 2-part displaced fracture of surgical neck of unspecified humerus
      - **HAC** 7th characters A & B see Appendix B for HAC conditional logic
    - **CC MCC +7th S42.224** 2-part nondisplaced fracture of surgical neck of right humerus
      - **HAC** 7th characters A & B see Appendix B for HAC conditional logic
    - **CC MCC +7th S42.225** 2-part nondisplaced fracture of surgical neck of left humerus
      - **HAC** 7th characters A & B see Appendix B for HAC conditional logic
    - **CC MCC +7th S42.226** 2-part nondisplaced fracture of surgical neck of unspecified humerus
      - **HAC** 7th characters A & B see Appendix B for HAC conditional logic
  - **+ S42.23** 3-part fracture of surgical neck of humerus
    - **CC MCC +7th S42.231** 3-part fracture of surgical neck of right humerus
      - **HAC** 7th characters A & B see Appendix B for HAC conditional logic
    - **CC MCC +7th S42.232** 3-part fracture of surgical neck of left humerus
      - **HAC** 7th characters A & B see Appendix B for HAC conditional logic
    - **CC MCC +7th S42.239** 3-part fracture of surgical neck of unspecified humerus
      - **HAC** 7th characters A & B see Appendix B for HAC conditional logic
  - **+ S42.24** 4-part fracture of surgical neck of humerus
    - **CC MCC +7th S42.241** 4-part fracture of surgical neck of right humerus
      - **HAC** 7th characters A & B see Appendix B for HAC conditional logic
    - **CC MCC +7th S42.242** 4-part fracture of surgical neck of left humerus
      - **HAC** 7th characters A & B see Appendix B for HAC conditional logic
    - **CC MCC +7th S42.249** 4-part fracture of surgical neck of unspecified humerus
      - **HAC** 7th characters A & B see Appendix B for HAC conditional logic
  - **+ S42.25** Fracture of greater tuberosity of humerus
    - **CC MCC +7th S42.251** Displaced fracture of greater tuberosity of right humerus
      - **HAC** 7th characters A & B see Appendix B for HAC conditional logic
    - **CC MCC +7th S42.252** Displaced fracture of greater tuberosity of left humerus
      - **HAC** 7th characters A & B see Appendix B for HAC conditional logic
    - **CC MCC +7th S42.253** Displaced fracture of greater tuberosity of unspecified humerus
      - **HAC** 7th characters A & B see Appendix B for HAC conditional logic
    - **CC MCC +7th S42.254** Nondisplaced fracture of greater tuberosity of right humerus
      - **HAC** 7th characters A & B see Appendix B for HAC conditional logic
    - **CC MCC +7th S42.255** Nondisplaced fracture of greater tuberosity of left humerus
      - **HAC** 7th characters A & B see Appendix B for HAC conditional logic
    - **CC MCC +7th S42.256** Nondisplaced fracture of greater tuberosity of unspecified humerus
      - **HAC** 7th characters A & B see Appendix B for HAC conditional logic

+ S42.26 Fracture of lesser tuberosity of humerus

- CC MCC +7th **S42.261** Displaced fracture of lesser tuberosity of right humerus
  - HAC 7th characters A & B see Appendix B for HAC conditional logic
- CC MCC +7th **S42.262** Displaced fracture of lesser tuberosity of left humerus
  - HAC 7th characters A & B see Appendix B for HAC conditional logic
- CC MCC +7th **S42.263** Displaced fracture of lesser tuberosity of unspecified humerus
  - HAC 7th characters A & B see Appendix B for HAC conditional logic
- CC MCC +7th **S42.264** Nondisplaced fracture of lesser tuberosity of right humerus
  - HAC 7th characters A & B see Appendix B for HAC conditional logic
- CC MCC +7th **S42.265** Nondisplaced fracture of lesser tuberosity of left humerus
  - HAC 7th characters A & B see Appendix B for HAC conditional logic
- CC MCC +7th **S42.266** Nondisplaced fracture of lesser tuberosity of unspecified humerus
  - HAC 7th characters A & B see Appendix B for HAC conditional logic

+ S42.27 Torus fracture of upper end of humerus

> The appropriate 7th character is to be added to all codes in subcategory S42.27
> A initial encounter for closed fracture
> D subsequent encounter for fracture with routine healing
> G subsequent encounter for fracture with delayed healing
> K subsequent encounter for fracture with nonunion
> P subsequent encounter for fracture with malunion
> S sequela

- CC +7th **S42.271** Torus fracture of upper end of right humerus
  - HAC 7th character A see Appendix B for HAC conditional logic
- CC +7th **S42.272** Torus fracture of upper end of left humerus
  - HAC 7th character A see Appendix B for HAC conditional logic
- CC +7th **S42.279** Torus fracture of upper end of unspecified humerus
  - HAC 7th character A see Appendix B for HAC conditional logic

+ S42.29 Other fracture of upper end of humerus
  Fracture of anatomical neck of humerus
  Fracture of articular head of humerus

- CC MCC +7th **S42.291** Other displaced fracture of upper end of right humerus
  - HAC 7th characters A & B see Appendix B for HAC conditional logic
- CC MCC +7th **S42.292** Other displaced fracture of upper end of left humerus
  - HAC 7th characters A & B see Appendix B for HAC conditional logic
- CC MCC +7th **S42.293** Other displaced fracture of upper end of unspecified humerus
  - HAC 7th characters A & B see Appendix B for HAC conditional logic
- CC MCC +7th **S42.294** Other nondisplaced fracture of upper end of right humerus
  - HAC 7th characters A & B see Appendix B for HAC conditional logic
- CC MCC +7th **S42.295** Other nondisplaced fracture of upper end of left humerus
  - *AHA CC: 1Q, 2019, 18-19*
  - HAC 7th characters A & B see Appendix B for HAC conditional logic
- CC MCC +7th **S42.296** Other nondisplaced fracture of upper end of unspecified humerus
  - HAC 7th characters A & B see Appendix B for HAC conditional logic

+ S42.3 Fracture of shaft of humerus
  Fracture of humerus NOS
  Fracture of upper arm NOS
  Excludes2: *physeal fractures of upper end of humerus (S49.0-)*
  physeal fractures of lower end of humerus (S49.1-)

+ S42.30 Unspecified fracture of shaft of humerus

- CC MCC +7th **S42.301** Unspecified fracture of shaft of humerus, right arm
  - HAC 7th characters A & B see Appendix B for HAC conditional logic
- CC MCC +7th **S42.302** Unspecified fracture of shaft of humerus, left arm
  - HAC 7th characters A & B see Appendix B for HAC conditional logic
- CC MCC +7th **S42.309** Unspecified fracture of shaft of humerus, unspecified arm
  - HAC 7th characters A & B see Appendix B for HAC conditional logic

+ S42.31 Greenstick fracture of shaft of humerus

> The appropriate 7th character is to be added to all codes in subcategory S42.31
> A initial encounter for closed fracture
> D subsequent encounter for fracture with routine healing
> G subsequent encounter for fracture with delayed healing
> K subsequent encounter for fracture with nonunion
> P subsequent encounter for fracture with malunion
> S sequela

- CC +7th **S42.311** Greenstick fracture of shaft of humerus, right arm
  - HAC 7th character A see Appendix B for HAC conditional logic
- CC +7th **S42.312** Greenstick fracture of shaft of humerus, left arm
  - HAC 7th character A see Appendix B for HAC conditional logic
- CC +7th **S42.319** Greenstick fracture of shaft of humerus, unspecified arm
  - HAC 7th character A see Appendix B for HAC conditional logic

+ S42.32 Transverse fracture of shaft of humerus

- CC MCC +7th **S42.321** Displaced transverse fracture of shaft of humerus, right arm
  - HAC 7th characters A & B see Appendix B for HAC conditional logic
- CC MCC +7th **S42.322** Displaced transverse fracture of shaft of humerus, left arm
  - HAC 7th characters A & B see Appendix B for HAC conditional logic
- CC MCC +7th **S42.323** Displaced transverse fracture of shaft of humerus, unspecified arm
  - HAC 7th characters A & B see Appendix B for HAC conditional logic
- CC MCC +7th **S42.324** Nondisplaced transverse fracture of shaft of humerus, right arm
  - HAC 7th characters A & B see Appendix B for HAC conditional logic
- CC MCC +7th **S42.325** Nondisplaced transverse fracture of shaft of humerus, left arm
  - HAC 7th characters A & B see Appendix B for HAC conditional logic
- CC MCC +7th **S42.326** Nondisplaced transverse fracture of shaft of humerus, unspecified arm
  - HAC 7th characters A & B see Appendix B for HAC conditional logic

+ S42.33 Oblique fracture of shaft of humerus

- CC MCC +7th **S42.331** Displaced oblique fracture of shaft of humerus, right arm
  - HAC 7th characters A & B see Appendix B for HAC conditional logic
- CC MCC +7th **S42.332** Displaced oblique fracture of shaft of humerus, left arm
  - HAC 7th characters A & B see Appendix B for HAC conditional logic
- CC MCC +7th **S42.333** Displaced oblique fracture of shaft of humerus, unspecified arm
  - HAC 7th characters A & B see Appendix B for HAC conditional logic
- CC MCC +7th **S42.334** Nondisplaced oblique fracture of shaft of humerus, right arm
  - HAC 7th characters A & B see Appendix B for HAC conditional logic

| CC MCC +7th S42.335 | Nondisplaced oblique fracture of shaft of humerus, left arm
HAC 7th characters A & B see Appendix B for HAC conditional logic
| CC MCC +7th S42.336 | Nondisplaced oblique fracture of shaft of humerus, unspecified arm
HAC 7th characters A & B see Appendix B for HAC conditional logic

+ **S42.34** Spiral fracture of shaft of humerus

| CC MCC +7th S42.341 | Displaced spiral fracture of shaft of humerus, right arm
HAC 7th characters A & B see Appendix B for HAC conditional logic
| CC MCC +7th S42.342 | Displaced spiral fracture of shaft of humerus, left arm
HAC 7th characters A & B see Appendix B for HAC conditional logic
| CC MCC +7th S42.343 | Displaced spiral fracture of shaft of humerus, unspecified arm
HAC 7th characters A & B see Appendix B for HAC conditional logic
| CC MCC +7th S42.344 | Nondisplaced spiral fracture of shaft of humerus, right arm
HAC 7th characters A & B see Appendix B for HAC conditional logic
| CC MCC +7th S42.345 | Nondisplaced spiral fracture of shaft of humerus, left arm
HAC 7th characters A & B see Appendix B for HAC conditional logic
| CC MCC +7th S42.346 | Nondisplaced spiral fracture of shaft of humerus, unspecified arm
HAC 7th characters A & B see Appendix B for HAC conditional logic

+ **S42.35** Comminuted fracture of shaft of humerus

| CC MCC +7th S42.351 | Displaced comminuted fracture of shaft of humerus, right arm
HAC 7th characters A & B see Appendix B for HAC conditional logic
| CC MCC +7th S42.352 | Displaced comminuted fracture of shaft of humerus, left arm
HAC 7th characters A & B see Appendix B for HAC conditional logic
| CC MCC +7th S42.353 | Displaced comminuted fracture of shaft of humerus, unspecified arm
HAC 7th characters A & B see Appendix B for HAC conditional logic
| CC MCC +7th S42.354 | Nondisplaced comminuted fracture of shaft of humerus, right arm
HAC 7th characters A & B see Appendix B for HAC conditional logic
| CC MCC +7th S42.355 | Nondisplaced comminuted fracture of shaft of humerus, left arm
HAC 7th characters A & B see Appendix B for HAC conditional logic
| CC MCC +7th S42.356 | Nondisplaced comminuted fracture of shaft of humerus, unspecified arm
HAC 7th characters A & B see Appendix B for HAC conditional logic

+ **S42.36** Segmental fracture of shaft of humerus

| CC MCC +7th S42.361 | Displaced segmental fracture of shaft of humerus, right arm
HAC 7th characters A & B see Appendix B for HAC conditional logic
| CC MCC +7th S42.362 | Displaced segmental fracture of shaft of humerus, left arm
HAC 7th characters A & B see Appendix B for HAC conditional logic
| CC MCC +7th S42.363 | Displaced segmental fracture of shaft of humerus, unspecified arm
HAC 7th characters A & B see Appendix B for HAC conditional logic
| CC MCC +7th S42.364 | Nondisplaced segmental fracture of shaft of humerus, right arm
HAC 7th characters A & B see Appendix B for HAC conditional logic
| CC MCC +7th S42.365 | Nondisplaced segmental fracture of shaft of humerus, left arm
HAC 7th characters A & B see Appendix B for HAC conditional logic
| CC MCC +7th S42.366 | Nondisplaced segmental fracture of shaft of humerus, unspecified arm
HAC 7th characters A & B see Appendix B for HAC conditional logic

+ **S42.39** Other fracture of shaft of humerus

| CC MCC +7th S42.391 | Other fracture of shaft of right humerus
HAC 7th characters A & B see Appendix B for HAC conditional logic
| CC MCC +7th S42.392 | Other fracture of shaft of left humerus
HAC 7th characters A & B see Appendix B for HAC conditional logic
| CC MCC +7th S42.399 | Other fracture of shaft of unspecified humerus
HAC 7th characters A & B see Appendix B for HAC conditional logic

+ **S42.4** Fracture of lower end of humerus
Fracture of distal end of humerus
Excludes2: *fracture of shaft of humerus (S42.3-)*
physeal fracture of lower end of humerus (S49.1-)

+ **S42.40** Unspecified fracture of lower end of humerus
Fracture of elbow NOS

| CC MCC +7th S42.401 | Unspecified fracture of lower end of right humerus
HAC 7th characters A & B see Appendix B for HAC conditional logic
| CC MCC +7th S42.402 | Unspecified fracture of lower end of left humerus
HAC 7th characters A & B see Appendix B for HAC conditional logic
| CC MCC +7th S42.409 | Unspecified fracture of lower end of unspecified humerus
HAC 7th characters A & B see Appendix B for HAC conditional logic

+ **S42.41** Simple supracondylar fracture without intercondylar fracture of humerus

| CC MCC +7th S42.411 | Displaced simple supracondylar fracture without intercondylar fracture of right humerus
HAC 7th characters A & B see Appendix B for HAC conditional logic
| CC MCC +7th S42.412 | Displaced simple supracondylar fracture without intercondylar fracture of left humerus
HAC 7th characters A & B see Appendix B for HAC conditional logic
| CC MCC +7th S42.413 | Displaced simple supracondylar fracture without intercondylar fracture of unspecified humerus
HAC 7th characters A & B see Appendix B for HAC conditional logic
| CC MCC +7th S42.414 | Nondisplaced simple supracondylar fracture without intercondylar fracture of right humerus
HAC 7th characters A & B see Appendix B for HAC conditional logic
| CC MCC +7th S42.415 | Nondisplaced simple supracondylar fracture without intercondylar fracture of left humerus
HAC 7th characters A & B see Appendix B for HAC conditional logic
| CC MCC +7th S42.416 | Nondisplaced simple supracondylar fracture without intercondylar fracture of unspecified humerus
HAC 7th characters A & B see Appendix B for HAC conditional logic

+ **S42.42** Comminuted supracondylar fracture without intercondylar fracture of humerus

| CC MCC +7th S42.421 | Displaced comminuted supracondylar fracture without intercondylar fracture of right humerus
HAC 7th characters A & B see Appendix B for HAC conditional logic
| CC MCC +7th S42.422 | Displaced comminuted supracondylar fracture without intercondylar fracture of left humerus
HAC 7th characters A & B see Appendix B for HAC conditional logic
| CC MCC +7th S42.423 | Displaced comminuted supracondylar fracture without intercondylar fracture of unspecified humerus
HAC 7th characters A & B see Appendix B for HAC conditional logic
| CC MCC +7th S42.424 | Nondisplaced comminuted supracondylar fracture without intercondylar fracture of right humerus
HAC 7th characters A & B see Appendix B for HAC conditional logic
| CC MCC +7th S42.425 | Nondisplaced comminuted supracondylar fracture without intercondylar fracture of left humerus
HAC 7th characters A & B see Appendix B for HAC conditional logic

CC MCC +7th S42.426 Nondisplaced comminuted supracondylar fracture without intercondylar fracture of unspecified humerus
  HAC 7th characters A & B see Appendix B for HAC conditional logic

+ **S42.43** Fracture (avulsion) of lateral epicondyle of humerus

CC MCC +7th S42.431 Displaced fracture (avulsion) of lateral epicondyle of right humerus
  HAC 7th characters A & B see Appendix B for HAC conditional logic

CC MCC +7th S42.432 Displaced fracture (avulsion) of lateral epicondyle of left humerus
  HAC 7th characters A & B see Appendix B for HAC conditional logic

CC MCC +7th S42.433 Displaced fracture (avulsion) of lateral epicondyle of unspecified humerus
  HAC 7th characters A & B see Appendix B for HAC conditional logic

CC MCC +7th S42.434 Nondisplaced fracture (avulsion) of lateral epicondyle of right humerus
  HAC 7th characters A & B see Appendix B for HAC conditional logic

CC MCC +7th S42.435 Nondisplaced fracture (avulsion) of lateral epicondyle of left humerus
  HAC 7th characters A & B see Appendix B for HAC conditional logic

CC MCC +7th S42.436 Nondisplaced fracture (avulsion) of lateral epicondyle of unspecified humerus
  HAC 7th characters A & B see Appendix B for HAC conditional logic

+ **S42.44** Fracture (avulsion) of medial epicondyle of humerus

CC MCC +7th S42.441 Displaced fracture (avulsion) of medial epicondyle of right humerus
  HAC 7th characters A & B see Appendix B for HAC conditional logic

CC MCC +7th S42.442 Displaced fracture (avulsion) of medial epicondyle of left humerus
  HAC 7th characters A & B see Appendix B for HAC conditional logic

CC MCC +7th S42.443 Displaced fracture (avulsion) of medial epicondyle of unspecified humerus
  HAC 7th characters A & B see Appendix B for HAC conditional logic

CC MCC +7th S42.444 Nondisplaced fracture (avulsion) of medial epicondyle of right humerus
  HAC 7th characters A & B see Appendix B for HAC conditional logic

CC MCC +7th S42.445 Nondisplaced fracture (avulsion) of medial epicondyle of left humerus
  HAC 7th characters A & B see Appendix B for HAC conditional logic

CC MCC +7th S42.446 Nondisplaced fracture (avulsion) of medial epicondyle of unspecified humerus
  HAC 7th characters A & B see Appendix B for HAC conditional logic

CC MCC +7th S42.447 Incarcerated fracture (avulsion) of medial epicondyle of right humerus
  HAC 7th characters A & B see Appendix B for HAC conditional logic

CC MCC +7th S42.448 Incarcerated fracture (avulsion) of medial epicondyle of left humerus
  HAC 7th characters A & B see Appendix B for HAC conditional logic

CC MCC +7th S42.449 Incarcerated fracture (avulsion) of medial epicondyle of unspecified humerus
  HAC 7th characters A & B see Appendix B for HAC conditional logic

+ **S42.45** Fracture of lateral condyle of humerus
  Fracture of capitellum of humerus

CC MCC +7th S42.451 Displaced fracture of lateral condyle of right humerus
  HAC 7th characters A & B see Appendix B for HAC conditional logic

CC MCC +7th S42.452 Displaced fracture of lateral condyle of left humerus
  HAC 7th characters A & B see Appendix B for HAC conditional logic

CC MCC +7th S42.453 Displaced fracture of lateral condyle of unspecified humerus
  HAC 7th characters A & B see Appendix B for HAC conditional logic

CC MCC +7th S42.454 Nondisplaced fracture of lateral condyle of right humerus
  HAC 7th characters A & B see Appendix B for HAC conditional logic

CC MCC +7th S42.455 Nondisplaced fracture of lateral condyle of left humerus
  HAC 7th characters A & B see Appendix B for HAC conditional logic

CC MCC +7th S42.456 Nondisplaced fracture of lateral condyle of unspecified humerus
  HAC 7th characters A & B see Appendix B for HAC conditional logic

+ **S42.46** Fracture of medial condyle of humerus
  Trochlea fracture of humerus

CC MCC +7th S42.461 Displaced fracture of medial condyle of right humerus
  HAC 7th characters A & B see Appendix B for HAC conditional logic

CC MCC +7th S42.462 Displaced fracture of medial condyle of left humerus
  HAC 7th characters A & B see Appendix B for HAC conditional logic

CC MCC +7th S42.463 Displaced fracture of medial condyle of unspecified humerus
  HAC 7th characters A & B see Appendix B for HAC conditional logic

CC MCC +7th S42.464 Nondisplaced fracture of medial condyle of right humerus
  HAC 7th characters A & B see Appendix B for HAC conditional logic

CC MCC +7th S42.465 Nondisplaced fracture of medial condyle of left humerus
  HAC 7th characters A & B see Appendix B for HAC conditional logic

CC MCC +7th S42.466 Nondisplaced fracture of medial condyle of unspecified humerus
  HAC 7th characters A & B see Appendix B for HAC conditional logic

+ **S42.47** Transcondylar fracture of humerus

CC MCC +7th S42.471 Displaced transcondylar fracture of right humerus
  HAC 7th characters A & B see Appendix B for HAC conditional logic

CC MCC +7th S42.472 Displaced transcondylar fracture of left humerus
  HAC 7th characters A & B see Appendix B for HAC conditional logic

CC MCC +7th S42.473 Displaced transcondylar fracture of unspecified humerus
  HAC 7th characters A & B see Appendix B for HAC conditional logic

CC MCC +7th S42.474 Nondisplaced transcondylar fracture of right humerus
  HAC 7th characters A & B see Appendix B for HAC conditional logic

CC MCC +7th S42.475 Nondisplaced transcondylar fracture of left humerus
  HAC 7th characters A & B see Appendix B for HAC conditional logic

CC MCC +7th S42.476 Nondisplaced transcondylar fracture of unspecified humerus
  HAC 7th characters A & B see Appendix B for HAC conditional logic

+ **S42.48** Torus fracture of lower end of humerus

> The appropriate 7th character is to be added to all codes in subcategory **S42.48**
> A initial encounter for closed fracture
> D subsequent encounter for fracture with routine healing
> G subsequent encounter for fracture with delayed healing
> K subsequent encounter for fracture with nonunion
> P subsequent encounter for fracture with malunion
> S sequela

CC +7th S42.481 Torus fracture of lower end of right humerus
  HAC 7th character A see Appendix B for HAC conditional logic

S42.482–S43.149 — Chapter 19: Injury, Poisoning and Certain Other Consequences of External Causes

CC +7th S42.482 Torus fracture of lower end of left humerus
- **HAC** 7th character A see Appendix B for HAC conditional logic

CC +7th S42.489 Torus fracture of lower end of unspecified humerus
- **HAC** 7th character A see Appendix B for HAC conditional logic

+ S42.49 Other fracture of lower end of humerus

CC MCC +7th S42.491 Other displaced fracture of lower end of right humerus
- **HAC** 7th characters A & B see Appendix B for HAC conditional logic

CC MCC +7th S42.492 Other displaced fracture of lower end of left humerus
- **HAC** 7th characters A & B see Appendix B for HAC conditional logic

CC MCC +7th S42.493 Other displaced fracture of lower end of unspecified humerus
- **HAC** 7th characters A & B see Appendix B for HAC conditional logic

CC MCC +7th S42.494 Other nondisplaced fracture of lower end of right humerus
- **HAC** 7th characters A & B see Appendix B for HAC conditional logic

CC MCC +7th S42.495 Other nondisplaced fracture of lower end of left humerus
- **HAC** 7th characters A & B see Appendix B for HAC conditional logic

CC MCC +7th S42.496 Other nondisplaced fracture of lower end of unspecified humerus
- **HAC** 7th characters A & B see Appendix B for HAC conditional logic

+ S42.9 Fracture of shoulder girdle, part unspecified
Fracture of shoulder NOS

CC MCC X+7th S42.90 Fracture of unspecified shoulder girdle, part unspecified
- **HAC** 7th characters A & B see Appendix B for HAC conditional logic

CC MCC X+7th S42.91 Fracture of right shoulder girdle, part unspecified
- **HAC** 7th characters A & B see Appendix B for HAC conditional logic

CC MCC X+7th S42.92 Fracture of left shoulder girdle, part unspecified
- **HAC** 7th characters A & B see Appendix B for HAC conditional logic

S43 Dislocation and sprain of joints and ligaments of shoulder girdle

Includes:
- avulsion of joint or ligament of shoulder girdle
- laceration of cartilage, joint or ligament of shoulder girdle
- sprain of cartilage, joint or ligament of shoulder girdle
- traumatic hemarthrosis of joint or ligament of shoulder girdle
- traumatic rupture of joint or ligament of shoulder girdle
- traumatic subluxation of joint or ligament of shoulder girdle
- traumatic tear of joint or ligament of shoulder girdle

Code also any associated open wound
Excludes2: strain of muscle, fascia and tendon of shoulder and upper arm (S46.-)

The appropriate 7th character is to be added to each code from category S43
- A initial encounter
- D subsequent encounter
- S sequela

+ S43.0 Subluxation and dislocation of shoulder joint
Dislocation of glenohumeral joint
Subluxation of glenohumeral joint

+ S43.00 Unspecified subluxation and dislocation of shoulder joint
Dislocation of humerus NOS
Subluxation of humerus NOS

- **+7th S43.001** Unspecified subluxation of right shoulder joint
- **+7th S43.002** Unspecified subluxation of left shoulder joint
- **+7th S43.003** Unspecified subluxation of unspecified shoulder joint
- **+7th S43.004** Unspecified dislocation of right shoulder joint
- **+7th S43.005** Unspecified dislocation of left shoulder joint
- **+7th S43.006** Unspecified dislocation of unspecified shoulder joint

+ S43.01 Anterior subluxation and dislocation of humerus
- **+7th S43.011** Anterior subluxation of right humerus
- **+7th S43.012** Anterior subluxation of left humerus
- **+7th S43.013** Anterior subluxation of unspecified humerus
- **+7th S43.014** Anterior dislocation of right humerus
- **+7th S43.015** Anterior dislocation of left humerus
- **+7th S43.016** Anterior dislocation of unspecified humerus

+ S43.02 Posterior subluxation and dislocation of humerus
- **+7th S43.021** Posterior subluxation of right humerus
- **+7th S43.022** Posterior subluxation of left humerus
- **+7th S43.023** Posterior subluxation of unspecified humerus
- **+7th S43.024** Posterior dislocation of right humerus
- **+7th S43.025** Posterior dislocation of left humerus
- **+7th S43.026** Posterior dislocation of unspecified humerus

+ S43.03 Inferior subluxation and dislocation of humerus
- **+7th S43.031** Inferior subluxation of right humerus
- **+7th S43.032** Inferior subluxation of left humerus
- **+7th S43.033** Inferior subluxation of unspecified humerus
- **+7th S43.034** Inferior dislocation of right humerus
- **+7th S43.035** Inferior dislocation of left humerus
- **+7th S43.036** Inferior dislocation of unspecified humerus

+ S43.08 Other subluxation and dislocation of shoulder joint
- **+7th S43.081** Other subluxation of right shoulder joint
- **+7th S43.082** Other subluxation of left shoulder joint
- **+7th S43.083** Other subluxation of unspecified shoulder joint
- **+7th S43.084** Other dislocation of right shoulder joint
- **+7th S43.085** Other dislocation of left shoulder joint
- **+7th S43.086** Other dislocation of unspecified shoulder joint

+ S43.1 Subluxation and dislocation of acromioclavicular joint

+ S43.10 Unspecified dislocation of acromioclavicular joint
- **+7th S43.101** Unspecified dislocation of right acromioclavicular joint
- **+7th S43.102** Unspecified dislocation of left acromioclavicular joint
- **+7th S43.109** Unspecified dislocation of unspecified acromioclavicular joint

+ S43.11 Subluxation of acromioclavicular joint
- **+7th S43.111** Subluxation of right acromioclavicular joint
- **+7th S43.112** Subluxation of left acromioclavicular joint
- **+7th S43.119** Subluxation of unspecified acromioclavicular joint

+ S43.12 Dislocation of acromioclavicular joint, 100%-200% displacement
- **+7th S43.121** Dislocation of right acromioclavicular joint, 100%-200% displacement
- **+7th S43.122** Dislocation of left acromioclavicular joint, 100%-200% displacement
- **+7th S43.129** Dislocation of unspecified acromioclavicular joint, 100%-200% displacement

+ S43.13 Dislocation of acromioclavicular joint, greater than 200% displacement
- **+7th S43.131** Dislocation of right acromioclavicular joint, greater than 200% displacement
- **+7th S43.132** Dislocation of left acromioclavicular joint, greater than 200% displacement
- **+7th S43.139** Dislocation of unspecified acromioclavicular joint, greater than 200% displacement

+ S43.14 Inferior dislocation of acromioclavicular joint
- **+7th S43.141** Inferior dislocation of right acromioclavicular joint
- **+7th S43.142** Inferior dislocation of left acromioclavicular joint
- **+7th S43.149** Inferior dislocation of unspecified acromioclavicular joint

- **S43.15** Posterior dislocation of acromioclavicular joint
  - +7th **S43.151** Posterior dislocation of right acromioclavicular joint
  - +7th **S43.152** Posterior dislocation of left acromioclavicular joint
  - +7th **S43.159** Posterior dislocation of unspecified acromioclavicular joint
- **S43.2** Subluxation and dislocation of sternoclavicular joint
  - **S43.20** Unspecified subluxation and dislocation of sternoclavicular joint
    - CC +7th **S43.201** Unspecified subluxation of right sternoclavicular joint
      - HAC 7th character A see Appendix B for HAC conditional logic
    - CC +7th **S43.202** Unspecified subluxation of left sternoclavicular joint
      - HAC 7th character A see Appendix B for HAC conditional logic
    - CC +7th **S43.203** Unspecified subluxation of unspecified sternoclavicular joint
      - HAC 7th character A see Appendix B for HAC conditional logic
    - CC +7th **S43.204** Unspecified dislocation of right sternoclavicular joint
      - HAC 7th character A see Appendix B for HAC conditional logic
    - CC +7th **S43.205** Unspecified dislocation of left sternoclavicular joint
      - HAC 7th character A see Appendix B for HAC conditional logic
    - CC +7th **S43.206** Unspecified dislocation of unspecified sternoclavicular joint
      - HAC 7th character A see Appendix B for HAC conditional logic
  - **S43.21** Anterior subluxation and dislocation of sternoclavicular joint
    - CC +7th **S43.211** Anterior subluxation of right sternoclavicular joint
      - HAC 7th character A see Appendix B for HAC conditional logic
    - CC +7th **S43.212** Anterior subluxation of left sternoclavicular joint
      - HAC 7th character A see Appendix B for HAC conditional logic
    - CC +7th **S43.213** Anterior subluxation of unspecified sternoclavicular joint
      - HAC 7th character A see Appendix B for HAC conditional logic
    - CC +7th **S43.214** Anterior dislocation of right sternoclavicular joint
      - HAC 7th character A see Appendix B for HAC conditional logic
    - CC +7th **S43.215** Anterior dislocation of left sternoclavicular joint
      - HAC 7th character A see Appendix B for HAC conditional logic
    - CC +7th **S43.216** Anterior dislocation of unspecified sternoclavicular joint
      - HAC 7th character A see Appendix B for HAC conditional logic
  - **S43.22** Posterior subluxation and dislocation of sternoclavicular joint
    - CC +7th **S43.221** Posterior subluxation of right sternoclavicular joint
      - HAC 7th character A see Appendix B for HAC conditional logic
    - CC +7th **S43.222** Posterior subluxation of left sternoclavicular joint
      - HAC 7th character A see Appendix B for HAC conditional logic
    - CC +7th **S43.223** Posterior subluxation of unspecified sternoclavicular joint
      - HAC 7th character A see Appendix B for HAC conditional logic
    - CC +7th **S43.224** Posterior dislocation of right sternoclavicular joint
      - HAC 7th character A see Appendix B for HAC conditional logic
    - CC +7th **S43.225** Posterior dislocation of left sternoclavicular joint
      - HAC 7th character A see Appendix B for HAC conditional logic
    - CC +7th **S43.226** Posterior dislocation of unspecified sternoclavicular joint

- **S43.3** Subluxation and dislocation of other and unspecified parts of shoulder girdle
  - **S43.30** Subluxation and dislocation of unspecified parts of shoulder girdle
    - Dislocation of shoulder girdle NOS
    - Subluxation of shoulder girdle NOS
    - +7th **S43.301** Subluxation of unspecified parts of right shoulder girdle
    - +7th **S43.302** Subluxation of unspecified parts of left shoulder girdle
    - +7th **S43.303** Subluxation of unspecified parts of unspecified shoulder girdle
    - +7th **S43.304** Dislocation of unspecified parts of right shoulder girdle
    - +7th **S43.305** Dislocation of unspecified parts of left shoulder girdle
    - +7th **S43.306** Dislocation of unspecified parts of unspecified shoulder girdle
  - **S43.31** Subluxation and dislocation of scapula
    - +7th **S43.311** Subluxation of right scapula
    - +7th **S43.312** Subluxation of left scapula
    - +7th **S43.313** Subluxation of unspecified scapula
    - +7th **S43.314** Dislocation of right scapula
    - +7th **S43.315** Dislocation of left scapula
    - +7th **S43.316** Dislocation of unspecified scapula
  - **S43.39** Subluxation and dislocation of other parts of shoulder girdle
    - +7th **S43.391** Subluxation of other parts of right shoulder girdle
    - +7th **S43.392** Subluxation of other parts of left shoulder girdle
    - +7th **S43.393** Subluxation of other parts of unspecified shoulder girdle
    - +7th **S43.394** Dislocation of other parts of right shoulder girdle
    - +7th **S43.395** Dislocation of other parts of left shoulder girdle
    - +7th **S43.396** Dislocation of other parts of unspecified shoulder girdle
- **S43.4** Sprain of shoulder joint
  - **S43.40** Unspecified sprain of shoulder joint
    - +7th **S43.401** Unspecified sprain of right shoulder joint
    - +7th **S43.402** Unspecified sprain of left shoulder joint
    - +7th **S43.409** Unspecified sprain of unspecified shoulder joint
  - **S43.41** Sprain of coracohumeral (ligament)
    - +7th **S43.411** Sprain of right coracohumeral (ligament)
    - +7th **S43.412** Sprain of left coracohumeral (ligament)
    - +7th **S43.419** Sprain of unspecified coracohumeral (ligament)
  - **S43.42** Sprain of rotator cuff capsule
    - *Excludes1:* rotator cuff syndrome (complete) (incomplete), not specified as traumatic (M75.1-)
    - *Excludes2:* injury of tendon of rotator cuff (S46.0-)
    - +7th **S43.421** Sprain of right rotator cuff capsule
    - +7th **S43.422** Sprain of left rotator cuff capsule
    - +7th **S43.429** Sprain of unspecified rotator cuff capsule
  - **S43.43** Superior glenoid labrum lesion
    - SLAP lesion
    - *AHA CC: 2Q, 2019, 26-27*
    - +7th **S43.431** Superior glenoid labrum lesion of right shoulder
    - +7th **S43.432** Superior glenoid labrum lesion of left shoulder
    - +7th **S43.439** Superior glenoid labrum lesion of unspecified shoulder
  - **S43.49** Other sprain of shoulder joint
    - **S43.491** Other sprain of right shoulder joint
    - **S43.492** Other sprain of left shoulder joint
    - **S43.499** Other sprain of unspecified shoulder joint
- **S43.5** Sprain of acromioclavicular joint
  - Sprain of acromioclavicular ligament
  - X+7th **S43.50** Sprain of unspecified acromioclavicular joint
  - X+7th **S43.51** Sprain of right acromioclavicular joint
  - X+7th **S43.52** Sprain of left acromioclavicular joint

- **+ S43.6 Sprain of sternoclavicular joint**
  - X+7th S43.60 Sprain of unspecified sternoclavicular joint
  - X+7th S43.61 Sprain of right sternoclavicular joint
  - X+7th S43.62 Sprain of left sternoclavicular joint
- **+ S43.8 Sprain of other specified parts of shoulder girdle**
  - X+7th S43.80 Sprain of other specified parts of unspecified shoulder girdle
  - X+7th S43.81 Sprain of other specified parts of right shoulder girdle
  - X+7th S43.82 Sprain of other specified parts of left shoulder girdle
- **+ S43.9 Sprain of unspecified parts of shoulder girdle**
  - X+7th S43.90 Sprain of unspecified parts of unspecified shoulder girdle
    - Sprain of shoulder girdle NOS
  - X+7th S43.91 Sprain of unspecified parts of right shoulder girdle
  - X+7th S43.92 Sprain of unspecified parts of left shoulder girdle

S44 Injury of nerves at shoulder and upper arm level

Code also any associated open wound (S41.-)
Excludes2: *injury of brachial plexus (S14.3-)*

The appropriate 7th character is to be added to each code from category S44
- A initial encounter
- D subsequent encounter
- S sequela

- **+ S44.0 Injury of ulnar nerve at upper arm level**
  - **Excludes1:** *ulnar nerve NOS (S54.0)*
  - X+7th S44.00 Injury of ulnar nerve at upper arm level, unspecified arm
  - X+7th S44.01 Injury of ulnar nerve at upper arm level, right arm
  - X+7th S44.02 Injury of ulnar nerve at upper arm level, left arm
- **+ S44.1 Injury of median nerve at upper arm level**
  - **Excludes1:** *median nerve NOS (S54.1)*
  - X+7th S44.10 Injury of median nerve at upper arm level, unspecified arm
  - X+7th S44.11 Injury of median nerve at upper arm level, right arm
  - X+7th S44.12 Injury of median nerve at upper arm level, left arm
- **+ S44.2 Injury of radial nerve at upper arm level**
  - **Excludes1:** *radial nerve NOS (S54.2)*
  - X+7th S44.20 Injury of radial nerve at upper arm level, unspecified arm
  - X+7th S44.21 Injury of radial nerve at upper arm level, right arm
  - X+7th S44.22 Injury of radial nerve at upper arm level, left arm
- **+ S44.3 Injury of axillary nerve**
  - X+7th S44.30 Injury of axillary nerve, unspecified arm
  - X+7th S44.31 Injury of axillary nerve, right arm
  - X+7th S44.32 Injury of axillary nerve, left arm
- **+ S44.4 Injury of musculocutaneous nerve**
  - X+7th S44.40 Injury of musculocutaneous nerve, unspecified arm
  - X+7th S44.41 Injury of musculocutaneous nerve, right arm
  - X+7th S44.42 Injury of musculocutaneous nerve, left arm
- **+ S44.5 Injury of cutaneous sensory nerve at shoulder and upper arm level**
  - X+7th S44.50 Injury of cutaneous sensory nerve at shoulder and upper arm level, unspecified arm
  - X+7th S44.51 Injury of cutaneous sensory nerve at shoulder and upper arm level, right arm
  - X+7th S44.52 Injury of cutaneous sensory nerve at shoulder and upper arm level, left arm
- **+ S44.8 Injury of other nerves at shoulder and upper arm level**
  - **+ S44.8X Injury of other nerves at shoulder and upper arm level**
    - +7th S44.8X1 Injury of other nerves at shoulder and upper arm level, right arm
    - +7th S44.8X2 Injury of other nerves at shoulder and upper arm level, left arm
    - +7th S44.8X9 Injury of other nerves at shoulder and upper arm level, unspecified arm

- **+ S44.9 Injury of unspecified nerve at shoulder and upper arm level**
  - X+7th S44.90 Injury of unspecified nerve at shoulder and upper arm level, unspecified arm
  - X+7th S44.91 Injury of unspecified nerve at shoulder and upper arm level, right arm
  - X+7th S44.92 Injury of unspecified nerve at shoulder and upper arm level, left arm

S45 Injury of blood vessels at shoulder and upper arm level

Code also any associated open wound (S41.-)
Excludes2: *injury of subclavian artery (S25.1)*
injury of subclavian vein (S25.3)

The appropriate 7th character is to be added to each code from category S45
- A initial encounter
- D subsequent encounter
- S sequela

- **+ S45.0 Injury of axillary artery**
  - **+ S45.00 Unspecified injury of axillary artery**
    - MCC +7th S45.001 Unspecified injury of axillary artery, right side
    - MCC +7th S45.002 Unspecified injury of axillary artery, left side
    - MCC +7th S45.009 Unspecified injury of axillary artery, unspecified side
  - **+ S45.01 Laceration of axillary artery**
    - MCC +7th S45.011 Laceration of axillary artery, right side
    - MCC +7th S45.012 Laceration of axillary artery, left side
    - MCC +7th S45.019 Laceration of axillary artery, unspecified side
  - **+ S45.09 Other specified injury of axillary artery**
    - MCC +7th S45.091 Other specified injury of axillary artery, right side
    - MCC +7th S45.092 Other specified injury of axillary artery, left side
    - MCC +7th S45.099 Other specified injury of axillary artery, unspecified side
- **+ S45.1 Injury of brachial artery**
  - **+ S45.10 Unspecified injury of brachial artery**
    - CC +7th S45.101 Unspecified injury of brachial artery, right side
    - CC +7th S45.102 Unspecified injury of brachial artery, left side
    - CC +7th S45.109 Unspecified injury of brachial artery, unspecified side
  - **+ S45.11 Laceration of brachial artery**
    - CC +7th S45.111 Laceration of brachial artery, right side
    - CC +7th S45.112 Laceration of brachial artery, left side
    - CC +7th S45.119 Laceration of brachial artery, unspecified side
  - **+ S45.19 Other specified injury of brachial artery**
    - CC +7th S45.191 Other specified injury of brachial artery, right side
    - CC +7th S45.192 Other specified injury of brachial artery, left side
    - CC +7th S45.199 Other specified injury of brachial artery, unspecified side
- **+ S45.2 Injury of axillary or brachial vein**
  - **+ S45.20 Unspecified injury of axillary or brachial vein**
    - CC +7th S45.201 Unspecified injury of axillary or brachial vein, right side
    - CC +7th S45.202 Unspecified injury of axillary or brachial vein, left side
    - CC +7th S45.209 Unspecified injury of axillary or brachial vein, unspecified side
  - **+ S45.21 Laceration of axillary or brachial vein**
    - CC +7th S45.211 Laceration of axillary or brachial vein, right side
    - CC +7th S45.212 Laceration of axillary or brachial vein, left side
    - CC +7th S45.219 Laceration of axillary or brachial vein, unspecified side
  - **+ S45.29 Other specified injury of axillary or brachial vein**
    - CC +7th S45.291 Other specified injury of axillary or brachial vein, right side
    - CC +7th S45.292 Other specified injury of axillary or brachial vein, left side
    - CC +7th S45.299 Other specified injury of axillary or brachial vein, unspecified side

- **+ S45.3 Injury of superficial vein at shoulder and upper arm level**
  - **+ S45.30** Unspecified injury of superficial vein at shoulder and upper arm level
    - CC +7th S45.301 Unspecified injury of superficial vein at shoulder and upper arm level, right arm
    - CC +7th S45.302 Unspecified injury of superficial vein at shoulder and upper arm level, left arm
    - CC +7th S45.309 Unspecified injury of superficial vein at shoulder and upper arm level, unspecified arm
  - **+ S45.31** Laceration of superficial vein at shoulder and upper arm level
    - CC +7th S45.311 Laceration of superficial vein at shoulder and upper arm level, right arm
    - CC +7th S45.312 Laceration of superficial vein at shoulder and upper arm level, left arm
    - CC +7th S45.319 Laceration of superficial vein at shoulder and upper arm level, unspecified arm
  - **+ S45.39** Other specified injury of superficial vein at shoulder and upper arm level
    - CC +7th S45.391 Other specified injury of superficial vein at shoulder and upper arm level, right arm
    - CC +7th S45.392 Other specified injury of superficial vein at shoulder and upper arm level, left arm
    - CC +7th S45.399 Other specified injury of superficial vein at shoulder and upper arm level, unspecified arm
- **+ S45.8 Injury of other specified blood vessels at shoulder and upper arm level**
  - **+ S45.80** Unspecified injury of other specified blood vessels at shoulder and upper arm level
    - CC +7th S45.801 Unspecified injury of other specified blood vessels at shoulder and upper arm level, right arm
    - CC +7th S45.802 Unspecified injury of other specified blood vessels at shoulder and upper arm level, left arm
    - CC +7th S45.809 Unspecified injury of other specified blood vessels at shoulder and upper arm level, unspecified arm
  - **+ S45.81** Laceration of other specified blood vessels at shoulder and upper arm level
    - CC +7th S45.811 Laceration of other specified blood vessels at shoulder and upper arm level, right arm
    - CC +7th S45.812 Laceration of other specified blood vessels at shoulder and upper arm level, left arm
    - CC +7th S45.819 Laceration of other specified blood vessels at shoulder and upper arm level, unspecified arm
  - **+ S45.89** Other specified injury of other specified blood vessels at shoulder and upper arm level
    - CC +7th S45.891 Other specified injury of other specified blood vessels at shoulder and upper arm level, right arm
    - CC +7th S45.892 Other specified injury of other specified blood vessels at shoulder and upper arm level, left arm
    - CC +7th S45.899 Other specified injury of other specified blood vessels at shoulder and upper arm level, unspecified arm
- **+ S45.9 Injury of unspecified blood vessel at shoulder and upper arm level**
  - **+ S45.90** Unspecified injury of unspecified blood vessel at shoulder and upper arm level
    - CC +7th S45.901 Unspecified injury of unspecified blood vessel at shoulder and upper arm level, right arm
    - CC +7th S45.902 Unspecified injury of unspecified blood vessel at shoulder and upper arm level, left arm
    - CC +7th S45.909 Unspecified injury of unspecified blood vessel at shoulder and upper arm level, unspecified arm
  - **+ S45.91** Laceration of unspecified blood vessel at shoulder and upper arm level
    - CC +7th S45.911 Laceration of unspecified blood vessel at shoulder and upper arm level, right arm
    - CC +7th S45.912 Laceration of unspecified blood vessel at shoulder and upper arm level, left arm
    - CC +7th S45.919 Laceration of unspecified blood vessel at shoulder and upper arm level, unspecified arm
  - **+ S45.99** Other specified injury of unspecified blood vessel at shoulder and upper arm level
    - CC +7th S45.991 Other specified injury of unspecified blood vessel at shoulder and upper arm level, right arm
    - CC +7th S45.992 Other specified injury of unspecified blood vessel at shoulder and upper arm level, left arm
    - CC +7th S45.999 Other specified injury of unspecified blood vessel at shoulder and upper arm level, unspecified arm

S46 Injury of muscle, fascia and tendon at shoulder and upper arm level

Code also any associated open wound (S41.-)
Excludes2: injury of muscle, fascia and tendon at elbow (S56.-)
sprain of joints and ligaments of shoulder girdle (S43.9)

The appropriate 7th character is to be added to each code from category S46
A initial encounter
D subsequent encounter
S sequela

- **+ S46.0 Injury of muscle(s) and tendon(s) of the rotator cuff of shoulder**
  - **+ S46.00** Unspecified injury of muscle(s) and tendon(s) of the rotator cuff of shoulder
    - +7th S46.001 Unspecified injury of muscle(s) and tendon(s) of the rotator cuff of right shoulder
    - +7th S46.002 Unspecified injury of muscle(s) and tendon(s) of the rotator cuff of left shoulder
    - +7th S46.009 Unspecified injury of muscle(s) and tendon(s) of the rotator cuff of unspecified shoulder
  - **+ S46.01** Strain of muscle(s) and tendon(s) of the rotator cuff of shoulder
    - +7th S46.011 Strain of muscle(s) and tendon(s) of the rotator cuff of right shoulder
    - +7th S46.012 Strain of muscle(s) and tendon(s) of the rotator cuff of left shoulder
    - +7th S46.019 Strain of muscle(s) and tendon(s) of the rotator cuff of unspecified shoulder
  - **+ S46.02** Laceration of muscle(s) and tendon(s) of the rotator cuff of shoulder
    - CC +7th S46.021 Laceration of muscle(s) and tendon(s) of the rotator cuff of right shoulder
    - CC +7th S46.022 Laceration of muscle(s) and tendon(s) of the rotator cuff of left shoulder
    - CC +7th S46.029 Laceration of muscle(s) and tendon(s) of the rotator cuff of unspecified shoulder
  - **+ S46.09** Other injury of muscle(s) and tendon(s) of the rotator cuff of shoulder
    - +7th S46.091 Other injury of muscle(s) and tendon(s) of the rotator cuff of right shoulder
    - +7th S46.092 Other injury of muscle(s) and tendon(s) of the rotator cuff of left shoulder
    - +7th S46.099 Other injury of muscle(s) and tendon(s) of the rotator cuff of unspecified shoulder
- **+ S46.1 Injury of muscle, fascia and tendon of long head of biceps**
  - **+ S46.10** Unspecified injury of muscle, fascia and tendon of long head of biceps
    - +7th S46.101 Unspecified injury of muscle, fascia and tendon of long head of biceps, right arm
    - +7th S46.102 Unspecified injury of muscle, fascia and tendon of long head of biceps, left arm
    - +7th S46.109 Unspecified injury of muscle, fascia and tendon of long head of biceps, unspecified arm

- **+ S46.11** Strain of muscle, fascia and tendon of long head of biceps
  AHA CC: 2Q, 2019, 27
  - **+7th S46.111** Strain of muscle, fascia and tendon of long head of biceps, right arm
  - **+7th S46.112** Strain of muscle, fascia and tendon of long head of biceps, left arm
  - **+7th S46.119** Strain of muscle, fascia and tendon of long head of biceps, unspecified arm
- **+ S46.12** Laceration of muscle, fascia and tendon of long head of biceps
  - **CC +7th S46.121** Laceration of muscle, fascia and tendon of long head of biceps, right arm
  - **CC +7th S46.122** Laceration of muscle, fascia and tendon of long head of biceps, left arm
  - **CC +7th S46.129** Laceration of muscle, fascia and tendon of long head of biceps, unspecified arm
- **+ S46.19** Other injury of muscle, fascia and tendon of long head of biceps
  - **+7th S46.191** Other injury of muscle, fascia and tendon of long head of biceps, right arm
  - **+7th S46.192** Other injury of muscle, fascia and tendon of long head of biceps, left arm
  - **+7th S46.199** Other injury of muscle, fascia and tendon of long head of biceps, unspecified arm
- **+ S46.2** Injury of muscle, fascia and tendon of other parts of biceps
  - **+ S46.20** Unspecified injury of muscle, fascia and tendon of other parts of biceps
    - **+7th S46.201** Unspecified injury of muscle, fascia and tendon of other parts of biceps, right arm
    - **+7th S46.202** Unspecified injury of muscle, fascia and tendon of other parts of biceps, left arm
    - **+7th S46.209** Unspecified injury of muscle, fascia and tendon of other parts of biceps, unspecified arm
  - **+ S46.21** Strain of muscle, fascia and tendon of other parts of biceps
    - **+7th S46.211** Strain of muscle, fascia and tendon of other parts of biceps, right arm
    - **+7th S46.212** Strain of muscle, fascia and tendon of other parts of biceps, left arm
    - **+7th S46.219** Strain of muscle, fascia and tendon of other parts of biceps, unspecified arm
  - **+ S46.22** Laceration of muscle, fascia and tendon of other parts of biceps
    - **CC +7th S46.221** Laceration of muscle, fascia and tendon of other parts of biceps, right arm
    - **CC +7th S46.222** Laceration of muscle, fascia and tendon of other parts of biceps, left arm
    - **CC +7th S46.229** Laceration of muscle, fascia and tendon of other parts of biceps, unspecified arm
  - **+ S46.29** Other injury of muscle, fascia and tendon of other parts of biceps
    - **+7th S46.291** Other injury of muscle, fascia and tendon of other parts of biceps, right arm
    - **+7th S46.292** Other injury of muscle, fascia and tendon of other parts of biceps, left arm
    - **+7th S46.299** Other injury of muscle, fascia and tendon of other parts of biceps, unspecified arm
- **+ S46.3** Injury of muscle, fascia and tendon of triceps
  - **+ S46.30** Unspecified injury of muscle, fascia and tendon of triceps
    - **+7th S46.301** Unspecified injury of muscle, fascia and tendon of triceps, right arm
    - **+7th S46.302** Unspecified injury of muscle, fascia and tendon of triceps, left arm
    - **+7th S46.309** Unspecified injury of muscle, fascia and tendon of triceps, unspecified arm
  - **+ S46.31** Strain of muscle, fascia and tendon of triceps
    - **+7th S46.311** Strain of muscle, fascia and tendon of triceps, right arm
    - **+7th S46.312** Strain of muscle, fascia and tendon of triceps, left arm
    - **+7th S46.319** Strain of muscle, fascia and tendon of triceps, unspecified arm
  - **+ S46.32** Laceration of muscle, fascia and tendon of triceps
    - **CC +7th S46.321** Laceration of muscle, fascia and tendon of triceps, right arm
    - **CC +7th S46.322** Laceration of muscle, fascia and tendon of triceps, left arm
    - **CC +7th S46.329** Laceration of muscle, fascia and tendon of triceps, unspecified arm
  - **+ S46.39** Other injury of muscle, fascia and tendon of triceps
    - **+7th S46.391** Other injury of muscle, fascia and tendon of triceps, right arm
    - **+7th S46.392** Other injury of muscle, fascia and tendon of triceps, left arm
    - **+7th S46.399** Other injury of muscle, fascia and tendon of triceps, unspecified arm
- **+ S46.8** Injury of other muscles, fascia and tendons at shoulder and upper arm level
  - **+ S46.80** Unspecified injury of other muscles, fascia and tendons at shoulder and upper arm level
    - **+7th S46.801** Unspecified injury of other muscles, fascia and tendons at shoulder and upper arm level, right arm
    - **+7th S46.802** Unspecified injury of other muscles, fascia and tendons at shoulder and upper arm level, left arm
    - **+7th S46.809** Unspecified injury of other muscles, fascia and tendons at shoulder and upper arm level, unspecified arm
  - **+ S46.81** Strain of other muscles, fascia and tendons at shoulder and upper arm level
    - **+7th S46.811** Strain of other muscles, fascia and tendons at shoulder and upper arm level, right arm
    - **+7th S46.812** Strain of other muscles, fascia and tendons at shoulder and upper arm level, left arm
    - **+7th S46.819** Strain of other muscles, fascia and tendons at shoulder and upper arm level, unspecified arm
  - **+ S46.82** Laceration of other muscles, fascia and tendons at shoulder and upper arm level
    - **CC +7th S46.821** Laceration of other muscles, fascia and tendons at shoulder and upper arm level, right arm
    - **CC +7th S46.822** Laceration of other muscles, fascia and tendons at shoulder and upper arm level, left arm
    - **CC +7th S46.829** Laceration of other muscles, fascia and tendons at shoulder and upper arm level, unspecified arm
  - **+ S46.89** Other injury of other muscles, fascia and tendons at shoulder and upper arm level
    - **+7th S46.891** Other injury of other muscles, fascia and tendons at shoulder and upper arm level, right arm
    - **+7th S46.892** Other injury of other muscles, fascia and tendons at shoulder and upper arm level, left arm
    - **+7th S46.899** Other injury of other muscles, fascia and tendons at shoulder and upper arm level, unspecified arm
- **+ S46.9** Injury of unspecified muscle, fascia and tendon at shoulder and upper arm level
  - **+ S46.90** Unspecified injury of unspecified muscle, fascia and tendon at shoulder and upper arm level
    - **+7th S46.901** Unspecified injury of unspecified muscle, fascia and tendon at shoulder and upper arm level, right arm
    - **+7th S46.902** Unspecified injury of unspecified muscle, fascia and tendon at shoulder and upper arm level, left arm
    - **+7th S46.909** Unspecified injury of unspecified muscle, fascia and tendon at shoulder and upper arm level, unspecified arm

Injury to Growth Plate (Salter-Harris Classification, Rang Modification)

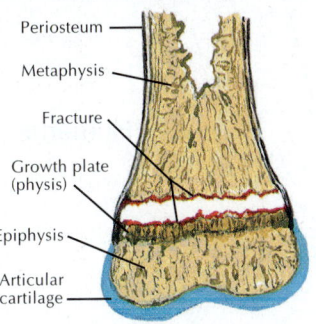

Type I. Complete separation of epiphysis from shaft through calcified cartilage (growth zone) of growth plate. No bone actually fractured; periosteum may remain intact. Most common in newborns and young children

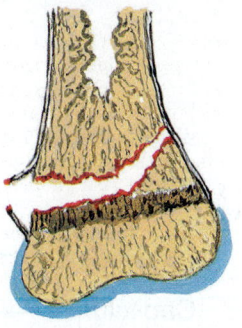

Type II. Most common. Line of separation extends partially across deep layer of growth plate and extends through metaphysis, leaving triangular portion of metaphysis attached to epiphyseal fragment

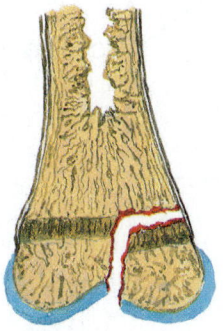

Type III. Uncommon. Intra-articular fracture through hepiphysis, across deep zone of growth plate to periphery. Open reduction and fixation often necessary

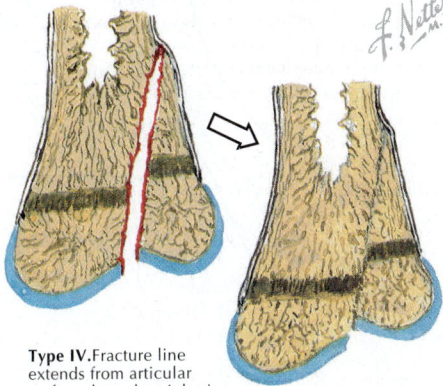

Type IV. Fracture line extends from articular surface through epiphysis, growth plate, and metaphysis. If fractured segment not perfectly realigned with open reduction, osseous bridge across growth plate may occur, resulting in partial growth arrest and joint angulation

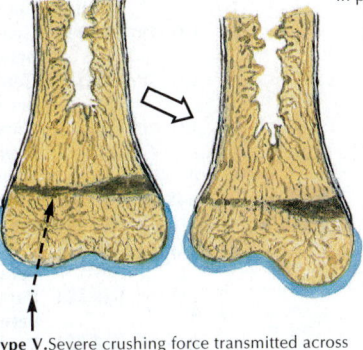

Type V. Severe crushing force transmitted across epiphysis to portion of growth plate by abduction or adduction stress or axial load. Minimal or no displacement makes radiographic diagnosis difficult; growth plate may nevertheless be damaged, resulting in partial growth arrest or shortening and angular deformity

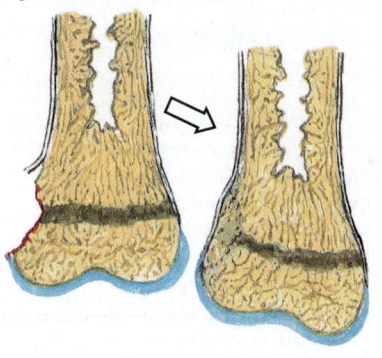

Type VI. Portion of growth plate sheared or cut off. Raw surface heals by forming bone bridge across growth plate, limiting growth on injured side and resulting in angular deformity

© 2002 Elsevier Inc. All rights reserved. www.netterimages.com

---

+ **S46.91** Strain of unspecified muscle, fascia and tendon at shoulder and upper arm level
 +7th **S46.911** Strain of unspecified muscle, fascia and tendon at shoulder and upper arm level, right arm
 +7th **S46.912** Strain of unspecified muscle, fascia and tendon at shoulder and upper arm level, left arm
 +7th **S46.919** Strain of unspecified muscle, fascia and tendon at shoulder and upper arm level, unspecified arm
+ **S46.92** Laceration of unspecified muscle, fascia and tendon at shoulder and upper arm level
 CC +7th **S46.921** Laceration of unspecified muscle, fascia and tendon at shoulder and upper arm level, right arm
 CC +7th **S46.922** Laceration of unspecified muscle, fascia and tendon at shoulder and upper arm level, left arm
 CC +7th **S46.929** Laceration of unspecified muscle, fascia and tendon at shoulder and upper arm level, unspecified arm
+ **S46.99** Other injury of unspecified muscle, fascia and tendon at shoulder and upper arm level
 +7th **S46.991** Other injury of unspecified muscle, fascia and tendon at shoulder and upper arm level, right arm
 +7th **S46.992** Other injury of unspecified muscle, fascia and tendon at shoulder and upper arm level, left arm
 +7th **S46.999** Other injury of unspecified muscle, fascia and tendon at shoulder and upper arm level, unspecified arm

Elbow

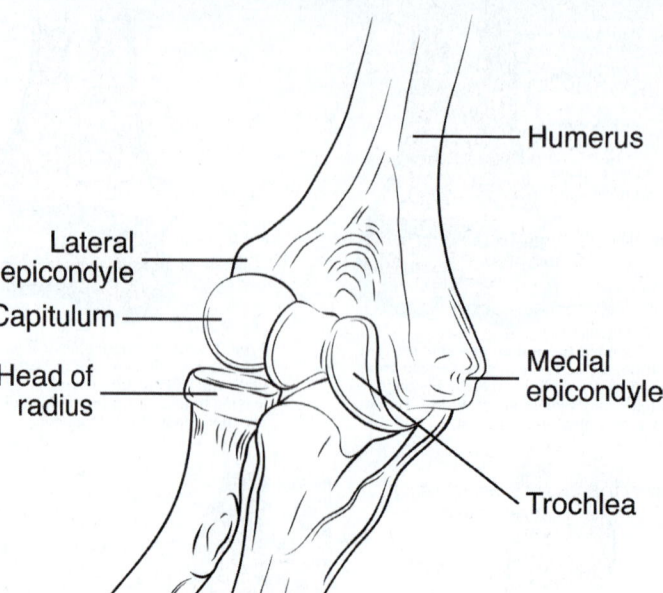

©AHIMA

S47 Crushing injury of shoulder and upper arm
  Use additional code for all associated injuries
  Excludes2: crushing injury of elbow (S57.0-)

  The appropriate 7th character is to be added to each code from category S47
  A initial encounter
  D subsequent encounter
  S sequela

X+7th S47.1 Crushing injury of right shoulder and upper arm
X+7th S47.2 Crushing injury of left shoulder and upper arm
X+7th S47.9 Crushing injury of shoulder and upper arm, unspecified arm

S48 Traumatic amputation of shoulder and upper arm
  An amputation not identified as partial or complete should be coded to complete
  Excludes1: traumatic amputation at elbow level (S58.0)

  The appropriate 7th character is to be added to each code from category S48
  A initial encounter
  D subsequent encounter
  S sequela

+ S48.0 Traumatic amputation at shoulder joint
  + S48.01 Complete traumatic amputation at shoulder joint
    CC +7th S48.011 Complete traumatic amputation at right shoulder joint
    CC +7th S48.012 Complete traumatic amputation at left shoulder joint
    CC +7th S48.019 Complete traumatic amputation at unspecified shoulder joint
  + S48.02 Partial traumatic amputation at shoulder joint
    CC +7th S48.021 Partial traumatic amputation at right shoulder joint
    CC +7th S48.022 Partial traumatic amputation at left shoulder joint
    CC +7th S48.029 Partial traumatic amputation at unspecified shoulder joint

+ S48.1 Traumatic amputation at level between shoulder and elbow
  + S48.11 Complete traumatic amputation at level between shoulder and elbow
    CC +7th S48.111 Complete traumatic amputation at level between right shoulder and elbow
    CC +7th S48.112 Complete traumatic amputation at level between left shoulder and elbow
    CC +7th S48.119 Complete traumatic amputation at level between unspecified shoulder and elbow
  + S48.12 Partial traumatic amputation at level between shoulder and elbow
    CC +7th S48.121 Partial traumatic amputation at level between right shoulder and elbow
    CC +7th S48.122 Partial traumatic amputation at level between left shoulder and elbow
    CC +7th S48.129 Partial traumatic amputation at level between unspecified shoulder and elbow
+ S48.9 Traumatic amputation of shoulder and upper arm, level unspecified
  + S48.91 Complete traumatic amputation of shoulder and upper arm, level unspecified
    CC +7th S48.911 Complete traumatic amputation of right shoulder and upper arm, level unspecified
    CC +7th S48.912 Complete traumatic amputation of left shoulder and upper arm, level unspecified
    CC +7th S48.919 Complete traumatic amputation of unspecified shoulder and upper arm, level unspecified
  + S48.92 Partial traumatic amputation of shoulder and upper arm, level unspecified
    CC +7th S48.921 Partial traumatic amputation of right shoulder and upper arm, level unspecified
    CC +7th S48.922 Partial traumatic amputation of left shoulder and upper arm, level unspecified
    CC +7th S48.929 Partial traumatic amputation of unspecified shoulder and upper arm, level unspecified

S49 Other and unspecified injuries of shoulder and upper arm

> The appropriate 7th character is to be added to each code from subcategories **S49.0** and **S49.1**
> A initial encounter for closed fracture
> D subsequent encounter for fracture with routine healing
> G subsequent encounter for fracture with delayed healing
> K subsequent encounter for fracture with nonunion
> P subsequent encounter for fracture with malunion
> S sequela

Review coding guideline C.19.c

- **S49.0 Physeal fracture of upper end of humerus**
  - **S49.00 Unspecified physeal fracture of upper end of humerus**
    - CC +7th **S49.001** Unspecified physeal fracture of upper end of humerus, right arm
      - HAC 7th character A see Appendix B for HAC conditional logic
    - CC +7th **S49.002** Unspecified physeal fracture of upper end of humerus, left arm
      - HAC 7th character A see Appendix B for HAC conditional logic
    - CC +7th **S49.009** Unspecified physeal fracture of upper end of humerus, unspecified arm
      - HAC 7th character A see Appendix B for HAC conditional logic
  - **S49.01 Salter-Harris Type I physeal fracture of upper end of humerus**
    - CC +7th **S49.011** Salter-Harris Type I physeal fracture of upper end of humerus, right arm
      - HAC 7th character A see Appendix B for HAC conditional logic
    - CC +7th **S49.012** Salter-Harris Type I physeal fracture of upper end of humerus, left arm
      - HAC 7th character A see Appendix B for HAC conditional logic
    - CC +7th **S49.019** Salter-Harris Type I physeal fracture of upper end of humerus, unspecified arm
      - HAC 7th character A see Appendix B for HAC conditional logic
  - **S49.02 Salter-Harris Type II physeal fracture of upper end of humerus**
    - CC +7th **S49.021** Salter-Harris Type II physeal fracture of upper end of humerus, right arm
      - HAC 7th character A see Appendix B for HAC conditional logic
    - CC +7th **S49.022** Salter-Harris Type II physeal fracture of upper end of humerus, left arm
      - HAC 7th character A see Appendix B for HAC conditional logic
    - CC +7th **S49.029** Salter-Harris Type II physeal fracture of upper end of humerus, unspecified arm
      - HAC 7th character A see Appendix B for HAC conditional logic
  - **S49.03 Salter-Harris Type III physeal fracture of upper end of humerus**
    - CC +7th **S49.031** Salter-Harris Type III physeal fracture of upper end of humerus, right arm
      - HAC 7th character A see Appendix B for HAC conditional logic
    - CC +7th **S49.032** Salter-Harris Type III physeal fracture of upper end of humerus, left arm
      - HAC 7th character A see Appendix B for HAC conditional logic
    - CC +7th **S49.039** Salter-Harris Type III physeal fracture of upper end of humerus, unspecified arm
      - HAC 7th character A see Appendix B for HAC conditional logic
  - **S49.04 Salter-Harris Type IV physeal fracture of upper end of humerus**
    - CC +7th **S49.041** Salter-Harris Type IV physeal fracture of upper end of humerus, right arm
      - HAC 7th character A see Appendix B for HAC conditional logic
    - CC +7th **S49.042** Salter-Harris Type IV physeal fracture of upper end of humerus, left arm
      - HAC 7th character A see Appendix B for HAC conditional logic
    - CC +7th **S49.049** Salter-Harris Type IV physeal fracture of upper end of humerus, unspecified arm
      - HAC 7th character A see Appendix B for HAC conditional logic
  - **S49.09 Other physeal fracture of upper end of humerus**
    - CC +7th **S49.091** Other physeal fracture of upper end of humerus, right arm
      - HAC 7th character A see Appendix B for HAC conditional logic
    - CC +7th **S49.092** Other physeal fracture of upper end of humerus, left arm
      - HAC 7th character A see Appendix B for HAC conditional logic
    - CC +7th **S49.099** Other physeal fracture of upper end of humerus, unspecified arm
      - HAC 7th character A see Appendix B for HAC conditional logic

- **S49.1 Physeal fracture of lower end of humerus**
  - **S49.10 Unspecified physeal fracture of lower end of humerus**
    - CC +7th **S49.101** Unspecified physeal fracture of lower end of humerus, right arm
      - HAC 7th character A see Appendix B for HAC conditional logic
    - CC +7th **S49.102** Unspecified physeal fracture of lower end of humerus, left arm
      - HAC 7th character A see Appendix B for HAC conditional logic
    - CC +7th **S49.109** Unspecified physeal fracture of lower end of humerus, unspecified arm
      - HAC 7th character A see Appendix B for HAC conditional logic
  - **S49.11 Salter-Harris Type I physeal fracture of lower end of humerus**
    - CC +7th **S49.111** Salter-Harris Type I physeal fracture of lower end of humerus, right arm
      - HAC 7th character A see Appendix B for HAC conditional logic
    - CC +7th **S49.112** Salter-Harris Type I physeal fracture of lower end of humerus, left arm
      - HAC 7th character A see Appendix B for HAC conditional logic
    - CC +7th **S49.119** Salter-Harris Type I physeal fracture of lower end of humerus, unspecified arm
      - HAC 7th character A see Appendix B for HAC conditional logic
  - **S49.12 Salter-Harris Type II physeal fracture of lower end of humerus**
    - CC +7th **S49.121** Salter-Harris Type II physeal fracture of lower end of humerus, right arm
      - HAC 7th character A see Appendix B for HAC conditional logic
    - CC +7th **S49.122** Salter-Harris Type II physeal fracture of lower end of humerus, left arm
      - HAC 7th character A see Appendix B for HAC conditional logic
    - CC +7th **S49.129** Salter-Harris Type II physeal fracture of lower end of humerus, unspecified arm
      - HAC 7th character A see Appendix B for HAC conditional logic
  - **S49.13 Salter-Harris Type III physeal fracture of lower end of humerus**
    - CC +7th **S49.131** Salter-Harris Type III physeal fracture of lower end of humerus, right arm
      - HAC 7th character A see Appendix B for HAC conditional logic
    - CC +7th **S49.132** Salter-Harris Type III physeal fracture of lower end of humerus, left arm
      - HAC 7th character A see Appendix B for HAC conditional logic
    - CC +7th **S49.139** Salter-Harris Type III physeal fracture of lower end of humerus, unspecified arm
      - HAC 7th character A see Appendix B for HAC conditional logic
  - **S49.14 Salter-Harris Type IV physeal fracture of lower end of humerus**
    - CC +7th **S49.141** Salter-Harris Type IV physeal fracture of lower end of humerus, right arm
      - HAC 7th character A see Appendix B for HAC conditional logic

S49.142–S50.919

CC +7th S49.142 Salter-Harris Type IV physeal fracture of lower end of humerus, left arm
  HAC 7th character A see Appendix B for HAC conditional logic

CC +7th S49.149 Salter-Harris Type IV physeal fracture of lower end of humerus, unspecified arm
  HAC 7th character A see Appendix B for HAC conditional logic

+ S49.19 Other physeal fracture of lower end of humerus

CC +7th S49.191 Other physeal fracture of lower end of humerus, right arm
  HAC 7th character A see Appendix B for HAC conditional logic

CC +7th S49.192 Other physeal fracture of lower end of humerus, left arm
  HAC 7th character A see Appendix B for HAC conditional logic

CC +7th S49.199 Other physeal fracture of lower end of humerus, unspecified arm
  HAC 7th character A see Appendix B for HAC conditional logic

+ S49.8 Other specified injuries of shoulder and upper arm

> The appropriate 7th character is to be added to each code in subcategory **S49.8**
> A initial encounter
> D subsequent encounter
> S sequela

X+7th S49.80 Other specified injuries of shoulder and upper arm, unspecified arm
X+7th S49.81 Other specified injuries of right shoulder and upper arm
X+7th S49.82 Other specified injuries of left shoulder and upper arm

+ S49.9 Unspecified injury of shoulder and upper arm

> The appropriate 7th character is to be added to each code in subcategory **S49.9**
> A initial encounter
> D subsequent encounter
> S sequela

X+7th S49.90 Unspecified injury of shoulder and upper arm, unspecified arm
X+7th S49.91 Unspecified injury of right shoulder and upper arm
X+7th S49.92 Unspecified injury of left shoulder and upper arm

Injuries to the elbow and forearm (S50-S59)

Excludes2: burns and corrosions (T20-T32)
frostbite (T33-T34)
injuries of wrist and hand (S60-S69)
insect bite or sting, venomous (T63.4)

S50 Superficial injury of elbow and forearm

Excludes2: superficial injury of wrist and hand (S60.-)

> The appropriate 7th character is to be added to each code from category S50
> A initial encounter
> D subsequent encounter
> S sequela

+ S50.0 Contusion of elbow
  X+7th S50.00 Contusion of unspecified elbow
  X+7th S50.01 Contusion of right elbow
  X+7th S50.02 Contusion of left elbow

+ S50.1 Contusion of forearm
  X+7th S50.10 Contusion of unspecified forearm
  X+7th S50.11 Contusion of right forearm
  X+7th S50.12 Contusion of left forearm

+ S50.3 Other superficial injuries of elbow
  + S50.31 Abrasion of elbow
    +7th S50.311 Abrasion of right elbow
    +7th S50.312 Abrasion of left elbow
    +7th S50.319 Abrasion of unspecified elbow
  + S50.32 Blister (nonthermal) of elbow
    +7th S50.321 Blister (nonthermal) of right elbow
    +7th S50.322 Blister (nonthermal) of left elbow
    +7th S50.329 Blister (nonthermal) of unspecified elbow

+ S50.34 External constriction of elbow
  +7th S50.341 External constriction of right elbow
  +7th S50.342 External constriction of left elbow
  +7th S50.349 External constriction of unspecified elbow

+ S50.35 Superficial foreign body of elbow
  Splinter in the elbow
  +7th S50.351 Superficial foreign body of right elbow
  +7th S50.352 Superficial foreign body of left elbow
  +7th S50.359 Superficial foreign body of unspecified elbow

+ S50.36 Insect bite (nonvenomous) of elbow
  +7th S50.361 Insect bite (nonvenomous) of right elbow
  +7th S50.362 Insect bite (nonvenomous) of left elbow
  +7th S50.369 Insect bite (nonvenomous) of unspecified elbow

+ S50.37 Other superficial bite of elbow
  Excludes1: open bite of elbow (S51.04)
  +7th S50.371 Other superficial bite of right elbow
  +7th S50.372 Other superficial bite of left elbow
  +7th S50.379 Other superficial bite of unspecified elbow

+ S50.8 Other superficial injuries of forearm
  + S50.81 Abrasion of forearm
    +7th S50.811 Abrasion of right forearm
    +7th S50.812 Abrasion of left forearm
    +7th S50.819 Abrasion of unspecified forearm
  + S50.82 Blister (nonthermal) of forearm
    +7th S50.821 Blister (nonthermal) of right forearm
    +7th S50.822 Blister (nonthermal) of left forearm
    +7th S50.829 Blister (nonthermal) of unspecified forearm
  + S50.84 External constriction of forearm
    +7th S50.841 External constriction of right forearm
    +7th S50.842 External constriction of left forearm
    +7th S50.849 External constriction of unspecified forearm
  + S50.85 Superficial foreign body of forearm
    Splinter in the forearm
    +7th S50.851 Superficial foreign body of right forearm
    +7th S50.852 Superficial foreign body of left forearm
    +7th S50.859 Superficial foreign body of unspecified forearm
  + S50.86 Insect bite (nonvenomous) of forearm
    +7th S50.861 Insect bite (nonvenomous) of right forearm
    +7th S50.862 Insect bite (nonvenomous) of left forearm
    +7th S50.869 Insect bite (nonvenomous) of unspecified forearm
  + S50.87 Other superficial bite of forearm
    Excludes1: open bite of forearm (S51.84)
    +7th S50.871 Other superficial bite of right forearm
    +7th S50.872 Other superficial bite of left forearm
    +7th S50.879 Other superficial bite of unspecified forearm

+ S50.9 Unspecified superficial injury of elbow and forearm
  + S50.90 Unspecified superficial injury of elbow
    +7th S50.901 Unspecified superficial injury of right elbow
    +7th S50.902 Unspecified superficial injury of left elbow
    +7th S50.909 Unspecified superficial injury of unspecified elbow
  + S50.91 Unspecified superficial injury of forearm
    S50.911 Unspecified superficial injury of right forearm
    S50.912 Unspecified superficial injury of left forearm
    S50.919 Unspecified superficial injury of unspecified forearm

S51 Open wound of elbow and forearm
  Code also any associated wound infection
  Excludes1: open fracture of elbow and forearm (S52.- with open fracture 7th character)
    traumatic amputation of elbow and forearm (S58.-)
  Excludes2: open wound of wrist and hand (S61.-)

  The appropriate 7th character is to be added to each code from category S51
  A initial encounter
  D subsequent encounter
  S sequela

+ **S51.0 Open wound of elbow**
  + **S51.00 Unspecified open wound of elbow**
    +7th S51.001 Unspecified open wound of right elbow
      AHA CC: 4Q, 2012, 108
    +7th S51.002 Unspecified open wound of left elbow
    +7th S51.009 Unspecified open wound of unspecified elbow
      Open wound of elbow NOS
  + **S51.01 Laceration without foreign body of elbow**
    +7th S51.011 Laceration without foreign body of right elbow
    +7th S51.012 Laceration without foreign body of left elbow
    +7th S51.019 Laceration without foreign body of unspecified elbow
  + **S51.02 Laceration with foreign body of elbow**
    +7th S51.021 Laceration with foreign body of right elbow
    +7th S51.022 Laceration with foreign body of left elbow
    +7th S51.029 Laceration with foreign body of unspecified elbow
  + **S51.03 Puncture wound without foreign body of elbow**
    +7th S51.031 Puncture wound without foreign body of right elbow
    +7th S51.032 Puncture wound without foreign body of left elbow
    +7th S51.039 Puncture wound without foreign body of unspecified elbow
  + **S51.04 Puncture wound with foreign body of elbow**
    +7th S51.041 Puncture wound with foreign body of right elbow
    +7th S51.042 Puncture wound with foreign body of left elbow
    +7th S51.049 Puncture wound with foreign body of unspecified elbow
  + **S51.05 Open bite of elbow**
      Bite of elbow NOS
      Excludes1: superficial bite of elbow (S50.36, S50.37)
    +7th S51.051 Open bite, right elbow
    +7th S51.052 Open bite, left elbow
    +7th S51.059 Open bite, unspecified elbow
+ **S51.8 Open wound of forearm**
  Excludes2: open wound of elbow (S51.0-)
  + **S51.80 Unspecified open wound of forearm**
    +7th S51.801 Unspecified open wound of right forearm
    +7th S51.802 Unspecified open wound of left forearm
    +7th S51.809 Unspecified open wound of unspecified forearm
      Open wound of forearm NOS
  + **S51.81 Laceration without foreign body of forearm**
    +7th S51.811 Laceration without foreign body of right forearm
    +7th S51.812 Laceration without foreign body of left forearm
    +7th S51.819 Laceration without foreign body of unspecified forearm
  + **S51.82 Laceration with foreign body of forearm**
    +7th S51.821 Laceration with foreign body of right forearm
    +7th S51.822 Laceration with foreign body of left forearm
    +7th S51.829 Laceration with foreign body of unspecified forearm
  + **S51.83 Puncture wound without foreign body of forearm**
    +7th S51.831 Puncture wound without foreign body of right forearm
    +7th S51.832 Puncture wound without foreign body of left forearm
    +7th S51.839 Puncture wound without foreign body of unspecified forearm
  + **S51.84 Puncture wound with foreign body of forearm**
    +7th S51.841 Puncture wound with foreign body of right forearm
    +7th S51.842 Puncture wound with foreign body of left forearm
    +7th S51.849 Puncture wound with foreign body of unspecified forearm
  + **S51.85 Open bite of forearm**
      Bite of forearm NOS
      Excludes1: superficial bite of forearm (S50.86, S50.87)
    +7th S51.851 Open bite of right forearm
    +7th S51.852 Open bite of left forearm
    +7th S51.859 Open bite of unspecified forearm

S52 Fracture of forearm
  NOTE A fracture not indicated as displaced or nondisplaced should be coded to displaced
    A fracture not indicated as open or closed should be coded to closed
    The open fracture designations are based on the Gustilo open fracture classification
  Excludes1: traumatic amputation of forearm (S58.-)
  Excludes2: fracture at wrist and hand level (S62.-)
    periprosthetic fracture around internal prosthetic elbow joint (M97.4)

  The appropriate 7th character is to be added to all codes from category S52
  A initial encounter for closed fracture
  B initial encounter for open fracture type I or II initial encounter for open fracture NOS
  C initial encounter for open fracture type IIIA, IIIB, or IIIC
  D subsequent encounter for closed fracture with routine healing
  E subsequent encounter for open fracture type I or II with routine healing
  F subsequent encounter for open fracture type IIIA, IIIB, or IIIC with routine healing
  G subsequent encounter for closed fracture with delayed healing
  H subsequent encounter for open fracture type I or II with delayed healing
  J subsequent encounter for open fracture type IIIA, IIIB, or IIIC with delayed healing
  K subsequent encounter for closed fracture with nonunion
  M subsequent encounter for open fracture type I or II with nonunion
  N subsequent encounter for open fracture type IIIA, IIIB, or IIIC with nonunion
  P subsequent encounter for closed fracture with malunion
  Q subsequent encounter for open fracture type I or II with malunion
  R subsequent encounter for open fracture type IIIA, IIIB, or IIIC with malunion
  S sequela

  Review coding guideline C.19.c
+ **S52.0 Fracture of upper end of ulna**
    Fracture of proximal end of ulna
    Excludes2: fracture of elbow NOS (S42.40-)
      fractures of shaft of ulna (S52.2-)
  + **S52.00 Unspecified fracture of upper end of ulna**
    CC MCC +7th S52.001 Unspecified fracture of upper end of right ulna
      HAC 7th characters B & C see Appendix B for HAC conditional logic
    CC MCC +7th S52.002 Unspecified fracture of upper end of left ulna
      HAC 7th characters B & C see Appendix B for HAC conditional logic
    CC MCC +7th S52.009 Unspecified fracture of upper end of unspecified ulna
      HAC 7th characters B & C see Appendix B for HAC conditional logic

+ S52.01 Torus fracture of upper end of ulna

> The appropriate 7th character is to be added to all codes in subcategory **S52.01**
> A initial encounter for closed fracture
> D subsequent encounter for fracture with routine healing
> G subsequent encounter for fracture with delayed healing
> K subsequent encounter for fracture with nonunion
> P - subsequent encounter for fracture with malunion
> S - sequela

CC +7th **S52.011** Torus fracture of upper end of right ulna
> HAC 7th character A see Appendix B for HAC conditional logic

CC +7th **S52.012** Torus fracture of upper end of left ulna
> HAC 7th character A see Appendix B for HAC conditional logic

CC +7th **S52.019** Torus fracture of upper end of unspecified ulna
> HAC 7th character A see Appendix B for HAC conditional logic

+ S52.02 Fracture of olecranon process without intraarticular extension of ulna

CC MCC +7th **S52.021** Displaced fracture of olecranon process without intraarticular extension of right ulna
> HAC 7th characters B & C see Appendix B for HAC conditional logic

CC MCC +7th **S52.022** Displaced fracture of olecranon process without intraarticular extension of left ulna
> HAC 7th characters B & C see Appendix B for HAC conditional logic

CC MCC +7th **S52.023** Displaced fracture of olecranon process without intraarticular extension of unspecified ulna
> HAC 7th characters B & C see Appendix B for HAC conditional logic

CC MCC +7th **S52.024** Nondisplaced fracture of olecranon process without intraarticular extension of right ulna
> HAC 7th characters B & C see Appendix B for HAC conditional logic

CC MCC +7th **S52.025** Nondisplaced fracture of olecranon process without intraarticular extension of left ulna
> HAC 7th characters B & C see Appendix B for HAC conditional logic

CC MCC +7th **S52.026** Nondisplaced fracture of olecranon process without intraarticular extension of unspecified ulna
> HAC 7th characters B & C see Appendix B for HAC conditional logic

+ S52.03 Fracture of olecranon process with intraarticular extension of ulna

CC MCC +7th **S52.031** Displaced fracture of olecranon process with intraarticular extension of right ulna
> HAC 7th characters B & C see Appendix B for HAC conditional logic

CC MCC +7th **S52.032** Displaced fracture of olecranon process with intraarticular extension of left ulna
> HAC 7th characters B & C see Appendix B for HAC conditional logic

CC MCC +7th **S52.033** Displaced fracture of olecranon process with intraarticular extension of unspecified ulna
> HAC 7th characters B & C see Appendix B for HAC conditional logic

CC MCC +7th **S52.034** Nondisplaced fracture of olecranon process with intraarticular extension of right ulna
> HAC 7th characters B & C see Appendix B for HAC conditional logic

CC MCC +7th **S52.035** Nondisplaced fracture of olecranon process with intraarticular extension of left ulna
> HAC 7th characters B & C see Appendix B for HAC conditional logic

CC MCC +7th **S52.036** Nondisplaced fracture of olecranon process with intraarticular extension of unspecified ulna
> HAC 7th characters B & C see Appendix B for HAC conditional logic

+ S52.04 Fracture of coronoid process of ulna

CC MCC +7th **S52.041** Displaced fracture of coronoid process of right ulna
> HAC 7th characters B & C see Appendix B for HAC conditional logic

CC MCC +7th **S52.042** Displaced fracture of coronoid process of left ulna
> HAC 7th characters B & C see Appendix B for HAC conditional logic

CC MCC +7th **S52.043** Displaced fracture of coronoid process of unspecified ulna
> HAC 7th characters B & C see Appendix B for HAC conditional logic

CC MCC +7th **S52.044** Nondisplaced fracture of coronoid process of right ulna
> HAC 7th characters B & C see Appendix B for HAC conditional logic

CC MCC +7th **S52.045** Nondisplaced fracture of coronoid process of left ulna
> HAC 7th characters B & C see Appendix B for HAC conditional logic

CC MCC +7th **S52.046** Nondisplaced fracture of coronoid process of unspecified ulna
> HAC 7th characters B & C see Appendix B for HAC conditional logic

+ S52.09 Other fracture of upper end of ulna

CC MCC +7th **S52.091** Other fracture of upper end of right ulna
> HAC 7th characters B & C see Appendix B for HAC conditional logic

CC MCC +7th **S52.092** Other fracture of upper end of left ulna
> HAC 7th characters B & C see Appendix B for HAC conditional logic

CC MCC +7th **S52.099** Other fracture of upper end of unspecified ulna
> HAC 7th characters B & C see Appendix B for HAC conditional logic

+ S52.1 Fracture of upper end of radius

Fracture of proximal end of radius

Excludes2: physeal fractures of upper end of radius (S59.2-)
fracture of shaft of radius (S52.3-)

+ S52.10 Unspecified fracture of upper end of radius

CC MCC +7th **S52.101** Unspecified fracture of upper end of right radius
> HAC 7th characters B & C see Appendix B for HAC conditional logic

CC MCC +7th **S52.102** Unspecified fracture of upper end of left radius
> HAC 7th characters B & C see Appendix B for HAC conditional logic

CC MCC +7th **S52.109** Unspecified fracture of upper end of unspecified radius
> HAC 7th characters B & C see Appendix B for HAC conditional logic

+ S52.11 Torus fracture of upper end of radius

> The appropriate 7th character is to be added to all codes in subcategory **S52.11**
> A initial encounter for closed fracture
> D subsequent encounter for fracture with routine healing
> G subsequent encounter for fracture with delayed healing
> K subsequent encounter for fracture with nonunion
> P subsequent encounter for fracture with malunion
> S sequela

CC +7th **S52.111** Torus fracture of upper end of right radius
> HAC 7th character A see Appendix B for HAC conditional logic

CC +7th **S52.112** Torus fracture of upper end of left radius
> HAC 7th character A see Appendix B for HAC conditional logic

CC +7th **S52.119** Torus fracture of upper end of unspecified radius
> HAC 7th character A see Appendix B for HAC conditional logic

+ S52.12 Fracture of head of radius

CC MCC +7th **S52.121** Displaced fracture of head of right radius
> HAC 7th characters B & C see Appendix B for HAC conditional logic

CC MCC +7th S52.122 Displaced fracture of head of left radius
 HAC 7th characters B & C see Appendix B for HAC conditional logic

CC MCC +7th S52.123 Displaced fracture of head of unspecified radius
 HAC 7th characters B & C see Appendix B for HAC conditional logic

CC MCC +7th S52.124 Nondisplaced fracture of head of right radius
 HAC 7th characters B & C see Appendix B for HAC conditional logic

CC MCC +7th S52.125 Nondisplaced fracture of head of left radius
 HAC 7th characters B & C see Appendix B for HAC conditional logic

CC MCC +7th S52.126 Nondisplaced fracture of head of unspecified radius
 HAC 7th characters B & C see Appendix B for HAC conditional logic

+ S52.13 Fracture of neck of radius

CC MCC +7th S52.131 Displaced fracture of neck of right radius
 HAC 7th characters B & C see Appendix B for HAC conditional logic

CC MCC +7th S52.132 Displaced fracture of neck of left radius
 HAC 7th characters B & C see Appendix B for HAC conditional logic

CC MCC +7th S52.133 Displaced fracture of neck of unspecified radius
 HAC 7th characters B & C see Appendix B for HAC conditional logic

CC MCC +7th S52.134 Nondisplaced fracture of neck of right radius
 HAC 7th characters B & C see Appendix B for HAC conditional logic

CC MCC +7th S52.135 Nondisplaced fracture of neck of left radius
 HAC 7th characters B & C see Appendix B for HAC conditional logic

CC MCC +7th S52.136 Nondisplaced fracture of neck of unspecified radius
 HAC 7th characters B & C see Appendix B for HAC conditional logic

+ S52.18 Other fracture of upper end of radius

CC MCC +7th S52.181 Other fracture of upper end of right radius
 HAC 7th characters B & C see Appendix B for HAC conditional logic

CC MCC +7th S52.182 Other fracture of upper end of left radius
 HAC 7th characters B & C see Appendix B for HAC conditional logic

CC MCC +7th S52.189 Other fracture of upper end of unspecified radius
 HAC 7th characters B & C see Appendix B for HAC conditional logic

+ S52.2 Fracture of shaft of ulna

+ S52.20 Unspecified fracture of shaft of ulna
 Fracture of ulna NOS

CC MCC +7th S52.201 Unspecified fracture of shaft of right ulna
 HAC 7th characters A - C see Appendix B for HAC conditional logic

CC MCC +7th S52.202 Unspecified fracture of shaft of left ulna
 HAC 7th characters A - C see Appendix B for HAC conditional logic

CC MCC +7th S52.209 Unspecified fracture of shaft of unspecified ulna
 HAC 7th characters A - C see Appendix B for HAC conditional logic

+ S52.21 Greenstick fracture of shaft of ulna

> The appropriate 7th character is to be added to all codes in subcategory **S52.21**
> A   initial encounter for closed fracture
> D   subsequent encounter for fracture with routine healing
> G   subsequent encounter for fracture with delayed healing
> K   subsequent encounter for fracture with nonunion
> P   subsequent encounter for fracture with malunion
> S   sequela

CC +7th S52.211 Greenstick fracture of shaft of right ulna
 HAC 7th character A see Appendix B for HAC conditional logic

CC +7th S52.212 Greenstick fracture of shaft of left ulna
 HAC 7th character A see Appendix B for HAC conditional logic

CC +7th S52.219 Greenstick fracture of shaft of unspecified ulna
 HAC 7th character A see Appendix B for HAC conditional logic

+ S52.22 Transverse fracture of shaft of ulna

CC MCC +7th S52.221 Displaced transverse fracture of shaft of right ulna
 HAC 7th characters A - C see Appendix B for HAC conditional logic

CC MCC +7th S52.222 Displaced transverse fracture of shaft of left ulna
 HAC 7th characters A - C see Appendix B for HAC conditional logic

CC MCC +7th S52.223 Displaced transverse fracture of shaft of unspecified ulna
 HAC 7th characters A - C see Appendix B for HAC conditional logic

CC MCC +7th S52.224 Nondisplaced transverse fracture of shaft of right ulna
 HAC 7th characters A - C see Appendix B for HAC conditional logic

CC MCC +7th S52.225 Nondisplaced transverse fracture of shaft of left ulna
 HAC 7th characters A - C see Appendix B for HAC conditional logic

CC MCC +7th S52.226 Nondisplaced transverse fracture of shaft of unspecified ulna
 HAC 7th characters A - C see Appendix B for HAC conditional logic

+ S52.23 Oblique fracture of shaft of ulna

CC MCC +7th S52.231 Displaced oblique fracture of shaft of right ulna
 HAC 7th characters A - C see Appendix B for HAC conditional logic

CC MCC +7th S52.232 Displaced oblique fracture of shaft of left ulna
 HAC 7th characters A - C see Appendix B for HAC conditional logic

CC MCC +7th S52.233 Displaced oblique fracture of shaft of unspecified ulna
 HAC 7th characters A - C see Appendix B for HAC conditional logic

CC MCC +7th S52.234 Nondisplaced oblique fracture of shaft of right ulna
 HAC 7th characters A - C see Appendix B for HAC conditional logic

CC MCC +7th S52.235 Nondisplaced oblique fracture of shaft of left ulna
 HAC 7th characters A - C see Appendix B for HAC conditional logic

CC MCC +7th S52.236 Nondisplaced oblique fracture of shaft of unspecified ulna
 HAC 7th characters A - C see Appendix B for HAC conditional logic

+ S52.24 Spiral fracture of shaft of ulna

CC MCC +7th S52.241 Displaced spiral fracture of shaft of ulna, right arm
 HAC 7th characters A - C see Appendix B for HAC conditional logic

CC MCC +7th S52.242 Displaced spiral fracture of shaft of ulna, left arm
 HAC 7th characters A - C see Appendix B for HAC conditional logic

CC MCC +7th	S52.243	Displaced spiral fracture of shaft of ulna, unspecified
		HAC 7th characters A - C see Appendix B for HAC conditional logic
CC MCC +7th	S52.244	Nondisplaced spiral fracture of shaft of ulna, right arm
		HAC 7th characters A - C see Appendix B for HAC conditional logic
CC MCC +7th	S52.245	Nondisplaced spiral fracture of shaft of ulna, left arm
		HAC 7th characters A - C see Appendix B for HAC conditional logic
CC MCC +7th	S52.246	Nondisplaced spiral fracture of shaft of ulna, unspecified arm
		HAC 7th characters A - C see Appendix B for HAC conditional logic
+	S52.25	Comminuted fracture of shaft of ulna
CC MCC +7th	S52.251	Displaced comminuted fracture of shaft of ulna, right arm
		HAC 7th characters A - C see Appendix B for HAC conditional logic
CC MCC +7th	S52.252	Displaced comminuted fracture of shaft of ulna, left arm
		HAC 7th characters A - C see Appendix B for HAC conditional logic
CC MCC +7th	S52.253	Displaced comminuted fracture of shaft of ulna, unspecified arm
		HAC 7th characters A - C see Appendix B for HAC conditional logic
CC MCC +7th	S52.254	Nondisplaced comminuted fracture of shaft of ulna, right arm
		HAC 7th characters A - C see Appendix B for HAC conditional logic
CC MCC +7th	S52.255	Nondisplaced comminuted fracture of shaft of ulna, left arm
		HAC 7th characters A - C see Appendix B for HAC conditional logic
CC MCC +7th	S52.256	Nondisplaced comminuted fracture of shaft of ulna, unspecified arm
		HAC 7th characters A - C see Appendix B for HAC conditional logic
+	S52.26	Segmental fracture of shaft of ulna
CC MCC +7th	S52.261	Displaced segmental fracture of shaft of ulna, right arm
		HAC 7th characters A - C see Appendix B for HAC conditional logic
CC MCC +7th	S52.262	Displaced segmental fracture of shaft of ulna, left arm
		HAC 7th characters A - C see Appendix B for HAC conditional logic
CC MCC +7th	S52.263	Displaced segmental fracture of shaft of ulna, unspecified arm
		HAC 7th characters A - C see Appendix B for HAC conditional logic
CC MCC +7th	S52.264	Nondisplaced segmental fracture of shaft of ulna, right arm
		HAC 7th characters A - C see Appendix B for HAC conditional logic
CC MCC +7th	S52.265	Nondisplaced segmental fracture of shaft of ulna, left arm
		HAC 7th characters A - C see Appendix B for HAC conditional logic
CC MCC +7th	S52.266	Nondisplaced segmental fracture of shaft of ulna, unspecified arm
		HAC 7th characters A - C see Appendix B for HAC conditional logic
+	S52.27	Monteggia's fracture of ulna
		Fracture of upper shaft of ulna with dislocation of radial head
CC MCC +7th	S52.271	Monteggia's fracture of right ulna
		HAC 7th characters B & C see Appendix B for HAC conditional logic
CC MCC +7th	S52.272	Monteggia's fracture of left ulna
		HAC 7th characters B & C see Appendix B for HAC conditional logic
CC MCC +7th	S52.279	Monteggia's fracture of unspecified ulna
		HAC 7th characters B & C see Appendix B for HAC conditional logic
+	S52.28	Bent bone of ulna
CC MCC +7th	S52.281	Bent bone of right ulna
		HAC 7th characters A - C see Appendix B for HAC conditional logic
CC MCC +7th	S52.282	Bent bone of left ulna
		HAC 7th characters A - C see Appendix B for HAC conditional logic
CC MCC +7th	S52.283	Bent bone of unspecified ulna
		HAC 7th characters A - C see Appendix B for HAC conditional logic
+	S52.29	Other fracture of shaft of ulna
CC MCC +7th	S52.291	Other fracture of shaft of right ulna
		HAC 7th characters A - C see Appendix B for HAC conditional logic
CC MCC +7th	S52.292	Other fracture of shaft of left ulna
		HAC 7th characters A - C see Appendix B for HAC conditional logic
CC MCC +7th	S52.299	Other fracture of shaft of unspecified ulna
		HAC 7th characters A - C see Appendix B for HAC conditional logic
+ S52.3		Fracture of shaft of radius
+	S52.30	Unspecified fracture of shaft of radius
CC MCC +7th	S52.301	Unspecified fracture of shaft of right radius
		HAC 7th characters A - C see Appendix B for HAC conditional logic
CC MCC +7th	S52.302	Unspecified fracture of shaft of left radius
		HAC 7th characters A - C see Appendix B for HAC conditional logic
CC MCC +7th	S52.309	Unspecified fracture of shaft of unspecified radius
		HAC 7th characters A - C see Appendix B for HAC conditional logic
+	S52.31	Greenstick fracture of shaft of radius

> The appropriate 7th character is to be added to all codes in subcategory S52.31
> A initial encounter for closed fracture
> D subsequent encounter for fracture with routine healing
> G subsequent encounter for fracture with delayed healing
> K subsequent encounter for fracture with nonunion
> P subsequent encounter for fracture with malunion
> S sequela

CC +7th	S52.311	Greenstick fracture of shaft of radius, right arm
		HAC 7th character A see Appendix B for HAC conditional logic
CC +7th	S52.312	Greenstick fracture of shaft of radius, left arm
		HAC 7th character A see Appendix B for HAC conditional logic
CC +7th	S52.319	Greenstick fracture of shaft of radius, unspecified arm
		HAC 7th character A see Appendix B for HAC conditional logic
+	S52.32	Transverse fracture of shaft of radius
CC MCC +7th	S52.321	Displaced transverse fracture of shaft of right radius
		HAC 7th characters A - C see Appendix B for HAC conditional logic
CC MCC +7th	S52.322	Displaced transverse fracture of shaft of left radius
		HAC 7th characters A - C see Appendix B for HAC conditional logic
CC MCC +7th	S52.323	Displaced transverse fracture of shaft of unspecified radius
		HAC 7th characters A - C see Appendix B for HAC conditional logic
CC MCC +7th	S52.324	Nondisplaced transverse fracture of shaft of right radius
		HAC 7th characters A - C see Appendix B for HAC conditional logic
CC MCC +7th	S52.325	Nondisplaced transverse fracture of shaft of left radius
		HAC 7th characters A - C see Appendix B for HAC conditional logic
CC MCC +7th	S52.326	Nondisplaced transverse fracture of shaft of unspecified radius
		HAC 7th characters A - C see Appendix B for HAC conditional logic

+ S52.33 Oblique fracture of shaft of radius
- CC MCC +7th **S52.331** Displaced oblique fracture of shaft of right radius
  - HAC 7th characters A - C see Appendix B for HAC conditional logic
- CC MCC +7th **S52.332** Displaced oblique fracture of shaft of left radius
  - HAC 7th characters A - C see Appendix B for HAC conditional logic
- CC MCC +7th **S52.333** Displaced oblique fracture of shaft of unspecified radius
  - HAC 7th characters A - C see Appendix B for HAC conditional logic
- CC MCC +7th **S52.334** Nondisplaced oblique fracture of shaft of right radius
  - HAC 7th characters A - C see Appendix B for HAC conditional logic
- CC MCC +7th **S52.335** Nondisplaced oblique fracture of shaft of left radius
  - HAC 7th characters A - C see Appendix B for HAC conditional logic
- CC MCC +7th **S52.336** Nondisplaced oblique fracture of shaft of unspecified radius
  - HAC 7th characters A - C see Appendix B for HAC conditional logic

+ S52.34 Spiral fracture of shaft of radius
- CC MCC +7th **S52.341** Displaced spiral fracture of shaft of radius, right arm
  - HAC 7th characters A - C see Appendix B for HAC conditional logic
- CC MCC +7th **S52.342** Displaced spiral fracture of shaft of radius, left arm
  - HAC 7th characters A - C see Appendix B for HAC conditional logic
- CC MCC +7th **S52.343** Displaced spiral fracture of shaft of radius, unspecified arm
  - HAC 7th characters A - C see Appendix B for HAC conditional logic
- CC MCC +7th **S52.344** Nondisplaced spiral fracture of shaft of radius, right arm
  - HAC 7th characters A - C see Appendix B for HAC conditional logic
- CC MCC +7th **S52.345** Nondisplaced spiral fracture of shaft of radius, left arm
  - HAC 7th characters A - C see Appendix B for HAC conditional logic
- CC MCC +7th **S52.346** Nondisplaced spiral fracture of shaft of radius, unspecified arm
  - HAC 7th characters A - C see Appendix B for HAC conditional logic

+ S52.35 Comminuted fracture of shaft of radius
- CC MCC +7th **S52.351** Displaced comminuted fracture of shaft of radius, right arm
  - HAC 7th characters A - C see Appendix B for HAC conditional logic
- CC MCC +7th **S52.352** Displaced comminuted fracture of shaft of radius, left arm
  - HAC 7th characters A - C see Appendix B for HAC conditional logic
- CC MCC +7th **S52.353** Displaced comminuted fracture of shaft of radius, unspecified arm
  - HAC 7th characters A - C see Appendix B for HAC conditional logic
- CC MCC +7th **S52.354** Nondisplaced comminuted fracture of shaft of radius, right arm
  - HAC 7th characters A - C see Appendix B for HAC conditional logic
- CC MCC +7th **S52.355** Nondisplaced comminuted fracture of shaft of radius, left arm
  - HAC 7th characters A - C see Appendix B for HAC conditional logic
- CC MCC +7th **S52.356** Nondisplaced comminuted fracture of shaft of radius, unspecified arm
  - HAC 7th characters A - C see Appendix B for HAC conditional logic

+ S52.36 Segmental fracture of shaft of radius
- CC MCC +7th **S52.361** Displaced segmental fracture of shaft of radius, right arm
  - HAC 7th characters A - C see Appendix B for HAC conditional logic
- CC MCC +7th **S52.362** Displaced segmental fracture of shaft of radius, left arm
  - HAC 7th characters A - C see Appendix B for HAC conditional logic
- CC MCC +7th **S52.363** Displaced segmental fracture of shaft of radius, unspecified arm
  - HAC 7th characters A - C see Appendix B for HAC conditional logic
- CC MCC +7th **S52.364** Nondisplaced segmental fracture of shaft of radius, right arm
  - HAC 7th characters A - C see Appendix B for HAC conditional logic
- CC MCC +7th **S52.365** Nondisplaced segmental fracture of shaft of radius, left arm
  - HAC 7th characters A - C see Appendix B for HAC conditional logic
- CC MCC +7th **S52.366** Nondisplaced segmental fracture of shaft of radius, unspecified arm
  - HAC 7th characters A - C see Appendix B for HAC conditional logic

+ S52.37 Galeazzi's fracture
  Fracture of lower shaft of radius with radioulnar joint dislocation
- CC MCC +7th **S52.371** Galeazzi's fracture of right radius
  - HAC 7th characters A - C see Appendix B for HAC conditional logic
- CC MCC +7th **S52.372** Galeazzi's fracture of left radius
  - HAC 7th characters A - C see Appendix B for HAC conditional logic
- CC MCC +7th **S52.379** Galeazzi's fracture of unspecified radius
  - HAC 7th characters A - C see Appendix B for HAC conditional logic

+ S52.38 Bent bone of radius
- CC MCC +7th **S52.381** Bent bone of right radius
  - HAC 7th characters A - C see Appendix B for HAC conditional logic
- CC MCC +7th **S52.382** Bent bone of left radius
  - HAC 7th characters A - C see Appendix B for HAC conditional logic
- CC MCC +7th **S52.389** Bent bone of unspecified radius
  - HAC 7th characters A - C see Appendix B for HAC conditional logic

+ S52.39 Other fracture of shaft of radius
- CC MCC +7th **S52.391** Other fracture of shaft of radius, right arm
  - HAC 7th characters A - C see Appendix B for HAC conditional logic
- CC MCC +7th **S52.392** Other fracture of shaft of radius, left arm
  - HAC 7th characters A - C see Appendix B for HAC conditional logic
- CC MCC +7th **S52.399** Other fracture of shaft of radius, unspecified arm
  - HAC 7th characters A - C see Appendix B for HAC conditional logic

+ S52.5 Fracture of lower end of radius
  Fracture of distal end of radius
  Excludes2: *physeal fractures of lower end of radius (S59.2-)*

+ S52.50 Unspecified fracture of the lower end of radius
- CC MCC +7th **S52.501** Unspecified fracture of the lower end of right radius
  - HAC 7th characters A - C see Appendix B for HAC conditional logic
- CC MCC +7th **S52.502** Unspecified fracture of the lower end of left radius
  - HAC 7th characters A - C see Appendix B for HAC conditional logic
- CC MCC +7th **S52.509** Unspecified fracture of the lower end of unspecified radius
  - HAC 7th characters A - C see Appendix B for HAC conditional logic

+ S52.51 Fracture of radial styloid process
- CC MCC +7th **S52.511** Displaced fracture of right radial styloid process
  - HAC 7th characters A - C see Appendix B for HAC conditional logic
- CC MCC +7th **S52.512** Displaced fracture of left radial styloid process
  - HAC 7th characters A - C see Appendix B for HAC conditional logic
- CC MCC +7th **S52.513** Displaced fracture of unspecified radial styloid process
  - HAC 7th characters A - C see Appendix B for HAC conditional logic
- CC MCC +7th **S52.514** Nondisplaced fracture of right radial styloid process
  - HAC 7th characters A - C see Appendix B for HAC conditional logic

CC MCC +7th S52.515 Nondisplaced fracture of left radial styloid process
- **HAC** 7th characters A - C see Appendix B for HAC conditional logic

CC MCC +7th S52.516 Nondisplaced fracture of unspecified radial styloid process
- **HAC** 7th characters A - C see Appendix B for HAC conditional logic

+ S52.52 Torus fracture of lower end of radius

> The appropriate 7th character is to be added to all codes in subcategory **S52.52**
> - A initial encounter for closed fracture
> - D subsequent encounter for fracture with routine healing
> - G subsequent encounter for fracture with delayed healing
> - K subsequent encounter for fracture with nonunion
> - P subsequent encounter for fracture with malunion
> - S sequela

CC +7th S52.521 Torus fracture of lower end of right radius
- **HAC** 7th character A see Appendix B for HAC conditional logic

CC +7th S52.522 Torus fracture of lower end of left radius
- **HAC** 7th character A see Appendix B for HAC conditional logic

CC +7th S52.529 Torus fracture of lower end of unspecified radius
- **HAC** 7th character A see Appendix B for HAC conditional logic

+ S52.53 Colles' fracture

CC MCC +7th S52.531 Colles' fracture of right radius
- **HAC** 7th characters A - C see Appendix B for HAC conditional logic

CC MCC +7th S52.532 Colles' fracture of left radius
- *AHA CC: 2Q, 2016, 4-5*
- **HAC** 7th characters A - C see Appendix B for HAC conditional logic

CC MCC +7th S52.539 Colles' fracture of unspecified radius
- **HAC** 7th characters A - C see Appendix B for HAC conditional logic

+ S52.54 Smith's fracture

CC MCC +7th S52.541 Smith's fracture of right radius
- **HAC** 7th characters A - C see Appendix B for HAC conditional logic

CC MCC +7th S52.542 Smith's fracture of left radius
- **HAC** 7th characters A - C see Appendix B for HAC conditional logic

CC MCC +7th S52.549 Smith's fracture of unspecified radius
- **HAC** 7th characters A - C see Appendix B for HAC conditional logic

+ S52.55 Other extraarticular fracture of lower end of radius

CC MCC +7th S52.551 Other extraarticular fracture of lower end of right radius
- **HAC** 7th characters A - C see Appendix B for HAC conditional logic

CC MCC +7th S52.552 Other extraarticular fracture of lower end of left radius
- **HAC** 7th characters A - C see Appendix B for HAC conditional logic

CC MCC +7th S52.559 Other extraarticular fracture of lower end of unspecified radius
- **HAC** 7th characters A - C see Appendix B for HAC conditional logic

+ S52.56 Barton's fracture

CC MCC +7th S52.561 Barton's fracture of right radius
- **HAC** 7th characters A - C see Appendix B for HAC conditional logic

CC MCC +7th S52.562 Barton's fracture of left radius
- **HAC** 7th characters A - C see Appendix B for HAC conditional logic

CC MCC +7th S52.569 Barton's fracture of unspecified radius
- **HAC** 7th characters A - C see Appendix B for HAC conditional logic

+ S52.57 Other intraarticular fracture of lower end of radius

CC MCC +7th S52.571 Other intraarticular fracture of lower end of right radius
- **HAC** 7th characters A - C see Appendix B for HAC conditional logic

CC MCC +7th S52.572 Other intraarticular fracture of lower end of left radius
- **HAC** 7th characters A - C see Appendix B for HAC conditional logic

CC MCC +7th S52.579 Other intraarticular fracture of lower end of unspecified radius
- **HAC** 7th characters A - C see Appendix B for HAC conditional logic

+ S52.59 Other fractures of lower end of radius

CC MCC +7th S52.591 Other fractures of lower end of right radius
- *AHA CC: 3Q, 2019, 9-10*
- **HAC** 7th characters A - C see Appendix B for HAC conditional logic

CC MCC +7th S52.592 Other fractures of lower end of left radius
- **HAC** 7th characters A - C see Appendix B for HAC conditional logic

CC MCC +7th S52.599 Other fractures of lower end of unspecified radius
- **HAC** 7th characters A - C see Appendix B for HAC conditional logic

+ S52.6 Fracture of lower end of ulna

+ S52.60 Unspecified fracture of lower end of ulna

CC MCC +7th S52.601 Unspecified fracture of lower end of right ulna
- **HAC** 7th characters A - C see Appendix B for HAC conditional logic

CC MCC +7th S52.602 Unspecified fracture of lower end of left ulna
- **HAC** 7th characters A - C see Appendix B for HAC conditional logic

CC MCC +7th S52.609 Unspecified fracture of lower end of unspecified ulna
- **HAC** 7th characters A - C see Appendix B for HAC conditional logic

+ S52.61 Fracture of ulna styloid process

CC MCC +7th S52.611 Displaced fracture of right ulna styloid process
- **HAC** 7th characters A - C see Appendix B for HAC conditional logic

CC MCC +7th S52.612 Displaced fracture of left ulna styloid process
- **HAC** 7th characters A - C see Appendix B for HAC conditional logic

CC MCC +7th S52.613 Displaced fracture of unspecified ulna styloid process
- **HAC** 7th characters A - C see Appendix B for HAC conditional logic

CC MCC +7th S52.614 Nondisplaced fracture of right ulna styloid process
- **HAC** 7th characters A - C see Appendix B for HAC conditional logic

CC MCC +7th S52.615 Nondisplaced fracture of left ulna styloid process
- **HAC** 7th characters A - C see Appendix B for HAC conditional logic

CC MCC +7th S52.616 Nondisplaced fracture of unspecified ulna styloid process
- **HAC** 7th characters A - C see Appendix B for HAC conditional logic

+ S52.62 Torus fracture of lower end of ulna

> The appropriate 7th character is to be added to all codes in subcategory **S52.62**
> - A initial encounter for closed fracture
> - D subsequent encounter for fracture with routine healing
> - G subsequent encounter for fracture with delayed healing
> - K subsequent encounter for fracture with nonunion
> - P subsequent encounter for fracture with malunion
> - S sequela

CC +7th S52.621 Torus fracture of lower end of right ulna
- **HAC** 7th character A see Appendix B for HAC conditional logic

CC +7th	S52.622	Torus fracture of lower end of left ulna
		HAC 7th character A see Appendix B for HAC conditional logic
CC +7th	S52.629	Torus fracture of lower end of unspecified ulna
		HAC 7th character A see Appendix B for HAC conditional logic
+ S52.69		Other fracture of lower end of ulna
CC MCC +7th	S52.691	Other fracture of lower end of right ulna
		AHA CC: 3Q, 2019, 9-10
		HAC 7th characters A - C see Appendix B for HAC conditional logic
CC MCC +7th	S52.692	Other fracture of lower end of left ulna
		HAC 7th characters A - C see Appendix B for HAC conditional logic
CC MCC +7th	S52.699	Other fracture of lower end of unspecified ulna
		HAC 7th characters A - C see Appendix B for HAC conditional logic
+ S52.9		Unspecified fracture of forearm
CC MCC X+7th	S52.90	Unspecified fracture of unspecified forearm
		HAC 7th characters A - C see Appendix B for HAC conditional logic
CC MCC X+7th	S52.91	Unspecified fracture of right forearm
		HAC 7th characters A - C see Appendix B for HAC conditional logic
CC MCC X+7th	S52.92	Unspecified fracture of left forearm
		HAC 7th characters A - C see Appendix B for HAC conditional logic

S53 Dislocation and sprain of joints and ligaments of elbow

Includes: avulsion of joint or ligament of elbow
laceration of cartilage, joint or ligament of elbow
sprain of cartilage, joint or ligament of elbow
traumatic hemarthrosis of joint or ligament of elbow
traumatic rupture of joint or ligament of elbow
traumatic subluxation of joint or ligament of elbow
traumatic tear of joint or ligament of elbow

Code also any associated open wound

Excludes2: strain of muscle, fascia and tendon at forearm level (S56.-)

The appropriate 7th character is to be added to each code from category S53
A initial encounter
D subsequent encounter
S sequela

+ **S53.0 Subluxation and dislocation of radial head**
Dislocation of radiohumeral joint
Subluxation of radiohumeral joint
Excludes1: Monteggia's fracture-dislocation (S52.27-)
+ **S53.00 Unspecified subluxation and dislocation of radial head**
+7th S53.001 Unspecified subluxation of right radial head
+7th S53.002 Unspecified subluxation of left radial head
+7th S53.003 Unspecified subluxation of unspecified radial head
+7th S53.004 Unspecified dislocation of right radial head
+7th S53.005 Unspecified dislocation of left radial head
+7th S53.006 Unspecified dislocation of unspecified radial head
+ **S53.01 Anterior subluxation and dislocation of radial head**
Anteriomedial subluxation and dislocation of radial head
+7th S53.011 Anterior subluxation of right radial head
+7th S53.012 Anterior subluxation of left radial head
+7th S53.013 Anterior subluxation of unspecified radial head
+7th S53.014 Anterior dislocation of right radial head
+7th S53.015 Anterior dislocation of left radial head
+7th S53.016 Anterior dislocation of unspecified radial head

+ **S53.02 Posterior subluxation and dislocation of radial head**
Posteriolateral subluxation and dislocation of radial head
+7th S53.021 Posterior subluxation of right radial head
+7th S53.022 Posterior subluxation of left radial head
+7th S53.023 Posterior subluxation of unspecified radial head
+7th S53.024 Posterior dislocation of right radial head
+7th S53.025 Posterior dislocation of left radial head
+7th S53.026 Posterior dislocation of unspecified radial head
+ **S53.03 Nursemaid's elbow**
+7th S53.031 Nursemaid's elbow, right elbow
AHA CC: 1Q, 2015, 3-21
+7th S53.032 Nursemaid's elbow, left elbow
+7th S53.033 Nursemaid's elbow, unspecified elbow
+ **S53.09 Other subluxation and dislocation of radial head**
+7th S53.091 Other subluxation of right radial head
+7th S53.092 Other subluxation of left radial head
+7th S53.093 Other subluxation of unspecified radial head
+7th S53.094 Other dislocation of right radial head
+7th S53.095 Other dislocation of left radial head
+7th S53.096 Other dislocation of unspecified radial head
+ **S53.1 Subluxation and dislocation of ulnohumeral joint**
Subluxation and dislocation of elbow NOS
Excludes1: dislocation of radial head alone (S53.0-)
+ **S53.10 Unspecified subluxation and dislocation of ulnohumeral joint**
+7th S53.101 Unspecified subluxation of right ulnohumeral joint
+7th S53.102 Unspecified subluxation of left ulnohumeral joint
+7th S53.103 Unspecified subluxation of unspecified ulnohumeral joint
+7th S53.104 Unspecified dislocation of right ulnohumeral joint
+7th S53.105 Unspecified dislocation of left ulnohumeral joint
+7th S53.106 Unspecified dislocation of unspecified ulnohumeral joint
+ **S53.11 Anterior subluxation and dislocation of ulnohumeral joint**
+7th S53.111 Anterior subluxation of right ulnohumeral joint
+7th S53.112 Anterior subluxation of left ulnohumeral joint
+7th S53.113 Anterior subluxation of unspecified ulnohumeral joint
+7th S53.114 Anterior dislocation of right ulnohumeral joint
AHA CC: 4Q, 2012, 108
+7th S53.115 Anterior dislocation of left ulnohumeral joint
+7th S53.116 Anterior dislocation of unspecified ulnohumeral joint
+ **S53.12 Posterior subluxation and dislocation of ulnohumeral joint**
+7th S53.121 Posterior subluxation of right ulnohumeral joint
+7th S53.122 Posterior subluxation of left ulnohumeral joint
+7th S53.123 Posterior subluxation of unspecified ulnohumeral joint
+7th S53.124 Posterior dislocation of right ulnohumeral joint
+7th S53.125 Posterior dislocation of left ulnohumeral joint
+7th S53.126 Posterior dislocation of unspecified ulnohumeral joint
+ **S53.13 Medial subluxation and dislocation of ulnohumeral joint**
+7th S53.131 Medial subluxation of right ulnohumeral joint
+7th S53.132 Medial subluxation of left ulnohumeral joint

- +7th S53.133 Medial subluxation of unspecified ulnohumeral joint
- +7th S53.134 Medial dislocation of right ulnohumeral joint
- +7th S53.135 Medial dislocation of left ulnohumeral joint
- +7th S53.136 Medial dislocation of unspecified ulnohumeral joint
- + S53.14 Lateral subluxation and dislocation of ulnohumeral joint
  - +7th S53.141 Lateral subluxation of right ulnohumeral joint
  - +7th S53.142 Lateral subluxation of left ulnohumeral joint
  - +7th S53.143 Lateral subluxation of unspecified ulnohumeral joint
  - +7th S53.144 Lateral dislocation of right ulnohumeral joint
  - +7th S53.145 Lateral dislocation of left ulnohumeral joint
  - +7th S53.146 Lateral dislocation of unspecified ulnohumeral joint
- + S53.19 Other subluxation and dislocation of ulnohumeral joint
  - +7th S53.191 Other subluxation of right ulnohumeral joint
  - +7th S53.192 Other subluxation of left ulnohumeral joint
  - +7th S53.193 Other subluxation of unspecified ulnohumeral joint
  - +7th S53.194 Other dislocation of right ulnohumeral joint
  - +7th S53.195 Other dislocation of left ulnohumeral joint
  - +7th S53.196 Other dislocation of unspecified ulnohumeral joint
- + S53.2 Traumatic rupture of radial collateral ligament
  - **Excludes1:** sprain of radial collateral ligament NOS (S53.43-)
  - X+7th S53.20 Traumatic rupture of unspecified radial collateral ligament
  - X+7th S53.21 Traumatic rupture of right radial collateral ligament
  - X+7th S53.22 Traumatic rupture of left radial collateral ligament
- + S53.3 Traumatic rupture of ulnar collateral ligament
  - **Excludes1:** sprain of ulnar collateral ligament (S53.44-)
  - X+7th S53.30 Traumatic rupture of unspecified ulnar collateral ligament
  - X+7th S53.31 Traumatic rupture of right ulnar collateral ligament
  - X+7th S53.32 Traumatic rupture of left ulnar collateral ligament
- + S53.4 Sprain of elbow
  - **Excludes2:** traumatic rupture of radial collateral ligament (S53.2-)
    traumatic rupture of ulnar collateral ligament (S53.3-)
  - + S53.40 Unspecified sprain of elbow
    - +7th S53.401 Unspecified sprain of right elbow
    - +7th S53.402 Unspecified sprain of left elbow
    - +7th S53.409 Unspecified sprain of unspecified elbow
      Sprain of elbow NOS
  - + S53.41 Radiohumeral (joint) sprain
    - +7th S53.411 Radiohumeral (joint) sprain of right elbow
    - +7th S53.412 Radiohumeral (joint) sprain of left elbow
    - +7th S53.419 Radiohumeral (joint) sprain of unspecified elbow
  - + S53.42 Ulnohumeral (joint) sprain
    - +7th S53.421 Ulnohumeral (joint) sprain of right elbow
    - +7th S53.422 Ulnohumeral (joint) sprain of left elbow
    - +7th S53.429 Ulnohumeral (joint) sprain of unspecified elbow
  - + S53.43 Radial collateral ligament sprain
    - +7th S53.431 Radial collateral ligament sprain of right elbow
    - +7th S53.432 Radial collateral ligament sprain of left elbow
    - +7th S53.439 Radial collateral ligament sprain of unspecified elbow
  - + S53.44 Ulnar collateral ligament sprain
    - +7th S53.441 Ulnar collateral ligament sprain of right elbow
    - +7th S53.442 Ulnar collateral ligament sprain of left elbow
    - +7th S53.449 Ulnar collateral ligament sprain of unspecified elbow
  - + S53.49 Other sprain of elbow
    - +7th S53.491 Other sprain of right elbow
    - +7th S53.492 Other sprain of left elbow
    - +7th S53.499 Other sprain of unspecified elbow

S54 Injury of nerves at forearm level
Code also any associated open wound (S51.-)
Excludes2: injury of nerves at wrist and hand level (S64.-)

The appropriate 7th character is to be added to each code from category S54
A initial encounter
D subsequent encounter
S sequela

- + S54.0 Injury of ulnar nerve at forearm level
  Injury of ulnar nerve NOS
  - X+7th S54.00 Injury of ulnar nerve at forearm level, unspecified arm
  - X+7th S54.01 Injury of ulnar nerve at forearm level, right arm
  - X+7th S54.02 Injury of ulnar nerve at forearm level, left arm
- + S54.1 Injury of median nerve at forearm level
  Injury of median nerve NOS
  - X+7th S54.10 Injury of median nerve at forearm level, unspecified arm
  - X+7th S54.11 Injury of median nerve at forearm level, right arm
  - X+7th S54.12 Injury of median nerve at forearm level, left arm
- + S54.2 Injury of radial nerve at forearm level
  Injury of radial nerve NOS
  - X+7th S54.20 Injury of radial nerve at forearm level, unspecified arm
  - X+7th S54.21 Injury of radial nerve at forearm level, right arm
  - X+7th S54.22 Injury of radial nerve at forearm level, left arm
- + S54.3 Injury of cutaneous sensory nerve at forearm level
  - X+7th S54.30 Injury of cutaneous sensory nerve at forearm level, unspecified arm
  - X+7th S54.31 Injury of cutaneous sensory nerve at forearm level, right arm
  - X+7th S54.32 Injury of cutaneous sensory nerve at forearm level, left arm
- + S54.8 Injury of other nerves at forearm level
  - + S54.8X Injury of other nerves at forearm level
    - +7th S54.8X1 Injury of other nerves at forearm level, right arm
    - +7th S54.8X2 Injury of other nerves at forearm level, left arm
    - +7th S54.8X9 Injury of other nerves at forearm level, unspecified arm
- + S54.9 Injury of unspecified nerve at forearm level
  - X+7th S54.90 Injury of unspecified nerve at forearm level, unspecified arm
  - X+7th S54.91 Injury of unspecified nerve at forearm level, right arm
  - X+7th S54.92 Injury of unspecified nerve at forearm level, left arm

S55 Injury of blood vessels at forearm level

Code also any associated open wound (S51.-)

Excludes2: injury of blood vessels at wrist and hand level (S65.-)
injury of brachial vessels (S45.1-S45.2)

The appropriate 7th character is to be added to each code from category S55
- A initial encounter
- D subsequent encounter
- S sequela

- + **S55.0** Injury of ulnar artery at forearm level
  - + **S55.00** Unspecified injury of ulnar artery at forearm level
    - CC +7th **S55.001** Unspecified injury of ulnar artery at forearm level, right arm
    - CC +7th **S55.002** Unspecified injury of ulnar artery at forearm level, left arm
    - CC +7th **S55.009** Unspecified injury of ulnar artery at forearm level, unspecified arm
  - + **S55.01** Laceration of ulnar artery at forearm level
    - CC +7th **S55.011** Laceration of ulnar artery at forearm level, right arm
    - CC +7th **S55.012** Laceration of ulnar artery at forearm level, left arm
    - CC +7th **S55.019** Laceration of ulnar artery at forearm level, unspecified arm
  - + **S55.09** Other specified injury of ulnar artery at forearm level
    - CC +7th **S55.091** Other specified injury of ulnar artery at forearm level, right arm
    - CC +7th **S55.092** Other specified injury of ulnar artery at forearm level, left arm
    - CC +7th **S55.099** Other specified injury of ulnar artery at forearm level, unspecified arm
- + **S55.1** Injury of radial artery at forearm level
  - + **S55.10** Unspecified injury of radial artery at forearm level
    - CC +7th **S55.101** Unspecified injury of radial artery at forearm level, right arm
    - CC +7th **S55.102** Unspecified injury of radial artery at forearm level, left arm
    - CC +7th **S55.109** Unspecified injury of radial artery at forearm level, unspecified arm
  - + **S55.11** Laceration of radial artery at forearm level
    - CC +7th **S55.111** Laceration of radial artery at forearm level, right arm
    - CC +7th **S55.112** Laceration of radial artery at forearm level, left arm
    - CC +7th **S55.119** Laceration of radial artery at forearm level, unspecified arm
  - + **S55.19** Other specified injury of radial artery at forearm level
    - CC +7th **S55.191** Other specified injury of radial artery at forearm level, right arm
    - CC +7th **S55.192** Other specified injury of radial artery at forearm level, left arm
    - CC +7th **S55.199** Other specified injury of radial artery at forearm level, unspecified arm
- + **S55.2** Injury of vein at forearm level
  - + **S55.20** Unspecified injury of vein at forearm level
    - CC +7th **S55.201** Unspecified injury of vein at forearm level, right arm
    - CC +7th **S55.202** Unspecified injury of vein at forearm level, left arm
    - CC +7th **S55.209** Unspecified injury of vein at forearm level, unspecified arm
  - + **S55.21** Laceration of vein at forearm level
    - CC +7th **S55.211** Laceration of vein at forearm level, right arm
    - CC +7th **S55.212** Laceration of vein at forearm level, left arm
    - CC +7th **S55.219** Laceration of vein at forearm level, unspecified arm
  - + **S55.29** Other specified injury of vein at forearm level
    - CC +7th **S55.291** Other specified injury of vein at forearm level, right arm
    - CC +7th **S55.292** Other specified injury of vein at forearm level, left arm
    - CC +7th **S55.299** Other specified injury of vein at forearm level, unspecified arm
- + **S55.8** Injury of other blood vessels at forearm level
  - + **S55.80** Unspecified injury of other blood vessels at forearm level
    - CC +7th **S55.801** Unspecified injury of other blood vessels at forearm level, right arm
    - CC +7th **S55.802** Unspecified injury of other blood vessels at forearm level, left arm
    - CC +7th **S55.809** Unspecified injury of other blood vessels at forearm level, unspecified arm
  - + **S55.81** Laceration of other blood vessels at forearm level
    - CC +7th **S55.811** Laceration of other blood vessels at forearm level, right arm
    - CC +7th **S55.812** Laceration of other blood vessels at forearm level, left arm
    - CC +7th **S55.819** Laceration of other blood vessels at forearm level, unspecified arm
  - + **S55.89** Other specified injury of other blood vessels at forearm level
    - CC +7th **S55.891** Other specified injury of other blood vessels at forearm level, right arm
    - CC +7th **S55.892** Other specified injury of other blood vessels at forearm level, left arm
    - CC +7th **S55.899** Other specified injury of other blood vessels at forearm level, unspecified arm
- + **S55.9** Injury of unspecified blood vessel at forearm level
  - + **S55.90** Unspecified injury of unspecified blood vessel at forearm level
    - CC +7th **S55.901** Unspecified injury of unspecified blood vessel at forearm level, right arm
    - CC +7th **S55.902** Unspecified injury of unspecified blood vessel at forearm level, left arm
    - CC +7th **S55.909** Unspecified injury of unspecified blood vessel at forearm level, unspecified arm
  - + **S55.91** Laceration of unspecified blood vessel at forearm level
    - CC +7th **S55.911** Laceration of unspecified blood vessel at forearm level, right arm
    - CC +7th **S55.912** Laceration of unspecified blood vessel at forearm level, left arm
    - CC +7th **S55.919** Laceration of unspecified blood vessel at forearm level, unspecified arm
  - + **S55.99** Other specified injury of unspecified blood vessel at forearm level
    - CC +7th **S55.991** Other specified injury of unspecified blood vessel at forearm level, right arm
    - CC +7th **S55.992** Other specified injury of unspecified blood vessel at forearm level, left arm
    - CC +7th **S55.999** Other specified injury of unspecified blood vessel at forearm level, unspecified arm

S56 Injury of muscle, fascia and tendon at forearm level

Code also any associated open wound (S51.-)

Excludes2: injury of muscle, fascia and tendon at or below wrist (S66.-)
sprain of joints and ligaments of elbow (S53.4-)

The appropriate 7th character is to be added to each code from category S56
- A initial encounter
- D subsequent encounter
- S sequela

- + **S56.0** Injury of flexor muscle, fascia and tendon of thumb at forearm level
  - + **S56.00** Unspecified injury of flexor muscle, fascia and tendon of thumb at forearm level
    - +7th **S56.001** Unspecified injury of flexor muscle, fascia and tendon of right thumb at forearm level
    - +7th **S56.002** Unspecified injury of flexor muscle, fascia and tendon of left thumb at forearm level
    - +7th **S56.009** Unspecified injury of flexor muscle, fascia and tendon of unspecified thumb at forearm level

- **+ S56.01** Strain of flexor muscle, fascia and tendon of thumb at forearm level
  - **+7th S56.011** Strain of flexor muscle, fascia and tendon of right thumb at forearm level
  - **+7th S56.012** Strain of flexor muscle, fascia and tendon of left thumb at forearm level
  - **+7th S56.019** Strain of flexor muscle, fascia and tendon of unspecified thumb at forearm level
- **+ S56.02** Laceration of flexor muscle, fascia and tendon of thumb at forearm level
  - **CC +7th S56.021** Laceration of flexor muscle, fascia and tendon of right thumb at forearm level
  - **CC +7th S56.022** Laceration of flexor muscle, fascia and tendon of left thumb at forearm level
  - **CC +7th S56.029** Laceration of flexor muscle, fascia and tendon of unspecified thumb at forearm level
- **+ S56.09** Other injury of flexor muscle, fascia and tendon of thumb at forearm level
  - **+7th S56.091** Other injury of flexor muscle, fascia and tendon of right thumb at forearm level
  - **+7th S56.092** Other injury of flexor muscle, fascia and tendon of left thumb at forearm level
  - **+7th S56.099** Other injury of flexor muscle, fascia and tendon of unspecified thumb at forearm level
- **+ S56.1** Injury of flexor muscle, fascia and tendon of other and unspecified finger at forearm level
  - **+ S56.10** Unspecified injury of flexor muscle, fascia and tendon of other and unspecified finger at forearm level
    - **+7th S56.101** Unspecified injury of flexor muscle, fascia and tendon of right index finger at forearm level
    - **+7th S56.102** Unspecified injury of flexor muscle, fascia and tendon of left index finger at forearm level
    - **+7th S56.103** Unspecified injury of flexor muscle, fascia and tendon of right middle finger at forearm level
    - **+7th S56.104** Unspecified injury of flexor muscle, fascia and tendon of left middle finger at forearm level
    - **+7th S56.105** Unspecified injury of flexor muscle, fascia and tendon of right ring finger at forearm level
    - **+7th S56.106** Unspecified injury of flexor muscle, fascia and tendon of left ring finger at forearm level
    - **+7th S56.107** Unspecified injury of flexor muscle, fascia and tendon of right little finger at forearm level
    - **+7th S56.108** Unspecified injury of flexor muscle, fascia and tendon of left little finger at forearm level
    - **+7th S56.109** Unspecified injury of flexor muscle, fascia and tendon of unspecified finger at forearm level
  - **+ S56.11** Strain of flexor muscle, fascia and tendon of other and unspecified finger at forearm level
    - **+7th S56.111** Strain of flexor muscle, fascia and tendon of right index finger at forearm level
    - **+7th S56.112** Strain of flexor muscle, fascia and tendon of left index finger at forearm level
    - **+7th S56.113** Strain of flexor muscle, fascia and tendon of right middle finger at forearm level
    - **+7th S56.114** Strain of flexor muscle, fascia and tendon of left middle finger at forearm level
    - **+7th S56.115** Strain of flexor muscle, fascia and tendon of right ring finger at forearm level
    - **+7th S56.116** Strain of flexor muscle, fascia and tendon of left ring finger at forearm level
    - **+7th S56.117** Strain of flexor muscle, fascia and tendon of right little finger at forearm level
    - **+7th S56.118** Strain of flexor muscle, fascia and tendon of left little finger at forearm level
    - **+7th S56.119** Strain of flexor muscle, fascia and tendon of finger of unspecified finger at forearm level
  - **+ S56.12** Laceration of flexor muscle, fascia and tendon of other and unspecified finger at forearm level
    - **CC +7th S56.121** Laceration of flexor muscle, fascia and tendon of right index finger at forearm level
    - **CC +7th S56.122** Laceration of flexor muscle, fascia and tendon of left index finger at forearm level
    - **CC +7th S56.123** Laceration of flexor muscle, fascia and tendon of right middle finger at forearm level
    - **CC +7th S56.124** Laceration of flexor muscle, fascia and tendon of left middle finger at forearm level
    - **CC +7th S56.125** Laceration of flexor muscle, fascia and tendon of right ring finger at forearm level
    - **CC +7th S56.126** Laceration of flexor muscle, fascia and tendon of left ring finger at forearm level
    - **CC +7th S56.127** Laceration of flexor muscle, fascia and tendon of right little finger at forearm level
    - **CC +7th S56.128** Laceration of flexor muscle, fascia and tendon of left little finger at forearm level
    - **CC +7th S56.129** Laceration of flexor muscle, fascia and tendon of unspecified finger at forearm level
  - **+ S56.19** Other injury of flexor muscle, fascia and tendon of other and unspecified finger at forearm level
    - **+7th S56.191** Other injury of flexor muscle, fascia and tendon of right index finger at forearm level
    - **+7th S56.192** Other injury of flexor muscle, fascia and tendon of left index finger at forearm level
    - **+7th S56.193** Other injury of flexor muscle, fascia and tendon of right middle finger at forearm level
    - **+7th S56.194** Other injury of flexor muscle, fascia and tendon of left middle finger at forearm level
    - **+7th S56.195** Other injury of flexor muscle, fascia and tendon of right ring finger at forearm level
    - **+7th S56.196** Other injury of flexor muscle, fascia and tendon of left ring finger at forearm level
    - **+7th S56.197** Other injury of flexor muscle, fascia and tendon of right little finger at forearm level
    - **+7th S56.198** Other injury of flexor muscle, fascia and tendon of left little finger at forearm level
    - **+7th S56.199** Other injury of flexor muscle, fascia and tendon of unspecified finger at forearm level
- **+ S56.2** Injury of other flexor muscle, fascia and tendon at forearm level
  - **+ S56.20** Unspecified injury of other flexor muscle, fascia and tendon at forearm level
    - **+7th S56.201** Unspecified injury of other flexor muscle, fascia and tendon at forearm level, right arm
    - **+7th S56.202** Unspecified injury of other flexor muscle, fascia and tendon at forearm level, left arm
    - **+7th S56.209** Unspecified injury of other flexor muscle, fascia and tendon at forearm level, unspecified arm

- **+ S56.21** Strain of other flexor muscle, fascia and tendon at forearm level
  - **+7th S56.211** Strain of other flexor muscle, fascia and tendon at forearm level, right arm
  - **+7th S56.212** Strain of other flexor muscle, fascia and tendon at forearm level, left arm
  - **+7th S56.219** Strain of other flexor muscle, fascia and tendon at forearm level, unspecified arm
- **+ S56.22** Laceration of other flexor muscle, fascia and tendon at forearm level
  - **CC +7th S56.221** Laceration of other flexor muscle, fascia and tendon at forearm level, right arm
  - **CC +7th S56.222** Laceration of other flexor muscle, fascia and tendon at forearm level, left arm
  - **CC +7th S56.229** Laceration of other flexor muscle, fascia and tendon at forearm level, unspecified arm
- **+ S56.29** Other injury of other flexor muscle, fascia and tendon at forearm level
  - **+7th S56.291** Other injury of other flexor muscle, fascia and tendon at forearm level, right arm
  - **+7th S56.292** Other injury of other flexor muscle, fascia and tendon at forearm level, left arm
  - **+7th S56.299** Other injury of other flexor muscle, fascia and tendon at forearm level, unspecified arm
- **+ S56.3** Injury of extensor or abductor muscles, fascia and tendons of thumb at forearm level
  - **+ S56.30** Unspecified injury of extensor or abductor muscles, fascia and tendons of thumb at forearm level
    - **+7th S56.301** Unspecified injury of extensor or abductor muscles, fascia and tendons of right thumb at forearm level
    - **+7th S56.302** Unspecified injury of extensor or abductor muscles, fascia and tendons of left thumb at forearm level
    - **+7th S56.309** Unspecified injury of extensor or abductor muscles, fascia and tendons of unspecified thumb at forearm level
  - **+ S56.31** Strain of extensor or abductor muscles, fascia and tendons of thumb at forearm level
    - **+7th S56.311** Strain of extensor or abductor muscles, fascia and tendons of right thumb at forearm level
    - **+7th S56.312** Strain of extensor or abductor muscles, fascia and tendons of left thumb at forearm level
    - **+7th S56.319** Strain of extensor or abductor muscles, fascia and tendons of unspecified thumb at forearm level
  - **+ S56.32** Laceration of extensor or abductor muscles, fascia and tendons of thumb at forearm level
    - **CC +7th S56.321** Laceration of extensor or abductor muscles, fascia and tendons of right thumb at forearm level
    - **CC +7th S56.322** Laceration of extensor or abductor muscles, fascia and tendons of left thumb at forearm level
    - **CC +7th S56.329** Laceration of extensor or abductor muscles, fascia and tendons of unspecified thumb at forearm level
  - **+ S56.39** Other injury of extensor or abductor muscles, fascia and tendons of thumb at forearm level
    - **+7th S56.391** Other injury of extensor or abductor muscles, fascia and tendons of right thumb at forearm level
    - **+7th S56.392** Other injury of extensor or abductor muscles, fascia and tendons of left thumb at forearm level
    - **+7th S56.399** Other injury of extensor or abductor muscles, fascia and tendons of unspecified thumb at forearm level
- **+ S56.4** Injury of extensor muscle, fascia and tendon of other and unspecified finger at forearm level
  - **+ S56.40** Unspecified injury of extensor muscle, fascia and tendon of other and unspecified finger at forearm level
    - **+7th S56.401** Unspecified injury of extensor muscle, fascia and tendon of right index finger at forearm level
    - **+7th S56.402** Unspecified injury of extensor muscle, fascia and tendon of left index finger at forearm level
    - **+7th S56.403** Unspecified injury of extensor muscle, fascia and tendon of right middle finger at forearm level
    - **+7th S56.404** Unspecified injury of extensor muscle, fascia and tendon of left middle finger at forearm level
    - **+7th S56.405** Unspecified injury of extensor muscle, fascia and tendon of right ring finger at forearm level
    - **+7th S56.406** Unspecified injury of extensor muscle, fascia and tendon of left ring finger at forearm level
    - **+7th S56.407** Unspecified injury of extensor muscle, fascia and tendon of right little finger at forearm level
    - **+7th S56.408** Unspecified injury of extensor muscle, fascia and tendon of left little finger at forearm level
    - **+7th S56.409** Unspecified injury of extensor muscle, fascia and tendon of unspecified finger at forearm level
  - **+ S56.41** Strain of extensor muscle, fascia and tendon of other and unspecified finger at forearm level
    - **+7th S56.411** Strain of extensor muscle, fascia and tendon of right index finger at forearm level
    - **+7th S56.412** Strain of extensor muscle, fascia and tendon of left index finger at forearm level
    - **+7th S56.413** Strain of extensor muscle, fascia and tendon of right middle finger at forearm level
    - **+7th S56.414** Strain of extensor muscle, fascia and tendon of left middle finger at forearm level
    - **+7th S56.415** Strain of extensor muscle, fascia and tendon of right ring finger at forearm level
    - **+7th S56.416** Strain of extensor muscle, fascia and tendon of left ring finger at forearm level
    - **+7th S56.417** Strain of extensor muscle, fascia and tendon of right little finger at forearm level
    - **+7th S56.418** Strain of extensor muscle, fascia and tendon of left little finger at forearm level
    - **+7th S56.419** Strain of extensor muscle, fascia and tendon of finger, unspecified finger at forearm level
  - **+ S56.42** Laceration of extensor muscle, fascia and tendon of other and unspecified finger at forearm level
    - **CC +7th S56.421** Laceration of extensor muscle, fascia and tendon of right index finger at forearm level
    - **CC +7th S56.422** Laceration of extensor muscle, fascia and tendon of left index finger at forearm level
    - **CC +7th S56.423** Laceration of extensor muscle, fascia and tendon of right middle finger at forearm level
    - **CC +7th S56.424** Laceration of extensor muscle, fascia and tendon of left middle finger at forearm level
    - **CC +7th S56.425** Laceration of extensor muscle, fascia and tendon of right ring finger at forearm level
    - **CC +7th S56.426** Laceration of extensor muscle, fascia and tendon of left ring finger at forearm level

- **CC +7th S56.427** Laceration of extensor muscle, fascia and tendon of right little finger at forearm level
- **CC +7th S56.428** Laceration of extensor muscle, fascia and tendon of left little finger at forearm level
- **CC +7th S56.429** Laceration of extensor muscle, fascia and tendon of unspecified finger at forearm level

+ **S56.49** Other injury of extensor muscle, fascia and tendon of other and unspecified finger at forearm level
  - **+7th S56.491** Other injury of extensor muscle, fascia and tendon of right index finger at forearm level
  - **+7th S56.492** Other injury of extensor muscle, fascia and tendon of left index finger at forearm level
  - **+7th S56.493** Other injury of extensor muscle, fascia and tendon of right middle finger at forearm level
  - **+7th S56.494** Other injury of extensor muscle, fascia and tendon of left middle finger at forearm level
  - **+7th S56.495** Other injury of extensor muscle, fascia and tendon of right ring finger at forearm level
  - **+7th S56.496** Other injury of extensor muscle, fascia and tendon of left ring finger at forearm level
  - **+7th S56.497** Other injury of extensor muscle, fascia and tendon of right little finger at forearm level
  - **+7th S56.498** Other injury of extensor muscle, fascia and tendon of left little finger at forearm level
  - **+7th S56.499** Other injury of extensor muscle, fascia and tendon of unspecified finger at forearm level

+ **S56.5** Injury of other extensor muscle, fascia and tendon at forearm level
  + **S56.50** Unspecified injury of other extensor muscle, fascia and tendon at forearm level
    - **+7th S56.501** Unspecified injury of other extensor muscle, fascia and tendon at forearm level, right arm
    - **+7th S56.502** Unspecified injury of other extensor muscle, fascia and tendon at forearm level, left arm
    - **+7th S56.509** Unspecified injury of other extensor muscle, fascia and tendon at forearm level, unspecified arm
  + **S56.51** Strain of other extensor muscle, fascia and tendon at forearm level
    - **+7th S56.511** Strain of other extensor muscle, fascia and tendon at forearm level, right arm
    - **+7th S56.512** Strain of other extensor muscle, fascia≈and tendon at forearm level, left arm
    - **+7th S56.519** Strain of other extensor muscle, fascia and tendon at forearm level, unspecified arm
  + **S56.52** Laceration of other extensor muscle, fascia and tendon at forearm level
    - **CC +7th S56.521** Laceration of other extensor muscle, fascia and tendon at forearm level, right arm
    - **CC +7th S56.522** Laceration of other extensor muscle, fascia and tendon at forearm level, left arm
    - **CC +7th S56.529** Laceration of other extensor muscle, fascia and tendon at forearm level, unspecified arm
  + **S56.59** Other injury of other extensor muscle, fascia and tendon at forearm level
    - **+7th S56.591** Other injury of other extensor muscle, fascia and tendon at forearm level, right arm
    - **+7th S56.592** Other injury of other extensor muscle, fascia and tendon at forearm level, left arm
    - **+7th S56.599** Other injury of other extensor muscle, fascia and tendon at forearm level, unspecified arm

+ **S56.8** Injury of other muscles, fascia and tendons at forearm level
  + **S56.80** Unspecified injury of other muscles, fascia and tendons at forearm level
    - **+7th S56.801** Unspecified injury of other muscles, fascia and tendons at forearm level, right arm
    - **+7th S56.802** Unspecified injury of other muscles, fascia and tendons at forearm level, left arm
    - **+7th S56.809** Unspecified injury of other muscles, fascia and tendons at forearm level, unspecified arm
  + **S56.81** Strain of other muscles, fascia and tendons at forearm level
    - **+7th S56.811** Strain of other muscles, fascia and tendons at forearm level, right arm
    - **+7th S56.812** Strain of other muscles, fascia and tendons at forearm level, left arm
    - **+7th S56.819** Strain of other muscles, fascia and tendons at forearm level, unspecified arm
  + **S56.82** Laceration of other muscles, fascia and tendons at forearm level
    - **CC +7th S56.821** Laceration of other muscles, fascia and tendons at forearm level, right arm
    - **CC +7th S56.822** Laceration of other muscles, fascia and tendons at forearm level, left arm
    - **CC +7th S56.829** Laceration of other muscles, fascia and tendons at forearm level, unspecified arm
  + **S56.89** Other injury of other muscles, fascia and tendons at forearm level
    - **+7th S56.891** Other injury of other muscles, fascia and tendons at forearm level, right arm
    - **+7th S56.892** Other injury of other muscles, fascia and tendons at forearm level, left arm
    - **+7th S56.899** Other injury of other muscles, fascia and tendons at forearm level, unspecified arm

+ **S56.9** Injury of unspecified muscles, fascia and tendons at forearm level
  + **S56.90** Unspecified injury of unspecified muscles, fascia and tendons at forearm level
    - **+7th S56.901** Unspecified injury of unspecified muscles, fascia and tendons at forearm level, right arm
    - **+7th S56.902** Unspecified injury of unspecified muscles, fascia and tendons at forearm level, left arm
    - **+7th S56.909** Unspecified injury of unspecified muscles, fascia and tendons at forearm level, unspecified arm
  + **S56.91** Strain of unspecified muscles, fascia and tendons at forearm level
    - **+7th S56.911** Strain of unspecified muscles, fascia and tendons at forearm level, right arm
    - **+7th S56.912** Strain of unspecified muscles, fascia and tendons at forearm level, left arm
    - **+7th S56.919** Strain of unspecified muscles, fascia and tendons at forearm level, unspecified arm
  + **S56.92** Laceration of unspecified muscles, fascia and tendons at forearm level
    - **CC +7th S56.921** Laceration of unspecified muscles, fascia and tendons at forearm level, right arm
    - **CC +7th S56.922** Laceration of unspecified muscles, fascia and tendons at forearm level, left arm
    - **CC +7th S56.929** Laceration of unspecified muscles, fascia and tendons at forearm level, unspecified arm

- **+ S56.99** Other injury of unspecified muscles, fascia and tendons at forearm level
  - **+7th S56.991** Other injury of unspecified muscles, fascia and tendons at forearm level, right arm
  - **+7th S56.992** Other injury of unspecified muscles, fascia and tendons at forearm level, left arm
  - **+7th S56.999** Other injury of unspecified muscles, fascia and tendons at forearm level, unspecified arm

S57 Crushing injury of elbow and forearm

Use additional code(s) for all associated injuries
Excludes2: crushing injury of wrist and hand (S67.-)

The appropriate 7th character is to be added to each code from category S57
- A initial encounter
- D subsequent encounter
- S sequela

- **+ S57.0** Crushing injury of elbow
  - **X+7th S57.00** Crushing injury of unspecified elbow
  - **X+7th S57.01** Crushing injury of right elbow
  - **X+7th S57.02** Crushing injury of left elbow
- **+ S57.8** Crushing injury of forearm
  - **X+7th S57.80** Crushing injury of unspecified forearm
  - **X+7th S57.81** Crushing injury of right forearm
  - **X+7th S57.82** Crushing injury of left forearm

S58 Traumatic amputation of elbow and forearm

An amputation not identified as partial or complete should be coded to complete
Excludes1: traumatic amputation of wrist and hand (S68.-)

The appropriate 7th character is to be added to each code from category S58
- A initial encounter
- D subsequent encounter
- S sequela

- **+ S58.0** Traumatic amputation at elbow level
  - **+ S58.01** Complete traumatic amputation at elbow level
    - **CC +7th S58.011** Complete traumatic amputation at elbow level, right arm
    - **CC +7th S58.012** Complete traumatic amputation at elbow level, left arm
    - **CC +7th S58.019** Complete traumatic amputation at elbow level, unspecified arm
  - **+ S58.02** Partial traumatic amputation at elbow level
    - **CC +7th S58.021** Partial traumatic amputation at elbow level, right arm
    - **CC +7th S58.022** Partial traumatic amputation at elbow level, left arm
    - **CC +7th S58.029** Partial traumatic amputation at elbow level, unspecified arm
- **+ S58.1** Traumatic amputation at level between elbow and wrist
  - **+ S58.11** Complete traumatic amputation at level between elbow and wrist
    - **CC +7th S58.111** Complete traumatic amputation at level between elbow and wrist, right arm
    - **CC +7th S58.112** Complete traumatic amputation at level between elbow and wrist, left arm
    - **CC +7th S58.119** Complete traumatic amputation at level between elbow and wrist, unspecified arm
  - **+ S58.12** Partial traumatic amputation at level between elbow and wrist
    - **CC +7th S58.121** Partial traumatic amputation at level between elbow and wrist, right arm
    - **CC +7th S58.122** Partial traumatic amputation at level between elbow and wrist, left arm
    - **CC +7th S58.129** Partial traumatic amputation at level between elbow and wrist, unspecified arm
- **+ S58.9** Traumatic amputation of forearm, level unspecified
  Excludes1: traumatic amputation of wrist (S68.-)
  - **+ S58.91** Complete traumatic amputation of forearm, level unspecified
    - **CC +7th S58.911** Complete traumatic amputation of right forearm, level unspecified
    - **CC +7th S58.912** Complete traumatic amputation of left forearm, level unspecified
    - **CC +7th S58.919** Complete traumatic amputation of unspecified forearm, level unspecified
  - **+ S58.92** Partial traumatic amputation of forearm, level unspecified
    - **CC +7th S58.921** Partial traumatic amputation of right forearm, level unspecified
    - **CC +7th S58.922** Partial traumatic amputation of left forearm, level unspecified
    - **CC +7th S58.929** Partial traumatic amputation of unspecified forearm, level unspecified

S59 Other and unspecified injuries of elbow and forearm

Excludes2: other and unspecified injuries of wrist and hand (S69.-)

The appropriate 7th character is to be added to each code from subcategories **S59.0, S59.1,** and **S59.2**
- A initial encounter for closed fracture
- D subsequent encounter for fracture with routine healing
- G subsequent encounter for fracture with delayed healing
- K subsequent encounter for fracture with nonunion
- P subsequent encounter for fracture with malunion
- S sequela

Review coding guideline C.19.c

- **+ S59.0** Physeal fracture of lower end of ulna
  - **+ S59.00** Unspecified physeal fracture of lower end of ulna
    - **CC +7th S59.001** Unspecified physeal fracture of lower end of ulna, right arm
      - **HAC** 7th character A see Appendix B for HAC conditional logic
    - **CC +7th S59.002** Unspecified physeal fracture of lower end of ulna, left arm
      - **HAC** 7th character A see Appendix B for HAC conditional logic
    - **CC +7th S59.009** Unspecified physeal fracture of lower end of ulna, unspecified arm
      - **HAC** 7th character A see Appendix B for HAC conditional logic
  - **+ S59.01** Salter-Harris Type I physeal fracture of lower end of ulna
    - **CC +7th S59.011** Salter-Harris Type I physeal fracture of lower end of ulna, right arm
      - **HAC** 7th character A see Appendix B for HAC conditional logic
    - **CC +7th S59.012** Salter-Harris Type I physeal fracture of lower end of ulna, left arm
      - **HAC** 7th character A see Appendix B for HAC conditional logic
    - **CC +7th S59.019** Salter-Harris Type I physeal fracture of lower end of ulna, unspecified arm
      - **HAC** 7th character A see Appendix B for HAC conditional logic
  - **+ S59.02** Salter-Harris Type II physeal fracture of lower end of ulna
    - **CC +7th S59.021** Salter-Harris Type II physeal fracture of lower end of ulna, right arm
      - **HAC** 7th character A see Appendix B for HAC conditional logic
    - **CC +7th S59.022** Salter-Harris Type II physeal fracture of lower end of ulna, left arm
      - **HAC** 7th character A see Appendix B for HAC conditional logic
    - **CC +7th S59.029** Salter-Harris Type II physeal fracture of lower end of ulna, unspecified arm
      - **HAC** 7th character A see Appendix B for HAC conditional logic
  - **+ S59.03** Salter-Harris Type III physeal fracture of lower end of ulna
    - **CC +7th S59.031** Salter-Harris Type III physeal fracture of lower end of ulna, right arm
      - **HAC** 7th character A see Appendix B for HAC conditional logic
    - **CC +7th S59.032** Salter-Harris Type III physeal fracture of lower end of ulna, left arm
      - **HAC** 7th character A see Appendix B for HAC conditional logic
    - **CC +7th S59.039** Salter-Harris Type III physeal fracture of lower end of ulna, unspecified arm
      - **HAC** 7th character A see Appendix B for HAC conditional logic

- **+ S59.04 Salter-Harris Type IV physeal fracture of lower end of ulna**
  - **CC +7th S59.041** Salter-Harris Type IV physeal fracture of lower end of ulna, right arm
    - HAC 7th character A see Appendix B for HAC conditional logic
  - **CC +7th S59.042** Salter-Harris Type IV physeal fracture of lower end of ulna, left arm
    - HAC 7th character A see Appendix B for HAC conditional logic
  - **CC +7th S59.049** Salter-Harris Type IV physeal fracture of lower end of ulna, unspecified arm
    - HAC 7th character A see Appendix B for HAC conditional logic
- **+ S59.09 Other physeal fracture of lower end of ulna**
  - **CC +7th S59.091** Other physeal fracture of lower end of ulna, right arm
    - HAC 7th character A see Appendix B for HAC conditional logic
  - **CC +7th S59.092** Other physeal fracture of lower end of ulna, left arm
    - HAC 7th character A see Appendix B for HAC conditional logic
  - **CC +7th S59.099** Other physeal fracture of lower end of ulna, unspecified arm
    - HAC 7th character A see Appendix B for HAC conditional logic
- **+ S59.1 Physeal fracture of upper end of radius**
  - **+ S59.10 Unspecified physeal fracture of upper end of radius**
    - **CC +7th S59.101** Unspecified physeal fracture of upper end of radius, right arm
    - **CC +7th S59.102** Unspecified physeal fracture of upper end of radius, left arm
    - **CC +7th S59.109** Unspecified physeal fracture of upper end of radius, unspecified arm
  - **+ S59.11 Salter-Harris Type I physeal fracture of upper end of radius**
    - **CC +7th S59.111** Salter-Harris Type I physeal fracture of upper end of radius, right arm
    - **CC +7th S59.112** Salter-Harris Type I physeal fracture of upper end of radius, left arm
    - **CC +7th S59.119** Salter-Harris Type I physeal fracture of upper end of radius, unspecified arm
  - **+ S59.12 Salter-Harris Type II physeal fracture of upper end of radius**
    - **CC +7th S59.121** Salter-Harris Type II physeal fracture of upper end of radius, right arm
    - **CC +7th S59.122** Salter-Harris Type II physeal fracture of upper end of radius, left arm
    - **CC +7th S59.129** Salter-Harris Type II physeal fracture of upper end of radius, unspecified arm
  - **+ S59.13 Salter-Harris Type III physeal fracture of upper end of radius**
    - **CC +7th S59.131** Salter-Harris Type III physeal fracture of upper end of radius, right arm
    - **CC +7th S59.132** Salter-Harris Type III physeal fracture of upper end of radius, left arm
    - **CC +7th S59.139** Salter-Harris Type III physeal fracture of upper end of radius, unspecified arm
  - **+ S59.14 Salter-Harris Type IV physeal fracture of upper end of radius**
    - **CC +7th S59.141** Salter-Harris Type IV physeal fracture of upper end of radius, right arm
    - **CC +7th S59.142** Salter-Harris Type IV physeal fracture of upper end of radius, left arm
    - **CC +7th S59.149** Salter-Harris Type IV physeal fracture of upper end of radius, unspecified arm
  - **+ S59.19 Other physeal fracture of upper end of radius**
    - **CC +7th S59.191** Other physeal fracture of upper end of radius, right arm
    - **CC +7th S59.192** Other physeal fracture of upper end of radius, left arm
    - **CC +7th S59.199** Other physeal fracture of upper end of radius, unspecified arm
- **+ S59.2 Physeal fracture of lower end of radius**
  - **+ S59.20 Unspecified physeal fracture of lower end of radius**
    - **CC +7th S59.201** Unspecified physeal fracture of lower end of radius, right arm
      - HAC 7th character A see Appendix B for HAC conditional logic
    - **CC +7th S59.202** Unspecified physeal fracture of lower end of radius, left arm
      - HAC 7th character A see Appendix B for HAC conditional logic
    - **CC +7th S59.209** Unspecified physeal fracture of lower end of radius, unspecified arm
      - HAC 7th character A see Appendix B for HAC conditional logic
  - **+ S59.21 Salter-Harris Type I physeal fracture of lower end of radius**
    - **CC +7th S59.211** Salter-Harris Type I physeal fracture of lower end of radius, right arm
      - HAC 7th character A see Appendix B for HAC conditional logic
    - **CC +7th S59.212** Salter-Harris Type I physeal fracture of lower end of radius, left arm
      - HAC 7th character A see Appendix B for HAC conditional logic
    - **CC +7th S59.219** Salter-Harris Type I physeal fracture of lower end of radius, unspecified arm
      - HAC 7th character A see Appendix B for HAC conditional logic
  - **+ S59.22 Salter-Harris Type II physeal fracture of lower end of radius**
    - **CC +7th S59.221** Salter-Harris Type II physeal fracture of lower end of radius, right arm
      - HAC 7th character A see Appendix B for HAC conditional logic
    - **CC +7th S59.222** Salter-Harris Type II physeal fracture of lower end of radius, left arm
      - HAC 7th character A see Appendix B for HAC conditional logic
    - **CC +7th S59.229** Salter-Harris Type II physeal fracture of lower end of radius, unspecified arm
      - HAC 7th character A see Appendix B for HAC conditional logic
  - **+ S59.23 Salter-Harris Type III physeal fracture of lower end of radius**
    - **CC +7th S59.231** Salter-Harris Type III physeal fracture of lower end of radius, right arm
      - HAC 7th character A see Appendix B for HAC conditional logic
    - **CC +7th S59.232** Salter-Harris Type III physeal fracture of lower end of radius, left arm
      - HAC 7th character A see Appendix B for HAC conditional logic
    - **CC +7th S59.239** Salter-Harris Type III physeal fracture of lower end of radius, unspecified arm
      - HAC 7th character A see Appendix B for HAC conditional logic
  - **+ S59.24 Salter-Harris Type IV physeal fracture of lower end of radius**
    - **CC +7th S59.241** Salter-Harris Type IV physeal fracture of lower end of radius, right arm
      - HAC 7th character A see Appendix B for HAC conditional logic
    - **CC +7th S59.242** Salter-Harris Type IV physeal fracture of lower end of radius, left arm
      - HAC 7th character A see Appendix B for HAC conditional logic
    - **CC +7th S59.249** Salter-Harris Type IV physeal fracture of lower end of radius, unspecified arm
      - HAC 7th character A see Appendix B for HAC conditional logic

Wrist

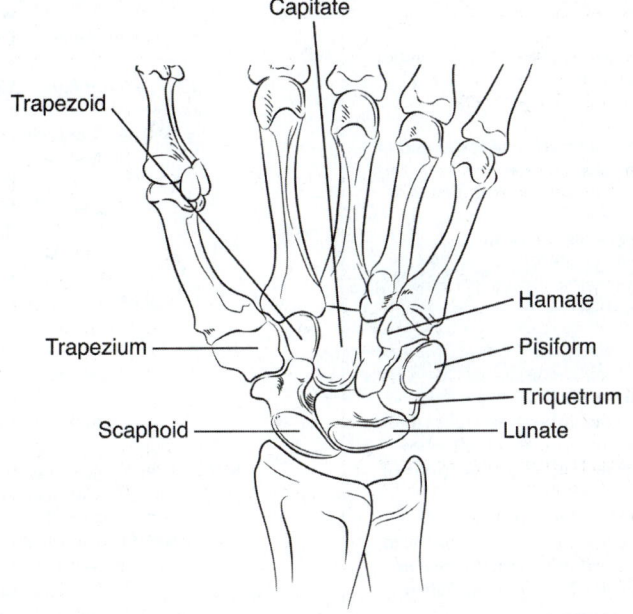

Bones of the Hand

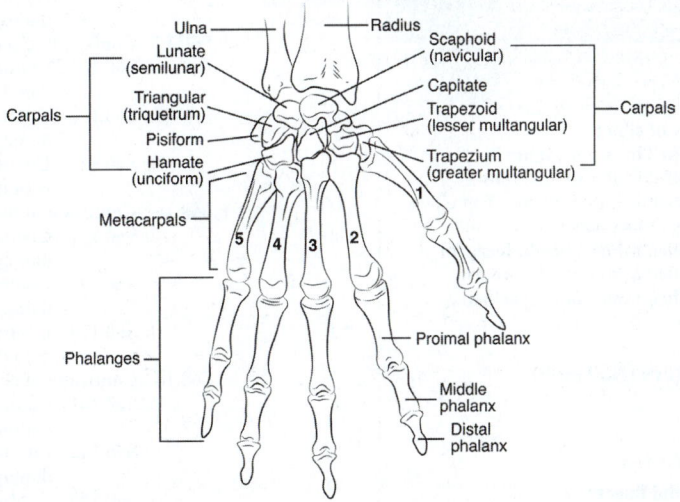

Muscles of the Hand

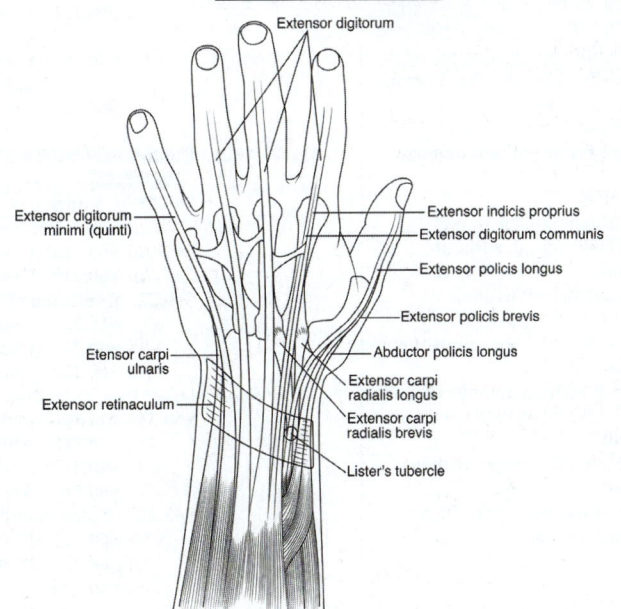

- **+ S59.29 Other physeal fracture of lower end of radius**
  - **CC +7th S59.291 Other physeal fracture of lower end of radius, right arm**
    - **HAC** 7th character A see Appendix B for HAC conditional logic
  - **CC +7th S59.292 Other physeal fracture of lower end of radius, left arm**
    - **HAC** 7th character A see Appendix B for HAC conditional logic
  - **CC +7th S59.299 Other physeal fracture of lower end of radius, unspecified arm**
    - **HAC** 7th character A see Appendix B for HAC conditional logic
- **+ S59.8 Other specified injuries of elbow and forearm**

  The appropriate 7th character is to be added to each code in subcategory **S59.8**
  A   initial encounter
  D   subsequent encounter
  S   sequela

  - **+ S59.80 Other specified injuries of elbow**
    - **+7th S59.801 Other specified injuries of right elbow**
    - **+7th S59.802 Other specified injuries of left elbow**
    - **+7th S59.809 Other specified injuries of unspecified elbow**
  - **+ S59.81 Other specified injuries of forearm**
    - **+7th S59.811 Other specified injuries right forearm**
    - **+7th S59.812 Other specified injuries left forearm**
    - **+7th S59.819 Other specified injuries unspecified forearm**
- **+ S59.9 Unspecified injury of elbow and forearm**

  The appropriate 7th character is to be added to each code in subcategory **S59.9**
  A   initial encounter
  D   subsequent encounter
  S   sequela

  - **+ S59.90 Unspecified injury of elbow**
    - **+7th S59.901 Unspecified injury of right elbow**
    - **+7th S59.902 Unspecified injury of left elbow**
    - **+7th S59.909 Unspecified injury of unspecified elbow**
  - **+ S59.91 Unspecified injury of forearm**
    - **+7th S59.911 Unspecified injury of right forearm**
    - **+7th S59.912 Unspecified injury of left forearm**
    - **+7th S59.919 Unspecified injury of unspecified forearm**

Injuries to the wrist, hand and fingers (S60-S69)

Excludes2: *burns and corrosions (T20-T32)*
frostbite (T33-T34)
insect bite or sting, venomous (T63.4)

S60 Superficial injury of wrist, hand and fingers

The appropriate 7th character is to be added to each code from category **S60**
A   initial encounter
D   subsequent encounter
S   sequela

- **+ S60.0 Contusion of finger without damage to nail**
  - **Excludes1:** *contusion involving nail (matrix) (S60.1)*
  - **X+7th S60.00 Contusion of unspecified finger without damage to nail**
    - Contusion of finger(s) NOS
  - **+ S60.01 Contusion of thumb without damage to nail**
    - **+7th S60.011 Contusion of right thumb without damage to nail**
    - **+7th S60.012 Contusion of left thumb without damage to nail**
    - **+7th S60.019 Contusion of unspecified thumb without damage to nail**
  - **+ S60.02 Contusion of index finger without damage to nail**
    - **+7th S60.021 Contusion of right index finger without damage to nail**
    - **+7th S60.022 Contusion of left index finger without damage to nail**
    - **+7th S60.029 Contusion of unspecified index finger without damage to nail**
  - **+ S60.03 Contusion of middle finger without damage to nail**
    - **+7th S60.031 Contusion of right middle finger without damage to nail**
    - **+7th S60.032 Contusion of left middle finger without damage to nail**
    - **+7th S60.039 Contusion of unspecified middle finger without damage to nail**
  - **+ S60.04 Contusion of ring finger without damage to nail**
    - **+7th S60.041 Contusion of right ring finger without damage to nail**
    - **+7th S60.042 Contusion of left ring finger without damage to nail**
    - **+7th S60.049 Contusion of unspecified ring finger without damage to nail**
  - **+ S60.05 Contusion of little finger without damage to nail**
    - **+7th S60.051 Contusion of right little finger without damage to nail**
    - **+7th S60.052 Contusion of left little finger without damage to nail**
    - **+7th S60.059 Contusion of unspecified little finger without damage to nail**
- **+ S60.1 Contusion of finger with damage to nail**
  - **X+7th S60.10 Contusion of unspecified finger with damage to nail**
  - **+ S60.11 Contusion of thumb with damage to nail**
    - **+7th S60.111 Contusion of right thumb with damage to nail**
    - **+7th S60.112 Contusion of left thumb with damage to nail**
    - **+7th S60.119 Contusion of unspecified thumb with damage to nail**
  - **+ S60.12 Contusion of index finger with damage to nail**
    - **+7th S60.121 Contusion of right index finger with damage to nail**
    - **+7th S60.122 Contusion of left index finger with damage to nail**
    - **+7th S60.129 Contusion of unspecified index finger with damage to nail**
  - **+ S60.13 Contusion of middle finger with damage to nail**
    - **+7th S60.131 Contusion of right middle finger with damage to nail**
    - **+7th S60.132 Contusion of left middle finger with damage to nail**
    - **+7th S60.139 Contusion of unspecified middle finger with damage to nail**
  - **+ S60.14 Contusion of ring finger with damage to nail**
    - **+7th S60.141 Contusion of right ring finger with damage to nail**
    - **+7th S60.142 Contusion of left ring finger with damage to nail**
    - **+7th S60.149 Contusion of unspecified ring finger with damage to nail**
  - **+ S60.15 Contusion of little finger with damage to nail**
    - **+7th S60.151 Contusion of right little finger with damage to nail**
    - **+7th S60.152 Contusion of left little finger with damage to nail**
    - **+7th S60.159 Contusion of unspecified little finger with damage to nail**
- **+ S60.2 Contusion of wrist and hand**
  - **Excludes2:** *contusion of fingers (S60.0-, S60.1-)*
  - **+ S60.21 Contusion of wrist**
    - **+7th S60.211 Contusion of right wrist**
    - **+7th S60.212 Contusion of left wrist**
    - **+7th S60.219 Contusion of unspecified wrist**
  - **+ S60.22 Contusion of hand**
    - **+7th S60.221 Contusion of right hand**
    - **+7th S60.222 Contusion of left hand**
    - **+7th S60.229 Contusion of unspecified hand**
- **+ S60.3 Other superficial injuries of thumb**
  - **+ S60.31 Abrasion of thumb**
    - **+7th S60.311 Abrasion of right thumb**
    - **+7th S60.312 Abrasion of left thumb**
    - **+7th S60.319 Abrasion of unspecified thumb**
  - **+ S60.32 Blister (nonthermal) of thumb**
    - **+7th S60.321 Blister (nonthermal) of right thumb**
    - **+7th S60.322 Blister (nonthermal) of left thumb**
    - **+7th S60.329 Blister (nonthermal) of unspecified thumb**

- **S60.34** **External constriction of thumb**
  Hair tourniquet syndrome of thumb
  Use additional cause code to identify the constricting item (W49.0-)
  - +7th **S60.341** External constriction of right thumb
  - +7th **S60.342** External constriction of left thumb
  - +7th **S60.349** External constriction of unspecified thumb
- **S60.35** **Superficial foreign body of thumb**
  Splinter in the thumb
  - +7th **S60.351** Superficial foreign body of right thumb
  - +7th **S60.352** Superficial foreign body of left thumb
  - +7th **S60.359** Superficial foreign body of unspecified thumb
- **S60.36** **Insect bite (nonvenomous) of thumb**
  - +7th **S60.361** Insect bite (nonvenomous) of right thumb
  - +7th **S60.362** Insect bite (nonvenomous) of left thumb
  - +7th **S60.369** Insect bite (nonvenomous) of unspecified thumb
- **S60.37** **Other superficial bite of thumb**
  Excludes1: open bite of thumb (S61.05-, S61.15-)
  - +7th **S60.371** Other superficial bite of right thumb
  - +7th **S60.372** Other superficial bite of left thumb
  - +7th **S60.379** Other superficial bite of unspecified thumb
- **S60.39** **Other superficial injuries of thumb**
  - +7th **S60.391** Other superficial injuries of right thumb
  - +7th **S60.392** Other superficial injuries of left thumb
  - +7th **S60.399** Other superficial injuries of unspecified thumb
- **S60.4** **Other superficial injuries of other fingers**
  - **S60.41** **Abrasion of fingers**
    - +7th **S60.410** Abrasion of right index finger
    - +7th **S60.411** Abrasion of left index finger
    - +7th **S60.412** Abrasion of right middle finger
    - +7th **S60.413** Abrasion of left middle finger
    - +7th **S60.414** Abrasion of right ring finger
    - +7th **S60.415** Abrasion of left ring finger
    - +7th **S60.416** Abrasion of right little finger
    - +7th **S60.417** Abrasion of left little finger
    - +7th **S60.418** Abrasion of other finger
      Abrasion of specified finger with unspecified laterality
    - +7th **S60.419** Abrasion of unspecified finger
  - **S60.42** **Blister (nonthermal) of fingers**
    - +7th **S60.420** Blister (nonthermal) of right index finger
    - +7th **S60.421** Blister (nonthermal) of left index finger
    - +7th **S60.422** Blister (nonthermal) of right middle finger
    - +7th **S60.423** Blister (nonthermal) of left middle finger
    - +7th **S60.424** Blister (nonthermal) of right ring finger
    - +7th **S60.425** Blister (nonthermal) of left ring finger
    - +7th **S60.426** Blister (nonthermal) of right little finger
    - +7th **S60.427** Blister (nonthermal) of left little finger
    - +7th **S60.428** Blister (nonthermal) of other finger
      Blister (nonthermal) of specified finger with unspecified laterality
    - +7th **S60.429** Blister (nonthermal) of unspecified finger
  - **S60.44** **External constriction of fingers**
    Hair tourniquet syndrome of finger
    Use additional cause code to identify the constricting item (W49.0-)
    - +7th **S60.440** External constriction of right index finger
    - +7th **S60.441** External constriction of left index finger
    - +7th **S60.442** External constriction of right middle finger
    - +7th **S60.443** External constriction of left middle finger
    - +7th **S60.444** External constriction of right ring finger
    - +7th **S60.445** External constriction of left ring finger
    - +7th **S60.446** External constriction of right little finger
    - +7th **S60.447** External constriction of left little finger
    - +7th **S60.448** External constriction of other finger
      External constriction of specified finger with unspecified laterality
    - +7th **S60.449** External constriction of unspecified finger
  - **S60.45** **Superficial foreign body of fingers**
    Splinter in the finger(s)
    - +7th **S60.450** Superficial foreign body of right index finger
    - +7th **S60.451** Superficial foreign body of left index finger
    - +7th **S60.452** Superficial foreign body of right middle finger
    - +7th **S60.453** Superficial foreign body of left middle finger
    - +7th **S60.454** Superficial foreign body of right ring finger
    - +7th **S60.455** Superficial foreign body of left ring finger
    - +7th **S60.456** Superficial foreign body of right little finger
    - +7th **S60.457** Superficial foreign body of left little finger
    - +7th **S60.458** Superficial foreign body of other finger
      Superficial foreign body of specified finger with unspecified laterality
    - +7th **S60.459** Superficial foreign body of unspecified finger
  - **S60.46** **Insect bite (nonvenomous) of fingers**
    - +7th **S60.460** Insect bite (nonvenomous) of right index finger
    - +7th **S60.461** Insect bite (nonvenomous) of left index finger
    - +7th **S60.462** Insect bite (nonvenomous) of right middle finger
    - +7th **S60.463** Insect bite (nonvenomous) of left middle finger
    - +7th **S60.464** Insect bite (nonvenomous) of right ring finger
    - +7th **S60.465** Insect bite (nonvenomous) of left ring finger
    - +7th **S60.466** Insect bite (nonvenomous) of right little finger
    - +7th **S60.467** Insect bite (nonvenomous) of left little finger
    - +7th **S60.468** Insect bite (nonvenomous) of other finger
      Insect bite (nonvenomous) of specified finger with unspecified laterality
    - +7th **S60.469** Insect bite (nonvenomous) of unspecified finger
  - **S60.47** **Other superficial bite of fingers**
    Excludes1: open bite of fingers (S61.25-, S61.35-)
    - +7th **S60.470** Other superficial bite of right index finger
    - +7th **S60.471** Other superficial bite of left index finger
    - +7th **S60.472** Other superficial bite of right middle finger
    - +7th **S60.473** Other superficial bite of left middle finger
    - +7th **S60.474** Other superficial bite of right ring finger
    - +7th **S60.475** Other superficial bite of left ring finger
    - +7th **S60.476** Other superficial bite of right little finger
    - +7th **S60.477** Other superficial bite of left little finger
    - +7th **S60.478** Other superficial bite of other finger
      Other superficial bite of specified finger with unspecified laterality
    - +7th **S60.479** Other superficial bite of unspecified finger
- **S60.5** **Other superficial injuries of hand**
  Excludes2: superficial injuries of fingers (S60.3-, S60.4-)
  - **S60.51** **Abrasion of hand**
    - +7th **S60.511** Abrasion of right hand
    - +7th **S60.512** Abrasion of left hand
    - +7th **S60.519** Abrasion of unspecified hand
  - **S60.52** **Blister (nonthermal) of hand**
    - +7th **S60.521** Blister (nonthermal) of right hand

- +7th S60.522 Blister (nonthermal) of left hand
- +7th S60.529 Blister (nonthermal) of unspecified hand
- + S60.54 External constriction of hand
  - +7th S60.541 External constriction of right hand
  - +7th S60.542 External constriction of left hand
  - +7th S60.549 External constriction of unspecified hand
- + S60.55 Superficial foreign body of hand
  - Splinter in the hand
  - +7th S60.551 Superficial foreign body of right hand
  - +7th S60.552 Superficial foreign body of left hand
  - +7th S60.559 Superficial foreign body of unspecified hand
- + S60.56 Insect bite (nonvenomous) of hand
  - +7th S60.561 Insect bite (nonvenomous) of right hand
  - +7th S60.562 Insect bite (nonvenomous) of left hand
  - +7th S60.569 Insect bite (nonvenomous) of unspecified hand
- + S60.57 Other superficial bite of hand
  - **Excludes1:** open bite of hand (S61.45-)
  - +7th S60.571 Other superficial bite of hand of right hand
  - +7th S60.572 Other superficial bite of hand of left hand
  - +7th S60.579 Other superficial bite of hand of unspecified hand
- + S60.8 Other superficial injuries of wrist
  - + S60.81 Abrasion of wrist
    - +7th S60.811 Abrasion of right wrist
    - +7th S60.812 Abrasion of left wrist
    - +7th S60.819 Abrasion of unspecified wrist
  - + S60.82 Blister (nonthermal) of wrist
    - +7th S60.821 Blister (nonthermal) of right wrist
    - +7th S60.822 Blister (nonthermal) of left wrist
    - +7th S60.829 Blister (nonthermal) of unspecified wrist
  - + S60.84 External constriction of wrist
    - +7th S60.841 External constriction of right wrist
    - +7th S60.842 External constriction of left wrist
    - +7th S60.849 External constriction of unspecified wrist
  - + S60.85 Superficial foreign body of wrist
    - Splinter in the wrist
    - +7th S60.851 Superficial foreign body of right wrist
    - +7th S60.852 Superficial foreign body of left wrist
    - +7th S60.859 Superficial foreign body of unspecified wrist
  - + S60.86 Insect bite (nonvenomous) of wrist
    - +7th S60.861 Insect bite (nonvenomous) of right wrist
    - +7th S60.862 Insect bite (nonvenomous) of left wrist
    - +7th S60.869 Insect bite (nonvenomous) of unspecified wrist
  - + S60.87 Other superficial bite of wrist
    - **Excludes1:** open bite of wrist (S61.55)
    - +7th S60.871 Other superficial bite of right wrist
    - +7th S60.872 Other superficial bite of left wrist
    - +7th S60.879 Other superficial bite of unspecified wrist
- + S60.9 Unspecified superficial injury of wrist, hand and fingers
  - + S60.91 Unspecified superficial injury of wrist
    - +7th S60.911 Unspecified superficial injury of right wrist
    - +7th S60.912 Unspecified superficial injury of left wrist
    - +7th S60.919 Unspecified superficial injury of unspecified wrist
  - + S60.92 Unspecified superficial injury of hand
    - +7th S60.921 Unspecified superficial injury of right hand
    - +7th S60.922 Unspecified superficial injury of left hand
    - +7th S60.929 Unspecified superficial injury of unspecified hand
  - + S60.93 Unspecified superficial injury of thumb
    - +7th S60.931 Unspecified superficial injury of right thumb
    - +7th S60.932 Unspecified superficial injury of left thumb
    - +7th S60.939 Unspecified superficial injury of unspecified thumb
  - + S60.94 Unspecified superficial injury of other fingers
    - +7th S60.940 Unspecified superficial injury of right index finger
    - +7th S60.941 Unspecified superficial injury of left index finger
    - +7th S60.942 Unspecified superficial injury of right middle finger
    - +7th S60.943 Unspecified superficial injury of left middle finger
    - +7th S60.944 Unspecified superficial injury of right ring finger
    - +7th S60.945 Unspecified superficial injury of left ring finger
    - +7th S60.946 Unspecified superficial injury of right little finger
    - +7th S60.947 Unspecified superficial injury of left little finger
    - +7th S60.948 Unspecified superficial injury of other finger
      - Unspecified superficial injury of specified finger with unspecified laterality
    - +7th S60.949 Unspecified superficial injury of unspecified finger

S61 Open wound of wrist, hand and fingers

Code also any associated wound infection
Excludes1: open fracture of wrist, hand and finger (S62.- with 7th character B)
traumatic amputation of wrist and hand (S68.-)

The appropriate 7th character is to be added to each code from category S61
A initial encounter
D subsequent encounter
S sequela

- + S61.0 Open wound of thumb without damage to nail
  - **Excludes1:** open wound of thumb with damage to nail (S61.1-)
  - + S61.00 Unspecified open wound of thumb without damage to nail
    - +7th S61.001 Unspecified open wound of right thumb without damage to nail
    - +7th S61.002 Unspecified open wound of left thumb without damage to nail
    - +7th S61.009 Unspecified open wound of unspecified thumb without damage to nail
  - + S61.01 Laceration without foreign body of thumb without damage to nail
    - +7th S61.011 Laceration without foreign body of right thumb without damage to nail
    - +7th S61.012 Laceration without foreign body of left thumb without damage to nail
    - +7th S61.019 Laceration without foreign body of unspecified thumb without damage to nail
  - + S61.02 Laceration with foreign body of thumb without damage to nail
    - +7th S61.021 Laceration with foreign body of right thumb without damage to nail
    - +7th S61.022 Laceration with foreign body of left thumb without damage to nail
    - +7th S61.029 Laceration with foreign body of unspecified thumb without damage to nail
  - + S61.03 Puncture wound without foreign body of thumb without damage to nail
    - +7th S61.031 Puncture wound without foreign body of right thumb without damage to nail
    - +7th S61.032 Puncture wound without foreign body of left thumb without damage to nail
    - +7th S61.039 Puncture wound without foreign body of unspecified thumb without damage to nail
  - + S61.04 Puncture wound with foreign body of thumb without damage to nail
    - +7th S61.041 Puncture wound with foreign body of right thumb without damage to nail
    - +7th S61.042 Puncture wound with foreign body of left thumb without damage to nail
    - +7th S61.049 Puncture wound with foreign body of unspecified thumb without damage to nail

- **+ S61.05** **Open bite of thumb without damage to nail**
  Bite of thumb NOS
  Excludes1: superficial bite of thumb (S60.36-, S60.37-)
  - +7th **S61.051** Open bite of right thumb without damage to nail
  - +7th **S61.052** Open bite of left thumb without damage to nail
  - +7th **S61.059** Open bite of unspecified thumb without damage to nail
- **+ S61.1** **Open wound of thumb with damage to nail**
  - **+ S61.10** Unspecified open wound of thumb with damage to nail
    - +7th **S61.101** Unspecified open wound of right thumb with damage to nail
    - +7th **S61.102** Unspecified open wound of left thumb with damage to nail
    - +7th **S61.109** Unspecified open wound of unspecified thumb with damage to nail
  - **+ S61.11** Laceration without foreign body of thumb with damage to nail
    - +7th **S61.111** Laceration without foreign body of right thumb with damage to nail
    - +7th **S61.112** Laceration without foreign body of left thumb with damage to nail
    - +7th **S61.119** Laceration without foreign body of unspecified thumb with damage to nail
  - **+ S61.12** Laceration with foreign body of thumb with damage to nail
    - +7th **S61.121** Laceration with foreign body of right thumb with damage to nail
    - +7th **S61.122** Laceration with foreign body of left thumb with damage to nail
    - +7th **S61.129** Laceration with foreign body of unspecified thumb with damage to nail
  - **+ S61.13** Puncture wound without foreign body of thumb with damage to nail
    - +7th **S61.131** Puncture wound without foreign body of right thumb with damage to nail
    - +7th **S61.132** Puncture wound without foreign body of left thumb with damage to nail
    - +7th **S61.139** Puncture wound without foreign body of unspecified thumb with damage to nail
  - **+ S61.14** Puncture wound with foreign body of thumb with damage to nail
    - +7th **S61.141** Puncture wound with foreign body of right thumb with damage to nail
    - +7th **S61.142** Puncture wound with foreign body of left thumb with damage to nail
    - +7th **S61.149** Puncture wound with foreign body of unspecified thumb with damage to nail
  - **+ S61.15** Open bite of thumb with damage to nail
    Bite of thumb with damage to nail NOS
    Excludes1: superficial bite of thumb (S60.36-, S60.37-)
    - +7th **S61.151** Open bite of right thumb with damage to nail
    - +7th **S61.152** Open bite of left thumb with damage to nail
    - +7th **S61.159** Open bite of unspecified thumb with damage to nail
- **+ S61.2** **Open wound of other finger without damage to nail**
  Excludes1: open wound of finger involving nail (matrix) (S61.3-)
  Excludes2: open wound of thumb without damage to nail (S61.0-)
  - **+ S61.20** Unspecified open wound of other finger without damage to nail
    - +7th **S61.200** Unspecified open wound of right index finger without damage to nail
    - +7th **S61.201** Unspecified open wound of left index finger without damage to nail
    - +7th **S61.202** Unspecified open wound of right middle finger without damage to nail
    - +7th **S61.203** Unspecified open wound of left middle finger without damage to nail
    - +7th **S61.204** Unspecified open wound of right ring finger without damage to nail
    - +7th **S61.205** Unspecified open wound of left ring finger without damage to nail
    - +7th **S61.206** Unspecified open wound of right little finger without damage to nail
    - +7th **S61.207** Unspecified open wound of left little finger without damage to nail
    - +7th **S61.208** Unspecified open wound of other finger without damage to nail
      Unspecified open wound of specified finger with unspecified laterality without damage to nail
    - +7th **S61.209** Unspecified open wound of unspecified finger without damage to nail
  - **+ S61.21** Laceration without foreign body of finger without damage to nail
    - +7th **S61.210** Laceration without foreign body of right index finger without damage to nail
    - +7th **S61.211** Laceration without foreign body of left index finger without damage to nail
    - +7th **S61.212** Laceration without foreign body of right middle finger without damage to nail
    - +7th **S61.213** Laceration without foreign body of left middle finger without damage to nail
    - +7th **S61.214** Laceration without foreign body of right ring finger without damage to nail
    - +7th **S61.215** Laceration without foreign body of left ring finger without damage to nail
    - +7th **S61.216** Laceration without foreign body of right little finger without damage to nail
    - +7th **S61.217** Laceration without foreign body of left little finger without damage to nail
    - +7th **S61.218** Laceration without foreign body of other finger without damage to nail
      Laceration without foreign body of specified finger with unspecified laterality without damage to nail
    - +7th **S61.219** Laceration without foreign body of unspecified finger without damage to nail
  - **+ S61.22** Laceration with foreign body of finger without damage to nail
    - +7th **S61.220** Laceration with foreign body of right index finger without damage to nail
    - +7th **S61.221** Laceration with foreign body of left index finger without damage to nail
    - +7th **S61.222** Laceration with foreign body of right middle finger without damage to nail
    - +7th **S61.223** Laceration with foreign body of left middle finger without damage to nail
    - +7th **S61.224** Laceration with foreign body of right ring finger without damage to nail
    - +7th **S61.225** Laceration with foreign body of left ring finger without damage to nail
    - +7th **S61.226** Laceration with foreign body of right little finger without damage to nail
    - +7th **S61.227** Laceration with foreign body of left little finger without damage to nail
    - +7th **S61.228** Laceration with foreign body of other finger without damage to nail
      Laceration with foreign body of specified finger with unspecified laterality without damage to nail
    - +7th **S61.229** Laceration with foreign body of unspecified finger without damage to nail
  - **+ S61.23** Puncture wound without foreign body of finger without damage to nail
    - +7th **S61.230** Puncture wound without foreign body of right index finger without damage to nail
    - +7th **S61.231** Puncture wound without foreign body of left index finger without damage to nail

+7th S61.232 Puncture wound without foreign body of right middle finger without damage to nail
+7th S61.233 Puncture wound without foreign body of left middle finger without damage to nail
+7th S61.234 Puncture wound without foreign body of right ring finger without damage to nail
+7th S61.235 Puncture wound without foreign body of left ring finger without damage to nail
+7th S61.236 Puncture wound without foreign body of right little finger without damage to nail
+7th S61.237 Puncture wound without foreign body of left little finger without damage to nail
+7th S61.238 Puncture wound without foreign body of other finger without damage to nail
Puncture wound without foreign body of specified finger with unspecified laterality without damage to nail
+7th S61.239 Puncture wound without foreign body of unspecified finger without damage to nail
+ S61.24 Puncture wound with foreign body of finger without damage to nail
+7th S61.240 Puncture wound with foreign body of right index finger without damage to nail
+7th S61.241 Puncture wound with foreign body of left index finger without damage to nail
+7th S61.242 Puncture wound with foreign body of right middle finger without damage to nail
+7th S61.243 Puncture wound with foreign body of left middle finger without damage to nail
+7th S61.244 Puncture wound with foreign body of right ring finger without damage to nail
+7th S61.245 Puncture wound with foreign body of left ring finger without damage to nail
+7th S61.246 Puncture wound with foreign body of right little finger without damage to nail
+7th S61.247 Puncture wound with foreign body of left little finger without damage to nail
+7th S61.248 Puncture wound with foreign body of other finger without damage to nail
Puncture wound with foreign body of specified finger with unspecified laterality without damage to nail
+7th S61.249 Puncture wound with foreign body of unspecified finger without damage to nail
+ S61.25 Open bite of finger without damage to nail
Bite of finger without damage to nail NOS
Excludes1: *superficial bite of finger (S60.46-, S60.47-)*
+7th S61.250 Open bite of right index finger without damage to nail
+7th S61.251 Open bite of left index finger without damage to nail
+7th S61.252 Open bite of right middle finger without damage to nail
+7th S61.253 Open bite of left middle finger without damage to nail
+7th S61.254 Open bite of right ring finger without damage to nail
+7th S61.255 Open bite of left ring finger without damage to nail
+7th S61.256 Open bite of right little finger without damage to nail
+7th S61.257 Open bite of left little finger without damage to nail
+7th S61.258 Open bite of other finger without damage to nail
Open bite of specified finger with unspecified laterality without damage to nail
+7th S61.259 Open bite of unspecified finger without damage to nail

+ S61.3 Open wound of other finger with damage to nail
+ S61.30 Unspecified open wound of finger with damage to nail
+7th S61.300 Unspecified open wound of right index finger with damage to nail
+7th S61.301 Unspecified open wound of left index finger with damage to nail
+7th S61.302 Unspecified open wound of right middle finger with damage to nail
+7th S61.303 Unspecified open wound of left middle finger with damage to nail
+7th S61.304 Unspecified open wound of right ring finger with damage to nail
+7th S61.305 Unspecified open wound of left ring finger with damage to nail
+7th S61.306 Unspecified open wound of right little finger with damage to nail
+7th S61.307 Unspecified open wound of left little finger with damage to nail
+7th S61.308 Unspecified open wound of other finger with damage to nail
Unspecified open wound of specified finger with unspecified laterality with damage to nail
+7th S61.309 Unspecified open wound of unspecified finger with damage to nail
+ S61.31 Laceration without foreign body of finger with damage to nail
+7th S61.310 Laceration without foreign body of right index finger with damage to nail
+7th S61.311 Laceration without foreign body of left index finger with damage to nail
+7th S61.312 Laceration without foreign body of right middle finger with damage to nail
+7th S61.313 Laceration without foreign body of left middle finger with damage to nail
+7th S61.314 Laceration without foreign body of right ring finger with damage to nail
+7th S61.315 Laceration without foreign body of left ring finger with damage to nail
+7th S61.316 Laceration without foreign body of right little finger with damage to nail
+7th S61.317 Laceration without foreign body of left little finger with damage to nail
+7th S61.318 Laceration without foreign body of other finger with damage to nail
Laceration without foreign body of specified finger with unspecified laterality with damage to nail
+7th S61.319 Laceration without foreign body of unspecified finger with damage to nail
+ S61.32 Laceration with foreign body of finger with damage to nail
+7th S61.320 Laceration with foreign body of right index finger with damage to nail
+7th S61.321 Laceration with foreign body of left index finger with damage to nail
+7th S61.322 Laceration with foreign body of right middle finger with damage to nail
+7th S61.323 Laceration with foreign body of left middle finger with damage to nail
+7th S61.324 Laceration with foreign body of right ring finger with damage to nail
+7th S61.325 Laceration with foreign body of left ring finger with damage to nail
+7th S61.326 Laceration with foreign body of right little finger with damage to nail
+7th S61.327 Laceration with foreign body of left little finger with damage to nail
+7th S61.328 Laceration with foreign body of other finger with damage to nail
Laceration with foreign body of specified finger with unspecified laterality with damage to nail
+7th S61.329 Laceration with foreign body of unspecified finger with damage to nail
+ S61.33 Puncture wound without foreign body of finger with damage to nail
+7th S61.330 Puncture wound without foreign body of right index finger with damage to nail

- +7th S61.331 Puncture wound without foreign body of left index finger with damage to nail
- +7th S61.332 Puncture wound without foreign body of right middle finger with damage to nail
- +7th S61.333 Puncture wound without foreign body of left middle finger with damage to nail
- +7th S61.334 Puncture wound without foreign body of right ring finger with damage to nail
- +7th S61.335 Puncture wound without foreign body of left ring finger with damage to nail
- +7th S61.336 Puncture wound without foreign body of right little finger with damage to nail
- +7th S61.337 Puncture wound without foreign body of left little finger with damage to nail
- +7th S61.338 Puncture wound without foreign body of other finger with damage to nail
    - Puncture wound without foreign body of specified finger with unspecified laterality with damage to nail
- +7th S61.339 Puncture wound without foreign body of unspecified finger with damage to nail
- + S61.34 Puncture wound with foreign body of finger with damage to nail
    - +7th S61.340 Puncture wound with foreign body of right index finger with damage to nail
    - +7th S61.341 Puncture wound with foreign body of left index finger with damage to nail
    - +7th S61.342 Puncture wound with foreign body of right middle finger with damage to nail
    - +7th S61.343 Puncture wound with foreign body of left middle finger with damage to nail
    - +7th S61.344 Puncture wound with foreign body of right ring finger with damage to nail
    - +7th S61.345 Puncture wound with foreign body of left ring finger with damage to nail
    - +7th S61.346 Puncture wound with foreign body of right little finger with damage to nail
    - +7th S61.347 Puncture wound with foreign body of left little finger with damage to nail
    - +7th S61.348 Puncture wound with foreign body of other finger with damage to nail
        - Puncture wound with foreign body of specified finger with unspecified laterality with damage to nail
    - +7th S61.349 Puncture wound with foreign body of unspecified finger with damage to nail
- + S61.35 Open bite of finger with damage to nail
    - Bite of finger with damage to nail NOS
    - **Excludes1:** *superficial bite of finger (S60.46-, S60.47-)*
    - +7th S61.350 Open bite of right index finger with damage to nail
    - +7th S61.351 Open bite of left index finger with damage to nail
    - +7th S61.352 Open bite of right middle finger with damage to nail
    - +7th S61.353 Open bite of left middle finger with damage to nail
    - +7th S61.354 Open bite of right ring finger with damage to nail
    - +7th S61.355 Open bite of left ring finger with damage to nail
    - +7th S61.356 Open bite of right little finger with damage to nail
    - +7th S61.357 Open bite of left little finger with damage to nail
    - +7th S61.358 Open bite of other finger with damage to nail
        - Open bite of specified finger with unspecified laterality with damage to nail
    - +7th S61.359 Open bite of unspecified finger with damage to nail
- + S61.4 Open wound of hand
    - + S61.40 Unspecified open wound of hand
        - +7th S61.401 Unspecified open wound of right hand
        - +7th S61.402 Unspecified open wound of left hand
        - +7th S61.409 Unspecified open wound of unspecified hand
    - + S61.41 Laceration without foreign body of hand
        - +7th S61.411 Laceration without foreign body of right hand
        - +7th S61.412 Laceration without foreign body of left hand
        - +7th S61.419 Laceration without foreign body of unspecified hand
    - + S61.42 Laceration with foreign body of hand
        - +7th S61.421 Laceration with foreign body of right hand
        - +7th S61.422 Laceration with foreign body of left hand
        - +7th S61.429 Laceration with foreign body of unspecified hand
    - + S61.43 Puncture wound without foreign body of hand
        - +7th S61.431 Puncture wound without foreign body of right hand
        - +7th S61.432 Puncture wound without foreign body of left hand
        - +7th S61.439 Puncture wound without foreign body of unspecified hand
    - + S61.44 Puncture wound with foreign body of hand
        - +7th S61.441 Puncture wound with foreign body of right hand
        - +7th S61.442 Puncture wound with foreign body of left hand
        - +7th S61.449 Puncture wound with foreign body of unspecified hand
    - + S61.45 Open bite of hand
        - Bite of hand NOS
        - **Excludes1:** *superficial bite of hand (S60.56-, S60.57-)*
        - +7th S61.451 Open bite of right hand
        - +7th S61.452 Open bite of left hand
        - +7th S61.459 Open bite of unspecified hand
- + S61.5 Open wound of wrist
    - + S61.50 Unspecified open wound of wrist
        - +7th S61.501 Unspecified open wound of right wrist
        - +7th S61.502 Unspecified open wound of left wrist
        - +7th S61.509 Unspecified open wound of unspecified wrist
    - + S61.51 Laceration without foreign body of wrist
        - +7th S61.511 Laceration without foreign body of right wrist
        - +7th S61.512 Laceration without foreign body of left wrist
        - +7th S61.519 Laceration without foreign body of unspecified wrist
    - + S61.52 Laceration with foreign body of wrist
        - +7th S61.521 Laceration with foreign body of right wrist
        - +7th S61.522 Laceration with foreign body of left wrist
        - +7th S61.529 Laceration with foreign body of unspecified wrist
    - + S61.53 Puncture wound without foreign body of wrist
        - +7th S61.531 Puncture wound without foreign body of right wrist
        - +7th S61.532 Puncture wound without foreign body of left wrist
        - +7th S61.539 Puncture wound without foreign body of unspecified wrist
    - + S61.54 Puncture wound with foreign body of wrist
        - +7th S61.541 Puncture wound with foreign body of right wrist
        - +7th S61.542 Puncture wound with foreign body of left wrist
        - +7th S61.549 Puncture wound with foreign body of unspecified wrist
    - + S61.55 Open bite of wrist
        - Bite of wrist NOS
        - **Excludes1:** *superficial bite of wrist (S60.86-, S60.87-)*
        - +7th S61.551 Open bite of right wrist
        - +7th S61.552 Open bite of left wrist
        - +7th S61.559 Open bite of unspecified wrist

S62 Fracture at wrist and hand level

NOTE A fracture not indicated as displaced or nondisplaced should be coded to displaced
A fracture not indicated as open or closed should be coded to closed

Excludes1: traumatic amputation of wrist and hand (S68.-)
Excludes2: fracture of distal parts of ulna and radius (S52.-)

The appropriate 7th character is to be added to each code from category S62
- A initial encounter for closed fracture
- B initial encounter for open fracture
- D subsequent encounter for fracture with routine healing
- G subsequent encounter for fracture with delayed healing
- K subsequent encounter for fracture with nonunion
- P subsequent encounter for fracture with malunion
- S sequela

Review coding guideline C.19.c

- **+ S62.0 Fracture of navicular [scaphoid] bone of wrist**
  - **+ S62.00 Unspecified fracture of navicular [scaphoid] bone of wrist**
    - CC +7th **S62.001** Unspecified fracture of navicular [scaphoid] bone of right wrist
      - HAC 7th character B see Appendix B for HAC conditional logic
    - CC +7th **S62.002** Unspecified fracture of navicular [scaphoid] bone of left wrist
      - AHA CC: 4Q, 2012, 106
      - HAC 7th character B see Appendix B for HAC conditional logic
    - CC +7th **S62.009** Unspecified fracture of navicular [scaphoid] bone of unspecified wrist
      - HAC 7th character B see Appendix B for HAC conditional logic
  - **+ S62.01 Fracture of distal pole of navicular [scaphoid] bone of wrist**
    Fracture of volar tuberosity of navicular [scaphoid] bone of wrist
    - CC +7th **S62.011** Displaced fracture of distal pole of navicular [scaphoid] bone of right wrist
      - HAC 7th character B see Appendix B for HAC conditional logic
    - CC +7th **S62.012** Displaced fracture of distal pole of navicular [scaphoid] bone of left wrist
      - HAC 7th character B see Appendix B for HAC conditional logic
    - CC +7th **S62.013** Displaced fracture of distal pole of navicular [scaphoid] bone of unspecified wrist
      - HAC 7th character B see Appendix B for HAC conditional logic
    - CC +7th **S62.014** Nondisplaced fracture of distal pole of navicular [scaphoid] bone of right wrist
      - HAC 7th character B see Appendix B for HAC conditional logic
    - CC +7th **S62.015** Nondisplaced fracture of distal pole of navicular [scaphoid] bone of left wrist
      - HAC 7th character B see Appendix B for HAC conditional logic
    - CC +7th **S62.016** Nondisplaced fracture of distal pole of navicular [scaphoid] bone of unspecified wrist
      - HAC 7th character B see Appendix B for HAC conditional logic
  - **+ S62.02 Fracture of middle third of navicular [scaphoid] bone of wrist**
    - CC +7th **S62.021** Displaced fracture of middle third of navicular [scaphoid] bone of right wrist
      - HAC 7th character B see Appendix B for HAC conditional logic
    - CC +7th **S62.022** Displaced fracture of middle third of navicular [scaphoid] bone of left wrist
      - HAC 7th character B see Appendix B for HAC conditional logic
    - CC +7th **S62.023** Displaced fracture of middle third of navicular [scaphoid] bone of unspecified wrist
      - HAC 7th character B see Appendix B for HAC conditional logic
    - CC +7th **S62.024** Nondisplaced fracture of middle third of navicular [scaphoid] bone of right wrist
      - HAC 7th character B see Appendix B for HAC conditional logic
    - CC +7th **S62.025** Nondisplaced fracture of middle third of navicular [scaphoid] bone of left wrist
      - HAC 7th character B see Appendix B for HAC conditional logic
    - CC +7th **S62.026** Nondisplaced fracture of middle third of navicular [scaphoid] bone of unspecified wrist
      - HAC 7th character B see Appendix B for HAC conditional logic
  - **+ S62.03 Fracture of proximal third of navicular [scaphoid] bone of wrist**
    - CC +7th **S62.031** Displaced fracture of proximal third of navicular [scaphoid] bone of right wrist
      - HAC 7th character B see Appendix B for HAC conditional logic
    - CC +7th **S62.032** Displaced fracture of proximal third of navicular [scaphoid] bone of left wrist
      - HAC 7th character B see Appendix B for HAC conditional logic
    - CC +7th **S62.033** Displaced fracture of proximal third of navicular [scaphoid] bone of unspecified wrist
      - HAC 7th character B see Appendix B for HAC conditional logic
    - CC +7th **S62.034** Nondisplaced fracture of proximal third of navicular [scaphoid] bone of right wrist
      - HAC 7th character B see Appendix B for HAC conditional logic
    - CC +7th **S62.035** Nondisplaced fracture of proximal third of navicular [scaphoid] bone of left wrist
      - HAC 7th character B see Appendix B for HAC conditional logic
    - CC +7th **S62.036** Nondisplaced fracture of proximal third of navicular [scaphoid] bone of unspecified wrist
      - HAC 7th character B see Appendix B for HAC conditional logic
- **+ S62.1 Fracture of other and unspecified carpal bone(s)**
  Excludes2: fracture of scaphoid of wrist (S62.0-)
  - **+ S62.10 Fracture of unspecified carpal bone**
    Fracture of wrist NOS
    - CC +7th **S62.101** Fracture of unspecified carpal bone, right wrist
      - HAC 7th character B see Appendix B for HAC conditional logic
    - CC +7th **S62.102** Fracture of unspecified carpal bone, left wrist
      - AHA CC: 4Q, 2012, 95-96
      - HAC 7th character B see Appendix B for HAC conditional logic
    - CC +7th **S62.109** Fracture of unspecified carpal bone, unspecified wrist
      - HAC 7th character B see Appendix B for HAC conditional logic
  - **+ S62.11 Fracture of triquetrum [cuneiform] bone of wrist**
    - CC +7th **S62.111** Displaced fracture of triquetrum [cuneiform] bone, right wrist
      - HAC 7th character B see Appendix B for HAC conditional logic
    - CC +7th **S62.112** Displaced fracture of triquetrum [cuneiform] bone, left wrist
      - HAC 7th character B see Appendix B for HAC conditional logic
    - CC +7th **S62.113** Displaced fracture of triquetrum [cuneiform] bone, unspecified wrist
      - HAC 7th character B see Appendix B for HAC conditional logic
    - CC +7th **S62.114** Nondisplaced fracture of triquetrum [cuneiform] bone, right wrist
      - HAC 7th character B see Appendix B for HAC conditional logic
    - CC +7th **S62.115** Nondisplaced fracture of triquetrum [cuneiform] bone, left wrist
      - HAC 7th character B see Appendix B for HAC conditional logic

CC +7th S62.116 Nondisplaced fracture of triquetrum [cuneiform] bone, unspecified wrist
    HAC 7th character B see Appendix B for HAC conditional logic

+ S62.12 Fracture of lunate [semilunar]
  CC +7th S62.121 Displaced fracture of lunate [semilunar], right wrist
    HAC 7th character B see Appendix B for HAC conditional logic
  CC +7th S62.122 Displaced fracture of lunate [semilunar], left wrist
    HAC 7th character B see Appendix B for HAC conditional logic
  CC +7th S62.123 Displaced fracture of lunate [semilunar], unspecified wrist
    HAC 7th character B see Appendix B for HAC conditional logic
  CC +7th S62.124 Nondisplaced fracture of lunate [semilunar], right wrist
    HAC 7th character B see Appendix B for HAC conditional logic
  CC +7th S62.125 Nondisplaced fracture of lunate [semilunar], left wrist
    HAC 7th character B see Appendix B for HAC conditional logic
  CC +7th S62.126 Nondisplaced fracture of lunate [semilunar], unspecified wrist
    HAC 7th character B see Appendix B for HAC conditional logic

+ S62.13 Fracture of capitate [os magnum] bone
  CC +7th S62.131 Displaced fracture of capitate [os magnum] bone, right wrist
    HAC 7th character B see Appendix B for HAC conditional logic
  CC +7th S62.132 Displaced fracture of capitate [os magnum] bone, left wrist
    HAC 7th character B see Appendix B for HAC conditional logic
  CC +7th S62.133 Displaced fracture of capitate [os magnum] bone, unspecified wrist
    HAC 7th character B see Appendix B for HAC conditional logic
  CC +7th S62.134 Nondisplaced fracture of capitate [os magnum] bone, right wrist
    HAC 7th character B see Appendix B for HAC conditional logic
  CC +7th S62.135 Nondisplaced fracture of capitate [os magnum] bone, left wrist
    HAC 7th character B see Appendix B for HAC conditional logic
  CC +7th S62.136 Nondisplaced fracture of capitate [os magnum] bone, unspecified wrist
    HAC 7th character B see Appendix B for HAC conditional logic

+ S62.14 Fracture of body of hamate [unciform] bone
  Fracture of hamate [unciform] bone NOS
  CC +7th S62.141 Displaced fracture of body of hamate [unciform] bone, right wrist
    HAC 7th character B see Appendix B for HAC conditional logic
  CC +7th S62.142 Displaced fracture of body of hamate [unciform] bone, left wrist
    HAC 7th character B see Appendix B for HAC conditional logic
  CC +7th S62.143 Displaced fracture of body of hamate [unciform] bone, unspecified wrist
    HAC 7th character B see Appendix B for HAC conditional logic
  CC +7th S62.144 Nondisplaced fracture of body of hamate [unciform] bone, right wrist
    HAC 7th character B see Appendix B for HAC conditional logic
  CC +7th S62.145 Nondisplaced fracture of body of hamate [unciform] bone, left wrist
    HAC 7th character B see Appendix B for HAC conditional logic
  CC +7th S62.146 Nondisplaced fracture of body of hamate [unciform] bone, unspecified wrist
    HAC 7th character B see Appendix B for HAC conditional logic

+ S62.15 Fracture of hook process of hamate [unciform] bone
  Fracture of unciform process of hamate [unciform] bone
  CC +7th S62.151 Displaced fracture of hook process of hamate [unciform] bone, right wrist
    HAC 7th character B see Appendix B for HAC conditional logic
  CC +7th S62.152 Displaced fracture of hook process of hamate [unciform] bone, left wrist
    HAC 7th character B see Appendix B for HAC conditional logic
  CC +7th S62.153 Displaced fracture of hook process of hamate [unciform] bone, unspecified wrist
    HAC 7th character B see Appendix B for HAC conditional logic
  CC +7th S62.154 Nondisplaced fracture of hook process of hamate [unciform] bone, right wrist
    HAC 7th character B see Appendix B for HAC conditional logic
  CC +7th S62.155 Nondisplaced fracture of hook process of hamate [unciform] bone, left wrist
    HAC 7th character B see Appendix B for HAC conditional logic
  CC +7th S62.156 Nondisplaced fracture of hook process of hamate [unciform] bone, unspecified wrist
    HAC 7th character B see Appendix B for HAC conditional logic

+ S62.16 Fracture of pisiform
  CC +7th S62.161 Displaced fracture of pisiform, right wrist
    HAC 7th character B see Appendix B for HAC conditional logic
  CC +7th S62.162 Displaced fracture of pisiform, left wrist
    HAC 7th character B see Appendix B for HAC conditional logic
  CC +7th S62.163 Displaced fracture of pisiform, unspecified wrist
    HAC 7th character B see Appendix B for HAC conditional logic
  CC +7th S62.164 Nondisplaced fracture of pisiform, right wrist
    HAC 7th character B see Appendix B for HAC conditional logic
  CC +7th S62.165 Nondisplaced fracture of pisiform, left wrist
    HAC 7th character B see Appendix B for HAC conditional logic
  CC +7th S62.166 Nondisplaced fracture of pisiform, unspecified wrist
    HAC 7th character B see Appendix B for HAC conditional logic

+ S62.17 Fracture of trapezium [larger multangular]
  CC +7th S62.171 Displaced fracture of trapezium [larger multangular], right wrist
    HAC 7th character B see Appendix B for HAC conditional logic
  CC +7th S62.172 Displaced fracture of trapezium [larger multangular], left wrist
    HAC 7th character B see Appendix B for HAC conditional logic
  CC +7th S62.173 Displaced fracture of trapezium [larger multangular], unspecified wrist
    HAC 7th character B see Appendix B for HAC conditional logic
  CC +7th S62.174 Nondisplaced fracture of trapezium [larger multangular], right wrist
    HAC 7th character B see Appendix B for HAC conditional logic
  CC +7th S62.175 Nondisplaced fracture of trapezium [larger multangular], left wrist
    HAC 7th character B see Appendix B for HAC conditional logic
  CC +7th S62.176 Nondisplaced fracture of trapezium [larger multangular], unspecified wrist
    HAC 7th character B see Appendix B for HAC conditional logic

+ S62.18 Fracture of trapezoid [smaller multangular]
  CC +7th S62.181 Displaced fracture of trapezoid [smaller multangular], right wrist
    HAC 7th character B see Appendix B for HAC conditional logic

CC +7th S62.182 Displaced fracture of trapezoid [smaller multangular], left wrist
　　HAC 7th character B see Appendix B for HAC conditional logic

CC +7th S62.183 Displaced fracture of trapezoid [smaller multangular], unspecified wrist
　　HAC 7th character B see Appendix B for HAC conditional logic

CC +7th S62.184 Nondisplaced fracture of trapezoid [smaller multangular], right wrist
　　HAC 7th character B see Appendix B for HAC conditional logic

CC +7th S62.185 Nondisplaced fracture of trapezoid [smaller multangular], left wrist
　　HAC 7th character B see Appendix B for HAC conditional logic

CC +7th S62.186 Nondisplaced fracture of trapezoid [smaller multangular], unspecified wrist
　　HAC 7th character B see Appendix B for HAC conditional logic

+ S62.2 Fracture of first metacarpal bone
　+ S62.20 Unspecified fracture of first metacarpal bone

CC +7th S62.201 Unspecified fracture of first metacarpal bone, right hand
　　HAC 7th character B see Appendix B for HAC conditional logic

CC +7th S62.202 Unspecified fracture of first metacarpal bone, left hand
　　HAC 7th character B see Appendix B for HAC conditional logic

CC +7th S62.209 Unspecified fracture of first metacarpal bone, unspecified hand
　　HAC 7th character B see Appendix B for HAC conditional logic

+ S62.21 Bennett's fracture

CC +7th S62.211 Bennett's fracture, right hand
　　HAC 7th character B see Appendix B for HAC conditional logic

CC +7th S62.212 Bennett's fracture, left hand
　　HAC 7th character B see Appendix B for HAC conditional logic

CC +7th S62.213 Bennett's fracture, unspecified hand
　　HAC 7th character B see Appendix B for HAC conditional logic

+ S62.22 Rolando's fracture

CC +7th S62.221 Displaced Rolando's fracture, right hand
　　HAC 7th character B see Appendix B for HAC conditional logic

CC +7th S62.222 Displaced Rolando's fracture, left hand
　　HAC 7th character B see Appendix B for HAC conditional logic

CC +7th S62.223 Displaced Rolando's fracture, unspecified hand
　　HAC 7th character B see Appendix B for HAC conditional logic

CC +7th S62.224 Nondisplaced Rolando's fracture, right hand
　　HAC 7th character B see Appendix B for HAC conditional logic

CC +7th S62.225 Nondisplaced Rolando's fracture, left hand
　　HAC 7th character B see Appendix B for HAC conditional logic

CC +7th S62.226 Nondisplaced Rolando's fracture, unspecified hand
　　HAC 7th character B see Appendix B for HAC conditional logic

+ S62.23 Other fracture of base of first metacarpal bone

CC +7th S62.231 Other displaced fracture of base of first metacarpal bone, right hand
　　HAC 7th character B see Appendix B for HAC conditional logic

CC +7th S62.232 Other displaced fracture of base of first metacarpal bone, left hand
　　HAC 7th character B see Appendix B for HAC conditional logic

CC +7th S62.233 Other displaced fracture of base of first metacarpal bone, unspecified hand
　　HAC 7th character B see Appendix B for HAC conditional logic

CC +7th S62.234 Other nondisplaced fracture of base of first metacarpal bone, right hand
　　HAC 7th character B see Appendix B for HAC conditional logic

CC +7th S62.235 Other nondisplaced fracture of base of first metacarpal bone, left hand
　　HAC 7th character B see Appendix B for HAC conditional logic

CC +7th S62.236 Other nondisplaced fracture of base of first metacarpal bone, unspecified hand
　　HAC 7th character B see Appendix B for HAC conditional logic

+ S62.24 Fracture of shaft of first metacarpal bone

CC +7th S62.241 Displaced fracture of shaft of first metacarpal bone, right hand
　　HAC 7th character B see Appendix B for HAC conditional logic

CC +7th S62.242 Displaced fracture of shaft of first metacarpal bone, left hand
　　HAC 7th character B see Appendix B for HAC conditional logic

CC +7th S62.243 Displaced fracture of shaft of first metacarpal bone, unspecified hand
　　HAC 7th character B see Appendix B for HAC conditional logic

CC +7th S62.244 Nondisplaced fracture of shaft of first metacarpal bone, right hand
　　HAC 7th character B see Appendix B for HAC conditional logic

CC +7th S62.245 Nondisplaced fracture of shaft of first metacarpal bone, left hand
　　HAC 7th character B see Appendix B for HAC conditional logic

CC +7th S62.246 Nondisplaced fracture of shaft of first metacarpal bone, unspecified hand
　　HAC 7th character B see Appendix B for HAC conditional logic

+ S62.25 Fracture of neck of first metacarpal bone

CC +7th S62.251 Displaced fracture of neck of first metacarpal bone, right hand
　　HAC 7th character B see Appendix B for HAC conditional logic

CC +7th S62.252 Displaced fracture of neck of first metacarpal bone, left hand
　　HAC 7th character B see Appendix B for HAC conditional logic

CC +7th S62.253 Displaced fracture of neck of first metacarpal bone, unspecified hand
　　HAC 7th character B see Appendix B for HAC conditional logic

CC +7th S62.254 Nondisplaced fracture of neck of first metacarpal bone, right hand
　　HAC 7th character B see Appendix B for HAC conditional logic

CC +7th S62.255 Nondisplaced fracture of neck of first metacarpal bone, left hand
　　HAC 7th character B see Appendix B for HAC conditional logic

CC +7th S62.256 Nondisplaced fracture of neck of first metacarpal bone, unspecified hand
　　HAC 7th character B see Appendix B for HAC conditional logic

+ S62.29 Other fracture of first metacarpal bone

CC +7th S62.291 Other fracture of first metacarpal bone, right hand
　　HAC 7th character B see Appendix B for HAC conditional logic

CC +7th S62.292 Other fracture of first metacarpal bone, left hand
　　HAC 7th character B see Appendix B for HAC conditional logic

CC +7th S62.299 Other fracture of first metacarpal bone, unspecified hand
　　HAC 7th character B see Appendix B for HAC conditional logic

+ S62.3 Fracture of other and unspecified metacarpal bone
　Excludes2: fracture of first metacarpal bone (S62.2-)
　+ S62.30 Unspecified fracture of other metacarpal bone

CC +7th S62.300 Unspecified fracture of second metacarpal bone, right hand
　　HAC 7th character B see Appendix B for HAC conditional logic

CC +7th S62.301 Unspecified fracture of second metacarpal bone, left hand
　　HAC 7th character B see Appendix B for HAC conditional logic

CC +7th	S62.302	Unspecified fracture of third metacarpal bone, right hand
		HAC 7th character B see Appendix B for HAC conditional logic
CC +7th	S62.303	Unspecified fracture of third metacarpal bone, left hand
		HAC 7th character B see Appendix B for HAC conditional logic
CC +7th	S62.304	Unspecified fracture of fourth metacarpal bone, right hand
		HAC 7th character B see Appendix B for HAC conditional logic
CC +7th	S62.305	Unspecified fracture of fourth metacarpal bone, left hand
		HAC 7th character B see Appendix B for HAC conditional logic
CC +7th	S62.306	Unspecified fracture of fifth metacarpal bone, right hand
		HAC 7th character B see Appendix B for HAC conditional logic
CC +7th	S62.307	Unspecified fracture of fifth metacarpal bone, left hand
		HAC 7th character B see Appendix B for HAC conditional logic
CC +7th	S62.308	Unspecified fracture of other metacarpal bone
		Unspecified fracture of specified metacarpal bone with unspecified laterality
		HAC 7th character B see Appendix B for HAC conditional logic
CC +7th	S62.309	Unspecified fracture of unspecified metacarpal bone
		HAC 7th character B see Appendix B for HAC conditional logic
+	S62.31	Displaced fracture of base of other metacarpal bone
CC +7th	S62.310	Displaced fracture of base of second metacarpal bone, right hand
		HAC 7th character B see Appendix B for HAC conditional logic
CC +7th	S62.311	Displaced fracture of base of second metacarpal bone, left hand
		HAC 7th character B see Appendix B for HAC conditional logic
CC +7th	S62.312	Displaced fracture of base of third metacarpal bone, right hand
		HAC 7th character B see Appendix B for HAC conditional logic
CC +7th	S62.313	Displaced fracture of base of third metacarpal bone, left hand
		HAC 7th character B see Appendix B for HAC conditional logic
CC +7th	S62.314	Displaced fracture of base of fourth metacarpal bone, right hand
		HAC 7th character B see Appendix B for HAC conditional logic
CC +7th	S62.315	Displaced fracture of base of fourth metacarpal bone, left hand
		HAC 7th character B see Appendix B for HAC conditional logic
CC +7th	S62.316	Displaced fracture of base of fifth metacarpal bone, right hand
		HAC 7th character B see Appendix B for HAC conditional logic
CC +7th	S62.317	Displaced fracture of base of fifth metacarpal bone, left hand
		HAC 7th character B see Appendix B for HAC conditional logic
CC +7th	S62.318	Displaced fracture of base of other metacarpal bone
		Displaced fracture of base of specified metacarpal bone with unspecified laterality
		HAC 7th character B see Appendix B for HAC conditional logic
CC +7th	S62.319	Displaced fracture of base of unspecified metacarpal bone
		HAC 7th character B see Appendix B for HAC conditional logic
+	S62.32	Displaced fracture of shaft of other metacarpal bone
CC +7th	S62.320	Displaced fracture of shaft of second metacarpal bone, right hand
		HAC 7th character B see Appendix B for HAC conditional logic
CC +7th	S62.321	Displaced fracture of shaft of second metacarpal bone, left hand
		HAC 7th character B see Appendix B for HAC conditional logic
CC +7th	S62.322	Displaced fracture of shaft of third metacarpal bone, right hand
		HAC 7th character B see Appendix B for HAC conditional logic
CC +7th	S62.323	Displaced fracture of shaft of third metacarpal bone, left hand
		HAC 7th character B see Appendix B for HAC conditional logic
CC +7th	S62.324	Displaced fracture of shaft of fourth metacarpal bone, right hand
		HAC 7th character B see Appendix B for HAC conditional logic
CC +7th	S62.325	Displaced fracture of shaft of fourth metacarpal bone, left hand
		HAC 7th character B see Appendix B for HAC conditional logic
CC +7th	S62.326	Displaced fracture of shaft of fifth metacarpal bone, right hand
		HAC 7th character B see Appendix B for HAC conditional logic
CC +7th	S62.327	Displaced fracture of shaft of fifth metacarpal bone, left hand
		HAC 7th character B see Appendix B for HAC conditional logic
CC +7th	S62.328	Displaced fracture of shaft of other metacarpal bone
		Displaced fracture of shaft of specified metacarpal bone with unspecified laterality
		HAC 7th character B see Appendix B for HAC conditional logic
CC +7th	S62.329	Displaced fracture of shaft of unspecified metacarpal bone
		HAC 7th character B see Appendix B for HAC conditional logic
+	S62.33	Displaced fracture of neck of other metacarpal bone
CC +7th	S62.330	Displaced fracture of neck of second metacarpal bone, right hand
		HAC 7th character B see Appendix B for HAC conditional logic
CC +7th	S62.331	Displaced fracture of neck of second metacarpal bone, left hand
		HAC 7th character B see Appendix B for HAC conditional logic
CC +7th	S62.332	Displaced fracture of neck of third metacarpal bone, right hand
		HAC 7th character B see Appendix B for HAC conditional logic
CC +7th	S62.333	Displaced fracture of neck of third metacarpal bone, left hand
		HAC 7th character B see Appendix B for HAC conditional logic
CC +7th	S62.334	Displaced fracture of neck of fourth metacarpal bone, right hand
		HAC 7th character B see Appendix B for HAC conditional logic
CC +7th	S62.335	Displaced fracture of neck of fourth metacarpal bone, left hand
		HAC 7th character B see Appendix B for HAC conditional logic
CC +7th	S62.336	Displaced fracture of neck of fifth metacarpal bone, right hand
		HAC 7th character B see Appendix B for HAC conditional logic
CC +7th	S62.337	Displaced fracture of neck of fifth metacarpal bone, left hand
		HAC 7th character B see Appendix B for HAC conditional logic
CC +7th	S62.338	Displaced fracture of neck of other metacarpal bone
		Displaced fracture of neck of specified metacarpal bone with unspecified laterality
		HAC 7th character B see Appendix B for HAC conditional logic
CC +7th	S62.339	Displaced fracture of neck of unspecified metacarpal bone
		HAC 7th character B see Appendix B for HAC conditional logic

+ **S62.34** Nondisplaced fracture of base of other metacarpal bone

CC +7th **S62.340** Nondisplaced fracture of base of second metacarpal bone, right hand
  HAC 7th character B see Appendix B for HAC conditional logic

CC +7th **S62.341** Nondisplaced fracture of base of second metacarpal bone, left hand
  HAC 7th character B see Appendix B for HAC conditional logic

CC +7th **S62.342** Nondisplaced fracture of base of third metacarpal bone, right hand
  HAC 7th character B see Appendix B for HAC conditional logic

CC +7th **S62.343** Nondisplaced fracture of base of third metacarpal bone, left hand
  HAC 7th character B see Appendix B for HAC conditional logic

CC +7th **S62.344** Nondisplaced fracture of base of fourth metacarpal bone, right hand
  HAC 7th character B see Appendix B for HAC conditional logic

CC +7th **S62.345** Nondisplaced fracture of base of fourth metacarpal bone, left hand
  HAC 7th character B see Appendix B for HAC conditional logic

CC +7th **S62.346** Nondisplaced fracture of base of fifth metacarpal bone, right hand
  HAC 7th character B see Appendix B for HAC conditional logic

CC +7th **S62.347** Nondisplaced fracture of base of fifth metacarpal bone, left hand
  HAC 7th character B see Appendix B for HAC conditional logic

CC +7th **S62.348** Nondisplaced fracture of base of other metacarpal bone
  Nondisplaced fracture of base of specified metacarpal bone with unspecified laterality
  HAC 7th character B see Appendix B for HAC conditional logic

CC +7th **S62.349** Nondisplaced fracture of base of unspecified metacarpal bone
  HAC 7th character B see Appendix B for HAC conditional logic

+ **S62.35** Nondisplaced fracture of shaft of other metacarpal bone

CC +7th **S62.350** Nondisplaced fracture of shaft of second metacarpal bone, right hand
  HAC 7th character B see Appendix B for HAC conditional logic

CC +7th **S62.351** Nondisplaced fracture of shaft of second metacarpal bone, left hand
  HAC 7th character B see Appendix B for HAC conditional logic

CC +7th **S62.352** Nondisplaced fracture of shaft of third metacarpal bone, right hand
  HAC 7th character B see Appendix B for HAC conditional logic

CC +7th **S62.353** Nondisplaced fracture of shaft of third metacarpal bone, left hand
  HAC 7th character B see Appendix B for HAC conditional logic

CC +7th **S62.354** Nondisplaced fracture of shaft of fourth metacarpal bone, right hand
  HAC 7th character B see Appendix B for HAC conditional logic

CC +7th **S62.355** Nondisplaced fracture of shaft of fourth metacarpal bone, left hand
  HAC 7th character B see Appendix B for HAC conditional logic

CC +7th **S62.356** Nondisplaced fracture of shaft of fifth metacarpal bone, right hand
  HAC 7th character B see Appendix B for HAC conditional logic

CC +7th **S62.357** Nondisplaced fracture of shaft of fifth metacarpal bone, left hand
  HAC 7th character B see Appendix B for HAC conditional logic

CC +7th **S62.358** Nondisplaced fracture of shaft of other metacarpal bone
  Nondisplaced fracture of shaft of specified metacarpal bone with unspecified laterality
  HAC 7th character B see Appendix B for HAC conditional logic

CC +7th **S62.359** Nondisplaced fracture of shaft of unspecified metacarpal bone
  HAC 7th character B see Appendix B for HAC conditional logic

+ **S62.36** Nondisplaced fracture of neck of other metacarpal bone

CC +7th **S62.360** Nondisplaced fracture of neck of second metacarpal bone, right hand
  HAC 7th character B see Appendix B for HAC conditional logic

CC +7th **S62.361** Nondisplaced fracture of neck of second metacarpal bone, left hand
  HAC 7th character B see Appendix B for HAC conditional logic

CC +7th **S62.362** Nondisplaced fracture of neck of third metacarpal bone, right hand
  HAC 7th character B see Appendix B for HAC conditional logic

CC +7th **S62.363** Nondisplaced fracture of neck of third metacarpal bone, left hand
  HAC 7th character B see Appendix B for HAC conditional logic

CC +7th **S62.364** Nondisplaced fracture of neck of fourth metacarpal bone, right hand
  HAC 7th character B see Appendix B for HAC conditional logic

CC +7th **S62.365** Nondisplaced fracture of neck of fourth metacarpal bone, left hand
  HAC 7th character B see Appendix B for HAC conditional logic

CC +7th **S62.366** Nondisplaced fracture of neck of fifth metacarpal bone, right hand
  HAC 7th character B see Appendix B for HAC conditional logic

CC +7th **S62.367** Nondisplaced fracture of neck of fifth metacarpal bone, left hand
  HAC 7th character B see Appendix B for HAC conditional logic

CC +7th **S62.368** Nondisplaced fracture of neck of other metacarpal bone
  Nondisplaced fracture of neck of specified metacarpal bone with unspecified laterality
  HAC 7th character B see Appendix B for HAC conditional logic

CC +7th **S62.369** Nondisplaced fracture of neck of unspecified metacarpal bone
  HAC 7th character B see Appendix B for HAC conditional logic

+ **S62.39** Other fracture of other metacarpal bone

CC +7th **S62.390** Other fracture of second metacarpal bone, right hand
  HAC 7th character B see Appendix B for HAC conditional logic

CC +7th **S62.391** Other fracture of second metacarpal bone, left hand
  HAC 7th character B see Appendix B for HAC conditional logic

CC +7th **S62.392** Other fracture of third metacarpal bone, right hand
  HAC 7th character B see Appendix B for HAC conditional logic

CC +7th **S62.393** Other fracture of third metacarpal bone, left hand
  HAC 7th character B see Appendix B for HAC conditional logic

CC +7th **S62.394** Other fracture of fourth metacarpal bone, right hand
  HAC 7th character B see Appendix B for HAC conditional logic

CC +7th **S62.395** Other fracture of fourth metacarpal bone, left hand
  HAC 7th character B see Appendix B for HAC conditional logic

CC +7th **S62.396** Other fracture of fifth metacarpal bone, right hand
  HAC 7th character B see Appendix B for HAC conditional logic

- **S62.5 Fracture of thumb**
  - **S62.50 Fracture of unspecified phalanx of thumb**
    - CC +7th **S62.397** Other fracture of fifth metacarpal bone, left hand
      - HAC 7th character B see Appendix B for HAC conditional logic
    - CC +7th **S62.398** Other fracture of other metacarpal bone
      Other fracture of specified metacarpal bone with unspecified laterality
      - HAC 7th character B see Appendix B for HAC conditional logic
    - CC +7th **S62.399** Other fracture of unspecified metacarpal bone
      - HAC 7th character B see Appendix B for HAC conditional logic

- **+ S62.5 Fracture of thumb**
  - **+ S62.50 Fracture of unspecified phalanx of thumb**
    - CC +7th **S62.501** Fracture of unspecified phalanx of right thumb
      - HAC 7th character B see Appendix B for HAC conditional logic
    - CC +7th **S62.502** Fracture of unspecified phalanx of left thumb
      - HAC 7th character B see Appendix B for HAC conditional logic
    - CC +7th **S62.509** Fracture of unspecified phalanx of unspecified thumb
      - HAC 7th character B see Appendix B for HAC conditional logic
  - **+ S62.51 Fracture of proximal phalanx of thumb**
    - CC +7th **S62.511** Displaced fracture of proximal phalanx of right thumb
      - HAC 7th character B see Appendix B for HAC conditional logic
    - CC +7th **S62.512** Displaced fracture of proximal phalanx of left thumb
      - HAC 7th character B see Appendix B for HAC conditional logic
    - CC +7th **S62.513** Displaced fracture of proximal phalanx of unspecified thumb
      - HAC 7th character B see Appendix B for HAC conditional logic
    - CC +7th **S62.514** Nondisplaced fracture of proximal phalanx of right thumb
      - HAC 7th character B see Appendix B for HAC conditional logic
    - CC +7th **S62.515** Nondisplaced fracture of proximal phalanx of left thumb
      - HAC 7th character B see Appendix B for HAC conditional logic
    - CC +7th **S62.516** Nondisplaced fracture of proximal phalanx of unspecified thumb
      - HAC 7th character B see Appendix B for HAC conditional logic
  - **+ S62.52 Fracture of distal phalanx of thumb**
    - CC +7th **S62.521** Displaced fracture of distal phalanx of right thumb
      - HAC 7th character B see Appendix B for HAC conditional logic
    - CC +7th **S62.522** Displaced fracture of distal phalanx of left thumb
      - HAC 7th character B see Appendix B for HAC conditional logic
    - CC +7th **S62.523** Displaced fracture of distal phalanx of unspecified thumb
      - HAC 7th character B see Appendix B for HAC conditional logic
    - CC +7th **S62.524** Nondisplaced fracture of distal phalanx of right thumb
      - HAC 7th character B see Appendix B for HAC conditional logic
    - CC +7th **S62.525** Nondisplaced fracture of distal phalanx of left thumb
      - HAC 7th character B see Appendix B for HAC conditional logic
    - CC +7th **S62.526** Nondisplaced fracture of distal phalanx of unspecified thumb
      - HAC 7th character B see Appendix B for HAC conditional logic

- **+ S62.6 Fracture of other and unspecified finger(s)**
  - *Excludes2:* fracture of thumb (S62.5-)
  - **+ S62.60 Fracture of unspecified phalanx of finger**
    - CC +7th **S62.600** Fracture of unspecified phalanx of right index finger
      - HAC 7th character B see Appendix B for HAC conditional logic
    - CC +7th **S62.601** Fracture of unspecified phalanx of left index finger
      - HAC 7th character B see Appendix B for HAC conditional logic
    - CC +7th **S62.602** Fracture of unspecified phalanx of right middle finger
      - HAC 7th character B see Appendix B for HAC conditional logic
    - CC +7th **S62.603** Fracture of unspecified phalanx of left middle finger
      - HAC 7th character B see Appendix B for HAC conditional logic
    - CC +7th **S62.604** Fracture of unspecified phalanx of right ring finger
      - HAC 7th character B see Appendix B for HAC conditional logic
    - CC +7th **S62.605** Fracture of unspecified phalanx of left ring finger
      - HAC 7th character B see Appendix B for HAC conditional logic
    - CC +7th **S62.606** Fracture of unspecified phalanx of right little finger
      - HAC 7th character B see Appendix B for HAC conditional logic
    - CC +7th **S62.607** Fracture of unspecified phalanx of left little finger
      - HAC 7th character B see Appendix B for HAC conditional logic
    - CC +7th **S62.608** Fracture of unspecified phalanx of other finger
      Fracture of unspecified phalanx of specified finger with unspecified laterality
      - HAC 7th character B see Appendix B for HAC conditional logic
    - CC +7th **S62.609** Fracture of unspecified phalanx of unspecified finger
      - HAC 7th character B see Appendix B for HAC conditional logic
  - **+ S62.61 Displaced fracture of proximal phalanx of finger**
    - CC +7th **S62.610** Displaced fracture of proximal phalanx of right index finger
      - HAC 7th character B see Appendix B for HAC conditional logic
    - CC +7th **S62.611** Displaced fracture of proximal phalanx of left index finger
      - HAC 7th character B see Appendix B for HAC conditional logic
    - CC +7th **S62.612** Displaced fracture of proximal phalanx of right middle finger
      - HAC 7th character B see Appendix B for HAC conditional logic
    - CC +7th **S62.613** Displaced fracture of proximal phalanx of left middle finger
      - HAC 7th character B see Appendix B for HAC conditional logic
    - CC +7th **S62.614** Displaced fracture of proximal phalanx of right ring finger
      - HAC 7th character B see Appendix B for HAC conditional logic
    - CC +7th **S62.615** Displaced fracture of proximal phalanx of left ring finger
      - HAC 7th character B see Appendix B for HAC conditional logic
    - CC +7th **S62.616** Displaced fracture of proximal phalanx of right little finger
      - HAC 7th character B see Appendix B for HAC conditional logic
    - CC +7th **S62.617** Displaced fracture of proximal phalanx of left little finger
      - HAC 7th character B see Appendix B for HAC conditional logic
    - CC +7th **S62.618** Displaced fracture of proximal phalanx of other finger
      Displaced fracture of proximal phalanx of specified finger with unspecified laterality
      - HAC 7th character B see Appendix B for HAC conditional logic
    - CC +7th **S62.619** Displaced fracture of proximal phalanx of unspecified finger
      - HAC 7th character B see Appendix B for HAC conditional logic
  - **+ S62.62 Displaced fracture of middle phalanx of finger**
    - CC +7th **S62.620** Displaced fracture of middle phalanx of right index finger
      - HAC 7th character B see Appendix B for HAC conditional logic

CC +7th S62.621 Displaced fracture of middle phalanx of left index finger
  HAC 7th character B see Appendix B for HAC conditional logic
CC +7th S62.622 Displaced fracture of middle phalanx of right middle finger
  HAC 7th character B see Appendix B for HAC conditional logic
CC +7th S62.623 Displaced fracture of middle phalanx of left middle finger
  HAC 7th character B see Appendix B for HAC conditional logic
CC +7th S62.624 Displaced fracture of middle phalanx of right ring finger
  HAC 7th character B see Appendix B for HAC conditional logic
CC +7th S62.625 Displaced fracture of middle phalanx of left ring finger
  HAC 7th character B see Appendix B for HAC conditional logic
CC +7th S62.626 Displaced fracture of middle phalanx of right little finger
  HAC 7th character B see Appendix B for HAC conditional logic
CC +7th S62.627 Displaced fracture of middle phalanx of left little finger
  HAC 7th character B see Appendix B for HAC conditional logic
CC +7th S62.628 Displaced fracture of middle phalanx of other finger
  Displaced fracture of middle phalanx of specified finger with unspecified laterality
  HAC 7th character B see Appendix B for HAC conditional logic
CC +7th S62.629 Displaced fracture of middle phalanx of unspecified finger
  HAC 7th character B see Appendix B for HAC conditional logic

+ S62.63 **Displaced fracture of distal phalanx of finger**
CC +7th S62.630 Displaced fracture of distal phalanx of right index finger
  HAC 7th character B see Appendix B for HAC conditional logic
CC +7th S62.631 Displaced fracture of distal phalanx of left index finger
  HAC 7th character B see Appendix B for HAC conditional logic
CC +7th S62.632 Displaced fracture of distal phalanx of right middle finger
  HAC 7th character B see Appendix B for HAC conditional logic
CC +7th S62.633 Displaced fracture of distal phalanx of left middle finger
  HAC 7th character B see Appendix B for HAC conditional logic
CC +7th S62.634 Displaced fracture of distal phalanx of right ring finger
  HAC 7th character B see Appendix B for HAC conditional logic
CC +7th S62.635 Displaced fracture of distal phalanx of left ring finger
  HAC 7th character B see Appendix B for HAC conditional logic
CC +7th S62.636 Displaced fracture of distal phalanx of right little finger
  HAC 7th character B see Appendix B for HAC conditional logic
CC +7th S62.637 Displaced fracture of distal phalanx of left little finger
  HAC 7th character B see Appendix B for HAC conditional logic
CC +7th S62.638 Displaced fracture of distal phalanx of other finger
  Displaced fracture of distal phalanx of specified finger with unspecified laterality
  HAC 7th character B see Appendix B for HAC conditional logic
CC +7th S62.639 Displaced fracture of distal phalanx of unspecified finger
  HAC 7th character B see Appendix B for HAC conditional logic

+ S62.64 **Nondisplaced fracture of proximal phalanx of finger**
CC +7th S62.640 Nondisplaced fracture of proximal phalanx of right index finger
  HAC 7th character B see Appendix B for HAC conditional logic
CC +7th S62.641 Nondisplaced fracture of proximal phalanx of left index finger
  HAC 7th character B see Appendix B for HAC conditional logic
CC +7th S62.642 Nondisplaced fracture of proximal phalanx of right middle finger
  HAC 7th character B see Appendix B for HAC conditional logic
CC +7th S62.643 Nondisplaced fracture of proximal phalanx of left middle finger
  HAC 7th character B see Appendix B for HAC conditional logic
CC +7th S62.644 Nondisplaced fracture of proximal phalanx of right ring finger
  HAC 7th character B see Appendix B for HAC conditional logic
CC +7th S62.645 Nondisplaced fracture of proximal phalanx of left ring finger
  HAC 7th character B see Appendix B for HAC conditional logic
CC +7th S62.646 Nondisplaced fracture of proximal phalanx of right little finger
  HAC 7th character B see Appendix B for HAC conditional logic
CC +7th S62.647 Nondisplaced fracture of proximal phalanx of left little finger
  HAC 7th character B see Appendix B for HAC conditional logic
CC +7th S62.648 Nondisplaced fracture of proximal phalanx of other finger
  Nondisplaced fracture of proximal phalanx of specified finger with unspecified laterality
  HAC 7th character B see Appendix B for HAC conditional logic
CC +7th S62.649 Nondisplaced fracture of proximal phalanx of unspecified finger
  HAC 7th character B see Appendix B for HAC conditional logic

+ S62.65 **Nondisplaced fracture of middle phalanx of finger**
CC +7th S62.650 Nondisplaced fracture of middle phalanx of right index finger
  HAC 7th character B see Appendix B for HAC conditional logic
CC +7th S62.651 Nondisplaced fracture of middle phalanx of left index finger
  HAC 7th character B see Appendix B for HAC conditional logic
CC +7th S62.652 Nondisplaced fracture of middle phalanx of right middle finger
  HAC 7th character B see Appendix B for HAC conditional logic
CC +7th S62.653 Nondisplaced fracture of middle phalanx of left middle finger
  HAC 7th character B see Appendix B for HAC conditional logic
CC +7th S62.654 Nondisplaced fracture of middle phalanx of right ring finger
  HAC 7th character B see Appendix B for HAC conditional logic
CC +7th S62.655 Nondisplaced fracture of middle phalanx of left ring finger
  HAC 7th character B see Appendix B for HAC conditional logic
CC +7th S62.656 Nondisplaced fracture of middle phalanx of right little finger
  HAC 7th character B see Appendix B for HAC conditional logic
CC +7th S62.657 Nondisplaced fracture of middle phalanx of left little finger
  HAC 7th character B see Appendix B for HAC conditional logic

CC +7th	S62.658	**Nondisplaced fracture of middle phalanx of other finger** Nondisplaced fracture of middle phalanx of specified finger with unspecified laterality **HAC** 7th character B see Appendix B for HAC conditional logic
CC +7th	S62.659	**Nondisplaced fracture of middle phalanx of unspecified finger** **HAC** 7th character B see Appendix B for HAC conditional logic
+	S62.66	**Nondisplaced fracture of distal phalanx of finger**
CC +7th	S62.660	**Nondisplaced fracture of distal phalanx of right index finger** **HAC** 7th character B see Appendix B for HAC conditional logic
CC +7th	S62.661	**Nondisplaced fracture of distal phalanx of left index finger** **HAC** 7th character B see Appendix B for HAC conditional logic
CC +7th	S62.662	**Nondisplaced fracture of distal phalanx of right middle finger** **HAC** 7th character B see Appendix B for HAC conditional logic
CC +7th	S62.663	**Nondisplaced fracture of distal phalanx of left middle finger** **HAC** 7th character B see Appendix B for HAC conditional logic
CC +7th	S62.664	**Nondisplaced fracture of distal phalanx of right ring finger** **HAC** 7th character B see Appendix B for HAC conditional logic
CC +7th	S62.665	**Nondisplaced fracture of distal phalanx of left ring finger** **HAC** 7th character B see Appendix B for HAC conditional logic
CC +7th	S62.666	**Nondisplaced fracture of distal phalanx of right little finger** **HAC** 7th character B see Appendix B for HAC conditional logic
CC +7th	S62.667	**Nondisplaced fracture of distal phalanx of left little finger** **HAC** 7th character B see Appendix B for HAC conditional logic
CC +7th	S62.668	**Nondisplaced fracture of distal phalanx of other finger** Nondisplaced fracture of distal phalanx of specified finger with unspecified laterality **HAC** 7th character B see Appendix B for HAC conditional logic
CC +7th	S62.669	**Nondisplaced fracture of distal phalanx of unspecified finger** **HAC** 7th character B see Appendix B for HAC conditional logic
+	S62.9	**Unspecified fracture of wrist and hand**
CC X+7th	S62.90	**Unspecified fracture of unspecified wrist and hand** **HAC** 7th character B see Appendix B for HAC conditional logic
CC X+7th	S62.91	**Unspecified fracture of right wrist and hand** **HAC** 7th character B see Appendix B for HAC conditional logic
CC X+7th	S62.92	**Unspecified fracture of left wrist and hand** **HAC** 7th character B see Appendix B for HAC conditional logic

S63 Dislocation and sprain of joints and ligaments at wrist and hand level

Includes: avulsion of joint or ligament at wrist and hand level
laceration of cartilage, joint or ligament at wrist and hand level
sprain of cartilage, joint or ligament at wrist and hand level
traumatic hemarthrosis of joint or ligament at wrist and hand level
traumatic rupture of joint or ligament at wrist and hand level
traumatic subluxation of joint or ligament at wrist and hand level
traumatic tear of joint or ligament at wrist and hand level

Code also any associated open wound

Excludes2: *strain of muscle, fascia and tendon of wrist and hand (S66.-)*

The appropriate 7th character is to be added to each code from category S63
A   initial encounter
D   subsequent encounter
S   sequela

+ S63.0		**Subluxation and dislocation of wrist and hand joints**
+ S63.00		**Unspecified subluxation and dislocation of wrist and hand** Dislocation of carpal bone NOS Dislocation of distal end of radius NOS Subluxation of carpal bone NOS Subluxation of distal end of radius NOS
+7th	S63.001	Unspecified subluxation of right wrist and hand
+7th	S63.002	Unspecified subluxation of left wrist and hand
+7th	S63.003	Unspecified subluxation of unspecified wrist and hand
+7th	S63.004	Unspecified dislocation of right wrist and hand
+7th	S63.005	Unspecified dislocation of left wrist and hand
+7th	S63.006	Unspecified dislocation of unspecified wrist and hand
+ S63.01		**Subluxation and dislocation of distal radioulnar joint**
+7th	S63.011	Subluxation of distal radioulnar joint of right wrist
+7th	S63.012	Subluxation of distal radioulnar joint of left wrist
+7th	S63.013	Subluxation of distal radioulnar joint of unspecified wrist
+7th	S63.014	Dislocation of distal radioulnar joint of right wrist
+7th	S63.015	Dislocation of distal radioulnar joint of left wrist
+7th	S63.016	Dislocation of distal radioulnar joint of unspecified wrist
+ S63.02		**Subluxation and dislocation of radiocarpal joint**
+7th	S63.021	Subluxation of radiocarpal joint of right wrist
+7th	S63.022	Subluxation of radiocarpal joint of left wrist
+7th	S63.023	Subluxation of radiocarpal joint of unspecified wrist
+7th	S63.024	Dislocation of radiocarpal joint of right wrist
+7th	S63.025	Dislocation of radiocarpal joint of left wrist
+7th	S63.026	Dislocation of radiocarpal joint of unspecified wrist
+ S63.03		**Subluxation and dislocation of midcarpal joint**
+7th	S63.031	Subluxation of midcarpal joint of right wrist
+7th	S63.032	Subluxation of midcarpal joint of left wrist
+7th	S63.033	Subluxation of midcarpal joint of unspecified wrist
+7th	S63.034	Dislocation of midcarpal joint of right wrist
+7th	S63.035	Dislocation of midcarpal joint of left wrist
+7th	S63.036	Dislocation of midcarpal joint of unspecified wrist
+ S63.04		**Subluxation and dislocation of carpometacarpal joint of thumb** **Excludes2:** *interphalangeal subluxation and dislocation of thumb (S63.1-)*
+7th	S63.041	Subluxation of carpometacarpal joint of right thumb
+7th	S63.042	Subluxation of carpometacarpal joint of left thumb
+7th	S63.043	Subluxation of carpometacarpal joint of unspecified thumb
+7th	S63.044	Dislocation of carpometacarpal joint of right thumb
+7th	S63.045	Dislocation of carpometacarpal joint of left thumb
+7th	S63.046	Dislocation of carpometacarpal joint of unspecified thumb
+ S63.05		**Subluxation and dislocation of other carpometacarpal joint** **Excludes2:** *subluxation and dislocation of carpometacarpal joint of thumb (S63.04-)*
+7th	S63.051	Subluxation of other carpometacarpal joint of right hand

- +7th **S63.052** Subluxation of other carpometacarpal joint of left hand
- +7th **S63.053** Subluxation of other carpometacarpal joint of unspecified hand
- +7th **S63.054** Dislocation of other carpometacarpal joint of right hand
- +7th **S63.055** Dislocation of other carpometacarpal joint of left hand
- +7th **S63.056** Dislocation of other carpometacarpal joint of unspecified hand
- \+ **S63.06** Subluxation and dislocation of metacarpal (bone), proximal end
  - +7th **S63.061** Subluxation of metacarpal (bone), proximal end of right hand
  - +7th **S63.062** Subluxation of metacarpal (bone), proximal end of left hand
  - +7th **S63.063** Subluxation of metacarpal (bone), proximal end of unspecified hand
  - +7th **S63.064** Dislocation of metacarpal (bone), proximal end of right hand
  - +7th **S63.065** Dislocation of metacarpal (bone), proximal end of left hand
  - +7th **S63.066** Dislocation of metacarpal (bone), proximal end of unspecified hand
- \+ **S63.07** Subluxation and dislocation of distal end of ulna
  - +7th **S63.071** Subluxation of distal end of right ulna
  - +7th **S63.072** Subluxation of distal end of left ulna
  - +7th **S63.073** Subluxation of distal end of unspecified ulna
  - +7th **S63.074** Dislocation of distal end of right ulna
  - +7th **S63.075** Dislocation of distal end of left ulna
  - +7th **S63.076** Dislocation of distal end of unspecified ulna
- \+ **S63.09** Other subluxation and dislocation of wrist and hand
  - +7th **S63.091** Other subluxation of right wrist and hand
  - +7th **S63.092** Other subluxation of left wrist and hand
  - +7th **S63.093** Other subluxation of unspecified wrist and hand
  - +7th **S63.094** Other dislocation of right wrist and hand
  - +7th **S63.095** Other dislocation of left wrist and hand
  - +7th **S63.096** Other dislocation of unspecified wrist and hand
- \+ **S63.1** Subluxation and dislocation of thumb
  - \+ **S63.10** Unspecified subluxation and dislocation of thumb
    - +7th **S63.101** Unspecified subluxation of right thumb
    - +7th **S63.102** Unspecified subluxation of left thumb
    - +7th **S63.103** Unspecified subluxation of unspecified thumb
    - +7th **S63.104** Unspecified dislocation of right thumb
    - +7th **S63.105** Unspecified dislocation of left thumb
    - +7th **S63.106** Unspecified dislocation of unspecified thumb
  - \+ **S63.11** Subluxation and dislocation of metacarpophalangeal joint of thumb
    - +7th **S63.111** Subluxation of metacarpophalangeal joint of right thumb
    - +7th **S63.112** Subluxation of metacarpophalangeal joint of left thumb
    - +7th **S63.113** Subluxation of metacarpophalangeal joint of unspecified thumb
    - +7th **S63.114** Dislocation of metacarpophalangeal joint of right thumb
    - +7th **S63.115** Dislocation of metacarpophalangeal joint of left thumb
    - +7th **S63.116** Dislocation of metacarpophalangeal joint of unspecified thumb
  - \+ **S63.12** Subluxation and dislocation of interphalangeal joint of thumb
    - +7th **S63.121** Subluxation of interphalangeal joint of right thumb
    - +7th **S63.122** Subluxation of interphalangeal joint of left thumb
    - +7th **S63.123** Subluxation of interphalangeal joint of unspecified thumb
    - +7th **S63.124** Dislocation of interphalangeal joint of right thumb
    - +7th **S63.125** Dislocation of interphalangeal joint of left thumb
    - +7th **S63.126** Dislocation of interphalangeal joint of unspecified thumb
- \+ **S63.2** Subluxation and dislocation of other finger(s)
  - **Excludes2:** subluxation and dislocation of thumb (S63.1-)
  - \+ **S63.20** Unspecified subluxation of other finger
    - +7th **S63.200** Unspecified subluxation of right index finger
    - +7th **S63.201** Unspecified subluxation of left index finger
    - +7th **S63.202** Unspecified subluxation of right middle finger
    - +7th **S63.203** Unspecified subluxation of left middle finger
    - +7th **S63.204** Unspecified subluxation of right ring finger
    - +7th **S63.205** Unspecified subluxation of left ring finger
    - +7th **S63.206** Unspecified subluxation of right little finger
    - +7th **S63.207** Unspecified subluxation of left little finger
    - +7th **S63.208** Unspecified subluxation of other finger
      Unspecified subluxation of specified finger with unspecified laterality
    - +7th **S63.209** Unspecified subluxation of unspecified finger
  - \+ **S63.21** Subluxation of metacarpophalangeal joint of finger
    - +7th **S63.210** Subluxation of metacarpophalangeal joint of right index finger
    - +7th **S63.211** Subluxation of metacarpophalangeal joint of left index finger
    - +7th **S63.212** Subluxation of metacarpophalangeal joint of right middle finger
    - +7th **S63.213** Subluxation of metacarpophalangeal joint of left middle finger
    - +7th **S63.214** Subluxation of metacarpophalangeal joint of right ring finger
    - +7th **S63.215** Subluxation of metacarpophalangeal joint of left ring finger
    - +7th **S63.216** Subluxation of metacarpophalangeal joint of right little finger
    - +7th **S63.217** Subluxation of metacarpophalangeal joint of left little finger
    - +7th **S63.218** Subluxation of metacarpophalangeal joint of other finger
      Subluxation of metacarpophalangeal joint of specified finger with unspecified laterality
    - +7th **S63.219** Subluxation of metacarpophalangeal joint of unspecified finger
  - \+ **S63.22** Subluxation of unspecified interphalangeal joint of finger
    - +7th **S63.220** Subluxation of unspecified interphalangeal joint of right index finger
    - +7th **S63.221** Subluxation of unspecified interphalangeal joint of left index finger
    - +7th **S63.222** Subluxation of unspecified interphalangeal joint of right middle finger
    - +7th **S63.223** Subluxation of unspecified interphalangeal joint of left middle finger
    - +7th **S63.224** Subluxation of unspecified interphalangeal joint of right ring finger
    - +7th **S63.225** Subluxation of unspecified interphalangeal joint of left ring finger
    - +7th **S63.226** Subluxation of unspecified interphalangeal joint of right little finger
    - +7th **S63.227** Subluxation of unspecified interphalangeal joint of left little finger
    - +7th **S63.228** Subluxation of unspecified interphalangeal joint of other finger
      Subluxation of unspecified interphalangeal joint of specified finger with unspecified laterality
    - +7th **S63.229** Subluxation of unspecified interphalangeal joint of unspecified finger

- +S63.23 **Subluxation of proximal interphalangeal joint of finger**
  - +7th S63.230 Subluxation of proximal interphalangeal joint of right index finger
  - +7th S63.231 Subluxation of proximal interphalangeal joint of left index finger
  - +7th S63.232 Subluxation of proximal interphalangeal joint of right middle finger
  - +7th S63.233 Subluxation of proximal interphalangeal joint of left middle finger
  - +7th S63.234 Subluxation of proximal interphalangeal joint of right ring finger
  - +7th S63.235 Subluxation of proximal interphalangeal joint of left ring finger
  - +7th S63.236 Subluxation of proximal interphalangeal joint of right little finger
  - +7th S63.237 Subluxation of proximal interphalangeal joint of left little finger
  - +7th S63.238 Subluxation of proximal interphalangeal joint of other finger
    - Subluxation of proximal interphalangeal joint of specified finger with unspecified laterality
  - +7th S63.239 Subluxation of proximal interphalangeal joint of unspecified finger
- +S63.24 **Subluxation of distal interphalangeal joint of finger**
  - +7th S63.240 Subluxation of distal interphalangeal joint of right index finger
  - +7th S63.241 Subluxation of distal interphalangeal joint of left index finger
  - +7th S63.242 Subluxation of distal interphalangeal joint of right middle finger
  - +7th S63.243 Subluxation of distal interphalangeal joint of left middle finger
  - +7th S63.244 Subluxation of distal interphalangeal joint of right ring finger
  - +7th S63.245 Subluxation of distal interphalangeal joint of left ring finger
  - +7th S63.246 Subluxation of distal interphalangeal joint of right little finger
  - +7th S63.247 Subluxation of distal interphalangeal joint of left little finger
  - +7th S63.248 Subluxation of distal interphalangeal joint of other finger
    - Subluxation of distal interphalangeal joint of specified finger with unspecified laterality
  - +7th S63.249 Subluxation of distal interphalangeal joint of unspecified finger
- +S63.25 **Unspecified dislocation of other finger**
  - +7th S63.250 Unspecified dislocation of right index finger
  - +7th S63.251 Unspecified dislocation of left index finger
  - +7th S63.252 Unspecified dislocation of right middle finger
  - +7th S63.253 Unspecified dislocation of left middle finger
  - +7th S63.254 Unspecified dislocation of right ring finger
  - +7th S63.255 Unspecified dislocation of left ring finger
  - +7th S63.256 Unspecified dislocation of right little finger
  - +7th S63.257 Unspecified dislocation of left little finger
  - +7th S63.258 Unspecified dislocation of other finger
    - Unspecified dislocation of specified finger with unspecified laterality
  - +7th S63.259 Unspecified dislocation of unspecified finger
    - Unspecified dislocation of unspecified finger with unspecified laterality

- +S63.26 **Dislocation of metacarpophalangeal joint of finger**
  - +7th S63.260 Dislocation of metacarpophalangeal joint of right index finger
  - +7th S63.261 Dislocation of metacarpophalangeal joint of left index finger
  - +7th S63.262 Dislocation of metacarpophalangeal joint of right middle finger
  - +7th S63.263 Dislocation of metacarpophalangeal joint of left middle finger
  - +7th S63.264 Dislocation of metacarpophalangeal joint of right ring finger
  - +7th S63.265 Dislocation of metacarpophalangeal joint of left ring finger
  - +7th S63.266 Dislocation of metacarpophalangeal joint of right little finger
  - +7th S63.267 Dislocation of metacarpophalangeal joint of left little finger
  - +7th S63.268 Dislocation of metacarpophalangeal joint of other finger
    - Dislocation of metacarpophalangeal joint of specified finger with unspecified laterality
  - +7th S63.269 Dislocation of metacarpophalangeal joint of unspecified finger
- +S63.27 **Dislocation of unspecified interphalangeal joint of finger**
  - +7th S63.270 Dislocation of unspecified interphalangeal joint of right index finger
  - +7th S63.271 Dislocation of unspecified interphalangeal joint of left index finger
  - +7th S63.272 Dislocation of unspecified interphalangeal joint of right middle finger
  - +7th S63.273 Dislocation of unspecified interphalangeal joint of left middle finger
  - +7th S63.274 Dislocation of unspecified interphalangeal joint of right ring finger
  - +7th S63.275 Dislocation of unspecified interphalangeal joint of left ring finger
  - +7th S63.276 Dislocation of unspecified interphalangeal joint of right little finger
  - +7th S63.277 Dislocation of unspecified interphalangeal joint of left little finger
  - +7th S63.278 Dislocation of unspecified interphalangeal joint of other finger
    - Dislocation of unspecified interphalangeal joint of specified finger with unspecified laterality
  - +7th S63.279 Dislocation of unspecified interphalangeal joint of unspecified finger
    - Dislocation of unspecified interphalangeal joint of unspecified finger without specified laterality
- +S63.28 **Dislocation of proximal interphalangeal joint of finger**
  - +7th S63.280 Dislocation of proximal interphalangeal joint of right index finger
  - +7th S63.281 Dislocation of proximal interphalangeal joint of left index finger
  - +7th S63.282 Dislocation of proximal interphalangeal joint of right middle finger
  - +7th S63.283 Dislocation of proximal interphalangeal joint of left middle finger
  - +7th S63.284 Dislocation of proximal interphalangeal joint of right ring finger
  - +7th S63.285 Dislocation of proximal interphalangeal joint of left ring finger
  - +7th S63.286 Dislocation of proximal interphalangeal joint of right little finger
  - +7th S63.287 Dislocation of proximal interphalangeal joint of left little finger
  - +7th S63.288 Dislocation of proximal interphalangeal joint of other finger
    - Dislocation of proximal interphalangeal joint of specified finger with unspecified laterality
  - +7th S63.289 Dislocation of proximal interphalangeal joint of unspecified finger

- **S63.29** Dislocation of distal interphalangeal joint of finger
  - +7th **S63.290** Dislocation of distal interphalangeal joint of right index finger
  - +7th **S63.291** Dislocation of distal interphalangeal joint of left index finger
  - +7th **S63.292** Dislocation of distal interphalangeal joint of right middle finger
  - +7th **S63.293** Dislocation of distal interphalangeal joint of left middle finger
  - +7th **S63.294** Dislocation of distal interphalangeal joint of right ring finger
  - +7th **S63.295** Dislocation of distal interphalangeal joint of left ring finger
  - +7th **S63.296** Dislocation of distal interphalangeal joint of right little finger
  - +7th **S63.297** Dislocation of distal interphalangeal joint of left little finger
  - +7th **S63.298** Dislocation of distal interphalangeal joint of other finger
    Dislocation of distal interphalangeal joint of specified finger with unspecified laterality
  - +7th **S63.299** Dislocation of distal interphalangeal joint of unspecified finger
- + **S63.3** Traumatic rupture of ligament of wrist
  - + **S63.30** Traumatic rupture of unspecified ligament of wrist
    - +7th **S63.301** Traumatic rupture of unspecified ligament of right wrist
    - +7th **S63.302** Traumatic rupture of unspecified ligament of left wrist
    - +7th **S63.309** Traumatic rupture of unspecified ligament of unspecified wrist
  - + **S63.31** Traumatic rupture of collateral ligament of wrist
    - +7th **S63.311** Traumatic rupture of collateral ligament of right wrist
    - +7th **S63.312** Traumatic rupture of collateral ligament of left wrist
    - +7th **S63.319** Traumatic rupture of collateral ligament of unspecified wrist
  - + **S63.32** Traumatic rupture of radiocarpal ligament
    - +7th **S63.321** Traumatic rupture of right radiocarpal ligament
    - +7th **S63.322** Traumatic rupture of left radiocarpal ligament
    - +7th **S63.329** Traumatic rupture of unspecified radiocarpal ligament
  - + **S63.33** Traumatic rupture of ulnocarpal (palmar) ligament
    - +7th **S63.331** Traumatic rupture of right ulnocarpal (palmar) ligament
    - +7th **S63.332** Traumatic rupture of left ulnocarpal (palmar) ligament
    - +7th **S63.339** Traumatic rupture of unspecified ulnocarpal (palmar) ligament
  - + **S63.39** Traumatic rupture of other ligament of wrist
    - +7th **S63.391** Traumatic rupture of other ligament of right wrist
    - +7th **S63.392** Traumatic rupture of other ligament of left wrist
    - +7th **S63.399** Traumatic rupture of other ligament of unspecified wrist
- + **S63.4** Traumatic rupture of ligament of finger at metacarpophalangeal and interphalangeal joint(s)
  - + **S63.40** Traumatic rupture of unspecified ligament of finger at metacarpophalangeal and interphalangeal joint
    - +7th **S63.400** Traumatic rupture of unspecified ligament of right index finger at metacarpophalangeal and interphalangeal joint
    - +7th **S63.401** Traumatic rupture of unspecified ligament of left index finger at metacarpophalangeal and interphalangeal joint
    - +7th **S63.402** Traumatic rupture of unspecified ligament of right middle finger at metacarpophalangeal and interphalangeal joint
    - +7th **S63.403** Traumatic rupture of unspecified ligament of left middle finger at metacarpophalangeal and interphalangeal joint
    - +7th **S63.404** Traumatic rupture of unspecified ligament of right ring finger at metacarpophalangeal and interphalangeal joint
    - +7th **S63.405** Traumatic rupture of unspecified ligament of left ring finger at metacarpophalangeal and interphalangeal joint
    - +7th **S63.406** Traumatic rupture of unspecified ligament of right little finger at metacarpophalangeal and interphalangeal joint
    - +7th **S63.407** Traumatic rupture of unspecified ligament of left little finger at metacarpophalangeal and interphalangeal joint
    - +7th **S63.408** Traumatic rupture of unspecified ligament of other finger at metacarpophalangeal and interphalangeal joint
      Traumatic rupture of unspecified ligament of specified finger with unspecified laterality at metacarpophalangeal and interphalangeal joint
    - +7th **S63.409** Traumatic rupture of unspecified ligament of unspecified finger at metacarpophalangeal and interphalangeal joint
  - + **S63.41** Traumatic rupture of collateral ligament of finger at metacarpophalangeal and interphalangeal joint
    - +7th **S63.410** Traumatic rupture of collateral ligament of right index finger at metacarpophalangeal and interphalangeal joint
    - +7th **S63.411** Traumatic rupture of collateral ligament of left index finger at metacarpophalangeal and interphalangeal joint
    - +7th **S63.412** Traumatic rupture of collateral ligament of right middle finger at metacarpophalangeal and interphalangeal joint
    - +7th **S63.413** Traumatic rupture of collateral ligament of left middle finger at metacarpophalangeal and interphalangeal joint
    - +7th **S63.414** Traumatic rupture of collateral ligament of right ring finger at metacarpophalangeal and interphalangeal joint
    - +7th **S63.415** Traumatic rupture of collateral ligament of left ring finger at metacarpophalangeal and interphalangeal joint
    - +7th **S63.416** Traumatic rupture of collateral ligament of right little finger at metacarpophalangeal and interphalangeal joint
    - +7th **S63.417** Traumatic rupture of collateral ligament of left little finger at metacarpophalangeal and interphalangeal joint
    - +7th **S63.418** Traumatic rupture of collateral ligament of other finger at metacarpophalangeal and interphalangeal joint
      Traumatic rupture of collateral ligament of specified finger with unspecified laterality at metacarpophalangeal and interphalangeal joint
    - +7th **S63.419** Traumatic rupture of collateral ligament of unspecified finger at metacarpophalangeal and interphalangeal joint

- **S63.42** Traumatic rupture of palmar ligament of finger at metacarpophalangeal and interphalangeal joint
  - +7th **S63.420** Traumatic rupture of palmar ligament of right index finger at metacarpophalangeal and interphalangeal joint
  - +7th **S63.421** Traumatic rupture of palmar ligament of left index finger at metacarpophalangeal and interphalangeal joint
  - +7th **S63.422** Traumatic rupture of palmar ligament of right middle finger at metacarpophalangeal and interphalangeal joint
  - +7th **S63.423** Traumatic rupture of palmar ligament of left middle finger at metacarpophalangeal and interphalangeal joint
  - +7th **S63.424** Traumatic rupture of palmar ligament of right ring finger at metacarpophalangeal and interphalangeal joint
  - +7th **S63.425** Traumatic rupture of palmar ligament of left ring finger at metacarpophalangeal and interphalangeal joint
  - +7th **S63.426** Traumatic rupture of palmar ligament of right little finger at metacarpophalangeal and interphalangeal joint
  - +7th **S63.427** Traumatic rupture of palmar ligament of left little finger at metacarpophalangeal and interphalangeal joint
  - +7th **S63.428** Traumatic rupture of palmar ligament of other finger at metacarpophalangeal and interphalangeal joint
    - Traumatic rupture of palmar ligament of specified finger with unspecified laterality at metacarpophalangeal and interphalangeal joint
  - +7th **S63.429** Traumatic rupture of palmar ligament of unspecified finger at metacarpophalangeal and interphalangeal joint
- **S63.43** Traumatic rupture of volar plate of finger at metacarpophalangeal and interphalangeal joint
  - +7th **S63.430** Traumatic rupture of volar plate of right index finger at metacarpophalangeal and interphalangeal joint
  - +7th **S63.431** Traumatic rupture of volar plate of left index finger at metacarpophalangeal and interphalangeal joint
  - +7th **S63.432** Traumatic rupture of volar plate of right middle finger at metacarpophalangeal and interphalangeal joint
  - +7th **S63.433** Traumatic rupture of volar plate of left middle finger at metacarpophalangeal and interphalangeal joint
  - +7th **S63.434** Traumatic rupture of volar plate of right ring finger at metacarpophalangeal and interphalangeal joint
  - +7th **S63.435** Traumatic rupture of volar plate of left ring finger at metacarpophalangeal and interphalangeal joint
  - +7th **S63.436** Traumatic rupture of volar plate of right little finger at metacarpophalangeal and interphalangeal joint
  - +7th **S63.437** Traumatic rupture of volar plate of left little finger at metacarpophalangeal and interphalangeal joint
  - +7th **S63.438** Traumatic rupture of volar plate of other finger at metacarpophalangeal and interphalangeal joint
    - Traumatic rupture of volar plate of specified finger with unspecified laterality at metacarpophalangeal and interphalangeal joint
  - +7th **S63.439** Traumatic rupture of volar plate of unspecified finger at metacarpophalangeal and interphalangeal joint
- **S63.49** Traumatic rupture of other ligament of finger at metacarpophalangeal and interphalangeal joint
  - +7th **S63.490** Traumatic rupture of other ligament of right index finger at metacarpophalangeal and interphalangeal joint
  - +7th **S63.491** Traumatic rupture of other ligament of left index finger at metacarpophalangeal and interphalangeal joint
  - +7th **S63.492** Traumatic rupture of other ligament of right middle finger at metacarpophalangeal and interphalangeal joint
  - +7th **S63.493** Traumatic rupture of other ligament of left middle finger at metacarpophalangeal and interphalangeal joint
  - +7th **S63.494** Traumatic rupture of other ligament of right ring finger at metacarpophalangeal and interphalangeal joint
  - +7th **S63.495** Traumatic rupture of other ligament of left ring finger at metacarpophalangeal and interphalangeal joint
  - +7th **S63.496** Traumatic rupture of other ligament of right little finger at metacarpophalangeal and interphalangeal joint
  - +7th **S63.497** Traumatic rupture of other ligament of left little finger at metacarpophalangeal and interphalangeal joint
  - +7th **S63.498** Traumatic rupture of other ligament of other finger at metacarpophalangeal and interphalangeal joint
    - Traumatic rupture of ligament of specified finger with unspecified laterality at metacarpophalangeal and interphalangeal joint
  - +7th **S63.499** Traumatic rupture of other ligament of unspecified finger at metacarpophalangeal and interphalangeal joint
- **S63.5** Other and unspecified sprain of wrist
  - **S63.50** Unspecified sprain of wrist
    - +7th **S63.501** Unspecified sprain of right wrist
    - +7th **S63.502** Unspecified sprain of left wrist
    - +7th **S63.509** Unspecified sprain of unspecified wrist
  - **S63.51** Sprain of carpal (joint)
    - +7th **S63.511** Sprain of carpal joint of right wrist
    - +7th **S63.512** Sprain of carpal joint of left wrist
    - +7th **S63.519** Sprain of carpal joint of unspecified wrist
  - **S63.52** Sprain of radiocarpal joint
    - **Excludes1:** traumatic rupture of radiocarpal ligament (S63.32-)
    - +7th **S63.521** Sprain of radiocarpal joint of right wrist
    - +7th **S63.522** Sprain of radiocarpal joint of left wrist
    - +7th **S63.529** Sprain of radiocarpal joint of unspecified wrist
  - **S63.59** Other specified sprain of wrist
    - +7th **S63.591** Other specified sprain of right wrist
    - +7th **S63.592** Other specified sprain of left wrist
    - +7th **S63.599** Other specified sprain of unspecified wrist

- **S63.6 Other and unspecified sprain of finger(s)**
  - **Excludes1:** *traumatic rupture of ligament of finger at metacarpophalangeal and interphalangeal joint(s) (S63.4-)*
  - **S63.60 Unspecified sprain of thumb**
    - +7th S63.601 Unspecified sprain of right thumb
    - +7th S63.602 Unspecified sprain of left thumb
    - +7th S63.609 Unspecified sprain of unspecified thumb
  - **S63.61 Unspecified sprain of other and unspecified finger(s)**
    - +7th S63.610 Unspecified sprain of right index finger
    - +7th S63.611 Unspecified sprain of left index finger
    - +7th S63.612 Unspecified sprain of right middle finger
    - +7th S63.613 Unspecified sprain of left middle finger
    - +7th S63.614 Unspecified sprain of right ring finger
    - +7th S63.615 Unspecified sprain of left ring finger
    - +7th S63.616 Unspecified sprain of right little finger
    - +7th S63.617 Unspecified sprain of left little finger
    - +7th S63.618 Unspecified sprain of other finger
      Unspecified sprain of specified finger with unspecified laterality
    - +7th S63.619 Unspecified sprain of unspecified finger
  - **S63.62 Sprain of interphalangeal joint of thumb**
    - +7th S63.621 Sprain of interphalangeal joint of right thumb
    - +7th S63.622 Sprain of interphalangeal joint of left thumb
    - +7th S63.629 Sprain of interphalangeal joint of unspecified thumb
  - **S63.63 Sprain of interphalangeal joint of other and unspecified finger(s)**
    - +7th S63.630 Sprain of interphalangeal joint of right index finger
    - +7th S63.631 Sprain of interphalangeal joint of left index finger
    - +7th S63.632 Sprain of interphalangeal joint of right middle finger
    - +7th S63.633 Sprain of interphalangeal joint of left middle finger
    - +7th S63.634 Sprain of interphalangeal joint of right ring finger
    - +7th S63.635 Sprain of interphalangeal joint of left ring finger
    - +7th S63.636 Sprain of interphalangeal joint of right little finger
    - +7th S63.637 Sprain of interphalangeal joint of left little finger
    - +7th S63.638 Sprain of interphalangeal joint of other finger
    - +7th S63.639 Sprain of interphalangeal joint of unspecified finger
  - **S63.64 Sprain of metacarpophalangeal joint of thumb**
    - +7th S63.641 Sprain of metacarpophalangeal joint of right thumb
    - +7th S63.642 Sprain of metacarpophalangeal joint of left thumb
    - +7th S63.649 Sprain of metacarpophalangeal joint of unspecified thumb
  - **S63.65 Sprain of metacarpophalangeal joint of other and unspecified finger(s)**
    - +7th S63.650 Sprain of metacarpophalangeal joint of right index finger
    - +7th S63.651 Sprain of metacarpophalangeal joint of left index finger
    - +7th S63.652 Sprain of metacarpophalangeal joint of right middle finger
    - +7th S63.653 Sprain of metacarpophalangeal joint of left middle finger
    - +7th S63.654 Sprain of metacarpophalangeal joint of right ring finger
    - +7th S63.655 Sprain of metacarpophalangeal joint of left ring finger
    - +7th S63.656 Sprain of metacarpophalangeal joint of right little finger
    - +7th S63.657 Sprain of metacarpophalangeal joint of left little finger
    - +7th S63.658 Sprain of metacarpophalangeal joint of other finger
      Sprain of metacarpophalangeal joint of specified finger with unspecified laterality
    - +7th S63.659 Sprain of metacarpophalangeal joint of unspecified finger
  - **S63.68 Other sprain of thumb**
    - +7th S63.681 Other sprain of right thumb
    - +7th S63.682 Other sprain of left thumb
    - +7th S63.689 Other sprain of unspecified thumb
  - **S63.69 Other sprain of other and unspecified finger(s)**
    - +7th S63.690 Other sprain of right index finger
    - +7th S63.691 Other sprain of left index finger
    - +7th S63.692 Other sprain of right middle finger
    - +7th S63.693 Other sprain of left middle finger
    - +7th S63.694 Other sprain of right ring finger
    - +7th S63.695 Other sprain of left ring finger
    - +7th S63.696 Other sprain of right little finger
    - +7th S63.697 Other sprain of left little finger
    - +7th S63.698 Other sprain of other finger
      Other sprain of specified finger with unspecified laterality
    - +7th S63.699 Other sprain of unspecified finger
- **S63.8 Sprain of other part of wrist and hand**
  - **S63.8X Sprain of other part of wrist and hand**
    - +7th S63.8X1 Sprain of other part of right wrist and hand
    - +7th S63.8X2 Sprain of other part of left wrist and hand
    - +7th S63.8X9 Sprain of other part of unspecified wrist and hand
- **S63.9 Sprain of unspecified part of wrist and hand**
  - X+7th S63.90 Sprain of unspecified part of unspecified wrist and hand
  - X+7th S63.91 Sprain of unspecified part of right wrist and hand
  - X+7th S63.92 Sprain of unspecified part of left wrist and hand

S64 Injury of nerves at wrist and hand level

Code also any associated open wound (S61.-)

> The appropriate 7th character is to be added to each code from category S64
> A initial encounter
> D subsequent encounter
> S sequela

- **S64.0 Injury of ulnar nerve at wrist and hand level**
  - X+7th S64.00 Injury of ulnar nerve at wrist and hand level of unspecified arm
  - X+7th S64.01 Injury of ulnar nerve at wrist and hand level of right arm
  - X+7th S64.02 Injury of ulnar nerve at wrist and hand level of left arm
- **S64.1 Injury of median nerve at wrist and hand level**
  - X+7th S64.10 Injury of median nerve at wrist and hand level of unspecified arm
  - X+7th S64.11 Injury of median nerve at wrist and hand level of right arm
  - X+7th S64.12 Injury of median nerve at wrist and hand level of left arm
- **S64.2 Injury of radial nerve at wrist and hand level**
  - X+7th S64.20 Injury of radial nerve at wrist and hand level of unspecified arm
  - X+7th S64.21 Injury of radial nerve at wrist and hand level of right arm
  - X+7th S64.22 Injury of radial nerve at wrist and hand level of left arm
- **S64.3 Injury of digital nerve of thumb**
  - X+7th S64.30 Injury of digital nerve of unspecified thumb
  - X+7th S64.31 Injury of digital nerve of right thumb
  - X+7th S64.32 Injury of digital nerve of left thumb
- **S64.4 Injury of digital nerve of other and unspecified finger**
  - X+7th S64.40 Injury of digital nerve of unspecified finger
  - **S64.49 Injury of digital nerve of other finger**
    - +7th S64.490 Injury of digital nerve of right index finger
    - +7th S64.491 Injury of digital nerve of left index finger
    - +7th S64.492 Injury of digital nerve of right middle finger

+7th S64.493 Injury of digital nerve of left middle finger
+7th S64.494 Injury of digital nerve of right ring finger
+7th S64.495 Injury of digital nerve of left ring finger
+7th S64.496 Injury of digital nerve of right little finger
+7th S64.497 Injury of digital nerve of left little finger
+7th S64.498 Injury of digital nerve of other finger
Injury of digital nerve of specified finger with unspecified laterality

+ S64.8 Injury of other nerves at wrist and hand level
  + S64.8X Injury of other nerves at wrist and hand level
    +7th S64.8X1 Injury of other nerves at wrist and hand level of right arm
    +7th S64.8X2 Injury of other nerves at wrist and hand level of left arm
    +7th S64.8X9 Injury of other nerves at wrist and hand level of unspecified arm

+ S64.9 Injury of unspecified nerve at wrist and hand level
  X+7th S64.90 Injury of unspecified nerve at wrist and hand level of unspecified arm
  X+7th S64.91 Injury of unspecified nerve at wrist and hand level of right arm
  X+7th S64.92 Injury of unspecified nerve at wrist and hand level of left arm

S65 Injury of blood vessels at wrist and hand level
Code also any associated open wound (S61.-)

> The appropriate 7th character is to be added to each code from category S65
> A initial encounter
> D subsequent encounter
> S sequela

+ S65.0 Injury of ulnar artery at wrist and hand level
  + S65.00 Unspecified injury of ulnar artery at wrist and hand level
    CC +7th S65.001 Unspecified injury of ulnar artery at wrist and hand level of right arm
    CC +7th S65.002 Unspecified injury of ulnar artery at wrist and hand level of left arm
    CC +7th S65.009 Unspecified injury of ulnar artery at wrist and hand level of unspecified arm
  + S65.01 Laceration of ulnar artery at wrist and hand level
    CC +7th S65.011 Laceration of ulnar artery at wrist and hand level of right arm
    CC +7th S65.012 Laceration of ulnar artery at wrist and hand level of left arm
    CC +7th S65.019 Laceration of ulnar artery at wrist and hand level of unspecified arm
  + S65.09 Other specified injury of ulnar artery at wrist and hand level
    CC +7th S65.091 Other specified injury of ulnar artery at wrist and hand level of right arm
    CC +7th S65.092 Other specified injury of ulnar artery at wrist and hand level of left arm
    CC +7th S65.099 Other specified injury of ulnar artery at wrist and hand level of unspecified arm

+ S65.1 Injury of radial artery at wrist and hand level
  + S65.10 Unspecified injury of radial artery at wrist and hand level
    CC +7th S65.101 Unspecified injury of radial artery at wrist and hand level of right arm
    CC +7th S65.102 Unspecified injury of radial artery at wrist and hand level of left arm
    CC +7th S65.109 Unspecified injury of radial artery at wrist and hand level of unspecified arm
  + S65.11 Laceration of radial artery at wrist and hand level
    CC +7th S65.111 Laceration of radial artery at wrist and hand level of right arm
    CC +7th S65.112 Laceration of radial artery at wrist and hand level of left arm
    CC +7th S65.119 Laceration of radial artery at wrist and hand level of unspecified arm
  + S65.19 Other specified injury of radial artery at wrist and hand level
    CC +7th S65.191 Other specified injury of radial artery at wrist and hand level of right arm
    CC +7th S65.192 Other specified injury of radial artery at wrist and hand level of left arm
    CC +7th S65.199 Other specified injury of radial artery at wrist and hand level of unspecified arm

+ S65.2 Injury of superficial palmar arch
  + S65.20 Unspecified injury of superficial palmar arch
    CC +7th S65.201 Unspecified injury of superficial palmar arch of right hand
    CC +7th S65.202 Unspecified injury of superficial palmar arch of left hand
    CC +7th S65.209 Unspecified injury of superficial palmar arch of unspecified hand
  + S65.21 Laceration of superficial palmar arch
    CC +7th S65.211 Laceration of superficial palmar arch of right hand
    CC +7th S65.212 Laceration of superficial palmar arch of left hand
    CC +7th S65.219 Laceration of superficial palmar arch of unspecified hand
  + S65.29 Other specified injury of superficial palmar arch
    CC +7th S65.291 Other specified injury of superficial palmar arch of right hand
    CC +7th S65.292 Other specified injury of superficial palmar arch of left hand
    CC +7th S65.299 Other specified injury of superficial palmar arch of unspecified hand

+ S65.3 Injury of deep palmar arch
  + S65.30 Unspecified injury of deep palmar arch
    CC +7th S65.301 Unspecified injury of deep palmar arch of right hand
    CC +7th S65.302 Unspecified injury of deep palmar arch of left hand
    CC +7th S65.309 Unspecified injury of deep palmar arch of unspecified hand
  + S65.31 Laceration of deep palmar arch
    CC +7th S65.311 Laceration of deep palmar arch of right hand
    CC +7th S65.312 Laceration of deep palmar arch of left hand
    CC +7th S65.319 Laceration of deep palmar arch of unspecified hand
  + S65.39 Other specified injury of deep palmar arch
    CC +7th S65.391 Other specified injury of deep palmar arch of right hand
    CC +7th S65.392 Other specified injury of deep palmar arch of left hand
    CC +7th S65.399 Other specified injury of deep palmar arch of unspecified hand

+ S65.4 Injury of blood vessel of thumb
  + S65.40 Unspecified injury of blood vessel of thumb
    CC +7th S65.401 Unspecified injury of blood vessel of right thumb
    CC +7th S65.402 Unspecified injury of blood vessel of left thumb
    CC +7th S65.409 Unspecified injury of blood vessel of unspecified thumb
  + S65.41 Laceration of blood vessel of thumb
    CC +7th S65.411 Laceration of blood vessel of right thumb
    CC +7th S65.412 Laceration of blood vessel of left thumb
    CC +7th S65.419 Laceration of blood vessel of unspecified thumb
  + S65.49 Other specified injury of blood vessel of thumb
    CC +7th S65.491 Other specified injury of blood vessel of right thumb
    CC +7th S65.492 Other specified injury of blood vessel of left thumb
    CC +7th S65.499 Other specified injury of blood vessel of unspecified thumb

+ S65.5 Injury of blood vessel of other and unspecified finger
  + S65.50 Unspecified injury of blood vessel of other and unspecified finger
    CC +7th S65.500 Unspecified injury of blood vessel of right index finger
    CC +7th S65.501 Unspecified injury of blood vessel of left index finger
    CC +7th S65.502 Unspecified injury of blood vessel of right middle finger
    CC +7th S65.503 Unspecified injury of blood vessel of left middle finger

- CC +7th **S65.504** Unspecified injury of blood vessel of right ring finger
- CC +7th **S65.505** Unspecified injury of blood vessel of left ring finger
- CC +7th **S65.506** Unspecified injury of blood vessel of right little finger
- CC +7th **S65.507** Unspecified injury of blood vessel of left little finger
- CC +7th **S65.508** Unspecified injury of blood vessel of other finger
  - Unspecified injury of blood vessel of specified finger with unspecified laterality
- CC +7th **S65.509** Unspecified injury of blood vessel of unspecified finger
- + **S65.51** Laceration of blood vessel of other and unspecified finger
  - CC +7th **S65.510** Laceration of blood vessel of right index finger
  - CC +7th **S65.511** Laceration of blood vessel of left index finger
  - CC +7th **S65.512** Laceration of blood vessel of right middle finger
  - CC +7th **S65.513** Laceration of blood vessel of left middle finger
  - CC +7th **S65.514** Laceration of blood vessel of right ring finger
  - CC +7th **S65.515** Laceration of blood vessel of left ring finger
  - CC +7th **S65.516** Laceration of blood vessel of right little finger
  - CC +7th **S65.517** Laceration of blood vessel of left little finger
  - CC +7th **S65.518** Laceration of blood vessel of other finger
    - Laceration of blood vessel of specified finger with unspecified laterality
  - CC +7th **S65.519** Laceration of blood vessel of unspecified finger
- + **S65.59** Other specified injury of blood vessel of other and unspecified finger
  - CC +7th **S65.590** Other specified injury of blood vessel of right index finger
  - CC +7th **S65.591** Other specified injury of blood vessel of left index finger
  - CC +7th **S65.592** Other specified injury of blood vessel of right middle finger
  - CC +7th **S65.593** Other specified injury of blood vessel of left middle finger
  - CC +7th **S65.594** Other specified injury of blood vessel of right ring finger
  - CC +7th **S65.595** Other specified injury of blood vessel of left ring finger
  - CC +7th **S65.596** Other specified injury of blood vessel of right little finger
  - CC +7th **S65.597** Other specified injury of blood vessel of left little finger
  - CC +7th **S65.598** Other specified injury of blood vessel of other finger
    - Other specified injury of blood vessel of specified finger with unspecified laterality
  - CC +7th **S65.599** Other specified injury of blood vessel of unspecified finger
- + **S65.8** Injury of other blood vessels at wrist and hand level
  - + **S65.80** Unspecified injury of other blood vessels at wrist and hand level
    - CC +7th **S65.801** Unspecified injury of other blood vessels at wrist and hand level of right arm
    - CC +7th **S65.802** Unspecified injury of other blood vessels at wrist and hand level of left arm
    - CC +7th **S65.809** Unspecified injury of other blood vessels at wrist and hand level of unspecified arm
  - + **S65.81** Laceration of other blood vessels at wrist and hand level
    - CC +7th **S65.811** Laceration of other blood vessels at wrist and hand level of right arm
    - CC +7th **S65.812** Laceration of other blood vessels at wrist and hand level of left arm
    - CC +7th **S65.819** Laceration of other blood vessels at wrist and hand level of unspecified arm
  - + **S65.89** Other specified injury of other blood vessels at wrist and hand level
    - CC +7th **S65.891** Other specified injury of other blood vessels at wrist and hand level of right arm
    - CC +7th **S65.892** Other specified injury of other blood vessels at wrist and hand level of left arm
    - CC +7th **S65.899** Other specified injury of other blood vessels at wrist and hand level of unspecified arm
- + **S65.9** Injury of unspecified blood vessel at wrist and hand level
  - + **S65.90** Unspecified injury of unspecified blood vessel at wrist and hand level
    - CC +7th **S65.901** Unspecified injury of unspecified blood vessel at wrist and hand level of right arm
    - CC +7th **S65.902** Unspecified injury of unspecified blood vessel at wrist and hand level of left arm
    - CC +7th **S65.909** Unspecified injury of unspecified blood vessel at wrist and hand level of unspecified arm
  - + **S65.91** Laceration of unspecified blood vessel at wrist and hand level
    - CC +7th **S65.911** Laceration of unspecified blood vessel at wrist and hand level of right arm
    - CC +7th **S65.912** Laceration of unspecified blood vessel at wrist and hand level of left arm
    - CC +7th **S65.919** Laceration of unspecified blood vessel at wrist and hand level of unspecified arm
  - + **S65.99** Other specified injury of unspecified blood vessel at wrist and hand level
    - CC +7th **S65.991** Other specified injury of unspecified blood vessel at wrist and hand of right arm
    - CC +7th **S65.992** Other specified injury of unspecified blood vessel at wrist and hand of left arm
    - CC +7th **S65.999** Other specified injury of unspecified blood vessel at wrist and hand of unspecified arm

S66 Injury of muscle, fascia and tendon at wrist and hand level

Code also any associated open wound (S61.-)

Excludes2: sprain of joints and ligaments of wrist and hand (S63.-)

The appropriate 7th character is to be added to each code from category S66
- A initial encounter
- D subsequent encounter
- S sequela

- + **S66.0** Injury of long flexor muscle, fascia and tendon of thumb at wrist and hand level
  - + **S66.00** Unspecified injury of long flexor muscle, fascia and tendon of thumb at wrist and hand level
    - +7th **S66.001** Unspecified injury of long flexor muscle, fascia and tendon of right thumb at wrist and hand level
    - +7th **S66.002** Unspecified injury of long flexor muscle, fascia and tendon of left thumb at wrist and hand level
    - +7th **S66.009** Unspecified injury of long flexor muscle, fascia and tendon of unspecified thumb at wrist and hand level
  - + **S66.01** Strain of long flexor muscle, fascia and tendon of thumb at wrist and hand level
    - +7th **S66.011** Strain of long flexor muscle, fascia and tendon of right thumb at wrist and hand level
    - +7th **S66.012** Strain of long flexor muscle, fascia and tendon of left thumb at wrist and hand level
    - +7th **S66.019** Strain of long flexor muscle, fascia and tendon of unspecified thumb at wrist and hand level

- **+ S66.02** Laceration of long flexor muscle, fascia and tendon of thumb at wrist and hand level
  - CC +7th **S66.021** Laceration of long flexor muscle, fascia and tendon of right thumb at wrist and hand level
  - CC +7th **S66.022** Laceration of long flexor muscle, fascia and tendon of left thumb at wrist and hand level
  - CC +7th **S66.029** Laceration of long flexor muscle, fascia and tendon of unspecified thumb at wrist and hand level
- **+ S66.09** Other specified injury of long flexor muscle, fascia and tendon of thumb at wrist and hand level
  - +7th **S66.091** Other specified injury of long flexor muscle, fascia and tendon of right thumb at wrist and hand level
  - +7th **S66.092** Other specified injury of long flexor muscle, fascia and tendon of left thumb at wrist and hand level
  - +7th **S66.099** Other specified injury of long flexor muscle, fascia and tendon of unspecified thumb at wrist and hand level
- **+ S66.1** Injury of flexor muscle, fascia and tendon of other and unspecified finger at wrist and hand level
  - *Excludes2:* Injury of long flexor muscle, fascia and tendon of thumb at wrist and hand level (S66.0-)
  - **+ S66.10** Unspecified injury of flexor muscle, fascia and tendon of other and unspecified finger at wrist and hand level
    - +7th **S66.100** Unspecified injury of flexor muscle, fascia and tendon of right index finger at wrist and hand level
    - +7th **S66.101** Unspecified injury of flexor muscle, fascia and tendon of left index finger at wrist and hand level
    - +7th **S66.102** Unspecified injury of flexor muscle, fascia and tendon of right middle finger at wrist and hand level
    - +7th **S66.103** Unspecified injury of flexor muscle, fascia and tendon of left middle finger at wrist and hand level
    - +7th **S66.104** Unspecified injury of flexor muscle, fascia and tendon of right ring finger at wrist and hand level
    - +7th **S66.105** Unspecified injury of flexor muscle, fascia and tendon of left ring finger at wrist and hand level
    - +7th **S66.106** Unspecified injury of flexor muscle, fascia and tendon of right little finger at wrist and hand level
    - +7th **S66.107** Unspecified injury of flexor muscle, fascia and tendon of left little finger at wrist and hand level
    - +7th **S66.108** Unspecified injury of flexor muscle, fascia and tendon of other finger at wrist and hand level
      Unspecified injury of flexor muscle, fascia and tendon of specified finger with unspecified laterality at wrist and hand level
    - +7th **S66.109** Unspecified injury of flexor muscle, fascia and tendon of unspecified finger at wrist and hand level
  - **+ S66.11** Strain of flexor muscle, fascia and tendon of other and unspecified finger at wrist and hand level
    - +7th **S66.110** Strain of flexor muscle, fascia and tendon of right index finger at wrist and hand level
    - +7th **S66.111** Strain of flexor muscle, fascia and tendon of left index finger at wrist and hand level
    - +7th **S66.112** Strain of flexor muscle, fascia and tendon of right middle finger at wrist and hand level
    - +7th **S66.113** Strain of flexor muscle, fascia and tendon of left middle finger at wrist and hand level
    - +7th **S66.114** Strain of flexor muscle, fascia and tendon of right ring finger at wrist and hand level
    - +7th **S66.115** Strain of flexor muscle, fascia and tendon of left ring finger at wrist and hand level
    - +7th **S66.116** Strain of flexor muscle, fascia and tendon of right little finger at wrist and hand level
    - +7th **S66.117** Strain of flexor muscle, fascia and tendon of left little finger at wrist and hand level
    - +7th **S66.118** Strain of flexor muscle, fascia and tendon of other finger at wrist and hand level
      Strain of flexor muscle, fascia and tendon of specified finger with unspecified laterality at wrist and hand level
    - +7th **S66.119** Strain of flexor muscle, fascia and tendon of unspecified finger at wrist and hand level
  - **+ S66.12** Laceration of flexor muscle, fascia and tendon of other and unspecified finger at wrist and hand level
    - CC +7th **S66.120** Laceration of flexor muscle, fascia and tendon of right index finger at wrist and hand level
    - CC +7th **S66.121** Laceration of flexor muscle, fascia and tendon of left index finger at wrist and hand level
    - CC +7th **S66.122** Laceration of flexor muscle, fascia and tendon of right middle finger at wrist and hand level
    - CC +7th **S66.123** Laceration of flexor muscle, fascia and tendon of left middle finger at wrist and hand level
    - CC +7th **S66.124** Laceration of flexor muscle, fascia and tendon of right ring finger at wrist and hand level
    - CC +7th **S66.125** Laceration of flexor muscle, fascia and tendon of left ring finger at wrist and hand level
    - CC +7th **S66.126** Laceration of flexor muscle, fascia and tendon of right little finger at wrist and hand level
    - CC +7th **S66.127** Laceration of flexor muscle, fascia and tendon of left little finger at wrist and hand level
    - CC +7th **S66.128** Laceration of flexor muscle, fascia and tendon of other finger at wrist and hand level
      Laceration of flexor muscle, fascia and tendon of specified finger with unspecified laterality at wrist and hand level
    - CC +7th **S66.129** Laceration of flexor muscle, fascia and tendon of unspecified finger at wrist and hand level
  - **+ S66.19** Other injury of flexor muscle, fascia and tendon of other and unspecified finger at wrist and hand level
    - +7th **S66.190** Other injury of flexor muscle, fascia and tendon of right index finger at wrist and hand level
    - +7th **S66.191** Other injury of flexor muscle, fascia and tendon of left index finger at wrist and hand level
    - +7th **S66.192** Other injury of flexor muscle, fascia and tendon of right middle finger at wrist and hand level
    - +7th **S66.193** Other injury of flexor muscle, fascia and tendon of left middle finger at wrist and hand level
    - +7th **S66.194** Other injury of flexor muscle, fascia and tendon of right ring finger at wrist and hand level
    - +7th **S66.195** Other injury of flexor muscle, fascia and tendon of left ring finger at wrist and hand level
    - +7th **S66.196** Other injury of flexor muscle, fascia and tendon of right little finger at wrist and hand level
    - +7th **S66.197** Other injury of flexor muscle, fascia and tendon of left little finger at wrist and hand level

- +7th **S66.198** Other injury of flexor muscle, fascia and tendon of other finger at wrist and hand level
  - Other injury of flexor muscle, fascia and tendon of specified finger with unspecified laterality at wrist and hand level
- +7th **S66.199** Other injury of flexor muscle, fascia and tendon of unspecified finger at wrist and hand level

+ **S66.2** Injury of extensor muscle, fascia and tendon of thumb at wrist and hand level
  + **S66.20** Unspecified injury of extensor muscle, fascia and tendon of thumb at wrist and hand level
    - +7th **S66.201** Unspecified injury of extensor muscle, fascia and tendon of right thumb at wrist and hand level
    - +7th **S66.202** Unspecified injury of extensor muscle, fascia and tendon of left thumb at wrist and hand level
    - +7th **S66.209** Unspecified injury of extensor muscle, fascia and tendon of unspecified thumb at wrist and hand level
  + **S66.21** Strain of extensor muscle, fascia and tendon of thumb at wrist and hand level
    - +7th **S66.211** Strain of extensor muscle, fascia and tendon of right thumb at wrist and hand level
    - +7th **S66.212** Strain of extensor muscle, fascia and tendon of left thumb at wrist and hand level
    - +7th **S66.219** Strain of extensor muscle, fascia and tendon of unspecified thumb at wrist and hand level
  + **S66.22** Laceration of extensor muscle, fascia and tendon of thumb at wrist and hand level
    - CC +7th **S66.221** Laceration of extensor muscle, fascia and tendon of right thumb at wrist and hand level
    - CC +7th **S66.222** Laceration of extensor muscle, fascia and tendon of left thumb at wrist and hand level
    - CC +7th **S66.229** Laceration of extensor muscle, fascia and tendon of unspecified thumb at wrist and hand level
  + **S66.29** Other specified injury of extensor muscle, fascia and tendon of thumb at wrist and hand level
    - +7th **S66.291** Other specified injury of extensor muscle, fascia and tendon of right thumb at wrist and hand level
    - +7th **S66.292** Other specified injury of extensor muscle, fascia and tendon of left thumb at wrist and hand level
    - +7th **S66.299** Other specified injury of extensor muscle, fascia and tendon of unspecified thumb at wrist and hand level

+ **S66.3** Injury of extensor muscle, fascia and tendon of other and unspecified finger at wrist and hand level
  Excludes2: *Injury of extensor muscle, fascia and tendon of thumb at wrist and hand level (S66.2-)*
  + **S66.30** Unspecified injury of extensor muscle, fascia and tendon of other and unspecified finger at wrist and hand level
    - +7th **S66.300** Unspecified injury of extensor muscle, fascia and tendon of right index finger at wrist and hand level
    - +7th **S66.301** Unspecified injury of extensor muscle, fascia and tendon of left index finger at wrist and hand level
    - +7th **S66.302** Unspecified injury of extensor muscle, fascia and tendon of right middle finger at wrist and hand level
    - +7th **S66.303** Unspecified injury of extensor muscle, fascia and tendon of left middle finger at wrist and hand level
    - +7th **S66.304** Unspecified injury of extensor muscle, fascia and tendon of right ring finger at wrist and hand level
    - +7th **S66.305** Unspecified injury of extensor muscle, fascia and tendon of left ring finger at wrist and hand level
    - +7th **S66.306** Unspecified injury of extensor muscle, fascia and tendon of right little finger at wrist and hand level
    - +7th **S66.307** Unspecified injury of extensor muscle, fascia and tendon of left little finger at wrist and hand level
    - +7th **S66.308** Unspecified injury of extensor muscle, fascia and tendon of other finger at wrist and hand level
      - Unspecified injury of extensor muscle, fascia and tendon of specified finger with unspecified laterality at wrist and hand level
    - +7th **S66.309** Unspecified injury of extensor muscle, fascia and tendon of unspecified finger at wrist and hand level
  + **S66.31** Strain of extensor muscle, fascia and tendon of other and unspecified finger at wrist and hand level
    - +7th **S66.310** Strain of extensor muscle, fascia and tendon of right index finger at wrist and hand level
    - +7th **S66.311** Strain of extensor muscle, fascia and tendon of left index finger at wrist and hand level
    - +7th **S66.312** Strain of extensor muscle, fascia and tendon of right middle finger at wrist and hand level
    - +7th **S66.313** Strain of extensor muscle, fascia and tendon of left middle finger at wrist and hand level
    - +7th **S66.314** Strain of extensor muscle, fascia and tendon of right ring finger at wrist and hand level
    - +7th **S66.315** Strain of extensor muscle, fascia and tendon of left ring finger at wrist and hand level
    - +7th **S66.316** Strain of extensor muscle, fascia and tendon of right little finger at wrist and hand level
    - +7th **S66.317** Strain of extensor muscle, fascia and tendon of left little finger at wrist and hand level
    - +7th **S66.318** Strain of extensor muscle, fascia and tendon of other finger at wrist and hand level
      - Strain of extensor muscle, fascia and tendon of specified finger with unspecified laterality at wrist and hand level
    - +7th **S66.319** Strain of extensor muscle, fascia and tendon of unspecified finger at wrist and hand level
  + **S66.32** Laceration of extensor muscle, fascia and tendon of other and unspecified finger at wrist and hand level
    - CC +7th **S66.320** Laceration of extensor muscle, fascia and tendon of right index finger at wrist and hand level
    - CC +7th **S66.321** Laceration of extensor muscle, fascia and tendon of left index finger at wrist and hand level
    - CC +7th **S66.322** Laceration of extensor muscle, fascia and tendon of right middle finger at wrist and hand level
    - CC +7th **S66.323** Laceration of extensor muscle, fascia and tendon of left middle finger at wrist and hand level
    - CC +7th **S66.324** Laceration of extensor muscle, fascia and tendon of right ring finger at wrist and hand level
    - CC +7th **S66.325** Laceration of extensor muscle, fascia and tendon of left ring finger at wrist and hand level
    - CC +7th **S66.326** Laceration of extensor muscle, fascia and tendon of right little finger at wrist and hand level
    - CC +7th **S66.327** Laceration of extensor muscle, fascia and tendon of left little finger at wrist and hand level

CC +7th	S66.328	Laceration of extensor muscle, fascia and tendon of other finger at wrist and hand level
		Laceration of extensor muscle, fascia and tendon of specified finger with unspecified laterality at wrist and hand level
CC +7th	S66.329	Laceration of extensor muscle, fascia and tendon of unspecified finger at wrist and hand level

+ **S66.39** Other injury of extensor muscle, fascia and tendon of other and unspecified finger at wrist and hand level
- +7th **S66.390** Other injury of extensor muscle, fascia and tendon of right index finger at wrist and hand level
- +7th **S66.391** Other injury of extensor muscle, fascia and tendon of left index finger at wrist and hand level
- +7th **S66.392** Other injury of extensor muscle, fascia and tendon of right middle finger at wrist and hand level
- +7th **S66.393** Other injury of extensor muscle, fascia and tendon of left middle finger at wrist and hand level
- +7th **S66.394** Other injury of extensor muscle, fascia and tendon of right ring finger at wrist and hand level
- +7th **S66.395** Other injury of extensor muscle, fascia and tendon of left ring finger at wrist and hand level
- +7th **S66.396** Other injury of extensor muscle, fascia and tendon of right little finger at wrist and hand level
- +7th **S66.397** Other injury of extensor muscle, fascia and tendon of left little finger at wrist and hand level
- +7th **S66.398** Other injury of extensor muscle, fascia and tendon of other finger at wrist and hand level
  - Other injury of extensor muscle, fascia and tendon of specified finger with unspecified laterality at wrist and hand level
- +7th **S66.399** Other injury of extensor muscle, fascia and tendon of unspecified finger at wrist and hand level

+ **S66.4** Injury of intrinsic muscle, fascia and tendon of thumb at wrist and hand level
+ **S66.40** Unspecified injury of intrinsic muscle, fascia and tendon of thumb at wrist and hand level
- +7th **S66.401** Unspecified injury of intrinsic muscle, fascia and tendon of right thumb at wrist and hand level
- +7th **S66.402** Unspecified injury of intrinsic muscle, fascia and tendon of left thumb at wrist and hand level
- +7th **S66.409** Unspecified injury of intrinsic muscle, fascia and tendon of unspecified thumb at wrist and hand level

+ **S66.41** Strain of intrinsic muscle, fascia and tendon of thumb at wrist and hand level
- +7th **S66.411** Strain of intrinsic muscle, fascia and tendon of right thumb at wrist and hand level
- +7th **S66.412** Strain of intrinsic muscle, fascia and tendon of left thumb at wrist and hand level
- +7th **S66.419** Strain of intrinsic muscle, fascia and tendon of unspecified thumb at wrist and hand level

+ **S66.42** Laceration of intrinsic muscle, fascia and tendon of thumb at wrist and hand level
- CC +7th **S66.421** Laceration of intrinsic muscle, fascia and tendon of right thumb at wrist and hand level
- CC +7th **S66.422** Laceration of intrinsic muscle, fascia and tendon of left thumb at wrist and hand level
- CC +7th **S66.429** Laceration of intrinsic muscle, fascia and tendon of unspecified thumb at wrist and hand level

+ **S66.49** Other specified injury of intrinsic muscle, fascia and tendon of thumb at wrist and hand level
- +7th **S66.491** Other specified injury of intrinsic muscle, fascia and tendon of right thumb at wrist and hand level
- +7th **S66.492** Other specified injury of intrinsic muscle, fascia and tendon of left thumb at wrist and hand level
- +7th **S66.499** Other specified injury of intrinsic muscle, fascia and tendon of unspecified thumb at wrist and hand level

+ **S66.5** Injury of intrinsic muscle, fascia and tendon of other and unspecified finger at wrist and hand level

Excludes2: *injury of intrinsic muscle, fascia and tendon of thumb at wrist and hand level (S66.4-)*

+ **S66.50** Unspecified injury of intrinsic muscle, fascia and tendon of other and unspecified finger at wrist and hand level
- +7th **S66.500** Unspecified injury of intrinsic muscle, fascia and tendon of right index finger at wrist and hand level
- +7th **S66.501** Unspecified injury of intrinsic muscle, fascia and tendon of left index finger at wrist and hand level
- +7th **S66.502** Unspecified injury of intrinsic muscle, fascia and tendon of right middle finger at wrist and hand level
- +7th **S66.503** Unspecified injury of intrinsic muscle, fascia and tendon of left middle finger at wrist and hand level
- +7th **S66.504** Unspecified injury of intrinsic muscle, fascia and tendon of right ring finger at wrist and hand level
- +7th **S66.505** Unspecified injury of intrinsic muscle, fascia and tendon of left ring finger at wrist and hand level
- +7th **S66.506** Unspecified injury of intrinsic muscle, fascia and tendon of right little finger at wrist and hand level
- +7th **S66.507** Unspecified injury of intrinsic muscle, fascia and tendon of left little finger at wrist and hand level
- +7th **S66.508** Unspecified injury of intrinsic muscle, fascia and tendon of other finger at wrist and hand level
  - Unspecified injury of intrinsic muscle, fascia and tendon of specified finger with unspecified laterality at wrist and hand level
- +7th **S66.509** Unspecified injury of intrinsic muscle, fascia and tendon of unspecified finger at wrist and hand level

+ **S66.51** Strain of intrinsic muscle, fascia and tendon of other and unspecified finger at wrist and hand level
- +7th **S66.510** Strain of intrinsic muscle, fascia and tendon of right index finger at wrist and hand level
- +7th **S66.511** Strain of intrinsic muscle, fascia and tendon of left index finger at wrist and hand level
- +7th **S66.512** Strain of intrinsic muscle, fascia and tendon of right middle finger at wrist and hand level
- +7th **S66.513** Strain of intrinsic muscle, fascia and tendon of left middle finger at wrist and hand level
- +7th **S66.514** Strain of intrinsic muscle, fascia and tendon of right ring finger at wrist and hand level
- +7th **S66.515** Strain of intrinsic muscle, fascia and tendon of left ring finger at wrist and hand level
- +7th **S66.516** Strain of intrinsic muscle, fascia and tendon of right little finger at wrist and hand level
- +7th **S66.517** Strain of intrinsic muscle, fascia and tendon of left little finger at wrist and hand level

- +7th **S66.518** Strain of intrinsic muscle, fascia and tendon of other finger at wrist and hand level
  - Strain of intrinsic muscle, fascia and tendon of specified finger with unspecified laterality at wrist and hand level
- +7th **S66.519** Strain of intrinsic muscle, fascia and tendon of unspecified finger at wrist and hand level
- + **S66.52** Laceration of intrinsic muscle, fascia and tendon of other and unspecified finger at wrist and hand level
  - CC +7th **S66.520** Laceration of intrinsic muscle, fascia and tendon of right index finger at wrist and hand level
  - CC +7th **S66.521** Laceration of intrinsic muscle, fascia and tendon of left index finger at wrist and hand level
  - CC +7th **S66.522** Laceration of intrinsic muscle, fascia and tendon of right middle finger at wrist and hand level
  - CC +7th **S66.523** Laceration of intrinsic muscle, fascia and tendon of left middle finger at wrist and hand level
  - CC +7th **S66.524** Laceration of intrinsic muscle, fascia and tendon of right ring finger at wrist and hand level
  - CC +7th **S66.525** Laceration of intrinsic muscle, fascia and tendon of left ring finger at wrist and hand level
  - CC +7th **S66.526** Laceration of intrinsic muscle, fascia and tendon of right little finger at wrist and hand level
  - CC +7th **S66.527** Laceration of intrinsic muscle, fascia and tendon of left little finger at wrist and hand level
  - CC +7th **S66.528** Laceration of intrinsic muscle, fascia and tendon of other finger at wrist and hand level
    - Laceration of intrinsic muscle, fascia and tendon of specified finger with unspecified laterality at wrist and hand level
  - CC +7th **S66.529** Laceration of intrinsic muscle, fascia and tendon of unspecified finger at wrist and hand level
- + **S66.59** Other injury of intrinsic muscle, fascia and tendon of other and unspecified finger at wrist and hand level
  - +7th **S66.590** Other injury of intrinsic muscle, fascia and tendon of right index finger at wrist and hand level
  - +7th **S66.591** Other injury of intrinsic muscle, fascia and tendon of left index finger at wrist and hand level
  - +7th **S66.592** Other injury of intrinsic muscle, fascia and tendon of right middle finger at wrist and hand level
  - +7th **S66.593** Other injury of intrinsic muscle, fascia and tendon of left middle finger at wrist and hand level
  - +7th **S66.594** Other injury of intrinsic muscle, fascia and tendon of right ring finger at wrist and hand level
  - +7th **S66.595** Other injury of intrinsic muscle, fascia and tendon of left ring finger at wrist and hand level
  - +7th **S66.596** Other injury of intrinsic muscle, fascia and tendon of right little finger at wrist and hand level
  - +7th **S66.597** Other injury of intrinsic muscle, fascia and tendon of left little finger at wrist and hand level
  - +7th **S66.598** Other injury of intrinsic muscle, fascia and tendon of other finger at wrist and hand level
    - Other injury of intrinsic muscle, fascia and tendon of specified finger with unspecified laterality at wrist and hand level
  - +7th **S66.599** Other injury of intrinsic muscle, fascia and tendon of unspecified finger at wrist and hand level

- + **S66.8** Injury of other specified muscles, fascia and tendons at wrist and hand level
  - + **S66.80** Unspecified injury of other specified muscles, fascia and tendons at wrist and hand level
    - +7th **S66.801** Unspecified injury of other specified muscles, fascia and tendons at wrist and hand level, right hand
    - +7th **S66.802** Unspecified injury of other specified muscles, fascia and tendons at wrist and hand level, left hand
    - +7th **S66.809** Unspecified injury of other specified muscles, fascia and tendons at wrist and hand level, unspecified hand
  - + **S66.81** Strain of other specified muscles, fascia and tendons at wrist and hand level
    - +7th **S66.811** Strain of other specified muscles, fascia and tendons at wrist and hand level, right hand
    - +7th **S66.812** Strain of other specified muscles, fascia and tendons at wrist and hand level, left hand
    - +7th **S66.819** Strain of other specified muscles, fascia and tendons at wrist and hand level, unspecified hand
  - + **S66.82** Laceration of other specified muscles, fascia and tendons at wrist and hand level
    - CC +7th **S66.821** Laceration of other specified muscles, fascia and tendons at wrist and hand level, right hand
    - CC +7th **S66.822** Laceration of other specified muscles, fascia and tendons at wrist and hand level, left hand
    - CC +7th **S66.829** Laceration of other specified muscles, fascia and tendons at wrist and hand level, unspecified hand
  - + **S66.89** Other injury of other specified muscles, fascia and tendons at wrist and hand level
    - +7th **S66.891** Other injury of other specified muscles, fascia and tendons at wrist and hand level, right hand
    - +7th **S66.892** Other injury of other specified muscles, fascia and tendons at wrist and hand level, left hand
    - +7th **S66.899** Other injury of other specified muscles, fascia and tendons at wrist and hand level, unspecified hand
- + **S66.9** Injury of unspecified muscle, fascia and tendon at wrist and hand level
  - + **S66.90** Unspecified injury of unspecified muscle, fascia and tendon at wrist and hand level
    - +7th **S66.901** Unspecified injury of unspecified muscle, fascia and tendon at wrist and hand level, right hand
    - +7th **S66.902** Unspecified injury of unspecified muscle, fascia and tendon at wrist and hand level, left hand
    - +7th **S66.909** Unspecified injury of unspecified muscle, fascia and tendon at wrist and hand level, unspecified hand
  - + **S66.91** Strain of unspecified muscle, fascia and tendon at wrist and hand level
    - +7th **S66.911** Strain of unspecified muscle, fascia and tendon at wrist and hand level, right hand
    - +7th **S66.912** Strain of unspecified muscle, fascia and tendon at wrist and hand level, left hand
    - +7th **S66.919** Strain of unspecified muscle, fascia and tendon at wrist and hand level, unspecified hand
  - + **S66.92** Laceration of unspecified muscle, fascia and tendon at wrist and hand level
    - CC +7th **S66.921** Laceration of unspecified muscle, fascia and tendon at wrist and hand level, right hand
    - CC +7th **S66.922** Laceration of unspecified muscle, fascia and tendon at wrist and hand level, left hand
    - CC +7th **S66.929** Laceration of unspecified muscle, fascia and tendon at wrist and hand level, unspecified hand

S66.99 Other injury of unspecified muscle, fascia and tendon at wrist and hand level
- +7th **S66.991** Other injury of unspecified muscle, fascia and tendon at wrist and hand level, right hand
- +7th **S66.992** Other injury of unspecified muscle, fascia and tendon at wrist and hand level, left hand
- +7th **S66.999** Other injury of unspecified muscle, fascia and tendon at wrist and hand level, unspecified hand

S67 Crushing injury of wrist, hand and fingers

Use additional code for all associated injuries, such as:
fracture of wrist and hand (S62.-)
open wound of wrist and hand (S61.-)

The appropriate 7th character is to be added to each code from category S67
- A initial encounter
- D subsequent encounter
- S sequela

+ **S67.0** Crushing injury of thumb
- X+7th **S67.00** Crushing injury of unspecified thumb
- X+7th **S67.01** Crushing injury of right thumb
- X+7th **S67.02** Crushing injury of left thumb

+ **S67.1** Crushing injury of other and unspecified finger(s)
  Excludes2: crushing injury of thumb (S67.0-)
- X+7th **S67.10** Crushing injury of unspecified finger(s)
- + **S67.19** Crushing injury of other finger(s)
  - +7th **S67.190** Crushing injury of right index finger
  - +7th **S67.191** Crushing injury of left index finger
  - +7th **S67.192** Crushing injury of right middle finger
  - +7th **S67.193** Crushing injury of left middle finger
  - +7th **S67.194** Crushing injury of right ring finger
  - +7th **S67.195** Crushing injury of left ring finger
  - +7th **S67.196** Crushing injury of right little finger
  - +7th **S67.197** Crushing injury of left little finger
  - +7th **S67.198** Crushing injury of other finger
    Crushing injury of specified finger with unspecified laterality

+ **S67.2** Crushing injury of hand
  Excludes2: crushing injury of fingers (S67.1-)
  crushing injury of thumb (S67.0-)
- X+7th **S67.20** Crushing injury of unspecified hand
- X+7th **S67.21** Crushing injury of right hand
- X+7th **S67.22** Crushing injury of left hand

+ **S67.3** Crushing injury of wrist
- X+7th **S67.30** Crushing injury of unspecified wrist
- X+7th **S67.31** Crushing injury of right wrist
- X+7th **S67.32** Crushing injury of left wrist

+ **S67.4** Crushing injury of wrist and hand
  Excludes1: crushing injury of hand alone (S67.2-)
  crushing injury of wrist alone (S67.3-)
  Excludes2: crushing injury of fingers (S67.1-)
  crushing injury of thumb (S67.0-)
- X+7th **S67.40** Crushing injury of unspecified wrist and hand
- X+7th **S67.41** Crushing injury of right wrist and hand
- X+7th **S67.42** Crushing injury of left wrist and hand

+ **S67.9** Crushing injury of unspecified part(s) of wrist, hand and fingers
- X+7th **S67.90** Crushing injury of unspecified part(s) of unspecified wrist, hand and fingers
- X+7th **S67.91** Crushing injury of unspecified part(s) of right wrist, hand and fingers
- X+7th **S67.92** Crushing injury of unspecified part(s) of left wrist, hand and fingers

S68 Traumatic amputation of wrist, hand and fingers

An amputation not identified as partial or complete should be coded to complete

The appropriate 7th character is to be added to each code from category S68
- A initial encounter
- D subsequent encounter
- S sequela

+ **S68.0** Traumatic metacarpophalangeal amputation of thumb
  Traumatic amputation of thumb NOS
  + **S68.01** Complete traumatic metacarpophalangeal amputation of thumb
  - +7th **S68.011** Complete traumatic metacarpophalangeal amputation of right thumb
  - +7th **S68.012** Complete traumatic metacarpophalangeal amputation of left thumb
  - +7th **S68.019** Complete traumatic metacarpophalangeal amputation of unspecified thumb
  + **S68.02** Partial traumatic metacarpophalangeal amputation of thumb
  - +7th **S68.021** Partial traumatic metacarpophalangeal amputation of right thumb
  - +7th **S68.022** Partial traumatic metacarpophalangeal amputation of left thumb
  - +7th **S68.029** Partial traumatic metacarpophalangeal amputation of unspecified thumb

+ **S68.1** Traumatic metacarpophalangeal amputation of other and unspecified finger
  Traumatic amputation of finger NOS
  Excludes2: traumatic metacarpophalangeal amputation of thumb (S68.0-)
  + **S68.11** Complete traumatic metacarpophalangeal amputation of other and unspecified finger
  - +7th **S68.110** Complete traumatic metacarpophalangeal amputation of right index finger
  - +7th **S68.111** Complete traumatic metacarpophalangeal amputation of left index finger
  - +7th **S68.112** Complete traumatic metacarpophalangeal amputation of right middle finger
  - +7th **S68.113** Complete traumatic metacarpophalangeal amputation of left middle finger
  - +7th **S68.114** Complete traumatic metacarpophalangeal amputation of right ring finger
  - +7th **S68.115** Complete traumatic metacarpophalangeal amputation of left ring finger
  - +7th **S68.116** Complete traumatic metacarpophalangeal amputation of right little finger
  - +7th **S68.117** Complete traumatic metacarpophalangeal amputation of left little finger
  - +7th **S68.118** Complete traumatic metacarpophalangeal amputation of other finger
    Complete traumatic metacarpophalangeal amputation of specified finger with unspecified laterality
  - +7th **S68.119** Complete traumatic metacarpophalangeal amputation of unspecified finger
  + **S68.12** Partial traumatic metacarpophalangeal amputation of other and unspecified finger
  - +7th **S68.120** Partial traumatic metacarpophalangeal amputation of right index finger
  - +7th **S68.121** Partial traumatic metacarpophalangeal amputation of left index finger
  - +7th **S68.122** Partial traumatic metacarpophalangeal amputation of right middle finger
  - +7th **S68.123** Partial traumatic metacarpophalangeal amputation of left middle finger

- **+7th S68.124** Partial traumatic metacarpophalangeal amputation of right ring finger
- **+7th S68.125** Partial traumatic metacarpophalangeal amputation of left ring finger
- **+7th S68.126** Partial traumatic metacarpophalangeal amputation of right little finger
- **+7th S68.127** Partial traumatic metacarpophalangeal amputation of left little finger
- **+7th S68.128** Partial traumatic metacarpophalangeal amputation of other finger
  - Partial traumatic metacarpophalangeal amputation of specified finger with unspecified laterality
- **+7th S68.129** Partial traumatic metacarpophalangeal amputation of unspecified finger
- **+ S68.4** Traumatic amputation of hand at wrist level
  - Traumatic amputation of hand NOS
  - Traumatic amputation of wrist
  - **+ S68.41** Complete traumatic amputation of hand at wrist level
    - **CC +7th S68.411** Complete traumatic amputation of right hand at wrist level
    - **CC +7th S68.412** Complete traumatic amputation of left hand at wrist level
    - **CC +7th S68.419** Complete traumatic amputation of unspecified hand at wrist level
  - **+ S68.42** Partial traumatic amputation of hand at wrist level
    - **CC +7th S68.421** Partial traumatic amputation of right hand at wrist level
    - **CC +7th S68.422** Partial traumatic amputation of left hand at wrist level
    - **CC +7th S68.429** Partial traumatic amputation of unspecified hand at wrist level
- **+ S68.5** Traumatic transphalangeal amputation of thumb
  - Traumatic interphalangeal joint amputation of thumb
  - **+ S68.51** Complete traumatic transphalangeal amputation of thumb
    - **+7th S68.511** Complete traumatic transphalangeal amputation of right thumb
    - **+7th S68.512** Complete traumatic transphalangeal amputation of left thumb
    - **+7th S68.519** Complete traumatic transphalangeal amputation of unspecified thumb
  - **+ S68.52** Partial traumatic transphalangeal amputation of thumb
    - **+7th S68.521** Partial traumatic transphalangeal amputation of right thumb
    - **+7th S68.522** Partial traumatic transphalangeal amputation of left thumb
    - **+7th S68.529** Partial traumatic transphalangeal amputation of unspecified thumb
- **+ S68.6** Traumatic transphalangeal amputation of other and unspecified finger
  - **+ S68.61** Complete traumatic transphalangeal amputation of other and unspecified finger(s)
    - **+7th S68.610** Complete traumatic transphalangeal amputation of right index finger
    - **+7th S68.611** Complete traumatic transphalangeal amputation of left index finger
    - **+7th S68.612** Complete traumatic transphalangeal amputation of right middle finger
    - **+7th S68.613** Complete traumatic transphalangeal amputation of left middle finger
    - **+7th S68.614** Complete traumatic transphalangeal amputation of right ring finger
    - **+7th S68.615** Complete traumatic transphalangeal amputation of left ring finger
    - **+7th S68.616** Complete traumatic transphalangeal amputation of right little finger
    - **+7th S68.617** Complete traumatic transphalangeal amputation of left little finger
    - **+7th S68.618** Complete traumatic transphalangeal amputation of other finger
      - Complete traumatic transphalangeal amputation of specified finger with unspecified laterality
    - **+7th S68.619** Complete traumatic transphalangeal amputation of unspecified finger

- **+ S68.62** Partial traumatic transphalangeal amputation of other and unspecified finger
  - **+7th S68.620** Partial traumatic transphalangeal amputation of right index finger
  - **+7th S68.621** Partial traumatic transphalangeal amputation of left index finger
  - **+7th S68.622** Partial traumatic transphalangeal amputation of right middle finger
  - **+7th S68.623** Partial traumatic transphalangeal amputation of left middle finger
  - **+7th S68.624** Partial traumatic transphalangeal amputation of right ring finger
  - **+7th S68.625** Partial traumatic transphalangeal amputation of left ring finger
  - **+7th S68.626** Partial traumatic transphalangeal amputation of right little finger
  - **+7th S68.627** Partial traumatic transphalangeal amputation of left little finger
  - **+7th S68.628** Partial traumatic transphalangeal amputation of other finger
    - Partial traumatic transphalangeal amputation of specified finger with unspecified laterality
  - **+7th S68.629** Partial traumatic transphalangeal amputation of unspecified finger
- **+ S68.7** Traumatic transmetacarpal amputation of hand
  - **+ S68.71** Complete traumatic transmetacarpal amputation of hand
    - **CC +7th S68.711** Complete traumatic transmetacarpal amputation of right hand
    - **CC +7th S68.712** Complete traumatic transmetacarpal amputation of left hand
    - **CC +7th S68.719** Complete traumatic transmetacarpal amputation of unspecified hand
  - **+ S68.72** Partial traumatic transmetacarpal amputation of hand
    - **CC +7th S68.721** Partial traumatic transmetacarpal amputation of right hand
    - **CC +7th S68.722** Partial traumatic transmetacarpal amputation of left hand
    - **CC +7th S68.729** Partial traumatic transmetacarpal amputation of unspecified hand

S69 Other and unspecified injuries of wrist, hand and finger(s)

> The appropriate 7th character is to be added to each code from category S69
> A initial encounter
> D subsequent encounter
> S sequela

- **+ S69.8** Other specified injuries of wrist, hand and finger(s)
  - **X+7th S69.80** Other specified injuries of unspecified wrist, hand and finger(s)
  - **X+7th S69.81** Other specified injuries of right wrist, hand and finger(s)
  - **X+7th S69.82** Other specified injuries of left wrist, hand and finger(s)
- **+ S69.9** Unspecified injury of wrist, hand and finger(s)
  - **X+7th S69.90** Unspecified injury of unspecified wrist, hand and finger(s)
  - **X+7th S69.91** Unspecified injury of right wrist, hand and finger(s)
  - **X+7th S69.92** Unspecified injury of left wrist, hand and finger(s)

Injuries to the hip and thigh (S70-S79)

Excludes2: *burns and corrosions (T20-T32)*
frostbite (T33-T34)
snake bite (T63.0-)
venomous insect bite or sting (T63.4-)

S70 Superficial injury of hip and thigh

> The appropriate 7th character is to be added to each code from category S70
> A initial encounter
> D subsequent encounter
> S sequela

- **+ S70.0** Contusion of hip
  - **X+7th S70.00** Contusion of unspecified hip
  - **X+7th S70.01** Contusion of right hip
  - **X+7th S70.02** Contusion of left hip

- **+ S70.1   Contusion of thigh**
  - X+7th S70.10   Contusion of unspecified thigh
  - X+7th S70.11   Contusion of right thigh
  - X+7th S70.12   Contusion of left thigh
- **+ S70.2   Other superficial injuries of hip**
  - + S70.21   Abrasion of hip
    - +7th S70.211   Abrasion, right hip
    - +7th S70.212   Abrasion, left hip
    - +7th S70.219   Abrasion, unspecified hip
  - + S70.22   Blister (nonthermal) of hip
    - +7th S70.221   Blister (nonthermal), right hip
    - +7th S70.222   Blister (nonthermal), left hip
    - +7th S70.229   Blister (nonthermal), unspecified hip
  - + S70.24   External constriction of hip
    - +7th S70.241   External constriction, right hip
    - +7th S70.242   External constriction, left hip
    - +7th S70.249   External constriction, unspecified hip
  - + S70.25   Superficial foreign body of hip
    - Splinter in the hip
    - +7th S70.251   Superficial foreign body, right hip
    - +7th S70.252   Superficial foreign body, left hip
    - +7th S70.259   Superficial foreign body, unspecified hip
  - + S70.26   Insect bite (nonvenomous) of hip
    - +7th S70.261   Insect bite (nonvenomous), right hip
    - +7th S70.262   Insect bite (nonvenomous), left hip
    - +7th S70.269   Insect bite (nonvenomous), unspecified hip
  - + S70.27   Other superficial bite of hip
    - **Excludes1:** *open bite of hip (S71.05-)*
    - +7th S70.271   Other superficial bite of hip, right hip
    - +7th S70.272   Other superficial bite of hip, left hip
    - +7th S70.279   Other superficial bite of hip, unspecified hip
- **+ S70.3   Other superficial injuries of thigh**
  - + S70.31   Abrasion of thigh
    - +7th S70.311   Abrasion, right thigh
    - +7th S70.312   Abrasion, left thigh
    - +7th S70.319   Abrasion, unspecified thigh
  - + S70.32   Blister (nonthermal) of thigh
    - +7th S70.321   Blister (nonthermal), right thigh
    - +7th S70.322   Blister (nonthermal), left thigh
    - +7th S70.329   Blister (nonthermal), unspecified thigh
  - + S70.34   External constriction of thigh
    - +7th S70.341   External constriction, right thigh
    - +7th S70.342   External constriction, left thigh
    - +7th S70.349   External constriction, unspecified thigh
  - + S70.35   Superficial foreign body of thigh
    - Splinter in the thigh
    - +7th S70.351   Superficial foreign body, right thigh
    - +7th S70.352   Superficial foreign body, left thigh
    - +7th S70.359   Superficial foreign body, unspecified thigh
  - + S70.36   Insect bite (nonvenomous) of thigh
    - +7th S70.361   Insect bite (nonvenomous), right thigh
    - +7th S70.362   Insect bite (nonvenomous), left thigh
    - +7th S70.369   Insect bite (nonvenomous), unspecified thigh
  - + S70.37   Other superficial bite of thigh
    - **Excludes1:** *open bite of thigh (S71.15)*
    - +7th S70.371   Other superficial bite of right thigh
    - +7th S70.372   Other superficial bite of left thigh
    - +7th S70.379   Other superficial bite of unspecified thigh
- **+ S70.9   Unspecified superficial injury of hip and thigh**
  - + S70.91   Unspecified superficial injury of hip
    - +7th S70.911   Unspecified superficial injury of right hip
    - +7th S70.912   Unspecified superficial injury of left hip
    - +7th S70.919   Unspecified superficial injury of unspecified hip
  - + S70.92   Unspecified superficial injury of thigh
    - +7th S70.921   Unspecified superficial injury of right thigh
    - +7th S70.922   Unspecified superficial injury of left thigh
    - +7th S70.929   Unspecified superficial injury of unspecified thigh

S71   Open wound of hip and thigh

Code also any associated wound infection
Excludes1: *open fracture of hip and thigh (S72.-)*
traumatic amputation of hip and thigh (S78.-)
Excludes2: *bite of venomous animal (T63.-)*
open wound of ankle, foot and toes (S91.-)
open wound of knee and lower leg (S81.-)

The appropriate 7th character is to be added to each code from category S71
- A   initial encounter
- D   subsequent encounter
- S   sequela

- **+ S71.0   Open wound of hip**
  - + S71.00   Unspecified open wound of hip
    - +7th S71.001   Unspecified open wound, right hip
    - +7th S71.002   Unspecified open wound, left hip
    - +7th S71.009   Unspecified open wound, unspecified hip
  - + S71.01   Laceration without foreign body of hip
    - +7th S71.011   Laceration without foreign body, right hip
    - +7th S71.012   Laceration without foreign body, left hip
    - +7th S71.019   Laceration without foreign body, unspecified hip
  - + S71.02   Laceration with foreign body of hip
    - +7th S71.021   Laceration with foreign body, right hip
    - +7th S71.022   Laceration with foreign body, left hip
    - +7th S71.029   Laceration with foreign body, unspecified hip
  - + S71.03   Puncture wound without foreign body of hip
    - +7th S71.031   Puncture wound without foreign body, right hip
    - +7th S71.032   Puncture wound without foreign body, left hip
    - +7th S71.039   Puncture wound without foreign body, unspecified hip
  - + S71.04   Puncture wound with foreign body of hip
    - +7th S71.041   Puncture wound with foreign body, right hip
    - +7th S71.042   Puncture wound with foreign body, left hip
    - +7th S71.049   Puncture wound with foreign body, unspecified hip
  - + S71.05   Open bite of hip
    - Bite of hip NOS
    - **Excludes1:** *superficial bite of hip (S70.26, S70.27)*
    - +7th S71.051   Open bite, right hip
    - +7th S71.052   Open bite, left hip
    - +7th S71.059   Open bite, unspecified hip
- **+ S71.1   Open wound of thigh**
  - + S71.10   Unspecified open wound of thigh
    - +7th S71.101   Unspecified open wound, right thigh
    - +7th S71.102   Unspecified open wound, left thigh
    - +7th S71.109   Unspecified open wound, unspecified thigh
  - + S71.11   Laceration without foreign body of thigh
    - +7th S71.111   Laceration without foreign body, right thigh
    - +7th S71.112   Laceration without foreign body, left thigh
    - +7th S71.119   Laceration without foreign body, unspecified thigh
  - + S71.12   Laceration with foreign body of thigh
    - +7th S71.121   Laceration with foreign body, right thigh
    - +7th S71.122   Laceration with foreign body, left thigh
    - +7th S71.129   Laceration with foreign body, unspecified thigh
  - + S71.13   Puncture wound without foreign body of thigh
    - +7th S71.131   Puncture wound without foreign body, right thigh
    - +7th S71.132   Puncture wound without foreign body, left thigh
    - +7th S71.139   Puncture wound without foreign body, unspecified thigh

- **S71.14** Puncture wound with foreign body of thigh
  - +7th **S71.141** Puncture wound with foreign body, right thigh
  - +7th **S71.142** Puncture wound with foreign body, left thigh
  - +7th **S71.149** Puncture wound with foreign body, unspecified thigh
- **S71.15** Open bite of thigh
  Bite of thigh NOS
  Excludes1: superficial bite of thigh (S70.37-)
  - +7th **S71.151** Open bite, right thigh
  - +7th **S71.152** Open bite, left thigh
  - +7th **S71.159** Open bite, unspecified thigh

S72 Fracture of femur

NOTE A fracture not indicated as displaced or nondisplaced should be coded to displaced
A fracture not indicated as open or closed should be coded to closed
The open fracture designations are based on the Gustilo open fracture classification

Excludes1: traumatic amputation of hip and thigh (S78.-)
Excludes2: fracture of lower leg and ankle (S82.-)
fracture of foot (S92.-)
periprosthetic fracture of prosthetic implant of hip (M97.0-)

The appropriate 7th character is to be added to all codes from category S72
- A initial encounter for closed fracture
- B initial encounter for open fracture type I or II
     initial encounter for open fracture NOS
- C initial encounter for open fracture type IIIA, IIIB, or IIIC
- D subsequent encounter for closed fracture with routine healing
- E subsequent encounter for open fracture type I or II with routine healing
- F subsequent encounter for open fracture type IIIA, IIIB, or IIIC with routine healing
- G subsequent encounter for closed fracture with delayed healing
- H subsequent encounter for open fracture type I or II with delayed healing
- J subsequent encounter for open fracture type IIIA, IIIB, or IIIC with delayed healing
- K subsequent encounter for closed fracture with nonunion
- M subsequent encounter for open fracture type I or II with nonunion
- N subsequent encounter for open fracture type IIIA, IIIB, or IIIC with nonunion
- P subsequent encounter for closed fracture with malunion
- Q subsequent encounter for open fracture type I or II with malunion
- R subsequent encounter for open fracture type IIIA, IIIB, or IIIC with malunion
- S sequela

Review coding guideline C.19.c

- **S72.0** Fracture of head and neck of femur
  Excludes2: physeal fracture of lower end of femur (S79.1-)
  physeal fracture of upper end of femur (S79.0-)
  - **S72.00** Fracture of unspecified part of neck of femur
    Fracture of hip NOS
    Fracture of neck of femur NOS
    - CC MCC +7th **S72.001** Fracture of unspecified part of neck of right femur
      - HAC 7th characters A - C see Appendix B for HAC conditional logic
    - CC MCC +7th **S72.002** Fracture of unspecified part of neck of left femur
      - HAC 7th characters A - C see Appendix B for HAC conditional logic
      - AHA CC: 1Q, 2015, 3-21; 4Q, 2015, 36-37
    - CC MCC +7th **S72.009** Fracture of unspecified part of neck of unspecified femur
      - HAC 7th characters A - C see Appendix B for HAC conditional logic
  - **S72.01** Unspecified intracapsular fracture of femur
    Subcapital fracture of femur
    - CC +7th **S72.011** Unspecified intracapsular fracture of right femur
      - HAC 7th characters A - C see Appendix B for HAC conditional logic
    - CC +7th **S72.012** Unspecified intracapsular fracture of left femur
      - HAC 7th characters A - C see Appendix B for HAC conditional logic
    - CC +7th **S72.019** Unspecified intracapsular fracture of unspecified femur
      - HAC 7th characters A - C see Appendix B for HAC conditional logic
  - **S72.02** Fracture of epiphysis (separation) (upper) of femur
    Transepiphyseal fracture of femur
    Excludes1: capital femoral epiphyseal fracture (pediatric) of femur (S79.01-)
    Salter-Harris Type I physeal fracture of upper end of femur (S79.01-)
    - CC MCC +7th **S72.021** Displaced fracture of epiphysis (separation) (upper) of right femur
      - HAC 7th characters A - C see Appendix B for HAC conditional logic
    - CC MCC +7th **S72.022** Displaced fracture of epiphysis (separation) (upper) of left femur
      - HAC 7th characters A - C see Appendix B for HAC conditional logic
    - CC MCC +7th **S72.023** Displaced fracture of epiphysis (separation) (upper) of unspecified femur
      - HAC 7th characters A - C see Appendix B for HAC conditional logic
    - CC MCC +7th **S72.024** Nondisplaced fracture of epiphysis (separation) (upper) of right femur
      - HAC 7th characters A - C see Appendix B for HAC conditional logic
    - CC MCC +7th **S72.025** Nondisplaced fracture of epiphysis (separation) (upper) of left femur
      - HAC 7th characters A - C see Appendix B for HAC conditional logic
    - CC MCC +7th **S72.026** Nondisplaced fracture of epiphysis (separation) (upper) of unspecified femur
      - HAC 7th characters A - C see Appendix B for HAC conditional logic
  - **S72.03** Midcervical fracture of femur
    Transcervical fracture of femur NOS
    - CC MCC +7th **S72.031** Displaced midcervical fracture of right femur
      - HAC 7th characters A - C see Appendix B for HAC conditional logic
    - CC MCC +7th **S72.032** Displaced midcervical fracture of left femur
      - HAC 7th characters A - C see Appendix B for HAC conditional logic
    - CC MCC +7th **S72.033** Displaced midcervical fracture of unspecified femur
      - HAC 7th characters A - C see Appendix B for HAC conditional logic
    - CC MCC +7th **S72.034** Nondisplaced midcervical fracture of right femur
      - HAC 7th characters A - C see Appendix B for HAC conditional logic
    - CC MCC +7th **S72.035** Nondisplaced midcervical fracture of left femur
      - HAC 7th characters A - C see Appendix B for HAC conditional logic
    - CC MCC +7th **S72.036** Nondisplaced midcervical fracture of unspecified femur
      - HAC 7th characters A - C see Appendix B for HAC conditional logic
  - **S72.04** Fracture of base of neck of femur
    Cervicotrochanteric fracture of femur
    - CC MCC +7th **S72.041** Displaced fracture of base of neck of right femur
      - HAC 7th characters A - C see Appendix B for HAC conditional logic
    - CC MCC +7th **S72.042** Displaced fracture of base of neck of left femur
      - HAC 7th characters A - C see Appendix B for HAC conditional logic
    - CC MCC +7th **S72.043** Displaced fracture of base of neck of unspecified femur
      - HAC 7th characters A - C see Appendix B for HAC conditional logic
    - CC MCC +7th **S72.044** Nondisplaced fracture of base of neck of right femur
      - HAC 7th characters A - C see Appendix B for HAC conditional logic

CC MCC +7th **S72.045** Nondisplaced fracture of base of neck of left femur
: HAC 7th characters A - C see Appendix B for HAC conditional logic

CC MCC +7th **S72.046** Nondisplaced fracture of base of neck of unspecified femur
: HAC 7th characters A - C see Appendix B for HAC conditional logic

+ **S72.05** Unspecified fracture of head of femur
Fracture of head of femur NOS

CC MCC +7th **S72.051** Unspecified fracture of head of right femur
: HAC 7th characters A - C see Appendix B for HAC conditional logic

CC MCC +7th **S72.052** Unspecified fracture of head of left femur
: HAC 7th characters A - C see Appendix B for HAC conditional logic

CC MCC +7th **S72.059** Unspecified fracture of head of unspecified femur
: HAC 7th characters A - C see Appendix B for HAC conditional logic

+ **S72.06** Articular fracture of head of femur

CC MCC +7th **S72.061** Displaced articular fracture of head of right femur
: HAC 7th characters A - C see Appendix B for HAC conditional logic

CC MCC +7th **S72.062** Displaced articular fracture of head of left femur
: HAC 7th characters A - C see Appendix B for HAC conditional logic

CC MCC +7th **S72.063** Displaced articular fracture of head of unspecified femur
: HAC 7th characters A - C see Appendix B for HAC conditional logic

CC MCC +7th **S72.064** Nondisplaced articular fracture of head of right femur
: HAC 7th characters A - C see Appendix B for HAC conditional logic

CC MCC +7th **S72.065** Nondisplaced articular fracture of head of left femur
: HAC 7th characters A - C see Appendix B for HAC conditional logic

CC MCC +7th **S72.066** Nondisplaced articular fracture of head of unspecified femur
: HAC 7th characters A - C see Appendix B for HAC conditional logic

+ **S72.09** Other fracture of head and neck of femur

CC MCC +7th **S72.091** Other fracture of head and neck of right femur
: HAC 7th characters A - C see Appendix B for HAC conditional logic

CC MCC +7th **S72.092** Other fracture of head and neck of left femur
: HAC 7th characters A - C see Appendix B for HAC conditional logic

CC MCC +7th **S72.099** Other fracture of head and neck of unspecified femur
: HAC 7th characters A - C see Appendix B for HAC conditional logic

+ **S72.1** Pertrochanteric fracture

+ **S72.10** Unspecified trochanteric fracture of femur
Fracture of trochanter NOS

CC MCC **S72.101** Unspecified trochanteric fracture of right femur
: HAC 7th characters A - C see Appendix B for HAC conditional logic

CC MCC **S72.102** Unspecified trochanteric fracture of left femur
: HAC 7th characters A - C see Appendix B for HAC conditional logic

CC MCC **S72.109** Unspecified trochanteric fracture of unspecified femur
: HAC 7th characters A - C see Appendix B for HAC conditional logic

+ **S72.11** Fracture of greater trochanter of femur

CC +7th **S72.111** Displaced fracture of greater trochanter of right femur
: HAC 7th characters A - C see Appendix B for HAC conditional logic

CC +7th **S72.112** Displaced fracture of greater trochanter of left femur
: HAC 7th characters A - C see Appendix B for HAC conditional logic

CC +7th **S72.113** Displaced fracture of greater trochanter of unspecified femur
: HAC 7th characters A - C see Appendix B for HAC conditional logic

CC +7th **S72.114** Nondisplaced fracture of greater trochanter of right femur
: HAC 7th characters A - C see Appendix B for HAC conditional logic

CC +7th **S72.115** Nondisplaced fracture of greater trochanter of left femur
: HAC 7th characters A - C see Appendix B for HAC conditional logic

CC +7th **S72.116** Nondisplaced fracture of greater trochanter of unspecified femur
: HAC 7th characters A - C see Appendix B for HAC conditional logic

+ **S72.12** Fracture of lesser trochanter of femur

CC +7th **S72.121** Displaced fracture of lesser trochanter of right femur
: HAC 7th characters A - C see Appendix B for HAC conditional logic

CC +7th **S72.122** Displaced fracture of lesser trochanter of left femur
: HAC 7th characters A - C see Appendix B for HAC conditional logic

CC +7th **S72.123** Displaced fracture of lesser trochanter of unspecified femur
: HAC 7th characters A - C see Appendix B for HAC conditional logic

CC +7th **S72.124** Nondisplaced fracture of lesser trochanter of right femur
: HAC 7th characters A - C see Appendix B for HAC conditional logic

CC +7th **S72.125** Nondisplaced fracture of lesser trochanter of left femur
: HAC 7th characters A - C see Appendix B for HAC conditional logic

CC +7th **S72.126** Nondisplaced fracture of lesser trochanter of unspecified femur
: HAC 7th characters A - C see Appendix B for HAC conditional logic

+ **S72.13** Apophyseal fracture of femur
Excludes1: *chronic (nontraumatic) slipped upper femoral epiphysis (M93.0-)*

CC +7th **S72.131** Displaced apophyseal fracture of right femur
: HAC 7th characters A - C see Appendix B for HAC conditional logic

CC +7th **S72.132** Displaced apophyseal fracture of left femur
: HAC 7th characters A - C see Appendix B for HAC conditional logic

CC +7th **S72.133** Displaced apophyseal fracture of unspecified femur
: HAC 7th characters A - C see Appendix B for HAC conditional logic

CC +7th **S72.134** Nondisplaced apophyseal fracture of right femur
: HAC 7th characters A - C see Appendix B for HAC conditional logic

CC +7th **S72.135** Nondisplaced apophyseal fracture of left femur
: HAC 7th characters A - C see Appendix B for HAC conditional logic

CC +7th **S72.136** Nondisplaced apophyseal fracture of unspecified femur
: HAC 7th characters A - C see Appendix B for HAC conditional logic

+ **S72.14** Intertrochanteric fracture of femur

CC +7th **S72.141** Displaced intertrochanteric fracture of right femur
AHA CC: 4Q, 2013, 128-129; 3Q, 2016, 16-17
: HAC 7th characters A - C see Appendix B for HAC conditional logic

CC +7th **S72.142** Displaced intertrochanteric fracture of left femur
: HAC 7th characters A - C see Appendix B for HAC conditional logic

CC +7th **S72.143** Displaced intertrochanteric fracture of unspecified femur
: HAC 7th characters A - C see Appendix B for HAC conditional logic

CC +7th **S72.144** Nondisplaced intertrochanteric fracture of right femur
: HAC 7th characters A - C see Appendix B for HAC conditional logic

CC +7th **S72.145** Nondisplaced intertrochanteric fracture of left femur
    HAC 7th characters A - C see Appendix B for HAC conditional logic

CC +7th **S72.146** Nondisplaced intertrochanteric fracture of unspecified femur
    HAC 7th characters A - C see Appendix B for HAC conditional logic

+ **S72.2** Subtrochanteric fracture of femur

CC X+7th **S72.21** Displaced subtrochanteric fracture of right femur
    HAC 7th characters A - C see Appendix B for HAC conditional logic

CC X+7th **S72.22** Displaced subtrochanteric fracture of left femur
    HAC 7th characters A - C see Appendix B for HAC conditional logic

CC X+7th **S72.23** Displaced subtrochanteric fracture of unspecified femur
    HAC 7th characters A - C see Appendix B for HAC conditional logic

CC X+7th **S72.24** Nondisplaced subtrochanteric fracture of right femur
    HAC 7th characters A - C see Appendix B for HAC conditional logic

CC X+7th **S72.25** Nondisplaced subtrochanteric fracture of left femur
    HAC 7th characters A - C see Appendix B for HAC conditional logic

CC X+7th **S72.26** Nondisplaced subtrochanteric fracture of unspecified femur
    HAC 7th characters A - C see Appendix B for HAC conditional logic

+ **S72.3** Fracture of shaft of femur

+ **S72.30** Unspecified fracture of shaft of femur

CC +7th **S72.301** Unspecified fracture of shaft of right femur
    AHA CC: 2Q, 2018, 12
    HAC 7th characters A - C see Appendix B for HAC conditional logic

CC +7th **S72.302** Unspecified fracture of shaft of left femur
    HAC 7th characters A - C see Appendix B for HAC conditional logic

CC +7th **S72.309** Unspecified fracture of shaft of unspecified femur
    HAC 7th characters A - C see Appendix B for HAC conditional logic

+ **S72.32** Transverse fracture of shaft of femur

CC MCC +7th **S72.321** Displaced transverse fracture of shaft of right femur
    HAC 7th characters A - C see Appendix B for HAC conditional logic

CC MCC +7th **S72.322** Displaced transverse fracture of shaft of left femur
    HAC 7th characters A - C see Appendix B for HAC conditional logic

CC MCC +7th **S72.323** Displaced transverse fracture of shaft of unspecified femur
    HAC 7th characters A - C see Appendix B for HAC conditional logic

CC MCC +7th **S72.324** Nondisplaced transverse fracture of shaft of right femur
    HAC 7th characters A - C see Appendix B for HAC conditional logic

CC MCC +7th **S72.325** Nondisplaced transverse fracture of shaft of left femur
    HAC 7th characters A - C see Appendix B for HAC conditional logic

CC MCC +7th **S72.326** Nondisplaced transverse fracture of shaft of unspecified femur
    HAC 7th characters A - C see Appendix B for HAC conditional logic

+ **S72.33** Oblique fracture of shaft of femur

CC MCC +7th **S72.331** Displaced oblique fracture of shaft of right femur
    HAC 7th characters A - C see Appendix B for HAC conditional logic

CC MCC +7th **S72.332** Displaced oblique fracture of shaft of left femur
    HAC 7th characters A - C see Appendix B for HAC conditional logic

CC MCC +7th **S72.333** Displaced oblique fracture of shaft of unspecified femur
    HAC 7th characters A - C see Appendix B for HAC conditional logic

CC MCC +7th **S72.334** Nondisplaced oblique fracture of shaft of right femur
    HAC 7th characters A - C see Appendix B for HAC conditional logic

CC MCC +7th **S72.335** Nondisplaced oblique fracture of shaft of left femur
    HAC 7th characters A - C see Appendix B for HAC conditional logic

CC MCC +7th **S72.336** Nondisplaced oblique fracture of shaft of unspecified femur
    HAC 7th characters A - C see Appendix B for HAC conditional logic

+ **S72.34** Spiral fracture of shaft of femur

CC MCC +7th **S72.341** Displaced spiral fracture of shaft of right femur
    HAC 7th characters A - C see Appendix B for HAC conditional logic

CC MCC +7th **S72.342** Displaced spiral fracture of shaft of left femur
    HAC 7th characters A - C see Appendix B for HAC conditional logic

CC MCC +7th **S72.343** Displaced spiral fracture of shaft of unspecified femur
    HAC 7th characters A - C see Appendix B for HAC conditional logic

CC MCC +7th **S72.344** Nondisplaced spiral fracture of shaft of right femur
    HAC 7th characters A - C see Appendix B for HAC conditional logic

CC MCC +7th **S72.345** Nondisplaced spiral fracture of shaft of left femur
    HAC 7th characters A - C see Appendix B for HAC conditional logic

CC MCC +7th **S72.346** Nondisplaced spiral fracture of shaft of unspecified femur
    HAC 7th characters A - C see Appendix B for HAC conditional logic

+ **S72.35** Comminuted fracture of shaft of femur

CC MCC +7th **S72.351** Displaced comminuted fracture of shaft of right femur
    HAC 7th characters A - C see Appendix B for HAC conditional logic

CC MCC +7th **S72.352** Displaced comminuted fracture of shaft of left femur
    HAC 7th characters A - C see Appendix B for HAC conditional logic

CC MCC +7th **S72.353** Displaced comminuted fracture of shaft of unspecified femur
    HAC 7th characters A - C see Appendix B for HAC conditional logic

CC MCC +7th **S72.354** Nondisplaced comminuted fracture of shaft of right femur
    HAC 7th characters A - C see Appendix B for HAC conditional logic

CC MCC +7th **S72.355** Nondisplaced comminuted fracture of shaft of left femur
    HAC 7th characters A - C see Appendix B for HAC conditional logic

CC MCC +7th **S72.356** Nondisplaced comminuted fracture of shaft of unspecified femur
    HAC 7th characters A - C see Appendix B for HAC conditional logic

+ **S72.36** Segmental fracture of shaft of femur

CC MCC +7th **S72.361** Displaced segmental fracture of shaft of right femur
    HAC 7th characters A - C see Appendix B for HAC conditional logic

CC MCC +7th **S72.362** Displaced segmental fracture of shaft of left femur
    HAC 7th characters A - C see Appendix B for HAC conditional logic

CC MCC +7th **S72.363** Displaced segmental fracture of shaft of unspecified femur
    HAC 7th characters A - C see Appendix B for HAC conditional logic

CC MCC +7th **S72.364** Nondisplaced segmental fracture of shaft of right femur
    HAC 7th characters A - C see Appendix B for HAC conditional logic

CC MCC +7th **S72.365** Nondisplaced segmental fracture of shaft of left femur
    HAC 7th characters A - C see Appendix B for HAC conditional logic

CC MCC +7th	**S72.366**	Nondisplaced segmental fracture of shaft of unspecified femur
		HAC 7th characters A - C see Appendix B for HAC conditional logic

+ **S72.39** Other fracture of shaft of femur

CC MCC +7th	**S72.391**	Other fracture of shaft of right femur
		HAC 7th characters A - C see Appendix B for HAC conditional logic
CC MCC +7th	**S72.392**	Other fracture of shaft of left femur
		HAC 7th characters A - C see Appendix B for HAC conditional logic
CC MCC +7th	**S72.399**	Other fracture of shaft of unspecified femur
		HAC 7th characters A - C see Appendix B for HAC conditional logic

+ **S72.4** Fracture of lower end of femur
    Fracture of distal end of femur
    Excludes2: *fracture of shaft of femur (S72.3-)*
                   physeal fracture of lower end of femur (S79.1-)

+ **S72.40** Unspecified fracture of lower end of femur

CC MCC +7th	**S72.401**	Unspecified fracture of lower end of right femur
		AHA CC: 4Q, 2016, 42-43
		HAC 7th characters A - C see Appendix B for HAC conditional logic
CC MCC +7th	**S72.402**	Unspecified fracture of lower end of left femur
		HAC 7th characters A - C see Appendix B for HAC conditional logic
CC MCC +7th	**S72.409**	Unspecified fracture of lower end of unspecified femur
		HAC 7th characters A - C see Appendix B for HAC conditional logic

+ **S72.41** Unspecified condyle fracture of lower end of femur
    Condyle fracture of femur NOS

CC MCC +7th	**S72.411**	Displaced unspecified condyle fracture of lower end of right femur
		HAC 7th characters A - C see Appendix B for HAC conditional logic
CC MCC +7th	**S72.412**	Displaced unspecified condyle fracture of lower end of left femur
		HAC 7th characters A - C see Appendix B for HAC conditional logic
CC MCC +7th	**S72.413**	Displaced unspecified condyle fracture of lower end of unspecified femur
		HAC 7th characters A - C see Appendix B for HAC conditional logic
CC MCC +7th	**S72.414**	Nondisplaced unspecified condyle fracture of lower end of right femur
		HAC 7th characters A - C see Appendix B for HAC conditional logic
CC MCC +7th	**S72.415**	Nondisplaced unspecified condyle fracture of lower end of left femur
		HAC 7th characters A - C see Appendix B for HAC conditional logic
CC MCC +7th	**S72.416**	Nondisplaced unspecified condyle fracture of lower end of unspecified femur
		HAC 7th characters A - C see Appendix B for HAC conditional logic

+ **S72.42** Fracture of lateral condyle of femur

CC MCC +7th	**S72.421**	Displaced fracture of lateral condyle of right femur
		HAC 7th characters A - C see Appendix B for HAC conditional logic
CC MCC +7th	**S72.422**	Displaced fracture of lateral condyle of left femur
		HAC 7th characters A - C see Appendix B for HAC conditional logic
CC MCC +7th	**S72.423**	Displaced fracture of lateral condyle of unspecified femur
		HAC 7th characters A - C see Appendix B for HAC conditional logic
CC MCC +7th	**S72.424**	Nondisplaced fracture of lateral condyle of right femur
		HAC 7th characters A - C see Appendix B for HAC conditional logic
CC MCC +7th	**S72.425**	Nondisplaced fracture of lateral condyle of left femur
		HAC 7th characters A - C see Appendix B for HAC conditional logic
CC MCC +7th	**S72.426**	Nondisplaced fracture of lateral condyle of unspecified femur
		HAC 7th characters A - C see Appendix B for HAC conditional logic

+ **S72.43** Fracture of medial condyle of femur

CC MCC +7th	**S72.431**	Displaced fracture of medial condyle of right femur
		HAC 7th characters A - C see Appendix B for HAC conditional logic
CC MCC +7th	**S72.432**	Displaced fracture of medial condyle of left femur
		HAC 7th characters A - C see Appendix B for HAC conditional logic
CC MCC +7th	**S72.433**	Displaced fracture of medial condyle of unspecified femur
		HAC 7th characters A - C see Appendix B for HAC conditional logic
CC MCC +7th	**S72.434**	Nondisplaced fracture of medial condyle of right femur
		HAC 7th characters A - C see Appendix B for HAC conditional logic
CC MCC +7th	**S72.435**	Nondisplaced fracture of medial condyle of left femur
		HAC 7th characters A - C see Appendix B for HAC conditional logic
CC MCC +7th	**S72.436**	Nondisplaced fracture of medial condyle of unspecified femur
		HAC 7th characters A - C see Appendix B for HAC conditional logic

+ **S72.44** Fracture of lower epiphysis (separation) of femur
    Excludes1: *Salter-Harris Type I physeal fracture of lower end of femur (S79.11-)*

CC MCC +7th	**S72.441**	Displaced fracture of lower epiphysis (separation) of right femur
		HAC 7th characters A - C see Appendix B for HAC conditional logic
CC MCC +7th	**S72.442**	Displaced fracture of lower epiphysis (separation) of left femur
		HAC 7th characters A - C see Appendix B for HAC conditional logic
CC MCC +7th	**S72.443**	Displaced fracture of lower epiphysis (separation) of unspecified femur
		HAC 7th characters A - C see Appendix B for HAC conditional logic
CC MCC +7th	**S72.444**	Nondisplaced fracture of lower epiphysis (separation) of right femur
		HAC 7th characters A - C see Appendix B for HAC conditional logic
CC MCC +7th	**S72.445**	Nondisplaced fracture of lower epiphysis (separation) of left femur
		HAC 7th characters A - C see Appendix B for HAC conditional logic
CC MCC +7th	**S72.446**	Nondisplaced fracture of lower epiphysis (separation) of unspecified femur
		HAC 7th characters A - C see Appendix B for HAC conditional logic

+ **S72.45** Supracondylar fracture without intracondylar extension of lower end of femur
    Supracondylar fracture of lower end of femur NOS
    Excludes1: *supracondylar fracture with intracondylar extension of lower end of femur (S72.46-)*

CC MCC +7th	**S72.451**	Displaced supracondylar fracture without intracondylar extension of lower end of right femur
		HAC 7th characters A - C see Appendix B for HAC conditional logic
CC MCC +7th	**S72.452**	Displaced supracondylar fracture without intracondylar extension of lower end of left femur
		HAC 7th characters A - C see Appendix B for HAC conditional logic
CC MCC +7th	**S72.453**	Displaced supracondylar fracture without intracondylar extension of lower end of unspecified femur
		HAC 7th characters A - C see Appendix B for HAC conditional logic

CC MCC +7th S72.454 Nondisplaced supracondylar fracture without intracondylar extension of lower end of right femur
 HAC 7th characters A - C see Appendix B for HAC conditional logic

CC MCC +7th S72.455 Nondisplaced supracondylar fracture without intracondylar extension of lower end of left femur
 HAC 7th characters A - C see Appendix B for HAC conditional logic

CC MCC +7th S72.456 Nondisplaced supracondylar fracture without intracondylar extension of lower end of unspecified femur
 HAC 7th characters A - C see Appendix B for HAC conditional logic

+ S72.46 Supracondylar fracture with intracondylar extension of lower end of femur
 Excludes1: supracondylar fracture without intracondylar extension of lower end of femur (S72.45-)

CC MCC +7th S72.461 Displaced supracondylar fracture with intracondylar extension of lower end of right femur
 HAC 7th characters A - C see Appendix B for HAC conditional logic

CC MCC +7th S72.462 Displaced supracondylar fracture with intracondylar extension of lower end of left femur
 HAC 7th characters A - C see Appendix B for HAC conditional logic

CC MCC +7th S72.463 Displaced supracondylar fracture with intracondylar extension of lower end of unspecified femur
 HAC 7th characters A - C see Appendix B for HAC conditional logic

CC MCC +7th S72.464 Nondisplaced supracondylar fracture with intracondylar extension of lower end of right femur
 HAC 7th characters A - C see Appendix B for HAC conditional logic

CC MCC +7th S72.465 Nondisplaced supracondylar fracture with intracondylar extension of lower end of left femur
 HAC 7th characters A - C see Appendix B for HAC conditional logic

CC MCC +7th S72.466 Nondisplaced supracondylar fracture with intracondylar extension of lower end of unspecified femur
 HAC 7th characters A - C see Appendix B for HAC conditional logic

+ S72.47 Torus fracture of lower end of femur

> The appropriate 7th character is to be added to all codes in subcategory **S72.47**
> A   initial encounter for closed fracture
> D   subsequent encounter for fracture with routine healing
> G   subsequent encounter for fracture with delayed healing
> K   subsequent encounter for fracture with nonunion
> P   subsequent encounter for fracture with malunion
> S   sequela

CC +7th S72.471 Torus fracture of lower end of right femur
 HAC 7th character A see Appendix B for HAC conditional logic

CC +7th S72.472 Torus fracture of lower end of left femur
 HAC 7th character A see Appendix B for HAC conditional logic

CC +7th S72.479 Torus fracture of lower end of unspecified femur
 HAC 7th character A see Appendix B for HAC conditional logic

+ S72.49 Other fracture of lower end of femur

CC MCC +7th S72.491 Other fracture of lower end of right femur
 HAC 7th characters A - C see Appendix B for HAC conditional logic

CC MCC +7th S72.492 Other fracture of lower end of left femur
 HAC 7th characters A - C see Appendix B for HAC conditional logic

CC MCC +7th S72.499 Other fracture of lower end of unspecified femur
 HAC 7th characters A - C see Appendix B for HAC conditional logic

MCC + S72.8 Other fracture of femur
 HAC 7th characters A - C see Appendix B for HAC conditional logic

+ S72.8X Other fracture of femur
 +7th S72.8X1 Other fracture of right femur
 +7th S72.8X2 Other fracture of left femur
 +7th S72.8X9 Other fracture of unspecified femur

+ S72.9 Unspecified fracture of femur
 Fracture of thigh NOS
 Fracture of upper leg NOS
 Excludes1: fracture of hip NOS (S72.00-, S72.01-)

CC MCC X+7th S72.90 Unspecified fracture of unspecified femur
 AHA CC: 4Q, 2012, 93-94
 HAC 7th characters A - C see Appendix B for HAC conditional logic

CC MCC X+7th S72.91 Unspecified fracture of right femur
 HAC 7th characters A - C see Appendix B for HAC conditional logic

CC MCC X+7th S72.92 Unspecified fracture of left femur
 HAC 7th characters A - C see Appendix B for HAC conditional logic

S73 Dislocation and sprain of joint and ligaments of hip

Includes: avulsion of joint or ligament of hip
 lacervw ation of cartilage, joint or ligament of hip
 sprain of cartilage, joint or ligament of hip
 traumatic hemarthrosis of joint or ligament of hip
 traumatic rupture of joint or ligament of hip
 traumatic subluxation of joint or ligament of hip
 traumatic tear of joint or ligament of hip

Code also any associated open wound
Excludes2: strain of muscle, fascia and tendon of hip and thigh (S76.-)

> The appropriate 7th character is to be added to each code from category S73
> A   initial encounter
> D   subsequent encounter
> S   sequela

+ S73.0 Subluxation and dislocation of hip
 Excludes2: dislocation and subluxation of hip prosthesis (T84.020, T84.021)

+ S73.00 Unspecified subluxation and dislocation of hip
 Dislocation of hip NOS
 Subluxation of hip NOS

CC +7th S73.001 Unspecified subluxation of right hip
 HAC 7th character A see Appendix B for HAC conditional logic

CC +7th S73.002 Unspecified subluxation of left hip
 HAC 7th character A see Appendix B for HAC conditional logic

CC +7th S73.003 Unspecified subluxation of unspecified hip
 HAC 7th character A see Appendix B for HAC conditional logic

CC +7th S73.004 Unspecified dislocation of right hip
 HAC 7th character A see Appendix B for HAC conditional logic

CC +7th S73.005 Unspecified dislocation of left hip
 HAC 7th character A see Appendix B for HAC conditional logic

CC +7th S73.006 Unspecified dislocation of unspecified hip
 HAC 7th character A see Appendix B for HAC conditional logic

+ S73.01 Posterior subluxation and dislocation of hip

CC +7th S73.011 Posterior subluxation of right hip
 HAC 7th character A see Appendix B for HAC conditional logic

CC +7th S73.012 Posterior subluxation of left hip
 HAC 7th character A see Appendix B for HAC conditional logic

CC +7th **S73.013** Posterior subluxation of unspecified hip
HAC 7th character A see Appendix B for HAC conditional logic

CC +7th **S73.014** Posterior dislocation of right hip
HAC 7th character A see Appendix B for HAC conditional logic

CC +7th **S73.015** Posterior dislocation of left hip
HAC 7th character A see Appendix B for HAC conditional logic

CC +7th **S73.016** Posterior dislocation of unspecified hip
HAC 7th character A see Appendix B for HAC conditional logic

+ **S73.02** Obturator subluxation and dislocation of hip

CC +7th **S73.021** Obturator subluxation of right hip
HAC 7th character A see Appendix B for HAC conditional logic

CC +7th **S73.022** Obturator subluxation of left hip
HAC 7th character A see Appendix B for HAC conditional logic

CC +7th **S73.023** Obturator subluxation of unspecified hip
HAC 7th character A see Appendix B for HAC conditional logic

CC +7th **S73.024** Obturator dislocation of right hip
HAC 7th character A see Appendix B for HAC conditional logic

CC +7th **S73.025** Obturator dislocation of left hip
HAC 7th character A see Appendix B for HAC conditional logic

CC +7th **S73.026** Obturator dislocation of unspecified hip
HAC 7th character A see Appendix B for HAC conditional logic

+ **S73.03** Other anterior subluxation and dislocation of hip

CC +7th **S73.031** Other anterior subluxation of right hip
HAC 7th character A see Appendix B for HAC conditional logic

CC +7th **S73.032** Other anterior subluxation of left hip
HAC 7th character A see Appendix B for HAC conditional logic

CC +7th **S73.033** Other anterior subluxation of unspecified hip
HAC 7th character A see Appendix B for HAC conditional logic

CC +7th **S73.034** Other anterior dislocation of right hip
HAC 7th character A see Appendix B for HAC conditional logic

CC +7th **S73.035** Other anterior dislocation of left hip
HAC 7th character A see Appendix B for HAC conditional logic

CC +7th **S73.036** Other anterior dislocation of unspecified hip
HAC 7th character A see Appendix B for HAC conditional logic

+ **S73.04** Central subluxation and dislocation of hip

CC +7th **S73.041** Central subluxation of right hip
HAC 7th character A see Appendix B for HAC conditional logic

CC +7th **S73.042** Central subluxation of left hip
HAC 7th character A see Appendix B for HAC conditional logic

CC +7th **S73.043** Central subluxation of unspecified hip
HAC 7th character A see Appendix B for HAC conditional logic

CC +7th **S73.044** Central dislocation of right hip
HAC 7th character A see Appendix B for HAC conditional logic

CC +7th **S73.045** Central dislocation of left hip
HAC 7th character A see Appendix B for HAC conditional logic

CC +7th **S73.046** Central dislocation of unspecified hip
HAC 7th character A see Appendix B for HAC conditional logic

+ **S73.1** Sprain of hip
+ **S73.10** Unspecified sprain of hip
+7th **S73.101** Unspecified sprain of right hip
+7th **S73.102** Unspecified sprain of left hip
+7th **S73.109** Unspecified sprain of unspecified hip
+ **S73.11** Iliofemoral ligament sprain of hip
+7th **S73.111** Iliofemoral ligament sprain of right hip
+7th **S73.112** Iliofemoral ligament sprain of left hip
+7th **S73.119** Iliofemoral ligament sprain of unspecified hip

+ **S73.12** Ischiocapsular (ligament) sprain of hip
+7th **S73.121** Ischiocapsular ligament sprain of right hip
+7th **S73.122** Ischiocapsular ligament sprain of left hip
+7th **S73.129** Ischiocapsular ligament sprain of unspecified hip

+ **S73.19** Other sprain of hip
+7th **S73.191** Other sprain of right hip
+7th **S73.192** Other sprain of left hip
  AHA CC: 4Q, 2014, 25
+7th **S73.199** Other sprain of unspecified hip

S74 Injury of nerves at hip and thigh level
Code also any associated open wound (S71.-)
Excludes2: *injury of nerves at ankle and foot level (S94.-)*
injury of nerves at lower leg level (S84.-)

The appropriate 7th character is to be added to each code from category S74
A initial encounter
D subsequent encounter
S sequela

+ **S74.0** Injury of sciatic nerve at hip and thigh level
X+7th **S74.00** Injury of sciatic nerve at hip and thigh level, unspecified leg
X+7th **S74.01** Injury of sciatic nerve at hip and thigh level, right leg
X+7th **S74.02** Injury of sciatic nerve at hip and thigh level, left leg

+ **S74.1** Injury of femoral nerve at hip and thigh level
X+7th **S74.10** Injury of femoral nerve at hip and thigh level, unspecified leg
X+7th **S74.11** Injury of femoral nerve at hip and thigh level, right leg
X+7th **S74.12** Injury of femoral nerve at hip and thigh level, left leg

+ **S74.2** Injury of cutaneous sensory nerve at hip and thigh level
X+7th **S74.20** Injury of cutaneous sensory nerve at hip and thigh level, unspecified leg
X+7th **S74.21** Injury of cutaneous sensory nerve at hip and high level, right leg
X+7th **S74.22** Injury of cutaneous sensory nerve at hip and thigh level, left leg

+ **S74.8** Injury of other nerves at hip and thigh level
+ **S74.8X** Injury of other nerves at hip and thigh level
+7th **S74.8X1** Injury of other nerves at hip and thigh level, right leg
+7th **S74.8X2** Injury of other nerves at hip and thigh level, left leg
+7th **S74.8X9** Injury of other nerves at hip and thigh level, unspecified leg

+ **S74.9** Injury of unspecified nerve at hip and thigh level
X+7th **S74.90** Injury of unspecified nerve at hip and thigh level, unspecified leg
X+7th **S74.91** Injury of unspecified nerve at hip and thigh level, right leg
X+7th **S74.92** Injury of unspecified nerve at hip and thigh level, left leg

S75 Injury of blood vessels at hip and thigh level
Code also any associated open wound (S71.-)
Excludes2: *injury of blood vessels at lower leg level (S85.-)*
injury of popliteal artery (S85.0)

The appropriate 7th character is to be added to each code from category S75
A initial encounter
D subsequent encounter
S sequela

+ **S75.0** Injury of femoral artery
+ **S75.00** Unspecified injury of femoral artery
MCC +7th **S75.001** Unspecified injury of femoral artery, right leg
MCC +7th **S75.002** Unspecified injury of femoral artery, left leg
MCC +7th **S75.009** Unspecified injury of femoral artery, unspecified leg

- **+ S75.01** Minor laceration of femoral artery
    - Incomplete transection of femoral artery
    - Laceration of femoral artery NOS
    - Superficial laceration of femoral artery
  - MCC +7th **S75.011** Minor laceration of femoral artery, right leg
  - MCC +7th **S75.012** Minor laceration of femoral artery, left leg
  - MCC +7th **S75.019** Minor laceration of femoral artery, unspecified leg
- **+ S75.02** Major laceration of femoral artery
    - Complete transection of femoral artery
    - Traumatic rupture of femoral artery
  - MCC +7th **S75.021** Major laceration of femoral artery, right leg
  - MCC +7th **S75.022** Major laceration of femoral artery, left leg
  - MCC +7th **S75.029** Major laceration of femoral artery, unspecified leg
- **+ S75.09** Other specified injury of femoral artery
  - MCC +7th **S75.091** Other specified injury of femoral artery, right leg
  - MCC +7th **S75.092** Other specified injury of femoral artery, left leg
  - MCC +7th **S75.099** Other specified injury of femoral artery, unspecified leg
- **+ S75.1** Injury of femoral vein at hip and thigh level
  - **+ S75.10** Unspecified injury of femoral vein at hip and thigh level
    - MCC +7th **S75.101** Unspecified injury of femoral vein at hip and thigh level, right leg
    - MCC +7th **S75.102** Unspecified injury of femoral vein at hip and thigh level, left leg
    - MCC +7th **S75.109** Unspecified injury of femoral vein at hip and thigh level, unspecified leg
  - **+ S75.11** Minor laceration of femoral vein at hip and thigh level
    - Incomplete transection of femoral vein at hip and thigh level
    - Laceration of femoral vein at hip and thigh level NOS
    - Superficial laceration of femoral vein at hip and thigh level
    - MCC +7th **S75.111** Minor laceration of femoral vein at hip and thigh level, right leg
    - MCC +7th **S75.112** Minor laceration of femoral vein at hip and thigh level, left leg
    - MCC +7th **S75.119** Minor laceration of femoral vein at hip and thigh level, unspecified leg
  - **+ S75.12** Major laceration of femoral vein at hip and thigh level
    - Complete transection of femoral vein at hip and thigh level
    - Traumatic rupture of femoral vein at hip and thigh level
    - MCC +7th **S75.121** Major laceration of femoral vein at hip and thigh level, right leg
    - MCC +7th **S75.122** Major laceration of femoral vein at hip and thigh level, left leg
    - MCC +7th **S75.129** Major laceration of femoral vein at hip and thigh level, unspecified leg
  - **+ S75.19** Other specified injury of femoral vein at hip and thigh level
    - MCC +7th **S75.191** Other specified injury of femoral vein at hip and thigh level, right leg
    - MCC +7th **S75.192** Other specified injury of femoral vein at hip and thigh level, left leg
    - MCC +7th **S75.199** Other specified injury of femoral vein at hip and thigh level, unspecified leg
- **+ S75.2** Injury of greater saphenous vein at hip and thigh level
    - **Excludes1:** *greater saphenous vein NOS (S85.3)*
  - **+ S75.20** Unspecified injury of greater saphenous vein at hip and thigh level
    - CC +7th **S75.201** Unspecified injury of greater saphenous vein at hip and thigh level, right leg
    - CC +7th **S75.202** Unspecified injury of greater saphenous vein at hip and thigh level, left leg
    - CC +7th **S75.209** Unspecified injury of greater saphenous vein at hip and thigh level, unspecified leg
- **+ S75.21** Minor laceration of greater saphenous vein at hip and thigh level
    - Incomplete transection of greater saphenous vein at hip and thigh level
    - Laceration of greater saphenous vein at hip and thigh level NOS
    - Superficial laceration of greater saphenous vein at hip and thigh level
  - CC +7th **S75.211** Minor laceration of greater saphenous vein at hip and thigh level, right leg
  - CC +7th **S75.212** Minor laceration of greater saphenous vein at hip and thigh level, left leg
  - CC +7th **S75.219** Minor laceration of greater saphenous vein at hip and thigh level, unspecified leg
- **+ S75.22** Major laceration of greater saphenous vein at hip and thigh level
    - Complete transection of greater saphenous vein at hip and thigh level
    - Traumatic rupture of greater saphenous vein at hip and thigh level
  - CC +7th **S75.221** Major laceration of greater saphenous vein at hip and thigh level, right leg
  - CC +7th **S75.222** Major laceration of greater saphenous vein at hip and thigh level, left leg
  - CC +7th **S75.229** Major laceration of greater saphenous vein at hip and thigh level, unspecified leg
- **+ S75.29** Other specified injury of greater saphenous vein at hip and thigh level
  - CC +7th **S75.291** Other specified injury of greater saphenous vein at hip and thigh level, right leg
  - CC +7th **S75.292** Other specified injury of greater saphenous vein at hip and thigh level, left leg
  - CC +7th **S75.299** Other specified injury of greater saphenous vein at hip and thigh level, unspecified leg
- **+ S75.8** Injury of other blood vessels at hip and thigh level
  - **+ S75.80** Unspecified injury of other blood vessels at hip and thigh level
    - CC +7th **S75.801** Unspecified injury of other blood vessels at hip and thigh level, right leg
    - CC +7th **S75.802** Unspecified injury of other blood vessels at hip and thigh level, left leg
    - CC +7th **S75.809** Unspecified injury of other blood vessels at hip and thigh level, unspecified leg
  - **+ S75.81** Laceration of other blood vessels at hip and thigh level
    - CC +7th **S75.811** Laceration of other blood vessels at hip and thigh level, right leg
    - CC +7th **S75.812** Laceration of other blood vessels at hip and thigh level, left leg
    - CC +7th **S75.819** Laceration of other blood vessels at hip and thigh level, unspecified leg
  - **+ S75.89** Other specified injury of other blood vessels at hip and thigh level
    - CC +7th **S75.891** Other specified injury of other blood vessels at hip and thigh level, right leg
    - CC +7th **S75.892** Other specified injury of other blood vessels at hip and thigh level, left leg
    - CC +7th **S75.899** Other specified injury of other blood vessels at hip and thigh level, unspecified leg
- **+ S75.9** Injury of unspecified blood vessel at hip and thigh level
  - **+ S75.90** Unspecified injury of unspecified blood vessel at hip and thigh level
    - CC +7th **S75.901** Unspecified injury of unspecified blood vessel at hip and thigh level, right leg
    - CC +7th **S75.902** Unspecified injury of unspecified blood vessel at hip and thigh level, left leg
    - CC +7th **S75.909** Unspecified injury of unspecified blood vessel at hip and thigh level, unspecified leg

- **+ S75.91** Laceration of unspecified blood vessel at hip and thigh level
  - CC +7th **S75.911** Laceration of unspecified blood vessel at hip and thigh level, right leg
  - CC +7th **S75.912** Laceration of unspecified blood vessel at hip and thigh level, left leg
  - CC +7th **S75.919** Laceration of unspecified blood vessel at hip and thigh level, unspecified leg
- **+ S75.99** Other specified injury of unspecified blood vessel at hip and thigh level
  - CC +7th **S75.991** Other specified injury of unspecified blood vessel at hip and thigh level, right leg
  - CC +7th **S75.992** Other specified injury of unspecified blood vessel at hip and thigh level, left leg
  - CC +7th **S75.999** Other specified injury of unspecified blood vessel at hip and thigh level, unspecified leg

S76 Injury of muscle, fascia and tendon at hip and thigh level

Code also any associated open wound (S71.-)

Excludes2: injury of muscle, fascia and tendon at lower leg level (S86)
sprain of joint and ligament of hip (S73.1)

> The appropriate 7th character is to be added to each code from category S76
> A initial encounter
> D subsequent encounter
> S sequela

- **+ S76.0** Injury of muscle, fascia and tendon of hip
  - **+ S76.00** Unspecified injury of muscle, fascia and tendon of hip
    - +7th **S76.001** Unspecified injury of muscle, fascia and tendon of right hip
    - +7th **S76.002** Unspecified injury of muscle, fascia and tendon of left hip
    - +7th **S76.009** Unspecified injury of muscle, fascia and tendon of unspecified hip
  - **+ S76.01** Strain of muscle, fascia and tendon of hip
    - +7th **S76.011** Strain of muscle, fascia and tendon of right hip
    - +7th **S76.012** Strain of muscle, fascia and tendon of left hip
    - +7th **S76.019** Strain of muscle, fascia and tendon of unspecified hip
  - **+ S76.02** Laceration of muscle, fascia and tendon of hip
    - CC +7th **S76.021** Laceration of muscle, fascia and tendon of right hip
    - CC +7th **S76.022** Laceration of muscle, fascia and tendon of left hip
    - CC +7th **S76.029** Laceration of muscle, fascia and tendon of unspecified hip
  - **+ S76.09** Other specified injury of muscle, fascia and tendon of hip
    - +7th **S76.091** Other specified injury of muscle, fascia and tendon of right hip
    - +7th **S76.092** Other specified injury of muscle, fascia and tendon of left hip
    - +7th **S76.099** Other specified injury of muscle, fascia and tendon of unspecified hip
- **+ S76.1** Injury of quadriceps muscle, fascia and tendon
  Injury of patellar ligament (tendon)
  - **+ S76.10** Unspecified injury of quadriceps muscle, fascia and tendon
    - +7th **S76.101** Unspecified injury of right quadriceps muscle, fascia and tendon
    - +7th **S76.102** Unspecified injury of left quadriceps muscle, fascia and tendon
    - +7th **S76.109** Unspecified injury of unspecified quadriceps muscle, fascia and tendon
  - **+ S76.11** Strain of quadriceps muscle, fascia and tendon
    - +7th **S76.111** Strain of right quadriceps muscle, fascia and tendon
    - +7th **S76.112** Strain of left quadriceps muscle, fascia and tendon
    - +7th **S76.119** Strain of unspecified quadriceps muscle, fascia and tendon
  - **+ S76.12** Laceration of quadriceps muscle, fascia and tendon
    - CC +7th **S76.121** Laceration of right quadriceps muscle, fascia and tendon
    - CC +7th **S76.122** Laceration of left quadriceps muscle, fascia and tendon
    - CC +7th **S76.129** Laceration of unspecified quadriceps muscle, fascia and tendon
  - **+ S76.19** Other specified injury of quadriceps muscle, fascia and tendon
    - +7th **S76.191** Other specified injury of right quadriceps muscle, fascia and tendon
    - +7th **S76.192** Other specified injury of left quadriceps muscle, fascia and tendon
    - +7th **S76.199** Other specified injury of unspecified quadriceps muscle, fascia and tendon
- **+ S76.2** Injury of adductor muscle, fascia and tendon of thigh
  - **+ S76.20** Unspecified injury of adductor muscle, fascia and tendon of thigh
    - +7th **S76.201** Unspecified injury of adductor muscle, fascia and tendon of right thigh
    - +7th **S76.202** Unspecified injury of adductor muscle, fascia and tendon of left thigh
    - +7th **S76.209** Unspecified injury of adductor muscle, fascia and tendon of unspecified thigh
  - **+ S76.21** Strain of adductor muscle, fascia and tendon of thigh
    - +7th **S76.211** Strain of adductor muscle, fascia and tendon of right thigh
    - +7th **S76.212** Strain of adductor muscle, fascia and tendon of left thigh
    - +7th **S76.219** Strain of adductor muscle, fascia and tendon of unspecified thigh
  - **+ S76.22** Laceration of adductor muscle, fascia and tendon of thigh
    - CC +7th **S76.221** Laceration of adductor muscle, fascia and tendon of right thigh
    - CC +7th **S76.222** Laceration of adductor muscle, fascia and tendon of left thigh
    - CC +7th **S76.229** Laceration of adductor muscle, fascia and tendon of unspecified thigh
  - **+ S76.29** Other injury of adductor muscle, fascia and tendon of thigh
    - +7th **S76.291** Other injury of adductor muscle, fascia and tendon of right thigh
    - +7th **S76.292** Other injury of adductor muscle, fascia and tendon of left thigh
    - +7th **S76.299** Other injury of adductor muscle, fascia and tendon of unspecified thigh
- **+ S76.3** Injury of muscle, fascia and tendon of the posterior muscle group at thigh level
  - **+ S76.30** Unspecified injury of muscle, fascia and tendon of the posterior muscle group at thigh level
    - +7th **S76.301** Unspecified injury of muscle, fascia and tendon of the posterior muscle group at thigh level, right thigh
    - +7th **S76.302** Unspecified injury of muscle, fascia and tendon of the posterior muscle group at thigh level, left thigh
    - +7th **S76.309** Unspecified injury of muscle, fascia and tendon of the posterior muscle group at thigh level, unspecified thigh
  - **+ S76.31** Strain of muscle, fascia and tendon of the posterior muscle group at thigh level
    - +7th **S76.311** Strain of muscle, fascia and tendon of the posterior muscle group at thigh level, right thigh
    - +7th **S76.312** Strain of muscle, fascia and tendon of the posterior muscle group at thigh level, left thigh
    - +7th **S76.319** Strain of muscle, fascia and tendon of the posterior muscle group at thigh level, unspecified thigh
  - **+ S76.32** Laceration of muscle, fascia and tendon of the posterior muscle group at thigh level
    - CC +7th **S76.321** Laceration of muscle, fascia and tendon of the posterior muscle group at thigh level, right thigh

- CC +7th **S76.322** Laceration of muscle, fascia and tendon of the posterior muscle group at thigh level, left thigh
- CC +7th **S76.329** Laceration of muscle, fascia and tendon of the posterior muscle group at thigh level, unspecified thigh
- \+ **S76.39** Other specified injury of muscle, fascia and tendon of the posterior muscle group at thigh level
  - +7th **S76.391** Other specified injury of muscle, fascia and tendon of the posterior muscle group at thigh level, right thigh
  - +7th **S76.392** Other specified injury of muscle, fascia and tendon of the posterior muscle group at thigh level, left thigh
  - +7th **S76.399** Other specified injury of muscle, fascia and tendon of the posterior muscle group at thigh level, unspecified thigh
- \+ **S76.8** Injury of other specified muscles, fascia and tendons at thigh level
  - \+ **S76.80** Unspecified injury of other specified muscles, fascia and tendons at thigh level
    - +7th **S76.801** Unspecified injury of other specified muscles, fascia and tendons at thigh level, right thigh
    - +7th **S76.802** Unspecified injury of other specified muscles, fascia and tendons at thigh level, left thigh
    - +7th **S76.809** Unspecified injury of other specified muscles, fascia and tendons at thigh level, unspecified thigh
  - \+ **S76.81** Strain of other specified muscles, fascia and tendons at thigh level
    - +7th **S76.811** Strain of other specified muscles, fascia and tendons at thigh level, right thigh
    - +7th **S76.812** Strain of other specified muscles, fascia and tendons at thigh level, left thigh
    - +7th **S76.819** Strain of other specified muscles, fascia and tendons at thigh level, unspecified thigh
  - \+ **S76.82** Laceration of other specified muscles, fascia and tendons at thigh level
    - CC +7th **S76.821** Laceration of other specified muscles, fascia and tendons at thigh level, right thigh
    - CC +7th **S76.822** Laceration of other specified muscles, fascia and tendons at thigh level, left thigh
    - CC +7th **S76.829** Laceration of other specified muscles, fascia and tendons at thigh level, unspecified thigh
  - \+ **S76.89** Other injury of other specified muscles, fascia and tendons at thigh level
    - +7th **S76.891** Other injury of other specified muscles, fascia and tendons at thigh level, right thigh
    - +7th **S76.892** Other injury of other specified muscles, fascia and tendons at thigh level, left thigh
    - +7th **S76.899** Other injury of other specified muscles, fascia and tendons at thigh level, unspecified thigh
- \+ **S76.9** Injury of unspecified muscles, fascia and tendons at thigh level
  - \+ **S76.90** Unspecified injury of unspecified muscles, fascia and tendons at thigh level
    - +7th **S76.901** Unspecified injury of unspecified muscles, fascia and tendons at thigh level, right thigh
    - +7th **S76.902** Unspecified injury of unspecified muscles, fascia and tendons at thigh level, left thigh
    - +7th **S76.909** Unspecified injury of unspecified muscles, fascia and tendons at thigh level, unspecified thigh
  - \+ **S76.91** Strain of unspecified muscles, fascia and tendons at thigh level
    - +7th **S76.911** Strain of unspecified muscles, fascia and tendons at thigh level, right thigh
    - +7th **S76.912** Strain of unspecified muscles, fascia and tendons at thigh level, left thigh
    - +7th **S76.919** Strain of unspecified muscles, fascia and tendons at thigh level, unspecified thigh
  - \+ **S76.92** Laceration of unspecified muscles, fascia and tendons at thigh level
    - CC +7th **S76.921** Laceration of unspecified muscles, fascia and tendons at thigh level, right thigh
    - CC +7th **S76.922** Laceration of unspecified muscles, fascia and tendons at thigh level, left thigh
    - CC +7th **S76.929** Laceration of unspecified muscles, fascia and tendons at thigh level, unspecified thigh
  - \+ **S76.99** Other specified injury of unspecified muscles, fascia and tendons at thigh level
    - +7th **S76.991** Other specified injury of unspecified muscles, fascia and tendons at thigh level, right thigh
    - +7th **S76.992** Other specified injury of unspecified muscles, fascia and tendons at thigh level, left thigh
    - +7th **S76.999** Other specified injury of unspecified muscles, fascia and tendons at thigh level, unspecified thigh

S77 Crushing injury of hip and thigh

Use additional code(s) for all associated injuries

Excludes2: crushing injury of ankle and foot (S97.-)
crushing injury of lower leg (S87.-)

The appropriate 7th character is to be added to each code from category S77
- A initial encounter
- D subsequent encounter
- S sequela

- \+ **S77.0** Crushing injury of hip
  - CC X+7th **S77.00** Crushing injury of unspecified hip
    - HAC 7th character A see Appendix B for HAC conditional logic
  - CC X+7th **S77.01** Crushing injury of right hip
    - HAC 7th character A see Appendix B for HAC conditional logic
  - CC X+7th **S77.02** Crushing injury of left hip
    - HAC 7th character A see Appendix B for HAC conditional logic
- \+ **S77.1** Crushing injury of thigh
  - CC X+7th **S77.10** Crushing injury of unspecified thigh
    - HAC 7th character A see Appendix B for HAC conditional logic
  - CC X+7th **S77.11** Crushing injury of right thigh
    - HAC 7th character A see Appendix B for HAC conditional logic
  - CC X+7th **S77.12** Crushing injury of left thigh
    - HAC 7th character A see Appendix B for HAC conditional logic
- \+ **S77.2** Crushing injury of hip with thigh
  - X+7th **S77.20** Crushing injury of unspecified hip with thigh
  - X+7th **S77.21** Crushing injury of right hip with thigh
  - X+7th **S77.22** Crushing injury of left hip with thigh

S78 Traumatic amputation of hip and thigh

An amputation not identified as partial or complete should be coded to complete

Excludes1: traumatic amputation of knee (S88.0-)

The appropriate 7th character is to be added to each code from category S78
- A initial encounter
- D subsequent encounter
- S sequela

+ S78.0 Traumatic amputation at hip joint
  + S78.01 Complete traumatic amputation at hip joint
    CC +7th S78.011 Complete traumatic amputation at right hip joint
    CC +7th S78.012 Complete traumatic amputation at left hip joint
    CC +7th S78.019 Complete traumatic amputation at unspecified hip joint
  + S78.02 Partial traumatic amputation at hip joint
    CC +7th S78.021 Partial traumatic amputation at right hip joint
    CC +7th S78.022 Partial traumatic amputation at left hip joint
    CC +7th S78.029 Partial traumatic amputation at unspecified hip joint
+ S78.1 Traumatic amputation at level between hip and knee
  Excludes1: traumatic amputation of knee (S88.0-)
  + S78.11 Complete traumatic amputation at level between hip and knee
    CC +7th S78.111 Complete traumatic amputation at level between right hip and knee
    CC +7th S78.112 Complete traumatic amputation at level between left hip and knee
    CC +7th S78.119 Complete traumatic amputation at level between unspecified hip and knee
  + S78.12 Partial traumatic amputation at level between hip and knee
    CC +7th S78.121 Partial traumatic amputation at level between right hip and knee
    CC +7th S78.122 Partial traumatic amputation at level between left hip and knee
    CC +7th S78.129 Partial traumatic amputation at level between unspecified hip and knee
+ S78.9 Traumatic amputation of hip and thigh, level unspecified
  + S78.91 Complete traumatic amputation of hip and thigh, level unspecified
    CC +7th S78.911 Complete traumatic amputation of right hip and thigh, level unspecified
    CC +7th S78.912 Complete traumatic amputation of left hip and thigh, level unspecified
    CC +7th S78.919 Complete traumatic amputation of unspecified hip and thigh, level unspecified
  + S78.92 Partial traumatic amputation of hip and thigh, level unspecified
    CC +7th S78.921 Partial traumatic amputation of right hip and thigh, level unspecified
    CC +7th S78.922 Partial traumatic amputation of left hip and thigh, level unspecified
    CC +7th S78.929 Partial traumatic amputation of unspecified hip and thigh, level unspecified

S79 Other and unspecified injuries of hip and thigh

> **NOTE** A fracture not indicated as open or closed should be coded to closed

> The appropriate 7th character is to be added to each code from subcategories **S79.0** and **S79.1**
> A initial encounter for closed fracture
> D subsequent encounter for fracture with routine healing
> G subsequent encounter for fracture with delayed healing
> K subsequent encounter for fracture with nonunion
> P subsequent encounter for fracture with malunion
> S sequela

Review coding guideline C.19.c

+ S79.0 Physeal fracture of upper end of femur
  Excludes1: apophyseal fracture of upper end of femur (S72.13-)
  nontraumatic slipped upper femoral epiphysis (M93.0-)
  + S79.00 Unspecified physeal fracture of upper end of femur
    CC MCC +7th S79.001 Unspecified physeal fracture of upper end of right femur
      HAC 7th character A see Appendix B for HAC conditional logic
    CC MCC +7th S79.002 Unspecified physeal fracture of upper end of left femur
      HAC 7th character A see Appendix B for HAC conditional logic
    CC MCC +7th S79.009 Unspecified physeal fracture of upper end of unspecified femur
      HAC 7th character A see Appendix B for HAC conditional logic
  + S79.01 Salter-Harris Type I physeal fracture of upper end of femur
    Acute on chronic slipped capital femoral epiphysis (traumatic)
    Acute slipped capital femoral epiphysis (traumatic)
    Capital femoral epiphyseal fracture
    Excludes1: chronic slipped upper femoral epiphysis(nontraumatic)(M93.02-)
    CC MCC +7th S79.011 Salter-Harris Type I physeal fracture of upper end of right femur
      HAC 7th character A see Appendix B for HAC conditional logic
    CC MCC +7th S79.012 Salter-Harris Type I physeal fracture of upper end of left femur
      HAC 7th character A see Appendix B for HAC conditional logic
    CC MCC +7th S79.019 Salter-Harris Type I physeal fracture of upper end of unspecified femur
      HAC 7th character A see Appendix B for HAC conditional logic
  + S79.09 Other physeal fracture of upper end of femur
    CC MCC +7th S79.091 Other physeal fracture of upper end of right femur
      HAC 7th character A see Appendix B for HAC conditional logic
    CC MCC +7th S79.092 Other physeal fracture of upper end of left femur
      HAC 7th character A see Appendix B for HAC conditional logic
    CC MCC +7th S79.099 Other physeal fracture of upper end of unspecified femur
      HAC 7th character A see Appendix B for HAC conditional logic
+ S79.1 Physeal fracture of lower end of femur
  + S79.10 Unspecified physeal fracture of lower end of femur
    CC +7th S79.101 Unspecified physeal fracture of lower end of right femur
      HAC 7th character A see Appendix B for HAC conditional logic
    CC +7th S79.102 Unspecified physeal fracture of lower end of left femur
      HAC 7th character A see Appendix B for HAC conditional logic
    CC +7th S79.109 Unspecified physeal fracture of lower end of unspecified femur
      HAC 7th character A see Appendix B for HAC conditional logic
  + S79.11 Salter-Harris Type I physeal fracture of lower end of femur
    CC +7th S79.111 Salter-Harris Type I physeal fracture of lower end of right femur
      HAC 7th character A see Appendix B for HAC conditional logic
    CC +7th S79.112 Salter-Harris Type I physeal fracture of lower end of left femur
      HAC 7th character A see Appendix B for HAC conditional logic
    CC +7th S79.119 Salter-Harris Type I physeal fracture of lower end of unspecified femur
      HAC 7th character A see Appendix B for HAC conditional logic
  + S79.12 Salter-Harris Type II physeal fracture of lower end of femur
    CC +7th S79.121 Salter-Harris Type II physeal fracture of lower end of right femur
      HAC 7th character A see Appendix B for HAC conditional logic
    CC +7th S79.122 Salter-Harris Type II physeal fracture of lower end of left femur
      HAC 7th character A see Appendix B for HAC conditional logic
    CC +7th S79.129 Salter-Harris Type II physeal fracture of lower end of unspecified femur
      HAC 7th character A see Appendix B for HAC conditional logic

+ **S79.13** Salter-Harris Type III physeal fracture of lower end of femur
- CC +7th **S79.131** Salter-Harris Type III physeal fracture of lower end of right femur
  - HAC 7th character A see Appendix B for HAC conditional logic
- CC +7th **S79.132** Salter-Harris Type III physeal fracture of lower end of left femur
  - HAC 7th character A see Appendix B for HAC conditional logic
- CC +7th **S79.139** Salter-Harris Type III physeal fracture of lower end of unspecified femur
  - HAC 7th character A see Appendix B for HAC conditional logic

+ **S79.14** Salter-Harris Type IV physeal fracture of lower end of femur
- CC +7th **S79.141** Salter-Harris Type IV physeal fracture of lower end of right femur
  - HAC 7th character A see Appendix B for HAC conditional logic
- CC +7th **S79.142** Salter-Harris Type IV physeal fracture of lower end of left femur
  - HAC 7th character A see Appendix B for HAC conditional logic
- CC +7th **S79.149** Salter-Harris Type IV physeal fracture of lower end of unspecified femur
  - HAC 7th character A see Appendix B for HAC conditional logic

+ **S79.19** Other physeal fracture of lower end of femur
- CC +7th **S79.191** Other physeal fracture of lower end of right femur
  - HAC 7th character A see Appendix B for HAC conditional logic
- CC +7th **S79.192** Other physeal fracture of lower end of left femur
  - HAC 7th character A see Appendix B for HAC conditional logic
- CC +7th **S79.199** Other physeal fracture of lower end of unspecified femur
  - HAC 7th character A see Appendix B for HAC conditional logic

+ **S79.8** Other specified injuries of hip and thigh

The appropriate 7th character is to be added to each code in subcategory **S79.8**
- A initial encounter
- D subsequent encounter
- S sequela

+ **S79.81** Other specified injuries of hip
  - +7th **S79.811** Other specified injuries of right hip
  - +7th **S79.812** Other specified injuries of left hip
  - +7th **S79.819** Other specified injuries of unspecified hip
+ **S79.82** Other specified injuries of thigh
  - +7th **S79.821** Other specified injuries of right thigh
  - +7th **S79.822** Other specified injuries of left thigh
  - +7th **S79.829** Other specified injuries of unspecified thigh

+ **S79.9** Unspecified injury of hip and thigh

The appropriate 7th character is to be added to each code in subcategory **S79.9**
- A - initial encounter
- D - subsequent encounter
- S - sequela

+ **S79.91** Unspecified injury of hip
  - +7th **S79.911** Unspecified injury of right hip
  - +7th **S79.912** Unspecified injury of left hip
  - +7th **S79.919** Unspecified injury of unspecified hip
+ **S79.92** Unspecified injury of thigh
  - +7th **S79.921** Unspecified injury of right thigh
  - +7th **S79.922** Unspecified injury of left thigh
  - +7th **S79.929** Unspecified injury of unspecified thigh

Injuries to the knee and lower leg (S80-S89)

Excludes2: burns and corrosions (T20-T32)
frostbite (T33-T34)
injuries of ankle and foot, except fracture of ankle and malleolus (S90-S99)
insect bite or sting, venomous (T63.4)

S80 Superficial injury of knee and lower leg

Excludes2: superficial injury of ankle and foot (S90.-)

The appropriate 7th character is to be added to each code from category S80
- A initial encounter
- D subsequent encounter
- S sequela

+ **S80.0** Contusion of knee
  - X+7th **S80.00** Contusion of unspecified knee
  - X+7th **S80.01** Contusion of right knee
  - X+7th **S80.02** Contusion of left knee
+ **S80.1** Contusion of lower leg
  - X+7th **S80.10** Contusion of unspecified lower leg
  - X+7th **S80.11** Contusion of right lower leg
  - X+7th **S80.12** Contusion of left lower leg
+ **S80.2** Other superficial injuries of knee
  + **S80.21** Abrasion of knee
    - +7th **S80.211** Abrasion, right knee
    - +7th **S80.212** Abrasion, left knee
    - +7th **S80.219** Abrasion, unspecified knee
  + **S80.22** Blister (nonthermal) of knee
    - +7th **S80.221** Blister (nonthermal), right knee
    - +7th **S80.222** Blister (nonthermal), left knee
    - +7th **S80.229** Blister (nonthermal), unspecified knee
  + **S80.24** External constriction of knee
    - +7th **S80.241** External constriction, right knee
    - +7th **S80.242** External constriction, left knee
    - +7th **S80.249** External constriction, unspecified knee
  + **S80.25** Superficial foreign body of knee
    Splinter in the knee
    - +7th **S80.251** Superficial foreign body, right knee
    - +7th **S80.252** Superficial foreign body, left knee
    - +7th **S80.259** Superficial foreign body, unspecified knee
  + **S80.26** Insect bite (nonvenomous) of knee
    - +7th **S80.261** Insect bite (nonvenomous), right knee
    - +7th **S80.262** Insect bite (nonvenomous), left knee
    - +7th **S80.269** Insect bite (nonvenomous), unspecified knee
  + **S80.27** Other superficial bite of knee
    Excludes1: open bite of knee (S81.05-)
    - +7th **S80.271** Other superficial bite of right knee
    - +7th **S80.272** Other superficial bite of left knee
    - +7th **S80.279** Other superficial bite of unspecified knee
+ **S80.8** Other superficial injuries of lower leg
  + **S80.81** Abrasion of lower leg
    - +7th **S80.811** Abrasion, right lower leg
    - +7th **S80.812** Abrasion, left lower leg
    - +7th **S80.819** Abrasion, unspecified lower leg
  + **S80.82** Blister (nonthermal) of lower leg
    - +7th **S80.821** Blister (nonthermal), right lower leg
    - +7th **S80.822** Blister (nonthermal), left lower leg
    - +7th **S80.829** Blister (nonthermal), unspecified lower leg
  + **S80.84** External constriction of lower leg
    - +7th **S80.841** External constriction, right lower leg
    - +7th **S80.842** External constriction, left lower leg
    - +7th **S80.849** External constriction, unspecified lower leg
  + **S80.85** Superficial foreign body of lower leg
    Splinter in the lower leg
    - +7th **S80.851** Superficial foreign body, right lower leg
    - +7th **S80.852** Superficial foreign body, left lower leg
    - +7th **S80.859** Superficial foreign body, unspecified lower leg

- **+ S80.86 Insect bite (nonvenomous) of lower leg**
  - +7th S80.861 Insect bite (nonvenomous), right lower leg
  - +7th S80.862 Insect bite (nonvenomous), left lower leg
  - +7th S80.869 Insect bite (nonvenomous), unspecified lower leg
- **+ S80.87 Other superficial bite of lower leg**
  - *Excludes1:* *open bite of lower leg (S81.85-)*
  - +7th S80.871 Other superficial bite, right lower leg
  - +7th S80.872 Other superficial bite, left lower leg
  - +7th S80.879 Other superficial bite, unspecified lower leg
- **+ S80.9 Unspecified superficial injury of knee and lower leg**
  - **+ S80.91 Unspecified superficial injury of knee**
    - +7th S80.911 Unspecified superficial injury of right knee
    - +7th S80.912 Unspecified superficial injury of left knee
    - +7th S80.919 Unspecified superficial injury of unspecified knee
  - **+ S80.92 Unspecified superficial injury of lower leg**
    - +7th S80.921 Unspecified superficial injury of right lower leg
    - +7th S80.922 Unspecified superficial injury of left lower leg
    - +7th S80.929 Unspecified superficial injury of unspecified lower leg

S81 Open wound of knee and lower leg

Code also any associated wound infection

Excludes1: open fracture of knee and lower leg (S82.-)
traumatic amputation of lower leg (S88.-)

Excludes2: open wound of ankle and foot (S91.-)

The appropriate 7th character is to be added to each code from category S81
- A   initial encounter
- D   subsequent encounter
- S   sequela

- **S81.0   Open wound of knee**
  - **S81.00   Unspecified open wound of knee**
    - +7th S81.001   Unspecified open wound, right knee
    - +7th S81.002   Unspecified open wound, left knee
    - +7th S81.009   Unspecified open wound, unspecified knee
  - **S81.01   Laceration without foreign body of knee**
    - +7th S81.011   Laceration without foreign body, right knee
    - +7th S81.012   Laceration without foreign body, left knee
    - +7th S81.019   Laceration without foreign body, unspecified knee
  - **S81.02   Laceration with foreign body of knee**
    - +7th S81.021   Laceration with foreign body, right knee
    - +7th S81.022   Laceration with foreign body, left knee
    - +7th S81.029   Laceration with foreign body, unspecified knee
  - **S81.03   Puncture wound without foreign body of knee**
    - +7th S81.031   Puncture wound without foreign body, right knee
    - +7th S81.032   Puncture wound without foreign body, left knee
    - +7th S81.039   Puncture wound without foreign body, unspecified knee
  - **S81.04   Puncture wound with foreign body of knee**
    - +7th S81.041   Puncture wound with foreign body, right knee
    - +7th S81.042   Puncture wound with foreign body, left knee
    - +7th S81.049   Puncture wound with foreign body, unspecified knee
  - **S81.05   Open bite of knee**
    Bite of knee NOS
    Excludes1: superficial bite of knee (S80.27-)
    - +7th S81.051   Open bite, right knee
    - +7th S81.052   Open bite, left knee
    - +7th S81.059   Open bite, unspecified knee

- **S81.8   Open wound of lower leg**
  - **S81.80   Unspecified open wound of lower leg**
    - +7th S81.801   Unspecified open wound, right lower leg
    - +7th S81.802   Unspecified open wound, left lower leg
    - +7th S81.809   Unspecified open wound, unspecified lower leg
  - **S81.81   Laceration without foreign body of lower leg**
    - +7th S81.811   Laceration without foreign body, right lower leg
    - +7th S81.812   Laceration without foreign body, left lower leg
    - +7th S81.819   Laceration without foreign body, unspecified lower leg
  - **S81.82   Laceration with foreign body of lower leg**
    - +7th S81.821   Laceration with foreign body, right lower leg
    - +7th S81.822   Laceration with foreign body, left lower leg
    - +7th S81.829   Laceration with foreign body, unspecified lower leg
  - **S81.83   Puncture wound without foreign body of lower leg**
    - +7th S81.831   Puncture wound without foreign body, right lower leg
    - +7th S81.832   Puncture wound without foreign body, left lower leg
    - +7th S81.839   Puncture wound without foreign body, unspecified lower leg
  - **S81.84   Puncture wound with foreign body of lower leg**
    - +7th S81.841   Puncture wound with foreign body, right lower leg
      AHA CC: 3Q, 2016, 24
    - +7th S81.842   Puncture wound with foreign body, left lower leg
    - +7th S81.849   Puncture wound with foreign body, unspecified lower leg
  - **S81.85   Open bite of lower leg**
    Bite of lower leg NOS
    Excludes1: superficial bite of lower leg (S80.86-, S80.87-)
    - +7th S81.851   Open bite, right lower leg
    - +7th S81.852   Open bite, left lower leg
    - +7th S81.859   Open bite, unspecified lower leg

S82 Fracture of lower leg, including ankle

NOTE   A fracture not indicated as displaced or nondisplaced should be coded to displaced
A fracture not indicated as open or closed should be coded to closed
The open fracture designations are based on the Gustilo open fracture classification

Includes: fracture of malleolus

Excludes1: traumatic amputation of lower leg (S88.-)

Excludes2: fracture of foot, except ankle (S92.-)
periprosthetic fracture around internal prosthetic ankle joint (M97.2)
periprosthetic fracture around internal prosthetic implant of knee joint (M97.1-)

The appropriate 7th character is to be added to all codes from category S82
- A   initial encounter for closed fracture
- B   initial encounter for open fracture type I or II
       initial encounter for open fracture NOS
- C   initial encounter for open fracture type IIIA, IIIB, or IIIC
- D   subsequent encounter for closed fracture with routine healing
- E   subsequent encounter for open fracture type I or II with routine healing
- F   subsequent encounter for open fracture type IIIA, IIIB, or IIIC with routine healing
- G   subsequent encounter for closed fracture with delayed healing
- H   subsequent encounter for open fracture type I or II with delayed healing
- J   subsequent encounter for open fracture type IIIA, IIIB, or IIIC with delayed healing
- K   subsequent encounter for closed fracture with nonunion
- M   subsequent encounter for open fracture type I or II with nonunion
- N   subsequent encounter for open fracture type IIIA, IIIB, or IIIC with nonunion
- P   subsequent encounter for closed fracture with malunion
- Q   subsequent encounter for open fracture type I or II with malunion
- R   subsequent encounter for open fracture type IIIA, IIIB, or IIIC with malunion
- S   sequela

Review coding guideline C.19.c

- **S82.0   Fracture of patella**
  Knee cap
  - **S82.00   Unspecified fracture of patella**
    - CC +7th S82.001   Unspecified fracture of right patella
      HAC 7th characters A - C see Appendix B for HAC conditional logic
    - CC +7th S82.002   Unspecified fracture of left patella
      HAC 7th characters A - C see Appendix B for HAC conditional logic
    - CC +7th S82.009   Unspecified fracture of unspecified patella
      HAC 7th characters A - C see Appendix B for HAC conditional logic

+ **S82.01 Osteochondral fracture of patella**
  CC +7th **S82.011** Displaced osteochondral fracture of right patella
  HAC 7th characters A - C see Appendix B for HAC conditional logic
  CC +7th **S82.012** Displaced osteochondral fracture of left patella
  HAC 7th characters A - C see Appendix B for HAC conditional logic
  CC +7th **S82.013** Displaced osteochondral fracture of unspecified patella
  HAC 7th characters A - C see Appendix B for HAC conditional logic
  CC +7th **S82.014** Nondisplaced osteochondral fracture of right patella
  HAC 7th characters A - C see Appendix B for HAC conditional logic
  CC +7th **S82.015** Nondisplaced osteochondral fracture of left patella
  HAC 7th characters A - C see Appendix B for HAC conditional logic
  CC +7th **S82.016** Nondisplaced osteochondral fracture of unspecified patella
  HAC 7th characters A - C see Appendix B for HAC conditional logic

+ **S82.02 Longitudinal fracture of patella**
  CC +7th **S82.021** Displaced longitudinal fracture of right patella
  HAC 7th characters A - C see Appendix B for HAC conditional logic
  CC +7th **S82.022** Displaced longitudinal fracture of left patella
  HAC 7th characters A - C see Appendix B for HAC conditional logic
  CC +7th **S82.023** Displaced longitudinal fracture of unspecified patella
  HAC 7th characters A - C see Appendix B for HAC conditional logic
  CC +7th **S82.024** Nondisplaced longitudinal fracture of right patella
  HAC 7th characters A - C see Appendix B for HAC conditional logic
  CC +7th **S82.025** Nondisplaced longitudinal fracture of left patella
  HAC 7th characters A - C see Appendix B for HAC conditional logic
  CC +7th **S82.026** Nondisplaced longitudinal fracture of unspecified patella
  HAC 7th characters A - C see Appendix B for HAC conditional logic

+ **S82.03 Transverse fracture of patella**
  CC +7th **S82.031** Displaced transverse fracture of right patella
  HAC 7th characters A - C see Appendix B for HAC conditional logic
  CC +7th **S82.032** Displaced transverse fracture of left patella
  HAC 7th characters A - C see Appendix B for HAC conditional logic
  CC +7th **S82.033** Displaced transverse fracture of unspecified patella
  HAC 7th characters A - C see Appendix B for HAC conditional logic
  CC +7th **S82.034** Nondisplaced transverse fracture of right patella
  HAC 7th characters A - C see Appendix B for HAC conditional logic
  CC +7th **S82.035** Nondisplaced transverse fracture of left patella
  HAC 7th characters A - C see Appendix B for HAC conditional logic
  CC +7th **S82.036** Nondisplaced transverse fracture of unspecified patella
  HAC 7th characters A - C see Appendix B for HAC conditional logic

+ **S82.04 Comminuted fracture of patella**
  CC +7th **S82.041** Displaced comminuted fracture of right patella
  HAC 7th characters A - C see Appendix B for HAC conditional logic
  CC +7th **S82.042** Displaced comminuted fracture of left patella
  HAC 7th characters A - C see Appendix B for HAC conditional logic
  CC +7th **S82.043** Displaced comminuted fracture of unspecified patella
  HAC 7th characters A - C see Appendix B for HAC conditional logic
  CC +7th **S82.044** Nondisplaced comminuted fracture of right patella
  HAC 7th characters A - C see Appendix B for HAC conditional logic
  CC +7th **S82.045** Nondisplaced comminuted fracture of left patella
  HAC 7th characters A - C see Appendix B for HAC conditional logic
  CC +7th **S82.046** Nondisplaced comminuted fracture of unspecified patella
  HAC 7th characters A - C see Appendix B for HAC conditional logic

+ **S82.09 Other fracture of patella**
  CC +7th **S82.091** Other fracture of right patella
  HAC 7th characters A - C see Appendix B for HAC conditional logic
  CC +7th **S82.092** Other fracture of left patella
  HAC 7th characters A - C see Appendix B for HAC conditional logic
  CC +7th **S82.099** Other fracture of unspecified patella
  HAC 7th characters A - C see Appendix B for HAC conditional logic

+ **S82.1 Fracture of upper end of tibia**
  Fracture of proximal end of tibia
  Excludes2: *fracture of shaft of tibia (S82.2-)*
  physeal fracture of upper end of tibia (S89.0-)

+ **S82.10 Unspecified fracture of upper end of tibia**
  CC MCC +7th **S82.101** Unspecified fracture of upper end of right tibia
  HAC 7th characters A - C see Appendix B for HAC conditional logic
  CC MCC +7th **S82.102** Unspecified fracture of upper end of left tibia
  HAC 7th characters A - C see Appendix B for HAC conditional logic
  CC MCC +7th **S82.109** Unspecified fracture of upper end of unspecified tibia
  HAC 7th characters A - C see Appendix B for HAC conditional logic

+ **S82.11 Fracture of tibial spine**
  CC MCC +7th **S82.111** Displaced fracture of right tibial spine
  HAC 7th characters A - C see Appendix B for HAC conditional logic
  CC MCC +7th **S82.112** Displaced fracture of left tibial spine
  HAC 7th characters A - C see Appendix B for HAC conditional logic
  CC MCC +7th **S82.113** Displaced fracture of unspecified tibial spine
  HAC 7th characters A - C see Appendix B for HAC conditional logic
  CC MCC +7th **S82.114** Nondisplaced fracture of right tibial spine
  HAC 7th characters A - C see Appendix B for HAC conditional logic
  CC MCC +7th **S82.115** Nondisplaced fracture of left tibial spine
  HAC 7th characters A - C see Appendix B for HAC conditional logic
  CC MCC +7th **S82.116** Nondisplaced fracture of unspecified tibial spine
  HAC 7th characters A - C see Appendix B for HAC conditional logic

- **S82.12 Fracture of lateral condyle of tibia**
  - CC MCC +7th **S82.121** Displaced fracture of lateral condyle of right tibia
    - HAC 7th characters A – C see Appendix B for HAC conditional logic
  - CC MCC +7th **S82.122** Displaced fracture of lateral condyle of left tibia
    - HAC 7th characters A – C see Appendix B for HAC conditional logic
  - CC MCC +7th **S82.123** Displaced fracture of lateral condyle of unspecified tibia
    - HAC 7th characters A – C see Appendix B for HAC conditional logic
  - CC MCC +7th **S82.124** Nondisplaced fracture of lateral condyle of right tibia
    - HAC 7th characters A – C see Appendix B for HAC conditional logic
  - CC MCC +7th **S82.125** Nondisplaced fracture of lateral condyle of left tibia
    - HAC 7th characters A – C see Appendix B for HAC conditional logic
  - CC MCC +7th **S82.126** Nondisplaced fracture of lateral condyle of unspecified tibia
    - HAC 7th characters A – C see Appendix B for HAC conditional logic
- **S82.13 Fracture of medial condyle of tibia**
  - CC MCC +7th **S82.131** Displaced fracture of medial condyle of right tibia
    - HAC 7th characters A – C see Appendix B for HAC conditional logic
  - CC MCC +7th **S82.132** Displaced fracture of medial condyle of left tibia
    - HAC 7th characters A – C see Appendix B for HAC conditional logic
  - CC MCC +7th **S82.133** Displaced fracture of medial condyle of unspecified tibia
    - HAC 7th characters A – C see Appendix B for HAC conditional logic
  - CC MCC +7th **S82.134** Nondisplaced fracture of medial condyle of right tibia
    - HAC 7th characters A – C see Appendix B for HAC conditional logic
  - CC MCC +7th **S82.135** Nondisplaced fracture of medial condyle of left tibia
    - HAC 7th characters A – C see Appendix B for HAC conditional logic
  - CC MCC +7th **S82.136** Nondisplaced fracture of medial condyle of unspecified tibia
    - HAC 7th characters A – C see Appendix B for HAC conditional logic
- **S82.14 Bicondylar fracture of tibia**
  - Fracture of tibial plateau NOS
  - CC MCC +7th **S82.141** Displaced bicondylar fracture of right tibia
    - HAC 7th characters A – C see Appendix B for HAC conditional logic
  - CC MCC +7th **S82.142** Displaced bicondylar fracture of left tibia
    - HAC 7th characters A – C see Appendix B for HAC conditional logic
  - CC MCC +7th **S82.143** Displaced bicondylar fracture of unspecified tibia
    - HAC 7th characters A – C see Appendix B for HAC conditional logic
  - CC MCC +7th **S82.144** Nondisplaced bicondylar fracture of right tibia
    - HAC 7th characters A – C see Appendix B for HAC conditional logic
  - CC MCC +7th **S82.145** Nondisplaced bicondylar fracture of left tibia
    - HAC 7th characters A – C see Appendix B for HAC conditional logic
  - CC MCC +7th **S82.146** Nondisplaced bicondylar fracture of unspecified tibia
    - HAC 7th characters A – C see Appendix B for HAC conditional logic
- **S82.15 Fracture of tibial tuberosity**
  - CC MCC +7th **S82.151** Displaced fracture of right tibial tuberosity
    - HAC 7th characters A – C see Appendix B for HAC conditional logic
  - CC MCC +7th **S82.152** Displaced fracture of left tibial tuberosity
    - HAC 7th characters A – C see Appendix B for HAC conditional logic
  - CC MCC +7th **S82.153** Displaced fracture of unspecified tibial tuberosity
    - HAC 7th characters A – C see Appendix B for HAC conditional logic
  - CC MCC +7th **S82.154** Nondisplaced fracture of right tibial tuberosity
    - HAC 7th characters A – C see Appendix B for HAC conditional logic
  - CC MCC +7th **S82.155** Nondisplaced fracture of left tibial tuberosity
    - HAC 7th characters A – C see Appendix B for HAC conditional logic
  - CC MCC +7th **S82.156** Nondisplaced fracture of unspecified tibial tuberosity
    - HAC 7th characters A – C see Appendix B for HAC conditional logic
- **S82.16 Torus fracture of upper end of tibia**

  > The appropriate 7th character is to be added to all codes in subcategory **S82.16**
  > A initial encounter for closed fracture
  > D subsequent encounter for fracture with routine healing
  > G subsequent encounter for fracture with delayed healing
  > K subsequent encounter for fracture with nonunion
  > P subsequent encounter for fracture with malunion
  > S sequela

  - CC +7th **S82.161** Torus fracture of upper end of right tibia
    - HAC 7th character A see Appendix B for HAC conditional logic
  - CC +7th **S82.162** Torus fracture of upper end of left tibia
    - HAC 7th character A see Appendix B for HAC conditional logic
  - CC +7th **S82.169** Torus fracture of upper end of unspecified tibia
    - HAC 7th character A see Appendix B for HAC conditional logic
- **S82.19 Other fracture of upper end of tibia**
  - CC MCC +7th **S82.191** Other fracture of upper end of right tibia
    - HAC 7th characters A – C see Appendix B for HAC conditional logic
  - CC MCC +7th **S82.192** Other fracture of upper end of left tibia
    - HAC 7th characters A – C see Appendix B for HAC conditional logic
  - CC MCC +7th **S82.199** Other fracture of upper end of unspecified tibia
    - HAC 7th characters A – C see Appendix B for HAC conditional logic
- **S82.2 Fracture of shaft of tibia**
  - **S82.20 Unspecified fracture of shaft of tibia**
    - Fracture of tibia NOS
    - CC MCC +7th **S82.201** Unspecified fracture of shaft of right tibia
      - HAC 7th characters A – C see Appendix B for HAC conditional logic
    - CC MCC +7th **S82.202** Unspecified fracture of shaft of left tibia
      - HAC 7th characters A – C see Appendix B for HAC conditional logic
    - CC MCC +7th **S82.209** Unspecified fracture of shaft of unspecified tibia
      - HAC 7th characters A – C see Appendix B for HAC conditional logic
  - **S82.22 Transverse fracture of shaft of tibia**
    - CC MCC +7th **S82.221** Displaced transverse fracture of shaft of right tibia
      - HAC 7th characters A – C see Appendix B for HAC conditional logic

CC MCC +7th S82.222 Displaced transverse fracture of shaft of left tibia
　　HAC 7th characters A - C see Appendix B for HAC conditional logic

CC MCC +7th S82.223 Displaced transverse fracture of shaft of unspecified tibia
　　HAC 7th characters A - C see Appendix B for HAC conditional logic

CC MCC +7th S82.224 Nondisplaced transverse fracture of shaft of right tibia
　　HAC 7th characters A - C see Appendix B for HAC conditional logic

CC MCC +7th S82.225 Nondisplaced transverse fracture of shaft of left tibia
　　HAC 7th characters A - C see Appendix B for HAC conditional logic

CC MCC +7th S82.226 Nondisplaced transverse fracture of shaft of unspecified tibia
　　HAC 7th characters A - C see Appendix B for HAC conditional logic

+ S82.23 Oblique fracture of shaft of tibia

CC MCC +7th S82.231 Displaced oblique fracture of shaft of right tibia
　　HAC 7th characters A - C see Appendix B for HAC conditional logic

CC MCC +7th S82.232 Displaced oblique fracture of shaft of left tibia
　　HAC 7th characters A - C see Appendix B for HAC conditional logic

CC MCC +7th S82.233 Displaced oblique fracture of shaft of unspecified tibia
　　HAC 7th characters A - C see Appendix B for HAC conditional logic

CC MCC +7th S82.234 Nondisplaced oblique fracture of shaft of right tibia
　　HAC 7th characters A - C see Appendix B for HAC conditional logic
　　AHA CC: 1Q, 2015, 3-21

CC MCC +7th S82.235 Nondisplaced oblique fracture of shaft of left tibia
　　HAC 7th characters A - C see Appendix B for HAC conditional logic

CC MCC +7th S82.236 Nondisplaced oblique fracture of shaft of unspecified tibia
　　HAC 7th characters A - C see Appendix B for HAC conditional logic

+ S82.24 Spiral fracture of shaft of tibia
　　Toddler fracture

CC MCC +7th S82.241 Displaced spiral fracture of shaft of right tibia
　　HAC 7th characters A - C see Appendix B for HAC conditional logic

CC MCC +7th S82.242 Displaced spiral fracture of shaft of left tibia
　　HAC 7th characters A - C see Appendix B for HAC conditional logic

CC MCC +7th S82.243 Displaced spiral fracture of shaft of unspecified tibia
　　HAC 7th characters A - C see Appendix B for HAC conditional logic

CC MCC +7th S82.244 Nondisplaced spiral fracture of shaft of right tibia
　　HAC 7th characters A - C see Appendix B for HAC conditional logic

CC MCC +7th S82.245 Nondisplaced spiral fracture of shaft of left tibia
　　HAC 7th characters A - C see Appendix B for HAC conditional logic

CC MCC +7th S82.246 Nondisplaced spiral fracture of shaft of unspecified tibia
　　HAC 7th characters A - C see Appendix B for HAC conditional logic

+ S82.25 Comminuted fracture of shaft of tibia

CC MCC +7th S82.251 Displaced comminuted fracture of shaft of right tibia
　　HAC 7th characters A - C see Appendix B for HAC conditional logic
　　AHA CC: 2Q, 2015, 6-7

CC MCC +7th S82.252 Displaced comminuted fracture of shaft of left tibia
　　HAC 7th characters A - C see Appendix B for HAC conditional logic

CC MCC +7th S82.253 Displaced comminuted fracture of shaft of unspecified tibia
　　HAC 7th characters A - C see Appendix B for HAC conditional logic

CC MCC +7th S82.254 Nondisplaced comminuted fracture of shaft of right tibia
　　HAC 7th characters A - C see Appendix B for HAC conditional logic

CC MCC +7th S82.255 Nondisplaced comminuted fracture of shaft of left tibia
　　HAC 7th characters A - C see Appendix B for HAC conditional logic

CC MCC +7th S82.256 Nondisplaced comminuted fracture of shaft of unspecified tibia
　　HAC 7th characters A - C see Appendix B for HAC conditional logic

+ S82.26 Segmental fracture of shaft of tibia

CC MCC +7th S82.261 Displaced segmental fracture of shaft of right tibia
　　HAC 7th characters A - C see Appendix B for HAC conditional logic

CC MCC +7th S82.262 Displaced segmental fracture of shaft of left tibia
　　HAC 7th characters A - C see Appendix B for HAC conditional logic

CC MCC +7th S82.263 Displaced segmental fracture of shaft of unspecified tibia
　　HAC 7th characters A - C see Appendix B for HAC conditional logic

CC MCC +7th S82.264 Nondisplaced segmental fracture of shaft of right tibia
　　HAC 7th characters A - C see Appendix B for HAC conditional logic

CC MCC +7th S82.265 Nondisplaced segmental fracture of shaft of left tibia
　　HAC 7th characters A - C see Appendix B for HAC conditional logic

CC MCC +7th S82.266 Nondisplaced segmental fracture of shaft of unspecified tibia
　　HAC 7th characters A - C see Appendix B for HAC conditional logic

+ S82.29 Other fracture of shaft of tibia

CC MCC +7th S82.291 Other fracture of shaft of right tibia
　　HAC 7th characters A - C see Appendix B for HAC conditional logic

CC MCC +7th S82.292 Other fracture of shaft of left tibia
　　HAC 7th characters A - C see Appendix B for HAC conditional logic

CC MCC +7th S82.299 Other fracture of shaft of unspecified tibia
　　HAC 7th characters A - C see Appendix B for HAC conditional logic

+ S82.3 Fracture of lower end of tibia
  Excludes1: bimalleolar fracture of lower leg (S82.84-)
  fracture of medial malleolus alone (S82.5-)
  Maisonneuve's fracture (S82.86-)
  pilon fracture of distal tibia (S82.87-)
  trimalleolar fractures of lower leg (S82.85-)

  + S82.30 Unspecified fracture of lower end of tibia
  CC +7th **S82.301** Unspecified fracture of lower end of right tibia
    HAC 7th characters B & C see Appendix B for HAC conditional logic
  CC +7th **S82.302** Unspecified fracture of lower end of left tibia
    HAC 7th characters B & C see Appendix B for HAC conditional logic
  CC +7th **S82.309** Unspecified fracture of lower end of unspecified tibia
    HAC 7th characters B & C see Appendix B for HAC conditional logic

  + S82.31 Torus fracture of lower end of tibia

  > The appropriate 7th character is to be added to all codes in subcategory S82.31
  > A initial encounter for closed fracture
  > D subsequent encounter for fracture with routine healing
  > G subsequent encounter for fracture with delayed healing
  > K subsequent encounter for fracture with nonunion
  > P subsequent encounter for fracture with malunion
  > S sequela

  CC +7th **S82.311** Torus fracture of lower end of right tibia
    HAC 7th character A see Appendix B for HAC conditional logic
  CC +7th **S82.312** Torus fracture of lower end of left tibia
    HAC 7th character A see Appendix B for HAC conditional logic
  CC +7th **S82.319** Torus fracture of lower end of unspecified tibia
    HAC 7th character A see Appendix B for HAC conditional logic

  + S82.39 Other fracture of lower end of tibia
  CC +7th **S82.391** Other fracture of lower end of right tibia
    HAC 7th characters B & C see Appendix B for HAC conditional logic
  CC +7th **S82.392** Other fracture of lower end of left tibia
    HAC 7th characters B & C see Appendix B for HAC conditional logic
    AHA CC: 1Q, 2015, 25
  CC +7th **S82.399** Other fracture of lower end of unspecified tibia
    HAC 7th characters B & C see Appendix B for HAC conditional logic

+ S82.4 Fracture of shaft of fibula
  Excludes2: fracture of lateral malleolus alone (S82.6-)

  + S82.40 Unspecified fracture of shaft of fibula
  CC MCC +7th **S82.401** Unspecified fracture of shaft of right fibula
    HAC 7th characters B & C see Appendix B for HAC conditional logic
  CC MCC +7th **S82.402** Unspecified fracture of shaft of left fibula
    HAC 7th characters B & C see Appendix B for HAC conditional logic
  CC MCC +7th **S82.409** Unspecified fracture of shaft of unspecified fibula
    HAC 7th characters B & C see Appendix B for HAC conditional logic

  + S82.42 Transverse fracture of shaft of fibula
  CC MCC +7th **S82.421** Displaced transverse fracture of shaft of right fibula
    HAC 7th characters B & C see Appendix B for HAC conditional logic
  CC MCC +7th **S82.422** Displaced transverse fracture of shaft of left fibula
    HAC 7th characters B & C see Appendix B for HAC conditional logic
  CC MCC +7th **S82.423** Displaced transverse fracture of shaft of unspecified fibula
    HAC 7th characters B & C see Appendix B for HAC conditional logic
  CC MCC +7th **S82.424** Nondisplaced transverse fracture of shaft of right fibula
    HAC 7th characters B & C see Appendix B for HAC conditional logic
  CC MCC +7th **S82.425** Nondisplaced transverse fracture of shaft of left fibula
    HAC 7th characters B & C see Appendix B for HAC conditional logic
  CC MCC +7th **S82.426** Nondisplaced transverse fracture of shaft of unspecified fibula
    HAC 7th characters B & C see Appendix B for HAC conditional logic

  + S82.43 Oblique fracture of shaft of fibula
  CC MCC +7th **S82.431** Displaced oblique fracture of shaft of right fibula
    HAC 7th characters B & C see Appendix B for HAC conditional logic
  CC MCC +7th **S82.432** Displaced oblique fracture of shaft of left fibula
    HAC 7th characters B & C see Appendix B for HAC conditional logic
  CC MCC +7th **S82.433** Displaced oblique fracture of shaft of unspecified fibula
    HAC 7th characters B & C see Appendix B for HAC conditional logic
  CC MCC +7th **S82.434** Nondisplaced oblique fracture of shaft of right fibula
    HAC 7th characters B & C see Appendix B for HAC conditional logic
  CC MCC +7th **S82.435** Nondisplaced oblique fracture of shaft of left fibula
    HAC 7th characters B & C see Appendix B for HAC conditional logic
  CC MCC +7th **S82.436** Nondisplaced oblique fracture of shaft of unspecified fibula
    HAC 7th characters B & C see Appendix B for HAC conditional logic

  + S82.44 Spiral fracture of shaft of fibula
  CC MCC +7th **S82.441** Displaced spiral fracture of shaft of right fibula
    HAC 7th characters B & C see Appendix B for HAC conditional logic
  CC MCC +7th **S82.442** Displaced spiral fracture of shaft of left fibula
    HAC 7th characters B & C see Appendix B for HAC conditional logic
  CC MCC +7th **S82.443** Displaced spiral fracture of shaft of unspecified fibula
    HAC 7th characters B & C see Appendix B for HAC conditional logic
  CC MCC +7th **S82.444** Nondisplaced spiral fracture of shaft of right fibula
    HAC 7th characters B & C see Appendix B for HAC conditional logic
  CC MCC +7th **S82.445** Nondisplaced spiral fracture of shaft of left fibula
    HAC 7th characters B & C see Appendix B for HAC conditional logic
  CC MCC +7th **S82.446** Nondisplaced spiral fracture of shaft of unspecified fibula
    HAC 7th characters B & C see Appendix B for HAC conditional logic

  + S82.45 Comminuted fracture of shaft of fibula
  CC MCC +7th **S82.451** Displaced comminuted fracture of shaft of right fibula
    HAC 7th characters B & C see Appendix B for HAC conditional logic
  CC MCC +7th **S82.452** Displaced comminuted fracture of shaft of left fibula
    HAC 7th characters B & C see Appendix B for HAC conditional logic
  CC MCC +7th **S82.453** Displaced comminuted fracture of shaft of unspecified fibula
    HAC 7th characters B & C see Appendix B for HAC conditional logic
  CC MCC +7th **S82.454** Nondisplaced comminuted fracture of shaft of right fibula
    HAC 7th characters B & C see Appendix B for HAC conditional logic

CC MCC +7th	S82.455	Nondisplaced comminuted fracture of shaft of left fibula
		HAC 7th characters B & C see Appendix B for HAC conditional logic
CC MCC +7th	S82.456	Nondisplaced comminuted fracture of shaft of unspecified fibula
		HAC 7th characters B & C see Appendix B for HAC conditional logic
+	S82.46	Segmental fracture of shaft of fibula
CC MCC +7th	S82.461	Displaced segmental fracture of shaft of right fibula
		HAC 7th characters B & C see Appendix B for HAC conditional logic
CC MCC +7th	S82.462	Displaced segmental fracture of shaft of left fibula
		HAC 7th characters B & C see Appendix B for HAC conditional logic
CC MCC +7th	S82.463	Displaced segmental fracture of shaft of unspecified fibula
		HAC 7th characters B & C see Appendix B for HAC conditional logic
CC MCC +7th	S82.464	Nondisplaced segmental fracture of shaft of right fibula
		HAC 7th characters B & C see Appendix B for HAC conditional logic
CC MCC +7th	S82.465	Nondisplaced segmental fracture of shaft of left fibula
		HAC 7th characters B & C see Appendix B for HAC conditional logic
CC MCC +7th	S82.466	Nondisplaced segmental fracture of shaft of unspecified fibula
		HAC 7th characters B & C see Appendix B for HAC conditional logic
+	S82.49	Other fracture of shaft of fibula
CC MCC +7th	S82.491	Other fracture of shaft of right fibula
		HAC 7th characters B & C see Appendix B for HAC conditional logic
CC MCC +7th	S82.492	Other fracture of shaft of left fibula
		HAC 7th characters B & C see Appendix B for HAC conditional logic
CC MCC +7th	S82.499	Other fracture of shaft of unspecified fibula
		HAC 7th characters B & C see Appendix B for HAC conditional logic
+	S82.5	**Fracture of medial malleolus**
		Excludes1: *pilon fracture of distal tibia (S82.87-)*
		Salter-Harris type III of lower end of tibia (S89.13-)
		Salter-Harris type IV of lower end of tibia (S89.14-)
CC X+7th	S82.51	Displaced fracture of medial malleolus of right tibia
		HAC 7th characters B & C see Appendix B for HAC conditional logic
CC X+7th	S82.52	Displaced fracture of medial malleolus of left tibia
		HAC 7th characters B & C see Appendix B for HAC conditional logic
CC X+7th	S82.53	Displaced fracture of medial malleolus of unspecified tibia
		HAC 7th characters B & C see Appendix B for HAC conditional logic
CC X+7th	S82.54	Nondisplaced fracture of medial malleolus of right tibia
		HAC 7th characters B & C see Appendix B for HAC conditional logic
CC X+7th	S82.55	Nondisplaced fracture of medial malleolus of left tibia
		HAC 7th characters B & C see Appendix B for HAC conditional logic
CC X+7th	S82.56	Nondisplaced fracture of medial malleolus of unspecified tibia
		HAC 7th characters B & C see Appendix B for HAC conditional logic

+	S82.6	**Fracture of lateral malleolus**
		Excludes1: *pilon fracture of distal tibia (S82.87-)*
CC X+7th	S82.61	Displaced fracture of lateral malleolus of right fibula
		HAC 7th characters B & C see Appendix B for HAC conditional logic
CC X+7th	S82.62	Displaced fracture of lateral malleolus of left fibula
		HAC 7th characters B & C see Appendix B for HAC conditional logic
CC X+7th	S82.63	Displaced fracture of lateral malleolus of unspecified fibula
		HAC 7th characters B & C see Appendix B for HAC conditional logic
CC X+7th	S82.64	Nondisplaced fracture of lateral malleolus of right fibula
		HAC 7th characters B & C see Appendix B for HAC conditional logic
CC X+7th	S82.65	Nondisplaced fracture of lateral malleolus of left fibula
		HAC 7th characters B & C see Appendix B for HAC conditional logic
CC X+7th	S82.66	Nondisplaced fracture of lateral malleolus of unspecified fibula
		HAC 7th characters B & C see Appendix B for HAC conditional logic
+	S82.8	**Other fractures of lower leg**
+	S82.81	Torus fracture of upper end of fibula

The appropriate 7th character is to be added to all codes in subcategory **S82.81**
A initial encounter for closed fracture
D subsequent encounter for fracture with routine healing
G subsequent encounter for fracture with delayed healing
K subsequent encounter for fracture with nonunion
P subsequent encounter for fracture with malunion
S sequela

CC +7th	S82.811	Torus fracture of upper end of right fibula
CC +7th	S82.812	Torus fracture of upper end of left fibula
CC +7th	S82.819	Torus fracture of upper end of unspecified fibula
+	S82.82	Torus fracture of lower end of fibula

The appropriate 7th character is to be added to all codes in subcategory **S82.82**
A initial encounter for closed fracture
D subsequent encounter for fracture with routine healing
G subsequent encounter for fracture with delayed healing
K subsequent encounter for fracture with nonunion
P subsequent encounter for fracture with malunion
S sequela

CC +7th	S82.821	Torus fracture of lower end of right fibula
CC +7th	S82.822	Torus fracture of lower end of left fibula
CC +7th	S82.829	Torus fracture of lower end of unspecified fibula
+	S82.83	Other fracture of upper and lower end of fibula
CC MCC +7th	S82.831	Other fracture of upper and lower end of right fibula
		HAC 7th characters B & C see Appendix B for HAC conditional logic
CC MCC +7th	S82.832	Other fracture of upper and lower end of left fibula
		HAC 7th characters B & C see Appendix B for HAC conditional logic
		AHA CC: 1Q, 2015, 25
CC MCC +7th	S82.839	Other fracture of upper and lower end of unspecified fibula
		HAC 7th characters B & C see Appendix B for HAC conditional logic

Tears of Meniscus

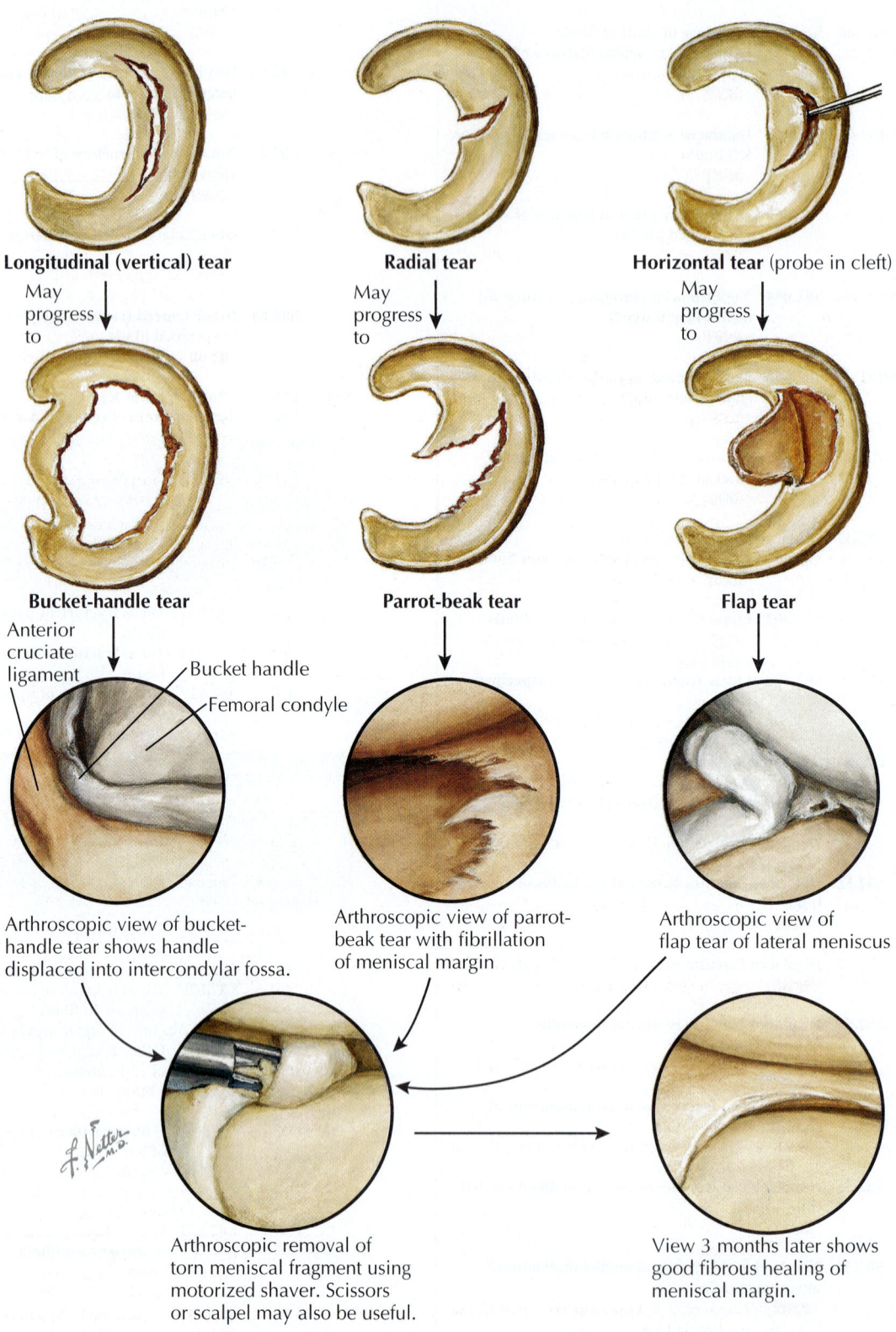

- **S82.84 Bimalleolar fracture of lower leg**
  - CC +7th **S82.841** Displaced bimalleolar fracture of right lower leg
    - HAC 7th characters B & C see Appendix B for HAC conditional logic
  - CC +7th **S82.842** Displaced bimalleolar fracture of left lower leg
    - HAC 7th characters B & C see Appendix B for HAC conditional logic
  - CC +7th **S82.843** Displaced bimalleolar fracture of unspecified lower leg
    - HAC 7th characters B & C see Appendix B for HAC conditional logic
  - CC +7th **S82.844** Nondisplaced bimalleolar fracture of right lower leg
    - HAC 7th characters B & C see Appendix B for HAC conditional logic
  - CC +7th **S82.845** Nondisplaced bimalleolar fracture of left lower leg
    - HAC 7th characters B & C see Appendix B for HAC conditional logic
  - CC +7th **S82.846** Nondisplaced bimalleolar fracture of unspecified lower leg
    - HAC 7th characters B & C see Appendix B for HAC conditional logic

- **S82.85 Trimalleolar fracture of lower leg**
  - CC +7th **S82.851** Displaced trimalleolar fracture of right lower leg
    - HAC 7th characters B & C see Appendix B for HAC conditional logic
  - CC +7th **S82.852** Displaced trimalleolar fracture of left lower leg
    - HAC 7th characters B & C see Appendix B for HAC conditional logic
  - CC +7th **S82.853** Displaced trimalleolar fracture of unspecified lower leg
    - HAC 7th characters B & C see Appendix B for HAC conditional logic
  - CC +7th **S82.854** Nondisplaced trimalleolar fracture of right lower leg
    - HAC 7th characters B & C see Appendix B for HAC conditional logic
  - CC +7th **S82.855** Nondisplaced trimalleolar fracture of left lower leg
    - HAC 7th characters B & C see Appendix B for HAC conditional logic
  - CC +7th **S82.856** Nondisplaced trimalleolar fracture of unspecified lower leg
    - HAC 7th characters B & C see Appendix B for HAC conditional logic

- **S82.86 Maisonneuve's fracture**
  - CC MCC +7th **S82.861** Displaced Maisonneuve's fracture of right leg
    - HAC 7th characters B & C see Appendix B for HAC conditional logic
  - CC MCC +7th **S82.862** Displaced Maisonneuve's fracture of left leg
    - HAC 7th characters B & C see Appendix B for HAC conditional logic
  - CC MCC +7th **S82.863** Displaced Maisonneuve's fracture of unspecified leg
    - HAC 7th characters B & C see Appendix B for HAC conditional logic
  - CC MCC +7th **S82.864** Nondisplaced Maisonneuve's fracture of right leg
    - HAC 7th characters B & C see Appendix B for HAC conditional logic
  - CC MCC +7th **S82.865** Nondisplaced Maisonneuve's fracture of left leg
    - HAC 7th characters B & C see Appendix B for HAC conditional logic
  - CC MCC +7th **S82.866** Nondisplaced Maisonneuve's fracture of unspecified leg
    - HAC 7th characters B & C see Appendix B for HAC conditional logic

- **S82.87 Pilon fracture of tibia**
  - CC +7th **S82.871** Displaced pilon fracture of right tibia
    - HAC 7th characters B & C see Appendix B for HAC conditional logic
  - CC +7th **S82.872** Displaced pilon fracture of left tibia
    - HAC 7th characters B & C see Appendix B for HAC conditional logic
  - CC +7th **S82.873** Displaced pilon fracture of unspecified tibia
    - HAC 7th characters B & C see Appendix B for HAC conditional logic
  - CC +7th **S82.874** Nondisplaced pilon fracture of right tibia
    - HAC 7th characters B & C see Appendix B for HAC conditional logic
  - CC +7th **S82.875** Nondisplaced pilon fracture of left tibia
    - HAC 7th characters B & C see Appendix B for HAC conditional logic
  - CC +7th **S82.876** Nondisplaced pilon fracture of unspecified tibia
    - HAC 7th characters B & C see Appendix B for HAC conditional logic

- **S82.89 Other fractures of lower leg**
  - Fracture of ankle NOS
  - CC +7th **S82.891** Other fracture of right lower leg
    - HAC 7th characters B & C see Appendix B for HAC conditional logic
  - CC +7th **S82.892** Other fracture of left lower leg
    - HAC 7th characters B & C see Appendix B for HAC conditional logic
  - CC +7th **S82.899** Other fracture of unspecified lower leg
    - HAC 7th characters B & C see Appendix B for HAC conditional logic

- **S82.9 Unspecified fracture of lower leg**
  - CC X+7th **S82.90** Unspecified fracture of unspecified lower leg
    - HAC 7th characters B & C see Appendix B for HAC conditional logic
  - CC X+7th **S82.91** Unspecified fracture of right lower leg
    - HAC 7th characters B & C see Appendix B for HAC conditional logic
  - CC X+7th **S82.92** Unspecified fracture of left lower leg
    - HAC 7th characters B & C see Appendix B for HAC conditional logic

S83 Dislocation and sprain of joints and ligaments of knee

Includes: avulsion of joint or ligament of knee
laceration of cartilage, joint or ligament of knee
sprain of cartilage, joint or ligament of knee
traumatic hemarthrosis of joint or ligament of knee
traumatic rupture of joint or ligament of knee
traumatic subluxation of joint or ligament of knee
traumatic tear of joint or ligament of knee

Code also any associated open wound

Excludes2: derangement of patella (M22.0-M22.3)
injury of patellar ligament (tendon) (S76.1-)
internal derangement of knee (M23.-)
old dislocation of knee (M24.36)
pathological dislocation of knee (M24.36)
recurrent dislocation of knee (M22.0)
strain of muscle, fascia and tendon of lower leg (S86.-)

The appropriate 7th character is to be added to each code from category S83
A initial encounter
D subsequent encounter
S sequela

- **S83.0 Subluxation and dislocation of patella**
  - **S83.00 Unspecified subluxation and dislocation of patella**
    - +7th **S83.001** Unspecified subluxation of right patella
    - +7th **S83.002** Unspecified subluxation of left patella
    - +7th **S83.003** Unspecified subluxation of unspecified patella
    - +7th **S83.004** Unspecified dislocation of right patella
    - +7th **S83.005** Unspecified dislocation of left patella
    - +7th **S83.006** Unspecified dislocation of unspecified patella

- **S83.01** Lateral subluxation and dislocation of patella
  - +7th **S83.011** Lateral subluxation of right patella
  - +7th **S83.012** Lateral subluxation of left patella
  - +7th **S83.013** Lateral subluxation of unspecified patella
  - +7th **S83.014** Lateral dislocation of right patella
  - +7th **S83.015** Lateral dislocation of left patella
  - +7th **S83.016** Lateral dislocation of unspecified patella
- **S83.09** Other subluxation and dislocation of patella
  - +7th **S83.091** Other subluxation of right patella
  - +7th **S83.092** Other subluxation of left patella
  - +7th **S83.093** Other subluxation of unspecified patella
  - +7th **S83.094** Other dislocation of right patella
  - +7th **S83.095** Other dislocation of left patella
  - +7th **S83.096** Other dislocation of unspecified patella
- **S83.1** Subluxation and dislocation of knee
  Excludes2: instability of knee prosthesis (T84.022, T84.023)
  - **S83.10** Unspecified subluxation and dislocation of knee
    - +7th **S83.101** Unspecified subluxation of right knee
    - +7th **S83.102** Unspecified subluxation of left knee
    - +7th **S83.103** Unspecified subluxation of unspecified knee
    - +7th **S83.104** Unspecified dislocation of right knee
    - +7th **S83.105** Unspecified dislocation of left knee
    - +7th **S83.106** Unspecified dislocation of unspecified knee
  - **S83.11** Anterior subluxation and dislocation of proximal end of tibia
    Posterior subluxation and dislocation of distal end of femur
    - +7th **S83.111** Anterior subluxation of proximal end of tibia, right knee
    - +7th **S83.112** Anterior subluxation of proximal end of tibia, left knee
    - +7th **S83.113** Anterior subluxation of proximal end of tibia, unspecified knee
    - +7th **S83.114** Anterior dislocation of proximal end of tibia, right knee
    - +7th **S83.115** Anterior dislocation of proximal end of tibia, left knee
    - +7th **S83.116** Anterior dislocation of proximal end of tibia, unspecified knee
  - **S83.12** Posterior subluxation and dislocation of proximal end of tibia
    Anterior dislocation of distal end of femur
    - +7th **S83.121** Posterior subluxation of proximal end of tibia, right knee
    - +7th **S83.122** Posterior subluxation of proximal end of tibia, left knee
    - +7th **S83.123** Posterior subluxation of proximal end of tibia, unspecified knee
    - +7th **S83.124** Posterior dislocation of proximal end of tibia, right knee
    - +7th **S83.125** Posterior dislocation of proximal end of tibia, left knee
    - +7th **S83.126** Posterior dislocation of proximal end of tibia, unspecified knee
  - **S83.13** Medial subluxation and dislocation of proximal end of tibia
    - +7th **S83.131** Medial subluxation of proximal end of tibia, right knee
    - +7th **S83.132** Medial subluxation of proximal end of tibia, left knee
    - +7th **S83.133** Medial subluxation of proximal end of tibia, unspecified knee
    - +7th **S83.134** Medial dislocation of proximal end of tibia, right knee
    - +7th **S83.135** Medial dislocation of proximal end of tibia, left knee
    - +7th **S83.136** Medial dislocation of proximal end of tibia, unspecified knee
  - **S83.14** Lateral subluxation and dislocation of proximal end of tibia
    - +7th **S83.141** Lateral subluxation of proximal end of tibia, right knee
    - +7th **S83.142** Lateral subluxation of proximal end of tibia, left knee
    - +7th **S83.143** Lateral subluxation of proximal end of tibia, unspecified knee
    - +7th **S83.144** Lateral dislocation of proximal end of tibia, right knee
    - +7th **S83.145** Lateral dislocation of proximal end of tibia, left knee
    - +7th **S83.146** Lateral dislocation of proximal end of tibia, unspecified knee
  - **S83.19** Other subluxation and dislocation of knee
    - +7th **S83.191** Other subluxation of right knee
    - +7th **S83.192** Other subluxation of left knee
    - +7th **S83.193** Other subluxation of unspecified knee
    - +7th **S83.194** Other dislocation of right knee
    - +7th **S83.195** Other dislocation of left knee
    - +7th **S83.196** Other dislocation of unspecified knee
- **S83.2** Tear of meniscus, current injury
  Excludes1: old bucket-handle tear (M23.2)
  - **S83.20** Tear of unspecified meniscus, current injury
    Tear of meniscus of knee NOS
    - +7th **S83.200** Bucket-handle tear of unspecified meniscus, current injury, right knee
    - +7th **S83.201** Bucket-handle tear of unspecified meniscus, current injury, left knee
    - +7th **S83.202** Bucket-handle tear of unspecified meniscus, current injury, unspecified knee
    - +7th **S83.203** Other tear of unspecified meniscus, current injury, right knee
    - +7th **S83.204** Other tear of unspecified meniscus, current injury, left knee
    - +7th **S83.205** Other tear of unspecified meniscus, current injury, unspecified knee
    - +7th **S83.206** Unspecified tear of unspecified meniscus, current injury, right knee
    - +7th **S83.207** Unspecified tear of unspecified meniscus, current injury, left knee
    - +7th **S83.209** Unspecified tear of unspecified meniscus, current injury, unspecified knee
  - **S83.21** Bucket-handle tear of medial meniscus, current injury
    - +7th **S83.211** Bucket-handle tear of medial meniscus, current injury, right knee
    - +7th **S83.212** Bucket-handle tear of medial meniscus, current injury, left knee
    - +7th **S83.219** Bucket-handle tear of medial meniscus, current injury, unspecified knee
  - **S83.22** Peripheral tear of medial meniscus, current injury
    - +7th **S83.221** Peripheral tear of medial meniscus, current injury, right knee
    - +7th **S83.222** Peripheral tear of medial meniscus, current injury, left knee
    - +7th **S83.229** Peripheral tear of medial meniscus, current injury, unspecified knee
  - **S83.23** Complex tear of medial meniscus, current injury
    - +7th **S83.231** Complex tear of medial meniscus, current injury, right knee
    - +7th **S83.232** Complex tear of medial meniscus, current injury, left knee
      AHA CC: 2Q, 2019, 26
    - +7th **S83.239** Complex tear of medial meniscus, current injury, unspecified knee
  - **S83.24** Other tear of medial meniscus, current injury
    - +7th **S83.241** Other tear of medial meniscus, current injury, right knee
    - +7th **S83.242** Other tear of medial meniscus, current injury, left knee
    - +7th **S83.249** Other tear of medial meniscus, current injury, unspecified knee

- **+ S83.25** Bucket-handle tear of lateral meniscus, current injury
  - +7th **S83.251** Bucket-handle tear of lateral meniscus, current injury, right knee
  - +7th **S83.252** Bucket-handle tear of lateral meniscus, current injury, left knee
  - +7th **S83.259** Bucket-handle tear of lateral meniscus, current injury, unspecified knee
- **+ S83.26** Peripheral tear of lateral meniscus, current injury
  - +7th **S83.261** Peripheral tear of lateral meniscus, current injury, right knee
  - +7th **S83.262** Peripheral tear of lateral meniscus, current injury, left knee
  - +7th **S83.269** Peripheral tear of lateral meniscus, current injury, unspecified knee
- **+ S83.27** Complex tear of lateral meniscus, current injury
  - +7th **S83.271** Complex tear of lateral meniscus, current injury, right knee
  - +7th **S83.272** Complex tear of lateral meniscus, current injury, left knee
  - +7th **S83.279** Complex tear of lateral meniscus, current injury, unspecified knee
- **+ S83.28** Other tear of lateral meniscus, current injury
  - +7th **S83.281** Other tear of lateral meniscus, current injury, right knee
  - +7th **S83.282** Other tear of lateral meniscus, current injury, left knee
  - +7th **S83.289** Other tear of lateral meniscus, current injury, unspecified knee
- **+ S83.3** Tear of articular cartilage of knee, current
  - X+7th **S83.30** Tear of articular cartilage of unspecified knee, current
  - X+7th **S83.31** Tear of articular cartilage of right knee, current
  - X+7th **S83.32** Tear of articular cartilage of left knee, current
- **+ S83.4** Sprain of collateral ligament of knee
  - **+ S83.40** Sprain of unspecified collateral ligament of knee
    - +7th **S83.401** Sprain of unspecified collateral ligament of right knee
    - +7th **S83.402** Sprain of unspecified collateral ligament of left knee
    - +7th **S83.409** Sprain of unspecified collateral ligament of unspecified knee
  - **+ S83.41** Sprain of medial collateral ligament of knee
    Sprain of tibial collateral ligament
    - +7th **S83.411** Sprain of medial collateral ligament of right knee
    - +7th **S83.412** Sprain of medial collateral ligament of left knee
    - +7th **S83.419** Sprain of medial collateral ligament of unspecified knee
  - **+ S83.42** Sprain of lateral collateral ligament of knee
    Sprain of fibular collateral ligament
    - +7th **S83.421** Sprain of lateral collateral ligament of right knee
    - +7th **S83.422** Sprain of lateral collateral ligament of left knee
    - +7th **S83.429** Sprain of lateral collateral ligament of unspecified knee
- **+ S83.5** Sprain of cruciate ligament of knee
  - **+ S83.50** Sprain of unspecified cruciate ligament of knee
    - +7th **S83.501** Sprain of unspecified cruciate ligament of right knee
    - +7th **S83.502** Sprain of unspecified cruciate ligament of left knee
    - +7th **S83.509** Sprain of unspecified cruciate ligament of unspecified knee
  - **+ S83.51** Sprain of anterior cruciate ligament of knee
    - +7th **S83.511** Sprain of anterior cruciate ligament of right knee
      AHA CC: 2Q, 2016, 3–4
    - +7th **S83.512** Sprain of anterior cruciate ligament of left knee
    - +7th **S83.519** Sprain of anterior cruciate ligament of unspecified knee
- **+ S83.52** Sprain of posterior cruciate ligament of knee
  - +7th **S83.521** Sprain of posterior cruciate ligament of right knee
  - +7th **S83.522** Sprain of posterior cruciate ligament of left knee
  - +7th **S83.529** Sprain of posterior cruciate ligament of unspecified knee
- **+ S83.6** Sprain of the superior tibiofibular joint and ligament
  - X+7th **S83.60** Sprain of the superior tibiofibular joint and ligament, unspecified knee
  - X+7th **S83.61** Sprain of the superior tibiofibular joint and ligament, right knee
  - X+7th **S83.62** Sprain of the superior tibiofibular joint and ligament, left knee
- **+ S83.8** Sprain of other specified parts of knee
  - **+ S83.8X** Sprain of other specified parts of knee
    - +7th **S83.8X1** Sprain of other specified parts of right knee
    - +7th **S83.8X2** Sprain of other specified parts of left knee
    - +7th **S83.8X9** Sprain of other specified parts of unspecified knee
- **+ S83.9** Sprain of unspecified site of knee
  - X+7th **S83.90** Sprain of unspecified site of unspecified knee
  - X+7th **S83.91** Sprain of unspecified site of right knee
  - X+7th **S83.92** Sprain of unspecified site of left knee

S84 Injury of nerves at lower leg level

Code also any associated open wound (S81.-)
Excludes2: injury of nerves at ankle and foot level (S94.-)

> The appropriate 7th character is to be added to each code from category S84
> A initial encounter
> D subsequent encounter
> S sequela

- **+ S84.0** Injury of tibial nerve at lower leg level
  - X+7th **S84.00** Injury of tibial nerve at lower leg level, unspecified leg
  - X+7th **S84.01** Injury of tibial nerve at lower leg level, right leg
  - X+7th **S84.02** Injury of tibial nerve at lower leg level, left leg
- **+ S84.1** Injury of peroneal nerve at lower leg level
  - X+7th **S84.10** Injury of peroneal nerve at lower leg level, unspecified leg
  - X+7th **S84.11** Injury of peroneal nerve at lower leg level, right leg
  - X+7th **S84.12** Injury of peroneal nerve at lower leg level, left leg
- **+ S84.2** Injury of cutaneous sensory nerve at lower leg level
  - X+7th **S84.20** Injury of cutaneous sensory nerve at lower leg level, unspecified leg
  - X+7th **S84.21** Injury of cutaneous sensory nerve at lower leg level, right leg
  - X+7th **S84.22** Injury of cutaneous sensory nerve at lower leg level, left leg
- **+ S84.8** Injury of other nerves at lower leg level
  - **+ S84.80** Injury of other nerves at lower leg level
    - +7th **S84.801** Injury of other nerves at lower leg level, right leg
    - +7th **S84.802** Injury of other nerves at lower leg level, left leg
    - +7th **S84.809** Injury of other nerves at lower leg level, unspecified leg
- **+ S84.9** Injury of unspecified nerve at lower leg level
  - X+7th **S84.90** Injury of unspecified nerve at lower leg level, unspecified leg
  - X+7th **S84.91** Injury of unspecified nerve at lower leg level, right leg
  - X+7th **S84.92** Injury of unspecified nerve at lower leg level, left leg

S85 Injury of blood vessels at lower leg level

Code also any associated open wound (S81.-)

Excludes2: injury of blood vessels at ankle and foot level (S95.-)

The appropriate 7th character is to be added to each code from category S85
- A   initial encounter
- D   subsequent encounter
- S   sequela

- **S85.0 Injury of popliteal artery**
  - **S85.00 Unspecified injury of popliteal artery**
    - MCC +7th S85.001 Unspecified injury of popliteal artery, right leg
    - MCC +7th S85.002 Unspecified injury of popliteal artery, left leg
    - MCC +7th S85.009 Unspecified injury of popliteal artery, unspecified leg
  - **S85.01 Laceration of popliteal artery**
    - MCC +7th S85.011 Laceration of popliteal artery, right leg
    - MCC +7th S85.012 Laceration of popliteal artery, left leg
    - MCC +7th S85.019 Laceration of popliteal artery, unspecified leg
  - **S85.09 Other specified injury of popliteal artery**
    - MCC +7th S85.091 Other specified injury of popliteal artery, right leg
    - MCC +7th S85.092 Other specified injury of popliteal artery, left leg
    - MCC +7th S85.099 Other specified injury of popliteal artery, unspecified leg

- **S85.1 Injury of tibial artery**
  - **S85.10 Unspecified injury of unspecified tibial artery**
    Injury of tibial artery NOS
    - CC +7th S85.101 Unspecified injury of unspecified tibial artery, right leg
    - CC +7th S85.102 Unspecified injury of unspecified tibial artery, left leg
    - CC +7th S85.109 Unspecified injury of unspecified tibial artery, unspecified leg
  - **S85.11 Laceration of unspecified tibial artery**
    - CC +7th S85.111 Laceration of unspecified tibial artery, right leg
    - CC +7th S85.112 Laceration of unspecified tibial artery, left leg
    - CC +7th S85.119 Laceration of unspecified tibial artery, unspecified leg
  - **S85.12 Other specified injury of unspecified tibial artery**
    - CC +7th S85.121 Other specified injury of unspecified tibial artery, right leg
    - CC +7th S85.122 Other specified injury of unspecified tibial artery, left leg
    - CC +7th S85.129 Other specified injury of unspecified tibial artery, unspecified leg
  - **S85.13 Unspecified injury of anterior tibial artery**
    - CC +7th S85.131 Unspecified injury of anterior tibial artery, right leg
    - CC +7th S85.132 Unspecified injury of anterior tibial artery, left leg
    - CC +7th S85.139 Unspecified injury of anterior tibial artery, unspecified leg
  - **S85.14 Laceration of anterior tibial artery**
    - CC +7th S85.141 Laceration of anterior tibial artery, right leg
    - CC +7th S85.142 Laceration of anterior tibial artery, left leg
    - CC +7th S85.149 Laceration of anterior tibial artery, unspecified leg
  - **S85.15 Other specified injury of anterior tibial artery**
    - CC +7th S85.151 Other specified injury of anterior tibial artery, right leg
    - CC +7th S85.152 Other specified injury of anterior tibial artery, left leg
    - CC +7th S85.159 Other specified injury of anterior tibial artery, unspecified leg
  - **S85.16 Unspecified injury of posterior tibial artery**
    - CC +7th S85.161 Unspecified injury of posterior tibial artery, right leg
    - CC +7th S85.162 Unspecified injury of posterior tibial artery, left leg
    - CC +7th S85.169 Unspecified injury of posterior tibial artery, unspecified leg
  - **S85.17 Laceration of posterior tibial artery**
    - CC +7th S85.171 Laceration of posterior tibial artery, right leg
    - CC +7th S85.172 Laceration of posterior tibial artery, left leg
    - CC +7th S85.179 Laceration of posterior tibial artery, unspecified leg
  - **S85.18 Other specified injury of posterior tibial artery**
    - CC +7th S85.181 Other specified injury of posterior tibial artery, right leg
    - CC +7th S85.182 Other specified injury of posterior tibial artery, left leg
    - CC +7th S85.189 Other specified injury of posterior tibial artery, unspecified leg

- **S85.2 Injury of peroneal artery**
  - **S85.20 Unspecified injury of peroneal artery**
    - CC +7th S85.201 Unspecified injury of peroneal artery, right leg
    - CC +7th S85.202 Unspecified injury of peroneal artery, left leg
    - CC +7th S85.209 Unspecified injury of peroneal artery, unspecified leg
  - **S85.21 Laceration of peroneal artery**
    - CC +7th S85.211 Laceration of peroneal artery, right leg
    - CC +7th S85.212 Laceration of peroneal artery, left leg
    - CC +7th S85.219 Laceration of peroneal artery, unspecified leg
  - **S85.29 Other specified injury of peroneal artery**
    - CC +7th S85.291 Other specified injury of peroneal artery, right leg
    - CC +7th S85.292 Other specified injury of peroneal artery, left leg
    - CC +7th S85.299 Other specified injury of peroneal artery, unspecified leg

- **S85.3 Injury of greater saphenous vein at lower leg level**
  Injury of greater saphenous vein NOS
  Injury of saphenous vein NOS
  - **S85.30 Unspecified injury of greater saphenous vein at lower leg level**
    - CC +7th S85.301 Unspecified injury of greater saphenous vein at lower leg level, right leg
    - CC +7th S85.302 Unspecified injury of greater saphenous vein at lower leg level, left leg
    - CC +7th S85.309 Unspecified injury of greater saphenous vein at lower leg level, unspecified leg
  - **S85.31 Laceration of greater saphenous vein at lower leg level**
    - CC +7th S85.311 Laceration of greater saphenous vein at lower leg level, right leg
    - CC +7th S85.312 Laceration of greater saphenous vein at lower leg level, left leg
    - CC +7th S85.319 Laceration of greater saphenous vein at lower leg level, unspecified leg
  - **S85.39 Other specified injury of greater saphenous vein at lower leg level**
    - CC +7th S85.391 Other specified injury of greater saphenous vein at lower leg level, right leg
    - CC +7th S85.392 Other specified injury of greater saphenous vein at lower leg level, left leg
    - CC +7th S85.399 Other specified injury of greater saphenous vein at lower leg level, unspecified leg

- **S85.4 Injury of lesser saphenous vein at lower leg level**
  - **S85.40 Unspecified injury of lesser saphenous vein at lower leg level**
    - CC +7th S85.401 Unspecified injury of lesser saphenous vein at lower leg level, right leg
    - CC +7th S85.402 Unspecified injury of lesser saphenous vein at lower leg level, left leg
    - CC +7th S85.409 Unspecified injury of lesser saphenous vein at lower leg level, unspecified leg
  - **S85.41 Laceration of lesser saphenous vein at lower leg level**
    - CC +7th S85.411 Laceration of lesser saphenous vein at lower leg level, right leg
    - CC +7th S85.412 Laceration of lesser saphenous vein at lower leg level, left leg
    - CC +7th S85.419 Laceration of lesser saphenous vein at lower leg level, unspecified leg

- **+ S85.49** Other specified injury of lesser saphenous vein at lower leg level
  - CC +7th **S85.491** Other specified injury of lesser saphenous vein at lower leg level, right leg
  - CC +7th **S85.492** Other specified injury of lesser saphenous vein at lower leg level, left leg
  - CC +7th **S85.499** Other specified injury of lesser saphenous vein at lower leg level, unspecified leg
- **+ S85.5** Injury of popliteal vein
  - **+ S85.50** Unspecified injury of popliteal vein
    - MCC +7th **S85.501** Unspecified injury of popliteal vein, right leg
    - MCC +7th **S85.502** Unspecified injury of popliteal vein, left leg
    - MCC +7th **S85.509** Unspecified injury of popliteal vein, unspecified leg
  - **+ S85.51** Laceration of popliteal vein
    - MCC +7th **S85.511** Laceration of popliteal vein, right leg
    - MCC +7th **S85.512** Laceration of popliteal vein, left leg
    - MCC +7th **S85.519** Laceration of popliteal vein, unspecified leg
  - **+ S85.59** Other specified injury of popliteal vein
    - MCC +7th **S85.591** Other specified injury of popliteal vein, right leg
    - MCC +7th **S85.592** Other specified injury of popliteal vein, left leg
    - MCC +7th **S85.599** Other specified injury of popliteal vein, unspecified leg
- **+ S85.8** Injury of other blood vessels at lower leg level
  - **+ S85.80** Unspecified injury of other blood vessels at lower leg level
    - CC +7th **S85.801** Unspecified injury of other blood vessels at lower leg level, right leg
    - CC +7th **S85.802** Unspecified injury of other blood vessels at lower leg level, left leg
    - CC +7th **S85.809** Unspecified injury of other blood vessels at lower leg level, unspecified leg
  - **+ S85.81** Laceration of other blood vessels at lower leg level
    - CC +7th **S85.811** Laceration of other blood vessels at lower leg level, right leg
    - CC +7th **S85.812** Laceration of other blood vessels at lower leg level, left leg
    - CC +7th **S85.819** Laceration of other blood vessels at lower leg level, unspecified leg
  - **+ S85.89** Other specified injury of other blood vessels at lower leg level
    - CC +7th **S85.891** Other specified injury of other blood vessels at lower leg level, right leg
    - CC +7th **S85.892** Other specified injury of other blood vessels at lower leg level, left leg
    - CC +7th **S85.899** Other specified injury of other blood vessels at lower leg level, unspecified leg
- **+ S85.9** Injury of unspecified blood vessel at lower leg level
  - **+ S85.90** Unspecified injury of unspecified blood vessel at lower leg level
    - CC +7th **S85.901** Unspecified injury of unspecified blood vessel at lower leg level, right leg
    - CC +7th **S85.902** Unspecified injury of unspecified blood vessel at lower leg level, left leg
    - CC +7th **S85.909** Unspecified injury of unspecified blood vessel at lower leg level, unspecified leg
  - **+ S85.91** Laceration of unspecified blood vessel at lower leg level
    - CC +7th **S85.911** Laceration of unspecified blood vessel at lower leg level, right leg
    - CC +7th **S85.912** Laceration of unspecified blood vessel at lower leg level, left leg
    - CC +7th **S85.919** Laceration of unspecified blood vessel at lower leg level, unspecified leg
  - **+ S85.99** Other specified injury of unspecified blood vessel at lower leg level
    - CC +7th **S85.991** Other specified injury of unspecified blood vessel at lower leg level, right leg
    - CC +7th **S85.992** Other specified injury of unspecified blood vessel at lower leg level, left leg
    - CC +7th **S85.999** Other specified injury of unspecified blood vessel at lower leg level, unspecified leg

S86 Injury of muscle, fascia and tendon at lower leg level

Code also any associated open wound (S81.-)

Excludes2: injury of muscle, fascia and tendon at ankle (S96.-)
injury of patellar ligament (tendon) (S76.1-)
sprain of joints and ligaments of knee (S83.-)

The appropriate 7th character is to be added to each code from category S86
- A initial encounter
- D subsequent encounter
- S sequela

- **+ S86.0** Injury of Achilles tendon
  - **+ S86.00** Unspecified injury of Achilles tendon
    - +7th **S86.001** Unspecified injury of right Achilles tendon
    - +7th **S86.002** Unspecified injury of left Achilles tendon
    - +7th **S86.009** Unspecified injury of unspecified Achilles tendon
  - **+ S86.01** Strain of Achilles tendon
    - +7th **S86.011** Strain of right Achilles tendon
    - +7th **S86.012** Strain of left Achilles tendon
    - +7th **S86.019** Strain of unspecified Achilles tendon
  - **+ S86.02** Laceration of Achilles tendon
    - CC +7th **S86.021** Laceration of right Achilles tendon
    - CC +7th **S86.022** Laceration of left Achilles tendon
    - CC +7th **S86.029** Laceration of unspecified Achilles tendon
  - **+ S86.09** Other specified injury of Achilles tendon
    - +7th **S86.091** Other specified injury of right Achilles tendon
    - +7th **S86.092** Other specified injury of left Achilles tendon
    - +7th **S86.099** Other specified injury of unspecified Achilles tendon
- **+ S86.1** Injury of other muscle(s) and tendon(s) of posterior muscle group at lower leg level
  - **+ S86.10** Unspecified injury of other muscle(s) and tendon(s) of posterior muscle group at lower leg level
    - +7th **S86.101** Unspecified injury of other muscle(s) and tendon(s) of posterior muscle group at lower leg level, right leg
    - +7th **S86.102** Unspecified injury of other muscle(s) and tendon(s) of posterior muscle group at lower leg level, left leg
    - +7th **S86.109** Unspecified injury of other muscle(s) and tendon(s) of posterior muscle group at lower leg level, unspecified leg
  - **+ S86.11** Strain of other muscle(s) and tendon(s) of posterior muscle group at lower leg level
    - +7th **S86.111** Strain of other muscle(s) and tendon(s) of posterior muscle group at lower leg level, right leg
    - +7th **S86.112** Strain of other muscle(s) and tendon(s) of posterior muscle group at lower leg level, left leg
    - +7th **S86.119** Strain of other muscle(s) and tendon(s) of posterior muscle group at lower leg level, unspecified leg
  - **+ S86.12** Laceration of other muscle(s) and tendon(s) of posterior muscle group at lower leg level
    - CC +7th **S86.121** Laceration of other muscle(s) and tendon(s) of posterior muscle group at lower leg level, right leg
    - CC +7th **S86.122** Laceration of other muscle(s) and tendon(s) of posterior muscle group at lower leg level, left leg
    - CC +7th **S86.129** Laceration of other muscle(s) and tendon(s) of posterior muscle group at lower leg level, unspecified leg
  - **+ S86.19** Other injury of other muscle(s) and tendon(s) of posterior muscle group at lower leg level
    - +7th **S86.191** Other injury of other muscle(s) and tendon(s) of posterior muscle group at lower leg level, right leg
    - +7th **S86.192** Other injury of other muscle(s) and tendon(s) of posterior muscle group at lower leg level, left leg
    - +7th **S86.199** Other injury of other muscle(s) and tendon(s) of posterior muscle group at lower leg level, unspecified leg

- **S86.2** Injury of muscle(s) and tendon(s) of anterior muscle group at lower leg level
  - **S86.20** Unspecified injury of muscle(s) and tendon(s) of anterior muscle group at lower leg level
    - +7th **S86.201** Unspecified injury of muscle(s) and tendon(s) of anterior muscle group at lower leg level, right leg
    - +7th **S86.202** Unspecified injury of muscle(s) and tendon(s) of anterior muscle group at lower leg level, left leg
    - +7th **S86.209** Unspecified injury of muscle(s) and tendon(s) of anterior muscle group at lower leg level, unspecified leg
  - **S86.21** Strain of muscle(s) and tendon(s) of anterior muscle group at lower leg level
    - +7th **S86.211** Strain of muscle(s) and tendon(s) of anterior muscle group at lower leg level, right leg
    - +7th **S86.212** Strain of muscle(s) and tendon(s) of anterior muscle group at lower leg level, left leg
    - +7th **S86.219** Strain of muscle(s) and tendon(s) of anterior muscle group at lower leg level, unspecified leg
  - **S86.22** Laceration of muscle(s) and tendon(s) of anterior muscle group at lower leg level
    - CC +7th **S86.221** Laceration of muscle(s) and tendon(s) of anterior muscle group at lower leg level, right leg
    - CC +7th **S86.222** Laceration of muscle(s) and tendon(s) of anterior muscle group at lower leg level, left leg
    - CC +7th **S86.229** Laceration of muscle(s) and tendon(s) of anterior muscle group at lower leg level, unspecified leg
  - **S86.29** Other injury of muscle(s) and tendon(s) of anterior muscle group at lower leg level
    - +7th **S86.291** Other injury of muscle(s) and tendon(s) of anterior muscle group at lower leg level, right leg
    - +7th **S86.292** Other injury of muscle(s) and tendon(s) of anterior muscle group at lower leg level, left leg
    - +7th **S86.299** Other injury of muscle(s) and tendon(s) of anterior muscle group at lower leg level, unspecified leg
- **S86.3** Injury of muscle(s) and tendon(s) of peroneal muscle group at lower leg level
  - **S86.30** Unspecified injury of muscle(s) and tendon(s) of peroneal muscle group at lower leg level
    - +7th **S86.301** Unspecified injury of muscle(s) and tendon(s) of peroneal muscle group at lower leg level, right leg
    - +7th **S86.302** Unspecified injury of muscle(s) and tendon(s) of peroneal muscle group at lower leg level, left leg
    - +7th **S86.309** Unspecified injury of muscle(s) and tendon(s) of peroneal muscle group at lower leg level, unspecified leg
  - **S86.31** Strain of muscle(s) and tendon(s) of peroneal muscle group at lower leg level
    - +7th **S86.311** Strain of muscle(s) and tendon(s) of peroneal muscle group at lower leg level, right leg
    - +7th **S86.312** Strain of muscle(s) and tendon(s) of peroneal muscle group at lower leg level, left leg
    - +7th **S86.319** Strain of muscle(s) and tendon(s) of peroneal muscle group at lower leg level, unspecified leg
  - **S86.32** Laceration of muscle(s) and tendon(s) of peroneal muscle group at lower leg level
    - CC +7th **S86.321** Laceration of muscle(s) and tendon(s) of peroneal muscle group at lower leg level, right leg
    - CC +7th **S86.322** Laceration of muscle(s) and tendon(s) of peroneal muscle group at lower leg level, left leg
    - CC +7th **S86.329** Laceration of muscle(s) and tendon(s) of peroneal muscle group at lower leg level, unspecified leg
- **S86.39** Other injury of muscle(s) and tendon(s) of peroneal muscle group at lower leg level
  - +7th **S86.391** Other injury of muscle(s) and tendon(s) of peroneal muscle group at lower leg level, right leg
  - +7th **S86.392** Other injury of muscle(s) and tendon(s) of peroneal muscle group at lower leg level, left leg
  - +7th **S86.399** Other injury of muscle(s) and tendon(s) of peroneal muscle group at lower leg level, unspecified leg
- **S86.8** Injury of other muscles and tendons at lower leg level
  - **S86.80** Unspecified injury of other muscles and tendons at lower leg level
    - +7th **S86.801** Unspecified injury of other muscle(s) and tendon(s) at lower leg level, right leg
    - +7th **S86.802** Unspecified injury of other muscle(s) and tendon(s) at lower leg level, left leg
    - +7th **S86.809** Unspecified injury of other muscle(s) and tendon(s) at lower leg level, unspecified leg
  - **S86.81** Strain of other muscles and tendons at lower leg level
    - +7th **S86.811** Strain of other muscle(s) and tendon(s) at lower leg level, right leg
    - +7th **S86.812** Strain of other muscle(s) and tendon(s) at lower leg level, left leg
    - +7th **S86.819** Strain of other muscle(s) and tendon(s) at lower leg level, unspecified leg
  - **S86.82** Laceration of other muscles and tendons at lower leg level
    - CC +7th **S86.821** Laceration of other muscle(s) and tendon(s) at lower leg level, right leg
    - CC +7th **S86.822** Laceration of other muscle(s) and tendon(s) at lower leg level, left leg
    - CC +7th **S86.829** Laceration of other muscle(s) and tendon(s) at lower leg level, unspecified leg
  - **S86.89** Other injury of other muscles and tendons at lower leg level
    - +7th **S86.891** Other injury of other muscle(s) and tendon(s) at lower leg level, right leg
    - +7th **S86.892** Other injury of other muscle(s) and tendon(s) at lower leg level, left leg
    - +7th **S86.899** Other injury of other muscle(s) and tendon(s) at lower leg level, unspecified leg
- **S86.9** Injury of unspecified muscle and tendon at lower leg level
  - **S86.90** Unspecified injury of unspecified muscle and tendon at lower leg level
    - +7th **S86.901** Unspecified injury of unspecified muscle(s) and tendon(s) at lower leg level, right leg
    - +7th **S86.902** Unspecified injury of unspecified muscle(s) and tendon(s) at lower leg level, left leg
    - +7th **S86.909** Unspecified injury of unspecified muscle(s) and tendon(s) at lower leg level, unspecified leg
  - **S86.91** Strain of unspecified muscle and tendon at lower leg level
    - +7th **S86.911** Strain of unspecified muscle(s) and tendon(s) at lower leg level, right leg
    - +7th **S86.912** Strain of unspecified muscle(s) and tendon(s) at lower leg level, left leg
    - +7th **S86.919** Strain of unspecified muscle(s) and tendon(s) at lower leg level, unspecified leg
  - **S86.92** Laceration of unspecified muscle and tendon at lower leg level
    - CC +7th **S86.921** Laceration of unspecified muscle(s) and tendon(s) at lower leg level, right leg
    - CC +7th **S86.922** Laceration of unspecified muscle(s) and tendon(s) at lower leg level, left leg
    - CC +7th **S86.929** Laceration of unspecified muscle(s) and tendon(s) at lower leg level, unspecified leg

+ **S86.99** Other injury of unspecified muscle and tendon at lower leg level
  +7th **S86.991** Other injury of unspecified muscle(s) and tendon(s) at lower leg level, right leg
  +7th **S86.992** Other injury of unspecified muscle(s) and tendon(s) at lower leg level, left leg
  +7th **S86.999** Other injury of unspecified muscle(s) and tendon(s) at lower leg level, unspecified leg

S87 Crushing injury of lower leg
Use additional code(s) for all associated injuries
Excludes2: crushing injury of ankle and foot (S97.-)

The appropriate 7th character is to be added to each code from category S87
- A initial encounter
- D subsequent encounter
- S sequela

+ **S87.0** Crushing injury of knee
  X+7th **S87.00** Crushing injury of unspecified knee
  X+7th **S87.01** Crushing injury of right knee
  X+7th **S87.02** Crushing injury of left knee
+ **S87.8** Crushing injury of lower leg
  X+7th **S87.80** Crushing injury of unspecified lower leg
  X+7th **S87.81** Crushing injury of right lower leg
  X+7th **S87.82** Crushing injury of left lower leg

S88 Traumatic amputation of lower leg
NOTE An amputation not identified as partial or complete should be coded to complete
Excludes1: traumatic amputation of ankle and foot (S98.-)

The appropriate 7th character is to be added to each code from category S88
- A initial encounter
- D subsequent encounter
- S sequela

+ **S88.0** Traumatic amputation at knee level
  + **S88.01** Complete traumatic amputation at knee level
    CC +7th **S88.011** Complete traumatic amputation at knee level, right lower leg
      AHA CC: 1Q, 2023, 27-30
    CC +7th **S88.012** Complete traumatic amputation at knee level, left lower leg
      AHA CC: 1Q, 2023, 27-30
    CC +7th **S88.019** Complete traumatic amputation at knee level, unspecified lower leg
  + **S88.02** Partial traumatic amputation at knee level
    CC +7th **S88.021** Partial traumatic amputation at knee level, right lower leg
    CC +7th **S88.022** Partial traumatic amputation at knee level, left lower leg
    CC +7th **S88.029** Partial traumatic amputation at knee level, unspecified lower leg
+ **S88.1** Traumatic amputation at level between knee and ankle
  + **S88.11** Complete traumatic amputation at level between knee and ankle
    CC +7th **S88.111** Complete traumatic amputation at level between knee and ankle, right lower leg
    CC +7th **S88.112** Complete traumatic amputation at level between knee and ankle, left lower leg
    CC +7th **S88.119** Complete traumatic amputation at level between knee and ankle, unspecified lower leg
  + **S88.12** Partial traumatic amputation at level between knee and ankle
    CC +7th **S88.121** Partial traumatic amputation at level between knee and ankle, right lower leg
    CC +7th **S88.122** Partial traumatic amputation at level between knee and ankle, left lower leg
    CC +7th **S88.129** Partial traumatic amputation at level between knee and ankle, unspecified lower leg
+ **S88.9** Traumatic amputation of lower leg, level unspecified
  + **S88.91** Complete traumatic amputation of lower leg, level unspecified
    CC +7th **S88.911** Complete traumatic amputation of right lower leg, level unspecified
    CC +7th **S88.912** Complete traumatic amputation of left lower leg, level unspecified
    CC +7th **S88.919** Complete traumatic amputation of unspecified lower leg, level unspecified
  + **S88.92** Partial traumatic amputation of lower leg, level unspecified
    CC +7th **S88.921** Partial traumatic amputation of right lower leg, level unspecified
    CC +7th **S88.922** Partial traumatic amputation of left lower leg, level unspecified
    CC +7th **S88.929** Partial traumatic amputation of unspecified lower leg, level unspecified

S89 Other and unspecified injuries of lower leg
NOTE A fracture not indicated as open or closed should be coded to closed
Excludes2: other and unspecified injuries of ankle and foot (S99.-)

The appropriate 7th character is to be added to each code from subcategories **S89.0**, **S89.1**, **S89.2**, and **S89.3**
- A initial encounter for closed fracture
- D subsequent encounter for fracture with routine healing
- G subsequent encounter for fracture with delayed healing
- K subsequent encounter for fracture with nonunion
- P subsequent encounter for fracture with malunion
- S sequela

Review coding guideline C.19.c
+ **S89.0** Physeal fracture of upper end of tibia
  + **S89.00** Unspecified physeal fracture of upper end of tibia
    CC +7th **S89.001** Unspecified physeal fracture of upper end of right tibia
      HAC 7th character A see Appendix B for HAC conditional logic
    CC +7th **S89.002** Unspecified physeal fracture of upper end of left tibia
      HAC 7th character A see Appendix B for HAC conditional logic
    CC +7th **S89.009** Unspecified physeal fracture of upper end of unspecified tibia
      HAC 7th character A see Appendix B for HAC conditional logic
  + **S89.01** Salter-Harris Type I physeal fracture of upper end of tibia
    CC +7th **S89.011** Salter-Harris Type I physeal fracture of upper end of right tibia
      HAC 7th character A see Appendix B for HAC conditional logic
    CC +7th **S89.012** Salter-Harris Type I physeal fracture of upper end of left tibia
      HAC 7th character A see Appendix B for HAC conditional logic
    CC +7th **S89.019** Salter-Harris Type I physeal fracture of upper end of unspecified tibia
      HAC 7th character A see Appendix B for HAC conditional logic
  + **S89.02** Salter-Harris Type II physeal fracture of upper end of tibia
    CC +7th **S89.021** Salter-Harris Type II physeal fracture of upper end of right tibia
      HAC 7th character A see Appendix B for HAC conditional logic
    CC +7th **S89.022** Salter-Harris Type II physeal fracture of upper end of left tibia
      HAC 7th character A see Appendix B for HAC conditional logic
    CC +7th **S89.029** Salter-Harris Type II physeal fracture of upper end of unspecified tibia
      HAC 7th character A see Appendix B for HAC conditional logic
  + **S89.03** Salter-Harris Type III physeal fracture of upper end of tibia
    CC +7th **S89.031** Salter-Harris Type III physeal fracture of upper end of right tibia
      HAC 7th character A see Appendix B for HAC conditional logic
    CC +7th **S89.032** Salter-Harris Type III physeal fracture of upper end of left tibia
      HAC 7th character A see Appendix B for HAC conditional logic
    CC +7th **S89.039** Salter-Harris Type III physeal fracture of upper end of unspecified tibia
      HAC 7th character A see Appendix B for HAC conditional logic

- **S89.04 Salter-Harris Type IV physeal fracture of upper end of tibia**
  - CC +7th **S89.041** Salter-Harris Type IV physeal fracture of upper end of right tibia
    - HAC 7th character A see Appendix B for HAC conditional logic
  - CC +7th **S89.042** Salter-Harris Type IV physeal fracture of upper end of left tibia
    - HAC 7th character A see Appendix B for HAC conditional logic
  - CC +7th **S89.049** Salter-Harris Type IV physeal fracture of upper end of unspecified tibia
    - HAC 7th character A see Appendix B for HAC conditional logic
- **S89.09 Other physeal fracture of upper end of tibia**
  - CC +7th **S89.091** Other physeal fracture of upper end of right tibia
    - HAC 7th character A see Appendix B for HAC conditional logic
  - CC +7th **S89.092** Other physeal fracture of upper end of left tibia
    - HAC 7th character A see Appendix B for HAC conditional logic
  - CC +7th **S89.099** Other physeal fracture of upper end of unspecified tibia
    - HAC 7th character A see Appendix B for HAC conditional logic
- **S89.1 Physeal fracture of lower end of tibia**
  - **S89.10 Unspecified physeal fracture of lower end of tibia**
    - CC +7th **S89.101** Unspecified physeal fracture of lower end of right tibia
    - CC +7th **S89.102** Unspecified physeal fracture of lower end of left tibia
    - CC +7th **S89.109** Unspecified physeal fracture of lower end of unspecified tibia
  - **S89.11 Salter-Harris Type I physeal fracture of lower end of tibia**
    - CC +7th **S89.111** Salter-Harris Type I physeal fracture of lower end of right tibia
    - CC +7th **S89.112** Salter-Harris Type I physeal fracture of lower end of left tibia
    - CC +7th **S89.119** Salter-Harris Type I physeal fracture of lower end of unspecified tibia
  - **S89.12 Salter-Harris Type II physeal fracture of lower end of tibia**
    - CC +7th **S89.121** Salter-Harris Type II physeal fracture of lower end of right tibia
    - CC +7th **S89.122** Salter-Harris Type II physeal fracture of lower end of left tibia
    - CC +7th **S89.129** Salter-Harris Type II physeal fracture of lower end of unspecified tibia
  - **S89.13 Salter-Harris Type III physeal fracture of lower end of tibia**
    - **Excludes1:** *fracture of medial malleolus (adult) (S82.5-)*
    - CC +7th **S89.131** Salter-Harris Type III physeal fracture of lower end of right tibia
    - CC +7th **S89.132** Salter-Harris Type III physeal fracture of lower end of left tibia
    - CC +7th **S89.139** Salter-Harris Type III physeal fracture of lower end of unspecified tibia
  - **S89.14 Salter-Harris Type IV physeal fracture of lower end of tibia**
    - **Excludes1:** *fracture of medial malleolus (adult) (S82.5-)*
    - CC +7th **S89.141** Salter-Harris Type IV physeal fracture of lower end of right tibia
    - CC +7th **S89.142** Salter-Harris Type IV physeal fracture of lower end of left tibia
    - CC +7th **S89.149** Salter-Harris Type IV physeal fracture of lower end of unspecified tibia
  - **S89.19 Other physeal fracture of lower end of tibia**
    - CC +7th **S89.191** Other physeal fracture of lower end of right tibia
    - CC +7th **S89.192** Other physeal fracture of lower end of left tibia
    - CC +7th **S89.199** Other physeal fracture of lower end of unspecified tibia

- **S89.2 Physeal fracture of upper end of fibula**
  - **S89.20 Unspecified physeal fracture of upper end of fibula**
    - CC +7th **S89.201** Unspecified physeal fracture of upper end of right fibula
    - CC +7th **S89.202** Unspecified physeal fracture of upper end of left fibula
    - CC +7th **S89.209** Unspecified physeal fracture of upper end of unspecified fibula
  - **S89.21 Salter-Harris Type I physeal fracture of upper end of fibula**
    - CC +7th **S89.211** Salter-Harris Type I physeal fracture of upper end of right fibula
    - CC +7th **S89.212** Salter-Harris Type I physeal fracture of upper end of left fibula
    - CC +7th **S89.219** Salter-Harris Type I physeal fracture of upper end of unspecified fibula
  - **S89.22 Salter-Harris Type II physeal fracture of upper end of fibula**
    - CC +7th **S89.221** Salter-Harris Type II physeal fracture of upper end of right fibula
    - CC +7th **S89.222** Salter-Harris Type II physeal fracture of upper end of left fibula
    - CC +7th **S89.229** Salter-Harris Type II physeal fracture of upper end of unspecified fibula
  - **S89.29 Other physeal fracture of upper end of fibula**
    - CC +7th **S89.291** Other physeal fracture of upper end of right fibula
    - CC +7th **S89.292** Other physeal fracture of upper end of left fibula
    - CC +7th **S89.299** Other physeal fracture of upper end of unspecified fibula
- **S89.3 Physeal fracture of lower end of fibula**
  - **S89.30 Unspecified physeal fracture of lower end of fibula**
    - CC +7th **S89.301** Unspecified physeal fracture of lower end of right fibula
    - CC +7th **S89.302** Unspecified physeal fracture of lower end of left fibula
    - CC +7th **S89.309** Unspecified physeal fracture of lower end of unspecified fibula
  - **S89.31 Salter-Harris Type I physeal fracture of lower end of fibula**
    - CC +7th **S89.311** Salter-Harris Type I physeal fracture of lower end of right fibula
    - CC +7th **S89.312** Salter-Harris Type I physeal fracture of lower end of left fibula
    - CC +7th **S89.319** Salter-Harris Type I physeal fracture of lower end of unspecified fibula
  - **S89.32 Salter-Harris Type II physeal fracture of lower end of fibula**
    - CC +7th **S89.321** Salter-Harris Type II physeal fracture of lower end of right fibula
    - CC +7th **S89.322** Salter-Harris Type II physeal fracture of lower end of left fibula
    - CC +7th **S89.329** Salter-Harris Type II physeal fracture of lower end of unspecified fibula
  - **S89.39 Other physeal fracture of lower end of fibula**
    - CC +7th **S89.391** Other physeal fracture of lower end of right fibula
    - CC +7th **S89.392** Other physeal fracture of lower end of left fibula
    - CC +7th **S89.399** Other physeal fracture of lower end of unspecified fibula
- **S89.8 Other specified injuries of lower leg**

  > The appropriate 7th character is to be added to each code in subcategory **S89.8**
  > A   initial encounter
  > D   subsequent encounter
  > S   sequela

  - X+7th **S89.80** Other specified injuries of unspecified lower leg
  - X+7th **S89.81** Other specified injuries of right lower leg
  - X+7th **S89.82** Other specified injuries of left lower leg
- **S89.9 Unspecified injury of lower leg**

  > The appropriate 7th character is to be added to each code in subcategory **S89.9**
  > A   initial encounter
  > D   subsequent encounter
  > S   sequela

  - X+7th **S89.90** Unspecified injury of unspecified lower leg
  - X+7th **S89.91** Unspecified injury of right lower leg
  - X+7th **S89.92** Unspecified injury of left lower leg

Injuries to the ankle and foot (S90-S99)

Excludes2: burns and corrosions (T20-T32)
fracture of ankle and malleolus (S82.-)
frostbite (T33-T34)
insect bite or sting, venomous (T63.4)

S90 Superficial injury of ankle, foot and toes

The appropriate 7th character is to be added to each code from category S90
A initial encounter
D subsequent encounter
S sequela

- **S90.0 Contusion of ankle**
  - S90.00 Contusion of unspecified ankle
  - S90.01 Contusion of right ankle
  - S90.02 Contusion of left ankle
- **S90.1 Contusion of toe without damage to nail**
  - **S90.11 Contusion of great toe without damage to nail**
    - S90.111 Contusion of right great toe without damage to nail
    - S90.112 Contusion of left great toe without damage to nail
    - S90.119 Contusion of unspecified great toe without damage to nail
  - **S90.12 Contusion of lesser toe without damage to nail**
    - S90.121 Contusion of right lesser toe(s) without damage to nail
    - S90.122 Contusion of left lesser toe(s) without damage to nail
    - S90.129 Contusion of unspecified lesser toe(s) without damage to nail
    Contusion of toe NOS
- **S90.2 Contusion of toe with damage to nail**
  - **S90.21 Contusion of great toe with damage to nail**
    - S90.211 Contusion of right great toe with damage to nail
    - S90.212 Contusion of left great toe with damage to nail
    - S90.219 Contusion of unspecified great toe with damage to nail
  - **S90.22 Contusion of lesser toe with damage to nail**
    - S90.221 Contusion of right lesser toe(s) with damage to nail
    - S90.222 Contusion of left lesser toe(s) with damage to nail
    - S90.229 Contusion of unspecified lesser toe(s) with damage to nail
- **S90.3 Contusion of foot**
  Excludes2: contusion of toes (S90.1-, S90.2-)
  - S90.30 Contusion of unspecified foot
    Contusion of foot NOS
  - S90.31 Contusion of right foot
  - S90.32 Contusion of left foot
- **S90.4 Other superficial injuries of toe**
  - **S90.41 Abrasion of toe**
    - S90.411 Abrasion, right great toe
    - S90.412 Abrasion, left great toe
    - S90.413 Abrasion, unspecified great toe
    - S90.414 Abrasion, right lesser toe(s)
    - S90.415 Abrasion, left lesser toe(s)
    - S90.416 Abrasion, unspecified lesser toe(s)
  - **S90.42 Blister (nonthermal) of toe**
    - S90.421 Blister (nonthermal), right great toe
    - S90.422 Blister (nonthermal), left great toe
    - S90.423 Blister (nonthermal), unspecified great toe
    - S90.424 Blister (nonthermal), right lesser toe(s)
    - S90.425 Blister (nonthermal), left lesser toe(s)
    - S90.426 Blister (nonthermal), unspecified lesser toe(s)
  - **S90.44 External constriction of toe**
    Hair tourniquet syndrome of toe
    - S90.441 External constriction, right great toe
    - S90.442 External constriction, left great toe
    - S90.443 External constriction, unspecified great toe
    - S90.444 External constriction, right lesser toe(s)
    - S90.445 External constriction, left lesser toe(s)
    - S90.446 External constriction, unspecified lesser toe(s)
  - **S90.45 Superficial foreign body of toe**
    Splinter in the toe
    - S90.451 Superficial foreign body, right great toe
    - S90.452 Superficial foreign body, left great toe
    - S90.453 Superficial foreign body, unspecified great toe
    - S90.454 Superficial foreign body, right lesser toe(s)
    - S90.455 Superficial foreign body, left lesser toe(s)
    - S90.456 Superficial foreign body, unspecified lesser toe(s)
  - **S90.46 Insect bite (nonvenomous) of toe**
    - S90.461 Insect bite (nonvenomous), right great toe
    - S90.462 Insect bite (nonvenomous), left great toe
    - S90.463 Insect bite (nonvenomous), unspecified great toe
    - S90.464 Insect bite (nonvenomous), right lesser toe(s)
    - S90.465 Insect bite (nonvenomous), left lesser toe(s)
    - S90.466 Insect bite (nonvenomous), unspecified lesser toe(s)
  - **S90.47 Other superficial bite of toe**
    Excludes1: open bite of toe (S91.15-, S91.25-)
    - S90.471 Other superficial bite of right great toe
    - S90.472 Other superficial bite of left great toe
    - S90.473 Other superficial bite of unspecified great toe
    - S90.474 Other superficial bite of right lesser toe(s)
    - S90.475 Other superficial bite of left lesser toe(s)
    - S90.476 Other superficial bite of unspecified lesser toe(s)
- **S90.5 Other superficial injuries of ankle**
  - **S90.51 Abrasion of ankle**
    - S90.511 Abrasion, right ankle
    - S90.512 Abrasion, left ankle
    - S90.519 Abrasion, unspecified ankle
  - **S90.52 Blister (nonthermal) of ankle**
    - S90.521 Blister (nonthermal), right ankle
    - S90.522 Blister (nonthermal), left ankle
    - S90.529 Blister (nonthermal), unspecified ankle
  - **S90.54 External constriction of ankle**
    - S90.541 External constriction, right ankle
    - S90.542 External constriction, left ankle
    - S90.549 External constriction, unspecified ankle
  - **S90.55 Superficial foreign body of ankle**
    Splinter in the ankle
    - S90.551 Superficial foreign body, right ankle
    - S90.552 Superficial foreign body, left ankle
    - S90.559 Superficial foreign body, unspecified ankle
  - **S90.56 Insect bite (nonvenomous) of ankle**
    - S90.561 Insect bite (nonvenomous), right ankle
    - S90.562 Insect bite (nonvenomous), left ankle
    - S90.569 Insect bite (nonvenomous), unspecified ankle
  - **S90.57 Other superficial bite of ankle**
    Excludes1: open bite of ankle (S91.05-)
    - S90.571 Other superficial bite of ankle, right ankle
    - S90.572 Other superficial bite of ankle, left ankle
    - S90.579 Other superficial bite of ankle, unspecified ankle
- **S90.8 Other superficial injuries of foot**
  - **S90.81 Abrasion of foot**
    - S90.811 Abrasion, right foot
    - S90.812 Abrasion, left foot
    - S90.819 Abrasion, unspecified foot
  - **S90.82 Blister (nonthermal) of foot**
    - S90.821 Blister (nonthermal), right foot
    - S90.822 Blister (nonthermal), left foot
    - S90.829 Blister (nonthermal), unspecified foot
  - **S90.84 External constriction of foot**
    - S90.841 External constriction, right foot
    - S90.842 External constriction, left foot
    - S90.849 External constriction, unspecified foot

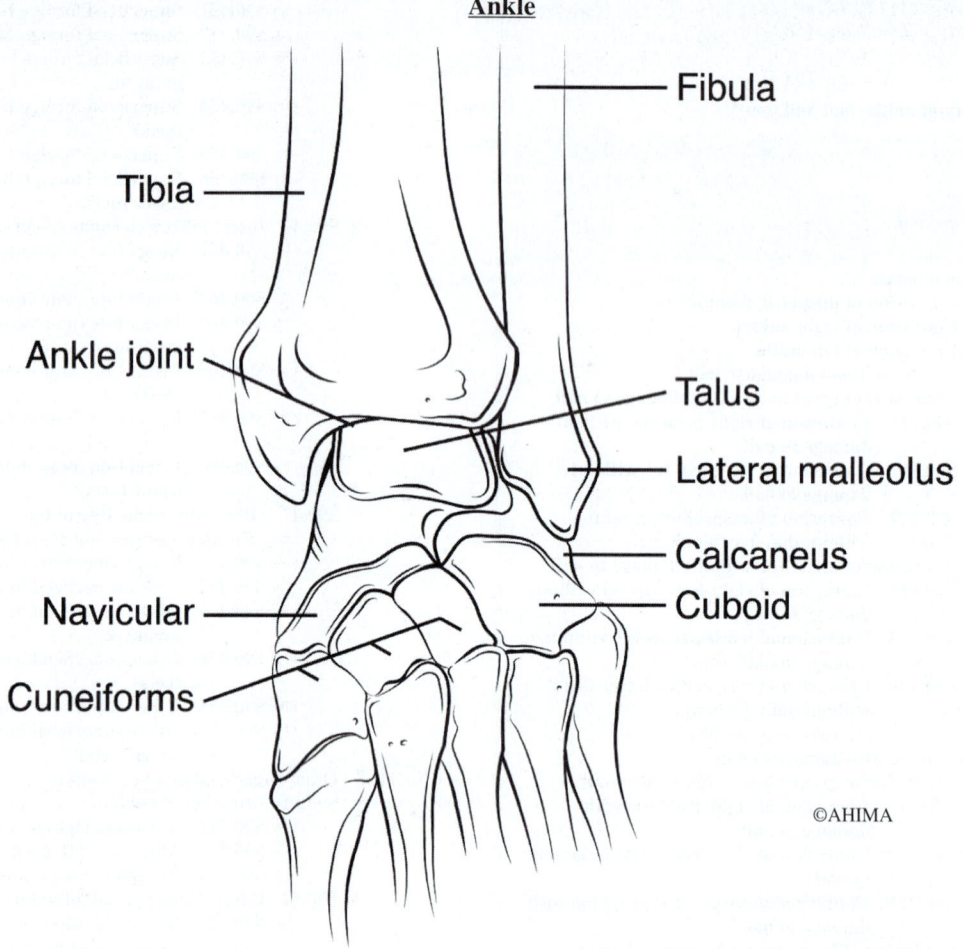

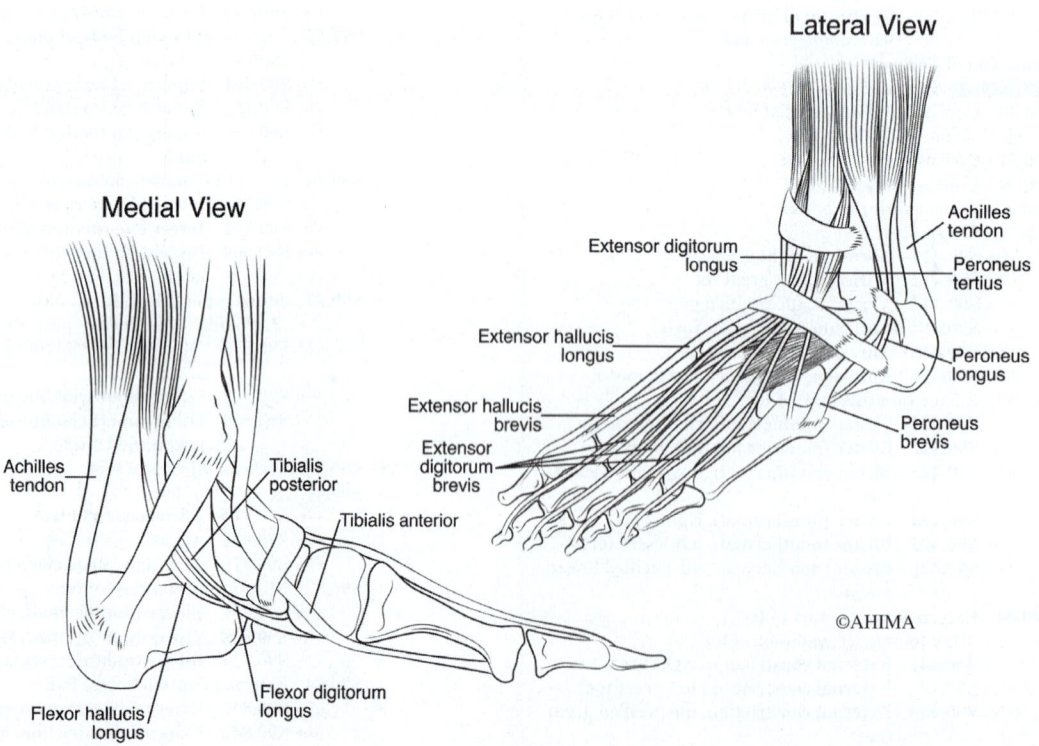

- **S90.85** Superficial foreign body of foot
  Splinter in the foot
  - +7th **S90.851** Superficial foreign body, right foot
  - +7th **S90.852** Superficial foreign body, left foot
  - +7th **S90.859** Superficial foreign body, unspecified foot
- **S90.86** Insect bite (nonvenomous) of foot
  - +7th **S90.861** Insect bite (nonvenomous), right foot
  - +7th **S90.862** Insect bite (nonvenomous), left foot
  - +7th **S90.869** Insect bite (nonvenomous), unspecified foot
- **S90.87** Other superficial bite of foot
  Excludes1: open bite of foot (S91.35-)
  - +7th **S90.871** Other superficial bite of right foot
  - +7th **S90.872** Other superficial bite of left foot
  - +7th **S90.879** Other superficial bite of unspecified foot
+ **S90.9** Unspecified superficial injury of ankle, foot and toe
  - **S90.91** Unspecified superficial injury of ankle
    - +7th **S90.911** Unspecified superficial injury of right ankle
    - +7th **S90.912** Unspecified superficial injury of left ankle
    - +7th **S90.919** Unspecified superficial injury of unspecified ankle
  - **S90.92** Unspecified superficial injury of foot
    - +7th **S90.921** Unspecified superficial injury of right foot
    - +7th **S90.922** Unspecified superficial injury of left foot
    - +7th **S90.929** Unspecified superficial injury of unspecified foot
  - **S90.93** Unspecified superficial injury of toes
    - +7th **S90.931** Unspecified superficial injury of right great toe
    - +7th **S90.932** Unspecified superficial injury of left great toe
    - +7th **S90.933** Unspecified superficial injury of unspecified great toe
    - +7th **S90.934** Unspecified superficial injury of right lesser toe(s)
    - +7th **S90.935** Unspecified superficial injury of left lesser toe(s)
    - +7th **S90.936** Unspecified superficial injury of unspecified lesser toe(s)

S91 Open wound of ankle, foot and toes

Code also any associated wound infection

Excludes1: open fracture of ankle, foot and toes (S92.-with 7th character B)
traumatic amputation of ankle and foot (S98.-)

> The appropriate 7th character is to be added to each code from category S91
> A initial encounter
> D subsequent encounter
> S sequela

+ **S91.0** Open wound of ankle
  - **S91.00** Unspecified open wound of ankle
    - +7th **S91.001** Unspecified open wound, right ankle
    - +7th **S91.002** Unspecified open wound, left ankle
    - +7th **S91.009** Unspecified open wound, unspecified ankle
  - **S91.01** Laceration without foreign body of ankle
    - +7th **S91.011** Laceration without foreign body, right ankle
    - +7th **S91.012** Laceration without foreign body, left ankle
      AHA CC: 1Q, 2021, 7-8
    - +7th **S91.019** Laceration without foreign body, unspecified ankle
  - **S91.02** Laceration with foreign body of ankle
    - +7th **S91.021** Laceration with foreign body, right ankle
    - +7th **S91.022** Laceration with foreign body, left ankle
    - +7th **S91.029** Laceration with foreign body, unspecified ankle
  - **S91.03** Puncture wound without foreign body of ankle
    - +7th **S91.031** Puncture wound without foreign body, right ankle
    - +7th **S91.032** Puncture wound without foreign body, left ankle
    - +7th **S91.039** Puncture wound without foreign body, unspecified ankle
  - **S91.04** Puncture wound with foreign body of ankle
    - +7th **S91.041** Puncture wound with foreign body, right ankle
    - +7th **S91.042** Puncture wound with foreign body, left ankle
    - +7th **S91.049** Puncture wound with foreign body, unspecified ankle
  - **S91.05** Open bite of ankle
    Excludes1: superficial bite of ankle (S90.56-, S90.57-)
    - +7th **S91.051** Open bite, right ankle
    - +7th **S91.052** Open bite, left ankle
    - +7th **S91.059** Open bite, unspecified ankle
+ **S91.1** Open wound of toe without damage to nail
  - **S91.10** Unspecified open wound of toe without damage to nail
    - +7th **S91.101** Unspecified open wound of right great toe without damage to nail
    - +7th **S91.102** Unspecified open wound of left great toe without damage to nail
    - +7th **S91.103** Unspecified open wound of unspecified great toe without damage to nail
    - +7th **S91.104** Unspecified open wound of right lesser toe(s) without damage to nail
    - +7th **S91.105** Unspecified open wound of left lesser toe(s) without damage to nail
    - +7th **S91.106** Unspecified open wound of unspecified lesser toe(s) without damage to nail
    - +7th **S91.109** Unspecified open wound of unspecified toe(s) without damage to nail
  - **S91.11** Laceration without foreign body of toe without damage to nail
    - +7th **S91.111** Laceration without foreign body of right great toe without damage to nail
    - +7th **S91.112** Laceration without foreign body of left great toe without damage to nail
    - +7th **S91.113** Laceration without foreign body of unspecified great toe without damage to nail
    - +7th **S91.114** Laceration without foreign body of right lesser toe(s) without damage to nail
    - +7th **S91.115** Laceration without foreign body of left lesser toe(s) without damage to nail
    - +7th **S91.116** Laceration without foreign body of unspecified lesser toe(s) without damage to nail
    - +7th **S91.119** Laceration without foreign body of unspecified toe without damage to nail
  - **S91.12** Laceration with foreign body of toe without damage to nail
    - +7th **S91.121** Laceration with foreign body of right great toe without damage to nail
    - +7th **S91.122** Laceration with foreign body of left great toe without damage to nail
    - +7th **S91.123** Laceration with foreign body of unspecified great toe without damage to nail
    - +7th **S91.124** Laceration with foreign body of right lesser toe(s) without damage to nail
    - +7th **S91.125** Laceration with foreign body of left lesser toe(s) without damage to nail
    - +7th **S91.126** Laceration with foreign body of unspecified lesser toe(s) without damage to nail
    - +7th **S91.129** Laceration with foreign body of unspecified toe(s) without damage to nail

- **+ S91.13** Puncture wound without foreign body of toe without damage to nail
  - +7th **S91.131** Puncture wound without foreign body of right great toe without damage to nail
  - +7th **S91.132** Puncture wound without foreign body of left great toe without damage to nail
  - +7th **S91.133** Puncture wound without foreign body of unspecified great toe without damage to nail
  - +7th **S91.134** Puncture wound without foreign body of right lesser toe(s) without damage to nail
  - +7th **S91.135** Puncture wound without foreign body of left lesser toe(s) without damage to nail
  - +7th **S91.136** Puncture wound without foreign body of unspecified lesser toe(s) without damage to nail
  - +7th **S91.139** Puncture wound without foreign body of unspecified toe(s) without damage to nail
- **+ S91.14** Puncture wound with foreign body of toe without damage to nail
  - +7th **S91.141** Puncture wound with foreign body of right great toe without damage to nail
  - +7th **S91.142** Puncture wound with foreign body of left great toe without damage to nail
  - +7th **S91.143** Puncture wound with foreign body of unspecified great toe without damage to nail
  - +7th **S91.144** Puncture wound with foreign body of right lesser toe(s) without damage to nail
  - +7th **S91.145** Puncture wound with foreign body of left lesser toe(s) without damage to nail
  - +7th **S91.146** Puncture wound with foreign body of unspecified lesser toe(s) without damage to nail
  - +7th **S91.149** Puncture wound with foreign body of unspecified toe(s) without damage to nail
- **+ S91.15** Open bite of toe without damage to nail
  Bite of toe NOS
  Excludes1: *superficial bite of toe (S90.46-,S90.47-)*
  - +7th **S91.151** Open bite of right great toe without damage to nail
  - +7th **S91.152** Open bite of left great toe without damage to nail
  - +7th **S91.153** Open bite of unspecified great toe without damage to nail
  - +7th **S91.154** Open bite of right lesser toe(s) without damage to nail
  - +7th **S91.155** Open bite of left lesser toe(s) without damage to nail
  - +7th **S91.156** Open bite of unspecified lesser toe(s) without damage to nail
  - +7th **S91.159** Open bite of unspecified toe(s) without damage to nail
- **+ S91.2** Open wound of toe with damage to nail
  - **+ S91.20** Unspecified open wound of toe with damage to nail
    - +7th **S91.201** Unspecified open wound of right great toe with damage to nail
    - +7th **S91.202** Unspecified open wound of left great toe with damage to nail
    - +7th **S91.203** Unspecified open wound of unspecified great toe with damage to nail
    - +7th **S91.204** Unspecified open wound of right lesser toe(s) with damage to nail
    - +7th **S91.205** Unspecified open wound of left lesser toe(s) with damage to nail
    - +7th **S91.206** Unspecified open wound of unspecified lesser toe(s) with damage to nail
    - +7th **S91.209** Unspecified open wound of unspecified toe(s) with damage to nail
  - **+ S91.21** Laceration without foreign body of toe with damage to nail
    - +7th **S91.211** Laceration without foreign body of right great toe with damage to nail
    - +7th **S91.212** Laceration without foreign body of left great toe with damage to nail
    - +7th **S91.213** Laceration without foreign body of unspecified great toe with damage to nail
    - +7th **S91.214** Laceration without foreign body of right lesser toe(s) with damage to nail
    - +7th **S91.215** Laceration without foreign body of left lesser toe(s) with damage to nail
    - +7th **S91.216** Laceration without foreign body of unspecified lesser toe(s) with damage to nail
    - +7th **S91.219** Laceration without foreign body of unspecified toe(s) with damage to nail
  - **+ S91.22** Laceration with foreign body of toe with damage to nail
    - +7th **S91.221** Laceration with foreign body of right great toe with damage to nail
    - +7th **S91.222** Laceration with foreign body of left great toe with damage to nail
    - +7th **S91.223** Laceration with foreign body of unspecified great toe with damage to nail
    - +7th **S91.224** Laceration with foreign body of right lesser toe(s) with damage to nail
    - +7th **S91.225** Laceration with foreign body of left lesser toe(s) with damage to nail
    - +7th **S91.226** Laceration with foreign body of unspecified lesser toe(s) with damage to nail
    - +7th **S91.229** Laceration with foreign body of unspecified toe(s) with damage to nail
  - **+ S91.23** Puncture wound without foreign body of toe with damage to nail
    - +7th **S91.231** Puncture wound without foreign body of right great toe with damage to nail
    - +7th **S91.232** Puncture wound without foreign body of left great toe with damage to nail
    - +7th **S91.233** Puncture wound without foreign body of unspecified great toe with damage to nail
    - +7th **S91.234** Puncture wound without foreign body of right lesser toe(s) with damage to nail
    - +7th **S91.235** Puncture wound without foreign body of left lesser toe(s) with damage to nail
    - +7th **S91.236** Puncture wound without foreign body of unspecified lesser toe(s) with damage to nail
    - +7th **S91.239** Puncture wound without foreign body of unspecified toe(s) with damage to nail
  - **+ S91.24** Puncture wound with foreign body of toe with damage to nail
    - +7th **S91.241** Puncture wound with foreign body of right great toe with damage to nail
    - +7th **S91.242** Puncture wound with foreign body of left great toe with damage to nail
    - +7th **S91.243** Puncture wound with foreign body of unspecified great toe with damage to nail
    - +7th **S91.244** Puncture wound with foreign body of right lesser toe(s) with damage to nail
    - +7th **S91.245** Puncture wound with foreign body of left lesser toe(s) with damage to nail
    - +7th **S91.246** Puncture wound with foreign body of unspecified lesser toe(s) with damage to nail
    - +7th **S91.249** Puncture wound with foreign body of unspecified toe(s) with damage to nail

- **S91.25** Open bite of toe with damage to nail
  Bite of toe with damage to nail NOS
  Excludes1: *superficial bite of toe (S90.46-, S90.47-)*
  - +7th **S91.251** Open bite of right great toe with damage to nail
  - +7th **S91.252** Open bite of left great toe with damage to nail
  - +7th **S91.253** Open bite of unspecified great toe with damage to nail
  - +7th **S91.254** Open bite of right lesser toe(s) with damage to nail
  - +7th **S91.255** Open bite of left lesser toe(s) with damage to nail
  - +7th **S91.256** Open bite of unspecified lesser toe(s) with damage to nail
  - +7th **S91.259** Open bite of unspecified toe(s) with damage to nail

- **S91.3** Open wound of foot
  - + **S91.30** Unspecified open wound of foot
    - +7th **S91.301** Unspecified open wound, right foot
    - +7th **S91.302** Unspecified open wound, left foot
    - +7th **S91.309** Unspecified open wound, unspecified foot
  - + **S91.31** Laceration without foreign body of foot
    - +7th **S91.311** Laceration without foreign body, right foot
    - +7th **S91.312** Laceration without foreign body, left foot
    - +7th **S91.319** Laceration without foreign body, unspecified foot
  - + **S91.32** Laceration with foreign body of foot
    - +7th **S91.321** Laceration with foreign body, right foot
    - +7th **S91.322** Laceration with foreign body, left foot
    - +7th **S91.329** Laceration with foreign body, unspecified foot
  - + **S91.33** Puncture wound without foreign body of foot
    - +7th **S91.331** Puncture wound without foreign body, right foot
    - +7th **S91.332** Puncture wound without foreign body, left foot
    - +7th **S91.339** Puncture wound without foreign body, unspecified foot
  - + **S91.34** Puncture wound with foreign body of foot
    - +7th **S91.341** Puncture wound with foreign body, right foot
    - +7th **S91.342** Puncture wound with foreign body, left foot
    - +7th **S91.349** Puncture wound with foreign body, unspecified foot
  - + **S91.35** Open bite of foot
    Excludes1: *superficial bite of foot (S90.86-, S90.87-)*
    - +7th **S91.351** Open bite, right foot
    - +7th **S91.352** Open bite, left foot
    - +7th **S91.359** Open bite, unspecified foot

S92 Fracture of foot and toe, except ankle

NOTE A fracture not indicated as displaced or nondisplaced should be coded to displaced
A fracture not indicated as open or closed should be coded to closed

Excludes2: *fracture of ankle (S82.-)*
fracture of malleolus (S82.-)
traumatic amputation of ankle and foot (S98.-)

The appropriate 7th character is to be added to each code from category S92
A initial encounter for closed fracture
B initial encounter for open fracture
D subsequent encounter for fracture with routine healing
G subsequent encounter for fracture with delayed healing
K subsequent encounter for fracture with nonunion
P subsequent encounter for fracture with malunion
S sequela

Review coding guideline C.19.c

- + **S92.0** Fracture of calcaneus
  Heel bone
  Os calcis
  Excludes2: *Physeal fracture of calcaneus (S99.0-)*
  - + **S92.00** Unspecified fracture of calcaneus
    - CC +7th **S92.001** Unspecified fracture of right calcaneus
      HAC 7th character B see Appendix B for HAC conditional logic
    - CC +7th **S92.002** Unspecified fracture of left calcaneus
      HAC 7th character B see Appendix B for HAC conditional logic
    - CC +7th **S92.009** Unspecified fracture of unspecified calcaneus
      HAC 7th character B see Appendix B for HAC conditional logic
  - + **S92.01** Fracture of body of calcaneus
    - CC +7th **S92.011** Displaced fracture of body of right calcaneus
      HAC 7th character B see Appendix B for HAC conditional logic
    - CC +7th **S92.012** Displaced fracture of body of left calcaneus
      HAC 7th character B see Appendix B for HAC conditional logic
    - CC +7th **S92.013** Displaced fracture of body of unspecified calcaneus
      HAC 7th character B see Appendix B for HAC conditional logic
    - CC +7th **S92.014** Nondisplaced fracture of body of right calcaneus
      HAC 7th character B see Appendix B for HAC conditional logic
    - CC +7th **S92.015** Nondisplaced fracture of body of left calcaneus
      HAC 7th character B see Appendix B for HAC conditional logic
    - CC +7th **S92.016** Nondisplaced fracture of body of unspecified calcaneus
      HAC 7th character B see Appendix B for HAC conditional logic
  - + **S92.02** Fracture of anterior process of calcaneus
    - CC +7th **S92.021** Displaced fracture of anterior process of right calcaneus
      HAC 7th character B see Appendix B for HAC conditional logic
    - CC +7th **S92.022** Displaced fracture of anterior process of left calcaneus
      HAC 7th character B see Appendix B for HAC conditional logic
    - CC +7th **S92.023** Displaced fracture of anterior process of unspecified calcaneus
      HAC 7th character B see Appendix B for HAC conditional logic
    - CC +7th **S92.024** Nondisplaced fracture of anterior process of right calcaneus
      HAC 7th character B see Appendix B for HAC conditional logic
    - CC +7th **S92.025** Nondisplaced fracture of anterior process of left calcaneus
      HAC 7th character B see Appendix B for HAC conditional logic
    - CC +7th **S92.026** Nondisplaced fracture of anterior process of unspecified calcaneus
      HAC 7th character B see Appendix B for HAC conditional logic

- **S92.03** Avulsion fracture of tuberosity of calcaneus
  - CC +7th **S92.031** Displaced avulsion fracture of tuberosity of right calcaneus
    - HAC 7th character B see Appendix B for HAC conditional logic
  - CC +7th **S92.032** Displaced avulsion fracture of tuberosity of left calcaneus
    - HAC 7th character B see Appendix B for HAC conditional logic
  - CC +7th **S92.033** Displaced avulsion fracture of tuberosity of unspecified calcaneus
    - HAC 7th character B see Appendix B for HAC conditional logic
  - CC +7th **S92.034** Nondisplaced avulsion fracture of tuberosity of right calcaneus
    - HAC 7th character B see Appendix B for HAC conditional logic
  - CC +7th **S92.035** Nondisplaced avulsion fracture of tuberosity of left calcaneus
    - HAC 7th character B see Appendix B for HAC conditional logic
  - CC +7th **S92.036** Nondisplaced avulsion fracture of tuberosity of unspecified calcaneus
    - HAC 7th character B see Appendix B for HAC conditional logic
- **S92.04** Other fracture of tuberosity of calcaneus
  - CC +7th **S92.041** Displaced other fracture of tuberosity of right calcaneus
    - HAC 7th character B see Appendix B for HAC conditional logic
  - CC +7th **S92.042** Displaced other fracture of tuberosity of left calcaneus
    - HAC 7th character B see Appendix B for HAC conditional logic
  - CC +7th **S92.043** Displaced other fracture of tuberosity of unspecified calcaneus
    - HAC 7th character B see Appendix B for HAC conditional logic
  - CC +7th **S92.044** Nondisplaced other fracture of tuberosity of right calcaneus
    - HAC 7th character B see Appendix B for HAC conditional logic
  - CC +7th **S92.045** Nondisplaced other fracture of tuberosity of left calcaneus
    - HAC 7th character B see Appendix B for HAC conditional logic
  - CC +7th **S92.046** Nondisplaced other fracture of tuberosity of unspecified calcaneus
    - HAC 7th character B see Appendix B for HAC conditional logic
- **S92.05** Other extraarticular fracture of calcaneus
  - CC +7th **S92.051** Displaced other extraarticular fracture of right calcaneus
    - HAC 7th character B see Appendix B for HAC conditional logic
  - CC +7th **S92.052** Displaced other extraarticular fracture of left calcaneus
    - HAC 7th character B see Appendix B for HAC conditional logic
  - CC +7th **S92.053** Displaced other extraarticular fracture of unspecified calcaneus
    - HAC 7th character B see Appendix B for HAC conditional logic
  - CC +7th **S92.054** Nondisplaced other extraarticular fracture of right calcaneus
    - HAC 7th character B see Appendix B for HAC conditional logic
  - CC +7th **S92.055** Nondisplaced other extraarticular fracture of left calcaneus
    - HAC 7th character B see Appendix B for HAC conditional logic
  - CC +7th **S92.056** Nondisplaced other extraarticular fracture of unspecified calcaneus
    - HAC 7th character B see Appendix B for HAC conditional logic

- **S92.06** Intraarticular fracture of calcaneus
  - CC +7th **S92.061** Displaced intraarticular fracture of right calcaneus
    - HAC 7th character B see Appendix B for HAC conditional logic
  - CC +7th **S92.062** Displaced intraarticular fracture of left calcaneus
    - HAC 7th character B see Appendix B for HAC conditional logic
  - CC +7th **S92.063** Displaced intraarticular fracture of unspecified calcaneus
    - HAC 7th character B see Appendix B for HAC conditional logic
  - CC +7th **S92.064** Nondisplaced intraarticular fracture of right calcaneus
    - HAC 7th character B see Appendix B for HAC conditional logic
  - CC +7th **S92.065** Nondisplaced intraarticular fracture of left calcaneus
    - HAC 7th character B see Appendix B for HAC conditional logic
  - CC +7th **S92.066** Nondisplaced intraarticular fracture of unspecified calcaneus
    - HAC 7th character B see Appendix B for HAC conditional logic
- **S92.1** Fracture of talus
  - Astragalus
  - **S92.10** Unspecified fracture of talus
    - CC +7th **S92.101** Unspecified fracture of right talus
      - HAC 7th character B see Appendix B for HAC conditional logic
    - CC +7th **S92.102** Unspecified fracture of left talus
      - HAC 7th character B see Appendix B for HAC conditional logic
    - CC +7th **S92.109** Unspecified fracture of unspecified talus
      - HAC 7th character B see Appendix B for HAC conditional logic
  - **S92.11** Fracture of neck of talus
    - CC +7th **S92.111** Displaced fracture of neck of right talus
      - HAC 7th character B see Appendix B for HAC conditional logic
    - CC +7th **S92.112** Displaced fracture of neck of left talus
    - CC +7th **S92.113** Displaced fracture of neck of unspecified talus
      - HAC 7th character B see Appendix B for HAC conditional logic
    - CC +7th **S92.114** Nondisplaced fracture of neck of right talus
      - HAC 7th character B see Appendix B for HAC conditional logic
    - CC +7th **S92.115** Nondisplaced fracture of neck of left talus
      - HAC 7th character B see Appendix B for HAC conditional logic
    - CC +7th **S92.116** Nondisplaced fracture of neck of unspecified talus
      - HAC 7th character B see Appendix B for HAC conditional logic
  - **S92.12** Fracture of body of talus
    - CC +7th **S92.121** Displaced fracture of body of right talus
      - HAC 7th character B see Appendix B for HAC conditional logic
    - CC +7th **S92.122** Displaced fracture of body of left talus
      - HAC 7th character B see Appendix B for HAC conditional logic
    - CC +7th **S92.123** Displaced fracture of body of unspecified talus
      - HAC 7th character B see Appendix B for HAC conditional logic
    - CC +7th **S92.124** Nondisplaced fracture of body of right talus
      - HAC 7th character B see Appendix B for HAC conditional logic
    - CC +7th **S92.125** Nondisplaced fracture of body of left talus
      - HAC 7th character B see Appendix B for HAC conditional logic
    - CC +7th **S92.126** Nondisplaced fracture of body of unspecified talus
      - HAC 7th character B see Appendix B for HAC conditional logic

- **S92.13** Fracture of posterior process of talus
  - CC +7th **S92.131** Displaced fracture of posterior process of right talus
    - HAC 7th character B see Appendix B for HAC conditional logic
  - CC +7th **S92.132** Displaced fracture of posterior process of left talus
    - HAC 7th character B see Appendix B for HAC conditional logic
  - CC +7th **S92.133** Displaced fracture of posterior process of unspecified talus
    - HAC 7th character B see Appendix B for HAC conditional logic
  - CC +7th **S92.134** Nondisplaced fracture of posterior process of right talus
    - HAC 7th character B see Appendix B for HAC conditional logic
  - CC +7th **S92.135** Nondisplaced fracture of posterior process of left talus
    - HAC 7th character B see Appendix B for HAC conditional logic
  - CC +7th **S92.136** Nondisplaced fracture of posterior process of unspecified talus
    - HAC 7th character B see Appendix B for HAC conditional logic
- **S92.14** Dome fracture of talus
  - *Excludes1:* osteochondritis dissecans (M93.2)
  - CC +7th **S92.141** Displaced dome fracture of right talus
    - HAC 7th character B see Appendix B for HAC conditional logic
  - CC +7th **S92.142** Displaced dome fracture of left talus
    - HAC 7th character B see Appendix B for HAC conditional logic
  - CC +7th **S92.143** Displaced dome fracture of unspecified talus
    - HAC 7th character B see Appendix B for HAC conditional logic
  - CC +7th **S92.144** Nondisplaced dome fracture of right talus
    - HAC 7th character B see Appendix B for HAC conditional logic
  - CC +7th **S92.145** Nondisplaced dome fracture of left talus
    - HAC 7th character B see Appendix B for HAC conditional logic
  - CC +7th **S92.146** Nondisplaced dome fracture of unspecified talus
    - HAC 7th character B see Appendix B for HAC conditional logic
- **S92.15** Avulsion fracture (chip fracture) of talus
  - CC +7th **S92.151** Displaced avulsion fracture (chip fracture) of right talus
    - HAC 7th character B see Appendix B for HAC conditional logic
  - CC +7th **S92.152** Displaced avulsion fracture (chip fracture) of left talus
    - HAC 7th character B see Appendix B for HAC conditional logic
  - CC +7th **S92.153** Displaced avulsion fracture (chip fracture) of unspecified talus
    - HAC 7th character B see Appendix B for HAC conditional logic
  - CC +7th **S92.154** Nondisplaced avulsion fracture (chip fracture) of right talus
    - HAC 7th character B see Appendix B for HAC conditional logic
  - CC +7th **S92.155** Nondisplaced avulsion fracture (chip fracture) of left talus
    - HAC 7th character B see Appendix B for HAC conditional logic
  - CC +7th **S92.156** Nondisplaced avulsion fracture (chip fracture) of unspecified talus
    - HAC 7th character B see Appendix B for HAC conditional logic
- **S92.19** Other fracture of talus
  - CC +7th **S92.191** Other fracture of right talus
    - HAC 7th character B see Appendix B for HAC conditional logic
  - CC +7th **S92.192** Other fracture of left talus
    - HAC 7th character B see Appendix B for HAC conditional logic
  - CC +7th **S92.199** Other fracture of unspecified talus
    - HAC 7th character B see Appendix B for HAC conditional logic
- **S92.2** Fracture of other and unspecified tarsal bone(s)
  - **S92.20** Fracture of unspecified tarsal bone(s)
    - CC +7th **S92.201** Fracture of unspecified tarsal bone(s) of right foot
      - HAC 7th character B see Appendix B for HAC conditional logic
    - CC +7th **S92.202** Fracture of unspecified tarsal bone(s) of left foot
      - HAC 7th character B see Appendix B for HAC conditional logic
    - CC +7th **S92.209** Fracture of unspecified tarsal bone(s) of unspecified foot
      - HAC 7th character B see Appendix B for HAC conditional logic
  - **S92.21** Fracture of cuboid bone
    - CC +7th **S92.211** Displaced fracture of cuboid bone of right foot
      - HAC 7th character B see Appendix B for HAC conditional logic
    - CC +7th **S92.212** Displaced fracture of cuboid bone of left foot
      - HAC 7th character B see Appendix B for HAC conditional logic
    - CC +7th **S92.213** Displaced fracture of cuboid bone of unspecified foot
      - HAC 7th character B see Appendix B for HAC conditional logic
    - CC +7th **S92.214** Nondisplaced fracture of cuboid bone of right foot
      - HAC 7th character B see Appendix B for HAC conditional logic
    - CC +7th **S92.215** Nondisplaced fracture of cuboid bone of left foot
      - HAC 7th character B see Appendix B for HAC conditional logic
    - CC +7th **S92.216** Nondisplaced fracture of cuboid bone of unspecified foot
      - HAC 7th character B see Appendix B for HAC conditional logic
  - **S92.22** Fracture of lateral cuneiform
    - CC +7th **S92.221** Displaced fracture of lateral cuneiform of right foot
      - HAC 7th character B see Appendix B for HAC conditional logic
    - CC +7th **S92.222** Displaced fracture of lateral cuneiform of left foot
      - HAC 7th character B see Appendix B for HAC conditional logic
    - CC +7th **S92.223** Displaced fracture of lateral cuneiform of unspecified foot
      - HAC 7th character B see Appendix B for HAC conditional logic
    - CC +7th **S92.224** Nondisplaced fracture of lateral cuneiform of right foot
      - HAC 7th character B see Appendix B for HAC conditional logic
    - CC +7th **S92.225** Nondisplaced fracture of lateral cuneiform of left foot
      - HAC 7th character B see Appendix B for HAC conditional logic
    - CC +7th **S92.226** Nondisplaced fracture of lateral cuneiform of unspecified foot
      - HAC 7th character B see Appendix B for HAC conditional logic

- **S92.23 Fracture of intermediate cuneiform**
  - CC +7th **S92.231** Displaced fracture of intermediate cuneiform of right foot
    - HAC 7th character B see Appendix B for HAC conditional logic
  - CC +7th **S92.232** Displaced fracture of intermediate cuneiform of left foot
    - HAC 7th character B see Appendix B for HAC conditional logic
  - CC +7th **S92.233** Displaced fracture of intermediate cuneiform of unspecified foot
    - HAC 7th character B see Appendix B for HAC conditional logic
  - CC +7th **S92.234** Nondisplaced fracture of intermediate cuneiform of right foot
    - HAC 7th character B see Appendix B for HAC conditional logic
  - CC +7th **S92.235** Nondisplaced fracture of intermediate cuneiform of left foot
    - HAC 7th character B see Appendix B for HAC conditional logic
  - CC +7th **S92.236** Nondisplaced fracture of intermediate cuneiform of unspecified foot
    - HAC 7th character B see Appendix B for HAC conditional logic
- **S92.24 Fracture of medial cuneiform**
  - CC +7th **S92.241** Displaced fracture of medial cuneiform of right foot
    - HAC 7th character B see Appendix B for HAC conditional logic
  - CC +7th **S92.242** Displaced fracture of medial cuneiform of left foot
    - HAC 7th character B see Appendix B for HAC conditional logic
  - CC +7th **S92.243** Displaced fracture of medial cuneiform of unspecified foot
    - HAC 7th character B see Appendix B for HAC conditional logic
  - CC +7th **S92.244** Nondisplaced fracture of medial cuneiform of right foot
    - HAC 7th character B see Appendix B for HAC conditional logic
  - CC +7th **S92.245** Nondisplaced fracture of medial cuneiform of left foot
    - HAC 7th character B see Appendix B for HAC conditional logic
  - CC +7th **S92.246** Nondisplaced fracture of medial cuneiform of unspecified foot
    - HAC 7th character B see Appendix B for HAC conditional logic
- **S92.25 Fracture of navicular [scaphoid] of foot**
  - CC +7th **S92.251** Displaced fracture of navicular [scaphoid] of right foot
    - HAC 7th character B see Appendix B for HAC conditional logic
  - CC +7th **S92.252** Displaced fracture of navicular [scaphoid] of left foot
    - HAC 7th character B see Appendix B for HAC conditional logic
  - CC +7th **S92.253** Displaced fracture of navicular [scaphoid] of unspecified foot
    - HAC 7th character B see Appendix B for HAC conditional logic
  - CC +7th **S92.254** Nondisplaced fracture of navicular [scaphoid] of right foot
    - HAC 7th character B see Appendix B for HAC conditional logic
  - CC +7th **S92.255** Nondisplaced fracture of navicular [scaphoid] of left foot
    - HAC 7th character B see Appendix B for HAC conditional logic
  - CC +7th **S92.256** Nondisplaced fracture of navicular [scaphoid] of unspecified foot
    - HAC 7th character B see Appendix B for HAC conditional logic

- **S92.3 Fracture of metatarsal bone(s)**
  - **Excludes2:** *Physeal fracture of metatarsal (S99.1-)*
  - **S92.30 Fracture of unspecified metatarsal bone(s)**
    - CC +7th **S92.301** Fracture of unspecified metatarsal bone(s), right foot
      - HAC 7th character B see Appendix B for HAC conditional logic
    - CC +7th **S92.302** Fracture of unspecified metatarsal bone(s), left foot
      - HAC 7th character B see Appendix B for HAC conditional logic
    - CC +7th **S92.309** Fracture of unspecified metatarsal bone(s), unspecified foot
  - **S92.31 Fracture of first metatarsal bone**
    - CC +7th **S92.311** Displaced fracture of first metatarsal bone, right foot
      - HAC 7th character B see Appendix B for HAC conditional logic
    - CC +7th **S92.312** Displaced fracture of first metatarsal bone, left foot
      - HAC 7th character B see Appendix B for HAC conditional logic
    - CC +7th **S92.313** Displaced fracture of first metatarsal bone, unspecified foot
      - HAC 7th character B see Appendix B for HAC conditional logic
    - CC +7th **S92.314** Nondisplaced fracture of first metatarsal bone, right foot
      - HAC 7th character B see Appendix B for HAC conditional logic
    - CC +7th **S92.315** Nondisplaced fracture of first metatarsal bone, left foot
      - HAC 7th character B see Appendix B for HAC conditional logic
    - CC +7th **S92.316** Nondisplaced fracture of first metatarsal bone, unspecified foot
      - HAC 7th character B see Appendix B for HAC conditional logic
  - **S92.32 Fracture of second metatarsal bone**
    - CC +7th **S92.321** Displaced fracture of second metatarsal bone, right foot
      - HAC 7th character B see Appendix B for HAC conditional logic
    - CC +7th **S92.322** Displaced fracture of second metatarsal bone, left foot
      - HAC 7th character B see Appendix B for HAC conditional logic
    - CC +7th **S92.323** Displaced fracture of second metatarsal bone, unspecified foot
      - HAC 7th character B see Appendix B for HAC conditional logic
    - CC +7th **S92.324** Nondisplaced fracture of second metatarsal bone, right foot
      - HAC 7th character B see Appendix B for HAC conditional logic
    - CC +7th **S92.325** Nondisplaced fracture of second metatarsal bone, left foot
      - HAC 7th character B see Appendix B for HAC conditional logic
    - CC +7th **S92.326** Nondisplaced fracture of second metatarsal bone, unspecified foot
      - HAC 7th character B see Appendix B for HAC conditional logic
  - **S92.33 Fracture of third metatarsal bone**
    - *AHA CC: 1Q, 2018, 3*
    - CC +7th **S92.331** Displaced fracture of third metatarsal bone, right foot
      - HAC 7th character B see Appendix B for HAC conditional logic
    - CC +7th **S92.332** Displaced fracture of third metatarsal bone, left foot
      - HAC 7th character B see Appendix B for HAC conditional logic
    - CC +7th **S92.333** Displaced fracture of third metatarsal bone, unspecified foot
      - HAC 7th character B see Appendix B for HAC conditional logic

CC +7th S92.334 Nondisplaced fracture of third metatarsal bone, right foot
  HAC 7th character B see Appendix B for HAC conditional logic
CC +7th S92.335 Nondisplaced fracture of third metatarsal bone, left foot
  HAC 7th character B see Appendix B for HAC conditional logic
CC +7th S92.336 Nondisplaced fracture of third metatarsal bone, unspecified foot
  HAC 7th character B see Appendix B for HAC conditional logic

+ **S92.34** Fracture of fourth metatarsal bone
  CC +7th S92.341 Displaced fracture of fourth metatarsal bone, right foot
    HAC 7th character B see Appendix B for HAC conditional logic
  CC +7th S92.342 Displaced fracture of fourth metatarsal bone, left foot
    HAC 7th character B see Appendix B for HAC conditional logic
  CC +7th S92.343 Displaced fracture of fourth metatarsal bone, unspecified foot
    HAC 7th character B see Appendix B for HAC conditional logic
  CC +7th S92.344 Nondisplaced fracture of fourth metatarsal bone, right foot
    HAC 7th character B see Appendix B for HAC conditional logic
  CC +7th S92.345 Nondisplaced fracture of fourth metatarsal bone, left foot
    HAC 7th character B see Appendix B for HAC conditional logic
  CC +7th S92.346 Nondisplaced fracture of fourth metatarsal bone, unspecified foot
    HAC 7th character B see Appendix B for HAC conditional logic

+ **S92.35** Fracture of fifth metatarsal bone
  CC +7th S92.351 Displaced fracture of fifth metatarsal bone, right foot
    HAC 7th character B see Appendix B for HAC conditional logic
  CC +7th S92.352 Displaced fracture of fifth metatarsal bone, left foot
    HAC 7th character B see Appendix B for HAC conditional logic
  CC +7th S92.353 Displaced fracture of fifth metatarsal bone, unspecified foot
    HAC 7th character B see Appendix B for HAC conditional logic
  CC +7th S92.354 Nondisplaced fracture of fifth metatarsal bone, right foot
    HAC 7th character B see Appendix B for HAC conditional logic
  CC +7th S92.355 Nondisplaced fracture of fifth metatarsal bone, left foot
    HAC 7th character B see Appendix B for HAC conditional logic
  CC +7th S92.356 Nondisplaced fracture of fifth metatarsal bone, unspecified foot
    HAC 7th character B see Appendix B for HAC conditional logic

+ **S92.4** Fracture of great toe
  Excludes2: *Physeal fracture of phalanx of toe (S99.2-)*
  + **S92.40** Unspecified fracture of great toe
    CC +7th S92.401 Displaced unspecified fracture of right great toe
    CC +7th S92.402 Displaced unspecified fracture of left great toe
    CC +7th S92.403 Displaced unspecified fracture of unspecified great toe
    CC +7th S92.404 Nondisplaced unspecified fracture of right great toe
    CC +7th S92.405 Nondisplaced unspecified fracture of left great toe
    CC +7th S92.406 Nondisplaced unspecified fracture of unspecified great toe

+ **S92.41** Fracture of proximal phalanx of great toe
  CC +7th S92.411 Displaced fracture of proximal phalanx of right great toe
  CC +7th S92.412 Displaced fracture of proximal phalanx of left great toe
  CC +7th S92.413 Displaced fracture of proximal phalanx of unspecified great toe
  CC +7th S92.414 Nondisplaced fracture of proximal phalanx of right great toe
  CC +7th S92.415 Nondisplaced fracture of proximal phalanx of left great toe
  CC +7th S92.416 Nondisplaced fracture of proximal phalanx of unspecified great toe

+ **S92.42** Fracture of distal phalanx of great toe
  CC +7th S92.421 Displaced fracture of distal phalanx of right great toe
  CC +7th S92.422 Displaced fracture of distal phalanx of left great toe
  CC +7th S92.423 Displaced fracture of distal phalanx of unspecified great toe
  CC +7th S92.424 Nondisplaced fracture of distal phalanx of right great toe
  CC +7th S92.425 Nondisplaced fracture of distal phalanx of left great toe
  CC +7th S92.426 Nondisplaced fracture of distal phalanx of unspecified great toe

+ **S92.49** Other fracture of great toe
  CC +7th S92.491 Other fracture of right great toe
  CC +7th S92.492 Other fracture of left great toe
  CC +7th S92.499 Other fracture of unspecified great toe

+ **S92.5** Fracture of lesser toe(s)
  Excludes2: *Physeal fracture of phalanx of toe (S99.2-)*
  + **S92.50** Unspecified fracture of lesser toe(s)
    CC +7th S92.501 Displaced unspecified fracture of right lesser toe(s)
    CC +7th S92.502 Displaced unspecified fracture of left lesser toe(s)
    CC +7th S92.503 Displaced unspecified fracture of unspecified lesser toe(s)
    CC +7th S92.504 Nondisplaced unspecified fracture of right lesser toe(s)
    CC +7th S92.505 Nondisplaced unspecified fracture of left lesser toe(s)
    CC +7th S92.506 Nondisplaced unspecified fracture of unspecified lesser toe(s)

+ **S92.51** Fracture of proximal phalanx of lesser toe(s)
  CC +7th S92.511 Displaced fracture of proximal phalanx of right lesser toe(s)
  CC +7th S92.512 Displaced fracture of proximal phalanx of left lesser toe(s)
  CC +7th S92.513 Displaced fracture of proximal phalanx of unspecified lesser toe(s)
  CC +7th S92.514 Nondisplaced fracture of proximal phalanx of right lesser toe(s)
  CC +7th S92.515 Nondisplaced fracture of proximal phalanx of left lesser toe(s)
  CC +7th S92.516 Nondisplaced fracture of proximal phalanx of unspecified lesser toe(s)

+ **S92.52** Fracture of middle phalanx of lesser toe(s)
  CC +7th S92.521 Displaced fracture of middle phalanx of right lesser toe(s)
  CC +7th S92.522 Displaced fracture of middle phalanx of left lesser toe(s)
  CC +7th S92.523 Displaced fracture of middle phalanx of unspecified lesser toe(s)
  CC +7th S92.524 Nondisplaced fracture of middle phalanx of right lesser toe(s)
  CC +7th S92.525 Nondisplaced fracture of middle phalanx of left lesser toe(s)
  CC +7th S92.526 Nondisplaced fracture of middle phalanx of unspecified lesser toe(s)

- **S92.53** Fracture of distal phalanx of lesser toe(s)
  - CC +7th **S92.531** Displaced fracture of distal phalanx of right lesser toe(s)
  - CC +7th **S92.532** Displaced fracture of distal phalanx of left lesser toe(s)
  - CC +7th **S92.533** Displaced fracture of distal phalanx of unspecified lesser toe(s)
  - CC +7th **S92.534** Nondisplaced fracture of distal phalanx of right lesser toe(s)
  - CC +7th **S92.535** Nondisplaced fracture of distal phalanx of left lesser toe(s)
  - CC +7th **S92.536** Nondisplaced fracture of distal phalanx of unspecified lesser toe(s)
- **S92.59** Other fracture of lesser toe(s)
  - CC +7th **S92.591** Other fracture of right lesser toe(s)
  - CC +7th **S92.592** Other fracture of left lesser toe(s)
  - CC +7th **S92.599** Other fracture of unspecified lesser toe(s)
- **S92.8** Other fracture of foot, except ankle
  - **S92.81** Other fracture of foot
    Sesamoid fracture of foot
    AHA CC: 4Q, 2016, 68
    - CC +7th **S92.811** Other fracture of right foot
      HAC 7th character B see Appendix B for HAC conditional logic
    - CC +7th **S92.812** Other fracture of left foot
      HAC 7th character B see Appendix B for HAC conditional logic
    - CC +7th **S92.819** Other fracture of unspecified foot
      HAC 7th character B see Appendix B for HAC conditional logic
- **S92.9** Unspecified fracture of foot and toe
  - **S92.90** Unspecified fracture of foot
    - CC +7th **S92.901** Unspecified fracture of right foot
      HAC 7th character B see Appendix B for HAC conditional logic
    - CC +7th **S92.902** Unspecified fracture of left foot
      HAC 7th character B see Appendix B for HAC conditional logic
    - CC +7th **S92.909** Unspecified fracture of unspecified foot
      HAC 7th character B see Appendix B for HAC conditional logic
  - **S92.91** Unspecified fracture of toe
    - CC +7th **S92.911** Unspecified fracture of right toe(s)
    - CC +7th **S92.912** Unspecified fracture of left toe(s)
    - CC +7th **S92.919** Unspecified fracture of unspecified toe(s)

S93 Dislocation and sprain of joints and ligaments at ankle, foot and toe level

Includes: avulsion of joint or ligament of ankle, foot and toe
laceration of cartilage, joint or ligament of ankle, foot and toe
sprain of cartilage, joint or ligament of ankle, foot and toe
traumatic hemarthrosis of joint or ligament of ankle, foot and toe
traumatic rupture of joint or ligament of ankle, foot and toe
traumatic subluxation of joint or ligament of ankle, foot and toe
traumatic tear of joint or ligament of ankle, foot and toe

Code also any associated open wound

Excludes2: strain of muscle and tendon of ankle and foot (S96.-)

The appropriate 7th character is to be added to each code from category S93
A initial encounter
D subsequent encounter
S sequela

- **S93.0** Subluxation and dislocation of ankle joint
  Subluxation and dislocation of astragalus
  Subluxation and dislocation of fibula, lower end
  Subluxation and dislocation of talus
  Subluxation and dislocation of tibia, lower end
  - X+7th **S93.01** Subluxation of right ankle joint
  - X+7th **S93.02** Subluxation of left ankle joint
  - X+7th **S93.03** Subluxation of unspecified ankle joint
  - X+7th **S93.04** Dislocation of right ankle joint
  - X+7th **S93.05** Dislocation of left ankle joint
  - X+7th **S93.06** Dislocation of unspecified ankle joint

- **S93.1** Subluxation and dislocation of toe
  - **S93.10** Unspecified subluxation and dislocation of toe
    Dislocation of toe NOS
    Subluxation of toe NOS
    - +7th **S93.101** Unspecified subluxation of right toe(s)
    - +7th **S93.102** Unspecified subluxation of left toe(s)
    - +7th **S93.103** Unspecified subluxation of unspecified toe(s)
    - +7th **S93.104** Unspecified dislocation of right toe(s)
    - +7th **S93.105** Unspecified dislocation of left toe(s)
    - +7th **S93.106** Unspecified dislocation of unspecified toe(s)
  - **S93.11** Dislocation of interphalangeal joint
    - +7th **S93.111** Dislocation of interphalangeal joint of right great toe
    - +7th **S93.112** Dislocation of interphalangeal joint of left great toe
    - +7th **S93.113** Dislocation of interphalangeal joint of unspecified great toe
    - +7th **S93.114** Dislocation of interphalangeal joint of right lesser toe(s)
    - +7th **S93.115** Dislocation of interphalangeal joint of left lesser toe(s)
    - +7th **S93.116** Dislocation of interphalangeal joint of unspecified lesser toe(s)
    - +7th **S93.119** Dislocation of interphalangeal joint of unspecified toe(s)
  - **S93.12** Dislocation of metatarsophalangeal joint
    - +7th **S93.121** Dislocation of metatarsophalangeal joint of right great toe
    - +7th **S93.122** Dislocation of metatarsophalangeal joint of left great toe
    - +7th **S93.123** Dislocation of metatarsophalangeal joint of unspecified great toe
    - +7th **S93.124** Dislocation of metatarsophalangeal joint of right lesser toe(s)
    - +7th **S93.125** Dislocation of metatarsophalangeal joint of left lesser toe(s)
    - +7th **S93.126** Dislocation of metatarsophalangeal joint of unspecified lesser toe(s)
    - +7th **S93.129** Dislocation of metatarsophalangeal joint of unspecified toe(s)
  - **S93.13** Subluxation of interphalangeal joint
    - +7th **S93.131** Subluxation of interphalangeal joint of right great toe
    - +7th **S93.132** Subluxation of interphalangeal joint of left great toe
    - +7th **S93.133** Subluxation of interphalangeal joint of unspecified great toe
    - +7th **S93.134** Subluxation of interphalangeal joint of right lesser toe(s)
    - +7th **S93.135** Subluxation of interphalangeal joint of left lesser toe(s)
    - +7th **S93.136** Subluxation of interphalangeal joint of unspecified lesser toe(s)
    - +7th **S93.139** Subluxation of interphalangeal joint of unspecified toe(s)
  - **S93.14** Subluxation of metatarsophalangeal joint
    - +7th **S93.141** Subluxation of metatarsophalangeal joint of right great toe
    - +7th **S93.142** Subluxation of metatarsophalangeal joint of left great toe
    - +7th **S93.143** Subluxation of metatarsophalangeal joint of unspecified great toe
    - +7th **S93.144** Subluxation of metatarsophalangeal joint of right lesser toe(s)
    - +7th **S93.145** Subluxation of metatarsophalangeal joint of left lesser toe(s)
    - +7th **S93.146** Subluxation of metatarsophalangeal joint of unspecified lesser toe(s)
    - +7th **S93.149** Subluxation of metatarsophalangeal joint of unspecified toe(s)

- **S93.3 Subluxation and dislocation of foot**
  - *Excludes2:* dislocation of toe (S93.1-)
  - **S93.30 Unspecified subluxation and dislocation of foot**
    - Dislocation of foot NOS
    - Sublocation of foot NOS
    - +7th S93.301 Unspecified subluxation of right foot
    - +7th S93.302 Unspecified subluxation of left foot
    - +7th S93.303 Unspecified subluxation of unspecified foot
    - +7th S93.304 Unspecified dislocation of right foot
    - +7th S93.305 Unspecified dislocation of left foot
    - +7th S93.306 Unspecified dislocation of unspecified foot
  - **S93.31 Subluxation and dislocation of tarsal joint**
    - +7th S93.311 Subluxation of tarsal joint of right foot
    - +7th S93.312 Subluxation of tarsal joint of left foot
    - +7th S93.313 Subluxation of tarsal joint of unspecified foot
    - +7th S93.314 Dislocation of tarsal joint of right foot
    - +7th S93.315 Dislocation of tarsal joint of left foot
    - +7th S93.316 Dislocation of tarsal joint of unspecified foot
  - **S93.32 Subluxation and dislocation of tarsometatarsal joint**
    - +7th S93.321 Subluxation of tarsometatarsal joint of right foot
    - +7th S93.322 Subluxation of tarsometatarsal joint of left foot
    - +7th S93.323 Subluxation of tarsometatarsal joint of unspecified foot
    - +7th S93.324 Dislocation of tarsometatarsal joint of right foot
    - +7th S93.325 Dislocation of tarsometatarsal joint of left foot
    - +7th S93.326 Dislocation of tarsometatarsal joint of unspecified foot
  - **S93.33 Other subluxation and dislocation of foot**
    - +7th S93.331 Other subluxation of right foot
    - +7th S93.332 Other subluxation of left foot
    - +7th S93.333 Other subluxation of unspecified foot
    - +7th S93.334 Other dislocation of right foot
    - +7th S93.335 Other dislocation of left foot
    - +7th S93.336 Other dislocation of unspecified foot
- **S93.4 Sprain of ankle**
  - *Excludes2:* injury of Achilles tendon (S86.0-)
  - **S93.40 Sprain of unspecified ligament of ankle**
    - Sprain of ankle NOS
    - Sprained ankle NOS
    - +7th S93.401 Sprain of unspecified ligament of right ankle
    - +7th S93.402 Sprain of unspecified ligament of left ankle
    - +7th S93.409 Sprain of unspecified ligament of unspecified ankle
  - **S93.41 Sprain of calcaneofibular ligament**
    - +7th S93.411 Sprain of calcaneofibular ligament of right ankle
    - +7th S93.412 Sprain of calcaneofibular ligament of left ankle
    - +7th S93.419 Sprain of calcaneofibular ligament of unspecified ankle
  - **S93.42 Sprain of deltoid ligament**
    - +7th S93.421 Sprain of deltoid ligament of right ankle
    - +7th S93.422 Sprain of deltoid ligament of left ankle
    - +7th S93.429 Sprain of deltoid ligament of unspecified ankle
  - **S93.43 Sprain of tibiofibular ligament**
    - +7th S93.431 Sprain of tibiofibular ligament of right ankle
    - +7th S93.432 Sprain of tibiofibular ligament of left ankle
    - +7th S93.439 Sprain of tibiofibular ligament of unspecified ankle
  - **S93.49 Sprain of other ligament of ankle**
    - Sprain of internal collateral ligament
    - Sprain of talofibular ligament
    - +7th S93.491 Sprain of other ligament of right ankle
    - +7th S93.492 Sprain of other ligament of left ankle
    - +7th S93.499 Sprain of other ligament of unspecified ankle

- **S93.5 Sprain of toe**
  - **S93.50 Unspecified sprain of toe**
    - +7th S93.501 Unspecified sprain of right great toe
    - +7th S93.502 Unspecified sprain of left great toe
    - +7th S93.503 Unspecified sprain of unspecified great toe
    - +7th S93.504 Unspecified sprain of right lesser toe(s)
    - +7th S93.505 Unspecified sprain of left lesser toe(s)
    - +7th S93.506 Unspecified sprain of unspecified lesser toe(s)
    - +7th S93.509 Unspecified sprain of unspecified toe(s)
  - **S93.51 Sprain of interphalangeal joint of toe**
    - +7th S93.511 Sprain of interphalangeal joint of right great toe
    - +7th S93.512 Sprain of interphalangeal joint of left great toe
    - +7th S93.513 Sprain of interphalangeal joint of unspecified great toe
    - +7th S93.514 Sprain of interphalangeal joint of right lesser toe(s)
    - +7th S93.515 Sprain of interphalangeal joint of left lesser toe(s)
    - +7th S93.516 Sprain of interphalangeal joint of unspecified lesser toe(s)
    - +7th S93.519 Sprain of interphalangeal joint of unspecified toe(s)
  - **S93.52 Sprain of metatarsophalangeal joint of toe**
    - +7th S93.521 Sprain of metatarsophalangeal joint of right great toe
    - +7th S93.522 Sprain of metatarsophalangeal joint of left great toe
    - +7th S93.523 Sprain of metatarsophalangeal joint of unspecified great toe
    - +7th S93.524 Sprain of metatarsophalangeal joint of right lesser toe(s)
    - +7th S93.525 Sprain of metatarsophalangeal joint of left lesser toe(s)
    - +7th S93.526 Sprain of metatarsophalangeal joint of unspecified lesser toe(s)
    - +7th S93.529 Sprain of metatarsophalangeal joint of unspecified toe(s)
- **S93.6 Sprain of foot**
  - *Excludes2:* sprain of metatarsophalangeal joint of toe (S93.52-) sprain of toe (S93.5-)
  - **S93.60 Unspecified sprain of foot**
    - +7th S93.601 Unspecified sprain of right foot
    - +7th S93.602 Unspecified sprain of left foot
    - +7th S93.609 Unspecified sprain of unspecified foot
  - **S93.61 Sprain of tarsal ligament of foot**
    - +7th S93.611 Sprain of tarsal ligament of right foot
    - +7th S93.612 Sprain of tarsal ligament of left foot
    - +7th S93.619 Sprain of tarsal ligament of unspecified foot
  - **S93.62 Sprain of tarsometatarsal ligament of foot**
    - +7th S93.621 Sprain of tarsometatarsal ligament of right foot
    - +7th S93.622 Sprain of tarsometatarsal ligament of left foot
    - +7th S93.629 Sprain of tarsometatarsal ligament of unspecified foot
  - **S93.69 Other sprain of foot**
    - +7th S93.691 Other sprain of right foot
    - +7th S93.692 Other sprain of left foot
    - +7th S93.699 Other sprain of unspecified foot

S94 Injury of nerves at ankle and foot level

Code also any associated open wound (S91.-)

The appropriate 7th character is to be added to each code from category S94
- A initial encounter
- D subsequent encounter
- S sequela

- **S94.0 Injury of lateral plantar nerve**
  - X+7th S94.00 Injury of lateral plantar nerve, unspecified leg
  - X+7th S94.01 Injury of lateral plantar nerve, right leg
  - X+7th S94.02 Injury of lateral plantar nerve, left leg
- **S94.1 Injury of medial plantar nerve**
  - X+7th S94.10 Injury of medial plantar nerve, unspecified leg
  - X+7th S94.11 Injury of medial plantar nerve, right leg
  - X+7th S94.12 Injury of medial plantar nerve, left leg

- **S94.2** Injury of deep peroneal nerve at ankle and foot level
  Injury of terminal, lateral branch of deep peroneal nerve
  - X+7th **S94.20** Injury of deep peroneal nerve at ankle and foot level, unspecified leg
  - X+7th **S94.21** Injury of deep peroneal nerve at ankle and foot level, right leg
  - X+7th **S94.22** Injury of deep peroneal nerve at ankle and foot level, left leg
- **S94.3** Injury of cutaneous sensory nerve at ankle and foot level
  - X+7th **S94.30** Injury of cutaneous sensory nerve at ankle and foot level, unspecified leg
  - X+7th **S94.31** Injury of cutaneous sensory nerve at ankle and foot level, right leg
  - X+7th **S94.32** Injury of cutaneous sensory nerve at ankle and foot level, left leg
- **S94.8** Injury of other nerves at ankle and foot level
  - **S94.8X** Injury of other nerves at ankle and foot level
    - +7th **S94.8X1** Injury of other nerves at ankle and foot level, right leg
    - +7th **S94.8X2** Injury of other nerves at ankle and foot level, left leg
    - +7th **S94.8X9** Injury of other nerves at ankle and foot level, unspecified leg
- **S94.9** Injury of unspecified nerve at ankle and foot level
  - X+7th **S94.90** Injury of unspecified nerve at ankle and foot level, unspecified leg
  - X+7th **S94.91** Injury of unspecified nerve at ankle and foot level, right leg
  - X+7th **S94.92** Injury of unspecified nerve at ankle and foot level, left leg

S95 Injury of blood vessels at ankle and foot level

Code also any associated open wound (S91.-)
Excludes2: injury of posterior tibial artery and vein (S85.1-, S85.8-)

The appropriate 7th character is to be added to each code from category S95
- A initial encounter
- D subsequent encounter
- S sequela

- **S95.0** Injury of dorsal artery of foot
  - **S95.00** Unspecified injury of dorsal artery of foot
    - CC +7th **S95.001** Unspecified injury of dorsal artery of right foot
    - CC +7th **S95.002** Unspecified injury of dorsal artery of left foot
    - CC +7th **S95.009** Unspecified injury of dorsal artery of unspecified foot
  - **S95.01** Laceration of dorsal artery of foot
    - CC +7th **S95.011** Laceration of dorsal artery of right foot
    - CC +7th **S95.012** Laceration of dorsal artery of left foot
    - CC +7th **S95.019** Laceration of dorsal artery of unspecified foot
  - **S95.09** Other specified injury of dorsal artery of foot
    - CC +7th **S95.091** Other specified injury of dorsal artery of right foot
    - CC +7th **S95.092** Other specified injury of dorsal artery of left foot
    - CC +7th **S95.099** Other specified injury of dorsal artery of unspecified foot
- **S95.1** Injury of plantar artery of foot
  - **S95.10** Unspecified injury of plantar artery of foot
    - CC +7th **S95.101** Unspecified injury of plantar artery of right foot
    - CC +7th **S95.102** Unspecified injury of plantar artery of left foot
    - CC +7th **S95.109** Unspecified injury of plantar artery of unspecified foot
  - **S95.11** Laceration of plantar artery of foot
    - CC +7th **S95.111** Laceration of plantar artery of right foot
    - CC +7th **S95.112** Laceration of plantar artery of left foot
    - CC +7th **S95.119** Laceration of plantar artery of unspecified foot
  - **S95.19** Other specified injury of plantar artery of foot
    - CC +7th **S95.191** Other specified injury of plantar artery of right foot
    - CC +7th **S95.192** Other specified injury of plantar artery of left foot
    - CC +7th **S95.199** Other specified injury of plantar artery of unspecified foot
- **S95.2** Injury of dorsal vein of foot
  - **S95.20** Unspecified injury of dorsal vein of foot
    - CC +7th **S95.201** Unspecified injury of dorsal vein of right foot
    - CC +7th **S95.202** Unspecified injury of dorsal vein of left foot
    - CC +7th **S95.209** Unspecified injury of dorsal vein of unspecified foot
  - **S95.21** Laceration of dorsal vein of foot
    - CC +7th **S95.211** Laceration of dorsal vein of right foot
    - CC +7th **S95.212** Laceration of dorsal vein of left foot
    - CC +7th **S95.219** Laceration of dorsal vein of unspecified foot
  - **S95.29** Other specified injury of dorsal vein of foot
    - CC +7th **S95.291** Other specified injury of dorsal vein of right foot
    - CC +7th **S95.292** Other specified injury of dorsal vein of left foot
    - CC +7th **S95.299** Other specified injury of dorsal vein of unspecified foot
- **S95.8** Injury of other blood vessels at ankle and foot level
  - **S95.80** Unspecified injury of other blood vessels at ankle and foot level
    - CC +7th **S95.801** Unspecified injury of other blood vessels at ankle and foot level, right leg
    - CC +7th **S95.802** Unspecified injury of other blood vessels at ankle and foot level, left leg
    - CC +7th **S95.809** Unspecified injury of other blood vessels at ankle and foot level, unspecified leg
  - **S95.81** Laceration of other blood vessels at ankle and foot level
    - CC +7th **S95.811** Laceration of other blood vessels at ankle and foot level, right leg
    - CC +7th **S95.812** Laceration of other blood vessels at ankle and foot level, left leg
    - CC +7th **S95.819** Laceration of other blood vessels at ankle and foot level, unspecified leg
  - **S95.89** Other specified injury of other blood vessels at ankle and foot level
    - CC +7th **S95.891** Other specified injury of other blood vessels at ankle and foot level, right leg
    - CC +7th **S95.892** Other specified injury of other blood vessels at ankle and foot level, left leg
    - CC +7th **S95.899** Other specified injury of other blood vessels at ankle and foot level, unspecified leg
- **S95.9** Injury of unspecified blood vessel at ankle and foot level
  - **S95.90** Unspecified injury of unspecified blood vessel at ankle and foot level
    - CC +7th **S95.901** Unspecified injury of unspecified blood vessel at ankle and foot level, right leg
    - CC +7th **S95.902** Unspecified injury of unspecified blood vessel at ankle and foot level, left leg
    - CC +7th **S95.909** Unspecified injury of unspecified blood vessel at ankle and foot level, unspecified leg
  - **S95.91** Laceration of unspecified blood vessel at ankle and foot level
    - CC +7th **S95.911** Laceration of unspecified blood vessel at ankle and foot level, right leg
    - CC +7th **S95.912** Laceration of unspecified blood vessel at ankle and foot level, left leg
    - CC +7th **S95.919** Laceration of unspecified blood vessel at ankle and foot level, unspecified leg
  - **S95.99** Other specified injury of unspecified blood vessel at ankle and foot level
    - CC +7th **S95.991** Other specified injury of unspecified blood vessel at ankle and foot level, right leg
    - CC +7th **S95.992** Other specified injury of unspecified blood vessel at ankle and foot level, left leg
    - CC +7th **S95.999** Other specified injury of unspecified blood vessel at ankle and foot level, unspecified leg

S96 Injury of muscle and tendon at ankle and foot level

Code also any associated open wound (S91.-)

Excludes2: injury of Achilles tendon (S86.0-)
sprain of joints and ligaments of ankle and foot (S93.-)

The appropriate 7th character is to be added to each code from category S96
- A initial encounter
- D subsequent encounter
- S sequela

- **S96.0 Injury of muscle and tendon of long flexor muscle of toe at ankle and foot level**
  - **S96.00 Unspecified injury of muscle and tendon of long flexor muscle of toe at ankle and foot level**
    - +7th S96.001 Unspecified injury of muscle and tendon of long flexor muscle of toe at ankle and foot level, right foot
    - +7th S96.002 Unspecified injury of muscle and tendon of long flexor muscle of toe at ankle and foot level, left foot
    - +7th S96.009 Unspecified injury of muscle and tendon of long flexor muscle of toe at ankle and foot level, unspecified foot
  - **S96.01 Strain of muscle and tendon of long flexor muscle of toe at ankle and foot level**
    - +7th S96.011 Strain of muscle and tendon of long flexor muscle of toe at ankle and foot level, right foot
    - +7th S96.012 Strain of muscle and tendon of long flexor muscle of toe at ankle and foot level, left foot
    - +7th S96.019 Strain of muscle and tendon of long flexor muscle of toe at ankle and foot level, unspecified foot
  - **S96.02 Laceration of muscle and tendon of long flexor muscle of toe at ankle and foot level**
    - CC +7th S96.021 Laceration of muscle and tendon of long flexor muscle of toe at ankle and foot level, right foot
    - CC +7th S96.022 Laceration of muscle and tendon of long flexor muscle of toe at ankle and foot level, left foot
    - CC +7th S96.029 Laceration of muscle and tendon of long flexor muscle of toe at ankle and foot level, unspecified foot
  - **S96.09 Other injury of muscle and tendon of long flexor muscle of toe at ankle and foot level**
    - +7th S96.091 Other injury of muscle and tendon of long flexor muscle of toe at ankle and foot level, right foot
    - +7th S96.092 Other injury of muscle and tendon of long flexor muscle of toe at ankle and foot level, left foot
    - +7th S96.099 Other injury of muscle and tendon of long flexor muscle of toe at ankle and foot level, unspecified foot
- **S96.1 Injury of muscle and tendon of long extensor muscle of toe at ankle and foot level**
  - **S96.10 Unspecified injury of muscle and tendon of long extensor muscle of toe at ankle and foot level**
    - +7th S96.101 Unspecified injury of muscle and tendon of long extensor muscle of toe at ankle and foot level, right foot
    - +7th S96.102 Unspecified injury of muscle and tendon of long extensor muscle of toe at ankle and foot level, left foot
    - +7th S96.109 Unspecified injury of muscle and tendon of long extensor muscle of toe at ankle and foot level, unspecified foot
  - **S96.11 Strain of muscle and tendon of long extensor muscle of toe at ankle and foot level**
    - +7th S96.111 Strain of muscle and tendon of long extensor muscle of toe at ankle and foot level, right foot
    - +7th S96.112 Strain of muscle and tendon of long extensor muscle of toe at ankle and foot level, left foot
    - +7th S96.119 Strain of muscle and tendon of long extensor muscle of toe at ankle and foot level, unspecified foot
  - **S96.12 Laceration of muscle and tendon of long extensor muscle of toe at ankle and foot level**
    - CC +7th S96.121 Laceration of muscle and tendon of long extensor muscle of toe at ankle and foot level, right foot
    - CC +7th S96.122 Laceration of muscle and tendon of long extensor muscle of toe at ankle and foot level, left foot
    - CC +7th S96.129 Laceration of muscle and tendon of long extensor muscle of toe at ankle and foot level, unspecified foot
  - **S96.19 Other specified injury of muscle and tendon of long extensor muscle of toe at ankle and foot level**
    - +7th S96.191 Other specified injury of muscle and tendon of long extensor muscle of toe at ankle and foot level, right foot
    - +7th S96.192 Other specified injury of muscle and tendon of long extensor muscle of toe at ankle and foot level, left foot
    - +7th S96.199 Other specified injury of muscle and tendon of long extensor muscle of toe at ankle and foot level, unspecified foot
- **S96.2 Injury of intrinsic muscle and tendon at ankle and foot level**
  - **S96.20 Unspecified injury of intrinsic muscle and tendon at ankle and foot level**
    - +7th S96.201 Unspecified injury of intrinsic muscle and tendon at ankle and foot level, right foot
    - +7th S96.202 Unspecified injury of intrinsic muscle and tendon at ankle and foot level, left foot
    - +7th S96.209 Unspecified injury of intrinsic muscle and tendon at ankle and foot level, unspecified foot
  - **S96.21 Strain of intrinsic muscle and tendon at ankle and foot level**
    - +7th S96.211 Strain of intrinsic muscle and tendon at ankle and foot level, right foot
    - +7th S96.212 Strain of intrinsic muscle and tendon at ankle and foot level, left foot
    - +7th S96.219 Strain of intrinsic muscle and tendon at ankle and foot level, unspecified foot
  - **S96.22 Laceration of intrinsic muscle and tendon at ankle and foot level**
    - CC +7th S96.221 Laceration of intrinsic muscle and tendon at ankle and foot level, right foot
    - CC +7th S96.222 Laceration of intrinsic muscle and tendon at ankle and foot level, left foot
    - CC +7th S96.229 Laceration of intrinsic muscle and tendon at ankle and foot level, unspecified foot
  - **S96.29 Other specified injury of intrinsic muscle and tendon at ankle and foot level**
    - +7th S96.291 Other specified injury of intrinsic muscle and tendon at ankle and foot level, right foot
    - +7th S96.292 Other specified injury of intrinsic muscle and tendon at ankle and foot level, left foot
    - +7th S96.299 Other specified injury of intrinsic muscle and tendon at ankle and foot level, unspecified foot
- **S96.8 Injury of other specified muscles and tendons at ankle and foot level**
  - **S96.80 Unspecified injury of other specified muscles and tendons at ankle and foot level**
    - +7th S96.801 Unspecified injury of other specified muscles and tendons at ankle and foot level, right foot
    - +7th S96.802 Unspecified injury of other specified muscles and tendons at ankle and foot level, left foot
    - +7th S96.809 Unspecified injury of other specified muscles and tendons at ankle and foot level, unspecified foot
  - **S96.81 Strain of other specified muscles and tendons at ankle and foot level**
    - +7th S96.811 Strain of other specified muscles and tendons at ankle and foot level, right foot
    - +7th S96.812 Strain of other specified muscles and tendons at ankle and foot level, left foot
    - +7th S96.819 Strain of other specified muscles and tendons at ankle and foot level, unspecified foot

- **S96.82** Laceration of other specified muscles and tendons at ankle and foot level
  - CC +7th **S96.821** Laceration of other specified muscles and tendons at ankle and foot level, right foot
  - CC +7th **S96.822** Laceration of other specified muscles and tendons at ankle and foot level, left foot
  - CC +7th **S96.829** Laceration of other specified muscles and tendons at ankle and foot level, unspecified foot
- **S96.89** Other specified injury of other specified muscles and tendons at ankle and foot level
  - +7th **S96.891** Other specified injury of other specified muscles and tendons at ankle and foot level, right foot
  - +7th **S96.892** Other specified injury of other specified muscles and tendons at ankle and foot level, left foot
  - +7th **S96.899** Other specified injury of other specified muscles and tendons at ankle and foot level, unspecified foot
- **+ S96.9** Injury of unspecified muscle and tendon at ankle and foot level
  - **+ S96.90** Unspecified injury of unspecified muscle and tendon at ankle and foot level
    - +7th **S96.901** Unspecified injury of unspecified muscle and tendon at ankle and foot level, right foot
    - +7th **S96.902** Unspecified injury of unspecified muscle and tendon at ankle and foot level, left foot
    - +7th **S96.909** Unspecified injury of unspecified muscle and tendon at ankle and foot level, unspecified foot
  - **+ S96.91** Strain of unspecified muscle and tendon at ankle and foot level
    - +7th **S96.911** Strain of unspecified muscle and tendon at ankle and foot level, right foot
    - +7th **S96.912** Strain of unspecified muscle and tendon at ankle and foot level, left foot
    - +7th **S96.919** Strain of unspecified muscle and tendon at ankle and foot level, unspecified foot
  - **+ S96.92** Laceration of unspecified muscle and tendon at ankle and foot level
    - CC +7th **S96.921** Laceration of unspecified muscle and tendon at ankle and foot level, right foot
    - CC +7th **S96.922** Laceration of unspecified muscle and tendon at ankle and foot level, left foot
    - CC +7th **S96.929** Laceration of unspecified muscle and tendon at ankle and foot level, unspecified foot
  - **+ S96.99** Other specified injury of unspecified muscle and tendon at ankle and foot level
    - +7th **S96.991** Other specified injury of unspecified muscle and tendon at ankle and foot level, right foot
    - +7th **S96.992** Other specified injury of unspecified muscle and tendon at ankle and foot level, left foot
    - +7th **S96.999** Other specified injury of unspecified muscle and tendon at ankle and foot level, unspecified foot

S97 Crushing injury of ankle and foot

Use additional code(s) for all associated injuries

The appropriate 7th character is to be added to each code from category S97
- A initial encounter
- D subsequent encounter
- S sequela

- **+ S97.0** Crushing injury of ankle
  - X+7th **S97.00** Crushing injury of unspecified ankle
  - X+7th **S97.01** Crushing injury of right ankle
  - X+7th **S97.02** Crushing injury of left ankle
- **+ S97.1** Crushing injury of toe
  - **+ S97.10** Crushing injury of unspecified toe(s)
    - +7th **S97.101** Crushing injury of unspecified right toe(s)
    - +7th **S97.102** Crushing injury of unspecified left toe(s)
    - +7th **S97.109** Crushing injury of unspecified toe(s)
      Crushing injury of toe NOS
  - **+ S97.11** Crushing injury of great toe
    - +7th **S97.111** Crushing injury of right great toe
    - +7th **S97.112** Crushing injury of left great toe
    - +7th **S97.119** Crushing injury of unspecified great toe
  - **+ S97.12** Crushing injury of lesser toe(s)
    - +7th **S97.121** Crushing injury of right lesser toe(s)
    - +7th **S97.122** Crushing injury of left lesser toe(s)
    - +7th **S97.129** Crushing injury of unspecified lesser toe(s)
- **+ S97.8** Crushing injury of foot
  - X+7th **S97.80** Crushing injury of unspecified foot
    Crushing injury of foot NOS
  - X+7th **S97.81** Crushing injury of right foot
  - X+7th **S97.82** Crushing injury of left foot

S98 Traumatic amputation of ankle and foot

NOTE An amputation not identified as partial or complete should be coded to complete

The appropriate 7th character is to be added to each code from category S98
- A initial encounter
- D subsequent encounter
- S sequela

- **+ S98.0** Traumatic amputation of foot at ankle level
  - **+ S98.01** Complete traumatic amputation of foot at ankle level
    - CC +7th **S98.011** Complete traumatic amputation of right foot at ankle level
    - CC +7th **S98.012** Complete traumatic amputation of left foot at ankle level
    - CC +7th **S98.019** Complete traumatic amputation of unspecified foot at ankle level
  - **+ S98.02** Partial traumatic amputation of foot at ankle level
    - CC +7th **S98.021** Partial traumatic amputation of right foot at ankle level
    - CC +7th **S98.022** Partial traumatic amputation of left foot at ankle level
    - CC +7th **S98.029** Partial traumatic amputation of unspecified foot at ankle level
- **+ S98.1** Traumatic amputation of one toe
  - **+ S98.11** Complete traumatic amputation of great toe
    - +7th **S98.111** Complete traumatic amputation of right great toe
    - +7th **S98.112** Complete traumatic amputation of left great toe
    - +7th **S98.119** Complete traumatic amputation of unspecified great toe
  - **+ S98.12** Partial traumatic amputation of great toe
    - +7th **S98.121** Partial traumatic amputation of right great toe
    - +7th **S98.122** Partial traumatic amputation of left great toe
    - +7th **S98.129** Partial traumatic amputation of unspecified great toe
  - **+ S98.13** Complete traumatic amputation of one lesser toe
    Traumatic amputation of toe NOS
    - +7th **S98.131** Complete traumatic amputation of one right lesser toe
    - +7th **S98.132** Complete traumatic amputation of one left lesser toe
    - +7th **S98.139** Complete traumatic amputation of one unspecified lesser toe
  - **+ S98.14** Partial traumatic amputation of one lesser toe
    - +7th **S98.141** Partial traumatic amputation of one right lesser toe
    - +7th **S98.142** Partial traumatic amputation of one left lesser toe
    - +7th **S98.149** Partial traumatic amputation of one unspecified lesser toe

- **S98.2 Traumatic amputation of two or more lesser toes**
  - **S98.21 Complete traumatic amputation of two or more lesser toes**
    - +7th **S98.211** Complete traumatic amputation of two or more right lesser toes
    - +7th **S98.212** Complete traumatic amputation of two or more left lesser toes
    - +7th **S98.219** Complete traumatic amputation of two or more unspecified lesser toes
  - **S98.22 Partial traumatic amputation of two or more lesser toes**
    - +7th **S98.221** Partial traumatic amputation of two or more right lesser toes
    - +7th **S98.222** Partial traumatic amputation of two or more left lesser toes
    - +7th **S98.229** Partial traumatic amputation of two or more unspecified lesser toes
- **S98.3 Traumatic amputation of midfoot**
  - **S98.31 Complete traumatic amputation of midfoot**
    - CC +7th **S98.311** Complete traumatic amputation of right midfoot
    - CC +7th **S98.312** Complete traumatic amputation of left midfoot
    - CC +7th **S98.319** Complete traumatic amputation of unspecified midfoot
  - **S98.32 Partial traumatic amputation of midfoot**
    - CC +7th **S98.321** Partial traumatic amputation of right midfoot
    - CC +7th **S98.322** Partial traumatic amputation of left midfoot
    - CC +7th **S98.329** Partial traumatic amputation of unspecified midfoot
- **S98.9 Traumatic amputation of foot, level unspecified**
  - **S98.91 Complete traumatic amputation of foot, level unspecified**
    - CC +7th **S98.911** Complete traumatic amputation of right foot, level unspecified
    - CC +7th **S98.912** Complete traumatic amputation of left foot, level unspecified
    - CC +7th **S98.919** Complete traumatic amputation of unspecified foot, level unspecified
  - **S98.92 Partial traumatic amputation of foot, level unspecified**
    - CC +7th **S98.921** Partial traumatic amputation of right foot, level unspecified
    - CC +7th **S98.922** Partial traumatic amputation of left foot, level unspecified
    - CC +7th **S98.929** Partial traumatic amputation of unspecified foot, level unspecified

S99 Other and unspecified injuries of ankle and foot

- **S99.0 Physeal fracture of calcaneus**
  AHA CC: 4Q, 2016, 68-69

  > The appropriate 7th character is to be added to each code in subcategory **S99.0**
  >
  > A initial encounter for closed fracture
  > B initial encounter for open fracture
  > D subsequent encounter for fracture with routine healing
  > G subsequent encounter for fracture with delayed healing
  > K subsequent encounter for fracture with nonunion
  > P subsequent encounter for fracture with malunion
  > S sequela

  - **S99.00 Unspecified physeal fracture of calcaneus**
    Unspecified physeal fracture of calcaneus
    - +7th **S99.001** Unspecified physeal fracture of right calcaneus
    - +7th **S99.002** Unspecified physeal fracture of left calcaneus
    - +7th **S99.009** Unspecified physeal fracture of unspecified calcaneus
  - **S99.01 Salter-Harris Type I physeal fracture of calcaneus**
    - +7th **S99.011** Salter-Harris Type I physeal fracture of right calcaneus
    - +7th **S99.012** Salter-Harris Type I physeal fracture of left calcaneus
    - +7th **S99.019** Salter-Harris Type I physeal fracture of unspecified calcaneus
  - **S99.02 Salter-Harris Type II physeal fracture of calcaneus**
    - +7th **S99.021** Salter-Harris Type II physeal fracture of right calcaneus
    - +7th **S99.022** Salter-Harris Type II physeal fracture of left calcaneus
    - +7th **S99.029** Salter-Harris Type II physeal fracture of unspecified calcaneus
  - **S99.03 Salter-Harris Type III physeal fracture of calcaneus**
    - +7th **S99.031** Salter-Harris Type III physeal fracture of right calcaneus
    - +7th **S99.032** Salter-Harris Type III physeal fracture of left calcaneus
    - +7th **S99.039** Salter-Harris Type III physeal fracture of unspecified calcaneus
  - **S99.04 Salter-Harris Type IV physeal fracture of calcaneus**
    - +7th **S99.041** Salter-Harris Type IV physeal fracture of right calcaneus
    - +7th **S99.042** Salter-Harris Type IV physeal fracture of left calcaneus
    - +7th **S99.049** Salter-Harris Type IV physeal fracture of unspecified calcaneus
  - **S99.09 Other physeal fracture of calcaneus**
    - +7th **S99.091** Other physeal fracture of right calcaneus
    - +7th **S99.092** Other physeal fracture of left calcaneus
    - +7th **S99.099** Other physeal fracture of unspecified calcaneus

- **S99.1 Physeal fracture of metatarsal**

  > The appropriate 7th character is to be added to each code in subcategory **S99.1**
  >
  > A initial encounter for closed fracture
  > B initial encounter for open fracture
  > D subsequent encounter for fracture with routine healing
  > G subsequent encounter for fracture with delayed healing
  > K subsequent encounter for fracture with nonunion
  > P subsequent encounter for fracture with malunion
  > S sequela

  - **S99.10 Unspecified physeal fracture of metatarsal**
    - +7th **S99.101** Unspecified physeal fracture of right metatarsal
    - +7th **S99.102** Unspecified physeal fracture of left metatarsal
    - +7th **S99.109** Unspecified physeal fracture of unspecified metatarsal
  - **S99.11 Salter-Harris Type I physeal fracture of metatarsal**
    - +7th **S99.111** Salter-Harris Type I physeal fracture of right metatarsal
    - +7th **S99.112** Salter-Harris Type I physeal fracture of left metatarsal
      AHA CC: 1Q, 2018, 3
    - +7th **S99.119** Salter-Harris Type I physeal fracture of unspecified metatarsal
  - **S99.12 Salter-Harris Type II physeal fracture of metatarsal**
    - +7th **S99.121** Salter-Harris Type II physeal fracture of right metatarsal
    - +7th **S99.122** Salter-Harris Type II physeal fracture of left metatarsal
    - +7th **S99.129** Salter-Harris Type II physeal fracture of unspecified metatarsal
  - **S99.13 Salter-Harris Type III physeal fracture of metatarsal**
    - +7th **S99.131** Salter-Harris Type III physeal fracture of right metatarsal
    - +7th **S99.132** Salter-Harris Type III physeal fracture of left metatarsal
    - +7th **S99.139** Salter-Harris Type III physeal fracture of unspecified metatarsal
  - **S99.14 Salter-Harris Type IV physeal fracture of metatarsal**
    - +7th **S99.141** Salter-Harris Type IV physeal fracture of right metatarsal
    - +7th **S99.142** Salter-Harris Type IV physeal fracture of left metatarsal
    - +7th **S99.149** Salter-Harris Type IV physeal fracture of unspecified metatarsal

- **S99.19 Other physeal fracture of metatarsal**
  - +7th S99.191 Other physeal fracture of right metatarsal
  - +7th S99.192 Other physeal fracture of left metatarsal
  - +7th S99.199 Other physeal fracture of unspecified metatarsal

- **S99.2 Phseal fracture of phalanx of toe**

  The appropriate 7th character is to be added to each code in subcategory **S99.2**
  - A initial encounter for closed fracture
  - B initial encounter for open fracture
  - D subsequent encounter for fracture with routine healing
  - G subsequent encounter for fracture with delayed healing
  - K subsequent encounter for fracture with nonunion
  - P subsequent encounter for fracture with malunion
  - S sequela

  - + **S99.20 Unspecified physeal fracture of phalanx of toe**
    - +7th S99.201 Unspecified physeal fracture of phalanx of right toe
    - +7th S99.202 Unspecified physeal fracture of phalanx of left toe
    - +7th S99.209 Unspecified physeal fracture of phalanx of unspecified toe
  - + **S99.21 Salter-Harris Type I physeal fracture of phalanx of toe**
    - +7th S99.211 Salter-Harris Type I physeal fracture of phalanx of right toe
    - +7th S99.212 Salter-Harris Type I physeal fracture of phalanx of left toe
    - +7th S99.219 Salter-Harris Type I physeal fracture of phalanx of unspecified toe
  - + **S99.22 Salter-Harris Type II physeal fracture of phalanx of toe**
    - +7th S99.221 Salter-Harris Type II physeal fracture of phalanx of right toe
    - +7th S99.222 Salter-Harris Type II physeal fracture of phalanx of left toe
    - +7th S99.229 Salter-Harris Type II physeal fracture of phalanx of unspecified toe
  - + **S99.23 Salter-Harris Type III physeal fracture of phalanx of toe**
    - +7th S99.231 Salter-Harris Type III physeal fracture of phalanx of right toe
    - +7th S99.232 Salter-Harris Type III physeal fracture of phalanx of left toe
    - +7th S99.239 Salter-Harris Type III physeal fracture of phalanx of unspecified toe
  - + **S99.24 Salter-Harris Type IV physeal fracture of phalanx of toe**
    - +7th S99.241 Salter-Harris Type IV physeal fracture of phalanx of right toe
    - +7th S99.242 Salter-Harris Type IV physeal fracture of phalanx of left toe
    - +7th S99.249 Salter-Harris Type IV physeal fracture of phalanx of unspecified toe
  - + **S99.29 Other physeal fracture of phalanx of toe**
    - +7th S99.291 Other physeal fracture of phalanx of right toe
    - +7th S99.292 Other physeal fracture of phalanx of left toe
    - +7th S99.299 Other physeal fracture of phalanx of unspecified toe

- + **S99.8 Other specified injuries of ankle and foot**

  The appropriate 7th character is to be added to each code from category **S99.8**
  - A initial encounter
  - D subsequent encounter
  - S sequela

  - + **S99.81 Other specified injuries of ankle**
    - +7th S99.811 Other specified injuries of right ankle
    - +7th S99.812 Other specified injuries of left ankle
    - +7th S99.819 Other specified injuries of unspecified ankle
  - + **S99.82 Other specified injuries of foot**
    - +7th S99.821 Other specified injuries of right foot
    - +7th S99.822 Other specified injuries of left foot
    - +7th S99.829 Other specified injuries of unspecified foot
- + **S99.9 Unspecified injury of ankle and foot**

  The appropriate 7th character is to be added to each code from category **S99.9**
  - A initial encounter
  - D subsequent encounter
  - S sequela

  - + **S99.91 Unspecified injury of ankle**
    - +7th S99.911 Unspecified injury of right ankle
    - +7th S99.912 Unspecified injury of left ankle
    - +7th S99.919 Unspecified injury of unspecified ankle
  - + **S99.92 Unspecified injury of foot**
    - +7th S99.921 Unspecified injury of right foot
    - +7th S99.922 Unspecified injury of left foot
    - +7th S99.929 Unspecified injury of unspecified foot

INJURY, POISONING AND CERTAIN OTHER CONSEQUENCES OF EXTERNAL CAUSES (T07-T88)

Injuries involving multiple body regions (T07)

Excludes1: burns and corrosions (T20-T32)
  frostbite (T33-T34)
  insect bite or sting, venomous (T63.4)
  sunburn (L55.-)

T07 Unspecified multiple injuries

The appropriate 7th character is to be added to each code from category T07
- A initial encounter
- D subsequent encounter
- S sequela

Excludes1: injury NOS (T14.90)
AHA CC: 4Q, 2017, 26
Review coding guideline C.19.b

Injury of unspecified body region (T14)

T14 Injury of unspecified body region

The appropriate 7th character is to be added to each code from category T14
- A initial encounter
- D subsequent encounter
- S sequela

Excludes1: multiple unspecified injuries (T07)
AHA CC: 4Q, 2017, 26

- **T14.8 Other injury of unspecified body region**
  - Abrasion NOS
  - Contusion NOS
  - Crush injury NOS
  - Fracture NOS
  - Skin injury NOS
  - Vascular injury NOS
  - Wound NOS
- + **T14.9 Unspecified injury**
  - **T14.90 Injury, unspecified**
    - Injury NOS
  - **T14.91 Suicide attempt**
    - Attempted suicide NOS

Effects of foreign body entering through natural orifice (T15-T19)

Use Additional code, if known, for foreign body entering into or through a natural orifice (W44.-)

Excludes2: *foreign body accidentally left in operation wound (T81.5-)*
foreign body in penetrating wound - See open wound by body region
residual foreign body in soft tissue (M79.5)
splinter, without open wound - See superficial injury by body region

T15 Foreign body on external eye

Excludes2: *foreign body in penetrating wound of orbit and eye ball (S05.4-, S05.5-)*
open wound of eyelid and periocular area (S01.1-)
retained foreign body in eyelid (H02.8-)
retained (old) foreign body in penetrating wound of orbit and eye ball (H05.5-, H44.6-, H44.7-)
superficial foreign body of eyelid and periocular area (S00.25-)

> The appropriate 7th character is to be added to each code from category T15
> A initial encounter
> D subsequent encounter
> S sequela

+ **T15.0** Foreign body in cornea
 X+7th **T15.00** Foreign body in cornea, unspecified eye
 X+7th **T15.01** Foreign body in cornea, right eye
 X+7th **T15.02** Foreign body in cornea, left eye
+ **T15.1** Foreign body in conjunctival sac
 X+7th **T15.10** Foreign body in conjunctival sac, unspecified eye
 X+7th **T15.11** Foreign body in conjunctival sac, right eye
 X+7th **T15.12** Foreign body in conjunctival sac, left eye
+ **T15.8** Foreign body in other and multiple parts of external eye
  Foreign body in lacrimal punctum
 X+7th **T15.80** Foreign body in other and multiple parts of external eye, unspecified eye
 X+7th **T15.81** Foreign body in other and multiple parts of external eye, right eye
 X+7th **T15.82** Foreign body in other and multiple parts of external eye, left eye
+ **T15.9** Foreign body on external eye, part unspecified
 X+7th **T15.90** Foreign body on external eye, part unspecified, unspecified eye
 X+7th **T15.91** Foreign body on external eye, part unspecified, right eye
 X+7th **T15.92** Foreign body on external eye, part unspecified, left eye

T16 Foreign body in ear

Includes: foreign body in auditory canal

> The appropriate 7th character is to be added to each code from category T16
> A initial encounter
> D subsequent encounter
> S sequela

X+7th **T16.1** Foreign body in right ear
X+7th **T16.2** Foreign body in left ear
X+7th **T16.9** Foreign body in ear, unspecified ear

T17 Foreign body in respiratory tract

> The appropriate 7th character is to be added to each code from category T17
> A initial encounter
> D subsequent encounter
> S sequela

X+7th **T17.0** Foreign body in nasal sinus
X+7th **T17.1** Foreign body in nostril
  Foreign body in nose NOS
+ **T17.2** Foreign body in pharynx
  Foreign body in nasopharynx
  Foreign body in throat NOS
 + **T17.20** Unspecified foreign body in pharynx
  +7th **T17.200** Unspecified foreign body in pharynx causing asphyxiation
  +7th **T17.208** Unspecified foreign body in pharynx causing other injury
 + **T17.21** Gastric contents in pharynx
  Aspiration of gastric contents into pharynx
  Vomitus in pharynx
  +7th **T17.210** Gastric contents in pharynx causing asphyxiation
  +7th **T17.218** Gastric contents in pharynx causing other injury
 + **T17.22** Food in pharynx
  Bones in pharynx
  Seeds in pharynx
  +7th **T17.220** Food in pharynx causing asphyxiation
  +7th **T17.228** Food in pharynx causing other injury
 + **T17.29** Other foreign object in pharynx
  +7th **T17.290** Other foreign object in pharynx causing asphyxiation
  +7th **T17.298** Other foreign object in pharynx causing other injury
+ **T17.3** Foreign body in larynx
 + **T17.30** Unspecified foreign body in larynx
  +7th **T17.300** Unspecified foreign body in larynx causing asphyxiation
  +7th **T17.308** Unspecified foreign body in larynx causing other injury
 + **T17.31** Gastric contents in larynx
  Aspiration of gastric contents into larynx
  Vomitus in larynx
  +7th **T17.310** Gastric contents in larynx causing asphyxiation
  +7th **T17.318** Gastric contents in larynx causing other injury
 + **T17.32** Food in larynx
  Bones in larynx
  Seeds in larynx
  +7th **T17.320** Food in larynx causing asphyxiation
  +7th **T17.328** Food in larynx causing other injury
 + **T17.39** Other foreign object in larynx
  +7th **T17.390** Other foreign object in larynx causing asphyxiation
  +7th **T17.398** Other foreign object in larynx causing other injury
+ **T17.4** Foreign body in trachea
 + **T17.40** Unspecified foreign body in trachea
  CC +7th **T17.400** Unspecified foreign body in trachea causing asphyxiation
  CC +7th **T17.408** Unspecified foreign body in trachea causing other injury
 + **T17.41** Gastric contents in trachea
  Aspiration of gastric contents into trachea
  Vomitus in trachea
  CC +7th **T17.410** Gastric contents in trachea causing asphyxiation
  CC +7th **T17.418** Gastric contents in trachea causing other injury
 + **T17.42** Food in trachea
  Bones in trachea
  Seeds in trachea
  CC +7th **T17.420** Food in trachea causing asphyxiation
  CC +7th **T17.428** Food in trachea causing other injury
 + **T17.49** Other foreign object in trachea
  CC +7th **T17.490** Other foreign object in trachea causing asphyxiation
  CC +7th **T17.498** Other foreign object in trachea causing other injury
+ **T17.5** Foreign body in bronchus
 + **T17.50** Unspecified foreign body in bronchus
  CC +7th **T17.500** Unspecified foreign body in bronchus causing asphyxiation
  CC +7th **T17.508** Unspecified foreign body in bronchus causing other injury
 + **T17.51** Gastric contents in bronchus
  Aspiration of gastric contents into bronchus
  Vomitus in bronchus
  CC +7th **T17.510** Gastric contents in bronchus causing asphyxiation
  CC +7th **T17.518** Gastric contents in bronchus causing other injury
 + **T17.52** Food in bronchus
  Bones in bronchus
  Seeds in bronchus
  CC +7th **T17.520** Food in bronchus causing asphyxiation
  CC +7th **T17.528** Food in bronchus causing other injury

- **+ T17.59 Other foreign object in bronchus**
  - CC +7th **T17.590** Other foreign object in bronchus causing asphyxiation
  - CC +7th **T17.598** Other foreign object in bronchus causing other injury
- **+ T17.8 Foreign body in other parts of respiratory tract**
  - Foreign body in bronchioles
  - Foreign body in lung
  - **+ T17.80** Unspecified foreign body in other parts of respiratory tract
    - CC +7th **T17.800** Unspecified foreign body in other parts of respiratory tract causing asphyxiation
    - CC +7th **T17.808** Unspecified foreign body in other parts of respiratory tract causing other injury
  - **+ T17.81** Gastric contents in other parts of respiratory tract
    - Aspiration of gastric contents into other parts of respiratory tract
    - Vomitus in other parts of respiratory tract
    - CC +7th **T17.810** Gastric contents in other parts of respiratory tract causing asphyxiation
    - CC +7th **T17.818** Gastric contents in other parts of respiratory tract causing other injury
  - **+ T17.82** Food in other parts of respiratory tract
    - Bones in other parts of respiratory tract
    - Seeds in other parts of respiratory tract
    - CC +7th **T17.820** Food in other parts of respiratory tract causing asphyxiation
    - CC +7th **T17.828** Food in other parts of respiratory tract causing other injury
  - **+ T17.89** Other foreign object in other parts of respiratory tract
    - CC +7th **T17.890** Other foreign object in other parts of respiratory tract causing asphyxiation
    - CC +7th **T17.898** Other foreign object in other parts of respiratory tract causing other injury
- **T17.9 Foreign body in respiratory tract, part unspecified**
  - **+ T17.90** Unspecified foreign body in respiratory tract, part unspecified
    - +7th **T17.900** Unspecified foreign body in respiratory tract, part unspecified causing asphyxiation
    - +7th **T17.908** Unspecified foreign body in respiratory tract, part unspecified causing other injury
  - **+ T17.91** Gastric contents in respiratory tract, part unspecified
    - Aspiration of gastric contents into respiratory tract, part unspecified
    - Vomitus in trachea respiratory tract, part unspecified
    - +7th **T17.910** Gastric contents in respiratory tract, part unspecified causing asphyxiation
    - +7th **T17.918** Gastric contents in respiratory tract, part unspecified causing other injury
  - **+ T17.92** Food in respiratory tract, part unspecified
    - Bones in respiratory tract, part unspecified
    - Seeds in respiratory tract, part unspecified
    - +7th **T17.920** Food in respiratory tract, part unspecified causing asphyxiation
    - +7th **T17.928** Food in respiratory tract, part unspecified causing other injury
  - **+ T17.99** Other foreign object in respiratory tract, part unspecified
    - +7th **T17.990** Other foreign object in respiratory tract, part unspecified in causing asphyxiation
    - +7th **T17.998** Other foreign object in respiratory tract, part unspecified causing other injury

T18 Foreign body in alimentary tract

Excludes2: *foreign body in pharynx (T17.2-)*

The appropriate 7th character is to be added to each code from category T18
- A initial encounter
- D subsequent encounter
- S sequela

- X +7th **T18.0** Foreign body in mouth
- **+ T18.1** Foreign body in esophagus
  - **Excludes2:** *foreign body in respiratory tract (T17.-)*
  - **+ T18.10** Unspecified foreign body in esophagus
    - +7th **T18.100** Unspecified foreign body in esophagus causing compression of trachea
      - Unspecified foreign body in esophagus causing obstruction of respiration
    - +7th **T18.108** Unspecified foreign body in esophagus causing other injury
  - **+ T18.11** Gastric contents in esophagus
    - Vomitus in esophagus
    - +7th **T18.110** Gastric contents in esophagus causing compression of trachea
      - Gastric contents in esophagus causing obstruction of respiration
    - +7th **T18.118** Gastric contents in esophagus causing other injury
  - **+ T18.12** Food in esophagus
    - Bones in esophagus
    - Seeds in esophagus
    - +7th **T18.120** Food in esophagus causing compression of trachea
      - Food in esophagus causing obstruction of respiration
    - +7th **T18.128** Food in esophagus causing other injury
  - **+ T18.19** Other foreign object in esophagus
    - +7th **T18.190** Other foreign object in esophagus causing compression of trachea
      - Other foreign body in esophagus causing obstruction of respiration
      - *AHA CC: 1Q, 2015, 23-24*
    - +7th **T18.198** Other foreign object in esophagus causing other injury
      - *AHA CC: 1Q, 2015, 23-24*
- X +7th **T18.2** Foreign body in stomach
- X +7th **T18.3** Foreign body in small intestine
- X +7th **T18.4** Foreign body in colon
- X +7th **T18.5** Foreign body in anus and rectum
  - Foreign body in rectosigmoid (junction)
- X +7th **T18.8** Foreign body in other parts of alimentary tract
- X +7th **T18.9** Foreign body of alimentary tract, part unspecified
  - Foreign body in digestive system NOS
  - Swallowed foreign body NOS

T19 Foreign body in genitourinary tract

Excludes2: *complications due to implanted mesh (T83.7-)*
mechanical complications of contraceptive device (intrauterine) (vaginal) (T83.3-)
presence of contraceptive device (intrauterine) (vaginal) (Z97.5)

The appropriate 7th character is to be added to each code from category T19
- A initial encounter
- D subsequent encounter
- S sequela

- X +7th **T19.0** Foreign body in urethra
- X +7th **T19.1** Foreign body in bladder
- ♀ X +7th **T19.2** Foreign body in vulva and vagina
- ♀ X +7th **T19.3** Foreign body in uterus
- ♂ X +7th **T19.4** Foreign body in penis
- X +7th **T19.8** Foreign body in other parts of genitourinary tract
- X +7th **T19.9** Foreign body in genitourinary tract, part unspecified

BURNS AND CORROSIONS (T20-T32)

Includes: burns (thermal) from electrical heating appliances
burns (thermal) from electricity
burns (thermal) from flame
burns (thermal) from friction
burns (thermal) from hot air and hot gases
burns (thermal) from hot objects
burns (thermal) from lightning
burns (thermal) from radiation
chemical burn [corrosion] (external) (internal)
scalds

Excludes2: *erythema [dermatitis] ab igne (L59.0)*
radiation-related disorders of the skin and subcutaneous tissue (L55-L59)
sunburn (L55.-)

Burns and corrosions of external body surface, specified by site (T20-T25)

Includes: burns and corrosions of first degree [erythema]
burns and corrosions of second degree [blisters][epidermal loss]
burns and corrosions of third degree [deep necrosis of underlying tissue] [full- thickness skin loss]

Use additional code from category T31 or T32 to identify extent of body surface involved
Review coding guideline C.19.d

T20 Burn and corrosion of head, face, and neck

Excludes2: *burn and corrosion of ear drum (T28.41, T28.91)*
burn and corrosion of eye and adnexa (T26.-)
burn and corrosion of mouth and pharynx (T28.0)

The appropriate 7th character is to be added to each code from category T20
A initial encounter
D subsequent encounter
S sequela

- **T20.0** Burn of unspecified degree of head, face, and neck
  Use additional external cause code to identify the source, place and intent of the burn (X00-X19, X75-X77, X96-X98, Y92)
  - X+7th **T20.00** Burn of unspecified degree of head, face, and neck, unspecified site
  - **T20.01** Burn of unspecified degree of ear [any part, except ear drum]
    Excludes2: *burn of ear drum (T28.41-)*
    - +7th **T20.011** Burn of unspecified degree of right ear [any part, except ear drum]
    - +7th **T20.012** Burn of unspecified degree of left ear [any part, except ear drum]
    - +7th **T20.019** Burn of unspecified degree of unspecified ear [any part, except ear drum]
  - X+7th **T20.02** Burn of unspecified degree of lip(s)
  - X+7th **T20.03** Burn of unspecified degree of chin
  - X+7th **T20.04** Burn of unspecified degree of nose (septum)
  - X+7th **T20.05** Burn of unspecified degree of scalp [any part]
  - X+7th **T20.06** Burn of unspecified degree of forehead and cheek
  - X+7th **T20.07** Burn of unspecified degree of neck
  - X+7th **T20.09** Burn of unspecified degree of multiple sites of head, face, and neck
- **T20.1** Burn of first degree of head, face, and neck
  Use additional external cause code to identify the source, place and intent of the burn (X00-X19, X75-X77, X96-X98, Y92)
  - X+7th **T20.10** Burn of first degree of head, face, and neck, unspecified site
  - **T20.11** Burn of first degree of ear [any part, except ear drum]
    Excludes2: *burn of ear drum (T28.41-)*
    - +7th **T20.111** Burn of first degree of right ear [any part, except ear drum]
    - +7th **T20.112** Burn of first degree of left ear [any part, except ear drum]
    - +7th **T20.119** Burn of first degree of unspecified ear [any part, except ear drum]
  - X+7th **T20.12** Burn of first degree of lip(s)
  - X+7th **T20.13** Burn of first degree of chin
  - X+7th **T20.14** Burn of first degree of nose (septum)
  - X+7th **T20.15** Burn of first degree of scalp [any part]
  - X+7th **T20.16** Burn of first degree of forehead and cheek
  - X+7th **T20.17** Burn of first degree of neck
  - X+7th **T20.19** Burn of first degree of multiple sites of head, face, and neck
- **T20.2** Burn of second degree of head, face, and neck
  Use additional external cause code to identify the source, place and intent of the burn (X00-X19, X75-X77, X96-X98, Y92)
  - X+7th **T20.20** Burn of second degree of head, face, and neck, unspecified site
  - **T20.21** Burn of second degree of ear [any part, except ear drum]
    Excludes2: *burn of ear drum (T28.41-)*
    - +7th **T20.211** Burn of second degree of right ear [any part, except ear drum]
    - +7th **T20.212** Burn of second degree of left ear [any part, except ear drum]
    - +7th **T20.219** Burn of second degree of unspecified ear [any part, except ear drum]
  - X+7th **T20.22** Burn of second degree of lip(s)
  - X+7th **T20.23** Burn of second degree of chin
  - X+7th **T20.24** Burn of second degree of nose (septum)
  - X+7th **T20.25** Burn of second degree of scalp [any part]
    AHA CC: 1Q, 2015, 3-21
  - X+7th **T20.26** Burn of second degree of forehead and cheek
  - X+7th **T20.27** Burn of second degree of neck
  - X+7th **T20.29** Burn of second degree of multiple sites of head, face, and neck
- **T20.3** Burn of third degree of head, face, and neck
  Use additional external cause code to identify the source, place and intent of the burn (X00-X19, X75-X77, X96-X98, Y92)
  - CC X+7th **T20.30** Burn of third degree of head, face, and neck, unspecified site
    HAC 7th character A see Appendix B for HAC conditional logic
  - **T20.31** Burn of third degree of ear [any part, except ear drum]
    Excludes2: *burn of ear drum (T28.41-)*
    - CC +7th **T20.311** Burn of third degree of right ear [any part, except ear drum]
      HAC 7th character A see Appendix B for HAC conditional logic
    - CC +7th **T20.312** Burn of third degree of left ear [any part, except ear drum]
      HAC 7th character A see Appendix B for HAC conditional logic
      AHA CC: 1Q, 2015, 3-21
    - CC +7th **T20.319** Burn of third degree of unspecified ear [any part, except ear drum]
      HAC 7th character A see Appendix B for HAC conditional logic
  - CC X+7th **T20.32** Burn of third degree of lip(s)
    HAC 7th character A see Appendix B for HAC conditional logic
  - CC X+7th **T20.33** Burn of third degree of chin
    HAC 7th character A see Appendix B for HAC conditional logic
  - CC X+7th **T20.34** Burn of third degree of nose (septum)
    HAC 7th character A see Appendix B for HAC conditional logic
  - CC X+7th **T20.35** Burn of third degree of scalp [any part]
    HAC 7th character A see Appendix B for HAC conditional logic
  - CC X+7th **T20.36** Burn of third degree of forehead and cheek
    HAC 7th character A see Appendix B for HAC conditional logic
  - CC X+7th **T20.37** Burn of third degree of neck
    HAC 7th character A see Appendix B for HAC conditional logic
  - CC X+7th **T20.39** Burn of third degree of multiple sites of head, face, and neck
    HAC 7th character A see Appendix B for HAC conditional logic
- **T20.4** Corrosion of unspecified degree of head, face, and neck
  Code first (T51-T65) to identify chemical and intent external cause code to identify place (Y92)
  - X+7th **T20.40** Corrosion of unspecified degree of head, face, and neck, unspecified site

- + T20.41 Corrosion of unspecified degree of ear [any part, except ear drum]
  - Excludes2: corrosion of ear drum (T28.91-)
  - +7th T20.411 Corrosion of unspecified degree of right ear [any part, except ear drum]
  - +7th T20.412 Corrosion of unspecified degree of left ear [any part, except ear drum]
  - +7th T20.419 Corrosion of unspecified degree of unspecified ear [any part, except ear drum]
- X+7th T20.42 Corrosion of unspecified degree of lip(s)
- X+7th T20.43 Corrosion of unspecified degree of chin
- X+7th T20.44 Corrosion of unspecified degree of nose (septum)
- X+7th T20.45 Corrosion of unspecified degree of scalp [any part]
- X+7th T20.46 Corrosion of unspecified degree of forehead and cheek
- X+7th T20.47 Corrosion of unspecified degree of neck
- X+7th T20.49 Corrosion of unspecified degree of multiple sites of head, face, and neck
- + T20.5 Corrosion of first degree of head, face, and neck
  - Code first (T51-T65) to identify chemical and intent
  - Use additional external cause code to identify place (Y92)
  - X+7th T20.50 Corrosion of first degree of head, face, and neck, unspecified site
  - + T20.51 Corrosion of first degree of ear [any part, except ear drum]
    - Excludes2: corrosion of ear drum (T28.91-)
    - +7th T20.511 Corrosion of first degree of right ear [any part, except ear drum]
    - +7th T20.512 Corrosion of first degree of left ear [any part, except ear drum]
    - +7th T20.519 Corrosion of first degree of unspecified ear [any part, except ear drum]
  - X+7th T20.52 Corrosion of first degree of lip(s)
  - X+7th T20.53 Corrosion of first degree of chin
  - X+7th T20.54 Corrosion of first degree of nose (septum)
  - X+7th T20.55 Corrosion of first degree of scalp [any part]
  - X+7th T20.56 Corrosion of first degree of forehead and cheek
  - X+7th T20.57 Corrosion of first degree of neck
  - X+7th T20.59 Corrosion of first degree of multiple sites of head, face, and neck
- + T20.6 Corrosion of second degree of head, face, and neck
  - Code first (T51-T65) to identify chemical and intent
  - Use additional external cause code to identify place (Y92)
  - X+7th T20.60 Corrosion of second degree of head, face, and neck, unspecified site
  - + T20.61 Corrosion of second degree of ear [any part, except ear drum]
    - Excludes2: corrosion of ear drum (T28.91-)
    - +7th T20.611 Corrosion of second degree of right ear [any part, except ear drum]
    - +7th T20.612 Corrosion of second degree of left ear [any part, except ear drum]
    - +7th T20.619 Corrosion of second degree of unspecified ear [any part, except ear drum]
  - X+7th T20.62 Corrosion of second degree of lip(s)
  - X+7th T20.63 Corrosion of second degree of chin
  - X+7th T20.64 Corrosion of second degree of nose (septum)
  - X+7th T20.65 Corrosion of second degree of scalp [any part]
  - X+7th T20.66 Corrosion of second degree of forehead and cheek
  - X+7th T20.67 Corrosion of second degree of neck
  - X+7th T20.69 Corrosion of second degree of multiple sites of head, face, and neck
- + T20.7 Corrosion of third degree of head, face, and neck
  - Code first (T51-T65) to identify chemical and intent
  - Use additional external cause code to identify place (Y92)
  - CC X+7th T20.70 Corrosion of third degree of head, face, and neck, unspecified site
    - HAC 7th character A see Appendix B for HAC conditional logic
  - + T20.71 Corrosion of third degree of ear [any part, except ear drum]
    - Excludes2: corrosion of ear drum (T28.91-)
    - CC +7th T20.711 Corrosion of third degree of right ear [any part, except ear drum]
      - HAC 7th character A see Appendix B for HAC conditional logic
    - CC +7th T20.712 Corrosion of third degree of left ear [any part, except ear drum]
      - HAC 7th character A see Appendix B for HAC conditional logic
    - CC +7th T20.719 Corrosion of third degree of unspecified ear [any part, except ear drum]
      - HAC 7th character A see Appendix B for HAC conditional logic
  - CC X+7th T20.72 Corrosion of third degree of lip(s)
    - HAC 7th character A see Appendix B for HAC conditional logic
  - CC X+7th T20.73 Corrosion of third degree of chin
    - HAC 7th character A see Appendix B for HAC conditional logic
  - CC X+7th T20.74 Corrosion of third degree of nose (septum)
    - HAC 7th character A see Appendix B for HAC conditional logic
  - CC X+7th T20.75 Corrosion of third degree of scalp [any part]
    - HAC 7th character A see Appendix B for HAC conditional logic
  - CC X+7th T20.76 Corrosion of third degree of forehead and cheek
    - HAC 7th character A see Appendix B for HAC conditional logic
  - CC X+7th T20.77 Corrosion of third degree of neck
    - HAC 7th character A see Appendix B for HAC conditional logic
  - CC X+7th T20.79 Corrosion of third degree of multiple sites of head, face, and neck
    - HAC 7th character A see Appendix B for HAC conditional logic

T21 Burn and corrosion of trunk

Includes: burns and corrosion of hip region
Excludes2: burns and corrosion of axilla (T22.- with fifth character 4)
burns and corrosion of scapular region (T22.- with fifth character 6)
burns and corrosion of shoulder (T22.- with fifth character 5)

The appropriate 7th character is to be added to each code from category T21
A initial encounter
D subsequent encounter
S sequela

- + T21.0 Burn of unspecified degree of trunk
  - Use external cause code to identify the source, place and intent of the burn (X00-X19, X75-X77, X96-X98, Y92)
  - X+7th T21.00 Burn of unspecified degree of trunk, unspecified site
  - X+7th T21.01 Burn of unspecified degree of chest wall
    - Burn of unspecified degree of breast
  - X+7th T21.02 Burn of unspecified degree of abdominal wall
    - Burn of unspecified degree of flank
    - Burn of unspecified degree of groin
  - X+7th T21.03 Burn of unspecified degree of upper back
    - Burn of unspecified degree of interscapular region
  - X+7th T21.04 Burn of unspecified degree of lower back
  - X+7th T21.05 Burn of unspecified degree of buttock
    - Burn of unspecified degree of anus
  - ♂ X+7th T21.06 Burn of unspecified degree of male genital region
    - Burn of unspecified degree of penis
    - Burn of unspecified degree of scrotum
    - Burn of unspecified degree of testis
  - ♀ X+7th T21.07 Burn of unspecified degree of female genital region
    - Burn of unspecified degree of labium (majus) (minus)
    - Burn of unspecified degree of perineum
    - Burn of unspecified degree of vulva
    - Excludes2: burn of vagina (T28.3)
  - X+7th T21.09 Burn of unspecified degree of other site of trunk

+ T21.1　Burn of first degree of trunk
　　Use external cause code to identify the source, place and intent of the burn (X00-X19, X75-X77, X96-X98, Y92)

- X+7th **T21.10** Burn of first degree of trunk, unspecified site
- X+7th **T21.11** Burn of first degree of chest wall
  - Burn of first degree of breast
- X+7th **T21.12** Burn of first degree of abdominal wall
  - Burn of first degree of flank
  - Burn of first degree of groin
- X+7th **T21.13** Burn of first degree of upper back
  - Burn of first degree of interscapular region
- X+7th **T21.14** Burn of first degree of lower back
- X+7th **T21.15** Burn of first degree of buttock
  - Burn of first degree of anus
- ♂ X+7th **T21.16** Burn of first degree of male genital region
  - Burn of first degree of penis
  - Burn of first degree of scrotum
  - Burn of first degree of testis
- ♀ X+7th **T21.17** Burn of first degree of female genital region
  - Burn of first degree of labium (majus) (minus)
  - Burn of first degree of perineum
  - Burn of first degree of vulva
  - **Excludes2:** *burn of vagina (T28.3)*
- X+7th **T21.19** Burn of first degree of other site of trunk

+ T21.2　Burn of second degree of trunk
　　Use external cause code to identify the source, place and intent of the burn (X00-X19, X75-X77, X96-X98, Y92)

- X+7th **T21.20** Burn of second degree of trunk, unspecified site
- X+7th **T21.21** Burn of second degree of chest wall
  - Burn of second degree of breast
- X+7th **T21.22** Burn of second degree of abdominal wall
  - Burn of second degree of flank
  - Burn of second degree of groin
- X+7th **T21.23** Burn of second degree of upper back
  - Burn of second degree of interscapular region
- X+7th **T21.24** Burn of second degree of lower back
- X+7th **T21.25** Burn of second degree of buttock
  - Burn of second degree of anus
- ♂ X+7th **T21.26** Burn of second degree of male genital region
  - Burn of second degree of penis
  - Burn of second degree of scrotum
  - Burn of second degree of testis
- ♀ X+7th **T21.27** Burn of second degree of female genital region
  - Burn of second degree of labium (majus) (minus)
  - Burn of second degree of perineum
  - Burn of second degree of vulva
  - **Excludes2:** *burn of vagina (T28.3)*
- X+7th **T21.29** Burn of second degree of other site of trunk

+ T21.3　Burn of third degree of trunk
　　Use additional external cause code to identify the source, place and intent of the burn (X00-X19, X75-X77, X96-X98, Y92)

- CC X+7th **T21.30** Burn of third degree of trunk, unspecified site
  - **HAC** 7th character A see Appendix B for HAC conditional logic
- CC X+7th **T21.31** Burn of third degree of chest wall
  - Burn of third degree of breast
  - *AHA CC: 2Q, 2016, 5-6*
  - **HAC** 7th character A see Appendix B for HAC conditional logic
- CC X+7th **T21.32** Burn of third degree of abdominal wall
  - Burn of third degree of flank
  - Burn of third degree of groin
  - **HAC** 7th character A see Appendix B for HAC conditional logic
- CC X+7th **T21.33** Burn of third degree of upper back
  - Burn of third degree of interscapular region
  - **HAC** 7th character A see Appendix B for HAC conditional logic
- CC X+7th **T21.34** Burn of third degree of lower back
  - **HAC** 7th character A see Appendix B for HAC conditional logic
- CC X+7th **T21.35** Burn of third degree of buttock
  - Burn of third degree of anus
  - **HAC** 7th character A see Appendix B for HAC conditional logic
- CC X+7th **T21.36** Burn of third degree of male genital region
  - Burn of third degree of penis
  - Burn of third degree of scrotum
  - Burn of third degree of testis
  - **HAC** 7th character A see Appendix B for HAC conditional logic
- CC X+7th **T21.37** Burn of third degree of female genital region
  - Burn of third degree of labium (majus) (minus)
  - Burn of third degree of perineum
  - Burn of third degree of vulva
  - **Excludes2:** *burn of vagina (T28.3)*
  - **HAC** 7th character A see Appendix B for HAC conditional logic
- CC X+7th **T21.39** Burn of third degree of other site of trunk
  - **HAC** 7th character A see Appendix B for HAC conditional logic

+ T21.4　Corrosion of unspecified degree of trunk
　　Code first (T51-T65) to identify chemical and intent
　　Use additional external cause code to identify place (Y92)

- X+7th **T21.40** Corrosion of unspecified degree of trunk, unspecified site
- X+7th **T21.41** Corrosion of unspecified degree of chest wall
  - Corrosion of unspecified degree of breast
- X+7th **T21.42** Corrosion of unspecified degree of abdominal wall
  - Corrosion of unspecified degree of flank
  - Corrosion of unspecified degree of groin
- X+7th **T21.43** Corrosion of unspecified degree of upper back
  - Corrosion of unspecified degree of interscapular region
- X+7th **T21.44** Corrosion of unspecified degree of lower back
- X+7th **T21.45** Corrosion of unspecified degree of buttock
  - Corrosion of unspecified degree of anus
- ♂ X+7th **T21.46** Corrosion of unspecified degree of male genital region
  - Corrosion of unspecified degree of penis
  - Corrosion of unspecified degree of scrotum
  - Corrosion of unspecified degree of testis
- ♀ X+7th **T21.47** Corrosion of unspecified degree of female genital region
  - Corrosion of unspecified degree of labium (majus) (minus)
  - Corrosion of unspecified degree of perineum
  - Corrosion of unspecified degree of vulva
  - **Excludes2:** *corrosion of vagina (T28.8)*
- X+7th **T21.49** Corrosion of unspecified degree of other site of trunk

+ T21.5　Corrosion of first degree of trunk
　　Code first (T51-T65) to identify chemical and intent
　　Use additional external cause code to identify place (Y92)

- X+7th **T21.50** Corrosion of first degree of trunk, unspecified site
- X+7th **T21.51** Corrosion of first degree of chest wall
  - Corrosion of first degree of breast
- X+7th **T21.52** Corrosion of first degree of abdominal wall
  - Corrosion of first degree of flank
  - Corrosion of first degree of groin
- X+7th **T21.53** Corrosion of first degree of upper back
  - Corrosion of first degree of interscapular region
- X+7th **T21.54** Corrosion of first degree of lower back
- X+7th **T21.55** Corrosion of first degree of buttock
  - Corrosion of first degree of anus
- ♂ X+7th **T21.56** Corrosion of first degree of male genital region
  - Corrosion of first degree of penis
  - Corrosion of first degree of scrotum
  - Corrosion of first degree of testis
- ♀ X+7th **T21.57** Corrosion of first degree of female genital region
  - Corrosion of first degree of labium (majus) (minus)
  - Corrosion of first degree of perineum
  - Corrosion of first degree of vulva
  - **Excludes2:** *corrosion of vagina (T28.8)*
- X+7th **T21.59** Corrosion of first degree of other site of trunk

- **T21.6 Corrosion of second degree of trunk**
  Code first (T51-T65) to identify chemical and intent
  Use additional external cause code to identify place (Y92)
  - X+7th **T21.60** Corrosion of second degree of trunk, unspecified site
  - X+7th **T21.61** Corrosion of second degree of chest wall
    Corrosion of second degree of breast
  - X+7th **T21.62** Corrosion of second degree of abdominal wall
    Corrosion of second degree of flank
    Corrosion of second degree of groin
  - X+7th **T21.63** Corrosion of second degree of upper back
    Corrosion of second degree of interscapular region
  - X+7th **T21.64** Corrosion of second degree of lower back
  - X+7th **T21.65** Corrosion of second degree of buttock
    Corrosion of second degree of anus
  - ♂ X+7th **T21.66** Corrosion of second degree of male genital region
    Corrosion of second degree of penis
    Corrosion of second degree of scrotum
    Corrosion of second degree of testis
  - ♀ X+7th **T21.67** Corrosion of second degree of female genital region
    Corrosion of second degree of labium (majus) (minus)
    Corrosion of second degree of perineum
    Corrosion of second degree of vulva
    Excludes2: corrosion of vagina (T28.8)
  - X+7th **T21.69** Corrosion of second degree of other site of trunk
- **T21.7 Corrosion of third degree of trunk**
  Code first (T51-T65) to identify chemical and intent
  Use additional external cause code to identify place (Y92)
  - CC X+7th **T21.70** Corrosion of third degree of trunk, unspecified site
    HAC 7th character A see Appendix B for HAC conditional logic
  - CC X+7th **T21.71** Corrosion of third degree of chest wall
    Corrosion of third degree of breast
    HAC 7th character A see Appendix B for HAC conditional logic
  - CC X+7th **T21.72** Corrosion of third degree of abdominal wall
    Corrosion of third degree of flank
    Corrosion of third degree of groin
    HAC 7th character A see Appendix B for HAC conditional logic
  - CC X+7th **T21.73** Corrosion of third degree of upper back
    Corrosion of third degree of interscapular region
    HAC 7th character A see Appendix B for HAC conditional logic
  - CC X+7th **T21.74** Corrosion of third degree of lower back
    HAC 7th character A see Appendix B for HAC conditional logic
  - CC X+7th **T21.75** Corrosion of third degree of buttock
    Corrosion of third degree of anus
    HAC 7th character A see Appendix B for HAC conditional logic
  - CC X+7th **T21.76** Corrosion of third degree of male genital region
    Corrosion of third degree of penis
    Corrosion of third degree of scrotum
    Corrosion of third degree of testis
    HAC 7th character A see Appendix B for HAC conditional logic
  - CC X+7th **T21.77** Corrosion of third degree of female genital region
    Corrosion of third degree of labium (majus) (minus)
    Corrosion of third degree of perineum
    Corrosion of third degree of vulva
    Excludes2: corrosion of vagina (T28.8)
    HAC 7th character A see Appendix B for HAC conditional logic
  - CC X+7th **T21.79** Corrosion of third degree of other site of trunk
    HAC 7th character A see Appendix B for HAC conditional logic

T22 Burn and corrosion of shoulder and upper limb, except wrist and hand

Excludes2: burn and corrosion of interscapular region (T21.-)
burn and corrosion of wrist and hand (T23.-)

The appropriate 7th character is to be added to each code from category T22
A   initial encounter
D   subsequent encounter
S   sequela

- **T22.0 Burn of unspecified degree of shoulder and upper limb, except wrist and hand**
  Use additional external cause code to identify the source, place and intent of the burn (X00-X19, X75-X77, X96-X98, Y92)
  - X+7th **T22.00** Burn of unspecified degree of shoulder and upper limb, except wrist and hand, unspecified site
  - **T22.01** Burn of unspecified degree of forearm
    - +7th **T22.011** Burn of unspecified degree of right forearm
    - +7th **T22.012** Burn of unspecified degree of left forearm
    - +7th **T22.019** Burn of unspecified degree of unspecified forearm
  - **T22.02** Burn of unspecified degree of elbow
    - +7th **T22.021** Burn of unspecified degree of right elbow
    - +7th **T22.022** Burn of unspecified degree of left elbow
    - +7th **T22.029** Burn of unspecified degree of unspecified elbow
  - **T22.03** Burn of unspecified degree of upper arm
    - +7th **T22.031** Burn of unspecified degree of right upper arm
    - +7th **T22.032** Burn of unspecified degree of left upper arm
    - +7th **T22.039** Burn of unspecified degree of unspecified upper arm
  - **T22.04** Burn of unspecified degree of axilla
    - +7th **T22.041** Burn of unspecified degree of right axilla
    - +7th **T22.042** Burn of unspecified degree of left axilla
    - +7th **T22.049** Burn of unspecified degree of unspecified axilla
  - **T22.05** Burn of unspecified degree of shoulder
    - +7th **T22.051** Burn of unspecified degree of right shoulder
    - +7th **T22.052** Burn of unspecified degree of left shoulder
    - +7th **T22.059** Burn of unspecified degree of unspecified shoulder
  - **T22.06** Burn of unspecified degree of scapular region
    - +7th **T22.061** Burn of unspecified degree of right scapular region
    - +7th **T22.062** Burn of unspecified degree of left scapular region
    - +7th **T22.069** Burn of unspecified degree of unspecified scapular region
  - **T22.09** Burn of unspecified degree of multiple sites of shoulder and upper limb, except wrist and hand
    - +7th **T22.091** Burn of unspecified degree of multiple sites of right shoulder and upper limb, except wrist and hand
    - +7th **T22.092** Burn of unspecified degree of multiple sites of left shoulder and upper limb, except wrist and hand
    - +7th **T22.099** Burn of unspecified degree of multiple sites of unspecified shoulder and upper limb, except wrist and hand
- **T22.1 Burn of first degree of shoulder and upper limb, except wrist and hand**
  Use additional external cause code to identify the source, place and intent of the burn (X00-X19, X75-X77, X96-X98, Y92)
  - X+7th **T22.10** Burn of first degree of shoulder and upper limb, except wrist and hand, unspecified site
  - **T22.11** Burn of first degree of forearm
    - +7th **T22.111** Burn of first degree of right forearm
    - +7th **T22.112** Burn of first degree of left forearm
    - +7th **T22.119** Burn of first degree of unspecified forearm
  - **T22.12** Burn of first degree of elbow
    - +7th **T22.121** Burn of first degree of right elbow
    - +7th **T22.122** Burn of first degree of left elbow
    - +7th **T22.129** Burn of first degree of unspecified elbow
  - **T22.13** Burn of first degree of upper arm
    - +7th **T22.131** Burn of first degree of right upper arm
    - +7th **T22.132** Burn of first degree of left upper arm
    - +7th **T22.139** Burn of first degree of unspecified upper arm

- **T22.14** Burn of first degree of axilla
  - +7th **T22.141** Burn of first degree of right axilla
  - +7th **T22.142** Burn of first degree of left axilla
  - +7th **T22.149** Burn of first degree of unspecified axilla
- **T22.15** Burn of first degree of shoulder
  - +7th **T22.151** Burn of first degree of right shoulder
  - +7th **T22.152** Burn of first degree of left shoulder
  - +7th **T22.159** Burn of first degree of unspecified shoulder
- **T22.16** Burn of first degree of scapular region
  - +7th **T22.161** Burn of first degree of right scapular region
  - +7th **T22.162** Burn of first degree of left scapular region
  - +7th **T22.169** Burn of first degree of unspecified scapular region
- **T22.19** Burn of first degree of multiple sites of shoulder and upper limb, except wrist and hand
  - +7th **T22.191** Burn of first degree of multiple sites of right shoulder and upper limb, except wrist and hand
  - +7th **T22.192** Burn of first degree of multiple sites of left shoulder and upper limb, except wrist and hand
  - +7th **T22.199** Burn of first degree of multiple sites of unspecified shoulder and upper limb, except wrist and hand
- **T22.2** Burn of second degree of shoulder and upper limb, except wrist and hand
  - Use additional external cause code to identify the source, place and intent of the burn (X00-X19, X75-X77, X96-X98, Y92)
  - X+7th **T22.20** Burn of second degree of shoulder and upper limb, except wrist and hand, unspecified site
  - **T22.21** Burn of second degree of forearm
    - +7th **T22.211** Burn of second degree of right forearm
    - +7th **T22.212** Burn of second degree of left forearm
    - +7th **T22.219** Burn of second degree of unspecified forearm
  - **T22.22** Burn of second degree of elbow
    - +7th **T22.221** Burn of second degree of right elbow
    - +7th **T22.222** Burn of second degree of left elbow
    - +7th **T22.229** Burn of second degree of unspecified elbow
  - **T22.23** Burn of second degree of upper arm
    - +7th **T22.231** Burn of second degree of right upper arm
    - +7th **T22.232** Burn of second degree of left upper arm
    - +7th **T22.239** Burn of second degree of unspecified upper arm
  - **T22.24** Burn of second degree of axilla
    - +7th **T22.241** Burn of second degree of right axilla
    - +7th **T22.242** Burn of second degree of left axilla
    - +7th **T22.249** Burn of second degree of unspecified axilla
  - **T22.25** Burn of second degree of shoulder
    - +7th **T22.251** Burn of second degree of right shoulder
    - +7th **T22.252** Burn of second degree of left shoulder
    - +7th **T22.259** Burn of second degree of unspecified shoulder
  - **T22.26** Burn of second degree of scapular region
    - +7th **T22.261** Burn of second degree of right scapular region
    - +7th **T22.262** Burn of second degree of left scapular region
    - +7th **T22.269** Burn of second degree of unspecified scapular region
  - **T22.29** Burn of second degree of multiple sites of shoulder and upper limb, except wrist and hand
    - +7th **T22.291** Burn of second degree of multiple sites of right shoulder and upper limb, except wrist and hand
    - +7th **T22.292** Burn of second degree of multiple sites of left shoulder and upper limb, except wrist and hand
    - +7th **T22.299** Burn of second degree of multiple sites of unspecified shoulder and upper limb, except wrist and hand

- **T22.3** Burn of third degree of shoulder and upper limb, except wrist and hand
  - Use additional external cause code to identify the source, place and intent of the burn (X00-X19, X75-X77, X96-X98, Y92)
  - CC X+7th **T22.30** Burn of third degree of shoulder and upper limb, except wrist and hand, unspecified site
    - HAC 7th character A see Appendix B for HAC conditional logic
  - **T22.31** Burn of third degree of forearm
    - CC +7th **T22.311** Burn of third degree of right forearm
      - HAC 7th character A see Appendix B for HAC conditional logic
    - CC +7th **T22.312** Burn of third degree of left forearm
      - HAC 7th character A see Appendix B for HAC conditional logic
    - CC +7th **T22.319** Burn of third degree of unspecified forearm
      - HAC 7th character A see Appendix B for HAC conditional logic
  - **T22.32** Burn of third degree of elbow
    - CC +7th **T22.321** Burn of third degree of right elbow
      - HAC 7th character A see Appendix B for HAC conditional logic
    - CC +7th **T22.322** Burn of third degree of left elbow
      - HAC 7th character A see Appendix B for HAC conditional logic
    - CC +7th **T22.329** Burn of third degree of unspecified elbow
      - HAC 7th character A see Appendix B for HAC conditional logic
  - **T22.33** Burn of third degree of upper arm
    - CC +7th **T22.331** Burn of third degree of right upper arm
      - HAC 7th character A see Appendix B for HAC conditional logic
    - CC +7th **T22.332** Burn of third degree of left upper arm
      - HAC 7th character A see Appendix B for HAC conditional logic
    - CC +7th **T22.339** Burn of third degree of unspecified upper arm
      - HAC 7th character A see Appendix B for HAC conditional logic
  - **T22.34** Burn of third degree of axilla
    - CC +7th **T22.341** Burn of third degree of right axilla
      - HAC 7th character A see Appendix B for HAC conditional logic
    - CC +7th **T22.342** Burn of third degree of left axilla
      - HAC 7th character A see Appendix B for HAC conditional logic
    - CC +7th **T22.349** Burn of third degree of unspecified axilla
      - HAC 7th character A see Appendix B for HAC conditional logic
  - **T22.35** Burn of third degree of shoulder
    - CC +7th **T22.351** Burn of third degree of right shoulder
      - HAC 7th character A see Appendix B for HAC conditional logic
    - CC +7th **T22.352** Burn of third degree of left shoulder
      - HAC 7th character A see Appendix B for HAC conditional logic
    - CC +7th **T22.359** Burn of third degree of unspecified shoulder
      - HAC 7th character A see Appendix B for HAC conditional logic
  - **T22.36** Burn of third degree of scapular region
    - CC +7th **T22.361** Burn of third degree of right scapular region
      - HAC 7th character A see Appendix B for HAC conditional logic
    - CC +7th **T22.362** Burn of third degree of left scapular region
      - HAC 7th character A see Appendix B for HAC conditional logic
    - CC +7th **T22.369** Burn of third degree of unspecified scapular region
      - HAC 7th character A see Appendix B for HAC conditional logic

---

+, +7th, X + 7th • Newborn • Pediatric • Maternity • Adult ♀ Female ♂ Male Manifestation Unacceptable PDX HCC CC MCC HAC

- **T22.39** Burn of third degree of multiple sites of shoulder and upper limb, except wrist and hand
  - CC +7th **T22.391** Burn of third degree of multiple sites of right shoulder and upper limb, except wrist and hand
    - HAC 7th character A see Appendix B for HAC conditional logic
  - CC +7th **T22.392** Burn of third degree of multiple sites of left shoulder and upper limb, except wrist and hand
    - HAC 7th character A see Appendix B for HAC conditional logic
  - CC +7th **T22.399** Burn of third degree of multiple sites of unspecified shoulder and upper limb, except wrist and hand
    - HAC 7th character A see Appendix B for HAC conditional logic

+ **T22.4** Corrosion of unspecified degree of shoulder and upper limb, except wrist and hand
  Code first (T51-T65) to identify chemical and intent
  Use additional external cause code to identify place (Y92)
  - X +7th **T22.40** Corrosion of unspecified degree of shoulder and upper limb, except wrist and hand, unspecified site
  - + **T22.41** Corrosion of unspecified degree of forearm
    - +7th **T22.411** Corrosion of unspecified degree of right forearm
    - +7th **T22.412** Corrosion of unspecified degree of left forearm
    - +7th **T22.419** Corrosion of unspecified degree of unspecified forearm
  - + **T22.42** Corrosion of unspecified degree of elbow
    - +7th **T22.421** Corrosion of unspecified degree of right elbow
    - +7th **T22.422** Corrosion of unspecified degree of left elbow
    - +7th **T22.429** Corrosion of unspecified degree of unspecified elbow
  - + **T22.43** Corrosion of unspecified degree of upper arm
    - +7th **T22.431** Corrosion of unspecified degree of right upper arm
    - +7th **T22.432** Corrosion of unspecified degree of left upper arm
    - +7th **T22.439** Corrosion of unspecified degree of unspecified upper arm
  - + **T22.44** Corrosion of unspecified degree of axilla
    - +7th **T22.441** Corrosion of unspecified degree of right axilla
    - +7th **T22.442** Corrosion of unspecified degree of left axilla
    - +7th **T22.449** Corrosion of unspecified degree of unspecified axilla
  - + **T22.45** Corrosion of unspecified degree of shoulder
    - +7th **T22.451** Corrosion of unspecified degree of right shoulder
    - +7th **T22.452** Corrosion of unspecified degree of left shoulder
    - +7th **T22.459** Corrosion of unspecified degree of unspecified shoulder
  - + **T22.46** Corrosion of unspecified degree of scapular region
    - +7th **T22.461** Corrosion of unspecified degree of right scapular region
    - +7th **T22.462** Corrosion of unspecified degree of left scapular region
    - +7th **T22.469** Corrosion of unspecified degree of unspecified scapular region
  - + **T22.49** Corrosion of unspecified degree of multiple sites of shoulder and upper limb, except wrist and hand
    - +7th **T22.491** Corrosion of unspecified degree of multiple sites of right shoulder and upper limb, except wrist and hand
    - +7th **T22.492** Corrosion of unspecified degree of multiple sites of left shoulder and upper limb, except wrist and hand
    - +7th **T22.499** Corrosion of unspecified degree of multiple sites of unspecified shoulder and upper limb, except wrist and hand

+ **T22.5** Corrosion of first degree of shoulder and upper limb, except wrist and hand
  Code first (T51-T65) to identify chemical and intent
  Use additional external cause code to identify place (Y92)
  - X +7th **T22.50** Corrosion of first degree of shoulder and upper limb, except wrist and hand unspecified site
  - + **T22.51** Corrosion of first degree of forearm
    - +7th **T22.511** Corrosion of first degree of right forearm
    - +7th **T22.512** Corrosion of first degree of left forearm
    - +7th **T22.519** Corrosion of first degree of unspecified forearm
  - + **T22.52** Corrosion of first degree of elbow
    - +7th **T22.521** Corrosion of first degree of right elbow
    - +7th **T22.522** Corrosion of first degree of left elbow
    - +7th **T22.529** Corrosion of first degree of unspecified elbow
  - + **T22.53** Corrosion of first degree of upper arm
    - +7th **T22.531** Corrosion of first degree of right upper arm
    - +7th **T22.532** Corrosion of first degree of left upper arm
    - +7th **T22.539** Corrosion of first degree of unspecified upper arm
  - + **T22.54** Corrosion of first degree of axilla
    - +7th **T22.541** Corrosion of first degree of right axilla
    - +7th **T22.542** Corrosion of first degree of left axilla
    - +7th **T22.549** Corrosion of first degree of unspecified axilla
  - + **T22.55** Corrosion of first degree of shoulder
    - +7th **T22.551** Corrosion of first degree of right shoulder
    - +7th **T22.552** Corrosion of first degree of left shoulder
    - +7th **T22.559** Corrosion of first degree of unspecified shoulder
  - + **T22.56** Corrosion of first degree of scapular region
    - +7th **T22.561** Corrosion of first degree of right scapular region
    - +7th **T22.562** Corrosion of first degree of left scapular region
    - +7th **T22.569** Corrosion of first degree of unspecified scapular region
  - + **T22.59** Corrosion of first degree of multiple sites of shoulder and upper limb, except wrist and hand
    - +7th **T22.591** Corrosion of first degree of multiple sites of right shoulder and upper limb, except wrist and hand
    - +7th **T22.592** Corrosion of first degree of multiple sites of left shoulder and upper limb, except wrist and hand
    - +7th **T22.599** Corrosion of first degree of multiple sites of unspecified shoulder and upper limb, except wrist and hand

+ **T22.6** Corrosion of second degree of shoulder and upper limb, except wrist and hand
  Code first (T51-T65) to identify chemical and intent
  Use additional external cause code to identify place (Y92)
  - X +7th **T22.60** Corrosion of second degree of shoulder and upper limb, except wrist and hand, unspecified site
  - + **T22.61** Corrosion of second degree of forearm
    - +7th **T22.611** Corrosion of second degree of right forearm
    - +7th **T22.612** Corrosion of second degree of left forearm
    - +7th **T22.619** Corrosion of second degree of unspecified forearm
  - + **T22.62** Corrosion of second degree of elbow
    - +7th **T22.621** Corrosion of second degree of right elbow
    - +7th **T22.622** Corrosion of second degree of left elbow
    - +7th **T22.629** Corrosion of second degree of unspecified elbow
  - + **T22.63** Corrosion of second degree of upper arm
    - +7th **T22.631** Corrosion of second degree of right upper arm
    - +7th **T22.632** Corrosion of second degree of left upper arm
    - +7th **T22.639** Corrosion of second degree of unspecified upper arm

- **+ T22.64 Corrosion of second degree of axilla**
  - +7th T22.641 Corrosion of second degree of right axilla
  - +7th T22.642 Corrosion of second degree of left axilla
  - +7th T22.649 Corrosion of second degree of unspecified axilla
- **+ T22.65 Corrosion of second degree of shoulder**
  - +7th T22.651 Corrosion of second degree of right shoulder
  - +7th T22.652 Corrosion of second degree of left shoulder
  - +7th T22.659 Corrosion of second degree of unspecified shoulder
- **+ T22.66 Corrosion of second degree of scapular region**
  - +7th T22.661 Corrosion of second degree of right scapular region
  - +7th T22.662 Corrosion of second degree of left scapular region
  - +7th T22.669 Corrosion of second degree of unspecified scapular region
- **+ T22.69 Corrosion of second degree of multiple sites of shoulder and upper limb, except wrist and hand**
  - +7th T22.691 Corrosion of second degree of multiple sites of right shoulder and upper limb, except wrist and hand
  - +7th T22.692 Corrosion of second degree of multiple sites of left shoulder and upper limb, except wrist and hand
  - +7th T22.699 Corrosion of second degree of multiple sites of unspecified shoulder and upper limb, except wrist and hand
- **+ T22.7 Corrosion of third degree of shoulder and upper limb, except wrist and hand**

  Code first (T51-T65) to identify chemical and intent external cause code to identify place (Y92)
  - CC X+7th T22.70 Corrosion of third degree of shoulder and upper limb, except wrist and hand, unspecified site
    - HAC 7th character A see Appendix B for HAC conditional logic
- **+ T22.71 Corrosion of third degree of forearm**
  - CC +7th T22.711 Corrosion of third degree of right forearm
    - HAC 7th character A see Appendix B for HAC conditional logic
  - CC +7th T22.712 Corrosion of third degree of left forearm
    - HAC 7th character A see Appendix B for HAC conditional logic
  - CC +7th T22.719 Corrosion of third degree of unspecified forearm
    - HAC 7th character A see Appendix B for HAC conditional logic
- **+ T22.72 Corrosion of third degree of elbow**
  - CC +7th T22.721 Corrosion of third degree of right elbow
    - HAC 7th character A see Appendix B for HAC conditional logic
  - CC +7th T22.722 Corrosion of third degree of left elbow
    - HAC 7th character A see Appendix B for HAC conditional logic
  - CC +7th T22.729 Corrosion of third degree of unspecified elbow
    - HAC 7th character A see Appendix B for HAC conditional logic
- **+ T22.73 Corrosion of third degree of upper arm**
  - CC +7th T22.731 Corrosion of third degree of right upper arm
    - HAC 7th character A see Appendix B for HAC conditional logic
  - CC +7th T22.732 Corrosion of third degree of left upper arm
    - HAC 7th character A see Appendix B for HAC conditional logic
  - CC +7th T22.739 Corrosion of third degree of unspecified upper arm
    - HAC 7th character A see Appendix B for HAC conditional logic
- **+ T22.74 Corrosion of third degree of axilla**
  - CC +7th T22.741 Corrosion of third degree of right axilla
    - HAC 7th character A see Appendix B for HAC conditional logic
  - CC +7th T22.742 Corrosion of third degree of left axilla
    - HAC 7th character A see Appendix B for HAC conditional logic
  - CC +7th T22.749 Corrosion of third degree of unspecified axilla
    - HAC 7th character A see Appendix B for HAC conditional logic
- **+ T22.75 Corrosion of third degree of shoulder**
  - CC +7th T22.751 Corrosion of third degree of right shoulder
    - HAC 7th character A see Appendix B for HAC conditional logic
  - CC +7th T22.752 Corrosion of third degree of left shoulder
    - HAC 7th character A see Appendix B for HAC conditional logic
  - CC +7th T22.759 Corrosion of third degree of unspecified shoulder
    - HAC 7th character A see Appendix B for HAC conditional logic
- **+ T22.76 Corrosion of third degree of scapular region**
  - CC +7th T22.761 Corrosion of third degree of right scapular region
    - HAC 7th character A see Appendix B for HAC conditional logic
  - CC +7th T22.762 Corrosion of third degree of left scapular region
    - HAC 7th character A see Appendix B for HAC conditional logic
  - CC +7th T22.769 Corrosion of third degree of unspecified scapular region
    - HAC 7th character A see Appendix B for HAC conditional logic
- **+ T22.79 Corrosion of third degree of multiple sites of shoulder and upper limb, except wrist and hand**
  - CC +7th T22.791 Corrosion of third degree of multiple sites of right shoulder and upper limb, except wrist and hand
    - HAC 7th character A see Appendix B for HAC conditional logic
  - CC +7th T22.792 Corrosion of third degree of multiple sites of left shoulder and upper limb, except wrist and hand
    - HAC 7th character A see Appendix B for HAC conditional logic
  - CC +7th T22.799 Corrosion of third degree of multiple sites of unspecified shoulder and upper limb, except wrist and hand
    - HAC 7th character A see Appendix B for HAC conditional logic

T23 Burn and corrosion of wrist and hand

The appropriate 7th character is to be added to each code from category T23
A initial encounter
D subsequent encounter
S sequela

- **+ T23.0 Burn of unspecified degree of wrist and hand**

  Use additional external cause code to identify the source, place and intent of the burn (X00-X19, X75-X77, X96-X98, Y92)
  - **+ T23.00 Burn of unspecified degree of hand, unspecified site**
    - +7th T23.001 Burn of unspecified degree of right hand, unspecified site
    - +7th T23.002 Burn of unspecified degree of left hand, unspecified site
    - +7th T23.009 Burn of unspecified degree of unspecified hand, unspecified site

- **T23.01** Burn of unspecified degree of thumb (nail)
  - +7th **T23.011** Burn of unspecified degree of right thumb (nail)
  - +7th **T23.012** Burn of unspecified degree of left thumb (nail)
  - +7th **T23.019** Burn of unspecified degree of unspecified thumb (nail)
- **T23.02** Burn of unspecified degree of single finger (nail) except thumb
  - +7th **T23.021** Burn of unspecified degree of single right finger (nail) except thumb
  - +7th **T23.022** Burn of unspecified degree of single left finger (nail) except thumb
  - +7th **T23.029** Burn of unspecified degree of unspecified single finger (nail) except thumb
- **T23.03** Burn of unspecified degree of multiple fingers (nail), not including thumb
  - +7th **T23.031** Burn of unspecified degree of multiple right fingers (nail), not including thumb
  - +7th **T23.032** Burn of unspecified degree of multiple left fingers (nail), not including thumb
  - +7th **T23.039** Burn of unspecified degree of unspecified multiple fingers (nail), not including thumb
- **T23.04** Burn of unspecified degree of multiple fingers (nail), including thumb
  - +7th **T23.041** Burn of unspecified degree of multiple right fingers (nail), including thumb
  - +7th **T23.042** Burn of unspecified degree of multiple left fingers (nail), including thumb
  - +7th **T23.049** Burn of unspecified degree of unspecified multiple fingers (nail), including thumb
- **T23.05** Burn of unspecified degree of palm
  - +7th **T23.051** Burn of unspecified degree of right palm
  - +7th **T23.052** Burn of unspecified degree of left palm
  - +7th **T23.059** Burn of unspecified degree of unspecified palm
- **T23.06** Burn of unspecified degree of back of hand
  - +7th **T23.061** Burn of unspecified degree of back of right hand
  - +7th **T23.062** Burn of unspecified degree of back of left hand
  - +7th **T23.069** Burn of unspecified degree of back of unspecified hand
- **T23.07** Burn of unspecified degree of wrist
  - +7th **T23.071** Burn of unspecified degree of right wrist
  - +7th **T23.072** Burn of unspecified degree of left wrist
  - +7th **T23.079** Burn of unspecified degree of unspecified wrist
- **T23.09** Burn of unspecified degree of multiple sites of wrist and hand
  - +7th **T23.091** Burn of unspecified degree of multiple sites of right wrist and hand
  - +7th **T23.092** Burn of unspecified degree of multiple sites of left wrist and hand
  - +7th **T23.099** Burn of unspecified degree of multiple sites of unspecified wrist and hand
- **T23.1** Burn of first degree of wrist and hand
  Use additional external cause code to identify the source, place and intent of the burn (X00-X19, X75-X77, X96-X98, Y92)
  - **T23.10** Burn of first degree of hand, unspecified site
    - +7th **T23.101** Burn of first degree of right hand, unspecified site
    - +7th **T23.102** Burn of first degree of left hand, unspecified site
    - +7th **T23.109** Burn of first degree of unspecified hand, unspecified site
  - **T23.11** Burn of first degree of thumb (nail)
    - +7th **T23.111** Burn of first degree of right thumb (nail)
    - +7th **T23.112** Burn of first degree of left thumb (nail)
    - +7th **T23.119** Burn of first degree of unspecified thumb (nail)
  - **T23.12** Burn of first degree of single finger (nail) except thumb
    - +7th **T23.121** Burn of first degree of single right finger (nail) except thumb
    - +7th **T23.122** Burn of first degree of single left finger (nail) except thumb
    - +7th **T23.129** Burn of first degree of unspecified single finger (nail) except thumb
  - **T23.13** Burn of first degree of multiple fingers (nail), not including thumb
    - +7th **T23.131** Burn of first degree of multiple right fingers (nail), not including thumb
    - +7th **T23.132** Burn of first degree of multiple left fingers (nail), not including thumb
    - +7th **T23.139** Burn of first degree of unspecified multiple fingers (nail), not including thumb
  - **T23.14** Burn of first degree of multiple fingers (nail), including thumb
    - +7th **T23.141** Burn of first degree of multiple right fingers (nail), including thumb
    - +7th **T23.142** Burn of first degree of multiple left fingers (nail), including thumb
    - +7th **T23.149** Burn of first degree of unspecified multiple fingers (nail), including thumb
  - **T23.15** Burn of first degree of palm
    - +7th **T23.151** Burn of first degree of right palm
    - +7th **T23.152** Burn of first degree of left palm
    - +7th **T23.159** Burn of first degree of unspecified palm
  - **T23.16** Burn of first degree of back of hand
    - +7th **T23.161** Burn of first degree of back of right hand
    - +7th **T23.162** Burn of first degree of back of left hand
    - +7th **T23.169** Burn of first degree of back of unspecified hand
  - **T23.17** Burn of first degree of wrist
    - +7th **T23.171** Burn of first degree of right wrist
    - +7th **T23.172** Burn of first degree of left wrist
    - +7th **T23.179** Burn of first degree of unspecified wrist
  - **T23.19** Burn of first degree of multiple sites of wrist and hand
    - +7th **T23.191** Burn of first degree of multiple sites of right wrist and hand
    - +7th **T23.192** Burn of first degree of multiple sites of left wrist and hand
    - +7th **T23.199** Burn of first degree of multiple sites of unspecified wrist and hand
- **T23.2** Burn of second degree of wrist and hand
  Use additional external cause code to identify the source, place and intent of the burn (X00-X19, X75-X77, X96-X98, Y92)
  - **T23.20** Burn of second degree of hand, unspecified site
    - +7th **T23.201** Burn of second degree of right hand, unspecified site
    - +7th **T23.202** Burn of second degree of left hand, unspecified site
    - +7th **T23.209** Burn of second degree of unspecified hand, unspecified site
  - **T23.21** Burn of second degree of thumb (nail)
    - +7th **T23.211** Burn of second degree of right thumb (nail)
    - +7th **T23.212** Burn of second degree of left thumb (nail)
    - +7th **T23.219** Burn of second degree of unspecified thumb (nail)
  - **T23.22** Burn of second degree of single finger (nail) except thumb
    - +7th **T23.221** Burn of second degree of single right finger (nail) except thumb
    - +7th **T23.222** Burn of second degree of single left finger (nail) except thumb
    - +7th **T23.229** Burn of second degree of unspecified single finger (nail) except thumb
  - **T23.23** Burn of second degree of multiple fingers (nail), not including thumb
    - +7th **T23.231** Burn of second degree of multiple right fingers (nail), not including thumb
    - +7th **T23.232** Burn of second degree of multiple left fingers (nail), not including thumb
    - +7th **T23.239** Burn of second degree of unspecified multiple fingers (nail), not including thumb

- **T23.24** Burn of second degree of multiple fingers (nail), including thumb
  - +7th **T23.241** Burn of second degree of multiple right fingers (nail), including thumb
  - +7th **T23.242** Burn of second degree of multiple left fingers (nail), including thumb
  - +7th **T23.249** Burn of second degree of unspecified multiple fingers (nail), including thumb
- **T23.25** Burn of second degree of palm
  - +7th **T23.251** Burn of second degree of right palm
  - +7th **T23.252** Burn of second degree of left palm
  - +7th **T23.259** Burn of second degree of unspecified palm
- **T23.26** Burn of second degree of back of hand
  - +7th **T23.261** Burn of second degree of back of right hand
  - +7th **T23.262** Burn of second degree of back of left hand
  - +7th **T23.269** Burn of second degree of back of unspecified hand
- **T23.27** Burn of second degree of wrist
  - +7th **T23.271** Burn of second degree of right wrist
  - +7th **T23.272** Burn of second degree of left wrist
  - +7th **T23.279** Burn of second degree of unspecified wrist
- **T23.29** Burn of second degree of multiple sites of wrist and hand
  - +7th **T23.291** Burn of second degree of multiple sites of right wrist and hand
  - +7th **T23.292** Burn of second degree of multiple sites of left wrist and hand
  - +7th **T23.299** Burn of second degree of multiple sites of unspecified wrist and hand
- **T23.3** Burn of third degree of wrist and hand
  Use additional external cause code to identify the source, place and intent of the burn (X00-X19, X75-X77, X96-X98, Y92)
- **T23.30** Burn of third degree of hand, unspecified site
  - CC +7th **T23.301** Burn of third degree of right hand, unspecified site
    AHA CC: 1Q, 2015, 3-21
    HAC 7th character A see Appendix B for HAC conditional logic
  - CC +7th **T23.302** Burn of third degree of left hand, unspecified site
    AHA CC: 2Q, 2016, 5
    HAC 7th character A see Appendix B for HAC conditional logic
  - CC +7th **T23.309** Burn of third degree of unspecified hand, unspecified site
    HAC 7th character A see Appendix B for HAC conditional logic
- **T23.31** Burn of third degree of thumb (nail)
  - CC +7th **T23.311** Burn of third degree of right thumb (nail)
    HAC 7th character A see Appendix B for HAC conditional logic
  - CC +7th **T23.312** Burn of third degree of left thumb (nail)
    HAC 7th character A see Appendix B for HAC conditional logic
  - CC +7th **T23.319** Burn of third degree of unspecified thumb (nail)
    HAC 7th character A see Appendix B for HAC conditional logic
- **T23.32** Burn of third degree of single finger (nail) except thumb
  - CC +7th **T23.321** Burn of third degree of single right finger (nail) except thumb
    HAC 7th character A see Appendix B for HAC conditional logic
  - CC +7th **T23.322** Burn of third degree of single left finger (nail) except thumb
    HAC 7th character A see Appendix B for HAC conditional logic
  - CC +7th **T23.329** Burn of third degree of unspecified single finger (nail) except thumb
    HAC 7th character A see Appendix B for HAC conditional logic

- **T23.33** Burn of third degree of multiple fingers (nail), not including thumb
  - CC +7th **T23.331** Burn of third degree of multiple right fingers (nail), not including thumb
    HAC 7th character A see Appendix B for HAC conditional logic
  - CC +7th **T23.332** Burn of third degree of multiple left fingers (nail), not including thumb
    HAC 7th character A see Appendix B for HAC conditional logic
  - CC +7th **T23.339** Burn of third degree of unspecified multiple fingers (nail), not including thumb
- **T23.34** Burn of third degree of multiple fingers (nail), including thumb
  - CC +7th **T23.341** Burn of third degree of multiple right fingers (nail), including thumb
    HAC 7th character A see Appendix B for HAC conditional logic
  - CC +7th **T23.342** Burn of third degree of multiple left fingers (nail), including thumb
    HAC 7th character A see Appendix B for HAC conditional logic
  - CC +7th **T23.349** Burn of third degree of unspecified multiple fingers (nail), including thumb
    HAC 7th character A see Appendix B for HAC conditional logic
- **T23.35** Burn of third degree of palm
  - CC +7th **T23.351** Burn of third degree of right palm
    HAC 7th character A see Appendix B for HAC conditional logic
  - CC +7th **T23.352** Burn of third degree of left palm
    HAC 7th character A see Appendix B for HAC conditional logic
  - CC +7th **T23.359** Burn of third degree of unspecified palm
    HAC 7th character A see Appendix B for HAC conditional logic
- **T23.36** Burn of third degree of back of hand
  - CC +7th **T23.361** Burn of third degree of back of right hand
    HAC 7th character A see Appendix B for HAC conditional logic
  - CC +7th **T23.362** Burn of third degree of back of left hand
    HAC 7th character A see Appendix B for HAC conditional logic
  - CC +7th **T23.369** Burn of third degree of back of unspecified hand
    HAC 7th character A see Appendix B for HAC conditional logic
- **T23.37** Burn of third degree of wrist
  - CC +7th **T23.371** Burn of third degree of right wrist
    HAC 7th character A see Appendix B for HAC conditional logic
  - CC +7th **T23.372** Burn of third degree of left wrist
    HAC 7th character A see Appendix B for HAC conditional logic
  - CC +7th **T23.379** Burn of third degree of unspecified wrist
    HAC 7th character A see Appendix B for HAC conditional logic
- **T23.39** Burn of third degree of multiple sites of wrist and hand
  - CC +7th **T23.391** Burn of third degree of multiple sites of right wrist and hand
    HAC 7th character A see Appendix B for HAC conditional logic
  - CC +7th **T23.392** Burn of third degree of multiple sites of left wrist and hand
    HAC 7th character A see Appendix B for HAC conditional logic
  - CC +7th **T23.399** Burn of third degree of multiple sites of unspecified wrist and hand
    HAC 7th character A see Appendix B for HAC conditional logic

+ **T23.4** Corrosion of unspecified degree of wrist and hand
  Code first (T51-T65) to identify chemical and intent
  Use additional external cause code to identify place (Y92)
  + **T23.40** Corrosion of unspecified degree of hand, unspecified site
    - +7th **T23.401** Corrosion of unspecified degree of right hand, unspecified site
    - +7th **T23.402** Corrosion of unspecified degree of left hand, unspecified site
    - +7th **T23.409** Corrosion of unspecified degree of unspecified hand, unspecified site
  + **T23.41** Corrosion of unspecified degree of thumb (nail)
    - +7th **T23.411** Corrosion of unspecified degree of right thumb (nail)
    - +7th **T23.412** Corrosion of unspecified degree of left thumb (nail)
    - +7th **T23.419** Corrosion of unspecified degree of unspecified thumb (nail)
  + **T23.42** Corrosion of unspecified degree of single finger (nail) except thumb
    - +7th **T23.421** Corrosion of unspecified degree of single right finger (nail) except thumb
    - +7th **T23.422** Corrosion of unspecified degree of single left finger (nail) except thumb
    - +7th **T23.429** Corrosion of unspecified degree of unspecified single finger (nail) except thumb
  + **T23.43** Corrosion of unspecified degree of multiple fingers (nail), not including thumb
    - +7th **T23.431** Corrosion of unspecified degree of multiple right fingers (nail), not including thumb
    - +7th **T23.432** Corrosion of unspecified degree of multiple left fingers (nail), not including thumb
    - +7th **T23.439** Corrosion of unspecified degree of unspecified multiple fingers (nail), not including thumb
  + **T23.44** Corrosion of unspecified degree of multiple fingers (nail), including thumb
    - +7th **T23.441** Corrosion of unspecified degree of multiple right fingers (nail), including thumb
    - +7th **T23.442** Corrosion of unspecified degree of multiple left fingers (nail), including thumb
    - +7th **T23.449** Corrosion of unspecified degree of unspecified multiple fingers (nail), including thumb
  + **T23.45** Corrosion of unspecified degree of palm
    - +7th **T23.451** Corrosion of unspecified degree of right palm
    - +7th **T23.452** Corrosion of unspecified degree of left palm
    - +7th **T23.459** Corrosion of unspecified degree of unspecified palm
  + **T23.46** Corrosion of unspecified degree of back of hand
    - +7th **T23.461** Corrosion of unspecified degree of back of right hand
    - +7th **T23.462** Corrosion of unspecified degree of back of left hand
    - +7th **T23.469** Corrosion of unspecified degree of back of unspecified hand
  + **T23.47** Corrosion of unspecified degree of wrist
    - +7th **T23.471** Corrosion of unspecified degree of right wrist
    - +7th **T23.472** Corrosion of unspecified degree of left wrist
    - +7th **T23.479** Corrosion of unspecified degree of unspecified wrist

+ **T23.49** Corrosion of unspecified degree of multiple sites of wrist and hand
  - +7th **T23.491** Corrosion of unspecified degree of multiple sites of right wrist and hand
  - +7th **T23.492** Corrosion of unspecified degree of multiple sites of left wrist and hand
  - +7th **T23.499** Corrosion of unspecified degree of multiple sites of unspecified wrist and hand

+ **T23.5** Corrosion of first degree of wrist and hand
  Code first (T51-T65) to identify chemical and intent
  Use additional external cause code to identify place (Y92)
  + **T23.50** Corrosion of first degree of hand, unspecified site
    - +7th **T23.501** Corrosion of first degree of right hand, unspecified site
    - +7th **T23.502** Corrosion of first degree of left hand, unspecified site
    - +7th **T23.509** Corrosion of first degree of unspecified hand, unspecified site
  + **T23.51** Corrosion of first degree of thumb (nail)
    - +7th **T23.511** Corrosion of first degree of right thumb (nail)
    - +7th **T23.512** Corrosion of first degree of left thumb (nail)
    - +7th **T23.519** Corrosion of first degree of unspecified thumb (nail)
  + **T23.52** Corrosion of first degree of single finger (nail) except thumb
    - +7th **T23.521** Corrosion of first degree of single right finger (nail) except thumb
    - +7th **T23.522** Corrosion of first degree of single left finger (nail) except thumb
    - +7th **T23.529** Corrosion of first degree of unspecified single finger (nail) except thumb
  + **T23.53** Corrosion of first degree of multiple fingers (nail), not including thumb
    - +7th **T23.531** Corrosion of first degree of multiple right fingers (nail), not including thumb
    - +7th **T23.532** Corrosion of first degree of multiple left fingers (nail), not including thumb
    - +7th **T23.539** Corrosion of first degree of unspecified multiple fingers (nail), not including thumb
  + **T23.54** Corrosion of first degree of multiple fingers (nail), including thumb
    - +7th **T23.541** Corrosion of first degree of multiple right fingers (nail), including thumb
    - +7th **T23.542** Corrosion of first degree of multiple left fingers (nail), including thumb
    - +7th **T23.549** Corrosion of first degree of unspecified multiple fingers (nail), including thumb
  + **T23.55** Corrosion of first degree of palm
    - +7th **T23.551** Corrosion of first degree of right palm
    - +7th **T23.552** Corrosion of first degree of left palm
    - +7th **T23.559** Corrosion of first degree of unspecified palm
  + **T23.56** Corrosion of first degree of back of hand
    - +7th **T23.561** Corrosion of first degree of back of right hand
    - +7th **T23.562** Corrosion of first degree of back of left hand
    - +7th **T23.569** Corrosion of first degree of back of unspecified hand
  + **T23.57** Corrosion of first degree of wrist
    - +7th **T23.571** Corrosion of first degree of right wrist
    - +7th **T23.572** Corrosion of first degree of left wrist
    - +7th **T23.579** Corrosion of first degree of unspecified wrist
  + **T23.59** Corrosion of first degree of multiple sites of wrist and hand
    - +7th **T23.591** Corrosion of first degree of multiple sites of right wrist and hand
    - +7th **T23.592** Corrosion of first degree of multiple sites of left wrist and hand
    - +7th **T23.599** Corrosion of first degree of multiple sites of unspecified wrist and hand

T23.6 Corrosion of second degree of wrist and hand
Code first (T51-T65) to identify chemical and intent
Use additional external cause code to identify place (Y92)

- **T23.60** Corrosion of second degree of hand, unspecified site
  - +7th **T23.601** Corrosion of second degree of right hand, unspecified site
  - +7th **T23.602** Corrosion of second degree of left hand, unspecified site
  - +7th **T23.609** Corrosion of second degree of unspecified hand, unspecified site
- **T23.61** Corrosion of second degree of thumb (nail)
  - +7th **T23.611** Corrosion of second degree of right thumb (nail)
  - +7th **T23.612** Corrosion of second degree of left thumb (nail)
  - +7th **T23.619** Corrosion of second degree of unspecified thumb (nail)
- **T23.62** Corrosion of second degree of single finger (nail) except thumb
  - +7th **T23.621** Corrosion of second degree of single right finger (nail) except thumb
  - +7th **T23.622** Corrosion of second degree of single left finger (nail) except thumb
  - +7th **T23.629** Corrosion of second degree of unspecified single finger (nail) except thumb
- **T23.63** Corrosion of second degree of multiple fingers (nail), not including thumb
  - +7th **T23.631** Corrosion of second degree of multiple right fingers (nail), not including thumb
  - +7th **T23.632** Corrosion of second degree of multiple left fingers (nail), not including thumb
  - +7th **T23.639** Corrosion of second degree of unspecified multiple fingers (nail), not including thumb
- **T23.64** Corrosion of second degree of multiple fingers (nail), including thumb
  - +7th **T23.641** Corrosion of second degree of multiple right fingers (nail), including thumb
  - +7th **T23.642** Corrosion of second degree of multiple left fingers (nail), including thumb
  - +7th **T23.649** Corrosion of second degree of unspecified multiple fingers (nail), including thumb
- **T23.65** Corrosion of second degree of palm
  - +7th **T23.651** Corrosion of second degree of right palm
  - +7th **T23.652** Corrosion of second degree of left palm
  - +7th **T23.659** Corrosion of second degree of unspecified palm
- **T23.66** Corrosion of second degree of back of hand
  - +7th **T23.661** Corrosion of second degree back of right hand
  - +7th **T23.662** Corrosion of second degree back of left hand
  - +7th **T23.669** Corrosion of second degree back of unspecified hand
- **T23.67** Corrosion of second degree of wrist
  - +7th **T23.671** Corrosion of second degree of right wrist
  - +7th **T23.672** Corrosion of second degree of left wrist
  - +7th **T23.679** Corrosion of second degree of unspecified wrist
- **T23.69** Corrosion of second degree of multiple sites of wrist and hand
  - +7th **T23.691** Corrosion of second degree of multiple sites of right wrist and hand
  - +7th **T23.692** Corrosion of second degree of multiple sites of left wrist and hand
  - +7th **T23.699** Corrosion of second degree of multiple sites of unspecified wrist and hand

T23.7 Corrosion of third degree of wrist and hand
Code first (T51-T65) to identify chemical and intent
Use additional external cause code to identify place (Y92)

- **T23.70** Corrosion of third degree of hand, unspecified site
  - CC +7th **T23.701** Corrosion of third degree of right hand, unspecified site
    - HAC 7th character A see Appendix B for HAC conditional logic
  - CC +7th **T23.702** Corrosion of third degree of left hand, unspecified site
    - HAC 7th character A see Appendix B for HAC conditional logic
  - CC +7th **T23.709** Corrosion of third degree of unspecified hand, unspecified site
    - HAC 7th character A see Appendix B for HAC conditional logic
- **T23.71** Corrosion of third degree of thumb (nail)
  - CC +7th **T23.711** Corrosion of third degree of right thumb (nail)
    - HAC 7th character A see Appendix B for HAC conditional logic
  - CC +7th **T23.712** Corrosion of third degree of left thumb (nail)
    - HAC 7th character A see Appendix B for HAC conditional logic
  - CC +7th **T23.719** Corrosion of third degree of unspecified thumb (nail)
    - HAC 7th character A see Appendix B for HAC conditional logic
- **T23.72** Corrosion of third degree of single finger (nail) except thumb
  - CC +7th **T23.721** Corrosion of third degree of single right finger (nail) except thumb
    - HAC 7th character A see Appendix B for HAC conditional logic
  - CC +7th **T23.722** Corrosion of third degree of single left finger (nail) except thumb
    - HAC 7th character A see Appendix B for HAC conditional logic
  - CC +7th **T23.729** Corrosion of third degree of unspecified single finger (nail) except thumb
    - HAC 7th character A see Appendix B for HAC conditional logic
- **T23.73** Corrosion of third degree of multiple fingers (nail), not including thumb
  - CC +7th **T23.731** Corrosion of third degree of multiple right fingers (nail), not including thumb
    - HAC 7th character A see Appendix B for HAC conditional logic
  - CC +7th **T23.732** Corrosion of third degree of multiple left fingers (nail), not including thumb
    - HAC 7th character A see Appendix B for HAC conditional logic
  - CC +7th **T23.739** Corrosion of third degree of unspecified multiple fingers (nail), not including thumb
    - HAC 7th character A see Appendix B for HAC conditional logic
- **T23.74** Corrosion of third degree of multiple fingers (nail), including thumb
  - CC +7th **T23.741** Corrosion of third degree of multiple right fingers (nail), including thumb
    - HAC 7th character A see Appendix B for HAC conditional logic
  - CC +7th **T23.742** Corrosion of third degree of multiple left fingers (nail), including thumb
    - HAC 7th character A see Appendix B for HAC conditional logic
  - CC +7th **T23.749** Corrosion of third degree of unspecified multiple fingers (nail), including thumb
    - HAC 7th character A see Appendix B for HAC conditional logic

- **T23.75** Corrosion of third degree of palm
  - CC +7th **T23.751** Corrosion of third degree of right palm
    - HAC 7th character A see Appendix B for HAC conditional logic
  - CC +7th **T23.752** Corrosion of third degree of left palm
    - HAC 7th character A see Appendix B for HAC conditional logic
  - CC +7th **T23.759** Corrosion of third degree of unspecified palm
    - HAC 7th character A see Appendix B for HAC conditional logic
- **T23.76** Corrosion of third degree of back of hand
  - CC +7th **T23.761** Corrosion of third degree of back of right hand
    - HAC 7th character A see Appendix B for HAC conditional logic
  - CC +7th **T23.762** Corrosion of third degree of back of left hand
    - HAC 7th character A see Appendix B for HAC conditional logic
  - CC +7th **T23.769** Corrosion of third degree back of unspecified hand
    - HAC 7th character A see Appendix B for HAC conditional logic
- **T23.77** Corrosion of third degree of wrist
  - CC +7th **T23.771** Corrosion of third degree of right wrist
    - HAC 7th character A see Appendix B for HAC conditional logic
  - CC +7th **T23.772** Corrosion of third degree of left wrist
    - HAC 7th character A see Appendix B for HAC conditional logic
  - CC +7th **T23.779** Corrosion of third degree of unspecified wrist
    - HAC 7th character A see Appendix B for HAC conditional logic
- **T23.79** Corrosion of third degree of multiple sites of wrist and hand
  - CC +7th **T23.791** Corrosion of third degree of multiple sites of right wrist and hand
    - HAC 7th character A see Appendix B for HAC conditional logic
  - CC +7th **T23.792** Corrosion of third degree of multiple sites of left wrist and hand
    - HAC 7th character A see Appendix B for HAC conditional logic
  - CC +7th **T23.799** Corrosion of third degree of multiple sites of unspecified wrist and hand
    - HAC 7th character A see Appendix B for HAC conditional logic

T24 Burn and corrosion of lower limb, except ankle and foot

Excludes2: burn and corrosion of ankle and foot (T25.-)
burn and corrosion of hip region (T21.-)

The appropriate 7th character is to be added to each code from category T24
- A initial encounter
- D subsequent encounter
- S sequela

- **T24.0** Burn of unspecified degree of lower limb, except ankle and foot
  Use additional external cause code to identify the source, place and intent of the burn (X00-X19, X75-X77, X96-X98, Y92)
  - **T24.00** Burn of unspecified degree of unspecified site of lower limb, except ankle and foot
    - +7th **T24.001** Burn of unspecified degree of unspecified site of right lower limb, except ankle and foot
    - +7th **T24.002** Burn of unspecified degree of unspecified site of left lower limb, except ankle and foot
    - +7th **T24.009** Burn of unspecified degree of unspecified site of unspecified lower limb, except ankle and foot
  - **T24.01** Burn of unspecified degree of thigh
    - +7th **T24.011** Burn of unspecified degree of right thigh
    - +7th **T24.012** Burn of unspecified degree of left thigh
    - +7th **T24.019** Burn of unspecified degree of unspecified thigh
  - **T24.02** Burn of unspecified degree of knee
    - +7th **T24.021** Burn of unspecified degree of right knee
    - +7th **T24.022** Burn of unspecified degree of left knee
    - +7th **T24.029** Burn of unspecified degree of unspecified knee
  - **T24.03** Burn of unspecified degree of lower leg
    - +7th **T24.031** Burn of unspecified degree of right lower leg
    - +7th **T24.032** Burn of unspecified degree of left lower leg
    - +7th **T24.039** Burn of unspecified degree of unspecified lower leg
  - **T24.09** Burn of unspecified degree of multiple sites of lower limb, except ankle and foot
    - +7th **T24.091** Burn of unspecified degree of multiple sites of right lower limb, except ankle and foot
    - +7th **T24.092** Burn of unspecified degree of multiple sites of left lower limb, except ankle and foot
    - +7th **T24.099** Burn of unspecified degree of multiple sites of unspecified lower limb, except ankle and foot
- **T24.1** Burn of first degree of lower limb, except ankle and foot
  Use additional external cause code to identify the source, place and intent of the burn (X00-X19, X75-X77, X96-X98, Y92)
  - **T24.10** Burn of first degree of unspecified site of lower limb, except ankle and foot
    - +7th **T24.101** Burn of first degree of unspecified site of right lower limb, except ankle and foot
    - +7th **T24.102** Burn of first degree of unspecified site of left lower limb, except ankle and foot
    - +7th **T24.109** Burn of first degree of unspecified site of unspecified lower limb, except ankle and foot
  - **T24.11** Burn of first degree of thigh
    - +7th **T24.111** Burn of first degree of right thigh
    - +7th **T24.112** Burn of first degree of left thigh
    - +7th **T24.119** Burn of first degree of unspecified thigh
  - **T24.12** Burn of first degree of knee
    - +7th **T24.121** Burn of first degree of right knee
    - +7th **T24.122** Burn of first degree of left knee
    - +7th **T24.129** Burn of first degree of unspecified knee
  - **T24.13** Burn of first degree of lower leg
    - +7th **T24.131** Burn of first degree of right lower leg
    - +7th **T24.132** Burn of first degree of left lower leg
    - +7th **T24.139** Burn of first degree of unspecified lower leg
  - **T24.19** Burn of first degree of multiple sites of lower limb, except ankle and foot
    - +7th **T24.191** Burn of first degree of multiple sites of right lower limb, except ankle and foot
    - +7th **T24.192** Burn of first degree of multiple sites of left lower limb, except ankle and foot
    - +7th **T24.199** Burn of first degree of multiple sites of unspecified lower limb, except ankle and foot

- **T24.2** **Burn of second degree of lower limb, except ankle and foot**
  Use additional external cause code to identify the source, place and intent of the burn (X00-X19, X75-X77, X96-X98, Y92)
  - **T24.20** Burn of second degree of unspecified site of lower limb, except ankle and foot
    - +7th **T24.201** Burn of second degree of unspecified site of right lower limb, except ankle and foot
    - +7th **T24.202** Burn of second degree of unspecified site of left lower limb, except ankle and foot
    - +7th **T24.209** Burn of second degree of unspecified site of unspecified lower limb, except ankle and foot
  - **T24.21** Burn of second degree of thigh
    - +7th **T24.211** Burn of second degree of right thigh
    - +7th **T24.212** Burn of second degree of left thigh
    - +7th **T24.219** Burn of second degree of unspecified thigh
  - **T24.22** Burn of second degree of knee
    - +7th **T24.221** Burn of second degree of right knee
    - +7th **T24.222** Burn of second degree of left knee
    - +7th **T24.229** Burn of second degree of unspecified knee
  - **T24.23** Burn of second degree of lower leg
    - +7th **T24.231** Burn of second degree of right lower leg
    - +7th **T24.232** Burn of second degree of left lower leg
    - +7th **T24.239** Burn of second degree of unspecified lower leg
  - **T24.29** Burn of second degree of multiple sites of lower limb, except ankle and foot
    - +7th **T24.291** Burn of second degree of multiple sites of right lower limb, except ankle and foot
    - +7th **T24.292** Burn of second degree of multiple sites of left lower limb, except ankle and foot
    - +7th **T24.299** Burn of second degree of multiple sites of unspecified lower limb, except ankle and foot
- **T24.3** **Burn of third degree of lower limb, except ankle and foot**
  Use additional external cause code to identify the source, place and intent of the burn (X00-X19, X75-X77, X96-X98, Y92)
  - **T24.30** Burn of third degree of unspecified site of lower limb, except ankle and foot
    - CC +7th **T24.301** Burn of third degree of unspecified site of right lower limb, except ankle and foot
      - HAC 7th character A see Appendix B for HAC conditional logic
    - CC +7th **T24.302** Burn of third degree of unspecified site of left lower limb, except ankle and foot
      - HAC 7th character A see Appendix B for HAC conditional logic
    - CC +7th **T24.309** Burn of third degree of unspecified site of unspecified lower limb, except ankle and foot
      - HAC 7th character A see Appendix B for HAC conditional logic
  - **T24.31** Burn of third degree of thigh
    - CC +7th **T24.311** Burn of third degree of right thigh
      - HAC 7th character A see Appendix B for HAC conditional logic
    - CC +7th **T24.312** Burn of third degree of left thigh
      - HAC 7th character A see Appendix B for HAC conditional logic
    - CC +7th **T24.319** Burn of third degree of unspecified thigh
      - HAC 7th character A see Appendix B for HAC conditional logic
  - **T24.32** Burn of third degree of knee
    - CC +7th **T24.321** Burn of third degree of right knee
      - HAC 7th character A see Appendix B for HAC conditional logic
    - CC +7th **T24.322** Burn of third degree of left knee
      - HAC 7th character A see Appendix B for HAC conditional logic
    - CC +7th **T24.329** Burn of third degree of unspecified knee
      - HAC 7th character A see Appendix B for HAC conditional logic
- **T24.33** Burn of third degree of lower leg
  - CC +7th **T24.331** Burn of third degree of right lower leg
    - HAC 7th character A see Appendix B for HAC conditional logic
  - CC +7th **T24.332** Burn of third degree of left lower leg
    - HAC 7th character A see Appendix B for HAC conditional logic
  - CC +7th **T24.339** Burn of third degree of unspecified lower leg
    - HAC 7th character A see Appendix B for HAC conditional logic
- **T24.39** Burn of third degree of multiple sites of lower limb, except ankle and foot
  - CC +7th **T24.391** Burn of third degree of multiple sites of right lower limb, except ankle and foot
    - *AHA CC: 2Q, 2016, 4*
    - HAC 7th character A see Appendix B for HAC conditional logic
  - CC +7th **T24.392** Burn of third degree of multiple sites of left lower limb, except ankle and foot
    - *AHA CC: 2Q, 2016, 4*
    - HAC 7th character A see Appendix B for HAC conditional logic
  - CC +7th **T24.399** Burn of third degree of multiple sites of unspecified lower limb, except ankle and foot
    - HAC 7th character A see Appendix B for HAC conditional logic
- **T24.4** **Corrosion of unspecified degree of lower limb, except ankle and foot**
  Code first (T51-T65) to identify chemical and intent
  Use additional external cause code to identify place (Y92)
  - **T24.40** Corrosion of unspecified degree of unspecified site of lower limb, except ankle and foot
    - +7th **T24.401** Corrosion of unspecified degree of unspecified site of right lower limb, except ankle and foot
    - +7th **T24.402** Corrosion of unspecified degree of unspecified site of left lower limb, except ankle and foot
    - +7th **T24.409** Corrosion of unspecified degree of unspecified site of unspecified lower limb, except ankle and foot
  - **T24.41** Corrosion of unspecified degree of thigh
    - +7th **T24.411** Corrosion of unspecified degree of right thigh
    - +7th **T24.412** Corrosion of unspecified degree of left thigh
    - +7th **T24.419** Corrosion of unspecified degree of unspecified thigh
  - **T24.42** Corrosion of unspecified degree of knee
    - +7th **T24.421** Corrosion of unspecified degree of right knee
    - +7th **T24.422** Corrosion of unspecified degree of left knee
    - +7th **T24.429** Corrosion of unspecified degree of unspecified knee
  - **T24.43** Corrosion of unspecified degree of lower leg
    - +7th **T24.431** Corrosion of unspecified degree of right lower leg
    - +7th **T24.432** Corrosion of unspecified degree of left lower leg
    - +7th **T24.439** Corrosion of unspecified degree of unspecified lower leg
  - **T24.49** Corrosion of unspecified degree of multiple sites of lower limb, except ankle and foot
    - +7th **T24.491** Corrosion of unspecified degree of multiple sites of right lower limb, except ankle and foot
    - +7th **T24.492** Corrosion of unspecified degree of multiple sites of left lower limb, except ankle and foot
    - +7th **T24.499** Corrosion of unspecified degree of multiple sites of unspecified lower limb, except ankle and foot

- **T24.5** Corrosion of first degree of lower limb, except ankle and foot
  Code first (T51-T65) to identify chemical and intent
  Use additional external cause code to identify place (Y92)
  - **T24.50** Corrosion of first degree of unspecified site of lower limb, except ankle and foot
    - +7th **T24.501** Corrosion of first degree of unspecified site of right lower limb, except ankle and foot
    - +7th **T24.502** Corrosion of first degree of unspecified site of left lower limb, except ankle and foot
    - +7th **T24.509** Corrosion of first degree of unspecified site of unspecified lower limb, except ankle and foot
  - **T24.51** Corrosion of first degree of thigh
    - +7th **T24.511** Corrosion of first degree of right thigh
    - +7th **T24.512** Corrosion of first degree of left thigh
    - +7th **T24.519** Corrosion of first degree of unspecified thigh
  - **T24.52** Corrosion of first degree of knee
    - +7th **T24.521** Corrosion of first degree of right knee
    - +7th **T24.522** Corrosion of first degree of left knee
    - +7th **T24.529** Corrosion of first degree of unspecified knee
  - **T24.53** Corrosion of first degree of lower leg
    - +7th **T24.531** Corrosion of first degree of right lower leg
    - +7th **T24.532** Corrosion of first degree of left lower leg
    - +7th **T24.539** Corrosion of first degree of unspecified lower leg
  - **T24.59** Corrosion of first degree of multiple sites of lower limb, except ankle and foot
    - +7th **T24.591** Corrosion of first degree of multiple sites of right lower limb, except ankle and foot
    - +7th **T24.592** Corrosion of first degree of multiple sites of left lower limb, except ankle and foot
    - +7th **T24.599** Corrosion of first degree of multiple sites of unspecified lower limb, except ankle and foot
- **T24.6** Corrosion of second degree of lower limb, except ankle and foot
  Code first (T51-T65) to identify chemical and intent
  Use additional external cause code to identify place (Y92)
  - **T24.60** Corrosion of second degree of unspecified site of lower limb, except ankle and foot
    - +7th **T24.601** Corrosion of second degree of unspecified site of right lower limb, except ankle and foot
    - +7th **T24.602** Corrosion of second degree of unspecified site of left lower limb, except ankle and foot
    - +7th **T24.609** Corrosion of second degree of unspecified site of unspecified lower limb, except ankle and foot
  - **T24.61** Corrosion of second degree of thigh
    - +7th **T24.611** Corrosion of second degree of right thigh
    - +7th **T24.612** Corrosion of second degree of left thigh
    - +7th **T24.619** Corrosion of second degree of unspecified thigh
  - **T24.62** Corrosion of second degree of knee
    - +7th **T24.621** Corrosion of second degree of right knee
    - +7th **T24.622** Corrosion of second degree of left knee
    - +7th **T24.629** Corrosion of second degree of unspecified knee
  - **T24.63** Corrosion of second degree of lower leg
    - +7th **T24.631** Corrosion of second degree of right lower leg
    - +7th **T24.632** Corrosion of second degree of left lower leg
    - +7th **T24.639** Corrosion of second degree of unspecified lower leg
  - **T24.69** Corrosion of second degree of multiple sites of lower limb, except ankle and foot
    - +7th **T24.691** Corrosion of second degree of multiple sites of right lower limb, except ankle and foot
    - +7th **T24.692** Corrosion of second degree of multiple sites of left lower limb, except ankle and foot
    - +7th **T24.699** Corrosion of second degree of multiple sites of unspecified lower limb, except ankle and foot
- **T24.7** Corrosion of third degree of lower limb, except ankle and foot
  Code first (T51-T65) to identify chemical and intent
  Use additional external cause code to identify place (Y92)
  - **T24.70** Corrosion of third degree of unspecified site of lower limb, except ankle and foot
    - CC +7th **T24.701** Corrosion of third degree of unspecified site of right lower limb, except ankle and foot
      - HAC 7th character A see Appendix B for HAC conditional logic
    - CC +7th **T24.702** Corrosion of third degree of unspecified site of left lower limb, except ankle and foot
      - HAC 7th character A see Appendix B for HAC conditional logic
    - CC +7th **T24.709** Corrosion of third degree of unspecified site of unspecified lower limb, except ankle and foot
      - HAC 7th character A see Appendix B for HAC conditional logic
  - **T24.71** Corrosion of third degree of thigh
    - CC +7th **T24.711** Corrosion of third degree of right thigh
      - HAC 7th character A see Appendix B for HAC conditional logic
    - CC +7th **T24.712** Corrosion of third degree of left thigh
      - HAC 7th character A see Appendix B for HAC conditional logic
    - CC +7th **T24.719** Corrosion of third degree of unspecified thigh
      - HAC 7th character A see Appendix B for HAC conditional logic
  - **T24.72** Corrosion of third degree of knee
    - CC +7th **T24.721** Corrosion of third degree of right knee
      - HAC 7th character A see Appendix B for HAC conditional logic
    - CC +7th **T24.722** Corrosion of third degree of left knee
      - HAC 7th character A see Appendix B for HAC conditional logic
    - CC +7th **T24.729** Corrosion of third degree of unspecified knee
      - HAC 7th character A see Appendix B for HAC conditional logic
  - **T24.73** Corrosion of third degree of lower leg
    - CC +7th **T24.731** Corrosion of third degree of right lower leg
      - HAC 7th character A see Appendix B for HAC conditional logic
    - CC +7th **T24.732** Corrosion of third degree of left lower leg
      - HAC 7th character A see Appendix B for HAC conditional logic
    - CC +7th **T24.739** Corrosion of third degree of unspecified lower leg
      - HAC 7th character A see Appendix B for HAC conditional logic
  - **T24.79** Corrosion of third degree of multiple sites of lower limb, except ankle and foot
    - CC +7th **T24.791** Corrosion of third degree of multiple sites of right lower limb, except ankle and foot
      - HAC 7th character A see Appendix B for HAC conditional logic

CC +7th **T24.792** Corrosion of third degree of multiple sites of left lower limb, except ankle and foot
HAC 7th character A see Appendix B for HAC conditional logic

CC +7th **T24.799** Corrosion of third degree of multiple sites of unspecified lower limb, except ankle and foot
HAC 7th character A see Appendix B for HAC conditional logic

T25 Burn and corrosion of ankle and foot

The appropriate 7th character is to be added to each code from category T25
A initial encounter
D subsequent encounter
S sequela

+ **T25.0** Burn of unspecified degree of ankle and foot
Use additional external cause code to identify the source, place and intent of the burn (X00-X19, X75-X77, X96-X98, Y92)
  + **T25.01** Burn of unspecified degree of ankle
    +7th **T25.011** Burn of unspecified degree of right ankle
    +7th **T25.012** Burn of unspecified degree of left ankle
    +7th **T25.019** Burn of unspecified degree of unspecified ankle
  + **T25.02** Burn of unspecified degree of foot
    Excludes2: burn of unspecified degree of toe(s) (nail) (T25.03-)
    +7th **T25.021** Burn of unspecified degree of right foot
    +7th **T25.022** Burn of unspecified degree of left foot
    +7th **T25.029** Burn of unspecified degree of unspecified foot
  + **T25.03** Burn of unspecified degree of toe(s) (nail)
    +7th **T25.031** Burn of unspecified degree of right toe(s) (nail)
    +7th **T25.032** Burn of unspecified degree of left toe(s) (nail)
    +7th **T25.039** Burn of unspecified degree of unspecified toe(s) (nail)
  + **T25.09** Burn of unspecified degree of multiple sites of ankle and foot
    +7th **T25.091** Burn of unspecified degree of multiple sites of right ankle and foot
    +7th **T25.092** Burn of unspecified degree of multiple sites of left ankle and foot
    +7th **T25.099** Burn of unspecified degree of multiple sites of unspecified ankle and foot

+ **T25.1** Burn of first degree of ankle and foot
Use additional external cause code to identify the source, place and intent of the burn (X00-X19, X75-X77, X96-X98, Y92)
  + **T25.11** Burn of first degree of ankle
    +7th **T25.111** Burn of first degree of right ankle
    +7th **T25.112** Burn of first degree of left ankle
    +7th **T25.119** Burn of first degree of unspecified ankle
  + **T25.12** Burn of first degree of foot
    Excludes2: burn of first degree of toe(s) (nail) (T25.13-)
    +7th **T25.121** Burn of first degree of right foot
    +7th **T25.122** Burn of first degree of left foot
    +7th **T25.129** Burn of first degree of unspecified foot
  + **T25.13** Burn of first degree of toe(s) (nail)
    +7th **T25.131** Burn of first degree of right toe(s) (nail)
    +7th **T25.132** Burn of first degree of left toe(s) (nail)
    +7th **T25.139** Burn of first degree of unspecified toe(s) (nail)
  + **T25.19** Burn of first degree of multiple sites of ankle and foot
    +7th **T25.191** Burn of first degree of multiple sites of right ankle and foot
    +7th **T25.192** Burn of first degree of multiple sites of left ankle and foot
    +7th **T25.199** Burn of first degree of multiple sites of unspecified ankle and foot

+ **T25.2** Burn of second degree of ankle and foot
Use additional external cause code to identify the source, place and intent of the burn (X00-X19, X75-X77, X96-X98, Y92)
  + **T25.21** Burn of second degree of ankle
    +7th **T25.211** Burn of second degree of right ankle
    +7th **T25.212** Burn of second degree of left ankle
    +7th **T25.219** Burn of second degree of unspecified ankle
  + **T25.22** Burn of second degree of foot
    Excludes2: burn of second degree of toe(s) (nail) (T25.23-)
    +7th **T25.221** Burn of second degree of right foot
    +7th **T25.222** Burn of second degree of left foot
    +7th **T25.229** Burn of second degree of unspecified foot
  + **T25.23** Burn of second degree of toe(s) (nail)
    +7th **T25.231** Burn of second degree of right toe(s) (nail)
    +7th **T25.232** Burn of second degree of left toe(s) (nail)
    +7th **T25.239** Burn of second degree of unspecified toe(s) (nail)
  + **T25.29** Burn of second degree of multiple sites of ankle and foot
    +7th **T25.291** Burn of second degree of multiple sites of right ankle and foot
    +7th **T25.292** Burn of second degree of multiple sites of left ankle and foot
    +7th **T25.299** Burn of second degree of multiple sites of unspecified ankle and foot

+ **T25.3** Burn of third degree of ankle and foot
Use external cause code to identify the source, place and intent of the burn (X00-X19, X75-X77, X96-X98, Y92)
  + **T25.31** Burn of third degree of ankle
    CC +7th **T25.311** Burn of third degree of right ankle
    HAC 7th character A see Appendix B for HAC conditional logic
    CC +7th **T25.312** Burn of third degree of left ankle
    HAC 7th character A see Appendix B for HAC conditional logic
    CC +7th **T25.319** Burn of third degree of unspecified ankle
    HAC 7th character A see Appendix B for HAC conditional logic
  + **T25.32** Burn of third degree of foot
    Excludes2: burn of third degree of toe(s) (nail) (T25.33-)
    CC +7th **T25.321** Burn of third degree of right foot
    HAC 7th character A see Appendix B for HAC conditional logic
    CC +7th **T25.322** Burn of third degree of left foot
    HAC 7th character A see Appendix B for HAC conditional logic
    CC +7th **T25.329** Burn of third degree of unspecified foot
    HAC 7th character A see Appendix B for HAC conditional logic
  + **T25.33** Burn of third degree of toe(s) (nail)
    CC +7th **T25.331** Burn of third degree of right toe(s) (nail)
    HAC 7th character A see Appendix B for HAC conditional logic
    CC +7th **T25.332** Burn of third degree of left toe(s) (nail)
    HAC 7th character A see Appendix B for HAC conditional logic
    CC +7th **T25.339** Burn of third degree of unspecified toe(s) (nail)
    HAC 7th character A see Appendix B for HAC conditional logic
  + **T25.39** Burn of third degree of multiple sites of ankle and foot
    CC +7th **T25.391** Burn of third degree of multiple sites of right ankle and foot
    HAC 7th character A see Appendix B for HAC conditional logic
    CC +7th **T25.392** Burn of third degree of multiple sites of left ankle and foot
    HAC 7th character A see Appendix B for HAC conditional logic

CC +7th **T25.399** Burn of third degree of multiple sites of unspecified ankle and foot
HAC 7th character A see Appendix B for HAC conditional logic

+ **T25.4 Corrosion of unspecified degree of ankle and foot**
Code first (T51-T65) to identify chemical and intent
Use additional external cause code to identify place (Y92)

+ **T25.41** Corrosion of unspecified degree of ankle
+7th **T25.411** Corrosion of unspecified degree of right ankle
+7th **T25.412** Corrosion of unspecified degree of left ankle
+7th **T25.419** Corrosion of unspecified degree of unspecified ankle

+ **T25.42** Corrosion of unspecified degree of foot
Excludes2: *corrosion of unspecified degree of toe(s) (nail) (T25.43-)*
+7th **T25.421** Corrosion of unspecified degree of right foot
+7th **T25.422** Corrosion of unspecified degree of left foot
+7th **T25.429** Corrosion of unspecified degree of unspecified foot

+ **T25.43** Corrosion of unspecified degree of toe(s) (nail)
+7th **T25.431** Corrosion of unspecified degree of right toe(s) (nail)
+7th **T25.432** Corrosion of unspecified degree of left toe(s) (nail)
+7th **T25.439** Corrosion of unspecified degree of unspecified toe(s) (nail)

+ **T25.49** Corrosion of unspecified degree of multiple sites of ankle and foot
+7th **T25.491** Corrosion of unspecified degree of multiple sites of right ankle and foot
+7th **T25.492** Corrosion of unspecified degree of multiple sites of left ankle and foot
+7th **T25.499** Corrosion of unspecified degree of multiple sites of unspecified ankle and foot

+ **T25.5 Corrosion of first degree of ankle and foot**
Code first (T51-T65) to identify chemical and intent
Use additional external cause code to identify place (Y92)

+ **T25.51** Corrosion of first degree of ankle
+7th **T25.511** Corrosion of first degree of right ankle
+7th **T25.512** Corrosion of first degree of left ankle
+7th **T25.519** Corrosion of first degree of unspecified ankle

+ **T25.52** Corrosion of first degree of foot
Excludes2: *corrosion of first degree of toe(s) (nail) (T25.53-)*
+7th **T25.521** Corrosion of first degree of right foot
+7th **T25.522** Corrosion of first degree of left foot
+7th **T25.529** Corrosion of first degree of unspecified foot

+ **T25.53** Corrosion of first degree of toe(s) (nail)
+7th **T25.531** Corrosion of first degree of right toe(s) (nail)
+7th **T25.532** Corrosion of first degree of left toe(s) (nail)
+7th **T25.539** Corrosion of first degree of unspecified toe(s) (nail)

+ **T25.59** Corrosion of first degree of multiple sites of ankle and foot
+7th **T25.591** Corrosion of first degree of multiple sites of right ankle and foot
+7th **T25.592** Corrosion of first degree of multiple sites of left ankle and foot
+7th **T25.599** Corrosion of first degree of multiple sites of unspecified ankle and foot

+ **T25.6 Corrosion of second degree of ankle and foot**
Code first (T51-T65) to identify chemical and intent
Use additional external cause code to identify place (Y92)

+ **T25.61** Corrosion of second degree of ankle
+7th **T25.611** Corrosion of second degree of right ankle
+7th **T25.612** Corrosion of second degree of left ankle
+7th **T25.619** Corrosion of second degree of unspecified ankle

+ **T25.62** Corrosion of second degree of foot
Excludes2: *corrosion of second degree of toe(s) (nail) (T25.63-)*
+7th **T25.621** Corrosion of second degree of right foot
+7th **T25.622** Corrosion of second degree of left foot
+7th **T25.629** Corrosion of second degree of unspecified foot

+ **T25.63** Corrosion of second degree of toe(s) (nail)
+7th **T25.631** Corrosion of second degree of right toe(s) (nail)
+7th **T25.632** Corrosion of second degree of left toe(s) (nail)
+7th **T25.639** Corrosion of second degree of unspecified toe(s) (nail)

+ **T25.69** Corrosion of second degree of multiple sites of ankle and foot
+7th **T25.691** Corrosion of second degree of right ankle and foot
+7th **T25.692** Corrosion of second degree of left ankle and foot
+7th **T25.699** Corrosion of second degree of unspecified ankle and foot

+ **T25.7 Corrosion of third degree of ankle and foot**
Code first (T51-T65) to identify chemical and intent
Use additional external cause code to identify place (Y92)

+ **T25.71** Corrosion of third degree of ankle
CC +7th **T25.711** Corrosion of third degree of right ankle
HAC 7th character A see Appendix B for HAC conditional logic
CC +7th **T25.712** Corrosion of third degree of left ankle
HAC 7th character A see Appendix B for HAC conditional logic
CC +7th **T25.719** Corrosion of third degree of unspecified ankle
HAC 7th character A see Appendix B for HAC conditional logic

+ **T25.72** Corrosion of third degree of foot
Excludes2: *corrosion of third degree of toe(s) (nail) (T25.73-)*
CC +7th **T25.721** Corrosion of third degree of right foot
HAC 7th character A see Appendix B for HAC conditional logic
CC +7th **T25.722** Corrosion of third degree of left foot
HAC 7th character A see Appendix B for HAC conditional logic
CC +7th **T25.729** Corrosion of third degree of unspecified foot
HAC 7th character A see Appendix B for HAC conditional logic

+ **T25.73** Corrosion of third degree of toe(s) (nail)
CC +7th **T25.731** Corrosion of third degree of right toe(s) (nail)
HAC 7th character A see Appendix B for HAC conditional logic
CC +7th **T25.732** Corrosion of third degree of left toe(s) (nail)
HAC 7th character A see Appendix B for HAC conditional logic
CC +7th **T25.739** Corrosion of third degree of unspecified toe(s) (nail)
HAC 7th character A see Appendix B for HAC conditional logic

+ **T25.79** Corrosion of third degree of multiple sites of ankle and foot
CC +7th **T25.791** Corrosion of third degree of multiple sites of right ankle and foot
HAC 7th character A see Appendix B for HAC conditional logic
CC +7th **T25.792** Corrosion of third degree of multiple sites of left ankle and foot
HAC 7th character A see Appendix B for HAC conditional logic
CC +7th **T25.799** Corrosion of third degree of multiple sites of unspecified ankle and foot
HAC 7th character A see Appendix B for HAC conditional logic

Burns and corrosions confined to eye and internal organs (T26-T28)

Review coding guideline C.19.d

T26 Burn and corrosion confined to eye and adnexa

The appropriate 7th character is to be added to each code from category T26
- A initial encounter
- D subsequent encounter
- S sequela

- **T26.0** Burn of eyelid and periocular area
  Use additional external cause code to identify the source, place and intent of the burn (X00-X19, X75-X77, X96-X98, Y92)
  - X+7th **T26.00** Burn of unspecified eyelid and periocular area
  - X+7th **T26.01** Burn of right eyelid and periocular area
  - X+7th **T26.02** Burn of left eyelid and periocular area
- **T26.1** Burn of cornea and conjunctival sac
  Use additional external cause code to identify the source, place and intent of the burn (X00-X19, X75-X77, X96-X98, Y92)
  - X+7th **T26.10** Burn of cornea and conjunctival sac, unspecified eye
  - X+7th **T26.11** Burn of cornea and conjunctival sac, right eye
  - X+7th **T26.12** Burn of cornea and conjunctival sac, left eye
- **T26.2** Burn with resulting rupture and destruction of eyeball
  Use additional external cause code to identify the source, place and intent of the burn (X00-X19, X75-X77, X96-X98, Y92)
  - CC X+7th **T26.20** Burn with resulting rupture and destruction of unspecified eyeball
    HAC 7th character A see Appendix B for HAC conditional logic
  - CC X+7th **T26.21** Burn with resulting rupture and destruction of right eyeball
    HAC 7th character A see Appendix B for HAC conditional logic
  - CC X+7th **T26.22** Burn with resulting rupture and destruction of left eyeball
    HAC 7th character A see Appendix B for HAC conditional logic
- **T26.3** Burns of other specified parts of eye and adnexa
  Use additional external cause code to identify the source, place and intent of the burn (X00-X19, X75-X77, X96-X98, Y92)
  - X+7th **T26.30** Burns of other specified parts of unspecified eye and adnexa
  - X+7th **T26.31** Burns of other specified parts of right eye and adnexa
  - X+7th **T26.32** Burns of other specified parts of left eye and adnexa
- **T26.4** Burn of eye and adnexa, part unspecified
  Use additional external cause code to identify the source, place and intent of the burn (X00-X19, X75-X77, X96-X98, Y92)
  - X+7th **T26.40** Burn of unspecified eye and adnexa, part unspecified
  - X+7th **T26.41** Burn of right eye and adnexa, part unspecified
  - X+7th **T26.42** Burn of left eye and adnexa, part unspecified
- **T26.5** Corrosion of eyelid and periocular area
  Code first (T51-T65) to identify chemical and intent

  Use additional external cause code to identify place (Y92)
  - X+7th **T26.50** Corrosion of unspecified eyelid and periocular area
  - X+7th **T26.51** Corrosion of right eyelid and periocular area
  - X+7th **T26.52** Corrosion of left eyelid and periocular area
- **T26.6** Corrosion of cornea and conjunctival sac
  Code first (T51-T65) to identify chemical and intent

  Use additional external cause code to identify place (Y92)
  - X+7th **T26.60** Corrosion of cornea and conjunctival sac, unspecified eye
  - X+7th **T26.61** Corrosion of cornea and conjunctival sac, right eye
  - X+7th **T26.62** Corrosion of cornea and conjunctival sac, left eye
- **T26.7** Corrosion with resulting rupture and destruction of eyeball
  Code first (T51-T65) to identify chemical and intent

  Use additional external cause code to identify place (Y92)
  - CC X+7th **T26.70** Corrosion with resulting rupture and destruction of unspecified eyeball
    HAC 7th character A see Appendix B for HAC conditional logic
  - CC X+7th **T26.71** Corrosion with resulting rupture and destruction of right eyeball
    HAC 7th character A see Appendix B for HAC conditional logic
  - CC X+7th **T26.72** Corrosion with resulting rupture and destruction of left eyeball
    HAC 7th character A see Appendix B for HAC conditional logic
- **T26.8** Corrosions of other specified parts of eye and adnexa
  Code first (T51-T65) to identify chemical and intent

  Use additional external cause code to identify place (Y92)
  - X+7th **T26.80** Corrosions of other specified parts of unspecified eye and adnexa
  - X+7th **T26.81** Corrosions of other specified parts of right eye and adnexa
  - X+7th **T26.82** Corrosions of other specified parts of left eye and adnexa
- **T26.9** Corrosion of eye and adnexa, part unspecified
  Code first (T51-T65) to identify chemical and intent

  Use additional external cause code to identify place (Y92)
  - X+7th **T26.90** Corrosion of unspecified eye and adnexa, part unspecified
  - X+7th **T26.91** Corrosion of right eye and adnexa, part unspecified
  - X+7th **T26.92** Corrosion of left eye and adnexa, part unspecified

T27 Burn and corrosion of respiratory tract

Use additional external cause code to identify the source and intent of the burn (X00-X19, X75-X77, X96-X98)

Use external cause code to identify place (Y92)

The appropriate 7th character is to be added to each code from category T27
- A initial encounter
- D subsequent encounter
- S sequela

- CC X+7th **T27.0** Burn of larynx and trachea
  HAC 7th character A see Appendix B for HAC conditional logic
- CC X+7th **T27.1** Burn involving larynx and trachea with lung
  HAC 7th character A see Appendix B for HAC conditional logic
- CC X+7th **T27.2** Burn of other parts of respiratory tract
  Burn of thoracic cavity
  HAC 7th character A see Appendix B for HAC conditional logic
- CC X+7th **T27.3** Burn of respiratory tract, part unspecified
  HAC 7th character A see Appendix B for HAC conditional logic
- CC X+7th **T27.4** Corrosion of larynx and trachea
  Code first (T51-T65) to identify chemical and intent
  HAC 7th character A see Appendix B for HAC conditional logic
- CC X+7th **T27.5** Corrosion involving larynx and trachea with lung
  Code first (T51-T65) to identify chemical and intent
  HAC 7th character A see Appendix B for HAC conditional logic
- CC X+7th **T27.6** Corrosion of other parts of respiratory tract
  Code first (T51-T65) to identify chemical and intent
  HAC 7th character A see Appendix B for HAC conditional logic
- CC X+7th **T27.7** Corrosion of respiratory tract, part unspecified
  Code first (T51-T65) to identify chemical and intent
  HAC 7th character A see Appendix B for HAC conditional logic

T28 Burn and corrosion of other internal organs

Use additional external cause code to identify the source and intent of the burn (X00-X19, X75-X77, X96-X98)

Use external cause code to identify place (Y92)

The appropriate 7th character is to be added to each code from category T28
- A initial encounter
- D subsequent encounter
- S sequela

- X+7th **T28.0** Burn of mouth and pharynx
- CC X+7th **T28.1** Burn of esophagus
  HAC 7th character A see Appendix B for HAC conditional logic
- CC X+7th **T28.2** Burn of other parts of alimentary tract
  HAC 7th character A see Appendix B for HAC conditional logic

- X+7th **T28.3** Burn of internal genitourinary organs
- + **T28.4** Burns of other and unspecified internal organs
  - X+7th **T28.40** Burn of unspecified internal organ
  - + **T28.41** Burn of ear drum
    - +7th **T28.411** Burn of right ear drum
    - +7th **T28.412** Burn of left ear drum
    - +7th **T28.419** Burn of unspecified ear drum
  - X+7th **T28.49** Burn of other internal organ
- X+7th **T28.5** Corrosion of mouth and pharynx
  - Code first (T51-T65) to identify chemical and intent
- CC X+7th **T28.6** Corrosion of esophagus
  - Code first (T51-T65) to identify chemical and intent
  - HAC 7th character A see Appendix B for HAC conditional logic
- CC X+7th **T28.7** Corrosion of other parts of alimentary tract
  - Code first (T51-T65) to identify chemical and intent
  - HAC 7th character A see Appendix B for HAC conditional logic
- X+7th **T28.8** Corrosion of internal genitourinary organs
  - Code first (T51-T65) to identify chemical and intent
- + **T28.9** Corrosions of other and unspecified internal organs
  - Code first (T51-T65) to identify chemical and intent
  - X+7th **T28.90** Corrosions of unspecified internal organs
  - + **T28.91** Corrosions of ear drum
    - +7th **T28.911** Corrosions of right ear drum
    - +7th **T28.912** Corrosions of left ear drum
    - +7th **T28.919** Corrosions of unspecified ear drum
  - X+7th **T28.99** Corrosions of other internal organs

Burns and corrosions of multiple and unspecified body regions (T30-T32)

T30 Burn and corrosion, body region unspecified
  Review coding guideline C.19.d.5
- **T30.0** Burn of unspecified body region, unspecified degree
  - This code is not for inpatient use. Code to specified site and degree of burns
  - Burn NOS
  - Multiple burns NOS
- **T30.4** Corrosion of unspecified body region, unspecified degree
  - This code is not for inpatient use. Code to specified site and degree of corrosion
  - Corrosion NOS
  - Multiple corrosion NOS

T31 Burns classified according to extent of body surface involved
  NOTE: This category is to be used as the primary code only when the site of the burn is unspecified. It should be used as a supplementary code with categories T20-T25 when the site is specified.
  Review coding guideline C.19.d.6
- **T31.0** Burns involving less than 10% of body surface
- + **T31.1** Burns involving 10-19% of body surface
  - CC **T31.10** Burns involving 10-19% of body surface with 0% to 9% third degree burns
    - Burns involving 10-19% of body surface NOS
    - HAC see Appendix B for HAC conditional logic
  - CC **T31.11** Burns involving 10-19% of body surface with 10-19% third degree burns
    - HAC see Appendix B for HAC conditional logic
- + **T31.2** Burns involving 20-29% of body surface
  - CC **T31.20** Burns involving 20-29% of body surface with 0% to 9% third degree burns
    - Burns involving 20-29% of body surface NOS
    - HAC see Appendix B for HAC conditional logic
  - MCC **T31.21** Burns involving 20-29% of body surface with 10-19% third degree burns
    - HAC see Appendix B for HAC conditional logic
  - MCC **T31.22** Burns involving 20-29% of body surface with 20-29% third degree burns
    - HAC see Appendix B for HAC conditional logic
- + **T31.3** Burns involving 30-39% of body surface
  - CC **T31.30** Burns involving 30-39% of body surface with 0% to 9% third degree burns
    - Burns involving 30-39% of body surface NOS
    - HAC see Appendix B for HAC conditional logic
  - MCC **T31.31** Burns involving 30-39% of body surface with 10-19% third degree burns
    - HAC see Appendix B for HAC conditional logic
  - MCC **T31.32** Burns involving 30-39% of body surface with 20-29% third degree burns
    - HAC see Appendix B for HAC conditional logic
  - MCC **T31.33** Burns involving 30-39% of body surface with 30-39% third degree burns
    - HAC see Appendix B for HAC conditional logic
- + **T31.4** Burns involving 40-49% of body surface
  - CC **T31.40** Burns involving 40-49% of body surface with 0% to 9% third degree burns
    - Burns involving 40-49% of body surface NOS
    - HAC see Appendix B for HAC conditional logic
  - MCC **T31.41** Burns involving 40-49% of body surface with 10-19% third degree burns
    - HAC see Appendix B for HAC conditional logic
  - MCC **T31.42** Burns involving 40-49% of body surface with 20-29% third degree burns
    - HAC see Appendix B for HAC conditional logic
  - MCC **T31.43** Burns involving 40-49% of body surface with 30-39% third degree burns
    - HAC see Appendix B for HAC conditional logic
  - MCC **T31.44** Burns involving 40-49% of body surface with 40-49% third degree burns
    - HAC see Appendix B for HAC conditional logic
- + **T31.5** Burns involving 50-59% of body surface
  - CC **T31.50** Burns involving 50-59% of body surface with 0% to 9% third degree burns
    - Burns involving 50-59% of body surface NOS
    - HAC see Appendix B for HAC conditional logic
  - MCC **T31.51** Burns involving 50-59% of body surface with 10-19% third degree burns
    - HAC see Appendix B for HAC conditional logic
  - MCC **T31.52** Burns involving 50-59% of body surface with 20-29% third degree burns
    - HAC see Appendix B for HAC conditional logic
  - MCC **T31.53** Burns involving 50-59% of body surface with 30-39% third degree burns
    - HAC see Appendix B for HAC conditional logic
  - MCC **T31.54** Burns involving 50-59% of body surface with 40-49% third degree burns
    - HAC see Appendix B for HAC conditional logic
  - MCC **T31.55** Burns involving 50-59% of body surface with 50-59% third degree burns
    - HAC see Appendix B for HAC conditional logic
- + **T31.6** Burns involving 60-69% of body surface
  - CC **T31.60** Burns involving 60-69% of body surface with 0% to 9% third degree burns
    - Burns involving 60-69% of body surface NOS
    - HAC see Appendix B for HAC conditional logic
  - MCC **T31.61** Burns involving 60-69% of body surface with 10-19% third degree burns
    - HAC see Appendix B for HAC conditional logic
  - MCC **T31.62** Burns involving 60-69% of body surface with 20-29% third degree burns
    - HAC see Appendix B for HAC conditional logic
  - MCC **T31.63** Burns involving 60-69% of body surface with 30-39% third degree burns
    - HAC see Appendix B for HAC conditional logic
  - MCC **T31.64** Burns involving 60-69% of body surface with 40-49% third degree burns
    - HAC see Appendix B for HAC conditional logic
  - MCC **T31.65** Burns involving 60-69% of body surface with 50-59% third degree burns
    - HAC see Appendix B for HAC conditional logic
  - MCC **T31.66** Burns involving 60-69% of body surface with 60-69% third degree burns
    - HAC see Appendix B for HAC conditional logic
- + **T31.7** Burns involving 70-79% of body surface
  - CC **T31.70** Burns involving 70-79% of body surface with 0% to 9% third degree burns
    - Burns involving 70-79% of body surface NOS
    - HAC see Appendix B for HAC conditional logic
  - MCC **T31.71** Burns involving 70-79% of body surface with 10-19% third degree burns
    - HAC see Appendix B for HAC conditional logic
  - MCC **T31.72** Burns involving 70-79% of body surface with 20-29% third degree burns
    - HAC see Appendix B for HAC conditional logic

MCC **T31.73** Burns involving 70-79% of body surface with 30-39% third degree burns
    HAC see Appendix B for HAC conditional logic

MCC **T31.74** Burns involving 70-79% of body surface with 40-49% third degree burns
    HAC see Appendix B for HAC conditional logic

MCC **T31.75** Burns involving 70-79% of body surface with 50-59% third degree burns
    HAC see Appendix B for HAC conditional logic

MCC **T31.76** Burns involving 70-79% of body surface with 60-69% third degree burns
    HAC see Appendix B for HAC conditional logic

MCC **T31.77** Burns involving 70-79% of body surface with 70-79% third degree burns
    HAC see Appendix B for HAC conditional logic

+ **T31.8** Burns involving 80-89% of body surface

CC **T31.80** Burns involving 80-89% of body surface with 0% to 9% third degree burns
    Burns involving 80-89% of body surface NOS
    HAC see Appendix B for HAC conditional logic

MCC **T31.81** Burns involving 80-89% of body surface with 10-19% third degree burns
    HAC see Appendix B for HAC conditional logic

MCC **T31.82** Burns involving 80-89% of body surface with 20-29% third degree burns
    HAC see Appendix B for HAC conditional logic

MCC **T31.83** Burns involving 80-89% of body surface with 30-39% third degree burns
    HAC see Appendix B for HAC conditional logic

MCC **T31.84** Burns involving 80-89% of body surface with 40-49% third degree burns
    HAC see Appendix B for HAC conditional logic

MCC **T31.85** Burns involving 80-89% of body surface with 50-59% third degree burns
    HAC see Appendix B for HAC conditional logic

MCC **T31.86** Burns involving 80-89% of body surface with 60-69% third degree burns
    HAC see Appendix B for HAC conditional logic

MCC **T31.87** Burns involving 80-89% of body surface with 70-79% third degree burns
    HAC see Appendix B for HAC conditional logic

MCC **T31.88** Burns involving 80-89% of body surface with 80-89% third degree burns
    HAC see Appendix B for HAC conditional logic

+ **T31.9** Burns involving 90% or more of body surface

CC **T31.90** Burns involving 90% or more of body surface with 0% to 9% third degree burns
    Burns involving 90% or more of body surface NOS
    HAC see Appendix B for HAC conditional logic

MCC **T31.91** Burns involving 90% or more of body surface with 10-19% third degree burns
    HAC see Appendix B for HAC conditional logic

MCC **T31.92** Burns involving 90% or more of body surface with 20-29% third degree burns
    HAC see Appendix B for HAC conditional logic

MCC **T31.93** Burns involving 90% or more of body surface with 30-39% third degree burns
    HAC see Appendix B for HAC conditional logic

MCC **T31.94** Burns involving 90% or more of body surface with 40-49% third degree burns
    HAC see Appendix B for HAC conditional logic

MCC **T31.95** Burns involving 90% or more of body surface with 50-59% third degree burns
    HAC see Appendix B for HAC conditional logic

MCC **T31.96** Burns involving 90% or more of body surface with 60-69% third degree burns
    HAC see Appendix B for HAC conditional logic

MCC **T31.97** Burns involving 90% or more of body surface with 70-79% third degree burns
    HAC see Appendix B for HAC conditional logic

MCC **T31.98** Burns involving 90% or more of body surface with 80-89% third degree burns
    HAC see Appendix B for HAC conditional logic

MCC **T31.99** Burns involving 90% or more of body surface with 90% or more third degree burns
    HAC see Appendix B for HAC conditional logic

T32 Corrosions classified according to extent of body surface involved

NOTE This category is to be used as the primary code only when the site of the corrosion is unspecified. It may be used as a supplementary code with categories T20-T25 when the site is specified.

Review coding guideline C.19.d.6

T32.0 Corrosions involving less than 10% of body surface

+ **T32.1** Corrosions involving 10-19% of body surface

CC **T32.10** Corrosions involving 10-19% of body surface with 0% to 9% third degree corrosion
    Corrosions involving 10-19% of body surface NOS
    HAC see Appendix B for HAC conditional logic

CC **T32.11** Corrosions involving 10-19% of body surface with 10-19% third degree corrosion
    HAC see Appendix B for HAC conditional logic

+ **T32.2** Corrosions involving 20-29% of body surface

CC **T32.20** Corrosions involving 20-29% of body surface with 0% to 9% third degree corrosion
    HAC see Appendix B for HAC conditional logic

MCC **T32.21** Corrosions involving 20-29% of body surface with 10-19% third degree corrosion
    HAC see Appendix B for HAC conditional logic

MCC **T32.22** Corrosions involving 20-29% of body surface with 20-29% third degree corrosion
    HAC see Appendix B for HAC conditional logic

+ **T32.3** Corrosions involving 30-39% of body surface

CC **T32.30** Corrosions involving 30-39% of body surface with 0% to 9% third degree corrosion
    HAC see Appendix B for HAC conditional logic

MCC **T32.31** Corrosions involving 30-39% of body surface with 10-19% third degree corrosion
    HAC see Appendix B for HAC conditional logic

MCC **T32.32** Corrosions involving 30-39% of body surface with 20-29% third degree corrosion
    HAC see Appendix B for HAC conditional logic

MCC **T32.33** Corrosions involving 30-39% of body surface with 30-39% third degree corrosion
    HAC see Appendix B for HAC conditional logic

+ **T32.4** Corrosions involving 40-49% of body surface

CC **T32.40** Corrosions involving 40-49% of body surface with 0% to 9% third degree corrosion
    HAC see Appendix B for HAC conditional logic

MCC **T32.41** Corrosions involving 40-49% of body surface with 10-19% third degree corrosion
    HAC see Appendix B for HAC conditional logic

MCC **T32.42** Corrosions involving 40-49% of body surface with 20-29% third degree corrosion
    HAC see Appendix B for HAC conditional logic

MCC **T32.43** Corrosions involving 40-49% of body surface with 30-39% third degree corrosion
    HAC see Appendix B for HAC conditional logic

MCC **T32.44** Corrosions involving 40-49% of body surface with 40-49% third degree corrosion
    HAC see Appendix B for HAC conditional logic

+ **T32.5** Corrosions involving 50-59% of body surface

CC **T32.50** Corrosions involving 50-59% of body surface with 0% to 9% third degree corrosion
    HAC see Appendix B for HAC conditional logic

MCC **T32.51** Corrosions involving 50-59% of body surface with 10-19% third degree corrosion
    HAC see Appendix B for HAC conditional logic

MCC **T32.52** Corrosions involving 50-59% of body surface with 20-29% third degree corrosion
    HAC see Appendix B for HAC conditional logic

MCC **T32.53** Corrosions involving 50-59% of body surface with 30-39% third degree corrosion
    HAC see Appendix B for HAC conditional logic

MCC **T32.54** Corrosions involving 50-59% of body surface with 40-49% third degree corrosion
    HAC see Appendix B for HAC conditional logic

MCC **T32.55** Corrosions involving 50-59% of body surface with 50-59% third degree corrosion
    HAC see Appendix B for HAC conditional logic

+ T32.6 Corrosions involving 60-69% of body surface
  CC T32.60 Corrosions involving 60-69% of body surface with 0% to 9% third degree corrosion
    HAC see Appendix B for HAC conditional logic
  MCC T32.61 Corrosions involving 60-69% of body surface with 10-19% third degree corrosion
    HAC see Appendix B for HAC conditional logic
  MCC T32.62 Corrosions involving 60-69% of body surface with 20-29% third degree corrosion
    HAC see Appendix B for HAC conditional logic
  MCC T32.63 Corrosions involving 60-69% of body surface with 30-39% third degree corrosion
    HAC see Appendix B for HAC conditional logic
  MCC T32.64 Corrosions involving 60-69% of body surface with 40-49% third degree corrosion
    HAC see Appendix B for HAC conditional logic
  MCC T32.65 Corrosions involving 60-69% of body surface with 50-59% third degree corrosion
    HAC see Appendix B for HAC conditional logic
  MCC T32.66 Corrosions involving 60-69% of body surface with 60-69% third degree corrosion
    HAC see Appendix B for HAC conditional logic
+ T32.7 Corrosions involving 70-79% of body surface
  CC T32.70 Corrosions involving 70-79% of body surface with 0% to 9% third degree corrosion
    HAC see Appendix B for HAC conditional logic
  MCC T32.71 Corrosions involving 70-79% of body surface with 10-19% third degree corrosion
    HAC see Appendix B for HAC conditional logic
  MCC T32.72 Corrosions involving 70-79% of body surface with 20-29% third degree corrosion
    HAC see Appendix B for HAC conditional logic
  MCC T32.73 Corrosions involving 70-79% of body surface with 30-39% third degree corrosion
    HAC see Appendix B for HAC conditional logic
  MCC T32.74 Corrosions involving 70-79% of body surface with 40-49% third degree corrosion
    HAC see Appendix B for HAC conditional logic
  MCC T32.75 Corrosions involving 70-79% of body surface with 50-59% third degree corrosion
    HAC see Appendix B for HAC conditional logic
  MCC T32.76 Corrosions involving 70-79% of body surface with 60-69% third degree corrosion
    HAC see Appendix B for HAC conditional logic
  MCC T32.77 Corrosions involving 70-79% of body surface with 70-79% third degree corrosion
    HAC see Appendix B for HAC conditional logic
+ T32.8 Corrosions involving 80-89% of body surface
  CC T32.80 Corrosions involving 80-89% of body surface with 0% to 9% third degree corrosion
    HAC see Appendix B for HAC conditional logic
  MCC T32.81 Corrosions involving 80-89% of body surface with 10-19% third degree corrosion
    HAC see Appendix B for HAC conditional logic
  MCC T32.82 Corrosions involving 80-89% of body surface with 20-29% third degree corrosion
    HAC see Appendix B for HAC conditional logic
  MCC T32.83 Corrosions involving 80-89% of body surface with 30-39% third degree corrosion
    HAC see Appendix B for HAC conditional logic
  MCC T32.84 Corrosions involving 80-89% of body surface with 40-49% third degree corrosion
    HAC see Appendix B for HAC conditional logic
  MCC T32.85 Corrosions involving 80-89% of body surface with 50-59% third degree corrosion
    HAC see Appendix B for HAC conditional logic
  MCC T32.86 Corrosions involving 80-89% of body surface with 60-69% third degree corrosion
    HAC see Appendix B for HAC conditional logic
  MCC T32.87 Corrosions involving 80-89% of body surface with 70-79% third degree corrosion
    HAC see Appendix B for HAC conditional logic
  MCC T32.88 Corrosions involving 80-89% of body surface with 80-89% third degree corrosion
    HAC see Appendix B for HAC conditional logic

+ T32.9 Corrosions involving 90% or more of body surface
  CC T32.90 Corrosions involving 90% or more of body surface with 0% to 9% third degree corrosion
    HAC see Appendix B for HAC conditional logic
  MCC T32.91 Corrosions involving 90% or more of body surface with 10-19% third degree corrosion
    HAC see Appendix B for HAC conditional logic
  MCC T32.92 Corrosions involving 90% or more of body surface with 20-29% third degree corrosion
    HAC see Appendix B for HAC conditional logic
  MCC T32.93 Corrosions involving 90% or more of body surface with 30-39% third degree corrosion
    HAC see Appendix B for HAC conditional logic
  MCC T32.94 Corrosions involving 90% or more of body surface with 40-49% third degree corrosion
    HAC see Appendix B for HAC conditional logic
  MCC T32.95 Corrosions involving 90% or more of body surface with 50-59% third degree corrosion
    HAC see Appendix B for HAC conditional logic
  MCC T32.96 Corrosions involving 90% or more of body surface with 60-69% third degree corrosion
    HAC see Appendix B for HAC conditional logic
  MCC T32.97 Corrosions involving 90% or more of body surface with 70-79% third degree corrosion
    HAC see Appendix B for HAC conditional logic
  MCC T32.98 Corrosions involving 90% or more of body surface with 80-89% third degree corrosion
    HAC see Appendix B for HAC conditional logic
  MCC T32.99 Corrosions involving 90% or more of body surface with 90% or more third degree corrosion
    HAC see Appendix B for HAC conditional logic

Frostbite (T33-T34)

Excludes2: hypothermia and other effects of reduced temperature (T68, T69.-)

T33 Superficial frostbite

Includes: frostbite with partial thickness skin loss

The appropriate 7th character is to be added to each code from category T33
- A initial encounter
- D subsequent encounter
- S sequela

+ T33.0 Superficial frostbite of head
  + T33.01 Superficial frostbite of ear
    CC +7th T33.011 Superficial frostbite of right ear
      HAC 7th character A see Appendix B for HAC conditional logic
    CC +7th T33.012 Superficial frostbite of left ear
      HAC 7th character A see Appendix B for HAC conditional logic
    CC +7th T33.019 Superficial frostbite of unspecified ear
      HAC 7th character A see Appendix B for HAC conditional logic
  CC X+7th T33.02 Superficial frostbite of nose
    HAC 7th character A see Appendix B for HAC conditional logic
  CC X+7th T33.09 Superficial frostbite of other part of head
    HAC 7th character A see Appendix B for HAC conditional logic
CC X+7th T33.1 Superficial frostbite of neck
  HAC 7th character A see Appendix B for HAC conditional logic
CC X+7th T33.2 Superficial frostbite of thorax
  HAC 7th character A see Appendix B for HAC conditional logic
CC X+7th T33.3 Superficial frostbite of abdominal wall, lower back and pelvis
  HAC 7th character A see Appendix B for HAC conditional logic
+ T33.4 Superficial frostbite of arm
  Excludes2: superficial frostbite of wrist and hand (T33.5-)
  CC X+7th T33.40 Superficial frostbite of unspecified arm
    HAC 7th character A see Appendix B for HAC conditional logic
  CC X+7th T33.41 Superficial frostbite of right arm
    HAC 7th character A see Appendix B for HAC conditional logic
  CC X+7th T33.42 Superficial frostbite of left arm
    HAC 7th character A see Appendix B for HAC conditional logic

- **T33.5 Superficial frostbite of wrist, hand, and fingers**
  - **T33.51 Superficial frostbite of wrist**
    - CC +7th **T33.511** Superficial frostbite of right wrist
      - HAC 7th character A see Appendix B for HAC conditional logic
    - CC +7th **T33.512** Superficial frostbite of left wrist
      - HAC 7th character A see Appendix B for HAC conditional logic
    - CC +7th **T33.519** Superficial frostbite of unspecified wrist
      - HAC 7th character A see Appendix B for HAC conditional logic
  - **T33.52 Superficial frostbite of hand**
    - *Excludes2:* superficial frostbite of fingers (T33.53-)
    - CC +7th **T33.521** Superficial frostbite of right hand
      - HAC 7th character A see Appendix B for HAC conditional logic
    - CC +7th **T33.522** Superficial frostbite of left hand
      - HAC 7th character A see Appendix B for HAC conditional logic
    - CC +7th **T33.529** Superficial frostbite of unspecified hand
      - HAC 7th character A see Appendix B for HAC conditional logic
  - **T33.53 Superficial frostbite of finger(s)**
    - CC +7th **T33.531** Superficial frostbite of right finger(s)
      - HAC 7th character A see Appendix B for HAC conditional logic
    - CC +7th **T33.532** Superficial frostbite of left finger(s)
      - HAC 7th character A see Appendix B for HAC conditional logic
    - CC +7th **T33.539** Superficial frostbite of unspecified finger(s)
      - HAC 7th character A see Appendix B for HAC conditional logic
- **T33.6 Superficial frostbite of hip and thigh**
  - CC X+7th **T33.60** Superficial frostbite of unspecified hip and thigh
    - HAC 7th character A see Appendix B for HAC conditional logic
  - CC X+7th **T33.61** Superficial frostbite of right hip and thigh
    - HAC 7th character A see Appendix B for HAC conditional logic
  - CC X+7th **T33.62** Superficial frostbite of left hip and thigh
    - HAC 7th character A see Appendix B for HAC conditional logic
- **T33.7 Superficial frostbite of knee and lower leg**
  - *Excludes2:* superficial frostbite of ankle and foot (T33.8-)
  - CC X+7th **T33.70** Superficial frostbite of unspecified knee and lower leg
    - HAC 7th character A see Appendix B for HAC conditional logic
  - CC X+7th **T33.71** Superficial frostbite of right knee and lower leg
    - HAC 7th character A see Appendix B for HAC conditional logic
  - CC X+7th **T33.72** Superficial frostbite of left knee and lower leg
    - HAC 7th character A see Appendix B for HAC conditional logic
- **T33.8 Superficial frostbite of ankle, foot, and toe(s)**
  - **T33.81 Superficial frostbite of ankle**
    - CC +7th **T33.811** Superficial frostbite of right ankle
      - HAC 7th character A see Appendix B for HAC conditional logic
    - CC +7th **T33.812** Superficial frostbite of left ankle
      - HAC 7th character A see Appendix B for HAC conditional logic
    - CC +7th **T33.819** Superficial frostbite of unspecified ankle
      - HAC 7th character A see Appendix B for HAC conditional logic
  - **T33.82 Superficial frostbite of foot**
    - CC +7th **T33.821** Superficial frostbite of right foot
      - HAC 7th character A see Appendix B for HAC conditional logic
    - CC +7th **T33.822** Superficial frostbite of left foot
      - HAC 7th character A see Appendix B for HAC conditional logic
    - CC +7th **T33.829** Superficial frostbite of unspecified foot
      - HAC 7th character A see Appendix B for HAC conditional logic
  - **T33.83 Superficial frostbite of toe(s)**
    - CC +7th **T33.831** Superficial frostbite of right toe(s)
      - HAC 7th character A see Appendix B for HAC conditional logic
    - CC +7th **T33.832** Superficial frostbite of left toe(s)
      - HAC 7th character A see Appendix B for HAC conditional logic
    - CC +7th **T33.839** Superficial frostbite of unspecified toe(s)
      - HAC 7th character A see Appendix B for HAC conditional logic
- **T33.9 Superficial frostbite of other and unspecified sites**
  - CC X+7th **T33.90** Superficial frostbite of unspecified sites
    - Superficial frostbite NOS
    - HAC 7th character A see Appendix B for HAC conditional logic
  - CC X+7th **T33.99** Superficial frostbite of other sites
    - Superficial frostbite of leg NOS
    - Superficial frostbite of trunk NOS
    - HAC 7th character A see Appendix B for HAC conditional logic

T34 Frostbite with tissue necrosis

The appropriate 7th character is to be added to each code from category T34
- A initial encounter
- D subsequent encounter
- S sequela

- **T34.0 Frostbite with tissue necrosis of head**
  - **T34.01 Frostbite with tissue necrosis of ear**
    - CC +7th **T34.011** Frostbite with tissue necrosis of right ear
      - HAC 7th character A see Appendix B for HAC conditional logic
    - CC +7th **T34.012** Frostbite with tissue necrosis of left ear
      - HAC 7th character A see Appendix B for HAC conditional logic
    - CC +7th **T34.019** Frostbite with tissue necrosis of unspecified ear
      - HAC 7th character A see Appendix B for HAC conditional logic
  - CC X+7th **T34.02** Frostbite with tissue necrosis of nose
    - HAC 7th character A see Appendix B for HAC conditional logic
  - CC X+7th **T34.09** Frostbite with tissue necrosis of other part of head
    - HAC 7th character A see Appendix B for HAC conditional logic
- CC X+7th **T34.1 Frostbite with tissue necrosis of neck**
  - HAC 7th character A see Appendix B for HAC conditional logic
- CC X+7th **T34.2 Frostbite with tissue necrosis of thorax**
  - HAC 7th character A see Appendix B for HAC conditional logic
- CC X+7th **T34.3 Frostbite with tissue necrosis of abdominal wall, lower back and pelvis**
  - HAC 7th character A see Appendix B for HAC conditional logic
- **T34.4 Frostbite with tissue necrosis of arm**
  - *Excludes2:* frostbite with tissue necrosis of wrist and hand (T34.5-)
  - CC X+7th **T34.40** Frostbite with tissue necrosis of unspecified arm
    - HAC 7th character A see Appendix B for HAC conditional logic
  - CC X+7th **T34.41** Frostbite with tissue necrosis of right arm
    - HAC 7th character A see Appendix B for HAC conditional logic
  - CC X+7th **T34.42** Frostbite with tissue necrosis of left arm
    - HAC 7th character A see Appendix B for HAC conditional logic
- **T34.5 Frostbite with tissue necrosis of wrist, hand, and finger(s)**
  - **T34.51 Frostbite with tissue necrosis of wrist**
    - CC +7th **T34.511** Frostbite with tissue necrosis of right wrist
      - HAC 7th character A see Appendix B for HAC conditional logic
    - CC +7th **T34.512** Frostbite with tissue necrosis of left wrist
      - HAC 7th character A see Appendix B for HAC conditional logic
    - CC +7th **T34.519** Frostbite with tissue necrosis of unspecified wrist
      - HAC 7th character A see Appendix B for HAC conditional logic

- **+ T34.52** Frostbite with tissue necrosis of hand
  - *Excludes2:* frostbite with tissue necrosis of finger(s) (T34.53-)
  - **CC +7th T34.521** Frostbite with tissue necrosis of right hand
    - HAC 7th character A see Appendix B for HAC conditional logic
  - **CC +7th T34.522** Frostbite with tissue necrosis of left hand
    - HAC 7th character A see Appendix B for HAC conditional logic
  - **CC +7th T34.529** Frostbite with tissue necrosis of unspecified hand
    - HAC 7th character A see Appendix B for HAC conditional logic
- **+ T34.53** Frostbite with tissue necrosis of finger(s)
  - **CC +7th T34.531** Frostbite with tissue necrosis of right finger(s)
    - HAC 7th character A see Appendix B for HAC conditional logic
  - **CC +7th T34.532** Frostbite with tissue necrosis of left finger(s)
    - HAC 7th character A see Appendix B for HAC conditional logic
  - **CC +7th T34.539** Frostbite with tissue necrosis of unspecified finger(s)
    - HAC 7th character A see Appendix B for HAC conditional logic
- **+ T34.6** Frostbite with tissue necrosis of hip and thigh
  - **CC X+7th T34.60** Frostbite with tissue necrosis of unspecified hip and thigh
    - HAC 7th character A see Appendix B for HAC conditional logic
  - **CC X+7th T34.61** Frostbite with tissue necrosis of right hip and thigh
    - HAC 7th character A see Appendix B for HAC conditional logic
  - **CC X+7th T34.62** Frostbite with tissue necrosis of left hip and thigh
    - HAC 7th character A see Appendix B for HAC conditional logic
- **+ T34.7** Frostbite with tissue necrosis of knee and lower leg
  - *Excludes2:* frostbite with tissue necrosis of ankle and foot (T34.8-)
  - **CC X+7th T34.70** Frostbite with tissue necrosis of unspecified knee and lower leg
    - HAC 7th character A see Appendix B for HAC conditional logic
  - **CC X+7th T34.71** Frostbite with tissue necrosis of right knee and lower leg
    - HAC 7th character A see Appendix B for HAC conditional logic
  - **CC X+7th T34.72** Frostbite with tissue necrosis of left knee and lower leg
    - HAC 7th character A see Appendix B for HAC conditional logic
- **+ T34.8** Frostbite with tissue necrosis of ankle, foot, and toe(s)
  - **+ T34.81** Frostbite with tissue necrosis of ankle
    - **CC +7th T34.811** Frostbite with tissue necrosis of right ankle
      - HAC 7th character A see Appendix B for HAC conditional logic
    - **CC +7th T34.812** Frostbite with tissue necrosis of left ankle
      - HAC 7th character A see Appendix B for HAC conditional logic
    - **CC +7th T34.819** Frostbite with tissue necrosis of unspecified ankle
      - HAC 7th character A see Appendix B for HAC conditional logic
  - **+ T34.82** Frostbite with tissue necrosis of foot
    - **CC +7th T34.821** Frostbite with tissue necrosis of right foot
      - HAC 7th character A see Appendix B for HAC conditional logic
    - **CC +7th T34.822** Frostbite with tissue necrosis of left foot
      - HAC 7th character A see Appendix B for HAC conditional logic
    - **CC +7th T34.829** Frostbite with tissue necrosis of unspecified foot
      - HAC 7th character A see Appendix B for HAC conditional logic
  - **+ T34.83** Frostbite with tissue necrosis of toe(s)
    - **CC +7th T34.831** Frostbite with tissue necrosis of right toe(s)
      - HAC 7th character A see Appendix B for HAC conditional logic
    - **CC +7th T34.832** Frostbite with tissue necrosis of left toe(s)
      - HAC 7th character A see Appendix B for HAC conditional logic
    - **CC +7th T34.839** Frostbite with tissue necrosis of unspecified toe(s)
      - HAC 7th character A see Appendix B for HAC conditional logic
- **+ T34.9** Frostbite with tissue necrosis of other and unspecified sites
  - **CC X+7th T34.90** Frostbite with tissue necrosis of unspecified sites
    - Frostbite with tissue necrosis NOS
    - HAC 7th character A see Appendix B for HAC conditional logic
  - **CC X+7th T34.99** Frostbite with tissue necrosis of other sites
    - Frostbite with tissue necrosis of leg NOS
    - Frostbite with tissue necrosis of trunk NOS
    - HAC 7th character A see Appendix B for HAC conditional logic

Poisoning by, adverse effects of and underdosing of drugs, medicaments and biological substances (T36-T50)

Includes: adverse effect of correct substance properly administered
poisoning by overdose of substance
poisoning by wrong substance given or taken in error
underdosing by (inadvertently) (deliberately) taking less substance than prescribed or instructed

Code first: for adverse effects, the nature of the adverse effect, such as:
adverse effect NOS (T88.7)
aspirin gastritis (K29.-)
blood disorders (D56-D76)
contact dermatitis (L23-L25)
dermatitis due to substances taken internally (L27.-)
nephropathy (N14.0-N14.2)

NOTE The drug giving rise to the adverse effect should be identified by use of codes from categories T36-T50 with fifth or sixth character 5.

Use additional: code(s) to specify:
manifestations of poisoning
underdosing or failure in dosage during medical and surgical care (Y63.6, Y63.8-Y63.9)
underdosing of medication regimen (Z91.12-, Z91.13-)

Excludes1: toxic reaction to local anesthesia in pregnancy (O29.3-)

Excludes2: abuse and dependence of psychoactive substances (F10-F19)
abuse of non-dependence-producing substances (F55.-)
drug reaction and poisoning affecting newborn (P00-P96)
immunodeficiency due to drugs (D84.821)
pathological drug intoxication (inebriation) (F10-F19)

Review coding guideline C.19.e

T36 Poisoning by, adverse effect of and underdosing of systemic antibiotics

Excludes1: antineoplastic antibiotics (T45.1-)
locally applied antibiotic NEC (T49.0)
topically used antibiotic for ear, nose and throat (T49.6)
topically used antibiotic for eye (T49.5)

The appropriate 7th character is to be added to each code from category T36
A initial encounter
D subsequent encounter
S sequela

- **+ T36.0** Poisoning by, adverse effect of and underdosing of penicillins
  - **+ T36.0X** Poisoning by, adverse effect of and underdosing of penicillins
    - **+7th T36.0X1** Poisoning by penicillins, accidental (unintentional)
      - Poisoning by penicillins NOS
    - **+7th T36.0X2** Poisoning by penicillins, intentional self-harm
    - **+7th T36.0X3** Poisoning by penicillins, assault
    - **+7th T36.0X4** Poisoning by penicillins, undetermined
    - **+7th T36.0X5** Adverse effect of penicillins
    - **+7th T36.0X6** Underdosing of penicillins

- **+ T36.1 Poisoning by, adverse effect of and underdosing of cephalosporins and other beta-lactam antibiotics**
  - **+ T36.1X Poisoning by, adverse effect of and underdosing of cephalosporins and other beta-lactam antibiotics**
    - +7th T36.1X1 Poisoning by cephalosporins and other beta-lactam antibiotics, accidental (unintentional)
      - Poisoning by cephalosporins and other beta-lactam antibiotics NOS
    - +7th T36.1X2 Poisoning by cephalosporins and other beta-lactam antibiotics, intentional self-harm
    - +7th T36.1X3 Poisoning by cephalosporins and other beta-lactam antibiotics, assault
    - +7th T36.1X4 Poisoning by cephalosporins and other beta-lactam antibiotics, undetermined
    - +7th T36.1X5 Adverse effect of cephalosporins and other beta-lactam antibiotics
    - +7th T36.1X6 Underdosing of cephalosporins and other beta-lactam antibiotics
- **+ T36.2 Poisoning by, adverse effect of and underdosing of chloramphenicol group**
  - **+ T36.2X Poisoning by, adverse effect of and underdosing of chloramphenicol group**
    - +7th T36.2X1 Poisoning by chloramphenicol group, accidental (unintentional)
      - Poisoning by chloramphenicol group NOS
    - +7th T36.2X2 Poisoning by chloramphenicol group, intentional self-harm
    - +7th T36.2X3 Poisoning by chloramphenicol group, assault
    - +7th T36.2X4 Poisoning by chloramphenicol group, undetermined
    - +7th T36.2X5 Adverse effect of chloramphenicol group
    - +7th T36.2X6 Underdosing of chloramphenicol group
- **+ T36.3 Poisoning by, adverse effect of and underdosing of macrolides**
  - **+ T36.3X Poisoning by, adverse effect of and underdosing of macrolides**
    - +7th T36.3X1 Poisoning by macrolides, accidental (unintentional)
      - Poisoning by macrolides NOS
    - +7th T36.3X2 Poisoning by macrolides, intentional self-harm
    - +7th T36.3X3 Poisoning by macrolides, assault
    - +7th T36.3X4 Poisoning by macrolides, undetermined
    - +7th T36.3X5 Adverse effect of macrolides
    - +7th T36.3X6 Underdosing of macrolides
- **+ T36.4 Poisoning by, adverse effect of and underdosing of tetracyclines**
  - **+ T36.4X Poisoning by, adverse effect of and underdosing of tetracyclines**
    - +7th T36.4X1 Poisoning by tetracyclines, accidental (unintentional)
      - Poisoning by tetracyclines NOS
    - +7th T36.4X2 Poisoning by tetracyclines, intentional self-harm
    - +7th T36.4X3 Poisoning by tetracyclines, assault
    - +7th T36.4X4 Poisoning by tetracyclines, undetermined
    - +7th T36.4X5 Adverse effect of tetracyclines
    - +7th T36.4X6 Underdosing of tetracyclines
- **+ T36.5 Poisoning by, adverse effect of and underdosing of aminoglycosides**
  - Poisoning by, adverse effect of and underdosing of streptomycin
  - **+ T36.5X Poisoning by, adverse effect of and underdosing of aminoglycosides**
    - +7th T36.5X1 Poisoning by aminoglycosides, accidental (unintentional)
      - Poisoning by aminoglycosides NOS
    - +7th T36.5X2 Poisoning by aminoglycosides, intentional self-harm
    - +7th T36.5X3 Poisoning by aminoglycosides, assault
    - +7th T36.5X4 Poisoning by aminoglycosides, undetermined
    - +7th T36.5X5 Adverse effect of aminoglycosides
    - +7th T36.5X6 Underdosing of aminoglycosides
- **+ T36.6 Poisoning by, adverse effect of and underdosing of rifampicins**
  - **+ T36.6X Poisoning by, adverse effect of and underdosing of rifampicins**
    - +7th T36.6X1 Poisoning by rifampicins, accidental (unintentional)
      - Poisoning by rifampicins NOS
    - +7th T36.6X2 Poisoning by rifampicins, intentional self-harm
    - +7th T36.6X3 Poisoning by rifampicins, assault
    - +7th T36.6X4 Poisoning by rifampicins, undetermined
    - +7th T36.6X5 Adverse effect of rifampicins
    - +7th T36.6X6 Underdosing of rifampicins
- **+ T36.7 Poisoning by, adverse effect of and underdosing of antifungal antibiotics, systemically used**
  - **+ T36.7X Poisoning by, adverse effect of and underdosing of antifungal antibiotics, systemically used**
    - +7th T36.7X1 Poisoning by antifungal antibiotics, systemically used, accidental (unintentional)
      - Poisoning by antifungal antibiotics, systemically used NOS
    - +7th T36.7X2 Poisoning by antifungal antibiotics, systemically used, intentional self-harm
    - +7th T36.7X3 Poisoning by antifungal antibiotics, systemically used, assault
    - +7th T36.7X4 Poisoning by antifungal antibiotics, systemically used, undetermined
    - +7th T36.7X5 Adverse effect of antifungal antibiotics, systemically used
    - +7th T36.7X6 Underdosing of antifungal antibiotics, systemically used
- **+ T36.8 Poisoning by, adverse effect of and underdosing of other systemic antibiotics**
  - **+ T36.8X Poisoning by, adverse effect of and underdosing of other systemic antibiotics**
    - +7th T36.8X1 Poisoning by other systemic antibiotics, accidental (unintentional)
      - Poisoning by other systemic antibiotics NOS
    - +7th T36.8X2 Poisoning by other systemic antibiotics, intentional self-harm
    - +7th T36.8X3 Poisoning by other systemic antibiotics, assault
    - +7th T36.8X4 Poisoning by other systemic antibiotics, undetermined
    - +7th T36.8X5 Adverse effect of other systemic antibiotics
      - *AHA CC: 1Q, 2017, 39*
    - +7th T36.8X6 Underdosing of other systemic antibiotics
- **+ T36.9 Poisoning by, adverse effect of and underdosing of unspecified systemic antibiotic**
  - X+7th T36.91 Poisoning by unspecified systemic antibiotic, accidental (unintentional)
    - Poisoning by systemic antibiotic NOS
  - X+7th T36.92 Poisoning by unspecified systemic antibiotic, intentional self-harm
  - X+7th T36.93 Poisoning by unspecified systemic antibiotic, assault
  - X+7th T36.94 Poisoning by unspecified systemic antibiotic, undetermined
  - X+7th T36.95 Adverse effect of unspecified systemic antibiotic
  - X+7th T36.96 Underdosing of unspecified systemic antibiotic

T37 Poisoning by, adverse effect of and underdosing of other systemic anti-infectives and antiparasitics

Excludes1: anti-infectives topically used for ear, nose and throat (T49.6-)
anti-infectives topically used for eye (T49.5-)
locally applied anti-infectives NEC (T49.0-)

The appropriate 7th character is to be added to each code from category T37
- A initial encounter
- D subsequent encounter
- S sequela

T37.0 Poisoning by, adverse effect of and underdosing of sulfonamides

- **T37.0X** Poisoning by, adverse effect of and underdosing of sulfonamides
  - **T37.0X1** Poisoning by sulfonamides, accidental (unintentional)
    - Poisoning by sulfonamides NOS
  - **T37.0X2** Poisoning by sulfonamides, intentional self-harm
  - **T37.0X3** Poisoning by sulfonamides, assault
  - **T37.0X4** Poisoning by sulfonamides, undetermined
  - **T37.0X5** Adverse effect of sulfonamides
  - **T37.0X6** Underdosing of sulfonamides

T37.1 Poisoning by, adverse effect of and underdosing of antimycobacterial drugs

Excludes1: rifampicins (T36.6-)
streptomycin (T36.5-)

- **T37.1X** Poisoning by, adverse effect of and underdosing of antimycobacterial drugs
  - **T37.1X1** Poisoning by antimycobacterial drugs, accidental (unintentional)
    - Poisoning by antimycobacterial drugs NOS
  - **T37.1X2** Poisoning by antimycobacterial drugs, intentional self-harm
  - **T37.1X3** Poisoning by antimycobacterial drugs, assault
  - **T37.1X4** Poisoning by antimycobacterial drugs, undetermined
  - **T37.1X5** Adverse effect of antimycobacterial drugs
  - **T37.1X6** Underdosing of antimycobacterial drugs

T37.2 Poisoning by, adverse effect of and underdosing of antimalarials and drugs acting on other blood protozoa

Excludes1: hydroxyquinoline derivatives (T37.8-)

- **T37.2X** Poisoning by, adverse effect of and underdosing of antimalarials and drugs acting on other blood protozoa
  - **T37.2X1** Poisoning by antimalarials and drugs acting on other blood protozoa, accidental (unintentional)
    - Poisoning by antimalarials and drugs acting on other blood protozoa NOS
  - **T37.2X2** Poisoning by antimalarials and drugs acting on other blood protozoa, intentional self-harm
  - **T37.2X3** Poisoning by antimalarials and drugs acting on other blood protozoa, assault
  - **T37.2X4** Poisoning by antimalarials and drugs acting on other blood protozoa, undetermined
  - **T37.2X5** Adverse effect of antimalarials and drugs acting on other blood protozoa
  - **T37.2X6** Underdosing of antimalarials and drugs acting on other blood protozoa

T37.3 Poisoning by, adverse effect of and underdosing of other antiprotozoal drugs

- **T37.3X** Poisoning by, adverse effect of and underdosing of other antiprotozoal drugs
  - **T37.3X1** Poisoning by other antiprotozoal drugs, accidental (unintentional)
    - Poisoning by other antiprotozoal drugs NOS
  - **T37.3X2** Poisoning by other antiprotozoal drugs, intentional self-harm
  - **T37.3X3** Poisoning by other antiprotozoal drugs, assault
  - **T37.3X4** Poisoning by other antiprotozoal drugs, undetermined
  - **T37.3X5** Adverse effect of other antiprotozoal drugs
  - **T37.3X6** Underdosing of other antiprotozoal drugs

T37.4 Poisoning by, adverse effect of and underdosing of anthelminthics

- **T37.4X** Poisoning by, adverse effect of and underdosing of anthelminthics
  - **T37.4X1** Poisoning by anthelminthics, accidental (unintentional)
    - Poisoning by anthelminthics NOS
  - **T37.4X2** Poisoning by anthelminthics, intentional self-harm
  - **T37.4X3** Poisoning by anthelminthics, assault
  - **T37.4X4** Poisoning by anthelminthics, undetermined
  - **T37.4X5** Adverse effect of anthelminthics
  - **T37.4X6** Underdosing of anthelminthics

T37.5 Poisoning by, adverse effect of and underdosing of antiviral drugs

Excludes1: amantadine (T42.8-)
cytarabine (T45.1-)

- **T37.5X** Poisoning by, adverse effect of and underdosing of antiviral drugs
  - **T37.5X1** Poisoning by antiviral drugs, accidental (unintentional)
    - Poisoning by antiviral drugs NOS
  - **T37.5X2** Poisoning by antiviral drugs, intentional self-harm
  - **T37.5X3** Poisoning by antiviral drugs, assault
  - **T37.5X4** Poisoning by antiviral drugs, undetermined
  - **T37.5X5** Adverse effect of antiviral drugs
  - **T37.5X6** Underdosing of antiviral drugs

T37.8 Poisoning by, adverse effect of and underdosing of other specified systemic anti-infectives and antiparasitics

Poisoning by, adverse effect of and underdosing of hydroxyquinoline derivatives

Excludes1: antimalarial drugs (T37.2-)

- **T37.8X** Poisoning by, adverse effect of and underdosing of other specified systemic anti-infectives and antiparasitics
  - **T37.8X1** Poisoning by other specified systemic anti-infectives and antiparasitics, accidental (unintentional)
    - Poisoning by other specified systemic anti-infectives and antiparasitics NOS
  - **T37.8X2** Poisoning by other specified systemic anti-infectives and antiparasitics, intentional self-harm
  - **T37.8X3** Poisoning by other specified systemic anti-infectives and antiparasitics, assault
  - **T37.8X4** Poisoning by other specified systemic anti-infectives and antiparasitics, undetermined
  - **T37.8X5** Adverse effect of other specified systemic anti-infectives and antiparasitics
  - **T37.8X6** Underdosing of other specified systemic anti-infectives and antiparasitics

T37.9 Poisoning by, adverse effect of and underdosing of unspecified systemic anti-infective and antiparasitics

- **T37.91** Poisoning by unspecified systemic anti-infective and antiparasitics, accidental (unintentional)
  - Poisoning by, adverse effect of and underdosing of systemic anti-infective and antiparasitics NOS
- **T37.92** Poisoning by unspecified systemic anti-infective and antiparasitics, intentional self-harm
- **T37.93** Poisoning by unspecified systemic anti-infective and antiparasitics, assault
- **T37.94** Poisoning by unspecified systemic anti-infective and antiparasitics, undetermined
- **T37.95** Adverse effect of unspecified systemic anti-infective and antiparasitic
- **T37.96** Underdosing of unspecified systemic anti-infectives and antiparasitics

T38 Poisoning by, adverse effect of and underdosing of hormones and their synthetic substitutes and antagonists, not elsewhere classified

> **Excludes1:** mineralocorticoids and their antagonists (T50.0-)
> oxytocic hormones (T48.0-)
> parathyroid hormones and derivatives (T50.9-)

The appropriate 7th character is to be added to each code from category T38
- A initial encounter
- D subsequent encounter
- S sequela

- **T38.0** Poisoning by, adverse effect of and underdosing of glucocorticoids and synthetic analogues
  > **Excludes1:** glucocorticoids, topically used (T49.-)
  - **T38.0X** Poisoning by, adverse effect of and underdosing of glucocorticoids and synthetic analogues
    - +7th **T38.0X1** Poisoning by glucocorticoids and synthetic analogues, accidental (unintentional)
      > Poisoning by glucocorticoids and synthetic analogues NOS
    - +7th **T38.0X2** Poisoning by glucocorticoids and synthetic analogues, intentional self-harm
    - +7th **T38.0X3** Poisoning by glucocorticoids and synthetic analogues, assault
    - +7th **T38.0X4** Poisoning by glucocorticoids and synthetic analogues, undetermined
    - +7th **T38.0X5** Adverse effect of glucocorticoids and synthetic analogues
    - +7th **T38.0X6** Underdosing of glucocorticoids and synthetic analogues

- **T38.1** Poisoning by, adverse effect of and underdosing of thyroid hormones and substitutes
  - **T38.1X** Poisoning by, adverse effect of and underdosing of thyroid hormones and substitutes
    - +7th **T38.1X1** Poisoning by thyroid hormones and substitutes, accidental (unintentional)
      > Poisoning by thyroid hormones and substitutes NOS
    - +7th **T38.1X2** Poisoning by thyroid hormones and substitutes, intentional self-harm
    - +7th **T38.1X3** Poisoning by thyroid hormones and substitutes, assault
    - +7th **T38.1X4** Poisoning by thyroid hormones and substitutes, undetermined
    - +7th **T38.1X5** Adverse effect of thyroid hormones and substitutes
    - +7th **T38.1X6** Underdosing of thyroid hormones and substitutes

- **T38.2** Poisoning by, adverse effect of and underdosing of antithyroid drugs
  - **T38.2X** Poisoning by, adverse effect of and underdosing of antithyroid drugs
    - +7th **T38.2X1** Poisoning by antithyroid drugs, accidental (unintentional)
      > Poisoning by antithyroid drugs NOS
    - +7th **T38.2X2** Poisoning by antithyroid drugs, intentional self-harm
    - +7th **T38.2X3** Poisoning by antithyroid drugs, assault
    - +7th **T38.2X4** Poisoning by antithyroid drugs, undetermined
    - +7th **T38.2X5** Adverse effect of antithyroid drugs
    - +7th **T38.2X6** Underdosing of antithyroid drugs

- **T38.3** Poisoning by, adverse effect of and underdosing of insulin and oral hypoglycemic [antidiabetic] drugs
  - **T38.3X** Poisoning by, adverse effect of and underdosing of insulin and oral hypoglycemic [antidiabetic] drugs
    - +7th **T38.3X1** Poisoning by insulin and oral hypoglycemic [antidiabetic] drugs, accidental (unintentional)
      > Poisoning by insulin and oral hypoglycemic [antidiabetic] drugs NOS

      Review coding guideline C.4.a.5.b
    - +7th **T38.3X2** Poisoning by insulin and oral hypoglycemic [antidiabetic] drugs, intentional self-harm
    - +7th **T38.3X3** Poisoning by insulin and oral hypoglycemic [antidiabetic] drugs, assault
    - +7th **T38.3X4** Poisoning by insulin and oral hypoglycemic [antidiabetic] drugs, undetermined
    - +7th **T38.3X5** Adverse effect of insulin and oral hypoglycemic [antidiabetic] drugs
    - +7th **T38.3X6** Underdosing of insulin and oral hypoglycemic [antidiabetic] drugs

      Review coding guideline C.4.a.5.a

- **T38.4** Poisoning by, adverse effect of and underdosing of oral contraceptives
  > Poisoning by, adverse effect of and underdosing of multiple- and single-ingredient oral contraceptive preparations
  - **T38.4X** Poisoning by, adverse effect of and underdosing of oral contraceptives
    - +7th **T38.4X1** Poisoning by oral contraceptives, accidental (unintentional)
      > Poisoning by oral contraceptives NOS
    - +7th **T38.4X2** Poisoning by oral contraceptives, intentional self-harm
    - +7th **T38.4X3** Poisoning by oral contraceptives, assault
    - +7th **T38.4X4** Poisoning by oral contraceptives, undetermined
    - +7th **T38.4X5** Adverse effect of oral contraceptives
    - +7th **T38.4X6** Underdosing of oral contraceptives

- **T38.5** Poisoning by, adverse effect of and underdosing of other estrogens and progestogens
  > Poisoning by, adverse effect of and underdosing of estrogens and progestogens mixtures and substitutes
  - **T38.5X** Poisoning by, adverse effect of and underdosing of other estrogens and progestogens
    - +7th **T38.5X1** Poisoning by other estrogens and progestogens, accidental (unintentional)
      > Poisoning by other estrogens and progestogens NOS
    - +7th **T38.5X2** Poisoning by other estrogens and progestogens, intentional self-harm
    - +7th **T38.5X3** Poisoning by other estrogens and progestogens, assault
    - +7th **T38.5X4** Poisoning by other estrogens and progestogens, undetermined
    - +7th **T38.5X5** Adverse effect of other estrogens and progestogens
    - +7th **T38.5X6** Underdosing of other estrogens and progestogens

- **T38.6** Poisoning by, adverse effect of and underdosing of antigonadotrophins, antiestrogens, antiandrogens, not elsewhere classified
  > Poisoning by, adverse effect of and underdosing of tamoxifen
  - **T38.6X** Poisoning by, adverse effect of and underdosing of antigonadotrophins, antiestrogens, antiandrogens, not elsewhere classified
    - +7th **T38.6X1** Poisoning by antigonadotrophins, antiestrogens, antiandrogens, not elsewhere classified, accidental (unintentional)
      > Poisoning by antigonadotrophins, antiestrogens, antiandrogens, not elsewhere classified NOS
    - +7th **T38.6X2** Poisoning by antigonadotrophins, antiestrogens, antiandrogens, not elsewhere classified, intentional self-harm
    - +7th **T38.6X3** Poisoning by antigonadotrophins, antiestrogens, antiandrogens, not elsewhere classified, assault
    - +7th **T38.6X4** Poisoning by antigonadotrophins, antiestrogens, antiandrogens, not elsewhere classified, undetermined
    - +7th **T38.6X5** Adverse effect of antigonadotrophins, antiestrogens, antiandrogens, not elsewhere classified
    - +7th **T38.6X6** Underdosing of antigonadotrophins, antiestrogens, antiandrogens, not elsewhere classified

- **T38.7 Poisoning by, adverse effect of and underdosing of androgens and anabolic congeners**
  - **T38.7X Poisoning by, adverse effect of and underdosing of androgens and anabolic congeners**
    - +7th **T38.7X1** Poisoning by androgens and anabolic congeners, accidental (unintentional)
      - Poisoning by androgens and anabolic congeners NOS
    - +7th **T38.7X2** Poisoning by androgens and anabolic congeners, intentional self-harm
    - +7th **T38.7X3** Poisoning by androgens and anabolic congeners, assault
    - +7th **T38.7X4** Poisoning by androgens and anabolic congeners, undetermined
    - +7th **T38.7X5** Adverse effect of androgens and anabolic congeners
    - +7th **T38.7X6** Underdosing of androgens and anabolic congeners
- **T38.8 Poisoning by, adverse effect of and underdosing of other and unspecified hormones and synthetic substitutes**
  - **T38.80 Poisoning by, adverse effect of and underdosing of unspecified hormones and synthetic substitutes**
    - +7th **T38.801** Poisoning by unspecified hormones and synthetic substitutes, accidental (unintentional)
      - Poisoning by unspecified hormones and synthetic substitutes NOS
    - +7th **T38.802** Poisoning by unspecified hormones and synthetic substitutes, intentional self-harm
    - +7th **T38.803** Poisoning by unspecified hormones and synthetic substitutes, assault
    - +7th **T38.804** Poisoning by unspecified hormones and synthetic substitutes, undetermined
    - +7th **T38.805** Adverse effect of unspecified hormones and synthetic substitutes
    - +7th **T38.806** Underdosing of unspecified hormones and synthetic substitutes
  - **T38.81 Poisoning by, adverse effect of and underdosing of anterior pituitary [adenohypophyseal] hormones**
    - +7th **T38.811** Poisoning by anterior pituitary [adenohypophyseal] hormones, accidental (unintentional)
      - Poisoning by anterior pituitary [adenohypophyseal] hormones NOS
    - +7th **T38.812** Poisoning by anterior pituitary [adenohypophyseal] hormones, intentional self-harm
    - +7th **T38.813** Poisoning by anterior pituitary [adenohypophyseal] hormones, assault
    - +7th **T38.814** Poisoning by anterior pituitary [adenohypophyseal] hormones, undetermined
    - +7th **T38.815** Adverse effect of anterior pituitary [adenohypophyseal] hormones
    - +7th **T38.816** Underdosing of anterior pituitary [adenohypophyseal] hormones
  - **T38.89 Poisoning by, adverse effect of and underdosing of other hormones and synthetic substitutes**
    - +7th **T38.891** Poisoning by other hormones and synthetic substitutes, accidental (unintentional)
      - Poisoning by other hormones and synthetic substitutes NOS
    - +7th **T38.892** Poisoning by other hormones and synthetic substitutes, intentional self-harm
    - +7th **T38.893** Poisoning by other hormones and synthetic substitutes, assault
    - +7th **T38.894** Poisoning by other hormones and synthetic substitutes, undetermined
    - +7th **T38.895** Adverse effect of other hormones and synthetic substitutes
    - +7th **T38.896** Underdosing of other hormones and synthetic substitutes

- **T38.9 Poisoning by, adverse effect of and underdosing of other and unspecified hormone antagonists**
  - **T38.90 Poisoning by, adverse effect of and underdosing of unspecified hormone antagonists**
    - +7th **T38.901** Poisoning by unspecified hormone antagonists, accidental (unintentional)
      - Poisoning by unspecified hormone antagonists NOS
    - +7th **T38.902** Poisoning by unspecified hormone antagonists, intentional self-harm
    - +7th **T38.903** Poisoning by unspecified hormone antagonists, assault
    - +7th **T38.904** Poisoning by unspecified hormone antagonists, undetermined
    - +7th **T38.905** Adverse effect of unspecified hormone antagonists
    - +7th **T38.906** Underdosing of unspecified hormone antagonists
  - **T38.99 Poisoning by, adverse effect of and underdosing of other hormone antagonists**
    - +7th **T38.991** Poisoning by other hormone antagonists, accidental (unintentional)
      - Poisoning by other hormone antagonists NOS
    - +7th **T38.992** Poisoning by other hormone antagonists, intentional self-harm
    - +7th **T38.993** Poisoning by other hormone antagonists, assault
    - +7th **T38.994** Poisoning by other hormone antagonists, undetermined
    - +7th **T38.995** Adverse effect of other hormone antagonists
    - +7th **T38.996** Underdosing of other hormone antagonists

T39 Poisoning by, adverse effect of and underdosing of nonopioid analgesics, antipyretics and antirheumatics

> The appropriate 7th character is to be added to each code from category T39
> A   initial encounter
> D   subsequent encounter
> S   sequela

- **T39.0 Poisoning by, adverse effect of and underdosing of salicylates**
  - **T39.01 Poisoning by, adverse effect of and underdosing of aspirin**
    - Poisoning by, adverse effect of and underdosing of acetylsalicylic acid
    - +7th **T39.011** Poisoning by aspirin, accidental (unintentional)
    - +7th **T39.012** Poisoning by aspirin, intentional self-harm
    - +7th **T39.013** Poisoning by aspirin, assault
    - +7th **T39.014** Poisoning by aspirin, undetermined
    - +7th **T39.015** Adverse effect of aspirin
      - *AHA CC: 1Q, 2016, 15*
    - +7th **T39.016** Underdosing of aspirin
  - **T39.09 Poisoning by, adverse effect of and underdosing of other salicylates**
    - +7th **T39.091** Poisoning by salicylates, accidental (unintentional)
      - Poisoning by salicylates NOS
    - +7th **T39.092** Poisoning by salicylates, intentional self-harm
    - +7th **T39.093** Poisoning by salicylates, assault
    - +7th **T39.094** Poisoning by salicylates, undetermined
    - +7th **T39.095** Adverse effect of salicylates
    - +7th **T39.096** Underdosing of salicylates
- **T39.1 Poisoning by, adverse effect of and underdosing of 4-Aminophenol derivatives**
  - **T39.1X Poisoning by, adverse effect of and underdosing of 4-Aminophenol derivatives**
    - +7th **T39.1X1** Poisoning by 4-Aminophenol derivatives, accidental (unintentional)
      - Poisoning by 4-Aminophenol derivatives NOS
    - +7th **T39.1X2** Poisoning by 4-Aminophenol derivatives, intentional self-harm
    - +7th **T39.1X3** Poisoning by 4-Aminophenol derivatives, assault

+7th T39.1X4 Poisoning by 4-Aminophenol derivatives, undetermined
+7th T39.1X5 Adverse effect of 4-Aminophenol derivatives
+7th T39.1X6 Underdosing of 4-Aminophenol derivatives

+ T39.2 Poisoning by, adverse effect of and underdosing of pyrazolone derivatives
  + T39.2X Poisoning by, adverse effect of and underdosing of pyrazolone derivatives
    +7th T39.2X1 Poisoning by pyrazolone derivatives, accidental (unintentional)
    Poisoning by pyrazolone derivatives NOS
    +7th T39.2X2 Poisoning by pyrazolone derivatives, intentional self-harm
    +7th T39.2X3 Poisoning by pyrazolone derivatives, assault
    +7th T39.2X4 Poisoning by pyrazolone derivatives, undetermined
    +7th T39.2X5 Adverse effect of pyrazolone derivatives
    +7th T39.2X6 Underdosing of pyrazolone derivatives

+ T39.3 Poisoning by, adverse effect of and underdosing of other nonsteroidal anti-inflammatory drugs [NSAID]
  + T39.31 Poisoning by, adverse effect of and underdosing of propionic acid derivatives
    Poisoning by, adverse effect of and underdosing of fenoprofen
    Poisoning by, adverse effect of and underdosing of flurbiprofen
    Poisoning by, adverse effect of and underdosing of ibuprofen
    Poisoning by, adverse effect of and underdosing of ketoprofen
    Poisoning by, adverse effect of and underdosing of naproxen
    Poisoning by, adverse effect of and underdosing of oxaprozin
    +7th T39.311 Poisoning by propionic acid derivatives, accidental (unintentional)
    +7th T39.312 Poisoning by propionic acid derivatives, intentional self-harm
    +7th T39.313 Poisoning by propionic acid derivatives, assault
    +7th T39.314 Poisoning by propionic acid derivatives, undetermined
    +7th T39.315 Adverse effect of propionic acid derivatives
    +7th T39.316 Underdosing of propionic acid derivatives
  + T39.39 Poisoning by, adverse effect of and underdosing of other nonsteroidal anti-inflammatory drugs [NSAID]
    +7th T39.391 Poisoning by other nonsteroidal anti-inflammatory drugs [NSAID], accidental (unintentional)
    Poisoning by other nonsteroidal anti-inflammatory drugs NOS
    +7th T39.392 Poisoning by other nonsteroidal anti-inflammatory drugs [NSAID], intentional self-harm
    +7th T39.393 Poisoning by other nonsteroidal anti-inflammatory drugs [NSAID], assault
    +7th T39.394 Poisoning by other nonsteroidal anti-inflammatory drugs [NSAID], undetermined
    +7th T39.395 Adverse effect of other nonsteroidal anti-inflammatory drugs [NSAID]
    +7th T39.396 Underdosing of other nonsteroidal anti-inflammatory drugs [NSAID]

+ T39.4 Poisoning by, adverse effect of and underdosing of antirheumatics, not elsewhere classified
  Excludes1: poisoning by, adverse effect of and underdosing of glucocorticoids (T38.0-)
  poisoning by, adverse effect of and underdosing of salicylates (T39.0-)
  + T39.4X Poisoning by, adverse effect of and underdosing of antirheumatics, not elsewhere classified
    +7th T39.4X1 Poisoning by antirheumatics, not elsewhere classified, accidental (unintentional)
    Poisoning by antirheumatics, not elsewhere classified NOS
    +7th T39.4X2 Poisoning by antirheumatics, not elsewhere classified, intentional self-harm
    +7th T39.4X3 Poisoning by antirheumatics, not elsewhere classified, assault
    +7th T39.4X4 Poisoning by antirheumatics, not elsewhere classified, undetermined
    +7th T39.4X5 Adverse effect of antirheumatics, not elsewhere classified
    +7th T39.4X6 Underdosing of antirheumatics, not elsewhere classified

+ T39.8 Poisoning by, adverse effect of and underdosing of other nonopioid analgesics and antipyretics, not elsewhere classified
  + T39.8X Poisoning by, adverse effect of and underdosing of other nonopioid analgesics and antipyretics, not elsewhere classified
    +7th T39.8X1 Poisoning by other nonopioid analgesics and antipyretics, not elsewhere classified, accidental (unintentional)
    Poisoning by other nonopioid analgesics and antipyretics, not elsewhere classified NOS
    +7th T39.8X2 Poisoning by other nonopioid analgesics and antipyretics, not elsewhere classified, intentional self-harm
    +7th T39.8X3 Poisoning by other nonopioid analgesics and antipyretics, not elsewhere classified, assault
    +7th T39.8X4 Poisoning by other nonopioid analgesics and antipyretics, not elsewhere classified, undetermined
    +7th T39.8X5 Adverse effect of other nonopioid analgesics and antipyretics, not elsewhere classified
    +7th T39.8X6 Underdosing of other nonopioid analgesics and antipyretics, not elsewhere classified

+ T39.9 Poisoning by, adverse effect of and underdosing of unspecified nonopioid analgesic, antipyretic and antirheumatic
  x+7th T39.91 Poisoning by unspecified nonopioid analgesic, antipyretic and antirheumatic, accidental (unintentional)
  Poisoning by nonopioid analgesic, antipyretic and antirheumatic NOS
  x+7th T39.92 Poisoning by unspecified nonopioid analgesic, antipyretic and antirheumatic, intentional self-harm
  x+7th T39.93 Poisoning by unspecified nonopioid analgesic, antipyretic and antirheumatic, assault
  x+7th T39.94 Poisoning by unspecified nonopioid analgesic, antipyretic and antirheumatic, undetermined
  x+7th T39.95 Adverse effect of unspecified nonopioid analgesic, antipyretic and antirheumatic
  x+7th T39.96 Underdosing of unspecified nonopioid analgesic, antipyretic and antirheumatic

T40 Poisoning by, adverse effect of and underdosing of narcotics and psychodysleptics [hallucinogens]
  Excludes2: drug dependence and related mental and behavioral disorders due to psychoactive substance use (F10.-F19.-)

The appropriate 7th character is to be added to each code from category T40
A initial encounter
D subsequent encounter
S sequela

+ T40.0 Poisoning by, adverse effect of and underdosing of opium
  + T40.0X Poisoning by, adverse effect of and underdosing of opium
    +7th T40.0X1 Poisoning by opium, accidental (unintentional)
    Poisoning by opium NOS

- +7th **T40.0X2** Poisoning by opium, intentional self-harm
- +7th **T40.0X3** Poisoning by opium, assault
- +7th **T40.0X4** Poisoning by opium, undetermined
- +7th **T40.0X5** Adverse effect of opium
- +7th **T40.0X6** Underdosing of opium
- + **T40.1** Poisoning by and adverse effect of heroin
  - + **T40.1X** Poisoning by and adverse effect of heroin
    - +7th **T40.1X1** Poisoning by heroin, accidental (unintentional)
      Poisoning by heroin NOS
    - +7th **T40.1X2** Poisoning by heroin, intentional self-harm
    - +7th **T40.1X3** Poisoning by heroin, assault
    - +7th **T40.1X4** Poisoning by heroin, undetermined
- + **T40.2** Poisoning by, adverse effect of and underdosing of other opioids
  - + **T40.2X** Poisoning by, adverse effect of and underdosing of other opioids
    - +7th **T40.2X1** Poisoning by other opioids, accidental (unintentional)
      Poisoning by other opioids NOS
    - +7th **T40.2X2** Poisoning by other opioids, intentional self-harm
    - +7th **T40.2X3** Poisoning by other opioids, assault
    - +7th **T40.2X4** Poisoning by other opioids, undetermined
    - +7th **T40.2X5** Adverse effect of other opioids
      AHA CC: 2Q, 2020, 24
    - +7th **T40.2X6** Underdosing of other opioids
- + **T40.3** Poisoning by, adverse effect of and underdosing of methadone
  - + **T40.3X** Poisoning by, adverse effect of and underdosing of methadone
    - +7th **T40.3X1** Poisoning by methadone, accidental (unintentional)
      Poisoning by methadone NOS
    - +7th **T40.3X2** Poisoning by methadone, intentional self-harm
    - +7th **T40.3X3** Poisoning by methadone, assault
    - +7th **T40.3X4** Poisoning by methadone, undetermined
    - +7th **T40.3X5** Adverse effect of methadone
    - +7th **T40.3X6** Underdosing of methadone
- + **T40.4** Poisoning by, adverse effect of and underdosing of other synthetic narcotics
  AHA CC: 4Q, 2020, 40
  - + **T40.41** Poisoning by, adverse effect of and underdosing of fentanyl or fentanyl analogs
    - +7th **T40.411** Poisoning by fentanyl or fentanyl analogs, accidental (unintentional)
    - +7th **T40.412** Poisoning by fentanyl or fentanyl analogs, intentional self-harm
    - +7th **T40.413** Poisoning by fentanyl or fentanyl analogs, assault
    - +7th **T40.414** Poisoning by fentanyl or fentanyl analogs, undetermined
    - +7th **T40.415** Adverse effect of fentanyl or fentanyl analogs
    - +7th **T40.416** Underdosing of fentanyl or fentanyl analogs
  - + **T40.42** Poisoning by, adverse effect of and underdosing of tramadol
    - +7th **T40.421** Poisoning by tramadol, accidental (unintentional)
    - +7th **T40.422** Poisoning by tramadol, intentional self-harm
    - +7th **T40.423** Poisoning by tramadol, assault
    - +7th **T40.424** Poisoning by tramadol, undetermined
    - +7th **T40.425** Adverse effect of tramadol
    - +7th **T40.426** Underdosing of tramadol
  - + **T40.49** Poisoning by, adverse effect of and underdosing of other synthetic narcotics
    - +7th **T40.491** Poisoning by other synthetic narcotics, accidental (unintentional)
    - +7th **T40.492** Poisoning by other synthetic narcotics, intentional self-harm
    - +7th **T40.493** Poisoning by other synthetic narcotics, assault
    - +7th **T40.494** Poisoning by other synthetic narcotics, undetermined
    - +7th **T40.495** Adverse effect of other synthetic narcotics
    - +7th **T40.496** Underdosing of other synthetic narcotics
- + **T40.5** Poisoning by, adverse effect of and underdosing of cocaine
  - + **T40.5X** Poisoning by, adverse effect of and underdosing of cocaine
    - +7th **T40.5X1** Poisoning by cocaine, accidental (unintentional)
      Poisoning by cocaine NOS
      AHA CC: 2Q, 2016, 8-9
    - +7th **T40.5X2** Poisoning by cocaine, intentional self-harm
    - +7th **T40.5X3** Poisoning by cocaine, assault
    - +7th **T40.5X4** Poisoning by cocaine, undetermined
    - +7th **T40.5X5** Adverse effect of cocaine
    - +7th **T40.5X6** Underdosing of cocaine
- + **T40.6** Poisoning by, adverse effect of and underdosing of other and unspecified narcotics
  - + **T40.60** Poisoning by, adverse effect of and underdosing of unspecified narcotics
    - +7th **T40.601** Poisoning by unspecified narcotics, accidental (unintentional)
      Poisoning by narcotics NOS
    - +7th **T40.602** Poisoning by unspecified narcotics, intentional self-harm
    - +7th **T40.603** Poisoning by unspecified narcotics, assault
    - +7th **T40.604** Poisoning by unspecified narcotics, undetermined
    - +7th **T40.605** Adverse effect of unspecified narcotics
    - +7th **T40.606** Underdosing of unspecified narcotics
  - + **T40.69** Poisoning by, adverse effect of and underdosing of other narcotics
    - +7th **T40.691** Poisoning by other narcotics, accidental (unintentional)
      Poisoning by other narcotics NOS
    - +7th **T40.692** Poisoning by other narcotics, intentional self-harm
    - +7th **T40.693** Poisoning by other narcotics, assault
    - +7th **T40.694** Poisoning by other narcotics, undetermined
    - +7th **T40.695** Adverse effect of other narcotics
    - +7th **T40.696** Underdosing of other narcotics
- + **T40.7** Poisoning by, adverse effect of and underdosing of cannabis (derivatives)
  AHA CC: 1Q, 2020, 8; 4Q, 2021, 30
  - + **T40.71** Poisoning by, adverse effect of and underdosing of cannabis (derivatives)
    - +7th **T40.711** Poisoning by cannabis, accidental (unintentional)
    - +7th **T40.712** Poisoning by cannabis, intentional self-harm
    - +7th **T40.713** Poisoning by cannabis, assault
    - +7th **T40.714** Poisoning by cannabis, undetermined
    - +7th **T40.715** Adverse effect of cannabis
    - +7th **T40.716** Underdosing of cannabis
  - + **T40.72** Poisoning by, adverse effect of and underdosing of synthetic cannabinoids
    - +7th **T40.721** Poisoning by synthetic cannabinoids, accidental (unintentional)
    - +7th **T40.722** Poisoning by synthetic cannabinoids, intentional self-harm
    - +7th **T40.723** Poisoning by synthetic cannabinoids, assault
    - +7th **T40.724** Poisoning by synthetic cannabinoids, undetermined
    - +7th **T40.725** Adverse effect of synthetic cannabinoids
    - +7th **T40.726** Underdosing of synthetic cannabinoids
- + **T40.8** Poisoning by and adverse effect of lysergide [LSD]
  - + **T40.8X** Poisoning by and adverse effect of lysergide [LSD]
    - +7th **T40.8X1** Poisoning by lysergide [LSD], accidental (unintentional)
      Poisoning by lysergide [LSD] NOS
    - +7th **T40.8X2** Poisoning by lysergide [LSD], intentional self-harm
    - +7th **T40.8X3** Poisoning by lysergide [LSD], assault
    - +7th **T40.8X4** Poisoning by lysergide [LSD], undetermined

- **T40.9 Poisoning by, adverse effect of and underdosing of other and unspecified psychodysleptics [hallucinogens]**
  - **T40.90 Poisoning by, adverse effect of and underdosing of unspecified psychodysleptics [hallucinogens]**
    - +7th T40.901 Poisoning by unspecified psychodysleptics [hallucinogens], accidental (unintentional)
    - +7th T40.902 Poisoning by unspecified psychodysleptics [hallucinogens], intentional self-harm
    - +7th T40.903 Poisoning by unspecified psychodysleptics [hallucinogens], assault
    - +7th T40.904 Poisoning by unspecified psychodysleptics [hallucinogens], undetermined
    - +7th T40.905 Adverse effect of unspecified psychodysleptics [hallucinogens]
    - +7th T40.906 Underdosing of unspecified psychodysleptics [hallucinogens]
  - **T40.99 Poisoning by, adverse effect of and underdosing of other psychodysleptics [hallucinogens]**
    - +7th T40.991 Poisoning by other psychodysleptics [hallucinogens], accidental (unintentional)
      Poisoning by other psychodysleptics [hallucinogens] NOS
    - +7th T40.992 Poisoning by other psychodysleptics [hallucinogens], intentional self-harm
    - +7th T40.993 Poisoning by other psychodysleptics [hallucinogens], assault
    - +7th T40.994 Poisoning by other psychodysleptics [hallucinogens], undetermined
    - +7th T40.995 Adverse effect of other psychodysleptics [hallucinogens]
    - +7th T40.996 Underdosing of other psychodysleptics [hallucinogens]

T41 Poisoning by, adverse effect of and underdosing of anesthetics and therapeutic gases

Excludes1: benzodiazepines (T42.4-)
cocaine (T40.5-)
complications of anesthesia during pregnancy (O29.-)
complications of anesthesia during labor and delivery (O74.-)
complications of anesthesia during the puerperium (O89.-)
opioids (T40.0-T40.2-)

> The appropriate 7th character is to be added to each code from category T41
> A initial encounter
> D subsequent encounter
> S sequela

- **T41.0 Poisoning by, adverse effect of and underdosing of inhaled anesthetics**
  Excludes1: oxygen (T41.5-)
  - **T41.0X Poisoning by, adverse effect of and underdosing of inhaled anesthetics**
    - +7th T41.0X1 Poisoning by inhaled anesthetics, accidental (unintentional)
      Poisoning by inhaled anesthetics NOS
    - +7th T41.0X2 Poisoning by inhaled anesthetics, intentional self-harm
    - +7th T41.0X3 Poisoning by inhaled anesthetics, assault
    - +7th T41.0X4 Poisoning by inhaled anesthetics, undetermined
    - +7th T41.0X5 Adverse effect of inhaled anesthetics
    - +7th T41.0X6 Underdosing of inhaled anesthetics
- **T41.1 Poisoning by, adverse effect of and underdosing of intravenous anesthetics**
  Poisoning by, adverse effect of and underdosing of thiobarbiturates
  - **T41.1X Poisoning by, adverse effect of and underdosing of intravenous anesthetics**
    - +7th T41.1X1 Poisoning by intravenous anesthetics, accidental (unintentional)
      Poisoning by intravenous anesthetics NOS
    - +7th T41.1X2 Poisoning by intravenous anesthetics, intentional self-harm
    - +7th T41.1X3 Poisoning by intravenous anesthetics, assault
    - +7th T41.1X4 Poisoning by intravenous anesthetics, undetermined
    - +7th T41.1X5 Adverse effect of intravenous anesthetics
    - +7th T41.1X6 Underdosing of intravenous anesthetics
- **T41.2 Poisoning by, adverse effect of and underdosing of other and unspecified general anesthetics**
  - **T41.20 Poisoning by, adverse effect of and underdosing of unspecified general anesthetics**
    - +7th T41.201 Poisoning by unspecified general anesthetics, accidental (unintentional)
      Poisoning by general anesthetics NOS
    - +7th T41.202 Poisoning by unspecified general anesthetics, intentional self-harm
    - +7th T41.203 Poisoning by unspecified general anesthetics, assault
    - +7th T41.204 Poisoning by unspecified general anesthetics, undetermined
    - +7th T41.205 Adverse effect of unspecified general anesthetics
      AHA CC: 4Q, 2016, 72-73
    - +7th T41.206 Underdosing of unspecified general anesthetics
  - **T41.29 Poisoning by, adverse effect of and underdosing of other general anesthetics**
    - +7th T41.291 Poisoning by other general anesthetics, accidental (unintentional)
      Poisoning by other general anesthetics NOS
    - +7th T41.292 Poisoning by other general anesthetics, intentional self-harm
    - +7th T41.293 Poisoning by other general anesthetics, assault
    - +7th T41.294 Poisoning by other general anesthetics, undetermined
    - +7th T41.295 Adverse effect of other general anesthetics
    - +7th T41.296 Underdosing of other general anesthetics
- **T41.3 Poisoning by, adverse effect of and underdosing of local anesthetics**
  Cocaine (topical)
  Excludes2: poisoning by cocaine used as a central nervous system stimulant (T40.5X1-T40.5X4)
  - **T41.3X Poisoning by, adverse effect of and underdosing of local anesthetics**
    - +7th T41.3X1 Poisoning by local anesthetics, accidental (unintentional)
      Poisoning by local anesthetics NOS
    - +7th T41.3X2 Poisoning by local anesthetics, intentional self-harm
    - +7th T41.3X3 Poisoning by local anesthetics, assault
    - +7th T41.3X4 Poisoning by local anesthetics, undetermined
    - +7th T41.3X5 Adverse effect of local anesthetics
    - +7th T41.3X6 Underdosing of local anesthetics
- **T41.4 Poisoning by, adverse effect of and underdosing of unspecified anesthetic**
  - X+7th T41.41 Poisoning by unspecified anesthetic, accidental (unintentional)
    Poisoning by anesthetic NOS
  - X+7th T41.42 Poisoning by unspecified anesthetic, intentional self-harm
  - X+7th T41.43 Poisoning by unspecified anesthetic, assault
  - X+7th T41.44 Poisoning by unspecified anesthetic, undetermined
  - X+7th T41.45 Adverse effect of unspecified anesthetic
  - X+7th T41.46 Underdosing of unspecified anesthetics
- **T41.5 Poisoning by, adverse effect of and underdosing of therapeutic gases**
  - **T41.5X Poisoning by, adverse effect of and underdosing of therapeutic gases**
    - +7th T41.5X1 Poisoning by therapeutic gases, accidental (unintentional)
      Poisoning by therapeutic gases NOS
    - +7th T41.5X2 Poisoning by therapeutic gases, intentional self-harm
    - +7th T41.5X3 Poisoning by therapeutic gases, assault
    - +7th T41.5X4 Poisoning by therapeutic gases, undetermined
    - +7th T41.5X5 Adverse effect of therapeutic gases
    - +7th T41.5X6 Underdosing of therapeutic gases

T42 Poisoning by, adverse effect of and underdosing of antiepileptic, sedative- hypnotic and antiparkinsonism drugs

Excludes2: drug dependence and related mental and behavioral disorders due to psychoactive substance use (F10.--F19.-)

The appropriate 7th character is to be added to each code from category T42
- A initial encounter
- D subsequent encounter
- S sequela

+ **T42.0 Poisoning by, adverse effect of and underdosing of hydantoin derivatives**
  + **T42.0X Poisoning by, adverse effect of and underdosing of hydantoin derivatives**
    - +7th T42.0X1 Poisoning by hydantoin derivatives, accidental (unintentional)
      - Poisoning by hydantoin derivatives NOS
    - +7th T42.0X2 Poisoning by hydantoin derivatives, intentional self-harm
    - +7th T42.0X3 Poisoning by hydantoin derivatives, assault
    - +7th T42.0X4 Poisoning by hydantoin derivatives, undetermined
    - +7th T42.0X5 Adverse effect of hydantoin derivatives
    - +7th T42.0X6 Underdosing of hydantoin derivatives

+ **T42.1 Poisoning by, adverse effect of and underdosing of iminostilbenes**
  Poisoning by, adverse effect of and underdosing of carbamazepine
  + **T42.1X Poisoning by, adverse effect of and underdosing of iminostilbenes**
    - +7th T42.1X1 Poisoning by iminostilbenes, accidental (unintentional)
      - Poisoning by iminostilbenes NOS
    - +7th T42.1X2 Poisoning by iminostilbenes, intentional self-harm
    - +7th T42.1X3 Poisoning by iminostilbenes, assault
    - +7th T42.1X4 Poisoning by iminostilbenes, undetermined
    - +7th T42.1X5 Adverse effect of iminostilbenes
    - +7th T42.1X6 Underdosing of iminostilbenes

+ **T42.2 Poisoning by, adverse effect of and underdosing of succinimides and oxazolidinediones**
  + **T42.2X Poisoning by, adverse effect of and underdosing of succinimides and oxazolidinediones**
    - +7th T42.2X1 Poisoning by succinimides and oxazolidinediones, accidental (unintentional)
      - Poisoning by succinimides and oxazolidinediones NOS
    - +7th T42.2X2 Poisoning by succinimides and oxazolidinediones, intentional self-harm
    - +7th T42.2X3 Poisoning by succinimides and oxazolidinediones, assault
    - +7th T42.2X4 Poisoning by succinimides and oxazolidinediones, undetermined
    - +7th T42.2X5 Adverse effect of succinimides and oxazolidinediones
    - +7th T42.2X6 Underdosing of succinimides and oxazolidinediones

+ **T42.3 Poisoning by, adverse effect of and underdosing of barbiturates**
  Excludes1: poisoning by, adverse effect of and underdosing of thiobarbiturates (T41.1-)
  + **T42.3X Poisoning by, adverse effect of and underdosing of barbiturates**
    - +7th T42.3X1 Poisoning by barbiturates, accidental (unintentional)
      - Poisoning by barbiturates NOS
    - +7th T42.3X2 Poisoning by barbiturates, intentional self-harm
    - +7th T42.3X3 Poisoning by barbiturates, assault
    - +7th T42.3X4 Poisoning by barbiturates, undetermined
    - +7th T42.3X5 Adverse effect of barbiturates
    - +7th T42.3X6 Underdosing of barbiturates

+ **T42.4 Poisoning by, adverse effect of and underdosing of benzodiazepines**
  + **T42.4X Poisoning by, adverse effect of and underdosing of benzodiazepines**
    - +7th T42.4X1 Poisoning by benzodiazepines, accidental (unintentional)
      - Poisoning by benzodiazepines NOS
    - +7th T42.4X2 Poisoning by benzodiazepines, intentional self-harm
    - +7th T42.4X3 Poisoning by benzodiazepines, assault
    - +7th T42.4X4 Poisoning by benzodiazepines, undetermined
    - +7th T42.4X5 Adverse effect of benzodiazepines
    - +7th T42.4X6 Underdosing of benzodiazepines

+ **T42.5 Poisoning by, adverse effect of and underdosing of mixed antiepileptics**
  + **T42.5X Poisoning by, adverse effect of and underdosing of antiepileptics**
    - +7th T42.5X1 Poisoning by mixed antiepileptics, accidental (unintentional)
      - Poisoning by mixed antiepileptics NOS
    - +7th T42.5X2 Poisoning by mixed antiepileptics, intentional self-harm
    - +7th T42.5X3 Poisoning by mixed antiepileptics, assault
    - +7th T42.5X4 Poisoning by mixed antiepileptics, undetermined
    - +7th T42.5X5 Adverse effect of mixed antiepileptics
    - +7th T42.5X6 Underdosing of mixed antiepileptics

+ **T42.6 Poisoning by, adverse effect of and underdosing of other antiepileptic and sedative-hypnotic drugs**
  Poisoning by, adverse effect of and underdosing of methaqualone
  Poisoning by, adverse effect of and underdosing of valproic acid
  Excludes1: poisoning by, adverse effect of and underdosing of carbamazepine (T42.1-)
  + **T42.6X Poisoning by, adverse effect of and underdosing of other antiepileptic and sedative-hypnotic drugs**
    - +7th T42.6X1 Poisoning by other antiepileptic and sedative-hypnotic drugs, accidental (unintentional)
      - Poisoning by other antiepileptic and sedative-hypnotic drugs NOS
    - +7th T42.6X2 Poisoning by other antiepileptic and sedative-hypnotic drugs, intentional self-harm
    - +7th T42.6X3 Poisoning by other antiepileptic and sedative-hypnotic drugs, assault
    - +7th T42.6X4 Poisoning by other antiepileptic and sedative-hypnotic drugs, undetermined
    - +7th T42.6X5 Adverse effect of other antiepileptic and sedative-hypnotic drugs
    - +7th T42.6X6 Underdosing of other antiepileptic and sedative-hypnotic drugs

+ **T42.7 Poisoning by, adverse effect of and underdosing of unspecified antiepileptic and sedative-hypnotic drugs**
  - X+7th T42.71 Poisoning by unspecified antiepileptic and sedative-hypnotic drugs, accidental (unintentional)
    - Poisoning by antiepileptic and sedative-hypnotic drugs NOS
  - X+7th T42.72 Poisoning by unspecified antiepileptic and sedative-hypnotic drugs, intentional self-harm
  - X+7th T42.73 Poisoning by unspecified antiepileptic and sedative-hypnotic drugs, assault
  - X+7th T42.74 Poisoning by unspecified antiepileptic and sedative-hypnotic drugs, undetermined
  - X+7th T42.75 Adverse effect of unspecified antiepileptic and sedative-hypnotic drugs
  - X+7th T42.76 Underdosing of unspecified antiepileptic and sedative-hypnotic drugs

- **T42.8 Poisoning by, adverse effect of and underdosing of antiparkinsonism drugs and other central muscle-tone depressants**
  Poisoning by, adverse effect of and underdosing of amantadine
  - **T42.8X Poisoning by, adverse effect of and underdosing of antiparkinsonism drugs and other central muscle-tone depressants**
    - +7th **T42.8X1** Poisoning by antiparkinsonism drugs and other central muscle-tone depressants, accidental (unintentional)
      Poisoning by antiparkinsonism drugs and other central muscle-tone depressants NOS
    - +7th **T42.8X2** Poisoning by antiparkinsonism drugs and other central muscle-tone depressants, intentional self-harm
    - +7th **T42.8X3** Poisoning by antiparkinsonism drugs and other central muscle-tone depressants, assault
    - +7th **T42.8X4** Poisoning by antiparkinsonism drugs and other central muscle-tone depressants, undetermined
    - +7th **T42.8X5** Adverse effect of antiparkinsonism drugs and other central muscle-tone depressants
    - +7th **T42.8X6** Underdosing of antiparkinsonism drugs and other central muscle-tone depressants

T43 Poisoning by, adverse effect of and underdosing of psychotropic drugs, not elsewhere classified

Excludes1: *appetite depressants (T50.5-)*
barbiturates (T42.3-)
benzodiazepines (T42.4-)
methaqualone (T42.6-)
psychodysleptics [hallucinogens] (T40.7-T40.9-)

Excludes2: *drug dependence and related mental and behavioral disorders due to psychoactive substance use (F10.-F19.-)*

The appropriate 7th character is to be added to each code from category T43
A initial encounter
D subsequent encounter
S sequela

- **T43.0 Poisoning by, adverse effect of and underdosing of tricyclic and tetracyclic antidepressants**
  - **T43.01 Poisoning by, adverse effect of and underdosing of tricyclic antidepressants**
    - +7th **T43.011** Poisoning by tricyclic antidepressants, accidental (unintentional)
      Poisoning by tricyclic antidepressants NOS
    - +7th **T43.012** Poisoning by tricyclic antidepressants, intentional self-harm
    - +7th **T43.013** Poisoning by tricyclic antidepressants, assault
    - +7th **T43.014** Poisoning by tricyclic antidepressants, undetermined
    - +7th **T43.015** Adverse effect of tricyclic antidepressants
    - +7th **T43.016** Underdosing of tricyclic antidepressants
  - **T43.02 Poisoning by, adverse effect of and underdosing of tetracyclic antidepressants**
    - +7th **T43.021** Poisoning by tetracyclic antidepressants, accidental (unintentional)
      Poisoning by tetracyclic antidepressants NOS
    - +7th **T43.022** Poisoning by tetracyclic antidepressants, intentional self-harm
    - +7th **T43.023** Poisoning by tetracyclic antidepressants, assault
    - +7th **T43.024** Poisoning by tetracyclic antidepressants, undetermined
    - +7th **T43.025** Adverse effect of tetracyclic antidepressants
    - +7th **T43.026** Underdosing of tetracyclic antidepressants

- **T43.1 Poisoning by, adverse effect of and underdosing of monoamine-oxidase-inhibitor antidepressants**
  - **T43.1X Poisoning by, adverse effect of and underdosing of monoamine-oxidase-inhibitor antidepressants**
    - +7th **T43.1X1** Poisoning by monoamine-oxidase-inhibitor antidepressants, accidental (unintentional)
      Poisoning by monoamine-oxidase-inhibitor antidepressants NOS
    - +7th **T43.1X2** Poisoning by monoamine-oxidase-inhibitor antidepressants, intentional self-harm
    - +7th **T43.1X3** Poisoning by monoamine-oxidase-inhibitor antidepressants, assault
    - +7th **T43.1X4** Poisoning by monoamine-oxidase-inhibitor antidepressants, undetermined
    - +7th **T43.1X5** Adverse effect of monoamine-oxidase-inhibitor antidepressants
    - +7th **T43.1X6** Underdosing of monoamine-oxidase-inhibitor antidepressants
- **T43.2 Poisoning by, adverse effect of and underdosing of other and unspecified antidepressants**
  - **T43.20 Poisoning by, adverse effect of and underdosing of unspecified antidepressants**
    - +7th **T43.201** Poisoning by unspecified antidepressants, accidental (unintentional)
      Poisoning by antidepressants NOS
    - +7th **T43.202** Poisoning by unspecified antidepressants, intentional self-harm
    - +7th **T43.203** Poisoning by unspecified antidepressants, assault
    - +7th **T43.204** Poisoning by unspecified antidepressants, undetermined
    - +7th **T43.205** Adverse effect of unspecified antidepressants
      Antidepressant discontinuation syndrome
    - +7th **T43.206** Underdosing of unspecified antidepressants
  - **T43.21 Poisoning by, adverse effect of and underdosing of selective serotonin and norepinephrine reuptake inhibitors**
    Poisoning by, adverse effect of and underdosing of SSNRI antidepressants
    - +7th **T43.211** Poisoning by selective serotonin and norepinephrine reuptake inhibitors, accidental (unintentional)
    - +7th **T43.212** Poisoning by selective serotonin and norepinephrine reuptake inhibitors, intentional self-harm
    - +7th **T43.213** Poisoning by selective serotonin and norepinephrine reuptake inhibitors, assault
    - +7th **T43.214** Poisoning by selective serotonin and norepinephrine reuptake inhibitors, undetermined
    - +7th **T43.215** Adverse effect of selective serotonin and norepinephrine reuptake inhibitors
    - +7th **T43.216** Underdosing of selective serotonin and norepinephrine reuptake inhibitors
  - **T43.22 Poisoning by, adverse effect of and underdosing of selective serotonin reuptake inhibitors**
    Poisoning by, adverse effect of and underdosing of SSRI antidepressants
    - +7th **T43.221** Poisoning by selective serotonin reuptake inhibitors, accidental (unintentional)
    - +7th **T43.222** Poisoning by selective serotonin reuptake inhibitors, intentional self-harm
    - +7th **T43.223** Poisoning by selective serotonin reuptake inhibitors, assault
    - +7th **T43.224** Poisoning by selective serotonin reuptake inhibitors, undetermined
    - +7th **T43.225** Adverse effect of selective serotonin reuptake inhibitors
      AHA CC: 2Q, 2022, 11-12
    - +7th **T43.226** Underdosing of selective serotonin reuptake inhibitors

- **T43.29 Poisoning by, adverse effect of and underdosing of other antidepressants**
  - +7th **T43.291** Poisoning by other antidepressants, accidental (unintentional)
    - Poisoning by other antidepressants NOS
  - +7th **T43.292** Poisoning by other antidepressants, intentional self-harm
  - +7th **T43.293** Poisoning by other antidepressants, assault
  - +7th **T43.294** Poisoning by other antidepressants, undetermined
  - +7th **T43.295** Adverse effect of other antidepressants
  - +7th **T43.296** Underdosing of other antidepressants
- + **T43.3 Poisoning by, adverse effect of and underdosing of phenothiazine antipsychotics and neuroleptics**
  - + **T43.3X Poisoning by, adverse effect of and underdosing of phenothiazine antipsychotics and neuroleptics**
    - +7th **T43.3X1** Poisoning by phenothiazine antipsychotics and neuroleptics, accidental (unintentional)
      - Poisoning by phenothiazine antipsychotics and neuroleptics NOS
    - +7th **T43.3X2** Poisoning by phenothiazine antipsychotics and neuroleptics, intentional self-harm
    - +7th **T43.3X3** Poisoning by phenothiazine antipsychotics and neuroleptics, assault
    - +7th **T43.3X4** Poisoning by phenothiazine antipsychotics and neuroleptics, undetermined
    - +7th **T43.3X5** Adverse effect of phenothiazine antipsychotics and neuroleptics
    - +7th **T43.3X6** Underdosing of phenothiazine antipsychotics and neuroleptics
- + **T43.4 Poisoning by, adverse effect of and underdosing of butyrophenone and thiothixene neuroleptics**
  - + **T43.4X Poisoning by, adverse effect of and underdosing of butyrophenone and thiothixene neuroleptics**
    - +7th **T43.4X1** Poisoning by butyrophenone and thiothixene neuroleptics, accidental (unintentional)
      - Poisoning by butyrophenone and thiothixene neuroleptics NOS
    - +7th **T43.4X2** Poisoning by butyrophenone and thiothixene neuroleptics, intentional self-harm
    - +7th **T43.4X3** Poisoning by butyrophenone and thiothixene neuroleptics, assault
    - +7th **T43.4X4** Poisoning by butyrophenone and thiothixene neuroleptics, undetermined
    - +7th **T43.4X5** Adverse effect of butyrophenone and thiothixene neuroleptics
    - +7th **T43.4X6** Underdosing of butyrophenone and thiothixene neuroleptics
- + **T43.5 Poisoning by, adverse effect of and underdosing of other and unspecified antipsychotics and neuroleptics**
  - **Excludes1:** *poisoning by, adverse effect of and underdosing of rauwolfia (T46.5-)*
  - + **T43.50 Poisoning by, adverse effect of and underdosing of unspecified antipsychotics and neuroleptics**
    - +7th **T43.501** Poisoning by unspecified antipsychotics and neuroleptics, accidental (unintentional)
      - Poisoning by antipsychotics and neuroleptics NOS
    - +7th **T43.502** Poisoning by unspecified antipsychotics and neuroleptics, intentional self-harm
    - +7th **T43.503** Poisoning by unspecified antipsychotics and neuroleptics, assault
    - +7th **T43.504** Poisoning by unspecified antipsychotics and neuroleptics, undetermined
    - +7th **T43.505** Adverse effect of unspecified antipsychotics and neuroleptics
      - *AHA CC: 4Q, 2022, 24*
    - +7th **T43.506** Underdosing of unspecified antipsychotics and neuroleptics
- + **T43.59 Poisoning by, adverse effect of and underdosing of other antipsychotics and neuroleptics**
  - +7th **T43.591** Poisoning by other antipsychotics and neuroleptics, accidental (unintentional)
    - Poisoning by other antipsychotics and neuroleptics NOS
  - +7th **T43.592** Poisoning by other antipsychotics and neuroleptics, intentional self-harm
    - *AHA CC: 1Q, 2017, 40*
  - +7th **T43.593** Poisoning by other antipsychotics and neuroleptics, assault
  - +7th **T43.594** Poisoning by other antipsychotics and neuroleptics, undetermined
  - +7th **T43.595** Adverse effect of other antipsychotics and neuroleptics
    - *AHA CC: 2Q, 2022, 11-12*
  - +7th **T43.596** Underdosing of other antipsychotics and neuroleptics
- + **T43.6 Poisoning by, adverse effect of and underdosing of psychostimulants**
  - **Excludes1:** *poisoning by, adverse effect of and underdosing of cocaine (T40.5-)*
  - + **T43.60 Poisoning by, adverse effect of and underdosing of unspecified psychostimulant**
    - +7th **T43.601** Poisoning by unspecified psychostimulants, accidental (unintentional)
      - Poisoning by psychostimulants NOS
    - +7th **T43.602** Poisoning by unspecified psychostimulants, intentional self-harm
    - +7th **T43.603** Poisoning by unspecified psychostimulants, assault
    - +7th **T43.604** Poisoning by unspecified psychostimulants, undetermined
    - +7th **T43.605** Adverse effect of unspecified psychostimulants
    - +7th **T43.606** Underdosing of unspecified psychostimulants
  - + **T43.61 Poisoning by, adverse effect of and underdosing of caffeine**
    - +7th **T43.611** Poisoning by caffeine, accidental (unintentional)
      - Poisoning by caffeine NOS
    - +7th **T43.612** Poisoning by caffeine, intentional self-harm
    - +7th **T43.613** Poisoning by caffeine, assault
    - +7th **T43.614** Poisoning by caffeine, undetermined
    - +7th **T43.615** Adverse effect of caffeine
    - +7th **T43.616** Underdosing of caffeine
  - + **T43.62 Poisoning by, adverse effect of and underdosing of amphetamines**
    - +7th **T43.621** Poisoning by amphetamines, accidental (unintentional)
      - Poisoning by amphetamines NOS
      - *AHA CC: 3Q, 2021, 8*
    - +7th **T43.622** Poisoning by amphetamines, intentional self-harm
    - +7th **T43.623** Poisoning by amphetamines, assault
    - +7th **T43.624** Poisoning by amphetamines, undetermined
    - +7th **T43.625** Adverse effect of amphetamines
    - +7th **T43.626** Underdosing of amphetamines
  - + **T43.63 Poisoning by, adverse effect of and underdosing of methylphenidate**
    - +7th **T43.631** Poisoning by methylphenidate, accidental (unintentional)
      - Poisoning by methylphenidate NOS
    - +7th **T43.632** Poisoning by methylphenidate, intentional self-harm
    - +7th **T43.633** Poisoning by methylphenidate, assault
    - +7th **T43.634** Poisoning by methylphenidate, undetermined
    - +7th **T43.635** Adverse effect of methylphenidate
    - +7th **T43.636** Underdosing of methylphenidate

- **+ T43.64 Poisoning by ecstasy**
  Poisoning by MDMA
  Poisoning by 3,4-methylenedioxymethamphetamine
  AHA CC: 4Q, 2018, 30-31
  - +7th **T43.641** Poisoning by ecstasy, accidental (unintentional)
    Poisoning by ecstasy NOS
    AHA CC: 4Q, 2018, 31
  - +7th **T43.642** Poisoning by ecstasy, intentional self-harm
  - +7th **T43.643** Poisoning by ecstasy, assault
  - +7th **T43.644** Poisoning by ecstasy, undetermined
- **+ T43.65 Poisoning by, adverse effect of and underdosing of methamphetamines**
  AHA CC: 4Q, 2022, 45-47
  - +7th **T43.651** Poisoning by methamphetamines accidental (unintentional)
    Poisoning by methamphetamines NOS
    AHA CC: 4Q, 2022, 46
  - +7th **T43.652** Poisoning by methamphetamines intentional self-harm
  - +7th **T43.653** Poisoning by methamphetamines, assault
  - +7th **T43.654** Poisoning by methamphetamines, undetermined
  - +7th **T43.655** Adverse effect of methamphetamines
    AHA CC: 4Q, 2022, 46-47
  - +7th **T43.656** Underdosing of methamphetamines
- **+ T43.69 Poisoning by, adverse effect of and underdosing of other psychostimulants**
  - +7th **T43.691** Poisoning by other psychostimulants, accidental (unintentional)
    Poisoning by other psychostimulants NOS
  - +7th **T43.692** Poisoning by other psychostimulants, intentional self-harm
  - +7th **T43.693** Poisoning by other psychostimulants, assault
  - +7th **T43.694** Poisoning by other psychostimulants, undetermined
  - +7th **T43.695** Adverse effect of other psychostimulants
  - +7th **T43.696** Underdosing of other psychostimulants
- **+ T43.8 Poisoning by, adverse effect of and underdosing of other psychotropic drugs**
  - **+ T43.8X Poisoning by, adverse effect of and underdosing of other psychotropic drugs**
    - +7th **T43.8X1** Poisoning by other psychotropic drugs, accidental (unintentional)
      Poisoning by other psychotropic drugs NOS
    - +7th **T43.8X2** Poisoning by other psychotropic drugs, intentional self-harm
    - +7th **T43.8X3** Poisoning by other psychotropic drugs, assault
    - +7th **T43.8X4** Poisoning by other psychotropic drugs, undetermined
    - +7th **T43.8X5** Adverse effect of other psychotropic drugs
    - +7th **T43.8X6** Underdosing of other psychotropic drugs
- **+ T43.9 Poisoning by, adverse effect of and underdosing of unspecified psychotropic drug**
  - X+7th **T43.91** Poisoning by unspecified psychotropic drug, accidental (unintentional)
    Poisoning by psychotropic drug NOS
  - X+7th **T43.92** Poisoning by unspecified psychotropic drug, intentional self-harm
  - X+7th **T43.93** Poisoning by unspecified psychotropic drug, assault
  - X+7th **T43.94** Poisoning by unspecified psychotropic drug, undetermined
  - X+7th **T43.95** Adverse effect of unspecified psychotropic drug
  - X+7th **T43.96** Underdosing of unspecified psychotropic drug

T44 Poisoning by, adverse effect of and underdosing of drugs primarily affecting the autonomic nervous system

> The appropriate 7th character is to be added to each code from category T44
> A   initial encounter
> D   subsequent encounter
> S   sequela

- **+ T44.0 Poisoning by, adverse effect of and underdosing of anticholinesterase agents**
  - **+ T44.0X Poisoning by, adverse effect of and underdosing of anticholinesterase agents**
    - +7th **T44.0X1** Poisoning by anticholinesterase agents, accidental (unintentional)
      Poisoning by anticholinesterase agents NOS
    - +7th **T44.0X2** Poisoning by anticholinesterase agents, intentional self-harm
    - +7th **T44.0X3** Poisoning by anticholinesterase agents, assault
    - +7th **T44.0X4** Poisoning by anticholinesterase agents, undetermined
    - +7th **T44.0X5** Adverse effect of anticholinesterase agents
    - +7th **T44.0X6** Underdosing of anticholinesterase agents
- **+ T44.1 Poisoning by, adverse effect of and underdosing of other parasympathomimetics [cholinergics]**
  - **+ T44.1X Poisoning by, adverse effect of and underdosing of other parasympathomimetics [cholinergics]**
    - +7th **T44.1X1** Poisoning by other parasympathomimetics [cholinergics], accidental (unintentional)
      Poisoning by other parasympathomimetics [cholinergics] NOS
    - +7th **T44.1X2** Poisoning by other parasympathomimetics [cholinergics], intentional self-harm
    - +7th **T44.1X3** Poisoning by other parasympathomimetics [cholinergics], assault
    - +7th **T44.1X4** Poisoning by other parasympathomimetics [cholinergics], undetermined
    - +7th **T44.1X5** Adverse effect of other parasympathomimetics [cholinergics]
    - +7th **T44.1X6** Underdosing of other parasympathomimetics [cholinergics]
- **+ T44.2 Poisoning by, adverse effect of and underdosing of ganglionic blocking drugs**
  - **+ T44.2X Poisoning by, adverse effect of and underdosing of ganglionic blocking drugs**
    - +7th **T44.2X1** Poisoning by ganglionic blocking drugs, accidental (unintentional)
      Poisoning by ganglionic blocking drugs NOS
    - +7th **T44.2X2** Poisoning by ganglionic blocking drugs, intentional self-harm
    - +7th **T44.2X3** Poisoning by ganglionic blocking drugs, assault
    - +7th **T44.2X4** Poisoning by ganglionic blocking drugs, undetermined
    - +7th **T44.2X5** Adverse effect of ganglionic blocking drugs
    - +7th **T44.2X6** Underdosing of ganglionic blocking drugs
- **+ T44.3 Poisoning by, adverse effect of and underdosing of other parasympatholytics [anticholinergics and antimuscarinics] and spasmolytics**
  Poisoning by, adverse effect of and underdosing of papaverine
  - **+ T44.3X Poisoning by, adverse effect of and underdosing of other parasympatholytics [anticholinergics and antimuscarinics] and spasmolytics**
    - +7th **T44.3X1** Poisoning by other parasympatholytics [anticholinergics and antimuscarinics] and spasmolytics, accidental (unintentional)
      Poisoning by other parasympatholytics [anticholinergics and antimuscarinics] and spasmolytics NOS
    - +7th **T44.3X2** Poisoning by other parasympatholytics [anticholinergics and antimuscarinics] and spasmolytics, intentional self-harm

- +7th **T44.3X3** Poisoning by other parasympatholytics [anticholinergics and antimuscarinics] and spasmolytics, assault
- +7th **T44.3X4** Poisoning by other parasympatholytics [anticholinergics and antimuscarinics] and spasmolytics, undetermined
- +7th **T44.3X5** Adverse effect of other parasympatholytics [anticholinergics and antimuscarinics] and spasmolytics
- +7th **T44.3X6** Underdosing of other parasympatholytics [anticholinergics and antimuscarinics] and spasmolytics

+ **T44.4** Poisoning by, adverse effect of and underdosing of predominantly alpha-adrenoreceptor agonists
  Poisoning by, adverse effect of and underdosing of metaraminol
  + **T44.4X** Poisoning by, adverse effect of and underdosing of predominantly alpha-adrenoreceptor agonists
    - +7th **T44.4X1** Poisoning by predominantly alpha-adrenoreceptor agonists, accidental (unintentional)
      Poisoning by predominantly alpha-adrenoreceptor agonists NOS
    - +7th **T44.4X2** Poisoning by predominantly alpha-adrenoreceptor agonists, intentional self-harm
    - +7th **T44.4X3** Poisoning by predominantly alpha-adrenoreceptor agonists, assault
    - +7th **T44.4X4** Poisoning by predominantly alpha-adrenoreceptor agonists, undetermined
    - +7th **T44.4X5** Adverse effect of predominantly alpha-adrenoreceptor agonists
    - +7th **T44.4X6** Underdosing of predominantly alpha-adrenoreceptor agonists

+ **T44.5** Poisoning by, adverse effect of and underdosing of predominantly beta-adrenoreceptor agonists
  Excludes1: poisoning by, adverse effect of and underdosing of beta-adrenoreceptor agonists used in asthma therapy (T48.6-)
  + **T44.5X** Poisoning by, adverse effect of and underdosing of predominantly beta-adrenoreceptor agonists
    - +7th **T44.5X1** Poisoning by predominantly beta-adrenoreceptor agonists, accidental (unintentional)
      Poisoning by predominantly beta-adrenoreceptor agonists NOS
    - +7th **T44.5X2** Poisoning by predominantly beta-adrenoreceptor agonists, intentional self-harm
    - +7th **T44.5X3** Poisoning by predominantly beta-adrenoreceptor agonists, assault
    - +7th **T44.5X4** Poisoning by predominantly beta-adrenoreceptor agonists, undetermined
    - +7th **T44.5X5** Adverse effect of predominantly beta-adrenoreceptor agonists
    - +7th **T44.5X6** Underdosing of predominantly beta-adrenoreceptor agonists

+ **T44.6** Poisoning by, adverse effect of and underdosing of alpha-adrenoreceptor antagonists
  Excludes1: poisoning by, adverse effect of and underdosing of ergot alkaloids (T48.0)
  + **T44.6X** Poisoning by, adverse effect of and underdosing of alpha-adrenoreceptor antagonists
    - +7th **T44.6X1** Poisoning by alpha-adrenoreceptor antagonists, accidental (unintentional)
      Poisoning by alpha-adrenoreceptor antagonists NOS
    - +7th **T44.6X2** Poisoning by alpha-adrenoreceptor antagonists, intentional self-harm
    - +7th **T44.6X3** Poisoning by alpha-adrenoreceptor antagonists, assault
    - +7th **T44.6X4** Poisoning by alpha-adrenoreceptor antagonists, undetermined
    - +7th **T44.6X5** Adverse effect of alpha-adrenoreceptor antagonists
    - +7th **T44.6X6** Underdosing of alpha-adrenoreceptor antagonists

+ **T44.7** Poisoning by, adverse effect of and underdosing of beta-adrenoreceptor antagonists
  + **T44.7X** Poisoning by, adverse effect of and underdosing of beta-adrenoreceptor antagonists
    - +7th **T44.7X1** Poisoning by beta-adrenoreceptor antagonists, accidental (unintentional)
      Poisoning by beta-adrenoreceptor antagonists NOS
    - +7th **T44.7X2** Poisoning by beta-adrenoreceptor antagonists, intentional self-harm
    - +7th **T44.7X3** Poisoning by beta-adrenoreceptor antagonists, assault
    - +7th **T44.7X4** Poisoning by beta-adrenoreceptor antagonists, undetermined
    - +7th **T44.7X5** Adverse effect of beta-adrenoreceptor antagonists
    - +7th **T44.7X6** Underdosing of beta-adrenoreceptor antagonists

+ **T44.8** Poisoning by, adverse effect of and underdosing of centrally-acting and adrenergic-neuron- blocking agents
  Excludes2: poisoning by, adverse effect of and underdosing of clonidine (T46.5)
  poisoning by, adverse effect of and underdosing of guanethidine (T46.5)
  + **T44.8X** Poisoning by, adverse effect of and underdosing of centrally-acting and adrenergic- neuron-blocking agents
    - +7th **T44.8X1** Poisoning by centrally-acting and adrenergic-neuron-blocking agents, accidental (unintentional)
      Poisoning by centrally-acting and adrenergic-neuron-blocking agents NOS
    - +7th **T44.8X2** Poisoning by centrally-acting and adrenergic-neuron-blocking agents, intentional self-harm
    - +7th **T44.8X3** Poisoning by centrally-acting and adrenergic-neuron-blocking agents, assault
    - +7th **T44.8X4** Poisoning by centrally-acting and adrenergic-neuron-blocking agents, undetermined
    - +7th **T44.8X5** Adverse effect of centrally-acting and adrenergic-neuron-blocking agents
    - +7th **T44.8X6** Underdosing of centrally-acting and adrenergic-neuron-blocking agents

+ **T44.9** Poisoning by, adverse effect of and underdosing of other and unspecified drugs primarily affecting the autonomic nervous system
  Poisoning by, adverse effect of and underdosing of drug stimulating both alpha and beta-adrenoreceptors
  + **T44.90** Poisoning by, adverse effect of and underdosing of unspecified drugs primarily affecting the autonomic nervous system
    - +7th **T44.901** Poisoning by unspecified drugs primarily affecting the autonomic nervous system, accidental (unintentional)
      Poisoning by unspecified drugs primarily affecting the autonomic nervous system NOS
    - +7th **T44.902** Poisoning by unspecified drugs primarily affecting the autonomic nervous system, intentional self-harm
    - +7th **T44.903** Poisoning by unspecified drugs primarily affecting the autonomic nervous system, assault
    - +7th **T44.904** Poisoning by unspecified drugs primarily affecting the autonomic nervous system, undetermined
    - +7th **T44.905** Adverse effect of unspecified drugs primarily affecting the autonomic nervous system
    - +7th **T44.906** Underdosing of unspecified drugs primarily affecting the autonomic nervous system
  + **T44.99** Poisoning by, adverse effect of and underdosing of other drugs primarily affecting the autonomic nervous system

- +7th **T44.991** Poisoning by other drug primarily affecting the autonomic nervous system, accidental (unintentional)
  - Poisoning by other drugs primarily affecting the autonomic nervous system NOS
- +7th **T44.992** Poisoning by other drug primarily affecting the autonomic nervous system, intentional self-harm
- +7th **T44.993** Poisoning by other drug primarily affecting the autonomic nervous system, assault
- +7th **T44.994** Poisoning by other drug primarily affecting the autonomic nervous system, undetermined
- +7th **T44.995** Adverse effect of other drug primarily affecting the autonomic nervous system
- +7th **T44.996** Underdosing of other drug primarily affecting the autonomic nervous system

T45 Poisoning by, adverse effect of and underdosing of primarily systemic and hematological agents, not elsewhere classified

> The appropriate 7th character is to be added to each code from category T45
> A initial encounter
> D subsequent encounter
> S sequela

- + **T45.0** Poisoning by, adverse effect of and underdosing of antiallergic and antiemetic drugs
  - **Excludes1:** poisoning by, adverse effect of and underdosing of phenothiazine-based neuroleptics (T43.3)
  - + **T45.0X** Poisoning by, adverse effect of and underdosing of antiallergic and antiemetic drugs
    - +7th **T45.0X1** Poisoning by antiallergic and antiemetic drugs, accidental (unintentional)
      - Poisoning by antiallergic and antiemetic drugs NOS
    - +7th **T45.0X2** Poisoning by antiallergic and antiemetic drugs, intentional self-harm
    - +7th **T45.0X3** Poisoning by antiallergic and antiemetic drugs, assault
    - +7th **T45.0X4** Poisoning by antiallergic and antiemetic drugs, undetermined
    - +7th **T45.0X5** Adverse effect of antiallergic and antiemetic drugs
    - +7th **T45.0X6** Underdosing of antiallergic and antiemetic drugs
- + **T45.1** Poisoning by, adverse effect of and underdosing of antineoplastic and immunosuppressive drugs
  - **Excludes1:** poisoning by, adverse effect of and underdosing of tamoxifen (T38.6)
  - + **T45.1X** Poisoning by, adverse effect of and underdosing of antineoplastic and immunosuppressive drugs
    - +7th **T45.1X1** Poisoning by antineoplastic and immunosuppressive drugs, accidental (unintentional)
      - Poisoning by antineoplastic and immunosuppressive drugs NOS
    - +7th **T45.1X2** Poisoning by antineoplastic and immunosuppressive drugs, intentional self-harm
    - +7th **T45.1X3** Poisoning by antineoplastic and immunosuppressive drugs, assault
    - +7th **T45.1X4** Poisoning by antineoplastic and immunosuppressive drugs, undetermined
    - +7th **T45.1X5** Adverse effect of antineoplastic and immunosuppressive drugs
      - Review coding guideline C.2.c.2
      - *AHA CC: 4Q, 2014, 22-23; 1Q, 2019, 17, 20-21; 2Q, 2019, 24-26, 28; 3Q, 2020, 22-23; 4Q, 2020, 11-12; 3Q, 2021, 4; 2Q, 2023, 10*
    - +7th **T45.1X6** Underdosing of antineoplastic and immunosuppressive drugs
- + **T45.2** Poisoning by, adverse effect of and underdosing of vitamins
  - **Excludes2:** poisoning by, adverse effect of and underdosing of nicotinic acid (derivatives) (T46.7)
    - poisoning by, adverse effect of and underdosing of iron (T45.4)
    - poisoning by, adverse effect of and underdosing of vitamin K (T45.7)
  - + **T45.2X** Poisoning by, adverse effect of and underdosing of vitamins
    - +7th **T45.2X1** Poisoning by vitamins, accidental (unintentional)
      - Poisoning by vitamins NOS
    - +7th **T45.2X2** Poisoning by vitamins, intentional self-harm
    - +7th **T45.2X3** Poisoning by vitamins, assault
    - +7th **T45.2X4** Poisoning by vitamins, undetermined
    - +7th **T45.2X5** Adverse effect of vitamins
    - +7th **T45.2X6** Underdosing of vitamins
      - **Excludes1:** vitamin deficiencies (E50-E56)
- + **T45.3** Poisoning by, adverse effect of and underdosing of enzymes
  - + **T45.3X** Poisoning by, adverse effect of and underdosing of enzymes
    - +7th **T45.3X1** Poisoning by enzymes, accidental (unintentional)
      - Poisoning by enzymes NOS
    - +7th **T45.3X2** Poisoning by enzymes, intentional self-harm
    - +7th **T45.3X3** Poisoning by enzymes, assault
    - +7th **T45.3X4** Poisoning by enzymes, undetermined
    - +7th **T45.3X5** Adverse effect of enzymes
    - +7th **T45.3X6** Underdosing of enzymes
- + **T45.4** Poisoning by, adverse effect of and underdosing of iron and its compounds
  - + **T45.4X** Poisoning by, adverse effect of and underdosing of iron and its compounds
    - +7th **T45.4X1** Poisoning by iron and its compounds, accidental (unintentional)
      - Poisoning by iron and its compounds NOS
    - +7th **T45.4X2** Poisoning by iron and its compounds, intentional self-harm
    - +7th **T45.4X3** Poisoning by iron and its compounds, assault
    - +7th **T45.4X4** Poisoning by iron and its compounds, undetermined
    - +7th **T45.4X5** Adverse effect of iron and its compounds
    - +7th **T45.4X6** Underdosing of iron and its compounds
      - **Excludes1:** iron deficiency (E61.1)
- + **T45.5** Poisoning by, adverse effect of and underdosing of anticoagulants and antithrombotic drugs
  - + **T45.51** Poisoning by, adverse effect of and underdosing of anticoagulants
    - +7th **T45.511** Poisoning by anticoagulants, accidental (unintentional)
      - Poisoning by anticoagulants NOS
    - +7th **T45.512** Poisoning by anticoagulants, intentional self-harm
    - +7th **T45.513** Poisoning by anticoagulants, assault
    - +7th **T45.514** Poisoning by anticoagulants, undetermined
    - +7th **T45.515** Adverse effect of anticoagulants
      - *AHA CC: 2Q, 2013, 34-35; 1Q, 2016, 14-15; 1Q, 2021, 4-5*
    - +7th **T45.516** Underdosing of anticoagulants
  - + **T45.52** Poisoning by, adverse effect of and underdosing of antithrombotic drugs
    - Poisoning by, adverse effect of and underdosing of antiplatelet drugs
    - **Excludes2:** poisoning by, adverse effect of and underdosing of aspirin (T39.01-)
      - poisoning by, adverse effect of and underdosing of acetylsalicylic acid (T39.01-)
    - +7th **T45.521** Poisoning by antithrombotic drugs, accidental (unintentional)
      - Poisoning by antithrombotic drug NOS
    - +7th **T45.522** Poisoning by antithrombotic drugs, intentional self-harm
    - +7th **T45.523** Poisoning by antithrombotic drugs, assault
    - +7th **T45.524** Poisoning by antithrombotic drugs, undetermined
    - +7th **T45.525** Adverse effect of antithrombotic drugs
      - *AHA CC: 1Q, 2016, 15*
    - +7th **T45.526** Underdosing of antithrombotic drugs

- **T45.6 Poisoning by, adverse effect of and underdosing of fibrinolysis-affecting drugs**
  - **T45.60 Poisoning by, adverse effect of and underdosing of unspecified fibrinolysis-affecting drugs**
    - +7th T45.601 Poisoning by unspecified fibrinolysis-affecting drugs, accidental (unintentional)
      - Poisoning by fibrinolysis-affecting drug NOS
    - +7th T45.602 Poisoning by unspecified fibrinolysis-affecting drugs, intentional self-harm
    - +7th T45.603 Poisoning by unspecified fibrinolysis-affecting drugs, assault
    - +7th T45.604 Poisoning by unspecified fibrinolysis-affecting drugs, undetermined
    - +7th T45.605 Adverse effect of unspecified fibrinolysis-affecting drugs
    - +7th T45.606 Underdosing of unspecified fibrinolysis-affecting drugs
  - **T45.61 Poisoning by, adverse effect of and underdosing of thrombolytic drugs**
    - +7th T45.611 Poisoning by thrombolytic drug, accidental (unintentional)
      - Poisoning by thrombolytic drug NOS
    - +7th T45.612 Poisoning by thrombolytic drug, intentional self-harm
    - +7th T45.613 Poisoning by thrombolytic drug, assault
    - +7th T45.614 Poisoning by thrombolytic drug, undetermined
    - +7th T45.615 Adverse effect of thrombolytic drugs
      - AHA CC: 2Q, 2017, 9-10
    - +7th T45.616 Underdosing of thrombolytic drugs
  - **T45.62 Poisoning by, adverse effect of and underdosing of hemostatic drugs**
    - +7th T45.621 Poisoning by hemostatic drug, accidental (unintentional)
      - Poisoning by hemostatic drug NOS
    - +7th T45.622 Poisoning by hemostatic drug, intentional self-harm
    - +7th T45.623 Poisoning by hemostatic drug, assault
    - +7th T45.624 Poisoning by hemostatic drug, undetermined
    - +7th T45.625 Adverse effect of hemostatic drug
    - +7th T45.626 Underdosing of hemostatic drugs
  - **T45.69 Poisoning by, adverse effect of and underdosing of other fibrinolysis-affecting drugs**
    - +7th T45.691 Poisoning by other fibrinolysis-affecting drugs, accidental (unintentional)
      - Poisoning by other fibrinolysis-affecting drug NOS
    - +7th T45.692 Poisoning by other fibrinolysis-affecting drugs, intentional self-harm
    - +7th T45.693 Poisoning by other fibrinolysis-affecting drugs, assault
    - +7th T45.694 Poisoning by other fibrinolysis-affecting drugs, undetermined
    - +7th T45.695 Adverse effect of other fibrinolysis-affecting drugs
    - +7th T45.696 Underdosing of other fibrinolysis-affecting drugs
- **T45.7 Poisoning by, adverse effect of and underdosing of anticoagulant antagonists, vitamin K and other coagulants**
  - **T45.7X Poisoning by, adverse effect of and underdosing of anticoagulant antagonists, vitamin K and other coagulants**
    - +7th T45.7X1 Poisoning by anticoagulant antagonists, vitamin K and other coagulants, accidental (unintentional)
      - Poisoning by anticoagulant antagonists, vitamin K and other coagulants NOS
    - +7th T45.7X2 Poisoning by anticoagulant antagonists, vitamin K and other coagulants, intentional self-harm
    - +7th T45.7X3 Poisoning by anticoagulant antagonists, vitamin K and other coagulants, assault
    - +7th T45.7X4 Poisoning by anticoagulant antagonists, vitamin K and other coagulants, undetermined
    - +7th T45.7X5 Adverse effect of anticoagulant antagonists, vitamin K and other coagulants
    - +7th T45.7X6 Underdosing of anticoagulant antagonist, vitamin K and other coagulants
      - **Excludes1:** vitamin K deficiency (E56.1)
- **T45.8 Poisoning by, adverse effect of and underdosing of other primarily systemic and hematological agents**
  - Poisoning by, adverse effect of and underdosing of liver preparations and other antianemic agents
  - Poisoning by, adverse effect of and underdosing of natural blood and blood products
  - Poisoning by, adverse effect of and underdosing of plasma substitute
  - **Excludes2:** poisoning by, adverse effect of and underdosing of immunoglobulin (T50.Z1)
    - poisoning by, adverse effect of and underdosing of iron (T45.4)
    - transfusion reactions (T80.-)
  - **T45.8X Poisoning by, adverse effect of and underdosing of other primarily systemic and hematological agents**
    - +7th T45.8X1 Poisoning by other primarily systemic and hematological agents, accidental (unintentional)
      - Poisoning by other primarily systemic and hematological agents NOS
    - +7th T45.8X2 Poisoning by other primarily systemic and hematological agents, intentional self-harm
    - +7th T45.8X3 Poisoning by other primarily systemic and hematological agents, assault
    - +7th T45.8X4 Poisoning by other primarily systemic and hematological agents, undetermined
    - +7th T45.8X5 Adverse effect of other primarily systemic and hematological agents
      - AHA CC: 4Q, 2016, 41-42
    - +7th T45.8X6 Underdosing of other primarily systemic and hematological agents
- **T45.9 Poisoning by, adverse effect of and underdosing of unspecified primarily systemic and hematological agent**
  - X+7th T45.91 Poisoning by unspecified primarily systemic and hematological agent, accidental (unintentional)
    - Poisoning by primarily systemic and hematological agent NOS
  - X+7th T45.92 Poisoning by unspecified primarily systemic and hematological agent, intentional self-harm
  - X+7th T45.93 Poisoning by unspecified primarily systemic and hematological agent, assault
  - X+7th T45.94 Poisoning by unspecified primarily systemic and hematological agent, undetermined
  - X+7th T45.95 Adverse effect of unspecified primarily systemic and hematological agent
  - X+7th T45.96 Underdosing of unspecified primarily systemic and hematological agent

T46 Poisoning by, adverse effect of and underdosing of agents primarily affecting the cardiovascular system

Excludes1: poisoning by, adverse effect of and underdosing of metaraminol (T44.4)

> The appropriate 7th character is to be added to each code from category T46
> A initial encounter
> D subsequent encounter
> S sequela

- **T46.0 Poisoning by, adverse effect of and underdosing of cardiac-stimulant glycosides and drugs of similar action**
  - **T46.0X Poisoning by, adverse effect of and underdosing of cardiac-stimulant glycosides and drugs of similar action**
    - +7th T46.0X1 Poisoning by cardiac-stimulant glycosides and drugs of similar action, accidental (unintentional)
      - Poisoning by cardiac-stimulant glycosides and drugs of similar action NOS

- +7th **T46.0X2** Poisoning by cardiac-stimulant glycosides and drugs of similar action, intentional self-harm
- +7th **T46.0X3** Poisoning by cardiac-stimulant glycosides and drugs of similar action, assault
- +7th **T46.0X4** Poisoning by cardiac-stimulant glycosides and drugs of similar action, undetermined
- +7th **T46.0X5** Adverse effect of cardiac-stimulant glycosides and drugs of similar action
- +7th **T46.0X6** Underdosing of cardiac-stimulant glycosides and drugs of similar action

+ **T46.1** Poisoning by, adverse effect of and underdosing of calcium-channel blockers
  + **T46.1X** Poisoning by, adverse effect of and underdosing of calcium-channel blockers
    - +7th **T46.1X1** Poisoning by calcium-channel blockers, accidental (unintentional)
      Poisoning by calcium-channel blockers NOS
    - +7th **T46.1X2** Poisoning by calcium-channel blockers, intentional self-harm
    - +7th **T46.1X3** Poisoning by calcium-channel blockers, assault
    - +7th **T46.1X4** Poisoning by calcium-channel blockers, undetermined
    - +7th **T46.1X5** Adverse effect of calcium-channel blockers
    - +7th **T46.1X6** Underdosing of calcium-channel blockers
      AHA CC: 1Q, 2022, 36; 1Q, 2023, 39

+ **T46.2** Poisoning by, adverse effect of and underdosing of other antidysrhythmic drugs, not elsewhere classified
  Excludes1: *poisoning by, adverse effect of and underdosing of beta-adrenoreceptor antagonists (T44.7-)*
  + **T46.2X** Poisoning by, adverse effect of and underdosing of other antidysrhythmic drugs
    - +7th **T46.2X1** Poisoning by other antidysrhythmic drugs, accidental (unintentional)
      Poisoning by other antidysrhythmic drugs NOS
    - +7th **T46.2X2** Poisoning by other antidysrhythmic drugs, intentional self-harm
    - +7th **T46.2X3** Poisoning by other antidysrhythmic drugs, assault
    - +7th **T46.2X4** Poisoning by other antidysrhythmic drugs, undetermined
    - +7th **T46.2X5** Adverse effect of other antidysrhythmic drugs
    - +7th **T46.2X6** Underdosing of other antidysrhythmic drugs

+ **T46.3** Poisoning by, adverse effect of and underdosing of coronary vasodilators
  Poisoning by, adverse effect of and underdosing of dipyridamole
  Excludes1: *poisoning by, adverse effect of and underdosing of calcium-channel blockers (T46.1)*
  + **T46.3X** Poisoning by, adverse effect of and underdosing of coronary vasodilators
    - +7th **T46.3X1** Poisoning by coronary vasodilators, accidental (unintentional)
      Poisoning by coronary vasodilators NOS
    - +7th **T46.3X2** Poisoning by coronary vasodilators, intentional self-harm
    - +7th **T46.3X3** Poisoning by coronary vasodilators, assault
    - +7th **T46.3X4** Poisoning by coronary vasodilators, undetermined
    - +7th **T46.3X5** Adverse effect of coronary vasodilators
    - +7th **T46.3X6** Underdosing of coronary vasodilators

+ **T46.4** Poisoning by, adverse effect of and underdosing of angiotensin-converting-enzyme inhibitors
  + **T46.4X** Poisoning by, adverse effect of and underdosing of angiotensin-converting-enzyme inhibitors
    - +7th **T46.4X1** Poisoning by angiotensin-converting-enzyme inhibitors, accidental (unintentional)
      Poisoning by angiotensin-converting-enzyme inhibitors NOS
    - +7th **T46.4X2** Poisoning by angiotensin-converting-enzyme inhibitors, intentional self-harm
    - +7th **T46.4X3** Poisoning by angiotensin-converting-enzyme inhibitors, assault
    - +7th **T46.4X4** Poisoning by angiotensin-converting-enzyme inhibitors, undetermined
    - +7th **T46.4X5** Adverse effect of angiotensin-converting-enzyme inhibitors
    - +7th **T46.4X6** Underdosing of angiotensin-converting-enzyme inhibitors

+ **T46.5** Poisoning by, adverse effect of and underdosing of other antihypertensive drugs
  Excludes2: *poisoning by, adverse effect of and underdosing of beta-adrenoreceptor antagonists (T44.7)*
  poisoning by, adverse effect of and underdosing of calcium-channel blockers (T46.1)
  poisoning by, adverse effect of and underdosing of diuretics (T50.0-T50.2)
  + **T46.5X** Poisoning by, adverse effect of and underdosing of other antihypertensive drugs
    - +7th **T46.5X1** Poisoning by other antihypertensive drugs, accidental (unintentional)
      Poisoning by other antihypertensive drugs NOS
    - +7th **T46.5X2** Poisoning by other antihypertensive drugs, intentional self-harm
    - +7th **T46.5X3** Poisoning by other antihypertensive drugs, assault
    - +7th **T46.5X4** Poisoning by other antihypertensive drugs, undetermined
    - +7th **T46.5X5** Adverse effect of other antihypertensive drugs
    - +7th **T46.5X6** Underdosing of other antihypertensive drugs
      AHA CC: 1Q, 2022, 36; 1Q, 2023, 39

+ **T46.6** Poisoning by, adverse effect of and underdosing of antihyperlipidemic and antiarteriosclerotic drugs
  + **T46.6X** Poisoning by, adverse effect of and underdosing of antihyperlipidemic and antiarteriosclerotic drugs
    - +7th **T46.6X1** Poisoning by antihyperlipidemic and antiarteriosclerotic drugs, accidental (unintentional)
      Poisoning by antihyperlipidemic and antiarteriosclerotic drugs NOS
    - +7th **T46.6X2** Poisoning by antihyperlipidemic and antiarteriosclerotic drugs, intentional self-harm
    - +7th **T46.6X3** Poisoning by antihyperlipidemic and antiarteriosclerotic drugs, assault
    - +7th **T46.6X4** Poisoning by antihyperlipidemic and antiarteriosclerotic drugs, undetermined
    - +7th **T46.6X5** Adverse effect of antihyperlipidemic and antiarteriosclerotic drugs
    - +7th **T46.6X6** Underdosing of antihyperlipidemic and antiarteriosclerotic drugs

+ **T46.7** Poisoning by, adverse effect of and underdosing of peripheral vasodilators
  Poisoning by, adverse effect of and underdosing of nicotinic acid (derivatives)
  Excludes1: *poisoning by, adverse effect of and underdosing of papaverine (T44.3)*
  + **T46.7X** Poisoning by, adverse effect of and underdosing of peripheral vasodilators
    - +7th **T46.7X1** Poisoning by peripheral vasodilators, accidental (unintentional)
      Poisoning by peripheral vasodilators NOS
    - +7th **T46.7X2** Poisoning by peripheral vasodilators, intentional self-harm
    - +7th **T46.7X3** Poisoning by peripheral vasodilators, assault
    - +7th **T46.7X4** Poisoning by peripheral vasodilators, undetermined
    - +7th **T46.7X5** Adverse effect of peripheral vasodilators
    - +7th **T46.7X6** Underdosing of peripheral vasodilators

- T46.8 Poisoning by, adverse effect of and underdosing of antivaricose drugs, including sclerosing agents
  - T46.8X Poisoning by, adverse effect of and underdosing of antivaricose drugs, including sclerosing agents
    - +7th T46.8X1 Poisoning by antivaricose drugs, including sclerosing agents, accidental (unintentional)
      - Poisoning by antivaricose drugs, including sclerosing agents NOS
    - +7th T46.8X2 Poisoning by antivaricose drugs, including sclerosing agents, intentional self-harm
    - +7th T46.8X3 Poisoning by antivaricose drugs, including sclerosing agents, assault
    - +7th T46.8X4 Poisoning by antivaricose drugs, including sclerosing agents, undetermined
    - +7th T46.8X5 Adverse effect of antivaricose drugs, including sclerosing agents
    - +7th T46.8X6 Underdosing of antivaricose drugs, including sclerosing agents
- T46.9 Poisoning by, adverse effect of and underdosing of other and unspecified agents primarily affecting the cardiovascular system
  - T46.90 Poisoning by, adverse effect of and underdosing of unspecified agents primarily affecting the cardiovascular system
    - +7th T46.901 Poisoning by unspecified agents primarily affecting the cardiovascular system, accidental (unintentional)
    - +7th T46.902 Poisoning by unspecified agents primarily affecting the cardiovascular system, intentional self-harm
    - +7th T46.903 Poisoning by unspecified agents primarily affecting the cardiovascular system, assault
    - +7th T46.904 Poisoning by unspecified agents primarily affecting the cardiovascular system, undetermined
    - +7th T46.905 Adverse effect of unspecified agents primarily affecting the cardiovascular system
    - +7th T46.906 Underdosing of unspecified agents primarily affecting the cardiovascular system
  - T46.99 Poisoning by, adverse effect of and underdosing of other agents primarily affecting the cardiovascular system
    - +7th T46.991 Poisoning by other agents primarily affecting the cardiovascular system, accidental (unintentional)
    - +7th T46.992 Poisoning by other agents primarily affecting the cardiovascular system, intentional self-harm
    - +7th T46.993 Poisoning by other agents primarily affecting the cardiovascular system, assault
    - +7th T46.994 Poisoning by other agents primarily affecting the cardiovascular system, undetermined
    - +7th T46.995 Adverse effect of other agents primarily affecting the cardiovascular system
    - +7th T46.996 Underdosing of other agents primarily affecting the cardiovascular system

T47 Poisoning by, adverse effect of and underdosing of agents primarily affecting the gastrointestinal system

> The appropriate 7th character is to be added to each code from category T47
> A initial encounter
> D subsequent encounter
> S sequela

- T47.0 Poisoning by, adverse effect of and underdosing of histamine H2-receptor blockers
  - T47.0X Poisoning by, adverse effect of and underdosing of histamine H2-receptor blockers
    - +7th T47.0X1 Poisoning by histamine H2-receptor blockers, accidental (unintentional)
      - Poisoning by histamine H2-receptor blockers NOS
    - +7th T47.0X2 Poisoning by histamine H2-receptor blockers, intentional self-harm
    - +7th T47.0X3 Poisoning by histamine H2-receptor blockers, assault
    - +7th T47.0X4 Poisoning by histamine H2-receptor blockers, undetermined
    - +7th T47.0X5 Adverse effect of histamine H2-receptor blockers
    - +7th T47.0X6 Underdosing of histamine H2-receptor blockers
- T47.1 Poisoning by, adverse effect of and underdosing of other antacids and anti-gastric-secretion drugs
  - T47.1X Poisoning by, adverse effect of and underdosing of other antacids and anti-gastric-secretion drugs
    - +7th T47.1X1 Poisoning by other antacids and anti-gastric-secretion drugs, accidental (unintentional)
      - Poisoning by other antacids and anti-gastric-secretion drugs NOS
    - +7th T47.1X2 Poisoning by other antacids and anti-gastric-secretion drugs, intentional self-harm
    - +7th T47.1X3 Poisoning by other antacids and anti-gastric-secretion drugs, assault
    - +7th T47.1X4 Poisoning by other antacids and anti-gastric-secretion drugs, undetermined
    - +7th T47.1X5 Adverse effect of other antacids and anti-gastric-secretion drugs
    - +7th T47.1X6 Underdosing of other antacids and anti-gastric-secretion drugs
- T47.2 Poisoning by, adverse effect of and underdosing of stimulant laxatives
  - T47.2X Poisoning by, adverse effect of and underdosing of stimulant laxatives
    - +7th T47.2X1 Poisoning by stimulant laxatives, accidental (unintentional)
      - Poisoning by stimulant laxatives NOS
    - +7th T47.2X2 Poisoning by stimulant laxatives, intentional self-harm
    - +7th T47.2X3 Poisoning by stimulant laxatives, assault
    - +7th T47.2X4 Poisoning by stimulant laxatives, undetermined
    - +7th T47.2X5 Adverse effect of stimulant laxatives
    - +7th T47.2X6 Underdosing of stimulant laxatives
- T47.3 Poisoning by, adverse effect of and underdosing of saline and osmotic laxatives
  - T47.3X Poisoning by and adverse effect of saline and osmotic laxatives
    - +7th T47.3X1 Poisoning by saline and osmotic laxatives, accidental (unintentional)
      - Poisoning by saline and osmotic laxatives NOS
    - +7th T47.3X2 Poisoning by saline and osmotic laxatives, intentional self-harm
    - +7th T47.3X3 Poisoning by saline and osmotic laxatives, assault
    - +7th T47.3X4 Poisoning by saline and osmotic laxatives, undetermined
    - +7th T47.3X5 Adverse effect of saline and osmotic laxatives
    - +7th T47.3X6 Underdosing of saline and osmotic laxatives

- T47.4 Poisoning by, adverse effect of and underdosing of other laxatives
  - T47.4X Poisoning by, adverse effect of and underdosing of other laxatives
    - +7th T47.4X1 Poisoning by other laxatives, accidental (unintentional)
      - Poisoning by other laxatives NOS
    - +7th T47.4X2 Poisoning by other laxatives, intentional self-harm
    - +7th T47.4X3 Poisoning by other laxatives, assault
    - +7th T47.4X4 Poisoning by other laxatives, undetermined
    - +7th T47.4X5 Adverse effect of other laxatives
    - +7th T47.4X6 Underdosing of other laxatives
- T47.5 Poisoning by, adverse effect of and underdosing of digestants
  - T47.5X Poisoning by, adverse effect of and underdosing of digestants
    - +7th T47.5X1 Poisoning by digestants, accidental (unintentional)
      - Poisoning by digestants NOS
    - +7th T47.5X2 Poisoning by digestants, intentional self-harm
    - +7th T47.5X3 Poisoning by digestants, assault
    - +7th T47.5X4 Poisoning by digestants, undetermined
    - +7th T47.5X5 Adverse effect of digestants
    - +7th T47.5X6 Underdosing of digestants
- T47.6 Poisoning by, adverse effect of and underdosing of antidiarrheal drugs
  - **Excludes2:** poisoning by, adverse effect of and underdosing of systemic antibiotics and other anti-infectives (T36-T37)
  - T47.6X Poisoning by, adverse effect of and underdosing of antidiarrheal drugs
    - +7th T47.6X1 Poisoning by antidiarrheal drugs, accidental (unintentional)
      - Poisoning by antidiarrheal drugs NOS
    - +7th T47.6X2 Poisoning by antidiarrheal drugs, intentional self-harm
    - +7th T47.6X3 Poisoning by antidiarrheal drugs, assault
    - +7th T47.6X4 Poisoning by antidiarrheal drugs, undetermined
    - +7th T47.6X5 Adverse effect of antidiarrheal drugs
    - +7th T47.6X6 Underdosing of antidiarrheal drugs
- T47.7 Poisoning by, adverse effect of and underdosing of emetics
  - T47.7X Poisoning by, adverse effect of and underdosing of emetics
    - +7th T47.7X1 Poisoning by emetics, accidental (unintentional)
      - Poisoning by emetics NOS
    - +7th T47.7X2 Poisoning by emetics, intentional self-harm
    - +7th T47.7X3 Poisoning by emetics, assault
    - +7th T47.7X4 Poisoning by emetics, undetermined
    - +7th T47.7X5 Adverse effect of emetics
    - +7th T47.7X6 Underdosing of emetics
- T47.8 Poisoning by, adverse effect of and underdosing of other agents primarily affecting gastrointestinal system
  - T47.8X Poisoning by, adverse effect of and underdosing of other agents primarily affecting gastrointestinal system
    - +7th T47.8X1 Poisoning by other agents primarily affecting gastrointestinal system, accidental (unintentional)
      - Poisoning by other agents primarily affecting gastrointestinal system NOS
    - +7th T47.8X2 Poisoning by other agents primarily affecting gastrointestinal system, intentional self-harm
    - +7th T47.8X3 Poisoning by other agents primarily affecting gastrointestinal system, assault
    - +7th T47.8X4 Poisoning by other agents primarily affecting gastrointestinal system, undetermined
    - +7th T47.8X5 Adverse effect of other agents primarily affecting gastrointestinal system
    - +7th T47.8X6 Underdosing of other agents primarily affecting gastrointestinal system
- T47.9 Poisoning by, adverse effect of and underdosing of unspecified agents primarily affecting the gastrointestinal system
  - X+7th T47.91 Poisoning by unspecified agents primarily affecting the gastrointestinal system, accidental (unintentional)
    - Poisoning by agents primarily affecting the gastrointestinal system NOS
  - X+7th T47.92 Poisoning by unspecified agents primarily affecting the gastrointestinal system, intentional self-harm
  - X+7th T47.93 Poisoning by unspecified agents primarily affecting the gastrointestinal system, assault
  - X+7th T47.94 Poisoning by unspecified agents primarily affecting the gastrointestinal system, undetermined
  - X+7th T47.95 Adverse effect of unspecified agents primarily affecting the gastrointestinal system
  - X+7th T47.96 Underdosing of unspecified agents primarily affecting the gastrointestinal system

T48 Poisoning by, adverse effect of and underdosing of agents primarily acting on smooth and skeletal muscles and the respiratory system

> The appropriate 7th character is to be added to each code from category T48
> A initial encounter
> D subsequent encounter
> S sequela

- T48.0 Poisoning by, adverse effect of and underdosing of oxytocic drugs
  - **Excludes1:** poisoning by, adverse effect of and underdosing of estrogens, progestogens and antagonists (T38.4-T38.6)
  - T48.0X Poisoning by, adverse effect of and underdosing of oxytocic drugs
    - +7th T48.0X1 Poisoning by oxytocic drugs, accidental (unintentional)
      - Poisoning by oxytocic drugs NOS
    - +7th T48.0X2 Poisoning by oxytocic drugs, intentional self-harm
    - +7th T48.0X3 Poisoning by oxytocic drugs, assault
    - +7th T48.0X4 Poisoning by oxytocic drugs, undetermined
    - +7th T48.0X5 Adverse effect of oxytocic drugs
    - +7th T48.0X6 Underdosing of oxytocic drugs
- T48.1 Poisoning by, adverse effect of and underdosing of skeletal muscle relaxants [neuromuscular blocking agents]
  - T48.1X Poisoning by, adverse effect of and underdosing of skeletal muscle relaxants [neuromuscular blocking agents]
    - +7th T48.1X1 Poisoning by skeletal muscle relaxants [neuromuscular blocking agents], accidental (unintentional)
      - Poisoning by skeletal muscle relaxants [neuromuscular blocking agents] NOS
    - +7th T48.1X2 Poisoning by skeletal muscle relaxants [neuromuscular blocking agents], intentional self-harm
    - +7th T48.1X3 Poisoning by skeletal muscle relaxants [neuromuscular blocking agents], assault
    - +7th T48.1X4 Poisoning by skeletal muscle relaxants [neuromuscular blocking agents], undetermined
    - +7th T48.1X5 Adverse effect of skeletal muscle relaxants [neuromuscular blocking agents]
    - +7th T48.1X6 Underdosing of skeletal muscle relaxants [neuromuscular blocking agents]
- T48.2 Poisoning by, adverse effect of and underdosing of other and unspecified drugs acting on muscles
  - T48.20 Poisoning by, adverse effect of and underdosing of unspecified drugs acting on muscles
    - +7th T48.201 Poisoning by unspecified drugs acting on muscles, accidental (unintentional)
      - Poisoning by unspecified drugs acting on muscles NOS
    - +7th T48.202 Poisoning by unspecified drugs acting on muscles, intentional self-harm

+7th **T48.203** Poisoning by unspecified drugs acting on muscles, assault
+7th **T48.204** Poisoning by unspecified drugs acting on muscles, undetermined
+7th T48.205 Adverse effect of unspecified drugs acting on muscles
+7th T48.206 Underdosing of unspecified drugs acting on muscles
+ T48.29 Poisoning by, adverse effect of and underdosing of other drugs acting on muscles
  +7th T48.291 Poisoning by other drugs acting on muscles, accidental (unintentional)
    Poisoning by other drugs acting on muscles NOS
  +7th **T48.292** Poisoning by other drugs acting on muscles, intentional self-harm
  +7th **T48.293** Poisoning by other drugs acting on muscles, assault
  +7th **T48.294** Poisoning by other drugs acting on muscles, undetermined
  +7th T48.295 Adverse effect of other drugs acting on muscles
  +7th T48.296 Underdosing of other drugs acting on muscles

+ **T48.3** Poisoning by, adverse effect of and underdosing of antitussives
  + **T48.3X** Poisoning by, adverse effect of and underdosing of antitussives
    +7th T48.3X1 Poisoning by antitussives, accidental (unintentional)
      Poisoning by antitussives NOS
    +7th **T48.3X2** Poisoning by antitussives, intentional self-harm
    +7th **T48.3X3** Poisoning by antitussives, assault
    +7th **T48.3X4** Poisoning by antitussives, undetermined
    +7th T48.3X5 Adverse effect of antitussives
    +7th T48.3X6 Underdosing of antitussives

+ **T48.4** Poisoning by, adverse effect of and underdosing of expectorants
  + **T48.4X** Poisoning by, adverse effect of and underdosing of expectorants
    +7th T48.4X1 Poisoning by expectorants, accidental (unintentional)
      Poisoning by expectorants NOS
    +7th **T48.4X2** Poisoning by expectorants, intentional self-harm
    +7th **T48.4X3** Poisoning by expectorants, assault
    +7th **T48.4X4** Poisoning by expectorants, undetermined
    +7th T48.4X5 Adverse effect of expectorants
    +7th T48.4X6 Underdosing of expectorants

+ **T48.5** Poisoning by, adverse effect of and underdosing of other anti-common-cold drugs
  Poisoning by, adverse effect of and underdosing of decongestants
  Excludes2: *poisoning by, adverse effect of and underdosing of antipyretics, NEC (T39.9-)*
  poisoning by, adverse effect of and underdosing of non-steroidal antiinflammatory drugs (T39.3-)
  poisoning by, adverse effect of and underdosing of salicylates (T39.0-)
  + **T48.5X** Poisoning by, adverse effect of and underdosing of other anti-common-cold drugs
    +7th T48.5X1 Poisoning by other anti-common-cold drugs, accidental (unintentional)
      Poisoning by other anti-common-cold drugs NOS
    +7th **T48.5X2** Poisoning by other anti-common-cold drugs, intentional self-harm
    +7th **T48.5X3** Poisoning by other anti-common-cold drugs, assault
    +7th **T48.5X4** Poisoning by other anti-common-cold drugs, undetermined
    +7th T48.5X5 Adverse effect of other anti-common-cold drugs
    +7th T48.5X6 Underdosing of other anti-common-cold drugs

+ **T48.6** Poisoning by, adverse effect of and underdosing of antiasthmatics, not elsewhere classified
  Poisoning by, adverse effect of and underdosing of beta-adrenoreceptor agonists used in asthma therapy
  Excludes1: *poisoning by, adverse effect of and underdosing of beta-adrenoreceptor agonists not used in asthma therapy (T44.5)*
  poisoning by, adverse effect of and underdosing of anterior pituitary [adenohypophyseal] hormones (T38.8)
  + **T48.6X** Poisoning by, adverse effect of and underdosing of antiasthmatics
    +7th T48.6X1 Poisoning by antiasthmatics, accidental (unintentional)
      Poisoning by antiasthmatics NOS
    +7th **T48.6X2** Poisoning by antiasthmatics, intentional self-harm
    +7th T48.6X3 Poisoning by antiasthmatics, assault
    +7th T48.6X4 Poisoning by antiasthmatics, undetermined
    +7th T48.6X5 Adverse effect of antiasthmatics
    +7th T48.6X6 Underdosing of antiasthmatics

+ **T48.9** Poisoning by, adverse effect of and underdosing of other and unspecified agents primarily acting on the respiratory system
  + **T48.90** Poisoning by, adverse effect of and underdosing of unspecified agents primarily acting on the respiratory system
    +7th T48.901 Poisoning by unspecified agents primarily acting on the respiratory system, accidental (unintentional)
    +7th **T48.902** Poisoning by unspecified agents primarily acting on the respiratory system, intentional self-harm
    +7th T48.903 Poisoning by unspecified agents primarily acting on the respiratory system, assault
    +7th T48.904 Poisoning by unspecified agents primarily acting on the respiratory system, undetermined
    +7th T48.905 Adverse effect of unspecified agents primarily acting on the respiratory system
    +7th T48.906 Underdosing of unspecified agents primarily acting on the respiratory system
  + **T48.99** Poisoning by, adverse effect of and underdosing of other agents primarily acting on the respiratory system
    +7th T48.991 Poisoning by other agents primarily acting on the respiratory system, accidental (unintentional)
    +7th **T48.992** Poisoning by other agents primarily acting on the respiratory system, intentional self-harm
    +7th T48.993 Poisoning by other agents primarily acting on the respiratory system, assault
    +7th T48.994 Poisoning by other agents primarily acting on the respiratory system, undetermined
    +7th T48.995 Adverse effect of other agents primarily acting on the respiratory system
    +7th T48.996 Underdosing of other agents primarily acting on the respiratory system

T49 **Poisoning by, adverse effect of and underdosing of topical agents primarily affecting skin and mucous membrane and by ophthalmological, otorhinolaryngological and dental drugs**

Includes: poisoning by, adverse effect of and underdosing of glucocorticoids, topically used

The appropriate 7th character is to be added to each code from category T49
A   initial encounter
D   subsequent encounter
S   sequela

- T49.0 Poisoning by, adverse effect of and underdosing of local antifungal, anti-infective and anti-inflammatory drugs
  - T49.0X Poisoning by, adverse effect of and underdosing of local antifungal, anti-infective and anti-inflammatory drugs
    - +7th T49.0X1 Poisoning by local antifungal, anti-infective and anti-inflammatory drugs, accidental (unintentional)
      - Poisoning by local antifungal, anti-infective and anti-inflammatory drugs NOS
    - +7th T49.0X2 Poisoning by local antifungal, anti-infective and anti-inflammatory drugs, intentional self-harm
    - +7th T49.0X3 Poisoning by local antifungal, anti-infective and anti-inflammatory drugs, assault
    - +7th T49.0X4 Poisoning by local antifungal, anti-infective and anti-inflammatory drugs, undetermined
    - +7th T49.0X5 Adverse effect of local antifungal, anti-infective and anti-inflammatory drugs
    - +7th T49.0X6 Underdosing of local antifungal, anti-infective and anti-inflammatory drugs
- T49.1 Poisoning by, adverse effect of and underdosing of antipruritics
  - T49.1X Poisoning by, adverse effect of and underdosing of antipruritics
    - +7th T49.1X1 Poisoning by antipruritics, accidental (unintentional)
      - Poisoning by antipruritics NOS
    - +7th T49.1X2 Poisoning by antipruritics, intentional self-harm
    - +7th T49.1X3 Poisoning by antipruritics, assault
    - +7th T49.1X4 Poisoning by antipruritics, undetermined
    - +7th T49.1X5 Adverse effect of antipruritics
    - +7th T49.1X6 Underdosing of antipruritics
- T49.2 Poisoning by, adverse effect of and underdosing of local astringents and local detergents
  - T49.2X Poisoning by, adverse effect of and underdosing of local astringents and local detergents
    - +7th T49.2X1 Poisoning by local astringents and local detergents, accidental (unintentional)
      - Poisoning by local astringents and local detergents NOS
    - +7th T49.2X2 Poisoning by local astringents and local detergents, intentional self-harm
    - +7th T49.2X3 Poisoning by local astringents and local detergents, assault
    - +7th T49.2X4 Poisoning by local astringents and local detergents, undetermined
    - +7th T49.2X5 Adverse effect of local astringents and local detergents
    - +7th T49.2X6 Underdosing of local astringents and local detergents
- T49.3 Poisoning by, adverse effect of and underdosing of emollients, demulcents and protectants
  - T49.3X Poisoning by, adverse effect of and underdosing of emollients, demulcents and protectants
    - +7th T49.3X1 Poisoning by emollients, demulcents and protectants, accidental (unintentional)
      - Poisoning by emollients, demulcents and protectants NOS
    - +7th T49.3X2 Poisoning by emollients, demulcents and protectants, intentional self-harm
    - +7th T49.3X3 Poisoning by emollients, demulcents and protectants, assault
    - +7th T49.3X4 Poisoning by emollients, demulcents and protectants, undetermined
    - +7th T49.3X5 Adverse effect of emollients, demulcents and protectants
    - +7th T49.3X6 Underdosing of emollients, demulcents and protectants
- T49.4 Poisoning by, adverse effect of and underdosing of keratolytics, keratoplastics, and other hair treatment drugs and preparations
  - T49.4X Poisoning by, adverse effect of and underdosing of keratolytics, keratoplastics, and other hair treatment drugs and preparations
    - +7th T49.4X1 Poisoning by keratolytics, keratoplastics, and other hair treatment drugs and preparations, accidental (unintentional)
      - Poisoning by keratolytics, keratoplastics, and other hair treatment drugs and preparations NOS
    - +7th T49.4X2 Poisoning by keratolytics, keratoplastics, and other hair treatment drugs and preparations, intentional self-harm
    - +7th T49.4X3 Poisoning by keratolytics, keratoplastics, and other hair treatment drugs and preparations, assault
    - +7th T49.4X4 Poisoning by keratolytics, keratoplastics, and other hair treatment drugs and preparations, undetermined
    - +7th T49.4X5 Adverse effect of keratolytics, keratoplastics, and other hair treatment drugs and preparations
    - +7th T49.4X6 Underdosing of keratolytics, keratoplastics, and other hair treatment drugs and preparations
- T49.5 Poisoning by, adverse effect of and underdosing of ophthalmological drugs and preparations
  - T49.5X Poisoning by, adverse effect of and underdosing of ophthalmological drugs and preparations
    - +7th T49.5X1 Poisoning by ophthalmological drugs and preparations, accidental (unintentional)
      - Poisoning by ophthalmological drugs and preparations NOS
    - +7th T49.5X2 Poisoning by ophthalmological drugs and preparations, intentional self-harm
    - +7th T49.5X3 Poisoning by ophthalmological drugs and preparations, assault
    - +7th T49.5X4 Poisoning by ophthalmological drugs and preparations, undetermined
    - +7th T49.5X5 Adverse effect of ophthalmological drugs and preparations
    - +7th T49.5X6 Underdosing of ophthalmological drugs and preparations
- T49.6 Poisoning by, adverse effect of and underdosing of otorhinolaryngological drugs and preparations
  - T49.6X Poisoning by, adverse effect of and underdosing of otorhinolaryngological drugs and preparations
    - +7th T49.6X1 Poisoning by otorhinolaryngological drugs and preparations, accidental (unintentional)
      - Poisoning by otorhinolaryngological drugs and preparations NOS
    - +7th T49.6X2 Poisoning by otorhinolaryngological drugs and preparations, intentional self-harm
    - +7th T49.6X3 Poisoning by otorhinolaryngological drugs and preparations, assault
    - +7th T49.6X4 Poisoning by otorhinolaryngological drugs and preparations, undetermined
    - +7th T49.6X5 Adverse effect of otorhinolaryngological drugs and preparations
    - +7th T49.6X6 Underdosing of otorhinolaryngological drugs and preparations
- T49.7 Poisoning by, adverse effect of and underdosing of dental drugs, topically applied
  - T49.7X Poisoning by, adverse effect of and underdosing of dental drugs, topically applied
    - +7th T49.7X1 Poisoning by dental drugs, topically applied, accidental (unintentional)
      - Poisoning by dental drugs, topically applied NOS
    - +7th T49.7X2 Poisoning by dental drugs, topically applied, intentional self-harm
    - +7th T49.7X3 Poisoning by dental drugs, topically applied, assault

+7th **T49.7X4** Poisoning by dental drugs, topically applied, undetermined
+7th **T49.7X5** Adverse effect of dental drugs, topically applied
+7th **T49.7X6** Underdosing of dental drugs, topically applied

+ **T49.8** Poisoning by, adverse effect of and underdosing of other topical agents
  Poisoning by, adverse effect of and underdosing of spermicides
  + **T49.8X** Poisoning by, adverse effect of and underdosing of other topical agents
    +7th **T49.8X1** Poisoning by other topical agents, accidental (unintentional)
      Poisoning by other topical agents NOS
    +7th **T49.8X2** Poisoning by other topical agents, intentional self-harm
    +7th **T49.8X3** Poisoning by other topical agents, assault
    +7th **T49.8X4** Poisoning by other topical agents, undetermined
    +7th **T49.8X5** Adverse effect of other topical agents
    +7th **T49.8X6** Underdosing of other topical agents

+ **T49.9** Poisoning by, adverse effect of and underdosing of unspecified topical agent
  X+7th **T49.91** Poisoning by unspecified topical agent, accidental (unintentional)
  X+7th **T49.92** Poisoning by unspecified topical agent, intentional self-harm
  X+7th **T49.93** Poisoning by unspecified topical agent, assault
  X+7th **T49.94** Poisoning by unspecified topical agent, undetermined
  X+7th **T49.95** Adverse effect of unspecified topical agent
  X+7th **T49.96** Underdosing of unspecified topical agent

T50 Poisoning by, adverse effect of and underdosing of diuretics and other and unspecified drugs, medicaments and biological substances

> The appropriate 7th character is to be added to each code from category T50
> A initial encounter
> D subsequent encounter
> S sequela

+ **T50.0** Poisoning by, adverse effect of and underdosing of mineralocorticoids and their antagonists
  + **T50.0X** Poisoning by, adverse effect of and underdosing of mineralocorticoids and their antagonists
    +7th **T50.0X1** Poisoning by mineralocorticoids and their antagonists, accidental (unintentional)
      Poisoning by mineralocorticoids and their antagonists NOS
    +7th **T50.0X2** Poisoning by mineralocorticoids and their antagonists, intentional self-harm
    +7th **T50.0X3** Poisoning by mineralocorticoids and their antagonists, assault
    +7th **T50.0X4** Poisoning by mineralocorticoids and their antagonists, undetermined
    +7th **T50.0X5** Adverse effect of mineralocorticoids and their antagonists
    +7th **T50.0X6** Underdosing of mineralocorticoids and their antagonists

+ **T50.1** Poisoning by, adverse effect of and underdosing of loop [high-ceiling] diuretics
  + **T50.1X** Poisoning by, adverse effect of and underdosing of loop [high-ceiling] diuretics
    +7th **T50.1X1** Poisoning by loop [high-ceiling] diuretics, accidental (unintentional)
      Poisoning by loop [high-ceiling] diuretics NOS
    +7th **T50.1X2** Poisoning by loop [high-ceiling] diuretics, intentional self-harm
    +7th **T50.1X3** Poisoning by loop [high-ceiling] diuretics, assault
    +7th **T50.1X4** Poisoning by loop [high-ceiling] diuretics, undetermined
    +7th **T50.1X5** Adverse effect of loop [high-ceiling] diuretics
    +7th **T50.1X6** Underdosing of loop [high-ceiling] diuretics

+ **T50.2** Poisoning by, adverse effect of and underdosing of carbonic-anhydrase inhibitors, benzothiadiazides and other diuretics
  Poisoning by, adverse effect of and underdosing of acetazolamide
  + **T50.2X** Poisoning by, adverse effect of and underdosing of carbonic-anhydrase inhibitors, benzothiadiazides and other diuretics
    +7th **T50.2X1** Poisoning by carbonic-anhydrase inhibitors, benzothiadiazides and other diuretics, accidental (unintentional)
      Poisoning by carbonic-anhydrase inhibitors, benzothiadiazides and other diuretics NOS
    +7th **T50.2X2** Poisoning by carbonic-anhydrase inhibitors, benzothiadiazides and other diuretics, intentional self-harm
    +7th **T50.2X3** Poisoning by carbonic-anhydrase inhibitors, benzothiadiazides and other diuretics, assault
    +7th **T50.2X4** Poisoning by carbonic-anhydrase inhibitors, benzothiadiazides and other diuretics, undetermined
    +7th **T50.2X5** Adverse effect of carbonic-anhydrase inhibitors, benzothiadiazides and other diuretics
    +7th **T50.2X6** Underdosing of carbonic-anhydrase inhibitors, benzothiadiazides and other diuretics

+ **T50.3** Poisoning by, adverse effect of and underdosing of electrolytic, caloric and water-balance agents
  Poisoning by, adverse effect of and underdosing of oral rehydration salts
  + **T50.3X** Poisoning by, adverse effect of and underdosing of electrolytic, caloric and water-balance agents
    +7th **T50.3X1** Poisoning by electrolytic, caloric and water-balance agents, accidental (unintentional)
      Poisoning by electrolytic, caloric and water-balance agents NOS
    +7th **T50.3X2** Poisoning by electrolytic, caloric and water-balance agents, intentional self-harm
    +7th **T50.3X3** Poisoning by electrolytic, caloric and water-balance agents, assault
    +7th **T50.3X4** Poisoning by electrolytic, caloric and water-balance agents, undetermined
    +7th **T50.3X5** Adverse effect of electrolytic, caloric and water-balance agents
      AHA CC: 2Q, 2022, 10-11
    +7th **T50.3X6** Underdosing of electrolytic, caloric and water-balance agents

+ **T50.4** Poisoning by, adverse effect of and underdosing of drugs affecting uric acid metabolism
  + **T50.4X** Poisoning by, adverse effect of and underdosing of drugs affecting uric acid metabolism
    +7th **T50.4X1** Poisoning by drugs affecting uric acid metabolism, accidental (unintentional)
      Poisoning by drugs affecting uric acid metabolism NOS
    +7th **T50.4X2** Poisoning by drugs affecting uric acid metabolism, intentional self-harm
    +7th **T50.4X3** Poisoning by drugs affecting uric acid metabolism, assault
    +7th **T50.4X4** Poisoning by drugs affecting uric acid metabolism, undetermined
    +7th **T50.4X5** Adverse effect of drugs affecting uric acid metabolism
    +7th **T50.4X6** Underdosing of drugs affecting uric acid metabolism

+ **T50.5** Poisoning by, adverse effect of and underdosing of appetite depressants
  + **T50.5X** Poisoning by, adverse effect of and underdosing of appetite depressants
    +7th **T50.5X1** Poisoning by appetite depressants, accidental (unintentional)
      Poisoning by appetite depressants NOS
    +7th **T50.5X2** Poisoning by appetite depressants, intentional self-harm
    +7th **T50.5X3** Poisoning by appetite depressants, assault
    +7th **T50.5X4** Poisoning by appetite depressants, undetermined

- +7th **T50.5X5** Adverse effect of appetite depressants
- +7th **T50.5X6** Underdosing of appetite depressants
+ **T50.6** Poisoning by, adverse effect of and underdosing of antidotes and chelating agents
  - *Poisoning by, adverse effect of and underdosing of alcohol deterrents*
  + **T50.6X** Poisoning by, adverse effect of and underdosing of antidotes and chelating agents
    - +7th **T50.6X1** Poisoning by antidotes and chelating agents, accidental (unintentional)
      - *Poisoning by antidotes and chelating agents NOS*
    - +7th **T50.6X2** Poisoning by antidotes and chelating agents, intentional self-harm
    - +7th **T50.6X3** Poisoning by antidotes and chelating agents, assault
    - +7th **T50.6X4** Poisoning by antidotes and chelating agents, undetermined
    - +7th **T50.6X5** Adverse effect of antidotes and chelating agents
    - +7th **T50.6X6** Underdosing of antidotes and chelating agents
+ **T50.7** Poisoning by, adverse effect of and underdosing of analeptics and opioid receptor antagonists
  + **T50.7X** Poisoning by, adverse effect of and underdosing of analeptics and opioid receptor antagonists
    - +7th **T50.7X1** Poisoning by analeptics and opioid receptor antagonists, accidental (unintentional)
      - *Poisoning by analeptics and opioid receptor antagonists NOS*
    - +7th **T50.7X2** Poisoning by analeptics and opioid receptor antagonists, intentional self-harm
    - +7th **T50.7X3** Poisoning by analeptics and opioid receptor antagonists, assault
    - +7th **T50.7X4** Poisoning by analeptics and opioid receptor antagonists, undetermined
    - +7th **T50.7X5** Adverse effect of analeptics and opioid receptor antagonists
    - +7th **T50.7X6** Underdosing of analeptics and opioid receptor antagonists
+ **T50.8** Poisoning by, adverse effect of and underdosing of diagnostic agents
  + **T50.8X** Poisoning by, adverse effect of and underdosing of diagnostic agents
    - +7th **T50.8X1** Poisoning by diagnostic agents, accidental (unintentional)
      - *Poisoning by diagnostic agents NOS*
    - +7th **T50.8X2** Poisoning by diagnostic agents, intentional self-harm
    - +7th **T50.8X3** Poisoning by diagnostic agents, assault
    - +7th **T50.8X4** Poisoning by diagnostic agents, undetermined
    - +7th **T50.8X5** Adverse effect of diagnostic agents
      - *AHA CC: 3Q, 2021, 9-10; 4Q, 2022, 33*
    - +7th **T50.8X6** Underdosing of diagnostic agents
+ **T50.A** Poisoning by, adverse effect of and underdosing of bacterial vaccines
  + **T50.A1** Poisoning by, adverse effect of and underdosing of pertussis vaccine, including combinations with a pertussis component
    - +7th **T50.A11** Poisoning by pertussis vaccine, including combinations with a pertussis component, accidental (unintentional)
    - +7th **T50.A12** Poisoning by pertussis vaccine, including combinations with a pertussis component, intentional self-harm
    - +7th **T50.A13** Poisoning by pertussis vaccine, including combinations with a pertussis component, assault
    - +7th **T50.A14** Poisoning by pertussis vaccine, including combinations with a pertussis component, undetermined
    - +7th **T50.A15** Adverse effect of pertussis vaccine, including combinations with a pertussis component
    - +7th **T50.A16** Underdosing of pertussis vaccine, including combinations with a pertussis component
  + **T50.A2** Poisoning by, adverse effect of and underdosing of mixed bacterial vaccines without a pertussis component
    - +7th **T50.A21** Poisoning by mixed bacterial vaccines without a pertussis component, accidental (unintentional)
    - +7th **T50.A22** Poisoning by mixed bacterial vaccines without a pertussis component, intentional self-harm
    - +7th **T50.A23** Poisoning by mixed bacterial vaccines without a pertussis component, assault
    - +7th **T50.A24** Poisoning by mixed bacterial vaccines without a pertussis component, undetermined
    - +7th **T50.A25** Adverse effect of mixed bacterial vaccines without a pertussis component
    - +7th **T50.A26** Underdosing of mixed bacterial vaccines without a pertussis component
  + **T50.A9** Poisoning by, adverse effect of and underdosing of other bacterial vaccines
    - +7th **T50.A91** Poisoning by other bacterial vaccines, accidental (unintentional)
    - +7th **T50.A92** Poisoning by other bacterial vaccines, intentional self-harm
    - +7th **T50.A93** Poisoning by other bacterial vaccines, assault
    - +7th **T50.A94** Poisoning by other bacterial vaccines, undetermined
    - +7th **T50.A95** Adverse effect of other bacterial vaccines
    - +7th **T50.A96** Underdosing of other bacterial vaccines
+ **T50.B** Poisoning by, adverse effect of and underdosing of viral vaccines
  + **T50.B1** Poisoning by, adverse effect of and underdosing of smallpox vaccines
    - +7th **T50.B11** Poisoning by smallpox vaccines, accidental (unintentional)
    - +7th **T50.B12** Poisoning by smallpox vaccines, intentional self-harm
    - +7th **T50.B13** Poisoning by smallpox vaccines, assault
    - +7th **T50.B14** Poisoning by smallpox vaccines, undetermined
    - +7th **T50.B15** Adverse effect of smallpox vaccines
    - +7th **T50.B16** Underdosing of smallpox vaccines
  + **T50.B9** Poisoning by, adverse effect of and underdosing of other viral vaccines
    - +7th **T50.B91** Poisoning by other viral vaccines, accidental (unintentional)
    - +7th **T50.B92** Poisoning by other viral vaccines, intentional self-harm
    - +7th **T50.B93** Poisoning by other viral vaccines, assault
    - +7th **T50.B94** Poisoning by other viral vaccines, undetermined
    - +7th **T50.B95** Adverse effect of other viral vaccines
      - *AHA CC: 1Q, 2021, 43-44*
    - +7th **T50.B96** Underdosing of other viral vaccines
+ **T50.Z** Poisoning by, adverse effect of and underdosing of other vaccines and biological substances
  + **T50.Z1** Poisoning by, adverse effect of and underdosing of immunoglobulin
    - +7th **T50.Z11** Poisoning by immunoglobulin, accidental (unintentional)
    - +7th **T50.Z12** Poisoning by immunoglobulin, intentional self-harm
    - +7th **T50.Z13** Poisoning by immunoglobulin, assault
    - +7th **T50.Z14** Poisoning by immunoglobulin, undetermined
    - +7th **T50.Z15** Adverse effect of immunoglobulin
    - +7th **T50.Z16** Underdosing of immunoglobulin
  + **T50.Z9** Poisoning by, adverse effect of and underdosing of other vaccines and biological substances
    - +7th **T50.Z91** Poisoning by other vaccines and biological substances, accidental (unintentional)
    - +7th **T50.Z92** Poisoning by other vaccines and biological substances, intentional self-harm
    - +7th **T50.Z93** Poisoning by other vaccines and biological substances, assault
    - +7th **T50.Z94** Poisoning by other vaccines and biological substances, undetermined

- +7th **T50.Z95** Adverse effect of other vaccines and biological substances
  - *AHA CC: 1Q, 2020, 18-19*
- +7th **T50.Z96** Underdosing of other vaccines and biological substances
- + **T50.9** Poisoning by, adverse effect of and underdosing of other and unspecified drugs, medicaments and biological substances
  - + **T50.90** Poisoning by, adverse effect of and underdosing of unspecified drugs, medicaments and biological substances
    - +7th **T50.901** Poisoning by unspecified drugs, medicaments and biological substances, accidental (unintentional)
      - *AHA CC: 1Q, 2015, 3-21*
    - +7th **T50.902** Poisoning by unspecified drugs, medicaments and biological substances, intentional self-harm
    - +7th **T50.903** Poisoning by unspecified drugs, medicaments and biological substances, assault
    - +7th **T50.904** Poisoning by unspecified drugs, medicaments and biological substances, undetermined
    - +7th **T50.905** Adverse effect of unspecified drugs, medicaments and biological substances
    - +7th **T50.906** Underdosing of unspecified drugs, medicaments and biological substances
  - + **T50.91** Poisoning by, adverse effect of and underdosing of multiple unspecified drugs, medicaments and biological substances
    - Multiple drug ingestion NOS
    - Code also any specific drugs, medicaments and biological substances
    - *AHA CC: 4Q, 2019, 17*
    - **T50.911** Poisoning by multiple unspecified drugs, medicaments and biological substances, accidental (unintentional)
    - **T50.912** Poisoning by multiple unspecified drugs, medicaments and biological substances, intentional self-harm
    - **T50.913** Poisoning by multiple unspecified drugs, medicaments and biological substances, assault
    - **T50.914** Poisoning by multiple unspecified drugs, medicaments and biological substances, undetermined
    - **T50.915** Adverse effect of multiple unspecified drugs, medicaments and biological substances
    - **T50.916** Underdosing of multiple unspecified drugs, medicaments and biological substance
  - + **T50.99** Poisoning by, adverse effect of and underdosing of other drugs, medicaments and biological substances
    - +7th **T50.991** Poisoning by other drugs, medicaments and biological substances, accidental (unintentional)
    - +7th **T50.992** Poisoning by other drugs, medicaments and biological substances, intentional self-harm
    - +7th **T50.993** Poisoning by other drugs, medicaments and biological substances, assault
    - +7th **T50.994** Poisoning by other drugs, medicaments and biological substances, undetermined
    - +7th **T50.995** Adverse effect of other drugs, medicaments and biological substances
    - +7th **T50.996** Underdosing of other drugs, medicaments and biological substances

Toxic effects of substances chiefly nonmedicinal as to source (T51-T65)

NOTE When no intent is indicated code to accidental. Undetermined intent is only for use when there is specific documentation in the record that the intent of the toxic effect cannot be determined.

Use additional code(s):
for all associated manifestations of toxic effect, such as: respiratory conditions due to external agents (J60-J70)

personal history of foreign body fully removed (Z87.821)
to identify any retained foreign body, if applicable (Z18.-)

Excludes1: contact with and (suspected) exposure to toxic substances (Z77.-)
Review coding guideline C.19.e

T51 Toxic effect of alcohol

> The appropriate 7th character is to be added to each code from category T51
> A initial encounter
> D subsequent encounter
> S sequela

- + **T51.0** Toxic effect of ethanol
  - Toxic effect of ethyl alcohol
  - **Excludes2:** acute alcohol intoxication or 'hangover' effects
    drunkenness (F10.129, F10.229, F10.929)
    pathological (F10.129, F10.229, F10.929)
    alcohol intoxication (F10.129, F10.229, F10.929)
  - + **T51.0X** Toxic effect of ethanol
    - +7th **T51.0X1** Toxic effect of ethanol, accidental (unintentional)
      - Toxic effect of ethanol NOS
    - +7th **T51.0X2** Toxic effect of ethanol, intentional self-harm
    - +7th **T51.0X3** Toxic effect of ethanol, assault
    - +7th **T51.0X4** Toxic effect of ethanol, undetermined
- + **T51.1** Toxic effect of methanol
  - Toxic effect of methyl alcohol
  - + **T51.1X** Toxic effect of methanol
    - +7th **T51.1X1** Toxic effect of methanol, accidental (unintentional)
      - Toxic effect of methanol NOS
    - +7th **T51.1X2** Toxic effect of methanol, intentional self-harm
    - +7th **T51.1X3** Toxic effect of methanol, assault
    - +7th **T51.1X4** Toxic effect of methanol, undetermined
- + **T51.2** Toxic effect of 2-Propanol
  - Toxic effect of isopropyl alcohol
  - + **T51.2X** Toxic effect of 2-Propanol
    - +7th **T51.2X1** Toxic effect of 2-Propanol, accidental (unintentional)
      - Toxic effect of 2-Propanol NOS
    - +7th **T51.2X2** Toxic effect of 2-Propanol, intentional self-harm
    - +7th **T51.2X3** Toxic effect of 2-Propanol, assault
    - +7th **T51.2X4** Toxic effect of 2-Propanol, undetermined
- + **T51.3** Toxic effect of fusel oil
  - Toxic effect of amyl alcohol
  - Toxic effect of butyl [1-butanol] alcohol
  - Toxic effect of propyl [1-propanol] alcohol
  - + **T51.3X** Toxic effect of fusel oil
    - +7th **T51.3X1** Toxic effect of fusel oil, accidental (unintentional)
      - Toxic effect of fusel oil NOS
    - +7th **T51.3X2** Toxic effect of fusel oil, intentional self-harm
    - +7th **T51.3X3** Toxic effect of fusel oil, assault
    - +7th **T51.3X4** Toxic effect of fusel oil, undetermined
- + **T51.8** Toxic effect of other alcohols
  - + **T51.8X** Toxic effect of other alcohols
    - +7th **T51.8X1** Toxic effect of other alcohols, accidental (unintentional)
      - Toxic effect of other alcohols NOS
    - +7th **T51.8X2** Toxic effect of other alcohols, intentional self-harm
    - +7th **T51.8X3** Toxic effect of other alcohols, assault
    - +7th **T51.8X4** Toxic effect of other alcohols, undetermined
- + **T51.9** Toxic effect of unspecified alcohol
  - X+7th **T51.91** Toxic effect of unspecified alcohol, accidental (unintentional)
  - X+7th **T51.92** Toxic effect of unspecified alcohol, intentional self-harm
  - X+7th **T51.93** Toxic effect of unspecified alcohol, assault
  - X+7th **T51.94** Toxic effect of unspecified alcohol, undetermined

T52 Toxic effect of organic solvents

Excludes1: halogen derivatives of aliphatic and aromatic hydrocarbons (T53.-)

The appropriate 7th character is to be added to each code from category T52
- A initial encounter
- D subsequent encounter
- S sequela

+ **T52.0 Toxic effects of petroleum products**
  - Toxic effects of gasoline [petrol]
  - Toxic effects of kerosene [paraffin oil]
  - Toxic effects of paraffin wax
  - Toxic effects of ether petroleum
  - Toxic effects of naphtha petroleum
  - Toxic effects of spirit petroleum
  - + **T52.0X Toxic effects of petroleum products**
    - +7th **T52.0X1** Toxic effect of petroleum products, accidental (unintentional)
      - Toxic effects of petroleum products NOS
    - +7th **T52.0X2** Toxic effect of petroleum products, intentional self-harm
    - +7th **T52.0X3** Toxic effect of petroleum products, assault
    - +7th **T52.0X4** Toxic effect of petroleum products, undetermined

+ **T52.1 Toxic effects of benzene**
  Excludes1: homologues of benzene (T52.2)
  nitroderivatives and aminoderivatives of benzene and its homologues (T65.3)
  - + **T52.1X Toxic effects of benzene**
    - +7th **T52.1X1** Toxic effect of benzene, accidental (unintentional)
      - Toxic effects of benzene NOS
    - +7th **T52.1X2** Toxic effect of benzene, intentional self-harm
    - +7th **T52.1X3** Toxic effect of benzene, assault
    - +7th **T52.1X4** Toxic effect of benzene, undetermined

+ **T52.2 Toxic effects of homologues of benzene**
  - Toxic effects of toluene [methylbenzene]
  - Toxic effects of xylene [dimethylbenzene]
  - + **T52.2X Toxic effects of homologues of benzene**
    - +7th **T52.2X1** Toxic effect of homologues of benzene, accidental (unintentional)
      - Toxic effects of homologues of benzene NOS
    - +7th **T52.2X2** Toxic effect of homologues of benzene, intentional self-harm
    - +7th **T52.2X3** Toxic effect of homologues of benzene, assault
    - +7th **T52.2X4** Toxic effect of homologues of benzene, undetermined

+ **T52.3 Toxic effects of glycols**
  - + **T52.3X Toxic effects of glycols**
    - +7th **T52.3X1** Toxic effect of glycols, accidental (unintentional)
      - Toxic effects of glycols NOS
    - +7th **T52.3X2** Toxic effect of glycols, intentional self-harm
    - +7th **T52.3X3** Toxic effect of glycols, assault
    - +7th **T52.3X4** Toxic effect of glycols, undetermined

+ **T52.4 Toxic effects of ketones**
  - + **T52.4X Toxic effects of ketones**
    - +7th **T52.4X1** Toxic effect of ketones, accidental (unintentional)
      - Toxic effects of ketones NOS
    - +7th **T52.4X2** Toxic effect of ketones, intentional self-harm
    - +7th **T52.4X3** Toxic effect of ketones, assault
    - +7th **T52.4X4** Toxic effect of ketones, undetermined

+ **T52.8 Toxic effects of other organic solvents**
  - + **T52.8X Toxic effects of other organic solvents**
    - +7th **T52.8X1** Toxic effect of other organic solvents, accidental (unintentional)
      - Toxic effects of other organic solvents NOS
    - +7th **T52.8X2** Toxic effect of other organic solvents, intentional self-harm
    - +7th **T52.8X3** Toxic effect of other organic solvents, assault
    - +7th **T52.8X4** Toxic effect of other organic solvents, undetermined

+ **T52.9 Toxic effects of unspecified organic solvent**
  - X+7th **T52.91** Toxic effect of unspecified organic solvent, accidental (unintentional)
  - X+7th **T52.92** Toxic effect of unspecified organic solvent, intentional self-harm
  - X+7th **T52.93** Toxic effect of unspecified organic solvent, assault
  - X+7th **T52.94** Toxic effect of unspecified organic solvent, undetermined

T53 Toxic effect of halogen derivatives of aliphatic and aromatic hydrocarbons

The appropriate 7th character is to be added to each code from category T53
- A initial encounter
- D subsequent encounter
- S sequela

+ **T53.0 Toxic effects of carbon tetrachloride**
  - Toxic effects of tetrachloromethane
  - + **T53.0X Toxic effects of carbon tetrachloride**
    - +7th **T53.0X1** Toxic effect of carbon tetrachloride, accidental (unintentional)
      - Toxic effects of carbon tetrachloride NOS
    - +7th **T53.0X2** Toxic effect of carbon tetrachloride, intentional self-harm
    - +7th **T53.0X3** Toxic effect of carbon tetrachloride, assault
    - +7th **T53.0X4** Toxic effect of carbon tetrachloride, undetermined

+ **T53.1 Toxic effects of chloroform**
  - Toxic effects of trichloromethane
  - + **T53.1X Toxic effects of chloroform**
    - +7th **T53.1X1** Toxic effect of chloroform, accidental (unintentional)
      - Toxic effects of chloroform NOS
    - +7th **T53.1X2** Toxic effect of chloroform, intentional self-harm
    - +7th **T53.1X3** Toxic effect of chloroform, assault
    - +7th **T53.1X4** Toxic effect of chloroform, undetermined

+ **T53.2 Toxic effects of trichloroethylene**
  - Toxic effects of trichloroethene
  - + **T53.2X Toxic effects of trichloroethylene**
    - +7th **T53.2X1** Toxic effect of trichloroethylene, accidental (unintentional)
      - Toxic effects of trichloroethylene NOS
    - +7th **T53.2X2** Toxic effect of trichloroethylene, intentional self-harm
    - +7th **T53.2X3** Toxic effect of trichloroethylene, assault
    - +7th **T53.2X4** Toxic effect of trichloroethylene, undetermined

- **T53.3 Toxic effects of tetrachloroethylene**
  - Toxic effects of perchloroethylene
  - Toxic effect of tetrachloroethene
  - + **T53.3X Toxic effects of tetrachloroethylene**
    - +7th T53.3X1 Toxic effect of tetrachloroethylene, accidental (unintentional)
      - Toxic effects of tetrachloroethylene NOS
    - +7th T53.3X2 Toxic effect of tetrachloroethylene, intentional self-harm
    - +7th T53.3X3 Toxic effect of tetrachloroethylene, assault
    - +7th T53.3X4 Toxic effect of tetrachloroethylene, undetermined
- **T53.4 Toxic effects of dichloromethane**
  - Toxic effects of methylene chloride
  - + **T53.4X Toxic effects of dichloromethane**
    - +7th T53.4X1 Toxic effect of dichloromethane, accidental (unintentional)
      - Toxic effects of dichloromethane NOS
    - +7th T53.4X2 Toxic effect of dichloromethane, intentional self-harm
    - +7th T53.4X3 Toxic effect of dichloromethane, assault
    - +7th T53.4X4 Toxic effect of dichloromethane, undetermined
- **T53.5 Toxic effects of chlorofluorocarbons**
  - + **T53.5X Toxic effects of chlorofluorocarbons**
    - +7th T53.5X1 Toxic effect of chlorofluorocarbons, accidental (unintentional)
      - Toxic effects of chlorofluorocarbons NOS
    - +7th T53.5X2 Toxic effect of chlorofluorocarbons, intentional self-harm
    - +7th T53.5X3 Toxic effect of chlorofluorocarbons, assault
    - +7th T53.5X4 Toxic effect of chlorofluorocarbons, undetermined
- **T53.6 Toxic effects of other halogen derivatives of aliphatic hydrocarbons**
  - + **T53.6X Toxic effects of other halogen derivatives of aliphatic hydrocarbons**
    - +7th T53.6X1 Toxic effect of other halogen derivatives of aliphatic hydrocarbons, accidental (unintentional)
      - Toxic effects of other halogen derivatives of aliphatic hydrocarbons NOS
    - +7th T53.6X2 Toxic effect of other halogen derivatives of aliphatic hydrocarbons, intentional self-harm
    - +7th T53.6X3 Toxic effect of other halogen derivatives of aliphatic hydrocarbons, assault
    - +7th T53.6X4 Toxic effect of other halogen derivatives of aliphatic hydrocarbons, undetermined
- **T53.7 Toxic effects of other halogen derivatives of aromatic hydrocarbons**
  - + **T53.7X Toxic effects of other halogen derivatives of aromatic hydrocarbons**
    - +7th T53.7X1 Toxic effect of other halogen derivatives of aromatic hydrocarbons, accidental (unintentional)
      - Toxic effects of other halogen derivatives of aromatic hydrocarbons NOS
    - +7th T53.7X2 Toxic effect of other halogen derivatives of aromatic hydrocarbons, intentional self-harm
    - +7th T53.7X3 Toxic effect of other halogen derivatives of aromatic hydrocarbons, assault
    - +7th T53.7X4 Toxic effect of other halogen derivatives of aromatic hydrocarbons, undetermined
- **T53.9 Toxic effects of unspecified halogen derivatives of aliphatic and aromatic hydrocarbons**
  - X+7th T53.91 Toxic effect of unspecified halogen derivatives of aliphatic and aromatic hydrocarbons, accidental (unintentional)
  - X+7th T53.92 Toxic effect of unspecified halogen derivatives of aliphatic and aromatic hydrocarbons, intentional self-harm
  - X+7th T53.93 Toxic effect of unspecified halogen derivatives of aliphatic and aromatic hydrocarbons, assault
  - X+7th T53.94 Toxic effect of unspecified halogen derivatives of aliphatic and aromatic hydrocarbons, undetermined

T54 Toxic effect of corrosive substances

The appropriate 7th character is to be added to each code from category T54
- A initial encounter
- D subsequent encounter
- S sequela

- + **T54.0 Toxic effects of phenol and phenol homologues**
  - + **T54.0X Toxic effects of phenol and phenol homologues**
    - +7th T54.0X1 Toxic effect of phenol and phenol homologues, accidental (unintentional)
      - Toxic effects of phenol and phenol homologues NOS
    - +7th T54.0X2 Toxic effect of phenol and phenol homologues, intentional self-harm
    - +7th T54.0X3 Toxic effect of phenol and phenol homologues, assault
    - +7th T54.0X4 Toxic effect of phenol and phenol homologues, undetermined
- + **T54.1 Toxic effects of other corrosive organic compounds**
  - + **T54.1X Toxic effects of other corrosive organic compounds**
    - +7th T54.1X1 Toxic effect of other corrosive organic compounds, accidental (unintentional)
      - Toxic effects of other corrosive organic compounds NOS
    - +7th T54.1X2 Toxic effect of other corrosive organic compounds, intentional self-harm
    - +7th T54.1X3 Toxic effect of other corrosive organic compounds, assault
    - +7th T54.1X4 Toxic effect of other corrosive organic compounds, undetermined
- + **T54.2 Toxic effects of corrosive acids and acid-like substances**
  - Toxic effects of hydrochloric acid
  - Toxic effects of sulfuric acid
  - + **T54.2X Toxic effects of corrosive acids and acid-like substances**
    - +7th T54.2X1 Toxic effect of corrosive acids and acid-like substances, accidental (unintentional)
      - Toxic effects of corrosive acids and acid-like substances NOS
    - +7th T54.2X2 Toxic effect of corrosive acids and acid-like substances, intentional self-harm
    - +7th T54.2X3 Toxic effect of corrosive acids and acid-like substances, assault
    - +7th T54.2X4 Toxic effect of corrosive acids and acid-like substances, undetermined
- + **T54.3 Toxic effects of corrosive alkalis and alkali-like substances**
  - Toxic effects of potassium hydroxide
  - Toxic effects of sodium hydroxide
  - + **T54.3X Toxic effects of corrosive alkalis and alkali-like substances**
    - +7th T54.3X1 Toxic effect of corrosive alkalis and alkali-like substances, accidental (unintentional)
      - Toxic effects of corrosive alkalis and alkali-like substances NOS
    - +7th T54.3X2 Toxic effect of corrosive alkalis and alkali-like substances, intentional self-harm
    - +7th T54.3X3 Toxic effect of corrosive alkalis and alkali-like substances, assault
    - +7th T54.3X4 Toxic effect of corrosive alkalis and alkali-like substances, undetermined
- + **T54.9 Toxic effects of unspecified corrosive substance**
  - X+7th T54.91 Toxic effect of unspecified corrosive substance, accidental (unintentional)
  - X+7th T54.92 Toxic effect of unspecified corrosive substance, intentional self-harm
  - X+7th T54.93 Toxic effect of unspecified corrosive substance, assault
  - X+7th T54.94 Toxic effect of unspecified corrosive substance, undetermined

T55 Toxic effect of soaps and detergents

The appropriate 7th character is to be added to each code from category T55
- A initial encounter
- D subsequent encounter
- S sequela

- **+ T55.0 Toxic effect of soaps**
  - **+ T55.0X Toxic effect of soaps**
    - +7th T55.0X1 Toxic effect of soaps, accidental (unintentional)
      Toxic effect of soaps NOS
    - +7th T55.0X2 Toxic effect of soaps, intentional self-harm
    - +7th T55.0X3 Toxic effect of soaps, assault
    - +7th T55.0X4 Toxic effect of soaps, undetermined
- **+ T55.1 Toxic effect of detergents**
  - **+ T55.1X Toxic effect of detergents**
    - +7th T55.1X1 Toxic effect of detergents, accidental (unintentional)
      Toxic effect of detergents NOS
    - +7th T55.1X2 Toxic effect of detergents, intentional self-harm
    - +7th T55.1X3 Toxic effect of detergents, assault
    - +7th T55.1X4 Toxic effect of detergents, undetermined

T56 Toxic effect of metals

Includes: toxic effects of fumes and vapors of metals
toxic effects of metals from all sources, except medicinal substances

Use additional code to identify any retained metal foreign body, if applicable (Z18.0-, T18.1-)

Excludes1: arsenic and its compounds (T57.0)
manganese and its compounds (T57.2)

The appropriate 7th character is to be added to each code from category T56
A   initial encounter
D   subsequent encounter
S   sequela

- **+ T56.0 Toxic effects of lead and its compounds**
  - **+ T56.0X Toxic effects of lead and its compounds**
    - +7th T56.0X1 Toxic effect of lead and its compounds, accidental (unintentional)
      Toxic effects of lead and its compounds NOS
    - +7th T56.0X2 Toxic effect of lead and its compounds, intentional self-harm
    - +7th T56.0X3 Toxic effect of lead and its compounds, assault
    - +7th T56.0X4 Toxic effect of lead and its compounds, undetermined
- **+ T56.1 Toxic effects of mercury and its compounds**
  - **+ T56.1X Toxic effects of mercury and its compounds**
    - +7th T56.1X1 Toxic effect of mercury and its compounds, accidental (unintentional)
      Toxic effects of mercury and its compounds NOS
    - +7th T56.1X2 Toxic effect of mercury and its compounds, intentional self-harm
    - +7th T56.1X3 Toxic effect of mercury and its compounds, assault
    - +7th T56.1X4 Toxic effect of mercury and its compounds, undetermined
- **+ T56.2 Toxic effects of chromium and its compounds**
  - **+ T56.2X Toxic effects of chromium and its compounds**
    - +7th T56.2X1 Toxic effect of chromium and its compounds, accidental (unintentional)
      Toxic effects of chromium and its compounds NOS
    - +7th T56.2X2 Toxic effect of chromium and its compounds, intentional self-harm
    - +7th T56.2X3 Toxic effect of chromium and its compounds, assault
    - +7th T56.2X4 Toxic effect of chromium and its compounds, undetermined
- **+ T56.3 Toxic effects of cadmium and its compounds**
  - **+ T56.3X Toxic effects of cadmium and its compounds**
    - +7th T56.3X1 Toxic effect of cadmium and its compounds, accidental (unintentional)
      Toxic effects of cadmium and its compounds NOS
    - +7th T56.3X2 Toxic effect of cadmium and its compounds, intentional self-harm
    - +7th T56.3X3 Toxic effect of cadmium and its compounds, assault
    - +7th T56.3X4 Toxic effect of cadmium and its compounds, undetermined
- **+ T56.4 Toxic effects of copper and its compounds**
  - **+ T56.4X Toxic effects of copper and its compounds**
    - +7th T56.4X1 Toxic effect of copper and its compounds, accidental (unintentional)
      Toxic effects of copper and its compounds NOS
    - +7th T56.4X2 Toxic effect of copper and its compounds, intentional self-harm
    - +7th T56.4X3 Toxic effect of copper and its compounds, assault
    - +7th T56.4X4 Toxic effect of copper and its compounds, undetermined
- **+ T56.5 Toxic effects of zinc and its compounds**
  - **+ T56.5X Toxic effects of zinc and its compounds**
    - +7th T56.5X1 Toxic effect of zinc and its compounds, accidental (unintentional)
      Toxic effects of zinc and its compounds NOS
    - +7th T56.5X2 Toxic effect of zinc and its compounds, intentional self-harm
    - +7th T56.5X3 Toxic effect of zinc and its compounds, assault
    - +7th T56.5X4 Toxic effect of zinc and its compounds, undetermined
- **+ T56.6 Toxic effects of tin and its compounds**
  - **+ T56.6X Toxic effects of tin and its compounds**
    - +7th T56.6X1 Toxic effect of tin and its compounds, accidental (unintentional)
      Toxic effects of tin and its compounds NOS
    - +7th T56.6X2 Toxic effect of tin and its compounds, intentional self-harm
    - +7th T56.6X3 Toxic effect of tin and its compounds, assault
    - +7th T56.6X4 Toxic effect of tin and its compounds, undetermined
- **+ T56.7 Toxic effects of beryllium and its compounds**
  - **+ T56.7X Toxic effects of beryllium and its compounds**
    - +7th T56.7X1 Toxic effect of beryllium and its compounds, accidental (unintentional)
      Toxic effects of beryllium and its compounds NOS
    - +7th T56.7X2 Toxic effect of beryllium and its compounds, intentional self-harm
    - +7th T56.7X3 Toxic effect of beryllium and its compounds, assault
    - +7th T56.7X4 Toxic effect of beryllium and its compounds, undetermined
- **+ T56.8 Toxic effects of other metals**
  - **+ T56.81 Toxic effect of thallium**
    - +7th T56.811 Toxic effect of thallium, accidental (unintentional)
      Toxic effect of thallium NOS
    - +7th T56.812 Toxic effect of thallium, intentional self-harm
    - +7th T56.813 Toxic effect of thallium, assault
    - +7th T56.814 Toxic effect of thallium, undetermined
  - **+ T56.82 Toxic effect of gadolinium**
    Excludes1: adverse effect of diagnostic agents (T50.8X5-)
    - X+7th T56.821 Toxic effect of gadolinium, accidental (unintentional)
      Toxic effect of gadolinium NOS
    - X+7th T56.822 Toxic effect of gadolinium, intentional self-harm
    - X+7th T56.823 Toxic effect of gadolinium, assault
    - X+7th T56.824 Toxic effect of gadolinium, undetermined
  - **+ T56.89 Toxic effects of other metals**
    - +7th T56.891 Toxic effect of other metals, accidental (unintentional)
      Toxic effects of other metals NOS
    - +7th T56.892 Toxic effect of other metals, intentional self-harm
    - +7th T56.893 Toxic effect of other metals, assault
    - +7th T56.894 Toxic effect of other metals, undetermined
- **+ T56.9 Toxic effects of unspecified metal**
  - X+7th T56.91 Toxic effect of unspecified metal, accidental (unintentional)

X+7th	T56.92	Toxic effect of unspecified metal, intentional self-harm
X+7th	T56.93	Toxic effect of unspecified metal, assault
X+7th	T56.94	Toxic effect of unspecified metal, undetermined

T57 Toxic effect of other inorganic substances

> The appropriate 7th character is to be added to each code from category T57
> A initial encounter
> D subsequent encounter
> S sequela

- **T57.0** Toxic effect of arsenic and its compounds
  - **T57.0X** Toxic effect of arsenic and its compounds
    - +7th **T57.0X1** Toxic effect of arsenic and its compounds, accidental (unintentional)
      - Toxic effect of arsenic and its compounds NOS
    - +7th **T57.0X2** Toxic effect of arsenic and its compounds, intentional self-harm
    - +7th **T57.0X3** Toxic effect of arsenic and its compounds, assault
    - +7th **T57.0X4** Toxic effect of arsenic and its compounds, undetermined
- **T57.1** Toxic effect of phosphorus and its compounds
  - *Excludes1:* organophosphate insecticides (T60.0)
  - **T57.1X** Toxic effect of phosphorus and its compounds
    - +7th **T57.1X1** Toxic effect of phosphorus and its compounds, accidental (unintentional)
      - Toxic effect of phosphorus and its compounds NOS
    - +7th **T57.1X2** Toxic effect of phosphorus and its compounds, intentional self-harm
    - +7th **T57.1X3** Toxic effect of phosphorus and its compounds, assault
    - +7th **T57.1X4** Toxic effect of phosphorus and its compounds, undetermined
- **T57.2** Toxic effect of manganese and its compounds
  - **T57.2X** Toxic effect of manganese and its compounds
    - +7th **T57.2X1** Toxic effect of manganese and its compounds, accidental (unintentional)
      - Toxic effect of manganese and its compounds NOS
    - +7th **T57.2X2** Toxic effect of manganese and its compounds, intentional self-harm
    - +7th **T57.2X3** Toxic effect of manganese and its compounds, assault
    - +7th **T57.2X4** Toxic effect of manganese and its compounds, undetermined
- **T57.3** Toxic effect of hydrogen cyanide
  - **T57.3X** Toxic effect of hydrogen cyanide
    - +7th **T57.3X1** Toxic effect of hydrogen cyanide, accidental (unintentional)
      - Toxic effect of hydrogen cyanide NOS
    - +7th **T57.3X2** Toxic effect of hydrogen cyanide, intentional self-harm
    - +7th **T57.3X3** Toxic effect of hydrogen cyanide, assault
    - +7th **T57.3X4** Toxic effect of hydrogen cyanide, undetermined
- **T57.8** Toxic effect of other specified inorganic substances
  - **T57.8X** Toxic effect of other specified inorganic substances
    - +7th **T57.8X1** Toxic effect of other specified inorganic substances, accidental (unintentional)
      - Toxic effect of other specified inorganic substances NOS
    - +7th **T57.8X2** Toxic effect of other specified inorganic substances, intentional self-harm
    - +7th **T57.8X3** Toxic effect of other specified inorganic substances, assault
    - +7th **T57.8X4** Toxic effect of other specified inorganic substances, undetermined
- **T57.9** Toxic effect of unspecified inorganic substance
  - X+7th **T57.91** Toxic effect of unspecified inorganic substance, accidental (unintentional)
  - X+7th **T57.92** Toxic effect of unspecified inorganic substance, intentional self-harm
  - X+7th **T57.93** Toxic effect of unspecified inorganic substance, assault
  - X+7th **T57.94** Toxic effect of unspecified inorganic substance, undetermined

T58 Toxic effect of carbon monoxide

> *Includes:* asphyxiation from carbon monoxide
> toxic effect of carbon monoxide from all sources

> The appropriate 7th character is to be added to each code from category T58
> A initial encounter
> D subsequent encounter
> S sequela

- **T58.0** Toxic effect of carbon monoxide from motor vehicle exhaust
  - Toxic effect of exhaust gas from gas engine
  - Toxic effect of exhaust gas from motor pump
  - X+7th **T58.01** Toxic effect of carbon monoxide from motor vehicle exhaust, accidental (unintentional)
  - X+7th **T58.02** Toxic effect of carbon monoxide from motor vehicle exhaust, intentional self-harm
  - X+7th **T58.03** Toxic effect of carbon monoxide from motor vehicle exhaust, assault
  - X+7th **T58.04** Toxic effect of carbon monoxide from motor vehicle exhaust, undetermined
- **T58.1** Toxic effect of carbon monoxide from utility gas
  - Toxic effect of acetylene
  - Toxic effect of gas NOS used for lighting, heating, cooking
  - Toxic effect of water gas
  - X+7th **T58.11** Toxic effect of carbon monoxide from utility gas, accidental (unintentional)
  - X+7th **T58.12** Toxic effect of carbon monoxide from utility gas, intentional self-harm
  - X+7th **T58.13** Toxic effect of carbon monoxide from utility gas, assault
  - X+7th **T58.14** Toxic effect of carbon monoxide from utility gas, undetermined
- **T58.2** Toxic effect of carbon monoxide from incomplete combustion of other domestic fuels
  - Toxic effect of carbon monoxide from incomplete combustion of coal, coke, kerosene, wood
  - **T58.2X** Toxic effect of carbon monoxide from incomplete combustion of other domestic fuels
    - +7th **T58.2X1** Toxic effect of carbon monoxide from incomplete combustion of other domestic fuels, accidental (unintentional)
    - +7th **T58.2X2** Toxic effect of carbon monoxide from incomplete combustion of other domestic fuels, intentional self-harm
    - +7th **T58.2X3** Toxic effect of carbon monoxide from incomplete combustion of other domestic fuels, assault
    - +7th **T58.2X4** Toxic effect of carbon monoxide from incomplete combustion of other domestic fuels, undetermined
- **T58.8** Toxic effect of carbon monoxide from other source
  - Toxic effect of carbon monoxide from blast furnace gas
  - Toxic effect of carbon monoxide from fuels in industrial use
  - Toxic effect of carbon monoxide from kiln vapor
  - **T58.8X** Toxic effect of carbon monoxide from other source
    - +7th **T58.8X1** Toxic effect of carbon monoxide from other source, accidental (unintentional)
    - +7th **T58.8X2** Toxic effect of carbon monoxide from other source, intentional self-harm
    - +7th **T58.8X3** Toxic effect of carbon monoxide from other source, assault
    - +7th **T58.8X4** Toxic effect of carbon monoxide from other source, undetermined
- **T58.9** Toxic effect of carbon monoxide from unspecified source
  - X+7th **T58.91** Toxic effect of carbon monoxide from unspecified source, accidental (unintentional)
  - X+7th **T58.92** Toxic effect of carbon monoxide from unspecified source, intentional self-harm
  - X+7th **T58.93** Toxic effect of carbon monoxide from unspecified source, assault
  - X+7th **T58.94** Toxic effect of carbon monoxide from unspecified source, undetermined

T59 Toxic effect of other gases, fumes and vapors

Includes: aerosol propellants
Excludes1: *chlorofluorocarbons (T53.5)*

The appropriate 7th character is to be added to each code from category T59
- A initial encounter
- D subsequent encounter
- S sequela

- **T59.0** Toxic effect of nitrogen oxides
  - **T59.0X** Toxic effect of nitrogen oxides
    - +7th T59.0X1 Toxic effect of nitrogen oxides, accidental (unintentional)
      - Toxic effect of nitrogen oxides NOS
    - +7th T59.0X2 Toxic effect of nitrogen oxides, intentional self-harm
    - +7th T59.0X3 Toxic effect of nitrogen oxides, assault
    - +7th T59.0X4 Toxic effect of nitrogen oxides, undetermined
- **T59.1** Toxic effect of sulfur dioxide
  - **T59.1X** Toxic effect of sulfur dioxide
    - +7th T59.1X1 Toxic effect of sulfur dioxide, accidental (unintentional)
      - Toxic effect of sulfur dioxide NOS
    - +7th T59.1X2 Toxic effect of sulfur dioxide, intentional self-harm
    - +7th T59.1X3 Toxic effect of sulfur dioxide, assault
    - +7th T59.1X4 Toxic effect of sulfur dioxide, undetermined
- **T59.2** Toxic effect of formaldehyde
  - **T59.2X** Toxic effect of formaldehyde
    - +7th T59.2X1 Toxic effect of formaldehyde, accidental (unintentional)
      - Toxic effect of formaldehyde NOS
    - +7th T59.2X2 Toxic effect of formaldehyde, intentional self-harm
    - +7th T59.2X3 Toxic effect of formaldehyde, assault
    - +7th T59.2X4 Toxic effect of formaldehyde, undetermined
- **T59.3** Toxic effect of lacrimogenic gas
  - Toxic effect of tear gas
  - **T59.3X** Toxic effect of lacrimogenic gas
    - +7th T59.3X1 Toxic effect of lacrimogenic gas, accidental (unintentional)
      - Toxic effect of lacrimogenic gas NOS
    - +7th T59.3X2 Toxic effect of lacrimogenic gas, intentional self-harm
    - +7th T59.3X3 Toxic effect of lacrimogenic gas, assault
    - +7th T59.3X4 Toxic effect of lacrimogenic gas, undetermined
- **T59.4** Toxic effect of chlorine gas
  - **T59.4X** Toxic effect of chlorine gas
    - +7th T59.4X1 Toxic effect of chlorine gas, accidental (unintentional)
      - Toxic effect of chlorine gas NOS
    - +7th T59.4X2 Toxic effect of chlorine gas, intentional self-harm
    - +7th T59.4X3 Toxic effect of chlorine gas, assault
    - +7th T59.4X4 Toxic effect of chlorine gas, undetermined
- **T59.5** Toxic effect of fluorine gas and hydrogen fluoride
  - **T59.5X** Toxic effect of fluorine gas and hydrogen fluoride
    - +7th T59.5X1 Toxic effect of fluorine gas and hydrogen fluoride, accidental (unintentional)
      - Toxic effect of fluorine gas and hydrogen fluoride NOS
    - +7th T59.5X2 Toxic effect of fluorine gas and hydrogen fluoride, intentional self-harm
    - +7th T59.5X3 Toxic effect of fluorine gas and hydrogen fluoride, assault
    - +7th T59.5X4 Toxic effect of fluorine gas and hydrogen fluoride, undetermined
- **T59.6** Toxic effect of hydrogen sulfide
  - **T59.6X** Toxic effect of hydrogen sulfide
    - +7th T59.6X1 Toxic effect of hydrogen sulfide, accidental (unintentional)
      - Toxic effect of hydrogen sulfide NOS
    - +7th T59.6X2 Toxic effect of hydrogen sulfide, intentional self-harm
    - +7th T59.6X3 Toxic effect of hydrogen sulfide, assault
    - +7th T59.6X4 Toxic effect of hydrogen sulfide, undetermined
- **T59.7** Toxic effect of carbon dioxide
  - **T59.7X** Toxic effect of carbon dioxide
    - +7th T59.7X1 Toxic effect of carbon dioxide, accidental (unintentional)
      - Toxic effect of carbon dioxide NOS
    - +7th T59.7X2 Toxic effect of carbon dioxide, intentional self-harm
    - +7th T59.7X3 Toxic effect of carbon dioxide, assault
    - +7th T59.7X4 Toxic effect of carbon dioxide, undetermined
- **T59.8** Toxic effect of other specified gases, fumes and vapors
  - **T59.81** Toxic effect of smoke
    - Smoke inhalation
    - **Excludes2:** *toxic effect of cigarette (tobacco) smoke (T65.22-)*
    - +7th T59.811 Toxic effect of smoke, accidental (unintentional)
      - Toxic effect of smoke NOS
    - +7th T59.812 Toxic effect of smoke, intentional self-harm
    - +7th T59.813 Toxic effect of smoke, assault
    - +7th T59.814 Toxic effect of smoke, undetermined
  - **T59.89** Toxic effect of other specified gases, fumes and vapors
    - +7th T59.891 Toxic effect of other specified gases, fumes and vapors, accidental (unintentional)
    - +7th T59.892 Toxic effect of other specified gases, fumes and vapors, intentional self-harm
    - +7th T59.893 Toxic effect of other specified gases, fumes and vapors, assault
    - +7th T59.894 Toxic effect of other specified gases, fumes and vapors, undetermined
- **T59.9** Toxic effect of unspecified gases, fumes and vapors
  - X+7th T59.91 Toxic effect of unspecified gases, fumes and vapors, accidental (unintentional)
  - X+7th T59.92 Toxic effect of unspecified gases, fumes and vapors, intentional self-harm
  - X+7th T59.93 Toxic effect of unspecified gases, fumes and vapors, assault
  - X+7th T59.94 Toxic effect of unspecified gases, fumes and vapors, undetermined

T60 Toxic effect of pesticides

Includes: toxic effect of wood preservatives

The appropriate 7th character is to be added to each code from category T60
- A initial encounter
- D subsequent encounter
- S sequela

- **T60.0** Toxic effect of organophosphate and carbamate insecticides
  - **T60.0X** Toxic effect of organophosphate and carbamate insecticides
    - +7th T60.0X1 Toxic effect of organophosphate and carbamate insecticides, accidental (unintentional)
      - Toxic effect of organophosphate and carbamate insecticides NOS
    - +7th T60.0X2 Toxic effect of organophosphate and carbamate insecticides, intentional self-harm
    - +7th T60.0X3 Toxic effect of organophosphate and carbamate insecticides, assault
    - +7th T60.0X4 Toxic effect of organophosphate and carbamate insecticides, undetermined
- **T60.1** Toxic effect of halogenated insecticides
  - **Excludes1:** *chlorinated hydrocarbon (T53.-)*
  - **T60.1X** Toxic effect of halogenated insecticides
    - +7th T60.1X1 Toxic effect of halogenated insecticides, accidental (unintentional)
      - Toxic effect of halogenated insecticides NOS
    - +7th T60.1X2 Toxic effect of halogenated insecticides, intentional self-harm
    - +7th T60.1X3 Toxic effect of halogenated insecticides, assault
    - +7th T60.1X4 Toxic effect of halogenated insecticides, undetermined

- **T60.2 Toxic effect of other insecticides**
  - **T60.2X Toxic effect of other insecticides**
    - +7th **T60.2X1** Toxic effect of other insecticides, accidental (unintentional)
      Toxic effect of other insecticides NOS
    - +7th **T60.2X2** Toxic effect of other insecticides, intentional self-harm
    - +7th **T60.2X3** Toxic effect of other insecticides, assault
    - +7th **T60.2X4** Toxic effect of other insecticides, undetermined
- **T60.3 Toxic effect of herbicides and fungicides**
  - **T60.3X Toxic effect of herbicides and fungicides**
    - +7th **T60.3X1** Toxic effect of herbicides and fungicides, accidental (unintentional)
      Toxic effect of herbicides and fungicides NOS
    - +7th **T60.3X2** Toxic effect of herbicides and fungicides, intentional self-harm
    - +7th **T60.3X3** Toxic effect of herbicides and fungicides, assault
    - +7th **T60.3X4** Toxic effect of herbicides and fungicides, undetermined
- **T60.4 Toxic effect of rodenticides**
  - **Excludes1:** strychnine and its salts (T65.1)
    thallium (T56.81-)
  - **T60.4X Toxic effect of rodenticides**
    - +7th **T60.4X1** Toxic effect of rodenticides, accidental (unintentional)
      Toxic effect of rodenticides NOS
    - +7th **T60.4X2** Toxic effect of rodenticides, intentional self-harm
    - +7th **T60.4X3** Toxic effect of rodenticides, assault
    - +7th **T60.4X4** Toxic effect of rodenticides, undetermined
- **T60.8 Toxic effect of other pesticides**
  - **T60.8X Toxic effect of other pesticides**
    - +7th **T60.8X1** Toxic effect of other pesticides, accidental (unintentional)
      Toxic effect of other pesticides NOS
    - +7th **T60.8X2** Toxic effect of other pesticides, intentional self-harm
    - +7th **T60.8X3** Toxic effect of other pesticides, assault
    - +7th **T60.8X4** Toxic effect of other pesticides, undetermined
- **T60.9 Toxic effect of unspecified pesticide**
  - X+7th **T60.91** Toxic effect of unspecified pesticide, accidental (unintentional)
  - X+7th **T60.92** Toxic effect of unspecified pesticide, intentional self-harm
  - X+7th **T60.93** Toxic effect of unspecified pesticide, assault
  - X+7th **T60.94** Toxic effect of unspecified pesticide, undetermined

T61 Toxic effect of noxious substances eaten as seafood

Excludes1: allergic reaction to food, such as:
  anaphylactic reaction or shock due to adverse food reaction (T78.0-)
  bacterial foodborne intoxications (A05.-)
  dermatitis (L23.6, L25.4, L27.2)
  food protein-induced enterocolitis syndrome (K52.21)
  food protein-induced enteropathy (K52.22)
  gastroenteritis (noninfective) (K52.29)
  toxic effect of aflatoxin and other mycotoxins (T64)
  toxic effect of cyanides (T65.0-)
  toxic effect of harmful algae bloom (T65.82-)
  toxic effect of hydrogen cyanide (T57.3-)
  toxic effect of mercury (T56.1-)
  toxic effect of red tide (T65.82-)

The appropriate 7th character is to be added to each code from category T61
A   initial encounter
D   subsequent encounter
S   sequela

- **T61.0 Ciguatera fish poisoning**
  - X+7th **T61.01** Ciguatera fish poisoning, accidental (unintentional)
  - X+7th **T61.02** Ciguatera fish poisoning, intentional self-harm
  - X+7th **T61.03** Ciguatera fish poisoning, assault
  - X+7th **T61.04** Ciguatera fish poisoning, undetermined

- **T61.1 Scombroid fish poisoning**
  Histamine-like syndrome
  - X+7th **T61.11** Scombroid fish poisoning, accidental (unintentional)
  - X+7th **T61.12** Scombroid fish poisoning, intentional self-harm
  - X+7th **T61.13** Scombroid fish poisoning, assault
  - X+7th **T61.14** Scombroid fish poisoning, undetermined
- **T61.7 Other fish and shellfish poisoning**
  - **T61.77 Other fish poisoning**
    - +7th **T61.771** Other fish poisoning, accidental (unintentional)
    - +7th **T61.772** Other fish poisoning, intentional self-harm
    - +7th **T61.773** Other fish poisoning, assault
    - +7th **T61.774** Other fish poisoning, undetermined
  - **T61.78 Other shellfish poisoning**
    - +7th **T61.781** Other shellfish poisoning, accidental (unintentional)
    - +7th **T61.782** Other shellfish poisoning, intentional self-harm
    - +7th **T61.783** Other shellfish poisoning, assault
    - +7th **T61.784** Other shellfish poisoning, undetermined
- **T61.8 Toxic effect of other seafood**
  - **T61.8X Toxic effect of other seafood**
    - +7th **T61.8X1** Toxic effect of other seafood, accidental (unintentional)
    - +7th **T61.8X2** Toxic effect of other seafood, intentional self-harm
    - +7th **T61.8X3** Toxic effect of other seafood, assault
    - +7th **T61.8X4** Toxic effect of other seafood, undetermined
- **T61.9 Toxic effect of unspecified seafood**
  - X+7th **T61.91** Toxic effect of unspecified seafood, accidental (unintentional)
  - X+7th **T61.92** Toxic effect of unspecified seafood, intentional self-harm
  - X+7th **T61.93** Toxic effect of unspecified seafood, assault
  - X+7th **T61.94** Toxic effect of unspecified seafood, undetermined

T62 Toxic effect of other noxious substances eaten as food

Excludes1: allergic reaction to food, such as:
  anaphylactic shock (reaction) due to adverse food reaction (T78.0-)
  bacterial food borne intoxications (A05.-)
  dermatitis (L23.6, L25.4, L27.2)
  food protein-induced enterocolitis syndrome (K52.21)
  food protein-induced enteropathy (K52.22)
  gastroenteritis (noninfective) (K52.29)
  toxic effect of aflatoxin and other mycotoxins (T64)
  toxic effect of cyanides (T65.0-)
  toxic effect of hydrogen cyanide (T57.3-)
  toxic effect of mercury (T56.1-)

The appropriate 7th character is to be added to each code from category T62
A   initial encounter
D   subsequent encounter
S   sequela

- **T62.0 Toxic effect of ingested mushrooms**
  - **T62.0X Toxic effect of ingested mushrooms**
    - +7th **T62.0X1** Toxic effect of ingested mushrooms, accidental (unintentional)
      Toxic effect of ingested mushrooms NOS
    - +7th **T62.0X2** Toxic effect of ingested mushrooms, intentional self-harm
    - +7th **T62.0X3** Toxic effect of ingested mushrooms, assault
    - +7th **T62.0X4** Toxic effect of ingested mushrooms, undetermined
- **T62.1 Toxic effect of ingested berries**
  - **T62.1X Toxic effect of ingested berries**
    - +7th **T62.1X1** Toxic effect of ingested berries, accidental (unintentional)
      Toxic effect of ingested berries NOS
    - +7th **T62.1X2** Toxic effect of ingested berries, intentional self-harm
    - +7th **T62.1X3** Toxic effect of ingested berries, assault
    - +7th **T62.1X4** Toxic effect of ingested berries, undetermined

- **+ T62.2 Toxic effect of other ingested (parts of) plant(s)**
  - **+ T62.2X Toxic effect of other ingested (parts of) plant(s)**
    - +7th T62.2X1 Toxic effect of other ingested (parts of) plant(s), accidental (unintentional)
      - Toxic effect of other ingested (parts of) plant(s) NOS
    - +7th T62.2X2 Toxic effect of other ingested (parts of) plant(s), intentional self-harm
    - +7th T62.2X3 Toxic effect of other ingested (parts of) plant(s), assault
    - +7th T62.2X4 Toxic effect of other ingested (parts of) plant(s), undetermined
- **+ T62.8 Toxic effect of other specified noxious substances eaten as food**
  - **+ T62.8X Toxic effect of other specified noxious substances eaten as food**
    - +7th T62.8X1 Toxic effect of other specified noxious substances eaten as food, accidental (unintentional)
      - Toxic effect of other specified noxious substances eaten as food NOS
    - +7th T62.8X2 Toxic effect of other specified noxious substances eaten as food, intentional self-harm
    - +7th T62.8X3 Toxic effect of other specified noxious substances eaten as food, assault
    - +7th T62.8X4 Toxic effect of other specified noxious substances eaten as food, undetermined
- **+ T62.9 Toxic effect of unspecified noxious substance eaten as food**
  - X+7th T62.91 Toxic effect of unspecified noxious substance eaten as food, accidental (unintentional)
    - Toxic effect of unspecified noxious substance eaten as food NOS
  - X+7th T62.92 Toxic effect of unspecified noxious substance eaten as food, intentional self-harm
  - X+7th T62.93 Toxic effect of unspecified noxious substance eaten as food, assault
  - X+7th T62.94 Toxic effect of unspecified noxious substance eaten as food, undetermined

T63 Toxic effect of contact with venomous animals and plants

Includes: bite or touch of venomous animal
pricked or stuck by thorn or leaf

Excludes2: ingestion of toxic animal or plant (T61.-, T62.-)

> The appropriate 7th character is to be added to each code from category T63
> A initial encounter
> D subsequent encounter
> S sequela

- **+ T63.0 Toxic effect of snake venom**
  - **+ T63.00 Toxic effect of unspecified snake venom**
    - +7th T63.001 Toxic effect of unspecified snake venom, accidental (unintentional)
      - Toxic effect of unspecified snake venom NOS
    - +7th T63.002 Toxic effect of unspecified snake venom, intentional self-harm
    - +7th T63.003 Toxic effect of unspecified snake venom, assault
    - +7th T63.004 Toxic effect of unspecified snake venom, undetermined
  - **+ T63.01 Toxic effect of rattlesnake venom**
    - +7th T63.011 Toxic effect of rattlesnake venom, accidental (unintentional)
      - Toxic effect of rattlesnake venom NOS
    - +7th T63.012 Toxic effect of rattlesnake venom, intentional self-harm
    - +7th T63.013 Toxic effect of rattlesnake venom, assault
    - +7th T63.014 Toxic effect of rattlesnake venom, undetermined
  - **+ T63.02 Toxic effect of coral snake venom**
    - +7th T63.021 Toxic effect of coral snake venom, accidental (unintentional)
      - Toxic effect of coral snake venom NOS
    - +7th T63.022 Toxic effect of coral snake venom, intentional self-harm
    - +7th T63.023 Toxic effect of coral snake venom, assault
    - +7th T63.024 Toxic effect of coral snake venom, undetermined
  - **+ T63.03 Toxic effect of taipan venom**
    - +7th T63.031 Toxic effect of taipan venom, accidental (unintentional)
      - Toxic effect of taipan venom NOS
    - +7th T63.032 Toxic effect of taipan venom, intentional self-harm
    - +7th T63.033 Toxic effect of taipan venom, assault
    - +7th T63.034 Toxic effect of taipan venom, undetermined
  - **+ T63.04 Toxic effect of cobra venom**
    - +7th T63.041 Toxic effect of cobra venom, accidental (unintentional)
      - Toxic effect of cobra venom NOS
    - +7th T63.042 Toxic effect of cobra venom, intentional self-harm
    - +7th T63.043 Toxic effect of cobra venom, assault
    - +7th T63.044 Toxic effect of cobra venom, undetermined
  - **+ T63.06 Toxic effect of venom of other North and South American snake**
    - +7th T63.061 Toxic effect of venom of other North and South American snake, accidental (unintentional)
      - Toxic effect of venom of other North and South American snake NOS
    - +7th T63.062 Toxic effect of venom of other North and South American snake, intentional self-harm
    - +7th T63.063 Toxic effect of venom of other North and South American snake, assault
    - +7th T63.064 Toxic effect of venom of other North and South American snake, undetermined
  - **+ T63.07 Toxic effect of venom of other Australian snake**
    - +7th T63.071 Toxic effect of venom of other Australian snake, accidental (unintentional)
      - Toxic effect of venom of other Australian snake NOS
    - +7th T63.072 Toxic effect of venom of other Australian snake, intentional self-harm
    - +7th T63.073 Toxic effect of venom of other Australian snake, assault
    - +7th T63.074 Toxic effect of venom of other Australian snake, undetermined
  - **+ T63.08 Toxic effect of venom of other African and Asian snake**
    - +7th T63.081 Toxic effect of venom of other African and Asian snake, accidental (unintentional)
      - Toxic effect of venom of other African and Asian snake NOS
    - +7th T63.082 Toxic effect of venom of other African and Asian snake, intentional self-harm
    - +7th T63.083 Toxic effect of venom of other African and Asian snake, assault
    - +7th T63.084 Toxic effect of venom of other African and Asian snake, undetermined
  - **+ T63.09 Toxic effect of venom of other snake**
    - +7th T63.091 Toxic effect of venom of other snake, accidental (unintentional)
      - Toxic effect of venom of other snake NOS
    - +7th T63.092 Toxic effect of venom of other snake, intentional self-harm
    - +7th T63.093 Toxic effect of venom of other snake, assault
    - +7th T63.094 Toxic effect of venom of other snake, undetermined
- **+ T63.1 Toxic effect of venom of other reptiles**
  - **+ T63.11 Toxic effect of venom of gila monster**
    - +7th T63.111 Toxic effect of venom of gila monster, accidental (unintentional)
      - Toxic effect of venom of gila monster NOS
    - +7th T63.112 Toxic effect of venom of gila monster, intentional self-harm
    - +7th T63.113 Toxic effect of venom of gila monster, assault
    - +7th T63.114 Toxic effect of venom of gila monster, undetermined

- **+ T63.12** Toxic effect of venom of other venomous lizard
  - +7th **T63.121** Toxic effect of venom of other venomous lizard, accidental (unintentional)
    Toxic effect of venom of other venomous lizard NOS
  - +7th **T63.122** Toxic effect of venom of other venomous lizard, intentional self-harm
  - +7th **T63.123** Toxic effect of venom of other venomous lizard, assault
  - +7th **T63.124** Toxic effect of venom of other venomous lizard, undetermined
- **+ T63.19** Toxic effect of venom of other reptiles
  - +7th **T63.191** Toxic effect of venom of other reptiles, accidental (unintentional)
    Toxic effect of venom of other reptiles NOS
  - +7th **T63.192** Toxic effect of venom of other reptiles, intentional self-harm
  - +7th **T63.193** Toxic effect of venom of other reptiles, assault
  - +7th **T63.194** Toxic effect of venom of other reptiles, undetermined
- **+ T63.2** Toxic effect of venom of scorpion
  - **+ T63.2X** Toxic effect of venom of scorpion
    - +7th **T63.2X1** Toxic effect of venom of scorpion, accidental (unintentional)
      Toxic effect of venom of scorpion NOS
    - +7th **T63.2X2** Toxic effect of venom of scorpion, intentional self-harm
    - +7th **T63.2X3** Toxic effect of venom of scorpion, assault
    - +7th **T63.2X4** Toxic effect of venom of scorpion, undetermined
- **+ T63.3** Toxic effect of venom of spider
  - **+ T63.30** Toxic effect of unspecified spider venom
    - +7th **T63.301** Toxic effect of unspecified spider venom, accidental (unintentional)
    - +7th **T63.302** Toxic effect of unspecified spider venom, intentional self-harm
    - +7th **T63.303** Toxic effect of unspecified spider venom, assault
    - +7th **T63.304** Toxic effect of unspecified spider venom, undetermined
  - **+ T63.31** Toxic effect of venom of black widow spider
    - +7th **T63.311** Toxic effect of venom of black widow spider, accidental (unintentional)
    - +7th **T63.312** Toxic effect of venom of black widow spider, intentional self-harm
    - +7th **T63.313** Toxic effect of venom of black widow spider, assault
    - +7th **T63.314** Toxic effect of venom of black widow spider, undetermined
  - **+ T63.32** Toxic effect of venom of tarantula
    - +7th **T63.321** Toxic effect of venom of tarantula, accidental (unintentional)
    - +7th **T63.322** Toxic effect of venom of tarantula, intentional self-harm
    - +7th **T63.323** Toxic effect of venom of tarantula, assault
    - +7th **T63.324** Toxic effect of venom of tarantula, undetermined
  - **+ T63.33** Toxic effect of venom of brown recluse spider
    - +7th **T63.331** Toxic effect of venom of brown recluse spider, accidental (unintentional)
    - +7th **T63.332** Toxic effect of venom of brown recluse spider, intentional self-harm
    - +7th **T63.333** Toxic effect of venom of brown recluse spider, assault
    - +7th **T63.334** Toxic effect of venom of brown recluse spider, undetermined
  - **+ T63.39** Toxic effect of venom of other spider
    - +7th **T63.391** Toxic effect of venom of other spider, accidental (unintentional)
    - +7th **T63.392** Toxic effect of venom of other spider, intentional self-harm
    - +7th **T63.393** Toxic effect of venom of other spider, assault
    - +7th **T63.394** Toxic effect of venom of other spider, undetermined

- **+ T63.4** Toxic effect of venom of other arthropods
  - **+ T63.41** Toxic effect of venom of centipedes and venomous millipedes
    - +7th **T63.411** Toxic effect of venom of centipedes and venomous millipedes, accidental (unintentional)
    - +7th **T63.412** Toxic effect of venom of centipedes and venomous millipedes, intentional self-harm
    - +7th **T63.413** Toxic effect of venom of centipedes and venomous millipedes, assault
    - +7th **T63.414** Toxic effect of venom of centipedes and venomous millipedes, undetermined
  - **+ T63.42** Toxic effect of venom of ants
    - +7th **T63.421** Toxic effect of venom of ants, accidental (unintentional)
    - +7th **T63.422** Toxic effect of venom of ants, intentional self-harm
    - +7th **T63.423** Toxic effect of venom of ants, assault
    - +7th **T63.424** Toxic effect of venom of ants, undetermined
  - **+ T63.43** Toxic effect of venom of caterpillars
    - +7th **T63.431** Toxic effect of venom of caterpillars, accidental (unintentional)
    - +7th **T63.432** Toxic effect of venom of caterpillars, intentional self-harm
    - +7th **T63.433** Toxic effect of venom of caterpillars, assault
    - +7th **T63.434** Toxic effect of venom of caterpillars, undetermined
  - **+ T63.44** Toxic effect of venom of bees
    - +7th **T63.441** Toxic effect of venom of bees, accidental (unintentional)
    - +7th **T63.442** Toxic effect of venom of bees, intentional self-harm
    - +7th **T63.443** Toxic effect of venom of bees, assault
    - +7th **T63.444** Toxic effect of venom of bees, undetermined
  - **+ T63.45** Toxic effect of venom of hornets
    - +7th **T63.451** Toxic effect of venom of hornets, accidental (unintentional)
    - +7th **T63.452** Toxic effect of venom of hornets, intentional self-harm
    - +7th **T63.453** Toxic effect of venom of hornets, assault
    - +7th **T63.454** Toxic effect of venom of hornets, undetermined
  - **+ T63.46** Toxic effect of venom of wasps
    Toxic effect of yellow jacket
    - +7th **T63.461** Toxic effect of venom of wasps, accidental (unintentional)
    - +7th **T63.462** Toxic effect of venom of wasps, intentional self-harm
    - +7th **T63.463** Toxic effect of venom of wasps, assault
    - +7th **T63.464** Toxic effect of venom of wasps, undetermined
  - **+ T63.48** Toxic effect of venom of other arthropod
    - +7th **T63.481** Toxic effect of venom of other arthropod, accidental (unintentional)
    - +7th **T63.482** Toxic effect of venom of other arthropod, intentional self-harm
    - +7th **T63.483** Toxic effect of venom of other arthropod, assault
    - +7th **T63.484** Toxic effect of venom of other arthropod, undetermined
- **+ T63.5** Toxic effect of contact with venomous fish
  Excludes2: *poisoning by ingestion of fish (T61.-)*
  - **+ T63.51** Toxic effect of contact with stingray
    - +7th **T63.511** Toxic effect of contact with stingray, accidental (unintentional)
    - +7th **T63.512** Toxic effect of contact with stingray, intentional self-harm
    - +7th **T63.513** Toxic effect of contact with stingray, assault
    - +7th **T63.514** Toxic effect of contact with stingray, undetermined

- +T63.59 Toxic effect of contact with other venomous fish
  - +7th T63.591 Toxic effect of contact with other venomous fish, accidental (unintentional)
  - +7th T63.592 Toxic effect of contact with other venomous fish, intentional self-harm
  - +7th T63.593 Toxic effect of contact with other venomous fish, assault
  - +7th T63.594 Toxic effect of contact with other venomous fish, undetermined
- +T63.6 Toxic effect of contact with other venomous marine animals
  - **Excludes1:** sea-snake venom (T63.09)
  - **Excludes2:** poisoning by ingestion of shellfish (T61.78-)
  - +T63.61 Toxic effect of contact with Portuguese Man-o-war
    - Toxic effect of contact with bluebottle
    - +7th T63.611 Toxic effect of contact with Portuguese Man-o-war, accidental (unintentional)
    - +7th T63.612 Toxic effect of contact with Portuguese Man-o-war, intentional self-harm
    - +7th T63.613 Toxic effect of contact with Portuguese Man-o-war, assault
    - +7th T63.614 Toxic effect of contact with Portuguese Man-o-war, undetermined
  - +T63.62 Toxic effect of contact with other jellyfish
    - +7th T63.621 Toxic effect of contact with other jellyfish, accidental (unintentional)
    - +7th T63.622 Toxic effect of contact with other jellyfish, intentional self-harm
    - +7th T63.623 Toxic effect of contact with other jellyfish, assault
    - +7th T63.624 Toxic effect of contact with other jellyfish, undetermined
  - +T63.63 Toxic effect of contact with sea anemone
    - +7th T63.631 Toxic effect of contact with sea anemone, accidental (unintentional)
    - +7th T63.632 Toxic effect of contact with sea anemone, intentional self-harm
    - +7th T63.633 Toxic effect of contact with sea anemone, assault
    - +7th T63.634 Toxic effect of contact with sea anemone, undetermined
  - +T63.69 Toxic effect of contact with other venomous marine animals
    - +7th T63.691 Toxic effect of contact with other venomous marine animals, accidental (unintentional)
    - +7th T63.692 Toxic effect of contact with other venomous marine animals, intentional self-harm
    - +7th T63.693 Toxic effect of contact with other venomous marine animals, assault
    - +7th T63.694 Toxic effect of contact with other venomous marine animals, undetermined
- +T63.7 Toxic effect of contact with venomous plant
  - +T63.71 Toxic effect of contact with venomous marine plant
    - +7th T63.711 Toxic effect of contact with venomous marine plant, accidental (unintentional)
    - +7th T63.712 Toxic effect of contact with venomous marine plant, intentional self-harm
    - +7th T63.713 Toxic effect of contact with venomous marine plant, assault
    - +7th T63.714 Toxic effect of contact with venomous marine plant, undetermined
  - +T63.79 Toxic effect of contact with other venomous plant
    - +7th T63.791 Toxic effect of contact with other venomous plant, accidental (unintentional)
    - +7th T63.792 Toxic effect of contact with other venomous plant, intentional self-harm
    - +7th T63.793 Toxic effect of contact with other venomous plant, assault
    - +7th T63.794 Toxic effect of contact with other venomous plant, undetermined

- +T63.8 Toxic effect of contact with other venomous animals
  - +T63.81 Toxic effect of contact with venomous frog
    - **Excludes1:** contact with nonvenomous frog (W62.0)
    - +7th T63.811 Toxic effect of contact with venomous frog, accidental (unintentional)
    - +7th T63.812 Toxic effect of contact with venomous frog, intentional self-harm
    - +7th T63.813 Toxic effect of contact with venomous frog, assault
    - +7th T63.814 Toxic effect of contact with venomous frog, undetermined
  - +T63.82 Toxic effect of contact with venomous toad
    - **Excludes1:** contact with nonvenomous toad (W62.1)
    - +7th T63.821 Toxic effect of contact with venomous toad, accidental (unintentional)
    - +7th T63.822 Toxic effect of contact with venomous toad, intentional self-harm
    - +7th T63.823 Toxic effect of contact with venomous toad, assault
    - +7th T63.824 Toxic effect of contact with venomous toad, undetermined
  - +T63.83 Toxic effect of contact with other venomous amphibian
    - **Excludes1:** contact with nonvenomous amphibian (W62.9)
    - +7th T63.831 Toxic effect of contact with other venomous amphibian, accidental (unintentional)
    - +7th T63.832 Toxic effect of contact with other venomous amphibian, intentional self-harm
    - +7th T63.833 Toxic effect of contact with other venomous amphibian, assault
    - +7th T63.834 Toxic effect of contact with other venomous amphibian, undetermined
  - +T63.89 Toxic effect of contact with other venomous animals
    - +7th T63.891 Toxic effect of contact with other venomous animals, accidental (unintentional)
    - +7th T63.892 Toxic effect of contact with other venomous animals, intentional self-harm
    - +7th T63.893 Toxic effect of contact with other venomous animals, assault
    - +7th T63.894 Toxic effect of contact with other venomous animals, undetermined
- +T63.9 Toxic effect of contact with unspecified venomous animal
  - X+7th T63.91 Toxic effect of contact with unspecified venomous animal, accidental (unintentional)
  - X+7th T63.92 Toxic effect of contact with unspecified venomous animal, intentional self-harm
  - X+7th T63.93 Toxic effect of contact with unspecified venomous animal, assault
  - X+7th T63.94 Toxic effect of contact with unspecified venomous animal, undetermined

T64 Toxic effect of aflatoxin and other mycotoxin food contaminants

The appropriate 7th character is to be added to each code from category T64
- A initial encounter
- D subsequent encounter
- S sequela

- +T64.0 Toxic effect of aflatoxin
  - X+7th T64.01 Toxic effect of aflatoxin, accidental (unintentional)
  - X+7th T64.02 Toxic effect of aflatoxin, intentional self-harm
  - X+7th T64.03 Toxic effect of aflatoxin, assault
  - X+7th T64.04 Toxic effect of aflatoxin, undetermined
- +T64.8 Toxic effect of other mycotoxin food contaminants
  - X+7th T64.81 Toxic effect of other mycotoxin food contaminants, accidental (unintentional)
  - X+7th T64.82 Toxic effect of other mycotoxin food contaminants, intentional self-harm
  - X+7th T64.83 Toxic effect of other mycotoxin food contaminants, assault
  - X+7th T64.84 Toxic effect of other mycotoxin food contaminants, undetermined

T65 Toxic effect of other and unspecified substances

The appropriate 7th character is to be added to each code from category T65
- A initial encounter
- D subsequent encounter
- S sequela

- **+ T65.0 Toxic effect of cyanides**
  - *Excludes1:* hydrogen cyanide (T57.3-)
  - **+ T65.0X Toxic effect of cyanides**
    - +7th T65.0X1 Toxic effect of cyanides, accidental (unintentional)
      - Toxic effect of cyanides NOS
    - +7th T65.0X2 Toxic effect of cyanides, intentional self-harm
    - +7th T65.0X3 Toxic effect of cyanides, assault
    - +7th T65.0X4 Toxic effect of cyanides, undetermined
- **+ T65.1 Toxic effect of strychnine and its salts**
  - **+ T65.1X Toxic effect of strychnine and its salts**
    - +7th T65.1X1 Toxic effect of strychnine and its salts, accidental (unintentional)
      - Toxic effect of strychnine and its salts NOS
    - +7th T65.1X2 Toxic effect of strychnine and its salts, intentional self-harm
    - +7th T65.1X3 Toxic effect of strychnine and its salts, assault
    - +7th T65.1X4 Toxic effect of strychnine and its salts, undetermined
- **+ T65.2 Toxic effect of tobacco and nicotine**
  - *Excludes2:* nicotine dependence (F17.-)
  - **+ T65.21 Toxic effect of chewing tobacco**
    - +7th T65.211 Toxic effect of chewing tobacco, accidental (unintentional)
      - Toxic effect of chewing tobacco NOS
    - +7th T65.212 Toxic effect of chewing tobacco, intentional self-harm
    - +7th T65.213 Toxic effect of chewing tobacco, assault
    - +7th T65.214 Toxic effect of chewing tobacco, undetermined
  - **+ T65.22 Toxic effect of tobacco cigarettes**
    - Toxic effect of tobacco smoke
    - Use additional code for exposure to second hand tobacco smoke (Z57.31, Z77.22)
    - +7th T65.221 Toxic effect of tobacco cigarettes, accidental (unintentional)
      - Toxic effect of tobacco cigarettes NOS
    - +7th T65.222 Toxic effect of tobacco cigarettes, intentional self-harm
    - +7th T65.223 Toxic effect of tobacco cigarettes, assault
    - +7th T65.224 Toxic effect of tobacco cigarettes, undetermined
  - **+ T65.29 Toxic effect of other tobacco and nicotine**
    - +7th T65.291 Toxic effect of other tobacco and nicotine, accidental (unintentional)
      - Toxic effect of other tobacco and nicotine NOS
    - +7th T65.292 Toxic effect of other tobacco and nicotine, intentional self-harm
    - +7th T65.293 Toxic effect of other tobacco and nicotine, assault
    - +7th T65.294 Toxic effect of other tobacco and nicotine, undetermined
- **+ T65.3 Toxic effect of nitroderivatives and aminoderivatives of benzene and its homologues**
  - Toxic effect of anilin [benzenamine]
  - Toxic effect of nitrobenzene
  - Toxic effect of trinitrotoluene
  - **+ T65.3X Toxic effect of nitroderivatives and aminoderivatives of benzene and its homologues**
    - +7th T65.3X1 Toxic effect of nitroderivatives and aminoderivatives of benzene and its homologues, accidental (unintentional)
      - Toxic effect of nitroderivatives and aminoderivatives of benzene and its homologues NOS
    - +7th T65.3X2 Toxic effect of nitroderivatives and aminoderivatives of benzene and its homologues, intentional self-harm
    - +7th T65.3X3 Toxic effect of nitroderivatives and aminoderivatives of benzene and its homologues, assault
    - +7th T65.3X4 Toxic effect of nitroderivatives and aminoderivatives of benzene and its homologues, undetermined
- **+ T65.4 Toxic effect of carbon disulfide**
  - **+ T65.4X Toxic effect of carbon disulfide**
    - +7th T65.4X1 Toxic effect of carbon disulfide, accidental (unintentional)
      - Toxic effect of carbon disulfide NOS
    - +7th T65.4X2 Toxic effect of carbon disulfide, intentional self-harm
    - +7th T65.4X3 Toxic effect of carbon disulfide, assault
    - +7th T65.4X4 Toxic effect of carbon disulfide, undetermined
- **+ T65.5 Toxic effect of nitroglycerin and other nitric acids and esters**
  - Toxic effect of 1,2,3-Propanetriol trinitrate
  - **+ T65.5X Toxic effect of nitroglycerin and other nitric acids and esters**
    - +7th T65.5X1 Toxic effect of nitroglycerin and other nitric acids and esters, accidental (unintentional)
      - Toxic effect of nitroglycerin and other nitric acids and esters NOS
    - +7th T65.5X2 Toxic effect of nitroglycerin and other nitric acids and esters, intentional self-harm
    - +7th T65.5X3 Toxic effect of nitroglycerin and other nitric acids and esters, assault
    - +7th T65.5X4 Toxic effect of nitroglycerin and other nitric acids and esters, undetermined
- **+ T65.6 Toxic effect of paints and dyes, not elsewhere classified**
  - **+ T65.6X Toxic effect of paints and dyes, not elsewhere classified**
    - +7th T65.6X1 Toxic effect of paints and dyes, not elsewhere classified, accidental (unintentional)
      - Toxic effect of paints and dyes NOS
    - +7th T65.6X2 Toxic effect of paints and dyes, not elsewhere classified, intentional self-harm
    - +7th T65.6X3 Toxic effect of paints and dyes, not elsewhere classified, assault
    - +7th T65.6X4 Toxic effect of paints and dyes, not elsewhere classified, undetermined
- **+ T65.8 Toxic effect of other specified substances**
  - **+ T65.81 Toxic effect of latex**
    - +7th T65.811 Toxic effect of latex, accidental (unintentional)
      - Toxic effect of latex NOS
    - +7th T65.812 Toxic effect of latex, intentional self-harm
    - +7th T65.813 Toxic effect of latex, assault
    - +7th T65.814 Toxic effect of latex, undetermined
  - **+ T65.82 Toxic effect of harmful algae and algae toxins**
    - Toxic effect of (harmful) algae bloom NOS
    - Toxic effect of blue-green algae bloom
    - Toxic effect of brown tide
    - Toxic effect of cyanobacteria bloom
    - Toxic effect of Florida red tide
    - Toxic effect of pfiesteria piscicida
    - Toxic effect of red tide
    - +7th T65.821 Toxic effect of harmful algae and algae toxins, accidental (unintentional)
      - Toxic effect of harmful algae and algae toxins NOS
    - +7th T65.822 Toxic effect of harmful algae and algae toxins, intentional self-harm
    - +7th T65.823 Toxic effect of harmful algae and algae toxins, assault
    - +7th T65.824 Toxic effect of harmful algae and algae toxins, undetermined

+ **T65.83** **Toxic effect of fiberglass**
- +7th **T65.831** Toxic effect of fiberglass, accidental (unintentional)
  - Toxic effect of fiberglass NOS
- +7th **T65.832** Toxic effect of fiberglass, intentional self-harm
- +7th **T65.833** Toxic effect of fiberglass, assault
- +7th **T65.834** Toxic effect of fiberglass, undetermined

+ **T65.89** **Toxic effect of other specified substances**
- +7th **T65.891** Toxic effect of other specified substances, accidental (unintentional)
  - Toxic effect of other specified substances NOS
  - *AHA CC: 1Q, 2018, 5*
- +7th **T65.892** Toxic effect of other specified substances, intentional self-harm
- +7th **T65.893** Toxic effect of other specified substances, assault
- +7th **T65.894** Toxic effect of other specified substances, undetermined

+ **T65.9** **Toxic effect of unspecified substance**
- X+7th **T65.91** Toxic effect of unspecified substance, accidental (unintentional)
  - Poisoning NOS
- X+7th **T65.92** Toxic effect of unspecified substance, intentional self-harm
- X+7th **T65.93** Toxic effect of unspecified substance, assault
- X+7th **T65.94** Toxic effect of unspecified substance, undetermined

Other and unspecified effects of external causes (T66-T78)

T66 Radiation sickness, unspecified
X+7th

Excludes1: specified adverse effects of radiation, such as:
- burns (T20-T31)
- leukemia (C91-C95)
- radiation gastroenteritis and colitis (K52.0)
- radiation pneumonitis (J70.0)
- radiation related disorders of the skin and subcutaneous tissue (L55-L59)
- sunburn (L55.-)

The appropriate 7th character is to be added to code T66
- A initial encounter
- D subsequent encounter
- S sequela

T67 Effects of heat and light

Excludes1: erythema [dermatitis] ab igne (L59.0)
malignant hyperpyrexia due to anesthesia (T88.3)
radiation-related disorders of the skin and subcutaneous tissue (L55-L59)

Excludes2: burns (T20-T31)
sunburn (L55.-)
sweat disorder due to heat (L74-L75)

The appropriate 7th character is to be added to each code from category T67
- A initial encounter
- D subsequent encounter
- S sequela

+ **T67.0** **Heatstroke and sunstroke**
Use additional code(s) to identify any associated complications of heatstroke, such as:
- coma and stupor (R40.-)
- rhabdomyolysis (M62.82)
- systemic inflammatory response syndrome (R65.1-)
AHA CC: 4Q, 2019, 17-18
HAC 7th character A see Appendix B for HAC conditional logic

- CC X+7th **T67.01** Heatstroke and sunstroke
  - Heat apoplexy
  - Heat pyrexia
  - Siriasis
  - Thermoplegia
  - HAC 7th character A see Appendix B for HAC conditional logic
- CC X+7th **T67.02** Exertional heatstroke
  - *AHA CC: 4Q, 2019, 17-18*
  - HAC 7th character A see Appendix B for HAC conditional logic
- CC X+7th **T67.09** Other heatstroke and sunstroke
  - HAC 7th character A see Appendix B for HAC conditional logic

- X+7th **T67.1** Heat syncope
  - Heat collapse
- X+7th **T67.2** Heat cramp
- X+7th **T67.3** Heat exhaustion, anhydrotic
  - Heat prostration due to water depletion
  - **Excludes1:** heat exhaustion due to salt depletion (T67.4)
- X+7th **T67.4** Heat exhaustion due to salt depletion
  - Heat prostration due to salt (and water) depletion
- X+7th **T67.5** Heat exhaustion, unspecified
  - Heat prostration NOS
- X+7th **T67.6** Heat fatigue, transient
- X+7th **T67.7** Heat edema
- X+7th **T67.8** Other effects of heat and light
- X+7th **T67.9** Effect of heat and light, unspecified

T68 Hypothermia
X+7th

Accidental hypothermia
Hypothermia NOS
Use additional code to identify source of exposure:
- Exposure to excessive cold of man-made origin (W93)
- Exposure to excessive cold of natural origin (X31)

Excludes1: hypothermia following anesthesia (T88.51)
hypothermia not associated with low environmental temperature (R68.0)
hypothermia of newborn (P80.-)

Excludes2: frostbite (T33-T34)

The appropriate 7th character is to be added to code T68
- A initial encounter
- D subsequent encounter
- S sequela

T69 Other effects of reduced temperature

Use additional code to identify source of exposure:
- Exposure to excessive cold of man-made origin (W93)
- Exposure to excessive cold of natural origin (X31)

Excludes2: frostbite (T33-T34)

The appropriate 7th character is to be added to each code from category T69
- A initial encounter
- D subsequent encounter
- S sequela

+ **T69.0** **Immersion hand and foot**
  + **T69.01** Immersion hand
    - +7th **T69.011** Immersion hand, right hand
    - +7th **T69.012** Immersion hand, left hand
    - +7th **T69.019** Immersion hand, unspecified hand
  + **T69.02** Immersion foot
    - Trench foot
    - CC +7th **T69.021** Immersion foot, right foot
      - HAC 7th character A see Appendix B for HAC conditional logic
    - CC +7th **T69.022** Immersion foot, left foot
      - HAC 7th character A see Appendix B for HAC conditional logic
    - CC +7th **T69.029** Immersion foot, unspecified foot
      - HAC 7th character A see Appendix B for HAC conditional logic

- X+7th **T69.1** Chilblains
- X+7th **T69.8** Other specified effects of reduced temperature
- X+7th **T69.9** Effect of reduced temperature, unspecified

T70 Effects of air pressure and water pressure

The appropriate 7th character is to be added to each code from category T70
- A initial encounter
- D subsequent encounter
- S sequela

- X+7th **T70.0** Otitic barotrauma
  - Aero-otitis media
  - Effects of change in ambient atmospheric pressure or water pressure on ears
- X+7th **T70.1** Sinus barotrauma
  - Aerosinusitis
  - Effects of change in ambient atmospheric pressure on sinuses

+ T70.2 Other and unspecified effects of high altitude
   Excludes2: polycythemia due to high altitude (D75.1)
   X+7th **T70.20** Unspecified effects of high altitude
   X+7th **T70.29** Other effects of high altitude
      Alpine sickness
      Anoxia due to high altitude
      Barotrauma NOS
      Hypobaropathy
      Mountain sickness
CC X+7th **T70.3** Caisson disease [decompression sickness]
   Compressed-air disease
   Diver's palsy or paralysis
   HAC 7th character A see Appendix B for HAC conditional logic
X+7th **T70.4** Effects of high-pressure fluids
   Hydraulic jet injection (industrial)
   Pneumatic jet injection (industrial)
   Traumatic jet injection (industrial)
X+7th **T70.8** Other effects of air pressure and water pressure
X+7th **T70.9** Effect of air pressure and water pressure, unspecified

T71 Asphyxiation
   Mechanical suffocation
   Traumatic suffocation
   Excludes1: acute respiratory distress (syndrome) (J80)
      anoxia due to high altitude (T70.2)
      asphyxia NOS (R09.01)
      asphyxia from carbon monoxide (T58.-)
      asphyxia from inhalation of food or foreign body (T17.-)
      asphyxia from other gases, fumes and vapors (T59.-)
      respiratory distress (syndrome) in newborn (P22.-)

   The appropriate 7th character is to be added to each code from category T71
   A   initial encounter
   D   subsequent encounter
   S   sequela

+ **T71.1 Asphyxiation due to mechanical threat to breathing**
   Suffocation due to mechanical threat to breathing
   + **T71.11 Asphyxiation due to smothering under pillow**
      CC +7th **T71.111** Asphyxiation due to smothering under pillow, accidental
         Asphyxiation due to smothering under pillow NOS
         HAC 7th character A see Appendix B for HAC conditional logic
      CC +7th **T71.112** Asphyxiation due to smothering under pillow, intentional self-harm
         HAC 7th character A see Appendix B for HAC conditional logic
      CC +7th **T71.113** Asphyxiation due to smothering under pillow, assault
         HAC 7th character A see Appendix B for HAC conditional logic
      CC +7th **T71.114** Asphyxiation due to smothering under pillow, undetermined
         HAC 7th character A see Appendix B for HAC conditional logic
   + **T71.12 Asphyxiation due to plastic bag**
      CC +7th **T71.121** Asphyxiation due to plastic bag, accidental
         Asphyxiation due to plastic bag NOS
         HAC 7th character A see Appendix B for HAC conditional logic
      CC +7th **T71.122** Asphyxiation due to plastic bag, intentional self-harm
         HAC 7th character A see Appendix B for HAC conditional logic
      CC +7th **T71.123** Asphyxiation due to plastic bag, assault
         HAC 7th character A see Appendix B for HAC conditional logic
      CC +7th **T71.124** Asphyxiation due to plastic bag, undetermined
         HAC 7th character A see Appendix B for HAC conditional logic

+ **T71.13 Asphyxiation due to being trapped in bed linens**
   CC +7th **T71.131** Asphyxiation due to being trapped in bed linens, accidental
      Asphyxiation due to being trapped in bed linens NOS
      HAC 7th character A see Appendix B for HAC conditional logic
   CC +7th **T71.132** Asphyxiation due to being trapped in bed linens, intentional self-harm
      HAC 7th character A see Appendix B for HAC conditional logic
   CC +7th **T71.133** Asphyxiation due to being trapped in bed linens, assault
      HAC 7th character A see Appendix B for HAC conditional logic
   CC +7th **T71.134** Asphyxiation due to being trapped in bed linens, undetermined
      HAC 7th character A see Appendix B for HAC conditional logic
+ **T71.14 Asphyxiation due to smothering under another person's body (in bed)**
   CC +7th **T71.141** Asphyxiation due to smothering under another person's body (in bed), accidental
      Asphyxiation due to smothering under another person's body (in bed) NOS
      HAC 7th character A see Appendix B for HAC conditional logic
   CC +7th **T71.143** Asphyxiation due to smothering under another person's body (in bed), assault
      HAC 7th character A see Appendix B for HAC conditional logic
   CC +7th **T71.144** Asphyxiation due to smothering under another person's body (in bed), undetermined
      HAC 7th character A see Appendix B for HAC conditional logic
+ **T71.15 Asphyxiation due to smothering in furniture**
   CC +7th **T71.151** Asphyxiation due to smothering in furniture, accidental
      Asphyxiation due to smothering in furniture NOS
      HAC 7th character A see Appendix B for HAC conditional logic
   CC +7th **T71.152** Asphyxiation due to smothering in furniture, intentional self-harm
      HAC 7th character A see Appendix B for HAC conditional logic
   CC +7th **T71.153** Asphyxiation due to smothering in furniture, assault
      HAC 7th character A see Appendix B for HAC conditional logic
   CC +7th **T71.154** Asphyxiation due to smothering in furniture, undetermined
      HAC 7th character A see Appendix B for HAC conditional logic
+ **T71.16 Asphyxiation due to hanging**
   Hanging by window shade cord
   Use additional code for any associated injuries, such as:
      crushing injury of neck (S17.-)
      fracture of cervical vertebrae (S12.0-S12.2-)
      open wound of neck (S11.-)
   CC +7th **T71.161** Asphyxiation due to hanging, accidental
      Asphyxiation due to hanging NOS
      Hanging NOS
      HAC 7th character A see Appendix B for HAC conditional logic
   CC +7th **T71.162** Asphyxiation due to hanging, intentional self-harm
      HAC 7th character A see Appendix B for HAC conditional logic
   CC +7th **T71.163** Asphyxiation due to hanging, assault
      HAC 7th character A see Appendix B for HAC conditional logic
   CC +7th **T71.164** Asphyxiation due to hanging, undetermined
      HAC 7th character A see Appendix B for HAC conditional logic

- **+ T71.19 Asphyxiation due to mechanical threat to breathing due to other causes**
  - CC +7th **T71.191** Asphyxiation due to mechanical threat to breathing due to other causes, accidental
    - Asphyxiation due to other causes NOS
    - *AHA CC: 4Q, 2016, 74-76*
    - HAC 7th character A see Appendix B for HAC conditional logic
  - CC +7th **T71.192** Asphyxiation due to mechanical threat to breathing due to other causes, intentional self-harm
    - HAC 7th character A see Appendix B for HAC conditional logic
  - CC +7th **T71.193** Asphyxiation due to mechanical threat to breathing due to other causes, assault
    - HAC 7th character A see Appendix B for HAC conditional logic
  - CC +7th **T71.194** Asphyxiation due to mechanical threat to breathing due to other causes, undetermined
    - HAC 7th character A see Appendix B for HAC conditional logic
- **+ T71.2 Asphyxiation due to systemic oxygen deficiency due to low oxygen content in ambient air**
  - Suffocation due to systemic oxygen deficiency due to low oxygen content in ambient air
  - CC X+7th **T71.20** Asphyxiation due to systemic oxygen deficiency due to low oxygen content in ambient air due to unspecified cause
    - HAC 7th character A see Appendix B for HAC conditional logic
  - CC X+7th **T71.21** Asphyxiation due to cave-in or falling earth
    - Use additional code for any associated cataclysm (X34-X38)
    - HAC 7th character A see Appendix B for HAC conditional logic
  - **+ T71.22 Asphyxiation due to being trapped in a car trunk**
    - CC +7th **T71.221** Asphyxiation due to being trapped in a car trunk, accidental
    - CC +7th **T71.222** Asphyxiation due to being trapped in a car trunk, intentional self-harm
    - CC +7th **T71.223** Asphyxiation due to being trapped in a car trunk, assault
    - CC +7th **T71.224** Asphyxiation due to being trapped in a car trunk, undetermined
  - **+ T71.23 Asphyxiation due to being trapped in a (discarded) refrigerator**
    - CC +7th **T71.231** Asphyxiation due to being trapped in a (discarded) refrigerator, accidental
    - CC +7th **T71.232** Asphyxiation due to being trapped in a (discarded) refrigerator, intentional self-harm
    - CC +7th **T71.233** Asphyxiation due to being trapped in a (discarded) refrigerator, assault
    - CC +7th **T71.234** Asphyxiation due to being trapped in a (discarded) refrigerator, undetermined
  - CC X+7th **T71.29** Asphyxiation due to being trapped in other low oxygen environment
    - HAC 7th character A see Appendix B for HAC conditional logic
- CC X+7th **T71.9 Asphyxiation due to unspecified cause**
  - Suffocation (by strangulation) due to unspecified cause
  - Suffocation NOS
  - Systemic oxygen deficiency due to low oxygen content in ambient air due to unspecified cause
  - Systemic oxygen deficiency due to mechanical threat to breathing due to unspecified cause
  - Traumatic asphyxia NOS
  - HAC 7th character A see Appendix B for HAC conditional logic

---

T73 Effects of other deprivation

The appropriate 7th character is to be added to each code from category T73
- A initial encounter
- D subsequent encounter
- S sequela

- X+7th **T73.0** Starvation
  - Deprivation of food
- X+7th **T73.1** Deprivation of water
- X+7th **T73.2** Exhaustion due to exposure
- X+7th **T73.3** Exhaustion due to excessive exertion
  - Exhaustion due to overexertion
- X+7th **T73.8** Other effects of deprivation
- X+7th **T73.9** Effect of deprivation, unspecified

T74 Adult and child abuse, neglect and other maltreatment, confirmed

Use additional code, if applicable, to identify any associated current injury.

Use additional external cause code to identify perpetrator, if known (Y07.-)

Excludes1: abuse and maltreatment in pregnancy (O9A.3-, O9A.4-, O9A.5-)
adult and child maltreatment, suspected (T76.-)

AHA CC: 4Q, 2018, 9; 1Q, 2023, 4

The appropriate 7th character is to be added to each code from category T74
- A initial encounter
- D subsequent encounter
- S sequela

Review coding guidelines C.5.c and C.19.f

- **+ T74.0 Neglect or abandonment, confirmed**
  - CC X+7th **T74.01** Adult neglect or abandonment, confirmed
  - CC X+7th **T74.02** Child neglect or abandonment, confirmed
- **+ T74.1 Physical abuse, confirmed**
  - **Excludes2:** sexual abuse (T74.2-)
  - CC X+7th **T74.11** Adult physical abuse, confirmed
  - CC X+7th **T74.12** Child physical abuse, confirmed
    - **Excludes2:** shaken infant syndrome (T74.4)
- **+ T74.2 Sexual abuse, confirmed**
  - Rape, confirmed
  - Sexual assault, confirmed
  - CC X+7th **T74.21** Adult sexual abuse, confirmed
  - CC X+7th **T74.22** Child sexual abuse, confirmed
- **+ T74.3 Psychological abuse, confirmed**
  - Bullying and intimidation, confirmed
  - Intimidation through social media, confirmed
  - Target of threatened harm, confirmed
  - Target of threatened physical violence, confirmed
  - Target of threatened sexual abuse, confirmed
  - X+7th **T74.31** Adult psychological abuse, confirmed
  - CC X+7th **T74.32** Child psychological abuse, confirmed
- CC X+7th **T74.4** Shaken infant syndrome
- **+ T74.5 Forced sexual exploitation, confirmed**
  - *AHA CC: 4Q, 2018, 32-33*
  - CC X+7th **T74.51** Adult forced sexual exploitation, confirmed
  - CC X+7th **T74.52** Child sexual exploitation, confirmed
- **+ T74.6 Forced labor exploitation, confirmed**
  - *AHA CC: 4Q, 2018, 32-33*
  - CC X+7th **T74.61** Adult forced labor exploitation, confirmed
  - CC X+7th **T74.62** Child forced labor exploitation, confirmed
- **+ T74.9 Unspecified maltreatment, confirmed**
  - CC X+7th **T74.91** Unspecified adult maltreatment, confirmed
  - CC X+7th **T74.92** Unspecified child maltreatment, confirmed
- **+ T74.A Financial abuse, confirmed**
  - X+7th **T74.A1** Adult financial abuse, confirmed
  - X+7th **T74.A2** Child financial abuse, confirmed

T75 Other and unspecified effects of other external causes

Excludes1: adverse effects NEC (T78.-)
Excludes2: burns (electric) (T20-T31)

The appropriate 7th character is to be added to each code from category T75
- A initial encounter
- D subsequent encounter
- S sequela

- **+ T75.0 Effects of lightning**
  - Struck by lightning

X+7th	T75.00	Unspecified effects of lightning	
		Struck by lightning NOS	
X+7th	T75.01	Shock due to being struck by lightning	
X+7th	T75.09	Other effects of lightning	

Use additional code for other effects of lightning

CC X+7th **T75.1** Unspecified effects of drowning and nonfatal submersion
Immersion
Excludes1: specified effects of drowning- code to effects
AHA CC: 1Q, 2023, 25-26
HAC 7th character A see Appendix B for HAC conditional logic

+ **T75.2** Effects of vibration
- X+7th T75.20 Unspecified effects of vibration
- X+7th T75.21 Pneumatic hammer syndrome
- X+7th T75.22 Traumatic vasospastic syndrome
- X+7th T75.23 Vertigo from infrasound
  - *Excludes1:* vertigo NOS (R42)
- X+7th T75.29 Other effects of vibration

X+7th **T75.3** Motion sickness
Airsickness
Seasickness
Travel sickness
Use additional external cause code to identify vehicle or type of motion (Y92.81-)

X+7th **T75.4** Electrocution
Shock from electric current
Shock from electroshock gun (taser)

+ **T75.8** Other specified effects of external causes
- X+7th T75.81 Effects of abnormal gravitation [G] forces
- X+7th T75.82 Effects of weightlessness
- X+7th T75.89 Other specified effects of external causes

T76 Adult and child abuse, neglect and other maltreatment, suspected
Use additional code, if applicable, to identify any associated current injury
Excludes1: adult and child maltreatment, confirmed (T74.-)
suspected abuse and maltreatment in pregnancy (O9A.3-, O9A.4-, O9A.5-)
suspected adult physical abuse, ruled out (Z04.71)
suspected adult sexual abuse, ruled out (Z04.41)
suspected child physical abuse, ruled out (Z04.72)
suspected child sexual abuse, ruled out (Z04.42)
AHA CC: 4Q, 2018, 9

The appropriate 7th character is to be added to each code from category T76
A initial encounter
D subsequent encounter
S sequela

Review coding guidelines C.5.c and C.19.f

+ **T76.0** Neglect or abandonment, suspected
- • CC X+7th T76.01 Adult neglect or abandonment, suspected
- • CC X+7th T76.02 Child neglect or abandonment, suspected
+ **T76.1** Physical abuse, suspected
- • CC X+7th T76.11 Adult physical abuse, suspected
- • CC X+7th T76.12 Child physical abuse, suspected
  - AHA CC: 2Q, 2019, 12
+ **T76.2** Sexual abuse, suspected
  Rape, suspected
  Excludes1: alleged abuse, ruled out (Z04.7)
- • CC X+7th T76.21 Adult sexual abuse, suspected
- • CC X+7th T76.22 Child sexual abuse, suspected
+ **T76.3** Psychological abuse, suspected
  Bullying and intimidation, suspected
  Intimidation through social medial, suspected
  Target of threatened harm, suspected
  Target of threatened physical violence, suspected
  Target of threatened sexual abuse, suspected
- • X+7th T76.31 Adult psychological abuse, suspected
- • CC X+7th T76.32 Child psychological abuse, suspected
+ **T76.5** Forced sexual exploitation, suspected
  AHA CC: 4Q, 2018, 32-33
- • CC X+7th T76.51 Adult forced sexual exploitation, suspected
- • CC X+7th T76.52 Child sexual exploitation, suspected
+ **T76.6** Forced labor exploitation, suspected
  AHA CC: 4Q, 2018, 32-33
- • CC X+7th T76.61 Adult forced labor exploitation, suspected
- • CC X+7th T76.62 Child forced labor exploitation, suspected
+ **T76.9** Unspecified maltreatment, suspected
- • CC X+7th T76.91 Unspecified adult maltreatment, suspected
- • CC X+7th T76.92 Unspecified child maltreatment, suspected
+ **T76.A** Financial abuse, suspected
- • X+7th T76.A1 Adult financial abuse, suspected
- • X+7th T76.A2 Child financial abuse, suspected

T78 Adverse effects, not elsewhere classified
Excludes2: complications of surgical and medical care NEC (T80-T88)

The appropriate 7th character is to be added to each code from category T78
A initial encounter
D subsequent encounter
S sequela

+ **T78.0** Anaphylactic reaction due to food
Anaphylactic reaction due to adverse food reaction
Anaphylactic shock or reaction due to nonpoisonous foods
Anaphylactoid reaction due to food
- CC X+7th T78.00 Anaphylactic reaction due to unspecified food
- CC X+7th T78.01 Anaphylactic reaction due to peanuts
- CC X+7th T78.02 Anaphylactic reaction due to shellfish (crustaceans)
- CC X+7th T78.03 Anaphylactic reaction due to other fish
- CC X+7th T78.04 Anaphylactic reaction due to fruits and vegetables
- CC X+7th T78.05 Anaphylactic reaction due to tree nuts and seeds
  Excludes2: anaphylactic reaction due to peanuts (T78.01)
- CC X+7th T78.06 Anaphylactic reaction due to food additives
- CC X+7th T78.07 Anaphylactic reaction due to milk and dairy products
- CC X+7th T78.08 Anaphylactic reaction due to eggs
- CC X+7th T78.09 Anaphylactic reaction due to other food products

X+7th **T78.1** Other adverse food reactions, not elsewhere classified
Use additional code to identify the type of reaction, if applicable
Excludes1: anaphylactic reaction or shock due to adverse food reaction (T78.0-)
anaphylactic reaction due to food (T78.0-)
bacterial food borne intoxications (A05.-)
Excludes2: allergic and dietetic gastroenteritis and colitis (K52.29)
allergic rhinitis due to food (J30.5)
dermatitis due to food in contact with skin (L23.6, L24.6, L25.4)
dermatitis due to ingested food (L27.2)
food protein-induced enterocolitis syndrome (K52.21)
food protein-induced enteropathy (K52.22)

CC X+7th **T78.2** Anaphylactic shock, unspecified
Allergic shock
Anaphylactic reaction
Anaphylaxis
Excludes1: anaphylactic reaction or shock due to adverse effect of correct medicinal substance properly administered (T88.6)
anaphylactic reaction or shock due to adverse food reaction (T78.0-)
anaphylactic reaction or shock due to serum (T80.5-)

X+7th **T78.3** Angioneurotic edema
Allergic angioedema
Giant urticaria
Quincke's edema
Excludes1: serum urticaria (T80.6-)
urticaria (L50.-)

+ **T78.4** Other and unspecified allergy
Excludes1: specified types of allergic reaction such as:
allergic diarrhea (K52.29)
allergic gastroenteritis and colitis (K52.29)
dermatitis (L23-L25, L27.-)
food protein-induced enterocolitis syndrome (K52.21)
food protein-induced enteropathy (K52.22)
hay fever (J30.1)
- X+7th T78.40 Allergy, unspecified
  Allergic reaction NOS
  Hypersensitivity NOS
- X+7th T78.41 Arthus phenomenon
  Arthus reaction
- X+7th T78.49 Other allergy
  AHA CC: 1Q, 2021, 42

X+7th **T78.8** Other adverse effects, not elsewhere classified

Certain early complications of trauma (T79)

T79 Certain early complications of trauma, not elsewhere classified

Excludes2: acute respiratory distress syndrome (J80)
complications occurring during or following medical procedures (T80-T88)
complications of surgical and medical care NEC (T80-T88)
newborn respiratory distress syndrome (P22.0)

The appropriate 7th character is to be added to each code from category T79
- A initial encounter
- D subsequent encounter
- S sequela

MCC X+7th T79.0 Air embolism (traumatic)
Excludes1: air embolism complicating abortion or ectopic or molar pregnancy (O00-O07, O08.2)
air embolism complicating pregnancy, childbirth and the puerperium (O88.0)
air embolism following infusion, transfusion, and therapeutic injection (T80.0)
air embolism following procedure NEC (T81.7-)

MCC X+7th T79.1 Fat embolism (traumatic)
Excludes1: fat embolism complicating:
abortion or ectopic or molar pregnancy (O00-O07, O08.2)
pregnancy, childbirth and the puerperium (O88.8)

CC X+7th T79.2 Traumatic secondary and recurrent hemorrhage and seroma

MCC X+7th T79.4 Traumatic shock
Shock (immediate) (delayed) following injury
Excludes1: anaphylactic shock due to adverse food reaction (T78.0-)
anaphylactic shock due to correct medicinal substance properly administered (T88.6)
anaphylactic shock due to serum (T80.5-)
anaphylactic shock NOS (T78.2)
electric shock (T75.4)
nontraumatic shock NEC (R57.-)
obstetric shock (O75.1)
postprocedural shock (T81.1-)
septic shock (R65.21)
shock complicating abortion or ectopic or molar pregnancy (O00-O07, O08.3)
shock due to anesthesia (T88.2)
shock due to lightning (T75.01)
shock NOS (R57.9)

MCC X+7th T79.5 Traumatic anuria
Crush syndrome
Renal failure following crushing

X+7th T79.6 Traumatic ischemia of muscle
Traumatic rhabdomyolysis
Volkmann's ischemic contracture
Excludes2: anterior tibial syndrome (M76.8)
compartment syndrome (traumatic) (T79.A-)
nontraumatic ischemia of muscle (M62.2-)

CC X+7th T79.7 Traumatic subcutaneous emphysema
Excludes2: emphysema NOS (J43)
emphysema (subcutaneous) resulting from a procedure (T81.82)

+ T79.A Traumatic compartment syndrome
Excludes1: fibromyalgia (M79.7)
nontraumatic compartment syndrome (M79.A-)
Excludes2: traumatic ischemic infarction of muscle (T79.6)

CC X+7th T79.A0 Compartment syndrome, unspecified
Compartment syndrome NOS

+ T79.A1 Traumatic compartment syndrome of upper extremity
Traumatic compartment syndrome of shoulder, arm, forearm, wrist, hand, and fingers

CC +7th T79.A11 Traumatic compartment syndrome of right upper extremity

CC +7th T79.A12 Traumatic compartment syndrome of left upper extremity

CC +7th T79.A19 Traumatic compartment syndrome of unspecified upper extremity

+ T79.A2 Traumatic compartment syndrome of lower extremity
Traumatic compartment syndrome of hip, buttock, thigh, leg, foot, and toes

CC +7th T79.A21 Traumatic compartment syndrome of right lower extremity

CC +7th T79.A22 Traumatic compartment syndrome of left lower extremity

CC +7th T79.A29 Traumatic compartment syndrome of unspecified lower extremity

CC X+7th T79.A3 Traumatic compartment syndrome of abdomen

CC X+7th T79.A9 Traumatic compartment syndrome of other sites

X+7th T79.8 Other early complications of trauma

X+7th T79.9 Unspecified early complication of trauma

Complications of surgical and medical care, not elsewhere classified (T80-T88)

Use additional code for adverse effect, if applicable, to identify drug (T36-T50 with fifth or sixth character 5)

Use additional code(s) to identify the specified condition resulting from the complication

Use additional code to identify devices involved and details of circumstances (Y62-Y82)

Excludes2: any encounters with medical care for postprocedural conditions in which no complications are present, such as:
artificial opening status (Z93.-)
closure of external stoma (Z43.-)
fitting and adjustment of external prosthetic device (Z44.-)
burns and corrosions from local applications and irradiation (T20-T32)
complications of surgical procedures during pregnancy, childbirth and the puerperium (O00-O9A)
mechanical complication of respirator [ventilator] (J95.850)
poisoning and toxic effects of drugs and chemicals (T36-T65 with fifth or sixth character 1-4 or 6)
postprocedural fever (R50.82)
specified complications classified elsewhere, such as:
cerebrospinal fluid leak from spinal puncture (G97.0)
colostomy malfunction (K94.0-)
disorders of fluid and electrolyte imbalance (E86-E87)
functional disturbances following cardiac surgery (I97.0-I97.1)
intraoperative and postprocedural complications of specified body systems (D78.-, E36.-, E89.-, G97.3-, G97.4, H59.3-, H59.-, H95.2-, H95.3, I97.4-, I97.5, J95.6-, J95.7, K91.6-, L76.-, M96.-, N99.-)
ostomy complications (J95.0-, K94.-, N99.5-)
postgastric surgery syndromes (K91.1)
postlaminectomy syndrome NEC (M96.1)
postmastectomy lymphedema syndrome (I97.2)
postsurgical blind-loop syndrome (K91.2)
ventilator associated pneumonia (J95.851)

T80 Complications following infusion, transfusion and therapeutic injection

Includes: complications following perfusion
Excludes2: bone marrow transplant rejection (T86.01)
febrile nonhemolytic transfusion reaction (R50.84)
fluid overload due to transfusion (E87.71)
posttransfusion purpura (D69.51)
transfusion associated circulatory overload (TACO) (E87.71)
transfusion (red blood cell) associated hemochromatosis (E83.111)
transfusion related acute lung injury (TRALI) (J95.84)

The appropriate 7th character is to be added to each code from category T80
- A initial encounter
- D subsequent encounter
- S sequela

MCC X+7th T80.0 Air embolism following infusion, transfusion and therapeutic injection
HAC 7th character A see Appendix B for HAC conditional logic

+, +7th, X + 7th • Newborn • Pediatric • Maternity • Adult ♀ Female ♂ Male Manifestation Unacceptable PDX HCC CC MCC HAC   1211

CC X+7th **T80.1** **Vascular complications following infusion, transfusion and therapeutic injection**
Use additional code to identify the vascular complication
Excludes2: extravasation of vesicant agent (T80.81-)
infiltration of vesicant agent (T80.81-)
vascular complications specified as due to prosthetic devices, implants and grafts (T82.8-, T83.8-, T84.8-, T85.8-)
postprocedural vascular complications (T81.7-)

+ **T80.2** **Infections following infusion, transfusion and therapeutic injection**
Use additional code to identify the specific infection, such as: sepsis (A41.9)
Use additional code (R65.2-) to identify severe sepsis, if applicable
Excludes2: infections specified as due to prosthetic devices, implants and grafts (T82.6-T82.7, T83.5-T83.6, T84.5-T84.7, T85.7)
postprocedural infections (T81.4-)
Review coding guideline C.1.d.5

+ **T80.21** **Infection due to central venous catheter**
Infection due to pulmonary artery catheter (Swan-Ganz catheter)

CC +7th **T80.211** **Bloodstream infection due to central venous catheter**
Catheter-related bloodstream infection (CRBSI) NOS
Central line-associated bloodstream infection (CLABSI)
Bloodstream infection due to Hickman catheter
Bloodstream infection due to peripherally inserted central catheter (PICC)
Bloodstream infection due to portacath (port-a-cath)
Bloodstream infection due to pulmonary artery catheter
Bloodstream infection due to triple lumen catheter
Bloodstream infection due to umbilical venous catheter
AHA CC: 4Q, 2018, 89; 1Q, 2019, 14
HAC 7th character A see Appendix B for HAC conditional logic

CC +7th **T80.212** **Local infection due to central venous catheter**
Exit or insertion site infection
Local infection due to Hickman catheter
Local infection due to peripherally inserted central catheter (PICC)
Local infection due to portacath (port-a-cath)
Local infection due to pulmonary artery catheter
Local infection due to triple lumen catheter
Local infection due to umbilical venous catheter
Port or reservoir infection
Tunnel infection
HAC 7th character A see Appendix B for HAC conditional logic

CC +7th **T80.218** **Other infection due to central venous catheter**
Other central line-associated infection
Other infection due to Hickman catheter
Other infection due to peripherally inserted central catheter (PICC)
Other infection due to portacath (port-a-cath)
Other infection due to pulmonary artery catheter
Other infection due to triple lumen catheter
Other infection due to umbilical venous catheter
HAC 7th character A see Appendix B for HAC conditional logic

CC +7th **T80.219** **Unspecified infection due to central venous catheter**
Central line-associated infection NOS
Unspecified infection due to Hickman catheter
Unspecified infection due to peripherally inserted central catheter (PICC)
Unspecified infection due to portacath (port-a-cath)
Unspecified infection due to pulmonary artery catheter
Unspecified infection due to triple lumen catheter
Unspecified infection due to umbilical venous catheter
HAC 7th character A see Appendix B for HAC conditional logic

CC X+7th **T80.22** **Acute infection following transfusion, infusion, or injection of blood and blood products**

CC X+7th **T80.29** **Infection following other infusion, transfusion and therapeutic injection**

+ **T80.3** **ABO incompatibility reaction due to transfusion of blood or blood products**
Excludes1: minor blood group antigens reactions (Duffy) (E) (K) (Kell) (Kidd) (Lewis) (M) (N) (P) (S) (T80.A-)

CC X+7th **T80.30** **ABO incompatibility reaction due to transfusion of blood or blood products, unspecified**
ABO incompatibility blood transfusion NOS
Reaction to ABO incompatibility from transfusion NOS
HAC 7th character A see Appendix B for HAC conditional logic

+ **T80.31** **ABO incompatibility with hemolytic transfusion reaction**

CC +7th **T80.310** **ABO incompatibility with acute hemolytic transfusion reaction**
ABO incompatibility with hemolytic transfusion reaction less than 24 hours after transfusion
Acute hemolytic transfusion reaction (AHTR) due to ABO incompatibility
HAC 7th character A see Appendix B for HAC conditional logic

CC +7th **T80.311** **ABO incompatibility with delayed hemolytic transfusion reaction**
ABO incompatibility with hemolytic transfusion reaction 24 hours or more after transfusion
Delayed hemolytic transfusion reaction (DHTR) due to ABO incompatibility
HAC 7th character A see Appendix B for HAC conditional logic

CC +7th **T80.319** **ABO incompatibility with hemolytic transfusion reaction, unspecified**
ABO incompatibility with hemolytic transfusion reaction at unspecified time after transfusion
Hemolytic transfusion reaction (HTR) due to ABO incompatibility NOS
HAC 7th character A see Appendix B for HAC conditional logic

CC X+7th **T80.39** **Other ABO incompatibility reaction due to transfusion of blood or blood products**
Delayed serologic transfusion reaction (DSTR) from ABO incompatibility
Other ABO incompatible blood transfusion
Other reaction to ABO incompatible blood transfusion
HAC 7th character A see Appendix B for HAC conditional logic

+	**T80.4**	**Rh incompatibility reaction due to transfusion of blood or blood products**	
		Reaction due to incompatibility of Rh antigens (C) (c) (D) (E) (e)	
CC X+7th	T80.40	**Rh incompatibility reaction due to transfusion of blood or blood products, unspecified**	
		Reaction due to Rh factor in transfusion NOS	
		Rh incompatible blood transfusion NOS	
+	**T80.41**	**Rh incompatibility with hemolytic transfusion reaction**	
CC +7th	T80.410	**Rh incompatibility with acute hemolytic transfusion reaction**	
		Acute hemolytic transfusion reaction (AHTR) due to Rh incompatibility	
		Rh incompatibility with hemolytic transfusion reaction less than 24 hours after transfusion	
CC +7th	T80.411	**Rh incompatibility with delayed hemolytic transfusion reaction**	
		Delayed hemolytic transfusion reaction (DHTR) due to Rh incompatibility	
		Rh incompatibility with hemolytic transfusion reaction 24 hours or more after transfusion	
CC +7th	T80.419	**Rh incompatibility with hemolytic transfusion reaction, unspecified**	
		Rh incompatibility with hemolytic transfusion reaction at unspecified time after transfusion	
		Hemolytic transfusion reaction (HTR) due to Rh incompatibility NOS	
CC X+7th	T80.49	**Other Rh incompatibility reaction due to transfusion of blood or blood products**	
		Delayed serologic transfusion reaction (DSTR) from Rh incompatibility	
		Other reaction to Rh incompatible blood transfusion	
+	**T80.A**	**Non-ABO incompatibility reaction due to transfusion of blood or blood products**	
		Reaction due to incompatibility of minor antigens (Duffy) (Kell) (Kidd) (Lewis) (M) (N) (P) (S)	
CC X+7th	T80.A0	**Non-ABO incompatibility reaction due to transfusion of blood or blood products, unspecified**	
		Non-ABO antigen incompatibility reaction from transfusion NOS	
+	**T80.A1**	**Non-ABO incompatibility with hemolytic transfusion reaction**	
CC +7th	T80.A10	**Non-ABO incompatibility with acute hemolytic transfusion reaction**	
		Acute hemolytic transfusion reaction (AHTR) due to non-ABO incompatibility	
		Non-ABO incompatibility with hemolytic transfusion reaction less than 24 hours after transfusion	
CC +7th	T80.A11	**Non-ABO incompatibility with delayed hemolytic transfusion reaction**	
		Delayed hemolytic transfusion reaction (DHTR) due to non-ABO incompatibility	
		Non-ABO incompatibility with hemolytic transfusion reaction 24 or more hours after transfusion	
CC +7th	T80.A19	**Non-ABO incompatibility with hemolytic transfusion reaction, unspecified**	
		Hemolytic transfusion reaction (HTR) due to non-ABO incompatibility NOS	
		Non-ABO incompatibility with hemolytic transfusion reaction at unspecified time after transfusion	
CC X+7th	T80.A9	**Other non-ABO incompatibility reaction due to transfusion of blood or blood products**	
		Delayed serologic transfusion reaction (DSTR) from non-ABO incompatibility	
		Other reaction to non-ABO incompatible blood transfusion	
+	**T80.5**	**Anaphylactic reaction due to serum**	
		Allergic shock due to serum	
		Anaphylactic shock due to serum	
		Anaphylactoid reaction due to serum	
		Anaphylaxis due to serum	
		Excludes1: ABO incompatibility reaction due to transfusion of blood or blood products (T80.3-)	
		allergic reaction or shock NOS (T78.2)	
		anaphylactic reaction or shock NOS (T78.2)	
		anaphylactic reaction or shock due to adverse effect of correct medicinal substance properly administered (T88.6)	
		other serum reaction (T80.6-)	
CC X+7th	T80.51	**Anaphylactic reaction due to administration of blood and blood products**	
CC X+7th	T80.52	**Anaphylactic reaction due to vaccination**	
		AHA CC: 1Q, 2021, 43	
CC X+7th	T80.59	**Anaphylactic reaction due to other serum**	
+	**T80.6**	**Other serum reactions**	
		Intoxication by serum	
		Protein sickness	
		Serum rash	
		Serum sickness	
		Serum urticaria	
		Excludes2: serum hepatitis (B16-B19)	
CC X+7th	T80.61	**Other serum reaction due to administration of blood and blood products**	
CC X+7th	T80.62	**Other serum reaction due to vaccination**	
		AHA CC: 1Q, 2021, 42	
CC X+7th	T80.69	**Other serum reaction due to other serum**	
		Code also, if applicable, arthropathy in hypersensitivity reactions classified elsewhere (M36.4)	
+	**T80.8**	**Other complications following infusion, transfusion and therapeutic injection**	
+	**T80.81**	**Extravasation of vesicant agent**	
		Infiltration of vesicant agent	
CC +7th	T80.810	**Extravasation of vesicant antineoplastic chemotherapy**	
		Infiltration of vesicant antineoplastic chemotherapy	
CC +7th	T80.818	**Extravasation of other vesicant agent**	
		Infiltration of other vesicant agent	
	T80.82	**Complication of immune effector cellular therapy**	
		Complication of chimeric antigen receptor (CAR-T) cell therapy	
		Complication of IEC therapy	
		Excludes2: complication of bone marrow transplant (T86.0)	
		complication of stem cell transplant (T86.5)	
		Use additional code to identify the specific complication, such as:	
		cytokine release syndrome (D89.83-)	
		immune effector cell-associated neurotoxicity syndrome (G92.0-)	
		AHA CC: 4Q, 2021, 31	
X+7th	T80.89	**Other complications following infusion, transfusion and therapeutic injection**	
		Delayed serologic transfusion reaction (DSTR), unspecified incompatibility	
		Use additional code to identify graft-versus-host reaction, if applicable, (D89.81-)	
		AHA CC: 4Q, 2020, 14-15	
+	**T80.9**	**Unspecified complication following infusion, transfusion and therapeutic injection**	
X+7th	T80.90	**Unspecified complication following infusion and therapeutic injection**	
+	**T80.91**	**Hemolytic transfusion reaction, unspecified incompatibility**	
		Excludes1: ABO incompatibility with hemolytic transfusion reaction (T80.31-)	
		Non-ABO incompatibility with hemolytic transfusion reaction (T80.A1-)	
		Rh incompatibility with hemolytic transfusion reaction (T80.41-)	
CC +7th	T80.910	**Acute hemolytic transfusion reaction, unspecified incompatibility**	
CC +7th	T80.911	**Delayed hemolytic transfusion reaction, unspecified incompatibility**	

1213

CC +7th **T80.919** Hemolytic transfusion reaction, unspecified incompatibility, unspecified as acute or delayed
  Hemolytic transfusion reaction NOS

X+7th **T80.92** Unspecified transfusion reaction
  Transfusion reaction NOS

T81 Complications of procedures, not elsewhere classified

Use additional code for adverse effect, if applicable, to identify drug (T36-T50 with fifth or sixth character 5)

Excludes2: complications following immunization (T88.0-T88.1)
  complications following infusion, transfusion and therapeutic injection (T80.-)
  complications of transplanted organs and tissue (T86.-)
  specified complications classified elsewhere, such as:
  complication of prosthetic devices, implants and grafts (T82-T85)
  dermatitis due to drugs and medicaments (L23.3, L24.4, L25.1, L27.0-L27.1)
  endosseous dental implant failure (M27.6-)
  floppy iris syndrome (IFIS) (intraoperative) H21.81
  intraoperative and postprocedural complications of specific body system (D78.-, E36.-, E89.-, G97.3-, G97.4, H59.3-, H59.-, H95.2-, H95.3, I97.4-, I97.5, J95, K91.-, L76.-, M96.-, N99.-)
  ostomy complications (J95.0-, K94.-, N99.5-)
  plateau iris syndrome (post-iridectomy) (postprocedural) (H21.82)
  poisoning and toxic effects of drugs and chemicals (T36-T65 with fifth or sixth character 1-4)

The appropriate 7th character is to be added to each code from category T81
A initial encounter
D subsequent encounter
S sequela

+ T81.1 Postprocedural shock
  Shock during or resulting from a procedure, not elsewhere classified
  Excludes1: anaphylactic shock NOS (T78.2)
    anaphylactic shock due to correct substance properly administered (T88.6)
    anaphylactic shock due to serum (T80.5-)
    electric shock (T75.4)
    obstetric shock (O75.1)
    shock due to anesthesia (T88.2)
    shock following abortion or ectopic or molar pregnancy (O00-O07, O08.3)
    traumatic shock (T79.4)

CC X+7th **T81.10** Postprocedural shock unspecified
  Collapse NOS during or resulting from a procedure, not elsewhere classified
  Postprocedural failure of peripheral circulation
  Postprocedural shock NOS

MCC X+7th **T81.11** Postprocedural cardiogenic shock

MCC X+7th **T81.12** Postprocedural septic shock
  Postprocedural endotoxic shock resulting from a procedure, not elsewhere classified
  Postprocedural gram-negative shock resulting from a procedure, not elsewhere classified
  Code first underlying infection
  Use additional code, to identify any associated acute organ dysfunction, if applicable
  Review coding guideline C.1.d.2 and C.1.d.5.c

MCC X+7th **T81.19** Other postprocedural shock
  Postprocedural hypovolemic shock
  AHA CC: 1Q, 2021, 13-14

+ T81.3 Disruption of wound, not elsewhere classified
  Disruption of any suture materials or other closure methods
  Excludes1: breakdown (mechanical) of permanent sutures (T85.612)
    displacement of permanent sutures (T85.622)
    disruption of cesarean delivery wound (O90.0)
    disruption of perineal obstetric wound (O90.1)
    mechanical complication of permanent sutures NEC (T85.692)
  AHA CC: 1Q, 2014, 23

CC X+7th **T81.30** Disruption of wound, unspecified
  Disruption of wound NOS

CC X+7th **T81.31** Disruption of external operation (surgical) wound, not elsewhere classified
  Dehiscence of operation wound NOS
  Disruption of operation wound NOS
  Disruption or dehiscence of closure of cornea
  Disruption or dehiscence of closure of mucosa
  Disruption or dehiscence of closure of skin and subcutaneous tissue
  Full-thickness skin disruption or dehiscence
  Superficial disruption or dehiscence of operation wound
  Excludes1: dehiscence of amputation stump (T87.81)
  AHA CC: 1Q, 2015, 3-21

CC X+7th **T81.32** Disruption of internal operation (surgical) wound, not elsewhere classified
  Deep disruption or dehiscence of operation wound NOS
  Disruption or dehiscence of closure of internal organ or other internal tissue
  Disruption or dehiscence of closure of muscle or muscle flap
  Disruption or dehiscence of closure of ribs or rib cage
  Disruption or dehiscence of closure of skull or craniotomy
  Disruption or dehiscence of closure of sternum or sternotomy
  Disruption or dehiscence of closure of tendon or ligament
  Disruption or dehiscence of closure of superficial or muscular fascia
  AHA CC: 3Q, 2017, 4; 2Q, 2020, 22-23

CC X+7th **T81.33** Disruption of traumatic injury wound repair
  Disruption or dehiscence of closure of traumatic laceration (external) (internal)

+ T81.4 Infection following a procedure
  Wound abscess following a procedure
  Use additional code to identify infection
  Use additional code (R65.2-) to identify severe sepsis, if applicable
  Excludes2: bleb associated endophthalmitis (H59.4-)
    infection due to infusion, transfusion and therapeutic injection (T80.2-)
    infection due to prosthetic devices, implants and grafts (T82.6-T82.7, T83.5-T83.6, T84.5-T84.7, T85.7)
    obstetric surgical wound infection (O86.0-)
    postprocedural fever NOS (R50.82)
    postprocedural retroperitoneal abscess (K68.11)
  AHA CC: 1Q, 2014, 23; 4Q, 2015, 37; 4Q, 2018, 33-34
  Review coding guidelines C.1.d.5.b and C.1.d.5

CC X+7th **T81.40** Infection following a procedure, unspecified
  HAC 7th character A see Appendix B for HAC conditional logic

CC X+7th **T81.41** Infection following a procedure, superficial incisional surgical site
  Subcutaneous abscess following a procedure
  Stitch abscess following a procedure
  HAC 7th character A see Appendix B for HAC conditional logic
  AHA CC: 4Q, 2018, 34

CC X+7th **T81.42** Infection following a procedure, deep incisional surgical site
  Intra-muscular abscess following a procedure
  HAC 7th character A see Appendix B for HAC conditional logic

CC X+7th **T81.43** Infection following a procedure, organ and space surgical site
  Intra-abdominal abscess following a procedure
  Subphrenic abscess following a procedure
  HAC 7th character A see Appendix B for HAC conditional logic

CC X+7th **T81.44** Sepsis following a procedure
  Use additional code to identify the sepsis
  HAC 7th character A see Appendix B for HAC conditional logic

CC X+7th **T81.49** Infection following a procedure, other surgical site
  HAC 7th character A see Appendix B for HAC conditional logic

- **+ T81.5 Complications of foreign body accidentally left in body following procedure**
  - **+ T81.50 Unspecified complication of foreign body accidentally left in body following procedure**
    - CC +7th **T81.500** Unspecified complication of foreign body accidentally left in body following surgical operation
      - HAC 7th character A see Appendix B for HAC conditional logic
    - CC +7th **T81.501** Unspecified complication of foreign body accidentally left in body following infusion or transfusion
      - HAC 7th character A see Appendix B for HAC conditional logic
    - CC +7th **T81.502** Unspecified complication of foreign body accidentally left in body following kidney dialysis
      - HAC 7th character A see Appendix B for HAC conditional logic
    - CC +7th **T81.503** Unspecified complication of foreign body accidentally left in body following injection or immunization
      - HAC 7th character A see Appendix B for HAC conditional logic
    - CC +7th **T81.504** Unspecified complication of foreign body accidentally left in body following endoscopic examination
      - HAC 7th character A see Appendix B for HAC conditional logic
    - CC +7th **T81.505** Unspecified complication of foreign body accidentally left in body following heart catheterization
      - HAC 7th character A see Appendix B for HAC conditional logic
    - CC +7th **T81.506** Unspecified complication of foreign body accidentally left in body following aspiration, puncture or other catheterization
      - HAC 7th character A see Appendix B for HAC conditional logic
    - CC +7th **T81.507** Unspecified complication of foreign body accidentally left in body following removal of catheter or packing
      - HAC 7th character A see Appendix B for HAC conditional logic
    - CC +7th **T81.508** Unspecified complication of foreign body accidentally left in body following other procedure
      - HAC 7th character A see Appendix B for HAC conditional logic
    - CC +7th **T81.509** Unspecified complication of foreign body accidentally left in body following unspecified procedure
      - HAC 7th character A see Appendix B for HAC conditional logic
  - **+ T81.51 Adhesions due to foreign body accidentally left in body following procedure**
    - CC +7th **T81.510** Adhesions due to foreign body accidentally left in body following surgical operation
      - HAC 7th character A see Appendix B for HAC conditional logic
    - CC +7th **T81.511** Adhesions due to foreign body accidentally left in body following infusion or transfusion
      - HAC 7th character A see Appendix B for HAC conditional logic
    - CC +7th **T81.512** Adhesions due to foreign body accidentally left in body following kidney dialysis
      - HAC 7th character A see Appendix B for HAC conditional logic
    - CC +7th **T81.513** Adhesions due to foreign body accidentally left in body following injection or immunization
      - HAC 7th character A see Appendix B for HAC conditional logic
    - CC +7th **T81.514** Adhesions due to foreign body accidentally left in body following endoscopic examination
      - HAC 7th character A see Appendix B for HAC conditional logic
    - CC +7th **T81.515** Adhesions due to foreign body accidentally left in body following heart catheterization
      - HAC 7th character A see Appendix B for HAC conditional logic
    - CC +7th **T81.516** Adhesions due to foreign body accidentally left in body following aspiration, puncture or other catheterization
      - HAC 7th character A see Appendix B for HAC conditional logic
    - CC +7th **T81.517** Adhesions due to foreign body accidentally left in body following removal of catheter or packing
      - HAC 7th character A see Appendix B for HAC conditional logic
    - CC +7th **T81.518** Adhesions due to foreign body accidentally left in body following other procedure
      - HAC 7th character A see Appendix B for HAC conditional logic
    - CC +7th **T81.519** Adhesions due to foreign body accidentally left in body following unspecified procedure
      - HAC 7th character A see Appendix B for HAC conditional logic
  - **+ T81.52 Obstruction due to foreign body accidentally left in body following procedure**
    - CC +7th **T81.520** Obstruction due to foreign body accidentally left in body following surgical operation
      - HAC 7th character A see Appendix B for HAC conditional logic
    - CC +7th **T81.521** Obstruction due to foreign body accidentally left in body following infusion or transfusion
      - HAC 7th character A see Appendix B for HAC conditional logic
    - CC +7th **T81.522** Obstruction due to foreign body accidentally left in body following kidney dialysis
      - HAC 7th character A see Appendix B for HAC conditional logic
    - CC +7th **T81.523** Obstruction due to foreign body accidentally left in body following injection or immunization
      - HAC 7th character A see Appendix B for HAC conditional logic
    - CC +7th **T81.524** Obstruction due to foreign body accidentally left in body following endoscopic examination
      - HAC 7th character A see Appendix B for HAC conditional logic
    - CC +7th **T81.525** Obstruction due to foreign body accidentally left in body following heart catheterization
      - HAC 7th character A see Appendix B for HAC conditional logic
    - CC +7th **T81.526** Obstruction due to foreign body accidentally left in body following aspiration, puncture or other catheterization
      - HAC 7th character A see Appendix B for HAC conditional logic
    - CC +7th **T81.527** Obstruction due to foreign body accidentally left in body following removal of catheter or packing
      - HAC 7th character A see Appendix B for HAC conditional logic
    - CC +7th **T81.528** Obstruction due to foreign body accidentally left in body following other procedure
      - HAC 7th character A see Appendix B for HAC conditional logic
    - CC +7th **T81.529** Obstruction due to foreign body accidentally left in body following unspecified procedure
      - HAC 7th character A see Appendix B for HAC conditional logic

+ T81.53 Perforation due to foreign body accidentally left in body following procedure

CC +7th T81.530 Perforation due to foreign body accidentally left in body following surgical operation
  HAC 7th character A see Appendix B for HAC conditional logic

CC +7th T81.531 Perforation due to foreign body accidentally left in body following infusion or transfusion
  HAC 7th character A see Appendix B for HAC conditional logic

+7th T81.532 Perforation due to foreign body accidentally left in body following kidney dialysis
  HAC 7th character A see Appendix B for HAC conditional logic

CC +7th T81.533 Perforation due to foreign body accidentally left in body following injection or immunization
  HAC 7th character A see Appendix B for HAC conditional logic

CC +7th T81.534 Perforation due to foreign body accidentally left in body following endoscopic examination
  HAC 7th character A see Appendix B for HAC conditional logic

CC +7th T81.535 Perforation due to foreign body accidentally left in body following heart catheterization
  HAC 7th character A see Appendix B for HAC conditional logic

CC +7th T81.536 Perforation due to foreign body accidentally left in body following aspiration, puncture or other catheterization
  HAC 7th character A see Appendix B for HAC conditional logic

CC +7th T81.537 Perforation due to foreign body accidentally left in body following removal of catheter or packing
  HAC 7th character A see Appendix B for HAC conditional logic

CC +7th T81.538 Perforation due to foreign body accidentally left in body following other procedure
  HAC 7th character A see Appendix B for HAC conditional logic

CC +7th T81.539 Perforation due to foreign body accidentally left in body following unspecified procedure
  HAC 7th character A see Appendix B for HAC conditional logic

+ T81.59 Other complications of foreign body accidentally left in body following procedure
  Excludes2: obstruction or perforation due to prosthetic devices and implants intentionally left in body (T82.0-T82.5, T83.0-T83.4, T83.7, T84.0-T84.4, T85.0-T85.6)

CC +7th T81.590 Other complications of foreign body accidentally left in body following surgical operation
  HAC 7th character A see Appendix B for HAC conditional logic
  AHA CC: 4Q, 2014, 24

CC +7th T81.591 Other complications of foreign body accidentally left in body following infusion or transfusion
  HAC 7th character A see Appendix B for HAC conditional logic

CC +7th T81.592 Other complications of foreign body accidentally left in body following kidney dialysis
  HAC 7th character A see Appendix B for HAC conditional logic

CC +7th T81.593 Other complications of foreign body accidentally left in body following injection or immunization
  HAC 7th character A see Appendix B for HAC conditional logic

CC +7th T81.594 Other complications of foreign body accidentally left in body following endoscopic examination
  HAC 7th character A see Appendix B for HAC conditional logic

CC +7th T81.595 Other complications of foreign body accidentally left in body following heart catheterization
  HAC 7th character A see Appendix B for HAC conditional logic

CC +7th T81.596 Other complications of foreign body accidentally left in body following aspiration, puncture or other catheterization
  HAC 7th character A see Appendix B for HAC conditional logic

CC +7th T81.597 Other complications of foreign body accidentally left in body following removal of catheter or packing
  HAC 7th character A see Appendix B for HAC conditional logic

CC +7th T81.598 Other complications of foreign body accidentally left in body following other procedure
  HAC 7th character A see Appendix B for HAC conditional logic

CC +7th T81.599 Other complications of foreign body accidentally left in body following unspecified procedure
  HAC 7th character A see Appendix B for HAC conditional logic

+ T81.6 Acute reaction to foreign substance accidentally left during a procedure
  Excludes2: complications of foreign body accidentally left in body cavity or operation wound following procedure (T81.5-)

CC X+7th T81.60 Unspecified acute reaction to foreign substance accidentally left during a procedure
  HAC 7th character A see Appendix B for HAC conditional logic

CC X+7th T81.61 Aseptic peritonitis due to foreign substance accidentally left during a procedure
  Chemical peritonitis
  HAC 7th character A see Appendix B for HAC conditional logic

CC X+7th T81.69 Other acute reaction to foreign substance accidentally left during a procedure
  HAC 7th character A see Appendix B for HAC conditional logic

+ T81.7 Vascular complications following a procedure, not elsewhere classified
  Air embolism following procedure NEC
  Phlebitis or thrombophlebitis resulting from a procedure
  Excludes1: embolism complicating abortion or ectopic or molar pregnancy (O00-O07, O08.2)
    embolism complicating pregnancy, childbirth and the puerperium (O88.-)
    traumatic embolism (T79.0)
  Excludes2: embolism due to prosthetic devices, implants and grafts (T82.8-, T83.81, T84.8-, T85.81-)
    embolism following infusion, transfusion and therapeutic injection (T80.0)

+ T81.71 Complication of artery following a procedure, not elsewhere classified

CC +7th T81.710 Complication of mesenteric artery following a procedure, not elsewhere classified

CC +7th T81.711 Complication of renal artery following a procedure, not elsewhere classified

CC +7th T81.718 Complication of other artery following a procedure, not elsewhere classified
  AHA CC: 2Q, 2019, 21-23

CC +7th T81.719 Complication of unspecified artery following a procedure, not elsewhere classified

CC X+7th T81.72 Complication of vein following a procedure, not elsewhere classified

+	**T81.8**	**Other complications of procedures, not elsewhere classified**
		Excludes2: *hypothermia following anesthesia (T88.51)*
		malignant hyperpyrexia due to anesthesia (T88.3)
X+7th	**T81.81**	**Complication of inhalation therapy**
X+7th	**T81.82**	**Emphysema (subcutaneous) resulting from a procedure**
CC X+7th	**T81.83**	**Persistent postprocedural fistula**
		Use Additional code, if known, for site of fistula such as:
		anal fistula (K60.3)
		anorectal fistula (K60.5)
		bladder fistula (N32.2)
		other female intestinal-genital tract fistulae (N82.4)
		AHA CC: 3Q, 2017, 3-5; 1Q, 2023, 30
X+7th	**T81.89**	**Other complications of procedures, not elsewhere classified**
		Use additional code to specify complication, such as:
		postprocedural delirium (F05)
		AHA CC: 1Q, 2014, 23
X+7th	**T81.9**	**Unspecified complication of procedure**

T82 Complications of cardiac and vascular prosthetic devices, implants and grafts

Excludes2: *failure and rejection of transplanted organs and tissue (T86.-)*

AHA CC: 3Q, 2020, 36

> The appropriate 7th character is to be added to each code from category T82
> A initial encounter
> D subsequent encounter
> S sequela

- **T82.0 Mechanical complication of heart valve prosthesis**
  Mechanical complication of artificial heart valve
  Excludes1: *mechanical complication of biological heart valve graft (T82.22-)*
  - CC X+7th **T82.01** Breakdown (mechanical) of heart valve prosthesis
  - CC X+7th **T82.02** Displacement of heart valve prosthesis
    Malposition of heart valve prosthesis
  - CC X+7th **T82.03** Leakage of heart valve prosthesis
  - CC X+7th **T82.09** Other mechanical complication of heart valve prosthesis
    Obstruction (mechanical) of heart valve prosthesis
    Perforation of heart valve prosthesis
    Protrusion of heart valve prosthesis
- **T82.1 Mechanical complication of cardiac electronic device**
  - **T82.11 Breakdown (mechanical) of cardiac electronic device**
    - CC +7th **T82.110** Breakdown (mechanical) of cardiac electrode
    - CC +7th **T82.111** Breakdown (mechanical) of cardiac pulse generator (battery)
    - CC +7th **T82.118** Breakdown (mechanical) of other cardiac electronic device
    - CC +7th **T82.119** Breakdown (mechanical) of unspecified cardiac electronic device
  - **T82.12 Displacement of cardiac electronic device**
    Malposition of cardiac electronic device
    - CC +7th **T82.120** Displacement of cardiac electrode
    - CC +7th **T82.121** Displacement of cardiac pulse generator (battery)
    - CC +7th **T82.128** Displacement of other cardiac electronic device
    - CC +7th **T82.129** Displacement of unspecified cardiac electronic device
  - **T82.19 Other mechanical complication of cardiac electronic device**
    Leakage of cardiac electronic device
    Obstruction of cardiac electronic device
    Perforation of cardiac electronic device
    Protrusion of cardiac electronic device
    - CC +7th **T82.190** Other mechanical complication of cardiac electrode
    - CC +7th **T82.191** Other mechanical complication of cardiac pulse generator (battery)
    - CC +7th **T82.198** Other mechanical complication of other cardiac electronic device
    - CC +7th **T82.199** Other mechanical complication of unspecified cardiac device
- **T82.2 Mechanical complication of coronary artery bypass graft and biological heart valve graft**
  Excludes1: *mechanical complication of artificial heart valve prosthesis (T82.0-)*
  - **T82.21 Mechanical complication of coronary artery bypass graft**
    - CC +7th **T82.211** Breakdown (mechanical) of coronary artery bypass graft
    - CC +7th **T82.212** Displacement of coronary artery bypass graft
      Malposition of coronary artery bypass graft
    - CC +7th **T82.213** Leakage of coronary artery bypass graft
    - CC +7th **T82.218** Other mechanical complication of coronary artery bypass graft
      Obstruction, mechanical of coronary artery bypass graft
      Perforation of coronary artery bypass graft
      Protrusion of coronary artery bypass graft
  - **T82.22 Mechanical complication of biological heart valve graft**
    - CC +7th **T82.221** Breakdown (mechanical) of biological heart valve graft
    - CC +7th **T82.222** Displacement of biological heart valve graft
      Malposition of biological heart valve graft
    - CC +7th **T82.223** Leakage of biological heart valve graft
    - CC +7th **T82.228** Other mechanical complication of biological heart valve graft
      Obstruction of biological heart valve graft
      Perforation of biological heart valve graft
      Protrusion of biological heart valve graft
- **T82.3 Mechanical complication of other vascular grafts**
  - **T82.31 Breakdown (mechanical) of other vascular grafts**
    - CC +7th **T82.310** Breakdown (mechanical) of aortic (bifurcation) graft (replacement)
      AHA CC: 3Q, 2020, 3-7
    - CC +7th **T82.311** Breakdown (mechanical) of carotid arterial graft (bypass)
    - CC +7th **T82.312** Breakdown (mechanical) of femoral arterial graft (bypass)
    - CC +7th **T82.318** Breakdown (mechanical) of other vascular grafts
    - CC +7th **T82.319** Breakdown (mechanical) of unspecified vascular grafts
  - **T82.32 Displacement of other vascular grafts**
    Malposition of other vascular grafts
    - CC +7th **T82.320** Displacement of aortic (bifurcation) graft (replacement)
    - CC +7th **T82.321** Displacement of carotid arterial graft (bypass)
    - CC +7th **T82.322** Displacement of femoral arterial graft (bypass)
    - CC +7th **T82.328** Displacement of other vascular grafts
    - CC +7th **T82.329** Displacement of unspecified vascular grafts
  - **T82.33 Leakage of other vascular grafts**
    - CC +7th **T82.330** Leakage of aortic (bifurcation) graft (replacement)
      AHA CC: 3Q, 2020, 4-7
    - CC +7th **T82.331** Leakage of carotid arterial graft (bypass)
    - CC +7th **T82.332** Leakage of femoral arterial graft (bypass)
    - CC +7th **T82.338** Leakage of other vascular grafts
    - CC +7th **T82.339** Leakage of unspecified vascular graft
  - **T82.39 Other mechanical complication of other vascular grafts**
    Obstruction (mechanical) of other vascular grafts
    Perforation of other vascular grafts
    Protrusion of other vascular grafts
    - CC +7th **T82.390** Other mechanical complication of aortic (bifurcation) graft (replacement)
      AHA CC: 3Q, 2020, 5
    - CC +7th **T82.391** Other mechanical complication of carotid arterial graft (bypass)
    - CC +7th **T82.392** Other mechanical complication of femoral arterial graft (bypass)
    - CC +7th **T82.398** Other mechanical complication of other vascular grafts
    - CC +7th **T82.399** Other mechanical complication of unspecified vascular grafts

- **T82.4 Mechanical complication of vascular dialysis catheter**
  Mechanical complication of hemodialysis catheter
  Excludes1: mechanical complication of intraperitoneal dialysis catheter (T85.62)
  - CC X+7th **T82.41** Breakdown (mechanical) of vascular dialysis catheter
  - CC X+7th **T82.42** Displacement of vascular dialysis catheter
    Malposition of vascular dialysis catheter
  - CC X+7th **T82.43** Leakage of vascular dialysis catheter
  - CC X+7th **T82.49** Other complication of vascular dialysis catheter
    Obstruction (mechanical) of vascular dialysis catheter
    Perforation of vascular dialysis catheter
    Protrusion of vascular dialysis catheter
- **T82.5 Mechanical complication of other cardiac and vascular devices and implants**
  Excludes2: mechanical complication of epidural and subdural infusion catheter (T85.61)
  - **T82.51** Breakdown (mechanical) of other cardiac and vascular devices and implants
    - CC +7th **T82.510** Breakdown (mechanical) of surgically created arteriovenous fistula
      AHA CC: 3Q, 2020, 36
    - CC +7th **T82.511** Breakdown (mechanical) of surgically created arteriovenous shunt
      AHA CC: 3Q, 2020, 37
    - CC +7th **T82.512** Breakdown (mechanical) of artificial heart
    - CC +7th **T82.513** Breakdown (mechanical) of balloon (counterpulsation) device
    - CC +7th **T82.514** Breakdown (mechanical) of infusion catheter
    - CC +7th **T82.515** Breakdown (mechanical) of umbrella device
    - CC +7th **T82.518** Breakdown (mechanical) of other cardiac and vascular devices and implants
    - CC +7th **T82.519** Breakdown (mechanical) of unspecified cardiac and vascular devices and implants
  - **T82.52** Displacement of other cardiac and vascular devices and implants
    Malposition of other cardiac and vascular devices and implants
    - CC +7th **T82.520** Displacement of surgically created arteriovenous fistula
    - CC +7th **T82.521** Displacement of surgically created arteriovenous shunt
    - CC +7th **T82.522** Displacement of artificial heart
    - CC +7th **T82.523** Displacement of balloon (counterpulsation) device
    - CC +7th **T82.524** Displacement of infusion catheter
      AHA CC: 3Q, 2019, 15-16; 2Q, 2020, 21-22
    - CC +7th **T82.525** Displacement of umbrella device
    - CC +7th **T82.528** Displacement of other cardiac and vascular devices and implants
    - CC +7th **T82.529** Displacement of unspecified cardiac and vascular devices and implants
  - **T82.53** Leakage of other cardiac and vascular devices and implants
    - CC +7th **T82.530** Leakage of surgically created arteriovenous fistula
    - CC +7th **T82.531** Leakage of surgically created arteriovenous shunt
    - CC +7th **T82.532** Leakage of artificial heart
    - CC +7th **T82.533** Leakage of balloon (counterpulsation) device
    - CC +7th **T82.534** Leakage of infusion catheter
    - CC +7th **T82.535** Leakage of umbrella device
    - CC +7th **T82.538** Leakage of other cardiac and vascular devices and implants
    - CC +7th **T82.539** Leakage of unspecified cardiac and vascular devices and implants
- **T82.59 Other mechanical complication of other cardiac and vascular devices and implants**
  Obstruction (mechanical) of other cardiac and vascular devices and implants
  Perforation of other cardiac and vascular devices and implants
  Protrusion of other cardiac and vascular devices and implants
  - CC +7th **T82.590** Other mechanical complication of surgically created arteriovenous fistula
  - CC +7th **T82.591** Other mechanical complication of surgically created arteriovenous shunt
  - CC +7th **T82.592** Other mechanical complication of artificial heart
  - CC +7th **T82.593** Other mechanical complication of balloon (counterpulsation) device
  - CC +7th **T82.594** Other mechanical complication of infusion catheter
  - CC +7th **T82.595** Other mechanical complication of umbrella device
  - CC +7th **T82.598** Other mechanical complication of other cardiac and vascular devices and implants
  - CC +7th **T82.599** Other mechanical complication of unspecified cardiac and vascular devices and implants
- CC X+7th **T82.6 Infection and inflammatory reaction due to cardiac valve prosthesis**
  Use additional code to identify infection
  HAC 7th character A see Appendix B for HAC conditional logic
- CC X+7th **T82.7 Infection and inflammatory reaction due to other cardiac and vascular devices, implants and grafts**
  Use additional code to identify infection
  HAC 7th character A see Appendix B for HAC conditional logic
  AHA CC: 1Q, 2015, 3-21; 4Q, 2018, 89; 1Q, 2019, 13-14
- **T82.8 Other specified complications due to cardiac and vascular prosthetic devices, implants and grafts**
  - **T82.81** Embolism due to cardiac and vascular prosthetic devices, implants and grafts
    - CC +7th **T82.817** Embolism due to cardiac prosthetic devices, implants and grafts
    - CC +7th **T82.818** Embolism due to vascular prosthetic devices, implants and grafts
  - **T82.82** Fibrosis due to cardiac and vascular prosthetic devices, implants and grafts
    - CC +7th **T82.827** Fibrosis due to cardiac prosthetic devices, implants and grafts
    - CC +7th **T82.828** Fibrosis due to vascular prosthetic devices, implants and grafts
  - **T82.83** Hemorrhage due to cardiac and vascular prosthetic devices, implants and grafts
    - CC +7th **T82.837** Hemorrhage due to cardiac prosthetic devices, implants and grafts
    - CC +7th **T82.838** Hemorrhage due to vascular prosthetic devices, implants and grafts
      AHA CC: 3Q, 2020, 36-37
  - **T82.84** Pain due to cardiac and vascular prosthetic devices, implants and grafts
    - CC +7th **T82.847** Pain due to cardiac prosthetic devices, implants and grafts
    - CC +7th **T82.848** Pain due to vascular prosthetic devices, implants and grafts
  - **T82.85** Stenosis due to cardiac and vascular prosthetic devices, implants and grafts
    - CC +7th **T82.855** Stenosis of coronary artery stent
      In-stent stenosis (restenosis) of coronary artery stent
      Restenosis of coronary artery stent
      AHA CC: 4Q, 2016, 69; 3Q, 2021, 6-8
    - CC +7th **T82.856** Stenosis of peripheral vascular stent
      In-stent stenosis (restenosis) of peripheral vascular stent
      Restenosis of peripheral vascular stent
      AHA CC: 4Q, 2016, 69
    - CC +7th **T82.857** Stenosis of other cardiac prosthetic devices, implants and grafts
    - CC +7th **T82.858** Stenosis of other vascular prosthetic devices, implants and grafts

- **+ T82.86** Thrombosis due to cardiac and vascular prosthetic devices, implants and grafts
  - **CC +7th T82.867** Thrombosis due to cardiac prosthetic devices, implants and grafts
    AHA CC: 2Q, 2019, 32-33
  - **CC +7th T82.868** Thrombosis due to vascular prosthetic devices, implants and grafts
    AHA CC: 2Q, 2023, 7
- **+ T82.89** Other specified complication of cardiac and vascular prosthetic devices, implants and grafts
  - **CC +7th T82.897** Other specified complication of cardiac prosthetic devices, implants and grafts
  - **CC +7th T82.898** Other specified complication of vascular prosthetic devices, implants and grafts
    AHA CC: 3Q, 2020, 3
- **CC X+7th T82.9** Unspecified complication of cardiac and vascular prosthetic device, implant and graft

T83 Complications of genitourinary prosthetic devices, implants and grafts

Excludes2: failure and rejection of transplanted organs and tissue (T86.-)

AHA CC: 4Q, 2016, 70-71

The appropriate 7th character is to be added to each code from category T83
- A initial encounter
- D subsequent encounter
- S sequela

- **+ T83.0** Mechanical complication of urinary catheter
  Excludes2: complications of stoma of urinary tract (N99.5-)
  - **+ T83.01** Breakdown (mechanical) of urinary catheter
    - **CC +7th T83.010** Breakdown (mechanical) of cystostomy catheter
    - **+7th T83.011** Breakdown (mechanical) of indwelling urethral catheter
    - **+7th T83.012** Breakdown (mechanical) of nephrostomy catheter
    - **+7th T83.018** Breakdown (mechanical) of other urinary catheter
      Breakdown (mechanical) of Hopkins catheter
      Breakdown (mechanical) of ileostomy catheter
      Breakdown (mechanical) of urostomy catheter
  - **+ T83.02** Displacement of urinary catheter
    Malposition of urinary catheter
    - **CC +7th T83.020** Displacement of cystostomy catheter
    - **+7th T83.021** Displacement of indwelling urethral catheter
    - **+7th T83.022** Displacement of nephrostomy catheter
    - **+7th T83.028** Displacement of other urinary catheter
      Displacement of Hopkins catheter
      Displacement of ileostomy catheter
      Displacement of urostomy catheter
  - **+ T83.03** Leakage of urinary catheter
    - **CC +7th T83.030** Leakage of cystostomy catheter
      AHA CC: 4Q, 2021, 18-19
    - **+7th T83.031** Leakage of indwelling urethral catheter
    - **+7th T83.032** Leakage of nephrostomy catheter
    - **+7th T83.038** Leakage of other urinary catheter
      Leakage of Hopkins catheter
      Leakage of ileostomy catheter
      Leakage of urostomy catheter
  - **+ T83.09** Other mechanical complication of urinary catheter
    Obstruction (mechanical) of urinary catheter
    Perforation of urinary catheter
    Protrusion of urinary catheter
    - **CC +7th T83.090** Other mechanical complication of cystostomy catheter
    - **+7th T83.091** Other mechanical complication of indwelling urethral catheter
    - **+7th T83.092** Other mechanical complication of nephrostomy catheter
    - **+7th T83.098** Other mechanical complication of other urinary catheter
      Other mechanical complication of Hopkins catheter
      Other mechanical complication of ileostomy catheter
      Other mechanical complication of urostomy catheter

- **+ T83.1** Mechanical complication of other urinary devices and implants
  - **+ T83.11** Breakdown (mechanical) of other urinary devices and implants
    - **CC +7th T83.110** Breakdown (mechanical) of urinary electronic stimulator device
      Excludes2: breakdown (mechanical) of electrode (lead) for sacral nerve neurostimulator (T85.111)
      breakdown (mechanical) of implanted electronic sacral neurostimulator, pulse generator or receiver (T85.113)
    - **CC +7th T83.111** Breakdown (mechanical) of implanted urinary sphincter
    - **CC +7th T83.112** Breakdown (mechanical) of indwelling ureteral stent
    - **CC +7th T83.113** Breakdown (mechanical) of other urinary stents
      Breakdown (mechanical) of ileal conduit stent
      Breakdown (mechanical) of nephroureteral stent
    - **CC +7th T83.118** Breakdown (mechanical) of other urinary devices and implants
  - **+ T83.12** Displacement of other urinary devices and implants
    Malposition of other urinary devices and implants
    - **CC +7th T83.120** Displacement of urinary electronic stimulator device
      Excludes2: displacement of electrode (lead) for sacral nerve neurostimulator (T85.121)
      displacement of implanted electronic sacral neurostimulator, pulse generator or receiver (T85.123)
    - **CC +7th T83.121** Displacement of implanted urinary sphincter
    - **CC +7th T83.122** Displacement of indwelling ureteral stent
    - **CC +7th T83.123** Displacement of other urinary stents
      Displacement of ileal conduit stent
      Displacement of nephroureteral stent
    - **CC +7th T83.128** Displacement of other urinary devices and implants
  - **+ T83.19** Other mechanical complication of other urinary devices and implants
    Leakage of other urinary devices and implants
    Obstruction (mechanical) of other urinary devices and implants
    Perforation of other urinary devices and implants
    Protrusion of other urinary devices and implants
    - **CC +7th T83.190** Other mechanical complication of urinary electronic stimulator device
      Excludes2: other mechanical complication of electrode (lead) for sacral nerve neurostimulator (T85.191)
      other mechanical complication of implanted electronic sacral neurostimulator, pulse generator or receiver (T85.193)
    - **CC +7th T83.191** Other mechanical complication of implanted urinary sphincter
    - **CC +7th T83.192** Other mechanical complication of indwelling ureteral stent
    - **CC +7th T83.193** Other mechanical complication of other urinary stent
      Other mechanical complication of ileal conduit stent
      Other mechanical complication of nephroureteral stent
    - **CC +7th T83.198** Other mechanical complication of other urinary devices and implants

+ T83.2 Mechanical complication of graft of urinary organ
- CC X+7th **T83.21** Breakdown (mechanical) of graft of urinary organ
- CC X+7th **T83.22** Displacement of graft of urinary organ
  - Malposition of graft of urinary organ
- CC X+7th **T83.23** Leakage of graft of urinary organ
- CC X+7th **T83.24** Erosion of graft of urinary organ
- CC X+7th **T83.25** Exposure of graft of urinary organ
- CC X+7th **T83.29** Other mechanical complication of graft of urinary organ
  - Obstruction (mechanical) of graft of urinary organ
  - Perforation of graft of urinary organ
  - Protrusion of graft of urinary organ

+ T83.3 Mechanical complication of intrauterine contraceptive device
- ♀ X+7th **T83.31** Breakdown (mechanical) of intrauterine contraceptive device
- ♀ X+7th **T83.32** Displacement of intrauterine contraceptive device
  - Malposition of intrauterine contraceptive device
  - Missing string of intrauterine contraceptive device
- ♀ X+7th **T83.39** Other mechanical complication of intrauterine contraceptive device
  - Leakage of intrauterine contraceptive device
  - Obstruction (mechanical) of intrauterine contraceptive device
  - Perforation of intrauterine contraceptive device
  - Protrusion of intrauterine contraceptive device

+ T83.4 Mechanical complication of other prosthetic devices, implants and grafts of genital tract
- **+ T83.41 Breakdown (mechanical) of other prosthetic devices, implants and grafts of genital tract**
  - ♂ CC +7th **T83.410** Breakdown (mechanical) of implanted penile prosthesis
    - Breakdown (mechanical) of penile prosthesis cylinder
    - Breakdown (mechanical) of penile prosthesis pump
    - Breakdown (mechanical) of penile prosthesis reservoir
  - CC +7th **T83.411** Breakdown (mechanical) of implanted testicular prosthesis
  - CC +7th **T83.418** Breakdown (mechanical) of other prosthetic devices, implants and grafts of genital tract
- **+ T83.42 Displacement of other prosthetic devices, implants and grafts of genital tract**
  - Malposition of other prosthetic devices, implants and grafts of genital tract
  - ♂ CC +7th **T83.420** Displacement of implanted penile prosthesis
    - Displacement of penile prosthesis cylinder
    - Displacement of penile prosthesis pump
    - Displacement of penile prosthesis reservoir
  - CC +7th **T83.421** Displacement of implanted testicular prosthesis
  - CC +7th **T83.428** Displacement of other prosthetic devices, implants and grafts of genital tract
    - *AHA CC: 1Q, 2018, 5-6*
- **+ T83.49 Other mechanical complication of other prosthetic devices, implants and grafts of genital tract**
  - Leakage of other prosthetic devices, implants and grafts of genital tract
  - Obstruction, mechanical of other prosthetic devices, implants and grafts of genital tract
  - Perforation of other prosthetic devices, implants and grafts of genital tract
  - Protrusion of other prosthetic devices, implants and grafts of genital tract
  - ♂ CC +7th **T83.490** Other mechanical complication of implanted penile prosthesis
    - Other mechanical complication of penile prosthesis cylinder
    - Other mechanical complication of penile prosthesis pump
    - Other mechanical complication of penile prosthesis reservoir
  - CC +7th **T83.491** Other mechanical complication of implanted testicular prosthesis
  - CC +7th **T83.498** Other mechanical complication of other prosthetic devices, implants and grafts of genital tract

+ T83.5 Infection and inflammatory reaction due to prosthetic device, implant and graft in urinary system
Use additional code to identify infection
- **+ T83.51 Infection and inflammatory reaction due to urinary catheter**
  - *Excludes2:* complications of stoma of urinary tract (N99.5-)
  - CC +7th **T83.510** Infection and inflammatory reaction due to cystostomy catheter
  - CC +7th **T83.511** Infection and inflammatory reaction due to indwelling urethral catheter
    - *AHA CC: 2Q, 2022, 7*
    - HAC 7th character A see Appendix B for HAC conditional logic
  - CC +7th **T83.512** Infection and inflammatory reaction due to nephrostomy catheter
  - CC +7th **T83.518** Infection and inflammatory reaction due to other urinary catheter
    - Infection and inflammatory reaction due to Hopkins catheter
    - Infection and inflammatory reaction due to ileostomy catheter
    - Infection and inflammatory reaction due to urostomy catheter
    - HAC 7th character A see Appendix B for HAC conditional logic
- **+ T83.59 Infection and inflammatory reaction due to prosthetic device, implant and graft in urinary system**
  - CC +7th **T83.590** Infection and inflammatory reaction due to implanted urinary neurostimulation device
    - *Excludes2:* infection and inflammatory reaction due to electrode lead of sacral nerve neurostimulator (T85.732)
      infection and inflammatory reaction due to pulse generator or receiver of sacralnerveneurostimulator (T85.734)
  - CC +7th **T83.591** Infection and inflammatory reaction due to implanted urinary sphincter
  - CC +7th **T83.592** Infection and inflammatory reaction due to indwelling ureteral stent
  - CC +7th **T83.593** Infection and inflammatory reaction due to other urinary stents
    - Infection and inflammatory reaction due to ileal conduit stents
    - Infection and inflammatory reaction due to nephroureteral stent
  - CC +7th **T83.598** Infection and inflammatory reaction due to other prosthetic device, implant and graft in urinary system
    - *AHA CC: 3Q, 2020, 25-26*

+ T83.6 Infection and inflammatory reaction due to prosthetic device, implant and graft in genital tract
Use additional code to identify infection
- CC X+7th **T83.61** Infection and inflammatory reaction due to implanted penile prosthesis
  - Infection and inflammatory reaction due to penile prosthesis cylinder
  - Infection and inflammatory reaction due to penile prosthesis pump
  - Infection and inflammatory reaction due to penile prosthesis reservoir
- CC X+7th **T83.62** Infection and inflammatory reaction due to implanted testicular prosthesis
- CC X+7th **T83.69** Infection and inflammatory reaction due to other prosthetic device, implant and graft in genital tract

- **T83.7 Complications due to implanted mesh and other prosthetic materials**
  - **T83.71 Erosion of implanted mesh and other prosthetic materials to surrounding organ or tissue**
    - ♀ +7th **T83.711** Erosion of implanted vaginal mesh to surrounding organ or tissue
      - Erosion of implanted vaginal mesh into pelvic floor muscles
    - CC +7th **T83.712** Erosion of implanted urethral mesh to surrounding organ or tissue
      - Erosion of implanted female urethral sling
      - Erosion of implanted male urethral sling
      - Erosion of implanted urethral mesh into pelvic floor muscles
    - CC +7th **T83.713** Erosion of implanted urethral bulking agent to surrounding organ or tissue
    - CC +7th **T83.714** Erosion of implanted ureteral bulking agent to surrounding organ or tissue
    - CC +7th **T83.718** Erosion of other implanted mesh to organ or tissue
    - CC +7th **T83.719** Erosion of other prosthetic materials to surrounding organ or tissue
  - **T83.72 Exposure of implanted mesh and other prosthetic materials into surrounding organ or tissue**
    - Extrusion of implanted mesh
    - ♀ +7th **T83.721** Exposure of implanted vaginal mesh into vagina
      - Exposure of implanted vaginal mesh through vaginal wall
    - CC +7th **T83.722** Exposure of implanted urethral mesh into urethra
      - Exposure of implanted female urethral sling
      - Exposure of implanted male urethral sling
      - Exposure of implanted urethral mesh through urethral wall
    - CC +7th **T83.723** Exposure of implanted urethral bulking agent into urethra
    - CC +7th **T83.724** Exposure of implanted ureteral bulking agent into ureter
    - CC +7th **T83.728** Exposure of other implanted mesh into organ or tissue
    - CC +7th **T83.729** Exposure of other prosthetic materials into organ or tissue
  - CC X+7th **T83.79** Other specified complications due to other genitourinary prosthetic materials
- **T83.8 Other specified complications of genitourinary prosthetic devices, implants and grafts**
  - CC X+7th **T83.81** Embolism due to genitourinary prosthetic devices, implants and grafts
  - CC X+7th **T83.82** Fibrosis due to genitourinary prosthetic devices, implants and grafts
  - CC X+7th **T83.83** Hemorrhage due to genitourinary prosthetic devices, implants and grafts
  - CC X+7th **T83.84** Pain due to genitourinary prosthetic devices, implants and grafts
  - CC X+7th **T83.85** Stenosis due to genitourinary prosthetic devices, implants and grafts
  - CC X+7th **T83.86** Thrombosis due to genitourinary prosthetic devices, implants and grafts
  - CC X+7th **T83.89** Other specified complication of genitourinary prosthetic devices, implants and grafts
    - *AHA CC: 3Q, 2022, 13*
- CC X+7th **T83.9** Unspecified complication of genitourinary prosthetic device, implant and graft

T84 Complications of internal orthopedic prosthetic devices, implants and grafts

Excludes2: failure and rejection of transplanted organs and tissues (T86.-)
fracture of bone following insertion of orthopedic implant, joint prosthesis or bone plate (M96.6)

The appropriate 7th character is to be added to each code from category T84
- A initial encounter
- D subsequent encounter
- S sequela

- **T84.0 Mechanical complication of internal joint prosthesis**
  - **T84.01 Broken internal joint prosthesis**
    - Breakage (fracture) of prosthetic joint
    - Broken prosthetic joint implant
    - **Excludes1:** periprosthetic joint implant fracture (M97.-)
    - CC +7th **T84.010** Broken internal right hip prosthesis
    - CC +7th **T84.011** Broken internal left hip prosthesis
    - CC +7th **T84.012** Broken internal right knee prosthesis
      - *AHA CC: 2Q, 2019, 27-28*
    - CC +7th **T84.013** Broken internal left knee prosthesis
    - CC +7th **T84.018** Broken internal joint prosthesis, other site
      - Use additional code to identify the joint (Z96.6-)
    - CC +7th **T84.019** Broken internal joint prosthesis, unspecified site
  - **T84.02 Dislocation of internal joint prosthesis**
    - Instability of internal joint prosthesis
    - Subluxation of internal joint prosthesis
    - CC +7th **T84.020** Dislocation of internal right hip prosthesis
    - CC +7th **T84.021** Dislocation of internal left hip prosthesis
    - CC +7th **T84.022** Instability of internal right knee prosthesis
    - CC +7th **T84.023** Instability of internal left knee prosthesis
    - CC +7th **T84.028** Dislocation of other internal joint prosthesis
      - Use additional code to identify the joint (Z96.6-)
    - CC +7th **T84.029** Dislocation of unspecified internal joint prosthesis
  - **T84.03 Mechanical loosening of internal prosthetic joint**
    - Aseptic loosening of prosthetic joint
    - CC +7th **T84.030** Mechanical loosening of internal right hip prosthetic joint
    - CC +7th **T84.031** Mechanical loosening of internal left hip prosthetic joint
    - CC +7th **T84.032** Mechanical loosening of internal right knee prosthetic joint
    - CC +7th **T84.033** Mechanical loosening of internal left knee prosthetic joint
    - CC +7th **T84.038** Mechanical loosening of other internal prosthetic joint
      - Use additional code to identify the joint (Z96.6-)
    - CC +7th **T84.039** Mechanical loosening of unspecified internal prosthetic joint
  - **T84.05 Periprosthetic osteolysis of internal prosthetic joint**
    - Use additional code to identify major osseous defect, if applicable (M89.7-)
    - CC +7th **T84.050** Periprosthetic osteolysis of internal prosthetic right hip joint
    - CC +7th **T84.051** Periprosthetic osteolysis of internal prosthetic left hip joint
    - CC +7th **T84.052** Periprosthetic osteolysis of internal prosthetic right knee joint
    - CC +7th **T84.053** Periprosthetic osteolysis of internal prosthetic left knee joint
    - CC +7th **T84.058** Periprosthetic osteolysis of other internal prosthetic joint
      - Use additional code to identify the joint (Z96.6-)
    - CC +7th **T84.059** Periprosthetic osteolysis of unspecified internal prosthetic joint

- **T84.06 Wear of articular bearing surface of internal prosthetic joint**
  - CC +7th **T84.060** Wear of articular bearing surface of internal prosthetic right hip joint
  - CC +7th **T84.061** Wear of articular bearing surface of internal prosthetic left hip joint
  - CC +7th **T84.062** Wear of articular bearing surface of internal prosthetic right knee joint
  - CC +7th **T84.063** Wear of articular bearing surface of internal prosthetic left knee joint
  - CC +7th **T84.068** Wear of articular bearing surface of other internal prosthetic joint
    Use additional code to identify the joint (Z96.6-)
  - CC +7th **T84.069** Wear of articular bearing surface of unspecified internal prosthetic joint
- **T84.09 Other mechanical complication of internal joint prosthesis**
  Prosthetic joint implant failure NOS
  - CC +7th **T84.090** Other mechanical complication of internal right hip prosthesis
    AHA CC: 1Q, 2019, 20
  - CC +7th **T84.091** Other mechanical complication of internal left hip prosthesis
  - CC +7th **T84.092** Other mechanical complication of internal right knee prosthesis
  - CC +7th **T84.093** Other mechanical complication of internal left knee prosthesis
  - CC +7th **T84.098** Other mechanical complication of other internal joint prosthesis
    Use additional code to identify the joint (Z96.6-)
  - CC +7th **T84.099** Other mechanical complication of unspecified internal joint prosthesis
- **T84.1 Mechanical complication of internal fixation device of bones of limb**
  Excludes2: mechanical complication of internal fixation device of bones of feet (T84.2-)
  mechanical complication of internal fixation device of bones of fingers (T84.2-)
  mechanical complication of internal fixation device of bones of hands (T84.2-)
  mechanical complication of internal fixation device of bones of toes (T84.2-)
  - **T84.11 Breakdown (mechanical) of internal fixation device of bones of limb**
    - CC +7th **T84.110** Breakdown (mechanical) of internal fixation device of right humerus
    - CC +7th **T84.111** Breakdown (mechanical) of internal fixation device of left humerus
    - CC +7th **T84.112** Breakdown (mechanical) of internal fixation device of bone of right forearm
    - CC +7th **T84.113** Breakdown (mechanical) of internal fixation device of bone of left forearm
    - CC +7th **T84.114** Breakdown (mechanical) of internal fixation device of right femur
    - CC +7th **T84.115** Breakdown (mechanical) of internal fixation device of left femur
    - CC +7th **T84.116** Breakdown (mechanical) of internal fixation device of bone of right lower leg
    - CC +7th **T84.117** Breakdown (mechanical) of internal fixation device of bone of left lower leg
    - CC +7th **T84.119** Breakdown (mechanical) of internal fixation device of unspecified bone of limb
  - **T84.12 Displacement of internal fixation device of bones of limb**
    Malposition of internal fixation device of bones of limb
    - CC +7th **T84.120** Displacement of internal fixation device of right humerus
    - CC +7th **T84.121** Displacement of internal fixation device of left humerus
    - CC +7th **T84.122** Displacement of internal fixation device of bone of right forearm
    - CC +7th **T84.123** Displacement of internal fixation device of bone of left forearm
    - CC +7th **T84.124** Displacement of internal fixation device of right femur
    - CC +7th **T84.125** Displacement of internal fixation device of left femur
    - CC +7th **T84.126** Displacement of internal fixation device of bone of right lower leg
    - CC +7th **T84.127** Displacement of internal fixation device of bone of left lower leg
    - CC +7th **T84.129** Displacement of internal fixation device of unspecified bone of limb
  - **T84.19 Other mechanical complication of internal fixation device of bones of limb**
    Obstruction (mechanical) of internal fixation device of bones of limb
    Perforation of internal fixation device of bones of limb
    Protrusion of internal fixation device of bones of limb
    - CC +7th **T84.190** Other mechanical complication of internal fixation device of right humerus
    - CC +7th **T84.191** Other mechanical complication of internal fixation device of left humerus
    - CC +7th **T84.192** Other mechanical complication of internal fixation device of bone of right forearm
    - CC +7th **T84.193** Other mechanical complication of internal fixation device of bone of left forearm
    - CC +7th **T84.194** Other mechanical complication of internal fixation device of right femur
    - CC +7th **T84.195** Other mechanical complication of internal fixation device of left femur
    - CC +7th **T84.196** Other mechanical complication of internal fixation device of bone of right lower leg
    - CC +7th **T84.197** Other mechanical complication of internal fixation device of bone of left lower leg
    - CC +7th **T84.199** Other mechanical complication of internal fixation device of unspecified bone of limb
- **T84.2 Mechanical complication of internal fixation device of other bones**
  - **T84.21 Breakdown (mechanical) of internal fixation device of other bones**
    - CC +7th **T84.210** Breakdown (mechanical) of internal fixation device of bones of hand and fingers
    - CC +7th **T84.213** Breakdown (mechanical) of internal fixation device of bones of foot and toes
    - CC +7th **T84.216** Breakdown (mechanical) of internal fixation device of vertebrae
    - CC +7th **T84.218** Breakdown (mechanical) of internal fixation device of other bones
  - **T84.22 Displacement of internal fixation device of other bones**
    Malposition of internal fixation device of other bones
    - CC +7th **T84.220** Displacement of internal fixation device of bones of hand and fingers
    - CC +7th **T84.223** Displacement of internal fixation device of bones of foot and toes
    - CC +7th **T84.226** Displacement of internal fixation device of vertebrae
    - CC +7th **T84.228** Displacement of internal fixation device of other bones

- T84.29 **Other mechanical complication of internal fixation device of other bones**
  - Obstruction (mechanical) of internal fixation device of other bones
  - Perforation of internal fixation device of other bones
  - Protrusion of internal fixation device of other bones
  - CC +7th **T84.290** Other mechanical complication of internal fixation device of bones of hand and fingers
  - CC +7th **T84.293** Other mechanical complication of internal fixation device of bones of foot and toes
  - CC +7th **T84.296** Other mechanical complication of internal fixation device of vertebrae
  - CC +7th **T84.298** Other mechanical complication of internal fixation device of other bones
- + T84.3 **Mechanical complication of other bone devices, implants and grafts**
  - *Excludes2:* other complications of bone graft (T86.83-)
  - + T84.31 **Breakdown (mechanical) of other bone devices, implants and grafts**
    - CC +7th **T84.310** Breakdown (mechanical) of electronic bone stimulator
    - CC +7th **T84.318** Breakdown (mechanical) of other bone devices, implants and grafts
  - + T84.32 **Displacement of other bone devices, implants and grafts**
    - Malposition of other bone devices, implants and grafts
    - CC +7th **T84.320** Displacement of electronic bone stimulator
    - CC +7th **T84.328** Displacement of other bone devices, implants and grafts
      - *AHA CC: 4Q, 2014, 28-29*
  - + T84.39 **Other mechanical complication of other bone devices, implants and grafts**
    - Obstruction (mechanical) of other bone devices, implants and grafts
    - Perforation of other bone devices, implants and grafts
    - Protrusion of other bone devices, implants and grafts
    - CC +7th **T84.390** Other mechanical complication of electronic bone stimulator
    - CC +7th **T84.398** Other mechanical complication of other bone devices, implants and grafts
- + T84.4 **Mechanical complication of other internal orthopedic devices, implants and grafts**
  - + T84.41 **Breakdown (mechanical) of other internal orthopedic devices, implants and grafts**
    - CC +7th **T84.410** Breakdown (mechanical) of muscle and tendon graft
    - CC +7th **T84.418** Breakdown (mechanical) of other internal orthopedic devices, implants and grafts
  - + T84.42 **Displacement of other internal orthopedic devices, implants and grafts**
    - Malposition of other internal orthopedic devices, implants and grafts
    - CC +7th **T84.420** Displacement of muscle and tendon graft
    - CC +7th **T84.428** Displacement of other internal orthopedic devices, implants and grafts
  - + T84.49 **Other mechanical complication of other internal orthopedic devices, implants and grafts**
    - Mechanical complication of other internal orthopedic devices, implants and grafts NOS
    - Obstruction (mechanical) of other internal orthopedic devices, implants and grafts
    - Perforation of other internal orthopedic devices, implants and grafts
    - Protrusion of other internal orthopedic devices, implants and grafts
    - CC +7th **T84.490** Other mechanical complication of muscle and tendon graft
    - CC +7th **T84.498** Other mechanical complication of other internal orthopedic devices, implants and grafts

- + T84.5 **Infection and inflammatory reaction due to internal joint prosthesis**
  - *Use additional code to identify infection*
  - CC X+7th **T84.50** Infection and inflammatory reaction due to unspecified internal joint prosthesis
  - CC X+7th **T84.51** Infection and inflammatory reaction due to internal right hip prosthesis
    - *AHA CC: 4Q, 2015, 36*
  - CC X+7th **T84.52** Infection and inflammatory reaction due to internal left hip prosthesis
    - *AHA CC: 1Q, 2015, 3-21*
  - CC X+7th **T84.53** Infection and inflammatory reaction due to internal right knee prosthesis
  - CC X+7th **T84.54** Infection and inflammatory reaction due to internal left knee prosthesis
  - CC X+7th **T84.59** Infection and inflammatory reaction due to other internal joint prosthesis
- + T84.6 **Infection and inflammatory reaction due to internal fixation device**
  - *Use additional code to identify infection*
  - CC X+7th **T84.60** Infection and inflammatory reaction due to internal fixation device of unspecified site
    - HAC 7th character A see Appendix B for HAC conditional logic
  - + T84.61 **Infection and inflammatory reaction due to internal fixation device of arm**
    - CC +7th **T84.610** Infection and inflammatory reaction due to internal fixation device of right humerus
      - HAC 7th character A see Appendix B for HAC conditional logic
    - CC +7th **T84.611** Infection and inflammatory reaction due to internal fixation device of left humerus
      - HAC 7th character A see Appendix B for HAC conditional logic
    - CC +7th **T84.612** Infection and inflammatory reaction due to internal fixation device of right radius
      - HAC 7th character A see Appendix B for HAC conditional logic
    - CC +7th **T84.613** Infection and inflammatory reaction due to internal fixation device of left radius
      - HAC 7th character A see Appendix B for HAC conditional logic
    - CC +7th **T84.614** Infection and inflammatory reaction due to internal fixation device of right ulna
      - HAC 7th character A see Appendix B for HAC conditional logic
    - CC +7th **T84.615** Infection and inflammatory reaction due to internal fixation device of left ulna
      - HAC 7th character A see Appendix B for HAC conditional logic
    - CC +7th **T84.619** Infection and inflammatory reaction due to internal fixation device of unspecified bone of arm
      - HAC 7th character A see Appendix B for HAC conditional logic
  - + T84.62 **Infection and inflammatory reaction due to internal fixation device of leg**
    - CC +7th **T84.620** Infection and inflammatory reaction due to internal fixation device of right femur
    - CC +7th **T84.621** Infection and inflammatory reaction due to internal fixation device of left femur
    - CC +7th **T84.622** Infection and inflammatory reaction due to internal fixation device of right tibia
    - CC +7th **T84.623** Infection and inflammatory reaction due to internal fixation device of left tibia
    - CC +7th **T84.624** Infection and inflammatory reaction due to internal fixation device of right fibula
    - CC +7th **T84.625** Infection and inflammatory reaction due to internal fixation device of left fibula
    - CC +7th **T84.629** Infection and inflammatory reaction due to internal fixation device of unspecified bone of leg

CC X+7th T84.63 Infection and inflammatory reaction due to internal fixation device of spine
  HAC 7th character A see Appendix B for HAC conditional logic

CC X+7th T84.69 Infection and inflammatory reaction due to internal fixation device of other site
  HAC 7th character A see Appendix B for HAC conditional logic

CC X+7th T84.7 Infection and inflammatory reaction due to other internal orthopedic prosthetic devices, implants and grafts
  Use additional code to identify infection
  HAC 7th character A see Appendix B for HAC conditional logic

+ **T84.8** Other specified complications of internal orthopedic prosthetic devices, implants and grafts

CC X+7th T84.81 Embolism due to internal orthopedic prosthetic devices, implants and grafts

CC X+7th T84.82 Fibrosis due to internal orthopedic prosthetic devices, implants and grafts

CC X+7th T84.83 Hemorrhage due to internal orthopedic prosthetic devices, implants and grafts

CC X+7th T84.84 Pain due to internal orthopedic prosthetic devices, implants and grafts

CC X+7th T84.85 Stenosis due to internal orthopedic prosthetic devices, implants and grafts

CC X+7th T84.86 Thrombosis due to internal orthopedic prosthetic devices, implants and grafts

CC X+7th T84.89 Other specified complication of internal orthopedic prosthetic devices, implants and grafts

CC X+7th T84.9 Unspecified complication of internal orthopedic prosthetic device, implant and graft

T85 Complications of other internal prosthetic devices, implants and grafts
  Excludes2: failure and rejection of transplanted organs and tissue (T86.-)
  AHA CC: 4Q, 2016, 71-72

> The appropriate 7th character is to be added to each code from category T85
> A initial encounter
> D subsequent encounter
> S sequela

+ **T85.0** Mechanical complication of ventricular intracranial (communicating) shunt

CC X+7th T85.01 Breakdown (mechanical) of ventricular intracranial (communicating) shunt

CC X+7th T85.02 Displacement of ventricular intracranial (communicating) shunt
  Malposition of ventricular intracranial (communicating) shunt

CC X+7th T85.03 Leakage of ventricular intracranial (communicating) shunt

CC X+7th T85.09 Other mechanical complication of ventricular intracranial (communicating) shunt
  Obstruction (mechanical) of ventricular intracranial (communicating) shunt
  Perforation of ventricular intracranial (communicating) shunt
  Protrusion of ventricular intracranial (communicating) shunt

+ **T85.1** Mechanical complication of implanted electronic stimulator of nervous system

+ **T85.11** Breakdown (mechanical) of implanted electronic stimulator of nervous system

CC +7th T85.110 Breakdown (mechanical) of implanted electronic neurostimulator of brain electrode (lead)

CC +7th T85.111 Breakdown (mechanical) of implanted electronic neurostimulator of peripheral nerve electrode (lead)
  Breakdown of electrode (lead) for cranial nerve neurostimulators
  Breakdown of electrode (lead) for gastric neurostimulators
  Breakdown of electrode (lead) for sacral nerve neurostimulators
  Breakdown of electrode (lead) for vagal nerve neurostimulators

CC +7th T85.112 Breakdown (mechanical) of implanted electronic neurostimulator of spinal cord electrode (lead)

CC +7th T85.113 Breakdown (mechanical) of implanted electronic neurostimulator, generator
  Breakdown (mechanical) of implanted electronic neurostimulator generator, brain, peripheral, gastric, spinal
  Breakdown (mechanical) of implanted electronic sacral neurostimulator, pulse generator receiver

CC +7th T85.118 Breakdown (mechanical) of other implanted electronic stimulator of nervous system

+ **T85.12** Displacement of implanted electronic stimulator of nervous system
  Malposition of implanted electronic stimulator of nervous system

CC +7th T85.120 Displacement of implanted electronic neurostimulator of brain electrode (lead)

CC +7th T85.121 Displacement of implanted electronic neurostimulator of peripheral nerve electrode (lead)
  Displacement of electrode (lead) for cranial nerve neurostimulators
  Displacement of electrode (lead) for gastric neurostimulators
  Displacement of electrode (lead) for sacral nerve neurostimulators
  Displacement of electrode (lead) for vagal nerve neurostimulators

CC +7th T85.122 Displacement of implanted electronic neurostimulator of spinal cord electrode (lead)

CC +7th T85.123 Displacement of implanted electronic neurostimulator, generator
  Displacement of implanted electronic neurostimulator generator, brain, peripheral, gastric, spinal
  Displacement of implanted electronic sacral neurostimulator, pulse generator receiver

CC +7th T85.128 Displacement of other implanted electronic stimulator of nervous system

+ **T85.19** Other mechanical complication of implanted electronic stimulator of nervous system
  Leakage of implanted electronic stimulator of nervous system
  Obstruction (mechanical) of implanted electronic stimulator of nervous system
  Perforation of implanted electronic stimulator of nervous system
  Protrusion of implanted electronic stimulator of nervous system

CC +7th T85.190 Other mechanical complication of implanted electronic neurostimulator of brain electrode (lead)

CC +7th T85.191 Other mechanical complication of implanted electronic neurostimulator of peripheral nerve electrode (lead)
  Other mechanical complication of electrode (lead) for cranial nerve neurostimulators
  Other mechanical complication of electrode (lead) for gastric neurostimulators
  Other mechanical complication of electrode (lead) for sacral nerve neurostimulators
  Other mechanical complication of electrode (lead) for vagal nerve neurostimulators

CC +7th T85.192 Other mechanical complication of implanted electronic neurostimulator of spinal cord electrode (lead)

- **CC +7th T85.193** Other mechanical complication of implanted electronic neurostimulator, generator
  - Other mechanical complication of implanted electronic neurostimulator generator, brain, peripheral, gastric, spinal
  - Other mechanical complication of implanted electronic sacral neurostimulator, pulse generator receiver
- **CC +7th T85.199** Other mechanical complication of other implanted electronic stimulator of nervous system
- **+ T85.2 Mechanical complication of intraocular lens**
  - **CC X+7th T85.21** Breakdown (mechanical) of intraocular lens
  - **CC X+7th T85.22** Displacement of intraocular lens
    - Malposition of intraocular lens
  - **CC X+7th T85.29** Other mechanical complication of intraocular lens
    - Obstruction (mechanical) of intraocular lens
    - Perforation of intraocular lens
    - Protrusion of intraocular lens
- **+ T85.3 Mechanical complication of other ocular prosthetic devices, implants and grafts**
  - *Excludes2:* other complications of corneal graft (T86.84-)
  - **+ T85.31** Breakdown (mechanical) of other ocular prosthetic devices, implants and grafts
    - **CC +7th T85.310** Breakdown (mechanical) of prosthetic orbit of right eye
    - **CC +7th T85.311** Breakdown (mechanical) of prosthetic orbit of left eye
    - **+7th T85.318** Breakdown (mechanical) of other ocular prosthetic devices, implants and grafts
  - **+ T85.32** Displacement of other ocular prosthetic devices, implants and grafts
    - Malposition of other ocular prosthetic devices, implants and grafts
    - **CC +7th T85.320** Displacement of prosthetic orbit of right eye
    - **CC +7th T85.321** Displacement of prosthetic orbit of left eye
    - **+7th T85.328** Displacement of other ocular prosthetic devices, implants and grafts
  - **+ T85.39** Other mechanical complication of other ocular prosthetic devices, implants and grafts
    - Obstruction (mechanical) of other ocular prosthetic devices, implants and grafts
    - Perforation of other ocular prosthetic devices, implants and grafts
    - Protrusion of other ocular prosthetic devices, implants and grafts
    - **CC +7th T85.390** Other mechanical complication of prosthetic orbit of right eye
    - **CC +7th T85.391** Other mechanical complication of prosthetic orbit of left eye
    - **+7th T85.398** Other mechanical complication of other ocular prosthetic devices, implants and grafts
- **+ T85.4 Mechanical complication of breast prosthesis and implant**
  - **CC X+7th T85.41** Breakdown (mechanical) of breast prosthesis and implant
  - **CC X+7th T85.42** Displacement of breast prosthesis and implant
    - Malposition of breast prosthesis and implant
  - **CC X+7th T85.43** Leakage of breast prosthesis and implant
  - **CC X+7th T85.44** Capsular contracture of breast implant
  - **CC X+7th T85.49** Other mechanical complication of breast prosthesis and implant
    - Obstruction (mechanical) of breast prosthesis and implant
    - Perforation of breast prosthesis and implant
    - Protrusion of breast prosthesis and implant

- **+ T85.5 Mechanical complication of gastrointestinal prosthetic devices, implants and grafts**
  - **+ T85.51** Breakdown (mechanical) of gastrointestinal prosthetic devices, implants and grafts
    - **CC +7th T85.510** Breakdown (mechanical) of bile duct prosthesis
    - **CC +7th T85.511** Breakdown (mechanical) of esophageal anti-reflux device
    - **CC +7th T85.518** Breakdown (mechanical) of other gastrointestinal prosthetic devices, implants and grafts
  - **+ T85.52** Displacement of gastrointestinal prosthetic devices, implants and grafts
    - Malposition of gastrointestinal prosthetic devices, implants and grafts
    - **CC +7th T85.520** Displacement of bile duct prosthesis
    - **CC +7th T85.521** Displacement of esophageal anti-reflux device
    - **CC +7th T85.528** Displacement of other gastrointestinal prosthetic devices, implants and grafts
  - **+ T85.59** Other mechanical complication of gastrointestinal prosthetic devices, implants and
    - Obstruction, mechanical of gastrointestinal prosthetic devices, implants and grafts
    - Perforation of gastrointestinal prosthetic devices, implants and grafts
    - Protrusion of gastrointestinal prosthetic devices, implants and grafts
    - **CC +7th T85.590** Other mechanical complication of bile duct prosthesis
    - **CC +7th T85.591** Other mechanical complication of esophageal anti-reflux device
    - **CC +7th T85.598** Other mechanical complication of other gastrointestinal prosthetic devices, implants and grafts
- **+ T85.6 Mechanical complication of other specified internal and external prosthetic devices, implants and grafts**
  - Review coding guidelines C.4.a.5.a and C.4.a.5.b
  - **+ T85.61** Breakdown (mechanical) of other specified internal prosthetic devices, implants and grafts
    - **CC +7th T85.610** Breakdown (mechanical) of cranial or spinal infusion catheter
      - Breakdown (mechanical) of epidural infusion catheter
      - Breakdown (mechanical) of intrathecal infusion catheter
      - Breakdown (mechanical) of subarachnoid infusion catheter
      - Breakdown (mechanical) of subdural infusion catheter
    - **CC +7th T85.611** Breakdown (mechanical) of intraperitoneal dialysis catheter
      - *Excludes1:* mechanical complication of vascular dialysis catheter (T82.4-)
    - **CC +7th T85.612** Breakdown (mechanical) of permanent sutures
      - *Excludes1:* mechanical complication of permanent (wire) suture used in bone repair (T84.1-T84.2)
    - **CC +7th T85.613** Breakdown (mechanical) of artificial skin graft and decellularized allodermis
      - Failure of artificial skin graft and decellularized allodermis
      - Non-adherence of artificial skin graft and decellularized allodermis
      - Poor incorporation of artificial skin graft and decellularized allodermis
      - Shearing of artificial skin graft and decellularized allodermis
    - **CC +7th T85.614** Breakdown (mechanical) of insulin pump
    - **CC +7th T85.615** Breakdown (mechanical) of other nervous system device, implant or graft
      - Breakdown (mechanical) of intrathecal infusion pump
    - **CC +7th T85.618** Breakdown (mechanical) of other specified internal prosthetic devices, implants and grafts

+ T85.62 Displacement of other specified internal prosthetic devices, implants and grafts
    Malposition of other specified internal prosthetic devices, implants and grafts

CC +7th **T85.620** Displacement of cranial or spinal infusion catheter
    Displacement of epidural infusion catheter
    Displacement of intrathecal infusion catheter
    Displacement of subarachnoid infusion catheter
    Displacement of subdural infusion catheter

CC +7th **T85.621** Displacement of intraperitoneal dialysis catheter
    Excludes1: *mechanical complication of vascular dialysis catheter (T82.4-)*

CC +7th **T85.622** Displacement of permanent sutures
    Excludes1: *mechanical complication of permanent (wire) suture used in bone repair (T84.1-T84.2)*

CC +7th **T85.623** Displacement of artificial skin graft and decellularized allodermis
    Dislodgement of artificial skin graft and decellularized allodermis

CC +7th **T85.624** Displacement of insulin pump

CC +7th **T85.625** Displacement of other nervous system device, implant or graft
    Displacement of intrathecal infusion pump

CC +7th **T85.628** Displacement of other specified internal prosthetic devices, implants and grafts
    AHA CC: 1Q, 2015, 3-21

+ T85.63 Leakage of other specified internal prosthetic devices, implants and grafts

CC +7th **T85.630** Leakage of cranial or spinal infusion catheter
    Leakage of epidural infusion catheter
    Leakage of intrathecal infusion catheter
    Leakage of subarachnoid infusion catheter
    Leakage of subdural infusion catheter
    AHA CC: 3Q, 2022, 24

CC +7th **T85.631** Leakage of intraperitoneal dialysis catheter
    Excludes1: *mechanical complication of vascular dialysis catheter (T82.4)*

CC +7th **T85.633** Leakage of insulin pump

CC +7th **T85.635** Leakage of other nervous system device, implant or graft
    Leakage of intrathecal infusion pump

CC +7th **T85.638** Leakage of other specified internal prosthetic devices, implants and grafts

+ T85.69 Other mechanical complication of other specified internal prosthetic devices, implants and grafts
    Obstruction, mechanical of other specified internal prosthetic devices, implants and grafts
    Perforation of other specified internal prosthetic devices, implants and grafts
    Protrusion of other specified internal prosthetic devices, implants and grafts

CC +7th **T85.690** Other mechanical complication of cranial or spinal infusion catheter
    Other mechanical complication of epidural infusion catheter
    Other mechanical complication of intrathecal infusion catheter
    Other mechanical complication of subarachnoid infusion catheter
    Other mechanical complication of subdural infusion catheter

CC +7th **T85.691** Other mechanical complication of intraperitoneal dialysis catheter
    Excludes1: *mechanical complication of vascular dialysis catheter (T82.4)*

CC +7th **T85.692** Other mechanical complication of permanent sutures
    Excludes1: *mechanical complication of permanent (wire) suture used in bone repair (T84.1-T84.2)*

CC +7th **T85.693** Other mechanical complication of artificial skin graft and decellularized allodermis

CC +7th **T85.694** Other mechanical complication of insulin pump

CC +7th **T85.695** Other mechanical complication of other nervous system device, implant or graft
    Other mechanical complication of intrathecal infusion pump

CC +7th **T85.698** Other mechanical complication of other specified internal prosthetic devices, implants and grafts
    Mechanical complication of nonabsorbable surgical material NOS

+ T85.7 Infection and inflammatory reaction due to other internal prosthetic devices, implants and grafts
    Use additional code to identify infection

CC X+7th **T85.71** Infection and inflammatory reaction due to peritoneal dialysis catheter

CC X+7th **T85.72** Infection and inflammatory reaction due to insulin pump

+ T85.73 Infection and inflammatory reaction due to nervous system devices, implants and graft

CC +7th **T85.730** Infection and inflammatory reaction due to ventricular intracranial (communicating) shunt

CC +7th **T85.731** Infection and inflammatory reaction due to implanted electronic neurostimulator of brain, electrode (lead)

CC +7th **T85.732** Infection and inflammatory reaction due to implanted electronic neurostimulator of peripheral nerve, electrode (lead)
    Infection and inflammatory reaction due to electrode (lead) for cranial nerve neurostimulators
    Infection and inflammatory reaction due to electrode (lead) for gastric neurostimulators
    Infection and inflammatory reaction due to electrode (lead) for sacral nerve neurostimulators
    Infection and inflammatory reaction due to electrode (lead) for vagal nerve neurostimulators

CC +7th **T85.733** Infection and inflammatory reaction due to implanted electronic neurostimulator of spinal cord, electrode (lead)

CC +7th **T85.734** Infection and inflammatory reaction due to implanted electronic neurostimulator, generator
    Generator pocket infection

CC +7th **T85.735** Infection and inflammatory reaction due to cranial or spinal infusion catheter
    Infection and inflammatory reaction due to epidural catheter
    Infection and inflammatory reaction due to intrathecal infsuion catheter
    Infection and inflammatory reaction due to subarachnoid catheter
    Infection and inflammatory reaction due to subdural catheter

CC +7th **T85.738** Infection and inflammatory reaction due to other nervous system device, implant or graft
    Infection and inflammatory reaction due to intrathecal infusion pump

- CC X+7th **T85.79** Infection and inflammatory reaction due to other internal prosthetic devices, implants and grafts
    - *AHA CC: 2Q, 2022, 7-8; 2Q, 2023, 27-28*
- + **T85.8** Other specified complications of internal prosthetic devices, implants and grafts, not elsewhere classified
    - + **T85.81** Embolism due to internal prosthetic devices, implants and grafts, not elsewhere classified
        - CC +7th **T85.810** Embolism due to nervous system prosthetic devices, implants and grafts
        - +7th **T85.818** Embolism due to other internal prosthetic devices, implants and grafts
    - + **T85.82** Fibrosis due to internal prosthetic devices, implants and grafts, not elsewhere classified
        - CC +7th **T85.820** Fibrosis due to nervous system prosthetic devices, implants and grafts
        - +7th **T85.828** Fibrosis due to other internal prosthetic devices, implants and grafts
    - + **T85.83** Hemorrhage due to internal prosthetic devices, implants and grafts, not elsewhere classified
        - CC +7th **T85.830** Hemorrhage due to nervous system prosthetic devices, implants and grafts
        - +7th **T85.838** Hemorrhage due to other internal prosthetic devices, implants and grafts
    - + **T85.84** Pain due to internal prosthetic devices, implants and grafts, not elsewhere classified
        - CC +7th **T85.840** Pain due to nervous system prosthetic devices, implants and grafts
        - +7th **T85.848** Pain due to other internal prosthetic devices, implants and grafts
    - + **T85.85** Stenosis due to internal prosthetic devices, implants and grafts, not elsewhere classified
        - CC +7th **T85.850** Stenosis due to nervous system prosthetic devices, implants and grafts
        - +7th **T85.858** Stenosis due to other internal prosthetic devices, implants and grafts
    - + **T85.86** Thrombosis due to internal prosthetic devices, implants and grafts, not elsewhere classified
        - CC +7th **T85.860** Thrombosis due to nervous system prosthetic devices, implants and grafts
        - +7th **T85.868** Thrombosis due to other internal prosthetic devices, implants and grafts
    - + **T85.89** Other specified complication of internal prosthetic devices, implants and grafts, not elsewhere classified
        - Erosion or breakdown of subcutaneous device pocket
        - CC +7th **T85.890** Other specified complication of nervous system prosthetic devices, implants and grafts
        - +7th **T85.898** Other specified complication of other internal prosthetic devices, implants and grafts
- X+7th **T85.9** Unspecified complication of internal prosthetic device, implant and graft
    - Complication of internal prosthetic device, implant and graft NOS

T86 Complications of transplanted organs and tissue
Use additional code to identify other transplant complications, such as:
graft-versus-host disease (D89.81-)
malignancy associated with organ transplant (C80.2)
post-transplant lymphoproliferative disorders (PTLD) (D47.Z1)
Review coding guideline C.2.r
Review coding guideline C.19.g.3

- + **T86.0** Complications of bone marrow transplant
    - CC **T86.00** Unspecified complication of bone marrow transplant
    - CC **T86.01** Bone marrow transplant rejection
    - CC **T86.02** Bone marrow transplant failure
    - CC **T86.03** Bone marrow transplant infection
    - CC **T86.09** Other complications of bone marrow transplant
- + **T86.1** Complications of kidney transplant
    - *Review coding guideline C.19.g.3.b*
    - CC **T86.10** Unspecified complication of kidney transplant
    - CC **T86.11** Kidney transplant rejection
    - CC **T86.12** Kidney transplant failure
        - *AHA CC: 1Q, 2014, 24*
    - CC **T86.13** Kidney transplant infection
        - Use additional code to specify infection
    - CC **T86.19** Other complication of kidney transplant
        - *AHA CC: 2Q, 2019, 7*
- + **T86.2** Complications of heart transplant
    - **Excludes1:** complication of:
        - artificial heart device (T82.5-)
        - heart-lung transplant (T86.3-)
    - CC **T86.20** Unspecified complication of heart transplant
    - CC **T86.21** Heart transplant rejection
    - CC **T86.22** Heart transplant failure
    - CC **T86.23** Heart transplant infection
        - Use additional code to specify infection
    - + **T86.29** Other complications of heart transplant
        - CC **T86.290** Cardiac allograft vasculopathy
            - **Excludes1:** atherosclerosis of coronary arteries (I25.75-, I25.76-, I25.81-)
        - CC **T86.298** Other complications of heart transplant
- + **T86.3** Complications of heart-lung transplant
    - CC **T86.30** Unspecified complication of heart-lung transplant
    - CC **T86.31** Heart-lung transplant rejection
    - CC **T86.32** Heart-lung transplant failure
    - CC **T86.33** Heart-lung transplant infection
        - Use additional code to specify infection
    - CC **T86.39** Other complications of heart-lung transplant
- + **T86.4** Complications of liver transplant
    - CC **T86.40** Unspecified complication of liver transplant
    - CC **T86.41** Liver transplant rejection
    - CC **T86.42** Liver transplant failure
    - CC **T86.43** Liver transplant infection
        - Use additional code to identify infection, such as: Cytomegalovirus (CMV) infection (B25.-)
    - CC **T86.49** Other complications of liver transplant
- CC **T86.5** Complications of stem cell transplant
    - Complications from stem cells from peripheral blood
    - Complications from stem cells from umbilical cord
    - *AHA CC: 4Q, 2020, 14*
- + **T86.8** Complications of other transplanted organs and tissues
    - + **T86.81** Complications of lung transplant
        - **Excludes1:** complication of heart-lung transplant (T86.3-)
        - CC **T86.810** Lung transplant rejection
        - CC **T86.811** Lung transplant failure
        - CC **T86.812** Lung transplant infection
            - Use additional code to specify infection
        - CC **T86.818** Other complications of lung transplant
            - *AHA CC: 2Q, 2019, 6-7*
        - CC **T86.819** Unspecified complication of lung transplant
    - + **T86.82** Complications of skin graft (allograft) (autograft)
        - **Excludes2:** complication of artificial skin graft (T85.693)
        - CC **T86.820** Skin graft (allograft) rejection
        - CC **T86.821** Skin graft (allograft) (autograft) failure
        - CC **T86.822** Skin graft (allograft) (autograft) infection
            - Use additional code to specify infection
        - CC **T86.828** Other complications of skin graft (allograft) (autograft)
        - CC **T86.829** Unspecified complication of skin graft (allograft) (autograft)
    - + **T86.83** Complications of bone graft
        - **Excludes2:** mechanical complications of bone graft (T84.3-)
        - CC **T86.830** Bone graft rejection
        - CC **T86.831** Bone graft failure
        - CC **T86.832** Bone graft infection
            - Use additional code to specify infection
        - CC **T86.838** Other complications of bone graft
            - *HA CC: 1Q, 2023, 30-31*
        - CC **T86.839** Unspecified complication of bone graft
    - + **T86.84** Complications of corneal transplant
        - **Excludes2:** mechanical complications of corneal graft (T85.3-)
        - *AHA CC: 4Q, 2020, 40*
        - + **T86.840** Corneal transplant rejection
            - CC **T86.8401** Corneal transplant rejection, right eye
            - CC **T86.8402** Corneal transplant rejection, left eye
            - CC **T86.8403** Corneal transplant rejection, bilateral

- CC T86.8409 Corneal transplant rejection, unspecified eye
- **+ T86.841 Corneal transplant failure**
  - CC T86.8411 Corneal transplant failure, right eye
  - CC T86.8412 Corneal transplant failure, left eye
  - CC T86.8413 Corneal transplant failure, bilateral
  - CC T86.8419 Corneal transplant failure, unspecified eye
- **+ T86.842 Corneal transplant infection**
  - CC T86.8421 Corneal transplant infection, right eye
  - CC T86.8422 Corneal transplant infection, left eye
  - CC T86.8423 Corneal transplant infection, bilateral
  - CC T86.8429 Corneal transplant infection, unspecified eye
  - *Use additional code to specify infection*
- **+ T86.848 Other complications of corneal transplant**
  - CC T86.8481 Other complications of corneal transplant, right eye
  - CC T86.8482 Other complications of corneal transplant, left eye
  - CC T86.8483 Other complications of corneal transplant, bilateral
  - CC T86.8489 Other complications of corneal transplant, unspecified eye
- **+ T86.849 Unspecified complication of corneal transplant**
  - CC T86.8491 Unspecified complication of corneal transplant, right eye
  - CC T86.8492 Unspecified complication of corneal transplant, left eye
  - CC T86.8493 Unspecified complication of corneal transplant, bilateral
  - CC T86.8499 Unspecified complication of corneal transplant, unspecified eye
- **+ T86.85 Complication of intestine transplant**
  - CC T86.850 Intestine transplant rejection
  - CC T86.851 Intestine transplant failure
  - CC T86.852 Intestine transplant infection
    - *Use additional code to specify infection*
  - CC T86.858 Other complications of intestine transplant
  - CC T86.859 Unspecified complication of intestine transplant
- **+ T86.89 Complications of other transplanted tissue**
  - Transplant failure or rejection of pancreas
  - CC T86.890 Other transplanted tissue rejection
  - CC T86.891 Other transplanted tissue failure
  - CC T86.892 Other transplanted tissue infection
    - *Use additional code to specify infection*
  - CC T86.898 Other complications of other transplanted tissue
  - CC T86.899 Unspecified complication of other transplanted tissue
- **+ T86.9 Complication of unspecified transplanted organ and tissue**
  - CC T86.90 Unspecified complication of unspecified transplanted organ and tissue
  - CC T86.91 Unspecified transplanted organ and tissue rejection
  - CC T86.92 Unspecified transplanted organ and tissue failure
  - CC T86.93 Unspecified transplanted organ and tissue infection
    - *Use additional code to specify infection*
  - CC T86.99 Other complications of unspecified transplanted organ and tissue

T87 Complications peculiar to reattachment and amputation

- **+ T87.0 Complications of reattached (part of) upper extremity**
  - **+ T87.0X Complications of reattached (part of) upper extremity**
    - CC T87.0X1 Complications of reattached (part of) right upper extremity
    - CC T87.0X2 Complications of reattached (part of) left upper extremity
    - CC T87.0X9 Complications of reattached (part of) unspecified upper extremity
- **+ T87.1 Complications of reattached (part of) lower extremity**
  - **+ T87.1X Complications of reattached (part of) lower extremity**
    - CC T87.1X1 Complications of reattached (part of) right lower extremity
    - CC T87.1X2 Complications of reattached (part of) left lower extremity
    - CC T87.1X9 Complications of reattached (part of) unspecified lower extremity
- CC **T87.2 Complications of other reattached body part**
- **+ T87.3 Neuroma of amputation stump**
  - T87.30 Neuroma of amputation stump, unspecified extremity
  - T87.31 Neuroma of amputation stump, right upper extremity
  - T87.32 Neuroma of amputation stump, left upper extremity
  - T87.33 Neuroma of amputation stump, right lower extremity
  - T87.34 Neuroma of amputation stump, left lower extremity
- **+ T87.4 Infection of amputation stump**
  - CC T87.40 Infection of amputation stump, unspecified extremity
  - CC T87.41 Infection of amputation stump, right upper extremity
  - CC T87.42 Infection of amputation stump, left upper extremity
  - CC T87.43 Infection of amputation stump, right lower extremity
  - CC T87.44 Infection of amputation stump, left lower extremity
- **+ T87.5 Necrosis of amputation stump**
  - T87.50 Necrosis of amputation stump, unspecified extremity
  - T87.51 Necrosis of amputation stump, right upper extremity
  - T87.52 Necrosis of amputation stump, left upper extremity
  - T87.53 Necrosis of amputation stump, right lower extremity
  - T87.54 Necrosis of amputation stump, left lower extremity
- **+ T87.8 Other complications of amputation stump**
  - T87.81 Dehiscence of amputation stump
  - T87.89 Other complications of amputation stump
    - Amputation stump contracture
    - Amputation stump contracture of next proximal joint
    - Amputation stump flexion
    - Amputation stump edema
    - Amputation stump hematoma
    - **Excludes2:** *phantom limb syndrome (G54.6-G54.7)*
    - *AHA CC: 3Q, 2022, 11*
- **T87.9 Unspecified complications of amputation stump**

T88 Other complications of surgical and medical care, not elsewhere classified

Excludes2: complication following infusion, transfusion and therapeutic injection (T80.-)
complication following procedure NEC (T81.-)
complications of anesthesia in labor and delivery (O74.-)
complications of anesthesia in pregnancy (O29.-)
complications of anesthesia in puerperium (O89.-)
complications of devices, implants and grafts (T82-T85)
complications of obstetric surgery and procedure (O75.4)
dermatitis due to drugs and medicaments (L23.3, L24.4, L25.1, L27.0-L27.1)
poisoning and toxic effects of drugs and chemicals (T36-T65 with fifth or sixth character 1-4)
specified complications classified elsewhere

AHA CC: 4Q, 2018, 89-90

> The appropriate 7th character is to be added to each code from category T88
> A initial encounter
> D subsequent encounter
> S sequela

CC X+7th T88.0 Infection following immunization
Sepsis following immunization
Review coding guideline C.1.d.5

CC X+7th T88.1 Other complications following immunization, not elsewhere classified
Generalized vaccinia
Rash following immunization
Excludes1: vaccinia not from vaccine (B08.011)
Excludes2: anaphylactic shock due to serum (T80.5-)
other serum reactions (T80.6-)
postimmunization arthropathy (M02.2)
postimmunization encephalitis (G04.02)
postimmunization fever (R50.83)

CC X+7th T88.2 Shock due to anesthesia
Use additional code for adverse effect, if applicable, to identify drug (T41.- with fifth or sixth character 5)
Excludes1: complications of anesthesia (in):
labor and delivery (O74.-)
pregnancy (O29.-)
puerperium (O89.-)
postprocedural shock NOS (T81.1-)

CC X+7th T88.3 Malignant hyperthermia due to anesthesia
Use additional code for adverse effect, if applicable, to identify drug (T41.- with fifth or sixth character 5)

X+7th T88.4 Failed or difficult intubation

+ T88.5 Other complications of anesthesia
Use additional code for adverse effect, if applicable, to identify drug (T41.- with fifth or sixth character 5)
AHA CC: 4Q, 2016, 72-73

X+7th T88.51 Hypothermia following anesthesia

X+7th T88.52 Failed moderate sedation during procedure
Failed conscious sedation during procedure
Excludes2: personal history of failed moderate sedation (Z92.83)

X+7th T88.53 Unintended awareness under general anesthesia during procedure
Excludes2: personal history of unintended awareness under general anesthesia (Z92.84)
AHA CC: 4Q, 2016, 72-73

X+7th T88.59 Other complications of anesthesia

CC X+7th T88.6 Anaphylactic reaction due to adverse effect of correct drug or medicament properly administered
Anaphylactic shock due to adverse effect of correct drug or medicament properly administered
Anaphylactoid reaction NOS
Use additional code for adverse effect, if applicable, to identify drug (T36-T50 with fifth or sixth character 5)
Excludes1: anaphylactic reaction due to serum (T80.5-)
anaphylactic shock or reaction due to adverse food reaction (T78.0-)
AHA CC: 1Q, 2020, 18-19

X+7th T88.7 Unspecified adverse effect of drug or medicament
Drug hypersensitivity NOS
Drug reaction NOS
Use additional code for adverse effect, if applicable, to identify drug (T36-T50 with fifth or sixth character 5)
Excludes1: specified adverse effects of drugs and medicaments (A00-R94 and T80-T88.6, T88.8)

X+7th T88.8 Other specified complications of surgical and medical care, not elsewhere classified
Use additional code to identify the complication
AHA CC: 2Q, 2022, 7-8

X+7th T88.9 Complication of surgical and medical care, unspecified

Chapter 20: External Causes of Morbidity (V00-Y99)

NOTE This chapter permits the classification of environmental events and circumstances as the cause of injury, and other adverse effects. Where a code from this section is applicable, it is intended that it shall be used secondary to a code from another chapter of the Classification indicating the nature of the condition. Most often, the condition will be classifiable to Chapter 19, Injury, poisoning and certain other consequences of external causes (S00-T88). Other conditions that may be stated to be due to external causes are classified in Chapters 1 to 18. For these conditions, codes from Chapter 20 should be used to provide additional information as to the cause of the condition.

AHA CC: 1Q, 2015, 3-21

This chapter contains the following category blocks:

V00-X58	Accidents
V00-V99	Transport accidents
V00-V09	Pedestrian injured in transport accident
V10-V19	Pedal cycle rider injured in transport accident
V20-V29	Motorcycle rider injured in transport accident
V30-V39	Occupant of three-wheeled motor vehicle injured in transport accident
V40-V49	Car occupant injured in transport accident
V50-V59	Occupant of pick-up truck or van injured in transport accident
V60-V69	Occupant of heavy transport vehicle injured in transport accident
V70-V79	Bus occupant injured in transport accident
V80-V89	Other land transport accidents
V90-V94	Water transport accidents
V95-V97	Air and space transport accidents
V98-V99	Other and unspecified transport accidents
W00-X58	Other external causes of accidental injury
W00-W19	Slipping, tripping, stumbling and falls
W20-W49	Exposure to inanimate mechanical forces
W50-W64	Exposure to animate mechanical forces
W65-W74	Accidental non-transport drowning and submersion
W85-W99	Exposure to electric current, radiation and extreme ambient air temperature and pressure
X00-X08	Exposure to smoke, fire and flames
X10-X19	Contact with heat and hot substances
X30-X39	Exposure to forces of nature
X50	Overexertion and strenuous or repetitive movements
X52-X58	Accidental exposure to other specified factors
X71-X83	Intentional self-harm
X92-Y09	Assault
Y21-Y33	Event of undetermined intent
Y35-Y38	Legal intervention, operations of war, military operations, and terrorism
Y62-Y84	Complications of medical and surgical care
Y62-Y69	Misadventures to patients during surgical and medical care
Y70-Y82	Medical devices associated with adverse incidents in diagnostic and therapeutic use
Y83-Y84	Surgical and other medical procedures as the cause of abnormal reaction of the patient, or of later complication, without mention of misadventure at the time of the procedure
Y90-Y99	Supplementary factors related to causes of morbidity classified elsewhere

C. Chapter-Specific Coding Guidelines

In addition to general coding guidelines, there are guidelines for specific diagnoses and/or conditions in the classification. Unless otherwise indicated, these guidelines apply to all health care settings. Please refer to Section II for guidelines on the selection of principal diagnosis.

20. Chapter 20: External Causes of Morbidity (V00-Y99)

The external causes of morbidity codes should never be sequenced as the first-listed or principal diagnosis.

External cause codes are intended to provide data for injury research and evaluation of injury prevention strategies. These codes capture how the injury or health condition happened (cause), the intent (unintentional or accidental; or intentional, such as suicide or assault), the place where the event occurred the activity of the patient at the time of the event, and the person's status (e.g., civilian, military).

There is no national requirement for mandatory ICD-10-CM external cause code reporting. Unless a provider is subject to a state-based external cause code reporting mandate or these codes are required by a particular payer, reporting of ICD-10-CM codes in Chapter 20, External Causes of Morbidity, is not required. In the absence of a mandatory reporting requirement, providers are encouraged to voluntarily report external cause codes, as they provide valuable data for injury research and evaluation of injury prevention strategies.

a. General External Cause Coding Guidelines

1) Used with any code in the range of A00.0-T88.9, Z00-Z99

An external cause code may be used with any code in the range of A00.0-T88.9, Z00-Z99, classification that represents a health condition due to an external cause. Though they are most applicable to injuries, they are also valid for use with such things as infections or diseases due to an external source, and other health conditions, such as a heart attack that occurs during strenuous physical activity.

2) External cause code used for length of treatment

Assign the external cause code, with the appropriate 7th character (initial encounter, subsequent encounter or sequela) for each encounter for which the injury or condition is being treated.

Most categories in chapter 20 have a 7th character requirement for each applicable code. Most categories in this chapter have three 7th character values: A, initial encounter, D, subsequent encounter and S, sequela. While the patient may be seen by a new or different provider over the course of treatment for an injury or condition, assignment of the 7th character for external cause should match the 7th character of the code assigned for the associated injury or condition for the encounter.

3) Use the full range of external cause codes

Use the full range of external cause codes to completely describe the cause, the intent, the place of occurrence, and if applicable, the activity of the patient at the time of the event, and the patient's status, for all injuries, and other health conditions due to an external cause.

4) Assign as many external cause codes as necessary

Assign as many external cause codes as necessary to fully explain each cause. If only one external code can be recorded, assign the code most related to the principal diagnosis.

5) The selection of the appropriate external cause code

The selection of the appropriate external cause code is guided by the Alphabetic Index of External Causes and by Inclusion and Exclusion notes in the Tabular List.

6) External cause code can never be a principal diagnosis

An external cause code can never be a principal (first-listed) diagnosis.

7) Combination external cause codes

Certain of the external cause codes are combination codes that identify sequential events that result in an injury, such as a fall which results in striking against an object. The injury may be due to either event or both. The combination external cause code used should correspond to the sequence of events regardless of which caused the most serious injury.

8) No external cause code needed in certain circumstances

No external cause code from Chapter 20 is needed if the external cause and intent are included in a code from another chapter (e.g. T36.0X1- Poisoning by penicillins, accidental (unintentional)).

b. Place of Occurrence Guideline

Codes from category Y92, Place of occurrence of the external cause, are secondary codes for use after other external cause codes to identify the location of the patient at the time of injury or other condition.

Generally, a place of occurrent code is assigned only once, at the initial encounter for treatment. However, in the rare instance that a new injury occurs during hospitalization, an additional place of occurrence code may be assigned. No 7th characters are used for Y92.

Do not use place of occurrence code Y92.9 if the place is not stated or is not applicable.

c. Activity Code

Assign a code from category Y93, Activity code, to describe the activity of the patient at the time the injury or other health condition occurred.

An activity code is used only once, at the initial encounter for treatment. Only one code from Y93 should be recorded on a medical record.

The activity codes are not applicable to poisonings, adverse effects, misadventures or sequela.

Do not assign Y93.9, Unspecified activity, if the activity is not stated.

A code from category Y93 is appropriate for use with external cause and intent codes if identifying the activity provides additional information about the event.

d. Place of Occurrence, Activity, and Status Codes Used with other External Cause Code

When applicable, place of occurrence, activity, and external cause status codes are sequenced after the main external cause code(s). Regardless of the number of external cause codes assigned, generally there should be only one place of occurrence code, one activity code, and one external cause status code assigned to an encounter. However, in the rare instance that a new injury occurs during hospitalization, an additional place of occurrence code may be assigned.

e. If the Reporting Format Limits the Number of External Cause Codes

If the reporting format limits the number of external cause codes that can be used in reporting clinical data, report the code for the cause/intent most related to the principal diagnosis. If the format permits capture of additional external cause codes, the cause/intent, including medical misadventures, of the additional events should be reported rather than the codes for place, activity, or external status.

f. Multiple External Cause Coding Guidelines

More than one external cause code is required to fully describe the external cause of an illness or injury. The assignment of external cause codes should be sequenced in the following priority:

If two or more events cause separate injuries, an external cause code should be assigned for each cause. The first-listed external cause code will be selected in the following order:

External codes for child and adult abuse take priority over all other external cause codes.

See Section I.C.19., Child and Adult abuse guidelines.

External cause codes for terrorism events take priority over all other external cause codes except child and adult abuse.

External cause codes for cataclysmic events take priority over all other external cause codes except child and adult abuse and terrorism.

External cause codes for transport accidents take priority over all other external cause codes except cataclysmic events, child and adult abuse and terrorism.

Activity and external cause status codes are assigned following all causal (intent) external cause codes.

The first-listed external cause code should correspond to the cause of the most serious diagnosis due to an assault, accident, or self-harm, following the order of hierarchy listed above.

g. Child and Adult Abuse Guideline

Adult and child abuse, neglect and maltreatment are classified as assault. Any of the assault codes may be used to indicate the external cause of any injury resulting from the confirmed abuse.

For confirmed cases of abuse, neglect and maltreatment, when the perpetrator is known, a code from Y07, Perpetrator of maltreatment and neglect, should accompany any other assault codes.

See Section I.C.19. Adult and child abuse, neglect and other maltreatment

h. Unknown or Undetermined Intent Guideline

If the intent (accident, self-harm, assault) of the cause of an injury or other condition is unknown or unspecified, code the intent as accidental intent. All transport accident categories assume accidental intent.

1) Use of undetermined intent

External cause codes for events of undetermined intent are only for use if the documentation in the record specifies that the intent cannot be determined.

i. Sequelae (Late Effects) of External Cause Guidelines

1) Sequelae external cause codes

Sequela are reported using the external cause code with the 7th character "S" for sequela. These codes should be used with any report of a late effect or sequela resulting from a previous injury.

See Section I.B.10 Sequela (Late Effects)

2) Sequela external cause code with a related current injury

A sequela external cause code should never be used with a related current nature of injury code.

3) Use of sequela external cause codes for subsequent visits

Use a late effect external cause code for subsequent visits when a late effect of the initial injury is being treated. Do not use a late effect external cause code for subsequent visits for follow- up care (e.g., to assess healing, to receive rehabilitative therapy) of the injury when no late effect of the injury has been documented.

j. Terrorism Guidelines

1) Cause of injury identified by the Federal Government (FBI) as terrorism

When the cause of an injury is identified by the Federal Government (FBI) as terrorism, the first-listed external cause code should be a code from category Y38, Terrorism. The definition of terrorism employed by the FBI is found at the inclusion note at the beginning of category Y38. Use additional code for place of occurrence (Y92.-). More than one Y38 code may be assigned if the injury is the result of more than one mechanism of terrorism.

2) Cause of an injury is suspected to be the result of terrorism

When the cause of an injury is suspected to be the result of terrorism a code from category Y38 should not be assigned. Suspected cases should be classified as assault.

3) Code Y38.9, Terrorism, secondary effects

Assign code Y38.9, Terrorism, secondary effects, for conditions occurring subsequent to the terrorist event. This code should not be assigned for conditions that are due to the initial terrorist act.

It is acceptable to assign code Y38.9 with another code from Y38 if there is an injury due to the initial terrorist event and an injury that is a subsequent result of the terrorist event.

k. External cause status

A code from category Y99, External cause status, should be assigned whenever any other external cause code is assigned for an encounter, including an Activity code, except for the events noted below. Assign a code from category Y99, External cause status, to indicate the work status of the person at the time the event occurred. The status code indicates whether the event occurred during military activity, whether a non-military person was at work, whether an individual including a student or volunteer was involved in a non-work activity at the time of the causal event.

A code from Y99, External cause status, should be assigned, when applicable, with other external cause codes, such as transport accidents and falls. The external cause status codes are not applicable to poisonings, adverse effects, misadventures or late effects. Do not assign a code from category Y99 if no other external cause codes (cause, activity) are applicable for the encounter.

An external cause status code is used only once, at the initial encounter for treatment. Only one code from Y99 should be recorded on a medical record.

Do not assign code Y99.9, Unspecified external cause status, if the status is not stated.

Accidents (V00-X58)

Transport accidents (V00-V99)

NOTE This section is structured in 12 groups. Those relating to land transport accidents (V00-V89) reflect the victim's mode of transport and are subdivided to identify the victim's 'counterpart' or the type of event. The vehicle of which the injured person is an occupant is identified in the first two characters since it is seen as the most important factor to identify for prevention purposes. A transport accident is one in which the vehicle involved must be moving or running or in use for transport purposes at the time of the accident.

Use additional code to identify:
Airbag injury (W22.1)
Type of street or road (Y92.4-)
Use of cellular telephone and other electronic equipment at the time of the transport accident (Y93.C-)

Excludes1: agricultural vehicles in stationary use or maintenance (W31.-)
assault by crashing of motor vehicle (Y03.-)
automobile or motor cycle in stationary use or maintenance- code to type of accident
crashing of motor vehicle, undetermined intent (Y32)
intentional self-harm by crashing of motor vehicle (X82)

Excludes2: transport accidents due to cataclysm (X34-X38)

NOTE Definitions related to transport accidents:

(a) A transport accident (V00-V99) is any accident involving a device designed primarily for, or used at the time primarily for, conveying persons or goods from one place to another.

(b) A public highway [trafficway] or street is the entire width between property lines (or other boundary lines) of land open to the public as a matter of right or custom for purposes of moving persons or property from one place to another. A roadway is that part of the public highway designed, improved and customarily used for vehicular traffic.

(c) A traffic accident is any vehicle accident occurring on the public highway [i.e. originating on, terminating on, or involving a vehicle partially on the highway]. A vehicle accident is assumed to have occurred on the public highway unless another place is specified, except i the case of accidents involving only off-road motor vehicles, which are classified as nontraffic accidents unless the contrary is stated.

(d) A nontraffic accident is any vehicle accident that occurs entirely in any place other than a public highway.

(e) A pedestrian is any person involved in an accident who was not at the time of the accident riding in or on a motor vehicle, railway train, streetcar or animal-drawn or other vehicle, or on a pedal cycle or animal. This includes, a person changing a tire, working on a parked care, or a person on foot. It also includes the user of a pedestrian conveyance such as a baby stroller, ice-skates, skis, sled, roller skates, a skateboard, nonmotorized or motorized wheelchair, motorized mobility scooter, or nonmotorized scooter.

(f) A driver is an occupant of a transport vehicle who is operating or intending to operate it.

(g) A passenger is any occupant of a transport vehicle other than the driver, except a person traveling on the outside of the vehicle.

(h) A person on the outside of a vehicle is any person being transported by a vehicle but not occupying the space normally reserved for the driver or passengers, or the space intended for the transport of property. This includes a person travailing on the bodywork, bumper, fender, roof, running board or step of a vehicle, as well as, hanging on the outside of the vehicle.

(i) A pedal cycle is any land transport vehicle operated solely by nonmotorized pedals including a bicycle or tricycle.

(j) A pedal cyclist is any person riding a pedal cycle or in a sidecar or trailer attached to a pedal cycle.

(k) A motorcycle is a two-wheeled motor vehicle with one or two riding saddles and sometimes with a third wheel for the support of a sidecar. The sidecar is considered part of the motorcycle. This includes a moped, motor scooter, or motorized bicycle.

(l) A motorcycle rider is any person riding a motorcycle or in a sidecar or trailer attached to the motorcycle.

(m) A three-wheeled motor vehicle is a motorized tricycle designed primarily for on-road use. This includes a motor-driven tricycle, a motorized rickshaw, or a three-wheeled motor car.

(n) A car [automobile] is a four-wheeled motor vehicle designed primarily for carrying up to 7 persons. A trailer being towed by the car is considered par of the car. It does not include a van or minivan - see definition (o)

(o) A pick-up truck or van is a four or six-wheeled motor vehicle designed for carrying passengers as well as property or cargo weighing less than the local limit for classification as a heavy goods vehicle, and not requiring a special driver's license. this includes a minivan and a sport-utility vehicle (SUV)

(p) A heavy transport vehicle is a motor vehicle designed primarily for carrying property, meeting local criteria for classification as a heavy goods vehicle in terms of weight and requiring a special driver's license.

(q) A bus (coach) is a motor vehicle designed or adapted primarily for carrying more than 10 passengers, and requiring a special driver's license.

(r) A railway train or railway vehicle is any device, with or without freight or passenger cars couple to it, designed for traffic on a railway track. This includes subterranean (subways) or elevated trains.

(s) A streetcar, is a device designed and used primarily for transporting passengers within a municipality, running on rails, usually subject to normal traffic control signals, and operated principally on a right-of-way that forms part of the roadway. This includes a tram or trolley that runs on rails. A trailer being towed by a streetcar is considered part of the streetcar.

(t) A special vehicle mainly used on industrial premises is a motor vehicle designed primarily for use within the building and premises of industrial or commercial establishments. This includes battery-powered airport passenger vehicles or baggage/mail trucks, forklifts, coal-cars in a coal min, logging cars and trucks used in mines or quarries.

(u) A special vehicle mainly used in agriculture is a motor vehicle designed specifically for use in farming and agriculture (horticulture), to work the land, tend and harvest crops and transport materials on the farm. This includes harvesters, farm machinery and tractor and trailers.

(v) A special construction vehicle is a motor vehicle designed specifically for use on construction and demolition sites. This includes bulldozers, diggers, earth levellers, dump trucks, backhoes, front-end loaders, pavers, and mechanical shovels.

(w) A special all-terrain vehicle is a motor vehicle of special design to enable it to negotiate over rough or soft terrain, snow or sand. Examples of special design are high construction, special wheels and tires, tracks, and support on a cushion of air. This includes snow mobiles, All terrain vehicles (ATV), and dune buggies. It does not include passenger vehicle designated as Sport Utility Vehicles (SUV).

(x) A water craft is any device designed for transporting passengers or goods on water. This includes motor or sail boats, ships, and hovercraft.

(y) An aircraft is any device for transporting passengers or goods in the air. This includes hot-air balloons, gliders, helicopters and airplanes.

(z) A military vehicle is any motorized vehicle operating on a public roadway owned by the military and being operated by a member of the military.

Pedestrian injured in transport accident (V00-V09)

Includes: person changing tire on transport vehicle
person examining engine of vehicle broken down in (on side of) road

Excludes1: *fall due to non-transport collision with other person (W03)*
pedestrian on foot falling (slipping) on ice and snow (W00.-)
struck or bumped by another person (W51)

AHA CC: 4Q, 2020, 41

V00 Pedestrian conveyance accident

Use additional place of occurrence and activity external cause codes, if known (Y92.-, Y93.-)

Excludes1: *collision with another person without fall (W51)*
fall due to person on foot colliding with another person on foot (W03)
fall from non-moving wheelchair, nonmotorized scooter and motorized mobility scooter without collision (W05.-)
pedestrian (conveyance) collision with other land transport vehicle (V01-V09)
pedestrian on foot falling (slipping) on ice and snow (W00.-)

The appropriate 7th character is to be added to each code from category V00
A initial encounter
D subsequent encounter
S sequela

+ **V00.0 Pedestrian on foot injured in collision with pedestrian conveyance**
  X+7th **V00.01 Pedestrian on foot injured in collision with roller-skater**
  X+7th **V00.02 Pedestrian on foot injured in collision with skateboarder**
  + **V00.03 Pedestrian on foot injured in collision with pedestrian conveyance**
    +7th **V00.031 Pedestrian on foot injured in collision with rider of standing electric scooter**
    +7th **V00.038 Pedestrian on foot injured in collision with rider of other standing micro-mobility pedestrian conveyance**
    Pedestrian on foot injured in collision with rider of hoverboard
    Pedestrian on foot injured in collision with rider of segway
  X+7th **V00.09 Pedestrian on foot injured in collision with other pedestrian conveyance**

+ **V00.1 Rolling-type pedestrian conveyance accident**
  Excludes1: *accident with baby stroller (V00.82-)*
  accident with wheelchair (powered) (V00.81-)
  accident with motorized mobility scooter (V00.83-)
  + **V00.11 In-line roller-skate accident**
    +7th **V00.111 Fall from in-line roller-skates**
    +7th **V00.112 In-line roller-skater colliding with stationary object**
    +7th **V00.118 Other in-line roller-skate accident**
      Excludes1: *roller-skater collision with other land transport vehicle(V01-V09 with 5th character 1)*
  + **V00.12 Non-in- line roller-skate accident**
    +7th **V00.121 Fall from non-in-line roller-skates**
    +7th **V00.122 Non-in-line roller-skater colliding with stationary object**
    +7th **V00.128 Other non-in-line roller-skating accident**
      Excludes1: *roller-skater collision with other land transport vehicle(V01-V09 with 5th character 1)*

- + **V00.13** Skateboard accident
  - +7th **V00.131** Fall from skateboard
  - +7th **V00.132** Skateboarder colliding with stationary object
  - +7th **V00.138** Other skateboard accident
    - *Excludes1:* *skateboarder collision with other land transport vehicle(V01-V09 with 5th character 2)*
- + **V00.14** Scooter (nonmotorized) accident
  - *Excludes1:* *motor scooter accident (V20-V29)*
  - +7th **V00.141** Fall from scooter (nonmotorized)
  - +7th **V00.142** Scooter (nonmotorized) colliding with stationary object
  - +7th **V00.148** Other scooter (nonmotorized) accident
    - *Excludes1:* *scooter (nonmotorized) collision with other land transport vehicle (V01-V09 with fifth character 9)*
- + **V00.15** Heelies accident
  - Rolling shoe
  - Wheeled shoe
  - Wheelies accident
  - +7th **V00.151** Fall from heelies
  - +7th **V00.152** Heelies colliding with stationary object
  - +7th **V00.158** Other heelies accident
- + **V00.18** Accident on other rolling-type pedestrian conveyance
  - +7th **V00.181** Fall from other rolling-type pedestrian conveyance
  - +7th **V00.182** Pedestrian on other rolling-type pedestrian conveyance colliding with stationary object
  - +7th **V00.188** Other accident on other rolling-type pedestrian conveyance
- + **V00.2** Gliding-type pedestrian conveyance accident
  - + **V00.21** Ice-skates accident
    - +7th **V00.211** Fall from ice-skates
    - +7th **V00.212** Ice-skater colliding with stationary object
    - +7th **V00.218** Other ice-skates accident
      - *Excludes1:* *ice-skater collision with other land transport vehicle(V01-V09 with 5th character 9)*
  - + **V00.22** Sled accident
    - +7th **V00.221** Fall from sled
    - +7th **V00.222** Sledder colliding with stationary object
    - +7th **V00.228** Other sled accident
      - *Excludes1:* *sled collision with other land transport vehicle (V01-V09 with 5th character 9)*
  - + **V00.28** Other gliding-type pedestrian conveyance accident
    - +7th **V00.281** Fall from other gliding-type pedestrian conveyance
    - +7th **V00.282** Pedestrian on other gliding-type pedestrian conveyance colliding with stationary object
    - +7th **V00.288** Other accident on other gliding-type pedestrian conveyance
      - *Excludes1:* *gliding-type pedestrian conveyance collision with other land transport vehicle(V01-V09 with 5th character 9)*
- + **V00.3** Flat-bottomed pedestrian conveyance accident
  - + **V00.31** Snowboard accident
    - +7th **V00.311** Fall from snowboard
    - +7th **V00.312** Snowboarder colliding with stationary object
    - +7th **V00.318** Other snowboard accident
      - *Excludes1:* *snowboarder collision with other land transport vehicle(V01-V09 with 5th character 9)*
  - + **V00.32** Snow-ski accident
    - +7th **V00.321** Fall from snow-skis
      - *AHA CC: 1Q, 2015, 3-21*
    - +7th **V00.322** Snow-skier colliding with stationary object
    - +7th **V00.328** Other snow-ski accident
      - *Excludes1:* *snow-skier collision with other land transport vehicle(V01-V09 with 5th character 9)*
  - + **V00.38** Other flat-bottomed pedestrian conveyance accident
    - +7th **V00.381** Fall from other flat-bottomed pedestrian conveyance
    - +7th **V00.382** Pedestrian on other flat-bottomed pedestrian conveyance colliding with stationary object
    - +7th **V00.388** Other accident on other flat-bottomed pedestrian conveyance
- + **V00.8** Accident on other pedestrian conveyance
  - + **V00.81** Accident with wheelchair (powered)
    - +7th **V00.811** Fall from moving wheelchair (powered)
      - *Excludes1:* *fall from non-moving wheelchair (W05.0)*
    - +7th **V00.812** Wheelchair (powered) colliding with stationary object
    - +7th **V00.818** Other accident with wheelchair (powered)
  - + **V00.82** Accident with baby stroller
    - +7th **V00.821** Fall from baby stroller
    - +7th **V00.822** Baby stroller colliding with stationary object
    - +7th **V00.828** Other accident with baby stroller
  - + **V00.83** Accident with motorized mobility scooter
    - +7th **V00.831** Fall from motorized mobility scooter
      - *Excludes1:* *fall from non-moving motorized mobility scooter (W05.2)*
    - +7th **V00.832** Motorized mobility scooter colliding with stationary object
    - +7th **V00.838** Other accident with motorized mobility scooter
  - + **V00.84** Accident with standing micro-mobility pedestrian conveyance
    - +7th **V00.841** Fall from standing electric scooter
    - +7th **V00.842** Pedestrian on standing electric scooter colliding with stationary object
    - +7th **V00.848** Other accident with standing micro-mobility pedestrian conveyance
      - Accident with hoverboard
      - Accident with segway
  - + **V00.89** Accident on other pedestrian conveyance
    - +7th **V00.891** Fall from other pedestrian conveyance
    - +7th **V00.892** Pedestrian on other pedestrian conveyance colliding with stationary object
    - +7th **V00.898** Other accident on other pedestrian conveyance
      - *Excludes1:* *other pedestrian (conveyance) collision with other land transport vehicle(V01-V09 with 5th character 9)*

V01 Pedestrian injured in collision with pedal cycle

> The appropriate 7th character is to be added to each code from category V01
> A   initial encounter
> D   subsequent encounter
> S   sequela

- + **V01.0** Pedestrian injured in collision with pedal cycle in nontraffic accident
  - X+7th **V01.00** Pedestrian on foot injured in collision with pedal cycle in nontraffic accident
    - Pedestrian NOS injured in collision with pedal cycle in nontraffic accident
  - X+7th **V01.01** Pedestrian on roller-skates injured in collision with pedal cycle in nontraffic accident
  - X+7th **V01.02** Pedestrian on skateboard injured in collision with pedal cycle in nontraffic accident
  - + **V01.03** Pedestrian on standing micro-mobility pedestrian conveyance injured in collision with pedal cycle in nontraffic accident
    - +7th **V01.031** Pedestrian on standing electric scooter injured in collision with pedal cycle in nontraffic accident

- **+7th V01.038** Pedestrian on other standing micro-mobility pedestrian conveyance injured in collision with pedal cycle in nontraffic accident
  - Pedestrian on hoverboard injured in collision with pedal cycle in nontraffic accident
  - Pedestrian on segway injured in collision with pedal cycle in nontraffic accident
- **X+7th V01.09** Pedestrian with other conveyance injured in collision with pedal cycle in nontraffic accident
  - Pedestrian with baby stroller injured in collision with pedal cycle in nontraffic accident
  - Pedestrian on ice-skates injured in collision with pedal cycle in nontraffic accident
  - Pedestrian on nonmotorized scooter injured in collision with pedal cycle in nontraffic accident
  - Pedestrian on sled injured in collision with pedal cycle in nontraffic accident
  - Pedestrian on snowboard injured in collision with pedal cycle in nontraffic accident
  - Pedestrian on snow-skis injured in collision with pedal cycle in nontraffic accident
  - Pedestrian in wheelchair (powered) injured in collision with pedal cycle in nontraffic accident
  - Pedestrian in motorized mobility scooter injured in collision with pedal cycle in nontraffic accident
- **+ V01.1** Pedestrian injured in collision with pedal cycle in traffic accident
  - **X+7th V01.10** Pedestrian on foot injured in collision with pedal cycle in traffic accident
    - Pedestrian NOS injured in collision with pedal cycle in traffic accident
  - **X+7th V01.11** Pedestrian on roller-skates injured in collision with pedal cycle in traffic accident
  - **X+7th V01.12** Pedestrian on skateboard injured in collision with pedal cycle in traffic accident
  - **+ V01.13** Pedestrian on standing micro-mobility pedestrian conveyance injured in collision with pedal cycle in traffic accident
    - **+7th V01.131** Pedestrian on standing electric scooter injured in collision with pedal cycle in traffic accident
    - **+7th V01.138** Pedestrian on other standing micro-mobility pedestrian conveyance injured in collision with pedal cycle in traffic accident
      - Pedestrian on hoverboard injured in collision with pedal cycle in traffic accident
      - Pedestrian on segway injured in collisiion with pedal cycle in traffic accident
  - **X+7th V01.19** Pedestrian with other conveyance injured in collision with pedal cycle in traffic accident
    - Pedestrian with baby stroller injured in collision with pedal cycle in traffic accident
    - Pedestrian on ice-skates injured in collision with pedal cycle in traffic accident
    - Pedestrian on nonmotorized scooter injured in collision with pedal cycle in traffic accident
    - Pedestrian on sled injured in collision with pedal cycle in traffic accident
    - Pedestrian on snowboard injured in collision with pedal cycle in traffic accident
    - Pedestrian on snow-skis injured in collision with pedal cycle in traffic accident
    - Pedestrian in wheelchair (powered) injured in collision with pedal cycle in traffic accident
    - Pedestrian in motorized mobility scooter injured in collision with pedal cycle in traffic accident
- **+ V01.9** Pedestrian injured in collision with pedal cycle, unspecified whether traffic or nontraffic accident
  - **X+7th V01.90** Pedestrian on foot injured in collision with pedal cycle, unspecified whether traffic or nontraffic accident
    - Pedestrian NOS injured in collision with pedal cycle, unspecified whether traffic or nontraffic accident
  - **X+7th V01.91** Pedestrian on roller-skates injured in collision with pedal cycle, unspecified whether traffic or nontraffic accident
  - **X+7th V01.92** Pedestrian on skateboard injured in collision with pedal cycle, unspecified whether traffic or nontraffic accident
  - **+ V01.93** Pedestrian on standing micro-mobility pedestrian conveyance injured in collision with pedal cycle, unspecified whether traffic or nontraffic accident
    - **+7th V01.931** Pedestrian on standing electric scooter injured in collision with pedal cycle, unspecified whether traffic or nontraffic accident
    - **+7th V01.938** Pedestrian on other standing micro-mobility pedestrian conveyance injured in collision with pedal cycle, unspecified whether traffic or nontraffic accident
      - Pedestrian on hoverboard injured in collision with pedal cycle, unspecified whether traffic or nontraffic accident
      - Pedestrian on segway injured in collision with pedal cycle, unspecified whether traffic or nontraffic accident
  - **X+7th V01.99** Pedestrian with other conveyance injured in collision with pedal cycle, unspecified whether traffic or nontraffic accident
    - Pedestrian with baby stroller injured in collision with pedal cycle, unspecified whether traffic or nontraffic accident
    - Pedestrian on ice-skates injured in collision with pedal cycle unspecified, whether traffic or nontraffic accident
    - Pedestrian on nonmotorized scooter injured in collision with pedal cycle, unspecified whether traffic or nontraffic accident
    - Pedestrian on sled injured in collision with pedal cycle unspecified, whether traffic or nontraffic accident
    - Pedestrian on snowboard injured in collision with pedal cycle, unspecified whether traffic or nontraffic accident
    - Pedestrian on snow-skis injured in collision with pedal cycle, unspecified whether traffic or nontraffic accident
    - Pedestrian in wheelchair (powered) injured in collision with pedal cycle, unspecified whether traffic or nontraffic accident
    - Pedestrian in motorized mobility scooter injured in collision with pedal cycle, unspecified whether traffic or nontraffic accident

V02 Pedestrian injured in collision with two- or three-wheeled motor vehicle

> The appropriate 7th character is to be added to each code from category V02
> A initial encounter
> D subsequent encounter
> S sequela

- **+ V02.0** Pedestrian injured in collision with two- or three-wheeled motor vehicle in nontraffic accident
  - **X+7th V02.00** Pedestrian on foot injured in collision with two- or three-wheeled motor vehicle in nontraffic accident
    - Pedestrian NOS injured in collision with two- or three-wheeled motor vehicle in nontraffic accident
  - **X+7th V02.01** Pedestrian on roller-skates injured in collision with two- or three-wheeled motor vehicle in nontraffic accident
  - **X+7th V02.02** Pedestrian on skateboard injured in collision with two- or three-wheeled motor vehicle in nontraffic accident
  - **+ V02.03** Pedestrian on standing micro-mobility pedestrian conveyance injured in collision with two- or three-wheeled motor vehicle in nontraffic accident
    - **+7th V02.031** Pedestrian on standing electric scooter injured in collision with two- or three-wheeled motor vehicle in nontraffic accident

+7th V02.038 Pedestrian on other standing micro-mobility pedestrian conveyance injured in collision with two- or three-wheeled motor vehicle in nontraffic accident
> Pedestrian on hoverboard injured in collision with two- or three-wheeled motor vehicle in nontraffic accident
> Pedestrian on segway injured in collision with two- or three-wheeled motor vehicle in nontraffic accident

X+7th V02.09 Pedestrian with other conveyance injured in collision with two- or three-wheeled motor vehicle in nontraffic accident
> Pedestrian with baby stroller injured in collision with two- or three-wheeled motor vehicle in nontraffic accident
> Pedestrian on ice-skates injured in collision with two- or three-wheeled motor vehicle in nontraffic accident
> Pedestrian on nonmotorized scooter injured in collision with two- or three-wheeled motor vehicle in nontraffic accident
> Pedestrian on sled injured in collision with two- or three-wheeled motor vehicle in nontraffic accident
> Pedestrian on snowboard injured in collision with two- or three-wheeled motor vehicle in nontraffic accident
> Pedestrian on snow-skis injured in collision with two- or three-wheeled motor vehicle in nontraffic accident
> Pedestrian in wheelchair (powered) injured in collision with two- or three-wheeled motor vehicle in nontraffic accident
> Pedestrian in motorized mobility scooter injured in collision with two- or three-wheeled motor vehicle in nontraffic accident

+ V02.1 Pedestrian injured in collision with two- or three-wheeled motor vehicle in traffic accident

X+7th V02.10 Pedestrian on foot injured in collision with two- or three-wheeled motor vehicle in traffic accident
> Pedestrian NOS injured in collision with two- or three-wheeled motor vehicle in traffic accident

X+7th V02.11 Pedestrian on roller-skates injured in collision with two- or three-wheeled motor vehicle in traffic accident

X+7th V02.12 Pedestrian on skateboard injured in collision with two- or three-wheeled motor vehicle in traffic accident

+ V02.13 Pedestrian on standing micro-mobility pedestrian conveyance injured in collision with two- or three-wheeled motor vehicle in traffic accident

X+7th V02.131 Pedestrian on standing electric scooter injured in collision with two- or three-wheeled motor vehicle in traffic accident

X+7th V02.138 Pedestrian on other standing micro-mobility pedestrian conveyance injured in collision with two- or three-wheeled motor vehicle in traffic accident
> Pedestrian on hoverboard injured in collision with two- or three-wheeled motor vehicle in traffic accident
> Pedestrian on segway injured in collision with two- or three-wheeled motor vehicle in traffic accident

X+7th V02.19 Pedestrian with other conveyance injured in collision with two- or three-wheeled motor vehicle in traffic accident
> Pedestrian with baby stroller injured in collision with two- or three-wheeled motor vehicle in traffic accident
> Pedestrian on ice-skates injured in collision with two- or three-wheeled motor vehicle in traffic accident
> Pedestrian on nonmotorized scooter injured in collision with two- or three-wheeled motor vehicle in traffic accident
> Pedestrian on sled injured in collision with two- or three-wheeled motor vehicle in traffic accident
> Pedestrian on snowboard injured in collision with two- or three-wheeled motor vehicle in traffic accident
> Pedestrian on snow-skis injured in collision with two- or three-wheeled motor vehicle in traffic accident
> Pedestrian in wheelchair (powered) injured in collision with two- or three-wheeled motor vehicle in traffic accident
> Pedestrian in motorized mobility scooter injured in collision with two- or three-wheeled motor vehicle in traffic accident

+ V02.9 Pedestrian injured in collision with two- or three-wheeled motor vehicle, unspecified whether traffic or nontraffic accident

X+7th V02.90 Pedestrian on foot injured in collision with two- or three-wheeled motor vehicle, unspecified whether traffic or nontraffic accident
> Pedestrian NOS injured in collision with two- or three-wheeled motor vehicle, unspecified whether traffic or nontraffic accident

X+7th V02.91 Pedestrian on roller-skates injured in collision with two- or three-wheeled motor vehicle, unspecified whether traffic or nontraffic accident

X+7th V02.92 Pedestrian on skateboard injured in collision with two- or three-wheeled motor vehicle, unspecified whether traffic or nontraffic accident

+ V02.93 Pedestrian on standing micro-mobility pedestrian conveyance injured in collision with two- or three wheeled motor vehicle, unspecified whether traffic or nontraffic accident

+7th V02.931 Pedestrian on standing electric scooter injured in collision with two- or three wheeled motor vehicle, unspecified whether traffic or nontraffic accident

+7th V02.938 Pedestrian on other standing micro-mobility pedestrian conveyance injured in collision with two- or three wheeled motor vehicle, unspecified whether traffic or nontraffic accident
> Pedestrian on hoverbaord injured in collision with two- or three wheeled motor vehicle, unspecified whether traffic or nontraffic accident
> Pedestrian on segway injured in collision with two- or three wheeled motor vehicle, unspecified whether traffic or nontraffic accident

X+7th V02.99 Pedestrian with other conveyance injured in collision with two- or three-wheeled motor vehicle, unspecified whether traffic or nontraffic accident
> Pedestrian with baby stroller injured in collision with two- or three-wheeled motor vehicle, unspecified whether traffic or nontraffic accident
> Pedestrian on ice-skates injured in collision with two- or three-wheeled motor vehicle, unspecified whether traffic or nontraffic accident
> Pedestrian on nonmotorized scooter injured in collision with two- or three-wheeled motor vehicle, unspecified whether traffic or nontraffic accident
> Pedestrian on sled injured in collision with two- or three-wheeled motor vehicle, unspecified whether traffic or nontraffic accident
> Pedestrian on snowboard injured in collision with two- or three-wheeled motor vehicle, unspecified whether traffic or nontraffic accident
> Pedestrian on snow-skis injured in collision with two- or three-wheeled motor vehicle, unspecified whether traffic or nontraffic accident
> Pedestrian in wheelchair (powered) injured in collision with two- or three-wheeled motor vehicle, unspecified whether traffic or nontraffic accident
> Pedestrian in motorized mobility scooter injured in collision with two- or three-wheeled motor vehicle, unspecified whether traffic or nontraffic accident

V03 Pedestrian injured in collision with car, pick-up truck or van

> The appropriate 7th character is to be added to each code from category V03
> A initial encounter
> D subsequent encounter
> S sequela

+ **V03.0 Pedestrian injured in collision with car, pick-up truck or van in nontraffic accident**

    X+7th **V03.00** Pedestrian on foot injured in collision with car, pick-up truck or van in nontraffic accident
        Pedestrian NOS injured in collision with car, pick-up truck or van in nontraffic accident

    X+7th **V03.01** Pedestrian on roller-skates injured in collision with car, pick-up truck or van in nontraffic accident

    X+7th **V03.02** Pedestrian on skateboard injured in collision with car, pick-up truck or van in nontraffic accident

    + **V03.03** Pedestrian on standing micro-mobility pedestrian conveyance injured in collision with car, pick-up or van in nontraffic accident

        +7th **V03.031** Pedestrian on standing electric scooter injured in collision with car, pick-up or van in nontraffic accident

        +7th **V03.038** Pedestrian on other standing micro-mobility pedestrian conveyance injured in collision with car, pick-up or van in nontraffic accident
            Pedestrian on hoverboard injured in collision with car, pick-up or van in nontraffic accident
            Pedestrian on segway injured in collision with car, pick-up or van in nontraffic accident

    X+7th **V03.09** Pedestrian with other conveyance injured in collision with car, pick-up truck or van in nontraffic accident
        Pedestrian with baby stroller injured in collision with car, pick-up truck or van in nontraffic accident
        Pedestrian on ice-skates injured in collision with car, pick-up truck or van in nontraffic accident
        Pedestrian on nonmotorized scooter injured in collision with car, pick-up truck or van in nontraffic accident
        Pedestrian on sled injured in collision with car, pick-up truck or van in nontraffic accident
        Pedestrian on snowboard injured in collision with car, pick-up truck or van in nontraffic accident
        Pedestrian on snow-skis injured in collision with car, pick-up truck or van in nontraffic accident
        Pedestrian in wheelchair (powered) injured in collision with car, pick-up truck or van in nontraffic accident
        Pedestrian in motorized mobility scooter injured in collision with car, pick-up truck or van in nontraffic accident

+ **V03.1 Pedestrian injured in collision with car, pick-up truck or van in traffic accident**

    X+7th **V03.10** Pedestrian on foot injured in collision with car, pick-up truck or van in traffic accident
        Pedestrian NOS injured in collision with car, pick-up truck or van in traffic accident

    X+7th **V03.11** Pedestrian on roller-skates injured in collision with car, pick-up truck or van in traffic accident

    X+7th **V03.12** Pedestrian on skateboard injured in collision with car, pick-up truck or van in traffic accident

    + **V03.13** Pedestrian on standing micro-mobility pedestrian conveyance injured in collision with car, pick-up or van in traffic accident

        +7th **V03.131** Pedestrian on standing electric scooter injured in collision with car, pick-up or van in traffic accident

        +7th **V03.138** Pedestrian on other standing micro-mobility pedestrian conveyance injured in collision with car, pick-up or van in traffic accident
            Pedestrian on hoverboard injured in collision with car, pick-up or van in traffic accident
            Pedestrian on segway injured in collision with car, pick-up or van in traffic accident

    X+7th **V03.19** Pedestrian with other conveyance injured in collision with car, pick-up truck or van in traffic accident
        Pedestrian with baby stroller injured in collision with car, pick-up truck or van in traffic accident
        Pedestrian on ice-skates injured in collision with car, pick-up truck or van in traffic accident
        Pedestrian on nonmotorized scooter injured in collision with car, pick-up truck or van in traffic accident
        Pedestrian on sled injured in collision with car, pick-up truck or van in traffic accident
        Pedestrian on snowboard injured in collision with car, pick-up truck or van in traffic accident
        Pedestrian on snow-skis injured in collision with car, pick-up truck or van in traffic accident
        Pedestrian in wheelchair (powered) injured in collision with car, pick-up truck or van in traffic accident
        Pedestrian in motorized mobility scooter injured in collision with car, pick-up truck or van in traffic accident

+ **V03.9 Pedestrian injured in collision with car, pick-up truck or van, unspecified whether traffic or nontraffic accident**

    X+7th **V03.90** Pedestrian on foot injured in collision with car, pick-up truck or van, unspecified whether traffic or nontraffic accident
        Pedestrian NOS injured in collision with car, pick-up truck or van, unspecified whether traffic or nontraffic accident

    X+7th **V03.91** Pedestrian on roller-skates injured in collision with car, pick-up truck or van, unspecified whether traffic or nontraffic accident

    X+7th **V03.92** Pedestrian on skateboard injured in collision with car, pick-up truck or van, unspecified whether traffic or nontraffic accident

    + **V03.93** Pedestrian on standing micro-mobility pedestrian conveyance injured in collision with car, pick-up or van, unspecified whether traffic or nontraffic accident

        +7th **V03.931** Pedestrian on standing electric scooter injured in collision with car, pick-up or van, unspecified whether traffic or nontraffic accident

        +7th **V03.938** Pedestrian on other standing micro-mobility pedestrian conveyance injured in collision with car, pick-up or van, unspecified whether traffic or nontraffic accident
            Pedestrian on hoverboard injured in collision with car, pick-up or van, unspecified whether traffic or nontraffic accident
            Pedestrian on segway injured in collision with car, pick-up or van, unspecified whether traffic or nontraffic accident

    X+7th **V03.99** Pedestrian with other conveyance injured in collision with car, pick-up truck or van, unspecified whether traffic or nontraffic accident
        Pedestrian with baby stroller injured in collision with car, pick-up truck or van, unspecified whether traffic or nontraffic accident
        Pedestrian on ice-skates injured in collision with car, pick-up truck or van, unspecified whether traffic or nontraffic accident
        Pedestrian on nonmotorized scooter injured in collision with car, pick-up truck or van, unspecified whether traffic or nontraffic accident
        Pedestrian on sled injured in collision with car, pick-up truck or van in nontraffic accident
        Pedestrian on snowboard injured in collision with car, pick-up truck or van, unspecified whether traffic or nontraffic accident

Pedestrian on snow-skis injured in collision with car, pick-up truck or van, unspecified whether traffic or nontraffic accident

Pedestrian in wheelchair (powered) injured in collision with car, pick-up truck or van, unspecified whether traffic or nontraffic accident

Pedestrian in motorized mobility scooter injured in collision with car, pick-up truck or van, unspecified whether traffic or nontraffic accident

V04 Pedestrian injured in collision with heavy transport vehicle or bus

Excludes1: pedestrian injured in collision with military vehicle (V09.01, V09.21)

> The appropriate 7th character is to be added to each code from category V04
> A initial encounter
> D subsequent encounter
> S sequela

+ **V04.0 Pedestrian injured in collision with heavy transport vehicle or bus in nontraffic accident**

  X+7th **V04.00 Pedestrian on foot injured in collision with heavy transport vehicle or bus in nontraffic accident**
     Pedestrian NOS injured in collision with heavy transport vehicle or bus in nontraffic accident

  X+7th **V04.01 Pedestrian on roller-skates injured in collision with heavy transport vehicle or bus in nontraffic accident**

  X+7th **V04.02 Pedestrian on skateboard injured in collision with heavy transport vehicle or bus in nontraffic accident**

  + **V04.03 Pedestrian on standing micro-mobility pedestrian conveyance injured in collision with heavy transport vehicle or bus in nontraffic accident**

    +7th **V04.031 Pedestrian on standing electric scooter injured in collision with heavy transport vehicle or bus in nontraffic accident**

    +7th **V04.038 Pedestrian on other standing micro-mobility pedestrian conveyance injured in collision with heavy transport vehicle or bus in nontraffic accident**
      Pedestrian on hoverboard injured in collision with heavy transport vehicle or bus in nontraffic accident
      Pedestrian on segway injured in collision with heavy transport vehicle or bus in nontraffic accident

  X+7th **V04.09 Pedestrian with other conveyance injured in collision with heavy transport vehicle or bus in nontraffic accident**
     Pedestrian with baby stroller injured in collision with heavy transport vehicle or bus in nontraffic accident
     Pedestrian on ice-skates injured in collision with heavy transport vehicle or bus in nontraffic accident
     Pedestrian on nonmotorized scooter injured in collision with heavy transport vehicle or bus in nontraffic accident
     Pedestrian on sled injured in collision with heavy transport vehicle or bus in nontraffic accident
     Pedestrian on snowboard injured in collision with heavy transport vehicle or bus in nontraffic accident
     Pedestrian on snow-skis injured in collision with heavy transport vehicle or bus in nontraffic accident
     Pedestrian in wheelchair (powered) injured in collision with heavy transport vehicle or bus in nontraffic accident
     Pedestrian in motorized mobility scooter injured in collision with heavy transport vehicle or bus in nontraffic accident

+ **V04.1 Pedestrian injured in collision with heavy transport vehicle or bus in traffic accident**

  X+7th **V04.10 Pedestrian on foot injured in collision with heavy transport vehicle or bus in traffic accident**
     Pedestrian NOS injured in collision with heavy transport vehicle or bus in traffic accident

  X+7th **V04.11 Pedestrian on roller-skates injured in collision with heavy transport vehicle or bus in traffic accident**

  X+7th **V04.12 Pedestrian on skateboard injured in collision with heavy transport vehicle or bus in traffic accident**

  + **V04.13 Pedestrian on standing micro-mobility pedestrian conveyance injured in collision with heavy transport vehicle or bus in traffic accident**

    +7th **V04.131 Pedestrian on standing electric scooter injured in collision with heavy transport vehicle or bus in traffic accident**

    +7th **V04.138 Pedestrian on other standing micro-mobility pedestrian conveyance injured in collision with heavy transport vehicle or bus in traffic accident**
      Pedestrian on hoverboard injured in collision with heavy transport vehicle or bus in traffic accident
      Pedestrian on segway injured in collision with heavy transport vehicle or bus in traffic accident

  X+7th **V04.19 Pedestrian with other conveyance injured in collision with heavy transport vehicle or bus in traffic accident**
     Pedestrian with baby stroller injured in collision with heavy transport vehicle or bus in traffic accident
     Pedestrian on ice-skates injured in collision with heavy transport vehicle or bus in traffic accident
     Pedestrian on nonmotorized scooter injured in collision with heavy transport vehicle or bus in traffic accident
     Pedestrian on sled injured in collision with heavy transport vehicle or bus in traffic accident
     Pedestrian on snowboard injured in collision with heavy transport vehicle or bus in traffic accident
     Pedestrian on snow-skis injured in collision with heavy transport vehicle or bus in traffic accident
     Pedestrian in wheelchair (powered) injured in collision with heavy transport vehicle or bus in traffic accident
     Pedestrian in motorized mobility scooter injured in collision with heavy transport vehicle or bus in traffic accident

+ **V04.9 Pedestrian injured in collision with heavy transport vehicle or bus, unspecified whether traffic or nontraffic accident**

  X+7th **V04.90 Pedestrian on foot injured in collision with heavy transport vehicle or bus, unspecified whether traffic or nontraffic accident**
     Pedestrian NOS injured in collision with heavy transport vehicle or bus, unspecified whether traffic or nontraffic accident

  X+7th **V04.91 Pedestrian on roller-skates injured in collision with heavy transport vehicle or bus, unspecified whether traffic or nontraffic accident**

  X+7th **V04.92 Pedestrian on skateboard injured in collision with heavy transport vehicle or bus, unspecified whether traffic or nontraffic accident**

  + **V04.93 Pedestrian on standing micro-mobility pedestrian conveyance injured in collision with heavy transport vehicle or bus, unspecified whether traffic or nontraffic accident**

    +7th **V04.931 Pedestrian on standing electric scooter injured in collision with heavy transport vehicle or bus, unspecified whether traffic or nontraffic accident**

    +7th **V04.938 Pedestrian on other standing micro-mobility pedestrian conveyance injured in collision with heavy transport vehicle or bus, unspecified whether traffic or nontraffic accident**
      Pedestrian on hoverboard injured in collision with heavy transport vehicle or bus, unspecified whether traffic or nontraffic accident
      Pedestrian on segway injured in collision with heavy transport vehicle or bus, unspecified whether traffic or nontraffic accident

X+7th V04.99 Pedestrian with other conveyance injured in collision with heavy transport vehicle or bus, unspecified whether traffic or nontraffic accident
- Pedestrian with baby stroller injured in collision with heavy transport vehicle or bus, unspecified whether traffic or nontraffic accident
- Pedestrian on ice-skates injured in collision with heavy transport vehicle or bus, unspecified whether traffic or nontraffic accident
- Pedestrian on nonmotorized scooter injured in collision with heavy transport vehicle or bus, unspecified whether traffic or nontraffic accident
- Pedestrian on sled injured in collision with heavy transport vehicle or bus, unspecified whether traffic or nontraffic accident
- Pedestrian on snowboard injured in collision with heavy transport vehicle or bus, unspecified whether traffic or nontraffic accident
- Pedestrian on snow-skis injured in collision with heavy transport vehicle or bus, unspecified whether traffic or nontraffic accident
- Pedestrian in wheelchair (powered) injured in collision with heavy transport vehicle or bus, unspecified whether traffic or nontraffic accident
- Pedestrian in motorized mobility scooter injured in collision with heavy transport vehicle or bus, unspecified whether traffic or nontraffic accident

V05 Pedestrian injured in collision with railway train or railway vehicle

> The appropriate 7th character is to be added to each code from category V05
> A initial encounter
> D subsequent encounter
> S sequela

+ V05.0 Pedestrian injured in collision with railway train or railway vehicle in nontraffic accident

X+7th V05.00 Pedestrian on foot injured in collision with railway train or railway vehicle in nontraffic accident
- Pedestrian NOS injured in collision with railway train or railway vehicle in nontraffic accident

X+7th V05.01 Pedestrian on roller-skates injured in collision with railway train or railway vehicle in nontraffic accident

X+7th V05.02 Pedestrian on skateboard injured in collision with railway train or railway vehicle in nontraffic accident

+ V05.03 Pedestrian on standing micro-mobility pedestrian conveyance injured in collision with railway train or railway vehicle in nontraffic accident

+7th V05.031 Pedestrian on standing electric scooter injured in collision with railway train or railway vehicle in nontraffic accident

+7th V05.038 Pedestrian on other standing micro-mobility pedestrian conveyance injured in collision with railway train or railway vehicle in nontraffic accident
- Pedestrian on hoverboard injured in collision with railway train or railway vehicle in nontraffic accident
- Pedestrian on segway injured in collision with railway train or railway vehicle in nontraffic accident

X+7th V05.09 Pedestrian with other conveyance injured in collision with railway train or railway vehicle in nontraffic accident
- Pedestrian with baby stroller injured in collision with railway train or railway vehicle in nontraffic accident
- Pedestrian on ice-skates injured in collision with railway train or railway vehicle in nontraffic accident
- Pedestrian on nonmotorized scooter injured in collision with railway train or railway vehicle in nontraffic accident
- Pedestrian on sled injured in collision with railway train or railway vehicle in nontraffic accident
- Pedestrian on snowboard injured in collision with railway train or railway vehicle in nontraffic accident
- Pedestrian on snow-skis injured in collision with railway train or railway vehicle in nontraffic accident
- Pedestrian in wheelchair (powered) injured in collision with railway train or railway vehicle in nontraffic accident
- Pedestrian in motorized mobility scooter injured in collision with railway train or railway vehicle in nontraffic accident

+ V05.1 Pedestrian injured in collision with railway train or railway vehicle in traffic accident

X+7th V05.10 Pedestrian on foot injured in collision with railway train or railway vehicle in traffic accident
- Pedestrian NOS injured in collision with railway train or railway vehicle in traffic accident

X+7th V05.11 Pedestrian on roller-skates injured in collision with railway train or railway vehicle in traffic accident

X+7th V05.12 Pedestrian on skateboard injured in collision with railway train or railway vehicle in traffic accident

+ V05.13 Pedestrian on standing micro-mobility pedestrian conveyance injured in collision with railway train or railway vehicle in traffic accident

+7th V05.131 Pedestrian on standing electric scooter injured in collision with railway train or railway vehicle in traffic accident

+7th V05.138 Pedestrian on other standing micro-mobility pedestrian conveyance injured in collision with railway train or railway vehicle in traffic accident
- Pedestrian on hoverboard injured in collision with railway train or railway vehicle in traffic accident
- Pedestrian on segway injured in collision with railway train or railway vehicle in traffic accident

X+7th V05.19 Pedestrian with other conveyance injured in collision with railway train or railway vehicle in traffic accident
- Pedestrian with baby stroller injured in collision with railway train or railway vehicle in traffic accident
- Pedestrian on ice-skates injured in collision with railway train or railway vehicle in traffic accident
- Pedestrian on nonmotorized scooter injured in collision with railway train or railway vehicle in traffic accident
- Pedestrian on sled injured in collision with railway train or railway vehicle in traffic accident
- Pedestrian on snowboard injured in collision with railway train or railway vehicle in traffic accident
- Pedestrian on snow-skis injured in collision with railway train or railway vehicle in traffic accident
- Pedestrian in wheelchair (powered) injured in collision with railway train or railway vehicle in traffic accident
- Pedestrian in motorized mobility scooter injured in collision with railway train or railway vehicle in traffic accident

+ V05.9 Pedestrian injured in collision with railway train or railway vehicle, unspecified whether traffic or nontraffic accident

X+7th V05.90 Pedestrian on foot injured in collision with railway train or railway vehicle, unspecified whether traffic or nontraffic accident
- Pedestrian NOS injured in collision with railway train or railway vehicle, unspecified whether traffic or nontraffic accident

X+7th V05.91 Pedestrian on roller-skates injured in collision with railway train or railway vehicle, unspecified whether traffic or nontraffic accident

X+7th V05.92 Pedestrian on skateboard injured in collision with railway train or railway vehicle, unspecified whether traffic or nontraffic accident

+ V05.93 Pedestrian on standing micro-mobility pedestrian conveyance injured in collision with railway train or railway vehicle, unspecified whether traffic or nontraffic accident

+7th V05.931 Pedestrian on standing electric scooter injured in collision with railway train or railway vehicle, unspecified whether traffic or nontraffic accident

+7th **V05.938** Pedestrian on other standing micro-mobility pedestrian conveyance injured in collision with railway train or railway vehicle, unspecified whether traffic or nontraffic accident
- Pedestrian on hoverboard injured in collision with railway train or railway vehicle, unspecified whether traffic or nontraffic accident
- Pedestrian on segway injured in collision with railway train or railway vehicle, unspecified whether traffic or nontraffic accident

X+7th **V05.99** Pedestrian with other conveyance injured in collision with railway train or railway vehicle, unspecified whether traffic or nontraffic accident
- Pedestrian with baby stroller injured in collision with railway train or railway vehicle, unspecified whether traffic or nontraffic
- Pedestrian on ice-skates injured in collision with railway train or railway vehicle, unspecified whether traffic or nontraffic
- Pedestrian on nonmotorized scooter injured in collision with railway train or railway vehicle, unspecified whether traffic or nontraffic
- Pedestrian on sled injured in collision with railway train or railway vehicle, unspecified whether traffic or nontraffic
- Pedestrian on snowboard injured in collision with railway train or railway vehicle, unspecified whether traffic or nontraffic
- Pedestrian on snow-skis injured in collision with railway train or railway vehicle, unspecified whether traffic or nontraffic
- Pedestrian in wheelchair (powered) injured in collision with railway train or railway vehicle, unspecified whether traffic or nontraffic
- Pedestrian in motorized mobility scooter injured in collision with railway train or railway vehicle, unspecified whether traffic or nontraffic

V06 **Pedestrian injured in collision with other nonmotor vehicle**

Includes: collision with animal-drawn vehicle, animal being ridden, nonpowered streetcar

Excludes1: pedestrian injured in collision with pedestrian conveyance (V00.0-)

> The appropriate 7th character is to be added to each code from category V06
> A initial encounter
> D subsequent encounter
> S sequela

+ **V06.0** Pedestrian injured in collision with other nonmotor vehicle in nontraffic accident
  X+7th **V06.00** Pedestrian on foot injured in collision with other nonmotor vehicle in nontraffic accident
  - Pedestrian NOS injured in collision with other nonmotor vehicle in nontraffic accident
  X+7th **V06.01** Pedestrian on roller-skates injured in collision with other nonmotor vehicle in nontraffic accident
  X+7th **V06.02** Pedestrian on skateboard injured in collision with other nonmotor vehicle in nontraffic accident
  + **V06.03** Pedestrian on standing micro-mobility pedestrian conveyance injured in collision with other nonmotor vehicle in nontraffic accident
    +7th **V06.031** Pedestrian on standing electric scooter injured in collision with other nonmotor vehicle in nontraffic accident
    +7th **V06.038** Pedestrian on other standing micro-mobility pedestrian conveyance injured in collision with other nonmotor vehicle in nontraffic accident
    - Pedestrian on hoverboard injured in collision with other nonmotor vehicle in nontraffic accident
    - Pedestrian on segway injured in collision with other nonmotor vehicle in nontraffic accident

X+7th **V06.09** Pedestrian with other conveyance injured in collision with other nonmotor vehicle in nontraffic accident
- Pedestrian with baby stroller injured in collision with other nonmotor vehicle in nontraffic accident
- Pedestrian on ice-skates injured in collision with other nonmotor vehicle in nontraffic accident
- Pedestrian on nonmotorized scooter injured in collision with other nonmotor vehicle in nontraffic accident
- Pedestrian on sled injured in collision with other nonmotor vehicle in nontraffic accident
- Pedestrian on snowboard injured in collision with other nonmotor vehicle in nontraffic accident
- Pedestrian on snow-skis injured in collision with other nonmotor vehicle in nontraffic accident
- Pedestrian in wheelchair (powered) injured in collision with other nonmotor vehicle in nontraffic accident
- Pedestrian in motorized mobility scooter injured in collision with other nonmotor vehicle in nontraffic accident

+ **V06.1** Pedestrian injured in collision with other nonmotor vehicle in traffic accident
  X+7th **V06.10** Pedestrian on foot injured in collision with other nonmotor vehicle in traffic accident
  - Pedestrian NOS injured in collision with other nonmotor vehicle in traffic accident
  X+7th **V06.11** Pedestrian on roller-skates injured in collision with other nonmotor vehicle in traffic accident
  X+7th **V06.12** Pedestrian on skateboard injured in collision with other nonmotor vehicle in traffic accident
  + **V06.13** Pedestrian on standing micro-mobility pedestrian conveyance injured in collision with other nonmotor vehicle in traffic accident
    +7th **V06.131** Pedestrian on standing electric scooter injured in collision with other nonmotor vehicle in traffic accident
    +7th **V06.138** Pedestrian on other standing micro-mobility pedestrian conveyance injured in collision with other nonmotor vehicle in traffic accident
    - Pedestrian on hoverboard injured in collision with other nonmotor vehicle in traffic accident
    - Pedestrian on segway injured in collision with other nonmotor vehicle in traffic accident

X+7th **V06.19** Pedestrian with other conveyance injured in collision with other nonmotor vehicle in traffic accident
- Pedestrian with baby stroller injured in collision with other nonmotor vehicle in nontraffic accident
- Pedestrian on ice-skates injured in collision with other nonmotor vehicle in traffic accident
- Pedestrian on nonmotorized scooter injured in collision with other nonmotor vehicle in traffic accident
- Pedestrian on sled injured in collision with other nonmotor vehicle in traffic accident
- Pedestrian on snowboard injured in collision with other nonmotor vehicle in traffic accident
- Pedestrian on snow-skis injured in collision with other nonmotor vehicle in traffic accident
- Pedestrian in wheelchair (powered) injured in collision with other nonmotor vehicle in traffic accident
- Pedestrian in motorized mobility scooter injured in collision with other nonmotor vehicle in traffic accident

+ **V06.9** Pedestrian injured in collision with other nonmotor vehicle, unspecified whether traffic or nontraffic accident
  X+7th **V06.90** Pedestrian on foot injured in collision with other nonmotor vehicle, unspecified whether traffic or nontraffic accident
  - Pedestrian NOS injured in collision with other nonmotor vehicle, unspecified whether traffic or nontraffic accident

X+7th V06.91 Pedestrian on roller-skates injured in collision with other nonmotor vehicle, unspecified whether traffic or nontraffic accident
X+7th V06.92 Pedestrian on skateboard injured in collision with other nonmotor vehicle, unspecified whether traffic or nontraffic accident
+ V06.93 Pedestrian on standing micro-mobility pedestrian conveyance injured in collision with other nonmotor vehicle, unspecified whether traffic or nontraffic accident
 +7th V06.931 Pedestrian on standing electric scooter injured in collision with other nonmotor vehicle, unspecified whether traffic or nontraffic accident
 +7th V06.938 Pedestrian on other standing micro-mobility pedestrian conveyance injured in collision with other nonmotor vehicle, unspecified whether traffic or nontraffic accident
  Pedestrian on hoverboard injured in collision with other nonmotor vehicle, unspecified whether traffic or nontraffic accident
  Pedestrian on other segway injured in collision with other nonmotor vehicle, unspecified whether traffic or nontraffic accident
X+7th V06.99 Pedestrian with other conveyance injured in collision with other nonmotor vehicle, unspecified whether traffic or nontraffic accident
 Pedestrian with baby stroller injured in collision with other nonmotor vehicle, unspecified whether traffic or nontraffic accident
 Pedestrian on ice-skates injured in collision with other nonmotor vehicle, unspecified whether traffic or nontraffic accident
 Pedestrian on nonmotorized scooter injured in collision with other nonmotor vehicle, unspecified whether traffic or nontraffic accident
 Pedestrian on sled injured in collision with other nonmotor vehicle, unspecified whether traffic or nontraffic accident
 Pedestrian on snowboard injured in collision with other nonmotor vehicle, unspecified whether traffic or nontraffic accident
 Pedestrian on snow-skis injured in collision with other nonmotor vehicle, unspecified whether traffic or nontraffic accident
 Pedestrian in wheelchair (powered) injured in collision with other nonmotor vehicle, unspecified whether traffic or nontraffic accident
 Pedestrian in motorized mobility scooter injured in collision with other nonmotor vehicle, unspecified whether traffic or nontraffic accident

V09 Pedestrian injured in other and unspecified transport accidents

> The appropriate 7th character is to be added to each code from category V09
> A initial encounter
> D subsequent encounter
> S sequela

+ V09.0 Pedestrian injured in nontraffic accident involving other and unspecified motor vehicles
 X+7th V09.00 Pedestrian injured in nontraffic accident involving unspecified motor vehicles
 X+7th V09.01 Pedestrian injured in nontraffic accident involving military vehicle
 X+7th V09.09 Pedestrian injured in nontraffic accident involving other motor vehicles
  Pedestrian injured in nontraffic accident by special vehicle
X+7th V09.1 Pedestrian injured in unspecified nontraffic accident
+ V09.2 Pedestrian injured in traffic accident involving other and unspecified motor vehicles
 X+7th V09.20 Pedestrian injured in traffic accident involving unspecified motor vehicles
 X+7th V09.21 Pedestrian injured in traffic accident involving military vehicle
 X+7th V09.29 Pedestrian injured in traffic accident involving other motor vehicles

X+7th V09.3 Pedestrian injured in unspecified traffic accident
X+7th V09.9 Pedestrian injured in unspecified transport accident

Pedal cycle rider injured in transport accident (V10-V19)

Includes: any non-motorized vehicle, excluding an animal-drawn vehicle, or a sidecar or trailer attached to the pedal cycle
Excludes2: rupture of pedal cycle tire (W37.0)

V10 Pedal cycle rider injured in collision with pedestrian or animal

> **Excludes1:** pedal cycle rider collision with animal-drawn vehicle or animal being ridden (V16.-)

> The appropriate 7th character is to be added to each code from category V10
> A initial encounter
> D subsequent encounter
> S sequela

X+7th V10.0 Pedal cycle driver injured in collision with pedestrian or animal in nontraffic accident
X+7th V10.1 Pedal cycle passenger injured in collision with pedestrian or animal in nontraffic accident
X+7th V10.2 Unspecified pedal cyclist injured in collision with pedestrian or animal in nontraffic accident
X+7th V10.3 Person boarding or alighting a pedal cycle injured in collision with pedestrian or animal
X+7th V10.4 Pedal cycle driver injured in collision with pedestrian or animal in traffic accident
X+7th V10.5 Pedal cycle passenger injured in collision with pedestrian or animal in traffic accident
X+7th V10.9 Unspecified pedal cyclist injured in collision with pedestrian or animal in traffic accident

V11 Pedal cycle rider injured in collision with other pedal cycle

> The appropriate 7th character is to be added to each code from category V11
> A initial encounter
> D subsequent encounter
> S sequela

X+7th V11.0 Pedal cycle driver injured in collision with other pedal cycle in nontraffic accident
X+7th V11.1 Pedal cycle passenger injured in collision with other pedal cycle in nontraffic accident
X+7th V11.2 Unspecified pedal cyclist injured in collision with other pedal cycle in nontraffic accident
X+7th V11.3 Person boarding or alighting a pedal cycle injured in collision with other pedal cycle
X+7th V11.4 Pedal cycle driver injured in collision with other pedal cycle in traffic accident
X+7th V11.5 Pedal cycle passenger injured in collision with other pedal cycle in traffic accident
X+7th V11.9 Unspecified pedal cyclist injured in collision with other pedal cycle in traffic accident

V12 Pedal cycle rider injured in collision with two- or three-wheeled motor vehicle

> The appropriate 7th character is to be added to each code from category V12
> A initial encounter
> D subsequent encounter
> S sequela

X+7th V12.0 Pedal cycle driver injured in collision with two- or three-wheeled motor vehicle in nontraffic accident
X+7th V12.1 Pedal cycle passenger injured in collision with two- or three-wheeled motor vehicle in nontraffic accident
X+7th V12.2 Unspecified pedal cyclist injured in collision with two- or three-wheeled motor vehicle in nontraffic accident
X+7th V12.3 Person boarding or alighting a pedal cycle injured in collision with two- or three-wheeled motor vehicle
X+7th V12.4 Pedal cycle driver injured in collision with two- or three-wheeled motor vehicle in traffic accident
X+7th V12.5 Pedal cycle passenger injured in collision with two- or three-wheeled motor vehicle in traffic accident
X+7th V12.9 Unspecified pedal cyclist injured in collision with two- or three-wheeled motor vehicle in traffic accident

V13 Pedal cycle rider injured in collision with car, pick-up truck or van

> The appropriate 7th character is to be added to each code from category V13
> A initial encounter
> D subsequent encounter
> S sequela

X+7th **V13.0** Pedal cycle driver injured in collision with car, pick-up truck or van in nontraffic accident
X+7th **V13.1** Pedal cycle passenger injured in collision with car, pick-up truck or van in nontraffic accident
X+7th **V13.2** Unspecified pedal cyclist injured in collision with car, pick-up truck or van in nontraffic accident
X+7th **V13.3** Person boarding or alighting a pedal cycle injured in collision with car, pick-up truck or van
X+7th **V13.4** Pedal cycle driver injured in collision with car, pick-up truck or van in traffic accident
X+7th **V13.5** Pedal cycle passenger injured in collision with car, pick-up truck or van in traffic accident
X+7th **V13.9** Unspecified pedal cyclist injured in collision with car, pick-up truck or van in traffic accident

V14 Pedal cycle rider injured in collision with heavy transport vehicle or bus

> **Excludes1:** *pedal cycle rider injured in collision with military vehicle (V19.81)*

> The appropriate 7th character is to be added to each code from category V14
> A initial encounter
> D subsequent encounter
> S sequela

X+7th **V14.0** Pedal cycle driver injured in collision with heavy transport vehicle or bus in nontraffic accident
X+7th **V14.1** Pedal cycle passenger injured in collision with heavy transport vehicle or bus in nontraffic accident
X+7th **V14.2** Unspecified pedal cyclist injured in collision with heavy transport vehicle or bus in nontraffic accident
X+7th **V14.3** Person boarding or alighting a pedal cycle injured in collision with heavy transport vehicle or bus
X+7th **V14.4** Pedal cycle driver injured in collision with heavy transport vehicle or bus in traffic accident
X+7th **V14.5** Pedal cycle passenger injured in collision with heavy transport vehicle or bus in traffic accident
X+7th **V14.9** Unspecified pedal cyclist injured in collision with heavy transport vehicle or bus in traffic accident

V15 Pedal cycle rider injured in collision with railway train or railway vehicle

> The appropriate 7th character is to be added to each code from category V15
> A initial encounter
> D subsequent encounter
> S sequela

X+7th **V15.0** Pedal cycle driver injured in collision with railway train or railway vehicle in nontraffic accident
X+7th **V15.1** Pedal cycle passenger injured in collision with railway train or railway vehicle in nontraffic accident
X+7th **V15.2** Unspecified pedal cyclist injured in collision with railway train or railway vehicle in nontraffic accident
X+7th **V15.3** Person boarding or alighting a pedal cycle injured in collision with railway train or railway vehicle
X+7th **V15.4** Pedal cycle driver injured in collision with railway train or railway vehicle in traffic accident
X+7th **V15.5** Pedal cycle passenger injured in collision with railway train or railway vehicle in traffic accident
X+7th **V15.9** Unspecified pedal cyclist injured in collision with railway train or railway vehicle in traffic accident

V16 Pedal cycle rider injured in collision with other nonmotor vehicle

> **Includes:** collision with animal-drawn vehicle, animal being ridden, streetcar

> The appropriate 7th character is to be added to each code from category V16
> A initial encounter
> D subsequent encounter
> S sequela

X+7th **V16.0** Pedal cycle driver injured in collision with other nonmotor vehicle in nontraffic accident
X+7th **V16.1** Pedal cycle passenger injured in collision with other nonmotor vehicle in nontraffic accident
X+7th **V16.2** Unspecified pedal cyclist injured in collision with other nonmotor vehicle in nontraffic accident
X+7th **V16.3** Person boarding or alighting a pedal cycle injured in collision with other nonmotor vehicle in nontraffic accident
X+7th **V16.4** Pedal cycle driver injured in collision with other nonmotor vehicle in traffic accident
X+7th **V16.5** Pedal cycle passenger injured in collision with other nonmotor vehicle in traffic accident
X+7th **V16.9** Unspecified pedal cyclist injured in collision with other nonmotor vehicle in traffic accident

V17 Pedal cycle rider injured in collision with fixed or stationary object

> The appropriate 7th character is to be added to each code from category V17
> A initial encounter
> D subsequent encounter
> S sequela

X+7th **V17.0** Pedal cycle driver injured in collision with fixed or stationary object in nontraffic accident
X+7th **V17.1** Pedal cycle passenger injured in collision with fixed or stationary object in nontraffic accident
X+7th **V17.2** Unspecified pedal cyclist injured in collision with fixed or stationary object in nontraffic accident
X+7th **V17.3** Person boarding or alighting a pedal cycle injured in collision with fixed or stationary object
X+7th **V17.4** Pedal cycle driver injured in collision with fixed or stationary object in traffic accident
X+7th **V17.5** Pedal cycle passenger injured in collision with fixed or stationary object in traffic accident
X+7th **V17.9** Unspecified pedal cyclist injured in collision with fixed or stationary object in traffic accident

V18 Pedal cycle rider injured in noncollision transport accident

> **Includes:** fall or thrown from pedal cycle (without antecedent collision)
> overturning pedal cycle NOS
> overturning pedal cycle without collision

> The appropriate 7th character is to be added to each code from category V18
> A initial encounter
> D subsequent encounter
> S sequela

X+7th **V18.0** Pedal cycle driver injured in noncollision transport accident in nontraffic accident
X+7th **V18.1** Pedal cycle passenger injured in noncollision transport accident in nontraffic accident
X+7th **V18.2** Unspecified pedal cyclist injured in noncollision transport accident in nontraffic accident
X+7th **V18.3** Person boarding or alighting a pedal cycle injured in noncollision transport accident
X+7th **V18.4** Pedal cycle driver injured in noncollision transport accident in traffic accident
X+7th **V18.5** Pedal cycle passenger injured in noncollision transport accident in traffic accident
X+7th **V18.9** Unspecified pedal cyclist injured in noncollision transport accident in traffic accident

V19 Pedal cycle rider injured in other and unspecified transport accidents

> The appropriate 7th character is to be added to each code from category V19
> A initial encounter
> D subsequent encounter
> S sequela

+ **V19.0** Pedal cycle driver injured in collision with other and unspecified motor vehicles in nontraffic accident
   X+7th **V19.00** Pedal cycle driver injured in collision with unspecified motor vehicles in nontraffic accident
   X+7th **V19.09** Pedal cycle driver injured in collision with other motor vehicles in nontraffic accident
+ **V19.1** Pedal cycle passenger injured in collision with other and unspecified motor vehicles in nontraffic accident
   X+7th **V19.10** Pedal cycle passenger injured in collision with unspecified motor vehicles in nontraffic accident
   X+7th **V19.19** Pedal cycle passenger injured in collision with other motor vehicles in nontraffic accident

- **+ V19.2** Unspecified pedal cyclist injured in collision with other and unspecified motor vehicles in nontraffic accident
  - **X+7th V19.20** Unspecified pedal cyclist injured in collision with unspecified motor vehicles in nontraffic accident
      Pedal cycle collision NOS, nontraffic
  - **X+7th V19.29** Unspecified pedal cyclist injured in collision with other motor vehicles in nontraffic accident
- **X+7th V19.3** Pedal cyclist (driver) (passenger) injured in unspecified nontraffic accident
    Pedal cycle accident NOS, nontraffic
    Pedal cyclist injured in nontraffic accident NOS
- **+ V19.4** Pedal cycle driver injured in collision with other and unspecified motor vehicles in traffic accident
  - **X+7th V19.40** Pedal cycle driver injured in collision with unspecified motor vehicles in traffic accident
  - **X+7th V19.49** Pedal cycle driver injured in collision with other motor vehicles in traffic accident
- **+ V19.5** Pedal cycle passenger injured in collision with other and unspecified motor vehicles in traffic accident
  - **X+7th V19.50** Pedal cycle passenger injured in collision with unspecified motor vehicles in traffic accident
  - **X+7th V19.59** Pedal cycle passenger injured in collision with other motor vehicles in traffic accident
- **+ V19.6** Unspecified pedal cyclist injured in collision with other and unspecified motor vehicles in traffic accident
  - **X+7th V19.60** Unspecified pedal cyclist injured in collision with unspecified motor vehicles in traffic accident
      Pedal cycle collision NOS (traffic)
  - **X+7th V19.69** Unspecified pedal cyclist injured in collision with other motor vehicles in traffic accident
- **+ V19.8** Pedal cyclist (driver) (passenger) injured in other specified transport accidents
  - **X+7th V19.81** Pedal cyclist (driver) (passenger) injured in transport accident with military vehicle
  - **X+7th V19.88** Pedal cyclist (driver) (passenger) injured in other specified transport accidents
- **X+7th V19.9** Pedal cyclist (driver) (passenger) injured in unspecified traffic accident
    Pedal cycle accident NOS

Motorcycle rider injured in transport accident (V20-V29)

Includes: electric bike
e-bike
e-bicycle
moped
motorcycle with sidecar
motorized bicycle
motor scooter

Excludes1: three-wheeled motor vehicle (V30-V39)
AHA CC: 4Q, 2022, 47

V20 Motorcycle rider injured in collision with pedestrian or animal

Excludes1: motorcycle rider collision with animal-drawn vehicle or animal being ridden (V26.-)

> The appropriate 7th character is to be added to each code from category V20
> A   initial encounter
> D   subsequent encounter
> S   sequela

- **+ V20.0** Motorcycle driver injured in collision with pedestrian or animal in nontraffic accident
  - **X+7th V20.01** Electric (assisted) bicycle driver injured in collision with pedestrian or animal in nontraffic accident
  - **X+7th V20.09** Other motorcycle driver injured in collision with pedestrian or animal in nontraffic accident
- **+ V20.1** Motorcycle passenger injured in collision with pedestrian or animal in nontraffic accident
  - **X+7th V20.11** Electric (assisted) bicycle passenger injured in collision with pedestrian or animal in nontraffic accident
  - **X+7th V20.19** Other motorcycle passenger injured in collision with pedestrian or animal in nontraffic accident
- **+ V20.2** Unspecified motorcycle rider injured in collision with pedestrian or animal in nontraffic accident
  - **X+7th V20.21** Unspecified electric (assisted) bicycle rider injured in collision with pedestrian or animal in nontraffic accident
  - **X+7th V20.29** Unspecified rider of other motorcycle injured in collision with pedestrian or animal in nontraffic accident
- **+ V20.3** Person boarding or alighting a motorcycle injured in collision with pedestrian or animal
  - **X+7th V20.31** Person boarding or alighting an electric (assisted) bicycle injured in collision with pedestrian or animal
  - **X+7th V20.39** Person boarding or alighting other motorcycle injured in collision with pedestrian or animal
- **+ V20.4** Motorcycle driver injured in collision with pedestrian or animal in traffic accident
  - **X+7th V20.41** Electric (assisted) bicycle driver injured in collision with pedestrian or animal in traffic accident
  - **X+7th V20.49** Other motorcycle driver injured in collision with pedestrian or animal in traffic accident
- **+ V20.5** Motorcycle passenger injured in collision with pedestrian or animal in traffic accident
  - **X+7th V20.51** Electric (assisted) bicycle passenger injured in collision with pedestrian or animal in traffic accident
  - **X+7th V20.59** Other motorcycle passenger injured in collision with pedestrian or animal in traffic accident
- **+ V20.9** Unspecified motorcycle rider injured in collision with pedestrian or animal in traffic accident
  - **X+7th V20.91** Unspecified electric (assisted) bicycle rider injured in collision with pedestrian or animal in traffic accident
  - **X+7th V20.99** Unspecified rider of other motorcycle injured in collision with pedestrian or animal in traffic accident

V21 Motorcycle rider injured in collision with pedal cycle

> The appropriate 7th character is to be added to each code from category V21
> A   initial encounter
> D   subsequent encounter
> S   sequela

- **+ V21.0** Motorcycle driver injured in collision with pedal cycle in nontraffic accident
  - **X+7th V21.01** Electric (assisted) bicycle driver injured in collision with pedal cycle in nontraffic accident
  - **X+7th V21.09** Other motorcycle driver injured in collision with pedal cycle in nontraffic accident
- **+ V21.1** Motorcycle passenger injured in collision with pedal cycle in nontraffic accident
  - **X+7th V21.11** Electric (assisted) bicycle passenger injured in collision with pedal cycle in nontraffic accident
  - **X+7th V21.19** Other motorcycle passenger injured in collision with pedal cycle in nontraffic accident
- **+ V21.2** Unspecified motorcycle rider injured in collision with pedal cycle in nontraffic accident
  - **X+7th V21.21** Unspecified electric (assisted) bicycle rider injured in collision with pedal cycle in nontraffic accident
  - **X+7th V21.29** Unspecified rider of other motorcycle injured in collision with pedal cycle in nontraffic accident
- **+ V21.3** Person boarding or alighting a motorcycle injured in collision with pedal cycle
  - **X+7th V21.31** Person boarding or alighting an electric (assisted) bicycle injured in collision with pedal cycle
  - **X+7th V21.39** Person boarding or alighting other motorcycle injured in collision with pedal cycle
- **+ V21.4** Motorcycle driver injured in collision with pedal cycle in traffic accident
  - **X+7th V21.41** Electric (assisted) bicycle driver injured in collision with pedal cycle in traffic accident
  - **X+7th V21.49** Other motorcycle driver injured in collision with pedal cycle in traffic accident
- **+ V21.5** Motorcycle passenger injured in collision with pedal cycle in traffic accident
  - **X+7th V21.51** Electric (assisted) bicycle passenger injured in collision with pedal cycle in traffic accident
  - **X+7th V21.59** Other motorcycle passenger injured in collision with pedal cycle in traffic accident
- **+ V21.9** Unspecified motorcycle rider injured in collision with pedal cycle in traffic accident
  - **X+7th V21.91** Unspecified electric (assisted) bicycle rider injured in collision with pedal cycle in traffic accident
  - **X+7th V21.99** Unspecified rider of other motorcycle injured in collision with pedal cycle in traffic accident

V22 Motorcycle rider injured in collision with two- or three-wheeled motor vehicle

> The appropriate 7th character is to be added to each code from category V22
> A initial encounter
> D subsequent encounter
> S sequela

- **V22.0 Motorcycle driver injured in collision with two- or three-wheeled motor vehicle in nontraffic accident**
  - X+7th V22.01 Electric (assisted) bicycle driver injured in collision with two- or three-wheeled motor vehicle in nontraffic accident
  - X+7th V22.09 Other motorcycle driver injured in collision with two- or three-wheeled motor vehicle in nontraffic accident
- **V22.1 Motorcycle passenger injured in collision with two- or three-wheeled motor vehicle in nontraffic accident**
  - X+7th V22.11 Electric (assisted) bicycle passenger injured in collision with two- or three-wheeled motor vehicle in nontraffic accident
  - X+7th V22.19 Other motorcycle passenger injured in collision with two- or three-wheeled motor vehicle in nontraffic accident
- **V22.2 Unspecified motorcycle rider injured in collision with two- or three-wheeled motor vehicle in nontraffic accident**
  - X+7th V22.21 Unspecified electric (assisted) bicycle rider injured in collision with two- or three-wheeled motor vehicle in nontraffic accident
  - X+7th V22.29 Unspecified rider of other motorcycle injured in collision with two- or three-wheeled motor vehicle in nontraffic accident
- **V22.3 Person boarding or alighting a motorcycle injured in collision with two- or three-wheeled motor vehicle**
  - X+7th V22.31 Person boarding or alighting an electric (assisted) bicycle injured in collision with two- or three-wheeled motor vehicle
  - X+7th V22.39 Person boarding or alighting other motorcycle injured in collision with two- or three-wheeled motor vehicle
- **V22.4 Motorcycle driver injured in collision with two- or three-wheeled motor vehicle in traffic accident**
  - X+7th V22.41 Electric (assisted) bicycle driver injured in collision with two- or three-wheeled motor vehicle in traffic accident
  - X+7th V22.49 Other motorcycle driver injured in collision with two- or three-wheeled motor vehicle in traffic accident
- **V22.5 Motorcycle passenger injured in collision with two- or three-wheeled motor vehicle in traffic accident**
  - X+7th V22.51 Electric (assisted) bicycle passenger injured in collision with two- or three-wheeled motor vehicle in traffic accident
  - X+7th V22.59 Other motorcycle passenger injured in collision with two- or three-wheeled motor vehicle in traffic accident
- **V22.9 Unspecified motorcycle rider injured in collision with two- or three-wheeled motor vehicle in traffic accident**
  - X+7th V22.91 Unspecified electric (assisted) bicycle rider injured in collision with two- or three-wheeled motor vehicle in traffic accident
  - X+7th V22.99 Unspecified rider of other motorcycle injured in collision with two- or three-wheeled motor vehicle in traffic accident

V23 Motorcycle rider injured in collision with car, pick-up truck or van

> The appropriate 7th character is to be added to each code from category V23
> A initial encounter
> D subsequent encounter
> S sequela

- **V23.0 Motorcycle driver injured in collision with car, pick-up truck or van in nontraffic accident**
  - X+7th V23.01 Electric (assisted) bicycle driver injured in collision with car, pick-up truck or van in nontraffic accident
  - X+7th V23.09 Other motorcycle driver injured in collision with car, pick-up truck or van in nontraffic accident
- **V23.1 Motorcycle passenger injured in collision with car, pick-up truck or van in nontraffic accident**
  - X+7th V23.11 Electric (assisted) bicycle passenger injured in collision with car, pick-up truck or van in nontraffic accident
  - X+7th V23.19 Other motorcycle passenger injured in collision with car, pick-up truck or van in nontraffic accident
- **V23.2 Unspecified motorcycle rider injured in collision with car, pick-up truck or van in nontraffic accident**
  - X+7th V23.21 Unspecified electric (assisted) bicycle rider injured in collision with car, pick-up truck or van in nontraffic accident
  - X+7th V23.29 Unspecified rider of other motorcycle injured in collision with car, pick-up truck or van in nontraffic accident
- **V23.3 Person boarding or alighting a motorcycle injured in collision with car, pick-up truck or van**
  - X+7th V23.31 Person boarding or alighting an electric (assisted) bicycle injured in collision with car, pick-up truck or van
  - X+7th V23.39 Person boarding or alighting other motorcycle injured in collision with car, pick-up truck or van
- **V23.4 Motorcycle driver injured in collision with car, pick-up truck or van in traffic accident**
  - X+7th V23.41 Electric (assisted) bicycle driver injured in collision with car, pick-up truck or van in traffic accident
  - X+7th V23.49 Other motorcycle driver injured in collision with car, pick-up truck or van in traffic accident
- **V23.5 Motorcycle passenger injured in collision with car, pick-up truck or van in traffic accident**
  - X+7th V23.51 Electric (assisted) bicycle passenger injured in collision with car, pick-up truck or van in traffic accident
  - X+7th V23.59 Other motorcycle passenger injured in collision with car, pick-up truck or van in traffic accident
- **V23.9 Unspecified motorcycle rider injured in collision with car, pick-up truck or van in traffic accident**
  - X+7th V23.91 Unspecified electric (assisted) bicycle rider injured in collision with car, pick-up truck or van in traffic accident
  - X+7th V23.99 Unspecified rider of other motorcycle injured in collision with car, pick-up truck or van in traffic accident

V24 Motorcycle rider injured in collision with heavy transport vehicle or bus

> **Excludes1:** *motorcycle rider injured in collision with military vehicle (V29.818)*

> The appropriate 7th character is to be added to each code from category V24
> A initial encounter
> D subsequent encounter
> S sequela

- **V24.0 Motorcycle driver injured in collision with heavy transport vehicle or bus in nontraffic accident**
  - X+7th V24.01 Electric (assisted) bicycle driver injured in collision with heavy transport vehicle or bus in nontraffic accident
  - X+7th V24.09 Other motorcycle driver injured in collision with heavy transport vehicle or bus in nontraffic accident
- **V24.1 Motorcycle passenger injured in collision with heavy transport vehicle or bus in nontraffic accident**
  - X+7th V24.11 Electric (assisted) bicycle passenger injured in collision with heavy transport vehicle or bus in nontraffic accident
  - X+7th V24.19 Other motorcycle passenger injured in collision with heavy transport vehicle or bus in nontraffic accident
- **V24.2 Unspecified motorcycle rider injured in collision with heavy transport vehicle or bus in nontraffic accident**
  - X+7th V24.21 Unspecified electric (assisted) bicycle rider injured in collision with heavy transport vehicle or bus in nontraffic accident
  - X+7th V24.29 Unspecified rider of other motorcycle injured in collision with heavy transport vehicle or bus in nontraffic accident

- + **V24.3** Person boarding or alighting a motorcycle injured in collision with heavy transport vehicle or bus
  - X+7th **V24.31** Person boarding or alighting an electric (assisted) bicycle injured in collision with heavy transport vehicle or bus
  - X+7th **V24.39** Person boarding or alighting other motorcycle injured in collision with heavy transport vehicle or bus
- + **V24.4** Motorcycle driver injured in collision with heavy transport vehicle or bus in traffic accident
  - X+7th **V24.41** Electric (assisted) bicycle driver injured in collision with heavy transport vehicle or bus in traffic accident
  - X+7th **V24.49** Other motorcycle driver injured in collision with heavy transport vehicle or bus in traffic accident
- + **V24.5** Motorcycle passenger injured in collision with heavy transport vehicle or bus in traffic accident
  - X+7th **V24.51** Electric (assisted) bicycle passenger injured in collision with heavy transport vehicle or bus in traffic accident
  - X+7th **V24.59** Other motorcycle passenger injured in collision with heavy transport vehicle or bus in traffic accident
- + **V24.9** Unspecified motorcycle rider injured in collision with heavy transport vehicle or bus in traffic accident
  - X+7th **V24.91** Unspecified electric (assisted) bicycle rider injured in collision with heavy transport vehicle or bus in traffic accident
  - X+7th **V24.99** Unspecified rider of other motorcycle injured in collision with heavy transport vehicle or bus in traffic accident

V25 Motorcycle rider injured in collision with railway train or railway vehicle

> The appropriate 7th character is to be added to each code from category V25
> A initial encounter
> D subsequent encounter
> S sequela

- + **V25.0** Motorcycle driver injured in collision with railway train or railway vehicle in nontraffic accident
  - X+7th **V25.01** Electric (assisted) bicycle driver injured in collision with railway train or railway vehicle in nontraffic accident
  - X+7th **V25.09** Other motorcycle driver injured in collision with railway train or railway vehicle in nontraffic accident
- + **V25.1** Motorcycle passenger injured in collision with railway train or railway vehicle in nontraffic accident
  - X+7th **V25.11** Electric (assisted) bicycle passenger injured in collision with railway train or railway vehicle in nontraffic accident
  - X+7th **V25.19** Other motorcycle passenger injured in collision with railway train or railway vehicle in nontraffic accident
- + **V25.2** Unspecified motorcycle rider injured in collision with railway train or railway vehicle in nontraffic accident
  - X+7th **V25.21** Unspecified electric (assisted) bicycle rider injured in collision with railway train or railway vehicle in nontraffic accident
  - X+7th **V25.29** Unspecified rider of other motorcycle injured in collision with railway train or railway vehicle in nontraffic accident
- + **V25.3** Person boarding or alighting a motorcycle injured in collision with railway train or railway vehicle
  - X+7th **V25.31** Person boarding or alighting an electric (assisted) bicycle injured in collision with railway train or railway vehicle
  - X+7th **V25.39** Person boarding or alighting other motorcycle injured in collision with railway train or railway vehicle
- + **V25.4** Motorcycle driver injured in collision with railway train or railway vehicle in traffic accident
  - X+7th **V25.41** Electric (assisted) bicycle driver injured in collision with railway train or railway vehicle in traffic accident
  - X+7th **V25.49** Other motorcycle driver injured in collision with railway train or railway vehicle in traffic accident
- + **V25.5** Motorcycle passenger injured in collision with railway train or railway vehicle in traffic accident
  - X+7th **V25.51** Electric (assisted) bicycle passenger injured in collision with railway train or railway vehicle in traffic accident
  - X+7th **V25.59** Other motorcycle passenger injured in collision with railway train or railway vehicle in traffic accident
- + **V25.9** Unspecified motorcycle rider injured in collision with railway train or railway vehicle in traffic accident
  - X+7th **V25.91** Unspecified electric (assisted) bicycle rider injured in collision with railway train or railway vehicle in traffic accident
  - X+7th **V25.99** Unspecified rider of other motorcycle injured in collision with railway train or railway vehicle in traffic accident

V26 Motorcycle rider injured in collision with other nonmotor vehicle

Includes: collision with animal-drawn vehicle, animal being ridden, streetcar

> The appropriate 7th character is to be added to each code from category V26
> A initial encounter
> D subsequent encounter
> S sequela

- + **V26.0** Motorcycle driver injured in collision with other nonmotor vehicle in nontraffic accident
  - X+7th **V26.01** Electric (assisted) bicycle driver injured in collision with other nonmotor vehicle in nontraffic accident
  - X+7th **V26.09** Other motorcycle driver injured in collision with other nonmotor vehicle in nontraffic accident
- + **V26.1** Motorcycle passenger injured in collision with other nonmotor vehicle in nontraffic accident
  - X+7th **V26.11** Electric (assisted) bicycle passenger injured in collision with other nonmotor vehicle in nontraffic accident
  - X+7th **V26.19** Other motorcycle passenger injured in collision with other nonmotor vehicle in nontraffic accident
- + **V26.2** Unspecified motorcycle rider injured in collision with other nonmotor vehicle in nontraffic accident
  - X+7th **V26.21** Unspecified electric (assisted) bicycle rider injured in collision with other nonmotor vehicle in nontraffic accident
  - X+7th **V26.29** Unspecified rider of other motorcycle injured in collision with other nonmotor vehicle in nontraffic accident
- + **V26.3** Person boarding or alighting a motorcycle injured in collision with other nonmotor vehicle
  - X+7th **V26.31** Person boarding or alighting an electric (assisted) bicycle injured in collision with other nonmotor vehicle
  - X+7th **V26.39** Person boarding or alighting other motorcycle injured in collision with other nonmotor vehicle
- + **V26.4** Motorcycle driver injured in collision with other nonmotor vehicle in traffic accident
  - X+7th **V26.41** Electric (assisted) bicycle driver injured in collision with other nonmotor vehicle in traffic accident
  - X+7th **V26.49** Other motorcycle driver injured in collision with other nonmotor vehicle in traffic accident
- + **V26.5** Motorcycle passenger injured in collision with other nonmotor vehicle in traffic accident
  - X+7th **V26.51** Electric (assisted) bicycle passenger injured in collision with other nonmotor vehicle in traffic accident
  - X+7th **V26.59** Other motorcycle passenger injured in collision with other nonmotor vehicle in traffic accident
- + **V26.9** Unspecified motorcycle rider injured in collision with other nonmotor vehicle in traffic accident
  - X+7th **V26.91** Unspecified electric (assisted) bicycle rider injured in collision with other nonmotor vehicle in traffic accident
  - X+7th **V26.99** Unspecified rider of other motorcycle injured in collision with other nonmotor vehicle in traffic accident

V27 Motorcycle rider injured in collision with fixed or stationary object

The appropriate 7th character is to be added to each code from category V27
- A initial encounter
- D subsequent encounter
- S sequela

+ **V27.0** Motorcycle driver injured in collision with fixed or stationary object in nontraffic accident
  - X+7th **V27.01** Electric (assisted) bicycle driver injured in collision with fixed or stationary object in nontraffic accident
  - X+7th **V27.09** Other motorcycle driver injured in collision with fixed or stationary object in nontraffic accident

+ **V27.1** Motorcycle passenger injured in collision with fixed or stationary object in nontraffic accident
  - X+7th **V27.11** Electric (assisted) bicycle passenger injured in collision with fixed or stationary object in nontraffic accident
  - X+7th **V27.19** Other motorcycle passenger injured in collision with fixed or stationary object in nontraffic accident

+ **V27.2** Unspecified motorcycle rider injured in collision with fixed or stationary object in nontraffic accident
  - X+7th **V27.21** Unspecified electric (assisted) bicycle rider injured in collision with fixed or stationary object in nontraffic accident
  - X+7th **V27.29** Unspecified rider of other motorcycle injured in collision with fixed or stationary object in nontraffic accident

+ **V27.3** Person boarding or alighting a motorcycle injured in collision with fixed or stationary object
  - X+7th **V27.31** Person boarding or alighting an electric (assisted) bicycle injured in collision with fixed or stationary object
  - X+7th **V27.39** Person boarding or alighting other motorcycle injured in collision with fixed or stationary object

+ **V27.4** Motorcycle driver injured in collision with fixed or stationary object in traffic accident
  - X+7th **V27.41** Electric (assisted) bicycle driver injured in collision with fixed or stationary object in traffic accident
  - X+7th **V27.49** Other motorcycle driver injured in collision with fixed or stationary object in traffic accident

+ **V27.5** Motorcycle passenger injured in collision with fixed or stationary object in traffic accident
  - X+7th **V27.51** Electric (assisted) bicycle passenger injured in collision with fixed or stationary object in traffic accident
  - X+7th **V27.59** Other motorcycle passenger injured in collision with fixed or stationary object in traffic accident

+ **V27.9** Unspecified motorcycle rider injured in collision with fixed or stationary object in traffic accident
  - X+7th **V27.91** Unspecified electric (assisted) bicycle rider injured in collision with fixed or stationary object in traffic accident
  - X+7th **V27.99** Unspecified rider of other motorcycle injured in collision with fixed or stationary object in traffic accident

V28 Motorcycle rider injured in noncollision transport accident

Includes: fall or thrown from motorcycle (without antecedent collision)
overturning motorcycle NOS
overturning motorcycle without collision

The appropriate 7th character is to be added to each code from category V28
- A initial encounter
- D subsequent encounter
- S sequela

+ **V28.0** Motorcycle driver injured in noncollision transport accident in nontraffic accident
  - X+7th **V28.01** Electric (assisted) bicycle driver injured in noncollision transport accident in nontraffic accident
  - X+7th **V28.09** Other motorcycle driver injured in noncollision transport accident in nontraffic accident

+ **V28.1** Motorcycle passenger injured in noncollision transport accident in nontraffic accident
  - X+7th **V28.11** Electric (assisted) bicycle passenger injured in noncollision transport accident in nontraffic accident
  - X+7th **V28.19** Other motorcycle passenger injured in noncollision transport accident in nontraffic accident

+ **V28.2** Unspecified motorcycle rider injured in noncollision transport accident in nontraffic accident
  - X+7th **V28.21** Unspecified electric (assisted) bicycle rider injured in noncollision transport accident in nontraffic accident
  - X+7th **V28.29** Unspecified rider of other motorcycle injured in noncollision transport accident in nontraffic accident

+ **V28.3** Person boarding or alighting a motorcycle injured in noncollision transport accident
  - X+7th **V28.31** Person boarding or alighting an electric (assisted) bicycle injured in noncollision transport accident
  - X+7th **V28.39** Person boarding or alighting other motorcycle injured in noncollision transport accident

+ **V28.4** Motorcycle driver injured in noncollision transport accident in traffic accident
  - X+7th **V28.41** Electric (assisted) bicycle driver injured in noncollision transport accident in traffic accident
  - X+7th **V28.49** Other motorcycle driver injured in noncollision transport accident in traffic accident

+ **V28.5** Motorcycle passenger injured in noncollision transport accident in traffic accident
  - X+7th **V28.51** Electric (assisted) bicycle passenger injured in noncollision transport accident in traffic accident
  - X+7th **V28.59** Other motorcycle passenger injured in noncollision transport accident in traffic accident

+ **V28.9** Unspecified motorcycle rider injured in noncollision transport accident in traffic accident
  - X+7th **V28.91** Unspecified electric (assisted) bicycle rider injured in noncollision transport accident in traffic accident
  - X+7th **V28.99** Unspecified rider of other motorcycle injured in noncollision transport accident in traffic accident

V29 Motorcycle rider injured in other and unspecified transport accidents

The appropriate 7th character is to be added to each code from category V29
- A initial encounter
- D subsequent encounter
- S sequela

+ **V29.0** Motorcycle driver injured in collision with other and unspecified motor vehicles in nontraffic accident
  + **V29.00** Motorcycle driver injured in collision with unspecified motor vehicles in nontraffic accident
    - +7th **V29.001** Electric (assisted) bicycle driver injured in collision with unspecified motor vehicles in nontraffic accident
    - +7th **V29.008** Other motorcycle driver injured in collision with unspecified motor vehicles in nontraffic accident
  + **V29.09** Motorcycle driver injured in collision with other motor vehicles in nontraffic accident
    - +7th **V29.091** Electric (assisted) bicycle driver injured in collision with other motor vehicles in nontraffic accident
    - +7th **V29.098** Other motorcycle driver injured in collision with other motor vehicles in nontraffic accident

+ **V29.1** Motorcycle passenger injured in collision with other and unspecified motor vehicles in nontraffic accident
  + **V29.10** Motorcycle passenger injured in collision with unspecified motor vehicles in nontraffic accident
    - +7th **V29.101** Electric (assisted) bicycle passenger injured in collision with unspecified motor vehicles in nontraffic accident
    - +7th **V29.108** Other motorcycle passenger injured in collision with unspecified motor vehicles in nontraffic accident

- **V29.19** Motorcycle passenger injured in collision with other motor vehicles in nontraffic accident
  - +7th **V29.191** Electric (assisted) bicycle passenger injured in collision with other motor vehicles in nontraffic accident
  - +7th **V29.198** Other motorcycle passenger injured in collision with other motor vehicles in nontraffic accident
- **V29.2** Unspecified motorcycle rider injured in collision with other and unspecified motor vehicles in nontraffic accident
  - **V29.20** Unspecified motorcycle rider injured in collision with unspecified motor vehicles in nontraffic accident
    - +7th **V29.201** Unspecified electric (assisted) bicycle rider injured in collision with unspecified motor vehicles in nontraffic accident
    - +7th **V29.208** Unspecified rider of other motorcycle injured in collision with unspecified motor vehicles in nontraffic accident
       Motorcycle collision NOS, nontraffic
  - **V29.29** Unspecified motorcycle rider injured in collision with other motor vehicles in nontraffic accident
    - +7th **V29.291** Unspecified electric (assisted) bicycle rider injured in collision with other motor vehicles in nontraffic accident
    - +7th **V29.298** Unspecified rider of other motorcycle injured in collision with other motor vehicles in nontraffic accident
- **V29.3** Motorcycle rider (driver) (passenger) injured in unspecified nontraffic accident
  - X+7th **V29.31** Electric (assisted) bicycle (driver) (passenger) injured in unspecified nontraffic accident
  - X+7th **V29.39** Other motorcycle (driver) (passenger) injured in unspecified nontraffic accident
     Motorcycle accident NOS, nontraffic
     Motorcycle rider injured in nontraffic accident NOS
- **V29.4** Motorcycle driver injured in collision with other and unspecified motor vehicles in traffic accident
  - **V29.40** Motorcycle driver injured in collision with unspecified motor vehicles in traffic accident
    - +7th **V29.401** Electric (assisted) bicycle driver injured in collision with unspecified motor vehicles in traffic accident
    - +7th **V29.408** Other motorcycle driver injured in collision with unspecified motor vehicles in traffic accident
  - **V29.49** Motorcycle driver injured in collision with other motor vehicles in traffic accident
    - +7th **V29.491** Electric (assisted) bicycle driver injured in collision with other motor vehicles in traffic accident
    - +7th **V29.498** Other motorcycle driver injured in collision with other motor vehicles in traffic accident
- **V29.5** Motorcycle passenger injured in collision with other and unspecified motor vehicles in traffic accident
  - **V29.50** Motorcycle passenger injured in collision with unspecified motor vehicles in traffic accident
    - +7th **V29.501** Electric (assisted) bicycle passenger injured in collision with unspecified motor vehicles in traffic accident
    - +7th **V29.508** Other motorcycle passenger injured in collision with unspecified motor vehicles in traffic accident
  - **V29.59** Motorcycle passenger injured in collision with other motor vehicles in traffic accident
    - +7th **V29.591** Electric (assisted) bicycle passenger injured in collision with other motor vehicles in traffic accident
    - +7th **V29.598** Other motorcycle passenger injured in collision with other motor vehicles in traffic accident
- **V29.6** Unspecified motorcycle rider injured in collision with other and unspecified motor vehicles in traffic accident
  - **V29.60** Unspecified motorcycle rider injured in collision with unspecified motor vehicles in traffic accident
    - +7th **V29.601** Unspecified electric (assisted) bicycle rider injured in collision with unspecified motor vehicles in traffic accident
    - +7th **V29.608** Unspecified rider of other motorcycle injured in collision with unspecified motor vehicles in traffic accident
       Motorcycle collision NOS (traffic)
  - **V29.69** Unspecified motorcycle rider injured in collision with other motor vehicles in traffic accident
    - +7th **V29.691** Unspecified electric (assisted) bicycle rider injured in collision with other motor vehicles in traffic accident
    - +7th **V29.698** Unspecified rider of other motorcycle injured in collision with other motor vehicles in traffic accident
- **V29.8** Motorcycle rider (driver) (passenger) injured in other specified transport accidents
  - **V29.81** Motorcycle rider (driver) (passenger) injured in transport accident with military vehicle
    - +7th **V29.811** Electric (assisted) bicycle rider (driver) (passenger) injured in transport accident with military vehicle
    - +7th **V29.818** Rider (driver) (passenger) of other motorcycle injured in transport accident with military vehicle
  - **V29.88** Motorcycle rider (driver) (passenger) injured in other specified transport accidents
    - +7th **V29.881** Electric (assisted) bicycle rider (driver) (passenger) injured in other specified transport accidents
    - +7th **V29.888** Rider (driver) (passenger) of other motorcycle injured in other specified transport accidents
- **V29.9** Motorcycle rider (driver) (passenger) injured in unspecified traffic accident
  - X+7th **V29.91** Electric (assisted) bicycle rider (driver) (passenger) injured in unspecified traffic accident
  - X+7th **V29.99** Rider (driver) (passenger) of other motorcycle injured in unspecified traffic accident
     Motorcycle accident NOS

Occupant of three-wheeled motor vehicle injured in transport accident (V30-V39)

Includes: motorized tricycle
motorized rickshaw
three-wheeled motor car

Excludes1: all-terrain vehicles (V86.-)
motorcycle with sidecar (V20-V29)
vehicle designed primarily for off-road use (V86.-)

V30 Occupant of three-wheeled motor vehicle injured in collision with pedestrian or animal

Excludes1: three-wheeled motor vehicle collision with animal-drawn vehicle or animal being ridden (V36.-)

The appropriate 7th character is to be added to each code from category V30
A   initial encounter
D   subsequent encounter
S   sequela

- X+7th **V30.0** Driver of three-wheeled motor vehicle injured in collision with pedestrian or animal in nontraffic accident
- X+7th **V30.1** Passenger in three-wheeled motor vehicle injured in collision with pedestrian or animal in nontraffic accident
- X+7th **V30.2** Person on outside of three-wheeled motor vehicle injured in collision with pedestrian or animal in nontraffic accident
- X+7th **V30.3** Unspecified occupant of three-wheeled motor vehicle injured in collision with pedestrian or animal in nontraffic accident
- X+7th **V30.4** Person boarding or alighting a three-wheeled motor vehicle injured in collision with pedestrian or animal
- X+7th **V30.5** Driver of three-wheeled motor vehicle injured in collision with pedestrian or animal in traffic accident
- X+7th **V30.6** Passenger in three-wheeled motor vehicle injured in collision with pedestrian or animal in traffic accident
- X+7th **V30.7** Person on outside of three-wheeled motor vehicle injured in collision with pedestrian or animal in traffic accident
- X+7th **V30.9** Unspecified occupant of three-wheeled motor vehicle injured in collision with pedestrian or animal in traffic accident

V31 Occupant of three-wheeled motor vehicle injured in collision with pedal cycle

> The appropriate 7th character is to be added to each code from category V31
> A initial encounter
> D subsequent encounter
> S sequela

X+7th **V31.0** Driver of three-wheeled motor vehicle injured in collision with pedal cycle in nontraffic accident
X+7th **V31.1** Passenger in three-wheeled motor vehicle injured in collision with pedal cycle in nontraffic accident
X+7th **V31.2** Person on outside of three-wheeled motor vehicle injured in collision with pedal cycle in nontraffic accident
X+7th **V31.3** Unspecified occupant of three-wheeled motor vehicle injured in collision with pedal cycle in nontraffic accident
X+7th **V31.4** Person boarding or alighting a three-wheeled motor vehicle injured in collision with pedal cycle
X+7th **V31.5** Driver of three-wheeled motor vehicle injured in collision with pedal cycle in traffic accident
X+7th **V31.6** Passenger in three-wheeled motor vehicle injured in collision with pedal cycle in traffic accident
X+7th **V31.7** Person on outside of three-wheeled motor vehicle injured in collision with pedal cycle in traffic accident
X+7th **V31.9** Unspecified occupant of three-wheeled motor vehicle injured in collision with pedal cycle in traffic accident

V32 Occupant of three-wheeled motor vehicle injured in collision with two- or three-wheeled motor vehicle

> The appropriate 7th character is to be added to each code from category V32
> A initial encounter
> D subsequent encounter
> S sequela

X+7th **V32.0** Driver of three-wheeled motor vehicle injured in collision with two- or three-wheeled motor vehicle in nontraffic accident
X+7th **V32.1** Passenger in three-wheeled motor vehicle injured in collision with two- or three-wheeled motor vehicle in nontraffic accident
X+7th **V32.2** Person on outside of three-wheeled motor vehicle injured in collision with two- or three-wheeled motor vehicle in nontraffic accident
X+7th **V32.3** Unspecified occupant of three-wheeled motor vehicle injured in collision with two- or three-wheeled motor vehicle in nontraffic accident
X+7th **V32.4** Person boarding or alighting a three-wheeled motor vehicle injured in collision with two- or three-wheeled motor vehicle
X+7th **V32.5** Driver of three-wheeled motor vehicle injured in collision with two- or three-wheeled motor vehicle in traffic accident
X+7th **V32.6** Passenger in three-wheeled motor vehicle injured in collision with two- or three-wheeled motor vehicle in traffic accident
X+7th **V32.7** Person on outside of three-wheeled motor vehicle injured in collision with two- or three-wheeled motor vehicle in traffic accident
X+7th **V32.9** Unspecified occupant of three-wheeled motor vehicle injured in collision with two- or three-wheeled motor vehicle in traffic accident

V33 Occupant of three-wheeled motor vehicle injured in collision with car, pick-up truck or van

> The appropriate 7th character is to be added to each code from category V33
> A initial encounter
> D subsequent encounter
> S sequela

X+7th **V33.0** Driver of three-wheeled motor vehicle injured in collision with car, pick-up truck or van in nontraffic accident
X+7th **V33.1** Passenger in three-wheeled motor vehicle injured in collision with car, pick-up truck or van in nontraffic accident
X+7th **V33.2** Person on outside of three-wheeled motor vehicle injured in collision with car, pick-up truck or van in nontraffic accident
X+7th **V33.3** Unspecified occupant of three-wheeled motor vehicle injured in collision with car, pick-up truck or van in nontraffic accident
X+7th **V33.4** Person boarding or alighting a three-wheeled motor vehicle injured in collision with car, pick-up truck or van
X+7th **V33.5** Driver of three-wheeled motor vehicle injured in collision with car, pick-up truck or van in traffic accident
X+7th **V33.6** Passenger in three-wheeled motor vehicle injured in collision with car, pick-up truck or van in traffic accident
X+7th **V33.7** Person on outside of three-wheeled motor vehicle injured in collision with car, pick-up truck or van in traffic accident
X+7th **V33.9** Unspecified occupant of three-wheeled motor vehicle injured in collision with car, pick-up truck or van in traffic accident

V34 Occupant of three-wheeled motor vehicle injured in collision with heavy transport vehicle or bus

> **Excludes1:** occupant of three-wheeled motor vehicle injured in collision with military vehicle (V39.81)

> The appropriate 7th character is to be added to each code from category V34
> A initial encounter
> D subsequent encounter
> S sequela

X+7th **V34.0** Driver of three-wheeled motor vehicle injured in collision with heavy transport vehicle or bus in nontraffic accident
X+7th **V34.1** Passenger in three-wheeled motor vehicle injured in collision with heavy transport vehicle or bus in nontraffic accident
X+7th **V34.2** Person on outside of three-wheeled motor vehicle injured in collision with heavy transport vehicle or bus in nontraffic accident
X+7th **V34.3** Unspecified occupant of three-wheeled motor vehicle injured in collision with heavy transport vehicle or bus in nontraffic accident
X+7th **V34.4** Person boarding or alighting a three-wheeled motor vehicle injured in collision with heavy transport vehicle or bus
X+7th **V34.5** Driver of three-wheeled motor vehicle injured in collision with heavy transport vehicle or bus in traffic accident
X+7th **V34.6** Passenger in three-wheeled motor vehicle injured in collision with heavy transport vehicle or bus in traffic accident
X+7th **V34.7** Person on outside of three-wheeled motor vehicle injured in collision with heavy transport vehicle or bus in traffic accident
X+7th **V34.9** Unspecified occupant of three-wheeled motor vehicle injured in collision with heavy transport vehicle or bus in traffic accident

V35 Occupant of three-wheeled motor vehicle injured in collision with railway train or railway vehicle

> The appropriate 7th character is to be added to each code from category V35
> A initial encounter
> D subsequent encounter
> S sequela

X+7th **V35.0** Driver of three-wheeled motor vehicle injured in collision with railway train or railway vehicle in nontraffic accident
X+7th **V35.1** Passenger in three-wheeled motor vehicle injured in collision with railway train or railway vehicle in nontraffic accident
X+7th **V35.2** Person on outside of three-wheeled motor vehicle injured in collision with railway train or railway vehicle in nontraffic accident
X+7th **V35.3** Unspecified occupant of three-wheeled motor vehicle injured in collision with railway train or railway vehicle in nontraffic accident
X+7th **V35.4** Person boarding or alighting a three-wheeled motor vehicle injured in collision with railway train or railway vehicle
X+7th **V35.5** Driver of three-wheeled motor vehicle injured in collision with railway train or railway vehicle in traffic accident
X+7th **V35.6** Passenger in three-wheeled motor vehicle injured in collision with railway train or railway vehicle in traffic accident
X+7th **V35.7** Person on outside of three-wheeled motor vehicle injured in collision with railway train or railway vehicle in traffic accident
X+7th **V35.9** Unspecified occupant of three-wheeled motor vehicle injured in collision with railway train or railway vehicle in traffic accident

V36 Occupant of three-wheeled motor vehicle injured in collision with other nonmotor vehicle

> **Includes:** collision with animal-drawn vehicle, animal being ridden, streetcar

> The appropriate 7th character is to be added to each code from category V36
> A initial encounter
> D subsequent encounter
> S sequela

V36.0–V39.81

X+7th	V36.0	Driver of three-wheeled motor vehicle injured in collision with other nonmotor vehicle in nontraffic accident
X+7th	V36.1	Passenger in three-wheeled motor vehicle injured in collision with other nonmotor vehicle in nontraffic accident
X+7th	V36.2	Person on outside of three-wheeled motor vehicle injured in collision with other nonmotor vehicle in nontraffic accident
X+7th	V36.3	Unspecified occupant of three-wheeled motor vehicle injured in collision with other nonmotor vehicle in nontraffic accident
X+7th	V36.4	Person boarding or alighting a three-wheeled motor vehicle injured in collision with other nonmotor vehicle
X+7th	V36.5	Driver of three-wheeled motor vehicle injured in collision with other nonmotor vehicle in traffic accident
X+7th	V36.6	Passenger in three-wheeled motor vehicle injured in collision with other nonmotor vehicle in traffic accident
X+7th	V36.7	Person on outside of three-wheeled motor vehicle injured in collision with other nonmotor vehicle in traffic accident
X+7th	V36.9	Unspecified occupant of three-wheeled motor vehicle injured in collision with other nonmotor vehicle in traffic accident

V37 Occupant of three-wheeled motor vehicle injured in collision with fixed or stationary object

> The appropriate 7th character is to be added to each code from category V37
> A   initial encounter
> D   subsequent encounter
> S   sequela

X+7th	V37.0	Driver of three-wheeled motor vehicle injured in collision with fixed or stationary object in nontraffic accident
X+7th	V37.1	Passenger in three-wheeled motor vehicle injured in collision with fixed or stationary object in nontraffic accident
X+7th	V37.2	Person on outside of three-wheeled motor vehicle injured in collision with fixed or stationary object in nontraffic accident
X+7th	V37.3	Unspecified occupant of three-wheeled motor vehicle injured in collision with fixed or stationary object in nontraffic accident
X+7th	V37.4	Person boarding or alighting a three-wheeled motor vehicle injured in collision with fixed or stationary object
X+7th	V37.5	Driver of three-wheeled motor vehicle injured in collision with fixed or stationary object in traffic accident
X+7th	V37.6	Passenger in three-wheeled motor vehicle injured in collision with fixed or stationary object in traffic accident
X+7th	V37.7	Person on outside of three-wheeled motor vehicle injured in collision with fixed or stationary object in traffic accident
X+7th	V37.9	Unspecified occupant of three-wheeled motor vehicle injured in collision with fixed or stationary object in traffic accident

V38 Occupant of three-wheeled motor vehicle injured in noncollision transport accident

> **Includes:** fall or thrown from three-wheeled motor vehicle
> overturning of three-wheeled motor vehicle NOS
> overturning of three-wheeled motor vehicle without collision

> The appropriate 7th character is to be added to each code from category V38
> A   initial encounter
> D   subsequent encounter
> S   sequela

X+7th	V38.0	Driver of three-wheeled motor vehicle injured in noncollision transport accident in nontraffic accident
X+7th	V38.1	Passenger in three-wheeled motor vehicle injured in noncollision transport accident in nontraffic accident
X+7th	V38.2	Person on outside of three-wheeled motor vehicle injured in noncollision transport accident in nontraffic accident
X+7th	V38.3	Unspecified occupant of three-wheeled motor vehicle injured in noncollision transport accident in nontraffic accident
X+7th	V38.4	Person boarding or alighting a three-wheeled motor vehicle injured in noncollision transport accident
X+7th	V38.5	Driver of three-wheeled motor vehicle injured in noncollision transport accident in traffic accident
X+7th	V38.6	Passenger in three-wheeled motor vehicle injured in noncollision transport accident in traffic accident
X+7th	V38.7	Person on outside of three-wheeled motor vehicle injured in noncollision transport accident in traffic accident
X+7th	V38.9	Unspecified occupant of three-wheeled motor vehicle injured in noncollision transport accident in traffic accident

V39 Occupant of three-wheeled motor vehicle injured in other and unspecified transport accidents

> The appropriate 7th character is to be added to each code from category V39
> A   initial encounter
> D   subsequent encounter
> S   sequela

+ **V39.0** Driver of three-wheeled motor vehicle injured in collision with other and unspecified motor vehicles in nontraffic accident

X+7th	V39.00	Driver of three-wheeled motor vehicle injured in collision with unspecified motor vehicles in nontraffic accident
X+7th	V39.09	Driver of three-wheeled motor vehicle injured in collision with other motor vehicles in nontraffic accident

+ **V39.1** Passenger in three-wheeled motor vehicle injured in collision with other and unspecified motor vehicles in nontraffic accident

X+7th	V39.10	Passenger in three-wheeled motor vehicle injured in collision with unspecified motor vehicles in nontraffic accident
X+7th	V39.19	Passenger in three-wheeled motor vehicle injured in collision with other motor vehicles in nontraffic accident

+ **V39.2** Unspecified occupant of three-wheeled motor vehicle injured in collision with other and unspecified motor vehicles in nontraffic accident

X+7th	V39.20	Unspecified occupant of three-wheeled motor vehicle injured in collision with unspecified motor vehicles in nontraffic accident
		Collision NOS involving three-wheeled motor vehicle, nontraffic
X+7th	V39.29	Unspecified occupant of three-wheeled motor vehicle injured in collision with other motor vehicles in nontraffic accident

X+7th **V39.3** Occupant (driver) (passenger) of three-wheeled motor vehicle injured in unspecified nontraffic accident
Accident NOS involving three-wheeled motor vehicle, nontraffic
Occupant of three-wheeled motor vehicle injured in nontraffic accident NOS

+ **V39.4** Driver of three-wheeled motor vehicle injured in collision with other and unspecified motor vehicles in traffic accident

X+7th	V39.40	Driver of three-wheeled motor vehicle injured in collision with unspecified motor vehicles in traffic accident
X+7th	V39.49	Driver of three-wheeled motor vehicle injured in collision with other motor vehicles in traffic accident

+ **V39.5** Passenger in three-wheeled motor vehicle injured in collision with other and unspecified motor vehicles in traffic accident

X+7th	V39.50	Passenger in three-wheeled motor vehicle injured in collision with unspecified motor vehicles in traffic accident
X+7th	V39.59	Passenger in three-wheeled motor vehicle injured in collision with other motor vehicles in traffic accident

+ **V39.6** Unspecified occupant of three-wheeled motor vehicle injured in collision with other and unspecified motor vehicles in traffic accident

X+7th	V39.60	Unspecified occupant of three-wheeled motor vehicle injured in collision with unspecified motor vehicles in traffic accident
		Collision NOS involving three-wheeled motor vehicle (traffic)
X+7th	V39.69	Unspecified occupant of three-wheeled motor vehicle injured in collision with other motor vehicles in traffic accident

+ **V39.8** Occupant (driver) (passenger) of three-wheeled motor vehicle injured in other specified transport accidents

X+7th	V39.81	Occupant (driver) (passenger) of three-wheeled motor vehicle injured in transport accident with military vehicle

X+7th V39.89 Occupant (driver) (passenger) of three-wheeled motor vehicle injured in other specified transport accidents

X+7th V39.9 Occupant (driver) (passenger) of three-wheeled motor vehicle injured in unspecified traffic accident
        Accident NOS involving three-wheeled motor vehicle

Car occupant injured in transport accident (V40-V49)

Includes: a four-wheeled motor vehicle designed primarily for carrying passengers
        automobile (pulling a trailer or camper)

Excludes1: bus (V50-V59)
        minibus (V50-V59)
        minivan (V50-V59)
        motorcoach (V70-V79)
        pick-up truck (V50-V59)
        sport utility vehicle (SUV) (V50-V59)

V40 Car occupant injured in collision with pedestrian or animal
    Excludes1: car collision with animal-drawn vehicle or animal being ridden (V46.-)

The appropriate 7th character is to be added to each code from category V40
A initial encounter
D subsequent encounter
S sequela

X+7th V40.0 Car driver injured in collision with pedestrian or animal in nontraffic accident
X+7th V40.1 Car passenger injured in collision with pedestrian or animal in nontraffic accident
X+7th V40.2 Person on outside of car injured in collision with pedestrian or animal in nontraffic accident
X+7th V40.3 Unspecified car occupant injured in collision with pedestrian or animal in nontraffic accident
X+7th V40.4 Person boarding or alighting a car injured in collision with pedestrian or animal
X+7th V40.5 Car driver injured in collision with pedestrian or animal in traffic accident
X+7th V40.6 Car passenger injured in collision with pedestrian or animal in traffic accident
X+7th V40.7 Person on outside of car injured in collision with pedestrian or animal in traffic accident
X+7th V40.9 Unspecified car occupant injured in collision with pedestrian or animal in traffic accident

V41 Car occupant injured in collision with pedal cycle

The appropriate 7th character is to be added to each code from category V41
A initial encounter
D subsequent encounter
S sequela

X+7th V41.0 Car driver injured in collision with pedal cycle in nontraffic accident
X+7th V41.1 Car passenger injured in collision with pedal cycle in nontraffic accident
X+7th V41.2 Person on outside of car injured in collision with pedal cycle in nontraffic accident
X+7th V41.3 Unspecified car occupant injured in collision with pedal cycle in nontraffic accident
X+7th V41.4 Person boarding or alighting a car injured in collision with pedal cycle
X+7th V41.5 Car driver injured in collision with pedal cycle in traffic accident
X+7th V41.6 Car passenger injured in collision with pedal cycle in traffic accident
X+7th V41.7 Person on outside of car injured in collision with pedal cycle in traffic accident
X+7th V41.9 Unspecified car occupant injured in collision with pedal cycle in traffic accident

V42 Car occupant injured in collision with two- or three-wheeled motor vehicle

The appropriate 7th character is to be added to each code from category V42
A initial encounter
D subsequent encounter
S sequela

X+7th V42.0 Car driver injured in collision with two- or three-wheeled motor vehicle in nontraffic accident
X+7th V42.1 Car passenger injured in collision with two- or three-wheeled motor vehicle in nontraffic accident
X+7th V42.2 Person on outside of car injured in collision with two- or three-wheeled motor vehicle in nontraffic accident
X+7th V42.3 Unspecified car occupant injured in collision with two- or three-wheeled motor vehicle in nontraffic accident
X+7th V42.4 Person boarding or alighting a car injured in collision with two- or three-wheeled motor vehicle
X+7th V42.5 Car driver injured in collision with two- or three-wheeled motor vehicle in traffic accident
X+7th V42.6 Car passenger injured in collision with two- or three-wheeled motor vehicle in traffic accident
X+7th V42.7 Person on outside of car injured in collision with two- or three-wheeled motor vehicle in traffic accident
X+7th V42.9 Unspecified car occupant injured in collision with two- or three-wheeled motor vehicle in traffic accident

V43 Car occupant injured in collision with car, pick-up truck or van

The appropriate 7th character is to be added to each code from category V43
A initial encounter
D subsequent encounter
S sequela

+ **V43.0** Car driver injured in collision with car, pick-up truck or van in nontraffic accident
    X+7th V43.01 Car driver injured in collision with sport utility vehicle in nontraffic accident
    X+7th V43.02 Car driver injured in collision with other type car in nontraffic accident
    X+7th V43.03 Car driver injured in collision with pick-up truck in nontraffic accident
    X+7th V43.04 Car driver injured in collision with van in nontraffic accident

+ **V43.1** Car passenger injured in collision with car, pick-up truck or van in nontraffic accident
    X+7th V43.11 Car passenger injured in collision with sport utility vehicle in nontraffic accident
    X+7th V43.12 Car passenger injured in collision with other type car in nontraffic accident
    X+7th V43.13 Car passenger injured in collision with pick-up truck in nontraffic accident
    X+7th V43.14 Car passenger injured in collision with van in nontraffic accident

+ **V43.2** Person on outside of car injured in collision with car, pick-up truck or van in nontraffic accident
    X+7th V43.21 Person on outside of car injured in collision with sport utility vehicle in nontraffic accident
    X+7th V43.22 Person on outside of car injured in collision with other type car in nontraffic accident
    X+7th V43.23 Person on outside of car injured in collision with pick-up truck in nontraffic accident
    X+7th V43.24 Person on outside of car injured in collision with van in nontraffic accident

+ **V43.3** Unspecified car occupant injured in collision with car, pick-up truck or van in nontraffic accident
    X+7th V43.31 Unspecified car occupant injured in collision with sport utility vehicle in nontraffic accident
    X+7th V43.32 Unspecified car occupant injured in collision with other type car in nontraffic accident
    X+7th V43.33 Unspecified car occupant injured in collision with pick-up truck in nontraffic accident
    X+7th V43.34 Unspecified car occupant injured in collision with van in nontraffic accident

+ **V43.4** Person boarding or alighting a car injured in collision with car, pick-up truck or van
    X+7th V43.41 Person boarding or alighting a car injured in collision with sport utility vehicle
    X+7th V43.42 Person boarding or alighting a car injured in collision with other type car

X+7th	V43.43	Person boarding or alighting a car injured in collision with pick-up truck
X+7th	V43.44	Person boarding or alighting a car injured in collision with van
+	V43.5	Car driver injured in collision with car, pick-up truck or van in traffic accident
X+7th	V43.51	Car driver injured in collision with sport utility vehicle in traffic accident
X+7th	V43.52	Car driver injured in collision with other type car in traffic accident
X+7th	V43.53	Car driver injured in collision with pick-up truck in traffic accident
X+7th	V43.54	Car driver injured in collision with van in traffic accident
+	V43.6	Car passenger injured in collision with car, pick-up truck or van in traffic accident
X+7th	V43.61	Car passenger injured in collision with sport utility vehicle in traffic accident
		AHA CC: 1Q, 2015, 3-21
X+7th	V43.62	Car passenger injured in collision with other type car in traffic accident
X+7th	V43.63	Car passenger injured in collision with pick-up truck in traffic accident
X+7th	V43.64	Car passenger injured in collision with van in traffic accident
+	V43.7	Person on outside of car injured in collision with car, pick-up truck or van in traffic accident
X+7th	V43.71	Person on outside of car injured in collision with sport utility vehicle in traffic accident
X+7th	V43.72	Person on outside of car injured in collision with other type car in traffic accident
X+7th	V43.73	Person on outside of car injured in collision with pick-up truck in traffic accident
X+7th	V43.74	Person on outside of car injured in collision with van in traffic accident
+	V43.9	Unspecified car occupant injured in collision with car, pick-up truck or van in traffic accident
X+7th	V43.91	Unspecified car occupant injured in collision with sport utility vehicle in traffic accident
X+7th	V43.92	Unspecified car occupant injured in collision with other type car in traffic accident
X+7th	V43.93	Unspecified car occupant injured in collision with pick-up truck in traffic accident
X+7th	V43.94	Unspecified car occupant injured in collision with van in traffic accident

V44 Car occupant injured in collision with heavy transport vehicle or bus

Excludes1: car occupant injured in collision with military vehicle (V49.81)

The appropriate 7th character is to be added to each code from category V44
- A initial encounter
- D subsequent encounter
- S sequela

X+7th	V44.0	Car driver injured in collision with heavy transport vehicle or bus in nontraffic accident
X+7th	V44.1	Car passenger injured in collision with heavy transport vehicle or bus in nontraffic accident
X+7th	V44.2	Person on outside of car injured in collision with heavy transport vehicle or bus in nontraffic accident
X+7th	V44.3	Unspecified car occupant injured in collision with heavy transport vehicle or bus in nontraffic accident
X+7th	V44.4	Person boarding or alighting a car injured in collision with heavy transport vehicle or bus
X+7th	V44.5	Car driver injured in collision with heavy transport vehicle or bus in traffic accident
X+7th	V44.6	Car passenger injured in collision with heavy transport vehicle or bus in traffic accident
X+7th	V44.7	Person on outside of car injured in collision with heavy transport vehicle or bus in traffic accident
X+7th	V44.9	Unspecified car occupant injured in collision with heavy transport vehicle or bus in traffic accident

V45 Car occupant injured in collision with railway train or railway vehicle

The appropriate 7th character is to be added to each code from category V45
- A initial encounter
- D subsequent encounter
- S sequela

X+7th	V45.0	Car driver injured in collision with railway train or railway vehicle in nontraffic accident
X+7th	V45.1	Car passenger injured in collision with railway train or railway vehicle in nontraffic accident
X+7th	V45.2	Person on outside of car injured in collision with railway train or railway vehicle in nontraffic accident
X+7th	V45.3	Unspecified car occupant injured in collision with railway train or railway vehicle in nontraffic accident
X+7th	V45.4	Person boarding or alighting a car injured in collision with railway train or railway vehicle
X+7th	V45.5	Car driver injured in collision with railway train or railway vehicle in traffic accident
X+7th	V45.6	Car passenger injured in collision with railway train or railway vehicle in traffic accident
X+7th	V45.7	Person on outside of car injured in collision with railway train or railway vehicle in traffic accident
X+7th	V45.9	Unspecified car occupant injured in collision with railway train or railway vehicle in traffic accident

V46 Car occupant injured in collision with other nonmotor vehicle

Includes: collision with animal-drawn vehicle, animal being ridden, streetcar

The appropriate 7th character is to be added to each code from category V46
- A initial encounter
- D subsequent encounter
- S sequela

X+7th	V46.0	Car driver injured in collision with other nonmotor vehicle in nontraffic accident
X+7th	V46.1	Car passenger injured in collision with other nonmotor vehicle in nontraffic accident
X+7th	V46.2	Person on outside of car injured in collision with other nonmotor vehicle in nontraffic accident
X+7th	V46.3	Unspecified car occupant injured in collision with other nonmotor vehicle in nontraffic accident
X+7th	V46.4	Person boarding or alighting a car injured in collision with other nonmotor vehicle
X+7th	V46.5	Car driver injured in collision with other nonmotor vehicle in traffic accident
X+7th	V46.6	Car passenger injured in collision with other nonmotor vehicle in traffic accident
X+7th	V46.7	Person on outside of car injured in collision with other nonmotor vehicle in traffic accident
X+7th	V46.9	Unspecified car occupant injured in collision with other nonmotor vehicle in traffic accident

V47 Car occupant injured in collision with fixed or stationary object

AHA CC: 4Q, 2016, 73

The appropriate 7th character is to be added to each code from category V47
- A initial encounter
- D subsequent encounter
- S sequela

X+7th	V47.0	Car driver injured in collision with fixed or stationary object in nontraffic accident
X+7th	V47.1	Car passenger injured in collision with fixed or stationary object in nontraffic accident
X+7th	V47.2	Person on outside of car injured in collision with fixed or stationary object in nontraffic accident
X+7th	V47.3	Unspecified car occupant injured in collision with fixed or stationary object in nontraffic accident
X+7th	V47.4	Person boarding or alighting a car injured in collision with fixed or stationary object
X+7th	V47.5	Car driver injured in collision with fixed or stationary object in traffic accident
X+7th	V47.6	Car passenger injured in collision with fixed or stationary object in traffic accident
X+7th	V47.7	Person on outside of car injured in collision with fixed or stationary object in traffic accident
X+7th	V47.9	Unspecified car occupant injured in collision with fixed or stationary object in traffic accident

V48 Car occupant injured in noncollision transport accident

Includes: overturning car NOS
overturning car without collision

> The appropriate 7th character is to be added to each code from category V48
> A initial encounter
> D subsequent encounter
> S sequela

X+7th **V48.0** Car driver injured in noncollision transport accident in nontraffic accident
X+7th **V48.1** Car passenger injured in noncollision transport accident in nontraffic accident
X+7th **V48.2** Person on outside of car injured in noncollision transport accident in nontraffic accident
X+7th **V48.3** Unspecified car occupant injured in noncollision transport accident in nontraffic accident
X+7th **V48.4** Person boarding or alighting a car injured in noncollision transport accident
X+7th **V48.5** Car driver injured in noncollision transport accident in traffic accident
X+7th **V48.6** Car passenger injured in noncollision transport accident in traffic accident
X+7th **V48.7** Person on outside of car injured in noncollision transport accident in traffic accident
X+7th **V48.9** Unspecified car occupant injured in noncollision transport accident in traffic accident

V49 Car occupant injured in other and unspecified transport accidents

> The appropriate 7th character is to be added to each code from category V49
> A initial encounter
> D subsequent encounter
> S sequela

+ **V49.0** Driver injured in collision with other and unspecified motor vehicles in nontraffic accident
  X+7th **V49.00** Driver injured in collision with unspecified motor vehicles in nontraffic accident
  X+7th **V49.09** Driver injured in collision with other motor vehicles in nontraffic accident
+ **V49.1** Passenger injured in collision with other and unspecified motor vehicles in nontraffic accident
  X+7th **V49.10** Passenger injured in collision with unspecified motor vehicles in nontraffic accident
  X+7th **V49.19** Passenger injured in collision with other motor vehicles in nontraffic accident
+ **V49.2** Unspecified car occupant injured in collision with other and unspecified motor vehicles in nontraffic accident
  X+7th **V49.20** Unspecified car occupant injured in collision with unspecified motor vehicles in nontraffic accident
  Car collision NOS, nontraffic
  X+7th **V49.29** Unspecified car occupant injured in collision with other motor vehicles in nontraffic accident
X+7th **V49.3** Car occupant (driver) (passenger) injured in unspecified nontraffic accident
  Car accident NOS, nontraffic
  Car occupant injured in nontraffic accident NOS
+ **V49.4** Driver injured in collision with other and unspecified motor vehicles in traffic accident
  X+7th **V49.40** Driver injured in collision with unspecified motor vehicles in traffic accident
  X+7th **V49.49** Driver injured in collision with other motor vehicles in traffic accident
+ **V49.5** Passenger injured in collision with other and unspecified motor vehicles in traffic accident
  X+7th **V49.50** Passenger injured in collision with unspecified motor vehicles in traffic accident
  X+7th **V49.59** Passenger injured in collision with other motor vehicles in traffic accident
+ **V49.6** Unspecified car occupant injured in collision with other and unspecified motor vehicles in traffic accident
  X+7th **V49.60** Unspecified car occupant injured in collision with unspecified motor vehicles in traffic accident
  Car collision NOS (traffic)
  X+7th **V49.69** Unspecified car occupant injured in collision with other motor vehicles in traffic accident

+ **V49.8** Car occupant (driver) (passenger) injured in other specified transport accidents
  X+7th **V49.81** Car occupant (driver) (passenger) injured in transport accident with military vehicle
  X+7th **V49.88** Car occupant (driver) (passenger) injured in other specified transport accidents
X+7th **V49.9** Car occupant (driver) (passenger) injured in unspecified traffic accident
  Car accident NOS
  AHA CC: 1Q, 2015, 3-21

Occupant of pick-up truck or van injured in transport accident (V50-V59)

Includes: a four or six wheel motor vehicle designed primarily for carrying passengers and property but weighing less than the local limit for classification as a heavy goods vehicle
minibus
minivan
sport utility vehicle (SUV)
truck
van

Excludes1: heavy transport vehicle (V60-V69)

V50 Occupant of pick-up truck or van injured in collision with pedestrian or animal

Excludes1: pick-up truck or van collision with animal-drawn vehicle or animal being ridden (V56.-)

> The appropriate 7th character is to be added to each code from category V50
> A initial encounter
> D subsequent encounter
> S sequela

X+7th **V50.0** Driver of pick-up truck or van injured in collision with pedestrian or animal in nontraffic accident
X+7th **V50.1** Passenger in pick-up truck or van injured in collision with pedestrian or animal in nontraffic accident
X+7th **V50.2** Person on outside of pick-up truck or van injured in collision with pedestrian or animal in nontraffic accident
X+7th **V50.3** Unspecified occupant of pick-up truck or van injured in collision with pedestrian or animal in nontraffic accident
X+7th **V50.4** Person boarding or alighting a pick-up truck or van injured in collision with pedestrian or animal
X+7th **V50.5** Driver of pick-up truck or van injured in collision with pedestrian or animal in traffic accident
X+7th **V50.6** Passenger in pick-up truck or van injured in collision with pedestrian or animal in traffic accident
X+7th **V50.7** Person on outside of pick-up truck or van injured in collision with pedestrian or animal in traffic accident
X+7th **V50.9** Unspecified occupant of pick-up truck or van injured in collision with pedestrian or animal in traffic accident

V51 Occupant of pick-up truck or van injured in collision with pedal cycle

> The appropriate 7th character is to be added to each code from category V51
> A initial encounter
> D subsequent encounter
> S sequela

X+7th **V51.0** Driver of pick-up truck or van injured in collision with pedal cycle in nontraffic accident
X+7th **V51.1** Passenger in pick-up truck or van injured in collision with pedal cycle in nontraffic accident
X+7th **V51.2** Person on outside of pick-up truck or van injured in collision with pedal cycle in nontraffic accident
X+7th **V51.3** Unspecified occupant of pick-up truck or van injured in collision with pedal cycle in nontraffic accident
X+7th **V51.4** Person boarding or alighting a pick-up truck or van injured in collision with pedal cycle
X+7th **V51.5** Driver of pick-up truck or van injured in collision with pedal cycle in traffic accident
X+7th **V51.6** Passenger in pick-up truck or van injured in collision with pedal cycle in traffic accident
X+7th **V51.7** Person on outside of pick-up truck or van injured in collision with pedal cycle in traffic accident
X+7th **V51.9** Unspecified occupant of pick-up truck or van injured in collision with pedal cycle in traffic accident

V52 Occupant of pick-up truck or van injured in collision with two- or three-wheeled motor vehicle

The appropriate 7th character is to be added to each code from category V52
- A initial encounter
- D subsequent encounter
- S sequela

X+7th **V52.0** Driver of pick-up truck or van injured in collision with two- or three-wheeled motor vehicle in nontraffic accident

X+7th **V52.1** Passenger in pick-up truck or van injured in collision with two- or three-wheeled motor vehicle in nontraffic accident

X+7th **V52.2** Person on outside of pick-up truck or van injured in collision with two- or three-wheeled motor vehicle in nontraffic accident

X+7th **V52.3** Unspecified occupant of pick-up truck or van injured in collision with two- or three-wheeled motor vehicle in nontraffic accident

X+7th **V52.4** Person boarding or alighting a pick-up truck or van injured in collision with two- or three-wheeled motor vehicle

X+7th **V52.5** Driver of pick-up truck or van injured in collision with two- or three-wheeled motor vehicle in traffic accident

X+7th **V52.6** Passenger in pick-up truck or van injured in collision with two- or three-wheeled motor vehicle in traffic accident

X+7th **V52.7** Person on outside of pick-up truck or van injured in collision with two- or three-wheeled motor vehicle in traffic accident

X+7th **V52.9** Unspecified occupant of pick-up truck or van injured in collision with two- or three-wheeled motor vehicle in traffic accident

V53 Occupant of pick-up truck or van injured in collision with car, pick-up truck or van

The appropriate 7th character is to be added to each code from category V53
- A initial encounter
- D subsequent encounter
- S sequela

X+7th **V53.0** Driver of pick-up truck or van injured in collision with car, pick-up truck or van in nontraffic accident

X+7th **V53.1** Passenger in pick-up truck or van injured in collision with car, pick-up truck or van in nontraffic accident

X+7th **V53.2** Person on outside of pick-up truck or van injured in collision with car, pick-up truck or van in nontraffic accident

X+7th **V53.3** Unspecified occupant of pick-up truck or van injured in collision with car, pick-up truck or van in nontraffic accident

X+7th **V53.4** Person boarding or alighting a pick-up truck or van injured in collision with car, pick-up truck or van

X+7th **V53.5** Driver of pick-up truck or van injured in collision with car, pick-up truck or van in traffic accident

X+7th **V53.6** Passenger in pick-up truck or van injured in collision with car, pick-up truck or van in traffic accident

X+7th **V53.7** Person on outside of pick-up truck or van injured in collision with car, pick-up truck or van in traffic accident

X+7th **V53.9** Unspecified occupant of pick-up truck or van injured in collision with car, pick-up truck or van in traffic accident

V54 Occupant of pick-up truck or van injured in collision with heavy transport vehicle or bus

Excludes1: occupant of pick-up truck or van injured in collision with military vehicle (V59.81)

The appropriate 7th character is to be added to each code from category V54
- A initial encounter
- D subsequent encounter
- S sequela

X+7th **V54.0** Driver of pick-up truck or van injured in collision with heavy transport vehicle or bus in nontraffic accident

X+7th **V54.1** Passenger in pick-up truck or van injured in collision with heavy transport vehicle or bus in nontraffic accident

X+7th **V54.2** Person on outside of pick-up truck or van injured in collision with heavy transport vehicle or bus in nontraffic accident

X+7th **V54.3** Unspecified occupant of pick-up truck or van injured in collision with heavy transport vehicle or bus in nontraffic accident

X+7th **V54.4** Person boarding or alighting a pick-up truck or van injured in collision with heavy transport vehicle or bus

X+7th **V54.5** Driver of pick-up truck or van injured in collision with heavy transport vehicle or bus in traffic accident

X+7th **V54.6** Passenger in pick-up truck or van injured in collision with heavy transport vehicle or bus in traffic accident

X+7th **V54.7** Person on outside of pick-up truck or van injured in collision with heavy transport vehicle or bus in traffic accident

X+7th **V54.9** Unspecified occupant of pick-up truck or van injured in collision with heavy transport vehicle or bus in traffic accident

V55 Occupant of pick-up truck or van injured in collision with railway train or railway vehicle

The appropriate 7th character is to be added to each code from category V55
- A initial encounter
- D subsequent encounter
- S sequela

X+7th **V55.0** Driver of pick-up truck or van injured in collision with railway train or railway vehicle in nontraffic accident

X+7th **V55.1** Passenger in pick-up truck or van injured in collision with railway train or railway vehicle in nontraffic accident

X+7th **V55.2** Person on outside of pick-up truck or van injured in collision with railway train or railway vehicle in nontraffic accident

X+7th **V55.3** Unspecified occupant of pick-up truck or van injured in collision with railway train or railway vehicle in nontraffic accident

X+7th **V55.4** Person boarding or alighting a pick-up truck or van injured in collision with railway train or railway vehicle

X+7th **V55.5** Driver of pick-up truck or van injured in collision with railway train or railway vehicle in traffic accident

X+7th **V55.6** Passenger in pick-up truck or van injured in collision with railway train or railway vehicle in traffic accident

X+7th **V55.7** Person on outside of pick-up truck or van injured in collision with railway train or railway vehicle in traffic accident

X+7th **V55.9** Unspecified occupant of pick-up truck or van injured in collision with railway train or railway vehicle in traffic accident

V56 Occupant of pick-up truck or van injured in collision with other nonmotor vehicle

Includes: collision with animal-drawn vehicle, animal being ridden, streetcar

The appropriate 7th character is to be added to each code from category V56
- A initial encounter
- D subsequent encounter
- S sequela

X+7th **V56.0** Driver of pick-up truck or van injured in collision with other nonmotor vehicle in nontraffic accident

X+7th **V56.1** Passenger in pick-up truck or van injured in collision with other nonmotor vehicle in nontraffic accident

X+7th **V56.2** Person on outside of pick-up truck or van injured in collision with other nonmotor vehicle in nontraffic accident

X+7th **V56.3** Unspecified occupant of pick-up truck or van injured in collision with other nonmotor vehicle in nontraffic accident

X+7th **V56.4** Person boarding or alighting a pick-up truck or van injured in collision with other nonmotor vehicle

X+7th **V56.5** Driver of pick-up truck or van injured in collision with other nonmotor vehicle in traffic accident

X+7th **V56.6** Passenger in pick-up truck or van injured in collision with other nonmotor vehicle in traffic accident

X+7th **V56.7** Person on outside of pick-up truck or van injured in collision with other nonmotor vehicle in traffic accident

X+7th **V56.9** Unspecified occupant of pick-up truck or van injured in collision with other nonmotor vehicle in traffic accident

V57 Occupant of pick-up truck or van injured in collision with fixed or stationary object

The appropriate 7th character is to be added to each code from category V57
- A initial encounter
- D subsequent encounter
- S sequela

X+7th **V57.0** Driver of pick-up truck or van injured in collision with fixed or stationary object in nontraffic accident

X+7th	V57.1	Passenger in pick-up truck or van injured in collision with fixed or stationary object in nontraffic accident
X+7th	V57.2	Person on outside of pick-up truck or van injured in collision with fixed or stationary object in nontraffic accident
X+7th	V57.3	Unspecified occupant of pick-up truck or van injured in collision with fixed or stationary object in nontraffic accident
X+7th	V57.4	Person boarding or alighting a pick-up truck or van injured in collision with fixed or stationary object
X+7th	V57.5	Driver of pick-up truck or van injured in collision with fixed or stationary object in traffic accident
X+7th	V57.6	Passenger in pick-up truck or van injured in collision with fixed or stationary object in traffic accident
X+7th	V57.7	Person on outside of pick-up truck or van injured in collision with fixed or stationary object in traffic accident
X+7th	V57.9	Unspecified occupant of pick-up truck or van injured in collision with fixed or stationary object in traffic accident

V58 Occupant of pick-up truck or van injured in noncollision transport accident

> **Includes:** overturning pick-up truck or van NOS
> overturning pick-up truck or van without collision

> The appropriate 7th character is to be added to each code from category V58
> A initial encounter
> D subsequent encounter
> S sequela

X+7th	V58.0	Driver of pick-up truck or van injured in noncollision transport accident in nontraffic accident
X+7th	V58.1	Passenger in pick-up truck or van injured in noncollision transport accident in nontraffic accident
X+7th	V58.2	Person on outside of pick-up truck or van injured in noncollision transport accident in nontraffic accident
X+7th	V58.3	Unspecified occupant of pick-up truck or van injured in noncollision transport accident in nontraffic accident
X+7th	V58.4	Person boarding or alighting a pick-up truck or van injured in noncollision transport accident
X+7th	V58.5	Driver of pick-up truck or van injured in noncollision transport accident in traffic accident
X+7th	V58.6	Passenger in pick-up truck or van injured in noncollision transport accident in traffic accident
X+7th	V58.7	Person on outside of pick-up truck or van injured in noncollision transport accident in traffic accident
X+7th	V58.9	Unspecified occupant of pick-up truck or van injured in noncollision transport accident in traffic accident

V59 Occupant of pick-up truck or van injured in other and unspecified transport accidents

> The appropriate 7th character is to be added to each code from category V59
> A initial encounter
> D subsequent encounter
> S sequela

+	V59.0	Driver of pick-up truck or van injured in collision with other and unspecified motor vehicles in nontraffic accident
X+7th	V59.00	Driver of pick-up truck or van injured in collision with unspecified motor vehicles in nontraffic accident
X+7th	V59.09	Driver of pick-up truck or van injured in collision with other motor vehicles in nontraffic accident
+	V59.1	Passenger in pick-up truck or van injured in collision with other and unspecified motor vehicles in nontraffic accident
X+7th	V59.10	Passenger in pick-up truck or van injured in collision with unspecified motor vehicles in nontraffic accident
X+7th	V59.19	Passenger in pick-up truck or van injured in collision with other motor vehicles in nontraffic accident
+	V59.2	Unspecified occupant of pick-up truck or van injured in collision with other and unspecified motor vehicles in nontraffic accident
X+7th	V59.20	Unspecified occupant of pick-up truck or van injured in collision with unspecified motor vehicles in nontraffic accident
		Collision NOS involving pick-up truck or van, nontraffic
X+7th	V59.29	Unspecified occupant of pick-up truck or van injured in collision with other motor vehicles in nontraffic accident
X+7th	V59.3	Occupant (driver) (passenger) of pick-up truck or van injured in unspecified nontraffic accident
		Accident NOS involving pick-up truck or van, nontraffic
		Occupant of pick-up truck or van injured in nontraffic accident NOS
+	V59.4	Driver of pick-up truck or van injured in collision with other and unspecified motor vehicles in traffic accident
X+7th	V59.40	Driver of pick-up truck or van injured in collision with unspecified motor vehicles in traffic accident
X+7th	V59.49	Driver of pick-up truck or van injured in collision with other motor vehicles in traffic accident
+	V59.5	Passenger in pick-up truck or van injured in collision with other and unspecified motor vehicles in traffic accident
X+7th	V59.50	Passenger in pick-up truck or van injured in collision with unspecified motor vehicles in traffic accident
X+7th	V59.59	Passenger in pick-up truck or van injured in collision with other motor vehicles in traffic accident
+	V59.6	Unspecified occupant of pick-up truck or van injured in collision with other and unspecified motor vehicles in traffic accident
X+7th	V59.60	Unspecified occupant of pick-up truck or van injured in collision with unspecified motor vehicles in traffic accident
		Collision NOS involving pick-up truck or van (traffic)
X+7th	V59.69	Unspecified occupant of pick-up truck or van injured in collision with other motor vehicles in traffic accident
+	V59.8	Occupant (driver) (passenger) of pick-up truck or van injured in other specified transport accidents
X+7th	V59.81	Occupant (driver) (passenger) of pick-up truck or van injured in transport accident with military vehicle
X+7th	V59.88	Occupant (driver) (passenger) of pick-up truck or van injured in other specified transport accidents
X+7th	V59.9	Occupant (driver) (passenger) of pick-up truck or van injured in unspecified traffic accident
		Accident NOS involving pick-up truck or van

Occupant of heavy transport vehicle injured in transport accident (V60-V69)

> **Includes:** 18 wheeler
> armored car
> panel truck

> **Excludes1:** bus
> motorcoach

V60 Occupant of heavy transport vehicle injured in collision with pedestrian or animal

> **Excludes1:** heavy transport vehicle collision with animal-drawn vehicle or animal being ridden (V66.-)

> The appropriate 7th character is to be added to each code from category V60
> A initial encounter
> D subsequent encounter
> S sequela

X+7th	V60.0	Driver of heavy transport vehicle injured in collision with pedestrian or animal in nontraffic accident
X+7th	V60.1	Passenger in heavy transport vehicle injured in collision with pedestrian or animal in nontraffic accident
X+7th	V60.2	Person on outside of heavy transport vehicle injured in collision with pedestrian or animal in nontraffic accident
X+7th	V60.3	Unspecified occupant of heavy transport vehicle injured in collision with pedestrian or animal in nontraffic accident
X+7th	V60.4	Person boarding or alighting a heavy transport vehicle injured in collision with pedestrian or animal
X+7th	V60.5	Driver of heavy transport vehicle injured in collision with pedestrian or animal in traffic accident
X+7th	V60.6	Passenger in heavy transport vehicle injured in collision with pedestrian or animal in traffic accident
X+7th	V60.7	Person on outside of heavy transport vehicle injured in collision with pedestrian or animal in traffic accident
X+7th	V60.9	Unspecified occupant of heavy transport vehicle injured in collision with pedestrian or animal in traffic accident

V61 Occupant of heavy transport vehicle injured in collision with pedal cycle

> The appropriate 7th character is to be added to each code from category V61
> A initial encounter
> D subsequent encounter
> S sequela

X+7th **V61.0** Driver of heavy transport vehicle injured in collision with pedal cycle in nontraffic accident
X+7th **V61.1** Passenger in heavy transport vehicle injured in collision with pedal cycle in nontraffic accident
X+7th **V61.2** Person on outside of heavy transport vehicle injured in collision with pedal cycle in nontraffic accident
X+7th **V61.3** Unspecified occupant of heavy transport vehicle injured in collision with pedal cycle in nontraffic accident
X+7th **V61.4** Person boarding or alighting a heavy transport vehicle injured in collision with pedal cycle while boarding or alighting
X+7th **V61.5** Driver of heavy transport vehicle injured in collision with pedal cycle in traffic accident
X+7th **V61.6** Passenger in heavy transport vehicle injured in collision with pedal cycle in traffic accident
X+7th **V61.7** Person on outside of heavy transport vehicle injured in collision with pedal cycle in traffic accident
X+7th **V61.9** Unspecified occupant of heavy transport vehicle injured in collision with pedal cycle in traffic accident

V62 Occupant of heavy transport vehicle injured in collision with two- or three-wheeled motor vehicle

> The appropriate 7th character is to be added to each code from category V62
> A initial encounter
> D subsequent encounter
> S sequela

X+7th **V62.0** Driver of heavy transport vehicle injured in collision with two- or three-wheeled motor vehicle in nontraffic accident
X+7th **V62.1** Passenger in heavy transport vehicle injured in collision with two- or three-wheeled motor vehicle in nontraffic accident
X+7th **V62.2** Person on outside of heavy transport vehicle injured in collision with two- or three-wheeled motor vehicle in nontraffic accident
X+7th **V62.3** Unspecified occupant of heavy transport vehicle injured in collision with two- or three-wheeled motor vehicle in nontraffic accident
X+7th **V62.4** Person boarding or alighting a heavy transport vehicle injured in collision with two- or three-wheeled motor vehicle
X+7th **V62.5** Driver of heavy transport vehicle injured in collision with two- or three-wheeled motor vehicle in traffic accident
X+7th **V62.6** Passenger in heavy transport vehicle injured in collision with two- or three-wheeled motor vehicle in traffic accident
X+7th **V62.7** Person on outside of heavy transport vehicle injured in collision with two- or three-wheeled motor vehicle in traffic accident
X+7th **V62.9** Unspecified occupant of heavy transport vehicle injured in collision with two- or three-wheeled motor vehicle in traffic accident

V63 Occupant of heavy transport vehicle injured in collision with car, pick-up truck or van

> The appropriate 7th character is to be added to each code from category V63
> A initial encounter
> D subsequent encounter
> S sequela

X+7th **V63.0** Driver of heavy transport vehicle injured in collision with car, pick-up truck or van in nontraffic accident
X+7th **V63.1** Passenger in heavy transport vehicle injured in collision with car, pick-up truck or van in nontraffic accident
X+7th **V63.2** Person on outside of heavy transport vehicle injured in collision with car, pick-up truck or van in nontraffic accident
X+7th **V63.3** Unspecified occupant of heavy transport vehicle injured in collision with car, pick-up truck or van in nontraffic accident
X+7th **V63.4** Person boarding or alighting a heavy transport vehicle injured in collision with car, pick-up truck or van
X+7th **V63.5** Driver of heavy transport vehicle injured in collision with car, pick-up truck or van in traffic accident
X+7th **V63.6** Passenger in heavy transport vehicle injured in collision with car, pick-up truck or van in traffic accident
X+7th **V63.7** Person on outside of heavy transport vehicle injured in collision with car, pick-up truck or van in traffic accident
X+7th **V63.9** Unspecified occupant of heavy transport vehicle injured in collision with car, pick-up truck or van in traffic accident

V64 Occupant of heavy transport vehicle injured in collision with heavy transport vehicle or bus

> **Excludes1:** occupant of heavy transport vehicle injured in collision with military vehicle (V69.81)

> The appropriate 7th character is to be added to each code from category V64
> A initial encounter
> D subsequent encounter
> S sequela

X+7th **V64.0** Driver of heavy transport vehicle injured in collision with heavy transport vehicle or bus in nontraffic accident
X+7th **V64.1** Passenger in heavy transport vehicle injured in collision with heavy transport vehicle or bus in nontraffic accident
X+7th **V64.2** Person on outside of heavy transport vehicle injured in collision with heavy transport vehicle or bus in nontraffic accident
X+7th **V64.3** Unspecified occupant of heavy transport vehicle injured in collision with heavy transport vehicle or bus in nontraffic accident
X+7th **V64.4** Person boarding or alighting a heavy transport vehicle injured in collision with heavy transport vehicle or bus while boarding or alighting
X+7th **V64.5** Driver of heavy transport vehicle injured in collision with heavy transport vehicle or bus in traffic accident
X+7th **V64.6** Passenger in heavy transport vehicle injured in collision with heavy transport vehicle or bus in traffic accident
X+7th **V64.7** Person on outside of heavy transport vehicle injured in collision with heavy transport vehicle or bus in traffic accident
X+7th **V64.9** Unspecified occupant of heavy transport vehicle injured in collision with heavy transport vehicle or bus in traffic accident

V65 Occupant of heavy transport vehicle injured in collision with railway train or railway vehicle

> The appropriate 7th character is to be added to each code from category V65
> A initial encounter
> D subsequent encounter
> S sequela

X+7th **V65.0** Driver of heavy transport vehicle injured in collision with railway train or railway vehicle in nontraffic accident
X+7th **V65.1** Passenger in heavy transport vehicle injured in collision with railway train or railway vehicle in nontraffic accident
X+7th **V65.2** Person on outside of heavy transport vehicle injured in collision with railway train or railway vehicle in nontraffic accident
X+7th **V65.3** Unspecified occupant of heavy transport vehicle injured in collision with railway train or railway vehicle in nontraffic accident
X+7th **V65.4** Person boarding or alighting a heavy transport vehicle injured in collision with railway train or railway vehicle
X+7th **V65.5** Driver of heavy transport vehicle injured in collision with railway train or railway vehicle in traffic accident
X+7th **V65.6** Passenger in heavy transport vehicle injured in collision with railway train or railway vehicle in traffic accident
X+7th **V65.7** Person on outside of heavy transport vehicle injured in collision with railway train or railway vehicle in traffic accident
X+7th **V65.9** Unspecified occupant of heavy transport vehicle injured in collision with railway train or railway vehicle in traffic accident

V66 Occupant of heavy transport vehicle injured in collision with other nonmotor vehicle

Includes: collision with animal-drawn vehicle, animal being ridden, streetcar

The appropriate 7th character is to be added to each code from category V66
- A initial encounter
- D subsequent encounter
- S sequela

- X+7th **V66.0** Driver of heavy transport vehicle injured in collision with other nonmotor vehicle in nontraffic accident
- X+7th **V66.1** Passenger in heavy transport vehicle injured in collision with other nonmotor vehicle in nontraffic accident
- X+7th **V66.2** Person on outside of heavy transport vehicle injured in collision with other nonmotor vehicle in nontraffic accident
- X+7th **V66.3** Unspecified occupant of heavy transport vehicle injured in collision with other nonmotor vehicle in nontraffic accident
- X+7th **V66.4** Person boarding or alighting a heavy transport vehicle injured in collision with other nonmotor vehicle
- X+7th **V66.5** Driver of heavy transport vehicle injured in collision with other nonmotor vehicle in traffic accident
- X+7th **V66.6** Passenger in heavy transport vehicle injured in collision with other nonmotor vehicle in traffic accident
- X+7th **V66.7** Person on outside of heavy transport vehicle injured in collision with other nonmotor vehicle in traffic accident
- X+7th **V66.9** Unspecified occupant of heavy transport vehicle injured in collision with other nonmotor vehicle in traffic accident

V67 Occupant of heavy transport vehicle injured in collision with fixed or stationary object

The appropriate 7th character is to be added to each code from category V67
- A initial encounter
- D subsequent encounter
- S sequela

- X+7th **V67.0** Driver of heavy transport vehicle injured in collision with fixed or stationary object in nontraffic accident
- X+7th **V67.1** Passenger in heavy transport vehicle injured in collision with fixed or stationary object in nontraffic accident
- X+7th **V67.2** Person on outside of heavy transport vehicle injured in collision with fixed or stationary object in nontraffic accident
- X+7th **V67.3** Unspecified occupant of heavy transport vehicle injured in collision with fixed or stationary object in nontraffic accident
- X+7th **V67.4** Person boarding or alighting a heavy transport vehicle injured in collision with fixed or stationary object
- X+7th **V67.5** Driver of heavy transport vehicle injured in collision with fixed or stationary object in traffic accident
- X+7th **V67.6** Passenger in heavy transport vehicle injured in collision with fixed or stationary object in traffic accident
- X+7th **V67.7** Person on outside of heavy transport vehicle injured in collision with fixed or stationary object in traffic accident
- X+7th **V67.9** Unspecified occupant of heavy transport vehicle injured in collision with fixed or stationary object in traffic accident

V68 Occupant of heavy transport vehicle injured in noncollision transport accident

Includes: overturning heavy transport vehicle NOS
overturning heavy transport vehicle without collision

The appropriate 7th character is to be added to each code from category V68
- A initial encounter
- D subsequent encounter
- S sequela

- X+7th **V68.0** Driver of heavy transport vehicle injured in noncollision transport accident in nontraffic accident
- X+7th **V68.1** Passenger in heavy transport vehicle injured in noncollision transport accident in nontraffic accident
- X+7th **V68.2** Person on outside of heavy transport vehicle injured in noncollision transport accident in nontraffic accident
- X+7th **V68.3** Unspecified occupant of heavy transport vehicle injured in noncollision transport accident in nontraffic accident
- X+7th **V68.4** Person boarding or alighting a heavy transport vehicle injured in noncollision transport accident
- X+7th **V68.5** Driver of heavy transport vehicle injured in noncollision transport accident in traffic accident
- X+7th **V68.6** Passenger in heavy transport vehicle injured in noncollision transport accident in traffic accident
- X+7th **V68.7** Person on outside of heavy transport vehicle injured in noncollision transport accident in traffic accident
- X+7th **V68.9** Unspecified occupant of heavy transport vehicle injured in noncollision transport accident in traffic accident

V69 Occupant of heavy transport vehicle injured in other and unspecified transport accidents

The appropriate 7th character is to be added to each code from category V69
- A initial encounter
- D subsequent encounter
- S sequela

- + **V69.0** Driver of heavy transport vehicle injured in collision with other and unspecified motor vehicles in nontraffic accident
  - X+7th **V69.00** Driver of heavy transport vehicle injured in collision with unspecified motor vehicles in nontraffic accident
  - X+7th **V69.09** Driver of heavy transport vehicle injured in collision with other motor vehicles in nontraffic accident
- + **V69.1** Passenger in heavy transport vehicle injured in collision with other and unspecified motor vehicles in nontraffic accident
  - X+7th **V69.10** Passenger in heavy transport vehicle injured in collision with unspecified motor vehicles in nontraffic accident
  - X+7th **V69.19** Passenger in heavy transport vehicle injured in collision with other motor vehicles in nontraffic accident
- + **V69.2** Unspecified occupant of heavy transport vehicle injured in collision with other and unspecified motor vehicles in nontraffic accident
  - X+7th **V69.20** Unspecified occupant of heavy transport vehicle injured in collision with unspecified motor vehicles in nontraffic accident
    Collision NOS involving heavy transport vehicle, nontraffic
  - X+7th **V69.29** Unspecified occupant of heavy transport vehicle injured in collision with other motor vehicles in nontraffic accident
- X+7th **V69.3** Occupant (driver) (passenger) of heavy transport vehicle injured in unspecified nontraffic accident
    Accident NOS involving heavy transport vehicle, nontraffic
    Occupant of heavy transport vehicle injured in nontraffic accident NOS
- + **V69.4** Driver of heavy transport vehicle injured in collision with other and unspecified motor vehicles in traffic accident
  - X+7th **V69.40** Driver of heavy transport vehicle injured in collision with unspecified motor vehicles in traffic accident
  - X+7th **V69.49** Driver of heavy transport vehicle injured in collision with other motor vehicles in traffic accident
- + **V69.5** Passenger in heavy transport vehicle injured in collision with other and unspecified motor vehicles in traffic accident
  - X+7th **V69.50** Passenger in heavy transport vehicle injured in collision with unspecified motor vehicles in traffic accident
  - X+7th **V69.59** Passenger in heavy transport vehicle injured in collision with other motor vehicles in traffic accident
- + **V69.6** Unspecified occupant of heavy transport vehicle injured in collision with other and unspecified motor vehicles in traffic accident
  - X+7th **V69.60** Unspecified occupant of heavy transport vehicle injured in collision with unspecified motor vehicles in traffic accident
    Collision NOS involving heavy transport vehicle (traffic)
  - X+7th **V69.69** Unspecified occupant of heavy transport vehicle injured in collision with other motor vehicles in traffic accident
- + **V69.8** Occupant (driver) (passenger) of heavy transport vehicle injured in other specified transport accidents
  - X+7th **V69.81** Occupant (driver) (passenger) of heavy transport vehicle injured in transport accidents with military vehicle
  - X+7th **V69.88** Occupant (driver) (passenger) of heavy transport vehicle injured in other specified transport accidents
- X+7th **V69.9** Occupant (driver) (passenger) of heavy transport vehicle injured in unspecified traffic accident
    Accident NOS involving heavy transport vehicle

Bus occupant injured in transport accident (V70-V79)

Includes: motorcoach

Excludes1: minibus (V50-V59)

V70 Bus occupant injured in collision with pedestrian or animal

The appropriate 7th character is to be added to each code from category V70
- A initial encounter
- D subsequent encounter
- S sequela

Excludes1: bus collision with animal-drawn vehicle or animal being ridden (V76.-)

- X+7th **V70.0** Driver of bus injured in collision with pedestrian or animal in nontraffic accident
- X+7th **V70.1** Passenger on bus injured in collision with pedestrian or animal in nontraffic accident
- X+7th **V70.2** Person on outside of bus injured in collision with pedestrian or animal in nontraffic accident
- X+7th **V70.3** Unspecified occupant of bus injured in collision with pedestrian or animal in nontraffic accident
- X+7th **V70.4** Person boarding or alighting from bus injured in collision with pedestrian or animal
- X+7th **V70.5** Driver of bus injured in collision with pedestrian or animal in traffic accident
- X+7th **V70.6** Passenger on bus injured in collision with pedestrian or animal in traffic accident
- X+7th **V70.7** Person on outside of bus injured in collision with pedestrian or animal in traffic accident
- X+7th **V70.9** Unspecified occupant of bus injured in collision with pedestrian or animal in traffic accident

V71 Bus occupant injured in collision with pedal cycle

The appropriate 7th character is to be added to each code from category V71
- A initial encounter
- D subsequent encounter
- S sequela

- X+7th **V71.0** Driver of bus injured in collision with pedal cycle in nontraffic accident
- X+7th **V71.1** Passenger on bus injured in collision with pedal cycle in nontraffic accident
- X+7th **V71.2** Person on outside of bus injured in collision with pedal cycle in nontraffic accident
- X+7th **V71.3** Unspecified occupant of bus injured in collision with pedal cycle in nontraffic accident
- X+7th **V71.4** Person boarding or alighting from bus injured in collision with pedal cycle
- X+7th **V71.5** Driver of bus injured in collision with pedal cycle in traffic accident
- X+7th **V71.6** Passenger on bus injured in collision with pedal cycle in traffic accident
- X+7th **V71.7** Person on outside of bus injured in collision with pedal cycle in traffic accident
- X+7th **V71.9** Unspecified occupant of bus injured in collision with pedal cycle in traffic accident

V72 Bus occupant injured in collision with two- or three-wheeled motor vehicle

The appropriate 7th character is to be added to each code from category V72
- A initial encounter
- D subsequent encounter
- S sequela

- X+7th **V72.0** Driver of bus injured in collision with two- or three-wheeled motor vehicle in nontraffic accident
- X+7th **V72.1** Passenger on bus injured in collision with two- or three-wheeled motor vehicle in nontraffic accident
- X+7th **V72.2** Person on outside of bus injured in collision with two- or three-wheeled motor vehicle in nontraffic accident
- X+7th **V72.3** Unspecified occupant of bus injured in collision with two- or three-wheeled motor vehicle in nontraffic accident
- X+7th **V72.4** Person boarding or alighting from bus injured in collision with two- or three-wheeled motor vehicle
- X+7th **V72.5** Driver of bus injured in collision with two- or three-wheeled motor vehicle in traffic accident
- X+7th **V72.6** Passenger on bus injured in collision with two- or three-wheeled motor vehicle in traffic accident
- X+7th **V72.7** Person on outside of bus injured in collision with two- or three-wheeled motor vehicle in traffic accident
- X+7th **V72.9** Unspecified occupant of bus injured in collision with two- or three-wheeled motor vehicle in traffic accident

V73 Bus occupant injured in collision with car, pick-up truck or van

The appropriate 7th character is to be added to each code from category V73
- A initial encounter
- D subsequent encounter
- S sequela

- X+7th **V73.0** Driver of bus injured in collision with car, pick-up truck or van in nontraffic accident
- X+7th **V73.1** Passenger on bus injured in collision with car, pick-up truck or van in nontraffic accident
- X+7th **V73.2** Person on outside of bus injured in collision with car, pick-up truck or van in nontraffic accident
- X+7th **V73.3** Unspecified occupant of bus injured in collision with car, pick-up truck or van in nontraffic accident
- X+7th **V73.4** Person boarding or alighting from bus injured in collision with car, pick-up truck or van
- X+7th **V73.5** Driver of bus injured in collision with car, pick-up truck or van in traffic accident
- X+7th **V73.6** Passenger on bus injured in collision with car, pick-up truck or van in traffic accident
- X+7th **V73.7** Person on outside of bus injured in collision with car, pick-up truck or van in traffic accident
- X+7th **V73.9** Unspecified occupant of bus injured in collision with car, pick-up truck or van in traffic accident

V74 Bus occupant injured in collision with heavy transport vehicle or bus

Excludes1: bus occupant injured in collision with military vehicle (V79.81)

The appropriate 7th character is to be added to each code from category V74
- A initial encounter
- D subsequent encounter
- S sequela

- X+7th **V74.0** Driver of bus injured in collision with heavy transport vehicle or bus in nontraffic accident
- X+7th **V74.1** Passenger on bus injured in collision with heavy transport vehicle or bus in nontraffic accident
- X+7th **V74.2** Person on outside of bus injured in collision with heavy transport vehicle or bus in nontraffic accident
- X+7th **V74.3** Unspecified occupant of bus injured in collision with heavy transport vehicle or bus in nontraffic accident
- X+7th **V74.4** Person boarding or alighting from bus injured in collision with heavy transport vehicle or bus
- X+7th **V74.5** Driver of bus injured in collision with heavy transport vehicle or bus in traffic accident
- X+7th **V74.6** Passenger on bus injured in collision with heavy transport vehicle or bus in traffic accident
- X+7th **V74.7** Person on outside of bus injured in collision with heavy transport vehicle or bus in traffic accident
- X+7th **V74.9** Unspecified occupant of bus injured in collision with heavy transport vehicle or bus in traffic accident

V75 Bus occupant injured in collision with railway train or railway vehicle

The appropriate 7th character is to be added to each code from category V75
- A initial encounter
- D subsequent encounter
- S sequela

- X+7th **V75.0** Driver of bus injured in collision with railway train or railway vehicle in nontraffic accident
- X+7th **V75.1** Passenger on bus injured in collision with railway train or railway vehicle in nontraffic accident
- X+7th **V75.2** Person on outside of bus injured in collision with railway train or railway vehicle in nontraffic accident
- X+7th **V75.3** Unspecified occupant of bus injured in collision with railway train or railway vehicle in nontraffic accident
- X+7th **V75.4** Person boarding or alighting from bus injured in collision with railway train or railway vehicle
- X+7th **V75.5** Driver of bus injured in collision with railway train or railway vehicle in traffic accident
- X+7th **V75.6** Passenger on bus injured in collision with railway train or railway vehicle in traffic accident
- X+7th **V75.7** Person on outside of bus injured in collision with railway train or railway vehicle in traffic accident
- X+7th **V75.9** Unspecified occupant of bus injured in collision with railway train or railway vehicle in traffic accident

V76 Bus occupant injured in collision with other nonmotor vehicle

Includes: collision with animal-drawn vehicle, animal being ridden, streetcar

The appropriate 7th character is to be added to each code from category V76
- A initial encounter
- D subsequent encounter
- S sequela

X+7th **V76.0** Driver of bus injured in collision with other nonmotor vehicle in nontraffic accident
X+7th **V76.1** Passenger on bus injured in collision with other nonmotor vehicle in nontraffic accident
X+7th **V76.2** Person on outside of bus injured in collision with other nonmotor vehicle in nontraffic accident
X+7th **V76.3** Unspecified occupant of bus injured in collision with other nonmotor vehicle in nontraffic accident
X+7th **V76.4** Person boarding or alighting from bus injured in collision with other nonmotor vehicle
X+7th **V76.5** Driver of bus injured in collision with other nonmotor vehicle in traffic accident
X+7th **V76.6** Passenger on bus injured in collision with other nonmotor vehicle in traffic accident
X+7th **V76.7** Person on outside of bus injured in collision with other nonmotor vehicle in traffic accident
X+7th **V76.9** Unspecified occupant of bus injured in collision with other nonmotor vehicle in traffic accident

V77 Bus occupant injured in collision with fixed or stationary object

The appropriate 7th character is to be added to each code from category V77
- A initial encounter
- D subsequent encounter
- S sequela

X+7th **V77.0** Driver of bus injured in collision with fixed or stationary object in nontraffic accident
X+7th **V77.1** Passenger on bus injured in collision with fixed or stationary object in nontraffic accident
X+7th **V77.2** Person on outside of bus injured in collision with fixed or stationary object in nontraffic accident
X+7th **V77.3** Unspecified occupant of bus injured in collision with fixed or stationary object in nontraffic accident
X+7th **V77.4** Person boarding or alighting from bus injured in collision with fixed or stationary object
X+7th **V77.5** Driver of bus injured in collision with fixed or stationary object in traffic accident
X+7th **V77.6** Passenger on bus injured in collision with fixed or stationary object in traffic accident
X+7th **V77.7** Person on outside of bus injured in collision with fixed or stationary object in traffic accident
X+7th **V77.9** Unspecified occupant of bus injured in collision with fixed or stationary object in traffic accident

V78 Bus occupant injured in noncollision transport accident

Includes: overturning bus NOS
overturning bus without collision

The appropriate 7th character is to be added to each code from category V78
- A initial encounter
- D subsequent encounter
- S sequela

X+7th **V78.0** Driver of bus injured in noncollision transport accident in nontraffic accident
X+7th **V78.1** Passenger on bus injured in noncollision transport accident in nontraffic accident
X+7th **V78.2** Person on outside of bus injured in noncollision transport accident in nontraffic accident
X+7th **V78.3** Unspecified occupant of bus injured in noncollision transport accident in nontraffic accident
X+7th **V78.4** Person boarding or alighting from bus injured in noncollision transport accident
X+7th **V78.5** Driver of bus injured in noncollision transport accident in traffic accident
X+7th **V78.6** Passenger on bus injured in noncollision transport accident in traffic accident
X+7th **V78.7** Person on outside of bus injured in noncollision transport accident in traffic accident
X+7th **V78.9** Unspecified occupant of bus injured in noncollision transport accident in traffic accident

V79 Bus occupant injured in other and unspecified transport accidents

The appropriate 7th character is to be added to each code from category V79
- A initial encounter
- D subsequent encounter
- S sequela

+ **V79.0** Driver of bus injured in collision with other and unspecified motor vehicles in nontraffic accident
  X+7th **V79.00** Driver of bus injured in collision with unspecified motor vehicles in nontraffic accident
  X+7th **V79.09** Driver of bus injured in collision with other motor vehicles in nontraffic accident
+ **V79.1** Passenger on bus injured in collision with other and unspecified motor vehicles in nontraffic accident
  X+7th **V79.10** Passenger on bus injured in collision with unspecified motor vehicles in nontraffic accident
  X+7th **V79.19** Passenger on bus injured in collision with other motor vehicles in nontraffic accident
+ **V79.2** Unspecified bus occupant injured in collision with other and unspecified motor vehicles in nontraffic accident
  X+7th **V79.20** Unspecified bus occupant injured in collision with unspecified motor vehicles in nontraffic accident
    Bus collision NOS, nontraffic
  X+7th **V79.29** Unspecified bus occupant injured in collision with other motor vehicles in nontraffic accident
X+7th **V79.3** Bus occupant (driver) (passenger) injured in unspecified nontraffic accident
  Bus accident NOS, nontraffic
  Bus occupant injured in nontraffic accident NOS
+ **V79.4** Driver of bus injured in collision with other and unspecified motor vehicles in traffic accident
  X+7th **V79.40** Driver of bus injured in collision with unspecified motor vehicles in traffic accident
  X+7th **V79.49** Driver of bus injured in collision with other motor vehicles in traffic accident
+ **V79.5** Passenger on bus injured in collision with other and unspecified motor vehicles in traffic accident
  X+7th **V79.50** Passenger on bus injured in collision with unspecified motor vehicles in traffic accident
  X+7th **V79.59** Passenger on bus injured in collision with other motor vehicles in traffic accident
+ **V79.6** Unspecified bus occupant injured in collision with other and unspecified motor vehicles in traffic accident
  X+7th **V79.60** Unspecified bus occupant injured in collision with unspecified motor vehicles in traffic accident
    Bus collision NOS (traffic)
  X+7th **V79.69** Unspecified bus occupant injured in collision with other motor vehicles in traffic accident
+ **V79.8** Bus occupant (driver) (passenger) injured in other specified transport accidents
  X+7th **V79.81** Bus occupant (driver) (passenger) injured in transport accidents with military vehicle
  X+7th **V79.88** Bus occupant (driver) (passenger) injured in other specified transport accidents
X+7th **V79.9** Bus occupant (driver) (passenger) injured in unspecified traffic accident
  Bus accident NOS

Other land transport accidents (V80-V89)

V80 Animal-rider or occupant of animal-drawn vehicle injured in transport accident

The appropriate 7th character is to be added to each code from category V80
- A initial encounter
- D subsequent encounter
- S sequela

+ **V80.0** Animal-rider or occupant of animal drawn vehicle injured by fall from or being thrown from animal or animal-drawn vehicle in noncollision accident
  + **V80.01** Animal-rider injured by fall from or being thrown from animal in noncollision accident
    +7th **V80.010** Animal-rider injured by fall from or being thrown from horse in noncollision accident
    +7th **V80.018** Animal-rider injured by fall from or being thrown from other animal in noncollision accident

V80.02–V81.89 Chapter 20: External Causes of Morbidity

- X+7th **V80.02** Occupant of animal-drawn vehicle injured by fall from or being thrown from animal-drawn vehicle in noncollision accident
  - Overturning animal-drawn vehicle NOS
  - Overturning animal-drawn vehicle without collision
+ **V80.1** Animal-rider or occupant of animal-drawn vehicle injured in collision with pedestrian or animal
  - *Excludes1:* animal-rider or animal-drawn vehicle collision with animal-drawn vehicle or animal being ridden (V80.7)
  - X+7th **V80.11** Animal-rider injured in collision with pedestrian or animal
  - X+7th **V80.12** Occupant of animal-drawn vehicle injured in collision with pedestrian or animal
+ **V80.2** Animal-rider or occupant of animal-drawn vehicle injured in collision with pedal cycle
  - X+7th **V80.21** Animal-rider injured in collision with pedal cycle
  - X+7th **V80.22** Occupant of animal-drawn vehicle injured in collision with pedal cycle
+ **V80.3** Animal-rider or occupant of animal-drawn vehicle injured in collision with two- or three-wheeled motor vehicle
  - X+7th **V80.31** Animal-rider injured in collision with two- or three-wheeled motor vehicle
  - X+7th **V80.32** Occupant of animal-drawn vehicle injured in collision with two- or three-wheeled motor vehicle
+ **V80.4** Animal-rider or occupant of animal-drawn vehicle injured in collision with car, pick-up truck, van, heavy transport vehicle or bus
  - *Excludes1:* animal-rider injured in collision with military vehicle (V80.910)
  - occupant of animal-drawn vehicle injured in collision with military vehicle (V80.920)
  - X+7th **V80.41** Animal-rider injured in collision with car, pick-up truck, van, heavy transport vehicle or bus
  - X+7th **V80.42** Occupant of animal-drawn vehicle injured in collision with car, pick-up truck, van, heavy transport vehicle or bus
+ **V80.5** Animal-rider or occupant of animal-drawn vehicle injured in collision with other specified motor vehicle
  - X+7th **V80.51** Animal-rider injured in collision with other specified motor vehicle
  - X+7th **V80.52** Occupant of animal-drawn vehicle injured in collision with other specified motor vehicle
+ **V80.6** Animal-rider or occupant of animal-drawn vehicle injured in collision with railway train or railway vehicle
  - X+7th **V80.61** Animal-rider injured in collision with railway train or railway vehicle
  - X+7th **V80.62** Occupant of animal-drawn vehicle injured in collision with railway train or railway vehicle
+ **V80.7** Animal-rider or occupant of animal-drawn vehicle injured in collision with other nonmotor vehicles
  - X+7th **V80.71** Animal-rider or occupant of animal-drawn vehicle injured in collision with animal being ridden
    - X+7th **V80.710** Animal-rider injured in collision with other animal being ridden
    - X+7th **V80.711** Occupant of animal-drawn vehicle injured in collision with animal being ridden
  - X+7th **V80.72** Animal-rider or occupant of animal-drawn vehicle injured in collision with other animal-drawn vehicle
    - X+7th **V80.720** Animal-rider injured in collision with animal-drawn vehicle
    - X+7th **V80.721** Occupant of animal-drawn vehicle injured in collision with other animal-drawn vehicle
  + **V80.73** Animal-rider or occupant of animal-drawn vehicle injured in collision with streetcar
    - X+7th **V80.730** Animal-rider injured in collision with streetcar
    - X+7th **V80.731** Occupant of animal-drawn vehicle injured in collision with streetcar
  - X+7th **V80.79** Animal-rider or occupant of animal-drawn vehicle injured in collision with other nonmotor vehicles
    - X+7th **V80.790** Animal-rider injured in collision with other nonmotor vehicles
    - X+7th **V80.791** Occupant of animal-drawn vehicle injured in collision with other nonmotor vehicles

+ **V80.8** Animal-rider or occupant of animal-drawn vehicle injured in collision with fixed or stationary object
  - X+7th **V80.81** Animal-rider injured in collision with fixed or stationary object
  - X+7th **V80.82** Occupant of animal-drawn vehicle injured in collision with fixed or stationary object
+ **V80.9** Animal-rider or occupant of animal-drawn vehicle injured in other and unspecified transport accidents
  + **V80.91** Animal-rider injured in other and unspecified transport accidents
    - +7th **V80.910** Animal-rider injured in transport accident with military vehicle
    - +7th **V80.918** Animal-rider injured in other transport accident
    - +7th **V80.919** Animal-rider injured in unspecified transport accident
      - Animal rider accident NOS
  + **V80.92** Occupant of animal-drawn vehicle injured in other and unspecified transport accidents
    - +7th **V80.920** Occupant of animal-drawn vehicle injured in transport accident with military vehicle
    - +7th **V80.928** Occupant of animal-drawn vehicle injured in other transport accident
    - +7th **V80.929** Occupant of animal-drawn vehicle injured in unspecified transport accident
      - Animal-drawn vehicle accident NOS

V81 Occupant of railway train or railway vehicle injured in transport accident
  - *Includes:* derailment of railway train or railway vehicle
  - person on outside of train
  - *Excludes1:* streetcar (V82.-)

  The appropriate 7th character is to be added to each code from category V81
  - A initial encounter
  - D subsequent encounter
  - S sequela

- X+7th **V81.0** Occupant of railway train or railway vehicle injured in collision with motor vehicle in nontraffic accident
  - *Excludes1:* Occupant of railway train or railway vehicle injured due to collision with military vehicle (V81.83)
- X+7th **V81.1** Occupant of railway train or railway vehicle injured in collision with motor vehicle in traffic accident
  - *Excludes1:* Occupant of railway train or railway vehicle injured due to collision with military vehicle (V81.83)
- X+7th **V81.2** Occupant of railway train or railway vehicle injured in collision with or hit by rolling stock
- X+7th **V81.3** Occupant of railway train or railway vehicle injured in collision with other object
  - Railway collision NOS
- X+7th **V81.4** Person injured while boarding or alighting from railway train or railway vehicle
- X+7th **V81.5** Occupant of railway train or railway vehicle injured by fall in railway train or railway vehicle
- X+7th **V81.6** Occupant of railway train or railway vehicle injured by fall from railway train or railway vehicle
- X+7th **V81.7** Occupant of railway train or railway vehicle injured in derailment without antecedent collision
+ **V81.8** Occupant of railway train or railway vehicle injured in other specified railway accidents
  - X+7th **V81.81** Occupant of railway train or railway vehicle injured due to explosion or fire on train
  - X+7th **V81.82** Occupant of railway train or railway vehicle injured due to object falling onto train
    - Occupant of railway train or railway vehicle injured due to falling earth onto train
    - Occupant of railway train or railway vehicle injured due to falling rocks onto train
    - Occupant of railway train or railway vehicle injured due to falling snow onto train
    - Occupant of railway train or railway vehicle injured due to falling trees onto train
  - X+7th **V81.83** Occupant of railway train or railway vehicle injured due to collision with military vehicle
  - X+7th **V81.89** Occupant of railway train or railway vehicle injured due to other specified railway accident

1258

X+7th V81.9 Occupant of railway train or railway vehicle injured in unspecified railway accident
  Railway accident NOS

V82 Occupant of powered streetcar injured in transport accident

  Includes: interurban electric car
  person on outside of streetcar
  tram (car)
  trolley (car)

  Excludes1: bus (V70-V79)
  motorcoach (V70-V79)
  nonpowered streetcar (V76.-)
  train (V81.-)

  The appropriate 7th character is to be added to each code from category V82
  A initial encounter
  D subsequent encounter
  S sequela

X+7th V82.0 Occupant of streetcar injured in collision with motor vehicle in nontraffic accident
X+7th V82.1 Occupant of streetcar injured in collision with motor vehicle in traffic accident
X+7th V82.2 Occupant of streetcar injured in collision with or hit by rolling stock
X+7th V82.3 Occupant of streetcar injured in collision with other object
  Excludes1: collision with animal-drawn vehicle or animal being ridden (V82.8)
X+7th V82.4 Person injured while boarding or alighting from streetcar
X+7th V82.5 Occupant of streetcar injured by fall in streetcar
  Excludes1: fall in streetcar:
  while boarding or alighting (V82.4)
  with antecedent collision (V82.0-V82.3)
X+7th V82.6 Occupant of streetcar injured by fall from streetcar
  Excludes1: fall from streetcar:
  while boarding or alighting (V82.4)
  with antecedent collision (V82.0-V82.3)
X+7th V82.7 Occupant of streetcar injured in derailment without antecedent collision
  Excludes1: occupant of streetcar injured in derailment with antecedent collision (V82.0-V82.3)
X+7th V82.8 Occupant of streetcar injured in other specified transport accidents
  Streetcar collision with military vehicle
  Streetcar collision with train or nonmotor vehicles
X+7th V82.9 Occupant of streetcar injured in unspecified traffic accident
  Streetcar accident NOS

V83 Occupant of special vehicle mainly used on industrial premises injured in transport accident

  Includes: battery-powered airport passenger vehicle
  battery-powered truck (baggage) (mail)
  coal-car in mine
  forklift (truck)
  logging car
  self-propelled industrial truck
  station baggage truck (powered)
  tram, truck, or tub (powered) in mine or quarry

  Excludes1: special construction vehicles (V85.-)
  special industrial vehicle in stationary use or maintenance (W31.-)

  The appropriate 7th character is to be added to each code from category V83
  A initial encounter
  D subsequent encounter
  S sequela

X+7th V83.0 Driver of special industrial vehicle injured in traffic accident
X+7th V83.1 Passenger of special industrial vehicle injured in traffic accident
X+7th V83.2 Person on outside of special industrial vehicle injured in traffic accident
X+7th V83.3 Unspecified occupant of special industrial vehicle injured in traffic accident
X+7th V83.4 Person injured while boarding or alighting from special industrial vehicle
X+7th V83.5 Driver of special industrial vehicle injured in nontraffic accident
X+7th V83.6 Passenger of special industrial vehicle injured in nontraffic accident
X+7th V83.7 Person on outside of special industrial vehicle injured in nontraffic accident
X+7th V83.9 Unspecified occupant of special industrial vehicle injured in nontraffic accident
  Special-industrial-vehicle accident NOS

V84 Occupant of special vehicle mainly used in agriculture injured in transport accident

  Includes: self-propelled farm machinery
  tractor (and trailer)

  Excludes1: animal-powered farm machinery accident (W30.8-)
  contact with combine harvester (W30.0)
  special agricultural vehicle in stationary use or maintenance (W30.-)

  The appropriate 7th character is to be added to each code from category V84
  A initial encounter
  D subsequent encounter
  S sequela

X+7th V84.0 Driver of special agricultural vehicle injured in traffic accident
X+7th V84.1 Passenger of special agricultural vehicle injured in traffic accident
X+7th V84.2 Person on outside of special agricultural vehicle injured in traffic accident
X+7th V84.3 Unspecified occupant of special agricultural vehicle injured in traffic accident
X+7th V84.4 Person injured while boarding or alighting from special agricultural vehicle
X+7th V84.5 Driver of special agricultural vehicle injured in nontraffic accident
X+7th V84.6 Passenger of special agricultural vehicle injured in nontraffic accident
X+7th V84.7 Person on outside of special agricultural vehicle injured in nontraffic accident
X+7th V84.9 Unspecified occupant of special agricultural vehicle injured in nontraffic accident
  Special-agricultural vehicle accident NOS

V85 Occupant of special construction vehicle injured in transport accident

  Includes: bulldozer
  digger
  dump truck
  earth-leveller
  mechanical shovel
  road-roller

  Excludes1: special industrial vehicle (V83.-)
  special construction vehicle in stationary use or maintenance (W31.-)

  The appropriate 7th character is to be added to each code from category V85
  A initial encounter
  D subsequent encounter
  S sequela

X+7th V85.0 Driver of special construction vehicle injured in traffic accident
X+7th V85.1 Passenger of special construction vehicle injured in traffic accident
X+7th V85.2 Person on outside of special construction vehicle injured in traffic accident
X+7th V85.3 Unspecified occupant of special construction vehicle injured in traffic accident
X+7th V85.4 Person injured while boarding or alighting from special construction vehicle
X+7th V85.5 Driver of special construction vehicle injured in nontraffic accident
X+7th V85.6 Passenger of special construction vehicle injured in nontraffic accident
X+7th V85.7 Person on outside of special construction vehicle injured in nontraffic accident
X+7th V85.9 Unspecified occupant of special construction vehicle injured in nontraffic accident
  Special-construction-vehicle accident NOS

V86 Occupant of special all-terrain or other off-road motor vehicle, injured in transport accident

  Excludes1: special all-terrain vehicle in stationary use or maintenance (W31.-)
  sport-utility vehicle (V50-V59)
  three-wheeled motor vehicle designed for on-road use (V30-V39)

  AHA CC: 4Q, 2017, 26

  The appropriate 7th character is to be added to each code from category V86
  A initial encounter
  D subsequent encounter
  S sequela

+ **V86.0 Driver of special all-terrain or other off-road motor vehicle injured in traffic accident**
  +7th **V86.01** Driver of ambulance or fire engine injured in traffic accident
  +7th **V86.02** Driver of snowmobile injured in traffic accident
  +7th **V86.03** Driver of dune buggy injured in traffic accident
  +7th **V86.04** Driver of military vehicle injured in traffic accident
  +7th **V86.05** Driver of 3- or 4- wheeled all-terrain vehicle (ATV) injured in traffic accident
  +7th **V86.06** Driver of dirt bike or motor/cross bike injured in traffic accident
  +7th **V86.09** Driver of other special all-terrain or other off-road motor vehicle injured in traffic accident
    Driver of go cart injured in traffic accident
    Driver of golf cart injured in traffic accident

+ **V86.1 Passenger of special all-terrain or other off-road motor vehicle injured in traffic accident**
  +7th **V86.11** Passenger of ambulance or fire engine injured in traffic accident
  +7th **V86.12** Passenger of snowmobile injured in traffic accident
  +7th **V86.13** Passenger of dune buggy injured in traffic accident
  +7th **V86.14** Passenger of military vehicle injured in traffic accident
  +7th **V86.15** Passenger of 3- or 4- wheeled all-terrain vehicle (ATV) injured in traffic accident
  +7th **V86.16** Passenger of dirt bike or motor/cross bike injured in traffic accident
  +7th **V86.19** Passenger of other special all-terrain or other off-road motor vehicle injured in traffic accident
    Passenger of go cart injured in traffic accident
    Passenger of golf cart injured in traffic accident

+ **V86.2 Person on outside of special all-terrain or other off-road motor vehicle injured in traffic accident**
  +7th **V86.21** Person on outside of ambulance or fire engine injured in traffic accident
  +7th **V86.22** Person on outside of snowmobile injured in traffic accident
  +7th **V86.23** Person on outside of dune buggy injured in traffic accident
  +7th **V86.24** Person on outside of military vehicle injured in traffic accident
  +7th **V86.25** Person on outside of 3- or 4- wheeled all-terrain vehicle (ATV) injured in traffic accident
  +7th **V86.26** Person on outside of dirt bike or motor/cross bike injured in traffic accident
  +7th **V86.29** Person on outside of other special all-terrain or other off-road motor vehicle injured in traffic accident
    Person on outside of go cart in traffic accident
    Person on outside of golf cart injured in traffic accident

+ **V86.3 Unspecified occupant of special all-terrain or other off-road motor vehicle injured in traffic accident**
  +7th **V86.31** Unspecified occupant of ambulance or fire engine injured in traffic accident
  +7th **V86.32** Unspecified occupant of snowmobile injured in traffic accident
  +7th **V86.33** Unspecified occupant of dune buggy injured in traffic accident
  +7th **V86.34** Unspecified occupant of military vehicle injured in traffic accident
  +7th **V86.35** Unspecified occupant of 3- or 4- wheeled all-terrain vehicle (ATV) injured in traffic accident
  +7th **V86.36** Unspecified occupant of dirt bike or motor/cross bike injured in traffic accident
  +7th **V86.39** Unspecified occupant of other special all-terrain or other off-road motor vehicle injured in traffic accident
    Unspecified occupant of go cart injured in traffic accident
    Unspecified occupant of golf cart injured in traffic accident

+ **V86.4 Person injured while boarding or alighting from special all-terrain or other off-road motor vehicle**
  +7th **V86.41** Person injured while boarding or alighting from ambulance or fire engine
  +7th **V86.42** Person injured while boarding or alighting from snowmobile
  +7th **V86.43** Person injured while boarding or alighting from dune buggy
  +7th **V86.44** Person injured while boarding or alighting from military vehicle
  +7th **V86.45** Person injured while boarding or alighting from a 3- or 4- wheeled all-terrain vehicle (ATV)
  +7th **V86.46** Person injured while boarding or alighting from a dirt bike or motor/cross bike
  +7th **V86.49** Person injured while boarding or alighting from other special all-terrain or other off-road motor vehicle
    Person injured while boarding or alighting from go cart
    Person injured while boarding or alighting from golf cart

+ **V86.5 Driver of special all-terrain or other off-road motor vehicle injured in nontraffic accident**
  +7th **V86.51** Driver of ambulance or fire engine injured in nontraffic accident
  +7th **V86.52** Driver of snowmobile injured in nontraffic accident
  +7th **V86.53** Driver of dune buggy injured in nontraffic accident
  +7th **V86.54** Driver of military vehicle injured in nontraffic accident
  +7th **V86.55** Driver of 3- or 4- wheeled all-terrain vehicle (ATV) injured in nontraffic accident
  +7th **V86.56** Driver of dirt bike or motor/cross bike injured in nontraffic accident, initial encounter
  +7th **V86.59** Driver of other special all-terrain or other off-road motor vehicle injured in nontraffic accident
    Driver of go cart injured in nontraffic accident
    Driver of golf cart injured in nontraffic accident

+ **V86.6 Passenger of special all-terrain or other off-road motor vehicle injured in nontraffic accident**
  +7th **V86.61** Passenger of ambulance or fire engine injured in nontraffic accident
  +7th **V86.62** Passenger of snowmobile injured in nontraffic accident
  +7th **V86.63** Passenger of dune buggy injured in nontraffic accident
  +7th **V86.64** Passenger of military vehicle injured in nontraffic accident
  +7th **V86.65** Passenger of 3- or 4- wheeled all-terrain vehicle (ATV) injured in nontraffic accident
  +7th **V86.66** Passenger of dirt bike or motor/cross bike injured in nontraffic accident
  +7th **V86.69** Passenger of other special all-terrain or other off-road motor vehicle injured in nontraffic accident
    Passenger of go cart injured in nontraffic accident
    Passenger of golf cart injured in nontraffic accident

+ **V86.7 Person on outside of special all-terrain or other off-road motor vehicle injured in nontraffic accident**
  +7th **V86.71** Person on outside of ambulance or fire engine injured in nontraffic accident
  +7th **V86.72** Person on outside of snowmobile injured in nontraffic accident
  +7th **V86.73** Person on outside of dune buggy injured in nontraffic accident
  +7th **V86.74** Person on outside of military vehicle injured in nontraffic accident
  +7th **V86.75** Person on outside of 3- or 4- wheeled all-terrain vehicle (ATV) injured in nontraffic accident
  +7th **V86.76** Person on outside of dirt bike or motor/cross bike injured in nontraffic accident

- **+7th V86.79** Person on outside of other special all-terrain or other off-road motor vehicles injured in nontraffic accident
  - Person on outside of go cart injured in nontraffic accident
  - Person on outside of golf cart injured in nontraffic accident
- **+ V86.9** Unspecified occupant of special all-terrain or other off-road motor vehicle injured in nontraffic accident
  - **+7th V86.91** Unspecified occupant of ambulance or fire engine injured in nontraffic accident
  - **+7th V86.92** Unspecified occupant of snowmobile injured in nontraffic accident
  - **+7th V86.93** Unspecified occupant of dune buggy injured in nontraffic accident
  - **+7th V86.94** Unspecified occupant of military vehicle injured in nontraffic accident
  - **+7th V86.95** Unspecified occupant of 3- or 4- wheeled all-terrain vehicle (ATV) injured in nontraffic accident
  - **+7th V86.96** Unspecified occupant of dirt bike or motor/cross bike injured in nontraffic accident
  - **+7th V86.99** Unspecified occupant of other special all-terrain or other off-road motor vehicle injured in nontraffic accident
    - Off-road motor-vehicle accident NOS
    - Other motor-vehicle accident NOS
    - Unspecified occupant of go cart injured in nontraffic accident
    - Unspecified occupant of golf cart injured in nontraffic accident

V87 Traffic accident of specified type but victim's mode of transport unknown

Excludes1: collision involving:
  pedal cycle (V10-V19)
  pedestrian (V01-V09)

The appropriate 7th character is to be added to each code from category V87
A initial encounter
D subsequent encounter
S sequela

- **X+7th V87.0** Person injured in collision between car and two- or three-wheeled powered vehicle (traffic)
- **X+7th V87.1** Person injured in collision between other motor vehicle and two- or three-wheeled motor vehicle (traffic)
- **X+7th V87.2** Person injured in collision between car and pick-up truck or van (traffic)
- **X+7th V87.3** Person injured in collision between car and bus (traffic)
- **X+7th V87.4** Person injured in collision between car and heavy transport vehicle (traffic)
- **X+7th V87.5** Person injured in collision between heavy transport vehicle and bus (traffic)
- **X+7th V87.6** Person injured in collision between railway train or railway vehicle and car (traffic)
- **X+7th V87.7** Person injured in collision between other specified motor vehicles (traffic)
- **X+7th V87.8** Person injured in other specified noncollision transport accidents involving motor vehicle (traffic)
- **X+7th V87.9** Person injured in other specified (collision)(noncollision) transport accidents involving nonmotor vehicle (traffic)

V88 Nontraffic accident of specified type but victim's mode of transport unknown

Excludes1: collision involving:
  pedal cycle (V10-V19)
  pedestrian (V01-V09)

The appropriate 7th character is to be added to each code from category V88
A initial encounter
D subsequent encounter
S sequela

- **X+7th V88.0** Person injured in collision between car and two- or three-wheeled motor vehicle, nontraffic
- **X+7th V88.1** Person injured in collision between other motor vehicle and two- or three-wheeled motor vehicle, nontraffic
- **X+7th V88.2** Person injured in collision between car and pick-up truck or van, nontraffic
- **X+7th V88.3** Person injured in collision between car and bus, nontraffic
- **X+7th V88.4** Person injured in collision between car and heavy transport vehicle, nontraffic
- **X+7th V88.5** Person injured in collision between heavy transport vehicle and bus, nontraffic
- **X+7th V88.6** Person injured in collision between railway train or railway vehicle and car, nontraffic
- **X+7th V88.7** Person injured in collision between other specified motor vehicle, nontraffic
- **X+7th V88.8** Person injured in other specified noncollision transport accidents involving motor vehicle, nontraffic
- **X+7th V88.9** Person injured in other specified (collision)(noncollision) transport accidents involving nonmotor vehicle, nontraffic

V89 Motor- or nonmotor-vehicle accident, type of vehicle unspecified

The appropriate 7th character is to be added to each code from category V89
A initial encounter
D subsequent encounter
S sequela

- **X+7th V89.0** Person injured in unspecified motor-vehicle accident, nontraffic
  - Motor-vehicle accident NOS, nontraffic
- **X+7th V89.1** Person injured in unspecified nonmotor-vehicle accident, nontraffic
  - Nonmotor-vehicle accident NOS (nontraffic)
- **X+7th V89.2** Person injured in unspecified motor-vehicle accident, traffic
  - Motor-vehicle accident [MVA] NOS
  - Road (traffic) accident [RTA] NOS
- **X+7th V89.3** Person injured in unspecified nonmotor-vehicle accident, traffic
  - Nonmotor-vehicle traffic accident NOS
- **X+7th V89.9** Person injured in unspecified vehicle accident
  - Collision NOS

Water transport accidents (V90-V94)

V90 Drowning and submersion due to accident to watercraft

Excludes1: civilian water transport accident involving military watercraft (V94.81-)
  fall into water not from watercraft (W16.-)
  military watercraft accident in military or war operations (Y36.0-, Y37.0-)
  water-transport-related drowning or submersion without accident to watercraft (V92.-)

The appropriate 7th character is to be added to each code from category V90
A initial encounter
D subsequent encounter
S sequela

- **+ V90.0** Drowning and submersion due to watercraft overturning
  - **X+7th V90.00** Drowning and submersion due to merchant ship overturning
  - **X+7th V90.01** Drowning and submersion due to passenger ship overturning
    - Drowning and submersion due to Ferry-boat overturning
    - Drowning and submersion due to Liner overturning
  - **X+7th V90.02** Drowning and submersion due to fishing boat overturning
  - **X+7th V90.03** Drowning and submersion due to other powered watercraft overturning
    - Drowning and submersion due to Hovercraft (on open water) overturning
    - Drowning and submersion due to Jet ski overturning
  - **X+7th V90.04** Drowning and submersion due to sailboat overturning
  - **X+7th V90.05** Drowning and submersion due to canoe or kayak overturning
  - **X+7th V90.06** Drowning and submersion due to (nonpowered) inflatable craft overturning
  - **X+7th V90.08** Drowning and submersion due to other unpowered watercraft overturning
    - Drowning and submersion due to windsurfer overturning

X+7th	V90.09	**Drowning and submersion due to unspecified watercraft overturning**
		Drowning and submersion due to boat NOS overturning
		Drowning and submersion due to ship NOS overturning
		Drowning and submersion due to watercraft NOS overturning
+	**V90.1**	**Drowning and submersion due to watercraft sinking**
X+7th	V90.10	**Drowning and submersion due to merchant ship sinking**
X+7th	V90.11	**Drowning and submersion due to passenger ship sinking**
		Drowning and submersion due to Ferry-boat sinking
		Drowning and submersion due to Liner sinking
X+7th	V90.12	**Drowning and submersion due to fishing boat sinking**
X+7th	V90.13	**Drowning and submersion due to other powered watercraft sinking**
		Drowning and submersion due to Hovercraft (on open water) sinking
		Drowning and submersion due to Jet ski sinking
X+7th	V90.14	**Drowning and submersion due to sailboat sinking**
X+7th	V90.15	**Drowning and submersion due to canoe or kayak sinking**
X+7th	V90.16	**Drowning and submersion due to (nonpowered) inflatable craft sinking**
X+7th	V90.18	**Drowning and submersion due to other unpowered watercraft sinking**
X+7th	V90.19	**Drowning and submersion due to unspecified watercraft sinking**
		Drowning and submersion due to boat NOS sinking
		Drowning and submersion due to ship NOS sinking
		Drowning and submersion due to watercraft NOS sinking
+	**V90.2**	**Drowning and submersion due to falling or jumping from burning watercraft**
X+7th	V90.20	**Drowning and submersion due to falling or jumping from burning merchant ship**
X+7th	V90.21	**Drowning and submersion due to falling or jumping from burning passenger ship**
		Drowning and submersion due to falling or jumping from burning Ferry-boat
		Drowning and submersion due to falling or jumping from burning Liner
X+7th	V90.22	**Drowning and submersion due to falling or jumping from burning fishing boat**
X+7th	V90.23	**Drowning and submersion due to falling or jumping from other burning powered watercraft**
		Drowning and submersion due to falling and jumping from burning Hovercraft (on open water)
		Drowning and submersion due to falling and jumping from burning Jet ski
X+7th	V90.24	**Drowning and submersion due to falling or jumping from burning sailboat**
X+7th	V90.25	**Drowning and submersion due to falling or jumping from burning canoe or kayak**
X+7th	V90.26	**Drowning and submersion due to falling or jumping from burning (nonpowered) inflatable craft**
X+7th	V90.27	**Drowning and submersion due to falling or jumping from burning water-skis**
X+7th	V90.28	**Drowning and submersion due to falling or jumping from other burning unpowered watercraft**
		Drowning and submersion due to falling and jumping from burning surf-board
		Drowning and submersion due to falling and jumping from burning windsurfer
X+7th	V90.29	**Drowning and submersion due to falling or jumping from unspecified burning watercraft**
		Drowning and submersion due to falling or jumping from burning boat NOS
		Drowning and submersion due to falling or jumping from burning ship NOS
		Drowning and submersion due to falling or jumping from burning watercraft NOS
+	**V90.3**	**Drowning and submersion due to falling or jumping from crushed watercraft**
X+7th	V90.30	**Drowning and submersion due to falling or jumping from crushed merchant ship**
X+7th	V90.31	**Drowning and submersion due to falling or jumping from crushed passenger ship**
		Drowning and submersion due to falling and jumping from crushed Ferry boat
		Drowning and submersion due to falling and jumping from crushed Liner
X+7th	V90.32	**Drowning and submersion due to falling or jumping from crushed fishing boat**
X+7th	V90.33	**Drowning and submersion due to falling or jumping from other crushed powered watercraft**
		Drowning and submersion due to falling and jumping from crushed Hovercraft
		Drowning and submersion due to falling and jumping from crushed Jet ski
X+7th	V90.34	**Drowning and submersion due to falling or jumping from crushed sailboat**
X+7th	V90.35	**Drowning and submersion due to falling or jumping from crushed canoe or kayak**
X+7th	V90.36	**Drowning and submersion due to falling or jumping from crushed (nonpowered) inflatable craft**
X+7th	V90.37	**Drowning and submersion due to falling or jumping from crushed water-skis**
X+7th	V90.38	**Drowning and submersion due to falling or jumping from other crushed unpowered watercraft**
		Drowning and submersion due to falling and jumping from crushed surf-board
		Drowning and submersion due to falling and jumping from crushed windsurfer
X+7th	V90.39	**Drowning and submersion due to falling or jumping from crushed unspecified watercraft**
		Drowning and submersion due to falling and jumping from crushed boat NOS
		Drowning and submersion due to falling and jumping from crushed ship NOS
		Drowning and submersion due to falling and jumping from crushed watercraft NOS
+	**V90.8**	**Drowning and submersion due to other accident to watercraft**
X+7th	V90.80	**Drowning and submersion due to other accident to merchant ship**
X+7th	V90.81	**Drowning and submersion due to other accident to passenger ship**
		Drowning and submersion due to other accident to Ferry-boat
		Drowning and submersion due to other accident to Liner
X+7th	V90.82	**Drowning and submersion due to other accident to fishing boat**
X+7th	V90.83	**Drowning and submersion due to other accident to other powered watercraft**
		Drowning and submersion due to other accident to Hovercraft (on open water)
		Drowning and submersion due to other accident to Jet ski
X+7th	V90.84	**Drowning and submersion due to other accident to sailboat**
X+7th	V90.85	**Drowning and submersion due to other accident to canoe or kayak**
X+7th	V90.86	**Drowning and submersion due to other accident to (nonpowered) inflatable craft**

X+7th	**V90.87**	**Drowning and submersion due to other accident to water-skis**
X+7th	**V90.88**	**Drowning and submersion due to other accident to other unpowered watercraft**

Drowning and submersion due to other accident to surf-board
Drowning and submersion due to other accident to windsurfer

X+7th	**V90.89**	**Drowning and submersion due to other accident to unspecified watercraft**

Drowning and submersion due to other accident to boat NOS
Drowning and submersion due to other accident to ship NOS
Drowning and submersion due to other accident to watercraft NOS

V91 Other injury due to accident to watercraft

Includes: any injury except drowning and submersion as a result of an accident to watercraft

Excludes1: civilian water transport accident involving military watercraft (V94.81-)
military watercraft accident in military or war operations (Y36, Y37.-)

Excludes2: drowning and submersion due to accident to watercraft (V90.-)

The appropriate 7th character is to be added to each code from category V91
- A initial encounter
- D subsequent encounter
- S sequela

+ **V91.0 Burn due to watercraft on fire**

Excludes1: burn from localized fire or explosion on board ship without accident to watercraft (V93.-)

X+7th	**V91.00**	**Burn due to merchant ship on fire**
X+7th	**V91.01**	**Burn due to passenger ship on fire**

Burn due to Ferry-boat on fire
Burn due to Liner on fire

X+7th	**V91.02**	**Burn due to fishing boat on fire**
X+7th	**V91.03**	**Burn due to other powered watercraft on fire**

Burn due to Hovercraft (on open water) on fire
Burn due to Jet ski on fire

X+7th	**V91.04**	**Burn due to sailboat on fire**
X+7th	**V91.05**	**Burn due to canoe or kayak on fire**
X+7th	**V91.06**	**Burn due to (nonpowered) inflatable craft on fire**
X+7th	**V91.07**	**Burn due to water-skis on fire**
X+7th	**V91.08**	**Burn due to other unpowered watercraft on fire**
X+7th	**V91.09**	**Burn due to unspecified watercraft on fire**

Burn due to boat NOS on fire
Burn due to ship NOS on fire
Burn due to watercraft NOS on fire

+ **V91.1 Crushed between watercraft and other watercraft or other object due to collision**

Crushed by lifeboat after abandoning ship in a collision

NOTE Select the specified type of watercraft that the victim was on at the time of the collision

X+7th	**V91.10**	**Crushed between merchant ship and other watercraft or other object due to collision**
X+7th	**V91.11**	**Crushed between passenger ship and other watercraft or other object due to collision**

Crushed between Ferry-boat and other watercraft or other object due to collision
Crushed between Liner and other watercraft or other object due to collision

X+7th	**V91.12**	**Crushed between fishing boat and other watercraft or other object due to collision**
X+7th	**V91.13**	**Crushed between other powered watercraft and other watercraft or other object due to collision**

Crushed between Hovercraft (on open water) and other watercraft or other object due to collision
Crushed between Jet ski and other watercraft or other object due to collision

X+7th	**V91.14**	**Crushed between sailboat and other watercraft or other object due to collision**
X+7th	**V91.15**	**Crushed between canoe or kayak and other watercraft or other object due to collision**
X+7th	**V91.16**	**Crushed between (nonpowered) inflatable craft and other watercraft or other object due to collision**
X+7th	**V91.18**	**Crushed between other unpowered watercraft and other watercraft or other object due to collision**

Crushed between surfboard and other watercraft or other object due to collision
Crushed between windsurfer and other watercraft or other object due to collision

X+7th	**V91.19**	**Crushed between unspecified watercraft and other watercraft or other object due to collision**

Crushed between boat NOS and other watercraft or other object due to collision
Crushed between ship NOS and other watercraft or other object due to collision
Crushed between watercraft NOS and other watercraft or other object due to collision

+ **V91.2 Fall due to collision between watercraft and other watercraft or other object**

Fall while remaining on watercraft after collision

NOTE Select the specified type of watercraft that the victim was on at the time of the collision

Excludes1: crushed between watercraft and other watercraft and other object due to collision (V91.1-)
drowning and submersion due to falling from crushed watercraft (V90.3-)

X+7th	**V91.20**	**Fall due to collision between merchant ship and other watercraft or other object**
X+7th	**V91.21**	**Fall due to collision between passenger ship and other watercraft or other object**

Fall due to collision between Ferry-boat and other watercraft or other object
Fall due to collision between Liner and other watercraft or other object

X+7th	**V91.22**	**Fall due to collision between fishing boat and other watercraft or other object**
X+7th	**V91.23**	**Fall due to collision between other powered watercraft and other watercraft or other object**

Fall due to collision between Hovercraft (on open water) and other watercraft or other object
Fall due to collision between Jet ski and other watercraft or other object

X+7th	**V91.24**	**Fall due to collision between sailboat and other watercraft or other object**
X+7th	**V91.25**	**Fall due to collision between canoe or kayak and other watercraft or other object**
X+7th	**V91.26**	**Fall due to collision between (nonpowered) inflatable craft and other watercraft or other object**
X+7th	**V91.29**	**Fall due to collision between unspecified watercraft and other watercraft or other object**

Fall due to collision between boat NOS and other watercraft or other object
Fall due to collision between ship NOS and other watercraft or other object
Fall due to collision between watercraft NOS and other watercraft or other object

+ **V91.3 Hit or struck by falling object due to accident to watercraft**

Hit or struck by falling object (part of damaged watercraft or other object) after falling or jumping from damaged watercraft

Excludes2: drowning or submersion due to fall or jumping from damaged watercraft (V90.2-, V90.3-)

X+7th	**V91.30**	**Hit or struck by falling object due to accident to merchant ship**
X+7th	**V91.31**	**Hit or struck by falling object due to accident to passenger ship**

Hit or struck by falling object due to accident to Ferry-boat
Hit or struck by falling object due to accident to Liner

X+7th	**V91.32**	**Hit or struck by falling object due to accident to fishing boat**
X+7th	**V91.33**	**Hit or struck by falling object due to accident to other powered watercraft**

Hit or struck by falling object due to accident to Hovercraft (on open water)
Hit or struck by falling object due to accident to Jet ski

X+7th	**V91.34**	**Hit or struck by falling object due to accident to sailboat**

X+7th V91.35 Hit or struck by falling object due to accident to canoe or kayak

X+7th V91.36 Hit or struck by falling object due to accident to (nonpowered) inflatable craft

X+7th V91.37 Hit or struck by falling object due to accident to water-skis
> Hit by water-skis after jumping off of waterskis

X+7th V91.38 Hit or struck by falling object due to accident to other unpowered watercraft
> Hit or struck by surf-board after falling off damaged surf-board
> Hit or struck by object after falling off damaged windsurfer

X+7th V91.39 Hit or struck by falling object due to accident to unspecified watercraft
> Hit or struck by falling object due to accident to boat NOS
> Hit or struck by falling object due to accident to ship NOS
> Hit or struck by falling object due to accident to watercraft NOS

+ V91.8 Other injury due to other accident to watercraft

X+7th V91.80 Other injury due to other accident to merchant ship

X+7th V91.81 Other injury due to other accident to passenger ship
> Other injury due to other accident to Ferry-boat
> Other injury due to other accident to Liner

X+7th V91.82 Other injury due to other accident to fishing boat

X+7th V91.83 Other injury due to other accident to other powered watercraft
> Other injury due to other accident to Hovercraft (on open water)
> Other injury due to other accident to Jet ski

X+7th V91.84 Other injury due to other accident to sailboat

X+7th V91.85 Other injury due to other accident to canoe or kayak

X+7th V91.86 Other injury due to other accident to (nonpowered) inflatable craft

X+7th V91.87 Other injury due to other accident to water-skis

X+7th V91.88 Other injury due to other accident to other unpowered watercraft
> Other injury due to other accident to surf-board
> Other injury due to other accident to windsurfer

X+7th V91.89 Other injury due to other accident to unspecified watercraft
> Other injury due to other accident to boat NOS
> Other injury due to other accident to ship NOS
> Other injury due to other accident to watercraft NOS

V92 Drowning and submersion due to accident on board watercraft, without accident to watercraft

> **Excludes1:** civilian water transport accident involving military watercraft (V94.81-)
> drowning or submersion due to accident to watercraft (V90-V91)
> drowning or submersion of diver who voluntarily jumps from boat not involved in an accident (W16.711, W16.721)
> fall into water without watercraft (W16.-)
> military watercraft accident in military or war operations (Y36, Y37)

> The appropriate 7th character is to be added to each code from category V92
> A initial encounter
> D subsequent encounter
> S sequela

+ V92.0 Drowning and submersion due to fall off watercraft
> Drowning and submersion due to fall from gangplank of watercraft
> Drowning and submersion due to fall overboard watercraft
> **Excludes2:** hitting head on object or bottom of body of water due to fall from watercraft (V94.0-)

X+7th V92.00 Drowning and submersion due to fall off merchant ship

X+7th V92.01 Drowning and submersion due to fall off passenger ship
> Drowning and submersion due to fall off Ferry-boat
> Drowning and submersion due to fall off Liner

X+7th V92.02 Drowning and submersion due to fall off fishing boat

X+7th V92.03 Drowning and submersion due to fall off other powered watercraft
> Drowning and submersion due to fall off Hovercraft (on open water)
> Drowning and submersion due to fall off Jet ski

X+7th V92.04 Drowning and submersion due to fall off sailboat

X+7th V92.05 Drowning and submersion due to fall off canoe or kayak

X+7th V92.06 Drowning and submersion due to fall off (nonpowered) inflatable craft

X+7th V92.07 Drowning and submersion due to fall off water-skis
> **Excludes1:** drowning and submersion due to falling off burning water-skis (V90.27)
> drowning and submersion due to falling off crushed water-skis (V90.37)
> hit by boat while water-skiing NOS (V94.-)

X+7th V92.08 Drowning and submersion due to fall off other unpowered watercraft
> Drowning and submersion due to fall off surf-board
> Drowning and submersion due to fall off windsurfer
> **Excludes1:** drowning and submersion due to fall off burning unpowered watercraft (V90.28)
> drowning and submersion due to fall off crushed unpowered watercraft (V90.38)
> drowning and submersion due to fall off damaged unpowered watercraft (V90.88)
> drowning and submersion due to rider of nonpowered watercraft being hit by other watercraft (V94.-)
> other injury due to rider of nonpowered watercraft being hit by other watercraft (V94.-)

X+7th V92.09 Drowning and submersion due to fall off unspecified watercraft
> Drowning and submersion due to fall off boat NOS
> Drowning and submersion due to fall off ship
> Drowning and submersion due to fall off watercraft NOS

+ V92.1 Drowning and submersion due to being thrown overboard by motion of watercraft
> **Excludes1:** drowning and submersion due to fall off surf-board (V92.08)
> drowning and submersion due to fall off water-skis (V92.07)
> drowning and submersion due to fall off windsurfer (V92.08)

X+7th V92.10 Drowning and submersion due to being thrown overboard by motion of merchant ship

X+7th V92.11 Drowning and submersion due to being thrown overboard by motion of passenger ship
> Drowning and submersion due to being thrown overboard by motion of Ferry-boat
> Drowning and submersion due to being thrown overboard by motion of Liner

X+7th V92.12 Drowning and submersion due to being thrown overboard by motion of fishing boat

X+7th V92.13 Drowning and submersion due to being thrown overboard by motion of other powered watercraft
> Drowning and submersion due to being thrown overboard by motion of Hovercraft

X+7th V92.14 Drowning and submersion due to being thrown overboard by motion of sailboat

X+7th V92.15 Drowning and submersion due to being thrown overboard by motion of canoe or kayak

X+7th V92.16 Drowning and submersion due to being thrown overboard by motion of (nonpowered) inflatable craft

X+7th V92.19 Drowning and submersion due to being thrown overboard by motion of unspecified watercraft
    Drowning and submersion due to being thrown overboard by motion of boat NOS
    Drowning and submersion due to being thrown overboard by motion of ship NOS
    Drowning and submersion due to being thrown overboard by motion of watercraft NOS

+ V92.2 Drowning and submersion due to being washed overboard from watercraft
    Code first any associated cataclysm (X37.0-)

X+7th V92.20 Drowning and submersion due to being washed overboard from merchant ship

X+7th V92.21 Drowning and submersion due to being washed overboard from passenger ship
    Drowning and submersion due to being washed overboard from Ferry-boat
    Drowning and submersion due to being washed overboard from Liner

X+7th V92.22 Drowning and submersion due to being washed overboard from fishing boat

X+7th V92.23 Drowning and submersion due to being washed overboard from other powered watercraft
    Drowning and submersion due to being washed overboard from Hovercraft (on open water)
    Drowning and submersion due to being washed overboard from Jet ski

X+7th V92.24 Drowning and submersion due to being washed overboard from sailboat

X+7th V92.25 Drowning and submersion due to being washed overboard from canoe or kayak

X+7th V92.26 Drowning and submersion due to being washed overboard from (nonpowered) inflatable craft

X+7th V92.27 Drowning and submersion due to being washed overboard from water-skis
    Excludes1: *drowning and submersion due to fall off water-skis (V92.07)*

X+7th V92.28 Drowning and submersion due to being washed overboard from other unpowered watercraft
    Drowning and submersion due to being washed overboard from surf-board
    Drowning and submersion due to being washed overboard from windsurfer

X+7th V92.29 Drowning and submersion due to being washed overboard from unspecified watercraft
    Drowning and submersion due to being washed overboard from boat NOS
    Drowning and submersion due to being washed overboard from ship NOS
    Drowning and submersion due to being washed overboard from watercraft NOS

V93 Other injury due to accident on board watercraft, without accident to watercraft
    Excludes1: *civilian water transport accident involving military watercraft (V94.81-)*
    other injury due to accident to watercraft (V91.-)
    military watercraft accident in military or war operations (Y36, Y37.-)
    Excludes2: *drowning and submersion due to accident on board watercraft, without accident to watercraft (V92.-)*

> The appropriate 7th character is to be added to each code from category V93
> A initial encounter
> D subsequent encounter
> S sequela

+ V93.0 Burn due to localized fire on board watercraft
    Excludes1: *burn due to watercraft on fire (V91.0-)*

X+7th V93.00 Burn due to localized fire on board merchant vessel

X+7th V93.01 Burn due to localized fire on board passenger vessel
    Burn due to localized fire on board Ferry-boat
    Burn due to localized fire on board Liner

X+7th V93.02 Burn due to localized fire on board fishing boat

X+7th V93.03 Burn due to localized fire on board other powered watercraft
    Burn due to localized fire on board Hovercraft
    Burn due to localized fire on board Jet ski

X+7th V93.04 Burn due to localized fire on board sailboat

X+7th V93.09 Burn due to localized fire on board unspecified watercraft
    Burn due to localized fire on board boat NOS
    Burn due to localized fire on board ship NOS
    Burn due to localized fire on board watercraft NOS

+ V93.1 Other burn on board watercraft
    Burn due to source other than fire on board watercraft
    Excludes1: *burn due to watercraft on fire (V91.0-)*

X+7th V93.10 Other burn on board merchant vessel

X+7th V93.11 Other burn on board passenger vessel
    Other burn on board Ferry-boat
    Other burn on board Liner

X+7th V93.12 Other burn on board fishing boat

X+7th V93.13 Other burn on board other powered watercraft
    Other burn on board Hovercraft
    Other burn on board Jet ski

X+7th V93.14 Other burn on board sailboat

X+7th V93.19 Other burn on board unspecified watercraft
    Other burn on board boat NOS
    Other burn on board ship NOS
    Other burn on board watercraft NOS

+ V93.2 Heat exposure on board watercraft
    Excludes1: *exposure to man-made heat not aboard watercraft (W92)*
    exposure to natural heat while on board watercraft (X30)
    exposure to sunlight while on board watercraft (X32)
    Excludes2: *burn due to fire on board watercraft (V93.0-)*

X+7th V93.20 Heat exposure on board merchant ship

X+7th V93.21 Heat exposure on board passenger ship
    Heat exposure on board Ferry-boat
    Heat exposure on board Liner

X+7th V93.22 Heat exposure on board fishing boat

X+7th V93.23 Heat exposure on board other powered watercraft
    Heat exposure on board hovercraft

X+7th V93.24 Heat exposure on board sailboat

X+7th V93.29 Heat exposure on board unspecified watercraft
    Heat exposure on board boat NOS
    Heat exposure on board ship NOS
    Heat exposure on board watercraft NOS

+ V93.3 Fall on board watercraft
    Excludes1: *fall due to collision of watercraft (V91.2-)*

X+7th V93.30 Fall on board merchant ship

X+7th V93.31 Fall on board passenger ship
    Fall on board Ferry-boat
    Fall on board Liner

X+7th V93.32 Fall on board fishing boat

X+7th V93.33 Fall on board other powered watercraft
    Fall on board Hovercraft (on open water)
    Fall on board Jet ski

X+7th V93.34 Fall on board sailboat

X+7th V93.35 Fall on board canoe or kayak

X+7th V93.36 Fall on board (nonpowered) inflatable craft

X+7th V93.38 Fall on board other unpowered watercraft

X+7th V93.39 Fall on board unspecified watercraft
    Fall on board boat NOS
    Fall on board ship NOS
    Fall on board watercraft NOS

+ V93.4 Struck by falling object on board watercraft
    Hit by falling object on board watercraft
    Excludes1: *struck by falling object due to accident to watercraft (V91.3)*

X+7th V93.40 Struck by falling object on merchant ship

X+7th V93.41 Struck by falling object on passenger ship
    Struck by falling object on Ferry-boat
    Struck by falling object on Liner

X+7th V93.42 Struck by falling object on fishing boat

X+7th V93.43 Struck by falling object on other powered watercraft
    Struck by falling object on Hovercraft

X+7th V93.44 Struck by falling object on sailboat

X+7th V93.48 Struck by falling object on other unpowered watercraft

X+7th V93.49 Struck by falling object on unspecified watercraft

+ V93.5 Explosion on board watercraft
    Boiler explosion on steamship
    Excludes2: *fire on board watercraft (V93.0-)*

X+7th	V93.50	Explosion on board merchant ship
X+7th	V93.51	Explosion on board passenger ship
		Explosion on board Ferry-boat
		Explosion on board Liner
X+7th	V93.52	Explosion on board fishing boat
X+7th	V93.53	Explosion on board other powered watercraft
		Explosion on board Hovercraft
		Explosion on board Jet ski
X+7th	V93.54	Explosion on board sailboat
X+7th	V93.59	Explosion on board unspecified watercraft
		Explosion on board boat NOS
		Explosion on board ship NOS
		Explosion on board watercraft NOS
+	V93.6	**Machinery accident on board watercraft**

Excludes1: machinery explosion on board watercraft (V93.4-)
machinery fire on board watercraft (V93.0-)

X+7th	V93.60	Machinery accident on board merchant ship
X+7th	V93.61	Machinery accident on board passenger ship
		Machinery accident on board Ferry-boat
		Machinery accident on board Liner
X+7th	V93.62	Machinery accident on board fishing boat
X+7th	V93.63	Machinery accident on board other powered watercraft
		Machinery accident on board Hovercraft
X+7th	V93.64	Machinery accident on board sailboat
X+7th	V93.69	Machinery accident on board unspecified watercraft
		Machinery accident on board boat NOS
		Machinery accident on board ship NOS
		Machinery accident on board watercraft NOS
+	V93.8	**Other injury due to other accident on board watercraft**
		Accidental poisoning by gases or fumes on watercraft
X+7th	V93.80	Other injury due to other accident on board merchant ship
X+7th	V93.81	Other injury due to other accident on board passenger ship
		Other injury due to other accident on board Ferry-boat
		Other injury due to other accident on board Liner
X+7th	V93.82	Other injury due to other accident on board fishing boat
X+7th	V93.83	Other injury due to other accident on board other powered watercraft
		Other injury due to other accident on board Hovercraft
		Other injury due to other accident on board Jet ski
X+7th	V93.84	Other injury due to other accident on board sailboat
X+7th	V93.85	Other injury due to other accident on board canoe or kayak
X+7th	V93.86	Other injury due to other accident on board (nonpowered) inflatable craft
X+7th	V93.87	Other injury due to other accident on board water-skis
		Hit or struck by object while waterskiing
X+7th	V93.88	Other injury due to other accident on board other unpowered watercraft
		Hit or struck by object while surfing
		Hit or struck by object while on board windsurfer
X+7th	V93.89	Other injury due to other accident on board unspecified watercraft
		Other injury due to other accident on board boat NOS
		Other injury due to other accident on board ship NOS
		Other injury due to other accident on board watercraft NOS

V94 Other and unspecified water transport accidents

Excludes1: military watercraft accidents in military or war operations (Y36, Y37)

The appropriate 7th character is to be added to each code from category V94
A initial encounter
D subsequent encounter
S sequela

X+7th	V94.0	**Hitting object or bottom of body of water due to fall from watercraft**

Excludes2: drowning and submersion due to fall from watercraft (V92.0-)

+	V94.1	**Bather struck by watercraft**
		Swimmer hit by watercraft
X+7th	V94.11	Bather struck by powered watercraft
X+7th	V94.12	Bather struck by nonpowered watercraft
+	V94.2	**Rider of nonpowered watercraft struck by other watercraft**
X+7th	V94.21	Rider of nonpowered watercraft struck by other nonpowered watercraft
		Canoer hit by other nonpowered watercraft
		Surfer hit by other nonpowered watercraft
		Windsurfer hit by other nonpowered watercraft
X+7th	V94.22	Rider of nonpowered watercraft struck by powered watercraft
		Canoer hit by motorboat
		Surfer hit by motorboat
		Windsurfer hit by motorboat
+	V94.3	**Injury to rider of (inflatable) watercraft being pulled behind other watercraft**
X+7th	V94.31	Injury to rider of (inflatable) recreational watercraft being pulled behind other watercraft
		Injury to rider of inner-tube pulled behind motor boat
X+7th	V94.32	Injury to rider of non-recreational watercraft being pulled behind other watercraft
		Injury to occupant of dingy being pulled behind boat or ship
		Injury to occupant of life-raft being pulled behind boat or ship
X+7th	V94.4	**Injury to barefoot water-skier**
		Injury to person being pulled behind boat or ship
+	V94.8	**Other water transport accident**
+	V94.81	Water transport accident involving military watercraft
+7th	V94.810	Civilian watercraft involved in water transport accident with military watercraft
		Passenger on civilian watercraft injured due to accident with military watercraft
+7th	V94.811	Civilian in water injured by military watercraft
+7th	V94.818	Other water transport accident involving military watercraft
X+7th	V94.89	Other water transport accident
X+7th	V94.9	**Unspecified water transport accident**
		Water transport accident NOS

Air and space transport accidents (V95-V97)

Excludes1: military aircraft accidents in military or war operations (Y36, Y37.-)

V95 Accident to powered aircraft causing injury to occupant

The appropriate 7th character is to be added to each code from category V95
A initial encounter
D subsequent encounter
S sequela

+	V95.0	**Helicopter accident injuring occupant**
X+7th	V95.00	Unspecified helicopter accident injuring occupant
X+7th	V95.01	Helicopter crash injuring occupant
X+7th	V95.02	Forced landing of helicopter injuring occupant
X+7th	V95.03	Helicopter collision injuring occupant
		Helicopter collision with any object, fixed, movable or moving
X+7th	V95.04	Helicopter fire injuring occupant
X+7th	V95.05	Helicopter explosion injuring occupant
X+7th	V95.09	Other helicopter accident injuring occupant
+	V95.1	**Ultralight, microlight or powered-glider accident injuring occupant**
X+7th	V95.10	Unspecified ultralight, microlight or powered-glider accident injuring occupant
X+7th	V95.11	Ultralight, microlight or powered-glider crash injuring occupant
X+7th	V95.12	Forced landing of ultralight, microlight or powered-glider injuring occupant
X+7th	V95.13	Ultralight, microlight or powered-glider collision injuring occupant
		Ultralight, microlight or powered-glider collision with any object, fixed, movable or moving
X+7th	V95.14	Ultralight, microlight or powered-glider fire injuring occupant

- X+7th V95.15 Ultralight, microlight or powered-glider explosion injuring occupant
- X+7th V95.19 Other ultralight, microlight or powered-glider accident injuring occupant
- + V95.2 Other private fixed-wing aircraft accident injuring occupant
  - X+7th V95.20 Unspecified accident to other private fixed-wing aircraft, injuring occupant
  - X+7th V95.21 Other private fixed-wing aircraft crash injuring occupant
  - X+7th V95.22 Forced landing of other private fixed-wing aircraft injuring occupant
  - X+7th V95.23 Other private fixed-wing aircraft collision injuring occupant
    - Other private fixed-wing aircraft collision with any object, fixed, movable or moving
  - X+7th V95.24 Other private fixed-wing aircraft fire injuring occupant
  - X+7th V95.25 Other private fixed-wing aircraft explosion injuring occupant
  - X+7th V95.29 Other accident to other private fixed-wing aircraft injuring occupant
- + V95.3 Commercial fixed-wing aircraft accident injuring occupant
  - X+7th V95.30 Unspecified accident to commercial fixed-wing aircraft injuring occupant
  - X+7th V95.31 Commercial fixed-wing aircraft crash injuring occupant
  - X+7th V95.32 Forced landing of commercial fixed-wing aircraft injuring occupant
  - X+7th V95.33 Commercial fixed-wing aircraft collision injuring occupant
    - Commercial fixed-wing aircraft collision with any object, fixed, movable or moving
  - X+7th V95.34 Commercial fixed-wing aircraft fire injuring occupant
  - X+7th V95.35 Commercial fixed-wing aircraft explosion injuring occupant
  - X+7th V95.39 Other accident to commercial fixed-wing aircraft injuring occupant
- + V95.4 Spacecraft accident injuring occupant
  - X+7th V95.40 Unspecified spacecraft accident injuring occupant
  - X+7th V95.41 Spacecraft crash injuring occupant
  - X+7th V95.42 Forced landing of spacecraft injuring occupant
  - X+7th V95.43 Spacecraft collision injuring occupant
    - Spacecraft collision with any object, fixed, moveable or moving
  - X+7th V95.44 Spacecraft fire injuring occupant
  - X+7th V95.45 Spacecraft explosion injuring occupant
  - X+7th V95.49 Other spacecraft accident injuring occupant
- X+7th V95.8 Other powered aircraft accidents injuring occupant
- X+7th V95.9 Unspecified aircraft accident injuring occupant
  - Aircraft accident NOS
  - Air transport accident NOS

V96 Accident to nonpowered aircraft causing injury to occupant

> The appropriate 7th character is to be added to each code from category V96
> A initial encounter
> D subsequent encounter
> S sequela

- + V96.0 Balloon accident injuring occupant
  - X+7th V96.00 Unspecified balloon accident injuring occupant
  - X+7th V96.01 Balloon crash injuring occupant
  - X+7th V96.02 Forced landing of balloon injuring occupant
  - X+7th V96.03 Balloon collision injuring occupant
    - Balloon collision with any object, fixed, moveable or moving
  - X+7th V96.04 Balloon fire injuring occupant
  - X+7th V96.05 Balloon explosion injuring occupant
  - X+7th V96.09 Other balloon accident injuring occupant
- + V96.1 Hang-glider accident injuring occupant
  - X+7th V96.10 Unspecified hang-glider accident injuring occupant
  - X+7th V96.11 Hang-glider crash injuring occupant
  - X+7th V96.12 Forced landing of hang-glider injuring occupant
  - X+7th V96.13 Hang-glider collision injuring occupant
    - Hang-glider collision with any object, fixed, moveable or moving
  - X+7th V96.14 Hang-glider fire injuring occupant
  - X+7th V96.15 Hang-glider explosion injuring occupant
  - X+7th V96.19 Other hang-glider accident injuring occupant
- + V96.2 Glider (nonpowered) accident injuring occupant
  - X+7th V96.20 Unspecified glider (nonpowered) accident injuring occupant
  - X+7th V96.21 Glider (nonpowered) crash injuring occupant
  - X+7th V96.22 Forced landing of glider (nonpowered) injuring occupant
  - X+7th V96.23 Glider (nonpowered) collision injuring occupant
    - Glider (nonpowered) collision with any object, fixed, moveable or moving
  - X+7th V96.24 Glider (nonpowered) fire injuring occupant
  - V96.25 Glider (nonpowered) explosion injuring occupant
  - X+7th V96.29 Other glider (nonpowered) accident injuring occupant
- X+7th V96.8 Other nonpowered-aircraft accidents injuring occupant
  - Kite carrying a person accident injuring occupant
- X+7th V96.9 Unspecified nonpowered-aircraft accident injuring occupant
  - Nonpowered-aircraft accident NOS

V97 Other specified air transport accidents

> The appropriate 7th character is to be added to each code from category V97
> A initial encounter
> D subsequent encounter
> S sequela

- X+7th V97.0 Occupant of aircraft injured in other specified air transport accidents
  - Fall in, on or from aircraft in air transport accident
  - **Excludes1:** *accident while boarding or alighting aircraft (V97.1)*
- X+7th V97.1 Person injured while boarding or alighting from aircraft
- + V97.2 Parachutist accident
  - X+7th V97.21 Parachutist entangled in object
    - Parachutist landing in tree
  - X+7th V97.22 Parachutist injured on landing
  - X+7th V97.29 Other parachutist accident
- + V97.3 Person on ground injured in air transport accident
  - X+7th V97.31 Hit by object falling from aircraft
    - Hit by crashing aircraft
    - Injured by aircraft hitting house
    - Injured by aircraft hitting car
  - X+7th V97.32 Injured by rotating propeller
  - X+7th V97.33 Sucked into jet engine
  - X+7th V97.39 Other injury to person on ground due to air transport accident
- + V97.8 Other air transport accidents, not elsewhere classified
  - **Excludes1:** *aircraft accident NOS (V95.9)*
    exposure to changes in air pressure during ascent or descent (W94.-)
  - + V97.81 Air transport accident involving military aircraft
    - +7th V97.810 Civilian aircraft involved in air transport accident with military aircraft
      - Passenger in civilian aircraft injured due to accident with military aircraft
    - +7th V97.811 Civilian injured by military aircraft
    - +7th V97.818 Other air transport accident involving military aircraft
  - X+7th V97.89 Other air transport accidents, not elsewhere classified
    - Injury from machinery on aircraft

Other and unspecified transport accidents (V98-V99)

Excludes1: *vehicle accident, type of vehicle unspecified (V89.-)*

V98 Other specified transport accidents

> The appropriate 7th character is to be added to each code from category V98
> A initial encounter
> D subsequent encounter
> S sequela

- X+7th V98.0 Accident to, on or involving cable-car, not on rails
  - Caught or dragged by cable-car, not on rails
  - Fall or jump from cable-car, not on rails
  - Object thrown from or in cable-car, not on rails
- X+7th V98.1 Accident to, on or involving land-yacht
- X+7th V98.2 Accident to, on or involving ice yacht

X+7th	V98.3	Accident to, on or involving ski lift
		Accident to, on or involving ski chair-lift
		Accident to, on or involving ski-lift with gondola
X+7th	V98.8	Other specified transport accidents
	V99	Unspecified transport accident

X+7th
The appropriate 7th character is to be added to code V99
- A initial encounter
- D subsequent encounter
- S sequela

Other external causes of accidental injury (W00-X58)

Slipping, tripping, stumbling and falls (W00-W19)

Excludes1: assault involving a fall (Y01-Y02)
fall from animal (V80.-)
fall (in) (from) machinery (in operation) (W28-W31)
fall (in) (from) transport vehicle (V01-V99)
intentional self-harm involving a fall (X80-X81)

Excludes2: at risk for fall (history of fall) (Z91.81)
fall (in) (from) burning building (X00.-)
fall into fire (X00-X04, X08)

W00 Fall due to ice and snow

Includes: pedestrian on foot falling (slipping) on ice and snow
Excludes1: fall on (from) ice and snow involving pedestrian conveyance (V00.-)
fall from stairs and steps not due to ice and snow (W10.-)

The appropriate 7th character is to be added to each code from category W00
- A initial encounter
- D subsequent encounter
- S sequela

X+7th **W00.0** Fall on same level due to ice and snow
AHA CC: 2Q, 2016, 4-5
X+7th **W00.1** Fall from stairs and steps due to ice and snow
X+7th **W00.2** Other fall from one level to another due to ice and snow
X+7th **W00.9** Unspecified fall due to ice and snow

W01 Fall on same level from slipping, tripping and stumbling

Includes: fall on moving sidewalk
Excludes1: fall due to bumping (striking) against object (W18.0-)
fall in shower or bathtub (W18.2-)
fall on same level NOS (W18.30)
fall on same level from slipping, tripping and stumbling due to ice or snow (W00.0)
fall off or from toilet (W18.1-)
slipping, tripping and stumbling NOS (W18.40)
slipping, tripping and stumbling without falling (W18.4-)

The appropriate 7th character is to be added to each code from category W01
- A initial encounter
- D subsequent encounter
- S sequela

X+7th **W01.0** Fall on same level from slipping, tripping and stumbling without subsequent striking against object
Falling over animal

+ **W01.1** Fall on same level from slipping, tripping and stumbling with subsequent striking against object

X+7th **W01.10** Fall on same level from slipping, tripping and stumbling with subsequent striking against unspecified object

+ **W01.11** Fall on same level from slipping, tripping and stumbling with subsequent striking against sharp object

+7th **W01.110** Fall on same level from slipping, tripping and stumbling with subsequent striking against sharp glass

+7th **W01.111** Fall on same level from slipping, tripping and stumbling with subsequent striking against power tool or machine

+7th **W01.118** Fall on same level from slipping, tripping and stumbling with subsequent striking against other sharp object

+7th **W01.119** Fall on same level from slipping, tripping and stumbling with subsequent striking against unspecified sharp object

+ **W01.19** Fall on same level from slipping, tripping and stumbling with subsequent striking against other object

+7th **W01.190** Fall on same level from slipping, tripping and stumbling with subsequent striking against furniture
AHA CC: 1Q, 2021, 4-5

+7th **W01.198** Fall on same level from slipping, tripping and stumbling with subsequent striking against other object

W03 Other fall on same level due to collision with another person
X+7th
Fall due to non-transport collision with other person
Excludes1: collision with another person without fall (W51)
crushed or pushed by a crowd or human stampede (W52)
fall involving pedestrian conveyance (V00-V09)
fall due to ice or snow (W00)
fall on same level NOS (W18.30)
AHA CC: 4Q, 2012, 108; 1Q, 2015, 3-21

The appropriate 7th character is to be added to code W03
- A initial encounter
- D subsequent encounter
- S sequela

W04 Fall while being carried or supported by other persons
X+7th
Accidentally dropped while being carried

The appropriate 7th character is to be added to code W04
- A initial encounter
- D subsequent encounter
- S sequela

W05 Fall from non-movitng wheelchair, nonmotorized scooter and motorized mobility scooter

Excludes1: fall from moving wheelchair (powered) (V00.811)
fall from moving motorized mobility scooter (V00.831)
fall from nonmotorized scooter (V00.141)
AHA CC: 2Q, 2019, 27-28

The appropriate 7th character is to be added to each code from category W05
- A initial encounter
- D subsequent encounter
- S sequela

X+7th **W05.0** Fall from non-moving wheelchair
X+7th **W05.1** Fall from non-moving nonmotorized scooter
X+7th **W05.2** Fall from non-moving motorized mobility scooter

W06 Fall from bed
X+7th
The appropriate 7th character is to be added to code W06
- A initial encounter
- D subsequent encounter
- S sequela

AHA CC: 4Q, 2020, 33

W07 Fall from chair
X+7th
The appropriate 7th character is to be added to code W07
- A initial encounter
- D subsequent encounter
- S sequela

W08 Fall from other furniture
X+7th
Fall from stool

The appropriate 7th character is to be added to code W08
- A initial encounter
- D subsequent encounter
- S sequela

W09 Fall on and from playground equipment
Excludes1: fall involving recreational machinery (W31)

The appropriate 7th character is to be added to each code from category W09
- A initial encounter
- D subsequent encounter
- S sequela

X+7th **W09.0** Fall on or from playground slide
X+7th **W09.1** Fall from playground swing
X+7th **W09.2** Fall on or from jungle gym
X+7th **W09.8** Fall on or from other playground equipment

W10 Fall on and from stairs and steps

Excludes1: Fall from stairs and steps due to ice and snow (W00.1)

The appropriate 7th character is to be added to each code from category W10
- A initial encounter
- D subsequent encounter
- S sequela

- X+7th **W10.0** Fall (on)(from) escalator
- X+7th **W10.1** Fall (on)(from) sidewalk curb
- X+7th **W10.2** Fall (on)(from) incline
  Fall (on) (from) ramp
- X+7th **W10.8** Fall (on) (from) other stairs and steps
- X+7th **W10.9** Fall (on) (from) unspecified stairs and steps

W11 Fall on and from ladder
X+7th

The appropriate 7th character is to be added to code W11
- A initial encounter
- D subsequent encounter
- S sequela

W12 Fall on and from scaffolding
X+7th

The appropriate 7th character is to be added to code W12
- A initial encounter
- D subsequent encounter
- S sequela

W13 Fall from, out of or through building or structure

The appropriate 7th character is to be added to each code from category W13
- A initial encounter
- D subsequent encounter
- S sequela

- X+7th **W13.0** Fall from, out of or through balcony
  Fall from, out of or through railing
- X+7th **W13.1** Fall from, out of or through bridge
- X+7th **W13.2** Fall from, out of or through roof
- X+7th **W13.3** Fall through floor
- X+7th **W13.4** Fall from, out of or through window

  Excludes2: fall with subsequent striking against sharp glass (W01.110-)
- X+7th **W13.8** Fall from, out of or through other building or structure
  Fall from, out of or through viaduct
  Fall from, out of or through wall
  Fall from, out of or through flag-pole
- X+7th **W13.9** Fall from, out of or through building, not otherwise specified

  Excludes1: collapse of a building or structure (W20.-)
  fall or jump from burning building or structure (X00.-)

W14 Fall from tree
X+7th

The appropriate 7th character is to be added to code W14
- A initial encounter
- D subsequent encounter
- S sequela

W15 Fall from cliff
X+7th

The appropriate 7th character is to be added to code W15
- A initial encounter
- D subsequent encounter
- S sequela

W16 Fall, jump or diving into water

Excludes1: accidental non-watercraft drowning and submersion not involving fall (W65-W74)
effects of air pressure from diving (W94.-)
fall into water from watercraft (V90-V94)
hitting an object or against bottom when falling from watercraft (V94.0)

Excludes2: striking or hitting diving board (W21.4)

The appropriate 7th character is to be added to each code from category W16
- A initial encounter
- D subsequent encounter
- S sequela

- + **W16.0** Fall into swimming pool
  Fall into swimming pool NOS
  Excludes1: fall into empty swimming pool (W17.3)
  - + **W16.01** Fall into swimming pool striking water surface
    - +7th **W16.011** Fall into swimming pool striking water surface causing drowning and submersion
      Excludes1: drowning and submersion while in swimming pool without fall (W67)
    - +7th **W16.012** Fall into swimming pool striking water surface causing other injury
  - + **W16.02** Fall into swimming pool striking bottom
    - +7th **W16.021** Fall into swimming pool striking bottom causing drowning and submersion
      Excludes1: drowning and submersion while in swimming pool without fall (W67)
    - +7th **W16.022** Fall into swimming pool striking bottom causing other injury
  - + **W16.03** Fall into swimming pool striking wall
    - +7th **W16.031** Fall into swimming pool striking wall causing drowning and submersion
      Excludes1: drowning and submersion while in swimming pool without fall (W67)
    - +7th **W16.032** Fall into swimming pool striking wall causing other injury
- + **W16.1** Fall into natural body of water
  Fall into lake
  Fall into open sea
  Fall into river
  Fall into stream
  - + **W16.11** Fall into natural body of water striking water surface
    - +7th **W16.111** Fall into natural body of water striking water surface causing drowning and submersion
      Excludes1: drowning and submersion while in natural body of water without fall (W69)
    - +7th **W16.112** Fall into natural body of water striking water surface causing other injury
  - + **W16.12** Fall into natural body of water striking bottom
    - +7th **W16.121** Fall into natural body of water striking bottom causing drowning and submersion
      Excludes1: drowning and submersion while in natural body of water without fall (W69)
    - +7th **W16.122** Fall into natural body of water striking bottom causing other injury
  - + **W16.13** Fall into natural body of water striking side
    - +7th **W16.131** Fall into natural body of water striking side causing drowning and submersion
      Excludes1: drowning and submersion while in natural body of water without fall (W69)
    - +7th **W16.132** Fall into natural body of water striking side causing other injury
- + **W16.2** Fall in (into) filled bathtub or bucket of water
  - + **W16.21** Fall in (into) filled bathtub
    Excludes1: fall into empty bathtub (W18.2)
    - +7th **W16.211** Fall in (into) filled bathtub causing drowning and submersion
      Excludes1: drowning and submersion while in filled bathtub without fall (W65)
    - +7th **W16.212** Fall in (into) filled bathtub causing other injury
  - + **W16.22** Fall in (into) bucket of water
    - +7th **W16.221** Fall in (into) bucket of water causing drowning and submersion
    - +7th **W16.222** Fall in (into) bucket of water causing other injury
- + **W16.3** Fall into other water
  Fall into fountain
  Fall into reservoir
  - + **W16.31** Fall into other water striking water surface
    - +7th **W16.311** Fall into other water striking water surface causing drowning and submersion
      Excludes1: drowning and submersion while in other water without fall (W73)
    - +7th **W16.312** Fall into other water striking water surface causing other injury

- **W16.32** Fall into other water striking bottom
  - +7th **W16.321** Fall into other water striking bottom causing drowning and submersion
    - *Excludes1:* *drowning and submersion while in other water without fall (W73)*
  - +7th **W16.322** Fall into other water striking bottom causing other injury
- **W16.33** Fall into other water striking wall
  - +7th **W16.331** Fall into other water striking wall causing drowning and submersion
    - *Excludes1:* *drowning and submersion while in other water without fall (W73)*
  - +7th **W16.332** Fall into other water striking wall causing other injury
- **W16.4** Fall into unspecified water
  - X+7th **W16.41** Fall into unspecified water causing drowning and submersion
  - X+7th **W16.42** Fall into unspecified water causing other injury
- **W16.5** Jumping or diving into swimming pool
  - **W16.51** Jumping or diving into swimming pool striking water surface
    - +7th **W16.511** Jumping or diving into swimming pool striking water surface causing drowning and submersion
      - *Excludes1:* *drowning and submersion while in swimming pool without jumping or diving (W67)*
    - +7th **W16.512** Jumping or diving into swimming pool striking water surface causing other injury
  - **W16.52** Jumping or diving into swimming pool striking bottom
    - +7th **W16.521** Jumping or diving into swimming pool striking bottom causing drowning and submersion
      - *Excludes1:* *drowning and submersion while in swimming pool without jumping or diving (W67)*
    - +7th **W16.522** Jumping or diving into swimming pool striking bottom causing other injury
  - **W16.53** Jumping or diving into swimming pool striking wall
    - +7th **W16.531** Jumping or diving into swimming pool striking wall causing drowning and submersion
      - *Excludes1:* *drowning and submersion while in swimming pool without jumping or diving (W67)*
    - +7th **W16.532** Jumping or diving into swimming pool striking wall causing other injury
- **W16.6** Jumping or diving into natural body of water
  - Jumping or diving into lake
  - Jumping or diving into open sea
  - Jumping or diving into river
  - Jumping or diving into stream
  - **W16.61** Jumping or diving into natural body of water striking water surface
    - +7th **W16.611** Jumping or diving into natural body of water striking water surface causing drowning and submersion
      - *Excludes1:* *drowning and submersion while in natural body of water without jumping or diving (W69)*
    - +7th **W16.612** Jumping or diving into natural body of water striking water surface causing other injury
  - **W16.62** Jumping or diving into natural body of water striking bottom
    - +7th **W16.621** Jumping or diving into natural body of water striking bottom causing drowning and submersion
      - *Excludes1:* *drowning and submersion while in natural body of water without jumping or diving (W69)*
    - +7th **W16.622** Jumping or diving into natural body of water striking bottom causing other injury
- **W16.7** Jumping or diving from boat
  - *Excludes1:* *Fall from boat into water -see watercraft accident (V90-V94)*
  - **W16.71** Jumping or diving from boat striking water surface
    - +7th **W16.711** Jumping or diving from boat striking water surface causing drowning and submersion
    - +7th **W16.712** Jumping or diving from boat striking water surface causing other injury
  - **W16.72** Jumping or diving from boat striking bottom
    - +7th **W16.721** Jumping or diving from boat striking bottom causing drowning and submersion
    - +7th **W16.722** Jumping or diving from boat striking bottom causing other injury
- **W16.8** Jumping or diving into other water
  - Jumping or diving into fountain
  - Jumping or diving into reservoir
  - **W16.81** Jumping or diving into other water striking water surface
    - +7th **W16.811** Jumping or diving into other water striking water surface causing drowning and submersion
      - *Excludes1:* *drowning and submersion while in other water without jumping or diving (W73)*
    - +7th **W16.812** Jumping or diving into other water striking water surface causing other injury
  - **W16.82** Jumping or diving into other water striking bottom
    - +7th **W16.821** Jumping or diving into other water striking bottom causing drowning and submersion
      - *Excludes1:* *drowning and submersion while in other water without jumping or diving (W73)*
    - +7th **W16.822** Jumping or diving into other water striking bottom causing other injury
  - **W16.83** Jumping or diving into other water striking wall
    - +7th **W16.831** Jumping or diving into other water striking wall causing drowning and submersion
      - *Excludes1:* *drowning and submersion while in other water without jumping or diving (W73)*
    - +7th **W16.832** Jumping or diving into other water striking wall causing other injury
- **W16.9** Jumping or diving into unspecified water
  - X+7th **W16.91** Jumping or diving into unspecified water causing drowning and submersion
  - X+7th **W16.92** Jumping or diving into unspecified water causing other injury

W17 Other fall from one level to another

> The appropriate 7th character is to be added to each code from category W17
> A   initial encounter
> D   subsequent encounter
> S   sequela

X+7th **W17.0 Fall into well**
X+7th **W17.1 Fall into storm drain or manhole**
X+7th **W17.2 Fall into hole**
           Fall into pit
X+7th **W17.3 Fall into empty swimming pool**
           Excludes1: fall into filled swimming pool (W16.0-)
X+7th **W17.4 Fall from dock**
  +   **W17.8 Other fall from one level to another**
X+7th   **W17.81 Fall down embankment (hill)**
X+7th   **W17.82 Fall from (out of) grocery cart**
               Fall due to grocery cart tipping over
X+7th   **W17.89 Other fall from one level to another**
               Fall from cherry picker
               Fall from lifting device
               Fall from mobile elevated work platform [MEWP]
               Fall from sky lift
               AHA CC: 2Q, 2015, 6-7

W18 Other slipping, tripping and stumbling and falls

> The appropriate 7th character is to be added to each code from category W18
> A   initial encounter
> D   subsequent encounter
> S   sequela

  +   **W18.0 Fall due to bumping against object**
           Striking against object with subsequent fall
           Excludes1: fall on same level due to slipping, tripping, or stumbling with subsequent striking against object (W01.1-)
X+7th   **W18.00 Striking against unspecified object with subsequent fall**
X+7th   **W18.01 Striking against sports equipment with subsequent fall**
X+7th   **W18.02 Striking against glass with subsequent fall**
X+7th   **W18.09 Striking against other object with subsequent fall**
  +   **W18.1 Fall from or off toilet**
X+7th   **W18.11 Fall from or off toilet without subsequent striking against object**
               Fall from (off) toilet NOS
X+7th   **W18.12 Fall from or off toilet with subsequent striking against object**
X+7th **W18.2 Fall in (into) shower or empty bathtub**
           Excludes1: fall in full bathtub causing drowning or submersion (W16.21-)
  +   **W18.3 Other and unspecified fall on same level**
X+7th   **W18.30 Fall on same level, unspecified**
X+7th   **W18.31 Fall on same level due to stepping on an object**
               Fall on same level due to stepping on an animal
               Excludes1: slipping, tripping and stumbling without fall due to stepping on animal (W18.41)
X+7th   **W18.39 Other fall on same level**
  +   **W18.4 Slipping, tripping and stumbling without falling**
           Excludes1: collision with another person without fall (W51)
X+7th   **W18.40 Slipping, tripping and stumbling without falling, unspecified**
X+7th   **W18.41 Slipping, tripping and stumbling without falling due to stepping on object**
               Slipping, tripping and stumbling without falling due to stepping on animal
               Excludes1: slipping, tripping and stumbling with fall due to stepping on animal (W18.31)
X+7th   **W18.42 Slipping, tripping and stumbling without falling due to stepping into hole or opening**
X+7th   **W18.43 Slipping, tripping and stumbling without falling due to stepping from one level to another**
X+7th   **W18.49 Other slipping, tripping and stumbling without falling**

W19 Unspecified fall
X+7th   Accidental fall NOS
           AHA CC: 4Q, 2012, 95-96; 2Q, 2021, 5; 4Q, 2022, 44-45

> The appropriate 7th character is to be added to code W19
> A   initial encounter
> D   subsequent encounter
> S   sequela

Exposure to inanimate mechanical forces (W20-W49)

Excludes1: assault (X92-Y09)
            contact or collision with animals or persons (W50-W64)
            exposure to inanimate mechanical forces involving military or war operations (Y36.-, Y37.-)
            intentional self-harm (X71-X83)

W20 Struck by thrown, projected or falling object

Code first any associated:
   cataclysm (X34-X39)
   lightning strike (T75.00)
Excludes1: falling object in machinery accident (W24, W28-W31)
            falling object in transport accident (V01-V99)
            object set in motion by explosion (W35-W40)
            object set in motion by firearm (W32-W34)
            struck by thrown sports equipment (W21.-)

> The appropriate 7th character is to be added to each code from category W20
> A   initial encounter
> D   subsequent encounter
> S   sequela

X+7th **W20.0 Struck by falling object in cave-in**
           Excludes2: asphyxiation due to cave-in (T71.21)
X+7th **W20.1 Struck by object due to collapse of building**
           Excludes1: struck by object due to collapse of burning building (X00.2, X02.2)
X+7th **W20.8 Other cause of strike by thrown, projected or falling object**
           Excludes1: struck by thrown sports equipment (W21.-)

W21 Striking against or struck by sports equipment
       Excludes1: assault with sports equipment (Y08.0-)
                   striking against or struck by sports equipment with subsequent fall (W18.01)

> The appropriate 7th character is to be added to each code from category W21
> A   initial encounter
> D   subsequent encounter
> S   sequela

  +   **W21.0 Struck by hit or thrown ball**
X+7th   **W21.00 Struck by hit or thrown ball, unspecified type**
X+7th   **W21.01 Struck by football**
X+7th   **W21.02 Struck by soccer ball**
X+7th   **W21.03 Struck by baseball**
X+7th   **W21.04 Struck by golf ball**
X+7th   **W21.05 Struck by basketball**
X+7th   **W21.06 Struck by volleyball**
X+7th   **W21.07 Struck by softball**
X+7th   **W21.09 Struck by other hit or thrown ball**
  +   **W21.1 Struck by bat, racquet or club**
X+7th   **W21.11 Struck by baseball bat**
X+7th   **W21.12 Struck by tennis racquet**
X+7th   **W21.13 Struck by golf club**
X+7th   **W21.19 Struck by other bat, racquet or club**
  +   **W21.2 Struck by hockey stick or puck**
    +   **W21.21 Struck by hockey stick**
        +7th **W21.210 Struck by ice hockey stick**
        +7th **W21.211 Struck by field hockey stick**
    +   **W21.22 Struck by hockey puck**
        X+7th **W21.220 Struck by ice hockey puck**
        X+7th **W21.221 Struck by field hockey puck**
  +   **W21.3 Struck by sports foot wear**
X+7th   **W21.31 Struck by shoe cleats**
               Stepped on by shoe cleats
X+7th   **W21.32 Struck by skate blades**
               Skated over by skate blades
X+7th   **W21.39 Struck by other sports foot wear**

1271

X+7th W21.4 Striking against diving board
   Use additional code for subsequent falling into water, if applicable (W16.-)
+ **W21.8 Striking against or struck by other sports equipment**
   X+7th **W21.81 Striking against or struck by football helmet**
   X+7th **W21.89 Striking against or struck by other sports equipment**
X+7th **W21.9 Striking against or struck by unspecified sports equipment**

W22 Striking against or struck by other objects
   Excludes1: striking against or struck by object with subsequent fall (W18.09)

   The appropriate 7th character is to be added to each code from category W22
   A   initial encounter
   D   subsequent encounter
   S   sequela

+ **W22.0 Striking against stationary object**
   Excludes1: striking against stationary sports equipment (W21.8)
   X+7th **W22.01 Walked into wall**
   X+7th **W22.02 Walked into lamppost**
   X+7th **W22.03 Walked into furniture**
   + **W22.04 Striking against wall of swimming pool**
      +7th **W22.041 Striking against wall of swimming pool causing drowning and submersion**
         Excludes1: drowning and submersion while swimming without striking against wall (W67)
      +7th **W22.042 Striking against wall of swimming pool causing other injury**
   X+7th **W22.09 Striking against other stationary object**
+ **W22.1 Striking against or struck by automobile airbag**
   X+7th **W22.10 Striking against or struck by unspecified automobile airbag**
   X+7th **W22.11 Striking against or struck by driver side automobile airbag**
   X+7th **W22.12 Striking against or struck by front passenger side automobile airbag**
   X+7th **W22.19 Striking against or struck by other automobile airbag**
X+7th **W22.8 Striking against or struck by other objects**
   Striking against or struck by object NOS
   Excludes1: struck by thrown, projected or falling object (W20.-)

W23 Caught, crushed, jammed or pinched in or between objects
   Excludes1: injury caused by cutting or piercing instruments (W25-W27)
   injury caused by firearms malfunction (W32.1, W33.1-, W34.1-)
   injury caused by lifting and transmission devices (W24.-)
   injury caused by machinery (W28-W31)
   injury caused by nonpowered hand tools (W27.-)
   injury caused by transport vehicle being used as a means of transportation (V01-V99)
   injury caused by struck by thrown, projected or falling object (W20.-)

   The appropriate 7th character is to be added to each code from category W23
   A   initial encounter
   D   subsequent encounter
   S   sequela

X+7th **W23.0 Caught, crushed, jammed, or pinched between moving objects**
X+7th **W23.1 Caught, crushed, jammed, or pinched between stationary objects**
X+7th **W23.2 Caught, crushed, jammed or pinched between a moving and stationary object**
   AHA CC: 4Q, 2022, 48

W24 Contact with lifting and transmission devices, not elsewhere classified
   Excludes1: transport accidents (V01-V99)

   The appropriate 7th character is to be added to each code from category W24
   A   initial encounter
   D   subsequent encounter
   S   sequela

X+7th **W24.0 Contact with lifting devices, not elsewhere classified**
   Contact with chain hoist
   Contact with drive belt
   Contact with pulley (block)
X+7th **W24.1 Contact with transmission devices, not elsewhere classified**
   Contact with transmission belt or cable

W25 Contact with sharp glass
X+7th
   Code first any associated:
      injury due to flying glass from explosion or firearm discharge (W32-W40)
      transport accident (V00-V99)
   Excludes1: fall on same level due to slipping, tripping and stumbling with subsequent striking against sharp glass (W01.110-)
   striking against sharp glass with subsequent fall (W18.02-)
   Excludes2: glass embedded in skin (W45.-)

   The appropriate 7th character is to be added to code W25
   A   initial encounter
   D   subsequent encounter
   S   sequela

W26 Contact with other sharp objects
   Excludes2: sharp object(s) embedded in skin (W45.-)
   AHA CC: 4Q, 2016, 73

   The appropriate 7th character is to be added to each code from category W26
   A   initial encounter
   D   subsequent encounter
   S   sequela

X+7th **W26.0 Contact with knife**
   Excludes1: contact with electric knife (W29.1)
X+7th **W26.1 Contact with sword or dagger**
X+7th **W26.2 Contact with edge of stiff paper**
   Paper cut
X+7th **W26.8 Contact with other sharp object(s), not elsewhere classified**
   Contact with tin can lid
X+7th **W26.9 Contact with unspecified sharp object(s)**

W27 Contact with nonpowered hand tool
   The appropriate 7th character is to be added to each code from category W27
   A   initial encounter
   D   subsequent encounter
   S   sequela

X+7th **W27.0 Contact with workbench tool**
   Contact with auger
   Contact with axe
   Contact with chisel
   Contact with handsaw
   Contact with screwdriver
X+7th **W27.1 Contact with garden tool**
   Contact with hoe
   Contact with nonpowered lawn mower
   Contact with pitchfork
   Contact with rake
X+7th **W27.2 Contact with scissors**
X+7th **W27.3 Contact with needle (sewing)**
   Excludes1: contact with hypodermic needle (W46.-)
X+7th **W27.4 Contact with kitchen utensil**
   Contact with fork
   Contact with ice-pick
   Contact with can-opener NOS

X+7th **W27.5** **Contact with paper-cutter**
X+7th **W27.8** **Contact with other nonpowered hand tool**
  Contact with nonpowered sewing machine
  Contact with shovel

W28 **Contact with powered lawn mower**
X+7th
  Powered lawn mower (commercial) (residential)
  Excludes1: *contact with nonpowered lawn mower (W27.1)*
  Excludes2: *exposure to electric current (W86.-)*

  The appropriate 7th character is to be added to code W28
  A initial encounter
  D subsequent encounter
  S sequela

W29 **Contact with other powered hand tools and household machinery**
  Excludes1: *contact with commercial machinery (W31.82)*
  contact with hot household appliance (X15)
  contact with nonpowered hand tool (W27.-)
  exposure to electric current (W86)

  The appropriate 7th character is to be added to each code from category W29
  A initial encounter
  D subsequent encounter
  S sequela

X+7th **W29.0** **Contact with powered kitchen appliance**
  Contact with blender
  Contact with can-opener
  Contact with garbage disposal
  Contact with mixer
X+7th **W29.1** **Contact with electric knife**
X+7th **W29.2** **Contact with other powered household machinery**
  Contact with electric fan
  Contact with powered dryer (clothes) (powered) (spin)
  Contact with washing-machine
  Contact with sewing machine
X+7th **W29.3** **Contact with powered garden and outdoor hand tools and machinery**
  Contact with chainsaw
  Contact with edger
  Contact with garden cultivator (tiller)
  Contact with hedge trimmer
  Contact with other powered garden tool
  Excludes1: *contact with powered lawn mower (W28)*
X+7th **W29.4** **Contact with nail gun**
X+7th **W29.8** **Contact with other powered hand tools and household machinery**
  Contact with do-it-yourself tool NOS

W30 **Contact with agricultural machinery**
  Includes: animal-powered farm machine
  Excludes1: *agricultural transport vehicle accident (V01-V99)*
  explosion of grain store (W40.8)
  exposure to electric current (W86.-)

  The appropriate 7th character is to be added to each code from category W30
  A initial encounter
  D subsequent encounter
  S sequela

X+7th **W30.0** **Contact with combine harvester**
  Contact with reaper
  Contact with thresher
X+7th **W30.1** **Contact with power take-off devices (PTO)**
X+7th **W30.2** **Contact with hay derrick**
X+7th **W30.3** **Contact with grain storage elevator**
  Excludes1: *explosion of grain store (W40.8)*
 + **W30.8** **Contact with other specified agricultural machinery**
  X+7th **W30.81** **Contact with agricultural transport vehicle in stationary use**
    Contact with agricultural transport vehicle under repair, not on public roadway
    Excludes1: *agricultural transport vehicle accident (V01-V99)*
  X+7th **W30.89** **Contact with other specified agricultural machinery**
X+7th **W30.9** **Contact with unspecified agricultural machinery**
  Contact with farm machinery NOS

W31 **Contact with other and unspecified machinery**
  Excludes1: *contact with agricultural machinery (W30.-)*
  contact with machinery in transport under own power or being towed by a vehicle (V01-V99)
  exposure to electric current (W86)

  The appropriate 7th character is to be added to each code from category W31
  A initial encounter
  D subsequent encounter
  S sequela

X+7th **W31.0** **Contact with mining and earth-drilling machinery**
  Contact with bore or drill (land) (seabed)
  Contact with shaft hoist
  Contact with shaft lift
  Contact with undercutter
X+7th **W31.1** **Contact with metalworking machines**
  Contact with abrasive wheel
  Contact with forging machine
  Contact with lathe
  Contact with mechanical shears
  Contact with metal drilling machine
  Contact with milling machine
  Contact with power press
  Contact with rolling-mill
  Contact with metal sawing machine
X+7th **W31.2** **Contact with powered woodworking and forming machines**
  Contact with band saw
  Contact with bench saw
  Contact with circular saw
  Contact with molding machine
  Contact with overhead plane
  Contact with powered saw
  Contact with radial saw
  Contact with sander
  Excludes1: *nonpowered woodworking tools (W27.0)*
X+7th **W31.3** **Contact with prime movers**
  Contact with gas turbine
  Contact with internal combustion engine
  Contact with steam engine
  Contact with water driven turbine
 + **W31.8** **Contact with other specified machinery**
  X+7th **W31.81** **Contact with recreational machinery**
    Contact with roller coaster
  X+7th **W31.82** **Contact with other commercial machinery**
    Contact with commercial electric fan
    Contact with commercial kitchen appliances
    Contact with commercial powered dryer (clothes) (powered) (spin)
    Contact with commercial washing-machine
    Contact with commercial sewing machine
    Excludes1: *contact with household machinery (W29.-)*
    contact with powered lawn mower (W28)
  X+7th **W31.83** **Contact with special construction vehicle in stationary use**
    Contact with special construction vehicle under repair, not on public roadway
    Excludes1: *special construction vehicle accident (V01-V99)*
  X+7th **W31.89** **Contact with other specified machinery**
X+7th **W31.9** **Contact with unspecified machinery**
  Contact with machinery NOS

W32 **Accidental handgun discharge and malfunction**
  Includes: accidental discharge and malfunction of gun for single hand use
  accidental discharge and malfunction of pistol
  accidental discharge and malfunction of revolver
  Handgun discharge and malfunction NOS
  Excludes1: *accidental airgun discharge and malfunction (W34.010, W34.110)*
  accidental BB gun discharge and malfunction (W34.010, W34.110)
  accidental pellet gun discharge and malfunction (W34.010, W34.110)
  accidental shotgun discharge and malfunction (W33.01, W33.11)

assault by handgun discharge (X93)
handgun discharge involving legal intervention (Y35.0-)
handgun discharge involving military or war operations (Y36.4-)
intentional self-harm by handgun discharge (X72)
Very pistol discharge and malfunction (W34.09, W34.19)

The appropriate 7th character is to be added to each code from category W32
- A initial encounter
- D subsequent encounter
- S sequela

X+7th W32.0 Accidental handgun discharge
X+7th W32.1 Accidental handgun malfunction
  Injury due to explosion of handgun (parts)
  Injury due to malfunction of mechanism or component of handgun
  Injury due to recoil of handgun
  Powder burn from handgun

W33 Accidental rifle, shotgun and larger firearm discharge and malfunction
  Includes: rifle, shotgun and larger firearm discharge and malfunction NOS
  Excludes1: accidental airgun discharge and malfunction (W34.010, W34.110)
  accidental BB gun discharge and malfunction (W34.010, W34.110)
  accidental handgun discharge and malfunction (W32.-)
  accidental pellet gun discharge and malfunction (W34.010, W34.110)
  assault by rifle, shotgun and larger firearm discharge (X94)
  firearm discharge involving legal intervention (Y35.0-)
  firearm discharge involving military or war operations (Y36.4-)
  intentional self-harm by rifle, shotgun and larger firearm discharge (X73)

The appropriate 7th character is to be added to each code from category W33
- A initial encounter
- D subsequent encounter
- S sequela

+ W33.0 Accidental rifle, shotgun and larger firearm discharge
  X+7th W33.00 Accidental discharge of unspecified larger firearm
    Discharge of unspecified larger firearm NOS
  X+7th W33.01 Accidental discharge of shotgun
    Discharge of shotgun NOS
  X+7th W33.02 Accidental discharge of hunting rifle
    Discharge of hunting rifle NOS
  X+7th W33.03 Accidental discharge of machine gun
    Discharge of machine gun NOS
  X+7th W33.09 Accidental discharge of other larger firearm
    Discharge of other larger firearm NOS

+ W33.1 Accidental rifle, shotgun and larger firearm malfunction
  Injury due to explosion of rifle, shotgun and larger firearm (parts)
  Injury due to malfunction of mechanism or component of rifle, shotgun and larger firearm
  Injury due to piercing, cutting, crushing or pinching due to (by) slide trigger mechanism, scope or other gun part
  Injury due to recoil of rifle, shotgun and larger firearm
  Powder burn from rifle, shotgun and larger firearm
  X+7th W33.10 Accidental malfunction of unspecified larger firearm
    Malfunction of unspecified larger firearm NOS
  X+7th W33.11 Accidental malfunction of shotgun
    Malfunction of shotgun NOS
  X+7th W33.12 Accidental malfunction of hunting rifle
    Malfunction of hunting rifle NOS
  X+7th W33.13 Accidental malfunction of machine gun
    Malfunction of machine gun NOS
  X+7th W33.19 Accidental malfunction of other larger firearm
    Malfunction of other larger firearm NOS

W34 Accidental discharge and malfunction from other and unspecified firearms and guns

The appropriate 7th character is to be added to each code from category W34
- A initial encounter
- D subsequent encounter
- S sequela

+ W34.0 Accidental discharge from other and unspecified firearms and guns
  X+7th W34.00 Accidental discharge from unspecified firearms or gun
    Discharge from firearm NOS
    Gunshot wound NOS
    Shot NOS
    AHA CC: 1Q, 2015, 3-21
  + W34.01 Accidental discharge of gas, air or spring-operated guns
    +7th W34.010 Accidental discharge of airgun
      Accidental discharge of BB gun
      Accidental discharge of pellet gun
    +7th W34.011 Accidental discharge of paintball gun
      Accidental injury due to paintball discharge
    +7th W34.018 Accidental discharge of other gas, air or spring-operated gun
  X+7th W34.09 Accidental discharge from other specified firearms
    Accidental discharge from Very pistol [flare]

+ W34.1 Accidental malfunction from other and unspecified firearms and guns
  X+7th W34.10 Accidental malfunction from unspecified firearms or gun
    Firearm malfunction NOS
  + W34.11 Accidental malfunction of gas, air or spring-operated guns
    +7th W34.110 Accidental malfunction of airgun
      Accidental malfunction of BB gun
      Accidental malfunction of pellet gun
    +7th W34.111 Accidental malfunction of paintball gun
      Accidental injury due to paintball gun malfunction
    +7th W34.118 Accidental malfunction of other gas, air or spring-operated gun
  X+7th W34.19 Accidental malfunction from other specified firearms
    Accidental malfunction from Very pistol [flare]

W35 Explosion and rupture of boiler
X+7th
  Excludes1: *explosion and rupture of boiler on watercraft (V93.4)*

The appropriate 7th character is to be added to code W35
- A initial encounter
- D subsequent encounter
- S sequela

W36 Explosion and rupture of gas cylinder

The appropriate 7th character is to be added to each code from category W36
- A initial encounter
- D subsequent encounter
- S sequela

X+7th W36.1 Explosion and rupture of aerosol can
X+7th W36.2 Explosion and rupture of air tank
X+7th W36.3 Explosion and rupture of pressurized-gas tank
X+7th W36.8 Explosion and rupture of other gas cylinder
X+7th W36.9 Explosion and rupture of unspecified gas cylinder

W37 Explosion and rupture of pressurized tire, pipe or hose

The appropriate 7th character is to be added to each code from category W37
- A initial encounter
- D subsequent encounter
- S sequela

X+7th W37.0 Explosion of bicycle tire
X+7th W37.8 Explosion and rupture of other pressurized tire, pipe or hose

W38 Explosion and rupture of other specified pressurized devices
X+7th

The appropriate 7th character is to be added to code W38
- A initial encounter
- D subsequent encounter
- S sequela

W39 Discharge of firework
X+7th

The appropriate 7th character is to be added to code W39
- A initial encounter
- D subsequent encounter
- S sequela

W40 Explosion of other materials

Excludes1: assault by explosive material (X96)
explosion involving legal intervention (Y35.1-)
explosion involving military or war operations (Y36.0-, Y36.2-)
intentional self-harm by explosive material (X75)

The appropriate 7th character is to be added to each code from category W40
- A initial encounter
- D subsequent encounter
- S sequela

X+7th W40.0 Explosion of blasting material
- Explosion of blasting cap
- Explosion of detonator
- Explosion of dynamite
- Explosion of explosive (any) used in blasting operations

X+7th W40.1 Explosion of explosive gases
- Explosion of acetylene
- Explosion of butane
- Explosion of coal gas
- Explosion in mine NOS
- Explosion of explosive gas
- Explosion of fire damp
- Explosion of gasoline fumes
- Explosion of methane
- Explosion of propane

X+7th W40.8 Explosion of other specified explosive materials
- Explosion in dump NOS
- Explosion in factory NOS
- Explosion in grain store
- Explosion in munitions

Excludes1: explosion involving legal intervention (Y35.1-)
explosion involving military or war operations (Y36.0-, Y36.2-)

X+7th W40.9 Explosion of unspecified explosive materials
- Explosion NOS

W42 Exposure to noise

The appropriate 7th character is to be added to each code from category W42
- A initial encounter
- D subsequent encounter
- S sequela

X+7th W42.0 Exposure to supersonic waves

X+7th W42.9 Exposure to other noise
- Exposure to sound waves NOS

W44 Foreign body entering into or through a natural orifice

Excludes2: contact with other sharp objects (W26)
contact with sharp glass (W25)
foreign body or object entering through skin (W45)

The appropriate 7th character is to be added to each code from category W44
- A initial encounter
- D subsequent encounter
- S sequela

+ W44.A Battery entering into or through a natural orifice
- **X+7th W44.A0** Battery unspecified, entering into or through a natural orifice
- **X+7th W44.A1** Button battery entering into or through a natural orifice
- **X+7th W44.A9** Other batteries entering into or through a natural orifice
  - Cylindrical battery

+ W44.B Plastic entering into or through a natural orifice
- **X+7th W44.B0** Plastic object unspecified, entering into or through a natural orifice
- **X+7th W44.B1** Plastic bead entering into or through a natural orifice
  - **Excludes2:** Plastic jewelry entering into or through a natural orifice (W44.B4)
- **X+7th W44.B2** Plastic coin entering into or through a natural orifice
- **X+7th W44.B3** Plastic toy and toy part entering into or through a natural orifice
- **X+7th W44.B4** Plastic jewelry entering into or through a natural orifice
  - **Excludes2:** Plastic bead entering into or through a natural orifice (W44.B1)
- **X+7th W44.B5** Plastic bottle entering into or through a natural orifice
- **X+7th W44.B9** Other plastic object entering into or through a natural orifice

+ W44.C Glass entering into or through a natural orifice
- **X+7th W44.C0** Glass unspecified, entering into or through a natural orifice
- **X+7th W44.C1** Sharp glass entering into or through a natural orifice
  - Glass shard entering into or through a natural orifice
- **X+7th W44.C2** Intact glass entering into or through a natural orifice
  - Intact glass bottle entering into or through a natural orifice

+ W44.D Magnetic metal entering into or through a natural orifice
- **X+7th W44.D0** Magnetic metal object unspecified, entering into or through a natural orifice
- **X+7th W44.D1** Magnetic metal bead entering into or through a natural orifice
- **X+7th W44.D2** Magnetic metal coin entering into or through a natural orifice
- **X+7th W44.D3** Magnetic metal toy entering into or through a natural orifice
- **X+7th W44.D4** Magnetic metal jewelry entering into or through a natural orifice
- **X+7th W44.D9** Other magnetic metal objects entering into or through a natural orifice

+ W44.E Non-magnetic metal entering into or through a natural orifice
- **X+7th W44.E0** Non-magnetic metal object unspecified, entering into or through a natural orifice
- **X+7th W44.E1** Non-magnetic metal bead entering into or through a natural orifice
- **X+7th W44.E2** Non-magnetic metal coin entering into or through a natural orifice
- **X+7th W44.E3** Non-magnetic metal toy entering into or through a natural orifice
- **X+7th W44.E4** Non-magnetic metal jewelry entering into or through a natural orifice
- **X+7th W44.E9** Other non-magnetic metal objects entering into or through a natural orifice
  - Bottle cap entering into or through a natural orifice
  - Can lid entering into or through a natural orifice
  - Pull tab entering into or through a natural orifice

+ W44.F Objects of natural or organic material entering into or through a natural orifice
- **X+7th W44.F0** Objects of natural or organic material unspecified, entering into or through a natural orifice
- **X+7th W44.F1** Bezoar entering into or through a natural orifice
- **X+7th W44.F2** Rubber band entering into or through a natural orifice
- **X+7th W44.F3** Food entering into or through a natural orifice
- **X+7th W44.F4** Insect entering into or through a natural orifice
- **X+7th W44.F9** Other object of natural or organic material, entering into or through a natural orifice

+ W44.G Other non-organic objects entering into or through a natural orifice
- **X+7th W44.G0** Other non-organic objects unspecified, entering into or through a natural orifice
- **X+7th W44.G1** Audio device entering into or through a natural orifice
  - Ear buds
  - Hearing aids
- **X+7th W44.G2** Combination metal and plastic toy and toy part entering into or through natural orifice
- **X+7th W44.G3** Combination metal and plastic jewelry entering into or through a natural orifice
- **X+7th W44.G9** Other non-organic objects entering into or through a natural orifice

- **W44.H Other sharp object entering into or through a natural orifice**
    - X+7th **W44.H0** Other sharp object unspecified, entering into or through a natural orifice
    - X+7th **W44.H1** Needle entering into or through a natural orifice
        Dart entering into or through a natural orifice
        Hypodermic needle entering into or through a natural orifice
        Safety pin entering into or through a natural orifice
        Sewing needle entering into or through a natural orifice
    - X+7th **W44.H2** Knife, sword or dagger entering into or through a natural orifice
- X+7th **W44.8** Other foreign body entering into or through a natural orifice
- X+7th **W44.9** Unspecified foreign body entering into or through a natural orifice
    Foreign body NOS entering into or through a natural orifice

W45 Foreign body or object entering through skin

Includes: foreign body or object embedded in skin
nail embedded in skin

Excludes2: contact with hand tools (nonpowered) (powered) (W27-W29)
contact with other sharp object(s) (W26.-)
contact with sharp glass (W25.-)
struck by objects (W20-W22)

The appropriate 7th character is to be added to each code from category W45
- A initial encounter
- D subsequent encounter
- S sequela

- X+7th **W45.0** Nail entering through skin
- X+7th **W45.8** Other foreign body or object entering through skin
    Splinter in skin NOS

W46 Contact with hypodermic needle

The appropriate 7th character is to be added to each code from category W46
- A initial encounter
- D subsequent encounter
- S sequela

- X+7th **W46.0** Contact with hypodermic needle
    Hypodermic needle stick NOS
- X+7th **W46.1** Contact with contaminated hypodermic needle

W49 Exposure to other inanimate mechanical forces

Includes: exposure to abnormal gravitational [G] forces
exposure to inanimate mechanical forces NEC

Excludes1: exposure to inanimate mechanical forces involving military or war operations (Y36.-, Y37.-)

The appropriate 7th character is to be added to each code from category W49
- A initial encounter
- D subsequent encounter
- S sequela

- + **W49.0** Item causing external constriction
    - X+7th **W49.01** Hair causing external constriction
    - X+7th **W49.02** String or thread causing external constriction
    - X+7th **W49.03** Rubber band causing external constriction
    - X+7th **W49.04** Ring or other jewelry causing external constriction
    - X+7th **W49.09** Other specified item causing external constriction
- X+7th **W49.9** Exposure to other inanimate mechanical forces

Exposure to animate mechanical forces (W50-W64)

Excludes1: Toxic effect of contact with venomous animals and plants (T63.-)

W50 Accidental hit, strike, kick, twist, bite or scratch by another person

Includes: hit, strike, kick, twist, bite, or scratch by another person NOS

Excludes1: assault by bodily force (Y04)
struck by objects (W20-W22)

The appropriate 7th character is to be added to each code from category W50
- A initial encounter
- D subsequent encounter
- S sequela

- X+7th **W50.0** Accidental hit or strike by another person
    Hit or strike by another person NOS
- X+7th **W50.1** Accidental kick by another person
    Kick by another person NOS
- X+7th **W50.2** Accidental twist by another person
    Twist by another person NOS
    AHA CC: 1Q, 2015, 3-21
- X+7th **W50.3** Accidental bite by another person
    Human bite
    Bite by another person NOS
- X+7th **W50.4** Accidental scratch by another person
    Scratch by another person NOS

W51 Accidental striking against or bumped into by another person

- X+7th **Excludes1:** assault by striking against or bumping into by another person (Y04.2)
    fall due to collision with another person (W03)

The appropriate 7th character is to be added to code W51
- A initial encounter
- D subsequent encounter
- S sequela

W52 Crushed, pushed or stepped on by crowd or human stampede

- X+7th Crushed, pushed or stepped on by crowd or human stampede with or without fall

The appropriate 7th character is to be added to code W52
- A initial encounter
- D subsequent encounter
- S sequela

+ W53 Contact with rodent

Includes: contact with saliva, feces or urine of rodent

The appropriate 7th character is to be added to each code from category W53
- A initial encounter
- D subsequent encounter
- S sequela

- + **W53.0** Contact with mouse
    - X+7th **W53.01** Bitten by mouse
    - X+7th **W53.09** Other contact with mouse
- + **W53.1** Contact with rat
    - X+7th **W53.11** Bitten by rat
    - X+7th **W53.19** Other contact with rat
- + **W53.2** Contact with squirrel
    - X+7th **W53.21** Bitten by squirrel
    - X+7th **W53.29** Other contact with squirrel
- + **W53.8** Contact with other rodent
    - X+7th **W53.81** Bitten by other rodent
    - X+7th **W53.89** Other contact with other rodent

W54 Contact with dog

Includes: contact with saliva, feces or urine of dog

The appropriate 7th character is to be added to each code from category W54
- A initial encounter
- D subsequent encounter
- S sequela

- X+7th **W54.0** Bitten by dog
    AHA CC: 4Q, 2017, 112-114
    Review coding guideline B.19.c
- X+7th **W54.1** Struck by dog
    Knocked over by dog
- X+7th **W54.8** Other contact with dog

W55 Contact with other mammals

Includes: contact with saliva, feces or urine of mammal

Excludes1: animal being ridden- see transport accidents
bitten or struck by dog (W54)
bitten or struck by rodent (W53.-)
contact with marine mammals (W56.-)

The appropriate 7th character is to be added to each code from category W55
- A initial encounter
- D subsequent encounter
- S sequela

- + **W55.0** Contact with cat
    - X+7th **W55.01** Bitten by cat
    - X+7th **W55.03** Scratched by cat
    - X+7th **W55.09** Other contact with cat

- **+ W55.1 Contact with horse**
  - X+7th W55.11 Bitten by horse
  - X+7th W55.12 Struck by horse
  - X+7th W55.19 Other contact with horse
- **+ W55.2 Contact with cow**
  - Contact with bull
  - X+7th W55.21 Bitten by cow
  - X+7th W55.22 Struck by cow
    - Gored by bull
  - X+7th W55.29 Other contact with cow
- **+ W55.3 Contact with other hoof stock**
  - Contact with goats
  - Contact with sheep
  - X+7th W55.31 Bitten by other hoof stock
  - X+7th W55.32 Struck by other hoof stock
    - Gored by goat
    - Gored by ram
  - X+7th W55.39 Other contact with other hoof stock
- **+ W55.4 Contact with pig**
  - X+7th W55.41 Bitten by pig
  - X+7th W55.42 Struck by pig
  - X+7th W55.49 Other contact with pig
- **+ W55.5 Contact with raccoon**
  - X+7th W55.51 Bitten by raccoon
  - X+7th W55.52 Struck by raccoon
  - X+7th W55.59 Other contact with raccoon
- **+ W55.8 Contact with other mammals**
  - X+7th W55.81 Bitten by other mammals
  - X+7th W55.82 Struck by other mammals
  - X+7th W55.89 Other contact with other mammals

W56 Contact with nonvenomous marine animal

Excludes1: contact with venomous marine animal (T63.-)

The appropriate 7th character is to be added to each code from category W56
- A initial encounter
- D subsequent encounter
- S sequela

- **+ W56.0 Contact with dolphin**
  - X+7th W56.01 Bitten by dolphin
  - X+7th W56.02 Struck by dolphin
  - X+7th W56.09 Other contact with dolphin
- **+ W56.1 Contact with sea lion**
  - X+7th W56.11 Bitten by sea lion
  - X+7th W56.12 Struck by sea lion
  - X+7th W56.19 Other contact with sea lion
- **+ W56.2 Contact with orca**
  - Contact with killer whale
  - X+7th W56.21 Bitten by orca
  - X+7th W56.22 Struck by orca
  - X+7th W56.29 Other contact with orca
- **+ W56.3 Contact with other marine mammals**
  - X+7th W56.31 Bitten by other marine mammals
  - X+7th W56.32 Struck by other marine mammals
  - X+7th W56.39 Other contact with other marine mammals
- **+ W56.4 Contact with shark**
  - X+7th W56.41 Bitten by shark
  - X+7th W56.42 Struck by shark
  - X+7th W56.49 Other contact with shark
- **+ W56.5 Contact with other fish**
  - X+7th W56.51 Bitten by other fish
  - X+7th W56.52 Struck by other fish
  - X+7th W56.59 Other contact with other fish
- **+ W56.8 Contact with other nonvenomous marine animals**
  - X+7th W56.81 Bitten by other nonvenomous marine animals
  - X+7th W56.82 Struck by other nonvenomous marine animals
  - X+7th W56.89 Other contact with other nonvenomous marine animals

W57 Bitten or stung by nonvenomous insect and other nonvenomous
X+7th arthropods

Excludes1: contact with venomous insects and arthropods (T63.2-, T63.3-, T63.4-)

The appropriate 7th character is to be added to code W57
- A initial encounter
- D subsequent encounter
- S sequela

W58 Contact with crocodile or alligator

The appropriate 7th character is to be added to each code from category W58
- A initial encounter
- D subsequent encounter
- S sequela

- **+ W58.0 Contact with alligator**
  - X+7th W58.01 Bitten by alligator
  - X+7th W58.02 Struck by alligator
  - X+7th W58.03 Crushed by alligator
  - X+7th W58.09 Other contact with alligator
- **+ W58.1 Contact with crocodile**
  - X+7th W58.11 Bitten by crocodile
  - X+7th W58.12 Struck by crocodile
  - X+7th W58.13 Crushed by crocodile
  - X+7th W58.19 Other contact with crocodile

W59 Contact with other nonvenomous reptiles

Excludes1: contact with venomous reptile (T63.0-, T63.1-)

The appropriate 7th character is to be added to each code from category W59
- A initial encounter
- D subsequent encounter
- S sequela

- **+ W59.0 Contact with nonvenomous lizards**
  - X+7th W59.01 Bitten by nonvenomous lizards
  - X+7th W59.02 Struck by nonvenomous lizards
  - X+7th W59.09 Other contact with nonvenomous lizards
    - Exposure to nonvenomous lizards
- **+ W59.1 Contact with nonvenomous snakes**
  - X+7th W59.11 Bitten by nonvenomous snake
  - X+7th W59.12 Struck by nonvenomous snake
  - X+7th W59.13 Crushed by nonvenomous snake
  - X+7th W59.19 Other contact with nonvenomous snake
- **+ W59.2 Contact with turtles**
  - **Excludes1:** contact with tortoises (W59.8-)
  - X+7th W59.21 Bitten by turtle
  - X+7th W59.22 Struck by turtle
  - X+7th W59.29 Other contact with turtle
    - Exposure to turtles
- **+ W59.8 Contact with other nonvenomous reptiles**
  - X+7th W59.81 Bitten by other nonvenomous reptiles
  - X+7th W59.82 Struck by other nonvenomous reptiles
  - X+7th W59.83 Crushed by other nonvenomous reptiles
  - X+7th W59.89 Other contact with other nonvenomous reptiles

W60 Contact with nonvenomous plant thorns and spines and sharp
X+7th leaves

Excludes1: Contact with venomous plants (T63.7-)

The appropriate 7th character is to be added to code W60
- A initial encounter
- D subsequent encounter
- S sequela

W61 Contact with birds (domestic) (wild)

Includes: contact with excreta of birds

The appropriate 7th character is to be added to each code from category W61
- A initial encounter
- D subsequent encounter
- S sequela

- **+ W61.0 Contact with parrot**
  - X+7th W61.01 Bitten by parrot
  - X+7th W61.02 Struck by parrot
  - X+7th W61.09 Other contact with parrot
    - Exposure to parrots
- **+ W61.1 Contact with macaw**
  - X+7th W61.11 Bitten by macaw
  - X+7th W61.12 Struck by macaw
  - X+7th W61.19 Other contact with macaw
    - Exposure to macaws
- **+ W61.2 Contact with other psittacines**
  - X+7th W61.21 Bitten by other psittacines
  - X+7th W61.22 Struck by other psittacines
  - X+7th W61.29 Other contact with other psittacines
    - Exposure to other psittacines

- **+ W61.3 Contact with chicken**
  - X+7th W61.32 Struck by chicken
  - X+7th W61.33 Pecked by chicken
  - X+7th W61.39 Other contact with chicken
    - Exposure to chickens
- **+ W61.4 Contact with turkey**
  - X+7th W61.42 Struck by turkey
  - X+7th W61.43 Pecked by turkey
  - X+7th W61.49 Other contact with turkey
- **+ W61.5 Contact with goose**
  - X+7th W61.51 Bitten by goose
  - X+7th W61.52 Struck by goose
  - X+7th W61.59 Other contact with goose
- **+ W61.6 Contact with duck**
  - X+7th W61.61 Bitten by duck
  - X+7th W61.62 Struck by duck
  - X+7th W61.69 Other contact with duck
- **+ W61.9 Contact with other birds**
  - X+7th W61.91 Bitten by other birds
  - X+7th W61.92 Struck by other birds
  - X+7th W61.99 Other contact with other birds
    - Contact with bird NOS

W62 Contact with nonvenomous amphibians

Excludes1: contact with venomous amphibians (T63.81-T63.83)

The appropriate 7th character is to be added to each code from category W62
- A initial encounter
- D subsequent encounter
- S sequela

- X+7th W62.0 Contact with nonvenomous frogs
- X+7th W62.1 Contact with nonvenomous toads
- X+7th W62.9 Contact with other nonvenomous amphibians

W64 Exposure to other animate mechanical forces
X+7th

Includes: exposure to nonvenomous animal NOS
Excludes1: contact with venomous animal (T63.-)

The appropriate 7th character is to be added to code W64
- A initial encounter
- D subsequent encounter
- S sequela

Accidental non-transport drowning and submersion (W65-W74)

Excludes1: accidental drowning and submersion due to fall into water (W16.-)
accidental drowning and submersion due to water transport accident (V90.-, V92.-)

Excludes2: accidental drowning and submersion due to cataclysm (X34-X39)

W65 Accidental drowning and submersion while in bath-tub
X+7th

Excludes1: accidental drowning and submersion due to fall in (into) bathtub (W16.211)

The appropriate 7th character is to be added to code W65
- A initial encounter
- D subsequent encounter
- S sequela

W67 Accidental drowning and submersion while in swimming-pool
X+7th

Excludes1: accidental drowning and submersion due to fall into swimming pool (W16.011, W16.021, W16.031)
accidental drowning and submersion due to striking into wall of swimming pool (W22.041)

The appropriate 7th character is to be added to code W67
- A initial encounter
- D subsequent encounter
- S sequela

W69 Accidental drowning and submersion while in natural water
X+7th

Accidental drowning and submersion while in lake
Accidental drowning and submersion while in open sea
Accidental drowning and submersion while in river
Accidental drowning and submersion while in stream

Excludes1: accidental drowning and submersion due to fall into natural body of water (W16.111, W16.121, W16.131)

The appropriate 7th character is to be added to code W69
- A initial encounter
- D subsequent encounter
- S sequela

W73 Other specified cause of accidental non-transport drowning and submersion
X+7th

Accidental drowning and submersion while in quenching tank
Accidental drowning and submersion while in reservoir

Excludes1: accidental drowning and submersion due to fall into other water (W16.311, W16.321, W16.331)

The appropriate 7th character is to be added to code W73
- A initial encounter
- D subsequent encounter
- S sequela

W74 Unspecified cause of accidental drowning and submersion
X+7th

Drowning NOS

The appropriate 7th character is to be added to code W74
- A initial encounter
- D subsequent encounter
- S sequela

Exposure to electric current, radiation and extreme ambient air temperature and pressure (W85-W99)

Excludes1: exposure to:
failure in dosage of radiation or temperature during surgical and medical care (Y63.2-Y63.5)
lightning (T75.0-)
natural cold (X31)
natural heat (X30)
natural radiation NOS (X39)
radiological procedure and radiotherapy (Y84.2)
sunlight (X32)

W85 Exposure to electric transmission lines
X+7th

Broken power line

The appropriate 7th character is to be added to code W85
- A initial encounter
- D subsequent encounter
- S sequela

W86 Exposure to other specified electric current

The appropriate 7th character is to be added to each code from category W86
- A initial encounter
- D subsequent encounter
- S sequela

- X+7th W86.0 Exposure to domestic wiring and appliances
- X+7th W86.1 Exposure to industrial wiring, appliances and electrical machinery
  - Exposure to conductors
  - Exposure to control apparatus
  - Exposure to electrical equipment and machinery
  - Exposure to transformers
- X+7th W86.8 Exposure to other electric current
  - Exposure to wiring and appliances in or on farm (not farmhouse)
  - Exposure to wiring and appliances outdoors
  - Exposure to wiring and appliances in or on public building
  - Exposure to wiring and appliances in or on residential institutions
  - Exposure to wiring and appliances in or on schools

W88 Exposure to ionizing radiation

Excludes1: exposure to sunlight (X32)

The appropriate 7th character is to be added to each code from category W88
- A initial encounter
- D subsequent encounter
- S sequela

- X+7th W88.0 Exposure to X-rays
- X+7th W88.1 Exposure to radioactive isotopes
- X+7th W88.8 Exposure to other ionizing radiation

W89 Exposure to man-made visible and ultraviolet light

Includes: exposure to welding light (arc)
Excludes2: exposure to sunlight (X32)

The appropriate 7th character is to be added to each code from category W89
- A initial encounter
- D subsequent encounter
- S sequela

X+7th W89.0 Exposure to welding light (arc)
X+7th W89.1 Exposure to tanning bed
X+7th W89.8 Exposure to other man-made visible and ultraviolet light
X+7th W89.9 Exposure to unspecified man-made visible and ultraviolet light

W90 Exposure to other nonionizing radiation
> **Excludes2:** exposure to sunlight (X32)
>
> The appropriate 7th character is to be added to each code from category W90
> A initial encounter
> D subsequent encounter
> S sequela

X+7th W90.0 Exposure to radiofrequency
X+7th W90.1 Exposure to infrared radiation
X+7th W90.2 Exposure to laser radiation
X+7th W90.8 Exposure to other nonionizing radiation

W92 Exposure to excessive heat of man-made origin
X+7th
> The appropriate 7th character is to be added to code W92
> A initial encounter
> D subsequent encounter
> S sequela

W93 Exposure to excessive cold of man-made origin
> The appropriate 7th character is to be added to each code from category W93
> A initial encounter
> D subsequent encounter
> S sequela

+ W93.0 Contact with or inhalation of dry ice
  X+7th W93.01 Contact with dry ice
  X+7th W93.02 Inhalation of dry ice
+ W93.1 Contact with or inhalation of liquid air
  X+7th W93.11 Contact with liquid air
    Contact with liquid hydrogen
    Contact with liquid nitrogen
  X+7th W93.12 Inhalation of liquid air
    Inhalation of liquid hydrogen
    Inhalation of liquid nitrogen
X+7th W93.2 Prolonged exposure in deep freeze unit or refrigerator
X+7th W93.8 Exposure to other excessive cold of man-made origin

W94 Exposure to high and low air pressure and changes in air pressure
> The appropriate 7th character is to be added to each code from category W94
> A initial encounter
> D subsequent encounter
> S sequela

X+7th W94.0 Exposure to prolonged high air pressure
+ W94.1 Exposure to prolonged low air pressure
  X+7th W94.11 Exposure to residence or prolonged visit at high altitude
  X+7th W94.12 Exposure to other prolonged low air pressure
+ W94.2 Exposure to rapid changes in air pressure during ascent
  X+7th W94.21 Exposure to reduction in atmospheric pressure while surfacing from deep-water diving
  X+7th W94.22 Exposure to reduction in atmospheric pressure while surfacing from underground
  X+7th W94.23 Exposure to sudden change in air pressure in aircraft during ascent
  X+7th W94.29 Exposure to other rapid changes in air pressure during ascent
+ W94.3 Exposure to rapid changes in air pressure during descent
  X+7th W94.31 Exposure to sudden change in air pressure in aircraft during descent
  X+7th W94.32 Exposure to high air pressure from rapid descent in water
  X+7th W94.39 Exposure to other rapid changes in air pressure during descent

W99 Exposure to other man-made environmental factors
X+7th
> The appropriate 7th character is to be added to code W99
> A initial encounter
> D subsequent encounter
> S sequela

Exposure to smoke, fire and flames (X00-X08)

Excludes1: arson (X97)
Excludes2: explosions (W35-W40)
  lightning (T75.0-)
  transport accident (V01-V99)

X00 Exposure to uncontrolled fire in building or structure
> **Includes:** conflagration in building or structure
> Code first any associated cataclysm
> **Excludes2:** Exposure to ignition or melting of nightwear (X05)
>   Exposure to ignition or melting of other clothing and apparel (X06.-)
>   Exposure to other specified smoke, fire and flames (X08.-)
>
> The appropriate 7th character is to be added to each code from category X00
> A initial encounter
> D subsequent encounter
> S sequela

X+7th X00.0 Exposure to flames in uncontrolled fire in building or structure
  AHA CC: 1Q, 2015, 3-21; 2Q, 2016, 5-6
X+7th X00.1 Exposure to smoke in uncontrolled fire in building or structure
X+7th X00.2 Injury due to collapse of burning building or structure in uncontrolled fire
  > **Excludes1:** injury due to collapse of building not on fire (W20.1)
X+7th X00.3 Fall from burning building or structure in uncontrolled fire
X+7th X00.4 Hit by object from burning building or structure in uncontrolled fire
X+7th X00.5 Jump from burning building or structure in uncontrolled fire
X+7th X00.8 Other exposure to uncontrolled fire in building or structure

X01 Exposure to uncontrolled fire, not in building or structure
> **Includes:** exposure to forest fire
>
> The appropriate 7th character is to be added to each code from category X01
> A initial encounter
> D subsequent encounter
> S sequela

X+7th X01.0 Exposure to flames in uncontrolled fire, not in building or structure
X+7th X01.1 Exposure to smoke in uncontrolled fire, not in building or structure
X+7th X01.3 Fall due to uncontrolled fire, not in building or structure
X+7th X01.4 Hit by object due to uncontrolled fire, not in building or structure
X+7th X01.8 Other exposure to uncontrolled fire, not in building or structure

X02 Exposure to controlled fire in building or structure
> **Includes:** exposure to fire in fireplace
>   exposure to fire in stove
>
> The appropriate 7th character is to be added to each code from category X02
> A initial encounter
> D subsequent encounter
> S sequela

X+7th X02.0 Exposure to flames in controlled fire in building or structure
X+7th X02.1 Exposure to smoke in controlled fire in building or structure
X+7th X02.2 Injury due to collapse of burning building or structure in controlled fire
  > **Excludes1:** injury due to collapse of building not on fire (W20.1)
X+7th X02.3 Fall from burning building or structure in controlled fire
X+7th X02.4 Hit by object from burning building or structure in controlled fire
X+7th X02.5 Jump from burning building or structure in controlled fire
X+7th X02.8 Other exposure to controlled fire in building or structure

X03 Exposure to controlled fire, not in building or structure

> **Includes:** exposure to bon fire
> exposure to camp-fire
> exposure to trash fire

> The appropriate 7th character is to be added to each code from category X03
> A initial encounter
> D subsequent encounter
> S sequela

X+7th **X03.0** Exposure to flames in controlled fire, not in building or structure
AHA CC: 1Q, 2015, 3-21

X+7th **X03.1** Exposure to smoke in controlled fire, not in building or structure

X+7th **X03.3** Fall due to controlled fire, not in building or structure

X+7th **X03.4** Hit by object due to controlled fire, not in building or structure

X+7th **X03.8** Other exposure to controlled fire, not in building or structure

X04 Exposure to ignition of highly flammable material
X+7th
> Exposure to ignition of gasoline
> Exposure to ignition of kerosene
> Exposure to ignition of petrol
>
> **Excludes2:** exposure to ignition or melting of nightwear (X05)
> exposure to ignition or melting of other clothing and apparel (X06)
>
> *AHA CC: 2Q, 2016, 4*

> The appropriate 7th character is to be added to code X04
> A initial encounter
> D subsequent encounter
> S sequela

X05 Exposure to ignition or melting of nightwear
X+7th
> **Excludes2:** exposure to uncontrolled fire in building or structure (X00.-)
> exposure to uncontrolled fire, not in building or structure (X01.-)
> exposure to controlled fire in building or structure (X02.-)
> exposure to controlled fire, not in building or structure (X03.-)
> exposure to ignition of highly flammable materials (X04.-)

> The appropriate 7th character is to be added to code X05
> A initial encounter
> D subsequent encounter
> S sequela

X06 Exposure to ignition or melting of other clothing and apparel

> **Excludes2:** exposure to uncontrolled fire in building or structure (X00.-)
> exposure to uncontrolled fire, not in building or structure (X01.-)
> exposure to controlled fire in building or structure (X02.-)
> exposure to controlled fire, not in building or structure (X03.-)
> exposure to ignition of highly flammable materials (X04.-)

> The appropriate 7th character is to be added to each code from category X06
> A initial encounter
> D subsequent encounter
> S sequela

X+7th **X06.0** Exposure to ignition of plastic jewelry
X+7th **X06.1** Exposure to melting of plastic jewelry
X+7th **X06.2** Exposure to ignition of other clothing and apparel
X+7th **X06.3** Exposure to melting of other clothing and apparel

X08 Exposure to other specified smoke, fire and flames

> The appropriate 7th character is to be added to each code from category X08
> A initial encounter
> D subsequent encounter
> S sequela

+ **X08.0** Exposure to bed fire
> Exposure to mattress fire

X+7th **X08.00** Exposure to bed fire due to unspecified burning material
X+7th **X08.01** Exposure to bed fire due to burning cigarette
AHA CC: 1Q, 2015, 3-21
X+7th **X08.09** Exposure to bed fire due to other burning material

+ **X08.1** Exposure to sofa fire
X+7th **X08.10** Exposure to sofa fire due to unspecified burning material
X+7th **X08.11** Exposure to sofa fire due to burning cigarette
X+7th **X08.19** Exposure to sofa fire due to other burning material

+ **X08.2** Exposure to other furniture fire
X+7th **X08.20** Exposure to other furniture fire due to unspecified burning material
X+7th **X08.21** Exposure to other furniture fire due to burning cigarette
X+7th **X08.29** Exposure to other furniture fire due to other burning material

X+7th **X08.8** Exposure to other specified smoke, fire and flames

Contact with heat and hot substances (X10-X19)

Excludes1: exposure to excessive natural heat (X30)
exposure to fire and flames (X00-X08)

X10 Contact with hot drinks, food, fats and cooking oils

> The appropriate 7th character is to be added to each code from category X10
> A initial encounter
> D subsequent encounter
> S sequela

X+7th **X10.0** Contact with hot drinks
X+7th **X10.1** Contact with hot food
X+7th **X10.2** Contact with fats and cooking oils

X11 Contact with hot tap-water

> **Includes:** contact with boiling tap-water
> contact with boiling water NOS
>
> **Excludes1:** contact with water heated on stove (X12)

> The appropriate 7th character is to be added to each code from category X11
> A initial encounter
> D subsequent encounter
> S sequela

X+7th **X11.0** Contact with hot water in bath or tub
> **Excludes1:** contact with running hot water in bath or tub (X11.1)

X+7th **X11.1** Contact with running hot water
> Contact with hot water running out of hose
> Contact with hot water running out of tap

X+7th **X11.8** Contact with other hot tap-water
> Contact with hot water in bucket
> Contact with hot tap-water NOS

X12 Contact with other hot fluids
X+7th
> Contact with water heated on stove
>
> **Excludes1:** hot (liquid) metals (X18)

> The appropriate 7th character is to be added to code X12
> A initial encounter
> D subsequent encounter
> S sequela

X13 Contact with steam and other hot vapors

> The appropriate 7th character is to be added to each code from category X13
> A initial encounter
> D subsequent encounter
> S sequela

X+7th **X13.0** Inhalation of steam and other hot vapors
X+7th **X13.1** Other contact with steam and other hot vapors

X14 Contact with hot air and other hot gases

> The appropriate 7th character is to be added to each code from category X14
> A initial encounter
> D subsequent encounter
> S sequela

X+7th **X14.0** Inhalation of hot air and gases
X+7th **X14.1** Other contact with hot air and other hot gases

X15 Contact with hot household appliances

Excludes1: contact with heating appliances (X16)
contact with powered household appliances (W29.-)
exposure to controlled fire in building or structure due to household appliance (X02.8)
exposure to household appliances electrical current (W86.0)

The appropriate 7th character is to be added to each code from category X15
- A initial encounter
- D subsequent encounter
- S sequela

X+7th X15.0 Contact with hot stove (kitchen)
X+7th X15.1 Contact with hot toaster
X+7th X15.2 Contact with hotplate
X+7th X15.3 Contact with hot saucepan or skillet
  Contact with hot cooking pan
  Contact with hot cooking pot
X+7th X15.8 Contact with other hot household appliances
  Contact with cooker
  Contact with kettle
  Contact with light bulbs

X16 Contact with hot heating appliances, radiators and pipes
X+7th
Excludes1: contact with powered appliances (W29.-)
exposure to controlled fire in building or structure due to appliance (X02.8)
exposure to industrial appliances electrical current (W86.1)

The appropriate 7th character is to be added to code X16
- A initial encounter
- D subsequent encounter
- S sequela

X17 Contact with hot engines, machinery and tools
X+7th
Excludes1: contact with hot heating appliances, radiators and pipes (X16)
contact with hot household appliances (X15)

The appropriate 7th character is to be added to code X17
- A initial encounter
- D subsequent encounter
- S sequela

X18 Contact with other hot metals
X+7th
Contact with liquid metal

The appropriate 7th character is to be added to code X18
- A initial encounter
- D subsequent encounter
- S sequela

X19 Contact with other heat and hot substances
X+7th
Excludes1: objects that are not normally hot, e.g., an object made hot by a house fire (X00-X08)

The appropriate 7th character is to be added to code X19
- A initial encounter
- D subsequent encounter
- S sequela

Exposure to forces of nature (X30-X39)

X30 Exposure to excessive natural heat
X+7th
Exposure to excessive heat as the cause of sunstroke
Exposure to heat NOS
Excludes1: excessive heat of man-made origin (W92)
exposure to man-made radiation (W89)
exposure to sunlight (X32)
exposure to tanning bed (W89)
AHA CC: 4Q, 2017, 112-114
Review coding guideline B.19.c

The appropriate 7th character is to be added to code X30
- A initial encounter
- D subsequent encounter
- S sequela

X31 Exposure to excessive natural cold
X+7th
Excessive cold as the cause of chilblains NOS
Excessive cold as the cause of immersion foot or hand
Exposure to cold NOS
Exposure to weather conditions
Excludes1: cold of man-made origin (W93.-)
contact with or inhalation of dry ice (W93.-)
contact with or inhalation of liquefied gas (W93.-)
AHA CC: 4Q, 2017, 112-114
Review coding guideline B.19.c

The appropriate 7th character is to be added to code X31
- A initial encounter
- D subsequent encounter
- S sequela

X32 Exposure to sunlight
X+7th
Excludes1: man-made radiation (tanning bed) (W89)
Excludes2: radiation-related disorders of the skin and subcutaneous tissue (L55-L59)

The appropriate 7th character is to be added to code X32
- A initial encounter
- D subsequent encounter
- S sequela

X34 Earthquake
X+7th
Excludes2: tidal wave (tsunami) due to earthquake (X37.41)

The appropriate 7th character is to be added to code X34
- A initial encounter
- D subsequent encounter
- S sequela

X35 Volcanic eruption
X+7th
Excludes2: tidal wave (tsunami) due to volcanic eruption (X37.41)

The appropriate 7th character is to be added to code X35
- A initial encounter
- D subsequent encounter
- S sequela

X36 Avalanche, landslide and other earth movements
X+7th
Includes: victim of mudslide of cataclysmic nature
Excludes1: earthquake (X34)
Excludes2: transport accident involving collision with avalanche or landslide not in motion (V01-V99)

The appropriate 7th character is to be added to each code from category X36
- A initial encounter
- D subsequent encounter
- S sequela

X36.0 Collapse of dam or man-made structure causing earth movement
AHA CC: 4Q, 2017, 112-114
Review coding guideline B.19.b
X36.1 Avalanche, landslide, or mudslide

X37 Cataclysmic storm

The appropriate 7th character is to be added to each code from category X37
- A initial encounter
- D subsequent encounter
- S sequela

X+7th X37.0 Hurricane
  Storm surge
  Typhoon
  AHA CC: 4Q, 2017, 112-114
  Review coding guideline B.19
X+7th X37.1 Tornado
  Cyclone
  Twister
X+7th X37.2 Blizzard (snow)(ice)
X+7th X37.3 Dust storm
+ X37.4 Tidalwave
  X+7th X37.41 Tidal wave due to earthquake or volcanic eruption
    Tidal wave NOS
    Tsunami
  X+7th X37.42 Tidal wave due to storm
  X+7th X37.43 Tidal wave due to landslide
X+7th X37.8 Other cataclysmic storms
  Cloudburst
  Torrential rain
  Excludes2: flood (X38)

X+7th X37.9 Unspecified cataclysmic storm
  Storm NOS
  Excludes1: collapse of dam or man-made structure causing earth movement (X36.0)

X38 Flood
X+7th
  Flood arising from remote storm
  Flood of cataclysmic nature arising from melting snow
  Flood resulting directly from storm
  Excludes1: collapse of dam or man-made structure causing earth movement (X36.0)
  tidal wave NOS (X37.41)
  tidal wave caused by storm (X37.42)
  AHA CC: 4Q, 2017, 112-114
  Review coding guideline B.19

  The appropriate 7th character is to be added to code X38
  A initial encounter
  D subsequent encounter
  S sequela

X39 Exposure to other forces of nature

  The appropriate 7th character is to be added to each code from category X39
  A initial encounter
  D subsequent encounter
  S sequela

  + X39.0 Exposure to natural radiation
  Excludes1: contact with and (suspected) exposure to radon and other naturally occurring radiation (Z77.123)
  exposure to man-made radiation (W88-W90)
  exposure to sunlight (X32)

  X+7th X39.01 Exposure to radon
  X+7th X39.08 Exposure to other natural radiation
X+7th X39.8 Other exposure to forces of nature

Overexertion and strenuous or repetitive movements (X50)

X50 Overexertion and strenuous or repetitive movements
  AHA CC: 4Q, 2016, 73-74

  The appropriate 7th character is to be added to each code from category X50
  A initial encounter
  D subsequent encounter
  S sequela

X+7th X50.0 Overexertion from strenuous movement or load
  Lifting heavy objects
  Lifting weights
X+7th X50.1 Overexertion from prolonged static or awkward postures
  Prolonged bending
  Prolonged kneeling
  Prolonged reaching
  Prolonged sitting
  Prolonged standing
  Prolonged twisting
  Static bending
  Static kneeling
  Static reaching
  Static sitting
  Static standing
  Static twisting
X+7th X50.3 Overexertion from repetitive movements
  Use of hand as hammer.
  Excludes2: Overuse from prolonged static or awkward postures (X50.1)
X+7th X50.9 Other and unspecified overexertion or strenuous movements or postures
  Contact pressure
  Contact stress

Accidental exposure to other specified factors (X52-X58)

X52 Prolonged stay in weightless environment
X+7th
  Weightlessness in spacecraft (simulator)

  The appropriate 7th character is to be added to code X52
  A initial encounter
  D subsequent encounter
  S sequela

X58 Exposure to other specified factors
X+7th
  Accident NOS
  Exposure NOS

  The appropriate 7th character is to be added to code X58
  A initial encounter
  D subsequent encounter
  S sequela

Intentional self-harm (X71-X83)
  Purposely self-inflicted injury
  Suicide (attempted)

X71 Intentional self-harm by drowning and submersion

  The appropriate 7th character is to be added to each code from category X71
  A initial encounter
  D subsequent encounter
  S sequela

X+7th X71.0 Intentional self-harm by drowning and submersion while in bathtub
X+7th X71.1 Intentional self-harm by drowning and submersion while in swimming pool
X+7th X71.2 Intentional self-harm by drowning and submersion after jump into swimming pool
X+7th X71.3 Intentional self-harm by drowning and submersion in natural water
X+7th X71.8 Other intentional self-harm by drowning and submersion
X+7th X71.9 Intentional self-harm by drowning and submersion, unspecified

X72 Intentional self-harm by handgun discharge
X+7th
  Intentional self-harm by gun for single hand use
  Intentional self-harm by pistol
  Intentional self-harm by revolver
  Excludes1: Very pistol (X74.8)

  The appropriate 7th character is to be added to code X72
  A initial encounter
  D subsequent encounter
  S sequela

X73 Intentional self-harm by rifle, shotgun and larger firearm
X+7th discharge
  Excludes1: airgun (X74.01)

  The appropriate 7th character is to be added to each code from category X73
  A initial encounter
  D subsequent encounter
  S sequela

X+7th X73.0 Intentional self-harm by shotgun discharge
X+7th X73.1 Intentional self-harm by hunting rifle discharge
X+7th X73.2 Intentional self-harm by machine gun discharge
X+7th X73.8 Intentional self-harm by other larger firearm discharge
X+7th X73.9 Intentional self-harm by unspecified larger firearm discharge

X74 Intentional self-harm by other and unspecified firearm and gun discharge

  The appropriate 7th character is to be added to each code from category X74
  A initial encounter
  D subsequent encounter
  S sequela

  + X74.0 Intentional self-harm by gas, air or spring-operated guns
  X+7th X74.01 Intentional self-harm by airgun
    Intentional self-harm by BB gun discharge
    Intentional self-harm by pellet gun discharge
  X+7th X74.02 Intentional self-harm by paintball gun
  X+7th X74.09 Intentional self-harm by other gas, air or spring-operated gun
X+7th X74.8 Intentional self-harm by other firearm discharge
  Intentional self-harm by Very pistol [flare] discharge
X+7th X74.9 Intentional self-harm by unspecified firearm discharge

X75 Intentional self-harm by explosive material
X+7th
  The appropriate 7th character is to be added to code X75
  A initial encounter
  D subsequent encounter
  S sequela

X76 Intentional self-harm by smoke, fire and flames

X+7th The appropriate 7th character is to be added to code X76
- A initial encounter
- D subsequent encounter
- S sequela

X77 Intentional self-harm by steam, hot vapors and hot objects

The appropriate 7th character is to be added to each code from category X77
- A initial encounter
- D subsequent encounter
- S sequela

X+7th **X77.0** Intentional self-harm by steam or hot vapors
X+7th **X77.1** Intentional self-harm by hot tap water
X+7th **X77.2** Intentional self-harm by other hot fluids
X+7th **X77.3** Intentional self-harm by hot household appliances
X+7th **X77.8** Intentional self-harm by other hot objects
X+7th **X77.9** Intentional self-harm by unspecified hot objects

X78 Intentional self-harm by sharp object

The appropriate 7th character is to be added to each code from category X78
- A initial encounter
- D subsequent encounter
- S sequela

X+7th **X78.0** Intentional self-harm by sharp glass
X+7th **X78.1** Intentional self-harm by knife
X+7th **X78.2** Intentional self-harm by sword or dagger
X+7th **X78.8** Intentional self-harm by other sharp object
        AHA CC: 1Q, 2022, 27-28
X+7th **X78.9** Intentional self-harm by unspecified sharp object

X79 Intentional self-harm by blunt object

X+7th The appropriate 7th character is to be added to code X79
- A initial encounter
- D subsequent encounter
- S sequela

X80 Intentional self-harm by jumping from a high place

X+7th Intentional fall from one level to another

The appropriate 7th character is to be added to code X80
- A initial encounter
- D subsequent encounter
- S sequela

X81 Intentional self-harm by jumping or lying in front of moving object

The appropriate 7th character is to be added to each code from category X81
- A initial encounter
- D subsequent encounter
- S sequela

X+7th **X81.0** Intentional self-harm by jumping or lying in front of motor vehicle
X+7th **X81.1** Intentional self-harm by jumping or lying in front of (subway) train
X+7th **X81.8** Intentional self-harm by jumping or lying in front of other moving object

X82 Intentional self-harm by crashing of motor vehicle

The appropriate 7th character is to be added to each code from category X82
- A initial encounter
- D subsequent encounter
- S sequela

X+7th **X82.0** Intentional collision of motor vehicle with other motor vehicle
X+7th **X82.1** Intentional collision of motor vehicle with train
X+7th **X82.2** Intentional collision of motor vehicle with tree
X+7th **X82.8** Other intentional self-harm by crashing of motor vehicle

X83 Intentional self-harm by other specified means

Excludes1: intentional self-harm by poisoning or contact with toxic substance- See Table of Drugs and Chemicals

The appropriate 7th character is to be added to each code from category X83
- A initial encounter
- D subsequent encounter
- S sequela

X+7th **X83.0** Intentional self-harm by crashing of aircraft
X+7th **X83.1** Intentional self-harm by electrocution
X+7th **X83.2** Intentional self-harm by exposure to extremes of cold
X+7th **X83.8** Intentional self-harm by other specified means

Assault (X92-Y09)

Includes: homicide
injuries inflicted by another person with intent to injure or kill, by any means

Excludes1: injuries due to legal intervention (Y35.-)
injuries due to operations of war (Y36.-)
injuries due to terrorism (Y38.-)

Review coding guideline C.19.f

X92 Assault by drowning and submersion

The appropriate 7th character is to be added to each code from category X92
- A initial encounter
- D subsequent encounter
- S sequela

X+7th **X92.0** Assault by drowning and submersion while in bathtub
X+7th **X92.1** Assault by drowning and submersion while in swimming pool
X+7th **X92.2** Assault by drowning and submersion after push into swimming pool
X+7th **X92.3** Assault by drowning and submersion in natural water
X+7th **X92.8** Other assault by drowning and submersion
X+7th **X92.9** Assault by drowning and submersion, unspecified

X93 Assault by handgun discharge

X+7th Assault by discharge of gun for single hand use
Assault by discharge of pistol
Assault by discharge of revolver

Excludes1: Very pistol (X95.8)

The appropriate 7th character is to be added to code X93
- A initial encounter
- D subsequent encounter
- S sequela

X94 Assault by rifle, shotgun and larger firearm discharge

Excludes1: airgun (X95.01)

The appropriate 7th character is to be added to each code from category X94
- A initial encounter
- D subsequent encounter
- S sequela

X+7th **X94.0** Assault by shotgun
X+7th **X94.1** Assault by hunting rifle
X+7th **X94.2** Assault by machine gun
X+7th **X94.8** Assault by other larger firearm discharge
X+7th **X94.9** Assault by unspecified larger firearm discharge

X95 Assault by other and unspecified firearm and gun discharge

The appropriate 7th character is to be added to each code from category X95
- A initial encounter
- D subsequent encounter
- S sequela

+ **X95.0** Assault by gas, air or spring-operated guns
  X+7th **X95.01** Assault by airgun discharge
       Assault by BB gun discharge
       Assault by pellet gun discharge
  X+7th **X95.02** Assault by paintball gun discharge
  X+7th **X95.09** Assault by other gas, air or spring-operated gun
X+7th **X95.8** Assault by other firearm discharge
       Assault by very pistol [flare] discharge
X+7th **X95.9** Assault by unspecified firearm discharge
       AHA CC: 3Q, 2016, 24

X96 Assault by explosive material

Excludes1: incendiary device (X97)
terrorism involving explosive material (Y38.2-)

The appropriate 7th character is to be added to each code from category X96
- A initial encounter
- D subsequent encounter
- S sequela

X+7th	**X96.0**	Assault by antipersonnel bomb
	Excludes1:	antipersonnel bomb use in military or war (Y36.2-)
X+7th	**X96.1**	Assault by gasoline bomb
X+7th	**X96.2**	Assault by letter bomb
X+7th	**X96.3**	Assault by fertilizer bomb
X+7th	**X96.4**	Assault by pipe bomb
X+7th	**X96.8**	Assault by other specified explosive
X+7th	**X96.9**	Assault by unspecified explosive

X97 **Assault by smoke, fire and flames**
X+7th

Assault by arson
Assault by cigarettes
Assault by incendiary device

The appropriate 7th character is to be added to code X97
- A initial encounter
- D subsequent encounter
- S sequela

X98 **Assault by steam, hot vapors and hot objects**

The appropriate 7th character is to be added to each code from category X98
- A initial encounter
- D subsequent encounter
- S sequela

X+7th	**X98.0**	Assault by steam or hot vapors
X+7th	**X98.1**	Assault by hot tap water
X+7th	**X98.2**	Assault by hot fluids
X+7th	**X98.3**	Assault by hot household appliances
X+7th	**X98.8**	Assault by other hot objects
X+7th	**X98.9**	Assault by unspecified hot objects

X99 **Assault by sharp object**

Excludes1: assault by strike by sports equipment (Y08.0-)

The appropriate 7th character is to be added to each code from category X99
- A initial encounter
- D subsequent encounter
- S sequela

X+7th	**X99.0**	Assault by sharp glass
X+7th	**X99.1**	Assault by knife
X+7th	**X99.2**	Assault by sword or dagger
X+7th	**X99.8**	Assault by other sharp object
X+7th	**X99.9**	Assault by unspecified sharp object
		Assault by stabbing NOS

Y00 **Assault by blunt object**
X+7th

Excludes1: assault by strike by sports equipment (Y08.0-)

The appropriate 7th character is to be added to code Y00
- A initial encounter
- D subsequent encounter
- S sequela

Y01 **Assault by pushing from high place**
X+7th

The appropriate 7th character is to be added to code Y01
- A initial encounter
- D subsequent encounter
- S sequela

Y02 **Assault by pushing or placing victim in front of moving object**

The appropriate 7th character is to be added to each code from category Y02
- A initial encounter
- D subsequent encounter
- S sequela

X+7th	**Y02.0**	Assault by pushing or placing victim in front of motor vehicle
X+7th	**Y02.1**	Assault by pushing or placing victim in front of (subway) train
X+7th	**Y02.8**	Assault by pushing or placing victim in front of other moving object

Y03 **Assault by crashing of motor vehicle**

The appropriate 7th character is to be added to each code from category Y03
- A initial encounter
- D subsequent encounter
- S sequela

X+7th	**Y03.0**	Assault by being hit or run over by motor vehicle
X+7th	**Y03.8**	Other assault by crashing of motor vehicle

Y04 **Assault by bodily force**

Excludes1: assault by:
submersion (X92.-)
use of weapon (X93-X95, X99, Y00)

The appropriate 7th character is to be added to each code from category Y04
- A initial encounter
- D subsequent encounter
- S sequela

X+7th	**Y04.0**	Assault by unarmed brawl or fight
X+7th	**Y04.1**	Assault by human bite
X+7th	**Y04.2**	Assault by strike against or bumped into by another person
X+7th	**Y04.8**	Assault by other bodily force
		Assault by bodily force NOS

Y07 **Perpetrator of assault, maltreatment and neglect**

NOTE Codes from this category are for use only in cases of confirmed abuse (T74.-)
Selection of the correct perpetrator code is based on the relationship between the perpetrator and the victim

Includes: perpetrator of abandonment
perpetrator of emotional neglect
perpetrator of mental cruelty
perpetrator of physical abuse
perpetrator of physical neglect
perpetrator of sexual abuse
perpetrator of torture
perpetrator of verbal abuse

Review coding guideline C.20.g
AHA CC: 4Q, 2018, 32-33

+ **Y07.0** Spouse or partner, perpetrator of maltreatment and neglect

Spouse or partner, perpetrator of maltreatment and neglect against spouse or partner
AHA CC: 1Q, 2023, 5

+ **Y07.01** Husband, perpetrator of maltreatment and neglect
- **Y07.010** Husband, current, perpetrator of maltreatment and neglect
- **Y07.011** Husband, former, perpetrator of maltreatment and neglect

+ **Y07.02** Wife, perpetrator of maltreatment and neglect
- **Y07.020** Wife, current, perpetrator of maltreatment and neglect
- **Y07.021** Wife, former, perpetrator of maltreatment and neglect

+ **Y07.03** Male partner, perpetrator of maltreatment and neglect
- **Y07.030** Male partner, current, perpetrator of maltreatment and neglect
- **Y07.031** Male partner, former, perpetrator of maltreatment and neglect

+ **Y07.04** Female partner, perpetrator of maltreatment and neglect
- **Y07.040** Female partner, current, perpetrator of maltreatment and neglect
- **Y07.041** Female partner, former, perpetrator of maltreatment and neglect

+ **Y07.05** Non-binary partner, current or former, perpetrator of maltreatment or neglect
Gender non-conforming partner, perpetrator of maltreatment and neglect
- **Y07.050** Non-binary partner, current, perpetrator of maltreatment and neglect
- **Y07.051** Non-binary partner, former, perpetrator of maltreatment and neglect

+ **Y07.1** Parent (adoptive) (biological), perpetrator of maltreatment and neglect
- **Y07.11** Biological father, perpetrator of maltreatment and neglect
- **Y07.12** Biological mother, perpetrator of maltreatment and neglect
- **Y07.13** Adoptive father, perpetrator of maltreatment and neglect
- **Y07.14** Adoptive mother, perpetrator of maltreatment and neglect

- **Y07.4 Other family member, perpetrator of maltreatment and neglect**
  - **Y07.41 Sibling, perpetrator of maltreatment and neglect**
    - *Excludes1:* stepsibling, perpetrator of maltreatment and neglect (Y07.435, Y07.436)
    - Y07.410 Brother, perpetrator of maltreatment and neglect
    - Y07.411 Sister, perpetrator of maltreatment and neglect
  - **Y07.42 Foster parent, perpetrator of maltreatment and neglect**
    - Y07.420 Foster father, perpetrator of maltreatment and neglect
    - Y07.421 Foster mother, perpetrator of maltreatment and neglect
  - **Y07.43 Stepparent or stepsibling, perpetrator of maltreatment and neglect**
    - Y07.430 Stepfather, perpetrator of maltreatment and neglect
    - Y07.432 Male friend of parent (co-residing in household), perpetrator of maltreatment and neglect
    - Y07.433 Stepmother, perpetrator of maltreatment and neglect
    - Y07.434 Female friend of parent (co-residing in household), perpetrator of maltreatment and neglect
    - Y07.435 Stepbrother, perpetrator or maltreatment and neglect
    - Y07.436 Stepsister, perpetrator of maltreatment and neglect
  - **Y07.44 Child, perpetrator of maltreatment and neglect**
    - Adopted child, perpetrator of maltreatment and neglect
    - Biological child, perpetrator of maltreatment and neglect
    - Daughter, perpetrator of maltreatment and neglect
    - Foster child, perpetrator of maltreatment and neglect
    - In-law child, perpetrator of maltreatment and neglect
    - Non-binary child, perpetrator of maltreatment and neglect
    - Son, perpetrator of maltreatment and neglect
    - Stepchild, perpetrator of maltreatment and neglect
  - **Y07.45 Grandchild, perpetrator of maltreatment and neglect**
    - Adopted grandchild, perpetrator of maltreatment and neglect
    - Biological grandchild, perpetrator of maltreatment and neglect
    - Foster grandchild, perpetrator of maltreatment and neglect
    - Granddaughter, perpetrator of maltreatment and neglect
    - Grandson, perpetrator of maltreatment and neglect
    - In-law grandchild, perpetrator of maltreatment and neglect
    - Non-binary grandchild, perpetrator of maltreatment and neglect
    - Step grandchild, perpetrator of maltreatment and neglect
  - **Y07.46 Grandparent, perpetrator of maltreatment and neglect**
    - Grandfather, perpetrator of maltreatment and neglect
    - Grandmother, perpetrator of maltreatment and neglect
    - Non-binary grandparent, perpetrator of maltreatment and neglect
  - **Y07.47 Parental sibling, perpetrator of maltreatment and neglect**
    - Aunt, perpetrator of maltreatment and neglect
    - Non-binary parental sibling, perpetrator of maltreatment and neglect
    - Uncle, perpetrator of maltreatment and neglect
  - **Y07.49 Other family member, perpetrator of maltreatment and neglect**
    - Y07.490 Male cousin, perpetrator of maltreatment and neglect
    - Y07.491 Female cousin, perpetrator of maltreatment and neglect
    - Y07.499 Other family member, perpetrator of maltreatment and neglect
- **Y07.5 Non-family member, perpetrator of maltreatment and neglect**
  - Y07.50 Unspecified non-family member, perpetrator of maltreatment and neglect
  - **Y07.51 Daycare provider, perpetrator of maltreatment and neglect**
    - Y07.510 At-home childcare provider, perpetrator of maltreatment and neglect
    - Y07.511 Daycare center childcare provider, perpetrator of maltreatment and neglect
    - Y07.512 At-home adultcare provider, perpetrator of maltreatment and neglect
    - Y07.513 Adultcare center provider, perpetrator of maltreatment and neglect
    - Y07.519 Unspecified daycare provider, perpetrator of maltreatment and neglect
  - **Y07.52 Healthcare provider, perpetrator of maltreatment and neglect**
    - Y07.521 Mental health provider, perpetrator of maltreatment and neglect
    - Y07.528 Other therapist or healthcare provider, perpetrator of maltreatment and neglect
      - Nurse perpetrator of maltreatment and neglect
      - Occupational therapist perpetrator of maltreatment and neglect
      - Physical therapist perpetrator of maltreatment and neglect
      - Speech therapist perpetrator of maltreatment and neglect
    - Y07.529 Unspecified healthcare provider, perpetrator of maltreatment and neglect
  - Y07.53 Teacher or instructor, perpetrator of maltreatment and neglect
    - Coach, perpetrator of maltreatment and neglect
  - Y07.54 Acquaintance or friend, perpetrator of maltreatment and neglect
  - Y07.59 Other non-family member, perpetrator of maltreatment and neglect
- **Y07.6 Multiple perpetrators of maltreatment and neglect**
  - *AHA CC: 4Q, 2018, 32-33*
- **Y07.9 Unspecified perpetrator of maltreatment and neglect**

Y08 Assault by other specified means

The appropriate 7th character is to be added to each code from category Y08
- A initial encounter
- D subsequent encounter
- S sequela

- **Y08.0 Assault by strike by sport equipment**
  - Y08.01 Assault by strike by hockey stick
  - Y08.02 Assault by strike by baseball bat
  - Y08.09 Assault by strike by other specified type of sport equipment
- **Y08.8 Assault by other specified means**
  - Y08.81 Assault by crashing of aircraft
  - Y08.89 Assault by other specified means

Y09 Assault by unspecified means

Assassination (attempted) NOS
Homicide (attempted) NOS
Manslaughter (attempted) NOS
Murder (attempted) NOS
Valid 3-character code, no further characters required

Event of undetermined intent (Y21-Y33)

Undetermined intent is only for use when there is specific documentation in the record that the intent of the injury cannot be determined. If no such documentation is present, code to accidental (unintentional)

Y21 Drowning and submersion, undetermined intent

The appropriate 7th character is to be added to each code from category Y21
- A initial encounter
- D subsequent encounter
- S sequela

- **X+7th Y21.0** Drowning and submersion while in bathtub, undetermined intent
- **X+7th Y21.1** Drowning and submersion after fall into bathtub, undetermined intent
- **X+7th Y21.2** Drowning and submersion while in swimming pool, undetermined intent
- **X+7th Y21.3** Drowning and submersion after fall into swimming pool, undetermined intent
- **X+7th Y21.4** Drowning and submersion in natural water, undetermined intent
- **X+7th Y21.8** Other drowning and submersion, undetermined intent
- **X+7th Y21.9** Unspecified drowning and submersion, undetermined intent

X+7th Y22 Handgun discharge, undetermined intent

Discharge of gun for single hand use, undetermined intent
Discharge of pistol, undetermined intent
Discharge of revolver, undetermined intent

Excludes2: very pistol (Y24.8)

The appropriate 7th character is to be added to code Y22
- A initial encounter
- D subsequent encounter
- S sequela

Y23 Rifle, shotgun and larger firearm discharge, undetermined intent

Excludes2: airgun (Y24.0)

The appropriate 7th character is to be added to each code from category Y23
- A initial encounter
- D subsequent encounter
- S sequela

- **X+7th Y23.0** Shotgun discharge, undetermined intent
- **X+7th Y23.1** Hunting rifle discharge, undetermined intent
- **X+7th Y23.2** Military firearm discharge, undetermined intent
- **X+7th Y23.3** Machine gun discharge, undetermined intent
- **X+7th Y23.8** Other larger firearm discharge, undetermined intent
- **X+7th Y23.9** Unspecified larger firearm discharge, undetermined intent

Y24 Other and unspecified firearm discharge, undetermined intent

The appropriate 7th character is to be added to each code from category Y24
- A initial encounter
- D subsequent encounter
- S sequela

- **X+7th Y24.0** Airgun discharge, undetermined intent
  BB gun discharge, undetermined intent
  Pellet gun discharge, undetermined intent
- **X+7th Y24.8** Other firearm discharge, undetermined intent
  Paintball gun discharge, undetermined intent
  Very pistol [flare] discharge, undetermined intent
- **X+7th Y24.9** Unspecified firearm discharge, undetermined intent

Y25 Contact with explosive material, undetermined intent
X+7th

The appropriate 7th character is to be added to code Y25
- A initial encounter
- D subsequent encounter
- S sequela

Y26 Exposure to smoke, fire and flames, undetermined intent
X+7th

The appropriate 7th character is to be added to code Y26
- A initial encounter
- D subsequent encounter
- S sequela

Y27 Contact with steam, hot vapors and hot objects, undetermined intent

The appropriate 7th character is to be added to each code from category Y27
- A initial encounter
- D subsequent encounter
- S sequela

- **X+7th Y27.0** Contact with steam and hot vapors, undetermined intent
- **X+7th Y27.1** Contact with hot tap water, undetermined intent
- **X+7th Y27.2** Contact with hot fluids, undetermined intent
- **X+7th Y27.3** Contact with hot household appliance, undetermined intent
- **X+7th Y27.8** Contact with other hot objects, undetermined intent
- **X+7th Y27.9** Contact with unspecified hot objects, undetermined intent

Y28 Contact with sharp object, undetermined intent

The appropriate 7th character is to be added to each code from category Y28
- A initial encounter
- D subsequent encounter
- S sequela

- **X+7th Y28.0** Contact with sharp glass, undetermined intent
- **X+7th Y28.1** Contact with knife, undetermined intent
- **X+7th Y28.2** Contact with sword or dagger, undetermined intent
- **X+7th Y28.8** Contact with other sharp object, undetermined intent
- **X+7th Y28.9** Contact with unspecified sharp object, undetermined intent

Y29 Contact with blunt object, undetermined intent
X+7th

The appropriate 7th character is to be added to code Y29
- A initial encounter
- D subsequent encounter
- S sequela

Y30 Falling, jumping or pushed from a high place, undetermined intent
X+7th

Victim falling from one level to another, undetermined intent

The appropriate 7th character is to be added to code Y30
- A initial encounter
- D subsequent encounter
- S sequela

Y31 Falling, lying or running before or into moving object, undetermined intent
X+7th

The appropriate 7th character is to be added to code Y31
- A initial encounter
- D subsequent encounter
- S sequela

Y32 Crashing of motor vehicle, undetermined intent
X+7th

The appropriate 7th character is to be added to code Y32
- A initial encounter
- D subsequent encounter
- S sequela

Y33 Other specified events, undetermined intent
X+7th

The appropriate 7th character is to be added to code Y33
- A initial encounter
- D subsequent encounter
- S sequela

Legal intervention, operations of war, military operations, and terrorism (Y35-Y38)

Y35 Legal intervention

Includes: any injury sustained as a result of an encounter with any law enforcement official, serving in any capacity at the time of the encounter, whether on-duty or off-duty. Includes: a injury to law enforcement official, suspect and bystander

The appropriate 7th character is to be added to each code from category Y35
- A initial encounter
- D subsequent encounter
- S sequela

AHA CC: 4Q, 2019, 18-19

- **+ Y35.0** Legal intervention involving firearm discharge
  - **+ Y35.00** Legal intervention involving unspecified firearm discharge
    Legal intervention involving gunshot wound
    Legal intervention involving shot NOS

- +7th **Y35.001** Legal intervention involving unspecified firearm discharge, law enforcement official injured
- +7th **Y35.002** Legal intervention involving unspecified firearm discharge, bystander injured
- +7th **Y35.003** Legal intervention involving unspecified firearm discharge, suspect injured
- +7th **Y35.009** Legal intervention involving unspecified firearm discharge, unspecified person injured
- + **Y35.01** Legal intervention involving injury by machine gun
  - +7th **Y35.011** Legal intervention involving injury by machine gun, law enforcement official injured
  - +7th **Y35.012** Legal intervention involving injury by machine gun, bystander injured
  - +7th **Y35.013** Legal intervention involving injury by machine gun, suspect injured
  - +7th **Y35.019** Legal intervention involving injury by machine gun, unspecified person injured
- + **Y35.02** Legal intervention involving injury by handgun
  - +7th **Y35.021** Legal intervention involving injury by handgun, law enforcement official injured
  - +7th **Y35.022** Legal intervention involving injury by handgun, bystander injured
  - +7th **Y35.023** Legal intervention involving injury by handgun, suspect injured
  - +7th **Y35.029** Legal intervention involving injury by handgun, unspecified person injured
- + **Y35.03** Legal intervention involving injury by rifle pellet
  - +7th **Y35.031** Legal intervention involving injury by rifle pellet, law enforcement official injured
  - +7th **Y35.032** Legal intervention involving injury by rifle pellet, bystander injured
  - +7th **Y35.033** Legal intervention involving injury by rifle pellet, suspect injured
  - +7th **Y35.039** Legal intervention involving injury by rifle pellet, unspecified person injured
- + **Y35.04** Legal intervention involving injury by rubber bullet
  - +7th **Y35.041** Legal intervention involving injury by rubber bullet, law enforcement official injured
  - +7th **Y35.042** Legal intervention involving injury by rubber bullet, bystander injured
  - +7th **Y35.043** Legal intervention involving injury by rubber bullet, suspect injured
  - +7th **Y35.049** Legal intervention involving injury by rubber bullet, unspecified person injured
- + **Y35.09** Legal intervention involving other firearm discharge
  - +7th **Y35.091** Legal intervention involving other firearm discharge, law enforcement official injured
  - +7th **Y35.092** Legal intervention involving other firearm discharge, bystander injured
  - +7th **Y35.093** Legal intervention involving other firearm discharge, suspect injured
  - +7th **Y35.099** Legal intervention involving injury other firearm discharge, unspecified person injured
- + **Y35.1** Legal intervention involving explosives
  - + **Y35.10** Legal intervention involving unspecified explosives
    - +7th **Y35.101** Legal intervention involving unspecified explosives, law enforcement official injured
    - +7th **Y35.102** Legal intervention involving unspecified explosives, bystander injured
    - +7th **Y35.103** Legal intervention involving unspecified explosives, suspect injured
    - +7th **Y35.109** Legal intervention involving unspecified explosives, unspecified person injured
  - + **Y35.11** Legal intervention involving injury by dynamite
    - +7th **Y35.111** Legal intervention involving injury by dynamite, law enforcement official injured
    - +7th **Y35.112** Legal intervention involving injury by dynamite, bystander injured
    - +7th **Y35.113** Legal intervention involving injury by dynamite, suspect injured
    - +7th **Y35.119** Legal intervention involving injury by dynamite, unspecified person injured
  - + **Y35.12** Legal intervention involving injury by explosive shell
    - +7th **Y35.121** Legal intervention involving injury by explosive shell, law enforcement official injured
    - +7th **Y35.122** Legal intervention involving injury by explosive shell, bystander injured
    - +7th **Y35.123** Legal intervention involving injury by explosive shell, suspect injured
    - +7th **Y35.129** Legal intervention involving injury by explosive shell, unspecified person injured
  - + **Y35.19** Legal intervention involving other explosives
    Legal intervention involving injury by grenade
    Legal intervention involving injury by mortar bomb
    - +7th **Y35.191** Legal intervention involving other explosives, law enforcement official injured
    - +7th **Y35.192** Legal intervention involving other explosives, bystander injured
    - +7th **Y35.193** Legal intervention involving other explosives, suspect injured
    - +7th **Y35.199** Legal intervention involving other explosives, unspecified person injured
- + **Y35.2** Legal intervention involving gas
  Legal intervention involving asphyxiation by gas
  Legal intervention involving poisoning by gas
  - + **Y35.20** Legal intervention involving unspecified gas
    - +7th **Y35.201** Legal intervention involving unspecified gas, law enforcement official injured
    - +7th **Y35.202** Legal intervention involving unspecified gas, bystander injured
    - +7th **Y35.203** Legal intervention involving unspecified gas, suspect injured
    - +7th **Y35.209** Legal intervention involving unspecified gas, unspecified person injured
  - + **Y35.21** Legal intervention involving injury by tear gas
    - +7th **Y35.211** Legal intervention involving injury by tear gas, law enforcement official injured
    - +7th **Y35.212** Legal intervention involving injury by tear gas, bystander injured
    - +7th **Y35.213** Legal intervention involving injury by tear gas, suspect injured
    - +7th **Y35.219** Legal intervention involving injury by tear gas, unspecified person injured
  - + **Y35.29** Legal intervention involving other gas
    - +7th **Y35.291** Legal intervention involving other gas, law enforcement official injured
    - +7th **Y35.292** Legal intervention involving other gas, bystander injured
    - +7th **Y35.293** Legal intervention involving other gas, suspect injured
    - +7th **Y35.299** Legal intervention involving other gas, unspecified person injured
- + **Y35.3** Legal intervention involving blunt objects
  Legal intervention involving being hit or struck by blunt object
  - + **Y35.30** Legal intervention involving unspecified blunt objects
    - +7th **Y35.301** Legal intervention involving unspecified blunt objects, law enforcement official injured
    - +7th **Y35.302** Legal intervention involving unspecified blunt objects, bystander injured
    - +7th **Y35.303** Legal intervention involving unspecified blunt objects, suspect injured
    - +7th **Y35.309** Legal intervention involving unspecified blunt objects, unspecified person injured

+ **Y35.31** Legal intervention involving baton
 +7th **Y35.311** Legal intervention involving baton, law enforcement official injured
 +7th **Y35.312** Legal intervention involving baton, bystander injured
 +7th **Y35.313** Legal intervention involving baton, suspect injured
 +7th **Y35.319** Legal intervention involving baton, unspecified person injured
+ **Y35.39** Legal intervention involving other blunt objects
 +7th **Y35.391** Legal intervention involving other blunt objects, law enforcement official injured
 +7th **Y35.392** Legal intervention involving other blunt objects, bystander injured
 +7th **Y35.393** Legal intervention involving other blunt objects, suspect injured
 +7th **Y35.399** Legal intervention involving other blunt objects, unspecified person injured
+ **Y35.4** Legal intervention involving sharp objects
  Legal intervention involving being cut by sharp objects
  Legal intervention involving being stabbed by sharp objects
 + **Y35.40** Legal intervention involving unspecified sharp objects
  +7th **Y35.401** Legal intervention involving unspecified sharp objects, law enforcement official injured
  +7th **Y35.402** Legal intervention involving unspecified sharp objects, bystander injured
  +7th **Y35.403** Legal intervention involving unspecified sharp objects, suspect injured
  +7th **Y35.409** Legal intervention involving unspecified sharp objects, unspecified person injured
 + **Y35.41** Legal intervention involving bayonet
  +7th **Y35.411** Legal intervention involving bayonet, law enforcement official injured
  +7th **Y35.412** Legal intervention involving bayonet, bystander injured
  +7th **Y35.413** Legal intervention involving bayonet, suspect injured
  +7th **Y35.419** Legal intervention involving bayonet, unspecified person injured
 + **Y35.49** Legal intervention involving other sharp objects
  +7th **Y35.491** Legal intervention involving other sharp objects, law enforcement official injured
  +7th **Y35.492** Legal intervention involving other sharp objects, bystander injured
  +7th **Y35.493** Legal intervention involving other sharp objects, suspect injured
  +7th **Y35.499** Legal intervention involving other sharp objects, unspecified person injured
+ **Y35.8** Legal intervention involving other specified means
 + **Y35.81** Legal intervention involving manhandling
  +7th **Y35.811** Legal intervention involving manhandling, law enforcement official injured
  +7th **Y35.812** Legal intervention involving manhandling, bystander injured
  +7th **Y35.813** Legal intervention involving manhandling, suspect injured
  +7th **Y35.819** Legal intervention involving manhandling, unspecified person injured
 + **Y35.83** Legal intervention involving a conducted energy device
  Electroshock device (taser)
  Stun gun
  +7th **Y35.831** Legal intervention involving a conducted energy device, law enforcement official injured
  +7th **Y35.832** Legal intervention involving a conducted energy device, bystander injured
  +7th **Y35.833** Legal intervention involving a conducted energy device, suspect injured
  +7th **Y35.839** Legal intervention involving a conducted energy device, unspecified person injured

+ **Y35.89** Legal intervention involving other specified means
 +7th **Y35.891** Legal intervention involving other specified means, law enforcement official injured
 +7th **Y35.892** Legal intervention involving other specified means, bystander injured
 +7th **Y35.893** Legal intervention involving other specified means, suspect injured
  AHA CC: 1Q, 2018, 5
 +7th **Y35.899** Legal intervention involving other specified means, unspecified person
  AHA CC: 4Q, 2021, 32
+ **Y35.9** Legal intervention, means unspecified
 X+7th **Y35.91** Legal intervention, means unspecified, law enforcement official injured
 X+7th **Y35.92** Legal intervention, means unspecified, bystander injured
 X+7th **Y35.93** Legal intervention, means unspecified, suspect injured
 X+7th **Y35.99** Legal intervention, means unspecified, unspecified person injured

Y36 Operations of war
  Includes: injuries to military personnel and civilians caused by war, civil insurrection, and peacekeeping missions
  Excludes1: injury to military personnel occurring during peacetime military operations (Y37.-)
  military vehicles involved in transport accidents with non-military vehicle during peacetime (V09.01, V09.21, V19.81, V29.818, V39.81, V49.81, V59.81, V69.81, V79.81)
  AHA CC: 3Q, 2014, 4-5

  The appropriate 7th character is to be added to each code from category Y36
  A initial encounter
  D subsequent encounter
  S sequela

+ **Y36.0** War operations involving explosion of marine weapons
 + **Y36.00** War operations involving explosion of unspecified marine weapon
  War operations involving underwater blast NOS
  +7th **Y36.000** War operations involving explosion of unspecified marine weapon, military personnel
  +7th **Y36.001** War operations involving explosion of unspecified marine weapon, civilian
 + **Y36.01** War operations involving explosion of depth-charge
  +7th **Y36.010** War operations involving explosion of depth-charge, military personnel
  +7th **Y36.011** War operations involving explosion of depth-charge, civilian
 + **Y36.02** War operations involving explosion of marine mine
  War operations involving explosion of marine mine, at sea or in harbor
  +7th **Y36.020** War operations involving explosion of marine mine, military personnel
  +7th **Y36.021** War operations involving explosion of marine mine, civilian
 + **Y36.03** War operations involving explosion of sea-based artillery shell
  +7th **Y36.030** War operations involving explosion of sea-based artillery shell, military personnel
  +7th **Y36.031** War operations involving explosion of sea-based artillery shell, civilian
 + **Y36.04** War operations involving explosion of torpedo
  +7th **Y36.040** War operations involving explosion of torpedo, military personnel
  +7th **Y36.041** War operations involving explosion of torpedo, civilian
 + **Y36.05** War operations involving accidental detonation of onboard marine weapons
  +7th **Y36.050** War operations involving accidental detonation of onboard marine weapons, military personnel
  +7th **Y36.051** War operations involving accidental detonation of onboard marine weapons, civilian

- **Y36.09** War operations involving explosion of other marine weapons
  - +7th **Y36.090** War operations involving explosion of other marine weapons, military personnel
  - +7th **Y36.091** War operations involving explosion of other marine weapons, civilian
- **Y36.1** War operations involving destruction of aircraft
  - **Y36.10** War operations involving unspecified destruction of aircraft
    - +7th **Y36.100** War operations involving unspecified destruction of aircraft, military personnel
    - +7th **Y36.101** War operations involving unspecified destruction of aircraft, civilian
  - **Y36.11** War operations involving destruction of aircraft due to enemy fire or explosives
    - War operations involving destruction of aircraft due to air to air missile
    - War operations involving destruction of aircraft due to explosive placed on aircraft
    - War operations involving destruction of aircraft due to rocket propelled grenade [RPG]
    - War operations involving destruction of aircraft due to small arms fire
    - War operations involving destruction of aircraft due to surface to air missile
    - +7th **Y36.110** War operations involving destruction of aircraft due to enemy fire or explosives, military personnel
    - +7th **Y36.111** War operations involving destruction of aircraft due to enemy fire or explosives, civilian
  - **Y36.12** War operations involving destruction of aircraft due to collision with other aircraft
    - +7th **Y36.120** War operations involving destruction of aircraft due to collision with other aircraft, military personnel
    - +7th **Y36.121** War operations involving destruction of aircraft due to collision with other aircraft, civilian
  - **Y36.13** War operations involving destruction of aircraft due to onboard fire
    - +7th **Y36.130** War operations involving destruction of aircraft due to onboard fire, military personnel
    - +7th **Y36.131** War operations involving destruction of aircraft due to onboard fire, civilian
  - **Y36.14** War operations involving destruction of aircraft due to accidental detonation of onboard munitions and explosives
    - +7th **Y36.140** War operations involving destruction of aircraft due to accidental detonation of onboard munitions and explosives, military personnel
    - +7th **Y36.141** War operations involving destruction of aircraft due to accidental detonation of onboard munitions and explosives, civilian
  - **Y36.19** War operations involving other destruction of aircraft
    - +7th **Y36.190** War operations involving other destruction of aircraft, military personnel
    - +7th **Y36.191** War operations involving other destruction of aircraft, civilian
- **Y36.2** War operations involving other explosions and fragments
  - *Excludes1:* war operations involving explosion of aircraft (Y36.1-)
    - war operations involving explosion of marine weapons (Y36.0-)
    - war operations involving explosion of nuclear weapons (Y36.5-)
    - war operations involving explosion occurring after cessation of hostilities (Y36.8-)
  - **Y36.20** War operations involving unspecified explosion and fragments
    - War operations involving air blast NOS
    - War operations involving blast NOS
    - War operations involving blast fragments NOS
    - War operations involving blast wave NOS
    - War operations involving blast wind NOS
    - War operations involving explosion NOS
    - War operations involving explosion of bomb NOS
    - +7th **Y36.200** War operations involving unspecified explosion and fragments, military personnel
    - +7th **Y36.201** War operations involving unspecified explosion and fragments, civilian
  - **Y36.21** War operations involving explosion of aerial bomb
    - +7th **Y36.210** War operations involving explosion of aerial bomb, military personnel
    - +7th **Y36.211** War operations involving explosion of aerial bomb, civilian
  - **Y36.22** War operations involving explosion of guided missile
    - +7th **Y36.220** War operations involving explosion of guided missile, military personnel
    - +7th **Y36.221** War operations involving explosion of guided missile, civilian
  - **Y36.23** War operations involving explosion of improvised explosive device [IED]
    - War operations involving explosion of person-borne improvised explosive device [IED]
    - War operations involving explosion of vehicle-borne improvised explosive device [IED]
    - War operations involving explosion of roadside improvised explosive device [IED]
    - +7th **Y36.230** War operations involving explosion of improvised explosive device [IED], military personnel
    - +7th **Y36.231** War operations involving explosion of improvised explosive device [IED], civilian
  - **Y36.24** War operations involving explosion due to accidental detonation and discharge of own munitions or munitions launch device
    - +7th **Y36.240** War operations involving explosion due to accidental detonation and discharge of own munitions or munitions launch device, military personnel
    - +7th **Y36.241** War operations involving explosion due to accidental detonation and discharge of own munitions or munitions launch device, civilian
  - **Y36.25** War operations involving fragments from munitions
    - +7th **Y36.250** War operations involving fragments from munitions, military personnel
    - +7th **Y36.251** War operations involving fragments from munitions, civilian
  - **Y36.26** War operations involving fragments of improvised explosive device [IED]
    - War operations involving fragments of person-borne improvised explosive device [IED]
    - War operations involving fragments of vehicle-borne improvised explosive device [IED]
    - War operations involving fragments of roadside improvised explosive device [IED]
    - +7th **Y36.260** War operations involving fragments of improvised explosive device [IED], military personnel
    - +7th **Y36.261** War operations involving fragments of improvised explosive device [IED], civilian
  - **Y36.27** War operations involving fragments from weapons
    - +7th **Y36.270** War operations involving fragments from weapons, military personnel
    - +7th **Y36.271** War operations involving fragments from weapons, civilian

- **Y36.29** War operations involving other explosions and fragments
  - War operations involving explosion of grenade
  - War operations involving explosions of land mine
  - War operations involving shrapnel NOS
  - +7th **Y36.290** War operations involving other explosions and fragments, military personnel
  - +7th **Y36.291** War operations involving other explosions and fragments, civilian
- **Y36.3** War operations involving fires, conflagrations and hot substances
  - War operations involving smoke, fumes, and heat from fires, conflagrations and hot substances
  - **Excludes1:** war operations involving fires and conflagrations aboard military aircraft (Y36.1-)
    - war operations involving fires and conflagrations aboard military watercraft (Y36.0-)
    - war operations involving fires and conflagrations caused indirectly by conventional weapons (Y36.2-)
    - war operations involving fires and thermal effects of nuclear weapons (Y36.53-)
  - **Y36.30** War operations involving unspecified fire, conflagration and hot substance
    - +7th **Y36.300** War operations involving unspecified fire, conflagration and hot substance, military personnel
    - +7th **Y36.301** War operations involving unspecified fire, conflagration and hot substance, civilian
  - **Y36.31** War operations involving gasoline bomb
    - War operations involving incendiary bomb
    - War operations involving petrol bomb
    - +7th **Y36.310** War operations involving gasoline bomb, military personnel
    - +7th **Y36.311** War operations involving gasoline bomb, civilian
  - **Y36.32** War operations involving incendiary bullet
    - +7th **Y36.320** War operations involving incendiary bullet, military personnel
    - +7th **Y36.321** War operations involving incendiary bullet, civilian
  - **Y36.33** War operations involving flamethrower
    - +7th **Y36.330** War operations involving flamethrower, military personnel
    - +7th **Y36.331** War operations involving flamethrower, civilian
  - **Y36.39** War operations involving other fires, conflagrations and hot substances
    - +7th **Y36.390** War operations involving other fires, conflagrations and hot substances, military personnel
    - +7th **Y36.391** War operations involving other fires, conflagrations and hot substances, civilian
- **Y36.4** War operations involving firearm discharge and other forms of conventional warfare
  - **Y36.41** War operations involving rubber bullets
    - +7th **Y36.410** War operations involving rubber bullets, military personnel
    - +7th **Y36.411** War operations involving rubber bullets, civilian
  - **Y36.42** War operations involving firearms pellets
    - +7th **Y36.420** War operations involving firearms pellets, military personnel
    - +7th **Y36.421** War operations involving firearms pellets, civilian
  - **Y36.43** War operations involving other firearms discharge
    - War operations involving bullets NOS
    - **Excludes1:** war operations involving munitions fragments (Y36.25-)
      - war operations involving incendiary bullets (Y36.32-)
    - +7th **Y36.430** War operations involving other firearms discharge, military personnel
    - +7th **Y36.431** War operations involving other firearms discharge, civilian
  - **Y36.44** War operations involving unarmed hand to hand combat
    - **Excludes1:** war operations involving combat using blunt or piercing object (Y36.45-)
      - war operations involving intentional restriction of air and airway (Y36.46-)
      - war operations involving unintentional restriction of air and airway (Y36.47-)
    - +7th **Y36.440** War operations involving unarmed hand to hand combat, military personnel
    - +7th **Y36.441** War operations involving unarmed hand to hand combat, civilian
  - **Y36.45** War operations involving combat using blunt or piercing object
    - +7th **Y36.450** War operations involving combat using blunt or piercing object, military personnel
    - +7th **Y36.451** War operations involving combat using blunt or piercing object, civilian
  - **Y36.46** War operations involving intentional restriction of air and airway
    - +7th **Y36.460** War operations involving intentional restriction of air and airway, military personnel
    - +7th **Y36.461** War operations involving intentional restriction of air and airway, civilian
  - **Y36.47** War operations involving unintentional restriction of air and airway
    - +7th **Y36.470** War operations involving unintentional restriction of air and airway, military personnel
    - +7th **Y36.471** War operations involving unintentional restriction of air and airway, civilian
  - **Y36.49** War operations involving other forms of conventional warfare
    - +7th **Y36.490** War operations involving other forms of conventional warfare, military personnel
    - +7th **Y36.491** War operations involving other forms of conventional warfare, civilian
- **Y36.5** War operations involving nuclear weapons
  - War operations involving dirty bomb NOS
  - **Y36.50** War operations involving unspecified effect of nuclear weapon
    - +7th **Y36.500** War operations involving unspecified effect of nuclear weapon, military personnel
    - +7th **Y36.501** War operations involving unspecified effect of nuclear weapon, civilian
  - **Y36.51** War operations involving direct blast effect of nuclear weapon
    - War operations involving blast pressure of nuclear weapon
    - +7th **Y36.510** War operations involving direct blast effect of nuclear weapon, military personnel
    - +7th **Y36.511** War operations involving direct blast effect of nuclear weapon, civilian
  - **Y36.52** War operations involving indirect blast effect of nuclear weapon
    - War operations involving being thrown by blast of nuclear weapon
    - War operations involving being struck or crushed by blast debris of nuclear weapon
    - +7th **Y36.520** War operations involving indirect blast effect of nuclear weapon, military personnel
    - +7th **Y36.521** War operations involving indirect blast effect of nuclear weapon, civilian
  - **Y36.53** War operations involving thermal radiation effect of nuclear weapon
    - War operations involving direct heat from nuclear weapon
    - War operation involving fireball effects from nuclear weapon
    - +7th **Y36.530** War operations involving thermal radiation effect of nuclear weapon, military personnel

- **+7th Y36.531** War operations involving thermal radiation effect of nuclear weapon, civilian
- **+ Y36.54** War operation involving nuclear radiation effects of nuclear weapon
  - War operation involving acute radiation exposure from nuclear weapon
  - War operation involving exposure to immediate ionizing radiation from nuclear weapon
  - War operation involving fallout exposure from nuclear weapon
  - War operation involving secondary effects of nuclear weapons
  - **+7th Y36.540** War operation involving nuclear radiation effects of nuclear weapon, military personnel
  - **+7th Y36.541** War operation involving nuclear radiation effects of nuclear weapon, civilian
- **+ Y36.59** War operation involving other effects of nuclear weapons
  - **+7th Y36.590** War operation involving other effects of nuclear weapons, military personnel
  - **+7th Y36.591** War operation involving other effects of nuclear weapons, civilian
- **+ Y36.6** War operations involving biological weapons
  - **+ Y36.6X** War operations involving biological weapons
    - **+7th Y36.6X0** War operations involving biological weapons, military personnel
    - **+7th Y36.6X1** War operations involving biological weapons, civilian
- **+ Y36.7** War operations involving chemical weapons and other forms of unconventional warfare
  - **Excludes1:** war operations involving incendiary devices (Y36.3-, Y36.5-)
  - **+ Y36.7X** War operations involving chemical weapons and other forms of unconventional warfare
    - **+7th Y36.7X0** War operations involving chemical weapons and other forms of unconventional warfare, military personnel
    - **+7th Y36.7X1** War operations involving chemical weapons and other forms of unconventional warfare, civilian
- **+ Y36.8** War operations occurring after cessation of hostilities
  - War operations classifiable to categories Y36.0-Y36.8 but occurring after cessation of hostilities
  - **+ Y36.81** Explosion of mine placed during war operations but exploding after cessation of hostilities
    - **+7th Y36.810** Explosion of mine placed during war operations but exploding after cessation of hostilities, military personnel
    - **+7th Y36.811** Explosion of mine placed during war operations but exploding after cessation of hostilities, civilian
  - **+ Y36.82** Explosion of bomb placed during war operations but exploding after cessation of hostilities
    - **+7th Y36.820** Explosion of bomb placed during war operations but exploding after cessation of hostilities, military personnel
    - **+7th Y36.821** Explosion of bomb placed during war operations but exploding after cessation of hostilities, civilian
  - **+ Y36.88** Other war operations occurring after cessation of hostilities
    - **+7th Y36.880** Other war operations occurring after cessation of hostilities, military personnel
    - **+7th Y36.881** Other war operations occurring after cessation of hostilities, civilian
  - **+ Y36.89** Unspecified war operations occurring after cessation of hostilities
    - **+7th Y36.890** Unspecified war operations occurring after cessation of hostilities, military personnel
    - **+7th Y36.891** Unspecified war operations occurring after cessation of hostilities, civilian
- **+ Y36.9** Other and unspecified war operations
  - **X+7th Y36.90** War operations, unspecified
  - **X+7th Y36.91** War operations involving unspecified weapon of mass destruction [WMD]
  - **X+7th Y36.92** War operations involving friendly fire

Y37 Military operations

Includes: injuries to military personnel and civilians occurring during peacetime on military property and during routine military exercises and operations

Excludes1: military aircraft involved in aircraft accident with civilian aircraft (V97.81-)
military vehicles involved in transport accident with civilian vehicle (V09.01, V09.21, V19.81, V29.818, V39.81, V49.81, V59.81, V69.81, V79.81)
military watercraft involved in water transport accident with civilian watercraft (V94.81-)
war operations (Y36.-)

The appropriate 7th character is to be added to each code from category Y37
- A initial encounter
- D subsequent encounter
- S sequela

- **+ Y37.0** Military operations involving explosion of marine weapons
  - **+ Y37.00** Military operations involving explosion of unspecified marine weapon
    - Military operations involving underwater blast NOS
    - **+7th Y37.000** Military operations involving explosion of unspecified marine weapon, military personnel
    - **+7th Y37.001** Military operations involving explosion of unspecified marine weapon, civilian
  - **+ Y37.01** Military operations involving explosion of depth-charge
    - **+7th Y37.010** Military operations involving explosion of depth-charge, military personnel
    - **+7th Y37.011** Military operations involving explosion of depth-charge, civilian
  - **+ Y37.02** Military operations involving explosion of marine mine
    - Military operations involving explosion of marine mine, at sea or in harbor
    - **+7th Y37.020** Military operations involving explosion of marine mine, military personnel
    - **+7th Y37.021** Military operations involving explosion of marine mine, civilian
  - **+ Y37.03** Military operations involving explosion of sea-based artillery shell
    - **+7th Y37.030** Military operations involving explosion of sea-based artillery shell, military personnel
    - **+7th Y37.031** Military operations involving explosion of sea-based artillery shell, civilian
  - **+ Y37.04** Military operations involving explosion of torpedo
    - **+7th Y37.040** Military operations involving explosion of torpedo, military personnel
    - **+7th Y37.041** Military operations involving explosion of torpedo, civilian
  - **+ Y37.05** Military operations involving accidental detonation of onboard marine weapons
    - **+7th Y37.050** Military operations involving accidental detonation of onboard marine weapons, military personnel
    - **+7th Y37.051** Military operations involving accidental detonation of onboard marine weapons, civilian
  - **+ Y37.09** Military operations involving explosion of other marine weapons
    - **+7th Y37.090** Military operations involving explosion of other marine weapons, military personnel
    - **+7th Y37.091** Military operations involving explosion of other marine weapons, civilian
- **+ Y37.1** Military operations involving destruction of aircraft
  - **+ Y37.10** Military operations involving unspecified destruction of aircraft
    - **+7th Y37.100** Military operations involving unspecified destruction of aircraft, military personnel

- +7th **Y37.101** Military operations involving unspecified destruction of aircraft, civilian
- + **Y37.11** Military operations involving destruction of aircraft due to enemy fire or explosives
    - Military operations involving destruction of aircraft due to air to air missile
    - Military operations involving destruction of aircraft due to explosive placed on aircraft
    - Military operations involving destruction of aircraft due to rocket propelled grenade [RPG]
    - Military operations involving destruction of aircraft due to small arms fire
    - Military operations involving destruction of aircraft due to surface to air missile
    - +7th **Y37.110** Military operations involving destruction of aircraft due to enemy fire or explosives, military personnel
    - +7th **Y37.111** Military operations involving destruction of aircraft due to enemy fire or explosives, civilian
- + **Y37.12** Military operations involving destruction of aircraft due to collision with other aircraft
    - +7th **Y37.120** Military operations involving destruction of aircraft due to collision with other aircraft, military personnel
    - +7th **Y37.121** Military operations involving destruction of aircraft due to collision with other aircraft, civilian
- + **Y37.13** Military operations involving destruction of aircraft due to onboard fire
    - +7th **Y37.130** Military operations involving destruction of aircraft due to onboard fire, military personnel
    - +7th **Y37.131** Military operations involving destruction of aircraft due to onboard fire, civilian
- + **Y37.14** Military operations involving destruction of aircraft due to accidental detonation of onboard munitions and explosives
    - +7th **Y37.140** Military operations involving destruction of aircraft due to accidental detonation of onboard munitions and explosives, military personnel
    - +7th **Y37.141** Military operations involving destruction of aircraft due to accidental detonation of onboard munitions and explosives, civilian
- + **Y37.19** Military operations involving other destruction of aircraft
    - +7th **Y37.190** Military operations involving other destruction of aircraft, military personnel
    - +7th **Y37.191** Military operations involving other destruction of aircraft, civilian
- + **Y37.2** Military operations involving other explosions and fragments
    - **Excludes1:** *military operations involving explosion of aircraft (Y37.1-)*
    - *military operations involving explosion of marine weapons (Y37.0-)*
    - *military operations involving explosion of nuclear weapons (Y37.5-)*
    - + **Y37.20** Military operations involving unspecified explosion and fragments
        - Military operations involving air blast NOS
        - Military operations involving blast NOS
        - Military operations involving blast fragments NOS
        - Military operations involving blast wave NOS
        - Military operations involving blast wind NOS
        - Military operations involving explosion NOS
        - Military operations involving explosion of bomb NOS
        - +7th **Y37.200** Military operations involving unspecified explosion and fragments, military personnel
        - +7th **Y37.201** Military operations involving unspecified explosion and fragments, civilian
    - + **Y37.21** Military operations involving explosion of aerial bomb
        - +7th **Y37.210** Military operations involving explosion of aerial bomb, military personnel
        - +7th **Y37.211** Military operations involving explosion of aerial bomb, civilian
    - + **Y37.22** Military operations involving explosion of guided missile
        - +7th **Y37.220** Military operations involving explosion of guided missile, military personnel
        - +7th **Y37.221** Military operations involving explosion of guided missile, civilian
    - + **Y37.23** Military operations involving explosion of improvised explosive device [IED]
        - Military operations involving explosion of person-borne improvised explosive device [IED]
        - Military operations involving explosion of vehicle-borne improvised explosive device [IED]
        - Military operations involving explosion of roadside improvised explosive device [IED]
        - +7th **Y37.230** Military operations involving explosion of improvised explosive device [IED], military personnel
        - +7th **Y37.231** Military operations involving explosion of improvised explosive device [IED], civilian
    - + **Y37.24** Military operations involving explosion due to accidental detonation and discharge of own munitions or munitions launch device
        - +7th **Y37.240** Military operations involving explosion due to accidental detonation and discharge of own munitions or munitions launch device, military personnel
        - +7th **Y37.241** Military operations involving explosion due to accidental detonation and discharge of own munitions or munitions launch device, civilian
    - + **Y37.25** Military operations involving fragments from munitions
        - +7th **Y37.250** Military operations involving fragments from munitions, military personnel
        - +7th **Y37.251** Military operations involving fragments from munitions, civilian
    - + **Y37.26** Military operations involving fragments of improvised explosive device [IED]
        - Military operations involving fragments of person-borne improvised explosive device [IED]
        - Military operations involving fragments of vehicle-borne improvised explosive device [IED]
        - Military operations involving fragments of roadside improvised explosive device [IED]
        - +7th **Y37.260** Military operations involving fragments of improvised explosive device [IED], military personnel
        - +7th **Y37.261** Military operations involving fragments of improvised explosive device [IED], civilian
    - + **Y37.27** Military operations involving fragments from weapons
        - +7th **Y37.270** Military operations involving fragments from weapons, military personnel
        - +7th **Y37.271** Military operations involving fragments from weapons, civilian
    - + **Y37.29** Military operations involving other explosions and fragments
        - Military operations involving explosion of grenade
        - Military operations involving explosions of land mine
        - Military operations involving shrapnel NOS
        - +7th **Y37.290** Military operations involving other explosions and fragments, military personnel
        - +7th **Y37.291** Military operations involving other explosions and fragments, civilian

+ **Y37.3** Military operations involving fires, conflagrations and hot substances

Military operations involving smoke, fumes, and heat from fires, conflagrations and hot substances

Excludes1: military operations involving fires and conflagrations aboard military aircraft (Y37.1-)
military operations involving fires and conflagrations aboard military watercraft (Y37.0-)
military operations involving fires and conflagrations caused indirectly by conventional weapons (Y37.2-)
military operations involving fires and thermal effects of nuclear weapons (Y36.53-)

+ **Y37.30** Military operations involving unspecified fire, conflagration and hot substance
 + 7th **Y37.300** Military operations involving unspecified fire, conflagration and hot substance, military personnel
 + 7th **Y37.301** Military operations involving unspecified fire, conflagration and hot substance, civilian
+ **Y37.31** Military operations involving gasoline bomb
 Military operations involving incendiary bomb
 Military operations involving petrol bomb
 + 7th **Y37.310** Military operations involving gasoline bomb, military personnel
 + 7th **Y37.311** Military operations involving gasoline bomb, civilian
+ **Y37.32** Military operations involving incendiary bullet
 + 7th **Y37.320** Military operations involving incendiary bullet, military personnel
 + 7th **Y37.321** Military operations involving incendiary bullet, civilian
+ **Y37.33** Military operations involving flamethrower
 + 7th **Y37.330** Military operations involving flamethrower, military personnel
 + 7th **Y37.331** Military operations involving flamethrower, civilian
+ **Y37.39** Military operations involving other fires, conflagrations and hot substances
 + 7th **Y37.390** Military operations involving other fires, conflagrations and hot substances, military personnel
 + 7th **Y37.391** Military operations involving other fires, conflagrations and hot substances, civilian

+ **Y37.4** Military operations involving firearm discharge and other forms of conventional warfare
 + **Y37.41** Military operations involving rubber bullets
  + 7th **Y37.410** Military operations involving rubber bullets, military personnel
  + 7th **Y37.411** Military operations involving rubber bullets, civilian
 + **Y37.42** Military operations involving firearms pellets
  + 7th **Y37.420** Military operations involving firearms pellets, military personnel
  + 7th **Y37.421** Military operations involving firearms pellets, civilian
 + **Y37.43** Military operations involving other firearms discharge
  Military operations involving bullets NOS
  Excludes1: military operations involving munitions fragments (Y37.25-)
  military operations involving incendiary bullets (Y37.32-)
  + 7th **Y37.430** Military operations involving other firearms discharge, military personnel
  + 7th **Y37.431** Military operations involving other firearms discharge, civilian
 + **Y37.44** Military operations involving unarmed hand to hand combat
  Excludes1: military operations involving combat using blunt or piercing object (Y37.45-)
  military operations involving intentional restriction of air and airway (Y37.46-)
  military operations involving unintentional restriction of air and airway (Y37.47-)
  + 7th **Y37.440** Military operations involving unarmed hand to hand combat, military personnel
  + 7th **Y37.441** Military operations involving unarmed hand to hand combat, civilian
 + **Y37.45** Military operations involving combat using blunt or piercing object
  + 7th **Y37.450** Military operations involving combat using blunt or piercing object, military personnel
  + 7th **Y37.451** Military operations involving combat using blunt or piercing object, civilian
 + **Y37.46** Military operations involving intentional restriction of air and airway
  + 7th **Y37.460** Military operations involving intentional restriction of air and airway, military personnel
  + 7th **Y37.461** Military operations involving intentional restriction of air and airway, civilian
 + **Y37.47** Military operations involving unintentional restriction of air and airway
  + 7th **Y37.470** Military operations involving unintentional restriction of air and airway, military personnel
  + 7th **Y37.471** Military operations involving unintentional restriction of air and airway, civilian
 + **Y37.49** Military operations involving other forms of conventional warfare
  + 7th **Y37.490** Military operations involving other forms of conventional warfare, military personnel
  + 7th **Y37.491** Military operations involving other forms of conventional warfare, civilian

+ **Y37.5** Military operations involving nuclear weapons
 Military operation involving dirty bomb NOS
 + **Y37.50** Military operations involving unspecified effect of nuclear weapon
  + 7th **Y37.500** Military operations involving unspecified effect of nuclear weapon, military personnel
  + 7th **Y37.501** Military operations involving unspecified effect of nuclear weapon, civilian
 + **Y37.51** Military operations involving direct blast effect of nuclear weapon
  Military operations involving blast pressure of nuclear weapon
  + 7th **Y37.510** Military operations involving direct blast effect of nuclear weapon, military personnel
  + 7th **Y37.511** Military operations involving direct blast effect of nuclear weapon, civilian
 + **Y37.52** Military operations involving indirect blast effect of nuclear weapon
  Military operations involving being thrown by blast of nuclear weapon
  Military operations involving being struck or crushed by blast debris of nuclear weapon
  + 7th **Y37.520** Military operations involving indirect blast effect of nuclear weapon, military personnel
  + 7th **Y37.521** Military operations involving indirect blast effect of nuclear weapon, civilian
 + **Y37.53** Military operations involving thermal radiation effect of nuclear weapon
  Military operations involving direct heat from nuclear weapon
  Military operation involving fireball effects from nuclear weapon
  + 7th **Y37.530** Military operations involving thermal radiation effect of nuclear weapon, military personnel
  + 7th **Y37.531** Military operations involving thermal radiation effect of nuclear weapon, civilian

- **Y37.54** Military operation involving nuclear radiation effects of nuclear weapon
    - Military operation involving acute radiation exposure from nuclear weapon
    - Military operation involving exposure to immediate ionizing radiation from nuclear weapon
    - Military operation involving fallout exposure from nuclear weapon
    - Military operation involving secondary effects of nuclear weapons
    - +7th **Y37.540** Military operation involving nuclear radiation effects of nuclear weapon, military personnel
    - +7th **Y37.541** Military operation involving nuclear radiation effects of nuclear weapon, civilian
- **Y37.59** Military operation involving other effects of nuclear weapons
    - +7th **Y37.590** Military operation involving other effects of nuclear weapons, military personnel
    - +7th **Y37.591** Military operation involving other effects of nuclear weapons, civilian
- **Y37.6** Military operations involving biological weapons
    - **Y37.6X** Military operations involving biological weapons
        - +7th **Y37.6X0** Military operations involving biological weapons, military personnel
        - +7th **Y37.6X1** Military operations involving biological weapons, civilian
- **Y37.7** Military operations involving chemical weapons and other forms of unconventional warfare
    - *Excludes1:* military operations involving incendiary devices (Y36.3-, Y36.5-)
    - **Y37.7X** Military operations involving chemical weapons and other forms of unconventional warfare
        - +7th **Y37.7X0** Military operations involving chemical weapons and other forms of unconventional warfare, military personnel
        - +7th **Y37.7X1** Military operations involving chemical weapons and other forms of unconventional warfare, civilian
- **Y37.9** Other and unspecified military operations
    - X+7th **Y37.90** Military operations, unspecified
    - X+7th **Y37.91** Military operations involving unspecified weapon of mass destruction [WMD]
    - X+7th **Y37.92** Military operations involving friendly fire

Y38 Terrorism

These codes are for use to identify injuries resulting from the unlawful use of force or violence against persons or property to intimidate or coerce a Government, the civilian population, or any segment thereof, in furtherance of political or social objective

Use additional code for place of occurrence (Y92.-)

The appropriate 7th character is to be added to each code from category Y38
A initial encounter
D subsequent encounter
S sequela

Review coding guideline C.20.j

- **Y38.0** Terrorism involving explosion of marine weapons
    - Terrorism involving depth-charge
    - Terrorism involving marine mine
    - Terrorism involving mine NOS, at sea or in harbor
    - Terrorism involving sea-based artillery shell
    - Terrorism involving torpedo
    - Terrorism involving underwater blast
    - **Y38.0X** Terrorism involving explosion of marine weapons
        - +7th **Y38.0X1** Terrorism involving explosion of marine weapons, public safety official injured
        - +7th **Y38.0X2** Terrorism involving explosion of marine weapons, civilian injured
        - +7th **Y38.0X3** Terrorism involving explosion of marine weapons, terrorist injured
- **Y38.1** Terrorism involving destruction of aircraft
    - Terrorism involving aircraft burned
    - Terrorism involving aircraft exploded
    - Terrorism involving aircraft being shot down
    - Terrorism involving aircraft used as a weapon
    - **Y38.1X** Terrorism involving destruction of aircraft
        - +7th **Y38.1X1** Terrorism involving destruction of aircraft, public safety official injured
        - +7th **Y38.1X2** Terrorism involving destruction of aircraft, civilian injured
        - +7th **Y38.1X3** Terrorism involving destruction of aircraft, terrorist injured
- **Y38.2** Terrorism involving other explosions and fragments
    - Terrorism involving antipersonnel (fragments) bomb
    - Terrorism involving blast NOS
    - Terrorism involving explosion NOS
    - Terrorism involving explosion of breech block
    - Terrorism involving explosion of cannon block
    - Terrorism involving explosion (fragments) of artillery shell
    - Terrorism involving explosion (fragments) of bomb
    - Terrorism involving explosion (fragments) of grenade
    - Terrorism involving explosion (fragments) of guided missile
    - Terrorism involving explosion (fragments) of land mine
    - Terrorism involving explosion of mortar bomb
    - Terrorism involving explosion of munitions
    - Terrorism involving explosion (fragments) of rocket
    - Terrorism involving explosion (fragments) of shell
    - Terrorism involving shrapnel
    - Terrorism involving mine NOS, on land
    - *Excludes1:* terrorism involving explosion of nuclear weapon (Y38.5)
      terrorism involving suicide bomber (Y38.81)
    - **Y38.2X** Terrorism involving other explosions and fragments
        - +7th **Y38.2X1** Terrorism involving other explosions and fragments, public safety official injured
        - +7th **Y38.2X2** Terrorism involving other explosions and fragments, civilian injured
        - +7th **Y38.2X3** Terrorism involving other explosions and fragments, terrorist injured
- **Y38.3** Terrorism involving fires, conflagration and hot substances
    - Terrorism involving conflagration NOS
    - Terrorism involving fire NOS
    - Terrorism involving petrol bomb
    - *Excludes1:* terrorism involving fire or heat of nuclear weapon (Y38.5)
    - **Y38.3X** Terrorism involving fires, conflagration and hot substances
        - +7th **Y38.3X1** Terrorism involving fires, conflagration and hot substances, public safety official injured
        - +7th **Y38.3X2** Terrorism involving fires, conflagration and hot substances, civilian injured
        - +7th **Y38.3X3** Terrorism involving fires, conflagration and hot substances, terrorist injured
- **Y38.4** Terrorism involving firearms
    - Terrorism involving carbine bullet
    - Terrorism involving machine gun bullet
    - Terrorism involving pellets (shotgun)
    - Terrorism involving pistol bullet
    - Terrorism involving rifle bullet
    - Terrorism involving rubber (rifle) bullet
    - **Y38.4X** Terrorism involving firearms
        - +7th **Y38.4X1** Terrorism involving firearms, public safety official injured
        - +7th **Y38.4X2** Terrorism involving firearms, civilian injured
        - +7th **Y38.4X3** Terrorism involving firearms, terrorist injured
- **Y38.5** Terrorism involving nuclear weapons
    - Terrorism involving blast effects of nuclear weapon
    - Terrorism involving exposure to ionizing radiation from nuclear weapon
    - Terrorism involving fireball effect of nuclear weapon
    - Terrorism involving heat from nuclear weapon
    - **Y38.5X** Terrorism involving nuclear weapons
        - +7th **Y38.5X1** Terrorism involving nuclear weapons, public safety official injured
        - +7th **Y38.5X2** Terrorism involving nuclear weapons, civilian injured
        - +7th **Y38.5X3** Terrorism involving nuclear weapons, terrorist injured

- **Y38.6 Terrorism involving biological weapons**
  Terrorism involving anthrax
  Terrorism involving cholera
  Terrorism involving smallpox
  - **Y38.6X Terrorism involving biological weapons**
    - +7th **Y38.6X1** Terrorism involving biological weapons, public safety official injured
    - +7th **Y38.6X2** Terrorism involving biological weapons, civilian injured
    - +7th **Y38.6X3** Terrorism involving biological weapons, terrorist injured
- **Y38.7 Terrorism involving chemical weapons**
  Terrorism involving gases, fumes, chemicals
  Terrorism involving hydrogen cyanide
  Terrorism involving phosgene
  Terrorism involving sarin
  - **Y38.7X Terrorism involving chemical weapons**
    - +7th **Y38.7X1** Terrorism involving chemical weapons, public safety official injured
    - +7th **Y38.7X2** Terrorism involving chemical weapons, civilian injured
    - +7th **Y38.7X3** Terrorism involving chemical weapons, terrorist injured
- **Y38.8 Terrorism involving other and unspecified means**
  - X+7th **Y38.80** Terrorism involving unspecified means
    Terrorism NOS
  - **Y38.81 Terrorism involving suicide bomber**
    - +7th **Y38.811** Terrorism involving suicide bomber, public safety official injured
    - +7th **Y38.812** Terrorism involving suicide bomber, civilian injured
  - **Y38.89 Terrorism involving other means**
    Terrorism involving drowning and submersion
    Terrorism involving lasers
    Terrorism involving piercing or stabbing instruments
    - +7th **Y38.891** Terrorism involving other means, public safety official injured
    - +7th **Y38.892** Terrorism involving other means, civilian injured
    - +7th **Y38.893** Terrorism involving other means, terrorist injured
- **Y38.9 Terrorism, secondary effects**
  NOTE This code is for use to identify conditions occurring subsequent to a terrorist attack not those that are due to the initial terrorist attack
  - **Y38.9X Terrorism, secondary effects**
    - +7th **Y38.9X1** Terrorism, secondary effects, public safety official injured
    - +7th **Y38.9X2** Terrorism, secondary effects, civilian injured

Complications of medical and surgical care (Y62-Y84)

Includes: complications of medical devices surgical and medical procedures as the cause of abnormal reaction of the patient, or of later complication, without mention of misadventure at the time of the procedure

Misadventures to patients during surgical and medical care (Y62-Y69)

Excludes1: surgical and medical procedures as the cause of abnormal reaction of the patient, without mention of misadventure at the time of the procedure (Y83-Y84)

Excludes2: breakdown or malfunctioning of medical device (during procedure) (after implantation) (ongoing use) (Y70-Y82)

- **Y62 Failure of sterile precautions during surgical and medical care**
  - **Y62.0** Failure of sterile precautions during surgical operation
  - **Y62.1** Failure of sterile precautions during infusion or transfusion
  - **Y62.2** Failure of sterile precautions during kidney dialysis and other perfusion
  - **Y62.3** Failure of sterile precautions during injection or immunization
  - **Y62.4** Failure of sterile precautions during endoscopic examination
  - **Y62.5** Failure of sterile precautions during heart catheterization
  - **Y62.6** Failure of sterile precautions during aspiration, puncture and other catheterization
  - **Y62.8** Failure of sterile precautions during other surgical and medical care
  - **Y62.9** Failure of sterile precautions during unspecified surgical and medical care

- **Y63 Failure in dosage during surgical and medical care**
  Excludes2: accidental overdose of drug or wrong drug given in error (T36-T50)
  - **Y63.0** Excessive amount of blood or other fluid given during transfusion or infusion
  - **Y63.1** Incorrect dilution of fluid used during infusion
  - **Y63.2** Overdose of radiation given during therapy
  - **Y63.3** Inadvertent exposure of patient to radiation during medical care
  - **Y63.4** Failure in dosage in electroshock or insulin-shock therapy
  - **Y63.5** Inappropriate temperature in local application and packing
  - **Y63.6** Underdosing and nonadministration of necessary drug, medicament or biological substance
    Review coding guideline C.19.e.5.c
  - **Y63.8** Failure in dosage during other surgical and medical care
    Review coding guideline C.19.e.5.c
  - **Y63.9** Failure in dosage during unspecified surgical and medical care
    Review coding guideline C.19.e.5.c

- **Y64 Contaminated medical or biological substances**
  - **Y64.0** Contaminated medical or biological substance, transfused or infused
  - **Y64.1** Contaminated medical or biological substance, injected or used for immunization
  - **Y64.8** Contaminated medical or biological substance administered by other means
  - **Y64.9** Contaminated medical or biological substance administered by unspecified means
    Administered contaminated medical or biological substance NOS

- **Y65 Other misadventures during surgical and medical care**
  - **Y65.0** Mismatched blood in transfusion
  - **Y65.1** Wrong fluid used in infusion
  - **Y65.2** Failure in suture or ligature during surgical operation
  - **Y65.3** Endotracheal tube wrongly placed during anesthetic procedure
  - **Y65.4** Failure to introduce or to remove other tube or instrument
  - **Y65.5 Performance of wrong procedure (operation)**
    - **Y65.51** Performance of wrong procedure (operation) on correct patient
      Wrong device implanted into correct surgical site
      Excludes1: performance of correct procedure (operation) on wrong side or body part (Y65.53)
    - **Y65.52** Performance of procedure (operation) on patient not scheduled for surgery
      Performance of procedure (operation) intended for another patient
      Performance of procedure (operation) on wrong patient
    - **Y65.53** Performance of correct procedure (operation) on wrong side or body part
      Performance of correct procedure (operation) on wrong side
      Performance of correct procedure (operation) on wrong site
  - **Y65.8** Other specified misadventures during surgical and medical care
    AHA CC: 2Q, 2019, 24; 1Q, 2022, 22

- **Y66 Nonadministration of surgical and medical care**
  Premature cessation of surgical and medical care
  Excludes1: DNR status (Z66)
  palliative care (Z51.5)
  Valid 3-character code, no further characters required

- **Y69 Unspecified misadventure during surgical and medical care**
  Valid 3-character code, no further characters required

Medical devices associated with adverse incidents in diagnostic and therapeutic use (Y70-Y82)

Includes: breakdown or malfunction of medical devices (during use) (after implantation) (ongoing use)

Excludes2: later complications following use of medical devices without breakdown or malfunctioning of device (Y83-Y84)
misadventure to patients during surgical and medical care, classifiable to (Y62-Y69)
surgical and other medical procedures as the cause of abnormal reaction of the patient, or of later complication, without mention of misadventure at the time of the procedure (Y83-Y84)

Y70 Anesthesiology devices associated with adverse incidents
- Y70.0 Diagnostic and monitoring anesthesiology devices associated with adverse incidents
- Y70.1 Therapeutic (nonsurgical) and rehabilitative anesthesiology devices associated with adverse incidents
- Y70.2 Prosthetic and other implants, materials and accessory anesthesiology devices associated with adverse incidents
- Y70.3 Surgical instruments, materials and anesthesiology devices (including sutures) associated with adverse incidents
- Y70.8 Miscellaneous anesthesiology devices associated with adverse incidents, not elsewhere classified

Y71 Cardiovascular devices associated with adverse incidents
- Y71.0 Diagnostic and monitoring cardiovascular devices associated with adverse incidents
- Y71.1 Therapeutic (nonsurgical) and rehabilitative cardiovascular devices associated with adverse incidents
- Y71.2 Prosthetic and other implants, materials and accessory cardiovascular devices associated with adverse incidents
- Y71.3 Surgical instruments, materials and cardiovascular devices (including sutures) associated with adverse incidents
- Y71.8 Miscellaneous cardiovascular devices associated with adverse incidents, not elsewhere classified

Y72 Otorhinolaryngological devices associated with adverse incidents
- Y72.0 Diagnostic and monitoring otorhinolaryngological devices associated with adverse incidents
- Y72.1 Therapeutic (nonsurgical) and rehabilitative otorhinolaryngological devices associated with adverse incidents
- Y72.2 Prosthetic and other implants, materials and accessory otorhinolaryngological devices associated with adverse incidents
- Y72.3 Surgical instruments, materials and otorhinolaryngological devices (including sutures) associated with adverse incidents
- Y72.8 Miscellaneous otorhinolaryngological devices associated with adverse incidents, not elsewhere classified

Y73 Gastroenterology and urology devices associated with adverse incidents
- Y73.0 Diagnostic and monitoring gastroenterology and urology devices associated with adverse incidents
- Y73.1 Therapeutic (nonsurgical) and rehabilitative gastroenterology and urology devices associated with adverse incidents
- Y73.2 Prosthetic and other implants, materials and accessory gastroenterology and urology devices associated with adverse incidents
- Y73.3 Surgical instruments, materials and gastroenterology and urology devices (including sutures) associated with adverse incidents
- Y73.8 Miscellaneous gastroenterology and urology devices associated with adverse incidents, not elsewhere classified

Y74 General hospital and personal-use devices associated with adverse incidents
- Y74.0 Diagnostic and monitoring general hospital and personal-use devices associated with adverse incidents
- Y74.1 Therapeutic (nonsurgical) and rehabilitative general hospital and personal-use devices associated with adverse incidents
- Y74.2 Prosthetic and other implants, materials and accessory general hospital and personal-use devices associated with adverse incidents
- Y74.3 Surgical instruments, materials and general hospital and personal-use devices (including sutures) associated with adverse incidents
- Y74.8 Miscellaneous general hospital and personal-use devices associated with adverse incidents, not elsewhere classified

Y75 Neurological devices associated with adverse incidents
- Y75.0 Diagnostic and monitoring neurological devices associated with adverse incidents
- Y75.1 Therapeutic (nonsurgical) and rehabilitative neurological devices associated with adverse incidents
- Y75.2 Prosthetic and other implants, materials and accessory neurological devices associated with adverse incidents
- Y75.3 Surgical instruments, materials and neurological devices (including sutures) associated with adverse incidents
- Y75.8 Miscellaneous neurological devices associated with adverse incidents, not elsewhere classified

Y76 Obstetric and gynecological devices associated with adverse incidents
- ♀ Y76.0 Diagnostic and monitoring obstetric and gynecological devices associated with adverse incidents
- ♀ Y76.1 Therapeutic (nonsurgical) and rehabilitative obstetric and gynecological devices associated with adverse incidents
- ♀ Y76.2 Prosthetic and other implants, materials and accessory obstetric and gynecological devices associated with adverse incidents
- ♀ Y76.3 Surgical instruments, materials and obstetric and gynecological devices (including sutures) associated with adverse incidents
- ♀ Y76.8 Miscellaneous obstetric and gynecological devices associated with adverse incidents, not elsewhere classified

Y77 Ophthalmic devices associated with adverse incidents
- Y77.0 Diagnostic and monitoring ophthalmic devices associated with adverse incidents
- + Y77.1 Therapeutic (nonsurgical) and rehabilitative ophthalmic devices associated with adverse incidents
  AHA CC: 4Q, 2020, 41
  - Y77.11 Contact lens associated with adverse incidents
    - Rigid gas permeable contact lens associated with adverse incidents
    - Soft (hydrophilic) contact lens associated with adverse incidents
  - Y77.19 Other therapeutic (nonsurgical) and rehabilitative ophthalmic devices associated with adverse incidents
- Y77.2 Prosthetic and other implants, materials and accessory ophthalmic devices associated with adverse incidents
- Y77.3 Surgical instruments, materials and ophthalmic devices (including sutures) associated with adverse incidents
- Y77.8 Miscellaneous ophthalmic devices associated with adverse incidents, not elsewhere classified

Y78 Radiological devices associated with adverse incidents
- Y78.0 Diagnostic and monitoring radiological devices associated with adverse incidents
- Y78.1 Therapeutic (nonsurgical) and rehabilitative radiological devices associated with adverse incidents
- Y78.2 Prosthetic and other implants, materials and accessory radiological devices associated with adverse incidents
- Y78.3 Surgical instruments, materials and radiological devices (including sutures) associated with adverse incidents
- Y78.8 Miscellaneous radiological devices associated with adverse incidents, not elsewhere classified

Y79 Orthopedic devices associated with adverse incidents
- Y79.0 Diagnostic and monitoring orthopedic devices associated with adverse incidents
- Y79.1 Therapeutic (nonsurgical) and rehabilitative orthopedic devices associated with adverse incidents
- Y79.2 Prosthetic and other implants, materials and accessory orthopedic devices associated with adverse incidents
- Y79.3 Surgical instruments, materials and orthopedic devices (including sutures) associated with adverse incidents
- Y79.8 Miscellaneous orthopedic devices associated with adverse incidents, not elsewhere classified

Y80 Physical medicine devices associated with adverse incidents
- Y80.0 Diagnostic and monitoring physical medicine devices associated with adverse incidents
- Y80.1 Therapeutic (nonsurgical) and rehabilitative physical medicine devices associated with adverse incidents
- Y80.2 Prosthetic and other implants, materials and accessory physical medicine devices associated with adverse incidents
- Y80.3 Surgical instruments, materials and physical medicine devices (including sutures) associated with adverse incidents
- Y80.8 Miscellaneous physical medicine devices associated with adverse incidents, not elsewhere classified

Y81 General- and plastic-surgery devices associated with adverse incidents
- Y81.0 Diagnostic and monitoring general- and plastic-surgery devices associated with adverse incidents
- Y81.1 Therapeutic (nonsurgical) and rehabilitative general- and plastic-surgery devices associated with adverse incidents

- **Y81.2** Prosthetic and other implants, materials and accessory general- and plastic-surgery devices associated with adverse incidents
- **Y81.3** Surgical instruments, materials and general- and plastic-surgery devices (including sutures) associated with adverse incidents
- **Y81.8** Miscellaneous general- and plastic-surgery devices associated with adverse incidents, not elsewhere classified

Y82 Other and unspecified medical devices associated with adverse incidents
- **Y82.8** Other medical devices associated with adverse incidents
- **Y82.9** Unspecified medical devices associated with adverse incidents

Surgical and other medical procedures as the cause of abnormal reaction of the patient, or of later complication, without mention of misadventure at the time of the procedure (Y83-Y84)

Excludes1: misadventures to patients during surgical and medical care, classifiable to (Y62-Y69)

Excludes2: breakdown or malfunctioning of medical device (after implantation) (during procedure) (ongoing use) (Y70-Y82)

Y83 Surgical operation and other surgical procedures as the cause of abnormal reaction of the patient, or of later complication, without mention of misadventure at the time of the procedure
- **Y83.0** Surgical operation with transplant of whole organ as the cause of abnormal reaction of the patient, or of later complication, without mention of misadventure at the time of the procedure
- **Y83.1** Surgical operation with implant of artificial internal device as the cause of abnormal reaction of the patient, or of later complication, without mention of misadventure at the time of the procedure
- **Y83.2** Surgical operation with anastomosis, bypass or graft as the cause of abnormal reaction of the patient, or of later complication, without mention of misadventure at the time of the procedure
- **Y83.3** Surgical operation with formation of external stoma as the cause of abnormal reaction of the patient, or of later complication, without mention of misadventure at the time of the procedure
- **Y83.4** Other reconstructive surgery as the cause of abnormal reaction of the patient, or of later complication, without mention of misadventure at the time of the procedure
- **Y83.5** Amputation of limb(s) as the cause of abnormal reaction of the patient, or of later complication, without mention of misadventure at the time of the procedure
- **Y83.6** Removal of other organ (partial) (total) as the cause of abnormal reaction of the patient, or of later complication, without mention of misadventure at the time of the procedure
- **Y83.8** Other surgical procedures as the cause of abnormal reaction of the patient, or of later complication, without mention of misadventure at the time of the procedure
  AHA CC: 2Q, 2023, 14
- **Y83.9** Surgical procedure, unspecified as the cause of abnormal reaction of the patient, or of later complication, without mention of misadventure at the time of the procedure

Y84 Other medical procedures as the cause of abnormal reaction of the patient, or of later complication, without mention of misadventure at the time of the procedure
- **Y84.0** Cardiac catheterization as the cause of abnormal reaction of the patient, or of later complication, without mention of misadventure at the time of the procedure
- **Y84.1** Kidney dialysis as the cause of abnormal reaction of the patient, or of later complication, without mention of misadventure at the time of the procedure
- **Y84.2** Radiological procedure and radiotherapy as the cause of abnormal reaction of the patient, or of later complication, without mention of misadventure at the time of the procedure
  AHA CC: 1Q, 2019, 21
  Review coding guideline C.2.c.2
- **Y84.3** Shock therapy as the cause of abnormal reaction of the patient, or of later complication, without mention of misadventure at the time of the procedure
- **Y84.4** Aspiration of fluid as the cause of abnormal reaction of the patient, or of later complication, without mention of misadventure at the time of the procedure
- **Y84.5** Insertion of gastric or duodenal sound as the cause of abnormal reaction of the patient, or of later complication, without mention of misadventure at the time of the procedure
- **Y84.6** Urinary catheterization as the cause of abnormal reaction of the patient, or of later complication, without mention of misadventure at the time of the procedure
- **Y84.7** Blood-sampling as the cause of abnormal reaction of the patient, or of later complication, without mention of misadventure at the time of the procedure
- **Y84.8** Other medical procedures as the cause of abnormal reaction of the patient, or of later complication, without mention of misadventure at the time of the procedure
  AHA CC: 4Q, 2014, 24; 1Q, 2021, 5-6; 2Q, 2023, 28
- **Y84.9** Medical procedure, unspecified as the cause of abnormal reaction of the patient, or of later complication, without mention of misadventure at the time of the procedure

Supplementary factors related to causes of morbidity classified elsewhere (Y90-Y99)

NOTE These categories may be used to provide supplementary information concerning causes of morbidity. They are not to be used for single-condition coding.

Y90 Evidence of alcohol involvement determined by blood alcohol level
Code first any associated alcohol related disorders (F10)
- **Y90.0** Blood alcohol level of less than 20 mg/100 ml
- **Y90.1** Blood alcohol level of 20-39 mg/100 ml
- **Y90.2** Blood alcohol level of 40-59 mg/100 ml
- **Y90.3** Blood alcohol level of 60-79 mg/100 ml
- **Y90.4** Blood alcohol level of 80-99 mg/100 ml
- **Y90.5** Blood alcohol level of 100-119 mg/100 ml
- **Y90.6** Blood alcohol level of 120-199 mg/100 ml
- **Y90.7** Blood alcohol level of 200-239 mg/100 ml
- **Y90.8** Blood alcohol level of 240 mg/100 ml or more
- **Y90.9** Presence of alcohol in blood, level not specified

Y92 Place of occurrence of the external cause
The following category is for use, when relevant, to identify the place of occurrence of the external cause. Use in conjunction with an activity code.
Place of occurrence should be recorded only at the initial encounter for treatment
Review coding guideline C.20.b

- **+ Y92.0** Non-institutional (private) residence as the place of occurrence of the external cause
  Excludes1: abandoned or derelict house (Y92.89)
  home under construction but not yet occupied (Y92.6-)
  institutional place of residence (Y92.1-)
  - **+ Y92.00** Unspecified non-institutional (private) residence as the place of occurrence of the external cause
    - **Y92.000** Kitchen of unspecified non-institutional (private) residence as the place of occurrence of the external cause
    - **Y92.001** Dining room of unspecified non-institutional (private) residence as the place of occurrence of the external cause
    - **Y92.002** Bathroom of unspecified non-institutional (private) residence as the place of occurrence of the external cause
    - **Y92.003** Bedroom of unspecified non-institutional (private) residence as the place of occurrence of the external cause
    - **Y92.007** Garden or yard of unspecified non-institutional (private) residence as the place of occurrence of the external cause
    - **Y92.008** Other place in unspecified non-institutional (private) residence as the place of occurrence of the external cause
    - **Y92.009** Unspecified place in unspecified non-institutional (private) residence as the place of occurrence of the external cause
      Home (NOS) as the place of occurrence of the external cause
      AHA CC: 2Q, 2021, 5

- **Y92.01** Single-family non-institutional (private) house as the place of occurrence of the external cause
  Farmhouse as the place of occurrence of the external cause
  Excludes1: barn (Y92.71)
  chicken coop or hen house (Y92.72)
  farm field (Y92.73)
  orchard (Y92.74)
  single family mobile home or trailer (Y92.02-)
  slaughter house (Y92.86)
  - Y92.010 Kitchen of single-family (private) house as the place of occurrence of the external cause
  - Y92.011 Dining room of single-family (private) house as the place of occurrence of the external cause
  - Y92.012 Bathroom of single-family (private) house as the place of occurrence of the external cause
  - Y92.013 Bedroom of single-family (private) house as the place of occurrence of the external cause
  - Y92.014 Private driveway to single-family (private) house as the place of occurrence of the external cause
  - Y92.015 Private garage of single-family (private) house as the place of occurrence of the external cause
  - Y92.016 Swimming-pool in single-family (private) house or garden as the place of occurrence of the external cause
  - Y92.017 Garden or yard in single-family (private) house as the place of occurrence of the external cause
  - Y92.018 Other place in single-family (private) house as the place of occurrence of the external cause
  - Y92.019 Unspecified place in single-family (private) house as the place of occurrence of the external cause
- **Y92.02** Mobile home as the place of occurrence of the external cause
  - Y92.020 Kitchen in mobile home as the place of occurrence of the external cause
  - Y92.021 Dining room in mobile home as the place of occurrence of the external cause
  - Y92.022 Bathroom in mobile home as the place of occurrence of the external cause
  - Y92.023 Bedroom in mobile home as the place of occurrence of the external cause
  - Y92.024 Driveway of mobile home as the place of occurrence of the external cause
  - Y92.025 Garage of mobile home as the place of occurrence of the external cause
  - Y92.026 Swimming-pool of mobile home as the place of occurrence of the external cause
  - Y92.027 Garden or yard of mobile home as the place of occurrence of the external cause
  - Y92.028 Other place in mobile home as the place of occurrence of the external cause
  - Y92.029 Unspecified place in mobile home as the place of occurrence of the external cause
- **Y92.03** Apartment as the place of occurrence of the external cause
  Condominium as the place of occurrence of the external cause
  Co-op apartment as the place of occurrence of the external cause
  - Y92.030 Kitchen in apartment as the place of occurrence of the external cause
  - Y92.031 Bathroom in apartment as the place of occurrence of the external cause
  - Y92.032 Bedroom in apartment as the place of occurrence of the external cause
  - Y92.038 Other place in apartment as the place of occurrence of the external cause
  - Y92.039 Unspecified place in apartment as the place of occurrence of the external cause
- **Y92.04** Boarding-house as the place of occurrence of the external cause
  - Y92.040 Kitchen in boarding-house as the place of occurrence of the external cause
  - Y92.041 Bathroom in boarding-house as the place of occurrence of the external cause
  - Y92.042 Bedroom in boarding-house as the place of occurrence of the external cause
  - Y92.043 Driveway of boarding-house as the place of occurrence of the external cause
  - Y92.044 Garage of boarding-house as the place of occurrence of the external cause
  - Y92.045 Swimming-pool of boarding-house as the place of occurrence of the external cause
  - Y92.046 Garden or yard of boarding-house as the place of occurrence of the external cause
  - Y92.048 Other place in boarding-house as the place of occurrence of the external cause
  - Y92.049 Unspecified place in boarding-house as the place of occurrence of the external cause
- **Y92.09** Other non-institutional residence as the place of occurrence of the external cause
  - Y92.090 Kitchen in other non-institutional residence as the place of occurrence of the external cause
  - Y92.091 Bathroom in other non-institutional residence as the place of occurrence of the external cause
  - Y92.092 Bedroom in other non-institutional residence as the place of occurrence of the external cause
  - Y92.093 Driveway of other non-institutional residence as the place of occurrence of the external cause
  - Y92.094 Garage of other non-institutional residence as the place of occurrence of the external cause
  - Y92.095 Swimming-pool of other non-institutional residence as the place of occurrence of the external cause
  - Y92.096 Garden or yard of other non-institutional residence as the place of occurrence of the external cause
  - Y92.098 Other place in other non-institutional residence as the place of occurrence of the external cause
    AHA CC: 2Q, 2017, 10-11
  - Y92.099 Unspecified place in other non-institutional residence as the place of occurrence of the external cause
- **Y92.1** Institutional (nonprivate) residence as the place of occurrence of the external cause
  - Y92.10 Unspecified residential institution as the place of occurrence of the external cause
  - **Y92.11** Children's home and orphanage as the place of occurrence of the external cause
    - Y92.110 Kitchen in children's home and orphanage as the place of occurrence of the external cause
    - Y92.111 Bathroom in children's home and orphanage as the place of occurrence of the external cause
    - Y92.112 Bedroom in children's home and orphanage as the place of occurrence of the external cause
    - Y92.113 Driveway of children's home and orphanage as the place of occurrence of the external cause
    - Y92.114 Garage of children's home and orphanage as the place of occurrence of the external cause
    - Y92.115 Swimming-pool of children's home and orphanage as the place of occurrence of the external cause
    - Y92.116 Garden or yard of children's home and orphanage as the place of occurrence of the external cause
    - Y92.118 Other place in children's home and orphanage as the place of occurrence of the external cause

- Y92.119 Unspecified place in children's home and orphanage as the place of occurrence of the external cause
- **+ Y92.12 Nursing home as the place of occurrence of the external cause**
  - Home for the sick as the place of occurrence of the external cause
  - Hospice as the place of occurrence of the external cause
  - Y92.120 Kitchen in nursing home as the place of occurrence of the external cause
  - Y92.121 Bathroom in nursing home as the place of occurrence of the external cause
  - Y92.122 Bedroom in nursing home as the place of occurrence of the external cause
    - *AHA CC: 4Q, 2020, 33*
  - Y92.123 Driveway of nursing home as the place of occurrence of the external cause
  - Y92.124 Garage of nursing home as the place of occurrence of the external cause
  - Y92.125 Swimming-pool of nursing home as the place of occurrence of the external cause
  - Y92.126 Garden or yard of nursing home as the place of occurrence of the external cause
  - Y92.128 Other place in nursing home as the place of occurrence of the external cause
  - Y92.129 Unspecified place in nursing home as the place of occurrence of the external cause
- **+ Y92.13 Military base as the place of occurrence of the external cause**
  - **Excludes1:** *military training grounds (Y92.83)*
  - Y92.130 Kitchen on military base as the place of occurrence of the external cause
  - Y92.131 Mess hall on military base as the place of occurrence of the external cause
  - Y92.133 Barracks on military base as the place of occurrence of the external cause
  - Y92.135 Garage on military base as the place of occurrence of the external cause
  - Y92.136 Swimming-pool on military base as the place of occurrence of the external cause
  - Y92.137 Garden or yard on military base as the place of occurrence of the external cause
  - Y92.138 Other place on military base as the place of occurrence of the external cause
  - Y92.139 Unspecified place military base as the place of occurrence of the external cause
- **+ Y92.14 Prison as the place of occurrence of the external cause**
  - Y92.140 Kitchen in prison as the place of occurrence of the external cause
  - Y92.141 Dining room in prison as the place of occurrence of the external cause
  - Y92.142 Bathroom in prison as the place of occurrence of the external cause
  - Y92.143 Cell of prison as the place of occurrence of the external cause
  - Y92.146 Swimming-pool of prison as the place of occurrence of the external cause
  - Y92.147 Courtyard of prison as the place of occurrence of the external cause
  - Y92.148 Other place in prison as the place of occurrence of the external cause
  - Y92.149 Unspecified place in prison as the place of occurrence of the external cause
- **+ Y92.15 Reform school as the place of occurrence of the external cause**
  - Y92.150 Kitchen in reform school as the place of occurrence of the external cause
  - Y92.151 Dining room in reform school as the place of occurrence of the external cause
  - Y92.152 Bathroom in reform school as the place of occurrence of the external cause
  - Y92.153 Bedroom in reform school as the place of occurrence of the external cause
  - Y92.154 Driveway of reform school as the place of occurrence of the external cause
  - Y92.155 Garage of reform school as the place of occurrence of the external cause
  - Y92.156 Swimming-pool of reform school as the place of occurrence of the external cause
  - Y92.157 Garden or yard of reform school as the place of occurrence of the external cause
  - Y92.158 Other place in reform school as the place of occurrence of the external cause
  - Y92.159 Unspecified place in reform school as the place of occurrence of the external cause
- **+ Y92.16 School dormitory as the place of occurrence of the external cause**
  - **Excludes1:** *reform school as the place of occurrence of the external cause (Y92.15-)*
    school buildings and grounds as the place of occurrence of the external cause (Y92.2-)
    school sports and athletic areas as the place of occurrence of the external cause (Y92.3-)
  - Y92.160 Kitchen in school dormitory as the place of occurrence of the external cause
  - Y92.161 Dining room in school dormitory as the place of occurrence of the external cause
  - Y92.162 Bathroom in school dormitory as the place of occurrence of the external cause
  - Y92.163 Bedroom in school dormitory as the place of occurrence of the external cause
  - Y92.168 Other place in school dormitory as the place of occurrence of the external cause
  - Y92.169 Unspecified place in school dormitory as the place of occurrence of the external cause
- **+ Y92.19 Other specified residential institution as the place of occurrence of the external cause**
  - Y92.190 Kitchen in other specified residential institution as the place of occurrence of the external cause
  - Y92.191 Dining room in other specified residential institution as the place of occurrence of the external cause
  - Y92.192 Bathroom in other specified residential institution as the place of occurrence of the external cause
  - Y92.193 Bedroom in other specified residential institution as the place of occurrence of the external cause
  - Y92.194 Driveway of other specified residential institution as the place of occurrence of the external cause
  - Y92.195 Garage of other specified residential institution as the place of occurrence of the external cause
  - Y92.196 Pool of other specified residential institution as the place of occurrence of the external cause
  - Y92.197 Garden or yard of other specified residential institution as the place of occurrence of the external cause
  - Y92.198 Other place in other specified residential institution as the place of occurrence of the external cause
  - Y92.199 Unspecified place in other specified residential institution as the place of occurrence of the external cause
- **+ Y92.2 School, other institution and public administrative area as the place of occurrence of the external cause**
  - Building and adjacent grounds used by the general public or by a particular group of the public
  - **Excludes1:** *building under construction as the place of occurrence of the external cause (Y92.6)*
    residential institution as the place of occurrence of the external cause (Y92.1)
    school dormitory as the place of occurrence of the external cause (Y92.16-)
    sports and athletics area of schools as the place of occurrence of the external cause (Y92.3-)
  - **+ Y92.21 School (private) (public) (state) as the place of occurrence of the external cause**
    - Y92.210 Daycare center as the place of occurrence of the external cause

- **Y92.211** Elementary school as the place of occurrence of the external cause
  - Kindergarten as the place of occurrence of the external cause
- **Y92.212** Middle school as the place of occurrence of the external cause
- **Y92.213** High school as the place of occurrence of the external cause
  - *AHA CC: 4Q, 2012, 108*
- **Y92.214** College as the place of occurrence of the external cause
  - University as the place of occurrence of the external cause
- **Y92.215** Trade school as the place of occurrence of the external cause
- **Y92.218** Other school as the place of occurrence of the external cause
- **Y92.219** Unspecified school as the place of occurrence of the external cause

Y92.22 Religious institution as the place of occurrence of the external cause
- Church as the place of occurrence of the external cause
- Mosque as the place of occurrence of the external cause
- Synagogue as the place of occurrence of the external cause

+ **Y92.23** Hospital as the place of occurrence of the external cause
  - **Excludes1:** ambulatory (outpatient) health services establishments (Y92.53-)
    home for the sick as the place of occurrence of the external cause (Y92.12-)
    hospice as the place of occurrence of the external cause (Y92.12-)
    nursing home as the place of occurrence of the external cause (Y92.12-)
  - **Y92.230** Patient room in hospital as the place of occurrence of the external cause
  - **Y92.231** Patient bathroom in hospital as the place of occurrence of the external cause
  - **Y92.232** Corridor of hospital as the place of occurrence of the external cause
  - **Y92.233** Cafeteria of hospital as the place of occurrence of the external cause
  - **Y92.234** Operating room of hospital as the place of occurrence of the external cause
  - **Y92.238** Other place in hospital as the place of occurrence of the external cause
  - **Y92.239** Unspecified place in hospital as the place of occurrence of the external cause

+ **Y92.24** Public administrative building as the place of occurrence of the external cause
  - **Y92.240** Courthouse as the place of occurrence of the external cause
  - **Y92.241** Library as the place of occurrence of the external cause
  - **Y92.242** Post office as the place of occurrence of the external cause
  - **Y92.243** City hall as the place of occurrence of the external cause
  - **Y92.248** Other public administrative building as the place of occurrence of the external cause

+ **Y92.25** Cultural building as the place of occurrence of the external cause
  - **Y92.250** Art Gallery as the place of occurrence of the external cause
  - **Y92.251** Museum as the place of occurrence of the external cause
  - **Y92.252** Music hall as the place of occurrence of the external cause
  - **Y92.253** Opera house as the place of occurrence of the external cause
  - **Y92.254** Theater (live) as the place of occurrence of the external cause
  - **Y92.258** Other cultural public building as the place of occurrence of the external cause

- **Y92.26** Movie house or cinema as the place of occurrence of the external cause
- **Y92.29** Other specified public building as the place of occurrence of the external cause
  - Assembly hall as the place of occurrence of the external cause
  - Clubhouse as the place of occurrence of the external cause

+ **Y92.3** Sports and athletics area as the place of occurrence of the external cause
  + **Y92.31** Athletic court as the place of occurrence of the external cause
    - **Excludes1:** tennis court in private home or garden (Y92.09)
    - **Y92.310** Basketball court as the place of occurrence of the external cause
    - **Y92.311** Squash court as the place of occurrence of the external cause
    - **Y92.312** Tennis court as the place of occurrence of the external cause
    - **Y92.318** Other athletic court as the place of occurrence of the external cause
  + **Y92.32** Athletic field as the place of occurrence of the external cause
    - **Y92.320** Baseball field as the place of occurrence of the external cause
    - **Y92.321** Football field as the place of occurrence of the external cause
    - **Y92.322** Soccer field as the place of occurrence of the external cause
    - **Y92.328** Other athletic field as the place of occurrence of the external cause
      - Cricket field as the place of occurrence of the external cause
      - Hockey field as the place of occurrence of the external cause
  + **Y92.33** Skating rink as the place of occurrence of the external cause
    - **Y92.330** Ice skating rink (indoor) (outdoor) as the place of occurrence of the external cause
    - **Y92.331** Roller skating rink as the place of occurrence of the external cause
  - **Y92.34** Swimming pool (public) as the place of occurrence of the external cause
    - **Excludes1:** swimming pool in private home or garden (Y92.016)
  - **Y92.39** Other specified sports and athletic area as the place of occurrence of the external cause
    - Golf-course as the place of occurrence of the external cause
    - Gymnasium as the place of occurrence of the external cause
    - Riding-school as the place of occurrence of the external cause
    - Stadium as the place of occurrence of the external cause

+ **Y92.4** Street, highway and other paved roadways as the place of occurrence of the external cause
  - **Excludes1:** private driveway of residence (Y92.014, Y92.024, Y92.043, Y92.093, Y92.113, Y92.123, Y92.154, Y92.194)
  + **Y92.41** Street and highway as the place of occurrence of the external cause
    - **Y92.410** Unspecified street and highway as the place of occurrence of the external cause
      - Road NOS as the place of occurrence of the external cause
    - **Y92.411** Interstate highway as the place of occurrence of the external cause
      - Freeway as the place of occurrence of the external cause
      - Motorway as the place of occurrence of the external cause
    - **Y92.412** Parkway as the place of occurrence of the external cause
    - **Y92.413** State road as the place of occurrence of the external cause
    - **Y92.414** Local residential or business street as the place of occurrence of the external cause

- Y92.415 Exit ramp or entrance ramp of street or highway as the place of occurrence of the external cause
+ Y92.48 Other paved roadways as the place of occurrence of the external cause
- Y92.480 Sidewalk as the place of occurrence of the external cause
- Y92.481 Parking lot as the place of occurrence of the external cause
- Y92.482 Bike path as the place of occurrence of the external cause
- Y92.488 Other paved roadways as the place of occurrence of the external cause

+ Y92.5 Trade and service area as the place of occurrence of the external cause
  Excludes1: *garage in private home (Y92.015)*
  schools and other public administration buildings (Y92.2-)

+ Y92.51 Private commercial establishments as the place of occurrence of the external cause
- Y92.510 Bank as the place of occurrence of the external cause
- Y92.511 Restaurant or café as the place of occurrence of the external cause
- Y92.512 Supermarket, store or market as the place of occurrence of the external cause
- Y92.513 Shop (commercial) as the place of occurrence of the external cause

+ Y92.52 Service areas as the place of occurrence of the external cause
- Y92.520 Airport as the place of occurrence of the external cause
- Y92.521 Bus station as the place of occurrence of the external cause
- Y92.522 Railway station as the place of occurrence of the external cause
- Y92.523 Highway rest stop as the place of occurrence of the external cause
- Y92.524 Gas station as the place of occurrence of the external cause
  Petroleum station as the place of occurrence of the external cause
  Service station as the place of occurrence of the external cause

+ Y92.53 Ambulatory health services establishments as the place of occurrence of the external cause
- Y92.530 Ambulatory surgery center as the place of occurrence of the external cause
  Outpatient surgery center, including that connected with a hospital as the place of occurrence of the external cause
  Same day surgery center, including that connected with a hospital as the place of occurrence of the external cause
- Y92.531 Health care provider office as the place of occurrence of the external cause
  Physician office as the place of occurrence of the external cause
- Y92.532 Urgent care center as the place of occurrence of the external cause
- Y92.538 Other ambulatory health services establishments as the place of occurrence of the external cause
  AHA CC: 1Q, 2019, 21

Y92.59 Other trade areas as the place of occurrence of the external cause
  Office building as the place of occurrence of the external cause
  Casino as the place of occurrence of the external cause
  Garage (commercial) as the place of occurrence of the external cause
  Hotel as the place of occurrence of the external cause
  Radio or television station as the place of occurrence of the external cause
  Shopping mall as the place of occurrence of the external cause
  Warehouse as the place of occurrence of the external cause

+ Y92.6 Industrial and construction area as the place of occurrence of the external cause
- Y92.61 Building [any] under construction as the place of occurrence of the external cause
- Y92.62 Dock or shipyard as the place of occurrence of the external cause
  Dockyard as the place of occurrence of the external cause
  Dry dock as the place of occurrence of the external cause
  Shipyard as the place of occurrence of the external cause
- Y92.63 Factory as the place of occurrence of the external cause
  Factory building as the place of occurrence of the external cause
  Factory premises as the place of occurrence of the external cause
  Industrial yard as the place of occurrence of the external cause
- Y92.64 Mine or pit as the place of occurrence of the external cause
  Mine as the place of occurrence of the external cause
- Y92.65 Oil rig as the place of occurrence of the external cause
  Pit (coal) (gravel) (sand) as the place of occurrence of the external cause
- Y92.69 Other specified industrial and construction area as the place of occurrence of the external cause
  Gasworks as the place of occurrence of the external cause
  Power-station (coal) (nuclear) (oil) as the place of occurrence of the external cause
  Tunnel under construction as the place of occurrence of the external cause
  Workshop as the place of occurrence of the external cause

+ Y92.7 Farm as the place of occurrence of the external cause
  Ranch as the place of occurrence of the external cause
  Excludes1: *farmhouse and home premises of farm (Y92.01-)*
- Y92.71 Barn as the place of occurrence of the external cause
- Y92.72 Chicken coop as the place of occurrence of the external cause
  Hen house as the place of occurrence of the external cause
- Y92.73 Farm field as the place of occurrence of the external cause
- Y92.74 Orchard as the place of occurrence of the external cause
- Y92.79 Other farm location as the place of occurrence of the external cause

+ Y92.8 Other places as the place of occurrence of the external cause
+ Y92.81 Transport vehicle as the place of occurrence of the external cause
  Excludes1: *transport accidents (V00-V99)*
- Y92.810 Car as the place of occurrence of the external cause
- Y92.811 Bus as the place of occurrence of the external cause
- Y92.812 Truck as the place of occurrence of the external cause
- Y92.813 Airplane as the place of occurrence of the external cause
- Y92.814 Boat as the place of occurrence of the external cause
- Y92.815 Train as the place of occurrence of the external cause
- Y92.816 Subway car as the place of occurrence of the external cause
- Y92.818 Other transport vehicle as the place of occurrence of the external cause

+ Y92.82 Wilderness area
- Y92.820 Desert as the place of occurrence of the external cause
- Y92.821 Forest as the place of occurrence of the external cause

Y92.828 Other wilderness area as the place of occurrence of the external cause
- Swamp as the place of occurrence of the external cause
- Mountain as the place of occurrence of the external cause
- Marsh as the place of occurrence of the external cause
- Prairie as the place of occurrence of the external cause

+ **Y92.83** Recreation area as the place of occurrence of the external cause

Y92.830 Public park as the place of occurrence of the external cause

Y92.831 Amusement park as the place of occurrence of the external cause

Y92.832 Beach as the place of occurrence of the external cause
- Seashore as the place of occurrence of the external cause

Y92.833 Campsite as the place of occurrence of the external cause

Y92.834 Zoological garden (Zoo) as the place of occurrence of the external cause

Y92.838 Other recreation area as the place of occurrence of the external cause

Y92.84 Military training ground as the place of occurrence of the external cause

Y92.85 Railroad track as the place of occurrence of the external cause

Y92.86 Slaughter house as the place of occurrence of the external cause

Y92.89 Other specified places as the place of occurrence of the external cause
- Derelict house as the place of occurrence of the external cause

Y92.9 Unspecified place or not applicable

Y93 Activity codes

NOTE Category Y93 is provided for use to indicate the activity of the person seeking healthcare for an injury or health condition, such as a heart attack while shoveling snow, which resulted from, or was contributed to, by the activity. These codes are appropriate for use for both acute injuries, such as those from chapter 19, and conditions that are due to the long-term, cumulative effects of an activity, such as those from chapter 13. They are also appropriate for use with external cause codes for cause and intent if identifying the activity provides additional information on the event. These codes should be used in conjunction with codes for external cause status (Y99) and place of occurrence (Y92).

This section contains the following broad activity categories:
- Y93.0 Activities involving walking and running
- Y93.1 Activities involving water and water craft
- Y93.2 Activities involving ice and snow
- Y93.3 Activities involving climbing, rappelling, and jumping off
- Y93.4 Activities involving dancing and other rhythmic movement
- Y93.5 Activities involving other sports and athletics played individually
- Y93.6 Activities involving other sports and athletics played as a team or group
- Y93.7 Activities involving other specified sports and athletics
- Y93.A Activities involving other cardiorespiratory exercise
- Y93.B Activities involving other muscle strengthening exercises
- Y93.C Activities involving computer technology and electronic devices
- Y93.D Activities involving arts and handcrafts
- Y93.E Activities involving personal hygiene and interior property and clothing maintenance
- Y93.F Activities involving caregiving
- Y93.G Activities involving food preparation, cooking and grilling
- Y93.H Activities involving exterior property and land maintenance, building and construction
- Y93.I Activities involving roller coasters and other types of external motion
- Y93.J Activities involving playing musical instrument
- Y93.K Activities involving animal care
- Y93.8 Activities, other specified
- Y93.9 Activity, unspecified

Review coding guideline C.20.c

+ **Y93.0** Activities involving walking and running
   Excludes1: activity, walking an animal (Y93.K1)
   activity, walking or running on a treadmill (Y93.A1)

   Y93.01 Activity, walking, marching and hiking
   Activity, walking, marching and hiking on level or elevated terrain
   Excludes1: activity, mountain climbing (Y93.31)

   Y93.02 Activity, running

+ **Y93.1** Activities involving water and water craft
   Excludes1: activities involving ice (Y93.2-)

   Y93.11 Activity, swimming
   Y93.12 Activity, springboard and platform diving
   Y93.13 Activity, water polo
   Y93.14 Activity, water aerobics and water exercise
   Y93.15 Activity, underwater diving and snorkeling
   Activity, SCUBA diving
   Y93.16 Activity, rowing, canoeing, kayaking, rafting and tubing
   Activity, canoeing, kayaking, rafting and tubing in calm and turbulent water
   Y93.17 Activity, water skiing and wake boarding
   Y93.18 Activity, surfing, windsurfing and boogie boarding
   Activity, water sliding
   Y93.19 Activity, other involving water and watercraft
   Activity involving water NOS
   Activity, parasailing
   Activity, water survival training and testing

+ **Y93.2** Activities involving ice and snow
   Excludes1: activity, shoveling ice and snow (Y93.H1)

   Y93.21 Activity, ice skating
   Activity, figure skating (singles) (pairs)
   Activity, ice dancing
   Excludes1: activity, ice hockey (Y93.22)

   Y93.22 Activity, ice hockey
   Y93.23 Activity, snow (alpine) (downhill) skiing, snowboarding, sledding, tobogganing and snow tubing
   Excludes1: activity, cross country skiing (Y93.24)

   Y93.24 Activity, cross country skiing
   Activity, nordic skiing
   Y93.29 Activity, other involving ice and snow
   Activity involving ice and snow NOS

+ **Y93.3** Activities involving climbing, rappelling and jumping off
   Excludes1: activity, hiking on level or elevated terrain (Y93.01)
   activity, jumping rope (Y93.56)
   activity, trampoline jumping (Y93.44)

   Y93.31 Activity, mountain climbing, rock climbing and wall climbing
   Y93.32 Activity, rappelling
   Y93.33 Activity, BASE jumping
   Activity, Building, Antenna, Span, Earth jumping
   Y93.34 Activity, bungee jumping
   Y93.35 Activity, hang gliding
   Y93.39 Activity, other involving climbing, rappelling and jumping off

+ **Y93.4** Activities involving dancing and other rhythmic movement
   Excludes1: activity, martial arts (Y93.75)

   Y93.41 Activity, dancing
   AHA CC: 4Q, 2012, 108
   Y93.42 Activity, yoga
   Y93.43 Activity, gymnastics
   Activity, rhythmic gymnastics
   Excludes1: activity, trampolining (Y93.44)
   Y93.44 Activity, trampolining
   Y93.45 Activity, cheerleading
   Y93.49 Activity, other involving dancing and other rhythmic movements

- **Y93.5** **Activities involving other sports and athletics played individually**
  - *Excludes1:* activity, dancing (Y93.41)
    activity, gymnastic (Y93.43)
    activity, trampolining (Y93.44)
    activity, yoga (Y93.42)
  - **Y93.51** Activity, roller skating (inline) and skateboarding
  - **Y93.52** Activity, horseback riding
  - **Y93.53** Activity, golf
  - **Y93.54** Activity, bowling
  - **Y93.55** Activity, bike riding
  - **Y93.56** Activity, jumping rope
  - **Y93.57** Activity, non-running track and field events
    - *Excludes1:* activity, running (any form) (Y93.02)
  - **Y93.59** Activity, other involving other sports and athletics played individually
    - *Excludes1:* activities involving climbing, rappelling, and jumping (Y93.3-)
      activities involving ice and snow (Y93.2-)
      activities involving walking and running (Y93.0-)
      activities involving water and watercraft (Y93.1-)
- **Y93.6** **Activities involving other sports and athletics played as a team or group**
  - *Excludes1:* activity, ice hockey (Y93.22)
    activity, water polo (Y93.13)
  - **Y93.61** Activity, american tackle football
    Activity, football NOS
  - **Y93.62** Activity, american flag or touch football
  - **Y93.63** Activity, rugby
  - **Y93.64** Activity, baseball
    Activity, softball
  - **Y93.65** Activity, lacrosse and field hockey
    AHA CC: 1Q, 2015, 3-21
  - **Y93.66** Activity, soccer
  - **Y93.67** Activity, basketball
    AHA CC: 4Q, 2019, 17-18
  - **Y93.68** Activity, volleyball (beach) (court)
  - **Y93.6A** Activity, physical games generally associated with school recess, summer camp and children
    Activity, capture the flag
    Activity, dodge ball
    Activity, four square
    Activity, kickball
  - **Y93.69** Activity, other involving other sports and athletics played as a team or group
    Activity, cricket
- **Y93.7** **Activities involving other specified sports and athletics**
  - **Y93.71** Activity, boxing
  - **Y93.72** Activity, wrestling
  - **Y93.73** Activity, racquet and hand sports
    Activity, handball
    Activity, racquetball
    Activity, squash
    Activity, tennis
  - **Y93.74** Activity, frisbee
    Activity, ultimate frisbee
  - **Y93.75** Activity, martial arts
    Activity, combatives
  - **Y93.79** Activity, other specified sports and athletics
    - *Excludes1:* sports and athletics activities specified in categories Y93.0-Y93.6
- **Y93.A** **Activities involving other cardiorespiratory exercise**
  Activities involving physical training
  - **Y93.A1** Activity, exercise machines primarily for cardiorespiratory conditioning
    Activity, elliptical and stepper machines
    Activity, stationary bike
    Activity, treadmill
  - **Y93.A2** Activity, calisthenics
    Activity, jumping jacks
    Activity, warm up and cool down
  - **Y93.A3** Activity, aerobic and step exercise
  - **Y93.A4** Activity, circuit training
  - **Y93.A5** Activity, obstacle course
    Activity, challenge course
    Activity, confidence course
  - **Y93.A6** Activity, grass drills
    Activity, guerilla drills
  - **Y93.A9** Activity, other involving cardiorespiratory exercise
    - *Excludes1:* activities involving cardiorespiratory exercise specified in categories Y93.0-Y93.7
- **Y93.B** **Activities involving other muscle strengthening exercises**
  - **Y93.B1** Activity, exercise machines primarily for muscle strengthening
  - **Y93.B2** Activity, push-ups, pull-ups, sit-ups
  - **Y93.B3** Activity, free weights
    Activity, barbells
    Activity, dumbbells
  - **Y93.B4** Activity, pilates
  - **Y93.B9** Activity, other involving muscle strengthening exercises
    - *Excludes1:* activities involving muscle strengthening specified in categories Y93.0-Y93.A
- **Y93.C** **Activities involving computer technology and electronic devices**
  - *Excludes1:* activity, electronic musical keyboard or instruments (Y93.J-)
  - **Y93.C1** Activity, computer keyboarding
    Activity, electronic game playing using keyboard or other stationary device
  - **Y93.C2** Activity, hand held interactive electronic device
    Activity, cellular telephone and communication device
    Activity, electronic game playing using interactive device
    - *Excludes1:* activity, electronic game playing using keyboard or other stationary device (Y93.C1)
  - **Y93.C9** Activity, other involving computer technology and electronic devices
- **Y93.D** **Activities involving arts and handcrafts**
  - *Excludes1:* activities involving playing musical instrument (Y93.J-)
  - **Y93.D1** Activity, knitting and crocheting
  - **Y93.D2** Activity, sewing
  - **Y93.D3** Activity, furniture building and finishing
    Activity, furniture repair
  - **Y93.D9** Activity, other involving arts and handcrafts
- **Y93.E** **Activities involving personal hygiene and interior property and clothing maintenance**
  - *Excludes1:* activities involving cooking and grilling (Y93.G-)
    activities involving exterior property and land maintenance, building and construction (Y93.H-)
    activities involving caregiving (Y93.F-)
    activity, dishwashing (Y93.G1)
    activity, food preparation (Y93.G1)
    activity, gardening (Y93.H2)
  - **Y93.E1** Activity, personal bathing and showering
  - **Y93.E2** Activity, laundry
  - **Y93.E3** Activity, vacuuming
  - **Y93.E4** Activity, ironing
  - **Y93.E5** Activity, floor mopping and cleaning
  - **Y93.E6** Activity, residential relocation
    Activity, packing up and unpacking involved in moving to a new residence
  - **Y93.E8** Activity, other personal hygiene
  - **Y93.E9** Activity, other interior property and clothing maintenance
- **Y93.F** **Activities involving caregiving**
  Activity involving the provider of caregiving
  - **Y93.F1** Activity, caregiving, bathing
  - **Y93.F2** Activity, caregiving, lifting
    AHA CC: 4Q, 2016, 73-74
  - **Y93.F9** Activity, other caregiving
- **Y93.G** **Activities involving food preparation, cooking and grilling**
  - **Y93.G1** Activity, food preparation and clean up
    Activity, dishwashing
  - **Y93.G2** Activity, grilling and smoking food
  - **Y93.G3** Activity, cooking and baking
    Activity, use of stove, oven and microwave oven
  - **Y93.G9** Activity, other involving cooking and grilling

+ **Y93.H** **Activities involving exterior property and land maintenance, building and construction**
    Y93.H1 Activity, digging, shoveling and raking
        Activity, dirt digging
        Activity, raking leaves
        Activity, snow shoveling
    Y93.H2 Activity, gardening and landscaping
        Activity, pruning, trimming shrubs, weeding
    Y93.H3 Activity, building and construction
    Y93.H9 Activity, other involving exterior property and land maintenance, building and construction

+ **Y93.I** **Activities involving roller coasters and other types of external motion**
    Y93.I1 Activity, roller coaster riding
    Y93.I9 Activity, other involving external motion

+ **Y93.J** **Activities involving playing musical instrument**
    Activity involving playing electric musical instrument
    Y93.J1 Activity, piano playing
        Activity, musical keyboard (electronic) playing
    Y93.J2 Activity, drum and other percussion instrument playing
    Y93.J3 Activity, string instrument playing
    Y93.J4 Activity, winds and brass instrument playing

+ **Y93.K** **Activities involving animal care**
    Excludes1: activity, horseback riding (Y93.52)
    Y93.K1 Activity, walking an animal
    Y93.K2 Activity, milking an animal
    Y93.K3 Activity, grooming and shearing an animal
    Y93.K9 Activity, other involving animal care

+ **Y93.8** **Activities, other specified**
    Y93.81 Activity, refereeing a sports activity
    Y93.82 Activity, spectator at an event
    Y93.83 Activity, rough housing and horseplay
        AHA CC: 1Q, 2015, 3-21
    Y93.84 Activity, sleeping
    Y93.85 Activity, choking game
        Activity, blackout game
        Activity, fainting game
        Activity, pass out game
        AHA CC: 4Q, 2016, 74-76

    Y93.89 Activity, other specified
  Y93.9 Activity, unspecified

Y95 **Nosocomial condition**
    Valid 3-character code, no further characters required
    AHA CC: 4Q, 2013, 119

Y99 **External cause status**
    NOTE A single code from category Y99 should be used in conjunction with the external cause code(s) assigned to a record to indicate the status of the person at the time the event occurred.
    Review coding guideline C.20.k
  Y99.0 Civilian activity done for income or pay
    Civilian activity done for financial or other compensation
    Excludes1: military activity (Y99.1)
        volunteer activity (Y99.2)
    AHA CC: 4Q, 2016, 73-74
  Y99.1 Military activity
    Excludes1: activity of off duty military personnel (Y99.8)
  Y99.2 Volunteer activity
    Excludes1: activity of child or other family member assisting in compensated work of other family member (Y99.8)
  Y99.8 Other external cause status
    Activity NEC
    Activity of child or other family member assisting in compensated work of other family member
    Hobby not done for income
    Leisure activity
    Off-duty activity of military personnel
    Recreation or sport not for income or while a student
    Student activity
    Excludes1: civilian activity done for income or compensation (Y99.0)
        military activity (Y99.1)
    AHA CC: 4Q, 2012, 108
  Y99.9 Unspecified external cause status

Chapter 21: Factors Influencing Health Status and Contact with Health Services (Z00-Z99)

NOTE Z codes represent reasons for encounters. A corresponding procedure code must accompany a Z code if a procedure is performed. Categories Z00-Z99 are provided for occasions when circumstances other than a disease, injury or external cause classifiable to categories A00-Y89 are recorded as 'diagnoses' or 'problems'. This can arise in two main ways:
(a) When a person who may or may not be sick encounters the health services for some specific purpose, such as to receive limited care or service for a current condition, to donate an organ or tissue, to receive prophylactic vaccination (immunization), or to discuss a problem which is in itself not a disease or injury.
(b) When some circumstance or problem is present which influences the person's health status but is not in itself a current illness or injury.

This chapter contains the following category blocks:

Z00-Z13	Persons encountering health services for examinations
Z14-Z15	Genetic carrier and genetic susceptibility to disease
Z16	Resistance to antimicrobial drugs
Z17	Estrogen receptor status
Z18	Retained foreign body fragments
Z19	Hormone sensitivity malignancy status
Z20-Z29	Persons with potential health hazards related to communicable diseases
Z30-Z39	Persons encountering health services in circumstances related to reproduction
Z40-Z53	Encounters for other specific health care
Z55-Z65	Persons with potential health hazards related to socioeconomic and psychosocial circumstances
Z66	Do not resuscitate status
Z67	Blood type
Z68	Body mass index (BMI)
Z69-Z76	Persons encountering health services in other circumstances
Z77-Z99	Persons with potential health hazards related to family and personal history and certain conditions influencing health status

C. Chapter-Specific Coding Guidelines

In addition to general coding guidelines, there are guidelines for specific diagnoses and/or conditions in the classification. Unless otherwise indicated, these guidelines apply to all health care settings. Please refer to Section II for guidelines on the selection of principal diagnosis.

21. Chapter 21: Factors Influencing Health Status and Contact with Health Services (Z00-Z99)

NOTE The chapter specific guidelines provide additional information about the use of Z codes for specified encounters.

a. Use of Z codes in any healthcare setting

Z codes are for use in any healthcare setting. Z codes may be used as either a first-listed (principal diagnosis code in the inpatient setting) or secondary code, depending on the circumstances of the encounter. Certain Z codes may only be used as first-listed or principal diagnosis.

b. Z Codes indicate a reason for an encounter or Provide Additional Information about a Patient Encounter

Z codes are not procedure codes. A corresponding procedure code must accompany a Z code to describe any procedure performed.

c. Categories of Z Codes

1) Contact/Exposure

Category Z20 indicates contact with, and suspected exposure to, communicable diseases. These codes are for patients who do not show any sign or symptom of a disease but are suspected to have been exposed to it by close personal contact with an infected individual or are in an area where a disease is epidemic.

Category Z77, Other contact with and (suspected) exposures hazardous to health, indicates contact with and suspected exposures hazardous to health.

Contact/exposure codes may be used as a first-listed code to explain an encounter for testing, or, more commonly, as a secondary code to identify a potential risk.

2) Inoculations and vaccinations

Code Z23 is for encounters for inoculations and vaccinations. It indicates that a patient is being seen to receive a prophylactic inoculation against a disease. Procedure codes are required to identify the actual administration of the injection and the type(s) of immunizations given. Code Z23 may be used as a secondary code if the inoculation is given as a routine part of preventive health care, such as a well-baby visit.

3) Status

Status codes indicate that a patient is either a carrier of a disease or has the sequelae or residual of a past disease or condition. This includes such things as the presence of prosthetic or mechanical devices resulting from past treatment. A status code is informative, because the status may affect the course of treatment and its outcome. A status code is distinct from a history code. The history code indicates that the patient no longer has the condition.

A status code should not be used with a diagnosis code from one of the body system chapters, if the diagnosis code includes the information provided by the status code. For example, code Z94.1, Heart transplant status, should not be used with a code from subcategory T86.2, Complications of heart transplant. The status code does not provide additional information. The complication code indicates that the patient is a heart transplant patient.

For encounters for weaning from a mechanical ventilator, assign a code from subcategory J96.1, Chronic respiratory failure, followed by code Z99.11, Dependence on respirator [ventilator] status.

The status Z codes/categories are:

Z14	Genetic carrier
	Genetic carrier status indicates that a person carries a gene, associated with a particular disease, which may be passed to offspring who may develop that disease. The person does not have the disease and is not at risk of developing the disease.
Z15	Genetic susceptibility to disease
	Genetic susceptibility indicates that a person has a gene that increases the risk of that person developing the disease.
	Codes from category Z15 should not be used as principal or first-listed codes. If the patient has the condition to which he/she is susceptible, and that condition is the reason for the encounter, the code for the current condition should be sequenced first. If the patient is being seen for follow-up after completed treatment for this condition, and the condition no longer exists, a follow-up code should be sequenced first, followed by the appropriate personal history and genetic susceptibility codes. If the purpose of the encounter is genetic counseling associated with procreative management, code Z31.5, Encounter for genetic counseling, should be assigned as the first-listed code, followed by a code from category Z15. Additional codes should be assigned for any applicable family or personal history.
Z16	Resistance to antimicrobial drugs
	This code indicates that a patient has a condition that is resistant to antimicrobial drug treatment. Sequence the infection code first.
Z17	Estrogen receptor status
Z18	Retained foreign body fragments
Z19	Hormone sensitivity malignancy status
Z21	Asymptomatic HIV infection status
	This code indicates that a patient has tested positive for HIV but has manifested no signs or symptoms of the disease.
Z22	Carrier of infectious disease
	Carrier status indicates that a person harbors the specific organisms of a disease without manifest symptoms and is capable of transmitting the infection.
Z28.3	Underimmunization status
	See Section I.B.14. for underimmunization documentation by clinicians other than the patient's provider.
Z33.1	Pregnant state, incidental
	This code is a secondary code only for use when the pregnancy is in no way complicating the reason for visit. Otherwise, a code from the obstetric chapter is required.
Z66	Do not resuscitate
	This code may be used when it is documented by the provider that a patient is on do not resuscitate status at any time during the stay.
Z67	Blood type
Z68	Body mass index (BMI)
	BMI codes should only be assigned when there is an associated, reportable diagnosis (such as obesity). Do not assign BMI codes during pregnancy.
	See Section I.B.14 for BMI documentation by clinicians other than the patient's provider.
Z74.01	Bed confinement status
Z76.82	Awaiting organ transplant status
Z78	Other specified health status
	Code Z78.1, Physical restraint status, may be used when it is documented by the provider that a patient has been put in restraints during the current encounter. Please note that this code should not be reported when it is documented by the provider that a patient is temporarily restrained during a procedure.

Z79	Long-term (current) drug therapy	

Codes from this category indicate a patient's continuous use of a prescribed drug (including such things as aspirin therapy) for the long-term treatment of a condition or for prophylactic use. It is not for use for patients who have addictions to drugs. This subcategory is not for use of medications for detoxification or maintenance programs to prevent withdrawal symptoms in patients with drug dependence (e.g., methadone maintenance for opiate dependence). Assign the appropriate code for the drug dependence instead.

Assign a code from Z79 if the patient is receiving a medication for an extended period as a prophylactic measure (such as for the prevention of deep vein thrombosis) or as treatment of a chronic condition (such as arthritis) or a disease requiring a lengthy course of treatment (such as cancer). Do not assign a code from category Z79 for medication being administered for a brief period of time to treat an acute illness or injury (such as a course of antibiotics to treat acute bronchitis).

Z88	Allergy status to drugs, medicaments and biological substances
	Except: Z88.9, Allergy status to unspecified drugs, medicaments and biological substances status
Z89	Acquired absence of limb
Z90	Acquired absence of organs, not elsewhere classified
Z91.0-	Allergy status, other than to drugs and biological substances
Z92.82	Status post administration of tPA (rtPA) in a different facility within the last 24 hours prior to admission to a current facility

Assign code Z92.82, Status post administration of tPA (rtPA) in a different facility within the last 24 hours prior to admission to current facility, as a secondary diagnosis when a patient is received by transfer into a facility and documentation indicates they were administered tissue plasminogen activator (tPA) within the last 24 hours prior to admission to the current facility.

This guideline applies even if the patient is still receiving the tPA at the time they are received into the current facility.

The appropriate code for the condition for which the tPA was administered (such as cerebrovascular disease or myocardial infarction) should be assigned first.

Code Z92.82 is only applicable to the receiving facility record and not to the transferring facility record.

Z93	Artificial opening status
Z94	Transplanted organ and tissue status
Z95	Presence of cardiac and vascular implants and grafts
Z96	Presence of other functional implants
Z97	Presence of other devices
Z98	Other postprocedural states

Assign code Z98.85, Transplanted organ removal status, to indicate that a transplanted organ has been previously removed. This code should not be assigned for the encounter in which the transplanted organ is removed. The complication necessitating removal of the transplant organ should be assigned for that encounter.

See section I.C19. for information on the coding of organ transplant complications.

Z99	Dependence on enabling machines and devices, not elsewhere classified

NOTE Categories Z89-Z90 and Z93-Z99 are for use only if there are no complications or malfunctions of the organ or tissue replaced, the amputation site or the equipment on which the patient is dependent.

4) History (of)

There are two types of history Z codes, personal and family. Personal history codes explain a patient's past medical condition that no longer exists and is not receiving any treatment, but that has the potential for recurrence, and therefore may require continued monitoring.

Family history codes are for use when a patient has a family member(s) who has had a particular disease that causes the patient to be at higher risk of also contracting the disease.

Personal history codes may be used in conjunction with follow-up codes and family history codes may be used in conjunction with screening codes to explain the need for a test or procedure. History codes are also acceptable on any medical record regardless of the reason for visit. A history of an illness, even if no longer present, is important information that may alter the type of treatment ordered. The reason for the encounter (for example, screening or counseling) should be sequenced first and the appropriate personal and/or family history code(s) should be assigned as additional diagnos(es).

The history Z code categories are:

Z80	Family history of primary malignant neoplasm
Z81	Family history of mental and behavioral disorders
Z82	Family history of certain disabilities and chronic diseases (leading to disablement)
Z83	Family history of other specific disorders
Z84	Family history of other conditions
Z85	Personal history of malignant neoplasm
Z86	Personal history of certain other diseases
Z87	Personal history of other diseases and conditions
Z91.4-	Personal history of psychological trauma, not elsewhere classified
Z91.5	Personal history of self-harm
Z91.81	History of falling
Z91.82	Personal history of military deployment
Z91.85	**Personal history of military service**
Z92	Personal history of medical treatment
	Except: Z92.0, Personal history of contraception Except: Z92.82, Status post administration of tPA (rtPA) in a different facility within the last 24 hours prior to admission to a current facility

5) Screening

Screening is the testing for disease or disease precursors in seemingly well individuals so that early detection and treatment can be provided for those who test positive for the disease (e.g., screening mammogram).

The testing of a person to rule out or confirm a suspected diagnosis because the patient has some sign or symptom is a diagnostic examination, not a screening. In these cases, the sign or symptom is used to explain the reason for the test.

A screening code may be a first-listed code if the reason for the visit is specifically the screening exam. It may also be used as an additional code if the screening is done during an office visit for other health problems. A screening code is not necessary if the screening is inherent to a routine examination, such as a pap smear done during a routine pelvic examination.

Should a condition be discovered during the screening then the code for the condition may be assigned as an additional diagnosis.

The Z code indicates that a screening exam is planned. A procedure code is required to confirm that the screening was performed.

The screening Z codes/categories:

Z11	Encounter for screening for infectious and parasitic diseases
Z12	Encounter for screening for malignant neoplasms
Z13	Encounter for screening for other diseases and disorders
	Except: Z13.9, Encounter for screening, unspecified
Z36	Encounter for antenatal screening for mother

6) Observation

There are three observation Z code categories. They are for use in very limited circumstances when a person is being observed for a suspected condition that is ruled out. The observation codes are not for use if an injury or illness or any signs or symptoms related to the suspected condition are present. In such cases the diagnosis/symptom code is used with the corresponding external cause code.

The observation codes are primarily to be used as principal/first-listed diagnosis. An observation code may be assigned as a secondary diagnosis code when the patient is being observed for a condition that is ruled out and is unrelated to the principal/first-listed diagnosis (e.g., patient presents for treatment following injuries sustained in a motor vehicle accident and is also observed for suspected COVID-19 infection that is subsequently ruled out). Also, when the principal diagnosis is required to be a code from category Z38, Liveborn infants according to place of birth and type of delivery, then a code form category Z05, Encounter for observation and evaluation of newborn for suspected diseases and conditions ruled out, is sequenced after the Z38 code. Additional codes may be used in addition to the observation code but only if they are unrelated to the suspected condition being observed.

Codes from subcategory Z03.7, Encounter for suspected maternal and fetal conditions ruled out, may either be used as a first-listed or as an additional code assignment depending on the case. They are for use in very limited circumstances on a maternal record when an encounter is for a suspected maternal or fetal condition that is ruled out during that encounter (for example, a maternal or fetal condition may be suspected due to an abnormal test result). These codes should not be used when the condition is confirmed. In those cases, the confirmed condition should be coded. In addition, these codes are not for use if an illness or any signs or symptoms related to the suspected condition or problem are present. In such cases the diagnosis/symptom code is used.

Additional codes may be used in addition to the code from subcategory Z03.7, but only if they are unrelated to the suspected condition being evaluated.

Codes from subcategory Z03.7 may not be used for encounters for antenatal screening of mother. *See Section I.C.21. Screening.*

For encounters for suspected fetal condition that are inconclusive following testing and evaluation, assign the appropriate code from category O35, O36, O40 or O41.

The observation Z code categories:

Z03	Encounter for medical observation for suspected diseases and conditions ruled out
Z04	Encounter for examination and observation for other reasons Except: Z04.9, Encounter for examination and observation for unspecified reason
Z05	Encounter for observation and evaluation of newborn for suspected diseases and conditions ruled out

7) Aftercare

Aftercare visit codes cover situations when the initial treatment of a disease has been performed and the patient requires continued care during the healing or recovery phase, or for the long-term consequences of the disease. The aftercare Z code should not be used if treatment is directed at a current, acute disease. The diagnosis code is to be used in these cases. Exceptions to this rule are codes Z51.0, Encounter for antineoplastic radiation therapy, and codes from subcategory Z51.1, Encounter for antineoplastic chemotherapy and immunotherapy. These codes are to be first-listed, followed by the diagnosis code when a patient's encounter is solely to receive radiation therapy, chemotherapy, or immunotherapy for the treatment of a neoplasm. If the reason for the encounter is more than one type of antineoplastic therapy, code Z51.0 and a code from subcategory Z51.1 may be assigned together, in which case one of these codes would be reported as a secondary diagnosis.

The aftercare Z codes should also not be used for aftercare for injuries. For aftercare of an injury, assign the acute injury code with the appropriate 7th character (for subsequent encounter).

The aftercare codes are generally first-listed to explain the specific reason for the encounter. An aftercare code may be used as an additional code when some type of aftercare is provided in addition to the reason for admission and no diagnosis code is applicable. An example of this would be the closure of a colostomy during an encounter for treatment of another condition.

Aftercare codes should be used in conjunction with other aftercare codes or diagnosis codes to provide better detail on the specifics of an aftercare encounter visit, unless otherwise directed by the classification. Should a patient receive multiple types of antineoplastic therapy during the same encounter, code Z51.0, Encounter for antineoplastic radiation therapy, and codes from subcategory Z51.1, Encounter for antineoplastic chemotherapy and immunotherapy, may be used together on a record. The sequencing of multiple aftercare codes depends on the circumstances of the encounter.

Certain aftercare Z code categories need a secondary diagnosis code to describe the resolving condition or sequelae. For others, the condition is included in the code title.

Additional Z code aftercare category terms include fitting and adjustment, and attention to artificial openings.

Status Z codes may be used with aftercare Z codes to indicate the nature of the aftercare. For example code Z95.1, Presence of aortocoronary bypass graft, may be used with code Z48.812, Encounter for surgical aftercare following surgery on the circulatory system, to indicate the surgery for which the aftercare is being performed. A status code should not be used when the aftercare code indicates the type of status, such as using Z43.0, Encounter for attention to tracheostomy, with Z93.0, Tracheostomy status.

The aftercare Z category/codes:

Z42	Encounter for plastic and reconstructive surgery following medical procedure or healed injury
Z43	Encounter for attention to artificial openings
Z44	Encounter for fitting and adjustment of external prosthetic device
Z45	Encounter for adjustment and management of implanted device
Z46	Encounter for fitting and adjustment of other devices
Z47	Orthopedic aftercare
Z48	Encounter for other postprocedural aftercare
Z49	Encounter for care involving renal dialysis
Z51	Encounter for other aftercare and medical care

8) Follow-up

The follow-up codes are used to explain continuing surveillance following completed treatment of a disease, condition, or injury. They imply that the condition has been fully treated and no longer exists. They should not be confused with aftercare codes, or injury codes with a 7th character for subsequent encounter, that explain ongoing care of a healing condition or its sequelae. Follow-up codes may be used in conjunction with history codes to provide the full picture of the healed condition and its treatment. The follow-up code is sequenced first, followed by the history code.

A follow-up code may be used to explain multiple visits. Should a condition be found to have recurred on the follow-up visit, then the diagnosis code for the condition should be assigned in place of the follow-up code.

The follow-up Z code categories:

Z08	Encounter for follow-up examination after completed treatment for malignant neoplasm
Z09	Encounter for follow-up examination after completed treatment for conditions other than malignant neoplasm

Codes Z08, Encounter for follow-up examination after completed treatment for malignant neoplasm, and Z09, Encounter for follow up examination after completed treatment for conditions other than malignant neoplasm, may be assigned following any type of completed treatment modality (including both medical and surgical treatments).

Z39	Encounter for maternal postpartum care and examination

9) Donor

Codes in category Z52, Donors of organs and tissues, are used for living individuals who are donating blood or other body tissue. These codes are only for individuals donating for others, not for self-donations. They are not used to identify cadaveric donations.

10) Counseling

Counseling Z codes are used when a patient or family member receives assistance in the aftermath of an illness or injury, or when support is required in coping with family or social problems.

The counseling Z codes/categories:

Z30.0-	Encounter for general counseling and advice on contraception
Z31.5	Encounter for procreative genetic counseling
Z31.6-	Encounter for general counseling and advice on procreation
Z32.2	Encounter for childbirth instruction
Z32.3	Encounter for childcare instruction
Z69	Encounter for mental health services for victim and perpetrator of abuse
Z70	Counseling related to sexual attitude, behavior and orientation
Z71	Persons encountering health services for other counseling and medical advice, not elsewhere classified

NOTE Code Z71.84, Encounter for health counseling related to travel, is to be used for health risk and safety counseling for future travel purposes.

Code Z71.85, Encounter for immunization safety counseling, is to be used for counseling of the patient or caregiver regarding the safety of a vaccine. This code should not be used for the provision of general information regarding risks and potential side effects during routine encounters for the administration of vaccines.

Code Z71.87, Encounter for pediatric-to-adult transition counseling, should be assigned when pediatric-to-adult transition counseling is the sole reason for the encounter or when this counseling is provided in addition to other services, such as treatment of a chronic condition. If both transition counseling and treatment of a medical condition are provided during the same encounter, the code(s) for the medical condition(s) treated and code Z71.87 should be assigned, with sequencing depending on the circumstances of the encounter.

Z76.81	Expectant mother prebirth pediatrician visit

11) Encounters for Obstetrical and Reproductive Services

See Section I.C.15. Pregnancy, Childbirth, and the Puerperium, for further instruction on the use of these codes.

Z codes for pregnancy are for use in those circumstances when none of the problems or complications included in the codes from the Obstetrics chapter exist (a routine prenatal visit or postpartum care). Codes in category Z34, Encounter for supervision of normal pregnancy, are always first-listed and are not to be used with any other code from the OB chapter.

Codes in category Z3A, Weeks of gestation, may be assigned to provide additional information about the pregnancy. Category Z3A codes should not be assigned for pregnancies with abortive outcomes (categories O00-O08), elective termination of pregnancy (code Z33.2), nor for postpartum conditions, as category Z3A is not applicable to these conditions. The date of the admission should be used to determine weeks of gestation for inpatient admissions that encompass more than one gestational week.

The outcome of delivery, category Z37, should be included on all maternal delivery records. It is always a secondary code. Codes in category Z37 should not be used on the newborn record.

Z codes for family planning (contraceptive) or procreative management and counseling should be included on an obstetric record either during the pregnancy or the postpartum stage, if applicable.

Z codes/categories for obstetrical and reproductive services:

Z30	Encounter for contraceptive management
Z31	Encounter for procreative management
Z32.2	Encounter for childbirth instruction
Z32.3	Encounter for childcare instruction
Z33	Pregnant state
Z34	Encounter for supervision of normal pregnancy
Z36	Encounter for antenatal screening of mother
Z3A	Weeks of gestation
Z37	Outcome of delivery
Z39	Encounter for maternal postpartum care and examination
Z76.81	Expectant mother prebirth pediatrician visit

12) Newborns and Infants

See Section I.C.16. Newborn (Perinatal) Guidelines, for further instruction on the use of these codes.

Newborn Z codes/categories:

Z76.1	Encounter for health supervision and care of foundling
Z00.1-	Encounter for routine child health examination
Z38	Liveborn infants according to place of birth and type of delivery

13) Routine and administrative examinations

The Z codes allow for the description of encounters for routine examinations, such as, a general check-up, or, examinations for administrative purposes, such as, a pre-employment physical. The codes are not to be used if the examination is for diagnosis of a suspected condition or for treatment purposes. In such cases the diagnosis code is used. During a routine exam, should a diagnosis or condition be discovered, it should be coded as an additional code. Pre-existing and chronic conditions and history codes may also be included as additional codes as long as the examination is for administrative purposes and not focused on any particular condition.

Some of the codes for routine health examinations distinguish between "with" and "without" abnormal findings. Code assignment depends on the information that is known at the time the encounter is being coded. For example, if no abnormal findings were found during the examination, but the encounter is being coded before test results are back, it is acceptable to assign the code for "without abnormal findings." When assigning a code for "with abnormal findings," additional code(s) should be assigned to identify the specific abnormal finding(s).

Pre-operative examination and pre-procedural laboratory examination Z codes are for use only in those situations when a patient is being cleared for a procedure or surgery and no treatment is given.

The Z codes/categories for routine and administrative examinations:

Z00	Encounter for general examination without complaint, suspected or reported diagnosis
Z01	Encounter for other special examination without complaint, suspected or reported diagnosis
Z02	Encounter for administrative examination Except: Z02.9, Encounter for administrative examinations, unspecified
Z32.0-	Encounter for pregnancy test

14) Miscellaneous Z codes

The miscellaneous Z codes capture a number of other health care encounters that do not fall into one of the other categories. Certain of these codes identify the reason for the encounter; others are for use as additional codes that provide useful information on circumstances that may affect a patient's care and treatment.

Prophylactic Organ Removal

For encounters specifically for prophylactic removal of an organ (such as prophylactic removal of breasts due to a genetic susceptibility to cancer or a family history of cancer), the principal or first-listed code should be a code from category Z40, Encounter for prophylactic surgery, followed by the appropriate codes to identify the associated risk factor (such as genetic susceptibility or family history).

If the patient has a malignancy of one site and is having prophylactic removal at another site to prevent either a new primary malignancy or metastatic disease, a code for the malignancy should also be assigned in addition to a code from subcategory Z40.0, Encounter for prophylactic surgery for risk factors related to malignant neoplasms. A Z40.0 code should not be assigned if the patient is having organ removal for treatment of a malignancy, such as the removal of the testes for the treatment of prostate cancer.

Miscellaneous Z codes/categories:

Z28	Immunization not carried out Except: Z28.3, Underimmunization status
Z29	Encounter for other prophylactic measures
Z40	Encounter for prophylactic surgery
Z41	Encounter for procedures for purposes other than remedying health state Except: Z41.9, Encounter for procedure for purposes other than remedying health state, unspecified
Z53	Persons encountering health services for specific procedures and treatment, not carried out
Z55	Problems related to education and literacy
Z56	Problems related to employment and unemployment
Z57	Occupational exposure to risk factors
Z58	Problems related to physical environment
Z59	Problems related to housing and economic circumstances
Z60	Problems related to social environment
Z62	Problems related to upbringing
Z63	Other problems related to primary support group, including family circumstances
Z64	Problems related to certain psychosocial circumstances
Z65	Problems related to other psychosocial circumstances
Z72	Problems related to lifestyle

Note: These codes should be assigned only when the documentation specifies that the patient has an associated problem.

Z73	Problems related to life management difficulty

NOTE These codes should be assigned only when the documentation specifies that the patient has an associated problem.

Z74	Problems related to care provider dependency Except: Z74.01, Bed confinement status
Z75	Problems related to medical facilities and other health care
Z76.0	Encounter for issue of repeat prescription
Z76.3	Healthy person accompanying sick person
Z76.4	Other boarder to healthcare facility
Z76.5	Malingerer [conscious simulation]
A91.A-	**Caregiver's noncompliance with patient's medical treatment and regimen**
Z91.1-	Patient's noncompliance with medical treatment and regimen
Z91.83	Wandering in diseases classified elsewhere
Z91.84-	Oral health risk factors
Z91.89	Other specified personal risk factors, not elsewhere classified

See Section I.B.14 for Z55-Z65 Persons with potential health hazards related to socioeconomic and psychosocial circumstances, documentation by clinicians other than the patient's provider.

15) Nonspecific Z codes

Certain Z codes are so non-specific, or potentially redundant with other codes in the classification, that there can be little justification for their use in the inpatient setting. Their use in the outpatient setting should be limited to those instances when there is no further documentation to permit more precise coding. Otherwise, any sign or symptom or any other reason for visit that is captured in another code should be used.

Nonspecific Z codes/categories:

Z02.9	Encounter for administrative examinations, unspecified
Z04.9	Encounter for examination and observation for unspecified reason
Z13.9	Encounter for screening, unspecified
Z41.9	Encounter for procedure for purposes other than remedying health state, unspecified
Z52.9	Donor of unspecified organ or tissue
Z86.59	Personal history of other mental and behavioral disorders
Z88.9	Allergy status to unspecified drugs, medicaments and biological substances status
Z92.0	Personal history of contraception

16) Z Codes That May Only be Principal/First-Listed Diagnosis

The following Z codes/categories may only be reported as the principal/first-listed diagnosis, except when there are multiple encounters on the same day and the medical records for the encounters are combined:

Z00	Encounter for general examination without complaint, suspected or reported diagnosis Except: Z00.6
Z01	Encounter for other special examination without complaint, suspected or reported diagnosis
Z02	Encounter for administrative examination
Z03	Encounter for medical observation for suspected diseases and conditions ruled out
Z04	Encounter for examination and observation for other reasons
Z33.2	Encounter for elective termination of pregnancy
Z31.81	Encounter for male factor infertility in female patient
Z31.83	Encounter for assisted reproductive fertility procedure cycle
Z31.84	Encounter for fertility preservation procedure
Z34	Encounter for supervision of normal pregnancy

Z39	Encounter for maternal postpartum care and examination
Z38	Liveborn infants according to place of birth and type of delivery
Z40	Encounter for prophylactic surgery
Z42	Encounter for plastic and reconstructive surgery following medical procedure or healed injury
Z51.0	Encounter for antineoplastic radiation therapy
Z51.1-	Encounter for antineoplastic chemotherapy and immunotherapy
Z52	Donors of organs and tissues Except: Z52.9, Donor of unspecified organ or tissue
Z76.1	Encounter for health supervision and care of foundling
Z76.2	Encounter for health supervision and care of other healthy infant and child
Z99.12	Encounter for respirator [ventilator] dependence during power failure

17) Social Determinants of Health

Social determinants of health (SDOH) codes describing social problems, conditions, or risk factors that influence a patient's health should be assigned when this information is documented in the patient's medical record. Assign as many SDOH codes as are necessary to describe all of the social problems, conditions, or risk factors documented during the current episode of care. For example, a patient who lives alone may suffer an acute injury temporarily impacting their ability to perform routine activities of daily living. When documented as such, this would support assignment of code Z60.2, Problems related to living alone. However, merely living alone, without documentation of a risk or unmet need for assistance at home, would not support assignment of code Z60.2. Documentation by a clinician (or patient-reported information that is signed off by a clinician) that the patient expressed concerns with access and availability of food would support assignment of code Z59.41, Food insecurity. Similarly, medical record documentation indicating the patient is homeless would support assignment of a code from subcategory Z59.0-, Homelessness.

For social determinants of health **classified to chapter 21**, such as information found in categories Z55-Z65, Persons with potential health hazards related to socioeconomic and psychosocial circumstances, code assignment may be based on medical record documentation from clinicians involved in the care of the patient who are not the patient's provider since this information represents social information, rather than medical diagnoses. For example, coding professionals may utilize documentation of social information from social workers, community health workers, case managers, or nurses, if their documentation is included in the official medical record.

Patient self-reported documentation may be used to assign codes for social determinants of health, as long as the patient self-reported information is signed-off by and incorporated into the medical record by either a clinician or provider.

Social determinants of health codes are located primarily in these Z code categories:

Z55	Problems related to education and literacy
Z56	Problems related to employment and unemployment
Z57	Occupational exposure to risk factors
Z58	Problems related to physical environment
Z59	Problems related to housing and economic circumstances
Z60	Problems related to social environment
Z62	Problems related to upbringing
Z63	Other problems related to primary support group, including family circumstances
Z64	Problems related to certain psychosocial circumstances
Z65	Problems related to other psychosocial circumstances

See Section I.B.14. Documentation by Clinicians Other than the Patient's Provider.

Persons encountering health services for examinations (Z00-Z13)

NOTE Nonspecific abnormal findings disclosed at the time of these examinations are classified to categories R70-R94.

Excludes1: examinations related to pregnancy and reproduction (Z30-Z36, Z39.-)

Z00 Encounter for general examination without complaint, suspected or reported diagnosis

> **Excludes1:** encounter for examination for administrative purposes (Z02.-)
> **Excludes2:** encounter for pre-procedural examinations (Z01.81-)
> special screening examinations (Z11-Z13)
> Review coding guidelines C.21.c.13 and C.21.c.16

+ **Z00.0 Encounter for general adult medical examination**
> Encounter for adult periodic examination (annual) (physical) and any associated laboratory and radiologic examinations
>
> **Excludes1:** encounter for examination of sign or symptom-code to sign or symptom
> general health check-up of infant orchild (Z00.12.-)

• **Z00.00 Encounter for general adult medical examination without abnormal findings**
> Encounter for adult health check-up NOS
> AHA CC: 1Q, 2016, 36-37; 4Q, 2017, 95-96

• **Z00.01 Encounter for general adult medical examination with abnormal findings**
> Use additional code to identify abnormal findings
> AHA CC: 1Q, 2016, 35-36

+ **Z00.1 Encounter for newborn, infant and child health examinations**
> Review coding guideline C.21.c.12

+ **Z00.11 Newborn health examination**
> Health check for child under 29 days old
> Use additional code to identify any abnormal findings
> **Excludes1:** health check for child over 28 days old (Z00.12.-)

• **Z00.110 Health examination for newborn under 8 days old**
> Health check for newborn under 8 days old

• **Z00.111 Health examination for newborn 8 to 28 days old**
> Health check for newborn 8 to 28 days old
> Newborn weight check

+ **Z00.12 Encounter for routine child health examination**
> Health check (routine) for child over 28 days old
> Immunizations appropriate for age
> Routine developmental screening of infant or child
> Routine vision and hearing testing
> **Excludes1:** health check for child under 29 days old (Z00.11-)
> health supervision of foundling or other healthy infant or child (Z76.1-Z76.2)
> newborn health examination (Z00.11-)

• **Z00.121 Encounter for routine child health examination with abnormal findings**
> Use additional code to identify abnormal findings
> AHA CC: 1Q, 2016, 34-35; 4Q, 2017, 95-96

• **Z00.129 Encounter for routine child health examination without abnormal findings**
> Encounter for routine child health examination NOS
> AHA CC: 1Q, 2016, 34-35

• **Z00.2 Encounter for examination for period of rapid growth in childhood**

• **Z00.3 Encounter for examination for adolescent development state**
> Encounter for puberty development state

Z00.5 Encounter for examination of potential donor of organ and tissue

Z00.6 Encounter for examination for normal comparison and control in clinical research program
> Examination of participant or control in clinical research program

+ **Z00.7 Encounter for examination for period of delayed growth in childhood**

• **Z00.70 Encounter for examination for period of delayed growth in childhood without abnormal findings**

• **Z00.71 Encounter for examination for period of delayed growth in childhood with abnormal findings**
> Use additional code to identify abnormal findings

Z00.8 Encounter for other general examination
> Encounter for health examination in population surveys

Z01 Encounter for other special examination without complaint, suspected or reported diagnosis

> **Includes:** routine examination of specific system
> **NOTE** Codes from category Z01 represent the reason for the encounter. A separate procedure code is required to identify any examinations or procedures performed
> **Excludes1:** encounter for examination for administrative purposes (Z02.-)
> encounter for examination for suspected conditions, proven not to exist (Z03.-)
> encounter for laboratory and radiologic examinations as a component of general medical examinations (Z00.0-)
> encounter for laboratory, radiologic and imaging examinations for sign(s) and symptom(s) - code to the sign(s) or symptom(s)
> **Excludes2:** screening examinations (Z11-Z13)
> Review coding guidelines C.21.c.13 and C.21.c.16

+ **Z01.0 Encounter for examination of eyes and vision**

Excludes1: examination for driving license (Z02.4)

Z01.00 Encounter for examination of eyes and vision without abnormal findings
　Encounter for examination of eyes and vision NOS

Z01.01 Encounter for examination of eyes and vision with abnormal findings
　Use additional code to identify abnormal findings
　AHA CC: 4Q, 2016, 21

+ Z01.02 Encounter for examination of eyes and vision following failed vision screening
　Excludes1: encounter for examination of eyes and vision with abnormal findings (Z01.01)
　　encounter for examination of eyes and vision without abnormal findings (Z01.00)
　AHA CC: 4Q, 2019, 20

　Z01.020 Examination for examination of eyes and vision following failed vision screening without abnormal findings

　Z01.021 Examination for examination of eyes and vision following failed vision screening with abnormal findings
　　Use additional code to identify abnormal findings

+ Z01.1 Encounter for examination of ears and hearing

　Z01.10 Encounter for examination of ears and hearing without abnormal findings
　　Encounter for examination of ears and hearing NOS
　　AHA CC: 4Q, 2016, 21

+ Z01.11 Encounter for examination of ears and hearing with abnormal findings

　Z01.110 Encounter for hearing examination following failed hearing screening
　　AHA CC: 3Q, 2016, 18-19

　Z01.118 Encounter for examination of ears and hearing with other abnormal findings
　　Use additional code to identify abnormal findings
　　AHA CC: 3Q, 2016, 17

　Z01.12 Encounter for hearing conservation and treatment

+ Z01.2 Encounter for dental examination and cleaning

　Z01.20 Encounter for dental examination and cleaning without abnormal findings
　　Encounter for dental examination and cleaning NOS

　Z01.21 Encounter for dental examination and cleaning with abnormal findings
　　Use additional code to identify abnormal findings

+ Z01.3 Encounter for examination of blood pressure

　Z01.30 Encounter for examination of blood pressure without abnormal findings
　　Encounter for examination of blood pressure NOS

　Z01.31 Encounter for examination of blood pressure with abnormal findings
　　Use additional code to identify abnormal findings

+ Z01.4 Encounter for gynecological examination
　Excludes2: pregnancy examination or test (Z32.0-)
　　routine examination for contraceptive maintenance (Z30.4-)

+ Z01.41 Encounter for routine gynecological examination
　　Encounter for general gynecological examination with or without cervical smear
　　Encounter for gynecological examination (general) (routine) NOS
　　Encounter for pelvic examination (annual) (periodic)
　　Use additional code:
　　　for screening for human papillomavirus, if applicable, (Z11.51)
　　　for screening vaginal pap smear, if applicable (Z12.72)
　　　to identify acquired absence of uterus, if applicable (Z90.71-)
　　Excludes1: gynecologic examination status-post hysterectomy for malignant condition (Z08)
　　　screening cervical pap smear not a part of a routine gynecological examination (Z12.4)

　♀ **Z01.411** Encounter for gynecological examination (general) (routine) with abnormal findings

　　Use additional code to identify abnormal findings

　♀ **Z01.419** Encounter for gynecological examination (general) (routine) without abnormal findings

　♀ **Z01.42** Encounter for cervical smear to confirm findings of recent normal smear following initial abnormal smear

+ Z01.8 Encounter for other specified special examinations

+ Z01.81 Encounter for preprocedural examinations
　　Encounter for preoperative examinations
　　Encounter for radiological and imaging examinations as part of preprocedural examination

　Z01.810 Encounter for preprocedural cardiovascular examination

　Z01.811 Encounter for preprocedural respiratory examination

　Z01.812 Encounter for preprocedural laboratory examination
　　Blood and urine tests prior to treatment or procedure
　　AHA CC: 3Q, 2020, 14-15; 1Q, 2021, 37-38; 2Q, 2023, 3-4

　Z01.818 Encounter for other preprocedural examination
　　Encounter for preprocedural examination NOS
　　Encounter for examinations prior to antineoplastic chemotherapy

Z01.82 Encounter for allergy testing
　Excludes1: encounter for antibody response examination (Z01.84)

Z01.83 Encounter for blood typing
　　Encounter for Rh typing

Z01.84 Encounter for antibody response examination
　　Encounter for immunity status testing
　Excludes1: encounter for allergy testing (Z01.82)
　AHA CC: 2Q, 2020, 11
　Review coding guideline C.1.g.1.k

Z01.89 Encounter for other specified special examinations

Z02 Encounter for administrative examination
　Review coding guidelines C.21.c.13 and C.21.c.16

Z02.0 Encounter for examination for admission to educational institution
　　Encounter for examination for admission to preschool (education)
　　Encounter for examination for re-admission to school following illness or medical treatment

Z02.1 Encounter for pre-employment examination

Z02.2 Encounter for examination for admission to residential institution
　Excludes1: examination for admission to prison (Z02.89)

Z02.3 Encounter for examination for recruitment to armed forces

Z02.4 Encounter for examination for driving license

Z02.5 Encounter for examination for participation in sport
　Excludes1: blood-alcohol and blood-drug test (Z02.83)

Z02.6 Encounter for examination for insurance purposes

+ Z02.7 Encounter for issue of medical certificate
　Excludes1: encounter for general medical examination (Z00-Z01, Z02.0-Z02.6, Z02.8-Z02.9)

Z02.71 Encounter for disability determination
　　Encounter for issue of medical certificate of incapacity
　　Encounter for issue of medical certificate of invalidity

Z02.79 Encounter for issue of other medical certificate

+ Z02.8 Encounter for other administrative examinations

Z02.81 Encounter for paternity testing

Z02.82 Encounter for adoption services

Z02.83 Encounter for blood-alcohol and blood-drug test
　　Use additional code for findings of alcohol or drugs in blood (R78.-)

Z02.84 Encounter for child welfare exam
　　Encounter for child welfare screening exam
　Excludes2: encounter for examination and observation for alleged child physical abuse (Z04.72)
　　encounter for examination and observation for alleged child rape (Z04.42)

Z02.89 Encounter for other administrative examinations
　　Encounter for examination for admission to prison
　　Encounter for examination for admission to summer camp

Encounter for immigration examination
Encounter for naturalization examination
Encounter for premarital examination
> **Excludes1:** *health supervision of foundling or other healthy infant or child (Z76.1-Z76.2)*

Z02.9 Encounter for administrative examinations, unspecified

Z03 Encounter for medical observation for suspected diseases and conditions ruled out

This category is to be used when a person without a diagnosis is suspected of having an abnormal condition, without signs or symptoms, which requires study, but after examination and observation, is ruled out. This category is also for use for administrative and legal observation status.

> **Excludes1:** *contact with and (suspected) exposures hazardous to health (Z77.-)*
> *encounter for observation and evaluation of newborn for suspected diseases and conditions, ruled out (Z05.-)*
> *person with feared complaint in whom no diagnosis is made (Z71.1)*
> *signs or symptoms under study- code to signs or symptoms*

AHA CC: 4Q, 2017, 27
Review coding guidelines C.21.c.6 and C.21.c.16

Z03.6 Encounter for observation for suspected toxic effect from ingested substance ruled out
Encounter for observation for suspected adverse effect from drug
Encounter for observation for suspected poisoning

+ Z03.7 Encounter for suspected maternal and fetal conditions ruled out
Encounter for suspected maternal and fetal conditions not found
> **Excludes1:** *known or suspected fetal anomalies affecting management of mother, not ruled out (O26.-, O35.-, O36.-, O40.-, O41.-)*

- ♀ **Z03.71** Encounter for suspected problem with amniotic cavity and membrane ruled out
Encounter for suspected oligohydramnios ruled out
Encounter for suspected polyhydramnios ruled out
- ♀ **Z03.72** Encounter for suspected placental problem ruled out
- ♀ **Z03.73** Encounter for suspected fetal anomaly ruled out
AHA CC: 4Q, 2016, 4-7
- ♀ **Z03.74** Encounter for suspected problem with fetal growth ruled out
- ♀ **Z03.75** Encounter for suspected cervical shortening ruled out
- ♀ **Z03.79** Encounter for other suspected maternal and fetal conditions ruled out
AHA CC: 4Q, 2016, 4-7

+ Z03.8 Encounter for observation for other suspected diseases and conditions ruled out
Z03.81 Encounter for observation for suspected exposure to biological agents ruled out
Z03.810 Encounter for observation for suspected exposure to anthrax ruled out
Z03.818 Encounter for observation for suspected exposure to other biological agents ruled out
AHA CC: 1Q, 2020, 34-36; 2Q, 2020, 8-9

+ Z03.82 Encounter for observation for suspected foreign body ruled out
> **Excludes1:** *retained foreign body (Z18.-)*
> *retained foreign body in eyelid (H02.81)*
> *residual foreign body in soft tissue (M79.5)*
> **Excludes2:** *confirmed foreign body ingestion or aspiration including*
> *foreign body in alimentary tract (T18)*
> *foreign body in ear (T16)*
> *foreign body on external eye (T15)*
> *foreign body in respiratory tract (T17)*

AHA CC: 4Q, 2020, 42
Z03.821 Encounter for observation for suspected ingested foreign body ruled out
Z03.822 Encounter for observation for suspected aspirated (inhaled) foreign body ruled out
Z03.823 Encounter for observation for suspected inserted (injected) foreign body ruled out
Encounter for observation for suspected inserted (injected) foreign body in eye ruled out
Encounter for observation for suspected inserted (injected) foreign body in orifice ruled out
Encounter for observation for suspected inserted (injected) foreign body in skin ruled out

Z03.83 Encounter for observation for suspected conditions related to home physiologic monitoring device ruled out
Encounter for observation for apnea alarm without findings
Encounter for observation for bradycardia alarm without findings
Encounter for observation for malfunction of home cardiorespiratory monitor
Encounter for observation for non-specific findings home physiologic monitoring device
Encounter for observation for pulse oximeter alarm without findings
> **Excludes1:** *apnea NOS (R06.81)*
> *neonatal bradycardia (P29.12)*
> *newborn apnea (P28.4-)*
> *primary sleep apnea of newborn (P28.3-)*
> *sleep apnea (G47.3-)*

AHA CC: 4Q, 2022, 51

Z03.89 Encounter for observation for other suspected diseases and conditions ruled out

Z04 Encounter for examination and observation for other reasons
Includes: encounter for examination for medicolegal reasons

This category is to be used when a person without a diagnosis is suspected of having an abnormal condition, without signs or symptoms, which requires study, but after examination and observation, is ruled-out. This category is also for use for administrative and legal observation status.

Review coding guidelines C.21.c.6 and C.21.c.16

Z04.1 Encounter for examination and observation following transport accident
> **Excludes1:** *encounter for examination and observation following work accident (Z04.2)*

AHA CC: 2Q, 2018, 8; 2Q, 2019, 11

Z04.2 Encounter for examination and observation following work accident

Z04.3 Encounter for examination and observation following other accident
AHA CC: 2Q, 2018, 7-8

+ Z04.4 Encounter for examination and observation following alleged rape
Encounter for examination and observation of victim following alleged rape
Encounter for examination and observation of victim following alleged sexual abuse

- **Z04.41** Encounter for examination and observation following alleged adult rape
Suspected adult rape, ruled out
Suspected adult sexual abuse, ruled out
Review coding guideline C.19.f

- **Z04.42** Encounter for examination and observation following alleged child rape
Suspected child rape, ruled out
Suspected child sexual abuse, ruled out
Review coding guideline C.19.f

Z04.6 Encounter for general psychiatric examination, requested by authority

+ Z04.7 Encounter for examination and observation following alleged physical abuse
- **Z04.71** Encounter for examination and observation following alleged adult physical abuse
Suspected adult physical abuse, ruled out
> **Excludes1:** *confirmed case of adult physical abuse (T74.-)*
> *encounter for examination and observation following alleged adult sexual abuse (Z04.41)*
> *suspected case of adult physical abuse, not ruled out (T76.-)*

Review coding guideline C.19.f

- **Z04.72** Encounter for examination and observation following alleged child physical abuse
Suspected child physical abuse, ruled out
> **Excludes1:** *confirmed case of child physical abuse (T74.-)*
> *encounter for examination and observation following alleged child sexual abuse (Z04.42)*

suspected case of child physical abuse, not ruled out (T76.-)
Review coding guideline C.19.f

+ Z04.8 Encounter for examination and observation for other specified reasons
Encounter for examination and observation for request for expert evidence
Review coding guideline C.19.f

Z04.81 Encounter for examination and observation of victim following forced sexual exploitation
AHA CC: 4Q, 2018, 32-33, 35

Z04.82 Encounter for examination and observation of victim following forced labor exploitation
AHA CC: 4Q, 2018, 32-33, 35

Z04.89 Encounter for examination and observation for other specified reasons
AHA CC: 4Q, 2018, 35

Z04.9 Encounter for examination and observation for unspecified reason
Encounter for observation NOS

Z05 Encounter for observation and evaluation of newborn for suspected diseases and conditions ruled out

NOTE This category is to be used for newborns, within the neonatal period (the first 28 days of life), who are suspected of having an abnormal condition, but without signs or symptoms, and which, after examination and observation, is ruled out.
Review coding guideline C.16.b
Review coding guideline C.21.c.6
AHA CC: 4Q, 2016, 77; 4Q, 2017, 27

- **Z05.0 Observation and evaluation of newborn for suspected cardiac condition ruled out**
- **Z05.1 Observation and evaluation of newborn for suspected infectious condition ruled out**
AHA CC: 2Q, 2019, 10-11
- **Z05.2 Observation and evaluation of newborn for suspected neurological condition ruled out**
- **Z05.3 Observation and evaluation of newborn for suspected respiratory condition ruled out**
+ Z05.4 Observation and evaluation of newborn for suspected genetic, metabolic or immunologic condition ruled out
  - **Z05.41 Observation and evaluation of newborn for suspected genetic condition ruled out**
  AHA CC: 4Q, 2016, 54-55
  - **Z05.42 Observation and evaluation of newborn for suspected metabolic condition ruled out**
  - **Z05.43 Observation and evaluation of newborn for suspected immunologic condition ruled out**
- **Z05.5 Observation and evaluation of newborn for suspected gastrointestinal condition ruled out**
- **Z05.6 Observation and evaluation of newborn for suspected genitourinary condition ruled out**
+ Z05.7 Observation and evaluation of newborn for suspected skin, subcutaneous, musculoskeletal and connective tissue condition ruled out
  - **Z05.71 Observation and evaluation of newborn for suspected skin and subcutaneous tissue condition ruled out**
  - **Z05.72 Observation and evaluation of newborn for suspected musculoskeletal condition ruled out**
  - **Z05.73 Observation and evaluation of newborn for suspected connective tissue condition ruled out**
+ Z05.8 Observation and evaluation of newborn for other specified suspected condition ruled out
  AHA CC: 1Q, 2022, 17
  - **Z05.81 Observation and evaluation of newborn for suspected condition related to home physiologic monitoring device ruled out**
    Encounter for observation of newborn for apnea alarm without findings
    Encounter for observation of newborn for bradycardia alarm without findings
    Encounter for observation of newborn for malfunction of home cardiorespiratory monitor
    Encounter for observation of newborn for non-specific findings home physiologic monitoring device
    Encounter for observation of newborn for pulse oximeter alarm without findings
    Excludes1: *encounter for observation for suspected conditions related to home physiologic monitoring device ruled out (Z03.83)*
    neonatal bradycardia (P29.12)
    other newborn apnea (P28.4-)
    primary sleep apnea of newborn (P28.3-)
  - **Z05.89 Observation and evaluation of newborn for other specified suspected condition ruled out**
- **Z05.9 Observation and evaluation of newborn for unspecified suspected condition ruled out**

Z08 Encounter for follow-up examination after completed treatment for malignant neoplasm
Medical surveillance following completed treatment
Use additional code to identify any acquired absence of organs (Z90.-)
Use additional code to identify the personal history of malignant neoplasm (Z85.-)
Excludes1: *aftercare following medical care (Z43-Z49, Z51)*
AHA CC: 3Q, 2020, 30
Review coding guideline C.21.c.8
Valid 3-character code, no further characters required

Z09 Encounter for follow-up examination after completed treatment for conditions other than malignant neoplasm
Medical surveillance following completed treatment
Use additional code to identify any applicable history of disease code (Z86.-, Z87.-)
Excludes1: *aftercare following medical care (Z43-Z49, Z51)*
surveillance of contraception (Z30.4-)
surveillance of prosthetic and other medical devices (Z44-Z46)
Review coding guideline C.1.g.1.j
Review coding guideline C.21.c.8
AHA CC: 1Q, 2017, 9; 2Q, 2020, 10-11; 1Q, 2021, 33-34; 3Q, 2022, 4
Valid 3-character code, no further characters required

Z11 Encounter for screening for infectious and parasitic diseases
Screening is the testing for disease or disease precursors in asymptomatic individuals so that early detection and treatment can be provided for those who test positive for the disease.
Excludes1: *encounter for diagnostic examination-code to sign or symptom*
Review coding guideline C.21.c.5

Z11.0 Encounter for screening for intestinal infectious diseases
Z11.1 Encounter for screening for respiratory tuberculosis
Encounter for screening for active tuberculosis disease
Z11.2 Encounter for screening for other bacterial diseases
Z11.3 Encounter for screening for infections with a predominantly sexual mode of transmission
Excludes2: *encounter for screening for human immunodeficiency virus [HIV] (Z11.4)*
encounter for screening for human papillomavirus (Z11.51)
Z11.4 Encounter for screening for human immunodeficiency virus [HIV]
Review coding guideline C.1.a.2.h
+ Z11.5 Encounter for screening for other viral diseases
Excludes2: *encounter for screening for viral intestinal disease (Z11.0)*
  Z11.51 Encounter for screening for human papillomavirus (HPV)
  Z11.52 Encounter for screening for COVID-19
  AHA CC: 1Q, 2021, 41-42; 2Q, 2023, 3-4
  Z11.59 Encounter for screening for other viral diseases
Z11.6 Encounter for screening for other protozoal diseases and helminthiases
Excludes2: *encounter for screening for protozoal intestinal disease (Z11.0)*
Z11.7 Encounter for testing for latent tuberculosis infection
AHA CC: 4Q, 2019, 20
Z11.8 Encounter for screening for other infectious and parasitic diseases
Encounter for screening for chlamydia
Encounter for screening for rickettsial
Encounter for screening for spirochetal
Encounter for screening for mycoses
Z11.9 Encounter for screening for infectious and parasitic diseases, unspecified

Z12 Encounter for screening for malignant neoplasms
Screening is the testing for disease or disease precursors in asymptomatic individuals so that early detection and treatment can be provided for those who test positive for the disease.
Use additional code to identify any family history of malignant neoplasm (Z80.-)

Excludes1: *encounter for diagnostic examination-code to sign or symptom*
Review coding guideline C.21.c.5

- **Z12.0** Encounter for screening for malignant neoplasm of stomach
- **+ Z12.1** Encounter for screening for malignant neoplasm of intestinal tract
  - **Z12.10** Encounter for screening for malignant neoplasm of intestinal tract, unspecified
  - **Z12.11** Encounter for screening for malignant neoplasm of colon
    Encounter for screening colonoscopy NOS
    AHA CC: 1Q, 2017, 8-9; 1Q, 2018, 6-7
  - **Z12.12** Encounter for screening for malignant neoplasm of rectum
  - **Z12.13** Encounter for screening for malignant neoplasm of small intestine
- **Z12.2** Encounter for screening for malignant neoplasm of respiratory organs
- **+ Z12.3** Encounter for screening for malignant neoplasm of breast
  - **Z12.31** Encounter for screening mammogram for malignant neoplasm of breast
    Excludes1: *inconclusive mammogram (R92.2)*
    AHA CC: 1Q, 2015, 24
  - **Z12.39** Encounter for other screening for malignant neoplasm of breast
- ♀ **Z12.4** Encounter for screening for malignant neoplasm of cervix
  Encounter for screening pap smear for malignant neoplasm of cervix
  Excludes1: *when screening is part of general gynecological examination (Z01.4-)*
  Excludes2: *encounter for screening for human papillomavirus (Z11.51)*
- ♂ **Z12.5** Encounter for screening for malignant neoplasm of prostate
- **Z12.6** Encounter for screening for malignant neoplasm of bladder
- **+ Z12.7** Encounter for screening for malignant neoplasm of other genitourinary organs
  - ♂ **Z12.71** Encounter for screening for malignant neoplasm of testis
  - ♀ **Z12.72** Encounter for screening for malignant neoplasm of vagina
    Vaginal pap smear status-post hysterectomy for non-malignant condition
    Use additional code to identify acquired absence of uterus (Z90.71-)
    Excludes1: *vaginal pap smear status-post hysterectomy for malignant conditions (Z08)*
  - ♀ **Z12.73** Encounter for screening for malignant neoplasm of ovary
  - **Z12.79** Encounter for screening for malignant neoplasm of other genitourinary organs
- **+ Z12.8** Encounter for screening for malignant neoplasm of other sites
  - **Z12.81** Encounter for screening for malignant neoplasm of oral cavity
  - **Z12.82** Encounter for screening for malignant neoplasm of nervous system
  - **Z12.83** Encounter for screening for malignant neoplasm of skin
  - **Z12.89** Encounter for screening for malignant neoplasm of other sites
    AHA CC: 1Q, 2021, 14-15
- **Z12.9** Encounter for screening for malignant neoplasm, site unspecified

Z13 Encounter for screening for other diseases and disorders

Screening is the testing for disease or disease precursors in asymptomatic individuals so that early detection and treatment can be provided for those who test positive for the disease.
Excludes1: *encounter for diagnostic examination-code to sign or symptom*
Review coding guideline C.21.c.5

- **Z13.0** Encounter for screening for diseases of the blood and blood-forming organs and certain disorders involving the immune mechanism
- **Z13.1** Encounter for screening for diabetes mellitus
- **+ Z13.2** Encounter for screening for nutritional, metabolic and other endocrine disorders
  - **Z13.21** Encounter for screening for nutritional disorder
  - **+ Z13.22** Encounter for screening for metabolic disorder
    - **Z13.220** Encounter for screening for lipoid disorders
      Encounter for screening for cholesterol level
      Encounter for screening for hypercholesterolemia
      Encounter for screening for hyperlipidemia
    - **Z13.228** Encounter for screening for other metabolic disorders
  - **Z13.29** Encounter for screening for other suspected endocrine disorder
    Excludes2: *encounter for screening for diabetes mellitus (Z13.1)*
- **+ Z13.3** Encounter for screening examination for mental health and behavioral disorders
  AHA CC: 4Q, 2018, 35-36
  - **Z13.30** Encounter for screening examination for mental health and behavioral disorders, unspecified
  - **Z13.31** Encounter for screening for depression
    Encounter for screening for depression, adult
    Encounter for screening for depression for child or adolescent
  - ♀ **Z13.32** Encounter for screening for maternal depression
    Encounter for screening for perinatal depression
  - **Z13.39** Encounter for screening examination for other mental health and behavioral disorders
    Encounter for screening for alcoholism
    Encounter for screening for intellectual disabilities
- **+ Z13.4** Encounter for screening for certain developmental disorders in childhood
  Encounter for development testing of infant or child
  Encounter for screening for developmental handicaps in early childhood
  Excludes2: *encounter for routine child health examination (Z00.12-)*
  AHA CC: 4Q, 2018, 36
  - **Z13.40** Encounter for screening for unspecified developmental delays
  - **Z13.41** Encounter for autism screening
  - **Z13.42** Encounter for screening for global developmental delays (milestones)
    Encounter for screening for developmental handicaps in early childhood
  - **Z13.49** Encounter for screening for other developmental delays
- **Z13.5** Encounter for screening for eye and ear disorders
  Excludes2: *encounter for general hearing examination (Z01.1-)*
  encounter for general vision examination (Z01.0-)
  AHA CC: 3Q, 2016, 17
- **Z13.6** Encounter for screening for cardiovascular disorders
- **+ Z13.7** Encounter for screening for genetic and chromosomal anomalies
  Excludes1: *genetic testing for procreative management (Z31.4-)*
  - **Z13.71** Encounter for nonprocreative screening for genetic disease carrier status
  - **Z13.79** Encounter for other screening for genetic and chromosomal anomalies
- **+ Z13.8** Encounter for screening for other specified diseases and disorders
  Excludes2: *screening for malignant neoplasms (Z12.-)*
  - **+ Z13.81** Encounter for screening for digestive system disorders
    - **Z13.810** Encounter for screening for upper gastrointestinal disorder
    - **Z13.811** Encounter for screening for lower gastrointestinal disorder
      Excludes1: *encounter for screening for intestinal infectious disease (Z11.0)*
    - **Z13.818** Encounter for screening for other digestive system disorders
  - **+ Z13.82** Encounter for screening for musculoskeletal disorder
    - **Z13.820** Encounter for screening for osteoporosis
    - **Z13.828** Encounter for screening for other musculoskeletal disorder

	Z13.83	Encounter for screening for respiratory disorder NEC
		Excludes1: *encounter for screening for respiratory tuberculosis (Z11.1)*
	Z13.84	Encounter for screening for dental disorders
+	Z13.85	Encounter for screening for nervous system disorders
	Z13.850	Encounter for screening for traumatic brain injury
	Z13.858	Encounter for screening for other nervous system disorders
	Z13.88	Encounter for screening for disorder due to exposure to contaminants
		Excludes1: *those exposed to contaminants without suspected disorders (Z57.-, Z77.-)*
	Z13.89	Encounter for screening for other disorder
		Encounter for screening for genitourinary disorders
	Z13.9	Encounter for screening, unspecified

Genetic carrier and genetic susceptibility to disease (Z14-Z15)

Z14 Genetic carrier
Review coding guideline C.21.c.3
+ **Z14.0 Hemophilia A carrier**
  - **Z14.01** Asymptomatic hemophilia A carrier
  - **Z14.02** Symptomatic hemophilia A carrier
- **Z14.1** Cystic fibrosis carrier
- **Z14.8** Genetic carrier of other disease

Z15 Genetic susceptibility to disease
  Includes: confirmed abnormal gene
  Use additional code, if applicable, for any associated family history of the disease (Z80-Z84)
  Excludes1: *chromosomal anomalies (Q90-Q99)*
  Review coding guideline C.21.c.3
+ **Z15.0 Genetic susceptibility to malignant neoplasm**
  Code first, if applicable, any current malignant neoplasm (C00-C75, C81-C96)
  Use additional code, if applicable, for any personal history of malignant neoplasm (Z85.-)
  - **Z15.01** Genetic susceptibility to malignant neoplasm of breast
  - ♀ **Z15.02** Genetic susceptibility to malignant neoplasm of ovary
  - ♂ **Z15.03** Genetic susceptibility to malignant neoplasm of prostate
  - ♀ **Z15.04** Genetic susceptibility to malignant neoplasm of endometrium
  - **Z15.09** Genetic susceptibility to other malignant neoplasm
    AHA CC: 1Q, 2021, 14-15
+ **Z15.8 Genetic susceptibility to other disease**
  - **Z15.81** Genetic susceptibility to multiple endocrine neoplasia [MEN]
    Excludes1: *multiple endocrine neoplasia [MEN] syndromes (E31.2-)*
  - **Z15.89** Genetic susceptibility to other disease

Resistance to antimicrobial drugs (Z16)

Z16 Resistance to antimicrobial drugs
  NOTE The codes in this category are provided for use as additional codes to identify the resistance and non-responsiveness of a condition to antimicrobial drugs.
  Code first the infection
  Excludes1: *Methicillin resistant Staphylococcus aureus infection (A49.02)*
  Methicillin resistant Staphylococcus aureus pneumonia (J15.212)
  Sepsis due to Methicillin resistant Staphylococcus aureus (A41.02)
  Review coding guideline C.1.c
  Review coding guideline C.21.c.3
+ **Z16.1 Resistance to beta lactam antibiotics**
  - CC **Z16.10** Resistance to unspecified beta lactam antibiotics
  - CC **Z16.11** Resistance to penicillins
    Resistance to amoxicillin
    Resistance to ampicillin
    Review coding guidelines C.1.e.1.a and C.1.e.1.b
  - CC **Z16.12** Extended spectrum beta lactamase (ESBL) resistance
  - CC **Z16.13** Resistance to carbapenem
    Excludes2: *Methicillin resistant Staphylococcus aureus infection in diseases classified elsewhere (B95.62)*
  - CC **Z16.19** Resistance to other specified beta lactam antibiotics
    Resistance to cephalosporins
+ **Z16.2 Resistance to other antibiotics**
  - CC **Z16.20** Resistance to unspecified antibiotic
    Resistance to antibiotics NOS
  - CC **Z16.21** Resistance to vancomycin
  - CC **Z16.22** Resistance to vancomycin related antibiotics
  - CC **Z16.23** Resistance to quinolones and fluoroquinolones
  - CC **Z16.24** Resistance to multiple antibiotics
  - CC **Z16.29** Resistance to other single specified antibiotic
    Resistance to aminoglycosides
    Resistance to macrolides
    Resistance to sulfonamides
    Resistance to tetracyclines
+ **Z16.3 Resistance to other antimicrobial drugs**
  Excludes1: *resistance to antibiotics (Z16.1-, Z16.2-)*
  - CC **Z16.30** Resistance to unspecified antimicrobial drugs
    Drug resistance NOS
  - CC **Z16.31** Resistance to antiparasitic drug(s)
    Resistance to quinine and related compounds
  - CC **Z16.32** Resistance to antifungal drug(s)
  - CC **Z16.33** Resistance to antiviral drug(s)
  + **Z16.34** Resistance to antimycobacterial drug(s)
    Resistance to tuberculostatics
    - CC **Z16.341** Resistance to single antimycobacterial drug
      Resistance to antimycobacterial drug NOS
    - CC **Z16.342** Resistance to multiple antimycobacterial drugs
  - CC **Z16.35** Resistance to multiple antimicrobial drugs
    Excludes1: *Resistance to multiple antibiotics only (Z16.24)*
  - CC **Z16.39** Resistance to other specified antimicrobial drug

Estrogen receptor status (Z17)

Z17 Estrogen receptor status
  Code first malignant neoplasm of breast (C50.-)
  Review coding guideline C.21.c.3
  - **Z17.0** Estrogen receptor positive status [ER+]
    AHA CC: 3Q, 2022, 14-15
  - **Z17.1** Estrogen receptor negative status [ER-]

Retained foreign body fragments (Z18)

Z18 Retained foreign body fragments
  Includes: embedded fragment (status)
  embedded splinter (status)
  retained foreign body status
  Excludes1: *artificial joint prosthesis status (Z96.6-)*
  foreign body accidentally left during a procedure (T81.5-)
  foreign body entering through orifice (T15-T19)
  in situ cardiac device (Z95.-)
  organ or tissue replaced by means other than transplant (Z96.-, Z97.-)
  organ or tissue replaced by transplant (Z94.-)
  personal history of retained foreign body fully removed (Z87.821)
  superficial foreign body (non-embedded splinter) - code to superficial foreign body, by site
  Review coding guideline C.21.c.3
+ **Z18.0 Retained radioactive fragments**
  - **Z18.01** Retained depleted uranium fragments
  - **Z18.09** Other retained radioactive fragments
    Other retained depleted isotope fragments
    Retained nontherapeutic radioactive fragments
+ **Z18.1 Retained metal fragments**
  Excludes1: *retained radioactive metal fragments (Z18.01-Z18.09)*
  - **Z18.10** Retained metal fragments, unspecified
    Retained metal fragment NOS
  - **Z18.11** Retained magnetic metal fragments
  - **Z18.12** Retained nonmagnetic metal fragments
- **Z18.2** Retained plastic fragments
  Acrylics fragments
  Diethylhexyl phthalates fragments
  Isocyanate fragments

+ **Z18.3** Retained organic fragments
    Z18.31 Retained animal quills or spines
    Z18.32 Retained tooth
    Z18.33 Retained wood fragments
    Z18.39 Other retained organic fragments
+ **Z18.8** Other specified retained foreign body
    Z18.81 Retained glass fragments
    Z18.83 Retained stone or crystalline fragments
        Retained concrete or cement fragments
    Z18.89 Other specified retained foreign body fragments
        AHA CC: 3Q, 2016, 24; 2Q, 2023, 27-28
  Z18.9 Retained foreign body fragments, unspecified material

Hormone sensitivity malignancy status (Z19)

Z19 Hormone sensitivity malignancy status
    Code first malignant neoplasm - see Table of Neoplasms, by site, malignant
    Review coding guideline C.21.c.3
    AHA CC: 4Q, 2016, 76
  Z19.1 Hormone sensitive malignancy status
  Z19.2 Hormone resistant malignancy status
    Castrate resistant prostate malignancy status

Persons with potential health hazards related to communicable diseases (Z20-Z29)

Z20 Contact with and (suspected) exposure to communicable diseases
    Excludes1: carrier of infectious disease (Z22.-)
        diagnosed current infectious or parasitic disease -see Alphabetic Index
    Excludes2: personal history of infectious and parasitic diseases (Z86.1-)
    Review coding guideline C.21.c.1
+ **Z20.0** Contact with and (suspected) exposure to intestinal infectious diseases
    Z20.01 Contact with and (suspected) exposure to intestinal infectious diseases due to Escherichia coli (E. coli)
    Z20.09 Contact with and (suspected) exposure to other intestinal infectious diseases
  Z20.1 Contact with and (suspected) exposure to tuberculosis
  Z20.2 Contact with and (suspected) exposure to infections with a predominantly sexual mode of transmission
  Z20.3 Contact with and (suspected) exposure to rabies
  Z20.4 Contact with and (suspected) exposure to rubella
  Z20.5 Contact with and (suspected) exposure to viral hepatitis
  Z20.6 Contact with and (suspected) exposure to human immunodeficiency virus [HIV]
    Excludes1: asymptomatic human immunodeficiency virus [HIV]
        HIV infection status (Z21)
  Z20.7 Contact with and (suspected) exposure to pediculosis, acariasis and other infestations
+ **Z20.8** Contact with and (suspected) exposure to other communicable diseases
    + **Z20.81** Contact with and (suspected) exposure to other bacterial communicable diseases
        Z20.810 Contact with and (suspected) exposure to anthrax
        Z20.811 Contact with and (suspected) exposure to meningococcus
        Z20.818 Contact with and (suspected) exposure to other bacterial communicable diseases
        AHA CC: 2Q, 2019, 10-11
    + **Z20.82** Contact with and (suspected) exposure to other viral communicable diseases
        AHA CC: 4Q, 2018, 35
        Z20.820 Contact with and (suspected) exposure to varicella
        Z20.821 Contact with and (suspected) exposure to Zika virus
        Review coding guideline C.1.f
        Z20.822 Contact with and (suspected) exposure to COVID-19
            Contact with and (suspected) exposure to SARS-CoV-2
        AHA CC: 1Q, 2021, 37-39, 41-42; 4Q, 2021, 109-110; 2Q, 2022, 28-29; 2Q, 2023, 3-4

    Z20.828 Contact with and (suspected) exposure to other viral communicable diseases
    AHA CC: 4Q, 2016, 4-7; 1Q, 2020, 34-36; 2Q, 2020, 4-5, 8-9; 3Q, 2020, 14-16; 1Q, 2021, 37-39; 3Q, 2022, 4
    Review coding guidelines C.1.g.1.e and C.1.g.1.g
  Z20.89 Contact with and (suspected) exposure to other communicable diseases
  Z20.9 Contact with and (suspected) exposure to unspecified communicable disease

Z21 Asymptomatic human immunodeficiency virus [HIV] infection status
    HIV positive NOS
    Code first Human immunodeficiency virus [HIV] disease complicating pregnancy, childbirth and the puerperium, if applicable (O98.7-)
    Excludes1: acquired immunodeficiency syndrome (B20)
        contact with human immunodeficiency virus [HIV] (Z20.6)
        exposure to human immunodeficiency virus [HIV] (Z20.6)
        human immunodeficiency virus [HIV] disease (B20)
        inconclusive laboratory evidence of human immunodeficiency virus [HIV] (R75)
    Review coding guidelines C.1.a.2.d, C.1.a.2.f and C.1.a.2.g
    Review coding guideline C.15.f
    Review coding guideline C.21.c.3
    AHA CC: 1Q, 2019, 10-11; 1Q, 2022, 36-37
    Valid 3-character code, no further characters required

Z22 Carrier of infectious disease
    Includes: colonization status
        suspected carrier
    Excludes2: carrier of viral hepatitis (B18.-)
    Review coding guideline C.21.c.3
  Z22.0 Carrier of typhoid
  Z22.1 Carrier of other intestinal infectious diseases
  Z22.2 Carrier of diphtheria
+ **Z22.3** Carrier of other specified bacterial diseases
    Z22.31 Carrier of bacterial disease due to meningococci
    + **Z22.32** Carrier of bacterial disease due to staphylococci
        Z22.321 Carrier or suspected carrier of Methicillin susceptible Staphylococcus aureus
            MSSA colonization
        Review coding guidelines C.1.e.1.c and C.1.e.1.d
        Z22.322 Carrier or suspected carrier of Methicillin resistant Staphylococcus aureus
            MRSA colonization
        Review coding guidelines C.1.e.1.c and C.1.e.1.d
    + **Z22.33** Carrier of bacterial disease due to streptococci
        Z22.330 Carrier of Group B streptococcus
        Excludes1: carrier of streptococcus group B (GBS) complicating pregnancy, childbirth and the puerperium (O99.82-)
        Z22.338 Carrier of other streptococcus
    + **Z22.34** Carrier of Acinetobacter baumannii
        Z22.340 Carrier of carbapenem-resistant Acinetobacter baumannii
        Z22.341 Carrier of carbapenem-sensitive Acinetobacter baumannii
        Z22.349 Carrier of Acinetobacter baumannii, unspecified
    + **Z22.35** Carrier of Enterobacterales
        Carrier of E. coli
        Carrier of K. pneumoniae
        Z22.350 Carrier of carbapenem-resistant Enterobacterales
        Z22.358 Carrier of other Enterobacterales
            Carrier of carbapenem-sensitive Enterobacterales
            Carrier of ESBL-producing Enterobacterales
            Carrier of extended-spectrum beta-lactamase producing Enterobacterales
        Z22.359 Carrier of Enterobacterales, unspecified
    Z22.39 Carrier of other specified bacterial diseases
  Z22.4 Carrier of infections with a predominantly sexual mode of transmission

Z22.6 Carrier of human T-lymphotropic virus type-1 [HTLV-1] infection

Z22.7 Latent tuberculosis
Latent tuberculosis infection (LTBI)
Excludes1: nonspecific reaction to cell mediated immunity measurement of gamma interferon antigen response without active tuberculosis (R76.12)
nonspecific reaction to tuberculin skin test without active tuberculosis (R76.11)
AHA CC: 4Q, 2019, 19

Z22.8 Carrier of other infectious diseases
Z22.9 Carrier of infectious disease, unspecified

Z23 Encounter for immunization
Code also, if applicable, encounter for immunization safety counseling (Z71.85)
Code first any routine childhood examination
NOTE Procedure codes are required to identify the types of immunizations given
AHA CC: 4Q, 2021, 34
Review coding guideline C.21.c.2
Valid 3-character code, no further characters required

Z28 Immunization not carried out and underimmunization status
Includes: vaccination not carried out
Code also, if applicable, encounter for immunization safety counseling (Z71.85)
AHA CC: 4Q, 2021, 34

+ **Z28.0** Immunization not carried out because of contraindication
  Z28.01 Immunization not carried out because of acute illness of patient
  Z28.02 Immunization not carried out because of chronic illness or condition of patient
  Z28.03 Immunization not carried out because of immune compromised state of patient
  Z28.04 Immunization not carried out because of patient allergy to vaccine or component
  Z28.09 Immunization not carried out because of other contraindication

Z28.1 Immunization not carried out because of patient decision for reasons of belief or group pressure
Immunization not carried out because of religious belief

+ **Z28.2** Immunization not carried out because of patient decision for other and unspecified reason
  Z28.20 Immunization not carried out because of patient decision for unspecified reason
  Z28.21 Immunization not carried out because of patient refusal
  Z28.29 Immunization not carried out because of patient decision for other reason

+ **Z28.3** Underimmunization status
Use additional code, if applicable, to identify:
immunization not carried out because of contraindication (Z28.0-)
immunization not carried out because of patient decision for other and unspecified reason
AHA CC: 4Q, 2021, 110; 1Q, 2022, 4-5
Review coding guideline C.21.c.3

+ **Z28.31** Underimmunization for COVID-19 status
NOTE These codes should not be used for individuals who are not eligible for the COVID-19 vaccines, as determined by the healthcare provider.
  Z28.310 Unvaccinated for COVID-19
  Z28.311 Partially vaccinated for COVID-19
  AHA CC: 1Q, 2022, 4-5

Z28.39 Other underimmunization status
Delinquent immunization status
Lapsed immunization schedule status

+ **Z28.8** Immunization not carried out for other reason
  Z28.81 Immunization not carried out due to patient having had the disease
  Z28.82 Immunization not carried out because of caregiver refusal
Immunization not carried out because of guardian refusal
Immunization not carried out because of parent refusal
Excludes1: immunization not carried out because of caregiver refusal because of religious belief (Z28.1)

Z28.83 Immunization not carried out due to unavailability of vaccine
Delay in delivery of vaccine
Lack of availability of vaccine
Manufacturer delay of vaccine
AHA CC: 4Q, 2018, 36

Z28.89 Immunization not carried out for other reason
Z28.9 Immunization not carried out for unspecified reason

Z29 Encounter for other prophylactic measures
Excludes1: desensitization to allergens (Z51.6)
prophylactic surgery (Z40.-)
Review coding guideline C.21.c.14
AHA CC: 4Q, 2016, 78-79

+ **Z29.1** Encounter for prophylactic immunotherapy
Encounter for administration of immunoglobulin
  Z29.11 Encounter for prophylactic immunotherapy for respiratory syncytial virus (RSV)
  Z29.12 Encounter for prophylactic antivenin
  Z29.13 Encounter for prophylactic Rho(D) immune globulin
  AHA CC: 3Q, 2019, 5
  Z29.14 Encounter for prophylactic rabies immune globin

Z29.3 Encounter for prophylactic fluoride administration

+ **Z29.8** Encounter for other specified prophylactic measures
AHA CC: 2Q, 2022, 27
  Z29.81 Encounter for HIV pre-exposure prophylaxis
Code also, if applicable, risk factors for HIV, such as:
contact with and (suspected) exposure to human immunodeficiency virus [HIV] (Z20.6)
high risk sexual behavior (Z72.5-)
Review coding guideline C.1.a.2.j
  Z29.89 Encounter for other specified prophylactic measures

Z29.9 Encounter for prophylactic measures, unspecified

Persons encountering health services in circumstances related to reproduction (Z30-Z39)

Z30 Encounter for contraceptive management
Review coding guideline C.21.c.11
AHA CC: 4Q, 2016, 78

+ **Z30.0** Encounter for general counseling and advice on contraception
Review coding guideline C.21.c.10

+ **Z30.01** Encounter for initial prescription of contraceptives
Excludes1: encounter for surveillance of contraceptives (Z30.4-)
  ♀ **Z30.011** Encounter for initial prescription of contraceptive pills
  ♀ **Z30.012** Encounter for prescription of emergency contraception
Encounter for postcoital contraception
  ♀ **Z30.013** Encounter for initial prescription of injectable contraceptive
  ♀ **Z30.014** Encounter for initial prescription of intrauterine contraceptive device
Excludes1: encounter for insertion of intrauterine contraceptive device (Z30.430, Z30.432)
  ♀ **Z30.015** Encounter for initial prescription of vaginal ring hormonal contraceptive
  Z30.016 Encounter for initial prescription of transdermal patch hormonal contraceptive device
  Z30.017 Encounter for initial prescription of implantable subdermal contraceptive
  ♀ **Z30.018** Encounter for initial prescription of other contraceptives
Encounter for initial prescription of barrier contraception
Encounter for initial prescription of diaphragm
  ♀ **Z30.019** Encounter for initial prescription of contraceptives, unspecified

Z30.02 Counseling and instruction in natural family planning to avoid pregnancy

Z30.09 Encounter for other general counseling and advice on contraception
Encounter for family planning advice NOS

Z30.2 Encounter for sterilization
 AHA CC: 3Q, 2021, 13

+ **Z30.4** Encounter for surveillance of contraceptives
   Z30.40 Encounter for surveillance of contraceptives, unspecified
   ♀ **Z30.41** Encounter for surveillance of contraceptive pills
     Encounter for repeat prescription for contraceptive pill
   ♀ **Z30.42** Encounter for surveillance of injectable contraceptive
   + **Z30.43** Encounter for surveillance of intrauterine contraceptive device
     ♀ **Z30.430** Encounter for insertion of intrauterine contraceptive device
     ♀ **Z30.431** Encounter for routine checking of intrauterine contraceptive device
     ♀ **Z30.432** Encounter for removal of intrauterine contraceptive device
     ♀ **Z30.433** Encounter for removal and reinsertion of intrauterine contraceptive device
       Encounter for replacement of intrauterine contraceptive device
   ♀ **Z30.44** Encounter for surveillance of vaginal ring hormonal contraceptive device
   ♀ **Z30.45** Encounter for surveillance of transdermal patch hormonal contraceptive device
   ♀ **Z30.46** Encounter for surveillance of implantable subdermal contraceptive
     Encounter for checking, reinsertion or removal of implantable subdermal contraceptive
   ♀ **Z30.49** Encounter for surveillance of other contraceptives
     Encounter for surveillance of barrier contraception
     Encounter for surveillance of diaphragm
 Z30.8 Encounter for other contraceptive management
    Encounter for postvasectomy sperm count
    Encounter for routine examination for contraceptive maintenance
    Excludes1: sperm count following sterilization reversal (Z31.42)
              sperm count for fertility testing (Z31.41)
 Z30.9 Encounter for contraceptive management, unspecified

Z31 Encounter for procreative management
   Excludes2: complications associated with artificial fertilization (N98.-)
             female infertility (N97.-)
             male infertility (N46.-)
   Review coding guideline C.21.c.11
 Z31.0 Encounter for reversal of previous sterilization
+ **Z31.4** Encounter for procreative investigation and testing
    Excludes1: postvasectomy sperm count (Z30.8)
   Z31.41 Encounter for fertility testing
     Encounter for fallopian tube patency testing
     Encounter for sperm count for fertility testing
   Z31.42 Aftercare following sterilization reversal
     Sperm count following sterilization reversal
   + **Z31.43** Encounter for genetic testing of female for procreative management
     Use additional code for recurrent pregnancy loss, if applicable (N96, O26.2-)
     Excludes1: nonprocreative genetic testing (Z13.7-)
     ♀ **Z31.430** Encounter of female for testing for genetic disease carrier status for procreative management
     ♀ **Z31.438** Encounter for other genetic testing of female for procreative management
   + **Z31.44** Encounter for genetic testing of male for procreative management
     Excludes1: nonprocreative genetic testing (Z13.7-)
     ♂ **Z31.440** Encounter of male for testing for genetic disease carrier status for procreative management
     ♂ **Z31.441** Encounter for testing of male partner of patient with recurrent pregnancy loss
     ♂ **Z31.448** Encounter for other genetic testing of male for procreative management
   Z31.49 Encounter for other procreative investigation and testing
 Z31.5 Encounter for procreative genetic counseling
    AHA CC: 4Q, 2017, 27
    Review coding guideline C.21.c.10
+ **Z31.6** Encounter for general counseling and advice on procreation
    Review coding guideline C.21.c.10
   Z31.61 Procreative counseling and advice using natural family planning
   Z31.62 Encounter for fertility preservation counseling
     Encounter for fertility preservation counseling prior to cancer therapy
     Encounter for fertility preservation counseling prior to surgical removal of gonads
   Z31.69 Encounter for other general counseling and advice on procreation
 ♀ **Z31.7** Encounter for procreative management and counseling for gestational carrier
    Excludes1: pregnant state, gestational carrier (Z33.3)
    AHA CC: 4Q, 2016, 78
+ **Z31.8** Encounter for other procreative management
   ♀ **Z31.81** Encounter for male factor infertility in female patient
     Review coding guideline C.21.c.16
   ♀ **Z31.82** Encounter for Rh incompatibility status
     Review coding guideline C.21.c.16
     AHA CC: 4Q, 2014, 17
   ♀ **Z31.83** Encounter for assisted reproductive fertility procedure cycle
     Patient undergoing in vitro fertilization cycle
     Use additional code to identify the type of infertility
     Excludes1: pre-cycle diagnosis and testing - code to reason for encounter
     AHA CC: 2Q, 2022, 15-16
     Review coding guideline C.21.c.16
   Z31.84 Encounter for fertility preservation procedure
     Encounter for fertility preservation procedure prior to cancer therapy
     Encounter for fertility preservation procedure prior to surgical removal of gonads
     Review coding guideline C.21.c.16
   Z31.89 Encounter for other procreative management
 Z31.9 Encounter for procreative management, unspecified

Z32 Encounter for pregnancy test and childbirth and childcare instruction
+ **Z32.0** Encounter for pregnancy test
    Review coding guideline C.21.c.13
   ♀ **Z32.00** Encounter for pregnancy test, result unknown
     Encounter for pregnancy test NOS
   • ♀ **Z32.01** Encounter for pregnancy test, result positive
   • ♀ **Z32.02** Encounter for pregnancy test, result negative
 Z32.2 Encounter for childbirth instruction
    Review coding guidelines C.21.c.10 and C.21.c.11
 Z32.3 Encounter for childcare instruction
    Encounter for prenatal or postpartum childcare instruction
    Review coding guidelines C.21.c.10 and C.21.c.11

Z33 Pregnant state
   Review coding guideline C.21.c.11
   AHA CC: 4Q, 2016, 78
 • ♀ **Z33.1** Pregnant state, incidental
    Pregnancy NOS
    Pregnant state NOS
    Excludes1: complications of pregnancy (O00-O9A)
              pregnant state, gestational carrier (Z33.3)
    Review coding guideline C.15.a.1
    Review coding guidelines C.21.c.3
 • ♀ **Z33.2** Encounter for elective termination of pregnancy
    Excludes1: early fetal death with retention of dead fetus (O02.1)
              late fetal death (O36.4)
              spontaneous abortion (O03)
    AHA CC: 2Q, 2023, 15-16
    Review coding guidelines C.15.q.1 and C.15.q.2
    Review coding guidelines C.21.c.16
 • ♀ **Z33.3** Pregnant state, gestational carrier
    Excludes1: encounter for procreative management and counseling for gestational carrier (Z31.7)

Z34 Encounter for supervision of normal pregnancy
   Excludes1: any complication of pregnancy (O00-O9A)
             encounter for pregnancy test (Z32.0-)
             encounter for supervision of high risk pregnancy (O09.-)
   Review coding guideline C.15.b.1
   Review coding guidelines C.21.c.11 and C.21.c.16
   AHA CC: 4Q, 2016, 4-7
+ **Z34.0** Encounter for supervision of normal first pregnancy
   • ♀ **Z34.00** Encounter for supervision of normal first pregnancy, unspecified trimester
   • ♀ **Z34.01** Encounter for supervision of normal first pregnancy, first trimester

- ♀ **Z34.02** Encounter for supervision of normal first pregnancy, second trimester
- ♀ **Z34.03** Encounter for supervision of normal first pregnancy, third trimester
+ **Z34.8** Encounter for supervision of other normal pregnancy
  - ♀ **Z34.80** Encounter for supervision of other normal pregnancy, unspecified trimester
  - ♀ **Z34.81** Encounter for supervision of other normal pregnancy, first trimester
  - ♀ **Z34.82** Encounter for supervision of other normal pregnancy, second trimester
  - ♀ **Z34.83** Encounter for supervision of other normal pregnancy, third trimester
    AHA CC: 4Q, 2014, 17
+ **Z34.9** Encounter for supervision of normal pregnancy, unspecified
  - ♀ **Z34.90** Encounter for supervision of normal pregnancy, unspecified, unspecified trimester
  - ♀ **Z34.91** Encounter for supervision of normal pregnancy, unspecified, first trimester
  - ♀ **Z34.92** Encounter for supervision of normal pregnancy, unspecified, second trimester
  - ♀ **Z34.93** Encounter for supervision of normal pregnancy, unspecified, third trimester

Z36 Encounter for antenatal screening of mother

Includes: Encounter for placental sample (taken vaginally)
Screening is the testing for disease or disease precursors in asymptomatic individuals so that early detection and treatment can be provided for those who test positive for the disease.

Excludes1: diagnostic examination- code to sign or symptom
encounter for suspected maternal and fetal conditions ruled out (Z03.7-)
suspected fetal condition affecting management of pregnancy - code to condition in Chapter 15

Excludes2: abnormal findings on antenatal screening of mother (O28.-)
genetic counseling and testing (Z31.43-, Z31.5)
routine prenatal care (Z34)

AHA CC: 4Q, 2017, 28
Review coding guidelines C.21.c.5 and C.21.c.11

- ♀ **Z36.0** Encounter for antenatal screening for chromosomal anomalies
- ♀ **Z36.1** Encounter for antenatal screening for raised alphafetoprotein level
  Encounter for antenatal screening for elevated maternal serum alphafetoprotein level
- ♀ **Z36.2** Encounter for other antenatal screening follow-up
  Non-visualized anatomy on a previous scan
- ♀ **Z36.3** Encounter for antenatal screening for malformations
  Screening for suspected anomaly
- ♀ **Z36.4** Encounter for antenatal screening for fetal growth retardation
  Intrauterine growth restriction (IUGR)/small-for-dates
- ♀ **Z36.5** Encounter for antenatal screening for isoimmunization
+ **Z36.8** Encounter for other antenatal screening
  - ♀ **Z36.81** Encounter for antenatal screening for hydrops fetalis
  - ♀ **Z36.82** Encounter for antenatal screening for nuchal translucency
  - ♀ **Z36.83** Encounter for antenatal screening for congenital cardiac abnormalities
  - ♀ **Z36.84** Encounter for antenatal screening for fetal lung maturity
  - ♀ **Z36.85** Encounter for antenatal screening for Streptococcus B
  - ♀ **Z36.86** Encounter for antenatal screening for for cervical length
    Screening for risk of pre-term labor
  - ♀ **Z36.87** Encounter for antenatal screening for uncertain dates
  - ♀ **Z36.88** Encounter for antenatal screening for fetal macrosomia
    Screening for large-for-dates
  - ♀ **Z36.89** Encounter for other specified antenatal screening
  - ♀ **Z36.8A** Encounter for antenatal screening for other genetic defects
- ♀ **Z36.9** Encounter for antenatal screening, unspecified

Z3A Weeks of gestation

NOTE Codes from category Z3A are for use, only on the maternal record, to indicate the weeks of gestation of the pregnancy, if known.
Code first obstetric condition or encounter for delivery (O09-O60, O80-O82)
AHA CC: 2Q, 2022, 3-4
Review coding guideline C.21.c.11 and C.15.a.7

+ **Z3A.0** Weeks of gestation of pregnancy, unspecified or less than 10 weeks
  - ♀ **Z3A.00** Weeks of gestation of pregnancy not specified
  - ♀ **Z3A.01** Less than 8 weeks gestation of pregnancy
  - ♀ **Z3A.08** 8 weeks gestation of pregnancy
  - ♀ **Z3A.09** 9 weeks gestation of pregnancy
+ **Z3A.1** Weeks of gestation of pregnancy, weeks 10-19
  - ♀ **Z3A.10** 10 weeks gestation of pregnancy
  - ♀ **Z3A.11** 11 weeks gestation of pregnancy
  - ♀ **Z3A.12** 12 weeks gestation of pregnancy
  - ♀ **Z3A.13** 13 weeks gestation of pregnancy
  - ♀ **Z3A.14** 14 weeks gestation of pregnancy
  - ♀ **Z3A.15** 15 weeks gestation of pregnancy
  - ♀ **Z3A.16** 16 weeks gestation of pregnancy
    AHA CC: 4Q, 2016, 4-7
  - ♀ **Z3A.17** 17 weeks gestation of pregnancy
  - ♀ **Z3A.18** 18 weeks gestation of pregnancy
    AHA CC: 2Q, 2019, 11
  - ♀ **Z3A.19** 19 weeks gestation of pregnancy
+ **Z3A.2** Weeks of gestation of pregnancy, weeks 20-29
  - ♀ **Z3A.20** 20 weeks gestation of pregnancy
    AHA CC: 4Q, 2016, 4-7
  - ♀ **Z3A.21** 21 weeks gestation of pregnancy
  - ♀ **Z3A.22** 22 weeks gestation of pregnancy
    AHA CC: 4Q, 2016, 4-7
  - ♀ **Z3A.23** 23 weeks gestation of pregnancy
  - ♀ **Z3A.24** 24 weeks gestation of pregnancy
  - ♀ **Z3A.25** 25 weeks gestation of pregnancy
  - ♀ **Z3A.26** 26 weeks gestation of pregnancy
  - ♀ **Z3A.27** 27 weeks gestation of pregnancy
  - ♀ **Z3A.28** 28 weeks gestation of pregnancy
  - ♀ **Z3A.29** 29 weeks gestation of pregnancy
+ **Z3A.3** Weeks of gestation of pregnancy, weeks 30-39
  - ♀ **Z3A.30** 30 weeks gestation of pregnancy
  - ♀ **Z3A.31** 31 weeks gestation of pregnancy
  - ♀ **Z3A.32** 32 weeks gestation of pregnancy
    AHA CC: 4Q, 2016, 4-7
  - ♀ **Z3A.33** 33 weeks gestation of pregnancy
  - ♀ **Z3A.34** 34 weeks gestation of pregnancy
  - ♀ **Z3A.35** 35 weeks gestation of pregnancy
  - ♀ **Z3A.36** 36 weeks gestation of pregnancy
  - ♀ **Z3A.37** 37 weeks gestation of pregnancy
  - ♀ **Z3A.38** 38 weeks gestation of pregnancy
    AHA CC: 2Q, 2016, 34
  - ♀ **Z3A.39** 39 weeks gestation of pregnancy
+ **Z3A.4** Weeks of gestation of pregnancy, weeks 40 or greater
  - ♀ **Z3A.40** 40 weeks gestation of pregnancy
    AHA CC: 2Q, 2014, 9
  - ♀ **Z3A.41** 41 weeks gestation of pregnancy
  - ♀ **Z3A.42** 42 weeks gestation of pregnancy
    AHA CC: 4Q, 2014, 23
  - ♀ **Z3A.49** Greater than 42 weeks gestation of pregnancy

Z37 Outcome of delivery

This category is intended for use as an additional code to identify the outcome of delivery on the mother's record. It is not for use on the newborn record.

Excludes1: *stillbirth (P95)*
Review coding guidelines C.15.b.5
Review coding guidelines C.15.n.3 and C.15.q.1
Review coding guidelines C.21.c.11

- ♀ **Z37.0** Single live birth
  AHA CC: 2Q, 2014, 9; 4Q, 2014, 17-18; 2Q, 2016, 34
- ♀ **Z37.1** Single stillbirth
- ♀ **Z37.2** Twins, both liveborn
- ♀ **Z37.3** Twins, one liveborn and one stillborn
- ♀ **Z37.4** Twins, both stillborn
+ **Z37.5** Other multiple births, all liveborn
  - ♀ **Z37.50** Multiple births, unspecified, all liveborn
  - ♀ **Z37.51** Triplets, all liveborn
  - ♀ **Z37.52** Quadruplets, all liveborn

- ♀ **Z37.53** Quintuplets, all liveborn
- ♀ **Z37.54** Sextuplets, all liveborn
- ♀ **Z37.59** Other multiple births, all liveborn
+ **Z37.6** Other multiple births, some liveborn
  - ♀ **Z37.60** Multiple births, unspecified, some liveborn
  - ♀ **Z37.61** Triplets, some liveborn
  - ♀ **Z37.62** Quadruplets, some liveborn
  - ♀ **Z37.63** Quintuplets, some liveborn
  - ♀ **Z37.64** Sextuplets, some liveborn
  - ♀ **Z37.69** Other multiple births, some liveborn
- ♀ **Z37.7** Other multiple births, all stillborn
- ♀ **Z37.9** Outcome of delivery, unspecified
  Multiple birth NOS
  Single birth NOS

Z38 Liveborn infants according to place of birth and type of delivery

This category is for use as the principal code on the initial record of a newborn baby. It is to be used for the initial birth record only. It is not to be used on the mother's record.
Review coding guideline C.16.a.2 and C.16.h
Review coding guideline C.17
Review coding guidelines C.21.c.6, C.21.c.12 and C.21.c.16
AHA CC: 2Q, 2015, 15; 4Q, 2016, 4-7, 54-55; 2Q, 2020, 13

+ **Z38.0** Single liveborn infant, born in hospital
  Single liveborn infant, born in birthing center or other health care facility
  AHA CC: 2Q, 2017, 5-7
  - **Z38.00** Single liveborn infant, delivered vaginally
    AHA CC: 4Q, 2018, 26; 4Q, 2020, 38; 4Q, 2021, 23
  - **Z38.01** Single liveborn infant, delivered by cesarean
    AHA CC: 3Q, 2016, 18
- **Z38.1** Single liveborn infant, born outside hospital
- **Z38.2** Single liveborn infant, unspecified as to place of birth
  Single liveborn infant NOS
+ **Z38.3** Twin liveborn infant, born in hospital
  - **Z38.30** Twin liveborn infant, delivered vaginally
  - **Z38.31** Twin liveborn infant, delivered by cesarean
- **Z38.4** Twin liveborn infant, born outside hospital
- **Z38.5** Twin liveborn infant, unspecified as to place of birth
+ **Z38.6** Other multiple liveborn infant, born in hospital
  - **Z38.61** Triplet liveborn infant, delivered vaginally
  - **Z38.62** Triplet liveborn infant, delivered by cesarean
  - **Z38.63** Quadruplet liveborn infant, delivered vaginally
  - **Z38.64** Quadruplet liveborn infant, delivered by cesarean
  - **Z38.65** Quintuplet liveborn infant, delivered vaginally
  - **Z38.66** Quintuplet liveborn infant, delivered by cesarean
  - **Z38.68** Other multiple liveborn infant, delivered vaginally
  - **Z38.69** Other multiple liveborn infant, delivered by cesarean
- **Z38.7** Other multiple liveborn infant, born outside hospital
- **Z38.8** Other multiple liveborn infant, unspecified as to place of birth

Z39 Encounter for maternal postpartum care and examination
Review coding guidelines C.21.c.8, C.21.c.11 and C.21.c.16
- ♀ **Z39.0** Encounter for care and examination of mother immediately after delivery
  Care and observation in uncomplicated cases when the delivery occurs outside a healthcare facility
  Excludes1: care for postpartum complication- see Alphabetic index
  AHA CC: 3Q, 2021, 13
  Review coding guideline C.15.o.4
- ♀ **Z39.1** Encounter for care and examination of lactating mother
  Encounter for supervision of lactation
  Excludes1: disorders of lactation (O92.-)
- ♀ **Z39.2** Encounter for routine postpartum follow-up

Encounters for other specific health care (Z40-Z53)

Categories Z40-Z53 are intended for use to indicate a reason for care. They may be used for patients who have already been treated for a disease or injury, but who are receiving aftercare or prophylactic care, or care to consolidate the treatment, or to deal with a residual state

Excludes2: follow-up examination for medical surveillance after treatment (Z08-Z09)

Z40 Encounter for prophylactic surgery
Excludes1: organ donations (Z52.-)
therapeutic organ removal-code to condition
Review coding guideline C.21.c.14 and C21.c.16

+ **Z40.0** Encounter for prophylactic surgery for risk factors related to malignant neoplasms
  Admission for prophylactic organ removal
  Use additional code to identify risk factor
  - **Z40.00** Encounter for prophylactic removal of unspecified organ
  - **Z40.01** Encounter for prophylactic removal of breast
  - ♀ **Z40.02** Encounter for prophylactic removal of ovary(s)
    Encounter for prophylactic removal of ovary(s) and fallopian tube(s)
  - ♀ **Z40.03** Encounter for prophylactic removal of fallopian tube(s)
    AHA CC: 4Q, 2017, 28
  - **Z40.09** Encounter for prophylactic removal of other organ
- **Z40.8** Encounter for other prophylactic surgery
- **Z40.9** Encounter for prophylactic surgery, unspecified

Z41 Encounter for procedures for purposes other than remedying health state
- **Z41.1** Encounter for cosmetic surgery
  Encounter for cosmetic breast implant
  Encounter for cosmetic procedure
  Excludes1: encounter for plastic and reconstructive surgery following medical procedure or healed injury (Z42.-)
  encounter for post-mastectomy breast implantation (Z42.1)
- ♂ **Z41.2** Encounter for routine and ritual male circumcision
  AHA CC: 3Q, 2018, 15
- **Z41.3** Encounter for ear piercing
- **Z41.8** Encounter for other procedures for purposes other than remedying health state
- **Z41.9** Encounter for procedure for purposes other than remedying health state, unspecified

Z42 Encounter for plastic and reconstructive surgery following medical procedure or healed injury
Excludes1: encounter for cosmetic plastic surgery (Z41.1)
encounter for plastic surgery for treatment of current injury - code to relevent injury
Review coding guidelines C.21.c.7 and C.21.c.16
- **Z42.1** Encounter for breast reconstruction following mastectomy
  Excludes1: deformity and disproportion of reconstructed breast (N65.1-)
- **Z42.8** Encounter for other plastic and reconstructive surgery following medical procedure or healed injury
  AHA CC: 1Q, 2017, 42-43

Z43 Encounter for attention to artificial openings
Includes: closure of artificial openings
passage of sounds or bougies through artificial openings
reforming artificial openings
removal of catheter from artificial openings
toilet or cleansing of artificial openings
Excludes1: complications of external stoma (J95.0-, K94.-, N99.5-)
Excludes2: fitting and adjustment of prosthetic and other devices (Z44-Z46)
Review coding guideline C.21.c.7
- **Z43.0** Encounter for attention to tracheostomy
- CC **Z43.1** Encounter for attention to gastrostomy
  Excludes2: artificial opening status only, without need for care (Z93.-)
- **Z43.2** Encounter for attention to ileostomy
  AHA CC: 3Q, 2016, 5
- **Z43.3** Encounter for attention to colostomy
- **Z43.4** Encounter for attention to other artificial openings of digestive tract
- **Z43.5** Encounter for attention to cystostomy
- **Z43.6** Encounter for attention to other artificial openings of urinary tract
  Encounter for attention to nephrostomy
  Encounter for attention to ureterostomy
  Encounter for attention to urethrostomy
- **Z43.7** Encounter for attention to artificial vagina
- **Z43.8** Encounter for attention to other artificial openings
- **Z43.9** Encounter for attention to unspecified artificial opening

Z44 Encounter for fitting and adjustment of external prosthetic device
Includes: removal or replacement of external prosthetic device
Excludes1: malfunction or other complications of device - see Alphabetical Index
presence of prosthetic device (Z97.-)
Review coding guideline C.21.c.7

Chapter 21: Factors Influencing Health Status and Contact with Health Services

- **+ Z44.0** Encounter for fitting and adjustment of artificial arm
  - **+ Z44.00** Encounter for fitting and adjustment of unspecified artificial arm
    - **Z44.001** Encounter for fitting and adjustment of unspecified right artificial arm
    - **Z44.002** Encounter for fitting and adjustment of unspecified left artificial arm
    - **Z44.009** Encounter for fitting and adjustment of unspecified artificial arm, unspecified arm
  - **+ Z44.01** Encounter for fitting and adjustment of complete artificial arm
    - **Z44.011** Encounter for fitting and adjustment of complete right artificial arm
    - **Z44.012** Encounter for fitting and adjustment of complete left artificial arm
    - **Z44.019** Encounter for fitting and adjustment of complete artificial arm, unspecified arm
  - **+ Z44.02** Encounter for fitting and adjustment of partial artificial arm
    - **Z44.021** Encounter for fitting and adjustment of partial artificial right arm
    - **Z44.022** Encounter for fitting and adjustment of partial artificial left arm
    - **Z44.029** Encounter for fitting and adjustment of partial artificial arm, unspecified arm
- **+ Z44.1** Encounter for fitting and adjustment of artificial leg
  - **+ Z44.10** Encounter for fitting and adjustment of unspecified artificial leg
    - **Z44.101** Encounter for fitting and adjustment of unspecified right artificial leg
    - **Z44.102** Encounter for fitting and adjustment of unspecified left artificial leg
    - **Z44.109** Encounter for fitting and adjustment of unspecified artificial leg, unspecified leg
  - **+ Z44.11** Encounter for fitting and adjustment of complete artificial leg
    - **Z44.111** Encounter for fitting and adjustment of complete right artificial leg
    - **Z44.112** Encounter for fitting and adjustment of complete left artificial leg
    - **Z44.119** Encounter for fitting and adjustment of complete artificial leg, unspecified leg
  - **+ Z44.12** Encounter for fitting and adjustment of partial artificial leg
    - **Z44.121** Encounter for fitting and adjustment of partial artificial right leg
    - **Z44.122** Encounter for fitting and adjustment of partial artificial left leg
    - **Z44.129** Encounter for fitting and adjustment of partial artificial leg, unspecified leg
- **+ Z44.2** Encounter for fitting and adjustment of artificial eye
  - *Excludes1:* mechanical complication of ocular prosthesis (T85.3)
  - **Z44.20** Encounter for fitting and adjustment of artificial eye, unspecified
  - **Z44.21** Encounter for fitting and adjustment of artificial right eye
  - **Z44.22** Encounter for fitting and adjustment of artificial left eye
- **+ Z44.3** Encounter for fitting and adjustment of external breast prosthesis
  - *Excludes1:* complications of breast implant (T85.4-)
    - encounter for adjustment or removal of breast implant (Z45.81-)
    - encounter for initial breast implant insertion for cosmetic breast augmentation (Z41.1)
    - encounter for breast reconstruction following mastectomy (Z42.1)
  - **Z44.30** Encounter for fitting and adjustment of external breast prosthesis, unspecified breast
  - **Z44.31** Encounter for fitting and adjustment of external right breast prosthesis
  - **Z44.32** Encounter for fitting and adjustment of external left breast prosthesis
- **Z44.8** Encounter for fitting and adjustment of other external prosthetic devices
- **Z44.9** Encounter for fitting and adjustment of unspecified external prosthetic device

---

Z45 Encounter for adjustment and management of implanted device
- *Includes:* removal or replacement of implanted device
- *Excludes1:* malfunction or other complications of device - see Alphabetical Index
- *Excludes2:* encounter for fitting and adjustment of non-implanted device (Z46.-)
- Review coding guideline C.21.c.7

- **+ Z45.0** Encounter for adjustment and management of cardiac device
  - **+ Z45.01** Encounter for adjustment and management of cardiac pacemaker
    - Encounter for adjustment and management of cardiac resynchronization therapy pacemaker (CRT-P)
    - *Excludes1:* encounter for adjustment and management of automatic implantable cardiac defibrillator with synchronous cardiac pacemaker (Z45.02)
    - **Z45.010** Encounter for checking and testing of cardiac pacemaker pulse generator [battery]
      - Encounter for replacing cardiac pacemaker pulse generator [battery]
    - **Z45.018** Encounter for adjustment and management of other part of cardiac pacemaker
      - *Excludes1:* presence of other part of cardiac pacemaker (Z95.0)
      - *Excludes2:* presence of prosthetic and other devices (Z95.1-Z95.5, Z95.811-Z97)
  - **Z45.02** Encounter for adjustment and management of automatic implantable cardiac defibrillator
    - Encounter for adjustment and management of automatic implantable cardiac defibrillator with synchronous cardiac pacemaker
    - Encounter for adjustment and management of cardiac resynchronization therapy defibrillator (CRT-D)
  - **Z45.09** Encounter for adjustment and management of other cardiac device
- **Z45.1** Encounter for adjustment and management of infusion pump
- **Z45.2** Encounter for adjustment and management of vascular access device
  - Encounter for adjustment and management of vascular catheters
  - *Excludes1:* encounter for adjustment and management of renal dialysis catheter (Z49.01)
  - AHA CC: 3Q, 2018, 20-21; 2Q, 2020, 21-22
- **+ Z45.3** Encounter for adjustment and management of implanted devices of the special senses
  - **Z45.31** Encounter for adjustment and management of implanted visual substitution device
  - **+ Z45.32** Encounter for adjustment and management of implanted hearing device
    - *Excludes1:* Encounter for fitting and adjustment of hearing aide (Z46.1)
    - **Z45.320** Encounter for adjustment and management of bone conduction device
    - **Z45.321** Encounter for adjustment and management of cochlear device
    - **Z45.328** Encounter for adjustment and management of other implanted hearing device
- **+ Z45.4** Encounter for adjustment and management of implanted nervous system device
  - **Z45.41** Encounter for adjustment and management of cerebrospinal fluid drainage device
    - Encounter for adjustment and management of cerebral ventricular (communicating) shunt
  - **Z45.42** Encounter for adjustment and management of neurostimulator
    - Encounter for adjustment and management of brain neurostimulator
    - Encounter for adjustment and management of gastric neurostimulator
    - Encounter for adjustment and management of peripheral nerve neurostimulator
    - Encounter for adjustment and management of sacral nerve neurostimulator

Encounter for adjustment and management of spinal cord neurostimulator
Encounter for adjustment and management of vagus nerve neurostimulator

Z45.49 Encounter for adjustment and management of other implanted nervous system device
AHA CC: 3Q, 2014, 19-20

+ **Z45.8** Encounter for adjustment and management of other implanted devices
  + **Z45.81** Encounter for adjustment or removal of breast implant
    Encounter for elective implant exchange (different material) (different size)
    Encounter for removal of tissue expander with or without synchronous insertion of permanent implant
    Excludes1: complications of breast implant (T85.4-)
    encounter for initial breast implant insertion for cosmetic breast augmentation (Z41.1)
    encounter for breast reconstruction following mastectomy (Z42.1)
    - **Z45.811** Encounter for adjustment or removal of right breast implant
    - **Z45.812** Encounter for adjustment or removal of left breast implant
    - **Z45.819** Encounter for adjustment or removal of unspecified breast implant
  - **Z45.82** Encounter for adjustment or removal of myringotomy device (stent) (tube)
  - **Z45.89** Encounter for adjustment and management of other implanted devices
    AHA CC: 4Q, 2014, 26-28

Z45.9 Encounter for adjustment and management of unspecified implanted device

Z46 Encounter for fitting and adjustment of other devices
Includes: removal or replacement of other device
Excludes1: malfunction or other complications of device - see Alphabetical Index
Excludes2: encounter for fitting and management of implanted devices (Z45.-)
issue of repeat prescription only (Z76.0)
presence of prosthetic and other devices (Z95-Z97)
Review coding guideline C.21.c.7

Z46.0 Encounter for fitting and adjustment of spectacles and contact lenses

Z46.1 Encounter for fitting and adjustment of hearing aid
Excludes1: encounter for adjustment and management of implanted hearing device (Z45.32-)

Z46.2 Encounter for fitting and adjustment of other devices related to nervous system and special senses
Excludes2: encounter for adjustment and management of implanted nervous system device (Z45.4-)
encounter for adjustment and management of implanted visual substitution device (Z45.31-)

Z46.3 Encounter for fitting and adjustment of dental prosthetic device
Encounter for fitting and adjustment of dentures

Z46.4 Encounter for fitting and adjustment of orthodontic device

+ **Z46.5** Encounter for fitting and adjustment of other gastrointestinal appliance and device
Excludes1: encounter for attention to artificial openings of digestive tract (Z43.1-Z43.4)
- **Z46.51** Encounter for fitting and adjustment of gastric lap band
- **Z46.59** Encounter for fitting and adjustment of other gastrointestinal appliance and device

Z46.6 Encounter for fitting and adjustment of urinary device
Excludes2: attention to artificial openings of urinary tract (Z43.5, Z43.6)

+ **Z46.8** Encounter for fitting and adjustment of other specified devices
  - **Z46.81** Encounter for fitting and adjustment of insulin pump
    Encounter for insulin pump titration
    Encounter for insulin pump instruction and training
  - **Z46.82** Encounter for fitting and adjustment of non-vascular catheter

  - **Z46.89** Encounter for fitting and adjustment of other specified devices
    Encounter for fitting and adjustment of wheelchair

Z46.9 Encounter for fitting and adjustment of unspecified device

Z47 Orthopedic aftercare
Excludes1: aftercare for healing fracture-code to fracture with 7th character D
Review coding guideline C.21.c.7

Z47.1 Aftercare following joint replacement surgery
Use additional code to identify the joint (Z96.6-)
AHA CC: 1Q, 2020, 23-24

Z47.2 Encounter for removal of internal fixation device
Excludes1: encounter for adjustment of internal fixation device for fracture treatment- code to fracture with appropriate 7th character
encounter for removal of external fixation device- code to fracture with 7th character D
infection or inflammatory reaction to internal fixation device (T84.6-)
mechanical complication of internal fixation device (T84.1-)

+ **Z47.3** Aftercare following explantation of joint prosthesis
Aftercare following explantation of joint prosthesis, staged procedure
Encounter for joint prosthesis insertion following prior explantation of joint prosthesis
AHA CC: 1Q, 2020, 23-24
- **Z47.31** Aftercare following explantation of shoulder joint prosthesis
Excludes1: acquired absence of shoulder joint following prior explantation of shoulder joint prosthesis (Z89.23-)
shoulder joint prosthesis explantation status (Z89.23-)
- **Z47.32** Aftercare following explantation of hip joint prosthesis
Excludes1: acquired absence of hip joint following prior explantation of hip joint prosthesis (Z89.62-)
hip joint prosthesis explantation status (Z89.62-)
AHA CC: 1Q, 2015, 16-17
- **Z47.33** Aftercare following explantation of knee joint prosthesis
Excludes1: acquired absence of knee joint following prior explantation of knee prosthesis (Z89.52-)
knee joint prosthesis explantation status (Z89.52-)

+ **Z47.8** Encounter for other orthopedic aftercare
- **Z47.81** Encounter for orthopedic aftercare following surgical amputation
Use additional code to identify the limb amputated (Z89.-)
- **Z47.82** Encounter for orthopedic aftercare following scoliosis surgery
- **Z47.89** Encounter for other orthopedic aftercare

Z48 Encounter for other postprocedural aftercare
Excludes1: encounter for aftercare following injury - code to Injury, by site, with appropriate 7th character for subsequent encounter
encounter for follow-up examination after completed treatment (Z08-Z09)
Excludes2: encounter for attention to artificial openings (Z43.-)
encounter for fitting and adjustment of prosthetic and other devices (Z44-Z46)
Review coding guideline C.21.c.7

+ **Z48.0** Encounter for attention to dressings, sutures and drains
Excludes1: encounter for planned postprocedural wound closure (Z48.1)
- **Z48.00** Encounter for change or removal of nonsurgical wound dressing
Encounter for change or removal of wound dressing NOS
- **Z48.01** Encounter for change or removal of surgical wound dressing
AHA CC: 4Q, 2015, 38; 2Q, 2019, 33
- **Z48.02** Encounter for removal of sutures
Encounter for removal of staples
- **Z48.03** Encounter for change or removal of drains

Z48.1 Encounter for planned postprocedural wound closure
  Excludes1: encounter for attention to dressings and sutures (Z48.0-)
+ **Z48.2** Encounter for aftercare following organ transplant
  CC **Z48.21** Encounter for aftercare following heart transplant
  CC **Z48.22** Encounter for aftercare following kidney transplant
  CC **Z48.23** Encounter for aftercare following liver transplant
  CC **Z48.24** Encounter for aftercare following lung transplant
  + **Z48.28** Encounter for aftercare following multiple organ transplant
    CC **Z48.280** Encounter for aftercare following heart-lung transplant
    Z48.288 Encounter for aftercare following multiple organ transplant
  + **Z48.29** Encounter for aftercare following other organ transplant
    CC **Z48.290** Encounter for aftercare following bone marrow transplant
    Z48.298 Encounter for aftercare following other organ transplant
  Z48.3 Aftercare following surgery for neoplasm
    Use additional code to identify the neoplasm
+ **Z48.8** Encounter for other specified postprocedural aftercare
  + **Z48.81** Encounter for surgical aftercare following surgery on specified body systems
    These codes identify the body system requiring aftercare. They are for use in conjunction with other aftercare codes to fully explain the aftercare encounter. The condition treated should also be coded if still present.
    Excludes1: aftercare for injury- code the injury with 7th character D
      aftercare following surgery for neoplasm (Z48.3)
    Excludes2: aftercare following organ transplant (Z48.2-)
      orthopedic aftercare (Z47.-)
    Z48.810 Encounter for surgical aftercare following surgery on the sense organs
    Z48.811 Encounter for surgical aftercare following surgery on the nervous system
      Excludes2: encounter for surgical aftercare following surgery on the sense organs (Z48.810)
    Z48.812 Encounter for surgical aftercare following surgery on the circulatory system
      AHA CC: 4Q, 2012, 96-97
    Z48.813 Encounter for surgical aftercare following surgery on the respiratory system
      AHA CC: 2Q, 2019, 33
    Z48.814 Encounter for surgical aftercare following surgery on the teeth or oral cavity
    Z48.815 Encounter for surgical aftercare following surgery on the digestive system
      AHA CC: 4Q, 2015, 38
    Z48.816 Encounter for surgical aftercare following surgery on the genitourinary system
      Excludes1: encounter for aftercare following sterilization reversal (Z31.42)
    Z48.817 Encounter for surgical aftercare following surgery on the skin and subcutaneous tissue
  Z48.89 Encounter for other specified surgical aftercare
Z49 Encounter for5 care involving renal dialysis
  Code also associated end stage renal disease (N18.6)
  Review coding guideline C.21.c.7
+ **Z49.0** Preparatory care for renal dialysis
  Encounter for dialysis instruction and training
  Z49.01 Encounter for fitting and adjustment of extracorporeal dialysis catheter
    Removal or replacement of renal dialysis catheter
    Toilet or cleansing of renal dialysis catheter

Z49.02 Encounter for fitting and adjustment of peritoneal dialysis catheter
+ **Z49.3** Encounter for adequacy testing for dialysis
  Z49.31 Encounter for adequacy testing for hemodialysis
  Z49.32 Encounter for adequacy testing for peritoneal dialysis
    Encounter for peritoneal equilibration test
Z51 Encounter for other aftercare and medical care
  Code also condition requiring care
  Excludes1: follow-up examination after treatment (Z08-Z09)
  Review coding guidelines C.2.a, C.2.e.2 and C.2.e.3
  Review coding guideline C.21.c.7
  Z51.0 Encounter for antineoplastic radiation therapy
    Review coding guidelines C.21.c.7 and C.21.c.16
+ **Z51.1** Encounter for antineoplastic chemotherapy and immunotherapy
    Excludes2: encounter for chemotherapy and immunotherapy for nonneoplastic condition- code to condition
    Review coding guidelines C.21.c.7 and C21.c.16
    Z51.11 Encounter for antineoplastic chemotherapy
      AHA CC: 3Q, 2015, 19-20; 1Q, 2022, 16-17
    Z51.12 Encounter for antineoplastic immunotherapy
  Z51.5 Encounter for palliative care
    AHA CC: 1Q, 2017, 48-49; 4Q, 2020, 98; 1Q, 2022, 18-19
  Z51.6 Encounter for desensitization to allergens
    AHA CC: 4Q, 2016, 77
+ **Z51.8** Encounter for other specified aftercare
    Excludes1: holiday relief care (Z75.5)
    Z51.81 Encounter for therapeutic drug level monitoring
      Code also any long-term (current) drug therapy (Z79.-)
      Excludes1: encounter for blood-drug test for administrative or medicolegal reasons (Z02.83)
    Z51.89 Encounter for other specified aftercare
      AHA CC: 4Q, 2012, 96-97
    NOTE Z51.89 is an acceptable PDX when reported with a secondary diagnosis.
Z52 Donors of organs and tissues
  Includes: autologous and other living donors
  Excludes1: cadaveric donor - omit code
    examination of potential donor (Z00.5)
  Review coding guidelines C.21.c.9 and C.21.c.16
+ **Z52.0** Blood donor
  + **Z52.00** Unspecified blood donor
    Z52.000 Unspecified donor, whole blood
    Z52.001 Unspecified donor, stem cells
    Z52.008 Unspecified donor, other blood
  + **Z52.01** Autologous blood donor
    Z52.010 Autologous donor, whole blood
    Z52.011 Autologous donor, stem cells
    Z52.018 Autologous donor, other blood
  + **Z52.09** Other blood donor
    Volunteer donor
    Z52.090 Other blood donor, whole blood
    Z52.091 Other blood donor, stem cells
    Z52.098 Other blood donor, other blood
+ **Z52.1** Skin donor
  Z52.10 Skin donor, unspecified
  Z52.11 Skin donor, autologous
  Z52.19 Skin donor, other
+ **Z52.2** Bone donor
  Z52.20 Bone donor, unspecified
  Z52.21 Bone donor, autologous
  Z52.29 Bone donor, other
  Z52.3 Bone marrow donor
  Z52.4 Kidney donor
  Z52.5 Cornea donor
  Z52.6 Liver donor
+ **Z52.8** Donor of other specified organs or tissues
  + **Z52.81** Egg (Oocyte) donor
    ♀ **Z52.810** Egg (Oocyte) donor under age 35, anonymous recipient
      Egg donor under age 35 NOS
    ♀ **Z52.811** Egg (Oocyte) donor under age 35, designated recipient

♀ **Z52.812** Egg (Oocyte) donor age 35 and over, anonymous recipient
Egg donor age 35 and over NOS
♀ **Z52.813** Egg (Oocyte) donor age 35 and over, designated recipient
♀ **Z52.819** Egg (Oocyte) donor, unspecified
Z52.89 Donor of other specified organs or tissues
Z52.9 Donor of unspecified organ or tissue
Donor NOS

Z53 Persons encountering health services for specific procedures and treatment, not carried out

+ **Z53.0** Procedure and treatment not carried out because of contraindication
  Z53.01 Procedure and treatment not carried out due to patient smoking
  Z53.09 Procedure and treatment not carried out because of other contraindication
Z53.1 Procedure and treatment not carried out because of patient's decision for reasons of belief and group pressure
+ **Z53.2** Procedure and treatment not carried out because of patient's decision for other and unspecified reasons
  Z53.20 Procedure and treatment not carried out because of patient's decision for unspecified reasons
  Z53.21 Procedure and treatment not carried out due to patient leaving prior to being seen by health care provider
  Z53.29 Procedure and treatment not carried out because of patient's decision for other reasons
+ **Z53.3** Procedure converted to open procedure
  AHA CC: 4Q, 2016, 79
  Z53.31 Laparoscopic surgical procedure converted to open procedure
  AHA CC: 4Q, 2016, 100-101
  Z53.32 Thoracoscopic surgical procedure converted to open procedure
  Z53.33 Arthroscopic surgical procedure converted to open procedure
  Z53.39 Other specified procedure converted to open procedure
Z53.8 Procedure and treatment not carried out for other reasons
Z53.9 Procedure and treatment not carried out, unspecified reason

Persons with potential health hazards related to socioeconomic and psychosocial circumstances (Z55-Z65)

AHA CC: 1Q, 2018, 18
Review coding guideline B.14

Z55 Problems related to education and literacy

Excludes1: disorders of psychological development (F80-F89)
Z55.0 Illiteracy and low-level literacy
Z55.1 Schooling unavailable and unattainable
Z55.2 Failed school examinations
Z55.3 Underachievement in school
Z55.4 Educational maladjustment and discord with teachers and classmates
Z55.5 Less than a high school diploma
No general equivalence degree (GED)
AHA CC: 4Q, 2021, 34-37
Z55.6 Problems related to health literacy
Difficulty understanding health related information
Difficulty understanding medication instructions
Problem completing medical forms
AHA CC: 1Q, 2023, 6
Z55.8 Other problems related to education and literacy
Problems related to inadequate teaching
Z55.9 Problems related to education and literacy, unspecified
Academic problems NOS

Z56 Problems related to employment and unemployment

Excludes2: occupational exposure to risk factors (Z57.-)
problems related to housing and economic circumstances (Z59.-)
Z56.0 Unemployment, unspecified
• **Z56.1** Change of job
Z56.2 Threat of job loss
Z56.3 Stressful work schedule
Z56.4 Discord with boss and workmates
Z56.5 Uncongenial work environment
Difficult conditions at work
Z56.6 Other physical and mental strain related to work
+ **Z56.8** Other problems related to employment
  Z56.81 Sexual harassment on the job
  Z56.82 Military deployment status
  Individual (civilian or military) currently deployed in theater or in support of military war, peacekeeping and humanitarian operations
  Z56.89 Other problems related to employment
Z56.9 Unspecified problems related to employment
Occupational problems NOS

Z57 Occupational exposure to risk factors

Z57.0 Occupational exposure to noise
Z57.1 Occupational exposure to radiation
Z57.2 Occupational exposure to dust
+ **Z57.3** Occupational exposure to other air contaminants
  Z57.31 Occupational exposure to environmental tobacco smoke
  Excludes2: exposure to environmental tobacco smoke (Z77.22)
  Z57.39 Occupational exposure to other air contaminants
Z57.4 Occupational exposure to toxic agents in agriculture
Occupational exposure to solids, liquids, gases or vapors in agriculture
Z57.5 Occupational exposure to toxic agents in other industries
Occupational exposure to solids, liquids, gases or vapors in other industries
Z57.6 Occupational exposure to extreme temperature
Z57.7 Occupational exposure to vibration
Z57.8 Occupational exposure to other risk factors
Z57.9 Occupational exposure to unspecified risk factor

Z58 Problems related to physical environment

AHA CC: 1Q, 2023, 6
Excludes2: occupational exposure (Z57.-)
Z58.6 Inadequate drinking-water supply
Lack of safe drinking water
Excludes2: deprivation of water (T73.1)
AHA CC: 4Q, 2021, 34-37
+ **Z58.8** Other problems related to physical environment
  Z58.81 Basic services unavailable in physical environment
  Unable to obtain internet service, due to unavailability in geographic area
  Unable to obtain telephone service, due to unavailability in geographic area
  Unable to obtain utilities, due to inadequate physical environment
  Z58.89 Other problems related to physical environment

Z59 Problems related to housing and economic circumstances

Excludes2: problems related to upbringing (Z62.-)
+ **Z59.0** Homelessness
  AHA CC: 4Q, 2017, 112-114; 4Q, 2021, 34-37
  Review coding guideline B.19.d
  CC **Z59.00** Homelessness unspecified
  CC **Z59.01** Sheltered homelessness
  Doubled up
  Living in a shelter such as: motel, scattered site housing, temporary or transitional living situation
  CC **Z59.02** Unsheltered homelessness
  Residing in place not meant for human inhabitation such as: abandoned buildings, cars, parks, sidewalk
  Residing on the street
+ **Z59.1** Inadequate housing
  Excludes1: problems related to the natural and physical environment (Z77.1-)
  AHA CC: 4Q, 2017, 112-114; 1Q, 2023, 6
  Review coding guideline B.19.d
  Z59.10 Inadequate housing, unspecified
  Inadequate housing NOS
  Z59.11 Inadequate housing environmental temperature
  Lack of air conditioning
  Lack of heating
  Z59.12 Inadequate housing utilities
  Lack of electricity services
  Lack of gas services
  Lack of oil services
  Lack of water services
  Excludes2: basic services unavailable in physical environment (Z58.81)

lack of adequate food (Z59.4-)
other problems related to housing and economic circumstances (Z59.8)

Z59.19 Other inadequate housing
  Pest infestation
  Restriction of space
  Technical defects in home preventing adequate care
  Unsatisfactory surroundings
Z59.2 Discord with neighbors, lodgers and landlord
Z59.3 Problems related to living in residential institution
  Boarding-school resident
  Excludes1: institutional upbringing (Z62.22)
+ **Z59.4 Lack of adequate food**
  Excludes2: deprivation of food (T73.0)
    effects of hunger (T73.0)
    inappropriate diet or eating habits (Z72.4)
    malnutrition (E40-E46)
  AHA CC: 4Q, 2021, 34-37
  Z59.41 Food insecurity
  Z59.48 Other specified lack of adequate food
    Inadequate food
    Lack of food
Z59.5 Extreme poverty
  AHA CC: 4Q, 2017, 112-114
  Review coding guideline B.19.d
Z59.6 Low income
Z59.7 Insufficient social insurance and welfare support
+ **Z59.8 Other problems related to housing and economic circumstances**
  AHA CC: 4Q, 2021, 34-37; 4Q, 2022, 52
  + **Z59.81 Housing instability, housed**
    Foreclosure on home loan
    Past due on rent or mortgage
    Unwanted multiple moves in the last 12 months
    Z59.811 Housing instability, housed, with risk of homelessness
      Imminent risk of homelessness
    Z59.812 Housing instability, housed, homelessness in past 12 months
    Z59.819 Housing instability, housed unspecified
      Excludes2: extreme poverty (Z59.5)
        financial security (Z59.86)
        low income (Z59.6)
        material hardship due to limited financial resources, not elsewhere classified (Z59.87)
  Z59.82 Transportation insecurity
    Excessive transportation time
    Inaccessible transportation
    Inadequate transportation
    Lack of transportation
    Unaffordable transportation
    Unreliable transportation
    Unsafe transportation
    Excludes2: unavailability and inaccessibility of healthcare facilities (Z75.3)
  Z59.86 Financial insecurity
    Bankruptcy
    Burdensome debt
    Economic strain
    Financial strain
    Money problems
    Running out of money
    Unable to make ends meet
    Excludes2: extreme poverty (Z59.5)
      low income (Z59.6)
      material hardship, not elsewhere classified (Z59.87)
  Z59.87 Material hardship due to limited financial resources, not elsewhere classified
    Material deprivation due to limited financial resources
    Unable to obtain adequate childcare due to limited financial resources
    Unable to obtain adequate clothing due to limited financial resources
    Unable to obtain adequate utilities due to limited financial resources
    Unable to obtain basic needs due to limited financial resources
    Excludes2: extreme poverty (Z59.5)

financial insecurity, not elsewhere classified (Z59.86)
low income (Z59.6)

  Z59.89 Other problems related to housing and economic circumstances
    Foreclosure on loan
    Isolated dwelling
    Problems with creditors
Z59.9 Problem related to housing and economic circumstances, unspecified

Z60 Problems related to social environment
  Z60.0 Problems of adjustment to life-cycle transitions
    Empty nest syndrome
    Phase of life problem
    Problem with adjustment to retirement [pension]
  Z60.2 Problems related to living alone
  Z60.3 Acculturation difficulty
    Problem with migration
    Problem with social transplantation
  Z60.4 Social exclusion and rejection
    Exclusion and rejection on the basis of personal characteristics, such as unusual physical appearance, illness or behavior.
    Social isolation
    Excludes1: target of adverse discrimination such as for racial or religious reasons (Z60.5)
  Z60.5 Target of (perceived) adverse discrimination and persecution
    Excludes1: social exclusion and rejection (Z60.4)
  Z60.8 Other problems related to social environment
    Inadequate social support
    Lack of emotional support
  Z60.9 Problem related to social environment, unspecified

Z62 Problems related to upbringing
  Includes: current and past negative life events in childhood
    current and past problems of a child related to upbringing
  Excludes2: maltreatment syndrome (T74.-)
    problems related to housing and economic circumstances (Z59.-)
  Z62.0 Inadequate parental supervision and control
  Z62.1 Parental overprotection
  + **Z62.2 Upbringing away from parents**
    Excludes1: problems with boarding school (Z59.3)
    • **Z62.21 Child in welfare custody**
      Child in foster care
      Child in welfare guardianship
    Z62.22 Institutional upbringing
      Child living in group home
      Child living in orphanage
      Code also, if applicable, child in welfare custody (Z62.21)
    Z62.23 Child in custody of non-parental relative
      Child in care of non-parental family member
      Child in custody of grandparent
      Child in kinship care
      Guardianship by non-parental relative
      Code also, if applicable, child in welfare custody (Z62.21)
    Z62.24 Child in custody of non-relative guardian
      Code also, if applicable, child in welfare custody (Z62.21)
    Z62.29 Other upbringing away from parents
  • **Z62.3 Hostility towards and scapegoating of child**
  Z62.6 Inappropriate (excessive) parental pressure
  + **Z62.8 Other specified problems related to upbringing**
    Code also, if applicable:
      absence of family member (Z63.3-)
      disappearance and death of family member (Z63.4)
      disruption of family by separation and divorce (Z63.5)
      other specified problems related to primary support group (Z63.8)
      other stressful life events affecting family and household (Z63.7-)
    + **Z62.81 Personal history of abuse in childhood**
      AHA CC: 1Q, 2023, 6
      Z62.810 Personal history of physical and sexual abuse in childhood
        Personal history of abuse in adolescence
        Excludes1: current child physical abuse (T74.12, T76.12)
          current child sexual abuse (T74.22, T76.22)

Z62.811 Personal history of psychological abuse in childhood
  Excludes1: current child psychological abuse (T74.32, T76.32)
Z62.812 Personal history of neglect in childhood
  Excludes1: current child neglect (T74.02, T76.02)
Z62.813 Personal history of forced labor or sexual exploitation in childhood
  AHA CC: 4Q, 2018, 32-33, 35
Z62.814 Personal history of child financial abuse
  Excludes1: current child financial abuse (T74.A2)
Z62.815 Personal history of intimate partner abuse in childhood
  Excludes2: adult and child abuse, neglect and other maltreatment, confirmed (T74-)
Z62.819 Personal history of unspecified abuse in childhood
  Excludes1: current child abuse NOS (T74.92, T76.92)

+ **Z62.82 Parent-child conflict**
  Z62.820 Parent-biological child conflict
    Parent-child problem NOS
  Z62.821 Parent-adopted child conflict
  Z62.822 Parent-foster child conflict
  Z62.823 Parent-step child conflict

+ **Z62.83 Non-parental relative or guardian-child conflict**
  Z62.831 Non-parental relative-child conflict
    Grandparent-child conflict
    Kinship-care child conflict
    Non-parental relative legal guardian-child conflict
    Other relative-child conflict
    Excludes1: group home staff-child conflict (Z62.833)
  Z62.832 Non-relative guardian-child conflict
    Excludes1: group home staff-child conflict (Z62.833)
  Z62.833 Group home staff-child conflict

+ **Z62.89 Other specified problems related to upbringing**
  Z62.890 Parent-child estrangement NEC
  Z62.891 Sibling rivalry
  Z62.892 Runaway [from current living environment]
    Child leaving living situation without permission
  Z62.898 Other specified problems related to upbringing

Z62.9 Problem related to upbringing, unspecified

Z63 Other problems related to primary support group, including family circumstances

Excludes2: maltreatment syndrome (T74.-, T76)
  parent-child problems (Z62.-)
  problems related to negative life events in childhood (Z62.-)
  problems related to upbringing (Z62.-)

Z63.0 Problems in relationship with spouse or partner
  Relationship distress with spouse or intimate partner
  Excludes1: counseling for spousal or partner abuse problems (Z69.1)
    counseling related to sexual attitude, behavior, and orientation (Z70.-)
Z63.1 Problems in relationship with in-laws
+ **Z63.3** Absence of family member
  Excludes1: absence of family member due to disappearance and death (Z63.4)
    absence of family member due to separation and divorce (Z63.5)
  Z63.31 Absence of family member due to military deployment
    Individual or family affected by other family member being on military deployment
    Excludes1: family disruption due to return of family member from military deployment (Z63.71)
  Z63.32 Other absence of family member

Z63.4 Disappearance and death of family member
  Assumed death of family member
  Bereavement
  AHA CC: 1Q, 2014, 25
Z63.5 Disruption of family by separation and divorce
  Marital estrangement
Z63.6 Dependent relative needing care at home
+ **Z63.7** Other stressful life events affecting family and household
  Z63.71 Stress on family due to return of family member from military deployment
    Individual or family affected by family member having returned from military deployment (current or past conflict)
  Z63.72 Alcoholism and drug addiction in family
  Z63.79 Other stressful life events affecting family and household
    Anxiety (normal) about sick person in family
    Health problems within family
    Ill or disturbed family member
    Isolated family
Z63.8 Other specified problems related to primary support group
  Family discord NOS
  Family estrangement NOS
  High expressed emotional level within family
  Inadequate family support NOS
  Inadequate or distorted communication within family
Z63.9 Problem related to primary support group, unspecified
  Relationship disorder NOS

Z64 Problems related to certain psychosocial circumstances

♀ **Z64.0** Problems related to unwanted pregnancy
♀ **Z64.1** Problems related to multiparity
Z64.4 Discord with counselors
  Discord with probation officer
  Discord with social worker

Z65 Problems related to other psychosocial circumstances

Z65.0 Conviction in civil and criminal proceedings without imprisonment
Z65.1 Imprisonment and other incarceration
Z65.2 Problems related to release from prison
Z65.3 Problems related to other legal circumstances
  Arrest
  Child custody or support proceedings
  Litigation
  Prosecution
Z65.4 Victim of crime and terrorism
  Victim of torture
Z65.5 Exposure to disaster, war and other hostilities
  Excludes1: target of perceived discrimination or persecution (Z60.5)
Z65.8 Other specified problems related to psychosocial circumstances
  At risk for feeling loneliness
  Religious or spiritual problem
Z65.9 Problem related to unspecified psychosocial circumstances

Do not resuscitate status (Z66)

Z66 Do not resuscitate
  DNR status
  Review coding guideline C.21.c.3
  Valid 3-character code, no further characters required

Blood type (Z67)

Z67 Blood type
  Review coding guideline C.21.c.3
  AHA CC: 3Q, 2015, 40
+ **Z67.1** Type A blood
  Z67.10 Type A blood, Rh positive
  Z67.11 Type A blood, Rh negative
+ **Z67.2** Type B blood
  Z67.20 Type B blood, Rh positive
  Z67.21 Type B blood, Rh negative
+ **Z67.3** Type AB blood
  Z67.30 Type AB blood, Rh positive
  Z67.31 Type AB blood, Rh negative
+ **Z67.4** Type O blood
  Z67.40 Type O blood, Rh positive
  Z67.41 Type O blood, Rh negative

+ **Z67.9** Unspecified blood type
  Z67.90 Unspecified blood type, Rh positive
  Z67.91 Unspecified blood type, Rh negative

Body mass index [BMI] (Z68)

Z68 Body mass index [BMI]
  Kilograms per meters squared
  NOTE BMI adult codes are for use for persons 20 years of age or older
  BMI pediatric codes are for use for persons 2-19 years of age. These percentiles are based on the growth charts published by the Centers for Disease Control and Prevention (CDC)
  Review coding guidelines B.14 and C.21.c.3
  AHA CC: 4Q, 2018, 77-83; 4Q, 2019, 19

- CC **Z68.1** Body mass index [BMI] 19.9 or less, adult
    AHA CC: 1Q, 2017, 39
+ **Z68.2** Body mass index [BMI] 20-29, adult
  - **Z68.20** Body mass index [BMI] 20.0-20.9, adult
  - **Z68.21** Body mass index [BMI] 21.0-21.9, adult
  - **Z68.22** Body mass index [BMI] 22.0-22.9, adult
  - **Z68.23** Body mass index [BMI] 23.0-23.9, adult
  - **Z68.24** Body mass index [BMI] 24.0-24.9, adult
  - **Z68.25** Body mass index [BMI] 25.0-25.9, adult
  - **Z68.26** Body mass index [BMI] 26.0-26.9, adult
  - **Z68.27** Body mass index [BMI] 27.0-27.9, adult
  - **Z68.28** Body mass index [BMI] 28.0-28.9, adult
  - **Z68.29** Body mass index [BMI] 29.0-29.9, adult
+ **Z68.3** Body mass index [BMI] 30-39, adult
  - **Z68.30** Body mass index [BMI] 30.0-30.9, adult
  - **Z68.31** Body mass index [BMI] 31.0-31.9, adult
  - **Z68.32** Body mass index [BMI] 32.0-32.9, adult
  - **Z68.33** Body mass index [BMI] 33.0-33.9, adult
  - **Z68.34** Body mass index [BMI] 34.0-34.9, adult
  - **Z68.35** Body mass index [BMI] 35.0-35.9, adult
    AHA CC: 3Q, 2022, 6-7
  - **Z68.36** Body mass index [BMI] 36.0-36.9, adult
  - **Z68.37** Body mass index [BMI] 37.0-37.9, adult
  - **Z68.38** Body mass index [BMI] 38.0-38.9, adult
  - **Z68.39** Body mass index [BMI] 39.0-39.9, adult
+ **Z68.4** Body mass index [BMI] 40 or greater, adult
  - CC **Z68.41** Body mass index [BMI] 40.0-44.9, adult
  - CC **Z68.42** Body mass index [BMI] 45.0-49.9, adult
  - CC **Z68.43** Body mass index [BMI] 50.0-59.9, adult
  - CC **Z68.44** Body mass index [BMI] 60.0-69.9, adult
  - CC **Z68.45** Body mass index [BMI] 70 or greater, adult
+ **Z68.5** Body mass index [BMI] pediatric
    AHA CC: 4Q, 2018, 81
  - **Z68.51** Body mass index [BMI] pediatric, less than 5th percentile for age
      AHA CC: 4Q, 2018, 82
  - **Z68.52** Body mass index [BMI] pediatric, 5th percentile to less than 85th percentile for age
  - **Z68.53** Body mass index [BMI] pediatric, 85th percentile to less than 95th percentile for age
  - **Z68.54** Body mass index [BMI] pediatric, greater than or equal to 95th percentile for age

Persons encountering health services in other circumstances (Z69-Z76)

Z69 Encounter for mental health services for victim and perpetrator of abuse

  Includes: counseling for victims and perpetrators of abuse
  Review coding guideline C.21.c.10

+ **Z69.0** Encounter for mental health services for child abuse problems
  + **Z69.01** Encounter for mental health services for parental child abuse
    - **Z69.010** Encounter for mental health services for victim of parental child abuse
        Encounter for mental health services for victim of child abuse by parent
        Encounter for mental health services for victim of child neglect by parent
        Encounter for mental health services for victim of child psychological abuse by parent
        Encounter for mental health services for victim of child sexual abuse by parent
    - **Z69.011** Encounter for mental health services for perpetrator of parental child abuse
        Encounter for mental health services for perpetrator of parental child neglect
        Encounter for mental health services for perpetrator of parental child psychological abuse
        Encounter for mental health services for perpetrator of parental child sexual abuse
      Excludes1: encounter for mental health services for non-parental child abuse (Z69.02-)
  + **Z69.02** Encounter for mental health services for non-parental child abuse
    - **Z69.020** Encounter for mental health services for victim of non-parental child abuse
        Encounter for mental health services for victim of non-parental child neglect
        Encounter for mental health services for victim of non-parental child psychological abuse
        Encounter for mental health services for victim of non-parental child sexual abuse
    - **Z69.021** Encounter for mental health services for perpetrator of non-parental child abuse
        Encounter for mental health services for perpetrator of non-parental child neglect
        Encounter for mental health services for perpetrator of non-parental child psychological abuse
        Encounter for mental health services for perpetrator of non-parental child sexual abuse
+ **Z69.1** Encounter for mental health services for spousal or partner abuse problems
  - **Z69.11** Encounter for mental health services for victim of spousal or partner abuse
      Encounter for mental health services for victim of spouse or partner neglect
      Encounter for mental health services for victim of spouse or partner psychological abuse
      Encounter for mental health services for victim of spouse or partner violence, physical
  - **Z69.12** Encounter for mental health services for perpetrator of spousal or partner abuse
      Encounter for mental health services for perpetrator of spouse or partner neglect
      Encounter for mental health services for perpetrator of spouse or partner psychological abuse
      Encounter for mental health services for perpetrator of spouse or partner violence, physical
+ **Z69.8** Encounter for mental health services for victim or perpetrator of other abuse
  - **Z69.81** Encounter for mental health services for victim of other abuse
      Encounter for mental health services for victim of non-spousal adult abuse
      Encounter for mental health services for victim of spouse or partner violence, sexual
      Encounter for rape victim counseling
  - **Z69.82** Encounter for mental health services for perpetrator of other abuse
      Encounter for mental health services for perpetrator of non-spousal adult abuse

Z70 Counseling related to sexual attitude, behavior and orientation
  Includes: encounter for mental health services for sexual attitude, behavior and orientation
  Excludes2: contraceptive or procreative counseling (Z30-Z31)
  Review coding guideline C.21.c.10

  Z70.0 Counseling related to sexual attitude
  Z70.1 Counseling related to patient's sexual behavior and orientation
      Patient concerned regarding impotence
      Patient concerned regarding non-responsiveness
      Patient concerned regarding promiscuity
      Patient concerned regarding sexual orientation

Z70.2 **Counseling related to sexual behavior and orientation of third party**
Advice sought regarding sexual behavior and orientation of child
Advice sought regarding sexual behavior and orientation of partner
Advice sought regarding sexual behavior and orientation of spouse

Z70.3 **Counseling related to combined concerns regarding sexual attitude, behavior and orientation**

Z70.8 **Other sex counseling**
Encounter for sex education

Z70.9 **Sex counseling, unspecified**

Z71 Persons encountering health services for other counseling and medical advice, not elsewhere classified

Excludes2: contraceptive or procreation counseling (Z30-Z31)
sex counseling (Z70.-)
Review coding guideline C.21.c.10

Z71.0 **Person encountering health services to consult on behalf of another person**
Person encountering health services to seek advice or treatment for non-attending third party
Excludes2: anxiety (normal) about sick person in family (Z63.7)
expectant (adoptive) parent(s) pre-birth pediatrician visit (Z76.81)

Z71.1 **Person with feared health complaint in whom no diagnosis is made**
Person encountering health services with feared condition which was not demonstrated
Person encountering health services in which problem was normal state
'Worried well'
Excludes1: medical observation for suspected diseases and conditions proven not to exist (Z03.-)
AHA CC: 4Q, 2016, 4-7

Z71.2 **Person consulting for explanation of examination or test findings**

Z71.3 **Dietary counseling and surveillance**
Use additional code for any associated underlying medical condition
Use additional code to identify body mass index (BMI), if known (Z68.-)

+ **Z71.4** **Alcohol abuse counseling and surveillance**
Use additional code for alcohol abuse or dependence (F10.-)

Z71.41 **Alcohol abuse counseling and surveillance of alcoholic**

Z71.42 **Counseling for family member of alcoholic**
Counseling for significant other, partner, or friend of alcoholic

+ **Z71.5** **Drug abuse counseling and surveillance**
Use additional code for drug abuse or dependence (F11-F16, F18-F19)

Z71.51 **Drug abuse counseling and surveillance of drug abuser**

Z71.52 **Counseling for family member of drug abuser**
Counseling for significant other, partner, or friend of drug abuser

Z71.6 **Tobacco abuse counseling**
Use additional code for nicotine dependence (F17.-)

Z71.7 **Human immunodeficiency virus [HIV] counseling**
Review coding guideline C.1.a.2.h

+ **Z71.8** **Other specified counseling**
Excludes2: counseling for contraception (Z30.0-)

Z71.81 **Spiritual or religious counseling**

Z71.82 **Exercise counseling**
AHA CC: 4Q, 2017, 27

Z71.83 **Encounter for nonprocreative genetic counseling**
Exludes1: counseling for procreative genetics (Z31.5)
counseling for procreative management (Z31.6)
AHA CC: 4Q, 2017, 27

Z71.84 **Encounter for health counseling related to travel**
Encounter for health risk and safety counseling for (international) travel
Code also, if applicable, encounter for immunization (Z23)
Excludes2: encounter for administrative examination (Z02.-)
encounter for other special examination without complaint, suspected or reported diagnosis (Z01.-)
AHA CC: 4Q, 2019, 20

Z71.85 **Encounter for immunization safety counseling**
Encounter for vaccine product safety counseling
Code also, if applicable, encounter for immunization (Z23)
Code also, if applicable, immunization not carried out (Z28.-)
Excludes1: encounter for health counseling related to travel (Z71.84)
AHA CC: 4Q, 2021, 34

Z71.87 **Encounter for pediatric-to-adult transition counseling**
Code also chronic condition, if applicable, such as:
autism spectrum disorder (F84.0)
congenital malformations of the circulatory system (Q20-Q28)
cystic fibrosis (E84.-)
sickle-cell disorder (D57-)
AHA CC: 4Q, 2022, 51

Z71.88 **Encounter for counseling for socioeconomic factors**
AHA CC: 4Q, 2022, 51

Z71.89 **Other specified counseling**

Z71.9 **Counseling, unspecified**
Encounter for medical advice NOS

Z72 Problems related to lifestyle

Excludes2: problems related to life-management difficulty (Z73.-)
problems related to socioeconomic and psychosocial circumstances (Z55-Z65)
Review coding guideline C.21.c.14

Z72.0 **Tobacco use**
Tobacco use NOS
Excludes1: history of tobacco dependence (Z87.891)
nicotine dependence (F17.2-)
tobacco dependence (F17.2-)
tobacco use during pregnancy (O99.33-)
Review coding guideline C.15.l.2

Z72.3 **Lack of physical exercise**

Z72.4 **Inappropriate diet and eating habits**
Excludes1: behavioral eating disorders of infancy or childhood (F98.2-F98.3)
eating disorders (F50.-)
lack of adequate food (Z59.48)
malnutrition and other nutritional deficiencies (E40-E64)

+ **Z72.5** **High risk sexual behavior**
Promiscuity
Excludes1: paraphilias (F65)

Z72.51 **High risk heterosexual behavior**

Z72.52 **High risk homosexual behavior**

Z72.53 **High risk bisexual behavior**

Z72.6 **Gambling and betting**
Excludes1: compulsive or pathological gambling (F63.0)

+ **Z72.8** **Other problems related to lifestyle**

+ **Z72.81** **Antisocial behavior**
Excludes1: conduct disorders (F91.-)

• **Z72.810** **Child and adolescent antisocial behavior**
Antisocial behavior (child) (adolescent) without manifest psychiatric disorder
Delinquency NOS
Group delinquency
Offenses in the context of gang membership
Stealing in company with others
Truancy from school

• **Z72.811** **Adult antisocial behavior**
Adult antisocial behavior without manifest psychiatric disorder

+ **Z72.82** Problems related to sleep
    Z72.820 Sleep deprivation
        Lack of adequate sleep
        Excludes1: insomnia (G47.0-)
    Z72.821 Inadequate sleep hygiene
        Bad sleep habits
        Irregular sleep habits
        Unhealthy sleep wake schedule
        Excludes1: insomnia (F51.0-, G47.0-)
    Z72.823 Risk of suffocation (smothering) under another while sleeping
        Child-caregiver co-sleeping
        Infant bed-sharing
        AHA CC: 4Q, 2022, 51
  Z72.89 Other problems related to lifestyle
    Self-damaging behavior
  Z72.9 Problem related to lifestyle, unspecified

Z73 Problems related to life management difficulty
  Excludes2: problems related to socioeconomic and psychosocial circumstances (Z55-Z65)
  Z73.0 Burn-out
  Z73.1 Type A behavior pattern
  Z73.2 Lack of relaxation and leisure
  Z73.3 Stress, not elsewhere classified
    Physical and mental strain NOS
    Excludes1: stress related to employment or unemployment (Z56.-)
  Z73.4 Inadequate social skills, not elsewhere classified
  Z73.5 Social role conflict, not elsewhere classified
  Z73.6 Limitation of activities due to disability
    Excludes1: care-provider dependency (Z74.-)
+ **Z73.8** Other problems related to life management difficulty
  + **Z73.81** Behavioral insomnia of childhood
    • **Z73.810** Behavioral insomnia of childhood, sleep-onset association type
    • **Z73.811** Behavioral insomnia of childhood, limit setting type
    • **Z73.812** Behavioral insomnia of childhood, combined type
    • **Z73.819** Behavioral insomnia of childhood, unspecified type
  Z73.82 Dual sensory impairment
  Z73.89 Other problems related to life management difficulty
  Z73.9 Problem related to life management difficulty, unspecified

Z74 Problems related to care provider dependency
  Excludes2: dependence on enabling machines or devices NEC (Z99.-)
+ **Z74.0** Reduced mobility
  Z74.01 Bed confinement status
    Bedridden
    Review coding guideline C.21.c.3
  Z74.09 Other reduced mobility
    Chairridden
    Reduced mobility NOS
    Excludes2: wheelchair dependence (Z99.3)
  Z74.1 Need for assistance with personal care
  Z74.2 Need for assistance at home and no other household member able to render care
  Z74.3 Need for continuous supervision
  Z74.8 Other problems related to care provider dependency
  Z74.9 Problem related to care provider dependency, unspecified

Z75 Problems related to medical facilities and other health care
  Z75.0 Medical services not available in home
    Excludes1: no other household member able to render care (Z74.2)
  Z75.1 Person awaiting admission to adequate facility elsewhere
    AHA CC: 4Q, 2017, 112-114
    Review coding guideline B.19.d
  Z75.2 Other waiting period for investigation and treatment
  Z75.3 Unavailability and inaccessibility of health-care facilities
    Excludes1: bed unavailable (Z75.1)
    AHA CC: 4Q, 2017, 112-114
    Review coding guideline B.19.d
  Z75.4 Unavailability and inaccessibility of other helping agencies
    AHA CC: 4Q, 2017, 112-114
    Review coding guideline B.19.d
  Z75.5 Holiday relief care

Z75.8 Other problems related to medical facilities and other health care
Z75.9 Unspecified problem related to medical facilities and other health care

Z76 Persons encountering health services in other circumstances
  Z76.0 Encounter for issue of repeat prescription
    Encounter for issue of repeat prescription for appliance
    Encounter for issue of repeat prescription for medicaments
    Encounter for issue of repeat prescription for spectacles
    Excludes2: issue of medical certificate (Z02.7)
        repeat prescription for contraceptive (Z30.4-)
  Z76.1 Encounter for health supervision and care of foundling
    Review coding guidelines C.21.c.12 and C.21.c.16
• **Z76.2** Encounter for health supervision and care of other healthy infant and child
    Encounter for medical or nursing care or supervision of healthy infant under circumstances such as adverse socioeconomic conditions at home
    Encounter for medical or nursing care or supervision of healthy infant under circumstances such as awaiting foster or adoptive placement
    Encounter for medical or nursing care or supervision of healthy infant under circumstances such as maternal illness
    Encounter for medical or nursing care or supervision of healthy infant under circumstances such as number of children at home preventing or interfering with normal care
    AHA CC: 4Q, 2017, 112-114
    Review coding guidelines B.19.d and C.21.c.16
  Z76.3 Healthy person accompanying sick person
  Z76.4 Other boarder to healthcare facility
    Excludes1: homelessness (Z59.0-)
  Z76.5 Malingerer [conscious simulation]
    Person feigning illness (with obvious motivation)
    Excludes1: factitious disorder (F68.1-, F68.A)
        peregrinating patient (F68.1-)
+ **Z76.8** Persons encountering health services in other specified circumstances
  Z76.81 Expectant parent(s) prebirth pediatrician visit
    Pre-adoption pediatrician visit for adoptive parent(s)
    Review coding guideline C.21.c.10
  Z76.82 Awaiting organ transplant status
    Patient waiting for organ availability
    Review coding guideline C.21.c.3
  Z76.89 Persons encountering health services in other specified circumstances
    Persons encountering health services NOS
    AHA CC: 2Q, 2014, 10

Persons with potential health hazards related to family and personal history and certain conditions influencing health status (Z77-Z99)

Code also any follow-up examination (Z08-Z09)

Z77 Other contact with and (suspected) exposures hazardous to health
  Includes: contact with and (suspected) exposures to potential hazards to health
  Excludes2: contact with and (suspected) exposure to communicable diseases (Z20.-)
    exposure to (parental) (environmental) tobacco smoke in the perinatal period (P96.81)
    newborn affected by noxious substances transmitted via placenta or breast milk (P04.-)
    occupational exposure to risk factors (Z57.-)
    retained foreign body (Z18.-)
    retained foreign body fully removed (Z87.821)
    toxic effects of substances chiefly nonmedicinal as to source (T51-T65)
  Review coding guideline C.21.c.1
+ **Z77.0** Contact with and (suspected) exposure to hazardous, chiefly nonmedicinal, chemicals
  + **Z77.01** Contact with and (suspected) exposure to hazardous metals
    Z77.010 Contact with and (suspected) exposure to arsenic
    Z77.011 Contact with and (suspected) exposure to lead

Z77.012 Contact with and (suspected) exposure to uranium
  Excludes1: retained depleted uranium fragments (Z18.01)
Z77.018 Contact with and (suspected) exposure to other hazardous metals
  Contact with and (suspected) exposure to chromium compounds
  Contact with and (suspected) exposure to nickel dust

+ **Z77.02** Contact with and (suspected) exposure to hazardous aromatic compounds
  Z77.020 Contact with and (suspected) exposure to aromatic amines
  Z77.021 Contact with and (suspected) exposure to benzene
  Z77.028 Contact with and (suspected) exposure to other hazardous aromatic compounds
    Aromatic dyes NOS
    Polycyclic aromatic hydrocarbons

+ **Z77.09** Contact with and (suspected) exposure to other hazardous, chiefly nonmedicinal, chemicals
  Z77.090 Contact with and (suspected) exposure to asbestos
  Z77.098 Contact with and (suspected) exposure to other hazardous, chiefly nonmedicinal, chemicals
    Dyes NOS

+ **Z77.1** Contact with and (suspected) exposure to environmental pollution and hazards in the physical environment
  + **Z77.11** Contact with and (suspected) exposure to environmental pollution
    Z77.110 Contact with and (suspected) exposure to air pollution
    Z77.111 Contact with and (suspected) exposure to water pollution
    Z77.112 Contact with and (suspected) exposure to soil pollution
    Z77.118 Contact with and (suspected) exposure to other environmental pollution
  + **Z77.12** Contact with and (suspected) exposure to hazards in the physical environment
    Z77.120 Contact with and (suspected) exposure to mold (toxic)
    Z77.121 Contact with and (suspected) exposure to harmful algae and algae toxins
      Contact with and (suspected) exposure to (harmful) algae bloom NOS
      Contact with and (suspected) exposure to blue-green algae bloom
      Contact with and (suspected) exposure to brown tide
      Contact with and (suspected) exposure to cyanobacteria bloom
      Contact with and (suspected) exposure to Florida red tide
      Contact with and (suspected) exposure to pfiesteria piscicida
      Contact with and (suspected) exposure to red tide
    Z77.122 Contact with and (suspected) exposure to noise
    Z77.123 Contact with and (suspected) exposure to radon and other naturally occurring radiation
      Excludes2: radiation exposure as the cause of a confirmed condition (W88-W90, X39.0-)
        radiation sickness NOS (T66)
    Z77.128 Contact with and (suspected) exposure to other hazards in the physical environment

+ **Z77.2** Contact with and (suspected) exposure to other hazardous substances
  Z77.21 Contact with and (suspected) exposure to potentially hazardous body fluids
  Z77.22 Contact with and (suspected) exposure to environmental tobacco smoke (acute) (chronic)
    Exposure to second hand tobacco smoke (acute) (chronic)
    Passive smoking (acute) (chronic)
    Excludes1: nicotine dependence (F17.-)
      tobacco use (Z72.0)
    Excludes2: occupational exposure to environmental tobacco smoke (Z57.31)
  Z77.29 Contact with and (suspected) exposure to other hazardous substances
    AHA CC: 2Q, 2016, 34

Z77.9 Other contact with and (suspected) exposures hazardous to health

Z78 Other specified health status
  Excludes2: asymptomatic human immunodeficiency virus [HIV] infection status (Z21)
    postprocedural status (Z93-Z99)
    sex reassignment status (Z87.890)
  Review coding guideline C.21.c.3
• ♀ **Z78.0** Asymptomatic menopausal state
    Menopausal state NOS
    Postmenopausal status NOS
    Excludes2: symptomatic menopausal state (N95.1)
  Z78.1 Physical restraint status
    Excludes1: physical restraint due to a procedure - omit code
  Z78.9 Other specified health status

Z79 Long term (current) drug therapy
  Includes: long term (current) drug use for prophylactic purposes
  Code also any therapeutic drug level monitoring (Z51.81)
  Excludes2: drug abuse and dependence (F11-F19)
    drug use complicating pregnancy, childbirth, and the puerperium (O99.32-)
  AHA CC: 1Q, 2021, 12-13
  Review coding guideline C.21.c.3
+ **Z79.0** Long term (current) use of anticoagulants and antithrombotics/antiplatelets
    Excludes2: long term (current) use of aspirin (Z79.82)
  Z79.01 Long term (current) use of anticoagulants
    AHA CC: 2Q, 2020, 20-21; 1Q, 2021, 4-5; 2Q, 2022, 17; 2Q, 2023, 28
  Z79.02 Long term (current) use of antithrombotics/antiplatelets
  Z79.1 Long term (current) use of non-steroidal anti-inflammatories (NSAID)
    Excludes2: long term (current) use of aspirin (Z79.82)
  Z79.2 Long term (current) use of antibiotics
  Z79.3 Long term (current) use of hormonal contraceptives
    Long term (current) use of birth control pill or patch
  Z79.4 Long term (current) use of insulin
    Excludes2: long-term (current) use of injectable non-insulin antidiabetic drugs (Z79.85)
      long term (current) use of oral antidiabetic drugs (Z79.84)
      long term (current) use of oral hypoglycemic drugs (Z79.84)
    AHA CC: 3Q, 2020, 31
    Review coding guidelines C.4.a.3 and C.4.a.6
    Review coding guidelines C.15.h and C.15.i
+ **Z79.5** Long term (current) use of steroids
  Z79.51 Long term (current) use of inhaled steroids
  Z79.52 Long term (current) use of systemic steroids
+ **Z79.6** Long term (current) use of immunomodulators and immunosuppressants
    Excludes2: long term (current) use of steroids (Z79.5-)
      long term (current) use of agents affecting estrogen receptors and estrogen levels (Z79.81-)
    AHA CC: 4Q, 2022, 50
  Z79.60 Long term (current) use of unspecified immunomodulators and immunosuppressants

Z79.61 Long term (current) use of immunomodulator
　Long term (current) use of apremilast
　Long term (current) use of immunomodulatory imide drug
　Long term (current) use of lenalidomide
　Long term (current) use of pomalidomide

+ **Z79.62** Long term (current) use of immunosuppressant
　Z79.620 Long term (current) use of immunosuppressive biologic
　　Long term (current) use of adalimumab
　　Long term (current) use of etanercept
　　Long term (current) use of infliximab
　　Long term (current) use of monoclonal antibodies
　Z79.621 Long term (current) use of calcineurin inhibitor
　　Long term (current) use of cyclosporine
　　Long term (current) use of tacrolimus
　Z79.622 Long term (current) use of Janus kinase inhibitor
　　Long term (current) use of tofacitinib
　Z79.623 Long term (current) use of mammalian target of rapamycin (mTOR) inhibitor
　　Long term (current) use of sirolimus
　Z79.624 Long term (current) use of inhibitors of nucleotide synthesis
　　Long term (current) use of azathioprine
　　Long term (current) use omycophenolate
　　Long term (current) use of purine synthesis (IMDH) inhibitors

+ **Z79.63** Long term (current) use of chemotherapeutic agent
　Z79.630 Long term (current) use of alkylating agent
　　Long term (current) use of chlorambucil
　　Long term (current) use of cisplatin
　　Long term (current) use of cyclophosphamide
　Z79.631 Long term (current) use of antimetabolite agent
　　Long term (current) use of 5-fluorouracil
　　Long term (current) use of 6-mercaptopurine
　　Long term (current) use of cytarabine
　　Long term (current) use of methotrexate
　Z79.632 Long term (current) use of antitumor antibiotic
　　Long term (current) use of bleomycin
　　Long term (current) use of doxorubicin
　　Long term (current) use of mitomycin C
　Z79.633 Long term (current) use of mitotic inhibitor
　　Long term (current) use of paclitaxel
　　Long term (current) use of plant alkaloids
　　Long term (current) use of vinblastine
　　Long term (current) use of vincristine
　Z79.634 Long term (current) use of topoisomerase inhibitor
　　Long term (current) use of etoposide
　　Long term (current) use of irinotecan
　　Long term (current) use of topotecan

Z79.64 Long term (current) use of myelosuppressive agent
　Long term (current) use of hydroxyurea

Z79.69 Long term (current) use of other immunomodulators and immunosuppressants

+ **Z79.8** Other long term (current) drug therapy
+ **Z79.81** Long term (current) use of agents affecting estrogen receptors and estrogen levels
　Code first if applicable:
　malignant neoplasm of breast (C50.-)
　malignant neoplasm of prostate (C61)

　Use additional code, if applicable, to identify:
　estrogen receptor positive status (Z17.0)
　family history of breast cancer (Z80.3)
　genetic susceptibility to malignant neoplasm (cancer) (Z15.0-)
　personal history of breast cancer (Z85.3)
　personal history of prostate cancer (Z85.46)
　postmenopausal status (Z78.0)
　Excludes1: hormone replacement therapy (Z79.890)

　Z79.810 Long term (current) use of selective estrogen receptor modulators (SERMs)
　　Long term (current) use of raloxifene (Evista)
　　Long term (current) use of tamoxifen (Nolvadex)
　　Long term (current) use of toremifene (Fareston)
　　AHA CC: 3Q, 2022, 14-15
　Z79.811 Long term (current) use of aromatase inhibitors
　　Long term (current) use of anastrozole (Arimidex)
　　Long term (current) use of exemestane (Aromasin)
　　Long term (current) use of letrozole (Femara)
　Z79.818 Long term (current) use of other agents affecting estrogen receptors and estrogen levels
　　Long term (current) use of estrogen receptor downregulators
　　Long term (current) use of fulvestrant (Faslodex)
　　Long term (current) use of gonadotropin-releasing hormone (GnRH) agonist
　　Long term (current) use of goserelin acetate (Zoladex)
　　Long term (current) use of leuprolide acetate (leuprorelin) (Lupron)
　　Long term (current) use of megestrol acetate (Megace)

Z79.82 Long term (current) use of aspirin
Z79.83 Long term (current) use of bisphosphonates
　AHA CC: 4Q, 2016, 21
Z79.84 Long term (current) use of oral hypoglycemic drugs
　Long term (current) use of oral antidiabetic drugs
　Excludes2: long-term (current) use of injectable non-insulin antidiabetic drugs (Z79.85)
　　long term (current) use of insulin (Z79.4)
　Review coding guidelines C.4.a.e and C.4.a.6
　Review coding guidelines C.15.h and C.15.i
　AHA CC: 4Q, 2016, 76; 3Q, 2020, 31
Z79.85 Long-term (current) use of injectable non-insulin antidiabetic drugs
　Excludes2: long term (current) use of insulin (Z79.4)
　　long term (current) use of oral hypoglycemic drugs (Z79.84)

+ **Z79.89** Other long term (current) drug therapy
　Z79.890 Hormone replacement therapy
　Z79.891 Long term (current) use of opiate analgesic
　　Long term (current) use of methadone for pain management
　　Excludes1: methodone use NOS (F11.9-)
　　　use of methodone for treatment of heroin addiction (F11.2-)
　Z79.899 Other long term (current) drug therapy
　　AHA CC: 3Q, 2015, 21-22; 4Q, 2015, 34; 2Q, 2020, 14-15; 3Q, 2020, 31; 4Q, 2020, 11-12
　　Review coding guideline C.4.a.3

Z80 Family history of primary malignant neoplasm
　Review coding guideline C.21.c.4
Z80.0 Family history of malignant neoplasm of digestive organs
　Conditions classifiable to C15-C26
　AHA CC: 1Q, 2018, 6-7
Z80.1 Family history of malignant neoplasm of trachea, bronchus and lung
　Conditions classifiable to C33-C34
Z80.2 Family history of malignant neoplasm of other respiratory and intrathoracic organs
　Conditions classifiable to C30-C32, C37-C39
Z80.3 Family history of malignant neoplasm of breast
　Conditions classifiable to C50.-

+ **Z80.4** Family history of malignant neoplasm of genital organs
　Conditions classifiable to C51-C63
　Z80.41 Family history of malignant neoplasm of ovary
　Z80.42 Family history of malignant neoplasm of prostate
　Z80.43 Family history of malignant neoplasm of testis
　Z80.49 Family history of malignant neoplasm of other genital organs

- **Z80.5** **Family history of malignant neoplasm of urinary tract**
    Conditions classifiable to C64-C68
    - **Z80.51** Family history of malignant neoplasm of kidney
    - **Z80.52** Family history of malignant neoplasm of bladder
    - **Z80.59** Family history of malignant neoplasm of other urinary tract organ
- **Z80.6** **Family history of leukemia**
    Conditions classifiable to C91-C95
- **Z80.7** **Family history of other malignant neoplasms of lymphoid, hematopoietic and related tissues**
    Conditions classifiable to C81-C90, C96.-
- **Z80.8** **Family history of malignant neoplasm of other organs or systems**
    Conditions classifiable to C00-C14, C40-C49, C69-C79
- **Z80.9** **Family history of malignant neoplasm, unspecified**
    Conditions classifiable to C80.1

Z81 Family history of mental and behavioral disorders
Review coding guideline C.21.c.4
- **Z81.0** **Family history of intellectual disabilities**
    Conditions classifiable to F70-F79
- **Z81.1** **Family history of alcohol abuse and dependence**
    Conditions classifiable to F10.-
- **Z81.2** **Family history of tobacco abuse and dependence**
    Conditions classifiable to F17.-
- **Z81.3** **Family history of other psychoactive substance abuse and dependence**
    Conditions classifiable to F11-F16, F18-F19
- **Z81.4** **Family history of other substance abuse and dependence**
    Conditions classifiable to F55
- **Z81.8** **Family history of other mental and behavioral disorders**
    Conditions classifiable elsewhere in F01-F99

Z82 Family history of certain disabilities and chronic diseases (leading to disablement)
Review coding guideline C.21.c.4
- **Z82.0** **Family history of epilepsy and other diseases of the nervous system**
    Conditions classifiable to G00-G99
- **Z82.1** **Family history of blindness and visual loss**
    Conditions classifiable to H54.-
- **Z82.2** **Family history of deafness and hearing loss**
    Conditions classifiable to H90-H91
- **Z82.3** **Family history of stroke**
    Conditions classifiable to I60-I64
- + **Z82.4** **Family history of ischemic heart disease and other diseases of the circulatory system**
    Conditions classifiable to I00-I5A, I65-I99
    - **Z82.41** Family history of sudden cardiac death
    - **Z82.49** Family history of ischemic heart disease and other diseases of the circulatory system
- **Z82.5** **Family history of asthma and other chronic lower respiratory diseases**
    Conditions classifiable to J40-J47
    Excludes2: family history of other diseases of the respiratory system (Z83.6)
- + **Z82.6** **Family history of arthritis and other diseases of the musculoskeletal system and connective tissue**
    Conditions classifiable to M00-M99
    - **Z82.61** Family history of arthritis
    - **Z82.62** Family history of osteoporosis
    - **Z82.69** Family history of other diseases of the musculoskeletal system and connective tissue
- + **Z82.7** **Family history of congenital malformations, deformations and chromosomal abnormalities**
    Conditions classifiable to Q00-Q99
    - **Z82.71** Family history of polycystic kidney
    - **Z82.79** Family history of other congenital malformations, deformations and chromosomal abnormalities
- **Z82.8** **Family history of other disabilities and chronic diseases leading to disablement, not elsewhere classified**

Z83 Family history of other specific disorders
Excludes2: contact with and (suspected) exposure to communicable disease in the family (Z20.-)
Review coding guideline C.21.c.4
- **Z83.0** **Family history of human immunodeficiency virus [HIV] disease**
    Conditions classifiable to B20
- **Z83.1** **Family history of other infectious and parasitic diseases**
    Conditions classifiable to A00-B19, B25-B94, B99
- **Z83.2** **Family history of diseases of the blood and blood-forming organs and certain disorders involving the immune mechanism**
    Conditions classifiable to D50-D89
- **Z83.3** **Family history of diabetes mellitus**
    Conditions classifiable to E08-E13
- + **Z83.4** **Family history of other endocrine, nutritional and metabolic diseases**
    Conditions classifiable to E00-E07, E15-E88
    - **Z83.41** Family history of multiple endocrine neoplasia [MEN] syndrome
    - **Z83.42** Family history of familial hypercholesterolemia
        AHA CC: 4Q, 2016, 77
    - + **Z83.43** Family history of other disorder of lipoprotein metabolism and other lipidemias
        AHA CC: 4Q, 2018, 6
        - **Z83.430** Family history of elevated lipoprotein(a)
            Family history of elevated Lp(a)
        - **Z83.438** Family history of other disorder of lipoprotein metabolism and other lipidemia
            Family history of familial combined hyperlipidemia
    - **Z83.49** Family history of other endocrine, nutritional and metabolic diseases
- + **Z83.5** **Family history of eye and ear disorders**
    - + **Z83.51** Family history of eye disorders
        Conditions classifiable to H00-H53, H55-H59
        Excludes2: family history of blindness and visual loss (Z82.1)
        - **Z83.511** Family history of glaucoma
        - **Z83.518** Family history of other specified eye disorder
    - **Z83.52** Family history of ear disorders
        Conditions classifiable to H60-H83, H92-H95
        Excludes2: family history of deafness and hearing loss (Z82.2)
- **Z83.6** **Family history of other diseases of the respiratory system**
    Conditions classifiable to J00-J39, J60-J99
    Excludes2: family history of asthma and other chronic lower respiratory diseases (Z82.5)
- + **Z83.7** **Family history of diseases of the digestive system**
    Conditions classifiable to D12, K00-K93
    - + **Z83.71** Family history of colonic polyps
        Excludes2: family history of malignant neoplasm of digestive organs (Z80.0)
        AHA CC: 1Q, 2021, 14-15
        - **Z83.710** Family history of adenomatous and serrated polyps
            Conditions classifiable to D12.-
            Family history of tubular adenoma polyps
            Family history of tubulovillous adenoma polyps
            Family history of villous adenoma polyps
        - **Z83.711** Family history of hyperplastic colon polyps
        - **Z83.718** Other family history of colon polyps
            Family history of inflammatory colon polyps
        - **Z83.719** Family history of colon polyps, unspecified
            Family history of colon polyps NOS
    - **Z83.79** Family history of other diseases of the digestive system

Z84 Family history of other conditions
Review coding guideline C.21.c.4
- **Z84.0** **Family history of diseases of the skin and subcutaneous tissue**
    Conditions classifiable to L00-L99
- **Z84.1** **Family history of disorders of kidney and ureter**
    Conditions classifiable to N00-N29
- **Z84.2** **Family history of other diseases of the genitourinary system**
    Conditions classifiable to N30-N99
- **Z84.3** **Family history of consanguinity**
- + **Z84.8** **Family history of other specified conditions**
    - **Z84.81** Family history of carrier of genetic disease
        AHA CC: 1Q, 2021, 14-15
    - **Z84.82** Family history of sudden infant death syndrome
        Family history of SIDS
        AHA CC: 4Q, 2016, 77
    - **Z84.89** Family history of other specified conditions

Z85 Personal history of malignant neoplasm

Code first any follow-up examination after treatment of malignant neoplasm (Z08)
Use additional code to identify:
alcohol use and dependence (F10.-)
exposure to environmental tobacco smoke (Z77.22)
history of tobacco dependence (Z87.891)
occupational exposure to environmental tobacco smoke (Z57.31)
tobacco dependence (F17.-)
tobacco use (Z72.0)

Excludes2: personal history of benign neoplasm (Z86.01-)
personal history of carcinoma-in-situ (Z86.00-)
Review coding guidelines C.2.d and C.2.m
Review coding guideline C.21.c.4

- **Z85.0** Personal history of malignant neoplasm of digestive organs
  - **Z85.00** Personal history of malignant neoplasm of unspecified digestive organ
  - **Z85.01** Personal history of malignant neoplasm of esophagus
    Conditions classifiable to C15
  - **Z85.02** Personal history of malignant neoplasm of stomach
    - **Z85.020** Personal history of malignant carcinoid tumor of stomach
      Conditions classifiable to C7A.092
    - **Z85.028** Personal history of other malignant neoplasm of stomach
      Conditions classifiable to C16
  - **Z85.03** Personal history of malignant neoplasm of large intestine
    - **Z85.030** Personal history of malignant carcinoid tumor of large intestine
      Conditions classifiable to C7A.022-C7A.025, C7A.029
    - **Z85.038** Personal history of other malignant neoplasm of large intestine
      Conditions classifiable to C18
  - **Z85.04** Personal history of malignant neoplasm of rectum, rectosigmoid junction, and anus
    - **Z85.040** Personal history of malignant carcinoid tumor of rectum
      Conditions classifiable to C7A.026
    - **Z85.048** Personal history of other malignant neoplasm of rectum, rectosigmoid junction, and anus
      Conditions classifiable to C19-C21
  - **Z85.05** Personal history of malignant neoplasm of liver
    Conditions classifiable to C22
  - **Z85.06** Personal history of malignant neoplasm of small intestine
    - **Z85.060** Personal history of malignant carcinoid tumor of small intestine
      Conditions classifiable to C7A.01-
    - **Z85.068** Personal history of other malignant neoplasm of small intestine
      Conditions classifiable to C17
  - **Z85.07** Personal history of malignant neoplasm of pancreas
    Conditions classifiable to C25
  - **Z85.09** Personal history of malignant neoplasm of other digestive organs
- **Z85.1** Personal history of malignant neoplasm of trachea, bronchus and lung
  - **Z85.11** Personal history of malignant neoplasm of bronchus and lung
    - **Z85.110** Personal history of malignant carcinoid tumor of bronchus and lung
      Conditions classifiable to C7A.090
    - **Z85.118** Personal history of other malignant neoplasm of bronchus and lung
      Conditions classifiable to C34
  - **Z85.12** Personal history of malignant neoplasm of trachea
    Conditions classifiable to C33
- **Z85.2** Personal history of malignant neoplasm of other respiratory and intrathoracic organs
  - **Z85.20** Personal history of malignant neoplasm of unspecified respiratory organ
  - **Z85.21** Personal history of malignant neoplasm of larynx
    Conditions classifiable to C32
  - **Z85.22** Personal history of malignant neoplasm of nasal cavities, middle ear, and accessory sinuses
    Conditions classifiable to C30-C31
  - **Z85.23** Personal history of malignant neoplasm of thymus
    - **Z85.230** Personal history of malignant carcinoid tumor of thymus
      Conditions classifiable to C7A.091
    - **Z85.238** Personal history of other malignant neoplasm of thymus
      Conditions classifiable to C37
  - **Z85.29** Personal history of malignant neoplasm of other respiratory and intrathoracic organs
- **Z85.3** Personal history of malignant neoplasm of breast
  Conditions classifiable to C50.-
  AHA CC: 3Q, 2020, 30
- **Z85.4** Personal history of malignant neoplasm of genital organs
  Conditions classifiable to C51-C63
  - ♀ **Z85.40** Personal history of malignant neoplasm of unspecified female genital organ
  - ♀ **Z85.41** Personal history of malignant neoplasm of cervix uteri
  - ♀ **Z85.42** Personal history of malignant neoplasm of other parts of uterus
  - ♀ **Z85.43** Personal history of malignant neoplasm of ovary
  - ♀ **Z85.44** Personal history of malignant neoplasm of other female genital organs
  - ♂ **Z85.45** Personal history of malignant neoplasm of unspecified male genital organ
  - ♂ **Z85.46** Personal history of malignant neoplasm of prostate
    AHA CC: 2Q, 2023, 5-6
  - ♂ **Z85.47** Personal history of malignant neoplasm of testis
  - ♂ **Z85.48** Personal history of malignant neoplasm of epididymis
  - ♂ **Z85.49** Personal history of malignant neoplasm of other male genital organs
- **Z85.5** Personal history of malignant neoplasm of urinary tract
  Conditions classifiable to C64-C68
  - **Z85.50** Personal history of malignant neoplasm of unspecified urinary tract organ
  - **Z85.51** Personal history of malignant neoplasm of bladder
  - **Z85.52** Personal history of malignant neoplasm of kidney
    Excludes1: personal history of malignant neoplasm of renal pelvis (Z85.53)
    - **Z85.520** Personal history of malignant carcinoid tumor of kidney
      Conditions classifiable to C7A.093
    - **Z85.528** Personal history of other malignant neoplasm of kidney
      Conditions classifiable to C64
  - **Z85.53** Personal history of malignant neoplasm of renal pelvis
  - **Z85.54** Personal history of malignant neoplasm of ureter
  - **Z85.59** Personal history of malignant neoplasm of other urinary tract organ
- **Z85.6** Personal history of leukemia
  Conditions classifiable to C91-C95
  Excludes1: leukemia in remission C91.0-C95.9 with 5th character 1
  Review coding guideline C.2.n
- **Z85.7** Personal history of other malignant neoplasms of lymphoid, hematopoietic and related tissues
  - **Z85.71** Personal history of Hodgkin lymphoma
    Conditions classifiable to C81
  - **Z85.72** Personal history of non-Hodgkin lymphomas
    Conditions classifiable to C82-C85
    AHA CC: 3Q, 2022, 28-29
  - **Z85.79** Personal history of other malignant neoplasms of lymphoid, hematopoietic and related tissues
    Conditions classifiable to C88-C90, C96
    Excludes1: multiple myeloma in remission (C90.01)
    plasma cell leukemia in remission (C90.11)
    plasmacytoma in remission (C90.21)
    Review coding guideline C.2.n
- **Z85.8** Personal history of malignant neoplasms of other organs and systems
  Conditions classifiable to C00-C14, C40-C49, C69-C75, C7A.098, C76-C79
  - **Z85.81** Personal history of malignant neoplasm of lip, oral cavity, and pharynx
    Conditions classifiable to C00-C14

Z85.810 Personal history of malignant neoplasm of tongue
Z85.818 Personal history of malignant neoplasm of other sites of lip, oral cavity, and pharynx
Z85.819 Personal history of malignant neoplasm of unspecified site of lip, oral cavity, and pharynx

+ Z85.82 Personal history of malignant neoplasm of skin
Z85.820 Personal history of malignant melanoma of skin
Conditions classifiable to C43
AHA CC: 3Q, 2022, 9
Z85.821 Personal history of Merkel cell carcinoma
Conditions classifiable to C4A
Z85.828 Personal history of other malignant neoplasm of skin
Conditions classifiable to C44

+ Z85.83 Personal history of malignant neoplasm of bone and soft tissue
Conditions classifiable to C40-C41; C45-C49
Z85.830 Personal history of malignant neoplasm of bone
Z85.831 Personal history of malignant neoplasm of soft tissue
Excludes2: *personal history of malignant neoplasm of skin (Z85.82-)*

+ Z85.84 Personal history of malignant neoplasm of eye and nervous tissue
Conditions classifiable to C69-C72
Z85.840 Personal history of malignant neoplasm of eye
Z85.841 Personal history of malignant neoplasm of brain
Z85.848 Personal history of malignant neoplasm of other parts of nervous tissue

+ Z85.85 Personal history of malignant neoplasm of endocrine glands
Conditions classifiable to C73-C75
Z85.850 Personal history of malignant neoplasm of thyroid
Z85.858 Personal history of malignant neoplasm of other endocrine glands

Z85.89 Personal history of malignant neoplasm of other organs and systems
Conditions classifiable to C7A.098, C76, C77-C79

Z85.9 Personal history of malignant neoplasm, unspecified
Conditions classifiable to C7A.00, C80.1

Z86 Personal history of certain other diseases
Code first any follow-up examination after treatment (Z09)
AHA CC: 4Q, 2019, 20
Review coding guideline C.21.c.4

+ Z86.0 Personal history of in-situ and benign neoplasms and neoplasms of uncertain behavior
Excludes2: *personal history of malignant neoplasms (Z85.-)*

+ Z86.00 Personal history of in-situ neoplasm
Conditions classifiable to D00-D09
Z86.000 Personal history of in-situ neoplasm of breast
Conditions classifiable to D05
♀ Z86.001 Personal history of in-situ neoplasm of cervix uteri
Conditions classifiable to D06
Personal history of cervical intraepithelial neoplasia III [CINIII]
Z86.002 Personal history of in-situ neoplasm of other and unspecified genital organs
Conditions classifiable to D07
Personal history of high-grade prostatic intraepithelial neoplasia III [HGPIN III]
Personal history of vaginal intraepithelial neoplasia III [VAIN III]
Personal history of vulvar intraepithelial neoplasia III [VAN III]
Z86.003 Personal history of in-situ neoplasm of oral cavity, esophagus and stomach
Conditions classifiable to D00
Z86.004 Personal history of in-situ neoplasm of other and unspecified digestive organs
Conditions classifiable to D01
Personal history of anal intraepithelial neoplasia III [AIN III]
Z86.005 Personal history of in-situ neoplasm of middle ear and respiratory system
Conditions classifiable to D02
Z86.006 Personal history of melanoma in-situ
Conditions classifiable to D03
Excludes2: *sites other than skin - code to personal history of in-situ neoplasm of the site*
Z86.007 Personal history of in-situ neoplasm of skin
Conditions classifiable to D04
Personal history of carcinoma in-situ of skin
Z86.008 Personal history of in-situ neoplasm of other site
Conditions classifiable to D09

+ Z86.01 Personal history of benign neoplasm
Z86.010 Personal history of colonic polyps
AHA CC: 1Q, 2017, 9; 1Q, 2021, 14-15
Z86.011 Personal history of benign neoplasm of the brain
Z86.012 Personal history of benign carcinoid tumor
Z86.018 Personal history of other benign neoplasm

Z86.03 Personal history of neoplasm of uncertain behavior

+ Z86.1 Personal history of infectious and parasitic diseases
Conditions classifiable to A00-B89, B99
Excludes1: *personal history of infectious diseases specific to a body system*
sequelae of infectious and parasitic diseases (B90-B94)
AHA CC: 4Q, 2016, 4-7
Z86.11 Personal history of tuberculosis
Z86.12 Personal history of poliomyelitis
Z86.13 Personal history of malaria
Z86.14 Personal history of Methicillin resistant Staphylococcus aureus infection
Personal history of MRSA infection
Z86.15 Personal history of latent tuberculosis infection
Z86.16 Personal history of COVID-19
Excludes1: *post COVID-19 condition (U09.9)*
AHA CC: 1Q, 2021, 33-35, 40-42; 4Q, 2021, 102-103, 107-108
Z86.19 Personal history of other infectious and parasitic diseases
AHA CC: 2Q, 2020, 10-12; 3Q, 2020, 13; 1Q, 2021, 33-35, 40-41; 3Q, 2022, 4
Review coding guideline C.1.g.1.i

Z86.2 Personal history of diseases of the blood and blood-forming organs and certain disorders involving the immune mechanism
Conditions classifiable to D50-D89

+ Z86.3 Personal history of endocrine, nutritional and metabolic diseases
Conditions classifiable to E00-E88
Z86.31 Personal history of diabetic foot ulcer
Excludes2: *current diabetic foot ulcer (E08.621, E09.621, E10.621, E11.621, E13.621)*
♀ Z86.32 Personal history of gestational diabetes
Personal history of conditions classifiable to O24.4-
Excludes1: *gestational diabetes mellitus in current pregnancy (O24.4-)*
Z86.39 Personal history of other endocrine, nutritional and metabolic disease
AHA CC: 1Q, 2020, 12-13

+ Z86.5 Personal history of mental and behavioral disorders
Conditions classifiable to F40-F59
• Z86.51 Personal history of combat and operational stress reaction
Z86.59 Personal history of other mental and behavioral disorders

+ Z86.6 Personal history of diseases of the nervous system and sense organs
Conditions classifiable to G00-G99, H00-H95

Z86.61 Personal history of infections of the central nervous system
Personal history of encephalitis
Personal history of meningitis

Z86.69 Personal history of other diseases of the nervous system and sense organs
AHA CC: 4Q, 2016, 21

+ Z86.7 Personal history of diseases of the circulatory system
Conditions classifiable to I00-I99
Excludes2: old myocardial infarction (I25.2)
personal history of anaphylactic shock (Z87.892)
postmyocardial infarction syndrome (I24.1)

+ Z86.71 Personal history of venous thrombosis and embolism

Z86.711 Personal history of pulmonary embolism

Z86.718 Personal history of other venous thrombosis and embolism
AHA CC: 2Q, 2020, 20-21

Z86.72 Personal history of thrombophlebitis

Z86.73 Personal history of transient ischemic attack (TIA), and cerebral infarction without residual deficits
Personal history of prolonged reversible ischemic neurological deficit (PRIND)
Personal history of stroke NOS without residual deficits
Excludes1: personal history of traumatic brain injury (Z87.820)
sequelae of cerebrovascular disease (I69.-)
Review coding guideline C.9.d.3

Z86.74 Personal history of sudden cardiac arrest
Personal history of sudden cardiac death successfully resuscitated

Z86.79 Personal history of other diseases of the circulatory system
AHA CC: 1Q, 2020, 12-13; 2Q, 2022, 14-15

Z87 Personal history of other diseases and conditions
Code first any follow-up examination after treatment (Z09)
AHA CC: 4Q, 2022, 50-51
Review coding guideline C.21.c.4

+ Z87.0 Personal history of diseases of the respiratory system
Conditions classifiable to J00-J99

Z87.01 Personal history of pneumonia (recurrent)

Z87.09 Personal history of other diseases of the respiratory system

+ Z87.1 Personal history of diseases of the digestive system
Conditions classifiable to K00-K93

Z87.11 Personal history of peptic ulcer disease

Z87.19 Personal history of other diseases of the digestive system
AHA CC: 1Q, 2017, 14-15

Z87.2 Personal history of diseases of the skin and subcutaneous tissue
Conditions classifiable to L00-L99
Excludes2: personal history of diabetic foot ulcer (Z86.31)

+ Z87.3 Personal history of diseases of the musculoskeletal system and connective tissue
Conditions classifiable to M00-M99
Excludes2: personal history of (healed) traumatic fracture (Z87.81)

+ Z87.31 Personal history of (healed) nontraumatic fracture

Z87.310 Personal history of (healed) osteoporosis fracture
Personal history of (healed) fragility fracture
Personal history of (healed) collapsed vertebra due to osteoporosis
Review coding guideline C.13.d.1

Z87.311 Personal history of (healed) other pathological fracture
Personal history of (healed) collapsed vertebra NOS
Excludes2: personal history of osteoporosis fracture (Z87.310)

Z87.312 Personal history of (healed) stress fracture
Personal history of (healed) fatigue fracture

Z87.39 Personal history of other diseases of the musculoskeletal system and connective tissue

+ Z87.4 Personal history of diseases of genitourinary system
Conditions classifiable to N00-N99

+ Z87.41 Personal history of dysplasia of the female genital tract
Excludes1: personal history of malignant neoplasm of female genital tract (Z85.40-Z85.44)
personal history of intraepithelial neoplasia III of female genital tract (Z86.001, Z86.008)

♀ **Z87.410 Personal history of cervical dysplasia**
♀ **Z87.411 Personal history of vaginal dysplasia**
♀ **Z87.412 Personal history of vulvar dysplasia**
♀ **Z87.42 Personal history of other diseases of the female genital tract**

+ Z87.43 Personal history of diseases of male genital organs
♂ **Z87.430 Personal history of prostatic dysplasia**
Excludes1: personal history of malignant neoplasm of prostate (Z85.46)
♂ **Z87.438 Personal history of other diseases of male genital organs**

+ Z87.44 Personal history of diseases of urinary system
Excludes1: personal history of malignant neoplasm of cervix uteri (Z85.41)

Z87.440 Personal history of urinary (tract) infections
Z87.441 Personal history of nephrotic syndrome
Z87.442 Personal history of urinary calculi
Personal history of kidney stones
Z87.448 Personal history of other diseases of urinary system

+ Z87.5 Personal history of complications of pregnancy, childbirth and the puerperium
Conditions classifiable to O00-O9A
Excludes2: recurrent pregnancy loss (N96)

♀ **Z87.51 Personal history of pre-term labor**
Excludes1: current pregnancy with history of pre-term labor (O09.21-)

♀ **Z87.59 Personal history of other complications of pregnancy, childbirth and the puerperium**
Personal history of trophoblastic disease

+ Z87.6 Personal history of certain (corrected) conditions arising in the perinatal period
Conditions classifiable to P00-P96
Excludes1: personal history of (corrected) congenital malformations (Z87.7-)

Z87.61 Personal history of (corrected) necrotizing enterocolitis of newborn

Z87.68 Personal history of other (corrected) conditions arising in the perinatal period

+ Z87.7 Personal history of (corrected) congenital malformations
Conditions classifiable to Q00-Q89 that have been repaired or corrected
Excludes1: congenital malformations that have been partially corrected or repair but which still require medical treatment - code to condition
Excludes2: other postprocedural states (Z98.-)
personal history of medical treatment (Z92.-)
presence of cardiac and vascular implants and grafts (Z95.-)
presence of other devices (Z97.-)
presence of other functional implants (Z96.-)
transplanted organ and tissue status (Z94.-)

+ **Z87.71** Personal history of (corrected) congenital malformations of genitourinary system
♂ **Z87.710** Personal history of (corrected) hypospadias
Z87.718 Personal history of other specified (corrected) congenital malformations of genitourinary system
+ **Z87.72** Personal history of (corrected) congenital malformations of nervous system and sense organs
Z87.720 Personal history of (corrected) congenital malformations of eye
Z87.721 Personal history of (corrected) congenital malformations of ear
Z87.728 Personal history of other specified (corrected) congenital malformations of nervous system and sense organs
+ **Z87.73** Personal history of (corrected) congenital malformations of digestive system
Z87.730 Personal history of (corrected) cleft lip and palate
Z87.731 Personal history of (corrected) tracheoesophageal fistula or atresia
Z87.732 Personal history of (corrected) persistent cloaca or cloacal malformations
Z87.738 Personal history of other specified (corrected) congenital malformations of digestive system
Z87.74 Personal history of (corrected) congenital malformations of heart and circulatory system
Z87.75 Personal history of (corrected) congenital malformations of respiratory system
+ **Z87.76** Personal history of (corrected) congenital malformations of integument, limbs and musculoskeletal system
Z87.760 Personal history of (corrected) congenital diaphragmatic hernia or other congenital diaphragm malformations
Z87.761 Personal history of (corrected) gastroschisis
Z87.762 Personal history of (corrected) prune belly malformation
Z87.763 Personal history of other (corrected) congenital abdominal wall malformations
Z87.768 Personal history of other specified (corrected) congenital malformations of integument, limbs and musculoskeletal system
+ **Z87.79** Personal history of other (corrected) congenital malformations
Z87.790 Personal history of (corrected) congenital malformations of face and neck
Z87.798 Personal history of other (corrected) congenital malformations
+ **Z87.8** Personal history of other specified conditions
Excludes2: *personal history of self harm (Z91.5-)*
Z87.81 Personal history of (healed) traumatic fracture
Excludes2: *personal history of (healed) nontraumatic fracture (Z87.31-)*
+ **Z87.82** Personal history of other (healed) physical injury and trauma
Conditions classifiable to S00-T88, except traumatic fractures
Z87.820 Personal history of traumatic brain injury
Excludes1: *personal history of transient ischemic attack (TIA), and cerebral infarction without residual deficits (Z86.73)*
Z87.821 Personal history of retained foreign body fully removed
Z87.828 Personal history of other (healed) physical injury and trauma
+ **Z87.89** Personal history of other specified conditions
Z87.890 Personal history of sex reassignment
Z87.891 Personal history of nicotine dependence
Excludes1: *current nicotine dependence (F17.2-)*
AHA CC: 2Q, 2017, 26-28
Z87.892 Personal history of anaphylaxis
Code also allergy status such as:
allergy status to drugs, medicaments and biological substances (Z88.-)
allergy status, other than to drugs and biological substances (Z91.0-)
Z87.898 Personal history of other specified conditions
AHA CC: 1Q, 2013, 21

Z88 **Allergy status to drugs, medicaments and biological substances**
Excludes2: *Allergy status, other than to drugs and biological substances (Z91.0-)*
Review coding guideline C.21.c.3
Z88.0 Allergy status to penicillin
Z88.1 Allergy status to other antibiotic agents
Z88.2 Allergy status to sulfonamides
AHA CC: 3Q, 2015, 23
Z88.3 Allergy status to other anti-infective agents
Z88.4 Allergy status to anesthetic agent
Z88.5 Allergy status to narcotic agent
Z88.6 Allergy status to analgesic agent
Z88.7 Allergy status to serum and vaccine
Z88.8 Allergy status to other drugs, medicaments and biological substances
Z88.9 Allergy status to unspecified drugs, medicaments and biological substances

Z89 **Acquired absence of limb**
Includes: amputation status
postprocedural loss of limb
post-traumatic loss of limb
Excludes1: *acquired deformities of limbs (M20-M21)*
congenital absence of limbs (Q71-Q73)
Review coding guideline C.21.c.3
+ **Z89.0** Acquired absence of thumb and other finger(s)
+ **Z89.01** Acquired absence of thumb
Z89.011 Acquired absence of right thumb
Z89.012 Acquired absence of left thumb
Z89.019 Acquired absence of unspecified thumb
+ **Z89.02** Acquired absence of other finger(s)
Excludes2: *acquired absence of thumb (Z89.01-)*
Z89.021 Acquired absence of right finger(s)
Z89.022 Acquired absence of left finger(s)
Z89.029 Acquired absence of unspecified finger(s)
+ **Z89.1** Acquired absence of hand and wrist
+ **Z89.11** Acquired absence of hand
Z89.111 Acquired absence of right hand
Z89.112 Acquired absence of left hand
Z89.119 Acquired absence of unspecified hand
+ **Z89.12** Acquired absence of wrist
Disarticulation at wrist
Z89.121 Acquired absence of right wrist
Z89.122 Acquired absence of left wrist
Z89.129 Acquired absence of unspecified wrist
+ **Z89.2** Acquired absence of upper limb above wrist
+ **Z89.20** Acquired absence of upper limb, unspecified level
Z89.201 Acquired absence of right upper limb, unspecified level
Z89.202 Acquired absence of left upper limb, unspecified level
Z89.209 Acquired absence of unspecified upper limb, unspecified level
Acquired absence of arm NOS
+ **Z89.21** Acquired absence of upper limb below elbow
Z89.211 Acquired absence of right upper limb below elbow
Z89.212 Acquired absence of left upper limb below elbow
Z89.219 Acquired absence of unspecified upper limb below elbow
+ **Z89.22** Acquired absence of upper limb above elbow
Disarticulation at elbow
Z89.221 Acquired absence of right upper limb above elbow
Z89.222 Acquired absence of left upper limb above elbow

Z89.229 Acquired absence of unspecified upper limb above elbow
+ Z89.23 Acquired absence of shoulder
Acquired absence of shoulder joint following explantation of shoulder joint prosthesis, with or without presence of antibiotic-impregnated cement spacer
Z89.231 Acquired absence of right shoulder
Z89.232 Acquired absence of left shoulder
Z89.239 Acquired absence of unspecified shoulder
+ Z89.4 Acquired absence of toe(s), foot, and ankle
+ Z89.41 Acquired absence of great toe
Z89.411 Acquired absence of right great toe
Z89.412 Acquired absence of left great toe
Z89.419 Acquired absence of unspecified great toe
+ Z89.42 Acquired absence of other toe(s)
Excludes2: acquired absence of great toe (Z89.41-)
Z89.421 Acquired absence of other right toe(s)
Z89.422 Acquired absence of other left toe(s)
Z89.429 Acquired absence of other toe(s), unspecified side
+ Z89.43 Acquired absence of foot
Z89.431 Acquired absence of right foot
Z89.432 Acquired absence of left foot
Z89.439 Acquired absence of unspecified foot
+ Z89.44 Acquired absence of ankle
Disarticulation of ankle
Z89.441 Acquired absence of right ankle
Z89.442 Acquired absence of left ankle
Z89.449 Acquired absence of unspecified ankle
+ Z89.5 Acquired absence of leg below knee
+ Z89.51 Acquired absence of leg below knee
Z89.511 Acquired absence of right leg below knee
Z89.512 Acquired absence of left leg below knee
Z89.519 Acquired absence of unspecified leg below knee
+ Z89.52 Acquired absence of knee
Acquired absence of knee joint following explantation of knee joint prosthesis, with or without presence of antibiotic-impregnated cement spacer
Z89.521 Acquired absence of right knee
Z89.522 Acquired absence of left knee
Z89.529 Acquired absence of unspecified knee
+ Z89.6 Acquired absence of leg above knee
+ Z89.61 Acquired absence of leg above knee
Acquired absence of leg NOS
Disarticulation at knee
Z89.611 Acquired absence of right leg above knee
Z89.612 Acquired absence of left leg above knee
Z89.619 Acquired absence of unspecified leg above knee
+ Z89.62 Acquired absence of hip
Acquired absence of hip joint following explantation of hip joint prosthesis, with or without presence of antibiotic-impregnated cement spacer
Disarticulation at hip
Z89.621 Acquired absence of right hip joint
Z89.622 Acquired absence of left hip joint
Z89.629 Acquired absence of unspecified hip joint
Z89.9 Acquired absence of limb, unspecified

Z90 **Acquired absence of organs, not elsewhere classified**
Includes: postprocedural or post-traumatic loss of body part NEC
Excludes1: congenital absence - see Alphabetical Index
Excludes2: postprocedural absence of endocrine glands (E89.-)
Review coding guideline C.21.c.3
+ Z90.0 Acquired absence of part of head and neck
Z90.01 Acquired absence of eye
Z90.02 Acquired absence of larynx
Z90.09 Acquired absence of other part of head and neck
Acquired absence of nose
Excludes2: teeth (K08.1)
+ Z90.1 Acquired absence of breast and nipple
Z90.10 Acquired absence of unspecified breast and nipple
Z90.11 Acquired absence of right breast and nipple
Z90.12 Acquired absence of left breast and nipple
Z90.13 Acquired absence of bilateral breasts and nipples
AHA CC: 3Q, 2022, 8
Z90.2 Acquired absence of lung [part of]
Z90.3 Acquired absence of stomach [part of]
+ Z90.4 Acquired absence of other specified parts of digestive tract
+ Z90.41 Acquired absence of pancreas
Code also exocrine pancreatic insufficiency (K86.81)
Use additional code to identify any associated: diabetes mellitus, postpancreatectomy (E13.-) insulin use (Z79.4)
Review coding guideline C.4.a.6.b.i
Z90.410 Acquired total absence of pancreas
Acquired absence of pancreas NOS
Z90.411 Acquired partial absence of pancreas
Z90.49 Acquired absence of other specified parts of digestive tract
Z90.5 Acquired absence of kidney
Z90.6 Acquired absence of other parts of urinary tract
Acquired absence of bladder
+ Z90.7 Acquired absence of genital organ(s)
Excludes1: personal history of sex reassignment (Z87.890)
Excludes2: female genital mutilation status (N90.81-)
+ Z90.71 Acquired absence of cervix and uterus
♀ Z90.710 Acquired absence of both cervix and uterus
Acquired absence of uterus NOS
Status post total hysterectomy
♀ Z90.711 Acquired absence of uterus with remaining cervical stump
Status post partial hysterectomy with remaining cervical stump
♀ Z90.712 Acquired absence of cervix with remaining uterus
+ Z90.72 Acquired absence of ovaries
♀ Z90.721 Acquired absence of ovaries, unilateral
♀ Z90.722 Acquired absence of ovaries, bilateral
Z90.79 Acquired absence of other genital organ(s)
AHA CC: 2Q, 2023, 5-6
+ Z90.8 Acquired absence of other organs
Z90.81 Acquired absence of spleen
Z90.89 Acquired absence of other organs

Z91 **Personal risk factors, not elsewhere classified**
Excludes2: contact with and (suspected) exposures hazardous to health (Z77.-)
exposure to pollution and other problems related to physical environment (Z77.1-)
female genital mutilation status (N90.81-)
personal history of physical injury and trauma (Z87.81, Z87.82-)
occupational exposure to risk factors (Z57.-)
AHA CC: 4Q, 2022, 49
+ Z91.0 Allergy status, other than to drugs and biological substances
Excludes2: Allergy status to drugs, medicaments, and biological substances (Z88.-)
Review coding guideline C.21.c.3
+ Z91.01 Food allergy status
Excludes2: food additives allergy status (Z91.02)
Z91.010 Allergy to peanuts
Z91.011 Allergy to milk products
Excludes1: lactose intolerance (E73.-)
Z91.012 Allergy to eggs
Z91.013 Allergy to seafood
Allergy to shellfish
Allergy to octopus or squid ink
Z91.014 Allergy to mammalian meats
Allergy to beef
Allergy to lamb
Allergy to pork
Allergy to red meats
AHA CC: 4Q, 2021, 33
Z91.018 Allergy to other foods
Allergy to nuts other than peanuts
Z91.02 Food additives allergy status
+ Z91.03 Insect allergy status
Z91.030 Bee allergy status
Z91.038 Other insect allergy status
+ Z91.04 Nonmedicinal substance allergy status
Z91.040 Latex allergy status
Latex sensitivity status
Z91.041 Radiographic dye allergy status
Allergy status to contrast media used for diagnostic X-ray procedure
Z91.048 Other nonmedicinal substance allergy status

Z91.09 Other allergy status, other than to drugs and biological substances

+ **Z91.1** Patient's noncompliance with medical treatment and regimen
  Code also: if applicable, to identify underdosing of specific drug (T36-T50 with final character 6)
  Excludes2: *caregiver noncompliance with patient's medical treatment and regimen (Z91.A-)*
  AHA CC: 1Q, 2023, 7

+ **Z91.11** Patient's noncompliance with dietary regimen
  Code also, if applicable, food insecurity (Z59.4-)
  Z91.110 Patient's noncompliance with dietary regimen due to financial hardship
  Z91.118 Patient's noncompliance with dietary regimen for other reason
  Inability to comply with dietary regimen
  Z91.119 Patient's noncompliance with dietary regimen due to unspecified reason

+ **Z91.12** Patient's intentional underdosing of medication regimen
  Code first underdosing of medication (T36-T50) with fifth or sixth character 6
  Excludes1: *adverse effect of prescribed drug taken as directed- code to adverse effect*
  poisoning (overdose) -code to poisoning
  Review coding guideline C.19.e.5.c
  Z91.120 Patient's intentional underdosing of medication regimen due to financial hardship
  Z91.128 Patient's intentional underdosing of medication regimen for other reason

+ **Z91.13** Patient's unintentional underdosing of medication regimen
  Code first underdosing of medication (T36-T50) with fifth or sixth character 6
  Excludes1: *adverse effect of prescribed drug taken as directed- code to adverse effect*
  poisoning (overdose) -code to poisoning
  Review coding guideline C.19.e.5.c
  Z91.130 Patient's unintentional underdosing of medication regimen due to age-related debility
  Z91.138 Patient's unintentional underdosing of medication regimen for other reason

+ **Z91.14** Patient's other noncompliance with medication regimen
  Patient's underdosing of medication NOS
  Review coding guideline C.19.e.5.c
  Z91.141 Patient's other noncompliance with medication regimen due to financial hardship
  Z91.148 Patient's other noncompliance with medication regimen for other reason

+ **Z91.15** Patient's noncompliance with renal dialysis
  Z91.151 Patient's noncompliance with renal dialysis sue to financial hardship
  Z91.158 Patient's noncompliance with renal dialysis for other reason

+ **Z91.19** Patient's noncompliance with other medical treatment and regimen
  Patient's nonadherence to medical treatment
  Z91.190 Patient's noncompliance with other medical treatment and regimen due to financial hardship
  Z91.198 Patient's noncompliance with other medical treatment and regimen for other reason
  Z91.199 Patient's noncompliance with other medical treatment and regimen due to unspecified reason

+ **Z91.A** Caregiver's noncompliance with patient's medical treatment and regimen
  + **Z91.A1** Caregiver's noncompliance with patient's dietary regimen
    Caregiver's inability to comply with patient's dietary regimen
    Code also, if applicable, food insecurity (Z59.4-)
    Z91.A10 Caregiver's noncompliance with patient's dietary regimen due to financial hardship
    Z91.A18 Caregiver's noncompliance with patient's dietary regimen for other reason

+ **Z91.A2** Caregiver's intentional underdosing of patient's medication regimen
  Code first underdosing of medication (T36-T50) with fifth or sixth character 6
  Z91.A20 Caregiver's intentional underdosing of patient's medication regimen due to financial hardship
  Z91.A28 Caregiver's intentional underdosing of medication regimen for other reason

Z91.A3 Caregiver's unintentional underdosing of patient's medication regimen
  Code first underdosing of medication (T36-T50) with fifth or sixth character 6

+ **Z91.A4** Caregiver's other noncompliance with patient's medication regimen
  Caregiver's underdosing of patient's medication NOS
  Caregiver's underdosing with patient's medication NOS
  Z91.A41 Caregiver's other noncompliance with patient's medication regimen due to financial hardship
  Z91.A48 Caregiver's other noncompliance with patient's medication regimen for other reason

+ **Z91.A5** Caregiver's noncompliance with patient's renal dialysis
  Z91.A51 Caregiver's noncompliance with patient's renal dialysis due to financial hardship
  Z91.A58 Caregiver's noncompliance with patient's renal dialysis for other reason

+ **Z91.A9** Caregiver's noncompliance with patient's other medical treatment and regimen
  Caregiver's nonadherence to patient's medical treatment
  Z91.A91 Caregiver's noncompliance with patient's other medical treatment and regimen due to financial hardship
  Z91.A98 Caregiver's noncompliance with patient's other medical treatment and regimen for other reason

+ **Z91.4** Personal history of psychological trauma, not elsewhere classified
  Review coding guideline C.21.c.4
  AHA CC: 1Q, 2023, 7

+ **Z91.41** Personal history of adult abuse
  Excludes2: *personal history of abuse in childhood (Z62.81-)*
  • **Z91.410** Personal history of adult physical and sexual abuse
    Excludes1: *current adult physical abuse (T74.11, T76.11)*
    current adult sexual abuse (T74.21-T76.11)
  • **Z91.411** Personal history of adult psychological abuse
  • **Z91.412** Personal history of adult neglect
    Excludes1: *current adult neglect (T74.01, T76.01)*
  • **Z91.413** Personal history of adult financial abuse
  • **Z91.414** Personal history of adult intimate partner abuse
  • **Z91.419** Personal history of unspecified adult abuse

Z91.42 Personal history of forced labor or sexual exploitation
  AHA CC: 4Q, 2018, 32-33, 35

Z91.49 Other personal history of psychological trauma, not elsewhere classified

+ **Z91.5** Personal history of self-harm
  Code also mental health disorder, if known.
  AHA CC: 4Q, 2021, 33
  Review coding guideline C.21.c.4
  Z91.51 Personal history of suicidal behavior
    Personal history of parasuicide
    Personal history of self-poisoning
    Personal history of suicide attempt
  Z91.52 Personal history of nonsuicidal self-harm
    Personal history of nonsuicidal self-injury
    Personal history of self-inflicted injury without suicidal intent
    Personal history of self-mutilation

- **Z91.8** Other specified personal risk factors, not elsewhere classified
  Review coding guideline C.21.c.4
  - **Z91.81** History of falling
    At risk for falling
    Review coding guideline C.18.d and C21.c.4
  - • **Z91.82** Personal history of military deployment
    Individual (civilian or military) with past history of military war, peacekeeping and humanitarian deployment (current or past conflict)
    Returned from military deployment
    Excludes2: personal history of military service (Z91.85)
    Review coding guideline C.21.c.4
  - **Z91.83** Wandering in diseases classified elsewhere
    Code first underlying disorder such as:
    Alzheimer's disease (G30.-)
    autism or pervasive developmental disorder (F84.-)
    intellectual disabilities (F70-F79)
    unspecified dementia with behavioral disturbance (F03.9-, F03.A-, F03.B-, F03.C-)
  - + **Z91.84** Oral health risk factors
    AHA CC: 4Q, 2017, 29
    Review coding guideline C.21.c.14
    - **Z91.841** Risk for dental caries, low
    - **Z91.842** Risk for dental caries, moderate
    - **Z91.843** Risk for dental caries, high
    - **Z91.849** Unspecified risk for dental caries
  - **Z91.85** Personal history of military service
    Personal history of serving in the armed forces
    Personal history of veteran
    Excludes2: personal history of military deployment (Z91.82)
  - **Z91.89** Other specified personal risk factors, not elsewhere classified
    Increased risk for social isolation
    AHA CC: 1Q, 2017, 45-46

Z92 Personal history of medical treatment
Excludes2: postprocedural states (Z98.-)
Review coding guideline C.21.c.4
- **Z92.0** Personal history of contraception
  Excludes1: counseling or management of current contraceptive practices (Z30.-)
  long term (current) use of contraception (Z79.3)
  presence of (intrauterine) contraceptive device (Z97.5)
- + **Z92.2** Personal history of drug therapy
  Excludes2: long term (current) drug therapy (Z79.-)
  - **Z92.21** Personal history of antineoplastic chemotherapy
  - **Z92.22** Personal history of monoclonal drug therapy
  - **Z92.23** Personal history of estrogen therapy
  - + **Z92.24** Personal history of steroid therapy
    - **Z92.240** Personal history of inhaled steroid therapy
    - **Z92.241** Personal history of systemic steroid therapy
    Personal history of steroid therapy NOS
  - **Z92.25** Personal history of immunosuppression therapy
    Excludes2: personal history of steroid therapy (Z92.24)
  - **Z92.29** Personal history of other drug therapy
- **Z92.3** Personal history of irradiation
  Personal history of exposure to therapeutic radiation
  Excludes1: exposure to radiation in the physical environment (Z77.12)
  occupational exposure to radiation (Z57.1)
- + **Z92.8** Personal history of other medical treatment
  AHA CC: 4Q, 2021, 33-34
  - **Z92.81** Personal history of extracorporeal membrane oxygenation (ECMO)
  - **Z92.82** Status post administration of tPA (rtPA) in a different facility within the last 24 hours prior to admission to current facility
    Code first condition requiring tPA administration, such as:
    acute cerebral infarction (I63.-)
    acute myocardial infarction (I21.-, I22.-)
    AHA CC: 4Q, 2013, 124
    Review coding guideline C.21.c.3
  - **Z92.83** Personal history of failed moderate sedation
    Personal history of failed conscious sedation
    Excludes2: failed moderate sedation during procedure (T88.52)
  - **Z92.84** Personal history of unintended awareness under general anesthesia
    Excludes2: unintended awareness under general anesthesia during procedure (T88.53)
    AHA CC: 4Q, 2016, 72-73, 77
  - + **Z92.85** Personal history of cellular therapy
    - **Z92.850** Personal history of Chimeric Antigen Receptor T-cell therapy
      Personal history of CAR-T cell therapy
    - **Z92.858** Personal history of other cellular therapy
    - **Z92.859** Personal history of cellular therapy, unspecified
  - **Z92.86** Personal history of gene therapy
  - **Z92.89** Personal history of other medical treatment
    AHA CC: 1Q, 2020, 18

Z93 Artificial opening status
Excludes1: artificial openings requiring attention or management (Z43.-)
complications of external stoma (J95.0-, K94.-, N99.5-)
Review coding guideline C.21.c.3
- **Z93.0** Tracheostomy status
  AHA CC: 4Q, 2013, 129
- **Z93.1** Gastrostomy status
- **Z93.2** Ileostomy status
- **Z93.3** Colostomy status
- **Z93.4** Other artificial openings of gastrointestinal tract status
- + **Z93.5** Cystostomy status
  - **Z93.50** Unspecified cystostomy status
  - **Z93.51** Cutaneous-vesicostomy status
  - **Z93.52** Appendico-vesicostomy status
  - **Z93.59** Other cystostomy status
- **Z93.6** Other artificial openings of urinary tract status
  Nephrostomy status
  Ureterostomy status
  Urethrostomy status
- **Z93.8** Other artificial opening status
- **Z93.9** Artificial opening status, unspecified

Z94 Transplanted organ and tissue status
Includes: organ or tissue replaced by heterogenous or homogenous transplant
Excludes1: complications of transplanted organ or tissue - see Alphabetical Index
Excludes2: presence of vascular grafts (Z95.-)
Review coding guideline C.21.c.3
- CC **Z94.0** Kidney transplant status
  Review coding guideline C.14.a.2
- CC **Z94.1** Heart transplant status
  Excludes1: artificial heart status (Z95.812)
  heart-valve replacement status (Z95.2-Z95.4)
- CC **Z94.2** Lung transplant status
- CC **Z94.3** Heart and lungs transplant status
- CC **Z94.4** Liver transplant status
- **Z94.5** Skin transplant status
  Autogenous skin transplant status
- **Z94.6** Bone transplant status
- **Z94.7** Corneal transplant status
- + **Z94.8** Other transplanted organ and tissue status
  - CC **Z94.81** Bone marrow transplant status
  - CC **Z94.82** Intestine transplant status
  - CC **Z94.83** Pancreas transplant status
  - CC **Z94.84** Stem cells transplant status
  - **Z94.89** Other transplanted organ and tissue status
- **Z94.9** Transplanted organ and tissue status, unspecified

Z95 Presence of cardiac and vascular implants and grafts

Excludes2: complications of cardiac and vascular devices, implants and grafts (T82.-)

Review coding guideline C.21.c.3

- **Z95.0 Presence of cardiac pacemaker**
  - Presence of cardiac resynchronization therapy (CRT-P) pacemaker
  - *Excludes1:* adjustment or management of cardiac device (Z45.0-)
    - adjustment or management of cardiac pacemaker (Z45.0)
    - presence of automatic (implantable) cardiac defibrillator with synchronous cardiac pacemaker (Z95.810)
  - AHA CC: 1Q, 2019, 33-34
- **Z95.1 Presence of aortocoronary bypass graft**
  - Presence of coronary artery bypass graft
- **Z95.2 Presence of prosthetic heart valve**
  - Presence of heart valve NOS
- **Z95.3 Presence of xenogenic heart valve**
- **Z95.4 Presence of other heart-valve replacement**
- **Z95.5 Presence of coronary angioplasty implant and graft**
  - *Excludes1:* coronary angioplasty status without implant and graft (Z98.61)
- + **Z95.8 Presence of other cardiac and vascular implants and grafts**
  - + **Z95.81 Presence of other cardiac implants and grafts**
    - **Z95.810 Presence of automatic (implantable) cardiac defibrillator**
      - Presence of automatic (implantable) cardiac defibrillator with synchronous cardiac pacemaker
      - Presence of cardiac resynchronization therapy defibrillator (CRT-D)
      - Present of cardioverter-defibrillator (ICD)
      - AHA CC: 2Q, 2022, 14-15
    - CC **Z95.811 Presence of heart assist device**
    - CC **Z95.812 Presence of fully implantable artificial heart**
    - **Z95.818 Presence of other cardiac implants and grafts**
  - + **Z95.82 Presence of other vascular implants and grafts**
    - **Z95.820 Peripheral vascular angioplasty status with implants and grafts**
      - *Excludes1:* peripheral vascular angioplasty without implant and graft (Z98.62)
    - **Z95.828 Presence of other vascular implants and grafts**
      - Presence of intravascular prosthesis NEC
- **Z95.9 Presence of cardiac and vascular implant and graft, unspecified**

Z96 Presence of other functional implants

Excludes2: complications of internal prosthetic devices, implants and grafts (T82-T85)
fitting and adjustment of prosthetic and other devices (Z44-Z46)

Review coding guideline C.21.c.3

- **Z96.0 Presence of urogenital implants**
- **Z96.1 Presence of intraocular lens**
  - Presence of pseudophakia
- + **Z96.2 Presence of otological and audiological implants**
  - **Z96.20 Presence of otological and audiological implant, unspecified**
  - **Z96.21 Cochlear implant status**
  - **Z96.22 Myringotomy tube(s) status**
  - **Z96.29 Presence of other otological and audiological implants**
    - Presence of bone-conduction hearing device
    - Presence of eustachian tube stent
    - Stapes replacement
- **Z96.3 Presence of artificial larynx**
- + **Z96.4 Presence of endocrine implants**
  - **Z96.41 Presence of insulin pump (external) (internal)**
  - **Z96.49 Presence of other endocrine implants**
- **Z96.5 Presence of tooth-root and mandibular implants**
- + **Z96.6 Presence of orthopedic joint implants**
  - **Z96.60 Presence of unspecified orthopedic joint implant**
  - + **Z96.61 Presence of artificial shoulder joint**
    - **Z96.611 Presence of right artificial shoulder joint**
    - **Z96.612 Presence of left artificial shoulder joint**
    - **Z96.619 Presence of unspecified artificial shoulder joint**
  - + **Z96.62 Presence of artificial elbow joint**
    - **Z96.621 Presence of right artificial elbow joint**
    - **Z96.622 Presence of left artificial elbow joint**
    - **Z96.629 Presence of unspecified artificial elbow joint**
  - + **Z96.63 Presence of artificial wrist joint**
    - **Z96.631 Presence of right artificial wrist joint**
    - **Z96.632 Presence of left artificial wrist joint**
    - **Z96.639 Presence of unspecified artificial wrist joint**
  - + **Z96.64 Presence of artificial hip joint**
    - Hip-joint replacement (partial) (total)
    - **Z96.641 Presence of right artificial hip joint**
      - AHA CC: 3Q, 2016, 16-17
    - **Z96.642 Presence of left artificial hip joint**
      - AHA CC: 1Q, 2015, 16-17
    - **Z96.643 Presence of artificial hip joint, bilateral**
    - **Z96.649 Presence of unspecified artificial hip joint**
  - + **Z96.65 Presence of artificial knee joint**
    - **Z96.651 Presence of right artificial knee joint**
    - **Z96.652 Presence of left artificial knee joint**
      - AHA CC: 3Q, 2019, 16-17
    - **Z96.653 Presence of artificial knee joint, bilateral**
    - **Z96.659 Presence of unspecified artificial knee joint**
  - + **Z96.66 Presence of artificial ankle joint**
    - **Z96.661 Presence of right artificial ankle joint**
    - **Z96.662 Presence of left artificial ankle joint**
    - **Z96.669 Presence of unspecified artificial ankle joint**
  - + **Z96.69 Presence of other orthopedic joint implants**
    - **Z96.691 Finger-joint replacement of right hand**
    - **Z96.692 Finger-joint replacement of left hand**
    - **Z96.693 Finger-joint replacement, bilateral**
    - **Z96.698 Presence of other orthopedic joint implants**
- **Z96.7 Presence of other bone and tendon implants**
  - Presence of skull plate
- + **Z96.8 Presence of other specified functional implants**
  - **Z96.81 Presence of artificial skin**
  - **Z96.82 Presence of neurostimulator**
    - Presence of brain neurostimulator
    - Presence of gastric neurostimulator
    - Presence of peripheral nerve neurostimulator
    - Presence of sacral nerve neurostimulator
    - Presence of spinal cord neurostimulator
    - Presence of vagus nerve neurostimulator
    - AHA CC: 4Q, 2019, 19
  - **Z96.89 Presence of other specified functional implants**
- **Z96.9 Presence of functional implant, unspecified**

Z97 Presence of other devices

Excludes1: complications of internal prosthetic devices, implants and grafts (T82-T85)
Excludes2: fitting and adjustment of prosthetic and other devices (Z44-Z46)
presence of cerebrospinal fluid drainage device (Z98.2)

Review coding guideline C.21.c.3

- **Z97.0 Presence of artificial eye**
- + **Z97.1 Presence of artificial limb (complete) (partial)**
  - **Z97.10 Presence of artificial limb (complete) (partial), unspecified**
  - **Z97.11 Presence of artificial right arm (complete) (partial)**
  - **Z97.12 Presence of artificial left arm (complete) (partial)**
  - **Z97.13 Presence of artificial right leg (complete) (partial)**
  - **Z97.14 Presence of artificial left leg (complete) (partial)**
  - **Z97.15 Presence of artificial arms, bilateral (complete) (partial)**
  - **Z97.16 Presence of artificial legs, bilateral (complete) (partial)**
- **Z97.2 Presence of dental prosthetic device (complete) (partial)**
  - Presence of dentures (complete) (partial)
- **Z97.3 Presence of spectacles and contact lenses**

Z97.4 Presence of external hearing-aid
♀ **Z97.5** Presence of (intrauterine) contraceptive device
  Excludes1: checking, reinsertion or removal of implantable subdermal contraceptive (Z30.46)
  checking, reinsertion or removal of intrauterine contraceptive device (Z30.43-)
Z97.8 Presence of other specified devices

Z98 Other postprocedural states
  Excludes2: aftercare (Z43-Z49, Z51)
  follow-up medical care (Z08-Z09)
  postprocedural complication - see Alphabetical Index
  Review coding guideline C.21.c.3

Z98.0 Intestinal bypass and anastomosis status
  Excludes2: bariatric surgery status (Z98.84)
  gastric bypass status (Z98.84)
  obesity surgery status (Z98.84)
Z98.1 Arthrodesis status
Z98.2 Presence of cerebrospinal fluid drainage device
  Presence of CSF shunt
Z98.3 Post therapeutic collapse of lung status
  Code first underlying disease
+ **Z98.4** Cataract extraction status
  Use additional code to identify intraocular lens implant status (Z96.1)
  Excludes1: aphakia (H27.0)
  Z98.41 Cataract extraction status, right eye
  Z98.42 Cataract extraction status, left eye
  Z98.49 Cataract extraction status, unspecified eye
+ **Z98.5** Sterilization status
  Excludes1: female infertility (N97.-)
  male infertility (N46.-)
  ♀ **Z98.51** Tubal ligation status
  ● ♂ **Z98.52** Vasectomy status
+ **Z98.6** Angioplasty status
  Z98.61 Coronary angioplasty status
    Excludes1: coronary angioplasty status with implant and graft (Z95.5)
    AHA CC: 4Q, 2022, 21-22
  Z98.62 Peripheral vascular angioplasty status
    Excludes1: peripheral vascular angioplasty status with implant and graft (Z95.820)
+ **Z98.8** Other specified postprocedural states
  AHA CC: 4Q, 2016, 76
  + **Z98.81** Dental procedure status
    Z98.810 Dental sealant status
    Z98.811 Dental restoration status
      Dental crown status
      Dental fillings status
    Z98.818 Other dental procedure status
  Z98.82 Breast implant status
    Excludes1: breast implant removal status (Z98.86)
    AHA CC: 3Q, 2022, 8
  Z98.83 Filtering (vitreous) bleb after glaucoma surgery status
    Excludes1: Inflammation (infection) of postprocedural bleb (H59.4-)
    AHA CC: 3Q, 2020, 29
  Z98.84 Bariatric surgery status
    Gastric banding status
    Gastric bypass status for obesity
    Obesity surgery status
    Excludes1: bariatric surgery status complicating pregnancy, childbirth, or the puerperium (O99.84)
    Excludes2: intestinal bypass and anastomosis status (Z98.0)
    AHA CC: 1Q, 2020, 12
  Z98.85 Transplanted organ removal status
    Transplanted organ previously removed due to complication, failure, rejection or infection
    Excludes1: encounter for removal of transplanted organ -code to complication of transplanted organ (T86.-)
  Z98.86 Personal history of breast implant removal

+ **Z98.87** Personal history of in utero procedure
  ♀ **Z98.870** Personal history of in utero procedure during pregnancy
    Excludes2: complications from in utero procedure for current pregnancy (O35.7)
    supervision of current pregnancy with history of in utero procedure during previous pregnancy (O09.82-)
  Z98.871 Personal history of in utero procedure while a fetus
+ **Z98.89** Other specified postprocedural states
  Z98.890 Other specified postprocedural states
    Personal history of surgery, note elsewhere classified
  ♀ **Z98.891** History of uterine scar from previous surgery
    Excludes1: Maternal care due to uterine scar from previous surgery (O34.2-)
    AHA CC: 4Q, 2016, 51-52

Z99 Dependence on enabling machines and devices, not elsewhere classified
  AHA CC: 1Q, 2020, 11
  Review coding guideline C.21.c.3
Z99.0 Dependence on aspirator
+ **Z99.1** Dependence on respirator
  Dependence on ventilator
  CC **Z99.11** Dependence on respirator [ventilator] status
    AHA CC: 1Q, 2015, 21
  CC **Z99.12** Encounter for respirator [ventilator] dependence during power failure
    Excludes1: mechanical complication of respirator [ventilator] (J95.850)
    AHA CC: 4Q, 2017, 112-114
    Review coding guidelines B19.d and C.21.c.16
Z99.2 Dependence on renal dialysis
  Hemodialysis status
  Peritoneal dialysis status
  Presence of arteriovenous shunt for dialysis
  Renal dialysis status NOS
  Excludes1: encounter for fitting and adjustment of dialysis catheter (Z49.0-)
  Excludes2: noncompliance with renal dialysis (Z91.15-)
  AHA CC: 3Q, 2022, 15-16
Z99.3 Dependence on wheelchair
  Wheelchair confinement status
  Code first cause of dependence, such as:
  muscular dystrophy (G71.0-)
  obesity (E66.-)
+ **Z99.8** Dependence on other enabling machines and devices
  Z99.81 Dependence on supplemental oxygen
    Dependence on long-term oxygen
    AHA CC: 4Q, 2013, 129
  Z99.89 Dependence on other enabling machines and devices
    Dependence on machine or device NOS

Chapter 22: Codes for Special Purposes (U00-U85)

This chapter contains the following blocks:
    U00-U49 Provisional assignment of new diseases of uncertain etiology or emergency use

C. Chapter-Specific Coding Guidelines

In addition to general coding guidelines, there are guidelines for specific diagnoses and/or conditions in the classification. Unless otherwise indicated, these guidelines apply to all health care settings. Please refer to Section II for guidelines on the selection of the principal diagnosis.

22. Chapter 22: Codes for Special Purposes (U00-U85)
    U07.0 Vaping-related disorder (*see Section I.C.10.e, Vaping-related disorders*)
    U07.1 COVID-19 (*see Section I.C.1.g.1., COVID-19 infection*)
    U09.9 Post COVID-19 condition, unspecified (see Section I.C.1.g.1.m)

Provisional assignment of new diseases of uncertain etiology or emergency use (U00-U49)

U07 Emergency use of U07

U07.0 Vaping related disorder (*see Section I.C.10.e, Vaping-related disorders*)
    Dabbing related lung damage
    Dabbing related lung injury
    E-cigarette, or vaping, product use associated lung injury [EVALI]
    Electronic cigarette related lung damage
    Electronic cigarette related lung injury
    Use additional code to identify manifestations, such as:
        abdominal pain (R10.84)
        acute respiratory distress syndrome (J80)
        diarrhea (R19.7)
        drug-induced interstitial lung disorder (J70.4)
        lipoid pneumonia (J69.1)
        weight loss (R63.4)
        AHA CC: 1Q, 2020, 3-4
        Review coding guideline C.11.3

MCC U07.1 COVID-19 (*see Section I.C.1.g.1., COVID-19 infection*)
    Use additional code to identify pneumonia or other manifestations, such as: pneumonia due to COVID-19 (J12.82)

    Use Additional code, if applicable, for associated conditions such as:
        COVID-19 associated coagulopathy (D68.8)
        disseminated intravascular coagulation (D65)
        hypercoagulable states (D68.69)
        thrombophilia (D68.69)

    Excludes2: *coronavirus as the cause of diseases classified elsewhere (B97.2-)*
        pneumonia due to SARS-associated coronavirus (J12.81)
    AHA CC: 2Q, 2020, 3-13; 3Q, 2020, 9-16; 4Q, 2020, 14; 1Q, 2021, 31-33, 36-40, 46-49; 4Q, 2021, 107-110; 2Q, 2022, 28-29
    Review coding guideline C.15.s
    Review coding guideline C.16.h

U09 Post COVID-19 condition

U09.9 Post COVID-19 condition, unspecified
    NOTE This code enables establishment of a link with COVID-19.
    This code is not to be used in cases that are still presenting with active COVID-19.
    However, an exception is made in cases of re-infection with COVID-19, occurring with a condition related to prior COVID-19.
    Post-acute sequela of COVID-19

    Code first the specific condition related to COVID-19 if known, such as:
        chronic respiratory failure (J96.1-)
        loss of smell (R43.8)
        loss of taste (R43.8)
        multisystem inflammatory syndrome (M35.81)
        pulmonary embolism (I26.-)
        pulmonary fibrosis (J84.10)
    AHA CC: 4Q, 2021, 31-32, 102-104, 106-108

Appendix A: CC/MCC Principal Diagnosis Collections and Exclusion Lists

Appendix A is provided online in a format suitable for spreadsheet and/or database use. Go to https://my.ahima.org/learningcenter and follow the directions listed on the inside front cover of this textbook to download the files.

Appendix B: Hospital-Acquired Conditions (HAC) List

Appendix B is provided online in a format suitable for spreadsheet and/or database use. Go to https://my.ahima.org/learningcenter and follow the directions listed on the inside front cover of this textbook to download the files.

Appendix C: New ICD-10-CM Codes FY2024

Appendix C is provided online in a format suitable for spreadsheet and/or database use. Go to https://my.ahima.org/learningcenter and follow the directions listed on the inside front cover of this textbook to download the files.

Appendix D: Deleted ICD-10-CM Codes FY2024

Appendix D is provided online in a format suitable for spreadsheet and/or database use. Go to https://my.ahima.org/learningcenter and follow the directions listed on the inside front cover of this textbook to download the files.